Veterinary pathology

Veterinary

Thomas Carlyle Jones
B.S., D.V.M., D.Sc.

Professor of Comparative Pathology, Emeritus
New England Regional Primate Research Center
Harvard Medical School

Ronald Duncan Hunt
B.S., D.V.M.

Professor of Comparative Pathology
Director, New England Regional Primate Research Center
Harvard Medical School

Norval William King
B.S., D.V.M.

Associate Professor of Comparative Pathology
New England Regional Primate Research Center
Harvard Medical School

pathology

Sixth Edition

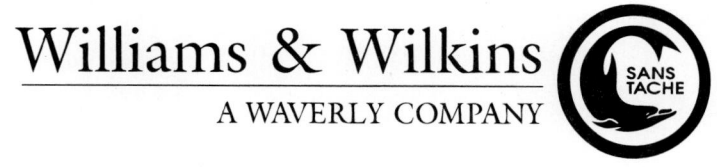

Williams & Wilkins

A WAVERLY COMPANY

SANS TACHE

BALTIMORE • PHILADELPHIA • LONDON • PARIS • BANGKOK
BUENOS AIRES • HONG KONG • MUNICH • SYDNEY • TOKYO • WROCLAW

Editor: Carroll Cann
Managing Editor: Susan Hunsberger
Production Coordinator: Cindy Park
Book Project Editor: Robert D. Magee
Designer: Arlene Putterman
Illustration Planner: Cindy Park
Cover Designer: Arlene Putterman
Typesetter: Maple Vail Composition
Printer: Maple Vail Press
Digitized Illustrations: Maple Vail Composition
Binder: Maple Vail Press

Copyright © 1997 Williams & Wilkins

351 West Camden Street
Baltimore, Maryland 21201-2436 USA

Rose Tree Corporate Center
1400 North Providence Road
Building II, Suite 5025
Media, Pennsylvania 19063-2043 USA

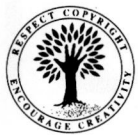

Accurate indications, adverse reactions and dosage schedules for drugs are provided in this book, but it is possible that they may change. The reader is urged to review the package information data of the manufacturers of the medications mentioned.

Printed in the United States of America

Library of Congress Cataloging-in-Publication Data

Jones, Thomas Carlyle.
   Veterinary pathology / Thomas Carlyle Jones, Ronald Duncan Hunt,
Norval W. King. — 6th ed.
      p. cm.
   Includes index.
   ISBN 0-683-04481-8
   1. Veterinary pathology. I. Hunt, Ronald Duncan. II. King,
Norval W. III. Title.
SF769.J65 1996
636.089'607—dc20   96-32932
                                               CIP

The publishers have made every effort to trace the copyright holders for borrowed material. If they have inadvertently overlooked any, they will be pleased to make the necessary arrangements at the first opportunity.

To purchase additional copies of this book, call our customer service department at **(800) 638-0672** or fax orders to **(800) 447-8438**. For other book services, including chapter reprints and large quantity sales, ask for the Special Sales department.

Canadian customers should call **(800) 268-4178**, or fax **(905) 470-6780**. For all other calls originating outside of the United States, please call **(410) 528-4223** or fax us at **(410) 528-8550**.

Visit Williams & Wilkins on the Internet: http://www.wwilkins.com or contact our customer service department at **custserv@wwilkins.com**. Williams & Wilkins customer service representatives are available from 8:30 am to 6:00 pm, EST, Monday through Friday, for telephone access.

97 98 99
1 2 3 4 5 6 7 8 9 10

Preface

This, the sixth edition of *Veterinary Pathology*, comes out forty years since the original publication of this text by Lea and Febiger of Philadelphia, who continued its publication through five editions. Fourteen years have elapsed since the fifth edition was published in 1983. The wealth of new information that has appeared in the literature during these intervening years is overwhelming. This is not stated as a disclaimer, but rather as a simple truth. It has become virtually impossible for any one individual to keep fully abreast of the medical literature, even in one specialty, such as veterinary pathology. To partially meet this demanding effort, we welcome to this edition, Norval W. King as a third co-author, and for the first time, we are pleased to include several chapters contributed by invited experts.

Our intent has been to maintain the original twofold objective, that is; *to serve as a textbook of pathology for both the veterinary student and advanced trainee who is preparing for a career in pathology, and to serve as a reference book to the veterinary or comparative pathologist and anyone else interested in this field.* We hope that this edition continues to meet these goals. Our presentations must be concise if we are to embrace the spectrum ranging from basic concepts of pathology to pathogenetic mechanisms of a myriad of specific diseases that affect animals. Emphasis remains on anatomic pathology.

While we attempted to incorporate as much knowledge on mechanisms of disease as possible, and to include ideas coming from applications of molecular pathology, we have, as in previous editions, sought to restrict discussions to those ideas and theories that appear solid enough to endure.

We are indebted to all those individuals who have contributed to the realization of this edition. These individuals include contributing authors, individuals who have furnished photographs, and those who have made helpful comments and suggestions for improvement. We especially acknowledge the large number of individuals who have contributed to the growing body of scientific literature upon which we relied. These persons are recognized by the list of references to their published work.

Special thanks go to Miss Beverly Blake for her talented editorial assistance.

We are grateful that the Waverly Company is willing to produce and promote this book, using the resources of its subsidiaries, Williams and Wilkins and Lea and Febiger. The support of Carroll C. Cann, Susan Hunsberger, and Cindy Park at Williams and Wilkins is also gratefully acknowledged.

Santa Fe, New Mexico
Southborough, Massachusetts

T.C. Jones
R.D. Hunt
N.W. King

Contributor list

DOUGLAS J. RINGLER, V.M.D.

Vice President of Pharmaceutical Development
Levkosite Incorporated
Cambridge, Massachusetts

JOSEPH ALROY, D.V.M.

Associate Professor of Pathology
Department of Pathology
Tufts University
Boston, Massachusetts

JOHN F. VAN VLEET, D.V.M., Ph.D.

Professor of Veterinary Pathology
Department of Veterinary Pathobiology
School of Veterinary Medicine
Purdue University
West Lafayette, Indiana

JAMES CARROLL WOODARD, D.V.M., Ph.D.

Professor of Pathology
Department of Pathology
College of Veterinary Medicine
University of Florida
Gainesville, Florida

ADALBERT KOESTNER, D.V.M., Ph.D.

Professor and Dean Emeritus
Department of Veterinary Biosciences
College of Veterinary Medicine
Ohio State University
Columbus, Ohio

Contents

Veterinary pathology

Introduction: Cells: death of cells and tissues

Pathology is the study of the derangement of molecules, cells, tissues, and function that occur in living organisms in response to injurious agents or deprivations. Many of these agents are chemical compounds that often include the products of other organisms, the most common of which are the pathogenic (disease-producing) microorganisms. Other injurious agents are various forms of energy, such as heat, radiation, and mechanical forces applied in excessive amounts. While most pathologic conditions result from the exposure of body tissues to injurious substances, deprivation of essential nutrients, such as proteins, minerals, vitamins, water, and oxygen may have an equally harmful effect. Genetic factors may also play an important role in pathology.

The key word in the definition of pathology is **response,** a spectrum of reactions ranging from reversible injury to irreversible injury and death to malignant transformation. When response impairs the health or well-being of the individual, it is regarded as disease.

The body is also subjected to many normal stimuli to which it responds in much the same, if not identical, manner as it does to abnormal or deleterious stimuli. For example, the processes of atrophy and necrosis that occur in normal involution of the thymus are not dissimilar from the atrophy and necrosis that occur when the normal blood supply of an organ or tissue is impaired. Certain responses, such as death of a cell following anoxia, are passive, but most responses, such as inflammations, are active and in most cases represent normal lifesaving defense mechanisms. In some cases, these protective mechanisms neutralize or eliminate the injurious agent early and clinically detectable disease does not develop. In other cases, these reactions are less efficient and consequently often more severe; in these cases, the patient may experience a variety of systemic abnormalities (**symptoms**) as well as visible manifestations (**signs**) as a consequence of the response. When this occurs, the patient has a clinical illness, which may be fatal. In some instances, these normally protective mechanisms go awry and result in further damage to the host. Thus, host defense reactions may vary widely in their effectiveness and intensity, may go unrecognized or be associated with varying degrees of clinical illness, may be beneficial or result in further injury, and may be lifesaving or fatal.

Pathologists must be able to recognize that all such reactions are real, consistent, and recognizable, and they must be aware of both the benefits and disadvantages of these reactions in the host. Animals have not completely adapted to their environment and, as the environment is constantly changing, there is little chance that they will.

As the late Dr. Hilton Smith wrote so eloquently in the first edition of this text: "To the extent that our knowledge permits any biologic science to be precise, pathology is that branch of medicine which attempts to relate morphologic changes to specific causes. When our understanding of the laws of nature becomes perfect, then it will be possible to predict the effect of a disease-producing agent with as much certainty as it is to measure the force of gravity and predict the course of a falling body. Under what appear to be entirely comparable conditions, one animal survives an infection and one succumbs, one person develops a malignant neoplasm and another does not. We tend to dismiss such biologic variations as differences in individual susceptibility and such irregularities must be expected even in carefully controlled biologic experiments. However, let no one suppose that each unexplained event is, in reality, without adequate cause; it is only because of our incomplete understanding and knowledge of pertinent facts that we tend to group such variable outcomes according to the laws of chance. Too much time has been wasted in considering pathology as a long list of separate observations on diseased animals and tissues. The conditions that occur in health and disease are fully related to each other and are based on chemical and physical laws as constant as any in science."

The study of pathologic processes may be approached at any of several different levels. At the **popu-lation** level, the interaction of organisms to each other and to the environment under various adverse conditions may contribute to pathologic states. At the level of the **organism,** pathologic states are made manifest by obvious clinical signs or by symptoms subjectively recognized by the human patient and are the result of changes in one or more organ systems. Specific pathologic changes in organs or tissues may be recognized by examination of the **gross** specimen or by study of tissue sections under the light microscope. At the **cellular** level, some pathologic states may be recognized with the light microscope; others, involving **intracellular** organelles, can be visualized only with the electron microscope. At the **molecular** level, detection of the chemical reactions that underlie all pathologic processes may require use of an extensive array of analytical biochemical and molecular biologic techniques. The rapid development and application of increasingly more sophisticated molecular biologic tools over the last few years holds great promise for unraveling the biochemical basis of disease.

Throughout medical history, detailed studies of gross and microscopic tissue specimens (**pathologic anatomy**) have contributed information regarding the nature of disease processes, and even today these studies continue to be key elements in the diagnosis of many diseases. Despite the increasing sophistication of modern molecular diagnostic tools, pathologic anatomy is still the principal means by which most diagnoses are made, or at least by which differential diagnosis proceeds. For this reason, gross and pathologic anatomy are emphasized in this text and, where possible, an attempt has been made to provide the reader with the current fundamental biochemical and molecular bases of disease.

THE NORMAL CELL

Our understanding of the biology of the cell and its complex interactions with cells of the same or different type has vastly improved since the preceding edition of this text. These advances have been made possible by the development of sophisticated investigative techniques applicable at both the cellular and molecular levels, including immunocytochemistry; immunoelectronmicroscopy; enzyme-linked immunoabsorbent assays (ELISA); flow cytometry and cell sorting techniques; efficient RNA and DNA sequencing and hybridization techniques; Northern, Southern, and Western blot procedures; and the polymerase chain reaction (PCR) for amplifying miniscule quantities of genetic material. Knowledge gained from the application of these techniques to the study of cells and tissues and their secretory products has markedly advanced our understanding of cell biology (Fig. 1-1).

Ultrastructure and function of cells

THE PLASMA MEMBRANE

The outer membrane of cells, commonly referred to as the **plasma membrane** or **plasmalemma,** has a re-

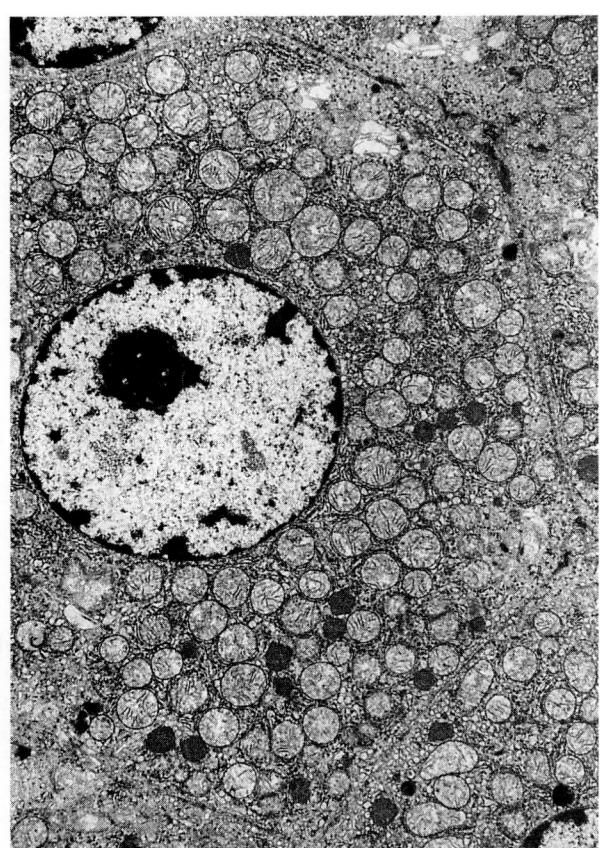

FIG. 1-1 The cell. Electron micrograph of portions of four liver cells from a cynomolgus monkey (*Macaca fascicularis*). Note nucleus containing a prominent nucleolus; cytoplasm containing numerous mitochondria; scattered darker staining peroxisomes; sparse lamellae of rough endoplasmic reticulum; and cell membranes separating adjacent cells (× 7000).

markably uniform ultrastructure consisting of two electron-dense layers, each about 30 Å in diameter and separated by a less dense layer of approximately the same thickness. Chemically, the plasma membrane consists of a double layer of amphipathic lipid molecules in which various proteins are embedded. Depending on the cell, the lipid component consists of various proportions of phospholipids, cholesterol, and glycolipids. These lipids characteristically have a hydrophilic polar end and a hydrophobic non-polar end that, when the lipids are exposed to water (such as extracellular fluid and cytosol), causes them to spontaneously orient themselves with the hydrophilic ends facing the aqueous medium and the hydrophobic ends facing each other. This property creates the bilayer of the plasma membrane. In addition, these lipids move freely within their respective layers, thus imparting a fluidity to the membrane. Various proteins embedded in or spanning the full thickness of the lipid bilayer (**transmembrane proteins**) also have hydrophilic and hydrophobic ends that account for their orientation within the membrane, and they are also capable of movement within the cell membrane. These proteins mediate many functions of the cell membrane, including (1) transporting specific molecules into and out of cells; (2) functioning as enzymes that catalyze membrane-associated reactions; (3) serving as structural links between the extracellular matrix and the cell cytoskeleton; and 4) functioning as receptors for receiving and transducing chemical signals from the cell's exterior. Hence, despite its seemingly simple appearance, the plasma membrane is in fact the site of a vast array of complex chemical reactions involved in maintaining normal cellular homeostasis as well as responsiveness to numerous extracelluar signals involved in cell division, differentiation, and function.

The plasma membrane is not always smooth; it may be altered to form specialized structures, such as microvilli, which increase absorptive surfaces on cells such as enterocytes of the intestine, and proximal convoluted tubular epithelial cells of the kidney. The cell membrane may also invaginate into the cytoplasm to form large **phagocytic vacuoles** or smaller **pinocytotic vesicles** that function in the uptake of particulate and fluid materials from the extracellular space by processes known as phagocytosis and pinocytosis. Pinocytosis results in the active uptake of minute droplets of fluid from the interstitium. This fluid contains inorganic ions such as sodium and potassium which, if allowed to increase in concentration in the cytosol, would exert increased oncotic pressure, causing the cell to swell. In addition, the plasma membrane is semipermeable, thus permitting the passive transfer of certain substances, depending on their molecular size, chemical composition, and electrical charge, from the interstitial fluid into the cytosol of the cell. To counteract the oncotic pressure exerted by colloidal proteins and ions within the cytosol, which, if unregulated, would promote cellular swelling and eventual bursting, an active membrane transport system termed the **sodium-potassium ion pump** exists within the plasma membrane. This pump is highly energy-dependent and requires generation of large amounts of adenosine triphosphate (ATP) by mitochondrial and glycolytic phosphorylations. Any permanent disruption in the function of these pumps or in the generation of ATP required to fuel them leads to sudden cellular swelling and eventual death of the cell. Cells are not at equilibrium with the interstitial fluid surrounding them; sodium, calcium, and water must be actively pumped out and potassium and magnesium pumped in against the forces of Donnan's equilibrium exerted by negatively-charged, nondiffusible, intracellular macromolecules, mainly proteins.

THE CYTOPLASM

The **cytoplasm** of normal cells consists of a protein-rich colloid known as **cytosol,** in which an amazing array of organelles are suspended. The number and kind of organelles vary with the type of cell and its function (Fig. 1-2). A brief review of the structure and function of the principal cellular organelles follows.

Mitochondria Mitochondria are among the most conspicuous of the organelles; they generate energy needed by the cell in the form of ATP. They are round to ovoid, bacteria-like organelles with a diameter of 0.5 to 1.0 μm. There are hundreds or thousands of mitochondria per cell, depending on the energy requirements of each particular cell. They are located in cer-

tain cells near the sites of highest ATP consumption. In cardiac muscle, for example, they are located adjacent to myofibrils; in spermatozoa, they are tightly wrapped around the flagellum; and in other cell types, they are near the microtubules of the cytoskeleton.

Mitochondria are bound by a pair of highly specialized membranes separated by a narrow intermembrane space. The outer membrane contains many transport proteins that form large aqueous channels permeable to all molecules of 10,000 d or less. The inner membrane is usually folded into structures referred to as **cristae,** which protrude into the mitochondrion matrix. The inner membrane contains (1) a high proportion of cardiolipin, which makes it unusually impermeable to ions; (2) a variety of transport proteins for small molecules, which are metabolized by mitochondrial enzymes present in the inner matrix; and (3) an enzyme complex (ATP synthetase), which produces ATP in the matrix.

Mitochondria produce ATP by a process known as oxidative phosphorylation (OXPHOS). In human cells and presumably in other mammalian cells as well, this process involves approximately 100 polypeptides, most of which are encoded in Mendelian inherited nuclear genes, and 13 of which are encoded in the maternally inherited mitochondrial DNA (mtDNA). Mitochondria, unlike many organelles, are not synthesized *de novo* but divide by binary fission. They contain their own mtDNA, which can be transcribed and translated to form proteins. Human mtDNA is a small (16.5 kb), circular, double-stranded molecule containing 13 structural genes, 22 transfer RNA genes, and 2 genes encoding the 165 and 125 mitochondrial ribosomal RNAs. All 13 peptides encoded by mtDNA are components of respiratory-chain complexes. Because all the mitochondria of a cell are contributed by the ovum during formation of the zygote, the mitochondrial genome is transmitted by maternal non-Mendelian inheritance. mtDNA has a mutation rate 10 to 20 times higher than nuclear DNA that functions in the same enzyme complex. Accordingly, mutations of mtDNA are transmitted by maternal inheritance. An affected mother passes the disease to all her offspring, but only her daughters transmit the trait in subsequent generations. Following mutation in mtDNA, the cytoplasm may contain a mixture of mutant and normal mtDNAs. Tissues, such as brain and skeletal muscle, requiring a high mitochondrial energy output are more severely affected by mutations of mtDNA than tissues having lower energy requirements.

Most OXPHOS genes are encoded by nuclear DNA (nDNA), and the polypeptides they encode are synthesized on "free" ribosomes in the cytosol and imported into the mitochondria after translation. These polypeptides cannot cross the mitochondrial membrane in their native conformation. The protein import machinery includes cytosolic "antifolding" proteins, "import factors," and "import receptors," which participate in preventing premature entry of the polypeptides into the mitochondria. Mutation in any of these steps may result in inherited mitochondrial disease. Mitochondria segregate randomly during cell division. Once the mu-

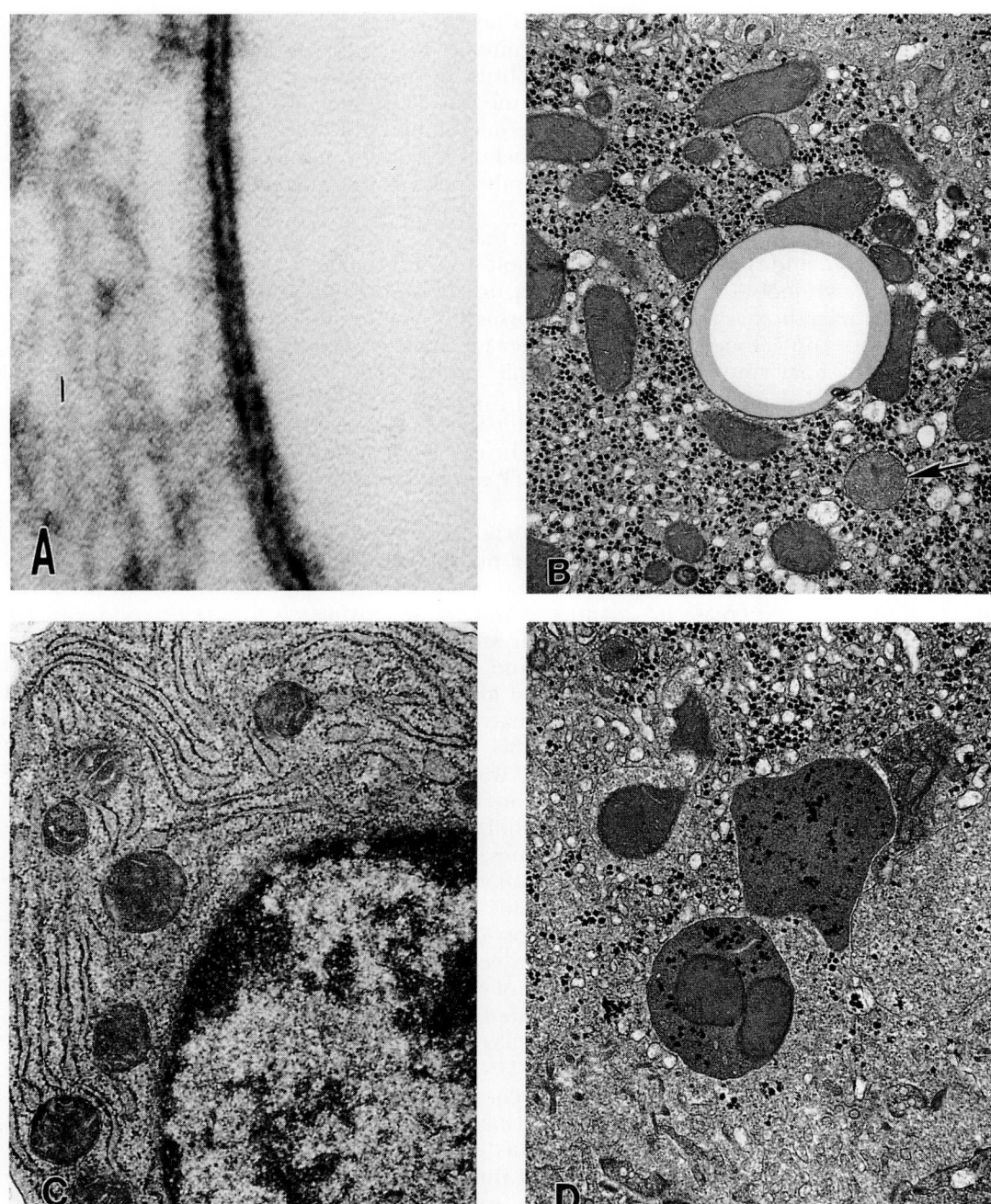

FIG. 1-2 Ultrastructure of cellular organelles. **A.** Section of a cell membrane consisting of an inner and outer electron-dense layer separated by an electron-lucent zone (× 600,000). **B.** Portion of the cytoplasm of an hepatocyte containing several mitochondria, numerous glycogen particles, dilated profiles of smooth endoplasmic reticulum, a single spherical lipid droplet, and a peroxisome *(arrow)* (× 18,000). **C.** Rough endoplasmic reticulum in a plasma cell (× 22,500). **D.** Two phagolysosomes (secondary lysosomes) in the liver containing glycogen particles and effete mitochondria (× 18,000).

tant mtDNA reaches a certain threshold, the cell begins to express the mutant phenotype.

Mitochondrial diseases are both inherited and acquired; they include myopathies, encephalomyopathies, and multisystem disorders. Clinically, animals with these diseases present with a history of weakness, exercise intolerance, and encephalopathy. Biochemical abnormali-

ties of the mitochondria (Fig. 1-3), such as lactic acidosis, the presence of "ragged red fibers" in muscle biopsies stained with modified Gomori trichrome stain (Fig. 1-4), and the ultrastructural demonstration of aggregates of mitochondria containing cystalloids (Fig. 1-5) are useful in their diagnosis. Mitochondrial myopathies have been recognized in horses, cattle, and in spe-

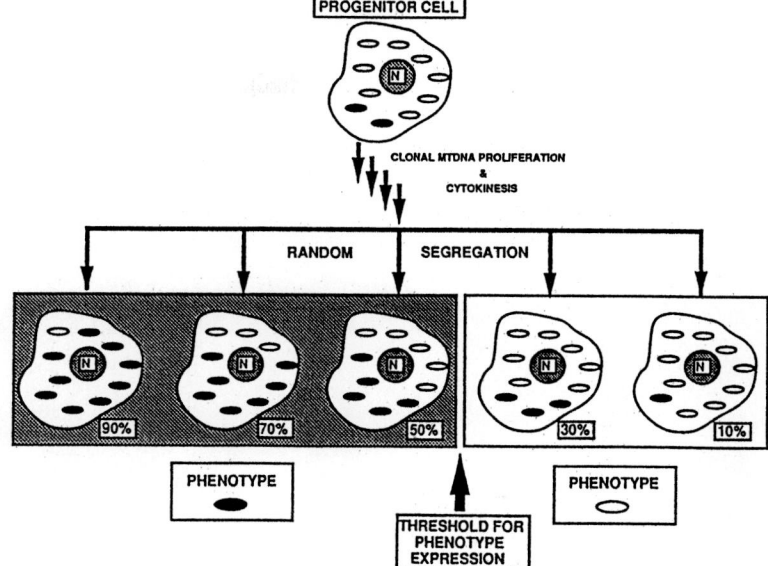

FIG. 1-3 Schematic illustrating replicative segregation of mtDNA. Mitochondria segregate randomly during cell division. When the number of mitochondria containing mutant mtDNA reaches a critical threshold, the cell begins to express the mutant phenotype. Mutant mitochondria *(solid ovals)*; normal mitochondria *(open ovals)*; nucleus *(N)*. (With permission of Dr. John M. Shoffner IV and Advances in Human Genetics 19).

cific breeds of dogs, i.e., Old English sheepdogs and Clumber and Sussex spaniels.

The Endoplasmic Reticulum A complex system of membranes, which traverses the cytoplasm to form canaliculi, cisternae, vesicles, or parallel arrays, is known as the **endoplasmic reticulum.** The endoplasmic reticulum corresponds to cytoplasmic structures described by light microscopy as basophilic bodies, Nissl substance, chromophilic substance, or the ergastoplasm. Some of

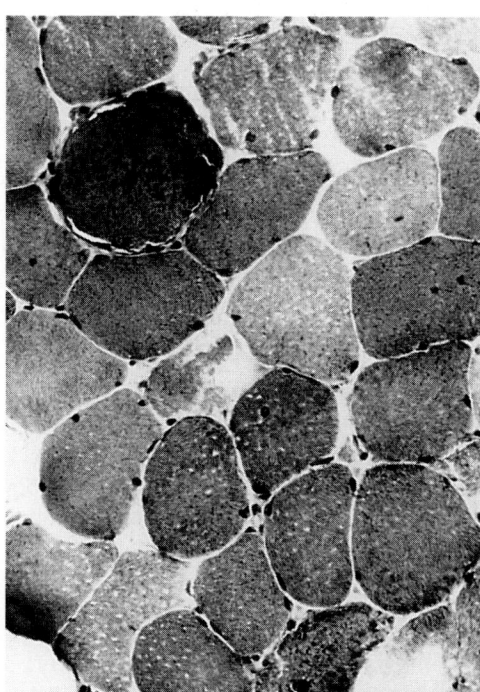

FIG. 1-4 Cross-section of skeletal muscle (Gomori trichrome stain). Note two "ragged red myofibers," which appear more granular and stain more intensely than the adjacent normal fibers (× 600). (Courtesy of Dr. Joseph Alroy, Tufts University School of Veterinary Medicine.)

these membranes have smooth outer surfaces and are referred to as the **smooth endoplasmic reticulum (SER)**; others have regularly spaced granules of RNA, known as **ribosomes,** on their outer surfaces and are referred to as **rough endoplasmic reticulum (RER).** The latter is highly developed in cells that produce large quantities of protein-rich secretion, such as plasma cells and pancreatic acinar cells. However, synthesis of protein is known to be associated with individual or clusters of ribosomes suspended in the cytosol unassociated with the endoplasmic reticulum (**free ribosomes** or **polyribosomes**).

The RER appears in electron micrographs as thin profiles of paired membranes having a granular outer surface and a smooth inner surface that surrounds flat or saccular spaces, called cisternae. The cisternae function as channels that isolate newly synthesized secretory products from the rest of the cell and transport it to the Golgi complex, where it is packaged and stored before being secreted. The RER may appear as single or, more often, aggregated profiles within the cell. Sometimes the cisternae of the RER become markedly distended by secretion and can be seen by light microscopy as distinct eosinophilic globules in the cytoplasm. The classic example is the massive accumulations of immunoglobulin, known as Russell bodies, within the RER of plasma cells.

The SER is continuous with the RER, differing only in the absence of ribosomes. SER is present in abundance in steroid-secreting cells of endocrine organs and may proliferate dramatically in liver cells following administration of certain chemicals and drugs, such as barbiturates. SER is known to be involved in the production of hormones from lipid precursors and in the detoxification of certain drugs and chemicals.

The Golgi Complex The **Golgi complex** (or Golgi apparatus) is typically located near the nucleus and, in secretory cells, at the apical pole of the nucleus. Ultrastructurally, the Golgi complex consists of parallel,

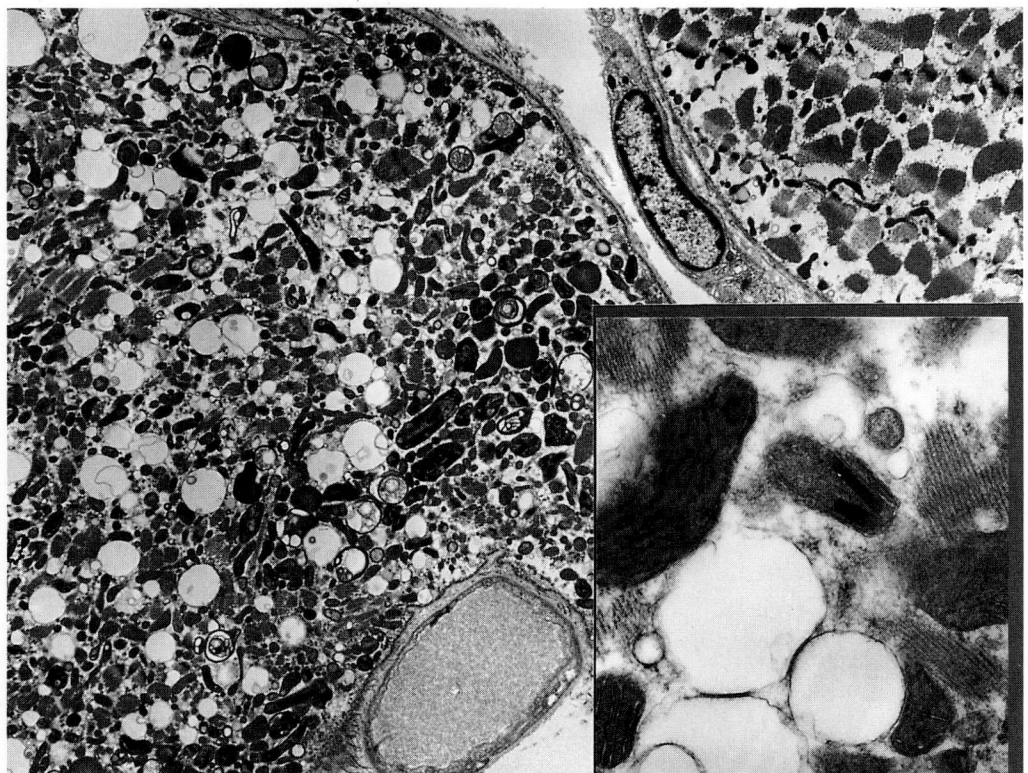

FIG. 1-5 Electron micrograph of two myofibers; one *(left)* contains fewer contractile elements, numerous abnormal mitochondria and vacuoles (× 3700.) Inset: Higher magnification of several abnormal mitochondria, one of which contains two crystalloids (× 23,300). (Courtesy of Dr. Joseph Alroy, Tufts University School of Veterinary Medicine.)

slightly curved arrays of stacked membrane-bound channels that vary in length and are usually about 150 Å wide. Clustered around the ends of these channels are numerous small vesicles, 400 to 800 Å in diameter. The cisternae may be distended with secretory product. Membrane-bound sacs containing secretion and referred to as **secretory granules** bud from the Golgi and accumulate in close proximity to it. The functions of the Golgi complex are not entirely known, but it is believed that it assembles secretory products brought to it through the endoplasmic reticulum after synthesis by the ribosomes. Polysaccharides may be added by the Golgi complex to the protein transported to it. Lipid absorbed by cells of the small intestine may accumulate in the Golgi complex of intestinal epithelial cells, but the exact nature of the chemical events at this site is unknown.

Lysosomes Lysosomes are a heterogeneous group of membrane-bound, enzyme-containing organelles found in the cytoplasm of all eukaryotic cells. They occur in two forms.

PRIMARY LYSOSOMES Primary lysosomes are round, approximately 50 μm, membrane-bound bodies with a dense core that contains many hydrolytic enzymes, including proteases, nucleases, glycosidases, lipases, phospholipases, phosphatases, and sulfatases. These lysosomal enzymes are used by the cell for controlled intracellular digestion of various macromolecules and, because they function optimally at pH 5 (the internal pH of lysosomes), they are termed acid hydrolases. They are synthesized on the RER, transported to its cisterna, and packaged in the Golgi apparatus, from which they pinch off as clathrin-coated vesicles. When they are released into the cytoplasm, the clathrin coat dissociates from the vesicles and they become primary lysosomes. After their formation, the fate of primary lysosomes is essentially 2-fold: Either they move to and fuse with the plasma membrane and discharge (secrete) their contents into the extracellular space by exocytosis, or they fuse with other vesicular organelles in the cytoplasm and discharge their contents into the lumens of the latter. The vesicular organelles include **phagocytic vacuoles, autophagic vacuoles,** and **pinocytotic vesicles,** which contain a variety of phagocytized or endocytosed material, including microorganisms and nutrients of various kinds as well as effete organelles.

SECONDARY LYSOSOMES When primary lysosomes fuse with these structures, they form what are known as ·**secondary lysosomes** or **phagolysosomes,** which can be highly variable in size and shape depending on their content. The membranes of primary and secondary lysosomes in normal cells are uniquely resistant to the digestive action of enzymes, which they surround and, thus, prevent leakage of these enzymes into the cytosol.

The specific granules of neutrophils and eosinophils contain acid hydrolases and are therefore examples of lysosomes.

Peroxisomes Peroxisomes are membrane-bound organelles which carry out a diverse set of metabolic functions. They measure from 0.1 μm in diameter (in brain or fibroblasts) to 1.5 μm in diameter (in liver or kidney) and sometimes contain a crystalline core. The single-membrane phospholipid of peroxisomes is synthesized by and buds from the smooth endoplasmic reticulum. Their matrix, crystalloid core proteins, and some major integral proteins are synthesized by free polyribosomes in the cytosol and then delivered to the peroxisomes. Peroxisomes have a nonpermeable membrane, with energy-requiring uptake systems for both small molecules and proteins. Current studies have demonstrated that a carboxy terminal, such as serine-lysine-leucine tripeptide, is necessary and sufficient for peroxisomal targeting.

Peroxisomes participate in the following processes (1) respiration based on H_2O_2-forming oxidases and catalase; (2) fatty acid β oxidation, similar to what occurs in mitochondria, but using different enzymes; (3) plasmalogen biosynthesis; (4) transamination; (5) purine catabolism; (6) glyconeogenesis; and (7) bile acid synthesis.

Centrioles Centrioles appear, by light microscopy, as pairs of deeply stained short rods, often adjacent to the nucleus in a zone known as the centrosome, or cell center. Cytologists often refer to a line through the nucleus and the centrosome as the "cell axis." In some cells, the centrioles are surrounded by the Golgi complex; in others, they are located immediately beneath the plasma membrane. One to forty pairs may occupy a single cell. Although their functions are not fully understood, they are clearly involved with organization of the cell, particularly during cell division. Their position after replication at opposite poles of the nucleus during mitosis facilitates the movement of chromosomes to opposite poles of the cytoplasm. The chromosomes are connected to dense bodies (satellites) adjacent to the centriole by means of the spindle fibers, which consist of **microtubules.** In ciliated cells, reduplicated centrioles form "basal bodies" that give rise to the cilia and serve as their kinetic centers.

Ultrastructurally, centrioles consist of a hollow cylinder, 0.15 in diameter and up to 0.5μm long. One end of the cylinder is open, the other closed. The pair is often arranged with their long axes perpendicular to each other. The wall of the cylinder is made up of nine evenly spaced hollow fibrils or tubules, each in triplicate. In some cells, ill-defined spherical bodies up to 700 Å in diameter are seen adjacent to the centriole. These pericentriolar structures are the satellites to which the mitotic "spindle fibers" are attached.

THE NUCLEUS

The **nucleus** houses the majority of cellular DNA and is the principal site of DNA replication, transcription, and RNA synthesis and processing. It is surrounded by a **nuclear envelope** consisting of two membranes, each about 75 Å thick, separated by a space about 400 to 700 Å wide, called the **perinuclear cisterna.** The outer membrane of the envelope is studded with ribosomes and often is continuous with the endoplasmic reticulum of the cytoplasm. The nuclear envelope derives its origin from these membranes. Inner and outer membranes of the nuclear envelope converge at intervals around circular structures known as **nuclear pores.** These are not open pores, but are fenestrations covered by a characteristic membrane. Through these structures materials are transferred to and from the cytoplasm of the cell.

Most of the nuclear content is made up of basophilic granular material called **chromatin** suspended in an aqueous medium known as the **nucleoplasm.** The distribution and structure of chromatin depends on the type of cell, its functional state, and the fixation and staining procedures used. The most dense granular component, called **heterochromatin,** which forms masses of various sizes, is considered to be relatively inactive metabolically. One specific mass of chromatin, located adjacent to the nuclear envelope in cells of females, is the **sex chromatin, or Barr body,** representing the inactivated X chromosome. The more loosely arranged chromatin granules are termed **euchromatin** and are considered to be in the metabolically active state. The principal cellular component of chromatin is DNA.

The Nucleolus The **nucleolus,** easily recognized by light microscopy, also has a characteristic ultrastructure (Fig. 1-6). This organelle plays a key role in the ribosomal RNA synthesis and assembly required for the synthesis of protein. The nucleolus consists of a rounded, usually basophilic mass located within the nucleoplasm, which disappears during mitosis, but in interphase has three distinct ultrastructural components: (1) an electron-lucent component, containing DNA from the nucleolar organizing region of a chromosome (**pars amorpha**); (2) a finely granular component, containing particles 15 nm in diameter, consisting of the most mature ribosomal precursor particles; and 3) a dense fibrillar component (**nucleolonema**), consisting of many fine 5-nm fibers composed of RNA transcripts.

The nucleus is not essential for the life of some cells, such as mature erythrocytes, platelets, and epithelial cells in the interior of the lens, but it is necessary for cell division and most complex metabolic functions.

OTHER CELL INCLUSIONS

Many other types of **cell inclusions** characterize different cell types. These include membrane-bound secretory products (**secretory granules**), found in various endocrine cells of the anterior pituitary and pancreatic islets. Similar inclusions are found in the secretory epithelium of exocrine glands, such as salivary, mucous, pancreatic acinar, and Brunner's gland cells. **Neurosecretory granules** characterize specialized neuroendocrine cells, such as those present in the hypothalamus. **Pigments** (i.e., melanin and lipofuscin) also appear as cytoplasmic inclusions, as do glycogen and lipid. These are described in detail in the appropriate chapters.

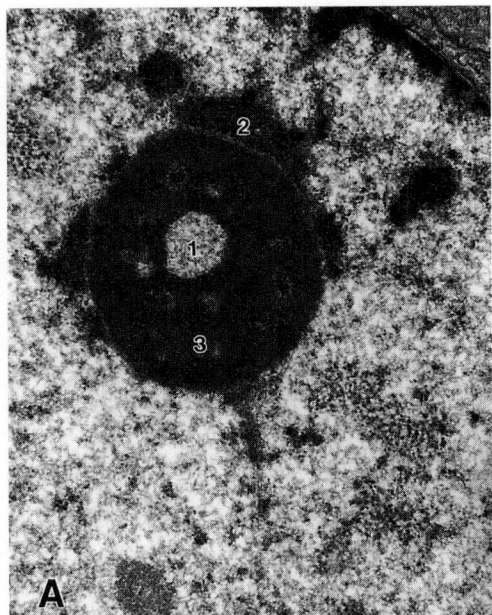
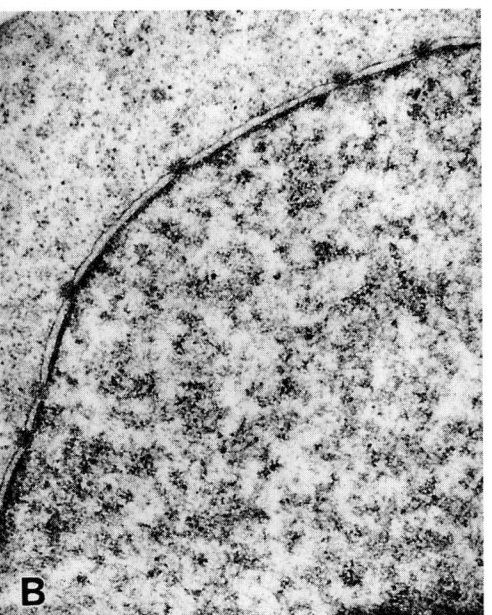

FIG. 1-6 Hepatocyte. **A.** Portion of the nucleus and entire nucleolus of a hepatocyte. The nucleolus has three parts: (1) Pars amorpha; (2) granular component; and (3) nucleonema (× 25,000). **B.** Portion of the nuclear membrane of a hepatocyte. Note inner and outer leaflets separated by perinuclear cisterna and the prominent nuclear pores (× 31,250).

CELL INJURY, CELL DEATH, AND NECROSIS

Before discussing these topics, it is important to define the precise meaning of the terms involved. **Cell injury** refers to any biochemical or structural alteration that impairs the ability of a cell to function normally. Such an injury may be mild, transient, and reversible, or it may be of such severity and duration that it becomes irreversible. **Cell death** is defined as that point when cell injury becomes irreversible, or has passed the **"point of no return."** Cell death occurs in two biochemically and morphologically distinct ways, **"accidental cell death"** and **apoptosis.** Finally, the term **necrosis** refers to the characteristic light microscopic changes resulting from enzymatic degradation of the nucleus and cytoplasm that define cell death. Typically, these changes cannot be seen for 12 to 18 hours after a cell has died. Thus, there is a period of time when a dead cell appears microscopically identical to a living cell. For example, a 10% solution of formalin, a commonly used fixative for histology, promptly kills living cells by immersion, but because this solution also inactivates hydrolytic enzymes contained in the dead cells, the cells do not undergo the characteristic microscopic changes of necrosis. Hence, it is customary in microscopic pathology to refer to a cell or tissue as living if it appears identical to living cells that have been placed in a fixative and as dead if it has any of the changes associated with necrosis.

Causes of Cell Injury and Death

The causes of cell injury and death are numerous and include: (1) forms of kinetic injury (mechanical, thermal, and radiation); (2) exposure to reactive forms of exogenous chemicals (poisonous compounds, toxins of plant and microbiologic origin) and endogenous chemicals(toxic products of metabolism, peroxides, and free radicals); (3) deprivation of essential nutrients (water, oxygen, and foodstuffs); and (4) immunologic reactions and genetic disorders.

Of the two distinct types of cell death, accidental cell death (formerly referred to simply as necrosis), is the most often recognized type and, although it has numerous causes, is typified by biochemical and morphologic alterations resulting from anoxia (**ischemia**). The other type, often referred to as "programmed cell death," but more appropriately termed **apoptosis,** results from activation and transcription of specific genes, commonly referred to as "suicide genes," that are found in all cells. In certain situations, activation of these genes occurs normally and accounts for the normal turnover of cells in the body. For example, during normal embryonic development, certain cells die at prescribed times, while others continue to proliferate. This phenomenon contributes to the normal sculpting of anatomic structures, such as digits on the limbuds. In adults, this mechanism allows involution of the thymus. However, under certain pathologic conditions, these genes can be activated prematurely or activated in cells where they are normally suppressed; this leads to premature senescence or atrophy of affected organs. Examples of this can be seen in (1) thymic atrophy, induced experimentally by corticosteroids and radiation; (2) cachexia, induced by tumor necrosis factor α (TNF-α); (3) in the lymphoid depletion that occurs in human and simian acquired immunodeficiency syndrome (AIDS), and (4) in the elimination of foreign or virally infected cells, when such death is mediated by cytotoxic T-lymphocytes (CTLs). Unlike accidental cell death, where large numbers of diversified cells in a tissue or organ are often affected, apoptosis tends to affect individual cells of a highly specific type, which suggests that certain cells have different threshholds for apoptosis.

Biochemical and Ultrastructural Changes of Cell Death

ACCIDENTAL CELL DEATH

Despite the many causes of accidental cell injury, certain basic mechanisms and alterations appear to be operant following most insults. Only a few forms of cell injury have been studied in detail; these include hypoxic cell injury, injury induced by free radicals, and selected forms of chemical injury. After each type of injury, a series of events unfold that ultimately lead to loss of cellular membrane integrity and acute cellular swelling. Of the three forms of accidental cell injury, injury due to hypoxia has been studied most extensively. Finally, a discussion of virus-induced cell injury is included.

Hypoxic cell injury

ACUTE CELLULAR SWELLING. Swelling of cells is one of the earliest recognizable microscopic changes following cellular injury (Fig. 1-7). If severe, it is visible by light microscopy and is known as **hydropic, or vacuolar, degeneration.** The cause is failure of the sodium-potassium ion pump mechanism necessary to maintain appropriate osmotic pressure inside the cell. Cells are not at equilibrium with their environment, thus an energy-dependent active process (ion pump) is required to counteract diffusion of sodium and water into and potassium out of the cell through the permeable cell membrane. Any failure in the pump results in an influx of cations and water in an attempt to reach equilibrium with the environment, an event that ultimately leads to rupture of the cell.

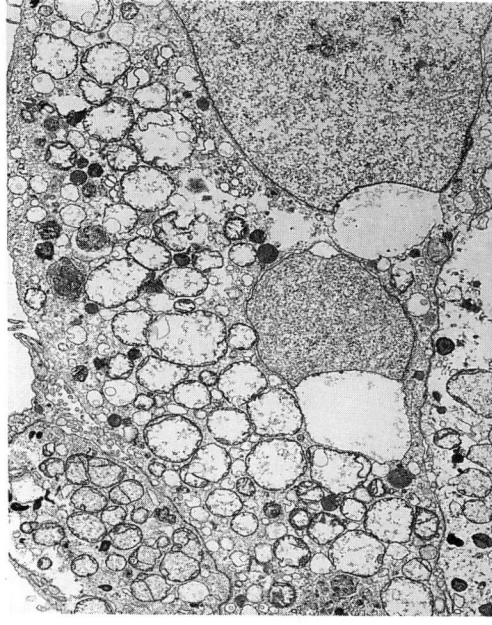

FIG. 1-7 Acute cellular swelling in a hepatocyte with irreversible cell injury. Note the pallor of nuclear chromatin, swelling and saccular dilatation of the perinuclear cysterna, cytosol, mitochondria and RER due to influx of extracellular water (hydropic change) ($\times$ 12,000).

In cases of hypoxia and other forms of injury, mitochondrial function is disrupted, curtailing the availability of ATP, without which the ion pumps fail. Temporarily, the anaerobic glycolytic pathway supplies ATP, but the release of lactic and other organic acids and the drop in intracellular pH results in enzyme inhibition, especially of the enzyme phosphofructokinase, further curtailing the ATP production. Glycolysis results in a **decrease in cellular glycogen,** which is one of the earliest recognizable events in all cell injury. The decrease in cellular pH causes clumping of nuclear chromatin and inactivation of nuclear RNA synthesis.

Diminished activity of the ion pump is followed by an influx of sodium and calcium into the cell and diffusion of potassium and magnesium out of the cell. The increased water content causes dilation of the cysternae of endoplasmic reticulum, disruption of the cell membrane from the cytoskeleton, and progressive swelling of the cell. Structures, such as microvilli, become distorted and form fluid-filled **blebs.** The decrease in ATP also results in decreased protein synthesis, further augmented by the loss of potassium. Mitochondrial membranes become more permeable, allowing water to diffuse into their matrix, causing them to swell. The change in mitochondrial and lysosomal membrane permeability results in leakage of enzymes into the cytosol, through the altered cell membrane into the extracellular space, and ultimately, into the blood. For certain tissues, elevated serum levels of specific soluble enzymes provide a clinical diagnostic measurement that confirms the existence of cell injury and, because of the tissue specificity of certain of their isozymes, often identifies the affected organ.

Calcium enters the injured cell and precipitates with phosphate on internal cell membranes, and activates endogenous phospholipase, an enzyme involved in the normal turnover of cell membranes. This, in turn, degrades phospholipids from the cell membrane, resulting in further damage and dysfunction. Unesterified free fatty acids that accumulate in the cytosol as the result of the breakdown of membrane phospholipids further damage the cell membranes by their detergent effect. The increase in cytosolic free calcium resulting from membrane damage is thought to be the most critical factor in determining cell death. A number of enzymes involved in degrading various components of the cell are known to be calcium-dependent and, hence, may be activated by the increased concentration of this cation.

At this stage, the cell has become irreversibly damaged (i.e., reached the "point of no return") and is dead. The interval between initiation of cell injury and the point of no return varies tremendously depending on the cause of injury and the metabolic rate and function of the affected cells. For example, in neurons deprived of oxygen this interval is as short as 5 minutes, whereas for fibroblasts deprived of oxygen it may be many hours.

Changes in Organelles. After cell death, lysosomes begin to swell and hydrolytic enzymes diffuse through their membranes, initiating the process of **autolysis**

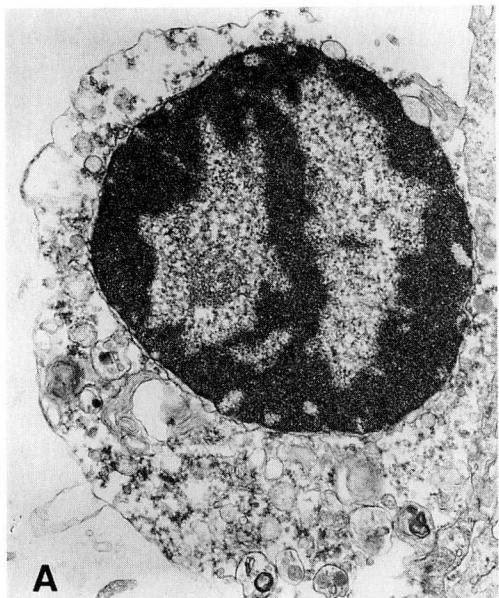
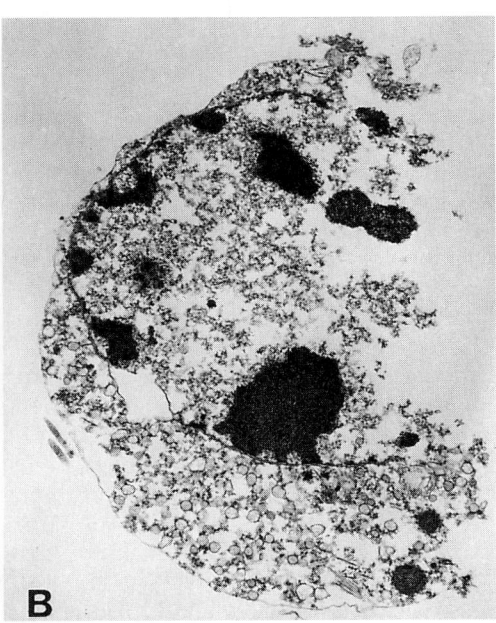

FIG. 1-8 Ultrastructural changes of necrosis. **A.** Pyknosis. Nucleus is shrunken, chromatin is more electron-dense than normal, and cytoplasm shows hydropic change and myelin figures (× 12,000). **B.** Karyorrhexis. Nuclear and cell membranes are disrupted. Note fragmentation of the chromatin into irregular electron-dense masses (× 12,000).

(self-digestion) and resulting in further coagulation and degradation of cellular proteins and nucleic acids in the nucleus and cytosol (Fig. 1-8). In the past, it was postulated that this form of cell death was the result of lysosomal enzyme release (the suicide-bag hypothesis); however, it is now accepted that enzyme release occurs subsequent to cell death.

Several other morphologic changes occur at or about this point: (1) ribosomes become detached from the RER membranes; (2) mitochondria and other organelles swell; (3) large fluid-filled blebs devoid of organelles protrude from the plasma membrane; (4) breaks eventually occur in the nuclear and plasma membranes, causing these structures to rupture; (5) nuclear chromatin loses its density; (6) dense inclusions representing calcium deposits appear in the swollen mitochondria; and (7) myelin figures may form. Myelin figures occur when hydrophilic phospholipids released from cell membranes into the aqueous medium of the cytosol form concentric lamellar whorls of membranes resembling myelin.

These events appear to be common to most forms of cell injury. A partial exception is direct damage to the cell membrane by blunt force or trauma, by certain chemical agents, or by certain forms of immunologic injury. Here, the loss of membrane integrity is immediate and cellular swelling more rapid, both occurring before a decrease in ATP.

When these morphologic changes occur in cells or tissues of a living organism, the process is termed **necrosis** and the cells or tissues are referred to as **necrotic.** However, when similar morphologic changes occur diffusely in tissues and organs after death of an organism, the processes are referred to as **postmortem autolysis.**

Products of putrefactive bacteria can result in further decomposition of tissues after somatic death. The challenge to the pathologist is in distinguishing antemortem from postmortem tissue changes.

During the course of becoming necrotic, dead cells leak various chemical substances, known collectively as **mediators of inflammation,** into the interstitial fluid. These mediators are highly chemotactic for neutrophils circulating in venules of the adjacent living tissues. Sensing the presence of these mediators through their action on endothelial cells, neutrophils initially stick to the endothelium, then migrate out of the vessels, and following a concentration gradient of the mediator, migrate toward the necrotic cells by a process known as **leukotaxis** (see inflammation discussion for further details regarding the biochemical mechanisms involved in this process). The presence of neutrophils in and around cells with morphologic changes consistent with necrosis distinguishes necrotic cells from cells that have undergone postmortem autolysis. Neutrophils indicate that the organism was alive at the time of and for at least 12 hours after the death of the cells or tissues occurred.

Cell injury induced by free radicals Tissue injury and death induced by free radicals occur by means of chemical and radiation injury, oxygen toxicity, and the aging process and during killing of microbial agents and tumor cells by phagocytic inflammatory cells. Free radicals are chemical species having a single unpaired electron in an outer orbit. The unpaired electron makes them unstable and extremely reactive with many inorganic and organic chemicals, particularly membrane lipids and proteins and nucleotides of DNA. Free radicals are notorious for initiating autocatalytic reactions, in which the chemicals with which free radicals react are, in turn, converted to free radicals and thus are made available to propagate cell injury. These highly reactive chemicals are generated within cells by exposure to radiation, by intracellular oxidative reactions that occur with normal metabolic processes, and by enzymatic degradation of exogenous chemicals and drugs. Most free radicals that are important in the induction of biologic injury are toxic intermediates derived from oxygen. The three most important are: (1) superoxide (O_2-), generated by autooxidative and oxidase reactions in the mitochondria and cytoplasm respectively, and neutralized by the enzyme superoxide dismutase; (2) hydrogen peroxide (H_2O_2), generated by dismutation of O_2- by superoxide dismutase and by catalase reactions occurring in peroxisomes; and (3) hydroxyl ions ($OH\cdot$), resulting from hydrolysis of water by ionizing radiation and interaction of hydrogen peroxide with certain metals, especially iron and copper. All of these compounds are capable of causing peroxidation of cell and organelle membranes, inactivation of critical cellular enzymes, and damage to DNA. The net result is that the cell becomes irreversibly damaged as a consequence of influx of water, electrolytes, and calcium into the cytosol; the cell swells, passes the point of no return, and undergoes changes similar, if not identical, to those seen in hypoxic cell injury, and eventually becomes necrotic.

Cell injury induced by chemicals Exogenous chemicals that induce cell injury and death do so by one of two methods: (1) binding directly to critical structural or reactive chemicals of cellular organelles and thereby damaging cell membranes or the ability of the cell to generate the ATP and energy that are required for maintenance of normal homeostasis and function; or (2) by being chemically transformed to more reactive metabolites that are capable of generating free radicals, which subsquently cause permanent membrane damage and cell death as previously described.

Cell injury induced by viruses Two types of viruses cause cell injury and death. **Cytolytic viruses** cause cell death by: (1) interfering with the ability of a cell to synthesize proteins and other macromolecules essential to maintaining cell life; (2) redirecting organelles of the cell to preferentially synthesize viral RNA, DNA, and structural proteins needed for replication and assembly of the virus; (3) mechanically damaging cellular organelles and disrupting the cytoskeleton with accumulations of large amounts of viral nucleic acids and proteins (**viral inclusion bodies**), some of which are themselves cytotoxic; and (4) inserting viral-encoded proteins in cell membranes, causing them to malfunction and leak.

Viruses that are **noncytolytic** in cell cultures may indirectly cause cell death *in vivo* by stimulating the host's immune response to viral antigens expressed on the surface of infected cells. In these situations, cell killing can be mediated either by a humoral or cellular immune response. In the humoral immune response, antibody directed toward viral antigens on the surfaces of cells acting in concert with the complement system (**complement-dependent cytolysis**) generates a membrane attack complex that causes infected cells to leak and swell as in accidental cell death. In addition, the Fc fragment of antibody bound to infected cells can also interact with leukocytes, such as macrophages, neutrophils, eosinophils, and natural killer (NK) cells, to cause death of virally infected cells (**antibody-dependent cell-mediated cytotoxicity**). Finally, virally infected cells may also be killed by **cell-mediated cytoxicity,** in which sensitized cytotoxic T-lymphocytes or NK cells bind to cells expressing specific viral antigens on their membranes. The mechanism by which virally infected cells are killed by cell-mediated cytotoxicity is different from antibody-mediated killing and is termed **apoptosis.**

APOPTOSIS Unlike accidental cell death caused by hypoxia, apoptosis tends to involve individual or small clusters of cells of a specific type. The precise biochemical and molecular events involved in this form of cell death are not yet fully elucidated. Although apoptosis is often referred to as genetically mediated or programmed cell death, the cytoplasmic changes that characterize apoptosis have been experimentally induced in cells from which the nuclei have been removed. This finding suggests that transcription of new genes and synthesis of their products are not essential for induction of apoptosis under all circumstances. Other evidence indicates that the protein molecules involved in the induction of apoptosis are constitutively expressed in mammalian cells but are normally rendered inactive by other proteins referred to as **antiapoptotic proteins,** which are synthesized by the same cell, possibly in response to so-called survival signals received from neighboring cells, the extracellular substrates, or fluid. These survival signals include growth factors, the extracellular matrix, and a variety of hormones. Loss of these factors spontaneously initiates apoptosis.

As previously mentioned, apoptosis may be physiologic and represent a mechanism by which a balance between cell growth and cell death is maintained, or it may be pathologic and deleterious to the host. Evidence is mounting that inhibition of apoptosis may be as important as amplified oncogene expression in the pathogenesis of certain neoplastic diseases. Although apoptosis may be initiated by many different extrinsic and intrinsic signals, these signal pathways converge at some point to activate a common genetically controlled apoptotic program. The genes and gene products responsible for apoptosis are presumed to be constitutively expressed in all cells and are tightly regulated by products of other genes. In mammalian species, proteins encoded by the *Bcl-2* family of genes are known to be potent inhibitors of apoptosis and, thus, are referred to as **antiapoptotic genes.** The first gene of this family was shown to be overexpressed in B-cell lymphomas (hence its name) as a consequence of the 14–18 chromosomal translocation that occurs in this neoplasm. Related genes have been found and studied extensively in animal species as low as the fruit fly (*Drosophila* species) and the nematode (*Caenorhabditis elegans*). Conservation of genes that regulate apoptosis over such a wide range of phylogenetic species attests to their vital importance in biology.

CELL SHRINKAGE In contrast to the acute swelling of cytoplasm and organelles that characterizes accidental cell death caused by hypoxia, apoptosis is characterized by **cell shrinkage.** The sodium-potassium ion pumps are not affected initially in this form of cell death and membranes remain intact. The proteins responsible for apoptosis, when released from the inhibitory effects of the antiapoptotic proteins, cause activation of cellular proteases that disrupt the cytoskeleton and cause the cell to shrink.

CHANGES IN ORGANELLES Cellular endonucleases are also activated early in apoptosis. Although not seen microscopically, these enzymes cleave the cell's DNA between nucleosomes, giving rise to fragments consisting of 180 to 200 base pairs. These fragments migrate in a characteristic ladder pattern when separated on agarose gel, in contrast to the heterogeneous fragments of degraded DNA that occur with accidental cell death.

Ultrastructurally, the nucleus of an apoptotic cell undergoes several characteristic alterations. The chromatin of apoptotic cells becomes markedly electron-dense and often assumes a half-moon configuration just beneath the intact nuclear membrane. The nuclei may also break up into multiple dense, membrane-bound masses, in contrast to the karyorrhexis seen in accidental death in which the nuclear membrane is disrupted (Figs. 1-9, 1-10, 1-11).

During the shrinkage process, the plasma membrane of an apoptotic cell emits small pseuopodia referred to as buds, rather than the blebs seen in hypoxic death. These pinch off from the shrunken remains of the apoptotic cell and give rise to **apoptotic bodies,**

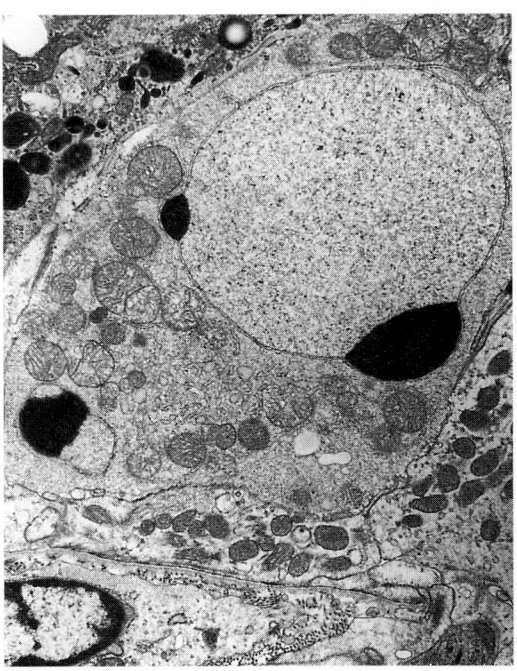

FIG. 1-10 An apoptotic epithelial cell at the tip of an intestinal villus. Characteristic nuclear changes: dense clumping of chromatin in crescent-shaped masses beneath intact nuclear membrane; fragmentation of nucleus into multiple nuclear membrane-bound chromatin (apoptotic) bodies ($\times$ 9600).

which are membrane-bound and contain organelles including mitochondria and intact lysosomes as well as masses of condensed chromatin surrounded by a nuclear membrane. Many of the same tinctorial changes seen in the nuclei and cytoplasm of necrotic cells are

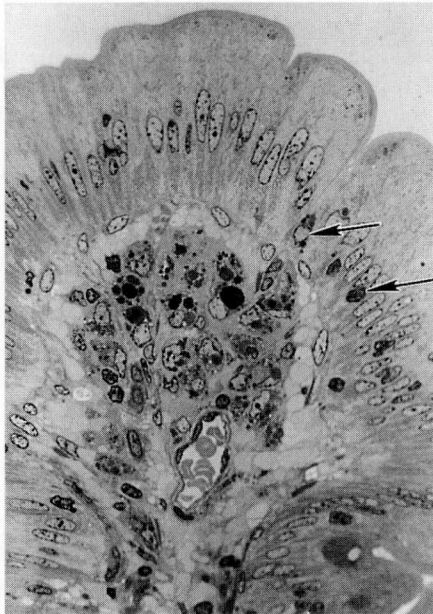

FIG. 1-9 One-micron plastic-embedded section of the tip of an intestinal villus. Note several apoptotic cells in the epithelium (*arrow*) and multiple macrophages in the lamina propria containing phagocytized apoptotic bodies ($\times$ 800). (Toluidine blue stain)

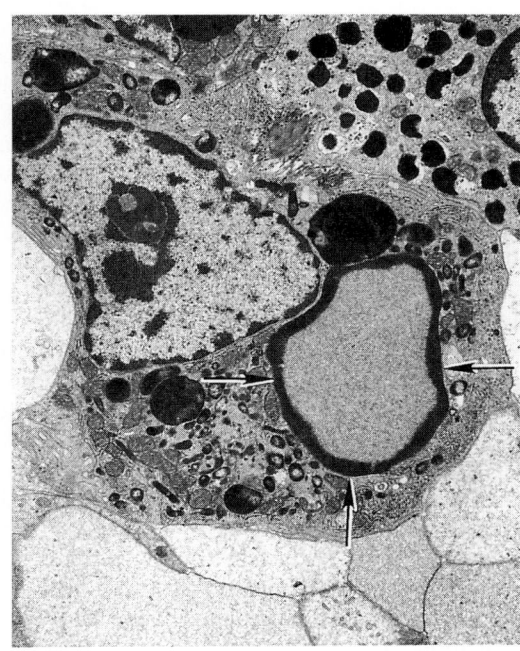

FIG. 1-11 Tingible-body macrophages in lamina propria of intestinal villus containing multiple phagocytized apoptotic bodies. Note characteristic apoptotic changes in one phagocytized nuclear body (*arrows*) ($\times$ 7200).

also seen in the bits of degraded chromatin and cytoplasm found in apoptotic bodies. Because the usual mediators of inflammation do not leak from these bodies, they do not evoke a perceptible inflammatory reaction. Instead they are picked up, much like any foreign particle would be, by scavenger macrophages and degraded within their phagolysosomes. Occasionally, apoptotic bodies are ingested by and degraded within neighboring parenchymal cells. Hence, the remains of cells that have died of these two forms of cell death differ substantially.

CHARACTERISTICS OF NECROTIC CELLS AND TISSUES

As previously stated, a cell may be beyond the point of no return, and therefore dead, before it can be recognized as such by routine microscopic examination. The microscopic changes that occur in dead tissue as a consequence of antemortem autolysis are collectively known as necrosis. Cells and tissues exhibiting these changes are referred to as **necrotic.**

Microscopic features of necrosis

We have chosen to present the microscopic changes associated with necrosis before presenting the gross changes in order to emphasize that, if the microscopic appearance is known, the gross picture may usually be deduced with some degree of accuracy, whereas the converse is not necessarily true.

CHANGES IN THE NUCLEUS

There are a variety of light microscopic changes that indicate cell necrosis in the nucleus of a dead cell. These changes are referred to by terms that describe specific microscopic appearances of the affected nuclei. However, it should not automatically be assumed that every nucleus goes through each of these stages before finally disappearing from the tissue. The nuclear changes include the following processes.

Pyknosis This is one of the more common nuclear alterations seen in dead cells, but it is not seen in all dead cells. The pyknotic nucleus is **decreased in size, round,** and homogeneously dark blue to black (**hyperchromatic**) when stained with hematoxylin and eosin. These changes occur because the nucleic acid component of chromatin has been enzymatically stripped of its associated nucleoproteins, is thus more acidic, and attracts more of the basic hematoxylin. The chromatin of a pyknotic nucleus is condensed; it is confined by a damaged nuclear membrane and lacks separation into euchromatin and heterochromatin components. The nucleolus is no longer visible. Pyknosis is seen best in dead epithelial cells, mononuclear inflammatory cells, and nerve cells. The elongated nuclei of connective tissue and muscle cells usually do not become round, but the loss of internal structure, condensation, and hyperchromasia of chromatin are obvious indicators that they are necrotic.

Karyorrhexis The term karyorrhexis is used to describe fragmentation of chromatin into tiny basophilic granules as a consequence of rupture of the nuclear membrane. It may occur *de novo,* or succeed pyknosis. The fragmented bits of chromatin may remain in the original position of the nucleus or be scattered throughout the cytoplasm of the necrotic cell and adjacent areas. Karyorrhexis is a prominent finding in abcesses and purulent exudates, in which the segmented nuclei of neutrophils readily break up into fragments indicating death of the cell.

Karyolysis Karyolysis is dissolution, or lysis, of the nuclear chromatin by nucleases released from leaking lysosomes of dead cells. The solubilized chromatin diffuses out of the leaky nuclear membrane into cytosol and interstitial fluids. When karyolysis is complete, the nuclear membrane disappears, but the term karyolysis is used to refer to the earlier stages, in which the nucleus appears as a hollow sphere surrounded by a faint outline, or ghost, of the nuclear membrane.

Loss of the nucleus All of the nuclear changes described above are hallmarks of a dead cell and eventually lead to loss of the nucleus. Platelets and erythrocytes are exceptions in that these cells are generally regarded as alive, even though they lack a nucleus, the ability to divide, and other characteristics of life (Fig. 1-12).

CHANGES IN THE CYTOPLASM

In some cases, the cytoplasm of a dead cell may not appear altered, but if its nucleus has any of the changes described above, the cell is dead. The following cytoplasmic alterations may be seen in necrotic cells.

Depletion of cytoplasmic glycogen One of the earliest events in hypoxic cell injury is depletion of intracellular glycogen caused by the switch from aerobic to anaerobic glycolysis. In normal cells, glycogen, a water-soluble carbohydrate, is dissolved during formalin fixation, leaving irregularly shaped empty spaces in the cytoplasm. In cells that have metabolically depleted glycogen before fixation, the cytosol and cytoplasmic organelles move into spaces previously occupied by glycogen so that the cytoplasm appears homogeneous rather than irregularly vacuolated after fixation. This change occurs before death of a cell and therefore may be reversible; it obviously persists after death of the cell and, thus, precedes the nuclear and cytoplasmic changes of necrosis.

Increased eosinophilia of cytoplasm The cytoplasm of a necrotic cell is often more eosinophilic than is the cytoplasm of a living cell. This is, in part, because of the enzymatic degradation of cytoplasmic RNA, which usually imparts a degree of basophilia to the cytoplasm. In addition, denaturation of cytoplasmic proteins gives rise to polypeptide chains having increased numbers of reactive sites for eosin. Together these factors account for the increased eosinophilia of the cytoplasm of a necrotic cell. This sign of necrosis is prominent when highly specialized epithelial cells, such as those of renal tubules and liver, undergo coagulation necrosis. The cytoplasm of necrotic neutrophils comprising pus often appears more red than normal.

Cytoplasmolysis As the changes characteristic of necrosis progress, the cytoplasm tends to become less

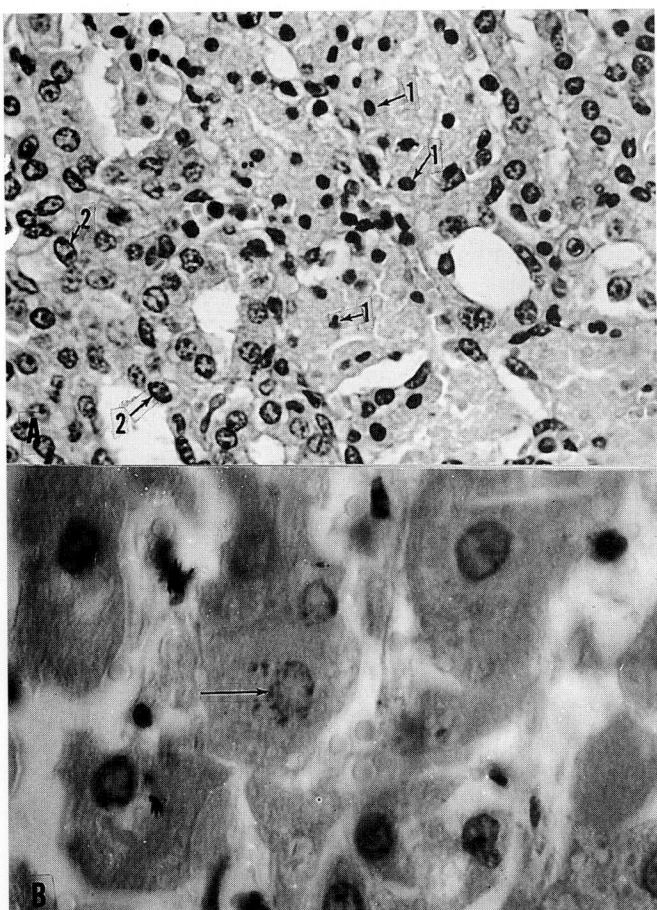

FIG. 1-12 Pyknosis and karyorrhexis. **A.** Pyknosis. Small, round, densely stained nuclei (1) at the margin of infarct in the pig kidney. Compare with the nuclei (2) of unaffected renal tubules (× 490). **B.** Karyorrhexis. Fragmentation of nuclear chromatin (*arrow*) in canine liver cell (× 800). (Courtesy of Lt. Col. F.D. Mauer, Armed Forces Institute of Pathology.)

and less dense and ultimately disappears completely. In some cases, it is possible for much of the cytoplasm to disappear while the cell remains alive, and therefore, the decision as to whether the cell is living or dead should depend on the appearance of the nucleus.

CHANGES IN THE WHOLE CELL

Loss of cell outline When the changes of necrosis are well advanced, it may be impossible to see the form and outline of the cells, although the material of which they are made obviously remains. In applying this criterion, pathologists should not be misled by failure to identify cell outlines, such as those in stratified squamous epithelium and smooth muscle, which are often indistinct in normal histologic specimens. This may be illustrated by the cells of an inflammatory exudate in which the nucleus or its remains is still visible but the shape and nature of the cell are quite unidentifiable. Complete loss of cell outline is seen in caseous necrosis of a tubercle.

Loss of differential staining Situations occur in which tissue can still be seen, but the nuclear and cytoplasmic colors, as well as those characteristic of different histologic tissues, cannot be distinguished. Chromatolysis is an important component of this process. The mucosa of an intestine involved either in necrosis or postmortem autolysis is an example: There is a stage in which the villi and glands are fairly well outlined, but no single individual cell or structure can be identified. This is an example of loss of both differential staining and cell outline.

Loss of cells If there is a detectable loss of cells in an organ or tissue, it must be assumed that they died and were removed by the combined processes of antemortem autolysis and heterolysis or by, as in the case of apoptosis, ingestion by macrophages or other phagocytic cells. Loss of cells from an organ or tissue has diagnostic significance if it involves the parenchyma as well as their surfaces. On surfaces of organs, such as the intestine and skin, where there is normally a high turnover of cells, dead cells lose their attachment to underlying structures and simply fall off the surface by a process termed **desquamation,** or sloughing. For example, enterocytes that reach the tips of villi undergo apoptosis, die, and desquamate into the lumen. Similarly, once keratinocytes reach the surface of the epidermis, they lose their nucleus, become keratinized, and desquamate as dried scales known as dander, or dandruff. The desquamated cells are rapidly replaced by others destined for the same fate. These cells have none of the changes that indicate necrosis; in such cases, the interval between cell death and desquamation is not sufficient for microscopic changes of necrosis to develop. However, cells often desquamate prematurely from an epithelium as the consequence of an underlying pathologic process, leaving the underlying basement membrane exposed. In these cases, the cells are regarded as necrotic. This occurs commonly in many forms of infectious bronchopneumonia and in enteric disorders in which the the mucosa often becomes denuded (of normal epithelium), eroded, or ulcerated.

Gross characteristics of dead tissue

LOSS OF COLOR

Dead tissue is typically paler than healthy tissue, except if it is filled with increased amounts of blood: then it may appear to be black. The pallor is caused by hemolysis of erythrocytes in areas of necrotic tissue in which normal amounts of blood were present and by diffusion of normally pigmented substances, such as myoglobin (present in striated muscle), from the cytosol of necrotic cells as a result of breakdown of cell membranes. However, if a large amount of hemolyzed blood is present in the necrotic tissue, it will impart a blackish-red color to the affected area.

LOSS OF STRENGTH

Necrotic tissue has less tensile strength than nonnecrotic tissue, because of the enzymatic digestion of the cytoskeleton, cell membranes, and intercellular connections. Sometimes, in removing the intestine from a cadaver at autopsy, a length of intestine that is necrotic because of obstruction or infarction or the entire intestine that is damaged by advanced postmortem autolysis may be too weak to support its own weight and may pull apart as it is raised. A finger may be easily thrust into a liver or lung that has undergone these changes.

ODORS

Odors of putrefaction may emanate from dead tissue colonized by saprophytic bacteria after gangrene or postmortem autolysis occur. This is because foul-smelling compounds, such as hydrogen sulfide, ammonia, and mercaptans (all by-products of bacterial fermentation of organic tissues, especially proteins) have formed.

NECROSIS

Although gross changes in physical consistency, such as coagulation, caseation, and liquefaction, often characterize necrotic tissue, these changes may sometimes be a result of postmortem autolysis. For example, brains sent to the laboratory without first being preserved by fixation or freezing often arrive in a state of complete liquefaction. This results from extensive postmortem hydrolysis of nervous tissue, the membranes of which contain high concentrations of lipids (Fig. 1-13).

DIFFERENTIATION OF NECROSIS AND POSTMORTEM AUTOLYSIS

Microscopic appearance

The following observations permit differentiation of tissues that died while the patient was still alive (i.e., necrotic tissue) from tissues that have undergone nonspecific biochemical degradation that occurs in all tissues

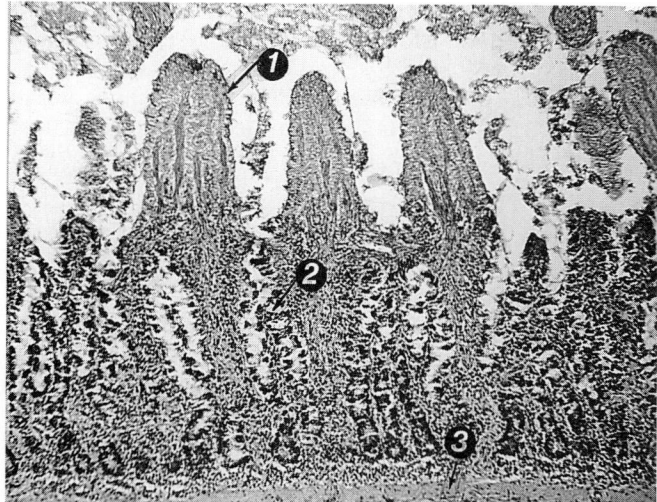

FIG. 1-13 Postmortem autolysis, canine small intestine. Villi (1) are denuded of epithelium, which is still present in crypts (2). Muscularis mucosae (3) (× 90). (Courtesy of Dr. R. O. Delano, Armed Forces Institute of Pathology)

not promptly preserved after the patient's death (i.e., the process of postmortem autolysis).

If tissue of healthy appearance is found along with degenerating tissue in the same section, the degenerate area represents necrosis and not postmortem autolysis; however, things are not always so simple. Postmortem autolysis sometimes has a decidedly patchy distribution, which can be deceiving and justifies reliance on other criteria to distinguish antemortem from postmortem death of tissue.

Erythrocytes within the blood vessels should be examined for sharpness of outline and for the degree to which they absorb the stain. The presence of hemolyzed erythrocytes in blood vessels of both apparently normal and abnormal areas of the tissue section is highly suggestive of some degree of postmortem autolysis, as such erythrocytes are not normally not found in the circulation. Formalin-fixed erythrocytes stained with hematoxylin and eosin should stain a bright copper-red; with mercuric chloride fixation, they should be rose-red. Alcohol fixation, however, hemolyzes erythrocytes, causing them to appear as empty circles, regardless of the stain used. Erythrocytes separated by hemorrhage from the circulation and their source of oxygen also undergo hemolysis within the living body, thus indicating the importance of examining both apparently normal and abnormal areas of tissue.

Dead tissue leaks chemical mediators of inflammation that cause local vasodilatation and vascular engorgement and attract inflammatory cells to the site. Thus, infiltration of inflammatory cells, mainly neutrophils, at the junction between living and necrotic tissue is a useful finding in identifying necrosis.

Knowledge of the relative rates at which postmortem autolysis affects different tissues also may be of assistance in distinguishing necrosis from postmortem autolysis. The mucosa of the intestine, gallbladder, and parenchyma of the pancreas undergo postmortem changes early because the usual intracellular autolysis is abetted by the action of the now uninhibited digestive juices. The adrenal medulla undergoes early postmortem liquefaction, so that it is not unusual to examine an otherwise rather well-preserved adrenal gland and find only a collapsed space where the medulla should be. Neurons are probably the next tissue to show changes of postmortem autolysis; connective tissue is among the last to do so. In the kidney, autolysis proceeds more rapidly in the (metabolically more active) epithelium of the proximal convoluted tubules than in the (less active) distal tubules.

Gross appearance

A common problem at autopsy is determining how long the animal has been dead. Enzymatic reactions that occur with autolysis and putrefaction are greatly inhibited by the low temperatures of refrigerators, but are vastly accelerated by high ambient environmental temperatures. Sheep have serious postmortem changes very early because the insulating effect of fleece prevents dissipation of body heat; the same is true of large swine, as a result of the insulating layer of fat. Postmortem changes proceed with unusual rapidity if the body temperature is very high at the time of death (e.g., heat stroke), if it continues to rise even after death (e.g., tetanus), or if potentially putrefactive organisms, such as *Clostridium septicum,* are disseminated through the blood at the time of, or possibly before, death. The latter phenomenon has, at times, resulted in a postmortem picture so startling as to be called "black disease," a name attributed to the almost universal blackish discoloration of congested, autolyzed tissues seen on removal of the animal's skin. "Pulpy-kidney disease" has been described in sheep when autolytic and putrefactive softening have especially involved the kidneys. Whether or not pathologists observe other specific changes in these animals, they have found that kidneys in such a state are severely congested amd contain large numbers of clostridial organisms.

If the digestive tract of herbivorous animals is filled with ingesta, fermentation and gas formation may cause great distention of the digestive tract within a few hours and concordant distention of the torso, pressing bloody foam out of the nostrils and causing the rectal lining to protrude in a pseudoprolapse. Distention caused by postmortem fermentation must be distinguished from that occuring with antemortem bloating (tympanites), a frequent cause of death in ruminants. Signs of anoxia usually accompany bloating that occurred during life.

When postmortem changes are well advanced, the muscles are softened, pale red, watery, and resemble meat that has been cooked slightly. An indication that postmortem autolysis is only moderately advanced is **postmortem imbibition,** which results from the hemolysis of erythrocytes in blood vessels. The hemoglobin that is released goes into solution in the blood plasma and, at the same time, the walls of the blood vessels become more permeable to fluids as the result of postmortem autolysis. Consequently, the red-tinged plasma diffuses out into surrounding tissues and is "imbibed" by them. The result is a distinct, dark red fringe along the course of blood vessels, which is seen most readily in white tissues, such as the mesentery or omentum. "Imbibition of bile" is a similar leaking of bile through the autolyzed wall of the gallbladder, staining adjacent liver tissue a greenish hue to a variable depth.

Additional clues may be gained on opening the heart. Ordinarily, rigor mortis contracts the left ventricle strongly and empties it of blood. The right ventricle remains more or less filled with blood and, when this blood is hemolyzed a few hours after death, the ventricular lining assumes an intense red color that does not wash off. If the left ventricle contains unclotted blood, rigor mortis has not yet occurred and death was recent. However, after a lapse of 24 to 72 hours (depending on the ambient temperature), the rigor has come and gone, allowing dark, hemolyzed blood from the disintegrating clot to run back into the left ventricle; this indicates prolonged postmortem autolysis. If the left ventricle contains clotted blood, the contractile forces of the myocardium were too low at the time of death for rigor mortis to develop, as is often the case with lingering illnesses.

In the rumen, reticulum, and omasum of ruminants, an impressive sign of postmortem autolysis is desquamation of the epithelium. Within a surprisingly short time after death, this comparatively thick surface layer is completely displaced by the slightest touch.

The cause of postmortem autolysis is obvious. The goals of pathologists are (1) to avoid it or at least minimize it, if at all possible, and (2) to distinguish it correctly from necrosis.

Forms of NECROSIS
Coagulation necrosis

Coagulation necrosis results when denaturation of cellular protein proceeds to denaturation of hydrolytic enzymes as well, thus halting the process of autolysis. Loss of water also favors denaturation without further decomposition. The remaining coagulated tissue ultimately is slowly liquefied through the process of heterolysis. Coagulation necrosis may not be evident in animals that died from diseases in which large numbers of neutrophils liquify dead tissues by means of heterolysis.

MICROSCOPIC APPEARANCE
The normal architecture of tissue with its cellular components is still recognizable, but the nuclei and cytoplasm exhibit characteristic changes. The nuclei appear karyolytic, pyknotic, or karyorrhectic or they may be absent. The cytoplasm is often strongly acidophilic.

GROSS APPEARANCE
The necrotic tissue is gray or white (unless filled with blood), firm, dense, and often depressed compared with surrounding living tissue.

CAUSES
Causes that especially tend to produce this variety of necrosis include: (1) local ischemia, as in infarcts; (2) toxic products of certain bacteria, as in calf diphtheria, necrophorus enteritis, and other forms of necrobacillosis; (3) certain locally acting poisons, such as mercuric chloride; (4) mild burns, whether produced by heat, electricity, or x-rays; and (5) Zenker's necrosis of muscle.

Caseous necrosis

Caseous necrosis occurs as part of the typical lesions of tuberculosis, syphilis (in humans), ovine caseous lymphadenitis, and other granulomas. This type of necrosis results from a mixture of coagulated protein and lipid. Once the cause is resolved, the caseous material is slowly liquefied and removed.

MICROSCOPIC APPEARANCE
Microscopically, there is loss of cell outline and a loss of differential staining. Cell walls and other histologic structures disappear, and the tissue disintegrates to form a finely granular mass that has a purplish color

(hematoxylin and eosin stain), resulting from the mixture of blue chromatin material with red material derived from the cytoplasm. The normal architectural pattern of the tissue is totally obliterated in affected areas.

GROSS APPEARANCE

The gross appearance is white, grayish, or yellowish and is suggestive of "milk curds" or cottage cheese, hence the name caseous. The necrotic tissue is dry, slightly greasy, and firm, without any cohesive strength, rendering it easily separable into granular fragments with a blunt instrument.

CAUSE

Caseous necrosis is caused by locally acting toxins of specific microorganisms of the characteristic diseases described above.

Liquefactive necrosis

While most necrotic tissue slowly disappears by a process of insidious and imperceptible liquefaction, there are situations in which this change proceeds rapidly with accumulation of measurable amounts of fluid and without any noticeable precursory change in the dying cells. This process is known as liquefaction necrosis.

The two principal sites for noticeable liquefaction of dying tissue are the central nervous system and abscesses. Areas of liquefactive necrosis sometimes occur in tuberculous lungs, producing cavities of considerable size.

MICROSCOPIC APPEARANCE

The necrotic area, large or small, appears as an empty space that not only is without any definitive lining but also has frayed and irregular edges and, usually, cells on the edge that may show some features of necrosis. A pink-staining proteinaceous precipitate may or may not remain from the liquid. The water is removed in the process of tissue dehydration preparatory to sectioning. In the case of an abscess, the liquid contains large numbers of neutrophils whose hydrolytic enzymes have liquified areas of dead tissue as well as themselves, leaving a liquified mass of cellular debris commonly referred to as pus.

GROSS APPEARANCE

The lesion is a cavity, small or large, containing fluid that is usually yellow-white and opaque. If the process is still in progress, the walls of the cavity are frayed and irregular and more or less softened. Such a fluid-filled space is not generally considered a cyst, since a true cyst involves the accumulation of fluid, usually a secretion, in a cavity that has a natural and permanent type of lining, usually epithelial. In liquefactive necrosis, the liquid usually is drained away by the lymphatics and the wall is merely the preexisting tissue in the process of disintegration. In an abscess, the liquefaction is a minor aspect compared with the accumulation of inflammatory exudate, which is of transcendent importance.

CAUSES

Liquefactive necrosis is caused by the same processes that cause general necrosis. The reason tissue liquefies in the brain and spinal cord almost as soon as it dies is thought to be the high lipid content and the low coagulable protein content of these tissues. Also, an acid reaction of the tissue is essential. Once neutrophils arrive at the necrotic tissue site, they extrude their primary granules (lysosomes) containing hydrolytic enzymes, which further degrade and liquify the remains of the necrotic cells as well as themselves. This digestion process by other cells is known as **heterolysis.** At this point, the coagulated remains of necrotic cells (**coagulation necrosis**) begin to undergo **liquefaction necrosis,** so that the liquified breakdown products can drain away via the circulation. In the case of abscesses, the liquefaction of tissue is attributable to liquefying toxins (lysins), which have been demonstrated for most of the bacteria responsible. The leukocytes, which comprise most of the inflammatory exudate, also produce hydrolytic enzymes that liquify dead cells. The liquefaction of old pulmonary tubercles may be regarded as an end stage of the type of caseous necrosis typically encountered, since all necrotic tissue tends ultimately to disappear by a slow process of liquefaction. However, secondary pyogenic infection and lytic substances produced by the bacteria probably play an important part in liquefaction necrosis in these tubercles (Fig. 1-14).

Necrosis of fat

When adipose tissue undergoes necrosis, the fat is often decomposed (perhaps slowly) into its two constituent radicals, fatty acid and glycerin. The fatty acid then combines in various proportions with metallic ions, chiefly sodium, potassium, and calcium, to form soaplike compounds. These compounds are not dissolved by the solvents used to remove fat from tissue during processing, hence the compounds persist.

MICROSCOPIC APPEARANCE

Sheets of lipocytes that are similar to those seen in normal adipose tissues may be observed; however, the lipid is replaced by solid, opaque material that is nearly homogeneous, but sometimes contains tiny, clear slits marking the site of dissolved fatty-acid crystals. The material takes on a bluish or a pinkish tinge, depending on the presence of sodium or potassium respectively, or purple, if calcium has been deposited. The nuclei tend to be pyknotic, but histologically are not of the ideal type to show this change clearly.

GROSS APPEARANCE

Adipose tissue that has undergone fat necrosis loses its shiny and semitranslucent appearance and becomes opaque, whitish, and solid or slightly granular.

CAUSES

Two causative mechanisms are recognized. The traditional **pancreatic necrosis of fat** occurs only in the abdominal cavity and is the result of the fat-splitting action of pancreatic lipase, which escapes from its proper

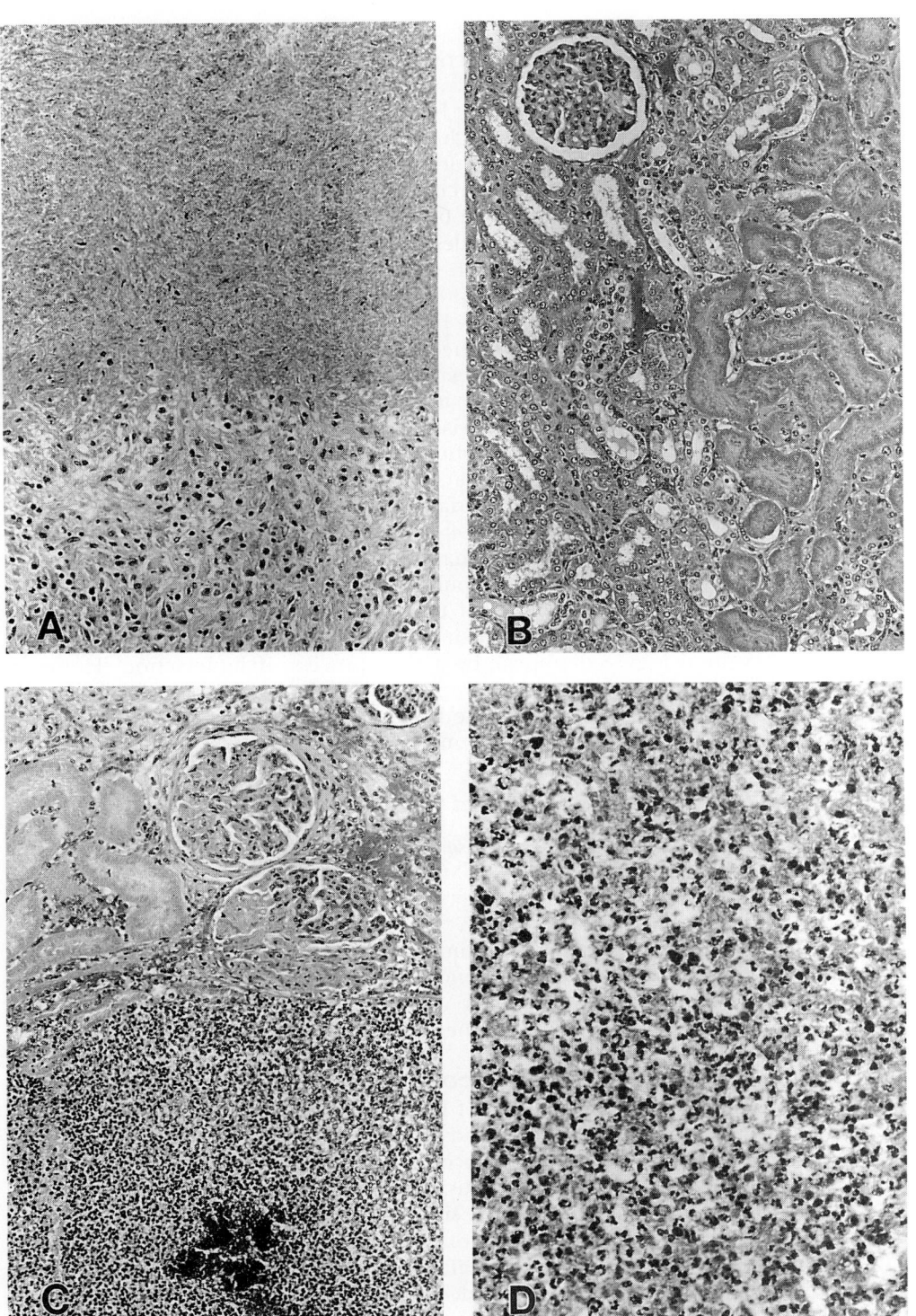

FIG. 1-14 Forms of necrosis. **A.** Caseation necrosis in center of tubercle in liver of rhesus monkey *(Macaca mulatta)* infected with *Mycobacterium tuberculosis.* The caseous exudate *(top)* is acellular and surrounded by a wall of epithelioid histiocytes *(bottom)* (× 200). **B.** Coagulation necrosis in renal infarct in rhesus monkey. Cells lining necrotic tubules *(right)* are devoid of stainable nuclei; viable tubules *(left)* contain nuclei (× 200). **C.** Liquefactive necrosis in staphylococcal abscess in kidney of rhesus monkey. Note coagulative necrosis of tubules *(upper left)* and total liquefaction of renal parenchyma by neutrophils in abscess (× 200). **D.** Higher magnification of area of liquefaction necrosis. Note numerous pyknotic and karyorrhectic nuclei of necrotic neutrophils (× 350).

ducts and channnels because of some other lesion in the ductal system of the pancreas, such as inflammation or invasion by a neoplasm (Fig. 1-15). However, the same type of change occurs outside the abdominal cavity as a result of pressure and mechamical trauma of subcutaneous adipose tissue. This is termed **traumatic necrosis of fat** and is best exemplified in the subcutaneous and intermuscular fat of the sternal region of a cow that has spent a prolonged period in sternal recum-

bency. Another form of fat necrosis that occurs in animals (most often in cattle) is characterized by large masses or nodules of necrotic adipose tissue, particularly in the abdominal cavity or retroperitoneal tissue, in the absence of pancreatic disease. The resemblance of this lesion to tumors has resulted in the synonym **lipomatosis.** If extensive, the lesions can lead to intestinal stenosis. It has been suggested that the disease is the result of crystallization of fatty acids and their soaps

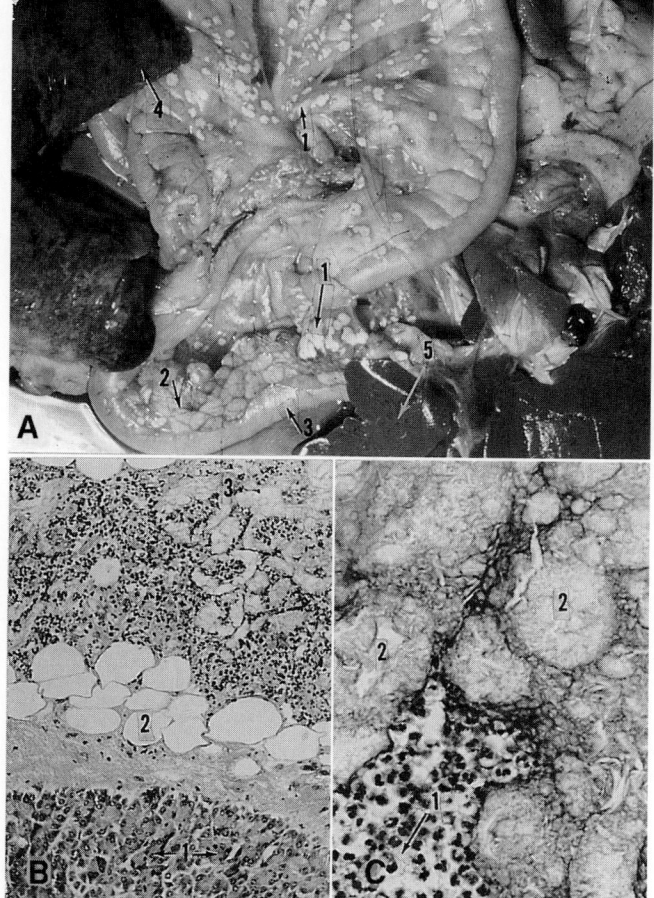

FIG. 1-15 Pancreatic necrosis of fat in mesentery of dog. **A.**Chalky appearing plaques (1), pancreas (2), duodenum (3), lung (4), and liver (5). **B.** Pancreas (1), normal fat cells (2) and necrotic fat (3) surrounded by leukocytes (× 165). **C.** Higher magnification of polymorphonuclear leukocytes (1) and necrotic (saponified) fat (2) (× 440). (**B.**and **C.,** Courtesy of Dr. Samuel Pollock, Armed Forces Institute of Pathology.)

when lipolysis exceeds the rate of fatty acid transport; thus, it differs from pancreatic or traumatic necrosis of fat.

SIGNIFICANCE

The presence of foci of fat necrosis in the abdominal cavity should prompt the pathologist to search for a related pancreatic lesion, although the nonpancreatic type can be found in this location as well (Fig. 1-15).

Zenker's necrosis

This condition, also known as **Zenker's degeneration,** occurs only in striated muscle. It is essentially coagulation of proteins of the sarcoplasm.

MICROSCOPIC APPEARANCE

The individual fibers are swollen and have a homo-

geneous hyaline or glassy appearance. The sarcoplasm is more eosinophilic than normal, devoid of characteristic cross-striations and obvious myofibrils, and nuclei are small and dark.

GROSS APPEARANCE

If the involved area is large enough to be recognized grossly, the muscle is pale tan to white, somewhat shiny and variably swollen.

CAUSES

The usual causes of Zenker's necrosis are toxins produced by pathogenic microorganisms, since this necrosis is often seen in conjunction with certain systemic or localized infections, but white-muscle diseases caused by certain nutritional deficiencies may present a similar change.

Disposition of necrotic tissue

Under exceptional circumstances, necrotic tissue may persist in the body for some time, but ultimately its disposal occurs by one of the following mechanisms.

1. Liquefaction by autolysis and heterolysis, and removal of the fluid by way of the blood and lymph. This is common when the number of dead cells in a given area at a given time is small; larger masses may gradually follow the same course. As previously stated, this is the rule in the central nervous system.
2. Liquefaction and formation of cystlike accumulations of fluid occur occasionally; the fluid accumulates faster than it is drained away.
3. Liquefaction with abscess formation occurs when necrosis is part of the damage inflicted by pyogenic bacteria. It is accompanied by formation of a purulent exudate. The tendency is for abscesses to rupture, the pus making its way to the nearest free surface along a path of subsequently developing necrosis in the overlying tissue.
4. Encapsulation without liquefaction. When there is little moisture, dead tissue may remain with little change, usually in the form of caseous or coagulative necrosis. The dead tissue acts as an irritant to the surrounding living tissue and incites a cellular (leukocytic) inflammatory reaction around it. Before many days pass, the reaction involves fibrosis and the formation of a fibrous capsule. Enclosed in this fibrous capsule, it may persist for a long time, causing the patient little or no harm. In addition to tubercles, dead helminth parasites within tissues are commonly encapsulated in this manner.
5. Desquamation or sloughing. Cells on an external or internal body surface regularly lose their attachment to underlying living tissue. Thin layers, such as an epithelial covering, desquamate (come off in flat, scalelike sheets). Larger and deeper masses of tissue "slough." Desquamated epithelial cells are often seen clumped together in the lumen of glands, ducts, bronchi, renal tubules, or intestine. The endothelial cells lining blood vessels behave similarly. Postmortem sloughing must be excluded.

6. Replacement by scar tissue is ultimately the terminal stage of abscesses, encapsulated areas, cystic cavities, infarcts, or diffuse tissue loss, such as occurs in the kidney and liver.
7. Calcification converts the dead tissue into a gritty mass. It is thus rendered inert and harmless, unless it is in a location where the hard and irregular material interferes mechanically with movement or the function of nearby structures.
8. Gangrene supervenes if areas become necrotic and are exposed directly or indirectly to external air and saprophytic bacteria.
9. Atrophy of the organ, tissue, or part naturally accompanies necrosis and the considerable loss of cells.
10. Regeneration, the formation of new cells like those lost, is a fortunate outcome in some cases. The regenerated cells are produced by mitosis of remaining cells that escaped or withstood the original necrotizing event. This is seen commonly on epithelial surfaces, in the lining cells of pulmonary alveoli and bronchi, and in the parenchymal cells of the liver and kidneys.

CHOLESTEROL CLEFTS

Cholesterol clefts may occur as by-products of necrosis, appearing as empty spaces left by crystals of cholesterol dissolved by solvents used in the preparation of the histologic specimen. The crystals have a characteristic shape: a flat, thin rhomboid plate with one corner cut out along lines parallel to the outer edges of the crystal. These spaces appear similar to shards of glass. The length and breadth of the space commonly falls between 50 and 100 mm with a thickness of 5 to 10 mm. In frozen sections where the cholesterol crystals are still present, they are anisotropic (birefringent) when viewed under polarized light.

Cholesterol is not usually grossly apparent, but in large amounts it is visible as shiny, yellowish, granular, or flaky material. Because the cholesterol that crystallizes in tissue comes from the decomposed cytoplasm and membranes of dead cells, these clefts are found in regions where considerable necrosis of cells relatively rich in that substance has occurred. Such regions include sites of old hemorrhages, old abscesses, and atheromas (Fig. 1-16).

Gangrene

Moist gangrene is a condition in which necrotic tissue is invaded by saprophytic and, usually, putrefactive bacteria. Necrotic tissue accessible to airborne bacteria is readily invaded; hence, we seldom speak of necrosis of limbs, ears, tails, lungs, intestines, or udder but rather of gangrene of these organs. **Microscopically,** the condition is recognized as a mixture of coagulation and liquefactive necrosis in which **large bacilli** (rod-shaped bacteria) are demonstrated. They need not be numerous. By ordinary hematoxylin and eosin stain, the bacteria are bluish, but much less so than nuclei, and hazy in outline as compared with results using specific stains

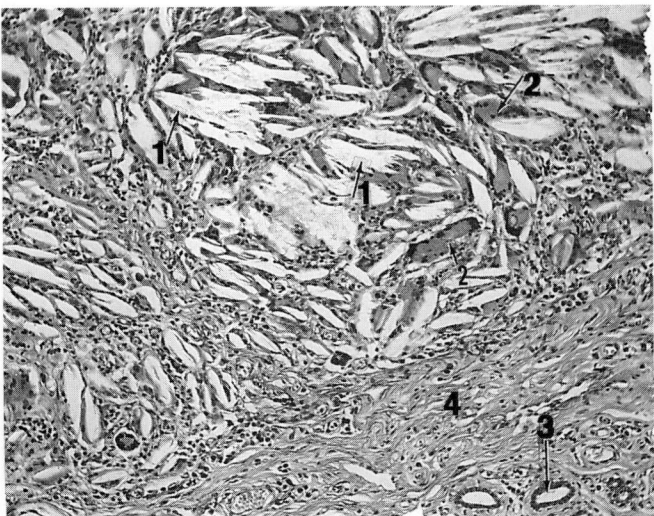

FIG. 1-16 Cholesterol clefts (1) at site of old hemorrhage and necrosis in canine mammary gland. Giant cells of foreign body type (2), mammary acini (3), connective tissue (4) (× 115). (Courtesy of Dr. W.H. Riser, Armed Forces Institute of Pathology)

for bacteria. Since many species of saprophytic bacteria are gas-formers, the gangrenous tissue may contain gas bubbles, recognizable as empty spaces of variable size having no wall of their own and tending to be spherical, but subject to distortion by the pressure of adjoining histologic structures.

The affected part, whether a limb or an area of lung or intestine, is swollen, soft, pulpy, and usually dark or black in color. It may have a foul, putrefactive odor, depending on the type of bacteria present. During life, an affected limb is cold and insensitive to touch or pain. This, the more frequent type of gangrene, occurs in tissues that are well-filled with blood at the time necrosis begins.

Dry gangrene occurs in tissues that have a limited content of blood and fluid or in tissues in which necrosis has developed slowly, with retardation of the natural circulation. Since dry tissue is not a favorable culture medium, the multiplication and spread of the bacteria is slow. The tissue becomes denatured or coagulated, and the part becomes cool, shrivelled, leathery, and discolored.

All areas of gangrene (moist and dry) are separated from the adjoining living tissue by **a sharp line of demarcation,** which is readily seen grossly, either during life or after death, as a swollen, reddish or bluish zone of hyperemia and inflammation.

CAUSES

The causes of gangrene are the causes of necrosis plus exposure to saprophytic bacteria. In the extremities and in the intestine, interference with the blood supply is the dominant cause. In the lungs and udder, toxic products of highly lethal bacteria are the usual causes. Irritant medicines intended for oral administration, but inadvertently inhaled, also set the stage in the lungs for the growth of both pathogenic and saprophytic microorganisms.

SIGNIFICANCE AND EFFECT

The principal therapeutic strategies are usually directed toward stopping the spread of the gangrenous process, which involves stopping the spread of cell death and necrosis, whatever the cause. Highly toxic substances are produced during bacterial decomposition of proteins in gangrenous tissue and elsewhere. These substances tend to be absorbed into the circulation of the adjoining living tissues, with disastrous consequences to the patient. Indeed, in a weakened and moribund patient, **sapremia** may occur: In this condition, saprophytic bacteria, which normally only grow in dead organic matter, are able to survive in the bloodstream and be disseminated throughout the living patient. For all of these reasons, amputation of a gangrenous extremity, even the udder, is often necessary to preserve the patient's life. In the intestine, early surgical removal of the gangrenous portion with anastomosis of healthy segments is the only hope for survival.

Nature also has its own way of dealing with gangrene in a patient with good resistance. As previously mentioned, the line of demarcation between viable and gangrenous tissue is an intense zone of inflammatory activity directed towards preventing bacterial colonization and killing of the healthy tissue. This involves recruitment of neutrophils as well as cellular and humoral immune reactions. These reactions are often successful, in which case separation of the dead tissue, even bone, eventually causes the gangrenous extremity to drop off, and the stump slowly heals. In dry gangrene, this is the usual outcome, and the process may involve no serious change in the general health of the individual (Fig. 1-17).

GAS GANGRENE

Several species of anaerobic spore-forming bacteria, classified in the genus *Clostridium,* have the capacity to grow in both dead and living tissues. Hence, they are both saprophytes and pathogens. They are able to kill animal tissue and to continue to multiply in it as saprophytes. They produce gas from constituents of the dead tissue, which appears as bubbles in the affected tissue. The group of diseases they produce are known as gas gangrenes, including specifically malignant edema and blackleg in animals and nonspecific wound infections in humans. They constitute examples of gangrene and necrosis occurring without the previous action of some other necrotizing agent.

Infarcts

An **infarct** is a localized area of tissue necrosis resulting from sudden obstruction of the blood supply to the affected area (**infarction**). It constitutes the most common naturally occurring example of hypoxic cell injury and death described earlier in this chapter. The necrosis is coagulative in type, but the affected tissue eventually passes through the entire sequence of changes described for removal of dead tissue. The area involved is ordinarily one supplied by a single "end artery" whose flow has been arrested, and the boundaries are, therefore, sharply delimited.

As the tissue dies, its capillary bed dies with it; thus, there is a reasonably well-circumscribed line with dead capillaries on one side and living on the other. A certain amount of blood diffuses back from the living into the dead capillaries, and these latter, being dead and without normal strength and resistance, permit the escape of blood into the surrounding necrotic tissue. Blood in the efferent veins doubtless flows back into the necrotic area in a similar way. Consequently, recent in-

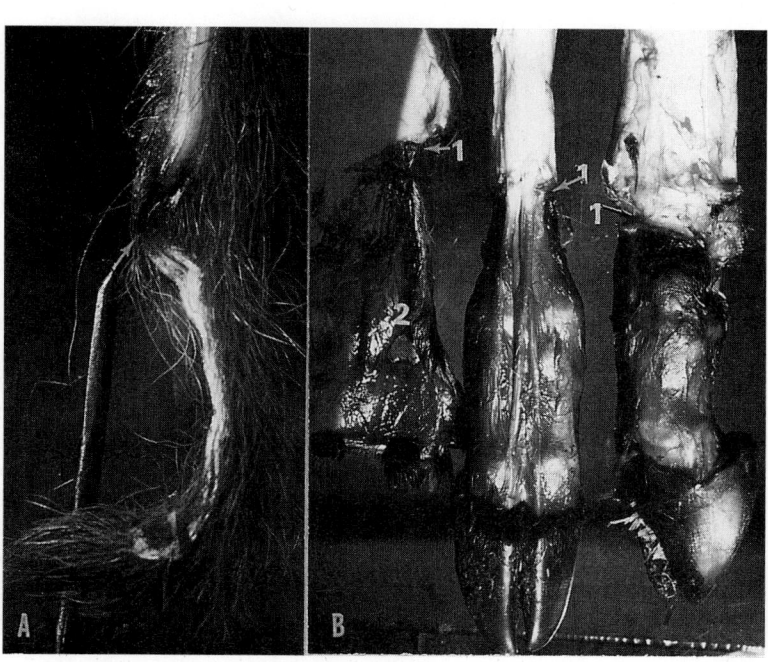

FIG. 1-17 Gangrene. **A.** Dry gangrene, ear (longitudinal section) of calf *(arrow)* following ergot poisoning. **B.** Moist gangrene, feet of same calf. Note sharp line of demarcation between black gangrenous and white living tissue (1); the skin, inside out, after removal (2).

farcts in some organs (e.g., spleen, lung) tend to fill with blood and thus are referred to as **hemorrhagic** or **red infarcts.** Other infarcts that occur in solid tissues, such as the kidney, appear paler than normal (**anemic** or **pale infarcts**) and are delineated by a peripheral rim of hemorrhage and congestion at the interface between necrotic and viable tissues.

MICROSCOPIC APPEARANCE

The picture is that of coagulative necrosis with or without the tissue spaces filled with blood, as just described. The shape of the necrotic area is that of the part supplied by the obstructed vessel beyond the point of obstruction. In sections of most organs, this is a triangular or wedge-shaped area with its apex near the point of obstruction and its base at or just beneath the organ's wall or capsule, which may have a sufficient blood supply of its own. Since necrotic tissue regularly releases a variety of mediators of inflammation into the adjacent viable tissues, an infarct more than 12 hours old is regularly surrounded by a zone of acute inflammation (hyperemia and neutrophil infiltration). Unfortunately for the diagnostician, this is sometimes mild. The smaller leukocytes must be carefully distinguished from the dark, angular fragments of nuclei of preexisting parenchymal cells, which, in the peripheral zone of an infarct, may remain for some time in a state of karyorrhexis rather than disappearing promptly by karyolysis. Old infarcts are chiefly fibrous. In the event that a small amount of blood continues to flow, any structure having previous access to it may survive as a living oasis in the necrotic desert. Renal glomeruli, for instance, may persist indefinitely, although other microscopic components of the kidney have long since disappeared (Fig. 1-18).

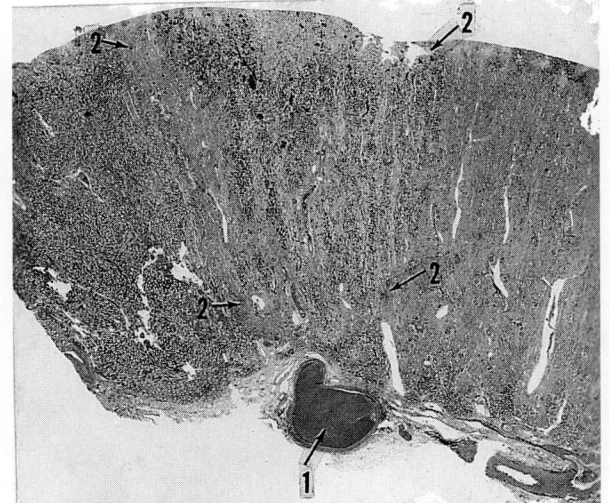

FIG. 1-18 Infarct in pig kidney infected experimentally with hog cholera virus. Note thrombus in arciform artery (1); margins of infarct *(arrows)* (2) (× 6). (Courtesy of Lt. Col. F.D. Maurer, Armed Forces Institute of Pathology)

GROSS APPEARANCE

The red or white color has already been described. Hemorrhagic infarcts may protrude slightly above the surrounding tissues; the pale ones tend to be slightly depressed. Old infarcts are decidedly sunken on the surface of the affected organ. In all cases they are sharply demarcated. In a three-dimensional view, the triangular shape seen microscopically is pyramidal or conical; the affected area, as seen on the surface of the organ, is likely to be irregular. The pale infarct is slightly denser and always tougher than the surrounding tissue; the hemorrhagic one may be softer.

CAUSE

By definition, an infarct is a localized area of coagulation necrosis resulting from obstruction of the blood supply to all or a portion of the affected organ. Most infarcts result from obstruction of arteries or arterioles that provide the only source of oxygenated blood to discrete portions of an organ, i.e., so-called end arteries. Examples of these include coronary arteries, renal arteries and their branches, and certain arteries of the brain. The most common cause of arterial occlusion in most animal species is a thrombus or embolus; in human beings, arterial damage from atherosclerosis is a major predisposing factor. Infarcts can also result secondarily from occlusion of the venous drainage of portions of an organ.

Possibly, there is some lack of precision in applying the term infarct to areas that become filled with blood because of external pressure sufficient to prevent the organ's venous outflow but not sufficient to obstruct completely the thicker-walled arteries. However, if the outflow of blood is obstructed, the accumulated blood soon becomes stagnant. In such cases, no more oxygen or other nutrients can be brought in and necrosis ensues. This is particularly common in segments of intestine in which the venous drainage becomes obstructed mechanically. In these instances, necrosis must be shown to be present in addition to tissues engorged with static blood in order to make it a true infarct, since it is the death of the tissue, rather than the filling with blood, that is of principal significance to the patient.

SPECIAL TYPES AND DIAGNOSIS

Infarcts of the kidney are typically conical with the apex near the corticomedullary junction and the path of the arcuate arteries. In dogs and pigs, an accompanying chronic valvular endocarditis is often demonstrable and may well be the source of the causative embolus. Infarcts of the kidney are rather frequent and typically are anemic, may be multiple, and often heal leaving only a narrow, fibrous scar.

Infarcts of the spleen are almost always hemorrhagic. Many shallow, subcapsular infarcts, difficult to distinguish from small subcapsular hematomas, are seen in hog cholera. Arterioles become obstructed because of swelling and hyperplasia of endothelial cells as a result of hog cholera virus infection.

Infarcts of the myocardium, far more rare in ani-

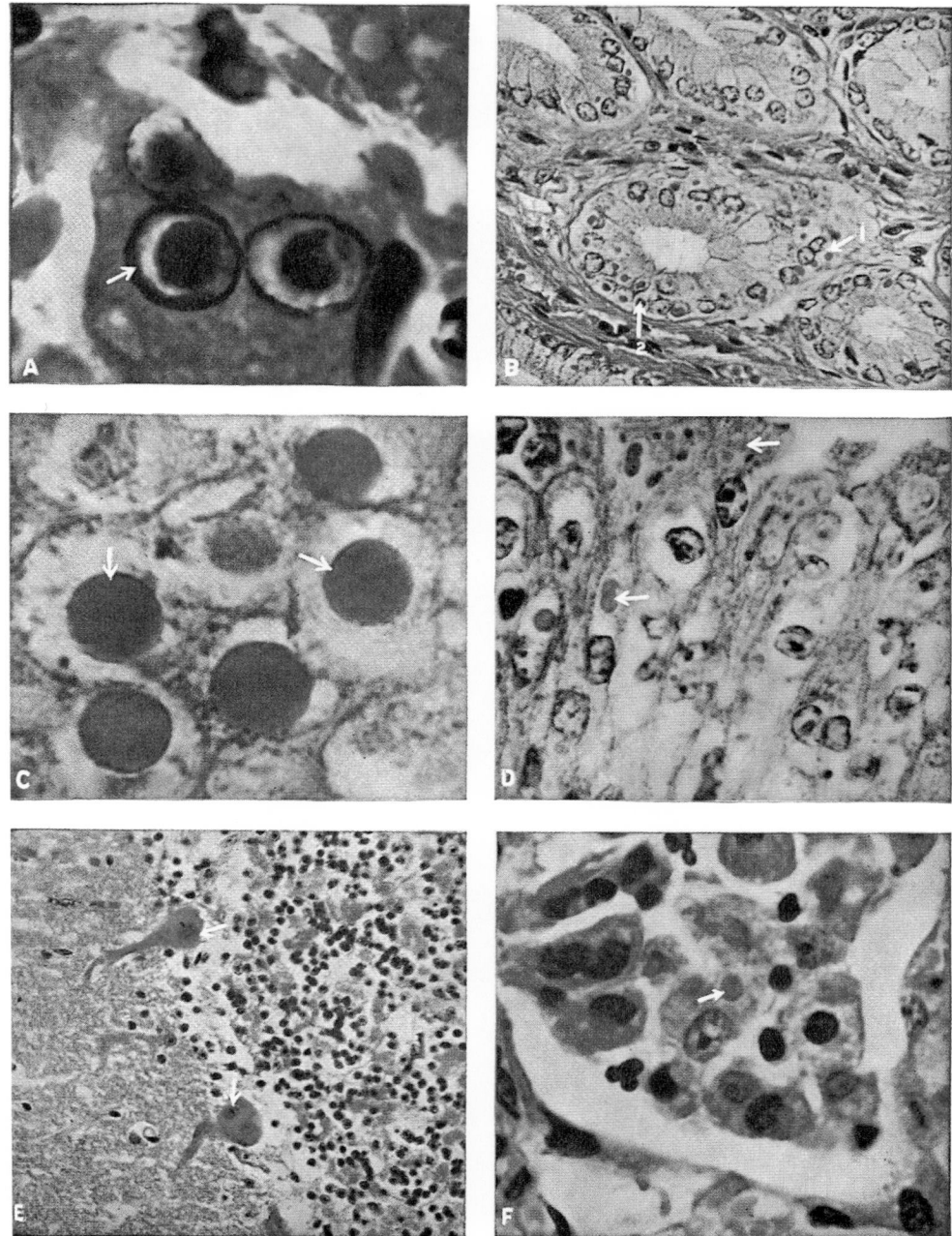

PLATE I

A. Infectious canine hepatitis, intranuclear inclusions in liver cells. (H & E, × 1850.) Note margination of nuclear chromatin (arrow) surrounding a clear halo around the inclusion body.

B. Canine distemper, cytoplasmic (1) and intranuclear (2) inclusion bodies in gastric epithelium. (H & E, × 470.)

C. Fowl pox, Bollinger bodies (arrows) in cytoplasm of epidermal cells. (H & E, × 1300.)

D. Canine distemper, cytoplasmic inclusions (arrows) in epithelial cells of urinary bladder. (Shorr's S-3 stain, × 525.)

E. Rabies, cytoplasmic inclusions (arrows) in Purkinje cells, cerebellum of cow. (Schleifstein modification of Wilhite stain, × 350.)

F. Canine distemper, cytoplasmic inclusion (arrow) in cells from pulmonary alveolar wall. (H & E, × 825.)

mals than in humans and usually from different causes, are either red or gray at the time they are discovered.

Infarcts of the brain are usually anemic and quickly reach a state of liquefaction necrosis in accordance with the susceptibility of nervous tissue to that outcome. The animal may survive, the infarcted area being represented by a hole in the brain parenchyma. These infarcts are rare in animals.

Intestinal infarcts usually involve a considerable length of the bowel. They are always hemorrhagic, and large amounts of blood diffuse into the lumen through the necrotic tissue. They are ordinarily caused by strangulation of the bowel caught in a hernial sac, an intussusception, or in a twisted loop of mesentery. In spite of the frequency of thrombotic injury to the anterior mesenteric artery by strongyle worms in the horse, emboli of sufficient importance to compromise the rather efficient system of arterial anastomosis are rare. Intestinal infarctions, unless promptly treated by surgical resection, develop gangrene that is fatal to the organism through invasion of saprophytic bacteria from the intestinal lumen. Obstruction of the lumen of the bowel by some foreign body is frequent in the dog and, if complete, produces the same type of lesion.

Infarcts may occur in the lung despite the (only moderately effective) circulation of the bronchial arteries as a secondary source of supply, but apparently they occur only when that circulation is also compromised by abnormally low blood pressure or perfusion. Emboli, single or multiple, occluding the pulmonary artery are the usual cause. Because of the secondary bronchial circulation as well as the extensive capillary network and the sponge-like nature of lung tissue, pulmonary infarcts are always hemorrhagic: the alveolar spaces in the necrotic area are filled with blood.

In animals, infarction of the lung is not common. It is probable that some areas of lung, filled with blood in a lobular distribution, have been called infarcts without meeting the criteria of necrosis and certainly without an apparent embolus. In the lung, it is not always easy to distinguish hemorrhagic infarction from simple hemorrhage or a localized hemorrhagic exudate.

True infarcts of the liver are almost nonexistent because both the portal vein and the hepatic artery supply large amounts of blood to this organ. If an infarct does occur, it is the result of obstruction of a branch of the hepatic artery; obstruction of the portal vein does not cause infarction.

References

Alberts B, Bray D, Lewis J, Raff M, Roberts K, Watson JD, eds. Molecular biology of the cell. New York/London:Garland, 1983.

Breitschwerdt EB, Kornegay JN, Wheeler SJ, Stevens JB, Baty CJ. Episodic weakness associated with exertional lactic acidosis and my-opathy in Old English sheepdog littermates. J Am Vet Med Assoc 1992;201:731–736.

Cheung JY, Benventre JV, Malis CD, Leaf A. Calcium and ischemic injury. N Engl J Med 1986;314:1670–1676.

de Duve C. The lysosome. Sci Am 1963;28:64–67.

Duke RC, Chervenak R, Cohen JJ. Endogenous endonuclease-induced DNA fragmentation: an early event in cell-mediated cytolysis. Proc Natl Acad Sci USA 1983;80:6361–6365.

Farber J L, El-Mofty S K. The biochemical pathology of liver cell necrosis. Am J Pathol 1975;81: 237–250.

Farber J. Membrane injury and calcium homeostasis in the pathogenesis of coagulative necrosis. Lab Invest 1982;47:114–123.

Finnie JW, Smith K, Mukherjee TM. Mitochondrial alterations in skeletal muscle in a bovine encephalopathy. Vet Rec 1991;129:384–385.

Herrtage ME, Houlton JEF. Collapsing Clumber spaniels. Vet Rec 1979;105:223.

Hockenberry D. Defining apoptosis. Am J Pathol 1995;146:16–19.

Houlton JEF, Herrtage ME. Mitochondrial myopathy in the Sussex spaniel. Vet Rec 1980;106:206.

Ito T. A pathological study on fat necrosis in swine. Jpn J Vet Sci 1973;35:299–310.

Ito T, Miura S, Ohshima K, Numakunai S. Pathological studies of fat necrosis (lipomatosis) in cattle. Jpn J Vet Sci 1968;30:141–150.

Jennings RB, Gnoti C E, Reiner KA. Ischemic tissue injury. Am J Pathol 1975; 81:179–198.

Kane AB. Commentary: redefining cell death. Am J Pathol 1995;146:1–2.

King DW, Paulson SR, Hannaford NC, et al. Cell death. I. The effect of injury on the proteins amd deoxyribonucleic acid of Ehrlich tumor cells. II. The effect of injury on the enzymatic protein of Ehrlich tumor cells. III. The effect of injury on water and electrolytes of Ehrlich tumor cells. IV. The effects of injury on the entrance of vital dye in Ehrlich tumor cells. Am J Pathol 1959;35:369–381, 575–589, 835–849, 1067–1079.

Majno G, Joris I. Apoptosis, oncosis, and necrosis. An overview of cell death. Am J Pathol 1995;146:3–15.

Majno G, LaGattula M, Thompson TE. Cellular death and necrosis: chemical, physical and morphologic changes in rat liver. Virchows Arch [Pathol Anat] 1960;333:421–465.

Scholte HR, Verduin MH, Ross JD, et al. Equine exertional rhadomyolysis: activity of the mitochondrial respiratory chain and carnitine system in skeletal muscle. Equine Vet J 1991;23:142–144.

Shoffner JM IV, Wallace DC. Oxidative phosphorylation diseases. Disorders of two genomes. Adv Hum Genet 1990;19:267–330.

Steller H. Apoptosis: mechanisms and genes of cellular suicide. Science 1995;267:1445–1449.

Steenbergen C, Murphy E, Levy L, London RE. Elevation in cytosolic free calcium concentration early in myocardial ischemia in perfused rat heart. Circ Res 1987;60:700–707.

Thompson CB. Apoptosis in the pathogenesis and treatment of disease. Science 1995,**267**:1456–1462.

Tosteson DC: Regulation of cell volume by sodium and potassium transport. In: Hoffman JF, ed. The cellular function of membrane transport. Englewood Cliffs, NJ:Prentice-Hall, 1964;3–22.

Trump BF, Goldblatt PJ, Stowell RE: et al. An electron microscopic study of mouse liver during necrosis in vivo (autolysis). Lab Invest 1962;**11**:986–1016.

Trump BF, Mergner WJ. Cell injury. In: Zweifach BW, Grant L, McCluskey RT, eds. The inflammatory process. New York:Academic Press 1974;1:115–257.

Vitovec J., Proks C., amd Valvoda V. Lipomatosis (fat necrosis) in canines and pigs. J Comp Pathol 1975;85:53–59.

Vogt MT, Farber E. On the molecular pathology of ischemic renal cell death: reversible and irreversible cellular and mitochondrial alterations. Am J Pathol 1968;53:1–26.

Intracellular and extracellular depositions; degenerations

In addition to the causes of cell injury and death described in Chapter 1, cells may undergo reversible or irreversible cell injury as a consequence of metabolic disturbances that result in the accumulation of abnormal amounts of endogenous substances within their cytoplasm, nucleus, or surrounding extracellular space. These metabolic defects may be present in cells directly affected by the deposits or, in some cases, in cells distantly removed from the site of deposition.

FATTY CHANGE

Fatty change is the term used to indicate the accumulation of discrete droplets of **neutral lipids (triglycerides)** within the cytoplasm of parenchymal cells. Fatty change occurs most often in the liver, kidney, and heart, and it may be caused by many disturbances in the normal synthesis and transport of fats to and from affected cells.

Causes

Fatty change results from either (1) the transport of lipids to affected cells in amounts that exceed their capacity to metabolize it or (2) from impairment of the cell's ability to synthesize proteins and lipoproteins required for transport of physiologic levels of lipid out of affected cells. The liver plays a central role in fat metabolism. To understand the pathogenesis of fatty change, knowledge of the normal processes involved in the transport of fats to and from the liver is helpful. Fats are normally transported to hepatocytes in the form of free fatty acids mobilized from triglycerides stored in lipocytes of the body's adipose tissue, and from water-soluble short-chain fatty acids that enter the portal circulation directly from the gut. Triglycerides absorbed from the intestine are in the form of **chylomicrons;** they enter the systemic circulation via the intestinal lacteals and thoracic duct rather than via the portal circulation. Chylomicrons are spherical particles composed of a central core of triglycerides surrounded by a layer of phospholipids, cholesterol, and apolipoproteins. They

are converted in capillaries of skeletal and cardiac muscle and adipose tissue by the enzyme endothelial lipoprotein lipase into free fatty acids, which are used by these tissues as well as by the liver as primary sources of energy. In the liver, all fatty acids are either oxidized directly for energy or are esterified to triglycerides. Normally, most hepatic triglycerides are coupled to specific apoprotein molecules made by the liver to form lipoproteins. These lipoproteins, i.e., low-density lipoproteins (LDL), very low-density lipoproteins (VLDL), and high-density lipoproteins (HDL), are secreted back into the circulation and used as the preferred sources of energy by other tissues. Some of the basic mechanisms involved in the pathogenesis of fatty change follow.

1. **Excessive release of free fatty acids** from adipose tissue results in delivery of increased amounts of these acids to the liver, heart, or kidney, where they may not be utilized as rapidly as they accumulate and, thus, are stored as triglycerides. This is the mechanism involved in fatty change from starvation or severe caloric restriction, in which free fatty acids are mobilized from the body's fat stores and transported to the liver for synthesis of glucose (**gluconeogenesis**) as a source of energy. This form of fatty change occurs often in cats with **idiopathic hepatic lipidosis,** a poorly understood condition associated with unexplained anorexia in obese cats and obese macaque monkeys.

2. **Decreased utilization or oxidation of fatty acids** may result from interference with cofactors such as carnitine, which is essential for oxidation of long-chain fatty acids. Bacterial toxins (e.g., diphtheria toxin) produce fatty change in this manner.

3. **Lipotrope deficiency** results in decreased phospholipid synthesis. Deficiency of methionine or choline decreases phospholipid synthesis and leads to esterification of diglycerides to triglycerides.

4. **Fatty acids preferentially esterified to triglycerides** may result from increased levels of α glycerophosphate. This is one of several mechanisms involved

in fatty change that occurs with excessive alcohol consumption.

5. **Impairment of apoprotein synthesis** interferes with the hepatocyte's ability to synthesize lipoproteins, the form in which triglycerides are excreted from the liver. A variety of poisons, including ethionine, carbon tetrachloride, puromycin, and yellow phosphorus, damage the cell's rough endoplasmic reticulum (RER) and interfere with protein synthesis. Dietary protein deficiency can also lead to fatty change because of insufficient amino acid substrates required for protein synthesis.

6. **Impairment of lipoprotein secretion** from the liver also results in the accumulation of triglycerides within hepatocytes. This mechanism is involved in experimental orotic acid intoxication.

Gross appearance

The gross appearance of organs with fatty change depends on the amount of lipid present within its parenchymal cells. If the amount of stored lipid is minimal, there may be no alterations in the gross appearance of the affected organ. Organs containing large quantities of lipid typically appear yellow-tan and paler than normal. They are often also larger than normal. The **liver,** in particular, may have rounded rather than sharp edges, and its capsular and cut surfaces may have a prominent, yellow, reticular pattern separated by thin, branching, red septa that correspond to the fat-laden hepatic cords and vasculature in the centrilobular and portal areas. In extreme cases, the liver floats when immersed in formalin, and small droplets of fat from the cut surface of the organ may be seen floating on the surface of fixative.

In the **heart,** fatty change appears as a yellow-tan streaking of the myocardium. This change has been compared to the appearance of a "thrush breast." When severe, the affected heart may also have a flabby consistency.

Fatty change in the **kidney** appears as a radial, yellow-tan streaking of the cortex and medulla that corresponds to the regions of the proximal convoluted tubules and medullary rays.

Microscopic appearance

In routine sections of **liver** stained with hematoxylin and eosin, the cytoplasm of affected cells contains either a single large or multiple small round empty vacuoles that distend the cell cytoplasm and displace the nucleus to the periphery (Fig. 2-1 and 2-2). In the **heart,** the lipid occurs in the sarcoplasm of myocytes in the form of numerous fine vacuoles rather than single large droplets. In the **kidney** with fatty change, the lipid occurs in multiple variable-sized droplets within the cytoplasm of epithelial cells of the proximal convoluted tubules and ascending loops of Henle. It should be noted that cat kidneys normally contain moderate to large amounts of lipid in their proximal tubular epithelium.

Lipids are extracted by the organic solvents used in routine paraffin embedding procedures but can be preserved for demonstration with special fat stains by preparing sections of either frozen or formalin-fixed tissue. Stains commonly used to demonstrate fats in frozen tissue sections are: oil red-O; Sudan III; Sudan IV (also known as scarlet red or scharlach red); osmic acid; and Nile blue sulfate.

Accumulation of neutral fat within cells causes them to expand and, in the liver, compress the lumens of sinusoids. Cells may become so distended that they rupture, spilling fat droplets into the surrounding tissues. Clinically, this may be associated with slight elevations in the liver enzymes aspartate aminotransferase

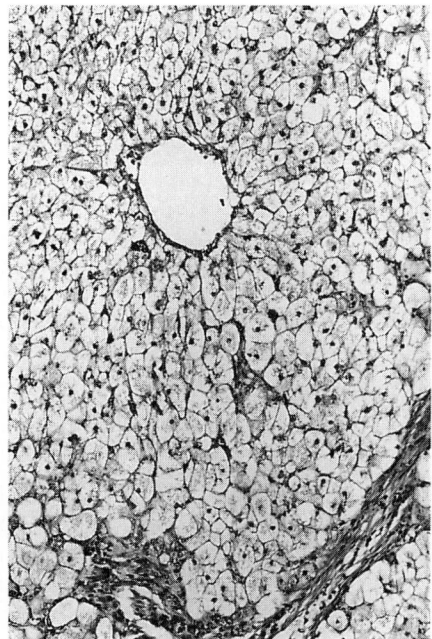

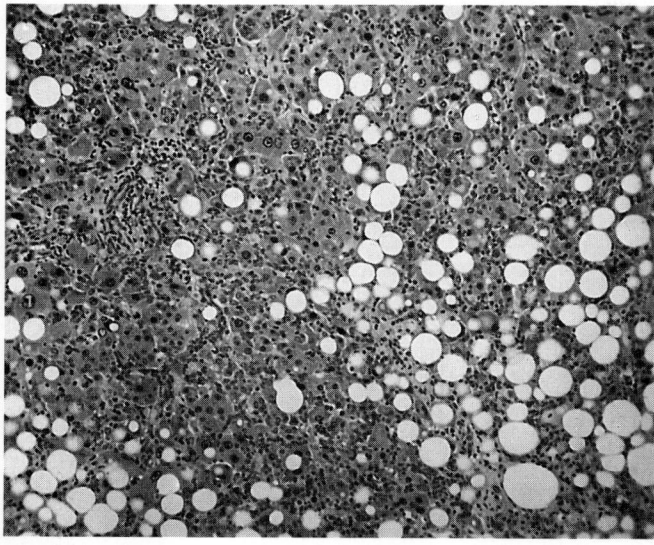

FIG. 2-1 Fatty change. **A.** Liver from a cat with idiopathic hepatic lipidosis. In this condition the fat is present in microdroplet form. **B.** Liver from a rat that received a diet deficient in choline and methionine.

(AST) and alanine aminotransferase (ALT), indicating mild hepatic necrosis. Microscopically, the released neutral lipids may be phagocytized by macrophages, resulting in the formation of widely scattered aggregates of lipid-laden macrophages (**lipogranulomas**).

Fatty change is generally regarded as a reversible form of cell injury, since removal of the basic cause results in return of the fatty liver to a normal state. If the cause is not corrected, affected cells become irreversibly damaged and die.

EXTRACELLULAR ACCUMULATION OF LIPIDS

In some situations, lipids may accumulate outside of cells. Rupture of cells with severe fatty change may release triglycerides or phospholipids into extracellular spaces, where pooling and phagocytosis by macrophages may make them visible. Cholesterol is released from cells or pooled from lipoproteins in crystalline

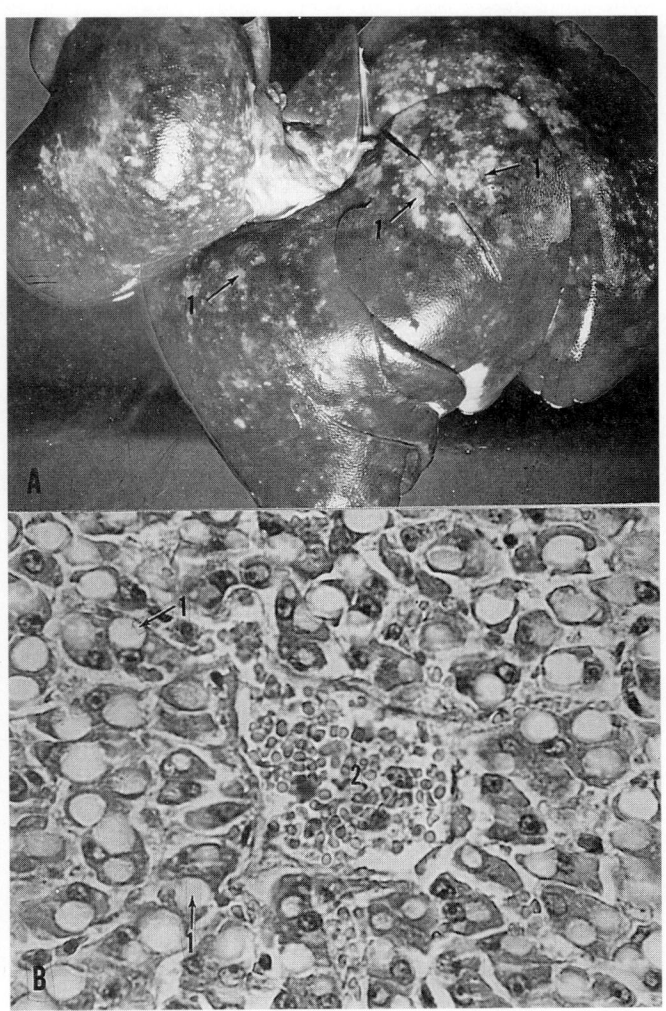

FIG. 2-2 Fatty change in liver of a dog given 200 mL of olive oil and cream 6 hours before (unexpected) death. **A.** Deposits of fat (1) are seen in all lobes. **B.** Fat droplets (1) in liver cells surrounding a central vein (2). (Courtesy of Dr. Melvin G. Rhoades and Armed Forces Institute of Pathology)

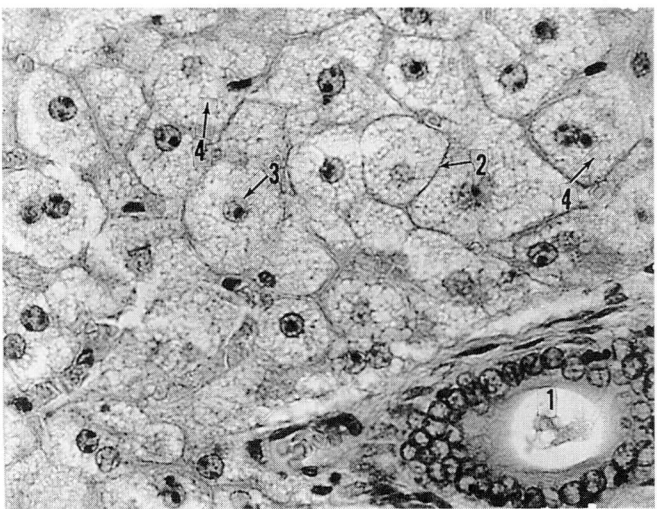

FIG. 2-3 Glycogen in liver cells of a dog; a normal finding in well-nourished animals; it disappears rapidly in many diseased states. Bile duct (1), distinct walls of liver cells (2), centrally located nuclei (3) of hepatic cells, and fine droplets of glycogen (4), which fill the cytoplasm of these cells (× 500). (Courtesy of Dr. Lester Barto and Armed Forces Institute of Pathology)

form (**cholesterol clefts**) as the result of hemorrhage. Fat may be seen in blood vessels in the form of **fat emboli** from traumatically injured adipose tissue or from bone marrow as a complication of bone fractures. Renal tubular epithelium with fatty change may rupture, spilling lipid droplets into the lumen to produce **fatty casts.**

FATTY INFILTRATION

Fatty infiltration, in contrast to fatty change, describes infiltration by normal-appearing lipocytes into the interstitial connective tissues of organs that do not normally contain appreciable quantities of adipose tissue. It occurs commonly in the heart and pancreas and is often found along with obesity.

FATTY DEGENERATION OF MYELIN

This condition, in which myelin is destroyed and stainable fat is produced as a product of degeneration, is discussed in more detail in Chapter 27, The Nervous System.

References

Abraham EP, Robb-Smith AHT. Degenerative changes and some of their consequences. In: Florey HW, ed. General pathology. 4th ed. Philadelphia:WB Saunders 1970;413–430.

Gordon ER, Lough J. Ultrastructural and biochemical aspects during the regression of an ethanol-induced fatty liver. Lab Invest 1972;26:154–162.

Isselbacher KJ, Greenberger NJ. Metabolic effects of alcohol on the liver. N Engl J Med 1964;270:351–371.

Johnson SE. Diseases of the liver. In: Ettinger SJ, Feldman EC, ed. Textbook of veterinary internal medicine. 4th ed. Philadelphia: WB Saunders 1995;2:1350–1353.

Lombardi B. Considerations on the pathogenesis of fatty liver. Lab Invest 1966;15:1–20.

Longnecker DS, Skinozuka H, Farber E. Molecular pathology of in vivo inhibition of protein synthesis. Am J Pathol 1968;52:891–915.

Kumar V, Deo MG, Ramalingaswami V. Mechanism of fatty liver in protein deficiency: an experimental study in the rhesus monkey. Gastroenterology 1972;62:445–451.

Meldolesi J, Clementi F, Chiesara E, et al. Cytoplasmic changes in rat liver after prolonged treatment with low doses of ethionine and adenine: an ultrastructural and biochemical study. Lab Invest 1967;17:265–275.

Meldolesi J, Vincenzi L, Bassan P, et al. Effects of carbon tetrachloride on the synthesis of liver endoplasmic reticulum membranes. Lab Invest 1968;19:315–323.

Reynolds ES, Yee AG. Liver parenchymal cell injury. VI. Significance of early glucose-6–phosphatase suppression and transient calcium influx following poisoning. Lab Invest 1968;19:273–281.

Rubin E, Lieber CS. The effects of ethanol on the liver. Int Rev Exp Pathol 1972;11:177–232.

Schlunk FF, Lombardi B. Liver liposomes. 1. Isolation and chemical characterization. Lab Invest 1967;17:30–38.

Schlunk FF, Lombardi B. On the ethionine-induced fatty liver in male and female rats. Lab Invest 1967;17:299–307.

GLYCOGEN DEPOSITION

Glycogen is sometimes called animal starch, since its chemical formula resembles those of the true starches in that it is a multiple of $C_6H_{10}O_5$. Carbohydrates of all kinds are normally carried in the blood as glucose (dextrose) and are stored as glycogen, mainly in the liver and skeletal muscle. Hence it is normal to have considerable amounts of glycogen in these tissues.

Occurrence

Excessive accumulations of glycogen may occur pathologically in the cytoplasm of epithelial cells of the liver and kidneys, leukocytes, cardiac muscle, and, less often, in smooth muscle, spleen, lymph nodes, and brain.

Gross appearance

Abnormal accumulations of glycogen are generally not associated with grossly visible changes in affected organs.

Microscopic appearance

Whether glycogen is deposited normally or abnormally, it appears as irregular, clear spaces within the cytoplasm of cells. This is because glycogen is water-soluble and readily dissolved by ordinary methods of tissue preparation, leaving empty spaces in the protein-rich cytosol. In contrast to the round vacuoles left in the cytoplasm when lipid is extracted from cells with fatty change, the extraction of glycogen deposits leaves irregularly shaped, clear spaces with indistinct outlines. This feature is helpful in distinguishing glycogen deposition from fatty change and from hydropic change. In addition, glycogen deposits usually do not displace the nucleus to the periphery of the cell as do severe fatty changes (Fig. 2-3). An exception to this occurs in dogs with **steroid-induced hepatopathy,** where the glycogen deposits in mid-zonal hepatocytes become so massive

that the nucleus and cytoplasmic organelles are often displaced to the periphery of the cell (Fig. 2-4).

The ultrastructural appearance of glycogen is characteristic. The method of fixation influences its appearance, but usually electron microscopy reveals its smallest unit as roughly isodiametric, slightly irregular particles, 150 to 300 Å in diameter. These **beta** particles usually coalesce to form aggregates called **alpha particles** or **rosettes.** The number of particles or rosettes varies greatly, as is to be expected, and may be present in such numbers as to obscure most intracellular organelles (Fig. 2-5).

The hepatocytes of well-nourished animals normally contain considerable glycogen, enough to give the cytoplasm a finely foamy appearance, varying with the amount of carbohydrate consumed and the interval between fixation of the liver and carbohydrate consumption.

Positive identification or differentiation necessitates special techniques. Tissues must be fixed in alcohol, and alcoholic-based stains are used so that no water comes in contact with the tissue. Best's carmine, one of the most useful stains for glycogen, colors the glycogen a bright pink.

Causes

The most frequent cause of excessive glycogen deposition in animal tissues is hyperglycemia, as occurs in diabetes mellitus. It is also seen with some frequency in the livers of dogs with hyperadrenocorticism or dogs receiving corticosteroid therapy (**steroid-induced**

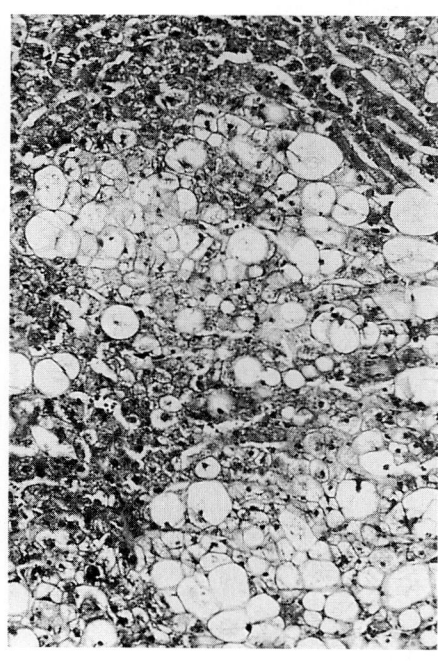

FIG. 2-4 Liver from a dog with steroid-induced hepatopathy. Marked swelling and vacuolar change of hepatocytes is caused by massive glycogen deposits that displace the nuclei and organelles of hepatocytes to the periphery (hematoxylin and eosin stain) (× 200).

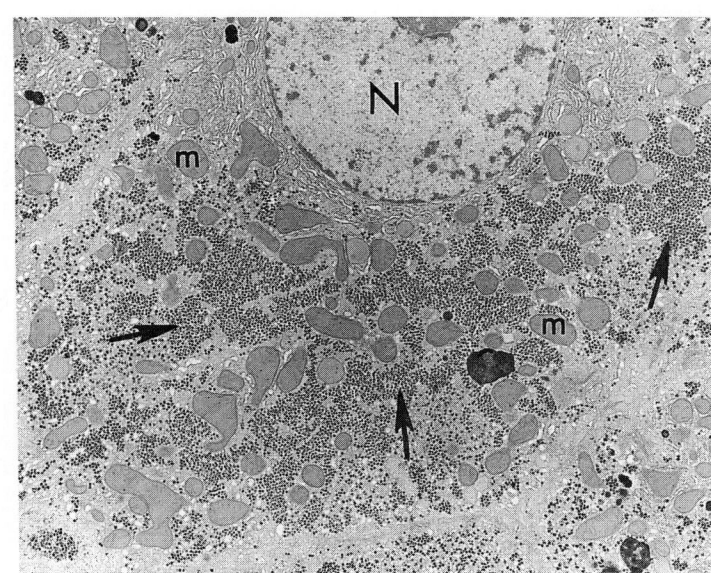

FIG. 2-5 Glycogen in a hepatocyte of an owl monkey (*Aotus trivirgatus*). It appears as numerous small electron-dense granules (*arrows*). *N,* nucleus; *m,* mitochondria.

hepatopathy). Other causes include the so-called **glycogen storage diseases (glycogenoses).** These are autosomal recessive inherited disorders characterized by deficiencies of various enzymes involved in the synthesis or degradation of glycogen. At least eight distinct types of glycogen storage diseases have been described in human beings; these are designated as types I through VIII. Four of these have also been reported in animals.

Type II glycogenosis, also known as **Pompe's disease,** is caused by a deficiency of lysosomal acid maltase (α1,4 glucosidase). It has been reported in an apparently healthy cat, in calves, and in a Japanese quail, all with muscular weakness. Unlike other glycogenoses, in this disease the **glycogen accumulates within lysosomes** of most cells of the body, but especially in the brain, muscles, and liver. This condition is more fully discussed under lysosomal storage diseases.

Type III glycogenosis, or **Cori's disease,** results from a deficiency of the **glycogen debranching enzyme,** amylo-1, 6-glucosidase, an enzyme involved in the breakdown of glycogen to glucose. The deficiency leads to the accumulation of large quantities of free glycogen particles in the cytosol of hepatocytes in particular, but also in myocardium, skeletal muscle, smooth muscle, and nerve cells. Hepatomegaly and hypoglycemia develop in animals with this disease. This condition has been described in German Shepherd dogs.

Type IV glycogenosis has recently been described in Norwegian Forest cats. As in human beings, kittens homozygous for this trait have a deficiency of the **glycogen branching enzyme,** which leads to storage of large quantities of abnormal glycogen in many tissues, but particularly in skeletal and cardiac muscle. Affected kittens may be stillborn or die soon after birth. Kittens that survive may appear normal for 5 to 7 months, after which progressive skeletal and cardiac muscle degeneration and atrophy develop, and they die at 12 to 14 months of age.

Type VII glycogenosis is caused by a deficiency of the M (muscle) type of phosphofructokinase (PFK) and has been described in English springer spaniel dogs. It is inherited as an autosomal recessive trait. Affected dogs have a persistent compensated hemolytic anemia and episodes of intravascular hemolysis with hemoglobinuria. Clinical signs include exercise intolerance, muscle wasting, and rarely, muscle cramping. Affected dogs have only 1% to 6% of normal muscle PFK activity and 10% to 20% of normal erythrocyte PFK activity. (Erythrocyte PFK is composed of 80% to 90% M-type PFK subunits). Muscle glycogen concentrations are approximately twice normal levels. Microscopically, affected muscle fibers stain paler than normal fibers and contain deposits of a PAS-positive amylopectin-like polysaccharide just beneath the sarcolemma.

References

Ceh L, Hauge JG, Svenkerud R, et al. Glycogenosis type III in the dog. Acta Vet Scand 1976;17:210–222.

Edwards JR, Richards RB. Bovine generalized glycogenosis type II: a clinico-pathological study. Br Vet J 1979;135:338–348.

Fittschen C, Bellamy JEC. Prednisone-induced morphologic and chemical changes in the livers of dogs. Vet Pathol 1984;21:399–406.

Fyfe JC, Van Winkle TJ, Haskins ME, et al. Glycogen storage disease type IV. Comp Pathol Bull 1994;26(3):3,6.

Harvey JW, Giger U. Muscle-type phosphofructokinase deficiency (glycogen storage disease type VII). Comp Pathol Bull 1991;23(4):3–4.

Harvey JW, Mays MBC, Gropp KE, et al. Polysaccharide storage myopathy in canine phosphofructokinase deficiency (Type VII glycogen storage disease). Vet Pathol 1990;27:1–8.

Matsui T, Kuroda S, Mizutani M, et al. Generalized glycogen storage disease in Japanese quail (*Coturnix coturnix japonica*). Vet Pathol 1983;20:312–321.

Rafiquzzaman, M, Svenkerud R, Strande A, et al. Glycogenosis in the dog. Acta Vet Scand 1976;17:196–209.

Sandstrom B, Westman J, Ockerman PA. Glycogenosis of the central nervous system in the cat. Acta Neuropathol (Berl) 1969;14:194–200.

Hydropic Change (Acute Cellular Swelling)

Hydropic change, synonymous with **hydropic degeneration** and **acute cellular swelling** (Chapter 1), describes increased intracellular water causing the cytoplasm and organelles to appear swollen and vacuolated. Any factor that impairs the ability of cell membranes to actively transport sodium out of cells leads to influx of excessive amounts of water into the cell. The increased intracellular water causes swelling of the cell, its mitochondria, and RER. Hydropic change is a frequent prelude to most forms of cell death, except apoptosis. Distinguishing hydropic change from glycogen deposition, in which cells fixed in formalin also appear vacuolated, may be difficult. As in glycogen deposition, the nuclei of cells with hydropic change are usually not displaced to the periphery of the cell (which is the case with fatty change).

Intracellular Accumulation of Protein

The accumulation of protein in the cytoplasm of cells, usually in the form of discrete eosinophilic droplets, is termed **hyaline droplet formation.** In the older literature it was often referred to erroneously as hyaline droplet degeneration, but it is not a degenerative change at all; it simply reflects increased absorption of protein by particular cells. It is seen most often in the cytoplasm of epithelial cells of the proximal convoluted tubules of the kidney. Plasma proteins leak from abnormal glomerular capillaries and are resorbed by pinocytosis from the lumens of the tubules. Upon entry into the cell, the pinocytotic vesicles fuse with lysosomes, and the protein is digested. If resorption exceeds the rate of digestion, microscopically visible, highly eosinophilic droplets of up to 10 nm in diameter accumulate in the cytoplasm of the cells. If protein leakage exceeds the absorptive capacity of these cells, eosinophilic albuminous or hyaline casts are present in the tubular lumens.

Lysosomal Storage Diseases

The lysosome is the primary disposal and recycling center of cells. It catabolizes cellular and extracellular macromolecules, providing amino acids, fatty acids, nucleic acids, and sugars for reuse in cellular synthesis. The degradation of all four classes of biologic macromolecules is mediated by large arrays of acid hydrolases. These enzymes, along with secretory and plasma membrane proteins, are synthesized and glycosylated in the RER and translocated to the Golgi apparatus (Fig. 2-6). In the Golgi, all the hydrolases, with the exceptions of glucocerebrosidase and acid phosphatase, are segregated from the rest of the newly synthesized proteins by the addition of a terminal mannose-6-phosphate residue. This residue serves as a recognition marker for specific receptors located on the plasma membrane as well as on membranes of the endoplasmic reticulum and Golgi. After the enzyme binds to the membrane receptor in the Golgi, the enzyme receptor complex exits the Golgi via coated vesicles and is transported either to the outside of the cell, where it is recaptured by pinocytosis after binding the plasma membrane, or to membrane-bound vesicles that become primary lysosomes. In the primary lysosome, the hydrolase is released from its mannose-6-phospate marker by acidification of the compartment and thus becomes reactive. The receptor then shuttles back to the Golgi and picks up and transfers another enzyme to the primary lysosome. Extracellular and intracellular constituents are transported by phagocytosis, endocytosis, craniophagy, and autophagy to be catabolized in the lysosomes. Once the macromolecules are catabolized, the degradation products are transferred to the cytosol and probably reused for synthesis. The catabolism of macromolecules in lysosomes may be regarded as a linear sequence of reactions in which the product of one reaction serves as substrate for the next (Fig. 2-6). Normally, most lysosomal hydrolases are present at sufficiently high levels of activity, and accumulation of substrate occurs only when the residual activity is below the critical threshold of 10% of normal enzyme activity.

About three dozen genetically determined, heterogeneous, metabolic, and acquired lysosomal disorders are classified as lysosomal storage diseases. The mode of inheritance in most of these conditions is autosomal recessive. Table 2-1 summarizes lysosomal storage disorders, their eponyms, and their characteristics, including primary deficiency, storage substrates, major organs involved, and corresponding disease in animals. Eight different mechanisms are currently known to cause lysosomal storage disease (Table 2-2). The majority of these conditions feature deficient activity of lysosomal enzymes resulting from mutation of the gene coding for specific hydrolase. The clinical heterogeneity of any one lysosomal enzyme is caused by multiplicity of mutant alleles, which leads to differences in the properties of residual enzymes or absence of enzymes. Usually, residual enzymes characterize juvenile or adult onset of disease, and absence of enzymes, the more severe infantile onset. The third mechanism is mutation resulting in a defective key enzyme, 6-phospho-N-acetyl-glucosamine transferase, leading to absence of the recognition marker on the lysosomal enzyme and, as a consequence, enzymes are not transported to the lysosome but are instead secreted from the cells. In the absence of functional protective protein, rapid degradation ensues of several lysosomal enzymes, such as β galactosidase and neuraminidase, thus resulting in deficient activity of these enzymes. Lysosomal degradation of several sphingolipids by acid hydrolases requires activator proteins (saposins), which are small nonenzymatic cofactors that assist the enzymes in attacking sphingolipids. Mutation in any one of these cofactors leads to storage disease. Acquired lysosomal storage diseases occur after intake of certain drugs, such as cationic amphophilic molecules, which elevate the lysosomal pH

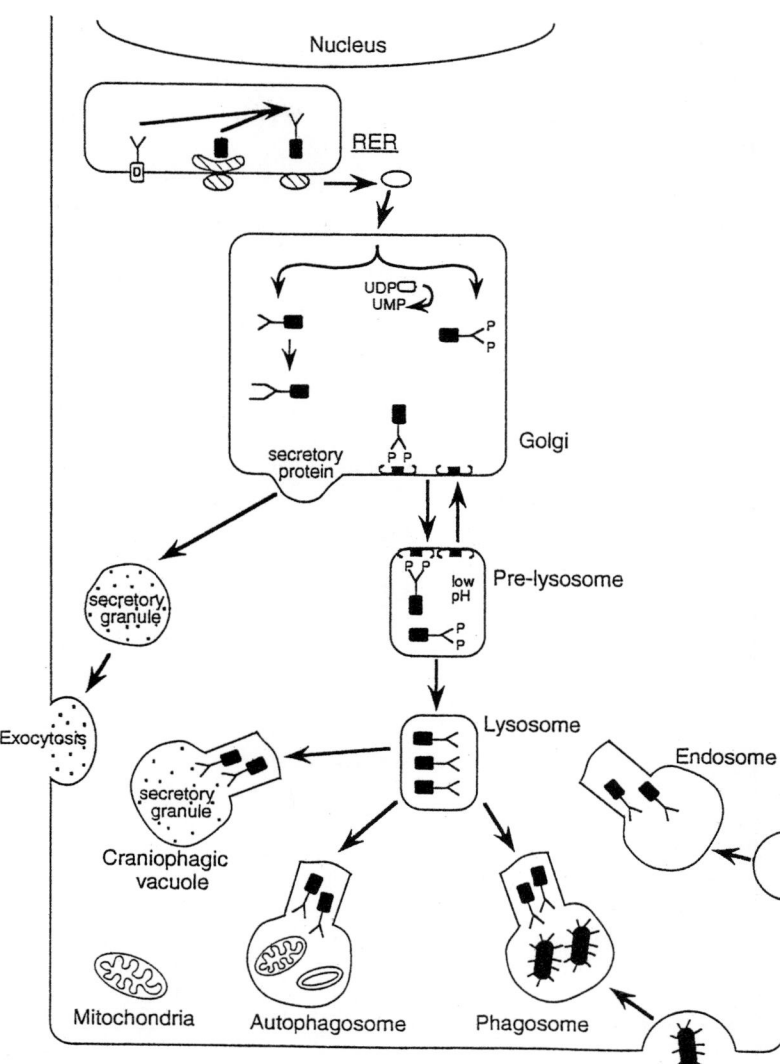

FIG. 2-6 Schematic illustration of synthesis and targeting of lysosomal hydrolases to lysosomes and mechanisms for transferring substrates to lysosomes for degradation. Nascent lysosomal hydrolase, secretory, and membrane proteins are glycosylated in the RER by transferance of preformed oligosaccharide from dolichol-P-P-oligosaccharide (D). These glycosylated glycoproteins are translocated to Golgi apparatus, where secretory and membrane glycoproteins are further modified and oligosaccharides of lysosomal hydrolases are phosphorylated (P). All but two lysosomal enzymes bind to M-P-receptors and are transported to prelysosome, where enzymes are released and receptor shuttles back to Golgi apparatus. In primary lysosome, prohydrolase is cleaved. Finally, secondary lysosome is formed by fusion of primary lysosome with phagosome.

and result in reduced enzyme activity, or after ingestion of certain alkaloids, such as swainsonine, which inhibits acid α mannosidase. Some acquired conditions are reversible. In general, it is assumed that the breakdown products in the lysosome, such as monosaccharides and amino acids, diffuse across the lysosomal membrane to the cytosol for reuse. Lysosomal storage of free sialic acid and cystine results from a defect in the efflux system of the lysosomal membrane. Oversupply of substrate resulting in abnormal lysosomal storage is observed in several hematologic disorders, including myeloid and lymphoblastic leukemias. Microscopically enlarged macrophages that simulate Gaucher's cells are seen in these conditions. There are additional lysosomal storage disorders in which the causal mechanisms are unknown.

Lysosomal storage diseases are classified according to their "major" stored material; the classifications are mucopolysaccharidosis, sphingolipidosis (glycolipid), lipidosis, glycoprotein and glycogen storage diseases,

and mucolipidosis. However, in many of these disorders there is a lysosomal accumulation of more than one type of undegraded compound; for example, in GM_1 and GM_2 gangliosidoses (Sandhoff's diseases), there is an accumulation of both glycolipid and glycoproteins. One reason for this is that the same hydrolases degrade more than one class of substrate that may include both glycolipids and glycoproteins.

The consequence of these defects is the abnormal accumulation of catabolites in lysosomes leading to severe impairment of cellular structure and function. Genetic defects are thought to occur in all cells of affected individuals. Morphologic manifestations in particular cell types depend on the extent to which these cells ordinarily make use of the enzyme impaired by the disease. Two types of changes (lesions) are seen in lysosomal storage disorders. Primary lesions consist of increased size and number of secondary lysosomes in affected cells. Secondary lesions are likely to be the consequence of disrupted recycling, and they are mani-

TABLE 2-1 **Lysosomal storage diseases**

Disease	Deficient hydrolase(s)	Nature of defect in human	Storage product(s)	Major organs involved	Corresponding disease in animals
Mucopolysaccharidoses					
MPS I (Hurler and Schele syndromes)	α-iduronidase		Dermatan sulfate, heparan sulfate	CNS, connective tissue, heart, skeleton, cornea	DSH cats; Plott hounds
MPS II (Hunter syndrome)	Iduronate sulfatase		Dermatan sulfate, heparan sulfate	CNS, connective tissue, heart, skeleton, cornea	Adult form in Pointer dogs
MPS III (Sanfilippo syndrome)					
Subtype A	Heparin N-sulfatase		Heparan sulfate	CNS	
Subtype B	N-acetyl-α-glucosaminidase		Heparan sulfate	CNS	
Subtype C	Acetyl CoA (α-glucosaminide N-acetyltransferase)		Heparan sulfate	CNS	
Subtype D	N-acetylglucosamine 6-sulfatase		Heparan sulfate	CNS	Nubian Goats
MPS IV (Morquio syndrome)					
Type A	N-acetylgalactosamine 6-sulfatase		Chondroitin-4-sulfate, keratin sulfate	Cartilage, skeleton, cornea, heart	
Type B	β-galactosidase	Mature β-galactosidase has reduced activity and aggregates poorly	Keratin sulfate	Cartilage, bone, cornea	
MPS VI (Maroteaux-Lamy syndrome)	Arylsulfatase B (N-acetylgalactosamine 4-sulfatase)	Mature arylsulfatase B (form 1) is inactive and is rapidly degraded. In cat, the mature arylsulfatase is stucturally abnormal	Dermatan sulfate, chondroitin-6-sulfate	Skeleton, cornea, heart	Siamese cats; rats

TABLE 2-1 (continued)

Disease	Deficient hydrolase(s)	Nature of defect in human	Storage product(s)	Major organs involved	Corresponding disease in animals
MPS VII (Sly's syndrome)	β-glucuronidase		Chondroitin-4 and 6 sulfates, dermatan sulfate, heparin sulfate	CNS, connective tissue, skeleton, heart	Dog, cat, mice
Sphingolipidoses					
Gaucher's Disease Infantile type 2	β-glucocerebrosidase	Maturation of precursor of β-glucocerebrosidase impaired	Glucosylceramide	Brain, spleen, liver, bone marrow	Silky terrier dog, sheep dog
Juvenile type 3				Brain, spleen, liver, bone marrow	
Adult type 1				Spleen, liver, bone marrow	
Fabry's disease	α-galactosidase		Trihexosylceramide	Blood vessels of skin, kidney and brain	
Schindler disease	α-N-acetylgalactosaminidase			Nervous system	
Metachromatic leukodystrophy Late infantile form	Arylsulfatase A	1) No precursors of arylsulphatase A formed 2) Enzyme rapidly degraded	Galactosylsulphatide	CNS, liver, kidney, gall bladder	Hawaiian Geese

(continued)

TABLE 2-1 (continued)

Disease	Deficient hydrolase(s)	Nature of defect in human	Storage product(s)	Major organs involved	Corresponding disease in animals
Metachromatic leukodystrophy Late onset form	Arylsulfatase A	Arylsulfatase A rapidly degraded in lysosomes			
Pseudodeficiency of arylsulfatase A	Arylsulfatase A	Synthesis of precursor reduced in size and with attested properties			
Metachromatic leukodystropy (variant form)	Arylsulfatase A activity	Absence of factors required for hydrolysis of galactosyl sulfatide	galactosyl sulfatide and other lipids containing this moiety		
Multiple sulfatase deficiency	At least 6 lysosomal sulfatases and a microsomal sulfatase	Lack of a cotranslational or posttranslational modification of all sulfatases		CNS, visceral organs, and skeleton	
Niemann-Pick diseases Type A (acute neuropathic)	Sphingomyelinase		Sphingomyelin	Brain, liver, spleen bone marrow	Miniature poodle; (spm/spm) mutant of C57BL/KsJ mice, BALB/c mice
Type B (chronic, without nervous system involvement)					
Type C (chronic neuropathic form)	Unknown		Long-chain, cholesterol	Brain, liver, spleen	Mice DSH & Siamese cats
GM$_1$-gangliosidosis Infantile form	β-galactosidase	Mature β-galactosidase polypeptide reduced in amount, inactive, and does not aggregate	GM$_1$-ganglioside, oligosaccharides	CNS, skeleton, viscera	English springer spaniel, Portuguese water dog

TABLE 2-1 (Continued)

Disease	Deficient hydrolase(s)	Nature of defect in human	Storage product(s)	Major organs involved	Corresponding disease in animals
Juvenile form	β-galactosidase		GM$_1$-ganglioside, oligosaccharides	CNS, viscera	Friesian calves; DSH, Siamese cats; Beagle dogs; Suffolk cross-bred sheep
Adult form	β-galactosidase				
GM$_2$-gangliosidosis Tay-Sachs' disease, A Variant	β-hexosaminidase A	1) No synthesis of precursor 2) Insoluble precursor found 3) Reduced synthesis of precursor 4) Defective association of one precursor with another	GM$_2$-ganglioside	CNS	Muntjac Deer
Sandhoff's disease	β-hexosaminidase A and B	The synthesis of β precursor; reduced maturation of precursor	GM$_2$-ganglioside	CNS	DSH cats; German Shorthair Pointer dogs; Yorkshire pigs
AB variant	Deficiency in GM$_2$ activator protein			CNS	Japanese spaniel
Gangliosidosis (unclassified)					Emu; black bear
Krabbe's disease Globoid cell leukodystrophy	Galactosylcerebroside β-galactosidase		Galactosylsphingosine	CNS	Cairn & West Highland white terriers; poodle, beagle and blue tick hound; Twitcher mice; polled Dorset sheep; DSH cats; rhesus monkeys
Farber's disease	Ceramidase		Ceramide	Subcutaneous nodules, joints, larynx	

(continued)

TABLE 2-1 (Continued)

Disease	Deficient hydrolase(s)	Nature of defect in human	Storage product(s)	Major organs involved	Corresponding disease in animals
Lipidoses					
Wolman's Disease	Acid lipase/cholesteryl esterase	Triglycerides, cholesteryl esters		Liver, spleen, adrenal	Shell parakeets
Cholesteryl ester storage disease	Acid lipase/cholesteryl esterase		Triglycerides, cholesteryl esters	Liver, spleen, heart	
Neuronal ceroid-lipofuscinosis (NCL)					
Infantile NCL	Palmitoyl protein thioesterase	Inactive mutated enzyme	Protein	CNS and heart	Swedish sheep
Late infantile NCL	Unknown	Unknown	Unknown	CNS and heart, endothelial cells	Rambouillet, South-Hampshire sheep; English setter and Blue Heeler dogs; Devon cattle
Juvenile and Adult NCL	Unknown	Unknown	Unknown	CNS and heart, endothelial cells	
Glycoprotein storage disease					
Aspartylglycosaminuria	Aspartylglycosaminidase		Fragments of glycoprotein, aspartyl-2-deoxyl-2- acetamide glycosylamine, N-linked oligosaccharides	CNS, connective tissue, bone marrow	
Mannosidosis	α-mannosidase	Precursor of α-mannosidase is not synthesized	Fragments of glycoprotein, N-linked oligosaccharides	CNS, skeleton, liver, spleen	Red Angus, Shorthorn, Galloway, Murray Grey cattle; DSH and Persian cats
	β-mannosidase		Fragments of glycoprotein	CNS, skeleton, liver, spleen	Anglo-Nubian Goats; cattle

TABLE 2-1 (Continued)

Disease	Deficient hydrolase(s)	Nature of defect in human	Storage product(s)	Major organs involved	Corresponding disease in animals
Fucosidosis	α-fucosidase		oligosaccharides, fragments of glycoprotein and glycolipids	CNS, spleen, liver	English springer Spaniel dogs
Sialidosis (mucolipidosis I)	Oligosaccharide neuraminidase		Fragments of glycoprotein	CNS, spleen, liver, skeleton	
Galactosialidosis	β-galactosidase and membrane-bound neuraminidase	Protective protein not synthesized; β-galactosidase degraded in lysosomes	Fragments of glycoprotein	CNS, spleen, liver, skeleton	Schipperke dogs
Glycogen storage disease (I–VIII)					
Pompe's disease, type II Early onset	α-glucosidase	1) No precursor synthesized 2) Enzymatically inactive prosynthesized	Glycogen	CNS, muscle, heart	Brahman and Shorthorn cattle, Arian, Lapland dogs; cats; and Corriedale sheep
Late onset	α-glucosidase	1) Reduced maturation of cosidase 2) Precursor of α-glucosidase rapidly degraded in prelysosomal compartment	Glycogen	CNS, muscle, heart	
Disorders of enzyme location					
Mucolipidosis II (I-cell disease)	Several	N-acetylglucosaminyl-phosphotransferase deficiency	Mucopolysaccharides, lipids, glycoproteins	CNS, connective tissue, skeleton, heart, kidney	
Mucolipidosis III (Pseudo-Hurler polydystrophy)	Several	1) N-acetylglucosaminyl-phosphotransferase partially deficient 2) N-acetylglucosaminyl phosphotransferase with reduced activity towards lysosomal enzymes	Mucopolysaccharides, lipids, glycoproteins	Joint and connective tissue predominantly	

(continued)

TABLE 2-1 (Continued)

Disease	Deficient hydrolase(s)	Nature of defect in human	Storage product(s)	Major organs involved	Corresponding disease in animals
Mucolipidosis IV	Unknown		Lipids	CNS, connective tissue	
Disorders of lysosomal efflux					
Cystinosis	Cystine efflux mediator		Cystine	Kidney	
Salla's disease	Sialic acid efflux mediator		Free sialic acid	CNS	
Infantile sialuria	Sialic acid efflux mediator		Free sialic acid	CNS, kidney, liver	

CNS, central nervous system; MPS, mucopolysaccharidosis; DSH, domestic shorthair.

TABLE 2-2 **Mechanisms Involved in lysosomal storage diseases**

Mechanism	*Examples*
Disorders in which no immunologically detectable enzyme is synthesized. This includes conditions with grossly abnormal structural genes.	Hurler's, Tay-Sachs', Sandhoff's, and Pompe's disease
Disorders in which a catalytically inactive polypeptide is synthesized. The mutation may also affect the stability or transport of the polypeptide.	GM_1-gangliosidosis, mucopolysaccharidosis VI, Pompe's and Tay-Sachs' diseases
Disorders in which a catalytically active enzyme is synthesized, but the enzyme is not segregated into lysosomes.	I cell disease, pseudo-Hurler polydystrophy
Disorders in which a catalytically active enzyme is synthesized; however, the enzyme is unstable in prelysosomal or lysosomal compartments.	Metachromatic leukodystrophy of late onset, multiple sulfatase deficiency, Pompe's disease of late onset, neuraminidase β-galactosidase deficiency
Disorders in which activator proteins (saposins) of lipid-degrading hydrolases are missing.	AB variant of GM_2-gangliosidosis, variants of Gaucher's and Farber's diseases, juvenile variant of metachromatic leukodystrophy
Disorders in which the structural gene for the hydrolases is normal, but there is a mutation in the gene(s) that code for posttranslation modification of the hydrolases.	Multiple sulfatase deficiencies
Disorders in which lysosomal enzyme deficiencies result from intoxication with natural or synthetic inhibitors of lysosomal enzymes.	Indolizidine alkaloid (i.e., swainsonine) disease, disease induced by cationic amphophilic drugs (i.e., amiodarone, chloroquine)
Disorders caused by a decrease in transport of degradation end product (i.e., free sialic acid, free cystine) out of the lysosomes	Salla disease, infantile sialidosis, cystinosis
Disorders caused by oversupply of substrate	Some leukemias that are associated with Gaucher's cells

fested as abnormal cellular and extracellular products, such as dysmyelinogenesis or dysostosis multiplex (Fig. 2-7).

Preliminary diagnosis is made by means of microscopic examination of blood smears (Fig. 2-8) and ultrastructural examination of skin biopsies. Diagnosis of mucopolysaccharidosis and diseases with interrupted catabolism of oligosaccharides may be determined by urinalysis. Specific diagnoses of the majority of lysosomal storage diseases may be determined by means of assay of the lysosomal hydrolase activity in white blood cells, cultured fibroblasts, and serum. Postmortem diagnosis is established by both morphologic and biochemical examination of specimens. Enlargement and vacuolization of neurons (Fig. 2-9) may be an indicator of lysosomal storage disease. Staining of frozen and paraffin sections with PAS, PAS-diastase, alcian-blue, or colloidal-iron, both with and without pretreatment with hyaluronidase and various lectins, is useful in identification of carbohydrate residue in glycolipid and oligosaccharides respectively. Sudan black and luxol fast blue stains are helpful in characterization of lipid storage. Storage of autofluorescent material is associated with neuronal ceroid lipofuscinosis and other storage diseases (Fig. 2-10). Ultrastructural analysis of affected cells may indicate the nature of the storage material. The presence of secondary lysosomes containing fine, lamellated membrane structures is suggestive of gangliosides (Fig. 2-11); coarse lamellated structures are seen in sphingomyelin storage; and twisted microtubules are

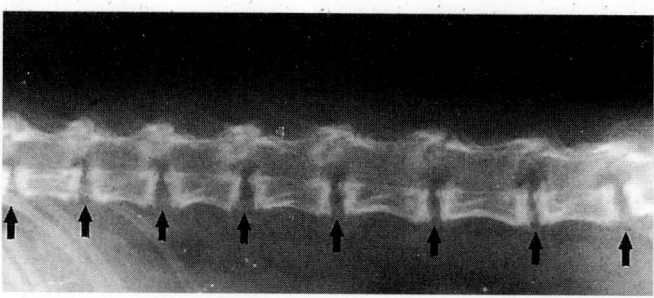

FIG. 2-7 Lumbar spine, lateral view, from 5-month-old Russian blue female cat with mucopolysaccharidosis VI. Intervertebral discs *(arrow)* are deformed, irregular, and abnormally wide.

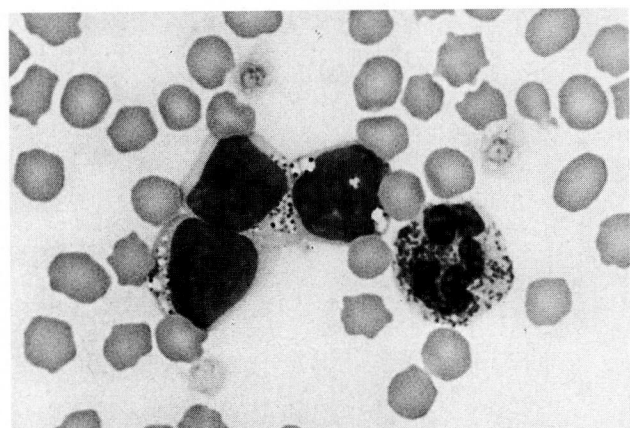

FIG. 2-8 Neutrophil and three lymphocytes from 7-month-old cat with mucopolysaccharidosis VI. Neutrophil contains numerous fine, but irregular metachromatic granules. Lymphocytes contain vacuoles containing metachromatic granules (Wright-Giemsa stain) (×750).

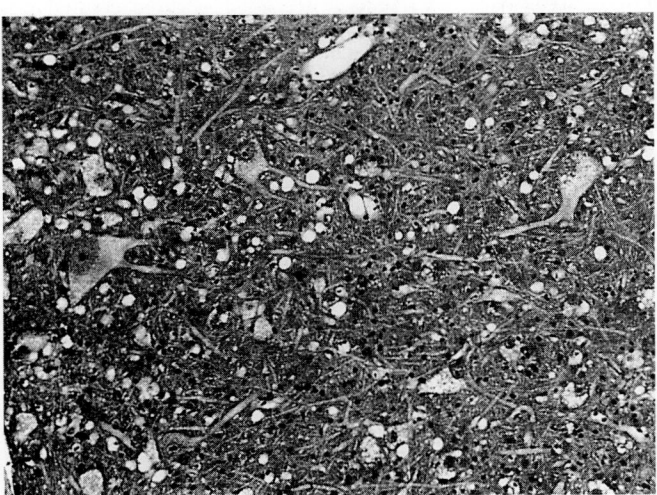

FIG. 2-9 Brainstem of 7-month-old female Persian cat with α mannosidosis. Note enlarged vacuolated neurons and astrocytes (hematoxylin and eosin stain) (×125).

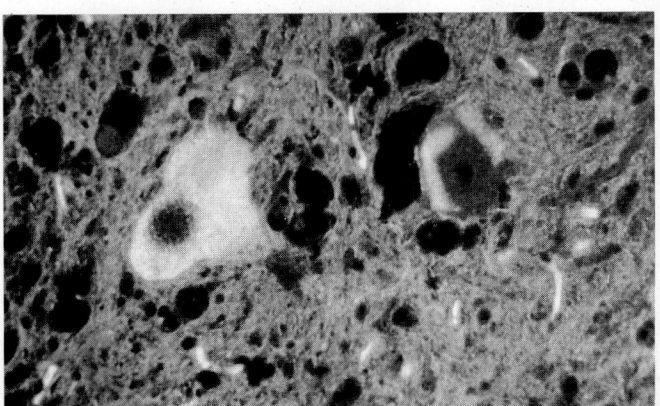

FIG. 2-10 Unstained paraffin section of spinal cord of 5-year-old spayed female Schipperke dog, with galactasidosis. Note autofluorescence in neuron under polarized light (×600).

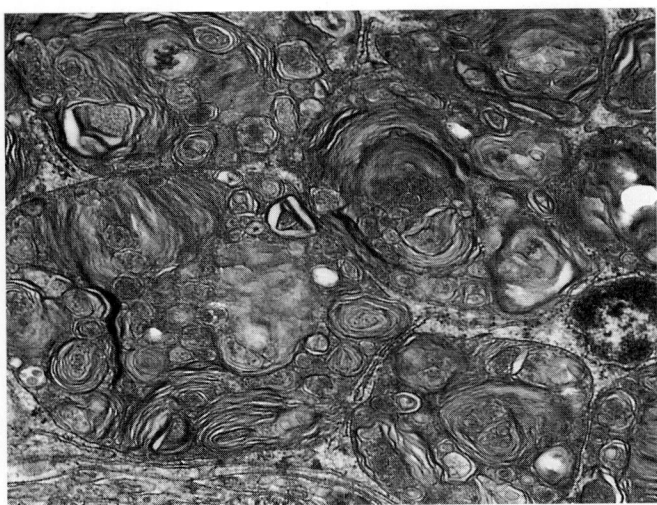

FIG. 2-11 Purkinje cell from cerebellum of 6-month-old female Portuguese water dog with GM_1 gangliosidosis. Note the lamellated membrane-structures characteristic of gangliosides (×18,000).

observed in storage of cerebrosides (Fig. 2-12). Fine, fibrillar material or empty-appearing vacuoles indicate storage of mucopolysaccharides or oligosaccharides (Fig. 2-13). Storage of fine fibrils and lamellated membrane structures within the same lysosome is often observed in mucopolysaccharidosis (Fig. 2-14). A finding of lysosomes containing curvilinear bodies is diagnostic for the late infantile, juvenile, and adult forms of neuronal ceroid lipofuscinosis (Fig. 2-15). Fresh frozen tissue can be used for assay of lysosomal enzymes and for extraction of stored lipids and oligosaccharides. Lipids also can be extracted from formalin-fixed tissues.

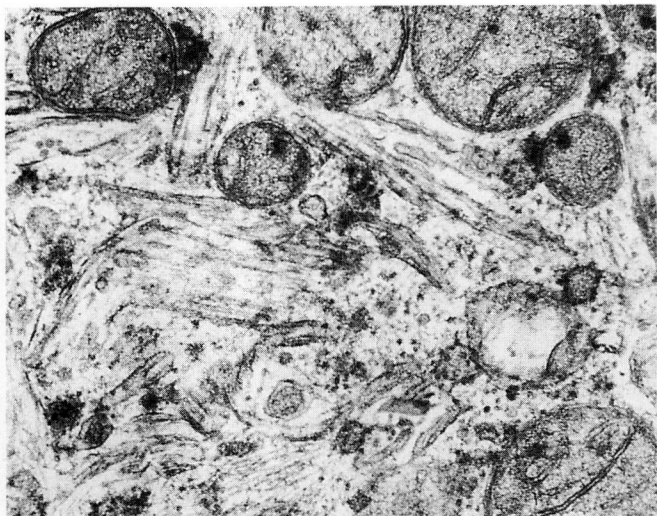

FIG. 2-12 Electron micrograph of globoid-cell from white matter of a 3-month-old rhesus monkey with Krabbe's disease. Numerous twisted microtubules are present, indicating storage of galactocerebrosides (×41,000).

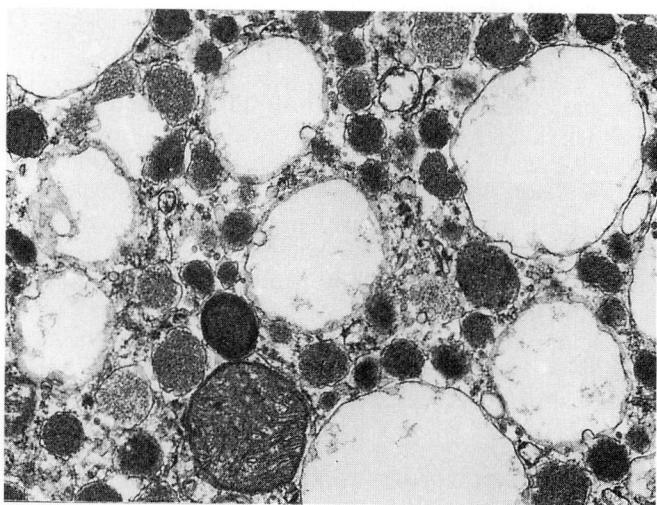

FIG. 2-13 Corticotropin-secreting cell from pituitary of a 7-month-old female Persian cat with α mannosidosis. Note secretory granules and large, empty-appearing secondary lysosomes, some containing few fine fibrils ($\times$ 18,000).

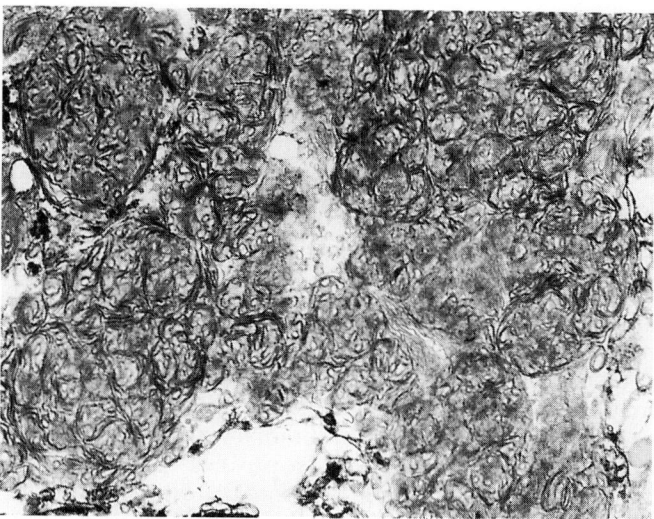

FIG. 2-15 Purkinje cell of cerebellum from 2-year-old Blue Heeler dog. Cytoplasm contains large secondary lysosomes laden with curvilinear bodies, which are diagnostic for late infantile, juvenile, and adult forms of neuronal ceroid-lipofuscinosis (X 21,800).

References

Alroy J, DeGasperi R, Warren CD. Application of lectin histochemistry and carbohydrate analysis to the characterization of lysosomal storage diseases. Carbohydrate Res 1991;213:229–250.

Alroy J, Kolodny EH. Lysosomal metabolism and its relevance to skeletal muscle. In: Engel AG, Franzini-Armstrong C, ed. Myology. 2nd ed. New York:McGraw-Hill 1944;708–735.

Alroy J, Knowles K, Schelling SH, et al. Retarded bone formation in GM_1-gangliosidosis: a study of the infantile form and comparison to two canine models. Virchows Arch 426:141–148. 1995.

Alroy J, Lee RE. Lysosomal storage diseases. In: Rosenberg AE, Schiller AL, ed. Orthopaedic Pathology. Philadelphia:WB Saunders (in press). 1997.

Castagnaro M, Alroy J, Ucci AA, et al. Lectin histochemistry and ultrastructure of feline kidneys from six different storage diseases. Virchows Arch B 1987;54:16–26.

Dorling PR. Lysosomal storage diseases in animals. In: Dingle JT, Den RT, Sly W, ed. Lysosomes in biology and pathology. Amsterdam:Elsevier 1984;347–379.

Elleder M. The spleen and storage disorders. In: Cuschieri A, Forbes CD, ed. Disorders of the spleen. Oxford:Blackwell Scientific 1995;151–190.

Glew RH, Basu A, Prence EM, et al. Lysosomal storage diseases. Lab Invest 1985;53:250–269.

Hansen HG, Graucob E. Hematologic cytology of storage diseases. Berlin: Springer-Verlag 1985.

Hruban Z. Pulmonary and generalized lysosomal storage induced by amphophilic drugs. Environ Health Perspect 1984;55:53–76.

Kay EM, Alroy J, Raghaven SS, et al. Dysmyelinogenesis in animal model of GM_1 gangliosidosis. Pediatr Neurol 1992;8:255–261.

Lake BD. Lysosomal and peroxisomal disorders. In: Adams JH, Duchen LW, ed. Greenfield's neuropathology. 5th ed. New York: Oxford Univ Press 1992;709–810.

Lovell KL. Caprine beta-mannosidosis: development of glial and myelin abnormalities in optic nerve and corpus callosum. Glia 1990;3:26–32.

Murnane RD, Prieur DJ, Ahern-Rindell AJ, et al. The lesions of an ovine lysosomal storage disease: initial characterization. Am J Pathol 1989;134:263–270.

Murnane RD, Hartley WJ, Prieur DJ. Similarity of lectin histochemistry of a lysosomal storage disease in a New Zealand lamb to that of ovine GM_1 gangliosidosis. Vet Pathol 1991;28:332–335.

Nanto-Salonen K, Larjava H, Saamanen AM, et al. Abnormal dermal proteoglycan in aspartylglucosaminuria: a possible mechanism for ultrastructural changes of collagen fibrils in a glycoprotein storage disorder. Conn Tissue Res 1987;16:367–376.

Scriver CR, Beaudet AL, Sly WS, et al. The metabolic basis of inherited disease, 7th ed. New York: McGraw-Hill 1995; Vol. II, pp. 2427–2879, Vol. III, pp. 3763–3797.

Walkley SU. Pathobiology of neuronal storage disease. Int Rev Neurobiol 1988;29:191–244.

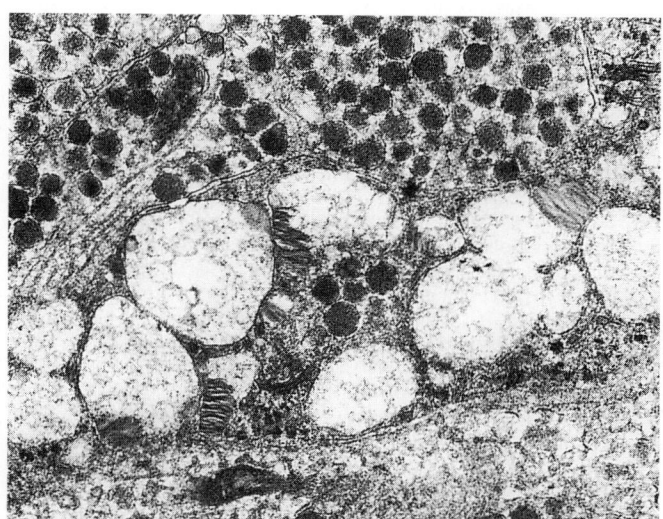

FIG. 2-14 Corticotropin-secreting cell from pituitary of a 6-month-old male Russian blue cat with mucopolysaccharidosis. Note secretory granules and secondary lysosomes containing fine fibrils and some lamellated membrane structures ($\times$ 18,000).

MUCOPOLYSACCHARIDOSES (MPS)

These diseases result from deficiency of one or more enzymes necessary for catabolism of mucopolysaccharides (glycosaminoglycans). Chondroitin sulfate, dermatan sulfate, heparin sulfate, and keratin sulfate are the major constituents of the glycosaminoglycan portion of proteoglycan (PG). There are three groups of proteoglycans: cell surface PG; small intracellular PG; and extracellular PG. The majority of PGs are located in the extracellular matrix, interacting with or binding to collagen, elastin, fibronectin, laminin, and plasma membrane. Their roles are, in part, resilience, binding water, maintenance of viscosity, regulation of fibrillogenesis and fibril diameter, cell recognition, cell attachment, and permeability. In mucopolysaccharidosis, mesenchymal cells, such as fibroblasts, chondrocytes, and bone cells that actively participate in recycling extracellular matrix, are most severely affected. In general, the Berry spot test is very useful in preliminary diagnosis of these conditions, although both false-positive and false-negative results occur, particularly in MPS III and MPS IV diseases. The presence of vacuoles containing metachromatic granules in white blood cells is indicative of mucopolysaccharidosis (Fig. 2-8). Ultrastructurally, affected cells contain secondary lysosomes with fine fibrils or appear empty, indicative of the storage of large or small mucopolysaccharides. In these conditions, the neurons often contain glycosphingolipids that appear as zebra bodies or lamellated membrane structures.

Mucopolysaccharidosis-I (MPS-I)

This category of disease has three manifestations identified with the eponyms Hurler, Hurler-Scheie, and Scheie syndromes.

Mucopolysaccharidosis-I is caused by the deficient activity of α L-iduronidase, resulting in lysosomal storage and urinary excretion of dermatan sulfate and heparin sulfate. Clinically, Hurler syndrome is the most severe manifestation of this enzyme deficiency; Hurler-Scheie syndrome is a slightly milder form; and Scheie syndrome is the mildest form. Deficient activity of α L-iduronidase occurs in domestic short-haired cats and Plott hounds. In both species, mesenchymal cells are most severely affected, resulting in facial and skeletal dysmorphia, corneal clouding, and cardiac valve insufficiency. Most affected cells store mucopolysaccharides, which are stainable with alcian blue and colloidal iron and are metachromatic with toluidine blue stain. Affected neurons store GM_1, GM_2 and GM_3, stainable with luxol fast blue and Sudan black.

Mucopolysaccharidosis-III (MPS-III)

This disease is also called Sanfilippo syndrome. The group of four different syndromes (designated as subtypes A to D) is characterized by deficient activity of one of four enzymes required for the degradation of heparin sulfate.

Only one subtype (D) has been identified in animal species. Deficient activity of N-acetylglucosamine 6-sulfatase has been identified in a Nubian goat with delayed motor development, growth retardation, and normal behavior. Histologic and biochemical studies of the liver and brain revealed lysosomal accumulation of glycosaminoglycans and GM_3 ganglioside.

Mucopolysaccharidosis-VI (MPS-VI)

This category of disease is also known as Maroteaux-Lamy syndrome. Mucopolysaccharidosis VI is caused by deficient activity of N-acetylgalactosamine 4-sulfatase (arylsulfatase B), which causes lysosomal storage and urinary excretion of dermatan sulfate. It has been described in Siamese cats and the Ishibashi hairless rat strain. Affected animals in both species are small and short with short tails and display facial dysmorphism and an abnormal skeleton (Fig. 2-7). Cloudy corneas and thickened atrioventricular valves occur in the cats, but not in the rats. The mesenchymal cells are vacuolated, but the neurons are not affected as they are in MPS-I.

Mucopolysacchridosis-VII (MPS-VII)

This disease is also called Sly's syndrome. Deficient activity of lysosomal β glucuronidase has been described in domestic short-haired cats, mixed-breed dogs, and mice. In all species, affected animals were small and had facial dysmorphism, retarded growth, and deformed axial and appendicular skeletons. Cloudy corneas and seizures were noted only in the cat. Most tissue storage and urinary excretion is of chondroitin-4 and chondroitin-6 sulfates, but storage and excretion of small amounts of dermatan and heparin sulfates also occur. Mesenchymal cells are most severely affected, and the lysosomes (vacuoles) either appear empty or contain fine fibrils. In contrast, the neurons contain lysosomes laden with lamellated membrane structures.

References

Alroy J, Freden GO, Goyal V, et al. Morphology of leukocytes from cats affected with α mannosidosis and mucopolysaccharidosis VI (MPS VI). Vet Pathol 1989;26:294–302.

Gitzelmann R, Bossard NU, Superti-Furga A, et al. Feline mucopolysaccharidosis VII due to β-glucuronidase deficiency. Vet Pathol 1994;31:435–443.

Haskins ME, Aguirre GD, Jezyk PF, et al. The pathology of the feline model of mucopolysaccharidosis I. Am J Pathol 1983;112:27–36.

Haskins ME, Bingel SA, Northington JW, et al. Spinal cord compression and hind limb paresis in cats with mucopolysaccharidosis VI. J Am Vet Med Assoc 1983;182:983–985.

Haskins ME, Desnick RT, DiFerrante N, et al. β Glucuronidase deficiency in a dog: a model of human mucopolysaccharidosis VII. Pediatr Res 1984;18:980–984.

Thompson JN, Jones MZ, Dawson G, et al. N-acetylglucosamine 6-sulphatase deficiency in a Nubian goat: a model of Sanfillipo syndrome type D (mucopolysaccharidosis IIID). J Inher Metab Dis 1992;15:760–768.

Vogler C, Berkenmeier EH, Sly WS, et al. A murine model of mucopolysaccharidosis VII. Gross and microscopic findings in β glucuronidase-deficient mice. Am J Pathol 1990;136:207–217.

Yoshida M, Ikadai H, Maekawa A, et al. Pathological characteristics of mucopolysaccharidosis VI in the rat. J Comp Pathol 1993; 109:141–153.

SPHINGOLIPIDOSES (LIPID STORAGE DISEASES)

Sphingolipidosis refers to a group of disorders caused by deficient activity of lysosomal hydrolases, which are involved in the degradation of lipids that contain sphingosine as the basic molecular unit.

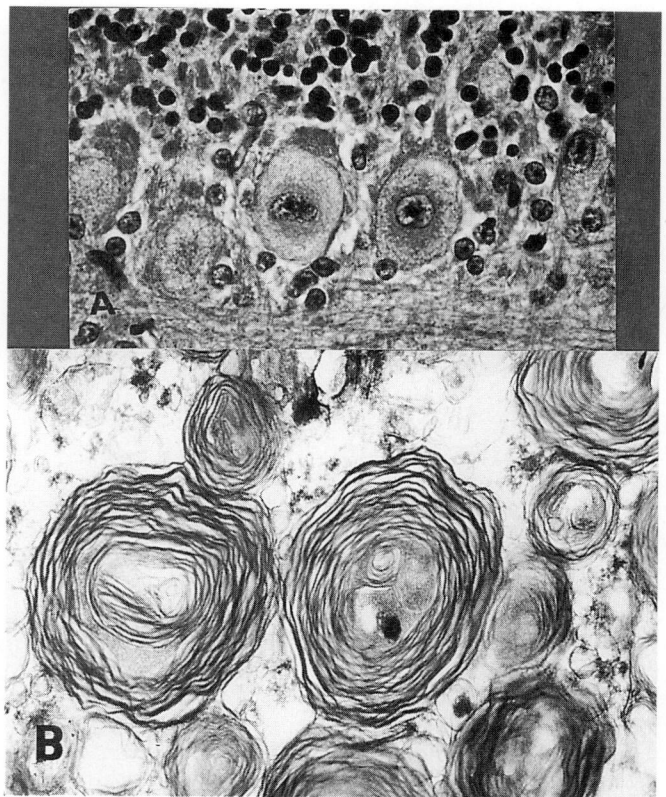

FIG. 2-16 GM₁ gangliosidosis in a cat. **A.** Glycoside-laden Purkinje cells. **B.** Ultrastructure of membranous inclusions in neuronal cytoplasm. (Courtesy of Dr. Henry J. Baker)

GM₁ Gangliosidosis

GM₁ gangliosidosis is caused by deficient activity of acid β galactosidase, resulting in storage of glycolipids, oligosaccharides, and glycosaminoglycans, with a nonreducing terminal β galactosidic linkage in various tissues and abnormal excretion of various compounds in the urine. Nonreducing terminal β galactosyl residues are found in glycolipids, glycoproteins, and glycosaminoglycans, which are the major constituents of the cell membrane and extracellular matrix; therefore, almost all cell types are affected. Neurons contain numerous enlarged lysosomes laden with lamellated membrane, because neuronal membrane is rich in gangliosides (Fig. 2-16), whereas other cell types store oligosaccharides or glycosaminoglycans. Early onset (**infantile form**) of GM₁ gangliosidosis occurs in English springer spaniels and Portuguese water dogs and is manifested by progressive neurologic impairment and skeletal dysplasia. In Friesian calves, Siamese and domestic short-haired cats, Beagle dogs, and Suffolk cross-bred sheep, the clinical onset is delayed. Affected animals have neurologic impairment, but no macroscopic skeletal involvement and, thus, clinically, manifestation is similar to the **juvenile form** of the disease in human beings.

GM₂ Gangliosidosis

The GM₂ gangliosidoses include five disorders that are characterized by primary or secondary deficient activity of lysosomal β hexosaminidase, resulting in lysosomal storage of GM₂ gangliosides. Normally, the β hexosaminidase α and β subunits form two catalytically active isozymes, β hexosaminidase A, which contains α and β subunits, and β hexosaminidase B, which contains two β subunits. In addition, an activator protein (saposin), which binds the glycolipid (GM₂ ganglioside) to the enzyme, is required. Deficient activity of β hexosaminidase A, caused by a mutated α subunit (Tay-Sachs' disease), or of activator protein results in abnormal storage of glycolipids. Deficient activity of β hexosaminidase A and B (Sandhoff's disease), causedby a mutated a β subunit, leads to abnormal storage of glycolipids, oligosaccharides, and glycosaminoglycans.

GM₂ gangliosidoses have been reported in domestic and Korat cats, in German shorthair pointers, Japanese spaniels, and Yorkshire pigs. In both breeds of cats, deficient activity of β hexosaminidase A and B leads to abnormal storage in numerous cell types. Their neurons are packed with lamellated membrane structures (glycolipids), whereas other cell types have empty-appearing vacuoles. In both breeds of dogs and in pigs, the major changes were in neuronal tissue. Morphologically, the storage compounds appeared as lamellated membrane structures. Deficient activity of hexosaminidase A, which is equivalent to human Tay-Sacs', has been reported in a Muntjac deer. Deficient activity of activator protein was found to be the cause of GM₂ gangliosidosis in a Japanese spaniel.

References

Alroy J, Orgood U, De Gasperi R, et al. G_{M1}-gangliosidosis: a clinical, morphologic, histochemical, and biochemical comparison of two different models. Am J Pathol 1992;140:675–689.

Bermudoz AJ, Johnson GC, Vanier MT, et al. Gangliosidosis in emus (*Dromaius novaehollandise* Avian Dis 1995;39:292–303.

Cork LC, Munnell JF, Lorenz MD. The pathology of feline GM₂-gangliosidosis. Am J Pathol 1978;90:723–734.

Cummings JF, Wood PA, Walkley SU, et al. GM₂-gangliosidosis in a Japanese spaniel. Acta Neuropathol 1985;67:247–253.

Donnelly WJC, Sheahan BJ. GM₁-gangliosidosis of Friesian calves: a review. Irish Vet J 1981;35:45–55.

Farrell DF, Baker HJ, Herndon RM, et al. Feline GM₁ gangliosidosis: biochemical and ultrastructural comparisons with the disease in man. J Neuropathol Exp Neurol 1973;32:1–18.

Fox J. Homer B, Alleman A, et al. GM₂ gangliosidosis in a Muntjac deer. Vet Pathol 1995;32:577.

Ishikawa Y, Li S-C, Wood PA, et al. Biochemical basis of type AB GM₂-gangliosidosis in a Japanese spaniel. J Neurochem 1987;48:860–864.

Karbe E. Gangliosidosis and other neuronal lipodystrophies with amaurosis in dogs. A comparative histopathological, histochemical, electron microscopical, and biochemical study. Arch Exp Vet Med 1971;25:1–48.

Kosanke SD, Pierce KR, Read WK. Morphogenesis of light and electron microscopic lesions in porcine GM₂-gangliosidosis. Vet Pathol 1979;16:6–17.

Murnane RD, Prieur DJ, Ahern-Rindell AJ, et al. The lesions of an ovine lysosomal storage disease: initial characterization. Am J Pathol 1989;134:263–270.

Neuwelt EA, Johnson WG, Blank NK, et al. Characterization of a new model of GM₂-gangliosidosis (Sandhoff's disease) in Korat cats. J Clin Invest 1985;76:482–490.

Rodriguez M, O'Brien JS, Garrett RS, et al. Canine GM₁-gangliosidosis: an ultrastructural and biochemical study. J Neuropathol Exp Neurol 1982;41:618–629.

Saunders GK, Wood PA, Myers RK, et al. GM₁ gangliosidosis in Portuguese water dogs: pathologic and biochemical findings. Vet Pathol 1988;25:265–269.

Shell LG, Pathoff AI, Carithers R, et al.: Neuronal-Visceral GM₁ gangliosidosis in Portuguese water dogs. J Vet Int Med 1989; 3:1–7.

Singer HS, Cork LC. Canine GM₂ gangliosidosis: morphological and biochemical analysis. Vet Pathol 1989;26:114–120.

Galactosialidosis

Galactosialidosis is characterized by deficient activity of both β galactosidase and α neuraminidase caused by mutation of protective protein, which results in accumulation of sialylated oligosaccharides and glycolipids. Adult onset of progressive neurologic signs has been described in a Schipperke dog. Morphologic findings indicated neuronal storage of glycolipids and storage of oligosaccharides in other cell types. Biochemical findings were consistent with those observed in galactosialidosis.

Glucosylceramide-lipidosis (Gaucher's disease)

Gaucher's disease is characterized primarily by deficient activity of glucocerebrosidase and abnormal accumulations of glucocerebrosides and polylactosaminoglycans. Rarely, deficient activity of activator protein may cause a similar condition. Since the major stored substrate originates from the plasma membrane of red and white blood cells, reticuloendothelial cells are the most severely affected. Adult type 1 Gaucher's disease, most common in human beings, is characterized by hepatosplenomegaly and bone marrow involvement. Infantile acute neuropathic type 2 and juvenile subacute neuropathic type 2 also occur.

The characteristic feature of Gaucher's disease is the presence of lipid-laden reticuloendothelial cells (Gaucher cells) within affected tissues such as the spleen, liver, and bone marrow. Gaucher cells have abundant striated cytoplasm, the appearance of which has been compared with that of wrinkled cigarette paper. Ultrastructurally, Gaucher cells have enlarged secondary lysosomes containing twisted tubular structures that indicate the presence of glucocerebrosides. Neurovisceral manifestation of Gaucher's disease has been described in a Sydney silky dog, and suspected visceral forms of the disease have been described in a pig and a sheep.

Gaucher-like cells are often observed in conditions in which there is an oversupply of substrate, such as myelogenous leukemia, lymphoma, and various types of hemolytic anemia, e.g., β thalassemia. In these conditions, there is an oversupply of plasma membrane from white or red blood cells, which must be catabolized by the reticuloendothelial cells.

Galactosylceramide-lipidosis

This disease is also known as globoid-cell leukodystrophy or Krabbe's disease. Galactosylceramide lipidosis is characterized by deficient activity of lysosomal galactosylcerebroside β galactosidase and the abnormal accumulation of galactosylsphingosine (psychosine). It has been found in "twitcher" mice, Cairn and West Highland white terri-

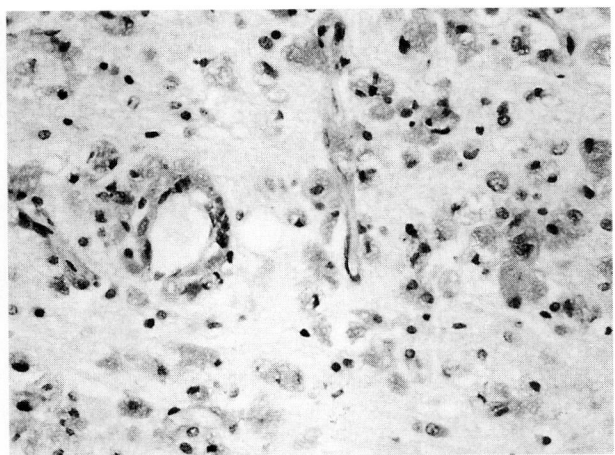

FIG. 2-17 Paraffin section through the corpus callosum of a 3-month-old rhesus monkey with galactosylceramide-lipidosis. Note massive infiltration by numerous histiocytes with enlarged globoid-shaped cytoplasm that stains PAS-positive.

ers, beagles, blue tick hounds, miniature poodles, domestic short-haired cats, polled Dorset sheep, and rhesus monkeys. Morphologically, lesions observed in all five species are the same. Myelinated tissues in the central and peripheral nerve systems are most severely affected, since galactosylceramide is found almost exclusively in myelin. Brain lesions include destruction of myelin and oligodendroglia, glial scarring, and abnormal infiltration throughout the white matter of distinctive epithelioid cells (globoid cells) (Fig. 2-17). The globoid cells are macrophages of mesodermal origin preferentially localized adjacent to blood vessels. Globoid-cell cytoplasm is stained with luxol fast-blue, Sudan black, Sudan IV, and PAS, and the cells contain enlarged secondary lysosomes filled with twisted tubules (Fig. 2-12).

References

Alroy J, Ucci AA, Goyal V, et al. Histochemical similarities between human and animal globoid cells in Krabbe's disease: a lectin study. Acta Neuropathol 1986;71:26–31.

Baskin G, Alroy J, Li Y-T, et al. Galactosylceramide-lipidosis in rhesus monkey. Lab Invest 1989;60:7A.

Beaudet AL. Gaucher's disease. N Engl J Med 1987;316:619–621.

Boysen BG, Tryphonas L, Harries NW. Globoid cell leukodystrophy in the blue tick hound dog. Can Vet J 1974;15:303–308.

DeGasperi R, Alroy J, Richard R, et al. Glycoprotein storage in Gaucher disease: lectin histochemistry and biochemical studies. Lab Invest 1990;63:385–393.

Duchen LW, Eicher EM, Jacobs JM, et al. Hereditary leukodystrophy in the mouse: the new mutant Twitcher. Brain 1980;103:695–710.

Fankhauser R, Luginbuhl H, Hartley WJ. Leukodystrophy of Krabbe's type in the dog.Vet Bull 1964;34(325):41.

Glew RH, Basu A, LaMarco KL, et al. Mammalian glucocerebrosidase: implications for Gaucher's disease. Lab Invest 1988;58:5–25.

Hartley WJ, Blakemore WF. Neurovisceral glucocerebroside storage (Gaucher's disease) in a dog. Vet Pathol 1973;10:191–201.

Johnson KH. Globoid leukodystrophy in the cat. J Am Vet Med Assoc 1970;157:2057–2064.

Johnson GR, Oliver JE Jr, Selcer R. Globoid cell leukodystrophy in a beagle. J Am Vet Med Assoc 1975;167:380–384.

Knowles K, Alroy J, Castagnaro M, et al. Adult-onset lysosomal storage disease in a Schipperke dog: clinical and biochemical studies. Acta Neuropathol 1993;86:306–312.

Laws L, Saal JR. Lipidosis of the hepatic reticuloendothelial cell in a sheep. Aust Vet J 1968;44:416–417.

Pritchard DH, Napthine DV, Sinclair AJ. Globoid cell leukodystrophy in polled Dorset sheep. Vet Pathol 1980;17:399–405.

Sandison AJ, Anderson LJ. Histiocytosis in two pigs and a cow: conditions resembling lipid storage disorders in man. J Pathol 1970;100:207–210.

Zaki FA, Kay WJ. Globoid cell leukodystrophy in a Miniature Poodle. J Am Vet Med Assoc 1973;163:248–250.

Sphingomyelin-Cholesterol Lipidoses

These disorders are also termed Niemann-Pick diseases. This group of diseases is divided into two types on the basis of etiology, and each type is subdivided into three different clinical manifestations.

Types A and B are caused by deficient activity of lysosomal sphingomyelinase and lysosomal accumulation of mostly sphingomyelin and cholesterol. The acute neuropathic form of type A has its counterpart in Balinese and Siamese cats and miniature poodles.

The primary cause of the type C disease is unknown, but it is characterized by decreased in vitro esterification of exogenous cholesterol, reduced sphingomyelinase activity, and lysosomal storage of sphingomyelin, cholesterol, and glycolipids. The acute neuropathic form of type C has been observed in domestic shorthaired cats, Boxer dogs, and mutant mouse strains C57BL/KsJ and NCTR-BALB/c.

In both type A and type B, the reticuloendothelial cells in various organs are affected. Neurons and hepatocytes are more severely affected in type A. The storage material is stained with Sudan black and oil red O and with PAS after digestion with diastase. Ultrastructurally, the lysosomes contain coarse lamellated membrane structures.

References

Baker HJ, Wood PA, Wenger DA, et al. Sphingomyelin lipidosis in a cat. Vet Pathol 1987;24:386–391.

Bundza A, Lowden JA, Charlton KM. Niemann-Pick disease in a poodle dog. Vet Pathol 1979;16:530–538.

Kuwamura M, Awakura T, Shimada A, et al. Type C Niemann-Pick disease in a boxer dog. Acta Neuropathol 1993;85:345–348.

Lowenthal AC, Cummings JF, Wenger DA, et al. Feline sphingolipidosis resembling Niemann-Pick diseases type C. Acta Neuropathol 1989;81:189–197.

Miyawaki S, Yoshida H, Mitsuoka S, et al. A mouse model for Niemann-Pick disease. Influence of genetic background on disease expression in spm/spm mice. J Hered 1986;77:379–384.

Pentchev PG, Gal AE, Boothe AD, et al. A lysosomal storage disorder in mice characterized by a dual deficiency of sphingomyelinase and glucocerebrosidase. Biochim Biophys Acta 1980;619:669–679.

Pentchev PG, Boothe AD, Kruth HS, et al. A genetic storage disorder in BALB/c mice with a metabolic block in esterification of exogenous cholesterol. J Biol Chem 1984;259:5784–5791.

Shio H, Fowler S, Bhuvaneswaran C, et al. Lysosomal lipid storage disorder in NCTR-BALB/c mice. II. Morphologic and cytochemical studies. Am J Pathol 1982;108:150–159.

GLYCOPROTEIN STORAGE DISEASES

In this group of storage disorders, oligosaccharides are the major storage compounds, although in some of the conditions a small amount of glycolipid compounds are stored as well. Glycoprotein molecules contain oligosaccharide chains covalently attached to a peptide backbone. There are two major types of glycoproteins, those that are linked through hydroxyl groups of serine or threonine (O-linked glycoproteins) and those that are linked through the free amino group of asparagine (N-linked glycoproteins). Glycoproteins are major constituents of cellular membranes and extracellular matrix, including proteoglycan and collagen. Thus, deficient activity of α fucosidase, β endo-N-acetylglucosaminidase, aspartylglucosaminidase, α neuraminidase (sialidase), β hexosaminidase A and B, α mannosidase, and β mannosidase, which participate in the degradation of oligosaccharides, is morphologically manifested in many cell types.

α Mannosidosis

Deficient activity of lysosomal α mannosidase results in cellular storage and urinary excretion of partially degraded N-linked oligosaccharides containing α mannosyl residues. The disease is inherited as an autosomal recessive trait and has been found in Red Angus, Murray Grey, Galloway, and Shorthorn cattle and in domestic short-haired and Persian cats. Acquired forms of α mannosidosis can result from prolonged ingestion of *Swainsona* species (i.e., *S. canescens, S. galegifolia*) or locoweed (*Astragalus lentiginosus*) or both, which contain indolizidine alkaloid, by inhibiting lysosomal acid α mannosidase. This also interferes with normal synthesis of N-linked glycoprotein by inhibiting Golgi α mannosidase II. The affected cells are vacuolated (Fig. 2-9) and contain numerous enlarged secondary lysosomes, which often appear empty or contain a few fine fibrils and a few small membrane fragments.

β Mannosidosis

An autosomal recessive inherited deficiency of β mannosidase activity has been described in Salers calves and newborn goats. The disease is characterized by stillbirth and neurologic impairment in these species. Histologically, affected individuals have extensive vacuolization of a wide variety of cells throughout the body, particularly the thyroid follicular and renal tubular epithelia, neurons, and macrophages. Hypomyelination is also a common feature of this disease, since thyroid hormone plays a major role in regulating myelination. The vacuolated cells contain a water-soluble oligosaccharide within lysosomes that dissolves during routine tissue processing.

α Fucosidosis

Fucosidosis is a lysosomal storage disease caused by a deficiency of α fucosidase that has been described in human patients and in English springer spaniels. This enzyme deficiency results principally in the accumulation of oligosaccharides, although some storage of glycolipids and glycopeptides also occurs. Although both species have a similar enzyme deficiency, studies indicate that human and canine fucosidosis differ in their lectin-binding patterns as well as in cell and organ involvement. Affected cells include reticuloendothelial cells, epithelial cells in various organs, fibroblasts, smooth muscle cells, neurons, and glial cells. Ultrastructural studies of most cell types revealed enlarged secondary lysosomes, which appear empty, indicating accumulation of oligosaccharides. In neurons, the lysosomes contain lamellated membrane structures suggestive of glycolipids.

References

Alroy J, Ucci AA, Warren CD. Human and canine fucosidosis. A comparative lectin histochemistry study. Acta Neuropathol (Berl) 1985;67:265–271.

Boyer PJ, Jones MZ, Nachreiner RF, et al. Caprine-mannosidosis. Abnormal thyroid structure and function in a lysosomal storage disease. Lab Invest 1990;63:100–106.

Bryan L, Schmutz S, Hodges SD, et al. Bovine-mannosidosis: pathologic and genetic findings in Salers calves. Vet Pathol 1993;30:130–139.

Dorling PR, Huxtable CR, Vogel P. Lysosomal storage in *Swainsona* spp. toxicosis: an induced mannosidosis. Neuropathol Appl Neurobiol 1978;4:285–295.

Embury DH, Jerrett IV. Mannosidosis in Galloway calves. Vet Pathol 1985;22:548–551.

Hartley WJ, Canfield PJ, Donnelly TM. A suspected new canine storage disease. Acta Neuropathol (Berl) 1982;56:225–232.

Jolly RD, Thompson KG. The pathology of bovine mannosidosis. Vet Pathol 1978;15:141–152.

Jolly RD, Thompson KG, Bayliss SL, et al. β-Mannosidosis in a Salers calf: a new storage disease of cattle. NZ Vet J 1990;38:102–105.

Jones MZ, Cunningham JG, Dade AW, et al. Caprine-mannosidosis: clinical and pathological features. J Neuropathol Exp Neurol 1983;42:268–285.

Kelly WR, Clague AE, Barns RJ, et al. Canine α fucosidosis: a storage disease of Springer Spaniels. Acta Neuropathol (Berl) 1983;60:9–13.

Molyneaux RJ, James LF. Loco intoxication: indolizidine alkaloids of spotted locoweed (*Astragalus lentiginosus*). Science 1983;216:190–191.

Render JA, Lovell KL, Jones MZ, et al. Ocular pathology of caprine-mannosidosis. Vet Pathol 1989;26:444–446.

Tulsiani DRP, Touster O. Swainsonine causes the production of hybrid glycoproteins by human skin fibroblasts and rat liver Golgi preparations. J Biol Chem 1983;258:7578–7585.

Vandevelde M, Frankhauser R, Bischel P, et al. Hereditary neurovisceral mannosidosis associated with α mannosidase deficiency in a family of Persian cats. Acta Neuropathol 1982;58:64–68.

Walkley SU, Blakemore WF, Purpura DP. Alterations in neuron morphology in feline mannosidosis. Acta Neuropathol 1981;53:75–79.

Warner TG, O'Brien JS. Genetic defects in glycoprotein metabolism. Annu Rev Genet 1983;17:395–441.

Neuronal Glycoproteinosis

This disease is also referred to as myoclonic epilepsy or LaFora's disease. This is a rare **nonlysosomal** storage disease of human beings, which has also been reported in Basset hounds and poodles. The signs include clonic twitching of muscles, somnolence, incoordination, convulsions, and progressive deterioration. Adult and aged dogs are more apt to be affected.

The distinguishing feature is the accumulation of glucoproteins (polyglucosans) in the form of microscopic bodies (LaFora bodies) in neurons and skeletal muscle cells (Fig. 2-18). These bodies are not membrane-bound and do not involve lysosomes, and there-

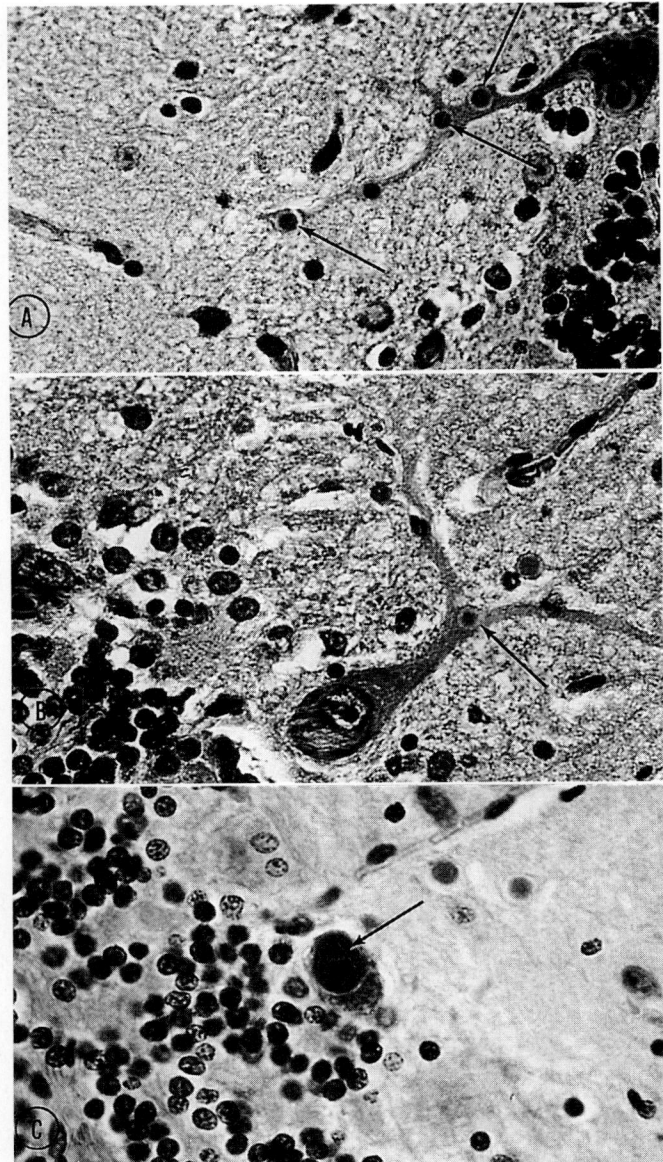

FIG. 2-18 Neuronal glycoproteinosis (Lafora's disease) in a dog. **A.** and **B.** Purkinje cells containing discrete Lafora bodies. **C.** Single large Lafora body displacing nucleus of Purkinje cell. (Courtesy Dr. James M. Holland and *American Journal of Pathology* 1970;58:509–530.

fore, this disease does not qualify as a lysosomal storage disease; it is a purely understood form of cellular degeneration. The inclusion bodies in this disease do not impart a vacuolated microscopic appearance to affected cells but appear as discrete basophilic, PAS-positive cytoplasmic inclusions. The inclusions are most frequent in the perikaya of Purkinje cells or in dendrites and, rarely, occur in peripheral neurons. They are also found in skeletal muscles between myofibrils or beneath the sarcolemma. Similar inclusion bodies have been described in unaffected, aged human patients but in much fewer numbers than in patients with myoclonic epilepsy.

Several forms of these inclusion bodies have been described, including (1) very small homogeneous PAS-

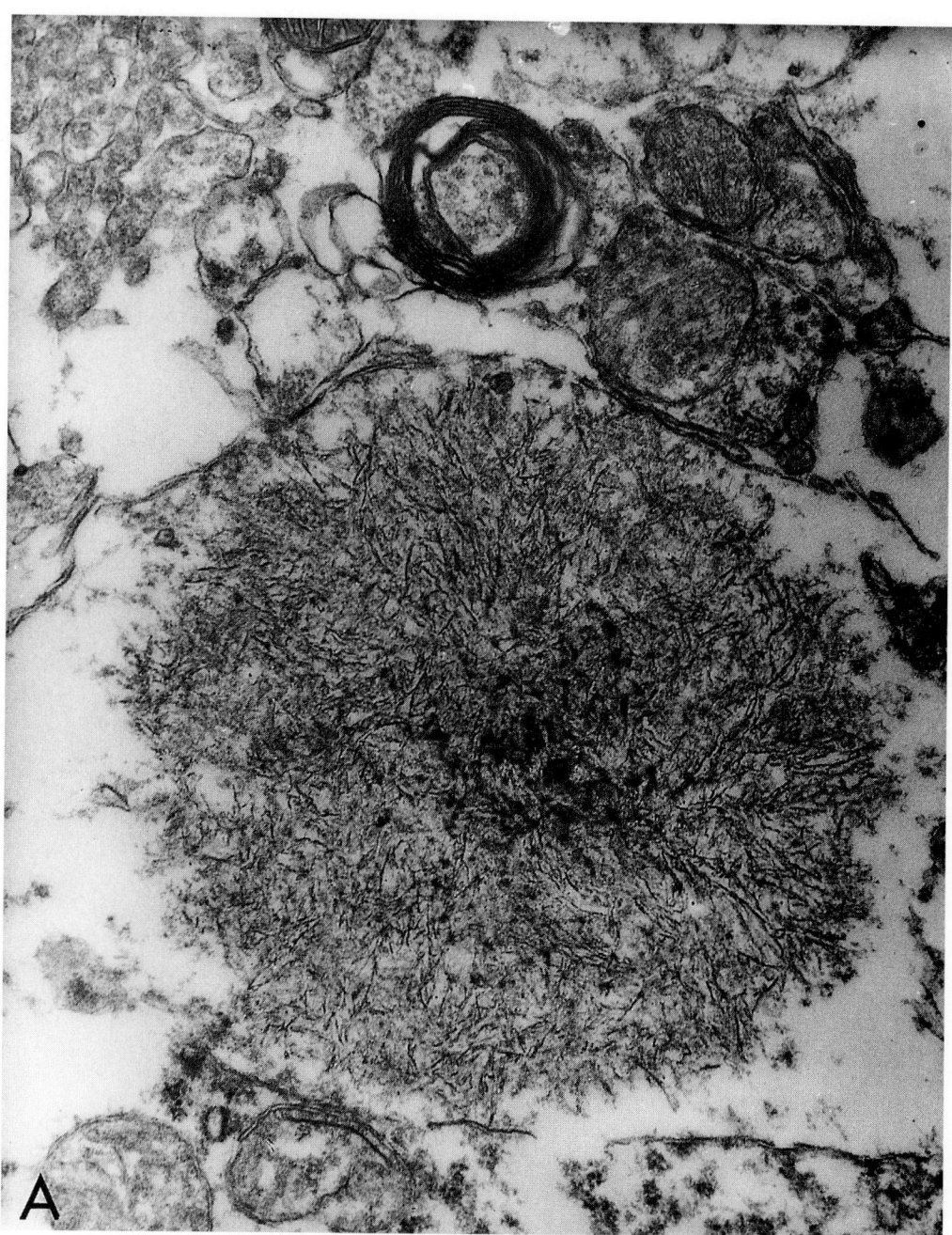

FIG. 2-19 Neuronal glyco-proteinosis (Lafora's disease). **A.** Fibrillar form of inclusion.

positive bodies; (2) bodies made up of aggregates of PAS-positive particles; (3) bodies with a smooth outer radial zone and concentric internal structure; and (4) bodies with a homogeneous center, concentric layering, light intermediate zone, and a smooth outer zone. These bodies are round, laminated, and basophilic if stained with hematoxylin and eosin and may be as large as 32 μm in diameter.

Ultrastructurally, these bodies consist of an electron-dense core surrounded by a fibrillar periphery without a limiting membrane (Fig. 2-19). The histochemical and ultrastructural features of these bodies in dogs suggest support for the thesis that the bodies consist of complex glycoproteins essentially similar to that reported in the human disease.

References

Busard HL, Span JP, Renkawek K, et al. Polyglucosan bodies in brain tissue: a systematic study. Clin Neuropathol 1994;13:60–63.
Kaiser E, Krauser K, Schwartz-Porsche D [LaFora's disease (progressive myoclonic epilepsy) in the Bassett hound—possibility of early diagnosis using muscle biopsy?] Tierarzl Prax 1991;19: 290–295.

GLYCOGEN STORAGE DISEASES

Glycogen is found in moderate amounts in all cells, where it serves as a readily available glycolytic fuel. In humans, at least ten different glycogen storage disorders are recognized. They result from either a deficiency of the enzymes or transporters that participate in glycogen metabolism, leading to storage of glycogen

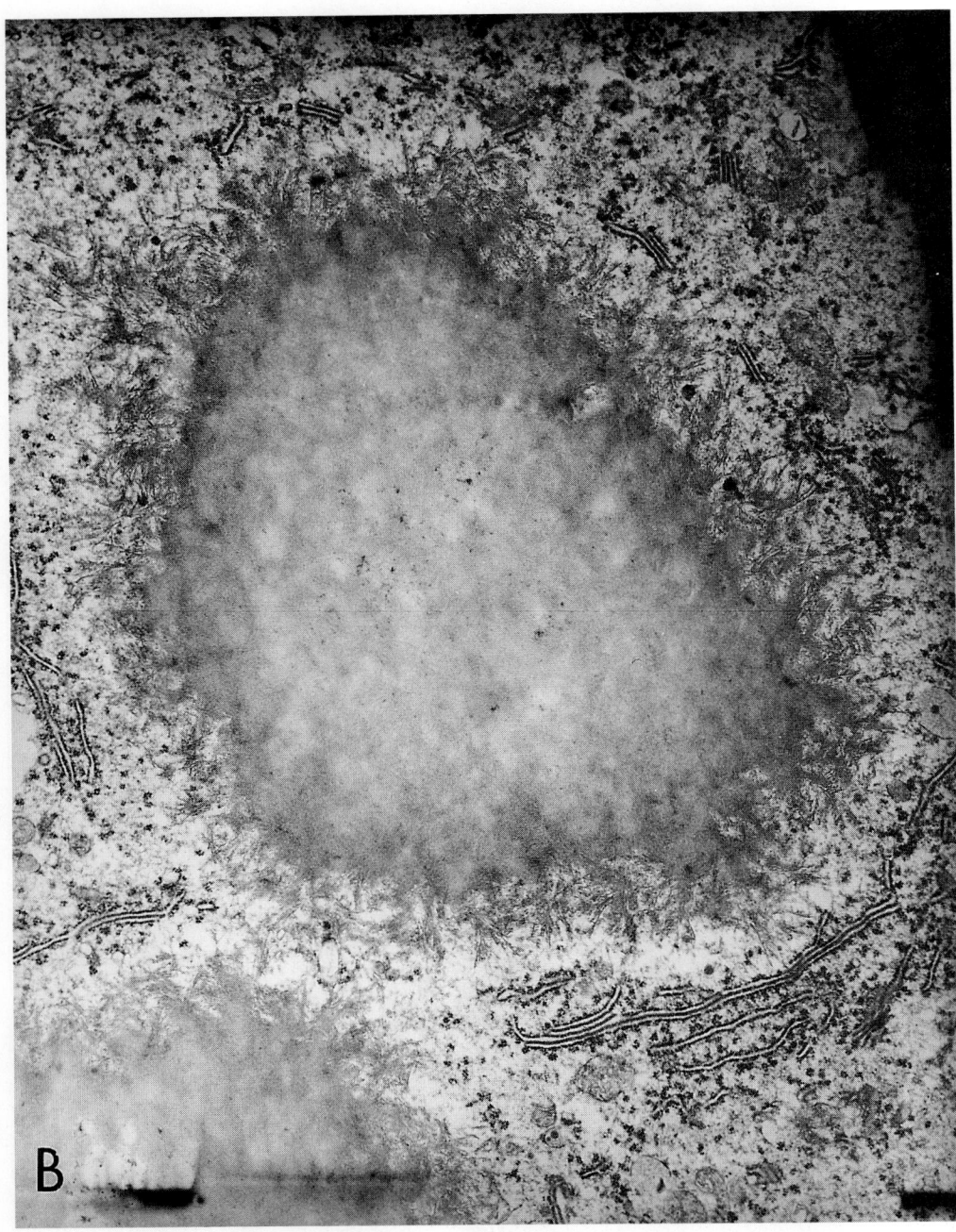

FIG. 2-19 (Cont) **B.** Homogeneous form of inclusion. (Courtesy of Dr. W.C. Davis)

in abnormal quantities or with an abnormal structure. Only glycogen storage type II, or Pompe's disease, is a lysosomal storage disorder.

Type II Glycogenosis

Type II glycogenosis, also known as Pompe's disease or acid maltase deficiency, is a lysosomal storage disease caused by a deficiency of $\alpha 1$, 4-glucosidase (acid maltase) activity and is characterized by storage of glycogen and acid polysaccharides. However, there are several reports of lysosomal storage of glycogen with normal activity of acid maltase. Type II glycogen storage disorders have been reported in several animal species. The Lapland dog has an infantile form of this disease; Shorthorn cattle have both infantile and late-onset forms; and Japanese quail and Brahman cattle have only the late-onset type. In addition, the disease has been reported in cats, Corriedale sheep, and Broad-Breasted White turkeys. Type II glycosidosis can be experimentally induced in rats by repeated intraperitoneal injections of acarbose, a pseudo-tetrasaccharide that competitively inhibits acid maltase. Stored glycogen can be demonstrated in all cell types by examining either frozen sections or ethanol-fixed, paraffin-embedded sections stained with PAS or Best's carmine. Pretreatment of the sections with diastase before staining abolishes the PAS reaction and thus confers greater specificity to the reaction.

It has been proposed that the abnormal accumulation of metachromatic alcian blue-positive material is an acid polysaccharide that contains phosphate groups and is removed by salivary gland amylase. Ultrastructurally, glycogen that appears as irregular A and B type, electron-dense particles accumulates in three different intracellular compartments: (1) as aggregates free in the cytosol; (2) in membrane-bound structures that contain only glycogen; and (3) in lysosomes along with heterogenous degradation products.

References

Czarnecki CM, Jegers A, Jankus EF. Characterization of glycogen in selected tissues of turkey poults with spontaneous round heart disease and furazolidone-induced cardiomyopathy. Acta Anat 1978;102:33–39.

DiMauro S, Tsujino S. Nonlysosomal glycogenoses. In: Engel AG, Franzini-Armstrong C, ed. Myology. 2nd ed. New York: McGraw-Hill 1994;1554–1576.

Engel AG, Hirschhorn R. Acid maltase deficiency. In: Engel AG, Franzini-Armstrong C, ed. Myology. 2nd ed. New York: McGraw-Hill 1994;1533–1553.

Hers H-G, Van Hoof F, de Barsy T. Glycogen storage diseases. Lysosomal enzymes. In: Scriver CR, Beaudet AL, Sly WS, Valle D, ed. The metabolic basis of inherited disease. 6th ed. New York: McGraw-Hill 1989;425–452.

Howell J McC, Dorling PR, Cook RD, et al. Infantile and late onset form of generalized glycogenosis type II in cattle. J Pathol 1981;134:266–277.

Manktelov BW, Hartley WJ. Generalized glycogen storage disease in sheep. J Comp Pathol 1975;85:139–145.

Murakami H, Takagi A, Nanaka S, et al. Glycogenosis II in a Japanese quail. Exp Anim (Tokyo) 1980;29:475–485.

Sandstrom B, Westman J, Ockerman PA. Glycosinosis of central nervous system in the cat. Acta Neuropathol 1969;14:194–200.

Ullrich K, Hermans MM, Visser WJ, et al. Lysosomal glycogen storage disease without deficiency of acid alpha glucosidase. In: Bartsocas CS, ed. Genetics of neuromuscular disorders. New York: Wiley 1989;163–171.

Walvoort HC. Glycogen storage diseases in animals and their potential value as models of human disease. J Inher Metab Dis 1983;6:3–16.

Walvoort HC, Dormans JA, Van den Ingh TS. Comparative pathology of the canine model of glycogen storage disease type II (Pompe's disease). J Inher Metab Dis 1985;8:38–46.

Wisselaar HA, Hermans MN, Visser WJ, et al. Biochemical genetics of glycogenosis type II in Brahman cattle. Biochem Biophys Res Commun 1993;190:941–947.

Neuronal ceroid-lipofuscinosis

Neuronal ceroid-lipofuscinosis (NCL), called Batten disease in human beings, is probably the most common group of lysosomal storage diseases. The natures of the deficient enzyme(s) or of the major storage compound(s) are unknown. NCL is used to describe these diseases because the stored substance is stainable with luxol fast blue and Sudan black, is autofluorescent, and is not extractable with lipid solvent; it is, however, distinguishable from lipofuscin (aging pigment). The disorder is classified in terms of age of onset and clinical manifestation into infantile, late infantile, juvenile, and adult forms. In all forms, partially degraded substrates are observed in neurons, but have a multisystemic cellular distribution. Ultrastructurally, in the infantile form, the storage material is granular and osmiophilic. In contrast, the storage material in the late infantile, juvenile, and adult forms has a characteristic curvilinear appearance (Fig. 2-10). Numerous conditions in animals have been diagnosed as neuronal ceroid-lipofuscinosis, although in only very few of these cases (i.e., sheep, Blue heeler [Australian] cattle, dogs) is the storage material similar to that described in human beings.

References

Appleby EC, Longsaffe JA, Bell FR Ceroid-lipofuscinosis in two Saluki dogs. J Comp Pathol 1982;92:375–380.

Armstrong D, Koppang N, Jolly RD. Ceroid-lipofuscinosis. Comp Pathol Bull 1980;12(2):2–4.

Bronson RT, Lake BD, Cook S, et al. Motor neuron degeneration of mice is a model of neuronal ceroid lipofuscinosis (Batten's disease). Ann Neurol 1992;33:381–385.

Edwards JF, Storts RW, Joyce JR, et al. Juvenile-onset neuronal ceroid-lipofuscinosis in Rambouillet sheep. Vet Pathol 1994;31:48–54.

Goebel HH, Ikeda K, Armstrong D, et al. Ultrastructural studies on lymphocytes in canine neuronal ceroid lipofuscinosis. Vet Pathol 1981;18:690–692.

Green PD, Little PB. Neuronal ceroid-lipofuscin storage in Siamese cats. Can J Comp Med 1974;38:207–212.

Harper PAW, Walker KH, Healy PJ, et al. Neurovisceral ceroid-lipofuscinosis in blind Devon cattle. Acta Neuropathol 1988;75:632–636.

Hoover DM, Little PB, Cole WD. Neuronal ceroid-lipofuscinosis in a mature dog. Vet Pathol 1984;21:359–361.

Jarplid B, Halita M. An animal model of the infantile type of neuronal ceroid-lipofuscinosis. J Inher Metab Dis 1993;16:274–277.

Jasty V, Kowalski RL, Fonseca EH, et al. An unusual case of generalized ceroid-lipofuscinosis in a cynomolgus monkey. Vet Pathol 1984;21:46–50.

Jolly RD, Shimada A, Dopfmer I, et al. Ceroid-lipofuscinosis (Batten's disease): pathogenesis and sequential neuropathological changes in ovine model. Neuropathol Appl Neurobiol 1989;15:371–383.

Koppang N. English Setter model and juvenile ceroid lipofuscinosis in man. Am J Med Genet 1992;42:599–604.

Martin JJ. Adult type of neuronal ceroid lipofuscinosis. Dev Neurosci 1991;13:331–338.

Nimmo Wilkie JS, Hudson EB. Neuronal and generalized ceroid-lipofuscinosis in a cocker spaniel. Vet Pathol 1982;19:623–628.

Rapola J. Neuronal ceroid-lipofuscinoses in childhood. Perspect Pediatr Pathol 1993;17:7–44.

Riis RC, Cummings JF, Loew ER, et al. Tibetan Terrier model of ceroid lipofuscinosis. Am J Med Genet 1992;42:615–621.

Sisk DB, Levesque DC, Wood PA, et al. Clinical and pathologic features of ceroid lipofuscinosis in two Australian Cattle Dogs. J Am Vet Med Assoc 1990;197:361–364.

Taylor RM, Farrow BRH. Ceroid-lipofuscinosis in Border Collie dogs. Acta Neuropathol 1988;75:627–631.

Vandevelde M, Fatzer R. Neuronal ceroid-lipofuscinosis in older Dachsunds. Vet Pathol 1980;17:686–692.

Wilkie JSN, Hudson EB. Neuronal and generalized ceroid-lipofuscinosis in a cocker spaniel. Vet Pathol 1982;19:623–628.

Wood PA, Sisk DB, Styer E, et al. Ceroidosis (ceroid-lipofuscinosis) in Australian cattle dogs. Am J Med Genet 1987;26:891–898.

DRUG-INDUCED LYSOSOMAL STORAGE DISEASE

There are numerous compounds which induce lysosomal storage, including certain therapeutic drugs. Some drugs, such as suramin (a trypanocidal and antifilarial drug), cause mucopolysaccharidosis by inhibition of iduronate sulfatase and β glucuronidase. Others, such as amiodarone (an antiarrhythmic drug), inhibit phospholipase A1 and A2 and result in phospholipidosis. Cationic amphophilic drugs, such as chloroquine, are suspected to alter membrane fluidity and thus result in inhibition of enzyme activity.

EXTRACELLULAR DEPOSITION OF PROTEINS

Amyloidosis

Amyloidosis is not a single disease, but a diverse group of diseases all characterized by the **extracelluar deposition of ultrastructurally similar, but biochemically distinct, proteins** (known as amyloid) in various organs and tissues. While the term amyloid means starchlike, the types of amyloid consist principally of fibrillar protein substances and small separate components of glycoprotein. The name evolved from the early observation that the cut surface of organs containing amyloid, when painted with an iodine solution and rinsed with dilute sulfuric acid, turned blue-violet, a positive test result for starch.

Gross appearance

Small amounts of amyloid are not visible. When accumulations become sufficiently large to be grossly visible, they appear as firm, white, opaque, lardlike deposits. In the spleen, discrete nodules of firm, white material resembling tapioca grains correspond to extensive deposits localized to splenic follicles. As a rule, amyloid deposition in organs other than the spleen results in a diffuse alteration in the overall appearance of the organ rather than in discrete deposits. The liver, for instance, when extensively involved, appears larger, paler, and firmer than normal.

Microscopic appearance

By light microscopy, amyloid appears as irregular globular or linear masses of an eosinophilic hyaline material if stained with hematoxylin and eosin (Fig. 2-20). In some locations, it may also appear faintly fibrillar. As it accumulates in the extracellular spaces, it compresses the adjacent parenchymal cells causing them to atrophy or die as a result of pressure or impairment of their blood supply. Several histochemical staining techniques can be used to distinguish amyloid from other eosinophilic extracellular deposits, such as collagen, fibrin, and immune complexes. The most common of these stains is Congo red, which stains amyloid orange-red if viewed under ordinary light but imparts a distinctive apple-green birefringence to the material when viewed with polarized light. The amyloid-associated (AA), amyloid light chain (AL), and transthyretin forms of amyloid (chemical properties discussed below) may be distinguished from one another on tissue section. Pretreatment of tissue sections containing AA protein with potassium permanganate abolishes its affinity for Congo red, whereas pretreatment of the other two forms does not. Although the Congo red stain is an excellent method to identify amyloid, it is not absolutely specific, especially if the tissues have been preserved with fixatives other than formalin. Thioflavin-T or S staining imparts fluorescence to amyloid with equal or

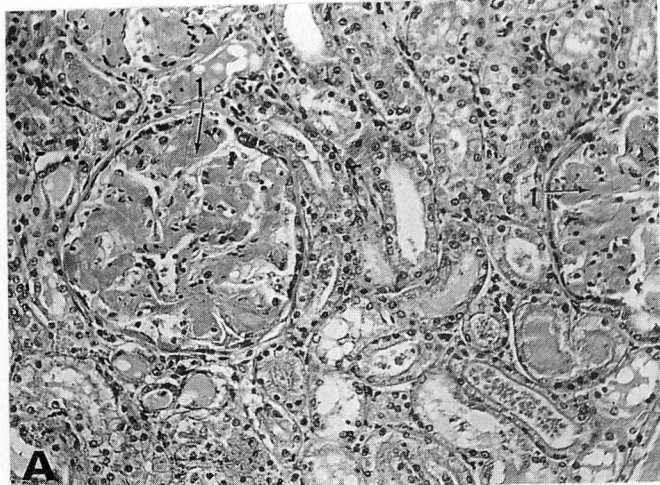

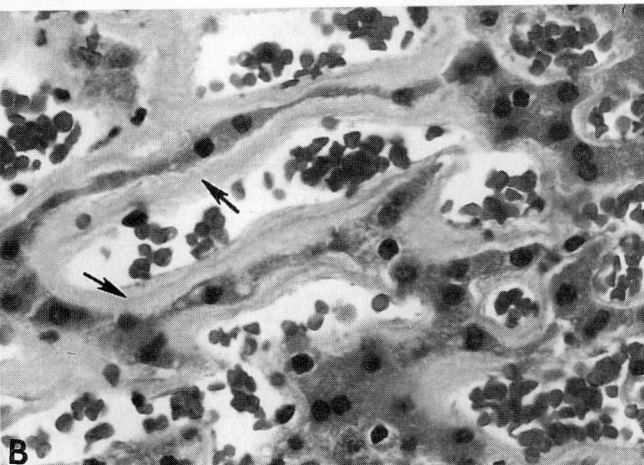

FIG. 2-20 Amyloidosis. **A.** Kidney of dog. Amyloid (1) is deposited in the glomerular tufts ($\times$ 175). (Courtesy of Dr. C.L. Davis and Armed Forces Institute of Pathology) **B.** Liver of monkey. Amyloid *(arrows)* is deposited in space of Disse between hepatocytes and endothelial lining of sinusoids. Hepatocytes are atrophic.

greater specificity than Congo red birefringence. Toluidine blue staining of amyloid results in a reddish polarization color that is not affected by fixation. Immunohistochemistry using specific antisera to the different forms of amyloid can also be a valuable tool in differentiating the forms.

PHYSICAL PROPERTIES

All forms of amyloid have an identical ultrastructure when viewed by transmission electron microscopy. The deposits consist of two distinct components, the major one being masses of nonbranching filaments of variable length with a diameter of 7.5 to 10.0 nm. These fibrils are oriented in a several patterns, including in individual units, side-by-side within bundles, and in an interlacing meshwork (Fig. 2-21). The second, closely associated, but minor component of amyloid consists of groups of pentagonal, toroid-shaped structures having an external diameter of approximately 9 nm and an internal diameter of 4 nm. These structures, known as the

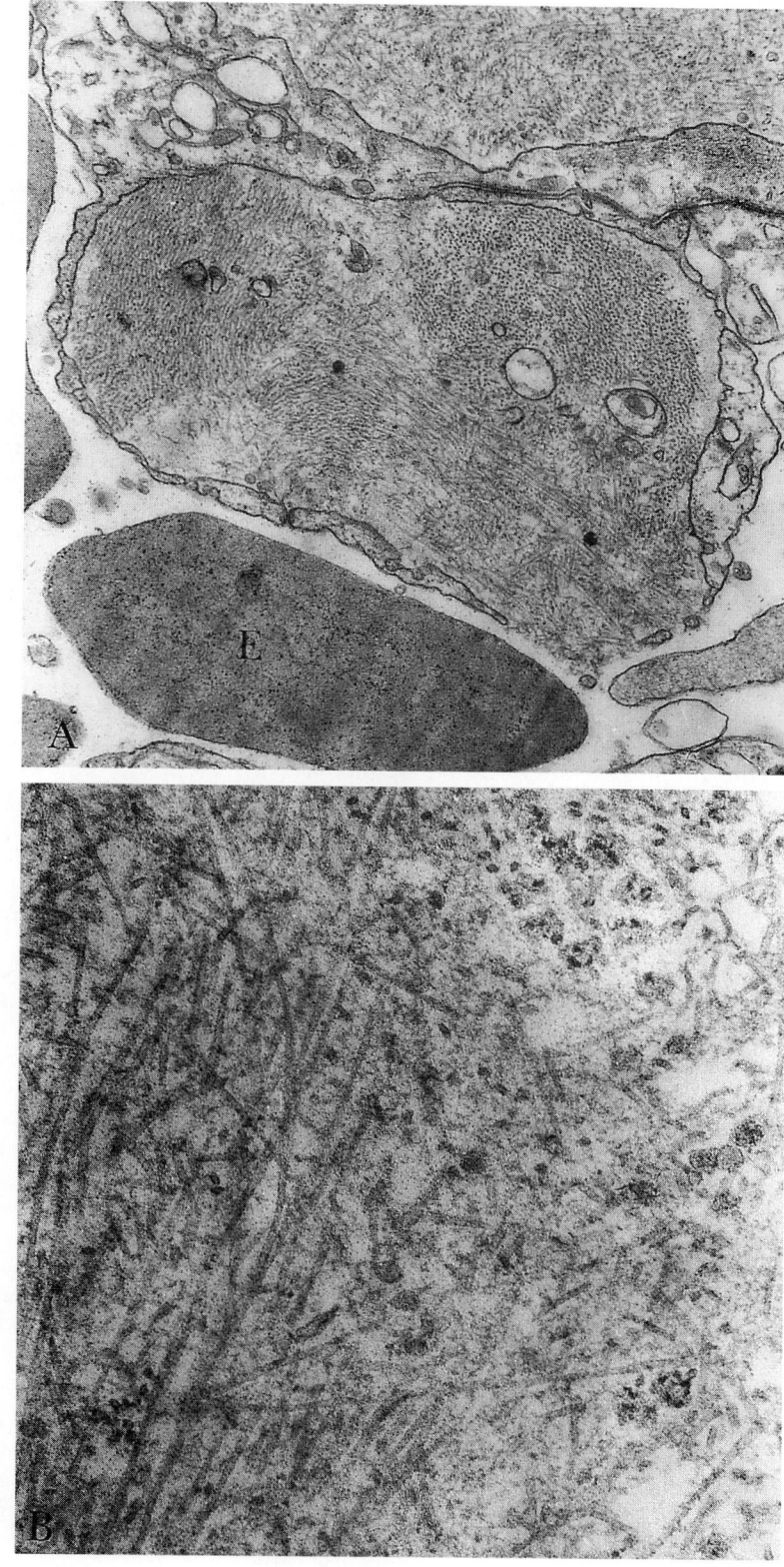

FIG. 2-21   Bovine renal amyloidosis.   **A.** Electromicrograph of subendothelial amyloid encircled by endothelial cytoplasm. *E,* erythrocyte. (Courtesy of Dr. E. Gruys and *Veterinary Pathology* 1975;12:94–110. **B.** Ultrastructure of amyloid fibrils in longitudinal and cross section. (Courtesy of Dr. E. Gruys)

P-components, constitute only 10% or less of the total amyloid deposits.

The classic apple-green birefringent property of amyloid when stained with Congo red is caused by a consistently repeating pattern in which the fibrils of amyloid are arranged. X-ray crystallography has revealed that the polymerized protein fibrils are arranged in a specific biophysical pattern known as a b-pleated sheet. The repeated order and regularity with which the Congo red molecules bind to this crystal-like array of amyloid fibrils confers the distinctive birefringence to the stained proteins.

CHEMICAL PROPERTIES.

Our admittedly incomplete knowledge regarding the pathogenesis of the various forms of amyloidosis has come from analyses of the chemical nature of these substances. As previously mentioned, the principal component of amyloid consists of fibrillar proteins, the remainder being the P-component, which is a glycoprotein identical to a normal a-1 serum glycoprotein. Chemically, there are two basic types of fibrillar proteins found in the various forms of amyloidosis. One of these, termed **amyloid light chain** (**AL**) protein, is derived from plasma cells and contains amino-terminal fragments of immunoglobulin light chains. The other, known as **amyloid-associated** (**AA**) protein, is not an immunoglobulin but is derived from a precursor protein known as **serum amyloid-associated** (**SAA**) protein synthesized by the liver. SAA is one of several acute phase proteins secreted by the liver in response to tissue damage. Hepatocytes are stimulated to secrete and release SAA in response to various cytokines (interleukin-1, interleukin-6, and TNF) released from macrophages after tissue injury. In the circulation, SAA binds to the high-density lipoprotein 3 (HDL3) subclass of lipoproteins and displaces other apolipoproteins.

The **P-component** of amyloid has a remarkable structural homology with **C-reactive protein,** another acute phase reactant secreted by the liver in response to chronic inflammatory processes or tissue destruction.

Other proteins that have been found in amyloid deposits associated with less frequent types of amyloidosis include: (1) mutant forms of transthyretin, a serum protein that binds and transports thyroxine and retinol in plasma; (2) β_2-microglobulin, a normal serum component of the MHC class I molecules; (3) β_2-amyloid protein (also known as A_4), a substance with properties of a transmembrane glycoprotein; and (4) certain hormone precursors (procalcitonin and proinsulin).

Classification.

Table 2-3 depicts the current classification of the various forms of amyloidosis, diseases with which they have been associated, precursor proteins, and the final type of amyloid found in each. Historically, amyloidosis has been divided into two basic types, i.e., primary and secondary. **Primary amyloidosis** occurs as a consequence of various forms of plasma cell dyscrasias, including multiple myeloma and other forms of monoclonal proliferation of B lymphocytes. **Secondary amyloidosis,** on the other hand, occurs in association with chronic inflammatory diseases, such as tuberculosis and long-standing suppurative processes. It also occurs with some frequency in horses that have been used for antisera production and can be induced experimentally by repeated injections of antigenic substances, such as casein and certain drugs. It can also be produced experimentally in mice by repeated subcutaneous injections of silver nitrate, which induces a chronic inflammatory reaction. Amyloidosis also occurs naturally as a complication of aging, in which case it is termed **senile amyloidosis.** Familial forms of amyloidosis have been found in human beings, some strains of mice, and certain breeds of dogs (Shar-Pei) and cats (Abyssinian).

Pathogenesis.

The pathogenesis of amyloidosis is still not fully understood, but it is thought to involve inadequate or defective degradation of the soluble precursors present in the circulation by cells of the mononuclear-phagocyte system. This defect leads to extracellular deposition of **insoluble forms** of the protein, often immediately adjacent to the resident mononuclear phagocytes of affected organs. These insoluble forms are relatively resistant to proteolysis *in vivo*.

Amyloidosis associated with plasma cell dyscrasias (**primary amyloidosis**) is the most common form of human amyloidosis in the United States, but it is uncommon in animals. In human beings, it is most often associated with multiple myeloma, a systemic neoplastic disease of plasma cells, but may be seen in other plasma cell abnormalities, such as Waldenstrom's macroglobulinemia, heavy chain disease, solitary plasmacytoma, and other types of B-cell lymphoma. In all of these conditions, the amyloid is of the AL type. With these disorders, the abnormal plasma cells secrete large quantities of whole immunoglobulin molecules of a single idiotype (monoclonal gammopathies) that can be detected by serum electrophoresis. In addition, these cells may secrete only the light chains of either the κ or λ type in serum. These circulating immunoglobulin light chains, known as **Bence-Jones protein,** are often excreted in the urine of patients with multiple myeloma, but do not necessarily imply that the patient also has amyloidosis. Since l VI light chains are the most frequent precursor of AL amyloid, it is thought that they may be more amyloidogenic than k light chains. Because amyloidosis does not develop in all patients with elevated levels of circulating light chains, there would appear to be differences in the proteolytic activity of mononuclear-phagocytes of those patients in whom the disease develops compared with those in whom it does not, but this has not been confirmed.

Amyloidosis associated with chronic inflammatory processes (**secondary or reactive amyloidosis**) is characterized by deposition of AA protein, an insoluble derivative of SAA. SAA is a soluble acute-phase protein synthesized and released by the liver in response to cytokines (IL-1, IL-6 and TNF) secreted by activated macrophages at sites of inflammation or tissue damage. In normal patients, SAA concentrations in plasma increase several hundredfold within 24 hours after an episode of acute inflammation. The normal biological function of SAA has not been identified, but since in plasma it binds to HDLs, the same molecules to which endotoxin binds, it has been speculated that one of its roles may be to enhance the clearance of endotoxin and other products of cell injury from the body. Another possible function of SAA is to direct HDLs to sites of tissue damage so that cholesterol released from dying cells may be recycled. An additional factor that plays an essential role in the pathogenesis of this type of amyloidosis is a glyco-

TABLE 2-3　**Types of amyloidosis**

Clinicopathologic Category	Associated disorders	Major fibril protein	Precursor protein	Species affected
Systemic amyloidosis				
Plasma cell dyscrasias with amyloid deposits (**primary amyloidosis**)	Multiple myeloma, plasmacytoma, and other monoclonal B-cell proliferations	AL	Immunoglobulin light chains, principally λ type	Human, dog, cat
Reactive systemic amyloidosis (**secondary amyloidosis**)	Chronic inflammatory diseases (rheumatoid arthritis, ulcerative colitis)	AA	SAA	Human, dog, cat, horse, nonhuman primates
Hemodialysis-associated amyloidosis	Chronic renal failure	β_2-microglobulin	β_2-microglobulin	Human
Hereditary amyloidosis Mediterranean fever	—	AA	SAA	Human
Hereditary familial amyloidosis	—	AA	SAA	Human, Shar Pei dogs, Abyssynian cats
Amyloidotic neuropathies	—	Transthyretin	Transthyretin	Human
Localized amyloidosis				
Cardiac	Senescence	Transthyretin	Transthyretin	Human, dog
Lung vasculature	Senescence	Apolipoprotein A-1	?	Human, dog
Cerebral	Alzheimer's disease, senescence, spongiform encephalopathies	A4 (β-protein) Prion protein	? ?	Human, sheep, cattle, goat, mink, cat
Endocrine Thyroid	Medullary carcinoma	Procalcitonin	Calcitonin	Human
Pancreatic islet	Non-insulin dependent diabetes mellitus; islet-cell tumors	Islet amyloid	Calcitonin Pancreatic islet polypeptide (IAPP)	Human, cat

protein termed **amyloid-enhancing factor (AEF).** It is distinct from the P component of amyloid, which is also a glycoprotein. In experimental mouse models of inflammation-induced amyloidosis, AEF appears in the spleen and liver 48 hours before the appearance of amyloid deposits in these organs. Moreover, if AEF is administered simultaneously with the inflammatory stimulus in this model, amyloid deposits occur much more rapidly than with the inflammatory stimulus alone. The mechanism by which AEF enhances amyloid deposition has not been identified.

Genetic factors may also be involved in the pathogenesis of amyloidosis. Monocyte-macrophages have cell surface-associated serine proteases capable of degrading SAA to AA-like intermediates and ultimately to soluble peptides. A genetic defect in this proteolytic capacity could conceivably lead to deposition of insoluble forms of AA proteins. In addition, patients with chronic inflammatory disease may also secrete other acute-phase proteins with protease-inhibiting activity, such as antitrypsin and antichymotrypsin, that could diminish the capacity of mononuclear phagocytes to degrade SAA to peptides. Normal serum is also known to have amyloid A degrading activity that correlates with the concentration of albumin in serum. Since patients with renal amyloidosis often lose serum proteins, especially albumin, in the urine, this could conceivably also reduce the AA protein degradative capacity of the patient's serum, causing AA amyloid to accumulate.

Organs affected.

Amyloidosis may affect only a single organ or involve multiple organs. The kidneys, liver, and spleen are common sites for amyloid deposition, but other organs, including lymph nodes, adrenals, pancreatic islets, and the gastrointestinal tract, may also be affected. Clinically, amyloidosis is a slowly progressive, insidious disease that often goes undetected until the deposits become so extensive that the affected organs cease to function normally.

In the **kidney,** amyloid usually appears first in the glomeruli (Fig. 2-20), although it may be restricted to the peritubular connective tissue of the medulla, a common finding in cats. The deposits in the glomeruli begin in the mesangium, spread progressively into the subendothelial portions of the capillary basement membranes, and eventually become so massive that they obliterate capillary lumens and the urinary space. Affected glomeruli become converted into solid, globular masses of amyloid. In some tissues, including the kidney, spleen, and liver, amyloid deposits favor the immediate vicinity or the actual wall of small blood vessels.

In the **spleen,** amyloid occurs in the germinal centers near the follicular dendritic cells of Malpighian corpuscles or along the sinuses adjacent to the fixed mononuclear phagocytes.

The deposits in the **liver** begin in the spaces of Disse between the Kupffer cells and the hepatocytes and ultimately may cause atrophy and necrosis of the hepatic parenchyma (Fig. 2-20).

Significance.

Most examples of amyloidosis are encountered at autopsy incidental to those diseases found in Table 2-3. However, if death from other causes does not intervene, amyloidosis progresses to the point where organ dysfunction alone may be fatal.

References

Anderson GA, Cullor JS. Generalized amyloidosis and peritonitis in a raccoon. J Am Vet Med Assoc 1982;181:1407.

Axelrad MA, Kisilevsky R, Willmer J, et al. Further characterization of amyloid-enhancing factor. Lab Invest 1982;47:139–146.

Barth W, Gordon JK, Willerson JT. Amyloidosis induced in mice by *Escherichia coli* endotoxin. Science 1968;162:694–695.

Benson MD, Dwulet FE, DiBartola SP. Identification and characterization of amyloid protein AA in spontaneous canine amyloidosis. Lab Invest 1985;52:448–452.

Blanchard JL, Baskin GB, Watson EA. Generalized amyloidosis in rhesus monkeys. Vet Pathol 1986;23:425–430.

Bowles MH, Mosier DA. Renal amyloidosis in a family of beagles. J Am Vet Med Assoc 1992;201:569–574.

Boyce JT, DiBartola SP, Chen DJ, et al. Familial renal amyloidosis in Abyssinian cats. Vet Pathol 1984;21:33–38.

Carothers MA, Johnson GC, DiBartola SP, et al. Extramedullary plasmacytoma and immunoblobulin-associated amyloidosis in a cat. J Am Vet Med Assoc 1989;195:1593–1597.

Clark L, Seawright AA. Generalized amyloidosis in seven cats. Pathol Vet 1969;6:117–134.

Cohen AS, Connors LH. The pathogenesis and biochemistry of amyloidosis. J Pathol 1987;151:1–10.

Cooper JH. Selective amyloid staining as a function of amyloid composition and structure. Histochemical analysis of the alkaline Congo red, standardized toluidine blue, and iodine methods. Lab Invest 1974;31:232–238.

Cornelius EA. Amyloidosis and renal papillary necrosis in male hybrid mice. Am J Pathol 1970;59:317–326.

DiBartola SP, Benson MD, Dwulet FE, et al. Isolation and characterization of amyloid protein AA in the Abyssinian cat. Lab Invest 1985;52:485–489.

DiBartola SP, Tarr MJ, Webb TM, et al. Tissue distribution of amyloid deposits in Abyssinian cats with familial amyloidosis. J Comp Pathol 1986;96:387–398.

DiBartola SP, Tarr MJ, Parker AT, et al. Clinicopathologic findings in dogs with renal amyloidosis: 59 cases (1976–1986). J Am Vet Med Assoc 1989;195:358–364.

DiBartola, Tarr MJ, Benson, MD, et al: Familial renal amyloidosis in Chinese Shar Pei dogs. J Am Vet Med Assoc 1990;197:483–487.

Geisel O, Linke RP. Generalized AA-amyloidosis in two hares (*Lepus europaeus*) immunohistochemically identified using poly- and monoclonal antibodies. Vet Pathol 1988;25:391–393.

Giesel O, Stiglmair-Herb M, Linke RP. Myeloma associated with immunoglobulin lambda-light chain derived amyloid in a dog. Vet Pathol 1990;27:375–376.

Glenner GG. Amyloid deposits and amyloidosis: the β-fibrilloses (Parts 1 and 2). N Engl J Med 1980;302:1283–1292, 1333–1343.

Gruys E. Ultrastructural and enzyme histochemical aspects of amyloidosis in the bovine renal medulla. Vet Pathol 1975;12:94–110.

Gueft B, Ghidoni JJ. The site of formation and ultrastructure of amyloid. Am J Pathol 1963;43:837–854.

Gueft B, Kikkawa Y, Hirschl S. An electron-microscopic study of amyloidosis from different species. In: Mandema E, Ruinen L, Schalten JH, Cohen AS,ed. Amyloidosis. Amsterdam: Elsevier 1968.

Ishihara T, Gondo T, Takahashi M, et al. Immunohistochemical and immunoelectron microscopical characterization of cerebrovascular and senile plaque amyloid in aged dogs' brains. Brain Res 1991;548:196–205.

Jakob W. Spontaneous amyloidosis of mammals. Vet Pathol 1971;8:292–306.

Janigan DT. Pathogenic mechanisms in protein-induced amyloidosis. Am J Pathol 1969;55:379–393.

Johnson KH, Sletten K, Hayden DW, et al. Pulmonary vascular amyloidosis in aged dogs: a new form of spontaneously occurring amyloidosis derived from apolipoprotein AI. Am J Pathol 1992;141:1013–1019.

Johnson KH, Westermark P, Nilsson G, et al. Feline insular amyloid: immunohistochemical and immunochemical evidence that the amyloid is insulin-related. Vet Pathol 1985;22:463–468.

Johnson R, Jamison K. Amyloidosis in six dairy cows. J Am Vet Med Assoc 1984;185:1538–1543.

Kisilevsky R. Amyloidosis: a familiar problem in the light of current pathogenetic developments. Lab Invest 1983;49:381–390.

Kisilevsky R, Axelrod M, Brunet S, et al. Effects of amyloid induction on plasma protein turnover, and its implication. Am J Pathol 1976;83:299–318.

Kisilevsky R, Subrahmanyan L. Serum amyloid A changes high density lipoprotein's cellar affinity: a clue to serum amyloid A's principal function. Lab Invest 1992;66:778–785.

Kitamoto T, Ogomori K, Tateishi J, et al. Formic acid pretreatment enhances immunostaining of cerebral and systemic amyloids. Lab Invest 1987;57:230–236.

Klatskin G Nonspecific green birefringence in Congo red-stained tissues. Am J Pathol 1969;56:1–13.

Linke RP, Hol PR, Geisel O. Immunohistochemical identification of generalized AA-amyloidosis in a mountain gazelle (*Gazella gazella*). Vet Pathol 1986;23:63–67.

Linker A, Carney HC. Presence and role of glycosaminoglycans in amyloidosis. Lab Invest 1987;57:297–305.

Murray M, Rushton A, Selman I. Bovine renal amyloidosis: a clinicopathological study. Vet Rec 1972;90:210–216.

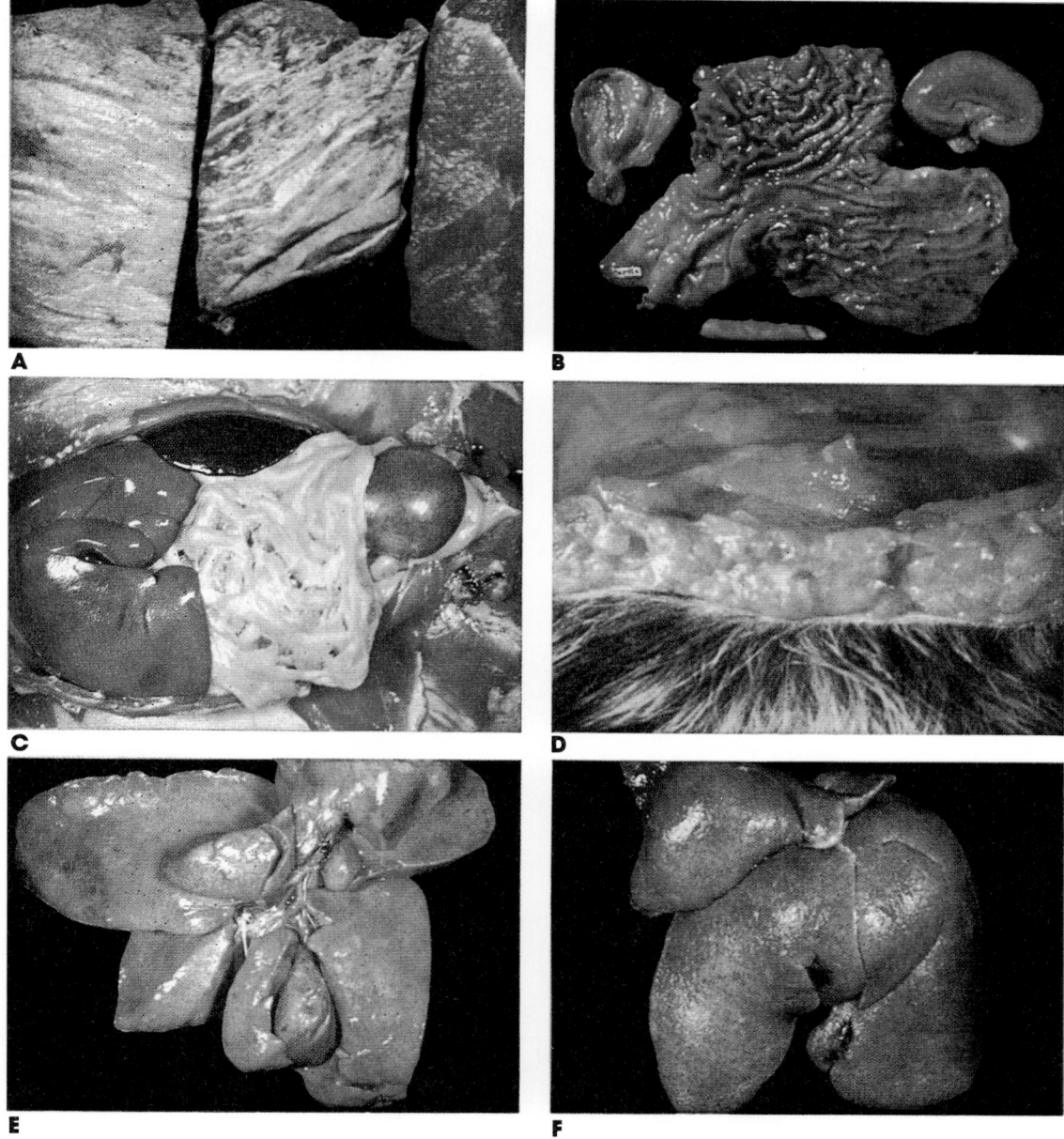

PLATE II

A. Azoturia in a yearling Palomino colt which became entangled in a halter rope and was unable to rise from a recumbent position. The colt was sacrificed after three days. Specimens of biceps femoris and latissimus dorsi muscles are illustrated, with normal muscle for comparison. (Case from Iowa School Vet. Med.)

B. Icterus due to acute leptospirosis in a male Springer Spaniel, nine months old. The yellow color is pronounced in tissues that are naturally pale (aorta, gastric and bladder mucosa) and is discernible in darker tissues (kidney, prostate)

C. Acute hemolytic icterus and hemolytic anemia due to *Hemabartonella felis*, affecting a two-year-old male cat. Note the yellow-colored omentum contrasting with the white intestines, the pale and swollen liver, and the enlarged, congested spleen. Most of this splenic enlargement is due to extramedullary

hematopoiesis. The bluish object is the urinary bladder filled with hemoglobin-stained urine. (Courtesy of Angell Memorial Animal Hospital)

D. Steatitis involving the subcutaneous fat of a one-year-old spayed female cat. This cat's diet consisted almost exclusively of canned red tuna. (Courtesy of Angell Memorial Animal Hospital)

E. Severe fatty infiltration of the liver, secondary to diabetes mellitus in a spayed female terrier, age 12 years. (Courtesy of Angell Memorial Animal Hospital)

F. Toxic hepatitis, following exposure to benzene, in a 12-year-old castrated male cat. Microscopic sections revealed severe focal necrosis, fatty degeneration and bile retention. The greenish color in the gross specimen results from oxidation of bilirubin to biliverdin. (Courtesy of Angell Memorial Animal Hospital)

O'Brien TD, Westermark P, Johnson KH. Islet amyloid polypeptide and calcitonin gene-related peptide immunoreactivity in amyloid and tumor cells of canine pancreatic endocrine tumors. Vet Pathol 1990;27:194–198.

Rodgers DR. Screening for amyloid with the thioflavin-T fluorescent method. Am J Clin Pathol 1965;44:59–61.

Rowland PH, Valentine BA, Stebbibs KE, et al. Cutaneous plasmacytomas with amyloid in six dogs. Vet Pathol 1991;28:125–130.

Saeed SM, Fine G. Thioflavin-T for amyloid detection. Am J Clin Pathol 1967;47:588–593.

Schuh JC. Primary amyloidosis in a dog. Vet Pathol 1988;25:102–104.

Schwartzman RM. Cutaneous amyloidosis associated with a monoclonal gammopathy in a dog. J Am Vet Med Assoc 1984;185:102–104.

Selkoe DJ. Amyloid protein and Alzheimer's disease. Sci Am 1991;265(5):68–78.

Shaw DP, Gunson DE, Evans LH. Nasal amyloidosis in four horses. Vet Pathol 1987;24:183–185.

Shirahama T, Cohen AS. Ultrastructural studies on renal peritubular amyloid experimentally induced in guinea pigs. 1. General aspects. Lab Invest 1968;19:122–131.

Shirahama T, Skinner M, Cohen AS, et al. Histochemical and immunohistochemical characterization of amyloid associated with chronic hemodialysis as β-2 microglobulin. Lab Invest 1985;53:705–709.

Shirahama T, Miurak, Ju S-T, et al. Amyloid enhancing factor-loaded macrophages in amyloid fibril formation. Lab Invest 1990;62:61–68.

Slauson DO, Gribble DH, Russell SW. A clinicopathological study of renal amyloidosis in dogs. J Comp Pathol 1970;80:335–343.

Stunzi H, Ehrensperger F, Wild P, et al. Systemic cutaneous and subcutaneous amyloidosis in the horse. Vet Pathol 1975;12:405–414.

Teilum G. Amyloidosis: origin from fixed periodic acid-Schiff positive reticuloendothelial cells in loco and basic factors in pathogenesis. Lab Invest 1966;15:98–110.

Trautwein G. Vergleichende Untersuchungen über das Amyloid und Paramyloid verschiedener Tierarten. I. Histomorphologie und fäberische Eigenschaften des amyloids und paramyloids. II. Histochemie des amyloids und paramyloids. Pathol Vet 1965;2:297–327, 493–513.

Wolman M. Amyloid, its nature and molecular structure. Comparison of a new toluidine blue polarized light method with traditional procedures. Lab Invest 1971;25:104–110.

Wolman M, Buber IJ. The cause of the green polarization color of amyloid stained with Congo red. Histochemie 1965;4:351–356.

Wright JR, Calkins E, Humphrey RL. Potassium permanganate reaction in amyloidosis. A histologic method to assist in differentiating forms of this disease. Lab Invest 1977;36:274–281.

Yano BL, Johnson KH, Hayden DW. Feline insular amyloid: histochemical distinction from secondary systemic amyloidosis. Vet Pathol 1981;18:181–187.

Yano BL, Hayden DW, Johnson KH. Feline insular amyloid: association with diabetes mellitus. Vet Pathol 1981;18:621–627.

Zuber RM. Systemic amyloidosis in Oriental and Siamese cats. Aust Vet Pract 1993;23:66–70.

Zucker-Franklin D, Franklin EC. Intracellular localization of human amyloid by fluorescence and electron microscopy. Am J Pathol 1970;59:23–41.

Albumins and Albuminous Fluids

It is customary in pathology to refer to nonspecific protein substances by what is almost always their principal constituent, albumin. Pathologically or otherwise, these substances are often encountered in microscopic sections as precipitates arising from body fluids. These situations include the following:

1. The lumen of a blood vessel may be filled with a pink-staining, homogeneous material. This is merely dehydrated plasma, with serum albumin as its visible component, the cells having settled after death to some other part of the vessel.
2. A similar precipitate is often seen in the renal tubules. In this case, it is albumin (and other proteins) precipitated and coagulated from the excreted urine; the diagnosis is albuminuria or proteinuria. Sometimes, the concentration may be so great that precipitation occurs during life, forming albuminous casts of the tubular lumens, which are recognizable in the voided urine. In sections of kidney, these are usually dense and deep-staining.
3. Most cysts are filled with albumin-containing fluid. The liquor folliculi, the "colloid" of the thyroid acini, and the salivary secretions are physiologic examples of similar fluids.
4. In the case of serous inflammatory exudates or the transudate of edema, the only visible substance remaining is the precipitate of albumin and related proteins. These are seen, for example, filling the alveoli of the lung, as well as in tissue spaces anywhere.

Microscopic appearance.

Albumin precipitated as just outlined is usually smoothly homogeneous, although occasionally it is seen (with high magnification) in the form of uniformly fine granules. It stains a bright, clear pink by the usual techniques. This purity of tint helps to distinguish albumin from amyloid and from fibrin, both of which have an opaque appearance because they give impure hues derived from a variety of wave-lengths.

Gross appearance.

All these substances look like a watery fluid unless, of course, the fluid is mixed with other substances, such as blood or pus.

Fibrin

Fibrin is another proteinaceous substance, physiologic or pathologic, which pathologists must learn to recognize.

Occurrence.

Fibrin is seen in the following: (1) wherever blood clots, as in internal hemorrhages and intravascular clots, either antemortem (thrombi) or postmortem; (2) the rare clotting of lymph; and (3) in fibrinous inflammatory exudates.

Gross appearance.

Fibrin, as seen in clots from which the blood cells have been removed by washing, is a dull white stringy material, the strands of which form a tangled mass. In fibrinous exudates, it is likely to be mixed with other exudative components, such as dead tissue and inflammatory cells (fibrinopurulent exudate) or fecal material (fibrinous enteritis), that modify its form and color.

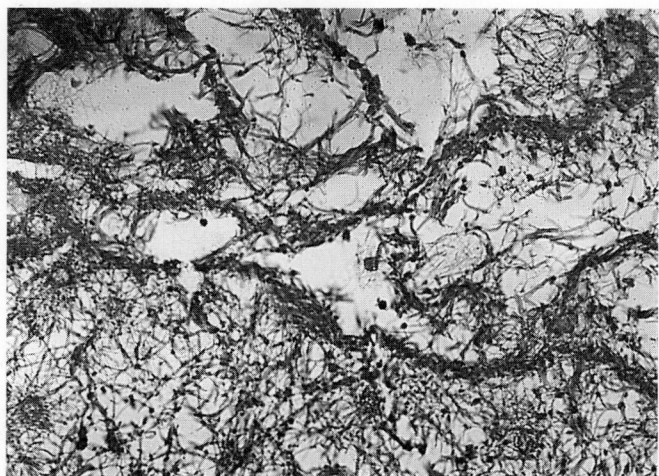

FIG. 2-22 Microscopic appearance of fibrin in blood clot in canine pulmonary vein. Note thin interlacing fibrils.

Microscopic appearance.

Fibrin stains pink, but usually it is a "dirty" or smudgy pink. Ordinarily, it is in the form of minute, tangled fibrils (Fig. 2-22), readily visible with a magnification of 400 or 500 diameters (high, dry lens), but in some cases it forms a solid and practically homogeneous mass. One of the best examples of this is fibrinous exudate in the pulmonary alveoli, which must be distinguished from the albumin of a serous exudate or inflammatory edema. If karyolysis has occurred in its vicinity, fibrin, being sponge-like, absorbs the released chromatin, thereby becoming endowed with the blue staining (by hematoxylin andeosin) characteristic of nuclei.

Causes

Are discussed in the respective discussions of clotting and exudates.

Significance.

Fibrin is formed from polymerization of fibrinogen, hence its source is blood, either directly or through the process of exudation. Fibrin is not innately a harmful substance: as an exudate upon mucous or serous surfaces, it forms a valuable protective coating; by closing an opened blood vessel, it terminates the loss of blood that might otherwise be fatal. However, in many situations, its ultimate effect is harmful, if not disastrous. Clots within the cardiovascular system (thrombi) all too often develop within major vessels, stopping the supply of blood to certain parts ofthe body with the consequences described in the discussion of necrosis. In the pulmonary alveoli, it prevents the entrance of air. While covering and protecting a surface, it interferes with normal functioning of the surface cells.

As to the fate of fibrin, there are two possibilities. The fibrin may be completely liquified by plasmin or hydrolytic enzymes of leukocytes. On the other hand, the mere presence of fibrin appears to act as a stimulus for the proliferation of nearby fibroblasts, with the result that the latter grow into it and, in the course of some days, the fibrin disappears and fibrous connective tissue takes its place, a process that is called **organization.** Thrombi are thus made permanent, as is also the solidification of the pulmonary alveoli. When fibrin is deposited on pleural and peritoneal surfaces, there is a strong probability that the opposing surfaces of organs may be permanently bound together by fibrous **adhesions,** as discussed in the section on fibrinous inflammation.

3

Mineral deposits and pigments

This chapter is about the pathologic deposits of minerals encountered in tissues on gross or microscopic examination; general metabolism of minerals is treated elsewhere. Some mineral substances are detected because they are also pigments, which have an intrinsic color. Also discussed here are pigments of organic origin, both endogenous and exogenous, which are encountered in tissues as normal components or as pathologic deposits.

PATHOLOGIC CALCIFICATION

Pathologic calcification is the deposition of calcium salts in tissues other than bone and teeth. The calcium is usually deposited as calcium phosphate and calcium carbonate, and may occur in the form of hydroxyapatite, which is similar to normal bone. Often, the salts are not chemically pure but rather accompanied by other ions, such as iron, which has led some pathologists to prefer the noncommittal term of mineralization.

Pathologic calcification may be divided into dystrophic calcification, metastatic calcification, and calcinosis circumscripta. The first two are discussed here; calcinosis circumscripta is discussed separately in the discussion of skin.

Dystrophic calcification

Dystrophic calcification is the deposition of calcium salts in dead or degenerating tissues. It is not related to calcium content of blood, which normally is approximately 10 mg/100 dL, and may occur in practically any tissue or organ. Dystrophic calcification, which is the type that occurs most often, involves tissues of the patient, but it can also occur in tissues of metazoan parasites that wander into various tissues of the host and die there, as in trichinosis.

MICROSCOPIC APPEARANCE.

Calcium carbonate or phosphate deposits usually occur in irregular granules of microscopic or slightly larger size. They typically exhibit a characteristic purplish color when stained with hematoxylin and eosin, although occasionally, with minor variations in technique, the eosin may predominate. The depth of color in the small particles encountered in microscopic sections depends on the thickness of the particle, and this often varies from point to point, as if the mineral were deposited in layers that progressively decrease in thickness toward the edge of the calcified granule. The form and structure of the granules or clump of granules are entirely irregular and unpredictable from tissue to tissue, although they may be confined to a given histologic structure, such as the wall of a small artery.

Calcium salts can be shown to greater advantage with special staining methods, such as the von Kossa and alizarin red S techniques. However, certain calcium salts, such as calcium oxalate, do not stain with hematoxylin nor do they react with the usual histochemical stains for calcium salts.

GROSS APPEARANCE.

Calcium particles, if separated from the surrounding tissue, would be white or gray, irregularly rounded, and often honeycombed. The material is less dense than ordinary limestone; small deposits often yield to the microtome knife with about an equal degree of fragmentation of stone and steel.

The most common method of detecting calcification grossly is to slice though the suspected area with a knife in search of a grating sound and gritty feeling. This is done routinely by meat inspectors examining for tuberculosis and other conditions in which calcification (Fig. 3-1) is a more or less constant feature.

Causes. The presence of dead or dying animal tissue is the fundamental cause of calcium deposition of this type; it is not related to an increased concentration of calcium in the blood. What local factors initiate the precipitation of calcium are unknown, but it has been suggested that local alkalinity in dead tissue favors the precipitation (Fig. 3-2). However, there is little evidence to support this hypothesis. Another suggestion is that fatty

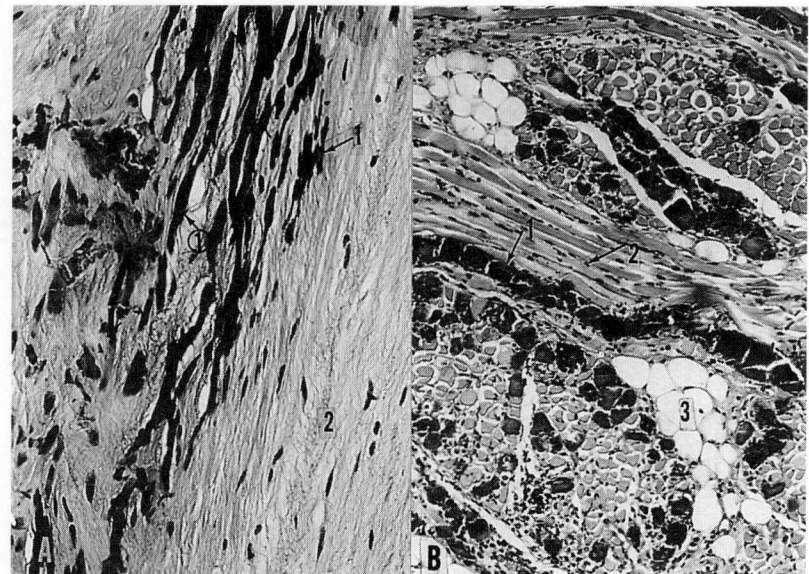

FIG. 3-1 Calcification. **A.** Deposits of calcium salts (1) in the myocardium of a cow (X 300), (Courtesy of Dr. J. F. Ryff, Armed Forces Institute of Pathology) **B.** Calcium deposition in skeletal muscles in tongue of foal possibly as result of vitamin E deficiency. Calcium salt (1) replaces the sarcoplasm in many muscle bundles. A few unaffected bundles (2) remain. Normal fat cells (3) are present (X 114). (Courtesy of Dr. W. O. Reed, and Armed Forces Institute of Pathology)

acids formed in necrotic tissue combine with calcium, forming soaps that are later replaced by phosphates and carbonates. No doubt this is important in fat necrosis, but again there is little evidence to indicate this mechanism is involved in dystrophic calcification. Increased levels of alkaline phosphatase have been demonstrated within sites of dystrophic calcification, but whether this enzyme is involved in the deposition of calcium salts is unknown, since the enzyme cannot be demonstrated consistently.

Among the sites where calcification is prone to develop are (1) the caseous centers of tubercles in tuberculosis (except avian) and caseous areas in other granulomatous diseases; (2) the rosettes and ensheathed colonies of actinomycotic and staphylococcal granulomas (botryomycosis), old thrombi, degenerating tumors, and old areas of scarring, including the degenerate walls of atheromatous blood vessels; and (3) the remains of parasites, such as trichinae, trematodes, encysted tapeworm larvae, demodectic mites, and others, which have been unable to complete their life cycles and have died in the tissues.

SIGNIFICANCE.

Calcium deposits are relatively permanent, but are harmless unless, by virtue of their location, they interfere mechanically with some function or reduce the strength of a tissue. Calcification has been listed as one of the ways by which the body disposes of dead tissue, since calcified material is functionally inert. Occasionally, calcification in certain locations may accompany and possibly be causally related to pathologic ossification.

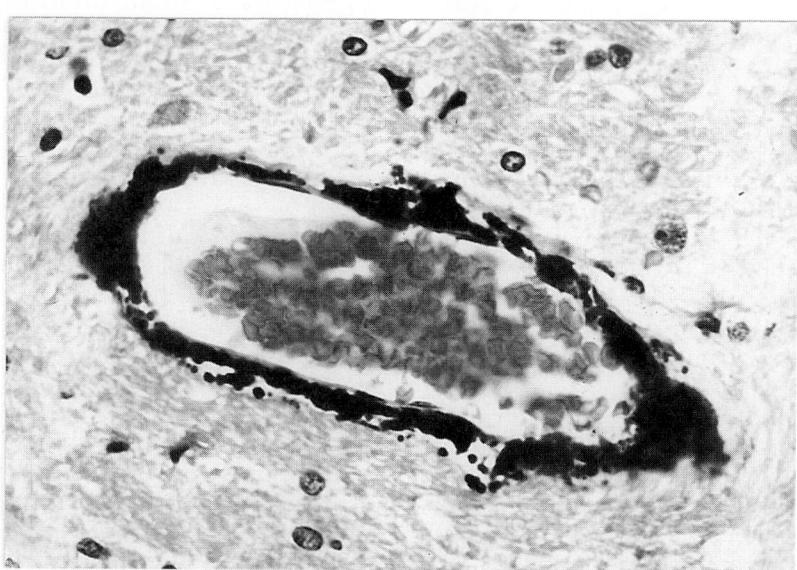

FIG. 3-2 Cerebrovascular siderosis in tamarin (*Saguinus oedipus*). Iron-positive and calcium-positive material in wall of cerebral arteriole. (Courtesy of New England Regional Primate Research Center, Harvard Medical School)

Metastatic calcification

Metastatic calcification is the precipitation of calcium salts as the result of a persistently high concentration of calcium in the blood. The tissues affected need not have been previously damaged. The staining qualities and gross appearance of the calcium salts do not differ from those described for dystrophic calcification.

CAUSES.

Metastatic calcification may result from the following: (1) primary hyperparathyroidism (this condition is exceedingly rare, especially in animals); (2) renal failure, in which the excretion of phosphate is reduced, resulting in increased serum levels of inorganic phosphate (Secondary hyperparathyroidism may develop in this situation, which accentuates calcium deposition, making it difficult to differentiate "dystrophic" from "metastatic" calcification caused by the presence of degenerative lesions of uremia.); 3) widespread calcification of the walls of arteries and other tissues from hypercalcemia produced by large excesses of vitamin D in the diet (Fig. 3-3). This may be encountered in livestock fed excessive amounts of artificial vitamins. There is evidence that ultrastructural lesions precede renal calcification in hypervitaminosis D in rats. By definition, the use of the term metastatic should be reassessed if similar findings are encountered in other tissues and other forms of metastatic calcification.

Widespread calcification of tissues has been ob-served in several species (i.e., cattle, sheep, goats) in different parts of the world. Evidence now indicates that certain plants containing the active principle of vitamin D (25-hydroxycholecalciferol) are responsible. **Enzootic calcinosis** is the term applied in Germany, Austria, South Africa, and India. One plant, yellow oat (*Trisetum flavescens,*) has been incriminated in Germany. A similar, if not identical disease, described in Argentina and Brazil designated **Enteque seco** has been reproduced experimentally by ingestion of a plant, *Solanum malacoxylon.* **Manchester wasting disease** described in Jamaica, and **Naalehu disease** reported from Hawaii, have similar features and recently also have been related to the consumption of *Solanum malacoxylon.* Calcinosis with associated hypercalcemia has been identified in Florida in horses that have ingested leaves of the shrub *Cestrum diurnam.*

The deposition of calcium salts is primary and most extensive in the elastica of the heart, aorta, and muscular arteries. Calcification also involves elastic fibers in the pulmonary parenchyma, trachea, bronchial cartilage, and heart valves. In severe cases in cattle and sheep, the flexor tendons of the forelimbs are calcified; the bones are hard and dense; osteoarthritis is present in carpal and tarsal joints; and the blood level of inorganic phosphorus is elevated. Calcification in the septa of the lungs may lead to ossification (Fig. 3-4).

In hyperadrenocorticism in dogs, calcification may occur in a variety of tissues, but especially in skin, lungs, and skeletal muscle. The mechanisms of this type of calcification are not understood.

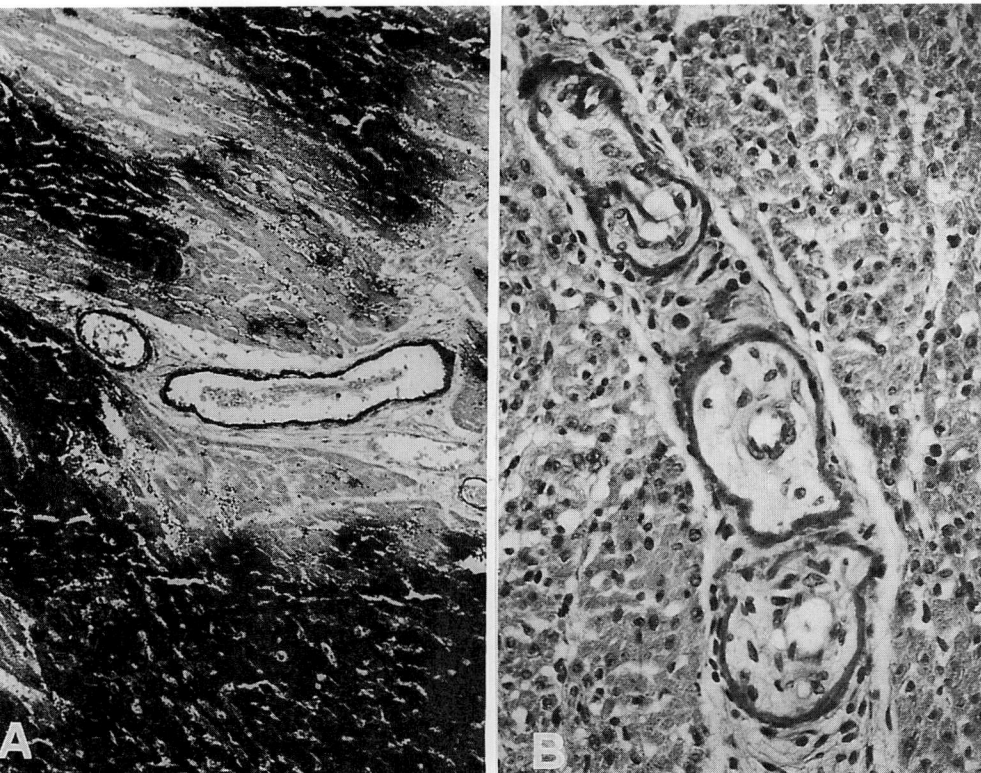

FIG. 3-3 Calcinosis in young swine caused by large doses of vitamin D₃. **A.** Myocardium; severe calcification in muscle cells and elastica of arteries, Von Kossa stain. **B.** Myocardium of same piglet; calcium in elastica of small artery, hematoxylin and eosin stain. (Courtesy of Prof. Dr. H. Luginbühl and Dr. H. Häni, with permission of the Schweizer Archiv für Tierheilkunde)

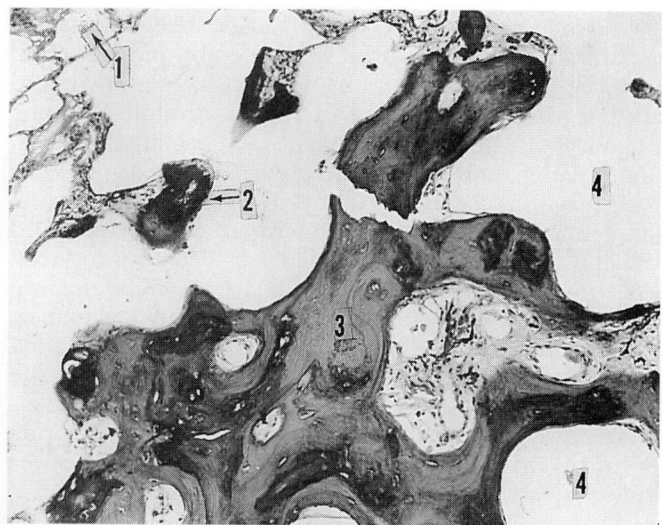

FIG. 3-4 Pathologic ossification of a bovine lung: seen in enzootic calcinosis. Alveoli (1), early calcification (2), and osteoid (3). Dilated alveolar spaces (4) are partially surrounded by bone (×250). (Courtesy of Dr. W. S. Bailey and Armed Forces Institute of Pathology).

PATHOLOGIC OSSIFICATION

Under most circumstances, pathologic ossification is abnormal and represents a form of metaplasia of nonosseous tissues (Chapter 4).

OCCURRENCE.

This syndrome a feature of the normal ontogeny of turkeys, in which, as they approach maturity, the tendons of their leg muscles turn to bone. In limited and variable degrees, a similar change is not unknown in other species. **Ossification of the lateral cartilages** of the horse's foot is an important cause of lameness. It occurs in large draft breeds, in older horses, and in those that have worked extensively on hard pavements, appearing in the forefeet, which bear the most weight. Rarely in old horses and old people, there is partial ossification of tracheal or laryngeal cartilages, especially if these have been exposed to stresses or have had inflammatory processes nearby. Additionally, widespread formation of bony spicules in the interalveolar septa of the lung is not rare. Chronically injured muscle is also prone to ossification, a condition referred to as **myositis ossificans.**

MICROSCOPIC APPEARANCE.

Small bits of ossified tissue are best distinguished from calcification by the presence of cells (osteocytes) and lacunae within bone; calcium deposits are acellular. Functioning marrow may also be found in areas of pathologic ossification.

CAUSES.

It appears that ossification is a response in older individuals to prolonged irritation; there is an heredi-

tary tendency in this direction. Heterotopic bone formation is also not infrequent at sites of dystrophic and metastatic calcification. Under these circumstances, fibroblasts differentiate to osteoblasts, forming osteoid, which calcifies to become bone in an identical manner to normal membranous bone formation.

SIGNIFICANCE.

Metaplastic bone at these ectopic sites may interfere with movement of tissue, such as muscle and lung, and interfere with the exchange of oxygen in the lungs as well.

References

de Barros S, Pohlenz J, Santigo C. Zur Kalzinose beim Schaf. Dtsch Tieraerztl Wochenschr 1970;77:346–349.

Dammrich K, Dirksen G, Plank P. Üer eine enzootische "Kalzinose" beim Rind. 3. Skelettveranderungen. Dtsch Tieraerztl Wochenschr 1970;77:342–346.

Dirksen G, Plank P, Spiess A, et al. Üer eine enzootische "Kalzinose" beim Rind. 1. Klinische Beobactungen und Untersuchen. Dtsch Tieraerztl Wochenschr 1970;77:321–338.

Dirksen G, Plank P, Hanichen T, Spiess A, Über eine enzootische "Kalzinose" beim Rind. 5. Experimentelle Untersucherungen an Kaninchen mit selektiver Verf'utterung von Knaufgras (*Dactylis glomerata*), Goldhafer (*Trisetum flavescens*) und einer Grasergemisch. Dtsch Tieraerztl Wochenschr 1972;79:77–79.

Gill BS, Singh M, Chopra AK. Enzootic calcinosis in sheep: clinical signs and pathology. Am J Vet Res 1976;37:545–552.

Gilka F, Corner AH, Sugden EA, et al. Heterotopic calcification in swine. Vet Pathol 1978;15:213–222.

Hani H, Thomann J, Schafer H. Zur calcinose des jungferkels. I. Beschreibung der spontanfalle. Schweiz Arch Tierheilkd 1975;117:9–18.

Hani H, Rossi GL. Zur calcinose des jungferkels. II. Pathogenese. Schweiz Arch Tierheilkd 1975;117:19–30.

Hanichen T, Plank P, Dirksen G. Ger eine enzootisch "Kalzinose" beim Rind. 2. Histomorphologische befunde an den weichgeweben. Dtsch Tieraerztl Wochenschr 1970;77:338–342.

Krook L, Wasserman RH, Shively JN, et al. Hypercalcemia and calcinosis in Florida horses: implication of the shrub *Cestrum diurnum,* as the causative agent. Cornell Vet 1975;65:26–56.

Pool RR, Williams JR, Bulgin M. Disseminated calcinosis cutis in a dog. J Am Vet Med Assoc 1972;**161:**291–292.

Singh G, Gill BS, Randhawa NS. Enzootic calcinosis in sheep: soil-plant-animal relationship. Am J Vet Res 1976;37:553–556.

Tustin RC, Pienar CH, Schmidt JM, et al. Enzootic calcinosis of sheep in South Africa. J S Afr Vet Assoc 1973;44:383–395.

Weidmann SM. Calcification of skeletal tissues. Int Rev Connect Tissue Res 1963;1:339–377.

GOUT

Gout is a condition in which crystals of uric acid or urates are deposited in tissues.

OCCURRENCE.

The disorder occurs in humans, birds, and reptiles, but has not been definitively recognized in other species. In human beings, common sites of involvement include articular and periarticular tissues, where the urate crystals attract and are phagocytized by neutrophils and macrophages. These cells release lysosomal enzymes and mediators of inflammation, which, in turn, exacerbate the acute inflammation and cause intense pain. Ultimately, a foreign body reaction to the

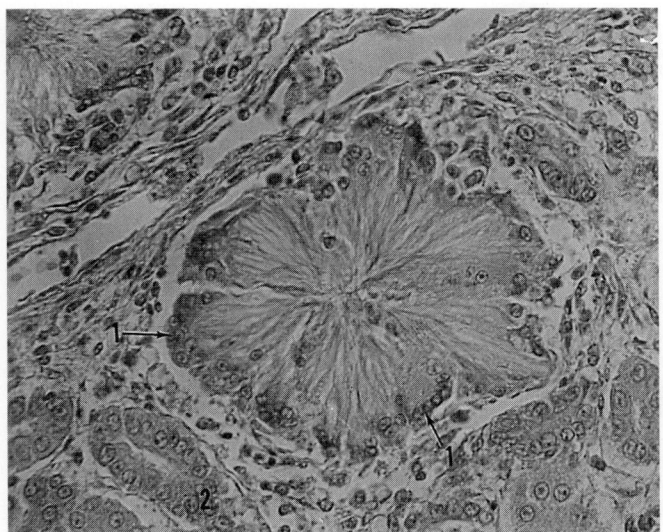

FIG. 3-5 Gout. Deposit of urate crystals in kidney of turkey. The urates are surrounded by multinucleated giant cells (1). Renal tubules (2) ($\times$ 425). (Courtesy of Dr. J. F. Olney and Armed Forces Institute of Pathology)

crystals (tophi) occurs at the site. The acute inflammation that characterizes gout waxes and wanes, despite the fact that the deposits persist.

In birds and reptiles, two forms of gout are recognized, a rare articular form similar to that just described and a visceral form that commonly affects serous membranes of visceral organs and the kidney (Fig. 3-5).

MICROSCOPIC APPEARANCE.

Inflammatory infiltrations, which include many neutrophils, macrophages, and foreign-body giant cells, in conjunction with clusters of sharp acicular, birefringent crystals or spaces left after they dissolve, located in an articular surface, joint capsule, or adjacent tissues are diagnostic of articular gout. Renal gout in birds and reptiles is characterized by the presence of urate deposits and associated inflammatory reactions in renal tubules and ureters. In the visceral form in these species, various serous surfaces are covered with finely crystalline or granular material that does not stain.

GROSS APPEARANCE.

Although relatively rare in animals, the gross appearance of a gouty joint is rather characteristic. The amount of precipitated urates may be so great as to form grossly visible white, chalky nodules known as "tophi" in the tissues. These may occur in subcutaneous tissues other than at joints and may ulcerate but seemingly without the severe pain that characterizes joint involvement.

In visceral gout, the serous surfaces of visceral organs, especially the parietal surface of the pericardium, are encrusted by a thin layer of grayish granular material that may have a metallic sheen. This appearance is enough to make a diagnosis.

CAUSES.

Uric acid and urates are end products of purine metabolism. In human patients where there are multiple forms and causes of gout, the concentration of uric acid in the blood is generally elevated (hyperuricemia). Causes include: (1) deficiency or increased activity of specific enzymes involved in purine metabolism; (2) impaired renal excretion of urates caused by renal disease or nephrotoxic drugs and chemicals; (3) genetic factors; and (4) environmental influences. In birds and reptiles, the kidneys eliminate semisolid urates rather than urine and uric acid. Factors associated with gout in these species include: impaired renal function and clearance of urates; nephrotoxic drugs; various dietary excesses (protein and calcium) and deficiencies (vitamin A); and dehydration.

SIGNIFICANCE.

Visceral gout in birds is seen only at necropsy. It is unknown whether birds or reptiles can recover from gout if the cause is removed. Articular gout is stubbornly recurrent in human patients and presumably so in those rare cases in animals.

Pseudogout

Lesions with clinical and radiographic features resembling articular gout, but caused by deposition of calcium pyrophosphate dihydrate or basic calcium phosphate (hydroxyapatite), are referred to as **pseudogout** or **chondrocalcinosis**. Similar lesions have been described in a dog and macaque monkeys. In the dog, a slowly enlarging radiopaque mass involved the joint of the fifth digit of one rear leg. The surgical specimen revealed a chalky-white mass attached to the joint, not the joint capsule. Microscopically, the mass contained aggregates of crystalline material separated by islands of connective tissue, not cartilage. The chemical nature of the deposited material clearly differentiates this lesion from gout, but the pathogenesis of pseudogout (Fig. 3-6) has not been established.

References

Austic RE, Cole RK. Impaired renal clearance of uric acid in chickens having hyperuricemia and articular gout. Am J Physiol 1972;223:525–530.

Christen P, Peacock WC, Christen AE, et al. Urate oxidase in primate phylogenesis. Eur J Biochem 1970;12:3–5.

Gibson JP, Roenigk WJ. Pseudogout in a dog. J Am Vet Med Assoc 1972;161:912–915.

Phelps P, McCarry DJ Jr. Crystal-induced inflammation in canine joints. II. Importance of polymorphonuclear leukocytes. J Exp Med 1966;124:115–127.

Schlotthauer CE, Bollman JL. Spontaneous gout in turkeys. J Am Vet Med Assoc 1934;85:98–103.

Schlumberger HG. Synovial gout in the parakeet. Lab Invest 1959;8:1304–1318.

Shirahama T, Cohen AS. Ultrastructural evidence for leakage of lysosomal contents after phagocytosis of monosodium urate crystals. Am J Pathol 1974;76:501–520.

Siller WG. Avian nephritis and visceral gout. Lab Invest 1959;8:1319–1357.

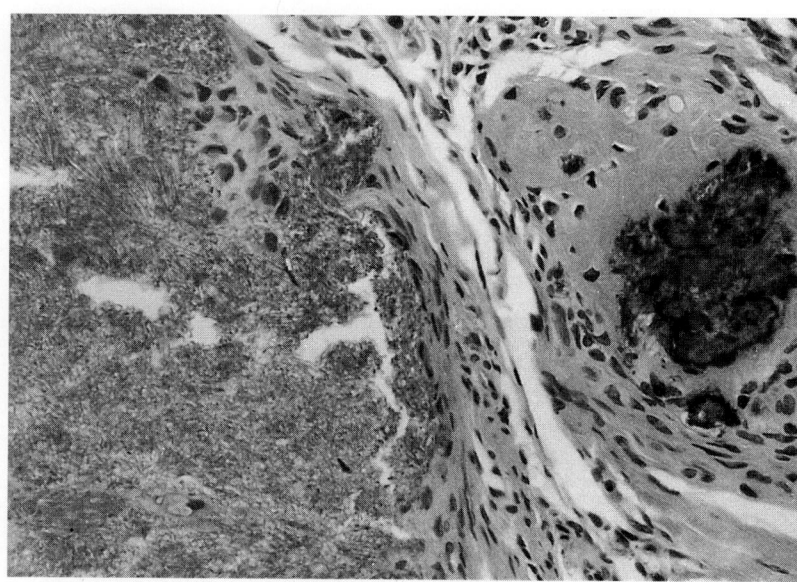

FIG. 3-6 Pseudogout. Mass of needle-shaped crystals and island of cartilage in skin of dog. (Courtesy of Dr. J. P. Gibson)

Spilberg I. Urate crystal arthritis in animals lacking Hageman factor. Arthritis Rheum 1974;17:143–148.

Wacker WEC. Man: sapient but gouty. N Engl J Med 1970;283:151–152.

Weissmann G, Rita GA. Molecular basis of gouty inflammation: interaction of monosodium urate crystals with lysosomes and liposomes. Nature New Biol 1972;240:167–172.

PIGMENTS

There is nothing logical about considering together the diverse and unrelated substances customarily grouped as pigments, except that in surveying the various abnormalities encountered in anatomic pathology, it is convenient to consider together substances with their own innate color, which renders artificial staining unnecessary.

A large number of pigments can be found in animal tissues. Some are normal; others are important components of specific diseases. The characteristics of the various types of pigments encountered in tissue sections are summarized in Table 3–1. For purposes of this discussion, pigments are classified as follows:

I. Exogenous (formed outside the body)
   A. Carbon
   B. Dusts
   C. Metals
   D. Tattoos
   E. Kaolin
   F. Carotenoids
II. Endogenous (formed inside the body)
   A. Phenolic pigments
   B. Hematogenous pigments
     1. Hemoglobins
     2. Hematins
     3. Parasitic pigments
     4. Hemosiderins
     5. Bile pigments
     6. Porphyrins (photosensitizing pigments)
   C. Lipogenic pigments
     1. Tissue lipofuscins

     2. Ceroid
     3. Vitamin E deficiency pigment
   D. Miscellaneous pigments
     1. Ochronosis pigment
     2. Dubin-Johnson pigment
     3. Cloisonné kidney

Carbon-anthracosis

Anthracosis is the condition in which carbon particles are found as a black pigment in the tissues (Figs. 3-7 and 3-8). Carbon is foremost among the exogenous pigments.

OCCURRENCE.

Carbon appears in the lungs and the lymph nodes that drain them and, rarely, in other organs if carried there by macrophages. It is common in humans and animals that live in smoky cities and in persons that work in coal mines.

MICROSCOPIC APPEARANCE.

Carbon appears as minute black granules, either between cells or in their cytoplasm. In the lungs, it is in the alveolar walls and the connective tissue septa, usually within macrophages. In lymph nodes, carbon is chiefly found between the lymphoid cells, but it is often phagocytized by large mononuclear cells and carried to other organs. Carbon can be distinguished from other pigments by its black color and, histochemically, by its resistance to all solvents and bleaching agents.

GROSS APPEARANCE.

Moderate or large amounts of carbon impart a mottling or speckling with black or gray to the lungs, the ventral portions of the lobes being affected more than the dorsal. Lymph nodes are likewise blackened. Anthracosis should not be confused with the black or brown color that almost invariably affects the medullary

TABLE 3-1   **Characteristics of common pigments as seen in tissue sections**

Pigment	Hematoxylin and eosin	Polaroscopy	Iron stains	Fat stains	Acid fast stains	Other distinguishing characteristics
Carbon	Black	Isotropic	—	—	—	Resistant to all stains and bleaching agents and microincineration
Melanin	Yellow-brown to black	Isotropic	—	—	—	Reduce silver; bleached by $KMnO_4$; combusted by microincineration
Hemosiderin	Yellow-brown	Isotropic	+	—	—	Nonfluorescent
Acid hematins	Brown	Anisotropic	—	—	—	Removed by saturated alcoholic picric acid
Porphyrin	Usually not visible except in rodent Harderian gland	Slightly anisotropic	—	—	—	Fluorescent at 365 mμ
Bilirubin	Bright yellow	Anisotropic if crystaline	—	—	—	Gmelin's test positive; nonfluorescent
Lipofuscins (wear and tear pigments and ceroid)	Yellow to brown	Isotropic	—	+	+	Fluorescent 365 mμ

region of bovine lymph nodes. This discoloration is due to a soluble pigment presumed to come from recently hemolyzed blood. Since the pigment is soluble, it is not seen in routinely prepared microscopic tissue sections. The presence of this pigment does not reflect any disease condition.

CAUSES AND SIGNIFICANCE.

Anthracosis is due to repeated and continued inhalation of coal dust or smoke as a consequence of living in cities. Coal miners are commonly afflicted, so that the heavily blackened lung is called "miner's lung" or

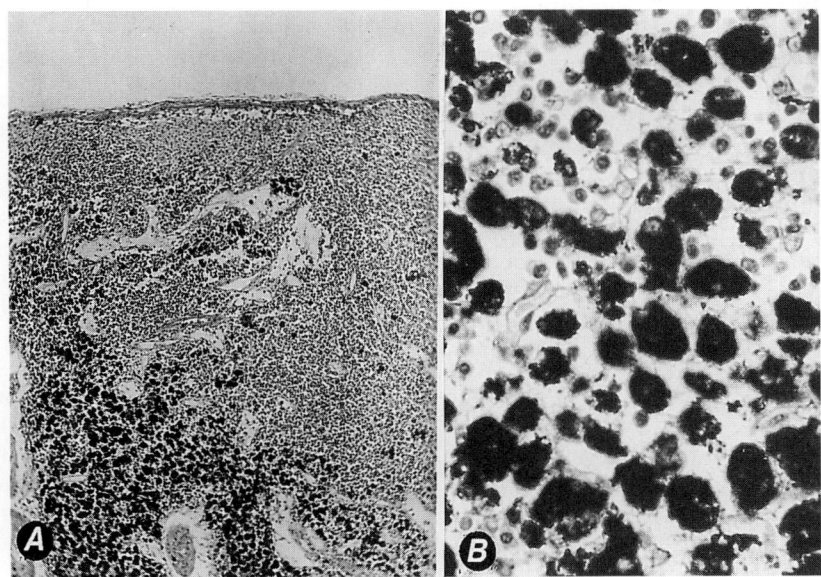

FIG. 3-7 Anthracosis in bronchial lymph node of aged dog. **A.** Low power view (X 67), macrophages laden with carbon, concentrated in medulla. **B.** Higher power (X 594) of medulla, same lymph node. (Courtesy of Armed Forces Institute of Pathology)

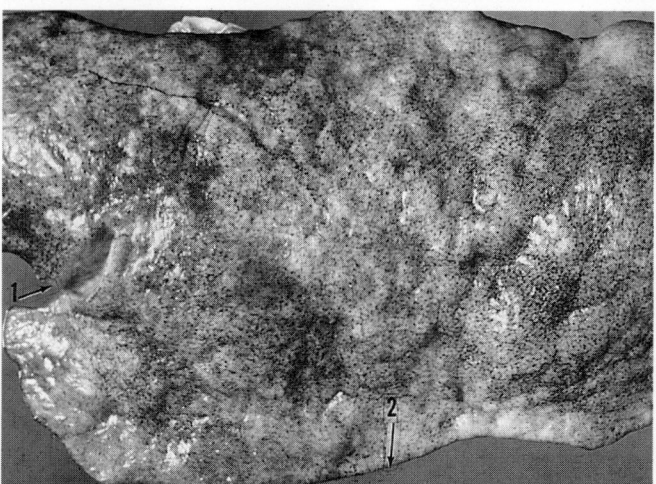

FIG. 3-8 Anthracosis, lung of dog. Finely particulate collections of carbon are visible from pleural surface. Cardiac notch (1) and ventral margin of lung (2).

"black lung disease." Reasonable amounts of anthracotic pigment do little harm and cause no symptoms but remain in the tissues for life; excessive amounts may cause slight pulmonary fibrosis and are suspected of predisposing to lung infections.

When dust is inhaled, the organic particles are short-lived, owing to clearance mechanisms of the body. Several kinds of mineral dusts, however, leave visible particles in the pulmonary tissues. Collectively, dust retained in the lung is termed **pneumoconiosis.** Anthracosis is a specialized form of pneumoconiosis in which the dust particles consist of carbon. Several other mineral dusts are important causes of pneumoconiosis, some of which induce life-threatening pulmonary disease.

Silicosis.

Silicon dioxide is inhaled in rock quarries and mines or in any other conditions in which rock is being cut or sandblasted. Microscopically, silicon dioxide occurs in the tissues as fine, anisotropic crystals, visualized only with polarized light. The crystals incite collagenous connective tissue proliferation, which takes the form of dense sclerotic nodules that often coalesce. The mechanism of action is damage to lysosomes. Following phagocytosis and fusion with lysosomes, the lysosomal membrane is damaged through a hydrogen-bonding reaction between silicic acid and the membrane. Released lysosomal enzymes in turn kill the macrophage, freeing the silica particles, which are engulfed again to repeat the same cycle. This may go on for life. Grossly, the lungs are nodular and firm, and may be pigmented as a result of concomitant anthracosis.

Siderosis.

Iron dust is inhaled chiefly as hematite or iron oxide from mines. The mineral does not incite fibrosis or an inflammatory reaction and is, therefore, of little significance. However, siderosis is often accompanied by silicosis. Microscopically, hematite and iron oxide appear as red crystals of varying size. They are anisotropic, appearing orange with polarized light, and iron can be specifically demonstrated with the Prussian blue reaction. Certain other iron salts and complexes may be black, blue, green, gray, or brown, and all do not react with the Prussian blue stain. In the gross specimen, hematite and iron oxide impart a brick-red color to the lungs.

Asbestosis.

Asbestos is widely used in the manufacture of fire-retardant insulating materials. Exposure of man or animals may result under many circumstances, but the most significant hazard to man occurs during manufacture, fabrication, or installation of products containing asbestos. Recognition of this hazard has led to changes in methods of manufacture of these products and serious restrictions in their use. Under microscopic examination, asbestos occurs as fine, white anisotropic fibers and as asbestos bodies. Asbestos bodies are long beaded rods with rounded ends, which are yellow-brown as a result of encrustations of iron that can be demonstrated with the Prussian blue reaction. Asbestos bodies are isotropic (dark under polarized light). Asbestos incites fibrous scarring of the pleura, around bronchioles and alveolar ducts and within alveolar septa. Discrete nodules, as in silicosis, do not develop. Foreign body giant cells may form adjacent to the asbestos particles. In human beings, asbestosis has been associated with bronchogenic carcinoma and mesothelioma of the pleura and peritoneum. Grossly, the pleura is thickened and the lungs are firm.

OTHER METALS AND EXOGENOUS PIGMENTS

Silver.

The disorder known as argyria is of historical interest only. Formerly, certain infections were commonly treated with various organic silver compounds, of which argyrol is about the only present day survivor. When large amounts were administered to human patients, silver was sometimes precipitated in the skin in amounts sufficient to impart to it an unsightly gray color. This was a permanent cosmetic injury of considerable importance to the victim. Obviously, the same would scarcely be true in animals.

Microscopically, silver occurs as an insoluble albuminate that is brown to black. It is deposited principally extracellularly between connective tissue fibers in the upper dermis. Only a small amount may be found within macrophages. In some cases, deposits may also occur extracellularly in the liver and kidney. Silver is not injurious to cells nor does it incite a cellular reaction.

Lead.

In chronic poisoning caused by the prolonged ingestion or assimilation of small amounts of lead compounds, a blue-black discoloration is imparted to the gums. Of considerable diagnostic importance, it is most pronounced immediately adjacent to the teeth, and is called the **lead line.** Chronic lead poisoning has occurred in animals as the result of grazing pastures contaminated by fumes and of smoke from smelters, or by drinking water similarly polluted. Ruminants and horses may ingest paint containing lead by chewing on painted wood surfaces. Puppies and children may chew on such surfaces or may eat pieces of paint that have flaked from old painted surfaces.

Bismuth.

Occasionally, in examining microscopic sections from the edge of a fistulous tract or sinus, such as might have been left by a penetrating foreign body, a faint gray-black pigment in the form of minute granules in and between cells is seen. Investigation reveals that this residue is from a bismuth-containing paste or powder injected into the tract for visualization by radiographic examination; bismuth salts are opaque to x-rays. This and similar delicate pigments should be sought via low magnification with a strong light directed down upon the slide and reflected back into the microscope, rather than by the usual light transmitted through the section.

Tattoos

A variety of pigments are used to produce tattoos, including India ink, China ink, Bismark brown, cinnabar, and kurkuma. These pigments are inert and produce no tissue reaction. Microscopically, they are seen extracellularly between connective tissue fibers of the dermis and within macrophages.

Kaolin

Also known as China clay or Fuller's earth, kaolin is a kind of clay derived by disintegration of an aluminous material, such as feldspar or mica. The essential mineral constituent is hydrated aluminum silicate (kaolinite), but the following chemical oxides may also be present: silicon (SiO_2); aluminum (Al_2O_3); iron (Fe_2O_3); titanium (TiO_2); calcium (CaO); magnesium (MgO); potassium (K_2O); sodium (Na_2O); manganese (MnO); copper (CuO); and sulfur (SO_3); along with water, carbon, and organic matter.

Kaolin has been incriminated as a cause of pneumoconiosis (kaolinosis), which leads to dense pulmonary scarring in man and nonhuman primates. It has also produced extensive subcutaneous granulomas in the pharyngeal and neck tissues of animals following overzealous administration of various kaolin-containing medications for gastrointestinal disease. Kaolin accidentally introduced into the subcutaneous tissue incites a striking influx of macrophages, producing dense nodules that displace adjacent tissues. The kaolin is visible as a homogeneous, faintly basophilic material and as fine anisotropic crystals within macrophages.

References

Hartley WJ, Mullins J, Lawson BM. Nutritional siderosis in the bovine. NZ Vet J 1959;7:99–105.
Heppleston AG. Changes in the lungs of rabbits and ponies inhaling coal dust underground. J Pathol 1954;67:349–359.
Higginson J, Gerritsen T, Walker ARP. Siderosis in the Bantu of Southern Africa. Am J Pathol 1953;29:779–815.
Kilburn KH, ed. Pulmonary reactions to organic materials. Ann NY Acad Sci 1974;221.
Kleckner MS, Baggenstross AH, Weir JF. Iron-storage diseases. Am J Clin Pathol 1955;25:915–931.
Lord GH, Willson JE. Foreign body granuloma in a rhesus monkey. J Am Vet Med Assoc 1968;153:910–913.
Lynch KM, McIver FA. Pneumoconiosis from exposure to kaolin dust: kaolinosis. Am J Pathol 1954;30:1117–1127.
Selikoff IJ. Lung cancer and mesothelioma during prospective surveillance of 1249 asbestos workers, 1953–1974. Ann NY Acad Sci 1976;271:448–456.
Selikoff IJ, Hammond EC. Asbestos associated disease in United States shipyards. CA 1978;28:87–99.
Smith BL, Poole WSH, Martinovich D. Pneumoconiosis in the captive New Zealand Kiwi. Vet Pathol 1973;10:94–101.
Suzuki Y, Churg J. Structure and development of the asbestos body. Am J Pathol 1969;55:79–107.
Taylor FA. Pigment of anthracosis. Proc Soc Exp Biol Med 1941;48:70–72.
Taylor KE. Ham discoloration due to iron injections. J Am Vet Med Assoc 1964;145:470–471.
Webster I. The ingestion of asbestos fibers. Environ Health Perspect 1974;9:199–202.
Weller W, Ulmer WT. Inhalation studies of organic coal-quartz dust mixture. Ann NY Acad Sci 1972;200:142–154.
Zaidi SH, Shanker R, Dogra RKS. Experimental infective pneumoconiosis: effect of asbestos dust and *Candida albicans* infection on lungs of rhesus monkeys. Environ Res 1973;6:274–286.

Carotenoid pigments

Carotenoid pigments are fat-soluble pigments of plant origin. They include α-carotene, β-carotene (the precursor of vitamin A) and xanthophyll, all of which are greenish-yellow. They are classed as **lipochrome pigments,** which are not to be confused with the endogenous lipofuscin pigments.

OCCURRENCE.

Pigments of this group occur normally in epithelial cells of the adrenal gland, lutein cells of the corpus luteum, epithelium of the testis and seminal vesicle, Kupffer cells of the liver, ganglion cells, the yolks of eggs, butter fat, and the adipose cells of animals such as horses and Jersey and Guernsey cattle, which have a markedly yellow body fat. The amount of carotenoid pigments in tissues varies between species, owing to their relative efficiency in converting β-carotene to vitamin A and rejecting carotenoids in the ingesta that are not required for vitamin A synthesis. The efficiency of these two functions is low in such species as fowl, horses, cattle, humans, and nonhuman primates.

Pathologically, the same type of pigment occurs in small tumors known as xanthomas. These tumors are not true neoplasms, but appear to be disorders of the mononuclear-phagocyte system.

Lipochrome pigments are only seen grossly, since the material is soluble in organic solvents used in tissue preparation.

HEPATIC CAROTENOSIS.

Bovine livers sometimes appear brilliant yellow or perhaps slightly reddish, but not however, with the greenish tinge characteristic of jaundice and bile retention or the pale yellow of fatty change. The pigment in this case is carotene, which in itself is harmless, but affected livers also show toxic changes consisting chiefly of focal or **centrilobular** necrosis and limited fatty change. These changes progress to varying degrees of portal cirrhosis and even to almost complete replacement of the liver tissue by fibrous tissue; mild lymphocytic infiltrations are also present. Feeding such livers experimentally to rats produces similar toxic changes in the livers of the rats, but not accumulation of carotene. It is presumed that the carotene remains unconverted and unmetabolized because of toxic injury to the liver cells, but this appears to be a peculiarity of the bovine species only. Investigators working with material obtained at meat inspection suspected some unidentified toxic plant as the cause.

Livers filled with retained bile pigment in obstructive jaundice, in spite of their usual greenish tinge, may be confused with hepatic carotenosis. The two can be differentiated by extracting a sample of minced liver with ether and water. After thorough shaking, the lighter ether will rise to the top with the yellow color of the carotene, if present. The water below will be colored yellow by bilirubin, the pigment of icterus, if such is present. Fatty liver not only has a lighter yellow color, but greater swelling if the condition is pronounced, and a lighter specific gravity, often floating in water or formalin.

Melanin

Passing to the **endogenous** group of pigments, the most important in the **autogenous** subgroup is melanin. Melanin is the pigment that gives color to the skin, hair, and iris, and provides the black, reflection-proof choroid layer of the eye.

While the complete chemistry of melanin is unknown, it is considered to be formed from the amino acid tyrosine, which differs from phenylalanine (β-phenyl, a-amino propionic acid) by having one hydroxy group attached to the phenyl group and therefore is also called hydroxyphenylalanine. Although the oxidative steps necessary to convert tyrosine to melanin are unknown, the copper-containing enzyme tyrosinase is required. There also exists, by artificial production, the substance dihydroxyphenylalanine, which has one more hydroxy group attached to the phenyl ring. This is further discussed in subsequent pages.

The mechanisms that control melanin formation are also poorly understood. It has been established in man and some animals that the pituitary produces two melanocyte-stimulating hormones; a-MSH and b-MSH. Although their function is not clear, they are believed to be important in the increased pigmentation seen in Addison's disease of human beings and in pregnancy. Corticotropin also has melanocyte-stimulating potential, but to a significantly lesser degree than MSH. Hydrocortisone decreases MSH release from the pituitary.

OCCURRENCE.

Normal physiologic deposits of melanin occur in the epidermis of animals and humans; there is a small amount in light-colored individuals and more in darker ones. The melanin exists as minute brown or black granules in the cytoplasm of epithelial cells, chiefly or entirely in the basal layer, the stratum germinativum. In black animals and human beings, some pigment extends into cells of the intermediate layers. It is produced by specialized dendritic cells known as melanocytes, which embryologically are derived from the neural crest. Melanocytes transfer melanin to neighboring keratinocytes by way of their dendritic processes. Hair partakes of the same pigmentation to a degree somewhat proportional to that of the skin. In hair, the melanin is in the cortical substance, having been derived from the epithelium of the hair follicle. It is reported that the melanin granules are large in dark hairs, smaller in lighter hairs. Bay, brown, and even sorrel horses have black skin, as do red and fawn cattle and red swine. In dogs and cats, this may not be the case, depending on breed. In animals with white spots, both hair and skin are nonpigmented at these sites. Gray horses owe their color to a mixture of white and black hairs over a black skin. White rabbits, rats, mice, and occasional individuals of any species are true **albinos,** having no pigment in hair, skin, or elsewhere, except the retina, which is not entirely devoid of pigment.

In some breeds of cattle (especially Jerseys) and dogs(e.g., Chows), the mucous membrane of the mouth shares the pigmentation of the adjacent skin. The same is true of hooves, e.g.,white hoof tissue growing from white skin, and is largely true of horns.

Melanin gives color to the iris, and a thick, black zone of melanin is deposited in a layer of cells where the retina joins the choroid, which totally blackens the interior of the uveal space.

In some people and especially in sheep, melanin is found here and there in certain dendritic cells of the pia-arachnoid. In sheep, this is common over the anterior part of the brain, but may be found even over the spinal cord. In some species, the substantia nigra of the brain is black because of melanin-containing nerve cells.

Melanin occurs pathologically or at least abnormally (1) in tumors known as melanomas, (2) in melanosis, (3) acanthosis nigricans, (4) abnormalities of human skin, such as freckles, (5) hyperpigmentation of skin associated with hyperadrenalism, (6) a rare inherited disease in man (Dubin-Johnson syndrome), and (7) mutant Corriedale sheep in which a hepatic excretory defect results in accumulation of melanin pigment in hepatocytes.

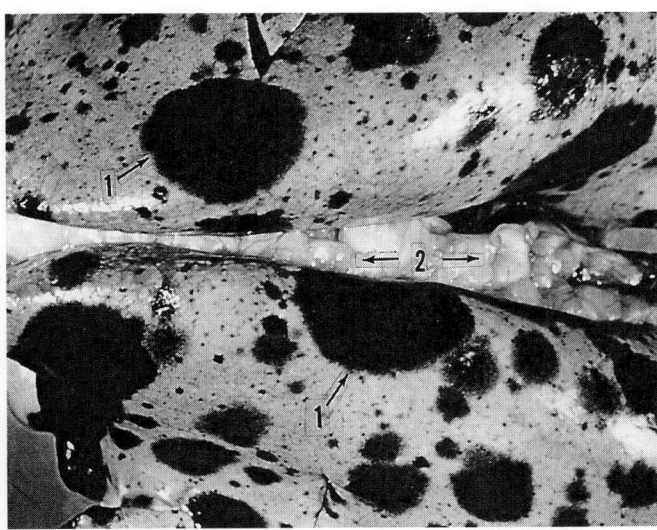

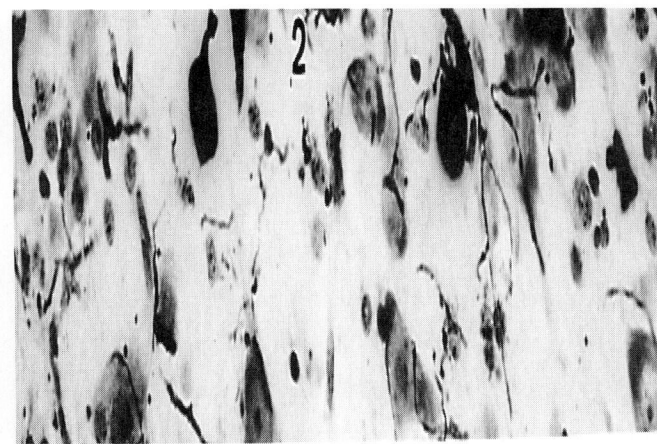

FIG. 3-10 Melanosis, thalamus of a goat. (1) Melanin-laden melanocytes with elongate processes; (2) melanophagic neurons (Luxol blue stain). (Courtesy of Dr. G. Bestetti, Prof. Dr. R. Fankhauser, and Prof. Dr. H. Luginbohl)

FIG. 3-9 Melanosis, lung of sheep. Large deposits of melanin (1), mediastinum (2). (Courtesy of Dr. C. L. Davis)

Melanosis (Fig. 3-9) is a deposition of melanin in various organs, especially lungs and aorta, as rather spectacular black or brown spots of irregular shape, often a centimeter or more in diameter. There is no change in texture, consistency, or form of the tissue and no tendency toward neoplasia. It is most often encountered by meat inspectors in animals in normal health.

Albinism represents a pathologic absence of melanin thought to result from an inability of melanocytes to synthesize sufficient functionally active tyrosinase. Melanocytes that are present in albinism are structurally identical to normal melanocytes. Inability to form melanin occurs with the development of **achromotrichia** in copper deficiency in several animal species, copper being an essential component of tyrosinase. Focal depigmentation may occur in scars and radiation burns.

MICROSCOPIC APPEARANCE.

Melanin takes the form of minute, rounded granules of light or dark brown color located in the cell cytoplasm. Ultrastructurally, the granules, known as melanosomes, are extremely dense, ellipsoid, and measure 0.3 by 0.7 μm. Melanin is produced in specialized dendritic cells known as **melanocytes** (Fig. 3-10) located in the basal aspect of the epidermis. These cells transfer melanin to adjacent keratinocytes via their long dendritic processes. Although in some other locations the presence of melanin may be attributable solely to dendritic cells of more or less similar morphology, it does not appear that all melanin formation can be accredited to cells of this type (for instance, in the substantia nigra), and it is difficult to reconcile this view with what one sees in day-to-day observations of skin sections. It is clear, however, that melanin does escape from its intracellular position, is seen extracellularly, is excreted in the urine in cases of great overproduction (malignant melanomas), and is frequently phagocytized by macrophages. When laden with melanin, these macrophages are called **melanophores (melanophages)**. Melanophores are often seen in the dermis beneath pigmented epithelium and not infrequently migrate in great numbers to regional lymph nodes, where they are appear as large, round cells filled with pigment composed of finer granules than those of hemosiderin, with which melanin can be confused. The **dopa reaction** can be used to distinguish melanocytes from melanophores; "dopa" is an acronym derived from the key letters of dioxyphenylalanine, an older equivalent of dihydroxyphenylalanine. If a section of fresh tissue is incubated with a solution of this substance, melanin-producing cells develop a black granular precipitate in their cytoplasm. This is pigment formed by the action of these cells on dihydroxyphenylalanine. Such cells have the same action on (mono) hydroxyphenylalanine (tyrosine). The reaction is caused by the action of an enzyme termed dopa-oxydase (tyrosinase), which is present in melanin-producing cells. The dopa reaction, then, is not a test for melanin but for the ability of cells to produce melanin. Since it must be performed on frozen sections of unfixed or slightly fixed tissue, precise localization of the enzyme is not easy, but in general, dopa-oxydase occurs where melanin occurs, except in the case of phagocytized and transported melanin. One may test for the actual presence of melanin granules by using Fontana's silver solution, which turns such granules black.

SIGNIFICANCE.

Melanin itself is not harmful, although melanomas, in which it may be extremely abundant, are often life-threatening; nor is melanosis harmful. In the skin, the amount of pigment increases with increased exposure to sunlight (or artificial ultraviolet rays) and is regarded as a protective mechanism against ultraviolet damage to the skin (discussed under photosensitization).

References

Fawcett DW. An atlas of fine structure. The cell, its organelles and inclusions. Philadelphia: WB Saunders 1966.

Flatt RE, Nelson LR, Middleton CC. Melanotic lesions in the internal organs of miniature swine. Arch Pathol 1972;93:71–75.

Gjesdal F. Investigations on the melanin granules with special consideration of the hair pigment. Acta Pathol Microbiol Scand Suppl 1959;133:112.

Kaliner G, Frese K, Fatzer R, et al. Thalamic melanosis in goats. Schweiz Arch Tierheilkd 1974;116:405–411.

Okum MR, Donnellan B, Pearson SH, et al. Melanin: a normal component of human eosinophils. Lab Invest 1974;30:681–685.

Hematogenous pigments

A variety of pigments are derivatives of hemoglobin metabolism. Certain pigments are normal physiologic components, which may accumulate to excess, such as hemosiderin and bilirubin, and others are pathologic, such as methemoglobin and hematins formed by protozoan and metazoan parasites.

HEMOGLOBIN

Hemoglobin, the normal pigment of erythrocytes, is in solution or colloidal state within those cells. It consists of a pigment, heme, plus the protein, globin. Heme is divisible into ferrous iron and a porphyrin (protoporphyrin III). The various porphyrins consist principally of four pyrrol rings with various hydrocarbon radicals attached (porphyrins are discussed later). The empirical formula of hemoglobin has been estimated to be approximately $C_{112}H_{1130}N_{214}S_2FeO_{245}$. It is noteworthy, however, that hemoglobin does not react in the usual tests for iron compounds.

Hemoglobin grossly imparts to individual erythrocytes a straw-yellow color, which deepens to crimson red when a thick layer of erythrocytes is viewed in the fresh state. It ordinarily is not seen microscopically; however, its presence is responsible for the eosinophilia of erythrocytes. Hemoglobin can be more specifically demonstrated by several histochemical techniques.

The gross tinctorial properties and chemistry of hemoglobin may be slightly altered under certain conditions, as in some poisonings and as a result of postmortem changes. In normal hemoglobin, iron is in the ferrous state and is either loosely oxygenated (not oxidized) and referred to as **oxyhemoglobin** or has given up its oxygen store and is referred to as **reduced hemoglobin.** The bright red of arterial blood is caused by the presence of oxyhemoglobin; the dark red of venous blood is caused by reduced hemoglobin.

Methemoglobin is a true oxide of hemoglobin (ferric iron) and is reddish-brown, often referred to as chocolate brown in contrast to the bright red oxyhemoglobin. It is produced by poisonings with nitrites, chlorates, and some organic compounds. **Sulfhemoglobin** is a combination of reduced hemoglobin and inorganic sulfide and is dark brown. It results from the action of nitrites and coal tar preparations (aniline, acetophenetidin, acetanilid) in the presence of excessive amounts of sulfur. A **sulfur methemoglobin** can form after death and cause greenish discoloration to abdominal structures. **Carboxyhemoglobin,** which is bright cherry-red, is the result of a combination of carbon monoxide with hemoglobin.

When erythrocytes undergo hemolysis, whether in the vessels after death, in an external or internal hemorrhage, or in a flask of blood for some laboratory purpose, the anoxic hemoglobin slowly escapes and carries its dark color to the surrounding fluids and tissues. Such discolored perivascular tissues after death represent **postmortem imbibition.**

HEMATINS

Hematins, more properly termed **acid hematins,** are pigments formed by the action of acids on hemoglobin. They are not normal breakdown products. The most familiar acid hematin is **acid formalin hematin,** which is formed when acid aqueous solutions of formaldehyde act on blood-rich tissues. It appears in tissue sections as a dark brown, finely granular, anisotropic pigment that does not stain with iron stains and may be seen both in vascular spaces and within or on top of various cellular elements. Acid formalin hematin is of no pathologic significance, but its presence can be annoying in that it must be differentiated from other pigments. It can be removed from tissue sections with saturated alcoholic picric acid. The use of neutral (pH 7.0) buffered formalin prevents its occurrence. A similar pigment may develop in extremely alkaline (above pH 8.0) formalin solutions. Other acid hematins that closely resemble acid formalin hematin can form from the action of acetic acid and hydrochloric acid. **Hydrochloric acid hematin** is often seen within and adjacent to gastric ulcers. It apparently forms from the action of gastric acid with hemoglobin.

Several parasitic diseases are associated with the deposition of hematin pigments in tissues. In **malaria,** hematins are present in parasitized erythrocytes and in the cytoplasm of reticuloendothelial cells in the spleen, lymph nodes, liver, and bone marrow. At each site, the pigment is yellow to dark brown and iron-negative. In erythrocytes, the pigment is anisotropic, whereas in reticuloendothelial cells, it is isotropic. The pigment is formed by the malarial parasites from the host's hemoglobin. Several species of trematodes also produce pigments believed to be hematins. *Fascioloides magna* in the ruminant liver deposits grossly visible pigment that accumulates adjacent to the parasite within macrophages. Various species of schistosomes produce anisotropic, iron-negative hematins, which accumulate in macrophages of the liver, spleen, bone marrow, and lymph nodes.

Pneumonyssus simicola (Fig. 3-11), the common lung mite of macaque monkeys, is associated with two pigments. One occurs as light brown to colorless, needle-like, brightly anisotropic crystals and the other as finely granular brown to black granules that are variably anisotropic. Both pigments are believed to be derived from hemoglobin metabolized by the mite. In contrast to hematins, most of the pigment stains with the usual iron stains, although isolated crystals and granules may be negative.

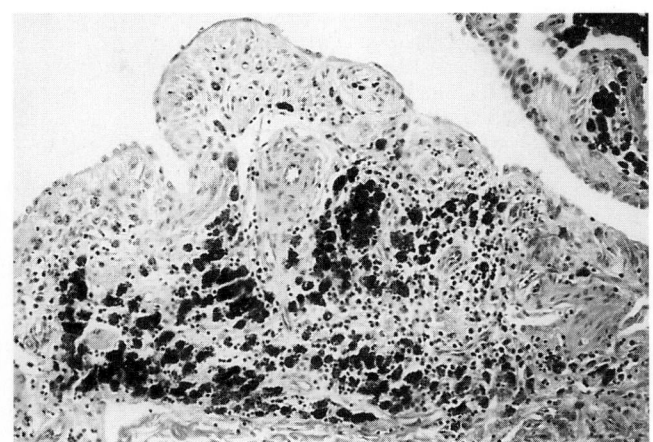

FIG. 3-11. *Pneumonyssus simicola* infestation of the lung of a rhesus monkey *(Macaca mulatta)*. Note parasitic hematin pigments within macrophages adjacent to bronchiole. *(Courtesy of New England Regional Primate Research Center, Harvard Medical School)*

HEMOSIDERIN

Hemosiderin is a shiny, golden yellow or golden brown pigment derived from hemoglobin (Fig. 3-12). It is usually seen within macrophages and responds to the usual tests for iron; chemically, it is the same as ferritin.

Occurrence. Hemosiderin occurs principally in the red pulp of the spleen and in other places where there has been extensive disintegration of erythrocytes. Such sites include old hemorrhages into the tissues, regressing ovarian corpora hemorrhagica, and chronically congested lungs. Rarely, large amounts accumulate within the epithelial cells of the liver, spleen, and kidneys. These are discussed separately under hemochromatosis.

Microscopic appearance. Hemosiderin takes the form of glittering golden-colored spherules, 2 or 3 μm in diameter, packed into round to oval macrophages. These hemosiderinophages are commonly so packed with pigment that the nucleus is obscured, but it is easy to surmise that the yellow, granular body is within a cell because of its size, shape, and rounded outline. At times, the color tends more toward brown, and the arrangement in spherical granules is less evident. The presence of hemosiderin in tissues is determined readily by an ordinary chemical test for its component iron, the **Prussian-blue reaction.** The application of a solution of potassium ferrocyanide to the microscopic section following treatment with an acid turns hemosiderin a strong greenish-blue, the potassium having been replaced by Fe to form ferric ferrocyanide, which, incidentally, is the common pigment of blue paints that are called Prussian blue. The same test can also be applied to fresh tissue; the whole area takes a diffuse bluish tinge if large amounts of hemosiderin are present.

Gross appearance. Small amounts of hemosiderin are not detected grossly, but large accumulations impart a brownish color to organs or tissues in which they occur.

Causes and special considerations. The cause of the formation of hemosiderin is the destruction or hemolysis of erythrocytes to an excessive degree. This occurs locally when there has been hemorrhage into the tissues.

Hemosiderin accumulates in mononuclear phagocytes of the spleen as the result of excessive hemolysis within the circulating blood, as in hemolytic anemia. It may also be present in Kupffer cells and hepatocytes of the liver, and in the tubular epithelium and interstitium of the kidney.

Hemosiderin accumulates in the spleen, lungs, and other organs as the result of chronic passive congestion. Chronic congestion of the spleen is most often the result of cirrhosis, along with congestion of the entire portal circulation.

Chronic passive congestion of the lungs is ordinarily caused by abnormalities of the heart, valvular insufficiency, or stenosis of the left side. The consequence of this is leakage of erythrocytes from alveolar capillaries into the adjacent alveolar spaces. These erythrocytes are phagocytized by alveolar macrophages, which transforms the hemoglobin into a golden-brown pigment. These hemosiderin-laden alveolar macrophages are termed **"heart failure cells."** Grossly, a brownish tinge is imparted to the lung tissue when the accumulation of hemosiderin is extensive. As a reaction to the constant pressure of blood in the distended capillaries, there is a diffuse increase of connective tissue throughout the alveolar walls, which tends to make the whole lung leathery and somewhat firm (**indurated**). On the basis of these two changes, it is common to refer to the condition as a whole as **brown induration** of the lungs.

Significance. The significance of hemosiderosis (deposition of hemosiderin in tissue) is merely that one of the foregoing disorders is present. The pigment itself is not harmful nor is it indestructible. In spite of the

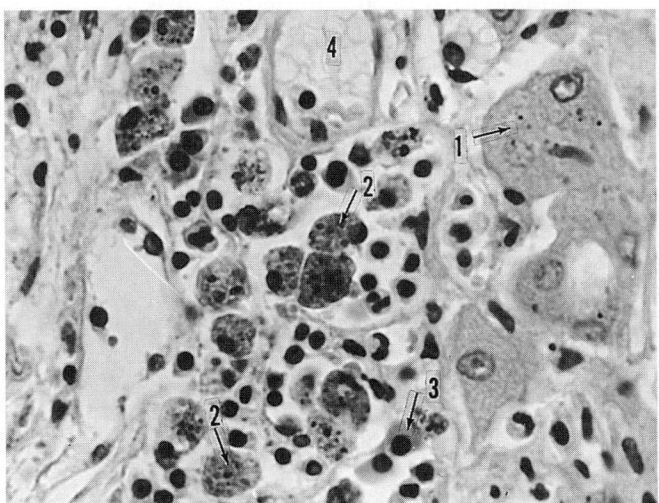

FIG. 3-12 Hemosiderin in portal area, liver of dog. Liver cell (1) with distended bile canaliculus, macrophages (2) with engulfed granules of brown staining hemosiderin, plasma cells (3), and branch of portal vein (4) (X 650). (Courtesy of Dr. D. J. Carren and Armed Forces Institute of Pathology)

possibility that chronic passive congestion may be responsible for its presence in the spleen, the presence of large amounts in this organ almost always indicates hemolytic anemia. Hemosiderosis is related to, but has a different pathogenesis than hemochromatosis.

HEMOCHROMATOSIS

Hemochromatosis is a rare condition in human beings in which a pigment indistinguishable from hemosiderin is deposited in tremendous amounts in the cytoplasm of epithelial cells of the liver and in lesser amounts in several other organs. It is accompanied by cirrhosis, apparently resulting from irritation by the pigment; by diabetes, probably causally related to the deposited pigment, although the islets are not destroyed; and by melanin pigmentation of the skin. On the basis of this triad of lesions, the name **bronze diabetes** has been in common use clinically. The cause is thought to be an inborn metabolic defect. In view of the fact that the body normally limits its absorption of iron to its scanty needs and eliminates the element slowly or not at all, evidence suggests that the pathogenesis may involve excessive absorption of dietary iron. It is agreed that this iron-containing pigment does not result from hemolysis; hence, it is different from hemosiderosis.

The syndrome has not been reported in animals, but in some instances heavy depositions of what appears to be the same pigment is found in livers and kidneys of animals. It is reported to occur in equine infectious anemia, without the spleen being similarly involved. It also occurs in anemias caused by deficiency of accessory hemoglobin-forming elements, i.e., copper and cobalt. Apparently, in those forms of anemia in which the hematopoietic tissue is active but unable to metabolize iron, iron accumulates in the tissues and is phagocytized in a form indistinguishable from hemosiderin. In all probability, increased amounts of iron are also absorbed.

A condition has been reported in goats grazing the mountains of northern Iraq (inaccessible to other animals) in which 3.6% of 700 goats had brown or blackish kidneys as a result of heavy deposition of a hemosiderin-like pigment in the epithelium of the proximal convoluted tubules, sometimes with evidence of mild injury to the cells, apparently caused by a deficiency of cobalt. Lesser amounts of this pigment were found in the Kupffer's (rarely the epithelial) cells of the liver and in reticuloendothelial cells of the spleen and lymph nodes. The testes had extensive necrosis of the seminiferous epithelium and had a positive Prussian-blue reaction. Other organs were normal. Affected goats were not clinically ill. The soil contained as much as 4% copper and 30% iron but was deficient in cobalt.

References

Hartley WJ, Mullins J, Lawson BM. Nutritional siderosis in the bovine. NZ Vet J 1959;7:99–105.

Higginson J, Gerritsen T, Walker ARP. Siderosis in the Bantu of Southern Africa. Am J Pathol 1953;29:779–815.

Kleckner MS, Baggenstross AH, Weir JF. Iron-storage diseases. Am J Clin Pathol 1955;25:915–931.

Plummer PJG. Three cases of osteohaemochromatosis in cattle. Can J Comp Med 1949;13:64–65.

Rimington C. Pigments of blood and bile. Lancet 1951;261:551–556.

Rimington C. Haems and porphyrins in health and disease. Acta Med Scand 1952;143:161–196.

Sheldon JH. Haemochromatosis. London: Oxford University Press 1935.

Zahawi S. Symmetrical cortical siderosis of the kidney in goats. Am J Vet Res 1957;18:861–867.

Bile pigments

Since older erythrocytes are normally destroyed in substantial numbers each day, a certain amount of hemoglobin is continually being metabolized. The iron and globin are recycled by the body, and the porphyrin is changed to a soluble pigment, **bilirubin,** by fixed macrophages in the bone marrow, spleen, and elsewhere. In the normal course of events, bilirubin circulates in the blood until it reaches the liver, where it is excreted in the bile and colors the excreted product. It accumulates pathologically whenever and wherever the disintegration of erythrocytes becomes excessive. Its further fate is discussed later in connection with icterus.

Although bilirubin ordinarily is a soluble substance, occasionally a bright yellow pigment, commonly called **hematoidin,** is encountered, especially at the sites of old hemorrhage. This is now believed to be the same as bilirubin, although it appears as a precipitate presumably because the solution becomes locally or temporarily supersaturated. Neither bilirubin nor hematoidin react positively to the usual tests for iron. This, and the fact that it remains as angular, yellow crystals and is seldom phagocytized, are the principal features that distinguish hematoidin from hemosiderin. Both are formed under the same conditions and have the same significance.

Biliverdin is an intermediary product in the formation of bilirubin; it is of similar chemical structure, but is green rather than yellow. Biliverdin is not ordinarily seen in tissue sections, but it is responsible in part for the blue-green discoloration of bruises.

In addition to their common presence at sites of hemorrhage, bile pigments are often seen in tissue sections under other circumstances. They may normally be observed in the bile ducts and gallbladder as bright orange-yellow masses. In obstructive jaundice, bile pigments may be seen in distended bile canaliculi, Kupffer cells, hepatocytes, and occasionally in epithelial cells of proximal convoluted tubules and portions of the loops of Henle in the kidney.

HYPERBILIRUBINEMIA (ICTERUS, JAUNDICE).

The formation of bilirubin from hemoglobin released from destroyed erythrocytes and its normal transport to the liver have already been referred to; however, before considering icterus, we examine these events more closely. In the breakdown of hemoglobin in the mononuclear phagocyte system, the cyclic structure of the iron-porphyrin compound (heme) is opened and the iron is removed and reusd by the body, as is the globin. The open-chained porphyrin is converted to a green pigment called **biliverdin.** Biliverdin is then reduced by biliverdin reductase to **bilirubin,** an orange-yellow pigment. Bound to albumin, bilirubin is then transported from the mononuclear phagocytic cells to the liver via the circulation. In the hepatocyte, the pigment is cleaved from albumin, conjugated with glucuronic acid, and excreted in the bile as **bilirubin-diglucuronide.** The enzyme involved at this point is uridine diphosphoglucose glucuronyl transferase. The conjugated bilirubin in the intestine is reduced by bacteria to urobilinogen (mesobilirubinogen and stercobilinogen). Some urobilinogen is reabsorbed into the portal circulation and carried to the liver (enterohepatic circulation), where most of it is converted to a bilirubin-like compound and re-excreted into the bile. A small amount of the absorbed urobilinogen enters the general circulation and is excreted in the urine. The urobilinogen that is not reabsorbed from the intestine is oxidized in the lower intestine to **urobilin and stercobilin,** which are normal pigments of feces.

Three pigments in this scheme are of primary importance to the diagnosis of icterus: (1) bilirubin diglucuronide, also called **conjugated bilirubin or direct-reacting bilirubin** (direct reaction to the Van den Bergh test) and cholebilirubin; (2) **nonconjugated bilirubin,** which is also called **indirect-reacting bilirubin** (indirect reaction to the Van den Bergh test), bilirubin, and hemobilirubin; and (3) **urobilinogen.**

Gross and microscopic appearance. Icterus is an important disorder clinically and postmortem in which the levels of bilirubin reach such a high concentration in the blood that all tissues of the body have a yellow tinge. However, since yellow is a weaker color than red, one must look for it where the tissues normally are white or pale, such as the sclera of the eye, the omentum, and mesentery. In considering the color of adipose tissue as a basis for diagnosis, the natural color of fat in the particular species and breed must be considered. The fat of horses, Jersey and Guernsey cattle, and certain nonhuman primates is normally yellow from carotenoid pigments. Mucous membranes and other tissues that are normally reddish may display a yellowish tinge if the icterus is severe. Since the bilirubin is in solution and not sufficiently concentrated to form a visible precipitate in tissue sections, icterus is seen only grossly. However, when the concentration of bile pigment (bilirubin) in the circulating blood is extremely high, it sometimes can be seen in microscopic sections of the kidney as a brownish precipitate or bile-stained albumin in the lumens of the tubules and by a brownish tinge in the ordinarily pink-staining (hematoxylin and eosin stain) cytoplasm of the epithelial lining cells. If the icterus is of the obstructive type, microscopic sections of the liver may contain accumulations of bile pigment in the distended bile canaliculi and ducts.

Causes. Depending on the causative mechanism, icterus or jaundice, hyperbilirubinemia is divided into three types; hemolytic, toxic, and obstructive.

Hemolytic jaundice results from excessive hemolysis of erythrocytes, ordinarily in the circulating blood. The more important disease conditions in which this type of icterus is pronounced are piroplasmosis, anaplasmosis, leptospirosis (partially hemolytic), and equine infectious anemia. A similar destruction of erythrocytes occurs in infections with hemolytic streptococci, *Clostridium hemolyticum bovis,* and *Bacillus anthracis,* but in these cases other aspects of the disease usually overshadow the jaundice. Indeed, these bacterial infections may progress so rapidly that the patient does not survive the two or three days necessary for the development of icterus. Ricin, saponin, and possibly other plant poisons; potassium or sodium chlorate; pyrogallic acid; nitrobenzene; and lead (if chronically ingested) are hemolytic poisons that may or may not produce visible icterus. The lethality of most snake venoms is caused by their hemolytic action, so that icterus is often seen after a lapse of a few days. Massive internal, usually intraperitoneal, hemorrhages result in icterus because of absorption of bilirubin from disintegrating erythrocytes of the free blood. Icterus neonatorum is a form of hemolytic jaundice; it is discussed in connection with hemolytic anemia. Congenital hyperbilirubinemia, inherited as a single recessive gene in the Gunn rat, results in icterus and kernicterus. The basic enzyme defect is the virtual absence of uridine diphosphoglucose (UDP) glucuronyl transferase, which results in the accumulation of unconjugated bilirubin in the blood.

Toxic jaundice is caused by toxic substances acting on cells of the liver and producing hydropic change, fatty change, and necrosis. Jaundice can result from these destructive changes in the liver in two ways. First, the hepatocytes may be damaged to such an extent that they cannot perform their excretory function. Hemobilirubin (unconjugated bilirubin) then remains in the blood, as in hemolytic jaundice. Secondly, the swelling of the hepatocytes may be sufficiently severe so as to block the outflow of bile from bile canaliculi. The bile is excreted from the cell, but its course to the gallbladder and intestine become obstructed. In this case, bilirubin diglucuronide, or posthepatic bilirubin, accumulates in the liver, from whence it is reabsorbed into the blood. As a rule, both these processes go on simultaneously, so that both kinds of bilirubin accumulate in the blood.

The causes of this hepatic damage are, in general, those that cause acute toxic hepatitis. They include hepatic toxins developed in the course of certain infections and extraneous poisons. Outstanding in veterinary medicine are poisonings by lupines and vetches, by plants of the genus *Senecio* (ragwort, groundsel), the genus *Amsinckia* (tarweed), and others. Several inorganic poisons are capable of causing jaundice, but chronic copper poisoning is the one most often reported as being accompanied by icterus. Numerous infectious diseases are accompanied by severe hepatic injury, but leptospirosis is outstanding in its ability to produce toxic (as well as hemolytic) icterus.

Obstructive jaundice results from obstruction of the normal flow of bile. Retained anywhere in the biliary passageways, much of the bile is reabsorbed into the blood stream. Some of it becomes dehydrated and is precipitated in the tissue as bile pigment. The obstruction may be caused by (1) blockage of bile canaliculi by swollen hepatocytes, (2) obstruction of the ducts (either inside or outside the liver) by flukes, fimbriated tapeworms (*Thysanosoma actinioides*) or ascarids, (3) compression of the intrahepatic ducts by the contracting fibrous tissue of biliary cirrhosis, (4) cholangitis, with swelling of the duct walls, (5) gallstones, (6) pressure on any part of the ductal system by neoplasms, granulomas, or abscesses, or (7) pressure of inflammatory swelling on the slanting orifice of the bile duct as it enters the duodenum at the papilla duodeni in duodenitis. The acute angle at which the duct passes through the duodenal wall subjects it to easy closure by the compression of inflammatory swelling.

Diagnosis of Icterus. In mild cases, the clinical discoloration may be equivocal; therefore, laboratory tests are often required to establish a definitive diagnosis of jaundice. The **icterus index** is determined merely by comparing the color of the serum with the yellow tint of a solution of toxic potassium dichromate of standard strength. The **Van den Bergh reaction** depends on the addition of sulfanilic acid and sodium nitrite to the serum, and the change in color is a quantitative indication of the presence of bilirubin diglucuronide. This is the **direct** Van den Bergh reaction. If alcohol is added to the mixture, hemobilirubin also reacts, constituting the **indirect** Van den Bergh reaction. Thus, hemolytic jaundice gives the indirect reaction and obstructive jaundice the direct reaction, a valuable aid in differentiation. Toxic jaundice usually gives both direct and indirect reactions. When the bile reaches the intestinal lumen, bacteria change it by chemical reduction into urobilinogen. Much of the urobilinogen is reabsorbed into the portal blood, carried to the liver, and normally excreted in the bile, but if hepatocytes have suffered the types of injury that accompany toxic hepatitis, the urobilinogen is incompletely removed from the blood and is excreted by the kidneys. Furthermore, the capacity of the liver to eliminate urobilinogen, as has also been pointed out with respect to bilirubin, is not unlimited. Thus, in hemolytic jaundice large amounts of urobilinogen are found in the feces and urine, because the amount of cholebilirubin originally excreted is maximal, contributing much urobilinogen to the feces, and the considerable excess above what the liver can degrade goes into the urine. In toxic jaundice, the amount in the urine is considerable, varying with the relative ability of the liver to excrete bilirubin and to decompose the resorbed urobilinogen. In obstructive jaundice, the amount of urobilinogen in the feces and urine is reduced, sometimes to zero. The actual test is usually made on urine, but feces can also be tested.

It is also common to perform certain simple tests for urine bilirubin (bile), the presence of which is called choluria. Since the kidneys are able to excrete bilirubin diglucuronide but not hemobilirubin, the urine is acholuric in hemolytic icterus but contains much bilirubin in obstructive jaundice. Because of its dual causative mechanism, toxic jaundice again falls between the two extremes, but some choluria is usually found.

In summary, a high icterus index indicates the presence of icterus. A positive direct Van den Bergh reaction indicates obstructive jaundice or at least the presence of bilirubin-diglucuronide, which may result from toxic and obstructive jaundice. A positive indirect Van den Bergh test indicates the presence of hemobilirubin, which signifies either hemolytic jaundice or toxic jaundice along with inability of the hepatic cells to function. With respect to urobilinogen in the urine, a certain amount is normal; smaller amounts or its absence indicate obstructive jaundice (no bile reaching the intestine); large amounts indicate hemolytic icterus with a normal degree of hepatic secretion or, in the absence of hemolytic disease, toxic jaundice with an impairment of the excretory function of the liver. With respect to the mere presence or absence of urinary bilirubin, obstructive icterus is choluric, hemolytic icterus is acholuric.

Other laboratory tests are available for determining the degree of icterus as well as general hepatic functions. If hemoglobinuria accompanies the icterus, a diagnosis of hemolytic jaundice is substantiated.

Significance. Jaundice is an important clue to any one of several different disorders. For jaundice to be meaningful diagnostically, the clinician must first be able to recognize it, then have access to the appropriate laboratory tests and, finally, have a thorough understanding of the pathogenetic mechanism involved in its occurrence. Bilirubin itself ordinarily is not a seriously harmful substance, although it may be directly responsible for some subjective symptoms that humans feel, such as itching on urination. It may also contribute to the development of necrosis of the renal epithelium in the poorly understood "hepatorenal" syndrome. The most noteworthy harmful effect of bilirubin *per se* is seen in newborn animals and infants with **kernicterus.** In this disorder, most often associated with erythroblastosis fetalis, the hippocampus, basal ganglia, midbrain, medulla, and floor of the fourth ventricle are grossly yellow, and there is microscopic evidence of neuronal degeneration. Although the accumulation of bilirubin to high levels in blood and tissues does not appear particularly harmful in the adult human or animal, it does seriously affect the developing neonatal brain. One example in which kernicterus develops as a natural disease in animals is the congenital hyperbilirubinemia that is hereditary in the Gunn strain of rats. If the cause can be overcome, the accumulated bilirubin promptly disappears.

References

Arias IM. Inheritable and congenital hyperbilirubinemia. Models for the study of drug metabolism. N Engl J Med 1971;285:1416–1421.

Butcher RE, Vorhees CV, Kindt CW, Keenan WJ. An experimental evaluation of phototherapy for hyperbilirubinemia in the Gunn rat. Am J Dis Child 1972;123:575–578.

Campbell CB, Burgess P, Roberts SA, et al. The use of rhesus monkeys to study biliary secretion with an intact enterohepatic circulation. Aust NZ J Med 1972;2:49–56.

Cornelius CE. Dubin-Johnson syndrome. Comp Pathol Bull 1970;2:2.

Cornelius CE, Arias IM: Crigler-Najjar syndrome—animal model: hereditary nonhemolytic unconjugated hyperbilirubinemia in Gunn rats. Am J Pathol 1972;69:369–371.

Dowling RH, Mack E, Small DM. Biliary lipid secretion and bile composition after acute and chronic interruption of the enterohepatic circulation in the rhesus monkey. IV. Primate biliary physiology. J Clin Invest 1971;50:1917–1926.

Ford EJH, Gopinath C. The excretion of phylloerythrin and bilirubin by the horse. Res Vet Sci 1974;16:186–198.

Johnson L, Sarmiento F, Blanc WA. Kernicterus in rats with an inherited deficiency of glucuronyl transferase. Am J Dis Child 1959;97:591–608.

Lester R, Schmid R. Bilirubin metabolism. N Engl J Med 1964;270:779–786.

Sawasaki Y, Yamada N, Nakajima H. Studies on kernicterus. I. Gunn rat: an animal model of human kernicterus with marked cerebellar hypoplasia. Proc Jpn Acad 1973;49:840–845.

Schaffner F, Scharnbeck HH, Hutterer F, et al. Mechanisms of cholestasis. VII. αNaphthylisothiocyanate-induced jaundice. Lab Invest 1973;28:321–331.

Schutta HS, Johnson L. Electron microscopic observations on acute bilirubin encephalopathy in Gunn rats induced by sulfadimethoxine. Lab Invest 1971;24:82–89.

Sherwood LM, Parris EE: Inheritable and congenital hyperbilirubinemia. N Engl J Med 1971;285:1416–1421.

Shimada K, Bricknell KS, Finegold SM. Deconjugation of bile acids by intestinal bacteria. Review of literature and additional studies. J Infect Dis 1969;119:273–281.

Snell AM. Fundamentals in the diagnosis of jaundice. JAMA, 1948;138:274–279.

Yearly RA, Grothaus RH. The Gunn rat as an animal model in comparative medicine. Lab Anim Sci 1971;21:362–366.

Porphyrins, photosensitizing pigments: photosensitization

The condition known as photosensitization, or more appropriately photosensitizational dermatitis, has been recognized in cattle, sheep, goats, pigs, and occasionally horses for many decades. The clinical manifestations, which appear several hours after exposure to strong sunlight, include burning or itching sensations, erythema, and pronounced inflammatory edema, the cardinal signs of inflammation. Often, the inflammation is so severe that the affected areas of skin become necrotic and slough within a few days. These changes are strictly confined to areas of the body surface that are directly exposed to sunlight and are unprotected by pigmentation, hair, or fleece. In **cattle** and **goats,** the thinly haired and usually nonpigmented teats, udder, and perineum are most often affected. In **sheep,** the muzzle, head, and ears are the most vulnerable areas, and edema is the most prominent inflammatory change, leading to the colloquial term **bighead,** or **geeldikkop,** a South African term meaning "thick, yellow head." In New Zealand, an equivalent term is **facial eczema.** The ears of affected sheep become so swollen that they droop; the face is swollen and the mandibular area so edematous that it resembles the edema of "bottle-jaw" caused by hypoproteinemia from severe gastrointestinal colonization by parasites. In **horses,** the face, lower portions of the limbs, and nonpigmented areas of the skin are most often affected. The cutaneous lesions usually heal after days or weeks, depending on the degree of severity, but shock and disturbances in overall body functions may be evident from the outset. Death is an occasional outcome as a result of secondary bacterial infections and gangrene at sites of cutaneous ulceration.

The lesion of photosensitization is more severe than that resulting from simple sunburn. Photosensitizational dermatitis results from the direct action of light on a photodynamic or fluorescent pigment of some type present in the skin. A photodynamic substance is one that absorbs specific wavelengths of ultraviolet and visible light known as the action spectrum and that transforms them into light of a longer wavelength. For most photodynamic chemicals, the action spectrum lies beyond the UV-B range. The resulting color often is red, since this is the color of the longest wavelength; undoubtedly some of the resulting energy is in the infrared portion of the spectrum. The energy absorbed from light by these photoactive pigments is either transferred directly to oxygen in the cytosol of the cell, resulting in the formation of oxygen free radicals, or indirectly through activation of xanthine oxidase by calcium-dependent proteases. The oxygen free radicals cause peroxidation of cell membranes, rupture of mitochondria and lysosomes, and degranulation of cutaneous mast cells, thereby accounting for the severe inflammation that characterizes photodermatitis. In nature, the fluorescent sensitizing pigments appear under three different and unrelated sets of circumstances, but the pigments, as far as they have been studied chemically, are relatives of hemoglobin and chlorophyll, being hematoporphyrins or the related phylloerythrin, a degradation product of chlorophyll. Both chlorophyll and hemoglobin molecules have as their basic components four pyrrole radicals tied together by methene groups (the basic structure of porphyrin).

Three major types of photosensitization are recognized: **type I, or primary photosensitization,** in which innately photodynamic plant pigments or drugs are ingested, absorbed, and enter the systemic circulation (Fig. 3-13); **type II, or congenital erythropoietic por-**

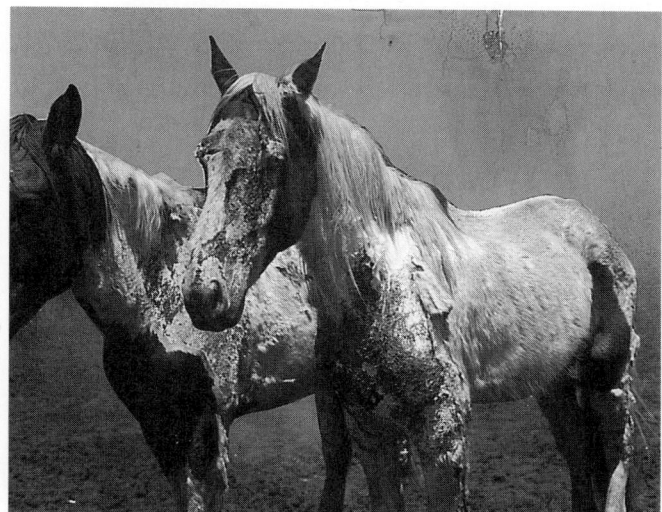

FIG. 3-13 Photosensitization of skin of horses. Note that lesions are in white skin and not in black areas of these spotted horses. (Courtesy of Dr. Rue Jensen) (From: Durrell LW, Jensen R, Klinger B. Poisonous and injurious plants in Colorado. Bulletin 412A. Colorado State University 1950.)

phyria or protophyria in which there is an inherited metabolic defect in porphyrin metabolism; and **type III, also referred to as secondary or hepatotoxic photosensitization,** in which there is interference with the excretion of phylloerythrin, a metabolic product of chlorophyll. In none of these conditions is the pigment seen in routine microscopic preparations. The pigment in porphyria is grossly visible. In certain rodents (mice, rats, hamsters), the Harderian gland, an intraorbital lacrimal gland, normally secretes a porphyrin pigment, which accounts for the red or brown tears seen in these species. This pigment can be seen microscopically in the gland as variably sized yellow to reddish granules.

PRIMARY PHOTOSENSITIZATION.

Primary photosensitization occurs in the absence of liver disease, icterus, or porphyrinemia and results from the ingestion and absorption into the systemic circulation of specific plant pigments, which themselves are innately photodynamic. The anthelmintic drug, phenothiazine, also has been associated with this type of photosensitization. Plant pigments responsible for primary photosensitization belong to two distinct families, the **helianthrones** and **furocoumarins.**

Helianthrones. Two important photodynamic agents, **hypericin** and **fagopyrin,** are included in this family; both are red fluorescent pigments that can be demonstrated in the plant as well as in the blood of affected animals. The diseases they cause are referred to as **hypericism** and **fagopyrism,** respectively.

Fagopyrism, resulting from eating buckwheat *(Fagopyrum esculentum),* affects sheep, goats, pigs, cattle, and horses. Hypericism, from ingestion of St. John's wort *(Hypericum perforatum)* or other closely related species, including goatweed, Tipton weed, amber, cammock, and Klamath weed, has been described in horses, cattle, sheep, and goats. In both conditions, the offending plant is ingested as a contaminant of foodstuffs or when pastures are poor.

In both conditions, the helianthrone pigment sensitizes the skin to sunlight in a manner similar to that caused by phylloerythrin and other porphyrins.

Furocoumarins. The principal photodynamic agents in this family of pigments are the **psoralens.** Interestingly, psoralen treatment coupled with ultraviolet irradiation has been used effectively in controlling psoriasis in humans. Plants containing photosensitizing psoralens include: spring parsley *(Cymopterus watsoni),* bishop's weed *(Ammi majus),* and Dutchman's breeches *(Thamnosma texana).* Photosensitizing dermatitis caused by ingestion of these plants has been described in cattle, sheep, and white chickens and ducks. In addition, the furocoumarin compounds also induce corneal edema and keratojunctivitis, presumably through excretion of the compounds in lacrimal secretions.

Finally, certain fungus-infected plants especially develop psoralen compounds that can induce photodermatitis by direct adsorption onto the skin followed by exposure to sunlight. A vesicular skin disease of this type affecting snouts of pigs from contact with fungus-infected celery *(Apium graveolens)* or fungus-infected

parsnips *(Pastinaca sativa)* has been described in New Zealand.

Phenothiazine. This commonly used anthelmintic may also cause primary photosensitization dermatitis. The drug is oxidized in the intestinal tract to phenothiazine sulfoxide, a photosensitive pigment normally metabolized by the liver. However, if it escapes the liver and enters the general circulation, dermatitis develops on exposure to sunlight. A damaged liver or the liver of young animals is less efficient in eliminating the sulfoxide. In addition to dermatitis, keratitis is a usual finding, owing to the excretion of phenothiazine sulfoxide in the tears and its entry into the aqueous humor. Photosensitization by this drug occurs most readily in swine, but cattle are also affected. Sheep are more resistant, apparently because of a greater efficiency of the sheep liver to reduce phenothiazine sulfoxide to phenothiazine sulfate.

References

Athar M, Elmets CA, Bickers DR, et al. A novel mechanism for the generation of superoxide anions in hematoporphrin derivative-mediated cutaneous photosensitization. J Clin Invest 1989;83:1137–1143.
Betty RC, Trikojus VM. Hypericin and a non-fluorescent photosensitive pigment from St. John's Wort *(Hypericum perforatum).* Aust J Exp Biol Med Sci 1943;21:175–182.
Binn W, James LF, Brooksby W. Cymopterus watsoni: A photosensitizing plant for sheep. Vet Med Small Anim Clin 1964;59:375–379.
Clare NT. Photosensitized keratitis in young cattle following the use of phenothiazine as an anthelmintic. II. The metabolism of phenothiazine in ruminants. Aust Vet J 1947;23:340–344.
Galitzer SJ, Oehme FW. Photosensitization: A literature review. Vet Sci Commun 1978;2:217–230.
Glastonbury JRW, Boal GK. Geeldikkop in goats. Aust Vet J 1985;62:62.
Gordon H McL, Green RJ. Phenothiazine photosensitization in sheep. Aust Vet J 1951;27:51–52.
Jha GJ, Iyer PKR. Pathology of photosensitizahon caused by experimental phenothiazine intoxication in cattle and sheep. Indian Vet J 1966;43:1078–1084.
Kirksen G, Tammen C. Keratitis in young cattle resultng from photosensitizaton after prolonged medication. Dtsch Tierarztl Wochenschr 1964;71:545–548.
Montogomery JF, Oliver RE, Poole WSH. A vesiculo-bullous disease in pigs resembling foot and mouth disease. I. Field cases. N Z Vet J 1987;38:21–26.
Montogomery JF, Oliver RE, Poole WSH. A vesiculo-bullous disease in pigs resembling foot and mouth disease. II. Experimental reproduction of the lesion. N Z Vet J 1987;38:27–30.
Pace N. The etiology of hypericism, a photosensitivity produced by St. John's wort. Am J Physiol 1942;136:650–656.
Shlosberg A, Egyed MN, Eilat A. The comparative photosensitizing properties of *Ammi majus* and *Ammi visnaga* in goslings. Avian Dis 1974;18:544–550.
Rowe LD. Photosensitization problems in livestock. Vet Clin North Am 1989;5:301–323.
Wender SH. Action of photosensitizing agents isolated from buckwheat. Am J Vet Res 1946;7:486–489.
Witzel DA, Dollahite JW, Jones LP. Photosensitization in sheep fed *Ammi majus* (bishop's weed) seed. Am J Vet Res 1978;39:319–320.

Congenital erythropoietic porphyria. Congenital erythropoietic porphyria has been described in humans, several breeds of cattle, swine, and in domestic shorthair and Siamese cats as a metabolic defect in the synthesis of the normal heme pigment, ferroprotoporphyrin. In cattle, the disease is inherited as an autosomal recessive trait, whereas in swine and cats it is an autosomal dominant disorder. The enzymatic defect in humans and cattle is a partial deficiency of uroporphyrinogen III cosynthetase, an important enzyme in the synthesis of heme. Deficiency of this enzyme results in failure of heme feedback suppression and, consequently, the overproduction of the photodynamic agents uroporphyrin I, coproporphyrin I, and protoporphyrin III, which accumulate in the tissues. These porphyrins, especially uroporphyrin I, absorb UV-A radiation from sunlight and, either directly or indirectly, through the activation of xanthine oxidase in the skin, generate oxygen free radicals which damage the membranes of cells and their organelles.

In cattle, the accumulation of porphyrins results in photosensitization dermatitis if the animal is exposed to strong sunlight. Interestingly, photosensitization dermatitis has not been reported in swine or cats with congenital porphyria, even in those with a white haircoat. The accumulation of porphyrins in dentine and bone gives rise to a red color, which has often gone by the misnomer, "osteohemochromatosis," or by the more colorful term, "pink tooth." Affected bones and teeth emit a strong reddish fluorescence with ultraviolet light, a useful aid to clinical and postmortem diagnosis. Because of increased renal excretion of porphyrin (porphyrinuria), the urine is amber-brown, becomes darker on standing, and emits a bright red fluorescence when exposed to ultraviolet light. The brownish color must be differentiated from that of hemoglobinuria and myoglobinuria. Discoloration of soft tissues caused by the accumulation of porphyrin is less obvious but may be encountered in the lungs or kidneys, which also fluoresce. Fluorescence also may be demonstrated in unstained tissue sections as well as in blood smears, in which the erythrocytes fluoresce. Except for its photosensitizing effect, this primary erythropoietic porphyria is generally harmless clinically.

Anemia has been reported in cattle and cats with porphyria, apparently resulting from inability to produce normal amounts of hemoglobin and a shortened life span of the erythrocyte.

Congenital Erythropoietic Protoporphyria. This autosomal recessive disorder has been described in Limousin cattle. Unlike in bovine congenital porphyria, affected cattle do not have discolored teeth or anemia or porphuria but develop only a photodermatitis. Animals homozygous for this trait have a deficiency of the enzyme ferrochelatase, which leads to the accumulation of protoporphyrin IX in the circulation and tissues; heterozygotes have approximately half the normal enzyme activity.

References

Clare NT, Stephens EH. Congenital porphyria in pigs. Nature (Lond) 1944;153:752–753.

Cornelius CE, Gronwall RR. Congenital photosensitivity and hyperbilirubinemia in Southdown sheep in the United States. Am J Vet Res 1968;29:291–295.

Flygers V, Levin EY. Congenital erythropoietic porphyria. Am J Pathol 1977;87:269–272.

Giddens WE, Labbe RF, Swango LJ, Padgett GA. Feline congenital erythropoietic porphyria associated with severe anemia and renal disease. Am J Pathol 1975;80:367–386.

Glenn BL, Glenn HG, Omtvedt IT. Congenital porphyria in the domestic cat (*Felis catus*): preliminary investigations on inheritance pattern. Am J Vet Res 1968;29:1653–1657.

Glenn BL. Feline porphyria. Comp Pathol Bull 1970;2(2):2–3.

Haydon M. Inherited congenital porphyria in calves. Can Vet J 1975;16:118–120.

Joergensen SK. Congenital porphyria in pigs. Br Vet J 1959;115:160–175.

Johnson LW, Schwartz S. Isotopic studies of erythrocyte survival in normal and porphyric cattle: influence of light exposure, blood withdrawal and splenectomy. Am J Vet Res 1970;31:2167–2178.

Kaneko JJ. Erythrokinetics and iron metabolism in bovine porphyria erythropoietica. Ann NY Acad Sci 1963;104:689–700.

Kaneko JJ, Zinkl JG, Keeton KS. Erythrocyte porphyrin and erythrocyte survival in bovine erythropoietic porphyria. Am J Vet Res 1971;32:1981–1986.

Meyer UA, Schmid R. Hereditary hepatic porphyrias. Fed Proc 1973;32:1649–1655.

Moore WE. Metabolic acidosis in bovine erythropoietic porphyria during the neonatal period. Am J Vet Res 1970;31:1561–1567.

Owen LN, Stevenson DE, Keilin J. Abnormal pigmentation and fluorescence in canine teeth. Res Vet Sci 1962;3:139–146.

Rimington C. Some cases of congenital porphyrinuria in cattle: chemical studies upon the living animals and post-mortem material. Onderstepoort J Vet Sci 1936;7:567–609.

Roe DA, Krook L, Wilkie BN. Hepatic porphyria in weaning pigs. J Invest Dermatol 1970;54:53–64.

Romeo G, Glenn BL, Levin EY. Uroporphyrinogen III. Cosynthetase in asymptomatic carriers of congenital erythropoietic porphyria. Biochem Genet 1970;4:719–726.

Rudolph WG, Kaneko JJ. Kinetics of erythroid bone marrow cells of normal and porphyric calves in vitro. Acta Haematol (Basel) 1971;45:330–335.

Scott DW, Mort JD, Tennant BC. Dermatohistopathologic changes in bovine congenital porphyria. Cornell Vet 1979;69:145–158.

Tobias G. Congenital porphyria in a cat. J Am Vet Med Assoc 1964;145:462–463.

Wass WM, Hoyt HH. Bovine congenital porphyria: studies on heredity; hematologic studies, including porphyrin analyses. Am J Vet Res 1965;26:654–658.

Hepatogenous photosensitization. The great majority of photosensitizations in animals are not derived from hemoglobin but are caused by a derivative of the plant kingdom's counterpart of hemoglobin, namely chlorophyll. Furthermore, these compounds only cause photosensivity if there is toxic injury to the liver. When the chlorophyll passes through the digestive tract of ruminants, one of the breakdown products is the pigment **phylloerythrin.** It differs from phylloporphyrin in that it has a ketone group attached to the sixth carbon atom, but for practical purposes it can be classed with the porphyrins. Normally, this phylloerythrin is removed from the circulation by the liver and is excreted in the bile. When the liver or its ductal system is injured in a way that interrupts this excretory function, the phylloerythrin, with its photosensitizing properties, reaches the skin by way of the circulating blood and the results are the same as those from the presence of hematogenous porphyrins.

There is usually no specific microscopic pattern of liver injury, although the changes described for acute toxic hepatitis are usually present. Often, but not always, icterus may be present as a consequence of the liver damage, and occasionally there are central nervous system disturbances and other signs of hepatic dysfunction. In two forms of hepatogenous photosensitization, more specific hepatic lesions are seen. "Facial eczema" of sheep and alfalfa-associated photosensitization produces a pericholangitis, which leads to occlusion of small bile ducts.

The causes of photosensitizing hepatitis are generally among those listed for acute toxic hepatitis, but it must be emphasized that only a small percentage of toxic hepatitides are accompanied by photosensitization. There may be several reasons for this, but the outstanding one is that the animal must be on a diet containing liberal amounts of chlorophyll (usually green pasture). Clare (1952), in his comprehensive monograph on photosensitization, listed the following agents as causing poisoning accompanied by photosensitization, hepatic dysfunction, and icterus: *Tribulus terrestris* plants grown for forage in parts of South Africa, causing geeldikkop, also known as "thick, yellow head," "thick ear," and geelsiekte; a mycotoxin from the fungus *Pithomyces chartarum*, growing on perennial ryegrass and other pastures, causing facial eczema of sheep in New Zealand; *Lippia rehmanni*, a South African plant; *Lantana camara*, a verbena-like plant that occurs in the United States as well as in South Africa and Ceylon; sacahuiste *(Nolina texana)*, found in western Texas; lechuguilla *(Agave lechuguilla)*, also a native of western Texas and nearby arid areas; second growth from stumps of the Brazilian tree called alecrim *(Holocalyx glaziovii)*; panick grasses *(Panicum miliaceum* and other species) in Australia and South Africa; leaves of the ngaio tree of New Zealand *(Myoporum laetum)*, which affects horses as well as ruminants; the Australian grass *Brachiaria brizantha*; the American morenita *(Kochia scoparia)*; *Tetradymia glabrata*, known as "coal-oil brush" in Utah and as "spring rabbit brush" in Nevada and *Tetradymia canescens*, the "spineless horse-brush" of Utah; *Microcystis flosaquae*, a blue-green alga that grows as a scum on lakes; the plant *Northecium ossifragum*, which causes the Norwegian disease of lambs called "alveld"; and *Kochia scoparia*, to which "black fever" is attributed. Other plants include the seeds of *Stryphnodendron obovatum*, *Erodium circutorium*, and Bermuda grass. A similar disorder is "yellowses," a disease of lambs in Scotland of uncertain cause (discussed under poisons).

Other plants, valuable as pasture or cured forage, have also been incriminated or suspected in outbreaks of photosensitization dermatitis, among them are: some of the trefoils and bur clovers *(Medicago* species); Alsike or Swedish clover *(Trifolium hybridum);* some plants of the cabbage family (rape, *Brassica rapa,* and kale, *Medicago denticulata)*; and the common perennial ryegrass, which forms so many winter pastures. Outbreaks of photosensitization occur at highly variable periods, often seasonal, and various explanations have been offered. Investigators in New Zealand discovered that under certain conditions of growth, temperature, and humidity, fields producing these forages became heavily overgrown with a fungus known either as *Sporidesmium bakeri* or *Pithomyces chartarum*. The fungal growth, when first noticed, was so heavy that mowing machines were blackened by its dark spores. In these cases, mycotoxin was discovered to be the active toxic principal responsible for the photosensitization, rather than the plants themselves. A similar mechanism has been suggested for photosensitization dermatitis resulting from ingestion of Bermuda grass in the southern United States and also for a hepatogenous photosensitivity caused by feeding flood-damaged alfalfa. Numerous other plants have been suspected of causing photosensitization if eaten by livestock.

In addition to these causes, cases of photosensitization accompanied by toxic hepatic injury and icterus have occurred in cattle treated with phenanthridinium, a trypanocidal drug. Carbon tetrachloride poisoning, hepatic fascioliasis (liver flukes), and Rift Valley fever can also lead to hepatogenous photosensitization.

In Southdown sheep, a **hereditary defect in hepatic excretion of phylloerythrin** resulting in photosensitivity has been described. This disease, which is also associated with hyperbilirubinemia, has been described in New Zealand and the United States. In this disorder, the livers appear histologically normal. A second syndrome, similar to the Dubin-Johnson syndrome in humans, has been described in Corriedale sheep in which there is also a failure to excrete phylloerythrin; it also is associated with photosensitivity dermatitis.

In summary, photosensitization as most often encountered in veterinary medicine involves a triad of hepatotoxic plants, fresh green feed in the diet, and exposure to direct sunlight. Exceptions exist (1) in the form of plants that supply a sensitizing pigment of their own, apparently involving no hepatic injury; (2) in certain animals that form porphyrins in their daily metabolism as a result of a hereditary metabolic defect, only sunlight being required to produce the characteristic dermatitis; and (3) certain drugs that have a direct photosensitizing effect.

References

Allison AC, Magnus IA, Young MR. Role of lysosomes and of cell membranes in photosensitization. Nature (Lond) 1966;209:874–878.

Arias I, Bernstein L, Toffler R, et al. Black liver disease in Corriedale sheep: a new mutant affecting hepatic excretory function. J Clin Invest 1964;43:1249–1250.

Blum HF. Photodynamic action and diseases caused by light. New York: Reinhold 1941.

Brown JMM. Advances in "geeldikkop" *(Tribulosis ovis)* research. J S Afr Vet Med Assoc 1959;30:97–111 and 1960;31:179–193.

Brown JMM. Biochemical lesions in the pathogenesis of "geeldikkop" *(Tribulosis ovis)* and enzootic icterus in sheep in South Africa. Ann NY Acad Sci 1963;104:504–538.

Clare NT. Photosensitivity in diseases of domestic animals. Commonwealth Bureau Animal Health Revue Series 1952;3.

Clare NT. Photosensitization in animals. Adv Vet Sci 1955;2:182–211.

Egyed MN, Schlosberg A, Eilat A. The susceptibility of young chickens, ducks, and turkeys to the photosensitizing effect of *Ammivisnaga* seeds. Avian Dis 1975;19:830–833.

Ford GE. Photosensitivity due to *Erodium* spp. Aust Vet J 1965;41:56.

Fowler ME, Berry LJ, Bushnell R, et al. *Sphenosciadium capitellatum* (whiteheads) toxicosis of cattle and horses. J Am Vet Med Assoc 1970;157:1187–1192.

Glenn BL, Monlux AW, Panciera RJ. A hepatogenous photosensitivity disease of cattle. I. Experimental production and clinical aspects of the disease. Pathol Vet 1964;1:469–484.

Glenn BL, Panciera RJ, Monlux AW. A hepatogenous photosensitivity disease of cattle. II. Histopathology and pathogenesis of the hepatic lesions. Pathol Vet 1965;2:49–57.

Johnson AE. Experimental photosensitization and toxicity in sheep produced by *Tetradymia glabrata*. Can J Comp Med 1974;38:406–410.

Mathews FP. Photosensitization and the photodynamic diseases of man and the lower animals. Arch Pathol 1937;23:399–429.

McFarlane D, Evans JV, Reid CSW. Photosensitivity diseases in New Zealand. XIV. The pathogenesis of facial eczema. NZ J Agric Res 1959;2:194–200.

McGavin MD, Gronwall RR, Cornelius CE, et al. Renal radial fibrosis in mutant Southdown sheep with congenital hyperbilirubinemia. Am J Pathol 1972;67:601–612.

Mia AS, Gronwall RR, Cornelius CE. Bilirubin C turnover studies in mutant Southdown sheep with congenital hyperbilirubinemia. Proc Soc Exp Biol Med 1970;133:955–959.

Mia AS, Cornelius CE, Gronwall RR. Increased bilirubin production from sources other than circulating erythrocytes in mutant Southdown sheep. Proc Soc Exp Biol Med 1971;136:227–230.

Mia AS, Gronwall RR, McGavin MD, et al. Renal function defect in mutant Southdown sheep with congenital hyperbilirubinemia. Proc Soc Exp Biol Med 1971;137:1237–1241.

Mortimer PH. The experimental intoxication of sheep with sporodesmin, a metabolic product of *Pithomyces chartarum*. III. Some changes in cellular components and coagulation properties of the blood, in serum proteins and in liver function. Res Vet Sci 1962;3:269–286.

Slater TF, Riley PA. Photosensitization and lysosomal damage. Nature 1966;209:151–154.

Synge RLM, White EP. Photosensitivity diseases in New Zealand. XXIII. Isolation of sporodesmin, a substance causing lesions characteristic of facial eczema from *Sporidesmium bakeri*. NZ J Agric Res 1960;3:907–921.

Thornton RH, Percival JC. A hepatotoxin from *Sporidesmium bakeri* (*Stemphylium botryosum*) capable of producing facial eczema disease in sheep. Nature 1959;183:63.

Van Tonder EM, Basson PA, van Rensburg IBJ. Geeldikkop: experimental induction by feeding the plant *Tribulus terrestris* L. (Zygophyllaceae). J S Afr Vet Assoc 1972;43:363–375.

Witzel DA, Dollahite JW, Jones LP. Photosensitization in sheep fed *Ammi majus* (Bishop's Weed) seed. Am J Vet Res 1978;39:319–322.

Lipogenic pigments

Lipogenic pigments constitute a group of colored substances derived mainly or partly from lipids; they are not the same as lipochrome or carotenoid pigments. Numerous tissue pigments have been classified as lipogenic, and the list of names applied to them is extensive, despite the fact that their individuality is not established.

Two pigments from the group are encountered with frequency or are of special pathologic significance. These are lipofuscin and ceroid.

LIPOFUSCIN

Synonyms include wear-and-tear pigment, the German abnutzen pigment, hemofuscin, and pigment of brown atrophy (Fig. 3-14). The multiple synonyms for lipofuscin suggests the confusion that exists with respect to this pigment. Lipofuscin represents a homogeneous group of intralysosomal pigments formed by the peroxidation and polymerization of unsaturated fatty acids derived from membranes of autophagocytized organelles. It occurs in a variety of tissues and cell types, but especially in postmitotic cells of organs such as the brain, heart (Fig. 3-14), and skeletal and smooth muscle. Lipo-

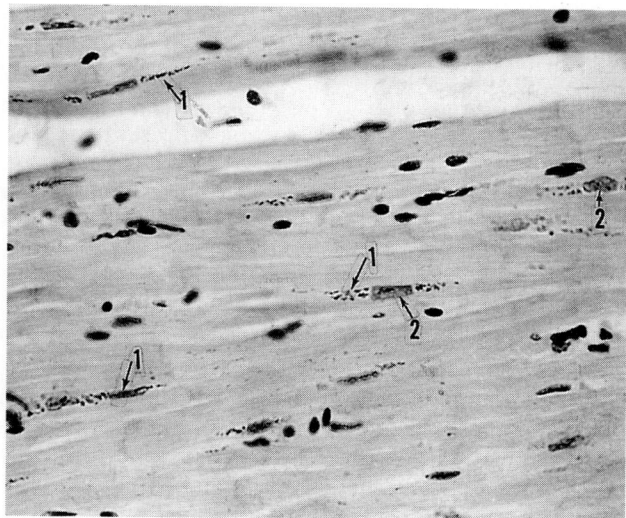

FIG. 3-14 Pigment of "brown atrophy" in bovine heart. Granules of lipofuscin (1) in cardiac muscle cells at poles of nuclei (2) (X 440). (Courtesy of Barnes General Hospital and Armed Forces Institute of Pathology)

fuscin is resistant to fat solvents and is sudanophilic (stains with fat stains), even after paraffin embedding procedures. It is usually acid-fast but negative for iron.

Lipofuscin occurs most often in certain cells of aging organisms and is seen in greatest quantity in organs undergoing cachectic or senile atrophy. Because it imparts a brown color to tissues, it has been referred to as the **pigment of brown atrophy.** However, lipofuscin may be seen in tissues from animals that are not cachectic or aged, necessitating caution in interpreting its significance.

Neuronal lipofuscin has received particular attention because of a possible relation to aging in humans and other species. It is thought that accumulation of lipofuscin in a neuron eventually interferes with its function and finally results in its destruction. This view is contested, but it is established that in one rare inherited disease, **neuronal ceroid-lipofuscinosis** (discussed in the previous chapter), pigment does accumulate excessively and produces neurologic deficit and death. The use of this name underlines the problem in distinguishing between ceroid and lipofuscin.

Microscopic appearance. The pigment takes the form of minute yellowish or darker brown granules. In heart muscle cells, it is located near the poles of the nucleus; in skeletal muscle, it is found in any part of the fiber; and in most parenchymatous organs, such as the liver or adrenal gland, it is distributed throughout the cytoplasm. In neurons, lipofuscin granules are seen in the cytoplasm forming a diffuse halo around the nucleus, clustered at one side of the nucleus, or aggregated at one or both poles of the nucleus in a polar or bipolar configuration.

Ultrastructure. Neuronal lipofuscin is osmiophilic but also is demonstrable following potassium permanganate and potassium bichromate fixation. The granule forms, in order of frequency, are as follows: (1) homogeneous or uniformly electron-dense; (2) finely granular; (3) vacuolated; (4) lamellated or banded; (5) coarse granular; or (6) compound or heterogeneous (combinations of types). These different forms are present within autophagolysosomes and represent the nondegradable end product of fatty acid peroxidation. Chemically, lipofuscin has been compared to linoleum which, is made by oxidation of the essential unsaturated fatty acids, linoleic and linolenic acids, found in various vegetable oils.

Gross appearance. If present in significant quantity, lipofuscin may impart a brownish tinge to cardiac and skeletal muscle.

Significance. The significance of lipofuscin cannot always be established, but it often indicates the presence of a wasting disease, senility, or emaciation. Atrophy of most cells, particularly skeletal muscle cells, is characterized by increased autophagy of intracellular organelles and, thus, formation of increased amounts of lipofuscin. This is the mechanism by which the cytoplasmic volume of individual cells is reduced. Old dairy cows that display the pigment in their skeletal musculature are usually those that go to slaughter when their usefulness as milk-producers is at an end; the condition is found by the veterinary meat inspector. These animals are always more or less emaciated, and the brownish discoloration is one of the grounds for condemning them as cachectic.

Unclassified lipofuscins. A blackish pigment is often seen grossly and microscopically in bovine lymph nodes, chiefly but not exclusively in the medullae of thoracic, mesenteric, and supramammary nodes. This pigment is finely granular, intracellular (in fixed mononuclear phagocytes), and has histochemical properties and reactions that appear to place it with the "lipofuscins." It increases with the age of the animal; it is absent in calves; it can hardly be considered pathologic, since it is commonly encountered in perfectly healthy cattle at meat inspection.

Apparently limited to certain regions of Australia, a diffuse, blackish pigmentation of the livers of sheep has been called melanosis. Almost 100% of the sheep show the pigment, beginning a few weeks after being brought into the given area. There is strong suspicion that it results from ingestion, perhaps only at certain seasons, of foliage of the Mulga tree (*Acacia aneura*), a widely used forage for sheep in these semiarid areas, but limited experimentation has not confirmed this. Cattle, which consume the plant less often, develop the pigmentation only occasionally. The livers may be slightly darkened or appear uniformly dark gray. Microscopically, the pigment takes the form of minute granules, first in the cytoplasm of hepatocytes, later in the Kupffer cells, reaching the portal lymph nodes via macrophages or as free particles. The first particles seen in the cytoplasm of liver cells are yellow; later they become black (from oxidation) and resemble granules of melanin. Histochemical studies have shown that the pigment is not melanin, but has the characteristics of "lipofuscin."

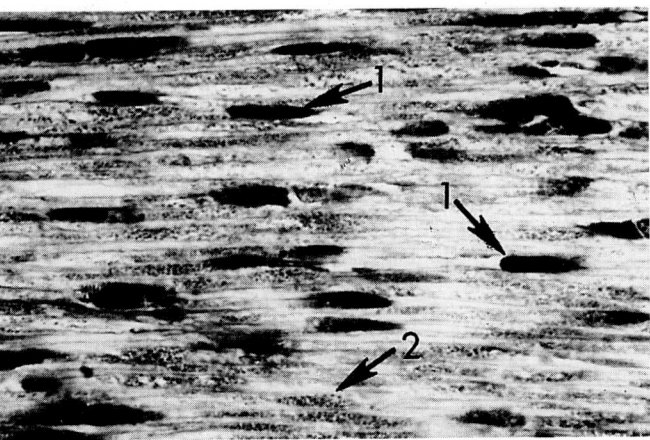

FIG. 3-15 Vitamin E deficiency pigment (ceroid). Large aggregates (1) and fine granules (2) of pigment in smooth muscle cells of the small intestine of a dog (PAS stain). (Courtesy of Dr. K. C. Hayes)

CEROID
Ceroid was first described by Lillie (1941) as a pigment that developed in the liver of rats with experimentally-induced cirrhosis. It has since also been produced in the livers of cattle, horses, dogs, pigs, rats, and guinea pigs. Its development is related to choline deficiency and, as with other lipofuscins, forms from unsaturated lipids. It occurs principally within macrophages, but also within hepatocytes.

An essentially identical pigment occurs with **vitamin E deficiency** in a variety of animal species. This form of ceroid is not restricted to the liver, but also occurs within macrophages throughout the body, fat cells, cardiac muscle, smooth muscle (Fig. 3-15) of the spleen and intestine (so called "leiomyometaplasts"), and ganglion cells. Often, the pigment is so abundant that it is visible grossly, giving rise to names such as "yellow fat disease" and "brown dog gut." Microscopically, both forms of ceroid are isotropic, granular to homogeneous, and yellow to brown. They are resistant to fat solvents, are sudanophilic even after paraffin embedding procedures, are acid-fast, and respond negatively to iron stains. Ceroid is indistinguishable histochemically from lipofuscin; however, its occurrence in differing situations probably justifies, for the present, the continued use of traditional terminology.

References
Bourne GH. Lipofuscin. Prog Brain Res 1973;40:187–201.
Brizzee KR. Ultrastructural studies on regional differences in lipofuscin accumulation in neuroglia of brain in nonhuman primates. Gerontologist 1974;14:36.
Casselman WGB. The in vitro preparation and histochemical properties of substances resembling ceroid. J Exp Med 1951;94:549–562.
Graham CE: Distribution of lipofuscin in the squirrel monkey *Saimiri sciurea*. Histochem J 1970;2:521–525.
Green PD, Little PB. Neuronal ceroid-lipofuscin storage in Siamese cats. Can J Comp Med 1974;38:207–212.

Hasan M, Glees P. Electron microscopical appearance of neuronal lipofuscin using different preparative techniques including freeze-etching. Exp Gerontol 1972;7:345–351.

Hasan M, Glees P. Genesis and possible dissolution of neuronal lipofuscin. Gerontologia 1972;18:217–236.

Hasan M, Glees P. Lipofuscin in monkey lateral geniculate body— electron microscope study. Acta Anat (Basel) 1973;84:85–95.

Koppang N. Canine ceroid-lipofuscinosis—a model for human neuronal ceroid-lipofuscinosis and ageing. Mech Ageing Dev 1973–1974;2:421–445.

Lee CS. Histochemical studies of the ceroid pigments of rats and mice and its relation to necrosis. JNCI 1950;11:339–349.

Lillie RD, Daft FS, Sebrell WH Jr. Cirrhosis of the liver in rats on a deficient diet and the effect of alcohol. Publ Health Rep 1941;56:1255–1258.

Mason KE, Hartsough GR. "Steatitis" or "yellow fat" in mink, and its relation to dietary fats and inadequacy of vitamin E. J Am Vet Med Assoc 1951;119:72–75.

Oliver C, Essner E, Zimring A, et al. Age-related accumulation of ceroid-like pigment in mice with Chediak-Higashi syndrome. Am J Pathol 1976;84:225–238.

Sharma SP, Manocha SL. Lipofuscin formation in developing nervous system of squirrel monkeys consequent to maternal dietary protein deficiency during gestation. Mech Ageing Dev 1977;6:1–14.

Trautwein GW: The occurrence of acid-fast lipopigments in animals. Am J Vet Res 1962;23:134–145.

von Wyler R. Ger die pigmentierung der Rinderlymphknoten [Pigmentation of lymph nodes in cattle]. Acta Anat 1952;14:365–382.

Whitehair CK, Schaefer AE, Elvehjem CA. Nutritional deficiencies in mink with special reference to hemorrhagic gastroenteritis, "yellow fat" and anemia. J Am Vet Med Assoc 1949;115:54–58.

Winter H. An environmental lipofuscin pigmentation of livers. Studies on the pigmentation affecting the sheep and other animals in certain districts of Australia. Papers presented by Faculty of Veterinary Science, University of Queensland, Australia. 1961;1:1–66.

Winter H. "Black kidneys" in cattle—a lipofuscinosis. J Pathol Bacteriol 1963;86:253–258.

Miscellaneous pigments

OCHRONOSIS PIGMENT.

Ochronosis is a feature of a rare hereditary disease of humans known as alkaptonuria (urinary excretion of homogentisic acid), in which there is a deficiency of the enzyme homogentisic acid oxidase. Homogentisic acid is a product formed during the metabolism of phenylalanine and tyrosine. The urine in alkaptonuria turns dark upon standing, as the acid is oxidized to a melanin-like product. A pigment is also deposited within tissues, especially in the walls of blood vessels, cartilage, tendons, and ligaments, and within other dense collagenous connective tissues, endocrine glands, kidneys, and lung. The pigment is believed to be a polymer derived from homogentisic acid and has similarities to melanin. Microscopically, it is yellow to brown, isotropic, and iron-negative. A similar syndrome has been reported in a chimpanzee and an orangutan.

DUBIN-JOHNSON PIGMENT.

The Dubin-Johnson syndrome, or chronic idiopathic jaundice, was first described as a disease in humans in 1954. The disorder, which is probably hereditary, is characterized by chronic icterus and an unidentified pigment in liver cells, which may be a lipofuscin but also shares many properties with melanin. An abnormality in the excretion of conjugated bilirubin is responsible for chronic icterus, but the mechanism of pigment formation is unknown. A similar disorder has been described in Corriedale sheep. In addition to chronic icterus (also caused by failure to excrete conjugated bilirubin) and hepatic pigmentation, photosensitivity occurred as a result of accumulation of phylloerythrin in serum. It was suggested that the pigment was melanin and that the disorder appeared to be functionally identical to the Dubin-Johnson syndrome of man.

CLOISONNÉ KIDNEY.

First described in Angora goats by Zahawi (1957), Cloisonné kidney is a dark brown, iron-negative pigmentation that occurs in the basement membranes of proximal convoluted tubules of the kidney, which imparts an appearance, in tissue section, reminiscent of enameled jewelry (cloisonné). It has also been described by Light (1960) in castrated male Angora goats. Light did not see the condition in female or noncastrated male goats. More recently, this condition has also been described in an adult male horse. The nature and significance of the condition is not known.

References

Arias I, Bernstein L, Toffler R, et al. Black liver disease in Corriedale sheep: a new mutation affecting hepatic excretory function. J Clin Invest 1964;43:1249–1250.

Cornelius CE, Arias IM, Osburn BI. Hepatic pigmentation with photosensitivity: a syndrome in Corriedale sheep resembling Dubin-Johnson syndrome in man. J Am Vet Med Assoc 1965;146:709–713.

Grossman IW, Altman NH. Caprine Cloisonné renal lesion. Arch Pathol 1969;88:609–612.

Light FW Jr. Pigmented thickening of the basement membranes of the renal tubules of the goat ("Cloisonné kidney"). Lab Invest 1960;9:228–238.

Marcato PS, Simoni P. Pigmentation of renal cortical tubules in horses. Vet Pathol 1982;19:572–573.

Zahawi SA. Symmetrical cortical siderosis of the kidneys in goats. Am J Vet Res 1957;18:861–867.

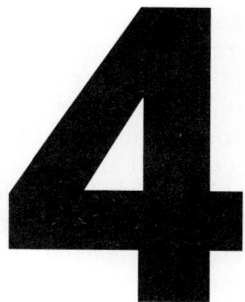

Disturbances of growth: aplasia to neoplasia

Disturbances of growth range from complete absence (aplasia) to uncontrolled proliferation (neoplasia). These two extremes always represent pathologic states that are deleterious to the patient, but many stages between these extremes occur under normal physiologic conditions or represent beneficial responses to various insults (although these conditions and responses are classified as disease). Thus, disturbances of growth are similar to the responses discussed under inflammation (Chapter 5) and immune-mediated diseases (Chapter 7).

APLASIA (AGENESIS)

Aplasia, or agenesis, is the complete failure of an organ or anatomic structure to form during embryogenesis. The term aplasia is also applied to the failure to form certain adult tissues that require continued replenishment, as in aplastic anemia. Pathologically, the organ or part is missing. If the part is vital for survival, the embryo or fetus may not survive gestation. Most examples in this category do not come to the pathologist's attention as a result of loss from early abortion or resorption. Other organisms may have types of aplasia that make them unable to survive extrauterine life. As a result, the most commonly seen examples involve paired structures (such as kidneys or gonads) or nonvital parts (such as limbs or a tail).

Causes

The causes of aplasia are generally not determined, but they may include inherited genetic defects, such as the absence of a tail in Manx cats or the absence of the thymus in nude mice. Poisons may cause aplasia, such as thalidomide, which causes absence of limbs (amelia) and *Veratrum californicum,* which causes (among other abnormalities) absence of the palate and gross facial deformities; various chemical agents and drugs may cause aplstic anemia. Some prenatal viral infections may also result in aplasia.

HYPOPLASIA

Hypoplasia is the failure of an organ or part to develop to normal size. It differs from atrophy in that the atrophic organ has shrunk from its previously normal size, whereas the hypoplastic organ never attained normal size. The disorder occurs during the period of growth, usually before birth but also during periods of postnatal growth. As with aplasia, the causes are often obscure; genetic defects, specific hormone deficiencies, certain infectious agents, and certain poisons may result in hypoplasia.

ATROPHY

Atrophy is a shrinking or reduction of an organ or tissue to less than its former or less than its normal size. It may be a normal physiologic phenomenon or a pathologic process. Atrophy may occur in two ways, both of which may occur simultaneously in the same organ: (1) through death of a portion of the constituent cells, or **numerical atrophy**; and (2) by a decrease in size of each constituent cell, or **quantitative atrophy.** Typically, it is the parenchymal cells rather than the stromal cells that undergo atrophy. Although atrophic cells have reduced function, they are not dead.

Microscopic appearance

Within an atrophic organ or tissue, cells of one or more histologic types may be fewer in number than normal (numerical atrophy) or present in normal numbers but individually smaller than normal size (quantitative atrophy). If the atrophic organ has a capsule, it may be wrinkled or undulating, reflecting the loss of volume of the underlying parenchyma. In addition, the components of the organ that are not affected may appear more prominent than usual. In the spleen, for example, the trabeculae may occupy a greater portion than usual of a given microscopic field because the volume of the intervening parenchyma has been reduced.

For the same reason, the glomeruli of an atrophic kidney appear more numerous as a result of a reduction in the number and size of intervening tubules. The pathologist should not be misled in the case of a very young animal's kidney, which has many small, uniform glomeruli and some incompletely developed tubules.

In atrophic muscle, the sarcoplasm of myocytes becomes variably reduced in amount and may not be discernible, leaving only the sarcolemma and endomysium, which may resemble fibrous tissue. In the atrophic liver, the hepatic cords may be intact but become extremely narrow.

Gross appearance

The organ or part is smaller than normal, which may be determined by visual inspection, by measuring, or by weighing. If a paired organ is in question, it should be compared with the size of its counterpart.

Causes

The causes of numerical atrophy are essentially the same as those of cell death, because this form of atrophy involves the loss of cells through either accidental death or apoptosis.

Starvation and malnutrition cause atrophy of almost all parenchymal tissues of the body and are primarily forms of quantitative atrophy. In starvation, the lipid contained in adipose tissue is first depleted to produce the energy necessary to sustain life. When this source of energy becomes exhausted, the proteins contained in the cytoplasm of muscular and glandular tissues are depleted as they are catabolized into an alternate source of energy. Practically all organs suffer some degree of atrophy with severe malnutrition.

Inadequate blood supply results in a deficiency of oxygen that causes quantitative atrophy of individual cells or numerical atrophy of the organ through death of a large proportion of the cells. For example, the stasis of blood associated with chronic passive congestion of the liver causes narrowing of the hepatic cords to half their normal width and, ultimately, their disappearance.

Lack of proper innervation has already been mentioned as causing muscle necrosis in "sweeney" of the horse's shoulder. However, some of the muscle cells remain alive, undergoing only quantitative atrophy through loss of their sarcoplasm. It is these cells that regenerate most successfully when recovery supervenes.

Disuse is a causative mechanism not encountered in the study of necrosis, but one of considerable importance with respect to atrophy. The wasting that occurs in an immobilized limb results from atrophy of both muscle and bone. Denervation may also cause disuse atrophy.

Prolonged **pressure** leads to atrophy, at first quantitative and later numerical with necrosis. A striking example is when a neoplasm invades the liver; the tumor eventually replaces most of the hepatic tissue. Another illustration is the slight depression of a healthy tissue under the area of the collar or the saddle of a horse, which signals that the animal has been working regularly.

Loss of hormonal stimulation produces atrophy of organs dependent on such secretions. Examples include atrophy of the prostate following orchiectomy or of the uterus after ovariectomy and atrophy of the opposite testis in a dog with a functional Sertoli cell tumor resulting from suppression of pituitary gonadotropin secretion.

Prolonged **overstimulation** leads exceptionally to atrophy, as in the thyroid exhaustion after proprolonged exophthalmic goiter.

Physiologic atrophy occurs under a variety of circumstances; a classic example is the resorption of a tadpole's tail in metamorphosis. In a similar way, the thymus almost disappears (involutes) as an organism approaches sexual maturity. Other examples are involution of the uterus and mammary glands after pregnancy and lactation, respectively, and atrophy of the endometrium during anestrus.

Classification of atrophy

It is sometimes useful to divide atrophy into several classes on the basis of special accompanying features. **Simple atrophy** needs no explanation; the term is used when none of the other classifying adjectives apply. In **fatty atrophy,** the missing cells have been replaced by adipose tissue. This occurs, for example, in physiologic atrophy of the thymus. In **fibrous atrophy,** sometimes called **"scirrhous"** atrophy, proliferating fibrous connective tissue fills in the space left by the dying cells. The proliferation of new connective tissue, in these cases, constitutes a form of chronic inflammation. **Pigment atrophy** is is accompanied by deposition of the pigment lipofuscin, also known as the pigment of brown atrophy. **Serous atrophy of fat** occurs with severe starvation when adipose tissue becomes depleted of lipid and somewhat mucinous in consistency.

Mechanisms

The mechanism of numerical atrophy involves apoptosis or individual cell death, necrosis, and heterolysis, all of which are discussed in Chapter 1. Quantitative atrophy, however, is accomplished by a process known as autophagy, which involves controlled sequestration of cellular organelles and components of the cytosol in membrane-bound vacuoles called autophagic vacuoles, in which they are degraded by lysosomal enzymes and their chemical constituents are recycled. Cole and colleagues (1971) demonstrated that autophagic vacuoles form within 5 to 10 minutes after occlusion of the portal blood supply to the liver, a process that leads to atrophy. What initiates atrophy is not known, but glucagon has beeen shown to stimulate the process.

HYPERTROPHY

An increase in size of an organ or tissue to more than its former size or more than its normal size is known as **organ hypertrophy.** It may be caused by an increase in the size of individual cells comprising the organ, in which case it is called **cellular hypertrophy,** or by an increase in the number of the constituent cells, which is termed **hyperplasia.** Hyperplasia is restricted to organs and tissues in which the cells retain the capacity to divide, a feature absent in many adult tissues. In general, hyperplasia is more effective in meeting increased functional demands than hypertrophy.

Hypertrophy of most tissues and organs results from a combination of cellular hypertrophy and hyperplasia. Pure hypertrophy (without hyperplasia) occurs only in organs in which cells have generally lost the ability to divide; for example, skeletal and cardiac muscle. However, even in muscle, limited cell division may accompany hypertrophy. Cellular hypertrophy results from an increase in the amount of new cytoplasm and its constituent organelles. Grossly, the organ is enlarged; microscopically, the appearance is unchanged except that the cells are larger, but this may be difficult to appreciate.

Classification

Two types of hypertrophy, not always distinguishable from one another, are recognized on the basis of their origin and probable cause. These are compensatory and hormonal hypertrophy.

COMPENSATORY OR ADAPTIVE HYPERTROPHY

This form of hypertrophy (Fig. 4-1) may represent a physiologic or pathologic response. It is often a consequence of impaired function of an organ system. For example, loss of one kidney, for any reason, results in gradual enlargement of the remaining kidney to compensate for the loss of function of the missing organ. Another example is found in the myocardium, which as a result of valvular deformities or hypertension, undergoes remarkable enlargement. Stenosis of the lumen of the pylorus of the stomach leads to hypertrophy of the

gastric musculature; similar partial obstruction of the intestinal or urethral lumen leads to hypertrophy of the intestinal or bladder smooth muscle, respectively. The enlargement of skeletal muscle as a result of repeated exercise is a physiologic form of compensatory hypertrophy.

HORMONAL HYPERTROPHY

This most often is a physiologic phenomenon, but in some instances, it may be pathologic. The enlargement of the mammary gland before the onset of lactation involves hypertrophy as well as hyperplasia (to be discussed), as does the great increase in size of the testes in birds and some mammals during the mating season.

Significance

Hypertrophy is an adaptive mechanism and a response to a need for increased function. Occasionally, the enlarged organ may constitute a mechanical hindrance to some other function, as in enlargement of the heart muscle that causes distortion of the valves and heart failure resulting from inadequate blood supply. While the increase in size occasioned by hypertrophy may be considerable, there are always definite limits to the maximum size that can be attained. Once the stimulus for hypertrophy is withdrawn, the hypertrophic process regresses, although the hypertrophied organ rarely returns to its previous size.

HYPERPLASIA

Hyperplasia is an absolute increase in number of cells in response to functional demands or other stimuli, leading to hypertrophy of the involved organ or tissue (Fig. 4-2). Usually, only a single cell type in any given tissue is affected. As stated earlier, hyperplasia is limited to cells capable of mitosis. For example, the number of pulmonary alveoli or renal nephrons cannot be increased nor can those lost to disease be replaced, despite hypertrophy and hyperplasia of individual cells. This greatly limits the potential for increased function for these organs.

Gross and microscopic appearance

Gross and microscopic appearances vary with the tissue affected and the cause. Hyperplasia of a glandular organ usually involves an increase in the height of the acinar epithelium and, at the same time, an increase in the number of its cells. In the same way that more hills of corn may be planted in a crooked row than a straight one, hyperplasia causes the contours of the acinar lining to become crooked, wavy, and folded, often to the extent that papillary projections protrude into the lumen. Indeed, the acinus may be more or less filled with papillary infoldings of an acinar lining that originally was a smoothly contoured circle. This is seen especially well in hyperplasia of the thyroid or prostate. In some instances, huge acini are formed at the expense of surrounding structures, as in **cystic hyperplasia** of the en-

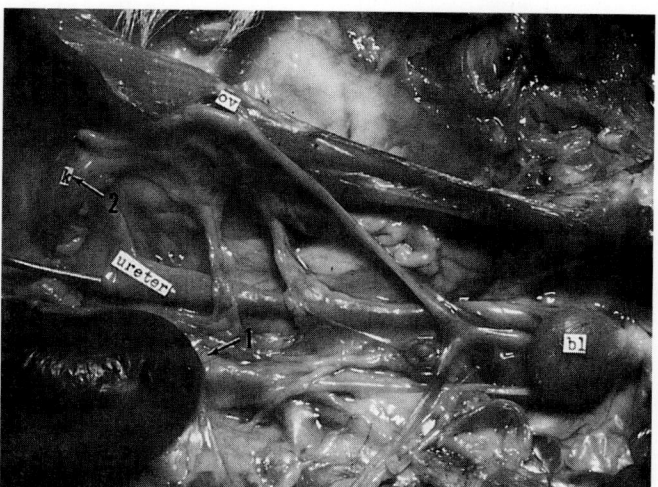

FIG. 4-1 Compensatory hypertrophy of right kidney *(1),* resulting from congenital hypoplasia of left kidney *(k, 2).* Left ovary *(ov)* and bladder *(bl).* From 5 1/2–month-old female terrier; died of canine distemper.

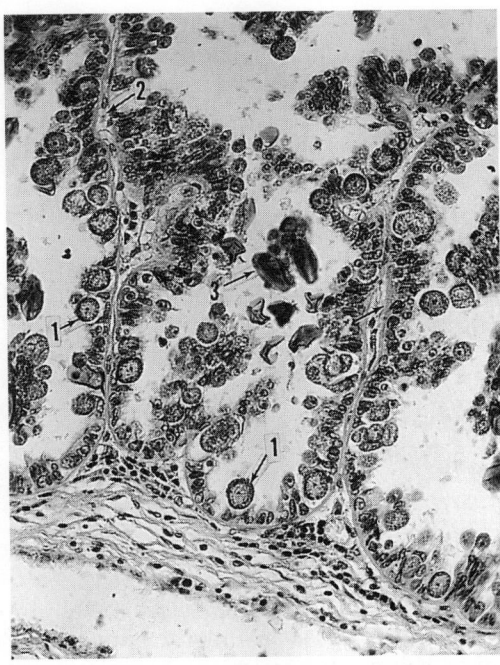

FIG. 4-2 Hyperplasia of intrahepatic biliary epithelium in liver of rabbit infected with *Eimeria stiedae*. Gametocytes *(1)* and oocysts *(3)*. Note long fronds of hyperplastic epithelial cells supported by delicate stroma *(2)* (X 250). (Courtesy of Dr. C.L. Davis and Armed Forces Institute of Pathology)

dometrium or mammary gland. Hyperplastic conditions of the epidermis may take the form of increased thickness of the prickle-cell layer (stratum spinosum), which is known as **acanthosis,** or of the cornified layer, which is called **hyperkeratosis.** Hyperplasia, which accompanies many forms of chronic inflammation with its associated fibrosis, as in hepatic cirrhosis, may result in the formation of large numbers of circumscribed, expanding nodules of proliferating cells. Hyperplastic cells usually have an increased nuclear to cytoplasmic ratio, although the number of cytoplasmic organelles may be increased. As expected, mitoses are more frequent.

Classification

As with hypertrophy, hyperplasia may be classified into two principal types, although multiple underlying stimuli may be operant in each.

COMPENSATORY OR ADAPTIVE HYPERPLASIA

This may be a physiologic or a pathologic response. After removal of a kidney or a partial hepatectomy, there occurs a physiologic hyperplasia of the opposite kidney or the remaining lobes of the liver. Pathologic destruction of one kidney initiates the same physiologic hyperplasia. Similarly, loss of blood or reduced atmospheric oxygen tension causes erythroid hyperplasia; the term regenerative hyperplasia is sometimes applied in these circumstances.

Other pathologic stimuli initiate a type of hyperplasia that is considered adaptive or compensatory, but the

nature of the stimulus or the true value of the response is usually unknown. Examples include lymphoid hyperplasia in response to infections (clearly of value), hyperplasia of the ducts of glands, and the protruded epithelium in hepatic coccidiosis (of uncertain value), epithelial or mesenchymal hyperplasia in pox viral infections, and epithelial hyperplasia associated with chronic irritation, as seen in corns.

HORMONAL HYPERPLASIA

Hormonal hyperplasia may also be physiologic or pathologic. Hyperplasia of the mammary glands or uterus associated with puberty or pregnancy are physiologic phenomena. In contrast, cystic hyperplasia of either of these tissues associated with malfunction of the ovaries is a pathologic change. The hyperplastic goiter of Graves' disease is another example of pathologic hormonal hyperplasia, as is iodine deficiency goiter.

Significance

In most respects, the significance of hyperplasia seems obvious. It sometimes appears to be only a short step from hyperplasia to the much more serious neoplasia. Still, there are comparatively few conditions in which a progression from hyperplasia to neoplasia is evident (exceptions; thyroid, parathyroid, and pancreatic islets). However, differentiation of hyperplasia from many benign neoplasms and even some malignant ones may be difficult. As in hypertrophy, hyperplasia ceases and regresses when the causative stimulus is withdrawn, but the organ may never completely return to its original size.

METAPLASIA

Metaplasia is the replacement of one type of fully differentiated tissue by one of another fully differentiated type; it is a substitution and not a true transformation. The new mature cell types are derived from reserve cells, which are capable of differentiating along several lines (Fig. 4-3). Metaplasia is usually considered an adaptive protective response, but its value is not always clear.

Occurrence

Metaplastic change of columnar or cuboidal epithelium into stratified squamous epithelium, usually cornifying, occurs in the trachea, bronchi, and bronchioles in response to chemical irritation and certain viral infections; in the gallblader when irritated by gall stones; in the ducts of glands; and in the protruded parts of prolapsed organs such as the cervix. In vitamin A deficiency, squamous metaplasia of the lining epithelium occurs in a variety of other locations, including the lacrimal ducts and renal pelves.

Connective tissue undergoes metaplasia to cartilage or bone, and cartilage changes to bone in a variety of situations. In cattle, the formation of large numbers of bony spicules in thickened alveolar septa of the lung is not a rare finding. Bony and cartilaginous metaplasia in adenocarcinomas and mixed tumors of the canine

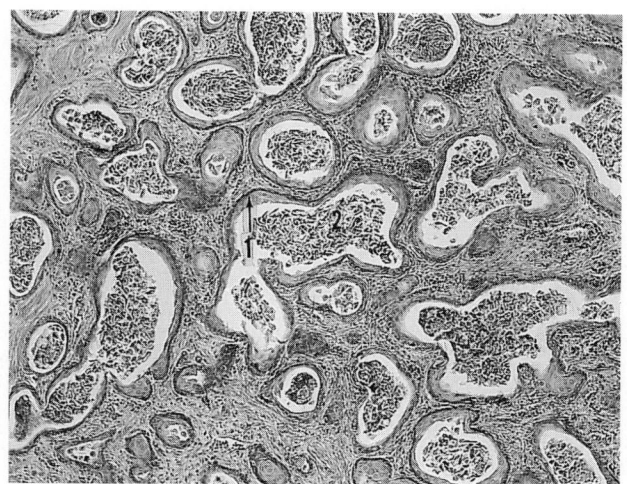

FIG. 4-3 Squamous metaplasia of prostate of dog, resulting from estrogen production of Sertoli cell tumor of testis. Prostatic acini are lined with squamous epithelium *(1)* and filled with keratin debris *(2)* (× 70). (Courtesy of Dr. W.H. Riser, and Armed Forces Institute of Pathology)

mammary gland is often found and may be so extensive that the major part of the neoplasm consists of bone. The ossification of tendons and cartilage is a form of metaplasia that has already been described. Rarely, the scars of abdominal wounds develop metaplastic bone.

Cause

The fundamental cause of metaplasia is a demand for a different kind of function, often for protection against chronic irritation. The exact mechanisms are essentially unknown.

Significance

Squamous metaplasia is almost always reversible, but it may precede neoplastic transformation. Most squamous cell carcinomas of the human lung and cervix arise from metaplastic squamous epithelium present in the normally mucus-secreting lining epithelium.

Dysplasia

Dysplasia (from *dys* = disordered and *plassein* = to form) is disordered or abnormal development of cells and tissues. It may occur during fetal or neonatal development or in adult tissues that are continuously replaced. Dystrophia is sometimes used as a synonym, but this is incorrect (*trophe* = nourishment). Dystrophy is a retrogressive change in a tissue after it has reached a stable adult state, as in nutritional muscular dystrophy.

Microscopic and gross appearance

Dysplasia occurring during development may or may not be reflected in a disordered microscopic appearance. In chondrodysplasia (chondrodystrophy), which causes abnormal endochondrial bone growth and

dwarfism, the cartalaginous growth plate is highly disorganized; whereas, in hip dysplasia, the acetabulum is grossly misshapen, but microscopically not remarkable. In renewable adult tissues, dysplasia occurs predominantly in epithelia, especially the skin, mucous membranes, and mucosae of the gastrointestinal tract, cervix, and vagina. Microscopically, dysplasia is characterized by disruption of orientational relationships, variation in size and shape of cells (pleomorphism), hyperchromasia of nuclei, increase in nuclear to cytoplasmic ratio, and increased mitotic activity.

Cause

Dysplasia occurring during development is probably caused by the same types of phenomena that cause aplasia and hypoplasia. In renewable adult tissues, dysplasia is generally believed to result from chronic irritation and is regarded as reversible. It may, however, be the hallmark of neoplastic transformation, as in dysplasia of metaplastic squamous epithelium of the human cervix. Dysplasia may be difficult to discern from anaplasia.

Anaplasia

Anaplasia is a reversion of cells to a more primitive and less differentiated type. Synonyms include dedifferentiation and undifferentiation. There is extensive pleomorphism, with some cells becoming very large (giant) with hyperchromatic nuclei and increased mitotic activity. Anaplasia is considered reversible and a precursor of neoplasia; it is also a feature of neoplastic tissue.

Developmental anomalies and malformations

Developmental anomalies ordinarily have their origins during embryonic life, when the development of most body structures begins. There are, however, exceptions. For example, if the epiphyseal cartilages of the femur of a child or an animal are severely damaged, as might occur with chronic osteomyelitis, the bone grows no more and the organism has a shortened and deformed leg, a malformation.

Forms of maldevelopment

The frequency of prenatal malformations is surprising; their wide variety is unbelievable. Most types have been given names, but these are omitted here. Reflection on the various forms reveals that they depend on one of several different errors in the developmental mechanism (Figs.4-4 through 4-8). Outstanding among these forms are the following.

ARREST OF DEVELOPMENT

This may occur in a certain part of the embryo, so that a certain structure is absent (aplasia) or too small (hypoplasia).

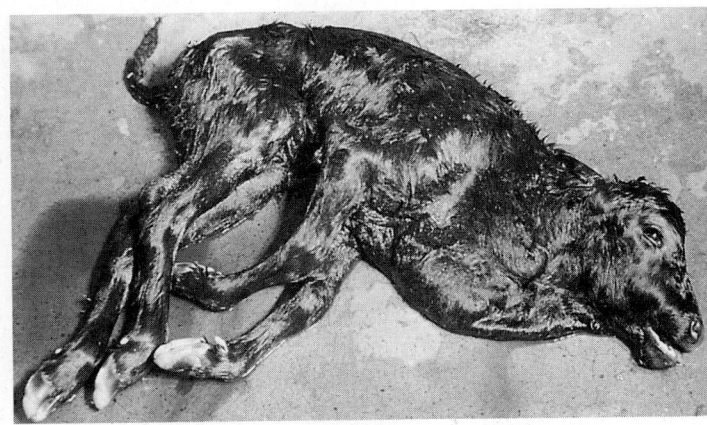

FIG. 4-4 *Ectopia cordis* in newborn Angus calf, full-term twin to normal calf. Diaphragm is absent; abdominal viscera in thorax; heart in subcutis of neck. Some calves with this anomaly have lived several months or years.

FAILURE OF A STRUCTURE TO DISAPPEAR

There are many examples of the failure of a certain embryonic or fetal structure to disappear when it should, such as the persistence of the ductus arteriosus or the thyroglossal duct. Atresia ani is a rather commmon malformation that results from failure of the skin overlying the anal opening to disappear.

ABERRANT STRUCTURES

Aberrant structures may be ectopic (Fig. 4-4) or heterotopic. It is not highly extraordinary to find islands of pancreatic tissue in the wall of the stomach or ectopic adrenal tissue in the kidney, testis, or pelvic tissues. Displacement of cutaneous and mucosal tissues into deeper areas is considered the proper explanation for the rather frequent appearance of dermoid cysts located near the exterior of the body, as well as for dentigerous cysts occurring in the head and neck. However, it is difficult to say just when such malformations become sufficiently complicated to be suspected of resulting from imperfect duplication.

DUPLICATIONS

Each cell or group of cells of the early embryo is destined to produce, as it multiplies, a particular adult

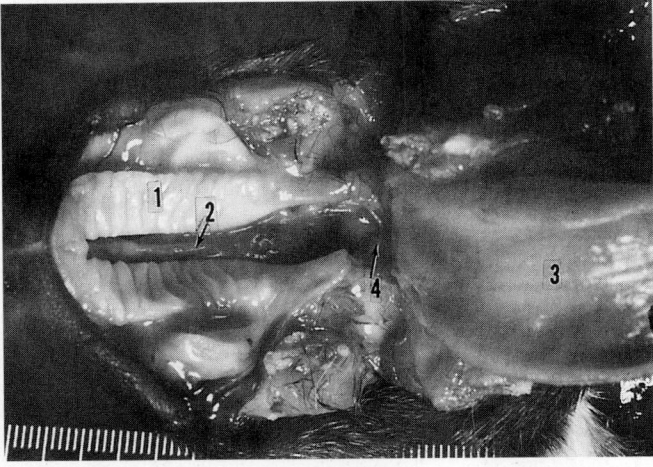

FIG. 4-5 Congenital anomaly. Cleft palate in 1–week-old bull dog. Hard palate *(1)*, cleft opening into nasal cavity *(2)*, deflected tongue *(3)*, and posterior nares *(4)*.

structure. If such a cell were to undergo division without further differentiation toward a particular organ or tissue, two cells with identical potential would be produced, each destined to form identical body structures, thus resulting in a duplication of organs or tissues. If the cell involved were the recently fertilized ovum, there would be two complete and identical individuals derived from the same zygote, i.e., monozygotic twins.

The work of experimental embryologists indicates that a slightly different process occurs. The fertilized ovum normally divides into two blastomeres, or primitive daughter cells.. In some simple animal species, these two blastomeres have been experimentally separated and each develops into a complete individual, an identical or uniovular twin. What must be almost complete separations of the two blastomeres has been accomplished by shaking or inverting the ovum at this two-cell stage, with the resulting formation of double monsters, i.e., twins like Siamese twins, almost but not completely separated. In other experiments with certain amphibian species, monsters with two heads or anterior ends have been produced by constricting the developing embryo at a somewhat later stage (during gastrulation). This procedure involves not only the separation of groups of cells, but a division of the supply of certain chemical hormones called "organizers." These organizers form in the appropriate region of the embryo and supply the necessary stimulus for the involved cells to differentiate into the particular types and structures needed, in this case, a head. If the plane of constriction is not exactly median, one of the heads is normal and the other is incomplete and imperfect in one way or another; usually it has only one eye. Double monsters and other radical malformations have also been produced by experimental embryologists in amphibian and similar lower animal species through such means as depriving the very early embryo of sufficient oxygen, applying minute amounts of certain toxic chemicals, or lowering the temperature unduly.

There may be any degree of duplication: two separate and perfect twins or two twins that are perfectly formed but joined together by more or less unduplicated tissue, such as abdomen to abdomen, back to back, or head to head. In such cases, the vital organs may or may not be duplicated. There may be duplica-

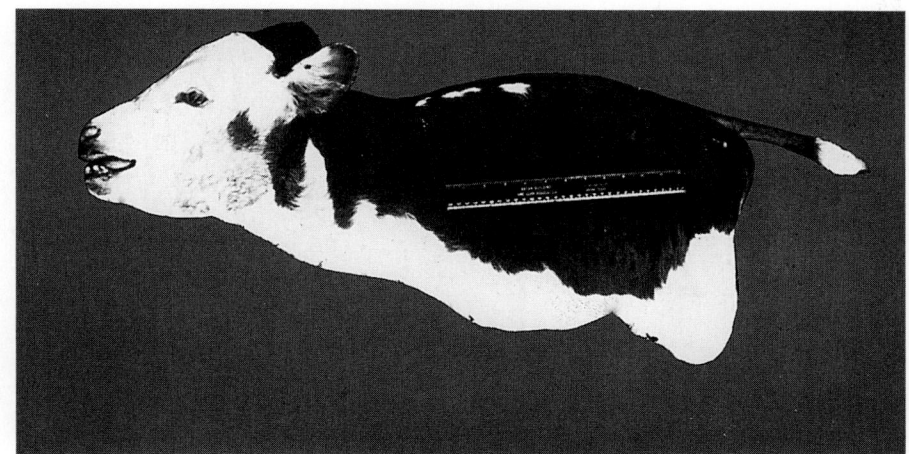

FIG. 4-6 Congenital anomaly, calf born alive but without legs (amelia) lived 3 days without nourishment and was given euthanasia. Similar anomaly in pigs is reported by Hutt to be caused by single recessive gene.

tion of almost any part of the animal's body; the muzzle, head, cephalothorax, tail, hindquarters, and/or others. Double pairs of fore or hind limbs may also occur; the latter are common.

As might be anticipated from the experimental results recorded above, duplicated parts are not necessar-ily equal, especially when the duplication is not a matter of right and left counterparts. The inequality is often such that one set of organs is more or less normal and perhaps functional, while the other recedes to a purely accessory status. We have seen a lamb that was born with two mouths, one in the normal place and one,

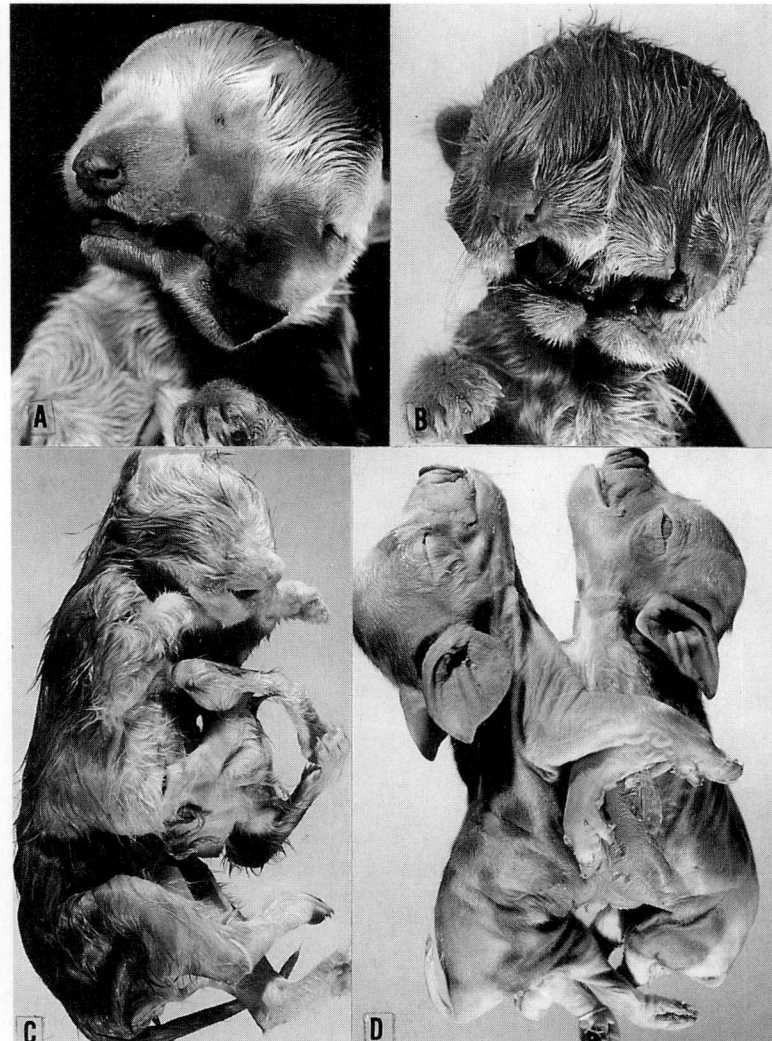

FIG. 4-7 Congenital anomalies. **A.** Partial dupli-cation of head (diprosopia) in fox-terrier puppy; lived for 2 days. **B.** Diprosopia in kitten. **C.** Twin kittens joined at abdomen; one is only partially de-veloped (heteradelphia). (Courtesy of Major A.C. Gi-rard and Armed Forces Institute of Pathology) **D.** Twin pigs joined at the thorax (thoracopagus).

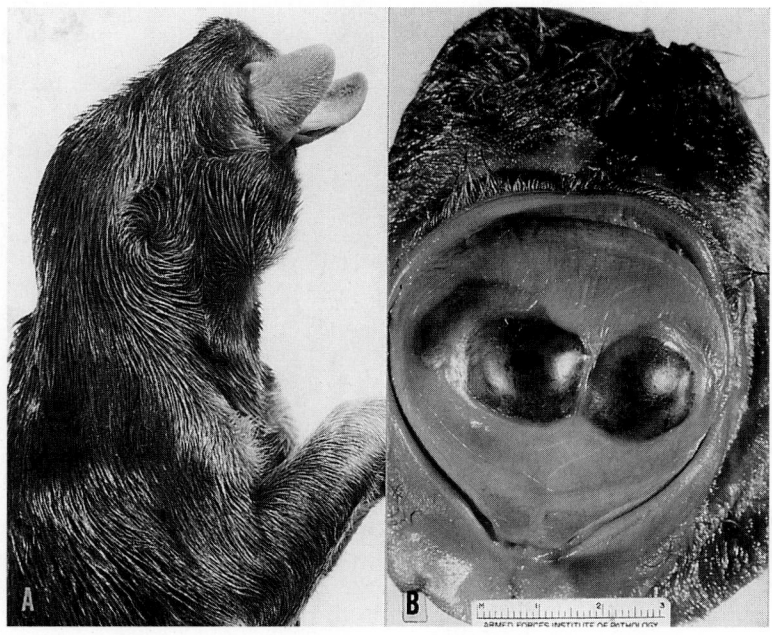

FIG. 4-8 Congenital anomalies. **A.** Absence of eyes (anophthalmia) and lower jaw in newborn puppy. **B.** Partially fused eyes (synophthalmia or cyclopegia) in newborn colt.

considerably smaller, in the right subparotid region. The accessory mouth chewed when the main mouth chewed, secreted saliva, and had three rudimentary teeth, but it did not have an opening into the pharynx. The lamb was raised to well past a year of age (dying of an accident) and, in the course of the animal's normal growth, the accessory mouth became relatively less and less prominent, since it grew very little.

Supernumerary parts, usually of minor nature, occur in some situations where the concept of duplication is less obvious, but probably still applicable, e.g., in the case of supernumerary digits in humans or animal. The extra digits are usually bilaterally symmetrical, but practically always imperfect and purely accessory. Supernumerary breasts are described in the human female and male. Supernumerary (and rudimentary) teats are common in the cow. However, in porcine and even canine species, a somewhat variable number of pairs of mammary glands is considered normal. Likewise, the number of vertebrae and ribs is subject to normal variation in some species.

ETIOLOGY

The causes of many congenital anomalies are essentially unknown; these are discussed in the appropriate chapters concerning organ systems. The important known causes of anomalies follow.

1. Prenatal viral infections, e.g., panleukopenia (cerebellar hypoplasia); Newcastle disease of chickens (ocular or auditory anomalies); bovine viral diarrhea infection of calves; blue tongue of sheep; and rickettsial infection. Most of these are associated with anomalies of the central nervous system.
2. Intrauterine exposure to poisons ingested by the mother, e.g., the plant *Veratrum californicum;* thalidomide; selenium; molybdenum; trypan blue; and sodium salicylate.
3. Vitamin deficiencies, e g., vitamin A and folic acid.
4. Experimentally, hyperthermia has induced congenital defects in many animals species, but its role in naturally occurring malformations is not known.
5. Genetic factors, i.e., the recombination of mutant genes, inherited from one or (usually) both parents.

References

Baker CA, Hendrickx AG, Cooper RW. Spontaneous malformations in squirrel monkey *(Saimiri sciureus)* fetuses with emphasis on cleft lip and palate. J Med Primatol 1977;6:13–22.

Berry CL, Beveridge BIB, Done JT, et al. Non-mendelian developmental defects: animal models and implications for research into human disease. Bull WHO 1977;55:475–487.

Blattner RJ, Williamson AP. Developmental abnormalities in the chick embryo following infection with Newcastle disease virus. Proc Soc Exp Biol Med 1951;77:619–621.

Cole S, Matter A, Karnovsky MJ. Autophagic vacuoles in experimental atrophy. Exp Mol Pathol 1971;14:158–175.

Dennis SM, Leipold HW. Syndactylism in a neonatal lamb. Cornell Vet 1970;60:23–27.

Dennis SM, Leipold HW. Aprosopia (facelessness) in lambs. Vet Rec 1972;90:365–367.

Goss RJ. Hypertrophy versus hyperplasia. Science 1966;153:1615–1620.

Hughes KL, Haughey KG, Hartley WJ. Spontaneous congenital developmental abnormalities observed at necropsy in a large survey of newly born dead lambs. Teratology 1972;5:5–10.

Kalter H, Warkany J. Experimental production of congenital malformations in mammals by metabolic procedure. Physiol Rev 1959;39:69–115.

Landtman B. Relationship between maternal conditions during pregnancy and congenital malformations. Arch Dis Child 1948;23:237–246.

Selby LA, Khalili A, Stewart RW, et al. Pathology and epidemiology of conjoined twinning in swine. Teratology 1973;8:1–9.

Shelburne JD, Arstila AV, Trump BF. Studies on cellular autophagocytosis. Cyclic AMP- and dibutyryl cyclic AMP-stimulated autophagy in rat liver. Am J Pathol 1973;72:521–540.

Thomson RG. Congenital bronchial hypoplasia in calves. Path Vet 1966;3:89–109.

NEOPLASIA

A neoplasm is a new growth of cells that (1) proliferates autonomously without control; (2) resembles to varying degrees the normal cells from which it arises both morphologically and functionally; (3) has no orderly pattern of growth; (4) serves no useful function for its host; and (5) stems from a variety of causes that alter the molecular events involved in the control of normal cell proliferation and differentiation. The term "cancer" is commonly used to refer to any malignant neoplasm without reference to a specific cell type. The even more general term "tumor," once used for inflammatory swellings, is now used almost exclusively as a synonym for any neoplasm, benign or malignant.

The key elements of any definition of neoplasia are "uncontrolled proliferation" and "no useful function." For most of the pathologic processes discussed in previous chapters, the mechanisms controlling the tissue responses are understood, and although these processes are considered disease, they generally are reactions that serve some useful purpose, in some cases life-saving, e.g., abscess, granuloma, hypertrophy, or hyperplasia.

Nomenclature

All neoplasms are composed of two basic tissue elements: (1) a **parenchyma,** consisting of the neoplastically-transformed, proliferating cells of epithelial or mesenchymal origin; and (2) a non-neoplastic, fibrovascular **stroma** that provides the framework for growth and the blood and nutrients required to sustain the neoplastic cells. The stroma of a neoplasm is an extension of the stroma of the adjacent normal tissue that is stimulated to proliferate and grow into the tumor by factors secreted by neoplastic cells. These mitogenic substances, commonly referred to as growth factors, are described in more detail in the discussion of tumor growth. The amount of stroma within a given neoplasm varies considerably depending on the nature of the neoplastic cells. Highly cellular neoplasms, such as lymphomas and seminomas, typically have very little stroma, whereas certain epithelial tumors, such as basal cell tumors, Sertoli cell tumors, and certain mammary adenocarcinomas, have a prominent stroma. Other adenocarcinomas are characterized by the formation of a dense collagenous connective tissue stroma provoked by the invading neoplastic epithelial cells. This phenomenon is referred to as a **desmoplastic reaction** and the neoplasm as a **scirrhous** (meaning hard) **adenocarcinoma** (Fig. 4-9) or **carcinoma.** Typical examples include certain carcinomas of the canine mammary gland and uterine adenocarcinomas in cows.

All neoplasms can be classified into one of four basic categories, i.e., benign and malignant neoplasms of epithelial origin and benign and malignant neoplasms of mesenchymal origin. A standardized system of nomenclature for neoplasms is necessary because certain types of neoplasms have relatively predictable clinical behaviors that respond most effectively to certain forms of therapy. Tumors are named according to their cell

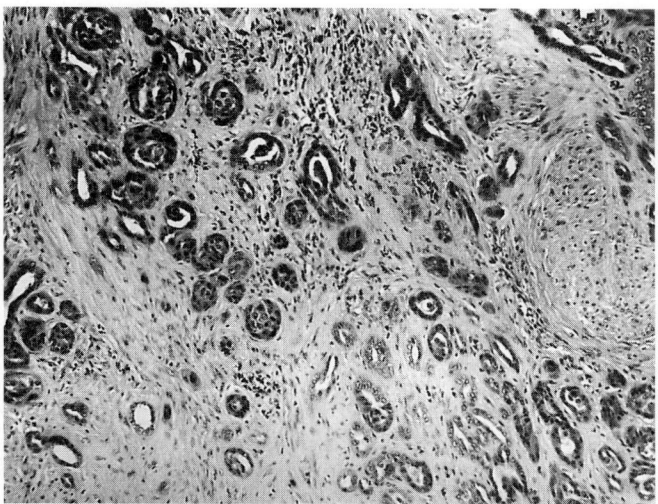

FIG. 4-9 Desmoplasia. Scirrhous adenocarcinoma of canine mammary gland. Many epithelial neoplasms incite proliferation of collagenous connective tissue (scirrhous tumors). Scirrhous adenocarcinomas also occur in stomach, bovine uterus, and other locations.

and tissue of origin, pattern of growth, and biologic behavior, which is deduced from known historical relationships between certain morphologic characteristics and clinical outcome. The names of most tumors end with the suffix "-oma," which simply means tumor. When "-oma" is coupled with a prefix denoting a particular cell type, such as fibroma, lipoma, leiomyoma, or pattern of growth, such as adenoma (gland) or papilloma (papilla), the terms indicate a **benign neoplasm.** If, in contrast, "-oma" is combined with the qualifier "carcino-" (crab-like), as in **carcinoma,** or "sarc-" (fleshy), as in **sarcoma,** the terms signify a **malignant neoplasm of epithelial cells** or a **malignant neoplasm of mesenchymal cells,** respectively, without reference to cell type or pattern of growth. As with benign neoplasms, cell types and patterns of growth of malignant neoplasms are indicated by adding the appropriate prefix (i.e., fibrosarcoma, liposarcoma, leiomyosarcoma) to indicate the malignant variants of the benign mesenchymal tumors listed above and adenocarcinoma or squamous cell carcinoma to indicate the malignant counterparts of adenoma and papilloma. Some important exceptions to this system of classification exist: Two neoplasms, **lymphoma** and **melanoma,** are both malignant despite the connotation of their names. Sometimes, the term malignant lymphoma is used to compensate for this disparity, but in reality this is a redundancy, since there are no benign lymphomas. Lymphosarcoma is a more appropriate label. Similarly, the term melanocytoma has been invoked recently to refer to the benign form of melanomas, which in the past have been classified as various forms of nevi.

A **teratoma** is a neoplasm that contains a haphazardly arranged mixture of tissue elements derived from all three germ cell layers, i.e., endoderm, mesoderm, and ectoderm. They may contain skin, hair, teeth, respiratory epithelium, nervous tissue, skeletal muscle, bone, cartilage, gastrointestinal epithelium, and/or other material. Teratomas arise from germ cells, either in the gonads or occasionally from germ cells that mistakenly wandered to ectopic sites during migration from the yolk sac to the genital ridges during embryonic development. Although in animals most teratomas are benign, in human beings malignant teratomas are encountered with some frequency. In the latter neoplasms, tissues derived from one or more germ cell layers exhibit features of malignancy.

The term **polyp** refers to a benign growth, either hyperplastic or neoplastic, that protrudes from the surface of a mucous membrane. Polyps may have a broad base of attachment (**sessile polyp**) or be attached by a narrow stalk or pedicle (**pedunculated polyp**). They are encountered most often in the upper respiratory tract, i.e., nasal passages, eustachian tubes, gastrointestinal tracts, and lower female genital tracts. The nomenclature of neoplasms derived from various types of tissue is presented in Table 4-1.

TABLE 4-1 **Nomenclature of selected neoplasms**

Tissue	Benign tumor	Malignant tumor
Connective Tissue		
Mature fibrous tissue	Fibroma	Fibrosarcoma
Embryonic fibrous tissue	Myxoma	Myxosarcoma
Cartilage	Chondroma	Chondrosarcoma
Bone	Osteoma	Osteosarcoma
Adipose tissue	Lipoma	Liposarcoma
Histiocytes	Histiocytoma	Malignant histiocytoma
Mast cells	Mast cell tumor	Malignant mast cell tumor
Endothelium		
Blood vessels	Hemangioma	Hemangiosarcoma
Lymphatics	Lymphangioma	Lymphangiosarcoma
Muscle		
Smooth muscle	Leiomyoma	Leiomyosarcoma
Striated muscle	Rhabdomyoma	Rhabdomyosarcoma
Hematopoietic Tissue		
Erythroblasts	None	Erythroid leukemia
Myeloblasts	None	Myeloid leukemia
Lymphatic Tissue		
Lymph nodes, spleen, thymus	None	Malignant lymphoma (lymphosarcoma)
Lymphoblasts	None	Lymphocytic (blastic) leukemia
Neural Tissue		
Glia	Glioma	Glioblastoma
Neurons	Ganglioneuroma	Neuroblastoma
Nerve sheath	Neurofibroma (Neurilemmoma)	Neurofibrosarcoma (Neurogenic sarcoma)
Melanocytes	Melanocytoma	Malignant melanoma
Epithelium		
Squamous epithelium	Papilloma	Squamous cell carcinoma
Transitional epithelium	Papilloma	Transitional cell carcinoma
Glandular epithelium	Adenoma	Adenocarcinoma
Tumors with Multiple Neoplastic Cell Types		
Ovary	Teratoma	Malignant teratoma
Kidney	—	Embryonal nephroma
Mammary gland	Benign mixed tumor	Malignant mixed tumor
	Complex adenoma	Complex adenocarcinoma
Salivary gland	Complex adenoma	Mixed tumor of salivary gland
Apocrine gland	Complex adenoma	Mixed tumor of apocrine gland

TABLE 4-2 **Comparison of benign and malignant neoplasms**

Characteristic	Benign	Malignant
Growth rate	Slow	Rapid
Growth limits	Circumscribed	Unrestricted
Mode of growth	Expansion	Invasion
Differentiation	Good	Anaplastic
Stroma	Usually abundant	Usually scant
Metastasis	None	Frequent
Recurrence	Rare	Frequent

MICROSCOPIC FEATURES OF BENIGN AND MALIGNANT NEOPLASMS

In vivo properties of tumor cells

Table 4-2 summarizes the biological differences between benign and malignant neoplasms (Fig. 4-10 through 4-17). These features include:

DEGREE OF DIFFERENTIATION

As mentioned earlier, the clinical behavior of most neoplasms can be predicted from their microscopic characteristics; however, there are exceptions. One of the most useful features for predicting the biologic behavior of a neoplasm is its degree of differentiation. The term **differentiation** refers to the degree to which the neoplastic cells resemble their normal counterparts, both in microscopic appearance and function. A well-differentiated neoplasm is composed of cells that bear a close resemblance to the normal tissue from which it arose, in terms of the appearance and pattern of growth of the neoplastic cells. A poorly differentiated neoplasm (often termed **undifferentiated** or **anaplastic**) is, in contrast, composed of primitive-appearing cells bearing only a remote or even no resemblance to the normal cell type and pattern of growth of the tissue from which it arose. As a rule, benign neoplasms tend to be well-differentiated. In contrast, malignant neoplasms vary tremendously in their degree of differentiation; some are well-differentiated and closely resemble the cell and tissue of origin, others are extremely undifferentiated and have an unidentifiable cell or tissue of origin. The terms **anaplasia** and its adjective form **anaplastic,** when applied to a neoplasm, literally imply a reversion to a more primitive state. In fact, such tumors are not composed of cells that have reverted to a more primitive state, but instead represent neoplasms that arise from malignant transformation of normal progenitor cells, such as basal or reserve cells, that simply fail to differentiate after the transforming event. This lack of differentiation results from the failure of the trans-

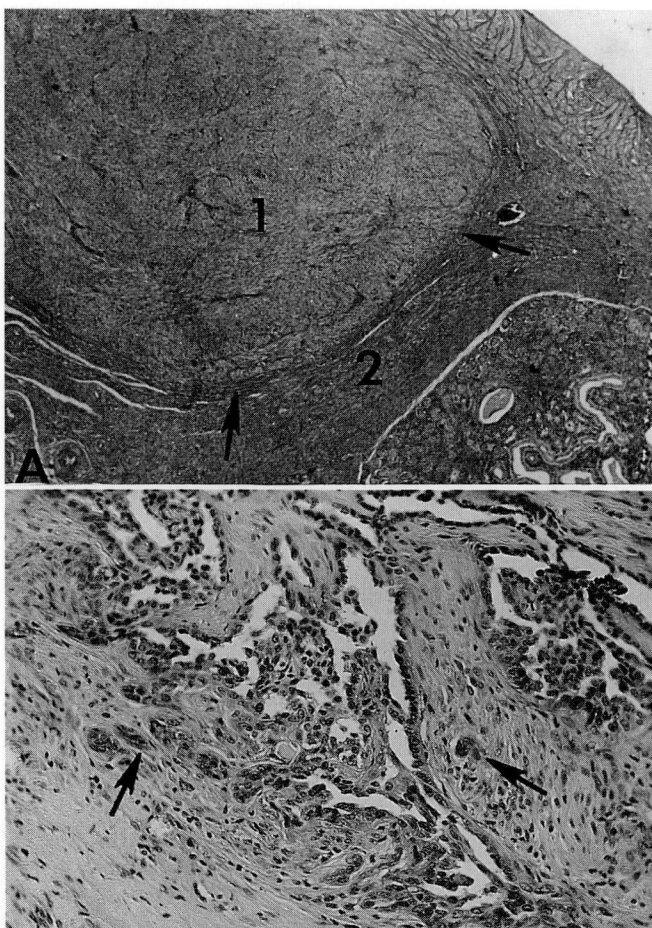

FIG. 4-10 Manner of growth of benign and malignant neoplasms. **A.** Leiomyoma of canine uterus. Growth by expansion and compression of adjacent tissue. Note smooth junction *(arrows)* between neoplasm *(1)* and normal tissue *(2)*. **B.** Adenocarcinoma of apocrine gland of canine skin. Growth by invasion. Note extension of cells from neoplasm into stroma *(arrows)*. (Courtesy of Armed Forces Institute of Pathology)

formed precursor cells to express those genes involved in normal cell differentiation and maturation rather than a reversion to a more primitive state.

CYTOLOGIC FEATURES

There are certain cytologic features of neoplastic cells that correlate with their degree of differentiation. The size and shape of the nuclei and cytoplasm of poorly differentiated neoplastic cells tend to vary more than those of normal cells (Fig. 4-18), a feature termed **pleomorphism.** In addition, the chromatin of poorly differentiated neoplastic cells stains more intensely than that of most normal cells, a feature termed **hyperchromasia.** Anaplastic cells also tend to have an **increased nuclear-cytoplasmic ratio,** which means an increased volume of the nucleus in proportion to the volume of the cytoplasm of the same cell. Since these cells are often actively proliferating and synthesizing in-

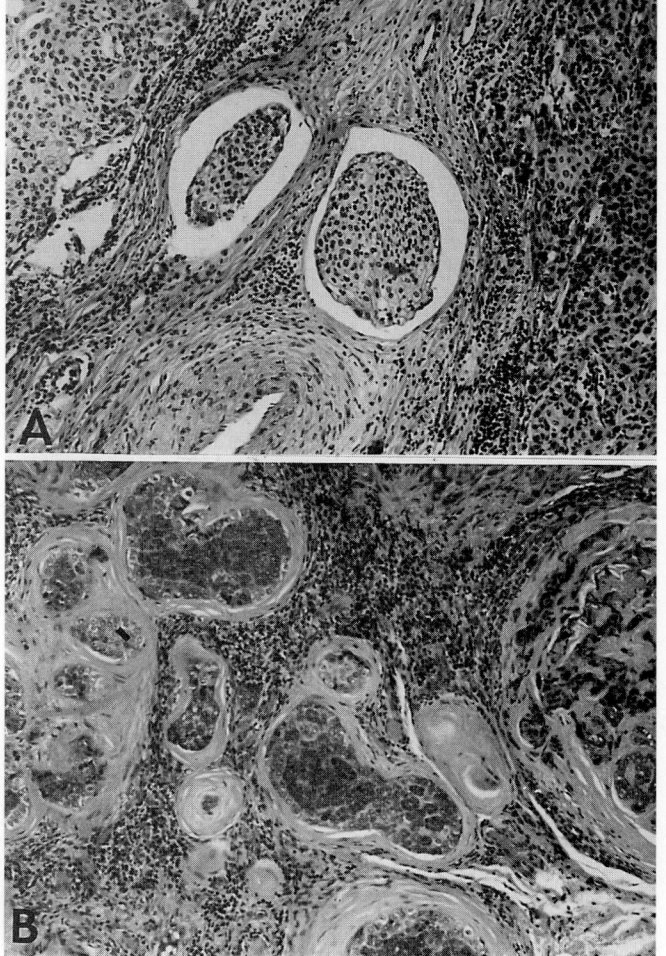

FIG. 4-11 Metastasis by way of lymphatics. **A.** Squamous cell carcinoma of cervix in lymphatics. (Courtesy of Harvard Medical School). **B.** Tumor cells growing within sclerotic lymphatics adjacent to adenocarcinoma of canine mammary gland.

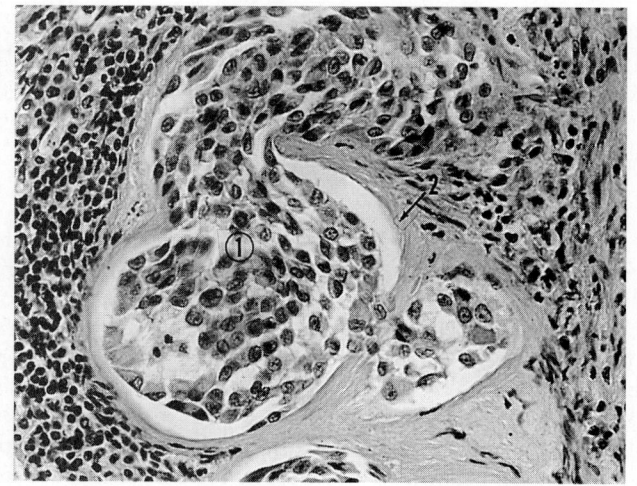

FIG. 4-12 Tumor embolus in small splenic artery of dog. Primary site of this undifferentiated carcinoma *(1)* was not determined. Note artery wall *(2)*. Infarct resulted from this embolus (×350). (Courtesy of Dr. David E. Lawrence and Armed Forces Institute of Pathology)

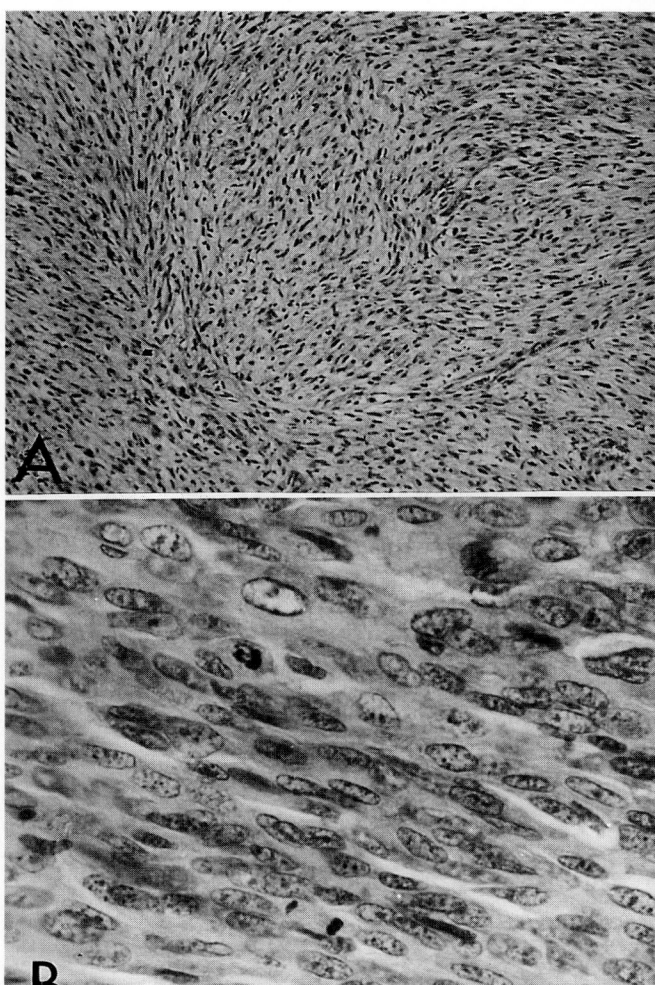

FIG. 4-13 Fibrosarcoma. Tissue and cells bear resemblance to normal fibrous connective tissue, except pattern of growth is disorganized *(A)*, cells *(B)* are more plump, and nuclei of cells more vesicular. (Courtesy of Armed Forces Institute of Pathology)

creased amounts of protein, their nucleoli tend to be larger and more prominent than those of their normal counterparts. Some extremely anaplastic neoplasms also contain **tumor giant cells,** which are large neoplastic cells with one or more strangely shaped, often hyperchromatic nuclei. Since anaplastic neoplasms tend to grow more rapidly than better-differentiated tumors, mitotic activity can achieve a high rate and mitotic figures may be abnormal, sometimes assuming tripolar and multipolar configurations. Because of their rapid proliferation, the parenchymal cells of a highly malignant neoplasm may actually exceed the growth of its stromal blood supply, thereby resulting in areas of infarction or ischemic necrosis of portions of the neoplasm.

RATE AND MANNER OF GROWTH

In general, benign neoplasms tend to grow slowly over a period of months or even years as well-circumscribed nodular masses, and their growth is usually by expansion rather than invasion. Consequently, they

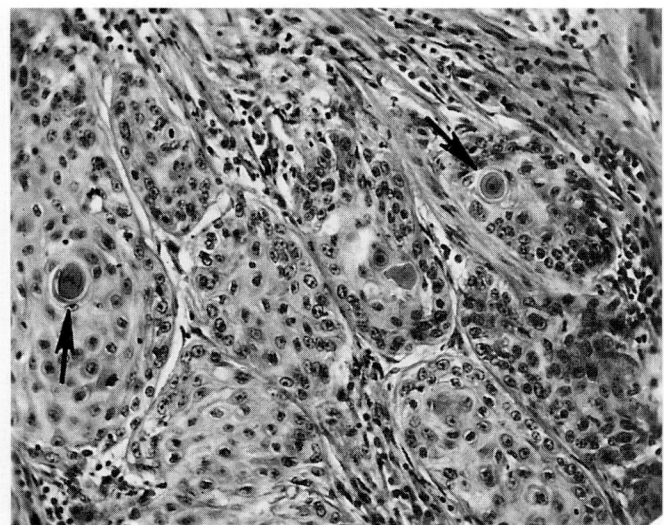

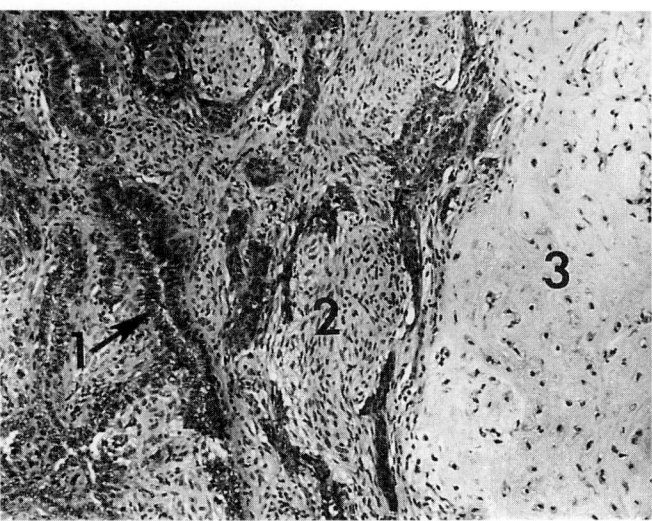

FIG. 4-14 Squamous cell carcinoma. Cells resemble normal squamous epithelium and mature from basal layer through keratinization. Note keratin pearls *(arrows)*. Pattern of growth is disorganized. (Courtesy of Armed Forces Institute of Pathology)

FIG. 4-15 Mixed tumor of mammary gland from dog. Some neoplasms contain more than one type of neoplastic cell. Note epithelial *(1)*, myoepithelial *(2)*, and cartilaginous *(3)* components.

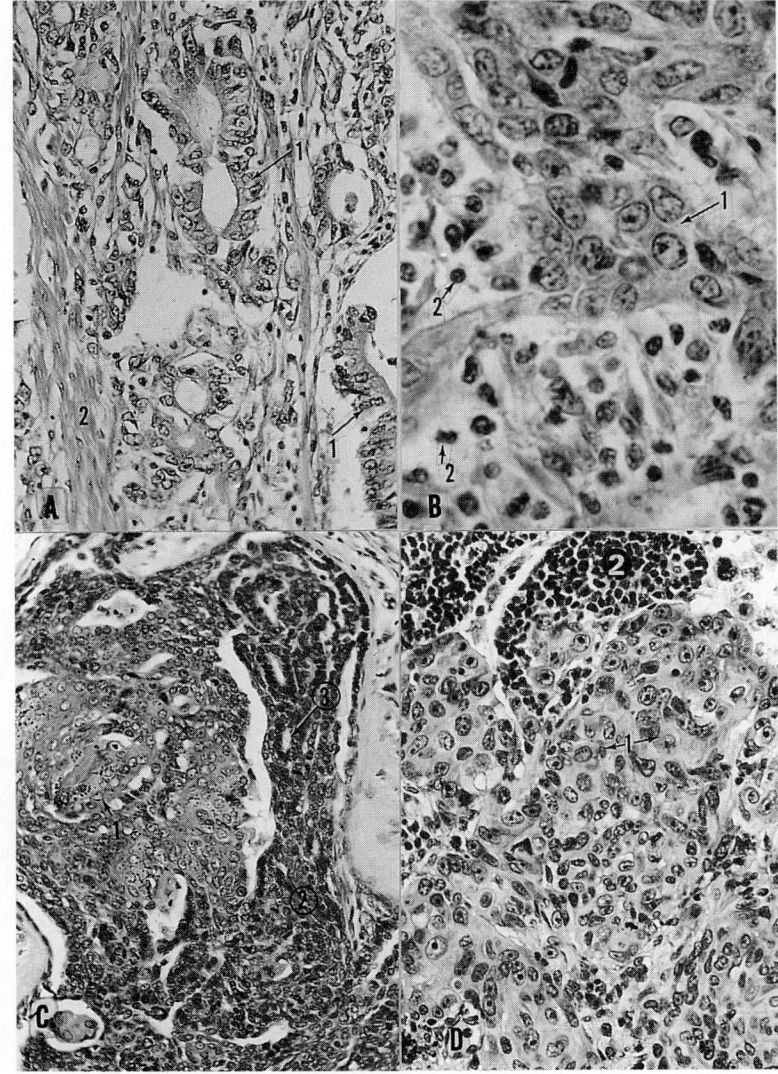

FIG. 4-16 Differences in microscopic appearance of adenocarcinoma. **A.** Adenocarcinoma arising in gastric mucosa and invading stomach wall of 8-year-old female Boston terrier. Neoplastic cells *(1)* form irregular acini as they invade muscularis *(2)*. (Courtesy of Dr. A. E. Rappoport) **B.** Undifferentiated cells *(1)* and lymphocytes *(2)* in adenocarcinoma in mammary gland of 25-year-old mare (x 750). (Courtesy of Dr. C. L. Davis) **C.** Squamous cells *(1)*, solid nests *(2)*, and acini *(3)* in adenocarcinoma of mammary gland of 6-year-old female English setter. (Courtesy of Angell Memorial Animal Hospital) **D.** Medullary carcinoma. Solid nests of carcinoma cells *(1)* in a lymph node *(2)* metastasis of primary adenocarcinoma of bile ducts of 15-year-old beagle. (Courtesy of Dr. D.N. Bader and Armed Forces Institute of Pathology)

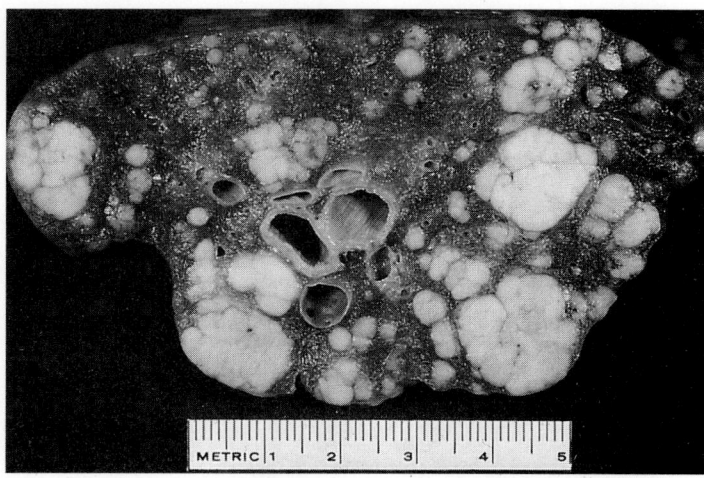

FIG. 4-17 Metastases in lung from adenocarcinoma of thyroid of 8-year-old male Irish setter. Note single and confluent nodules are not all equal in size. (Courtesy of Angell Memorial Animal Hospital.)

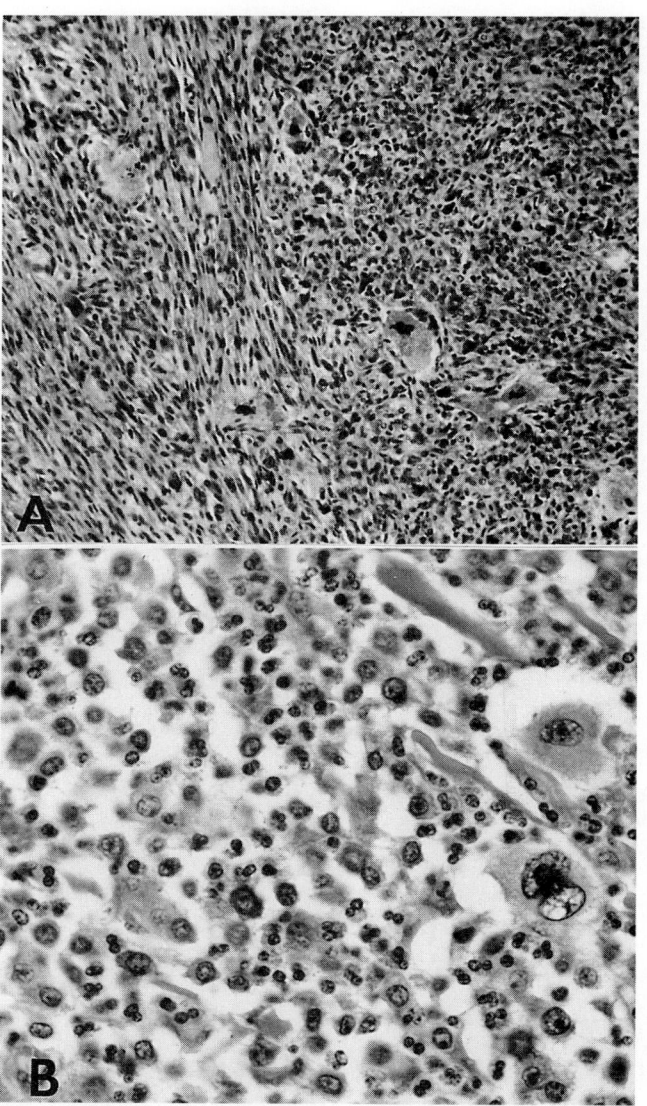

FIG. 4-18 Pleomorphism and tumor giant cells are often features of malignancy. **A.** Fibrosarcoma with disorderly pattern of growth and cellular pleomorphism. (Courtesy of Harvard Medical School.) **B.** Tumor giant cells in canine mast-cell tumor. (Courtesy of Armed Forces Institute of Pathology)

tend to compress the surrounding normal tissues, causing the latter to undergo atrophy or necrosis. Although tumors exhibiting these characteristics are referred to as benign, they are not harmless. Depending on their location and degree of function, benign tumors can, in some instances, be a more serious problem than certain malignant tumors. For example, a meningioma arising within the cranial cavity or spinal canal, if left untreated, can cause severe neurologic impairment and even death resulting from compression of adjacent vital neurologic structures. Similarly, a functional adenoma of pancreatic islet cells (insulinoma) or thyroid follicular epithelial cells may cause death from hypoglycemia or cardiac failure resulting from hyperthyroidism, respectively. Certain benign tumors may appear suddenly and grow more rapidly than some malignant neoplasms, but because of their location, the benign tumors cause very little in the way of clinical problems. Classic examples of this are the canine cutaneous histiocytoma and viral papillomas of many different species, both of which also undergo spontaneous regression.

Malignant neoplasms vary widely in their rate of growth; some are extremely slow-growing, but others, if left untreated, reach mammoth proportions rapidly. Unlike benign tumors, most malignant neoplasms are invasive and progressively replace the surrounding normal parenchyma of the affected organ. The pattern of growth of malignant tumors is haphazard, random, and remarkably uncoordinated. Small nests of tumor cells often break away from the main mass of the primary neoplasm and autonomously invade surrounding tissues, including venules and lymphatics, to become tumor cell emboli. These small nests of intravascular neoplastic cells may then be transported by blood or lymph to other sites within the same or different organs or to regional lymph nodes, where they continue to grow. This means of dissemination of a neoplasm is referred to as **metastasis.** Benign neoplasms do not metastasize.

METASTASIS

The term metastasis refers to the spread of portions of a malignant neoplasm to sites away from the primary tumor and growth at the new location: It constitutes the most definitive evidence of malignancy (Fig. 4-11). Metastasis occurs by one of three basic routes: (1) by direct exfoliation of tumor cells from a primary neoplasm into a body cavity with subsequent implantation and growth of the cells on mesothelial surfaces, a process referred to as seeding; (2) by invasion of lymphatics and transport of the tumor cells as emboli in the lymph (Fig. 4-11); and (3) by direct invasion of blood vessels with dissemination of the neoplastic emboli via the bloodstream (Fig. 4-12). Tumors noted for seeding of body cavities include carcinomas of the ovary and mesotheliomas. As a general rule, carcinomas initially tend to metastasize via lymphatics and spread to the regional lymph nodes where they lodge and continue to grow or, in rare instances, are destroyed by the host's immune system. Adenocarcinoma of the canine mammary gland and squamous cell carcinoma of the oral cavity of cats often metastasize to regional lymph nodes before they become widely disseminated. Carcinomas can also directly invade blood vessels and be disseminated by the blood. Since most lymph is eventually returned to the bloodstream, secondary hematogenous spread of carcinomas is not unusual. Sarcomas, on the other hand, have a greater propensity to initially spread via blood vessels, but they too are capable of lymphatic invasion and dissemination. Hemangiosarcomas and osteosarcomas are classic examples of neoplasms that often metastasize by means of the hematogenous route. Once tumor cells enter the bloodstream, they are often surrounded by masses of adherent platelets that enhance their survival and capacity to colonize new sites.

INVASIVENESS

In order for a neoplasm to metastasize, it must have the capacity to invade and degrade the extracellular matrix at its site of origin, penetrate the basement membranes of vascular walls to enter the lumen of the vessel, and after lodging at a new location, reverse these processes so as to emigrate from capillaries to invade the tissues at its new location. These processes involve cell surface receptors reacting with components of the extracellular matrix and basement membranes, including collagen, laminin, and fibronectin. In addition, tumor cells having a propensity for metastasis also secrete various enzymes involved in degrading the collagen component of basement membranes and extracellular matrix as well as various glycoprotein elements. These enzymes include: collagenases, elastases, proteinases, peptidases, and plasmin. The hydrolytic action of these enzymes cleaves a path for the migration of neoplastic cells into the interstitial connective tissue at the new sites, which they may or may not colonize. Very little is known regarding the motility of tumor cells in such circumstances.

Factors determining whether or not a cluster of tumor cells that has been transported to another site by the circulation survives at the new site are not well understood. Experimental evidence suggests that interactions between receptors on the surface of tumor cells and those in different organs may partially explain the homing mechanism that certain metastatic tumors have for particular organs or tissues.

GENETIC PROPERTIES OF TUMOR CELLS

Most neoplasms of human beings are of monoclonal origin, which means that all of its parenchymal cells are derived from a single neoplastically transformed cell. Although this issue has not been examined as thoroughly in neoplasms of domestic animals as in humans, it is very likely true in these species as well. Monoclonal tumors often arise from a single genetic mutation that renders the cell neoplastically transformed and thus not responsive to the genetic control mechanisms that regulate normal cell proliferation and differentiation. Given the appropriate circumstances, this single transformed cell survives in the tissue from which it arose, escapes the host's immune surveillance system designed to eliminate such abnormal cells, and divides *in situ* to produce daughter cells with similar properties. This process is known as **initiation** of tumorigenesis. The progeny of these transformed daughter cells, after many rounds of division, give rise to a sufficient number of descendants to produce a clinically detectable mass or neoplasm. During the course of this clonal expansion, individual tumor cells may undergo further random genetic mutations that confer properties of greater or lesser survivability of the progeny of that cell, a process known as **progression.** Therefore, even though a neoplasm is spoken of as being monoclonal in terms of its transforming mutation, by the time it becomes large enough to be recognized, it is usually composed of heterogeneous, subclonal populations of cells with distinctly different biologic properties. In these cases, the bulk of the tumor cells usually display properties that confer a selective advantage over the host's ability to cope with them. Such advantages might include the requirement for less oxygen and nutrients than normal cells, less immunogenicity, and the properties of invasiveness and metastasis.

In vitro properties of tumor cells

Since the advent of tissue culture in the 1950s, an enormous effort has been made to determine the biologic differences between neoplastically transformed cells and their normal counterparts using *in vitro* techniques. These studies have led to the discovery of significant differences between neoplastic and normal cells, which include the following.

FAILURE TO UNDERGO CONTACT (DENSITY-DEPENDENT) INHIBITION

Most normal epithelial and mesenchymal cells, when placed in culture, attach to the surface of the flask; flatten and divide until they form a confluent monolayer that covers the surface available to them; and then cease dividing. The *in vivo* correlate of this phenomenon occurs in normal wound healing when the epidermal and mesenchymal cells of the skin stop dividing once the edges of a surgical incision or wound have been joined. Neoplastically transformed cells, on the other hand, do not stop growing when the monolayer reaches confluency, but instead grow on top of one another to form multiple layers. This phenomenon results from failure of such cells to respond to the normal cell membrane signaling mechanisms that stop cells from dividing once they become coupled to or in contact with one another. This leads to the formation of jumbled masses of cells with no orderly pattern of growth, a feature also seen in neoplasms *in vivo*.

DIMINISHED COHESIVENESS

Transformed cells do not bind to one another as avidly as normal cells because of alterations in the glycoprotein components of their cell membranes.

DECREASED REQUIREMENT FOR SERUM CONTAINING EXOGENOUS GROWTH FACTORS

Many neoplastically transformed cells grow well in culture medium containing less serum than is required for growth of nontransformed cells of the same type. *In vivo*, this gives them a decided advantage over the normal cells from which they were derived and leads to invasion and replacement of the latter. These cells often have an enhanced expression of growth factor receptors on their surface membranes and also continuously secrete growth factors that bind to these receptors on the same or adjacent cells in an autocrine or paracrine type of growth stimulation.

LACK OF ANCHORAGE DEPENDENCE

Most normal cells when placed in cell culture must adhere to the surface of the container before they begin to divide. This is not a characteristic of neoplastic cells, which can grow well even in soft agar.

FAILURE TO UNDERGO TERMINAL DIFFERENTIATION

Neoplastic cells generally do not become fully differentiated when grown in culture, whereas normal cells often do. Once a cell becomes terminally differentiated, it loses its capacity to divide and is destined to die. This is not true of most neoplastic cells, which do not undergo terminal differentiation and thus retain their ability to survive and multiply, again giving them a decided advantage over normal cells.

IMMORTALIZATION

Normal cells grown in culture undergo a finite number of cell divisions and die. This process is thought to result from progressive loss of nucleotides from the terminal ends, or telomeres, of chromosomes until the cell can no longer divide. Cells that have reached this critical degree of telomeric shortening can no longer be maintained in culture, even when subcultured in fresh medium. In contrast, transformed cells can be passaged indefinitely. This property of transformed cells has been exploited in the establishment of numerous continuous cell lines. Recently, it has been shown that many types of transformed cells do not undergo the progressive telomeric shortening that occurs in normal cells with each cell division. Amazingly, these cells contain active repair mechanisms that replace nucleotides lost during cell division. One such mechanism involves the activity of an enzyme called telomerase This enzyme is expressed in many cells during embryologic development, but becomes inactive in most cells after birth.

FORMATION OF TRANSPLANTABLE TUMORS

Unlike their normal counterparts, neoplastically transformed cells that have been maintained in culture are able to form tumors when inoculated into animals of the same species and strain.

References

Aaronson SA, Tronick SR. Growth factors. In: Holland JF, Frei E, Bast RC, et al., ed. Cancer medicine. 3rd ed. Philadelphia:Lea & Febiger 1993;33–48.

Bishop JM. Molecular themes in oncogenesis. Cell 1991;64:235–248.

Boon T. Teaching the immune sytem to fight cancer. Sci Am 1993;268:82–89.

Cantley LC, Auger KR, Carpenter C, et al. Oncogenes and signal transduction. Cell 1991;64:281–302.

Cordon-Cardo C. Mutation of cell cycle regulators; biological and clinical implications for human neoplasia. Am J Pathol 1995;147:545–560.

Cross M, Dexter TM. Growth factors in development, transformation, and tumorigenesis. Cell 1991;64:271–280.

Donehower LA, Harvey M, Slagle BL, et al. Mice deficient for p53 are developmentally normal but susceptible to spontaneous tumors. Nature 1992;356:215–217.

Fearon ER, Vogelstein B. Tumor suppressor genes and cancer. In: Holland JF, Frei, E, Bast, RC, et al, ed. Cancer medicine. 3rd ed. Philadelphia: Lea & Febiger 1993;77–90.

Feig L. The many roads that lead to *Ras*. Science 1993;260:767–768.

Goodrich DW, Lee W. Abrogation by c-*myc* of G1 phase arrest induced by RB protein but not by p53. Nature 1992;360:177–179.

Greider CW, Blackburn EH. Telomeres, telomerase and cancer. Sci Am 1996;274:92–99.

Harris CC, Hollstein M. Clinical implications of the p53 tumor suppressor gene. N Engl J Med 1993;329:1318–1327.

Hockenberry DM, Oltvai ZN, Yin X-M, et al. *Bcl-2* functions in an antioxidant pathway to prevent apoptosis. Cell 1993;75:241–251.

Hunter T. Cooperation between oncogenes. Cell 1991;64:249–270.

Klein G. Oncogenes. In: Holland JF, Frei, E, Bast, RC, et al., ed. Cancer medicine. 3rd ed. Philadelphia:Lea & Febiger 1993;65–77.

Lane DP. A death in the life of p53. Nature 1993;362:786–787.

Lewin B. Oncogene conversion by regulatory changes in transcription factors. Cell 1991;64:303–312.

Marshall CJ. Tumor suppressor genes. Cell 1991;64:313–326.

McCormick F. How receptors turn *Ras* on. Nature 1993;363:15–16.

Priester WA, Mantel N. Occurrence of tumors in domestic animals, data from 12 United States and Canadian colleges of veterinary medicine. JNCI 1971;17:1333–1344.

Pusztal L, Lewis CE, Lorenzen J, et al. Growth factors: regulation of normal and neoplastic growth. J Pathol 1993;169:191–201.

Schwartz RS. Another look at immunologic surveillance. N Engl J Med 1975;293:181–184.

Vogelstein B, Kinzler KW. Carcinogens leave fingerprints. Nature 1992;355:209–210.

Weinberg RA. Oncogenes, antioncogenes and the molecular basis of multistep carcinogenesis. Cancer Res 1989;49:3713–3721.

Zaldivar R. Incidence of spontaneous neoplasms in beagles. J Am Vet Med Assoc 1967;151:1319–1321.

CAUSES OF NEOPLASIA

The causes of neoplasia are numerous and diverse, but the common denominator linking them all is the induction of mutations in those portions of a cell's genome that control mitotic division and differentiation. The causes of these mutations include: (1) spontaneous errors in DNA replication, including chromosomal translocations; (2) various forms of radiation; (3) chemical carcinogens; and (4) oncogenic viruses. Before discussing the mechanisms by which each of these agents causes neoplasia, a basic understanding of the molecular events involved in normal cell division and maturation is necessary.

When normal cells become detached from one another they undergo mitotic division until contact with one another recurs. The signals that initiate and terminate cell division emanate from the cell surface and are transmitted to the nucleus by means of a series of primary and secondary chemical messages that take place in the cell membrane and cytosol, respectively. These messages involve the generation of a cascade of enzymatic reactions involving specific molecules within the plasma membrane, including phospholipids, guanine-binding proteins, transmembrane proteins with specific growth factor receptor activity on their extracellular terminus and a specific phosphokinase activity on their intracellular terminus, and several cytoplasmic protein kinases. The culmination of this cascade of enzymatic reactions is the phophorylation of certain proteins, which then enter the cell nucleus, bind to specific portions of the cell's DNA, and initiate or terminate cell division. Those genes involved in normal cell division and differentiation are termed **proto-oncogenes.** This name derives from the fact that they represent the cellular precursors of **viral oncogenes,** a topic discussed later in this chapter. There are now more than 30 known cellular proto-oncogenes and this list continues to expand (Table 4-3). The protein products of proto-oncogenes can be conveniently divided into four major categories on the basis of their functional activity: These categories are (1) protein kinases, (2) proteins that bind with glutamyl transpeptidase (GTP), (3) growth factors, and (4) nuclear transcriptional proteins. The activation and suppression of transcription of these proto-oncogenes is controlled by other genes referred to as **regulatory genes,** which are located immediately upstream from the respective proto-oncogenes (towards the 5' end of the genome). The products of these regulatory genes either initiate or terminate DNA synthesis and transcription of genes involved with cell growth and differentiation. The phosphorylated proteins generated by the signal transduction pathways activate or inactivate these regulatory genes, which "turn on" or "turn off" proto-oncogene expression and cell division. Hence, mutations responsible for neoplastic transformation may involve proto-oncogenes directly or the genes that regulate their expression. Such mutations lead to the formation of abnormal gene products that fail to respond to the cell's normal feedback mechanisms. The effect of this is continuous and unregulated cell division and neoplasia.

Neoplasms resulting from spontaneous genetic mutations

Neoplasms arising from spontaneous genetic mutations may be difficult or impossible to distinguish from those caused by known environmental carcinogens (e.g., radiation, chemicals), especially in the absence of a history of exposure to the latter. Fortunately, DNA replication is a relatively error-free phenomenon, but in those rare instances where errors do occur, cells have sophisticated proofreading and repair mechanisms that identify and usually eliminate them. In addition, certain spontaneous mutations may not be compatible with survival, in which case the cell containing the mutation dies. On extremely rare occasions, however, a cell containing a transforming mutation escapes the cell's normal DNA error recognition and repair system, survives, continues to divide, and gives rise to clones of cells containing the same mutation that escape the body's immune surveillance system. This compounding set of circumstances results in the generation of a monoclonal neoplasm. Spontaneous genetic mutations that result in neoplastic transformation may involve one or more proto-oncogenes or genes that control their expression. When a mutated proto-oncogene results in neoplastic transformation, the altered gene is referred to as a **cellular** or **c-oncogene.**

Occasionally, during cell division, a portion of one chromosome becomes translocated to the arm of another chromosome; this may lead to neoplastic transormation. The best-studied example of this occurs in Burkitt's lymphoma of humans, a neoplastic disease associated with polyclonal mitogenic stimulation of B lymphocytes by Epstein-Barr virus and possibly by malarial parasites. Occasionally during the course of this B lymphocyte stimulation, a portion of chromosome 8 containing the proto-oncogene c-*myc* becomes translocated to chromosome 14 immediately adjacent to the constitutively-expressed gene for the immuglobulin heavy chain (IgH). This translocation removes c-*myc* from the control of its own regulatory genes and places it under the influence of the promotor genes for IgH, a gene which is expressed more or less continuously. This results in the continuous, rather than regulated, expression of c-*myc*, the product of which is a DNA-binding protein thought to interact with genes associated with cell proliferation. Hence, when translocations occur that disrupt the normal association of proto-oncogenes with their regulatory genes, neoplastic transformation may result.

Radiation-induced neoplastic transformation

Two types of radiant energy have been strongly linked with neoplastic diseases, i.e., ultraviolet radiation and various forms of ionizing radiation. The mechanisms involved in the induction of neoplasia with these two forms of energy are different and, therefore, are discussed separately.

Ultraviolet (UV) radiation from sunlight has been associated with skin cancers in both humans and animals. Light-skinned people with a history of prolonged exposure to intense sunlight have an increased incidence of squamous cell carcinomas, basal cell carcinomas, and malignant melanomas of the skin. In animals, the best-documented examples of UV radiation-induced cancer are squamous cell carcinomas that occur on the cornea and white skin of the eyelids of Hereford cattle

TABLE 4-3 **Proto-oncogenes and their biologic characteristics**

Proto-oncogenes by category	Retroviruses containing homologous v-oncogenes	Human tumors expressing gene product	Cellular localization of protein product	Function of oncogene protein
Protein kinases				
src	Rous sarcoma virus	—	Plasma membrane	Tyrosine kinase
yes	Avian sarcoma virus	—	Plasma membrane	Tyrosine kinase
abl	Abelson murine leukemia virus	Chronic myelogenous leukemia (9 to 22 translocation)	Plasma membrane	Tyrosine kinase
fes	Feline sarcoma virus	Acute myelogenous leukemia (15;17 translocation)	Plasma membrane	Tyrosine kinase
met	—	Osteosarcoma		Tyrosine kinase
erb-B	Avian erythroblastosis virus	Amplified in quamous cell carcinomas	Transmembrane	EGF receptor/tyrosine kinase
neu (erb-B2)	—	Amplified in breast carcinoma	Transmembrane	EGF receptor/tyrosine kinase
fms	Feline sarcoma virus	—	Transmembrane	CSF-1 receptor/tyrosine kinase
ros	Avian sarcoma virus	—	Transmembrane	Growth factor receptor/tyrosine kinase
mos	Moloney murine sarcoma virus	Acute myelogenous leukemia (8;21 translocation)	Cytoplasm	Serine/threonine kinase
GTP-binding proteins				
H-ras	Harvey murine sarcoma virus	Wide variety of human cancers	Plasma membrane	GTP-binding proteins with GTPase activity
K-ras	Kirsten murine sarcoma virus	Wide variety of human cancers	Plasma membrane	GTP-binding proteins with GTPase activity
N-ras	—	Neuroblastomas	Plasma membrane	GTP-binding proteins with GTPase activity
Growth factors				
sis	Simian sarcoma virus	—	Secreted	Similar to PDGF
int-2	Mouse mammary tumor virus	—	Secreted	Related to FGF
Nuclear Transcription proteins				
myc	Avian myelocytoma virus	Burkitt's lymphoma (8;14 translocation), also amplified in small cell carcinoma of lung	Nucleus	Nuclear binding protein
L-myc	—	Amplified in small cell carcinoma of lung	Nucleus	?

(continued)

TABLE 4-3 continued)

Proto-oncogenes by category	Retroviruses containing homologous v-oncogenes	Human tumors expressing gene product	Cellular localization of protein product	Function of oncogene protein
N-myc	—	Amplified in neuro-blastomas	Nucleus	?
myb	—	Amplified in colon cancer cell lines	Nucleus	?
fos	Murine osteosarcoma virus	—	Nucleus	?
Unclassified proteins				
bcl-2	—	Follicular lymphoma (14;18 translocation)	?	Anti-apoptosis protein

and on the pinnae of white cats. The pathogenesis of UV radiation-induced neoplasia is multifactorial and involves DNA damage and the generation of pyrimidine dimers; failure to repair this damage results in further transcriptional errors and, ultimately, in neoplasia. Suppression of cell-mediated immunity by UV radiation is also thought to contribute to the progression of the neoplastically tranformed cells.

Ionizing radiation is caused by electromagnetic forms of energy, such as x-rays and gamma rays; by charged particles, such as protons and electrons; and by high energy-emitting neutral particles, known as neutrons. Depending on the type of radiation, dose, duration of exposure, nature of the target tissue, and an assortment of host factors, including the efficiency of DNA repair mechanisms, ionizing radiation may have no effect on cells, be directly lethal to cells, or cause genetic mutations that lead to neoplastic transformation. Mutations that occur in the DNA of irradiated cells may be a direct effect of the ionizing radiation or be induced indirectly by the generation of highly charged free radicals from water and oxygen in the cytosol, which in turn damages DNA. The precise mutations that lead to neoplastic transformation have not been well documented, but it would seem logical to assume that they probably involve either direct mutations of proto-oncogenes, giving rise to **cellular oncogenes (c-oncogenes)**, which fail to respond to the cell's own regulatory mechanisms, or possibly alterations in the genes that regulate proto-oncogene expression, i.e., **suppressor genes (anti-oncogenes)**, rendering them no longer effective. As a general rule, actively growing tissues are more susceptible to ionizing radiation-induced damage and neoplastic transformation than tissues having a low mitotic rate. Accordingly, the tissues of fetuses and young, growing organisms are more affected by ionizing radiation than those of adults. Likewise, in adults those tissues with a high rate of mitotic activity (e.g., bone marrow, testes, intestinal mucosa) are more

susceptible to damage and neoplastic transformation than those with a low rate of mitotic activity (e.g., brain, muscle). In veterinary medicine, neoplastic disorders confirmed as resulting from ionizing radiation are rare, and most examples involve experimental exposure to known forms of radiation. In human beings, accidental or even intentional exposure to ionizing radiation occurs as a consequence of certain occupations, such as mining radioactive materials, or as the result of radiation therapy for other forms of neoplasia.

Chemical-induced neoplasms

The earliest evidence suggesting that certain chemical substances might cause cancer was published in 1775 by Sir Percivall Pott who reported a high incidence of carcinoma of the scrotum in chimney sweeps from London. This type of neoplasm was almost unheard of in other men. The carcinogenic nature of soot and tars resulting from incomplete combustion of fossil fuels was unknown at that time, so these unusual cancers at first were thought to be caused by chronic irritation. As various hydrocarbons and other organic chemicals were increasingly used during the industrial age, the suspicion arose that neoplasms might result from contact with them. In 1915, Yamagiwa and Ichikawa succeeded in producing cutaneous papillomas and carcinomas of the skin of rabbits after repeated applications of coal tar over a period of several months. Subsequently, similar experiments by others demonstrated that mice are even more susceptible to tar-induced cancer than rabbits, whereas other common laboratory animals are more resistant. Armed with this data, chemists set out to identify the chemicals in coal tar that exert the carcinogenic effect. In 1930, the first carcinogenic substance was identified as dibenzanthracene, a polycyclic aromatic hydrocarbon of which there are a number of derivatives. Since then, literally hundreds of additional chemicals have been shown to transform cells *in vitro* and to

TABLE 4-4 **Classification of chemical carcinogens**

Direct-acting carcinogens

Alkylating agents
β-Propriolactone
Dimethyl sulfate
Diepoxbutane and other epoxides
Ethyl methanesulfonate
Nitrogen mustard
Cancer therapeutic drugs (chlorambucil, cyclophospha-mide, methyl nitrosurea)

Acylating agents
1-Acetyl-imidazole
Dimethylcarbamyl chloride

Indirect-acting carcinogens

Polycyclic and heterocyclic aromatic hydrocarbons
Benzanthracene
Benzopyrene
Dibenzanthracene
3-Methylcholanthrene
7,12-Dimethylbenzanthracene
Cigarette smoke, tars, soot

Aromatic amines, amides, and azo dyes
2-Naphthylamine
Benzidine
2-Acetylaminofluorene
Dimethylaminobenzene
4-Aminophenol
3-Hydroxyanthranilic acid
3-Hydroxyzanthine

Plant and microbial products
Aflatoxin B_1
Betel nuts
Cycasin
Griseofulvin
Pyrrolizidine alkaloids
Safrole (Sassafras)

Other chemicals
Nitrosamine and amides
Vinyl chloride and polychlorinated biphenyls (PCBs)
Insecticides and fungicides

induce neoplasms *in vivo.* As illustrated in Table 4-4, these chemicals fall into two broad categories, those that are directly carcinogenic (**direct-acting carcinogens**) and those which are carcinogenic only after being metabolized to highly reactive metabolites (**indirect-acting carcinogens**). There are only a few direct-acting chemical carcinogens; these are highly reactive electrophiles (chemicals that react with negatively charged centers of other compounds, including DNA). Most chemical carcinogens are of the indirect-acting type. These compounds, although inert themselves, if metabolized by enzymes of the cytochrome P-450 detoxifying system in the liver, generate highly carcinogenic metabolites. Through these oxidation-reduction reactions,

fat-soluble organic compounds that have an affinity for body fat and lipid-rich cell membranes are converted to water-soluble metabolites that can be coupled with glucuronides and excreted in the bile. Some of these secondary metabolites, however, are highly electrophilic and cause mutations in cellular proto-oncogenes, thus generating cellular oncogenes that do not respond to the normal signals that regulate gene transcription; thus, these metabolites of indirect-acting carcinogens cause neoplasia in a manner similar to direct-acting carcinogens.

The pathogenesis of chemical-induced neoplasia has been investigated extensively by the application of known carcinogens to the skin of mice and in *in vitro* cellular transformation assays. These studies have revealed that chemical carcinogenesis is a multistep process involving two distinct phases referred to as **initiation** and **promotion.** Initiation involves the rapid induction of chemically-induced, permanent mutation in a cell's DNA that alone is not transforming, but which renders the altered cell and its progeny irreversibly susceptible to subsequent transforming events caused by either the same or different chemicals. Chemicals responsible for these two types of alterations are referred to as initiators and promoters, respectively. Some chemicals can act as both initiators and promoters in the genesis of certain neoplasms. Interestingly, exposure to an initiating agent must precede exposure to a promoter if neoplastic transformation is to occur; in the reverse order, or even if exposure to one agent is administered alone, neoplasia does not occur. Unlike initiation, which occurs rapidly and sometimes after only a single exposure to a highly reactive electrophilic substance, promotion generally requires multiple exposures (sometimes referred to as "hits") to either the same or different chemical at critical doses over a period of weeks or months. Promoters are not electrophilic compounds nor do they alter a cell's DNA: They act by interfering with the normal signal transduction pathways that control cell proliferation and differentiation. The prototyical tumor promoters are chemicals known as phorbol esters. Structurally, these compounds resemble certain degradative products of membrane phospholipids involved in the normal signal transduction process. Cells exposed to promoters *in vitro* often develop an altered phenotype but do not become transformed, unless they have been previously exposed to an initiating agent. Hence, exposure to chemicals that only function as promoters does not alter a cell's genome. In fact, studies with the mouse skin model and *in vitro* transformation assays have shown that the effects of promoting agents may be reversible if exposure to the agent is terminated or if the interval between successive exposures is sufficiently long. When malignant transformation does occur, the cell becomes irreversibly altered and may develop into a neoplasm *in vivo,* or in the case of *in vitro* transformed cells, a neoplasm that grows progressively when inoculated into immunodeficient ("nude") mice. Promoters thus amplify the effects of initiators.

References

Farber E, Sarma DSR. Hepatocarcinogenesis: a dynamic cellular perspective. Lab Invest 1987;56:4–22.

Pott P. Chirurgical observations relative to the cancer of the scrotum London, 1775. Reprinted in: Natl Cancer Inst Monogr 1963;10:7–13.

Yamagiwa K, Ichikawa K. Experimentelle Studie uber die Pathogenese der Epithelialgeschwulste. Mitt Med Fak Tokio 1915;15:295–344.

Virus-induced neoplasms

Viruses affecting animals and humans are classified into 22 distinct taxonomic families. On the basis of their nuclei acid content, they can be grouped into two broad families; 7 contain DNA and 15 contain RNA. Of the 22 families, 5 of the 7 DNA-containing families and only 1 of the 15 RNA-containing families include certain viruses that produce neoplasms (i.e., are oncogenic), either naturally or under experimental conditions, or both. However, not all viruses in these 6 families are oncogenic. Those families containing oncogenic agents are as follows

DNA-containing families
Poxviridae (poxviruses)
Herpesviridae (herpesviruses)
Adenoviridae (adenoviruses)
Papovaviridae (papovaviruses)
Hepadnaviridae (hepatitis B virus)

RNA-containing family
Retroviridae (oncornaviruses)

Oncogenic viruses cause neoplasms (1) by interfering with the normal regulation and expression of proto-oncogenes and anti-oncogenes in infected cells or (2) by introducing viral-encoded homologs of proto-oncogenes (**viral oncogenes**) into the host cell genome. Since the mechanisms vary for different families, they will be discussed by family groups.

ONCOGENIC DNA VIRUSES

Poxviruses It is arguable whether poxviruses should be regarded as oncogenic, since the proliferative epidermal and, occasionally, mesenchymal lesions caused by the majority of the agents in this family are self-limiting and undergo spontaneous regression. This same argument, however, can be applied to papillomaviruses, which many writers on the subject regard as oncogenic, even though most agents in this family also cause benign epithelial lesions that often regress. Certain papillomaviruses in humans have also been strongly linked to speciific types of carcinomas; this bolsters the argument for the oncogenicity of papillomaviruses. Table 4-5 lists poxviruses that produce benign and, occasionally, fatal malignant tumors in various animal species and humans.

Poxviruses are the largest of the DNA-containing viruses in terms of virion size. They are transmitted by direct contact, by arthropod vectors, and by fomites and, with few exceptions, undergo replication in epithelial cells, principally in the epidermis, but occasionally in other types of epithelia (fowlpox sometimes infects respiratory epithelium) and mesenchymal connective tissue. Poxvirus virions are large, complex, brick-shaped or ovoid-shaped structures with an external envelope containing lipid and tubular or globular proteins that encompass one or two lateral bodies and a core, which contains a single large molecule of double-stranded DNA. Within the virion are more than 30 dif-

TABLE 4-5 **Poxvirus-induced tumors or tumor-like lesions**

Virus	Host(s)	Lesion and clinical outcome
Myxomatosis virus	Sylvilagus (cottontail) rabbits Oryctolagus (domestic) rabbits	Benign fibromas the regress Malignant mesenchymal tumors of dermis and other organs
Shope rabbit fibroma virus	Sylvilagus (cottontail) rabbits Oryctolagus (domestic) rabbits	Dermal fibromas that regress
Hare fibroma virus	Hares	Dermal fibromas that regress
Squirrel fibroma virus	Grey squirrel, woodchucks	Dermal fibromas that regress; rarely fibrosarcomas that metastasize
Yaba virus	Rhesus, cynomolgus and African green monkeys, humans	Benign, mesenchymal tumors of the dermis that regress
Molluscum contagiosum	Humans, horses	Benign epidermal, papilloma-like lesions that regress
Genital (papilloma) virus of swine [a misnomer]	Male and female swine	Papillomatous lesions of the mucosa of the vagina, vulva, penis, and prepuce that regress

TABLE 4-6 **Oncogenic herpesviruses**

Virus	Host(s)	Neoplasm and clinical outcome
Lucke renal adenocarcinoma virus	*Rana pipiens* (leopard frog)	Renal adenocarcinoma with death from renal failure
Marek's disease virus	Chickens	Neural lymphoma with or without visceral involvement leading to paralysis and death
Herpesvirus samiri	*Saimiri sciureus* (squirrel monkey)	Latent, subclinical infection
	Saguinus oedipus (cotton-top tamarin); *Aotus trivirgatus* (owl monkey); *Ateles spp.* (spider monkeys); domestic rabbits	Rapidly fatal, generalized T-cell lymphoma with or without leukemia
Herpesvirus ateles	*Ateles geofroyii* (spider monkey)	Latent, subclinical infection
	Saguinus oedipus (cotton-top tamarin)	Rapidly fatal, generalized T-cell lymphoma
Herpesvirus sylvilagus	Sylvilagus (cottontail) rabbits	Lymphoid hyperplasia and lymphoma
Epstein Barr virus	Humans	Infectious mononucleosis, Burkitt's (B-cell) lymphoma, nasopharyngeal carcinoma
	Saguinus oedipus (cotton-top tamarin)	Fatal B cell lymphoma

ferent structural proteins and several enzymes, including a DNA-dependent RNA polymerase. Interestingly, one of the genes of the poxvirus genome has extensive sequence homology with the proto-oncogene for **epidermal growth factor** and its product has similar activity. Unlike the other oncogenic DNA viruses, poxvirus replication takes place in the cytoplasm of infected cells and their genetic material is not integrated into the host-cell genome. The pronounced proliferative response of cells infected with poxviruses is thought to be caused by the accumulation of large quantities of viral-encoded, epidermal growth factor-like protein in the cytoplasm of cells, causing them to undergo excessive mitotic division, which leads to nodular proliferations known clinically as "pocks" or, in some cases, fibromas. In rare instances, infected mesenchymal cells undergo malignant transformation and produce fibrosarcomas or primitive mesenchymal sarcomas that kill the host. This has been documented for myxomatosis virus of rabbits and deer fibroma virus.

Herpesviruses The family Herpesviridae encompasses a large number of ubiquitous viruses that, on the basis of distinct biologic properties, may be further divided into three subfamilies: Alphaherpesvirinae (cytolytic herpesviruses), Betaherpesvirinae (cytomegaloviruses), and Gammaherpesvirinae (lymphotropic herpesvirinae). With the exception of Lucke renal adenocarcinoma virus, all oncogenic herpesviruses are classifed in the subfamily Gammaherpesvirinae; these

are listed in Table 4-6. Unlike the poxviruses, herpesviruses replicate in the nucleus of infected cells. The viral genome remains in the nucleus as nonintegrated molecules of circular DNA. Different herpesviruses cause malignant transformation by different mechanisms.

Epstein-Barr virus (EBV), the prototypic lymphotropic herpesvirus, is the cause of infectious mononucleosis, a benign lymphoproliferative disease with worldwide distribution in juvenile and young adult humans. This virus has also been strongly linked to two forms of human neoplastic disease in different parts of the world. In regions of Africa where malaria is endemic, EBV plays a major role in the pathogenesis of Burkitt's lymphoma, a disease of young children. Burkitt's lymphoma is a neoplastic disease of B lymphocytes and has a predilection for the maxilla, the mandible, and occasionally, the gonads. The neoplastic lymphoid cells in this disease have a characteristic chromosomal translocation in which a portion of chromosome 8 bearing the proto-oncogene *myc* becomes translocated immediately adjacent to the gene for the heavy chain of immunoglobulin (IgH) on chromosome 14. Because the latter gene is more or less continuously expressed in B cells under the influence of its own enhancer/promoter sequences, this translocation causes the *myc* gene to also be continuously transcribed, leading to unregulated synthesis of the *myc* product, a nuclear binding protein normally involved in the regulation of cell division. Additionally, EBV is capable of immortalizing human as well as certain nonhuman primate B lympho-cytes *in vitro*. The accessory role played by malarial organisms in this multifactorial disease likely involves impairment of the host's immune system with failure to eliminate the EBV-transformed B lymphocytes. EBV encodes several proteins, which are not related to the products of cellular proto-oncogenes, but are important for transformation. One of these, termed latency mem-brane protein-1 (LMP-1), is a transmembrane protein that interacts with another molecule known as tumor necrosis receptor-associated factor (TRAF). This protein binds to the intracellular domain of the tumor necrosis factor receptor (TNFr), causing activation of nuclear factor kappa B (NFkB), a pivotal molecule in many cell functions. NFkB then moves from the cytoplasm into the nucleus and initiates DNA transcription and cell proliferation. The second EBV-encoded protein im-portant in neoplastic transformation is LMP-2. It is also a transmembrane protein, but is not related to LMP-1. LMP-2 binds to and inactivates two molecules known as syk and lyn, the result being inactivation of the major B-cell tyrosine kinase. This action blocks EBV replica-tion and thus prevents infected cells from undergoing virus-induced lysis. The third protein encoded for by EBV is known as EBV nuclear antigen (EBNA). EBNA is a transcriptional protein required for viral replica-tion. EBV-associated B-cell lymphomas occur with some frequency in patients receiving immunosuppressive therapy after organ transplantation and in patients with AIDS. This observation strongly suggests that im-paired cell-mediated immunity contributes to the pathogenesis of this virus-associated neoplasm.

EBV has also been associated with another neo-plasm referred to as nasopharyngeal carcinoma, a tu-mor seen with some frequency in the southern prov-inces of China and in areas of the Caribbean. It is composed of neoplastic nasopharyngeal epithelial cells and prominent infiltrates of lymphocytes that are not neoplastic. The mechanisms involved in transformation of these cells have not been as well studied as those involved in Burkitt's lymphoma. Whether the mecha-nism is the same or different from that involved in the other herpesvirus-associated epithelial neoplasm, Lucke renal adenocarcinoma, is unknown.

Another lymphotropic herpesvirus that causes lymphoma is *Herpesvirus saimiri*. This virus occurs com-monly as a latent infection of squirrel monkeys without clinical disease. If the virus is inoculated into several other nonhuman primate species, including tamarins (*Saguinus oedipus, S. fuscicollis, S. nigricollis, S. mystax*), marmosets (*Callithrix jacchus*), owl monkeys (*Aotus trivir-gatus*), howler monkeys (*Aloutta caraya*), spider monkeys (*Ateles geoffroyi*), and African green monkeys (*Cercopi-thecus aethiops*), it causes lymphoma and leukemias de-rived from T lymphocytes. *H. saimiri* encodes for two proteins important in cellular transformation. Neither of these has homology with known cellular proto-onco-gene products. One is an oncoprotein termed saimiri-transforming protein (STP). It, like the oncoproteins of EBV, is a transmembrane protein, but it functions by interacting with the cell's normal *ras* oncoprotein in a

way that inactivates the protein's GTPase activity and thus causes the infected T lymphocytes to become transformed. The other important protein encoded by this virus is termed tyrosine-like interacting protein (TIP), which interacts with lymphocyte cell kinase, the major T cell tyrosine kinase, and prevents viral replica-tion and associated cytolysis. Thus, its action is similar to that of LMP-2 of EBV.

Similarly, *Herpesvirus ateles*, which occurs as a latent, subclinical infection of spider monkeys (*Ateles spp.*), causes a T-cell lymphoma and leukemia when experi-mentally inoculated into tamarins, marmosets, and owl monkeys. The molecular basis of its transforming ability has not been investigated.

Herpesvirus sylvilagus, although commonly listed as an oncogenic herpesvirus, causes a nonfatal lympho-proliferative disease of cottontail rabbits, which on close scrutiny resembles infectious mononucleosis rather than lymphoma. The phenotype of the proliferating cells and the mechanisms involved in its pathogenesis have not been studied.

Adenoviruses Adenoviruses are nonenveloped DNA viruses that occur commonly as clinical and sub-clinical infections of the respiratory and alimentary tracts of animals and humans. Although ubiquitous in nature, they have never been confirmed as the cause of any naturally occurring neoplasm in any species. Exper-imentally, however, some serotypes of adenoviruses have been shown to be highly oncogenic if inoculated into newborn hamsters, mice, and rats. There are at least 35 serotypes of human and 24 serotypes of simian adeno-viruses. Simian and avian adenoviruses have also been shown to be oncogenic under similar experimental con-ditions. on the basis of their biologic properties *in vivo* and *in vitro,* the human serotypes have been classified as highly oncogenic (serotypes 12, 18, and 31), weakly oncogenic (serotypes 3, 7, 11, 14, 16, and 21), or non-oncogenic *in vivo,* but capable of transforming hamster cells *in vitro* (serotypes 1, 2, 5, 6, 9, 10, 13, 15, 17, 19 and 26). Transformed cells and neoplasms induced by adenoviruses contain copies of the viral DNA integrated into their genome so that only early genes of the virus are transcribed, not the late genes required for com-plete virus replication. Some of these early genes en-code intranuclear proteins, referred to as a T proteins or antigens (T = tumor). These early adenovirus pro-teins (E1A and E1B) bind to a normal cellular protein known as p53, which is the product of a cell cycle regu-latory gene or anti-oncogene. In normal cells, p53 has many functions, one of which is to interact with an-other protein (p21) to arrest cells in G1 phase of the cell cycle. Inactivation of p53 by virus-encoded T pro-teins results in uncontrolled expression of cellular proto-oncogenes and neoplastic transformation. A simi-lar mechanism underlies the neoplastic transformation caused by the papovaviruses.

Papovaviruses Papovaviruses are nonenveloped vi-ruses containing a single circular strand of DNA. The name is an acronym derived from the first two letters of three words: **pa**pilloma, **po**lyoma, and **va**cuolating agent (a synonym for simian virus 40), the three major groups of agents encompassed by this family. The family is divided into two genera: *Papillomavirus* and *Polyomavirus*. These are listed in Table 4-7.

Papillomaviruses cause benign, solitary or multiple, papillary neoplasms known as papillomas or "warts" on the skin and oral and genital mucous membranes of animals and humans. A few papillomaviruses (deer fibroma virus and bovine papilloma virus) produce tumors of fibrous connective tissue rather than papillomas. In humans, specific virus types have also been associated with squamous cell carcinomas. Papillomaviruses are relatively host-specific and are unique in that they have not been successfully propagated in tissue culture. There are numerous types of papillomaviruses in both animals and humans, and these viruses often have their own unique biologic properties. In human beings alone, more than 50 distinct types have been identified. Papillomaviruses are generally transmitted by direct contact and less often by insect vectors. After entering the nucleus of a susceptible cell, the viral DNA occurs in one of two forms, episomally as molecules of circular DNA or integrated into the host-cell DNA. Viral replica-

TABLE 4-7 **Oncogenic papovaviruses**

Virus	Neoplasm(s)	Risk factors
Genus: *Papillomavirus* (all naturally occurring)		
Human papilloma viruses (50 different types)	Cutaneous, laryngeal, and genital papillomas	Solar radiation, immunosuppressive states, and sexual promiscuity
Bovine papilloma viruses	**Cattle:** Cutaneous and alimentary papillomas; genital fibropapillomas and esophageal carcinomas **Horses:** Equine sarcoid	Immunosuppressive states and possibly bracken fern ingestion
Canine papilloma viruses	Cutaneous and oral papillomas	?
Equine papilloma viruses	Cutaneous papillomas	?
Ovine papilloma viruses	Cutaneous papillomas	?
Rabbit papilloma viruses	Cutaneous and oral papillomas	?
Hamster papilloma virus	Cutaneous papillomas	?
Mouse papilloma virus	Cutaneous papillomas	?
Nonhuman primate papilloma viruses (chimpanzee, rhesus and colobus monkeys)	Cutaneous papillomas	?
Deer fibroma virus	Cutaneous fibromas	?
Parrot papilloma virus	Cutaneous papillomas	?
Genus: *Polyomavirus* (all experimentally-induced only)		
Polyomavirus maccacae (SV40; "vacuolating agent"; macaque monkey polyomavirus)	Sarcomas, lymphomas, and ependymomas in young mice, hamsters	Immature or compromised immune system
Polyomavirus muris 1 (mouse polyomavirus)	Sarcomas and carcinomas in young mice, rats, hamsters, and guinea pigs	Immature or compromised immune system
Polyomavirus hominis 1 (BK virus; human polyomavirus 1)	Ependymomas, pancreatic islet cell tumors, and osteosarcomas in young hamsters	Immature or compromised immune system
Polyomavirus hominis 2 (JC virus; human polyomavirus 2)	Neuroglial tumors, ependymomas, and meningiomas in young hamsters and owl monkeys	Immature or compromised immune system

tion only occurs in those cells in which the viral genome exists in the episomal form. The replicative cycle of papillomaviruses is intricately linked to the stages of differentiation of squamous epithelial cells. Early during the course of infection, cells at the basal aspect of the epithelium undergo extensive proliferation, leading to the formation of papillary projections of the epithelium and underlying fibrovascular connective tissue, a typical papilloma or wart. It has been shown that the human papillomaviruses encode two early proteins, E6 and E7, which bind to and inactivate cellular p53 and pRb respectively. Inactivation of these cell cycle regulators results in pronounced papillary proliferation of the undifferentiated squamous cells early in the course of infection. At this stage, there is no active transcription of the late structural genes of the virus, hence no virions can be found in infected cells. As the proliferating cells become progressively more differentiated through the accumulation of cytokeratin and keratohyaline granules, transcription of late genes of the virus occurs, and the nuclei develop basophilic inclusion bodies composed of numerous mature papillomavirus virions. At this stage, the cytoplasm of inclusion body-bearing cells becomes progressively swollen and vacuolated and the cell dies. This releases mature virions that can be transmitted to other susceptible individuals. Most benign papillomas in animals and humans eventually undergo spontaneous regression through the combined cytotoxic action of the replicating virus and the host's cell-mediated immune response. Individual animals or humans become immune to that specific type.

In human beings, papillomaviruses types 16 and 18 have been associated with several forms of anogenital cancer, particularly cervical carcinoma. An extremely high percentage of patients with precancerous lesions of the cervix, as well as patients with invasive carcinoma of the cervix, have integrated copies of one of these two papillomaviral genomes in the DNA of the abnormal cells. In these cases, the viral genome is integrated in a manner that only allows the early (transforming) genes of the virus (E6 and E7) to be transcribed, hence no viral replication or cytolytic effect occurs. This results in malignant transformation and carcinoma, in contrast to the benign, self-limiting nature of virally permissive papillomas.

Polyomavirus virions are smaller than papillomaviruses, usually cause latent infections in their respective hosts, and have only revealed their oncogenic potential under experimental conditions. Two such agents have been studied extensively, polyomavirus of mice and simian virus 40 (SV 40).

Murine polyomavirus occurs commonly as a latent infection of wild mice but is rare in commercially raised mice. The virus is excreted in the saliva, urine, and feces of infected mice. It can cause a wasting and paralytic syndrome in immunodeficient nude mice. Interest in this polyomavirus stems from its ability to cause a wide variety of neoplasms (hence the name polyoma) in newborn or suckling mice, rats, guinea pigs, hamsters, rabbits, and ferrets. Adult animals are resistant to tumor induction. The tumors include carcinomas and sarcomas of the salivary gland, mammary gland, skin, kidney, thryoid, blood vessels, thymus, bone, and cartilage.

Three types of cytopathology occur in cells infected with polyomavirus *in vitro* and presumably *in vivo* as well. Cells permissive to polyomavirus replication go through two phases: an early phase, during which viral and cellular proteins are synthesized, inducing the cell to move from G0 or G1 phase of the cell cycle to the S phase; and a late phase, during which both viral and cellular DNA are replicated, viral structural proteins are made, and mature virions are assembled. Such a permissive infection results in the formation of amphophilic, intranuclear inclusion bodies in the infected cell and cell death. This is termed a **lytic infection.** Thus, permissive cells do not become transformed; they die.

Cells from a number of nonrodent species can be infected by polyomavirus but do not permit viral replication. Such cells are induced to enter the S phase of the cell cycle by the viral and cellular proteins synthesized during the early phase, but because of viral and cellular enzyme incompatibility cannot synthesize viral DNA and thus no viral replication or lysis occurs. These cells continue to divide (transformed) as long as the early viral and cellular proteins are synthesized but eventually revert to normal after the original viral DNA is diluted by successive cell divisions. This constitutes a **transient** or **abortive type of transformation.**

As with certain adenovirus and papillomavirus infections, polyomavirus can also become integrated into the host-cell DNA and cause **nonpermissive, permanently transforming infection.** This occurs when polyomavirus DNA becomes integrated into the host-cell DNA so that only the early proteins become constitutively expressed through the action of the viruses' own promoter sequences. In such cases, the complete viral genome and late structural genes of the virus are integrated upstream from the viral promoter sequences and therefore are not transcribed. When this occurs, viral replication cannot occur and only the early genes of the virus are expressed. Polyomavirus encodes for three early proteins (oncoproteins) referred to as large, middle, and small T proteins. Cultured rodent cells that express only the large T protein become immortalized and can grow in medium with minimal to no serum, but such cells do not assume the complete transformed phenotype, since they do not form tumors when inoculated into nude mice. The presence of both the large and middle-sized T proteins of polyomavirus are necessary to acquire the malignant phenotype. The large T protein of polyomavirus is a nuclear DNA-binding protein that plays an important role in enhancing both viral and DNA transcription during a lytic cycle. The pattern of integration of the viral DNA into the host-cell genome does not allow viral DNA replication but only cellular DNA replication: this forces the cell to continue to divide. The middle T protein is a membrane-bound protein that interacts with *src*, a normal cellular proto-oncogene product with tyrosine-kinase activity. The interaction of middle T with *src* causes a fifty-fold or greater increase in the enzyme activity of this oncoprotein, thus providing the second step required for transformation. The small T protein also appears to have a role in the induction of complete transformation, but this is less well defined.

Simian virus 40 (SV 40 or vacuolating agent) occurs commonly as a latent infection of rhesus and cynomolgus monkeys, and only causes disease in these species if the animal becomes immunocompromised. Under the latter circumstance, SV 40 causes nephritis and pneumonia and neurologic lesions similar to progressive multifocal leukoencephalopathy of humans. SV 40 is highly oncogenic when inoculated into newborn hamsters; it causes a variety of sarcomas including lymphosarcoma, osteosarcoma, and anaplastic sarcomas. When inoculated intracerebrally, it has caused ependymomas. Similar to infection with murine polyomavirus, infection by SV 40 can be permissive and lytic or nonpermissive and transforming, depending on whether the viral DNA is present in the nucleus in episomal or integrated form. The permissiveness of the infected cell plays a major role in determining whether or not the cell is killed as a consequence of viral replication or transformed as a result of integration of the viral genome into nonpermissive cells.

The basic biology and transforming capacity of SV 40 is similar to murine polyomavirus, except that SV 40 encodes two, rather than three, early proteins. These are referred to as large T and small T. The large T protein is a nuclear binding protein that functions much the same way as the analagous protein of murine polyomavirus: It binds to and inactivates p53 and pRB, both of which are products of anti-oncogenes (tumor suppressor genes). However, it also has a component that binds to the plasma membrane and functions much like the middle T protein of murine polyomavirus.

Hepadnaviruses The term hepadnavirus is an acronym derived from **hepa**titis **DNA virus.** There are four members of this family that have been associated with spontaneously occurring hepatitis and hepatocellular carcinoma in their respective host species. These are human **hepatitis virus B (HBV), woodchuck hepatitis virus, ground squirrel hepatitis virus,** and **duck hepatitis virus.** In their respective host species, these viruses are significant causes of chronic perisistent hepatitis, which may progress to cirrhosis and liver cancer. As with a number of the DNA-containing oncogenic viruses, infection can be permissive, with the production of large amounts of infectious virus, or the virus can become integrated into the liver-cell DNA and cause malignant transformation. The precise molecular mechanism involved in malignant transformation caused by the hepadnaviruses has not been fully elucidated. It is known, however, that the chronic hepatitis resulting from infection by this family of viruses is accompanied by extensive regeneration of hepatocytes, thus increasing the pool of mitotic cells subject to spontaneous mutations or mutations induced by chemicals, such as aflatoxin. Aflatoxin is known to be an important co-factor in the pathogenesis of hepatocellular carcinoma in those parts of the world where HBV-associated hepatocellular carcinoma is endemic. Mutations of the anti-oncogene p53 are one mutation type that occurs with increased frequency in liver cancers of patients in these areas. In addition, HBV encodes a regulatory protein termed Hbx, which interferes with growth control of infected cells by activating certain host-cell proto-oncogenes. Hbx protein also activates protein kinase C, an important element of several signal transduction pathways, and in this way, resembles the action of certain tumor promoters mentioned in the discussion of chemical carcinogenesis.

ONCOGENIC RNA VIRUSES

Retroviruses Retroviruses constitute the only family of RNA tumor viruses. This family is divided into three subfamilies: (1) the **oncoviruses** or RNA tumor viruses; (2) the **lentiviruses;** and (3) the **foamy viruses,** or **spumaviruses.** We shall only be concerned with the oncovirus subfamily. Retroviruses are approximately 100 nm in diameter and have a glycoprotein envelope that surrounds a capsid containing the viral RNA genome. Contained within the virions of all members of this family is an enzyme known as RNA-dependent DNA polymerase, commonly referred to as **"reverse transcriptase."** This enzyme catalyzes the transcription of an RNA molecule into a molecule of DNA; the reverse of what occurs in most biologic systems. This phenomenon of reverse transcription is reflected in the family name. The retrovirus genome consists of two identical strands of single-stranded, positive RNA. After entering a cell, the reverse transciptase copies the viral RNA into a single strand of negative DNA and catalyzes the synthesis of a complemenatary strand of positive DNA. This covalently linked circle of double-stranded DNA, referred to as a provirus, is then randomly integrated into the host-cell DNA by a virally encoded enzyme known as **integrase.** After integration, the proviral DNA is transcribed by the cell's own machinery to form viral messenger RNA and genomic RNA that is incorporated into new virions. The envelope of retroviruses is acquired by budding through cell membranes.

The envelope, core shell, and nucleocapsid of oncoviruses are arranged concentrically. The virion contains six proteins, two of which are glycoproteins that form peplomeres on the viral envelope. Protein p30 (mammalian oncoviruses) or p27 (avian oncoviruses), which form the core shell, exhibit shared interspecies antigenicity, an important factor in delineating mammalian from avian types. Interestingly, proviral DNA of retroviruses can be found in the cellular DNA of a number of species. These are referred to as endogenous retrovirus sequences. Although they are often not expressed, they can occasionally be activated by physical or chemical agents or by superinfection with other oncoviruses. Many of the oncogenic retroviruses are defective in their ability to replicate but may be rescued via complementation by helper viruses. The group is very large and contains many agents that cause leukemias or sarcomas in a variety of animal species.

Figure 4-19 depicts the gene sequence of the proviral DNA of a standard replicatively competent retrovirus.

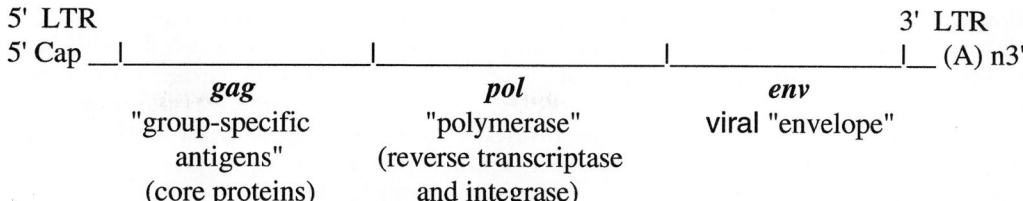

FIG. 4-19 Graphic illustration of the genomic organization of a prototypic oncogenic retrovirus. Note that the three constitutive genes *gag, pol,* and *env* are flanked by long terminal repeat (LTR) sequences that contain elements that promote and enhance transcription of the viral genome.

Three constitutive genes are required for viral replication (*gag, pol,* and *env*) and are flanked on the 5′ and 3′ ends of the genome by sequences referred to as **long terminal repeats,** or **LTRs.** These LTRs contain identical sequences, but the left 5′ LTR enhances and promotes transcription of the viral genome, whereas the right 3′ LTR specifies the site of polyadenylation of the mRNA transcript, which prevents it from being rapidly degraded in the cytoplasm. The *gag* (core protein) transcript contains a protease, whereas the *gag-pol* polyprotein is eventually cleaved and processed to form the reverse transcriptase and integrase required for integra-

TABLE 4-8   **Oncogenic retroviruses**

Virus type	V-oncogene	Species affected
Rapidly transforming viruses		
Murine viruses		
Abelson murine leukemia virus	abl	Mouse
Moloney murine sarcoma virus	mos	Mouse
Harvey murine sarcoma virus	H-ras	Rat
Kirsten murine sarcoma virus	K-ras	Rat
FBJ murine osteosarcoma virus	fos	Mouse
Mouse mammary tumor virus	int-1, int-2	Mouse
3611 murine sarcoma virus	raf (mil)	Mouse
Other mammalian viruses		
Simian sarcoma virus	sis	Wooly monkey, gibbons
Feline sarcoma virus	fes	Cats
Avian viruses		
Rous sarcoma virus	src	Chicken
Avian myeloblastosis	myb	Chicken
Avian myelocytomatosis virus	myc	Chicken
Avian erythroblastosis virus	erb-A, erb-B	Chicken
Reticuloendotheliosis virus	rel	Turkey
Yamaguchi-Esh sarcoma virus	yes	Chicken
Fujinami sarcoma virus	fps (fes)	Chicken
UR 2 avian sarcoma virus	ros	Chicken
Avian SKV770 virus	ski	Chicken
Slowly transforming viruses		
Murine viruses		
Gross murine leukemia virus	—	Mouse
Graffi murine leukemia virus	—	Mouse
Kaplan and Rich sarcoma virus	—	Mouse
Other mammalian viruses		
Feline leukemia virus	—	Cat
Bovine leukemia virus	—	Cattle
Simian T cell leukemia virus	?	Old world primates
Human T cell leukemia virus	tat, tax	Humans

tion into host-cell DNA. These final processing events involving the *gag* and *gag-pol* proteins is mediated by the virally encoded protease after the virions have been assembled.

The oncogenic retroviruses can be divided into two distinct types based on the efficiency and rapidity with which they transform cells. These are referred to as **rapidly transforming retroviruses** and **slowly transforming retroviruses** (Table 4-8). The mechanisms by which they cause neoplastic transformation are different and are discussed separately.

RAPIDLY TRANSFORMING RETROVIRUSES These viruses, which produce tumors rapidly and with a high level of efficiency, are responsible for naturally occurring tumors of animals as well as experimentally induced tumors in laboratory animals. They transform cells *in vitro*. Each virus in this group contains a **viral oncogene** (v-oncogene), which was acquired originally from a host-cell proto-oncogene by recombinant events at some earlier time in evolution of the virus. Although the nucleotide sequence of v-oncogenes may differ slightly from their parent proto-oncogenes as a result of the acquisition of point mutations, their activity is similar to that of their parent gene. At present, there are approximately 30 known retrovirus oncogenes that have genetic homology with avian and mammalian proto-oncogenes. The spectrum of neoplastic diseases produced by this group of viruses reflects the expression of the particular v-oncogene. All except one of the oncogene-containing retroviruses are "defective" in that they have acquired the oncogene at the expense of all or a portion of one of the three genes essential for viral replication. Therefore, these agents require a helper virus to replicate. The helper retrovirus, when it infects a

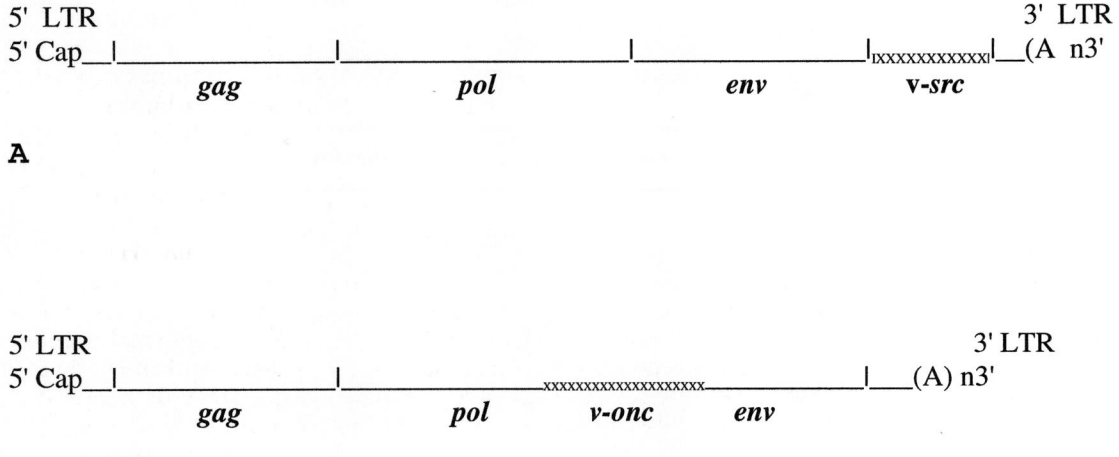

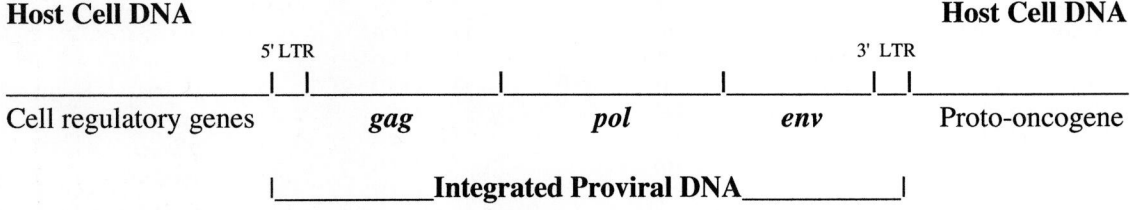

FIG.4-20 A. Diagram of the genomic organization of Rous sarcoma virus, the only replicatively competent rapidly transforming retrovirus. Note that the virus has a full complement of constitutive genes, *gag, pol* and *env,* but in addition has acquired the oncogene *v-src,* derived from the proto-oncogene src. **B.** Diagram of the genomic organization of a typical "defective" rapidly transforming retrovirus. These agents have acquired a v-oncogene from a proto-oncogene but in doing so have lost a portion of one or more of the constitutive genes, *pol* or *env* that are required for viral replication. **C.** Diagram of the integrated proviral DNA of a slowly transforming retrovirus into the host cell DNA. Note that the proviral DNA is inserted at a site between a normal cell proto-oncogene and its regulatory sequences. This results in the proto-oncogene coming under the control of the promoting and enhancing sequences of the 3'LTR of the virus thereby resulting in unregulated production of the proto-oncogene product and malignant transformation.

cell containing a defective retroviral genome, provides the missing gene product needed for the defective oncogenic retrovirus to replicate. The Schmidt-Rubin strain of Rous sarcoma virus is the only rapidly transforming retrovirus that is not defective. It contains all three constitutive genes required for replication of the virus plus a viral oncogene known as *src* (sarcoma). The genome of the nondefective Schmidt-Rubin strain of Rous sarmoma virus is depicted in the following diagram.

Figure 4-20 depicts the proviral genome of all other "defective" acutely transforming retroviruses.

The transforming capacity of the rapidly transforming retroviruses is not dependent on the proviral DNA integrating at a specific site within the host-cell DNA, as is true for the slowly transforming retroviruses. In fact, every cell that is infected with an acutely transforming virus becomes transformed, because transcription of the integrated proviral DNA is under the control of the left LTR of the provirus, not the host-cell regulatory genes. Consequently, transcription of the viral genome occurs more or less continuously in the infected cell with the accumulation of large quanities of viral oncogene product within the cell. There are no negative feed-back mechanisms that control v-oncogene expression, as in proto-oncogene expression in unaffected cells. The unregulated synthesis of viral oncoprotein causes infected cells to divide continuously and become immortalized. Because many cells in an *in vitro* culture system or in a host animal are transformed shortly after infection, the tumors caused by this group of viruses are polyclonal in origin. This means that the proviral DNA is integrated at random sites within the host-cell DNA in the populations of cells making up the transformed culture or neoplasm, in contrast to what is found in cells transformed by slowly transformed retroviruses.

SLOW TRANSFORMING RETROVIRUSES Retroviruses included in this group **do not contain viral oncogenes.** This group of agents includes many of the avian leukosis viruses, wild-type mouse leukemia viruses, feline leukemia viruses, bovine leukemia viruses, and gibbon ape leukemia virus. These agents produce a wide spectrum of diseases, usually after a **long latent period.** They have a full complement of *gag, pol,* and *env* genes and, therefore, are capable of replicating on their own. They **do not transform cells in vitro.** The agents included in this group cause neoplastic transformation by the phenomenon of "insertional mutagenesis" or "downstream promotion" of a proto-oncogene. For neoplastic transformation to occur with this group of viruses, integration of the proviral DNA has to be immediately upstream of a normal cellular proto-oncogene. Integration at such a specific site is purely a chance event and thus occurs in a small number of infected cells. This accounts for the long latent period between infection and the development of a neoplasm. The consequences of integration of a provirus DNA molecule upstream from a cellular proto-oncogene are two-fold. First, the insertion of the provirus immediately adjacent to a proto-oncogene effectively removes the proto-onco-

gene from control by its normal host-cell regulatory genes. Secondly, the promoting and enhancing sequences of the 3' LTR of the proviral DNA cause continuous and unregulated expression of the neighboring proto-oncogene, leading to increased synthesis of gene product. This results in uncontrolled proliferation and malignant transformation.

Tumors caused by slowly transforming retroviruses, because they result from the progeny of a single transformed cell, are monoclonal in origin. This means that all cells comprising the neoplasm have the proviral DNA integrated at precisely the same site within the tumor-cell DNA.

Certain slowly oncogenic retroviruses appear to cause leukemias by yet another mechanism involving oncogenes that are not derived from cellular proto-oncogenes. These include **human** and **simian T-cell leukemia viruses (HTLV-1 and HTLV-2 and STLV-1)** and **bovine leukemia viruses (BLV).** These viruses have been associated with lymphoproliferative disorders and leukemias and lymphomas in humans, Old World nonhuman primates, and cattle, respectively. The first isolates of HTLV-1 and HTLV-2 were from human patients with aggressive forms of cutaneous lymphoma known as mycosis fungoides and Sezary's syndrome, or hairy cell leukemia. Isolates of the same or similar virus have also been obtained from patients on the islands of Kyushu and Shikoku in southwestern Japan, where there is a high incidence of adult T-cell leukemia. HTLV-1 is closely related to STLV-1 and more distantly related to BLV. HTLV-1 is an exogenous human virus, since its sequences are not present in the DNA of normal human patients. In those patients with T-cell leukemia, HTLV sequences are present only in the DNA of neoplastic T-cell lines, not in the DNA of normal T cells and B cells, thus indicating that the virus was not transmitted in the germ-cell line of the patient. The tumor cells are specifically of the T4 positive subset of T lymphocytes.

The genomes of HTLV-I and STLV-1 have been characterized and found to resemble those of other nondefective, leukemogenic retroviruses, such as murine leukemia virus, bovine leukemia virus, and avian lymphoma virus, in that they do not contain a cell-derived oncogene. In addition to *gag, pol* and *env,* they contain several additional genes that are clearly involved in their ability to transform T cells *in vitro* and which probably play a role in their oncogenicity *in vivo.* One of these genes, known at *tax,* codes for a protein that stimulates transcription of viral mRNA by acting on the 5' LTR of proviral DNA. In addition to stimulating the 5'LTR, *tax* genes may activate host genes responsible for controlling T-lymphocyte proliferation, including c-*fos*, c-*sis*, and the genes that encode IL-2, IL-2r, (IL-2 receptor) and GM-CSF (granulocyte-macrophage colony-stimulating factor) thereby causing a polyclonal proliferation of T cells or a lymphoproliferative disorder. It has been suggested that other unidentified events are probably involved in monoclonal neoplastic transformation. Co-infection with other viral agents may promote neoplastic transformation.

Parasite-induced neoplasia

Certain helminthic parasites have been associated with the occurrence of specific types of neoplasms, but the mechanisms involved in tumor induction are not well defined. Most such tumors simply have been ascribed to chronic irritation, but no systematic effort has been made to define the molecular basis for tumor formation in such cases. Bilharziasis, better known as schistosomiasis *(Schistosoma hematobium)*, has been considered a cause of carcinoma of the human bladder, especially since the two conditions occur together and the incidence of carcinoma of the bladder is high in those populations (e.g., Egypt) that are heavily parasitized. The blood flukes produce extensive, chronic cystitis, but they are not universally accepted as the primary cause of this cancer.

Cysticercus fasciolaris, the cystic or larval stage of the cat tapeworm, *Taenia taeniaeformis,* found in the liver of rats, has been associated both naturally and experimentally with what some investigators have considered fibrosarcomas in the connective tissue wall surrounding the cyst.

In the dog, *Spirocerca lupi,* a nematode that invades the wall of the lower esophagus, produces 1 to 2 cm spherical, nodular masses having the histologic features of fibrosarcomas or osteosarcomas. These tumors commonly extend into the mediastinal tissues and result in ulceration of the esophageal mucosa. Such tumors have been reported as metastasizing to the lungs and other visceral organs. Evidence is strong that this parasite has a causal relationship to the surrounding neoplasm, but the mechanism involved is not known.

Similarly, *Heterakis isolonche* has been associated with fibrosarcomatous tumors of the cecal wall of the pheasant.

Chronic inflammation-induced neoplasms

Recently, there have been a number of reports describing the occurrence of fibrosarcomas and malignant fibrous histiocytomas in the subcutis of the neck and interscapular regions and in the skeletal musculature of the thigh of cats vaccinated with feline leukemia virus and rabies virus, alone or in combination. These sites are favored for vaccination of cats. The neoplasms are very often preceded by a granulomatous panniculitis induced by components of the vaccine at the site of injection. A small percentage of these granulomas progress to neoplasia. The pathogenesis of neoplastic transformation in these cases has not been determined. In particular, it is not known if feline sarcoma virus plays a role in tumor induction in these cases or if cytokines released by macrophages, histiocytes, and other inflammatory cells at the site of vaccination are responsible for neoplastic transformation of fibroblasts. Similar tumors have been associated with various surgically implanted foreign bodies, especially orthopedic devices, such as metallic plates and pins.

Heredity factors associated with neoplasia

The vast amount of experimentation in this aspect of neoplasia, conducted chiefly on mice, has shown that whether one of the recognized carcinogens actually produces a tumor depends on the relative susceptibility of the individual organism. In inbred mice, the susceptibility or lack thereof is transmitted from one generation to the next. For instance, certain strains of mice are highly susceptible to carcinoma of the skin, while others are resistant. Other strains, which have a high susceptibility to mammary adenocarcinoma, have been bred. Some families have a high resistance to all forms of neoplasia. These characteristics are thus to be considered hereditary, although neoplasms themselves are not inherited. Hereditary factors play a significant role in determining the susceptibility of an individual animal to various carcinogens. This may be as simple as the inheritance of light-colored skin, which predisposes to skin cancer induced by ultraviolet light, or the susceptibility to a known oncogenic virus; more often than not, the fundamental basis for decreased or increased susceptibility is not known.

TUMOR IMMUNITY

The subject of the immunogenicity of naturally occurring tumors of animals and humans is controversial. It is clear from experimental studies, however, that viral and certain chemically induced tumors in laboratory animals do elicit a demonstrable immune response that, in some cases, can be passively transferred. In these cases, the immune response may involve either the cellular (Fig. 4-21) or humoral immune system or both, and be directed towards new (and therefore foreign) antigens expressed on the surface of the transformed cells. Such studies have led to the concept of immunologic surveillance, which theorizes that an im-

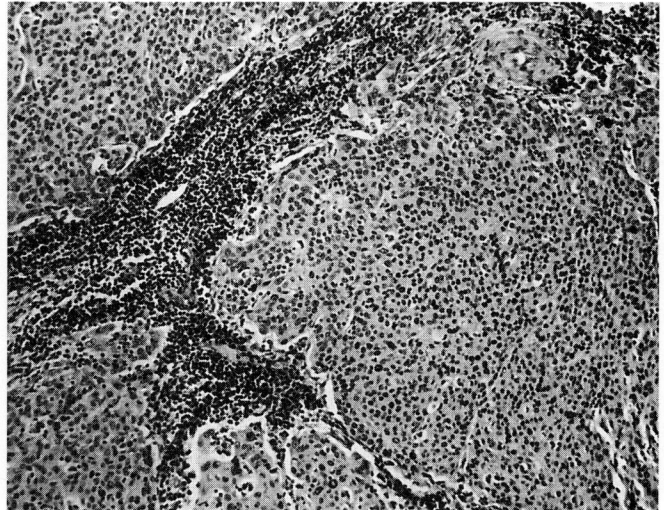

FIG. 4-21 Infiltration of lymphocytes within squamous cell carcinoma may represent a cellular immune response.

mune response destroys most cancer cells during the early stage of tumor formation, and only transformed cells that escape this surveillance system become clinically apparent. Data supporting this theory is largely derived from experimental studies; evidence to the contrary includes the fact that in animals and human beings with immunodeficiency disease, especially of cellular immunity (e.g., athymic nude mice), and in immunosuppressed animals and human beings, there is not a general increase in neoplasia except of the immune system, i.e, lymphomas and leukemias. Others have interpreted the increase in neoplasia of the immune system in these cases as a failure to terminate lymphoproliferation stimulated by an antigen and not a failure of immunologic surveillance.

Experimentally, however, animals can be protected against certain forms of neoplasia, and treatment by immunotherapy (directing the immune system to specifically attack tumor cells bearing certain antigens) can cause tumor regression. These observations provide hope for the improvement of cancer treatment.

The immune response to neoplastic cells targets new or unmasked antigens in or on tumor cells. These are termed **tumor-specific antigens (TSAs),** which are only found on tumor cells, and **tumor-associated antigens (TAAs),** which are present on tumor cells but also on some normal cells.

Tumor-specific antigens.

TSAs may be induced by chemical carcinogens and by various oncogenic viruses. The antigens in tumors induced by chemical carcinogens are distinct for each tumor, even when they are within the same animal and caused by the same chemical; whereas tumors induced by the same virus, even if of different histogenetic origin, share tumor-associated antigens. The chemically-induced TSAs are, in fact, mutant forms of normal cellular proteins, and in many cases are the products of mutated proto-oncogenes, anti-oncogenes, or other cellular proteins. In normal cells, when peptides derived from these gene products are transported to the surface of the cell bound to a cleft in the class I major histocompatibility complex (MHC) molecule, they are recognized as "self" and thus do not evoke an immune response. On the other hand, when peptides derived from mutated forms of these proteins are presented on the cell surface by the same MHC molecules they are recognized as non-self or "foreign" and thus evoke a cellular immune response. Because chemically-induced genetic mutations are random events and do not involve the same mutation in every transformed cell, multiple monoclonal tumors caused by the same chemical, even in the same animal, may express different tumor-specific antigens. In contrast, TSAs expressed on the surfaces of cells transformed by oncogenic viruses represent peptides derived from viral encoded proteins, not cellular proteins, and thus are truely foreign antigens. TSAs are capable of eliciting both a cellular and a humoral immune response.

Tumor-associated antigens.

TAAs are antigens that are expressed on certain neoplastic cells, but are also expressed by normal cells. They include **oncofetal antigens,** such as alpha-fetoprotein and carcinoembryonic antigen, which are proteins expressed during embryonic development, but are normally not expressed postnatally. Their expression on tumor cells is thought to represent a disturbance in the program that normally keeps their synthesis repressed. Other forms of TAAs include **tumor-associated carbohydrate antigens,** which represent mutated forms of glycoprotein and glycolipid molecules including poorly glycosylated mucins, and **differentiation antigens.** The latter include antigens expressed only during certain stages of normal cell differentiation and in transformed cells arrested at a comparable stage of differentiation. Tumor-associated antigens being expressed in certain normal cells generally do not evoke an immune response but, when detected, can be useful in the diagnosis of certain cancers.

Mechanisms of tumor immunity

TSAs induce both a humoral and a cellular immune response, but the latter is most effective in destroying cancer cells. **CD8 + lymphocytes (cytotoxic T lymphocytes)** occur in and around many tumors. but their role in killing tumor cells appears to be most effective against virally induced neoplasms to which they have become sensitized. **Natural killer (NK) cells,** another population of lymphocytes, are capable after activation by interleukin 2 (IL-2) of killing tumor cells without previous antigen sensitization. The antigens responsible for NK cell targeting of tumor cells have not been identified. NK cells may also act in conjunction with antibodies to tumor-specific antigens to kill tumor cells by the **antibody-dependent cellular cytotoxicity (ADCC) reaction.** Finally, macrophages, operating in concert with T lymphocytes, may also kill tumor cells by the generation of oxygen free radicals and secretion of cytokines, such as tumor necrosis factor α (TNF-α). Despite the immunogenicity of tumors, it appears that in many cases the host's defense mechanisms are incapable of halting the progression of most neoplasms. Proposed explanations for this failure include the following: (1) all tumors do not bear foreign antigens; (2) the immune response is inadequate; and (3) soluble blocking factors (antigen-antibody complexes) interfere with cellular immunity.

References

Bittner JJ. Some possible effects of nursing on the mammary gland tumor incidence in mice. Science 1936;84:162.
Cook RH, Olson C Jr. Experimental transmission of cutaneous papilloma of the horse. Am J Pathol 1951;27:1087–1097.
DeMonbreun WA, Goodpasture EW. Infectious oral papillomatosis of dogs. Am J Pathol 1932;8:43–56.
Dunning WF, Curtis MR. Malignancy induced by *Cysticercus fasciolaris:* its independence of age of the host when infested. Am J Cancer 1939;37:312–328.

Dunning WF, Curtis MR. Multiple peritoneal sarcoma in rats from injection of washed ground, *Taenia* larvae. Cancer Res 1946;6:668–670.

Ellermann V, Bang O. Experimentelle leukaemie bei Huhnern. Zentralbl Bakt 1908;46:595–609.

Finkel MP, Biskis BO, Jinkins PB. Virus-induction of osteosarcomas in mice. Science 1966;151:689–701.

Friend C. Cell-free transmission in adult Swiss mice of a disease having the character of a leukemia. J Exp Med 1967;105:307–318.

Furth J. Observations with a new transmissible strain of the leucosis (leucemia) of fowls. J Exp Med 1931;53:243–267.

Furth J. Lymphomatosis, myelomatosis and endothelioma of chickens caused by a filterable agent. 1. Transmission experiments. J Exp Med 1933;58:253–275.

Gross L. "Spontaneous" leukemia developing in C3H mice following inoculation, in infancy, with AK-leukemic extracts, or Akembryos. Proc Soc Exp Biol Med 1951;76:27–32.

Gross L. A filterable agent recovered from AK-leukemic extracts causing salivary gland car-cinomas in C3H mice. Proc Soc Exp Biol Med 1953;83:414–421.

Gross L. Viral etiology of "spontaneous" mouse leukemia: a review. Cancer Res 1958;18:371–381.

Harvey JJ. An unidentified virus which causes the rapid production of tumours in mice. Nature 1964;204:1104–1105.

Hendrick MJ, Goldschmidt MH, Shofer FS, et al. Postvaccinal sarcomas in the cat: epidemiology and electron probe microanalytical identification of aluminum. Cancer Res 1992;52:5391–5394.

Huebner RJ, Todaro GG. Oncogenes of RNA tumor viruses as determinants of cancer. Proc Natl Acad Sci USA 1969;64:1087–1094.

Jarrett WFH, Martin WB, Crighton GW, et al. Leukemia in the cat. Transmission experiments with leukemia (lymphosarcoma). Nature 1964;202:566–568.

Kass PH, Barnes WG, Spangler WL, et al. Epidemiologic evidence for a causal relation between vaccination and fibrosarcoma tumorgenesis in cats. J Am Vet Med Assoc 1993;203:396–405.

Kilham L, Herman CM, Fisher ER. Naturally occurring fibromas of grey squirrels related to Shope's rabbit fibroma. Proc Soc Exp Biol Med 1953;82:298–301.

Lucke B. Carcinoma in the leopard frog. Its probable causation by a virus. J Exp Med 1938;68:457–468.

Melendez LV, Hunt RD, Daniel MD, et al. Herpesvirus saimiri. II. Experimentally induced malignant lymphoma in primates. Lab Anim Care 1969;19:378–386.

Opler SR. Observations on a new virus associated with guinea pig leukemia: preliminary note. JNCI 1967;38:797–800.

Parsons RJ, Kidd JG. Oral papillomatosis of rabbits. A virus disease. J Exp Med 1943;77:233–250.

Rous P. A transmissible avian neoplasm (sarcoma of the common fowl). J Exp Med 1910;12:697–705.

Rous P. The virus tumors and the tumor problem. Am J Cancer 1936;28:233–272.

Seibold HR, Bailey WS, Hoerlein BF, et al. Observations on the possible relations of malignant esophageal tumors and *Spirocerca lupi* lesions in the dog. Am J Vet Res 1955;16:5–14.

Shope RE. Infectious papillomatosis of rabbits. J Exp Med 1933;58:607–624.

Shope RE. A transmissible tumor-like condition in rabbits. J Exp Med 1932;56:793–802.

Shope RE. An infectious fibroma of deer. Proc Soc Exp Biol Med 1955;88:533–535.

Snyder SP, Theilen GH. Transmissible feline fibrosarcoma. Nature 1969;221:1074–1075.

Theilen GH, Gould D, Fowler M, et al. C-type virus in tumor tissue of a woolly monkey *(Lagothrix spp.)* with fibrosarcoma. JNCI 1971;47:881–889.

5

Inflammation and repair

Douglas J. Ringler

A pathologic phenomenon known and studied from ancient times, inflammation has long been defined as **the reaction of the tissues to an irritant.** Although, owing to its simplicity, this definition is difficult to surpass, two important characteristics are omitted. First, inflammation is a dynamic process and not a state, and secondly, the process depends on viable tissue. The definition proposed by Ebert (Zweifach and colleagues, 1965), though more cumbersome, is more complete: "Inflammation is a process which begins following sublethal injury to tissue and ends with complete healing." This definition also includes the end result of inflammation, i.e., healing, which is a part of the dynamic process and not a distinct entity unto itself. The basic meaning of the verb "to inflame" is to "set fire to." Many who have suffered the agonies of a severe, acute inflammatory reaction in a tender spot will attest to the aptness of the word.

The clinical signs that characterize inflammation are, as stated by Celsus (30 BC–38 AD) in the first century and by every medical writer since that time, *rubor et tumor cum calore et dolore,* which translated means "redness and swelling with heat and pain." These signs and symptoms are known as the **cardinal signs** of inflammation. The redness is caused by a great increase of blood in the inflamed part. The swelling comes from the increase of blood and the additional presence of substances which, like sap from a tree, have exuded from the blood vessels into the surrounding tissues and are called exudates. The heat, objective rather than subjective, also results from the increased flow of blood, carrying warmth to the periphery from the higher interior temperatures of the body. The pain is often attributed to increased pressure on nerve endings, but the irritating effects of toxic products and certain mediators of the process may be of greater significance, since the degree of pain that accompanies inflammations of apparently equal extent and severity may be highly variable. Rudolf Virchow (1821–1905), a German pathologist, later added loss of function as a fifth cardinal sign

of inflammation in 1858, although the Greek physician Galen (130–300 AD) is often given credit for it. Pain-initiated reflex inhibition of muscle movements, mechanical swelling, and tissue destruction all contribute to loss of function.

Inflammation is both a beneficial phenomenon, i.e., it leads to healing, and a random series of events, seemingly without purpose, i.e., it continues as a prolonged, unending process. It occurs in all the more complex forms of animal life. Without its protection, animals and humans could not have survived their enemies, a fact which appears to have been first perceived by John Hunter (1728–1793) about 200 years ago. Hunter recognized inflammation not as a deleterious response but as a beneficial process by demonstrating that the rubor and calore of the response are secondary to increased blood flow through dilated vascular channels. He also found that "small globules" (leukocytes) and fluid (plasma) within inflamed tissues originated from these swollen vessels. The effect of these hyperemic and leaky vascular changes is to bring the humoral and cellular components of the immune system into immediate contact with the inciting irritant or the cells that have been injured by it. By this means, the causative irritant, if still present, can often be destroyed or at least confined, which is the first prerequisite to recovery from injury.

Hunter was the first to recognize the importance of the microvasculature in the inflammatory reaction; however, it was Virchow's student Julius Cohnheim (1839–1884), who studied the vascular events in detail using a frog's tongue and foot-web. He was the first to recognize and describe the sequence of vascular events, i.e., dilation, stasis of blood, and margination and emigration of leukocytes, that today are the foundation for the study of the inflammatory process.

Without inflammation, survival is not possible, but like other vital processes, inflammation may become aberrant and harmful. Diseases thought to be immunologic in origin, such as rheumatic fever, rheumatoid arthritis, glomerulonephritis, and disseminated lupus erythematosus, are associated with inflammatory reactions that provide no obvious benefit, but rather inflict harm upon the host.

NATURE AND TYPES OF IRRITANTS CAUSING INFLAMMATION

It may be advantageous to review here, before proceeding to a study of the inflammatory process itself, the **causes of inflammation:**

1. **Pathogenic organisms** or, more precisely, the toxic and injurious substances produced by them. Included in this group are bacteria, viruses, fungi, protozoa, and parasitic metazoa. More is said later about the effects of each class.
2. **Chemical poisons,** which are of endless variety. As explained under the heading of necrosis (which also is produced by many chemical poisons), poisons may act either on the tissues with which they come in immediate contact or on more distant cells, such as those of the liver, kidney, and brain, which are often susceptible to highly diluted poisons in blood. Some poisons, such as cyanides and strychnine, kill without causing either inflammation or necrosis.
3. **Mechanical and thermal injuries.** Prominent among these are burns by heat, electricity, light, or other radiant energy. Excessive cold, as well as blows and lacerations, are also included.
4. **Immune reactions.** An inflammatory reaction is often associated with antigen-antibody and cellular interactions that occur under various circumstances. Included are delayed hypersensitivity, the Arthus reaction, the Shwartzman reaction, serum sickness, and certain autoimmune diseases.

References

Hurley JV. Acute inflammation. New York: Churchill Livingstone 1983.
Movat HZ. The inflammatory reaction. New York: Elsevier 1985.
Ryan GB, Majno G. Acute inflammation: a review. Am J Pathol 1977;86:185–276.
Thomas L. Adaptive aspects of inflammation. Keynote address at Third Symposium, Intl Inflammation Club, Brook Lodge, Michigan, June 1–3, 1970.
Virchow R. Die cellularpathologie in ihrer begrundung auf physiologische und pathologische gewebelehre. Berlin: August Hirschwald 1858;1–440.
Zweifach BW, Grant L, McClusky RI, eds. The inflammatory process. New York: Academic Press 1965.

THE INFLAMMATORY PROCESS

Although sometimes thought of as a dynamic single entity, the inflammatory process is composed of many interacting parts, each seemingly unrelated to one another, but each functioning to create the morphologic signs associated with this reaction. Inflammatory changes in tissues result from the complicated interplay of these components. How these components react independently and with one another, with host cells, and with foreign noxious material is ultimately the essence of the inflammatory reaction. It is not our intention to discuss each of these components in depth, but rather to concentrate on morphologic changes and present the more accepted or plausible explanations for their development. The discussion of inflammation in this chapter is meant to provide a foundation on which the student of pathology can build.

There are four major components of the inflammatory process. **Plasma proteins** leak into the perivascular space at an inflammatory site, accounting for the tumor or swelling. Included with albumin, immunoglobulins, and various other proteins are zymogens, which are inactive proteases that, after enzymatic activation, cause the initiation and functioning of the complement, fibrinolytic, coagulation, and kinin systems. These systems each have independent functions and create a cascade of enzymatic reactions. However, in an inflammatory reaction, specific proteins elaborated in these enzymatic cascades are important in triggering or mediating specific inflammatory sequelae. These systems are discussed in greater detail later.

Fixed tissue cells, such as mast cells, fibroblasts, and endothelium, are particularly important in the initiation of inflammation, because they are either the target of the primary irritant or the most affected by the damage caused to adjacent cells. These cells, particularly endothelium, are very important in maintaining the reaction through phenotypic alterations and by the production of soluble inflammatory mediators.

Leukocytes and platelets arrive at the site of inflammation by way of the bloodstream. Leukocytes migrate to the perivascular space to phagocytize and degrade organisms or debris. Conversely, platelets exert their influence while remaining within the vascular space, but as leukocytes do, elaborate inflammatory mediators.

Mediators of the inflammatory reaction consist of proteins, acidic lipids, and vasoactive amines that, as alluded to previously, are produced and elaborated by the three other components of the inflammatory reaction described above. Newly discovered mediators and the morphologic effects of these as well as those discovered years ago represent an area of intense research interest. It is beyond the scope of this book to address each one, but many of the well characterized mediators are discussed in this chapter.

THE CELLS IN INFLAMMATION

Before describing the inflammatory process, let us consider the cells comprising the inflammatory exudate.

Neutrophil leukocytes

These cells, sometimes known as polymorphs, polys, polymorphonuclear cells, and granulocytes, but for which the most popular designation is neutrophils, are the characteristic component of pus, or **purulent exudate,** and represent key cells in the earliest events in the inflammatory reaction. They are particularly important in host defense against bacterial and fungal infections; however, they also may damage host tissues in the process and are sometimes instrumental in inciting inflammation in some noninfectious diseases. The term **heterophil** is used to describe the functional counterpart of the neutrophil in certain species, such as the rabbit and guinea pig, in which the granules of the cells are eosinophilic. The less desirable term, pseudoeosinophil, has also been applied to the neutrophil of these species.

Formed in the bone marrow from granulocytic stem cells, the mature neutrophil, when released into the circulation, has a multilobed nucleus and numerous cytoplasmic granules (Fig. 5–1). When observed by electron microscopy, the nuclear lobes appear disconnected as a result of ultrathin sectioning. The chroma-

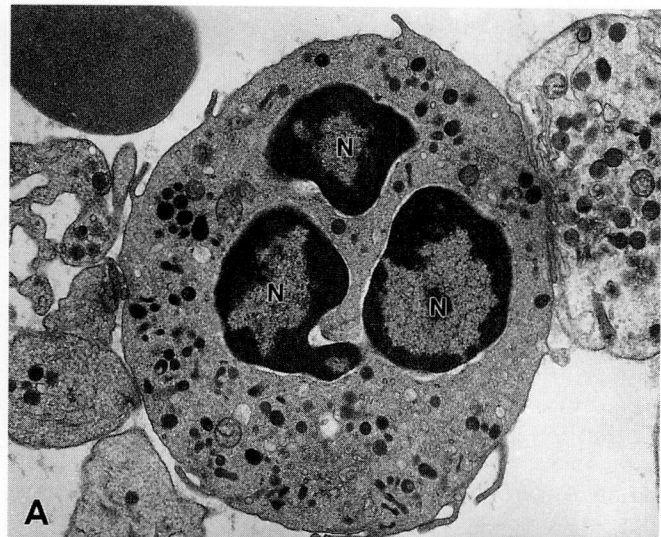

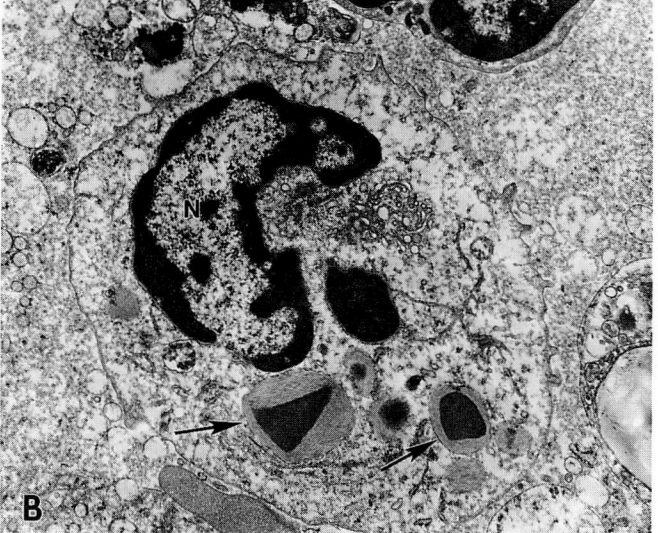

FIG. 5-1 A. Electron photomicrograph of a neutrophil from the peripheral blood of a rhesus monkey *(Macaca mulatta)*. The lobes of the nucleus *(N)* appear separate as a result of thin sectioning. There are multiple round to oval electron-dense granules within the cytoplasm. **B.** Electron photomicrograph of an eosinophil from the peripheral blood of a marmoset *(Saguinus nigricollis)*. The nucleus *(N)* is polymorphonuclear like the neutrophil; but unlike the neutrophil, the cytoplasmic granules *(arrows)* contain dense crystalline bodies. (Courtesy of Dr. N.W. King)

tin is concentrated near the nuclear membrane. Mitochondria are generally few, and little or no endoplasmic reticulum is present. A Golgi apparatus is usually evident. There is a paucity of organized cytoplasmic structures other than the granules.

There are two types of cytoplasmic granules. **Azurophil granules** contain myeloperoxidase and are generally larger and more dense than the **neutrophil-specific** granules. They are surrounded by a membrane and have a moderately electron-dense matrix. Both types are lysosome-like in that they fuse with phagosomes (phagocytic vacuoles) to form phagolysosomes. Inside these granules are an elaborate repertoire of degradative enzymes, which include acid hydrolases, lysozyme, neutral proteases, and cationic proteins. The specific granules are more numerous than the azurophil granules and contain components that are usually not found in the azurophil granules, such as lactoferrin, vitamin B_{12}-binding proteins, receptors for chemoattractants, and reactive oxygen metabolites. During cellular activation, specific and azurophil granules fuse with phagosomes, but specific granules also fuse with the plasma membrane, which causes the contents of specific granules to be extruded into the extracellular milieu. The presence of these granular enzymes in the cellular microenvironment may elicit considerable tissue damage and be the nidus for subsequent inflammatory disease, even in the absence of bacterial or fungal organisms. The presence of the granular enzymes inside the phagosomes serves to kill and/or degrade the phagocytized organism or material.

The half-life of neutrophils is approximately 6 hours, so their continual replenishment is required to both the circulation and inflammatory exudates, as neutrophils are fully differentiated and incapable of division. It is not certain what constitutes the graveyard for dying neutrophils, but probably most either exit the body through mucosal surfaces, such as the intestinal tract, or senescent cells are removed by the reticuloendothelial system.

Neutrophils, like other leukocytes, leave the blood in response to tissue damage; but neutrophils, in particular, are attracted to foci of infections with pyogenic bacteria. They reach these areas quickly, within a few hours, and primarily function by engulfing small particles, a process known as **phagocytosis.** They may ingest foreign matter, such as carbon, pigments, cellular debris, and most importantly, organisms such as bacteria. Certain serum proteins called **opsonins** facilitate phagocytosis, although some foreign organisms can be phagocytized without previous opsonization. There are essentially two classes of opsonins: immunoglobulin proteins and complement components. Opsonins function by first coating the foreign material. The phagocytic cell then recognizes the opsonin-coated material via specific receptors for the opsonin. These include Fc receptors for IgG and C3b receptors for complement. The interaction of the leukocyte with the opsonin triggers the events that lead to total engulfment of the opsonized foreign material. The next step in the process is the destruction of the phagocytized material (covered in detail later in this chapter). If, however, the material, such as a carbon particle, cannot be degraded by the cell, it is released upon the cell's death, to be engulfed again by another phagocytic cell. Recognition of opsonized material by a neutrophil activates the cell and causes: (1) degranulation of specific granules to the outside, (2) production of superoxide anions, and (3) release of arachidonic acid metabolites, which participate in proinflammatory activities in their own right. Additional functions ascribed to neutrophils are presented in this chapter.

Neutrophils have no ability to multiply at an inflammatory site. Replacement for the large numbers of cells killed on the inflammatory battleground must come from the original source, the myeloid tissue in the bone marrow. Thus, it is not surprising that, as an acute suppurative inflammatory reaction develops, the number of neutrophils in the circulating blood is perceptibly, often markedly, increased. Moderate increases in the numbers of these cells may also accompany certain toxemias, pregnancy, severe blood loss, and certain neoplastic processes.

References

Belcher RW, Carney JF, Monahan FG. An electron microscopic study of phagocytosis of *Candida albicans* by polymorphonuclear leukocytes. Lab Invest 1973;29:620–627.

Malech HL, Gallin JI. Neutrophils in human diseases. N Engl J Med 1987;317:687–694.

Normann SJ. Kinetics of phagocytosis: III. Two colloid reactions, competitive inhibition, and degree of inhibition between similar and dissimilar foreign particles. Lab Invest 1974;31:286–293.

Stossel TP. Phagocytosis (parts I, II, and III). N Engl J Med 1974;290:717–723, 774–780, 833–839.

Weissmann G, Smolen JE, Korchak HM. Release of inflammatory mediators from stimulated neutrophils. N Engl J Med 1980;303:27–34.

Wetzel BK, Horn RG, Spicer SS. Fine structural studies on the development of heterophil, eosinophil, and basophil in rabbits. Lab Invest 1967;16:349–382.

Eosinophil leukocytes

The functions of the eosinophil leukocyte in the battle against disease have been a matter of speculation and study ever since the cell was first described by Paul Ehrlich in 1879. However, eosinophils are known to be increased in number and must play an important part in atopic disease, such as asthma, and in the invasions by many (but not all) parasitic helminths and arthopods.

The mature circulating eosinophil, produced in the bone marrow, varies in appearance between species. In most, the nucleus is slightly lobed, but rarely to the extent of the mature neutrophil. As seen in humans, dogs, and horses, the nucleus consists of two tear-drop lobes connected by a thin strand; whereas in the rat, the nucleus is usually an annular ring without distinct lobes. The cytoplasmic granules also vary in the different species, being unusually large in the horse; rod-like in the cat; ovoid in the sheep, cow, and pig; and round but variable in size in the dog. The ultrastructure of the eosinophil nucleus is similar to that of neutrophils (Fig. 5-1). The cytoplasmic granules are distinct and have attracted attention because of their uptake of stains of acid pH, which makes them acidophilic. They are membrane-bound structures with a moderately dense matrix in which is embedded a very dense structure of crystalline appearance. The predominant protein in this crystalloid is major basic protein (MBP), and this protein has been shown to be directly toxic for a number of helminth and protozoal parasites. This crystalloid varies in shape from round (dog) to square (humans) to rectangular (cat, rat). Other cytoplasmic organelles are not numerous; mitchondria are few and the endoplasmic reticulum is sparse. Eosinophils contain a complement of enzymes similar to those of the neutrophil, but lack detectable lysozyme, phagocytin, and neutrophil basic protein. Instead, they have a host of degradative and oxidative eosinophil-specific proteins, such as MBP, eosinophil cationic protein, eosinophil peroxidase, and eosinophil-derived neurotoxin. Furthermore, the eosinophil contains enzymes that are, in contrast, anti-inflammatory in nature, such as histaminase, kinase, arylsulfatase, and the membrane-associated enzyme, lysophospholipase, which is responsible for Charcot-Leyden crystal protein. However, the importance of these modulating proteins in the control of the inflammatory reaction has yet to be substantiated.

Like neutrophils, eosinophils have a short life span (a few days) and are end-stage cells incapable of division. Although the normal number in the circulating blood in most species is small, vast reserves are present in the bone marrow and in the walls of the intestines, lungs, skin, and vagina. Rapid changes can occur in the circulating number, apparently from interchanges with the tissue pool. Adrenal corticosteroids induce a swift reduction or disappearance of eosinophils in the blood (eosinopenia), which accounts for the eosinopenia in shock or the "alarm" reaction. Experimental injection of histamine also induces eosinopenia.

As indicated, the function of eosinophils is likely related to, but not limited to, hypersensitivity reactions and some parasitic infections. In fact, current opinion defines multiple roles for the eosinophil, which include: (1) limited phagocytic capabilities, (2) cytotoxicity of nonphagocytosable targets (particularly helminth parasites), (3) augmentation of the inflammatory reaction during an immediate hypersensitivity reaction, and (4) the modulation of allergic reactions by inhibiting potent proinflammatory products from mast cells, but currently there is very little *in vivo* data to support this hypothesis.

In terms of phagocytosis, eosinophils have the capability to engulf bacteria, mycoplasma, yeast, protozoa, antigen-antibody complexes, and a number of inert materials. However, when compared to neutrophils, eosinophils are less efficient at both phagocytosis and killing.

If unable to phagocytize the target, the eosinophil is, nevertheless, able to function as a cytotoxic leukocyte, particularly in many parasitic helminth infections, including schistosomiasis, fascioliasis, trichinellosis, nippostrongylosis, onchocerciasis, dipetalonemiasis, and trypanosomiasis. The eosinophil is able to recognize its target after it is coated with complement (C3b), IgG, or even IgE by way of specific membrane receptors for these molecules. Adhesion ensues between the target and eosinophil through these receptor-ligand interactions. The target is then killed by eosinophil degranulation at the site of adhesion and, as previously mentioned, the eosinophil-related granule contents such as MBP, eosinophil cationic protein, and eosinophil-derived neurotoxin are directly cytotoxic to some cells and parasites.

In addition to these functions, eosinophils are now thought to be responsible for significant tissue damage and therefore play an important role in the augmentation of the inflammatory response, particularly in hypersensitivity reactions. The deleterious effects are largely related to the toxic and damaging effects of extruded granule contents, oxygen-free radical production, and the capacity to produce proinflammatory products, such as leukotrienes. Therefore, when attracted to an inflammatory focus by eosinophil chemoattractants, which can be produced by many different cell types, including mast cells, lymphocytes, neutrophils, and macrophages, eosinophils congregate in the area and increase the severity of the inflammatory reaction. The exact nature of the stimuli responsible for preferential elaboration of eosinophil chemoattractants over other leukocyte chemoattractants, however, is not understood.

It was once thought that eosinophils were able to modulate immediate hypersensitivity reactions by the elaboration of products that could inhibit mast-cell derived proinflammatory products. These anti-inflammatory products in eosinophil granules include histaminase, kininase, arylsulfatase B, and lysophospholipase. While no one disputes the existence of these anti-inflammatory products in eosinophils, their importance in modulation of the inflammatory response *in vivo* has not been definitively documented to date. Therefore, instead of perceiving eosinophils as inflammatory modulators, it is probably more accurate to consider them as producers of inflammatory injury.

References

Butterworth AE, David JR. Eosinophil function. N Engl J Med 1981;304:154–156.

Cohen SG. The eosinophil and eosinophilia. N Engl J Med 1974;290:457–459.

David JR, Vadas MA, Butterworth AE, et al. Enhanced helminthotoxic capacity of eosinophils from patients with eosinophilia. N Engl J Med 1980;303:1147–1152.

Hung KS. Electron microscopic observations on eosinophil leukocyte granules in dog blood. Anat Rec 1972;174:165–174.

Nutman TB, Cohen SG, Ottesen EA. The eosinophil, eosinophilia, and eosinophil-related disorders. I. Structure and development. II. Eosinophil infiltration and function. Allergy Proc 1988;9:641–647.

Olsson I, Venge P, Spitznagel JK, et al. Arginine-rich cationic proteins of human eosinophil granules: comparison of the constituents of eosinophilic and neutrophilic leukocytes. Lab Invest 1977;36:493–500.

Sullivan TJ. The role of eosinophils in inflammatory reactions. Prog Hematol 1979;11:65–82.

Walls PS, Beeson PB. Mechanism of eosinophilia. VIII. Importance of local cellular reactions in stimulating eosinophil production. Clin Exp Immunol 1972;12:111–119.

Mast cells

Although mast cells are not usually looked upon as a cellular component of the inflammatory exudate, accumulating evidence has begun to solidify their role in the initiation of the vascular and cellular responses in inflammatory reactions. Like eosinophils, mast cells were identified more than a century ago by Paul Ehrlich, and they have been the target of much debate and intrigue since that time. They are derived from bone marrow precursors and are found in all organs rich in connective tissue. They are particularly abundant in tissues at the host-environmental junction, such as the skin, gastrointestinal mucosa, and respiratory tract. In virtually all instances in these tissues, the mast cell is located adjacent to small venules. In this strategic location, they can serve as "gatekeepers of the microvasculature" (Klein and associates, 1989) by providing rapid delivery of preformed inflammatory mediators capable of influencing the vascular tone and leukocyte adhesive quality of endothelium.

Mast cells vary in shape and size within and between species. The nucleus is round or oval and contains a prominent nucleolus. The cytoplasm is distinctive, containing many spherical basophilic and metachromatic granules. The ultrastructure of the granule varies from finely granular to concentric lamellae of filaments presenting a whorled or scrolled pattern (Fig. 5-2). Mitochondria, Golgi, and endoplasmic reticulum are also found in the cytoplasm, although often obscured by the multitude of granules.

It is precisely these granules that give mast cells their ability to influence the inflammatory reaction. Upon appropriate stimulation, mast cells degranulate,

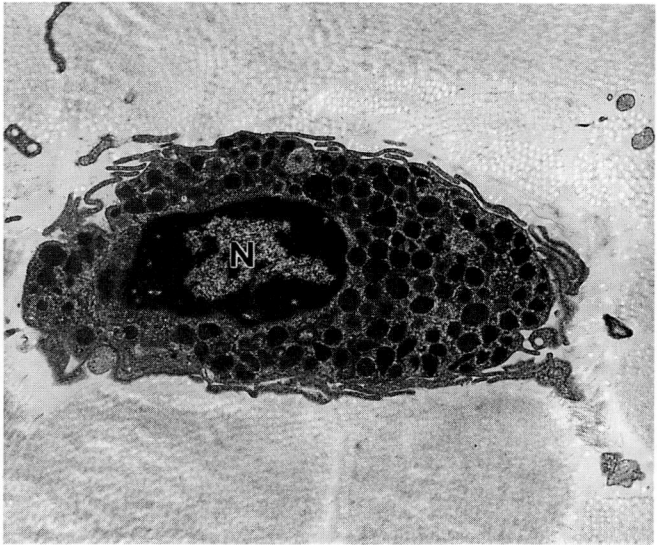

FIG. 5-2 Transmission electron photomicrograph of a human dermal mast cell. Multiple round electron-dense, membrane-bound granules of uniform size are present within the cytoplasm. Each mast cell typically contains between 20 to 40 of these cytoplasmic granules. *N*, nucleus. (Courtesy of Dr. G.F. Murphy)

resulting in the elaboration of a number of preformed proinflammatory products. Foremost is histamine, a vasoactive amine that enhances vascular permeability for serum proteins by creating gaps between endothelial cells. Similarly, heparin, released from mast cell granules, acts as a physiologic anticoagulant and stimulates the migration of capillary endothelial cells to the area. In addition, on degranulation, other enzymes and damaging oxygen metabolites are released from the confines of the granule into the local microenvironment, initiating local injury to surrounding cells. The mast cell is also capable of manufacturing inflammatory mediators *de novo* upon stimulation, such as prostaglandins and leukotrienes. Collectively, the results of stimulation and degranulation are somewhat dependent on the site but in general terms include increased vascular permeability, vasodilation, anticoagulation, tissue destruction, smooth-muscle spasm, mucus secretion, and attraction of other leukocytes, particularly eosinophils. A more complete discussion of granule contents of mast cells appears later in this chapter.

Degranulation can be induced by a number of mechanisms: (1) the cross-linking of surface IgE molecules by antigen on the mast cell surface membrane; (2) the presence of complement fragments, C3a, C4a, and C5a, termed **anaphylatoxins,** which bind to membrane receptors and trigger degranulation; (3) in some individuals, physical stimuli, including trauma, cold, heat, and light, elicits release of granule contents; (4) substance P, which is released from unmyelinated nerve endings and induces mast cell degranulation; and (5) cytokines, the effects of which, in the initiation of the inflammatory response through mast cell degranulation, are now being investigated. Because mast cells respond immediately by degranulation through antigen recognition via IgE surface receptors and because many mast cell mediators such as histamine are preformed and ready for immediate release, mast cells are intimately involved in **type I immediate hypersensitivity (anaphylactic) reactions,** such as allergic rhinitis, allergic asthma, and urticaria.

However, recent investigations into mast cell physiology have revealed that mast cells may be involved in the initiation of delayed inflammatory phenomena not normally associated with immediate hypersensitivity disease. Klein and colleagues (1989), Gordon and Galli (1990), and others have found that mast cells also contain a potent inflammatory protein once thought to be made only by macrophages and their related cells. This protein cytokine, **TNF-α,** is associated with mast cell granules, released upon degranulation, and primarily affects endothelium by making it adhesive for leukocytes. Therefore, in addition to its effects on vascular permeability, mast cells are also capable of triggering the early inflammatory events associated with leukocytic infiltration of the tissues.

References

Benditt EP, Lagunoff D. The mast cell. Its structure and function. Prog Allergy 1964;8:195–202.
Bienenstock J, Tomioka M, Stead R, et al. Mast cell involvement in various inflammatory processes. Am Rev Respir Dis 1987;135:S5–S8.
Dexter TM, Stoddart RW, Quazzaz STA. What are mast cells for? Nature 1981;291:110–111.
Galli SJ. New approaches for the analysis of mast cell maturation, heterogeneity, and function. Fed Proc 1987;46:1906–1914.
Gordon JR, Galli SJ. Mast cells as a source of both preformed and immunologically inducible TNF-α/cachectin. Nature 1990;346:274–276.
Ishizaka T, Conrad DH, Schulman ES, et al. IgE-mediated triggering signals for mediator release from human mast cells and basophils. Fed Proc 1984;43:2840–2851.
Kaliner MA. The mast cell a fascinating riddle. N Engl J Med 1979;301:498–499.
Klein LM, Lavker RM, Matis WL, et al. Degranulation of human mast cells induces an endothelial antigen central to leukocyte adhesion. Proc Natl Acad Sci USA 1989;86:8972–8976.

Basophil leukocytes

Basophils are found in very low numbers in the circulating blood. They have a lobed nucleus, and the cytoplasm contains deeply basophilic and metachromatic granules, which, like mast cells, contain histamine and heparin. It comes as no surprize, therefore, that basophils and mast cells have similar functions. Both cell types have high affinity receptors for IgE antibodies on their cell surface, both degranulate when a multivalent antigen bridges two IgE molecules on the surface membrane, and thus both cell types function in hypersensitivity reactions by the release of granular contents into the extracellular environment.

References

Dvorak AM, Galli SJ, Morgan E, et al. Anaphylactic degranulation of guinea pig basophilic leukocytes: II. Evidence for regranulation of mature basophils during recovery from degranulation *in vitro.* Lab Invest 1982;46:461–475.
Hastie R. A study of the ultrastructure of human basophil leukocytes. Lab Invest 1974;31:223–231.
Murata F, Spicer SS. Ultrastructural comparison of basophilic leukocytes and mast cells in the guinea pig. Am J Anat 1974;139:335–352.

Mononuclear phagocytes

The mononuclear phagocyte system represents several different cell types found in a variety of organs, each related by common lineage and/or function. **Macrophages** are the prototypic mononuclear phagocyte, a name, still used today, that was coined more than a century ago by Elie Metchnikoff in his descriptions of large phagocytic cells in multiple organs. Macrophages are found throughout most of the organs of the body, some of which are specialized, fully differentiated cells specific for their resident organ. These include the Kupffer cells of the liver, alveolar macrophages of the lung, pleural and peritoneal macrophages, free and fixed macrophages in lymphoid and mucosal tissues, microgliacytes of the central nervous system, osteoclasts of bone, and histiocytes of connective tissue. All of these cells, however, are derived from a common precursor, the blood **monocyte.**

Monocytes are derived from bone marrow, and morphologically have indented nuclei and relatively

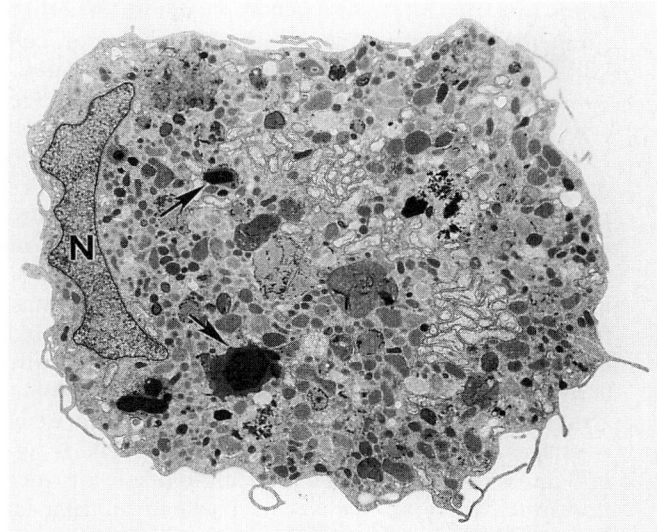

FIG. 5-3 Transmission electron photomicrograph of a pulmonary alveolar macrophage from a rhesus monkey. The nucleus *(N)* is eccentrically located within the cell. The cytoplasm is crowded with a heterogeneous population of membrane-bound lysosomal and secretory granules and phagocytic vacuoles, some of which contain crystalline structures *(arrows)*.

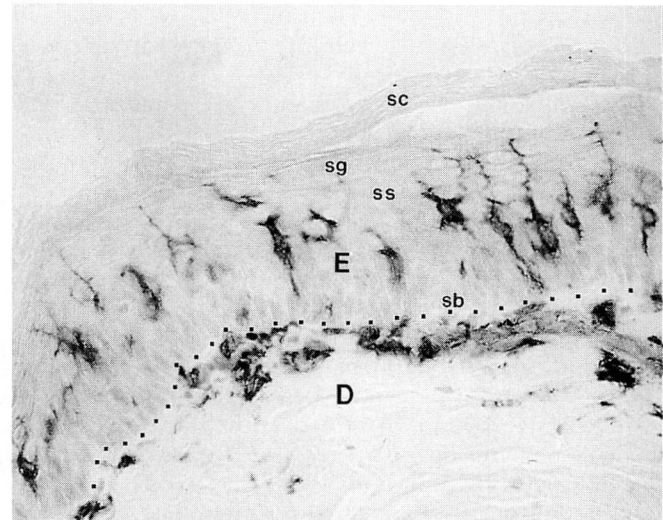

FIG. 5-4 Photomicrograph of a frozen section of skin from a rhesus monkey immunohistochemically stained using a monoclonal antibody against CD1 antigen, which detects epidermal Langerhans cells, the antigen-presenting dendritic cell of the skin. The dotted line represents the location of the basement membrane, which separates the epidermis *(E)* from the underlying dermis *(D)*. The approximate locations of the stratum basale *(sb)*, stratum spinosum *(ss)*, stratum granulosum *(sg)*, and stratum corneum *(sc)* within the epidermis are shown. Within the epidermis are multiple Langerhans cells, each having delicate dendritic processes that traverse throughout the epidermis and occasionally reach the cutaneous surface.

abundant cytoplasm. Contained within the cytoplasm are multiple mitochondria, a well-formed Golgi apparatus, and rough and smooth endoplasmic reticulum, sometimes appearing as vesicles. The tissue macrophage (Fig. 5-3) has a similar structure to the monocyte but is different in a number of respects. It is typically much larger and irregularly shaped, measuring between 20 and 80 μm in diameter. The cytoplasm is voluminous, sometimes with multiple vacuoles. The nuclei are usually centrally or slightly eccentrically located within the cell, and they contain prominent nucleoli. Ultrastructurally, macrophages contain many cytoplasmic membrane-bound granules (both secretory and lysosomal), vacuoles, and endocytotic vesicles.

Recently, a number of laboratories have provided evidence that **dendritic cells** (Fig. 5-4) should be included as members of the mononuclear phagocyte system (Murphy and colleagues, 1986; King and Katz, 1990). Like macrophages, dendritic cells are found in numerous organs in the body but are distinct because of their unique dendritic morphology. Dendritic cells include Langerhans cells of the epidermis, follicular dendritic cells of nodal and splenic follicles, and interdigitating dendritic cells within the T-lymphocyte areas of lymph node and spleen, although there are dendritic cells in most organs that have not yet been studied in detail. Their relatedness to other mononuclear phagocytes is largely based on their ability to function as potent **antigen-presenting cells**, because they are relatively poor at phagocytosis. Like other mononuclear phagocytes, they are derived from the bone marrow, but their precise ontogenic relationship to macrophages has not been definitively established to date.

Macrophages and related cells perform varied essential roles, many of which are involved in the inflammatory process. Essentially, these roles can be divided into six different areas:

1. *Phagocytosis: originally, the fundamental raison d'etre.* Macrophages remove foreign material or organisms, necrotic tissue debris, and senescent cells by way of engulfment and digestion; this mechanism represents one of the first host defenses against pathogenic microorganisms. Like neutrophils, macrophages recognize foreign organisms or material through opsonins that bind to specific sites on both the macrophage and the foreign invader. Internalization of the material with subsequent destruction is triggered by these receptor-ligand events.

2. *Accessory cell function.* One of the primary functions of macrophages and dendritic cells is to initiate cell-mediated immune responses by presenting antigen to lymphocytes (thus their functional name as antigen-presenting cells). Antigen presentation actually involves "processing" the antigen first, which encompasses internalization and degradation of the antigen into smaller fragments. These smaller peptide fragments are then incorporated into the plasma membrane, complexed to major histocompatibility complex (MHC) molecules. It is generally accepted that T cells only recognize antigens when they are complexed with MHC molecules on the

surface of antigen-presenting cells. As mentioned previously, dendritic cells are particularly potent as antigen-presenting cells.

3. *Secretory function.* Macrophages are capable of the production and secretion of a large repertoire of proinflammatory, procoagulatory, and immune regulatory products. Procoagulatory products include coagulation factors V and VII, and thromboplastin, or tissue factor, which activates the extrinsic coagulation cascade. Proinflammatory products include IL-1, tumor necrosis factor, platelet activating factor, prostaglandins, and complement components. Additionally, macrophage-derived soluble mediators such as IL-1 and tumor necrosis factor are required to induce T-lymphocyte activation after the initial T cell recognition of antigen on the surface of the macrophage. Macrophages are also capable of the elaboration of enzymes, such as lysozyme, proteases, and lipases, which not only have the capability of killing organisms, but facilitate the digestion and subsequent removal of injured or dead tissue.

4. *Wound healing.* Macrophages play pivotal roles in wound repair. First, the macrophage functions as a phagocyte, engulfing and destroying opportunistic bacterial organisms and necrotic tissue debris. Second, it serves to orchestrate the wound healing process by producing locally acting factors that stimulate the growth of new vessels to the area and induce fibroblasts to migrate to the area, divide, and produce collagen, the primary component of scar tissue.

5. *Regulation of granulocyte and monocyte pools.* In the steady state, there is a uniform turnover of mononuclear phagocytes and granulocytes between the bone marrow, blood, and tissues. However, after tissue injury and during the inflammatory response to that injury, the rate of production of these cells increases in the bone marrow, and increased numbers of monocytes and/or granulocytes (usually neutrophils) may be detected in the peripheral circulation. The enhanced production of these cells in the bone marrow is controlled by hormonal-like factors secreted by macrophages at the site of tissue injury. These factors travel to the bone marrow via the blood stream, where they stimulate specific bone marrow stem cells to divide and differentiate to mature effector cells. Some of these factors include macrophage colony stimulating factor (M-CSF), granulocyte-macrophage colony stimulating factor (GM-CSF), granulocyte colony stimulating factor (G-CSF), and interleukin-3 (IL-3).

6. *Modulation of tumor cell growth.* Macrophages are often found within a variety of tumors. Although their function in these neoplastic tissues is not fully understood, they are, in the laboratory, able to recognize tumor cells and either inhibit their growth or kill them. The mechanisms by which macrophages are able to subserve this function likely involve the production of soluble toxic mediators, such as tumor necrosis factor and/or direct cell-to-cell contact with release of macrophage granular constit-

uents into the intercellular compartment. Whether these mechanisms mediate substantial tumor cell killing *in vivo,* however, has yet to be substantiated.

Macrophages are fully differentiated end-stage cells that do not, under normal circumstances, divide. Compared to neutrophils, macrophages live relatively long lives, having turnover times in tissues between 1 and 2 weeks. On the other hand, **multinucleate giant cells** (Fig. 5-5) have a life span of only a few days. These cells arise from the fusion of macrophages, usually in the setting of **granulomatous inflammation,** which is described later in this chapter. Multinucleate giant cells are metabolically active and produce comparable quantities of enzymes and other proteins as do single-nucleate macrophages; however, their phagocytic potential is significantly reduced. Three morphologically distinct multinucleate giant cells can be seen in tissues. **Langhans' giant cell** has many spherical nuclei arranged in a more or less complete wreath just inside its hazy and indefinite periphery. A **Touton giant cell** is similar to a Langhans' giant cell in that the nuclei are arranged in a circle, but Touton giant cells are two-toned; there is a rim of cytoplasm peripherally that is foamy, while the cytoplasm centrally is eosinophilic. These giant cells are sometimes found in settings of granulomatous inflammation involving large quantities of lipid. On the other hand, a **foreign-body giant cell** contains nuclei that are piled up in a jumbled mass at the center of the cell.

References

Adams DO. The granulomatous inflammatory response: a review. Am J Pathol 1976;84:164–191.

Chambers TJ. Multinucleate giant cells. J Pathol 1978;126:125–148.

Foucar K, Foucar E. The mononuclear phagocyte and immunoregulatory effector (M-PIRE) system: evolving concepts. Semin Diagn Pathol 1990;7:4–18.

Geppert TD, Lipsky PE. Antigen presentation at the inflammatory site. Crit Rev Immunol 1989;9:313–362.

King PD, Katz DR. Mechanisms of dendritic cell function. Immunol Today 1990;11:206–211.

Knighton DR, Fiegel VD. Macrophage-derived growth factors in wound healing: regulation of growth factor production by the oxygen microenvironment. Am Rev Respir Dis 1989;140:1108–1111.

Murphy GF, Messadi D, Fonferko E, et al. Phenotypic transformation of macrophages to Langerhans cells in the skin. Am J Pathol 1986;123:401–406.

North RJ. The concept of the activated macrophage. J Immunol 1978;121:806–809.

Papadimitriou JM, Ashman RB. Macrophages: current views on their differentiation, structure, and function. Ultrastruct Pathol 1989;13:343–372.

Unanue ER. Secretory function of mononuclear phagocytes. A review. Am J Pathol 1976;83:396–418.

Lymphocytes

The inflammatory cells described previously are similar in that they can respond to literally a limitless number of infectious organisms and foreign antigens; their specificity is not related to the cell itself, but instead to opsonization of the foreign material (for the phagocytic

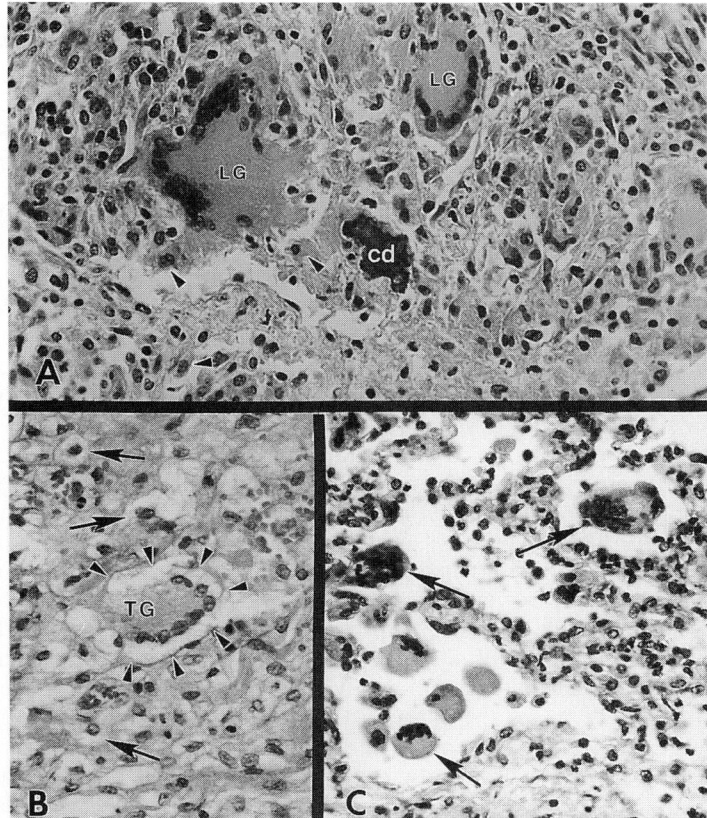

FIG. 5-5 Tissues containing multinucleate giant cells. **A.** Granulomatous inflammation in tuberculosis of an equine lung. Macrophages *(arrowheads)*, Langhans giant cells *(LG)*, and calcareous debris *(cd)* are present (× 435) (Courtesy of Dr. J.R.M. Innes and Armed Forces Institute of Pathology) **B.** Xanthomatosis, subcutis of a cat. There is granulomatous inflammation with numerous lipid-containing macrophages *(arrows)* and a Touton giant cell *(TG)*, which is characterized by a peripheral rim of foamy cytoplasm and a central core of eosinophilic cytoplasm. Arrowheads mark the cytoplasmic borders of the giant cell. (Courtesy of Laboratory of Pathology, School of Veterinary Medicine, University of Pennsylvania and the Armed Forces Institute of Pathology) **C.** Granulomatous pneumonia in a rhesus monkey infected with simian immunodeficiency virus. Multiple foreign-body giant cells *(arrows)* are present in alveolar spaces.

cells) or IgE (for the mast cells). Therefore, each granulocyte or macrophage can respond by chemoattraction, activation, phagocytosis, and killing of most foreign material, regardless of the antigenic determinants of the material. Lymphocytes, however, are unique in that they are committed from their inception to respond to specific antigens. Each lymphocyte is preprogrammed during its maturation to recognize only a single antigen; thus, there are lymphocytes circulating in the blood which together can recognize more than 10^8 antigens, most of which have never even been in contact with the host. For those antigens that the immune system has never seen, there are very few antigen-specific lymphocytes in the body. These rare circulating cells act as sentinels and can respond quickly by clonal expansion and differentiation upon antigenic challenge. The host's ability to respond, therefore, to virtually a limitless number of antigens is achieved by the circulation of large numbers of lymphocytes that each differ in their antigenic receptors. On the other hand, during an active infection with a particular organism, there is clonal expansion of lymphocytes specific for the antigens of the foreign organism, and it is only these lymphocytes that are activated to differentiate into effector cells; the other lymphocytes are passive observers.

Functionally, lymphocytes can be categorized into two broad classes. B lymphocytes are responsible for **humoral immunity,** while T lymphocytes control **cellular or cell-mediated immunity.** Morphologically, they can-

not be distinguished from each other. Resting lymphocytes are approximately 8 to 10 μm in diameter and contain a round nucleus and a narrow rim of cytoplasm (Fig. 5-6). A smaller number of lymphocytes have larger nuclei with more prominent nucleoli and a greater amount of a more basophilic cytoplasm; these are

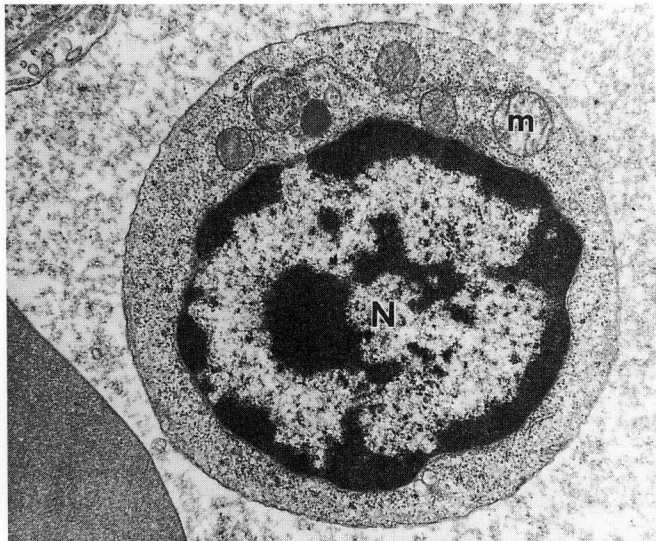

FIG. 5-6 Transmission electron photomicrograph of a lymphocyte in the peripheral blood of a marmoset *(Saguinus oedipus). N,* nucleus; *m,* mitochondria.

lymphoblasts and represent lymphocytes that have been activated to divide by antigenic stimulation. The cytoplasm of resting lymphocytes contains only mitochondria and a few small vesicles, whereas lymphoblasts contain, in addition, a prominent Golgi apparatus and endoplasmic reticulum.

B cells are specialized to make antibodies, and it is this characteristic that is used to distinguish them from T cells. They are manufactured independent of antigens in the bone marrow of mammals and in the **bursa of Fabricius** in birds, a structure in the wall of the cloaca. Although the bone marrow (and bursa in birds) is important for the *de novo* synthesis of B cells, B cells can also be made in peripheral lymphoid organs, e.g., the spleen, lymph nodes, and the gut-associated lymphoid tissue from existing B cells that divide in response to antigenic challenge. B cells represent approximately 10% of the lymphocytes in the peripheral circulation, and all of them express immunoglobulins on their cell surface. Under appropriate antigenic stimulation and signals from T cells, B cells differentiate in the tissues to **plasma cells,** which are fully differentiated cells that secrete immunoglobulins into the local microenvironment. These cells are smoothly spherical or elliptical, with much more cytoplasm (and therefore somewhat larger) than a lymphocyte (Fig. 5-7). The nucleus resembles that of a lymphocyte in being spherical, but it is almost always eccentrically placed in the cell. The cytoplasm appears homogeneous and as a rule, but not invariably, is slightly more basophilic in its staining reaction than most cytoplasm, taking a nearly magenta shade of purplish red. Often the cytoplasm contains a distinct hyaline sphere called a **Russell body.** The electron microscopic features of the nucleus are not distinctive; however, the cytoplasm, in addition to distinct Golgi bodies and mitochondria, is filled with an abundant amount of rough endoplasmic reticulum, reflecting its high capability to produce protein. Within the cisternae of the endoplasmic reticulum, homogeneous material (immunoglobulin) is found which, as it

increases in amount, dilates the cisterna and gives the Russell body its characteristic microscopic appearance. Because of the high protein production of the plasma cell, the cytoplasm is rich in messenger and transfer RNA, which imparts a positive reaction on a methyl green pyronine histochemical stain.

After differentiation, the mature B cell circulates in the blood and lymph vasculature with a half-life of probably about 2 days; however, antigen primed cells have a much longer functional life span. They can be found in strategic locations within lymphoid organs, specifically in cortical follicles of lymph nodes, follicles of the Peyer's patches in the gut (or gut-associated lymphoid tissue), or follicles of the splenic white pulp.

Immunoglobulins on the surface membranes of B cells act as receptors for antigens. The vast array of immunoglobulins produced by B cells and plasma cells, an array so diverse that virtually all natural and synthetic antigens can be recognized by a circulating pre-programmed cell, represents one of the wonders of nature, particularly since the genome used to construct these different immunoglobulins is finite in size. The method used to make such a diverse spectrum of different immunoglobulin molecules from germ-line DNA is called **gene rearrangement.** An immunoglobulin molecule is composed of two identical heavy chain subunits and two identical light chain subunits (either kappa or lambda). Each subunit is composed of variable and constant regions, and the variability of the amino acids within the variable regions is what confers the specificity of antigen binding. For example, the gene for the heavy chain in nonhematopoietic (somatic) cells is characterized by separate coding regions, termed variable (V), diversity (D), joining (J), and constant (C). Within each region (except the C region), there are multiple copies of individual segments, each differing to varying degrees one from the other. The variable region of the immunoglobulin molecule is encoded by the V, D, and J coding regions, while the constant region is encoded by the C coding region. Early in lymphocyte develop-

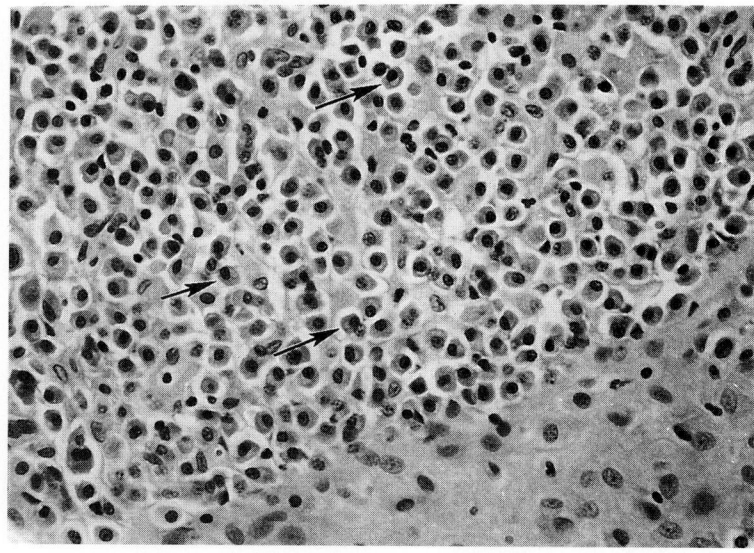

FIG. 5-7 Plasma-cell pododermatitis in a cat. There is a dense infiltrate of plasma cells within the adipose and subcutaneous connective tissue of the foot pad. Plasma cells with juxtanuclear rarefaction of cytoplasmic staining, representing the Golgi apparatus, are depicted by arrows. (Courtesy of Dr. M. Simon)

ment and apparently only in lymphocytes, one segment from the D region is brought together with one segment from the J region followed by one segment from the V region. The copy of the C region is then added, and it is the C region DNA that confers antibody isotype, so that the C_μ DNA imparts the identity of the immunoglobulin as being of the IgM isotype. With multiple combinations of gene segments possible, a large number of different genes can be constructed in the lymphocyte population, each different in size and structure and each a specific marker for an individual lymphocyte or its daughter cells. The same process occurs for light chains, except that no D region is present in these genes. The idea that all cells in the body contain the same DNA, therefore, is not true; only somatic cells containing the germ-line (all gene segments) configuration are identical. If a group of lymphocytes have identical immunoglobulin genes, then they must have arisen from one cell and thus represent a **monoclonal** or neoplastic proliferation. If a group of lymphocytes have different immunoglobulin genes, then they represent a **polyclonal** proliferation, seen for example in inflammatory reactions. It is now possible to determine this information using Southern blot analysis of DNA from lymphocytes in tissue, exudates, or blood.

B cells can be activated by two different mechanisms. Firstly, the T-independent mechanism involves antigens that have repeating epitopes, such as polysaccharides, which cross-link adjacent surface immunoglobulins on the B cell. The cross-linking of surface antibody signals the B cell to proliferate and differentiate. The second mechanism is dependent on the help of T cells and generally involves protein fragment antigens. The B cell recognizes the antigen by its surface antibody and internalizes it, processes it (a mechanism similarly done by antigen-presenting cells), and presents it on the surface bound to MHC class II molecules. The antigen is then presented to a T cell, which becomes activated and makes particular growth factors (mediators) for the B cell, directing it to divide to make memory cells or causing it to terminally differentiate to a plasma cell.

Using either mechanism, B cells are able to recognize free, unbound antigen on their cell surface. Thus, B cells represent an arm of the immune system that serves to recognize foreign antigen located in the extracellular compartment. T lymphocytes, on the other hand, are adapted to protect the host against antigens that are trapped or incorporated on or within the surface of other cells. Unlike B cells, T cells do not generally respond to free antigens. They must be presented to the T cell by antigen-presenting cells in context with MHC molecules, and these MHC molecules must be recognized as self molecules by the T cell before the T cell recognizes the antigen. This dual recognition of antigen only in context with MHC molecules is known as **MHC restriction.** MHC molecules are generally of two types: class I molecules, expressed on virtually all nucleated cells; and class II molecules (sometimes referred to as Ia antigens), only found on specialized antigen-presenting cells. MHC molecules are highly poly-

morphic and are contained within the immunoglobulin superfamily and thus have variable regions that are capable of binding antigens.

By far, the vast majority of T cells arise from precursors within the thymus. It is there that the thymocytes gain their MHC restriction and cell surface expression of accessory glycoproteins. Mature postthymic T cells constitute the majority of the lymphocytes in the peripheral blood and likely live for several months. They are not resident in any one lymphoid organ. Instead, they traverse from one lymphoid organ to another and constitute the **"recirculating lymphocyte pool."** In lymphoid organs, however, they can be found within the paracortex of lymph nodes or the nonfollicular regions of the splenic white pulp. Here they search for bloodborne antigens removed by the spleen or antigens carried to regional lymph nodes from a localized site of infection.

T cells can be essentially divided into two subsets based on their surface expression of accessory molecules and binding of MHC molecules. The CD4 molecule (cluster designation 4) is a glycoprotein found on a group of T cells that only recognize antigen when it is complexed with MHC class II self molecules, found on the surface of antigen-presenting cells (APCs). Typical APCs include Langerhans cells of the epidermis, dendritic cells of lymph node and other tissues, and macrophages. B cells and sometimes endothelial cells can also present antigen to CD4$^+$ T cells. The CD8 molecule is found on most of the other T cells so that expression of both CD4 and CD8 is mutually exclusive (except during development in the thymus). CD8$^+$ T cells only recognize antigen when it is complexed with MHC class I molecules. Both CD8 and CD4 molecules bind to the nonpolymorphic regions of their respective MHC molecules.

The T cell recognizes antigen and thus derives its tremendous specificity by virtue of its T cell receptor (TCR). It is composed of two chains of proteins, each belonging to the immunoglobulin superfamily and each undergoing gene rearrangement to form a single exon by joining segments of the V, J, D, and C regions, similar to immunoglobulins. Therefore, like immunoglobulins, the TCR has remarkable diversity between different lymphocyte clones and can recognize a tremendous number of antigens. The TCR, once bound to antigen and MHC molecules, forms a trimolecular complex that activates the cell. This activation induces the T cell to express new surface molecules, secrete cytokines, proliferate, and differentiate into effector cells. The signalling and triggering necessary for T cell activation are mediated through a set of molecules called CD3, which is complexed and in close association with the TCR. Only T cells express CD3; thus, it is a useful marker in tissues and cell suspensions for cells of the T cell lineage.

Once activated, T cells are induced to proliferate and differentiate into effector cells. T cell effector function can be classified to those functions associated either with direct cell contact with other cells or the release of soluble cytokine mediators. T cells expressing the CD4 molecule generally differentiate into cells that produce mediators that augment the functioning of, or provide help to, other immune cells, thus defining CD4$^+$ cells as **helpers/inducers.** For example, for a B cell to differentiate to a plasma cell in response to a protein antigen, T cell help from CD4$^+$ cells is crucial. This help is likely in the form of T cell-derived B cell growth factors, or cytokines, such as interleukin-4 and interleukin-5. CD8$^+$ effector cells, on the other hand, are usually engaged in the active lysis of target cells bearing foreign antigens. These **cytotoxic lymphocytes (CTLs)** are antigen-specific and MHC class I restricted, in that they only kill target cells that express both the foreign antigen (recognized by the TCR) in context with self MHC I molecules. Therefore, one animal's CTLs can only lyse target cells derived from the same animal. It should be emphasized that both types of T cells are triggered by antigen in a MHC-restricted manner, but only CD8$^+$ T cells are restricted in their effector function. That is, CTLs only kill targets expressing self MHC class I molecules, while CD4$^+$ effector cells that manufacture mediators have the potential to influence both cells expressing MHC class II and those that do not.

In the early 1970's, it was discovered that some CD8$^+$ cells, under certain laboratory conditions, can down-regulate immune reactions. The term **T suppressors** was used to describe the CD8$^+$ cells observed doing this. However, because of the difficulty in isolating and studying these cells *in vivo*, they represent something of a black box, and until their ontogeny and characterization is substantiated, the use of the term "T suppressors" should be avoided.

In addition, it should be noted that resting T lymphocytes recognize their antigen from APCs, and during antigen exposure of the host, these T cells are held up in lymphoid organs by T cell-APC binding. Once primed by antigen, these T cells, after undergoing several rounds of replication in lymphoid tissues and differentiation into effector cells, are released into the circulation. However, unlike resting T cells, they quickly leave the lymphocyte recirculating pool and migrate randomly throughout mucosal tissues, scanning the tissues for their specific antigen. They also congregate at inflammatory sites, and these preferential migratory patterns are likely controlled by endothelial-lymphocyte adhesion interactions, which are described subsequently in this chapter.

Furthermore, there is a cell in the peripheral blood of uncertain lineage that, unlike CTLs, can kill cell targets without regard to antigen recognition or MHC I expression. Therefore, they are capable of MHC-unrestricted cytotoxicity. These cells, referred to as natural killer cells (NK cells), do not express the TCR and do not rearrange the genes associated with the TCR. They may or may not express CD8 molecules. Large granular lymphocytes (LGLs) represent a subset of NK cells, but not all NK cells are LGLs. Therefore, NK cells may, in fact, represent a heterogenous group of cells composed of cells from different lineages. Thus, for the present,

they are defined only by their functional attributes and not their histogenesis.

References

Beverley PCL. Human T-cell memory. Curr Top Microbiol Immunol 1990;159:111–122.

Gray D, Leanderson T. Expansion, selection and maintenance of memory B-cell clones. Curr Top Microbiol Immunol 1990;159:1–17.

Hansson M. Growth and differentiation factors for B and T cells. Leuk Res 1990;14:705–710.

Marrack P, Kappler JW. The T cell receptors. Chem Immunol 1990;49:69–81.

Melief CJM. T cell differentiation and function. Curr Probl Dermatol 1990;19:1–8.

Paul, WE. Fundamental immunology. 2nd ed. New York: Raven Press 1989.

van der Valk P, Herman CJ. Leukocyte functions. Lab Invest 1987;57:127–137.

Whitacre CC. Immunology: a state of the art lecture. Ann NY Acad Sci 1990;594:1–16.

Young LHY. How lymphocytes kill. Annu Rev Med 1990;41:45–51.

NORMAL VASCULAR ANATOMY AND FLUID EXCHANGE

The inflammatory process, particularly when acute, is primarily a circulatory phenomenon involving changes in the amount and quality of blood reaching the affected area. These changes have already been alluded to in describing the cardinal signs of inflammation. Regardless of the nature of the injurious agent or the location of the insult, the basic character of the initial vascular response is remarkably constant. Changes in endothelial structure and metabolism, whether elicited directly by the primary insulting irritant or secondarily by mediators, are largely responsible for the circulatory events that herald inflammatory reactions. Thus, before describing this vascular response, it is important to review normal endothelial anatomy and how it functions in the steady state.

Normal vascular anatomy

The endothelial lining of small vessels (i.e., the microcirculation) varies both structurally and functionally in different organs. Endothelium can be classified into four major categories, each differentiated from one another on the basis of the continuity (or lack thereof) of the endothelial barrier.

Continuous endothelium is the most widely distributed type. It is found in arteries, arterioles, venules, veins and capillaries of most tissues, including skin, heart, lung, brain, smooth and skeletal muscle, and loose connective tissue. Adjacent endothelial cells are connected to one another through pleomorphic intercellular junctions ranging from gap junctions in muscle (15 to 20 nm separation of endothelial cell membranes) to tight junctions (in brain), where the fusion of adjacent cell membranes accounts for the blood-brain barrier. The basement membrane beneath the endothelial cells completely surrounds the vessel without interruption.

The second type of endothelium is the **fenestrated** type, which occurs in the capillaries of endocrine and exocrine glands, intestinal mucosa, and renal glomeruli. These vessels have fenestrae or openings ranging in size from 0.5 to 1.0 μm in diameter where the endothelial lining is either entirely missing, (e.g., glomerular capillaries) or is reduced to an endothelial cell membrane. The basement membrane is complete, as in continuous endothelium.

Sinusoidal vessels are the third type and are found in liver and spleen. In these vessels, the endothelial cells have numerous large deficiencies, seemingly within the cytoplasm of the cells rather than in the junctions between them. These "holes" permit the efflux of even the largest molecules from the vascular lumen. The underlying basement membrane is incomplete or entirely absent.

Lastly, a specialized endothelium is found within the postcapillary venules of lymphoid tissues. These endothelial cells are particularly large and columnar, thus accounting for their status as **"high endothelium,"** and are specialized for lymphocyte traffic from the blood to lymphoid compartments.

Normal fluid exchange

Under normal circumstances, there is a constant exchange of nutrients (i.e., glucose) and cellular by-products (i.e., CO_2) between the blood and interstitium. This essential process occurs predominantly within the capillaries, and indeed, each cell of the body is usually less than 30 μm away from a capillary loop. The exchange of substances between the vascular and extravascular compartments is normally highly regulated in each type of tissue so that the fluid escaping from the vascular bed equals the fluid that eventually returns. This precise regulation of fluid exchange is mediated by changes in pressure and flow in the capillaries. Neural and humoral factors, oxygen tension, and locally released products of metabolic activity affect pressure and flow by altering the intrinsic contractility of precapillary sphincters and the smooth muscle walls of arterioles and veins.

It is easy to understand how plasma components cross fenestrated and discontinuous endothelium. However, most tissues of the body contain continuous endothelium, and the movement of material across these vessels is not as easily understood. By far, the most important means by which plasma components cross continuous endothelium barriers is by the process of **diffusion.** Solutes diffuse across the vascular wall because of the random thermal motion of these materials back and forth across the wall. If a concentration difference exists between each side of the barrier, more of the solute crosses the barrier by chance from the more concentrated side than from the more dilute side. The result is a net "flow" from the side containing the greater concentration of the solute to the side containing the lower concentration. If there is no concentration difference, then the amount of the solute that crosses into the extracellular compartment equals the amount that enters the intracellular compartment. Lipid-soluble materials and water diffuse fairly rapidly by directly crossing the endothelial membrane. Larger molecules that are not lipid soluble cannot pass directly through the lipid bilayer of endothelial cell walls; they must use capillary intercellular slits (6 to 7 nm in diameter) or a system of "endothelial pores." The exact anatomic features of endothelial pores has not been completely elucidated, but it is clear that the passage of plasma components across the endothelium cannot be explained entirely by the direct passage of lipids and water across the endothelial membrane and/or through the intercellular slits. Whether the pore system actually involves micropinocytotic vesicles that shuttle solutes across the endothelial cell, transient transendothelial channels, transient endothelial cell discontinuities, or a combination of these is still a subject of academic debate and controversy.

Fluids and solutes also pass across the vascular wall by a process called **bulk flow.** Although more solute and fluid passes by way of diffusion, bulk flow is important because it is most affected by physiologic changes in flow and pressure. Overall, bulk transfer occurs largely because of a difference in **hydrostatic pressure** on one side of the vessel wall versus the other; usually materials travel from the area of high pressure to the area of low pressure. There is usually greater hydrostatic pressure within the intravascular space. Therefore, under normal circumstances, the passage of fluid and solute occurs *en bloc* from the intravascular space, through the capillary pores and slits, and into the interstitial space.

Normal fluid balance between the intravascular and interstitial spaces is maintained by two sets of opposing forces, each using diffusion and bulk transfer as the means to accomplish this balance. The interplay of these forces was first described by Starling in 1896 in what is now classically referred to as **Starling's law.** Briefly, E.H. Starling pointed out that under normal conditions, the amount of fluid filtered out of the arterial capillaries roughly equals the fluid returned to the venous capillaries. There are four forces responsible for this near equilibrium. **Capillary hydrostatic pressure** moves fluid out of the capillaries. At the arterial end, this pressure approximates 30 mm Hg above atmospheric pressure, while at the venous end, it roughly equals 10 mm Hg. A number of indirect measurements of capillary pressure have resulted in a figure of 17 mm Hg for mean capillary pressure. **Hydrostatic pressure of the interstitial space** represents the actual pressure exerted by the fluid entrapped between reticular fibers in the extravascular space. Although direct measurement of this pressure is difficult, indirect methods have shown it to be slightly subatmospheric, except in tissues surrounded by capsules (e.g., kidney, eye) or bone (e.g., brain), where it is slightly greater than atmospheric pressure. However, for most tissues in the body, this pressure is approximately -5.3 mm Hg, which, because of its negativity, causes the suction of fluid from vascular lumena into the interstitial space. **Plasma colloid on-**

cotic pressure is exerted when substances of high molecular weight are impeded from passing through the endothelial intercellular slits or pores. Therefore, these molecules, which consist predominantly of plasma proteins, are more concentrated in the blood than in the interstitial space. Their presence in the blood causes an oncotic pressure of approximately 28 mm Hg to be exerted on water to pass from the interstitium into the vascular space. **Interstitial fluid colloid oncotic pressure** exists because some protein from the plasma escapes into the interstitium via transport across the endothelium by transient channels, pinocytosis, or by the presence of large pores. Although the number of these molecules in the interstitium is small compared to the vascular space (and therefore, the oncotic pressure gradient is proportionally smaller), they still exert a small pressure gradient for the flow of fluid out of the vessel, which approximates 6 mm Hg.

Figure 5-8 illustrates the four forces responsible for fluid exchange in the capillary and interstitial space. As depicted, if mean pressures are used in the calculations, there is a small net outward force of fluid into the interstitial space. This **net filtration,** in the steady state, is picked up by lymphatic vessels and returned to the circulation. If actual hydrostatic pressures are used in the calculations, there is a net **outward** force of fluid at the arterial capillary and a smaller net **inward** force at the venous capillary. The effect of these resultant pressures is the flow of plasma fluid through the tissues from the

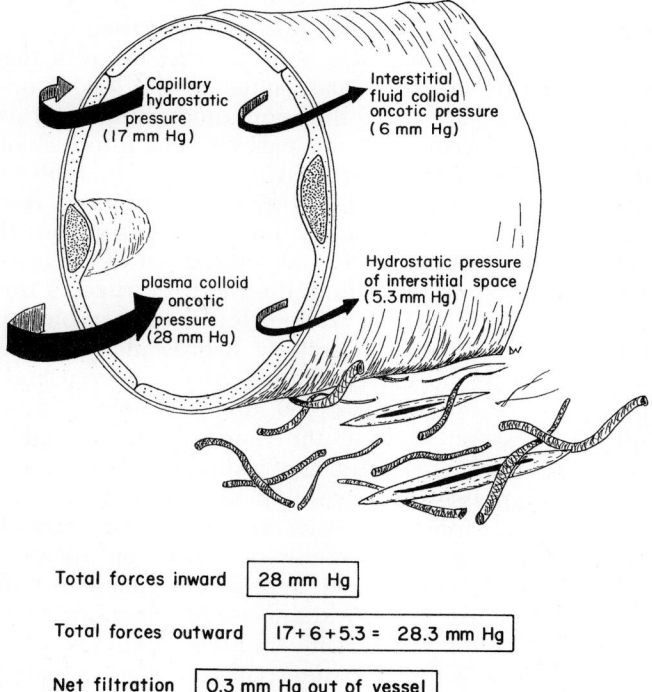

Total forces inward	28 mm Hg
Total forces outward	17 + 6 + 5.3 = 28.3 mm Hg
Net filtration	0.3 mm Hg out of vessel

FIG. 5-8 Schematic drawing of forces responsible for fluid exchange in the capillary and interstitial space. If mean pressures are used for the four forces, there is a small net outward force of fluid from the capillary lumen to the extravascular space. This remaining fluid is generally transported back into the circulation by the lymphatic vasculature.

arterial ends of the capillaries to the venous ends of the capillaries, where 90% of the fluid is normally reabsorbed by the capillary. The remaining 10% is transported back into the circulation by the lymphatic vasculature.

Because plasmic fluid exchange involves the precise balancing of these forces, perturbations in this delicate system can have significant consequences for the tissue. These perturbations and subsequent tissue changes are best exemplified during the inflammatory process.

VASCULAR ANATOMY AND FLUID EXCHANGE IN INFLAMMATION
Changes in blood flow in inflammation

When a tissue is initially injured, the amount and quality of blood reaching the damaged site is significantly altered. After mechanical stroking of skin, for example, changes in blood flow are manifested by pallor (decreased flow) or redness (increased flow). These gross tissue changes each have a microscopic correlate.

The first response to injury involves a **transient constriction** of arterioles. Cohnheim in 1889 was the first to realize that this change does not always occur, but when it does, many capillaries that once carried blood collapse as a result of decreased capillary hydrostatic pressure and flow. Apparently, this arteriolar constriction results from smooth muscle contraction of the arteriolar wall, which is mediated directly by the damaging stimulus. The result at the gross tissue level is localized, transient pallor.

The next response is **widespread dilation** of arterioles and venules. Capillaries that were collapsed are opened, and the tissue becomes hyperemic, red (rubor) and warm (calor). Chemical mediators, most notably prostaglandins, are responsible for the relaxation of arteriolar smooth muscle and the subsequent dilation and increased capillary blood flow. Initially, blood flows very rapidly through the dilated vasculature, and this flow rate can last minutes or hours depending on the severity and nature of the inciting noxious event. After the primary dilation of vessels at the injured site, a more extensive halo or flare develops and radiates peripherally from the area. This hyperemia, likewise, results from dilation of arterioles and veins. However, the cause of this flare results, in part, from the axon reflex, a direct neuronal effect.

Because of arteriolar dilation, blood flow increases rapidly and hydrostatic pressure increases in all vessels. The forces maintaining normal fluid exchange (Starling's law) are perturbed, and the increase in vascular hydrostatic pressure results in the exudation of protein-rich fluid into the interstitial space. (In reality, increased hydrostatic force is not the only mechanism accounting for vascular leakage, as discussed later.) Consequently, tissue swelling or edema (tumor) ensues. The loss of vascular fluid without concomitant loss of cells results in the increase of blood viscosity, and more force is necessary to push the viscous blood through the venules and capillaries. Because the pressure driving this flow remains the same, the blood slows and, in some cases, stops altogether, resulting in **vascular stasis.** If flow doesn't begin again, the tissue perfused by these capillaries dies.

As the blood slows, erythrocytes, leucocytes, and platelets begin to distribute themselves more evenly throughout the vascular lumen, i.e., blood flow becomes **nonlaminar.** Under normal, noninflammatory circumstances, heavier solid elements of the blood are drawn to the center of the flow. However, when flow slows, the axial congregation of cells becomes less pronounced and more cells are found nearer to the endothelial wall. This nonlaminar flow is beneficial for the eventual emigration of these cells through the vascular wall into the interstitial space.

Changes in vascular permeability in inflammation

Increased vascular permeability to proteinacious fluid is one of the most noticeable changes that occur during the inflammatory reaction, and, as previously mentioned, it is this phenomenon that accounts for the stasis of venous and capillary blood flow. In addition, the leakage of fluid into the interstitial space leads to tissue swelling (tumor) or edema. Collection of fluid within the tissues occurs because removal of this fluid by the lymphatics cannot keep pace with the volume leaking from the vessels.

There are three patterns of vascular leakage associated with acute inflammation. The **immediate transient response** occurs just after mild tissue injury and lasts for 30 minutes or less. Chemical mediators, such as histamine from degranulated mast cell granules, leukotrienes from leukocytes, bradykinin and other activated proteins in the serum, and acetyl-glyceryl-ether-phosphorycholine (AGEPC) or platelet activating factor (PAF) are responsible for this effect. Leakage of this type almost exclusively occurs in the postcapillary venules, as shown by Majno and colleagues (1961), who followed intravenously injected colloidal carbon through the vasculature of the rat cremaster muscle after exposure to histamine. They found that venules between 20 and 30 μm in diameter became black with intramural collections of carbon while arterioles and smaller capillaries were spared. In a companion study, Majno and Palade (1961), demonstrated that colloidal carbon within these venules was deposited near widened endothelial intercellular gap junctions and between the endothelium and basement membrane. These results (subsequently confirmed by others) suggested that the increased permeability of this response was caused by the presence of transiently widened gaps between individual endothelial cell membranes, which allowed plasma containing larger proteins that were normally prevented from traversing through the vascular wall to easily escape through the endothelial barrier. Apparently, the unaltered basement membrane provided some degree of filtration capacity to the escaping protein-rich fluid.

Just how do these endothelial gaps form? In a later

study, Majno and colleagues (1969), found morphologic changes to endothelial nuclei that suggested contraction of the cell. They hypothesized that if sufficient hydrostatic pressure was available in the venule when this contraction occurred, then intercellular gaps would form (Fig. 5-9). Supporting this hypothesis was the finding by Becker and Murphy (1969) that endothelial cells contain cytoplasmic contractile actin filaments. The result is that endothelial contraction with concurrent increased hydrostatic pressure (from arteriolar dilation) act synergistically to culminate in increased vascular permeability. Although these two processes can act independently, the effect of either one on vascular permeability is significantly smaller than the combined effect of both acting together (Fig. 5-9).

The **immediate-sustained** reaction also occurs immediately after tissue injury, but lasts from several hours to several days. It usually occurs after especially severe injuries, and leakage of vessels results from direct damage to the endothelial cells. All vessels, including arterioles, capillaries, and venules are affected by this nonspecific insult.

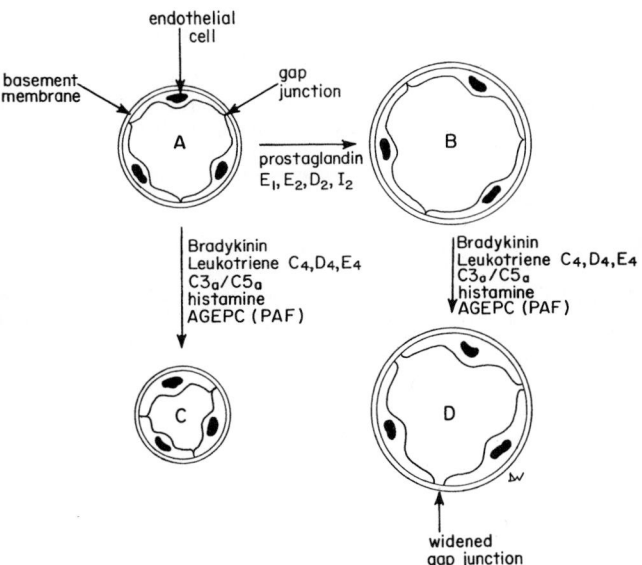

FIG. 5-9 The immediate-transient response. Diagrammatic representation of a post-capillary venule *(PCV)*, demonstrating the synergistic action of vasodilation and endothelial contraction on vascular permeability. **A.** Normal PCV. **B.** Response to prostaglandins, arterioles dilate, resulting in increased hydrostatic pressure in PCVs. The PCV is stretched, but the endothelium remains fixed in relation to basement membrane. Very little widening of gap junctions occurs. **C.** Response to certain mediators (i.e., bradykinin, leukotrienes, complement components, among others); the endothelium contracts, but the hydrostatic pressure in the PCV may not be sufficient to keep vessel dilated. Subsequently, very little widening of the gap junctions occurs: increased permeability is partially dependent on increased hydrostatic pressure. **D.** When prostaglandins and other mediators work in concert, the endothelium contracts in relation to the basement membrane while the vessel remains dilated as a result of increased hydrostatic pressure. The result is widening of the gap junctions and subsequent leakage of plasma proteins from the PCV.

The **delayed-prolonged** response usually occurs some time after the initial inciting injury, peaks in 2 to 4 hours, and then gradually subsides by 6 to 8 hours after tissue injury. Many of us have experienced this response in our own skin by sunbathing; 3 hours after intense sun exposure, the skin is red, hot, and swollen. In contrast to the immediate-transient response in which leakage occurs almost exclusively from venules, Cotran and Majno (1964) have shown that, in the delayed-prolonged response, leakage occurs from venules and capillaries. Whether this leakage occurs through intercellular gaps or directly damaged endothelium is still a topic of debate.

References

Becker CG, Murphy GE. Demonstrations of contractile protein in endothelium and cells of the heart valves, endocardium, intima, arteriosclerotic plaques, and Aschoff bodies of rheumatic heart disease. Am J Pathol 1969;55:1–37.

Cotran RS. The delayed and prolonged vascular leakage in inflammation: II. An electron microscopic study of the vascular response after thermal injury. Am J Pathol 1965;46:589–620.

Cotran RS, Majno G. The delayed and prolonged vascular leakage in inflammation: I. Topography of the leaking vessels after thermal injury. Am J Pathol 1964;45:261–281.

Ham KN, Hurley JV. An electron-microscope study of the vascular response to mild thermal injury in the rat. J Pathol Bacteriol 1968;95:175–183.

Hay JB, Hobbs BB, Johnston MG, et al. The role of hyperemia in cellular hypersensitivity reactions. Int Arch Allergy Appl Immunol 1977;55:324–331.

Hurley JV. An electron microscopic study of leucocytic emigration and vascular permeability in rat skin. Aust J Exp Biol 1963;41:171–186.

Majno G, Joris I. Endothelium 1977: a review. Adv Exp Med 1978;104:169–225, 481–526.

Majno G, Palade GE. Studies on inflammation. I. The effect of histamine and serotonin on vascular permeability: an electron microscopic study. J Biophys Biochem Cytol 1961;11:571–605.

Majno G, Gilmore V, Leventhal M. On the mechanism of vascular leakage caused by histamine-type mediators. Circ Res 1967;21:833–847.

Majno G, Palade GE, Schoefl GI. Studies on inflammation. II. The site of action of histamine and serotonin along the vascular tree: a topographic study. J Biophys Biochem Cytol 1961;11:607–627.

Majno G, Shea SM, Leventhal M. Endothelial contraction induced by histamine-type mediators. J Cell Biol 1969;42:647–672.

Pappenheimer JR, Renkin EM, Borrero LM. Filtration, diffusion and molecular sieving through peripheral capillary membranes. Am J Physiol 1951;167:13–46.

Simionescu N, Simionescu M, Palade GE. Permeability of muscle capillaries to small hemepeptides: evidence for the existence of patent transendothelial channels. J Cell Biol 1975;64:586–607.

Vane J, Botting R. Inflammation and the mechanism of action of anti-inflammatory drugs. FASEB J 1987;1:89–96.

CELLULAR EVENTS IN THE ACUTE INFLAMMATORY REACTION

Aside from hyperemia and an increase in vascular permeability, the influx of leukocytes (primarily neutrophils and monocytes) from the peripheral circulation to the extracellular space represents one of the most important manifestations of the acute inflammatory reaction. These cells are primarily responsible for the engulfment (a process referred to as **phagocytosis**) and killing of bacteria and the removal of tissue debris and immune complexes. In addition, these cells manufacture important cytokines, enzymes, and oxidizing reagents that serve to either regulate the severity of the inflammatory response or facilitate the removal of necrotic tissue so that the process of repair can begin. For example, prostaglandins and leukotrienes, two important classes of mediators produced by leukocytes either during the process of migration to the extracellular space or after reaching the perivascular domain, can largely account for the heightened vascular leakage previously described. Therefore, perturbations in fluid balance that occur in the inflammatory response are for the most part cell-dependent, since depletion of neutrophils in experimental animals abrogates the development of dilated, leaky vessels (Issekutz, 1981; Cybulsky and others, 1988). In addition to being the source of important immunoregulatory molecules, leukocytes and neutrophils (in particular) can cause considerable damage to fixed tissue cells by the production of damaging oxygen radicals and enzymes. These oxygen metabolites and enzymes can damage endothelium directly, resulting in leakage independent of that from mediator influence.

The process of migration of leukocytes to an area of tissue damage can be explained in principal by the interaction of cell-surface proteins that control adherence and chemoattractant concentration differences that control migration (Springer, 1990). This process in the acute inflammatory reaction can be temporally divided into four stages:

Margination This event is the first step in the complicated process of cell migration from the intravascular space to the extravascular compartment. As described previously, when fluid dynamics and flow in the vessel are perturbed so that fluid is lost into the interstitial space, the normal axial flow of cells in the vessel is lost. Flow becomes nonlaminar, and instead of traveling in the central axis of the vessel, the cells **marginate** along the periphery of the vessel, closest to the endothelial surface. This event facilitates the next step in the migratory process.

Adhesion At sites of acute inflammation, neutrophils and later, monocytes and lymphocytes, stick to the luminal endothelial surface. This process only occurs in postcapillary venules and small veins and was first noticed by Cohnheim in his now classic frog tongue experiments. The mechanisms responsible for leukocyte adhesion are complex, and many intriguing questions remain to be answered. However, it is clear that the process of adhesion is explained by the modulation of receptor and ligand proteins on both endothelium and leukocytes. Therefore, adhesion involves both endothelial-dependent and leukocyte-dependent mechanisms.

Endothelial-dependent mechanisms have been proposed to explain leukocyte adhesion largely because endothelial cells of postcapillary venules in sites of inflammation hypertrophy (become plump) and synthesize new proteins normally absent or found only sparingly in resting vascular beds (Fig. 5-10). Endothelial cells in culture can be stimulated or activated with macrophage-related cytokines, such as IL-I or TNF-α

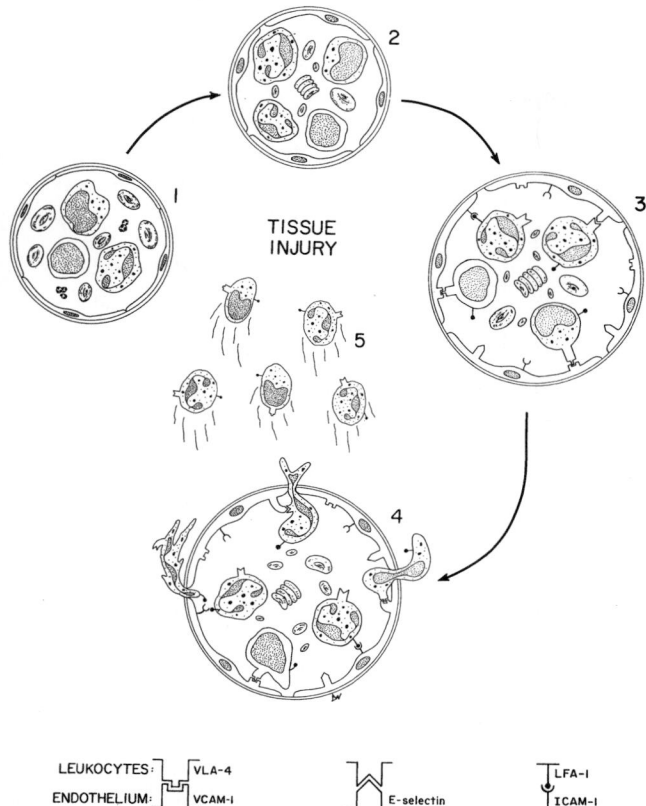

LEUKOCYTES: ⊢ VLA-4   ⊤ LFA-I
ENDOTHELIUM: ⊢ VCAM-I   ⋀ E-selectin   ⊥ ICAM-I

FIG. 5-10 Evolving leukocyte margination, adhesion, emigration, and chemotaxis in and around a post-capillary venule *(PCV)* near a site of tissue injury. (1) Normal PCV. (2) Margination. In response to mediators released from fixed cells at the site of injury, endothelial cells contract, creating gap junctions between them. Vascular permeability increases, plasma escapes into the extravascular space, and the blood in the vessel becomes more viscous. The normal axial flow of the blood becomes nonlaminar, so the leukocytes marginate along the endothelial surface. (3) Adhesion. The mediators released from local fixed cells induce the expression of new protein receptors on the endothelial and leukocyte surface. Complementary receptor-ligand interactions between leukocytes and endothelium cause the leukocytes to stick to the endothelial cell surface. (4) Emigration. Adherent leukocytes force pseudopodia through endothelial intercellular gap junctions and squeeze through to the extracellular space. (5) Chemotaxis. The leukocytes are attracted to the area of tissue injury by following a concentration gradient of a soluble attractant. See text for some representative attractants.

(Table 5-1), which induce the adhesion of neutrophils, monocytes, lymphocytes, and some leukocyte cell lines to the endothelial surface (Munro and others, 1989; Bevilacqua and others, 1985; Pober and others, 1986; Rice and others, 1990). Cytokine-mediated activation of endothelium involves the *de novo* production of receptor proteins on the endothelial cell membrane, which interact with complementary proteins on leukocytes. Adhesion then involves receptor-ligand interactions between the membranes of leukocytes and endothelium.

There are principally three classes of adhesion molecules: (1) the **immunoglobulin superfamily;** (2) the **in-**

tegrin family; and (3) the **selectin family** (Chapter 7). These three families include many different molecules that are important in cell-to-cell interactions in the immune response, but for the purposes of this chapter, only those involved in leukocyte-endothelial interactions are discussed.

There are four major endothelial adhesion proteins that have been isolated and characterized. In the selectin family is **E-selectin** (originally referred to as **ELAM-1**). E-selectin is the first endothelial adhesion molecule induced by certain cytokines such as IL-1 and TNF-α and peaks between 2 and 4 hours after exposure to cytokine (Munro and others, 1989). It is present, however, only transiently and begins to disappear within 12 to 24 hours without repeated stimulation (Fig. 5-11). It has been shown to mediate, at least in part, the adhesion of polymorphonuclear cells to the endothelial surface.

Another selectin believed to mediate endothelial adhesion of polymorphonuclear cells very early in the inflammatory reaction is P-selectin (once referred to as GMP-140 or PADGEM). This protein differs from E-selectin in that it is found constitutively in cytoplasmic Weibel-Palade bodies of resting endothelial cells. However, during endothelial activation and within minutes, it is redistributed to the endothelial cell membrane where it mediates neutrophil adherence.

Therefore, because of these two selectins, the cell type first seen in the inflammatory exudate is the neutrophil. In the immunoglobulin superfamily are two endothelial adhesion proteins: **intercellular adhesion molecule 1 (ICAM-1)** and most recently, **vascular cell adhesion molecule 1 (VCAM-1)** (Rice and colleagues, 1990; Osborn and colleagues, 1989). ICAM-1 contributes to the endothelial adhesion of most leukocyte cell types, including neutrophils, monocytes, and lymphocytes. However, ICAM-l-dependent binding of lymphocytes may play only a minor role in lymphocyte recognition of endothelial markers. Probably more important in lymphocyte and monocyte adhesion to endothelium is involvement of the newly described endothelial protein, VCAM-1 (also referred to as INCAM-110). Like E-selectin, both ICAM-1 and VCAM-1 appear on the endothelial cell membrane in response to cytokines such as IL-1 and TNF-α, but they appear later than E-selectin and persist for longer periods of time (Fig. 5-11). The temporal expression of these four endothelium adhesion proteins in response to cytokine stimulation provides a mechanism for what pathologists have described for decades: the first cell to arrive at a site of tissue damage is the neutrophil followed later by lymphocytes and monocytes.

In contrast to the effects of IL-1, which only acts on endothelium to induce adhesion molecules, other mediators increase leukocyte adhesion to endothelium by either acting principally on leukocytes or on both leukocytes and endothelium. Complement components and TNF-α, in particular, induce a family of cell surface glycoproteins on leukocytes designated **β2 integrins.** These molecules are a trio of heterodimers, one of which is termed **lymphocyte function-related antigen-1** (LFA-1 or CD11/CD18). LFA-1 serves as the leukocyte

TABLE 5-1 **Summary of cytokines and their functions**

Cytokine	Source	Effects
IL-1 α/β	Predominantly activated macrophages, but other cell types, including endothelium, epithelium, and fibroblasts	1. T-cell activation/proliferation; induces cytokine release from lymphocytes, induces IL-2 receptor on lymphocytes 2. Endogenous pyrogen 3. Causes mobilization of neutrophils from bone marrow; chemoattractant 4. Activation of endothelium 5. Induces cartilage and bone resorption, and muscle proteolysis 6. Activation of macrophages and chemoattractant 7. Mitogenic effect for fibroblasts 8. Membrane perturbation and activation of phospholipase A_2 and release of arachidonic acid 9. Partly responsible for hepatocyte acute phase reaction 10. Stimulates collagenase from fibroblasts 11. Activates B cells (cofactor in proliferation) 12. Enhances natural killer (NK) cell activity
IL-2	Activated T lymphocytes	1. Cofactor in replication and differentiation of T and B cells and NK cells
IL-3 (multi-colongy stimulating factor or multi-CSF)	Activated T lymphocytes	1. Supports viability and differentiation of hematopoietic progenitors in bone marrow (including granulocytes, macrophages, megakaryocytes, mast cells, erythroid cells, and T and B cells)
IL-4	Activated T lymphocytes	1. Costimulant for B cell proliferation 2. Increases MHC class II expression 3. Induces T cell activation 4. Stimulatory effect on hematopoietic progenitors 5. Inhibits macrophage cytokine production under special circumstances
IL-5	Activated T lymphocytes	1. Stimulates proliferation of activated B cells (in mice) 2. Induces eosinophil differentiation 3. Differentiation of cytotoxic T cells 4. Upregulation of IL-2 receptors on T cells
IL-6	Many different activated cell types, including fibroblasts, macrophages, endothelium, T and B cells, mesangial cells, keratinocytes	1. B-cell growth and differentiation 2. Synergizes with IL-1 for induction of T cell proliferation 3. Induces generation of cytotoxic T cells 4. Induction of hepatocellular acute phase response 5. Endogenous pyrogen 6. Enhances NK cell cytotoxicity
IL-7	Unknown cells in spleen, thymus, and bone marrow	1. Promotion of B-cell precursor differentiation 2. Proliferation of mitogen-activated T cells
IL-8	Activated T lymphocytes and monocytes, endothelial cells, fibroblasts	1. Leukocyte-endothelial adhesion inhibitor 2. Activates neutrophils by increasing superoxide anion production, degranulation, and arachidonic acid metabolites 3. Potent neutrophil chemoattractant

(continued)

TABLE 5-1 (continued)

Cytokine	Source	Effects
IL-9	Activated T lymphocytes	1. T cell growth factor 2. Supports growth of erythroid progenitors 3. Stimulates mast cells
IL-10	Activated T lymphocytes	1. Inhibits cytokine synthesis from other T cells (cytokine synthesis inhibitory factor)
TNF-α (Cachectin)	Activated macrophages; possibly mast cells	1. Mimics most effects of IL-1, except for lymphocyte activation 2. Inhibits hematopoietic precursor growth 3. Hemorrhagic necrosis of some tumors 4. Stimulates GM-CSF from lung fibroblasts and endothelium 5. Suppresses lipoprotein lipase 6. Principal mediator in gram-negative shock (endocrine role) 7. Activation of neutrophils (CD 18 induction, chemotaxis, degranulation) 8. Activation of endothelium 9. Enhances macrophage cytotoxic potential (autocrine role) 10. Inhibits thrombomodulin 11. Stimulates production of other cytokines and arachidonic acid metabolites in some cells (paracrine role) 12. Mitogenic for fibroblasts 13. Induces bone and cartilage resorption
Monocyte chemotactic and activating factor (MCAF)	Activated T lymphocytes and monocytes; activated endothelial cells, fibroblasts	1. Potent monocyte chemoattractant 2. Activates monocytes
Tumor necrosis factor-β (lymphotoxin)	Activated lymphocytes	1. Same as TNF-α
Interferon-γ	Activated lymphocytes	1. Suppresses hematopoietic colony formation 2. Induces MHC class I and class II molecules on multiple cell types 3. Increases numbers of TNF-α receptors on certain cell lines 4. Activates macrophages and induces cytokine production 5. Antiviral activity 6. Activates endothelium (induces ICAM-1 molecules)
Granulocyte macrophage colony-stimulating factor (GM-CSF)	T cells, endothelium, fibroblasts	1. Promotes neutrophilic, eosinophilic, macrophage bone marrow colonies 2. Activates mature granulocytes and macrophages
Granulocyte colony-stimulating factor (G-CSF)	Monocytes, fibroblasts	1. Promotes neutrophilic colonies 2. Activates mature granulocytes
Macrophage colony-stimulating factor (M-CSF, or CSF-1)	Monocytes, fibroblasts, endothelium	1. Promotes macrophage colonies 2. Activates mature macrophages

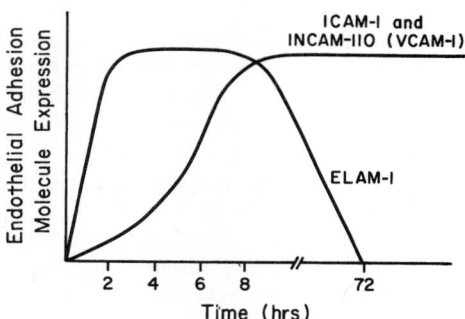

FIG. 5-11 Patterns of expression of adhesion molecules on endothelium after cytokine stimulation. E-selectin appears first, but begins to disappear within 12 to 24 hours. ICAM-1 and VCAM-1, on the other hand, increase later than E-selectin and persist for longer periods of time. Moderate ICAM-1 expression is found in normal resting endothelial cells before stimulation.

receptor for the endothelial ICAM-1 protein described above. The importance of LFA-1 to adhesion and the subsequent mounting of an inflammatory response is emphasized by the recently described human congenital disease, leukocyte adhesion deficiency (LAD), whereby afflicted patients have mutations in the $\beta2$ chain of the LFA-1 molecule (Springer, 1985). Subsequently, these patients are less able to localize inflammatory cells to areas of tissue damage and thus are susceptible to life-threatening infections and impaired wound healing. The **$\beta1$ integrins** are composed of a group of six adhesion proteins called **very late antigen (VLA)** proteins, so named because the first two proteins isolated from this group were induced on lymphocytes weeks after primary antigenic stimulation. VLA-4 is constitutively expressed on resting lymphocytes and monocytes, and this protein is the ligand for VCAM-1. The leukocyte-associated ligand for the other endothelial molecules, E-selectin and P-selectin, have yet to be fully characterized. How these molecules interrelate during an acute inflammatory response in the vascular bed is diagrammatically represented in Fig. 5-10. For a more complete discussion of adhesion molecules, the reader is encouraged to see the relevant sections of Chapter 7.

Emigration Adherent leukocytes migrate along the endothelial surface until they reach an intercellular junction. They force pseudopodia through the intercellular junction, squeeze through the endothelium, and then break through the basement membrane into the extracellular space (Fig. 5-10). The mechanisms by which leukocytes traverse the basement membrane is unkown but may involve an active enzymatic digestion of the basement membrane. Often erythrocytes follow leukocytes across the endothelial barrier, but in contrast to the active process of leukocyte emigration, erythrocyte **diapedesis** is a passive process, requires no energy, no ameboid movement, or adherence to endothelium. The erythrocytes are not considered as having any effect on the inflammatory process. In some cases, their number increases, leading to the designation **hemorrhagic**

inflammation. Although leukocyte emigration and increased vascular permeability often occur simultaneously, they are separate phenomena and one can, under special circumstances, occur without the other.

Chemotaxis The force that attracts leukocytes into inflamed or damaged tissues is called **chemotaxis** and is defined as directed cellular migration along a concentration gradient of a soluble attractant. Therefore, migrating leukocytes travel toward the source of the attractant or in the direction of increasing concentration. The mechanism by which cells "sense" concentration gradients is multiple receptors for the attractant on the cell surface and comparison of the concentration at different locations on the cell membrane. Thus, ameboid movement occurs towards the side of the cell with the greatest concentration of the attractant. Leukocytes only travel along surfaces and cannot move in the fluid phase. Often the surface that is used is fibrin, which forms from the exudation of plasma proteins, but any surface suffices. Of the many factors isolated and tested, those that appear most important as chemotactic factors include soluble bacterial products; complement components, especially C5a; byproducts of the arachidonic acid lipoxygenase pathways (p. 137) such as leukotriene B4 and 5–HETE; and factors and cytokines (e.g., IL-8) (Table 5-1) released from activated lymphocytes (lymphokines), macrophages, neutrophils, mast cells, and basophils. Once at the site of tissue damage, leukocytes are prepared to subserve their function.

In addition to chemotaxis, whether lymphocytes and monocytes remain at an inflammatory site partly depends on the other VLA proteins. To date, six of these proteins have been characterized, and five (VLA-1,2,4,5,6) either increase in quantity on mononuclear leukocytes or increase their avidity for their respective ligand in response to activation stimuli. As previously mentioned, VLA-4 serves as the ligand for the endothelial adhesion molecule, VCAM-1. All six represent receptors for either one or more of the extracellular matrix components fibronectin, laminin, and collagen. Modulation of VLA proteins on lymphocytes and monocytes thus define the affinity of these cells for its extravascular microenvironmental milieu. In simple terms, the expression of these cell membrane proteins in response to antigen, cytokine, or other activation signals make the leukocyte "stickier" once it has traversed out of the vascular space.

References

Bevilacqua MP, Pober JS, Mendrick DL, et al. Identification of an inducible endothelial-leukocyte adhesion molecule. Proc Natl Acad Sci USA 1987;84:9238–9242.

Bevilacqua MP, Pober JS, Wheeler ME, et al. Interleukin 1 acts on cultured human vascular endothelium to increase the adhesion of polymorphonuclear leukocytes, monocytes, and related leukocyte cell lines. J Clin Invest 1985;76:2003–2011.

Cotran RS. American Association of Pathologists President's Address: New roles for the endothelium in inflammation and immunity. Am J Pathol 1987;129:407–413.

Cybulsky MI, Chan MKW, Movat HZ. Acute inflammation and microthrombosis induced by endotoxin, interleukin-1, and tumor necrosis factor and their implication in gram-negative infection. Lab Invest 1988;58:365–378.

Issekutz AC. Vascular responses during acute neutrophilic inflammation: their relationship to *in vivo* neutrophil emigration. Lab Invest 1981;45:435–441.

Jalkanen S, Steere AC, Fox RI, et al. A distinct endothelial cell recognition system that controls lymphocyte traffic into inflamed synovium. Science 233:556–558.

Kelley JL, Rozek MM, Suenram CA, et al. Activation of human peripheral blood monocytes by lipoproteins. Am J Pathol 1988;130:223–231.

Kramer N, Perez HD, Goldstein IM. An immunoglobulin (IgG) inhibitor of polymorphonuclear leukocyte motility in a patient with recurrent infection. N Engl J Med 1980;303:1253–1258.

Marchesi VT, Gowans JL. The migration of lymphocytes through the endothelium of venules in lymph nodes: an electron microscope study. Proc R Soc Biol Med 1963;159:283–290.

Movat HZ, Burrowes CE, Cybulsky MI, et al. Acute inflammation and a Shwartzman-like reaction induced by interleukin-1 and tumor necrosis factor: synergistic action of the cytokines in the induction of inflammation and microvascular injury. Am J Pathol 1987;129:463–476.

Munro JM, Pober JS, Cotran RS. Tumor necrosis factor and interferon-γ induce distinct patterns of endothelial activation and associated leukocyte accumulation in skin of *Papio anubis*. Am J Pathol 1989;135:121–133.

Nightingale G, Hurley JV. Relationship between lymphocyte emigration and vascular endothelium in chronic inflammation. Pathology 1978;10:27–44.

Osborn L, Hession C, Tizard R, et al. Direct expression cloning of vascular cell adhesion molecule 1, a cytokine-induced endothelial protein that binds to lymphocytes. Cell 1989;59:1203–1211.

Paz RA, Spector WG. The mononuclear-cell response to injury. J Pathol Bacteriol 1962;84:85–103.

Pober JS, Bevilacqua MP, Mendrick DL, et al. Two distinct monokines, interleukin 1 and tumor necrosis factor, each independently induce biosynthesis and transient expression of the same antigen on the surface of cultured human vascular endothelial cells. J Immunol 1986;136:1680–1687.

Rice GE, Bevilacqua MP. An inducible endothelial cell surface glycoprotein mediates melanoma adhesion. Science 1989;246:1303–1306.

Rice GE, Munro JM, Bevilacqua MP. Inducible cell adhesion molecule 110 (INCAM-110) is an endothelial receptor for lymphocytes: a CD11/CD184–independent adhesion mechanism. J Exp Med 1990;171:1369–1374.

Schoefl GI. The migration of lymphocytes across the vascular endothelium in lymphoid tissue: a reexamination. J Exp Med 1972;136:568–588.

Spada CS, Woodward DF, Hawley SB, et al. Synergistic effects of LTB$_4$ and LTD$_4$ on leukocyte emigration into the guinea pig conjunctiva. Am J Pathol 1988;130:354–368.

Springer TA. The LFA-1, Mac-1 glycoprotein family and its deficiency in an inherited disease. Fed Proc 1985;44:2660–2677.

Springer TA. Adhesion receptors of the immune system. Nature 1990;346:425–434.

Springer TA, Dustin ML, Kishimoto TK, et al. The lymphocyte function-associated LFA-1, CD2, and LFA-3 molecules: cell adhesion receptors of the immune system. Annu Rev Immunol 1987;5:223–252.

Zigmond SH. Mechanisms of sensing chemical gradients by polymorphonuclear leukocytes. Nature 1974;249:250–252.

CONSEQUENCES OF VASCULAR PERMEABILITY CHANGES AND CELLULAR EVENTS

Because of increased hydrostatic pressure in postcapillary venules and increased vascular permeability, serum escapes into the extravascular space. This fluid flow results in **edema,** or swelling of the inflamed tissues. The separation of endothelial gap junctions allows large protein molecules, such as albumin, to escape into the interstitium. Therefore, the specific gravity of this exudate approaches that of the blood plasma itself, and all of the proteins in the plasma appear in the exudate. This is a beneficial situation. In the first place, the fluid greatly dilutes toxic substances formed within the body or introduced from without. In such conditions as bee stings and snake bites, this dilution process is of primary importance. An even more important benefit in infectious inflammations is the fact that plasma brings with it antibodies against the pathogen, if the victim had developed a humoral immune response against the organism. Lastly, plasma brings with it all the components of the plasma enzyme systems, which are uniquely integrated into the initiation, control, and resolution of the inflammatory process.

These enzyme systems are a complex interrelating process that produce biologically active molecules and peptide fragments. Although they are interrelated (Fig. 5-12), the four enzyme systems are considered separately.

The Coagulation Cascade. The clotting system is described in detail in Chapter 6. Briefly, clotting may be initiated by activation of either the intrinsic or extrinsic pathway. The intrinsic pathway is initiated by activation of the Hageman factor (Factor XII) by contact with negatively charged surfaces (e.g., a vascular wall with denuded endothelium). The extrinsic pathway begins when tissue thromboplastin (tissue factor), a hydrophobic protein manufactured by normal and activated macrophages, endothelium, fibroblasts, and other fixed cells, activates Factor VII. Both pathways converge at the activation of Factor X, which ultimately results in the production of thrombin and the conversion of fibrinogen to fibrin. Thus, a fibrin clot forms at the site of plasma leakage, and fibrin gel formation is often seen in histologic sections of inflamed tissues. Fibrin is very important in the inflammatory process, because it provides a matrix for the chemotactic migration of leukocytes into the area. Leukocytes cannot "swim" in a pool of liquid plasma; thus, the fibrin gel provides a substrate for leukocyte migration, and furthermore, provides a limited barrier to motile foreign organisms.

The Kinin System. Activated Hageman factor (Factor XIIa, sometimes referred to as prekallikrein activator), while participating in the intrinsic coagulation cascade, also serves another function. Activated Hageman factor initiates the cleavage of prekallikrein, a plasma protein, to kallikrein (Fig. 5-12). Kallikrein, in turn, digests another plasma protein zymogen, high molecular weight kininogen (HMW-kininogen), to generate the vasoactive peptide **bradykinin.** Prekallikrein and HMW-kininogen circulate as a bimolecular complex. Bradykinin has potent pharmacologic effects. First, it induces endothelial contraction, thus widening endothelial gap junctions and increasing vascular permeability. Second, it causes vasodilation, thus amplifying the increased vasopermeability effects. Third, it activates phospholipase A$_2$, which in turn liberates arachidonic acid and arachidonic metabolites that have profound vasopermeability effects in their own right. Lastly, bradykinin induces local pain.

Fibrinolytic System. The fibrinolytic system serves as

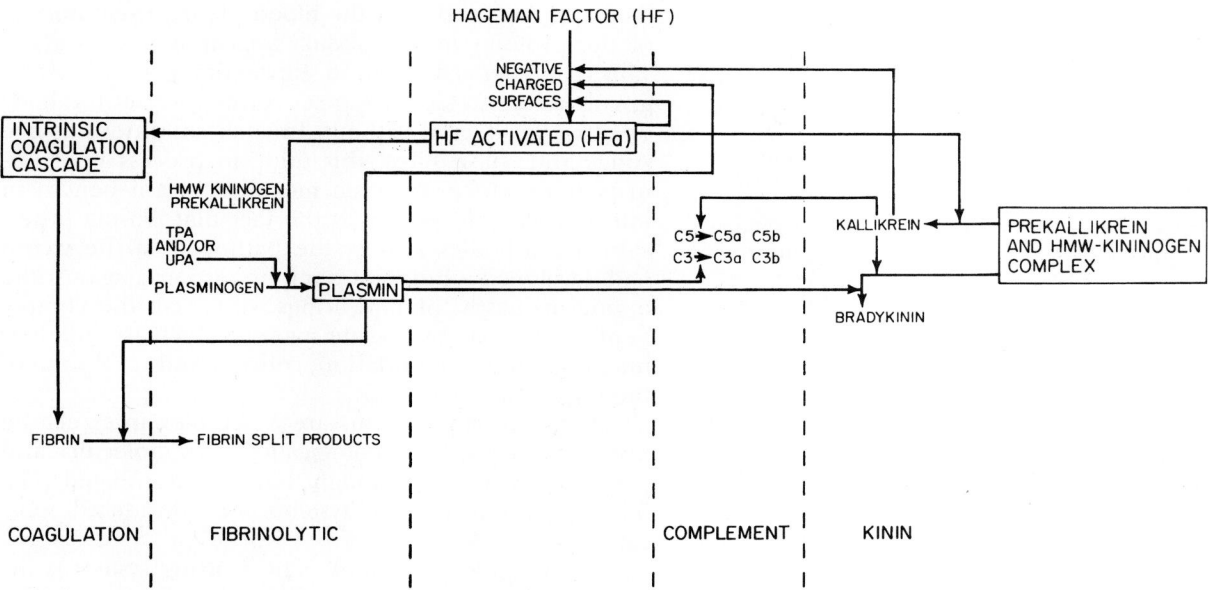

FIG. 5-12 Interrelationship between the coagulation, fibrinolytic, complement, and kinin plasma enzyme systems.

an important mechanism in the dissolution of the fibrin clot. There are actually three different mechanisms to remove fibrin. The least complicated involves the direct degradation of fibrin by fibrinolytic enzymes released from living and dead leukocytes in the area of inflammation. The second involves the direct removal of fibrin by leukocytes capable of phagocytosis or engulfment, especially macrophages. The third, and probably the most important, is mediated by **plasmin.** Plasmin degrades fibrin to fibrin split products, which are soluble, removed via the lymphatics, and can be detected in the serum of patients with coagulative disorders or severe inflammatory disease. Moreover, fibrin-split products are chemotactic for neutrophils. Plasmin is derived from the digestion of the plasma zymogen, plasminogen. This conversion can be initiated in a number of ways (Fig. 5-12). First, activated Hageman factor (Factor XIIa), along with HMW-kininogen and prekallikrein, can initiate the conversion of plasminogen to plasmin (Factor XII-dependent pathway). Second, there are a number of **plasminogen activators,** some found in plasma, such as urokinase-like plasminogen activator (UPA), and another made predominantly by endothelium and macrophages, (tissue-type; TPA), which can directly initiate the conversion of plasminogen to plasmin. In addition to augmenting fibrin degradation, plasmin can directly initiate the conversion of HMW-kininogen to bradykinin, which has powerful vasoactive and proinflammatory functions.

The Complement Cascade. Another important plasma-derived system in inflammation is the complement system. During its step-by-step sequence, molecules are released which directly influence vasopermeability and leukocyte activation and function, and its endpoint serves to "complement" humoral immune responses by forming a **membrane attack complex (MAC)** that lyses

bacteria, parasitic organisms, or foreign cells. Like the other pathways, the complement system is composed of plasma-derived zymogens, which undergo limited proteolysis of specific peptide bonds to form active proteases (Fig. 5-13). Activation can occur by two different mechanisms. The **classical pathway,** initiated by complexes of antibody with antigen, begins with C1, which is actually composed of three subunits, C1q, C1r, C1s. Except for C4, the reaction proceeds in order through C9. The **alternate pathway** is triggered by plant, fungal, or bacterial polysaccharides in the presence of Factor D, Factor B, and magnesium. Both pathways converge at the activation of C5, which results in the formation of C5b-9, a complex of complement components comprising MAC. MAC is unique because it has the ability to insert itself into membranes, thus destroying membrane integrity and causing cell lysis.

Aside from its membrane destructive properties, the complement cascade generates the potent inflammatory peptides C3a, C4a, and C5a. These peptides, termed **anaphylatoxins,** induce degranulation of mast cells with release of histamine, which causes increased vascular permeability and smooth muscle contraction similar to that occurring during anaphylaxis. C5a also is chemotactic for leukocytes.

C3b is important for two reasons: first, it is a component of C5 convertase in both the classical and alternate pathways; and second, it acts as an **opsonin,** promoting phagocytosis of C3b-coated material by way of C3b receptors on macrophages, neutrophils, and eosinophils.

Lastly, the complement system is not entirely autonomous. Other enzymes from the fibrinolytic and kinin systems can activate complement components by themselves. Kallikrein can initiate the conversion of C5 to C5a, while another function of plasmin is the direct ac-

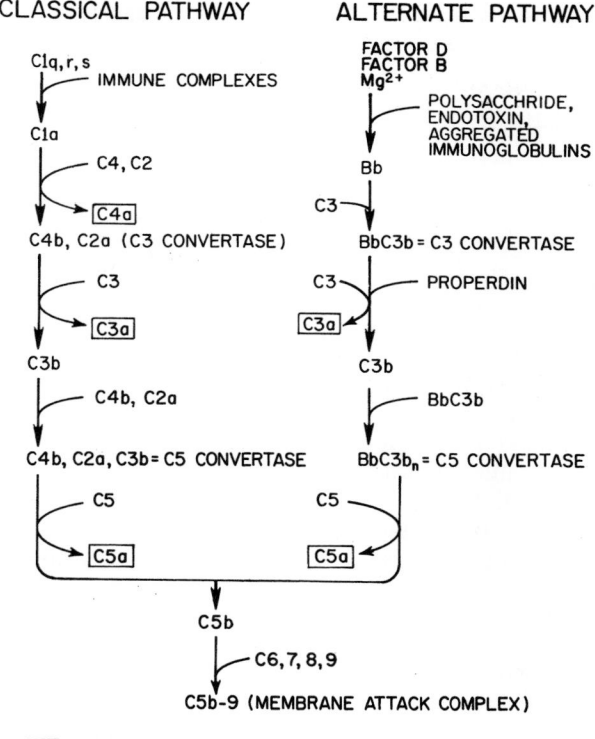

FIG. 5-13 The complement system.

tivation of C3 to the important inflammatory components, C3a and C3b (Fig. 5-12).

Thus, these four enzyme systems collectively and interdependently are responsible for the elaboration of plasma protein-derived inflammatory mediators. However, as previously mentioned, there are other inflammatory mediators that are derived principally from cells, both those fixed at the site of tissue damage and those that have migrated to the site from a nearby vessel. Some of these chemicals are preformed within cytoplasmic membrane-bound compartments (e.g., the vasoactive amines and lysosomal enzymes), while others are manufactured rapidly *de novo* at the time of cellular activation. There are six principal classes of cell-associated inflammatory mediators:

1. Cytokines
2. Arachidonic acid (AA) metabolites
3. Acetyl-glyceryl-ether-phosphorylcholine (AGEPC) or platelet activating factor (PAF)
4. Vasoactive amines
5. Granular constituents other than vasoactive amines
6. Oxidizing reagents

Cell-associated inflammatory mediators

CYTOKINES

Cytokines represent a class of polypeptides that provide the necessary means for cells to communicate with one another. These proteins, which cells manufacture on appropriate stimulation, have the capability to in-

fluence the function and activity of other cells. If the cytokine is released into the extracellular environment and influences the same cell that manufactures it, it has an **autocrine** effect. If it influences cells in the immediate vicinity of its release, it has a **paracrine** effect, and if it is able to exert a systemic influence, it has an **endocrine** effect identical to hormone function.

Because cytokines represent the communicative link between many different cells, they play crucial roles in immunity, inflammation, and hematopoiesis. During the last 20 years, it became evident that communication between a number of different cells was necessary for the proper development of an immune response; thus, many of the cytokines isolated so far are important in the initiation and control of immune responses, including the inflammatory response. However, the list of biologic activities for each cytokine grows constantly, and new cytokines are being isolated and studied at an exciting and accelerating pace. Therefore, in all likelihood, more cytokines will be found, and even though some cytokines are only known to play roles in certain events at the present time, they are probably plurifunctional and modulate many different biologic processes. In 1979, the name "interleukin" (IL) was chosen by a number of prominent immunologists to designate mediators that serve as communication signals between leukocytes. Unfortunately, not all of the cytokines have been given an "interleukin" designation. It is entirely reasonable, therefore, that in the days ahead, the names of most, if not all, of the cytokines will change. Table 5-1 is a list of many of the cytokines isolated to date and their functions.

Cytokine elaboration from cells affects the nature of the inflammatory response predominantly by influencing the activation state of other cells. The cytokines believed to be most involved in this process are IL-1 and TNF-α, which are, themselves, predominantly elaborated by activated macrophages, and interferon-γ and TNF-β, factors produced by activated lymphocytes. These proteins activate a number of cells, either fixed cells, such as endothelium, or other inflammatory cells. **Activation** has been defined for endothelial cells as "quantitative changes in the level of expression of specific gene products (i.e., proteins) that, in turn, endow endothelial cells with new capacities that cumulatively allow endothelial cells to perform new functions" (Pober, 1988). This definition can be applied to other cells involved in the inflammatory response as well.

The consequences of cellular activation in the inflammatory response depends upon the type of cell being activated. Generally, endothelial cells respond to cytokine activation signals by hypertrophy (becoming more plump) and the generation of E-selectin, ICAM-1, and VCAM-1 adhesion molecules, as previously described. These cell-membrane proteins in turn mediate leukocyte adhesion to the endothelial surface, a prerequisite for subsequent emigration into the perivascular space. In addition, endothelium increases its expression of MHC molecules (both class I and class II), which facilitate the recognition of antigens between immune cells (Chapter 7) and, in this case, endothelium. Furthermore, upon activation, the endothelial surface becomes more **thrombogenic;** thus, clotting is more easily induced. This phenomenon is largely caused by: (1) the increased production of **tissue factor** or **thromboplastin** by the endothelial cell, which activates the extrinsic coagulation cascade; and (2) the decreased production of **thrombomodulin,** a membrane protein that keeps coagulation in check by inactivating thrombin, on the endothelial surface. In response to specific cytokines, such as TNF-α and IFN-γ, endothelial cells also produce their own cytokines. Especially noted in this regard is IL-1, a requisite protein in the activation and clonal expansion of antigen-primed lymphocytes.

Leukocytes are also activated by cytokines. First, leukocytes respond to cytokine influence by producing and incorporating more LFA-1 molecules in their cell membrane, thereby making them more efficient in their attachment to ICAM-l-expressing endothelium. Second, leukocytes require cytokines to reach their full functional potential. For example, lymphocytes require IL-1 to proliferate and differentiate into effector cells in response to antigen. Macrophages and neutrophils are able to phagocytize and kill foreign organisms much more efficiently in response to certain cytokines, especially IFN-γ for macrophages and TNF-α for neutrophils. Additionally, both cytokine-primed macrophages and neutrophils are able to increase their biosynthesis and/or release of lysosomal enzymes, granule contents (neutrophils), cytokines, and reactive oxygen intermediates. Third, cytokines generally increase intracellular calcium in the leukocyte, which activates cellular **phospholipase A$_2$.** This enzyme, when activated, liberates arachidonic acid from the phospholipid bilayer of the cell membrane. Arachidonic acid represents the building block for two important classes of lipid cellular mediators, the prostaglandins and leukotrienes.

Cytokines also influence the fixed structural cells of tissue, generally in a way that is beneficial for healing and repair. For example, fibroblasts are induced to divide and produce more collagen and proteolytic enzymes in response to certain cytokines. A more detailed account of healing and repair is addressed at the end of this chapter.

Lastly, cytokines have an endocrine effect, which largely accounts for the systemic signs of inflammation, defined collectively as the **acute phase response.** Table 5-2 list the 5 components of the acute phase response. First and foremost is **fever.** It is now well established that IL-1 and TNF-α are at least partly responsible for fever, which explains why IL-1 was once called the endogenous pyrogen. Although the exact mechanism has not been entirely elucidated, the circulating cytokines increase production of prostaglandin E$_2$ (PGE$_2$) in the anterior hypothalamus. This lipid mediator affects hypothalamic control of sympathetic stimulation of cutaneous vessels, effectively decreasing cutaneous flow and heat dissipation, thereby resulting in higher core temperatures.

Second, the liver is stimulated to produce a number of proteins that can be detected in elevated amounts in patients with inflammatory disease. Table 5-3 lists many of these acute phase proteins. Beside IL-1 and TNF-α,

TABLE 5-2 **Characteristics of acute phase response**

Fever
Hepatocyte acute-phase protein production
Leukocytosis
Catabolic processes
Increases in plasma copper and decreases in plasma iron and zinc

which are partly responsible for this effect, it has been recently shown that IL-6 is probably the most important mediator of this reaction. Hepatocytes have large numbers of IL-6 receptors on their surface, and they begin producing acute phase proteins *de novo* immediately after stimulation with IL-6.

Third, during the acute phase response, changes in certain heavy metals can be detected in the plasma. Specifically, there is an increase in copper, while concomitantly, there is a decrease in iron and zinc. These changes can be considered a unique protective host mechanism, because it has been shown that the host and the invading microbe are in competition for iron and zinc. Therefore, decreased availability of iron and zinc, along with increased temperatures associated with fever, can limit microbial growth. Decreases in iron are likely related to cytokine degranulation of neutrophils, which releases the iron-binding compound, lactoferrin. Lactoferrin-iron complexes are then phagocytized by mononuclear phagocytes and effectively removed from the circulation. Copper is required for proper immune functioning, and increases in copper are likely secondary to increases in plasma concentrations of the copper-binding protein, ceruloplasmin. This protein is one of the acute phase proteins manufactured in the liver in response to cytokine stimulation.

Fourth, during the acute phase response, there is an increase in the number of leukocytes in the peripheral circulation, termed **leukocytosis.** In the acute inflammatory reaction, the increase in neutrophils, the common cell involved, is largely caused by an accelerated release of mature and immature neutrophils from pools within the bone marrow. IL-1 and TNF-α are largely responsible for this effect. Immature neutrophils, often referred to as "bands" or "stabs," do not have accentuated lobulations of their nucleus. When they are detected in elevated numbers in the blood, the finding is frequently expressed as a "shift to the left."

TABLE 5-3 **Acute phase proteins**

Fibrinogen
Haptoglobin
Ceruloplasmin
Serum amyloid A
C-reactive protein
α 2-macrofetoprotein
Complement proteins
Coagulation proteins

Immature granulocytes are usually detected in the blood during an active pyogenic inflammatory reaction. Occasionally, if an acute inflammatory reaction is particularly severe, the absolute leukocyte count in the blood increases to extraordinarily high levels, such as 30,000 to 50,000/μL. At this point, this leukocytosis is termed a **leukemoid reaction** and must be differentiated from **leukemia,** which is a neoplastic production of one type of leukocyte. **Leukopenia,** on the other hand, refers to a marked decrease in the white cell count as is seen in some infections, most notably viral.

Fifth, if the inciting inflammatory stimulus is not removed and the acute phase response is long-lasting, then **catabolism** becomes clinically evident in the form of muscle wasting, weight loss, and weakness. One of the most potent effects TNF-α is its ability to suppress synthesis of lipoprotein lipase, an enzyme required for the utilization of serum triglycerides. Kawakami and Cerami (1981) originally noted this effect in animals with chronic wasting parasitic disease and named **cachectin** for the effector protein responsible for the resultant lipemia and weight loss. However, nearly a century ago, Coley (1893) recognized that there was a factor in patients with artificially-induced inflammatory disease that was capable of causing hemorrhagic necrosis of some tumors. This factor was subsequently named tumor necrosis factor (Carswell and others, 1975; Mannel and others, 1980). It was not until 1985 that cachectin and TNF-α were recognized to be the same molecule (Beutler and colleagues, 1985). IL-1 also has a minor effect in lipid utilization, thus having a contributory role in the catabolic state of the patient with chronic inflammatory disease.

Thus, cytokines represent a large and diverse group of protein messengers that are capable of influencing a multitude of biologic effects. From local inflammatory effects that control the nature and extent of leukocyte infiltration to systemic clinical manifestations like fever and weight loss, cytokines are crucial in mediating responses to cellular injury. With such a large role in host defense, it is particularly interesting that some viruses, like HIV-1 and the related SIV, have evolved adaptive mechanisms that utilize host-derived cytokines to their advantage. For example, one mechanism both viruses have to escape immune surveillance is to use TNF-α manufactured by the host to boost viral replication within an infected cell. This mechanism is indeed very effective, because TNF-α is of course the same molecule the host uses to incite an inflammatory reaction to rid itself of the invading pathogen and therefore in abundant supply. However, there are other cell-derived mediators of inflammation that are important and deserving of description, some of which are produced in response to cytokine stimulation of the cell.

ARACHIDONIC ACID (AA) METABOLITES

The vasoactive metabolites of arachidonic acid (**eicosanoids**) represent a fascinating group of lipid mediators that are synthesized *de novo* and released by many cells, including activated leukocytes, platelets, and mast cells. They are all derived from essential polyunsaturated fatty acids, such as linoleic acid, that have been esterified in the liver to produce arachidonic acid and incorporated into various phospholipids within cell membranes. Before production into vasoactive AA metabolites, arachidonic acid must be liberated from the lipid bilayer of the membrane and used in one of the production pathways. This step appears to be the rate-limiting step in the process and likely represents a way to control production. Arachidonic acid is made available from the membrane when the bilayer is perturbed by insult (e.g., complement activation) or appropriate antigenic or mediator stimulation (e.g., bradykinin, TNF-α), causing an influx of calcium from the extracellular space into the cytoplasmic compartment. This sudden rise in cytoplasmic calcium activates the enzyme **phospholipase A$_2$,** which directly hydrolyzes arachidonic acid from the lipid membrane. Platelets may use phospholipase C and diacylglycerol lipase to remove arachidonic acid from the cell membrane, but the net effect of either system is an increase in the intracellular concentration of arachidonic acid.

Free intracellular arachidonic acid may be metabolized by two major pathways: the **cyclo-oxygenase pathway** results in the formation of **prostaglandins** and **thromboxane A$_2$,** while the **lipoxygenase pathway** produces **leukotrienes** and **lipoxins** (Fig. 5-14). The mediators produced from the metabolism of arachidonic acid have been described as **autocoids,** because they are produced quickly, tend to act only in their local microenvironment, and are only active for a short period of time. However, it is probably more accurate to think of them as mediators similar to cytokines that have only a paracrine or autocrine effect.

Leukotrienes have potent effects on many different cells, including endothelium and leukocytes. The sulfidopeptide leukotrienes, LTC$_4$, LTD$_4$, and LTE$_4$, are collectively known as the **slow-reacting substance of anaphylaxis (SRS-A),** because their biologic effects are characteristic of immediate hypersensitivity reactions. These include a contractile effect on smooth muscle (inducing bronchospasm), increased vascular permeability (through endothelial contraction), and vasoconstrictive effects. These three sulfidopeptide leukotrienes are actually much more potent than histamine in inducing these effects, and it is believed that these mediators play a key role in the pathogenesis of bronchial asthma. On the other hand, LTB$_4$ has fewer of the hypersensitivity characteristics. LTB$_4$ primarily stimulates a number of leukocyte functions, including chemotaxis, phagocytosis, degranulation, digestion, and production of reactive oxygen intermediates. It also increases leukocyte adhesion to endothelium by influencing adhesion molecules on both endothelium and leukocytes. LTB$_4$ increases microvascular permeability, but this effect is more insidious than the quick and dramatic effect produced by sulfidopeptide leukotrienes.

Initial lipoxygenation of AA at a different carbon position (C-15 instead of C-5) can lead to the formation of two biologically active compounds, **lipoxin A** and **lipoxin B.** From data from *in vitro* experiments, these compounds stimulate granulocytes and cause chemotaxis (like LTB$_4$), but unlike LTB$_4$, have no effect on

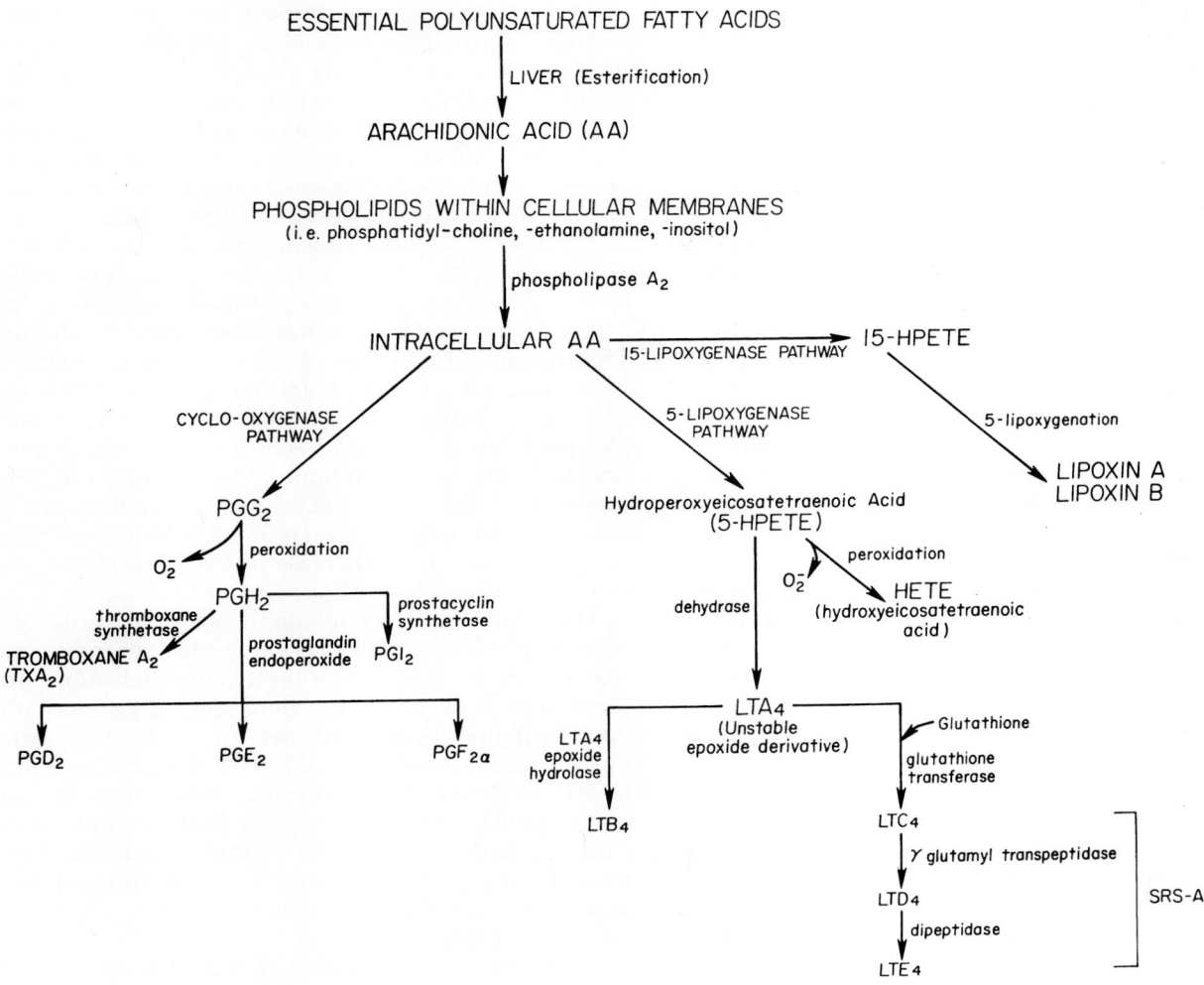

FIG. 5-14 Arachidonic acid metabolism to prostaglandins, leukotrienes, thromboxane A₂, and lipoxins.

vascular permeability or leukocyte adherence to endothelium.

Metabolism of AA via the cyclo-oxygenase pathway leads to the formation of prostaglandins and thromboxane A₂ (TXA₂). Thromboxane is a prominent metabolite made by activated platelets, and it induces pulmonary vasoconstriction, platelet aggregation, and neutrophil adherence to endothelium. Endothelium is a key source of prostacyclin, or prostaglandin I₂ (PGI₂), which appears to counter the effects of thromboxane in that it causes vasodilatation, inhibits platelet aggregation, and suppresses neutrophil adherence to endothelium. The other prostaglandins, PGD₂ and PGE₂, are made by a number of different cell types and are particularly known for their vasodilatative properties. Figure 5-9 depicts how prostaglandins and leukotrienes can work synergistically to influence vascular permeability during an inflammatory response.

ACETYL-GLYCERYL-ETHER-PHOSPHORYLCHOLINE (AGEPC) OR PLATELET ACTIVATING FACTOR (PAF)

AGEPC or platelet activating factor (PAF) is a lipid mediator that is manufactured *de novo* after stimulation by a variety of cells involved in the inflammatory process, including neutrophils, monocyte/macrophages, lymphocytes, basophils, mast cells, endothelial cells, and platelets. Like leukotrienes, it has a wide spectrum of proinflammatory effects. Indeed, PAF and leukotrienes may be synthesized simultaneously from similar lipid building blocks. Therefore, the inflammatory inductive effects of PAF and leukotrienes in tissue overlap and may serve to augment each other *in vivo*. The proinflammatory effects induced by PAF include vasodilatation, increased vascular permeability (many thousand times more potent than LTC₄ and its derivatives), chemotaxis and stimulation of granulocytes, platelet aggregation, and induction of local inflammatory cells to produce other mediators.

VASOACTIVE AMINES

In contrast to the *de novo* synthesis of protein and lipid mediators previously described, the vasoactive amines represent mediators that are **preformed** and stored in **secretory granules. Histamine** is the prototypic vasoactive amine found in the granules of mast cells, basophils, eosinophils, and platelets; **serotonin** is a similar amine found predominantly in mast cells and platelets, and although most species store and respond to serotonin, it is likely more important in rodents than in other animals. Because of their storage within cytoplasmic granules, these amines are available for immediate use. Therefore, upon appropriate stimulation, degranulation ensues and releases these vasoactive amines into the extracellular environment, where they can profoundly affect the functioning of endothelium, smooth muscle, and leukocytes. Because of this immediate availability, vasoactive amines are the principle mediators in **immediate hypersensitivity reactions (type I)** or **anaphylactic** reactions as well as the immediate transient vascular permeability response in an acute inflammatory reaction. Thus, these amines are involved in the earliest changes in response to tissue and cellular injury. In a general sense, they induce vasodilatation, increased venular permeability, and smooth muscle contraction, including that of the respiratory and gastrointestinal tract, but their effect is very short-lived (only minutes). Therefore, if the inflammatory response is to be maintained, other more long-lasting mediators, such as cytokines and vasoactive lipids, are needed at the site.

As previously discussed, degranulation and release of vasoactive amines may be induced primarily by the cross-linking of surface IgE molecules by antigen on mast cells and basophils or by the presence of complement fragments.

GRANULAR CONSTITUENTS OTHER THAN VASOACTIVE AMINES

Mast cell granules contain a wide array of preformed compounds that contribute to the immediate response associated with degranulation. These include: (1) proteases, such as tryptase and chymase, that digest the basement membranes of blood vessels, effectively increasing vascular permeability; (2) proteoglycans, such as heparin and chondroitin sulfate, which serve to stabilize and protect the proteases from antiproteases; and (3) chemotactic factors, such as **eosinophil chemotactic factor of anaphylaxis (ECF-A),** which recruits eosinophils to the area and represents a group of preformed peptides, and **neutrophil chemotactic factor,** which is presumed to selectively attract neutrophils.

In contrast, granulocytes and macrophages contain lysosomal granules in the cytoplasm that are primarily for release into phagocytic vacuoles rather than the extracellular space. When lysosomal granules fuse with phagocytic vacuoles, a **phagolysosome** is formed; this process represents the cell's first step in the ultimate killing of phagocytized foreign organisms. These lysosomal granules contain a number of proteases and enzymes that can kill bacteria, fungi, and protozoal organisms, but if released into the extracellular environment, they create tissue damage and contribute to the initiation and evolution of the inflammatory response. Table 5-4 is a partial list of lysosomal contents from granulocytes and macrophages. Small quantities of lysosomal contituents, however, are released (or regurgitated) into the extracellular space during the process of

TABLE 5-4 **Lysosomal contents**

Acid hydrolases

Acid phosphatase
β-glucuronidase

Cationic proteins

Defensins*
Bactericidal/permeability-increasing protein*
Major basic protein (MBP) (eosinophils)*
Eosinophil cationic protein (ECP)
Eosinophil-derived neurotoxin
Alkaline phosphatase
Neutrophil basic protein (NBP)*
Eosinophil peroxidase*

Esterases

Phospholipase B
Lysophospholipase (Charcot-Leyden crystal protein)+

Proteases

Cathepsins
Collagenase
Elastase
Plasminogen activator (macrophages)
Aminopeptidase
Kininase+

Nonenzymatic molecules

Phagocytin*
Plasminogen
Lactoferrin

Nucleases

Ribonuclease
Deoxyribonuclease

Other hydrolases

Lysozyme*
Amylase
Arylsulfatase B+

Oxidoreductases

Myeloperoxidase*
Coenzyme Q
Histaminase+

*Antimicrobial; + anti-inflammatory.

phagocytosis, and significantly larger quantities are released after the cell dies and lyses. Therefore, lysosomal contents are associated with mediation of the inflammatory response, even if only in an indirect fashion.

OXIDIZING REAGENTS

During the process of phagocytosis, neutrophils and macrophages are stimulated to quickly produce a number of very reactive oxygen intermediates. The metabolism of oxygen during phagocytosis and killing is covered later in discussions dealing with cell functions in the inflammatory response. Suffice it to say here, that during phagocytosis, these reactive oxygen metabolites are released into the surrounding tissues where, similar to released lysosomal contents, they create tissue damage in their own right. Hence, just by their presence outside the cell, they contribute to the progression and the severity of the inflammatory response.

References

Beutler B, Cerami A. Cachectin: more than a tumor necrosis factor. N Engl J Med 1987;316:379–385.

Beutler B, Greenwald D, Hulmes JD, et al. Identity of tumour necrosis factor and the macrophage-secreted factor cachectin. Nature 1985;316:552–554.

Carlson GP, Kaneko JJ. Intravascular granulocyte kinetics in developing calves. Am J Vet Res 1975;36:421–425.

Carswell EA, Old IJ, Kassel RL, et al. An endotoxin-induced serum factor that causes necrosis of tumors. Proc Natl Acad Sci USA 1975;72:3666–3670.

Clark SC, Kamen R. The human hematopoietic colony-stimulating factors. Science 1987;236:1229–1237.

Coley WB. The treatment of malignant tumors by repeated inoculations of erysipelas; with a report of ten original cases. Am J Med Sci 1893;105:487–511.

Dinarello CA. Interleukin-1. Rev Infect Dis 1984;6:51–95.

Dinarello CA, Mier JW. Lymphokines. N Engl J Med 1987;317:940–945.

Donahue RE, Yang Y-C, Clark SC. Human P40 T-cell growth factor (interleukin-9) supports erythroid colony formation. Blood 1990;75:2271–2275.

Durum SK, Schmidt JA, Oppenheim JJ. Interleukin 1: an immunological perspective. Annu Rev Immunol 1985;3:263–287.

Ebertz JM, Hirshman CA, Kettelkamp NS, et al. Substance P-induced histamine release in human cutaneous mast cells. J Invest Dermatol 1987;88:682–685.

Feuerstein G, Hallenbeck JM. Leukotrienes in health and disease. FASEB J 1987;1:186–192.

Ford-Hutchinson AW. Leukotrienes: their formation and role as inflammatory mediators. Fed Proc 1985;44:25–29.

Furie B, Furie BC. The molecular basis of blood coagulation. Cell 1988;53:505–518.

Gimbrone MA Jr, Obin MS, Brock AF, et al. Endothelial interleukin-8: a novel inhibitor of leukocyte-endothelial interactions. Science 1989;246:1601–1603.

Goetzl EJ, Payan DG, Goldman DW. Immunopathogenetic roles of leukotrienes in human diseases. J Clin Immunol 1984;4:79–84.

Hansen B. Leukotrienes: biology and role in disease. J Vet Intern Med 1989;3:59–72.

Hugli TE. Complement and cellular triggering reactions: introductory remarks. Fed Proc 1984;43:2540–2542.

Issekutz AC, Szpejda M. Evidence that platelet activating factor may mediate some acute inflammatory responses. Lab Invest 1986;54:275–281.

Joris I, Majno G, Corey EJ, et al. The mechanism of vascular leakage induced by leukotriene E$_4$: endothelial contraction. Am J Pathol 1987;126:19–24.

Kaplan AP. Hageman factor-dependent pathways: mechanism of initiation and bradykinin formation. Fed Proc 1983;42:3123–3127.

Kawakami M, Cerami A. Studies of endotoxin-induced decrease in lipoprotein lipase activity. J Exp Med 1981;154:631–639.

Koeffler HP, Gasson J, Ranyard J, et al. Recombinant human TNF$_\alpha$ stimulates production of granulocyte colony-stimulating factor. Blood 1987;70:55–59.

Le J, Vilcek J. Tumor necrosis factor and interleukin 1: Cytokines with multiple overlapping biological activities. Lab Invest 1987;56:234–248.

Lee TH, Hoover RL, Williams JD, et al. Effect of dietary enrichment with eicosapentaenoic and docosahexaenoic acids on in vitro neutrophil and monocyte leukotriene generation and neutrophil function. N Engl J Med 1985;312:1217–1224.

Lewis RA, Austen KF. The biologically active leukotrienes: biosynthe-sis, matabolism, receptors, functions, and pharmacology. J Clin Invest 1984;73:889–897.

Malik AB, Perlman MB, Cooper JA, et al. Pulmonary microvascular effects of arachidonic acid metabolites and their role in lung vascular injury. Fed Proc 1985;44:36–42.

Mannel DN, Moore RN, Mergenhagen SE. Macrophages as a source of tumoricidal activity (tumor-necrotizing factor). Infect Immun 1980;30:523–530.

Michel L, Mencia-Huerta J-M, Benveniste J, et al. Biologic properties of LTB$_4$ and Paf-acether in vivo in human skin. J Invest Dermatol 1987;88:675–681.

Mizel SB. The interleukins. FASEB J 1989;3:2379–2388.

Moore KW, Vieira P, Fiorentino DF, et al. Homology of cytokine synthesis inhibitory factor (IL-10) to the Epstein-Barr virus gene BCRFI. Science 1990;248:1230–1234.

Oppenheim JJ, Stadler BM, Siraganian RP, et al. Lymphokines: their role in lymphocyte responses. Properties of interleukin 1. Fed Proc 1982;41:257–268.

Pinckard RN. The "new" chemical mediators of inflammation. In: Majno G, Cotran RS, eds. Current topics in inflammation and infection. Baltimore: Williams and Wilkins 1982;3:38–53.

Pober JS. Cytokine-mediated activation of vascular endothelium. Am J Pathol 1988;133:426–433.

Prasse KW, Kaeberle ML, Ramsey FK. Blood neutrophilic granulocyte kinetics in cats. Am J Vet Res 1973;34:1021–1025.

Renauld JC, Goethals A, Houssiau F, et al. Human P40/IL-9: expression in activated CD4$^+$ T cells, genomic organization, and comparison with the mouse gene. J Immunol 1990;144:4235–4241.

Samuelsson B, Dahlen S-E, Lindgren JA, et al. Leukotrienes and lipox-ins: structures, biosynthesis, and biological effects. Science 1987;237:1171–1176.

Schroder J-M: The monocyte-derived neutrophil activating peptide (nap/interleukin 8) stimulates human neutrophil arachidonate-5-lipoxygenase, but not the release of cellular arachidonate. J Exp Med 1989;170:847–863.

Serafin WE, Austen KF. Mediators of immediate hypersensitivity reactions. N Engl J Med 1987;317:30–34.

Sherry B, Cerami A. Cachectin/tumor necrosis factor exerts endocrine, paracrine, and autocrine control of inflammatory responses. J Cell Biol 1988;107:1269–1277.

Sieff CA. Hematopoietic growth factors. J Clin Invest 1987;79:1549–1557.

Strober W, James SP. The interleukins. Pediatr Res 1988;24:549–557.

Williams JD, Czop JK, Austen KF. Release of leukotrienes by human monocytes on stimulation of their phagocytic receptor for particulate activators. J Immunol 1984;132:3034–3040.

Zachariae COC, Anderson AO, Thompson HL, et al. Properties of monocyte chemotactic and activating factor (MCAF) purified from a human fibrosarcoma cell line. J Exp Med 1990;171:2177–2182.

CELLULAR FUNCTIONS IN THE ACUTE INFLAMMATORY REACTION

Once a leukocyte has arrived at a site of tissue injury and emigrated from the microvasculature, it is prepared to serve its function. The precise role that each cell assumes during the evolution of an inflammatory exudate depends partly on cell type, on whether the inciting injurious agent has been removed, and on whether the inflammatory process is still active or diminishing. However, leukocytes can respond in only a limited number of ways in an inflammatory setting; some of these general functions are outlined below.

Lymphocytes

At the beginning of this chapter, we stated that lymphocytes respond to their predetermined antigen, whether present on the surface of antigen-presenting cells or on the cell membrane of potential targets of attack. Following this recognition, lymphocytes respond by clonal expansion and differentiation to either CTLs that bear CD8 antigen or helper/inducers that bear CD4 antigen. Helper/inducer lymphocytes augment the functioning and/or differentiation of other immune cells by the elaboration of specific mediators, such as interferon-γ, IL-2, or B-cell growth factors, such as IL-4 and IL-5. However, CTLs are specific in their effector function by destroying antigen-expressing target cells (Chapter 7).

Phagocytes (granulocytes and macrophages)

Granulocytes and macrophages are phagocytes, able to first recognize and attach to particulate foreign or necrotic debris (via opsonins), engulf it using a process called phagocytosis, and then kill and/or degrade it using specialized mechanisms. As previously indicated, granulocytes and macrophages have a large repertoire of degrading enzymes within cytoplasmic membrane-bound granules. These granules can fuse with phagosomes to form phagolysosomes, thereby beginning the proteolytic digestion of the engulfed foreign material or tissue debris, a process that does not require the additional use of oxygen. However, over evolutionary time, these cells have developed oxygen-using mechanisms that are extremely damaging to and ultimately kill foreign organisms. In fact, during phagocytosis, phagocytes exhibit a "burst" of oxygen consumption (appropriately coined the **respiratory burst**), and the extra oxygen consumed by the cell is used for the generation of reactive oxygen metabolites. These reactive oxygen molecules may then be used for killing phagocytized organisms; however, they are also implicated in tissue injury in their own right and possibly are involved in the modulation of certain cell functions.

The respiratory burst begins by the activation of a membrane-bound oxidase that uses NADPH (generated from the hexose-monophosphate shunt) to reduce two molecules of oxygen into the form of two molecules of superoxide (O_2):

$$2O_2 + NADPH \rightarrow 2O_2^- + NADP^+ + H^-$$

This reaction begins at the site on the plasma membrane where phagocytosis has been initiated, and the generation of superoxide, a free radical, can be damaging to an organism being engulfed as well as the surrounding microenvironment. Its role in phagocyte-mediated tissue injury results from the ability of superoxide to oxidize metal ion complexes or organic substrates. However, superoxide can be removed from the site by dismutation, which may occur spontaneously in aqueous solution or may be catalyzed by the cytoplasmic enzyme, superoxide dismutase, at neutral or alkaline pH levels:

$$2O_2^- + 2H^+ \rightarrow H_2O_2 + O_2$$

The resultant product, hydrogen peroxide (H_2O_2), is also irritating to tissues but to a lesser extent than superoxide radicals. However, the formation of hydrogen peroxide is essential for the ultimate formation of two other very potent antimicrobial agents. Each of these antimicrobial products are generated by two different mechanisms, one by a myeloperoxidase-dependent pathway, and one by a myeloperoxidase-independent pathway.

Myeloperoxidase-dependent pathway (the H_2O_2-myeloperoxidase-halide system)

Neutrophils and monocytes contain cytoplasmic granules containing myeloperoxidase, an enzyme that, in the presence of hydrogen peroxide, catalyzes the oxidation of halides (either chloride, iodide, or bromide) to generate an oxidized halide and water:

$$H_2O_2 + Cl^- (or\ I^-, Br^-) \rightarrow ClOH + H_2O$$

The oxidized halide (in this case, hypochlorous acid) is a potent oxidant that can react with many biologically important compounds.

Myeloperoxidase-independent pathway. For some phagocytes, such as macrophages, that often contain little myeloperoxidase, another mechanism exists whereby hydrogen peroxide can be used without myeloperoxidase to form another reactive antimicrobial compound. This reaction (Haber-Weiss reaction) is catalyzed by metal ions and involves the interaction of superoxide with hydrogen peroxide to form the highly reactive hydroxyl radical (OH):

$$O_2^- + H_2O_2 \rightarrow OH^{\cdot} + OH^- + O_2$$

Thus, phagocytes have a significant armamentarium of oxygen-derived metabolites and lysosomal constituents that can be used in combat against foreign organisms or even tumor cells. The hydroxy radical, in particular, is so reactive that it essentially combines with almost any molecule it touches. However, the other oxygen species and enzymes encased within phagocytes underscore the multiplicity of mechanisms and functions of phagocytes during an inflammatory response.

References

Brune K, Schmid L, Glatt M, et al. Correlation between antimicrobial activity and peroxidase content of leukocytes. Nature 1973;245: 209–210.

Halliwell B, Hoult JR, Blake DR. Oxidants, inflammation, and anti-inflammatory drugs. FASEB J 1988;2:2867–2873.

Weiss SJ, LoBuglio AF. Phagocyte-generated oxygen metabolites and cellular injury. Lab Invest 1982;47:5–18.

TYPES OF INFLAMMATION

We have described the early microscopic changes that typify an inflammatory reaction, specifically: (1) vascular dilatation, (2) plasma leakage from the vascular bed, and (3) leukocyte migration from the vascular lumen to the perivascular space. Moreover, we have attempted to explain these alterations mechanistically. These early responses are hallmarks of the inflammatory reaction, so that one or more of these changes can be found in most inflamed tissues. Thus, tissues have a limited number of ways that they can respond to injury. However, the morphologic appearance of inflammation under the microscope can vary somewhat depending on anatomic site, nature of the inflammatory stimulus, and immunocompetence of the host. In the most general sense, two types of inflammation exist: **acute** and **chronic.**

Acute inflammation

Acute inflammation arises suddenly, often within minutes or hours of injury, and progresses rather rapidly to either resolution or chronic inflammation. The terms, acute and chronic, similar to their descriptive use in clinical conditions, refer solely to the duration of the inflammatory process. Therefore, acute inflammation is traditionally defined as inflammation which has a course of hours to days, while the course for chronic inflammation is more protracted and generally measured in weeks, months, or even years. However, even though, by their strictest definitions, these terms refer only to time course, it is probably more meaningful to think of them in relation to the morphologic patterns that typify each. In this sense, acute inflammation is characterized by the presence of an **exudate,** a protein-rich fluid (specific gravity of more than 1.017) formed outside the blood vessel that usually contains cells and cell debris. Thus, acute inflammation is typically exudative, an example being an abscess, which is a cavity containing pus (a **purulent** exudate containing large numbers of neutrophils). **Suppurative inflammation** is another name for acute inflammatory responses that result in the formation of pus. Chronic inflammation, on the other hand, is productive or proliferative rather than exudative. Resident cells at the sites of chronic inflammation proliferate and produce additional matrix substances; the cell type is usually, but not exclusively, mononuclear. It should be noted, however, that exudation and proliferation are not mutually exclusive. Changes ascribed to both acute and chronic inflammation are found in a number of inflammatory lesions. For example, repeated active bouts of bacterial otitis externa (infection of the external ear canal and/or pinna) of a dog may have foci of neutrophil extravasation and exudation in the wall of the canal (acute inflammation) in conjunction with increased collagen deposition and a mononuclear cell infiltrate (chronic inflammation). Therefore, although the time frame defining acute and chronic inflammation is absolute, the histologic appearance of each are often seen concurrently in the same specimen.

A helpful way to categorize different types of acute inflammation is by the nature of the exudate. While only a fluid, strictly speaking, can exude, leukocytes and erythrocytes may or may not leave the blood as part of the exudate. In addition, the character of the fluid component is at least partly dependent on anatomic site and inciting stimulus. Thus, exudates can vary considerably.

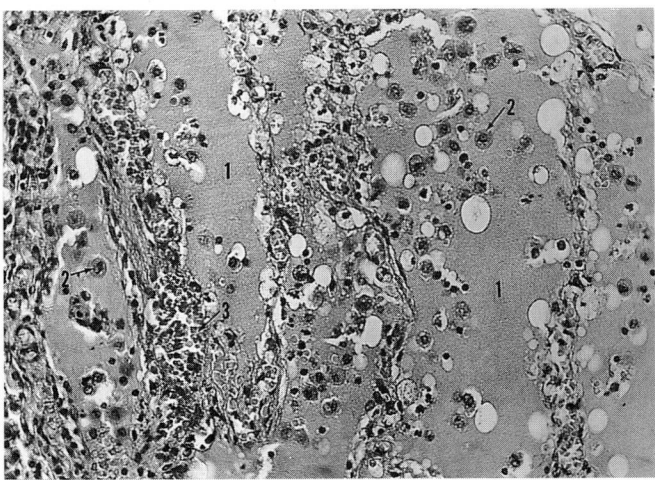

FIG. 5-15 Inflammatory edema of the lungs of an elephant with pulmonary tuberculosis. Albuminous fluid *(1)*, mononuclear cells *(2)*, and congested capillaries *(3)*. (× 300.) (Courtesy of National Zoological Park and Armed Forces Institute of Pathology)

Serous inflammation

Serous inflammation is characterized by the exudation of blood serum, a clear, albuminous fluid. This is the form which is equivalent to **inflammatory edema** (Figs. 5-15 and 5-16). Serous inflammation is a common manifestation early in the acute inflammatory reaction and often occurs when the inciting tissue injury is relatively mild.

OCCURRENCE

This type of inflammation is especially common in serous cavities, doubtless because of the large areas of well-vascularized surfaces that line these cavities and the

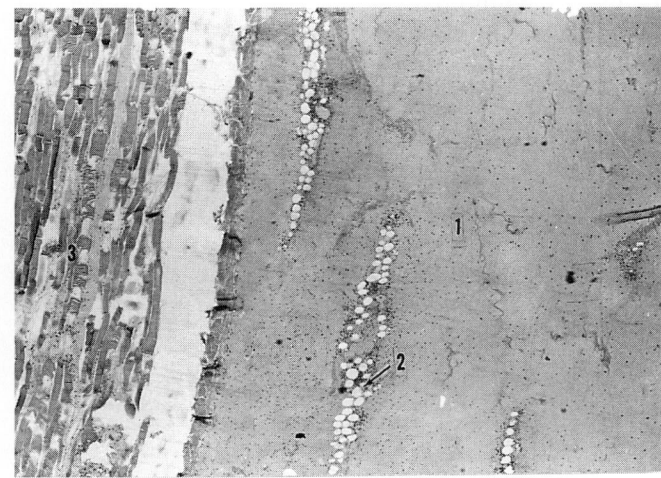

FIG. 5-16 Inflammatory edema in subcutaneous musculature of a horse with purpura hemorrhagica. Albuminous material *(1)* containing cells and fibrin; leukocytes accumulated around fat cells *(2)*, and skeletal muscle *(3)* with fibers separated by edema fluid. (Courtesy of Army Veterinary Research Laboratory, Armed Forces Institute of Pathology)

thinness of the surface mesothelium. Serous inflammation also occurs in the lungs, as the first stage in certain pneumonias, in response to various inhaled chemical irritants, and as the result of at least one irritant that is ingested and presumably eliminated through the lungs, namely, alpha-naphthyl-thiourea (the rat poison, ANTU). Blisters or vesicles, such as those that form in the skin after a bee sting or a second-degree burn, or affect the mucosa, in such diseases as aphthous fever, vesicular stomatitis, and vesicular exanthema, are examples of localized serous inflammation.

MICROSCOPIC APPEARANCE

Microscopically, a homogeneous, pink-staining precipitate is seen; natural spaces are distended by it and artificial ones are created, as in the case of vesicles. With the precipitated fluid, there are usually a few scattered leukocytes of various kinds and traces of fibrin. The hyperemic and congested vessels are conspicuous.

GROSS APPEARANCE

A watery fluid fills the body cavities or tissue spaces; this differs little from the plasma of the blood. Neither is it easily distinguished from the fluid of true edema. The presence of small amounts of fibrin clinging to involved surfaces or of a cloudiness caused by the presence of a few leukocytes indicates an inflammatory origin. Other than by the gross appearance, the fluid can often, but not always, be differentiated from edema arising from circulatory disturbances by characterization of the fluid as a transudate or exudate. Typically, an acute transudate arising from circulatory disturbances has a specific gravity of less than 1.017, while an inflammatory exudate contains a more elevated specific gravity of more than 1.017.

CAUSES

This type of inflammation may be caused by a number of irritants, many of which are transient. In the serous cavities, this is practically always an infection. Joint cavities constitute an exception in that a serous exudate, or excess of synovia, often results from trauma. In the peritoneal, pleural, and pericardial cavities, enteric bacterial organisms are often responsible; rarely the actinobacillus and the virus of bovine encephalitis may cause the infection. In the spinal canal and cerebral cavity, an inflammatory increase of fluid accompanies most of the viral and bacterial infections that attack these nervous tissues, with a typical group of symptoms resulting from increased intracranial pressure.

In the lungs, the usual cause is a bacterial or viral infection that commonly goes on to produce the more severe purulent or fibrinous reactions some hours later. In fact, most pneumonias begin with a serous exudate, the so-called inflammatory edema. Various chemical irritants produce serous exudation in the lungs. Ordinarily they are chemicals that reach the lungs by inhalation and include many irritant gases, including chloroform and even ether.

In addition, the bites from many venomous animals ranging from ants to serpents can induce serous inflammation. The usual effect of a bite of the American rattlesnake (*Crotalus* species) is a tremendous local inflammatory edema and a serous exudate, even to the extent that the fluid passes through the overlying intact skin. Moreover, simple cutaneous abrasions, if of the right depth and severity, induce an exudate of this type. These are abrasions not quite deep enough to cause bleeding. An hour after the injury is inflicted, drops of yellowish fluid appear on the surface, where they dry and form a scab.

SIGNIFICANCE AND EFFECT

The first effect of serous exudation is to dilute any material with which it mixes. This is advantageous if a toxin is present, because the most effective means of weakening the local effectiveness of a toxin is to dilute it a thousandfold. In case the host animal has antibodies to the toxin, the serous exudate is useful in bringing the toxin, in a diluted form, in contact with antibodies in the serum.

The pressure of exuded serum produces swelling of the part and interferes with its function, but any pain that is present usually must be attributed to other factors, judging from the sensations of persons who suffer from accumulations of noninflammatory fluids. Indeed, in pleuritis, the severe pain disappears when the serous exudate arrives to lubricate and separate the hyperemic and severely irritated surfaces of visceral and parietal pleural membranes. Summarizing, it may be said that as long as an inflammation remains serous, it is comparatively mild. The fluid is promptly resorbed if the cause is overcome.

Fibrinous inflammation

This type of inflammation is characterized by an exudate containing large amounts of fibrinogen (Fig. 5-17), which clots to form fibrin, the most conspicuous component. However, the other constituents of acute inflammatory exudates are also present in some degree.

OCCURRENCE

Fibrinous inflammation occurs chiefly on mucous and serous membranes and is particularly frequent in the pericardial sac. The respiratory mucous membranes (from pharynx to lung alveoli), the pleura and peritoneum, synovial membranes, and the lower intestinal mucous membrane are also locations where this type of inflammation is prone to occur.

MICROSCOPIC APPEARANCE.

Fibrin is seen adherent to the surface that produced it, detached fibrin seldom remains as a part of the microscopic section. The fibrils may sometimes be traced into the epithelial or mesothelial cells of the parent surface. These latter cells, as a result of the toxic action of the irritant responsible for the fibrin, are sometimes necrotic. Coagulative necrosis is typical, but ultimately the cells pass through the various changes that are characteristic of dead tissue. With the fibrin, there are small but variable amounts of precipitated se-

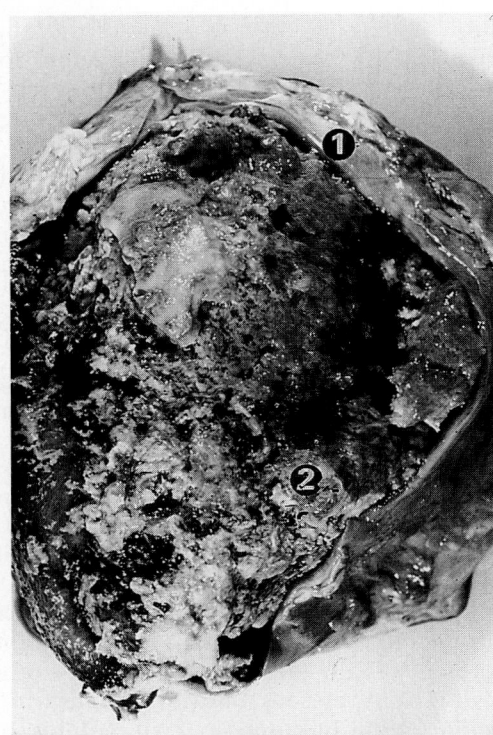

FIG. 5-17 Fibrinous exudate. Pericardium *(1)* and epicardium are covered by thick yellow fibrillar exudate with some hemorrhage *(2)*. Young pig with streptococcal infection. (Courtesy of Prof. Dr. H. Luginbühl.)

rum (protein), leukocytes, and even erythrocytes. The underlying viable tissue is hyperemic. The amount of exudate may be minute or massive. The exudate is sometimes formed in recurrent surges, or waves, so that one zone of exudate may be thin and lacelike, a second zone dense and deep-staining, and a third heavily sprinkled with leukocytes. In the pulmonary alveoli and less commonly in other places, the fibrin may be so densely packed as to form a solid, nonfibrillar mass. Since many leukocytes often accompany the fibrin and die in its vicinity, the already mentioned tendency of fibrin to suffer a blue-staining discoloration from karyolysis and chromatolysis is often pronounced, more so in one area than in another.

GROSS APPEARANCE

In the earliest stages, a dull and cloudy haze on a surface that should be smooth and shiny (serous membranes especially) is all that discloses the presence of a fibrinous exudate, but as the condition advances, a conspicuous covering of whitish fuzzy or stringy material develops. This may increase to a thickness of a centimeter with a shaggy outer surface, shreds of fibrin hanging here and there. The fibrin is sometimes reddened with blood, or it may be mingled with the fluid of a serous exudate, which may accompany the fibrinous variety. The layer of fibrin is at times dense and tough, and is then aptly called a **pseudomembrane** (false membrane), for it forms a white or yellowish sheet like a piece of thick paper.

A **diphtheritic membrane,** in contrast, is one in which the fibrinous exudate is so firmly attached to the underlying surface that it cannot be removed unless it is torn off along with a superficial layer of bleeding tissue. This diphtheritic membrane is characteristic of human diphtheria, hence the name. Calf diphtheria has an entirely different cause (the necrophorus organism), but the lesion is often much the same as that of human diphtheria.

Fibrinous exudates are sometimes voluminous in amount and retain the shape of the structure in which they were molded, thus forming a **fibrinous cast.** Most astonishing fibrinous casts, several inches long and having the exact form of a bronchus and its branches, are sometimes coughed up by animals, commonly bovines, which may not appear very ill before or after the event. Hollow casts lining an intestine may be several feet in length. When voided with the feces, it may at first seem that the animal has passed a segment of its intestine. These are seen at least in horses and cattle.

CAUSES

Fibrinous inflammation usually arises in response to the colonization of certain microorganisms. Prominent among these are the diphtheria bacillus, which attacks humans only, *Clostridium difficile, Salmonella, Clostridium,* and *Shigella* species, and the virus of avian laryngotracheitis. The viruses of feline infectious enteritis (panleukopenia), malignant catarrhal fever, and feline infectious peritonitis are somewhat less notable for production of fibrinous exudates.

Many fibrinous exudates are mixed with the serous variety and are called serofibrinous; others are combined with purulent inflammation (to be described shortly), constituting a fibrinopurulent type. In these combined forms, we may list many causes of serous and purulent inflammations as causes of the fibrinous inflammations as well. This applies most frequently to the pyogenic organisms, to which the reaction is usually purulent.

In such cases, the part of the body involved appears to be an important factor in determining whether the exudate is fibrinous. It has been stated that fibrinous inflammation occurs chiefly on mucous and serous surfaces. This is so true that it seems proper to accord to the anatomic location a causative role. For example, any acute inflammation of the pericardium is almost sure to be fibrinous, serofibrinous, or fibrinopurulent. The same is likely to be true of inflammations of the pleura, peritoneum, and even the meninges. Burns are at times followed by a fibrinous reaction, apparently without infection.

SIGNIFICANCE AND EFFECT

As far as the inflamed area is concerned, the fibrin probably serves a number of useful purposes. It may prevent blood loss (erythrocytes) through the dead and unprotected surface that usually underlies it (coagulative necrosis), and it protects the underlying tissues from further irritation. Certainly a "sore throat" coated with a layer of exudate is less painful than it is after the coating has been removed. The strands of fibrin serve also to form a framework useful in supporting leukocytes as they migrate through the inflamed zone.

If the inflammation terminates with reasonable promptness, the underlying surface is regenerated and the fibrin is dissolved. On a free mucous surface, it may be sloughed, as in the case of the bronchial and intestinal casts previously mentioned. But on the serous surfaces and in the pulmonary alveoli, fibrin remaining for some days is likely to undergo **organization** by fibrous tissue. The fibroblasts build into the zone of fibrin by proliferation of those in the underlying tissue. Such fibrous tissue is permanent. It is especially unfortunate on serous surfaces, such as those of the pleura, pericardium, and peritoneum, for it tends to build across from one opposing surface to another, forming permanent **adhesions** that tie them together and prevent movement and function. Barring this contingency, the organized layer on a surface becomes, as the inflammation subsides, covered with mesothelial cells that form a surface similar to that which existed previously. If fibrin in the alveoli of the lung is organized, that portion of the lung is permanently converted into fibrous tissue, a process known as **carnification** (*carneus* = flesh).

Purulent inflammation

Purulent inflammation is characterized by the formation of large quantities of **pus** (Fig. 5-18). Pus is a purulent exudate, typically a liquid of creamy color and consistency, but it may be thin and almost watery, or inspissated and semisolid. Its creamy yellow color is changed to bluish or greenish if *Pseudomonas aeruginosa* is among the infecting bacteria. It carries a blackish discoloration if it comes from black hoofs of horses, the color reportedly being due to sulfides. The definitive characteristic of pus is the presence of numerous neutrophilic polymorphonuclear granulocytes. These "neutrophils," living or necrotic, together with necrotic cells of the preexisting tissue, more or less liquefied, and minor amounts of the other constituents of inflammatory exudates, including serum, constitute the ingredients of pus. When pus is present in major or minor degree, the inflammatory process is said to be purulent.

The term suppurative inflammation or **suppuration** is a variant of the general term and implies that considerable amounts of pus are produced; usually it runs from a surface or fills cavities.

An **abscess** is defined as a circumscribed collection of pus. When well developed, it has a wall or capsule of fibrous tissue separating it from the surrounding tissue. In size, abscesses vary from microscopic to almost unlimited dimensions.

MICROSCOPIC APPEARANCE

The appearance of considerable numbers of neutrophilic leukocytes in or on a tissue justifies a diagnosis of purulent inflammation. Usually these are seen in great numbers, but they do not need to be more numerous than accompanying lymphocytes for the purulent designation to be employed. It should be noted

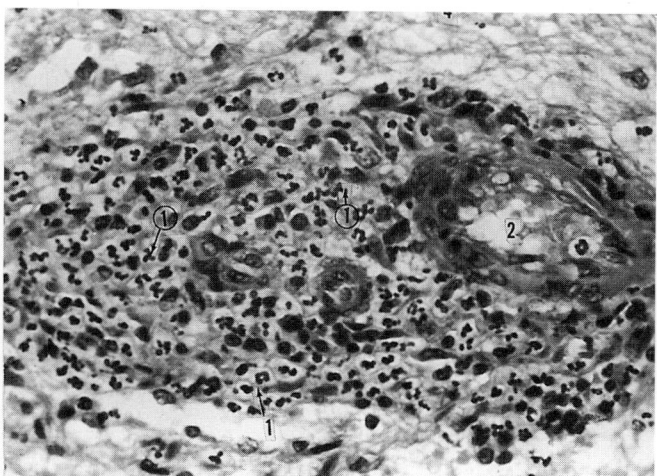

FIG. 5-18   Purulent inflammation. Polymorphonuclear neutrophilic leukocytes ("neutrophils" or "polymorphs") *(1)* adjacent to an artery *(2)* in the brain of a horse with generalized infection with *Streptococcus pyogenes*. Grossly visible abscesses were found elsewhere in the cerebrum (× 600.) (Courtesy of Army Veterinary Research Laboratory, Armed Forces Institute of Pathology)

that lymphocytes, as well as plasma cells and macrophages, are present in varying numbers in many inflammatory reactions. Many of the neutrophils undergo necrosis and are recognized by their small size, dark and irregularly shaped nuclei, and acidophilic cytoplasm. In addition to hyperemia or congestion, a minor amount of fibrin; serum (as a pink-staining precipitate); and various other leukocytes, fixed; and wandering cells are seen in conjunction with the neutrophils.

GROSS APPEARANCE

The purulent exudate consists of pus, the general appearance of which has been described as viscous, cream-colored fluid with possible variations extending from a watery consistency, such as results from some streptococcal infections, to a material that is practically a solid as the result of resorption of fluid. The red discoloration resulting from hemorrhage, the blue-green color coming from the pigment-forming *Pseudomonas* organisms, and the black color from disintegrating hoof material have also been described. Pus may be seen exuding from an infected wound or mucous membrane. It may be confined within abscesses or the body cavities. Its presence in the pulmonary alveoli, a phase of pneumonia called gray hepatization, is demonstrated by incising the lung and pressing it out from the cut surfaces. The beginning student is familiar with it, if nowhere else, as the thick yellow and sometimes foulsmelling fluid that is expectorated or blown from the nose in the late stages of a "cold."

CAUSES

Purulent or suppurative inflammations are caused by **pyogenic bacteria;** the word pyogenic means "pus forming." The principal members of this group of bacteria are the pyogenic bacilli, *Corynebacterium pyogenes,* and its relatives, *C. renale* and *C. equi*, *Pseudomonas aeruginosa*, and rarely, *Escherichia coli*. Pyogenic cocci include *Staphylococcus* and *Streptococcus* species. The tubercle bacillus is a pus-former in the very earliest stages of infection, and tuberculous meningitis may be purulent simply because the patient dies before the usual type of tuberculous lesion becomes established. The reaction in several of the infectious granulomas tends to be purulent in the immediate vicinity of the invading organisms. Chief among these granulomas are actinomycosis, actinobacillosis, the form of staphylococcal granuloma formerly called botryomycosis, coccidioidomycosis, blastomycosis, glanders, and chronic tularemia.

SIGNIFICANCE AND EFFECT

The liquefactive necrosis of tissue that is a feature of pus formation illustrates the fact that purulent inflammation is a prompt and violent reaction against irritant organisms. The vigorous microphagic and other activities of the neutrophils are often accompanied by effective production of humoral antibodies (immune bodies) as well as fever; all of these are potent defenses. These organisms also happen to be among the most vulnerable to available therapeutic agents.

Pus usually contains large numbers of the causative bacteria, living or dead, and the various toxic products of their metabolism. Confined pus is a source for absorption of toxic substances or organisms into the circulation, often with harmful results. When pyogenic bacteria or their toxins enter the bloodstream, systemic disease called sepsis or **septicemia** results. Typically, fever and other constitutional signs are present, and the condition is quite serious because of the potential for colonization of parenchymatous organs and the central nervous system. For these reasons it is of the utmost importance that an abscess or other suppurative lesion have free drainage to the outside; surgical intervention sometimes is necessary.

Abscesses, however, may become sterile; the body defenses may have killed all of the causative bacteria. The accumulated pus, with no way to escape, commonly remains for some time before being slowly absorbed and organized.

Hemorrhagic inflammation

Hemorrhagic inflammation and hemorrhagic exudates are characterized by large numbers of erythrocytes that leave their normal channels by diapedesis to exude from a body surface or into nearby tissues. With them are any or all of the components of other types of exudates, e.g., serum, leukocytes, and especially fibrin, so that the whole exudate bears some resemblance to clotted or unclotted blood.

OCCURRENCE

While this type of inflammation occurs within the tissues in such diseases as blackleg, anthrax, pasteurellosis, and purpura hemorrhagica, it is especially likely to involve mucous surfaces. The lungs may also develop this type of inflammation. Hemorrhagic gastritis and enteritis are among the most common manifestations of this type of exudate.

MICROSCOPIC APPEARANCE

Distinguishing hemorrhagic exudate from simple hemorrhage may be a problem. However, the various components of the blood are present in other than their normal proportions, and the constituents of exudates, such as fibrin, leukocytes, or both, are always more plentiful than in normal blood. Also, the exudate is diffuse in distribution, having come from an area, not from one or a few points, as would be the case with a simple hemorrhage.

GROSS APPEARANCE

Blood-colored material, sometimes fluid or semi-fluid, but usually clotted and of gelatinous consistency, appears on a surface or in tissue spaces. It is likely to be somewhat streaked or varying in color and consistency, revealing that the material is not pure clotted blood. The inflamed surface is deep red. It may be confused with the type of catarrhal inflammation in which the principal changes are severe hyperemia and loss of epithelium, but usually in the latter type, bloody fluid has not escaped from the tissue and the reddening of the surface is not quite so pronounced. Blood, whether as an exudate or as a hemorrhage, coming from any but the most posterior part of the gastrointestinal tract, colors the feces black. Coming from the lungs, it is foamy from admixed air, but when it comes from the respiratory passages this is not the case.

CAUSES

The causes of hemorrhagic inflammation are highly virulent microorganisms and acute poisoning by certain chemicals when in contact, in concentrated form, with digestive or other mucous membranes, or when such substances are eliminated by way of mucous membranes, especially those of the lower bowel, bladder, or gallbladder. Among these substances are phenol, arsenic, and phosphorus. The clotted exudate of laryngotracheitis of chickens has been mentioned as fibrinous. It is also hemorrhagic, with individual cases varying as to which type predominates. The pathogenic leptospirae and the virus of canine hepatitis are pathogens notable for causing hemorrhagic inflammation, doubtless the direct result of injury to vascular endothelium.

SIGNIFICANCE AND EFFECT

Hemorrhagic inflammation arises quickly and is all too likely to presage an early fatality, although in some instances it subsides with almost equal rapidity upon removal of the cause.

Catarrhal or mucous inflammation

The characteristic component of this type of inflammatory exudate is mucus, which comes from cells rather than from the blood. Mucus is produced by epithelial cells, either the mucous glands that open on mucous membranes or the one-celled mucous glands called goblet cells. For this reason, the occurrence of mucous or catarrhal inflammation is limited to mucous membranes. The number of goblet cells in a given mucous membrane may vary, and it is possible for epithelia not normally equipped with them to develop mucus-secreting cells.

MICROSCOPIC APPEARANCE

Commonly, the excessive mucus is readily visible as pale bluish or grayish strands of mucin clinging to the mucous membrane that produced it. The increased number of goblet cells may be conspicuously apparent. In many cases, however, another important feature is loss by necrosis and desquamation of much of the surface epithelium. Rather often this becomes the predominant feature of catarrhal inflammation, leaving the affected mucous membrane denuded of its epithelial covering, somewhat hyperemic, and containing slight or moderate infiltrations of lymphocytes. The hyperemia and the presence of reactive cells usually suffice to differentiate this condition from postmortem desquamation of the epithelium.

GROSS APPEARANCE

The predominantly mucous forms of catarrhal inflammation are recognized by the presence of the clear, slimy, mucin-containing fluid that has already been described as mucus. This is readily recognized on postmortem examination. During life, it may even drip from the nostrils if the nasal mucosa is involved. Mucous colitis, a fairly common condition, can often be recognized clinically by opaque white shreds or patches of semidehydrated mucus adhering to the formed feces or mixed with the excrement if it is softer.

When the inflammation is characterized less by mucus than by hyperemia and loss of epithelium, the inflamed surface shows little but the red color of raw meat with slight swelling. Limited amounts of mucus or of fibrinous or purulent material may or may not be present. Sometimes there is such an admixture of pus that the term mucopurulent is used. In mucous cholecystitis, the mucus may be seen imperfectly mixed with bile or it may not be discernible.

CAUSES

The irritants that cause this type of inflammation are mild in character or of short duration. They include bacterial and viral infections of low virulence or in their early stages. A "cold," as seen most often in humans and poultry, forms a good example in its earlier stages of catarrhal inflammation. Later the mucous exudate may become purulent.

Mildly or transiently irritating chemicals cause mucous inflammation. Inhaled formalin, chlorine, bromine, and chlorpicrin (tear gas) fall in this category, as do many antiseptics used in too great a concentration on delicate mucous membranes. There is considerable difference in what can be endured by the columnar epithelium of the cervix and uterus in comaprison with what can be endured by the squamous lining of the mouth.

Irritating foods in the digestive tract can set up catarrhal inflammation. In some cases, it is difficult to say whether a case of transient catarrhal gastroenteritis is caused directly by the food or by microorganisms in it, but mild forms are often caused by foods of improper quality for the species concerned or foods consumed excessively or consumed at a time when the nervous or other status of the digestive tract is not compatible with them (equine spasmodic colics, excessive horse meat in dogs). Along with the mild inflammation of the digestive mucosa, there is usually an increase of intraintestinal fluid and diarrhea, which can be viewed as a serous exudate.

The inhalation of ordinary dust, in considerable amounts, is sufficient to initiate a mucous reaction in the air passages. Inhalation of substances containing foreign proteins to which the patient is hypersensitive causes copious mucous exudation in "hay fever" of humans.

SIGNIFICANCE AND EFFECT

The flow of mucus is protective in that it tends to wash away the irritating substance. If the cause is removed, the flow of mucus subsides and the lost epithelium is quickly restored by proliferation of a few cells that survive here and there. If the injurious agent continues to act, especially if it is a microorganism, the inflammation appears to lead to hypersensitivity and hyperactivity of mucous glands and a chronic catarrh, especially in the respiratory passages.

These five forms complete the list of acute exudative inflammations as they are usually classified. It is evident that a given case may represent a mixture of two or more types, and also that a reaction may change from a mild to a more severe form. Likewise, the severe forms may subside gradually, assuming a catarrhal character, not to mention gradual change to chronic forms, which are yet to be considered. On the whole, however, the type of reaction encountered is likely to give a useful clue to the cause of the condition.

Chronic inflammation

Chronic inflammation represents a process that characterizes numerous disorders, many of known cause and many in which the cause has yet to be determined. Like acute inflammation, chronic inflammation represents a host response to an inciting stimulus. However, there are a number of differences. First, rather than typically being exudative, chronic inflammatory reactions are usually productive or proliferative. Cells at the site proliferate and produce matrix substances that add structural (i.e., collagen) and nutritional support (i.e., new blood vessels) to the lesion. Many of these changes represent components of the **repair** process, which will be described in subsequent pages. Second, many of the inciting stimuli are not harmful to the host tissues. For example, chronic inflammatory reactions are often observed in autoimmune diseases, where the host's immune system is directed against self antigens. In this case, the inciting stimulus is nothing more than a host component, certainly not a potentially injurious agent. In this respect, as we shall see, many of the chronic inflammatory reactions are induced more by the host's sensitivity to the inciting agent than by the tissue injury actually induced by the inciting agent/stimulus. Third, in most cases, chronic inflammatory reactions contain different inflammatory cells than those seen in the acute inflammatory reaction.

OCCURRENCE

Chronic inflammation can arise in a number of specific circumstances. It can follow a long-term (weeks, months, or years) acute inflammatory reaction. Particularly in the instance where the inciting stimulus is persistent, chronic inflammation would reside together with acute inflammation. If acute inflammatory reactions are repeated at the same anatomic site, then chronic inflammation might ensue. Histologic evidence of chronic inflammation would likely be observed in many tissues subjected to frequent acute inflammatory reactions, some examples being recurrent infections of the anal sacs in dogs or urinary bladder of cats or dogs. Lastly, chronic inflammation occurs in response to a number of specific inflammatory stimuli.

MICROSCOPIC APPEARANCE

The histologic hallmark of chronic inflammation is the infiltration of tissues with mononuclear inflammatory cells, specifically, macrophages, lymphocytes, and plasma cells. In addition, resident parenchymal cells proliferate. Fibroblasts become more numerous and produce more collagen, the single largest component of connective (scar) tissue. Endothelial cells divide and make new blood vessels. Tissues containing epithelium often have hyperplastic epithelial structures, a direct result of an increased mitotic rate of epithelial cells. Additionally, if the chronic inflammatory reaction is particularly severe and persistent, normal structures, which were once present, are replaced by connective tissue, with or without mononuclear inflammatory cells. This loss accounts for the functional impairment of particular organs after continued insult from chronic inflammatory reactions. For this reason, chronic inflammatory disease can be life-threatening when localized in parenchymal organs. When exclusively at other sites, such as skin and joints, chronic inflammation can be severely debilitating and painful, but rarely is it solely responsible for death of the host.

It should be stressed that despite this description of chronic inflammation, its microscopic appearance is quite heterogeneous. Certain examples of chronic inflammatory reactions are characterized by infiltrates comprised mostly of lymphocytes; most notable among these are viral infections of the central nervous system. Perivascular lymphocytic infiltration of the brain is the typical and often only visible expression of such infections such as rabies, Aujeszky's disease, lymphocytic choriomeningitis, equine encephalomyelitis, and Teschen disease. In contrast, infiltrates consisting almost exclusively of macrophages are typical for Johne's disease of cattle, a debilitating infection of the intestinal tract with *Mycobacterium paratuberculosis*. Additional examples include plasma cell pododermatitis of cats (Fig. 5-7), where the inflammation is almost entirely composed of plasma cells. However, in the vast majority of cases of chronic inflammatory disease, a mixture of these cell types are present. In fact, as mentioned previously, signs attributed to both acute and chronic inflammation may be present simultaneously. Although purulent exudation is not a typical finding in chronic inflammatory reactions, it may be present multifocally and interspersed between chronic inflammatory foci.

GROSS APPEARANCE

If the inflammation is not particularly severe or longstanding or if the proliferative component is not profound, it may not be noticed grossly. If, however, there is a large component of connective tissue, the inflammatory focus is indurated and tan and occasionally feels gritty upon cutting with a scalpel. If the connective tissue has yet to develop, the only gross change may be tinctorial, the tissue being more white to tan than normal.

CAUSES

As mentioned previously, chronic inflammation can arise from a setting of persistent acute inflammation or repeated bouts of acute inflammation, but chronic inflammation is typically associated with some forms of inflammatory stimuli. Stimuli that cannot be removed by the host defenses fall into this category. These can include organisms, such as mycobacterial species and some retroviruses, which, either because of their high replicative capacity or the host's inability to kill them, cannot be effectively removed. Also included are nondegradeable compounds, such as talc, carbon, silica, asbestos, and hydrophobic organic materials such as oil. Phagocytic cells have great difficulty digesting these materials; thus, they continue to be passed from phagocyte to phagocyte, never being eliminated and acting as a nidus for continued inflammatory disease.

Probably the most important factor in inducing chronic inflammation is the nature of the host's immune response to the stimulus. If the response from the host to an antigen is particularly exuberant or longlasting, that response will likely be in the form of chronic inflammation. In these cases, chronic inflammation usually arises slowly, without acute inflammation and, at first, without symptoms. Over time, these chronic inflammatory reactions induce significant tissue damage and profound debilitation. All of the autoimmune diseases of animals and humans fall within this category. Lymphocytes are usually a component in these inflammatory reactions, because they provide the antigenic specificity to both antibody and cell-mediated immune reactions at the tissue level.

SIGNIFICANCE AND EFFECT

Chronic inflammation underlies the basis for some of the most debilitating and fatal diseases known. Lentiviral diseases of ungulates (caprine arthritis-encephalitis virus, ovine maedi-visna), autoimmune glomerulonephritis or rheumatoid arthritis, viral encephalitides, or pulmonary asbestosis all represent chronic inflammatory disorders that are typically progressive, uniformly crippling, and often result in death.

Granulomatous inflammation

A type of chronic inflammation that is ubiquitous in nature, yet still to some degree mysterious, is granulomatous inflammation. As a type of chronic inflammation, granulomatous inflammation is a manifestation of some of the most debilitating chronic diseases of humans and animals. In the strictest sense, it is defined as chronic inflammation with the presence of **granulomas.** However, over the years, significant liberty has been taken by pathologists in their classification of granulomatous inflammation, so that any chronic inflammatory infiltrate comprised predominantly of cells of the mononuclear phagocyte system, such as macrophages, has often been categorized as granulomatous inflammation. Using either definition, infiltration of monocyte-derived cells is critical for the development of granulomatous inflammation.

A granuloma is a focally discreet chronic inflammatory reaction comprised predominantly, but not exclusively, of macrophages (Fig. 5-19). In order to be classified as a granuloma, the macrophages must be **organized,** or aggregated, in closely packed collections or sheets. Studies of the cells obtained from granulomas suggests that **activation** of macrophages within these lesions is a fairly universal feature. Similar to endothelial activation defined previously, macrophage activation implies that new functions are gained after appropriate stimulation. Thus, macrophages comprising a granuloma typically are more efficient at killing intracellular microorganisms; are more productive in extracellular secretion, particularly of cytokines and certain degradative enzymes; have enhanced phagocytic capabilities; and can recognize and kill tumor cell targets more effectively. However, differences in granulomas exist, depending on the inciting stimulus and host response, and functional changes of macrophages in these lesions do not always change in tandem. Macrophages from one granuloma may be comprised of macrophages with enhanced killing abilities that are poorly phagocytic, while cells from another granuloma may have the reverse functional profile.

In many if not most granulomas, macrophages differentiate into cells called **epithelioid macrophages.** These cells are found exclusively within granulomatous infiltrates, and their presence is a histologic hallmark of granulomatous inflammation. They have abundant, finely granular eosinophilic cytoplasm, vesicular nuclei, and indistinct cell boundaries, similar to some epithelial cells; hence their name. Ultrastructurally, these cells have very closely applied and interdigitated cell membranes, which explains why their cell boundaries are difficult to discern under the light microscope. The cytoplasm contains numerous mitochondria, an elaborate Golgi apparatus, and abundant rough endoplasmic reticulum. Interestingly, the cells have a paucity of endo-

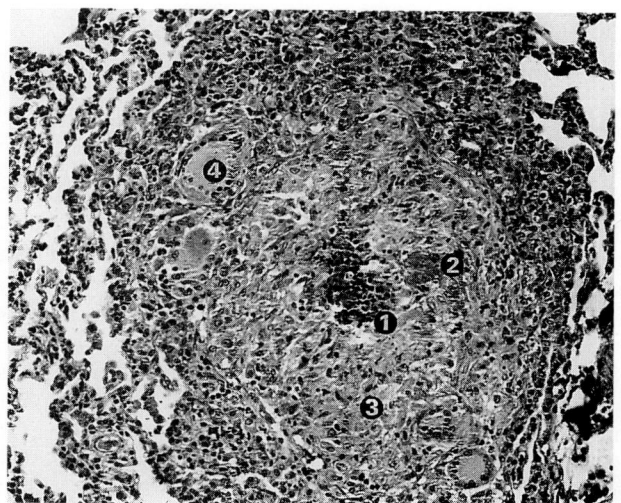

FIG. 5-19 Granulomatous inflammation. Tubercle in the lung of a rhesus monkey. In center of granuloma are neutrophils *(1)* and coagulation necrosis *(2)*. Macrophages *(3)* make up most of the lesion. Langhans' giant cell *(4)*. The periphery contains lymphocytes, plasma cells, monocytes, and few fibroblasts. (Courtesy of Prof. Dr. H. Luginbühl)

cytosed material and phagocytic vacuoles. Collectively, these morphologic characteristics suggest that the epithelioid macrophage is specialized for biosynthesis and protein secretion, rather than phagocytosis and killing.

Besides macrophages and epithelioid macrophages, other cell types may or may not be present within granulomatous infiltrates. Most notable are the multinucleate giant cells. As depicted in Fig. 5-5, there are three types of multinucleate giant cells: the foreign body type, the Langhans type, and the Touton giant cell. All are formed by the fusion of macrophages within the lesion, rather than nuclear mitosis without cytoplasmic division. Similar to epithelioid macrophages, these giant cells have important secretory functions. However, compared to other macrophages, these cells are relatively short-lived and generally die within days after formation. Lymphocytes, plasma cells, fibroblasts, and occasional granulocytes can also be found in many granulomas. Fibroblasts make collagen, the supporting building blocks of scar (connective) tissue, and it is this connective tissue that accounts for the induration of longstanding granulomas. The formation of permanent connective tissue at the site of a granuloma is particularly prominent when necrosis and tissue destruction are a significant component of the granuloma.

The central role of granulomatous inflammation is to defend the host against persistent irritants, whether from endogenous or exogenous sources. If a particular irritant cannot be removed by typical acute and chronic inflammatory reactions, then an attempt is made to wall off, sequester, phagocytize, and destroy the inciting agent by a granulomatous inflammatory response. In this regard, irritants that are poorly soluble, persistent, and not easily degradable by macrophages are typical stimuli that incite a granulomatous response; certain mycobacterial organisms, silica, barium sulphate, beryllium, and *Schistosoma* parasites are just a few examples.

Another factor important in the genesis of granulomatous inflammation is the host immune response to the offending inciting agent. Granulomas can be divided into "high turnover" and "low turnover" granulomas. High turnover granulomas are characterized by significant macrophage death within the lesion and are usually seen when a hypersensitivity to the inciting agent is present. Macrophages within these granulomas are replaced by recruitment of emigrating monocytes from the peripheral circulation as well as local mitotic division of macrophages within the granuloma. These granulomas typically, but not always, contain epithelioid macrophages, lymphocytes, and giant cells. The presence of the inciting agent is often scarce and difficult to find. Agents that induce this type of granuloma include mycobacteria, fungi, helminths and their ova, and many organisms that replicate intracellularly (e.g., *Brucella* species). In contrast, low turnover granulomas have little macrophage death, and the macrophage infiltrate is generally maintained by longevity of the macrophage population, rather than replacement by vascular emigration and cell division. Epithelioid macrophages may not be present, and the inciting agent is often found within the majority of the macrophages in the lesion. A hypersensitivity reaction is usually not a component; thus, lymphocytes are uncommon. This type of granuloma is typically formed in response to agents that are inert, nontoxic, and fail to evoke an immune response, such as silk sutures, oil, carrageenan, and barium sulphate. It should be clear from the previous discussion that the nature of the stimulus as well as the immune response from the host are probably the two most important factors in the development of granulomatous inflammation in tissues.

References

Adams DO. The structure of mononuclear phagocytes differentiating *in vivo*: I. Sequential fine and histologic studies of the effect of Bacillus Calmette-Guerin (BCG). Am J Pathol 1974;76:17–48.

Adams DO. The granulomatous inflammatory response: a review. Am J Pathol 1976;84:164–191.

Adams DO, Hamilton TA. The activated macrophage and granulomatous inflammation. Curr Top Pathol 1989;79:151–167.

Kunkel SL, Chensue SW, Strieter RM, et al. Cellular and molecular aspects of granulomatous inflammation. Am J Respir Cell Mol Biol 1989;1:439–447.

Montali RJ. Comparative pathology of inflammation in the higher vertebrates (reptiles, birds and mammals). J Comp Pathol 1988;99:1–26.

Sheffield EA. The granulomatous inflammatory response. J Pathol 1990;160:1–2.

Spector WG, Lykke AWJ. The cellular evolution of inflammatory granulomata. J Pathol Bacteriol 1966;92:163–177.

Tanaka A, Emori K, Nagao S, et al. Epithelioid granuloma formation requiring no T-cell function. Am J Pathol 1982;106:165–170.

Williams GT, Williams WJ. Granulomatous inflammation—a review. J Clin Pathol 1983;36:723–733.

RESOLUTION AND REPAIR

Concurrent with the inflammatory response and continuing after inflammation has resolved, repair processes attempt to restore the anatomic and functional integrity of the tissue. Some types of tissue, such as epithelial surfaces, regenerate fairly well after tissue injury. However, in many types of tissues in mammals, regeneration does not occur; instead, repair processes fill in the damaged area with a simple yet resilient extracellular matrix, the connective tissue scar. The process of repair is not nearly as restorative as regeneration. For example, a salamander has regenerative mechanisms with the capacity to completely replace an amputated limb: by comparison, repair of damaged mammalian tissue is crude. Nonetheless, the mechanisms involved in the events leading to scar formation are complex and indeed vital for the survival of the animal. In this section, we describe the mechanisms and morphologic appearance of the healing wound, a healing process that is one of the most common and fundamental encountered by both clinicians and pathologists.

Wound healing is a complex cascade of biochemical and cellular events in response to tissue injury. If wound healing is to be successful, these events must be instituted in proper sequence, and the final outcome (generally a connective tissue scar) represents the collective summation of all of these events. Moreover, the processes involved in wound repair must be precisely controlled; otherwise, repair processes might run rampant with deleterious consequences. An example of inadequate control of the repair process is a **keloid**, an exuberant connective tissue scar in response to a cutaneous wound. In this instance, the scar contains excessive quantities of collagen, which results in a tumor-like projection above the skin surface.

There has been an explosion of knowledge on the cellular and biochemical events in wound repair. For the sake of simplicity, these events can be temporally divided into three phases: (1) **inflammation,** (2) **fibroblastic phase,** and (3) **maturation and remodeling.** Although it is useful to think of repair in terms of these phases, in reality, they overlap with each other, and components of each may often be found in the same tissue.

Inflammation phase

As previously described, inflammation is the body's response to tissue injury. Whether the insult is thermal, chemical, traumatic, or biologic, in most cases the vascular integrity of the insulted area is disrupted. Blood vessel disruption leads to the extravasation of blood (or sometimes only plasma, if the damage is minor) into the surrounding tissue. The earliest events in the healing process are those directed at preventing any further loss of blood. Injured vessels constrict. Platelet adhesion and aggregation occur at the site, and activation of the coagulation cascade ensues. The result is the formation of a **thrombus,** which serves two purposes. First, it limits further blood loss (**hemostasis**). Secondly, it provides a preliminary matrix, which sets the stage for further repair processes.

Extravasated platelets adhere to the collagen in the perivascular space, using platelet cell membrane receptors specific for extracellular matrix proteins. Contact with fibrillar collagen activates the platelets, so that specific adhesion proteins on the platelet membrane are induced. One such protein is platelet glycoprotein IIb/IIIa, a $\beta3$ integrin (Table 7-2). Once bound to collagen or other extracellular matrix proteins, the platelets release the contents of their alpha granules, which contain fibrinogen, fibronectin, von Willebrand factor, and thrombospondin. These additional extracellular matrix molecules add to the aggregated mass of platelets and fibrin, and they interact with adhesion molecules on platelets via platelet glycoprotein IIb/IIIa. These interactions stabilize and strengthen the new provisional matrix. Moreover, the fibrinogen from the plasma escaping from the damaged vasculature, as well as the fibrinogen released from platelets, is induced to polymerize by way of the extrinsic (tissue factor-induced) or intrinsic (activated by negatively charged surfaces) coagulation pathways. Thus, the extravascular gel that provisionally fills the cavity created by the initial wound is composed of material from the coagulation cascade (fibrin), aggregated platelets from the blood, and a weak extracellular matrix, consisting of fibrinogen, fibronectin, and von Willebrand factor, much of which originated from activated entrapped platelets within the thrombus.

This initial sequence of events after vascular injury provides all the stimuli necessary for the induction of an acute inflammatory reaction. The plasma-derived coagulation molecule, activated Hageman factor (factor XII), initiates the kinin system to generate the vasoactive peptide, bradykinin. Aside from its vasoactive properties, it induces the production of arachidonic metabolites, which are potent proinflammatory molecules. Additionally, the fibrinolytic system degrades fibrin to fibrin-split products, which are chemotactic for neutrophils. Cleaved complement components also participate in the primary induction of inflammation by the production of anaphylatoxins, which degranulate mast cells and provide important chemotactic substances for leukocytes. The interrelationship of the four plasma enzyme system is reviewed in Figure 5-12.

Neutrophils and macrophages rapidly respond to this new rich source of chemoattractants and activating stimuli. The newly formed extracellular matrix also provides a substrate for subsequent leukocyte migration. The first leukocytes to arrive at the wound site are neutrophils. Their function is to phagocytize and kill any bacteria in the area. The prevention of bacterial colonization of the wound is important for the expedient repair of the area; however, neutrophil emigration to the site is not essential for repair processes to take place. Neutrophil depletion experiments failed to abrogate healing in experimental studies (Simpson and Ross, 1972). This purulent infiltrate resolves after the first few days, provided bacterial contamination and colonization of the area do not occur.

In contrast to the role neutrophils play in repair processes, the subsequent influx of macrophages into the wound area is the single most critical element in the induction of repair mechanisms. Monocyte-derived macrophages begin to accumulate at the wound site between 2 and 5 days after injury. Their roles include assisting neutrophils in phagocytosis of organisms and tissue debris, as well as the removal of effete neutrophils. More importantly, macrophages release a number of growth factors and cytokines, which are important in the maintenance of the inflammatory reaction and in the initiation, maturation, and control of the wound healing process (Table 5-5).

The signals responsible for macrophage production of repair growth factors are uniquely governed by the local microenvironment. With damage to the microvasculature at the wound site and formation of an avascular thrombus, tissue at the center of the wound is ischemic. Moreover, the presence of activated neutrophils and macrophages further increases the metabolic demand for oxygen in the area. Consequently, oxygen tension falls and lactic acid increases as cells utilize anaerobic glycolysis for energy, and thus, pH decreases in the wound space. It is this combination of hypoxia, acidity, and lactate concentration that activates the wound macrophages to send out distress signals. These distress signals are manifested by the elaboration of specific growth factors from the wound macrophages. These macrophage-derived growth factors (Table 5-5) are collectively responsible for the next sequence of changes that characterize the fibroblastic phase of wound repair.

Fibroblastic phase

With the activation of wound macrophages and elaboration of specific growth factors, the extracellular matrix can begin to be replaced by stronger and more resilient connective tissue. The major component of a mature connective tissue scar is collagen; thus, in the healing wound, collagen-producing fibroblasts are recruited from the wound edge and induced to make collagen, a collective process referred to as **fibroplasia. Neovascularization** occurs concurrently with fibroplasia, so that new capillaries sprout from viable vessels at the wound edge and migrate into the wound space. **Wound contraction** begins to bring the wound edges closer together, and if the original tissue was covered by an epithelial surface, **reepithelialization** begins to cover the healing wound.

Fibroplasia begins by the formation of **granulation tissue** within the wound space. This tissue consists of a loose matrix of collagen, fibronectin, and hyaluronic acid with macrophages, fibroblasts, and leaky, newly formed vessels. The fibroblasts, which are its principal component, are elongated fibrillar cells with plump, ovoid, hyperchromatic nuclei. Mitoses are common. These cells often form bundles or fasciculi. The new capillaries have plump endothelial nuclei and often run in parallel arrays perpendicular to the surface (Fig. 5-20). The tissue is edematous and characterized by multiple empty spaces, as a result of the immaturity of the new capillaries, which tend to leak fluid. The surfaces, when seen with the naked eye, appear to bear many red "granules," which are actually the blunt ends of these loops of new capillaries coursing perpendicular to the

TABLE 5-5 **Protein growth factors involved in tissue repair**

Factor	Source	Effects on repair processes
Platelet-derived growth factor (PDGF)	Platelets, macrophages, endothelial cells	1. Chemotactic for fibroblasts, monocytes, polymorphonuclear cells, smooth muscle cells 2. Mitogenic for fibroblasts 3. Increases fibroblast production of extracellular matrix
Transforming growth factor-β (TGF-β)	Platelets, T cells, macrophages	1. Chemotactic for fibroblasts and leukocytes 2. Regulation of cell proliferation (inhibits replication of keratinocytes, lymphocytes, endothelium, and some epithelium, but stimulates proliferation of fibroblasts and osteoblasts) 3. Stimulates production of extracellular matrix 4. Induces production of other factors 5. Stimulates angiogenesis *in vivo* (but inhibits *in vitro*)
Fibroblast growth factors (FGF) (basic and acidic)	Many different cell types in most organs	1. Stimulates angiogenesis (chemotactic and mitogenic) 2. Mitogenic for endothelium, smooth muscle, fibroblasts, skeletal myocytes, chondrocytes 3. Affects differentiation of many cell types
Epidermal growth factor (EGF, or urogastrone)	Platelets, macrophages	1. Increases proliferation of epithelium, endothelium and fibroblasts 2. Increases production of glycosaminoglycans 3. Decreases collagen synthesis
Insulin-like growth factors (somatomedins)	fibroblasts, hepatocytes	1. Mitogenic for fibroblasts
IL-1	Predominantly macrophages and endothelium	1. Chemotactic for leukocytes and some epithelial cells 2. Stimulates proliferation of keratinocytes, fibroblasts, smooth muscle, and endothelium 3. Enhances fibroblast production of extracellular matrix
TNF-α	Macrophages	1. Mitogenic for fibroblasts 2. Angiogenic *in vivo* (but inhibits *in vitro*) 3. Stimulates collagenase production from many cell types 4. Bone/cartilage resorption
Interferon-γ	Lymphocytes	1. Inhibits fibroblast proliferation 2. Inhibits collagen synthesis

surface. The tissue is typically deep red and bleeds very easily.

The signals responsible for the formation of granulation tissue are varied. First, as mentioned previously, growth factors likely play a crucial role in the cell migration and differentiation required for granulation tissue development. Although the requisite peptide growth factors can originate from a number of cell types, wound macrophages and entrapped platelets in the thrombus are probably the major contributors involved (Table 5-5). Second, the extracellular matrix, formed by plasma constituents, platelets, macrophages, and the incoming fibroblasts, provide a medium for adhesion, migration, and guidance of the cells that will comprise the developing granulation tissue. Third, the anatomic nature of the wound itself provides a stimulus for cell migration and proliferation into the wound space ("free-edge effect"). Normal cells have controls on their proliferative capacity through their interactions with adjacent cells by a process referred to as **contact inhibition.** That is, by their close association with their neighbors, cells gain "environmental cues" that favor the inhibition of mitotic activity. In contrast, neoplastic cells have lost all contact inhibition and proliferate relentlessly. In the wound, the cells residing at the wound edge have lost the normal contact inhibition signals present before injury. Thus, they tend to proliferate in the direction of the wound space.

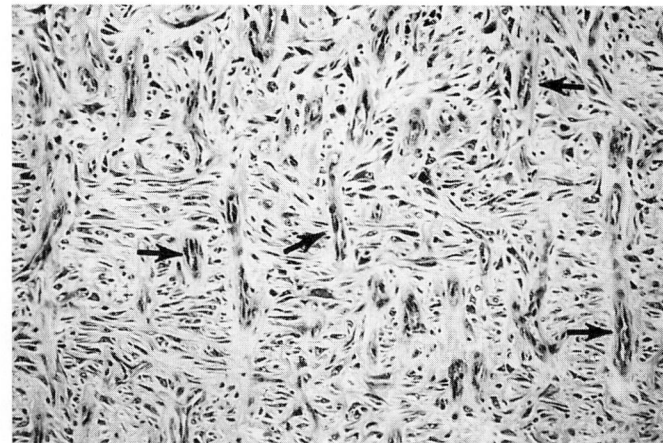

FIG. 5-20 Fibrous granulation tissue at the base of a healing ulcer of the rectum of a cow. The organization of new blood vessels *(arrows)* perpendicular to fibroblasts and collagen is typical and allows differentiation from fibroma. (Courtesy of Dr. C. L. Davis)

Neovascularization (**angiogenesis**) occurs simultaneously with the ingrowth of fibroblasts from the wound edge. Endothelial cells within intact capillaries at the wound edge break through the basement membrane of the vessel wall by secreting collagenase and plasminogen activator. They then migrate toward the wound space using the wound extracellular matrix as a substratum. These migrating cells differentiate into a new capillary tube; most, if not all, of the neovascularization that occurs in the wound is secondary to differentiation of migrating endothelial cells. Proliferation of endothelial cells generally occurs only in the parent vessel to replace the migrating cells. The capillary sprout joins the parent capillary to establish blood flow. Macrophages within the wound space are responsible for the elaboration of angiogenic substances, most notably **fibroblast growth factors (FGFs).** As mentioned previously, hypoxia is the driving force behind macrophage elaboration of factors that favor both fibroblast migration and angiogenesis.

There is continual rebuilding and change in the constituents of the extracellular matrix during the process of wound repair. Initially, the extracellular matrix comprising the wound space was composed of proteins largely derived from platelets and plasma. With the migration of macrophages into the wound and subsequent formation of granulation tissue, the extracellular matrix components (Table 5-6) are manufactured from cells *in situ*. In particular, fibroblasts deposit large quantities of **fibronectin** in the wound. Fibronectin serves a number of functions; in particular, it acts as a necessary substratum for cell attachment. In contrast, the other major component of extracellular matrix at this time, **hyaluronic acid,** a glycosaminoglycan polysaccharide,

TABLE 5-6 **Extracellular matrix components**

Component	Source	Roles
Fibronectin	Platelets, macrophages, fibroblasts, hepatocytes, epithelial cells, endothelial cells, smooth muscle cells	1. Chemotactic for macrophages 2. Stimulation of endothelial and fibroblast movement 3. Substratum for cell movement 4. Opsonin for phagocytes 5. Acts as a scaffold for new matrix deposition (i.e., collagen) 6. Facilitates fibroblast proliferation 7. Ligand for adhesion molecules (integrins) on cells
Proteoglycans (protein core with glycosaminoglycan polysaccharide chain; i.e., heparin, heparan sulfate, chondroitin-4-sulfate, keratin sulfate, dermatan sulfate)	Fibroblasts	1. Strengthens cell attachment to substratum 2. Contributes to tissue resilience 3. May regulate collagen fibrillogensis 4. Heparin stimulates endothelial migration *in vitro*
Hyaluronic acid (glycosaminoglycan polysaccharide)	Fibroblasts	1. Important in cell motility (facilitates cell-substratum adhesion-disadhesion) 2. May promote cell division
Collagen	Fibroblasts	1. Major component of mature scar tissue 2. Provides tensile strength of healing wounds
Elastin	Fibroblasts	1. Provides elasticity to matrix
Laminin	Epithelial cells, endothelial cells, monocytes	1. Attaches cells to basement membranes 2. Promotes adherence of cells to type IV collagen

weakens cell attachment to the substratum. The combination of these two matrix components provides an efficient microenvironment for cell movement, which involves the continual attachment, dislodgement, and reattachment of cells from the wound matrix. Indeed, fibronectin, along with hyaluronic acid, are the predominant matrix components during the earliest phases of wound repair, which largely involve cell migration. As the wound heals, hyaluronic acid decreases in concentration, and sulfated glycosaminoglycans, or proteoglycans (such as heparin sulfate, dermatan sulfate, and chondroitin-4-sulfate) increase. This change in proteoglycan composition favors cell attachment and immobility. With the cessation of movement, cells differentiate into more mature (and functional) phenotypes. Endothelial cells mature into cells lining functional capillaries, and fibroblasts begin to manufacture collagen. Fibronectin is used as a template for fibroblast production and deposition of collagen, so as the wound matures, proteoglycans and fibronectin are increasingly replaced by collagen, the major structural component of the scar.

With the change in the composition of the extracellular matrix, fibroblasts undergo some dramatic phenotypic changes, from those of immature, replicating, migratory cells to collagen-producing factories. The cytoplasm becomes more voluminous and contains abundant rough endoplasmic reticulum, as might be expected from a cell actively engaged in protein synthesis. Collagen is the most common protein found in animals, and its production involves a number of post-translational events. Each collagen molecule is composed of three polypeptide chains wrapped around each other in a helix. The biochemical composition of the individual chains and the combination of these chains that comprise the collagen molecule account for the multiple types of collagen found in the tissues (Table 5-7). Each collagen molecule, however, is similar in that the polypeptide chains have the amino acid glycine in every third position, with proline and lysine often in the other positions. The polypeptide chains are manufactured in the cytoplasm of the fibroblast on ribosomes. From there, they pass into the cisternae of the rough endoplasmic reticulum, where the three chains are assembled into a helix. Critical to helix formation is the hydroxylation of proline and lysine residues to form hydroxyproline and hydroxylysine, respectively. Hydroxylation of lysine and proline is necessary for helical stability and subsequent release from the cell. After helix formation, the molecule is referred to as **procollagen.** Once outside the cell, the procollagen molecule is cleaved of its terminal globular nonhelical domains by specific procollagen peptidases. Now referred to as **tropocollagen,** without the terminal nonhelical domains, these molecules can polymerize to form fibrils, which make up collagen fibers, the structural backbone of mature collagen. Collagen types I to III are fibrillar; types IV and V fail to undergo proteolytic cleaving of the terminal procollagen domains, and these globular domains prevent polymerization into fibrils.

Even though low oxygen tension in the wound is

TABLE 5-7 **Types of Collagen**

Type	Form	Distribution
I	Fibrillar	Skin, tendons, ligaments, bone, scar tissue
II	Fibrillar	Cartilage, nucleus pulposus
III	Fibrillar	Blood vessels, skin, early wounds
IV	Nonfibrillar	Basement membranes
V	Nonfibrillar	Pericellular in multiple tissues, blood vessels
VI, VII, VIII, IX, X	Unknown	Unknown

the stimulus for macrophage elaboration of vital growth factors, hypoxia is detrimental to a number of normal physiologic processes; in particular, collagen synthesis by fibroblasts. Oxygen is required for the hydroxylation of proline and lysine residues in the polypeptide chains assembled in the cytoplasm of the fibroblast. Without enough oxygen, the helical procollagen molecule is not formed and is not subsequently released into the extracellular space. In addition to oxygen, vitamin C is also required for these hydroxylations to take place. The source of this higher oxygen demand in the wound is the new blood vasculature arriving from the wound edge. There is, thus, a delicate balance in gas permeability in the healing wound, with hypoxia driving cell migration and angiogenesis early on, and higher oxygen levels supplying the metabolic demands associated with collagen synthesis later.

At the same time that collagen is being produced, some fibroblasts differentiate into contractile cells called **myofibroblasts.** As described by Gabbiani and Majno (1972), fibroblasts in granulation tissue begin to develop structural and functional features similar to smooth muscle cells. Ultrastructurally, there is retraction of the endoplasmic reticulum and Golgi apparatus to perinuclear positions, and cytoplasmic actin filaments become oriented parallel to the cell's long axis. It has been postulated that these cells are responsible for the phenomenon of **wound contraction,** a process whereby the size of the wound space is decreased by bringing the wound edges closer together. This process minimizes the area to be healed and thus is truly beneficial, in most cases. According to the hypothesis, myofibroblasts align themselves along the border of the wound and then provide contractile forces transmitted to the surrounding tissue through cell-cell and cell-matrix linkages. However, other investigators feel that wound contraction can be explained entirely by tractional forces generated by fibroblasts when they migrate on the substratum of the extracellular matrix (Grierson and others, 1988). This hypothesis contends that a healing wound contracts because of distortion of the extracellular matrix caused by the shearing forces generated by the forward propulsion of migrating fibroblasts. Regardless of the mechanism involved, wound contraction decreases the time necessary for a gaping wound to heal.

Within hours after cutaneous injury, **reepithelialization** begins by migration of epithelial cells from the wound edge. The stimuli responsible for this migration are the same as those for fibroblasts, i.e. growth factors, particularly the peptide, epidermal growth factor (EGF), and the "free edge effect." Concurrent with migration, epithelial cells undergo specific phenotypic alterations, including retraction of intracellular tonofilaments, dissolution of intercellular desmosomes, and the formation of peripheral cytoplasmic actin filaments. The underlying basement membrane is dissolved, presumably by proteases made by the epithelial cells. These alterations free the cells from the underlying basement membrane and adjacent epithelial cells and give them the capacity to move laterally. The cells migrate on a the provisional extracellular matrix, with a significant proportion of fibronectin produced by the migrating epithelial cells themselves. Epithelial migration occurs most rapidly when the wound surface is moist and well oxygenated. If a scab or eschar is overlying the wound, the migrating cells dissect between the matrix and overlying debris, but the process is impeded somewhat. Once reepithelialization is complete across the wound surface, the epithelial cells revert back to their normal phenotype, the basement membrane is reconstituted by the new epithelium, and hemidesmosomes and desmosomes are reformed. As with collagen synthesis, reepithelialization is affected by oxygen tension. Reepithelialization occurs best when oxygen tension is high from a combination of previous angiogenic activity within the wound and exposure to air. Such conditions create a dilemma for clinicians who continue to search for wound dressings that are oxygen-permeable yet prevent wound desiccation.

Maturation and remodelling

The final phase of wound healing is maturation and remodelling of the extracellular matrix. It is during this phase that the wound scar gains its maximum strength, but this process is a slow one. For a scar to reach its maximum tensile strength, many months or even years of remodelling are required; yet, a fully mature cutaneous scar is only approximately 70% as strong as normal intact skin.

The strength of a fibrous connective scar can be attributed to: (1) accruing collagen deposition and (2) remodelling of the collagen fibrils so that larger collagen bundles with more covalent cross-linking between collagen fibrils are formed. Initially, tropocollagen polymerizes extracellularly into fibrils using weak electro-static forces and hydrogen bonds. However, under the control of the enzyme lysyl oxidase, lysines, hydroxylysines, or glycosylated lysines within the tropocollagen molecule are oxidized to aldehydes. The aldehydes then form links with either other aldehyde groups or with unoxidized lysine residues. These cross-links form between tropocollagen molecules within a fibril and between fibrils themselves, so that larger collagen fibers composed of many fibrils are formed. The formation of these larger collagen fibers with significant cross-linking between fibrils accounts for the great tensile strength inherent in a scar.

However, the process of scar remodelling involves the continual production, digestion, aggregation, and orientation of the collagen fibrils and fibers. A steady balance between collagen production and breakdown is reached, so that even though collagen production remains high in the scar, the scar does not grow in size. Collagen is initially deposited on the fibronectin template in a somewhat haphazard fashion. Depending on the nature and direction of the stresses placed upon the tissue, these collagen fibers are subsequently digested by the enzyme, collagenase, and deposited again in arrangements similar to the adjacent unaffected tissue. For example, a healing tendon first forms a connective tissue scar with a disorderly array of collagen fibers. This immature scar will not withstand even normal day-to-day stresses placed upon it. However, as the scar remodels, the collagen fibers become oriented parallel to the directional forces placed upon it, similar to the collagen fibers comprising the tendon. By so doing, the scar gains tensile strength and, thus, functional integrity. Collagenase is produced by a number of cell types within the wound, including leukocytes, macrophages, fibroblasts, and epithelial cells. While collagen synthesis is oxygen dependent, collagen degradation with collagenase is not. Thus, a wound scar without proper vascular support and oxygenation becomes progressively smaller and weaker from the catabolic processes associated with collagen lysis without concomitant synthesis.

From the preceding discussion, wound healing can be regarded as a complicated interplay of cells, growth factors, extracellular matrix components, and oxygen, with dynamic, often reciprocal, relationships existing between them. For example, hypoxia, through macrophage stimulation and elaboration of growth factors, drives cell migration and angiogenesis in the wound space. With restoration of blood flow and increased oxygen levels in the area once again, collagen synthesis and cell proliferation are favored, and angiogenesis and cell migration are inhibited. The presence of growth factors influences fibroblast production of extracellular matrix components, while the composition of the extracellular matrix can influence cellular function. Moreover, despite the attempt to present the processes of healing and repair as specific phases comprised of precise mechanisms, there is significant overlap between the repair phases. In addition, there is significant variation in the nature, composition, and duration of the phases in different wounds depending on the tissue site, degree of bacterial contamination and infection, blood supply, and extent of tissue damage.

References

Baird A, Walicke PA. Fibroblast growth factors. Br Med Bull 1989;45:438–452.

Barbul A. Immune aspects of wound repair. Clin Plast Surg 1990;17:433–442.

Barnes D. Growth factors involved in repair processes: an overview. Methods Enzymol 1988;163:707–715.

Clark RAF. Cutaneous tissue repair: basic biologic considerations. I J Am Acad Dermatol 1985;13:701–725.

Clark RAF. Potential roles of fibronectin in cutaneous wound repair. Arch Dermatol 1988;124:201–206.

Clark RAF. Wound repair. Curr Opin Cell Biol 1989;1:1000–1008.

Fujikawa LS, Foster CS, Harrist TJ, et al. Fibronectin in healing rabbit corneal wounds. Lab Invest 1981;45:120–129.

Gabbiani G, Majno G. Dupuytren's contracture: fibroblast contraction? Am J Pathol 1972;66:131–146.

Grierson I, Joseph J, Miller M, et al. Wound repair: the fibroblast and the inhibition of scar formation. Eye 1988;2:135–148.

Grotendorst GR. Growth factors as regulators of wound repair. Int J Tissue React 1988;10:337–344.

Hardy MA. The biology of scar formation. Phys Ther 1989;69:1014–1024.

Hunt TK. The physiology of wound healing. Ann Emerg Med 1988;17:1265–1273.

Knighton DR, Fiegel VD. The macrophages: effector cell wound repair. Prog Clin Biol Res 1989;299:217–226.

Knighton DR, Fiegel VD. Macrophage-derived growth factors in wound healing: regulation of growth factor production by the oxygen microenvironment. Am Rev Respir Dis 1989;140:1108–1111.

LaVan FB, Hunt TK. Oxygen and wound healing. Clin Plast Surg 1990;17:463–472.

Leibovich SJ, Ross R. The role of the macrophage in wound repair: a study with hydrocortisone and antimacrophage serum. Am J Pathol 1975;78:71–100.

Martin BM, Gimbrone MA, Unanue ER, et al. Stimulation of non-lymphoid mesenchymal cell proliferation by a macrophage-derived growth factor. J Immunol 1981;126:1510–1515.

Pessa ME, Bland KI, Copeland EM. Growth factors and determinants of wound repair. J Surg Res 1987;42:207–217.

Reed BR, Clark RAF. Cutaneous tissue repair: practical implications of current knowledge. II. J Am Acad Dermatol 1985;13:919–941.

Rothe M, Falanga V. Growth factors: their biology and promise in dermatologic diseases and tissue repair. Arch Dermatol 1989;125:1390–1398.

Ryan GB, Cliff WJ, Gabbiani G, et al. Myofibroblasts in human granulation tissue. Hum Pathol 1974;5:55–67.

Simpson DM, Ross R. The neutrophilic leukocyte in wound repair. A study with antineutrophil serum. J Clin Invest 1972;51:2009–2023.

Sprugel KH, McPherson JM, et al. Effects of growth factors in vivo: I. Cell ingrowth into porous subcutaneous chambers. Am J Pathol 1987;129:601–613.

Trabucchi E, Radaelli E, Marazzi M, et al. The role of mast cells in wound healing. Int J Tissue React 1988;10:367–372.

Wahl SM, Wong H, McCartney-Francis N. Role of growth factors in inflammation and repair. J Cell Biochem 1989;40:193–199.

FEVER

Fever has been occasionally noted as being a part of inflammation for centuries (Celsus, 30 BC–38 AD), and was for a long time thought to be a disease itself. The first experiments designed to establish a relationship between inflammation and fever were carried out by Billroth and Frese, about 100 years ago, but the experiments were not conclusive (Atkins and Bodel, 1972).

Currently, fever is distinguished from other hyperthermias (discussed later) on the basis of several characteristics:

1. The elevation in body temperature is generated by thermoregulation only, resulting from the action of inflammatory cytokines on the preoptic anterior hypothalamic areas of the brain.
2. The increase in the thermopreferendum is evident, particularly at the outset of fever. Humans and animals seek a warmer, more comfortable temperature during a "chill."
3. The higher temperature is maintained by a fully functional thermoregulatory system. The "set point" on the body "thermostat" is simply put at a higher temperature.
4. Antipyretic drugs, such as aspirin, can intervene in the febrile process to reduce the body temperature.

None of the foregoing criteria applies to the other hyperthermias.

Fever occurs in representative species of several phyla (Kluger, 1979). Live and dead bacteria have been used to produce fever in fishes, amphibians, reptiles, birds, and mammals. Antipyretic drugs have been shown to reduce the experimental fever in all of these species, except amphibians. Studies to establish the effect of endogenous pyrogens (to be discussed) have not been completed on representative species of all of these phyla.

Newborn mammals (humans, sheep, guinea pigs) do not manifest fever in the presence of infections. Neonatal lambs and guinea pigs are refractory to bacterial pyrogens administered experimentally. Large doses of bacterial endotoxins, administered intravenously, produce fever in the guinea pig, however. This apparent resistance to fever in the neonate is postulated to be caused by immaturity of the mechanisms in the central nervous system or to an effect of circulating antipyretic substances. Such substances have been shown in the blood of lambs and ewes close to the time of parturition (Cooper and others, 1979).

The central system of temperature regulation is located in the preoptic anterior hypothalamus. Obliterative lesions at this site remove the ability to regulate body temperature.

It is now well established that fever is a systemic sign of inflammation and, thus, a component of the acute phase response. Moreover, elevated circulating levels of macrophage-derived cytokines, particularly IL-1 and TNF-α, are at least partly responsible for fever induction. Thus, exogenous agents, such as bacteria endotoxin, are believed to cause fever by the activation of resident tissue macrophages with the subsequent production and release of IL-1, TNF-α, and probably other related macrophage-derived cytokines.

The value of fever to the diseased host is still not clearly demonstrated, although some deleterious effects upon survival have been shown to occur experimentally when fever is abated by use of antipyretics. Philosophically, it seems that the ability to respond to infection by elevated temperature must have some beneficial effects;

otherwise, it would not have survived as a function in so many animal species.

References

Atkins E, Bodel P. Fever. N Engl J Med. 1972;286:27–34.

Atkins E, Bodel P. Clinical fever: Its history, manifestations and pathogenesis. Fed Proc 1979;38:57–63.

Bernheim HA, Kluger MJ. Fever: effect of drug-induced antipyresis in survival. Science 1976;193:237–239.

Bernheim HA, Block LH, Atkins E. Fever: pathogenesis, pathophysiology, and purpose. Ann Intern Med 1979;91:261–270.

Cranston WI. Central mechanisms of fever. Fed Proc. 1979;38:49–51.

Cooper KE, Veale WL, Kasting N, et al. Ontogeny of fever. Fed Proc 1979;38:35–38.

Dinarello CA. Production of endogenous pyrogen. Fed Proc 1979;38:52–56.

Greaves MW. Prostaglandins and inflammation. In: S. M. M. Karim, ed. Prostaglandins: physiological, pharmacological and pathological aspects. Baltimore: University Park Press 1976;293–302.

Kluger MJ. Phylogeny of fever. Fed Proc 1979;38:30–34.

Pickering GW. Fever. In: H. W. Florey, ed. General pathology. 4th ed. London: Lloyd-Luke 1970;394–412.

Robinson S, ed. Problems in temperature regulation and exercise. Fed Proc 1973;32:1563–1622.

OTHER HYPERTHERMIAS

The body temperature is increased in several other conditions that do not conform to the definition of fever. Among those presently known are certain pathologic and pharmacologic states in humans and animals, including: (1) **malignant hyperthermia** of humans and swine (discussed in the chapter on skeletal muscle); an inherited predisposition, triggered by certain drugs, with usually fatal hyperthermia; (2) **hypothalamic lesions,** natural or experimental, which destroy or disturb the temperature-regulating center; (3) metabolic disease associated with **thyrotoxicosis** (hyperthyroidism) or with **pheochromocytoma** of the adrenal gland; (4) disturbance of **monoamine metabolism** in the central nervous system; (5) prolonged administration of **atropine.**

Hyperthermia of exercise is also recognized as a situation featuring elevated temperature. In this case, dissipation of heat is inadequate to dispose of heat generated by the exercise. Elevated temperature persists as long as the exercise continues. The physiologic mechanisms are not completely understood.

Heat exhaustion (heat prostration, heat stroke)

Under certain conditions, animals are unable to eliminate sufficient heat to maintain body temperature at a level compatible with life. In the absence of adequate clinical study or a satisfactory history, the pathologist may have difficulty recognizing this syndrome and be at a loss for an adequate explanation of the animal's death. In those instances in which an adequate history is available, it is found that the animal has been exposed to unusually high heat and humidity, a confined space, and some psychologic stress (fear, excitement).

The essential signs are high fever (106°F to 110°F), which may be lowered by cold water or other cooling methods, severe hyperpnea and respiratory distress, severe discomfort, congested mucosae, tachycardia, excitement, collapse, and sudden death. Fetuses in pregnant animals may die in utero and be delivered or retained, resulting in severe metritis.

GROSS APPEARANCE

Generalized hyperemia is most severe in the respiratory tract, especially in the lungs and tracheal and bronchial mucosae. Lungs may also be edematous and occasionally contain focal consolidations of bronchopneumonia. Other organs, such as the heart, kidneys, meninges, lymph nodes, and muscles, may also be severely congested. Preexisting cardiac disease (e.g., dirofilariasis) or pulmonary disease (focal pneumonia) may accentuate the effect of heat and may contribute to the death of the animal. Unexpectedly extensive autolysis is often evident, particularly in dogs and swine.

MICROSCOPIC APPEARANCE

The lesions are compatible with those seen grossly. The vasculature of the lungs is severely engorged and edema is evident in alveoli. Centrilobular necrosis, disassociation of hepatocytes, and congestion are often found in the liver. Subendocardial and subepicardial hemorrhages are found in the heart. Capillary congestion is evident in kidneys, meninges, lymph nodes, and other structures.

DIAGNOSIS

The diagnosis of heat exhaustion depends upon consideration of several factors. The persistent high fever, distress, and sudden death of an animal that could have been exposed to high temperature and humidity should arouse suspicion. The gross hyperemia, especially of the respiratory system; unusually rapid autolysis; and absence of lesions of other specific infectious diseases are helpful factors in arriving at a diagnosis.

References

Busey WM, Coate WB, Badger DW. Histopathologic effects of nitrogen dioxide exposure and heat stress in cynomolgus monkeys. Toxicol Appl Pharmacol 1974;29:130.

Clowes GHA Jr, O'Donnell TF Jr. Heat stroke. N Engl J Med. 1974;291:564–567.

Hickey TE, Kelly WA. Heatstroke in a colony of squirrel monkeys. J Am Vet Med Assoc 1972;161:700–703.

Krum SH, Osborne CA. Heatstroke in the dog: A polysystemic disorder. J Am Vet Med Assoc 1977;170:531–535.

Musacchia XJ. Fever and hyperthermia. Fed Proc 1979;38:27–29.

Stitt JT. Fever versus hyperthermia. Fed Proc 1979;38:39–43.

6

Disturbances of circulation

Interference with circulation and, therefore, with blood supply to vital organs may arise from a variety of mechanisms. The hemodynamic changes of concern in this chapter are thrombosis, hemorrhage, hyperemia, edema, and shock. Circulatory changes are also a principal manifestation of other entities, such as heart failure, primary vascular disease, and anemia, which are reviewed in other chapters; and changes in circulation are an integral component of the inflammatory process, discussed in the preceding chapter.

COAGULATION

Blood must remain fluid, yet at the same time be able to coagulate to arrest hemorrhage in the event of damage to blood vessels. Normally these two opposing forces are in balance; however, under some circumstances, the forces that maintain fluidity or that allow for coagulation become aberrant. When this occurs, blood may fail to clot, resulting in uncontrolled hemorrhage or, conversely, blood may unnecessarily clot, which sets the stage for thrombosis and its consequences. The mechanisms controlling fluidity and coagulation are highly complex interactions of endothelium, platelets, and the coagulation system. Only key features are highlighted here.

Endothelium

The normal endothelium serves to prevent coagulation by (1) serving as a mechanical barrier to the highly thrombogenic subendothelial connective tissue, which contains tissue factor; and (2) by producing a number of factors, which (a) inhibit platelet aggregation, (b) constrain the coagulation system, and (c) favor dissolution of clots. Endothelial cells inhibit the aggregation of platelets in several ways. In the presence of endothelial cell damage and initiation of coagulation, endothelial cells release prostacyclin (PGI_2), which inhibits further platelet aggregation and is also a vasodilator. In addition, endothelial cells inhibit platelet aggregation by enzymatically destroying adenosine diphosphate (ADP), which is released from platelets and promotes platelet aggregation. ADP released from platelets as well as thrombin formed in the coagulation cascade, stimulate the endothelial cells to release nitric oxide, which, in addition to being an important vasodilator, inhibits the adhesion, activation, and aggregation of platelets. Endothelial cells suppress coagulation through the elaboration of protein C (a vitamin K-dependent protein), which, along with its cofactor protein S (another vitamin K-dependent protein), is an anticoagulant that inactivates the active cofactor forms of factors VIII and V. Release of protein C is initiated when thrombin combines with the endothelial-membrane receptor, thrombomodulin. Further, on the surface of endothelial cells, a heparin-like molecule serves to emphasize the activity of antithrombin III, a plasma protein that inactivates thrombin. Dissolution of clots (fibrin) is aided by endothelial cells through elaboration of plasminogen activators promoting fibrinolysis.

While possessing the ability to suppress coagulation, endothelial cells simultaneously have the capacity to stimulate clotting. When damaged, endothelial cells elaborate thromboplastin (tissue factor), which initiates the coagulation cascade. They also secrete von Willebrand factor (vWF), which is necessary for the adherence of platelets. vWF also serves as a carrier protein for factor VIII and is an inhibitor of plasminogen activator; it is synthesized in endothelial cells (and in megakaryocytes) in rod-shaped organelles known as Weibel-Palade bodies.

Platelets

Platelets serve to prevent hemorrhage through their ability to plug small rents in vascular integrity and to promote coagulation. When a vessel wall is injured and its protective endothelium is disrupted, platelets **adhere** almost immediately to the subendothelial collagen at the site of injury. Glycoprotein 1b receptors on the platelet membrane bind to vWF, which is synthesized by endothelial cells and secreted into the subendothelium, where it binds to collagen. Genetic deficiency of either vWF or platelet receptors results in hemorrhagic disease. Adherence of platelets is facilitated by their peripheral position in the laminar flow of blood. Once adhered, platelets become **activated** and release several factors that promote **aggregation** of platelets to form a **temporary hemostatic plug** and contribute to initiation of the coagulation sequence. ADP released from dense bodies of platelets and thromboxane A_2 (TxA_2) formed by activated platelets serve to promote further aggregation through other glycoproteins on the platelet membrane (glycoproteins IIb and IIIa), which also bind to fibrinogen. TxA_2 also serves as a potent vasoconstrictor. Additionally, serotonin and epinephrine, also released from platelets, serve as platelet agonists. These additional platelets recruited to the hemostatic plug bind to receptors on the surface of platelets rather than to vWF. Further, on the platelet surface, receptors are expressed for factor VIII, factor V, and calcium, which serve to activate factor X and the formation of thrombin. Under the influence of ADP, TxA_2, and thrombin, aggregated platelets undergo what is termed viscous metamorphosis, forming the **secondary hemostatic plug** within which fibrin is ultimately deposited.

Coagulation cascade.

Blood coagulation involves a sequence of events that converts, by cleavage of peptide bonds, a group of proenzymes and proteins that normally circulate in the blood in an inactive form, culminating in the formation of thrombin and its conversion of soluble fibrinogen to insoluble fibrin. The various factors are listed in Table 6-1. Classically, the generation of thrombin is described in two separate pathways, the **intrinsic pathway** and the **extrinsic pathway,** neither of which are considered to represent the *in vivo* physiologic pathway. These are depicted in Figure 6-1, based on schemes presented by McFarlane (1964), Roberts and Lozier (1992), Luchtman-Jones and Broze (1995), and Furie and Furie (1992). The intrinsic pathway, which is measured by the activated partial thromboplastin time, is initiated by the activation of factor XII on contact with (1) glass in a test tube (blood does not clot in a paraffin-lined tube), (2) prekallikrein, or (3) high molecular weight kininogen. Activated factor XII activates factor XI, which in turn activates factor IX. Activated factor IX in a complex with activated factor VIII, along with calcium and phospholipids (platelet factor 3 or PF-3) from platelets, activates factor X. Activated factor X in a complex with activated factor V, calcium, and phospholipids converts prothrombin to thrombin, which then converts fibrinogen to fibrin. The extrinsic pathway, which is measured by the prothrombin time, begins with binding between tissue factor and factor VII. This activated complex, in the presence of calcium and phospholipids, activates factor X, which in turn converts prothrombin to thrombin, as in the instrinsic pathway. Cross-over between the two pathways occurs with the activation of factor IX (in addition to factor X) by tissue-factor-activated factor VII complex. Physiologically, coagulation probably is initiated by activation of factor IX by activated factor VII-tissue-factor complex, as shown by the dotted line in Figure 6-1. This is supported by observations that severe bleeding disorders occur when there is

TABLE 6-1	**Partial listing of major coagulation factors**
Factor I	Fibrinogen
Factor II	Prothrombin
Factor III	Tissue factor (tissue thromboplastin)
Factor IV	Calcium
Factor V	Proaccelerin, labile factor
Factor VII	Proconvertin, precursor of serum prothrombin conversion accelerator (Pro-SPCA)
Factor VIII	Antihemophilic factor A, antihemophilic globulin
Factor IX	Christmas factor, plasma thromboplastin component (PTC), antihemophilic factor B
Factor X	Stuart-Prower factor
Factor XI	Plasma thromboplastin antecedent (PTA)
Factor XII	Hageman factor
Factor XIII	Fibrin stabilizing factor

deficiency of either factor VIII, IX, or VII and that deficiency of factor XII is not associated with bleeding. Thus, physiologically coagulation represents a combination of both pathways. Once fibrin is formed, it spontaneously polymerizes, forming a clot, further strengthened by cross-linking through the action of factor XIII.

Amplification and prevention of coagulation

In addition to the factors depicted in the schematic in Figure 6-1, other compounds interact with clotting factors to regulate coagulation and feedback mechanisms that ensure that coagulation is kept in balance by either amplifying or inhibiting the process. The role of platelets in the amplification of coagulation has already been mentioned, as have the various functions of endothelial cells, including the release of protein C, which inactivates factors V and VIII. Endothelial cells also elaborate agents that serve to retard aggregation of platelets. Dilution of clotting factors in the bloodstream and their degradation by macrophages and the liver also serve to control and prevent coagulation. **Tissue factor pathway inhibitor (TFPI)** is a factor that binds to and inactivates factor X and inhibits activated factor VII-tissue-factor complex. A plasma glycoprotein, termed **antithrombin** or **antithrombin III,** also serves to control coagulation. This protein combines with and inactivates thrombin. By itself it is not highly active; however, its function is greatly enhanced by heparin, which is believed to come

INTRINSIC PATHWAY　　　**EXTRINSIC PATHWAY**

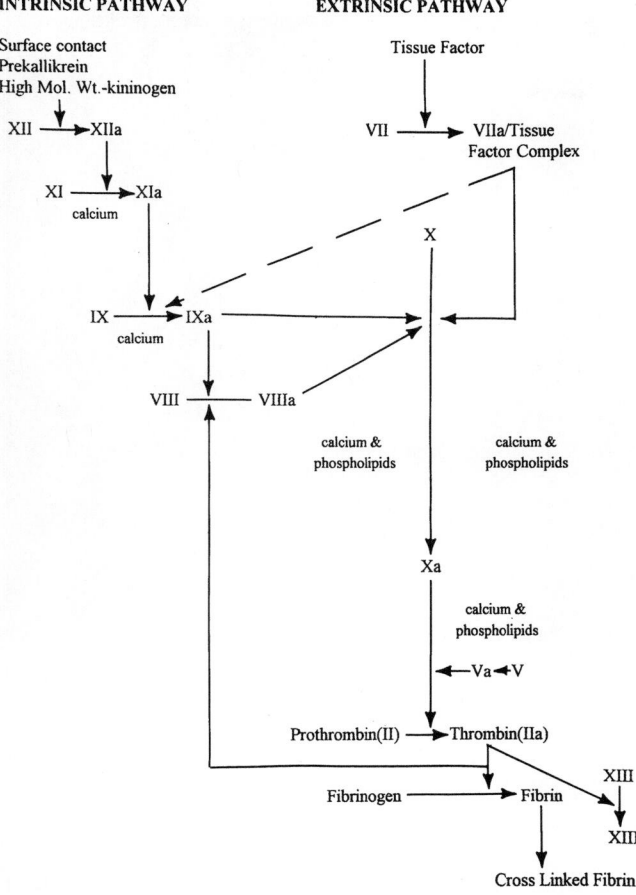

FIG. 6-1 Classically, generation of thrombin is described in two separate pathways, the **intrinsic pathway** and the **extrinsic pathway,** neither of which are considered to represent the *in vivo* physiologic pathway. These are depicted in here, based on schemes presented by McFarlane (1964), Roberts and Lozier (1962), Luchtman-Jones and Broze (1995), and Furie and Furie (1992).

from the vascular wall. Antithrombin also inhibits activated factor X, as well as activated factors IX, XI, XII; and kallikrein has also been shown to inhibit plasmin as well.

Dissolution of clots

In addition to factors that prevent coagulation, a system termed the **fibrinolytic system** exists for the dissolution of clots. This is effected by the fibrinolytic protease, **plasmin.** Plasmin is formed from its precursor, **plasminogen,** which circulates in the plasma. This conversion requires **tissue plasminogen activator (TPA)** or **urokinase.** The system is kept in check through **plasminogen activator inhibitor-1 (PAI-1),** released by endothelial cells, and **α-2 plasmin inhibitor,** which binds and inactivates plasmin. Plasmin is also capable of digesting fibrinogen and factors V and VIII.

References

Braunwald E. Regulation of the circulation. N Engl J Med 1974;290:1124–1129.

Davie EW, Ratnoff OD. Waterfall sequence for intrinsic blood clotting. Science 1964;145:1310–1312.
Deykin D. Emerging concepts of platelet function. N Engl J Med 1974;290:144–151.
Fiore LD, Deykin D. Mechanisms of hemostasis and arterial thrombosis. Cardiol Clin 1994;12:399–409.
Frelier PF, Lewis RM. Hematologic and coagulation abnormalities in acute bovine sarcocystosis. Am J Vet Res 1984;45:40–48.
Furie B, Furie BC. Molecular and cellular biology of blood coagulation. N Engl J Med 1992;326:800–806.
Goldberg ID, Stemerman MB, Handin RI. Vascular permeation of platelet factor 4 after endothelial injury. N Engl J Med 1980;209:611–612.
High KA, Roberts HR, ed. Molecular basis of thrombosis and hemostasis. New York: Marcel Dekker 1995;(xii) 669.
Lindahl AK. Tissue factor inhibitor: a potent inhibitor of in-vitro coagulation and in-vivo thrombus formation. Curr Opin Lipidol 1994;5:434–439.
Luchtman-Jones L, Broze GJ Jr. The current status of coagulation. Ann Med 1995;27:47–52.
MacFarlane RG. An enzyme cascade in the blood clotting mechanism, and its function as a biochemical amplifier. Nature (Lond) 1964;202:498–499.
Mann KG. The coagulation explosion. Ann NY Acad Sci 1994;714:265–269.
Packham MA. Role of platelets in thrombosis and hemostasis. Can J Physiol Pharmacol 1994;72(3):278–284.
Roberts HR, Lozier JN. New perspectives on the coagulation cascade. J Hosp Practice 1992;27:97–105, 109–112.
Rowsell HC. The hemostatic mechanisms of mammals and birds in health and disease. Adv Vet Sci 1968;12:337–410.
Ruf W, Edgington TS. Structural biology of tissue factor, the initiator of thrombogenesis in vivo. FASEB J 1994;8:385–390.
Shearer MJ. Vitamin K. Lancet 1995;345:229–234.
Slappendel RJ. Disseminated intravascular coagulation. Vet Clin North Am Small Anim Pract 1988;18:169–184.
Stubbs MT, Bode W. Coagulation factors and their inhibitors. Curr Opin Struct Biol 1994;4:823–832.
Troy GC. An overview of hemostasis. Vet Clin North Am Small Anim Pract 1988;8:5–20.

THROMBOSIS (ANTEMORTEM CLOTS)

Thrombosis is the pathologic formation of a clot, termed a **thrombus,** within the cardiovascular system (Figs. 6-2 and 6-3). Depending on their location and size, thrombi may lead to serious interference with the flow of blood, resulting in infarction or passive congestion; may give rise to emboli with their sequelae; and may serve as sites for growth of bacteria.

Causes

There are three principal causes of thrombosis: (1) **endothelial injury;** (2) **disruption in regular flow of blood;** and (3) **hypercoagulability.**

INJURY TO ENDOTHELIAL CELLS

Such injury initiates coagulation, leading to thrombosis. Endothelial cells may be damaged through trauma, toxemias, metabolic disorders, and inflammatory disease of vessel walls initiated by infectious agents or immunologic injury. A specific example would be thrombosis of the anterior mesenteric artery caused by invasion of larvae of *Strongylus vulgaris* and other worms. This is so common that every equine autopsy should include examination of this artery. Thrombosis of the iliac arteries in horses, causing intermittent lameness and pain in both hind legs, is not infrequent in

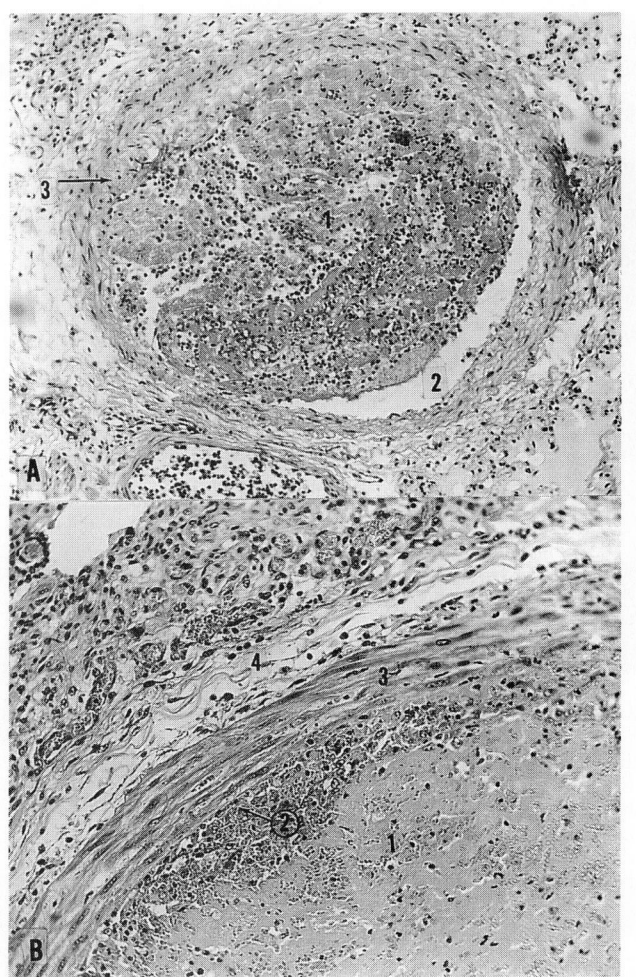

FIG. 6-2 Pulmonary artery thrombosis. **A.** Thrombosis of branch of pulmonary artery, lung of 5-year-old cocker spaniel with pyometra. Thrombus *(1),* lumen of artery *(2),* attachment of thrombus to intima *(3)* (×115). (Courtesy of Dr. Samuel Pollock and Armed Forces Institute of Pathology) **B.** Thrombosis of branch of pulmonary artery in an 11-year-old Scottish terrier with chronic valvular endocarditis. Hyaline material in the thrombus *(1),* proliferation of endothelium *(2),* media of distended artery *(3),* and edema in the adventitia *(4)* (×185). (Courtesy of Dr. Elihu Bond and Armed Forces Institute of Pathology)

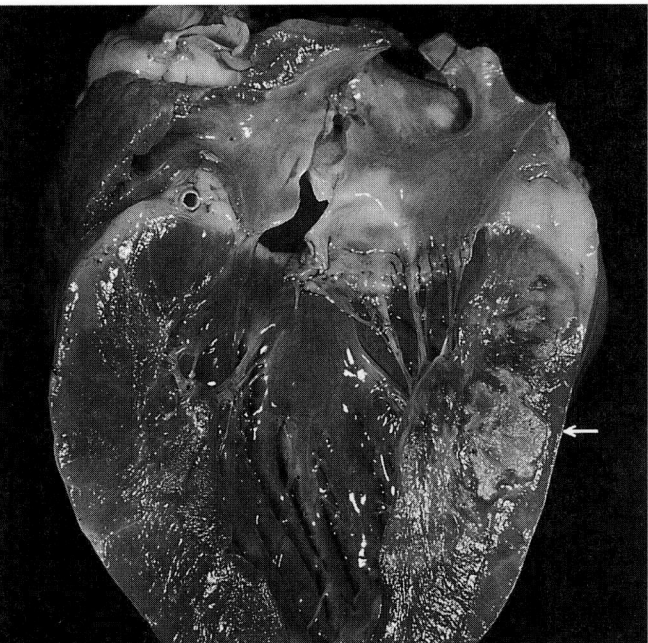

FIG. 6-3 Infarction of myocardium of left ventricle of heart of 8-year-old male Airedale dog with malignant lymphoma. The infarction is believed to be the result of occlusion of a branch of the left coronary artery by tumor growth. (Courtesy of Angell Memorial Animal Hospital)

horses and also is ascribed to strongyle larvae *via* thromboembolism. Injury by heartworms, *Dirofilaria immitis,* occasionally causes thrombosis of pulmonary arteries in dogs. The various causes of endocarditis (i.e., uremia, *Streptococcus* species, and *Erysipelothrix* species) may lead to the formation of thrombi on the endocardium or heart valves. Endothelial damage associated with cardiomyopathies often results in mural thrombi. These are particularly frequent in the left atrium of cats with cardiomyopathy.

DISRUPTION OF BLOOD FLOW

Disruption of the regular flow of blood interferes with the normal laminar flow, which is characterized by red and white blood cells occupying the central portion of the stream with platelets at the periphery but separated from the endothelium by plasma. Disorders that may cause turbulence in the arterial circulation or stasis in the venous circulation disrupt this flow and bring platelets into contact with the endothelium, encouraging coagulation. Once coagulation is initiated, the turbulence or stasis impedes the clearance of clotting factors through dilution. Turbulence may also damage endothelium. Thrombosis resulting from disrupted blood flow is seen in aneurysms, cardiac anomalies, and venous stasis resulting from almost any cause, e.g., cardiac insufficiency, inactivity, or increased viscosity caused by such disorders as polycythemia. Thrombosis of veins of the legs resulting from venous stasis is a particularly common form of thrombosis in humans and is the most common cause of pulmonary embolism.

HYPERCOAGULABILITY OF BLOOD

This is a recognized predisposing factor to thrombosis in humans but less well studied in animals. Even in humans the mechanisms are not always clear but are ascribed to either increased levels of activated clotting factors or decreased levels of inhibitors. A hereditary deficiency of antithrombin III and of protein C is recognized in humans and is associated with hypercoagulability. In dogs, deficiency of antithrombin III has been seen in association with glomerular disease and liver disease.

Gross appearance

Grossly, a thrombus occurring within arteries or the heart is seen as a friable mass with a dull, irregularly roughened or somewhat stringy surface. The color is a mixture of red and gray, usually in irregular layers or laminations (**lines of Zahn**). On at least one side, the thrombus is attached to the wall of the blood vessel. Arterial thrombi are often referred to as grey thrombi. In contrast, venous thrombi are usually red and often have a shiny surface, closely resembling a postmortem clot. On close inspection, however, some degree of lamination is usually evident, as is an attachment to the wall of the vein. If a thrombus totally obstructs the lumen, it is termed an **occlusive** or **occluding thrombus**. The thrombus may sometimes have a free end trailing downstream, often attaining a surprising length, and this type is termed an **obturating thrombus**. Thrombi forming in the heart are termed **mural thrombi** when on the wall and **vegetative thrombi** when on the valves.

Microscopic appearance

Microscopically, thrombi are composed of admixtures of the formed elements of blood along with fibrin (Fig. 6-2). Arterial thrombi are seen as alternating zones of homogeneous platelets (lines of Zahn) and tangled strands of fibrin mixed with varying numbers of erythrocytes and leukocytes. These often appear as regular laminations, but more often are rather disorganized. Venous thrombi contain larger numbers of erythrocytes

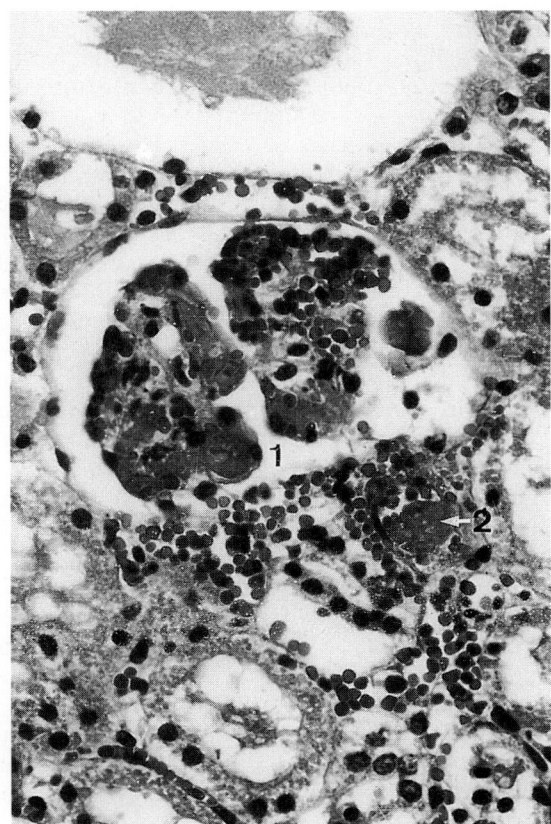

FIG. 6-4 DIC. Fibrinous emboli in capillaries *(1)* and afferent arteriole *(2)* of renal glomerulus of a pig with streptococcal sepsis. Streptococci were demonstrated by culture and by special stains in the emboli. (Courtesy of Prof. Dr. H. Luginbühl.)

admixed with the fibrin, and zones of platelets are usually not apparent.

Outcome

Thrombi may continue to enlarge, but simultaneously undergo resolution. They may be removed through fibrinolytic activity, but more usually are organized through dissolution by the action of leukocytes and their gradual replacement by the ingrowth of fibrovascular connective tissue. If nonocclusive, their surface is re-endothelialized. Blood channels also develop within the organized thrombus, some of which may restore circulation, in which case the thrombus is termed a **canalized thrombus**.

Differentiation from postmortem clots is of importance in certain septicemias and anoxic conditions, in which (except when death results) the greater part of the blood coagulates. This clotted blood must be differentiated from thrombi, especially venous thrombi. Postmortem clots are dark red, smooth, and shiny on the outside and molded to the vessel in which they are formed, like jelly in a container. They are of uniform texture and unattached to the vessel wall. Because of these characteristics, they are sometimes called **currant-jelly clots**. Settling and separation of red cells from the fluid phase of the blood before coagulation results in what is termed a **chicken-fat clot**. This type of postmortem clot is often found in the chambers of the heart. Microscopically, postmortem clots are composed of erythrocytes, leukocytes, and very fine strands of fibrin, in contrast to the coarser fibrin strands of thrombi. They lack zones of homogeneous platelets.

DISSEMINATED INTRAVASCULAR COAGULATION

Disseminated intravascular coagulation (DIC) is characterized by the appearance of myriads of fibrin thrombi within the small blood vessels, including capillaries and sinusoids(Fig. 6-4). It is not a primary disease; rather, it is precipitated by other events. In humans, most examples are associated with obstetric complications. In animals, it is seen in severe systemic infections, septic (endotoxic) shock, neoplastic diseases, extensive trauma or burns, and following extensive surgery. Viral diseases associated with DIC include hog cholera, infectious canine hepatitis, blue tongue, Aleutian disease, and epizootic hemorrhagic disease of deer. DIC has also been seen in cattle with acute sarcocystosis, presumably resulting from endothelial damage by schizonts. The pathogenesis is believed to be the release of tissue factor, factors from damaged endothelium, or the direct activation of clotting factors by substances released into the circulation in these various disorders. The thrombi may be encountered in any organ or tissue, but are particularly common in the lungs, kidneys, liver, spleen, adrenal gland, heart, and brain, where they may lead to infarction, dysfunction, and diverse clinical signs. The generation of extensive thrombosis depletes the circulation of platelets and the various clotting factors and simultaneously activates plasminogen, which not only digests fibrin but also digests fibrinogen and factors V and VIII. The net effect of this loss of platelets and clotting factors leads to failure of further coagulation, and severe bleeding becomes one of the principal clinical findings. Hemolytic anemia also develops, resulting from fragmentation of red blood cells as they traverse the fibrin clogged vasculature (microangiopathic hemolytic anemia).

EMBOLISM

Emboli are foreign bodies floating in the blood. Several kinds are recognized. The most common and important are **thromboemboli** (fibrin emboli), pieces of thrombi that have broken loose. In microscopic and gross appearance, they resemble thrombi. They are almost always found lodged in an arterial bifurcation (Fig. 6-5) or in a place where the lumen of the artery becomes too small to permit their passage. Thromboemboli arising from venous thrombi most often lodge in the pulmonary arterial tree; they may cause pulmonary infarction or right-sided heart failure. Emboli arising from arterial or cardiac thrombi that lodge in arteries in the systemic circulation are termed systemic embolism; they invariably cause infarction. Saddle thrombi at the termination of the aorta often arise from thromboemboli from the left atrium in cats with cardiomyopathy.

Fat emboli are droplets of endogenous fat that have entered the circulation (Fig. 6-6A). While not detected grossly, they are readily visible microscopically as sharply defined clear vacuoles of various sizes lodged within arterioles or capillaries. A fracture (or fractures) of bone is the most common cause of fat embolism; the mechanical trauma frees fat from the marrow's adipose cells. Less easily, fat embolism may occur from severe trauma of subcutaneous fat and occasionally from metabolic diseases, such as diabetes. In experimental animals, fat embolism can occur in the extreme hepatic fatty change seen with deficiency of choline, methionine, or cystine.

Fat emboli are usually numerous and are carried

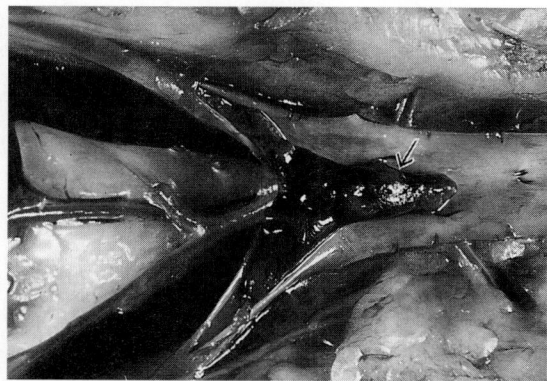

FIG. 6-5 Saddle embolus *(arrow)* at bifurcation of the aorta of an 8-year-old spayed female cat. This embolus presumably originated in the left atrium. (Courtesy of Angell Memorial Animal Hospital)

through the heart to lodge in pulmonary arterioles and capillaries. Extensive fat emboli can be fatal because of interference with pulmonary circulation, causing unexpected death rapidly after a traumatic incident. Some fat emboli may pass through the lungs and enter the systemic circulation. In humans, fat emboli have been associated with a complex syndrome characterized by severe respiratory distress. It is ascribed to either toxic injury to the pulmonary vasculature from fatty acids or activation of the coagulation system causing DIC.

Gas emboli, most commonly air, cause bubbles in the blood that may coalesce and obstruct the flow of blood, resulting in infarction. Gas embolism is not common but may occur when traumatic or surgical wounds rupture large blood vessels and the pumping action of muscles or respiration sucks air into the bloodstream. In humans, gas embolism is seen following a rapid change in atmospheric pressure, i.e., in scuba and deep sea divers and in construction workers emerging from underwater compartments (caissons) in which the air pressure has been raised to several times that of normal atmospheric pressure. When atmospheric pressure rapidly returns to normal, the gases dissolved in the blood under high pressure return to their gaseous state, becoming gas emboli. Oxygen in the blood remains in solution or is utilized, but nitrogen and helium (often substituted for nitrogen in compressed gas) do not. The result is termed **decompression sickness,** which occurs in an acute form termed the **bends** and in a chronic form termed **caisson disease.** The bends is characterized by acute pain (from occlusion of vessels in the muscles and joints), respiratory distress, and coma (from occlusion of pulmonary and cerebral vessels). Caisson disease is characterized by ischemic necrosis of bone, the pathogenesis of which is not clear.

Bacterial emboli are clumps of bacteria (Fig. 6-6B), which sometimes are mechanically sloughed into the venous flow from heavily infected tissues. The result is multiple sites of infection when the emboli lodge in capillaries. Most often, bacterial emboli are infected thromboemboli from bacterial endocarditis.

Parasitic emboli may include fragments of adult canine heartworms, *Dirofilaria immitis,* usually in branches of the pulmonary artery; clumps of blood flukes, *Schistosoma* species; and groups of agglutinated trypanosomes.

Emboli made up of neoplastic cells are occasionally seen and must occur often in patients with cancer, since it is by tumor cells carried in the bloodstream that malignant neoplasms are able to metastasize (Fig. 6–7).

Other types of emboli include red bone marrow emboli resulting from fractures, amniotic fluid emboli, hepatic emboli following trauma to the liver, clumps of agglutinated red blood cells (spodogenous emboli), foreign bodies such as broken needles or hair introduced in venipuncture, and trophoblastic emboli, which occur in the chinchilla and in primates.

References

Badimon L, Meyer BJ, Badimon JJ. Thrombin in arterial thrombosis. Haemostasis 1994;24:69–80.

Dahlbäck B. Inherited resistance to activated protein C, a major cause

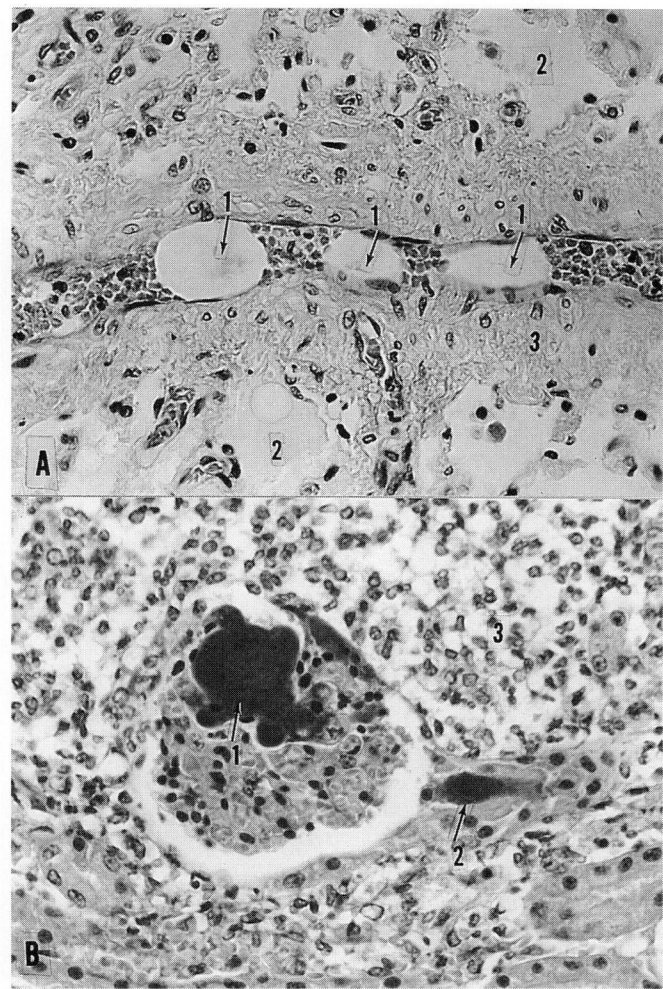

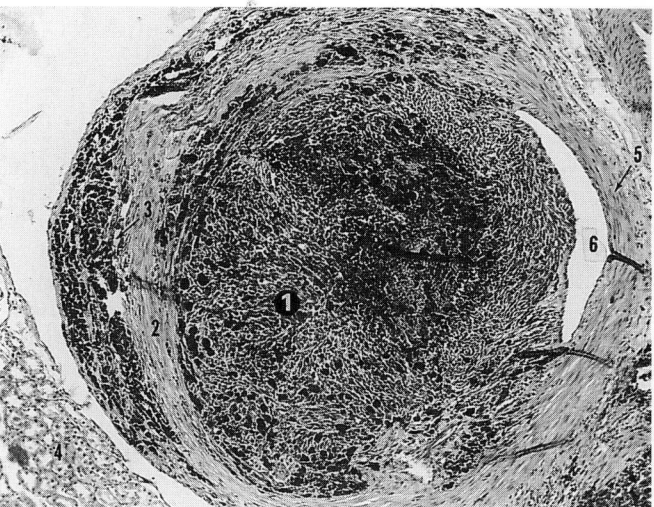

FIG. 6-7 Thrombosis of renal artery by implantation of tumor embolus. The neoplasm was malignant melanoma, primary in the oral mucosa of a 9-year-old dog. Tumor *(1)* attached to artery wall *(2)*, which has been penetrated by tumor cells *(3)*. Renal tubules *(4)*, uninvolved artery wall *(5)*, and lumen of the artery *(6)* (× 70). (Courtesy of Dr. F. L. Povar and Armed Forces Institute of Pathology)

FIG. 6-6 Emboli. **A.** Fatty emboli in a branch of the pulmonary artery of a dog hit and killed by an automobile. Globules of fat *(1)* expand the arterial wall and displace blood cells. Pulmonary alveoli *(2)* are present in the section (×395). (Courtesy of Dr. Elihu Bond and Armed Forces Institute of Pathology) **B.** Bacterial emboli in a renal glomerulus of a foal infected with *Shigella equuli*. A bacterial colony is seen in the glomerulus *(1)* and in the efferent tubule *(2)*; leukocytes have accumulated around the glomerulus *(3)* (×315). (Courtesy of Army Veterinary Research Laboratory and Armed Forces Institute of Pathology)

of venous thrombosis, is due to a mutation in the factor V gene. Haemostasis 1994;24:139–151.

Garner R, Chater BV, Brown DL. The role of complement in endotoxic shock and disseminated intravascular coagulation: experimental observations in the dog. Br J Haematol 1974;28:393–401.

Gerrity RG, Richardson M, Caplan BA, et al. Endotoxin-induced vascular endothelial injury and repair. II. Focal injury, en face morphology, (³H) thymidine uptake and circulating endothelial cells in the dog. Exp Mol Pathol 1976;24:59–69.

Green RA. Pathophysiology of antithrombin III deficiency. Vet Clin North Am Small Anim Clin 1988;18:95–104.

Jacobs RR, Wheeler EJ, Jelenko C, et al. Fat embolism: a microscopic and ultrastructure evaluation of two animal models. Trauma 1973;13:980–993.

Johnstone IB, Physick-Sheard P, Crane S. Breed, age, and gender differences in plasma antithrombin-III activity in clinically normal young horses. Am J Vet Res 1989;50:1571–1573.

Legendre AM, Krehbiel JD. Disseminated intravascular coagulation in a dog with hemothorax and hemangiosarcoma. J Am Vet Med Assoc 1977;171:1070–1071.

McKay DG, Margaretten W. Disseminated intravascular coagulation in virus diseases. Arch Intern Med 1967;120:129.

Morris DD, Beech J. Disseminated intravascular coagulation in six horses. J Am Vet Med Assoc 1983;183:1067–1072.

Robboy SJ, Major MC, Colman RW, et al. Pathology of disseminated intravascular coagulation. Hum Pathol 1972;3:327–343.

Schafer AI. Hypercoagulable states: molecular genetics to clinical practice. Lancet 1994;344:1739–1742.

Schiefer B, Searcy G. Disseminated intravascular coagulation and consumption coagulopathy. Can Vet J 1975;16:151–159.

Schoendorf TH, Rosenberg M, Beller FK. Endotoxin-induced disseminated intravascular coagulation in nonpregnant rats. Am J Pathol 1971;65:51–58.

Thomson GW, McSherry BJ, Valli VEO. Endotoxin induced disseminated intravascular coagulation in cattle. Can J Comp Med 1974;38:457–466.

Tvedten HW, Langham RF. Trophoblastic emboli in a chinchilla. J Am Vet Med Assoc 1974;165:828–829.

Weiss RC, Dodds WJ, Scott FW. Disseminated intravascular coagulation in experimentally induced feline infectious peritonitis. Am J Vet Res 1980;41:663–671.

Wheeler A, Rubenstein EB. Current management of disseminated intravascular coagulation. Oncology 1994;8(9):69–79.

Wingfield WE, Corley EA. Fatal air embolism associated with pneumourethrography and pneumocystography in a dog. J Am Vet Med Assoc 1972;160:1616–1618.

FAILURE TO CLOT

A number of acquired and congenital disorders result in interference with the normal coagulation process and are characterized by spontaneous hemorrhage or excessive hemorrhage after traumatic injury.

Inherited coagulation factor deficiences

Factor I (fibrinogen) deficiency has been reported in dogs and goats. In dogs, the disorder is manifested by severe bleeding episodes and low fibrinogen levels in the plasma. The disease has been described in Saint Bernard dogs but has also been observed in other breeds.

Hereditary afibrinogenemia has been studied in a family of Saanen goats (Breukink and colleagues, 1972). This is a severe hemorrhagic disorder in newborn and young goats, characterized by bleeding from the mucous membranes and umbilicus and bleeding into joints and subcutaneous tissues. The inheritance pattern is compatible with a single autosomal incompletely dominant gene. Fibrinogen levels in heterozygotes were recorded as a trace or completely absent.

Factor II (prothrombin) deficiency has been reported in puppies with severe bleeding tendencies and in adult dogs with more moderate signs. In boxers, it is inherited as an autosomal recessive trait.

Factor VII (proconvertin) deficiency is described in beagles, Alaskan malamutes, and miniature schnauzers, where it is inherited as an autosomal recessive trait. The effects of this deficiency are usually mild; hemorrhages following surgery and bruises are the essential manifestations.

Factor VIII deficiency (hemophilia A) is the classic hemophilia of historical fame as the tragic affliction of many male members of the European and Russian royal families. The same disorder was first identified in dogs and is now recognized in many different breeds as well as in cats, horses, and Hereford cattle. It is the most commonly reported coagulopathy of animals and is inherited as a sex-linked recessive gene. Carrier females have reduced levels of factor VIII but do not show signs of disease unless homozygous for the trait, which is rare. The severity of bleeding in affected males is highly variable, being most severe in larger breeds of dogs and horses. Hemorrhage may appear to be spontaneous or may follow even minor trauma. As with the disorder in humans, hemarthrosis causing lameness is a common occurrence.

Factor IX deficiency, also known as **hemophilia B,** or **Christmas disease,** is seen in several breeds of dogs (e.g., Cairn terriers, Black and Tan coonhounds, Saint Bernard dogs, Alaskan malamutes) and cats. It is inherited as a sex-linked recessive trait. Bleeding is often severe. A combination of both hemophilia A and B has been described in a family of French bulldogs.

Factor X (Stuart-Prower factor) deficiency has been reported in Cocker spaniel dogs (Dodds, 1973). In this report, the disease was manifested in newborn or young adult dogs by severe bleeding and in adult animals by a mild bleeding disorder, usually prolonged estrual bleeding or bleeding following surgery. Inheritance is by an autosomal dominant trait.

Factor XI (plasma thromboplastin antecedent) deficiency is recognized in Holstein cattle, Great Pyrenee dogs, English springer spaniels, and Kerry blue terriers.

In cattle, the disease is inherited as an autosomal recessive trait; this appears to be similar to the inheritance in dogs. Bleeding is usually not severe, except following surgery.

Factor XII (Hageman factor) deficiency has been reported in dogs and cats as an autosomal recessive trait. It is not associated with bleeding. Further evidence that factor XII is not essential for normal hemostasis is its complete absence in marine mammals (i.e., dolphins, killer whales, and porpoises), in fowl (i.e., ducks, geese, chickens, turkeys, and pigeons), and in most reptiles (i.e., lizards, turtles, and tiger snakes). Factor XII deficiency and defective plasma thromboplastin formation have been described in horses, but none of them had any bleeding tendency.

Von Willebrand's disease, or deficiency of vWF, is recognized in many different breeds of dogs (e.g., German shepherds, golden retrievers, miniature schnauzers, Scottish terriers, Doberman pinschers, and Pembroke Welsh corgis) and has been described in Poland China and Yorkshire-Hampshire swine, cats, horses, and rabbits. The inheritance is autosomal, which appears to be recessive in some breeds and species and dominant in others. In dogs, most examples are of dominant inheritance pattern, but in Scottish terriers and Chesapeake Bay retrievers it is seen as a recessive trait. In humans, both recessively transmitted and dominantly transmitted forms of the disease exist with differing quantitative and qualitative defects. vWF is actually a series of oligomers, referred to as multimers, which range in molecular weight from 500 to 10,000 kd with varying ability to bind platelets. The inherited deficiencies may be characterized by an absolute deficiency of all multimers to qualitative defects. The primary result of reduced levels of vWF is a failure of platelet adhesion to the walls of damaged blood vessels. This step is critical to hemostasis as platelets form the primary plug in vascular rents and participate in coagulation. The severity of bleeding is, however, highly variable. Since vWF serves as a carrier protein for factor VIII, this factor may also be deficient, thus exacerbating the disease. **Acquired deficiency of vWF** is seen in association with hypothyroidism.

Prekallikrein (Fletcher factor) deficiency has been described in horses and a dog, as well as in humans. The deficiency is not associated with bleeding, but it does result in a prolonged activated partial thromboplastin time. Prekallikrein is important to the initiation of the intrinsic coagulation pathway but not to *in vivo* coagulation.

DISORDERS OF THROMBOCYTES

Thrombocytopenia, a decrease in numbers of platelets, or **defective function of platelets** are important causes of defective hemostasis in animals. Most are acquired disorders that may be primary or secondary to other diseases. The principal mechanisms are listed in Table 6–2.

Inherited defects in thrombocyte function (throm-

TABLE 6-2 Disorders of thrombocytes

Defective function

    Inherited

        Defect in membrane glycoproteins preventing adhesion
            or aggregation

        Defect in release of ADP and other platelet factors

    Acquired

        Drug induced, e.g., aspirin

        Uremia

Thrombocytopenia

    Increased destruction or consumption

        Autoimmune (idiopathic) thrombocytopenia

        Isoimmune thrombocytopenia

        Drug-induced thrombocytopenia

        Disseminated intravascular coagulation (DIC)

        Thrombotic thrombocytopenic purpura

    Decreased production

        Defective megakaryopoiesis

            Aplastic and myelophthisic anemias

            Infectious disease (canine ehrlichiosis)

            Drug-induced

    Sequestration of thrombocytes

---

bopathia) may involve surface glycoproteins or the synthesis and/or release of platelet factors. Defective or deficient surface glycoprotein GPIb, which precludes platelets from adhering to vWF/collagen (thus resembling von Willebrand's disease), is known as Bernard-Soulier syndrome in humans. With defective or deficient surface glycoprotein GPIIb and GPIIIa, known as Glanzmann's disease of humans, there is failure of platelet aggregation with ADP, thrombin, and fibrin. A third defect is characterized by failure of platelets to release ADP and other constituents of their granules or failure to synthesize these compounds, thus interfering with aggregation. These disorders are sometimes referred to as "storage pool disease." In otterhounds, a hereditary autosomal dysfunction of platelets has been described, in which there is a failure of platelet aggregation, in comparison with thrombasthenia or Glanzmann's disease of humans resulting from a lack of GPIIb and GPIIIa. What is suggested as a similar abnormality has been described in a horse. Qualitative hereditary dysfunction of platelets, which are also autosomal traits, has also been observed in Simmental cattle, American foxhounds, Basset hounds, Spitz dogs, cats, and fawn-hooded rats. The basic defect in these species appears to be failure to synthesize or release platelet granule factors. The disorder in Simmental cattle and Basset hounds appears to be similar. In both, GPIIb and GPIIIa appear to be normal. Platelets from affected Simmental cattle fail to aggregate and secrete in response to ADP. One feature of Chediak-Higashi syndrome in Aleutian mink, cattle, Persian cats, and humans is prolonged bleeding caused by a defect in platelet storage of ADP. **Acquired platelet dysfunction** is

seen in association with certain drugs, most notably aspirin and other nonsteroidal anti-inflammatory agents, as well as phenylbutazone. Aspirin inhibits the enzyme cyclooxygenase, which is necessary for the production of thromboxane A_2 (TXA_2), prostacyclin (PGI_2), and prostaglandins that are involved in platelet aggregation. Its effect on platelets is permanent, because platelets lack the biosynthetic capacity to synthesize new protein. Other drugs that may produce platelet dysfunction include estrogens, sulfonamides, penicillins, and phenothiazines. Uremia also results in platelet dysfunction.

Thrombocytopenia can result from several different mechanisms, either as primary disorders of platelets or secondary to other diseases. As indicated in Table 6-2, a decrease in absolute numbers of platelets may result from (1) increased destruction or consumption, (2) decreased production, or (3) sequestration. Regardless of mechanism, thrombocytopenia is characterized by spontaneous bleeding that is most easily visible on mucous membranes, subcutaneous hematomas, and bleeding from the gastrointestinal tract and urogenital system. Those examples resulting from increased destruction of thrombocytes can be differentiated from other mechanisms by the presence of large numbers of mature and immature megakaryocytes in the bone marrow.

Increased destruction or consumption

Autoimmune (idiopathic) thrombocytopenia is recognized in dogs and horses, but probably occurs in all species. It is generally considered a primary autoimmune disease, as the precipitating event is not identified. The autoimmune destruction of platelets results from autoantibodies that bind to platelet surface glycoproteins, causing their ingestion by macrophages, which bind to the Fc portion of the antibody. In humans, it is usually the glycoproteins IIb and IIIa that are targeted. It may well be the result of viral infections as with certain other "autoimmune" diseases. This also occurs in conjunction with autoimmune hemolytic anemia. It may also occur as a secondary immune-mediated destruction of platelets, as for example in conjunction with immune-mediated hemolytic anemias after repeated blood transfusions. Thrombocytopenia is a regular feature of equine infectious anemia; is seen in tick-borne fever; and is also reportedly a feature in cats infected with feline immunodeficiency virus, but the mechanism is not known. What precipitates an autoimmune reaction against platelets, as with other autoimmune diseases, is poorly understood.

Isoimmune thrombocytopenia, recognized in baby pigs, is caused by maternal isoimmunization. The disorder, described in Norway, Sweden, Finland, England, and Canada, is analogous to isoimmune hemolytic anemias (e.g., erythroblastosis fetalis, hemolytic disease of the newborn). After numerous pregnancies, antibodies against platelets of the offspring are developed in the sow during gestation, as a result of mating with a boar possessing platelet antigens different from those of the sow. Piglets recieving antithrombocyte antibodies in the colostrum develop purpura within 8 to 72 hours after birth, which may lead to death.

Drug-induced thrombocytopenia is associated with a number of different types of drugs in humans, but it is less well studied in animals. Quinidine, thiazide diuretics, heparin, various antibiotics (e.g., streptomycin, penicillin), and sulfonamides are examples. In some cases of drug-induced thrombocytopenia, the destruction of platelets is believed to be immune-mediated. Heparin-induced thrombocytopenia is complement-mediated.

Disseminated intravascular coagulation (DIC), previously discussed, results in consumption of platelets (and clotting factors) that leads to the paradoxical hemorrhage associated with this condition. **Thrombotic thrombocytopenic purpura** is also associated with a consumption thrombocytopenia. Here, the mechanism is not understood, but it is not the result of activation of coagulation mechanisms, as in DIC. This disorder is characterized by myriads of platelet aggregates in arterioles and capillaries that appear as hyaline obstructions. Hypotheses regarding their development include immune-mediated endothelial damage and release of an abnormal platelet agglutinating factor through the factor VIII-von Willebrand complex.

Decreased production of thrombocytes is seen in association with generalized diseases of the bone marrow. These include the various causes of aplastic and myelophthisic anemias as well as infectious diseases and certain poisons and drugs that have a predilection for destruction of the bone marrow. Thus, thrombocytopenia is seen in such diseases as leukemia and lymphoma, which replace the marrow and erhlichiosis that causes a pancytopenia. Drugs may affect thrombopoiesis through myelosuppression, direct toxicity to megakaryocytes, or by initiating an immune destruction of megakaryocytes. Some of the many drugs included are chloramphenicol, streptomycin, estrogen, chlorothiazide, azothioprine, cyclophosphamide, and vincristine. Poisons such as bracken fern cause severe hypoplasia of hematopoietic tissues with thrombocytopenia.

Sequestration of thrombocytes may occur in conditions characterized by splenomegaly. The spleen, which normally sequesters a large number of platelets, may when enlarged isolate such a high percentage of thrombocytes that hemostasis is affected.

Acquired coagulopathies

The best known of the acquired coagulopathies is poisoning by **vitamin K antagonists.** This is seen in sweet clover poisoning, which contains coumarin, and in poisoning by rodenticides containing warfarin. Sulfaquinoxaline is another vitamin K antagonist. The poisoning is also seen in humans receiving coumarin as a therapeutic anticoagulant. Vitamin K is a required cofactor for the hepatic enzyme gamma-glutamyl-carboxylase, which is required for function of factors II, VII, IX, and X and proteins C and S. Vitamin K deficiency itself results in the same hemorrhagic disease, but this is rare. A vitamin K-dependent coagulopathy characterized by deficiencies of factors II, VII, IX, and X has been de-

scribed in British Devon Rex cats. The disorder, which was responsive to oral vitamin K therapy, was shown to result from defective gamma-glutamyl-carboxylase binding with vitamin K. This most likely is an inherited disorder and not acquired. **Hepatic disease** may affect the production of many different coagulation factors. Factors I, II, V, VII, IX, X, XI, XII, and XIII, as well as proteins C and S, antithrombin III, and plasminogen are synthesized by hepatocytes. As previously discussed, DIC causes depletion of most clotting factors and hemorrhage.

HEMORRHAGE

Hemorrhage is the escape of blood from a vessel, whether it be to the outside of the body, into a body cavity, or into adjacent tissues. The ordinary rapid flow of blood through a break or cut in a vessel wall is called **hemorrhage by rhexis** (break or bursting). Considerable amounts of blood may also be lost by a slow oozing of fluid and the escape of blood cells one by one through minute or imperceptible imperfections in the vessel walls. This is called **hemorrhage by diapedesis.**

Tiny hemorrhages that leave dots of blood not much larger than the point of a pin are called **petechiae** (Fig. 6-8A). Slightly larger hemorrhages are termed **purpura.** Somewhat larger hemorrhagic spots, about 1 cm in diameter, on a body surface or in the tissues are called **ecchymoses** (Fig. 6-8B). **Extravasation** refers to hemorrhages in the tissues spread over considerable areas. Hemorrhage into a body cavity is referred to as **hemothorax, hemopericardium, hemoperitoneum,** and so on.

When blood escapes into the tissues and produces a tumor-like enlargement, the mass usually goes by the term **hematoma,** although **hematocyst** is more appropriate. A simple example is the common "blood blister," familiar to all who have aimed a hammer blow at a nail but somehow had it strike the thumb.

Causes

Hemorrhage may result from a wide variety of causes. It is a feature of so many different diseases that no attempt is made to review them here. All the disorders discussed earlier under failure to clot are characterized by hemorrhage. Any **mechanical trauma,** cutting or breaking a blood vessel, necrosis, **destruction of vessel walls** as by an ulcer or spreading neoplasm, rupture of a vessel weakened by an aneurysm, or other degenerative disease of a vessel wall may result in hemorrhage (Fig. 6-9). Passive congestion is often associated with hemorrhage caused by rupture of capillaries. Several **deficiency diseases,** such as vitamin C deficiency, or **scurvy,** are characterized by hemorrhage. Although most animals synthesize adequate vitamin C, scurvy is seen in guinea pigs and nonhuman primates, which require an exogenous source of this vitamin. The essential role of vitamin K in producing clotting factors has already been discussed. In some species, hemorrhage is a feature of vitamin E deficiency. Hemorrhage is seen in many poi-

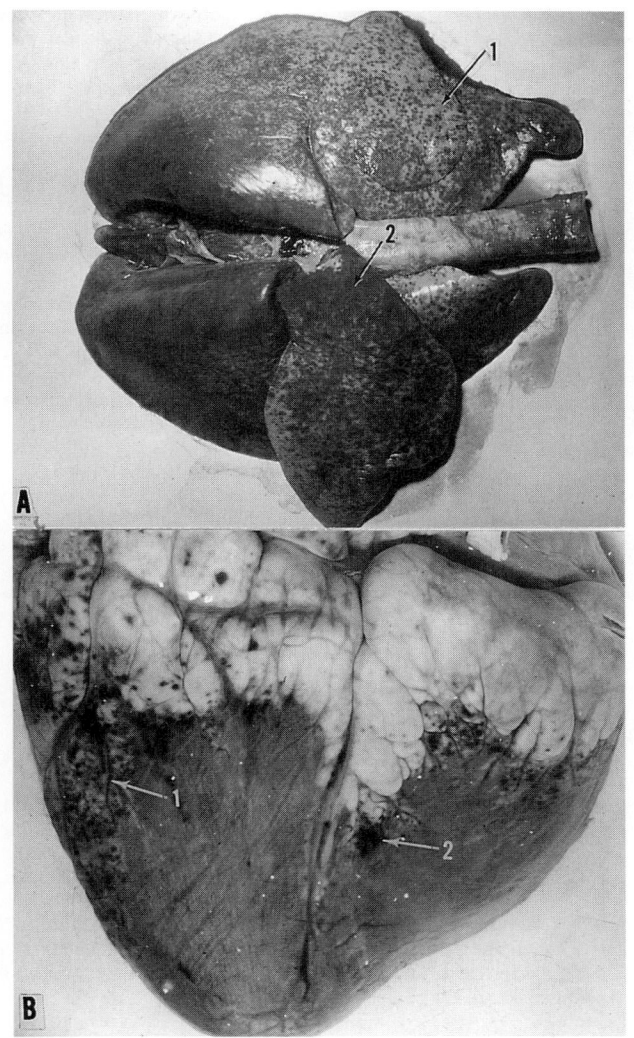

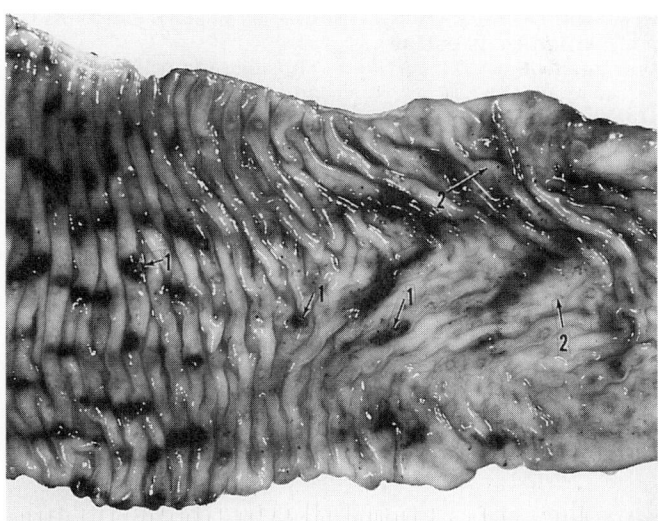

FIG. 6-10 Hemorrhages in the colon of a dog with rickettsiosis of "salmon poisoning." Ecchymoses *(1)* and petechiae *(2)*. (Courtesy of Dr. Wm. J. Hadlow)

sonings. Mechanisms include interference with coagulation (sweet clover poisoning, warfarin); disruption of hematopoiesis (bracken fern, trichlorethylene-extracted soybean meal); or necrosis with associated hemorrhage (arsenic). Exposure to high levels of **ionizing radiation** causes hemorrhage through its direct effect on hematopoiesis as well as vascular integrity. Hemorrhage accompanies many **infectious diseases** including hog cholera, canine infectious hepatitis, anthrax, blackleg, leptospirosis, and "salmon poisoning" (Fig. 6-10).

References

Ainsworth DM, Dodds WJ, Brown CM. Deficiency of the contact phase of intrinsic coagulation in a horse. J Am Vet Med Assoc 1985;187:71–72.

Archer RK, Allen BV. True haemophilia in horses. Vet Rec 1972;91:655–656.

FIG. 6-8 Hemorrhage. **A.** Petechiae *(1)* and extravasations *(2)* of blood in the pleura of a dog dying of fulminant leptospirosis. **B.** Petechiae *(1)* and ecchymoses *(2)* in epicardium of the heart of a Hereford cow after intravenous injection of formalin solution.

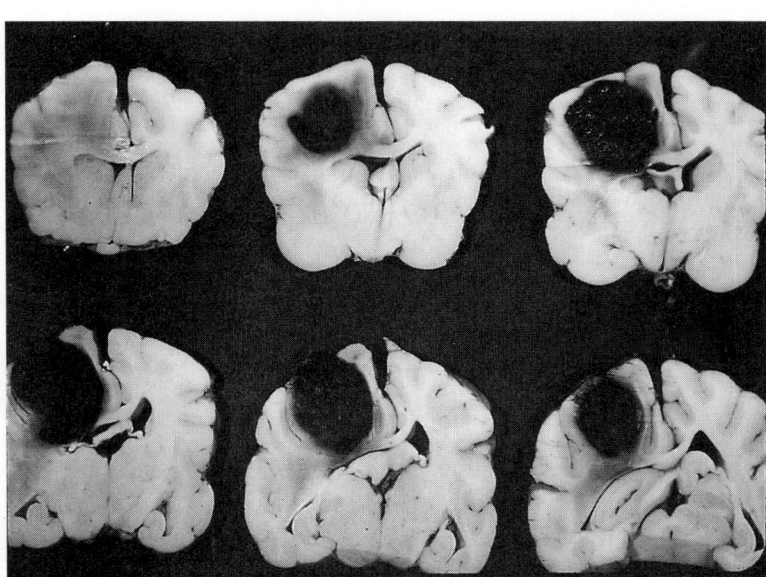

FIG. 6-9 Hemorrhage into brain as a complication of arteriosclerosis in a 12-year-old male Spitz dog. The brain has been sectioned at 1 cm intervals. (Courtesy of Angell Memorial Animal Hospital)

Archer RK, Bowden RST. A case of true haemophilia in a Labrador dog. Vet Rec 1959;71:560.

Avgeris S, Lothrop CD Jr, McDonald TP. Plasma von Willebrand factor concentration and thyroid function in dogs. J Am Vet Med Assoc 1990;196:921–924.

Badylak SF, Dodds WJ, Van Vleet JF. Plasma coagulation factor abnormalities in dogs with naturally occurring hepatic disease. Am J Vet Res 1983;44:2336–2341.

Bell TG, Padgett GA, Patterson WR, et al. Prolonged bleeding time in Aleutian mink associated with a cyclo-oxygenase-independent aggregation defect and nucleotide deficit in blood platelets. Am J Vet Res 1980;41:910–914.

Benson RE, Dodds WJ. Autosomal factor VIII deficiency in rabbits: size variations of rabbit factor VIII. Thromb Haemost 1977;38:380–383.

Bogart R, Muhrer ME. The inheritance of a hemophilia-like condition in swine. J Hered 1942;33:59–64.

Boudreau MK, Crager C, Dillon AR, et al. Identification of an intrinsic platelet function defect in Spitz dogs. J Vet Intern Med 1994;8:93–98.

Bowie EJW, Hart HC, von Arkel C, et al. Tests of hemostasis in swine: normal values and values in pigs affected with von Willebrand's disease. Am J Vet Res 1973;34:1405–1408.

Breukink HJ, Owen CA Jr, Zollman PE, et al. Congenital afibrinogenemia in goats. Zentralbl Veterinaermed 1972;19A:661–676.

Brinkhous KM, Graham JB. Hemophilia in the female dog. Science 1950;111:723–724.

Brooks M, Dodds WJ, Raymond SL. Epidemiologic features of von Willebrand's disease in Doberman Pinschers, Scottish Terriers, and Shetland Sheepdogs: 260 cases (1984–1988). J Am Vet Med Assoc 1992;200:1123–1127.

Capel-Edwards A, Hall DE. Factor VII deficiency in the Beagle dog. Lab Anim 1968;2:105–112.

Catalfamo JL, Dodds WJ. Hereditary and acquired thrombopathias. Vet Clin North Am Small Anim Pract 1988;18:185–193.

Chinn DR, Dodds WJ, Selcer BA. Prekallikrein deficiency in a dog. J Am Vet Med Assoc 1986;188:69–71.

Cines DB, Kaywin P, Bina M, et al. Heparin-associated thrombocytopenia. N Engl J Med 1980;303:788–795.

Cotter SM, Brenner RM, Dodds WJ. Hemophilia A in three unrelated cats. J Am Vet Med Assoc 1978;172:166–168.

Dodds WJ. Familial canine thrombocytopathy. Thromb Diath Haemorrh 1967;26(Suppl):241–248.

Dodds WJ. Current concepts of hereditary coagulation disorders in dogs. Experimentation Animale 1969;1:243–252.

Dodds WJ: Canine von Willebrand's disease. J Lab Clin Med 1970;76:713–721.

Dodds WJ. Canine factor X (Stuart-Prower factor) deficiency. J Lab Clin Med 1973;82:560–566.

Dodds WJ. Further studies of canine von Willebrand's disease. Blood 1975;45:221–230.

Dodds WJ, Kull JE. Canine factor XI (plasma thromboplastin antecedent) deficiency. J Lab Clin Med 1971;78:746–752.

Fass DN, Brockway WJ, Owen CA Jr, et al. Factor VIII (Willebrand) antigen and ristocetin-Willebrand factor in pigs with von Willebrand's disease. Thromb Res 1976;8:319–327.

Feldman BF, Thomason KJ, Jain NC. Quantitative platelet disorders. Vet Clin North Am Small Anim Pract 1988;18:35–49.

Fogh JM. A study of hemophilia A in German Shepherd dogs in Denmark. Vet Clin North Am Small Anim Pract 1988;18:245–254.

Fogh JM, Fogh IT. Inherited coagulation disorders. Vet Clin North Am Small Anim Pract 1988;18:231–243.

Gentry PA, Crane S, Lotz F. Factor XI (plasma thromboplastin antecedent) deficiency in cattle. Can Vet J 1975;16:118–120.

Gralnick HR, Sultan Y, Coller BS. Von Willebrand's disease: combined qualitative and quantitative abnormalities. N Engl J Med 1977;296:1024–1030.

Green RA, White R. Feline factor XII (Hageman) deficiency. Am J Vet Res 1977;38:893–896.

Handagama P, Feldman BF. Thrombocytopenia and drugs. Vet Clin North Am Small Anim Pract 1988;18:51–65.

Hargis AM, Feldman BF. Evaluation of hemostatic defects secondary to vascular tumors in dogs: 11 cases (1983–1988). J Am Vet Med Assoc 1991;198:891–894.

Hart SW, Nolte I. Hemostatic disorders in feline immunodeficiency virus-seropositive cats. J Vet Intern Med 1994;8(5):355–362.

Howell J McC, Lambert PS. A case of haemophilia A in a dog. Vet Rec 1964;76:1103–1105.

Hoyer LW. Hemophilia A. N Engl J Med 1994;330:38–47.

Hutchins DR, Lepherd EE, Crook IG. A case of equine haemophilia. Aust Vet J 1967;43:83–87.

Hutt FB, Rickard CG, Field RA. Sex-linked hemophilia in dogs. J Hered 1948;39:2–9.

Johnson GS, Lees GE, Benson RE, et al. A bleeding disease (von Willebrand's disease) in a Chesapeake Bay Retriever. J Am Vet Med Assoc 1980;176:1261–1263.

Johnson GS, Turrentine MA, Kraus KH. Canine von Willebrand's disease: a heterogeneous group of bleeding disorders. Vet Clin North Am Small Anim Pract 1988;18:195–229.

Joshi BC, Jain NC. Detection of antiplatelet antibody on serum and megakaryocytes of dogs with autoimmune thrombocytopenia. Am J Vet Res 1976;37:681–685.

Kaneko JJ, Cordy DR, Carlson G. Canine hemophilia resembling classic hemophilia A. J Am Vet Med Assoc 1967;150:15–21.

Knowler C, Giger U, Dodds WJ, et al. Factor XI deficiency in Kerry Blue Terriers. J Am Vet Med Assoc 1994;205:1557–1561.

Lewis EF, Holman HH. Haemophilia in a Saint Bernard dog. Vet Rec 1951;63:666–667.

Littlewood JD, Shaw SC, Coombes LM. Vitamin K-dependent coagulopathy in a British Devon Rex cat. J Small Anim Pract 1995;36:115–118.

Maddison JE, Watson AD, Eade IG, et al. Vitamin K-dependent multifactor coagulopathy in Devon Rex cats. J Am Vet Med Assoc 1990;197:1495–1497.

Mattson JC, Estry DW, Bell TG, et al. Defective contact activation of platelets from dogs with basset hound hereditary thrombopathy. Thromb Res 1986;44:23–38.

Menard M, Meyers KM. Storage pool deficiency in cattle with Chediak-Higashi syndrome results from an absence of dense granule precursors in their megakaryocytes. Blood 1988;72:1726–1734.

Miura N, Senba H, Ogawa H, et al. A case of equine thrombasthenia. Nippon Juigaku Zasshi 1987;49:155–158.

Mustard JF. Canine factor VII deficiency. Br J Haematol 1962;8:43–47.

Nolte I, Heyde P, Mischke R, et al. A study on the efficiency of a phospholipid solution in dogs with aspirin-induced thrombocytopathy. Zentralbl Veterinaermed 1994;[A]41(5):385–395.

O'Keefe DA, Couto CG. Coagulation abnormalities associated with neoplasia. Vet Clin North Am Small Anim Pract 1988;18:157–168.

Patrono C. Aspirin as an antiplatelet drug. N Engl J Med 1994;330:1287–1294.

Patterson WR, Padgett GA, Bell TG. Abnormal release of storage pool adenine nucleotides from platelets of dogs affected with basset hound hereditary thrombopathy. Thromb Res 1985;37:61–71.

Patterson WR, Kunicki TJ, Bell TG. Two-dimensional electrophoretic studies of platelets from dogs affected with basset hound hereditary thrombopathy: a thrombasthenia-like aggregation defect. Thromb Res 1986;42(2):195–203.

Patterson WR, Estry DW, Schwartz KA, et al. Absent platelet aggregation with normal fibrinogen binding in basset hound hereditary thrombopathy. Thromb Haemost 1989;62:1011–1015.

Prieur DJ, Meyers KM. Genetics of the fawn-hooded rat strain. The coat color dilution and platelet storage pool deficiency are pleiotropic effects of the autosomal recessive red-eyed dilution gene. J Hered 1984;75:349–352.

Rackear DG. Drugs that alter the hemostatic mechanism. Vet Clin North Am Small Anim Pract 1988;18:67–77.

Rowsell HC, Mustard JF. Blood coagulation disorders in some common laboratory animals. Lab Anim Care 1963;13:752–762.

Rowsell HC. The hemostatic mechanism of mammals and birds in health and disease. Adv Vet Sci 1968;12:337–410.

Sanger VL, Mairs RE, Trapp AL. Hemophilia in a foal. J Am Vet Med Assoc 1964;144:259–264.

Schulman A, Lusk R, Lippincott CL, et al. Diphacinone-induced coagulopathy in the dog. J Am Vet Med Assoc 1986;188:402–405.

Searcy GP, Sheridan D, Dobson KA. Preliminary studies of a platelet function disorder in Simmental cattle. Can J Vet Res 1990;54:394–396.

Searcy GP, Frojmovic MM, McNicol A, et al. Platelets from bleeding Simmental cattle mobilize calcium, phosphorylate myosin light chain and bind normal numbers of fibrinogen molecules but have abnormal cytoskeletal assembly and aggregation in response to ADP. Thromb Haemost 1994;71:240–246.

Sherding RG, DiBartola SP. Hemophilia B (factor IX deficiency) in an Old English Sheepdog. J Am Vet Med Assoc 1980;176:141–142.

Soute BA, Ulrich MM, Watson AD, et al. Congenital deficiency of all vitamin K-dependent blood coagulation factors due to a defective vitamin K-dependent carboxylase in Devon Rex cats. Thromb Haemost 1992;68:521–525.

Spurling NW, Burton LK, Peacock R, et al. Hereditary factor-VII deficiency in the Beagle. Br J Haematol 1972;23:59–67.

Steficek BA, Thomas JS, Baker JC, et al. Hemorrhagic diathesis associated with a hereditary platelet disorder in Simmental cattle. J Vet Diagn Invest 1993;5(2):202–207.

Sutherland RJ, Cambridge H, Bolton JR. Functional and morphological studies on blood platelets in a thrombasthenic horse. Aust Vet J 1989;66:366–370.

Turrentine MA, Sculley PW, Green EM, et al. Prekallikrein deficiency in a family of miniature horses. Am J Vet Res 1986;47:2464–2467.

HYPEREMIA AND CONGESTION

Both terms denote an excess of blood in the vessels of a given part. This can occur in either of two ways: too much blood being brought in by the arteries with dilation of arteries and arterioles or too little being drained out by the veins. The term **active hyperemia** indicates the increased volume of blood is of arterial origin and the term **passive hyperemia,** or more often **passive congestion** or simply **congestion,** results from interference with venous drainage.

Active hyperemia

This condition is usually associated with the inflammatory process as discussed in Chapter 5. It may also follow exposure to heat, either locally or total body. It is mediated by vasoactive amines and neurogenic mechanisms.

GROSS APPEARANCE

Grossly, to a greater or lesser extent depending on the original color, the part takes on the bright red color of arterial blood. The part is also warmer than usual, and pulsating arteries, which are not usually perceptible, may be felt.

MICROSCOPIC APPEARANCE

Microscopically, arterioles and capillaries are dilated and filled with blood. They also appear to be more numerous. If the cause is inflammatory (as it usually is), the other morphologic features of inflammation are apparent.

Passive congestion

This condition results from obstruction of venous return, which may be a local event or a generalized phenomenon. **Local passive congestion** may develop as a consequence of complete or partial obstruction of veins draining a part. Bandages applied too tightly, venous thrombosis, and pressure from neoplasms are examples of causes. Gravity is the cause of **hypostatic congestion.** This is a congestion, often quite noticeable, of the organs and tissues on the lower side of a recumbent animal. Especially in large animals, there is a strong tendency for blood to gravitate to the lower side of the body. This may cause death in an otherwise healthy horse confined for some hours in an unnatural position from which it cannot rise. Heart failure (Chapter 21) causes more **generalized passive congestion.** With combined right and left failure all systems are affected. With left-sided failure, the congestion is principally evident in the pulmonary vasculature, and with right-sided failure, the pulmonary vessels are spared, but passive congestion occurs throughout the rest of the body, being particularly conspicuous in the liver, spleen, and dependent parts (Fig. 6-11).

GROSS APPEARANCE

Grossly, the congested part is slightly swollen and tends to have a bluish-red tinge **(cyanosis).** The part is usually more wet than normal as a result of edema and, if the congestion is chronic, may be firm because of fibrosis. During life, the temperature of the part may be discernibly lower than normal.

MICROSCOPIC APPEARANCE

Microscopically, the capillaries and veins are dilated and full of blood; likewise, the sinusoidal blood spaces of the liver and spleen are filled with blood when these organs are involved. Edema may be extensive, particularly in passive congestion of the lungs, in which the alveoli become filled with fluid. Small hemorrhages are present

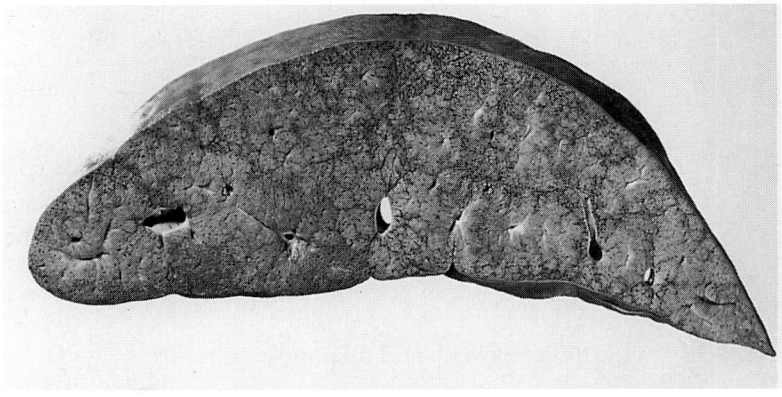

FIG. 6-11 Chronic passive congestion of liver of 8-month-old Hereford steer. The underlying lesions were large firm "vegetative" masses on the leaflets of the tricuspid valve. (Courtesy of Dr. W. J. Hadlow)

from ruptured capillaries. In the lung, extravasated red blood cells become engulfed by alveolar macrophages and are converted to hemosiderin (the so-called "heart failure cells"). The hypoxia resulting from congestion leads to necrosis of parenchymal tissue, which in acute cardiac failure may cause extensive centrilobular necrosis of the liver (nutmeg liver). With **chronic passive congestion,** loss of parenchymal tissue is more insidious, and fibrous connective tissue surrounds veins and replaces lost parenchyma. This results in cirrhosis of the liver and what is termed **brown induration of the lung** resulting from fibrosis of alveolar septae and presence of heart failure cells. Similar fibrosis occurs along the sinusoids in the chronically congested spleen.

EDEMA

Edema is the accumulation of fluid in the interstitium (intercellular spaces) (Figs. 6-12 and 6-13) or body cavities. Excessive fluid within cells is termed acute cellular swelling or hydropic degeneration (Chapter 2). Edema may be general or local. It may also be inflammatory (discussed in Chapter 5) or noninflammatory. Edema of most organs and tissues is generally termed edema, and the organ or tissue is edematous. Extensive edema of subcutaneous tissues is termed **anasarca;** within body cavities, **hydrothorax, hydropericardium, ascites** (peritoneal cavity); in the scrotum, **hydrocele;** and in the amniotic sac, **hydrops amnii.** Certain diseases characterized by edema have been given names, such as *brisket disease* (accumulation of fluid in the sternal region).

Gross appearance

Grossly, edematous organs and tissues are swollen and wet and may ooze fluid when cut. The fluid is pale yellowish and may clot, but usually it drips from the cut

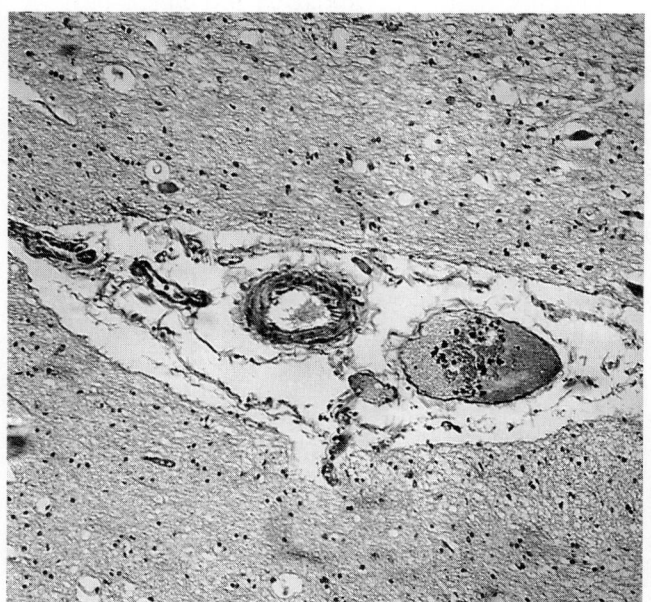

FIG. 6-12 Perivascular edema, brain of a horse (hematoxylin and eosin stain, × 200)

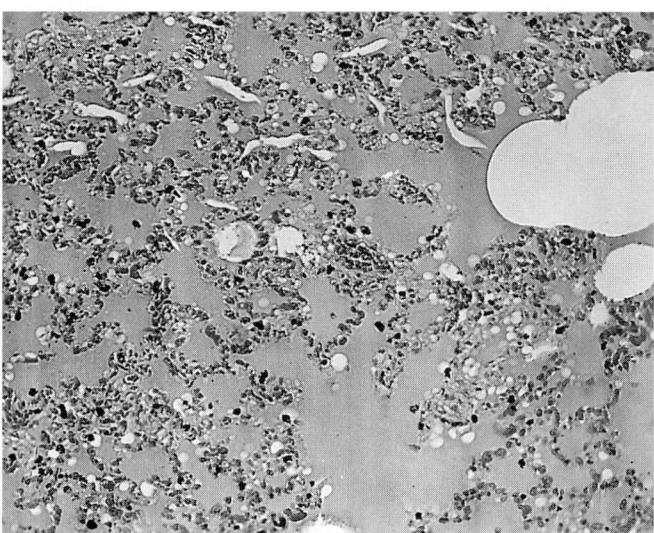

FIG. 6-13 Edema of lung of dog. Note homogeneous protein material fills alveoli (hematoxylin and eosin stain, × 170) (Courtesy of Armed Forces Institute of Pathology)

surface; if pressure is applied, a much larger amount of fluid may be squeezed from the tissue. During life, the edematous part, if external, is cool. There is no redness and no sign of pain. Affected tissues have a firm but doughy consistency. The tissue "pits on pressure," meaning that if a finger is pressed into the edematous tissue, the fluid is dispersed into nearby tissue spaces. When the finger is removed, the pit remains for a moment or two (Fig. 6-14).

Edematous swelling along the ventral abdominal wall (**dependent edema**) is often several centimeters thick and rather sharply delimited so that a conspicuous longitudinal ridge marks its boundaries along each side. The swelling commonly diffuses into the preputial region in males and fades out anteriorly in the sternal region. In other examples ("brisket disease" of cattle), the swelling is most pronounced in the sternal region. Sometimes the edema is conspicuous externally only as a sagging protrusion of the submandibular tissues. This is especially true in sheep suffering from gastrointestinal parasitism, the condition called "bottle-jaw" among stockmen.

Microscopic appearance

Microscopically, the spaces between adjacent cells, fibrils, and other structures are enlarged. During life they were, of course, filled with fluid; in the microscopic section, a faint, pink-staining residue of precipitated albumin may or may not remain, depending on the amount of proteins in the edema fluid. Considerable judgment must be employed in interpreting empty intercellular spaces. A certain, but variable, amount of space is left between cells by shrinkage that occurs in the preparation of sections by the paraffin or similar techniques. These artificial spaces tend to be less numerous, less uniform in size, and less evenly distrib-

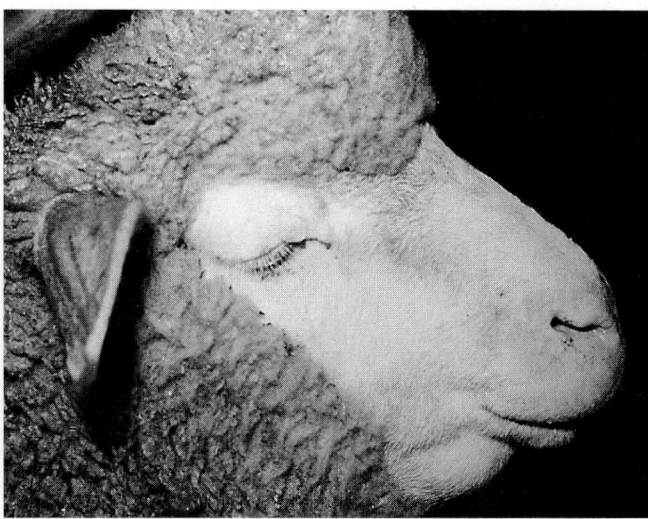

FIG. 6-14 Edema, subcutis, inframandibular region. Sheep with severe trichostrongylosis. Swollen tissue was doughy in consistency and pitted on digital pressure. (Courtesy of Dr A. Tontis and Prof Dr H. Luginbühl)

uted than the spaces that result from edema. Shrinkage follows natural lines of cleavage, which usually lie between one kind of tissue and another, although they do not separate epithelium from its connective tissue base. A few erythrocytes, leukocytes, or fibrils of fibrin may be present, but any considerable number of the last two indicates inflammation. Edema of long standing becomes organized by fibrous connective tissue.

Edema of the brain betrays itself first by distention of the perivascular and even the perineuronal spaces, but excessive shrinkage may be deceptive. The sulci are compressed and the convolutions flattened by pressure against the cranium, a situation more easily noticed grossly than microscopically. In edema of the lungs, the alveoli are filled with fluid. There is usually enough protein present to render the condition noticeable microscopically.

Causes

Edema results from a disruption of the normal balance between the fluid compartments of the blood, interstitium, and lymphatics. Normally, there is a continuous flow of fluid from the blood into the interstitium and then back to the bloodstream. Fluid leaves the bloodstream at the arteriolar end of the microcirculation as a result of the greater hydrostatic pressure in the arterioles than in the interstitium. The force of hydrostatic pressure is opposed by the osmotic pressure from plasma proteins (chiefly albumin); however, the hydrostatic pressure exceeds the osmotic force. At the venous side of the microcirculation, the hydrostatic pressure has decreased and the osmotic pressure of the blood increased such that most of the interstitial fluid is drawn back into the bloodstream. Fluid which does not re-enter the venules is conveyed by lymphatics back to the bloodstream. This fluid exchange is described in detail in Chapter 5.

Mechanisms

Four basic mechanisms lead to disruption of this balance, resulting in edema: (1) increased hydrostatic pressure; (2) decreased plasma osmotic pressure; (3) lymphatic obstruction; and (4) retention of sodium. These four mechanisms are, however, not always independent from one another.

INCREASED HYDROSTATIC PRESSURE

This mechanism has its effect by increasing the flow of fluid from the blood to the interstitium and decreasing the flow from the interstitium back to the blood. The edema of passive congestion is caused by increased venular blood pressure and may be localized or generalized. **Localized edema** resulting from increased hydrostatic pressure occurs when the flow of blood in veins is obstructed due to thrombosis, external pressure, or disorders such as cirrhosis. **Generalized edema** caused by increased hydrostatic pressure results from impaired cardiac function leading to congestive heart failure and **cardiac edema.** Cardiac edema is further complicated by a series of events, culminating in retention of sodium and aggravation of cardiac function (Chapter 21, Heart Failure).

DECREASED PLASMA OSMOTIC PRESSURE

This mechanism results from hypoproteinemia, which lowers the osmotic force necessary for movement of fluid from the interstitium into venules. Hypoproteinemia may result from (1) renal disease characterized by proteinuria (**renal edema**), (2) dietary protein deficiency (**nutritional edema, cachectic edema**), (3) decreased synthesis of plasma proteins caused by liver disease, or (4) loss of plasma proteins caused by heavy infestations with intestinal parasites such as trichostrongyles (**parasitic edema**). Each of these can result in loss of blood volume and contribute to the development of congestive heart failure, thus further contributing to edema as well as other problems.

LYMPHATIC OBSTRUCTION

This mechanism, which is similar to localized venous stasis, leads to **lymphedema.** Conditions that place external pressure on veins also affect lymphatics. Several infectious diseases of animals primarily affect lymph nodes and lymphatics and, in addition to their inflammatory lesions, may cause obstruction and edema (e.g., bovine farcy, ulcerative lymphangitis, epizootic lymphangitis). In humans and animals in tropical countries, filarids of the genera *Brugia* and *Wuchereria* inhabit lymphatics, causing obstruction and edema. **Congenital hereditary lymphedema** (Fig. 6-15) is a rare disorder characterized by discontinuity or absence of lymph vessels. The condition, described in children, dogs, cattle, and swine, may be characterized by generalized edema or edema restricted to the limbs.

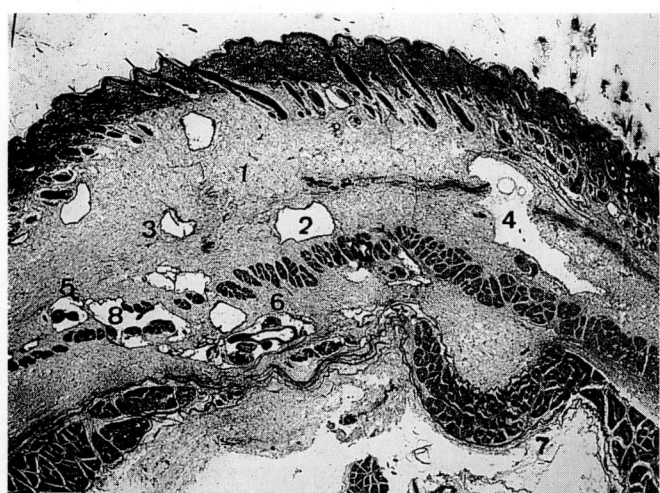

FIG. 6-15 Congenital hereditary lymphedema, 1-day-old puppy. Section of skin of thorax. The subcutis *(1)* is thickened and contains edema of low protein content. Blood vessels are irregularly dilated *(2,4)*, some vascular valves *(3)* appear ruptured, some lymph vessels surround thick-walled veins *(5)* or arteries *(6)*. The panniculus muscle bundles are separated by edematous stroma *(7)* and by dilated lymph vessels *(8)*. (Courtesy of Prof Dr H. Luginbühl and Journal of Medical Genetics)

RETENTION OF SODIUM

Excessive consumption of either salt or water by a normal individual does not cause edema. However, failure to excrete sodium and its associated retention of water does lead to generalized edema. This is seen in renal disorders in which there is increased reabsorption of sodium, as in glomerulonephritis. As mentioned, congestive heart failure also leads to reduced urinary sodium excretion.

References

Davies AP, Hardy R, Larsen R, et al. Primary lymphedema in three dogs. J Am Vet Med Assoc 1979;174:1316–1320.

Frank MM, Gelfand JA, Atkinson JP. Hereditary angioedema. The clinical syndrome and its management. Ann Intern Med 1976;84:580–593.

Ladds PW, Dennis SM, Leipold HW. Lethal congenital edema in Bulldog pups. J Am Vet Med Assoc 1971;159:81–86.

Leighton RL, Suter PF. Primary lymphedema of the hind limb in the dog. J Am Vet Med Assoc 1970;175:369–374.

Lieberman AH. Current status of aldosterone in the etiology of edema. Arch Intern Med 1958;102:990–997.

Luginbühl H, Chacko SK, Patterson DF, et al: Congenital hereditary lymphoedema in the dog. J Med Genet 1967;4:153–165.

Mulei CM, Atwell RB. Congenital lymphoedema in an Ayrshire-Friesian crossbred female calf. Aust Vet J 1989;66:227–228.

van der Patte SCJ. The pathogenesis of congenital hereditary lymphedema in the pig. Lymphology 1978;11:10–21.

Shock

Shock is the result of a relatively sudden generalized inability of the circulatory system to perfuse cells and tissues with adequate oxygen and nutrients to meet metabolic requirements. It is often defined as **circulatory collapse** and is characterized by marked hypotension. If not corrected very early, the absence of oxygen and nutrients leads to anaerobic metabolism, lactic acidosis, cellular and organic dysfunction, cell death, and ultimately death of the patient. The control of blood pressure for adequate perfusion is essentially regulated by two factors: peripheral vascular resistance and cardiac output, which are both under the control of a myriad of interactive complex physiologic mechanisms including vasoactive amines, autonomic control of vascular smooth muscle, epinephrine, the renin-angiotensin system, and many others. In shock, these mechanisms attempt to compensate for the reduced perfusion, but may be inadequate or, as with some of the compensatory mechanisms involved in heart failure, actually exacerbate shock by causing vasoconstriction in certain organs and tissues, further reducing perfusion of already ischemic cells and tissues.

Causes

The **causes** of shock are any insult that dramatically reduces cardiac output or peripheral resistance. On the basis of the cause, shock can be classified as **(1) hypovolemic (oligemic), (2) cardiogenic, (3) septic or endotoxic, (4) neurogenic (traumatic),** or **(5) anaphylactic.** The latter three are often referred to as **distributive shock.**

HYPOVOLEMIC SHOCK

This type of shock is the simplest to understand. It results from a large loss of fluid, as for example with extensive hemorrhage, vomiting, diarrhea, or severe burns. Certain infections that affect the vasculature can also lead to substantial fluid loss resulting in shock (e.g., equine viral arteritis, hemorrhagic fevers, African swine fever). The result of these insults is a marked reduction in blood volume and therefore cardiac output.

CARDIOGENIC SHOCK

This results from inadequate cardiac systolic output caused by primary cardiac disease in the presence of adequate intravascular blood volume. It is much more common in humans than animals because of the higher frequency of myocardial infarction; however, other diseases that affect left ventricular performance may also result in cardiogenic shock. These include infectious diseases that affect the myocardium, valvular disease, pericardial tamponade (obstructive shock), and certain nutritional deficiencies, all of which occur in animals.

In both hypovolemic and cardiogenic shock, a variety of neuroendocrine compensatory responses are initiated to compensate for the hypotension and the real or perceived hypovolemia. These are comparable to those compensatory responses induced in congestive heart failure (Chapter 21). Baroreceptors and chemoreceptors trigger the sympathetic nervous system to vasoconstriction, increased heart rate, and contractility. The adrenal medulla is stimulated to release norepinephrine and epinephrine, which increases vasoconstriction and increased heart rate. Activation of the renin-angiotensin system produces increased levels of angiotensin II with further vasoconstriction, and aldosterone secretion causes retention of sodium and water. These mechanisms may be adequate to prevent death, but if blood or fluid loss or the primary cardiac defect is not corrected, death from shock results. Vasoconstriction, while essential to maintain blood pressure, further contributes to tissue anoxia, which can aggravate the situation. This is partially compensated for by redistribution of blood toward the brain, heart, and kidneys and away from the skin, intestines, and skeletal muscle.

SEPTIC (ENDOTOXIC) SHOCK

This type of shock is caused by a marked decrease in peripheral vascular resistance caused by arteriolar dilation and pooling (and leaking) of blood in dilated capillaries and venules, which effectively reduces blood volume. This functional hypovolemia leads to hypotension and a reduction in cardiac output, further contributing to hypotension and shock. Septic shock results from an infection, most usually with gram-negative bacteria, such as strains of *Escherichia coli*, *Klebsiella* species and *Pseudomonas* species, although gram-positive bacteria, such as *Streptococcus* species, may also be an offender. The infection, either localized or septicemic, leads to the release of potent mediators that initiate a series of events leading to circulatory collapse. Lipopolysaccharides (endotoxic lipopolysaccharides, endotoxin) are the offending mediators released by gram-negative bacteria which, when introduced experimentally, have been shown to cause shock. The peptidoglycans and lipoteichoic acids of gram-positive bacteria initiate the events. These endotoxins interact with and damage endothelial cells and leukocytes (principally monocytes and neutrophils), stimulating the release of a number of humoral mediators, either directly or indirectly, which affect circulation, initiate coagulation, and activate complement. These include, among others, TNFα, interleukin-β (IL-1β), prostaglandins, thromboxanes, platelet activating factor, tissue factor, kinins, histamine, endorphins, and nitric oxide. It is TNFα and IL-1β that appear to be the most important factors in mediating shock. While certain of these mediators promote vasoconstriction, many cause peripheral vasodilation, which is the principal mechanism causing functional hypovolemia. DIC, a common accompaniment to septic shock, results from activation of platelets and the release of tissue factor and plasminogen activator inhibitor. The net effect of hypovolemia, endothelial damage, DIC, and acidosis is tissue damage, organ dysfunction, and, if not corrected, death.

NEUROGENIC SHOCK

This may follow severe trauma, pain, or restraint. These incidents somehow cause an inhibition of vasomotor control, allowing arteriolar dilation and pooling of blood in capillaries and venules.

ANAPHYLACTIC SHOCK

Anaphylactic shock (Chapter 7) also results from pooling of blood in capillaries and venules resulting from arteriolar dilation. This is mediated through the release of histamine and other mediators. Anaphylaxis is further complicated by increased vascular permeability and fluid loss.

LESIONS OF SHOCK

Lesions seen in shock are primarily the result of hypoxia caused by the combination of reduced blood volume, hypotension, and compensatory vasoconstriction, coupled with those lesions of the precipitating event. They are characterized by cellular degeneration and necrosis which, in shock, are particularly evident in the liver, kidneys, heart, and gastrointestinal tract. In septic shock, necrotizing lesions are usually more extensive because of the considerable endothelial damage and DIC. In all types, except shock following massive hemorrhage, there is severe congestion of most organs and tissues, especially the liver, gastrointestinal tract, adrenal glands, and sometimes the kidneys. Hemorrhage usually occurs in the gastrointestinal tract, endocardium, and adrenal cortices. Cellular degeneration and necrosis is particularly evident in the kidney in the form of acute tubular necrosis, which particularly affects the proximal convoluted tubules, although the distal tubules may also show damage. Acute tubular necrosis is associated with renal failure and, in the living animal with shock, oliguria. Multiple small foci of necrosis are present throughout the myocardium. Foci of necrosis occur throughout the gastrointestinal mucosa. There is also necrosis of hepatocytes, particularly in the centrilobular zone. The lungs are edematous and, in septic shock, the alveolar capillaries are often plugged with aggregated platelets. Varying degrees of adrenal cortical necrosis are usually present. The brain may contain lesions of ischemic injury comparable to that seen from other causes of anoxia (laminar necrosis).

References

Allen DA, Schertel ER. Pathogenic aspects of circulatory shock. Vet Clin North Am Equine Pract 1994;10(3):495–501.

Balis JU, Rappaport ES, Gerber L, et al. Development of lung lesions in endotoxin shock. Am J Pathol 1972;66:53a.

Balis JU, Rappaport ES, Gerber L, et al. A primate model for prolonged endotoxin shock: blood-vascular reactions and effects of glucocorticoid treatment. Lab Invest 1978;38:511–523.

Califf RM, Bengtson JR. Cardiogenic shock. N Engl J Med 1994;330:1724–1730.

Chang J, Hackel DB. Comparative study of myocardial lesions in hemorrhagic shock. Lab Invest 1973;28:641–647.

Coalson JJ, Hinshaw LB, Guenter CA, et al. Pathophysiologic responses of the subhuman primate in experimental septic shock. Lab Invest 1975;32:561–569.

Cox E, Schrauwen E, Cools V, et al. Experimental induction of diarrhoea in newly-weaned piglets. Zentralbl Veterinarmed [A] 1991;38:418–426.

Dupe R, Bywater RJ, Goddard M. A hypertonic infusion in the treatment of experimental shock in calves and clinical shock in dogs and cats. Vet Rec 1993;133:585–590.

Houston MC. Pathophysiology of shock. Crit Care Nurs Clin North Am 1990;2(2):143–149.

Ogata M, Ago K, Ago M, et al. [A case of death due to neurogenic

shock.] Nippon Hoigaku Zasshi [Jpn J Legal Med] 1992;
46(2):152–158.

Pingleton WW, Coalson JJ, Guenter CA. Significance of leukocytes in endotoxic shock. Exp Mol Pathol 1975;22:183–194.

Rudloff E, Kirby R. Hypovolemic shock and resuscitation. Vet Clin North Am Small Anim Pract 1994;24:1015–1039.

Rutherford RB, Trow RS. Pathophysiology of irreversible hemorrhagic shock in monkeys. J Surg Res 1973;14:538–550.

Selkurt EE. Physiological basis of circulatory shock. Status of investigative aspects of hemorrhagic shock. Fed Proc 1970;29:1832–1835.

Stickles LE Jr. Shock. Part 1. Basic origins and causes. Canine Pract 1975;2:48–52.

Villeda CJ, Williams SM, Wilkinson PJ, et al. Consumption coagulopathy associated with shock in acute African swine fever. Arch Virol 1993;133:467–475.

7
Immunopathology

Immunity, or the resistance to disease, particularly infectious disease, occurs in two basic types, **natural (innate or native)** and **acquired (adaptive or specific).** The mechanisms involved in these two distinct but complementary forms of immunity are different and are discussed separately.

NATURAL IMMUNITY

The best form of immunity results from individual species variation in susceptibility to infectious diseases. For example, horses, swine, and cattle are resistant to infection with canine distemper virus, a highly pathogenic agent for dogs. Similarly, feline panleukopenia virus affects a variety of feline species, but ruminants and a number of other species are totally resistant. This form of immunity is genetically determined and results from basic biologic incompatibilities between a given species and an infectious agent that do not allow infection to occur. In the case of viral infections, such resistance may result from lack of an appropriate receptor molecule required for the agent to gain entrance to host cells.

In addition to these absolute forms of immunity, relative degrees of resistance occur with other infectious agents. For example, *Bacillus anthracis* causes an acute fatal disease in cattle, whereas in dogs and horses the disease is relatively mild. Even within a species, certain breeds are more resistant to certain infectious agents than others. Zebu cattle *(Bos indicus),* for instance, are more resistant to piroplasmosis than domestic cattle *(Bos taurus).* Similarly, the many strains of laboratory rodents differ markedly in their resistance to disease.

Certain elements of acquired immunity may be responsible for some of these differences, but most are thought to be genetically determined. Age, sex, hormonal status, nutritional status, and environment influence natural as well as acquired immunity. Only female mice that have had one or more pregnancies develop carcinoma of the mammary gland caused by mouse mammary tumor virus, despite the fact that males and virgin females are also infected. Rats defi-

cient in iron are significantly more susceptible to salmonellosis than nondeficient rats.

Aside from these species-specific forms of resistance, other factors are also involved in innate resistance. The skin and mucous membranes, when intact, serve as effective mechanical barriers that prevent many organisms from gaining entrance to the host. The layer of mucus that covers the respiratory epithelium entraps inhaled particles, including microorganisms, which are propelled by the cilia to the oropharynx, where they are swallowed. Saliva, gastric acid, and intestinal enzymes offer protection by destroying many organisms.

Cells involved in natural immunity

Neutrophils and **macrophages** are important cellular elements in natural immunity because they are capable of phagocytizing, killing, and enzymatically degrading a wide variety of microorganisms in nonimmune hosts. However, phagocytosis by these cells is greatly enhanced if the microorganism is coated (opsonized) with acquired antibodies. The microbicidal action of these phagocytic cells is primarily the result of the generation of hydrogen peroxide and superoxide through myeloperoxidase in neutrophils and catalase in macrophages. Other bacteriocidal molecules, such as cationic proteins and lactoferrin, are present in neutrophils. The hydrolytic enzymes of lysosomes do not kill bacteria but are responsible for digestion and elimination of dead organisms after they have been killed by these other mechanisms. This is not a perfect system; many bacteria are not killed after being phagocytized but instead actively multiply within the phagocyte and eventually kill it by the production of toxins.

Chemical substances involved in natural immunity

Natural antibodies, which are identical to acquired IgM and IgG antibodies, are also regarded as components of natural immunity. The majority of natural antibodies are low-affinity, anticarbohydrate antibodies that are thought to be generated against polysaccharides pres-

177

ent in the cell walls of enteric bacteria. These are thymus-independent antigens: B lymphocytes do not require the cognate help of CD4+ (helper) T lymphocytes to generate antibodies against them.

The cellular production of several proteins, known as **interferons,** provides a defense mechanism against viruses and possibly other microbes. The action of interferons falls somewhere between natural immunity and acquired immunity, resembling the former because it is nonspecific and without memory, but similar to acquired immunity because its production depends on infection with an invading organism. Although the production of interferons is also stimulated by certain bacterial, protozoan, and mycotic organisms, the antimicrobial activity of these proteins appears to be most effective in limiting viral infections, particularly in nonimmune individuals.

The complement system is an important component of both natural and acquired immunity: it can act alone (**alternate pathway**) or in concert with the humoral immune system (**classic pathway**) to cause microbial killing. The term **complement** originally referred to a heat-labile substance present in normal plasma that "complements," or enhances, the lytic action of antibodies bound to bacteria and other cells. The activity of this substance could be destroyed by heating the se-

rum to 560°C before applying it to the target cells. It is now known that this important defense mechanism does not result from a single substance, but instead from the action of nine separate soluble proteins, designated C1 through C9; these, in turn, give rise to an additional nine proteins that interact with one another to effect cell lysis. The complement system amplifies the protective functions of antibodies as well as certain hypersensitivity reactions. We will not attempt to describe the details of this complex system, but will mention only a few of the important steps involved in its function. For an in-depth discussion of this system, the student is referred to Abbas, Lichtman, and Pober, 1994.

The **classic complement activation pathway** is initiated when the C1 molecule binds to an antigen-antibody complex, whereas the **alternative pathway** is initiated by contact of the C3 molecule with certain activating surfaces, such as bacterial cell walls. Both of these pathways eventually converge and produce what is known as the membrane attack complex (MAC). The MAC is a complex of molecules composed of C5–C9. This complex creates pores in the membrane to which it is bound and causes osmotic lysis of the coated cell. These pathways are depicted diagramatically in Figure 7-1.

Viral interference is a phenomenon in which an an-

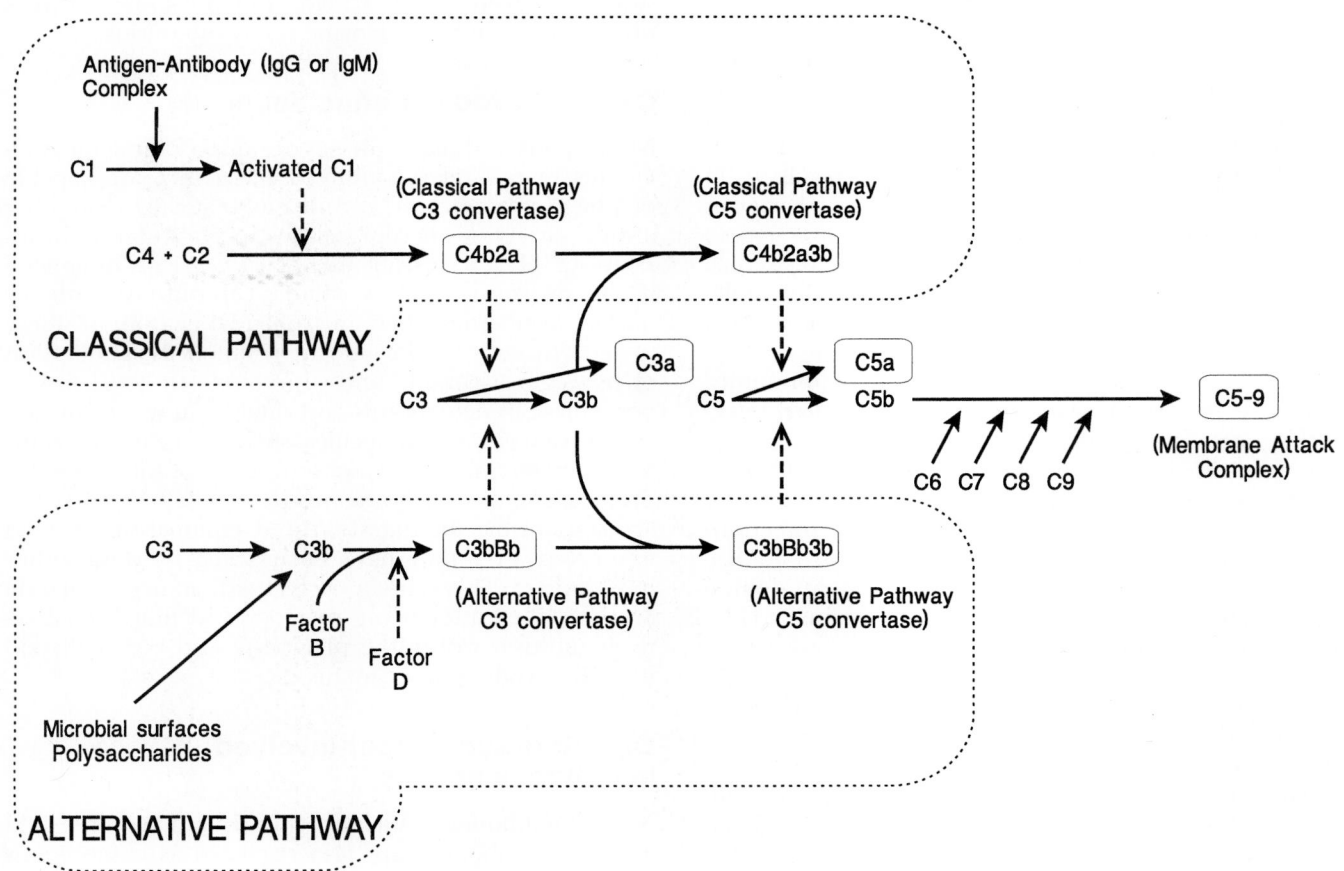

FIG. 7-1 The complement system. Note that the classic and alternate pathways converge into a common pathway after the cleavage of C5, which causes generation of the membrane attack complex, C5–9.

imal or tissue infected with one virus is rendered resistant to simultaneous infection with a second virus. It is now known that most viruses, on infecting a cell, stimulate the production and release of proteins known as interferons, which prevent or interfere with the replication of the same or different virus in adjacent noninfected cells. Interferon is not virus-specific, but it is specific to a species or host. Its mode of action appears to be paracrine in nature: its secretion from infected cells interferes with the synthesis of viral nucleic acid and proteins in subsequently infected cells and thus limits replication and spread of the virus. Interferon is not in itself antiviral, but apparently induces newly infected cells to produce other substances that interfere with viral replication. Attempts have been made to administer exogenous interferon or to stimulate its endogenous secretion as a means of treating viral diseases, but this has met with limited success to date.

ACQUIRED IMMUNITY

Acquired immunity, also referred to as **specific immunity,** is only one component of the highly integrated host defense system, in which many different kinds of cells and molecules function cooperatively (Fig. 7-2). Three features distinguish acquired immunity from in-

nate or natural immunity: (1) acquired immunity requires previous exposure to the microorganism or antigen to become active; (2) acquired immunity is highly specific for certain antigens; and (3) acquired immunity has memory.

Cells involved in acquired immunity

The ultimate target of all acquired immune responses is an **antigen,** which is usually a foreign molecule derived from a wide variety of microbial agents and environmental sources.

Specialized **antigen-presenting cells (APCs),** known as **macrophages,** roam the body in search of foreign antigens, which they phagocytize and degrade into antigenic peptides. Other APCs include **Langerhan's cells** of the skin; **interdigitating dendritic cells** present in areas of T-cell-rich lymph nodes, spleen, and interstitial tissues of many organs; and **follicular dendritic cells** found in the germinal centers of lymph nodes, spleen, and mucosa-associated lymphoid tissues. During the course of processing foreign antigens, APCs couple these antigenic peptides to **major histocompatibility complex (MHC) molecules** and present the MHC-peptide complex on the surface of the cell in a form that can be recognized by other cells (Fig. 7-2). MHC mole-

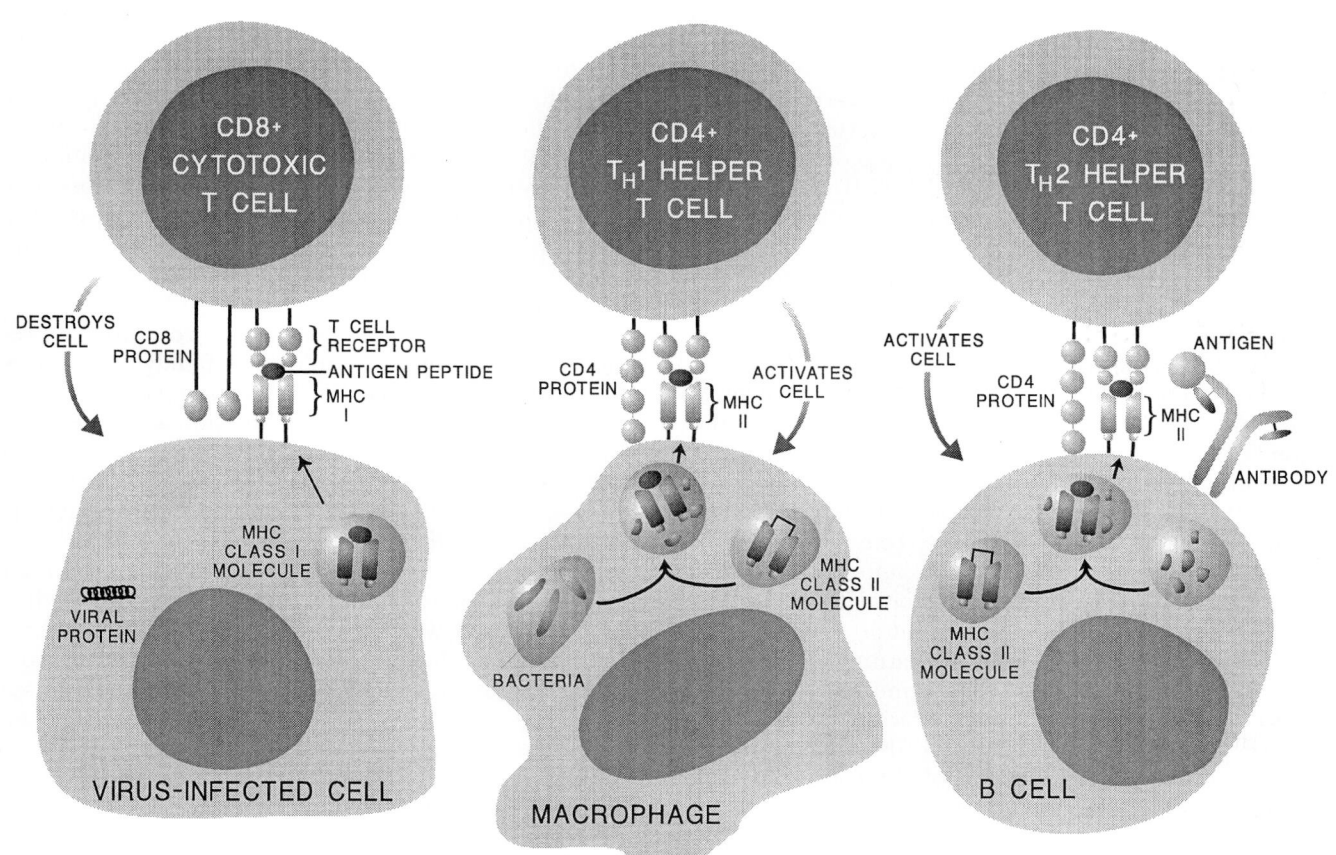

FIG. 7-2 T-lymphocyte interactions with other cells of the acquired immune system.

cules occur in two classes, class I and class II, each having a cleft that binds antigenic peptides for presentation. The two different classes of MHC molecules present peptides that arise from different places within cells.

MHC class I molecules are constitutively expressed on the plasma membranes of virtually all nucleated cells; class I molecules bind peptides that originate in the cytoplasm of the cell. If the peptide happens to be foreign, such as those produced by a virus, they are complexed to the MHC class I molecule and transported to the surface of the infected cell, where they are recognized by CD8+ cytotoxic T cells (Fig. 7-2). The latter cells, in turn, secrete chemicals that kill the infected cell.

MHC class II molecules are primarily expressed on the surface of B lymphocytes, macrophages, and dendritic and endothelial cells. Peptides that bind to class II molecules for presentation on the surfaces of cells are those that are produced within phagolysosomes of macrophages. These include degradative products of bacteria that have been phagocytized by macrophages and peptides derived from circulating foreign antigens that have been internalized and processed by B lymphocytes after binding to the B-cell receptor. Macrophages presenting peptides bound to MHC class II molecules are recognized and become bound to a subset of CD4+ lymphocytes, known as T_{H1} cells. Unlike cytotoxic T cells, T_{H1} cells do not kill the infected macrophage but, instead, secrete chemicals that activate the macrophage, signaling it to destroy organisms within its phagosomes. B lymphocytes presenting MHC class II peptide complexes on their surface are recognized by and become bound to a subset of CD4+ T lymphocytes known as T_{H2}, or helper T cells. The T-cell receptors (TCR) of the T_{H2} cells bind to the antigen MHC II complex on the surface of B lymphocytes, which signals the B cell to proliferate and begin making antibody.

Another very important class of cells involved in the acquired immune response are the thymus-derived **T lymphocytes.** These cells, often referred to simply as **T cells,** can be further divided into specific subsets based on their function and phenotype. Probably the most important cells of the acquired immune system are the **helper T cells,** which can be distinguished from other subsets of T cells by the presence of a distinctive molecule on their surface referred to as CD4 (cluster designation 4). These CD4+ T cells secrete a number of chemical substances, known as cytokines, that orchestrate the functional activity of effector cells involved in both the cellular and humoral immune systems (Fig. 7-2). Those cells involved with regulating the function of effector cells of the cellular immune system are termed T_{H1} cells, while those regulating the humoral immune system are termed T_{H2} cells. Their specific roles in regulating the function of these two immune systems have been discussed above.

Another distinctive subset of T cells are the **cytolytic (cytotoxic) T lymphocytes,** or **CTLs.** These cells also have a distinctive membrane marker, known as CD8, that allows them to be differentiated from other T cells. CD8+ cells are responsible for killing virus-infected cells and cells expressing foreign antigens on their surfaces, such as mismatched MHC molecules on the surfaces of transplanted allogeneic cells or organs. A counterpart to the helper function of CD4+ lymphocytes exists in the CD8+ class of T lymphocytes. A proportion of the population of CD8+ lymphocytes secretes cytokines that suppress the activity of B cells and CTLs. These so-called **suppressor T cells** are antigen-specific and therefore dampen the immune response of cells responding to the same antigen. The precise mechanism by which this suppression is exerted is the subject of controversy.

Adhesion molecules involved in the immune system

For effective immune surveillance, it is critical that competent immune cells be able to circulate freely in the blood and lymph vasculature, acting as sentinels in search of foreign organisms or tissue injury. To be successful, this patrolling of the body by immune cells must, at some point, become directed to a particular site where they perform some function. This targeting of cells to certain tissues can be explained by: (1) chemoattractant concentration gradients; and/or (2) by the differential expression of specific adhesion molecules among immune cells, between immune cells and fixed cells, and between immune cells and the substances comprising the extravascular matrix. The study of intercellular adhesion molecules involved in inflammatory and immunologic reactions is a rapidly advancing field of scientific investigation; hence, only the basic adhesion molecules involved in an immune response and how they interact to (1) direct trafficking and localization of immune cells from the vasculature to the tissues, and (2) work in concert to enhance antigen-receptor dependent T lymphocyte functions will be discussed.

Three groups of adhesion surface receptors are recognized. The **immunoglobulin superfamily** is composed of two types of proteins. The first group, i.e., CD2, CD3, CD4, CD8, LFA-3 (lymphocyte function-associated antigen), ICAM-1 (intercellular adhesion molecules), and MHC molecules, is important for the adhesion of T lymphocytes to other cells, primarily antigen-presenting cells. As discussed in Chapter 5, CD3 is complexed to the TCR, which is responsible for the antigen specificity of the T cell. It recognizes antigen as a peptide fragment associated with MHC molecules. T cells bearing CD4 (helper-inducers) only recognize antigen presented in context with MHC class II molecules, whereas cells bearing CD8 (cytotoxic cells) only recognize antigen presented in context with MHC class I proteins. MHC class I proteins recognize antigen fragments that have been synthesized by the cell, such as viral proteins, while MHC class II molecules recognize fragments that have been first phagocytized and degraded ("processed") by the cell, usually an antigen-presenting cell.

Therefore, cells bearing MHC class I antigen complexes tend to be recognized as target cells and eliminated by cytotoxic CD8+ cells, whereas those cells presenting MHC class II antigen complexes are usually recognized as antigen-presenting cells by CD4+ T cells. Both of these cell-to-cell interactions (cytotoxicity and antigen presentation) depend on the close adhesion of the effector and target cells. The necessary adhesive forces involved are supplied by the TCR-antigen-MHC trimolecular complex, with stabilizing forces supplied by other receptor-ligand interactions. These include CD4-MHC class II (in the case of antigen-presentation), CD8-MHC class I (in the case of cytotoxicity), CD2-LFA-3, and LFA-19(a β_2 integrin)-ICAM-1/2 interactions.

CD3 is closely associated with the TCR and is thought to supply a necessary signal from the TCR that initiates the activation cascade for the T cell in terms of clonal proliferation and subsequent differentiation. The second group of immunoglobulin superfamilies of adhesion proteins, ICAM-1/2 and VCAM-1 (vascular cellular adhesion molecule), are largely expressed on endothelial cells, and the differential expression of these proteins on the surface of endothelial cells can affect the adhesion of leukocytes within the vascular bed at sites of inflammation.

Integrins comprise the second major group of adhesion receptor molecules. Integrins are heterodimers composed of α and β peptide chains; there are three subfamilies of integrins, each differing from the other on the basis of their β chains. β_1 integrins are represented by the very late activation (VLA) proteins, which are expressed on a wide variety of cells. VLA proteins, as a group, recognize matrix components of tissue, such as collagen, laminin and fibronectin. Therefore, qualitative and/or quantitative changes in VLA expresson on leukocytes represent an important means of controlling changes in VLA-matrix interactions, thereby influencing the adhesiveness of leukocytes for their local environment. The end result of increasing the expresson of VLA proteins on the surfaces of leukocytes is their retention at the site of inflammation or tissue damage. β_3 integrins are functionally similar to VLA proteins in terms of their affinity for matrix components. The β_2 integrins, including LFA-1 (CD11aCD18), Mac-1, also known as complement receptor 3 (CR3; CD11b/CD18), and CR4 (CD11c/CD18), on the other hand, are only expressed on leukocytes and are involved in the adherence of leukocytes to each other, to endothelial cells via ICAM-1, or to plasma inflammatory products that have leaked from nearby vessels, such as fibrinogen and the inactivated complement byproduct, iC3b.

The third group of adhesion receptors, **selectins,** are structurally similar to lectins at their N terminus. All three members of this group help regulate lymphocyte and neutrophil adherence to endothelium at sites of inflammation. The molecule L-selectin (CD62L), formerly LAM-1, is present on the surface of all circulating leukocytes, except for a small subpopulation of memory lymphocytes. It helps lymphocytes bind to high endothelial venules present in lymphoid organs and is important in their recirculation through lymph nodes from the blood. L-selectin is shed from the surface of leukocytes once the cell is activated and begins to migrate into the extravascular space. This suggests that it is only important in the early events of neutrophil and lymphocyte adherence to endothelium. Its loss or downregulation permits leukocytes to escape the force of adhesion to endothelium and to move into the extravascular space. E-selectin (formerly ELAM-1) is only transiently expressed on the surface of endothelial cells in response to various cytokines, including interleukin-1 (IL-1), tumor necrosis factor (TNF), and lipopolysaccharide. It is synthesized *de novo* in response to such stimuli.

When considering these adhesion molecules in an immune response, it is helpful to classify them temporally during leukocyte migration from the microvasculature and by leukocyte type. As described in Chapter 5, the migration of leukocytes from blood can be divided into four stages: (1) margination; (2) adhesion; (3) emigration; and (4) chemotaxis-tissue localization. The process of margination is not cell-type specific, because margination results from vascular leakage of plasma and a subsequent increase in blood viscosity, followed by margination of the larger solid components of the blood along the endothelial surface. Therefore, this step does not involve the action of adhesion molecules. However, the other stages of leukocyte migration from the vasculature are dependent on the expression of specific adhesion molecules on leukocytes, fixed cells, and matrix proteins.

Humoral immunity

The adjective "humoral" is a holdover from the teachings of Hippocrates. In the view of this renowned Greek physician, the body contained four humors or fluids (blood, phlegm, black bile, and yellow bile), and diseases resulted from disorders of those humors (fluids). In modern medicine, **antibodies** are glycoprotein substances present in body fluids (humors), especially in the blood, which combat disease. Antibodies are formed in the body, and thus are acquired as the result of exposure to foreign substances, including inanimate chemicals as well as nonpathogenic and pathogenic microorganisms and their toxic products. Collectively, those substances that stimulate the production of antibodies are known as **antigens** or **immunogens.**

ANTIGENS

Antigens, with few exceptions, are substances that are foreign to the host. The most immunogenic antigens (those that induce the greatest antibody response) are high molecular weight proteins. Less complex polypeptides, polysaccharides, and nucleic acids may also be immunogenic, but most simple chemicals are not. However, if certain simple chemicals are coupled to a carrier protein, they can create a new antigenic site on that protein and induce antibodies to that reactive site. Antibodies induced in this way bind to the smaller molecule in the absence of the carrier protein. Chemicals with these properties are referred to as **haptens.**

Antibodies to antigens that are chemically similar may cross-react, a feature which may confer partial immunity to similar microorganisms, but which can also complicate definitive diagnosis by serologic tests. Most natural antigens have several antigenic determinants or recognition sites, each capable of stimulating an antibody against itself. Thus, for a given antigen, there is a group of antibodies (not a single antibody), each with an affinity for a specific antigenic determinant on the same molecule.

The antibody response to an antigen can be greatly enhanced if the antigen is presented in a vehicle that causes the antigen to be released to the body slowly. Such vehicles are known as **adjuvants**; these include oils, waxes, killed tubercle bacilli, alum, and aluminum hydroxide.

ANTIBODIES

Antibodies are glycoproteins that react specifically with the antigenic determinant that induced their formation. They are part of the globulins of serum, and collectively are termed **immunoglobulins.** Five classes of immunoglobulins are recognized: IgG, IgA, IgM, IgD, and IgE (Table 7-1). IgG is the most abundant immunoglobulin in serum and is the principal antibody that combats microorganisms and also mediates many of the immediate type hypersensitivity reactions. IgM, the largest immunoglobulin molecule, is the first antibody formed after antigen exposure. IgM functions in the same manner as IgG. IgA is the major immunoglobulin in external secretions. It is produced locally by plasma cells in tissues, such as the mucosa of the gastrointestinal and respiratory tracts, and serves as a first line of defense at these sites. It also is believed to be important in local immediate hypersensitivity reactions, although IgE is the principal antibody in such hypersensitivities.

IgE, which is abundant in respiratory and intestinal mucosae, binds to the surface of mast cells and basophils and, when it comes in contact with its specific antigen, causes the mast cell to release a number of chemical mediators of inflammation (histamine, eosinophil chemotactic factor, and others). This action results in vasodilation and vascular leakage, permitting circulating antibodies and leukocytes to accumulate at the site of the offending organism or antigen. However, if the antigen is some relatively innocuous environmental allergen, such as pollen, the reaction would seem to serve no useful purpose and is thus considered an allergic reaction or disease. The classic example of this is the rhinitis and nasal congestion that characterizes "hay fever." IgE is also important in providing protection against intestinal helminths. The function of IgD, other than as an antigen receptor, is not known; it is present only in trace amounts.

Antibodies also may be classified on the basis of their function or *in vitro* properties. These classifications include: (1) **antitoxins,** which chemically and quantitatively neutralize specific bacterial exotoxins (tetanus, diphtheria, botulism); (2) **agglutinins,** which cause agglutination of bacteria into large clumps, making their dissemination more difficult; (3) **precipitins,** which precipitate soluble proteins, thus limiting their dissemination and chemical activity; (4) **lysins,** which lyse cells and gram-negative bacteria by activating the complement system; and (5) **opsonins,** which coat bacteria and thereby promote their phagocytosis by neutrophils and macrophages.

The role played by antibodies in such hypersensitivity reactions as anaphylaxis, the Arthus phenomenon, and immune complex diseases are described later in the discussions of those entities. The simple binding of an antibody to a microbial agent does not usually result in its destruction but may facilitate its phagocytosis and killing by macrophages and neutrophils. To be effective in killing microbes, antibodies bound to the surface of

TABLE 7-1 **Characteristics of immunoglobulins**

Immunoglobulin	*Molecular weight*	*Approx. total % immunoglobulin in serum*	*Normal functions*
IgG	160,000	75%	Principal antiviral, antibacterial, and antitoxin
IgA	170,000	16%	Immunoglobulin of external secretions
IgM	900,000	7%	Initial antibody; functions as IgG
IgD	180,000	0.2%	Unknown
IgE	200,000	0.01%	Mediates vascular events of inflammation

microbial agents must also bind complement, a group of plasma proteins that interact with antigen-antibody complexes to form chemicals that perforate the membrane of the organism. Such antibodies are referred to as **complement-fixing antibodies.** Antibodies that destroy the agent are termed **neutralizing antibodies.**

After exposure to an antigen, there is a latent period of 4 to 6 days before antibodies to that antigen are detectable in the serum. The response peaks around 14 days after exposure and slowly declines after about 21 days. The principal component of this primary response is IgM. On second exposure, the latent period is shorter, the level of antibody is higher and is maintained longer, and the response is predominantly by IgG. This hastened and enhanced response is a function of the memory of the immune reaction and is referred to as an **anamnestic response.** It results from a rapid activation and expansion of that population of lymphocytes specific for that particular antigen.

Before being recognized by a B lymphocyte, most antigens are processed by macrophages. Much of the antigen is catabolized by the macrophages, but some antigenic peptides derived from it are presented by the antigen-presenting cells (APCs) to B lymphocytes having receptors on their cell membrane specific for the peptide. These B-cell receptors are IgM molecules identical to those subsequently secreted by the more differentiated B cells. On antigenic stimulation, B lymphocytes become larger and are termed immunoblasts. They undergo proliferation and differentiation into antibody-forming plasma cells and, presumably, long-lived lymphocytes, which serve as memory cells. Although B lymphocytes can produce antibody in the absence of T cells, in most instances there is participation by a particular class of T cells, known as **helper T cells.**

T lymphocytes have molecules on their surfaces, known as T-cell receptors (TCRs), that enable each cell of this type to recognize and bind to a specific MHC-peptide combination. The CD4+ helper T cells, when activated by this binding process, undergo an autocrine type of clonal proliferation and secrete cytokines, which mobilize other elements of the immune system, including macrophages, B lymphocytes, and cytotoxic T lymphocytes (CTLs). One group of cells that responds to cytokines elaborated by the T_{H2} subset of helper T cells are B lymphocytes that have immunoglobulin receptor molecules of a single antigenic specificity on their surface. Unlike the receptors on T lymphocytes, the B-cell receptors can recognize pieces of antigens free in solution without these antigens being presented in association with MHC molecules. Antigens can be of two basic types; proteins, which are referred to as thymus-dependent antigens, and carbohydrates and lipids, which are thymus-independent antigens. When activated by their specific antigen, B lymphocytes proliferate and differentiate into plasma cells that synthesize and secrete immunoglobulins specific for that particular antigen. By binding to antigens, the secreted immunoglobulins can neutralize them or initiate their destruction by complement enzymes or by circulating phagocytic cells (neutrophils, macrophages). During this process, some of

the T and B lymphocytes become memory cells that persist in the circulation for life, and thus enhance the immune system's readiness to eliminate the same antigen on subsequent exposures. Because the genes for immunoglobulins present in B cells mutate frequently, the antibody response actually becomes increasingly more effective with repeated immunizations or exposures.

In the spleen and lymph nodes, B lymphocytes, which are of bone marrow origin (in birds, bursa of Fabricius origin), are predominantly located in lymphocytic follicles around germinal centers. They account for about 15% of circulating lymphocytes. In contrast, T lymphocytes in lymph nodes and spleen are located in interfollicular or paracortical areas. They account for about 85% of circulating lymphocytes. B lymphocytes have immunoglobulin molecules on their cell membranes, a feature that distinguishes them from T cells. When antigen is presented to B cells, it binds to the immunoglobulin receptors, which coalesce to form a single polar cap that is taken in by the cell. There follows a period of 6 to 8 hours, when the cell does not have surface receptors.

Morphologically, stimulation of the humoral immune system is characterized by development of germinal centers in lymph nodes and spleen and the appearance of large numbers of plasma cells. Plasma cells also appear locally in mucosae, probably reflecting local IgA and possibly other immunoglobulin synthesis.

To explain recognition of self and nonself, Burnet (1972) advanced the **selective (or clonal) theory** of antibody production. This theory proposes that clones of cells exist that have the inherent capacity to produce antibody on stimulation by the proper antigen and that this clone is stimulated to reproduce more cells with the same capacity. The theory suggests that, for every possible antigen (including self), a cell or clone of cells exists that has the genetically endowed ability to produce a specific antibody to that specific antigen and that the antigen must find (select) the proper cell or cells with which to interact. To explain self-recognition and immunologic tolerance before birth, it is theorized that self-antigens of the host interact with self-reactive cells before birth, and before these cells have the ability to proliferate, they are eliminated from the host.

Cell-mediated (cellular) immunity

The **cell-mediated immune response** does not involve circulating antibodies and cannot be passively transferred with serum. It is, however, a form of acquired immunity and, like humoral immunity, it requires a stimulus, is highly specific, and has a memory. Cell-mediated immunity accounts for the resistance and reaction associated with tuberculosis and the efficacy of the tuberculin reaction. Probably most organisms causing granulomatous diseases (Chapter 12) elicit a cell-mediated immune response, including some of the simple bacteria (e.g., *Listeria* species, *Brucella* species), higher bacteria (e.g., *Mycobacterium* species), protozoa, and metazoan parasites. Cell-mediated immunity is also the major mechanism of graft rejection and the destruction (or attempted destruction) of neoplasms. The lesions associated with certain viral diseases also result from cell-mediated immunity. An example is lymphocytic choriomeningitis virus, which leads to the appearance of new (and foreign) membrane antigens on affected cells. In this disease, the lymphocytic reaction can be prevented by suppressing the cellular immune response. In many other viral infections, the cytolytic T-cell response to new membrane antigens is of key importance in eliminating virus-infected cells from the body. The delayed hypersensitivity diseases are also mediated through cell-mediated immune mechanisms.

The cell-mediated immune response results from the interaction of thymus-derived lymphocytes (T lymphocytes) and antigen-presenting cells (APCs), such as macrophages. The latent period requires several days to 2 weeks to reach its peak. On second exposure, rather than an immediate response, the reaction begins slowly, peaking at 24 to 72 hours. The fact that cells must be brought to the antigen (rather than circulating antibodies) explains this delayed reaction. Antigen is first processed by APCs and presented to T cells by macrophages, similar to what occurs in the humoral immune system. Sensitized T cells in turn release chemicals referred to as **chemokines,** which call forth additional macrophages that accumulate at the reaction site. Macrophages are the principal effector cells in the cell-mediated immune response.

Microscopically, the delayed reaction is characterized by proliferation of large lymphocytes in the paracortical regions of lymph nodes. Some of these sensitized T cells enter the circulation and make contact with the stimulating antigen on first or second exposure. It is believed that contact occurs by chance, rather than by a specific chemotactic event. On recognition of the specific antigen(s), the T lymphocytes release chemokines, which attract monocytes (macrophages) from the bloodstream. The sensitized lymphocytes may participate directly in destroying the antigen, especially in lysis of cells, but the macrophages attracted to the site also elaborate cytotoxic substances as well as possess enhanced phagocytic ability. The macrophages, however, require activation by cytokines, such as interferon-γ, released from the activated T cells. This is a specific reaction, but once activated, the macrophages are nonspecifically cytotoxic. If sensitized or activated T cells lyse cells directly, they are called **cytotoxic or cytolytic T cells (CTLs).** These play a role in eliminating cells bearing new membrane antigens, as occurs in viral diseases and on some tumor cells. The killing by CTLs requires intimate contact between the effector cell and its target and is restricted to those cells in which the foreign antigen is presented in association with a self MHC class I molecule. The subsequent killing of the target cell by a CTL is accomplished through one of two mechanisms: (1) release of cytoplasmic granules containing a protein known as **perforin,** which causes pores to form in cell membranes, resulting in osmotic lysis of cells; and (2) signalling transcription of the target cell's own

apoptosis genes. Certain cytokines released from activated T cells also cause degranulation of mast cells and basophils, initiating the classic inflammatory reaction.

In certain granulomatous reactions, but especially in tuberculosis, activated macrophages differentiate into epithelioid cells, large polygonal cells with eosinophilic cytoplasm. These cells have ruffled cell membranes that interdigitate, causing them to resemble epithelial cells. Fusion of macrophages results in the formation of multinucleated giant cells, which are conspicuous in many granulomatous diseases, but are not a feature of the cellular immune responses to tissue grafts and delayed hypersensitivity reactions. If elicited by the injection of tuberculin, this mononuclear cellular response is primarily perivenular, but in granulomatous diseases this is not the case.

Neutrophils may be present in small numbers but are not an essential component of delayed immunity. Complement also is not involved.

Humoral and cellular immunity work in concert. Although some reactions are purely humoral (lysis of foreign erythrocytes) and others are apparently purely cellular (tuberculin reaction), both often operate simultaneously.

In summary, cellular immunity mediated through T lymphocytes: (1) regulates B cells as helper T cells or suppressor T cells; (2) provides resistance to certain bacteria, viruses, and other organisms; (3) is involved in transplantation and tumor immunity; and (4) is responsible for delayed hypersensitivity reactions.

Lysis of cells can be mediated through either antibody and complement or cytolytic T cells. The third major class of lymphocytes does not express surface markers for T or B cells and were once termed **null cells.** This class of lymphocytes contains prominent cytoplasmic granules, and the cells are now known as **large granular lymphocytes** or **natural killer (NK) cells.** These cells are capable of destroying some, but not all, tumor cells and some, but not all, virus-infected cells. They lack a specific T-cell receptor, and their killing ability is not specific for a particular viral antigenic determinant nor are they MHC-restricted. As such, they are part of the natural, rather than the acquired, immune system. NK cells express the CD2 molecule on their surfaces and a low-affinity receptor for Fc component of IgG, known as CD16. They bind to cells coated with IgG, resulting in their lysis, a reaction termed **antibody-dependent cell cytotoxicity.** NK cells are the principal cellular mediator of this form of killing.

The humoral and cellular immune systems and their interaction are depicted schematically in Figure 7-2.

References

Abbas AK, Lichtman AH, Pober JS. Cellular and molecular immunology. 2nd ed. Philadelphia: WB Saunders 1994.

Ahmed R, Gray D. Immunological memory and protective immunity: understanding their relation. Science 1996;272:54–59.

Burnet FM. A reassessment of the forbidden clone hypothesis of autoimmune disease. Aust J Exp Biol Med Sci 1972;50:1–9.

Butcher EC, Picker LJ. Lymphocyte homing and homeostasis. Science 1996;272:60–66.

Dvorak AM, Mihm MC Jr, Dvorak HF. Morphology of delayed-type hypersensitivity reactions in humans. II. Ultrastructural alterations affecting the microvasculature and the tissue mast cells. Lab Invest 1976;34:179–191.

Fearon DT, Locksley RM. The instructive role of innate immunity in the acquired immune response. Science 1996;272:50–53.

Nossal GJV. Life, death and the immune system. Sci Am 1993;269: 53–62.

Janeway CA Jr. How the immune system recognizes invaders. Sci Am 1993;269:73–79.

Marrack P, Kappler JW. How the immune system recognizes the body. Sci Am 1993;269:81–89.

Springer TA. Traffic signals for lymphocyte recirculation and leukocyte emigration: the multistep paradigm. Cell 1994;76:301–314.

Paul WE: Infectious diseases and the immune system. Sci Am **269**:91–97, 1993.

Weissman IL, Cooper MD: How the immune system develops. Sci Am **269**:65–71, 1993.

IMMUNE REACTIONS AND HYPERSENSITIVITY

In recent years, much attention has been directed to diseases resulting from reactions on the part of the immune system, which are grouped under the term hypersensitivity diseases, allergic diseases, or broadly under immunopathology (Table 7-2). However, the specific hypersensitivity diseases are not the usual outcome of immune reactions. The immune system affords each individual higher animal protection from invasion by other organisms, thus preserving both individuality and the species. Deficiencies in the immune system, such as hypogammaglobulinemia and thymic aplasia, which are on the opposite end of the spectrum from hypersensitivity, clearly emphasize the importance of the immune system for survival. The immune system, however, is not perfect. It appears still to be in the process of evolving, as complete immunity to infectious disease is rarely achieved. Aside from natural or innate immunity, a significant time lag is required to produce protective levels of antibodies or to generate cellular immune responses, such that these systems do not afford the individual protection from highly virulent organisms, e.g., the anthrax bacillus in cattle. Various hypersensitivity disorders also illustrate the imperfections of the system. Although most of the experimentally induced hypersensitivity diseases have naturally occurring counterparts, these are not common, and some may even be iatrogenic in origin. For example, the injection of large quantities of horse serum containing antibodies to the diptheria toxin into humans, as done during the early part of this century for the treatment of diptheria, leads to an immune-complex disorder known as serum sickness. Glomerulonephritis, resulting from the deposition of antigen-antibody complexes, occurs commonly in certain infectious diseases with no obvious benefit to the host. A number of autoimmune diseases that result

---

TABLE 7-2 **Hypersensitivity diseases**

Classification	*Principal immunoglobulin*	*Manifestations*	*Mechanism of damage*
Immediate Type			
I a. Generalized anaphylaxis	IgE	Anaphylaxis	Mediators from reagin-sensitized cells
b. Acute allergic reactions (localized anaphylaxis)	IgE	Urticaria, hives, asthma, GI allergy	Mediators from reagin-sensitized cells
II Cytotoxic hypersensitivity (cytotoxic anaphylaxis)	IgG, IgM, and Complement	Transfusion reactions, hemolytic anemia, thrombocytopenia	Complement
III Arthus reaction or immune-complex disease	IgG, IgM and Complement	Serum sickness, glomerulonephritis, vasculitis	Complement and polymorphonuclear leukocytes
Delayed Type			
IV Delayed hypersensitivity	None Sensitized T lymphocytes	Contact dermatitis (drugs, poison ivy), tuberculosis, tuberculin reaction, graft rejection	Lymphokines from antigen-sensitized lymphocytes

from the immune system attacking the tissues of its host are well documented in animals and humans, again with no known advantage to the host.

IMMUNODEFICIENCIES

A number of genetic and congenitally acquired defects in innate and acquired immune systems render affected individuals more susceptible to infectious agents and, in some cases, neoplasms. Those involving the innate immune system affect neutrophil and macrophage numbers and function, the complement system, and NK cells, while those affecting the acquired immune system impair the host's ability to make antibodies or develop a cell-mediated immune response. These have been described in humans and a number of animal species. Most often these disorders are first recognized by the increased susceptibility of the affected individual to infection. Those associated with neutrophil and B-cell or humoral defects generally result in increased susceptibility to bacterial infections; those with T-cell defects, in increased susceptibility to certain opportunistic organisms or agents that often exist as latent infections in immunocompetent hosts. In some of these immunodeficient states, both humoral and cellular immunity are compromised. In several, there is also an increased incidence of certain neoplastic diseases, especially lymphomas, suggesting the importance of immune surveillance in eliminating transformed cells. Immunodeficiencies are divided into primary and secondary disorders.

Primary immunodeficiency disorders

NEUTROPHIL DISORDERS

Canine cyclic neutropenia is a genetic disorder of grey collies in which there is a defect in bone marrow stem-cell maturation, leading to cyclic neutropenia every 8 to 12 days. The neutropenia lasts for 2 to 4 days, during which affected animals are predisposed to bacterial infections of the respiratory and gastrointestinal tracts. In addition to decreased numbers, the neutrophils of affected dogs also have a myeloperoxidase deficiency and a defect in iodination, both of which impair the microbicidal function of these cells. Affected dogs, as a rule, do not survive beyond 3 years of age.

Pelger-Huët anomaly, an autosomal recessive disorder, is characterized by hyposegmentation of the nuclei of neutrophils and other granulocytes. It has been described in humans, rabbits, dogs, and domestic shorthair cats. The nuclei of granulocytes of individuals with Pelger-Huët anomaly remain round, ovoid, or bean-shaped and resemble normal band neutrophils. Most of the canine and feline cases have been in clinically healthy individuals who are heterozygous for the trait. These individuals usually present with a blood picture that suggests a persistent left shift in the absence of a bacterial infection. In most cases, it is an incidental finding in animals that are ill from other causes. Recent studies suggest that heterozygous forms of the anomaly in dogs and cats are benign and do not predispose affected individuals to infection. The homozygous form

of the anomaly has been described in a single stillborn kitten that also had chondrodysplasia. In people and rabbits, the homozygous form is lethal.

References

Latimer KS, Kircher IM, Lindl PA et al. Leukocyte function in Pelger-Huët anomaly of dogs. J Leukocyte Biol 1989;45:301–310.
Latimer KS, Rakich PM, Thompson DF. Pelger-Huët anomaly in cats. Vet Pathol 1985;22:370–374.
Latimer KS, Rowland GN, Mahaffey MB. Homozygous Pelger-Huët anomaly and chondrodysplasia in a stillborn kitten. Vet Pathol 1988;25:325–328.
Nachtsheim H. The Pelger-anomaly in man and rabbits. J Hered 1950;41:131–137.

Chediak-Higashi disease (CHD) syndrome is an autosomal recessive disorder characterized by partial albinism or hair color dilution, increased susceptibility to bacterial infections, and a tendency to hemorrhage. It is a rare disorder in humans, cattle (Brangus, Hereford, and Japanese Black), Persian cats, and killer whales but affects all mink of the Aleutian strain and all beige mice, i.e., all mice homozygous for the bg (beige) gene. The disorder is characterized by the presence of large granules in the cytoplasm of a variety of different cell types. Cells affected include neutrophils and macrophages that contain abnormally large lysosomes and melanocytes that contain large melanosomes, which result in the dilution of haircoat color and light-colored irises, nerve cells, and platelets. These abnormally large cytoplasmic granules result from an increased membrane fluidity and a tendency of membrane-bound vesicles of many different types to fuse. This abnormality is also thought to cause defects in cell motility and microtubule function, which affect neutrophil, macrophage, and NK cell function. Cats heterozygous for the trait also manifest some impairment of neutrophil migration when compared with normal controls.

References

Colgan SP, Blancquaert A-MB, Thrall MA, et al. Defective in vitro mobility of polymorphonuclear leukocytes of homozygote and heterozygote Chediak-Higashi cats. Vet Immunol Immunopathol 1992;31:205–227.
Klein M, Roder J, Haliotis T, et al. Chediak-Higashi gene in humans. II. The selectivity of the defect in natural killer and antibody-dependent cell mediated cytotoxicity function. J Exp Med 1980;151:1049–1058.
Padgett GA, Holland JM, Prieur DJ, et al. The Chediak-Higashi Syndrome: a review of the disease in man, mink, cattle and mice. In: Animal models for biomedical research III. Washington, DC: National Academy of Sciences 1970;1–12.
Roder JC. The beige mutation in the mouse. I. A stem cell predetermined impairment in natural killer cell function. J Immunol 1979;123:2168–2173.

ADHESION MOLECULE DEFICIENCIES

Leukocyte adhesion deficiency syndromes (LAD-1, LAD-2) are rare autosomal recessive disorders characterized by recurrent bacterial and fungal infections, often beginnning at an early age. LAD-1 is characterized by a deficiency or mutation of the ß chain of the $ß_2$ integrin molecules, LFA-1, Mac-1 (CR3), and CR4. These molecules are normally present on the surface of neutrophils, monocytes, and lymphocytes and are responsible for the adhesion of these cells to each other, to endothelial cells via ICAM-1, or to plasma inflammatory products that have leaked from nearby vessels, such as fibrinogen and the opsonizing complement byproduct, iC3b. LAD-1 syndromes have been described in humans, Holstein cattle, and Irish setter dogs. In the latter two species, the syndrome was originally referred to as bovine and canine granulocytopathy syndromes, respectvely. The β_2 integrins are critically important for the adhesion of leukocytes to the endothelial-cell ligand ICAM-1, an essential step for the emigration of these cells from venules. Affected individuals often have pronounced neutrophilic leukocytosis, but these circulating neutrophils cannot extravasate at sites of infection. In addition to impaired neutrophil emigration, macrophage and cytotoxic T-cell emigration may also be impaired.

References

Kehrli ME Jr, Ackermann MR, Shuster DE, et al. Animal model of human disease: Bovine leukocyte adhesion deficiency: β_2 integrin deficiency in young Holstein cattle. Am J Pathol 1992;140:1489–1492.

Kehril ME, Schmalstieg FC, Anderson DC, et al. Molecular definition of the bovine granulocytopathy syndrome: identification of deficiency of the Mac-1 (CD11b/CD18) glycoprotein. Am J Vet Res 1990;51:1826–1836.

COMPLEMENT DEFICIENCIES

Complement deficiencies have been recognized in humans, dogs, guinea pigs, mice, and rabbits. C3 and C5 deficiency in humans has been linked with recurrent infections, as has C3 deficiency in dogs, but not in all patients. Affected individuals are unable to opsonize and destroy bacterial organisms. Deficiency of C4 in guinea pigs, C5 in mice, and C6 in rabbits has not been associated with increased incidence of infections. Apparently, normal levels of C3 are sufficiently protective.

B-LYMPHOCYTE DEFICIENCIES

Agammaglobulinemia and **hypogammaglobulinemia** may result from defective synthesis, increased catabolism, or **excessive loss of immunoglobulins.** In humans, defective synthesis occurs in several disorders, many of which are transmitted genetically. In some, such as the human disease **X-linked agammaglobulinemia (Bruton disease)** and its equine counterpart **equine agammaglobulinemia,** B cells are lacking in tissues and in the circulation and the disorder manifests itself early in life. There is no detectable IgM, IgA, IgD, or IgE in serum, and IgG levels are less than 10% of normal. Affected individuals have normal numbers of T lymphocytes. The transplacental transfer of maternal IgG affords some protection for affected infant boys and foals during the first few months of life. In contrast, a condition known as **common, variable, unclassified immunodeficiency** ("acquired" hypogammaglobulinemia) may occur at any age and be characterized by either a total lack of B cells or normal or increased numbers of B cells. The B cells, however, fail to differentiate into immunoglobulin-secreting cells. Both sexes are affected in this disorder.

Other conditions exist in which there is a selective deficiency in a single class of immunoglobulins. **Selective IgA deficiencies** have been described in the German shepherd, beagle, and shar-pei breeds of dogs. **Selective IgM deficiencies** have been reported in Arabian and Quarter House breeds of horses and in Doberman Pinscher dogs, and a **selective IgG2 deficiency** has been documented in Red Danish cattle. With all of these immunoglobulin deficiencies, affected individuals are predisposed to infections, particularly bacterial infections.

Transient hypogammaglobulinemia of infancy is a rare condition in which there is an apparent delay in B-cell maturation, and passively acquired maternal IgG levels decline before immunoglobulin synthesis by the infant. It has also been described in Samoyed puppies, lambs, and Arabian foals that have an increased susceptibility to bacterial infections of various types. This disease is self-limiting, since affected individuals generally have normal levels of immunoglobulin by 6 months of age.

Hypercatabolism of immunoglobulins that leads to deficiency has been described in several forms in humans but not in other animals. These include familial idiopathic hypercatabolic hypoproteinemia, Wiskott-Aldrich syndrome, and myotonic dystrophy.

Excessive loss of immunoglobulins (and other serum proteins) can occur in certain forms of renal and gastrointestinal disease. Both glomerular and tubular damage can lead to losses, but intact immunoglobulin loss is greatest with glomerular disease. Gastrointestinal loss of immunoglobulins in humans and animals is linked to diseases that affect lymphatic drainage, such as intestinal lymphangiectasia (protein-losing enteropathy).

T-LYMPHOCYTE DEFICIENCIES

Deficiencies of T cells generally result in more serious susceptibility to infection than defects involving B cells, owing to the essential contributions of T cells to normal B-cell function.

Severe combined immunodeficiency (SCID) is an inherited disorder characterized by abnormal development of B and T lymphocytes from stem cells in the bone marrow. In humans, SCID occurs as an autosomal recessive and an X-linked recessive disorder. The autosomal recessive disorders result from a deficiency of either adenosine deaminase (ADA) or purine nucleoside phophorylase (PNP); deficiency of either leads to an accumalation of catabolites that are toxic to B and T lymphocytes. Another autosomal recessive form of SCID in humans, termed **bare lymphocyte syndrome,** results from deficient expression of MHC class II molecules. This deficiency causes lack of antigen presentation to CD4+ T lymphocytes, impaired delayed type hypersensitivity responses, and deficient antibody responses to thymus-dependent protein antigens. Affected patients are highly susceptible to infections, particularly viral infections, and may die before 2 years of age. The X-linked form of SCID in humans results from mutations in the gene that encodes for the γ chain of the interleukin-2 receptor (IL-2rγ), a chain critical for binding of IL-2, IL-4, IL-7, IL-9, and IL-15. This results in a deficiency of B and T lymphocytes, because IL-7 and perhaps other interleukins serve as a critical growth factor for B and T lymphocyte progenitor cells. The involvement of this critical molecule in multiple cytokine receptors explains the extreme severity of this X-linked form of SCID.

In **horses,** a SCID syndrome identical to the autosomal recessive form of the human disease has been described in the Arabian and Appaloosa breeds only. As in humans, there are no T or B cells; affected foals cannot synthesize immunoglobulins and lack cell-mediated immunity. They may be normal for the first few months of life, but as circulating maternal IgG acquired through colostrum diminishes, the foal become increasingly more susceptible to infections. The disease is characterized by lack of immunoglobulins, lymphopenia, and death before 5 months of age. The most common lethal opportunistic infections in these foals are pneumonias caused by viral (adenovirus), bacterial *(Rhodococcus equi),* fungal *(Pneumocystis carinii),* or protozoal *(Cryptosporidium)* organisms. The important pathologic features focus on lymphoid organs. The thymus is aplastic or extremely hypoplastic, with only the epithelial components present. Lymph nodes contain few lymphocytes and totally lack follicles or germinal centers; there are no plasma cells. The spleen has a similar appearance. The disease is inherited as an autosomal recessive trait that causes defective B and T lymphocyte stem-cell maturation.

A similar disease occurs in so-called **scid** mice, which lack both B and T lymphocytes as a result of a block in the maturation of bone marrow precursor cells. Affected mice are homozygous for the mutant autosomal recessive gene, *scid,* located on chromosome 16. This deficiency of B and T lymphocytes is caused by an abnormality in the DNA repair mechanisms essential for rearrangements of the T-cell receptor and immunoglobulin genes. The cells lack antigen receptors and consequently are eliminated during embryonic development. These mice have few or no antibodies in their serum, and lymph nodes and spleen are devoid of lymphocytes. The thymuses are extremely small and consist primarily of medullary tissue. Macrophage activation and function are not impaired, nor is NK-cell function. Affected mice are very susceptible to microbial infections, especially *Pneumocystis carinii* pneumonia, and must be maintained in a pathogen-free environment. Affected mice also have a high incidence of thymic lymphomas, emphasizing once again the importance of an immunocompetent immune system in preventing lymphoid malignancies.

A canine X-linked form of SCID similar to that in humans has been described in Basset Hound puppies and Bassett Hound crosses. Affected male pups develop infections of the skin, oral cavity, and ears during the first few weeks of life. Shortly after birth, affected pups have few if any circulating T cells and increased numbers of circulating B cells, similar to young boys with the comparable disease. Unlike the human disorder, however, at 5 to 7 weeks of age T cells begin to appear in the circulation of approximately one half of the affected dogs, but the absolute number of T cells never reaches that of normal dogs. Affected pups have depressed T-lymphocyte function and low levels of circulating IgA and IgG; circulating levels of IgM are reported to be variable. As in humans, affected pups have mutations in the gene for the common γ chains of IL2r, IL-4r, IL-7r, IL-9r, and IL-15r.

References

Felsburg PJ, Somberg RL, Perryman LE. Domestic animal models of severe combined immunodeficiency: canine X-linked severe combined immundeficiency and severe combined immunodeficiency in horses. Immunodefic Rev 1992;3:277–303.

Jezyk PF, Felsburg PJ, Haskins ME, et al. X-linked severe combined immundeficiency in the dog. Clin Immunol Immunopathol 1989;52:173–179.

McGuire TC, Banks KL, Davis WC. Alterations of the thymus and other lymphoid tissues in young horses with combined immunodeficiency. Am J Pathol 1976;84:39–54.

McGuire TC, Banks KL, Evans DR, et al. Agammaglobulinemia in a horse with evidence of functional T lymphocytes. Am J Vet Res 1976;37:41–46.

McGuire TC, Banks KL, Poppie MJ. Animal model of human disease: Combined immunodeficiency (severe), Swiss-type agammaglobulinemia: combined immunodeficiency in horses. Am J Pathol 1975;80:551–554.

McGuire TC, Poppie MJ. Primary hypogammaglobulinemia and thymic hypoplasia in horses. Fed Proc 1973;32:821.

McGuire TC, Poppie MJ, Banks KL. Combined (B and T lymphocyte) immunodeficiency: a fatal genetic disease in Arabian foals. J Vet Med Assoc 1974;164:70–76.

McGuire TC, Poppie MJ, Banks KL. Hypogammaglobulinemia predisposing to infection in foals. J Am Vet Med Assoc 1975;166:71–75.

Muscoplat CC, Johnson DW, Pomeroy KA, et al. Lymphocyte subpopulations and immunodeficiency in calves with acute lymphocytic leukemia. Am J Vet Res 1974;35:1571–1574.

Perryman LE, Boreson CR, Conaway MW, et al. Combined immunodeficiency in an Appaloosa foal. Vet Pathol 1984;21:547–548.

Poppie MJ, McGuire TC. Combined immunodeficiency in foals of Arabian breeding: evaluation of mode of inheritance and estimation of prevalence of affected foals and carrier mares and stallions. J Am Vet Med Assoc 1977;170:31–33.

Somberg RL, Tipold A, Hartnett BJ, et al. Postnatal development of T cells in dogs with X-linked severe combined immunodeficiency. J Immunol 1996;156:1431–1435.

Snyder PW, Kazacos EA, Felsburg PJ. Histologic characterization of the thymus in canine X-linked severe combined immunodeficiency. Clin Immunol Immunopathol 1993;67:55–67.

Congenital thymic aplasia or **DiGeorge syndrome** results from a failure of normal embryogenesis of the thymus and parathyroid glands, which are derived from the third and fourth pharyngeal clefts. In humans, the disease is often associated with anomalies of the heart and major blood vessels and mental retardation. The thymus may be entirely aplastic or hypoplastic. In many children, T-cell function improves with age, but if the cell-mediated immune response is severely impaired, death results from recurrent infections.

The **nude athymic mouse and rat** are counterparts to congenital thymic aplasia of humans. The hairlessness that characterizes homozygous animals is inherited as an autosomal recessive trait, which has nothing to do with thymic aplasia except that the latter is linked to this genetic trait. There are no T cells, but B cells with surface immunoglobulin receptors are present. Unless precautions are taken, the mice die within a few months of birth. Neonatally thymectomized mice are not as severely impaired, apparently as a result of migration of some T cells from the thymus before birth. Severe **thymic hypoplasia,** referred to as **A-46 lethal trait,** has also been described in calves of the Black-pied Danish and Holstein breeds. Affected calves develop severe cutaneous exanthema, parakeratosis, and alopecia that begins on the face between 4 to 8 weeks of age. The cutaneous lesions become secondarily infected by bacterial organisms and death usually occurs by 4 months of age. These animals have a marked reduction in T lymphocytes and impaired cell-mediated immune responses. Interestingly, the condition appears to result from a genetic inability to absorb zinc, as zinc therapy results in recovery of the skin lesions and restores T cells to lymphoid tissues. A condition, termed **lethal acrodermatitis in bull terriers,** has a number of clinical and pathologic similarities to the A-46 lethal trait of cattle, except that affected pups do not respond to zinc therapy.

Two strains of **dwarf mice** have a T-cell defect resulting from autosomal recessive traits; these include the **Snell-Bagg mouse** with the mutant gene *dw* (dwarf) and the **Ames mouse** with the mutant gene *df* (Ames dwarf). After weaning, individuals homozygous for these traits experience: (1) growth retardation caused by lack of growth hormone and prolactin-producing cells in the pituitary, (2) progressive thymic atrophy, (3) loss of T-cell function, and (4) predisposition to infections.

References

Brummerstedt E, Andresen E, Basse A, et al. Lethal trait A46 in cattle. Nord Vet Med 1974;26:279.
Pelletier M, Montplaisir S. The nude mouse: a model of deficient T cell function. Methods Achiev Exp Pathol 1975;7:149–166.

Other T-Cell deficiency states occur in humans that have not been described in animals. In immunodeficiency with ataxia telangiectasia, B-cell and T-cell function is defective, with the latter usually being more severe. Patients with this disorder have increased susceptibility to infection, experience multiple autoimmune disorders, have a high incidence of neoplasia later in life, and are extremely susceptible to ionizing radiation, probably as a result of a defect in DNA repair mechanisms. **Wiskott-Aldrich syndrome** is an X-linked recessive disorder with variable degrees of T-cell and B-cell dysfunction. Patients with this disorder experience eczematous lesions of the skin, thrombocytopenia, and increased susceptibility to bacterial infections, especially encapsulated pyogenic organisms. There is a defect in the ability to respond to thymus-independent antigens, such as polysaccharide antigens found in bacterial cell walls.

Secondary immunodeficiency disorders

FAILURE OF PASSIVE TRANSFER OF MATERNAL IMMUNOGLOBULINS

One of the most common acquired forms of immunodeficiency in veterinary medicine is failure of a neonatal animal to acquire maternal antibodies through the ingestion of colostrum. This is a particular problem in foals, calves, lambs, kids, and piglets.

VIRUS-INDUCED IMMUNOSUPPRESSION

A large number of viral infections of humans and animals have been implicated in cases of transient immunosuppression and even permanent immunodeficiency. Many of these viral agents exert their effects by directly infecting cells of the immune system, especially lymphocytes and macrophages. Depending on the nature of the virus, the infection may be subclinical or latent, such as occurs with certain leukemia viruses. Immunosuppression may also accompany such diseases as canine distemper, hog cholera, bovine virus diarrhea, feline immunodeficiency virus, and others. These are discussed in Chapter 8.

Immunosuppression may also result from certain nutrient deficiencies and exposure to toxic inorganic and organic chemicals (Chapter 16, zinc).

References

Perryman LE, Hoover EA, Yohn DS. Immunologic reactivity in the cat: immunosuppression in experimental feline leukemia. J Natl Cancer Inst 1972;49:1357–1365.
Stevens DR, Osburn BI. Immune deficiency in a dog with distemper. J Am Vet Med Assoc 1976;168:493–498.

HYPERSENSITIVITY REACTIONS AND DISEASES

Hypersensitivity represents an accelerated or accentuated immune response to a degree that is often detrimental rather than beneficial. This is especially true when violent reactions, which may be fatal, develop in response to exposure to ordinarily innocuous substances. The terms allergic (**allergy**) and atopic (**atopy**) are synonyms use to describe this type of reaction.

Hypersensitivity reactions are classically divided into **immediate** and **delayed types.** The immediate reactions include anaphylaxis (systemic anaphylaxis), acute allergic reactions (local anaphylaxis), cytotoxic hypersensitivity (cytotoxic anaphylaxis), and immune-complex disease, which includes the Arthus reaction and serum sickness. Delayed reactions are classically represented by the positive tuberculin reaction, organ transplant rejection, and contact dermatitis. Autoimmunity, a special form of hypersensitivity, is discussed separately.

Immediate hypersensitivities

ANAPHYLAXIS

Anaphylaxis can be experimentally induced by injecting an animal intravenously with a sensitizing dose of a protein, such as albumin or serum from another species. After a latent period of approximately 10 to 14 days, a second injection of the same protein is given by the same route. The dose and nature of the protein are such that they would be harmless to a normal animal, as in the case of the first injection, but in an animal that has already been sensitized in this way, a violent and usually fatal reaction ensues often within minutes.

This reaction is referred to as **acute (systemic) anaphylaxis.**

Signs of anaphylaxis vary between species, owing to differences in the target organ and relative sensitivities to chemical mediators of the reaction. The fundamental reaction is constriction of smooth muscle. In the guinea pig, contraction of the smooth muscle of bronchioles is the outstanding effect, with dyspnea and partial or complete suffocation. In the dog, contraction of venous passages, especially the hepatic veins, is the principal manifestation, with severe congestion of the liver and other visceral organs, leading to hypotension or shock. Horses, cats, and mice respond in a manner similar to guinea pigs. Cutaneous edema and dyspnea have been reported in cattle. In rats, the findings are increased vascular permeability and hemorrhage in the small intestine. In rabbits, constriction of pulmonary arteries and dilation of the right side of the heart occur. In contrast to other species, in rabbits, antigen-antibody complexes precipitate in pulmonary capillaries accompanied by platelet and leukocyte clumping, which cause pulmonary hypertension and death.

Pathologic findings are not dramatic in any species. Pulmonary edema, congestion, and emphysema are characteristic of bronchiolar constriction. Visceral congestion and hemorrhage are seen in the rat and dog. The absence or reduction in the number of mast cells (indicative of degranulation or disruption) is a usual feature but often difficult to assess.

Anaphylaxis and other immediate (not delayed) hypersensitivities depend on circulating serum antibodies, which can be transferred to another individual. The combination of antibody with specific antigen results in the release of various chemical mediators of the reaction. Two types of interaction may lead to the release of mediators: (1) **cytotropic anaphylaxis** and (2) **aggregate anaphylaxis.** A third reaction, which may lead to an anaphylactic-type response, is considered separately under cytotoxic hypersensitivity.

Cytotropic anaphylaxis is the usual mechanism of anaphylaxis. In this type, the antibodies (cytotropic antibodies) become fixed to receptors on specific target cells, which include mast cells and basophils. IgE antibodies are the most important class of immunoglobulins involved in this form of hypersensitivity. The combination of antigen with antibody fixed on the surface of mast cells and basophils rapidly triggers the release of preformed biogenic (vasoactive) and newly synthesized chemical mediators of inflammation from the target cells. Complement is not essential for this reaction. If cytotropic antibodies are passively transferred from a sensitized to a nonsensitized individual, a day or two is required before the antibodies become fixed to the target cells, and anaphylaxis can be induced in the nonsensitized individual by antigen exposure.

In aggregate anaphylaxis, antigen and antibody combine in the serum, and this immune complex reacts with complement to release the polypeptides cleaved from C3 and C5 (C3a and C5a), once called anaphylatoxin. C3a and C5a cause the release of mediators of inflammation from target cells, chiefly histamine from mast cells. Because fixation of antibodies to effector cells is not required in this type of anaphylaxis, it can be induced immediately after passive transfer of antibodies. Aggregate anaphylaxis is not a common form of anaphylaxis and requires large amounts of circulating antibody.

The mediators released from target cells, ultimately to cause constriction of smooth muscle, have been the subject of considerable investigation. The more important mediators include the vasoactive amines, histamine and serotonin, which are present in the granules of mast cells and basophils, and various lipid mediators of inflammation synthesized *de novo* in mast cells and basophils after antigen binding. These lipid mediators include three classes of compounds derived from enzymatic degradation of arachidonic acid from membrane phospholipids of mast cells. These are: prostaglandin D_2, resulting from the action of cyclooxygenase; three leukotrienes (LTC_4, LTD_4 and LTE_4), resulting from the action of 5–lipoxygenase and other enzymes; and platelet-activating factor (PAF), resulting from the action of phopholipase A_2. Leukotrienes were previously referred to as the slow-reactive substance of anaphylaxis (SRS-A). The action of these amines and lipid mediators differs depending on the target tissue affected. Histamine, for example, causes contraction of endothelial cells and relaxation of vascular smooth muscle, causing vascular engorgement and leakage. Its effect on bronchial and intestinal smooth muscle, on the other hand, is constriction. Prostaglandins have been identified in anaphylaxis and are known to cause contraction of smooth muscle. A substance termed eosinophil chemotactic factor of anaphylaxis (ECF-A) has been identified in anaphylaxis and in mast cells. The release of this substance is believed to attract eosinophils to sites of hypersensitivity reactions.

ACUTE ALLERGIC REACTIONS

An acute allergic reaction called **local anaphylaxis** is a localized immediate hypersensitivity reaction. The reaction is usually localized to the skin and, hence, is often known also as **cutaneous anaphylaxis.** The reaction, however, need not be confined to the skin; the nasal mucosa or lung is often the target organ. For many decades (if not centuries), it has been recognized that certain humans, and occasionally animals, suffer from hypersensitivity to organic substances of great variety. If the offending substance is a particular food, the hypersensitivity is shown by digestive disturbances or cutaneous rashes (hives). If the object of the hypersensitivity is an inhaled substance, the result is "hay fever," a seromucous inflammation of the upper air passages; asthma, a spasmodic and hypertropic narrowing of the bronchioles; or hypersensitivity pneumonitis. These allergic diseases are often called **atopy** or **atopic allergy.** These types of reaction require previous sensitization, although the offending substance and time of sensitization are often unknown and may be difficult to determine. The number and types of allergens (antigens) in these reactions are exhaustive, including pollens and other plant products, foods, molds, animal and bird dander, parasitic organisms, and parenterally injected substances, such as vaccines, antibiotics, and any other substance containing foreign proteins. The mechanism is believed to be the same as described for cytotropic anaphylaxis. The reaction depends on the production of specific IgE antibody to the offending antigen. IgE becomes fixed to tissue mast cells, which release their contents on subsequent attachment of antigen. Before identification, the IgE antibodies were referred to as **reagins**, a term still used occasionally.

In addition to fixed IgE antibodies, there are also circulating antibodies (predominantly IgG) specific for the antigen. These are also known as blocking antibodies, because they compete for the antigen and, if present in high enough levels, block the hypersensitivity reaction. Injection of repeated small doses of antigen (small enough to avoid systemic anaphylaxis) raises the level of blocking antibodies, a procedure used to immunize or desensitize individuals with atopic allergies, though often without great prophylactic value.

In humans, localized anaphylaxis most often presents itself as hives, hay fever, or asthma. In dogs, the reaction is usually characterized by dermatitis, regardless of route of entry of the antigen. Another example of this form of hypersensitivity is atypical interstitial pneumonia of cattle (hypersensitivity pneumonitis; pulmonary emphysema-adenomatous syndrome), a disease resembling farmer's lung of humans.

Reference

Wilkie BN. Hypersensitivity pneumonitis: experimental production in calves with antigens of *Micropolyspora faeni*. Can J Comp Med 1976;40:221–227.

CYTOTOXIC HYPERSENSITIVITY

Also called cytotoxic anaphylaxis, this form of hypersensitivity is characterized by an antigen-antibody reaction on the surface of a cell, which activates the complement system and results in cell lysis. It occurs in transfusion reactions, erythroblastosis fetalis, autoimmune hemolytic anemia, certain forms of thrombocytopenia, and some viral anemias, such as equine infectious anemia. If the reaction does not fix complement, lysis does not occur, but the affected cells, if they are erythrocytes, agglutinate or are phagocytized by the reticuloendothelial system (erythrophagocytosis). Immune cytolysis may also be important in the lysis of cells altered by viruses and cancer cells (leukemia cells), both of which may bear foreign surface antigens.

IMMUNE-COMPLEX DISEASES

These diseases result from the interaction of antibody with soluble or fixed antigens and complement, leading to an inflammatory reaction. Immune-complex diseases include the *Arthus reaction, serum sickness,* and *chronic immune-complex disease.* The latter group constitutes the most important form in animals. Offending antigens may be iatrogenically introduced foreign proteins; bacterial, parasitic, and viral proteins; autologous antigens; or unknown antigens.

The **Arthus reaction** is an expression of immediate hypersensitivity, principally characterized by vasculitis. As with anaphylaxis, it depends on circulating antibody. An experimentally initiated Arthus reaction consists of a focal area of inflammation and necrosis at the site of antigen injection in a previously sensitized animal. The injected antigen combines with and precipitates antibody and complement in vessel walls. The release of chemotactic complement components (C5a and C5b) attracts neutrophils, which infiltrate and surround the vessel. Participation of neutrophils is necessary for the necrosis, edema, hemorrhage, and thrombosis that accompany the reaction. If neutrophil infiltration is blocked, the Arthus reaction does not develop. Tissue damage results from the release of lysosomal enzymes from neutrophils attracted to the site and activation of other processes of the acute inflammatory response.

Serum sickness is similar to the Arthus reaction in some respects, but classically, it develops in individuals not previously sensitized to the responsible antigen. Instead, when a large amount of antigen, such as horse serum, is injected, some remains in circulation after the specific antibody response becomes evident, which is generally in 6 to 12 days. The resulting circulating antigen-antibody complex leads to the development of serum sickness. Although most of this complex is removed from circulation by the fixed mononuclear phagocyte system, some is deposited in vessel walls along with complement. Released chemotactic factors from complement cause an infiltration of neutrophils into the vessel wall, resulting in a necrotizing vasculitis. Many vessels may be affected, but lesions are seen particularly in major arteries, the endocardium, and renal glomeruli. This form of "immediate" hypersensitivity is referred to as acute serum sickness.

Chronic serum sickness results from the continuous (or repeated) exposure to antigen causing the formation of immune complexes in blood. This form, also known as **chronic immune-complex disease,** is important in the pathogenesis of many diseases of humans and animals. The antigen may be: (1) an autoantigen, as in autoimmune diseases, such as systemic lupus erythematosus (SLE) in humans, autoimmune disease of New Zealand Black mice, and SLE of dogs; (2) viral antigens, as in lymphocytic choriomeningitis, equine infectious anemia, or Aleutian disease; or (3) bacterial antigens, as seen in poststreptococcal glomerulonephritis of humans. Although other lesions and other immune reactions may occur in some of these diseases (e.g., cytotropic hemolytic anemia in SLE dogs or delayed hypersensitivity in lymphocytic choriomeningitis), the most outstanding lesion results from the deposition of immune complexes as irregular, electron-dense granular deposits on the epithelial side of the basement membrane. These may or may not contain complement. The deposits ultimately lead to immune complex glomerulonephritis and chronic renal insufficiency. Deposition in vessel walls leads to vasculitis, as described for serum sickness and the Arthus reaction.

There are many forms of glomerular disease and vasculitis in which immunoglobulin, with or without complement, can be demonstrated by immunofluorescence and which morphologically resemble known immune-complex diseases. However, the antigens responsible for the formation of the complexes are usually unknown.

Delayed hypersensitivity

Most features of delayed hypersensitivity have been presented in our previous discussion of **cell-mediated immunity.** The mechanisms and morphologic features are the same as those of the protective aspects of delayed immunity. Delayed hypersensitivity is a component of the tuberculin reaction, tuberculosis and probably most other granulomatous diseases, graft rejection, graft-versus-host reaction, contact dermatitides, and some autoimmune diseases. The essential microscopic feature of most forms of delayed hypersensitivity is perivenular accumulation of mononuclear cells, which ultimately extends into adjacent tissues. As in the immediate hypersensitivity reaction, the "allergens" are numerous and often not identified. Details of the histopathology of granulomatous diseases are described in Chapter 11.

TRANSPLANT REJECTION

Transplant rejection is characterized by cellular infiltrates composed of cytotoxic T lymphocytes and macrophages (attracted by mediators released from sensitized T cells). These cells, which surround and infiltrate the foreign tissue, are stimulated by foreign MHC molecules located on cell membranes of such tissues. Humoral antibodies are also elicited, but are not believed to play a major role in rejection.

CONTACT DERMATITIS

This reaction is characterized by a slow onset (from 1 to 10 days, depending on whether exposure is primary or secondary) after exposure to a sensitizing antigen. The best known examples are poison ivy dermatitis in humans and flea-allergy dermatitis in dogs and cats. Histologically, the superficial dermis is infiltrated with lymphocytes, macrophages, and variable numbers of eosinophils. Hyperemia and edema of the dermis occur, and vesicles may form in the epidermis.

AUTOIMMUNITY

In hypersensitivity reactions, a normal process can become aberrant or overreactive and thus more harmful than the noxious stimuli initiating the reaction. Autoimmunity represents another aberrant reaction on the part of immunologic mechanisms that harm the host and for which no advantage can be found. As defined by Burnet (1972), autoimmunity is "a condition in which structural or functional damage is produced by the reaction of immunocytes or antibodies with normal components of the body." How can antibodies form against one's own tissues? What happens to self-recognition? Using Burnet's clonal theory of antibody formation, several conceivable mechanisms have been set

forth to explain autoimmunity; however, the underlying cause in all cases is essentially unknown.

Anatomic segregation of antigen

If, during maturation of the immune system, a particular antigen is anatomically segregated or not formed until later in life, this antigen will not be recognized as self, as it will never have had the opportunity to inactivate immunologically competent clones capable of reacting to it. For all practical purposes, the antigen is foreign. This mechanism has been postulated for **Hashimoto's disease** of humans and similar forms of **lymphocytic thyroiditis** in dogs. Spermatozoa and the lens of the eye are other examples of locations of isolated antigens.

Alteration of antigens

If tissues are altered so that new and foreign reactive antigenic sites are present, they will stimulate antibody formation. It is postulated that radiation-induced mutations, infections, and certain chemicals might produce antigenic alteration of tissue proteins.

Cross reactions between antigens

If foreign antigens possess reactive sites in common with tissue proteins, antibodies to the foreign antigen might react with tissue proteins. Rheumatic fever and glomerulonephritis in humans may be the result of this type of cross reaction between tissue proteins and certain strains of streptococci.

Forbidden clones

It has been postulated that autoimmunity might be caused by alteration of immunocytes, with the appearance of new clones, or by a failure of the normal suppression mechanisms allowing clones to persist or reappear. These forbidden clones, as Burnet has called them, would then be capable of producing antibodies to tissue proteins. It is not known why new, forbidden, or abnormal clones appear, but it is believed that a genetic predisposition exists in certain individuals. Remember that the clonal selection theory of Burnet is itself hypothetical and not proven.

Whatever the mechanism, autoimmunity represents a failure to recognize self, and serious and often fatal diseases develop from this reaction for which no satisfactory treatment exists.

Both humoral and cellular immunity contribute to autoimmune disease. Two humoral mechanisms may participate. In one, the antibody is directed against a specific fixed-tissue antigen restricted to a specific tissue. Examples include thyroiditis, encephalitis, and orchitis. In the second form, antibody reacts with antigen, forming immune complexes, which are deposited in glomeruli or vessels and result in disease at these sites. The process (but not the antigen) is essentially the same as described previously for immune-complex hypersensitivity diseases and is appropriately termed **autologous immune-complex disease.** There is also little tolerance for intracellular components, and their release is followed by production of autoantibodies and/or immune T lymphocytes. This regularly follows tissue necrosis. However, the presence of such an autoimmune response does not imply disease that causes tissue injury, because antibody does not penetrate cell membranes.

TYPES OF AUTOIMMUNE DISEASES

In humans, a variety of diseases are thought to be autoimmune in origin, whereas the examples are fewer in animals. The following are the most important of these.

Antiglomerular Basement Membrane Nephritis (Anti-GBM Nephritis, Goodpasture's Syndrome)

This is a rare disease in which autoantibodies are made against a noncollagen domain of the type IV collagen present in glomerular basement membrane. A similar antigen is found in the basement membranes of pulmonary alveoli. In contrast to that form of glomerulonephritis caused by the deposition of circulating immune complexes, the autoantibodies in anti-GBM nephritis are deposited in a smooth linear pattern along the GBM rather than in globular deposits. Patients with Goodpasture's syndrome have both pulmonary hemorrhage and gomerulonephritis. Complement binds to these antibody-GBM complexes, initiating the classical pathway of complement activation and the formation of C5a, which is highly chemotactic for neutrophils. Hydrolytic enzymes from the neutrophils are responsible for much of the tissue damage that occurs in this disease.

A spontaneously occurring anti-GBM nephropathy has also been described in 6 of 53 horses without clinical evidence of renal disease. Affected horses had thickened glomerular basement membranes containing IgG and complement, but no evidence of neutrophil infiltration. Horses did not have autoimmune deposits in their lungs.

Anti-GBM nephritis can be produced experimentally in several laboratory animal species by immunization with foreign GBM. Likewise, an interstitial nephritis can be induced by immunization with tubular basement membrane (**antitubular basement membrane nephritis**). Spontaneous antitubular basement membrane nephritis is a rare disease of humans and probably of animals.

References

Banks KL, Henson JB. Immunologically mediated glomerulonephritis of horses. II. Anti-glomerular basement membrane antibody and other mechanisms in spontaneous disease. Lab Invest 1972;26:708–716.

Burnet FM. A reassessment of the forbidden clone hypothesis of autoimmune disease. Aust J Exp Biol Med Sci 1972;50:1–9.

van Zweiten MJ, Bhan AK, McCluskey RT, et al. Studies on the pathogenesis of experimental antitubular basement membrane nephritis in the guinea pig. Am J Pathol 1976;83:531–541.

Autoimmune Hemolytic Anemia (AIHA)

In this disease, antibodies are produced against an individual's own red blood cells, which accelerate their destruction by hemolysis and removal by the liver and spleen. Mice of the New Zealand Black (NZB) strain almost invariably develop autoimmune hemolytic anemia, as well as other immunologic lesions. AIHA also occurs in dogs, cats, horses, and cattle, often in conjunction with other immunologic abnormalities. In dogs, all ages are susceptible, but AIHA occurs most often between 2 to 8 years of age; females are affected three to four times more often than males. The anemia may be severe in dogs and is associated with hepatosplenomegaly and often with thrombocytopenia. Five classes of AIHA are recognized in dogs: in three of these (classes I, III, and IV), hemolysis occurs extravascularly; and in two (classes II and V), it occurs intravascularly. Class I is mediated by IgG or IgM, which coats erythrocytes so that they agglutinate and are removed from the circulation by fixed mononuclear phagocytes of the spleen and liver. Class III, which is the most common form in dogs, results from IgG coating of red blood cells, resulting in incomplete complement activation, but allowing opsonization of the cells for phagocytosis by cells of the fixed mononuclear phagocyte system. Class IV (also known as cold agglutinin disease) is mediated by IgM autoantibodies, which are optimally active at 4°C to 10°C, well below normal body temperature. Cells agglutinated by this mechanism are also removed from the circulation by fixed mononuclear phagocytes. Classes II and V AIHA are mediated by IgM antierythrocytic antibodies, which, when bound to red blood cells, intrinsically activate the complement system with formation of the membrane attack complex, causing cell lysis. Hence, hemolysis occurs intravascularly. Autoantibodies on red blood cells of patients with AIHA can be demonstrated by the direct Coombs' test.

Allergic encephalomyelitis

This disease can be produced by injection of central nervous system tissue from individuals of the same or different species. The responsible antigen is a protein of myelinated tissue termed **myelin basic protein.** The lesions are those of vasculitis and destruction and demyelination of white matter, accompanied by infiltration of mononuclear cells. Humoral autoantibodies and sensitized T cells are demonstrable. Post-rabies vaccination encephalitis is an example of this disorder; vaccines derived from tissue culture rather than rabbit-brain suspension now preclude its development. The pathogenesis of demyelinating encephalitis associated with neurotropic viruses, such as canine distemper, also depend on an autoimmune response.

Lymphocytic thyroiditis

An autoimmune thyroiditis may be experimentally induce by immunization with heterologous thyroglobulin. The lesion is characterized by a chronic lymphocytic thyroiditis causing diffuse or focal infiltration of the thyroid gland with lymphocytes and the appearance of lymphocytic follicles with germinal centers, macrophages, and plasma cells accompanying the infiltrate. Lymphocytes and plasma cells invade between thyroid epithelial cells, resulting in destruction of the follicular epithelium and basement membrane and, ultimately, in fibrosis and hyperplasia of the follicular epithelium. The disease occurs spontaneously in rats, dogs, an obese strain of chickens, and humans, in whom it is known as Hashimoto's disease. The disease in chickens results in hypothyroidism and obesity. In other species, there is less severe hypothyroidism. Neonatal bursectomy, but not thymectomy, prevents or reduces the severity of the disease in chickens, indicating that the disorder is primarily the result of antithyroid antibodies. The pathogenesis in other species has not been clarified, but it is suspected that cell-mediated immunity may play an important role.

Lymphocytic orchitis in a closed colony of Beagle dogs has been associated with lymphocytic thyroiditis. Both are presumed to be autoimmune in origin and, in part, genetically influenced.

References

Bigazzi PE, Rose NR. Spontaneous autoimmune thyroiditis in animals as a model of human disease. Prog Allergy 1975;19:245–274.

Wick G, Sundick RS, Albine B. A review: the obese strain (OS) of chickens: an animal model with spontaneous autoimmune thyroiditis. Clin Immunol Immunopathol 1974;3:272–300.

Systemic lupus erythematosus (SLE)

This is a complex autoimmune disease of humans and dogs. A milder form of the disease has been termed **discoid lupus erythematosus.** Antibodies are formed against a variety of tissue components, including DNA, RNA, and other nucleoproteins (all collectively called antinuclear antibodies, or ANA); thyroglobulin; and erythrocyte-membrane antigens. Affected dogs often manifest some form of shifting leg lameness caused by polyarthritis or polymyositis. Lesions of the skin and mucocutaneous junctions may also occur in dogs with SLE (Chapter 17). The more significant (and life-threatening) pathology of SLE is related to the circulation of immune complexes. In humans and dogs, diagnosis is made on the basis of a combination of clinical signs accompanied by a positive LE and/or ANA test. The LE test is based on forcing a blood clot or bone marrow sample that has been incubated at 37°C for 1 hour through a fine mesh screen, which causes some of the cells damaged by this procedure to extrude their nuclei into the serum. The anti-DNA antibodies and C3 in the serum opsonizes the extruded nuclei, which are then engulfed by neutrophils in the serum. The phagocytized nucleus appears as a large pink-purple cytoplasmic mass, which pushes the nucleus of the neutrophil to the periphery of the cell. These LE cells can then be demonstrated in buffy-coat smears stained by the Wright-Giemsa method. The ANA test, on the other hand, is an indirect immunofluorescent test that demonstrates the presence of serum antibodies with specificity for nuclear antigens. It is thought to be more specific than the LE test, but both tests may yield false-positive or false-negative results.

The clinicopathologic picture is characterized by hemolytic anemia, thrombocytopenic purpura, leukopenia, fibrinoid degeneration of collagen, and arthritis. The antinuclear antibodies themselves cannot directly damage cells, as they cannot cross cell membranes. In the course of the normal turnover of cells, however, antinuclear antibodies form complexes with the released protein. These lead to autologous immune-complex disease, which is of major importance to the pathogenesis of the disease, causing vasculitis (Arthus phenomenon) and immune-complex glomerulonephritis. Renal failure is often the most serious concern in LE. The pathogenesis of the thrombocytopenia is not established. Antiplatelet antibodies have not been demonstrated. The cause of LE is unknown. It was suspected to be hereditary, but studies in dogs have not supported this hypothesis. Lewis and colleagues (1973) have presented evidence to suggest that a transmissible agent is associated with the canine disease. Beaucher and colleagues (1977) speculated that the disease in humans and dogs may be caused by a common environmental exposure, possibly an infectious agent.

References

Beaucher WN, Garman RH, Condemi IJ. Familial lupus erythematosus: antibodies to DNA in household dogs. N Engl J Med 1977;296:982–984.

Krum SH, Cardinet GH, Anderson BC, et al. Polymyositis and polyarthritis associated with systemic lupus erythematosus in a dog. J Am Vet Med Assoc 1977;170:61–64.

Lewis RM, Hathaway JE. Canine systemic lupus erythematosus presenting with symmetrical polyarthritis. Br J Small Anim Pract 1976;8:273–284.

Lewis RM, Henry WB, Thornton GW, et al A syndrome of autoimmune hemolytic anemia and thrombocytopenia in dogs. Soc Proc J Am Vet Med Assoc 1963;1:140–163.

Lewis RM, Schwartz RS. Canine systemic lupus erythematosus. Genetic analysis of an established breeding colony. J Exp Med 1971;134:417–438.

Lewis RM, André-Schwartz J, Harris GS, et al. Canine systemic lupus erythematosus. Transmission of serologic abnormalities by cell-free filtrates. J Clin Invest 1973;52:1893–1907.

New Zealand Black (NZB) mice disease

This spontaneous, complex polygenic inherited form of autoimmune disease bears some resemblance to SLE. Affected mice develop autoantibodies against erythrocyte membranes, DNA, and thymocytes and have circulating immune complexes. There are numerous genes that contribute to this disorder. Mice develop Coombs'-positive autoimmune hemolytic anemia and an autologous immune-complex glomerulonephritis. They also have abnormal T-cell and B-cell function, causing secretion of higher than normal levels of IgG immunoglobulins by 3 months of age. A high incidence of lymphoma also occurs in this strain.

References

Natl Res Council. Hereditary immunodeficiencies. In: Immunodeficient rodents: a guide to their immunobiology, husbandry and use. Washington, DC: National Academy Press 1989;36–139.

Talal N, Steinberg AD. The pathogenesis of autoimmunity in New Zealand Black mice. Curr Top Microbiol Immunol 1974;64:79–103.

Rheumatoid arthritis

Humans with rheumatoid arthritis and animals with a comparable arthritis have autoantibodies to immunoglobulins, principally IgM and IgG. These antibodies are called rheumatoid factor and are present in other disorders, such as SLE. The significance of rheumatoid factor in the pathogenesis of arthritis is not established, but in addition to its presence in serum, it is present in the form of an immune complex in synovial fluids.

References

Lewis RM, Borel Y. Canine rheumatoid arthritis: a case report. Arthritis Rheum 1971;14:67–72.

Pemphigus vulgaris

This autoimmune disease is characterized by bullae of the skin and mucous membranes that result in large ulcers. It results from the separation of epidermal cells from one another (acantholysis) caused by degeneration of intercellular space substance and the loss of intercellular bridges. The disease occurs in humans and has been described in dogs and cats. In this condition, autoantibodies directed against intercellular space substance cause the release of epithelial proteases that disrupt epithelial connections and result in suprabasal clefts and vesicle formation. A characteristic microscopic finding in this disease is the presence of isolated keratinocytes (acantholytic keratinocytes) floating free in the intraepidermal vesicle or pustule (Chapter 17).

Reference

Hurvitz AI, Feldman E. A disease in dogs resembling human pemphigus vulgaris. J Am Vet Med Assoc 1975;166:585–590.

Bullous pemphigoid

In this rare, vesiculobullous, autoimmune disease of the skin and/or oral mucosa of humans and dogs, autoantibodies are directed against a keratinocyte synthesized antigen that is found in the hemidesmisomes of basal cells of the epidermis and the upper portion of the lamina lucida of the basement membrane. Immunofluorescent or immunohistochemical procedures demonstrate the presence of immunoglobulin, either IgM or IgG, and complement along the basement membrane of the epidermis and/or oral mucosa. These antibody-antigen-complement complexes attract neutrophils and eosinophils, which release proteolytic enzymes that cause disruption of the dermal-epidermal junction and vesicle or bullae formation. The vesicles and bullae eventually become pustules as neutrophils and eosinophils accumulate within them. These eventually rupture leaving areas of ulceration (Chapter 17).

Orchitis

Orchitis can be induced by immunization with spermatozoa or their antigens. The lesion is characterized by focal or diffuse infiltration of the testes, vas deferens, and epididymis with lymphocytes and lesser numbers of other mononuclear cells. Naturally occurring lymphocytic orchitis has been speculated to be of autoimmune origin. The condition has been described in a closed colony of beagle dogs in which there was also a high incidence of lymphocytic thyroiditis. Orchitis or epididymitis of infectious or traumatic origin may be exacerbated by the release of spermatozoa to surrounding tissues.

Ophthalmitis

Immunization with lens protein, uveal antigen, and retinal antigens can induce an autoimmune ophthalmitis. The ensuing lesions are principally characterized by mononuclear cell infiltration of the uvea, often accompanied by multinucleated giant cells and granulomas. The role of autoantibodies in naturally occurring ophthalmitis is not clear, but circulating antibodies and cell-mediated immunity have been demonstrated in a high percentage of humans with noninfectious uveitis.

Other autoimmune disorders

Autoimmune inflammation of other organs and tissues has been recognized in humans and can be induced experimentally in laboratory animals. Examples include autoimmune insulitis, which results in transient diabetes mellitus; autoimmune adrenalitis; myasthenia gravis; aplastic anemia; "idiopathic" neutropenia; thrombocytopenia; parathyroiditis; and pernicious anemia in humans. Idiopathic polyneuritis (Coonhound paralysis; Guillain-Barré-like syndrome) of dogs has been speculated to be an autoimmune disease. Many organs and tissues share antigens, which may result in multiple organ disease after immunization with antigen from a single tissue. For example, the liver, kidney, duodenum, ileum, and colon have common antigens. This may explain the complexity of many autoimmune diseases.

Viruses and "autoimmunity"

Viral infections almost invariably elicit a humoral immune response, but in addition, they may stimulate a cell-mediated immune response that is crucial to the pathogenesis of the lesions and to resolution of the infection. This cell-mediated reaction, which has been variably termed a hypersensitivity reaction and an autoimmune response, is directed against viral-encoded cell membrane antigens, which are foreign to the host.

These are not viral capsid antigens, but new membrane antigens stimulated by the viral infection. Humoral antibodies are also formed against these antigens. The reaction is aimed at rejection of virus-infected tissue by the host, a process similar to that of transplant rejection. This reaction, of course, results in the destruction of infected host tissues or organs, which may lead to resolution of the infection or, if extensive, death of the host. In some examples, the suppression of cellular immunity prevents the reaction and the disease, suggesting that the responsible viral infection is essentially harmless.

This disease mechanism is best studied in lymphocytic choriomeningitis infection of mice, where, if infection occurs in mice more than a few days old, an intense lymphocytic inflammatory response occurs in almost all organs, causing death, elimination of the infection, or a persistent infection. If the mouse is infected *in utero* or at 1 day of age, an acute reaction does not occur; instead, a persistent infection is established. It was once thought that this represented a form of complete tolerance, but humoral and cell-mediated immune responses were found to be elicited. A chronic disease results, with destruction of cells as well as the formation of virus-antibody immune complexes, leading to vasculitis and glomerulonephritis. Other viral infections, in which similar mechanisms are important to their pathogenesis, include lactic dehydrogenase infection of mice, Moloney sarcoma virus of mice, Aleutian disease of mink, equine infectious anemia, hog cholera, virus-induced leukemias, and cytomegalovirus infection. Further study probably will demonstrate that most viral infections are associated with new membrane antigens and that certain unexplained autoimmune diseases are the result of previous viral infections.

Summarizing this account and earlier comments, viruses may induce several immunopathologic changes. These include: (1) **depression of humoral and cellular immune responses;** (2) **production of immune complexes with resultant associated disease;** and (3) **induction of new antigens on cell membranes, causing cell destruction through either antibody and complement binding or cell-mediated immune responses.** Less well characterized is the potentiation of the immune response by certain viruses, such as lactic dehydrogenase virus and Venezuelan equine encephalitis virus.

8

Diseases caused by viruses

Viruses are submicroscopic infectious agents that are among the smallest and simplest of all life forms. Their simplicity separates viruses from all other infectious agents. Other microorganisms, namely *Mycoplasma,* *Chlamydia,* and *Rickettsia* species, and bacteria and protozoa, are cells that multiply by binary fission. They all contain DNA, ribosomes, and organelles. Viruses, in contrast, are not cells; they contain only one type of nucleic acid, DNA or RNA, double-stranded or single-stranded; have no ribosomes; no organelles; and do not multiply by binary fission. Viruses are obligate intracellular parasites dependent on host-cell machinery for protein synthesis and replication. They are essentially nucleoprotein entities or genetic elements surrounded by a protective coat; they are capable of passing from one cell to another. Viruses affect almost all other life forms, including vertebrates, invertebrates, microorganisms (e.g., *Mycoplasma* species and bacteria), and plants.

The interaction between virus and host cell determines whether the relationship is deleterious (pathogenic) or not. Most virus infections are, in fact, subclinical, i.e., infection does not lead to overt disease. Viruses, however, are responsible for many of the most important and often fatal infections of animals, such as canine distemper, rinderpest, and hog cholera, as well as certain neoplastic diseases. The outcome of infection is dependent on many factors, which include the nature of the specific virus and its cell tropism, genetic resistance of the species or breed affected, and immune response, age, nutritional status, and hormone levels of the individual animal affected, to mention a few.

CLASSIFICATION AND NOMENCLATURE OF VIRUSES

In recent years, a significant body of information has been gathered concerning the biochemical, ultrastructural, and molecular characteristics of viruses that forms the basis for their classification. Many classification systems for viruses have been employed and their names and schemes for classification are still evolving.

The affinity (tropism) of viruses for specific tissues is one of the characteristics that was a reason for group-ing similar viruses, leading to their classification as neurotropic, epitheliotropic, pneumotropic, and other designations. This feature, however, is variable, as many viruses infect numerous types of tissue. Tropism may also vary depending on species affected, age of animal, and other circumstances. It is still, however, not only useful but necessary for the pathologist to be familiar with the effects of each virus as an aid in diagnosis.

The two principal characteristics used in the current classification system are virion morphology and nucleic acid type. These are supplemented with other characteristics, including mode of replication, susceptibility to physical and chemical agents, antigenicity (serologic relatedness), means of transmission, cell tropism, and clinical and pathologic effects. Using these parameters, viruses are grouped into families, subfamilies, genera, and species. Viral families are designated by terms ending in the suffix "**-viridae,**" subfamilies by "**-virinae,**" and genera by "**-virus.**" For the most part, there is no singly accepted convention for naming viral species; rather, historical custom prevails, using terms such as "hog cholera" or "canine distemper." Virus families, grouped on the basis of principal characteristics, are listed in Table 8-1 and represented schematically in Fig. 8-1.

ULTRASTRUCTURAL MORPHOLOGY OF VIRUSES

Each "virus-particle" (virion) has a central core of deoxyribonucleic acid (DNA) or ribonucleic acid (RNA) surrounded by a protein coat called the **capsid.** The capsid is composed of a large number of distinguishable morphologic units, called **capsomeres,** held together by noncovalent bonds. The nucleic acid core plus its capsid is referred to as the **nucleocapsid** (Fig. 8-2). The nucleocapsid may be surrounded by a lipoprotein **envelope (peplos)** or may lack this envelope ("naked"). The envelope is derived from nuclear or cytoplasmic membranes of the cell in which the virion is produced. The essential structure of the envelope is a phospholipid bilayer in which are embedded specific proteins. These phospholipids may be similar or identi-

TABLE 8-1 **Classification of viruses according to genetic characteristics**

Characteristics	Family	Example of virus
Double-stranded DNA		
Enveloped	Poxviridae	Cowpox, swinepox viruses
	Iridoviridae	African swine fever virus
	Herpesviridae	Pseudorabies, infectious bovine rhinotracheitis viruses
Non-enveloped	Adenoviridae	Bovine adenovirus
	Papovaviridae	Shope papilloma virus
	Hepadnaviridae	Woodchuck hepatitis virus
Single-stranded DNA		
Non-enveloped	Parvoviridae	Feline panleukopenia virus
Double-stranded RNA		
Non-enveloped	Reoviridae	Bluetongue virus
Bisegmented Double-stranded RNA Non-enveloped	Birnaviridae	Infectious pancreatic necrosis of fish
Single-stranded RNA		
Enveloped		
No DNA in replication		
Positive-sense genome	Togaviridae	Hog cholera virus
	Coronaviridae	Transmissible gastroenteritis virus
Negative-sense genome	Paramyxoviridae	Canine distemper virus
	Orthomyxoviridae	Influenze viruses
	Rhabdoviridae	Rabies virus (rhabdovirus)
	Bunyaviridae	Rift Valley fever
	Arenaviridae	Lymphocytic choriomeningitis virus
DNA step in replication	Retroviridae	Feline leukemia virus
Non-enveloped	Picornaviridae	Swine vesicular disease virus
	Caliciviridae	Vesicular exanthema virus

cal to those of the host cell. Radially arranged structures (**peplomers)** may project from the outer surface of the envelope. The envelope, therefore, is made up of an inner lipid layer, a protein coat, and peplomers as the outermost layer. Some virions may have more than one envelope.

The nucleocapsid of the virion contains the genome of the virus. The envelope contains the specific material that determines the viral antigenicity and interacts with receptor sites on the cell membrane of the host cell to initiate infection.

Virions range in size from the large poxvirus, measuring 300 nm by 250 nm by 100 nm, to the parvoviruses, which are only 20 nm in diameter. The shape of the virion is largely determined by the organization of the capsid and its relationship to the central core of nucleic acid. Two basic groups of structures or symmetries are recognized. One is **icosahedral** or **cubic** symmetry, in which condensed nucleic acid is surrounded by a capsid in the form of a 20-faceted icosahedron, each facet composed of a specific number of capsomeres, de-

pending on the virus group. The other basic shape is **helical, spiral,** or **screw** symmetry, in which the nucleic acid and capsomeres are bound together forming filamentous or rod-like particles.

MULTIPLICATION

Many of the pathologic effects of viral infections result from the process of viral multiplication. This involves a series of events beginning with entry of the virus into the host and the ultimate release of new virions. The intervening molecular events vary among viral families. **Entry** into the host may be by direct inoculation into the bloodstream, as is the case with arthropod-borne viruses (e.g., *Togaviridae),* but most viruses enter by penetrating the skin or mucosal barrier of the respiratory or gastrointestinal tract. If the portal of entry is the target organ, further transport is not necessary; however, many viruses must be transported to their ultimate site of replication and disease production. This may involve primary replication in cells at the portal of entry and

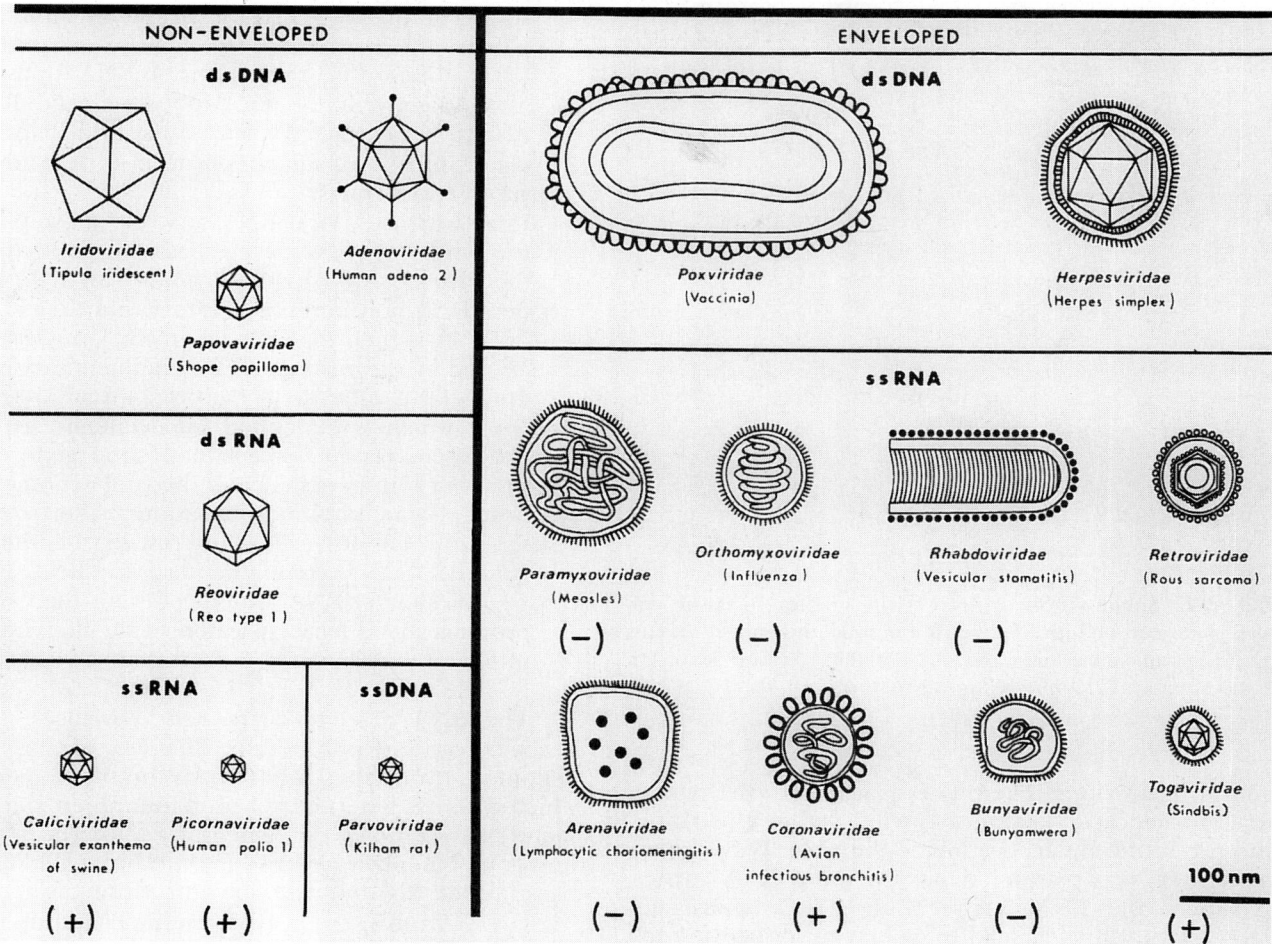

FIG. 8-1 Families of viruses that infect vertebrates. (Used with permission from Matthews REF and Intervirology. Basel/New York: S. Karger.

then spread via the lymphatics or the bloodstream (such as with certain herpesviruses), direct spread via lymphatics or bloodstream (such as with reoviruses), spread via infected lymphocytes (such as with cytomegaloviruses), or spread via neuronal axons (such as with rhabdoviruses, which cause rabies). Vertical transmission provides another mechanism of entry, where viruses may cross the placenta to the fetus (such as with cytomegalovirus) or be carried as part of the germ plasm (such as with certain retroviruses).

Attachment to cells involves specific binding of virus to the cell surface. The presence or absence of specific receptors accounts for the susceptibility of a given cell type or types, or the tissue tropism of the virus. Viral entry obviously does not imply infection, as certain species lack appropriate receptors for specific viruses. The absence of receptors, however, does not mean that a cell type is incapable of supporting viral multiplication. Experimental introduction of virus into a non-susceptible cell may lead to multiplication. Also, *in vitro* cell tropism may not be indicative of *in vivo* cell susceptibility. Certain cells, lacking receptors *in vivo*, may gain receptors in cell culture.

Penetration into the cell immediately follows attach-

ment. With enveloped viruses, the virion envelope fuses with the plasma membrane allowing entry of the nucleocapsid. Non-enveloped viruses enter by endocytosis (pinocytosis) of the virion or by translocation of the virion across the plasma membrane.

Following penetration the virion is **uncoated,** i.e., the viral RNA or DNA is exposed by removal of all or part of the capsid. For most viruses, the process is dependent on cellular enzymes. Uncoating is followed by what is termed the **eclipse phase,** when no virions are evident. Infection of a cell (attachment and penetration) does not necessarily lead to viral multiplication and cell damage, i.e., a productive infection. The cell must be **permissive** for a productive infection to ensue, and entry does not necessarily imply permissiveness. Nonproductive infection may also result from infection by defective viruses. Viruses may enter a cell and their RNA or DNA may persist in the cell (whether incorporated into the cell genome or not) without a productive infection. **Persistent infection** may, under appropriate and usually unknown circumstances, be activated to productive infection or lead to cell transformation. **Viral multiplication** involves expression of viral genes, leading to replication of the viral genome and produc-

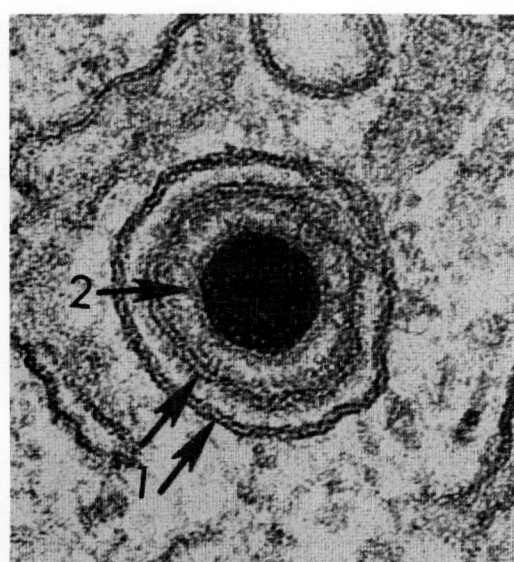

FIG. 8-2 Single virion of herpesvirus simplex in tissue culture of rat cerebellum. Note envelopes *(1)* and capsid *(2)* surrounding the dense nucleoid. (× 220,000.) (Courtesy of Dr. JE Leestma and *Laboratory Investigation.)*

tion of new virions. The process varies with the type of viral nucleic acid, enzymes carried within the virion, and the intracellular location of the virus. With the exception of single-stranded positive-sense RNA viruses, in which viral RNA can serve directly as messenger RNA, all viral nucleic acid must be transcribed to messenger RNA. DNA viruses that replicate in the nucleus use host RNA polymerase for transcription to messenger RNA, whereas all other viruses are dependent on transcriptases carried within the virion.

Several schemes are involved with RNA viruses. **Multiplication of single-stranded RNA viruses** involves one of three schemes, which are discussed in the following list.

1. **Picornaviruses and togaviruses are positive (+)** strand viruses; their RNA can serve directly as messenger RNA. After infecting a cell, viral RNA links to ribosomes and is directly translated to proteins, giving rise to a polymerase allowing direct synthesis of a complimentary negative (−) strand RNA from the parental (+) strand. The (−) strand then serves as a template for synthesis of additional (+) strands, which in turn can repeat the process and ultimately form viral progeny. Since replication is not dependent on any enzyme carried by the virion, RNA extracted from (+) strand RNA viruses is infectious.

2. **Orthomyxoviruses, paramyxoviruses, bunyaviruses, arenaviruses, and rhabdoviruses are negative (−)** strand viruses. The first step in multiplication requires that virion RNA be transcribed into a (+) messenger RNA, a step dependent on a transcriptase carried within the virion. Translation products of the messenger RNA then serve to allow transcription of (−) strand virion RNA into a complimentary (+) strand, which serves as a template for synthesis of (−) strand virion RNA for assembly into progeny. In contrast to (+) strand RNA viruses, RNA extracted from (−) strand RNA viruses is not infectious, since replication is dependent on virion transcriptase.

3. **In retroviruses, viral RNA** serves as a template for the synthesis of (viral) DNA, a step dependent on the enzyme reverse transcriptase (an RNA-dependent DNA polymerase) carried within the virion. Viral RNA is then digested by an RNA nuclease, also carried by the virion, and a complimentary copy of (viral) DNA is formed, resulting in double-stranded DNA, which is integrated into cellular DNA. The process may stop here, without viral gene expression, but with persistence of the viral genome in the host genome. Viral multiplication results from transcription (by host cell transcriptase) of integrated (viral) DNA into complimentary viral RNA. Positive (+) messenger RNA, which codes for the necessary proteins to be packaged along with the viral RNA into viral progeny, is also produced.

The RNA of double-stranded reoviruses is transcribed by virion polymerase. The (−) strand of the genome is transcribed into (+) strand messenger RNA, which is translated into viral proteins and enzymes. The same (+) strands serve as templates for transcription into complimentary negative (−) strands, yielding double-stranded RNA for assembly into virions.

DNA viruses also have several multiplication schemes. **The double-stranded DNA of papovavirus, adenovirus, and herpesvirus** is transported in the unenveloped virion to the nucleus, in which cellular enzymes are used for production of messenger RNA. Replication of DNA uses host-cell DNA polymerase in the case of papovaviruses, whereas herpesviruses and adenoviruses use virally coded polymerase. A large number of virally coded proteins, which are made in the cytoplasm, are involved in the multiplication and assembly process. **Poxvirus** multiplication occurs in the cytoplasm. The virion is probably uncoated by both cellular enzymes and enzyme products of an early transcribed messenger RNA. Cytoplasmic DNA replication is under the control of enzymes carried within the virion and translation products of early and late messenger RNA.

Single-stranded parvoviruses replicate in the nucleus and are comprised of three groups. The autonomous parvoviruses (genera parvovirus), which include most animal pathogens, are dependent on host-cell enzymes for synthesis of complimentary DNA to form double-stranded DNA. This in turn is transcribed to messenger RNA and genomic DNA. The dependovirus genus, or adeno-associated viruses, require coinfection with an adenovirus for replication to occur; the adenovirus apparently supplies DNA polymerase. Members of the third genus, densovirus, only infect arthropods.

The genome of **Hepadnaviridae** is partly double-stranded DNA and partly single-stranded DNA. The single-stranded region is first repaired by virion DNA polymerase, yielding complete circular double-stranded DNA. DNA is then transcribed by cellular enzymes into two classes of RNA, messenger RNA and genomic RNA. The genomic RNA serves as a template for synthesis of viral DNA by means of a reverse transcriptase coded in the viral genome. A portion of the genomic RNA, which remains after partial degradation, serves as the template for the incomplete complimentary strand of DNA of the mature virion.

Release of new virions

Most all non-enveloped viruses mature within the host cell, either in the nucleus or cytoplasm, and depend on cell lysis for their release. Enveloped viruses obtain their surrounding membranes by budding, which may result in release of virus without necessarily leading to cell lysis. All negative-strand RNA viruses, togaviruses, and retroviruses are released through budding, i.e., the virion is extruded through the cell membrane, which along with some viral proteins becomes the virion envelope. Retroviruses and arenaviruses bud, causing little cell damage, i.e., they are noncytolytic. Other budding viruses, such as togaviruses, paramyxoviruses, and rhabdoviruses, however, are cytolytic.

Poxviruses are released by both mechanisms. Intracellular virions develop a membrane and acquire an envelope presumably from Golgi apparatus, which fuses with the plasma membrane, releasing virions with a double-layered envelope. Most poxvirus virions, however, are released without an envelope on disruption of the cell. Both types of particles are infectious; however, those released by budding more readily attach to host cells. Herpesviruses, in contrast to all other enveloped viruses, acquire their envelope from the inner lamella of the nuclear membrane. The enveloped virions pass within cisternae, through and without contact with the cytoplasm, to the cell surface and are are released. This scheme would appear to allow viral release without cell disruption; however, productive herpesvirus infection is invariably cytolytic.

Cellular injury

Once a virus has entered a susceptible and permissive cell (a cell with appropriate receptors and one which can support replication), the effect on the cell varies with the nature of the interaction between virus and cell. Many different morphologic features can ensue, but there are essentially three types of interaction: (1) cytocidal; (2) infection without apparent pathologic effect; and (3) cell transformation.

Cytocidal viruses cause cell lysis or necrosis, a feature of many herpesviruses, picornaviruses, parvoviruses, adenoviruses, and flaviviruses. All the mechanisms that result in cell death are not understood, but they relate to alterations in host-cell metabolism. Viruses do not generate toxins in the way that bacteria do; however, protein products coded for and produced by the virus, such as capsid proteins, are often toxic. More importantly, the coding for viral proteins results in a shutdown of host protein synthesis and, ultimately, of host DNA and RNA synthesis, which is incompatible with cell survival.

Infection without apparent cytopathic effect (usually noncytocidal viruses) may take two forms, i.e., **persistent infection** and **latent infection.** In persistent infection, viral replication and release take place without killing the cell. This is the usual result of infection with arenaviruses and retroviruses; virions are released by budding without apparent cellular damage. Another form of persistent infection is that termed **chronic infection.** After recovery from acute disease, in which cellular lysis may be an important component of the host cell-virion interaction, virus is not eliminated from the host, but remains within selected populations of cells and continues to be reproduced at low levels. These chronic infections may result in: (1) infectious carriers, as is the case with foot and mouth disease; (2) chronic disease, as seen in African swine fever; or (3) disease years after initial infection, as seen in canine distemper encephalitis (old dog encephalitis).

Latent viral infection differs from persistent infection in that the virion genome resides in the cell, but there is no replication of virus. Almost all herpesviruses (alpha, beta, and gamma) establish latent infections following initial exposure. The **alpha** or **neurotropic herpesviruses,** such as infectious bovine rhinotracheitis virus and herpesvirus simplex, enter neurons in cranial or spinal ganglia via axons, in which they reside as episomal DNA, probably for the life of the host. Under appropriate circumstances the latent virus can be reactivated, in which case virions move down axons and enter a productive cycle in epithelial cells. This results in shedding of virus and, in some cases, overt lesions and disease. **Betaherpesviruses (cytomegaloviruses)** establish latent infections in epithelial cells of secretory glands, the kidney and lymphoreticular cells. **Gammaherpesviruses (lymphotropic herpesviruses)** usually establish latent infections in lymphoid cells.

The term **slow virus** infection represents a special form of persistent infection. Its use is restricted to viral infections with very long incubation periods that result in slowly progressive fatal disease, such as the lentiviruses (e.g., maedi/visna virus, HIV) and viruses causing scrapie, mink encephalopathy, and chronic wasting disease of captive mule deer and elk. Lentiviruses are retroviruses, whereas the other agents in this classification are most unconventional.

Cell lysis also follows an immune response to virus-infected cells. Most viruses, both cytocidal and noncytocidal, impart new antigens, recognized by the host as foreign, to the surface of infected cells. A cell-mediated response effected by specifically sensitized T lymphocytes leads to destruction of virus-infected cells. This represents one of the most important defense mechanisms in viral disease; the destruction of infected cells limits the release and spread of new virions (Chapter 7). Natural killer (NK) cells may also play a role in lysis of virus-infected cells, as may antibody and complement. The importance of these mechanisms in resistance to and recovery from viral infections is exemplified by the seriousness of viral diseases in immunodeficiencies, particularly those affecting T-cell functions (Chapter 7).

The immune response does not always result in beneficial effects. Certain noncytocidal viruses may infect cells without inflicting apparent harm. Lymphocytic choriomeningitis virus (LCMV) is the best studied example. Ordinarily, in mice the virus is transmitted horizontally (in utero), and there is immune tolerance to the virus and infected cells. However, when adult mice (and other species) are infected, serious disease results from a cytotoxic T-cell response. Immune complex disease also develops in these individuals.

A cytopathic effect of great diagnostic value is the formation of **inclusion bodies.** Although not a feature of all viral infections, they are characteristic of many. Inclusion bodies consist of aggregates of virions and viral proteins. In most replicating cycles, a great surplus of viral proteins do not assemble into virions. Inclusion bodies may be intranuclear, intracytoplasmic, basophilic, or eosinophilic. They are intranuclear in herpesvirus, adenovirus, and parvovirus infections; and intracytoplasmic in poxvirus, paramyxovirus, reovirus, and rhabdovirus infections. Certain viruses induce both intranuclear and intracytoplasmic inclusion bodies, such as the viruses causing canine distemper and measles and, often, cytomegaloviruses. The relative proportions of virions and proteins vary between viral infections. Adenovirus inclusion bodies are crystalline aggregates of virions. Poxvirus inclusions may be composed predominantly of either virions (basophilic) or of viral proteins (eosinophilic). Herpesvirus inclusion bodies contain a mixture of virions and protein with the latter predominating late in the replicative cycle.

Syncytial cell formation (e.g., multinucleated cells, polykaryocytes) is another cytopathic effect of certain viral infections. Such cells are a regular and often diagnostically important feature of herpesvirus and paramyxovirus lesions.

Certain viruses have the ability to transform cells in vitro from normal cells to cells with characteristics of cancer cells or to induce tumors in animals either naturally or experimentally. They are referred to as oncogenic viruses and include both DNA and RNA viruses. DNA viruses capable of inducing tumors include polyomaviruses, papillomaviruses, adenoviruses, herpesviruses, and hepatitis B-like viruses. Cell transformation by DNA viruses is nonproductive; viral progeny are not produced. Under appropriate in vitro and in vivo settings, however, oncogenic herpesviruses, polyomaviruses, and adenoviruses may induce productive infection, causing cell death. In transformed cells, the DNA of polyomaviruses, adenoviruses, and hepatitis virus is integrated into cellular DNA; the DNA of oncogenic herpesviruses and papillomaviruses is episomal. The RNA tumor viruses are members of the retrovirus family and are collectively known as **oncornaviruses** (page 330). In contrast to DNA tumor viruses, oncornaviruses simultaneously transform cells during a productive, but noncytocidal, infection. The viral genome becomes integrated into host-cell DNA as a DNA copy of viral RNA.

References

Brown F, Hull R. Comparative virology of the small RNA viruses. J Gen Virol 1973;20:43–60.

Brown F, Tinsley TW, ed. Comparative virology (symposium). J Gen Virol 1973;20(Suppl):1–130.

Dalton AJ, Haguenau F, ed. An atlas of ultrastructure of animal viruses and bacteriophages. Vol. 5. Ultrastructure in biological systems. New York: Academic Press 1973.

Fenner F, Bachmann PA, Gibbs EPJ, et al. Veterinary virology. 1st ed. New York: Academic Press 1987.

Fenner FJ, Gibbs EPJ, Murphy FA, et al. Veterinary virology, 2nd ed. New York: Academic Press 1993.

Fields BN, Knipe DM, ed. Virology. 2nd ed. Vol 1 and 2. New York: Raven Press 1990.

Francki RIB, Fauquet CM, Knudson DL, et al, ed. Classification and nomenclature of viruses. Arch Virol, Suppl 2, Report 5. New York: Springer-Verlag 1991.

Lwoff A. The concept of viruses. J Gen Microbiol 1957;17:239–253.

Maramorosch K, ed. The atlas of insect and plant viruses. Vol. 8. Ultrastructure in biological systems. New York, Academic Press 1977.

Matthews REF. Classification and nomenclature of viruses. Intervirology 1982;17:1–115.

Varmus H. Reverse transcription. Sci Am 1987;257(3):56–64.

White DO, Fenner F. Medical virology. 3rd ed. New York: Academic Press 1986.

Poxviridae

Viruses classified in this family, *Poxviridae,* are responsible for infections in humans, animals, birds, and insects. These viruses produce generalized disease with pustular (pock = pustule) lesions or benign tumors of the skin. The pox viruses are the largest animal viruses (Matthews, 1982); they have complex, brick-shaped virions up to 450 nm by 260 nm; contain single, linear molecules of double-stranded DNA; have a molecular weight of 85 to 240 million daltons; and multiply and mature in the cytoplasm of host cells. Sites of multiplication are visible by light microscopy as inclusion bodies. The virions contain several enzymes including a DNA-dependent transcriptase. Mature virions may be released by budding, in which case they are enveloped, or after cell lysis, in which case they lack an envelope. Five genera contain pathogens for animals, but several viruses have not been classified (Table 8-2).

Diseases caused by orthopoxviruses

SMALLPOX (VARIOLA)

This human disease, now extinct, was a highly contagious viral infection with a febrile onset followed in a few days by characteristic cutaneous eruptions. Beginning as macules, these soon became papules, then vesicles, and finally, within about 10 days, pustules, which underwent typical umbilication. The disease was observed in three clinical types: discrete, confluent, and hemorrhagic, in order of increasing mortality. A mild form of the disease, varioloid, was seen in persons who had been partially immunized by vaccination. A milder form of the disease, known as **alastrim** or **variola minor,** was caused by an immunologically indistinguishable, but less virulent, strain of virus.

The cutaneous lesion in smallpox begins as a circumscribed zone of congestion and lymphocytic infiltration in the dermal papillae underlying the affected epidermis. Epidermal cells swell, are isolated by extrusion of fluid between cell surfaces, and eventually become necrotic. Before necrosis occurs, the epithelial cells contain basophilic or eosinophilic cytoplasmic inclusions, **Guarnieri bodies,** composed of myriads of minute spherical granules, and **Borrel** or **Paschen bodies,** believed to be the elementary visible form of the virus. As necrosis occurs in the affected epithelium, a clear vesicle forms and soon fills with neutrophils. This pustular lesion, which is from 2 to 4 mm in diameter, appears grossly to be both elevated above the surface and embedded in the skin. The contents of the pustule become desiccated, producing an umbilicated lesion; healing follows; and a deep, pitted scar is left. Hemorrhagic pneumonia and cutaneous and renal hemorrhages have been observed in fatal cases.

Vaccinia Vaccinia is the virus used for immunization of humans against smallpox. The origin of the virus is obscure. Classically, it was considered to have been derived from cowpox, but continuous passage over many years through humans, laboratory animals, and tissue culture has resulted in the "creation" of a laboratory virus, which although infectious to a wide spectrum of animals, does not exist as a natural disease. Two major types of vaccinia occur, a dermatotropic strain and a neurotropic strain, properties developed on the basis of the method of propagating the virus in laboratory rabbits. The vaccinia virus, or closely related viruses, have been isolated from spontaneous diseases in several animal species, and certain of the pox diseases discussed in this section may not be distinct entities, but rather vaccinia infections. Vaccinia is known to be infectious for rabbits, mice, cattle, sheep, swine, monkeys, and humans. The lesions produced in each of these species is similar to those described for smallpox. (Table 8-2).

BUFFALOPOX

This contagious disease of water buffaloes, which has been reported from India, Indonesia, Pakistan, Egypt, Italy, and Russia, is caused by a virus similar to vaccinia virus and has been found to produce disease in guinea pigs, rabbits, and infant white Swiss mice. Lesions predominantly occur on the teats and udders of milking buffaloes. Infant mice experimentally infected with this virus developed hindquarter paralysis within 4 days after inoculation, followed by death. Postmortem lesions consisted of white necrotic nodules predominantly in the lungs of infected mice.

RABBITPOX

Outbreaks of pox in rabbits have been described as caused by a virus indistinguishable from vaccinia. The disease may become generalized, with necrotizing lesions in the oral mucous membranes, lungs, liver, adrenal glands, testicles, and lymph nodes, in addition to cutaneous pocks. The skin lesions lack the vesicular character seen in most other poxvirus infections. Inclusion bodies have not been reported.

TABLE 8-2 **Pox diseases of vertebrates _(Chordopoxvirinae)_ caused by _Poxviridae_ ***

Orthopoxvirus	_Parapoxvirus_	_Capripoxvirus_	_Avipoxvirus_	_Leporipoxvirus_	_Suipoxvirus_	_Unclassified_
Vaccinia (Type sp.)	Contagious ovine ecthyma, orf (Type sp.)	Sheep-pox (Type sp.)	Fowlpox (Type sp.)	Myxoma of rabbits (Type sp.)	Swinepox (Type sp.)	Carnivorepox (related to cowpox)
Variola (Smallpox)	Bovine pustular stomatitis	Goatpox	Canarypox	Hare fibroma		Elephantpox (related to cowpox)
Ectromelia (Mousepox)	Contagious ecthyma, chamois	Lumpy skin disease of cattle	Juncopox	Rabbit (Shope) fibroma		
Monkeypox	(Neethling)		Pigeonpox			Molluscum contagiosum of human
			Quailpox	Squirrel fibroma		
Cowpox	Pseudocowpox (Milkers' nodules)		Sparrowpox			Yaba monkey tumor pox
Buffalopox			Starlingpox			
	Sealpox					
Rabbitpox			Turkeypox			Tanapox (serologically related to Yaba pox
Camelpox						
Raccoonpox†						

*Subfamily _Entomopoxvirinae,_ or poxviruses of insects, is not included in this table.
†Probably orthopoxvirus (see R.E.F. Matthews, 1982).

References

Arita I, Henderson DA. Smallpox and monkeypox in primates. Primates Med 1969;3:122–123.

Baxby D. Poxvirus hosts and reservoirs: brief review. Arch Virol 1977;55:169–179.

Bras G. The morbid anatomy of smallpox. Documentia de Medicina Geographica et Tropica 1952;4:303–351.

Breman JG, Arita I. The confirmation and maintenance of smallpox eradication. N Engl J Med 1980;303:1263–1273.

Chandra R, Singh IP, Garg SK, et al. Experimental pathogenesis of buffalo-pox virus in rabbits: clinico-pathological studies. Arch Virol 1986;30:390–396.

Christensen LR, Bond E, Matanic B. "Pockless" rabbit pox. Lab Anim Care 1967;17:281–296.

Councilman WT, Magrath GB, Brinkerhoff WR. The pathological anatomy and histology of variola. J Med Res 1904;11:12–134.

Dogra SC, Sharma VK, Pandey R. Susceptibility of infant white Swiss mice to buffalo-pox virus. Vet Rec 1978;102:382–383.

Downie AW, Dumbell KR. Pox viruses. Ann Rev Microbiol 1956;10:237–252.

Fenner F, Burnet FM. A short description of the pox-virus group (vaccinia and related viruses). Virology 1957;4:305–314.

Fenner F. The biological characters of several strains of vaccinia, cowpox, and rabbitpox viruses. Virology. 1958;5:502–529.

Green HSN. Rabbitpox. I. Clinical manifestations and cause of the disease. II. Pathology of the epidemic disease. J Exp Med 1934;60:427–440, 441–456.

Jezek Z, Khodakevich LN, Wickett JF. Smallpox and its post-eradication surveillance. Bull WHO 1987;65:425–434.

Joklik WK. The poxviruses. Bacteriol Rev 1966;30:33–66.

Lal SM, Singh IP. Buffalopox-A review. Trop Anim Health Prod 1977;9:107–112.

Lillie RD. Smallpox and vaccinia. Arch Pathol. 1930;10:241–291.

Maqsood M. Generalised buffalo-pox. Vet Rec 1958;70:321–322.

Minnigan H, Moyer RW. Intracellular location of rabbit poxvirus nucleic acid within infected cells as determined by in situ hybridization. J Virol 1985;55:634–643.

Moyer RW, Graves RL, Rothe CT. The white pock. Mutants of rabbit poxvirus. III. Terminal DNA sequence duplication and transposition in rabbit poxvirus. Cell 1980;22:545–553.

Rana UVS, Garg SK, Chandra R, et al. Pathogenesis of buffalo-pox virus in buffalo calves. Int J Zoon 1985;12:156–162.

Rana UVS, Garg SK, Chandra R, et al. Immune response in buffalo calves experimentally infected with buffalo-pox virus. J Commun Dis 1986;18:193–197.

Wolman M. Pathologic findings in hemorrhagic smallpox (purpura variolosa): report of case with special reference to Feulgen's reaction in tissues. Am J Clin Pathol 1951;21:1127–1138.

Woodroofe GM, Fenner F. Serological relationships within the poxvirus group: an antigen common to all members of the group. Virology 1962;16:334–341.

MOUSEPOX (INFECTIOUS ECTROMELIA)

The pox virus causing this disease is also classified in the genus **orthopoxvirus** because of its immunologic relationship to others in the group. Mousepox occurs in Europe and has, at times, caused serious outbreaks in laboratories in the United States. The disease may result in cutaneous or disseminated lesions. The clinical disease has been described as occurring in two forms: a rapidly fatal form, with few or no cutaneous lesions; and a chronic form, characterized by ulceration of the skin, particularly the feet, tail, and snout. These are not dissimilar forms of the disease, but rather represent different stages in the pathogenesis of the infection. The infection begins with a primary lesion of the skin characterized by edema, ulceration, and later scarring, which releases virus to the lymphatics and the blood, enabling it to localize and multiply in the liver and spleen. Virus is released from these organs, localizes in other viscera (salivary gland, lung, pancreas, lymph nodes, Peyer's patches, the small intestine, kidney, and urinary bladder) and in the skin. The localization in the epidermis results in secondary skin lesions characterized by a generalized papular rash, which may progress to ulceration of the skin and gangrene of the extremities. If multiplication in the liver and spleen is exceptionally rapid, death may occur at this stage without premonitory clinical signs or a skin rash, except for the primary lesion, which may be small, absent, or overlooked. The lesions in this fulminating form of the disease are principally confined to the liver and spleen. In the liver, focal areas of necrosis are randomly distributed without any lobular pattern. The splenic lesions are also characterized by focal necrosis, which affects both the lymphoid follicles and the intervening reticuloendothelial tissue. Other visceral lesions may include focal necrosis of lymph nodes, Peyer's patches, mucosa of the small intestine, lung, kidney, urinary bladder, pancreas, and salivary gland. Eosinophilic, intracytoplasmic inclusion bodies may occur in all of these locations. The primary and secondary skin lesions are characterized by spongiosis and ballooning degeneration of the epidermis, followed by necrosis and ulceration with a lymphocytic infiltration of the dermis. Eosinophilic intracytoplasmic inclusion bodies occur in the ballooned epithelial cells. During the stage of the secondary skin rash, conjunctivitis and blepharitis are common, and ulcers may occur on the tongue and buccal mucous membranes. Mortality ranges from 50% to 100% and varies with the strain of mouse. If death does not occur in the stage of virus multiplication in the spleen and liver, recovery usually follows, unless the secondary cutaneous lesions are exceptionally severe or if gangrene occurs. In recovered mice, hairless scars may be present in the skin, and dense scars are usually present in the spleen.

The definitive diagnosis is based on the demonstration of antihemagglutinins to vaccinia in the sera of convalescent mice; or cross-immunization of mice with the agents of vaccinia and mousepox; or viral isolation and identification.

References

Bhatt PN, Jacoby RO. Mousepox in inbred mice innately resistant or susceptible to lethal infection with ectromelia virus. I. Clinical responses. Lab Anim Sci 1987;37:11–15.

Briody BA. The natural history of mousepox. In: Viruses of laboratory rodents. Nat Cancer Inst Monogr 1966;20:105–116.

Fenner F. Mousepox (infectious ectromelia of mice): a review. J Immunol 1949;63:341–373.

Fenner F. The clinical features and pathogenesis of mouse pox (infectious ectromelia of mice). J Pathol Bact 1948;60:529–552.

Jacoby RO, Bhatt PN. Mousepox in inbred mice innately resistant or susceptible to lethal infection with ectromelia virus. II. Pathogenesis. Lab Anim Sci 1987;37:16–22.

New AE. Ectromelia (mousepox) in the United States. Lab Anim Sci 1981;31(part II):549–635.

MONKEYPOX

Monkeypox was first identified in a colony of *Macaca fascicularis* in Denmark in 1958. Subsequently, several other outbreaks of monkeypox have occurred in Europe and the United States. Old World monkeys,

New World monkeys, and great apes are susceptible. The disease is especially severe in apes. The disease has also been recognized as a rare zoonosis, occurring sporadically in humans in West and Central Africa, particularly Zaire. Monkeypox virus is a distinct virus immunologically related to other members of the orthopoxvirus genus, including smallpox, from which it must be differentiated. The virus of monkeypox is clearly different from other poxviruses that infect monkeys, such as the Yaba and tanapox viruses discussed later in this chapter.

Monkeypox is characterized by a generalized cutaneous rash and pocks. These eruptions may be seen anywhere on the skin and on oral, pharyngeal, or tracheal mucous membranes, but are most common on the hands, feet, legs, and buttocks. Generalized fatal infection can occur, particularly in infants, with necrotizing lesions in many visceral organs, especially lymph nodes, spleen, and Peyer's patches.

Microscopically, the lesions resemble those already described for smallpox. The presence of intracytoplasmic inclusion bodies assists in the diagnosis.

References

Anonymous. The current status of human monkeypox: memorandum from a WHO meeting. Bull WHO 1984;62:703–713.
Arita I, Jezek Z, Khodakevich L, et al. Human monkeypox: a newly emerged zoonosis in the tropical rain forests of Africa. Am J Trop Med Hyg 1985;34:781–789.
Cho CT, Wenner HA. Monkeypox virus. Bacteriol Rev 1973;37:1–18.
Heberling RL, Kalter SS. Induction, course, and transmissibility of monkeypox in baboon (Papio cynocephalus). J Infect Dis 1971;124:33–38.
Lourie B, Bingham PG, Evans HH, et al. Human infection with monkey poxvirus. Laboratory investigations of six cases in West Africa. Bull WHO 1972;46:633–639.
Magnus P, von Anderson EK, Peterson KB. A pox-like disease in cynomologous monkeys. Acta Path Microbiol Scand 1959;46:156–176.
Marennikova SS, Gurvish EB, Shelukhina EM. Comparison of the properties of five pox virus strains isolated from monkeys. Arch Virol 1971;33:201–210.
Marennikova SS, Šeluhina EM, Mal'ceva NN, et al. Isolation and properties of the causal agent of a new variola-like disease (monkeypox) in humans. Bull WHO 1972;46:599–611.
Marennikova SS, Seluhina EM, Mal'ceva NN, et al. Poxviruses isolated from clinically ill and asymptomatically infected monkeys and a chimpanzee. Bull WHO 1972;46:613–620.
Mutombo WM, Arita I, Jezek Z. Human monkeypox transmitted by a chimpanzee in a tropical rain-forest area of Zaire. Lancet 1983;i:735–737.
Nicholas AH. Poxvirus of primates. I. Growth of virus in vitro and comparison with other poxviruses. II. Immunology J Natl Cancer Inst 1970;45:897–914.
Prier JE, Sauer RM, Malsberger RG, et al. Studies on a pox disease of monkeys. II. Isolation of the etiologic agent. Am J Vet Res. 1960;21:381–384.
Sauer RM, Prier JE, Buchanan RS, et al. Studies on a pox disease of monkeys. I. Pathology Am J Vet Res 1960;21:377–380.
Stagles MJ, Watson AA, Boyd JF, et al. The histopathology and electron microscopy of a human monkeypox lesion. Trans R Soc Trop Med Hyg 1985;79:192–202.

COWPOX

This disease in cattle is caused by a virus with an unusually wide host range. It is closely related to, but distinguishable from, variola and vaccinia. The disease, which is not common, is mild and self-limiting, and its lesions are found only on the teats and udder. Microscopically, the lesions resemble smallpox, with vesiculation and cytoplasmic inclusions. The disease is spread by milking. Human infection may occur, with lesions usually limited to the hands.

Cowpox, or a very similar virus, has also been recognized in domestic cats in Holland, Belgium, Great Britain, and Austria, causing a rash of varying distribution, lesions in the mouth, conjunctivitis, and in some cases, pneumonia. There are at least two reports of transmission from infected cats to humans. Cowpox virus has infected large cats (e.g., lions, cheetahs) and elephants in zoological gardens and circuses, where the virus often causes severe and fatal pneumonia. The reservoir host for cowpox virus is not known, but is believed to be wild rodents, which serve as the source of infection for other species.

The disease in cows must be differentiated from pseudocowpox and bovine herpesvirus 2 (bovine mammillitis).

Experimental infection can be induced in rabbits, guinea pigs, mice, cats, and monkeys. Cattle are also susceptible to vaccinia; infection usually results from exposure to a person recently vaccinated.

References

Anonymous. What's new pussycat? Cowpox. Lancet 1986;ii:668.
Baxby D, Ashton DG, Jones D, et al. Cowpox virus infection in unusual hosts. Vet Rec 1979;104:175.
Bennett M, Gaskell CJ, Baxby D, et al. Poxvirus infection in the domestic cat: some clinical and epidemiological observations. Vet Rec 1986;118:387–390.
Brown A, Bennett M, Gaskell CJ. Fatal poxvirus infection in association with FIV infection. Vet Rec 1989;124:19–20.
Downie AW, Haddock DW. A variant of cowpox virus. Lancet 1952;May 24:1049–1050.
Downie AW. A study of the lesions produced experimentally by cowpox virus. J Pathol Bact 1939;48:361–378.
Gaskell RM, Gaskell CJ, Evans HH, et al. Natural and experimental pox virus infection in the domestic cat. Vet Rec 1983;112:164–170.
Hester HR, Boley LE, Graham R. Studies on cowpox. I. An outbreak of natural cowpox and its relation to vaccinia. Cornell Vet 1941;31:360–378.
Maltseva NN, Akatova-Shelukhina EM, Yumasheva MA, et al. The aetiology of epizootics of certain smallpox like infections in cattle and methods of differentiating vaccinia, cowpox and swine pox viruses. J Hyg Epidemiol Microbiol Immunol. 1966;10:202–209.
Martland MF, Fowler S, Poulton GJ, et al. Pox virus infection of a domestic cat. Vet Rec 1983;112:171–172.
Pether JVS, Trevains PH, Harrison SRB, et al. Cowpox from cat to man. Lancet 1986;i:38–39.
Willemse A, Egberink HF. Transmission of cowpox virus infection from domestic cat to man. Lancet 1985;i:1515.

CAMELPOX

Occurring in Africa and southwestern Asia, camelpox is a debilitating, often fatal poxvirus infection of camels. Mortality may be high and the lesions generalized in young camels, as described for smallpox; a milder, localized form of the disease develops in older camels. The virus is distinct and humans are not susceptible.

References

Jezek Z, Kriz B, Rothbauer V. Camelpox and its risk to the human population. J Hyg Epidemiol Microbiol Immunol 1983;27:29-42 [Vet Bull 1984;54:97].
Kriz B. A study of camelpox in Somalia. J Comp Pathol 1982;92:1–8.

Diseases caused by avipoxviruses

The host antigen-related viruses known to affect avian species are in general species-specific (Fig. 8-3), but may infect hosts of other avian species. These pox diseases are known as **fowlpox** (avianpox, contagious epithelioma), **canarypox, pigeonpox,** and **turkeypox.** It was with the agent of fowlpox that Woodruff and Goodpasture (1930) demonstrated that a single elementary (Borrel) body separated from the inclusion (Bollinger) body was capable of inducing typical infection. The spontaneous lesions in chickens occur in the skin of the head, particularly the comb and wattles, or in the mucosa of the mouth or nasal passages, where a diphtheritic membrane forms. Lesions on the feet, legs, and body are less common.

References

Fitzner RE, Miller RA, Pierce CA, et al. Avian pox in a red-tailed hawk *(Buteo jamaicensis)*. J Wildl Dis 1985;21:298-301.

Giddens WE Jr, Swango LJ, Henderson JD, et al. Canary pox in sparrows and canaries (Fringillidae) and in weavers (Polceidae). Pathology and host specificity of the virus. Vet Pathol. 1971;8:260–280.

Hofstad MS, Miller RA, Pierce CA, et al, ed. Diseases of poultry. 8th ed. Ames, Iowa: Iowa State University Press 1984.

Sadasiv EC, Chang PW, Gulka G. Morphogenesis of canary poxvirus and its entrance into inclusion bodies. Am J Vet Res 1985;46:529–535.

Woodruff CE, Goodpasture EW. The infectivity of isolated inclusion bodies in fowl pox. Am J Pathol 1929;5:1–9.

Woodruff CE, Goodpasture EW. Relation of virus of fowl pox to specific cellular inclusions in the disease. Am J Pathol 1930;6:713–720.

Woodruff CE. Comparison of the lesions of fowl pox and vaccinia in the chick, with especial reference to the virus bodies. Am J Pathol 1930;6:169–173.

Diseases caused by capripoxviruses

Three diseases result from infection by viruses of this genus, capripoxvirus: **Sheep-pox, goatpox,** and **lumpy skin disease** (Neethling).

Whether they represent three distinct, but immunologically related, viruses is uncertain. They may be variants of a single virus with varying degrees of species pathogenicity. Different isolates from the same species also vary considerably in virulence. Mosquitoes and other arthropods may mechanically transmit the virus.

SHEEP-POX

Sheep-pox is prevalent in parts of North Africa, Asia, and Southern Europe, but is not known to occur in the United States. It is a serious disease with cutaneous lesions appearing particularly in areas devoid of wool, such as the cheeks, lips, and nostrils. Ulcerative lesions on the tongue, gums, and cheeks are common. The disease has a tendency to become generalized, resembling smallpox in this respect, and mortality may reach 50% in adults and approach 100% in lambs. There is variation in susceptibility by breed; Merino sheep are highly susceptible, whereas Algerian sheep are comparatively resistant.

The lesions in the epidermis are similar to those of other poxviruses, with localized acanthosis and hyperplasia followed by vesiculation, starting in the middle layers of epithelium. In addition, the edematous underlying dermis and subcutis contain many distinctive cells, called "cellules claveleuses" of Borrel or "sheep-pox cells." These cells, concentrated especially around blood vessels and between collagen bundles, have nuclei with marginated chromatin, nucleoli, and a large

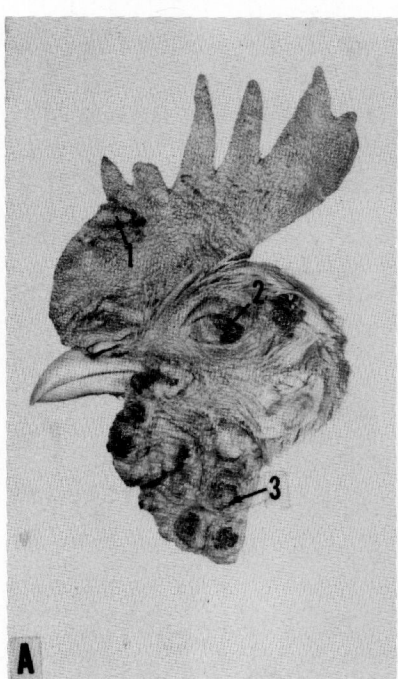 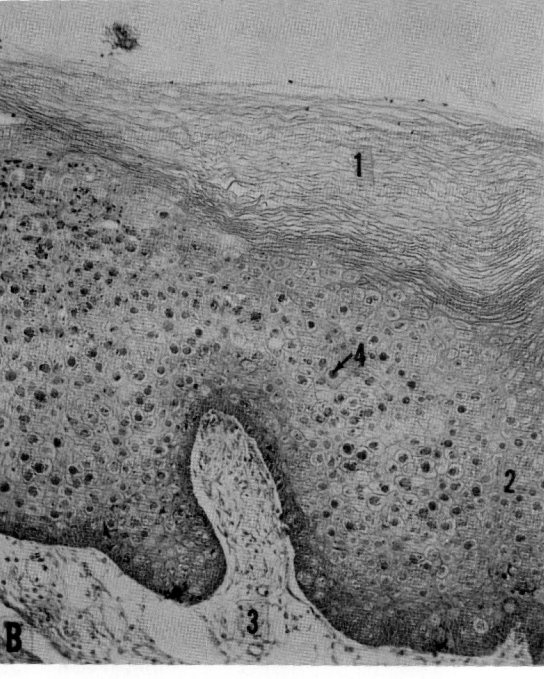

FIG. 8-3 Poxvirus. **A.** Fowl pox. Lesions on comb *(1)*, eyelid *(2)*, and wattle *(3)* of a chicken. (Contributed by Dr. CL Davis.) **B.** Canary pox. Lesions (× 100), skin of foot of canary. Wide layer of keratin *(1)*, hyperplastic epidermis *(2)*, edema in dermis *(3)*, and Bollinger bodies *(4)*. (Courtesy of Armed Forces Institute of Pathology; contributed by Dr. J. Andrade dos Santos.)

vacuole in the center of the nucleus. The cytoplasm of these cells varies in shape, some resembling monocytes, others resembling macrophages. Some cells are fusiform, with the appearance of fibroblasts. The cytoplasm of most of these cells contains eosinophilic inclusion bodies. These bodies, as seen under the electron microscope, are sites of viral replication, with a granular matrix and round developing virions as well as some characteristic ovoid-shaped mature pox virions. These mature virus particles are also seen elsewhere in the cytoplasm. Similar inclusions, of course, are seen in infected keratinocytes.

Severe necrotizing vasculitis involves dermal and subcutaneous blood vessels. This results in ischemic necrosis and intense infiltration by neutrophils in and around the affected blood vessels.

Pneumonia with "sheep-pox cells" and inclusion bodies in alveolar septal cells is the most important of the visceral lesions, but foci of necrosis and "sheep-pox cells" may also develop in the heart, liver, kidneys, adrenals, pancreas, and elsewhere.

GOATPOX

This disease exists in North Africa, the Middle East, parts of Europe, and India. The virus is immunologically related to and possibly the same as that of sheep-pox. It has been reported on rare occasions to infect men who are in close contact with goats. The disease has a somewhat longer incubation and is less severe than sheep-pox. The skin lesions are smaller in goatpox and are seldom hemorrhagic.

References

Bennett SCJ, Horgan ES, Mensur AH. The pox disease of sheep and goats. J Comp Pathol 1944;54:131–159.

Davies FG, Otema C. Relationships of capripox viruses found in Kenya with two Middle Eastern strains and some orthopox viruses. Res Vet Sci 1981;31:253–255.

Kitching RP, Taylor WP. Clinical and antigenic relationship between isolates of sheep and goat pox viruses. Trop Anim Health Prod 1985;17:64–74.

Kitching RP, Taylor WP. Transmission of capripoxvirus. Res Vet Sci 1985;39:196–199.

Kitching RP, McGrane JJ, Taylor WP. Capripox in the Yemen Arab Republic and the Sultanate of Oman. Trop Anim Health Prod 1986;18:115–122.

Krishnan E. Pathogenesis of sheep-pox. Indian Vet J 1968;45:297–302.

Murray M, Martin WB, Koylu A. Experimental sheep-pox: a histological and ultrastructural study. Res Vet Sci 1973;15:201–208.

Plowright W, MacLeod WG, Ferris RD. The pathogenesis of sheep-pox in the skin of sheep. J Comp Pathol 1959;69:400–413.

Sawhney AN, Singh AK, Malik BS. Goat-pox an anthropozoonosis. Indian J Med Res. 1972;60:683–684.

Sen DC. Immunobiological relationships of goat pox and sheep pox viruses. Indian J Med Res. 1968;56:1153–1156.

Sen KC, Datt NS. Studies on goat pox virus. I. Host range pathogenicity. II. Serological reactions. Indian J Vet Sci. 1968;38:388–393, 394–398.

Singh IP, Pandey R, Srivastava RN, et al. Sheep pox: a review. Vet Bull 1979;49:145–154.

Sharma SN, Dhanda MR. Studies on sheep and goat pox viruses: pathogenicity. Indian J. Animal Health. 1972;11:39–46.

Vigario JD, Ferraz FP. Study of sheep-pox virus synthesis by fluorescent antibody technique. Am J Vet Res. 1967;28:809–813.

LUMPY-SKIN DISEASE

Lumpy-skin disease is a disease of cattle and buffalo restricted to Africa, first seen in Northern Rhodesia (Zambia) in 1929. It is caused by a poxvirus (Neethling virus) related to the viruses of sheep-pox and goatpox. It is thought to be transmitted by insect vectors, principally flies. The disease is characterized by a generalized cutaneous eruption of round, firm nodules, varying from 0.5 cm to 5.0 cm in diameter. Nodules may also appear on oral, nasal, and genital mucous membranes, and there is enlargement of the superficial lymph nodes. The mortality rate is generally low, but may approach 10%. Microscopically, the nodule is characterized by the inflammatory reaction in the dermis; the nodule is composed of edema; perivascular collections of lymphocytes, macrophages, plasma cells, and neutrophils; and proliferating fibroblasts. There is acanthosis, parakeratosis, and hyperkeratosis of the epidermis followed by necrosis and vesicle formation. Eosinophilic cytoplasmic inclusion bodies form in keratinocytes, fibroblasts, and macrophages. Necrosis of the entire nodule precedes healing, which usually requires 3 to 5 weeks, but some nodules may persist for months. Rabbits, impalas, and giraffes are experimentally susceptible to the virus.

The disease may be differentiated from a herpesvirus infection (called Allerton virus), which is common in cattle in Kenya, by the microscopic lesions and by finding the characteristic pox virions in those lesions.

References

Ali AA, Esmat M, Attia H, et al. Clinical and pathological studies on lumpy skin disease in Egypt. Vet Rec 1990;127:549–550.

Ayre-Smith RA. The symptoms and clinical diagnosis of lumpy-skin disease. Vet Rec 1960;72:469–472.

Davies FG, Krauss H, Lund J, et al. The laboratory diagnosis of lumpy skin disease. Res Vet Sci 1971;12:123–127.

Munz EK, Owen NC. Electron microscopic studies on lumpy-skin disease virus type "neethling." Onderstepoort J Vet Res 1966;33:3–8.

Prozesky L, Barnard BJH. A study of the pathology of lumpy skin disease in cattle. Onderstepoort J Vet Res 1982;49:167–175.

Weiss KE. Lumpy skin disease. Virology Monographs 1968;3:109–131.

Woods JA. Lumpy skin disease—a review. Trop Anim Health Prod 1988;20:11–17.

Diseases caused by leporipoxviruses

INFECTIOUS MYXOMATOSIS OF RABBITS

The spontaneous occurrence of infectious myxomatosis in South American rabbits was first described by Sanarelli in 1898. During the intervening years the malady has been observed in many other parts of the world, where it has decimated the wild rabbit population and threatened the domesticated rabbit population. In *Oryctolagus* species, the disease is characterized by the appearance of firm, elevated nodules in the skin, particularly in the vicinity of the eyes, mouth, nose, ears, and genitalia. Purulent conjunctivitis is a rather constant feature. The disease runs a rapid, highly fatal course, with death occurring a week or two after onset of symptoms.

The causative agent is a poxvirus that can be readily

transmitted to susceptible rabbits but not to other animals. Its relation to the virus of the Shope fibroma is indicated by the immunity of rabbits against myxomatosis after infection with the fibroma virus. The virus exists in a natural state in wild rabbits in South America *(Sylvilagus braziliani)* and California *(Sylvilagus bachmani)*, occurring as an enzootic disease characterized by local cutaneous swelling without systemic lesions or mortality. The disease is exceptionally rare in hares *(Lepus* species), which are naturally resistant to the virus. In the European, or common laboratory rabbit *(Oryctolagus cuniculus)*, both wild and domestic, the virus produces a systemic disease with a mortality rate of more than 99%. In Australia and probably Europe, following the deliberate introduction of the virus into wild populations of *Oryctolagus cuniculus,* attenuated strains of myxoma virus have evolved, which are less virulent and result in a disease with a lower mortality rate. Also the extreme lethality of myxomatosis has resulted in the evolution of a population of rabbits in these geographic areas with genetic resistance to the disease. In contrast, the virulence of the virus can increase, especially in more resistant populations of rabbits. This has been seen in Great Britain, where myxomatosis was first identified in 1953. Mosquitoes and fleas serve as mechanical vectors for natural transmission of the virus.

Lesions The lesions in the skin are described by Rivers as numerous elevated, round, or ovoid masses that sometimes cause the skin to appear purplish. Most of these nodules are firm and solid, but those near the genitalia may be edematous. Vesiculation of the epidermis over the lesions is evident grossly, and the vesicles are replaced by crusts, if the animal survives long enough. On cut section, the consistency of the cutaneous nodules is firm and tough, the epidermis is thickened or vesiculated, and the corium and subcutis contain gelatinous material interspersed with numerous blood vessels. The nodules are sometimes attached to the underlying musculature. The lymph nodes become enlarged, solid, and uniform in consistency.

Microscopically (Figs. 8-4 and 8-5), the earliest change is increase in size and number of cells in the Malpighian layer, accompanied by the appearance of acidophilic granules, which increase in number and eventually fill the cytoplasm. Blue, rod-shaped bodies are sometimes seen among the acidophilic granules. The nuclei become swollen or vacuolated, and their chromatin is fragmented. The cells undergo dissolution to form vesicles in the epidermis, which subsequently coalesce into rather large bullae. In the underlying corium, large, stellate or polygonal cells appear along with much amorphous material, many neutrophils, and multinucleated cells. The nuclei of the stellate cells are swollen and contain some mitoses, and granules assumed to be ingested material are seen in the cytoplasm. These cells are often concentrated around blood vessels, and the endothelial cells of some vessels increase in number and size.

In the lymph nodes, hyperplasia of lymphoid cells occurs; the reticulum cells in the follicles increase in number and mix with a few neutrophils and eosino-phils. The medulla is edematous, especially around vessels, and contains collections of neutrophils, eosinophils, mononuclear cells, and fibroblasts. Edema appears around small vessels and fibrin thrombi may be seen in the sinuses. Later many lymphocytes are lost, and overgrowth of reticuloendothelial cells interspersed with islands of neutrophils replaces most of the node. Later the reticulum may undergo cystic degeneration.

Diagnosis Diagnosis is made on the basis of clinical features, along with the gross and microscopic lesions, which are characteristic of the disease. Confirmation can be obtained by transmission of the disease to susceptible rabbits or by virus isolation.

References

Fenner F, Ratcliffe FN. Myxomatosis. Cambridge: Cambridge Univ Press 1965.

Fenner F. Myxomatosis. Br Med Bull 1959;15:240–245.

Hurst EW. Myxoma and the Shope fibroma. I. Histology of myxoma. Br J Exp Pathol 1937;18:1–15.

Rivers TM. Observations on the pathological changes induced by virus myxomatosum (Sanarelli). J Exp Med. 1930;51:965–976.

Ross J, Sanders MF. Changes in the virulence of myxoma virus strains in Britain. Epidemiol Infect 1987;98:113–117.

Ross J, Tittensor AM. The establishment and spread of myxomatosis and its effect on rabbit populations. Philos Trans R Soc Lond B 1986;314:599–606.

Sanarelli G. Das myxomatogene virus; Beitrag zum Studium der Krankheitserreger ausserhalb des Sichtbaren. Zentralbl Bakt. 1898; 23:865–873.

Sellers RF. Possible windborne spread of myxomatosis to England in 1952. Epidemiol Infect 1987;98:119–125.

Stewart FW. The fundamental pathology of infectious myxomatosis. Am J Cancer 1931;15:2013–2028.

SHOPE FIBROMA

Fibromas occurring naturally in the skin of wild cottontail rabbits *(Sylvilagus)* were described by Shope in 1932 and shown to be caused by a filtrable virus, classified as a poxvirus. These lesions are also transmitted experimentally to domestic rabbits *(Oryctolagus)*, and the agent was demonstrated to be related to that of infectious myxomatosis. The fibroma virus produces an effective immunity to subsequent infection by myxomatosis, although in other respects there is no resemblance between the two diseases.

Lesions The lesions in the Shope fibroma are often multiple and are described as elevations of the skin by a fibrous mass; the overlying epidermis is thickened and sends bulbous, proliferating epithelium deep into the tumor. The tumors are benign proliferations of fibroblasts that eventually regress. Variant viruses, which cause invasive or generalized tumors, have been identified. One of these, termed malignant rabbit fibroma virus (malignant rabbit virus), was derived from a recombination of Shope fibroma virus and myxoma virus (Strayer and Sell, 1983; Strayer and others, 1983a). Large eosinophilic inclusions occur in the cytoplasm of the affected keratinocytes.

Viruses similar to the Shope fibroma virus have been reported to cause fibromas in brush rabbits *(Sylvilagus)* in California, fibromas in hares *(Lepus)* in Europe and Africa, and fibromas in gray squirrels in North America. A skin disease resembling a parapoxvirus in-

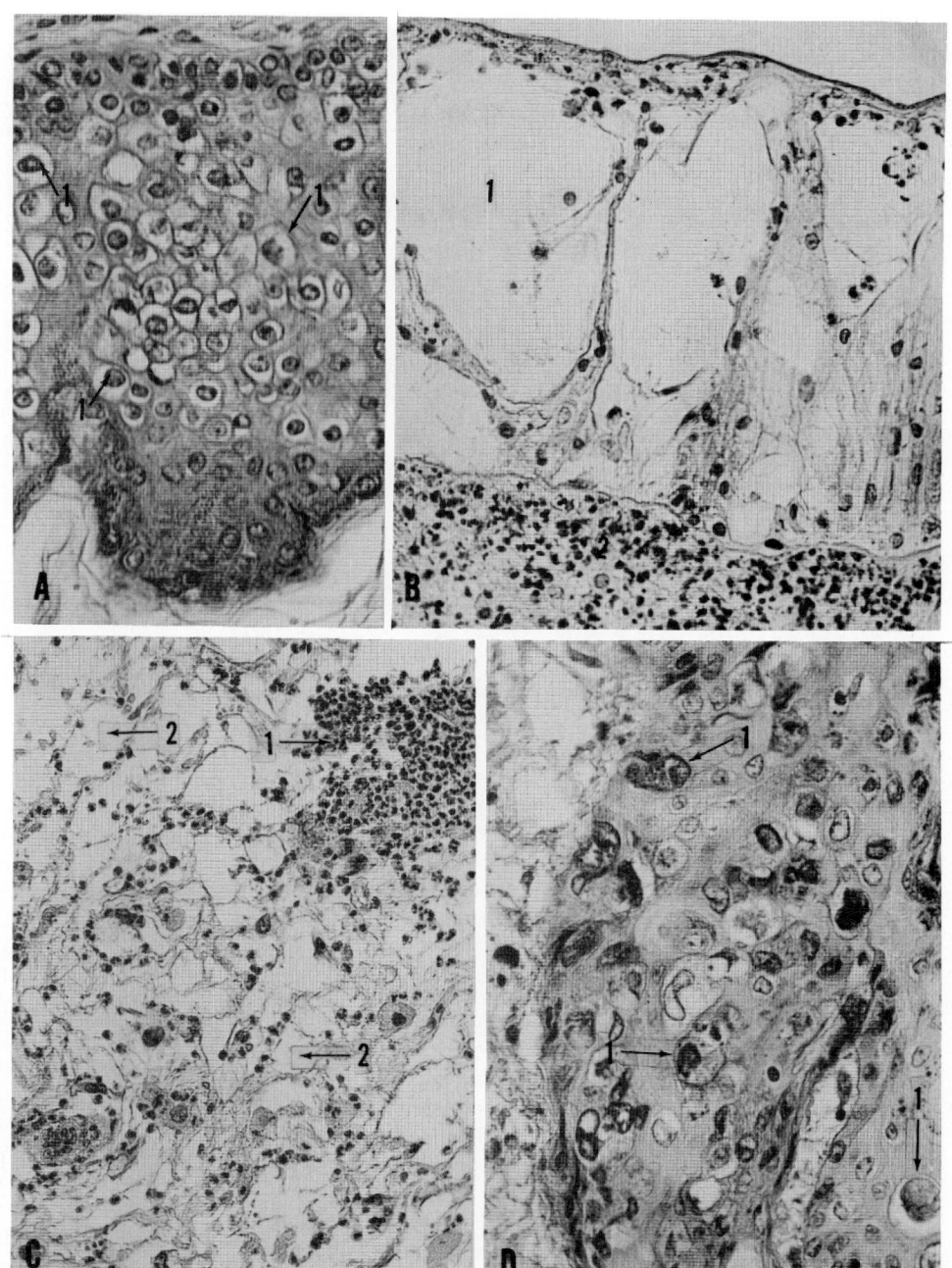

FIG. 8-4 Infectious myxomatosis of rabbits. **A.** Hyperplastic epidermis (× 365). Note large cells with vacuoles surrounding nuclei *(1)*. **B.** Large vesicle *(1)* in epidermis in a later stage (× 395). **C.** Microabscess *(1)* and edematous spaces *(2)* in dermis (× 235). **D.** Giant, distorted nuclei *(1)* in the epidermis (× 395). (Courtesy of Armed Forces Institute of Pathology; contributed by Dr. J. Andrade dos Santos.)

fection has also been seen in squirrels in California, Maryland, and Great Britain.

References

Cilli V. Aspetti Virologici del Fibroma di Shope e suoi Rapporti con il Mixoma di Sanarelli. G Mal Infet Parassit 1958;10:1017–1040.

Karstad L, Thorsen J, Davies G, et al. Poxvirus fibromas on African hares. J Wildl Dis 1977;13:245–247.

Novilla MN, Flyger V, Jacobson ER, et al. Systemic phycomycosis and multiple fibromas in a gray squirrel *(Sciurus carolinensis)*. J Wildl Dis 1981;17:89–95.

O'Connor DJ, Diters RW, Nielsen SW. Poxvirus and multiple tumors in an Eastern gray squirrel. J Am Vet Med Assoc 1980;177: 792–795.

Scott AC, Keymer IF, Labram J. Parapox infection of the red squirrel *(Sciurus vulgaris)*. Vet Rec 1981;109:202.

Shope RE. A transmissible tumor-like condition in rabbits. J Exp Med 1932;56:793–802.

Shope RE. A filterable virus causing a tumor-like condition in rabbits and its relationship to virus myxomatosum. J Exp Med 1932;56:803–833.

Strayer DS, Cabirac G, Sell S, et al. Malignant rabbit fibroma virus: observations on the culture and histopathologic characteristics of a new virus-induced rabbit tumor. JNCI 1983a;71:91–104.

Strayer DS, Corbeil LB, Cabirac GF, et al. Malignant rabbit fibroma virus: report of a new virus-induced tumor causing secondary immunodeficiency. Fed Proc 1982;41(809A):408.

Strayer DS, Skaletsky E, Cabirac GF, et al. Malignant rabbit fibroma virus causes secondary immunosuppression in rabbits. J Immunol 1983b;130:399–404.

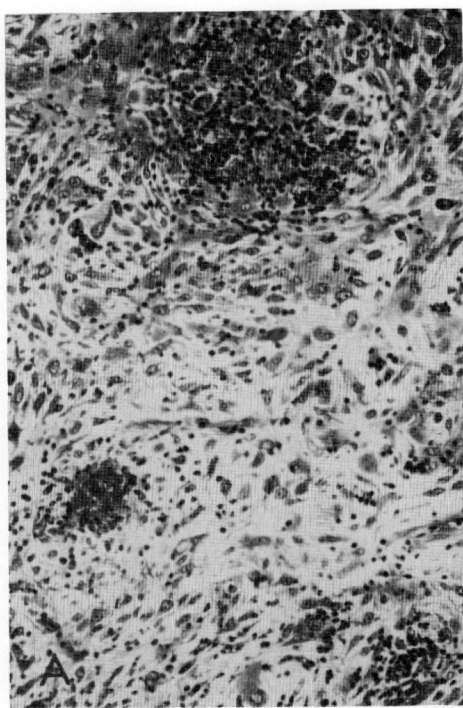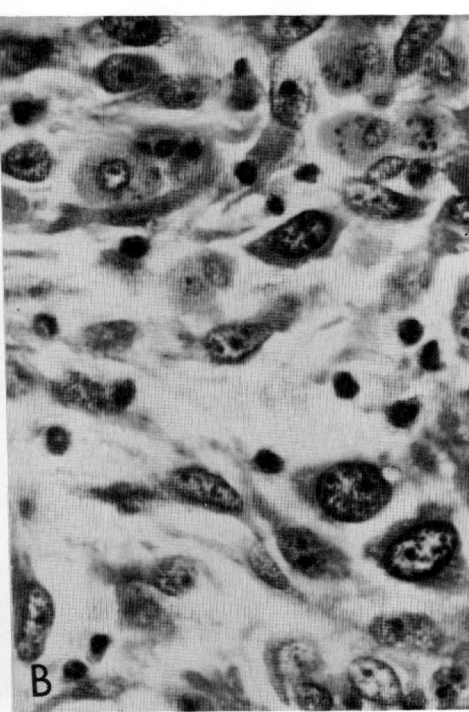

FIG. 8-5 Infectious myxomatosis, rabbit. **A.** Replacement of a lymph node by large "myxoma" cells. **B.** Higher magnification of "myxoma" cells in a lymph node. (Courtesy of Dr. F. Fenner.)

Upton C, McFadden G. Tumorigenic poxviruses: analysis of viral DNA sequences implicated in the tumorigenicity of Shope fibroma virus and malignant rabbit virus. Virology 1986;152:308–321.

Diseases caused by parapoxviruses

CONTAGIOUS OVINE ECTHYMA

Synonyms for the name of this disease are contagious pustular dermatitis, infectious labial dermatitis, "scabby mouth," "sore mouth," and "orf." Contagious ecthyma is an infectious poxvirus disease of sheep and goats in which vesicular or pustular lesions develop on the lips, oral mucous membranes, udder, and rarely, feet. It is also transmissible to humans, and there are rare reports of its occurrence in dogs. The virus is immunologically related to the viruses of bovine papular stomatitis (Fig. 8-6) and pseudocowpox. The virus also appears to be related to the virus of ulcerative dermatosis of sheep. Mild transitory pustular lesions, particularly on the forearm, characterize the human disease, which has occurred after contact with infected sheep. Infection has been reproduced in sheep with material taken from such human lesions. The disease is known in the United States, Europe, and Australia. Mortality is low unless complicated by screwworm larvae *(Callitroga hominivorax, Cochilomyia macellaria)* or bacterial infection *(Fusobacterium necrophorum)*. The disease is most severe in lambs and kids. Usually lesions resolve in 2 to 4 weeks, but there are reports of lesions persisting for several months.

Lesions The gross lesions appear as significantly raised papules, vesicles, and then pustules, with necrosis and eventual sloughing of the affected areas. Microscopically, the lesions are sharply delimited, with the affected epidermis overlying a densely cellular dermis, richly vascular, and infiltrated with leukocytes and edema. The epidermis proliferates, becoming several times normal thickness with long extensions into the dermis. Although hyperplasia of the epidermis is seen in most poxvirus infections, it is particularly striking in ecthyma. The epidermis undergoes degenerative changes consisting of vacuolation, ballooning, degeneration, vesiculation, and pustule formation. Eosinophilic cytoplasmic inclusion bodies are present in keratinocytes, but they are transitory.

Diagnosis The diagnosis of contagious ecthyma is based on the characteristic lesions and isolation and identification of the virus. The disease must be differentiated from sheep-pox and ulcerative dermatosis. The virus is immunologically distinct from sheep-pox virus, and although related, separable from the virus of ulcerative dermatosis. The downgrowth of the basal layer of epidermis into the dermis, which does not occur in sheep-pox or ulcerative dermatosis, is a distinctive feature. The widespread cutaneous distribution of the lesions of sheep-pox and the preputial lesions of ulcerative dermatosis also aid in differential diagnosis.

References

Abdussalam M. Contagious pustular dermatitis. 2. Pathological histology. J Comp Pathol. 1957;67:217–222.

Abdussalam M.. Contagious pustular dermatitis. 3. Experimental infection (rabbits). J Comp Pathol. 1957;67:305–319.

Ames TR, Robinson RA, O'Leary TP, et al. Tail lesions of contagious ecthyma associated with docking. J Am Vet Med Assoc 1984;184:88–90.

Boughton IB, Hardy WT. Contagious ecthyma (sore mouth) of sheep and goats. J Am Vet Med Assoc 1934;85:150–178.

Buddle BM, Dellers RW, Schurig GG. [1] Heterogeneity of contagious

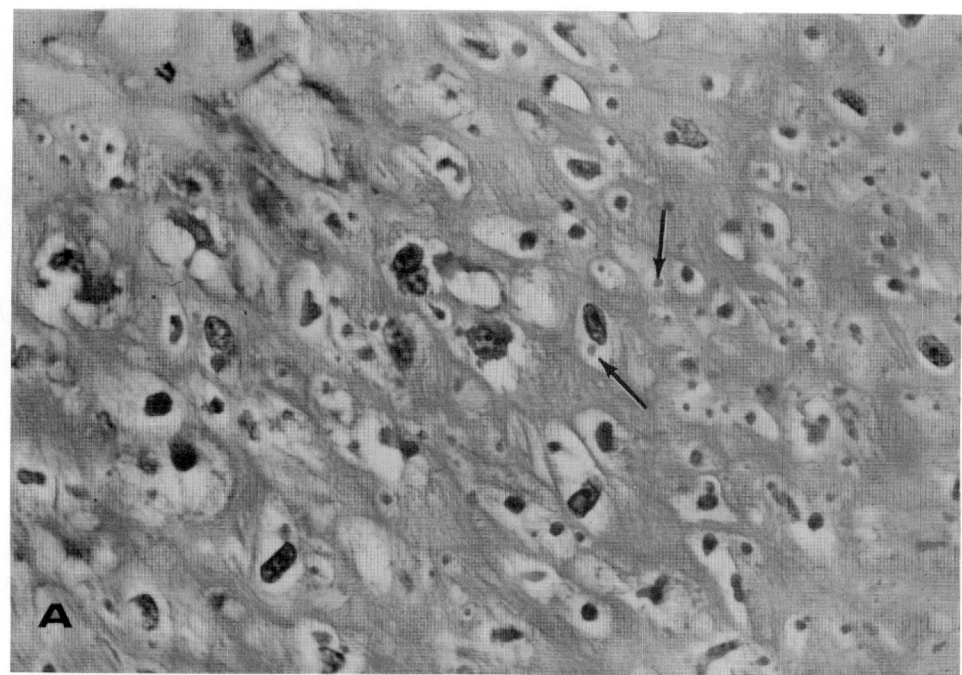

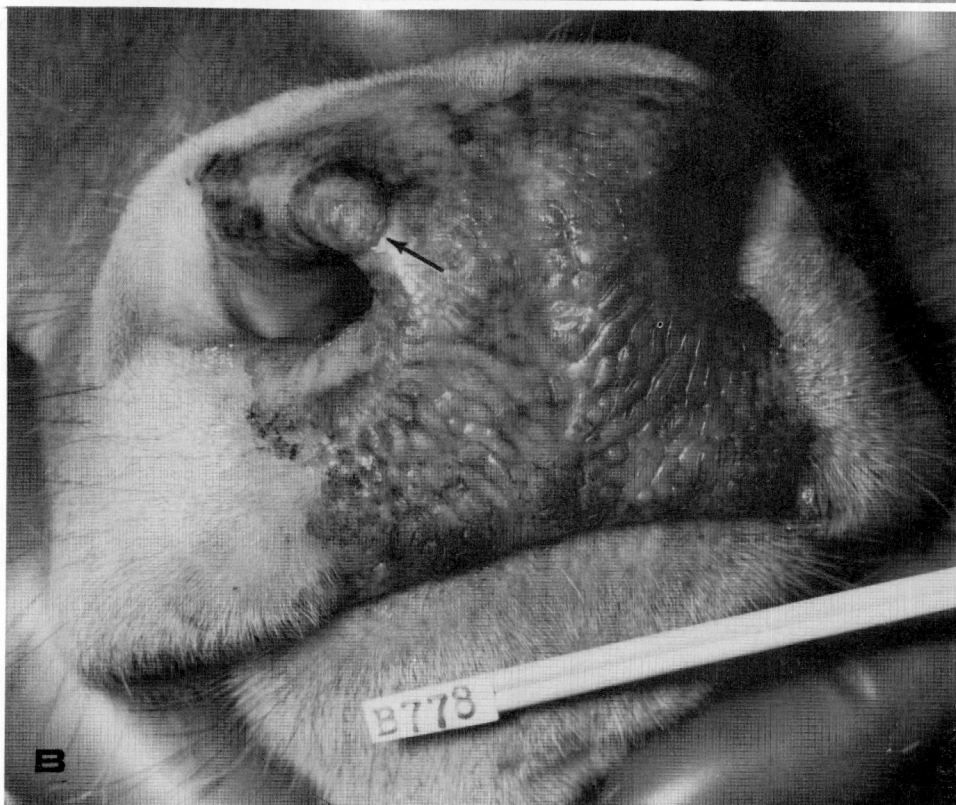

FIG. 8-6 Bovine papular stomatitis. **A.** Photomicrograph of epithelium containing eosinophilic inclusion bodies *(arrows).* **B.** Muzzle of a calf with an experimentally induced papular lesion of nostril *(arrow).* (Courtesy of Dr. Richard A. Griesemer, Ohio State University.)

ecthyma virus isolates. [2] Contagious ecthyma virus-vaccination failures. Am J Vet Res 1984;45:75–79, 263–266.

Clark RK, Jessup DA, Kock MD, et al. Survey of desert bighorn sheep in California for exposure to selected infectious diseases. J Am Vet Med Assoc 1985;187:1175–1179.

Dashtseren TS, Solovyev BV, Varejka F, et al. Camel contagious ecthyma (pustular dermatitis). Acta Virol 1984;28:122–127.

Greig A, Linklater KA, Clark WA. Persistent orf in a ram. Vet Rec 1984;115:149.

Lance WR, Hibler CP, DeMartini J. Experimental contagious ecthyma in mule deer, white-tailed deer, pronghorn and wapiti. J Wildl Dis 1983;19:165–169.

Moore DM, MacKenzie WF, Doepel F, et al. Contagious ecthyma in lambs and laboratory personnel. Lab Anim Sci 1983;33: 473–475.

Park VM, Mackerras IM, Sutherland AK, et al. Transmission of contagious ecthyma from sheep to man. Med J Aust. 1951;2:628–632.

Wheeler CE, Cawley EP. The microscopic picture of ecthyma contagiosum (orf) in sheep, rabbits, and men. Am J Pathol. 1956;32: 535–545.

Wilkinson GT, Prydie J, Scarnell J. Possible "orf" (contagious pustular dermatitis, contagious ecthyma of sheep) infection in the dog. Vet Rec 1970;87:766–767.

BOVINE PAPULAR STOMATITIS

Bovine papular stomatitis is a mild disease (also known as **infectious ulcerative stomatitis and esophagitis**) that causes lesions in and around the mouths of young cattle; it has been recognized from time to time in Europe and the United States. The disease does not cause serious illness, but simulates some features of certain important bovine diseases (aphthous fever, vesicular stomatitis, mucosal disease, and viral diarrhea).

The causative virus is closely related to and in fact may be the same as pseudocowpox virus (discussed next). It also infects humans, producing mild erythematous papules on the hands and arms, comparable to "milkers' nodules," which are associated with pseudocowpox virus.

The disease affects young calves for the most part; clinical signs are mild; and fever is not usually seen, although viremia evidently occurs.

Lesions Generally, the lesions are found on the lips, muzzle, nostrils, gingivae, tongue, and oral mucosa; in sacrificed animals, lesions are found in the esophagus, rumen, reticulum, and omasum. The earliest lesions are recognized grossly as small hyperemic foci of 2 to 4 mm in diameter, often on the lower margin of the nostrils and occasionally on the palate or inner surface of the lips. In about a day, the center of these foci become elevated from the surface to form a low, convex, whitish papule. At this time, the epidermis is focally hyperplastic and contains focal areas of hydropic degeneration. Nuclei in these zones are often pyknotic and occasionally undergo karyorrhexis. As the disease progresses, the hydropic lesions move toward the surface, and the affected keratinocytes often contain spherical cytoplasmic inclusion bodies that are 10 μ or more in diameter, homogeneous, and eosinophilic, and usually only one is found per cell. Congestion of the adjacent lamina propria usually gives the papular lesion a reddish or pink hue at this time. The lesions may become infiltrated with neutrophils and ultimately progress to erosions or ulcers. Healing is usually uneventful.

Diagnosis The diagnosis is usually based on the mild clinical course, the gross and histologic appearance of the lesions, and the isolation and identification of the virus.

References

Abraham A, Davidson M, Schclarek M. First isolation of bovine stomatitis papulosa virus in Israel. Vet Rec 1985;116:379.

Bohac JG, Yates WDG. Concurrent bovine virus diarrhea and bovine papular stomatitis infection in a calf. Can Vet J 1980;21:310–313.

Buttner D, et al. The fine structure of the virions of contagious pustular dermatitis and bovine papular stomatitis. Arch Ges Virusforsch 1964;14:657–673.

Carson CA, Kerr KM, Grumbles LC. Bovine papular stomatitis: experimental transmission from man. Am J Vet Res 1968;29:1783–1790.

Carson CA, Kerr KM. Bovine papular stomatitis with apparent transmission to man. J Am Vet Med Assoc 1967;151:183–187.

Chalmers GA. Papular stomatitis in beef calves. Can Vet J 1987;28:108.

Griesemer RA, Cole CR. Bovine papular stomatitis. I. Recognition in the United States. J Am Vet Med Assoc 1960;137:404–410.

Griesemer RA, Cole CR. Bovine papular stomatitis. II. The experimentally produced disease. Am J Vet Res 1961;22:473–481.

Griesemer RA, Cole CR. Bovine papillary stomatitis. III. Histopathology. Am J Vet Res 1961;22:482–486.

Plowright W, Ferris RD. Papular stomatitis of cattle in Kenya and Nigeria. Vet Rec 1959;71:718–722.

Pritchard WR, Claflin RM, Gustafson DP, et al. An infectious ulcerative stomatitis of cattle. J Am Vet Med Assoc 1958;132:273–278.

Schnurrenberger PR, Swango LJ, Bowman GM, et al. Bovine papular stomatitis incidence in veterinary students. Can J Comp Med 1980;44:239–243.

Snider TG III, McConnell S, Pierce KR. Increased incidence of bovine papular stomatitis in neonatal calves. Arch Virol 1982;71:251–258.

Pseudocowpox

The virus of pseudocowpox is called **paravaccinia,** but is not related to vaccinia or cowpox. It is closely related to contagious ovine ecthyma virus and bovine papular stomatitis virus. The lesions are limited to the teats and udders of milking cows and appear as red papules and vesicles. Microscopically, there is proliferation of the subepithelial capillary network, vesicular degeneration of the epithelium, and eosinophilic cytoplasmic inclusion bodies. Infection does not confer immunity. The disease is transmissible to humans as "milkers' nodules," and oral lesions may develop in suckling calves, which help to transmit the infection by cross-sucking.

References

Cheville NF, Shey DJ. Pseudocowpox in dairy cattle. Am Vet Med Assoc 1967;150:855–861.

Duncan AG. Milkers' nodules. Canad Med Assoc J 1957;77:339–342.

Francis PG. Teat skin lesions and mastitis. Br Vet J 1984;140:430–436.

Friedman-Keen AE, Rowe SP, Banfield WG. Milkers' nodules. Isolation of poxvirus from a human case. Science 1963;140:1335–1336.

Huck RA. A paravaccinia virus isolated from cows' teats. Vet Rec 1966;78:503–504.

Laurence B. Cowpox in humans and its relationship with milkers' nodules. Lancet 1955;268:764–766.

Liebermann H. Relationships between milkers' nodules, udder pox, papular stomatitis and contagious ecthyma. Zarztl Fortbildung 1967;61:447–448.

Mullowney PC. Dermatologic diseases of cattle. Part II. Infectious diseases. Compend Contin Educ Pract Vet 1982;4(1):S3–S10.

Nagington J, Lauder TM, Smith JS. Bovine papular stomatitis, pseudocowpox and milker's nodules. Vet Rec 1967;81:306–313.

Nagington J, Tee GH, Smith JS. Milker's nodule virus infection in Dorset and their similarity to orf. Nature 1965;208:505–507.

Neal EJE, Calvert HT. Milker's nodules. Some observations on true and false cowpox apropos an outbreak in a closed community. Br J Derm 1967;79:318–324.

Diseases Caused by Suipoxvirus

SWINEPOX

Swinepox virus is the only member of this genus. This common disease in the Corn Belt of the United States principally affects young swine (Fig. 8-7). The virus of swinepox is not related to that of vaccinia and may be transmitted by the swine louse, *Haematopinus*

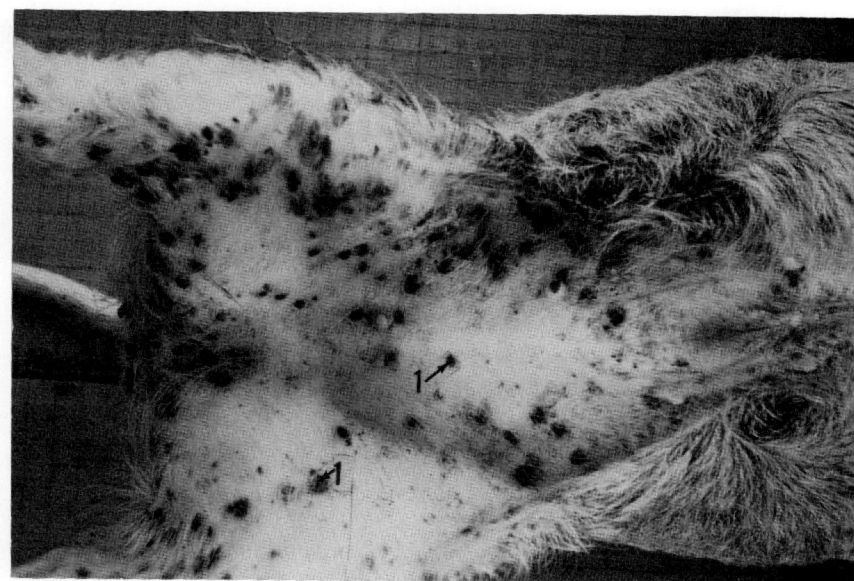

FIG. 8-7   Swine pox, abdomen of a pig. Note hemorrhagic appearance of pox lesions *(1)*.

suis, though a vector is not necessary for transmission. The incubation period is 5 to 7 days, after which erythematous areas and then papules, 4 to 5 mm in diameter, appear. These lesions usually are limited to the underside of the body but may involve the skin generally. In the vesicular and pustular stages, the lesions often escape observation and are detected only when they have become umbilicated. Eosinophilic cytoplasmic inclusion bodies develop in epithelial cells. Rare cases of congenital infection of newborn pigs with generalized pox lesions have been reported. Swine are also susceptible to vaccinia virus; this is the most common and severe form of pox in swine in Europe. True swinepox also occurs in Europe.

References

Blakemore F, Abdussalam M. Morphology of the elementary bodies and cell inclusions in swine pox. J Comp Pathol 1956;66: 373–377.

Borst GHA, Kimman TG, Gielkens ALJ, et al. Four sporadic cases of congenital swinepox. Vet Rec 1990;127:61–63.

Cheville NF. The cytopathology of swine pox in the skin of swine. Am J Pathol 1966;49:339–352.

Kasza L, Griesemer RA. Experimental swine pox. Am J Vet Res 1962;23:443–451.

McNutt SH, Murray C, Purwin P. Swine pox. J Am Vet Med Assoc 1929;74:752–761.

Murray C. Swine pox. J Am Vet Med Assoc 1937;90:326–330.

Nakamatsu M, Gogo M, Morita M. Electron microscopy of the inclusion bodies in pigpox. Jap J Vet Sci 1968;30:289–297.

Neufeld JL. Spontaneous pustular dermatitis in a newborn piglet associated with a poxvirus. Can Vet J 1981;22:156–158.

Diseases caused by unclassified poxviruses

Unclassified poxvirus diseases considered here include tanapox and benign epidermal monkey pox (Fig. 8-8), molluscum contagiosum, and ulcerative dermatosis.

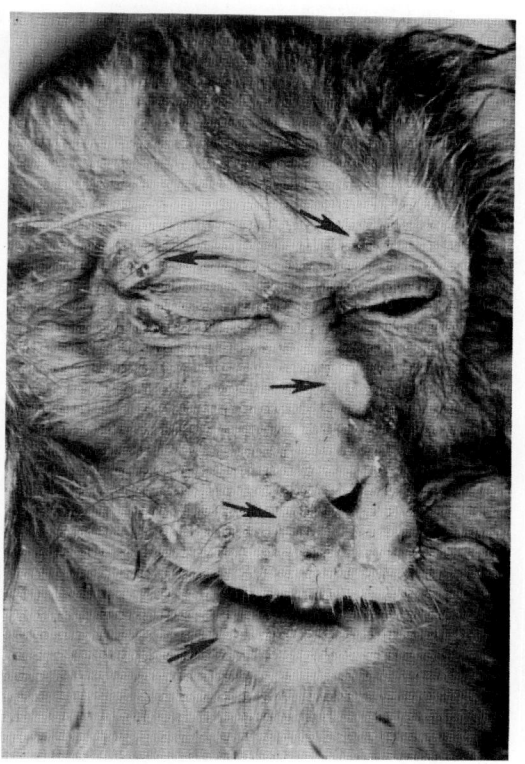

FIG. 8-8   Benign epidermal monkeypox. Numerous elevated pocks on the skin of the face of a macaque. (Courtesy of Dr. W. P. McNulty.)

TANAPOX AND BENIGN EPIDERMAL MONKEY POX

Tanapox, named after the Tana River in Kenya, is a poxvirus infection of humans in Eastern Africa to which macaques and African nonhuman primates are susceptible; these animals also serve as reservoirs of infection. A disease termed benign epidermal monkeypox, described in various captive macaques in Oregon, Texas,

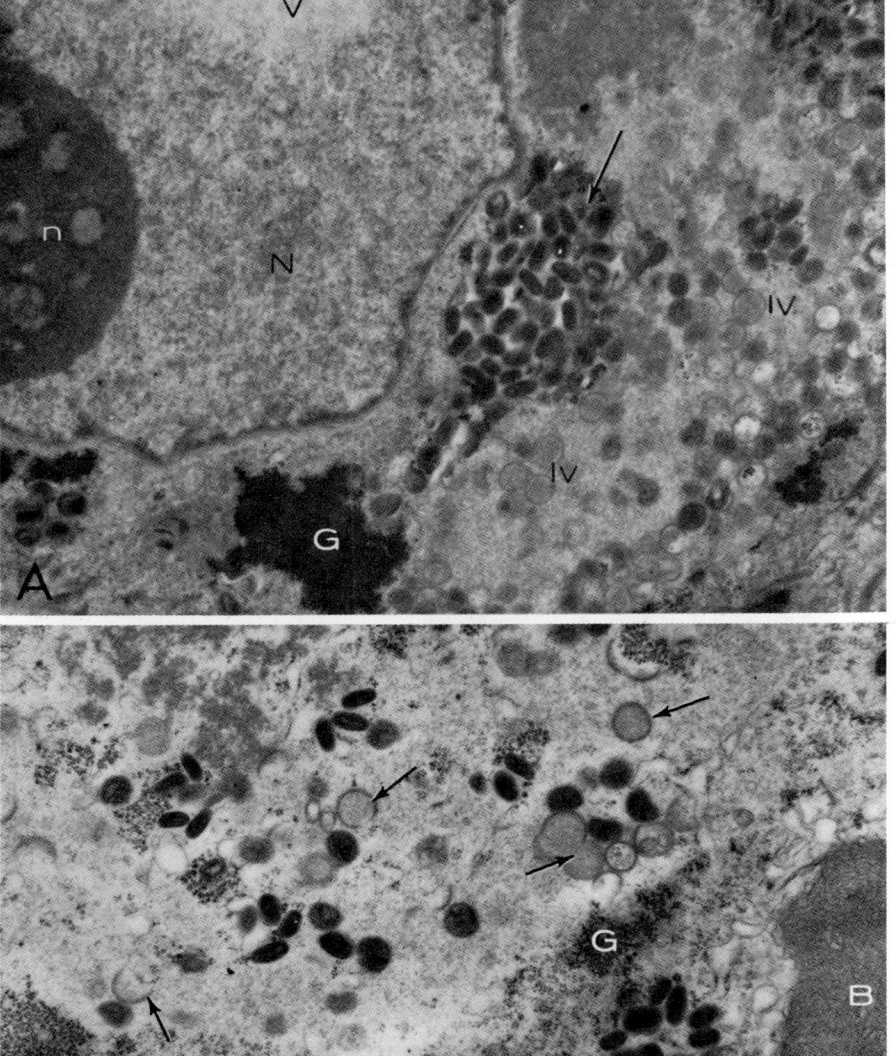

FIG. 8-9 Benign epidermal monkeypox. **A.** Portion of an epithelial cell with nuclear vacuolization *(V)*; abundant mature viral particles *(arrow)* surrounded by immature particles *(IV)*. *G*, glycogen; *N*, nucleus; *n*, nucleolus (× 17,000). **B.** Immature viral particles *(arrows)* and dense crystalloid bodies *(B)*. *G*, glycogen (× 26,000). (Courtesy of Dr. W. P. McNulty.)

and California and also called "Or Te Ca" poxvirus or Oregon poxvirus, is caused by the same virus as tanapox. In these outbreaks, animal handlers in contact with the monkeys became infected. The virus is immunologically related to Yaba monkey tumor virus (discussed later), but is not related to smallpox or vaccinia. The lesions consist of multiple large, crusted elevations of the skin, especially on the face, arms, and perineum. Microscopically (Fig. 8-9), there is marked hyperplasia of the epidermis and adnexae somewhat similar to contagious ovine ecthyma. Keratinocytes contain large, granular cytoplasmic inclusion bodies. There is necrosis of keratinocytes, but vesicles are usually not formed. A similar poxvirus infection has been described in the common marmoset (*Callithrix jacchus*), a New World species.

References

Casey HW, Woodruff JM, Butcher WI. Electron microscopy of a benign epidermal pox disease of rhesus monkeys. Am J Pathol 1967;51:431–446.

Cheville N, et al. Cytopathic changes in lesions of a pox disease in monkeys. Iowa State Univ Vet 1968;30:77–81 [Vet Bull 1969;39: 3328].

Downie AW, et al. Tanapox: a new disease caused by a pox virus. Br Med J 1971;1:363–368.

Downie AW, Espana C. Comparison of Tanapox virus and Yaba-like viruses causing epidemic disease in monkeys. J Hyg (Camb) 1972;70:23–33.

Downie AW, Espana C. A comparative study of Tanapox and Yaba viruses. J Gen Virol 1973;19:37–49.

Gough AW, Barsoum NJ, Gracon SI, et al. Poxvirus infection in a colony of common marmosets (Callithrix jacchus). Lab Anim Sci 1982;32:87–90.

Hall AS, McNulty WP Jr. A contagious pox disease in monkeys. J Am Vet Med Assoc 1967;151:833–838.

Jezek Z, Arita I, Szczeniowski M, et al. Human tanapox in Zaire: clinical and epidemiological observations on cases confirmed by laboratory studies. Bull WHO 1985;63:1027–1035.

Kupper JL, Casey HW, Johnson DK. Experimental Yaba and benign epidermal monkey pox in rhesus monkeys. Lab Anim Care 1970;20:979–988.

McNulty WP, et al. A pox disease in monkeys transmitted to man. Arch Dermatol 1968;97:286–293.

MOLLUSCUM CONTAGIOSUM

Molluscum contagiosum is a disease of humans caused by a distinct poxvirus. The lesions are characterized by epithelial hyperplasia and extremely large eosinophilic inclusion bodies (molluscum bodies), which enlarge to eventually occupy a whole cell.

A disease histologically similar to molluscum contagiosum has been described in chimpanzees, marsupials, South American sea lions, and horses. In horses, the lesions are microscopically identical to those seen in humans and have been described as localized about the muzzle, penis and prepuce; however, a report by Cooley and others (1987) describes a case with more generalized distribution.

References

Bagnall BG, Wilson GR. Molluscum contagiosum in a red kangaroo. Aust J Dermatol 1974;15:115–120.

Cooley AJ, Reinhard MK, Gross TL, et al. Molluscum contagiosum in a horse with granulomatous enteritis. J Comp Pathol 1987;97:29–34.

Douglas JD, et al. Molluscum contagiosum in chimpanzees. J Am Vet Med Assoc 1967;151:901–904.

Goodpasture WE, Woodruff CE. Molluscum contagiosum. Am J Pathol 1931;7:1–9.

Gribble D. Poxvirus infection in the horse resembling molluscum contagiosum: a case report. Proc 31st Annu Mtng Am Coll Vet Pathol 1980.

McKenzie RA, Fay FR, Prior HC. Poxvirus infection of the skin of an eastern grey kangaroo. Aust Vet J 1979;55:188–190.

Moens Y, Kombe AH. Molluscum contagiosum in a horse. Equine Vet J 1988;20:143–145.

Oriel JD. The increase in molluscum contagiosum. Br Med J 1987;294:74.

Rahaley RS, Mueller RE. Molluscum contagiosum in a horse. Vet Pathol 1983;20:247–250.

ULCERATIVE DERMATOSIS

Synonyms for ulcerative dermatosis are infectious balanoposthitis, ulcerative vulvitis, lip and leg ulcerations, and pesgras. Ulcerative dermatosis is a disease of sheep and goats characterized by an ulcerative dermatitis of the lips, legs, feet, prepuce, and vulva. The virus is a member of the poxvirus group and is immunologically related, but distantly, to the virus of contagious ovine ecthyma. The lesions are poorly studied but reportedly nonspecific in microscopic appearance and lack the hyperplasia of epidermis seen in contagious ecthyma.

References

Flook WH. An outbreak of venereal disease among sheep (ulcerative dermatosis). J Comp Pathol 1903;76:374–375.

McFadyean JA. A contagious disease of the generative organ of sheep. J Comp Pathol 1903;16:375–376.

Roberts RS, Bolton JFA. A venereal disease of sheep. Vet Rec 1945;57:686–687.

Trueblood MS. Relationship of ovine contagious ecthyma and ulcerative dermatosis. Cornell Vet 1966;56:521–526.

Tunnicliff EA. Ulcerative dermatosis of sheep. Am J Vet Res 1949;10:240–249.

YABA POXVIRUS

Yaba poxvirus affects many species of Asian and African monkeys, as well as humans. The virus is enzootic in Africa and has been responsible for lesions in laboratory-housed monkeys and, rarely, in their human attendants. The lesions are tumor-like masses in the subcutis, composed of proliferating, pleomorphic mononuclear cells (histiocytes that contain irregularly shaped, eosinophilic, cytoplasmic inclusion bodies). Neutrophils and lymphocytes infiltrate the lesion. This disease resembles lumpy skin disease of cattle. The lesions are not true tumors and eventually regress.

References

Ambrus JL, Strandstrom HV. Susceptibility of Old World monkeys to Yaba virus. Nature (London) 1966;211:876.

Ambrus JL, Strandstrom HV, Kawinski W. "Spontaneous" occurrence of Yaba tumor in a monkey colony. Experimentia 1969;25:64–65.

Behbehani AM, et al. Yaba tumor virus. I. Studies on pathogenesis and immunity. Proc Soc Exp Biol Med 1968;129:556–561.

Bruestle ME, Golden JG, Hall A III, et al. Naturally occurring Yaba tumor in a baboon (Papio papio). Lab Anim Sci 1981;31:292–294.

Grace JT, Mirand EA. Human susceptibility to a simian tumor virus. Ann NY Acad Sci 1963;108:1123–1128.

Grace JT Jr, Mirand EA. Yaba virus infection in humans. Exp Med Surg 1965;23:213–216.

Kupper JL, Casey HW, Johnson DK. Experimental Yaba and benign epidermal monkey pox in rhesus monkeys. Lab Anim Care 1970;20:979–988.

Nivan JSC, et al. Subcutaneous growths in monkeys produced by poxvirus. J Pathol Bacteriol 1961;81:1–14.

Rouhandeh H. Yaba virus. Dev Vet Virol 1988;6:1–15.

HORSEPOX

Apparently an ancient disease of horses, horsepox is known in Europe but not in the United States. It is believed to be caused by an immunologically distinct virus, but the relationship of the horsepox virus to other poxviruses is not known. Lesions may occur on the lips, nose, oral mucosa, and genitalia. "Grease-heel," papular dermatitis, and Uasin Gishu skin disease of the horse may represent other forms of horsepox.

References

Andrews C, Pereira HG. Viruses of vertebrates. 2nd ed. London: Bailliere, Tindal and Cassell 1967.

Eby CH. A note in the history of horse pox. J Am Vet Med Assoc 1958;132:420–422.

Jayo MJ, Jensen LA, Leipold HW, et al. Poxvirus infection in a donkey. Vet Pathol 1986;23:635–637.

Kaminjolo JS Jr, Winqvist G. Histopathology of skin lesions in Uasin Gishu skin disease of horses. J Comp Pathol 1975;85:391–395.

McIntyre RW. Virus papular dermatitis of the horse. Am J Vet Res 1949;10:229–232.

OTHER POXVIRUSES

Several other distinct poxvirus diseases have been described in a variety of animal species. Pox occurs in several different species of seals. Isolates have been classified in the parapoxvirus group. The lesions resemble those caused by other viruses in this group, and transmission to humans who handled infected seals has been documented. A probable orthopoxvirus disease has been reported in raccoons.

References

Hicks BD and Worthy GAJ. Sealpox in captive grey seals (*Halichoerus grypus*) and their handlers. J Wildl Dis 1987;23:1–6.

Parsons BL and Pickup DJ. Tandemly repeated sequences are present at the ends of the DNA of raccoonpox virus. Virology 1987;161:45–53.

Wilson TM and Poglayen-Neuwall I. Pox in South American sea lions (*Otaria byronia*). Can J Comp Med 1971;35:174–177.

HERPESVIRIDAE

The family **Herpesviridae** (herpes = creeping) is divided into three subfamilies: **Alphaherpesvirinae; Betaherpesvirinae;** and **Gammaherpesvirinae.**

Alphaherpesvirinae are cytocidal viruses with necrosis as the principal pathologic effect. These herpesviruses often have a broad host range and wide cell tropism. Disease may be localized and transient or generalized and fatal; the outcome depends on the species affected and the age and immune status of the host. Recovery is followed by lifelong latent infection, most usually in nerve ganglia. Recurrence of active disease is common.

The **Betaherpesvirinae** group is comprised of the cytomegaloviruses, which have a very restricted host range (Fig. 8-10). Infected cells become very large and bear intranuclear and sometimes cytoplasmic inclusion bodies (cytomegalic inclusion body disease). They ultimately undergo lysis through the effects of viral replication or host immune response. Recovery is followed by persistent or latent infection in a variety of tissues, including secretory glands (especially salivary glands), kidneys, and lymph nodes. As with alphaherpesviruses, recurrent infection is common.

Gammaherpesvirinae are lymphotropic herpesviruses tropic for either B or T lymphocytes. Their host range is narrow and infection is followed by lifelong latency in lymphocytes. Pathologic effects may vary from no discernible disease to lymphoma.

The nucleic acid of herpesviruses is double-stranded DNA, and ultrastructurally, the capsid is icosahedral in shape, about 100 nm to 200 nm in diameter with 162 capsomers. The virions are surrounded by an envelope acquired by budding through the inner lamella of the nuclear membrane.

Most of the herpesviruses have been given species names on the basis of their usual host. Table 8-3 presents a summary of the more important herpesviruses, their hosts, species names, and the diseases they cause. Several score of additional herpesviruses have been identified in other mammals, as well as in birds, reptiles, amphibia, insects, and even mollusks.

Reference

Roizman B, et al. Herpesviridae: definition, provisional nomenclature, and taxonomy. Intervirology 1981;16:201–217.

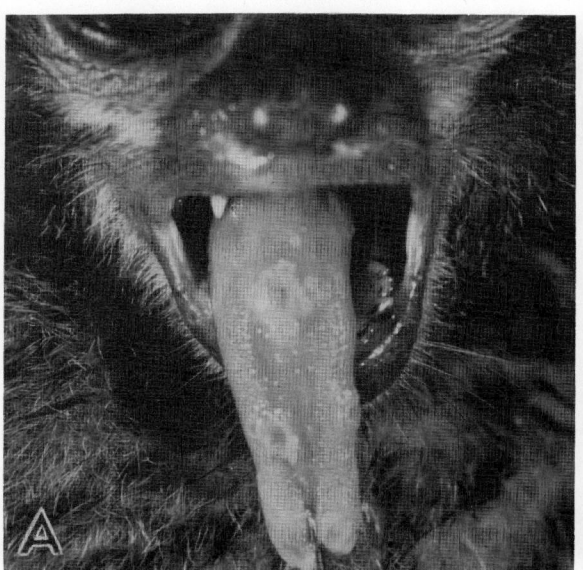
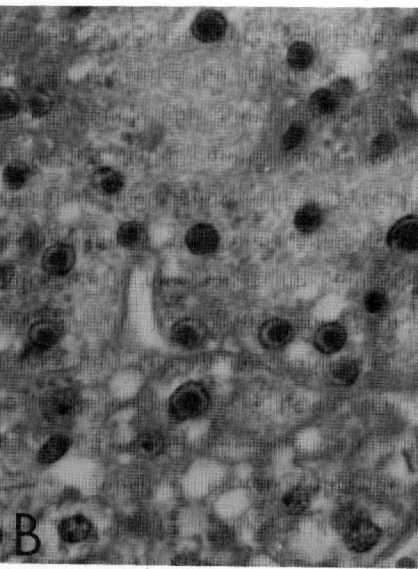

FIG. 8-10 Herpesvirus simplex infection of an owl monkey (*Aotus trivirgatus*). **A.** Ulcerative glossitis. **B.** Intranuclear inclusion bodies in hepatocytes. (Courtesy of New England Regional Primate Research Center, Harvard Medical School.)

TABLE 8-3 **Diseases caused by *Herpesviridae***

Virus	Host(s)	Disease
Alphaherpesviruses		
Herpesvirus simplex, type 1	Humans, apes, monkeys	Herpes simplex, usually oral; generalized in owl monkeys
H. simplex, type 2	Humans, apes, monkeys	Genital herpes
H. varicella-zoster	Humans	Varicella (chicken pox) and zoster (shingles)
Simian varicella	Macaques, African green monkeys, Patas monkeys	Simian varicella
H. simiae, "B-virus"	Nonhuman primates, humans	Herpesvirus B
H. canis	Canines	Canine herpes
H. suis	Swine, cattle	Pseudorabies, Aujeszky's disease
Bovine herpesvirus, type 1	Bovines	Infectious bovine rhinotracheitis, infectious pustular vulvovaginitis, infectious balanoposthitis, viral abortion
Bovine herpesvirus, type 2	Bovines	Herpesvirus mammillitis
Equine herpesvirus, type 1 (EHV-1, subtype 1)	Equines	Viral abortion, rhinopneumonitis, neonatal death, neurologic disease, enterocolitis
Equine herpesvirus, type 4 (EHV-1, subtype 2)	Equines	Rhinopneumonitis, viral abortion
Equine herpesvirus, type 3	Equines	Coital exanthema
H. felis	Felines	Infectious rhinotracheitis
Avian herpesvirus, type 1	Birds	Infectious laryngotracheitis
H. tamarinus	Squirrel monkeys, tamarins, marmosets, owl monkeys	Localized disease and carried by squirrel monkeys; generalized disease in marmosets, tamarins, and owl monkeys
Betaherpesviruses		
Porcine cytomegaloviruses (CMV)	Swine	Inclusion-body rhinitis, generalized CMV infection
Cytomegaloviruses of bovines, equines, apes, monkeys, guinea pigs, rats, and others	Host-specific	No discernable disease response to localized or generalized CMV infection
Gammaherpesviruses		
Epstein-Barr Virus	Humans	Infectious mononucleosis; probably Burkitt's lymphoma and nasopharyngeal carcinoma

(continued)

TABLE 8-3 (continued)

Virus	Host(s)	Disease
H. saimiri	Squirrel monkey (*Saimiri scuireus*)	Carried by squirrel monkeys; experimentally produces lymphoma in marmosets, tamarins, owl monkeys, and rabbits
H. ateles	Spider monkeys (*Ateles* spp.)	Carried by spider monkeys; experimentally produces lymphoma in marmosets, tamarins, owl monkeys, and rabbits
Marek's disease virus*	Chickens	Avian lymphomatosis, Marek's disease
Malignant catarrhal fever virus	Bovines	Malignant catarrhal fever
Unclassified Herpesvirus		
Lucké's virus	Frogs	Adenocarcinoma of kidney

*Although Marek's disease virus causes lymphoma, its genome more closely resembles an alphaherpesvirus.

Diseases caused by Alphaherpesviruses

Most **Alphaherpesviruses** produce localized cytolytic lesions on mucosal surfaces of the mouth, respiratory or genital tract, skin, or eye. Primary infection often goes unnoticed but may be characterized by vesicles, pustules, and ulcers. During this phase, progeny virus enter naked nerve endings in the epidermis and travel centripetally to sensory neurons in respective ganglia. Presumably by multiplying in ganglia, virions travel centrifugally down axons and (protected from humoral antibodies) enter epithelial cells at sites served by the ganglion; thereby extending the duration and extent of the acute primary infection. Following healing of the primary lesion by action of humoral and cellular immune mechanisms, viral DNA remains latent in neurons, presumably for life. Lesions may recur in response to a variety of stimuli; latent virus becomes active, spreading down axons (still protected from antibodies) to re-enter epithelial cells and repeat the lytic cycle.

In young animals, particularly neonates, primary infection may become widespread, with necrotizing lesions in many organs and tissues. Systemic spread is also seen in immunocompromised individuals and aberrant hosts (animals which have not evolved with the virus). Virus may also be transported by way of mononuclear cells to the placenta leading to abortion or neonatal infection.

Spread of alphaherpesviruses is by contact and droplets.

HERPESVIRUS SIMPLEX INFECTION IN PRIMATES (HERPESVIRUS HOMINIS)

Herpesvirus simplex infection is one of the oldest viral diseases known to humans. The use of the word herpes in medicine can be traced as far back as Hippocrates, and descriptions clearly related to the disease as it is now understood in humans were published in the seventeenth century. Many early reports describe experimental transmission of herpesvirus simplex to laboratory animals, such as rabbits, guinea pigs, mice, rats, and hamsters. Herpesvirus simplex is an important spontaneous disease of owl monkeys (*Aotus trivirgatus*), a New World species, and gibbons (*Hylobates lar*), an anthropoid ape.

The Disease in Humans Humans, the natural host and reservoir for herpesvirus simplex, assume a role similar to that of the rhesus monkey with herpesvirus B, the squirrel monkey with herpesvirus T, and swine with herpesvirus suis. Two antigenically different herpes simplex viruses infect humans. Type 1 usually affects the lips and oral mucosa; type 2 causes lesions on the genital mucosae of both sexes and is transmitted by coitus. Primary infection with type 1 virus occurs principally in young children, taking the form of an acute gingivostomatitis, which heals with no serious side effects. By adolescence or early adulthood, 90% to 95% of all individuals have become infected, as evidenced by the presence of serum-neutralizing antibodies. Many people, despite the presence of antibodies, suffer from periodic recurrence of secondary herpes simplex infection for much of their lives, often with several episodes occurring each year. Recurrent lesions are believed to be the result of activation of a latent infection that persists in all infected individuals for life. A variety of stimuli have been associated with activation, including fever (in which the lesion is called a "fever blister"), colds (in which the lesion is called a "cold sore"), fatigue, menstruation, emotional distress, and certain foods.

Lesions Primary recurrent lesions are characterized by small clusters of vesicles that rupture, leaving erosions or ulcers that heal in 5 to 10 days. Hyperesthesia and neuralgia often precede the lesions and may persist for variable periods of time after healing. The mucocutaneous junction of the lip is the most common site, but the external nares, oral mucosa, conjunctiva, skin, esophagus, external genitalia, vagina, and cervix are not uncommon locations.

Microscopic features are ballooning degeneration, necrosis, intracellular edema, multinucleated giant cells, and intranuclear inclusion bodies. Virus is readily isolated during the course and up to 3 weeks after recovery. Interestingly, virus can be recovered from a proportion of the population (7% to 20%) in the absence of visible lesions.

Herpes simplex infection in humans is not always a benign disease. In neonates and young children, primary infection (usually type 2) may lead to a fatal generalized disease affecting most organs and tissues, and in adults, fatal meningoencephalitis may develop. The lesions in both of these forms are characterized by focal necrosis and intranuclear inclusion bodies in the affected tissues. There is a strong association between type 2 genital infection and carcinoma of the cervix in women, but a causative role is not proven.

The disease in nonhuman primates In the chimpanzee (*Pan troglodytes* and *P. paniscus*), gibbon (*Hylobates lar*), and probably other apes, herpes simplex infection is analogous to that in humans, usually remaining localized and resolving. Recurrence of both oral and genital lesions has been described in chimpanzees. A relative high incidence of encephalitis in gibbons suggests a slightly less analogous host/virus relationship to that seen in humans. Experimentally, the infection in cebus monkeys (*Cebus apella*, *C. albifrons*) and baboons (*Papio cynocephalus*) is also analogous to the infection in humans. Natural infection in owl monkeys (*Aotus trivirgatus*), tree shrews (*Tupaia glis*), and lemurs (*Lemur catta*) and experimental infection in tamarins (*Saguinus oedipus*) occur as epizootics with rapid generalized dissemination of lesions and high mortality rates. Following an incubation period of about 7 days, a short clinical illness occurs, characterized by oral and labial ulceration, ulcerative dermatitis, conjunctivitis, anorexia, hyperesthesia, weakness and incoordination. Death is the usual outcome in 2 to 3 days.

DIAGNOSIS A presumptive diagnosis of herpes simplex infection in monkeys can be made on the basis of history and pathologic changes. However, generally the lesions cannot be distinguished from herpesvirus T infection in some species; therefore, definitive diagnosis requires viral isolation and identification.

References

Corey L and Spear PG. Infections with Herpes simplex viruses (Parts I and II). N Engl J Med 1986;314:686–691,749–757.

Hunt RD, Melendez LV. Herpes virus infections of non-human primates: a review. Lab Anim Care 1969;19:221–234.

Kalter SS, Felsburg PJ, Heberling RL, et al. Experimental *Herpesvirus hominis* type 2 infection in nonhuman primates. Proc Soc Exp Biol Med 1972;136:964–968.

Katzin DS, Connor JD, Wilson LA, et al. Experimental Herpes simplex infection in the Owl monkey. Proc Soc Exp Biol Med 1967;125:391–398.

Kemp GE, Losos GL, Causey OR, et al. Isolation of *Herpesvirus hominis* from lemurs: a naturally occurring epizootic at a zoological garden in Nigeria. Afr J Med Sci 1972;3:177–185.

Leestma JE, Bornstein MB, Sheppard RD, et al. Ultrastructural aspects of Herpes simplex virus infection in organized cultures of mammalian nervous tissue. Lab Invest 1969;20:70–78.

McClure HM, Keeling ME, Olberding B, et al. Natural *Herpesvirus hominis* infection of tree shrews (*Tupaia glis*). Lab Anim Sci 1972;22:517–521.

McClure HM, Swenson RB, Kalter SS, et al. Natural genital *Herpesvirus hominis* infection in chimpanzees (*Pan troglodytes* and *Pan paniscus*). Lab Anim Sci 1980;30:895–901.

Melendez LV, Espana C, Hunt RD, et al. Natural Herpes simplex infection in Owl monkey (*Aotus trivirgatus*). Lab Anim Care 1969;19:38–45.

Palmer AE, et al. A preliminary report on investigation of oncogenic potential of herpes simplex virus type 2 in cebus monkeys. Cancer Res 1976;36:807–809.

Olson LC, Buescher EL, Artenstein MS, et al. Herpesvirus infections of the human central nervous system. N Engl J Med 1967;277:1271–1277.

Smith PC, Yuill TM, Buchanan RD, et al. The gibbon (*Hylobates lar*), a new primate host for Herpesvirus hominis. I. A natural epizootic in a laboratory colony. J Infect Dis 1969;120:292–297.

Smith PC, Yuill TM, Buchanan RD. Natural and experimental infection of gibbons with Herpesvirus hominis. Ann Prog Report SEATO Med Res Lab and SEATO Clinical Res Cen, Bangkok, Thailand, 1958;258–261.

Wildy P. Herpesvirus. Intervirology 1986;25:117–140.

HERPESVIRUS B INFECTION OF MONKEYS (HERPES-B, HERPESVIRUS SIMIAE, B-VIRUS)

In 1934, Sabin and Wright isolated a virus from the brain of a human patient who died after being bitten by an apparently normal rhesus monkey (*Macaca mulatta*). The virus was shown subsequently to be carried by Old World monkeys of the genus *Macaca*, with little or no disease is evident in the carriers. On the basis of the presence of clinical disease, virus isolation, and/or serum-neutralizing antibodies, most species of macaques have been found to be natural reservoir hosts for the virus.

The disease in monkeys The bulk of our knowledge of herpesvirus B comes from studies with rhesus monkeys, in which the infection is very comparable to herpes simplex infection in humans. Following infection, clinical disease is characterized by vesicles and ulcers, particularly on the dorsal surface of the tongue and on the mucocutaneous junction of the lip, but it is not known whether lesions invariably follow infection. In addition to the oral mucous membranes, the skin may develop vesicles and ulcers, and the virus may cause conjunctivitis. These lesions heal uneventfully in 7 to 14 days. The disease is rarely fatal.

Microscopically, the lesions are characterized by ballooning degeneration and necrosis of epithelial cells and the presence of intranuclear inclusion bodies (Fig. 8-11). Multinucleated epithelial cells containing intranuclear inclusion bodies (Fig. 8-12) are also usually present. Inclusion bodies may also be found in macrophages and in endothelial cells. During the course of clinical disease in the rhesus and cynomolgus monkey, visceral lesions may also develop. These are characterized by foci of necrosis in the liver, associated with intra-

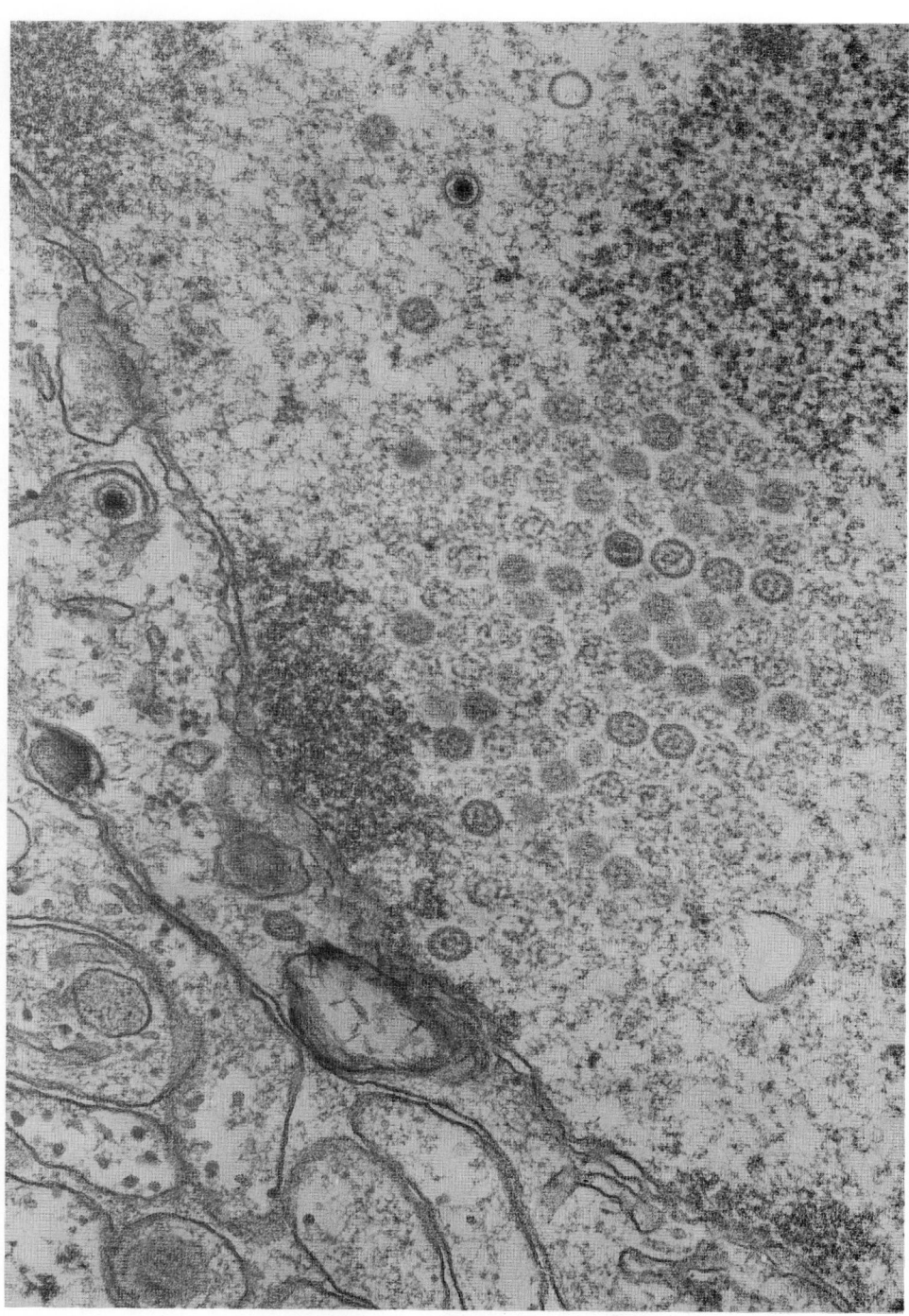

FIG. 8-11 Intranuclear inclusion body of herpesvirus simplex in tissue culture. Note crystalline array of viral particles within nucleus (× 50,000). (Courtesy of Dr. J. E. Leestma and *Laboratory Investigation.*

nuclear inclusion bodies. In the central nervous system, neuronal necrosis and gliosis associated with minimal perivascular cuffing with lymphocytes may be found. Intranuclear inclusion bodies occur in glial cells and neurons. The lesions are most common in the nucleus and tract of the descending branches of the trigeminal nerve, between the roots of origin of the facial and auditory nerves, and at the roots of the trigeminal and facial nerves.

The infection spreads within a colony of monkeys by means of direct contact, fomites, and probably aerosols, until nearly 100% of the colony has become infected, as determined by the presence of serum-neutralizing antibodies. Oral lesions are not encountered in every animal, which is explained in part by failure to observe them.

Once a monkey is infected with herpesvirus B, the animal should probably be considered infected for life with persistent or latent infection in ganglia. Recurrent lesions are not common, but the virus may be isolated from the oral cavity, vagina, blood, urine, and feces of animals without overt disease.

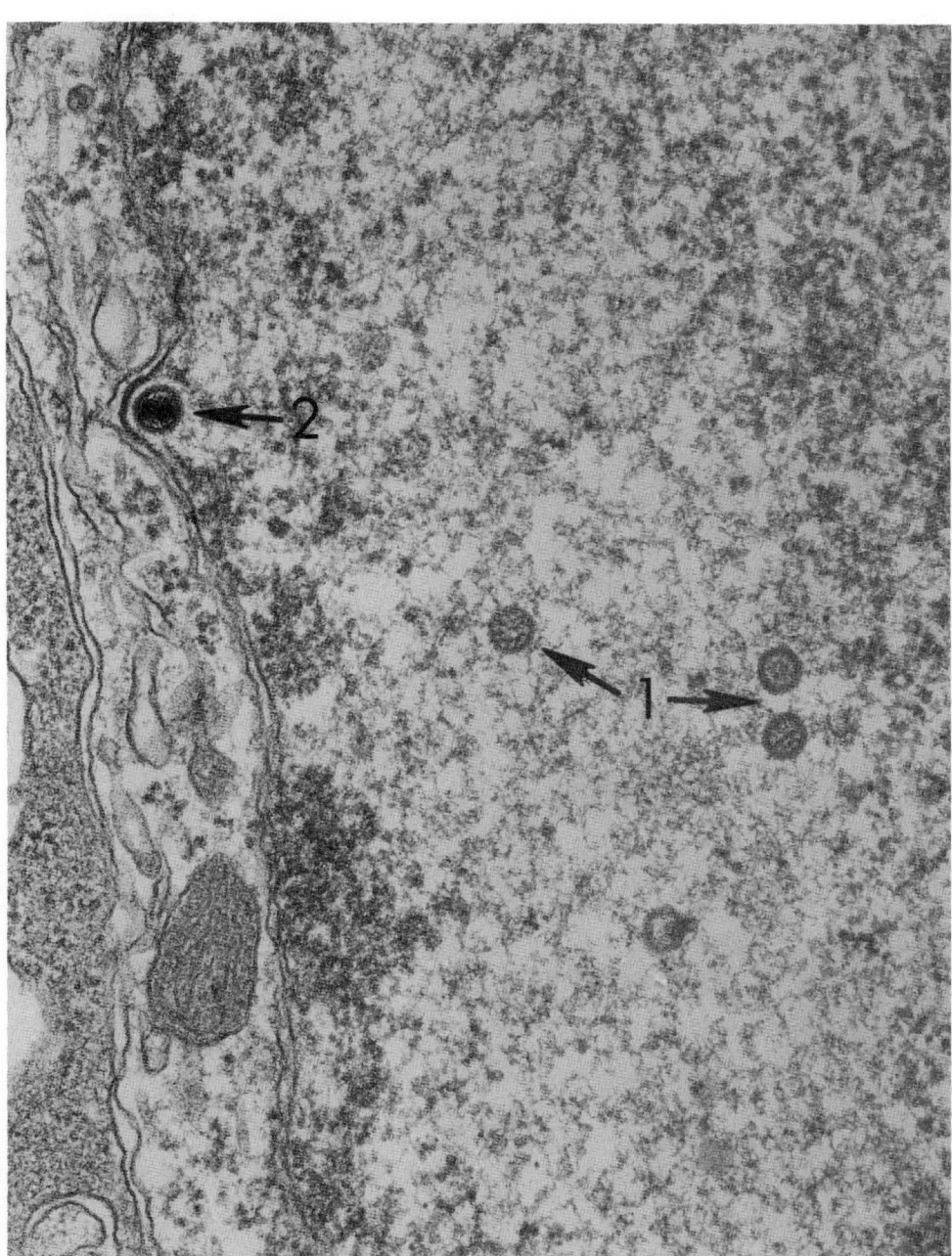

FIG. 8-12 Herpesvirus simplex infection in tissue culture of nervous tissue. Note unenveloped viral particles in the nucleus *(1)*. Single virion *(2)* is approaching bulging nuclear membrane, a stage preparatory to envelopment (× 40,000). (Courtesy of Dr. J. E. Leestma and *Laboratory Investigation.*)

The disease in humans The principal importance of herpesvirus B is not its hazards to the reservoir hosts but the fatal disease that the virus produces in humans. Although the rate of morbidity is low, most cases have proved fatal. Infections usually follow a monkey bite. The disease is characterized clinically and pathologically by encephalomyelitis. Focal necrosis may occur in the liver, spleen, lymph nodes, and adrenal glands. Intranuclear inclusion bodies may be found in any affected tissue but have not been demonstrated in all cases.

DIAGNOSIS A presumptive diagnosis can be made from the characteristic lesions. Because of the number of simian herpesviruses, definitive diagnosis requires isolation and identification of the virus. A rise in titer of serum-neutralizing antibodies may support the diagnosis.

References

Anderson DC, Swenson RB, Orkin JL, et al. Primary *Herpesvirus simiae* (B-virus) infection in infant macaques. Lab Anim Sci 1994;44: 526–530.

Davidson WL. B virus infection in man. Ann NY Acad Sci 1960;85: 970–979.

Holmes GP, et al. B virus *(Herpesvirus simiae)* infection of humans: epidemiologic investigation of a cluster. Ann Intern Med 1990; 112:833–839.

Hunt RD, Melendez LV. Herpes virus infections of non-human primates: a review. Lab Anim Care 1969;19:221–234.

Keeble SA. B virus infection in monkeys. Ann NY Acad Sci 1960;85: 960–969.

Keeble SA, Christofinis GJ, Wood W. Natural B-virus infection in rhesus monkeys. J Pathol Bact 1958;76:189–199.

Sabin AB, Wright AM. Acute ascending myelitis following a monkey bite, with isolation of a virus capable of reproducing the disease. J Exper Med 1934;59:115–136.

Sabin AB. Studies on the B virus. I. The immunological identity of a virus isolated from a human case of ascending myelitis associated with visceral necrosis. Br J Exp Pathol 1934;15:248–269.

Tribe GW. The pathogenesis and epidemiology of B-virus. Primate Supply 1982;7(1):18–24.

Weigler BJ. Biology of B virus in macaque and human hosts: a review. Clin Infect Dis 1992;14:555–567.

Wilson RB, Holscher MA, Chang T, et al. Fatal *Herpesvirus simiae* (B virus) infection in a patas monkey *(Erythrocebus patas).* J Vet Diagn Invest 1990;2:242–244.

Zwartouw HT, MacArthur JA, Boulter EA, et al. Transmission of B virus infection between monkeys especially in relation to breeding colonies. Lab Anim 1984;18:125–130.

Herpesvirus T infection of monkeys (herpesvirus M, herpesvirus platyrrhinae I)

Herpesvirus T infection has many similarities to herpesvirus B infection; however, the virus is distinct and the susceptible hosts are New World monkeys. Herpesvirus T is carried as a latent viral infection by the Squirrel monkey *(Saimiri sciureus).* On the basis of evidence derived from circulating serum-neutralizing antibodies, cinnamon ringtail monkeys*((Cebus albifrons),* and spider monkeys *(Ateles* species) are also likely natural reservoir hosts. Although the morbidity rate is high, clinical disease is rarely seen in the reservoir host, and has only been documented in the squirrel monkey, in which the lesions consist of vesicles and ulcers of the oral mucous membranes. The microscopic features are identical to herpesvirus B infection in the rhesus monkey. Visceral lesions or changes in the central nervous system are not known to occur. The disease in the reservoir hosts is not known to be fatal. Exacerbation of oral lesions is also not known to occur, but as with herpesvirus B infection, the virus can be excreted in the absence of visible lesions. All available evidence suggests that latent infection remains for life.

Marmosets *(Saguinus* species) and owl monkeys *(Aotus trivirgatus)* have a less fortunate relationship with herpesvirus T. In these hosts, herpesvirus T produces an epizootic disease of high morbidity and mortality rates. The clinical features, which develop following an incubation period of 7 to 10 days, are characterized by anorexia, lassitude, oral and labial vesicles and ulcers, ulcerative dermatitis (especially of the face), and occasionally conjunctivitis. Hyperesthesia, as evidenced by intense scratching, may be the most obvious sign. After a course of 2 to 3 days, most animals become moribund and die.

Gross lesions consist of vesicles and/or ulcers of the skin, lips, oral cavity, esophagus, small intestine, cecum, and colon. Hemorrhage is present in most lymph nodes, the adrenal cortices, and, occasionally, the lung. Microscopically, variable-sized foci of necrosis and intranuclear inclusion bodies are found in most organs and tissues of the body. Lesions are most common in the oral cavity, small and large intestine, liver, spleen, lymph nodes, adrenal cortex, and ganglia. Multinucleated giant cells are present in lesions of the oral cavity and skin. Encephalitis is not common, and, when present, it is not extensive.

DIAGNOSIS In either the reservoir or the fatally affected hosts, the characteristic lesions allow for a presumptive diagnosis. However, because other herpesviruses occur in New World monkeys, the virus should be isolated and identified. In owl monkeys, the lesions of herpesvirus T infection cannot be differentiated from those of herpesvirus simplex infection.

References

Daniel MD, Karpas A, Melendez LV, et al. Isolation of Herpes-T virus from a spontaneous disease in Squirrel monkeys (Saimiri sciureus). Arch Virusforsch 1967;22:324–331.

Holmes AW, Caldwell RG, Dedmon RE, et al. Isolation and characterization of a new Herpes virus. J Immunol1964;92:602–610.

Holmes AW, Devine JA, Nowakowski E, et al. The epidemiology of a Herpes virus infection of New World monkeys. J Immunol 1966;96:668–671.

Hunt RD, Melendez LV. Herpes virus infections of nonhuman primates: A review. Lab Anim Care 1969;19:221–234.

Hunt RD, Melendez LV. Spontaneous Herpes-T infection in the Owl monkey (Aotus trivirgatus). Path Vet 1966;3:1–26.

King NW, Hunt RD, Daniel MD, et al. Overt Herpes-T infection in Squirrel monkeys (Saimiri sciureus). Lab Anim Care 1967;17: 413–423.

Melendez LV, Hunt RD, Garcia FG, et al. A latent Herpes-T infection in Saimiri sciureus (Squirrel monkey). In: Fiennes RNTW, ed. Some recent developments in comparative medicine. London: Academic Press 1966;393–397.

HERPESVIRUS VARICELLA/ZOSTER

Varicella, or **chickenpox,** is one of the most common childhood infections. It is characterized by a papulovesicular rash beginning on the trunk and spreading centrifugally to the head and limbs. The virus is believed to enter via the respiratory mucosa and, after a phase of viremia, localize and replicate in reticuloendothelial tissues. After a second phase of viremia, virus localizes in dermal capillary endothelial cells and then spreads to the epidermis. Microscopically, the epidermal lesions are identical to those described for herpes simplex infection with the exception of the initial endothelial lesion. Generalization may occur with widespread vascular damage and parenchymal lesions in almost any organ.

Zoster, or **shingles,** represents activation of latent varicella infection and is characterized by vesicular dermatitis along the distribution of peripheral or cranial nerves. Although associated with severe pain and hyperesthesia, it usually resolves. Lesions in the skin resemble varicella. There is, in addition, lymphocytic inflammation and neuronal necrosis in associated ganglia. Dissemination may occur, especially in immunocompromised patients.

Simian varicella Although herpesvirus varicella/zoster cannot be transmitted to nonhuman primates (with the exception of the common marmoset, described by Provost and colleagues, 1987), a number of

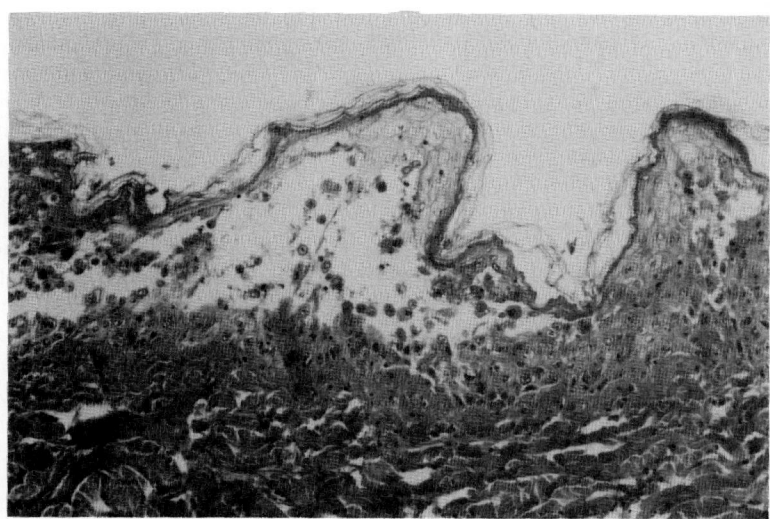

FIG. 8-13 Liverpool vervet monkey virus infection. Vesicular dermatitis of a vervet monkey *(Cercopithecus aethiops)*. (Courtesy of Dr. E. Thorpe.)

viruses of simian origin share characteristics with human varicella/zoster, yet are distinct and different. Three closely related simian viruses are recognized: **Liverpool Vervet monkey virus** from the African green monkey *(Cercopithecus aethiops)*; **Delta or Patas herpesvirus** from *Erythrocebus patas*; and **Medical Lake herpesvirus** from the pig-tailed macaque *(Macaca nemestrina)*, the Japanese macaque *(M fuscata)*, and the cynomolgus monkey *(M fascicularis)*. Simian varicella is a severe generalized infection with a high rate of mortality. Lesions are typical of alphaherpesviruses and are disseminated (Fig. 8-13). A mild form of varicella has been seen in chimpanzees (chimpanzee herpesvirus).

References

Blakely GA, Lourie B, Morton WG, et al. A varicella-like disease in macaque monkeys. J Infect Dis 1973;127:617–625.

Clarkson MJ, Thorpe E, McCarthy K. A virus disease of captive vervet monkeys *(Cercopithecus aethiops)* caused by a new herpesvirus. Arch Virusforsch 1967;22:219–234.

Heuschele WP. Varicella (chicken pox) in three young anthropoid apes. J Am Vet Med Assoc 1960;136:256–257.

Iltis JP, Aarons MC, Castellano GA, et al. Simian varicella virus (Delta herpesvirus) infection of patas monkeys leading to pneumonia and encephalitis. Proc Soc Exp Biol Med 1982;169:266–279.

McCarthy K, Thorpe E, Laursen AC, et al. Exanthematous disease in patas monkeys caused by a herpes virus. Lancet 1968;2:856–857.

Padovan D, Cantrell CA. Varicella-like herpesvirus infections of non-human primates. Lab Anim Sci 1986;36:7–13.

Provost PJ, Keller PM, Banker FS, et al. Successful infection of the common marmoset *(Callithrix jacchus)* with human varicella-zoster virus. J Virol 1987;61:2951–2955.

Roberts ED, Baskin GB, Soike K, et al. Pathologic changes of experimental simian varicella (Delta herpesvirus) infection in African green monkeys *(Cercopithecus aethiops)*. Am J Vet Res 1984;45: 523–530.

Weller TH. Varicella and herpes zoster. Changing concepts of the natural history, control, and importance of a not-so-benign virus (Parts I and II). N Engl J Med 1983;309:1362–1368, 1434–1440.

Wenner HA, Abel D, Barrick S, et al. Clinical and pathogenetic studies of Medical Lake macaque virus infections in cynomolgus monkeys (simian varicella). J Infect Dis 1977;135:611–622.

White RJ, Simmons L, Wilson RB. Chickenpox in young anthropoid apes: clinical and laboratory findings. J Am Vet Med Assoc 1972;161:690–692.

Wolf RH, Smetana HF, Allen WP, et al. Pathology and clinical history of Delta herpesvirus infection in patas monkeys. Lab Anim Sci 1974;24:218–221.

ADDITIONAL SIMIAN HERPESVIRUSES

Many other herpesviruses have been recovered from nonhuman primates, a few of which deserve mention.

An agent termed **spider monkey herpesvirus** was isolated from a young spider monkey that died of a generalized infection with oral and labial erosions and ulcers. Further examples of spontaneous disease have not been reported.

A virus named **SA8** was originally recovered from an African green monkey with myelitis. Asymptomatic latent infection is common in adult baboons, and serious infection, principally characterized by pneumonia, has been demonstrated in infant baboons.

Herpesviruses of uncertain classification have been recovered from both healthy and diseased tree shrews *(Tupaia glis)*. Recovered animals remain persistently infected. It has been suggested that the virus may cause lymphoma.

Herpesvirus saimiri is carried in latent form by squirrel monkeys *(Saimiri sciureus)*, but may be transmitted experimentally to owl monkeys *(Aotus* species), rabbits, or marmosets *(Saguinas* species), producing malignant lymphoma in these animals. Herpesvirus ateles is carried latently by spider monkeys *(Ateles* species) and also produces malignant lymphoma when inoculated into marmosets or owl monkeys. The malignant lymphoma caused by herpesvirus saimiri may result from contact between infected squirrel monkeys and normal owl monkeys.

References

Darai G, Koch H-G. Tree shrew herpesvirus: pathogenicity and latency. Curr Top Vet Med Anim Sci 1984;27:91–102.

Eichberg J, Kalter SS, Heberling RL, et al. Experimental herpesvirus infection of baboons *(Papio cynocephalus)* and African green monkeys *(Cercopithecus aethiops)* and recovery of virus by tissue explants. Arch Virusforsch 1973;43:304–314.

Hull RN, Dwyer AC, Holmes AW, et al. Recovery and characterization of a new simian herpesvirus from a fatally infected spider monkey. JNCI 1972;49:225–231.

Hunt RD, Melendez LV. Herpes virus infections of non-human primates: A review. Lab Anim Care 1969;19:221–234.

Lennette EH. Workshop on viral diseases which impede colonization of nonhuman primates. Natl Center for Primate Biology, Univ of California at Davis, May 22–24, 1968.

Loomis MR, O'Neill T, Bush M, et al. Fatal herpesvirus infection in patas monkeys and a black and white colobus monkey. J Am Vet Med Assoc 1981;179:1236–1239.

Malherbe H, Harwin R. Neurotropic virus in African monkeys. Lancet 1958;2:530.

Malherbe H, Harwin R, Ulrich M. The cytopathic effects of Vervet monkey viruses. S A Med J 1963;37:407–411.

Malherbe H, Strickland-Cholmley M. Virus from baboons. Lancet 1969;2:1300.

Ochoa R, Henk WG, Confer AW, et al. Herpesviral pneumonia and septicemia in two infant gelada baboons *(Theropithecus gelada).* J Med Primatol 1982;11:52–58.

Herpesvirus canis infection of dogs

Herpesvirus canis was first isolated, characterized, and identified as the cause of a fatal systemic infection of neonatal puppies in 1965. From available evidence, it appears that dogs are the natural and reservoir hosts for this herpesvirus, in a manner analogous to herpesvirus simplex in humans, herpesvirus B in monkeys, and herpesvirus suis in swine, although the incidence is lower. Most dogs become infected with the virus without a history of associated illness, and the virus can be isolated from puppies and adult dogs in the absence of recognizable disease. Although adult dogs carry the virus as a latent infection, it has been shown to cause a mild tracheobronchitis. The occurrence of fatal infections in neonatal puppies (Fig. 8-14) appears to be analogous to the parallel condition of fatal herpesvirus simplex in infants or fatal herpesvirus suis in piglets. These are each an example of fatal disease in the host that usually carries the virus as a latent infection.

Puppies are infected in utero or during birth by exposure to the virus in the vagina. The infection results in either stillbirth or an acute fatal disease in the first 3 weeks of life. After 3 to 5 weeks of age, infection is usually asymptomatic.

LESIONS The most striking gross pathologic change is hemorrhage, especially of the renal cortices and lungs, but the stomach, intestine, and adrenals may also sustain hemorrhages. Serosanguineous fluid is usually present in the thoracic and abdominal cavities, and splenomegaly and enlargement of lymph nodes are evident. Variably sized gray foci are often present in the lungs, kidneys, and liver.

Microscopically, the lesions in all tissues are characterized by focal necrosis and the presence of intranuclear inclusion bodies. These necrotizing lesions may be found in most organs and tissues, including the lung, kidneys, liver, spleen, lymph nodes, adrenal, intestines, eyes, and brain. Usually the lesions are most extensive in the kidneys and lungs. The lesions in the central nervous system are those of a disseminated, nonsuppurative encephalomyelitis with focal malacia of the cerebral cortex, cerebellar cortex, basal ganglia, and gray columns of the spinal cord. Secondary lesions appear later in the white matter. Infection in adult dogs is usually not associated with histopathologic changes, but the virus may produce a catarrhal tracheobronchitis with intranuclear inclusions in the lining epithelium. Inclusion bodies in both neonates and adults may be difficult to demonstrate, unless an acid fixative such as Zenker's fluid has been used.

DIAGNOSIS The characteristic necrotizing lesions and intranuclear inclusion bodies in neonatal or stillborn puppies allows for a presumptive diagnosis. Definitive diagnosis requires virus isolation and characterization. Dogs are natural hosts for this virus and subject to latent infection; therefore, virus isolation in the absence of characteristic histopathologic lesions must be interpreted with caution.

References

Albert DM, Lahav M, Carmichael LE, et al. Canine herpes-induced retinal dysplasia and associated ocular anomalies. Invest Ophthalmol 1976;15:267–278.

Carmichael LE, Strandberg JD, Barnes FD. Identification of a cytopathogenic agent infectious for puppies as a canine herpesvirus. Proc Soc Exp Biol Med 1966;120:644–650.

Carmichael LE, Squire RA, Krook L. Clinical and pathologic features of a fatal viral disease of newborn pups. Am J Vet Res 1965;26:803–814.

Cornwell HJC, Wright NG, Campbell RSF, et al. Neonatal disease in the dog associated with a Herpes-like virus. Vet Rec 1966;79:661–662.

Cornwell HJC, Wright NG. Neonatal canine herpesvirus infection: a review of present knowledge. Vet Rec 1969;84:2–6.

Hashimoto A, Hirai K, Yamaguchi T, et al. Experimental transplacental infection of pregnant dogs with canine herpesvirus. Am J Vet Res 1982;43:844–850.

Kakuk TJ, Conner GH. Experimental canine herpesvirus in the gnotobiotic dog. Lab Anim Care 1970;20:69–79.

Karpas A. Experimental production of canine tracheobronchitis (kennel cough) with canine herpesvirus isolated from naturally infected dogs. Am J Vet Res 1968;29:1251–1257.

Karpas A, et al. Canine tracheobronchitis: isolation and characterization of the agent with experimental reproduction of the disease. Proc Soc Exp Biol Med 1968;127:45–52.

Lundgren DL, Clapper WE. Neutralization of canine herpesvirus by dog and human serums: a survey. Am J Vet Res 1969;30:479–482.

Percy DH, Olander HJ, Carmichael LE. Encephalitis in the newborn pup due to a canine herpesvirus. Path Vet 1968;5:135–145.

Percy DH, et al. Pathogenesis of canine herpesvirus encephalitis. Am J Vet Res 1970;31:145–156.

Stewart SE, et al. Herpes-like virus isolated from neonatal and fetal dogs. Science 1965;148:1341–1343.

Wright NG, Cornwell HJC. Experimental herpes virus infection in young puppies. Res Vet Sci 1968;9:295–299.

Pseudorabies (infectious bulbar paralysis, Aujeszky's disease, mad itch)

Pseudorabies, a disease to which many species are susceptible, is caused by a virus of the herpes group termed herpesvirus suis. The disease was first described by Aujeszky (1902) in Hungary but is now known to occur in many parts of the world, including the United States. Natural infection occurs in swine, cattle, dogs,

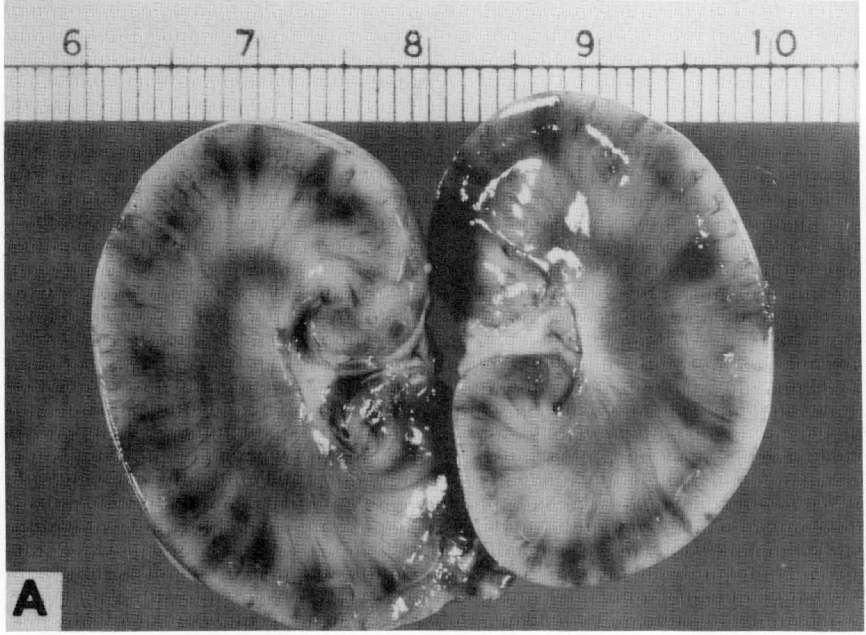

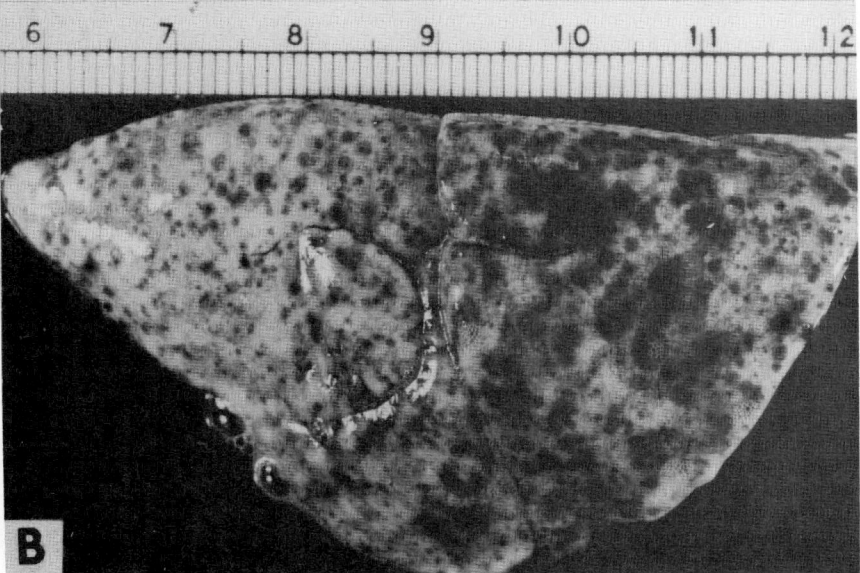

FIG. 8-14 Herpesvirus canis infection in a puppy. **A.** Hemorrhage and necrosis in renal cortex. **B.** Numerous petechiae, ecchymoses, and suffusion in lung. (Courtesy of Dr. T. J. Kakuk and *Laboratory Animal Care.*)

cats, sheep, rats, and mink, but it is of greatest importance in cattle, in which the disease is nearly always fatal. The infection is similar with respect to epizootiology, clinical signs, and pathologic changes to certain other herpesvirus infections, such as herpesvirus B and herpesvirus simplex.

Epizootiology and signs Swine and probably rats serve as the natural and reservoir hosts for herpesvirus suis. Swine are susceptible to infection, but adult animals rarely exhibit symptoms or die from the disease. In adult swine, a mild febrile, nonfatal disease may occur, but recovery is the rule. In piglets (Fig. 8-15), the infection is more severe, occurring as an acute illness that may lead to death in 24 to 48 hours without specific clinical signs. Piglets more than 4 weeks of age may

show signs of involvement of the central nervous system, usually as incoordination of the hindquarters, tremors, convulsions, and eventual paralysis. Disseminated lesions in other tissues may also occur. Although it is uncommon, older pigs may develop encephalitis and die of the infection. Intrauterine infection can occur, resulting in abortion and stillbirth.

Young and adult swine may excrete the virus in the absence of clinical disease, a situation analogous to herpesvirus simplex in humans. This may represent activation of a latent infection maintained in ganglia. Swine serve as the source of infection for cattle and sheep, usually when housed together, but transmission can take place even if the animals are separated by fencing.

Intense itching develops in the skin of the bovine

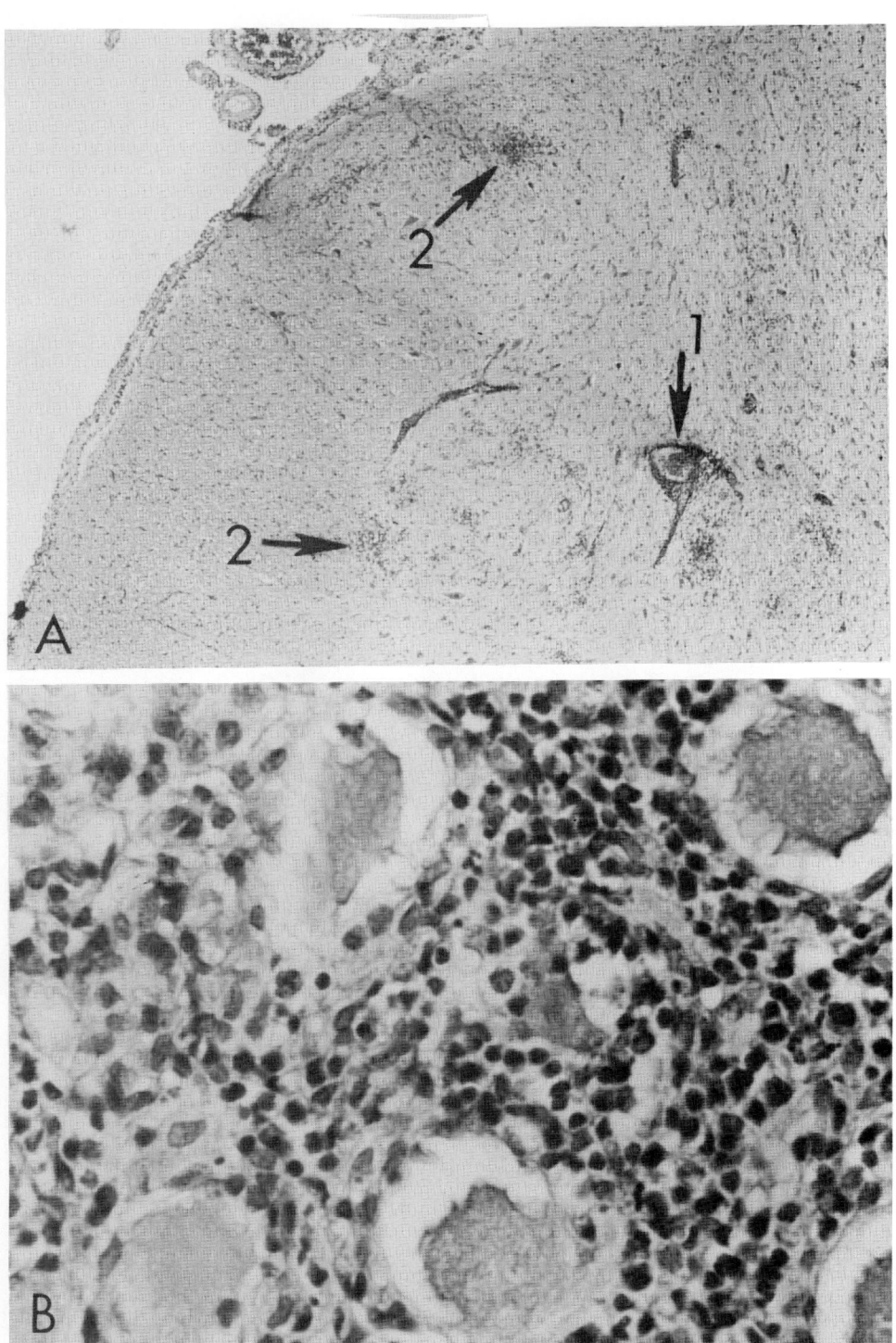

FIG. 8-15 Pseudorabies in a piglet. **A.** Encephalitis with perivascular cuffing *(1)* and glial nodules *(2)*. **B.** Semilunar ganglioneuritis with ganglion cell necrosis, capsule cell proliferation, and a pleomorphic cellular infiltrate. (Courtesy of Dr. H. J. Olander.)

at the point of contact after about 50 hours. Frenzied scratching of this area by the animal causes ulceration of the skin, and secondary infection ensues. Paralysis may develop, and cattle may die rather suddenly with indications of bulbar involvement. The disease affects cattle of all ages and is almost always fatal. The course in affected dogs and cats is similar and also rapidly fatal. Rabbits are particularly susceptible to artificial ex-

posure to this disease; guinea pigs, somewhat less so. Monkeys are also readily infected by experimental means.

Lesions After natural or experimental inoculation of animals, herpesvirus suis reaches their central nervous system by traveling up nerve fibers. Lesions occur in the nerve fibers, ganglia, and central nervous system in all species; the extent and distribution depends on the site of inoculation, duration of the illness, and species type. In general, central lesions are most extensive in the spinal ganglia, temporal cerebral cortex, and basal ganglia of the brain.

In the bovine and ovine, intense inflammation of paravertebral ganglia occurs (Fig. 8-16). Lesions in the brain are more variable. Moderate perivascular cuffing of lymphocytes and some foci of microglial proliferation are seen, but most neurons are normal or exhibit only mild chromatolysis. Intranuclear inclusion bodies are present in neurons and glial cells.

In swine, the lesions in the central nervous system may be very mild or unrecognizable. There are vascular, perivascular, and interstitial lesions with slight nerve cell degeneration. Inclusion bodies are present, but may be few in number. In addition to invasion of the nervous system, lesions are often present in other organs and tissues. Focal necrosis of pharyngeal mucosa, tonsils, lymph nodes, lungs, liver, and adrenal cortex associated with intranuclear inclusion bodies in both epithelial and mesenchymal cells are commonly encountered, especially in young piglets. Invasion of tissues outside the nervous system is unusual in other species, although adrenal cortical necrosis with inclusion bodies has been reported in experimental pseudorabies in sheep.

Necrotizing placentitis with intranuclear inclusion bodies in trophoblast and mesenchymal cells preceeds abortion in swine.

Diagnosis Pseudorabies may be suspected in disease outbreaks in which animals die shortly after showing severe pruritus limited to a specific area of the skin. Cattle or sheep with the disease have almost always been closely associating with swine or wild rats. The microscopic lesions in the skin and spinal ganglia are of some presumptive significance, but the final diagnosis of pseudorabies depends on reproduction of the disease in experimental animals. This is most readily accomplished by the subcutaneous injection of rabbits with suspensions of nervous tissue from diseased animals. These rabbits show intense, frenzied itching, with characteristic local inflammation of the skin. Death is caused by respiratory failure, and the chief pathologic manifestations are necrotic changes in ganglion cells.

References

Aujeszky A. Über eine Neue Infektionskrankheit bei Haustiere. Zentralbl f Bakt. Part I. (Orig) 1902;32:353–357.

Bergmann B, Becker C-H. Studies on the pathomorphology and pathogenesis of Aujeszky's disease. I. Histopathology of the spinal ganglia, spinal nerve roots and spinal cord of guinea pigs after experimental infection. Path Vet 1967;4:97–119.

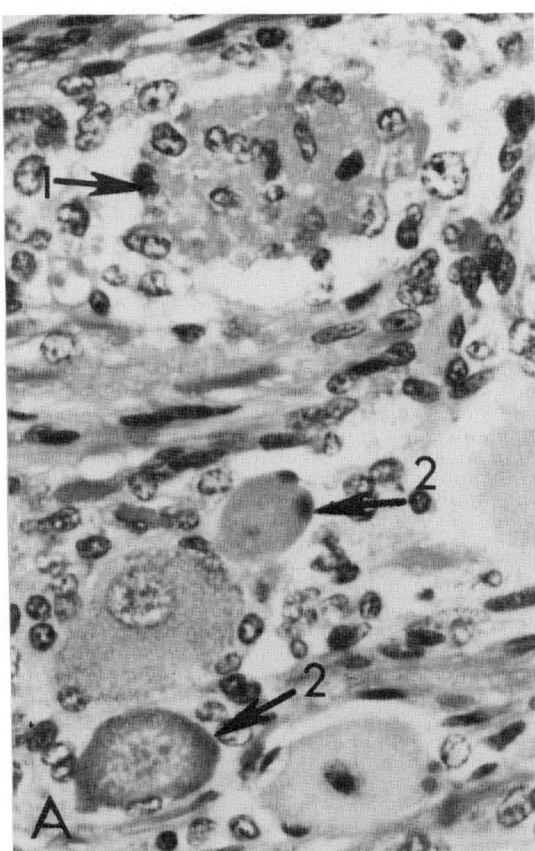 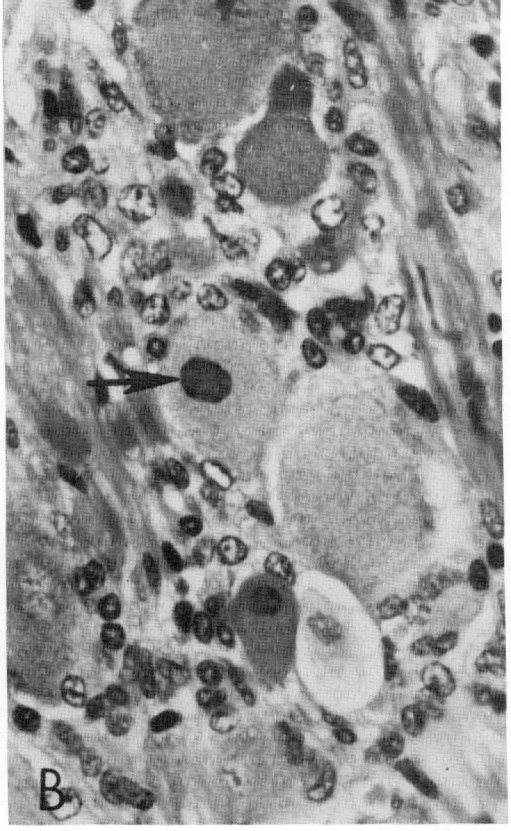

FIG. 8-16 Pseudorabies in a lamb. **A.** Dorsal root ganglioneuritis with a neuronophagic nodule *(1)* and neuron necrosis *(2)*. **B.** A neuron containing an intranuclear inclusion body. (Courtesy of Dr. R. M. McCraken and Dr. C. Dow.)

Cernovsky J. Histopathology of the central nervous system in Aujeszky's disease. Veterinárstvi 1965;15:176–178.

Corner AH. Pathology of experimental Aujeszky's disease in piglets. Res Vet Sci 1965;6:337–343.

Csontos L, Szeky A. Gross and microscopic lesions in the nasopharynx of pigs with Aujeszky's disease. Acta Vet Hung 1966;16:175–186.

Davies EB and Beran GW. Spontaneous shedding of pseudorabies virus from a clinically recovered postparturient sow. J Am Vet Med Assoc 1980;176:1345–1347.

Dow C, McFerran JB. Experimental Aujeszky's disease in sheep. Am J Vet Res 1964;25:461–468.

Dow C, McFerran JB. The neuropathology of Aujeszky's disease in the pig. Res Vet Sci 1962;3:436–442, VB 504–63.

Dow C, McFerran JB. The pathology of Aujeszky's disease in cattle. J Comp Pathol 1962;72:337–347, VB 827–63.

Dow C, McFerran JB. Aujeszky's disease in the dog and cat. Vet Rec 1963;75:1099–1102, VB 1288–64.

Dow C, McFerran JB. Experimental studies on Aujeszky's disease in cattle. J Comp Pathol. 1966;76:379–385.

Dow C, McFerran JB. Experimental studies on Aujeszky's disease in sheep. Br Vet J 1966;122:464–470.

Gutekunst DE, Pirtle EC, Miller LD, et al. Isolation of pseudorabies virus from trigeminal ganglia of a latently infected sow. Am J Vet Res 1980;41:1315–1316.

Hsu FS, Chu RM, Lee RCT, et al. Placental lesions caused by pseudorabies virus in pregnant sows. J Am Vet Med Assoc 1980;177:636–641.

Huck RA, et al. The isolation of Aujeszky's disease virus from dogs. Vet Rec 1969;84:232.

Hurst EW. Studies on pseudorabies. I. Histology of the disease, with a note on the symptomatology. J Exper Med 1933;58:415–433.

Knosel H. Zur Histopathologie der Aujeszky's Chen Krankheit bei Hund und Katze. Zentbl Vet Med 1968;12B:592–598.

Knosel H. Histopathology of Aujeszky's disease in pigs. Deutsch Tierarztl Wschr 1965;72:279–282.

Narita M, Kubo M, Fukusho A, et al. Necrotizing enteritis in piglets associated with Aujeszky's disease virus infection. Vet Pathol 1984;21:450–452.

Narita M, Shimizu M, Kawamura H, et al. Pathologic changes in pigs with prednisolone-induced recrudescence of herpesvirus infection. Am J Vet Res 1985;46:1506–1510.

Olander HJ, et al. Pathologic findings in swine affected with a virulent strain of Aujeszky's virus. Pathol Vet 1966;3:64–82.

Shope RE. Experiments on the epidemiology of pseudorabies. I. Mode of transmission of the disease in swine and their possible role in its spread to cattle. J Exp Med 1935;62:85–99.

Shope RE. Experiments on the epidemiology of pseudorabies. II. Prevalence of the disease among Middle Western swine and the possible role of rats in herd-to-herd infections. J Exp Med 1935;62:101–117.

Thawley DG, Wright JC, Solorzano RF. Epidemiologic monitoring following an episode of pseudorabies involving swine, sheep, and cattle. J Am Vet Med Assoc 1980;176:1001–1003.

INFECTIOUS BOVINE RHINOTRACHEITIS

This disease catagory includes a constellation of disease names, i.e., infectious pustular vulvovaginitis, coital exanthema, vesicular veneral disease, vesicular vaginitis, coital vesicular vaginitis, or coital vesicular exanthema. First isolated in Colorado in association with a respiratory disease of cattle, the virus of infectious bovine rhinotracheitis (IBR) is now recognized as a herpesvirus of bovines of worldwide distribution and termed bovine herpesvirus type 1. After recovery of the animal from active viral disease, the virus remains latent in sciatic and trigeminal ganglia and sheds periodically in a manner believed to be similar to that seen with herpesviruses of other species such as humans (herpesvirus simplex), monkeys (herpesvirus T and herpsvirus B), and dogs (herpesvirus canis). The virus is responsible for a variety of clinicopathologic manifestations in addition to upper respiratory disease, which include conjunctivitis, encephalitis, mastitis, infectious pustular vulvovaginitis and balanoposthitis, abortion, and systemic infection in calves. Currently, investigators doing in-depth studies of viral isolates are finding that differing viral strains are responsible for the varied clinicopathologic manifestations. Infectious bovine rhinotracheitis and infectious pustular vulvovaginitis are the most common manifestations.

Respiratory form Young cattle, assembled in large numbers such as in feedlots, are most susceptible to the disease. The disease is highly infectious, with morbidity rates often approaching 100% and mortality rates of up to 10% of infected animals. The symptoms begin with fever, anorexia, and a mucous nasal discharge, which later becomes mucopurulent and occasionally is tinged with blood. Respiratory distress is evidenced by dilated nostrils, mouth breathing, inspiratory dyspnea, and coughing. Conjunctivitis often accompanies the respiratory form of the disease, but may also occur independently. The course in most cases is about 10 days, but in approximately 10% of sick animals, it may be prolonged. Chronically affected animals lose much flesh and an estimated 3% die.

The gross lesions in cases of the rhinotracheitis form are usually limited to the nasal passages, paranasal sinuses, trachea, and bronchi. Thick mucopurulent exudate clings tenaciously to the congested, often edematous, nasal and turbinate mucosa. The lining of all paranasal sinuses is congested, glistens with excess mucus, and occasionally shows petechiae. The tracheal mucosa is similarly congested and covered with mucopurulent exudate. Severe edema in the wall of the trachea often extends into the walls of the major bronchi. In the trachea, the accumulation of edema between the mucosa and the cartilaginous rings may cause the wall to become as much as 2 cm thick, thereby decreasing the diameter of the lumen. Stenosis of the trachea contributes to the respiratory distress and may result in death from asphyxia or bronchopneumonia.

Microscopically, necrosis of the respiratory tract mucosa with intense neutrophilic and mononuclear inflammation of the submucosa is apparent. The mucosa becomes ulcerated and overlaid with fibrin and necrotic debris. Intranuclear inclusion bodies are present in epithelial cells.

Neonatal form During an outbreak of rhinotracheitis, the infection in very young calves may become generalized. The condition is acute and usually fatal, often with no signs of respiratory system involvement. Pathologically, the lesions in this form of the disease consist of widespread focal necrosis. In both natural and experimental cases, focal necrosis has been observed in the respiratory epithelium, liver, kidney, spleen, lymph nodes, and the mucosa of the oral cavity, esophagus, and forestomachs. Intranuclear inclusion bodies have been described in each of these tissues.

Genital form Gillespie and co-workers (1957) discovered that IBR virus also causes another bovine disease with quite dissimilar manifestations. This disease, infectious pustular vulvovaginitis, has been known for many years, often under other names, such as **coital exanthema, vesicular venereal disease, vesicular vaginitis, coital vesicular vaginitis,** or **coital vesicular exanthema.** It has often been reported in Europe and occasionally in North America. This infection involves principally the female genital tract, as the name implies, but lesions may occur on male genitalia as well. The manifestations of this disease in the cow are described as appearing suddenly 24 to 72 hours after coitus with an infected bull. The mucosa of the vulva becomes reddened with dark red punctate foci, which quickly grow to form vesicles and pustules. These lesions are less than 0.1 to 5.0 mm in diameter and may be water-clear to yellowish-red in color. The pustules may form a yellowish membrane by coalescence. The membrane soon becomes detached to reveal an underlying zone of ulceration. Some pain may be manifested during this stage, and the vulva may become obviously swollen. Affected bulls with similar lesions on the penis and prepuce usually have a small amount of preputial exudate and may be left with some adhesions, although they usually recover completely in about 2 weeks. Healing is usually complete in about 2 weeks, however, recurrent attacks may occur, which probably represent recurrence of latent infection as seen in herpes simplex type 2 genital infections in humans. Cows and bulls can carry the virus in the absence of visible lesions. Microscopically, the lesions consist of foci of necrosis of the mucosal epithelium with an associated inflammatory reaction. Intranuclear inclusion bodies develop within epithelial cells. Limited evidence suggests that the IBR virus may cause a similar disease in sows and boars.

Abortion   The IBR virus is also an important cause of abortion in cattle. The abortion generally occurs after the rhinotracheitis form of the disease or the use of modified live IBR vaccine. Two weeks to two months after the respiratory disease or vaccination, up to 60% of pregnant cows in a herd may abort. Although abortion may occur at any stage of pregnancy, it is most common in the third trimester. The critical period for exposure appears to be 4 1/2 to 6 1/2 months after conception. At the time of abortion, there is no recognizable clinical disease in the dam. Advanced postmortem autolysis is the most striking gross finding in the fetus, which is expelled 24 to 36 hours after intrauterine death. Microscopically characteristic lesions in the fetus consist of focal necrosis in the liver, lymph nodes, spleen, and kidney. Intranuclear inclusion bodies may be found in each of these tissues, but they may be difficult to demonstrate owing to the extensive autolysis. There is also necrotizing placentitis.

The pattern of IBR abortion and the fetal lesions are remarkably similar to equine rhinopneumonitis abortion in mares. Both diseases are caused by herpes viruses.

Other manifestations of IBR   Experimentally, IBR virus has caused mastitis characterized by focal necrosis and intranuclear inclusion bodies. The virus also causes conjunctivitis, which may occur in conjunction with or independently of the respiratory disease (Fig. 8-17). Encephalitis caused by IBR virus has been reported in calves in Australia and the United States. The virus most likely gains entry by way of nerve fibers. The lesions are characterized by neuronal necrosis and intranuclear inclusion bodies in neurons. Perivascular cuffing with lymphocytes and a mononuclear meningeal infiltration is also seen. In view of the neurotropism exhibited by most members of the herpesvirus group, this finding is not surprising.

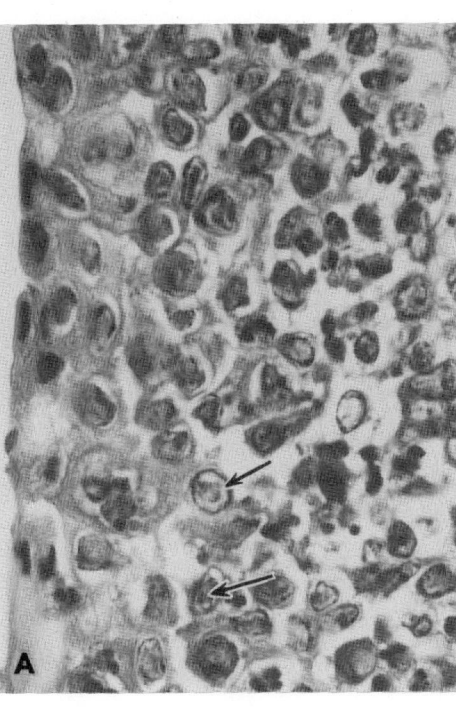
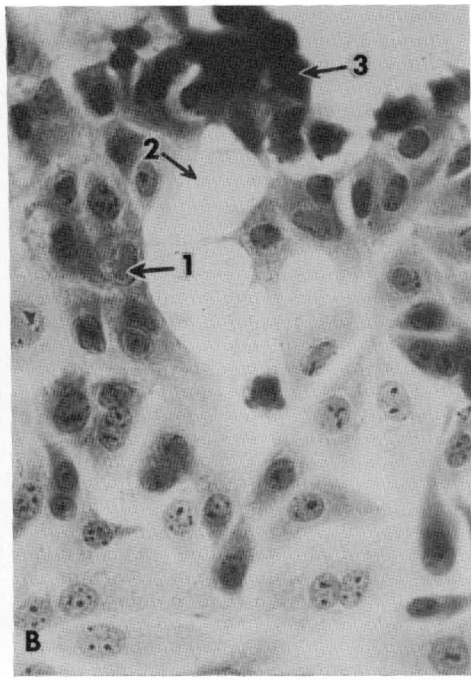

FIG. 8-17   Infectious bovine rhinotracheitis. **A.** Mucosa of nasal septum of a calf, 36 hr after infection. Intranuclear inclusions *(arrows).* (Hematoxylin and eosin stain, × 700.) **B.** Virally infected tissue culture of bovine renal cells. Effect of virus is indicated by intranuclear inclusion bodies *(1),* and cytopathogenic effect evidenced by vacuoles *(2)* and pyknotic nuclei *(3).* (Hematoxylin and eosin stain, × 390.) (Courtesy of Colonel Fred D. Maurer and the Armed Forces Institute of Pathology.)

Diagnosis A presumptive diagnosis of infectious bovine rhinotracheitis in any of its many forms may be made on the basis of characteristic clinical signs and demonstration of necrotizing lesions containing intranuclear inclusion bodies. The diagnosis may be confirmed by isolation and characterization of the virus.

References

Abinanti FR, Plumer GJ. The isolation of infectious bovine rhinotracheitis virus from cattle affected with conjunctivitis—observations on the experimental infection. Am J Vet Res 1961;22:13–17.

Baker JA, McEntee K, Gillespie JH. Effects of infectious bovine rhinotracheitis-infectious pustular vulvovaginitis (IBR-IPV) virus on newborn calves. Cornell Vet 1960;50:156–170.

Barenfus B, et al. Isolation of infectious bovine rhinotracheitis virus from calves with meningoencephalitis. J Am Vet Med Assoc 1963;143:725–728.

Chow TL, Davis RW. The susceptibility of mule deer to infectious bovine rhinotracheitis. Am J Vet Res 1964;25:518–519.

Corner AH, Greig AS, Hill DP. A histological study of the effects of the herpesvirus of infectious bovine rhinotracheitis in the lactating bovine mammary gland. Can J Comp Med Vet Sci 1967;31:320–330.

Crandell RA, Cheatham WJ, Maurer FD. Infectious bovine rhinotracheitis—the occurrence of intranuclear inclusion bodies in experimentally infected animals. Am J Vet Res 1959;20:505–509.

French EL. A specific virus encephalitis in calves: Isolation and characterization of the causal agent. Aust Vet J 1962;38:216–221.

French EL. Relationship between infectious bovine rhinotracheitis (IBR) virus and a virus isolated from calves with encephalitis. Aust Vet J 1962;38:555–556.

Gillespie JH, Lee KM, Baker JA. Infectious bovine rhinotracheitis. Am J Vet Res 1957;18:530–535.

Hall WTK, et al. The pathogenesis of encephalitis caused by the infectious bovine rhinotracheitis virus. Aust Vet J 1966;42:299–327.

Homan EJ, Easterday BC. Isolation of bovine herpesvirus-1 from trigeminal ganglia of clinically normal cattle. Am J Vet Res 1980;41:1212–1213.

Jensen R, Griner LA, Chow TL, et al. Infectious rhinotracheitis in feedlot cattle. I. Pathology and symptoms. Proc US Livestock San A 1955;189–199.

Kendrick JW, Gillespie JH, McEntee K. Infectious pustular vulvovaginitis of cattle. Cornell Vet 1958;48:458–495.

Kendrick JW, Straub OC. Infectious bovine rhinotracheitis infectious-pustular vulvovaginitis virus infection in pregnant cows. Am J Vet Res 1967;28:1269–1282.

Kennedy PC, Richards WPC. The pathology of abortion caused by the virus of infectious bovine rhinotracheitis. Path Vet 1964;1:7–17.

Madin SH, York CJ, McKercher DJ. Isolation of the infectious bovine rhinotracheitis virus. Science 1956;124:721–722.

McFeely RA, Merritt AM, Stearly EL. Abortion in a dairy herd vaccinated for infectious bovine rhinotracheitis. J Am Vet Med Assoc 1968;153:657–661.

McKercher DG. Infectious bovine rhinotracheitis. Adv Vet Sci 1959;5:299–328.

McKercher DG, Moulton JE, Madin SH, et al. A newly recognized virus disease in cattle. Am J Vet Res 1957;18:246–256.

McKercher DG, Straub OC, Saito JK, et al. Comparative studies of the etiological agents of infectious bovine rhinotracheitis and infectious pustular vulvovaginitis. Can J Comp Med 1959;23:320–328.

Molello JA, et al. Placental pathology. V. Placental lesions of cattle experimentally infected with infectious bovine rhinotracheitis virus. Am J Vet Res 1966;27:907–915.

Nelson RD. Effects of infectious bovine rhinotracheitis virus on bovine tracheal epithelium: a scanning electron microscopic study. Am J Vet Res 1974;35:831–833.

Owen NV, Chow TL, Molello JA. Bovine fetal lesions experimentally produced by infectious bovine rhinotracheitis virus. Am J Vet Res 1964;25:1617–1626.

Sattar SA, Bohl EH. Some studies of infectious bovine rhinotracheitis (IBR) virus infection in calves. Can J Comp Med 1968;32:587–592.

Saxegaard F, Onstad O. Isolation and identification of IBR IPV virus from cases of vaginitis and balanitis in swine and from healthy swine. Nord Vet Med 1967;19:54–57.

Snowdon WA. The IBR-IPV virus: reaction to infection and intermittent recovery of virus from experimentally infected cattle. Aust Vet J 1965;41:135–142.

Van Kruiningen HJ, Bartholomew RC. Infectious bovine rhinotracheitis diagnosed by lesions in a calf. J Am Vet Med Assoc 1964;144:1008–1012.

EQUINE ALPHAHERPESVIRUS INFECTIONS

Horses are subject to three alphaherpesviruses: equine herpesvirus type 1 (equine herpesvirus-1, subtype 1), which is an important cause of abortion, neonatal death, respiratory disease, and neurologic disease; equine herpesvirus type 4 (equine herpesvirus-1, subtype 2), which mainly causes acute respiratory disease in young horses, but may also cause abortion; and equine herpesvirus type 3, the cause of equine coital exanthema. Equine herpesvirus type 2 is a betaherpesvirus (cytomegalovirus).

The type 1 and type 4 viruses were formerly considered a single agent. It is now clear that, at the least, they represent distinct strains or subtypes with differing disease manifestations, although both may cause abortion and respiratory disease. Those isolates from epizootics of abortion are clearly different from those associated with respiratory disease. Here we present them as two separate but closely related viruses. The Syrian hamster is experimentally susceptible to both.

Virtually nothing is known concerning latency or recurrence of the equine herpesviruses.

Equine herpesvirus abortion A viral disease of the equine fetus orginally described by Dimock (1940), under the term equine virus abortion, has since become well-established as a cause of intrauterine death of near-term equine fetuses worldwide. It is a particular hazard in horse breeding establishments. It is caused by herpesvirus equi type 1.

SIGNS Infection of the fetus with the agent of virus abortion has some characteristic features on the basis of which a presumptive diagnosis may often be made. The disease almost exclusively affects the fetus during the eighth to eleventh months of pregnancy; the majority of abortions occur in the ninth and tenth months. The fetus is expelled from the uterus promptly after death or, in some cases, before the heartbeat stops, usually with no more difficulty than is experienced in normal parturition. Complications, such as retained placenta, delayed involution, and postparturient metritis, are seldom encountered after abortion caused by this viral agent. The mare usually recovers promptly, showing little more than a slight transitory fever. A storm of abortions may occur, as many as 90% of the pregnant mares in a band being affected, or the disease may be limited to only a small fraction of the susceptible mares. Neonatal infection may lead to fatal generalized disease.

LESIONS In the aborted fetus, the lesions are typically found in the lungs, liver, and lymph nodes, although some icteric discoloration, interlobular pulmonary edema, and excess peritoneal fluid are significant gross findings. The changes in the liver, which usually is congested, may be seen grossly as tiny gray subcapsular foci, usually from 2 to 5 mm in diameter, scattered throughout the lobules. Microscopically, these foci consist of sharply demarcated aggregations of necrotic liver cells. Liver cells surrounding the foci of necrosis often contain small eosinophilic intranuclear inclusions (Fig. 8-18). Enlargement of the nucleus or margination of the chromatin is seldom associated with these inclu-

sions, which usually are quite small, although large enough to replace most of the internal structure of the nucleus. In the lung, interlobular edema and excessive pleural fluid are constant gross lesions. The microscopic changes in the lung consist of cellular debris in the lumen of the bronchi and bronchioles, and partial or complete erosion of adjacent epithelium. In epithelial cells near the eroded areas, the nuclei contain eosinophilic inclusions similar to those in liver cells (Fig. 8-18). Similar intranuclear inclusions and foci of necrosis are found in the spleen and lymph nodes in many cases.

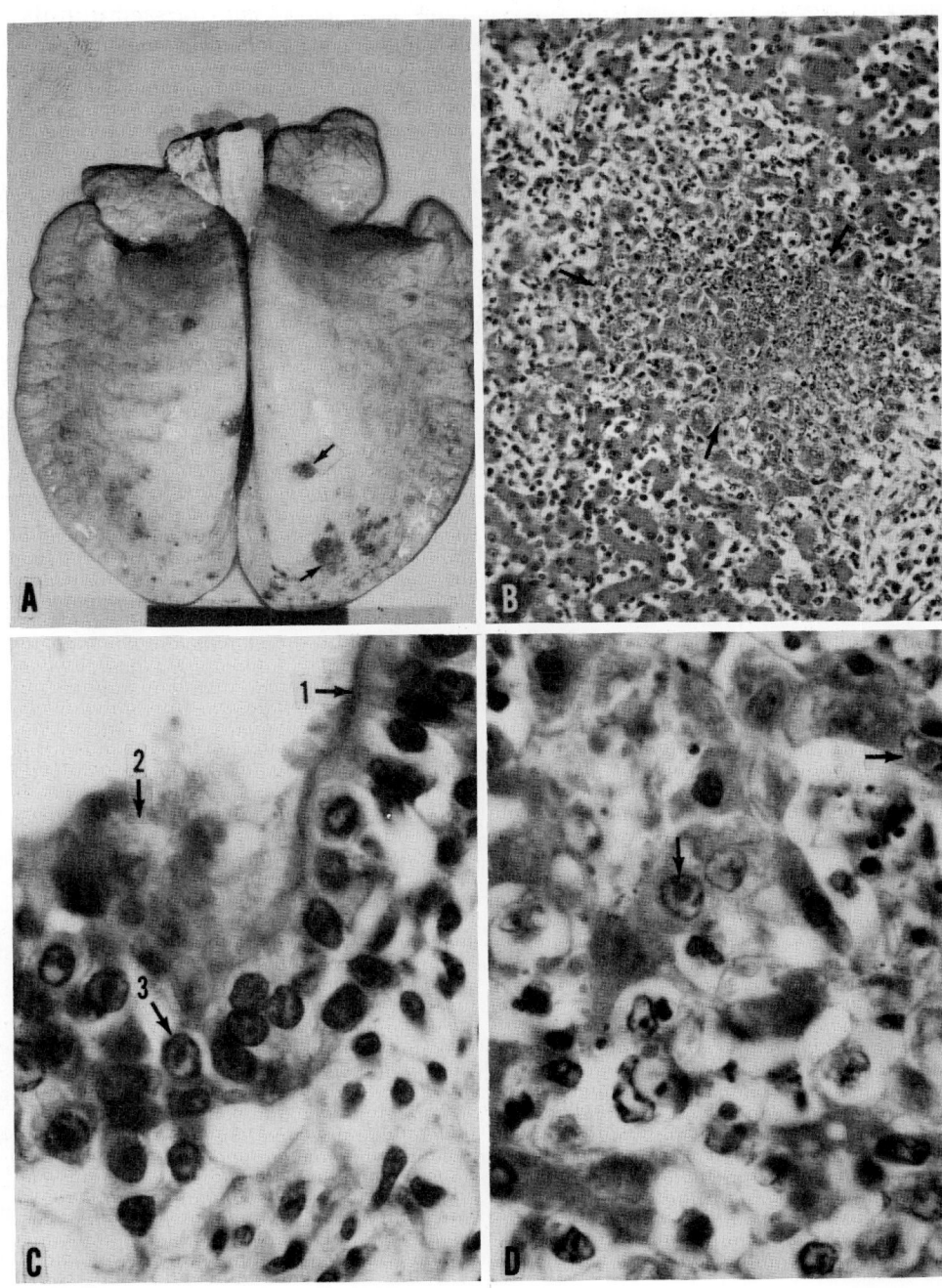

FIG. 8-18 Equine rhinopneumonitis. **A.** Hemorrhages in pleura, lung of an aborted fetus. **B.** Focal necrosis *(arrows)* in liver (× 145). **C.** Erosion and proliferation of bronchiolar epithelium (× 825). Bronchiolar epithelium *(1)*, which is desquamated and hyperplastic *(2)* and contains intranuclear inclusions *(3)*. **D.** Intranuclear inclusions *(arrows)* in liver cells (× 825). (Courtesy of Armed Forces Institute of Pathology; contributed by Dr. Rufus Humphrey.)

Equine viral rhinopneumonitis At about the same time that a virus was identified as a cause of abortion in horses, a virus was isolated by Jones and co-workers (1948) from young horses with a respiratory disease. This disease was responsible for a large number of deaths of horses in remount depots during World War II, usually from pneumonic complications. The disease was called equine influenza at the time, although no immunologic relationship could be demonstrated between this virus and that of swine or human influenza; furthermore, it has other characteristics quite different from those of the other influenza viruses. It is now recognized that the principal causative agent of rhinopneumonitis is **herpesvirus equi type 4,** a virus closely related to the herpesvirus of equine herpesvirus abortion.

SIGNS In young horses from 1 to 4 years of age, fever develops with abrupt onset about 3 days after intravenous or intranasal instillation of the virus. Slight congestion of nasal and conjunctival mucosae occurs, the animal is somewhat depressed, and a dry, hacking cough may develop; the fever usually subsides in 2 to 4 days, and the animal recovers promptly. In complicated cases observed in natural outbreaks in large groups of horses, however, severe respiratory symptoms may appear, particularly when beta-hemolytic streptococci are also involved. Death may result from pneumonia or, in a few cases, from purpura hemorrhagica or streptococcal septicemia. One late sequel is damage to the left recurrent laryngeal nerve, which produces paralysis of the vocal cords, causing characteristic sounds with each inspiration ("roaring"). The virus may also cause late abortion, but herpesvirus equi type 1 or subtype 1 (discussed previously) is much more commonly implicated.

LESIONS Most horses recover. In those that succumb, the lesions are often complicated by the effects of hemolytic streptococci and other bacteria that invade the respiratory system along with the virus. Hemorrhagic or purulent bronchopneumonia is the most common finding in fatal cases, but disseminated abscesses or purpura hemorrhagica may also be found. The virus attacks the respiratory epithelium, resulting in lysis and intranuclear inclusion bodies, which are usually scant at this stage of the disease. The dominant lesions are purulent rhinitis, tracheitis, and pneumonia.

Equine herpesvirus-associated meningoencephalomyelitis In the past two decades, an increasing number of reports have called attention to a possible relationship between equine herpesvirus 1 and a syndrome of ataxia and paralysis. Most often, but not invariably, this syndrome follows epizootics of herpesvirus abortion or respiratory disease. Clinically, there is sudden onset of unilateral or bilateral foreleg and/or hind leg lameness, causing ataxia. This may rapidly progress to fore or hind leg paralysis or complete quadriplegia and recumbency, often causing death. The nature of the meningoencephalomyelitis is not comparable to that caused by other alphaherpesviruses. Inclusion bodies are absent, and it is difficult to recover virus. The principle lesions, which may be present in the brain, spinal cord, meninges, and ganglia, consist of arteriolitis character-

ized by mononuclear cuffing and infiltration, medial necrosis, endothelial hyperplasia, and necrosis and thrombosis. Multinucleated giant cells may be present in the Virchow-Robin space, but the cells lack the inclusion bodies usually seen in alphaherpesvirus-induced polykaryocytes. Focal poliomalacia and leukomalacia are present and are thought to be secondary to vascular damage. There is no evidence of primary viral neurotropism. The pathogenesis of the vasculitis is not understood, but an immune complex-mediated disease has been suggested.

Enterocolitis Enterocolitis, characterized by viral replication in crypt epithelial cells, has been seen in a horse with neurologic equine herpesvirus type 1 infection and also has been seen in young foals experimentally infected with the virus.

Equine coital exanthema A disease reminiscent of infectious pustular vulvovaginitis of cattle is cased by **herpesvirus equi type 3,** an agent distinct from other equine herpesviruses (Fig. 8-18). The disease is characterized by vesicles, pustules, erosions,, and ulcers of the vagina, vulva, perineum, penis and prepuce and less often of the teats and lips. The lesions heal without complication. The virus does not cause abortion.

References

Allen GP, Yeargan MR, Turtinen LW, et al. A new field strain of equine abortion virus (equine herpesvirus-1) among Kentucky horses. Am J Vet Res 1985;46:138–140.

Carman S, Nagy I, Caldwell D, et al. Equine herpesvirus type 1 neurological disease and enterocolitis in mature standardbred horses. J Vet Diagn Invest 1993;5:261–265.

Charlton KM, Mitchell D, Girard A, et al. Meningoencephalomyelitis in horses associated with equine herpesvirus 1 infection. Vet Pathol 1976;13:59–68.

Chowdhury SI, Kubin G, Ludwig H. Equine herpesvirus type 1 (EHV-1) induced abortions and paralysis in a Lipizzaner stud: a contribution to the classification of equine herpesviruses. Arch Virol 1986;90:273–288.

Dimock WW. The diagnosis of virus abortion in mares. J Am Vet Med Assoc 1940;96:665–666.

Doll ER. Intrauterine and intrafetal inoculations with equine abortion virus in pregnant mares. Cornell Vet. 1953;43:112–121.

Doll ER, Wallace ME, Richards MG. Thermal, hematological, and serological responses of weanling horses following inoculation with equine abortion virus: its similarity to equine influenza. Cornell Vet 1954;44:181–190.

Doll ER, Bryans JT, McCollum WH, et al. Isolation of a filterable agent causing arteritis of horses and abortion by mares. Its differentiation from the equine abortion (influenza) virus. Cornell Vet 1957;47:3–41.

Girard A, Greig AS, Mitchell D. A virus associated with vulvitis and balanitis in the horse: a preliminary report. Can J Comp Med 1968;32:603–604.

Jackson TA, Osburn BI, Cordy DR, et al. Equine herpesvirus 1 infection of horses: studies on the experimentally induced neurologic disease. Am J Vet Res 1977;38:709–719.

Jones TC, Maurer FD. The pathology of equine influenza. Am J Vet Res 1943;4:15–31.

Jones TC, et al. Transmission and immunization studies on equine influenza. Am J Vet Res 1948;9:243–253.

Little PB and Thorsen J. Disseminated necrotizing myeloencephalitis: a herpes-associated neurological disease of horses. Vet Pathol 1976;13:161–171.

Pascoe RR, Spradbrow PB, Bagust TJ. An equine genital infection resembling coital exanthema associated with a virus. Aust Vet 1969;45:166–170.

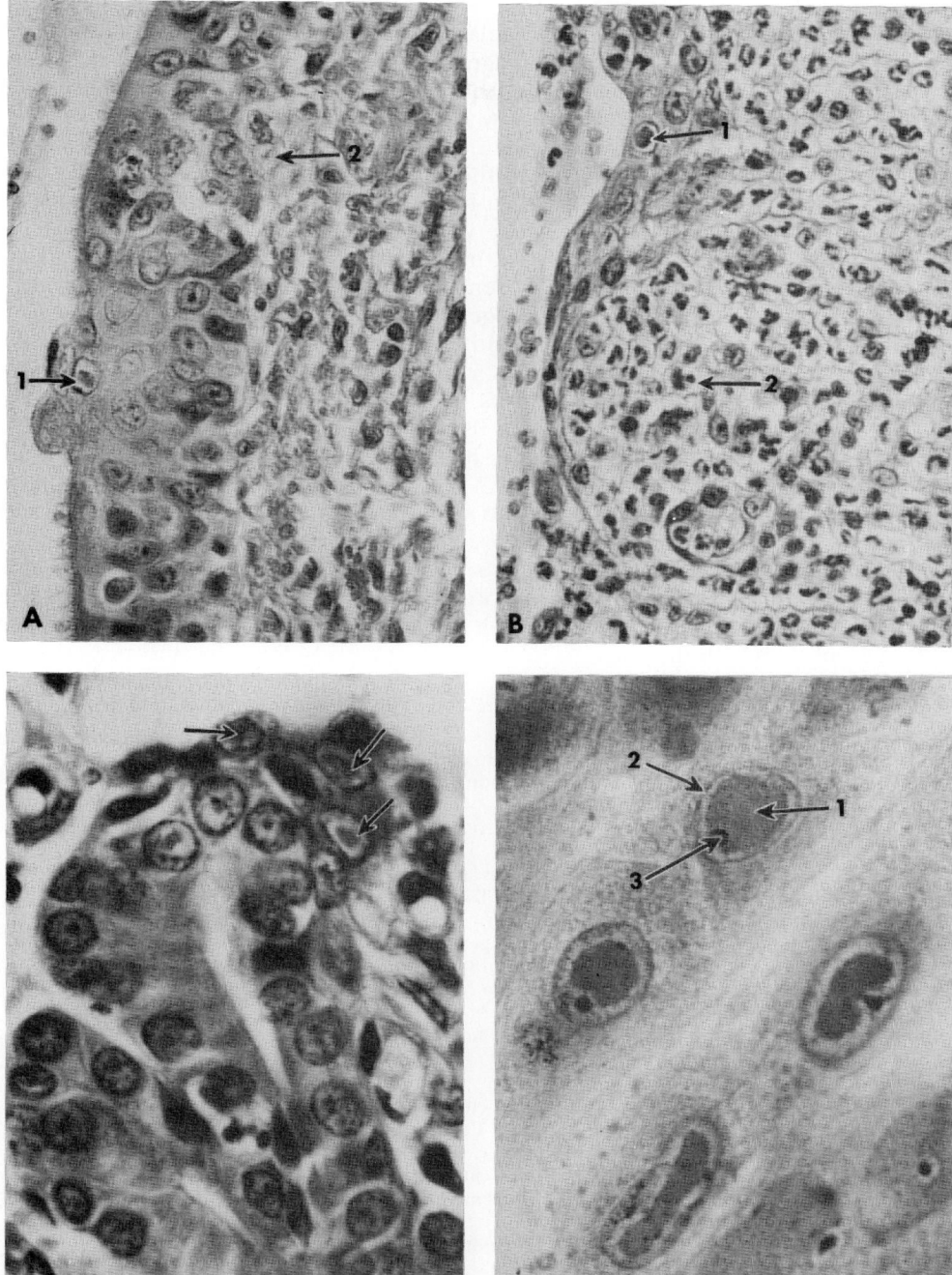

FIG. 8-19 Feline viral rhinotracheitis. **A.** Nasopharynx of cat infected with the virus. Intranuclear inclusion *(1)* and early necrosis *(2)* of the epithelium. (Hematoxylin and eosin stain, × 530.) **B.** Nasopharynx of cat, later stage of infection. Intranuclear inclusion *(1)* still present in mucosa, and neutrophils *(2)* invading the necrotic epithelium. (Hematoxylin and eosin stain, × 530.) **C.** Intranuclear inclusions in nasal epithelium. (Hematoxylin and eosin stain, × 1190.) **D.** Intranuclear inclusion *(1)* in cells of feline kidney tissue culture. Marginated nuclear chromatin *(2)* and nucleolus *(3)*. (Hematoxylin and eosin stain, × 1100.) (Courtesy of Colonel Fred D. Maurer and the Armed Forces Institute of Pathology.)

Plummer G, Bowling CP, Goodheart CR. Comparison of four horse herpesviruses. J Virol 1969;4:738–741.

Studdert MJ. Restriction endonuclease DNA fingerprinting of respiratory, foetal and perinatal foal isolates of equine herpesvirus type 1. Arch Virol 1983;77:249–258.

Westerfield C, Dimock WW. The pathology of equine virus abortion. J Am Vet Med Assoc 1946;109:101–111.

FELINE VIRAL RHINOTRACHEITIS

The isolation and identification, by Crandell and Maurer (1958), of a virus clearly related to an upper respiratory disease of cats is of particular significance because the agent has been shown to cause a widely disseminated disease of cats. Crandell and Maurer named this disease "feline viral rhinotracheitis," an apt designation that indicated its cause as well as the species and anatomic structures affected. The virus has been characterized as a herpesvirus named **feline herpesvirus 1.** The disease is manifested by sudden onset of sneezing and copious discharge of a mucous nasal exudate. This exudate may be seen clinging to the nostrils or on the forelegs as a result of the cat's efforts to clear its nose. Ulcerative glossitis often accompanies the respiratory signs. A transient fever occurs in the early stages. Young, recently weaned kittens are particularly susceptible, but the disease may affect cats of all ages. It is likely that this disease is responsible for much of the illness referred to as "coryza," which appears with such frequency in catteries and veterinary hospitals.

Lesions The lesions are confined to the nasal cavities, tongue, pharynx, larynx, and trachea for the most part, only rarely involving the lungs. The virus attacks the respiratory and oral epithelium, resulting in necrosis of cells and, in early stages, the presence of intranuclear inclusions (Fig. 8-19). This change in the epithelium is followed by ulceration and leukocytic infiltration. The intranuclear inclusions can also be demonstrated in tissue cultures of the virus, using feline kidney cells. The virus produces giant cells and has a significant necrotizing effect on the cells in the tissue culture.

The virus may also cause abortion and systemic disease of the neonate in a manner analogous to other herpesvirus infections such as herpesvirus simplex, herpesvirus canis, and infectious bovine rhinotracheitis. Viruses closely related to feline herpesvirus have been recovered from dogs with diarrhea.

References

Crandell RA, Ganaway JR, Niemann WH, et al. Comparative study of three isolates with the original feline viral rhinotracheitis. Am J Vet Res 1960;21:504–506.

Crandell RA, Madin SH. Experimental studies on a new feline virus. Am J Vet Res 1960;21:551–556.

Crandell RA, Maurer FD. Isolation of a feline virus associated with intranuclear inclusion bodies. Proc Soc Exp Biol Med 1958;97:487–490.

Crandell RA, Relzkemper JA, Niemann WH, et al. Experimental feline viral rhinotracheitis. J Am Vet Med Assoc 1961;138:191–196.

Ditchfield J, Grinyer I. Feline rhinotracheitis virus: a feline herpesvirus. Virology 1965;26:504–506.

Harbour DA, Howard PE, Gaskell RM. Isolation of feline calicivirus and feline herpesvirus from domestic cats 1980 to 1989. Vet Rec 1991;128:77–80.

Hoover EA, Rokovsky MW, Griesemer RA. Experimental feline viral rhinotracheitis in the germfree cat. Am J Pathol 1970;58:269–282.

Junge RE, Miller RE, Boever WJ, et al. Persistent cutaneous ulcers associated with feline herpesvirus type 1 infection in a cheetah. J Am Vet Med Assoc 1991;198:1057–1058.

Karpas A, Routledge JK. Feline herpes virus: isolations and experimental studies. Zbl Vet Med 1968;15:599–606.

Kramer JW, Evermann JF, Leathers CW, et al. Experimental infection of two dogs with a canine isolate of feline herpevirus type 1. Vet Pathol 1991;28:338–340.

Truyen U, Stockhofe-Zurwieden N, Kaaden OR, et al. A case report: encephalitis in lions. DTW [Dtsch Tierärztl Wochenschr] 1990;97:89–91 [Vet Bull 1991;61:6241].

BOVINE ULCERATIVE MAMILLITIS (BOVINE HERPESVIRUS MAMILLITIS)

Although recognized earlier, a specific ulcerative disease of the bovine teat caused by a herpesvirus was first reported by Martin, Martin, and Lauder (1964). The virus, known as bovine herpesvirus 2, which is a distinct member of the herpesvirus group, is not distinguishable from the Allerton virus, a herpesvirus causing a generalized skin disease in Africa called "pseudo-lumpyskin" disease (lumpy skin disease is a poxvirus infection of cattle).

Lesions The lesions of ulcerative mamillitis are usually confined to the teats (Fig. 8-20), although lesions may spread to the skin of the udder and perineum and to the face and oral cavity of nursing calves. In contrast, "pseudolumpyskin" disease is characterized by generalized skin lesions, particularly on the face, neck, back, and perineum. Beginning as local areas of erythema and edema, the lesions progress to vesicles, which rupture, leaving scab-covered ulcers. Healing without visible scarring generally occurs in 10 to 18 days, though lesions may persist up to 3 months. Microscopically (Figs. 8-20 and 8-21), the features resemble other localized herpesvirus-induced lesions (i.e., lesions of herpesvirus simplex, B, and T). In the epidermis, ballooning degeneration, intercellular edema, and necrosis lead to vesiculation. Multinucleated giant cells form within the epidermis. Intranuclear inclusion bodies are numerous in epithelial cells and giant cells. A cellular inflammatory response develops in the dermis.

Diagnosis The disease must be differentiated from cowpox, pseudocowpox, and lumpy skin disease. Histologically, the presence of giant cells and intranuclear inclusion bodies differentiates herpesvirus infections from poxvirus infections, which are characterized by cytoplasmic inclusions. Viral isolation and identification are enough for a definitive diagnosis.

References

Martin WB, James H, Lauder IM, et al. Pathogenesis of bovine mamillitis virus infection in cattle. Am J Vet Res 1969;30:2151–2166.

Martin WB, Martin B, Hay D, et al. Bovine ulcerative mamillitis caused by a herpesvirus. Vet Rec 1966;78:494–497.

Martin WB, Hay D, Crawford LV, et al. Characteristics of bovine mamillitis virus. J Gen Microbiol 1966;45:325–332.

Martin WB, Martin B, Lauder IM. Ulceration of cows' teats caused by a virus. Vet Rec 1964;76:15–16.

Reed DE, Langpap MS, Anson MA. Characterization of herpesviruses isolated from lactating cows with mammary pustular dermatitis. Am J Vet Res 1977;38:1631–1634.

Rweyemamu MM, Johnson RH, McCrea MR. Bovine herpes mamillitis virus. III. Observations on experimental infection. Br Vet J 1968;124:317–323.

Rweyemamu MM, Johnson RH, Tutt JB. Some observations on herpes virus mamillitis of bovine animals. Vet Rec 1966;79:810–811.

Rweyemamu MM, Osborne AD, Johnson RH. Observations on the histopathology of bovine herpes mamillitis. Res Vet Sci 1969;10:203–207.

Diseases caused by betaherpesviruses

CYTOMEGALIC INCLUSION DISEASES

Cytomegalic inclusion diseases, which affect a variety of animal species including humans, are caused by relatively host-specific viruses termed cytomegaloviruses, classified within the betaherpesvirus group. The viruses characteristically induce the formation of extremely large cells of up to 40 μ in diameter, which bear large intranuclear inclusion bodies.

In contrast to alphaherpesviruses, cytoplasmic inclusion bodies are also often present. These represent accumulations of mature virions in cytoplasmic vesicles. Most of the cytomegaloviruses have a particular affinity

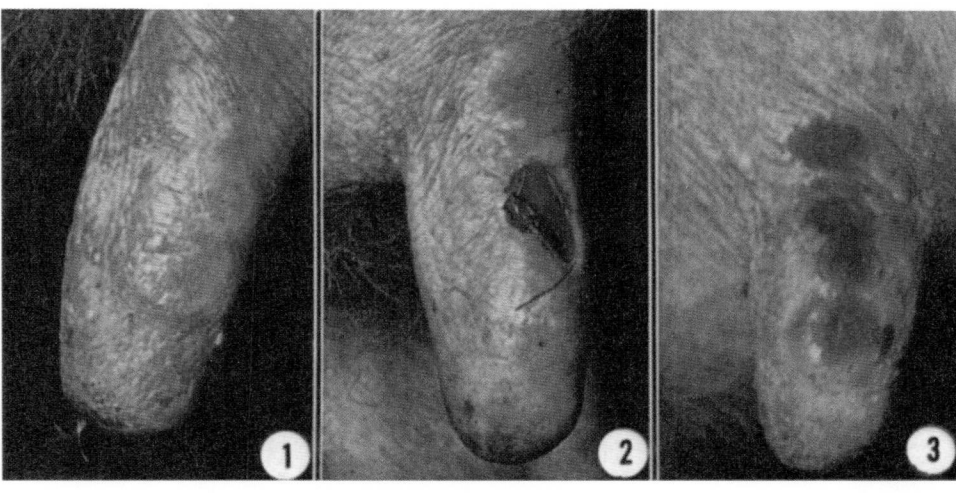

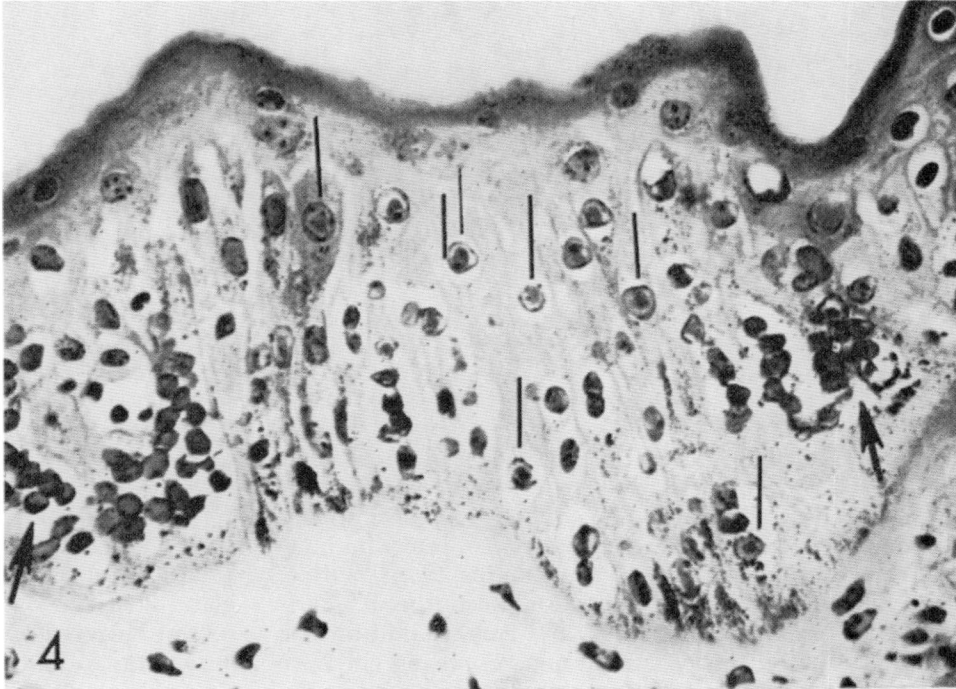

FIG. 8-20 Herpesvirus mamillitis. *(1)* Early raised plaque followed by *(2)* ulceration and *(3)* scab formation. *(4)* Epithelial cells of teat epithelium containing intranuclear inclusion bodies *(bars).* Multinucleated cells are also evident *(arrows).* (Courtesy of Dr. W. B. Martin, Dr. I. M. Lauder, and *American Journal of Veterinary Research 30: 2151–2166, 1969.*)

for salivary glands. The infection is most often latent or subclinical, but under proper circumstances, overwhelming generalized and often fatal infection may develop. Specific cytomegaloviruses have been isolated from humans, guinea pigs, mice, rats, African green monkeys *(Cercopithecus aethiops),* swine (inclusion body rhinitis), ground squirrels, cattle (**hovine herpesvirus 3**), horses (**equine herpesvirus 2**), and cats. Although viruses have not been isolated, lesions compatible with cytomegalovirus infection have been seen in the rhesus monkey *(Macaca mulatta),* cebus monkey, hamster, chimpanzee, gorilla, sheep, sand rat, and tarsier. As indicated, in most species the infection is of little concern; the principal task is in recognition and differential diagnosis. As with most other herpesviruses, incidence of infection is very high and remains latent for life with

periodic shedding; in this case, usually in the urine. As causes of disease, any of the manifestations seen in humans should be expected to occur in domestic animals. Three cytomegalic inclusion diseases will be considered here to illustrate the host-virus relationships.

Cytomegalic inclusion disease in humans (human herpesvirus 5) Detected on the basis of the presence of complement-fixing antibodies, cytomegalovirus infection is common in humans. Pathologically, the infection can be divided into two forms. In the localized form of the disease, inclusion-bearing megalocytes without associated tissue damage or inflammatory reaction are confined to the salivary gland or kidney. This is the most common expression of the disease in humans and in various animal cytomegalovirus infections. **Generalized** cytomegalic inclusion disease, although less com-

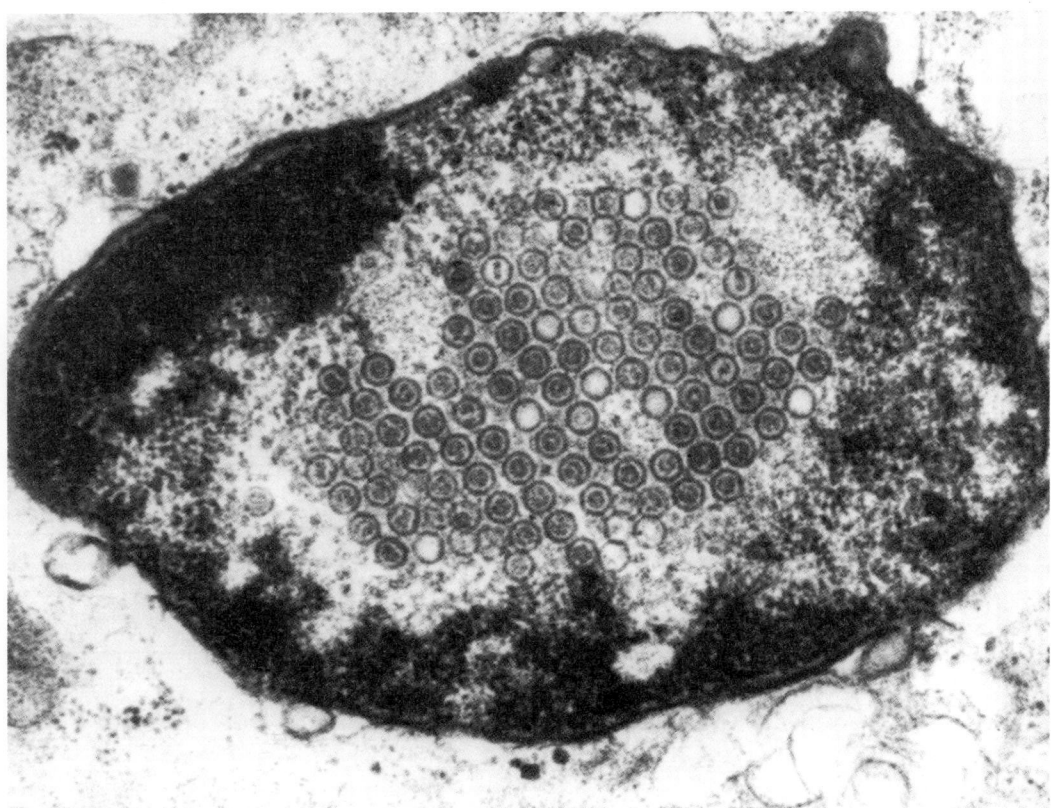

FIG. 8-21 Herpesvirus mamillitis. Numerous viral particles form an inclusion body in an epidermal cell (× 42,000). (Courtesy of Dr. W. B. Martin, Dr. I. M. Lauder, and *American Journal of Veterinary Research.*)

mon, is a serious and often fatal disorder. This form is most common in newborns, who are believed to have become infected *in utero*. Less often, it is seen in older children. Characteristic megalocytes and inclusion bodies may be found in the salivary glands, kidneys, liver, lungs, adrenals, thyroids, pancreas, thymus, and brain, often associated with necrosis and cellular infiltration. Often the child's size is subnormal. Surviving children may develop hydrocephalus, microcephaly, microphthalmia, and mental retardation. Generalized cytomegalic inclusion disease also occurs in adults, usually in association with neoplastic disease, immunosuppressive therapy, or infection with human immunodeficiency disease virus (which causes AIDS). Monkeys infected with simian immunodeficiency virus also often succumb to generalized cytomegalic inclusion disease.

Cytomegalic inclusion disease in guinea pigs This spontaneous viral disease of guinea pigs has been the subject of considerable investigation. The disease, although not uncommon, is usually occult, and it is most often recognized by a finding of large eosinophilic or basophilic inclusion bodies in the nuclei of ducts of salivary glands. Experimental serial passage of the agent through young guinea pigs enhances its virulence until it is able to produce illness and even death. The infection is of interest in comparison with a cytomegalic inclusion disease of infants, in which the inclusion bodies are similar (Fig. 8-22). The causative agents of the hu-

man and animal disease, however, are distinctly different.

The intranuclear inclusions in the guinea pig diseases (Fig. 8-23) are usually not accompanied by any specific necrotic or inflammatory changes. A salivary gland duct that otherwise appears normal may contain several enlarged epithelial nuclei, with margination of chromatin and a large central mass, which is either eosinophilic or slightly basophilic. The inclusion body has some resemblance to that of canine hepatitis.

The virus may disseminate through the body of the guinea pig, particularly when its virulence is enhanced by serial passage, but apparently it localizes in the submaxillary salivary gland, even when introduced into the subcutis. While the infection seldom causes much loss in colonies of laboratory animals, its presence makes the guinea pig unsuitable for research on other viruses whose lesions might be confused with those of the salivary gland virus.

Inclusion body rhinitis of swine (porcine herpesvirus 2) Inclusion body rhinitis of swine is a cytomegalovirus disease first described in Great Britain in 1955. The disease, known to occur in Europe and the United States, principally affects piglets aged 2 to 3 weeks, producing a mild catarrhal to purulent rhinitis (Fig. 8-24). Morbidity is high, but the disease has a low mortality rate, unless complicated by more serious secondary pathogens. As in humans, the porcine virus can cross the placenta

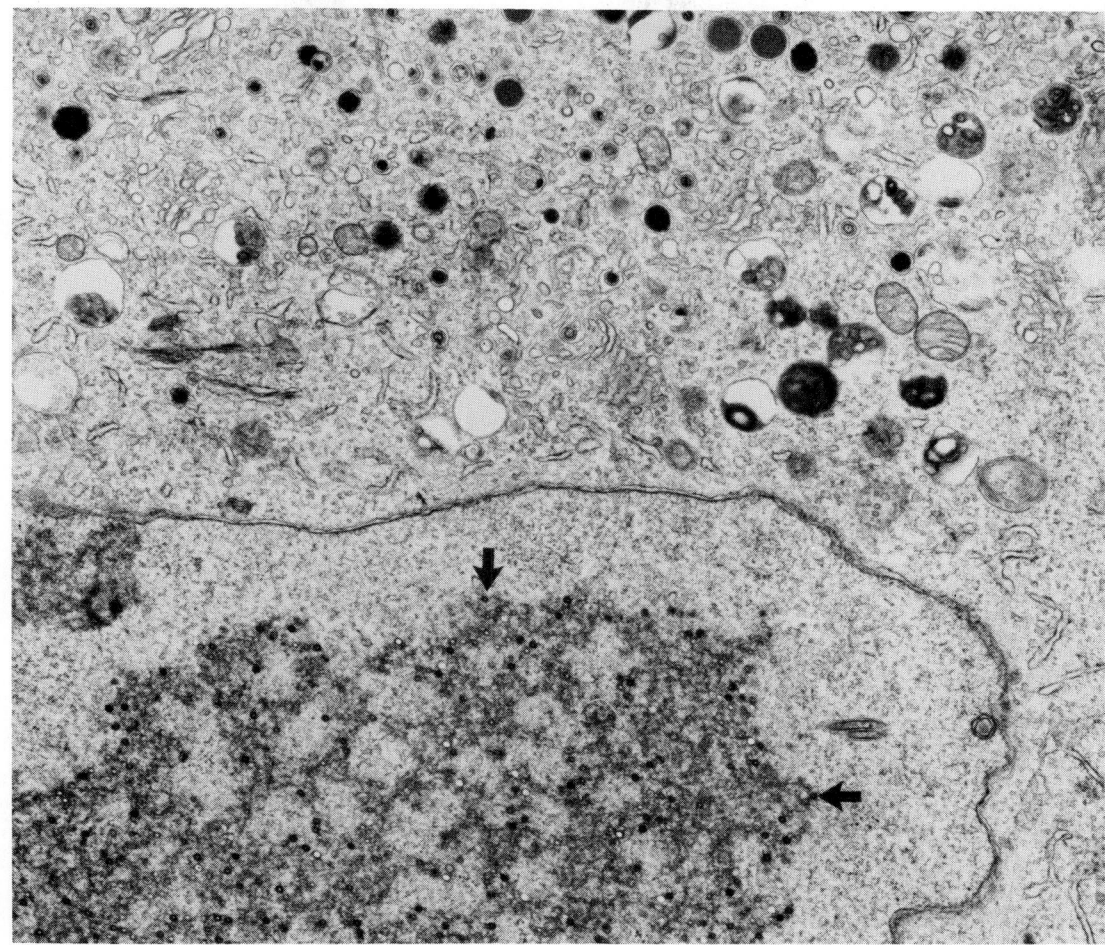

FIG. 8-22 Human cytomegalovirus in tissue culture of human fibroblast. Nucleus contains large inclusion body consisting of virions, viral structural protein, and DNA *(arrows).* (Courtesy of Dr. N. W. King, Jr.)

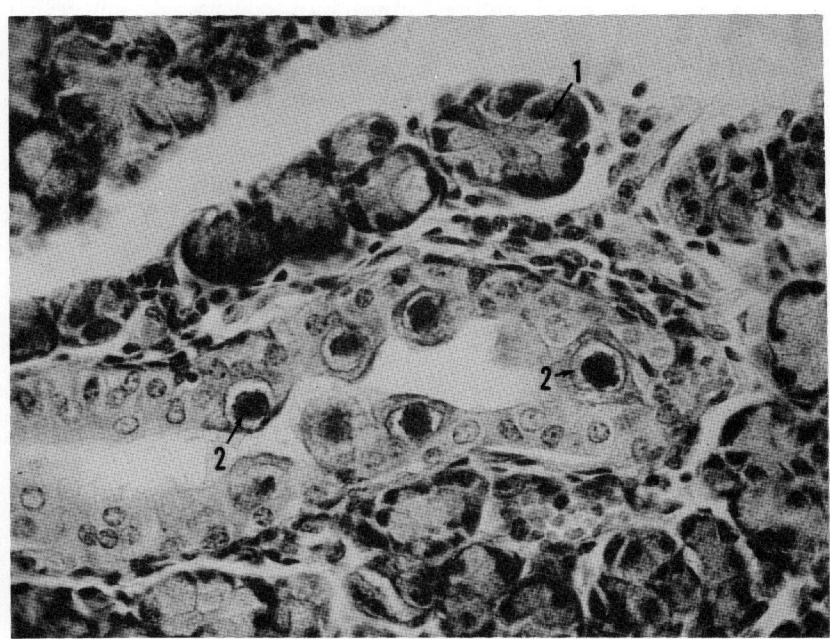

FIG. 8-23 Salivary gland virus disease in guinea pig (× 395). Salivary acinar epithelium *(1)*, intranuclear inclusions in epithelium of a duct *(2).* (Courtesy of Armed Forces Institute of Pathology; contributed by Major C. N. Barron.)

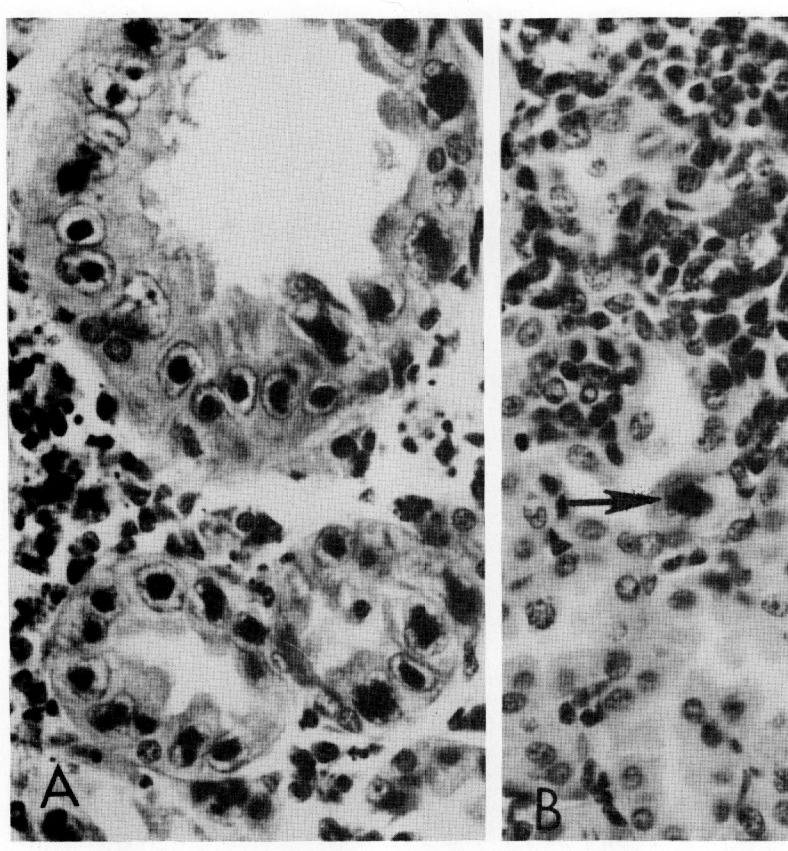

FIG. 8-24 Inclusion-body rhinitis of swine. **A.** Numerous intranuclear inclusion bodies in nasal glands. (Courtesy of Dr. J. R. Duncan.) **B.** Intranuclear inclusion body *(arrow)* in renal tubular epithelial cell and lymphocytic nephritis. (Courtesy of Dr. D. F. Kelly.)

and cause fetal death or generalized disease in neonates.

Microscopically, the picture is dominated by inclusion-bearing megalocytes in the glandular epithelium of the nasal cavity. Recovery is usually uneventful. In the experimentally induced disease, inclusion bodies are first seen 10 days after infection and are usually absent by 27 days postinfection. Inclusion-bearing megalocytes have also been described in the kidney and salivary gland.

Mouse thymic necrosis virus Mouse thymic necrosis virus, also termed TA and murid herpesvirus type 3, is a lymphotropic virus that causes extensive necrosis of the thymus, lymph nodes, and spleen and immunosuppression in newborn laboratory and wild mice. It is antigenically distinct from the mouse cytomegalovirus, murid herpesvirus type 2. Lesions apparently develop only if mice are infected within 24 to 48 hours after birth. Most infected animals recover; however, the virus establishes a persistent infection in salivary glands, lymph nodes, and spleen and is spread horizontally. Infection of adult mice leads to persistent infection without disease. The virus is tropic for CD4 T lymphocytes, which results in the presence of intranuclear inclusion bodies and ultimate necrosis. Necrosis is most severe in the thymus, which may be almost entirely ablated within a week of infection. This usually is not fatal, and the thymus is reconstituted within 4 to 6 weeks. The virus has been compared to human herpesvirus type 6, which is also a lymphotropic T cytolytic herpesvirus.

References

Baskin GB. Disseminated cytomegalovirus infection in immunodeficient rhesus monkeys. Am J Pathol 1987;129:345–352.

Black PH, Hartley JW, Rowe WP. Isolation of a cytomegalovirus from African green monkeys. Proc Soc Exp Biol Med 1963;112:601–605.

Cole R, Kuttner AG. A filterable virus present in the submaxillary glands of guinea pigs. J Exp Med 1926;44:855–873.

Cowdry EV, Scott GN. Nuclear inclusions suggestive of virus action in the salivary glands of the monkey, *Cebus fatuellus*. Am J Pathol 1935;11:647–658.

Cowdry EV, Scott GN. Nuclear inclusions in the kidneys of Macacus Rhesus monkeys. Am J Pathol 1935;11:659–668.

Craighead JE, Hanshaw JB, Carpenter CB. Cytomegalovirus infection after renal allotransplantation. J Am Med Assoc 1967;201:725–728.

Cross SS, Parker JC, Rowe WP, et al. Biology of mouse thymic virus, a herpesvirus of mice, and the antigenic relationship to mouse cytomegalovirus. Infect Immun 1979;26:1186–1195.

Diosi P, Babusceac L, David C. Recovery of cytomegalovirus from the submaxillary glands of ground squirrels. Arch Ges Virusforsch 1967;20:383–386.

Diosi P, et al. Incidence of cytomegalic infection in man. Pathologia et Microbiologia 1967;30:453–468.

Done TC. An "inclusion-body" rhinitis of pigs (preliminary report). Vet Rec 1955;67:525–527.

Duncan JR, Ramsey FK, Switzer WP. Electron microscopy of cytomegalic inclusion disease of swine (inclusion body rhinitis). Am J Vet Res 1965;26:939–947.

Fetterman GH, et al. Generalized cytomegalic inclusion disease of the newborn. Arch Pathol 1968;86:86–94.

Goodwin RFW, Whittleston P. Inclusion-body rhinitis of pigs: an experimental study of some factors that affect the incidence of inclusion bodies in the nasal mucosa. Res Vet Sci 1967;8:346–352.

Hanshaw JB. Cytomegaloviruses. Virology monographs. New York: Springer-Verlag 1968;3:1–23.

Harding JDJ. Inclusion body rhinitis of swine in Maryland. Am J Vet Res 1958;19:907–912.

Hoover DM, Thacker HL. Ovine pulmonary cytomegalovirus. Vet Pathol 1979;16:413–419.

Houff SA, London WT, Wallen WC, et al. Congenital cytomegalovirus virus infection in rhesus monkeys. Neurology 1980;30(Abstr PP54):397.

Hsiung GD, et al. Characterization of a cytomegalo-like virus isolated from spontaneously degenerated equine kidney cell culture. Proc Soc Exp Biol Med 1969;130:80–84.

Hunt RD, Melendez LV, King NW Jr. Cytomegalic inclusion disease in sand rats (Psammomys obesus): histopathologic evidence. Am J Vet Res 1967;28:1190–1193.

Johnson KP. Mouse cytomegalovirus: placental infection. J Infect Dis 1969;120:445–450.

Kelly DF. Pathology of extranasal lesions in experimental inclusion body rhinitis of pigs. Res Vet Sci 1967;8:472–478.

Kendall O, et al. Cytomegaloviruses as common adventitious contaminants in primary African green monkey kidney cell cultures. J Nat Cancer Inst 1969;42:489–496.

Kruger JM, Osborne CA, Goyal SM, et al. Clinicopathologic and pathologic findings of herpesvirus-induced urinary tract infection in conventionally reared cats. Am J Vet Res 1990;51:1649–1655.

Morse SS. Mouse thymic necrosis virus: a novel murine lymphotropic agent. Lab Anim Sci 1987;37:717–725.

Morse SS, Valinsky JE. Mouse thymic virus (MTLV): a mammalian herpesvirus cytolytic for CD4$^+$ (L3T4$^+$) T lymphocytes. J Exp Med 1989;169:591–596.

Naeye RL. Cytomegalic inclusion disease, the fetal disorder. Am J Clin Pathol 1967;47:738–744.

Rabson AS, et al. Isolation and growth of rat cytomegalovirus in vitro. Proc Soc Exp Biol Med 1969;131:923–927.

Rifkind D. Cytomegalovirus infection after renal transplantation. Arch Intern Med 1965;116:553–558.

Rinker CT, McGraw JP. Cytomegalic inclusion disease in childhood leukemia. Cancer 1967;20:36–39.

Rowe WP, Capps WI. A new mouse virus causing necrosis of the thymus in newborn mice. J Exp Med 1961;113:831–844.

Smith AA, McNulty WP Jr. Salivary gland inclusion disease in the tarsier. Lab Anim Care 1969;19:479–481.

Tsuchiya Y, Isshiki O, Yamada H. Generalized cytomegalovirus infection in gorilla. Jap J Med Sci Biol 1970;23:71–73.

Vogel FS, Pinkerton H. Spontaneous salivary gland virus disease in chimpanzees. Arch Pathol 1955;60:281–285.

Wood BA, Dutz W, Cross SS. Neonatal infection with mouse thymic virus: spleen and lymph node necrosis. J Gen Virol 1981;57:139–147.

Diseases caused by gammaherpesviruses

The lymphotropic herpesviruses are subject to extensive research owing to the demonstration that the Epstein-Barr virus (EBV) has been shown to cause infectious mononucleosis in humans and has a strong association with Burkitt's lymphoma and nasopharyngeal carcinoma. Other members of this class of viruses include two simian gammaherpesviruses, herpesvirus saimiri and herpesvirus ateles, which cause lymphoma experimentally in nonhuman primates and rabbits; herpesvirus sylvilagus, a cause of lymphoma and a syndrome resembling infectious mononucleosis in cottontail rabbits, to which domestic rabbits are not susceptible; the virus of malignant catarrhal fever; and a number of lymphotropic viruses related to EBV of Old World primates, but pathogenicity of these viruses has not been established. The virus of Marek's disease, or avian neurolymphomatosis in chickens, would appear to be a gammaherpesvirus on the basis of its lymphotropism, but its genome more closely resembles an alphaherpesvirus. The Lucké herpesvirus, the cause of renal carcinoma in leopard frogs, is not classified and has not been grown in cultured cells.

BOVINE MALIGNANT CATARRH (MALIGNANT CATARRHAL FEVER, SNOTSIEKTE)

Malignant catarrh is an infectious disease of cattle in which the principal manifestations are catarrhal and mucopurulent inflammation of the eyes and nostrils, erosions in the oral mucosa, rapid emaciation, enlargement of lymph nodes, corneal opacity, and nervous symptoms. The disease has a worldwide distribution, occurring in Europe, Africa, and the United States. In Africa, the causative herpesvirus is carried by wildebeest (Connochaetus gnu, C. taurinus), which serve as the source of infection for cattle. In the United States, sheep carry and are the source of this infectious agent. The disease is not transmissible between infected cattle. Rabbits are apparently the only laboratory animals that are experimentally susceptible.

Signs and course Experimental infection, after an incubation period of 14 to 60 days, is followed by high fever and catarrhal conjunctivitis and rhinitis, which are evidenced by mucopurulent discharge from the eyes and nose. This exudate characteristically streams from the eyes and nostrils, but soon dries and adheres. The eyes are sensitive to strong light; the cornea becomes opaque in the final stages. Emaciation develops rapidly. The skin of the muzzle is eroded, and the nasal passages are obstructed by mucopurulent exudate. At the start of the fever, the inside of the mouth is merely congested, but in some cases erosions develop inside the cheeks and on the roof of the mouth that are reported to be grossly indistinguishable from the erosive oral lesions of rinderpest. Diarrhea is common, and nervous manifestations are seen in the final stages. In mild forms of the disease, skin lesions may be observed. These consist of thickening and peeling, particularly of the skin of the neck, axillae, and perineum. The lymph nodes are swollen (an almost constant sign), and those that appear as small, subcutaneous nodules forming a chain along the jugular groove of the neck can be observed clinically. The disease is almost invariably fatal.

Lesions The most consistent lesion in almost all organs is a marked perivascular and intramural infiltration of mononuclear cells, chiefly lymphocytes. Arteries and arterioles in almost all organs are affected, and often there is medial necrosis and endothelial swelling. This change may be responsible for the inflammatory and necrotizing lesions seen grossly and microscopically.

Lymph nodes are invariably swollen; sometimes entire nodes or areas seen on cut section are cherry pink and the cut surface often appears granular. The principal microscopic changes in these lymph nodes are reported to be dilation of lymphatic channels and severe edema and proliferation of reticuloendothelial cells and lymphocytes. In the heart and skeletal muscles, perivascular infiltrations by lymphoid cells have been described.

In the nostrils, sharply demarcated, irregularly shaped erosions of the mucosa are covered with a tenacious mucopurulent exudate. Microscopically, these lesions are seen to be the result of necrosis of the epithelium and intense lymphocyte infiltration of the underlying stroma. Cellular exudate may cover the surface of the eroded area. Lesions that are essentially similar develop in the oral and pharyngeal mucosae.

Congestion, edema, and erosions have been found in the esophagus, rumen, reticulum, and omasum. In the abomasum, catarrhal inflammation of the mucosa occasionally develops, and an increase of eosinophils in the submucosa has been reported. Erosions and ulcers may be present in the abomasum. The small and large intestines both show submucous hyperemia, edema, and an occasional nonspecific increase in eosinophils. Goblet cells are often increased in the small intestine, but croupous membranes are rare.

In the eye, congestion and edema are severe, particularly at the limbus; the lamina propria of the cornea is often edematous, the fibers are swollen and separated, and the corneal epithelium occasionally exhibits ballooning and vesicle formation. The iris stroma is usually congested and contains some inflammatory cells. Fibrinous exudate in the anterior and posterior chambers and occasionally posterior and anterior synechiae with leukocytic infiltration indicate iridocyclitis.

The liver and kidneys are often grossly enlarged and mottled. Grossly, the renal cortex may contain gray to white foci which resemble infarcts. Microscopically, these lesions consist of collections of mononuclear cells. Similar infiltrates are found in the periportal tissues of the liver.

In the brain, a "cooked" gross appearance and an odor resembling that of broth have been described, but the basis for these observations is not clear. Microscopic lesions that have been reported include edema and lymphocytic infiltration in the meninges, especially in the pia mater, deep in the sulci. Perivascular edema and accumulation of lymphocytes are almost always noted and are particularly pronounced in the medulla, pons, olfactory bulb, corpus striatum, caudate nucleus, and hippocampus, as well as in the cerebrum, cerebellum, and spinal gray matter. Variable degenerative changes have been described in neurons, but are irregular in occurrence.

Although the condition is caused by a herpesvirus, the biologic behavior of this virus is unlike cytocidal herpesviruses, such as those of bovine viral rhinotracheitis, feline viral rhinotracheitis, or equine abortion. The behavior of the virus does, however, resemble lymphotropic herpesvirus, such as the Epstein-Barr virus or herpesvirus saimiri. As pointed out by Plowright (1968), Hunt and Billups (1979), and others: (1) no free virus is present in tissues of affected cattle, and virus cannot be recovered except by co-cultivation techniques; (2) the virus is associated with lymphocytes; (3) the virus induces classic herpetic cytopathogenic effects in vitro, but in affected cattle there is no herpetic necrosis, no inclusion body, and no syncytial giant cell formation; (4) the disease is not considered contagious

among cattle; (5) the incubation period is highly variable; and (6) the principal pathologic features are lymphocytic proliferation and infiltration and vasculitis. Exactly what is going on remains to be determined; it may be a lymphoproliferative disease on the order of infectious mononucleosis caused by EBV or an immune-mediated lymphoproliferation and vasculitis directed against viral antigens in infected cells.

Diagnosis The diagnosis of malignant catarrh is often difficult. It may be differentiated from rinderpest by the greater infectivity and shorter course of rinderpest and its more pronounced gross intestinal lesions. The microscopic changes in the mucosae and lymph nodes are also of value in differentiating these two diseases. Considerably more study of malignant catarrh is needed, as are better methods for its recognition.

References

Berkman RN, Barner RD, Morrill CC, et al. Bovine malignant catarrhal fever in Michigan. II. Pathology. Am J Vet Res 1960;21:1015–1027.

Castro AE, Heuschele WP, Schramke ML, et al. Ultrastructure of cellular changes in the replication of the alcelaphine herpesvirus-1 of malignant catarrhal fever. Am J Vet Res 1985;46:1231–1237.

Danskin D, Burdin ML. Bovine petechial fever. Vet Rec 1963;75:391–394, VB 3139–63.

Edington N, Patel J, Russell PH, et al. The nature of the acute lymphoid proliferation in rabbits infected with the herpes virus of bovine malignant catarrhal fever. Eur J Cancer 1979;15:1515–1522.

Fourie JM, Snyman PS. Blouwildebeestoog. J S Afr Vet Med Assoc 1942;13:43–47.

Hunt RD, Billups LH. Wildebeest-associated catarrhal fever in Africa: a neoplastic disease of cattle caused by an oncogenic Herpesvirus? Com Immun Microbiol Infect Dis 1979;2:275–283.

Liggitt HD, DeMartini JC. The pathomorphology of malignant catarrhal fever. I. Generalized lymphoid vasculitis. II. Multisystemic epithelial lesions. Vet Pathol 1980;17:58–72, 73–83.

Manjoer M. Renjakit Ingusan, a disease resembling malignant catarrhal fever in India. VB 1958;2144.

Milne EM, Reid HW. Recovery of a cow from malignant catarrhal fever. Vet Rec 1990;126:640–641.

Murray RB, Blood DC. An outbreak of bovine malignant catarrh in a dairy herd. I. Clinical and pathological observations. Can Vet J 1962;2:227–281, VB 1962;32:130.

Pierson RE, Hamdy FM, Dardiri AH, et al. Comparison of African and American forms of malignant catarrhal fever: transmission and clinical signs. Am J Vet Res 1979;40:1091–1095.

Plowright W. The blood leukocytes in infectious malignant catarrh of the ox and rabbit. J Comp Pathol Therap 1953;63:318–334.

Plowright W. Malignant catarrhal fever. J Am Vet Med Assoc 1968;152:795–804.

Stenius PI. Bovine malignant catarrh. A statistical histopathological and experimental study. Bull Inst Path Vet, Helsinki, 1952.

Unclassified herpesviruses

Lucké described a carcinoma of the kidney, in 1934, as a common spontaneous tumor of the leopard frog (*Rana pipiens*), particularly in northern New England states. He later suggested that the disease was caused by a transmissible virus. Present evidence suggests that the neoplasm is caused by a virus of the herpesvirus group. The tumors may occur in one or both kidneys as multiple white nodules.

Microscopically, they appear as typical carcinomas. A unique feature is the presence of intranuclear inclusion bodies and typical herpesvirus particles within tumor cells in winter months but not in summer months. If affected frogs are artificially exposed to cold temperatures for prolonged periods of time in the summer, virus particles are synthesized.

References

Gross L. Oncogenic viruses. Vol 1, 3rd ed. New York: Pergamon Press 1983.

Lucké B. A neoplastic disease of the kidney of the frog, *Rana pipiens*. Am J Cancer 1934;20:352–379, 1934.

Lucké B. Carcinoma in the leopard frog. Its probable causation by a virus. J Exp Med 1938;68:457–468.

ADENOVIRIDAE

Many adenoviruses (adeno = gland), distinguished from one another by immunologic methods, have been isolated from mammals. However, with the exception of canine hepatitis, most are not serious causes of disease in animals other than those that are immunocompromised. The family *Adenoviridae* contains two genera: mastadenovirus (masto = mammal) and aviadenovirus (avi = bird). All are unenveloped icosahedral viruses, 70 to 90 nm in diameter, with 252 capsomers, of which 240 are hexons (hexamers) and 12 at the vertices are pentons (pentamers). A fiber 20 to 50 nm long with a terminal knob projects from each pentamer. The pentons have been shown to be toxic to cells and may represent a viral "toxin." The nucleic acid consists of a single linear molecule of double-stranded DNA, which is replicated in the nucleus, where a characteristic inclusion body is produced. Experimentally, several adenoviruses have been shown to cause malignant neoplasms in newborn hamsters and other laboratory animals and to transform cells in tissue culture. These properties have been subject to extensive investigation, but a causal relationship to spontaneous neoplasms has not been established. Ordinarily adenoviruses are highly species specific. Adenoviruses of several serotypes have been recovered from many species, including bovine, ovine, porcine, equine, murine, and canine types. These viruses are currently identified by the species of origin and a number (e.g., bovine adenovirus type 3). They are most often associated with pneumonia or enteritis (Fig. 8–45D).

Diseases caused by mastadenoviruses

INFECTIOUS CANINE HEPATITIS

This disease is also called hepatitis contagiosa canis and canine adenovirus infection, and the virus is labeled canine adenovirus 1. Although certain lesions of infectious canine hepatitis have been recognized for many years, its clinical features, etiology, and identification as a separate disease were not established until the classic report of Rubarth appeared in 1947. Rubarth pointed out that fox encephalitis virus, shown by Green to be infective for dogs, undoubtedly was identical to the virus of canine hepatitis. This has since been confirmed.

Infectious canine hepatitis is principally disseminated by excretion of virus in the urine and acquired as a naso-oral infection, often leading to pharyngitis and tonsilitis as initial signs. It occurs worldwide, but in countries where widespread vaccination is practiced, overt disease is now rare. Coyotes, wolves, and raccoons are also susceptible.

Signs Canine hepatitis principally affects young dogs. The infection is common but most often goes unnoticed or is inapparent. When clinical disease is evident, its course is rather variable but often peracute, with the first signs manifested only a few hours before death. Commonly, however, the illness is apparent for several days before death or recovery occurs. The disease starts with apathy, followed by anorexia and, in many cases, intense thirst. Severe, disfiguring subcutaneous edema of the head, neck, and ventral aspects of the trunk is a striking but rare manifestation. Vomiting and diarrhea, the latter with hemorrhage, are common symptoms, and abdominal pain is often expressed by moaning sounds. Body temperature is elevated at onset, but it may fall abruptly to subnormal levels as death approaches.

Central nervous system signs are uncommon and, when seen, take the form of clonic spasms of the extremities and neck, paralysis of the hindquarters, or in a rare case, extreme agitation. The mucous membranes usually appear anemic, sometimes slightly icteric, but rarely deeply jaundiced. Petechiae may occur on the anemic membranes, particularly those of the gingiva. Generally the tonsils are reddened and swollen, with the result that tonsillitis is often the initial diagnosis. Copious lacrimation with hyperemic conjunctivae is rather common. Sometimes diffuse, opaque cloudiness in the cornea ("blue eye") develops 1 to 3 weeks after initial signs. This corneal cloudiness disappears spontaneously if the animal recovers. In the urine, albumin may be present in significant amounts, but that is usually its only abnormality. Other clinicopathologic findings include neutropenia and lymphopenia during the course, with a lymphocytosis during recovery; prolonged bleeding and coagulation times; and elevation of SGOT and SGPT.

Lesions The virus of canine hepatitis has an affinity for parenchymal and Kupffer cells of the liver and endothelial cells generally. Affected cells develop specific basophilic intranuclear inclusion bodies and become necrotic. Reticuloendothelial cells and occasionally other cells, such as renal tubular epithelium, may be affected. In experimentally infected animals, it is possible to produce intranuclear inclusions in other tissues. For example, in animals injected via the cisterna magna with fox encephalitis virus, intranuclear inclusions develop in ependymal cells; in foxes inoculated by the testicular route, inclusions develop in interstitial cells; in dogs inoculated intraperitoneally, inclusions develop in the lining cells of the peritoneum. Gross lesions are dominated by hemorrhage, particularly of the stomach and serosal surfaces, resulting from endothelial damage and loss of coagulation factors of hepatic origin. The spleen and lymph nodes are edematous and congested and may contain hemorrhage. The liver is usually congested and somewhat enlarged, and the gallbladder wall is edematous and thickened.

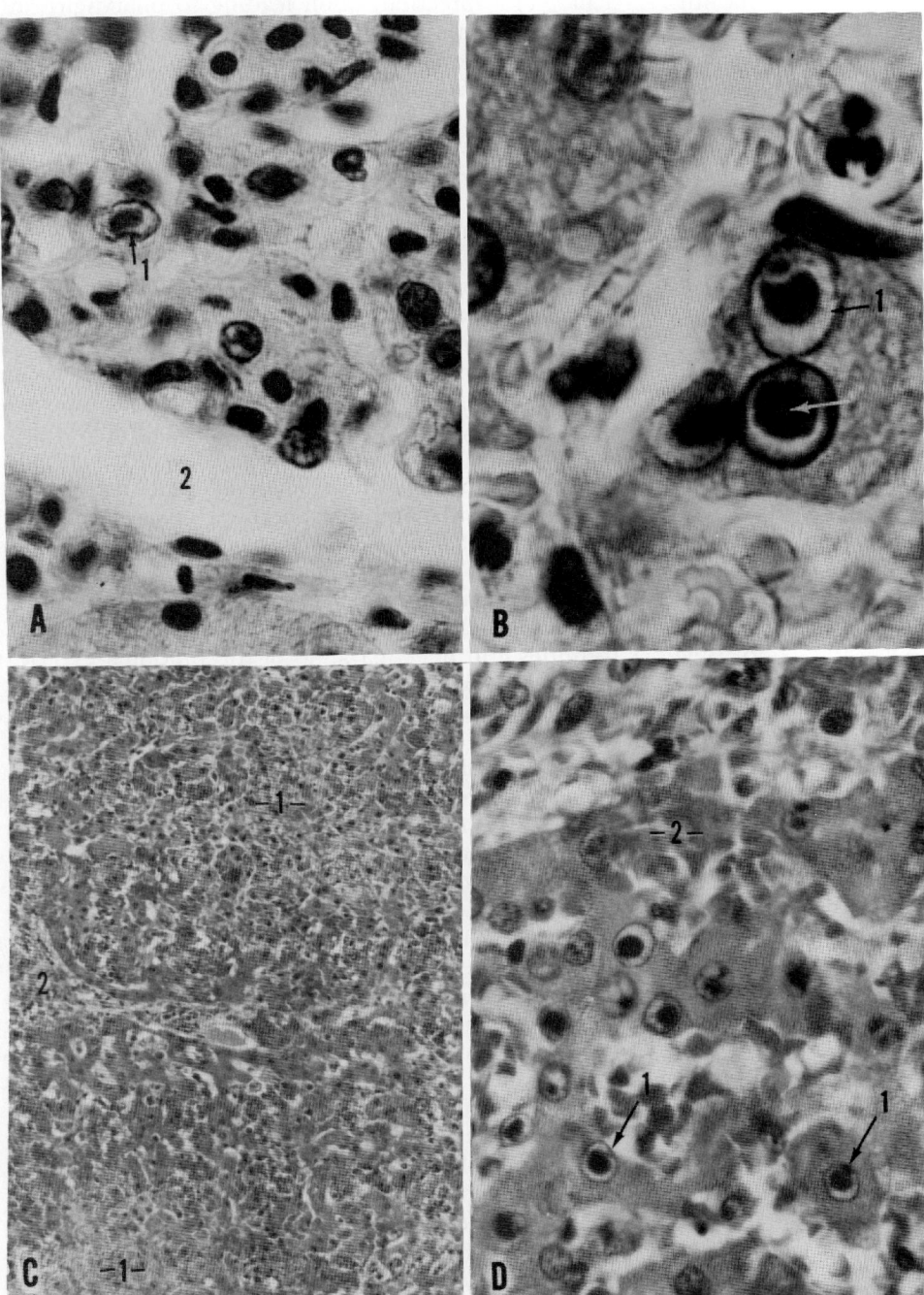

FIG. 8-25 Infectious canine hepatitis. **A.** Intranuclear inclusion *(1)* in endothelial cell of glomerular tuft, Bowman's space *(2)* (× 1080). **B.** Intranuclear inclusion in hepatic cells *(arrow)* (× 1850). Note margination of nuclear chromatin *(1).* (Contributed by Dr. N. Breslauer.) **C.** Foci of necrosis *(1)* in liver (× 125). Portal area *(2).* **D.** Intranuclear inclusion *(1)* in liver cells (× 615). Note lacunose dilation of sinusoids *(2).* (Courtesy of Armed Forces Institute of Pathology; contributed by Dr. W. J. Foster.)

The most characteristic microscopic lesion is focal hepatic necrosis, particularly in the periportal region of the lobules. Hepatocytes become acidophilic, lose their cellular outline, and ultimately disappear, to be replaced by dilated sinusoids.

Intranuclear inclusion bodies are prominent (Fig. 8-25), usually in partly degenerating cells adjacent to areas of necrosis (Fig. 8-26). The nucleus is greatly enlarged, and its chromatin is displaced to its peripheral margin (margination of chromatin). The inclusion, which almost fills the nucleus, has a rather indistinct spherical outline and usually takes a somewhat baso-

philic tint in sections stained with hematoxylin and eosin. Except for a fine granularity (Fig. 8-27), the inclusion body has little demonstrable internal structure. Similar inclusions may be found in endothelial cells and Kupffer cells. Recovery is followed by complete regeneration of the liver.

In a high percentage of cases, the gallbladder wall is edematous, usually grayish, and thickened to as much as 5 mm. Sometimes hemorrhage and edema cause the gallbladder to appear reddish black. Fine precipitation of fibrinous exudate is often seen on the serosa of the gallbladder. The hepatic lymph nodes are often edema-

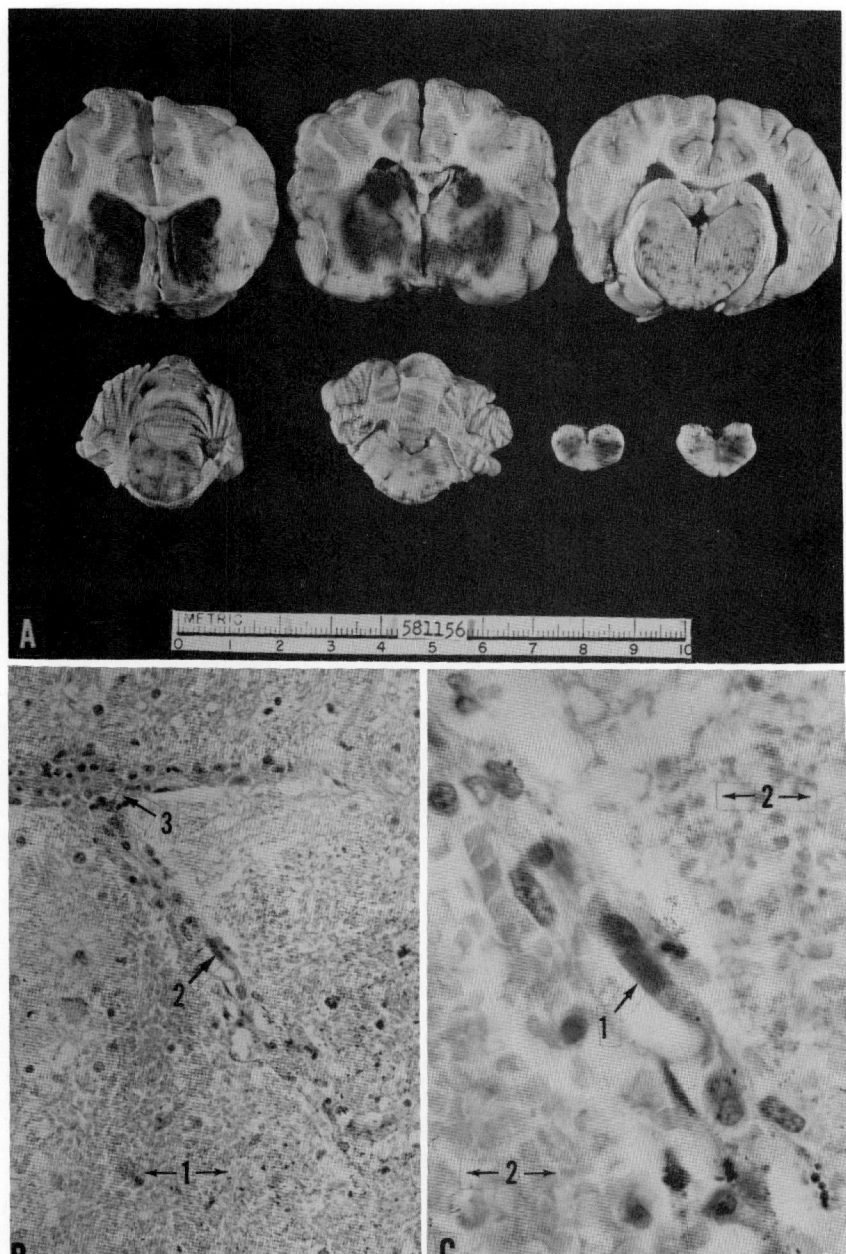

FIG. 8-26 Infectious canine hepatitis. Hemorrhages in the central nervous system. **A.** Bilaterally symmetrical hemorrhagic zones in the brain. **B.** One of the small hemorrhages (× 235) in the brain. Erythrocytes free in the brain parenchyma (1), originating in ruptured capillary with intranuclear inclusion (2) in endothelial cell near site of rupture. Vessel branches (3). **C.** Higher magnification of **B.** (× 1100), with inclusion body (1) in nucleus of endothelial cell. Note adjacent hemorrhage (2). (Courtesy of Armed Forces Institute of Pathology; contributed by Dr. D. L. Coffin.)

tous and occasionally contain petechiae. Capillary rupture with intranuclear inclusions in endothelium can be demonstrated microscopically in liver and gallbladder.

The spleen is usually enlarged and contains an abnormal amount of blood. Infarcts are seldom seen. Intranuclear inclusions may be found without difficulty in cells presumed to be reticuloendothelial cells as well as in endothelial cells.

Lesions in the other visceral organs are inconstant and, when present, are related to changes in vascular endothelium. Petechiae surround small capillaries, and intranuclear inclusions may be found in the endothelium of these vessels. Often, near the site of hemor-

rhage, the number of endothelial cells on the inner surface of the vessels is increased. These changes can produce edema as well as hemorrhage, particularly in lymph nodes, mesentery, tonsils, and under serous surfaces.

In the kidney, intranuclear inclusions may be found microscopically in endothelial cells of the glomerular tufts. These inclusions are limited to one or two in each glomerulus and are rarely associated with any demonstrable lesion in nephrons. Occasionally intranuclear inclusions are present in epithelial cells of collecting tubules. Focal nonsuppurative interstitial nephritis has been described in dogs in the convalescent stages of experimental infectious canine hepatitis.

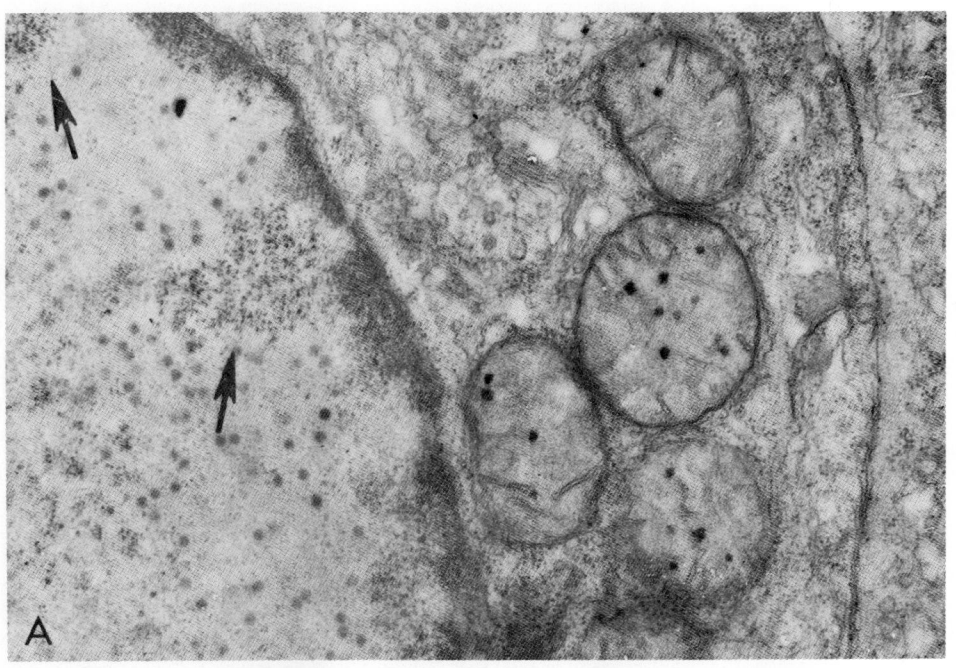

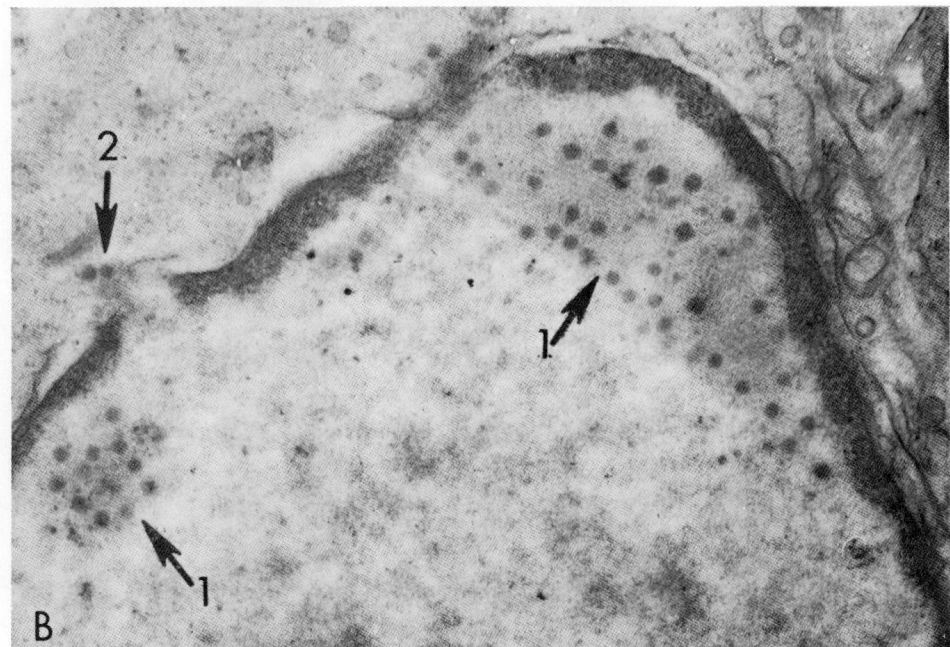

FIG. 8-27 Infectious canine hepatitis. **A.** Adenovirus particles *(arrows)* scattered throughout nucleus of a hepatocyte (× 23,700). **B.** Virus particles in hepatocyte nucleus in crystalline formations *(1)*. Virus particles *(2)* are also escaping from the nucleus (× 30,000). (Courtesy of Dr. K. F. Givan and *Laboratory Investigation.*)

The lesions in the brain are directly related to the changes in capillary endothelium. The involved endothelial cells are increased in number, and some contain elongated intranuclear inclusions conforming to the shape of the enlarged nucleus, in which the chromatin is marginated. Many of the capillaries are surrounded by a small collar of hemorrhage. These hemorrhages may be particularly prominent in the thalamus, midbrain, pons, and medulla oblongata, with grossly demonstrable bilateral symmetry, or they may be diffusely distributed throughout the brain and, for the most part, microscopic. In a few instances, necrosis, loss of

myelin, and occasional collections of glial cells are noted adjacent to affected vessels. These appear to be secondary to interference with circulation.

Carmichael (1964, 1965) has demonstrated that the ocular lesions that develop in dogs recovering from canine hepatitis are the result of an Arthus-type hypersensitivity reaction. Persistent virus within ocular tissues during the antibody response to the infection provides the proper prerequisites for an Arthus reaction. The principal lesion consists of iridocyclitis characterized by hyperemia, edema, and infiltration of plasma cells, neutrophils, and lymphocytes. The cornea is edematous and infiltrated with neutrophils, lymphocytes, and macrophages. Inclusion bodies are not present, although during the acute stages of the disease (before the hypersensitivity reaction), they may be numerous in the ciliary body and iris.

Interstitial nephritis and glomerular lesions are also reported as sequelae to infection. Their pathogenesis has not been elucidated. Virus may be excreted in the urine for as long as 30 days.

Diagnosis The diagnosis in the living animal is difficult because of the nonspecific nature of the symptoms. Microscopic demonstration of focal necrosis and intranuclear inclusions in surgically ablated tonsils or liver biopsy specimens is sufficient to confirm a presumptive clinical diagnosis. After death, the diagnosis is not a problem; it is established by the demonstration of typical lesions associated with characteristic intranuclear inclusions. Immunohistochemical techniques and viral isolation may be used, if necessary. This disease may occur in association with others, such as canine distemper or leptospirosis; hence, it may present a difficult but not insoluble diagnostic problem.

References

Appel M, Carmichael LE, Robson DS. Canine adenovirus type 2— induced immunity to two canine adenoviruses in pups with maternal antibody. Am J Vet Res 1975;36:1199–1202.

Carmichael LE. The pathogenesis of ocular lesions of infectious canine hepatitis. Pathol Vet 1964;1:73–95.

Carmichael LE. The pathogenesis of ocular lesions of infectious canine hepatitis. II. Experimental ocular hypersensitivity produced by the virus. Pathol Vet 1965;2:344–359.

Coffin DL. The pathology of so-called acute tonsilitis of dogs in relation to contagious canine hepatitis (Rubarth). J Am Vet Med Assoc 1948;112:355–362.

Fenner F, Bachmann PA, Gibbs EPJ, et al. Veterinary virology. New York: Academic Press 1987.

Fujimoto Y. Studies on infectious canine hepatitis. I. Histopathological studies on spontaneous cases. Jpn J Vet Res 1957;5:51–70.

Garg SP, Moulton JE, Sekhri KK. Histochemical and electron microscopic studies of dog kidney cells in the early stages of infection with infectious canine hepatitis virus. Am J Vet Res 1967;28:725–730.

Givan KF, Jezequel A-M. Infectious canine hepatitis: a virologic and ultrastructural study. Lab Invest 1969;20:36–45.

Green RG, Dewey ET. Fox encephalitis and canine distemper. Proc Soc Exp Biol Med 1929;27:129–130.

Green RG, Katter MS, Shillinger JE, et al. Epizoötic fox encephalitis. IV. The intranuclear inclusions. Am J Hyg 1933;18:462–481.

Green RG, Shillinger JE. Epizoötic fox encephalitis. VI. A description of the experimental infection in dogs. Am J Hyg 1934;19:362–391.

Innes JRM. Hepatitis contagiosa canis (Rubarth) in Great Britain. Vet Rec 1949;61:173–175.

Larin NM. Epidemiological studies of canine virus hepatitis (Rubarth's Disease). Vet Res 1958;70:295–297.

Lindblad G, Bjorkman N. Ultra-structural alterations in sinusoidal endothelium of liver and bone marrow in dogs with experimental *hepatitis contagiosa canis*. Acta Pathol Microbiol Scand 1964;62:155–163.

Poppensiek GC, Baker JA. Persistence of virus in urine as factor in spread of infectious hepatitis in dogs. Proc Soc Exp Biol Med 1951;77:279–281.

Rubarth S. An acute virus disease with liver lesions in dogs (hepatitis contagiosa canis). A pathologico-anatomical and etiological investigation. Acta Path Microbiol Scand (Suppl) 1947;69.

Sarma PS, et al. Induction of tumors in hamsters with infectious canine hepatitis virus. Nature 1967;215:293–294.

Wright NG, et al. Canine adenovirus respiratory disease: isolation of infectious canine hepatitis virus from natural cases and the experimental production of the disease. Vet Rec 1972;90:411–416.

Wright NG, Thompson H, Cornwell HJC, et al. Ultrastructure of the kidney and urinary excretion of renal antigens in experimental canine adenovirus infection. Res Vet Sci 1973;14:376–380.

CANINE ADENOVIRUS 2

Ditchfield and others (1962) isolated an adenovirus, distinct from the virus of infectious canine hepatitis, from dogs with laryngotracheitis. This virus is now recognized as a cause of conjunctivitis, upper respiratory disease, and less often, pneumonia, although inapparent or mild infection is usual. It has also been associated with enteritis. Canine adenovirus 2 may occur in conjunction with more serious diseases, such as canine distemper. It is considered to be one of the causes of kennel cough. Clinically, there may be fever, nasal discharge, coughing, and occasionally dyspnea. Mortality is very low. The mucosa of the pharynx, larynx, trachea and bronchi are hyperemic and occasionally ulcerated and covered with a purulent or fibrinous exudate. The principal microscopic features are necrosis of respiratory epithelium and the presence of typical adenoviral intranuclear inclusion bodies.

References

Binn LN, Eddy GA, Lazar EC, et al. Viruses recovered from laboratory dogs with respiratory disease. Proc Soc Exp Biol Med 1967;126:140–145.

Campbell RSF, Thompson H, Cornwall HJC, et al. Respiratory adenovirus infection in the dog. Vet Rec 1968;83:203–204.

Ditchfield J, Macpherson LW, Zbitnew A. Association of a canine adenovirus (Toronto A26/61) with an outbreak of laryngotracheitis (kennel cough). Can Vet J 1962;3:238–247.

Ducatelle R, Thoonen H, Coussement W, et al. Pathology of natural canine adenovirus pneumonia. Res Vet Sci 1981;31:207–212.

Hamelin C, Jouvenne P, Assaf R. Association of a type-2 canine adenovirus with an outbreak of diarrhoeal disease among a large dog congregation. J Diarrhoeal Dis Res 1985;3(2):84–87.

Swango LJ, Wooding WL, Binn LN. A comparison of the pathogenesis and antigenicity of infectious canine hepatitis virus and the A26/61 virus strain (Toronto). J Am Vet Med Assoc 1970;156:1687–1696.

BOVINE ADENOVIRAL INFECTIONS

Bovine adenoviruses of several serotypes have been isolated from cattle in several parts of the United States, Europe, Great Britain, Australia, and Japan. Some of them (types 3 and 5) appear to be more pathogenic than others to young calves, producing disease concentrated in the respiratory and gastrointestinal tracts of these animals. Surveys of the presence of antibodies in the serum of cattle indicate that infection is widespread, but rarely leads to overt disease.

Clinical signs usually focus on respiratory tract disease with fever and often keratoconjunctivitis or gastrointestinal tract involvement with tympanitis, colic, and diarrhea. Systemic infection, with edema and hemorrhage around joints, has been described as "weak calf syndrome." Morbidity is usually low, but as many as 80% of all calves in a large herd may eventually exhibit signs of the disease. Mortality is low.

Lesions The lesions may be generalized or limited to the respiratory or gastrointestinal tracts. The characteristic gross lesions in the respiratory tract start in nasal passages as mucinous exudate, which eventually becomes mucopurulent. Diffuse congestion and hemorrhage in the lungs lead to consolidation of entire lobules in parts of the lung. Hemorrhage and edema are evident in the lymph nodes related to the respiratory tract, and petechiae and edema may be seen in the kidneys, adrenal cortex, myocardium, and wall of the intestine. Petechiae and edema are especially conspicuous around major joints in outbreaks in which lameness is a common sign.

Microscopically, respiratory tract lesions are characterized by necrosis of respiratory epithelium with the presence of characteristic intranuclear inclusion bodies in epithelial and endothelial cells. The necrotizing lesions are associated with desquamation and inflammation and are followed by epithelial proliferation. Interstitial pneumonia may occur. In the gastrointestinal form, the virus invades enterocytes of villous epithelium leading to necrosis and blunting of villi (see Fig. 8–45D). Inclusion bodies occur within affected enterocytes. In some examples, inclusion bodies may be limited to endothelial cells of capillaries, arterioles, and venules in the lamina propria and submucosa or may also involve the epithelium. Systemic disease characteristically involves endothelial cells, particularly capillaries and small vessels, in which necrosis, edema, and hemorrhage are accompanied by characteristic intranuclear inclusion bodies, especially in the intestine, kidneys and joints.

In experimental cases following intranasal and intratracheal instillation of virus, viral inclusions appear in respiratory epithelium and endothelial cells, particularly in bronchioles and alveolar septa. The bronchiolar epithelium may become multilayered and the lumen filled with cellular debris. Thickening of interalveolar septa is a common feature. Pulmonary lobules that are not consolidated may become atelectatic.

References

Bulmer WW, Tsai KS, Little PB. Adenovirus infection in two calves. J Am Vet Med Assoc 1975;166:233–238.

Cutlip RC, McClurkin AW. Lesions and pathogenesis of disease in young calves experimentally induced by a bovine adenovirus type 5 isolated from a calf with weak calf syndrome. Am J Vet Res 1975;36:1095–1098.

Darbyshire JH, et al. The pathogenesis and pathology of infection in calves with a strain of bovine adenovirus type 3. Res Vet Sci 1966;7:81–93.

Darbyshire JH. Bovine adenoviruses. J Am Vet Med Assoc 1968;152:786–792.

Lehmkuhl HD, Smith MH, Dierks RE. A bovine adenovirus type 3: isolation, characterization, and experimental infection in calves. Arch Virol 1975;48:39–46.

Mattson DE. Adenovirus infection in cattle. J Am Vet Med Assoc 1973;163:894–896.

Mattson DE. Naturally occurring infection of calves with a bovine adenovirus. Am J Vet Res 1973;34:623–630.

Mohanty SB. Comparative study of bovine adenoviruses. Am J Vet Res 1971;32:1899–1905.

Smyth JA, Cush PF, Adair BM, et al. Adenovirus associated enterocolitis in a bullock. Vet Rec 1986;119:574–576.

OVINE ADENOVIRAL INFECTIONS

Several different species of ovine adenoviruses have been identified and associated with disease; bovine adenoviruses have also been recovered from sheep with respiratory tract disease. As in cattle, ovine adenoviruses are associated with conjunctivitis, respiratory tract disease, and enteritis. Respiratory lesions may involve the tract from the nasal cavity to the lungs and are characterized by epithelial necrosis and typical adenoviral inclusion bodies, which are followed by epithelial hyperplasia. Marked cytomegaly (nuclear and cytoplasmic) of infected respiratory epithelial cells is seen in sheep infected with ovine adenovirus type 6. Some strains are also known to cause focal hepatic necrosis with intranuclear inclusion bodies in hepatocytes (ovine adenovirus type 6 and untyped virus) or nephritis with intranuclear inclusion bodies in endothelial cells (ovine adenovirus type 5).

Ordinarily, morbidity and mortality are low, but there are reports of epizootics with morbidity rates of more than 10% and mortality rates of up to 4%, usually caused by pneumonia complicated by bacterial infection.

References

Adair BM, McKillop ER, McFerran JB. Serologic classification of two ovine adenovirus isolates from the central United States. Am J Vet Res 1985;46:945–946.

Cutlip RC, Lehmkuhl HD. Eperimental infection of lambs with ovine adenovirus isolate RTS-151: lesions. Am J Vet Res 1983;44:2395–2402.

Cutlip RC, Lehmkuhl HD. Pulmonary lesions in lambs experimentally infected with ovine adenovirus 5 strain RTS-42. Vet Pathol 1986;23:589–593.

LeaMaster BR, Evermann JF, Lehmkuhl HD. Identification of ovine adenovirus types five and six in an epizootic of respiratory tract disease in recently weaned lambs. J Am Vet Med Assoc 1987;190:1545–1547.

Lehmkuhl HD, Cutlip RC. Experimental infection of lambs with ovine adenovirus isolate RTS-151: clinical, microbiological, and serologic responses. Am J Vet Res 1984;45:260–262.

Lehmkuhl HD, Cutlip RC. Inoculation of lambs with ovine adenovirus 5 (Mastadenovirus ovi 5) strain RTS-42. Am J Vet Res 1986;47:724–726.

EQUINE ADENOVIRAL INFECTION

Adenovirus infection is associated with respiratory disease in foals, but as with other species, most often the infection is clinically inapparent. It is, however, a particularly important secondary infection and predominant cause of death in certain Arabian foals with inherited combined immunodeficiency disease.

The usual signs include sudden onset of fever with mucous to mucopurulent nasal discharge, cough, dyspnea, tachycardia, and increased respiratory rate, abnormal lung sounds, and in some instances, death.

The lesions are usually confined to the respiratory tract, with mucopurulent rhinitis, tracheitis, and coniform, prune-colored consolidation of dependent portions of the lungs. Bronchiolar thickening results from proliferation of the lining epithelial cells and accumulation of leukocytes around the bronchiole. Necrosis of cells results in cellular debris partially or completely filling the lumen. Basophilic intranuclear inclusions are located in epithelial cells along the entire respiratory tract. These inclusions may also be found in association with focal necrosis in epithelial cells lining the renal pelvis, ureter, urinary bladder, and urethra; epithelial cells also affected include those of the conjunctiva, lacrimal glands, salivary glands, and the pancreas. Occasionally focal lesions may be found in the gastrointestinal tract, particularly the small intestine.

Pulmonary consolidation is concentrated around affected bronchioles, with atelectasis, desquamation of alveolar lining cells, and thickening of the alveolar septa. Lymph nodes and splenic corpuscles are small, as is the thymus; these features are probably related to the inherited immunodeficiency.

References

Corrier DE, Montgomery D, Scutchfield WL. Adenovirus in the intestinal epithelium of a foal with prolonged diarrhea. Vet Pathol 1982;19:564–567.
England JJ, McChesney AE, Chow TL. Characterization of an equine adenovirus. Am J Vet Res 1973;34:1587–1590.
McChesney AE, et al. Adenoviral infection in suckling Arabian foals. Path Vet 1970;7:547–565.
McChesney AE, England JJ, Rich LJ. Adenoviral infection in foals. J Am Vet Med Assoc 1973;162:545–549.
McChesney AE, et al. Experimental transmission of equine adenovirus in Arabian and non-Arabian foals. Am J Vet Res 1974;35:1015–1024.
McChesney AE, England JJ. Adenoviral infection in foals. J Am Vet Med Assoc 1975;166:83–85.
McGuire TC, Poppie MJ. Hypogammaglobulinemia and thymic hypoplasia in horses: a primary combined immuno-deficiency disorder. Infect Immun 1973;8:272–277.
Studdert MJ, Wilks CR, Coggins L. Antigenic comparisons and serologic survey of equine adenoviruses. Am J Vet Res 1974;35:693–699.
Studdert MJ, Blackney MH. Isolation of an adenovirus antigenically distinct from equine adenovirus type 1 from diarrheic foal feces. Am J Vet Res 1982;43:543–544.
Whitlock RH, Dellers RW, Shively JN. Adenoviral pneumonia in a foal. Cornell Vet 1975;65:393–401.

PORCINE ADENOVIRUSES

Porcine adenovirus infection is widespread, and virus can be isolated with some regularity from feces. Clinical and pathologic changes are uncommon, but there are reports of spontaneous and experimentally induced disease, including pneumonia, enteritis, and encephalitis. Epithelial necrosis and intranuclear inclusion bodies in the respiratory tract and small intestine are the most usual findings. Generalized infection with particular involvement of endothelial cells, as seen in some other species, has been described in colostrum-deprived pigs.

References

Coussement W, Ducatelle R, Charlier G, et al. Adenovirus enteritis in pigs. Am J Vet Res 1981;42:1905–1911.
Derbyshire JB, Clarke MC, Collins AP. Serological and pathogenicity studies with some unclassified porcine adenoviruses. J Comp Pathol 1975;85:437–443.
Ducatelle R, Coussement W, Hoorens J. Sequential pathological study of experimental porcine adenovirus enteritis. Vet Pathol 1982;19:179–189.
Edington N, Kasza L, Christofinis GL. Meningoencephalitis in gnotobiotic pigs inoculated intranasally and orally with porcine adenovirus 4. Res Vet Sci 1972;13:289–291.
Kasza L. Isolation of an adenovirus from the brain of a pig. Am J Vet Res 1966;27:751–758.
Narita M, Imada T, Fukusho A. Pathologic changes caused by transplacental infection with an adenovirus-like agent in pigs. Am J Vet Res 1985;46:1126–1129.
Shadduck JA, Kasza L, Koestner A. Pathogenic properties of a porcine adenovirus. Lab Invest 1967;16:635.

SIMIAN ADENOVIRUSES

At least 27 distinct adenoviruses have been isolated from various species of nonhuman primates. Most were not recovered from diseased animals, although a few have been isolated from monkeys with upper respiratory disease, pneumonia, conjunctivitis, or gastroenteritis. Adenoviruses are important as secondary infections in immunosuppressed monkeys where necrotizing pancreatitis, nephritis, and pneumonia with intranuclear inclusion bodies in epithelial cells are the predominant lesions.

The fact that certain simian adenoviruses are oncogenic has attracted much more attention than has their role in spontaneous disease of monkeys. Thirteen simian adenoviruses have been shown to induce undifferentiated neoplasms when injected into newborn hamsters.

References

Chandler FW, Callaway CS, Adams SR. Pancreatitis associated with an adenovirus in a rhesus monkey. Vet Pathol 1974;11:165–171.
Heberling RL. The simian adenoviruses. In: T-W-Fiennes RN, ed. Pathology of simian primates. Part II. Basel: Karger 1972;572–591.
Merkow LP, Slifkin M. Simian adenoviruses. Prog Exp Tumor Res 1973;18:67–87.
Schoeb TR, DaRif CA. Deaths of newborn tree shrews. Lab Anim Sci 1987;37:453–454.

MURINE ADENOVIRAL INFECTIONS

A latent virus isolated by Hartley and Rowe (1960) from leukemic mice was shown to be a part of the *Adenoviridae* family. This agent is oncogenic in newborn hamsters, and under some conditions, it has a predilection for specific organs. Experimental infections may produce lesions concentrated in the central nervous system, or may result in severe necrotizing lesions in the adrenal cortex. This latter tissue affinity has evoked the idea that adenovirus infection might be an antecedent to adrenal cortical atrophy. An adenoviral pneumonia has been reported in guinea pigs.

References

Hartley JW, Rowe WP. A new mouse virus apparently related to the adenovirus group. Virology 1960;11:645–647.
Heck FC Jr, Sheldon WG, Gleiser CA. Pathogenesis of experimentally produced mouse adenovirus infection in mice. Am J Vet Res 1972;33:841–846.
Hoenig EM, Margolis G, Kilham L. Experimental adenovirus infection of the mouse adrenal gland II. Electron microscopic observations. Am J Pathol 1974;75:375–394.
Kunstyr I, Maess J, Naumann S, et al. Adenovirus pneumonia in guinea pigs: an experimental reproduction of the disease. Lab Anim 1984;18:55–60.
Margolis G, Kilham L, Hoenig EM. Experimental adenovirus infection of the mouse adrenal gland I. Light microscopic observations. Am J Pathol 1974;75:363–374.

HUMAN ADENOVIRAL INFECTIONS

The first human adenovirus was isolated from cultures of adenoidal tissue from infants (Rowe and others, 1953) and from military recruits with an acute respiratory illness (Hilleman and Werner, 1954). A large number of such adenoviruses have subsequently been isolated from human sources. Some of these viruses are responsible for respiratory disease, conjunctivitis, gastroenteritis, cystitis, and occasionally meningoencephalitis. They are also important in immunocompromised patients. Many of these viruses produce undifferentiated neoplasms in newborn hamsters, starting at the site of inoculation (Merkow and Slifkin, 1973). Some types of adenovirus are oncogenic in the central nervous system of newborn Sprague-Dawley rats. Intracerebral inoculation of human adenovirus type 12 results in numerous medulloepitheliomatous tumors along the ventricular system in the brain and spinal cord of these rats.

Some adenoviruses have been associated with the occurrence of ileocecal intussusception in young children (Yunis and others, 1975).

References

Hilleman MR, Werner JH. Recovery of a new agent from patients with acute respiratory illness. Proc Soc Exp Biol Med 1954;85:183–188.
Merkow LP, Slifkin M, ed. Oncogenic adenoviruses. Prog Exp Tumor Res 1973;18:1–293.
Mukai N, Kobayashi S. Human adenovirus-induced medulloepitheliomatous neoplasms in Sprague-Dawley rats. Am J Pathol 1973;73:671–690.
Rowe WP, et al. Isolation of a cytopathogenic agent from human adenoids undergoing spontaneous degeneration in tissue culture. Proc Soc Exp Biol Med 1953;84:570–573.

IRIDOVIRIDAE

African swine fever virus is the only member of the family *Iridoviridae* that affects mammals. Other member viruses infect insects, fish, and frogs. Iridovirus virions replicate in the cytoplasm of infected cells, although the nucleus is required for replication. *Poxviridae* are the only other DNA viruses that assemble in the cytoplasm. Virions are released either by budding, in which case they gain an envelope, or through cell lysis. The latter particles are unenveloped, but infectious. The nucleocapsid is icosahedral, 125 to 300 nm in diameter, and the single linear molecule of DNA is 100 to 250 million daltons.

Many of the viruses classified in this family reproduce in insects: Tipula iridescent virus, Sericesthis iridescent virus, Chilo iridescent virus, and Aedes iridescent virus. Vertebrate viruses include Gecko virus, lymphocystic virus of fish, frog virus 3, and African swine fever virus (Hess, 1971).

African Swine Fever (wart hog disease)

African swine fever was first recognized in domestic swine (*Sus scrofula*) taken to Africa by European settlers, who soon associated the disease with contact between domestic swine and wild wart hogs (*Phacochoerus africanus*), which are asymptomatic carriers of the virus. Bush pigs (*Potamochoerus pocus*) can also serve as asymptomatic carriers. Ticks of the genus *Ornithodoros* are biologic vectors, which serve as the primary means of maintaining the infection and spreading it to domestic swine. Transmission also follows ingestion of uncooked, infected pork products. Once introduced into domestic swine by ticks or infected meat, the virus readily spreads by contact. The disease spread, in 1957, to Lisbon, Portugal, presumably from Angola, by means of processed pork products and, by 1960, had spread to Spain. In 1971, a serious outbreak started in Cuba and subsequently spread to the Dominican Republic, Haiti, and Brazil. It has occurred in several European countries, most recently in Belgium in 1985. It is now thought to have been eradicated from all these areas, with the exception of Africa. Multiple strains of virus of varying virulence now exist.

CLINICAL MANIFESTATIONS

Only an acute clinical form of the disease was known in domestic swine until about 1947, when imported swine, allowed free range and in probable contact with wart hogs, developed a chronic form of the disease. This form of the disease made recognition more difficult. Acute African swine fever characteristically commences with a high fever that precedes the appearance of other symptoms by several days. During this febrile period, affected swine may appear well and have a hearty appetite; then, in their final 48 hours, they become depressed, weak, apathetic, and cyanotic; develop cough and dyspnea; and then die. With some strains of virus, vomiting and diarrhea may be observed, and there may be hemorrhage from the nose or anus. Pregnant sows may abort.

As indicated, a more protracted course of the disease is now recognized. Some domesticated swine recover and act as carriers of the virus.

LESIONS Changes grossly evident in African swine fever are similar in many respects to those of hog cholera but are generally more severe. Lymph nodes, especially adrenal, hepatic, and gastric, are usually diffusely hemorrhagic. Intralobular pulmonary edema is seen in about 40% of the swine that succumb; petechiae and ecchymoses are found in the pleura, pericardium, and peritoneum in most cases. Edema and congestion are common in the gallbladder and in the adjacent portions of the liver. Extensive perirenal, diffuse subcapsular, and pelvic hemorrhages are encountered in a few cases. Hemorrhages into the renal cortex, if found at all, are numerous. The spleen is engorged and swollen in about 10% of cases; gastric ulceration is severe in about 20%. Catarrhal enteritis is commonly found. The stomachs of about 80% of swine that die are full of feed, indicating the fulminant nature of the disease. Pneumonia is a rare complication.

The pathogenesis of the extensive hemorrhage is not entirely understood. African swine fever virus does not affect endothelial cells as does the virus of hog cholera. Marked thrombocytopenia as well as prolongation of activated partial thromboplastin time, 1-stage pro-thrombin time, thrombin clotting time, and an increase in factor VIII-related antigen have been demonstrated in experimentally infected pigs and are thought to contribute to the extensive hemorrhage. How these changes come about is not clear.

The microscopic lesions in African swine fever (Fig. 8-28) have been studied critically and been compared to those of hog cholera. The vascular lesions in African swine fever are similar to these of hog cholera, but result in more severe circulatory disturbances (e.g., edema, hemorrhages, infarction) (Fig. 8-29). Severe karyolysis of lymphocytes occurs in African swine fever in contrast to hog cholera, in which lymphopenia occurs but no severe destruction of lymphocytes is found in tissue sections. A particularly striking lesion in the African disease is found in the ellipsoids of the spleen, which become acellular and thus are clearly demonstrated in tissue sections (Fig. 8-28). There may be focal periportal necrosis in the liver accompanied by an infiltration of lymphocytes. Blood vessels in the brain are often infiltrated and surrounded by degenerating lymphocytes (Fig. 8-29D).

The lesions in natural cases of the chronic form of the disease have been described as consisting of pneumonia, fibrinous pericarditis and pleuritis, arthritis, and generalized enlargement of lymph nodes with hypoplasia of lymphocytic cells. Hypogammaglobulinemia accompanies these lesions. Pigs experimentally infected with virus of low virulence also exhibit pneumonia with some interstitial components, such as infiltration by lymphoid cells and thickening of alveolar walls, focal areas of consolidation with desquamation of alveolar lining cells, and localized zones of necrosis with organization around them. These lesions are equally evident in animals that received several challenges of virus, including some given intratracheally. Aside from focal proliferation of lymphocytes and plasma cells in many parenchymatous organs, lesions in other systems also appear essentially nonspecific. Lesions described in experimentally induced abortion include focal placentitis and hepatic necrosis and interstitial pneumonia in the fetus.

DIAGNOSIS The lesions and epizootiologic circumstances are helpful in acute cases of African swine fever. The prolonged cases and latent infections require isolation and identification of the virus in appropriate tissue culture. Immunochistochemical techniques have been used to identify viral antigens in tissues of affected swine with some degree of success.

References

Biront P, Castryck F, Leunen J. An epizootic of African swine fever in Belgium and its eradication. Vet Rec 1987;120:432–434.

Coggins L. African swine fever virus. Pathogenesis. Prog Med Virol 1974;18:48–63.

Edwards JF, Dodds WJ, Slauson DO. Coagulation changes in African swine fever virus infection. Am J Vet Res 1984;45:2414–2420.

Edwards JF, Dodds WJ, Slauson DO. Megakaryocytic infection and thrombocytopenia in African swine fever. Vet Pathol 1985;22:171–176.

Fenner F, Bachmann PA, Gibbs EPJ, et al. Veterinary virology. New York: Academic Press 1987.

Greig A. Pathogenesis of African swine fever in pigs naturally exposed to the disease. J Comp Pathol 1972;82:73–79.

Groocock CM, Hess WR, Gladney WJ. Experimental transmission of African swine fever virus by *Ornithodoros coriaceus*, an argasid tick indigenous to the United States. Am J Vet Res 1980;41:591–594.

Hess WR. African swine fever: a reassessment. Adv Vet Sci Comp Med 1981;25:39–69.

Hess WR. African swine fever virus. Virol Monogr 1971;9:1–33.

Konno S, Taylor WD, Dardiri AH. Acute African swine fever. Prolifera-

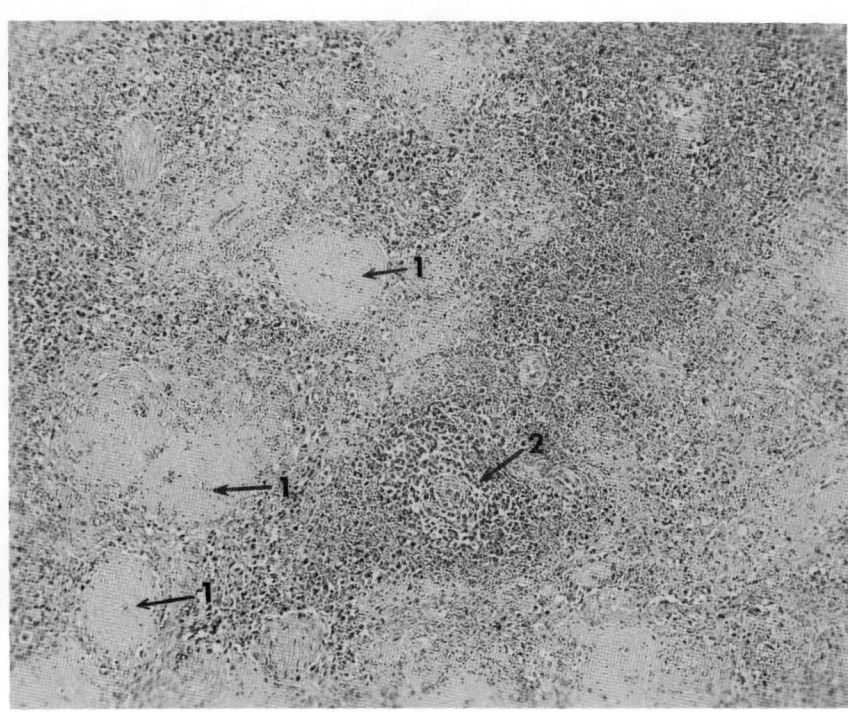

FIG. 8-28 Spleen of a pig with African swine fever. Splenic ellipsoids are enlarged and effaced by hyalin material *(1)*. Lymphocytes *(2)* are largely necrotic or absent. (Courtesy of Colonel Fred D. Maurer and the Armed Forces Institute of Pathology.)

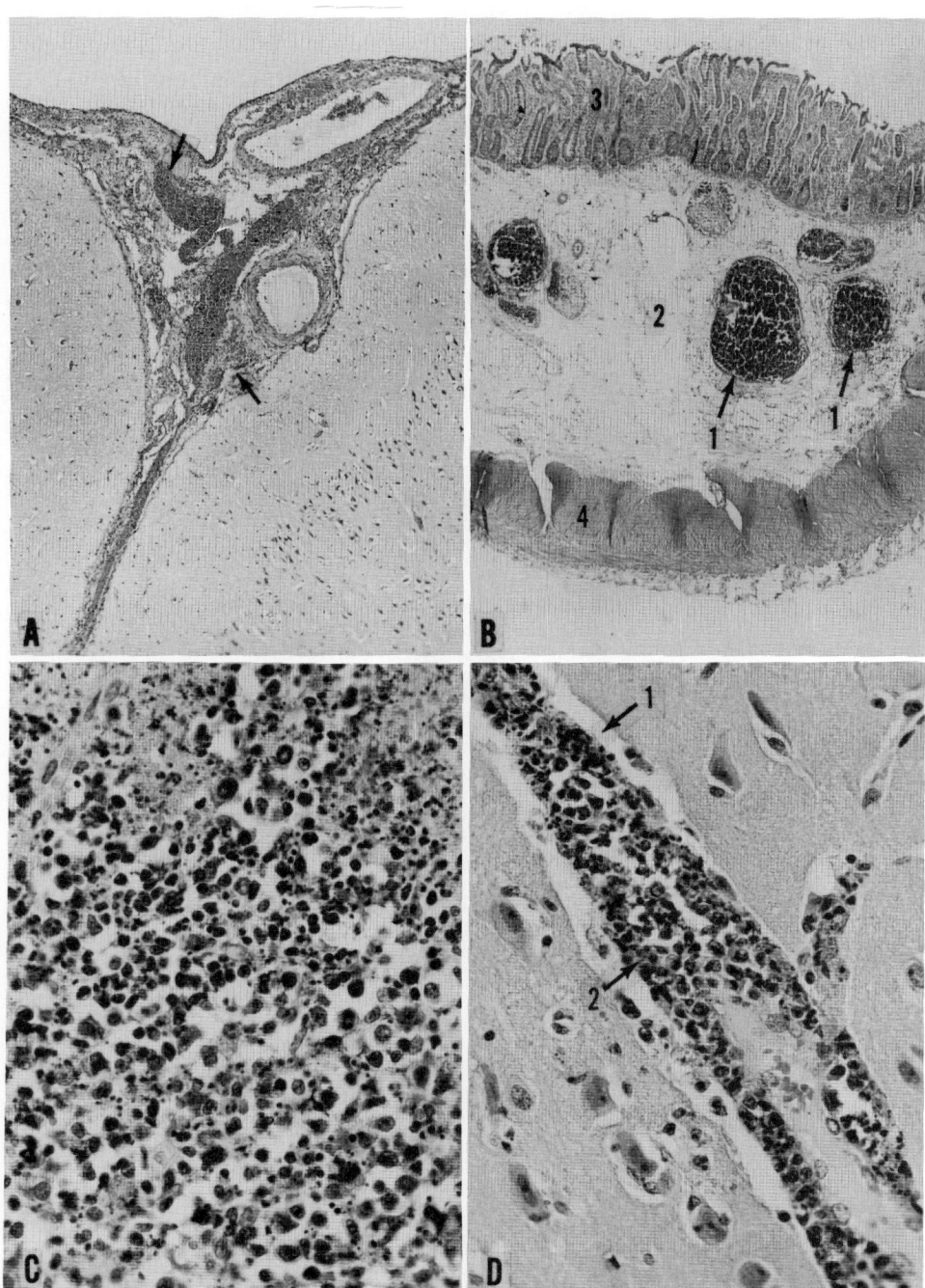

FIG. 8-29 African swine fever. **A.** Hemorrhages *(arrows)* in pia mater (× 50). **B.** Colon. Congested submucosal veins *(1)*, edema in submucosa *(2)*, hemorrhage in mucosa *(3)*(× 26). Note muscularis *(4)*. **C.** Severe karyorrhexis involving lymphoid cells in lymph node (× 395). **D.** Vein in cerebral cortex (× 305). Note Virchow-Robin space *(1)* is empty, but wall of vein *(2)* is infiltrated by lymphoid cells. (Courtesy of Lt. Col. F. D. Maurer.)

tive phase in lymphoreticular tissue and the reticuloendothelial system. Cornell Vet 1971;61:71–84.

Konno S, Taylor WD, Hess WR, et al. Liver pathology in African swine fever. Cornell Vet 1971;61:125–150.

Maurer FD, Griesemer RA, Jones TC. The pathology of African swine fever—a comparison with hog cholera. Am J Vet Res 1958;19: 517–539.

McVicar JW, Mebus CA, Becker HN, et al. Induced African swine fever in feral pigs. J Am Vet Med Assoc 1981;179:441–446.

Moulton J, Coggins L. Comparison of lesions in acute and chronic African swine fever. Cornell Vet 1968;58:364–388.

Moulton JE, Pan IC, Hess WR, et al. Pathologic features of chronic

pneumonia in pigs with experimentally induced African swine fever. Am J Vet Res 1975;36:27–32.

Pan IC, Hess WR. Virulence in African swine fever: its measurement and implications. Am J Vet Res 1984;45:361–366.

Pan IC, Hess WR. Diversity of African swine fever virus. Am J Vet Res 1985;46:314–320.

Schlafer DH, Mebus CA. Abortion in sows experimentally infected with African swine fever virus: pathogenesis studies. Am J Vet Res 1987;48:246–254.

Sierra MA, Bernabe A, Mozos E, et al. Ultrastructure of the liver in pigs with experimental African swine fever. Vet Pathol 1987;24: 460–462.

PAPOVAVIRIDAE

The family *Papovaviridae* (Table 8-4) was created by the grouping of three different viruses leading to the acronym "papova," derived from *pa*pilloma virus, *po*lyoma virus and *va*cuolating agent. Papovaviruses are small (45 to 55 nm in diameter), nonenveloped, icosahedral virions with 72 capsomers. The genome consists of one molecule of double-stranded DNA 3 to 5 million daltons in molecular weight. The family contains two genera, papillomavirus and polyomavirus, which are immunologically distinct.

The genus papillomavirus contains the viral agents responsible for benign papillomatosis (e.g., warts, verrucae vulgaris) in humans and other animals. The viruses are highly species specific with the exception of bovine papillomaviruses. Most also have a narrow tissue specificity; for example, oral papillomatosis in rabbits and dogs is produced by viruses that differ from those that infect cutaneous surfaces. Most animal species that have been adequately studied are afflicted by their own variety of papillomatosis. The list of known susceptible species is added to from time to time.

As with other oncogenic DNA viruses, viral replication does not occur in the transformed, rapidly dividing cells, and thus, viral particles and viral antigen are not demonstrable in cells of the germinal layer. Transformed cells do contain freely replicating episomal viral DNA. However, the cells of the upper layers, i.e., the epidermis, are permissive for viral replication and viral particles can be localized here. Basophilic intranuclear inclusion bodies may, on occasion, also be seen in the cells. The fibroblastic proliferation that accompanies many papillomas (e.g., bovine fibropapilloma, equine sarcoid) also lacks viral particles. Papillomaviruses have not been adapted to tissue culture, which has impeded study. Only human and bovine papillomaviruses have been characterized in any detail.

The genus polyomavirus (poly = many; oma = tumor) is made up of several viruses of considerable scien-

TABLE 8-4 **Diseases caused by Papillomaviruses**

Name of virus	Host(s)	Name of disease
Bovine type 1	Cattle Horses	Cutaneous fibropapilloma Equine sarcoid
Bovine type 2	Cattle Horses	Cutaneous fibropapilloma Equine sarcoid
Bovine type 3	Cattle	Cutaneous papilloma
Bovine type 4	Cattle	Alimentary tract papilloma
Bovine type 5	Cattle	Teat fibropapilloma (rice-grain papilloma)
Bovine type 6	Cattle	Teat papilloma (frond papilloma)
Equine papillomavirus	Horses	Cutaneous papilloma
Canine oral papillomavirus	Canines	Oral papilloma
Cottontail rabbit papillomavirus (Shope fibroma)	Cottontail rabbits, domestic rabbits, hares	Cutaneous papilloma (may progress to squamous cell carcinoma)
Rabbit oral papilloma	Domestic rabbits	Oral papilloma
Deer papillomavirus	Deer	Cutaneous fibroma
Ovine papillomavirus	Sheep	Cutaneous papilloma
Caprine papillomavirus	Goats	Cutaneous papilloma Mammary papilloma
Porcine papillomavirus	Swine	Genital papilloma

tific interest because of their oncogenic and transforming effects on cells in mammalian systems. Their pathogenicity in nature appears negligible. The specific viruses in this genus include SE polyoma virus of mice, K virus of rats, simian virus 40 (SV 40), rabbit vacuolating virus (plus others), and the viruses of progressive multifocal leukoencephalopathy of humans.

Papillomatosis (common warts, verrucae vulgaris)

The common wart that adorns the finger of the child has its counterpart in nearly every animal species; it was first described centuries ago. In some animals, these warts are precise lesions that fastidiously refuse to grow anywhere but in a selected type of epithelium, e.g., in the mouth. In other animals, massively huge and roughly keratinized warts indiscriminately involve large areas of the skin. Most warts are known from observation to be infectious by contact, and many have been shown by experiment to be transmissible. In cutaneous papillomas of the rabbit and goat, transformation of simple hyperplastic squamous epithelium to frankly malignant squamous cell carcinoma has been demonstrated. Thus it appears that papillomatoses represent infectious disease caused by viruses and characterized by benign hyperplasia of stroma and epithelium, which may, under certain circumstances, undergo malignant change. These viruses may therefore be considered among those which induce tumors.

BOVINE CUTANEOUS PAPILLOMATOSIS

In the bovine species, cutaneous papillomatosis is more common than in any other domestic animal. The disease affects young animals more often and more severely, but may affect cattle of all ages.

At least six distinct bovine papillomaviruses have been recognized (Table 8-4). The most usual form seen, caused by bovine papillomavirus types 1 and 2, differs from papillomas seen in other species in that there is a striking proliferation of connective tissue, giving rise to the term **fibropapilloma.** These are most commonly found about the head and neck (Figs. 8-30 and 8-31), but may also occur on the udder and external genitalia (Fig. 8-32). The disease is generally self-limiting and recovery without treatment is the usual course; but when lesions occur on the genitalia, they may interfere with reproduction.

The typical bovine fibropapilloma appears grossly as a rough, cauliflower-like mass of varying size and irregular shape, elevated above the skin surface and attached by either a narrow stalk or a broad base. The lesions are first seen as numerous, closely spaced elevations of the skin, which are round and smooth but soon become rough and horny (Figs. 8-30 and 8-31).

Microscopically, the lesions are made up of greatly thickened epidermis, which is both acanthotic and hyperkeratotic, supported in elongated fronds by a core of hyperplastic dermis. In some lesions, overgrowth of the connective tissue elements of the dermis is a dominant feature. Epithelial cells of the stratum spinosum

occasionally contain intranuclear eosinophilic, homogeneous structures, which may represent viral inclusion bodies.

More classical papillomas with only a modest connective tissue support are caused by bovine papillomaviruses type 3 (skin) and type 5 (teat). These tend to be smaller and less pedunculated. Bovine papillomavirus type 4 causes papillomas of the esophagus, forestomach, and urinary bladder, which, concomitant with the consumption of brake fern (bracken), may progress to squamous cell carcinoma.

Olson and associates (1959) experimentally demonstrated that the bovine papilloma virus can induce fibromas and polyps of the bovine urinary bladder similar to the naturally occurring tumors associated with chronic enzootic hematuria. The same team, in 1965, isolated a virus resembling the bovine papilloma virus from spontaneous urinary bladder tumors of cattle. Experimentally, the bovine papilloma virus has also been shown to induce fibromatous meningeal tumors in calves and hamsters and fibromatous tumors in the skin of horses, hamsters, and mice.

EQUINE SARCOID

The pathologic characteristics of this growth are presented in Chapter 18. The entity was first recognized by Jackson (1936) in South Africa, who found evidence suggesting that it was transferable from one part of the horse's body to another. He also thought that the abnormal proliferation was primarily epidermal, and that the underlying dermis later became affected and assumed a preponderant role. In these two respects, he perceived a resemblance to common warts (papillomas), which are known to have a viral origin.

Olson (1948) experimentally demonstrated what Jackson suspected and also that the lesion can be transplanted from one cutaneous site to another in the same horse (autotransplantation). Later, Olson and Cook (1951) were able to produce a lesion resembling equine sarcoid by inoculating the horse's skin with material from bovine papillomas (warts), a unique crossing of species boundaries. It is now generally accepted that bovine papillomaviruses 1 and 2 cause equine sarcoid.

EQUINE CUTANEOUS PAPILLOMATOSIS

Common warts are most often found on the nose, muzzle, and lips of horses during their first and second years of life. These lesions are experimentally transmissible to horses by exposure of scarified skin to triturated suspensions of warts, before or after filtration through bacteria-retaining filters; calves, lambs, dogs, rabbits, and guinea pigs are not susceptible. Natural transmission between horses appears to occur through simple contact. The incubation period is 2 to 3 months; the duration of the lesions is about 2 months; spontaneous regression has occurred in all reported cases. Reinfection is rarely observed in animals that have recovered from the disease.

The papillomas of this equine disease are usually small, discrete, and attached by a narrow stalk, but in some cases, they are very numerous and may be con-

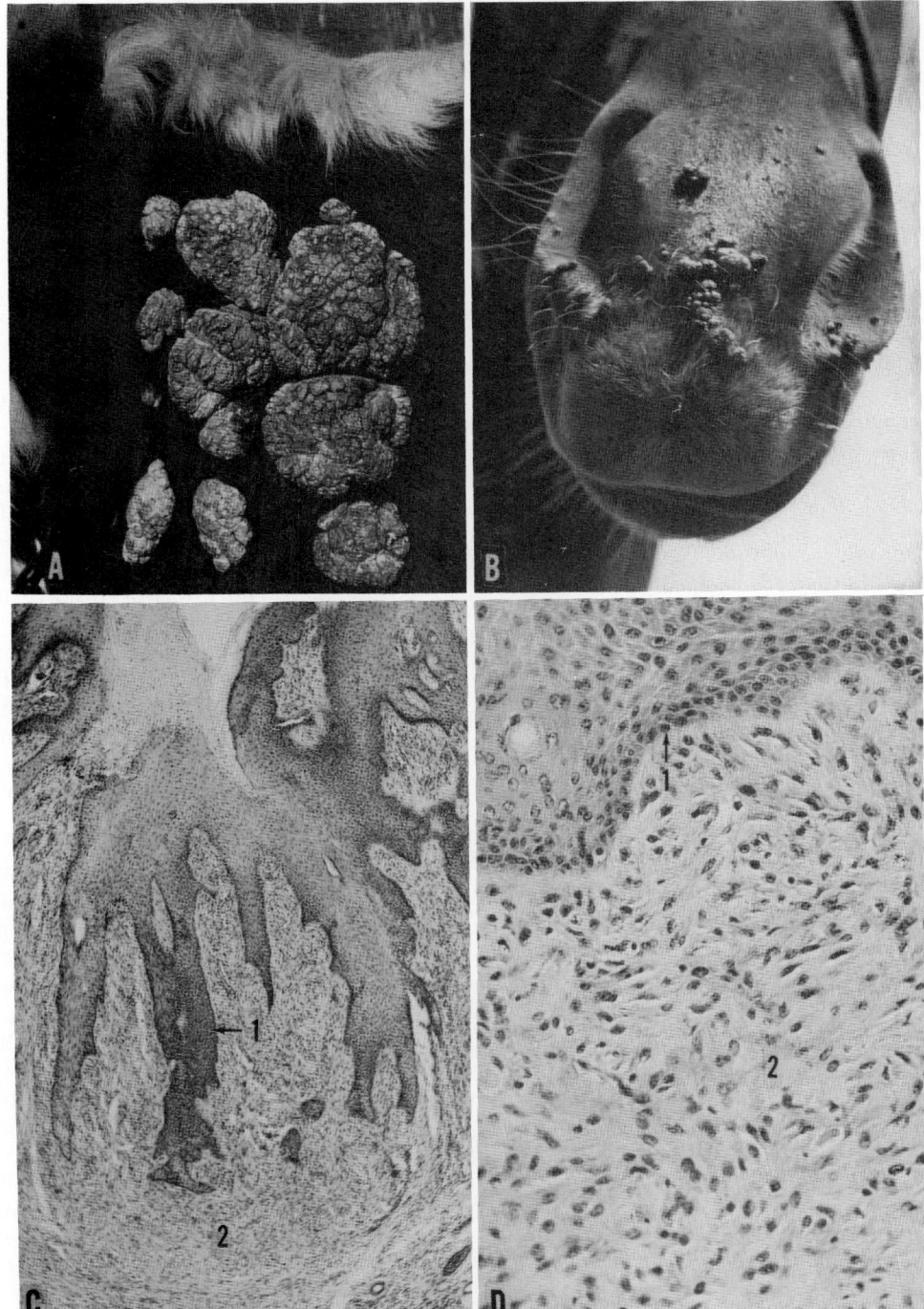

FIG. 8-30 Papillomatosis. **A.** Bovine papillomatosis (warts), neck of Hereford steer. **B.** Equine papillomatosis, nose of a horse. (Photographs courtesy of Dr. Carl Olson, Jr.) **C.** Experimentally transmitted bovine papillomatosis (× 35), 41 days after inoculation. Note elongated growth of epidermis *(1)* and cellular dermis *(2)*. **D.** Higher magnification (× 210), with hyperplastic but sharply demarcated epidermis *(1)* and richly cellular dermis *(2)*. (Courtesy of Armed Forces Institute of Pathology; contributed by Dr. Carl Olson, Jr.)

fluent. Small papillomas may appear as elongated, elevated nodules with a smooth surface, but larger ones have the rough surface characteristic of warts in other species.

Microscopically, hyperplastic, folded layers of squamous epithelium are supported by a thin core of connective tissue that is continuous with the dermis. Acanthosis and hyperkeratosis are prominent features in the affected epidermis. The outer layers of the acanthotic prickle cell layer exhibit so-called balloon degeneration, and aggregations of keratohyaline granules may be present in the cells. The lesions, in general, do not differ from those of papillomatosis in other species.

CANINE ORAL PAPILLOMATOSIS

Infectious papillomas have been known for many years (McFadyean and Hobday, 1898) to occur in the oral cavity of young dogs. These lesions are transmissible by contact or through injection of bacteria-free suspensions of wart material but will grow only on the oral mucosa. Skin and other epithelial surfaces are refractory to infection. Only dogs and other canines are sus-

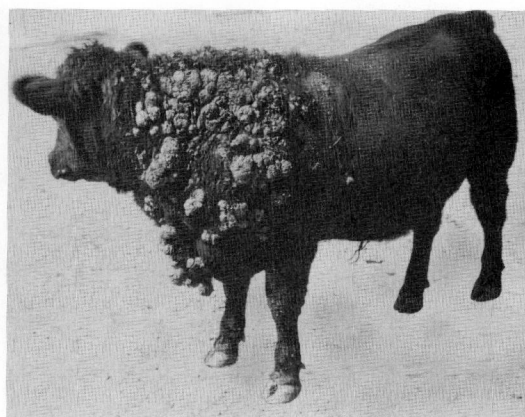

FIG. 8-31 Bovine cutaneous papillomatosis (warts). Aberdeen-Angus steer.

ceptible; attempts to infect guinea pigs, rabbits, rats, mice, monkeys, and kittens have been unsuccessful. Although cutaneous warts do occur in dogs, apparently they are not caused by the same virus that induces the oral lesions. The duration of oral papillomas is usually from 3 to 5 months.

Lesions The lesions may be single but more often are multiple, and in some dogs are so numerous as to interfere with mastication and deglutition. They occur anywhere on the oral mucosa, such as the cheeks, tongue, palate, or pharynx, but do not extend below the epiglottis or into the esophagus. The papillomas are sharply delimited, single or confluent, cauliflower-

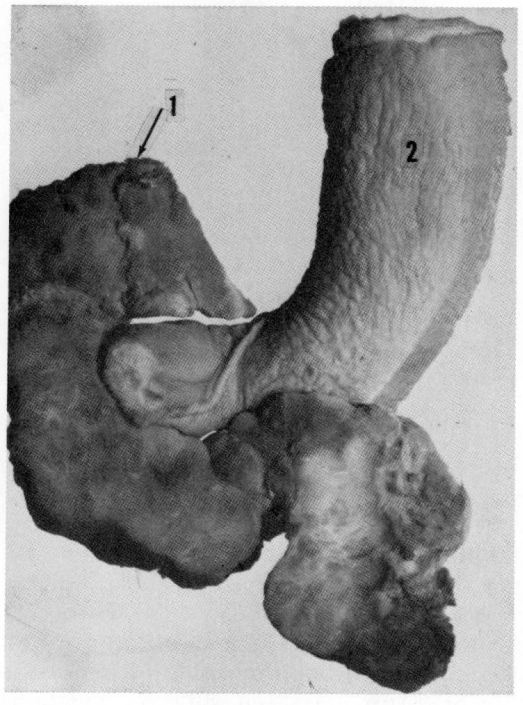

FIG. 8-32 Bovine fibropapillomatosis. Large roughly irregular mass *(1)* on glans penis *(2)* of bull.

shaped masses with a roughened surface, elevated from the oral mucosa.

Microscopically (Fig. 8-33), the earliest lesion is seen as a sharply circumscribed segment of hyperplastic epithelium in which mitotic figures are common. The prickle-cell layer becomes progressively thicker as the lesion grows; some cells lose their intercellular bridges, and there is beginning papillary formation. Hyperkeratosis becomes a prominent feature, and although cells of the malpighian layer remain normal in size, the squamous cells become larger; their cytoplasm is vacuolated or filled with albuminous material. The nuclei of the squamous cells either become greatly enlarged, or, in the outer layers, shrunken and distorted. The superficial cells apparently drop out, leaving a meshwork in the thick keratin layer. In older lesions, a few cytoplasmic inclusions, 1 to 5 μ in diameter, may be seen just under the keratin layer. These are interpreted as keratohyaline masses. In some sections basophilic inclusions fill nuclei of epithelial cells. Viral particles have been demonstrated in epithelial nuclei, and their presence has been correlated with the development of the basophilic inclusions. The underlying corium is relatively unchanged, but it sends out long vascular fronds to support the finger-like projections of hyperplastic epithelium. A few plasma cells and lymphocytes may be seen in the stroma underlying old lesions. There have been reports of squamous cell carcinoma at the site of inoculation in dogs vaccinated for oral papillomatosis.

CUTANEOUS PAPILLOMATOSIS OF RABBITS

An infectious papillomatosis of wild cottontail rabbits *(Sylvilagus floridanus)* was originally investigated by Shope (1933); hence, it is often referred to as the Shope papilloma. The warts in this disease are usually found in cases of natural infection involving the skin of the inner surface of the thighs, abdomen, or neck and shoulders. The lesions are black or gray, 0.5 to 1.0 cm in diameter and 1.0 to 1.5 cm in height, and are covered with a thick layer of keratin. They may become malignant. Domestic rabbits *(Oryctolagus cuniculus)* are rarely affected naturally, but can be experimentally infected, as can jackrabbits *(Lepus californicus)* and snowshoe hares *(L. americanus)*, in which the papillomas may also progress to squamous cell carcinoma and metastasize.

ORAL PAPILLOMATOSIS OF RABBITS

Spontaneous papillomatosis of the oral cavity of domestic rabbits *(Oryctolagus)* has been described by Parson and Kidd (1943) and demonstrated to be the result of a virus infection. The viral agent is distinct from the Shope papilloma virus, which affects the epithelium of the skin but not the mouth. These spontaneous papillomas are small, discrete, gray-white nodules, either sessile or pedunculated. Usually multiple and sometimes numerous, they are almost always situated on the undersurface of the tongue, occasionally on the gums, and rarely on the floor of the mouth. The lesions are pre-

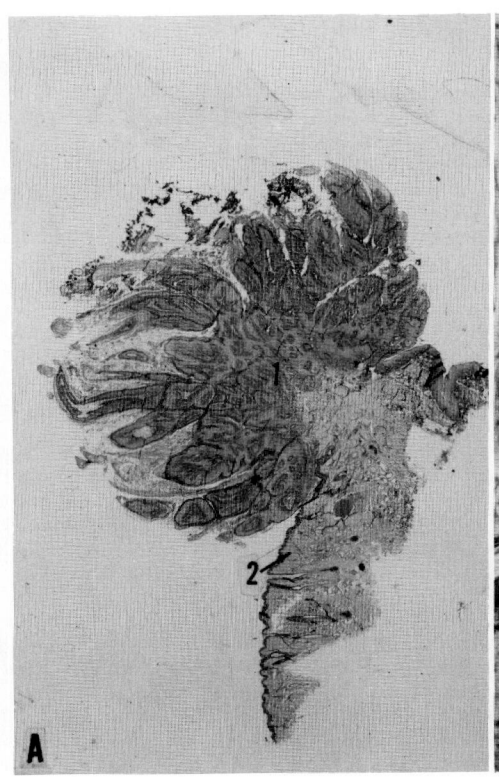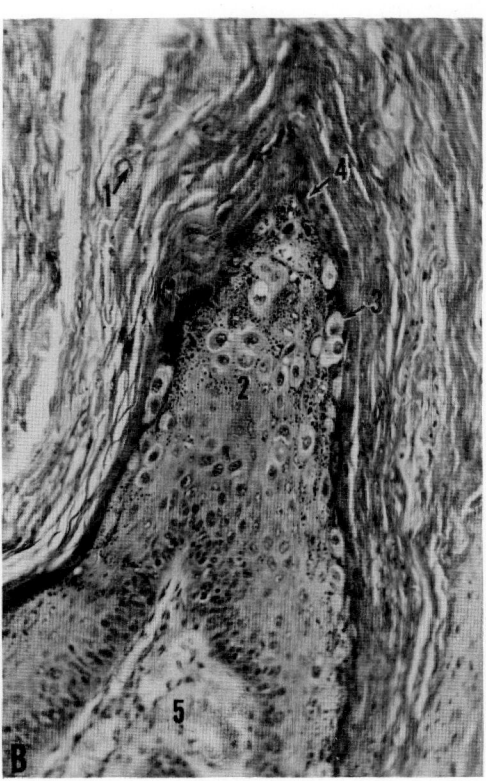

FIG. 8-33 Canine oral papillomatosis. **A.** A verrucous mass *(1)* arising from the junction of oral mucosa and skin *(2)* (× 7). **B.** Higher magnification (× 160). Note extensive layer of keratin *(1)*, long fronds of hyperplastic epidermis *(2)* containing some vacuoles *(3)* and eleidin granules *(4)* on a core of connective tissue stroma *(5)*. (Courtesy of the Armed Forces Institute of Pathology; contributed by Dr. S. Pollock.)

dominantly small, with a smooth dome-shaped surface, but occasionally are larger, sometimes attaining a diameter of 5 mm, with a rugose, cauliflower-like surface.

Microscopically, the lesions appear as discrete nodules of thickened, folded, hyperplastic epithelium, supported by sharply demarcated stroma that may form delicate papillae. In lesions of long standing, the prominent changes are seen in epithelial cells; those of the malpighian layer become large, coarsely vacuolated, and irregularly polyhedral in shape. The nuclei of all layers, particularly of the prickle cells, become enlarged, vesicular, and may contain eosinophilic or basophilic inclusion bodies. The inclusions contain viral particles. There is little tendency toward excessive keratinization of the affected epithelium; the outer layers merely appear denser and more eosinophilic in stained sections.

Experimentally, the virus causes fibromas when injected into newborn hamsters.

OVINE AND CAPRINE PAPILLOMATOSIS

There are few reports of papillomas in sheep and goats. In sheep, they may occur as fibropapillomas or squamous papillomas and are usually seen about the face and ears or forelimbs. Malignant transformation has been described.

In goats, most reports concern white Saanen or Angoras, however, Moulton (1954) described an outbreak that affected only black goats. Two forms have been described, one limited to the teats and udder, and a cutaneous form found especially about the head, face, shoulder, neck, and upper part of the forelimb. Malig-

nant transformation to squamous cell carcinoma may occur.

CUTANEOUS FIBROMA OF DEER

Cutaneous fibromas are reportedly the most common neoplasm of white-tailed deer (*Odocoileus virginianus*) and are also common in mule deer (*O. hemionus*). The tumors were shown to be transmissible more than 30 years ago and are now recognized as being caused by deer papillomavirus, an agent related to, but distinct from, bovine papillomavirus type 1. Tumors develop within several weeks following inoculation and most usually regress in about 2 to 3 months. Tumors contain viral genome, but are not permissive for viral replication.

PORCINE GENITAL PAPILLOMA

A transmissible papilloma of the genital tract of swine has been described, but it is an uncommon disease.

PAPILLOMATOSIS OF MONKEYS

Papillomas are not seen often in monkeys. They have been described in cebus, rhesus and colobus monkeys. The first report, by Lucké, Ratcliffe, and Breedis (1950), described a papilloma in a brown cebus monkey, which the investigators experimentally transmitted to another skin site on the same monkey and later to 11 of 13 other monkeys. Both Old and New World monkeys were included in the susceptible group, an unusual host range for a papillomavirus.

The incubation period was about 2 weeks; regres-

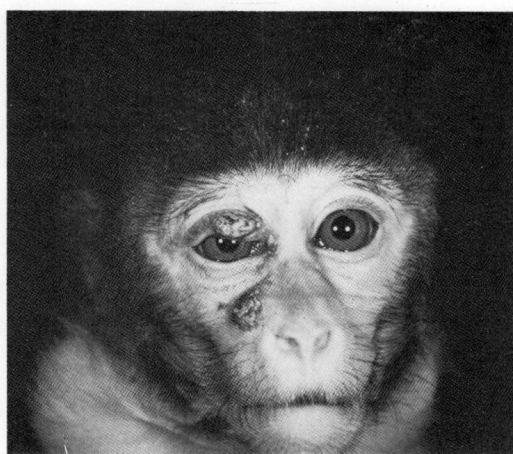

FIG. 8-34 Cutaneous papillomatosis of face of a rhesus monkey (*Macaca mulatta*). (Courtesy of New England Regional Primate Research Center, Harvard Medical School.)

sion of the lesions occurred between the fourth and eighth months (Fig. 8-34), and no evidence of malignancy was seen during a subsequent 8-month period of observation.

References

Bagdonas V, Olson C Jr. Observations on the epizootiology of cutaneous papillomatosis (warts) of cattle. J Am Vet Med Assoc 1953; 122:393–397.

Brobst DF, Dulac GC. Meningeal tumors induced in calves with the bovine cutaneous papilloma virus. Pathol Vet 1969;6:135–145.

Brobst DF, Hinsman EJ. Electron microscopy of the bovine cutaneous papilloma. Pathol Vet 1966;3:196–207.

Brobst DF, Olson C. Histopathology of urinary bladder tumors induced by bovine cutaneous papilloma agent. Cancer Res 1965; 25:12–19.

Campo MS, Moar MH, Laird HM, et al. Molecular heterogeneity and lesion site specificity of cutaneous bovine papillomaviruses. Virology 1981;113:323–335.

Cheville NF, Olson CL. Cytology of the canine oral papilloma. Am J Pathol 1964;45:848–872.

Cook RH, Olson C Jr. Experimental transmission of cutaneous papilloma of the horse. Am J Pathol 1951;27:1087–1097.

Davis CL, Kemper HE. Common warts (papillomata) in goats. J Am Vet Med Assoc 1936;88:175–179.

DeMonbreun WA, Goodpasture EW. Infectious oral papillomatosis of dogs. Am J Pathol 1932;8:43–56.

Fujimoto Y, Olson C. The fine structure of the bovine wart. Path Vet 1966;3:659–684.

Gordon DW, Olson C. Meningiomas and fibroblastic neoplasia in calves induced with the bovine papilloma virus. Cancer Res 1968;28:2423–2431.

Jarrett WFH, Murphy J, O'Neil RW, et al. Virus-induced papillomas of the alimentary tract of cattle. Int J Cancer 1980;22:323–328.

Jarrett WFH, Campo MS, O'Neil BW, et al. A novel bovine papillomavirus (BPV-6) causing true epithelial papillomas of the mammary gland skin: a member of a proposed new BPV subgroup. Virology 1984;136:255–264.

Lancaster W, Olson C. Animal papillomaviruses. Microbiol Rev 1982;46:191–207.

Lucké B, Ratcliffe H, Breedis C. Transmissible papilloma in monkeys. Fed Proc 1950;9:337.

McEntee K. Transmissible fibropapillomas of the external genitalia of cattle. Rep NY State Veterinary College, Cornell Univ, Ithaca, NY, 1950–51;28.

McEntee K. Fibropapillomas on the external genitalia of cattle. Cornell Vet 1950;40:304–312.

McFadyean J, Hobday F. Note on the experimental transmission of warts in the dog. J Comp Pathol Ther 1898;11:341–344.

Moulton JE. Cutaneous papillomas on the udders of milk goats. North Am Vet 1954;35:29–33.

O'Banion MK, Sundberg JP. Papillomavirus genomes in experimentally-induced fibromas in white-tailed deer. Am J Vet Res 1987;48:1453–1455.

Olson C Jr. Equine sarcoid; a cutaneous neoplasm. Am J Vet Res 1948;9:333–341.

Olson C, Cook RH. Cutaneous sarcoma-like lesions of the horse caused by the agent of bovine papilloma. Proc Soc Exp Biol Med 1951;77:281–284.

Olson C, et al. A urinary bladder tumor induced by a bovine cutaneous papilloma agent. Cancer Res 1959;19:779–782.

Olson C, Pamukcu AM, Brobst DF. Papilloma-like virus from bovine urinary bladder tumors. Cancer Res 1965;25:840–849.

Parish WE. A transmissible genital papilloma of the pig resembling condyloma acuminatum of humans. J Pathol Bacteriol 1961;81: 331–345.

Parsons RJ, Kidd JG. Oral papillomatosis of rabbits: a virus disease. J Exp Med 1943;77:233–250.

Penberthy J. Contagious warty tumors in dogs. J Comp Pathol Ther 1898;11:363–365.

Pfister H, Linz U, Gissmann L, et al. Partial characterization of a new type of bovine papilloma viruses. Virology 1979;96:1–8.

Ragland WL, Spencer GR. Attempts to relate bovine papilloma virus to the cause of equine sarcoid: Equidae inoculated intradermally with bovine papilloma virus. Am J Vet Res 1969;30:743–752.

Ragland WL, Spencer GR. Attempts to relate bovine papilloma virus to the cause of equine sarcoid: immunity to bovine papilloma virus. Am J Vet Res 1968;29:1363–1366.

Rangan SRS, Gutter A, Baskin GB, et al. Virus associated papillomas in colobus monkeys (*Colobus guereza*). Lab Anim Sci 1980;30: 885–889.

Rous P, Beart JW. The progression to carcinoma of virus-induced rabbit papillomas (Shope). J Exp Med 1935;62:523–548.

Shope RE. Infectious papillomatosis of rabbits. J Exp Med 1933;58: 607–624.

Shope RE. An infectious fibroma of deer. Proc Soc Exp Biol Med 1955;88:533–535.

Shope RE, Mangold R, MacNamara LG, et al. An infectious cutaneous fibroma of the Virginia white-tailed deer (*Odocoileus virginianus*). J Exp Med 1958;108:797–802.

Sundberg JP, Chiodini RJ, Nielsen SW. Transmission of the white-tailed deer cutaneous fibroma. Am J Vet Res 1985;46:1150–1154.

Sundberg JP, Junge RE, El Shazly MO. Oral papillomatosis in New Zealand white rabbits. Am J Vet Res 1985;46:664–668.

Sundberg JP, O'Banion MK, Schmidt-Didier E, et al. Cloning and characterization of a canine oral papillomavirus. Am J Vet Res 1986;47:1142–1144.

Sundberg JP, Reszka AA, Williams ES, et al. An oral papillomavirus that infected one coyote and three dogs. Vet Pathol 1991;28: 87–88.

Sundberg JP, Williams ES, Hill D, et al. Detection of papillomaviruses in cutaneous fibromas of white-tailed and mule deer. Am J Vet Res 1985;46:1145–1149.

Theilen G, Wheeldon EB, East N, et al. Goat papillomatosis. Am J Vet Res 1985;46:2519–2526.

Vanselow BA, Spradbrow PB, Jackson ARB. Papillomaviruses, papillomas and squamous cell carcinomas in sheep. Vet Rec 1982; 110:561–562.

Voss JL. Transmission of equine sarcoid. Am J Vet Res 1969;30: 183–191.

Watrach AM. The ultrastructure of canine cutaneous papilloma. Cancer Res 1969;29:2079–2084.

DISEASES CAUSED BY POLYOMAVIRUS

Polyomaviruses are species-specific and have been identified in mice, hamsters, rabbits, monkeys, cattle, and humans. Ordinarily, infection is inapparent; however, in immunocompromised individuals reactivation may occur and lead to disease; for example, JC virus infection causes progressive multifocal leukoencephalopathy in humans. In domestic animals, polyomaviruses appear to be of little to no significance.

The prototype of this genus is the **polyomavirus of mice,** first described by Sarah E. Stewart and Bernice E. Eddy. This virus normally causes an inapparent infection of wild mice and, less often, laboratory mice. Experimentally, the virus causes a variety of neoplasms in a spectrum of hosts, but there is little evidence that it is an important cause of spontaneous neoplasms. Suckling mice, rats, guinea pigs, hamsters, rabbits, and ferrets are among the susceptible species. Tumors include pleomorphic tumors of the salivary glands, renal cortical tumors, renal sarcomas, subcutaneous sarcomas, adenocarcinomas of the mammary glands, adrenal carcinomas, epithelial thymomas, epidermoid carcinomas, osteosarcomas, hemangioendotheliomas, mesotheliomas, adenocarcinomas of sweat glands, and thyroid adenocarcinomas. Viral DNA is integrated in transformed cells, which, as with other DNA tumor viruses, are not permissive for a productive infection. Rare cells may enter a productive cycle with virions visible in the nucleus.

Simian virus 40 (SV40) is a polyomavirus of rhesus monkeys *(Macaca mulatta),* which occurs as an inapparent infection of high incidence. Natural infection of other nonhuman primates occurs, probably through exposure to rhesus monkeys. In rhesus monkeys infected with simian immunodeficiency virus, SV40 may lead to overt disease, usually pneumonia with large intranuclear inclusion bodies in pneumocytes. Most interest in SV40 has focused on the virus being oncogenic when inoculated into suckling or young hamsters. Following subcutaneous inoculation of hamsters under 2 days of age, 95% develop tumors at the site of injection 2.5 to 3 months later. The neoplasms are highly undifferentiated sarcomas, usually containing multinucleated giant cells. Intracerebral injection leads to ependymomas. Hamsters become almost entirely resistant to infection after 3 weeks of age, unless inoculated via the intravenous route. If they are so inoculated, 4 to 6 months after injection, they develop anaplastic sarcomas as well as lymphoma and osteogenic sarcoma. The mastomys *(Rattus mastomys natalensis),* the only other susceptible host, develops ependymoma 111 to 225 days after subcutaneous inoculation of newborns. Millions of humans in the United States were exposed to SV40 as a contaminant of poliovirus vaccines prepared in monkey kidney cultures. There is no evidence that any ill effects followed.

K-virus, or **mouse pneumonitis virus,** (see also pneumonia virus of mice) is a polyomavirus carried as a latent infection by mice, unassociated with spontaneous disease. Experimentally, the virus has been shown to cause a fatal interstitial pneumonia when injected into suckling mice. The most striking lesion is hypertrophy and proliferation of endothelial and alveolar lining cells, both of which may contain basophilic intranuclear inclusion bodies. Virus also replicates in macrophages and Kupffer cells, which may also bear inclusion bodies.

References

Diamandopoulis GT. Leukemia, lymphoma and osteosarcoma induced in the Syrian golden hamster by simian virus 40. Science 1972;176:173–175.
Eddy BE. The polyoma virus (B). Adv Virus Res 1960;7:91–102.
Eddy BE. Polyoma virus. Virology Monographs 1969;7:1–114.
Fisher CR, Kilham L. Pathology of a pneumotropic virus recovered from C3H mice carrying the Bittner milk agent. Arch Pathol 1953;55:14–19.
Stewart SE. The polyoma virus (A). Adv Virus Res 1960;7:61–90.

*P*ARVOVIRIDAE

The family *Parvoviridae* (parvo = small) is made up of unique DNA viruses that have a genome consisting of single-stranded DNA. Three genera make up this family: **parvovirus,** which contains the viruses of interest as causes of disease in animals; **dependovirus** (adenovirus-associated virus), which contains defective viruses that are dependent on coinfection with another virus, usually an adenovirus, for replication; and **densovirus,** whose members only infect arthropods (Table 8-5).

Parvoviruses are the smallest viruses of vertebrates, measuring about 18 to 26 nm in diameter. They are believed to be of icosahedral symmetry with 32 capsomers and are nonenveloped. The genome is a single-stranded DNA of about 1.5 to 2.0×10^6 molecular weight, which is usually negative-sense, although positive-sense virions are also packaged. A unique feature of parvoviruses is their dependence on cell replication for viral DNA synthesis to occur. This restricts lesions to those tissues in which cells are undergoing mitosis and explains the difference in cell tropism seen in fetal, neonatal, and adult animals. The manifestations of most parvovirus infections of animals (Table 8-5) focus on their replication in the gastrointestinal tract, bone marrow, or fetus. A parvovirus of humans (B19) has been incriminated as a cause of polyarthritis.

Parvoviruses are highly stable, resistant to chemical and physical reagents, and are not affected seriously by heat at 60°C for an hour. Thus, the environment may remain contaminated long after diseased animals have been removed.

Diseases caused by parvoviruses

FELINE PANLEUKOPENIA (FELINE DISTEMPER, FELINE ENTERITIS, AGRANULOCYTOSIS)

Feline panleukopenia is a highly contagious and usually fatal febrile disease of domestic cats and other felidae, which has been recognized since the early twentieth century. Parvoviruses, which are very similar and often indistinguishable from the virus of feline panleukopenia, have been identified as causes of disease in mink, i.e., mink enteritis virus (MEV); raccoons, i.e., raccoon parvovirus; and foxes, i.e., fox parvovirus, blue fox parvovirus (Table 8-5). However, isolates may vary in their pathogenicity for these different species. In cats,

TABLE 8-5   **Diseases caused by *Parvoviridae***

Virus	*Disease*	*Species*
Feline panleukopenia*	Feline panleukopenia, cerebellar hypoplasia	Cats
Mink enteritis virus*	Mink enteritis	Mink
Raccoon parvovirus*	Enteritis	Raccoons
Canine parvovirus 2	Enteritis, myocarditis	Dogs
Bovine parvovirus	Diarrhea	Cattle
Porcine parvovirus	Infertility, fetal death and maceration	Swine
Rat virus and H-1	Experimentally: hepatitis, cerebellar hypoplasia, hemorrhagic encephalopathy	Rats
Minute virus of mice	Experimentally: Dwarfism Cerebellar hypoplasia	Hamsters Mice
Aleutian disease virus	Aleutian disease	Mink
Minute virus of canines	Usually none; abortion, infertility	Dogs
Fox parvovirus*	Enteritis, reproductive failure	Foxes

*All very closely related

the disease is characterized by severe panleukopenia, fever, and enteritis that results in extreme dehydration. The disease runs a rapid course. Its onset is marked by lassitude and abrupt elevation of temperature to between 104°F and 105°F. The fever is diphasic; it falls after about 24 hours and rises approximately 48 hours later. Severe leukopenia, involving all of the granulocytic series (agranulocytosis) and all other leukocytes, is a constant feature. Vomiting and intractable diarrhea also may be observed. Death often occurs shortly after the second peak of temperature.

Lesions   The gross lesions seen at necropsy usually consist of extreme dehydration and emaciation, with mucopurulent exudate on the nasal and lacrimal mucosae. The mucosa of the terminal part of the ileum is often covered with hemorrhagic exudate. The lymph nodes of the mesentery are edematous and somewhat enlarged. The bone marrow of the long bones often appears greasy, yellowish or white, and semifluid. The lack of hematopoietic marrow is obvious.

The principal microscopic lesions are found in the gastrointestinal tract (Fig. 8-35), where the virus replicates in dividing cells in the crypts (Fig. 8-45H). The superficial layers of the mucosa in the small intestine are eroded, and the remaining epithelium has undergone proliferation. The crypts are dilated with mucus and lined with irregular, hyperplastic epithelial cells. Here, inflammatory infiltration of the lamina propria occurs, but little change is seen in the submucosa. In some cases granular, eosinophilic intranuclear inclusions are seen in the lining epithelium remaining at the sites of erosion. These inclusions, when present, are helpful in diagnosis.

Lesions consistently occur in lymphoid organs, which are the site of initial viral replication before dissemination to gastrointestinal epithelium or other tissues. Early in the disease, lymph nodes are edematous and hyperemic, and histiocytes proliferate. This is soon followed by necrosis of lymphocytes in follicular and paracortical regions in lymph nodes, the malpighian corpuscles of the spleen, the cortex of the thymus, and Peyer's patches. Intranuclear inclusion bodies are occasionally present in what appear to be histiocytes. There is continued proliferation of histiocytes, which engulf lymphocytic debris as well as erythrocytes. Lymphocytic follicles ultimately become composed of eosinophilic debris and reticular cells. In animals surviving infection, marked regenerative hyperplasia of lymphocytes occurs.

The bone marrow is markedly hypocellular, resulting from necrosis of all stem-cell populations. This, too, is followed by hyperplasia in surviving animals. Inclusion body myocarditis, as seen in canine parvovirus infection, is not a frequent feature of feline panleukopenia; however, examples have been described in young kittens.

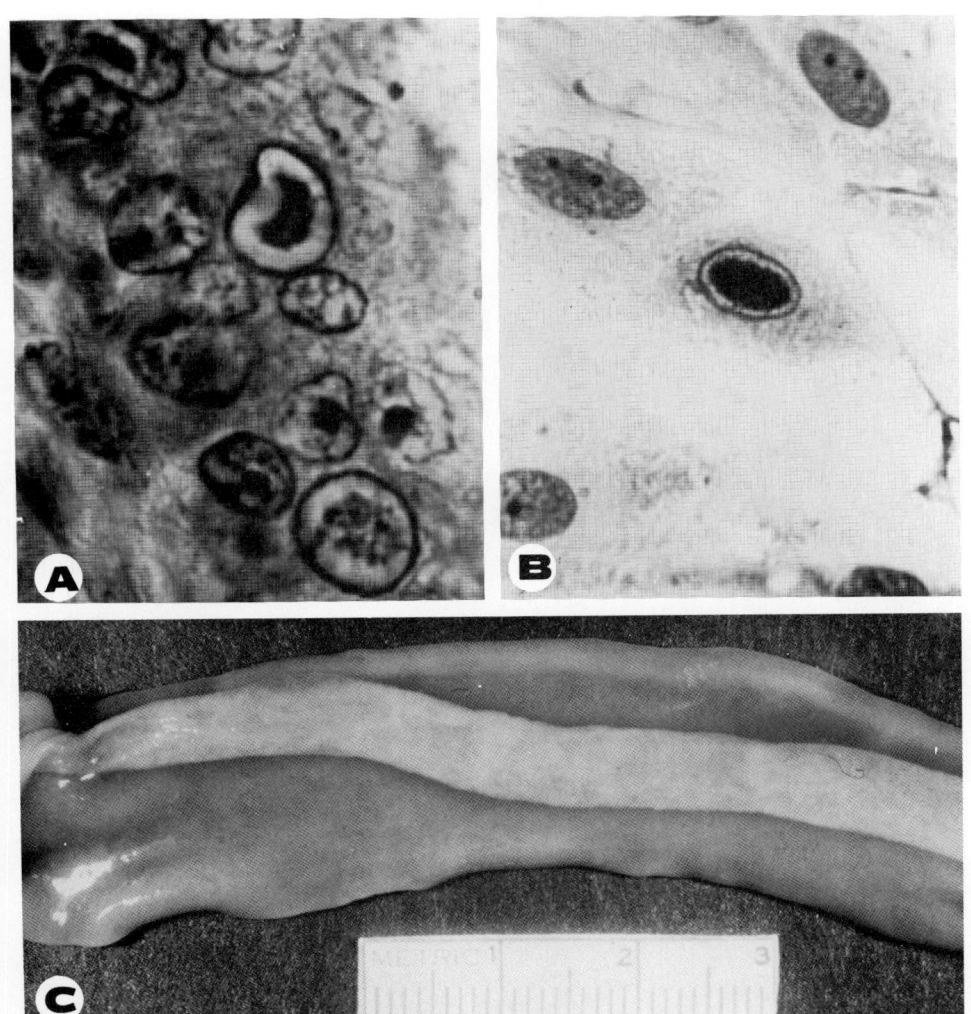

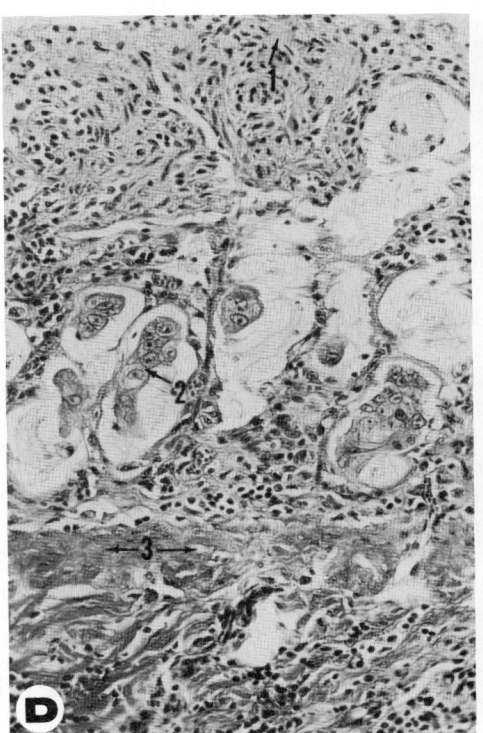
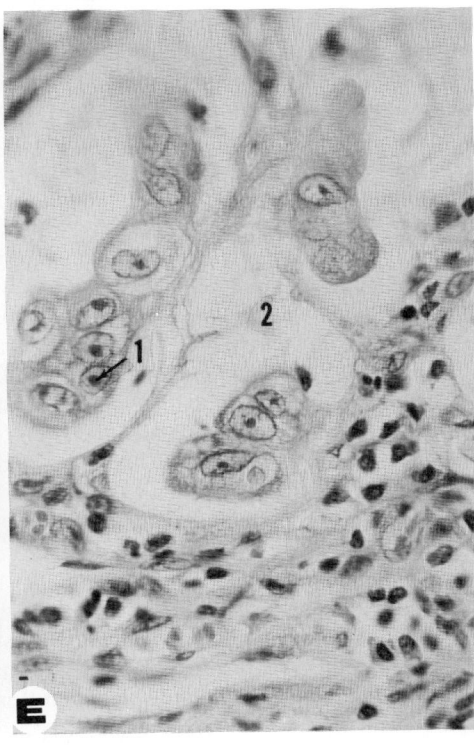

FIG. 8-35   Feline panleukopenia.
A. Intranuclear inclusions of panleukopenia (infectious feline enteritis) virus in intestinal epithelium of a cat, 5 days after inoculation with the virus.   **B.** Inclusion
in culture of feline kidney cells, 5
days after inoculation with virus.
(Courtesy of Dr. John R. Gorham,
Washington State University.)   **C.**
Fibrinous cast in lumen of a 7-
month-old male cat with panleukopenia. (Courtesy of Angell Memorial Animal Hospital.)   **D.** Wall of
feline small intestine (× 210).
Loss of epithelium at tips of villi
(1), disorganization and proliferation of epithelial cells in crypts (2).
Note collection of mucus. **E.**
Higher magnification (× 590) to
show intranuclear inclusions (1)
and collections of mucus (2); muscularis mucosa (3). (**D, E.** Courtesy
of the Armed Forces Institute of
Pathology; contributed by Dr. J. T.
Bryans.)

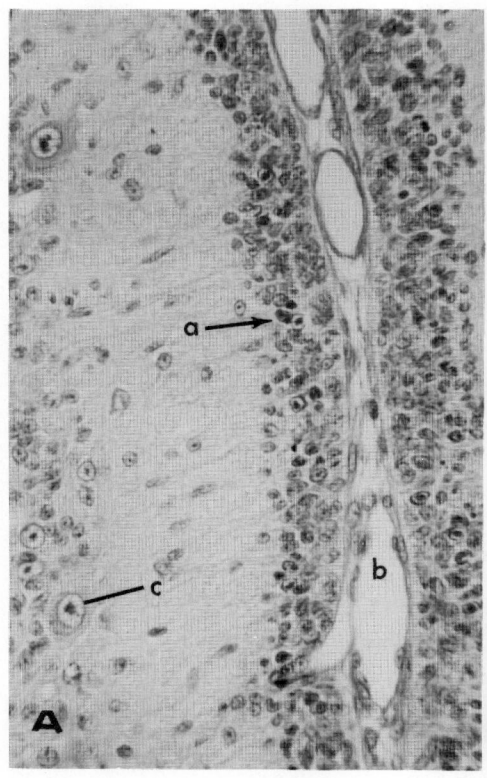 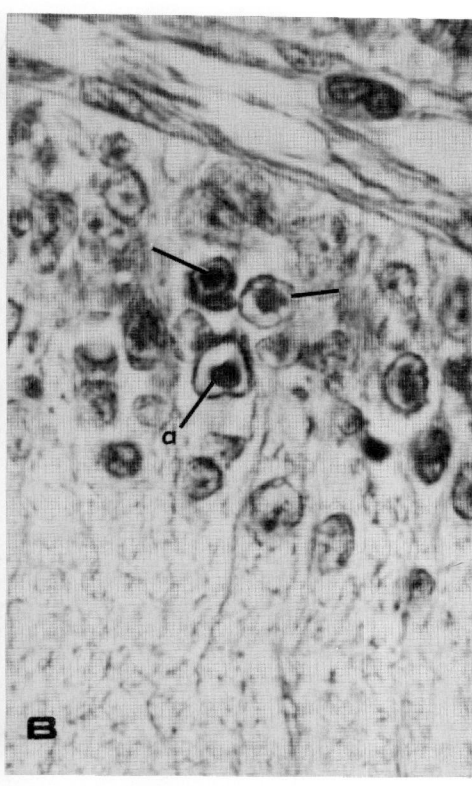

FIG. 8-36 Cerebellum of a 21-day-old kitten, which received panleukopenia virus at birth. **A.** Note intranuclear inclusions and necrotic cells in the cells of the germinal layer *(a)* adjacent to the vascular pia mater *(b)*, Purkinje cells *(c)*. **B.** Higher magnification. Note intranuclear inclusions *(a)* and margination of chromatin in affected nuclei. (Courtesy of Dr. George Margolis, Dartmouth Medical School.)

Diagnosis A presumptive diagnosis usually can be made on the basis of the symptoms and the agranulocytosis. Demonstration of intranuclear inclusions in the epithelial cells of the small intestine is helpful in postmortem diagnosis, but unfortunately inclusions are not always present.

Panleukopenia and cerebellar hypoplasia Kilham, Margolis, and Colby (1967) demonstrated that the virus of feline panleukopenia can produce cerebellar hypoplasia in kittens. The virus, when injected into the fetus or intravenously into a pregnant cat, invades cells of the external germinal layer of the fetal cerebellum, producing intranuclear inclusion bodies and necrosis, which leads to gross or microscopic "hypoplasia" of the cerebellum in the newborn kitten (Fig. 8-36). Inclusion bodies may persist to the early neonatal period, but usually are not evident after birth. Virus, however, may be isolated from various tissues, especially the kidney, for several months. The virus has also been isolated from natural cases of cerebellar hypoplasia in kittens. Kilham (1966) had previously demonstrated that rat virus can induce cerebellar hypoplasia in kittens, rats, and hamsters. Although it appears that panleukopenia virus is an important cause of cerebellar hypoplasia in kittens, the relative importance of rat virus is undetermined. These studies are of great significance in that a viral cause has been demonstrated for a disease accepted by many to represent a genetic abnormality.

Kilham's studies are also of interest because they demonstrated that feline panleukopenia virus could also induce cerebellar hypoplasia in ferrets, a species not considered susceptible to classic panleukopenia.

References

Bestetti G, Zwahlen R. Generalized parvovirus infection with inclusion-body myocarditis in two kittens. J Comp Pathol 1985;95:393–397.

Carlson JH, Scott FW, Duncan JR. Feline panleukopenia 1. Pathogenesis in germfree and specific pathogen free cats. Vet Pathol 1977;14:79–88.

Carlson JH, Scott FW. Feline panleukopenia II. The relationship of intestinal mucosal cell proliferation rates to viral infection and development of lesions. Vet Pathol 1977;14:173–181.

Csiza CK, de Lahunta A, Scott FW, et al. Pathogenesis of feline panleukopenia virus in susceptible newborn kittens. II. Pathology and immunofluorescence. Infect Immun 1971;3:838–846.

Csiza CK, Scott FW, de Lahunta A, et al. Immune carrier state of feline panleukopenia virus-infected cats. Am J Vet Res 1971;32:419–426.

Csiza CK, Scott FW, de Lahunta A, et al. Feline viruses. XIV. Transplacental infections in spontaneous panleukopenia of cats. Cornell Vet 1971;61:423–439.

Csiza CK, Scott FW, de Lahunta A, et al. Spontaneous feline ataxia. Cornell Vet 1972;62:300–322.

Farrell RK, Burger D, Hartsough GR, et al. Relationship of mink virus enteritis virus and feline panleukopenia virus: rapid onset of mink virus enteritis virus protection after feline panleukopenia virus infection. Am J Vet Res 1972;33:2351–2352.

Frelier PF, Leininger RW, Armstrong LD, et al. Suspected parvovirus infection in porcupines. J Am Vet Med Assoc 1984;185:1291–1294.

Hammon WD, Enders JF. A virus disease of cats principally characterized by aleucocytosis, enteric lesions and the presence of intranuclear inclusion bodies. J Exp Med 1939;69:327–351.

Johnson GR, Koestner A, Rohovsky MW. Experimental feline infectious enteritis in the germfree cat. Path Vet 1967;4:275–288.

Johnson RH, Margolis G, Kilham L. Identity of feline ataxia virus with feline panleucopenia virus. Nature Lond 1967;214:175–177.

Kilham L, Margolis G. Viral etiology of spontaneous ataxia of cats. Am J Pathol 1966;48:991–1011.

Kilham L, Margolis G, Colby ED. Congenital infections of cats and ferrets by feline panleukopenia virus manifested by cerebellar hypoplasia. Lab Invest 1967;17:465–480.

Kilham L, Margolis G, Colby ED. Cerebellar ataxia and its congenital transmission in cats by feline panleukopenia virus. J Am Vet Med Assoc 1971;158:888–901.

Krunajevic T. Experimental virus enteritis in mink. Acta Vet Scand (Suppl) 1970;30:1–88.

Langheinrich KA, Neilsen SW. Histopathology of feline panleukopenia. J Am Vet Med Assoc 1971;158:863–872.

Larson S, Flagstad A, Aalbaek B. Experimental feline panleucopenia in the conventional cat. Vet Pathol 1976;13:216–240.

Lawrence JS, Syverton JT, Shaw JS, et al. Infectious feline agranulocytosis. Am J Pathol 1940;16:333–354.

Lucas AM, Riser WH. Intranuclear inclusions in panleukopenia of cats. Am J Pathol 1945;21:435–465.

Nettles VF, Pearson JE, Gustafson GA, et al. Parvovirus infection in translocated raccoons. J Am Vet Med Assoc 1980;177:787–789.

Parrish CR, Gorham JR, Schwartz TM, et al. Characterization of antigenic variation among mink enteritis virus isolates. Am J Vet Res 1984;45:2591–2599.

Parrish CR, Leathers CW, Pearson R, et al. Comparisons of feline panleukopenia virus, canine parvovirus, raccoon parvovirus, and mink enteritis virus and their pathogenicity for mink and ferrets. Am J Vet Res 1987;48:1429–1435.

Percy DH, Scott FW, Albert DM. Retinal dysplasia due to feline panleukopenia virus infection. J Am Vet Med Assoc 1975;167:935–937.

Riser WH. The histopathology of panleucopenia (agranulocytosis) in the domestic cat. Am J Vet Res 1946;7:455–465.

Rohovsky MW, Griesemer RA. Experimental feline infectious enteritis in the germfree cat. Pathol Vet 1967;4:391–410.

CANINE PARVOVIRUS INFECTION

Although a parvovirus (called "minute virus of canines") was isolated from normal dogs in 1970, it was not until 1978 that a parvovirus was associated with a disease of dogs. In 1978, an apparently new or heretofore unrecognized disease entity suddenly appeared in several parts of the world. The virus is over 98% identical in DNA sequence to the virus of feline panleukopenia, mink enteritis virus, and the parvoviruses of raccoons and foxes. In contrast to these other parvoviruses, canine parvovirus appears to cause disease only in canines. It does not replicate in cats and does so only very poorly in mink or raccoons. Since its recognition in 1978, the canine virus has undergone two evolutionary changes such that the virus present worldwide today is distinct from the original virus.

The infection can lead to two distinct clinicopathologic presentations: an intestinal form, which is the main form in dogs older than 6 weeks; and a cardiac form, which occurs in younger dogs.

Intestinal form The intestinal form, which may occur in dogs of all ages but is most severe in young pups, is characterized by vomiting, diarrhea, and dehydration. There may be fever and leukopenia. Microscopically (Fig. 8-37), there is a necrotizing enteritis of the small intestine reminiscent of feline panleukopenia, with dilated crypts and, often, regeneration of epithelium. Intranuclear inclusion bodies are found in intestinal epithelial cells of dogs with this infection as often as they are in cats with panleukopenia. Lesions in lymphoid organs resemble those seen in feline panleukopenia. There is lymphopenia and neutropenia resulting from necrosis of precursor cells. These signs and lesions may occur in conjunction with the cardiac form.

Cardiac form The cardiac form is confined to puppies 2 to 8 weeks of age. This form may exist with or without signs or lesions in the small intestine. Clinically, death may be sudden or follow a brief period of dyspnea and sometimes signs of enteritis. Microscopically, there are multiple foci of myocardial necrosis associated with a mononuclear cellular infiltrate. Fibrosis may be evident in dogs surviving an acute episode. Intranuclear inclusion bodies are present in myofibers.

Less often, in neonates, canine parvovirus may lead to generalized infection with necrotizing lesions and inclusion bodies in tissues other than the gastrointestinal tract and heart, including brain, liver, lungs, kidneys, and adrenal cortex. Vascular endothelium is severely affected, causing the lesions at these sites to be hemorrhagic.

Diagnosis Diagnosis depends on the lesions and isolation of the virus. The myocardial form is unique, but the intestinal form may be confused with other causes of enteritis, such as coronavirus infections. The latter is not usually milder clinically and is not associated with leukopenia or significant necrosis of intestinal epithelium.

Minute virus of canines (MVC) This parvovirus was first recovered from dogs in 1967 (Binn and others, 1970). It is widespread in dog populations, but appears not to be a significant pathogen. Experimentally, inoculation of puppies has led to lymphocytic necrosis and mild duodenitis, but this has not been recorded as a spontaneous disease. Carmichael and associates (1991) have also demonstrated that, like other parvoviruses, the virus can infect the canine fetus and lead to fetal death or the birth of weak pups that die soon after.

References

Binn LN, Lazar EC, Eddy GA, et al. Recovery and characterization of a minute virus of canines. Infect Immun 1970;1:503–508.

Boosinger TR, Rebar AH, DeNicola DB, et al. Bone marrow alterations associated with canine parvoviral enteritis. Vet Pathol 1982;19:558–561.

Carman PS, Povey RC. Pathogenesis of canine parvovirus-2 in dogs: [1] Haematology, serology and virus recovery. [2] Histopathology and antigen identification in tissues. Res Vet Sci 1985;38:134–140, 141–150.

Carmichael LE, Schlafer DH, Hashimoto A. Pathogenicity of minute virus of canines (MVC) for the canine fetus. Cornell Vet 1991;81:151–171.

Carpenter JL, Roberts RM, Harpster NK, et al. Intestinal cardiopulmonary forms of parvovirus infection in a litter of pups. J Am Vet Med Assoc 1980;176:1269–1273.

Cooper BJ, Carmichael LE, Appel MJG, et al. Canine viral enteritis. II. Morphologic lesions in naturally occurring parovirus infection. Cornell Vet 1979;69:134–144.

Hayes MA, Russell RG, Babicek LA, et al. Sudden death in young dogs with myocarditis caused by parvovirus. J Am Vet Med Assoc 1979;174:1197–1203.

Johnson BJ, Castro AE. Isolation of canine parvovirus from a dog brain with severe necrotizing vasculitis and encephalomalacia. J Am Vet Med Assoc 1984;184:1398–1399.

Lenghaus C, Studdert MJ. Generalized parvovirus disease in neonatal pups. J Am Vet Med Assoc 1982;181:41–45.

Macartney L, McCandlish IAP, Thompson H, et al. Canine parvovirus enteritis 1: [1] Clinical, haematological and pathological features of experimental infection. [2] Pathogenesis. [3] Scanning electron microscopical features of experimental infection. Vet Rec 1984;115:201–210, 453–460, 533–537.

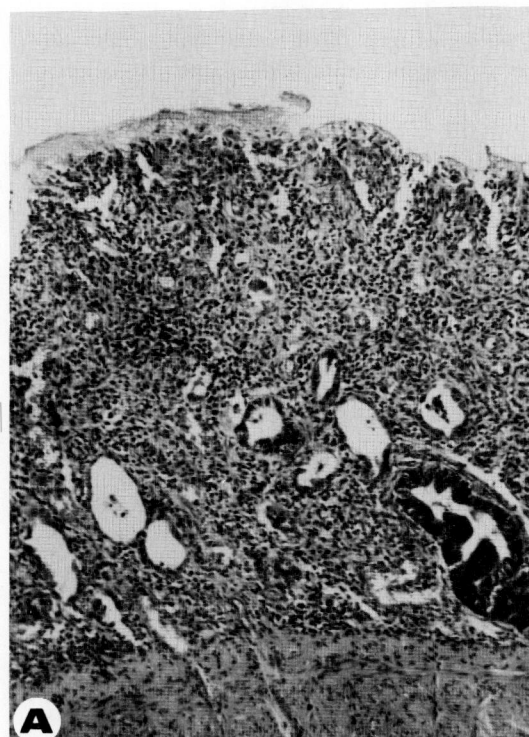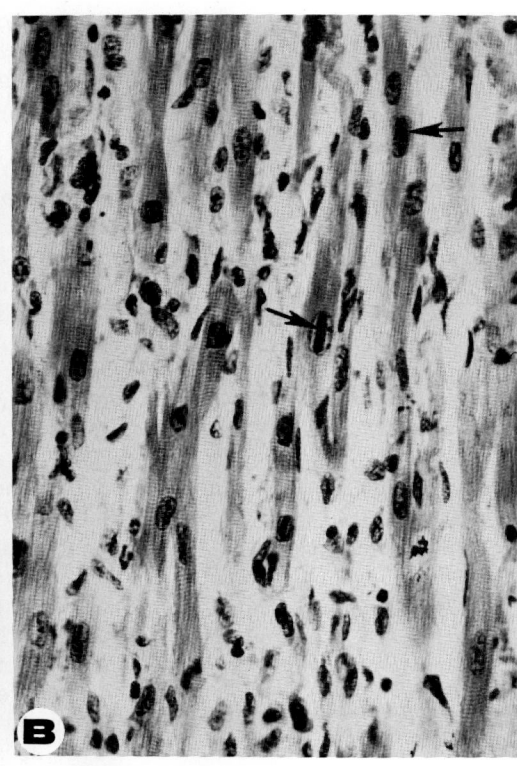

FIG. 8-37 Canine parvovirus infection. **A.** Necrotizing enteritis, ileum. Note extensive necrosis and loss of epithelial cells lining villi and crypts resulting in collapse and fusion of villi. Scattered crypts are dilated and lined by hypertrophic, regenerating epithelial cells. **B.** Myocarditis, characterized by interstitial edema, sparse mononuclear inflammatory cell infiltration, and basophilic intranuclear inclusion bodies in myofibers *(arrows)*. (Courtesy of Dr. Norval W. King.)

Macartney L, Parrish CR, Binn LN, et al. Characterization of minute virus of canines (MVC) and its pathogenicity for pups. Cornell Vet 1988;78:131–145.

Meunier PC, Cooper BJ, Appel MJG, et al. Experimental viral myocarditis: parvoviral infection of neonatal pups. Vet Pathol 1984; 21:509–515.

Meunier PC, Cooper BJ, Appel MJG, et al. Pathogenesis of canine parvovirus enteritis: the importance of viremia. Vet Pathol 1985;22:60–71.

Meunier PC, Cooper BJ, Appel MJG, et al. Pathogenesis of canine parvovirus enteritis: sequential virus distribution and passive immunization studies. Vet Pathol 1985;22:617–624.

Nelson DT, Eustis SL, McAdaragh JP, et al. Lesions of spontaneous canine viral enteritis. Vet Pathol 1979;16:680–686.

Parrish CR. The emergence and evolution of canine parvovirus—an example of recent host range mutation. Semin Virol 1994;5: 121–132.

Reed AP, Jones EV, Miller TJ. Nucleotide sequence and genome organization of canine parvovirus. J Virol 1988;62:266–276.

Robinson WF, Huxtable CR, Pass DA, et al. Canine parvoviral myocarditis: a morphologic description of the natural disease. Vet Pathol 1980;17:282–293.

Tratschin J-D, McMaster GK, Kronauer G, et al. Canine parvovirus: relationship to wild-type and vaccine strains of feline panleukopenia virus and mink enteritis virus. J Gen Virol 1982;61:33–41.

BOVINE PARVOVIRUS INFECTION

Bovine parvovirus has been isolated from the intestinal tract of young calves afflicted with a severe but transitory diarrhea. It appears that each of several isolates are closely related and are presumably the same agent, which is immunologically different from parvovirus derived from any other species.

Although the virus is widely distributed and infection common, bovine parvovirus rarely causes serious disease. Oral or intravenous administration of bovine parvovirus to newborn calves results in mucoid to watery diarrhea 24 to 48 hours later. Intestinal cells at all levels of the digestive tract become infected, but those of the small intestine appear to be most clearly involved. Viremia persists for 4 to 6 days, but virus may be isolated from feces for up to 11 days. The illness is usually transitory but may be severe if complicated by other viral or bacterial infections. Lesions are similar to those seen in feline panleukopenia, but less severe. The diagnosis depends on isolation and identification of the virus in cultures of bovine cells or on demonstration of specific immunofluorescence or ultrastructurally typical virions in affected cells.

References

Abinanti FR, Warfield MS. Recovery of a hemadsorbing virus (Haden) from the gastrointestinal tract of calves. Virology 1961;14: 288–289.

Bates RC, Storz J, Reed DE. Isolation and characterization of bovine parvoviruses. J Infect Dis 1972;126:531–536.

Durham PJK, Johnson RH, Isles H, et al. Epidemiological studies of parvovirus infections in calves on endemically infected properties. Res Vet Sci 1985;38:234–240.

Durham PJK, Lax A, Johnson RH. Pathological and virological studies of experimental parvoviral enteritis in calves. Res Vet Sci 1985; 38:209–219.

Storz J, Bates RC, Warren GS, et al. Distribution of antibodies against bovine parvovirus 1 in cattle and other animal species. Am J Vet Res 1972;33:269–272.

Storz J, Bates RC. Parvovirus infections in calves. J Am Vet Med Assoc 1973;163:884–886.

Woods GT. Bovine parvovirus 1, bovine syncytial virus, and bovine respiratory syncytial virus and their infections. Adv Vet Sci Comp Med 1974;18:273–286.

PORCINE PARVOVIRUS INFECTION

Parvovirus is widespread in swine populations, judging by the demonstration of antibodies and recovery of strains of the agent. The principal effects of the virus are on reproduction; it causes intrauterine death of fetuses. Abortion rarely occurs; infected swine fetuses undergo maceration or mummification but are not usually expelled prematurely. The only noticeable sign of infection may be infertility. Lesions of infected pig fetuses have not been described in detail, except to record the presence of virus in macerated or mummified fetuses. Virus is easily demonstrated with fluorescent antibody staining technique.

Porcine parvovirus is not known to cause disease in nonpregnant adult swine. Although it has been ascribed to causing weakness in neonates, experimental infection has failed to produce disease in neonatal swine.

References

Brown TT Jr, Paul PS, Mengeling WL. Response of conventionally raised weanling pigs to experimental infection with a virulent strain of porcine parvovirus. Am J Vet Res 1980;41:1211–1224.

Cartwright SF, Lucas M, Huck RA. A small hemagglutinating porcine DNA virus. I. Isolation and properties. J Comp Pathol 1969;79: 371–377.

Cartwright SF, Lucas M, Huck RA. A small hemagglutinating porcine DNA virus. II. Biological and serological studies. J Comp Pathol 1971;81:145–156.

Cutler RS, Molitor TW, Leman AD, et al. Farm studies of porcine parvovirus infection. J Am Vet Med Assoc 1983;182:592–594.

Cutlip RC, Mengeling WL. Experimentally induced infection of neonatal swine with porcine parvovirus. Am J Vet Res 1975;36:1179–1182.

Cutlip RC, Mengeling WL. Pathogenesis of in utero infection: experimental infection of eight and ten-week-old porcine fetuses with porcine parvovirus. Am J Vet Res 1975;36:1751–1754.

Koestner A, Kasga L, Kindig O, et al. Ultrastructure alterations of tissue cultures infected with a pathogenic porcine adenovirus. Am J Pathol 1968;53:651–665.

Lucas MH, Cartwright SF, Wrathall AE. Genital infection of pigs with porcine parvovirus. J Comp Pathol 1974;84:347–350.

Mengeling WL. Porcine parvovirus: frequency of naturally occurring transplacental infection and viral contamination of fetal porcine kidney cell cultures. Am J Vet Res 1975;36:41–44.

Mengeling WL, Cutlip RC. Pathogenesis of in utero infection: experimental infection of five-week-old porcine fetuses with porcine parvovirus. Am J Vet Res 1975;36:1173–1177.

Mengeling WL, Cutlip RC. Reproductive disease experimentally induced by exposing pregnant gilts to porcine parvovirus. Am J Vet Res 1976;37:1393–1400.

Mengeling WL, Paul PS. Interepizootic survival of porcine parvovirus. J Am Vet Med Assoc 1986;188:1293–1295.

Mengeling WL, Cutlip RC, Wilson RA, et al. Fetal mummification associated with porcine parvovirus infection. J Am Vet Med Assoc 1975;166:993–995.

Rodeffer HE, Leman AD, Dunne HW, et al. Reproductive failure in swine associated with maternal seroconversion for porcine parvovirus. J Am Vet Med Assoc 1975;166:991–992.

MURINE PARVOVIRUS INFECTIONS

Parvoviruses of rats and mice are common as latent infections in wild and laboratory rodents, but do not produce spontaneous disease. They have, however, been of interest as model systems for the study of parvoviruses. Experimentally, several syndromes have been induced. Kilham rat virus (RV) has been shown in rats to cause (1) fetal death and resorption; (2) neonatal hepatitis characterized by focal necrosis and basophilic intranuclear inclusion bodies in hepatocytes, Kupffer cells, endothelial cells, and biliary epithelium; (3) cerebellar hypoplasia resulting from necrosis of the external granular layer associated with intranuclear inclusion bodies; and (4) severe hemorrhagic encephalopathy in neonates, resulting from the effect of the virus on endothelium and proliferating cells in the neonatal brain. A similar encephalopathy has been produced by infection with a closely related rat parvovirus called H-1. RV has also been experimentally shown to cause cerebellar hypoplasia in cats. Both RV and H-1 are pathogenic for fetal and neonatal hamsters in which they have induced a variety of lesions that include disseminated disease in the fetus or neonate; cerebellar hypoplasia; and a "mongoloid" dwarfism resulting from viral replication in actively proliferating skeletal and dental progenitor cells. Weanling and adult hamsters are not susceptible. Minute virus of mice (MVM), which is also a common infection but doesn't cause natural disease, has also been experimentally shown to cause dwarfing in hamsters as well as cerebellar hypoplasia when inoculated into newborn mice. Because of their effect in the hamster, RV, H-1 and MVM have been referred to as **hamster osteolytic virus.**

References

Baringer JR, Nathanson N. Parvovirus hemorrhagic encephalopathy of rats. Electron microscopic observations of the vascular lesions. Lab Invest 1972;27:514–522.

Cole GA, Nathanson N, Rivet H. Viral hemorrhagic encephalopathy of rats. II. Pathogenesis of central nervous system lesions. Am J Epidemiol 1970;91:339–348.

Lipton H, Nathanson N, Hodous J. Enteric transmission of parvoviruses; pathogenesis of rat virus infection in adult rats. Am J Epidemiol 1972;96:443–446.

Margolis G, Kilham L. Parvovirus infection, vascular endothelium, and hemorrhagic encephalopathy. Lab Invest 1970;22:478–488.

Nathanson N, Cole GA, Santos GW, et al. Viral hemorrhagic encephalopathy of rats. I. Isolation, identification, and properties of the HER strain of rat virus. Am J Epidemiol 1970;91:328–338.

Siegl G, Bates RC, Berns KI, et al. Characteristics and taxonomy of Parvoviridae. Intervirology 1985;23:61–73.

ALEUTIAN DISEASE OF MINK

Aleutian disease is a parvovirus infection of mink that is particularly fatal to mink that are homozygous for a recessive gene that confers a distinctive blue color to the fur, which is called Aleutian. Mink heterozygous for this gene are less severely affected, and the disease has a much longer course. Mink lacking the gene (and ferrets) are susceptible to infection and may carry and excrete the virus for years without developing clinical signs. The unique susceptibility of Aleutian mink results from linkage of the Aleutian gene to a gene responsible for a lysosomal anomaly of granule-producing cells, termed **Chediak-Higashi syndrome.** Mink of the Aleutian color are thus affected by this syndrome, one feature of which is the inability of phagocytes to destroy immune complexes.

Although Aleutian disease virus is classified as a parvovirus, the pathogenesis of the disease and the histopathology are distinct from those parvoviruses discussed above, in which disease is based on replication and destruction of mitotic cells and the presence of intranuclear inclusion bodies. Aleutian disease, in contrast, is a virally induced immune complex disease. The virus establishes a persistent infection with continuous release of virions. Lymphocytes are believed to be the target cell. Although viral antigens are found in macrophages throughout the body, this probably represents phagocytized antigen-antibody complexes. The immune response to the continuous release of virus leads to hypergammaglobulinemia, a distinctive feature of infection. After a few months, total gammaglobulin levels in serum are five times normal levels and consist almost entirely of a monoclonal response to the virus. The immune response fails to eliminate the virus, and the failure to eliminate the resultant antigen-antibody complex leads to deposition throughout the vascular system, glomeruli, and other tissues, causing immune-complex disease. Even virus bound to antibody is not neutralized. Infectious virus is excreted in saliva, urine, and feces throughout the term of infection. "Vertical" transmission also occurs through the placenta to the fetus.

Signs The disease is manifested in affected mink by lethargy, anorexia, cachexia, and occasionally fever, which may reach 107°F. Thrombocytopenia and anemia are present. Blood often exudes from the mouth and sometimes from the anus. Young kits tend to die within a few days after signs of illness are seen, but most adults live for 3 to 5 weeks. Some may survive for many months, but among animals that show signs, 90% or more can be expected to die.

Lesions Grossly, mink dying of Aleutian disease are emaciated with marked lymphadenopathy, splenomegaly, and hepatomegaly. The kidneys are pale, and petechiae are widespread. Microscopically, the lesions are characterized by focal accumulations of plasma cells in several organs; hyaline and inflammatory changes in the walls of small arteries; dilation and proliferation of intrahepatic bile ducts; focal or diffuse interstitial fibrosis of the kidneys; glomerulonephritis; hemorrhages; and focal encephalomalacia with nonsuppurative leptomeningitis. Large numbers of plasma cells in the tissues is a consistent feature of the disease and is undoubtedly the source of the excessive gammaglobulins found in serum.

Plasma cell infiltration may be so extensive as to resemble multiple myeloma; however, the cells are quite well differentiated. The widespread arteritis and glomerulonephritis are typical of immune-complex disease.

An acute interstitial pneumonia has been described in young mink, which is thought to be caused by Aleutian disease virus. In this syndrome, intranuclear inclusion bodies were found in alveolar type-II cells and there was no evidence of immune-complex disease. This more closely resembles a classical cytocidal parvoviral infection than typical Aleutian disease.

References

Alexandersen S. Acute interstitial pneumonia in mink kits: experimental reproduction of the disease. Vet Pathol 1986;23:579–588.

Alexandersen S, Bloom ME, Wolfinbarger J. Evidence of restricted viral replication in adult mink infected with Aleutian disease of mink parvovirus. J Virol 1988;62:1495–1507.

Drommer W, Trautwein G. Pathogenesis of Aleutian disease in the mink. VII. Chronic hepatitis and proliferation of bile ducts. Vet Pathol 1975;12:77–93.

Eklund CM, Hadlow WJ, Kennedy RC, et al. Aleutian disease of mink: properties of the etiologic agent and the host responses. J Infect Dis 1968;118:510–526.

Hadlow WJ, Race RE, Jackson TA. Lymphoreticular proliferative disease in mink homozygous for the Aleutian gene. JNCI 1972; 49:1455–1457.

Hadlow WJ. Ocular lesions in mink affected with Aleutian disease. Vet Pathol 1982;19:5–15.

Helmboldt CF, Jungherr EL. The pathology of Aleutian disease in mink. Am J Vet Res 1958;19:212–222.

Henson JB, Leader RW, Gorham JR, et al. The sequential development of lesions in spontaneous Aleutian disease of mink. Pathol Vet 1966;3:289–314.

Henson JB, Leader RW, Gorham JR, et al. The sequential development of ultrastructural lesions in the glomeruli of mink with experimental Aleutian disease. Lab Invest 1968;19:153–162.

Henson JB, Gorham JR, Tanaka Y. Renal glomerular ultrastructure in mink affected by Aleutian disease. Lab Invest 1967;17:123–139.

Johnson MI, Henson JB, Gorham JR. The influence of genotype on the development of glomerular lesions in mink with Aleutian disease virus. Am J Pathol 1975;81:321–336.

Karstad L. Aleutian disease. A slowly progressive viral infection of mink. Curr Top Microbiol Immunol 1967;40:9–21.

Karstad L, Pridham TJ. Aleutian disease of mink. 1. Evidence of its viral etiology. Can J Comp Med Vet Sci 1962;26:97–102.

Larsen S, Alexandersen S, Lund E, et al. Acute interstitial pneumonitis caused by Aleutian disease virus in mink kits. Acta Pathol Microbiol Immunol Scand (A) 1984;92:391–393.

Obel A-L. Studies on a disease in mink with systemic proliferation of the plasma cells. Am J Vet Res 1959;20:384–393.

Padgett GA, Gorham JR, Henson JB. Epizootiologic studies of Aleutian disease. I. Transplacental transmission of the virus. J Infect Dis 1967;117:35–38.

Pan IC, Tsai KS, Karstad L. Glomerulonephritis in Aleutian disease of mink: histological and immunofluorescence studies. J Pathol 1970;101:119–127.

Pan IC, Tsai KS, Grinyer I, et al. Glomerulonephritis in Aleutian disease of mink: ultrastructural studies. J Pathol 1970;102:33–40.

Porter DD, Larsen AE, Porter HG. The pathogenesis of Aleutian disease of mink. III. Immune complex arteritis. Am J Pathol 1973;71:331–344.

Porter DD, Larsen AE. Aleutian disease of mink. Prog Med Virol 1974;18:32–47.

Roth S, Kaaden O-R, van Dawen S, et al. Aleutian disease virus in B and T lymphocytes from blood and spleen and in bone marrow cells from naturally infected mink. Intervirology 1984;22: 211–217.

PICORNAVIRIDAE

A large number of viruses (Table 8–6) are grouped in the family *Picornaviridae* (pico = small, rna = ribonucleic acid). These viruses are serologically distinct but similar in terms of their morphology and physical and

TABLE 8-6 **Diseases caused by *Picornaviridae***

Enterovirus

Poliomyelitis
Coxsackie viruses
Porcine polioencephalomyelitis
Poliomyelitis of mice
Bovine enterovirus infection
Swine vesicular disease
Avian encephalomyelitis
Duck hepatitis
Human hepatitis A

Cardiovirus

Encephalomyocarditis

Rhinovirus

Human rhinovirus infection
Bovine rhinovirus infection
Equine rhinovirus infection

Aphthovirus

Foot and mouth disease
(Aphthous fever)

chemical properties. They are responsible for a spectrum of illnesses in humans and animals.

Viruses grouped in the *Picornaviridae* have an icosahedral capsid 25 to 30 nm in diameter and are nonenveloped. The viral nucleic acid consists of a single linear molecule of positive-sense single-stranded RNA with a molecular weight of 2.6 daltons. The RNA extraced from the virion is infectious.

The family **Picornaviridae** is divided into four genera: enterovirus; cardiovirus; rhinovirus; and aphthovirus. Each genus contains animal pathogens that induce diseases with specific characteristics. The single physical distinction between the genera is their pH stability.

Enteroviruses initially invade the oropharynx and, because of their stability at a low pH, also pass through the stomach to the intestines, where replication also occurs. Initial replication occurs at these sites, most probably in lymphocytes. Subsequent viremia allows dissemination to other target organs, such as the central nervous system.

The aphthovirus genus only contains the virus (seven serotypes and 53 subtypes) of foot and mouth disease. These viruses are inactivated at a pH of less than 7. Primary replication occurs in the pharynx after inhalation of aerosols or ingestion of contaminated materials, with subsequent viremia and spread to other organs and tissues.

Members of the rhinovirus genus, which are also susceptible to low pH, include pathogens for humans, cattle, and horses and are highly species specific. These viruses replicate in the upper respiratory tract, which is their primary and definitive site of localization.

Encephalomyocarditis virus is the only member of

the cardiovirus genus. This agent's definitive tropism is either the central nervous system or the myocardium.

Diseases caused by enteroviruses

POLIOMYELITIS OF MICE (MOUSE ENCEPHALOMYELITIS, THEILER'S DISEASE)

A spontaneous disease of albino mice, characterized by progressive flaccid paralysis, particularly of the hind legs, was reported in 1934 by Theiler, who demonstrated its cause to be a filterable virus. The disease is not transmissible to other laboratory animals. Although in nature few mice exhibit symptoms, large numbers with no apparent illness may carry the virus in the intestinal tract. The virus can be demonstrated by the intracranial inoculation of normal mice with bacteria-free suspensions of intestinal contents taken from carrier animals. The epizootiologic characteristics, along with the selective distribution of the lesions in the central nervous system, are closely comparable with those of poliomyelitis in humans. The virus usually inhabits the digestive tract and only rarely involves the central nervous system.

Lesions Lesions of the murine disease are most often found in the substantia nigra, tegmentum, reticular formation, olivary nuclei, nuclei of the fifth and eighth nerves, and red and dentate nuclei. Changes in the caudate nuclei are not often observed. The anterior horns of the spinal cord are severely involved after the onset of paralysis. The lesions consist not only of vascular and perivascular changes, but also of neuronal degeneration, necrosis, and neuronophagia. The virus not only causes destruction of neurons but also results in primary demyelination, particularly in mice that survive the acute phase of the disease or that are not infected until 2 to 4 weeks of age. Demyelination has been shown to result from immunologic response to the virus, which can be negated with immunosuppressive measures, as well as from lytic infection of oligodendrocytes.

Diagnosis The diagnosis can be established by demonstrating the lesions and isolating the virus from infected animals. The virus can be identified by appropriate methods. Although apparently producing a disease analogous to human poliomyelitis, the virus is antigenically distinct from that of poliomyelitis.

References

Dal Canto MC, Lipton HL. Primary demyelination in Theiler's virus infection. An ultrastructural study. Lab Invest 1975;33:626–637.
Daniels JB, Pappenheimer AM, Richardson S. Observations on encephalomyelitis of mice, DA strain. J Exp Med 1952;96:517–530.
Lipton HL, Dal Canto MC. Theiler's virus-induced demyelination: Prevention by immunosuppression. Science 1976;192:62–64.
Olitsky PK, Schlesinger RW. Histopathology of CNS of mice infected with virus of Theiler's disease (spontaneous encephalomyelitis). Proc Soc Exp Biol Med 1941;47:79–83.
Rodriguez M, Leibowitz JL, Powell HC, et al. Neonatal infection with the Daniels strain of Theiler's murine encephalomyelitis virus. Lab Invest 1983;49:672–679.
Rosenthal A, Fujinami RS, Lampert PW. Mechanism of Theiler's virus-

induced demyelination in nude mice. Lab Invest 1986;54: 515–520.

Theiler M. Spontaneous encephalomyelitis of mice—a new virus disease. Science 1934;80:122.

Theiler M. Spontaneous encephalomyelitis of mice. J Exp Med 1937;65:705–719.

Theiler M, Gard S. Encephalomyelitis of mice. J Exp Med 1940;72: 49–67.

Theiler M, Gard S. Epidemiology of mouse encephalomyelitis. J Exp Med 1940;72:79–90.

POLIOMYELITIS IN PRIMATES

The virus responsible for poliomyelitis in humans is the type species for the genus enterovirus. The virus is a common, and apparently nonpathogenic, inhabitant of the digestive tract, and is also responsible for paralytic poliomyelitis of children and young adults. The virus, under natural conditions, may also be transmitted from human to nonhuman primates, such as the chimpanzee *(Pan troglodytes* or *P. paniscus)*, gorilla *(Gorilla gorilla)*, orangutan *(Pongo pygmaeus)*, and rhesus monkey *(Macaca mulatta)*. The virus may be carried in the intestines of these species and, in some instances, may cause paralytic poliomyelitis. The rhesus and crab-eating macaque monkey *(Macaca fascicularis)* have also been used extensively in testing poliomyelitis vaccines, which have been efficacious in reducing the frequency of paralytic poliomyelitis.

References

Allmond BW Jr, Froeschle JE, Guilloud NB. Paralytic poliomyelitis in large laboratory primates. Virologic investigation and report on the use of oral poliomyelitis virus (OPV) vaccine. Am J Epidemiol 1967;85:229–239.

Guilloud NB, Allmond BW, Froeschle JE, et al. Paralytic poliomyelitis in laboratory primates. J Am Vet Med Assoc 1969;155:1190–1193.

Douglas JD, Soike KF, Raynor J. The incidence of poliovirus in chimpanzees *(Pan troglodytes)*. Lab Anim Care 1970;20:265–268.

Suleman MA, Johnson BJ, Tarara R, et al. An outbreak of poliomyelitis caused by poliovirus type 1 in captive black and white colobus monkeys *(Colobus abyssinicus kikuyuensis)* in Kenya. Trans R Soc Trop Med Hyg 1984;78:665–669.

PORCINE ENCEPHALOMYELITIS

Several enteroviruses have been recovered from swine, one of which, termed porcine enterovirus 1, causes encephalomyelitis. Over the years, throughout the world, several outbreaks of porcine encephalomyelitis of varying severity have been described, many of which were given specific disease names. It is now recognized that they are caused by the same virus and are a single disease. The first of these was called **Teschen disease** (Bohemian pest), so named after the province of Czechoslovakia in which the first outbreak was identified. Other terms include **poliomyelitis suum, benign enzootic paresis, Talfan disease,** and **Canadian or North American viral encephalomyelitis** (also **Ontario encephalomyelitis**).

The disease is similar to poliomyelitis of humans in that the virus may be isolated from the intestinal tract, and the ventral columns of gray matter in the spinal cord (Fig 8-38) are consistently affected. However, in the porcine disease, the lesions in the cerebral cortex and cerebellum are much more extensive and indiscriminately located than in poliomyelitis (Fig 8-39).

Signs Following an incubation period of 10 to 20 days, the onset is usually accompanied by fever (104°F to 105°F), anorexia, lassitude, depression, and sometimes slight incoordination, particularly, of the rear limbs. Recovery may occur, or these symptoms may be followed within a few hours or, at most, 1 to 3 days by a stage of irritability, by stiffness of the extremities, and, in severe cases, by tremors, nystagmus, violent clonic convulsions, prostration, and coma. Convulsions accom-

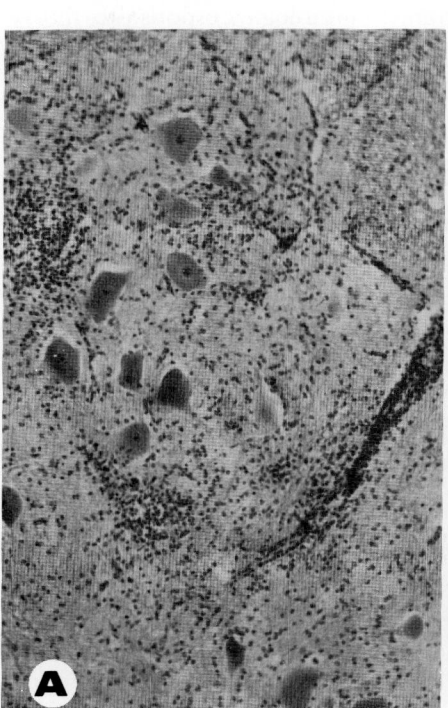 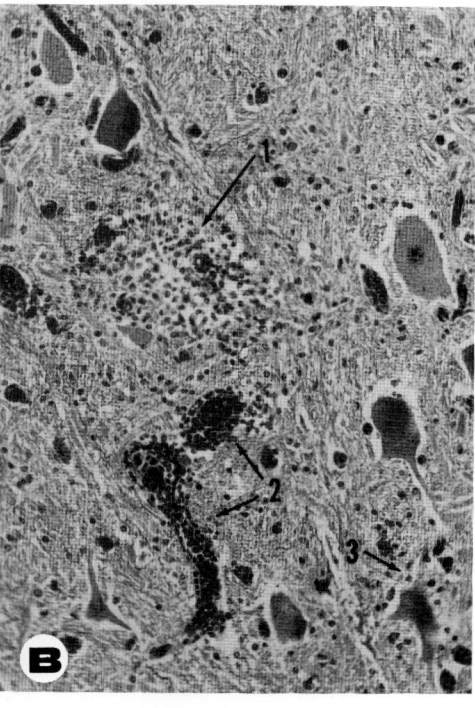

FIG. 8-38 Encephalomyelitis of swine. **A.** Ventral horn of spinal cord of a pig. (Hematoxylin and eosin stain, × 110.) (Courtesy of Dr. Aage Thordal-Christensen, Royal Veterinary and Agricultural College, Copenhagen.) **B.** Ventral horn of spinal cord of a pig (× 160). Nodule of inflammatory cells *(1)*, perivascular "cuffing" by lymphocytes *(2)*, neuronophagia *(3)*. (Courtesy of the Armed Forces Institute of Pathology; contributed by Dr. M. M. Kaplan.)

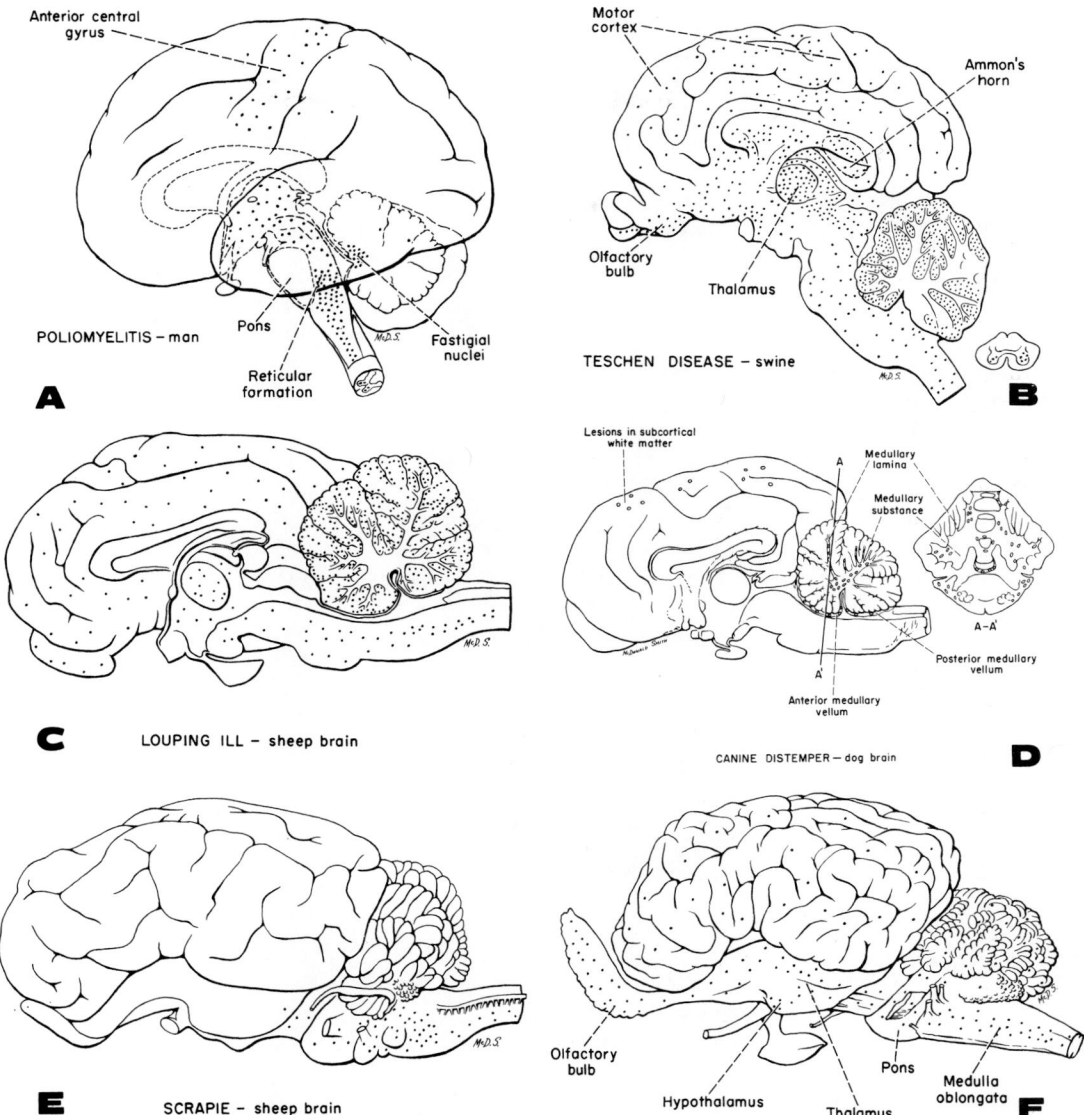

FIG. 8-39 Distribution of lesions in neurotropic viral diseases. **A.** Poliomyelitis in humans. **B.** Porcine encephalomyelitis. **C.** "Louping ill," sheep. **D.** Canine distemper. **E.** "Scrapie," brain of a sheep. **F.** Equine encephalomyelitis, brain of a horse. (Courtesy of the Armed Forces Institute of Pathology.)

panied by loud squealing can be set off by a stimulus, such as a sudden noise. Stiffness and opisthotonus are the most persistent symptoms in some cases. A sudden drop in temperature followed by paralysis and death 3 or 4 days after onset is the usual course, although some animals die within 24 hours. Others survive but are left with a flaccid posterior paralysis. Usually, if held up on their feet, these swine eat ravenously and may, in fact, be kept alive for long periods.

Swine of all ages are affected during epizootics, but once the disease is endemic, clinical disease is limited to newborn pigs and newly introduced pigs.

Lesions There are no specific gross lesions. Microscopic lesions are limited to the central nervous system

(Fig. 8-40). The virus attacks neurons of brain and cord, producing changes linked to the destruction of these nerve cells. The lesions have a specific distribution, a point that can be utilized to some extent in differential diagnosis. The spinal cord is constantly affected, the changes being principally limited to the ventral columns of the gray matter. The cerebellum also suffers rather intensely, with the Purkinje, molecular, and granular layers being involved, in order of decreasing severity. In some cases, the leptomeninges over the cerebellum are heavily infiltrated with lymphocytes. The thalamus also sustains considerable damage, and lesions of decreasing intensity occur in the basal nuclei, the base of the brain generally, olfactory bulbs, hippocam-

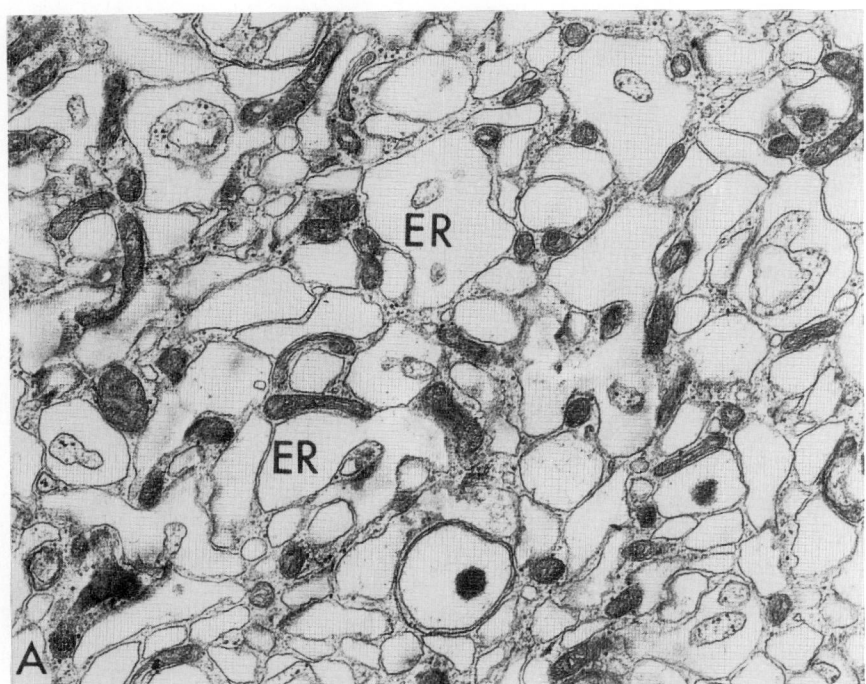

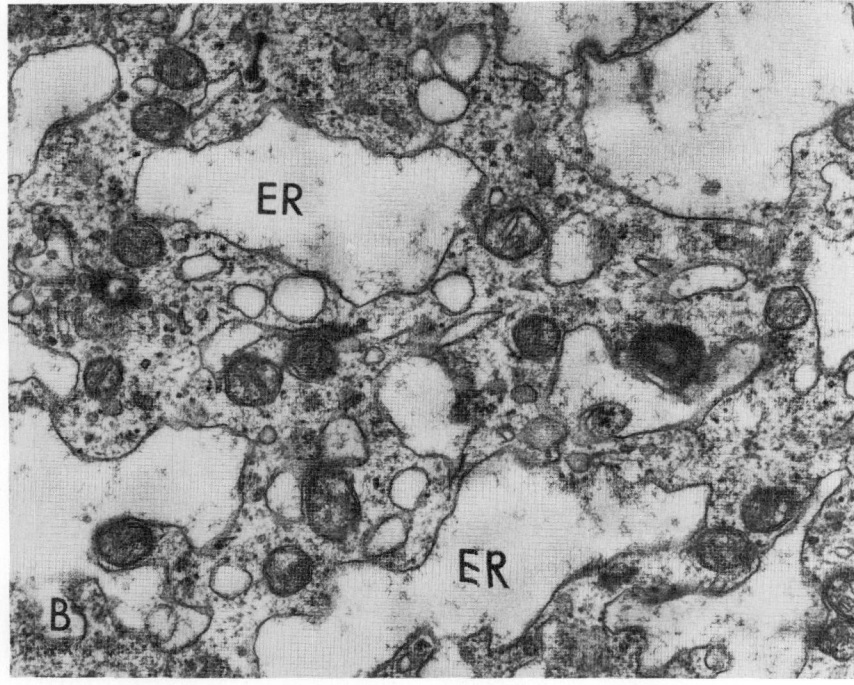

FIG. 8-40 Porcine encephalomyelitis. **A.** Extensive vesiculation of neuronal endoplasmic reticulum cisternae *(ER)*. (× 23,700.) **B.** Higher magnification of the dilated endoplasmic reticulum cisternae *(ER)*. Mitochondria are compressed (× 35,000). (Courtesy of Dr. A. Koestner and *American Journal of Pathology.*)

pal gyrus, and the pons and medulla. The motor cortex, although more vulnerable than the rest of the cerebral cortex, is not a site of predilection.

In affected sites, multipolar nerve cells undergo degeneration of varying degrees up to and including necrosis accompanied by neuronophagia, inflammatory or glial nodules, occasional hemorrhage, and rather diffuse infiltration of leukocytes, predominantly lymphocytes. Rarely are neutrophils a part of the exudate in this disease. Accumulations of lymphocytes in the peri-

vascular (Robin-Virchow) spaces are often seen. They are usually adjacent to lesions in the gray matter and may extend into the white matter; otherwise, the white matter is not involved.

Diagnosis The demonstration of typical microscopic lesions in the brain and spinal cord is sufficient for presumptive diagnosis. The preponderance of glial nodules; their distribution in the ventral columns of the spinal cord, the cerebral cortex, and cerebellum; and the intense lymphocytic infiltration of the cerebellar leptomeninges are important to this decision. The definitive diagnosis requires that the virus be isolated and identified or that specific antibodies be demonstrable in increased quantities in the serum of recovered swine.

References

Bück G, Guesnel JJ. Infectious paralysis of pigs (Teschen disease) in Madagascar. Bull Epizoot Dis Afr 1954;2:279–281.

Chaproniere DM, Done JT, Andrewes CH. Comparative serological studies on Talfan and Teschen diseases and similar conditions. Br J Exp Pathol 1958;39:74–77.

Dobberstein J. Histopathologie des Zentralnerven-systems bei der Poliomyelitis des Schweines. Ztschr Infektionskr 1942;59:54–80.

Done JT. The pathological differentiation of diseases of the central nervous system of the pig. (Proc 75th Ann Congr BVA, Cambridge, 1957) Vet Rec 1957;69:1341–1349.

Gardiner MR. Polio-encephalomyelitis of pigs in Western Australia. (VB 2266–62) Aust Vet J 1962;38:24–26.

Harding JDJ, Done JT, Kershaw GF. A transmissible polioencephalomyelitis of pigs (Talfan disease). Vet Rec 1957;69:824–832.

Horstmann DM. Experiments with Teschen disease (virus encephalomyelitis of swine). J Immunol 1952;69:379–394.

Ishitani B, et al. Studies on a swine virus disease with nervous symptoms which occurred in the winter of this year. II. Histopathological observations. Jpn J Vet Sci 1954;16:138–139.

Kaplan MM, Meranze DR. Porcine virus encephalomyelitis and its possible biological relationship to human poliomyelitis. Vet Med 1948;43:330–341.

Kasza L. Swine polioencephalomyelitis viruses isolated from the brains and intestines of pigs. Am J Vet Res 1965;26:131–137.

Kment A. Zur histopathologie des Zentralnerven-systems bei der Teschener Schweinelähmung. Wien Tierärztl Wochenschr 1940;27:361–362.

Koestner A, Kasza L, Holman JE. Electron microscopic evaluation of the pathogenesis of porcine polioencephalomyelitis. Am J Pathol 1966;49:325–327.

Koestner A, Long JF, Kasza L. Occurrence of viral polioencephalomyelitis in suckling pigs in Ohio. J Am Vet Med Assoc 1962;140:811–814.

Long JF, Koestner A, Kasza L. Pericarditis and myocarditis in germ-free and pathogen-free pigs experimentally infected with a porcine polioencephalomyelitis virus. Lab Invest 1966;15:1228.

Long JF, Koestner A, Liss L. Experimental porcine polioencephalomyelitis in germfree pigs. A silver carbonate study of neuronal degeneration and glial response. Pathologia Vet 1967;4:186–198.

Manuelidis EE, Sprinz H, Horstmann DM. Pathology of Teschen disease. Am J Pathol 1954;30:567–597.

Mills JHL, Nielsen SW. Porcine polioencephalomyelitides. Adv Vet Sci 1968;12:33–104.

Richards WPC, Savan M. Viral encephalomyelitis of pigs. A preliminary report on the tranmissibility and pathology of a disease observed in Ontario. Cornell Vet 1960;50:132–155.

Sasahara J, et al. Studies of a swine virus disease with nervous symptoms which occurred in the winter of this year. I. Isolation of the virus. Jpn J Vet Sci 1954;16:139.

Thordal-Christensen A. A study of benign enzootic paresis of pigs in Denmark. Copenhagen: Carl FR Mortensen 1959.

Treffny L. Massenerkrankungen von Schweinen in Teschner Land. Zverolekarsky Obzor 1930;23:235–236.

Watanabe H, Pospisil Z, Mensik J. Study on the pigs infected with virulent Teschen disease virus (KNM strain) with special reference to immunofluorescence. Jpn J Vet Res 1971;19:87–102.

SWINE VESICULAR DISEASE

Any disease outbreak that affects cloven-hoofed animals and has clinical features of foot and mouth disease (aphthous fever) is bound to attract a great deal of attention. This was the case when in 1966, in Italy, a febrile disease of swine was recognized in association with vesicles on the mouth, snout, and feet. Lameness and ulcerations followed the early vesiculation (Nardelli and associates, 1968). All these features are indistinguishable from the signs of foot and mouth disease. A distinctive enterovirus has been identified in association with swine vesicular disease, making it possible to differentiate this infection from vesicular exanthema (calicivirus), aphthous fever (enterovirus or aphthovirus), or vesicular stomatitis (vesiculovirus).

Swine vesicular disease now has been recognized in the United Kingdom, Hong Kong, Austria, France, Poland, and Italy. Some strains of the virus produce a disseminated encephalitis following natural or experimental exposure (Monlux and others, 1974, 1975). Also of interest is the close relationship, as determined by immunodiffusion tests, of the swine vesicular disease virus and coxsackievirus B, a common pathogen to humans. The swine virus also is suspected of infecting laboratory workers who have been in contact with it. It has been postulated (Brown, Talbot and Burrows, 1973) that the swine vesicular disease virus and coxsackie B virus may have had the same antecedents. Coxsackievirus B has been associated with aseptic meningitis, encephalitis, myositis, orchitis, myocarditis, diarrhea, respiratory disease, and vesicular and papular rash in humans. It also has been isolated from neonatal infants with a fulminating disease, which culminates in degenerative changes in many organs.

Lesions Changes in the stratified epithelium are most evident in the skin of the coronary band of the hoof, the metatarsus, and metacarpus. Coagulation necrosis in the malpighian layer results in vesiculation and sloughing and is followed by regenerative pseudoepitheliomatous hyperplasia. Similar lesions develop on the snout, lips, and tongue and over the tonsils in about 10% of affected swine. Epithelial cells in renal pelvis, bladder, tonsillar crypts, ducts of pancreas, and salivary glands undergo degenerative changes, with formation of periodic acid-Schiff-positive material in individual cells (Lenghaus and Mann, 1976). Mild meningoencephalitis may be seen, but signs of CNS disease are unusual.

References

Brown F, Talbot P, Burrows R. Antigenic differences between isolates of swine vesicular disease virus and their relationship to Coxsackie B5 virus. Nature (London) 1973;245:315–316.

Burrows R, Greig A, Goodridge D. Swine vesicular disease. Res Vet Sci 1973;15:141–144.

Graves JH. Serological relationship of swine vesicular disease virus and Coxsackie B virus. Nature (London) 1973;245:314–315.

Lai SS, McKercher PD, Moore DM, et al. Pathogenesis of swine vesicular disease in pigs. Am J Vet Res 1979;40:463–468.

Lenghaus C, Mann JA. General pathology of experimental swine vesicular disease. Vet Pathol 1976;13:186–196.

Lenghaus C, Mann JA, Done JT, et al. Neuropathology of experimental swine vesicular disease in pigs. Res Vet Sci 1976;21:19–27.

Monlux WS, Graves JH, McKercher PD. Brain and spinal cord lesions in pigs inoculated with swine vesicular disease virus (Hong Kong strain). Am J Vet Res 1974;35:615–617.

Monlux WS, McKercher PD, Graves JH. Brain and spinal cord lesions in pigs inoculated with swine vesicular disease (UKG Strain) virus and coxsackievirus B5. Am J Vet Res 1975;36:1745–1749.

Nardelli L, Lodetti E, Gualandi GL, et al. A foot and mouth disease syndrome in pigs caused by an enterovirus. Nature (London) 1968;219:1275–1276.

OTHER ENTEROVIRUSES

Many other enteroviruses have been identified in addition to those discussed above. The coxsackievirus and echovirus groups contain a number of agents associated with a diverse group of illnesses in humans to include febrile illness, meningitis, paralysis, myocarditis, and acute hemorrhagic conjunctivitis. Additional enteroviruses have been recovered from domestic animals and nonhuman primates, but are of uncertain pathologic significance. In swine, enteroviruses have been associated with a variety of reproductive disorders. These agents have been termed the SMEDI group of picornaviruses, which is an acronym for *s*tillbirths, *m*ummifications, *e*mbryonic *d*eaths, and *i*nfertility.

References

Dunne HW, Gobble JL, Hokanson JF, et al. Porcine reproductive failure associated with a newly identified "SMEDI" group of picornaviruses. Am J Vet Res 1965;26:1284–1297.

Huang J, Gentry RF, Zarkower A. Experimental infection of pregnant sows with porcine enteroviruses. Am J Vet Res 1980;41:469–473.

Diseases caused by cardioviruses

VIRAL ENCEPHALOMYOCARDITIS

A disease characterized chiefly by myocarditis, first described by Helwig and Schmidt (1945) in gibbons and chimpanzees, is now recognized as a viral infection of many animal species, which may lead to either encephalitis (Fig. 8-41) or myocarditis, depending on the host.

The virus is carried by rodents, chiefly wild rats, in which the infection is inapparent. As a spontaneous disease in animals, it is of greatest importance in nonhuman primates (Old and New World) and swine, in which the virus produces a fatal myocarditis and may occur as outbreaks with high rates of morbidity and mortality.

The principal lesion is interstitial myocarditis. The heart usually is dilated and there is some slightly blood-tinged pericardial effusion. Occasionally, bilateral hydrothorax and pulmonary edema are observed. Microscopically, there is necrosis of myocardial fibers and intense infiltration with polymorphonuclear and mononuclear cells. In baboons and swine, the virus has also been associated with abortion and stillbirth. Encephalitis, as well as necrosis of the acinar pancreas (discussed later), has been noted in experimentally infected squirrel monkeys. The experimentally induced disease in mice usually results in encephalomyelitis as well as myocarditis. Hamsters and rats have been reported to be susceptible, with the resultant disease similar to that seen in mice. The virus is reported to produce myelitis in horses and myocarditis in cattle. Rabbits and guinea pigs are somewhat refractory to experimental infection. Microscopic calcification of muscle bundles has been described in guinea pigs in which attempts had been made to induce the infection, but this change may not be due to the virus of encephalomyocarditis. In humans, the virus has been associated with central nervous system disease, but its causative role is uncertain.

Strains of encephalomyocarditis virus have been developed with differing tissue tropisms, including acinar pancreas and salivary and lacrimal glands. One which has been of considerable experimental interest pro-

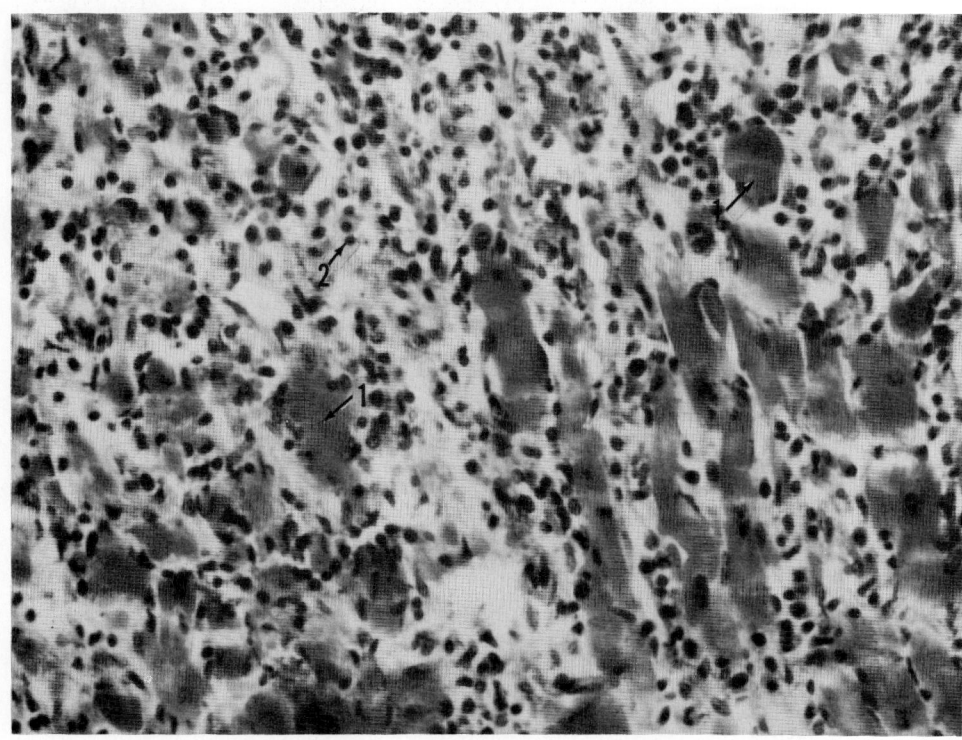

FIG. 8-41 Encephalomyocarditis, myocardium (× 350) of gibbon. Fragmented myocardial fibers *(1)* are separated by intense infiltration of lymphocytes *(2)* and plasma cells. (Courtesy of the Armed Forces Institute of Pathology; contributed by Lt. Col. F. C. Helwig.)

duces necrosis of the islets of Langerhans and diabetes mellitus.

References

Acland HM, Littlejohns IR. Encephalomyocarditis virus infection of pigs. 1. An outbreak in New South Wales. Aust Vet J 1975;51:409–415.

Blanchard JL, Soike K, Baskin GB. Encephalomyocarditis virus infection in African green and squirrel monkeys: comparison of pathologic effects. Lab Anim Sci 1987;37:635–639.

Craighead JE. Pathogenicity of the M and E variants of the encephalomyocarditis (EMC) virus. I. Myocardiotropic and neurotropic properties. II. Lesions of the pancreas, parotid and lacrimal glands. Am J Pathol 1966;48:333–345, 375–386.

Craighead JE, McLane MF. Diabetes mellitus: induction in mice by encephalomyocarditis virus. Science 1968;162:913–914.

Craighead JE, Kanich RE, Kessler JB. Lesions of the islets of Langerhans in encephalomyocarditis virus-infected mice with diabetes mellitus-like disease. Am J Pathol 1974;74:287–300.

Gainer JH, Sandefur JR, Bigler WJ. High mortality in a Florida swine herd infected with the encephalomyocarditis virus. An accompanying epizootiologic survey. Cornell Vet 1968;58:31–47.

Helwig FC, Schmidt ECH. A filter passing agent producing interstitial myocarditis in anthropoid apes and small animals. Science 1945;102:31–33.

Hubbard GB, Soike KF, Butler TM, et al. An encephalomyocarditis virus epizootic in a baboon colony. Lab Anim Sci 1992;42:233–239.

Kim HS, Christianson WT, Joo HS. Characterization of encephalomyocarditis virus isolated from aborted swine fetuses. Am J Vet Res 1991;52:1649–1652.

Littlejohns IR, Acland HM. Encephalomyocarditis virus infection of pigs. 2. Experimental disease. Aust Vet J 1975;51:416–422.

Roca-Garcia M, Sanmartin-Barberi C. The isolation of encephalomyocarditis virus from *Aotus* monkeys. Am J Trop Med Hyg 1957;6:840–852.

Schmidt ECH. Virus myocarditis. Pathologic and experimental studies. Am J Pathol 1948;24:97–117.

Tesh RB. The prevalence of encephalomyocarditis virus neutralizing antibodies among various human populations. Am J Trop Med Hyg 1978;27:144–149.

Tesh RB, Wallace GD. Observations on the natural history of encephalomyocarditis virus. Am J Trop Med Hyg 1978;27:133–143.

Watt DA, Spradbrow PB. Experimental encephalomyocarditis virus infection of pigs. Aust Vet J 1974;50:316–319.

Diseases Caused by Rhinoviruses

The rhinoviruses cause the common cold in humans. More than 100 distinct rhinoviruses have been identified from humans; however, very few have been recognized as causes of disease in domestic animals. The human isolates do not infect domestic animals, although great apes are susceptible but do not develop disease. Distinct rhinoviruses that cause mild respiratory disease in horses and cattle have been identified. The infection is of little consequence, although it could predispose the infected animal to other respiratory pathogens. The equine rhinovirus is reported to infect humans.

References

Bögel K. Bovine rhinoviruses. J Am Vet Med Assoc 1968;152:780–783.

Lupton HW, Smith MH, Frey ML. Identification and characterization of a bovine rhinovirus isolated from Iowa cattle with acute respiratory tract disease. Am J Vet Res 1980;41:1029–1034.

Mohanty SB, Lillie MG, Albert TF, et al Experimental exposure of calves to a bovine rhinovirus. Am J Vet Res 1969;30:1105–1111.

Plummer G. An equine respiratory enterovirus. Some biologic and physical properties. Arch Ges Verusforsch 1963;12:694–700.

Rosenquist BD. Rhinoviruses: isolation from cattle with acute respiratory disease. Am J Vet Res 1971;32:685–688.

Disease Caused by Aphthovirus

FOOT AND MOUTH DISEASE (APHTHOUS FEVER).

The several serotypes of foot and mouth disease virus are the only members of this genus, and foot and mouth disease is the only disease caused by this group. Foot and mouth disease has a special place in the history of virology, for it was the first animal virus to be recognized. Loeffler and Frosch demonstrated in 1897 that the causative agent passed through Berkefeld filters and, thus, recorded for the first time an infectious agent smaller than other known microorganisms (Brooksby, 1982). It was also with foot and mouth disease virus that different serotypes between strains of an animal virus were first recognized.

Aphthous fever is an important and widespread disease caused by a virus with strong epitheliotropic features. The disease occurs naturally in cloven-hoofed animals, the most important of which are cattle, sheep, goats, and swine. It may also affect ruminants, such as deer, goats, and antelope, and under some conditions, ruminants act as reservoirs for the infection. Guinea pigs, suckling mice, birds, and carnivores have been successfully inoculated with the virus. Natural infection may occur in humans, in whom the disease is usually mild and limited to acute fever associated with the appearance of vesicles on the hands, feet, and oral mucosae.

Although aphthous fever is prevalent in all of Europe, Africa, much of Asia, and in some countries of South America, the disease has been prevented from re-entering the United States since 1929, when a severe outbreak occurred in California. This and previous outbreaks were stamped out by stringent quarantine of infected areas and slaughter of exposed and infected animals. Important outbreaks have occurred in Mexico and Canada, but appear to have been controlled.

The virus occurs in seven principal antigenic types. These are designated in the international nomenclature as: O (from the department of Oise); A (from Allemagne); C (from a revised classification where O and A were termed A and B); SAT 1, SAT 2, SAT 3 (from South African territories); and Asia 1. Although the symptoms and lesions produced by each virus type are essentially similar, infection with one virus does not immunize against the others. In recent years numerous subtypes have been identified, which are also antigenically distinct.

Pathogenesis Features of particular significance in this disease are the extreme infectiousness of the virus and the ease with which it can be carried, not only by infected animals and their products but also mechanically by humans and other animals. The virus may be transported on the shoes or clothing of humans, in or on the bodies of migratory birds or animals, and in such products as raw hides, milk, bedding, and forage. Recovered cattle can carry the virus for periods of up to 2 years, and recovered sheep may carry it for up to 6 months. The virus apparently does not persist in recovered swine. Infection is spread principally by the airborne route. Primary viral replication occurs in the pharynx or respiratory tract, with subsequent viremia and dissemination throughout the body, which produces secondary lesions, chiefly in epithelial tissues.

Signs The signs are directly related to the lesions of the disease. Those in the oral mucosa produce excess salivation and make eating painful, thus causing the infected animal to refuse food and water. Smacking of the lips and tongue is characteristic. The epithelium of the dorsum of the tongue usually becomes eroded. Lesions of the feet may produce lameness. Aphthae may be detected on other parts of the body that are lightly haired, such as the skin of the udder, the vulva, and the conjunctiva.

In young animals (lambs and calves), acute gastroenteritis and myocarditis are common and the mortality rate is very high. In animal populations that have been exposed to the disease, the mortality rate is low, rarely more than 5% in adult animals, although certain virus strains can cause a mortality rate as high as 60%.

Lesions On cattle, the distribution of the vesicular lesions is characteristic. The oral mucosa over the lips, dorsum of the tongue, and palate is most severely involved. Lesions occur in the skin near the coronary band adjacent to the interdigital space and are also common in other areas in which the hair is sparse, such as the vulva, teats, and udder. The conjunctiva may be affected, as may be the part of the forestomach that is lined with squamous epithelium (rumen, reticulum, and omasum). Small epidermal vesicles may also occur in grossly normal skin of the brisket, abdomen, hock, carpus, and perineum. In addition to these specific vesicular lesions, punctate hemorrhages or diffuse edema of the mucosa may be observed in the abomasum and small intestine. The mucosa of the large intestine may be hyperemic and blue-red, and some animals may bear subpleural, subepithelial, or subepicardial hemorrhages. These, however, are not considered primary lesions.

The specific lesions in their early stages are microscopic and are limited to the epithelium at the sites of predilection. The lesion starts with localized "balloon" degeneration of cells in the middle of the stratum spinosum of the epithelium. Here, the intercellular prickles are lost; the epithelial cells become round and detached from one another; their cytoplasm takes an intensely eosinophilic stain; and their nuclei are pyknotic. Edematous fluid containing bits of fibrin accumulates between and separates the cells. Neutrophils infiltrate the epithelium at this stage. Liquefaction necrosis and an accumulation of serum and leukocytes produce vesicles roofed over by the compressed stratum corneum, lucidum, and granulosum, and extending down to the basal layer, which usually remains in place over the heavily congested dermis. These small vesicles (aphthae) coalesce to form bullae, which cause large areas of epithelium to be detached and easily shed or rubbed off. Loss of epithelium is most common on the dorsal surface of the anterior two-thirds of the bovine tongue,

which is separated by a transverse notch from a dorsal eminence occupying the posterior third of the tongue. The entire epithelium over the anterior area may be lost, leaving a raw, red surface that oozes blood. The pain from this denuded area explains the severe anorexia, which is often a sign. In addition to the virus, the vesicles contain necrotic epithelial cells, leukocytes, occasional erythrocytes, and, in the late stages, bacteria. Small pleomorphic bodies have been described in lymphocytes and epithelial cells, but these have not been established as virus particles or specific "inclusions."

Lesions in the myocardium are most common in the fatal disease in very young calves or lambs but also occur in pigs and young goats. The lesions observed in the wall and septum of the left ventricle (seldom in the atria) appear as small, grayish foci of irregular size, which may give the myocardium a somewhat striped appearance (so-called "tiger heart"). Microscopically, hyaline degeneration and necrosis of myocardial fibers are accompanied by an intense lymphocytic, occasionally neutrophilic, infiltration. The myocardial lesion is not strictly specific for infections with the virus of foot and mouth disease, but it is believed to be the one that most commonly causes death of newborn animals.

In the skeletal muscle, lesions similar to those in the myocardium may be observed. Sharply delimited areas of necrosis are seen grossly as gray foci of various sizes and microscopically as necrosis of muscle bundles associated with intense leukocytic infiltration. A similar, but much more severe, acute myositis occurs in suckling mice experimentally inoculated with the virus. Because of the susceptibility of their musculature, young mice are being used with increasing frequency in experimental study of the virus.

Diagnosis In differential diagnosis of aphthous fever (foot and mouth disease), it is necessary to consider all other so-called "vesicular diseases," such as vesicular exanthema, swine vesicular disease, and vesicular stomatitis. These cannot be differentiated with absolute certainty by their symptoms and lesions. It is necessary, therefore, to isolate and identify the virus or to demonstrate complement-fixing or virus-neutralizing antibodies in recovered animals. The agar gel diffusion reaction is also useful in detecting antigenic relationships. Immunofluorescent methods are used to detect viral antigen in cells (Mohanty and Cottral, 1970).

References

Brooksby JB. Portraits of viruses: Foot-and-mouth disease virus. Intervirology 1982;18:1–23.
Burrows R. Studies on the carrier state of cattle exposed to foot and mouth disease virus. J Hyg (Lond) 1966;64:81–90.
Burrows R, Mann JA, Garland AJM, et al. The pathogenesis of natural and simulated natural foot-and-mouth disease infection in cattle. J Comp Pathol 1981;91:599–609.
Capel-Edwards M. The susceptibility of small mammals to foot-and-mouth disease virus. Vet Bull 1971;41:815–823.
Fenner F, Bachmann PA, Gibbs EPJ, et al. Veterinary virology. New York: Academic Press 1987.
Frenkel HS. Histologic changes in explanted bovine epithelial tongue tissue infected with the virus of foot and mouth disease. Am J Vet Res 1949; 10:142–145.

Gailiunas P. Microscopic skin lesions in cattle with foot-and-mouth disease. Arch Ges Virus-forsch 1968;25:188–200.

Gailiunas P, Cottral GE, Seibold HR. Teat lesions in heifers experimentally infected with foot-and-mouth disease virus. Am J Vet Res 1964;25:1062–1069.

Galloway IA, Elford WJ. Filtration of the virus of foot-and-mouth disease through a new series of graded collodion membranes. Br J Exp Pathol 1931;12:407–425.

Mohanty GC, Cottral GE. Immunofluorescent detection of foot-and-mouth disease virus in the esophageal-pharyngeal fluids of inoculated cattle. Am J Vet Res 1970;31:1187–1196.

Planterose DN, Ryand JKO. A 65 S particle containing viral protein in cells infected with foot-and-mouth disease virus. Virology 1965;26:372–374.

Platt H. Observations on the pathology of experimental foot and mouth disease in adult guinea pigs. J Pathol Bact 1931;6:119–131.

Scott FW, Cottral GE, Gailiunas P. Persistence of foot-and-mouth disease virus in external lesions and saliva of experimentally infected cattle. Am J Vet Res 1966;27:1531–1536.

Seibold HR. The histopathology of foot and mouth disease in pregnant and lactating mice. Am J Vet Res 1960;21:870–877.

Skinner HH. Propagation of strains of foot and mouth disease virus in unweaned white mice. Proc Roy Soc Med 1951;44:1041–1044.

Terpstra C. Pathogenesis of foot-and-mouth disease in experimentally infected pigs. Bull Off Internat Epizoot 1972;77:859–874.

Yilma T. Morphogenesis of vesiculation in foot-and-mouth disease. Am J Vet Res 1980;41:1537–1542.

CALICIVIRIDAE

Viruses in this family were once included in *Picornaviridae;* however, they have enough distinguishing features to be classified as a separate group. Caliciviruses are slightly larger than picornaviruses, and the virion has 32 cup-shaped surface depressions giving rise to their name (Calix = cup). The more important viruses in this group are: the virus of vesicular exanthema of swine; feline calicivirus; viral hemorrhagic disease of rabbits; and San Miguel sea lion virus. Other caliciviruses have been isolated from dogs, cattle, swine, and a number of other mammalian species as well as fish. Some have been associated with enteric disease.

There are a number of other small RNA viruses whose classification is somewhat uncertain. These include the **Norwalk virus** and several other agents that cause outbreaks of gastrointestinal disease in humans and the **astroviruses,** so named because of a star-shaped ultrastructural appearance. The latter have been associated with outbreaks of gastroenteritis in humans (especially children), calves, lambs, piglets, dogs, and kittens. These are discussed later in this chapter.

Vesicular Exanthema

Vesicular exanthema of swine is characterized by fever and vesicle formation in the epithelium of the snout, lips, nostrils, tongue, feet, and mammary glands. It was first described in 1935, by Traum, whose observations were made on garbage-fed swine in California. The occurrence of this disease in a geographic area from which aphthous fever had been eliminated only with great economic loss and the similarity of the symptoms and lesions of the two diseases magnified its importance. Actually, vesicular exanthema runs a mild, rapid course of about 10 days and is almost never fatal. So

that proper measures for control can be adopted, it is essential that it be differentiated from aphthous fever, vesicular stomatitis, and swine vesicular disease, which produce similar manifestations.

In the early 1950s, vesicular exanthema had been recognized to be widespread in the United States, but by 1956 it was declared eradicated.

Epidemiologic evidence prompted Madin (1975) to postulate that the causative virus had its origin in some natural reservoir and was transmitted by feeding uncooked garbage to swine. This theory appears to be partially confirmed by the identification of the San Miguel sea lion virus from aborted sea lion fetuses on the island of San Miguel in California. This virus appears to be nearly identical to the calicivirus of vesicular exanthema. It seems likely that sea lion (*Zalophus c. californianus*) carcasses were fed to swine to cause the initial porcine infection and that the disease was spread widely by uncooked pork scraps taken from railroad dining cars and fed to other swine.

LESIONS

The lesions of vesicular exanthema appear 16 to 28 hours after experimental inoculation of vesicle fluid; they are slightly reddened areas at the sites of inoculation. An abrupt rise in temperature to as high as 107°F, is accompanied or followed shortly by the appearance of small vesicles filled with clear or straw-colored fluid. The vesicles occur in the epithelium of the snout, nose, lips, gums, and tongue and between digits, around the coronary band, on the ball of the foot, or even in the dew-claws. Vesicles may develop on the udder and teats of nursing sows. Vesicles sometimes coalesce. Spontaneous rupture of all vesicles occurs after a few days and is soon followed by healing. The covering of eroded areas becomes brown and dry and gradually sloughs off. After 7 to 10 days, only slightly scarred areas are left at the sites of vesiculation. Ulceration and presumably secondary bacterial infections of lesions on the feet may cause a few of the heavier animals to remain lame for some time. The cutaneous lesions are believed to be morphologically indistinguishable from the intraepithelial lesions of foot and mouth disease, but systemic lesions are not seen in vesicular exanthema.

DIAGNOSIS

The diagnosis of vesicular exanthema depends on complement-fixation tests, animal inoculations, or virus isolation and identification, which are necessary to distinguish it from foot-and-mouth disease, vesicular stomatitis, or swine vesicular disease.

References

Bankowski RA, Keith HB, Stuart EE, et al. Recovery of the fourth immunological type of vesicular exanthema virus in California. J Am Vet Med Assoc 1954;125:383–384.

Crawford AB. Experimental vesicular exanthema of swine. J Am Vet Med Assoc 1937;90:380–395.

Gelberg HB, Mebus CA, Lewis RM. Experimental vesicular exanthema of swine virus and San Miguel sea lion virus infection in phocid seals. Vet Pathol 1982;19:406–412.

Gelberg HB, Dieterich RA, Lewis RM. Vesicular exanthema of swine and San Miguel sea lion virus: experimental and field studies in otarid seals, feeding trials in swine. Vet Pathol 1982;19:413–423.

Gelberg HB, Lewis RM. The pathogenesis of vesicular exanthema of swine virus and San Miguel sea lion virus in swine. Vet Pathol 1982;19:424–443.

Madin SH. Vesicular exanthema. In: Dunne HW, Leman AD, ed. Disease of swine. 4th ed. Ames, Iowa: Iowa State Univ Press 1975.

Madin SH, Traum J. Experimental studies with vesicular exanthema of swine. Vet Med 1953;48:395–400.

Sawyer JC. Vesicular exanthema of swine and San Miguel sea lion virus. J Am Vet Med Assoc 1976;169:707–709.

Smith AW, Akers TG. Vesicular exanthema of swine. J Am Vet Med Assoc 1976;169:700–703.

Smith AW, Akers TG, Madin SH, et al. San Miguel sea lion virus isolation, preliminary characterization and relationship to vesicular exanthema of swine virus. Nature (London) 1973;244:108–109.

Traum J. Vesicular exanthema. J Am Vet Med Assoc 1936;88:316–334.

Feline calicivirus disease

Feline calicivirus causes an acute respiratory disease characterized by fever (often biphasic); depression; anorexia; dyspnea or polypnea; pulmonary rales; and vesicles resulting in ulcers of the nostrils, tongue, or hard palate. Sneezing may occur, but nasal or conjunctival discharge is not a significant feature.

LESIONS

The effects of caliciviruses on the tissues vary with virulence of the strain. The significant lesions include vesicles of the nostrils, tongue, oral mucosa, or hard palate. These vesicles are followed by further necrosis of cells in the epithelium, leaving sharply demarcated ulcers that heal slowly. Viral antigen may be demonstrated in cells at the margin of these ulcers by immunofluorescence technique (Holzinger and Kahn, 1970).

In the lung, the virus has a tropism for alveolar type I epithelial cells, which become necrotic and initiate a purulent inflammatory response. This is followed by adenomatous proliferation of type II alveolar lining cells, with eventual shedding of these cells into the alveoli. These changes result in sharply demarcated, irregularly outlined gross lesions in the lungs. These are solid dark purple, often located near the periphery of the lung. Sharply demarcated bands of congestion in about a fifth of inoculated cats have been described (Holzinger and Kahn, 1970), but the underlying reason for this change has not been recognized. Ultrastructurally, virions may be seen in relation to smooth endoplasmic reticulum, often in vesicles (Love and Sabine, 1975). Virions may also be seen in crystalline arrays, along membranous cisternae, and in fine fibrillar material.

Viral invasion of enterocytes of the small intestine is also a feature of infection leading to enteritis. Arthritis has also been attributed to feline calicivirus.

DIAGNOSIS

Diagnosis is made by identification of the virus by isolation or immunologic means. The disease may be differentiated from feline viral rhinotracheitis, which is generally more severe and in which typical herpesvirus intranuclear inclusions occur: The oral ulcers in calicivirus infections are significantly smaller than those seen in feline viral rhinotracheitis.

References

Flagstad A. Experimental picornavirus infection in cats. Acta Vet Scand 1973;14:501–510.

Holzinger EA, Kahn DE. Pathologic features of picornavirus infections in cats. Am J Vet Res 1970;31:1623–1630.

Hoover EA, Kahn DE. Lesions produced by feline picornaviruses of different virulence in pathogen-free cats. Vet Pathol 1973;10:307–322.

Hoover EA, Kahn DE. Experimentally induced feline calicivirus infection: clinical signs and lesions. J Am Vet Med Assoc 1975;166:463–468.

Kahn DE, Gillespie JH. Feline viruses. X. Characterization of a newly isolated picornavirus causing interstitial pneumonia and ulcerative stomatitis in the domestic cat. Cornell Vet 1970;60:669–683.

Kahn DE, Gillespie JH. Feline viruses: pathogenesis of picornavirus infection in the cat. Am J Vet Res 1971;32:521–531.

Kahn DE, Hoover EA, Bittle JL. Induction of immunity to feline caliciviral disease. Infect Immun 1975;511:1003–1009.

Love DN. Pathogenicity of a strain of feline calicivirus for domestic kittens. Aust Vet J 1975;51:541–546.

Pedersen NC, Laliberte L, Ekman S: A transient febrile "limping" syndrome of kittens caused by two different strains of feline calicivirus. Feline Pract 1983;13:26–35.

Povey RC, Wardley RC, Jessen H. Feline picornavirus infection: the in vivo carrier state. Vet Rec 1973;92:224–229.

Schaffer FL, et al: Caliciviridae. Intervirology 1980;14:1–6.

Studdert MJ, Martin MC, Peterson JE. Viral diseases of the respiratory tract of cats: isolation and properties of viruses tentatively classified as picornaviruses. Am J Vet Res 1970;31:1723–1732.

Viral hemorrhagic disease of rabbits (European brown hare syndrome)

What appears to be a new disease, first reported in Angora rabbits in China in 1984, is now recognized as occurring throughout Eastern and Western Europe, Asia, Northern Africa, and Mexico. In domestic rabbits (*Oryctolagus cuniculus*), the disease has been termed **viral hemorrhagic disease.** A very similar and possibly identical disease, which also occurs in European hares (*Lepus timidus*), is called **European brown hare syndrome.** Both diseases are caused by a closely related or identical calicivirus.

Although inapparent or mild clinical infection can occur, especially in young animals, the disease usually presents as a peracute or acute epizootic with high rates of morbidity and mortality, often approaching 100%. Peracute infection is characterized by animals found dead without premonitory signs, and the acute disease is characterized by animals dying within 12 to 48 hours after signs of anorexia, fever, epistaxis, dyspnea, prostration, and signs of central nervous system dysfunction (e.g., convulsions, ataxia, posterior paresis, opisthotonus). Animals surviving for longer periods develop severe icterus.

Pathologically, the striking characteristic lesion is extensive disseminated necrosis of the liver. Multiple, often coalescing collections of hepatocytes, particularly at the periphery of the lobules, become eosinophilic and their nuclei undergo karyorrhexis and pyknosis.

Mononuclear and polymorphonuclear leukocytes infiltrate the necrotic zones. Often there is calcification of hepatocytes within and adjacent to the lesions. Other findings include necrosis of lymphocytes in lymph nodes and spleen and extensive hemorrhages throughout the body. Hemorrhage and edema are particularly striking in the lung. Necrotizing lesions have also been reported in the pancreas, adrenals, and kidneys. Thrombi may be found in small blood vessels in many tissues, including the central nervous system. Nonsuppurative encephalomyelitis has also been reported.

References

Chasey D, Duff P. European brown hare syndrome and associated virus particles in the UK. Vet Rec 1990;126:623–624.

Granzow H, Schirrmeier H, Tews G. [Viral haemorrhagic septicaemia of rabbits: some properties of the causal agent.] Monatschrft Veterinaermed 1989;44:379–380. [Vet Bull 1990;60:2554]

Lee CS, Park CK, Shin TK, et al. An outbreak of rabbit sudden death in Korea suspected of a new viral hepatitis. Jpn J Vet Sci 1990;52:1135–1137. [Vet Bull 1991;61:3413]

Liu SJ, Xue HP, Pu BQ, et al. [A new viral disease in rabbits.] Anim Husb Vet Med (Xumu yu Shouyi) 1984;16:253–255. [Vet Bull 1985;55:5600]

Morisse J-P, coordinator. Viral haemorrhagic disease of rabbits and the European brown hare syndrome. Office Int Epizoot 1991;10(2):259–526.

Ohlinger VF, Haas B, Meyers G, et al. Identification and characterization of the virus causing rabbit hemorrhagic disease. J Virol 1990;64:3331–3336.

Smíd B, Valícek L, Rodák L, Stepánek J, Jurák E. Rabbit haemorrhagic disease: an investigation of some properties of the virus and evaluation of an inactivated vaccine. Vet Microbiol 1991;26:77–85. [Vet Bull 1991;61:2637]

Xu FN, Shen WP, Liu SJ. [Study of the pathology of viral haemorrhagic disease in rabbits.] Anim Husb Vet Med (Xumu yu Shouyi) 1985;17:153–155. [Vet Bull 198656:5261]

Other Caliciviruses

Caliciviruses have been recovered from puppies with oral vesicles, ulcers, and enteritis. Attempts to experimentally reproduce the disease have not been successful.

The causal relationship of bovine calicivirus (Newbury agent) to enteritis is much stronger. In affected calves, the virus invades enterocytes along the sides of villi of the anterior small intestine (Fig. 8-45E). Similar observations have been made with caliciviruses from piglets.

The San Miguel sea lion virus affects a variety of sea mammals as well as domestic mammals. In sea mammals, the virus is associated with vesicular lesions on the flippers.

References

Hall GA. Comparative pathology of infection by novel diarrhoea viruses. Ciba Found Symp 1987;128:192–217.

Hall GA. Mechanisms of mucosal injury: animal studies. In: Farthing MJG, ed. Viruses and the gut. Proc 9th BSG/SK&F Int Workshop. Section III. Pathogenesis of gut virus infections. London: Smith Kline & French Laboratories Ltd. 1988;27–29.

Mochizuki M, Kawanishi A, Sakamoto H, et al. A calicivirus isolated from a dog with fatal diarrhoea. Vet Rec 1993;132:221–222.

REOVIRIDAE

The family *Reoviridae* contains six genera, three of which infect animals: **orthoreovirus (reovirus), orbivirus,** and **rotavirus.** The original isolates were termed reovirus, an acronym for *respiratory enteric orphan virus*, because they were not associated with any disease. Indeed, most reoviruses of the genus orthoreovirus are considered nonpathogenic. The most important pathogens are in the orbivirus genus, which includes bluetongue virus (Fig. 8-42), African horse sickness virus, epizootic hemorrhagic disease of deer virus, equine encephalosis virus, and Ibaraki virus. The rotaviruses cause enteritis in many different species. All reoviruses are nonenveloped icosahedral virions of 60 to 80 nm in size, which contain segmented double-stranded RNA.

Diseases Caused by Orthoreoviruses

The term reovirus is ordinarily used for members of this genus, most of which are considered nonpathogenic. There are three serotypes (1, 2, and 3), distinguishable by hemagglutination-inhibition and antibody-neutralization tests. The reoviruses have been used extensively to study viral replication, viral genetics, and viral pathogenesis. Although experimental cytopathology and disease have been very well documented, the viruses as a group remain relatively unimportant as natural pathogens. Reovirus infection has, however, been demonstrated in most members of the animal kingdom. Reoviruses have been associated with gastrointestinal and respiratory disease in cats (type 3), dogs (types 1 and 2), and horses (type 3). Chronic respiratory disease and tenosynovitis can be caused by reoviruses in poultry. In mice, natural infection with type 3 reovirus can cause hepatitis and encephalitis. Experimentally, a great many lesions have been induced in mice, including encephalitis, ependymitis and hydrocephalus, necrosis of myocardial and skeletal muscle, pneumonia, and hepatitis.

References

Baskerville A, McFerran JB, Conner T. The pathology of experimental infection of pigs with type 1 *Reovirus* of porcine origin. Res Vet Sci 1971;12:172–174.

Binn LN, et al. Recovery of *Reovirus*, type 2 from an immature dog with respiratory tract disease. Am J Vet Res 1977;38:927–929.

Conner M, Gillespie J, Schiff E, et al. Experimental infection of horses and ponies by oral and intranasal routes with New York State reovirus type 3 and German reovirus types 1 and 3 equine isolates. Zentralbl Veterinarmed 1984;31:707–717.

Csiza CK. Characterization and serotyping of three feline *Reovirus* isolates. Infec Immun 1974;9:159–166.

Joklik WK, ed. The reoviridae. New York: Plenum Press 1983;571.

Lamont PH. Reoviruses. J Am Vet Med Assoc 1968;152:807–813.

Margolis G, Kilham L, Gonatas NK. *Reovirus* type III encephalitis: observations of virus-cell interactions in neural tissues. I. Light microscopy studies. Lab Invest 1971;24:91–100.

Massie EL, Shaw EO. *Reovirus* Type I in laboratory dogs. Am J Vet Res 1966;27:783–787.

Olson NO. Reovirus infections. In: Hofstad MS, et al, ed. Diseases of poultry. 7th ed. Ames, Iowa: Iowa State Univ Press, 1978.

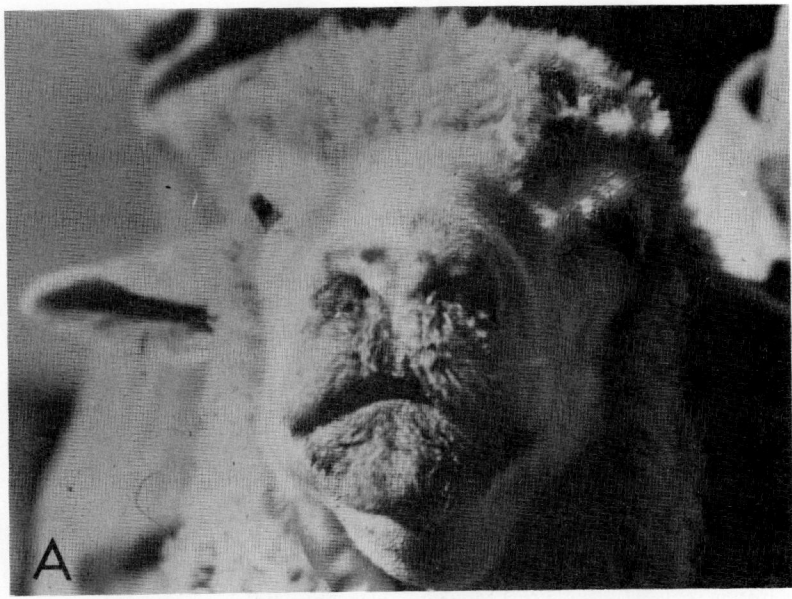

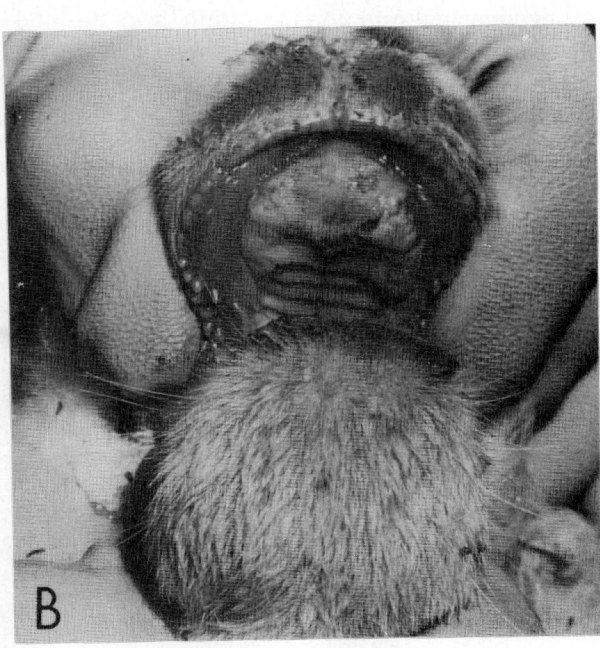

FIG. 8-42 Bluetongue, sheep (orbivirus). **A.** Edematous swelling of lips and nostrils. **B.** Ulcers of dental pad and swelling of lips and buccal mucosa. (Courtesy of Dr. J. G. Bowne and *Journal of the American Veterinary Medical Association.*)

Scott FW, Kahn DE, Gillespie JH. Feline viruses: isolation, characterization, and pathogenicity of a feline reovirus. Am J Vet Res 1970;31:11–20.

Walters MN-I, et al. Murine infection with *Reovirus*. III. Pathology of infection with types 1 and 2. Br J Exp Pathol 1965;46:200–212.

Diseases caused by orbiviruses

The genus orbivirus (orb = ring) contains viruses that multiply in arthropods as well as in vertebrates. In terms of biologic behavior, therefore, these are arboviruses (arbo = arthropodborne), a word that is no longer used in classification of viruses. Bluetongue virus is the type species. This virus has double-stranded RNA with a molecular weight of 15 million daltons, which occurs as ten separate pieces. The virion has an outer diffuse layer in which are found seven capsid polypeptides. The capsid is believed to be icosahedral, with 32 capsomeres, 8 to 11 nm in diameter. The inner core is about 55 nm in diameter. The virion is nonenveloped and contains a virus-specific transcriptase. The virions are assembled in the cytoplasm of host cells.

BLUETONGUE OF SHEEP (CATARRHAL FEVER OF SHEEP, "SOREMUZZLE")

Bluetongue is a viral disease of sheep, cattle, and goats transmitted by biting insects of the genus *Culicoides*. The disease was first recognized in South Africa in 1902. It was apparently confined to the African continent until the 1940s, when significant outbreaks subsequently occurred in Mediterranean countries. The disease was identified in the early 1950s in the western United States. It is now recognized to occur worldwide in tropical, subtropical, and temperate climates. There are 24 different serotypes of bluetongue virus, which are only variably cross-protective. Only four of these occur in the United States (types 10, 11, 13, and 17).

Bluetongue is most severe in sheep; the severity of the infection depends on the strain of virus and breed of sheep. Most domestic species are highly susceptible. Cattle, goats, and deer are also susceptible to infection. In cattle, the infection is usually not apparent (Fig. 8-43), although it may resemble a mild version of the disease in sheep. Cattle may carry the virus for protracted periods of time, with the development of sporadic viremia adequate for insect transmission. The virus has also been recovered from bovine semen. In Africa, the blesbok antelope is considered a reservoir host for the virus. In deer, the disease (and virus) is remarkably similar to epizootic **hemorrhagic disease** of deer.

Pathogenesis On entry into the host, viral replication is believed to initially occur in hematopoietic cells, resulting in viremia and subsequent replication in endothelial cells throughout the body. Endothelial cell damage is responsible for the widespread gross and microscopic lesions. Endothelial cells become swollen and later become necrotic, causing edema, hemorrhage, thrombosis, and infarction.

Signs High fever (105°F) is the first sign, with associated reddening of the nasal and oral mucosae and excessive salivation. A watery discharge from the nostrils later becomes mucous and may dry to form crusts. Edematous swellings arise in the lips, tongue, ears, face, and intermandibular space. Edema and cyanosis of the tongue are so striking that they have given the disease its name (Fig. 8-43), even though they are not always present. Petechiae soon appear on the oral and nasal mucosae, where the epithelium apparently becomes thickened and is shed, leaving excoriations and bleeding points. As the fever subsides, flushing of the skin and feet appears; the coronets become warm and tender, and later the pink periople band turns red. This results in stiffness and lameness. Hemorrhage into the medullary canals of the growing horn at the junction of skin and hoof leaves a "streaky zone" parallel to the periople. This irregular zone or line persists but is moved away from the coronet with growth of the hoof, and its color gradually changes from bright red to brown because of the breakdown of hemoglobin in the exudate. The presence of this zone is of distinct value in identifying a previous attack of the disease.

The disease may terminate in severe emaciation, prostration, and muscular weakness (occasionally with torticollis), which may last 3 weeks or more, followed by pulmonary edema and death from pneumonia. In prolonged cases, a "break" in the growth of wool may cause the fleece to be shed.

The morbidity rate in mild outbreaks is usually

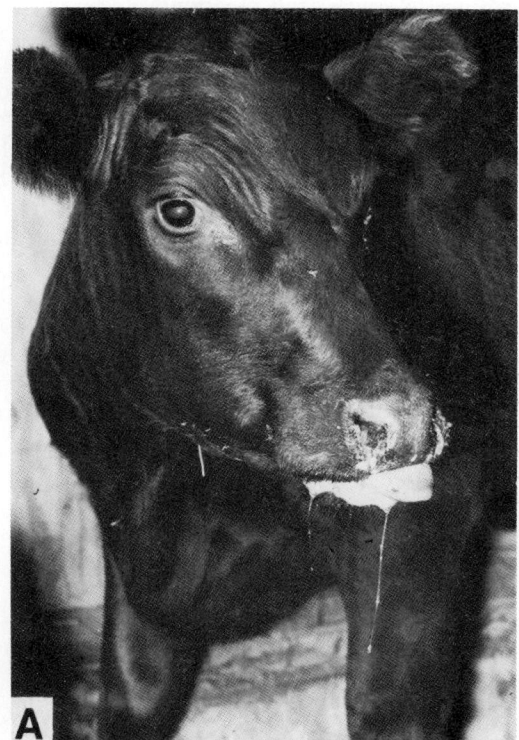

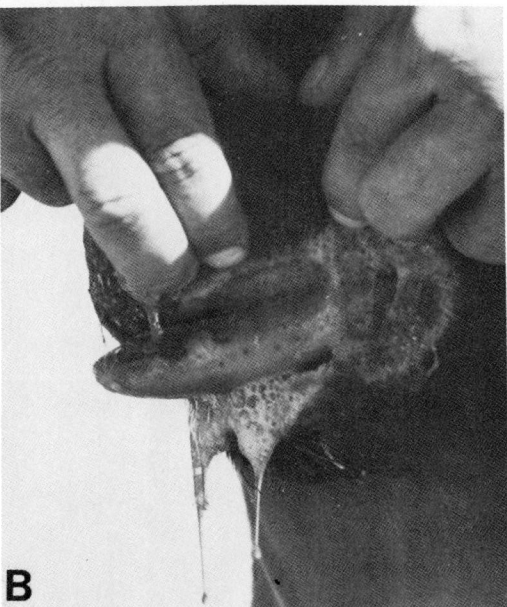

FIG. 8-43 Bluetongue, shorthorn heifer. **A.** The muzzle is dry and cracked and a mucopurulent exudate surrounds the nares. **B.** Erosions on the lateral surface of the tongue. (Courtesy of Dr. J. G. Bowne and *Journal of the American Veterinary Medical Association.*)

about 50% of a flock, and the mortality rate is about 7%. In severe outbreaks, however, losses from death may reach 50%. Sheep of all ages are susceptible, but in the United States, adults seem to be affected more often than lambs.

Lesions As indicated, the lesions of bluetongue emanate from replication of the virus in endothelial cells, and are characterized by edema, hyperemia, hemorrhage, and infarction. There is extensive edema of the subcutis, especially about the head and neck and in the intermuscular fascia. The changes around the mouth that characterize clinical disease consist of hyperemia, edema, cyanosis, and multiple hemorrhages, especially of the muzzle, tongue, and cheeks, with erosion and even ulceration of the epithelium. The dental pad, hard palate, gums, esophagus, reticulum, and rumen may have similar lesions.

Microscopic examination of the hoof and adjacent skin reveals intense hyperemia of the vascular corium, most concentrated at the tips of the dermal papillae (Fig. 8-44), associated with edema and infiltration with neutrophils. The red "streak," or zone, seen grossly in

the wall of the hoof is the result of the accumulation of erythrocytes as well as neutrophils in the hollow medullary canals of the horny wall, which continue as channels from the dermal papillae. At the periople, these channels may become dilated, although distal to the zone they are of capillary size.

The musculature usually contains foci of gross hemorrhage, which are associated with microscopic evidence of necrotic changes in muscle bundles. These changes have been described as hyalinization and loss of striations in the muscle bundles and as pyknosis of sarcolemmal nuclei, resulting in coagulation, irregular swelling, and fragmentation of sarcoplasm. Proliferation of sarcolemmal nuclei and occasional calcific stippling of sarcoplasm have been reported.

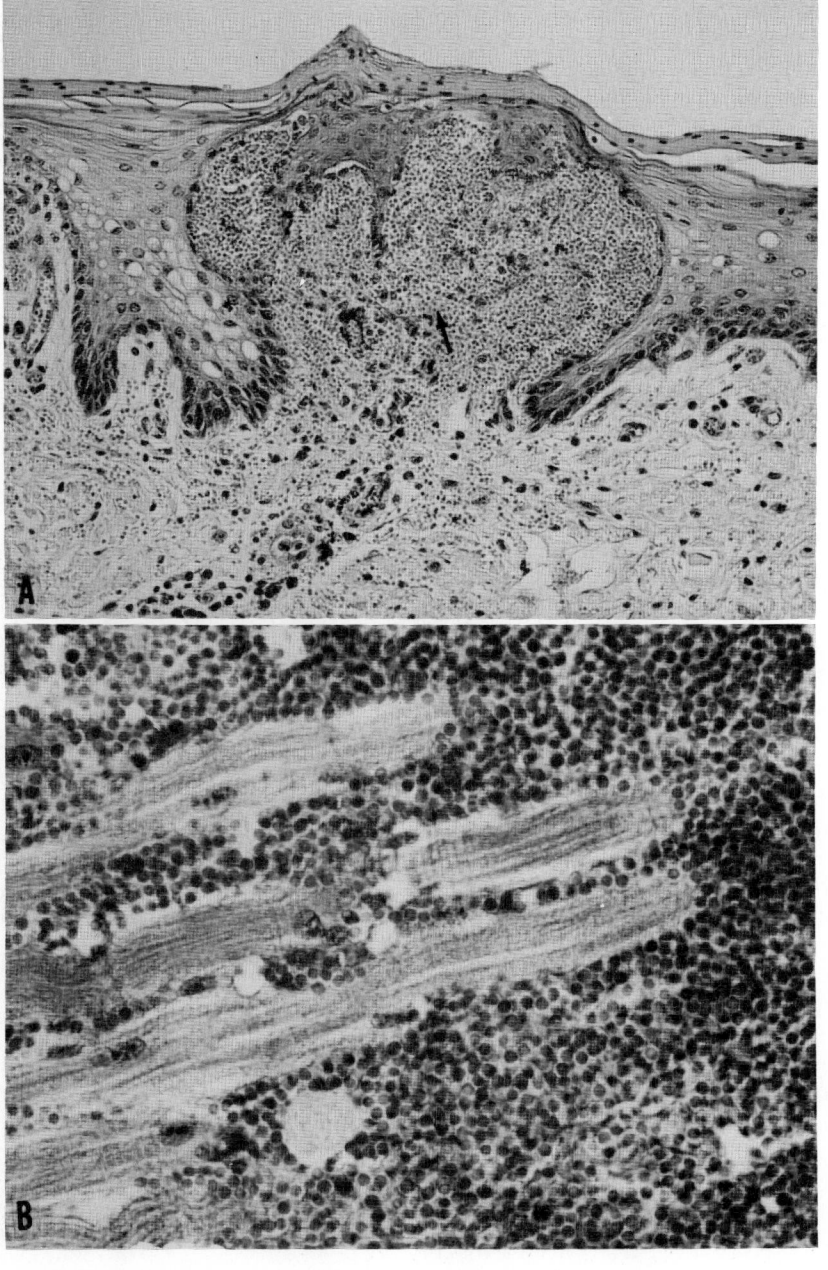

FIG. 8-44 Bluetongue. Hemorrhages in the tongue of a year-old ewe. **A.** Hemorrhage into a lingual papilla (arrow) ($\times$ 190). **B.** Severe hemorrhage isolating muscle bundles in the tongue ($\times$ 560). (Courtesy of the Armed Forces Institute of Pathology; contributed by Dr. W. S. Monlux.)

Hemorrhage and necrosis also occurs in the myocardium, particularly of the papillary muscles of the left ventricle. An almost constant lesion is hemorrhage emanating from the vasum vasorum in the wall of the base of the pulmonary artery. Similar hemorrhage may occur in the aorta and other large arteries. There is congestion and hemorrhage in lymph nodes and the spleen as well as in most other tissues.

Bluetongue virus infection during pregnancy may result in fetal infection, which causes severe cerebral abnormalities in both sheep and cattle. This may follow natural infection or use of attenuated vaccines. The nature and severity of the disease is dependent on the stage of pregnancy. In ewes exposed at 40 to 60 days of pregnancy and cattle at 60 to 120 days, a severe necrotizing encephalopathy occurs, which, at birth, is manifested as hydrocephaly. Later in pregnancy, focal necrotizing lesions develop, which is seen as porencephaly at birth. Lamb fetuses exposed after 100 days of gestation develop a focal encephalitis with glial nodules; a necrosis of the retina also develops, which causes lambs or calves to be born with retinal dysplasia in addition to the cerebral abnormalities. Experimentally, cerebral necrosis can be induced by inoculation of newborn mice.

Although the clinical and gross findings of swayback (enzootic ataxia) may be similar, the two processes may be differentiated, because swayback is a demyelinating disease in which inflammatory changes do not occur.

Diagnosis The clinical diagnosis may be made from the symptoms and gross lesions, but bluetongue must be differentiated from photosensitization, contagious ecthyma, foot-and-mouth disease, *Oestrus ovis* infestation, ulcerative dermatitis, and sheep-pox. In cattle, the disease must be differentiated from foot-and-mouth disease, rinderpest, vesicular stomatitis, infectious rhinotracheitis, mycotic stomatitis, and the bovine virus diarrhea-mucosal disease complex. At present, isolation and identification of the virus are necessary to confirm the diagnosis.

References

Bowne JG. Bluetongue disease. Adv Vet Sci Comp Med 1971;15:1–46.

Bowne JG, Luedke AJ, Jochim MM, et al. Bluetongue disease in cattle. J Am Vet Med Assoc 1968;153:662–668.

De Kock G, DuToit R, Neidtz WO. Observations on blue tongue in cattle and sheep. Onderstepoort J Vet Sci Anim Ind 1937;8:129–181.

Enright FM, Osburn BI. Ontogeny of host responses in ovine fetuses infected with bluetongue virus. Am J Vet Res 1980;41:224–229.

Gibbs EPJ. Bluetongue—an analysis of current problems, with particular reference to importation of ruminants to the United States. J Am Vet Med Assoc 1983;182:1190–1194.

Griner LA, et al. Bluetongue associated with abnormalities in newborn lambs. J Am Vet Med Assoc 1964;145:1013–1019.

Hardy WT, Price DA. Soremuzzle of sheep. J Am Vet Med Assoc 1952;120:23–25.

Luedke AJ, Bowne JG, Jochim MM, et al. Clinical and pathological features of bluetongue in sheep. Am J Vet Res 1964;25:963–970.

Luedke AJ, Jochim MM, Hones RH. Bluetongue in cattle: effects of *Culicoides varipennis*-transmitted bluetongue virus on pregnant heifers and their calves. Am J Vet Res 1977;38:1687–1695.

Luedke AJ, Jochim MM, Hones RH. Bluetongue in cattle: effects of vector-transmitted bluetongue virus on calves previously infected in utero. Am J Vet Res 1977;38:1697–1700.

MacLachlan NJ, Osburn BI. Bluetongue virus-induced hydranencephaly in cattle. Vet Pathol 1983;20:563–573.

MacLachlan NJ, Osburn BI, Ghalib HW, et al. Bluetongue virus-induced encephalopathy in fetal cattle. Vet Pathol 1985;22:415–417.

Mahrt CR, Osburn BI. Experimental bluetongue virus infection of sheep. [1] Effect of previous vaccination: clinical and immunologic studies. [2] Effect of vaccination: pathologic, immunofluorescent and ultrastructural studies. Am J Vet Res 1986;47:1191–1197, 1198–1203.

McGowan B. An epidemic resembling soremuzzle or blue tongue in California sheep. Cornell Vet 1953;43:213–216.

McKercher DG, McGowan B, Howarth JA, et al. A preliminary report on the isolation and identification of the blue tongue virus from sheep in California. J Am Vet Med Assoc 1953;122:300–301.

Moulton JE. Pathology of bluetongue of sheep. J Am Vet Med Assoc 1961;138:493–498.

Osburn BI, et al. Epizootiologic study of bluetongue: virologic and serologic results. Am J Vet Res 1981;42:884–887.

Phillips RM, Carnahan DL, Rademacher DJ. Virus isolation from semen of bulls serologically positive for bluetongue virus. Am J Vet Res 1986;47:84–85.

Ramsay EC, Rodgers SJ, Castro AE, et al. Perinatal bluetongue viral infection in exotic ruminants. J Am Vet Med Assoc 1985;187:1249–1251.

Richards WPC, Cordy DR. Bluetongue virus infection: pathologic responses of nervous systems in sheep and mice. Science 1967;156:530–531.

Richardson C, Taylor WP, Terlecki S, et al. Observations on transplacental infection with bluetongue virus in sheep. Am J Vet Res 1985;46:1912–1922.

Shultz G, Delay PD. Losses in newborn lambs associated with bluetongue vaccination of pregnant ewes. J Am Vet Med Assoc 1955;127:224–226.

Thomas AD, Neidtz WO. Further observations on the pathology of blue tongue in sheep. Onderstepoort J Vet Sci Anim Ind 1947;22:27–40.

Vosdingh RA, Trainer DO, Easterday BC. Experimental bluetongue disease in white-tailed deer. Can J Comp Med Vet Sci 1968;32:382–387.

Waldvogel AS, Anderson CA, Higgins RJ, et al. Neurovirulence of the UC-2 and UC-8 strains of bluetongue virus serotype 11 in newborn mice. Vet Pathol 1987;24:404–410.

Young S, Cordy DR. An ovine fetal encephalopathy caused by bluetongue vaccine virus. J Neuropath Exp Neurol 1964;23:635–659.

EPIZOOTIC HEMORRHAGIC DISEASE OF DEER AND IBARAKI DISEASE

A serious, widely distributed disease of white-tailed deer (*Odocoileus virginianus*) was described in New Jersey by Shope and associates (1955) and later demonstrated to be caused by a specific virus (Shope and associates, 1960), which has since been shown to infect other wild ruminants throughout much of the United States and Canada. A similar but milder disease of cattle, known as Ibaraki disease and first described in 1959 in Japan, is caused by a closely related virus. Sheep do not develop disease when exposed to either virus. *Culicoides* flies serve as vectors for the viruses.

The clinical and pathologic features of infection are essentially identical to bluetongue in sheep.

References

Campbell CH, Barker TL, Jochim MM. Antigenic relationship of Ibaraki, bluetongue, and epizootic hemorrhagic disease viruses. Vet Microbiol 1978;3:15–22.

Feldner TJ, Smith MH. Epizootic hemorrhagic disease virus in Montana: isolation and serologic survey. Am J Vet Res 1981;42:1198–1202.

Fletch AL, Karstad LH. Studies on the pathogenesis of experimental epizootic hemorrhagic disease of white-tailed deer. Can J Comp Med 1970;35:224–229.

Fosberg SA, Stauber EH, Renshaw HW. Isolation and characterization of epizootic hemorrhagic disease virus from white-tailed deer (Odocoileus virginianus) in eastern Washington. Am J Vet Res 1977;38:361–364.

Foster NM, Metcalf HE, Barber TL, et al. Bluetongue and epizootic hemorrhagic disease virus isolations from vertebrate and invertebrate hosts at a common geographic site. J Am Vet Med Assoc 1980;176:126–129.

Hoff GL, Trainer DO. Experimental infection in North American elk with epizootic hemorrhagic disease virus. J Wildl Dis 1973;9:129–132.

Hoff GL, Trainer DO. Observations on bluetongue and epizootic hemorrhagic disease viruses in white-tailed deer. I. Distribution of virus in the blood. II. Cross-challenge. J Wildl Dis 1974;10:25–31.

Karstad L, Winter A, Trainer DO. Pathology of epizootic hemorrhagic disease of deer. Am J Vet Res 1961;22:227–235.

Odiawa G, Blue JL, Tyler DE, et al. Bluetongue and epizootic hemorrhagic disease in ruminants in Georgia: survey by serotest and virologic isolation. Am J Vet Res 1985;46:2193–2196.

Prestwood AK, Kistner TP, Kellogg FE, et al. The 1971 outbreak of hemorrhagic disease among white-tailed deer of the southeastern United States. J Wildl Dis 1974;10:217–224.

Shope RE, MacNamara LG, Margold R. Report on the deer mortality; epizootic hemorrhagic disease of deer. New Jersey Outdoors 1955;6:16–21.

Shope RE, MacNamara LG, Margold R. A virus-induced epizootic hemorrhagic disease of the Virginia white-tailed deer (Odocoileus virginianus). J Exp Med 1960;111:155–170.

Thomas FC, Miller J. A comparison of bluetongue virus and EHD virus: electromicroscopy and serology. Can J Comp Med. 35:22–27, 1971.

Thompson LH, Mecham JO, Holbrook FR. Isolation and characterization of epizootic hemorrhagic disease virus from sheep and cattle in Colorado. Am J Vet Res 1988;49:1050–1052.

Wilhelm AR, Trainer DO. A comparison of several viruses of epizootic hemorrhagic disease of deer. J Inf Dis 1967;117:48–54.

AFRICAN HORSE SICKNESS

The apparently nonspecific name, African horse sickness, applies to a specific and important disease of Equidae caused by an an orbivirus that is transmitted by several species of Culicoides. The disease was apparently present in South Africa when the first European settlers brought their horses and mules into that country in the 18th century, and it has in recent years crossed the boundaries of other countries, including Egypt, Israel, West Pakistan, Afghanistan, Cyprus, Iraq, Syria, Lebanon, Turkey, India, Iran, Jordan, and Spain.

The etiologic agent is an orbivirus similar to the bluetongue virus. Several different serotypes have been identified, which are not entirely cross-protective. The host range includes horses, mules, donkeys, goats, dogs, and ferrets. Native horses are the most susceptible, and very high rates of morbidity and mortality occur. The disease in mules is somewhat less severe than in horses, but more severe than in donkeys. A variety of laboratory animals may be infected.

Signs The clinical features of African horse sickness usually are described as conforming to one of four types. The first is the least serious and is more often observed in partially immune animals, particularly don-keys. Mild fever, anorexia, dyspnea, and an accelerated heart rate may be all that is observed; rapid recovery follows. The acute pulmonary form of the disease is recognized by an incubation period of 3 to 5 days, sudden onset of high fever (105°F to 107°F), and severe dyspnea caused by pulmonary edema, often with frothy exudates in the nostrils. Sweating and coughing may occur, and death usually results within a few hours of onset of the pulmonary edema. This form has been described in dogs as well. A third clinical type of the disease is the subacute cardiac form, in which the incubation period and course are usually longer than in the pulmonary form. It is distinguished by the occurrence of edema of the head, neck, lips, eyelids, cheek, and tongue, and most characteristically, edematous bulging of the supraorbital fossa. Petechiae may appear on the ventral aspect of the tongue; abdominal pain and paralysis of the esophagus may be manifested; and death usually is caused by cardiac failure and hypoxia. In a fourth, mixed form of the disease, a combination of pulmonary and cardiac lesions are found at necropsy.

Lesions The lesions at necropsy usually can be correlated with the clinical form of the disease. The most striking changes are seen in the respiratory system. Hydrothorax usually accompanies the severe edema, which involves the subpleural and interlobular stroma and fills alveoli in many lobules. Frothy fluid usually fills the bronchi, trachea, and the rest of the upper respiratory tract. Fibrin and proteinaceous material are recognizable microscopically in the edematous tissues, and leukocytes may also be present. In some cases, these leukocytes may be present in sufficient numbers to suggest bronchopneumonia.

The cardiac lesions are also significant. Hydropericardium is usually present, along with petechiae and inflammatory edema in the epicardium. Disseminated foci of myocardial necrosis are seen microscopically and are often accentuated by hemorrhages, which may be recognized grossly. Sometimes edema may involve the adventitia of arterioles; but otherwise, small blood vessels do not contain identifiable lesions.

Depletion of lymphocytes is usually evident in the spleen and lymph nodes; reticuloendothelial and plasma cells are usually increased in number, although the spleen is not usually enlarged. Some lymph nodes may be grossly hemorrhagic. The gastrointestinal tract may be involved. Edema around the pharynx may account for the presumed paralysis of the esophagus noted in some descriptions of the clinical features. Hemorrhage is common in the gastric mucosa. The liver is usually only congested. Hemorrhage and edema may be found in the kidneys, particularly involving the peripelvic fat.

The **pathogenesis** of the lesions has not been elucidated. Endothelial cell damage, as seen in bluetongue and epizootic hemorrhagic disease, which serves as the basis for most tissue changes in the disorders, is not a feature of African horse sickness.

Diagnosis The diagnosis is usually made presumptively in enzootic regions from the clinical features and necropsy findings but should be confirmed by recovery and identification of the virus.

Differentiation from equine viral arteritis should be considered because both diseases are characterized by edema and hemorrhage in the subcutis, heart, and lungs. The specific lesions in the musculature of arterioles in arteritis would be useful, but isolation and identification of the virus should also be undertaken.

References

Breese SS Jr, Ozawa Y, Dardiri AH. Electron microscopic characterization of African horse-sickness virus. J Am Vet Med Assoc 1969;155:391–400.

Brown CC, Dardiri AH. African horse sickness: a continuing menace. J Am Vet Med Assoc 1990;196:2019–2021.

Henning MW. Animal diseases of South Africa. 3rd ed. Pretoria: Central News Agency 1956.

Howell PG. African horsesickness. FAO Agricult Studies 1963;61: 71–108.

Lecatsas G, Erasmus BJ. Electron microscopic study of the formation of African horse-sickness virus. Arch Ges Virusforsch 1967;22: 442–450.

Maurer FD, McCully RM. African horsesickness—with emphasis on pathology. Am J Vet Res 1963;24:235–266.

McCollum WH, Ozawa Y, Dardiri AH. Serologic differentiation between African horse-sickness and equine arteritis. Am J Vet Res 1970;31:1963–1966.

Newsholme SJ. A morphological study of the lesions of African horse-sickness. Onderstepoort J Vet Res 1983;50:7–24.

Piercy SE. Some observations on African horse-sickness including an account of an outbreak amongst dogs. East African Agric J. 1951;17:1–3.

Reid NR. African horse-sickness. Br Vet J 1961;118:137–142.

Tessler J. Detection of African horsesickness viral antigens in tissues by immunofluorescence. Can J Comp Med 1972;36:167–169.

Wetzel H, Nevill EM, Erasmus BJ. Studies on the transmission of African horsesickness. Onderstepoort J Vet Res 1970;37:165–168.

EQUINE ENCEPHALOSIS

Equine encephalosis virus was first identified in 1967 in South Africa. It is apparently limited to that country. Several serotypes have been recognized. The clinical disease may be peracute with alternating periods of hyperexcitement and depression (which gave rise to the name encephalosis), or be expressed as a mild febrile disease. The virus has also been recovered from equine abortions. Serologic surveys have revealed that the incidence of infection far exceeds clinical disease. Lesions described in the acute disease include generalized venous congestion, brain edema, catarrhal enteritis, and fatty liver. The pathogenesis is not understood and the lesions of little assistance in diagnosis. Diagnosis requires recovery of the virus, which is distinct from other animal orbiviruses.

Reference

Gorman BM, Taylor J, Walker PJ. Orbiviruses. In: Joklik WK, ed. The Reoviridae. New York: Plenum Press 1983;291–292, 306–307.

Diseases caused by rotaviruses

Members of the genus rotavirus are important causes of diarrhea in young animals and children throughout the world (Fig. 8-45). The virions have a distinctive appearance with a sharply defined outer capsid resembling a wheel (rota = L., wheel). They are icasohedral, about 70 nm in diameter. Most rotaviruses share common inner capsid antigens; however, recently, isolates that are serologically distinct have been obtained. These have been referred to as **pararotaviruses** or **novel rotaviruses** and have been recovered from swine, calves, rats, lambs, and children. Rotavirus diarrhea or enteritis is recognized in infant children, calves, mice, lambs, pigs, dogs, foals, and other animals and birds. Rotaviruses are not highly species specific. The pathogenesis and lesions are similar in each species. After ingestion, the low pH-stable rotaviruses infect epithelial cells of the small intestine, producing lesions initially in the anterior portion of the intestine that progress distally. Only differentiated columnar epithelial cells lining the apical halves of villi are susceptible. Entry and replication does not occur in immature or proliferating cells in the crypts (Fig. 8-45A). These cells may lack receptors for the virus. Lesions and signs follow an extremely short incubation period, developing within hours. Epithelial cells develop distended cisternae of the endoplasmic reticulum and swollen mitochondria with viral particles appearing in the distended cisternae and lysosomes. There is loss of microvilli. Epithelial cells become vacuolated and shed prematurely. Villi thus become atrophic and shortened. An additional change seen in infections with the pararotaviruses is the formation of syncytia or multinucleated cells formed by fusion of enterocytes on the surface of villi (Fig. 8-45B). In surviving animals, villi return to normal in 3 to 4 weeks.

Reduced levels of disaccharides have been described, which cause reduction in lactose digestion and promotion of bacterial growth, resulting in an osmotic effect that further contributes to diarrhea. Large numbers of viral particles are shed in the feces, which is the principal source for dissemination of the disease, either through direct contact or by contamination of water supplies and by airborne spread. The virions are highly resistant to drying, high temperatures and other environmental conditions and can remain infectious for months. In all species, rotaviral enteritis is significantly more severe when complicated by simultaneous infection with enterotoxigenic *Escherichia coli*.

References

Benfield DA, et al. Combined rotavirus and K99 *Escherichia coli* infection in gnotobiotic pigs. Am J Vet Res 1988;49:330–337.

Da Costa Mendes VM, De Beer MC, Goosen GH, et al. Isolation and preliminary characterization of a caprine rotavirus. Onderstepoort J Vet Res 1994;61:291–294.

Joklik WK, ed. The Reoviridae. New York: Plenum Press 1983.

LeBaron CW, et al. Annual rotavirus epidemic patterns in North America. Results of a 5–year retrospective survey of 88 centers in Canada, Mexico, and the United States. JAMA 1990;264:983–988.

Pedley S, Bridger JC, Chasey D, et al. Definition of two new groups of atypical rotaviruses. J Gen Virol 1986;67:131–137.

Snodgrass DR, Herring AJ, Campbell I, et al. Comparison of atypical rotaviruses from calves, piglets, lambs and man. J Gen Virol 1984;65:909–914.

Rotavirus

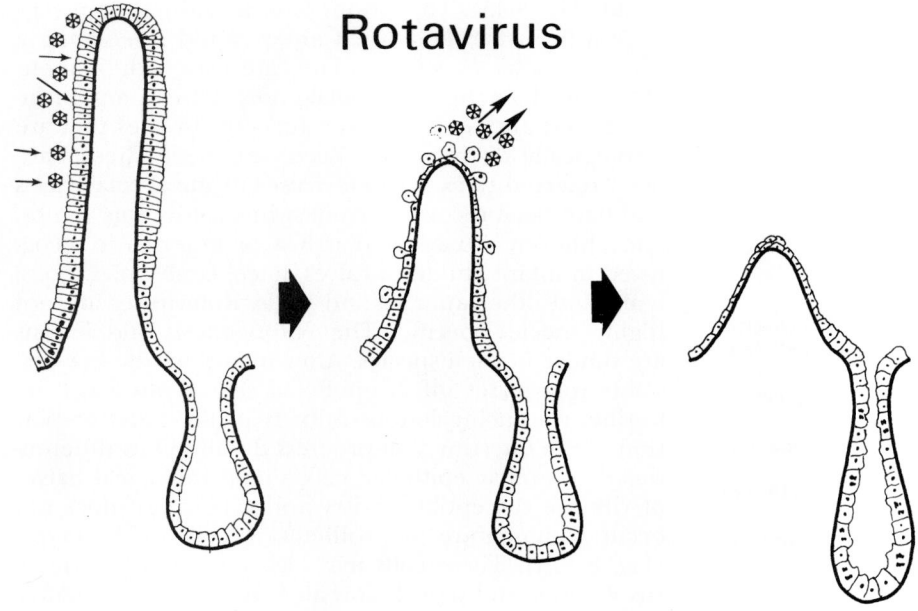

FIG. 8-45 Comparative features of pathogenesis of enteropathogenic viruses. **A.** Group A rotaviruses infect entire length of small intestine (usually proximal in calves and mid-to-distal in piglets). Mature enterocytes toward villous tip are preferentially infected, leading to necrosis, sloughing, stunted villi, and hypertrophy of enterocytes in crypts.

Novel rotavirus (group B)

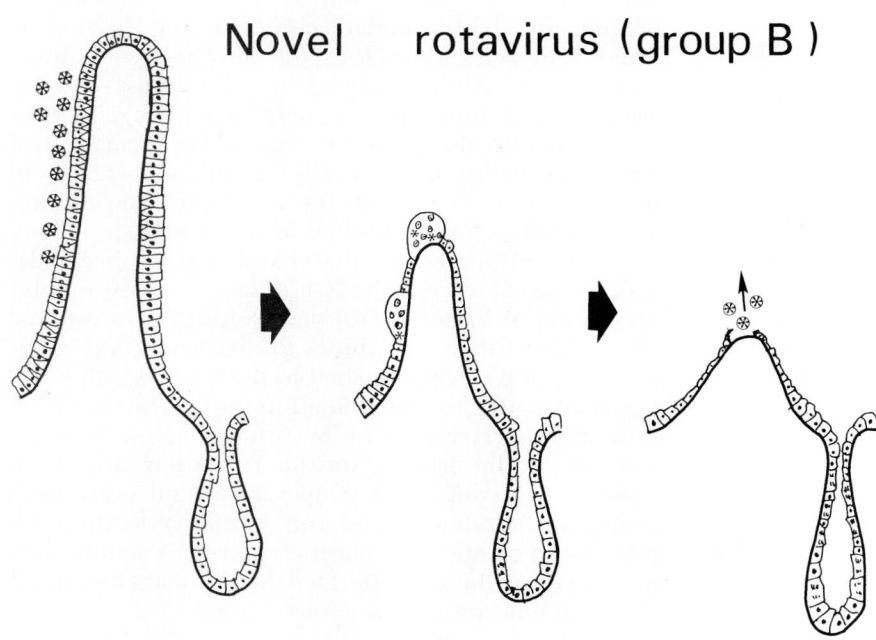

B. Group B rotaviruses have comparable pathogenesis to group A rotaviruses; but they are more often associated with multinucleated syncytia on surface of villi.

Torres-Medina A. [1] Effect of combined rotavirus and *Escherichia coli* in neonatal gnotobiotic calves. [2] Effect of rotavirus and/or *Escherichia coli* infection on the aggregated lymphoid follicles in the small intestine of neonatal gnotobiotic calves. Am J Vet Res 1984;45:643–651, 652–660.

NEONATAL CALF DIARRHEA (SCOURS)

This serious disease of calves appears during the first 2 weeks of life, affects most of the animals of the herd, and causes death of up to half of infected animals. The principal sign is the appearance of yellowish, watery feces, which soon leads to severe dehydration. This syndrome has been known for many years and had

usually been attributed to enteric bacteria, such as *Escherichia coli*. Although multiple factors may well be involved and are not clearly understood, it seems likely that rotaviruses are the essential etiologic factor (Figs. 8-46 and 8-47).

LESIONS

Lesions resemble those described on the previous page.

DIAGNOSIS

Diagnosis is greatly facilitated in clinical cases by the use of immunofluorescent staining of desquamated

Coronavirus

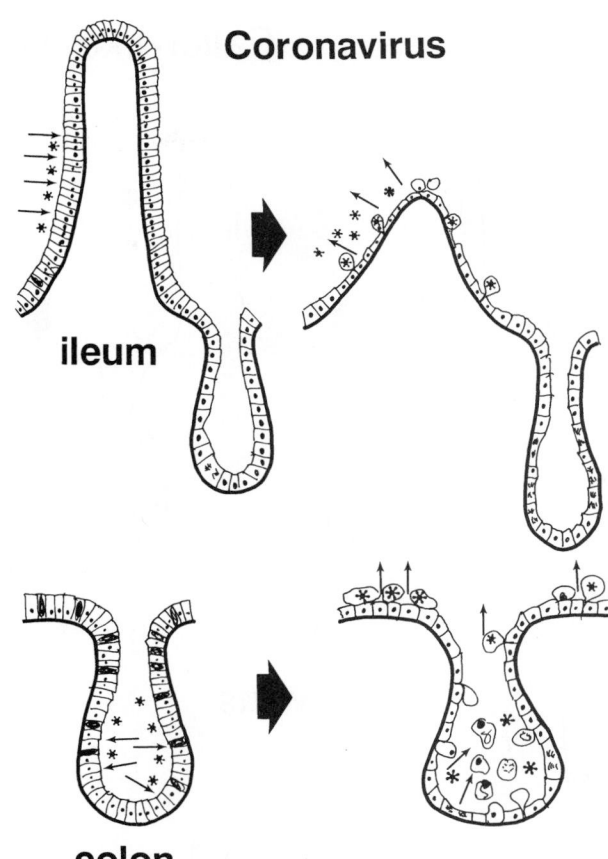

ileum

colon

C. Coronaviruses induce lesions that resemble rotavirus infection but mainly affect distal small intestine and may also infect surface and crypt cells of colon.

Adenovirus

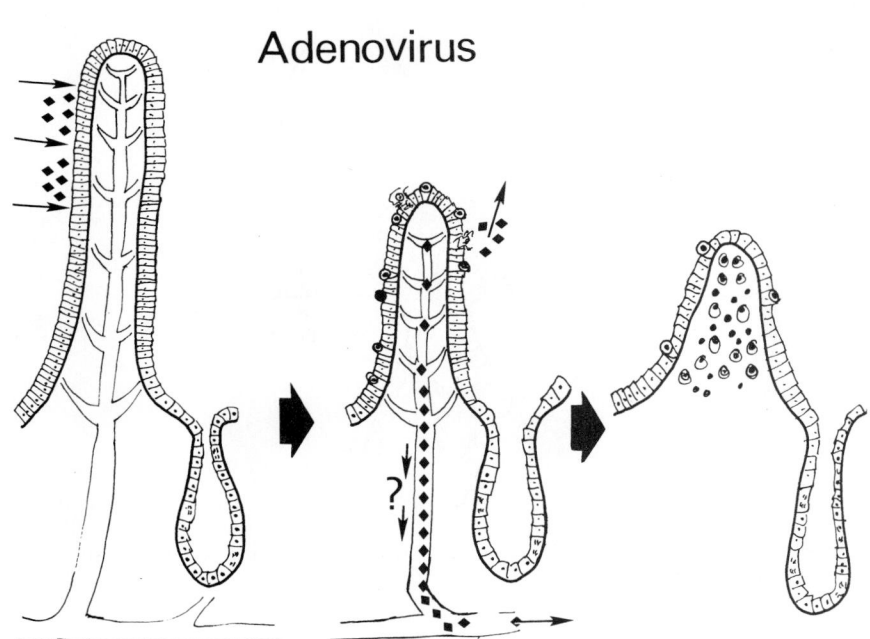

D. Adenoviruses also primarily affect villi, causing necrosis of enterocytes and blunting of villi. Large numbers of intranuclear inclusion bodies are usually present.

Calici-like virus

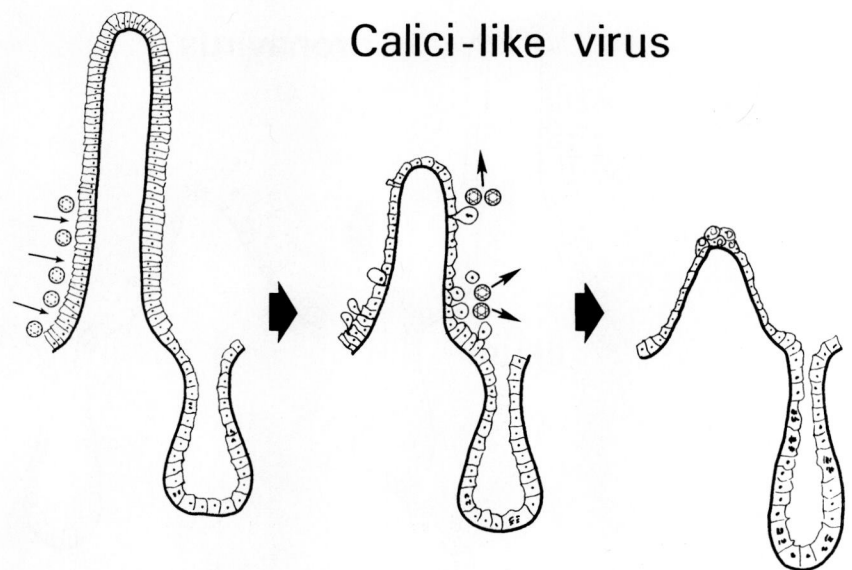

FIG. 8-45 E. Calici-like viruses, which have caused enteritis in calves (Newburg agent) and piglets, primarily invade enterocytes along sides of villi in small intestine. Infected cells swell, degenerate, and slough. Villi become stunted and fused.

Breda virus

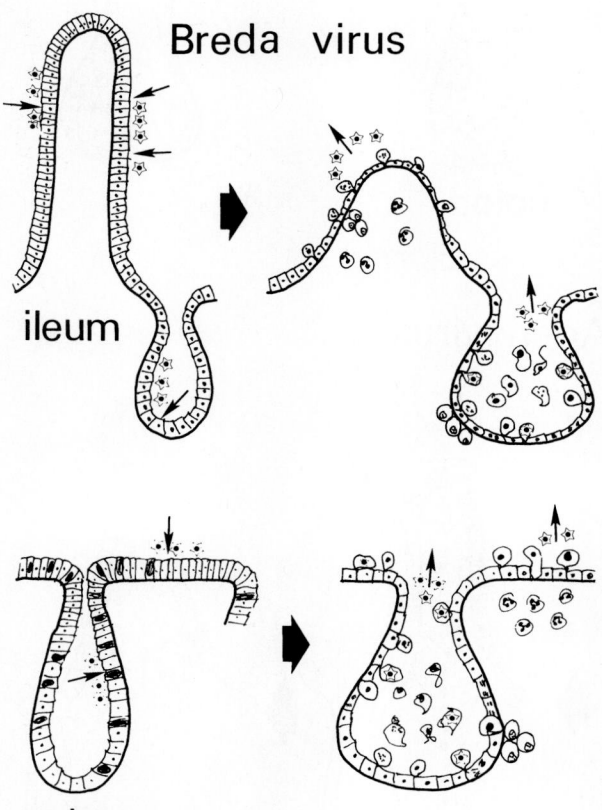

ileum

colon

F. Breda virus affects both villous and crypt enterocytes of small intestine, as well as surface and crypt cells in cecum and colon. Villi become stunted and fused and crypts dilated.

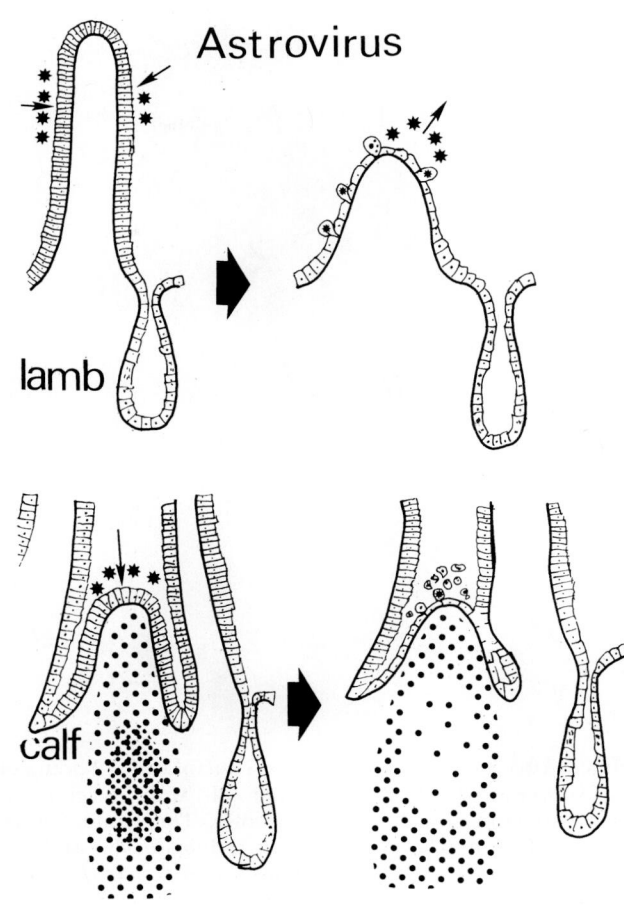

Astrovirus

lamb

calf

G. Astrovirus enteritis differs between lambs and calves. In lambs, mature enterocytes of villi are affected, causing stunting and fusion. In calves, dome M cells and absorptive cells are affected and exfoliate. Germinal centers of underlying lymphoid tissue become depleted.

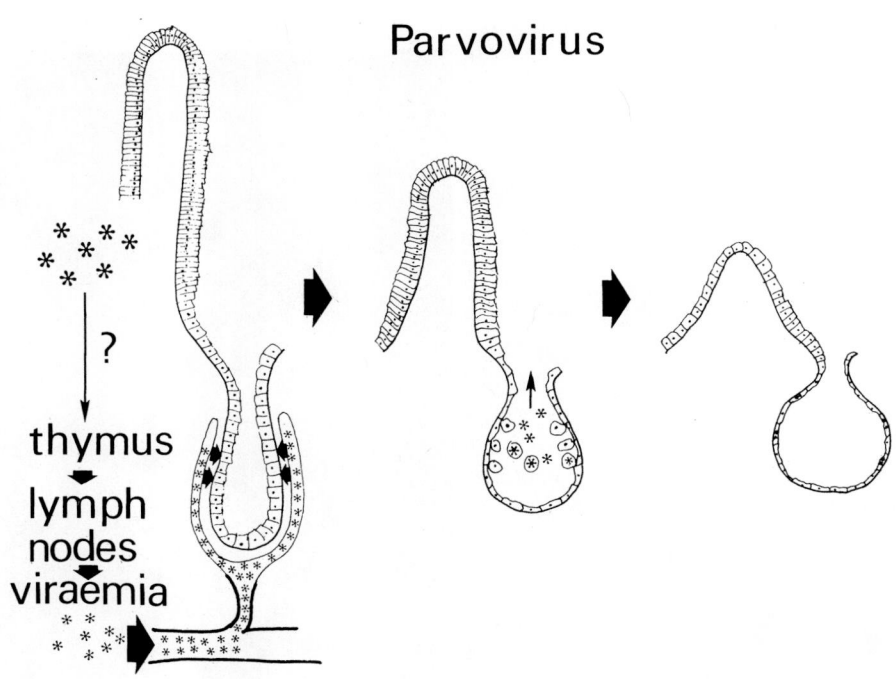

Parvovirus

thymus
lymph nodes
viraemia

H. Parvoviruses, which cause enteritis in cats and dogs, only infect and destroy dividing cells in crypts of small intestine. Villi become stunted and fused, and crypts dilate. (**A, C.** Courtesy of Dr. G. A. Hall, Institute for Animal Health, Agricultural and Food Research Council; **B, D-H.** Courtesy of Dr. G. A. Hall and *Ciba Foundation Symposium* 1987;128:192–217.)

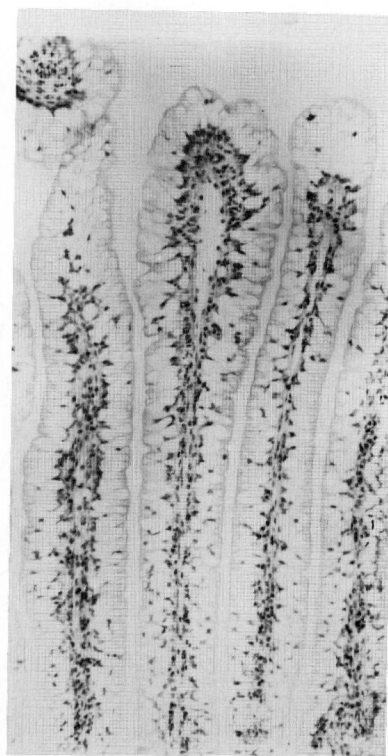

FIG. 8-46 Ileum of uninoculated control calf, 72 hours old. Villi are covered with tall columnar cells with nuclei at base, and cytoplasm contains clear vacuoles. The lamina propria contains lacteal and few other cells. (Hematoxylin and eosin stain.) (Courtesy of Dr. C. A. Mebus and *Veterinary Pathology.*)

epithelial cells in fecal specimens. This technique has demonstrated that the agent is widely distributed throughout the United States (White and others, 1970).

References

Bridger JC, Woode GN. Neonatal calf diarrhea: identification of the reovirus-like (rotavirus) agent in faeces by immunofluorescence and immune electron microscopy. Br Vet J 1975;131:528–535.

Fernelius AL, et al. Cell culture adaptation and propagation of a Reovirus-like agent of calf diarrhea from a field outbreak in Nebraska. Arch Virusforsch 1972;37:114–130.

Flewett TH, et al. Relation between viruses from acute gastroenteritis of children and newborn calves. Lancet 1974;2:61–63.

Mebus CA, Underdahl NR, Rhodes MB, et al. Calf diarrhea (scours): reproduced with a virus from a field outbreak. Univ Nebr Res Bull 1969;233:1–16.

Mebus CA, Stair EL, Underdahl NR, et al. Pathology of neonatal calf diarrhea induced by a reo-like virus. Vet Pathol 1971;8:490–505.

Reynolds DJ, Hall GA, Debney TG, et al. Pathology of natural rotavirus infection in clinically normal calves. Res Vet Sci 1985;38:264–269.

Stair EL, Mebus CA, Twiehaus MJ, et al. Neonatal calf diarrhea: electron microscopy of intestines infected with a reovirus-like agent. Vet Pathol 1973;10:155–170.

Stiglmair-Herb MT, Pospischil A, Hess RG, et al. Enzyme histochemistry of the small intestinal mucosa in experimental infections of calves with rotavirus and enterotoxigenic *Escherichia coli.* Vet Pathol 1986;23:125–131.

Vonderfecht SL, Eiden JJ, Torres A, et al. Identification of a bovine enteric syncytial virus as a nongroup A rotavirus. Am J Vet Res 1986;47:1913–1918.

White RG, Mebus CA, Twiehaus MJ. Incidence of herds infected with a neonatal calf diarrhea virus. Vet Med 1970;65:487–489.

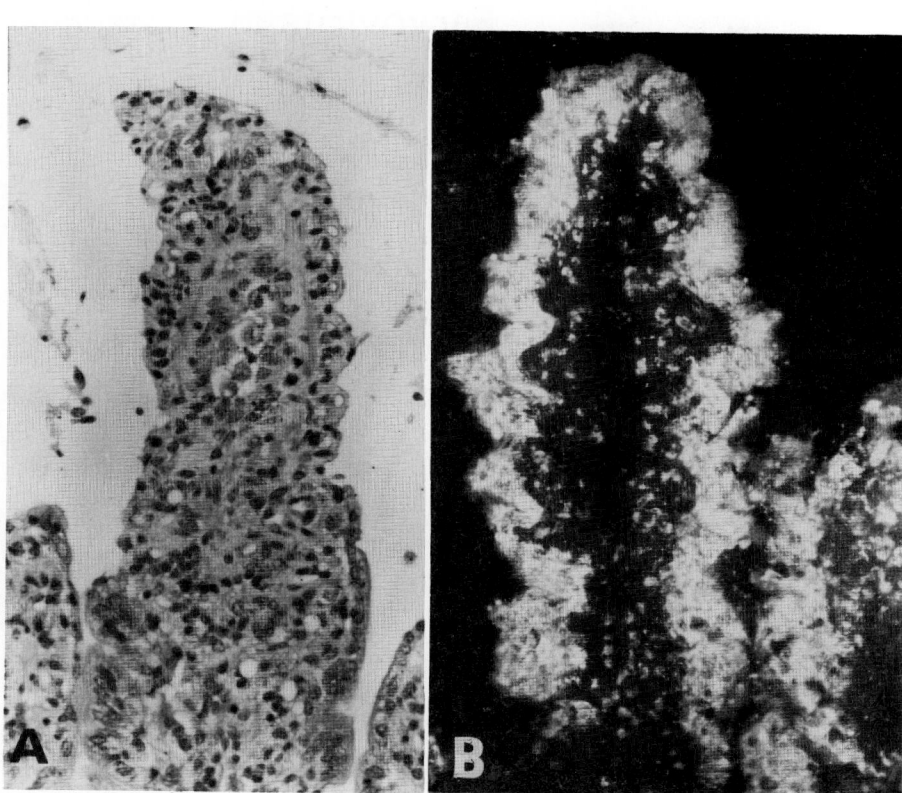

FIG. 8-47 A villus of ileum of calf infected with virus of neonatal calf enteritis (rotavirus). **A.** From calf killed 4.5 hours after onset of diarrhea. Epithelial cells are lost from distal two-thirds of villus. Cells are increased in lamina propria. **B.** From a calf killed one-half hour after onset of diarrhea. Immunofluorescence demonstrates presence of viral antigen in epithelial cells of distal two-thirds of villus. (Courtesy of Dr. C. A. Mebus and *Veterinary Pathology.*)

EPIDEMIC DIARRHEAL DISEASE OF MICE (EPIZOOTIC DIARRHEAL DISEASE OF INFANT MICE (EDIM))

This rotavirus infection often presents a serious problem in colonies of laboratory mice, because it is hard to control and has a very high mortality rate among suckling animals. Entire mouse colonies have been sacrificed in efforts to eliminate diseases.

Adult mice can become infected and eliminate the virus for varying periods of time in their feces; however, clinical disease does not occur.

The disease appears in suckling mice up to 15 days of age, but does not affect mice that have reached weaning age (22 days). Although the nursing females are ostensibly normal, their affected young appear somewhat shrunken or dehydrated, with dry whitish scales over the skin of the back and shoulder. Some mice have a cyanotic color, especially noticeable along the neck and between the shoulders. Diarrhea is evidenced by profuse soiling of the perineal region and tail with yellowish fecal material. Death often occurs soon after onset, but if mice survive more than 2 days, a tenacious, somewhat darker material often stains the perianal region, and in such cases, death may follow severe obstipation. In mild, uncomplicated cases, mice recover completely in 2 to 5 days, although the growth of some may be retarded.

The lesions are as described above, however, in contrast to most rotavirus infections, inclusion bodies may be seen in affected epithelial cells. The inclusion bodies, described originally by Pappenheimer and Enders (1947), are spherical, sharply outlined, 1 to 4 μ in diameter, and sometimes surrounded by a narrow clear halo. Laidlaw's acid fuchsin-phosphomolybdic acid-orange G stain reveals these inclusions to be intensely fuchsinophilic. They are eosinophilic with hematoxylin and eosin stain, and resemble the inclusion bodies of canine distemper.

References

Adams WR, Kraft LM. Epizootic diarrhea of infant mice: identification of the etiologic agent. Science 1963;141:359–360.
Adams WR, Kraft LM. Electron-microscopic study of the intestinal epithelium of mice infected with the agent of epizootic diarrhea of infant mice (EDIM virus). Am J Pathol 1967;51:39–60.
Banfield WG, Kasnic G, Blackwell JH. Further observations on the virus of epizootic diarrhea of infant mice. Virology 1968;36: 411–421.
Cheever FS, Mueller JH. Epidemic diarrheal disease of suckling mice. I. Manifestations, epidemiology and attempts to transmit the disease. J Exp Med 1947;85:405–416.
Cheever FS, Mueller JH. Epidemic diarrheal disease of suckling mice. III. The effect of strain, litter and season on the incidence of the disease. J Exp Med 1948;88:309–316.
Kraft LM. Two viruses causing diarrhea in infant mice. In: Harris RJC, ed. The problems of laboratory animal disease. New York: Academic Press 1962;115–130.
Kraft LM. Response of the mouse to the virus of epidemic diarrhea of infant mice. Neutralizing antibodies and carrier state. Lab Anim Care 1961;11:125–127.
Pappenheimer AM, Enders JF. An epidemic diarrheal disease of suckling mice. II. Inclusions in the intestinal epithelial cells. J Exp Med 1947;85:417–422.
Pappenheimer AM, Cheever FS. Epidemic diarrheal disease of suck-
ling mice. IV. Cytoplasmic inclusion bodies in intestinal epithelium in relation to the disease. J Exp Med 1948;88:317–324.
Rodriguez-Toro G. Natural epizootic diarrhea of infant mice (EDIM): a light and electron microscope study. Exp Mol Pathol 1980;32: 241–252.

PORCINE ROTAVIRAL ENTERITIS

A syndrome of enteric disease is recognized clinically in piglets 1 to 4 weeks of age. The principal signs are diarrhea, anorexia, depression, and occasional vomiting, with a mortality rate of from 7% to 20% of affected animals. This is often referred to as "milk scours," "white scours," or "three-week scours." One of the most likely causative agents in this clinical syndrome is a porcine rotavirus. This agent may be differentiated from the virus of transmissible gastroenteritis virus, porcine enterovirus, and enteropathogenic *Escherichia coli* (colibacillosis).

Lesions The lesions resemble typical rotaviral enteritis described above. In swine affected with pararotaviruses, syncytial cells may be seen.

Diagnosis The diagnosis may be established by identification of the rotavirus, achieved by isolation in tissue culture, or by direct demonstration of viral antigen in intestinal epithelial cells, using immunofluorescence methods. The differentiation from the virus of transmissible gastroenteritis (a coronavirus) is particularly critical.

References

Bohl EH, et al. Rotavirus as a cause of diarrhea in pigs. J Am Vet Med Assoc 1978;172:458–463.
Chasey D, Lucas M. Detection of rotavirus in experimentally infected piglets. Res Vet Sci 1977;22:124–125.
Gelberg HB, Hall WF, Woode GN, et al. Multinucleate enterocytes associated with experimental group A porcine rotavirus infection. Vet Pathol 1990;27:453–454.
Hall GA, Bridger IC, Chandler RL, et al. Gnotobiotic piglets experimentally infected with neonatal calf diarrhoea reovirus-like agent (rotavirus). Vet Pathol 1976;13:197–210.
Lecce JG, King MW, Mock R. Reovirus-like agent associated with fatal diarrhea in neonatal pigs. Infect Immun 1976;14:816–825.
McAdaragh JP, et al. Pathogenesis of rotaviral enteritis in gnotobiotic pigs: a microscopic study. Am J Vet Res 1980;41:1572–1581.
McNulty MS, et al. A reovirus-like agent (rotavirus) associated with diarrhea in neonatal pigs. Vet Microbiol 1976;1:55–63.
Pearson GR, McNulty MS. Pathological changes in the small intestine of neonatal pigs infected with a pig reovirus-like agent (rotavirus). J Comp Pathol 1977;87:363–375.
Saif LJ, Bohl EH, Kohler EM, et al. Immune electron microscopy of transmissible gastroenteritis virus and Rotavirus (reovirus-like agent) of swine. Am J Vet Res 1977;38:13–20.
Theil KW, Bohl EH, Agnes AG. Cell culture propagation of porcine rotavirus (Reovirus-like agent). Am J Vet Res 1977;38:1765–1768.
Theil KW, et al. Pathogenesis of porcine rotaviral infection in experimentally inoculated gnotobiotic pigs. Am J Vet Res 1978;39:213–220.
Theil KW, Saif LJ, Moorhead PD, et al. Porcine rotavirus-like virus (group B rotavirus): characterization and pathogenicity for gnotobiotic pigs. J Clin Microbiol 1985;21:340–345.

ROTAVIRAL INFECTION IN OTHER SPECIES

Viruses of the genus rotavirus are widely distributed among mammals. In addition to the more extensively studied diseases in children, calves, piglets, and mice, viral isolations have been reported from lambs, foals, dogs, deer, monkeys, rabbits, ferrets, raccoons, rats, chickens, and turkeys.

References

Conner ME, Darlington RW. Rotavirus infection in foals. Am J Vet Res 1980;41:1699–1703.

DiGiacomo RF, Thouless ME. Epidemiology of naturally occurring rotavirus infection in rabbits. Lab Anim Sci 1986;36:153–156.

England JJ, Poston RP. Electron microscopic identification and subsequent isolation of a rotavirus from a dog with fatal neonatal diarrhea. Am J Vet Res 1980;41:782–783.

Evans RH. Rotavirus-associated diarrhea in young raccoons (Procyon lotor), striped skunks (Mephitis mephitis) and red foxes (Vulpes vulpes). J Wildl Dis 1984;20:79–85.

Flewett TH, Bryden AS, Davies H. Virus diarrhea in foals and other animals. Vet Rec 1975;96:477.

Hoshino Y, Wyatt RG, Scott FW, et al. Isolation and characterization of a canine rotavirus. Arch Virol 1982;72:113–125.

Johnson CA, Snider TG III, Henk WG, et al. A scanning and transmission electron microscopic study of rotavirus-induced intestinal lesions in neonatal gnotobiotic dogs. Vet Pathol 1986;23:443–453.

McNulty MS, et al. Reovirus-like agent (Rotavirus) from lambs. Infect Immun 1976;14:1332–1338.

Schoeb TR, et al. Rotavirus-associated diarrhea in a commercial rabbitry. Lab Anim Sci 1986;36:149–152.

Snodgrass DR, Smith W, Gray EW, et al. A rotavirus in lambs with diarrhea. Res Vet Sci 1976;20:113–114.

Snodgrass DR, Herring JA, Gray EW. Experimental rotavirus infection in lambs. J Comp Pathol 1976;86:637–642.

Torres-Medina A. Isolation of an atypical rotavirus causing diarrhea in neonatal ferrets. Lab Anim Sci 1987;37:167–171.

Tzipori S, Caple IW, Butler R. Isolation of a rotavirus from deer. Vet Rec 1976;99:398.

TOGAVIRIDAE

The family **Togaviridae** (toga = cloak) is made up of a large number of viruses incorporating those agents formerly classified as arboviruses (ar = arthropod, bo = borne), as well as a number of related viruses that do not involve arthropod transmission cycles (Table 8-7). There is still some confusion about these classifications, but each agent in this family is a spherical single-stranded, positive-sense RNA virus, 40 to 70 nm in diameter.

Here we will consider this family as consisting of five genera: alphavirus, flavivirus, rubivirus, pestivirus and arterivirus, as well as some unclassified agents.

The genus **alphavirus** is made up of those viruses formerly known as group A arboviruses. It includes some 26 serologically related viruses, all of which are arthropodborne. Three of these are pathogens for horses as well as humans: Eastern equine encephalomyelitis; Western equine encephalomyelitis; and Venezuelan equine encephalomyelitis.

The genus **flavivirus** (flavi = yellow), made up of some 60 antigenically related viruses, includes those viruses formerly called group B arboviruses. Some viral classification schemes identify this group as a separate family, **Flaviviridae**. All flaviviruses of medical importance are arthropodborne. Table 8–7 lists some of the more significant diseases.

With rare exception, alphaviruses and flaviviruses are transmitted by the bites of arthropods, most usually mosquitoes and ticks. For each virus, there are specific arthropods necessary for perpetuation of the transmission cycle, a factor which restricts the geographical distribution of the disease. Arthropods become infected on biting a viremic vertebrate host. The virus replicates first in the arthropod's gut and ultimately passes via the hemolymph to other tissues, including the salivary gland, from which it can be passed to another vertebrate host. The arthropod remains infected through life, and although there is continuous viral replication, no harm is done to the arthropod. In some viral arthropod relationships, the virus can be transmitted from generation to generation. Certain of the diseases seen in domestic animals represent spillover from an arthropod-wild animal cycle. Such is the case with Eastern and Western equine encephalomyelitis and yellow fever. In these situations, the wild vertebrate hosts (often birds)

TABLE 8-7 **Diseases caused by *Togaviridae* ***

Alphavirus	Arterivirus	Flavivirus	Pestivirus	Rubivirus	Unclassified
(Group A arboviruses)	Equine viral arteritis	(Group B arboviruses)	Hog cholera	Rubella (humans)	Simian hemorragic fever
Equine encephalomyelitis	Porcine reproductive and respiratory syndrome virus	Yellow fever	Bovine viral diarrhea-mucosal disease		Lactic dehydrogenase virus
Western		Dengue type I	Border disease		
Eastern		St. Louis encephalitis			
Venezuelan		Japanese B encephalitis			
Semliki Forest virus		West Nile virus			
Chikungunya virus		Murray Valley encephalitis			
Sinbis virus		Russian tick-borne encephalitis			
		Louping-ill virus			
		Kyasanur Forest disease			
		Wesselsbron disease			
		Powassan viral encephalitis			

*The genera flavivirus and pestivirus are also classified as a separate family, the *Flaviviridae*.

do not develop disease, but do develop an adequate viremia to allow perpetuation of the cycle. In contrast, horses (and other susceptible species) develop disease, but typically there is not a significant viremia. Thus, usually they are dead-end hosts. The virus probably gains access to the nervous system via centripetal spread by way of peripheral and cranial nerves. As with many viral infections, most alphavirus and flavivirus infections are inapparent.

The remaining genera and unclassified togaviruses are not dependent on an arthropod transmission cycle. The **pestivirus** genus includes hog cholera virus and bovine viral diarrhea virus (mucosal disease, border disease). Some classifications place the genus pestivirus along with the **flaviviruses** in the family *Flaviviridae*. The **rubivirus** genus contains the human pathogen rubella virus. Equine arteritis virus and the recently recognized virus of the porcine reproductive and respiratory syndrome are the only members of the **arterivirus** genus. Unclassified togaviruses include simian hemorrhagic fever virus and lactic dehydrogenase virus of mice.

Diseases caused by alphaviruses (group A arboviruses)

EQUINE ENCEPHALOMYELITIS

A widespread disease of the central nervous system of horses was recognized in the United States as early as 1912 and was reported by Stange, who originally proposed the name "equine encephalomyelitis" (1948). The disease was the cause of serious losses, particularly in the central part of the country, during the 1920s and 1930s. It was variously known as forage poisoning, cerebral spinal meningitis, staggers, Borna disease, botulism, and Kansas horse plague. During the summer of 1930, equine encephalomyelitis virus was isolated by Meyer, Haring, and Howitt (1931) from an affected horse. This discovery was the forerunner of many significant advances in the understanding and control of viral encephalitis in many species, including humans. The virus isolated by Meyer and colleagues is now known as the "Western" strain of equine encephalomyelitis virus, to distinguish it from an antigenically different virus isolated from horses in the eastern part of the United States, the "Eastern" strain (Ten Broeck and Merrill, 1933). A third strain of virus that produces similar signs and lesions was isolated by Kubes and Rios (1939) from animals in Venezuela and is known as the "Venezuelan" strain. The Western strain occurs throughout most of the United States west of the Mississippi River, but also has been recognized in several states along the eastern seaboard and in Central and South America. In contrast, the Eastern strain is principally limited to the eastern seaboard. The Venezuelan strain occurs in several South American countries, e.g., Panama, Trinidad, and Mexico; it also exists in the Everglades region of Florida. In 1971, a serious epizootic occurred in Mexico and Texas (Johnson and Martin, 1974).

The demonstration by Kelser, in 1933, that mosquitoes may serve as vectors of the virus of equine encephalomyelitis provided an explanation for many of its epizootiologic features. Soon after, it was discovered that the equine encephalomyelitis viruses are infective for large numbers of animals, including humans. Although other species of domestic animals, such as dogs, pigs, goats, calves, and a variety of domestic fowl, can be infected, the infection is usually (but not always) inapparent. Many laboratory animals (e.g., guinea pigs, mice, hamsters, monkeys) are susceptible.

The enzootic cycles of these three encephalitic viruses involve mosquitoes, birds, reptiles, and rodents with occasional epizootic spillover into horses and humans. The cycles are still not completely understood. The Western strain infects a variety of passerine birds and is transmitted by *Culex tarsalis*, a mosquito that also feeds on mammals. The Eastern strain also infects passerine birds, but uses *Culiseta melanura*, a mosquito that rarely feeds on mammals. Presumably with amplification of the mosquito-bird cycle, other species of mosquitoes, such as *Aedes*, become infected and transmit the virus to horses. Reptiles and amphibians may also be infected and may play a role in perpetuation of the Western and Eastern strains. The infection in most avian species is asymptomatic; however, in certain birds, such as the ring-necked pheasant, the Eastern strain causes clinical disease with high mortality. The Venezuelan strain of encephalomyelitis, of which there are four subtypes of the virus, involves an enzootic cycle between rodents, birds, and *Culex melanconium* mosquitoes in swampy areas. Other species of mosquitoes, including *Aedes, Mansonia,* and *Psorophora,* can transmit the virus among horses and, owing to high levels of viremia, even mechanical insect transmission is believed possible. As a result of mosquito transmission, the diseases are seasonal, with the greatest incidence in summer and fall, and end abruptly with the first killing frost. How the virus lives through winter is not known.

Even though equine encephalomyelitis is an important disease in horses and humans, infection of these species is rather incidental to the perpetuation of the virus, in that viremia generally is not adequate to infect mosquitoes, with the exception of the Venezuelan strain, where viremia levels can be high. Since the signs and lesions caused by the three strains of virus are essentially the same, they are considered together.

Signs The signs of derangement of the central nervous system usually appear suddenly after an incubation period of 1 to 3 weeks. Affected animals lose awareness of their surroundings and wander about aimlessly, walk continuously in circles, are unresponsive to commands, and may collide with objects or crash through fences. High fever often occurs at the outset, but in some cases body temperature has returned to normal by the time nervous symptoms appear. As the disease advances, stupor is evident and paralysis of various groups of muscles sets in. This flaccid paralysis increases rapidly; the animal lies down, is unable to regain its footing, and soon succumbs. Approximately 50% of horses infected with the Western strain of virus die; in the Eastern strain, this figure reaches 90%; and in the Venezuelan strain, between 50% and 80% die.

Lesions No gross lesion can be considered characteristic of this disease. The viruses of equine encephalomyelitis attack neurons, hence the damage is to these cells. Affected neurons undergo various degenerative changes, culminating in necrosis. These changes are manifested by dissolution and loss of tigroid substance (tigrolysis) and chromatin (chromatolysis), fragmentation of the cell, and its removal by phagocytes (neuronophagia) (Fig. 8-48). This process attracts leukocytes and glial cells, which form small nodules around the injured neuron; such nodules may persist after all traces of the nerve cell are gone. The gray matter around affected neurons may also become edematous and diffusely infiltrated with lymphocytes, neutrophils, and small numbers of erythrocytes. Lymphocytes escaping from nearby arterioles are often trapped in the Virchow-Robin space to form a wide collar of densely packed cells around the blood vessel. This "perivascular cuffing" may extend into the white matter, where it is the only significant change. Perivascular cuffing is a striking microscopic finding, but it is not specific for equine encephalomyelitis; it occurs in numerous inflammatory lesions of the central nervous system.

The distribution of the lesions in the central nervous system varies, depending somewhat on the strain of virus. With the Eastern strain, the gray masses are diffusely involved, the lesions are numerous, and neutrophils are often a prominent component of the exudate. The presence of these neutrophils appears to be the result of the severity of the infection and the short fatal course of the disease; thus, it is not absolutely diagnostic of the Eastern type. Infection with any strain of virus may result in lesions in the gray matter of the cerebral or cerebellar cortex, but they are most numerous in the olfactory bulbs, thalamus, hypothalamus, brain stem, and in both dorsal and ventral gray columns of the spinal cord. The gasserian and other ganglia may contain an increased number of mononuclear cells.

In certain laboratory animals (rabbits, guinea pigs, mice) that have been experimentally infected, there is a tendency toward massive necrosis of certain olfactory centers (rhinencephalic cortex ventral to fissura rhinica and cornu Ammonis); however, other viruses may also affect these species in a similar manner. In monkeys, the Western strain has been shown to cross the placenta, infecting the fetus and leading to abortion or malformation of the brain. Studies on the pathogenesis of Venezuelan equine encephalitis virus in mice and hamsters have demonstrated viral replication in B-cell areas of lymphocytic organs, hepatocytes, and pancreatic acinar cells before invasion of the central nervous system. Experimentally infected hamsters died before encephalitis developed.

Diagnosis A presumptive diagnosis may be made on finding the microscopic lesions diffusely distributed through the gray matter of the central nervous system. A confirmed diagnosis can be made only on the basis of isolation and identification of the virus or through specific staining techniques.

References

Albrecht P. Pathogenesis of neurotropic arbovirus infections. Curr Top Microbiol Immunol 1968;43:44–91.

Bigler WJ, McLean RG. Wildlife as sentinels for Venezuelan equine encephalomyelitis. J Am Vet Med Assoc 1973;163:657–661.

Chamberlain RW. Vector relationships of the arthropod borne en-

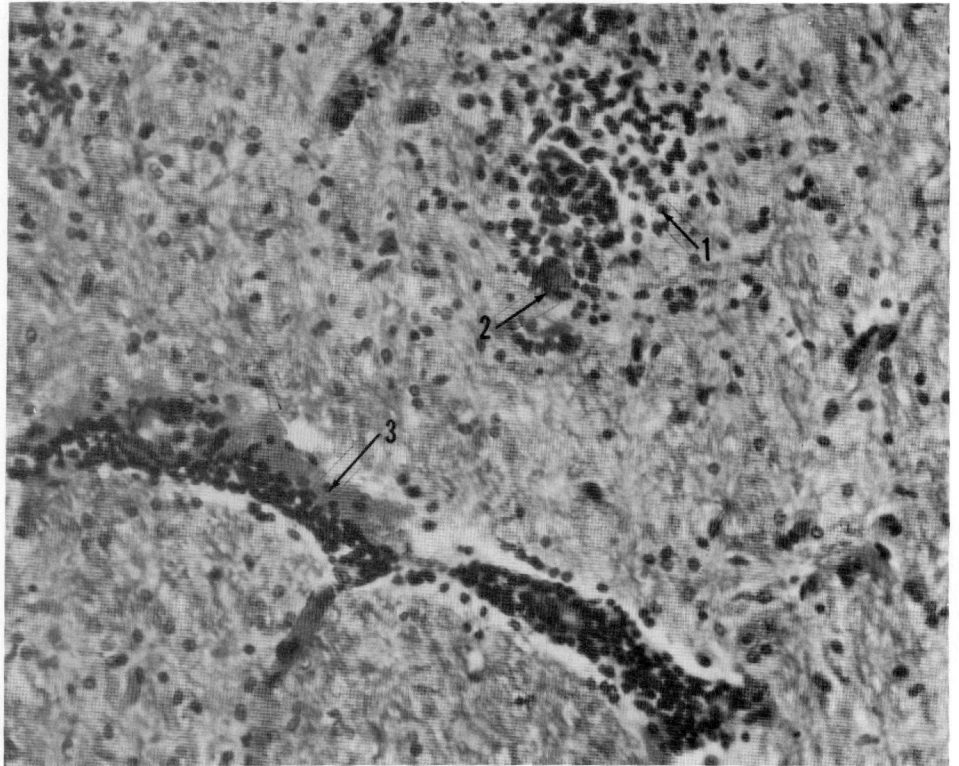

FIG. 8-48 Equine encephalomyelitis (Western strain), cerebrum of horse (× 280). Nodule of lymphoid cells *(1)* adjacent to neuron undergoing phagocytosis *(2)*. Lymphocytes *(3)* in wall of blood vessel and Virchow-Robin space. (Courtesy of the Armed Forces Institute of Pathology; contributed by Dr. L. T. Giltner.)

cephalitides in North America. Ann NY Acad Sci 1958;70: 312–319.

Editorial note. J Am Vet Med Assoc 1948;113:464.

Ehrenkranz NJ, et al. The natural occurrence of Venezuelan equine encephalitis in the United States. N Engl J Med 1970;282: 298–302.

Fothergill LD, Dingle JH, Farber S, et al. Human encephalitis caused by virus of Eastern variety of equine encephalomyelitis. N Engl J Med 1938;291:411.

Gleiser CA, et al. The comparative pathology of experimental Venezuelan equine encephalomyelitis infection in different animal hosts. J Infect Dis 1962;110:80–97 [VB 2271–62].

Gorelkin L, Jahrling PB. Pancreatic involvement by Venezuelan equine encephalitis virus in the hamster. Am J Pathol 1974;75: 349–362.

Habluetzel JE, Grimes JE, Pigott MB Jr. Serologic evidence of naturally occurring Venezuelan equine encephalomyelitis virus infection in a dog. J Am Vet Med Assoc 1973;162:461–462.

Hess AD, Holden P. The natural history of the arthropod-borne encephalitides in the United States. Ann NY Acad Sci 1958;70: 294–311.

Hurst EW. The histology of equine encephalomyelitis. J Exp Med 1934;59:529–542.

Jackson AC, SenGupta SK, Smith JF. Pathogenesis of Venezuelan equine encephalitis virus infection in mice and hamsters. Vet Pathol 1991;28:410–418.

Jahrling PB, Scherer WF. Histopathology and distribution of viral antigens in hamsters infected with virulent and benign Venezuelan encephalitis viruses. Am J Pathol 1973;72:25–38.

Jennings WL, Allen RH, Lewis AL. Western equine encephalomyelitis in a Florida horse. Am J Trop Med 1966;15:96–97.

Johnson KM, Martin DH. Venezuelan equine encephalitis. Adv Vet Sci Comp Med 1974;18:79–116.

Kelser RA. Mosquitoes as vectors of the virus of equine encephalomyelitis. J Am Vet Med Assoc 1933;82:767–771.

Kissling RE. Host relationship of the arthropod-borne encephalitides. Ann NY Acad Sci 1958;70:320–326.

Kubes V, Rios FA. Causative agent of infectious equine encephalomyelitis in Venezuela. Science 1939;90:20–21.

London WT, et al. Teratological effects of western equine encephalitis virus on the fetal nervous system of Macaca mulatta. Teratology 1982;25:71–79.

McGee ED, Littleton CH, Mapp JB, et al. Eastern equine encephalomyelitis in an adult cow. Vet Pathol 1992;29:361–363.

Meyer KF, Haring CM, Howitt B. The etiology of epizootic encephalomyelitis of horses in the San Joaquin Valley, 1930. Science 1931;74:227–228.

Monath TP. Arthropod-borne encephalitides in the Americas. Bull WHO 1979;57:513–533.

Monath TP, Cropp CB, Harrison AK. Mode of entry of a neurotropic arbovirus into the central nervous system. Reinvestigation of an old controversy. Lab Invest 1983;48:399–410.

Monath TP, McLean RG, Cropp CB, et al. Diagnosis of eastern equine encephalomyelitis by immunofluorescent staining of brain tissue. Am J Vet Res 1981;42:1418–1421.

Monlux WS, Luedke AJ. Brain and spinal cord lesions in horses inoculated with Venezuelan equine encephalomyelitis virus (epidemic American and Trinidad strains). Am J Vet Res 1973;34:465–473.

Pursell AR, et al. Naturally occurring and artificially induced Eastern encephalomyelitis in pigs. J Am Vet Med Assoc 1972;161: 1143–1147.

Pursell AR, Mitchell FE, Seibold HR. Naturally occurring and experimentally induced Eastern encephalomyelitis in calves. J Am Vet Med Assoc 1976;169:1101–1103.

Roberts ED, Sanmartin C, Payan J, et al. Neuropathologic changes in 15 horses with naturally occurring Venezuelan equine encephalomyelitis. Am J Vet Res 1970;31:1223–1229.

Weil A, Breslich PJ. Histopathology of the central nervous system in the North Dakota epidemic encephalitis. J Neuropath Exp Neurol 1942;1:49–58.

OTHER ALPHAVIRUSES

More than 20 additional members of the alphavirus group cause disease in humans but are not of impor-

tance to animal health. One agent, **Getah virus,** related to Ross River virus of humans, has been recovered from horses, pigs, and mosquitoes in Japan, Australia, and Southeast Asia. In Japan, the virus has been incriminated as the cause of a severe nonfatal enzootic disease of horses, characterized by fever, rash, and edema of the hind legs. Also in Japan, Getah virus has been associated with a peracute disease of newborn pigs characterized by fever, depression, tremor, and diarrhea.

References

Kamada M, et al. Equine Getah virus infection: isolation of the virus from racehorses during an enzootic in Japan. Am J Trop Med Hyg 1980;29:984–988.

Kumanomido T, Wada R, Kanemaru T, et al. Clinical and virological observations on swine experimentally infected with Getah virus. Vet Microbiol 1988;16:295–301.

Yago K, Hagiwara S, Kawamura H, et al. A fatal case in newborn piglets with Getah virus infection: isolation of the virus. Jpn J Vet Sci (Nippon Juigaku Zasshi) 1987;49:989–994.

Diseases caused by flaviviruses

JAPANESE B ENCEPHALITIS

Japanese encephalitis is a viral disease of humans, horses, swine, and cattle, which is most prevalent in Japan, China, and elsewhere in Asia. The disease is arthropodborne with an enzootic cycle involving *Culex tritaeniorhynchus* (and other *Culex* species), swine, and birds, principally ardeid species (egrets, herons) and ducks.

Infection is most important in humans when the virus causes encephalitis. Horses and other equines may also develop encephalitis; however, infection in cattle is almost always asymptomatic. In swine, the virus is an important cause of abortion and neonatal mortality. Adult swine do not develop disease but do serve as amplifiers of the infection.

Lesions In fatal infections in humans, neuronophagic nodules are observed in all parts of the gray matter; the thalamus, substantia nigra, nucleus basalis, and anterior horns of the spinal cord are most severely involved. In the spinal cord, the lesions tend to become confluent; whereas in the cerebral cortex and cerebellum, the lesions are generally discrete. The neuronophagic nodules indicate involvement of neurons.

In animals, including aborted and stillborn pigs, similar lesions are seen, particularly in the gray matter of the cerebral cortex and basal ganglia.

Diagnosis Although the presence of typical lesions may suggest Japanese B encephalitis, these lesions cannot with certainty be differentiated from those of louping ill, Teschen disease, or even equine encephalomyelitis. In order to make a definitive diagnosis, it is necessary to isolate the causative virus or demonstrate specific neutralizing antibody production after infection.

References

Burns KF. Congenital Japanese B encephalitis of swine. Proc Soc Exp Biol NY 1950;75:621–625.

Burns KF, Matumoto M. Japanese equine encephalomyelitis. J Am Vet Med Assoc 1949;115:112–115, 167–170.

Burns KF, Matumoto M. Survey of animals for inapparent infection with the virus of Japanese B encephalitis. Am J Vet Res 1949;10:146–149.

Monath TP. Flaviviruses. In; Fields BN, Knipe DM, eds. Virology. 2nd ed. Vol 1. Chapter 27. New York: Raven Press 1990;763–814.

Haymaker W, Sabin AB. Topographic distribution of lesions in the central nervous system in Japanese B encephalitis. Arch Neurol Psychiat 1947;57:673–692.

Webster LT. Japanese B encephalitis virus; its differentiation from St. Louis encephalitis virus and relationship to louping-ill virus. J Exp Med 1938;67:609–618.

Zimmerman HM. Pathology of Japanese B encephalitis. Am J Pathol 1946;22:965–991.

OVINE ENCEPHALOMYELITIS (LOUPING ILL)

Louping ill is a tickborne encephalitis, principally of sheep, which occurs in Scotland, Northern England, Wales, and Ireland. Humans are susceptible, but infection is usually mild. Encephalitis can also occur in horses, and sporadic cases have been described in cattle. The disease is of principal importance, however, in sheep.

Affected animals, usually lambs, exhibit a peculiar "louping" gait, which gives the disease its common name. The tick, *Ixodes ricinus*, transmits louping ill to sheep under natural conditions, which accounts for the seasonal occurrence of the disease.

Lesions Louping ill virus produces lesions associated with the destruction of neurons diffusely distributed throughout the gray matter. Although these neuronal lesions are found throughout the cerebral cortex, they are most concentrated in the cerebellum, where loss of Purkinje cells and focal glial or inflammatory nodules are also observed. In the ventral horn of the spinal cord and medulla, motor neurons are often, but not consistently, affected. The lesions are similar in intensity and distribution to those of Teschen disease (porcine encephalomyelitis). The experimental lesions in sheep are similar to those that occur in the natural disease.

Louping ill has been experimentally transmitted to mice, pigs, and monkeys. In mice, it produces a uniformly fatal disease in which the principal change is diffuse encephalomyelitis, with neutrophilic infiltration and perivascular cuffing as the prominent features. Necrosis in the hippocampus and granular layer of the cerebellum is also noted. In monkeys, symptoms of ataxia are produced and, while encephalomyelitis is less diffuse than in the mouse, the Purkinje cells in the cerebellum are largely destroyed and the anterior horn cells of the spinal cord are damaged. Cytoplasmic inclusion bodies in neurons have been described in mice and monkeys with experimentally induced louping ill; they have not been found in the natural infection in sheep. In pigs, only the clinical manifestations of the experimental disease are known. They include hyperesthesia, tremors of the head and limbs, incoordination of movement, and inability to stand. Pigs usually recover from the experimentally induced infection.

Diagnosis A presumptive diagnosis can be made on the basis of the microscopic lesions in the brain and spinal cord, but definitive diagnosis depends on isolation and identification of the virus.

References

Brownlee A, Wilson DR. Studies in the histopathology of louping-ill. J Comp Pathol Ther 1932;45:67–92.

Doherty PC, Reid HW. Experimental louping-ill in sheep and lambs. II. Neuropathology. J Comp Pathol 1971;81:331–336.

Doherty PC, Reid HW, Smith W. Louping-ill encephalomyelitis in the sheep. IV. Nature of the perivascular inflammatory reaction. J Comp Pathol 1971;81:545–549.

Doherty PC, Smith W, Reid HW. Louping-ill encephalomyelitis in the sheep. V. Histopathogenesis of the fatal disease. J Comp Pathol 1972;82:337–344.

Doherty PC, Vantsis JT, Hart R. Louping-ill encephalomyelitis in the sheep. VT. Infection of the 120 day foetus. J Comp Pathol 1972;82:385–392.

Dow C, McFerran JB. Experimental Aujeszky's disease in sheep. Am J Vet Res 1964;25:461–468.

MacLeod J, Gordon WS. Studies in louping-ill. II. Transmission by the sheep tick (Ixodes ricinus L.). J Comp Pathol Ther 1932;45:240–252.

Pool WA, Brownlee A, Wilson DR. The etiology of "louping-ill." J Comp Pathol Ther 1930;43:253–290.

Timoney PI, Donnelly WJC, Clements LO, et al. Encephalitis caused by louping ill virus in a group of horses in Ireland. Equine Vet Res J 1976;8:113–117.

Wood M. Intranuclear inclusion bodies in the brain of guinea-pigs infected with louping ill virus with special reference to the effect of treatment with cyclophosphamide. Br J Exp Pathol 1974;55:56–63.

KYASANUR FOREST DISEASE

This disease, caused by a pestivirus, is an infection of Old World monkeys (*M. radiata* and *Presbytis entellus*) and humans, transmitted by a tick, *Haemophysalis spinigera*. Kyasanur Forest disease has not been described outside India. The hemorrhagic tendencies are generally more severe in simian hemorrhagic fever than in Kyasanur Forest disease, and marked splenomegaly and lymphocytic necrosis are not features of the disease. Nonsuppurative encephalomyelitis may occur in Kyasanur Forest disease. Mice are susceptible to Kyasanur Forest disease, but the virus of simian hemorrhagic fever does not kill mice, a point that can aid differentiation. Definitive diagnosis of either infection requires virus isolation and identification.

References

Goverdhan MK, et al. Epizootiology of Kyasanur Forest disease in wild monkeys of Shimoga District, Mysore State (1957–1964). Indian J Med Res 1974;62:497–510.

Iyer CGS, et al. Kyasanur Forest disease. Part VII. Pathological findings in monkeys, Presbytis entellus and Macaca radiata, found dead in the forest. Indian J Med Res 1960;48:276–286.

Webb HE, Burston J. Clinical and pathological observations with special reference to the nervous system in Macaca radiata infected with Kyasanur Forest disease virus. Trans Royal Soc Trop Med Hyg 1966;60:325–331.

Webb HE. Kyasanur Forest disease virus infection in monkeys. Lab Anim Handb 1969;4:131–134.

Webb HE, Chatterjea JB. Clinico-pathological observations on monkeys infected with Kyasanur Forest disease virus, with special reference to the haemopoietic system. Br J Haemat 1962;8:401–413.

WESSELSBRON DISEASE

Wesselsbron disease is caused by a flavivirus transmitted by *Aedes* mosquitoes in sub-Saharan Africa. It is most important as an infection of sheep, in which it closely resembles and must be differentiated from Rift Valley fever (discussed under the *Bunyaviridae* family). Mild infection may occur in cattle and humans. The disease in sheep is characterized by fever, subcutaneous edema, and jaundice; the principal lesion is necrotizing hepatitis. Mortality may be high. Infection and vaccination can lead to abortion, hydrops amnii, prolonged gestation, and fetal malformations, particularly of the nervous system.

Reference

Weiss KE, Haig DA, Alexander RA. Wesselsbron virus—a virus not previously described, associated with abortion in domestic animals. Onderstepoort J Vet Res 1956;27:183–195.

POWASSAN VIRAL ENCEPHALITIS

Powassan virus, a member of the flavivirus genus, was first recovered from a child in the town of Powassan, Ontario, Canada. Although widely distributed in Canada and the United States, the virus rarely causes human disease, and disease is apparently restricted to Ontario, the eastern United States, and possibly the Soviet Union. The virus is maintained in a cycle involving *Ixodes* ticks and a variety of small mammals, including skunks, squirrels, and ground hogs, which do not develop any detectable illness. Antibodies to Powassan virus have also been detected in horses, cats, and snowshoe hares. Focal, necrotizing, nonsuppurative meningoencephalitis has been experimentally induced in horses, cats, and snowshoe hares. The virus is thought to cause disease naturally in horses, although the frequency is uncertain.

References

Keane DP, Parent J, Little PB. California serogroup and Powassan virus infection of cats. Can J Microbiol 1987;33:693–697.
Little PB, Thorsen J, Moore W, et al. Powassan viral encephalitis: a review and experimental studies in the horse and rabbit. Vet Pathol 1985;22:500–507.

YELLOW FEVER

Yellow fever, a serious viral disease of humans, has been recognized since the seventeenth century. It is included in this text as the virus in the prototype of the flavivirus genus; most species of nonhuman primates are not only susceptible to infection but also aid the perpetuation of the disease through what is known as jungle yellow fever, or the sylvatic cycle. The disease is principally found in Central and South America and Africa, but occurred in Europe in the eighteenth century and in the United States, as far north as Boston, as late as 1905. The **urban cycle** of yellow fever is human to human transmission via the mosquito *Aedes aegypti*. The **jungle cycle** is monkey to monkey transmission. In the New World, the mosquito *Haemagogus spergozzini* is the main vector, and in Africa, *Aedes africanus*. Crossover of the two cycles allows the virus to enter human populations from nonhuman primate "reservoirs." *Haemagogus* mosquitoes feed on humans who enter the forest, especially when trees are felled, as it is a tree mosquito. In Africa, the cross-over is effected by a third mosquito, *Aedes simpsoni*, which feeds on humans and monkeys.

After an incubation period of 3 to 10 days, clinical signs develop that vary from mild to fulminating disease. Mortality is about 10%. Signs include fever, aching muscles, headache, nausea, jaundice, and vomiting, which often contains blood ("black vomit"). Pathologic findings include icterus and hemorrhages but are dominated by hepatic necrosis, particularly of the midzone of the lobule. Necrotic hepatocytes undergo a peculiar hyalin change to form what is termed the "Councilman body." Small eosinophilic granular intranuclear inclusion bodies (Torres bodies) also develop. Neither body contains virions, only amorphous material.

Most species of nonhuman primates are highly susceptible, although there is some variation among species. The European hedgehog *(Erinaceus europaeus)* is also susceptible. Infant mice can be infected experimentally; in them, in contrast to the other species, the principal lesion is encephalitis, whether inoculated via the intraperitoneal or intracerebral route. There are many **other members of the flavivirus group** that are pathogens of humans, but not animals. These pathogens cause encephalitis (St. Louis encephalitis, Murray Valley encephalitis, tickborne encephalitis); rash and fever (Dengue fever, West Nile fever); and hemorrhagic fever (Omsk hemorrhagic fever).

The remaining genus of the *Togaviridae*, **rubivirus**, contains the human pathogen rubella virus.

References

Bearcroft WGC. The histopathology of the liver of yellow fever-infected rhesus monkeys. J Pathol Bacteriol 1957;74:295–303.
Felsenfeld AD. The arboviruses. In: T-W-Fiennes RN, ed. Pathology of simian primates. Part II. Basel: Karger 1972;523–536.
Rodhain F. The role of monkeys in the biology of dengue and yellow fever. Comp Immunol Microbiol Infect Dis 1991;14:9–19.
Smetana HF. The histopathology of experimental yellow fever. Virchows Arch Pathol Anat 1962;335:411–427.

Diseases caused by pestiviruses

The pestivirus genus in the family *Togaviridae* contains the viruses of hog cholera, bovine viral diarrhea-mucosal disease, and border disease. Each of these viruses conforms to the physical and biochemical characteristics accepted for the family *Togaviridae*, which are defined as having an RNA genome, packed into a capsidal shell with icosahedral symmetry and surrounded by an envelope of lipoprotein. The virions of these viuses are 40 to 70 nm in diameter and contain isometric cores. Frequent deviations of the spherical shape of the virions are believed to be caused by conformation of a loosely fitting envelope. Immunologic similarities have been demonstrated between the viruses of hog cholera and bovine mucosal disease. It is possible that the taxonomic arrangement of these viruses may be changed in the future, but it seems advantageous to consider together diseases caused by these related viruses.

References

Horzinek M, Maess J, Laufs R. Studies on the substructure of togaviruses, 11. Analysis of equine arteritis rubella, bovine viral diarrhea and hog cholera viruses. Arch Virusforsch 1971;33:307–318.

Spradbrow P. Arbovirus infections of domestic animals. Vet Bull 1966;36:55–61.

HOG CHOLERA (SWINE FEVER, SWINE PLAGUE)

Hog cholera is an acute, febrile, highly contagious, and often fatal disease of swine. First recognized as a separate entity by Salmon and Smith in 1885, its viral etiology was demonstrated by De Schweinitz and Dorset in 1903.

In 1962, a national program was instituted in the United States aimed at the eventual eradication of hog cholera. It was estimated at that time that 4000 to 5000 herds of swine were subject to outbreaks of the disease each year. The program, conducted by state and federal officials and practicing veterinarians, was aimed at total eradication of the disease. Steps were taken to identify outbreaks of the disease, to prevent its spread by slaughter of infected and exposed animals, and to prevent movement of animals from any potentially infected area. The manufacture and use of all vaccines containing live or modified live virus was halted in 1969, because the vaccines were shown to be a source of new outbreaks. By 1974, all 50 states were declared to be free of hog cholera.

As the disease was restricted by these eradication measures, the florid, typical disease that had always been expected was rarely seen. Smoldering atypical cases of the disease were identified as hog cholera only after careful laboratory work involving infection of susceptible swine or identification of the virus by immunologic means (Fig. 8-49).

All this may mean that current veterinary students in the United States will never encounter hog cholera as a disease problem or may not recognize the disease,

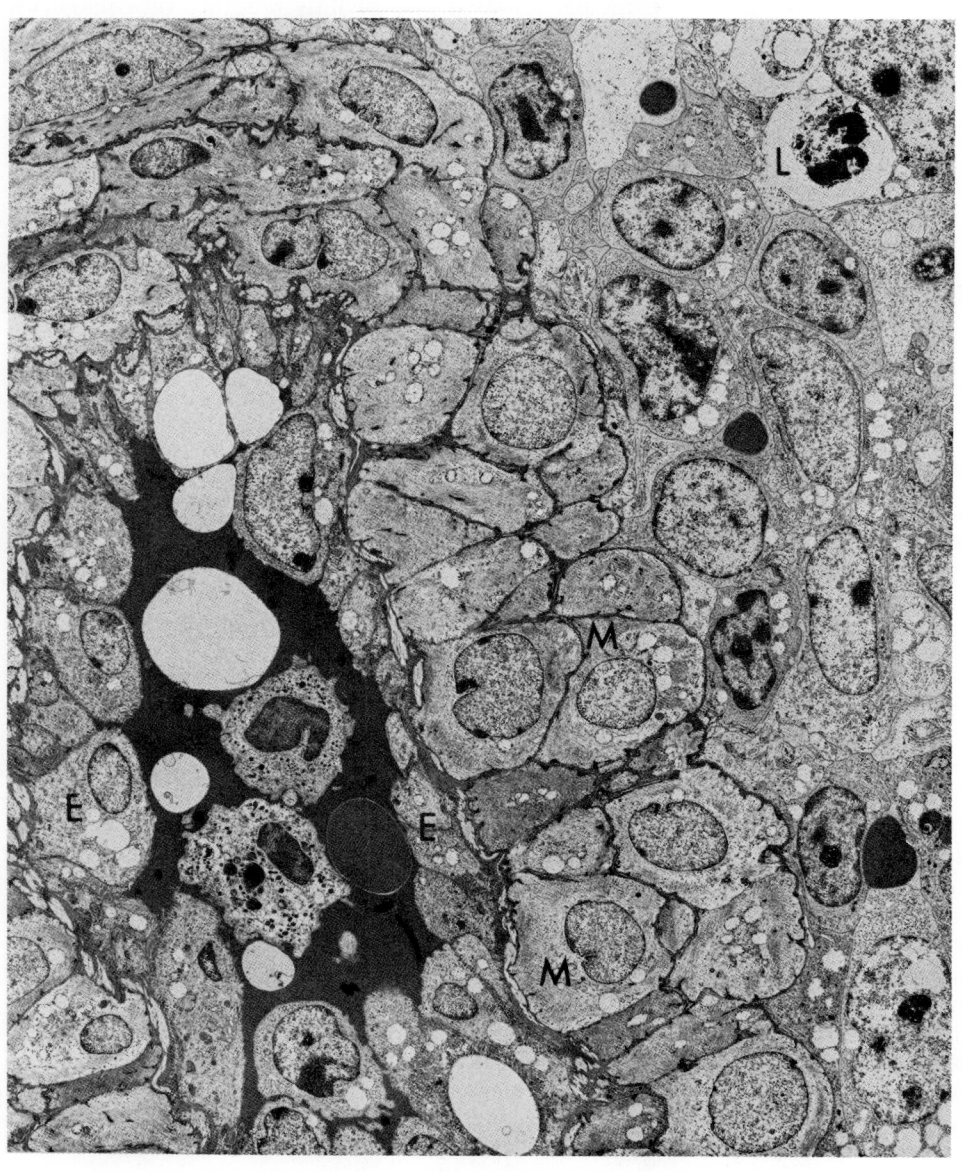

FIG. 8-49 Hog cholera. Swelling and degeneration of endothelial cells *(E)* and muscle cells *(M)* of central arteriole of spleen. Necrotic lymphocyte *(L)* is within macrophage. (Courtesy Dr. N. F. Cheville and *Laboratory Investigation*.)

if it should appear. If the disease is now nonexistent in this country and does not reappear, the following pages on hog cholera may not apply to the United States. However, it seems prudent to recount here the features of the disease, should it reappear.

Signs After an incubation period of about 3 days following experimental exposure or as many as 7 days after field exposure, depression and a high fever (106°F) are first manifested. These signs are accompanied by severe leukopenia, in which the total leukocyte count may be less than 4,000/mm^3 of blood. Although only a few animals in a herd may be infected initially, the disease spreads rapidly to all susceptible animals in contact with the disease. In addition to weakness and inappetence, nervous symptoms are commonly observed; these include lethargy, occasional convulsions, grinding of the teeth, and difficulty in locomotion. In swine with light skin, erythematous lesions appear, particularly on the skin of the abdomen, axillae, and inner surfaces of the legs. Most animals die less than 10 days after the onset of signs; in a few that live longer, evidence of intestinal and pulmonary involvement are more likely to be observed. In natural outbreaks, nearly 100% of susceptible animals in a herd may be expected to die. The disease in nature is limited to domestic and wild swine, but virus propagation can be accomplished experimentally in rabbits, after modification of the virus by repeated alternate passage between swine and rabbits.

Infection with hog cholera virus of reduced virulence can result in a more protracted course, which has been termed "chronic" hog cholera. Following an acute reaction and apparent remission, there is an exacerba-tion of the acute disease, resulting in death as late as 40 to 70 days after the initial signs of infection. Swine with chronic disease play an important role in the dissemination of hog cholera, because they excrete virus intermittently throughout the entire course of the infection. Swine vaccinated with live attenuated virus may also excrete virulent virus and serve as a source of infection to nonimmune swine.

A variety of fetal and neonatal abnormalities have been attributed to natural exposure to hog cholera virus or vaccination with modified live virus during pregnancy. The most critical period of exposure appears to be after 20 days of gestation; however, earlier infection may result in embryonic death and absorption. Abnormalities include mummification, anasarca, ascites, stillbirth, cerebellar hypoplasia, hypomyelinogenesis, congenital tremors, and neonatal death. Although the mechanism leading to these changes is not clear at present, virus crosses the placenta and invades fetal tissues and can be demonstrated or isolated from piglets. The immune status of the sow is not related to the development of fetal infection. Infection *in utero* can also lead to lesions resembling hog cholera in adult swine or to the birth of persistently infected swine that shed the virus.

Lesions The virus of hog cholera exerts a direct effect on the vascular system, and the signs and lesions result from changes in the capillaries (Fig. 8-50), precapillaries, arteries, and veins. For this reason, the gross lesions appear as areas of congestion, hemorrhage, or infarction, depending on the organs involved and the severity and duration of the vascular changes. In acute cases and in swine sacrificed early in the disease, gross

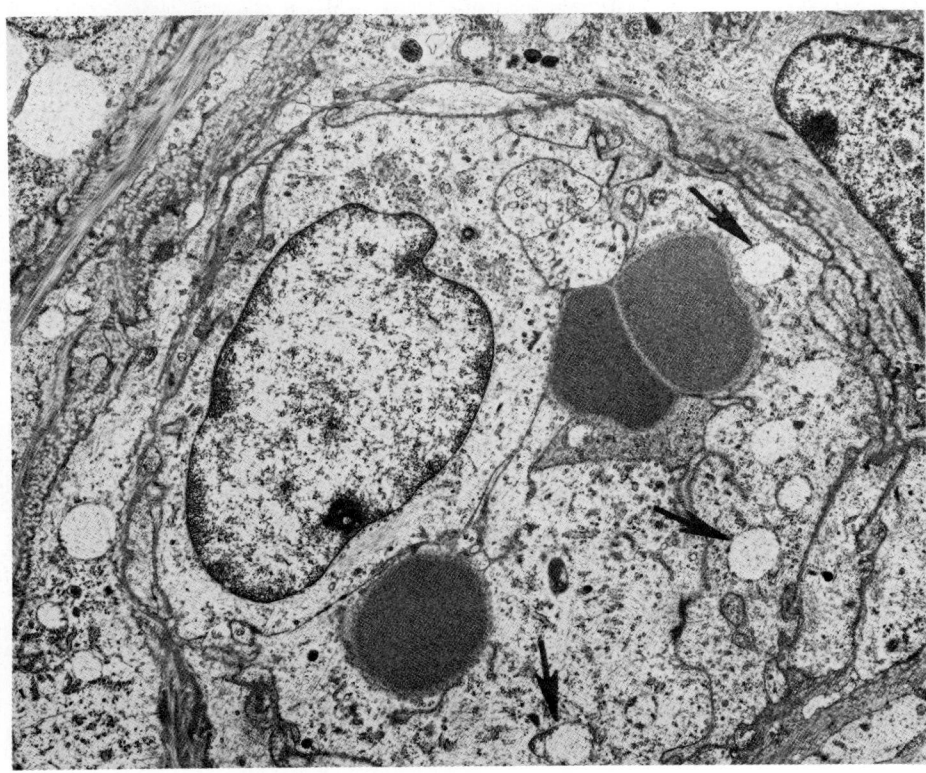

FIG. 8-50 Hog cholera. Swollen endothelial cells obliterating capillary lumen. Mitochondria *(arrows)* are swollen and have lost their cristae. (Courtesy of Dr. N. F. Cheville.)

lesions may be difficult to detect, but in cases of longer duration, they may be found in a wide variety of organs. According to Kernkamp (1939), gross lesions are seen in organs in the following order of frequency: kidney (Fig. 8-51), lymph nodes, urinary bladder, skin (in white-skinned animals), spleen, larynx, lungs, and large intestine. With less frequency, lesions are found in the heart, liver, small intestine, and stomach.

In the vascular system, the specific action of the virus is manifested grossly by petechiae and ecchymoses, but the nature of the lesions can be determined only by microscopic examination. The earliest and most pronounced lesions are found in the capillaries and pre-capillaries; some vessels are closed, others are dilated. The most constant change is swelling and proliferation of endothelial cells accompanied by a decrease in staining intensity. The endothelial nuclei are thus enlarged, increased in number, pale-staining, and may pile up to occlude the lumen or be desquamated and lost. The capillary basement membrane is pale, eosinophilic, hyaline, and homogeneous, and these changes may extend to the collagen and reticulum fibers that surround the vessel. The capillary wall may become completely hyalinized, resulting in partial or complete occlusion. Fat droplets may be seen in the capillary walls or in the surrounding area of necrosis. Thrombosis is rare in ar-

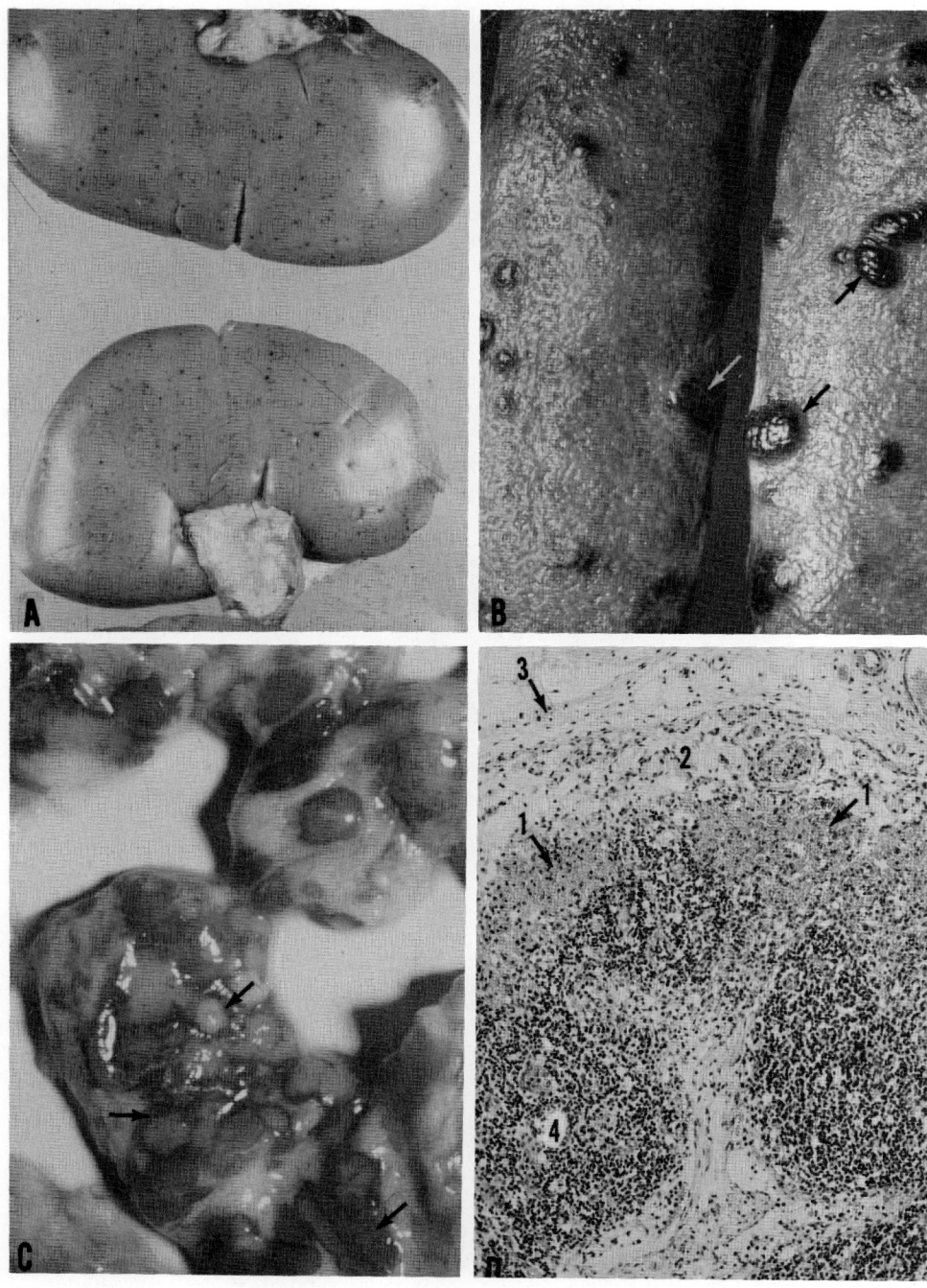

FIG. 8-51 Hog cholera. **A.** Petechiae in kidney. **B.** Infarcts (arrows) in spleen. **C.** Hemorrhages (arrows) in lymph nodes. **D.** Hemorrhages (1) in cell-poor substance of lymph node (× 90). Note that subcapsular sinusoids (2) and capsule (3) are not involved. Lymphoid follicle at (4). (Courtesy of the Armed Forces Institute of Pathology.)

terioles or smaller vessels. In small and medium-sized arteries, the lesions are similar to those in capillaries but are less frequent and more striking. In the larger of these arteries and in veins, swelling and proliferation of the endothelium are associated with separation and distention of fibers of the media and adventitia, perhaps by edema. The media and adventitia may be hyalinized, and occasionally, necrosis is seen, with an adventitial infiltrate of cells showing pyknosis and karyorrhexis. Thrombosis occasionally occurs in arteries involved in this manner. Similar lesions may be seen in veins but rarely in lymph vessels. Vascular changes are most severe in lymph nodes, spleen, and kidneys and less severe in the nervous system, liver, intestine, skin, and other organs.

In the central nervous system, the lesions are related to the vasculature and, therefore, may appear in any part of this system as early as 6 days after infection and before signs are observed. Aside from congestion of the vasculature, gross changes are not seen in the brain. The most striking microscopic lesion results from accumulation of lymphocytes in the perivascular (Virchow-Robin) spaces around arteries and veins (Fig. 8-52) and may be large enough to be detected in stained sections with very low magnification. This perivascular cuffing with lymphocytes, mononuclear cells,

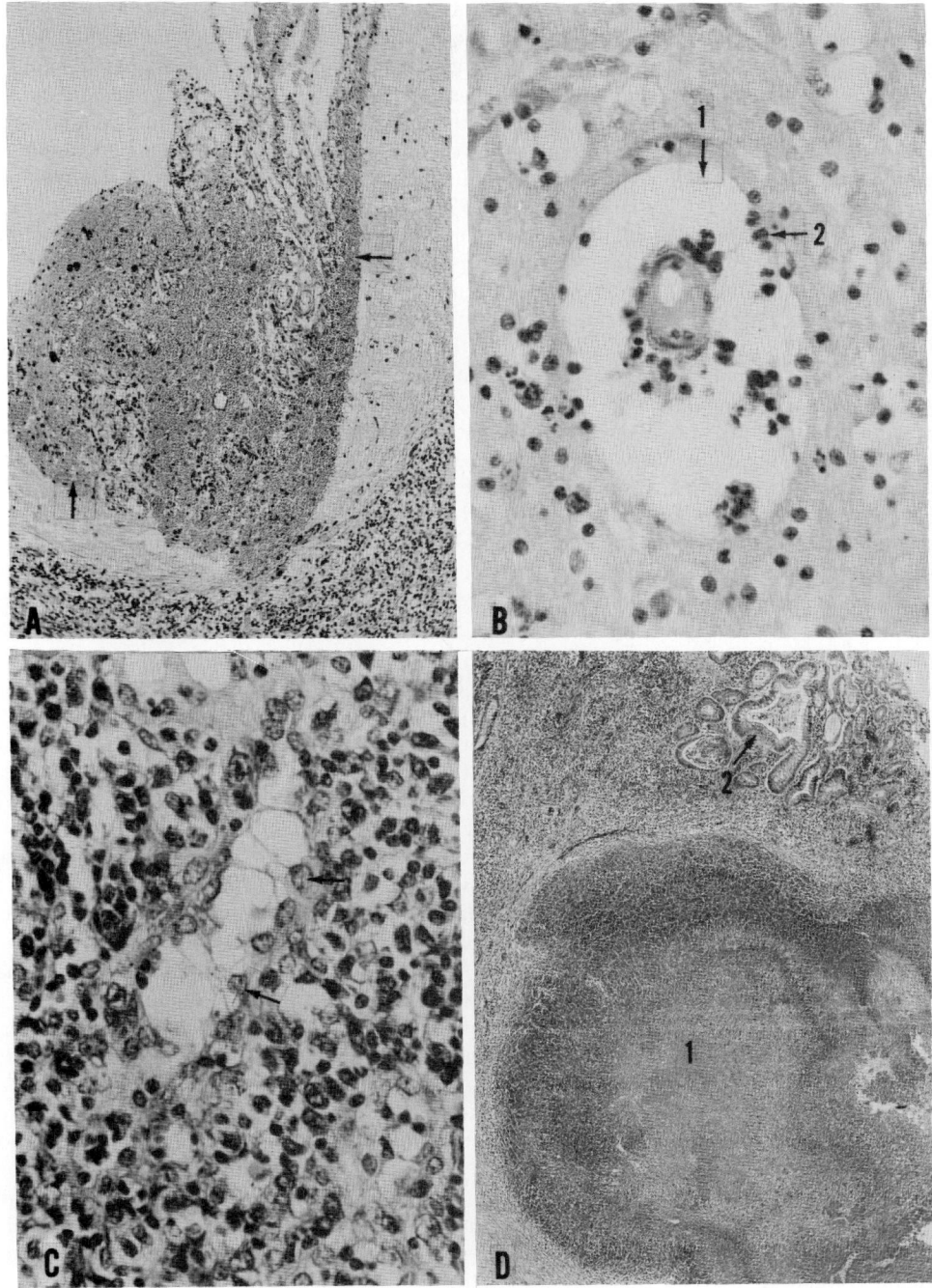

FIG. 8-52 Hog cholera. **A.** Hemorrhage *(arrows)* in pia mater (× 75). **B.** Edematous distention *(1)* of Virchow-Robin space and aggregation of a few leukocytes *(2)* in cerebrum (× 220). **C.** Proliferation of endothelial nuclei *(arrows)* in lymph node (× 410). (Contributed by Lt. Col. F. D. Maurer.) **D.** Sharply demarcated zone of necrosis *(1)* in colon (× 35). Epithelium *(2).* (Courtesy of the Armed Forces Institute of Pathology; contributed by Lt. Col. F. D. Maurer.)

plasma cells, and occasional eosinophils often outlines the vessel as it extends into the parenchyma from the pia-arachnoid. Neutrophils are not a part of the inflammatory exudate, but in severe cases, leukocytes may infiltrate the tissues surrounding the perivascular space. Hemorrhages may be observed around blood vessels, especially in the cerebellum and the spinal cord. Similarly, perivascular accumulations of mononuclear and red blood cells may be found in the choroid plexus. Conspicuously absent are thrombi, emboli, or patches of softening. Small nodules of proliferated microglia are present, particularly within white matter, but sometimes diffusely scattered through both white and gray matter. These small, sharply outlined nodules are made up chiefly of microglial cells but may include leukocytes. Such microglial nodules are rather subtle even in microscopic sections. Occasionally, Hortega cells containing many mitotic figures are seen in concentric arrangement around vessels. Of much less significance are the changes in the neurons, which are neither specific nor common, but a few affected nerve cells may be noted adjacent to or in areas of glial proliferation. The large pyramidal cells are more likely to be damaged than are multipolar cells of the cortex and gray nuclei. Some Purkinje cells may be affected. In the involved neuronal cells, the nucleus is swollen and located peripherally; its chromatin is fragmented and the nucleolus is absent. There may be tigrolysis of the cytoplasm, with vacuolation and loss of Nissl's granules. The cell membrane may be denticulated. Occasional neuronophagia and satellitosis are seen in the gray masses of the brain, cerebellum, and cord. There is no demyelination. Inclusion bodies, resembling those described by Joest and Degen in Borna disease and by Hurst in equine encephalomyelitis and poliomyelitis, are found in a few cases but are not considered specific. These inclusions are intranuclear, round, homogeneous, acidophilic or occasionally basophilic, and several may be found in a single neuron.

In the spleen, infarction caused by lesions in the arteries occurs in about 50% of cases. Grossly, the infarcts are sharply outlined, red in color, irregular in shape, and elevated (Fig. 8-51); some are definitely wedge-shaped. Microscopically, degenerative changes in the wall of follicular or trabecular arteries are characterized by proliferation of endothelium, hyalinization, and necrosis in the media and adventitia with resultant thrombosis. Hemorrhagic infarction related to these vascular lesions is demonstrable as sharply demarcated areas of necrosis.

Gross lesions are seen in one or more lymph nodes in more than 80% of animals that die of hog cholera. Even in nodes of the same animal, they vary from swelling and hyperemia with bright red, subcapsular hemorrhages outlining the periphery of the node to dense, dark-colored hemorrhages obscuring the entire nodal architecture. In the milder lesions, the fresh hemorrhage is confined to the cell-poor substance, which in porcine lymph nodes lies just beneath the cortical and adjacent to the trabecular sinuses. (The secondary follicles are located deep in the node near the trabeculae,

as reported by Seifried and Cain in 1932. This is the reverse of the anatomic arrangement in most other species.) The cortical sinuses, even in hemorrhagic nodes, seldom contain red blood cells. Pronounced changes are usually observed in the capillaries, arterioles, and venules, particularly in the cell-poor substance. Swelling and proliferation of endothelial nuclei are striking, and are accompanied by occlusion of the lumen and duplication of the vessels. Diffuse accumulation of erythrocytes may obscure most of the histologic features of nodes that are severely involved.

In the skin, erythematous areas resulting from cyanosis are the most common gross lesions. They usually appear as areas of purplish discoloration, 1 to 15 cm in diameter, on the ventral surface of the abdomen and the thorax, the medial surface of the thigh and leg, the ears, the medial surface of the forearm, the skin of the perineum, and the snout. Edema and necrosis with sloughing are rare. The cyanotic changes usually can be readily detected in white-skinned swine, less easily in brown-skinned swine, and rarely in the black breeds. The typical changes in the vascular system also are responsible for these cutaneous lesions.

In the kidney, sharply demarcated petechiae, from 1 to 5 mm in diameter, are visible grossly just beneath the capsule and deep in the renal cortex. These petechiae give the kidney a characteristic appearance, which has been likened to that of a turkey egg (Fig. 8-51). Microscopically, hemorrhages are found in the interstitial stroma and in Bowman's spaces, and from the latter, blood may flow into the convoluted tubules. These hemorrhages are related to the typical lesions in the vasculature.

The digestive system is most obviously affected in animals dying after a more prolonged course. Diffuse catarrhal inflammation may be seen but is not specific for hog cholera. The characteristic lesion is a spherical ulcer in the mucosa, particularly of the colon. These ulcers are sharply circumscribed, single or multiple; they originate as small congested areas with adherent fecal material and develop into encrusted button-shaped foci ("button ulcers") a few millimeters in diameter. Cut sections reveal a sharply demarcated zone of necrosis in the underlying mucosa and submucosa. This lesion develops after occlusion of a small artery by swelling and hydropic changes in its endothelium; thus, the "button ulcer" is the result of infarction and evolves through the same sequence of events as the infarcts in the spleen.

Diagnosis The diagnosis can usually be made on the basis of the clinical manifestations and gross and microscopic lesions. In the presence of fever without other symptoms, differentiation from acute systemic swine erysipelas may be a problem, but it can be solved by isolation of the organism of swine erysipelas from the bloodstream. Acute arthritis, common in erysipelas, has specific diagnostic value because it does not occur in hog cholera. Teschen disease can be differentiated by the microscopic lesions found in the central nervous system. Confirmation of the diagnosis of hog cholera is accomplished by injection of blood or tissue filtrates from suspected swine into cholera-susceptible pigs, with controls receiving a large simultaneous dose of anticholera immune serum. The pigs receiving antiserum should remain well, and the unprotected pigs should sicken and die of hog cholera. This method obviously is suitable only for herd diagnosis. The virus can be isolated in tissue culture, but unfortunately, most strains do not produce cytopathic effects. However, the presence of the virus can be demonstrated by the application of fluorescent antibody staining to infected cell cultures. This test has proven reliable and is replacing the older pig inoculation test. Fluorescent antibody staining may also be applied directly to tissue sections.

References

Baetz AL, Mengeling WL, Booth GD. Blood constituent changes associated with hog cholera virus infection of swine. Am J Vet Res 1971;32:1479–1490.

Carbrey EA, et al. Transmission of hog cholera by pregnant sows. J Am Vet Med Assoc 1966;149:23–30.

Carbrey EA, Stewart WC, Kresse JI, et al. Persistent hog cholera infection detected during virulence typing of 135 field isolates. Am J Vet Res 1980;41:946–949.

Cheville NF, Mengeling WL. The pathogenesis of chronic hog cholera (swine fever), histologic, immunofluorescent, and electron microscopic studies. Lab Invest 1969;20:261–274.

Cheville NF, Mengeling WL, Zinober MR. Ultrastructural and immunofluorescent studies of glomerulonephritis in chronic hog cholera. Lab Invest 1970;22:458–467.

De Schweinitz EA, Dorset M. A form of hog cholera not caused by the hog cholera bacillus. Circular 41, U.S.D.A., BAI, Washington, DC, September 28, 1903.

Dunne HW, Clark CD. Embryonic death, fetal mummification, stillbirth, and neonatal death in pigs of gilts vaccinated with attenuated live-virus hog cholera vaccine. Am J Vet Res 1968;29:787–796.

Dunne HW, et al. A study of an encephalitic strain of hog cholera virus. Am J Vet Res 1952;13:277–289.

Dunne HW, Smith EM, Runnells RA. The relation of infarction to the formation of button ulcers in hog cholera infected pigs. Proc Am Vet Med Assoc 1952;155–160.

Dunne HW, Reich CV, Hokanson JF, et al. Variations in the virus of hog cholera. A study of chronic cases. Proc Am Vet Med Assoc 1955;148–153.

Emerson JL, Delez AL. Cerebellar hypoplasia, hypomyelinogenesis, and congenital tremors of pigs, associated with prenatal hog cholera vaccination of sows. J Am Vet Med Assoc 1965;147:47–54.

Freeman A. All 50 states hog cholera free. J Am Vet Med Assoc 1974;165:158–162.

Helmboldt CF, Jungherr EL. Neuropathologic diagnosis of hog cholera. Am J Vet Res 1950;11:41–49.

Helmboldt CF, Jungherr EL. Further observations on the neuropathological diagnosis of hog cholera. Am J Vet Res 1952;13:309–317.

Johnson KP, Ferguson LC, Byington DP, et al. Multiple fetal malformations due to persistent viral infection. I. Abortion, intrauterine death, and gross abnormalities in fetal swine infected with hog cholera vaccine virus. Lab Invest 1974;30:608–617.

Jones RK, Doyle LP. A study of encephalitis in swine in relation to hog cholera. Am J Vet Res 1953;14:415–419.

Kernkamp HCH. Lesions of hog cholera: Their frequency of occurrence. J Am Vet Med Assoc 1939;95:159–166.

Loan RW, Storm MM. Propagation and transmission of hog cholera virus in nonporcine hosts. Am J Vet Res 1968;29:807–811.

Mengeling WL, Packer RA. Pathogenesis of chronic hog cholera: host response. Am J Vet Res 1969;30:409–417.

Plateau E, Vannier Ph, Tillon JP. Atypical hog cholera infection: viral isolation and clinical study of in utero transmission. Am J Vet Res 1980;41:2012–2015.

Roehrer H. Histologische Untersuchungen bei Schweinepest. I.

Lymphknotenveränderungen in akuten Fällen. Arch f Tierheilk 1930–1931;62:345–372.

Roehrer H. Histologische Untersuchungen bei Schweinepest. II. Veränderungen im Zentralner-vensystem in akuten Fällen. Arch Tierheilk 1930–1931;62:439–462.

Salmon DE, Smith T. Rep Comm Agr. Washington DC. 1885.

Saulmon EE. Final phase of hog cholera eradication. J Am Vet Med Assoc 1974;164:304–306.

Seifried O. Histological studies on hog cholera. I. Lesions in the central nervous system. J Exp Med 1931;53:277–289.

Seifried O. Cain CB. Histological studies on hog cholera. II. Lesions of the vascular system. J Exp Med 1932;56:345–349.

Seifried O. Cain CB. Histological studies on hog cholera. III. Lesions in the various organs. J Exp Med 1932;56:351–362.

Stewart WC, et al. Transmission of hog cholera virus by mosquitoes. Am J Vet Res 1975;36:611–614.

Tidwell Mac A, et al. Transmission of hog cholera virus by horseflies (Tabanidae: Diptera). Am J Vet Res 1972;33:615–622.

Van der Molen EJ, van Oirschot JT. Congenital persistent swine fever (hog cholera). I. Pathomorphological lesions in lymphoid tissues, kidney and adrenal. II. Further pathomorphological observations with special emphasis on epithelial, vascular, and nervous tissues. Zentralbl Veterinarmed (B) 1981;28:89–101, 190–204.

Vannier P, Plateau E, Tillon JP. Congenital tremor in pigs farrowed from sows given hog cholera virus during pregnancy. Am J Vet Res 1981;42:135–137.

BOVINE VIRUS DIARRHEA AND MUCOSAL DISEASE

A contagious disease of cattle in New York State was first described in 1946 by Olafson, McCallum, and Fox, who demonstrated its viral etiology and termed the infection virus diarrhea. The disease was characterized by high morbidity rates and low (4% to 8%) mortality rates. Also in 1946, Childs described a disease of cattle in Canada similar to virus diarrhea, which was more severe and had a high mortality rate, although herd morbidity rates were low. In 1953, Ramsey and Chivers, in Iowa, described a syndrome nearly identical to that described by Childs, and named the syndrome mucosal disease. Pritchard and associates, in 1954 and 1956, reported the occurrence of a disease in Indiana that closely resembled virus diarrhea in its clinical signs, morbidity and mortality rates, and gross and microscopic lesions. In the literature, this disease became known as **Indiana virus diarrhea.** Virus diarrhea and mucosal disease have since been described in other parts of the United States and are now known to occur worldwide (Fig. 8-53).

It is now recognized that each of these syndromes is caused by antigenically related viruses and that the variable clinical picture with respect to morbidity and mortality is determined by viral strain variations and mode of infection. Bovine viral diarrhea virus (BVDV) occurs in two biotypes, **cytopathogenic BVDV** (cpBVDV) and **noncytopathogenic BVDV** (noncpBVDV) on the basis of their effects on tissue culture cells. The two variants may also be distinguished by the presence of an 80-kDa protein, which is present in all cpBVDV strains but absent from all noncpBVDV strains. Virus diarrhea occurs sporadically as a transient acute infection with a high morbidity rate and is a highly contagious but usually mild disease in cattle exposed postnatally, usually between 6 months and 2 years of age, to cpBVDV. Although usually a mild disease, new strains of BVDV have caused outbreaks with high mortality rates.

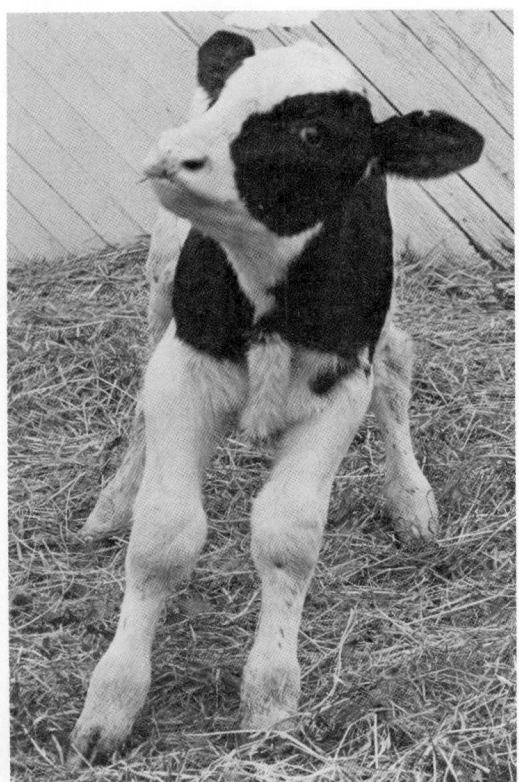

FIG. 8-53 Bovine viral diarrhea/mucosal disease. Cerebellar hypoplasia in 3-day-old Holstein calf. Virus was inoculated into dam at 150 days of gestation. Calf was blind and ataxic. (Courtesy of Dr. G. M. Ward and *Cornell Veterinarian.*)

Mucosal disease, on the other hand, develops in cattle that become infected *in utero* with noncpBVDV. These animals develop a persistent infection to which they are immunotolerant. Mucosal disease develops in these animals when the persistent noncpBVDV undergoes a transformation to cpBVDV through a process of RNA recombination. It generally appears in the animal between 6 months and 2 years of age and the result is inevitably fatal. Mucosal disease can be experimentally produced by superinfection of persistently infected animals with cpBVDV, but only if the virus matches the antigenic pattern of the persisting noncpBVDV. Antigenically different strains of cpBVDV are cleared.

Border disease of sheep (discussed later) is caused by the same virus or an essentially indistinguishable variant. The virus of hog cholera is also related. Swine can be infected with BVDV, but the virus ordinarily does not cause clinical disease. In pregnant swine, it may cause fetal death and resorption.

Signs The clinical signs include high fever (105°F to 108°F), anorexia, depression, and diarrhea accompanied by excessive salivation, with stringy mucus hanging from the muzzle to the ground. Severe leukopenia is observed rather constantly in the early stages of the disease. Ulcers develop in the mouth, nose, and muzzle of severely affected animals. Mucous or mucopurulent nasal discharges are conspicuous in some animals; others

cough throughout the course of the disease. Disturbances in distribution of body heat may be observed by touching; the ears, muzzle, and extremities may be cold, while other parts of the body may be very warm. The nasal and oral mucosae are congested, varying from pink to red. The conjunctiva may be congested, but the eye is not otherwise involved. Dehydration and suspension of milk secretion and rumination occur in severe infections, and the animals so affected are weak and tend to be recumbent. Abortions, stillbirths, and mummified fetuses are common after acute attacks, even in animals that appear to be recovering. Septic metritis after abortion may result in death. In the fetus, lesions similar to those of the adult may be seen in the gastrointestinal tract. Calves born alive may be persistently infected and later succumb to mucosal disease. Congenital cerebellar hypoplasia (Fig. 8-54), cataracts, retinal atrophy, microphthalmia, optic neuritis, and malformations of the choriocapillaries have been noted in calves born to naturally and experimentally infected dams.

Lesions At necropsy, except for general dehydration and emaciation of the carcass, the principal gross lesions are found in the gastrointestinal tract. Sharply delimited, irregularly-shaped ulcers or erosions of the mucosa are found on the dental pad, palate, lateral surfaces of the tongue, and inside of the cheeks. Ulcers may also occur on the muzzle and at the external nares, although usually the nasal mucosae are merely reddened. On the mucous membrane of the pharynx, irregularly shaped ulcers of varying size may be covered by a tenacious gray exudate. Necrotic lesions may be confined to the pharynx or may extend to the larynx. Some animals develop pneumonia.

In the esophagus, the entire mucous membrane may contain shallow erosions or ulcers with sharply delimited, irregular margins and a red base (Fig. 8-55). At times, these lesions coalesce to form elongated ulcers or erosions, with necrotic material adhering to some.

The abomasal mucosa may be diffusely reddened or may contain petechiae and a few ulcers. Hemorrhages may be present in the leaves of the omasum. The mucosa of the small intestine, cecum, and colon is reddened and may contain small hemorrhages and ulcers, particularly over Peyer's patches, where necrosis of intestinal glands and lymphoid tissue reminiscent of the lesions of rinderpest is often seen. There also may be necrosis in lymph nodes and the spleen, which may contribute to immunosuppression. Necrotizing arteritis, presumably immune-mediated, develops in many organs and tissues, including the gastrointestinal tract (Fig. 8-56).

In cattle with chronic mucosal disease, there is chronic ulceration of the oral cavity as well as the skin, particularly in the perineum, skin-horn junction, and around the hooves. Lameness and deformed hooves are a clinical feature.

A peculiar skeletal disorder of cattle, termed hyena disease because the affected animal's stance resembles a hyena, is thought to be caused by bovine viral diarrhea virus. The disease, which has been seen in several

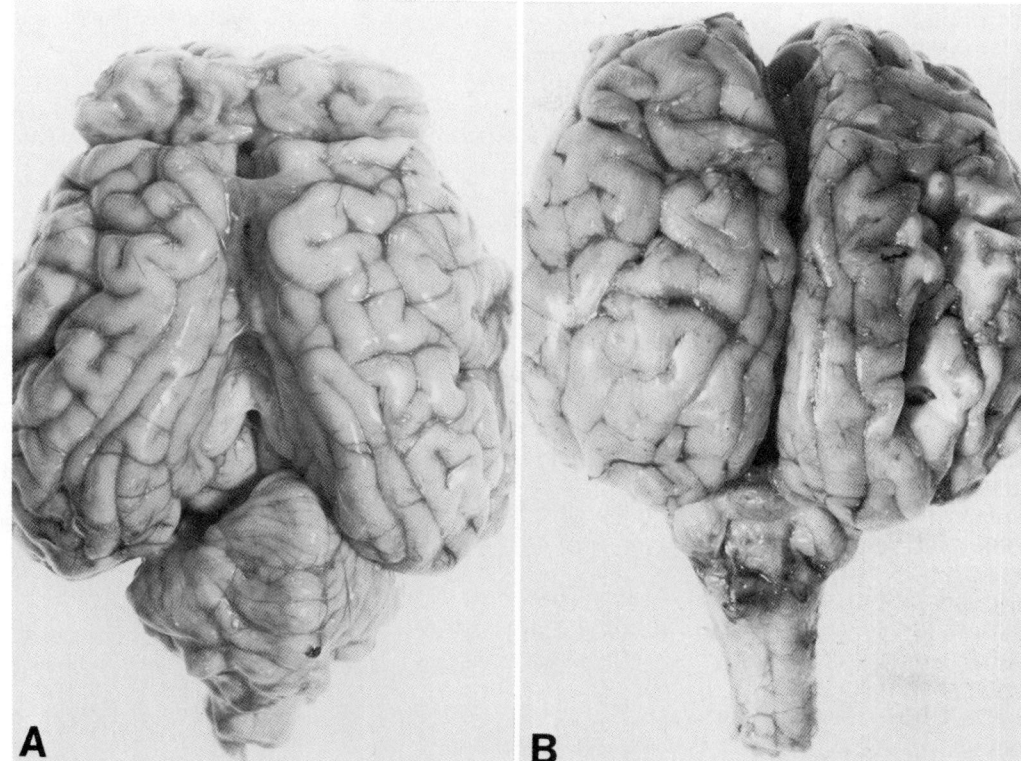

FIG. 8-54 Bovine viral diarrhea/mucosal disease. **A.** Brain of normal, uninoculated calf, 1 month old. **B.** Brain of 33-day-old blind and ataxic calf. Severe hypoplasia of cerebellum. (Courtesy of Dr. G. M. Ward and *Cornell Veterinarian.*)

countries, is characterized by reduced longitudinal growth rate of long bones, particularly the femur and tibia, resulting from failure of the cartilaginous growth plate to mature. Hemorrhages have been observed in the vaginal mucosa, subcutis generally, and the epicardium.

Diagnosis The resemblance of the lesions of virus diarrhea to the gastrointestinal lesions of rinderpest and the oral lesions of malignant catarrhal fever complicates the differential diagnosis. At present, cross-immunity and cross-serum neutralization tests can be used to distinguish rinderpest from virus diarrhea. Malignant catarrh can be differentiated by its slower spread and the characteristic ocular, nasal, and brain lesions that it produces. Viral isolation and identification provides the only precise means of diagnosis.

References

Baker JA, York CJ, Gillespie JH, et al. Virus diarrhea in cattle. Am J Vet Res 1954;15:525–531.

Baker JC. Bovine viral diarrhea virus: a review. J Am Vet Med Assoc 1987;190:1449–1458.

Bistner SI, Rubin LF, Saunders LZ. The ocular lesions of bovine viral diarrhea-mucosal disease. Pathol Vet 1970;7:275–286.

Brown TT, et al. Virus induced congenital anomalies of the bovine fetus. II. Histopathology of cerebellar degeneration (hypoplasia) induced by the virus of bovine viral diarrhea-mucosal disease. Cornell Vet 1973;63:561–578.

Brown TT, et al. Pathogenetic studies of infection of the bovine fetus with bovine viral diarrhea virus. I. Cerebellar atrophy. Vet Pathol 1974;11:486–505.

Brown TT, et al. Pathogenetic studies of infection of the bovine fetus with bovine viral diarrhea virus. II. Ocular lesions. Vet Pathol 1975;12:394–404.

Brownlie J. The pathogenesis of bovine virus diarrhoea virus infections. Rev Sci Tech 1990a;9:43–59.

Brownlie J. Pathogenesis of mucosal disease and molecular aspects of bovine virus diarrhoea virus. Vet Microbiol 1990b;23:371–382.

Brownlie J, Clarke MC. Experimental and spontaneous mucosal disease of cattle: a validation of Koch's postulates in the definition of pathogenesis. Intervirology 1993;51–59.

Carlson RG, Pritchard WR, Doyle LP. The pathology of virus diarrhea of cattle in Indiana. Am J Vet Res 1957;18:560–568.

Casaro APE, Kendrick JW, Kennedy PC. Response of the bovine fetus to bovine viral diarrhea-mucosal disease virus. Am J Vet Res 1971;32:1543–1562.

Childs T. X disease of cattle—Saskatchewan. Can J Comp Med Vet Sci 1970;10:316.

Ellis JA, Davis WC, Belden EL, et al. Flow cytofluorimetric analysis of lymphocyte subset alterations in cattle infected with bovine viral diarrhea virus. Vet Pathol 1988;25:231–236.

Espinasse J, Parodi AL, Constantin A, et al. Hyena disease in cattle: a review. Vet Rec 1986;118:328–330.

Hjerpe CA. Atypical bovine virus diarrhea. J Am Vet Med Assoc 1964;144:1278–1293.

Jewett CJ, Kelling CL, Frey ML, et al. Comparative pathogenicity of selected bovine viral diarrhea virus isolates in gnotobiotic lambs. Am J Vet Res 1990;51:1640–1644.

Kahrs RF, Scott FW, de Lahunta A. Bovine viral diarrhea-mucosa disease, abortion and congenital cerebellar hypoplasia in a dairy herd. J Am Vet Med Assoc 1970;156:851–857.

Kahrs RF, Scott FW, de Lahunta A. Congenital cerebellar hypoplasia and ocular defects in calves following bovine viral diarrhea-

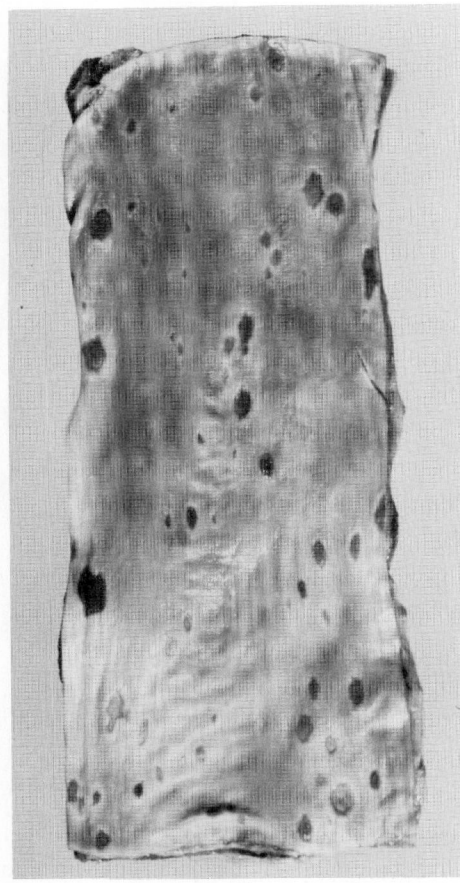

FIG. 8-55 Bovine viral diarrhea/mucosal disease. Esophageal ulcers in an Angus steer. (Courtesy of Dr. W. J. Hadlow.)

mucosal disease infection in pregnant cattle. J Am Vet Assoc 1970;156:1443–1450.

Kent TH, Moon HW. The comparative pathology of some enteric diseases. Vet Pathol 1973;10:414–469.

Lambert G, Fernelius AL, Cheville NF. Experimental bovine viral diarrhea in neonatal calves. J Am Vet Med Assoc 1969;154:181–189.

Olafson P, McCallum AD, Fox FH. An apparently new transmissible disease of cattle. Cornell Vet 1946;36:205–213.

Olafson P, Rickard CG. Further observations on the virus diarrhea (new transmissible disease) of cattle. Cornell Vet 1947;37:104–106.

Pellerin C, van den Hurk J, Lecomte J, et al. Identification of a new group of bovine viral diarrhea virus strains associated with severe outbreaks and high mortalities. Virology 1994;203:260–268.

Pritchard WR, Bunnell D, Moses HE, et al. Virus diarrhea of cattle in Indiana. Ann Rep Purdue Agric Exper Sta 1954.

Pritchard WR, Taylor DB, Moses HE, et al. A transmissible disease affecting the mucosae of cattle. J Am Vet Med Assoc 1956;128:1–5.

Ramsey FK, Chivers WH. Mucosal disease of cattle. North Am Vet 1953;34:629–633.

Ramsey FK. The pathology of a mucosal disease of cattle. Proc Am Vet Med Assoc 1954;162–167.

Riond J-L, Cullen JM, Godfrey VL, et al. Bovine viral virus-induced cerebellar disease in a calf. J Am Vet Med Assoc 1990;197:1631–1632.

Tarry DW, Bernal L, Edwards S. Transmission of bovine virus diarrhoea virus by blood feeding flies. Vet Rec 1991;128:82–84.

Tautz N, Thiel H-J, Dubovi EJ, et al. Pathogenesis of mucosal disease: a cytopathogenic pestivirus generated by an internal deletion. J Virol 1994;68:3289–3297.

Terpstra C, Wensvoort G. Natural infections of pigs with bovine viral diarrhoea virus associated with signs resembling swine fever. Res Vet Sci 1988;45:137–142.

Ward GM, et al. A study of experimentally induced bovine viral diarrhea-mucosal disease in pregnant cows and their progeny. Cornell Vet 1969;59:525–538.

Ward GM. Bovine cerebellar hypoplasia apparently caused by BVD-MD virus. A case report. Cornell Vet 1969;59:570–576.

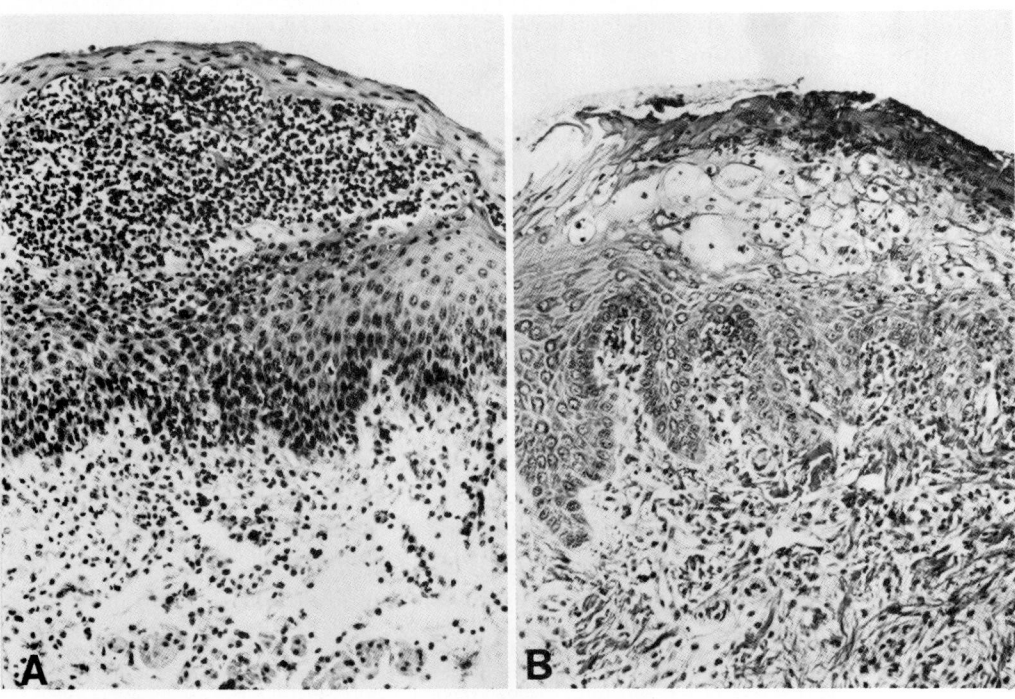

FIG. 8-56 Bovine viral diarrhea/mucosal disease. **A.** Esophagus of infected newborn calf. Necrosis of middle layers of epithelium with leukocytic infiltration. **B.** Buccal mucosa of infected premature calf with necrosis of stratum germinativum of epithelium. (Courtesy of Dr. G. M. Ward and *Cornell Veterinarian*.)

Ward GM. Experimental infection of pregnant sheep with bovine viral diarrhea-mucosal disease virus. Cornell Vet 1971;61:179–191.

Wensvoort G, Terpstra C. Bovine viral diarrhoea virus infections in piglets born to sows vaccinated against swine fever with contaminated vaccine. Res Vet Sci 1988;45:143–148.

Wilhelmsen CL, Bolin SR, Ridpath JF, et al. Lesions and localization of viral antigen in tissues of cattle with experimentally induced or naturally acquired mucosal disease, or with naturally acquired chronic bovine viral diarrhea. Am J Vet Res 1991;52:269–275.

BORDER DISEASE OF SHEEP (FUZZY LAMB, HAIRY-SHAKER LAMB, HYPOMYELINOSIS CONGENITA)

Border disease is a virally-induced congenital disease named after the Welsh Border Country, in which it was first recognized as a sporadic disease of lambs in 1959. It is characterized by birth of lambs with a hairy coat, severe tremors within a month of birth, and poor growth and viability. Border disease is now known to occur worldwide; goats are also susceptible. It is caused by a virus very similar to the pestiviruses of bovine viral diarrhea and hog cholera. The latter two viruses have been shown capable of infecting sheep and causing a border disease-like syndrome. Infection in adult sheep with border disease virus is subclinical and the virus is eventually eliminated; however, in pregnant ewes the virus crosses the placenta and infects the fetus, leading to several possible outcomes. Early *in utero* infection may result in immune tolerance and birth of lambs that are permanent carriers and shedders of the virus, serving as the main source of infection to other sheep. Early infection may also lead to embryonic death and abortion. Fetuses infected before 90 days gestation, which survive and do not develop immune tolerance, develop typical border disease. Affected lambs are born with an abnormally coarse, long, and straight birthcoat, described as "hairy." This is most evident in fine-fleeced and medium-fleeced breeds. Neurologic signs include continuous tremors, tonic-clonic contraction of skeletal muscles, and uncoordinated movements. The combination of abnormal fleece and neurologic signs has led affected lambs to be termed "hairy shakers." In lambs that survive, neurologic signs and fleece abnormalities gradually resolve in the first few months of life. These lambs eliminate the virus and do not become shedders.

Lesions Microscopically, the fleece changes result from an aberrant growth and differentiation of primary hair follicles. Primary follicles are enlarged, containing enlarged primary fibers, of which a high proportion are more heavily medullated than normal. There are fewer secondary follicles. The principal lesion in the central nervous system is hypomyelinogenesis in all parts of the brain and spinal cord, although the spinal cord is more consistently affected than the brain. There is an associated increase in the number of cells, particularly glial cells in the cerebral white matter, and accumulation of lipid between the fascicles. Glial nuclei are increased in number and, in myelin stains, nerve fibers are twisted, distorted, and swollen, giving them a beaded appearance. Gitter cells are not usually conspicuous, in spite of the apparent presence of lipid in the affected neuropil. It appears that border disease virus affects the differentiation of oligodendrocytes, precluding myelina-

tion of axons; myelin that is formed is also of an abnormal chemical composition. **Grossly,** there may be hydroencephaly, an undersized cerebral cortex, and the presence of cysts or cavities in the brain and spinal cord. Changes have also been described in cerebral arteries and arterioles, which are affected by what has been termed periarteritis, with an infiltration of lymphocytes and macrophages in the adventitia, occasionally extending to the media and intima. Placental necrosis may be extensive, contributing to retarded growth rate. Depressed levels of circulating thyroid hormones have also been noted, which also may contribute to the retardation of growth.

References

Anderson CA, Sawyer M, Higgins RJ, et al. Experimentally induced ovine border disease: extensive hypomyelination with minimal viral antigen in neonatal spinal cord. Am J Vet Res 1987;48:499–503.

Anderson CA, Higgins RJ, Waldvogel AS, et al. Tropism of border disease virus for oligodendrocytes in ovine fetal brain cell cultures. Am J Vet Res 1987;48:822–827.

Anderson CA, Higgins RJ, Smith ME, et al. Border disease. Virus-induced decrease in thyroid hormone levels with associated hypomyelination. Lab Invest 57:168–175, 1987.

Barlow RM, Dickinson AG. On the pathology and histochemistry of the central nervous system in border disease of sheep. Res Vet Sci. 6:230–237, 1965.

Barlow RM, Gardiner AC. Experiments in border disease. I. Transmission, pathology and some serological aspects of the experimental disease. J Comp Pathol Ther 1969;79:397–405.

Barlow RM, Gardiner AC, Storey IJ, et al. Experiments in border disease. II. Some aspects of the disease in the foetus. J Comp Pathol 1970;80:635–643.

Barlow RM. Experiments in border disease. IV. Pathological changes in ewes. J Comp Pathol 1972;82:151–157.

Clarke GL, Osburn BI. Transmissible congenital demyelinating encephalopathy of lambs. Vet Pathol 1978;15:68–82.

Derbyshire MB, Barlow RM. Experiments in Border disease. IX. The pathogenesis of the skin lesion. J Comp Pathol 1976;86:557–570.

Dickinson AG, Barlow RM. The demonstration of the transmissibility of border disease of sheep. Vet Rec 1967;81:114.

Durham PJK, Forbes-Faulkner JC, Poole WSH. Hairy shaker disease: preliminary studies on the nature of the agent, and the induced serological response. NZ Vet J 1975;23:236–240.

Gardiner AC, Barlow RM. Experiments in Border disease. III. Some epidemiological considerations with reference to the experimental disease. J Comp Pathol 1972;82:29–35.

Hamilton A, Timoney PJ. B.V.D. virus and border disease. Vet Rec 1972;91:468.

Hamilton A, Timoney PJ. Bovine virus diarrhea/mucosal disease virus and border disease. Res Vet Sci 1973;15:265–267.

Huck RA. Transmission of border disease in goats. Vet Rec 1973;92:151.

Hughes LE, Kershaw GF, Shaw IG. "B" or border disease: an undescribed disease of sheep. Vet Rec 1959;71:313–317.

Hussin AA, Woldehiwet Z. Border disease: a review. Vet Bull 1994;64:1131–1151.

Kelling CL, Kennedy JE, Stine LC, et al. Genetic comparison of ovine and bovine pestiviruses. Am J Vet Res 1990;51:2019–2024.

Orr MB, Barlow RM. Experiments in Border disease. X. The postnatal skin lesion in sheep and goats. J Comp Pathol 1978;88:295–302.

Orr MB, Barlow RM, Ryder ML. Histological and histochemical studies of fetal skin follicles in Border disease of sheep. Res Vet Sci 1977;22:56–61.

Plant JW, Acland HM, Gard GP. A mucosal disease virus as a cause of abortion, hairy birth coat and unthriftiness in sheep. I. Infection of pregnant ewes and observations on aborted foetuses and lambs dying before one week of age. Aust Vet J 1976;52:57–63.

Sawyer MM, Schore CE, Menzies PI, et al. Border disease in a flock of sheep: epidemiologic, laboratory, and clinical findings. J Am Vet Med Assoc 1986;189:61–65.

Stewart WC, Miller LD, Kresse JI, et al. Bovine viral diarrhea infection in pregnant swine. Am J Vet Res 1980;41:459–462.

Storey IJ, Barlow RM. Experiments in Border disease. VI. Lipid and enzyme histochemistry. J Comp Pathol 1972;82:163–170.

Terlecki S, Herbert CN, Done JT. Morphology of experimental Border disease of lambs. Res Vet Sci 1973;15:310–317.

Ward GM. Experimental infection of pregnant sheep with bovine viral diarrhea-mucosal disease virus. Cornell Vet 1971;61:179–185.

Zakarian B, Barlow RM, Rennie JC, et al. Periarteritis in experimental Border disease of sheep. II. Morphology and histochemistry of the lesion. J Comp Pathol 1976;86:477–489.

Diseases caused by arteriviruses

The arterivirus genus includes equine viral arteritis virus, porcine reproductive and respiratory syndrome virus, simian hemorrhagic fever virus, and lactic dehydrogenase virus.

EQUINE VIRAL ARTERITIS

An outbreak of an infectious disease of horses, characterized by depression, edematous swelling of the limbs, intense pink or red discoloration of the conjunctiva, palpebral edema, abortion of pregnant mares, enteritis, and pneumonic complications, was described by Doll, Knappenberger, and Bryans (1957). The filterable agent that they isolated from the affected animals produces panleukopenia, abortion, and death in experimentally infected horses. The principal lesions of the disease, described by Jones, Doll, and Bryans (1957), are degenerative and inflammatory changes in the endothelium and in the media of small arteries (Fig. 8-57). Some of the clinical features of equine viral arteritis are not unlike those described 50 or more years ago, called equine influenza ("epizootic cellulitis" or "pink eye"), or more recently, rhinopneumonitis. Early writers did not describe the microscopic lesions of epizootic cellulitis, nor did they identify the causative agent; thus, these important features cannot be compared with the lesions and virus of equine arteritis. However, equine rhinopneumonitis can be readily distinguished by its characteristic lesions and virus. The name **equine viral arteritis,** proposed for this disease, indicates both the nature of the etiologic agent and the lesions it produces.

The causative virus is generally classified as a togavirus; however, it has been recently shown to be related to the coronavirus group. Serologic surveys indicate that infection with equine viral arteritis virus is widespread, but clinical disease is not common, suggesting most infections are subclinical. The infection is rarely fatal, but up to 80% of pregnant mares may abort during or shortly after clinical disease. Spread is primarily via the respiratory route, although venereal transmission by carrier stallions can also occur.

Lesions The gross lesions in animals experimentally infected with the equine arteritis virus consist of congestion, edema, and petechiae in the conjunctiva, nasal mucosa, pharynx, larynx, and guttural pouches; edema of the subcutis of the legs and near sites of inoculation; hydrothorax and petechiae in the pleura; edema in the mediastinum, base of the heart, pericardium, and the interlobular pulmonary septa; edema and enlargement of the mediastinal lymph nodes; petechiae on the endocardium and epicardium; distention of the pericardial sac with fluid; and edema and petechiae in the mesentery, particularly along the course of the ileocecalcolic and anterior mesenteric arteries. In addition, the peritoneal cavity often contains an excessive amount of fluid, sometimes as much as 8 to 10 L; petechiae are commonly found on the visceral as well as the parietal peritoneum and omentum; the mesenteric lymph nodes are large and edematous, some contain hemorrhages; and the walls of the small intestine, cecum, and colon are often edematous and sometimes bloody in appearance. The distribution of edema in the intestine is characteristic; segments 1 to 3 feet long that are slightly to severely edematous alternate with segments of normal thickness. The mucosa over the edematous segments of intestine is rugose and the lumen is constricted. In the cecum, submucosal edema is often more severe at the apex than at the base or in other parts. Edema and petechiae may also be observed in the broad ligament and elsewhere. Hemorrhages into the adrenal cortex are frequently found.

The microscopic lesions confirm the presence of widespread edema, vascular dilation, and to a smaller extent, hemorrhages (Fig. 8-57). Generally, the veins are fully distended with blood and the lymphatic vessels with lymph, but otherwise they are not affected. The small arteries throughout the body, however, show severe changes, especially in those tissues that exhibit gross lesions.

The most severe arterial lesions are usually seen in the submucosa of the cecum and colon. The earliest change is manifested by replacement of small parts of the arterial media by homogeneous eosinophilic material. This displaces the nuclei and cytoplasm of the muscular coat of the artery and is usually accompanied by edema and some cellular infiltration in the adventitia. In more advanced lesions, tiny areas of necrosis appear in the media, either as small foci involving a segment of the muscular coat, or as more extensive, concentric zones of necrosis in the outer layers. This is accompanied by leukocytic infiltration into both the adventitia and the media. Scattered bits of nuclear chromatin are also in evidence in these areas.

Estes and Cheville (1970) have described the ultrastructure of the vascular lesions as predominantly endothelial cell damage characterized by dilation of cisternae, appearance of ribosome-like particles within cisternae of endoplasmic reticulum, and the presence of viral particles 58 nm in diameter within cytoplasmic vacuoles. Swelling of endothelial cells and platelet thrombi often obliterate capillary lumina. Edema appears to be the direct result of injury to capillaries. The investigators suggested that degeneration of smooth muscle cells was a secondary lesion not associated with direct viral injury.

No specific lesions are present in aborted fetuses; the abortion results from generalized vascular disease in the mare or necrotizing myometritis, which may occur independently of generalized vascular disease (Coignoul and Cheville, 1984).

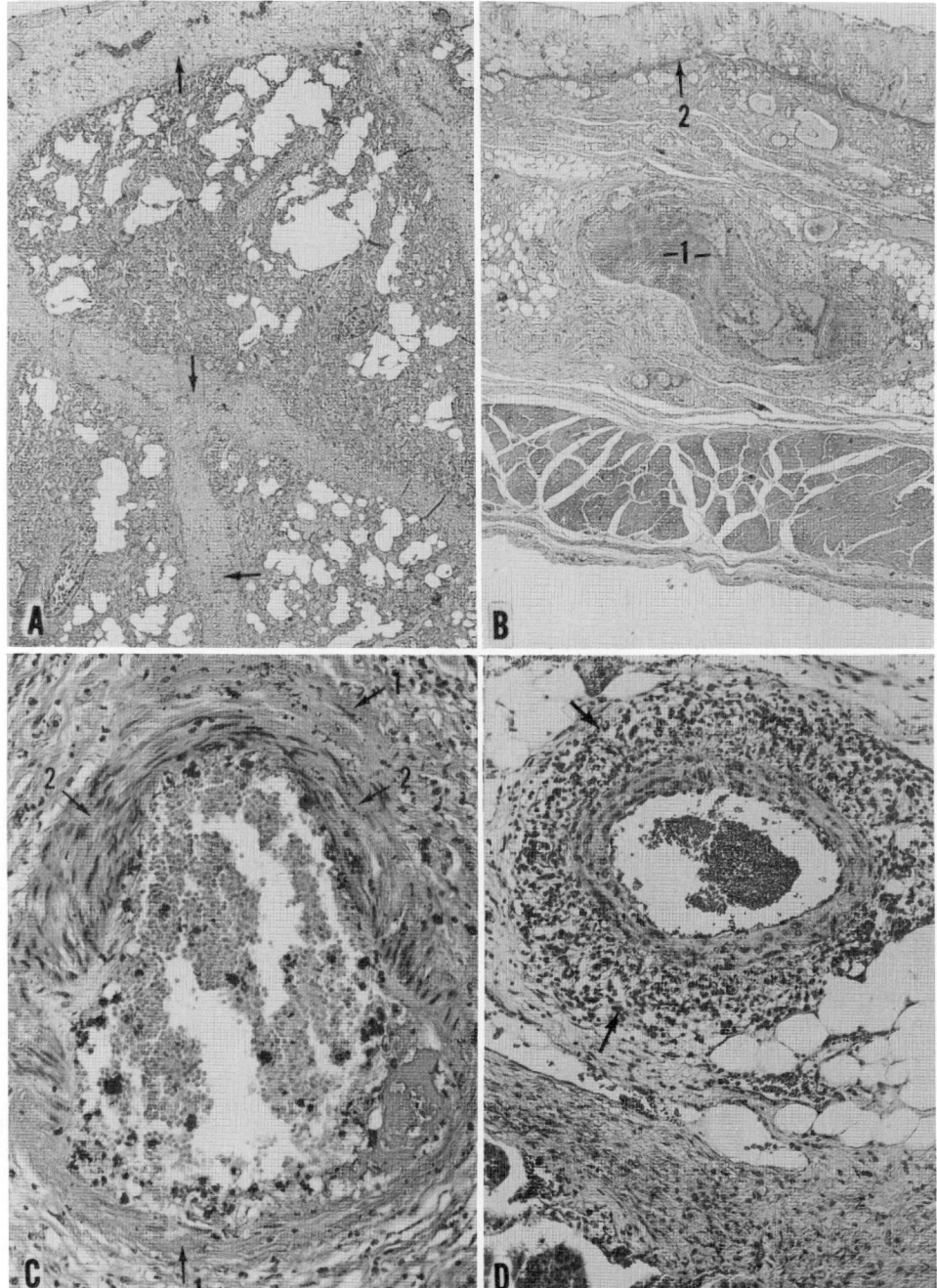

FIG. 8-57 Equine viral arteritis. **A.** Edema of pleura and interlobular septa *(arrows)* (× 15). **B.** Thrombosis *(1)* of submucosal artery in infarcted segment of small intestine. Muscularis mucosa *(2)* separates necrotic mucosa and the congested, edematous submucosa. **C.** Early necrotizing lesion in media of artery in submucosa of cecum. Cellular debris and homogeneous eosinophilic material replaces media *(2)*. **D.** Affected artery in adrenal capsule. Note intense infiltration of adventitia by lymphocytes *(arrows)*, and concentric loss of cells of media. (Courtesy of the Armed Forces Institute of Pathology; contributed by Dr. E. R. Doll.)

Diagnosis The microscopic lesions of equine viral arteritis are characteristic enough to distinguish the disease from equine rhinopneumonitis, in which the characteristic lesions include foci of necrosis in lung, liver, and lymph nodes, with intranuclear inclusion bodies.

The inflammatory lesions in the small arteries are observed in the adult horse in equine viral arteritis, but the necrotizing lesions and intranuclear inclusions of equine rhinopneumonitis are usually only found in the aborted fetus. The viruses of both diseases grow and produce cytopathogenic effects in monolayer cultures of renal cells of several species. This should permit more effective identification of the respective viruses in order to further confirm the specific diagnosis.

References

Bryans JT, Doll ER, Crowe EW, et al. The blood picture and thermal reaction in experimental, uncomplicated equine viral arteritis. Cornell Vet 1957;47:42–52.

Coignoul FL, Cheville NF. Pathology of maternal genital tract, placenta, and fetus in equine viral arteritis. Vet Pathol 1984;21:333–340.

Crawford TB, Henson JB. Viral arteritis of horses. Adv Exp Med Biol 1972;22:175–183.

den Boon JA, Snijder EJ, Chirnside ED, et al. Equine arteritis virus is not a togavirus but belongs to the coronaviruslike superfamily. J Virol 1991;65:2910–2920.

Doll ER, Bryans JT, McCollum WH, et al. Isolation of a filterable agent causing arteritis of horses and abortion by mares. Its differentiation from the equine abortion (influenza) virus. Cornell Vet 1957;47:3–41.

Doll ER, Knappenberger RE, Bryans JT. An outbreak of abortion caused by the virus of equine arteritis. Cornell Vet 1957;47: 69–75.

Estes PC, Cheville NF. The ultrastructure of vascular lesions in equine viral arteritis. Am J Pathol 1970;58:235–253.

Jones TC, Doll ER, Bryans JT. The lesions of equine viral arteritis. Cornell Vet 1957;47:52–68.

McCollum WH, Doll ER, Wilson JC, et al. Propagation of equine arteritis virus in monolayer cultures of equine kidney. Am J Vet Res 1961;22:731–735.

McCollum WH, Doll ER, Wilson JC, et al. Isolation and propagation of equine arteritis virus in monolayer cell cultures of rabbit kidney. Cornell Vet 1962;52:452–458.

McCollum WH, Prickett WH, Bryans JT. Temporal distribution of equine arteritis virus in respiratory mucosa, tissues and body fluids of horses infected by inhalation. Res Vet Sci 1971;12:459–464.

Timoney PJ, McCollum WH. Equine viral arteritis. Can Vet J 1987;28: 693–695.

Van der Zeijst BAM, Horzinek MC, Moennig V. The genome of equine arteritis virus. Virology 1975;68:418–425.

Wilson JC, Doll ER, McCollum WH, et al. Propagation of equine arteritis virus previously adapted to cell cultures of equine kidney in monolayer cultures of hamster kidney. Cornell Vet 1962;52: 200–205.

PORCINE REPRODUCTIVE AND RESPIRATORY SYNDROME

Porcine reproductive and respiratory syndrome (PRRS) is a newly recognized disease of pigs characterized by reproductive failure in sows, pneumonia in young swine, and preweaning mortality. It was first recognized in the United States in North Carolina, Iowa, and Minnesota in 1987 and 1988 and has since been recognized in England and several European countries. In the United States, it was first termed "**mystery swine disease**" and, in England, "**blue-eared pig disease.**" It has also been referred to as **porcine epidemic abortion and respiratory syndrome** (PEARS) and **swine infertility and respiratory syndrome** (SIRS). Viral isolates from differing outbreaks in the United States and Europe are related, but not antigenically identical. European isolates are often referred to as the **Lelystad virus,** after the first isolate by the Dutch Central Veterinary Institute. The agent is classified as an arterivirus.

The syndrome is still not well-defined; the clinical signs and severity of the infection have been variable. The principal manifestation is late-term abortion, stillbirths, premature farrowings, and the birth of weak piglets. The incidence can range from 3% to 80%. Affected sows may be slow to return to normal production. Other signs in sows and boars include fever, inappetence, lethargy, and labored breathing. In Britain, patchy bluish or reddish discoloration of the skin is seen. Mortality rates in adults are low. Clinical signs, particularly respiratory distress, are much more severe in young piglets, which also exhibit conjunctivitis, periorbital edema, and a poor growth rate. Mortality rates in piglets may approach 100%. In Britain, diarrhea is reportedly a feature of the disease.

A variety of pathologic features have been described, but the picture is not clearly defined. The exact basis for abortion is not clear. No specific lesions have been noted in the placenta or in fetuses. The consistent microscopic feature in field cases and experimentally infected piglets is an interstitial pneumonia characterized by extensive thickening of the alveolar septae with presence of mononuclear cells and interlobular edema. Exudation of lymphocytes, histiocytes, and plasma cells into alveoli has been described, but some reports describe a loss of alveolar macrophages. Hypertrophy and hyperplasia of type II pneumocytes has also been described in some reports. There may be necrosis and squamous metaplasia of airway epithelium with an associated mononuclear infiltration from the nasal passages through the lung. Lymphoid depletion in the thymus, spleen, and lymph nodes is also reported. Meningeal vasculitis, enteritis, and lymphocytic accumulations in the myocardium and kidney, as well as other lesions, have been seen, but it is not known whether they are specific for this disease. Secondary infections are common in young piglets and may contribute to mortality.

References

Collins JE, et al. Isolation of swine infertility and respiratory syndrome virus (isolate ATCC VR-2332) in North America and experimental reproduction of the disease in gnotobiotic pigs. J Vet Diagn Invest 1992;4:117–126.

Done SH, Paton DJ. Porcine reproductive and respiratory syndrome: clinical disease, pathology and immunosuppression. Vet Rec 1995;136:32–35.

Gordon SC. Effects of blue-eared pig disease on a breeding and fattening unit. Vet Rec 1992;130:513–514.

Goyal SM. Porcine reproductive and respiratory syndrome. J Vet Diagn Invest 1993;5:656–664.

Halbur PG, Paul PS, Vaughn EM, et al. Experimental reproduction of pneumonia in gnotobiotic pigs with porcine respiratory coronavirus isolate AR310. J Vet Diagn Invest 1993;5:184–188.

Hopper SA, White MEC, Twiddy N. An outbreak of blue-eared pig disease (porcine reproductive and respiratory syndrome) in four pig herds in Great Britain. Vet Rec 1992;131:140–144.

Kay RM, Done SH, Paton DJ. Effect of sequential porcine reproductive and respiratory syndrome and swine influenza on the growth and performance of finishing pigs. Vet Rec 1994;135:199–204.

Morrison RB, et al. Serologic evidence incriminating a recently isolated virus (ATCC VR-2332) as the cause of swine infertility and respiratory syndrome (SIRS). J Vet Diagn Invest 1992;4:186–188.

Anonymous. Porcine reproductive and respiratory syndrome (PRRS or blue-eared pig disease). Vet Rec 1992;130:87–89.

Sangar DV, Rowlands DJ, Brown F. Encephalomyocarditis virus antibodies in sera from apparently normal pigs. Vet Rec 1977;100:240–241.

Wensvoort G, Terpstra C, Pol J. "Blue ear" disease of pigs. [letter] Vet Rec 1991;128:574.

White M. "Blue ear" pig disease. [letter] Vet Rec 1991;128:574.

SIMIAN HEMORRHAGIC FEVER

Simian hemorrhagic fever is a highly fatal infectious disease of monkeys. The disease, which has only been reported in Old World primates of the genus *Macaca (M. mulatta, M. fascicularis, M. arctoides)*, has occurred in primate colonies in the United States, England, and Russia. The virus can be carried by patas monkeys (*Erythrocebus patas*), African green monkeys (*Cercopithecus aethiops*) and baboons (*Papio* species). Clinical signs include rapid onset, fever, facial edema, cyanosis, anorexia, dehydration, epistaxis, melena, and cutaneous, subcutaneous, and retrobulbar hemorrhage.

The course runs 10 to 15 days, and the mortality rate is high.

Lesions The gross and microscopic lesions are dominated by hemorrhage, which may be found in almost any organ or tissue, although most constantly in the skin, nasal mucosa, lung, gastrointestinal tract, perirenal tissues, renal capsule, adrenal gland, and periocular tissues. There is severe splenomegaly and necrosis of lymphocytic follicles of the spleen, lymph nodes, tonsils, and Peyer's patches. Thrombi are often seen in small veins and capillaries. Degenerative changes may occur in the liver, kidney, brain, and bone marrow; these changes are believed to be caused by blood stasis and hypoxia.

References

Abilgaard C, et al. Simian hemorrhagic fever: studies of coagulation and pathology. Am J Trop Med Hyg 1975;24:537–544.

Allen AM, et al. Simian hemorrhagic fever. II. Studies in pathology. Am J Trop Med 1968;17:413–421.

Giddens WE Jr, et al. The pathogenesis of simian hemorrhagic fever: hematologic and histopathologic studies. Lab Invest 1975;32:424.

Gravell M, Palmer AE, Rodriguez M, et al. Method to detect asymptomatic carriers of simian hemorrhagic fever virus. Lab Anim Sci 1980;30:988–991.

London WT. Epizootiology, transmission and approach to prevention of fatal simian hemorrhagic fever in rhesus monkeys. Nature 1977;268:344–345.

Palmer AE, et al. Simian hemorrhagic fever. I. Clinical and epizootiologic aspects of an outbreak among quarantined monkeys. Am J Trop Med 1968;17:404–412.

Tauraso NM, et al. Simian hemorrhagic fever. III. Isolation and characterization of a viral agent. Am J Trop Med Hyg 1968;17:422–431.

Tauraso NM, Kalter SS, Ratner JJ, et al. Simian hemorrhagic fever. In: Goldsmith EI, Moor-Jankowski J, ed. Medical primatology. Basel: Karger 1971.

Trousdale MD, Trent DW, Shelokov A. Simian hemorrhagic fever virus: a new togavirus (39111). Proc Soc Exp Biol Med 1975;150:707–711.

Wood O, Tauraso N, Liebhaber H. Electron microscopic study of tissue cultures infected with simian haemorrhagic fever virus. J Gen Virol 1970;7:129–136.

LACTIC DEHYDROGENASE VIRUS (LDV)

In mice, LDV causes a chronic subclinical infection with lifelong viremia. The only identifiable abnormality induced by infection is an up to tenfold increase in serum lactic dehydrogenase level and increases in levels of serum isocitric dehydrogenase, malic dehydrogenase, glutamic dehydrogenase, and glutathione reductase. The cause of the increased serum enzyme levels results from an interference with enzyme clearance systems. Serum enzyme levels fall to normal after about 2 weeks. Circulating virus antibody complexes lead to the development of immune-complex glomerulonephritis late in the infection. Some strains of the virus have been shown to cause polioencephalomeylitis or leukoencephalomyelitis in particular strains of mice.

References

Notkins AL. Lactic dehydrogenase virus. Bacteriol Rev 1965;29:143–160.

Notkins AL. Enzymatic and immunologic alterations in mice infected with lactic dehydrogenase virus. Am J Pathol 1971;64:733–746.

Riley V, Lilly F, Huerto E, et al. Transmissible agent associated with 26 types of experimental mouse neoplasms. Science 1960;132:545–547.

Stroop WG, Brinton MA. Mouse strain-specific central nervous system lesions associated with lactate dehydrogenase-elevating virus infection. Lab Invest 1983;49:334–345.

PARAMYXOVIRIDAE

Viruses classified in the family *Paramyxoviridae* (para = alongside, myxo = mucus) are pleomorphic, enveloped viruses, with RNA occurring as a single negative-sense molecule with a molecular weight of 5 to 7×10^6. The virions may be spherical or filamentous. The principal members of the family are listed in Table 8-8. The viruses grouped in the genus paramyxovirus all contain neuroaminidase, whereas viruses in the other genuses do not. Those in the genus morbillivirus are antigenically related and induce similar diseases. The family contains many important pathogens for domestic and wild animals and humans.

Diseases caused by paramyxoviruses

The genus paramyxovirus currently contains the viruses that cause mumps in children, Newcastle disease in chickens, and parainfluenza viruses, which infect several species.

PARAINFLUENZA

The parainfluenza viruses are important respiratory pathogens (Figs. 8-58, 8-59, and 8-60) of animals and humans, especially the young. The numerous isolates are subdivided into four types or groups, which contain many related viruses of varying virulence.

Parainfluenza-1 These viruses have been recovered from humans, rats, mice, rabbits, monkeys, and swine.

TABLE 8-8 *Paramyxoviridae*

Paramyxoviruses

Newcastle disease
Mumps
Parainfluenza-1 (human, murine) (Sendai)
Parainfluenza-2 (human, simian, canine)
Parainfluenza-3 (human, simian, bovine, ovine)
Parainfluenza-4 (human)
Avian paramyxoviruses (types 2–9)

Morbilliviruses

Measles
Canine distemper
Rinderpest
Peste-des-petits (ruminants)
Phocine distemper (seals)
Cetacean distemper (porpoises, dolphins)
Equine morbillivirus ?

Pneumoviruses

Respiratory syncytial virus (human)
Pneumonia virus of mice

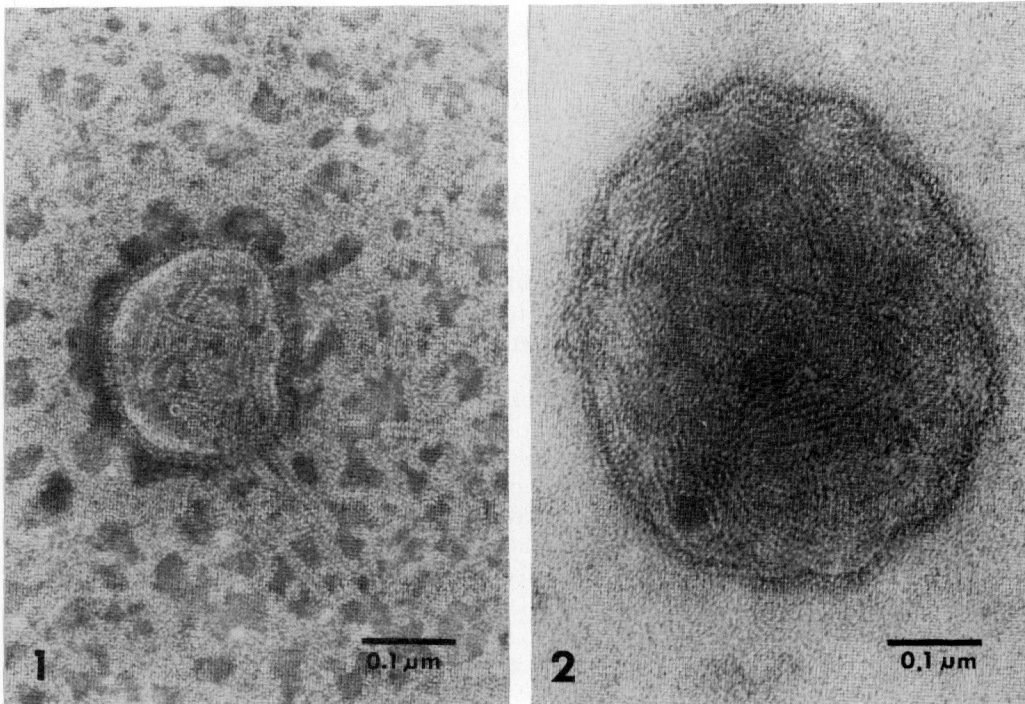

FIG. 8-58 Bovine parainfluenza-3 virus. *1* and *2,* Ultrastructure of virion containing filamentous nucleocapsids. (From McLean AM, Doane FW. The morphogenesis and cytopathology of bovine parainfluenza type 3 virus. J Gen Virol 1971;12:271. Courtesy of Cambridge University Press.)

In children, the three viruses, parainfluenza-1, parainfluenza-2, and parainfluenza-3, are a major cause of upper respiratory disease (croup) as well as pneumonia and bronchiolitis. The prototype virus (Sendai virus), or initial isolate, was recovered from a laboratory mouse. This agent is widespread in laboratory rats and mice, and although infection is usually subclinical, it can cause serious respiratory disease with high rates of mortality, especially when introduced into naive colonies. The virus invades respiratory epithelium from the nasal cavity to alveolar lining cells, resulting in necrosis. A lymphocytic inflammatory response, which may persist long after recovery, surrounds and infiltrates the airways. Regeneration and repair rapidly follows the acute stage and is characterized by marked hyperplasia and often squamous metaplasia of bronchial epithelium and of alveolar lining cells. Multinucleated cells may develop in the respiratory mucosa, and intranuclear and intracytoplasmic eosinophilic inclusion bodies may be present in bronchial epithelial cells.

References

Appell LH, Kovatch RM, Reddecliff JM, et al. Pathogenesis of Sendai virus infection in mice. Am J Vet Res 1971;32:1835–1841.

Burek JD, Zurcher C, Van Nunen MCJ, et al. A naturally occurring epizootic caused by Sendai virus in breeding and aging rodent colonies. II. Infection in the rat. Lab Anim Sci 1977;27:963–971.

Parker JC, Tennant RW, Ward TG, et al. Enzootic Sendai virus infections in mouse breeder colonies within the United States. Science 1964;146:936–938.

Rao GN, Haseman JK, Edmondson J. Influence of viral infections on body weight, survival, and tumor prevalence in Fischer 344/NCr rats on two-year studies. Lab Anim Sci 1989;39:389–393.

Zurcher C, Burek JD, Van Nunen MCJ, et al. A naturally occurring epizootic caused by Sendal virus in breeding and aging rodent colonies. I. Infection in the mouse. Lab Anim Sci 1977;27:955–962.

Parainfluenza-2 These viruses have been recovered from humans, monkeys, and dogs. The prototype of this group was recovered from a monkey and is called simian virus 5 (SV5). Canine parainfluenza-2 virus causes upper respiratory disease of dogs, especially in kennels, and is considered one of the key causes of the "kennel cough" syndrome. Infection is manifested by coughing associated with rhinitis, tracheitis, bronchitis, and less often, conjunctivitis and bronchopneumonia. Multinucleated giant cells and cytoplasmic inclusion bodies have been described in tissue culture (Crandell and others, 1968). An isolate of a canine parainfluenza virus from a dog with posterior paresis has been shown experimentally to cause encephalitis and hydrocephalus. Other parainfluenza viruses have also been shown to cause encephalitis and hydrocephalus if inoculated into experimental animals. One strain of mumps virus has been shown in suckling hamsters to affect ependymal and choroid plexus cells, causing aqueductal stenosis that results in hydrocephalus.

References

Appel MJC, Percy DH. SV 5–like parainfluenza virus in dogs. J Am Vet Med Assoc 1970;156:1778–1781.

Baumgärtner W, Krakowka S, Durchfeld B. In vitro cytopathogenicity

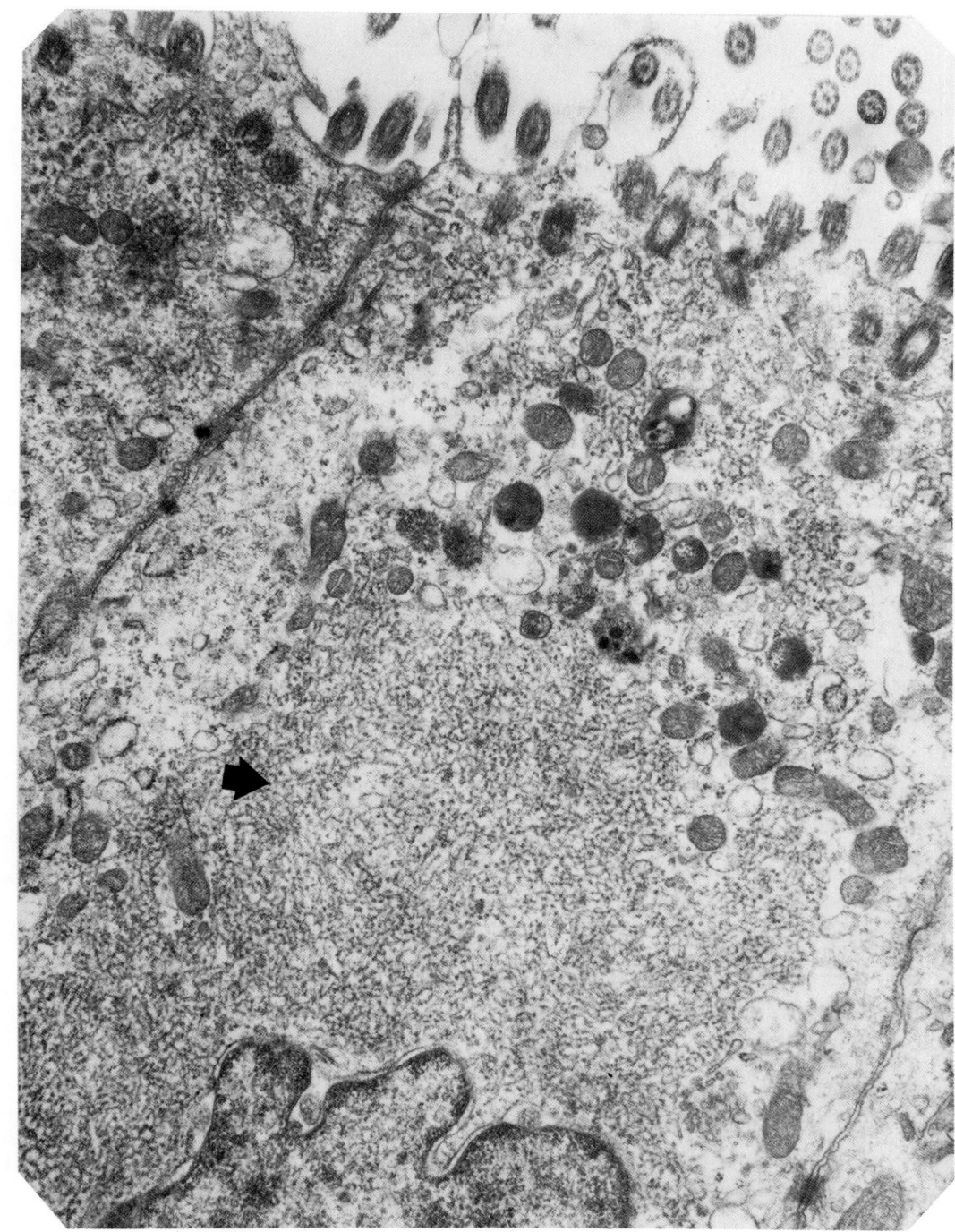

FIG. 8-59   Bovine parainfluenza-3 virus. Infected bovine ciliated cell; aggregate of viral nucleocapsids, filamentous structures about 18 nm in diameter *(arrow)*. (Courtesy of Dr. K-S, Tsai and *Infection and Immunity.)*

and in vivo virulence of two strains of canine parainfluenza virus. Vet Pathol 1991;28:324–331.

Baumgärtner WK, Krakowka S, Koestner A, et al. Acute encephalitis and hydrocephalus in dogs caused by canine parainfluenza virus. Vet Pathol 1982;19:79–92.

Binn LN, Lazar EC. Comments on epizootiology of parainfluenza SV5 in dogs. J Am Vet Med Assoc 1970;156:1774–1777.

Bittle JL, Emery JB. The epizootiology of canine parainfluenza. J Am Vet Med Assoc 1970;156:1771–1773.

Crandell RA, Brumlow WB, Davison VE. Isolation of a parainfluenza virus from sentry dogs with upper respiratory disease. Am J Vet Res 1968;29:2141–2147.

Cornwell HJC, et al. Isolation of parainfluenza virus SV5 from dogs with respiratory disease. Vet Rec 1976;98:301–302.

Evermann JF, Lincoln JD, McKiernan AJ. Isolation of a paramyxovirus from the cerebrospinal fluid of a dog with posterior paresis. J Am Vet Med Assoc 1980;177:1132–1134.

Parainfluenza-3   This virus infection (Figs. 8-58, 8-59, and 8-60) has been demonstrated in humans, cat-

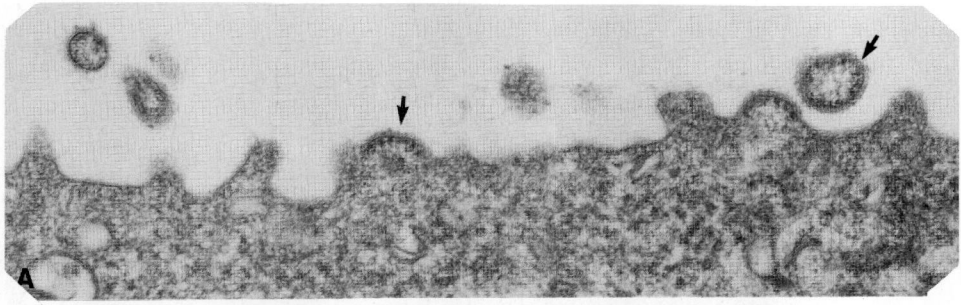

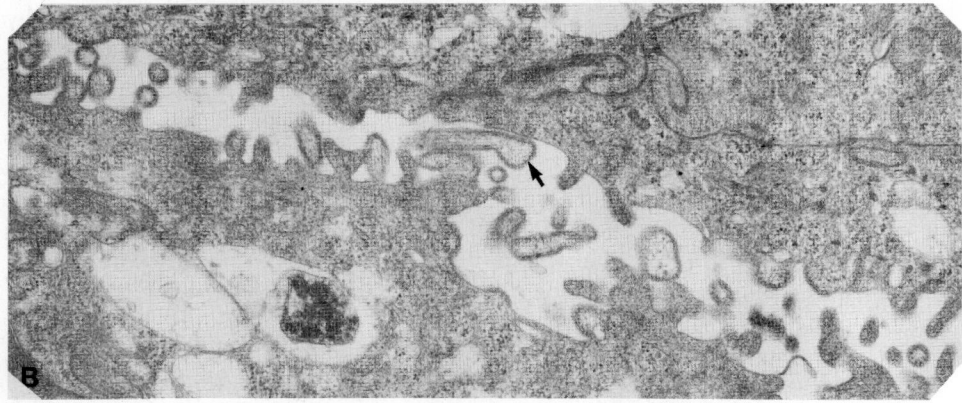

FIG. 8-60 Bovine parainfluenza-3 virus. Viral particles *(arrows)* and virus budding from cell membranes *(arrows)* in bovine cell from lining of small bronchiole. (Courtesy of Dr. K-S, Tsai and *Infection and Immunity.)*

tle, sheep, pigs, dogs, cats, monkeys, apes, guinea pigs, and rats. Infection in cattle and sheep is common, where uncomplicated disease is characterized by a short course of fever, rhinitis with nasal discharge, lacrimation, coughing, and dyspnea. Interstitial pneumonia with proliferation of septal cells and bronchiolar and alveolar epithelium, and multinucleated cells with both intranuclear and cytoplasmic eosinophilic inclusions may occur. The importance of bovine and ovine parainfluenza-3 infection is its predisposing to other respiratory pathogens, particularly *Pasteurella hemolytica,* which causes **shipping fever.**

References

Carter ME, Hunter R. Isolation of parainfluenza type 3 virus from sheep in New Zealand. NZ Vet J 1970;18:226–227.

Dawson PS, Darbyshire JH, Lamont PH. The inoculation of calves with parainfluenza 3 virus. Res Vet Sci 1965;6:108–113.

Frank GH, Marshall RG. Parainfluenza-3 virus infection of cattle. J Am Vet Med Assoc 1973;163:858–860.

Gale C. Role of parainfluenza-3 in cattle. J Dairy Sci 1970;53:621–625.

Hamdy AH. Association of myxo-virus parainfluenza-3 with pneumoenteritis of calves: virus isolation. Am J Vet Res 1966;27:981–986.

Hore DE, Stevenson RG. Respiratory infection of lambs with an ovine strain parainfluenza type 3. Res Vet Sci 1969;10:342–350.

Jones EE, Alford PL, Reingold AL, et al. Predisposition to invasive pneumococcal illness following parainfluenza type 3 virus infection in chimpanzees. J Am Vet Med Assoc 1984;185:1351–1353.

Martin DP, Kaye HS. Epizootic of parainfluenza-3 virus infection in gibbons. J Am Vet Med Assoc 1983;183:1185–1187.

McLean AM, Doane FW. The morphogenesis and cytopathology of bovine parainfluenza type 3 virus. J Gen Virol 1971;12:271–279.

Omar AR, Jennings AR, Betts AO. The experimental disease produced in calves by the J121 strain of parainfluenza virus type 3. Res Vet Sci 1966;7:379–388.

Parks JB, Post G, Thorne T, et al. Parainfluenza-3 virus infection in Rocky Mountain bighorn sheep. J Am Vet Med Assoc 1972;161:669–673.

Reisinger RC, Heddleston KI, Manthei CA. A myxovirus (SF-4) associated with shipping fever of cattle. J Am Vet Med Assoc 1959;135:147–152.

Stevenson RG, Hore DE. Comparative pathology of lambs and calves infected with parainfluenza virus type 3. J Comp Pathol 1970;80:613–618.

Timoney PJ. Recovery of parainfluenza-3 virus from acute respiratory infection in calves. Irish Vet J 1971;25:121–124.

Tsai K-S, Thomson RG. Bovine parainfluenza type 3 virus infection; ultrastructural aspects of viral pathogenesis in the bovine respiratory tract. Infect Immun 1975;11:783–803.

Woods GT, Sibinovic K, Marquis G. Experimental exposure of calves, lambs, and colostrum-deprived pigs to bovine myxovirus parainfluenza-3. Am J Vet Res 1965;26:52–56.

Parainfluenza-4 This virus has been recovered only from human patients, specifically from children and adults with mild upper respiratory disease.

Mumps Virus This virus is also a member of the paramyxovirus genus but is not a pathogen for domestic animals.

References

Hsiung GD. Parainfluenza-5 virus. Infection of humans and animal. Prog Med Virol 1972;14:241–274.

Diseases caused by morbilliviruses

The morbillivirus genus contains several very important pathogens of humans and animals (Table 8-8). Measles, canine distemper, and rinderpest are the three classic members of the group. These viruses are morphologically indistinguishable and antigenically closely related. A relationship between these three viruses was first suggested by Pinkerton, Smiley, and Anderson (1945) on the basis of pathologic similarities, before the immunologic relationship was demonstrated. The principal difference among canine distemper, rinderpest, and measles viruses is their natural hosts. Canine distemper (Figs. 8-61 and 8-62) causes natural disease in *Canidae* species (dog, wolf, fox), *Mustelidae* species (weasel, ferret, mink, badger), *Procyonidae* species (raccoon), and *Viveridae* species (Binturong). Rinderpest virus causes natural disease in species of the order *Artiodactyla* (cattle, water buffalo, camels, goats, sheep); and measles causes natural disease in primates (humans, apes, monkeys). More recently recognized morbilliviruses include phocine morbillivirus, which causes phocine distemper disease in seals; a morbillivirus that affects porpoises and dolphins (cetacean morbillivirus); and a morbillivi-

rus that caused a fatal disease in horses and humans in Australia. These latter three agents may represent newly evolved agents or the entry of previously unrecognized viruses into new hosts.

CANINE DISTEMPER

The common and serious disease of dogs, known as canine distemper, is caused by the virus originally described by Carré (1905), later studied extensively by Laidlaw and Duncan (1926), and now classified in the genus morbillivirus. The protean clinical manifestations of canine distemper have led to some confusion and difficulty in both clinical diagnosis and experimental investigation of the disease. Many febrile diseases simulate certain features of canine distemper; in fact, only

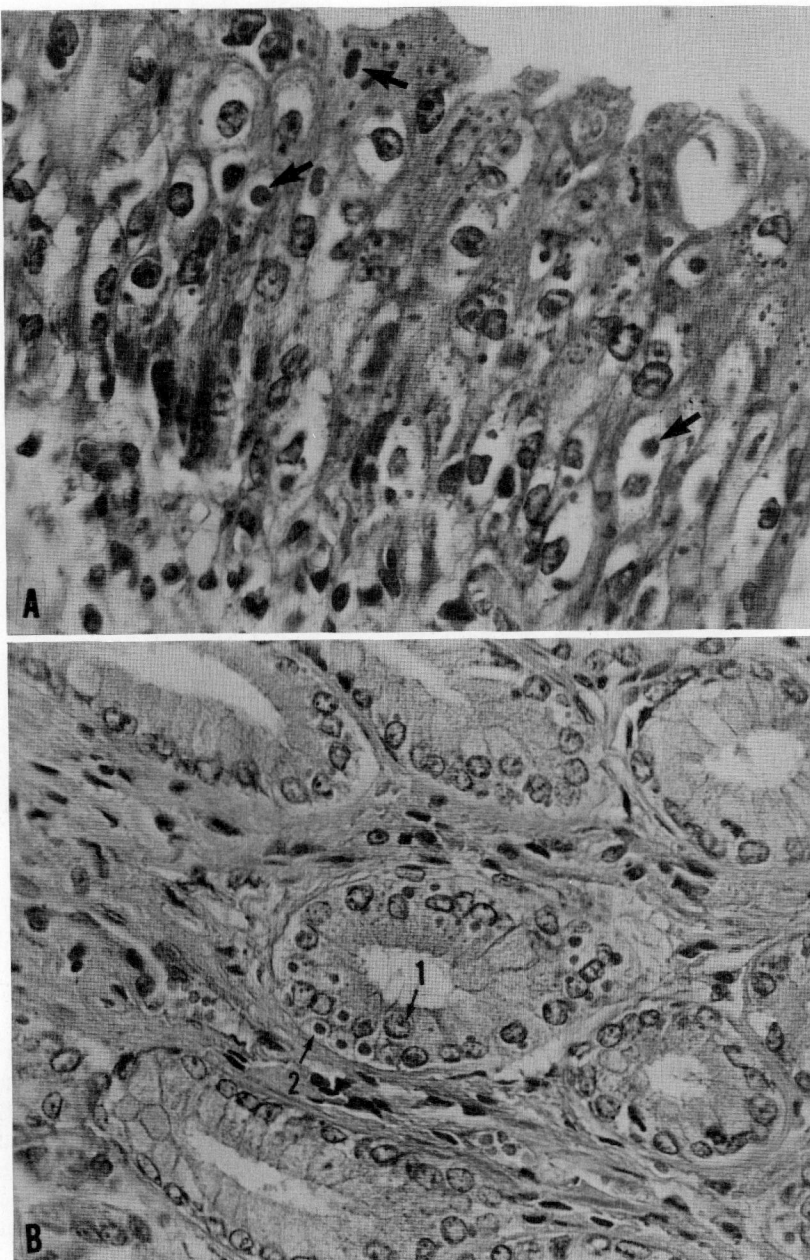

FIG. 8-61 Canine distemper. **A.** Inclusion bodies *(arrows)* in cytoplasm of epithelium of urinary bladder (× 525). (Contributed by Dr. C. L. Davis.) **B.** Intranuclear *(1)* and cytoplasmic *(2)* inclusion bodies in gastric epithelium (× 470). (Courtesy of the Armed Forces Institute of Pathology; contributed by Dr. E. E. Ruebush.)

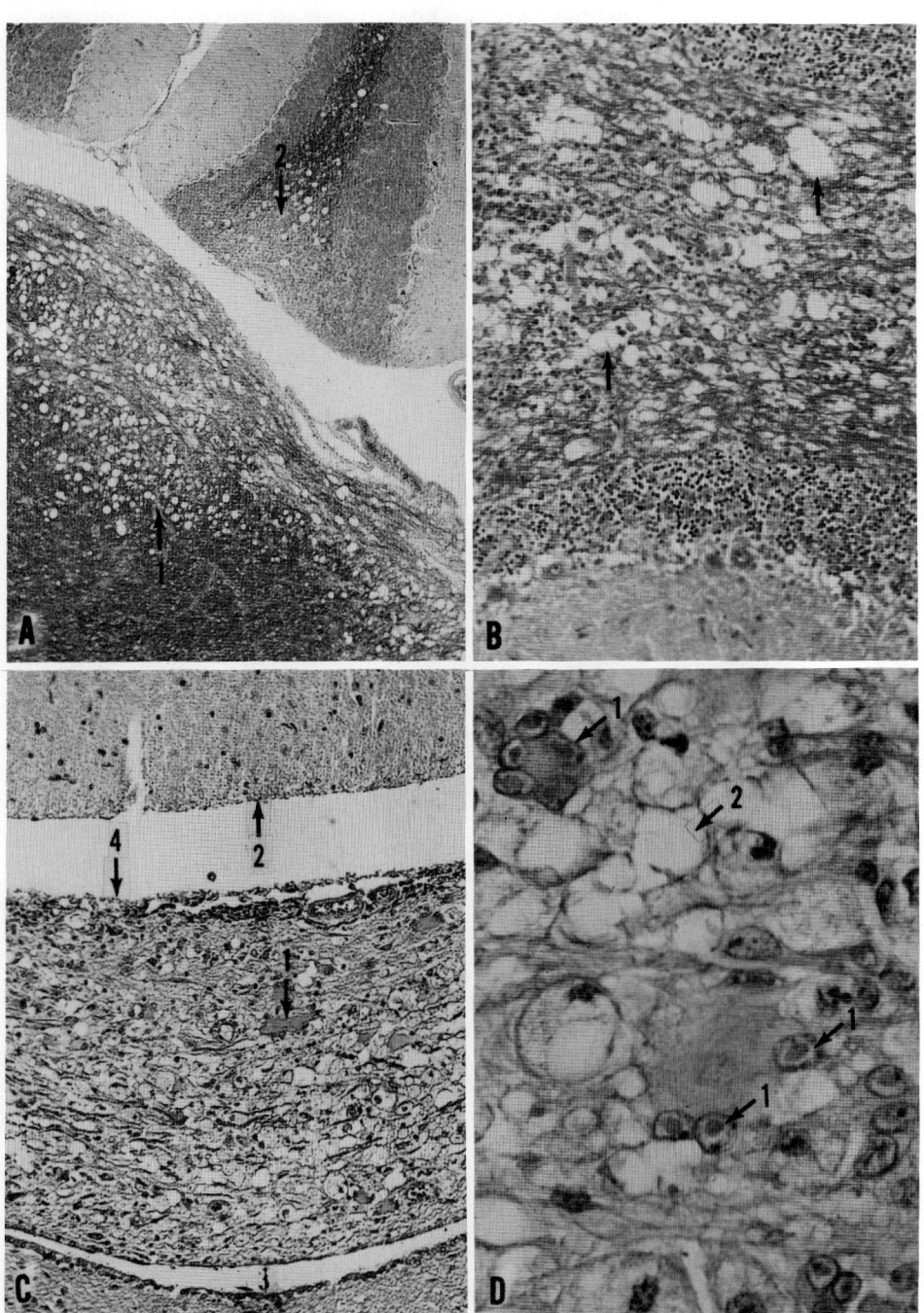

FIG. 8-62 Canine distemper. Lesions in central nervous system. **A.** Status spongiosus in brachium pontis *(1)* and medullary part of folium *(2)* of cerebellum (Weil's stain) (× 35). (Courtesy of the Armed Forces Institute of Pathology; contributed by Dr. J. R. M. Innes.) **B.** Spongy area in myelinated part of folium of cerebellum (hematoxylin and eosin stain; × 1.50). Note large irregular vacuoles *(arrows)* and increased number of cells. (Contributed by Dr. C. H. Beckman.) **C.** Lesion in anterior medullary velum (× 100). (Hematoxylin and eosin stain.) "Gemistocytic" astrocytes *(1)*, cerebellar cortex *(2)*, fourth ventricle *(3)*, and artifactually detached pia mater *(4)*. **D.** Higher magnification (× 600). Intranuclear inclusions *(1)* in gemistocytes with fused cytoplasm. Large droplets of lipid (myelin) *(2)*. (Courtesy of Armed Forces Institute of Pathology; contributed by Dr. Elihu Bond.)

in recent years has clinical differentiation of such diseases as canine hepatitis, herpesvirus, parainfluenza, and leptospirosis been possible. Not only dogs are susceptible to the virus; also susceptible are other members of the family *Canidae* (wolves, coyotes) as well as the families *Mustelidae* (ferrets, mink), *Viverridae* (Binturong), and *Procyonidae* (raccoon). Severe epizootics of a pathologically almost identical disease have been seen in harbour seals *(Phoca vitulina)* in the Baltic and North Seas. The virus recovered from seals is very similar to that of canine distemper, although not identical. It has been termed **phocid distemper virus**; dogs and mink

are susceptible. Another similar virus has been recovered from a porpoise. Squirrel monkeys have been infected by intracerebral inoculation with distemper virus.

Signs Exposure of susceptible dogs to the virus of Carré results in an acute fever, which appears after 7 or 8 days of incubation. Within 96 hours, body temperature usually drops rapidly to approximately normal levels, where it remains until the eleventh or twelfth day, when it climbs to a second peak. This diphasic fever curve is a characteristic feature of the disease. Coryza, purulent conjunctivitis, and bronchitis are manifested in varying degrees. Bronchopneumonia may occur. Very often, vesiculopustular lesions appear on the abdomen. In some cases, there is hyperkeratosis of the digital pads ("hard pad disease"). Usually, leukopenia and thrombocytopenia also develop. In many cases, diarrhea results in severe dehydration and emaciation. Manifestations of meningoencephalitis occur in about 50% of affected dogs; however, lesions are present in a much higher percentage (Fig. 8-62). Nervous signs may develop during the acute phase of the disease and continue after abatement of other signs, since they are not usually manifested until some days or weeks after the acute phase. Signs include chewing movements, excessive salivation, incoordination, circling, neuromuscular tics, continuous rhythmic movements, nystagmus, torticollis, and convulsions. Blindness and paralysis are less common nervous manifestations. Although the disease may occur in a mild, nonfatal form, most animals with severe nervous, respiratory, and enteric signs die of the infection.

In a small number of dogs which recover, the virus remains latent in the brain and may cause "old dog encephalitis" years later. This resembles the subacute sclerosing panencephalitis that occurs years after recovery from measles and is associated with the measles virus.

Pathogenesis Canine distemper virus is spread by the respiratory route with initial viral replication in respiratory epithelium and alveolar macrophages, soon spreading to the tonsils and bronchial lymph nodes. Before clinical signs appear, cell-associated virus (mostly associated with lymphocytes) circulates through the bloodstream to other organs and tissues, including the brain. Free virus (viremia) has also been demonstrated in the bloodstream. It is unclear whether the central nervous system is invaded as a result of true viremia or of invasion by cell-associated virus. Viral replication and direct damage to neurons and astrocytes occurs, as well as indirect damage to oligodendroglial cells, resulting in demyelination (Fig. 8-62). There is no evidence of direct damage to oligodendrogliocytes. The progression of the demyelinating encephalitis, however, owes its pathogenesis to the development of a local immune response similar to that of experimental allergic encephalomyelitis. The mechanism whereby "old dog encephalitis" develops is not clear. In measles-associated subacute sclerosing panencephalitis, suppressed virus remains in the central nervous system and, following some unknown stimulus, causes defective replication without development of complete viral particles but with spread of the "virus" from cell to cell. It is proposed that the suppressed virus does not express antigens on the surface of infected cells, thus allowing its persistence and escape from the immune system.

Lesions In the respiratory system, purulent or catarrhal exudate may be found over the nasal and pharyngeal mucosae. In microscopic sections, characteristic cytoplasmic and intranuclear inclusion bodies often are seen in cells associated with the exudate. These inclusions are eosinophilic when stained by hematoxylin and eosin and can be demonstrated distinctly by numerous other stains, particularly the Schorr S-3 stain. In the cytoplasm, they are round or ovoid and vary from 5 to 20 μ in diameter. They are usually homogeneous and sharply demarcated and occasionally lie in vacuoles adjacent to the nucleus. The intranuclear inclusions, which are similar to the cytoplasmic ones in appearance, cause only slight enlargement of the nucleus and little, if any, margination of the chromatin. The immunofluorescence technique may be used to demonstrate that these inclusions contain viral antigen.

In the lung, the lesions may be manifested by a purulent bronchopneumonia in which bronchi and adjacent alveoli are filled with neutrophils, mucin, and tissue debris. In early stages, the exudate may contain some blood, neutrophils, and mononuclear cells. In other cases, collections of mononuclear cells lining alveolar walls or partially filling alveoli are the only evidence of infection. In some examples of this type, multinucleated giant cells form in the bronchial lining, alveolar septa, and freely in alveoli. This form of giant-cell pneumonia is similar to that associated with measles in humans and monkeys. Cytoplasmic and, less often, intranuclear inclusions are found in these giant cells, in other mononuclear cells, and in cells of the bronchiolar and bronchial epithelium.

In the skin, particularly of the abdomen, a vesicular and pustular dermatitis may occur. The vesicles and pustules are confined to the malpighian layer of the epidermis, but some congestion of the underlying dermis is usual and lymphocytic infiltration is occasional. Nuclear or cytoplasmic inclusion bodies may be present within epithelial cells, especially those of sebaceous glands. On the foot pads, extensive proliferation of the keratin layer of the epidermis results in a clinically recognizable lesion, which is called "hard-pad disease." This lesion can develop in other diseases, e.g., toxoplasmosis, and therefore is not specific for canine distemper.

The urinary tract epithelium, particularly of the renal pelvis and bladder, may contain congested vessels and microscopically demonstrable cytoplasmic or intranuclear inclusion bodies (Fig. 8-61).

The stomach and intestines may contain large numbers of cytoplasmic and some intranuclear inclusions in the lining epithelium. Aside from these inclusions, few lesions are observed. In the large intestine, mucous exudate is often excessive; congestion and lymphocytic infiltration of the lamina propria may be demonstrable.

There is necrosis of both T-cell and B-cell areas in lymph nodes and the spleen. Rarely, multinucleated giant cells, which bear inclusion bodies, are present.

Of particular interest in the clinical diagnosis of distemper is the finding that cytoplasmic inclusions appear in some circulating neutrophils of affected dogs. The occurrence of these inclusions in leukocytes is evidence that the virus is present, but their absence is of little value in determining the absence of the virus. Less often, similar inclusions are found in circulating lymphocytes. In some cases, inclusion bodies can be demonstrated in conjunctival epithelium.

Distemper does not cause significant lesions in the liver, although inclusions may be present in biliary epithelium. The presence of viral antigen in these inclusions is demonstrable with specific immunofluorescence technique.

In the central nervous system, the canine distemper virus has an affinity for the myelinated portions of the brain and spinal cord; thus, in contrast to such infections as equine encephalomyelitis, Teschen disease, and poliomyelitis, the neurons are not primarily affected. The distribution and nature of the lesions in canine distemper, therefore, differ from those in most other viral encephalitides. The lesions of canine distemper in the nervous system were at one time thought to be caused by some other agent and were often referred to as "McIntyre's encephalitis." The lesions can be detected only by microscopic study. They vary in intensity and scope, usually in direct relation to the severity and duration of the clinical disease. The structures most constantly affected are the cerebellar peduncles (brachium pontis, brachium conjunctivum, and restiform body), the anterior medullary velum, the myelinated tracts of the cerebellum, and the white columns of the spinal cord. The subcortical white matter of the cerebrum is usually spared. The lesions are characterized by rather sharply delimited areas of destruction, particularly in the myelinated tracts of the areas mentioned. Under low-power microscopy, especially in tissue stained by Weil's method, sharply delimited holes of irregular size give the affected tracts a "spongy" appearance (status spongiosa). Increased numbers of microglia and astrocytes and, often, collections of lymphocytes in the Virchow-Robin spaces around nearby vessels are associated with this spongy appearance. Occasionally, "gitter" cells are gathered around areas of necrosis in the white matter. Gemistocytic astrocytes or "gemistocytes" figure prominently in the exudate at many points and there may be multinucleated astrocytes. Intranuclear inclusions within "gemistocytes" and certain microglia are a characteristic feature of this lesion. In the cerebrum, the lesion is somewhat similar, but the most prominent microscopic feature is the apparent increase in the number of capillaries. This appearance may result from proliferation of capillaries or, more likely, from distention and congestion of blood vessels and loss of surrounding parenchyma, causing the vasculature to appear more prominent. In many cases, lesions are limited to the cerebellar folia, the cerebellar peduncles, or the anterior medullary velum. In other cases, they are observed only in the anterior medullary velum, a delicate tract lying over the roof of the fourth ventricle.

Although overshadowed by the changes in the myelinated tracts, degenerative changes also develop in neurons, apparently resulting from both primary viral invasion and retrograde lesions secondary to axon damage. There is pyknosis, chromatolysis, gliosis, and neuronophagia. Rarely, cytoplasmic or nuclear inclusion bodies can be found in neurons. Neuronal necrosis may be present in the cerebral and cerebellar cortex, pontine and medullary nuclei, and spinal cord. In most cases, leptomeningitis, principally characterized by infiltrating lymphocytes, is present. Jubb, Saunders, and

Coates (1957) demonstrated that intraocular lesions occur in most cases of canine distemper.

In the retina, there is congestion, edema, perivascular cuffing with lymphocytes, degeneration of ganglion cells, and gliosis. Neuritis of the optic nerve with demyelination and gliosis may also be present. Intranuclear inclusions are present in glia of the retina and optic nerve. The lesions lead to retinal atrophy of all layers. Swelling and proliferation of retinal pigment epithelium is also usually present. An anterior uveitis characterized by mononuclear cell infiltration along with multinucleated giant cells is a common finding.

In so-called "old dog encephalitis", the most striking lesion in the central nervous system is marked perivascular cuffing with almost pure populations of lymphocytes. The very wide cuffs are present in both gray and white matter. There may be focal demyelination, and there is scattered necrosis of neurons. Intranuclear inclusion bodies may be found in glial cells and neurons. There is no lesion resembling canine distemper in any visceral organ. Dubielzig and associates (1981) demonstrated that the virus affects the enamel organ in developing teeth, leading to necrosis and multinucleated giant cells bearing cytoplasmic inclusion bodies. This tropism accounts for the defects in dental enamel seen in dogs that have recovered from canine distemper.

Diagnosis Postmortem diagnosis can be made on the basis of a history of the typical clinical disease and the demonstration of characteristic lesions and cytoplasmic and intranuclear viral inclusions. Immunologic staining techniques or viral isolation and identification confirms the diagnosis.

During life, clinical diagnosis can be confirmed by finding typical inclusion bodies in smears of cells of the respiratory epithelium or peripheral blood. Unfortunately, these inclusions are not present in all cases, hence their absence does not preclude the diagnosis of distemper. In dogs, toxoplasmosis often occurs in association with canine distemper. Lesions of both diseases should be sought if evidence of either infection is apparent.

References

Adams JM, et al. Old dog encephalitis and demyelinating diseases in man. Vet Pathol 1975;12:220–226.

Blixenkrone-Moller M, Svansson V, Örvell C, et al. Phocid distemper virus—a threat to terrestrial mammals? Vet Rec 1990;127:263–264.

Broadhurst J, MacLean ME, Saurino V. Nasal inclusion bodies in dog distemper. Cornell Vet 1938;28:9–15.

Cabasso VJ. Canine distemper and hardpad disease. Vet Med 1952; 47:417–423.

Carré H. Sur la maladie des jeunes chiens. Compt Rend Acad d Sc 1905;140:689–690.

Cello RM, Moulton JE, McFarland S. The occurrence of inclusion bodies in the circulating neutrophils of dogs with canine distemper. Cornell Vet 1959;49:127–146.

Cordy DR. Canine encephalomyelitis. Cornell Vet 1942;32:11–28.

Cornwell HJC, Campbell RSF, Vantsis JT, et al. Studies in experimental canine distemper. I. Clinico-pathological findings. J Comp Pathol 1965;75:3–17.

Cornwell HJC, Vantsis JT, Campbell RSF, et al. Studies in experimental canine distemper. II. Virology, inclusion body studies and haematology. J Comp Pathol Ther 1965;75:19–34.

Cosby SL, et al. Characterization of a seal morbillivirus. [letter] Nature (Lond) 1988;336:115–116.

Crook E, McNutt SH. Experimental distemper in mink and ferrets. II. Appearance and significance of histopathological changes. Am J Vet Res 1959;20:378–383.

De Monbreun WA. Histopathology of natural and experimental canine distemper. Am J Pathol 1937;13:187–212.

Dickson D. Canine distemper may be killing North Sea seals. Science 1988;241:1282.

Domingo M, et al. Morbillivirus in dolphins. [letter] Nature (Lond) 1990;348:21.

Dubielzig RR, Higgins RJ, Krakowka S. Lesions of the enamel organ of developing dog teeth following experimental inoculation of gnotobiotic puppies with canine distemper virus. Vet Pathol 1981;18:684–689.

Ducatelle R, Coussement W, Hoorens J. Demonstration of canine distemper viral antigen in paraffin sections, using an unlabeled antibody-enzyme method. Am J Vet Res 1980;41:1860–1862.

Ferry NS. Etiology of canine distemper. J Infect Dis 1911;8:399–420.

Gibson JP, Griesemer RA, Koestner A. Experimental distemper in the gnotobiotic dog. Path Vet 1965;2:1–19.

Grachev MA, et al. Distemper virus in Baikal seals. [letter] Nature (Lond) 1989;338:209.

Greene RG, Evans CA. A comparative study of distemper inclusions. Am J Hyg 1939;29:73–87.

Hartley WJ. A post-vaccinal inclusion body encephalitis in dogs. Vet Pathol 1975;11:301–312.

Hoff GL, Biglet WJ, Proctor SJ, et al. Epizootic of canine distemper virus infection among urban raccoons and gray foxes. J Wildl Dis 1974;10:423–428.

Imagawa DT. Relationships among measles, canine distemper and rinderpest viruses. Prog Med Virol 1968;10:160–193.

Johnson GC, Krakowka S, Axthelm MK. Prolonged viral antigen retention in the brain of a gnotobiotic dog experimentally infected with canine distemper virus. Vet Pathol 1987;24:87–89.

Johnson RT, et al. Measles encephalomyelitis—clinical and immunologic studies. N Engl J Med 1984;310:137–141.

Jubb KB, Saunders LZ, Coates HV. The intraocular lesions of canine distemper. J Comp Pathol Ther 1957;67:21–29.

Kennedy S. A review of the 1988 European seal morbillivirus epizootic. Vet Rec 1990;127:563–567.

Kennedy S, Smyth JA, McCullough SJ, et al. Confirmation of cause of recent seal deaths. [letter] Nature (Lond) 1988;335:404.

Kennedy S, et al. Histopathologic and immunocytochemical studies of distemper in seals. Vet Pathol 1989;26:97–103.

Kennedy S, Smyth JA, Cush PF, et al. Histopathologic and immunocytochemical studies of distemper in harbor porpoises. Vet Pathol 1991;28:1–7.

Köbl S, Schnabel H, Mikula M. [Distemper virus infection as cause of death of badgers in Austria.] Tierärztl Prax 1990;13:81–84. [Vet Bull 1991;61:5667.]

Koprowski H, et al. A study of canine encephalitis. Am J Hyg 1950;51:63–75.

Krakowka S, McCullough B, Koestner A, et al. Myelin-specific autoantibodies associated with central nervous system demyelination in canine distemper virus infection. Infect Immun 1973;8:819–827.

Krakowka S, Higgins RJ, Metzler AE. Plasma phase viremia in canine distemper virus infection. Am J Vet Res 1980;41:144–146.

Krakowka S, Higgins RJ, Koestner A. Canine distemper virus: review of structural and functional modulations in lymphoid tissues. Am J Vet Res 1980;41:284–292.

Kriesel HR. A comparative study of the manifestations and histopathology of canine distemper and experimental fox encephalitis infection in dogs. Cornell Vet 1938;28:324–330.

Laidlaw PP, Dunkin GW. Studies in dog distemper: III. The nature of the virus. J Comp Pathol Ther 1926;39:222–230.

Lincoln SD, Gorham JR, Ott RL, et al. Etiologic studies of old dog encephalitis. I. Demonstration of canine distemper viral antigen in the brain in two cases. Vet Pathol 1971;8:1–8.

Lincoln SD, Gorham JR, Davis WC, et al. Studies of old dog encephalitis. Vet Pathol 1973;10:124–129.

MacIntyre AB, Trevan DJ, Montgomerie RF. Observations on canine encephalitis. Vet Rec 1948;60:635–648.

Mahy BWJ, Barrett T, Evans S, et al. Characterization of a seal morbillivirus. [letter] Nature 1988;336:115.

McCullough B, Krakowka S, Koestner A. Experimental canine distemper virus-induced lymphoid depletion. Am J Pathol 1974;74:155–170.

McCullough B, Krakowka S, Koestner A. Experimental canine distemper virus-induced demyelination. Lab Invest 1974;31:216–222.

McGowan JP. Some observations on a laboratory epidemic principally among dogs and cats, in which the animals affected presented the symptoms of the disease called distemper. J Pathol Bact 1911;15:372–426.

Nagata T, Ochikubo F, Yoshikawa Y, et al. Encephalitis induced by a canine distemper virus in squirrel monkeys. J Med Primatol 1990;19:137–149.

Osterhaus ADME, Vedder EJ. Identification of virus causing recent seal deaths. [letter] Nature (Lond) 1988;335:20.

Osterhaus ADME, Green J, De Vries P, et al. Canine distemper virus in seals. [letter] Nature (Lond) 1988;335:403–404.

Osterhaus ADME, et al. Distemper virus in Baikal seals. [letter] Nature (Lond) 1989;338:209–210.

Perdrau JR, Pugh LP. The pathology of disseminated encephalomyelitis of the dog (the "nervous form of canine distemper"). J Pathol Bact 1930;33:79–91.

Pinkerton H, Smiley WL, Anderson WAD. Giant cell pneumonia with inclusions. A lesion common to Hecht's disease, distemper and measles. Am J Pathol 1945;21:1–23.

Richter WR, Moize SM. Ultrastructural nature of canine distemper inclusions in the urinary bladder. Pathol Vet 1970;7:346–352.

Sever JL. Persistent measles infection of the central nervous system: subacute sclerosing panencephalitis. Rev Infect Dis 1983;5:467–473.

Tajima M, Itabashi M, Motohashi T. Light and electron microscopic studies of lymph node of mink exposed to canine distemper virus. Am J Vet Res 1971;32:913–924.

Trudgett A, Lyons C, Welsh MJ, et al. Analysis of a seal and porpoise morbillivirus using monoclonal antibodies. Vet Rec 1991;128:61.

Vandevelde M, Kristensen B, Braund KG, et al. Chronic canine distemper virus encephalitis in mature dogs. Vet Pathol 1980;17:17–28.

Vandevelde M, Kristensen F, Kristensen B, et al. Immunological and pathological findings in demyelinating encephalitis associated with canine distemper virus infection. Acta Neuropathol (Berl) 1982;56:1–8. [Vet Bull 1986;56:3894.]

Warren J. The relationships of the viruses of measles, canine distemper and rinderpest. Adv Virus Res 1960;7:27–60.

Whittem JH, Blood DC. Canine encephalitis, pathological and clinical observations. Aust Vet J 1950;26:73–83.

Wisnicky W, Wipf L. Significance of inclusion bodies of distemper. Am J Vet Res 1942;3:285–288.

Wisniewski HC, Raine S, Kay WJ. Observations on viral demyelinating encephalomyelitis canine distemper. Lab Invest 1972;26:589–599.

Zurbriggen A, Vandevelde M, Dumas M. Secondary degeneration of oligodendrocytes in canine distemper virus infection in vitro. Lab Invest 1986;54:424–431.

RINDERPEST (CATTLE PLAGUE)

Rinderpest has been a serious disease of cattle from antiquity and is today the foremost cause of death in cattle in Africa and Asia; it is not present in the Western Hemisphere or in Europe. Mortality rates in cattle vary from 25% to 90%, depending on the strains of virus involved and the resistance of the animals. The incubation period is from 6 to 9 days after infection by contact, but only 2 or 3 days after experimental injection of the virus. Sheep, swine, goats, deer, camels, and buffalo are also susceptible to natural or artificial infection with rinderpest virus. The virus is immunologically and pathologically related to the viruses of canine distemper and measles. The virus is currently classified in the genus morbillivirus and family *Paramyxoviridae*.

Signs The onset of illness is indicated by a sharp rise in body temperature (104°F to 105°F) accompanied by restlessness, dryness of the muzzle, and constipation. Within a day or two, nasal and lacrimal discharges appear. Other manifestations are photophobia, depression, excessive thirst, starry coat, retarded rumination, anorexia, leukopenia, and excessive salivation. A maculopapular rash may develop on parts of the body where hair is fine. The fever usually reaches its peak on the third to the fifth day, but drops abruptly with the onset of diarrhea, even though other symptoms are intensified. Lesions in the oral mucosa may appear by the second or third day of fever, but usually do not become conspicuous until after the onset of diarrhea. As the diarrhea increases in severity, it is accompanied by abdominal pain, accelerated respiration, occasional cough, severe dehydration, and emaciation, after which prostration, subnormal temperature, and death occur, usually after a course of 6 to 12 days.

Lesions The rinderpest virus has a particular affinity for lymphoid tissue and for epithelial tissues of the gastrointestinal tract, in which it produces severe characteristic effects.

In lymphoid tissue, the virus causes necrosis of lymphocytes, which is striking in microscopic sections of lymph nodes, spleen, and Peyer's patches. The destruction of lymphocytes is first evidenced by a fragmentation of nuclei in the germinal centers, and, in a short time, most of the mature lymphocytes disappear. The lymph follicles are involved to various degrees, depending on the severity and stage of the disease. Multinucleated giant cells containing eosinophilic cytoplasmic inclusion bodies are often present. Rarely, intranuclear inclusions are seen in these cells. Edema and congestion of capillaries are also seen microscopically, but only the edema can be detected grossly. The destruction of lymphoid cells leaves a fibrillar, somewhat eosinophilic and acellular matrix in place of the lymphoid follicles. The matrix may be surrounded by lymphocytes, plasma cells, nuclear debris, and macrophages. Although these changes in lymphoid tissue are essentially the same in lymph nodes and in the Peyer's patches, grossly they are seen to better advantage in the latter, which may be darkened with hemorrhage and slough out, leaving deep craters in the intestinal wall.

In the experimental disease in the rabbit, this affinity for lymphocytes is particularly well demonstrated in the Peyer's patches, in the sacculus rotundus, and appendix, where characteristic lesions, grossly chalk-white, stand out individually in contrast to the adjacent flesh-colored tissues. When viewed from the serous surface, these collections of lymphoid follicles have the appearance of white hexagonal tile separated by dark cement.

In the digestive system of cattle, the rinderpest virus produces typical lesions in the epithelium, varying with the anatomic features of the parts of the digestive tract affected. Application of the virus to the oral mucosa does not readily produce infection, which suggests that the virus is carried to the oral mucosa by the blood-

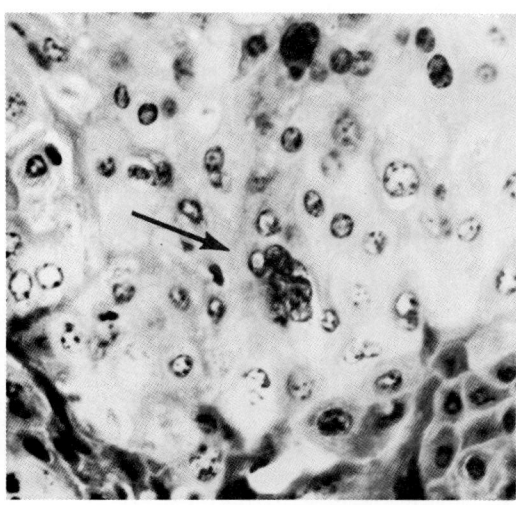

FIG. 8-63 Rinderpest. Multinucleated giant cell in lingual mucosa; small intranuclear inclusion body is evident. (Courtesy of Dr. W. Plowright.)

stream (Fig. 8-63). In the squamous epithelium of the oral cavity, the first evidence of the presence of the virus is necrosis of a few epithelial cells (Fig. 8-64) in the deep layers of the stratum malphigii. These affected cells have pyknotic and fragmented nuclei and irregular, eosinophilic cytoplasm; they appear shrunken and are separated from the adjoining epithelium by a clear space. As these necrotic areas increase in size and extend toward the surface, the cornified layer above them becomes elevated and causes them to appear grossly as tiny, grayish-white, slightly raised puncta. Multinucleated giant cells form in the stratum spinosum. Eosinophilic cytoplasmic inclusion bodies form in the mucosal epithelial cells and giant cells. Intranuclear inclusion bodies are reportedly rarely seen. Vesicles are not formed in this disease. The foci of necrosis in the epithelium usually remain discrete for a time, but later coalesce to form large areas of erosion. Since the basal layer of the squamous epithelium is rarely penetrated, ulcers seldom form. The erosions are shallow, with a red, raw-appearing floor, bounded by essentially normal epithelium, which provides a sharply demarcated margin. The lesions in the oral mucosa have a selective distribution: the inside of the lower lip, the adjacent gum, the cheeks near the commissures, and the ventral surface of the free portion of the tongue. In severe cases, lesions may extend from these sites to the hard palate and pharynx, and in fulminant cases, they may extend to all the mucous surfaces of the tongue with the singular exception of the anterior seven-eighths of its dorsal surface. The esophageal lesions, particularly those of its upper third, are similar to those in the mouth and pharynx, but usually less severe. The rumen, reticulum, and omasum rarely exhibit any lesions, although in a few instances small eroded foci are found in the omasal leaves.

The abomasum is one of the most common sites of the lesions of rinderpest. They are most severe and

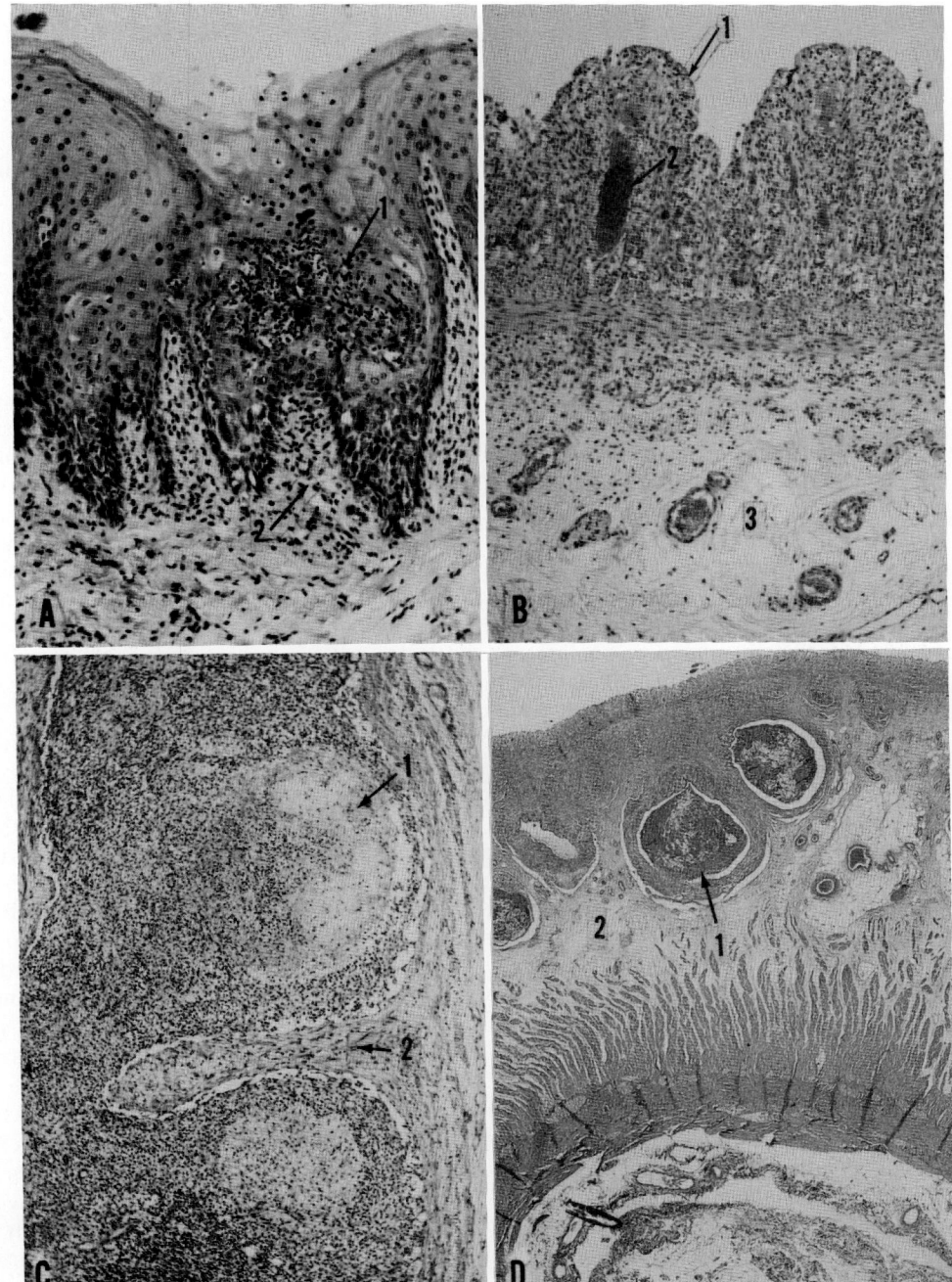

FIG. 8-64 Rinderpest. **A.** Early necrotizing lesion *(1)* in epithelium of cow's tongue. Some edema and leukocytic infiltration *(2)* of underlying stroma. **B.** Erosion of epithelium *(1)*, congestion of capillaries *(2)* in lamina propria of mucosa, and edema *(3)* of submucosa of cecum (× 75). **C.** Necrosis of lymphoid cells *(1)*, leaving only fibrillar and nuclear debris in lymphoid follicles. Cortical trabeculus *(2)* extends from capsule of this lymph node (× 48). **D.** Lesion (× 15) at ceco-colic junction. Infundibuli filled with necrotic debris *(1)*, edema in submucosa *(2)*, which separates bundles of inner muscularis. (Courtesy of the Armed Forces Institute of Pathology; contributed by Lt. Col. F. D. Maurer.)

consistent in the pyloric region, where necrotic foci of microscopic size in the epithelium are accompanied by capillary congestion and hemorrhage in the underlying lamina propria. This results in the gross appearance of irregularly outlined, superficial streaks of color, ranging from bright red to dark brown. The lesions tend to follow the edges of the broad plicae as streaks extending into the fundus, but become more numerous and diffuse in the flattened portion of the pylorus. Edema may be extensive in the submucosa of plicae, involving an entire fold and causing it to appear grossly thickened and gelatinous on cross section. As necrosis of the epithelium progresses, the infected areas become slate-colored and the epithelium sloughs away, leaving sharply outlined, irregular erosions with a red, raw floor oozing blood. In cases of relatively longer standing, black clotted blood may partially or completely fill these pits in the mucosa. Often the most tenacious portion of the clot is at the periphery of the erosion and clings to the edges, leaving the center open. Deep ulceration occasionally occurs, with microscopic evidence of penetration of the muscularis mucosae. In fatal cases, the lumen of the abomasum is usually empty, except for blood-tinged mucous material.

In the small intestine, severe lesions are less common than in the mouth, abomasum, or large intestine, but streaks of hemorrhage and, less often, erosions along the crest of the folds of mucous membrane may be found, particularly in the initial part of the duodenum and terminal ileum. Peyer's patches are exceptionally vulnerable, and even in the presence of relatively normal adjacent mucous membrane, the lymphoid tissue may become so necrotic that patches slough out, leaving deep, raw craters in the intestinal wall.

The large intestine, as a rule, is more seriously damaged than the small intestine, with prominent lesions around the ileocecal valve, at the cecocolic junction, and in the rectum. In the cecum, lesions may be confined to the region of the ileocecal valve. In well-developed cases of rinderpest, the crest of the folds of mucous membrane throughout the cecum are bright red because of the numerous petechiae. These may be interpreted as diffuse hemorrhages unless examined closely under a good light, when they are seen to be sharply demarcated spots, 0.5 to 1.0 mm in diameter, immediately beneath the most superficial layer of cells. In early lesions, the petechiae are bright red, but they become darker and tend to coalesce as the lesion ages. Microscopic examination reveals that most of the spots that grossly appear to be hemorrhages are, in fact, greatly distended capillaries, packed with erythrocytes, in the lamina propria. Streaks of congestion along the folds of mucosa produce a characteristic "barred" or "zebra-striped" appearance. As the disease progresses and the mucosa becomes eroded, diffuse congestion and bleeding from the raw surfaces may occur over large areas. When the intestine is opened, the mucosa is diffusely red and the lumen contains dark, partially clotted blood.

At the cecocolic junction, there is a segment of intestine about 4 inches long in which the wall is normally thickened and the mucosal rugae, which are broader than in either the cecum or colon, are arranged both transversely and longitudinally. This transverse arrangement is in contrast to that in the colon, where the rugae are longitudinal. Histologically, in this area, numerous tiny infundibula are formed by invaginations of epithelium through the muscularis mucosa. In the submucosa, these form goblet-shaped structures with collections of lymphocytes and sometimes lymphoid follicles along their base. These histologic characteristics influence both the gross and microscopic lesions that occur in this segment of the intestine. Since the virus invades both the epithelium and the lymphoid cells, the lesions are accentuated. Necrosis of the lymphoid tissues and closure of the orifice at the neck of the infundibula result in isolation of necrotic tissue in the submucosa. This attracts some leukocytic infiltrate, which contributes to the thickening of the wall. Erosion of epithelium, particularly at the opening of the infundibula, gives rise to small raw pits deeper than those elsewhere in the intestine. Congestion is likely to be greater in this segment, and the increased thickness of the wall is partly the result of edema in the submucosa and muscularis.

The changes in the colon and rectum vary in intensity from a few longitudinal streaks of congestion along the crest of the folds of the mucosa to erosions of the mucosal epithelium, which may be so extensive that only small islands of intact mucous membrane remain. The lumen is filled with dark, partially coagulated blood, which has oozed from the raw surfaces. The characteristic streaks of congestion and hemorrhage are more common and striking in the rectum than in the colon.

The liver is affected only secondarily in rinderpest, with chronic passive congestion resulting from cardiac and pulmonary complications as the usual lesion. In the gallbladder, however, the lesions appear to be related specifically to the virus; they are similar to those in the lower part of the intestinal tract, varying from scattered petechiae to diffuse blotches of hemorrhage with occasional free bleeding into the lumen.

In the respiratory system, the epithelium is susceptible to the virus. Petechiae may appear on the turbinates, and erosions as well as petechiae may occur in the larynx if the oral mucosa is severely involved. In the trachea, streaks of hemorrhage in the mucosa are almost invariably found in cases with well-developed lesions elsewhere. Most common are longitudinal streaks of rusty hemorrhage in the anterior third of the trachea, but the erosions usually associated with congestion and hemorrhage are rare. The lungs seem to be involved only secondarily. In animals that are killed early in the course of illness or that die after 2 or 3 days of illness, the lungs usually appear grossly normal. In longstanding cases in which diarrhea, dehydration, emaciation, and prolonged recumbence with labored respiration have been symptoms, necropsy may reveal both interlobular and alveolar emphysema accompanied by congestion and hemorrhage of varying degree and, occasionally, by small areas of consolidation. Microscopically, there is no evidence of cellular damage directly attributable to the virus, but interlobular and interalveolar as well as alveolar emphysema may be observed. Vascular congestion can usually be explained on the basis of hypostasis.

The lesions of the heart also appear to be secondary, and are seen only in cases of prolonged duration. The most nearly constant finding is subendocardial hemorrhage over the papillary muscles of the left ventricle; seldom is the right ventricle involved. The myocardium is often flaccid and bears streaks of light color, but microscopic examination rarely discloses significant changes.

In the urinary system, there may be evidence of edema around the renal pelvis and occasional desquamation of pelvic epithelium. The nephrons are affected in only a few instances, usually in cases of long duration. In the urinary bladder, the epithelium may be desquamated and the underlying stroma infiltrated with erythrocytes. The infiltrates are seen grossly as thin red blotches, measuring as much as 2 mm in diameter, with irregular and fading edges. Sometimes they become confluent.

Lesions in the skin, though not common, may be

seen as a maculopapular rash over the sparsely haired portions of the body, the vulva, and prepuce. Microscopically, they resemble those of the oral mucosa.

A virus very closely related to rinderpest and causing an acute, highly fatal disease of sheep and goats in West Africa is termed **Peste-des-petits-ruminants.** It does not naturally affect cattle, nor does experimental infection lead to disease in cattle; it does, however, confer immunity to rinderpest virus.

Diagnosis The clinical, gross, and microscopic features of the disease are adequate for a presumptive diagnosis, which should, however, be confirmed by immunologic or virologic diagnostic techniques. Differential diagnosis must include other acute gastroenteric infections such as viral diarrhea-mucosal disease and malignant catarrhal fever.

References

Brown CC, Mariner JC, Olander HJ. An immunohistochemical study of the pneumonia caused by pestes des petits ruminants virus. Vet Pathol 1991;28:166–170.
Imagawa DT. Relationships among measles, canine distemper and rinderpest viruses. Progr Med Virol 1968;10:160–193.
Maurer FD, Jones TC, Easterday B, et al. The pathology of rinderpest. Proc Am Vet Med Assoc 1955;201–211.
Plowright W. Rinderpest virus. Virology Monogr 1968;3:25–110.
Scott GR. Rinderpest. Adv Vet Sci 1964;9:113–224.
Tajima M, Ushijima T. The pathogenesis of rinderpest in the lymph nodes of cattle. Light and electron microscopic studies. Am J Pathol 1971;62:221–236.
Yamanouchi K, et al. Pathogenesis of rinderpest virus infection in rabbits. I. Clinical signs, immune response, histological changes, and virus growth patterns. Infect Immun 1974;9:199–205.
Yamanouchi K, et al. Pathogenesis of rinderpest virus infection in rabbits. II. Effect of rinderpest virus on the immune functions of rabbits. Infect Immun 1974;9:206–211.

MEASLES (RUBEOLA, MONKEY INTRANUCLEAR INCLUSION AGENT, MORBILLUS)

Measles is a highly infectious exanthematous viral disease of humans, principally children. The virus and its pathologic effects are closely related to canine distemper and rinderpest. In addition to the characteristic exanthematous rash, measles infection in humans may result in primary giant-cell pneumonia and encephalomyelitis. Secondary bronchopneumonia is an important complication. Microscopically, the rash is characterized by vesiculation and necrosis of epithelial cells with an associated inflammatory response in the dermis. Epithelial cells may contain intranuclear inclusion bodies, and multinucleated giant cells are often present. The most characteristic pathologic feature is the Warthin-Finkeldey lymphoid giant cell, which is found in lymph nodes, spleen, Peyer's patches, appendix, and tonsils. These cells contain up to 100 small, deeply basophilic nuclei, which only rarely bear inclusions. Primary pneumonia is also characterized by giant cells, but here the cells have fewer, more leptochromatic nuclei, and both intranuclear and cytoplasmic eosinophilic inclusion bodies are often present. In measles encephalomyelitis, there is congestion, hemorrhage, perivascular cuffing, and demyelination.

Measles is also known to be infectious for several species of monkeys, including rhesus (*Macaca mulatta*), cynomolgus (*M. fascicularis*), Taiwan macaque (*M. cyclopis*), baboons (*Papio* species), African green monkeys (*Ceropithecus aethiops*), colobus monkeys (*Colobus guereza*), squirrel monkeys (*Saimiri sciureus*), and marmosets (*Saguinus* and *Callithrix* species). Although measles is rare in their native habitats, few rhesus monkeys escape infection once they are brought into captivity. Clinical disease is rarely recorded, either because it is mild or initial infection occurred en route to the laboratory. However, monkeys may exhibit conjunctivitis and an exanthematous rash, which lasts for 3 to 4 days.

Encephalitis is a rather common occurrence in acute measles. Much less often, subacute sclerosing panencephalitis occurs, which develops months or years following recovery from the acute disease. In newly imported animals dying of other causes, or killed in the course of experimentation, visceral lesions resulting from measles infection are encountered with some frequency, even in the absence of a rash. Most often these are a result of by giant-cell pneumonia, with intranuclear and cytoplasmic inclusion bodies within giant cells and respiratory epithelial cells. Lymphoid giant cells are less common than in human measles, but may be present.

In marmosets and colobus monkeys, measles may be more serious. Epizootics with high mortality rates have occurred, apparently the result of variant viruses with greater virulence.

In addition to pneumonia, marmosets develop gastritis and enterocolitis, with thinning and sloughing of surface epithelium. Large syncytial cells are present near the eroded surface of mucosa and within the crypts. These large cells often contain eosinophilic intranuclear inclusions. Crypts are often dilated and contain neutrophils. Foci of necrosis, multinucleated giant cells, and inclusion bodies may also be present in the liver, kidney, uterus, pancreas, and salivary gland.

Diagnosis Presumptive diagnosis is established on the basis of the characteristic lesions. Definitive diagnosis requires viral isolation and identification.

References

Albrecht P, et al. Subacute sclerosing panencephalitis: experimental infection in primates. Science 1977;195:64–66.
Albrecht P, et al. Fatal measles infection in marmosets: pathogenesis and prophylaxis. Infect Immun 1980;27:969–978.
Barringer JR, Griffith JF. Experimental measles virus encephalitis. A light, phase, fluorescence, and electron microscopic study. Lab Invest 1970;23:335–346.
Byington DP, Johnson KP. Subacute sclerosing panencephalitis virus in immunosuppressed adult hamsters. Lab Invest 1975;32:91–97.
Covell WP. The occurrence of intranuclear inclusions in monkeys unaccompanied by specific signs of disease. Am J Pathol 1932;8:151–158.
Fraser CEO, et al. A paramyxovirus causing fatal gastroenterocolitis in marmoset monkeys. Prim Med 1978;10:261–270.
Hall WC, Kovatch RM, Herman PH, et al. Pathology of measles in Rhesus monkeys. Vet Pathol 1971;8:307–319.
Kamahora J. Experimental pathology of measles in monkeys. Jpn J Med Sci Biol 1965;18:51.
Kamahora J, Nii S. Pathological and immunological studies of mon-

keys infected with measles virus. Arch Ges Virusforsch 1965;16:161–167.

Levy BM, Mirkovic RR. An epizootic of measles in a marmoset colony. Lab Anim Sci 1971;21:33–39.

Lorenz D, Albrecht P. Susceptibility of tamarins *(Saguinus)* to measles virus. Lab Anim Sci 1980;30:661–665.

Manning PJ, Banks KL, Lehner NDM. Naturally occurring giant cell pneumonia in the Rhesus monkey (Macaca mulatta). J Am Vet Med Assoc 1968;153:899–904.

Meyer HM, Jr, Brooks BE, Douglas RD, Rogers NG. Ecology of measles in monkeys. Am J Dis Child 1962;103:307–313.

Örvell C, Norrby E. Further studies on the immunologic relationships among measles, distemper, and rinderpest viruses. J Immunol 1974;113:1850–1858.

Phillips LR, Colman G, Clarke M. Measles in monkeys. Vet Rec 1975;97:436.

Potkay S, Ganaway JR, Rogers NG, et al. An epizootic of measles in a colony of Rhesus monkeys (Macaca mulatta). Am J Vet Res 1966;27:331–334.

Raine CS, Byington DP, Johnson KP. Subacute sclerosing panencephalitis in the hamster: ultrastructure of the acute disease in newborns and weanlings. Lab Invest 1975;33:108–116.

Remfry J. Measles epizootic with five deaths in newly imported rhesus monkeys (Macaca mulatta). Lab Anim 1976;10:49–57.

Scott GBD, Keymer IF. The pathology of measles in Abyssinian colobus monkeys (Colobus guereza): a description of an outbreak. J Pathol 1975;117:229–233.

Sergiev PG, Ryazantseva NE, Shroit IG. The dynamics of pathological processes in experimental measles in monkeys. Acta Virol 1960;4:265–273.

Shishido A, Yamanouchi K. Encephalomyelitis induced by paramyxovirus in nonhuman primates with a special reference to possible viral etiology of multiple sclerosis. Neurology (Minneap) 1976;26:83–84.

Taniguchi T, Kamahora J, Kato S, et al. Pathology in monkeys experimentally infected with measles virus. Med J Osaka Univ 1954;5:367–379.

Ueda S, Otsuka T, Okuno Y. Experimental subacute sclerosing panencephalitis (SSPE) in a monkey by subcutaneous inoculation with a defective SSPE virus. Biken J 1975;18:179–181.

Yamanouchi K, et al. Giant cell formation in lymphoid tissues of monkeys inoculated with various strains of measles virus. Jpn J Med Sci Biol 1970;23:131–145.

PHOCINE AND CETACEAN MORBILLIVIRUSES

In 1988, an epizootic disease occurred in common seals *(Phoca vitullina)* in the seas of Northern Europe, and in the same year, in Siberian seals *(Phoca siberica)* in Lake Baikal in Siberia. Thousands of seals died during these apparently unrelated epizootics. Late in the same year, a comparable disease was observed in six porpoises *(Phocoena phocoena)* off the coast of County Down in Northern Ireland. In 1990, an epizootic killed hundreds of striped dolphins *(Stenella coeruleoalba)* in the Mediterranean Sea. Investigations of each of these epizootics revealed that the sea mammals died of a disease resembling canine distemper. The diseases have been termed phocine distemper, cetacean distemper, seal distemper, porpoise distemper, and dolphin distemper. Morbilliviruses were isolated, which, although related to known morbilliviruses, were demonstrated to be distinct. Comparisons of the viral isolates indicate that the seal or phocine virus is genetically distinct from the dolphin and porpoise virus. Thus, two previously unrecognized morbilliviruses appeared at about the same time. They most likely crossed from some other species to which they were confined. Mink have been demonstrated to be susceptible to the phocine virus. The diseases in sea mammals caused by phocine and cetacean viruses are similar and are discussed together.

Affected animals are weak and show respiratory signs, such as dyspnea, coughing, and serous or mucopurulent nasal and ocular discharge. Many develop subcutaneous emphysema around the neck and thorax. Nervous signs, which include altered behavior, twitching, and convulsions, are also seen. The pathologic findings resemble those of canine distemper. There is bronchiolo-interstitial pneumonia, with multinucleated giant cells (syncytial cells) and hyperplasia of type II alveolar epithelium. Eosinophilic nuclear and cytoplasmic inclusion bodies occur in syncytial cells, alveolar macrophages, and bronchial epithelium. Nonsuppurative encephalitis is common and consists of mild lymphocytic perivascular cuffing, neuronal necrosis (particularly of the cerebral cortex), focal gliosis, demyelination, and accumulations of gemastocytic astrocytes in white matter. Nuclear and cytoplasmic inclusion bodies occur within neurons. Syncytial cells are also described in white matter. There is depletion and necrosis of lymphocytes in lymphoid tissues, and syncytial cells may be present within the cortex of lymph nodes. As similarly seen in canine distemper, nuclear and cytoplasmic inclusion bodies may be found in other cells, such as the gastric mucosa and transitional epithelium of the urinary tract.

References

Barrett T, Visser IKG, Mamaev L, et al. Dolphin and porpoise morbilliviruses are genetically distinct from phocine distemper virus. Virology 1993;193:1010–1012.

Blixenkrone-Moller M. Biological properties of phocine distemper virus and canine distemper virus. APMIS Suppl 1993;36:1–51.

Bolt G, Blixenkrone-Moller M. Nucleic acid hybridization analyses confirm the presence of a hitherto unknown morbillivirus in Mediterranean dolphins. Vet Microbiol 1994;41:363–372.

Domingo M, et al. Pathologic and immunocytochemical studies of morbillivirus infection in striped dolphins (Stenella coeruleoalba). Vet Pathol 1992;29:1–10.

Kennedy S. A review of the 1988 European seal morbillivirus epizootic. Vet Rec 1990;127:563–567.

Kennedy S, Smyth JA, Cush PF, et al. Viral distemper now found in porpoises. Nature (Lond) 1988;336:21.

Pohlmeyer G, Pohlenz J, Wohlsein P. Intestinal lesions in experimental phocine distemper: light microscopy, immunohistochemistry and electron microscopy. J Comp Pathol 1993;109:57–69.

MORBILLIVIRUS PNEUMONIA OF HORSES

In the fall of 1994, an outbreak of respiratory disease occurred in a stable of horses in Hendra, a suburb of Brisbane, Queensland, Australia. Fourteen of 21 sick horses died or were killed. A trainer and a stable hand also became ill, and the trainer died after 6 days of intensive care. The disease in the horses and the trainer was characterized by interstitial pneumonia with marked pulmonary edema. Syncytial cells with cytoplasmic inclusion bodies were prominent in the walls and endothelium of pulmonary capillaries and arterioles as well as in blood vessels, lymph nodes, spleen, stomach, heart, kidneys, and brain. A morbillivirus was recovered, which, although related to other members of the genus, appears to be a newly recognized virus. Its origin is not known. No further occurrence of the disease has been noted.

References

Murray K, et al. A novel morbillivirus pneumonia of horses and its transmission to humans. Emerg Infect Dis 1995;1:31–33.
Murray K, et al. A morbillivirus that causes fatal disease in horses and humans. Science 1995;268:94–97.

Diseases caused by pneumoviruses

The genus *Pneumovirus* contains three important viruses: human respiratory syncytial virus, bovine respiratory syncytial virus, and pneumonia virus of mice. The two respiratory syncytial viruses are related antigenically to each other but not to pneumonia virus of mice.

HUMAN RESPIRATORY SYNCYTIAL VIRUS (HRSV)

Human RSV is the most important cause of lower respiratory tract infection in infants and children. The virus was first recovered from chimpanzees with upper respiratory disease and termed "chimpanzee coryzal agent," until it was recovered from children and its clinical pathologic significance was recognized. In children, the virus causes a proliferative interstitial pneumonia with necrosis of tracheal and bronchial epithelium. There are multinucleated giant cells, which contain intranuclear and intracytoplasmic eosinophilic inclusion bodies. Many species of nonhuman primates can be infected with HRSV, but clinical disease is usually absent except in chimpanzees, owl monkeys, and cebus monkeys.

BOVINE RESPIRATORY SYNCYTIAL VIRUS (BRSV)

Bovine RSV occurs worldwide and affects cattle and sheep, particularly the young, during the winter months. The incidence of infection is high, and the virus is one of the major causes of respiratory disease in cattle. The disease may be mild or severe, with a high morbidity rate but a low mortality rate. Clinically, there is fever, coughing, hyperpnea, serous oculonasal discharge, and lethargy. The virus causes an interstitial pneumonia with necrosis of bronchial, bronchiolar, and alveolar epithelium (Fig. 8-65): Inclusion-bearing multinucleated giant cells form at these sites. Epithelial hyperplasia and metaplasia ensue with healing. Infection with BRSV predisposes the respiratory tract to other viruses, such as parainfluenza-3, and bacterial pathogens, such as *Pasteurella haemolytica*, causing significantly more severe pneumonia. The lesions of BRSV closely resemble those caused by parainfluenza-3 virus, from which they must be differentiated.

PNEUMONIA VIRUS OF MICE (PVM)

PVM is a widely distributed infection of laboratory mice but not important as a cause of clinical disease under natural conditions. In fact, reports of naturally occurring disease are rare. Serologic evidence indicates that the infection is also common in rats, hamsters, gerbils, guinea pigs, and possibly rabbits and monkeys. Ex-

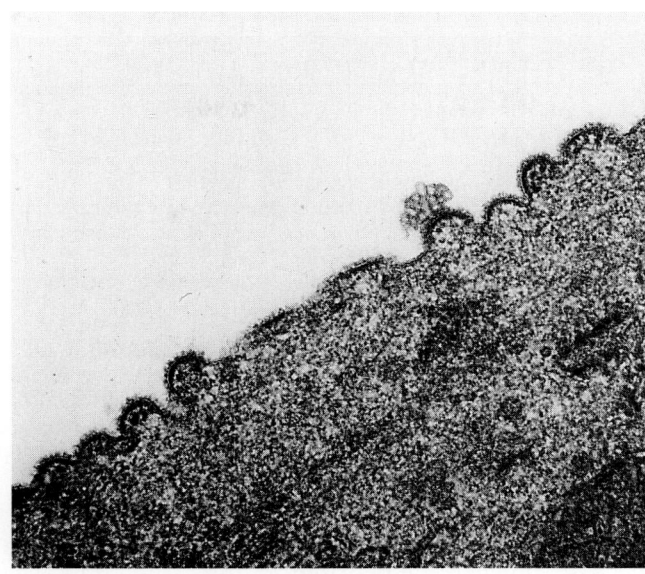

FIG. 8-65 Bovine respiratory syncytial virus infection, calf. Bronchial epithelium with multiple virions budding from the apical plasmalemma. (Courtesy of Dr. W.L. Castleman and *American Journal of Veterinary Research* 1985;46:554–560).

perimentally in mice, the virus can induce interstitial pneumonia and necrotizing bronchiolitis similar to Sendai virus infection.

References

Al-Darraji AM, Cutlip RC, Lehmkuhl HD, et al. Experimental infection of lambs with bovine respiratory syncytial virus and *Pasteurella haemolytica*: pathologic studies. Am J Vet Res 1982;43:224–229.
Belshe RB, et al. Experimental respiratory syncytial virus infection of four species of primates. J Med Virol 1977;1:157–162.
Bryson DG, McNulty MS, Logan EF, et al. Respiratory syncytial virus pneumonia in young calves: clinical and pathologic findings. Am J Vet Res 1983;44:1648–1655.
Bryson DG, McConnell S, McAliskey M, et al. Ultrastructural features of alveolar lesions in induced respiratory syncytial virus pneumonia of calves. Vet Pathol 1991;28:286–292.
Bryson DG, Platten MF, McConnell S, et al. Ultrastructural features of lesions in bronchiolar epithelium in induced respiratory syncytial virus pneumonia of calves. Vet Pathol 1991;28:293–299.
Castleman WL, Lay JC, Dubovi EJ, et al. Experimental bovine respiratory syncytial virus infection in conventional calves: light microscopic lesions, microbiology, and studies on lavaged lung cells. Am J Vet Res 1985;46:547–553.
Chanock RM, Parrott RH, Vargosko AJ, et al. Acute respiratory tract disease of viral etiology. IV. Respiratory syncytial virus. Am J Publ Health 1962;52:918–925.
Horsfall FL Jr, Curnen EC. Studies on pneumonia virus of mice (PVM). II. Immunological evidence of latent infection with the virus in numerous mammalian species. J Exp Med 1946;83:43–64.
Horsfall FL Hahn RG. A latent virus in normal mice capable of producing pneumonia in its natural host. J Exp Med 1940;71:391–408.
Kimman TG, Straver PJ, Zimmer GM. Pathogenesis of naturally acquired bovine respiratory syncytial virus infection in calves: morphologic and serologic findings. Am J Vet Res 1989;50:684–693.
Morris JA, Blount RE Jr, Savage RE. Recovery of cytopathogenic agent from chimpanzees with coryza. Proc Soc Exp Biol Med 1956;92:544–550.
Prince GA, et al. Respiratory syncytial virus infection in owl monkeys:

viral shedding, immunological response, and associated illness caused by wild-type virus and two temperature-sensitive mutants. Infect Immun 1979;26:1009–1013.

Richardson LS, et al. Experimental respiratory syncytial virus pneumonia in cebus monkeys. J Med Virol 1978;2:45–59.

Richter CB, Thigpen JE, Richter CS, et al. Fatal pneumonia with terminal emaciation in nude mice caused by pneumonia virus of mice. Lab Anim Sci 1988;38:255–261.

Trigo FJ, Breeze RG, Liggitt HD, et al. Interaction of bovine respiratory syncytial virus and *Pasteurella haemolytica* in the ovine lung. Am J Vet Res 1984;45:1671–1678.

Trigo FJ, Breeze RG, Evermann JF, et al. Pathogenesis of experimental bovine respiratory syncytial virus infection in sheep. Am J Vet Res 1984;45:1663–1670.

van den Ingh TSGAM, Verhoeff J, van Nieuwstadt APKMI. Clinical and pathological observations on spontaneous bovine respiratory syncytial virus infections in calves. Res Vet Sci 1982;33: 152–158.

ORTHOMYXOVIRIDAE

The family **Orthomyxoviridae** (ortho = correct, true; myxo = mucus) is comprised of the "true" influenza viruses, currently classified in one genus, influenzavirus. Based on antigenic characteristics, influenza viruses are subgrouped into three types: A, B and C. Only type A influenza viruses are of concern as causes of natural disease of animals; they cause equine, swine, and avian influenza. Additionally, nonhuman primates are susceptible to human influenza viruses, both naturally and experimentally.

The three virus types are about 120 nm in diameter and irregularly spherical, although they are often filamentous on initial isolation. The virion envelope is covered with a layer of two kinds of glycoprotein spikes (peplomers), which contain strain-specific antigens, either hemagglutinin or neuraminidase. The genome is negative-sense, single-stranded RNA, divided into eight separate segments (seven in type C). The virion contains a transcriptase, and multiplication occurs in the nucleus and cytoplasm of infected cells. Virions mature by budding from the plasma membrane.

Influenza viruses are spread by aerosols and establish infection in the respiratory tract, where they attach and replicate in respiratory epithelium from the nares to bronchioles. There has been considerable speculation as to the potential of influenza viruses as teratogenic agents. Experimentally, a variety of fetal abnormalities have been induced, but their role in natural disease is uncertain.

References

Anschutz W, Scholtissek C, Rott P. Genetic relationship between different influenza strains. Med Microbiol Immunol 1972;158: 26–31.

Fuccillo DA, Sever JL. Viral teratology. Bacteriol Rev 1973;37:19–31.

Krous HF, Altshuler G, London WT, et al. Congenital hydrocephalus produced by attenuated influenza A virus vaccine in rhesus monkeys. Am J Pathol 1978;92:317–320.

London WT, Fuccillo DA, Sever JL, et al. Influenza virus as a teratogen in rhesus monkeys. Nature (Lond) 1975;225:483–484.

Murphy BR, Sly DL, Hosier NT, et al. Evaluation of three strains of influenza A virus in humans and in owl, cebus and squirrel monkeys. Infect Immun 1980;28:688–691.

Paniker CKJ, Nair CMG. Experimental infection of animals with influenzavirus types A and B. Bull WHO 1972;47:461–463.

Tumova B, Schild GC. Antigenic relationships between type A influenzaviruses of human, porcine, equine and avian origin. Bull WHO 1972;47:453–460.

EQUINE INFLUENZA

The term influenza has been in use for centuries to describe respiratory diseases of humans and animals, often being used as a catch-all diagnosis for diseases of uncertain cause. Influenza should be restricted to those specific diseases caused by agents classified within the family *Orthomyxoviridae*, genus *Influenzavirus*. Equine influenza virus was first isolated and identified in 1958 in Czechoslovakia (A/Equi 1 serotype). A second serotype (A/Equi 2) was isolated in 1963 in Miami. Both serotypes are of worldwide distribution and cause similar syndromes, which are highly infectious and spread rapidly.

Signs Clinical signs include nasal discharge, cough, dyspnea, fever, depression, and reluctance to move. The illness lasts 2 to 7 days. The disease is rarely, if ever, fatal in adult horses, but death is reported in young foals. Secondary bacterial infection may complicate the disease in both adult and young animals.

Lesions The lesions of equine influenza have been studied histologically in a few instances. As summarized by Gerber (1970), erosions of mucosae have been noted in the nose, pharynx, larynx, and trachea. In the lung, the lesions have been described as peribronchitis, bronchitis with hyaline membranes in alveoli, periarteritis, and bronchopneumonia.

Diagnosis Positive diagnosis depends on: (1) demonstration of serum-neutralizing antibodies, (2) isolation and identification of the virus, or (3) demonstration of viral antigens with immunological staining techniques. The clinical disease must be differentiated from other respiratory diseases. Equine rhinopneumonitis may resemble influenza, but as a respiratory disease it is principally an infection of young horses. Differentiating features of equine viral arteritis include edema of the limbs, colic, diarrhea, conjunctivitis, and photophobia. Viral arteritis is also associated with abortion during the course or in early convalescence. Rhinovirus infections of horses produce respiratory illnesses that are indistinguishable from influenza except by identification of the specific virus involved.

References

Blaskovic D. Experimental infection of horses with equine influenza viruses. In: Bryans JT, Gerber H, ed. Proceedings of second international conference of equine infectious diseases. Paris, 1969. Basel: Karger 1970;111–117.

Gerber H. Clinical features, sequelae and epidemiology of equine influenza. In: Bryans JT, Gerber H, ed. Proceedings of second international conference of equine infectious disease. Paris, 1969. Basel: Karger 1970;63–80.

Hofer B, et al. An investigation of the etiology of viral respiratory disease in a remount depot. In: Bryans JT, Gerber H, ed. Equine infectious diseases III. Basel: Karger 1973.

McQueen JL, Steele JH, Robinson RQ. Influenza in animals. Adv Vet Sci 1968;12:285–336.

Powell DG, et al. The outbreak of equine influenza in England April/May, 1973. Vet Rec 1974;94:282–287.

Rose MA, Round MC, Beveridge WIB. Influenza in horses and donkeys in Britain, 1969. Vet Rec 1970;86:768–769.

Sinvinova O, et al. Isolation of a virus causing respiratory disease in horses. Acta Virol 1958;2:52–61.

Todd JD, Lief FS, Cohen D. Experimental infection of ponies with the Hong Kong variant of human influenza virus. Am J Epidemiol 1970;92:330–336.

Waddell GH, Teigland MB, Sigel MM. A new influenza virus associated with equine respiratory disease. J Am Vet Med Assoc 1963;143:587–590.

SWINE INFLUENZA

Swine influenza is an infectious respiratory disease of swine caused by a virus in the genus influenzavirus, family *Orthomyxoviridae,* acting in synergy with a gram-negative bacterial organism, *Hemophilus influenzae suis.* The swine influenza virus is closely related to the viruses of human influenza type A; in fact, its transmission to laboratory animals (mice, ferrets) by Shope was the opening step to extensive work with similar viruses to which humans are susceptible. Shope was also the first to postulate that swine influenza resulted from the infection of swine by the virus responsible for the 1918 pandemic of influenza. This view has been reinforced somewhat by the recent appearance of swine influenza A in the human population, fortunately not in pandemic form. In addition, Shope demonstrated that the swine lungworm can act as intermediate host and reservoir for the swine influenza virus during interenzoötic periods. The virus is introduced into susceptible pigs by lungworm larvae; infection is provoked by the presence of *H. influenzae suis*; then the disease can spread to other pigs in the herd by direct contact. Swine, ferrets, and mice are susceptible to the experimental disease. There is some experimental evidence to indicate that swine of 2 to 3 weeks of age undergo severe pneumonia when inoculated with swine influenza virus during the migration of *Ascaris suum* larvae through the lungs.

Signs The disease principally affects young pigs; after an incubation period of 24 to 48 hours, animals exhibit fever, rhinitis, cough, and inappetence. These symptoms usually abate after 3 to 5 days, but in some cases, transitory fever may recur within 3 weeks. Dyspnea associated with severe pulmonary involvement is observed in some cases, and death occurs after severe pneumonia. The mortality rate is usually not high (approximately 1%), but in some outbreaks may assume serious proportions. The morbidity rate may approach 100%.

Lesions The specific lesions of swine influenza are restricted to the trachea, bronchi, bronchioles, alveolar ducts, and alveoli. The gross evidence of pathologic changes in these structures consists in part of mucopurulent exudate, which lies over the tracheal and bronchial mucosae and fills smaller branches of the bronchi. Plugging of these bronchi and bronchioles results in sharply demarcated, prune-colored areas of atelectasis. Consolidation of lung parenchyma occurs around the bronchi, starting adjacent to their finer branches. Experimental intranasal exposure of swine to the virus alone results in atelectasis restricted to the pendant portions of the lung, especially in the cardiac, apical, and intermediate lobes. The addition of *H. influenzae suis* to the inoculum produces more extensive pulmonary involvement: atelectasis extends to include the pendant portions of the diaphragmatic lobes, and peribronchial consolidation of the upper portions of all lobes occurs. Mucopurulent exudate in the bronchial system is also more extensive. Frank pneumonic consolidation and fibrinous pleuritis develop in affected animals exposed concurrently to unfavorable conditions, such as cold, wet weather and shipping.

The microscopic changes that follow the intranasal instillation of swine influenza virus in mice, described by Dubin (1945), appear to parallel those that occur in swine. In mice, the virus produces necrosis of the lining cells of alveoli and bronchi and, to a smaller extent, those of the lower part of the trachea. Because of the loss of nuclei and hyalinization of cytoplasm of the epithelial cells, this necrotic process often appears as a hyaline membrane. Proliferation of the epithelial cells accompanies these necrotic changes and persists after changes have resolved. In the bronchi and bronchioles, the growth of epithelium progresses to such a remarkable degree that it fills the adjacent alveoli. These intra-alveolar plugs of epithelial cells begin to degenerate about the fourteenth day, and some alveoli are reopened. The epithelium of the bronchi and bronchioles is restored during the third week of convalescence. The pneumonia is characterized by necrosis of alveolar walls with formation of hyaline membranes lining the alveolar sacs, accompanied by congestion, focal hemorrhages, severe perivascular and intralobular edema, and infiltration with inflammatory leukocytes, principally mononuclear cells. Areas of collapsed lung parenchyma appear as early as the second day, as a result of obstruction of bronchi by pus, mucus, and desquamated cells. These areas of atelectasis may become heavily infiltrated with leukocytes. Peribronchiolar alveoli are often consolidated as the result of infiltration of mononuclear cells or the ingrowth of respiratory epithelium. Consolidated alveoli are restored to a functional state by necrosis and phagocytic removal of the cells with which they are filled.

Diagnosis The symptoms and gross and microscopic lesions provide a basis for the presumptive diagnosis of swine influenza. Definitive diagnosis depends on: (1) demonstration of a significant elevation of virus-neutralizing or antihemagglutinin antibodies in the sera of swine during the course of an infection, (2) isolation and identification of the swine influenza virus type A, or (3) demonstration of viral antigens with immunologic staining techniques.

References

Brown TT, Mengeling WL, Paul PS, et al. Porcine fetuses with pulmonary hypoplasia resulting from experimental swine influenza virus infection. Vet Pathol 1980;17:455–468.

Dubin IN. A pathological study of mice infected with the virus of swine influenza. Am J Pathol 1945;21:1121–1134.

Easterday BC. Influenza virus infection of the suckling pig. Acta Vet Brno 1971;40:33–42.

Kundin WD. Hong Kong A-2 influenza virus infection among swine during human epidemic in Taiwan. Nature 1970;228:857.

Kundin WD, Easterday BC. Hong Kong influenza infection in swine: experimental and field observation. Bull WHO 1972;47:489–491.

Pereira HG. Swine influenza. Nature 1976;261:10.

Popovici V, et al. Infection of pigs with an influenza virus related to the A2/Hong Kong/1/68 strain. Acta Virol 1972;16:363.

Schnurrenberger PR, Woods GT, Martin RJ. Serologic evidence of human infection with swine influenza virus. Am Rev Respir Dis 1970;102:356–361.

Shope RE. The etiology of swine influenza. Science 1931;73:214–215.

Shope RE. The swine lungworm as a reservoir and intermediate host for swine influenza virus. I. The presence of swine influenza virus in healthy and susceptible pigs. J Exp Med 1941;74:41–47.

Shope RE. Swine influenza. Experimental transmission and pathology. J Exp Med 1931;54:349–359.

Shope RE. The swine lungworm as a reservoir and intermediate host for swine influenza virus. II. The transmission of swine influenza virus by the swine lungworm. J Exp Med 1941;74:49–68.

Smith TF, et al. Isolation of swine influenza virus from autopsy lung tissue of man. N Engl J Med 1976;294:708–710.

Underdahl NR. The effect of Ascaris suum migration on the severity of swine influenza. J Am Vet Med Assoc 1958;133:380–383.

Urman HK, Underdahl NR, Young GA. Comparative histopathology of experimental swine influenza and virus pneumonia of pigs in disease-free swine. Am J Vet Res 1958;19:913–917.

Webster RG. On the origin of pandemic influenza viruses. Top Microbiol Immunol 1972;59:75–105.

RHABDOVIRIDAE

The family **Rhabdoviridae** (rhabdo = rod) contains a large number of enveloped, single-stranded, negative-sense RNA viruses (Table 8-9). They are all bullet-shaped, with a width of about 70 nm and a length of 180 nm. The lipoprotein envelope contains conspicuous peplomers that contain glycoprotein, which mediates attachment to the host-cell receptor. The virion contains a transcriptase essential to initiate replication. Both positive-strand and negative-strand viral RNA is replicated, but only the negative strand is packaged into virions.

The family contains a large number of different viruses infectious for humans, domestic animals, fish, invertebrates, and plants. Many, but not all, are transmitted by arthropods. There are two genera, vesiculovirus and lyssavirus. Additionally, there are a large number of rhabdoviruses that have yet to be classified. Table 8–9 lists these viruses.

Diseases caused by vesiculoviruses

The genus vesiculovirus contains several serotypes of vesicular stomatitis virus, the prototype virus of the rhabdovirus family, and three less well characterized viruses: Piry, Chandipura, and Isfahan. **Piry virus** was originally isolated from an opossum in Belem, Brazil, and has been associated with an acute nonfatal febrile illness of humans. **Chandipura virus** was first isolated in India from humans and may also cause an acute, nonfatal febrile illness. **Isfahan virus,** originally recovered from sandflies in Iran, infects humans and gerbils, but its significance as a pathogen is not clear.

VESICULAR STOMATITIS

The virus of vesicular stomatitis may naturally affect swine, cattle, horses, and humans, producing a disease that has close similarities to aphthous fever (foot and

TABLE 8-9 *Rhabdoviridae*

Vesiculovirus

Vesicular stomatitis virus
  New Jersey, Indiana, Argentina, Brazil

Lyssavirus

Rabies virus
Lagos bat virus
Mokola virus
Duvenhage virus
Obodhiang virus
Kotonkan virus

Unclassified

Bovine ephemeral fever virus
Flanders-Hart-Part virus
Mt. Elgon bat virus
Sigma virus
Hemorrhagic septicemia virus of trout (Egtved)
Infectious hematopoietic necrosis virus (trout, salmon)
Spring viremia of carp
Pike fry disease
Rhabdoviruses of eels

mouth disease) and vesicular exanthema. Sheep and goats are not affected. Several laboratory animals can be infected, including mice and guinea pigs. There are two principal strains of vesicular stomatitis virus in North America: the New Jersey strain, which is the most virulent and most common, and the Indian strain. Immunity to one strain does not confer immunity to the other. Other serotypes have been identified in South America.

Vesicular stomatitis is present only in the warm months of the year, appearing in the late spring and disappearing with the coming of freezing weather. It is most common in cattle and horses, but severe outbreaks have been reported in swine in serum-producing biologic plants. Insects are believed to be the principal vectors of transmission. Mosquitoes (Aedes species), black flies (Simulium species), phlebotomine sand flies, eye gnats (Hippelates), and midges (Culicoides species) have been identified as possible vectors. There is evidence that bats (Myotus lucifugus lucifugus) are susceptible to the virus of vesicular stomatitis and might serve to maintain the virus in winter months.

Lesions The lesions of vesicular stomatitis are most commonly found on the tongue and oral mucosa but may also occur on the teats and at the coronary band. Infection is by contact with or bites of insects, with lesions developing at the site. Viremic spread to other sites does not play a role.

Microscopically, there is intercellular edema in the stratum spinosum, eventually leading to cell dissociation and necrosis. Neutrophils and macrophages infiltrate the necrotic tissue, which sloughs, leaving erosions that are subject to secondary infection. Although the intraepithelial edema may become abundant enough to result in a vesicle, this occurs in less than 30% of the lesions. Healing usually occurs in 7 to 10 days and is followed by immunity to the specific strain of virus involved.

The ultrastructural features of the lesions of vesicular stomatitis (Proctor and Sherman, 1975) confirm the occurrence of intercellular edema and necrosis of superficial epithelial cells (keratinocytes). Virions bud from the plasma membrane and are seen in intracellular vesicles. Replication of desmosomes is a prominent feature at opposing cell membranes, and numerous free desmosomes accumulate in the cytoplasm. This phenomenon appears to be the result of endocytosis of the desmosomes after breaks occur in the related plasma membrane. Enlarging intracellular vesicles eventually isolate epithelial cells, especially keratinocytes, which undergo necrosis.

Diagnosis The lesions of vesicular stomatitis are essentially similar in distribution, location, and microscopic appearance to those of aphthous fever and vesicular exanthema. The lesions of these three diseases cannot be definitively distinguished on morphologic grounds, in spite of the less conspicuous vesiculation evident in vesicular stomatitis. Vesicular stomatitis, unlike aphthous fever, rarely causes myocarditis and is almost never fatal. The virus may be seen in ultramicroscopic sections or isolated for identification in tissue culture systems.

References

Chow TL, Hansen RR, McNutt SH. Pathology of vesicular stomatitis in cattle. Proc Am Vet Med Assoc 1951;119–124.

Chow TL, McNutt SH. Pathological changes of experimental vesicular stomatitis of swine. Am J Vet Res 1953;14:420–424.

Dal Canto MC, Rabinowitz SG, Johnson TC. An ultrastructural study of central nervous system disease produced by wild-type and temperature-sensitive mutants of vesicular stomatitis virus. Lab Invest 1976;35:185–196.

Fields BN, Hawkins K. Human infection with the virus of vesicular stomatitis during an epizootic. N Engl J Med 1967;277:989–994.

Goodger WJ, Thurmond M, Nehay H, et al. Economic impact of an epizootic of bovine vesicular stomatitis in California. J Am Vet Med Assoc 1985;186:370–373.

Hansen DE, Thurmond MC, Thorburn M. Factors associated with the spread of clinical vesicular stomatitis in California dairy cattle. Am J Vet Res 1985;46:789–795.

Proctor SJ, Sherman KC. Ultrastructural changes in bovine lingual epithelium infected with vesicular stomatitis virus. Vet Pathol 1975;12:362–377.

Ribelin WE. The cytopathogenesis of vesicular stomatitis virus infection in cattle. Am J Vet Res 1958;19:66–73.

Schnitzlein WM, Reichmann ME. Characterization of New Jersey vesicular stomatitis virus isolates from horses and black flies during the 1982 outbreak in Colorado. Virology 1985;142:426–431.

Seibold HR, Sharp JB Jr. A revised concept of the pathologic changes of the tongue in cattle with vesicular stomatitis. Am J Vet Res 1960;21:35–51.

Srihongse S. Vesicular stomatitis virus infection in Panamanian primates and other vertebrates. Am J Epidemiol 1969;90:69–76.

Sudia WD, Fields BN, Calisher CH. The isolation of vesicular stomatitis virus (Indian strain) and other viruses from mosquitoes in New Mexico, 1965. Am J Epidemiol 1967;86:598–602.

Tesh RB, Chaniotis BN, Johnson KM. Vesicular stomatitis virus (Indiana serotype): transmission by phlebotomine sandflies. Science 1972;175:1477–1479.

Tesh RB, Peralta PH, Johnson KM. Ecologic studies of vesicular stomatitis virus. I. Prevalence of infection among animals and humans living in an area of endemic VSV activity. Am J Epidemiol 1969;90:225–261.

Thurmond MC, Ardans AA, Picanso JP, et al. Vesicular stomatitis virus (New Jersey strain) infection in two California dairy herds: an epidemiologic study. J Am Vet Med Assoc 1987;191:965–970.

Walton TE, Webb PA, Kramer WL, et al. Epizootic vesicular stomatitis in Colorado, 1982: epidemiologic and entomologic studies. Am J Trop Med Hyg 1987;36:166–176.

Diseases caused by lyssaviruses

Rabies is the most important member of the lyssavirus genus and was once considered a unique virus with no antigenically related relatives. Several other viruses antigenically related to rabies virus have, however, been identified. Although to date these other viruses are geographically restricted to Africa, they have the potential to cause rabies-like disease. Some of the viruses cannot be distinguished from rabies virus with standard techniques, such as fluorescent antibody staining; however, they can be distinguished with the use of more precise methods using monoclonal antibodies. These agents are **Lagos bat virus, Mokola virus,** and **Duvenhage virus,** which are quite similar to rabies virus, and the **Obodhiang** and **Kotonkan viruses,** which are related to Mokola virus.

The Lagos bat virus was first isolated from frugivorous bats *(Eidolon helvum)* on Lagos Island in Nigeria (Boulger and Porterfield, 1958). It was subsequently shown to kill three-day-old mice by intracerebral inoculation but not by the intraperitoneal route. This virus does not kill guinea pigs, rabbits, or one species of African monkey *(Cerocebus torquatus).*

The Mokola virus was originally isolated from the brains of shrews *(Crocidura* species), collected in Nigeria, and subsequently from the brains of children succumbing to a neurologic disorder. The virus is pathogenic for mice, and neutralizing antibodies have been demonstrated in cattle, sheep, goats, swine, and birds in Nigeria. More recent studies indicate that both the Lagos bat and Mokola viruses produce fatal disease in dogs and monkeys *(M. mulatta)* when inoculated intracerebrally (Tignor and others, 1973; Percy and others, 1973).

Duvenhage virus was isolated in South Africa from the brain of a human who died of a rabies-like disease after the bite of a bat.

The Obodhiang virus was recovered from *Mansonia uniformis* mosquitoes in the Sudan. No disease has been associated with this virus.

Kotonkan virus was recovered from the brains of *Culicoides* species. Reactions to the complement-fixation and fluorescent antibody tests are similar to those of the Mokola virus but not the same if the neutralization test is used. Neutralizing antibodies to this virus have been demonstrated in the sera of humans, cattle, rodents, insectivores, sheep, and horses. In cattle, Kotonkan has been associated with a disease resembling bovine ephemeral fever (Shope and others, 1970; Kemp and others, 1972, 1973; Tignor and others, 1973).

RABIES (HYDROPHOBIA, LYSSA, RAGE, TOLLWUT)

Rabies is a viral encephalitis to which all warm-blooded animals, including humans, are susceptible. Rabies exists worldwide with the exception of England, Australia, Japan, Sweden, Hawaii, and certain other islands which are completely free of the disease. In the United States, Canada, and Western Europe (where rabies in dogs is controlled through vaccination), rabies is endemic in wildlife, particularly skunks, foxes, raccoons, and bats. Cats are the most often affected domestic animals in the United States. In Asia, Latin America, and Africa, rabies is endemic in dogs and wildlife and numerous cases occur each year in humans. Vampire bats are important in the spread of the disease, particularly to cattle in South America. Here, the disease occurs as paralytic rabies, known as **Derrienge.** As a rule, rabies in humans results from the bite of a rabid dog, cat, skunk, raccoon, fox, or wolf. These animals also transmit the disease to cattle, horses, and sheep, which, however, seldom spread it further. Insectivorous and frugivorous bats may also harbor and transmit the virus, often without clinical signs of disease. In humans, most bites by a rabid animal do not lead to infection; however, once disease is established, it is nearly always fatal. Bites to the head are much more likely to lead to rabies infection than those to the extremities. Contrary to what was once thought, all animals that become infected do not succumb to the disease. This is true in bats, which can harbor the virus for long intervals, either apparently not developing encephalitis or having recovered from encephalitis. Humans and dogs can recover from rabies, although it is not the rule. Inapparent infection can also occur in dogs, leaving them immune to challenge.

Pathogenesis Most infections with rabies virus occur after the bite of a rabid animal with virus-containing saliva. Virus may be in the saliva before the onset of clinical signs. Rare cases of rabies have occurred in humans from breathing the air in a cave where thousands of bats were living. After viral entry, there is a variable incubation period of 1 week to 1 year with a mean of 1 to 2 months. It is this long interval that makes post-exposure vaccination effective. Virus first replicates in myocytes and is shed into extracellular spaces, entering peripheral or cranial nerves and progressing up axons to enter spinal or cranial ganglia, where rapid replication and spread throughout the central nervous system occurs (Color Plate I, E). The form of the virus during its axoplasmic flow is unclear. Intact virions have not been demonstrated in axons during this phase of the infection. There is eventual centrifugal spread via nerves throughout the body to other tissues, including the salivary glands.

Rabies has occurred after the use of modified live virus vaccines in several animal species, especially cats.

Signs After the bite of a rabid animal or penetration of the virus through the skin by some other means, the incubation period varies from a few days to several months. The clinical symptoms usually appear in one of two forms: the "dumb" or the "furious." In the dumb form of rabies, the animal falls into a stupor and has the peculiar staring expression characteristic of paralysis of the muscles of mastication. In the "furious" form, the animal goes into rages, biting and slashing at any moving object or even inanimate objects, such as sticks and trees. The furious champing of the jaws is accompanied by excessive salivation; the saliva streams from the mouth or is churned into foam, which may adhere to the lips and face. A radical change in temperament occurs; wild animals that normally shun humans venture into the open and attack humans. The rabid dog, fox, or wolf tends particularly to attack a moving person or animal. Paralysis may follow either the "furious" or "dumb" stage of the disease. Death occurs within 10 days of the first symptoms.

Lesions The lesions of rabies are microscopic, limited to the central nervous system, and extremely variable in extent. They may be subtle and indiscernible, except for early necrosis of neurons with specific cytoplasmic inclusion bodies in the affected nerve cells. In some cases, diffuse encephalitis is demonstrated by perivascular cuffing, neuronophagic nodules, and other indications of destruction of neurons throughout the brain. These changes tend to be particularly prominent in the brain stem, the hippocampus, and the gasserian ganglia. According to Lapi, Davis, and Anderson (1952), specific lesions develop earlier and more constantly in the gasserian ganglia than elsewhere in the nervous system and may be present even before specific inclusion bodies can be demonstrated. These lesions consist of focal proliferation of the capsule cells surrounding the ganglion cells, mild infiltration of lymphocytes and plasma cells, and encroachment of proliferating glial cells on the neurons. These collections of proliferating glial cells replacing neurons are known as **Babès' nodules.** They may be seen in association with inclusion bodies in the cytoplasm of nearby ganglion cells.

In 1903, spherical cytoplasmic inclusion bodies with specific tinctorial characteristics were described by Negri in neurons of dogs, cats, and rabbits that were experimentally infected with rabies virus. These inclusion bodies have subsequently been called **Negri bodies,** and are accepted as specific indications of infection with rabies virus (Fig. 8-66). Electron microscopic observations (Fig. 8-67) indicate that Negri bodies represent well-defined electron-dense masses, which may or may not contain or be associated with rabies virions. The nature and significance of the matrix is not understood, but may represent a necessary component for viral replication or a reaction on the part of the infected neuron. Negri bodies are not always present in rabies, and certain strains of rabies virus do not produce inclusion bodies, indicating that Negri bodies are not necessary for viral replication. Negri bodies are always intracytoplasmic; in the rabid dog they are found most readily in the hippocampus, but in cattle they are more numerous in the Purkinje cells of the cerebellum (Color Plate I, E). It is possible for all neurons, even those of the ganglia, to contain these inclusions. Negri bodies have a distinct limiting membrane and may be encircled by a narrow, clear halo. In tissue sections, they usually

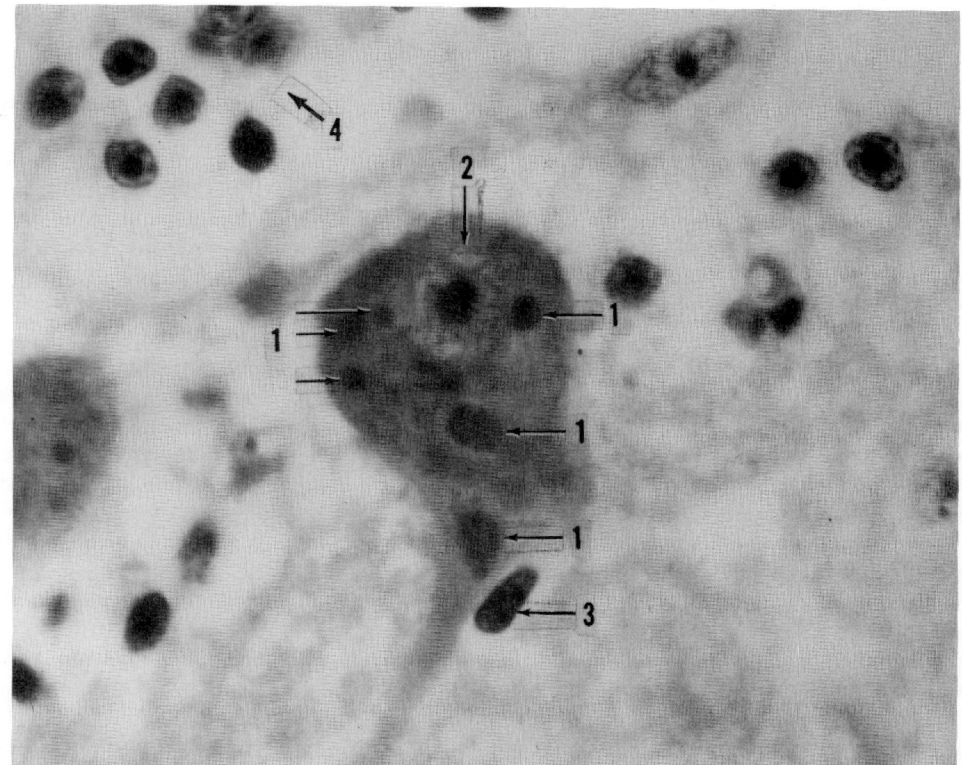

FIG. 8-66 Rabies, cerebellum of a cow (× 1350). An unusual number of Negri bodies *(1)* are present in a Purkinje cell. Nucleus of the Purkinje cell *(2)*, nucleus of a microglial cell *(3)*, and cells of a granular layer *(4)*. Schleifstein modification of the Wilhite stain. (Courtesy of the Armed Forces Institute of Pathology; contributed by Lt. Col. F. D. Maurer.)

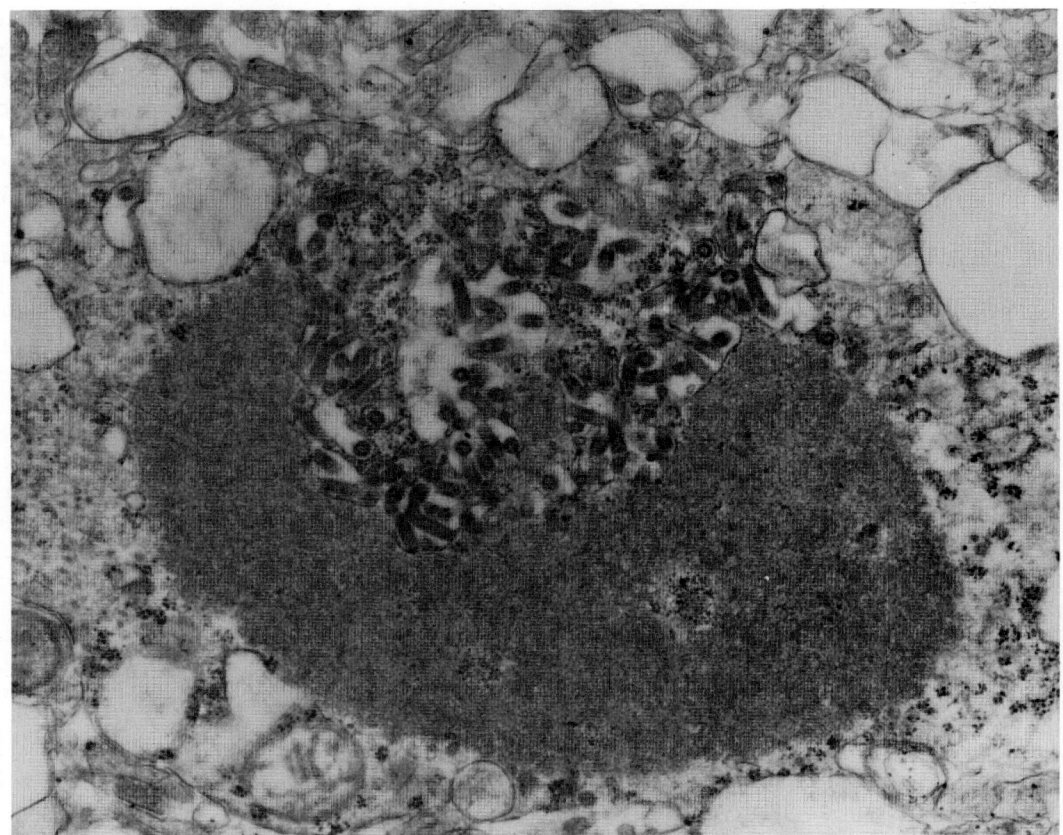

FIG. 8-67 Rabies, hippocampus of fox. Neuronal inclusion containing bullet-shaped and rod-shaped virus particles. (× 30,000.) (Courtesy of Dr. R. E. Dierks and *American Journal of Pathology*; electronmicrograph taken by Dr. F. A. Murphy.)

measure from 2 to 8 μ in diameter. One or several may be present in an affected nerve cell. These inclusions may be entirely within the cell body or they may occur in dendrites, where they are likely to be elongated, conforming to the shape of these processes. A granular, slightly basophilic internal structure can be demonstrated in preparations with Mann's stain.

The staining characteristics of the Negri body are of considerable interest. The hematoxylin and eosin method does not differentiate Negri bodies well. They become only a slightly darker shade of the color of the surrounding cytoplasm, but the clear halo may serve to delimit them. The Schleifstein modification of the Wilhite stain (Color Plate I, E) is particularly successful with tissue fixed in Zenker's solution. When stained by this method, Negri bodies are bright magenta, contrasting with the purplish cytoplasm of the neuron; red blood cells are somewhat yellowish or copper-colored. The Williams modification of the van Gieson's stain gives a similar effect. In impression smears, Seller's stain is effective; the inclusion body is bright red or magenta against the pale blue background of the neuronal cytoplasm. Mann's and Giemsa's stains are also useful, particularly in impression smears. No matter which stain is used, it is important that the person who examines material to confirm the diagnosis be thoroughly familiar with the characteristics of the stain and the appearance of Negri bodies. The final recognition of Negri bodies should not be left to the novice.

Spongiform lesions in the neuropil of the gray matter have been described in experimentally induced rabies in skunks, foxes, cows, horses, and cats (Charlton, 1984; Charlton and others, 1987). The lesions, primarily consisting of membrane-bound vacuoles 2 to 60 μm in diameter, are indistinguishable from other spongiform encephalopathies, such as scrapie, transmissible mink encephalopathy, the spongiform encephalopathies of elk and mule deer, and Creutzfeldt-Jakob disease.

When the virus centrifugally invades the salivary gland, degenerative changes leading to necrosis may be encountered in the acinar epithelium, principally affecting mucogenic cells of the mandibular salivary gland. Virus can readily be demonstrated within these cells by fluorescent antibody techniques and electron microscopy. A moderate infiltration of lymphocytes and plasma cells accompanies the degenerative changes.

Diagnosis The diagnosis of rabies can be based on the symptoms if they are typical, but should be confirmed by laboratory examination. Demonstration of typical Negri bodies is considered diagnostic; however, the brains of as many as 30% of infected animals may not contain demonstrable Negri bodies. Diagnosis should be confirmed using immunoflourescent or the newer peroxidase-antiperoxidase staining techniques. The latter procedure, which can be performed on paraffin-embedded tissue, has largely replaced reliance on the presence of Negri bodies or mouse inoculation.

Mice of all ages are susceptible to rabies virus, but newborn mice less than 3 days of age are most sensitive.

Following intracerebral inoculation, newborn mice usually succumb within 14 days, but should be examined daily for at least 4 weeks before the test is considered negative. The virus is demonstrated in the brains of mice that die (1) by finding Negri bodies, (2) by a neutralization test in other mice, or preferably, (3) by the fluorescent antibody identification of the virus. Rabies virus may also be isolated by injecting suspected brain suspensions into tissue culture. Positive results can be obtained in 24 hours, and the virus identified by the fluorescent antibody method.

In animals in which rabies is suspected but cannot be demonstrated, an attempt should be made to determine the cause of death or cause of encephalitis. Diseases to consider are canine hepatitis, toxoplasmosis, distemper in dogs, *Oestrus ovis* infestation in sheep, and listeriosis in sheep and cattle. The brain, spinal cord, or meninges may also be involved in diseases of unknown etiology. Differentiation of canine hepatitis and canine distemper are of considerable importance, since inclusion bodies may occur in both of these diseases. Both are also much more common in dogs than is rabies. In canine hepatitis involving the brain, intranuclear inclusions are found in endothelial cells in association with rupture of capillary walls and microscopic hemorrhages. The inclusions of canine distemper are most readily demonstrable in glial cells, particularly in the nuclei of gemistocytic astrocytes and microglia. Fluorescence antibody techniques show that distemper inclusions occur in neurons, but they are less readily demonstrable with other methods. Cytoplasmic inclusions are less commonly found in the brain in canine distemper.

Groups of tiny spherical bodies without a definite limiting membrane are encountered in the cytoplasm of neurons of nonrabid animals. Since at one time they were thought to be associated with rabies, they were given the name "Lyssa bodies." It now seems clear that they are not specific for rabies. They have been described in the dog, cat, skunk, fox, and laboratory white mouse. Although they can be easily confused with Negri bodies, they lack an internal structure, are more acidophilic, and are highly refractile. In the brains of normal cats, other cytoplasmic inclusions with tinctorial characteristics that are essentially the same as those of Negri bodies have been described. These feline inclusions cannot be differentiated morphologically from Negri bodies; therefore, it may be necessary to resort to animal inoculation or fluorescent antibody techniques when rabies is suspected in the cat.

References

Arko RJ, Schneider LG, Baer GM. Non-fatal canine rabies. Am J Vet Res 1973;34:937–938.

Baer GM, Olson HR. Recovery of pigs from rabies. J Am Vet Med Assoc 1972;160:1127–1128.

Beauregard M, Boulanger P, Webster WA. The use of fluorescent antibody staining in the diagnosis of rabies. Can J Comp Med 1965; 29:141–147.

Beck AM, Felser SR, Glickman LT. An epizootic of rabies in Maryland, 1982–1984. Am J Publ Health 1987;77:42–44.

Behymer DE, et al. Observations on the pathogenesis of rabies: experimental infection with a virus coyote origin. J Wildl Dis 1974; 10:197–203.

Bishop DHL, ed. Rhabdoviruses, Vol I. Boca Raton: CRC Press 1979.

Boulger LR. Natural rabies in a laboratory monkey. Lancet 1966;1:941–943.

Centers for Disease Control. Rabies in a llama—Oklahoma. MMWR 1990;39(12):203–204.

Charlton KM. Rabies: spongiform lesions in the brain. Acta Neuropathol (Berl) 1984;63:198–202.

Charlton KM, Casey GA, Webster WA, et al. Experimental rabies in skunks and foxes. Pathogenesis of the spongiform lesions. Lab Invest 1987;57:634–645.

Constantine DG, Emmons RW, Woodie JD. Rabies virus in nasal mucosa of naturally infected bats. Science 1972;175:1255–1256.

Covell WP, Danks WBC. Studies on the nature of the Negri body. Am J Pathol 1932;8:557–571.

Debbie JG. Rabies. Prog Med Virol 1974;18:241–256.

Dierks RE, Murphy FA, Harrison AK. Extraneural rabies virus infection. Virus development in fox salivary gland. Am J Pathol 1969;54:251–273.

Diesch SL, Hendricks SL, Currier RW. The role of cats in human rabies exposures. J Am Vet Med Assoc 1982;181:1510–1512.

Doege TC, Northrop RL. Evidence for inapparent rabies infection. Lancet 1974;2:826–829.

du Plessis JL. The topographical distribution of Negri bodies in the brain. J S Afr Vet Med Assoc 1965;36:203–207.

Esh JB, Cunningham JG, Wiktor TJ. Vaccine induced rabies in four cats. J Am Vet Med Assoc 1982;180:1336–1338.

Fekadu M. Asymptomatic non-fatal canine rabies. Lancet 1975;1:569.

Fekadu M, Baer GM. Recovery from clinical rabies of 2 dogs inoculated with a rabies virus strain from Ethiopia. Am J Vet Res 1980;41:1632–1634.

Fekadu M, Chandler FW, Harrison AK. Pathogenesis of rabies in dogs inoculated with an Ethiopian rabies virus strain. Immunofluorescence, histologic and ultrastructural studies of the central nervous system. Arch Virol 1982;71:109–126.

Fekadu M, Shadduck JH, Chandler FW, et al. Pathogenesis of rabies virus from a Danish bat (Eptesicus serotinus): neuronal changes suggestive of spongiosis. Arch Virol 1988;99:187–203.

Fischman HR, Schaeffer M. Pathogenesis of experimental rabies as revealed by immunofluorescence. Ann NY Acad Sci 1971;177:78–97.

Fischman HR, Strandberg JD. Inapparent rabies virus infection of the central nervous system. J Am Vet Med Assoc 1973;163:1050–1055.

Flamand A, Wiktor TJ, Koprowski H. Use of hybridoma monoclonal antibodies in the detection of antigenic differences between rabies and rabies-related virus proteins. I. The nucleocapsid protein. J Gen Virol 1980;48:97–104.

Goodpasture EW. Studies of rabies with reference to neural transmission of virus in rabbits and structure and significance of Negri bodies. Am J Pathol 1925;1:547–582.

Herzog E. Histologic diagnosis of rabies. Arch Pathol 1945;39:279–280.

Hottle GA, et al. Electron microscopy of rabies inclusion (Negri) bodies. Proc Soc Exp Biol 1951;77:721–723.

Kemp GE, et al. Mokola virus. Further studies on IbAn27377, a new rabies-related etiologic agent of zoonosis in Nigeria. Am J Trop Med Hyg 1972;21:356–359.

Kemp GE, et al. Kotonkan, a new rhabdovirus related to Mokola virus of the rabies serogroup. Am J Epidemiol 1973;98:43–49.

Lapi A, Davis CL, Anderson WA. The gasserian ganglion in animals dead of rabies. J Am Vet Med Assoc 1952;120:379–384.

Martell D, Montes FC, Alcocer BR. Transplacental transmission of bovine rabies after natural infection. J Infect Dis 1973;127:291–293.

Martell MA, et al. Experimental bovine paralytic rabies—"derriengue." Vet Rec 1974;95:527–530.

Murphy FA, Bauer SP, Harrison AK, et al. Comparative pathogenesis of rabies and rabies-like viruses: viral infection and transit from inoculation site to the central nervous system. Lab Invest 1973;28:361–376.

Murphy FA, Harrison AK, Winn WC, et al. Comparative pathogenesis of rabies and rabies-like viruses: infection of the central nervous

system and centrifugal spread of virus to peripheral tissues. Lab Invest 1973;29:1–16.

Negri A. Beitrag zum Studium der Aetiologie der Tollwuth. Ztschr Hyg Infektionskr 1903;43:507–528.

Palmer DG, Ossent P, Suter MM, et al. Demonstration of rabies viral antigen in paraffin tissue sections: comparison of the immunofluorescence technique with the unlabeled antibody enzyme method. Am J Vet Res 1985;46:283–286.

Percy DH, Bhatt PN, Tignor GH, et al. Experimental infection of dogs and monkeys with two rabies serogroup viruses, Lagos Bat and Mokola (IbAn 27377). Gross pathologic and histopathologic changes. Vet Pathol 1973;10:534–549.

Prins B, Loewen K. Bat rabies in British Columbia, 1971–1985. Can Vet J 1988;29:41–44.

Reid-Sanden FL, Dobbins JG, Smith JS, et al. Rabies surveillance in the United States during 1989. J Am Vet Med Assoc 1990;197:1571–1583.

Rupprecht CE, Dietzschold B. Perspectives on rabies virus pathogenesis. Lab Invest 1987;57:603–606.

Shope RE, et al. Two African viruses serologically and morphologically related to rabies virus. J Virol 1970;6:690–692.

Szlochta HL, Habel RE. Inclusions resembling Negri bodies in the brains of nonrabid cats. Cornell Vet 1953;43:207–212.

Tierkel ES. Rabies. Adv Vet Sci 1959;5:183–226.

Tignor GH, Shope RE, Bhatt PN, et al. Experimental infection of dogs and monkeys with two rabies serogroup viruses, Lagos bat and Mokalo (IbAn27377): clinical, serologic, virologic, and fluorescent antibody studies. J Infect Dis 1973;128:471–478.

Winkler WG, Baker EF Jr, Hopkins CC. An outbreak of non-bite transmitted rabies in a laboratory animal colony. Am J Epidemiol 1972;95:267–277.

BOVINE EPHEMERAL FEVER (BOVINE EPIZOOTIC FEVER, THREE-DAY SICKNESS, STIFF SICKNESS)

This subtle disease was apparently known in Africa as early as 1867, but its exact nature was obscure until 1967, when Westhuizen first isolated and identified the etiologic agent. The viral agent was identified as having features similar to those of vesicular stomatitis and rabies and is currently classified in the rhabdovirus family. The natural disease is characterized by transitory fever, inappetence, hyperpnea or dyspnea of short duration, mucous to purulent nasal discharge, shivering, and a shifting lameness. In some cases, rumination may cease for a few days and ruminal stasis, diarrhea, or constipation may occur. Occasional posterior paralysis has been described. Many animals become ill but few die from the disease.

Bovine ephemeral fever has been reported from Africa, Asia, and Australia. Epizootiologic features, such as seasonal appearance of the disease, failure of transmission by contact, apparent spread by leaps over long distances, and the tendency for outbreaks to occur during seasons of heavy rainfall, indicate that the virus is probably transmitted by biting insects. Experiments with stable flies and mosquitoes indicate that they are probably not responsible for transmission of this virus. *Culicoides* species are suspected to be the vectors, along with mosquitoes, but confirming evidence is lacking.

Lesions Gross lesions reported in natural and experimental cases include generalized vascular engorgement, edematous lymph nodes, congestion of abomasal mucosa, hydropericardium, hydrothorax, rhinitis, tracheitis, and pulmonary emphysema. Tendovaginitis, fasciculitis, and cellulitis and focal necrosis of muscle have also been described. Petechiae may be seen in epineurium of peripheral nerves.

Lesions noted with the light microscope appear to be limited to venules and capillaries, particularly in muscles, tendon sheaths, synovial membranes, fascia, and skin. Endothelial cells may be hyperplastic, and the vessels surrounded by edema and leukocytic infiltration. Some vessel walls are necrotic; others, thrombosed. Hemosiderosis of spleen and lymph nodes has also been associated with the disease.

Diagnosis Diagnosis may be confirmed by isolation and identification of the virus or by identifying viral antigens in tissues of affected animals by specific immunofluorescent techniques. Clinically, Kotonkan virus infection in Africa and Ibaraki disease (an orbivirus) in Japan resemble bovine ephemeral fever.

References

Basson PA, Pienaar JG, van der Westhuizen B. The pathology of ephemeral fever: a study of the experimental disease in cattle. J S Afr Vet Med Assoc 1969;40:385–397.

Burgess GW. Bovine ephemeral fever: a review. Vet Bull 1971;41:887–895.

Heuschele WP. Bovine ephemeral fever. I. Characteristics of the causative virus. Arch ges Virusforsch 1970;30:195–202.

Holmes IH, Doherty RL. Morphology and development of bovine ephemeral fever virus. J Virol 1970;5:91–96.

Lecatsas G. Further observations on the ultrastructure of ephemeral fever virus. Onderstepoort J Vet Res 1970;37:145–146.

Matumoto M, et al. Behavior of bovine ephemeral fever virus in laboratory animals and cell cultures. Jpn J Microbiol 1970;14:413–421.

Parsonson IM, Snowdon WA. Ephemeral fever virus. I. Excretion in semen of infected bulls and attempts to infect female cattle by the intrauterine inoculation of virus. II. Experimental infection of pregnant cattle. Aust Vet J 1974;50:329–337.

Snowdon WA. Bovine ephemeral fever: the reaction of cattle to different strains of ephemeral fever virus and the antigenic comparison of two strains of virus. Aust Vet J 1970;46:258–266.

Theodoridis A. Fluorescent antibody studies on ephemeral fever virus. Onderstepoort J Vet Res 1969;36:187–190.

Tzipori S, Spradbrow PB. Development and behaviour of a strain of bovine ephemeral fever virus with unusual host range. J Comp Pathol 1974;84:1–8.

Tzipori S. The susceptibility of young calves and newborn to bovine ephemeral fever virus. Aust Vet J 1975;51:254–255.

Young JS. Ephemeral fever and congenital deformities in calves. Aust Vet J 1969;45:574–576.

RETROVIRIDAE

The family *Retroviridae* contains a diverse group of RNA viruses that are divided into three subfamilies: oncornaviruses (oncos = tumor); lentiviruses (lente = slow); and spumaviruses (spuma = foam). Important members of each group are listed in Table 8-10.

The family derives its name from the presence of the enzyme reverse transcriptase (RNA-dependent DNA-polymerase), which is carried in the virion of all member viruses (retro = reverse). The genome of these viruses consists of two single-stranded positive-sense molecules of RNA (i.e., diploid). In contrast to other RNA viruses, the information stored in the virion nucleic acid is not directly translated; instead, a double-stranded DNA replica of viral RNA is generated by way of reverse transcription. This multistep process is de-

TABLE 8-10 *Retroviridae*

Lentivirinae (exogenous)

Visna/maedi virus
Caprine arthritis-encephalitis virus
Human immunodeficiency virus (HIV-1, HIV-2)
Simian immunodeficiency virus
Feline immunodeficiency virus
Bovine immunodeficiency virus

Oncovirinae (RNA tumor viruses)

Type C oncovirus group (most are exogenous)
  Feline leukemia virus
  Feline sarcoma virus
  Bovine leukemia virus
  Ovine leukemia virus
  Porcine leukemia virus
  Gibbon ape leukemia virus (Simian sarcoma virus)
  Murine sarcoma/leukemia viruses
  Human T cell leukemia virus (HTLV-1, HTLV-II)
  Simian T-cell leukemia virus (STLV-1)
  Rat type C oncovirus
  Baboon type C oncovirus
  Avian type C oncoviruses
Type B oncovirus group
  Mouse mammary tumor virus (endogenous)
Type D oncovirus group (exogenous)
  Jaagsiekte virus (pulmonary adenocarcinoma virus of sheep)
  Mason-Pfizer monkey virus group (simian retrovirus)

Spumavirinae (foamy viruses, inapparent infections)

Bovine syncytial virus
Feline syncytial virus
Hamster syncytial virus
Human foamy virus
Simian foamy virus (9 serotypes)

pendent on and catalyzed by virally encoded reverse transcriptase. The virally generated DNA is synthesized in the cytoplasm, but subsequently may be integrated into host-cell DNA and termed "provirus integrated DNA." Expression of provirus DNA can occur whether or not the viral DNA is integrated, but perpetuation of the virus is clearly most efficient if integration has occurred. The proviral DNA of certain retroviruses is integrated in germ cells and transmitted vertically (**genetic transmission**) with every cell thus containing proviral DNA. These viruses are known as **endogenous** and generally remain quiescent, not being expressed and of low or no pathogenicity. Vertical transmission can also occur by virion passage across the placenta (**congenital transmission**). Viruses transmitted by the horizontal route are termed **exogenous** and are the retroviruses of most importance as causes of disease.

Retroviruses characteristically cause a chronic cellular infection that does not lead to early cell lysis; in fact, with the oncoviruses, infection leads to uncontrolled cellular proliferation. This is in contrast to most other RNA viruses, for which infection and replication lead to cell death. All retroviruses contain three or four genes in common. Each bears genes for reverse transcriptase referred to as *pol* genes (polymerase), a gene for core proteins called the *gag* gene (group specific antigens), and a gene encoding for virion peplomer proteins called the *env* gene (envelope). Members of the oncovirus subfamily may contain a fourth gene responsible for cellular transformation. This is called the viral oncogene, or *v-onc*.

All retroviruses share a similar morphology, consisting of an inner core or nucleoid of RNA surrounded by an icosahedral capsid, which in turn is surrounded by a lipid-containing envelope bearing glycoprotein projections. Virions are 80 nm to 130 nm in diameter. There are differences between groups of retroviruses with respect to the shape of the nucleoid, the prominence of envelop projections, and the process of budding from cell membranes to produce mature virions. All lentiviruses, however, bud from cell membranes with a characteristic crescent at the cell membrane. This feature, originally noted with certain oncornaviruses, gave rise to the term type C virus. Replication of oncornaviruses only occurs in dividing cells, whereas lentiviruses can replicate in nondividing cells.

References

Fenner F, Bachmann PA, Gibbs EPJ, et al. Veterinary Virology. Academic Press, New York: 1987.

Hardy WD Jr. Naturally occurring retroviruses (RNA tumor viruses). (Parts I, II and II cont'd.) Cancer Invest 1983;1:67–83, 163–174, 333–343.

Varmus H. Reverse transcription. Sci Am 1987;257(3):56–64.

Diseases Caused by *Lentivirinae*

Lentiviruses have come from general obscurity into the forefront of viral pathology with the discovery that the cause of acquired immunodeficiency syndrome (AIDS) of humans is a lentivirus, human immunodeficiency virus (HIV). Lentiviruses affecting animals include the viruses of visna and maedi (which are nearly identical), caprine arthritis-encephalitis virus, equine infectious anemia virus, feline immunodeficiency virus, bovine immunodeficiency virus, and simian immunodeficiency virus. Lentiviruses establish a chronic persistent infection with a protracted incubation period. Sigurdsson (1954), studying visna and maedi, introduced the term "slow virus" infections to describe chronicity, a term now used for other lentiviruses as well as some other chronic, nonlentiviral diseases, such as scrapie. Lentiviral infections persist even though they initiate humoral and cellular immune responses. A number of hypotheses have been put forward to explain persistence, but the mechanism these viruses use to escape elimination is largely unclear. They share the characteristics described above with other retroviruses, but differ antigenically from one another and the members of the oncornavirus and spumavirus subfamilies. They also differ in their morphogenesis and have more genes. They do not require dividing cells for replication, and transcription and translation occurs from nonintegrated viral DNA. The

crescent formed in the cell membrane during budding is thicker than that of other retroviruses, and the nucleoid is cylindrical or rod-shaped.

Pathologically, lentiviruses establish themselves in macrophages and lymphocytes and interfere with immune functions. It is for this reason that the more recent isolates have been termed immunodeficiency viruses, following the nomenclature established for human immunodeficiency virus. The lesions associated with the different lentiviruses may vary, but most cause some combination of the following: (1) lymphadenopathy with marked follicular hyperplasia, which may progress to lymphoid depletion; (2) lymphocytic infiltrates, often nodular in any tissue; (3) interstitial pneumonia; (4) encephalomyelitis; or (4) arthritis. In severely immunodeficient animals, opportunistic infections may develop (especially true for HIV) and may dominate the pathologic findings and be the immediate cause of presenting signs or death.

VISNA/MAEDI (OVINE PROGRESSIVE PNEUMONIA, LYMPHOID INTERSTITIAL PNEUMONIA, CHRONIC VIRAL ENCEPHALOMYELITIS OF SHEEP)

A chronic viral encephalomyelitis of sheep was first reported in Iceland by Sigurdsson, Thormar, and Palsson in 1935. The name "visna," an Icelandic word for shrinkage or wasting, was used to indicate one clinical feature of the disease in the paralyzed sheep. A chronic progressive pneumonia in sheep was recognized in 1939 by Gislason (Guadnadottir, 1974) and named "maedi," an Icelandic word meaning dyspnea. It is now believed that visna and maedi are caused by the same virus. A disease similar to maedi, described in the Netherlands and named **zwoegerziekte,** is also caused by the same virus. The same or a similar virus appears to cause the progressive pneumonia (Marsh, 1923) described first in sheep in Montana (Kennedy and others, 1968). Infection with the virus can also lead to polyarthritis and mastitis.

Owing to the long interval between infection and development of clinical disease, which is usually 2 to 3 years but may be as long as 8 years, these disorders are seen only in adult sheep. Goats are susceptible, but they are subject to their own lentiviral infection, caprine arthritis-encephalitis. Infection is principally spread by the respiratory route with initial replication in macrophages, leading to a cell-associated viremia and dissemination of the virus to the brain and other organs. Although the incidence of infection in a flock can be high, the percentage of sheep developing clinical disease is low. Once clinical signs develop, however, the disease is invariably fatal.

Lesions of visna Although, when originally encountered, the virus appeared to affect either the lungs or the central nervous system, it now seems evident that both systems may be affected in the same animal. The lesions in the central nervous system consist of zones of demyelination with destruction of paraventricular white matter in the cerebellum and cerebrum. Similar lesions have a focal distribution in the spinal cord (Fig. 8-68). The demyelinated zones are surrounded by gliosis and

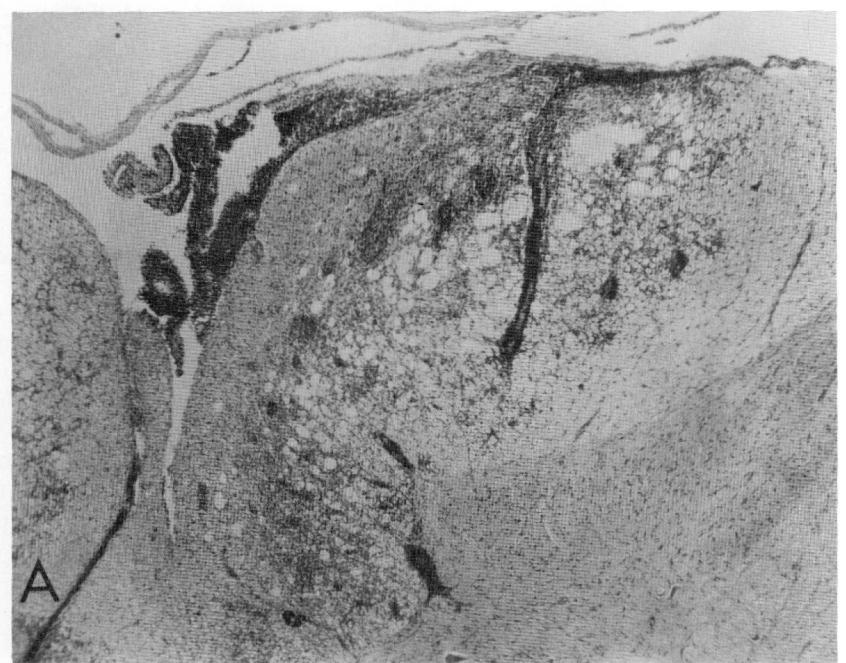

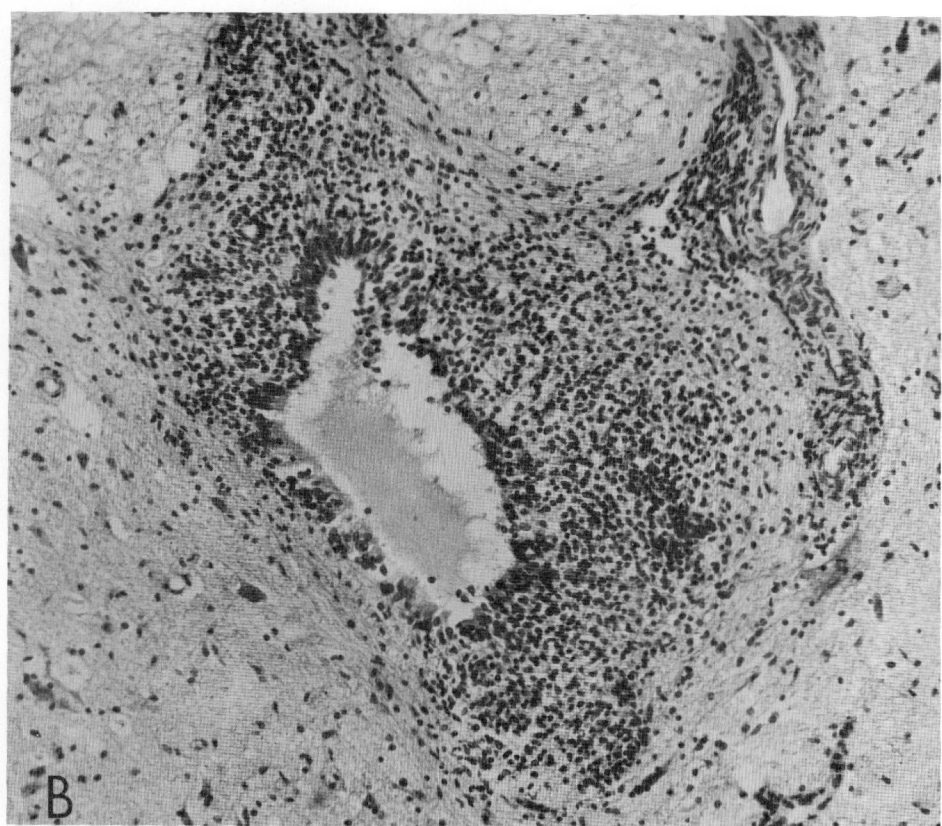

FIG. 8-68 Visna. **A.** Leptomeningeal infiltrate, perivascular cuffing, and microcavitation of lumbar spinal cord. **B.** Cellular infiltration surrounding central canal of cervical spinal cord. (Courtesy of Dr. Pall A. Palsson.)

lymphocytic infiltration. The meninges of both brain and spinal cord are usually infiltrated by lymphocytes and other mononuclear cells.

The lesions in the central nervous system result in severely increased numbers of cells in the cerebrospinal fluid (pleocytosis). This is of value in distinguishing the clinical disease from scrapie, which does not result in pleocytosis.

Lesions of maedi/progressive pneumonia The gross lesions of the pulmonary form of this infection (maedi) are quite characteristic. The lungs do not collapse fully when the thorax is opened. They have a

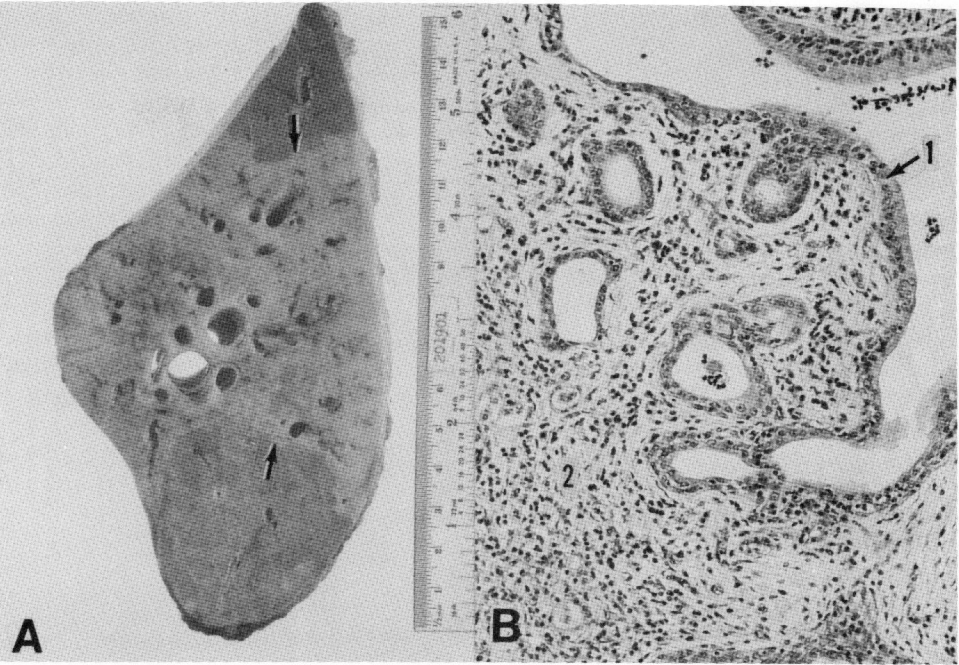

FIG. 8-69 Pneumonia. **A.** Ovine progressive pneumonia. Lung of a sheep. Note area of consolidation *(arrows)* in center of lung. **B.** The same lung (× 130). Note hyperplasia of epithelium of bronchioles *(1)* and alveolar ducts, and intense inflammation and fibrosis that obliterate the alveoli *(2)*. (Contributed by Dr. Hadleigh Marsh; courtesy of Armed Forces Institute of Pathology.)

dense, rubbery consistency but do not appear consolidated. All lobes have a uniform grayish-yellow to grayish-blue color and are of uniform consistency. This feature contrasts markedly with the sharp differences between normal and consolidated areas in lungs with the usual type of acute pneumonia. The lungs are distended, appear large, and actually weigh two to five times as much as normal adult sheep lungs (i.e., normally 300 to 500 g). The cut surface is dry and exudate cannot be expressed, except possibly some mucus from the large bronchi.

The microscopic lesions in the lung reveal that the loss of elasticity and compressibility as well as the grayish color are caused by a great increase in thickness of the alveolar walls. This thickening may be so great that the alveolar spaces are obliterated. The thickening is caused by proliferation and infiltration of reticuloendothelial or mesenchymal cells that invade the septa everywhere. As is the case in many types of reticuloendothelial proliferation, the cells vary from large round mononuclear forms, some of which appear to be macrophages, to short fibroblastic cells. Hyperemia of the interalveolar capillaries is a feature in early stages. The smooth muscle of the alveolar ducts (terminal bronchioles) is hyperplastic. Lymph nodules occur along the course of the bronchi and bronchioles. Alveolar lining cells in alveoli near the bronchi tend to become swollen and cuboid. A few large mononuclear cells contain one or more peculiar cytoplasmic inclusions, 1 to 3 μ in diameter, which take a soft bluish-gray color with Giemsa's stain. These are probably specific for the disease.

There is generalized follicular hyperplasia in lymph nodes and the spleen, and lymphoid infiltrates may be found in almost any organ. The polyarthritis is characterized by villous hyperplasia of the synovial membrane and an extensive lymphocytic and plasma-cell infiltration.

References

Boer GF de. Zwoegerziekte virus, the causative agent for progressive interstitial pneumonia (maedi) and meningo-leucoencephalitis (visna) in sheep. Res Vet Sci 1975;18:15–25.

Brahic M, Stowring L, Ventura P, et al. Gene expression in visna virus infection in sheep. Nature (Lond) 1981;292:240–242.

Cutlip RC, Lehmkuhl HD, Brogden KA, et al. Seroprevalence of ovine progressive pneumonia virus in various domestic and wild animal species, and species susceptibility to the virus. Am J Vet Res 1991;52:189–191.

Deng P, Cutlip RC, Lehmkuhl HD, et al. Ultrastructure and frequency of mastitis caused by ovine progressive pneumonia virus infection in sheep. Vet Pathol 1986;23:184–189.

Ellis JA, DeMartini JC. Immunomorphologic and morphometric changes in pulmonary lymph nodes of sheep with progressive pneumonia. Vet Pathol 1985;22:32–41.

Georgsson G, et al. The ultrastructure of early visna lesions. Acta Neuropathol 1977;37:127–135.

Gonda MA, Wong-Staal F, Gallo RC, et al. Sequence homology and morphologic similarity of HTLV-III and visna virus, a pathogenic lentivirus. Science 1985;227:173–177.

Gudnadottir M. Visna-maedi in sheep. Prog Med Virol 1974;18:336–349.

Haase AT. The slow infection caused by visna virus. Curr Top Microbiol Immunol 1975;72:101–156.

Haase AT, Stowring L, Narayan O, et al. Slow persistent infection caused by visna virus: role of host restriction. Science 1977;195:175–177.

Harter DH, Coward JE. Sheep progressive pneumonia viruses: "slow" cytolytic agents with tumor virus properties: a review. Tex Rep Biol Med 1974;32:649–664.

Kennedy RC, Eklund CM, Lopez C, et al. Isolation of a virus from the lungs of Montana sheep affected with progressive pneumonia. Virology 1968;35:483–484.

Kennedy-Stoskopf S, Narayan O. Neutralizing antibodies to visna lentivirus: mechanism of action and possible role in virus persistence. J Virol 1986;59:37–44.

Marsh H. Progressive pneumonia in sheep. J Am Vet Med Assoc 1923;62:458–473.

Narayan O, Silverstein AM, Price D, et al. Visna virus infection of American lambs. Science 1974;183:1202–1203.

Nobel TA, Neumann F, Klopfer U. Pathological changes in lungs of imported sheep with special reference to maedi. Refuah Veterinarith 1973;30:19–23.

Oldstone MBA, Lampert PW, Lee S, et al. Pathogenesis of the slow disease of the central nervous system associated with WM 1504 E virus. Am J Pathol 1977;88:193–212.

Oliver RE, Gorham JR, Parish SF, et al. Ovine progressive pneumonia: pathologic and virologic studies on the naturally occurring disease. Am J Vet Res 1981;42:1554–1559.

Oliver RE, Gorham JR, Perryman LE, et al. Ovine progressive pneumonia: experimental intrathoracic, intracerebral, and intra-articular infections. Am J Vet Res 1981;42:1560–1564.

Palsson PA, Georgsson G, Petursson G, et al. Experimental visna in Icelandic lambs. Acta Vet Scand 1977;18:122–128.

Petursson G, et al. Pathogenesis of visna. I. Sequential virologic, serologic and pathologic studies. Lab Invest 1976;35:402–412.

Ressang AA, Stam FC, DeBoer GF. A meningo-leucoencephalomyelitis resembling visna in Dutch Zwoeger sheep. Pathol Vet 1966;3:401–411.

Robinson WF, Ellis TM. The pathological features of an interstitial pneumonia of goats. J Comp Pathol 1984;94:55–64.

Sigurdsson B. Maedi, a slow progressive pneumonia of sheep: an epizootiological and pathological study. Br Vet J 1954;110:255–270.

Sigurdsson B, Grimsson H, Palsson PA. Maedi, a chronic progressive infection of sheeps' lungs. J Infect Dis 1952;90:233–241.

Sigurdsson B, Palsson PA. Visna of sheep. A slow demyelinating infection. Br J Exp Pathol 1958;39:519–528.

Sigurdsson B. Observations on three slow infections of sheep, with general remarks on infections which develop slowly and some of their special characteristics. Br Vet J 1954;110:341–354.

Sigurdsson B, Palsson PA, Grimsson H. Visna, a demyelinating transmissible disease of sheep. J Neuropathol Exp Neurol 1957;16:389–403.

Sigurdsson B, Palsson PA, van Bogaert L. Pathology of visna (transmissible demyelinating disease of sheep in Iceland). Acta Neuropath 1962;1:343–362.

CAPRINE ARTHRITIS-ENCEPHALITIS

Cork and associates first described a new disease of goats in 1974 that is now known as caprine arthritis-encephalitis (CAE) and recognized as one of the most important diseases of goats. It is caused by a lentivirus related to the visna/maedi virus, which is distributed worldwide with prevalence rates of up to 80% in some herds; however, the number of infected animals with clinical disease is usually 25% or less. Sheep can be infected with the virus.

The pathologic effects of the virus on goats are remarkably similar to those seen in visna/maedi of sheep; however, arthritis is paramount and pneumonia of lesser severity. The principal route of infection is via colostrum or milk.

Signs The encephalitic form of the disease is usually seen in young goats 1 to 4 months of age, in contrast to most lentiviral infections. Affected kids first have difficulty abducting the hind limbs and become ataxic. An ascending paralysis progresses to total posterior paralysis and ultimately tetraparesis. There may be torticollis, and the head is held upward or at another angle. There is only mild fever, if any, but interstitial pneumonia may accompany this stage and be evident clinically.

The arthritic form is seen in adult goats and is usually a chronic, slowly progressive disorder, developing over months. All joints are affected, but swelling of the carpal, hock, and stifle joints is most obvious.

Lesions Central nervous system lesions are confined to the white matter and characterized by disseminated perivascular accumulations of mononuclear cells and demyelination. The mononuclear cuffs are composed of lymphocytes, macrophages, and large reticulum cells. Reactive astrocytes and gitter cells are present. The lesions are most severe from the mesencephalon caudally. The leptomeninges are focally infiltrated with lymphocytes.

The articular lesions are characterized by a villous proliferative synovitis with extensive lymphocytic infiltration. Similar lesions are present in tendon sheaths and bursae.

In the lung, there is an interstitial pneumonia with pronounced lymphoid hyperplasia (Fig. 8-69).

References

Cheevers WP, Knowles DP, McGuire TC, et al. Chronic disease in goats orally infected with two isolates of the caprine arthritis-encephalitis lentivirus. Lab Invest 1988;58:510–517.

Cork LC, Hadlow WJ, Crawford TB, et al. Infectious leukoencephalomyelitis of young goats. J Infect Dis 1974;129:134–141.

Crawford TB, Adams DS, Cheevers WP, et al. Chronic arthritis in goats caused by a retrovirus. Science 1980;207:997–999.

East NE, Rowe JD, Madewell BR, et al. Serologic prevalence of caprine arthritis-encephalitis virus in California goat dairies. J Am Vet Med Assoc 1987;190:182–186.

Ellis TM, Robinson WF, Wilcox GE. The pathology and aetiology of lung lesions in goats infected with caprine arthiritis-encephalitis virus. Aust Vet J 1988;65:69–73.

Gazit A, Yaniv A, Dvir M, et al. The caprine arthritis-encephalitis virus is a distinct virus within the lentiviral group. Virology 1983;124:192–195.

Gogolewski RP, Adams DS, McGuire TC, et al. Antigenic cross-reactivity between caprine arthritis-encephalitis, visna and progressive pneumonia viruses involves all virion-associated proteins and glycoproteins. J Gen Virol 1985;66:1233–1240.

Lairmore MD, Poulson JM, Adducci TA, et al. Lentivirus-induced lymphoproliferative disease. Comparative pathogenicity of phenotypically distinct ovine lentivirus strains. Am J Pathol 1988;130:80–90.

Norman S, Smith MC. Caprine arthritis-encephalitis: review of the neurologic form in 30 cases. J Am Vet Med Assoc 1983;182:1342–1345.

Roberson SM, McGuire TC, Klevjer-Anderson P, et al. Caprine arthritis-encephalitis virus is distinct from visna and progressive pneumonia viruses as measured by genome sequence homology. J Virol 1982;44:755–758.

Smith MC, Cutlip R. Effects of infection with caprine arthritis-encephalitis virus on milk production in goats. J Am Vet Med Assoc 1988;193:63–67.

EQUINE INFECTIOUS ANEMIA (SWAMP FEVER)

Infectious anemia of equines, a lentiviral disease with worldwide distribution, first recognized and described in France in 1843 (Henson and McGuire, 1974), is not only a serious economic problem but also a model useful for the study of mechanisms involved in prolonged persistence of virus in the host and its pathogenic effects. Once the virus gains access to a susceptible animal, it can be demonstrated in the circulating blood as long as the animal lives; despite the immune response, the virus persists as with other lentiviral infections. The infection may be almost subclinical, or it may be acute with febrile manifestations and a rapidly fatal outcome. Infected horses have lived as long as 18 years with few signs; yet, at any time, minute amounts of their blood injected into normal horses induces acute infectious anemia. Horses that apparently have recovered from the acute disease may suddenly exhibit severe symptoms and die after exposure to some deleterious influence (hard work, for example, or injection of an additional, though minute, amount of infectious anemia virus). It would seem that host and parasite, under some conditions, maintain a delicate balance. Equines (horses, mules, asses) are the only species susceptible to natural or experimental exposure.

The virus is transmitted mechanically by the bite of a mosquito (*Nopheles psorophora* or *Culex pipiens quinquefasciatus*) or biting fly (*Stomoxys calcitrans, Tabanus fuscicostatus*) or by the transfer of a minute amount of blood from an infected horse to a normal one by the use of unsterilized hypodermic needles, tattoo needles, curry combs, or items of equipment, such as harness, bit, or saddle. The disease is not spread by ordinary contact.

Antigens in the virus of equine infectious anemia have been demonstrated by complement-fixation, complement-fixation-inhibition, precipitin, and immuno-fluorescence techniques. Humoral antibody response is not quantitatively deficient in infected animals; thus, loss of antibody response cannot be accepted as explanation of the life-long persistence of the virus in the equine host. Circulating virus-antibody complexes are demonstrable and may lead to immune complex disease. An agar-gel immunodiffusion test, developed by Coggins, has proved effective in detecting antibodies and the presence of virus in horses (Coggins and Norcross, 1970; Coggins and others, 1972).

Clinical manifestations For purposes of description, the **clinical disease** is usually divided into three types: acute, subacute, and chronic. Cases of the disease, however, often fall simultaneously into two or more of these groups and, in the various stages, may pass through all three. The pathologic manifestations within each clinical type are similar to those in the other two; nonetheless, this classification is convenient, and even though it is arbitrary, it will be followed in the discussion of clinical and pathologic features.

Acute equine infectious anemia is characterized by rapid onset of high fever (to 108°F) after an incubation period of 1 to 3 weeks. The fever is accompanied by extreme weakness, excessive thirst, inappetence, depression, edema of the lower abdomen, and sublingual or nasal hemorrhages. Such an attack leads to death (in less than a month) or survival, with the disease assuming the subacute or chronic form. Anemia is not a prominent feature at the onset, but there is a gradual reduction in circulating red blood cells The normal count of 8 million/mm³ drops to about 4 million/mm³ in most cases.

In the subacute form, the disease is manifested by relapsing fever and recurrence of other symptoms at irregular intervals. The symptoms during these exacerbations are similar to those of the acute type, but generally less severe. The attacks may increase in severity, with

gradual weight loss, debility, edema of dependent parts, and unsteady gait becoming increasingly evident. Death may supervene during any of these recurrent attacks. Pallor of mucous membranes usually indicates the loss of circulating erythrocytes, which may fall as low as 1.5 million/mm³, and as a rule, the sedimentation rate is greatly increased. Accentuation of symptoms may be brought about by hard work, starvation, "blood letting," or other unfavorable factors.

The chronic form of the disease may develop after the animal has passed through an acute infection, or it may occur in the absence of an obvious attack. Experimental injection of minute amounts of the virus often results in chronic infectious anemia. Some animals appear to be in good health except for transient febrile manifestations at intervals of a month or two. Others remain thin despite a good diet, occasionally show edema under the thorax and abdomen, and may become weak or uncoordinated. The red cell count is usually 2 to 3 million/mm³ below normal, but evidence of severe anemia is seldom observed.

Pathogenesis The anemia that appears intermittently in this disease seems to be caused principally by destruction of red blood cells by means of an immunologically mediated mechanism. Erythrocytes of infected horses are coated with antiviral antibodies and complement 3 (McGuire, Henson, and Quist, 1969a, b). This binding to the cell surface results in increased osmotic fragility, shortened half-life, and erythrophagocytosis. Plasma hemoglobin level increases and serum haptoglobin level decreases in infected animals. These findings point toward hemolysis as a key factor in genesis of the anemia. Another, probably less important factor is depression of the bone marrow during acute episodes, as indicated by a decrease in both plasma iron turnover and utilization of radioactive iron.

Renal glomeruli are affected in horses with active disease. The glomeruli have thickened basement membranes and mesangium, cells are increased in numbers, and neutrophils are present. Equine immunoglobulin (IgG) and complement 3 (C3) can be demonstrated in the mesangium and on basement membranes (Banks and others, 1972). It appears that this glomerulitis is the result of deposition of virus-antibody complexes that have been demonstrated in the peripheral circulation. The immunologic factors involved in lesions in other organs have not been studied adequately, but it appears likely that immunologic factors may also be involved in the induction of lesions in other organs, such as the liver.

Lesions The nature of the lesions found during necropsy of horses that died of infectious anemia or were sacrificed during its course depends to a great extent on the clinical type of disease and the duration of illness. In other words, an animal that dies during an attack after several exacerbations characteristic of the chronic disease exhibits different tissue changes than one that dies after a single acute attack. It is convenient, therefore, to describe the lesions in relation to the clinical type of the disease.

GENERAL LESIONS: ACUTE DISEASE Icterus, edema,

and hemorrhage are the principal gross findings at necropsy. Edema is most prominent in the subcutis of the ventral wall of the abdomen, at the base of the heart, and in the perirenal and sublumbar fat. The hemorrhages are petechial or, less often, ecchymotic and are found in the edematous areas or in serous membranes, particularly the pleura and peritoneum. Swelling of the parenchymatous organs is common and is more fully described in connection with each system.

GENERAL LESIONS: SUBACUTE TYPE Edema and hemorrhages may be features, but they are likely to be less conspicuous than anemia; swelling and pigmentation of the liver; enlargement of the spleen, lymph nodes, and kidneys; and hyperplasia of the bone marrow.

GENERAL LESIONS: CHRONIC DISEASE Hypertrophy of the spleen and bone marrow may be the only pathologic changes in a sacrificed animal (Fig. 8-70).

HEART: ACUTE DISEASE The heart is usually enlarged, the ventricles are increased in size, and the myocardium is pale and flabby. Hemorrhages and edema occur in the epicardium and pericardium, and the pericardial sac may contain excessive amounts of clear or sanguinous fluid. Microscopically, edema and hemorrhages are found, along with some lymphocytic infiltration of the adventitia of myocardial vessels.

HEART: SUBACUTE DISEASE In the myocardium, some muscle bundles have microscopically visible hyaline degeneration associated with varying degrees of leukocytic infiltration. The majority of the infiltrating cells are lymphocytes, which tend to concentrate around blood vessels.

HEART: CHRONIC DISEASE Little of specific significance can be found.

LIVER: ACUTE DISEASE The liver may be grossly enlarged, red to dark brown, and may occasionally exhibit

hemorrhages. Microscopic examination usually reveals edema and lymphocytic infiltration of Glisson's capsule; congestion and dilation of sinusoids; swelling of Kupffer's cells (some containing hemosiderin); macrophages containing hemosiderin in the sinusoids; and sometimes, loss of liver cells at the center of lobules.

LIVER: SUBACUTE DISEASE The liver is usually enlarged, dark brown, and firm, and on its cut surface, the lobular markings are more distinct than on that of the normal organ. The distended central veins and the adjacent sinusoids may be evident grossly as dark brown or red puncta in a meshwork of dark brown lines. The microscopic changes are often striking, although not every section of the liver is affected equally. The central veins are congested with blood; the sinusoids show lacunose dilation and are filled with lymphocytes, plasma cells, macrophages containing hemosiderin or erythrocytes, and reticuloendothelial cells. The reticuloendothelial cells often form small nodules of cells within the sinusoids and occasionally in portal areas. The Kupffer's cells are enlarged and often filled with hemosiderin. Stains for iron clearly demonstrate this hemosiderosis in affected livers. Liver cells are often compressed by the enlargement of sinusoids, contain some pigment, and may be reduced in number. Glisson's capsule usually contains many lymphocytes, plasma cells, and some histiocytes. Myeloid cells have been described in these portal areas by some observers in cases of prolonged duration, but megakaryocytes have not been seen.

LIVER: CHRONIC DISEASE The lesions are not constant or as striking as in the subacute type, although the same microscopic changes may be seen in lesser degree. The gross appearance of the liver is not distinctive.

SPLEEN: ACUTE DISEASE The spleen is nearly twice normal size. The capsule is tense and may bear pete-

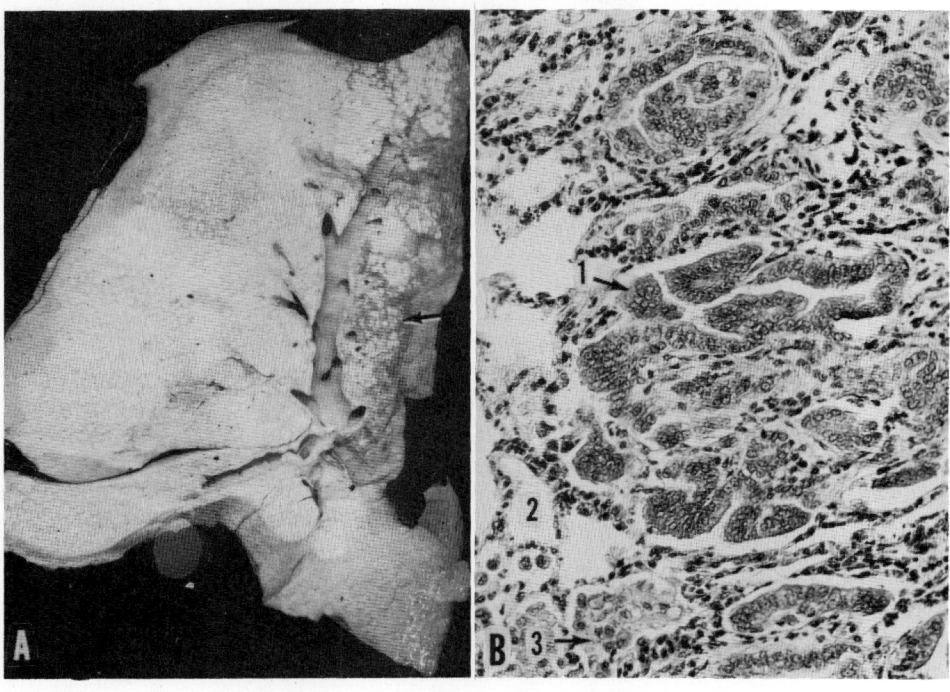

FIG. 8-70 *A*, Pulmonary adenomatosis (jaagsiekte). Lung of a sheep. Note nodules (arrow) of gray consolidation in some areas, diffuse solid zones in others. Contributor: Col. M. W. Hale. *B*, Pulmonary adenomatosis in a sheep lung (× 195). Note columnar cells *(1)* which fill alveoli. Some alveoli are intact *(2)*, others filled with macrophages *(3)*. Contributor: Dr. T. F. Shirlaw. (Courtesy of Armed Forces Institute of Pathology.)

chiae. The cut surface is turgid, cherry red or dark red, and somewhat granular, with little liquid component. Hemorrhagic infarcts have been reported but are inconstant. The splenic follicles may be less prominent and more widely separated than usual. Microscopically, the red pulp is increased in volume and very cellular, although in some sections severe congestion or hemorrhagic infarction of the splenic sinusoids obscures other details. This increase in volume of the red pulp, which widens the distance between the trabeculae and the splenic corpuscles, results from infiltration of the cords of Bilroth with mononuclear cells. These cells are individually discrete and have irregular, somewhat eosinophilic cytoplasm and round, hyperchromic nuclei. They are monotonously uniform in size and shape and often occur in aggregations around sinusoids. These cells are believed to arise in the reticuloendothelium and to be immature lymphoid cells. Myeloid cells, megakaryocytes, and erythroblasts are seldom found. Eosinophils (normal in the equine spleen) are still present, but hemosiderin (common in the equine spleen) is reduced in amount.

SPLEEN: SUBACUTE AND CHRONIC DISEASE The spleen may be the only visceral organ in which gross or microscopic evidence of this smouldering viral infection can be seen. The spleen is enlarged; its cut surface is light red or reddish brown and somewhat turgid and does not exude fluid. The trabeculae are usually widely separated, as are the splenic corpuscles, which are enlarged and clearly visible in some gross specimens. In older affected horses, the enlarged, soft, nonfibrous organ has more nearly the appearance of the spleen of colts under 1 year of age. Microscopic evidence of reticuloendothelial hyperplasia in the cords of Bilroth, similar to that described for the acute form, is the basis for its gross appearance. Hemosiderin is usually present in macrophages, but is not increased in amount.

LYMPH NODES: ACUTE DISEASE The changes in lymph nodes, which may be enlarged, mimic those described in the spleen. If death occurs early, there is atrophy and necrosis of lymphocytes. If acute disease is prolonged, the lesions are proliferative, characterized by replacement of the normal cytoarchitecture by diffuse sheets of mononuclear cells considered to be reticuloendothelial cells or immature lymphocytes. There may be cellular infiltration of the trabeculae, capsule, and perinodal fat.

LYMPH NODES: SUBACUTE AND CHRONIC DISEASE The proliferative response with replacement of normal structures by reticuloendothelial and lymphoid cells is generally more pronounced than in the acute type.

BONE MARROW: ACUTE DISEASE The normally fatty marrow usually contains red or yellowish-red areas which, on microscopic examination, are seen to be areas of active hematopoietic marrow.

BONE MARROW: SUBACUTE DISEASE The centers of long bones contain large areas of red, somewhat edematous, and occasionally hemorrhagic-appearing marrow.

BONE MARROW: CHRONIC DISEASE The marrow of the long bones, even in aged horses, is predominantly red rather than fatty. This hyperplasia of the hemato-poietic marrow is more obvious in the gross specimen than in microscopic sections, since the effect is quantitative. The microscopic picture is one of hematopoietic marrow with myeloid and erythroid elements in approximately normal proportion. It is obvious from these findings that hematopoiesis is not depressed but rather stimulated, probably as the result of destruction of erythrocytes. Large numbers of reticuloendothelial and lymphoid cells are interposed between the erythroid and myeloid elements.

KIDNEY: ACUTE DISEASE The kidneys are usually involved in the edema that affects the perirenal tissues, particularly in the region of the pelvis. Intense infiltration of immature lymphoid cells into the interstitial stroma of both cortex and medulla is especially prominent around blood vessels and occasionally around glomeruli. This lymphoid infiltration takes on a nodular distribution in some cases. There is generally an increased cellularity to the mesangium of the glomeruli. Immunoglobulins and complement have been demonstrated with immunofluorescent techniques.

KIDNEY: SUBACUTE AND CHRONIC DISEASE The lymphoid cells may be present in smaller numbers.

OTHER ORGANS It is possible for all organs and tissues of the body to show evidence of the reticuloendothelial hyperplasia described in spleen, lymph nodes, liver, and kidney, but these changes are not constant nor particularly distinctive. In the adrenal gland, lymphoid cell masses may separate parenchymal cells in much the same manner as in the liver. Endothelial cells of the adrenal have been reported to contain hemosiderin. Rarely, neurologic signs and granulomatous encephalomyelitis have been described. The frequency of this lesion in horses is not known, but equine infectious anemia should be suspected when granulomatous encephalitis is encountered, considering the frequency of encephalitis in other lentiviral diseases.

Hematologic Changes The anemia is characteristically normocytic and normochromic. Reticulocytosis or other evidence of increased erythropoiesis is not evident. The anemia appears to result from a combination of hemolysis, erythrophagocytosis, and a decreased production of erythrocytes. The response of the bone marrow has received little attention; although usually described as hyperplastic, there is little evidence of increased erythropoiesis. To the contrary, studies of Obara and Nakajima (1961) and McGuire and others (1969) indicate both a decrease in erythrocyte life span and production. Following an immediate lymphopenia, the disease is characterized by lymphocytosis and the appearance of iron-laden monocytes or siderocytes in the peripheral blood. Thrombocytopenia is a usual finding. Serum levels of gamma globulin are usually increased in the acute stages, and the Coombs' test results are reportedly positive.

Diagnosis A presumptive diagnosis can be made in the living animal during acute exacerbations of the disease or by recognizing characteristic gross and microscopic lesions at necropsy. Definitive diagnosis, however, depends on specific identification of the virus, either in the affected animal or after isolation in horse leukocyte cultures. The gel-diffusion test is particularly useful in detecting humoral antibodies in the serum of infected horses. The presence of these antibodies is consistently associated with virus, hence the test is a useful method to detect the virus. Fluorescein-labeled immunoglobulins are useful to demonstrate viral antigens in infected tissues.

References

Banks KL, Henson JB, McGuire TC. Immunologically mediated glomerulitis of horses. I. Pathogenesis in persistent infection by equine infectious anemia virus. Lab Invest 1972;26:701–707.

Cheevers WP, McGuire TC. Equine infectious anemia virus: immunopathogenesis and persistence. Rev Infect Dis 1985;7:83–88.

Coggins L, Norcross NL. Immunodiffusion reaction in equine infectious anemia. Cornell Vet 1970;60:330–335.

Coggins L, Norcross NL, Nusbaum SR. Diagnosis of equine infectious anemia by immunodiffusion test. Am J Vet Res 1972;33:11–18.

Coggins L. Mechanism of viral persistence in equine infectious anemia. Cornell Vet 1975;65:143–151.

Coggins L. Carriers of equine infectious anemia virus. J Am Vet Med Assoc 1984;184:279–281.

Evans KS, Carpenter SL, Sevoian M. Detection of equine infectious anemia virus in horse leukocyte cultures derived from horses in various stages of equine infectious anemia viral infection. Am J Vet Res 1984;45:20–25.

Hawkins JA, et al. Role of horse fly (Tabanus fuscicostatus Hine) and stable fly (Stomoxys calcitrans L.) in transmission of equine infectious anemia to ponies in Louisiana. Am J Vet Res 1973;34:1583–1586.

Hawkins JA., et al. Transmission of equine infectious anemia virus by Tabanus fuscicostatus. J Am Vet Med Assoc 1976;168:63–64.

Henson JB, McGuire TC. Immunopathology of equine infectious anemia. Am J Clin Pathol 1971;56:306–314.

Henson JB, McGuire TC. Equine infections anemia. Prog Med Virol 1974;18:352–354.

Issel CJ, Foil LD. Studies on equine infectious anemia virus transmission by insects. J Am Vet Med Assoc 1984;184:293–297.

Ito Y. Morphogenesis of equine infectious anaemia virus. Acta Virol (Praha). 1974;18:352–354.

Johnson AW. Equine infectious anemia: the literature 1966–1975. Vet Bull 1976;46:559–574.

Kemen MJ Jr, Coggins L. Equine infectious anemia: transmission from infected mares to foals. J Am Vet Med Assoc 1972;161:496–499.

Knowles RC. An overview of equine infectious anemia control and regulation in the United States. J Am Vet Med Assoc 1984;184:289–292.

Konno S, Yamamoto H. Pathology of equine infectious anemia. Proposed classification of pathologic types of disease. Cornell Vet 1970;60:393–449.

McClure JJ, Lindsay WA, Taylor W, et al. Ataxia in four horses with equine infectious anemia. J Am Vet Med Assoc 1982;180:279–283.

McGuire TC, Henson JB, Quist SE. Viral-induced hemolysis in equine infectious anemia. Am J Vet Res 1969;30:2091–2097.

McGuire TC, Henson JB, Quist SE. Impaired bone marrow response in equine infectious anemia. Am J Vet Res 1969;30:2099–2113.

McGuire TC, Henson JB, Keown GH. Equine infectious anaemia: the role of Heinz bodies in the pathogenesis of anaemia. Res Vet Sci 1970;11:354–357.

McGuire TC, Perryman LE, Henson JB. Immunoglobulin composition of the hypergammaglobulinemia of equine infectious anemia. Fed Proc 1970;29:435.

McGuire TC, Crawford TB, Henson JB. Immunofluorescent localization of equine infectious anemia virus in tissue. Am J Pathol 1971;62:283–294.

McGuire TC, Crawford TB. Demonstration of circulating infectious virus-antibody complexes in equine infectious anemia. Fed Proc 1972;31:635.

Obara J, Nakajima H. Kinetics of iron metabolism in equine infectious anemia. Jpn J Vet Sci 1961;23:247–252.

Obara J, Nakajima H. Lifespan of ^{31}Cr-labeled erythrocytes in equine infectious anemia. Jpn J Vet Sci 1961;23:207–209.

Perryman LE, McGuire TC, Banks KL, et al. Decreased C3 levels in a chronic virus infection: equine infectious anemia. J Immun 1971;106:1074–1078.

Stein CD, Osteen OL, Mort LO, et al. Experimental transmission of equine infectious anemia by contact and body secretions and excretions. Vet Med 1944;39:46–52.

Umphenour NW, Kemen MJ, Coggins L. Equine infectious anemia: a retrospective study of an epizootic. J Am Vet Med Assoc 1974;164:66–69.

Vallée H, Carré H. Nature infectieuse de l'anémie du cheval. CR Acad Sci 1904;139:331–33.

Yamamoto H, Yoshino T, Nakajima H, et al. Relationship between histopathological and serological findings in field cases of equine infectious anemia. Natl Inst Anim Health Q 1972;12: 193–200.

FELINE IMMUNODEFICIENCY VIRUS (FIV)

Feline immunodeficiency virus is a lentivirus that was first isolated in 1987 from domestic cats with an immunodeficiency syndrome (Pedersen and others). The virus has since been identified in cats throughout the world, and serologic surveys indicate its presence in several species of wild *Felidae* species. FIV bears many similarities to HIV. It is tropic for T lymphocytes, macrophages, and astrocytes. It is transmitted primarily by biting and, accordingly, the highest incidence is in male cats living outdoors. Very often FIV-infected cats are also infected with feline leukemia virus (FeLV). A variety of clinical and pathologic findings have been associated with FIV infection, especially when accompanied by FeLV infection in the same animal. It appears, however, that cats are more adapted to FIV than are humans to HIV and that FIV is less immunosuppressive than HIV. There is no evidence that an AIDS-like pandemic comparable to AIDS in humans is occurring in cats. Nevertheless, analogies have been drawn between the clinicopathologic course of FIV infection and HIV infection.

Primary infection may lead to low-grade fever, generalized lymphadenopathy, and on occasion, diarrhea. This is most often observed in young cats and usually persists for 2 to 4 weeks, although lymphadenopathy has been described as persisting for several months. This is followed by a clinically quiescent interval of 1 to 2 years during which there is depression of the CD4$^+$ to CD8$^+$ T-cell ratio. Subsequently, infected cats may develop recurrent fever, lymphadenopathy, anemia, diarrhea, and weight loss of protracted duration. Chronic secondary infections, especially gingivitis, dermatitis, and upper respiratory disease, and opportunistic infections are described as the final stages of infection. Opportunistic infections associated with FIV include toxoplasmosis, calicivirus infection, feline herpesvirus infection, cryptococcosis, candidiasis, mycobacteriosis, hemobartonellosis, and others. Several neurologic abnormalities have also been associated with FIV infection, including dementia, twitching, tremors, and convulsions.

Lesions Lesions in affected cats primarily reflect those of opportunistic infections. Encephalitis, characterized by perivascular mononuclear infiltrates and glial nodules, is seen in a high percentage of affected cats and most likely is a primary FIV lesion comparable to the encephalitis seen in AIDS. Care must be taken, however, to ensure that it is not the result of toxoplasmosis or other agents that can lead to encephalitis. Histologically, the lymphadenopathy is characterized by follicular hyperplasia early in the course of infection, which, over time, may progress to marked lymphoid depletion.

References

Davidson MG, Rottman JB, English RV, et al. Feline immunodeficiency virus predisposes cats to acute generalized toxoplasmosis. Am J Pathol 1993;143:1486–1497.
Egberink H, Horzinek MC. Animal immunodeficiency viruses. Vet Microbiol 1992;33:311–331.
George JW, Pedersen NC, Higgins J. The effect of age on the course of experimental feline immunodeficiency virus infection in cats. AIDS Res Hum Retroviruses 1993;9:897–905.
English RV, Nelson P, Johnson CM, et al. Development of clinical disease in cats experimentally infected with feline immunodeficiency virus. J Infect Dis 1994;170:543–552.
Matsumura S, Ishidat, Washizu T, et al. Pathologic features of acquired immunodeficiency-like syndrome in cats experimentally infected with feline immunodeficiency virus. J Vet Med Sci 1993;55:387–394.
Pedersen NC, Barlough JE. Clinical overview of feline immunodeficiency virus. J Am Vet Med Assoc 1991;199:1298–1305.
Pedersen NC, Ho EW, Brown ML, et al. Isolation of a T-lymphotropic virus from domestic cats with an immunodeficiency-like syndrome. Science 1987;235:790–793.
Yamamoto JK, Sparger E, Ho EW, et al. Pathogenesis of experimentally induced feline immunodeficiency virus infection in cats. Am J Vet Res 1988;49:1246–1258.

BOVINE IMMUNODEFICIENCY VIRUS

Bovine immunodeficiency virus (BIV), a lentivirus, is one of three bovine retroviruses; the others are bovine leukemia virus (a type C oncornavirus), and bovine spumavirus (a foamy virus). BIV was the first of the bovine retroviruses to be isolated, which occurred in the course of the search for the cause of bovine enzootic leukemia in the 1960s. Since BIV did not prove to be the cause of bovine leukemia, the virus, termed BIV R-29, remained unstudied until the recognition of HIV as the cause of AIDS in humans. BIV was the third of the lentiviruses to be discovered, preceded by equine infectious anemia virus and the ovine lentivirus of visna/maedi and ovine progressive pneumonia.

The original BIV isolate was recovered from an 8-year-old Holstein cow in Louisiana that had lymphocytosis and a gradually weakening condition. Since then, several additional isolates have been obtained. Based on experimental infection and observations of naturally infected cattle, the infection is lifelong and associated with lymphocytosis or lymphopenia, generalized lymphadenopathy, and multiple grossly visible subcutaneous nodules of lymphocytes. Lymphocytic cuffing in the brain and lymphocytic meningitis are described along with, in some examples, neuronal degeneration and lymphocytic infiltration of the neuropil. Studies of infected herds have associated infection with lethargy, mastitis, chronic pododermatitis, pneumonia, mycotic abomasitis, injection site myositis, and abscessation and lymphosarcoma. It has been speculated that persistent infection with BIV predisposes to the effects of bovine

leukemia virus. Further study is necessary to determine if the infection leads to a syndrome analogous to AIDS, but, owing to the usual short life span of cattle, the consequences of prolonged infection are difficult to assess. Serologic surveys indicate that about 4% of cattle from the southern United States are infected and that about 40% of beef herds and 68% of dairy herds are infected.

A closely related, but variant lentivirus has been recovered from cattle (*Bos javanicus*) in Bali with Jembrana disease, a disorder first recognized in 1964. This is an acute, severe disease characterized by fever, lymphadenopathy, and lymphopenia. In lymph nodes and the spleen, there is hyperplasia of lymphoblasts in parafollicular areas with follicular atrophy. The incubation period is 5 to 12 days with a mortality of about 17%. This acute behavior of a lentivirus is analogous to some isolates of simian immunodeficiency virus (SIVpbj).

References

Chadwick BJ, Coelen RJ, Sammels LM, et al. Genomic sequence analysis identifies Jembrana disease virus as a new bovine lentivirus. J Gen Virol 1995;76:189–192.
Gonda MA. Bovine immunodeficiency virus. AIDS 1992;6:759–776.
Gonda MA. The lentiviruses of cattle. In: Levy JA, ed. The retroviridae. Vol 3, Chapter 3. New York: Plenum Press 1994;83–109.
Gonda MA, Braun MJ, Carter SG, et al. Characterization and molecular cloning of a bovine lentivirus related to human immunodeficiency virus. Nature (Lond) 1987;330:388–391.
Gonda MA, Luther DG, Fong SE, et al. Bovine immunodeficiency virus: molecular biology and virus-host interactions. Virus Res 1994;32:155–181.
Van Der Maaten MJ, Boothe AD, Seger CL. Isolation of a virus from cattle with persistent lymphocytosis. JNCI 1972;49:1649–1657.

SIMIAN IMMUNODEFICIENCY VIRUS

Several lentiviruses called simian immunodeficiency virus (SIV) have been identified in Old World monkeys. They are related to human immunodeficiency virus (HIV) and serve as important models to study pathogenesis and strategies for vaccination and therapy for AIDS. Four groups of viruses are currently recognized. SIVagm is very prevalent in African green monkeys, but has not been associated with any disease in this species. SIVagm has about a 55% to 60% homology with the other three groups. SIVsmm is a common infection of sooty mangabey monkeys. No disease has been associated with infection in mangabeys, but this virus and SIVmac (the prototype SIV isolated from captive rhesus monkeys) causes a disease resembling AIDS in rhesus monkeys (*Macaca mulatta*) and pig-tailed macaques (*M. nemestrina*). SIVsmm, SIVmac, and HIV-2 are very closely related viruses. The third group, recovered from mandrills (*Mandrillus sphinx*), is termed SIVmnd. It also has a 55% to 60% homology with the other groups, and there is no data on its pathogenicity. The fourth group is HIV-1, the principal cause of AIDS in humans. A closely related SIV has been recovered from a healthy wild-caught chimpanzee (SIVcpz).

The immunodeficiency disease caused by SIVmac and SIVsmm in macaques is not common in captive monkeys and appears to result from cross-species infection of a virus carried by one species to another susceptible species. As with other lentiviral infections, the virus establishes a persistent infection with a prodromal period of months to years before clinical signs appear. The clinical and pathologic findings in the experimental disease as well as the few natural infections reported are remarkably similar to AIDS. The virus affects macrophages and CD4$^+$ lymphocytes, leading to immunodeficiency. Clinically, there is a rash, diarrhea, wasting, and enlargement of lymph nodes.

Pathologically, generalized lymphadenopathy characterized by hyperplasia is followed by lymphoid depletion in the terminal stages, nodular lymphocytic infiltrates in a variety of tissues, interstitial pneumonia with syncytial cells, and granulomatous encephalitis. Superimposed on these changes are a variety of opportunistic infections that influence the clinical signs and often account for death, which, once signs develop, is inevitable. These opportunistic infections, among others, include *Pneumocystis carinii* pneumonia, cytomegalic inclusion body disease, cryptosporidiosis, and *Mycobacterium avium/intracellulare* infection.

References

Baskin GB, Murphey-Corb M, Watson EA, et al. Necropsy findings in rhesus monkeys experimentally infected with cultured simian immunodeficiency virus (SIV)/Delta. Vet Pathol 1988;25:456–467.

Chalifoux LV, King NW, Letvin NL. Morphologic changes in lymph nodes of macaques with an immunodeficiency syndrome. Lab Invest 1984;51:22–26.

Daniel MD, Letvin NL, King NW, et al. Isolation of T-cell tropic HTLV-III-like retrovirus from macaques. Science 1985;228:1201–1204.

Desrosiers RC. The simian immunodeficiency viruses. Annu Rev Microbiol 1988;42:607–625.

Desrosiers RC. The simian immunodeficiency viruses. Annu Rev Immunol 1990;8:557–578.

Kanki PJ, Alroy J, Essex M. Isolation of T-lymphotropic retrovirus related to HTLV-III/LAV from wild-caught African green monkeys. Science 1985;230:951–954.

King NW. Simian models of acquired immunodeficiency syndrome (AIDS): a review. Vet Pathol 1986;23:345–353.

Li Y, Naidu YM, Daniel MD, et al. Extensive genetic variability of simian immunodeficiency virus from African green monkeys. J Virol 1989;63:1800–1802.

Ringler DJ, Hunt RD, Desrosiers RC, et al. Simian immunodeficiency virus-induced meningoencephalitis: natural history and retrospective study. Ann Neurol 1988;23(Suppl):S101–S107.

Ringler DJ, Wyand MS, Walsh DG, et al. Cellular localization of simian immunodeficiency virus in lymphoid tissues. I. Immunohistochemistry and electron microscopy. Am J Pathol 1989;134:373–383.

Schneider J, Hunsmann G. Simian lentiviruses - the SIV group. AIDS 1988;2:1–9.

Wyand MS, Ringler DJ, Naidu YM, et al. Cellular localization of simian immunodeficiency virus in lymphoid tissues. II. In situ hybridization. Am J Pathol 1989;134:385–393.

Diseases Caused by *Oncovirinae*

Ever since Ellerman and Bang demonstrated the cell-free transmission of fowl leukosis in 1908 and the subsequent demonstration of fowl leukosis viruses, the search for oncogenic viral causes of leukemia in humans and animals has been intense. A specific RNA virus was first discovered in mice by Ludwig Gross in 1951, and now several viruses of laboratory and domestic animals and

humans have been associated with lymphoma and leukemia. Most of these are oncoviruses.

The subfamily *oncovirinae* is the largest group of retroviruses and includes a number of oncogenic viruses. All members of the subfamily, however, have not been shown to be oncogenic. On the basis of morphology and the sequence in which they were originally described, retrovirus particles are classified into four types: A, B, C, and D.

A-type particles were originally identified as the immature nucleocapsids of mouse mammary tumor virus (MMTV), the mature enveloped virions of which became the prototype B$^-$ type particles. A-type particles appear as intracytoplasmic, hollow, 60–90 nm spherical structures with a double-contoured wall. Morphologically similar particles were subsequently recognized within the cisternae of the endoplasmic reticulum of rodent cell lines expressing provirus sequences of noninfectious, endogenous retroviruses. These were termed intracisternal A particles.

B-type retrovirus particles are represented by the mature extracellular enveloped virions of MMTV. These particles arise from introcytoplasmic A-type particles that bud through the cell membrane to acquire an envelope with prominent surface spikes. As the particles mature in the extracellular space, their A-type nucleocapsids are transformed into solid cores eccentrically situated within the envelope.

C-type particles comprise most of the avian and mammalian leukemia viruses. They do not develop from preformed, cytoplasmic A-type particles. Instead, their nucleocapsid formation occurs simultaneously with development of the viral envelope from the cell membrane. The initial stage of nucleocapsid assembly appears in the cytoplasm as a crescent-shaped object just beneath a slightly thickened, bulging segment of cell membrane that becomes the viral envelope. The fact that the developing nucleocapsid is crescent or C-shaped is purely coincidental to the scheme of classification. As development proceeds, the crescent-shaped nucleocapsid becomes spherical like an A-type particle, is totally surrounded by the cell membrane-derived envelope and eventually pinches off by a process known as "budding." In the extracellular space the nucleocapsids of these 80–110 nm virions condense into a solid, electron-dense core located centrally within the envelope. The envelope of mature C-type particles bears barely discernible surface spikes.

D-type retrovirus particles are represented by 5 different serotypes of Old World monkey viruses, including Mason-Pfizer monkey virus (MPMV), simian retroviruses 1 and 2 (SRV 1 and 2), and two additional agents termed SRV 4 and 5. Of these, MPMV and SRV 1 and 2 have been associated with immunodeficiency disorders of Old World monkeys. In addition, two endogenous retroviruses, one from squirrel monkeys (SMRV) and the other from langurs (PO-1-Lu), have type D morphology. Type D particles, like type B particles, develop from intracytoplasmic A-type nucleocapsids that bud through the cell membrane to acquire their envelope. Once in the extracellular space, however, the sperical nucleocapsids become condensed and conical or cylindrical in configuration. Their envelopes also has small spikes protruding from it.

Other retroviruses with distinctive morphology, but which have not yet been assigned a letter designation are the lentiviruses and spumaviruses (foamy viruses). The lentiviruses bud like type-C particles, but during maturation in the extracellular space the spherical nucleoid becomes a dense conical or cylindrical structure similar to that of mature type-D particles. The envelope bears small surface spikes. The spumaviruses, develop from cytoplasmic A-type nucleocapsids and during the course of budding through the cell membrane the envelope develops very prominent spikes on its surface. The nucleocapsid becomes condensed but often retains a hollow center.

TYPE C ONCOVIRUSES: FELINE LEUKEMIA VIRUS

Transmission of feline lymphoma was first demonstrated by Jarrett and associates (1964a) by inoculation of newborn kittens with a suspension from lymphomatous feline lymph nodes in which C-type particles (Figs. 8-71, 8-72, and 8-73) were demonstrated (Jarrett and others, 1964b). This virus is now termed feline leukemia virus (FeLV), a virus associated with a variety of disorders, which collectively represent the most important cause of death of cats. FeLV occurs worldwide with an incidence of up to 50% in densely populated areas. The virus is transmitted horizontally, primarily by means of salivary and nasal secretions of cats that have persistent and active FeLV infection having contact with susceptible cats. Two principal outcomes follow primary infec-

tion. **The first is a self-limiting infection** (sometimes termed "regressive" infection) in which the initial virus replication in lymphoid tissue is either totally eliminated by the immune system or may remain as provirus, which is contained through immune mechanisms. Approximately 60% of infected cats fall into this category and do not develop any FeLV-associated disease. Provirus can, however, become activated if there is immune dysfunction. In this event, infected cats may go on to become viremic and develop FeLV disease. **The second outcome is progressive infection with persistent viremia.** The initial viral replication in lymphoid tissues, usually in the oropharynx, is not contained and is followed by viremia and generalized viral infection of lymphocytes, macrophages, intestines, salivary glands, pancreas, and urinary bladder. These cats are infectious because virus is excreted through these sites.

Persistent infection and viremia is ultimately followed by any of several disease processes, which lead to death. This usually requires months or years following initial infection; however, some infections may result in illness or death within a few weeks. Most viremic cats die within 3 years of infection. Those disorders caused by FeLV are grouped into **cytoproliferative diseases** and **cytosuppressive diseases.** The particular outcome is, in part, determined by the specific FeLV viral subtype and the age of cat at time of infection (infection early in life is more likely to be followed by viremia), immune status of the cat, and probably the genetic makeup of the cat.

The principal disorders resulting from FeLV infection include the following:

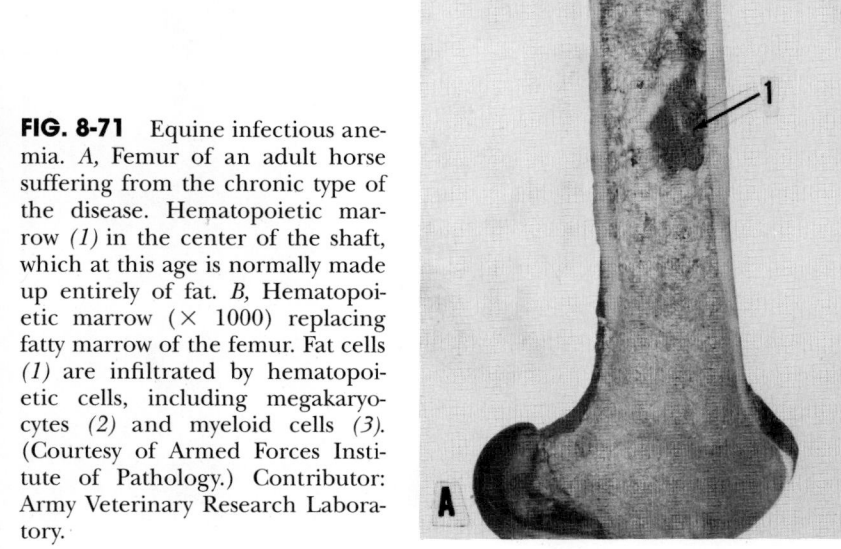
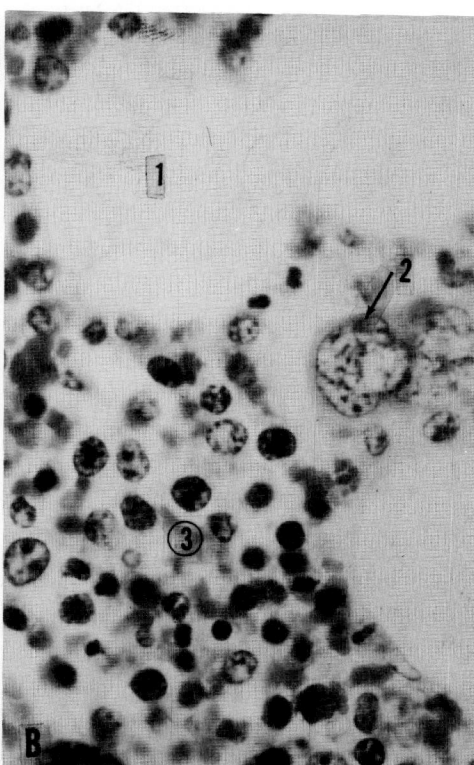

FIG. 8-71 Equine infectious anemia. *A,* Femur of an adult horse suffering from the chronic type of the disease. Hematopoietic marrow *(1)* in the center of the shaft, which at this age is normally made up entirely of fat. *B,* Hematopoietic marrow (× 1000) replacing fatty marrow of the femur. Fat cells *(1)* are infiltrated by hematopoietic cells, including megakaryocytes *(2)* and myeloid cells *(3).* (Courtesy of Armed Forces Institute of Pathology.) Contributor: Army Veterinary Research Laboratory.

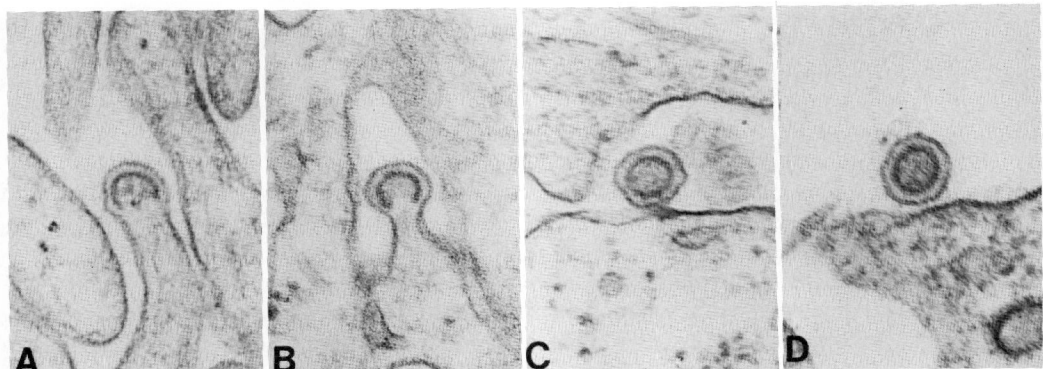

FIG. 8-72 Development of virions of *Retroviridae* (C-type particles). Progressive stages in the development of the virion on a cytoplasmic membrane are seen in A through D. (Courtesy of Dr. Norval W. King, Jr. and Proceedings of National Academy of Science.)

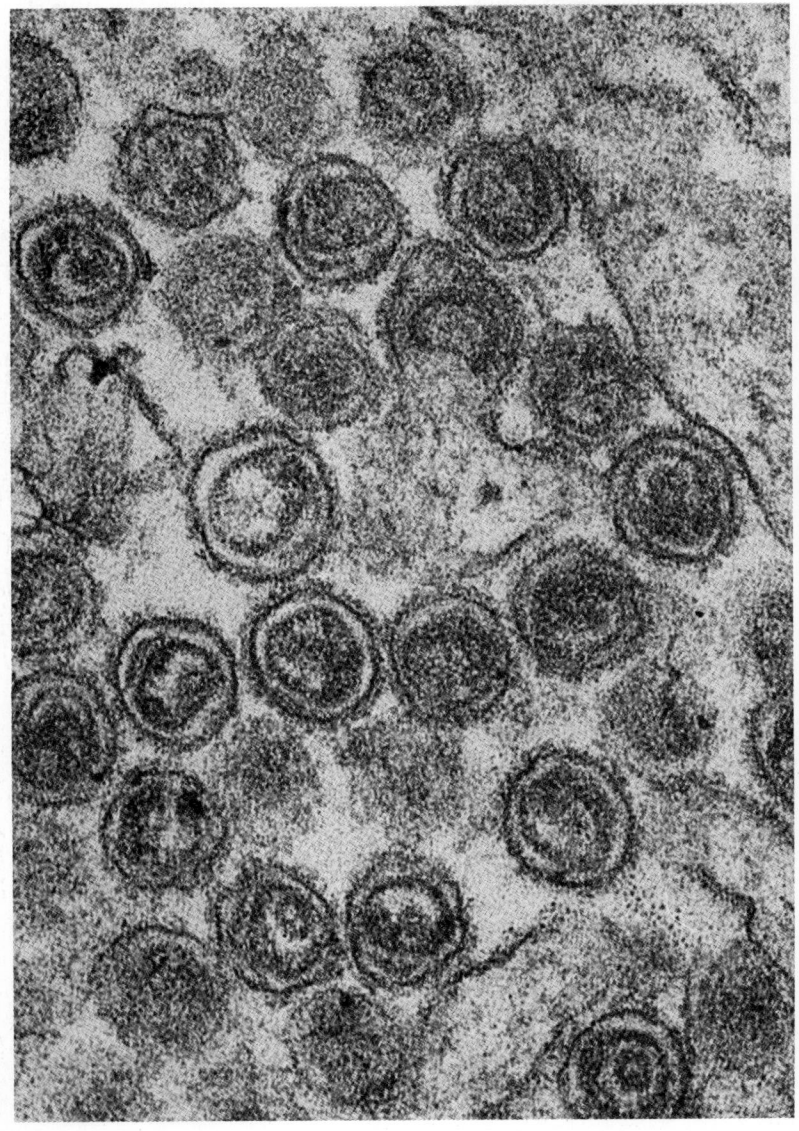

FIG. 8-73 Feline leukemia virus. Intracellular mature C-type viral particles (approximately × 150,000). (Courtesy of Dr. G. H. Theilen.)

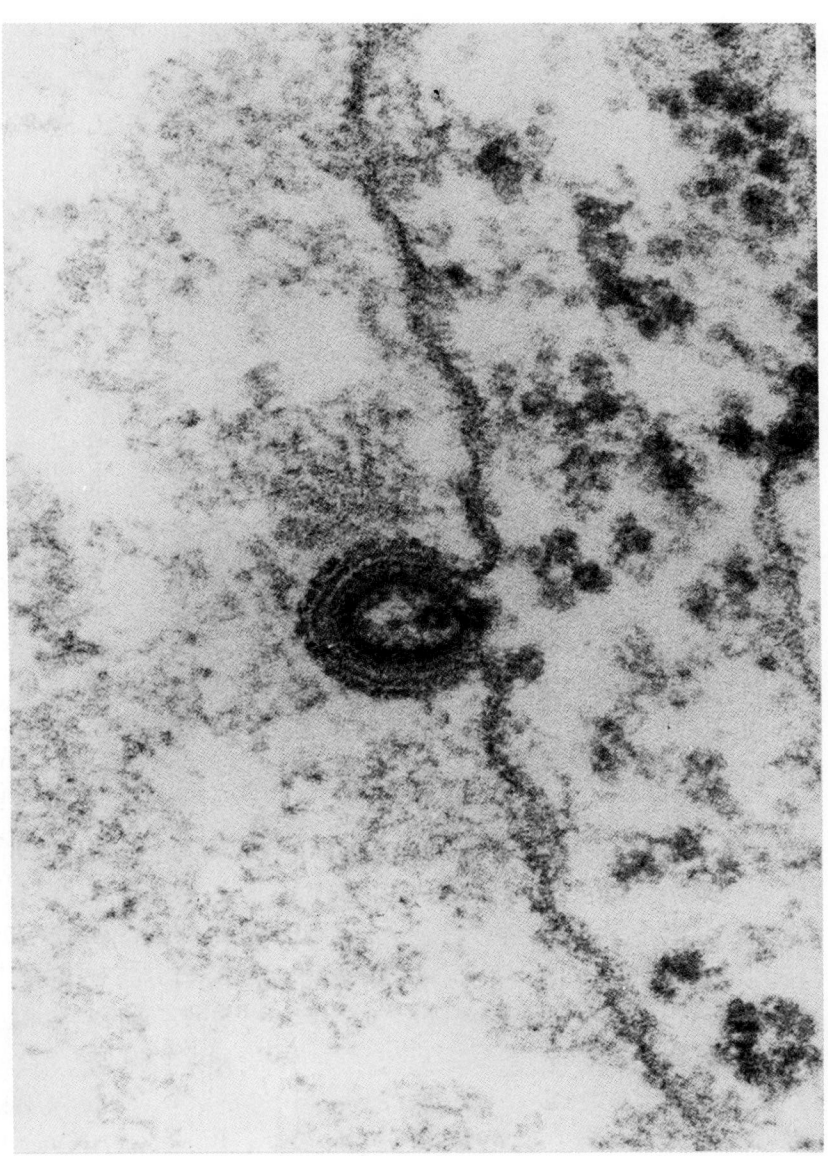

FIG. 8-74 Feline leukemia virus. Advanced stage of the budding process of the C-type virus from the cytoplasmic membrane of a lympho-cyte (approximately × 200,000). Courtesy of Dr. G. H. Theilen.)

1. **Malignant lymphoma** with or without leukemia is the most common malignancy in cats, and most (but not all) cases are caused by FeLV. It results from viral activation of cellular proto-oncogenes. On the basis of anatomic distribution, several forms are recognized: (1) **Thymic lymphoma** principally occurs in young cats (less than 3 years of age) and is characterized by a large tumor mass or masses originating in and replacing the thymus gland and filling the mediastinum; (2) **Alimentary lymphoma,** seen more in older cats, is characterized by solid tumors that infiltrate the gastrointestinal tract, abdominal lymph nodes, and, often, the liver, spleen, and kidneys; (3) **Multicentric lymphoma,** usually seen in mature cats, is characterized by generalized lymphoma affecting many organs and tissues; and (4) **Unclassified lymphoma,** which usually presents as isolated tumor masses in nonlymphoid tissues, such as the eye or central nervous system. Most ex-amples of lymphoma, with the exception of the alimentary form, are of T-cell origin.

2. **Lymphocytic leukemia,** which may occur in conjunction with malignant lymphoma.

3. **Erythroid and myeloid leukemias (myeloproliferative disorders),** which are the most common leukemias in cats and which may occur together. **Myelofibrosis,** is another outcome.

4. Fibrosarcoma results from infection with **feline sarcoma virus.** This virus is a defective mutant of FeLV that lacks part of the viral genome and is unable to replicate. In the presence of FeLV, however, virus replication can occur; the FeLV serves as a helper virus, providing the missing genes.

5. **Myelosuppression syndrome,** which is characterized by **anemia** and/or **leukopenia** (lymphopenia and neutropenia), is a frequent outcome of FeLV infection. It results from suppression of erythropoiesis and myelopoiesis. The anemia may become very se-

vere and is usually normocytic and normochromic (nonregenerative anemia). Regenerative anemia, characterized by macrocytosis and reticulocytosis and the appearance of nucleated red blood cells in peripheral circulation, can also occur; this may be hemolytic in origin and is not associated with myelosuppression.

6. **Immunosuppression** is seen at some stage in most cats infected with FeLV. In some infections, it is the dominant manifestation and is characterized by progressive loss of function and a decrease in numbers of both T and B lymphocytes as well as neutrophils. It is associated with secondary infections, particularly of the upper respiratory tract, gingivitis, chronic dermatitis, and enteritis. The role of the more recently identified **feline immunodeficiency virus** acting alone or in concert with FeLV in causing immunosuppression requires more study.

7. **Enteropathy,** characterized by chronic diarrhea and wasting, may result from FeLV infection of crypt cells of the intestinal epithelium. Pathologically, there is villus atrophy and fusion.

8. **Infertility** resulting from fetal death and resorption is ascribed to FeLV infection of the placenta and fetus.

9. **Neurologic disease** has been observed in FeLV-infected cats but not studied in detail. This could also represent a result of **feline immunodeficiency virus** infection, which is recognized as neurotropic.

Diagnosis The presence of the virus may be demonstrated by electron-microscopic photographs of replicating C-type particles (Figs. 8-71 to 8-73). A fluorescent antibody test is used to detect antigen in leukocytes in blood smears (Hardy and others, 1973). A third method is to isolate the virus in feline cell cultures from plasma or oral swabs of cats.

References

Boid R, McOrist S, Jones TW, et al. Isolation of FeLV from a wild felid *(Felis silvestris)*. Vet Rec 1991;128:256.

Essex M, Cotter SM, Carpenter JL. Feline virus-induced tumors and the immune response: recent developments. Am J Vet Res 1973;34:809–812.

Hardy WD Jr, et al. Feline leukemia virus: occurrence of viral antigen in the tissues of cats with lymphosarcoma and other diseases. Science 1969;166:1019–1021.

Hardy WD Jr, et al. Horizontal transmission of feline leukemia virus. Nature 1973;244:266–269.

Hinshaw VS, Blank H. Isolation of feline leukemia virus from clinical specimens. Am J Vet Res 1977;38:55–57.

Hoover EA, Mullins JI. Feline leukemia virus infection and disease. J Am Vet Med Assoc 1991;199:1287–1297.

Jarrett O. Overview of feline leukemia virus research. J Am Vet Med Assoc 1991;199:1279–1281.

Jarrett WFH, et al. Transmission experiments with leukemia. Nature 1964;202:566–567.

Jarrett WFH, Crawford EM, Marten WB, et al. A virus-like particle associated with leukaemia. Nature 1964;202:567–568.

Jarrett WFH, et al. Horizontal transmission of leukaemia virus and leukaemia in the cat. J Natl Cancer Inst 1973;51:833–841.

Jarrett O. Natural history of feline leukaemia virus. J Small Anim Pract 1975;16:409–413.

Kawakami TG, et al. C-type viral particles in plasma of cats with feline leukemia. Science 1967;158:1049–1050.

Mackey LJ, Jarrett WFH, Jarrett O, et al. An experimental study of virus leukemia in cats. J Natl Cancer Inst 1972;48:1663–1670.

McMichael JC, Stiers S, Coffin S. Prevalence of feline leukemia virus infection among adult cats at an animal control center: assocation of viremia with phenotype and season. Am J Vet Res 1986;47:765–768.

Reinacher M. Feline leukemia virus-associated enteritis - a condition with features of feline panleukopenia. Vet Pathol 1987;24:1–4.

Rojko JL, Kociba GJ. Pathogenesis of infection by the feline leukemia virus. J Am Vet Med Assoc 1991;199:1305–1310.

Sarma PS, et al. Differential host range of viruses of feline leukemia-sarcoma complex. Virology 1975;64:438–446.

Schrenzel MD, Higgins RJ, Hinrichs SH, et al. Type C retroviral expression in feline olfactory neuroblastomas. Acta Neuropathol 1990;80:547–553.

Weiser MG, Kociba GJ. Erythrocyte macrocytosis in feline leukemia virus associated anemia. Vet Pathol 1983;20:687–697.

OTHER TYPE C ONCOVIRUSES

A C-type oncovirus, **bovine leukemia virus,** first isolated in 1969, is recognized as the cause of malignant lymphoma in adult cattle. The virus affects B lymphocytes, leading to either persistent lymphocytosis or generalized lymphoma. Infection is spread horizontally. **Ovine leukemia virus** is a related virus recovered from sheep and associated with lymphoma in this species. **Porcine leukemia virus** is a C-type virus associated with lymphoma in young swine.

Another type C oncovirus is associated with granulocytic leukemia and lymphoma in gibbons. This is known as the **gibbon ape leukemia virus.** The same virus was first recovered from a fibrosarcoma in a woolly monkey and termed "simian sarcoma virus." Unrelated type C viruses that are related to human T-cell leukemia virus (HTLV-I, HTLV-II) have been recovered from macaque monkeys. These have been termed simian T-cell leukemia virus (STLV); however, they have not yet been shown to be oncogenic.

References

Evermann JF. Bovine leukemia virus infection. Mod Vet Pract 1983;64:103–105.

Frazier ME. Evidence for retrovirus in miniature swine with radiation-induced leukemia or metaplasia. Arch Virol 1985;83:83–97.

Ghysdael J, Bruck C, Kettmann R, et al. Bovine leukemia virus. Curr Top Microbiol Immunol 1984;112:1–19.

Heeney JL, Valli PJS, Jacobs RM, et al. Evidence for bovine leukemia virus infection of peripheral blood monocytes and limited antigen expression in bovine lymphoid tissue. Lab Invest 1992;66:608–617.

Johnsen EO, Wooding WL, Tanticharoenyos P, et al. Malignant lymphoma in the gibbon. J Am Vet Med Assoc 1971;159:563–566.

Kawakami TG, Huff SD, Buckley PM, et al. C-type virus associated with gibbon lymphosarcoma. Nature New Biol 1972;235:170–171.

Kawakami TG, McDowell TS. Factor regulating the onset of chronic myelogenous leukemia in gibbons. In: Essex M, Todaro G, zur Hausen H, ed. Viruses in naturally occurring cancers. Cold Spring Harbor Conferences on Cell Proliferation. Vol 7, Section 8. Cold Spring Harbor Laboratory 1980;719–727.

Kawakami TG, Kollias GV Jr, Holmberg C. Oncogenicity of gibbon type-C myelogenous leukemia virus. Int J Cancer 1980;25:641–646.

Kettmann R, Deschamps J, Cleuter Y, et al. Leukemogenesis of bovine leukemia virus: proviral DNA integration and lack of RNA expression of viral long terminal repeat and 3' proximate cellular sequences. Proc Natl Acad Sci USA 1982;79:2465–2469.

Lieber MM, Sherr CJ, Benveniste RE, et al. Biologic and immunologic properties of porcine type C viruses. Virology 1975;66:616–619.

Miller JM, Miller LD, Olson C, et al. Virus-like particles in phytohe-magglutinin-stimulated lymphocyte cultures with reference to bovine lymphosarcoma. JNCI 1969;43:1297–1305.

Rohde W, Pauli G, Paulsen J, et al. Bovine and ovine leukemia viruses. I. Characterization of viral antigens. J Virol 1978;26:159–164.

Suzuka I, Sekiguchi K, Kodama M. Some characteristics of a porcine retrovirus from a cell line derived from swine malignant lymphoma. FEBS Lett 1985;183:124–128.

Watanabe T, Seiki M, Tsujimoto H, et al. Sequence homology of the simian retrovirus genome with human T-cell leukemia virus type I. Virology 1985;144:59–65.

TYPE B ONCOVIRUSES: MAMMARY-TUMOR MILK VIRUS

It has been known for many years that the offspring of hybrid mice produced by pairs from two inbred strains have an increased incidence of certain mammary tumors if their mothers are descendants of strains in which the incidence of mammary tumors is high. Bittner demonstrated in 1936 that a factor in the milk of the mice from the affected strains is responsible for the production of these tumors, even though they do not appear until the offspring mature. The frequency of tumors could be sharply reduced in mice with the same genetic background by putting them to nurse on foster mothers that did not carry the factor. The mammary-tumor milk agent is known to be a virus. The virus, which is transmitted in milk, infects infant mice when nursing, whether or not the mother has mammary cancer, as infected mice may be "latently" infected and excrete virus in the absence of disease. Newly infected mice may similarly transmit the virus to their offspring without developing mammary tumors. Once infected, development of mammary tumors requires a genetic susceptibility and appropriate hormone influence, which is usually provided by pregnancy.

Not all mammary tumors in mice are related to this virus, for several transplantable tumors have been recognized in mice that are free of the milk agent. The murine mammary tumor associated with the milk agent is of much interest in experimental oncology, as it provides a link in the chain of evidence pointing toward a viral etiology for neoplasia.

References

Bentvelzen P, Hilgers J. Murine mammary tumor virus. In: Klein G, ed. Viral oncology. New York: Raven Press 1980;311–355.

Gross L. Oncogenic viruses. International Series of Monographs on Pure and Applied Biology. Vol. 11. New York: Pergamon Press 1961.

Gross L. Oncogenic viruses. 2nd ed. New York: Pergamon Press 1970;238–280.

TYPE D ONCOVIRUSES

Type D oncoviruses have been shown to be of pathologic significance only in sheep, in which a type D virus is associated with jaagsiekte, and in nonhuman primates. The prototype virus, Mason-Pfizer monkey virus, was originally isolated from an adenocarcinoma of the mammary gland of a rhesus monkey; however, no causal relationship has been demonstrated. Several additional related type D retroviruses have since been identified, principally in macaques, that have been termed simian retroviruses (SRV). Infection is common in macaques; the virus causes immunosuppression leading to opportunistic infections. An unusual lesion associated with infection, termed retroperitoneal fibromatosis, is characterized by marked fibroblastic proliferation surrounding abdominal and occasionally thoracic organs.

JAAGSIEKTE (OVINE PULMONARY ADENOMA, PULMONARY CARCINOMA OF SHEEP)

Derived from Afrikaans words meaning "drive" (jaagt) and "sickness," jaagsiekte is the South African name of a neoplastic disease of older sheep, which may first reveal its existence by dyspneic and anoxic symptoms after the stress of strenuous exertion, such as a long drive. The disease runs a progressive afebrile course of several months or longer. It has many points of similarity to Marsh's ovine progressive pneumonia, but one difference is the considerable catarrhal nasal discharge that is characteristic of jaagsiekte. The two diseases can occur simultaneously. Besides South Africa, the malady occurs in Europe, England, Iceland, Israel, and Peru.

It is well established that jaagsiekte is transmissible to susceptible sheep by contact, aerosol, and intratracheal or intrapulmonary injection of affected lung tissue from sheep with the disease. Over the years, several different viruses have been suggested as the cause of jaagsiekte; however, morphologic, biochemical, and immunologic findings have implicated a type D retrovirus as the cause. The agent has not yet been cultured.

Lesions The lesions of jaagsiekte consist of multiple foci of neoplastic alveolar type II cells in acinar and papillary patterns (Fig. 8-74). The result is a pronounced thickening of the alveolar walls and their interstices and partial obliteration of the alveolar spaces by small adenocarcinomas, although their malignancy is not clearly evident. Lymphocytes accompany the reticuloendothelial cells, but proliferated fibroblasts appear to be practically absent until the later stages, when fibrosis is extensive. A certain number of mononuclear cells and lymphocytes spill over into the alveoli and, accompanied by a few neutrophils, appear as an exudate in some of the bronchi. There is, however, never any exudate comparable to that seen in the acute exudative pneumonias. The peribronchiolar lymph nodules are also hyperplastic and markedly enlarged, as is true in Marsh's progressive pneumonia and other chronic inflammations of the lungs (Fig. 8–69). Metastatic lesions consisting of adenomatous foci in bronchial and mediastinal lymph nodes comparable to those seen in the lung have been reported by numerous authors. Less often, the metastases are associated with a desmoplastic reaction similar to that encountered in certain carcinomas. A few reports have described extrathoracic metastases to sites such as muscle and kidney. The proliferative nature of the pulmonary lesion coupled with metastases is strong evidence that jaagsiekte is neoplastic and malignant.

Diagnosis Both jaagsiekte and maedi/progressive pneumonia are chronic lung diseases with long incubation periods. Maedi/progressive pneumonia is not neoplastic and is characterized by interstitial pneumonia and marked lymphocytic nodular hyperplasia.

References

Chauhan HVS, Singh CM. Studies on the pathology of pulmonary adenomatosis complex of sheep and goats. II. Viral pneumonitis (a typical pneumonia). Indian J Anim Sci 1971;41:272–276.

Cowdry EV, Marsh H. Comparative pathology of South African jaagziekte and Montana progressive pneumonia of sheep. J Exper Med 1927;45:571–586.

Cuba-Caparo A. Adenomatosis Pulmonar de los Ovinos en el Peru. Bull Off Int Epiz 1961;56:840–849.

Cuba-Caparo A, De La Vega E, Copaira M. Pulmonary adenomatosis of sheep, metastasizing bronchiolar tumors. Am J Vet Res 1961;22:673–682.

de Kock G. The transformation of the lining of the pulmonary alveoli with special reference to adenomatosis in the lungs (jaagziekte) of sheep. Am J Vet Res 1958;19:261–269.

Duran-Reynals F, et al. The pulmonary adenomatosis complex in sheep. Ann NY Acad Sci 1958;70:726–742.

Hod I, Perk K, Nobel TA, et al. Lung carcinoma of sheep (jaagsiekte). III. Lymph node, blood, and immunoglobulin. J Natl Cancer Inst 1972;48:487–507.

MacKay JMK. Tissue culture studies of sheep pulmonary adenomatosis (jaagsiekte). J Comp Pathol 1969;79:141–146.

Malmquist WA, Krauss HH, Moulton JE, et al. Morphologic study of virus-infected lung cell cultures from sheep pulmonary adenomatosis. Lab Invest 1972;26:528–533.

Markson LM, Terlecki S. The experimental transmission of ovine pulmonary adenomatosis. Pathol Vet 1964;1:269–288.

Martin WB, et al. Experimental production of sheep pulmonary adenomatosis (jaagsiekte). Nature 1976;264:183–184.

Nisbet DI, MacKay JMK, Smith W, et al. Ultrastructure of sheep pulmonary adenomatosis (jaagsiekte). J Pathol 1971;103:157–162.

Nobel TA, Neumann F, Klopfer U. Histological patterns of the metastases in pulmonary adenomatosis of sheep (jaagsiekte). J Comp Pathol 1969;79:537–540.

Perk K, Hod I, Nobel TA. Pulmonary adenomatosis of sheep (jaagsiekte). I. Ultrastructure of the tumor. J Natl Cancer Inst 1971;46:525–537.

Perk K, Hod I, Presentey B, et al. Lung carcinoma of sheep (jaagsiekte). II. Histogenesis of the tumor. J Natl Cancer Inst 1971;47:197–205.

Perk K, Michalides R, Spiegelman S, et al. Biochemical and morphologic evidence for the presence of an RNA tumor virus in pulmonary carcinoma of sheep (jaagsiekte). J Natl Cancer Inst 1974;53:131–135.

Rosadio RH, Lairmore MD, Russell HI, et al. Retrovirus-associated ovine pulmonary carcinoma (sheep pulmonary adenomatosis) and lymphoid interstitial pneumonia. I. Lesion development and age susceptibility. Vet Pathol 1988;25:475–483.

Rosadio RH, Sharp JM, Lairmore MD, et al. Lesions and retroviruses associated with naturally occurring ovine pulmonary carcinoma (sheep pulmonary adenomatosis). Vet Pathol 1988;25:58–66.

Sharp JM, Angus KW, Gray EW, et al. Rapid transmission of sheep pulmonary adenomatosis (jaagsiekte) in young lambs. Arch Virol 1983;78:89–95.

Sharp JM, Herring AJ. Sheep pulmonary adenomatosis: demonstration of a protein which crossreacts with the major core proteins of Mason-Pfizer monkey virus and mouse mammary tumour virus. J Gen Virol 1983;64:2323–2327.

Sigurdsson B. Adenomatosis of sheep lungs. Experimental transmission. Arch ges Virus-forsch 1958;8:51–58.

Smith W, Mackay JMK. Morphological observations on a virus associated with sheep pulmonary adenomatosis (jaagsiekte). J Comp Pathol 1969;79:421–424.

Tustin RC, Geyer SM. Transmission of ovine jaagsiekte using neoplastic cells grown in tissue culture. J S Afr Vet Med Assoc 1971;42:181–182.

Verwoerd DW, Payne A, York DF, et al. Isolation and preliminary characterization of the jaagsiekte retrovirus (JRSV). Onderstepoort J Vet Res 1983;50:309–316.

Wandera JG. Sheep pulmonary adenomatosis (jaagsiekte). Adv Vet Sci Comp Med 1971;15:251–283.

Wandera JG, Krauss H. The ultrastructure of sheep pulmonary adenomatosis. Zentbl Vet Med 1971;18A:325–334.

Wandera JG. Experimental transmission of sheep pulmonary adenomatosis (jaagsiekte). Vet Rec 1968;83:478–482.

Spumavirinae

The Spumavirinae, or foamy viruses, are retroviruses that are endemic in a number of species of mammals including cats, cattle, nonhuman primates, humans, and hamsters. The infection persists for the lifetime of infected hosts, and the viruses are shed orally. The incidence of infection is high, but infection is asymptomatic. To date, no specific disease has been associated with the foamy viruses, but it has been suggested that they might be related to certain chronic neurologic disorders as well as some forms of thyroiditis. They are often recovered in tissue culture as annoying "contaminants" with typical retroviral characteristics, causing a foamy degeneration of cultured cells.

References

Aguzzi A. The foamy virus family: molecular biology, epidemiology and neuropathology. Biochim Biophys Acta 1993;1155:1–24.

Benveniste RE, Todaro GJ. Evolution of primate oncornaviruses: an endogenous virus from langurs (Presbytis spp.) with related virogene sequences in other Old World monkeys. Proc Natl Acad Sci USA 1977;74:4557–4561.

Benveniste RE, Stromberg K, Morton WR, et al. Association of retroperitoneal fibromatosis with type D retroviruses. In: Salzman LA, ed. Animal models of retrovirus infection and their relationship to AIDS. New York: Academic Press 1986;335–353.

Bouillant AMP, Becker SAWE. Ultrastructural comparison of Oncovirinae (type C), Spumavirinae, and Lentivirinae: three subfamilies of Retroviridae found in farm animals. JNCI 1984;72:1075–1084.

Chopra HC, Mason MM. A new virus in a spontaneous mammary tumor of a rhesus monkey. Cancer Res 1970;30:2081–2086.

Daniel MD, King NW, Letvin NL, et al. A new type D retrovirus isolated from macaques with an immunodenficiency syndrome. Science 1984;223:602–605.

Daniel MD, et al. Prevalence of antibodies to 3 retroviruses in a captive colony of macaque monkeys. Int J Cancer 1988;41:601–608.

Desrosiers RC, et al. Retrovirus D/New England and its relation to Mason-Pfizer monkey virus. J Virol 1985;54:552–560.

Fine DL, et al. Responses of infant rhesus monkeys to inoculation with Mason-Pfizer monkey virus materials. JNCI 1975;54:651–658.

Flügel RM. Spumaviruses: a group of complex retroviruses. J Acquir Immune Defic Syndr 1991;4:730–750.

Giddens WE Jr, et al. Idiopathic retroperitoneal fibrosis: an enzootic disease in the pigtail monkey (Macaca nemestrina). (abstr) Lab Invest 1979;40:294.

Giddens WE Jr, Morton WR, Hefti E, et al. Enzootic retroperitoneal fibromatosis in Macaca spp. Monogr Primatol 1983;2:249–253.

Giddens WE Jr, Tsai C-C, Morton WR, et al. Retroperitoneal fibromatosis and acquired immunodeficiency syndrome in macaques. Am J Pathol 1985;119:253–263.

Gravell M, London WT, Lecatsas G, et al. Transmission of simian acquired immunodeficiency syndrome (SAIDS) with type D retrovirus isolated from saliva or urine. Proc Soc Exp Biol Med 1984;177:491–494.

Hooks JJ, Gibbs CJ Jr. The foamy viruses. Bacteriol Rev 1975;39:169–185.

Kwang H-S, Pedersen NC, Lerche NW, et al. Viremia, antigenemia, and serum antibodies in rhesus macaques infected with simian retrovirus type 1 and their relationship to disease course. Lab Invest 1987;56:591–597.

Letvin NL, et al. Experimental infection of rhesus monkeys with type D retrovirus. J Virol 1984;52:683–686.

Marczynska B, Jones CJ, Wolfe LG. Syncytium-forming virus of common marmosets (Callithrix jacchus jacchus). Infect Immun 1981; 31:1261–1269.

Marx PA, et al. Simian AIDS: isolation of a type D retrovirus and transmission of the disease. Science 1984;223:1083–1086.

Marx PA, et al. Isolation of a new serotype of simian acquired immune deficiency syndrome type D retrovirus from Celebes black macaques (Macaca nigra) with immune deficiency and retroperitoneal fibromatosis. J Virol 1985;56:571–578.

Marx PA, et al. Prevention of simian acquired immune deficiency syndrome with a formalin-inactivated type D retrovirus vaccine. J Virol 1986;60:431–435.

Nagra RM, Burrola PG, Wiley CA. Development of spongiform encephalopathy in retroviral infected mice. Lab Invest 1992;66: 292–302.

Neumann-Haefelin D, Fleps U, Renne R, et al. Foamy viruses. Intervirology 1993;35:196–207.

Pedersen NC, Pool RR, O'Brien T. Feline chronic progressive polyarthritis. Am J Vet Res 1980;41:522–535.

Rhodes-Feuillette A, Saal F, Lasneret J, et al. Isolation and characterization of a new simian foamy virus serotype from lymphocytes of a Papio cynocephalus baboon. J Med Primatol 1979;8:308–320.

Schnitzer TJ. Characterization of a simian foamy virus isolated from a spontaneous primate lymphoma. J Med Primatol 1981;10: 312–328.

Shiigi SM, et al. Association of SAIDS/RF-related signs with current or past SAIDS type 2 retrovirus infection in a colony of Celebes black macaques. Lab Anim Sci 1986;36:20–23.

Stromberg K, et al. Characterization of exogenous type D retrovirus from a fibroma of a macaque with simian AIDS and fibromatosis. Science 1984;224:289–292.

Tsai C-C, Giddens WE Jr, Morton WR, et al. Retroperitoneal fibromatosis and acquired immunodeficiency syndrome in macaques: epidemiologic studies. Lab Anim Sci 1985;35:460–464.

Tsai C-C, Giddens WE Jr, Ochs HD, et al. Retroperitoneal fibromatosis and acquired immunodeficiency syndrome in macaques: clinical and immunologic studies. Lab Anim Sci 1986;36:119–125.

ARENAVIRIDAE

The family *Arenaviridae* contains several viruses that usually infect rodents but may spread to humans or other animals. The virions are spherical or pleomorphic, measuring 100 to 300 nm in diameter. The virions contain a variable number of electron-dense granules, 20 to 25 nm in diameter, which have a sandy appearance, giving the group its name (arenosus = sandy). These represent inactive host cell ribosomes that become incorporated during the process of budding. A dense, double-layer lipid membrane surrounds the virion, which contains a core made up of particles similar to ribosomes. The virion proteins include two glycopeptides and two polypeptides. The genome consists of a single-stranded RNA in several segments, differing in molecular weight. Most of the genome is negative-sense, but it is, in part, positive-sense, hence, the name ambisense for the family. Virions are readily inactivated by acid, heat, radiation, or lipid solvent. Their buoyant density in sucrose is 1.17 to 1.18 g/cm^3. Replication occurs in the cytoplasm of host cells. Transmission occurs by means of contaminated food, water, air, or inoculation. This group of viruses causes several important hemorrhagic fevers of humans (Lassa, Machupo, and Juniri viruses). The family at present contains one genus, arenavirus; the type species is the lymphocytic choriomeningitis virus (Fig. 8-75).

Diseases caused by arenaviruses

Arenaviruses are associated with several diseases, including lymphocytic choriomeningitis, Argentine and Bolivian hemorrhagic fever, and Lassa fever. The *Arenaviridae* contain a number of other viruses in the Tacaribe complex, which are either nonpathogenic or undefined.

LYMPHOCYTIC CHORIOMENINGITIS

Lymphocytic chloriomeningitis is a viral disease to which humans and many animals are susceptible. House mice and, to a smaller degree, other animals may harbor the virus without showing signs, except in the rare case in which fatal paralytic meningoencephalitis develops. The virus has been demonstrated in laboratory and house mice, monkeys, dogs, guinea pigs, roaches, ticks, and humans. Experimental infection has also been produced in most of these species, but in rabbits, young chickens, hamsters, and horses, few symptoms follow experimental exposure, although these animals may harbor the virus for several days.

The disease not only is capable of invalidating experimental results, it is also a hazard to laboratory workers, for it is believed that humans may become infected through intact skin and conjunctiva or by inhalation or ingestion of the virus. Blood sucking insects, such as mosquitoes and ticks, may also transmit the disease. The course in humans is usually 2 or 3 weeks, and fortunately, the disease is rarely fatal.

Infection is widespread in wild mice in the United States and Europe and colonies of laboratory mice, as well as hamsters, are likely to harbor the virus unless special precautions are taken. In mice, two patterns of infection may occur: persistent infection, which is common, or acute infection. In both, host immune responses are responsible for disease, the virus itself being noncytopathic. Intrauterine transmission is the principal means of spread, although virus is also shed in the urine and feces. Most mice, therefore, are either infected at birth or shortly thereafter, and they carry the virus throughout their lives as a persistent infection, which is passed on to the next generation. The infection is well tolerated, but complete tolerance is not always established. In some individuals a cellular and humoral immune response leads to a chronic immune-mediated disease. Circulating virus antibody complexes lead to immune complex glomerulonephritis and vasculitis. Splenic hyperplasia, lymphocytic infiltration in many tissues, and focal hepatic necrosis are believed to result from a cell-mediated immune response.

Acute lymphocytic choriomeningitis follows natural or experimental infection of adult mice or of mice 48 hours or more after birth. Infection is followed by viral replication in multiple tissues. The most striking lesion is marked lymphocytic infiltration of the meninges, which is most pronounced in the pia-arachnoid at the base of the brain, in the choroid plexus, and sometimes, in the perivascular spaces of the submeningeal and subependymal vessels. Encephalitis with neuronal necrosis is not a feature. Lymphocytic infiltrates are also present in other tissues, particularly the liver and

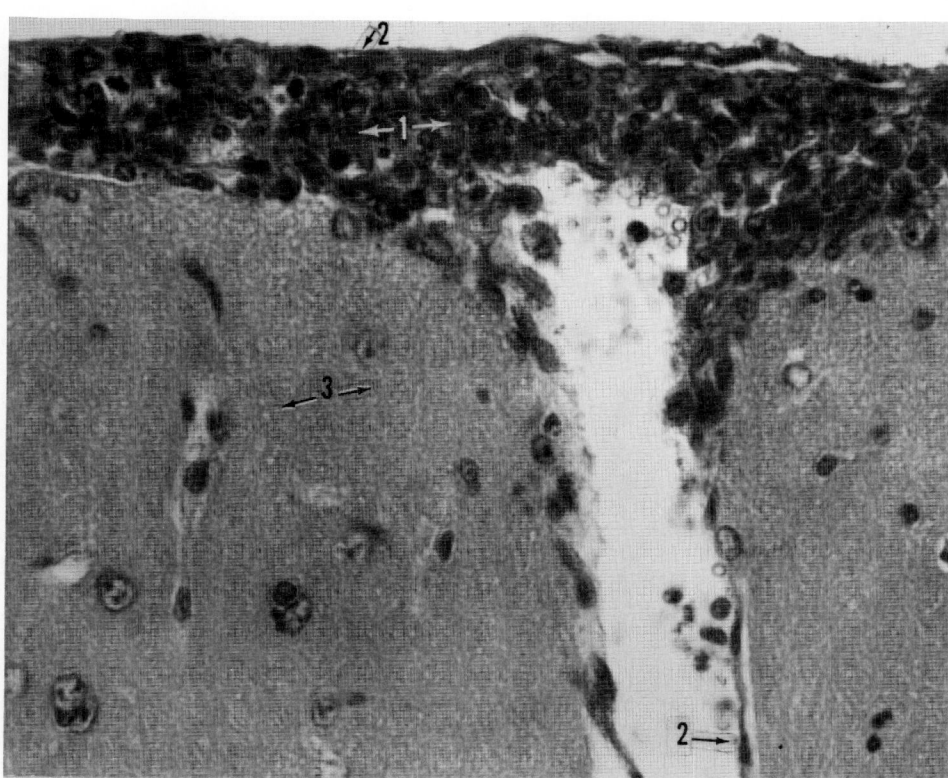

FIG. 8-75 Lymphocytic chorio-meningitis, cerebrum of a mouse (× 865). Lymphocytes *(1)* infiltrate and elevate the pia *(2)*. Cerebral cortex *(3)*. (Courtesy of the Armed Forces Institute of Pathology; contributed by the Army Medical School.)

lung, and are most often perivascular. There is hyperplasia of lymphocytes as well as necrosis of lymphocytes in the spleen and lymph nodes. Similar lesions dominate the microscopic picture in other species affected with the acute disease. The lesions result from a cellular immune response to virally induced antigens on the surface of infected cells, which the host recognizes as foreign. The lesions and disease can be prevented with immunosuppression. Acute lymphocytic choriomeningitis need not lead to death. The cellular immune response may successfully reject the infected tissues leaving the animal immune, or it may hold the acute infection in relative check but leave a persistent infection eventually leading to chronic lymphocytic meningitis as described above.

Experimentally, lymphocytic choriomeningitis virus has been shown to induce a variety of interesting lesions. Inoculation of suckling mice or rats can lead to cerebellar hypoplasia caused by an immune-mediated necrosis of the granular cell layer. An inflammatory retinopathy may also develop in rats. Two curious endocrinologic abnormalities can be caused by LCM virus. Persistent infection of the adenohypophysis or β cells in the pancreatic islets of Langerhans can lead to reduced secretion of growth hormone or insulin, resulting in either pituitary dwarfism or diabetes. Virus is demonstrable in these tissues, but no cell lysis or inflammatory reaction is present. Curiously, LCM virus has also been shown to prevent autoimmune type I diabetes in the nonobese diabetic mouse. Persistent infection of lymphocytes by the virus prevents their mounting the usual autoimmune disease seen in this strain of mouse, a most interesting observation with respect to the use of viruses as therapeutic tools and especially interesting with a virus whose usual disease is dependent on an immune response.

A strain of lymphocytic choriomeningitis virus has recently been identified as the cause of a highly fatal epizootic disease in new world primates in the family *Callitrichidae* (marmosets and tamarins) in North American zoos. The disease, which is contracted from infected mice, is primarily characterized by necrotizing hepatitis and has been designated callitrichid hepatitis. The hepatic lesions consist of random foci of degeneration and necrosis associated with a mild mononuclear and neutrophilic infiltration. Focal necrosis also occurs in the spleen, abdominal lymph nodes, adrenal cortex and intestinal tract.

References

Cole GA, Gilden DH, Monjan AA, et al. Lymphocytic choriomeningitis virus: pathogenesis of acute central nervous system disease. Fed Proc 1971;30:1831–1841.

Dalldorf G. Lymphocytic choriomeningitis of dogs. Cornell Vet 1943;33:347–350.

del Cerro M, Nathanson N, Monjan AA. Pathogenesis of cerebellar hypoplasia produced by lymphocytic choriomeningitis virus infection of neonatal rats. II. An ultrastructural study of the immune-mediated pathology. Lab Invest 1975;33:608–617.

Hotchin J. The contamination of laboratory animals with lymphocytic choriomeningitis virus. Am J Pathol 1971;64:747–769.

Hotchin J, et al. Lymphocytic choriomeningitis in a hamster colony causes infection of hospital personnel. Science 1974;185:1173–1174.

Lehmann-Grube F. Portraits of viruses: arenaviruses. Intervirology 1984;22:121–145.

Lehmann-Grube F, Löhler J. Immunopathologic alterations of lymphatic tissues of mice infected with lymphocytic choriomeningitis virus. II. Pathogenetic mechanism. Lab Invest 1981;44:205–213.

Lillie RD, Armstrong C. Pathology of lymphocytic choriomeningitis in mice. Arch Pathol 1945;40:141–152.

Mims CA. Effect on the fetus of maternal infection with lymphocytic choriomeningitis (LCM) virus. J Infect Dis 1969;120:582–597.

Löhler J, Lehmann-Grube F. Immunopathologic alterations of lymphatic tissues of mice infected with lymphocytic choriomeningitis virus. I. Histopathologic findings. Lab Invest 1981;44:193–204.

Monjan AA, Silverstein AM, Cole GA. Lymphocytic choriomeningitis virus-induced retinopathy in newborn rats. Invest Ophthalmol 1972;11:850–856.

Montali RJ, Connolly BM, Armstrong DL, et al. Pathology and Immunohistocytochemistry of Callitrichid hepatitis, an emerging disease of captive new world primates caused by lymphocytic choriomeningitis virus. Am J Path 1995;1441–1449.

Oldstone MBA. Prevention of type I diabetes in nonobese diabetic mice by virus infection. Science 1988;239:500–502.

Oldstone MB, Dixon FJ. Pathogenesis of chronic disease associated with persistent lymphocytic choriomeningitis viral infection. II. Relationship of the antilymphocytic choriomeningitis immune response to tissue injury in chronic lymphocytic choriomeningitis disease. J Exp Med 1970;131:1–19.

Oldstone MBA, et al. Virus-induced alterations in homeostasis: alterations in differentiated functions of infected cells in vivo. Science 1982;218:1125–1127.

Oldstone MBA, Southern P, Rodriguez M, et al. Virus persists in B cells of islets of Langerhans and is associated with chemical manifestations of diabetes. Science 1984;224:1440–1443.

Rodriguez M, von Wedel RJ, Garrett RS, et al. Pituitary dwarfism in mice persistently infected with lymphocytic choriomeningitis virus. Lab Invest 1983;49:48–53.

Traub E. An epidemic in a mouse colony due to lymphocytic choriomeningitis. J Exp Med 1936;63:533–546.

Walker DH, Murphy FA, Whitfield SG, et al. Lymphocytic choriomeningitis: ultrastructural pathology. Exp Mol Pathol 1975;23:245–265.

BOLIVIAN AND ARGENTINE HEMORRHAGIC FEVER

These are principally diseases of humans, but several species are susceptible, including rhesus monkeys (*Macaca mulatta*). Argentine hemorrhagic fever, which is restricted to Argentina, is caused by an arenavirus known as Junin virus, carried by rodents of the *Calomys* genus. The arenavirus called Machupo virus, also carried by *Calomys* species, is the cause of Bolivian hemorrhagic fever, a disease restricted to Bolivia. Junin and Machupo viruses are members of the Tacaribe complex. Both diseases are characterized by fever and hemorrhage. Pathologically, hemorrhage is the most prominent finding. There also may be hepatic necrosis with Councilman bodies, myocarditis, and lymphoid necrosis. The pathogenesis of the disease does not involve an immune-mediated mechanism as in lymphocytic choriomeningitis; however, experimentally, intracerebral inoculation of newborn mice can lead to cerebellar heterotopia or meningitis that is immune mediated.

In rhesus and African green monkeys, the experimental disease mimics that of humans.

References

Ambrosio AM, Enria DA, Maiztegui JI. Junin virus isolation from lympho-mononuclear cells of patients with Argentine hemorrhagic fever. Intervirology 1986;25:97–102.

Eddy GA, Scott SK, Wagner FS, et al. Pathogenesis of Machupo virus infection in primates. Bull WHO 1975;52:516–521.

Frigerio MJ, Rondinone SN, Callelo MA, et al. Junin virus infection of *Calithrix jacchus:* haematological findings. Acta Virol 1982;26:270–278.

Kenyon RH, Green DE, Maiztegui JI, et al. Viral strain dependent differences in experimental Argentine hemorrhagic fever (Junin virus) infection of guinea pigs. Intervirology 1988;29:133–143.

Laguens RM, Avila MM, Samoilovich SR, et al. Pathogenicity of an attenuated strain (XJCl3) of Junin virus: morphological and virological studies in experimentally infected guinea pigs. Intervirology 1983;20:195–201.

McLeod CG Jr, Stookey JL, Eddy GA, et al. Pathology of chronic Bolivian hemorrhagic fever in the rhesus monkey. Am J Pathol 1976;84:211–224.

McLeod CG Jr, Stookey JL, White JD, et al. Pathology of Bolivian hemorrhagic fever in the African green monkey. Am J Trop Med Hyg 1978;27:822–826.

Oubiña JR, Milei J, Bolomo NJ, et al. Experimental Argentine hemorrhagic fever: myocardial involvement in *Cebus* monkey. J Med Primatol 1986;15:391–397.

Terrell TG, Stookey JL, Eddy GA, et al. Pathology of Bolivian hemorrhagic fever in the rhesus monkey. Am J Pathol 1973;73:477–494.

Weissenbacher MC, et al. Induction of Junin virus persistence in adult athymic mice. Intervirology 1986;25:210–215.

Lassa fever

Lassa fever was first recognized as a new disease of humans in 1969 in the course of an outbreak on the Jos plateau of Nigeria in West Africa. The disease may be subclinical, but florid cases occur, with death in some instances within 4 weeks. Rhesus monkeys (*Macaca mulatta*), squirrel monkeys (*Saimiri sciureus*), guinea pigs, hamsters, mice, and rats have been experimentally infected with the virus, an arenavirus, resulting in a severe viremia and fatal outcome. Transfer of virus to African multimammate rats (*Mastomys natalensis*) resulted in persistent viremia at high titer but no obvious illness in these animals. This species is believed to provide the principal reservoir for the virus in nature.

The experimental infection in monkeys results in high viral titers and lesions in many organs at death. These lesions may be summarized as necrosis of lymphocytes in the spleen, necrosis of renal tubular epithelium, myocarditis, arteritis, and disseminated necrosis of hepatocytes. In animals with a survival time of 28 days or longer, choriomeningitis may be evident. The infection and its effects on the hosts are similar to that

TABLE 8-11 **Diseases Caused by *Coronaviridae* (Genus: *Coronavirus*)**

Avian infectious bronchitis virus
Human coronavirus
Porcine transmissible gastroenteritis virus
Rat coronavirus
Turkey bluecomb disease virus
Calf neonatal diarrhea coronavirus
Murine hepatitis virus
Porcine hemagglutinating encephalitis virus
Rat sialodacryoadenitis virus
Feline infectious peritonitis virus
Canine coronavirus

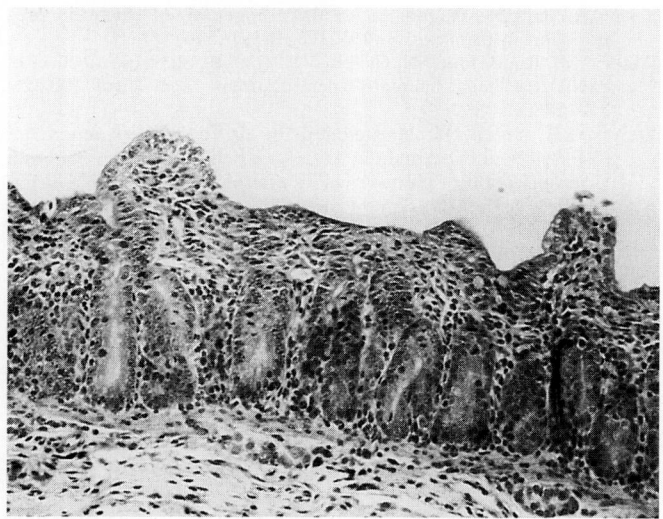

FIG. 8-76 Coronavirus enteritis in a piglet. Mid-jejunum with a flat avillous mucosa. (Courtesy of Drs. W. Coussement, J. Hoorens, and *Veterinary Pathology* 1982;19:46–56.)

seen in the type species: lymphocytic choriomeningitis viral infection.

References

Buckley SM, Casals J. Lassa fever, a new virus disease of man from West Africa. III. Isolation and characterization of the virus. Am J Trop Med Hyg 1970;19:680–691.

Frame JD, Baldwin JM, Gocke DJ, et al. Lassa fever, a new virus disease of man from West Africa. I. Clinical description and pathological findings. Am J Trop Med Hyg 1970;19:670–676.

Jahrling PB, Hesse RA, Eddy GA, et al. Lassa virus infection of rhesus monkeys: pathogenesis and treatment with ribavirin. J Infect Dis 1980;141:580–589.

Moe JB, Jahrling PB. Fatal arenavirus infection. Comp Pathol Bull 1984;16(3):3.

Walker DH, Wulff H, Lange JV, et al. Comparative pathology of Lassa virus infection in monkeys, guinea-pigs, and Mastomys natalensis. Bull WHO 1975;52:523–534.

Walker DH, Wulff H, Murphy FA. Experimental Lassa virus infection in the squirrel monkey. Am J Pathol 1975;80:261–278.

CORONAVIRIDAE

The virions of this family (Table 8-11) of viruses are pleomorphic enveloped particles averaging about 100 nm in diameter. Unique club-shaped peplomers, about 15 to 20 nm long, project from the envelope, giving the appearance of a crown in negatively stained electron micrographs (corona = crown). The genome consists of one molecule of single-stranded, positive-sense RNA with a molecular weight of 9 million daltons. Virion RNA acts as messenger RNA, first producing an RNA polymerase, which forms a full-length minus strand template that serves to make new positive-sense virion RNA. Replication occurs in the cytoplasm. The envelope is acquired by budding through internal cytoplasmic membranes of endoplasmic reticulum and the Golgi apparatus, and the virions are then transported in vesicles to the cell membrane for release.

Avian infectious bronchitis virus, the type species

for the single genus, coronavirus, is quite distinct immunologically. Several of the coronaviruses of mammals cross-react serologically. Some viruses of the group agglutinate the red blood cells of other species, e.g., human coronavirus and hemagglutinating encephalitis virus of piglets.

Along with rotaviruses, coronaviruses are important causes of gastroenteritis. They, [may] also [may] cause respiratory disease, hepatitis, encephalomyelitis, serositis, and other diseases in several animal species.

Diseases caused by coronavirus

A list of coronaviruses appears in Table 8-11. The name of each of these viruses identifies the disease with which it is associated.

TRANSMISSIBLE GASTROENTERITIS OF SWINE

First described by Doyle and Hutchings (1946), transmissible gastroenteritis (TGE) of swine is a highly contagious viral disease, especially in young pigs. It now is established that the causative agent is a coronavirus (Fig. 8-76) that meets the morphologic, physical, and chemical characteristics of this genus. This virus may be distinguished from another porcine coronavirus, the hemagglutinating encephalomyelitis virus of piglets, which agglutinates and hemabsorbs *in vitro* the red blood cells of chicks, hamsters, and rats. The transmissible gastroenteritis virus lacks these properties and also can be distinguished by the viral neutralization test. Another coronavirus, termed CV777, is antigenically different from the coronavirus of transmissible gastroenteritis but causes an essentially identical enteritis in piglets. The disease has been termed **porcine epidemic diarrhea.** The virus of TGE is antigenically related to feline infectious peritonitis virus and canine coronavirus.

Signs In pigs less than 10 days of age, the disease is characterized by acute diarrhea, vomiting, excessive thirst, weight loss, and dehydration, which lead to death in 2 to 5 days. Morbidity and mortality rates may approach 100%. In older piglets and adults, clinical signs may not be apparent or there may be profuse diarrhea, vomiting, depression, and failure to gain or maintain weight. The morbidity rate in older swine may also approach 100%, but the mortality rate is low.

Lesions In pigs dying of transmissible gastroenteritis, few gross findings are evident. The carcass is dehydrated and curdled milk is usually present in the stomach. The mucosa of the stomach and small intestine is congested and often contains petechiae. Microscopically, there is marked shortening and fusion of villi of the small intestine (Fig. 8-45C; 8-76). Villous length is reduced several fold, and villi are lined with flattened to cuboid epithelial cells rather than with the normal columnar cells. The brush border of the epithelium is irregularly absent, the cytoplasm vacuolated, and the nuclei small and often pyknotic. Ultrastructurally, microvilli are shortened and irregular; there is swelling and disruption of mitochondria and vacuolation of the endoplasmic reticulum. The lamina propria is infiltrated with mononuclear cells and neutrophils, but inflammatory exudation is not a striking feature. Thake (1968) has demonstrated that the villous atrophy is the combined effect of virally induced villous cell destruction and improper maturation of cells as they advance from the crypts to the villi. Focal necrosis of the gastric mucosa has been described. In most cases there is evidence of nephrosis. Hydropic and hyalin droplet degeneration are present in the epithelium of proximal convoluted tubules, and proteinaceous casts may be numerous. Okinawa and Maeda (1966) have described reticuloendothelial hyperplasia and loss of lymphocytes in lymph nodes and spleens of experimentally infected pigs.

Diagnosis Presumptive diagnosis can be made by means of the clinical signs and supported by finding the histopathologic lesions in the small intestine.

The virus of transmissible gastroenteritis may be identified by specific immunofluorescence or by neutralization in tissue culture systems. It may be distinguished from the hemagglutinating encephalomyelitis virus by its lack of hemagglutination of erythrocytes *in vitro*.

References

Bay WW, Doyle LP, Hutchings LM. The pathology and symptomatology of transmissible gastroenteritis. Am J Vet Res 1951;12: 215–218.

Butler DG, Gall DG, Kelly MH, et al.. Transmissible gastroenteritis. Mechanisms responsible for diarrhea in an acute viral enteritis in piglets. J Clin Invest 1974;53:1335–1342.

Chu RM, Glock RD, Ross RF. Changes in gut-associated lymphoid tissues of the small intestine of eight-week-old pigs infected with transmissible gastroenteritis virus. Am J Vet Res 1982;43:67–76.

Coussement W, Ducatelle R, Debouck P, et al. Pathology of experimental CV777 coronavirus enteritis in piglets. I. Histological and histochemical study. Vet Pathol 1982;19:46–56.

Debouck P, Pensaert M. Experimental infection of pigs with a new porcine enteric coronavirus, CV 777. Am J Vet Res 1980;41: 219–223.

Doyle LP, Hutchings LM. A transmissible gastroenteritis in pigs. J Am Vet Med Assoc 1946;108:257–259.

Ducatelle R, Coussement W, Debouck P, et al. Pathology of experimental CV777 coronavirus enteritis in piglets. II. Electron microscopic study. Vet Pathol 1982;19:57–66.

Hooper BE, Haelterman EO. Lesions of the gastrointestinal tract of pigs infected with transmissible gastroenteritis. Can J Comp Med 1969;33:29–36.

Horvath I, Mocsari E. Ultrastructural changes in the small intestinal epithelium of suckling pigs affected with a transmissible gastroenteritis (TGE)-like disease. Arch Virol 1981;68:103–113.

Moon HW, Norman JO, Lambert G. Age dependent resistance to transmissible gastroenteritis of swine (TGE). J. Clinical signs and some mucosal dimensions in small intestine. Can J Comp Med 1973;37:157–166.

Moon HW, et al. Age-dependent resistance to transmissible gastroenteritis of swine. III. Effects of epithelial cell kinetics on coronavirus production and on atrophy of intestinal villi. Vet Pathol 1975;12:434–445.

Morin M, Morehouse LG, Solorzano RF, et al. Transmissible gastroenteritis in feeder swine: clinical immunofluorescence and histopathological observations. Can J Comp Med 1973;37:239–248.

Morin M, Morehouse LG. Transmissible gastroenteritis in feeder pigs: observations on the jejunal epithelium of normal feeder pigs and feeder pigs infected with TGE virus. Can J Comp Med 1974;38:227–235.

Okinawa A, Maeda M. Histopathology of transmissible gastroenteritis in experimentally infected newborn piglets. I. Lesions in the digestive tract. Nat Inst Anim Health Q (Tokyo) 1965;5:190–201,

Okinawa A, Maeda M. Histopathology of transmissible gastroenteritis in experimentally infected newborn piglets. II. Lesions in organs other than digestive tract and pathologic features of TGE. Nat Inst Anim Health Q (Tokyo) 1966;6:64–72.

Olson DP, Waxler GL, Roberts AW. Small intestinal lesions of transmissible gastroenteritis in gnotobiotic pigs: A scanning electron microscopic study. Am J Vet Res 1973;34:1239–1245.

Pensaert M, Haelterman EO, Burnstein T. Transmissible gastroenteritis of swine: virus-intestinal cell interactions. I. Immunofluorescence, histopathology and virus production in the small intestine through the course of infection. Arch Ges Virusforsch 1970;31:321–334.

Pensaert M, Haelterman EO, Hinsman EJ. Transmissible gastroenteritis of swine: virus-intestinal cell interactions. II. Electron microscopy of the epithelium in isolated jejunal loops. Arch Ges Virusforsch 1970;31:335–351.

Saif LJ, Bohl EH, Kohler EM, et al. Immune electron microscopy of transmissible gastroenteritis virus and Rotavirus (reovirus-like agent) of swine. Am J Vet Res 1977;38:13–20.

Thake DC. Jejunal epithelium in transmissible gastroenteritis of swine. Am J Pathol 1968;53:149–168.

Thake DC, Moon HW, Lambert G. Epithelial cell dynamics in transmissible gastroenteritis of neonatal pigs. Vet Pathol 1973;10: 330–341.

Trapp AL, Sanger VL, Stalnaker E. Lesions of the small intestinal mucosa in transmissible gastroenteritis-infected germfree pigs. Am J Vet Res 1966;27:1695–1702.

Wagner JE, Beamer PD, Ristic M. Electron microscopy of intestinal epithelial cells of piglets infected with a transmissible gastroenteritis virus. Can J Comp Med 1973;37:177–188.

Waxler GL. Lesions of transmissible gastroenteritis in the pig as determined by scanning electron microscopy. Am J Vet Res 1972;33:1323–1328.

Woods RD, Cheville NF, Gallagher JE. Lesions in the small intestine of newborn pigs inoculated with porcine, feline, and canine coronaviruses. Am J Vet Res 1981;42:1163–1169.

PORCINE CORONAVIRAL ENCEPHALOMYELITIS

Two clinical entities in neonatal swine, both caused by coronaviruses, have been described. The first disease, manifested by encephalomyelitis, was reported by Alexander and associates (1959) in Canada. The etiologic agent was called "hemagglutinating encephalomyelitis virus." The second clinical entity, reported from England, was named after its clinical features, "vomiting and wasting disease of piglets" (Cartwright and colleagues, 1969). The causative agent of this disease proved to be a virus similar or identical to the hemagglutinating encephalomyelitis virus. Thus, it appears that similar viruses may produce different clinical pictures under differing conditions. The virus can also be recovered from clinically normal swine.

Signs Baby pigs usually manifest the first signs of the disease 4 to 7 days after birth; these signs are anorexia, lethargy, vomiting, and constipation, soon followed by signs of involvement of the central nervous system, which include hyperesthesia (squealing and paddling movements in response to a sudden noise), stilted gait, and progressive posterior paralysis. In advanced stages, the pigs lie prostrate; are dyspneic and blind; show nystagmus; and are in coma. The vomiting and wasting disease also starts within a few days after birth with vomiting and retching, inappetence, and excessive thirst (and impaired ability to drink). They fail to gain weight, become emaciated, and usually die within a week or two. A few surviving animals fail to grow normally.

Lesions The virus gains entry via the respiratory tract and spreads to the brain by way of peripheral nerves, with lesions first appearing in sensory nuclei. Nonsuppurative encephalomyelitis follows, with neuronal necrosis, glial nodules, diffuse gliosis, and perivascular aggregations of lymphocytes.

The pathogenesis of vomiting and wasting disease is less well understood, but is thought to represent both involvement of nerves and peripheral ganglia as well as the propensity of coronaviruses to infect the gastrointestinal tract.

Diagnosis Diagnosis is based presumptively on clinical signs and lesions but must be confirmed by identification of the virus. Not only must the infectious agent be distinguished from other coronaviruses but also from the Teschen disease group of enteroviruses.

References

Alexander TJL, Richards WPC, Roe CK. An encephalomyelitis of suckling pigs in Ontario. Can J Comp Med 1959;23:316–319.

Andries K, Pensaert MB. Virus isolation and immunofluorescence in different organs of pigs infected with hemagglutinating encephalomyelitis virus. Am J Vet Res 1980a;41:215–218.

Andries K, Pensaert MB. Immunofluorescence studies on the pathogenesis of hemagglutinating encephalomyelitis virus infection in pigs after oronasal inoculation. Am J Vet Res 1980b;41:1372–1378.

Appel M, Greig AS, Corner AH. Encephalomyelitis of swine caused by a hemagglutinating virus. IV. Transmission studies. Res Vet Sci 1965;6:482–489.

Cartwright SF, et al. Vomiting and wasting disease of piglets. Vet Rec 1969;84:175–176.

Cutlip RC, Mengeling WL. Lesions induced by hemagglutinating encephalomyelitis virus strain 67N in pigs. Am J Vet Res 1972;33:2003–2009.

Greig AS, et al. A hemagglutinating virus producing encephalomyelitis in baby pigs. Can J Comp Med Vet Sci 1962;26:49–56.

Greig AS. Hemagglutinating encephalomyelitis virus infection. In: Dunne HW, Lemon AD, ed. Diseases of swine. 4th ed. Chapter 17. Ames, Iowa: Iowa State Univ Press 1975;385–390.

Mengeling WL, Cutlip RC. Experimentally induced infection of newborn pigs with hemagglutinating encephalomyelitis virus strain 67N. Am J Vet Res 1972;33:953–956.

Mengeling WL, Coria MF. Buoyant density of hemagglutinating encephalomyelitis virus of swine. Comparison with avian infectious bronchitis virus. Am J Vet Res 1972;33:1359–1363.

Mengeling WL. Porcine coronaviruses: co-infection of cell cultures with transmissible gastroentritis virus and hemagglutinating encephalomyelitis virus. Am J Vet Res 1973;34:779–783.

Mitchell D. Encephalomyelitis of swine caused by a hemagglutinating virus. I. Case histories. Res Vet Sci 1963;4:506–510.

Phillips JIH, Cartwright SF, Scott AC. The size and morphology of T.G.E. and vomiting and wasting disease viruses of pigs. Vet Rec 1971;88:311–312.

Richards WPC, Savan M. Viral encephalomyelitis of pigs. A preliminary report on the transmissibility and pathology of a disease observed in Ontario. Cornell Vet 1960;50:132–155.

FELINE INFECTIOUS PERITONITIS

Feline infectious peritonitis, a disease of cats of worldwide distribution, is caused by a coronavirus. Cats of all ages are susceptible. The disease occurs with a sporadic incidence, yet serologic surveys suggest an infection rate approaching 90% in many populations. Several interpretations for this discrepancy between the incidence of infection versus clinical disease have been offered: Many infections may be subclinical; progression of disease may be facilitated by immunosuppression from concurrent infection with feline leukemia virus or feline immunodeficiency virus; positive serologic findings may represent cross-reactions with other feline coronaviruses or coronaviruses of other species (e.g., cats are susceptible to subclinical infection by transmissible gastroenteritis virus).

Signs Feline infectious peritonitis is a slowly progressive fatal disease with a course of one to several months. Signs vary with the distribution of lesions and the extent of peritoneal and/or pleural effusion. If effusion is extensive, the disease has been referred to as the effusive, or wet, form; and when effusion is not extensive, the disease is considered noneffusive, or dry. Affected cats are febrile, and there is chronic weight loss, anorexia, and depression. There may be gradual abdominal enlargement, dyspnea, vomiting, and diarrhea. In some cats, neurologic signs develop, which include ataxia, paresis, seizures, and blindness.

Lesions The abdominal cavity contains excessive fluid, often as much as 1 L (Fig. 8-77) The fluid is yellow, viscid, and transparent, though it may contain flakes of fibrin. A gray-white granular exudate is present over all serosal surfaces, and is especially thick over the liver and spleen. A similar inflammatory lesion and exudate may affect the pleural cavity and pericardium. Multiple granulomatous nodules are often present on the surface and throughout the liver, pancreas, kidney, lung, and other organs. The meninges may be opaque, and gross signs of panophthalmitis may be observable. In protracted cases, organization of fibrinous exudate can result in severe distortion of abdominal viscera. Microscopically, the peritonitis or pleuritis is a classic fibrinous inflammation, consisting of a layer of fibrin of varied thickness that contains cellular debris over a layer of neutrophils, lymphocytes, and macrophages. Fibroplasia and proliferation of capillaries may accompany the exudate in protracted cases. The inflammatory process may extend beneath the serosa into any of the affected tissues.

Throughout other organs, such as the liver, pancreas, kidney, lymph nodes, muscular layers of the gastrointestinal tract, meninges, and eye, the microscopic lesions consist of multiple foci of necrosis or granulomatous inflammation usually seen extending from and incorporating the wall of a blood vessel. The cellular infiltrate includes macrophages, lymphocytes, plasma cells, and neutrophils. The lesion appears to be a primary vasculitis, and evidence suggests that it is mediated through immune mechanisms. Circulating immune complexes have been demonstrated in affected cats, as has the presence of such complexes in renal glomeruli and the granulomatous lesions. Disseminated intravascular coagulation has also been demonstrated in affected cats, a feature seen in other viral immune complex diseases.

Diagnosis The clinical signs are usually sufficient for diagnosis of the disease in the living animal. The gross and microscopic features are not duplicated by other forms of peritonitis. Specific immunofluorescence may be demonstrated in tissues of cats infected with the virus.

FIG. 8-77 Feline infectious peritonitis. **A.** Organizing fibrinous peritonitis in a 4-year-old female cat. The exudate binds the intestines together *(1)* and covers and compresses the liver *(2)*. **B.** Chronic organizing peritonitis in a 15-year-old female cat. Cloudy fluid *(1)* distends the abdomen, the parietal peritoneum is thick and tough *(2)*, the mesentery *(3)* is short and thick, and the liver *(4)* is compressed and distorted in shape by the exudate covering capsule. **C.** Another view of the same liver with thick, tough fibrous exudate on the capsule, compressing and distorting the liver. (Courtesy of Angell Memorial Animal Hospital.)

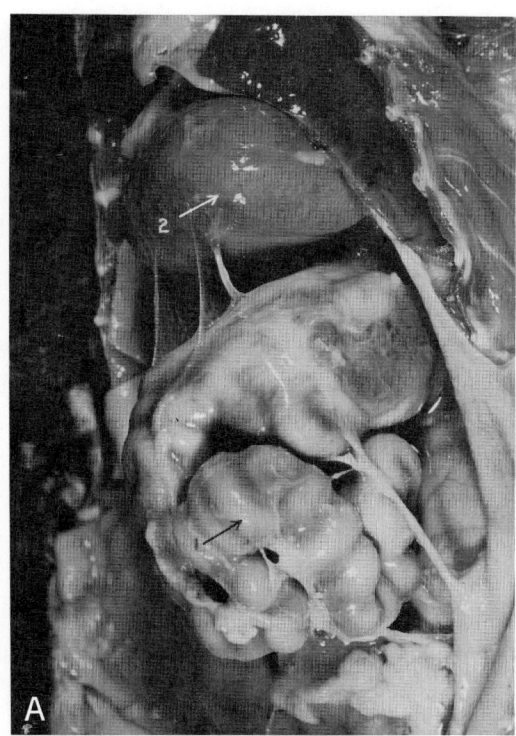

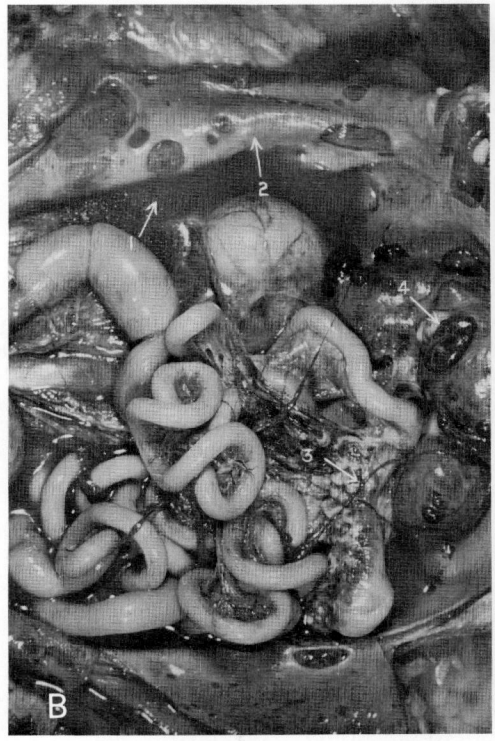

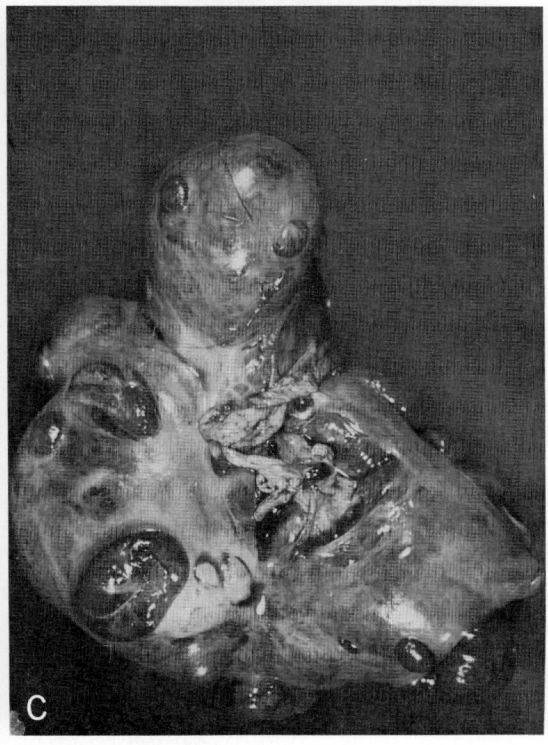

References

Doherty MJ. Ocular manifestations of feline infectious peritonitis. J Am Vet Med Assoc 1971;159:417–424.

Evermann JF, Baumgartener L, Ott RL, et al. Characterization of a feline infectious peritonitis virus isolate. Vet Pathol 1981;18:256–265.

Hardy WD Jr, Hurvitz AI. Feline infectious peritonitis: experimental studies. J Am Vet Med Assoc 1971;158:994–1002.

Hoshino Y, Scott FW. Immunofluorescent and electron microscopic studies of feline small intestinal organ cultures infected with feline infectious peritonitis virus. Am J Vet Res 1980;41:672–681.

Jacobse-Geels HEL, Daha MR, Horzinek MC. Antibody, immune complexes, and complement activity fluctuations in kittens with experimentally induced feline infectious peritonitis. Am J Vet Res 1982;43:666–670.

Krum S, Johnson K, Wilson J. Hydrocephalus associated with the noneffusive form of feline infectious peritonitis. J Am Vet Med Assoc 1975;167:746–748.

Montali RJ, Strandberg JD. Extraperitoneal lesions in feline infectious peritonitis. Vet Pathol 1972;9:109–121.

Pedersen NC, Boyle JF. Immunologic phenomena in the effusive form of feline infectious peritonitis. Am J Vet Res 1980;41:868–876.

Pedersen NC, Boyle JF, Floyd K. Infection studies in kittens, using feline infectious peritonitis virus propagated in cell culture. Am J Vet Res 1981;42:363–367.

Robison RL, Holzworth J, Gilmore CE. Naturally occurring feline infectious peritonitis: signs and clinical diagnosis. J Am Vet Med Assoc 1971;158:981–986.

Slauson DO, Finn JP. Meningoencephalitis and panophthalmitis in feline infectious peritonitis. J Am Vet Med Assoc 1972;160:729–734.

Ward JM, Gribble DH, Dungworth DL. Feline infectious peritonitis: experimental evidence for its multiphasic nature. Am J Vet Res 1974;35:1271–1275.

Watson ADJ, Huxtable CRR, Bennett AM. Feline infectious peritonitis. Aust Vet J 1974;50:393–397.

Weiss RC, Scott FW. Pathogenesis of feline infectious peritonitis: nature and development of viremia. Am J Vet Res 1981a;42:382–390.

Weiss RC, Scott FW. Pathogenesis of feline infectious peritonitis: pathologic changes and immunofluorescence. Am J Vet Res 1981b;42:2036–2048.

Wolfe LG and Griesemer RA. Feline infectious peritonitis. Pathol Vet 1966;3:255–270.

Zook BC, King NW, Robison RL, et al. Ultrastructural evidence for the viral etiology of feline infectious peritonitis. Pathol Vet 1968;5:91–95.

Sialodacryoadenitis Virus and Rat Coronavirus

Two coronaviruses can affect rats, sialodacryoadenitis virus and rat coronavirus. **Sialodacryoadenitis virus** (SDAV) causes a specific nonfatal inflammation of salivary and lacrimal glands (sialo = saliva; dacryo = lacrymal). The disease was first described by Innes and Stanton (1961) in rats housed in two different laboratories. The infection may occur as an epizootic in naive colonies, with a large number of rats developing lesions, or enzootically with only a few animals developing signs.

Signs The neck of affected rats is swollen, with the head sunk into the neck, giving the rats the short, "hunched head and neck appearance of guinea pigs." The thickening is caused by the enlarged submaxillary glands and surrounding edematous tissues. Gross edema may be seen at necropsy, involving the intermandibular space to the base of the neck. The submaxillary glands grossly appear swollen, tense, edematous, and congested.

Lesions Histopathologic changes, which may be found in the submandibular and parotid salivary glands and the exorbital and harderian lacrimal glands, consist of focal necrosis and acute inflammation affecting all parts of each gland. The lobules are separated from one another by edematous and fibrinous exudate plus infiltration by neutrophils, lymphocytes, histiocytes, and connective tissue cells. Hemorrhage is not conspicuous. Mast cells are present only in small numbers. The parenchyma of the gland is very much altered as a result of distortion and loss of acinar and ductal cells, with intense infiltration by inflammatory cells and edema. Loss of cells appears to progress by involving a few at a time with no massive necrosis. No specific cytologic features occur in the disease, distinguishing it from the greatly enlarged nuclei and inclusions that occur in cytomegalovirus infection.

In some instances, squamous metaplasia of duct epithelium occludes the lumen and results in changes in the gland caused by obstruction. Keratinization of these squamous cells is not a feature, however. The harderian gland may manifest similar lesions; the appearance of red tears on the cheek resulting from porphyrins in the lacrimal secretion may indicate involvement of this gland. Release of porphyrins is thought to contribute to persistence of lesions in the harderian gland after their resolution in the other glands.

Other lesions that have been associated with SDAV infection include keratoconjunctivitis, rhinotracheitis, interstitial pneumonia, and thymic necrosis.

Infection with **rat coronavirus** (Parker's coronavirus) is most often inapparent. In unweaned rats, the virus may cause rhinotracheitis and interstitial pneumonia.

References

Bhatt PN, Percy DH, Jonas AM. Characterization of the virus of sialodacryoadenitis of rats: a member of the coronavirus group. J Infect Dis 1972;126:123–130.

Hajjar AM, DiGiacomo RF, Carpenter JK, et al. Chronic sialodacryoadenitis virus (SDAV) infection in athymic rats. Lab Anim Sci 1991;41:22–25.

Hunt RD. Dacryoadenitis in the Sprague-Dawley rat. Am J Vet Res 1963;24:638–640.

Innes JRM, Stanton MF. Acute disease of the submaxillary and harderian glands (sialodacryoadenitis) of rats with cytomegaly and no inclusion bodies. Am J Pathol 1961;38:455–468.

Jacoby RO, Bhatt PN, Jonas AM. Pathogenesis of sialodacryoadenitis in gnotobiotic rats. Vet Pathol 1975;12:196–209.

Jacoby RO, Bhatt PN, Jonas AM. Viral diseases. In: Baker HJ, Lindsey JR, Weisbroth SH, ed. The laboratory rat. Vol I. Biology and diseases. New York: Academic Press 1979;271–306.

Jonas AM, et al. Sialodacryoadenitis in the rat. A light and electron microscopic study. Arch Pathol 1969;88:613–622.

Parker JC, Cross SS, Rowe WP. Rat coronavirus (RCV): a prevalent, naturally occurring pneumotropic virus of rats. Arch Virusforsch 1970;31:293–302.

Percy DH, Williams KL. Experimental Parker's coronavirus infection in Wistar rats. Lab Anim Sci 1990;40:603–607.

Percy DH, Wojcinski ZW, Schunk MK. Sequential changes in the Harderian and exorbital lacrimal glands in Wistar rats infected with sialodacryoadenitis virus. Vet Pathol 1989;26:238–245.

Wojcinski ZW, Percy DH. Sialodacryoadenitis virus-associated lesions in the lower respiratory tract of rats. Vet Pathol 1986;23:278–286.

CORONAVIRAL CALF DIARRHEA

Many organisms, i.e., bacteria, fungi, mycoplasma, chlamydia, or viruses, have been implicated in diseases of young calves in which the principal clinical manifestation is diarrhea. Rotaviruses are the most important cause of calf diarrhea; however, coronaviruses are also recognized as a cause of acute diarrhea in calves. Most often coronavirus diarrhea affects calves less than 3 weeks of age. The onset is acute and diarrhea lasts 4 to 5 days. Although usually less severe than rotavirus diarrhea, dehydration and electrolyte imbalance can lead to death. Coronavirus has also been associated with diarrhea (including winter dysentery) in adult cattle.

Lesions The virus has an affinity for the epithelial cells of the villi of the small intestine. Replication of the virus in these cells is accompanied by loss of epithelium and blunting and fusion of villi. In the colon, surface and crypt epithelial cells are attacked, with loss of surface cells and cystic dilation and accumulation of cellular debris in underlying crypts (Fig. 8-45C). The colonic lesions resemble those often described in **winter dysentery,** a diarrheal disease of more mature calves and adult cattle. A role for coronavirus as the cause has been proposed and evidence presented by Van Kruiningen and others (1987).

The virus can replicate in respiratory epithelium and has been recovered from calves with respiratory disease. Its significance as an important cause of respiratory disease is not clear.

Diagnosis The virus can be demonstrated by suitable immunofluorescent techniques in affected cells in the small and large intestine and in affected reactive lymph nodes of the mesentery. Virus can also be demonstrated specifically in intestinal epithelial cells shed into the intestinal lumen. Diagnosis depends on confirmed identification of the etiologic agent.

References

Langpap TJ, Bergeland ME, Reed DE. Coronaviral enteritis of young calves: virologic and pathologic findings in naturally occurring infections. Am J Vet Res 1979;40:1476–1478.

Mebus CA, Stair EL, Rhodes MB, et al. Neonatal calf diarrhea: propagation, attenuation, and characteristics of a coronavirus-like agent. Am J Vet Res 1973;34:145–150.

Mebus CA, Stair EL, Rhodes MB, et al. Pathology of neonatal calf diarrhea induced by a coronavirus-like agent. Vet Pathol 1973;10:45–64.

Mebus CA, Newman LE, Stair EL Jr. Scanning electron, light, and immunofluorescent microscopy of intestine of gnotobiotic calf infected with calf diarrheal coronavirus. Am J Vet Res 1975;36:1719–1726.

Saif LJ, Redman DR, Moorhead PD, et al. Experimentally induced coronavirus infections in calves: viral replication in the respiratory and intestinal tracts. Am J Vet Res 1986;47:1426–1432.

Saif LJ, Brock KV, Redman DR, et al. Winter dysentery in dairy herds: electron microscopic and serological evidence for an association with coronavirus infection. Vet Rec 1991;128:447–449.

Van Kruiningen HJ, Khairallah LH, Sasseville VG, et al. Calfhood coronavirus enterocolitis: a clue to the etiology of winter dysentery. Vet Pathol 1987;24:564–567.

MURINE HEPATITIS

A murine virus, originally isolated by Cheever and others (1949) in connection with disseminated encephalomyelitis and subsequently as a closely related strain from cases of hepatitis (Gledhill and others, 1951), is now recognized as the mouse hepatitis virus, a *Coronavirus.* More recently the same coronavirus has been identified as the cause of an enteritis originally described as lethal intestinal disease of infant mice (LIDIM) by Kraft in 1962. The nature of infection (e.g., hepatitis, encephalomyelitis, or enteritis) and its severity is dependent on the strain of virus as well as age and strain of mouse. The virus is highly contagious, but most often the infection is subclinical. Acute disease is often precipitated by experimental manipulation during active infection. The virus does not establish latency.

Lesions **Hepatitis** is characterized by multiple foci of hepatic necrosis and hemorrhage, which may be visible grossly. Both hepatocytes and Kupffer cells are affected. Syncytial cells may be present at the margins of the necrotic foci and on the serosal surfaces of the peritoneum and pleura.

The **encephalitic form** is principally characterized by a demyelinating encephalomyelitis, often with syncytial cells in the meninges. A unique mechanism has been proposed for the pathogenesis of demyelination. The virus has been shown to induce class I major histocompatibility antigens on oligodendrocytes and astrocytes, cells that normally do not express these antigens. Presumably this alteration allows the development of an immune-mediated demyelination. Experimentally, the virus can cause demyelinating encephalitis in rats.

The enteric form, lethal intestinal disease of infant mice (LIDIM), usually seen in mice from 16 to 20 days of age, is characterized by loss of intestinal epithelial cells, with blunting of villi and the occurrence of syncytial cells. The mortality rate is high. Few gross changes occur; the stomach is empty, the small intestine often distended with gas, and unformed feces is present in the colon.

Microscopically, multinucleated epithelial cells are present in the villi of the small intestine. These and other cells slough, leaving ulcers. The villi decrease in size and number, resembling the atrophic villi of transmissible gastroenteritis of swine. Eosinophilic cytoplasmic inclusion bodies have been reported in the epithelial giant cells, but their specificity is not established.

Diagnosis Diagnosis is confirmed by identification of the virus in the presence of compatible lesions. The enteric form must be differentiated from other viral causes of murine diarrhea, especially the rotavirus of EDIM and reovirus.

References

Barthold SW. Host age and genotypic effects on enterotropic mouse hepatitis virus infection. Lab Anim Sci 1987;37:36–40.

Biggers DC, Kraft LM, Sprinz H. Lethal intestinal virus infection of mice (LIVIM), an important new model for study of the response of the intestinal mucosa to injury. Am J Pathol 1964;45:413–422.

Cheever FS, Daniels JB, Pappenheimer AM, et al. A murine virus (JHM) causing disseminated encephalomyelitis with extensive destruction of myelin. J. Isolation and biologic properties of the virus. J Exp Med 1949;90:181–194.

Gledhill AW, Andrewes CH. A hepatitis virus of mice. Br J Exp Pathol 1951;32:559–568.

Gledhill AW, Dick GWA, Andrewes CH. Production of hepatitis in mice by the combined action of two filterable agents. Lancet 1952;2:509–511.

Hierholzer JC, Broderson JR, Murphy FA. New strain of mouse hepatitis virus as the cause of lethal enteritis in infant mice. Infect Immun 1979;24:508–522.

Kraft LM. An apparently new lethal virus disease of infant mice. Science 1962;137:182–183.

Lavi E, Fishman PS, Highkin MK, et al. Limbic encephalitis after inhalation of a murine coronavirus. Lab Invest 1988;58:31–36.

Suzumura A, Lavi E, Weiss SR, et al. Coronavirus infection induces H-2 antigen expression on oligodendrocytes and astrocytes. Science 1986;232:991–993.

Watanabe R, Wege H, ter Meulen V. Comparative analysis of coronavirus JHM-induced demyelinating encephalomyelitis in Lewis and Brown Norway rats. Lab Invest 1987;57:375–384.

CANINE CORONAVIRUS

A coronavirus, first recovered and associated with diarrhea in military dogs in 1971 (Binn and others, 1974), is now recognized as relatively widespread. The virus is related to those of transmissible gastroenteritis and feline infectious peritonitis. Infection is most severe in young dogs; signs include diarrhea, vomiting, and dehydration lasting about a week. Most animals recover. Infection also may be clinically inapparent.

The intestinal lesions resemble other enteric coronavirus infections, with marked shortening and fusion of intestinal villi.

References

Appel MJG, Cooper BJ, Greisen H, et al. Status report: canine viral enteritis. J Am Vet Med Assoc 1978;173:1516–1518.

Binn LN, Lazar EC, Keenan KP, et al. Recovery and characterization of a coronavirus from military dogs with diarrhea. Proc US Anim Health Assoc 1974(1975);78:359–366.

Carmichael LE. Infectious canine enteritis caused by a corona-like virus. Canine Pract 1978;5:25–27.

Keenan KP, Jervis HR, Marchwicki RH, et al. Intestinal infection of neonatal dogs with canine coronavirus 1–71: Studies by virologic, histologic, histochemical, and immunofluorescent techniques. Am J Vet Res 1976;37:247–256.

Woods RD, Cheville NF, Gallagher JE. Lesions in the small intestine of newborn pigs inoculated with porcine, feline, and canine coronaviruses. Am J Vet Res 1981;42:1163–1169.

BUNYAVIRIDAE

This family of viruses derives its name from Bunyamwera, a place in Uganda where the type species (Bunyamwera virus) was isolated. The family contains over 200 viruses divided into 5 genera, but only a few are important pathogens of animals. Most of the viruses are biologically arthropod borne, with mosquitoes, ticks, sandflies, or *Culicoides* species serving as vectors. Transovarial tranmission is known in some of them.

In the family *Bunyaviridae*, the virions are spherical and enveloped, 90 to 100 nm in diameter. The envelope contains at least one virus-specified glycopeptide. The internal ribonucleoprotein occurs in long strands 2.0 to 2.5 nm wide. The genome consists of a negative-sense single-stranded RNA in three pieces, with molecular weights of about 4, 2, and 0.8×10^6 daltons and a total molecular weight of 6 to 7×10^6 daltons. The virions develop in the cytoplasm of host cells and mature by budding into smooth-surfaced membranes in or adjacent to the Golgi region.

The three most important diseases of animals caused by members of the *Bunyaviridae* are **Rift Valley fever, Akabane,** and **Nairobi sheep disease,** none of which occur in the United States. **Cache Valley virus** has emerged as a cause of arthrogryposis-hydranencephaly complex in sheep.

Reference

Calisher CH. Evolutionary significance of the taxonomic data regarding bunyaviruses of the family Bunyaviridae. Intervirology 1988;29:268–276.

RIFT VALLEY FEVER

Rift Valley fever is an acute viral disease which, in nature, principally affects sheep and cattle, causing heavy mortality rates in young lambs and calves and abortion in pregnant ewes and cows. Humans may contract the infection during the course of an epizootic among domestic animals or by handling the virus in the laboratory. Sometimes human cases of an influenza type may provide the first indication of the existence of an epizootic of Rift Valley fever. Montgomery, in 1912, was the first to report the disease as an acute and highly fatal infection of lambs, and Stordy published similar observations the next year. Both reports were from Kenya, where the disease occurred on farms in the Rift Valley, a geologic depression that starts in Iran, continues through North and Central Africa, and ends in the eastern Transvaal. Like many other newly reported diseases of unknown etiology, this one was named for the location where it was first observed. Not until 1931 was it established as a distinct entity by Daubney, Hudson, and Garnham, who were the first to demonstrate that it could be transmitted to susceptible animals. Rift Valley fever has a wide distribution in Africa, but has not been recognized in domestic animals outside of that continent.

Although the virus may be transmitted to susceptible animals by inoculation of infected blood or serum (Fig. 8-78), in nature it is usually transmitted by arthropod vectors. The culicine mosquitoes, particularly *Eretmapodites chrysogastor,* have been shown experimentally to be capable of transmitting the disease. Experimental transmission of the virus to goats, mice, rats, wild rodents, and golden hamsters, as well as to its natural hosts, has been successful. The African buffalo, ferrets, and monkeys, both New and Old World, are susceptible, although some species of primates appear to have resistance. Cats merely exhibit transitory febrile symptoms, and dogs, guinea pigs, rabbits, mongooses, hedgehogs, tortoises, frogs, and birds are refractory to artificial infection. Humans are particularly susceptible and can easily become infected.

Signs After an extremely short incubation period, from 20 to 72 hours after infection, the course in young lambs is brief. They may be disinclined to move, refuse to eat, exhibit some form of abdominal pain, and shortly thereafter become recumbent and unable to rise. Death may occur within 24 hours. It is not unusual for lambs to die before symptoms are observed. In adult sheep also, the disease often is not recognized; the infected animal is found dead without having displayed any indication of illness. Vomiting may be observed as the only symptom, but pregnant ewes usually abort in the course of the illness or during convalescence. In cattle, the disease may appear as a storm of abortions; the symptoms also are often indefinite, being manifested by a brief febrile period with inappetence, profuse salivation, diarrhea, abdominal pain, roughened hair coat, and cessation of lactation. The mortality rate in cattle is not high, but erosions of the buccal mucosae, necrosis of the skin of the udder or scrotum, laminitis, and coronitis may occur.

In humans, the initial symptoms, after an incubation period of 4 to 6 days, are malaise, nausea, hyperthermia, epigastric pain, and a sensation of fullness over the region of the liver. There is usually complete anorexia, followed by rigors, violent headache, characteristic flushing of the face, injection of the conjunc-

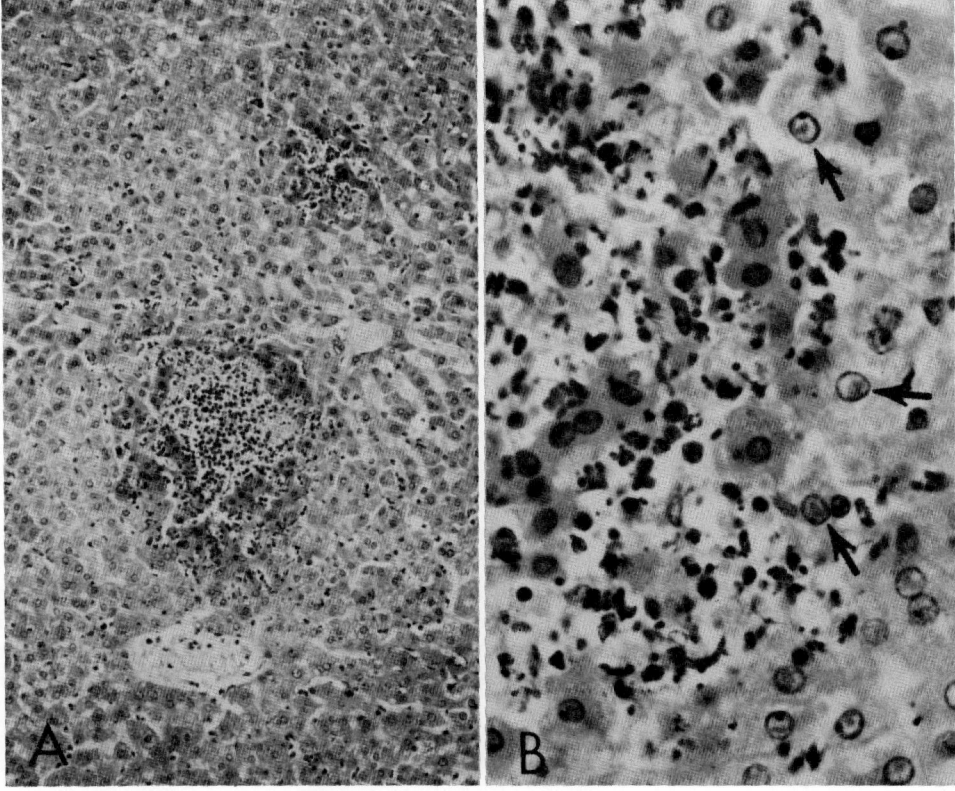

FIG. 8-78 Rift Valley fever, experimental infection in a hamster. **A.** Focal hepatic necrosis accompanied by purulent inflammation. **B.** Higher magnification, illustrating small eosinophilic intranuclear inclusion bodies *(arrows)* in hepatocytes.

tiva, photophobia, aching pains in the back and joints, vertigo, and sometimes epistaxis. The disease in humans is rarely fatal and immunity follows recovery, but serious sequelae, such as thrombophlebitis, retinopathy, and retinal detachment, have been reported.

Lesions The disagreement in the literature concerning the characteristic gross and microscopic changes in Rift Valley fever indicate the need for further study. Varying manifestations in the susceptible species also create problems. According to Schultz (1951) and others, the most constant and characteristic lesions are found in the liver. In sheep, the organ is grossly enlarged, its surface is mottled gray to grayish red or purple and bears numerous gray to white subcapsular, opaque loci. Microscopically, these foci are seen as areas of necrosis involving parenchymal cells near the central veins. The affected liver cells have swollen, eosinophilic, hyaline cytoplasm and pyknotic or fragmented nuclei; their appearance suggests the Councilman bodies of yellow fever. Findlay (1933) has described intranuclear inclusions, but their specificity is in doubt, since replication occurs in the cytoplasm of affected cells. They have also been seen in experimental animals, but inclusion bodies do not form in tissue culture. The studies of McGavran and Easterday (1963) suggest that the inclusion bodies present a degenerative change, in that they were not formed of viral particles. The common "paracentral" location of the liver lesion is suggestive of the changes associated with anoxia. In lambs, the liver usually is gray to reddish-brown, but sometimes ochre yellow, and the distribution of the

gray necrotic lesions is likely to be more diffuse than in adult sheep.

The gallbladder wall may be thickened by edema and contain subserosal hemorrhages, particularly near its attachment to the liver.

The visible mucosae are usually cyanotic and the vessels of the skin and subcutis are injected, particularly over the head and neck. The mammary gland may be grossly purple in color, but no mastitis is present. Hemorrhages may occur in the subcutis of the axillae and the medial and lower aspects of the limbs.

Hemorrhages may also be seen in the peritoneum of the gastrointestinal tract and diaphragm, as well as under the pleura, pericardium, and endocardium and in the myocardium. Similar hemorrhages may occur in the submucosa and muscularis of the gastrointestinal tract and in the pancreas, kidney, adrenal, lung, thymus, and lymph nodes (especially those of the mesentery). The lymph nodes are enlarged and appear moist and reddened, and the mesenteric and periportal nodes may contain numerous hemorrhages. Necrotic foci among lymphoid cells, with infiltration of neutrophils, vascular congestion, and edema, may be detected microscopically.

Ulceration of the intestinal mucosa may be seen in the terminal portion of the ileum, the cecum, and the initial part of the colon. Hemorrhagic lesions in some cases involve the entire gastrointestinal tract but may be caused by secondary factors.

The lungs are invariably hyperemic and edematous, often with subpleural and diffuse hemorrhages. Consolidation, particularly in the apical and cardiac lobes, may be fibrinous in character. In addition to bearing hemorrhages, the kidneys are usually slightly enlarged and show histologic evidence of nephrosis (swelling and loss of cell outline in tubular epithelium, albuminous casts in convoluted and collecting tubules, hemosiderin in tubular epithelium, congestion).

The spleen is usually enlarged and exhibits subcapsular petechiae. The malpighian bodies are indistinct because of reduction of lymphocytes. In the red pulp, hemorrhages with adjoining masses of pyknotic and fragmented nuclei may be seen, and sometimes collections of neutrophils may be seen.

Diagnosis Rift Valley fever should be suspected in outbreaks of highly fatal disease affecting both lambs and calves, especially if persons who are associated with the sick animals or who handle infective materials display mild febrile symptoms. In addition, the occurrence of abortion in adult animals and the presence of the gross and microscopic lesions, particularly those of the liver, are believed to permit a presumptive diagnosis. Neutralization of infective blood by immune serum, using mice as test animals, confirms the diagnosis. A serum neutralization test with mice may also be employed.

References

Alexander PA. Rift Valley fever in the Union. J S Afr Vet Med Assoc 1951;22:105–111.
Daubney R, Hudson JR, Garnham PC. Enzootic hepatitis or Rift Valley fever. An undescribed virus disease of sheep, cattle and man from East Africa. J Pathol Bact 1931;34:545–579.
Davies FG, Clausen B, Lund LJ. The pathogenicity of Rift Valley fever virus for the baboon. Trans R Soc Trop Med Hyg 1972;66:363–365.
Easterday BC. Rift Valley fever. Adv Vet Sci 1965;10:65–127.
Easterday BC, McGavran MH, Rooney JR, Murphy LC. The pathogenesis of Rift Valley fever in lambs. Am J Vet Res 1962;23:470–479.
Findlay GM. Rift Valley fever or enzootic hepatitis. Tr R Soc Trop Med Hyg 1932;25:229–265.
Findlay GM. Cytological changes in the liver in Rift Valley fever with special reference to the nuclear inclusions. Br J Exp Pathol 1933;14:207–219.
Hussein NA, Chizyuka RZ, Ksiazek TG, et al. Epizootic of Rift Valley fever in Zambia. Vet Rec 1987;121:111.
Ksiazek TG, et al. Rift Valley fever among domestic animals in the recent West African outbreak. Res Virol 1989;140:67–77.
McGavran MH, Easterday BC. Rift Valley fever virus hepatitis. Light and electron microscopic studies in the mouse. Am J Pathol 1963;42:587–607.
Sabin AB, Blumberg RW. Human infection with Rift Valley fever virus and immunity twelve years after single attack. Proc Soc Exp Biol Med 1947;64:385–389.
Schultz KCA. The pathology of Rift Valley fever or enzootic hepatitis in South Africa. J S Afr Vet Med Assoc 1951;22:113–120.
Schwentker FF, Rivers TM. Rift Valley fever in man. Report of a fatal laboratory infection complicated by thrombophlebitis. J Exp Med 1934;59:305–313.
Smithburn KC, Haddow AJ, Gillett JD. Rift Valley fever: isolation of the virus from wild mosquitoes. Br J Exp Pathol 1948;29:107–121.

AKABANE DISEASE (CONGENITAL ARTHROGRYPOSIS HYDRANENCEPHALY SYNDROME)

Akabane disease, caused by a bunyavirus termed Akabane virus, is an arbovirus infection of cattle, which leads to disease of the fetus without concurrent systemic lesions in the pregnant cow. No disease occurs in bulls. Natural disease also has been recently described in sheep. The virus is transmitted by mosquitoes (*Culex* and *Aedes* species) and the midge, *Culicoides brevitarsis*. The disease has occurred in Japan, Australia, Israel, and the Middle East.

In the fetus, the virus invades the brain and skeletal muscle, causing encephalomyelitis and polymyositis. Encephalitis occurs regardless of the age of the fetus when affected; however, myositis only occurs when the fetus is infected during the first half of gestation. The fetus may die and abort, be stillborn, or be born with deformities (Fig. 8-79). The nonsuppurative encephalomyelitis is characterized by extensive necrosis and endothelial proliferation, leading to formation of cysts, porencephaly, and hydranencephaly. Hydrocephalus is a common manifestation. There is loss of neurons in the ventral horn of the spinal cord. Myositis is accompanied by swelling and necrosis and fragmentation of myotubules or myofibers. At birth, muscles are smaller than normal and replaced by adipose tissue, giving rise to the designation **"runt-muscle disease"** (waishokinsho) and **"runt-muscle fiber"** (waishokinseni) (Fig. 8-80).

Arthrogryposis of any or all legs and twisting of the spinal column in various ways (e.g., scoliosis, torticollis, lordosis, kyphosis) are prominent in newborn calves (Fig. 8-79). These abnormalities are believed to be of neurogenic origin.

Fetal sheep and goats can be experimentally infected with Akabane virus as can young hamsters, mice. and guinea pigs, and certain features of the natural disease can be reproduced. Akabane disease must be differentiated from other forms of congenital arthrogryposis.

References

Haughey KG, Hartley WJ, Della-Porta AJ, et al. Akabane disease in sheep. Aust Vet J 1988;65:136–140.
Kirkland PD, Barry RD, Harper PAW, et al. The development of Akabane virus-induced congenital abnormalities in cattle. Vet Rec 1988;122:582–586.
Konno S, Nakagawa M. Akabane disease in cattle: congenital abnormalities caused by viral infection. Experimental disease. Vet Pathol 1982;19:267–279.
Konno S, Moriwaki M, Nakagawa M. Akabane disease in cattle: congenital abnormalities caused by viral infection. Spontaneous disease. Vet Pathol 1982;19:246–266.
Konno S, et al. Myopathy and encephalopathy in chick embryos experimentally infected with Akabane virus. Vet Pathol 1988;25:1–8.

OTHER *BUNYAVIRIDAE*

Of the scores of viruses in this family, only a few others are of interest here.

Nairobi sheep disease is a bunyavirus infection of sheep and goats, which occurs in Kenya. The disease is seen when animals are moved from the Nairobi area to market. The virus is transmitted by the tick *Rhipicephalus appendiculatus,* in which transovarian infection occurs. Affected sheep develop an acute hemorrhagic gastroenteritis with a high rate of mortality.

A group of related bunyaviruses referred to as the

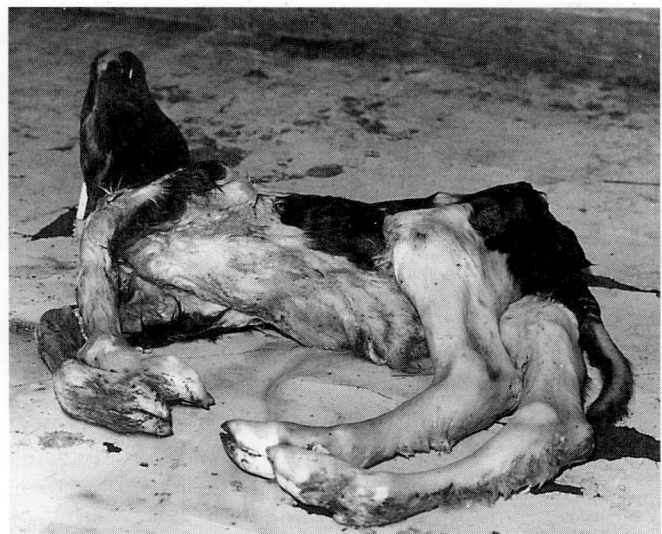

FIG. 8-79 Akabane disease in calf. Arthrogryposis in all four legs. (Courtesy of Dr. S Konno and *Veterinary Pathology* 1982; 19:246–266.)

California serogroup are important as causes of encephalitis in humans. The two best studied members are **La Crosse virus** and **snowshoe hare virus.** These agents are transmitted by mosquitoes, with *Aeda triseriatus* being the principal vector, and infect a wide variety of wild and domestic animals, resulting in viremia and viral amplification. Disease does not appear to occur in animals, but reports of encephalitis in horses exposed to these agents emphasizes diagnostic consideration of them after more traditional causes of encephalitis are ruled out.

Other bunyavirus diseases of humans, such as Cri-

mean-Congo hemorrhagic fever and rodentborne nephropathy or hemorrhagic fever (hemorrhagic fever with renal syndrome; Korean hemorrhagic fever; Hantaan virus), also infect a variety of animal species, but apparently do not cause disease.

Cache Valley virus is widespread throughout North America and capable of infecting a variety of species including domestic and wild ruminants, horses, pigs, and humans. For the most part, it appears that these infections are asymptomatic. The virus, however, has been associated with arthrogryposis, hydranencephaly, and other fetal abnormalities in sheep in Texas. Experimental *in utero* inoculation of pregnant sheep between 27 and 54 days of gestation has confirmed that Cache Valley virus infection can lead to arthrogryposis and hydranencephaly, as well as fetal mummification, reabsorption, and oligohydramnios.

References

Amundson TE, Yuill TM. Natural La Crosse virus infection in the red fox *(Vulpes fulva)*, gray fox *(Urocyon cinereoargenteus)*, raccoon *(Procyon lotor)*, and opossum *(Didelphis virginiana).* Am J Trop Med Hyg 1981;30:706–714.
Amundson TE, Yuill TM, DeFoliart GR. Experimental La Crosse virus infection of red fox *(Vulpes fulva)*, raccoon *(Procyon lotor)*, opossum *(Didelphis virginiana)*, and woodchuck *(Marmota monax).* Am J Trop Med Hyg 1985;34:586–595.
Bennett M, et al. Prevalence of antibody to hantavirus in some cat populations in Britain. Vet Rec 1990;127:548–549.
Bishop DHL, et al Bunyaviridae. Intervirology 1980;14:125–143.
Casals J, Tignor GH. The *Nairovirus* genus: serological relationships. Intervirology 1980;14:144–147.
Chung SI, Livingston CW Jr, Edwards JF, et al. Congenital malformations in sheep resulting from in utero inoculation of Cache Valley virus. Am J Vet Res 1990;51:1645–1648.
Chung SI, et al. Evidence that Cache Valley virus induces congenital malformations in sheep. Vet Microbiol 1990;21:297–307.
Dantas JR Jr, et al. Viruses of hemorrhagic fever with renal syndrome

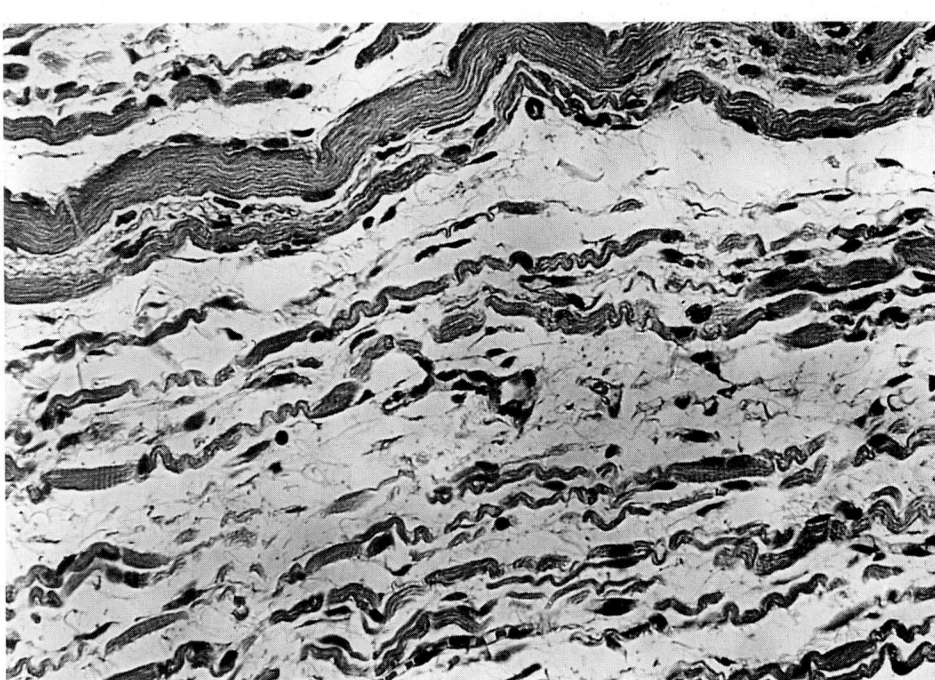

FIG. 8-80 Akabane disease. Muscular dysplasia, or "runt-muscle" disease. Note thinning and loss of myofibers; many lack transverse striations. (Courtesy of Dr. S. Konno and *Veterinary Pathology* 1982; 19: 246–266.)

(HFRS) grouped by immunoprecipitation and hemagglutination inhibition. Intervirology 1987;27:161–165.

Hantavirus disease. Lancet 1990;336:407–408.

Lynch JA, Binnington BD, Artsob H. California serogroup virus infection in a horse with encephalitis. J Am Vet Med Assoc 1985;186:389–390.

McLean RG, Calisher CH, Parham GL. Isolation of Cache Valley virus and detection of antibody for selected arboviruses in Michigan horses in 1980. Am J Vet Res 1987;48:1039–1041.

Seymour C, Amundson TE, Yuill TM, et al. Experimental infection of chipmunks and snowshoe hares with La Crosse and snowshoe hare viruses and four of their reassortants. Am J Trop Med Hyg 1983;32:1147–1153.

Tao H, Semao X, Zinyi C, et al. Morphology and morphogenesis of viruses of hemorrhagic fever with renal syndrome. II. Inclusion bodies - ultrastructural markers of hantavirus-infected cells. Intervirology 1987;27:45–52.

Terpstra C. Physical and biologic properties of Nairobi sheep disease virus. Vet Microbiol 1983;8:531–541.

PRIONS

Prions is the term applied to the agents that cause a group of diseases of humans and animals known as **spongiform encephalopathies.** These include **scrapie, bovine spongiform encephalopathy, transmissible mink encephalopathy, chronic wasting disease of mule deer and elk, spongiform encephalopathy of cats, Kuru, Creutzfeldt-Jakob disease, Gerstmann-Straussler syndrome,** and possibly other **neurologic disorders of humans** (Table 8-12). These diseases share many characteristics. The incubation period is long (months to years or decades), and the clinical course lasts for weeks to years, invariably slowly progressing to death. Thus they are "slow virus" diseases, but should not be confused with other slow viruses, such as visna. Lesions are, for the most part, restricted to the central nervous system and characteristically include neuronal degeneration with neuronal vacuolation (spongiform degeneration), reactive astrocytosis, and often "amyloid plaque" formation. Immunosuppression or immunopotentiation does not alter the incubation period, course, or duration of the disease. Immune B-cell and T-cell functions are intact.

Prions are most unconventional agents, differing in many important biologic, physical, and chemical features from viruses. Indeed, they might best be viewed as an entirely separate category. They are, however, filterable, and they do orchestrate cellular pathways for their replication. There is no evidence, however, that they contain nucleic acid, and they are not visible as recognizable virions by electron microscopy. They are resistant to most physical and chemical virucidal treatments including ultraviolet radiation, ionizing radiation, ultrasonication, proteases, nucleases, heat (to 80°C; they are incompletely inactivated at 100°C), formaldehyde, chloroform, and ether.

Prions appear to represent an abnormal isoform of a normal protein. Animals susceptible to prion disease(s) bear a gene (PrP gene), which encodes for normal protein termed the "prion protein" (PrP) or "cellular prion protein" (PrPc). This protein attaches itself to the outer leaflet of the plasma membrane lipid bilayer, but its function is not known. In the spongiform en-

---

TABLE 8-12 **Subacute spongiform encephalopathies**

Scrapie of sheep and goats
Bovine spongiform encephalopathy
Transmissible mink encephalopathy
Chronic wasting disease of captive mule deer and elk
Feline spongiform encephalopathy
Kuru of humans
Creutzfeldt-Jakob disease of humans
Gerstmann-Straussler syndrome of humans

---

cephalopathies, an abnormal isoform of PrP (usually termed "scrapie PrP" or "PrPsc", or "scrapie-associated fibril protein" [SAF]) is generated, which accumulates in and around neurons as large aggregates of polymerized macromolecular fibrils comparable to amyloid protein. These fibrils of PrPsc are resistant to proteases, whereas normal PrP is not. It is these paracrystalline arrays or fibrils of prion protein that make up the "amyloid plaques" seen in the spongiform encephalopathies.

It is not clear by what mechanism the infective prion agents alter the type of PrP transcribed. Both PrPc and PrPsc are transcribed from the same gene; therefore, the disease-linked modification of the protein is believed to be a post-transcriptional event. How the ingestion of PrPsc leads to its initiation and the development of one or the other of the spongiform encephalopathies is not understood.

Variations in such features as disease incidence, breed and species susceptibility, and incubation time have been recognized for several of the spongiform encephalopathies. These, in part, are explained by mutations and polymorphisms in the PrP gene as well as variants of or differing strains of PrPsc identified in the same host. Passage of a prion through an alternate host can also alter the prion. For example, with the passage of sheep scrapie through mink, the prion loses its pathogenicity for mice; and with passage of goat scrapie through monkeys, it loses its pathogenicity for sheep. At the same time, however, the prions of the various spongiform encephalopathies share a remarkably similar host range (Table 8-13). It may be that the various spongiform encephalopathies are each caused by a variant strain of the same agent, and it is hypothesized that they all may stem from scrapie. Bovine spongiform encephalopathy is believed to have resulted from the ingestion by cattle of meat and bone meal from scrapie-infected sheep. Transmissible mink encephalopathy is also thought to arise from feeding infected sheep parts to mink. There is no evidence that the consumption of infected animal products by humans is associated with any spongiform encephalopathy; however, it is hypothesized that the human spongiform encephalopathies arose from sheep through butchering and kitchen accidents.

In addition to being infectious diseases, certain of the spongiform encephalopathies in humans, such as Gerstmann-Straussler syndrome, can occur as familial diseases with a mendelian dominant inheritance pat-

TABLE 8-13 **Experimental transmission of the Spongiform Encephalopathies**

Disease	Partial listing of experimental animals									
	New World monkeys	Old World monkeys	Sheep	Goats	Pigs	Mink	Ferret	Mice	Hamsters	Guinea pigs
Scrapie	+		+	+		+		+	+	
TSE/mink	+	+	+	+		+	+	−	+	
BSE	+		+	+	+	+		+		
Kuru	+	+		+		+	+	+		
Creutzfeldt-Jakob	+	+	−	+				+	+	+

BSE = Bovine spongiform encephalopathy; TSE/mink = Transmissible mink encephalopathy
+, positive transmission; −, no transmission.

tern. This results from mutations within the PrP gene, different mutations giving rise to differing prion diseases.

References

Diener TO, McKinley MP, Prusiner SB. Viroids and prions. Proc Natl Acad Sci USA 1982;79:5220–5224.

Goldman W, Hunter N, Smith G, et al. PrP genotype and agent effects in scrapie: change in allelic interaction with different isolates of agent in sheep, a natural host of scrapie. J Gen Virol 1994;75(Pt 5):989–995.

Guiroy DC, Williams ES, Song KJ, et al. Fibrils in brain of Rocky Mountain elk with chronic wasting disease contain scrapie amyloid. Acta Neuropathol 1993;86:77–80.

Kitamoto T, Tateishi J. Human prion disease with variant prion protein. Philos Trans R Soc Lond (B) Biol Sci 1994;343:391–398.

Leggett MM, Dukes J, Pirie HM. A spongiform encephalopathy in a cat. Vet Rec 1990;127:586–588.

Liberski PP, Yanagihara R, Gibbs CJ Jr, et al. Tubulovesicular structures in experimental Creutzfeldt-Jakob disease and scrapie. Intervirology 1988;29:115–119.

Pearson GR, et al. Feline spongiform encephalopathy. (letter) Vet Rec 1991;128:532.

Prion disease—spongiform encephalopathies unveiled. Lancet 1990; 336:21–22.

Prusiner SB. Molecular biology and genetics of prion diseases. Philos Trans R Soc Lond (B) Biol Sci 1994;343:447–463.

Prusiner SB, DeArmond SJ. Prions causing nervous system degeneration. Lab Invest 1987;56:349–363.

Prusiner SB, DeArmond SJ. Prion diseases of the central nervous system. Monogr Pathol 1990;(32):86–122.

Prusiner SB, Torchia M, Westaway D. Molecular biology and genetics of prions — implications for sheep scrapie, "mad cows", and the BSE epidemic. Cornell Vet 1991;81:85–101.

Schrueder BE. General aspects of transmissible spongiform encephalopathies and hypotheses about the agents. Vet Q 1993;15: 164–174.

Snow AD, et al. Immunolocalization of heparin sulfate proteoglycans to the prion protein amyloid plaques of Gerstmann-Straussler syndrome, Creutzfeldt-Jakob disease and scrapie. Lab Invest 1990;63:601–611.

Stahl N, Prusiner SB. Prions and prion proteins. FASEB J 1991;5: 2799–2807.

Weissmann C: The prion's progress. Nature 1991;349:569–571.

Weissmann C, Bueler H, Fischer M, et al. Role of PrP gene in transmissible spongiform encephalopathies. Intervirology 1993;35: 164–175.

Wells GA. Pathology of nonhuman spongiform encephalopathies: variations and their implications for pathogenesis. Dev Biol Stand 1993;80:61–69.

Wells GA, McGill IS. Recently described scrapie-like encephalopathies of animals: case definitions. Res Vet Sci 1992;53:1–10.

"SCRAPIE" OF SHEEP (OVINE SPONGIFORM ENCEPHALOPATHY)

"Scrapie" is the colloquial name of a disease of sheep and goats, derived from the principal clinical manifestation, which is almost continuous scraping of the skin against any reasonably stationary object as a result of the intense pruritus the animal suffers. The disease has been known in Scotland for at least two centuries and is now recognized throughout Great Britain, Europe, and Asia. It was first recognized in the United States in 1947 and in Canada in 1938. Although scrapie has occurred in Australia, New Zealand, and South Africa, strict slaughter programs have eradicated the disease. In Iceland, scrapie is called **rida** and in France, **la tremblante.** Scrapie was the first of the prion subacute spongiform encephalopathies shown to be transmissible. The infectious agent, or prion, whose characteristics are described above, can be transmitted to mice and other species, and it has been suggested that the scrapie agent crossed species at some point (and may still be capable of doing so) to cause spongiform encephalopathies of other animals and humans. The principal means of transmission is from infected ewes to their lambs early in life. The placenta is infectious, suggesting prenatal transmission may also be important. Lateral transmission is also believed to occur between adult sheep. Owing to the resistance of prions to physical and chemical agents, environmental contamination probably persists for long periods. Sheep grazed on pastures previously occupied by infected sheep can become infected. Experimentally, scrapie can be transmitted to sheep through the oral, nasal, and parenteral routes. The prion first is identifiable in the tonsils and the pharyngeal and mesenteric lymph nodes. The incubation period is prolonged (from 1 to 5 years), restricting the clinical disease to adult sheep.

Signs The signs, which appear in adult sheep, are usually characterized at the outset by restlessness and a startled look; the eyes have a fixed and wild expression. The pupils are dilated. The sheep may hold its head down and wag it as if hunting a fly. Its movements are aimless, and stiffness of the forelegs results in a trotting gait, a characteristic that gives the disease its German name, trabberkrankheit. The animal usually grinds its teeth. Twitching, at first confined to the lips, soon involves the muscles of the shoulders and thighs as well. The voice may be altered. If startled, the animal may fall in an epileptiform seizure of brief duration. The skin irritation apparently starts in the lumbar region, then may involve the rest of the body surface. The intense pruritus causes the sheep to rub against objects continuously until the wool coat is almost completely lost. Scratching the back of an affected animal causes it to grind its teeth and show a characteristic rapid twitching of the lips. Incoordination may be followed by paralysis and inability to stand, and finally the animal dies.

Lesions No characteristic gross lesion is found in this disease; the specific tissue alterations are limited to microscopic changes in the medulla oblongata, pons, midbrain, and spinal cord. The most striking and diagnostic lesion is the presence of large vacuoles in the cytoplasm of neurons, associated with rather diffuse astrogliosis and occasional accumulation of lymphocytes in the Virchow-Robin spaces. These lesions are most numerous in nuclei of the medulla and are not found in the cerebral cortex or cerebellum. Sections taken just anterior to the calamus scriptorius are most likely to contain affected cells; therefore, these should be selected for microscopic examination aimed at establishing the diagnosis. The nuclear masses in the medulla most often involved are the reticular formation and the medial vestibular and lateral cuneate nuclei. Vacuolated neurons are found less often in the hypoglossal nuclei, the inferior olive, and the gray columns of the spinal cord. In experimentally transmitted cases, the lesions tend to be more widespread. In some cases, amyloid plaques consisting of prion protein are found in the molecular and granular layers of the cerebellum. Neutral fat can sometimes be demonstrated in the white matter, but otherwise demyelination is not obvious. The exact distribution of the tissue changes and the correlation between them and the symptoms are yet to be established. In the experimental disease in sheep, goats, and mice, in addition to the changes described, there is widespread status spongiosus. Lesions in muscles have been reported in some studies, but these changes may be the result of a concurrent disease.

Diagnosis The diagnosis is made on the basis of the clinical signs and is confirmed by histologic examination of the brain and spinal cord, with particular investigation of the medulla oblongata, pons, and midbrain. Special study should be given sections from that area of medulla immediately cranial to the calamus scriptorius.

Specific diagnosis is now feasible with antisera against purified prion protein or scrapie-associated fibril protein, either on tissue reaction or extracts of brain.

References

Adams DH, Field EJ. The infective process in scrapie. Lancet. 1968;2:714–716.

Barnett KC, Palmer AC. Retinopathy in sheep affected with natural scrapie. Res Vet Sci 1971;12:383–385.

Barry RA, McKinley MP, Bendheim PE, et al. Antibodies to the scrapie protein decorate prion rods. J Immunol 1985;135:603–613.

Bendheim PE, Barry RA, DeArmond SJ, et al. Antibodies to a scrapie prion protein. Nature 1984;310:418–421.

Bertrand I, Carré H, Lucam F. La tremblante du mouton. Rec Méd Vet 1937;113:586–603.

Bertrand I, Carré H, Lucam F. La tremblante du mouton. Rec Méd Vet 1937;113:540–561.

Bignami A, Parry HB. Electron microscopic studies of the brain of sheep with natural scrapie. I. The fine structure of neuronal vacuolation. Brain 1972;95:319–326.

Bignami A, Parry HB. Electron microscopic studies of the brain of sheep with natural scrapie. II. The small nerve processes in neuronal degeneration. Brain 1973;95:487–499.

Bolton DC, McKinley MP, Prusiner SB. Molecular characteristics of the major scrapie prion protein. Biochemistry 1984;23:5898–5906.

Brownlee A. Histopathological studies of scrapie, an obscure disease of sheep. Br Vet J 1940;96:254–259.

Bruce ME, Fraser H. Amyloid plaques in the brains of mice infected with scrapie: morphological variation and staining properties. Neuropathol Appl Neurobiol 1975;1:189–202.

Carp RI, Merz PA, Kascsak RJ, et al. Nature of the scrapie agent: current status of facts and hypotheses. J Gen Virol 1985;66:1357–1368.

Chandler RL. Encephalopathy in mice produced by inoculation with scrapie brain material. Lancet 1961;1:1378.

Cho HJ. Antibody to scrapie-associated fibril protein identifies a cellular antigen. J Gen Virol 1986;67:243–253.

Cuillé J, Chelle PL. La maladie dite tremblante du mouton est-elle inoculable? C R Acad Sci 1936;203:1552–1554.

DeArmond SJ, McKinley MP, Barry RA, et al. Identification of prion amyloid filaments in scrapie-infected brain. Cell 1985;41:221–235.

Dickinson AG. Scrapie. Nature 1974;252:179–180.

Dickinson AG, Fraser H, Outram GW. Scrapie incubation time can exceed natural lifespan. Nature 1975;256:732–733.

Gajdusek DC. Slow-virus infections of the nervous system. N Engl J Med 1967;276:392–400.

Gajdusek DC. Unconventional viruses and the origin and disappearance of kuru. Science 1977;197:943–960.

Gibbons RA, Hunter GD. Nature of the scrapie agent. Nature (Lond.) 1967;215:1041–1043.

Gibbs CJ Jr, Gajdusek DC. Transmission of scrapie to the cynomolgus monkey (Macaca fascicularis). Nature 1972;236:73–74.

Gibbs CJ Jr, Gajdusek DC. Experimental subacute spongiform virus encephalopathies in primates and other laboratory animals. Science 1973;182:67–68.

Hadlow WJ. Scrapie and kuru. Lancet 1959;2:289–290.

Hadlow WJ. The pathology of experimental scrapie in the dairy goat. Res Vet Sci 1961;2:289–314. [VB 549–562]

Hadlow WJ, Race RE. Cerebrocortical degeneration in goats inoculated with mink-passaged scrapie virus. Vet Pathol 1986;23:543–549.

Hadlow WJ, Kennedy RC, Race RE, et al. Virologic and neurohistologic findings in dairy goats affected with natural scrapie. Vet Pathol 1980;17:187–199.

Hanson RP, et al. Susceptibility of mink to sheep scrapie. Science 1971;172:859–861.

Harcourt RA, Anderson MA. Naturally-occurring scrapie in goats. Vet Rec 1974;94:504.

Holman HH, Pattison IH. Further evidence on the significance of vacuolated nerve cells in the medulla oblongata of sheep affected with scrapie. J Comp Pathol Ther 1940;1943;53:231–236.

Hunter GD. Scrapie. Prog Med Virol 1974;18:289–306.

Kimberlin RH. Scrapie agent: prions or virions? Nature 1982;297:107–108.

Kretzschmar HA, Prusiner SB, Stowring LE, et al. Scrapie prion proteins are synthesized in neurons. Am J Pathol 1986;122:1–5.

Lamar CH, Gustafson DP, Krasovich M, et al. Ultrastructural studies of spleen, brains, and brain cell cultures of mice with scrapie. Vet Pathol 1974;11:13–19.

Leader RW, Hurvitz AI. Interspecies patterns of slow virus diseases. Annu Rev Med 1972;23:191–200.

Marsh RF. Slow virus diseases of the central nervous system. Adv Vet Sci Comp Med 1974;18:155–178.

Marsh RF, Kimberlin RH. Comparison of scrapie and transmissible mink encephalopathy in hamster. II. Clinical signs, pathology and pathogenesis. J Infect Dis 1975;131:104–110.

Merz PA, Somerville RA, Wisniewski HM. Comparative ultrastructure of scrapie associated fibrils and CNS amyloid fibrils. J Neuropathol Exp Neurol 1982;41:359.

Merz PA, et al. Infection-specific particle from the unconventional slow virus diseases. Science 1984;225:437–440.

Morris JA, Gajdusek DC. Encephalopathy in mice following inoculation of scrapie sheep brain. Nature (London) 1963;197:1084–1086.

Palmer AC. Studies in scrapie. Vet Rec 1957;69:1318–1328.

Pattison IH, Jones KM. The possible nature of the transmissible agent of scrapie. Vet Rec 1967;80:2–9.

Pattison IH, Gordon WS, Millson GC. Experimental production of scrapie in goats. J Comp Pathol 1959;69:300–312.

Perry HB. Scrapie: A transmissible hereditary disease of sheep. Nature (Lond.) 1960;185:441–443.

Prusiner SB. Novel proteinaceous infectious particles cause scrapie. Science 1982;216:136–144.

Stockman S. Contribution to the study of the disease known as scrapie. J Comp Pathol Ther 1926;39:42–59.

Wiley CA, et al. Immuno-gold localization of prion filaments in scrapie-infected hamster brains. Lab Invest 1987;57:646–656.

Ward RL, Porter DD, Stevens JG. Nature of the scrapie agent: evidence against a viroid. J Virol 1974;14:1099–1103.

Wright PAL. The histopathology of the spinal cord in scrapie disease of sheep. J Comp Pathol 1960;70:70–83.

Zlotnik I. The histopathology of the brain stem of sheep affected with experimental scrapie. J Comp Pathol 1958;68:428–438.

Zlotnik I. The histopathology of the brain of goats affected with scrapie. J Comp Pathol 1961;71:440–448.

BOVINE SPONGIFORM ENCEPHALOPATHY

Bovine spongiform encephalopathy was first recognized in cattle in 1986 (Wilesmith and others, 1988) in England and rapidly emerged as an important disease of cattle in Great Britain. The data collected to date indicate that the disorder is caused by a prion similar to or identical with the cause of scrapie. It can be transmitted to mice; and fibrils comparable to scrapie-associated fibrils (SAF), which react with antisera to SAF, can be recovered from brains of affected cattle. It has been suggested that meat and bone meal from scrapie-infected sheep may have introduced the disease to cattle. Direct spread between cattle has not been documented, but the disease has been transferred to cattle by parenteral inoculation of brain homogenates from natural cases. The disease has apparently been transmitted to a pig by way of intracerebral inoculation of infective cattle brain. No natural example of spongiform encephalopathy has been described in pigs. Inoculation of calves with mink brain affected with transmissible mink encephalopathy led to spongiform encephalopathy 18

months later (Marsh and others, 1991). Strict control of food sources appears to have curtailed further spread of the disease. The occurrence of the disease in cattle has coincided with several examples of spongiform encephalopathy in exotic bovids in British zoos.

Affected animals develop slowly progressive behavioral and locomotor changes. They become excitable and exhibit apprehension and aggression when approached, handled, or disturbed. A hind-leg ataxia progresses to the point of animals stumbling or falling. These signs along with weakness and loss of good bodily condition progress over 1 to 4 months, leading to death or slaughter. The disorder has mainly been seen in dairy cows between 2 and 5 years of age.

Pathologically, lesions are confined to the nervous system and resemble the other subacute spongiform encephalopathies with vacuolation of neurons and neuropils, leading to a spongiform appearance of the gray matter (Fig. 8-81). Lesions are reportedly most pronounced in brain stem nuclei. There is mild gliosis. Amyloid plaques have not been described, but scrapie-associated fibrils have been recovered from affected brains.

Diagnosis is made by a combination of clinical and pathologic findings or, more specifically, through the use of antibodies to prion protein or scrapie-associated fibrils (Fig. 8-82).

Jeffrey and Wells (1988) have described a similar spongiform encephalopathy in a nyala *(Tragelaphus angasi)* bred and maintained in a wildlife park in England.

References

Andrews AH. Bovine spongiform encephalopathy. Vet Rec 1988;122:566–567.

Spongiform encephalopathy confirmed in a young kudu. Vet Rec 1990;127:606.

Baker HF, Ridley RM, Wells GAH. Experimental transmission of BSE and scrapie to the common marmoset. Vet Rec 1993;132:403–406.

Barlow RM, Middleton DJ. Dietary transmission of bovine spongiform encephalopathy to mice. Vet Rec 1990;126:111–112.

Bassett HF, Sheridan C. Case of BSE in the Irish Republic. Vet Rec 1989;124:151.

Cranwell MP, et al. Bovine spongiform encephalopathy. Vet Rec 1988;122:190.

Dawson M, Wells GAH, Parker BNJ. Preliminary evidence of the experimental transmissibility of bovine spongiform encephalopathy to cattle. Vet Rec 1990;126:112–113.

Encephalopathy found in pig experimental study. Vet Rec 1990;127:318.

Farquhar CF, Somerville RA, Ritchie LA. Post-mortem immunodiagnosis of scrapie and bovine spongiform encephalopathy. J Virol Methods 1989;24:215–222.

Fraser H, McConnell I, Wells GAH, et al. Transmission of bovine spongiform encephalopahy to mice. Vet Rec 1988;123:472.

Hope J, et al. Fibrils from brains of cows with new cattle disease contain scrapie-associated protein. Nature 1988;336:390–392.

Jeffrey M, Wells GAH. Spongiform encephalopathy in a nyala *(Tragelaphus angasi)*. Vet Pathol 1988;25:398–399.

Marsh RF, Bessen RA, Lehmann S, et al. Epidemiological and experimental studies on a new incident of transmissible mink encephalopathy. J Gen Virol 1991;72:589–594.

Scott PR, Aldridge BM, Holmes LA, et al. Bovine spongiform encephalopathy in an adult British Friesian cow. Vet Rec 1988;123:373–374.

Wells GAH, et al. A novel progressive spongiform encephalopathy in cattle. Vet Rec 1987;121:419–420.

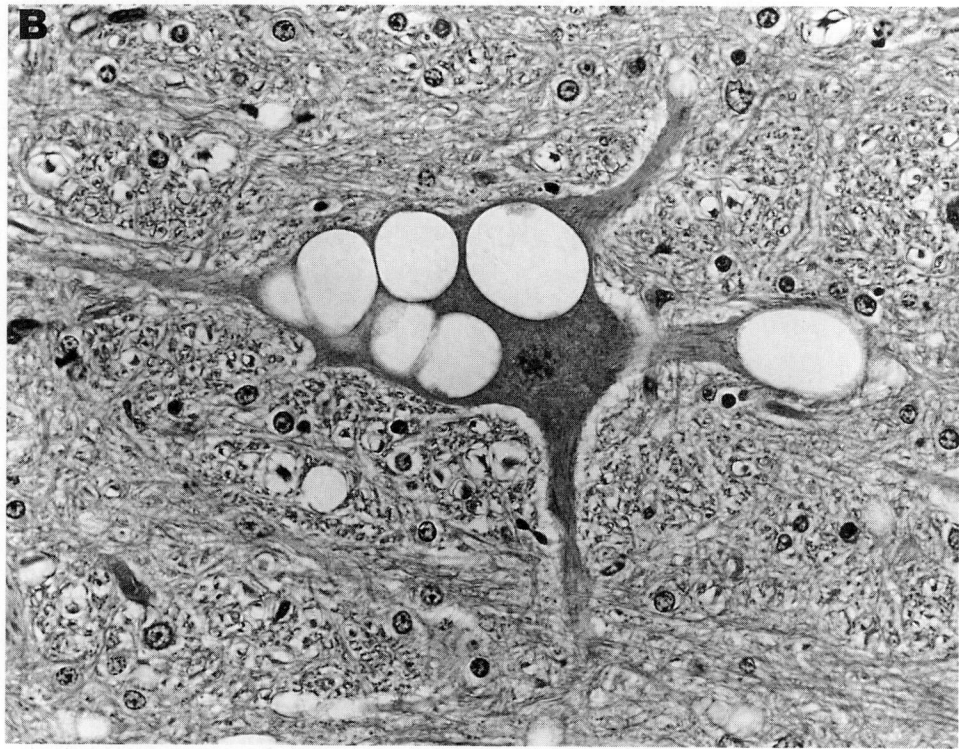

FIG. 8-81 Bovine spongiform encephalopathy. **A.** Vacuolation of gray-matter neuropil, solitary tract nucleus, medulla oblongata. **B.** Vacuoles in neuronal perikaryon and associated neurite, medulla oblongata. (Courtesy of Dr. G.A.H. Wells; Crown Copyright 1990; Ministry of Agriculture, Fisheries, and Food; Central Veterinary Laboratory.)

Wells GAH, Hancock RD, Cooley WA, et al. Bovine spongiform encephalopathy: diagnostic significance of vacuolar changes in selected nuclei of the medulla oblongata. Vet Rec 1989;125:521–524.

Wijeratne WVS, Curnow RN. A study of the inheritance of susceptibility to bovine spongiform encephalopathy. Vet Rec 1990;126:5–8.

Wilesmith JW. Bovine spongiform encephalopathy: epidemiological factors associated with the emergence of an important new animal pathogen in Great Britain. Semin Virol 1994;5:179–187.

Wilesmith JW, Wells GAH, Cranwell MP, et al. Bovine spongiform encephalopathy: epidemiological studies. Vet Rec 1988;123:638–644.

Winter MH, Aldridge BM, Scott PR, et al. Occurrence of 14 cases of

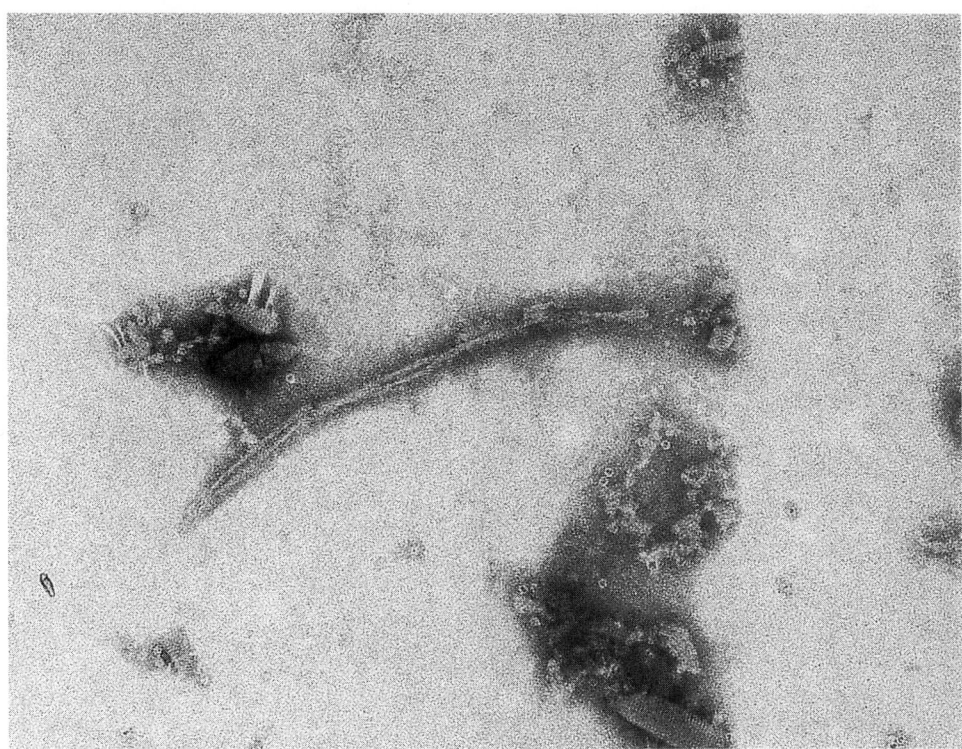

FIG. 8-82 Bovine spongiform encephalopathy, fresh brain extract. Electron micrograph of negatively stained fibril, which closely resembles scrapie fibrils. (Courtesy of Dr. G.A.H. Wells; Crown Copyright 1990; Ministry of Agriculture, Fisheries, and Food; Central Veterinary Laboratory.)

bovine spongiform encephalopathy in a closed dairy herd. Br Vet J 1989;145:191–194.

SPONGIFORM ENCEPHALOPATHY OF MULE DEER AND ELK

A disease termed wasting disease of captive mule deer *(Odocoileus hemionus)* was recognized in Colorado in 1978, and shortly thereafter a similar disorder was seen in captive elk *(Cervus elaphus nelsoni).* These are now recognized as spongiform encephalopathies that closely resemble scrapie pathologically. Amyloid plaques and scrapie-associated fibrils are present in affected brains.

References

Cunningham AA, Wells GAH, Scott AC, et al. Transmissible spongiform encephalopathy in greater kudu *(Tragelaphus strepsiceros).* Vet Rec 1993;132:68.
Guiroy DC, Williams ES, Song KJ, et al. Fibrils in brain of Rocky Mountain elk with chronic wasting disease contain scrapie amyloid. Acta Neuropathol 1993;86:77–80.
Williams ES, Young S. Chronic wasting disease of captive mule deer: a spongiform encephalopathy. J Wildl Dis 1980;16:89–98.
Williams ES, Young S. Spongiform encephalopathy of Rocky Mountain elk. J Wildl Dis 1982;18:465–471.
Williams ES, Young S. Neuropathology of chronic wasting disease of mule deer *(Odocoileus hemionus)* and elk *(Cervus elaphus nelsoni).* Vet Pathol 1993;30:36–45.

FELINE SPONGIFORM ENCEPHALOPATHY

A spongiform encephalopathy of cats was first recognized in England in 1990. The origin of the disease is not known, but it may have developed following consumption of bovine offal from cattle affected with bovine spongiform encephalopathy. The disease is seen in older cats, which present with various neurologic signs, such as behavioral changes, tremors, and ataxia. Pathologically, there is diffuse spongiform change in the grey matter characterized by vacuolation of the neuropil and within neurons. Fibrils and modified prion protein have been identified in affected brains, making the disorder comparable to other spongiform encephalopathies.

References

Leggett MM, Dukes J, Pirie HM. A spongiform encephalopathy in a cat. Vet Rec 1990;127:585–588.
Pearson GR, et al. Feline spongiform encephalopathy. Vet Rec 1991;128:532.
Pearson GR, et al. Feline spongiform encephalopathy: fibril and PrP studies. Vet Rec 1992;131:307–310.

TRANSMISSIBLE MINK ENCEPHALOPATHY

Transmissible mink encephalopathy (TME) is a spongiform encephalopathy of mink, which was first recognized in Wisconsin in 1947, and later in Idaho; Ontario, Canada; and East Germany. Brains of affected mink contain a modified prion protein, which is considered by most to be the same agent as the cause of scrapie. The disease arises from the feeding of affected sheep parts, and subsequently spreads among mink through fighting and cannibalism. Outbreaks of the disease, however, have occurred in the United States in the absence of feeding affected sheep parts. These are thought to have arisen from the feeding of cattle parts even though bovine spongiform encephalopathy has not been seen in the United States. Interestingly, the first occurrence of cattle-associated TME was recognized at about the same time that the bovine disease was first observed in England. Bovine spongiform encephalopathy has been experimentally transmitted to mink. The mink prion can infect most of the same species as the scrapie prion, except for mice.

The clinical signs are characterized by slowly progressive locomotor incoordination, excitability, late somnolence, and occasionally convulsions. Death follows a course of 3 to 8 weeks. Lesions are restricted to the central nervous system, where widespread neuronal degeneration and marked astrogliosis are found in the cerebrum, cerebellum, and brainstem. The gray matter may have a spongy appearance. Neurons, especially in the cerebellar peduncles, may contain cytoplasmic vacuoles similar to those seen in scrapie.

References

Burger D, Hartsough GR. Encephalopathy of mink. II. Experimental and natural transmission. J Infect Dis 1965;115:393–399.

Burger D, Hartsough GR. Transmissible encephalopathy of mink. Nat Inst Neurol Dis and Blindness Monograph No. 2. 1965;297–305.

Eckroade RJ, Zu Rhein GM, Marsh RF, et al. Transmissible mink encephalopathy: Experimental transmission to the squirrel monkey. Science 1970;169:1088–1090.

Eckroade RJ, ZuRhein GM, Hanson RP. Experimental transmissible mink encephalopathy: brain lesions and their sequential development in mink. In: Prusiner SB, Hadlow WJ, eds. Slow transmissible diseases of the nervous system. Vol. 1. New York: Academic Press 1979;409–449.

Grabow JD, et al. Transmissible mink encephalopathy agent in squirrel monkeys. Serial electroencephalographic, clinical and pathologic studies. Neurology (Minneap). 1973;23:820–832.

Hadlow WJ, Race RE, Kennedy RC. Experimental infection of sheep and goats with transmissible mink encephalopathy virus. Can J Vet Res 1987;51:135–144.

Hartsough GR, Burger D. Encephalopathy of mink. I. Epizoologic and clinical observations. J Infect Dis 1965;115:387–392.

Marsh RF, Bessen RA. Epidemiologic and experimental studies on transmissible mink encephalopathy. Dev Biol Stand 1993;80:111–118.

Marsh RF, Bessen RA. Physicochemical and biological characterizations of distinct strains of the transmissible mink encephalopathy agent. Philos Trans R Soc Lond (B) Biol Sci 1994;343:413–414.

Marsh RF, Miller JM, Hanson RP. Transmissible mink encephalopathy: studies on the peripheral lymphocyte. Infect Immun 1973;7:352–355.

Marsh RF, Hanson RP. On the origin of transmissible mink encephalopathy. In: Prusiner SB, Hadlow WJ, eds. Slow transmissible diseases of the nervous system. Vol. 1. New York: Academic Press 1979;451–460.

Robinson MM, et al. Experimental infection of mink with bovine spongiform encephalopathy. J Gen Virol 1994;75(Pt 9):2151–2155.

ZuRhein GM, Eckroade R, Marsh RF. Experimental transmissible mink encephalopathy (TME) in mink, monkey, and hamster. Electron microscopic studies. J Neuropathol Exp Neurol 1971;30:124.

KURU

Kuru is the name applied to a neurologic disease that afflicted certain primitive people of New Guinea. These people had a common language and observed ritualistic cannibalism of near relatives. The occurrence of kuru in families led to the assumption that the disease was hereditary. After a description of the lesions of kuru was published, Hadlow (1959) drew attention to the unique similarities of the lesions of kuru to those of scrapie, and pointed out that failures to transmit the disease to animals may have resulted from lack of anticipation of the prolonged incubation period. Hadlow's perception was correct; the first successful transmission of kuru was to a chimpanzee after an incubation period of many months (Gajdusek and Gibbs, 1971). Subsequently, the disease has been transmitted to Old and New World monkeys, mink, goats, mice, and ferrets. In humans, the disease is disappearing since the cannibalistic practice has been curtailed. The prion is not transmitted through the placenta, neonatally, or from affected adult to adult.

CREUTZFELDT-JAKOB DISEASE

This rare, presenile dementia of human patients is found worldwide and sometimes has a familial pattern, especially the variant form termed **Gerstmann-Straussler syndrome.** Using the experience gained with kuru, an infectious agent has been transmitted from human patients to chimpanzees, Old and New World monkeys, mice, hamsters, guinea pigs, and cats. This success has enlarged the possibilities of gaining a better understanding of the cause and nature of this disease and has stimulated the search for viruses in other human neuropathies such as multiple sclerosis, Alzheimer's disease, Parkinson's disease, and many others. Transmission can occur through transplantation, and the disease has developed after brain surgery and from injection of contaminated hormone preparations. The origin of most examples have not been identified; these may represent hereditary forms. Some examples of Creutzfeldt-Jakob disease in Great Britain have been associated with bovine spongiform encephalopathy.

References

Alter M, Frank Y, Doyne H, et al. Creutzfeldt-Jakob disease after eating ovine brains? N Engl J Med 1975;292:927.

Beck E, Daniel PM. Neuropathological studies in primates suffering from experimental kuru or Creutzfeldt-Jakob disease. Adv Neurol 1975;10:341–346.

Beck E, et al. Experimental kuru in the spider monkey: histopathological and ultrastructural studies of the brain during early stages of incubation. Brain 1975;98:595–620.

Bockman JM, Kingsbury DT, McKinley MP, et al. Creutzfeldt-Jakob disease prion proteins in human brains. N Engl J Med 1985;312:73–78.

Brownell B, Campbell MJ, Greenham LW. The experimental transmission of Creutzfeldt-Jakob disease. J Neuropathol Exp Neurol 1976;35:98.

Comte-Devolx J, et al. Experimental kuru in the rhesus monkey: a clinical study. J Med Primatol 1980;9:28–38.

Gajdusek DC, Gibbs CJ Jr. Transmission of two subacute spongiform encephalopathies of humans (kuru and Creutzfeldt-Jakob disease) to New World monkeys. Nature 1971;230:588–591.

Gajdusek DC, Gibbs CJ Jr. Transmission of kuru from man to rhesus monkey *(Macaca mulatta)* 8 1/2 years after inoculation. Nature 1972;240:351.

Gajdusek DC, Gibbs CJ Jr. Subacute and chronic diseases caused by atypical infections with unconventional viruses in aberrant hosts. Perspect Virol 1973;8:279–311.

Gajdusek DC, Gibbs CJ Jr, Alpers M, ed. Slow, latent, and temperate virus infections. National Institute of Neurological Diseases and Blindness Monographs, No 2. Washington, DC 1965.

Hadlow WJ. Scrapie and kuru. Lancet 1959;2:289–290.

Harrington MG, Merril CR, Asher DM, et al. Abnormal proteins in the cerebrospinal fluid of patients with Creutzfeldt-Jakob disease. N Engl J Med 1986;315:279–283.

Manuelidis EE. Transmission of Creutzfeldt-Jakob disease from man to the guinea pig. Science 1975;190:571–572.

Masters CL, et al. Experimental kuru in the gibbon and sooty mangabey and Creutzfeldt-Jakob disease in the pigtailed macaque: with a summary of the host range of the subacute spongiform virus encephalopathies. J Med Primatol 1976;5:205–209.

Peterson DA, et al. Transmission of kuru and Creutzfeldt-Jakob disease to marmoset monkeys. Intervirology 1973/1974;2:14–19.

HEPADNAVIRIDAE

Viral hepatitis is one of the most important diseases and infectious public health hazards of humans. Viral hepatitis is not a single entity, but rather can result from infection with one of several distinct viruses, some of which have only recently been identified and are yet to be precisely classified. The hepatitis viruses of humans include: **hepatitis A virus** (HAV), which is an enterovirus (family *Picornaviridae)*; **hepatitis B virus** (HBV), an hepadnavirus; **hepatitis Delta virus** (HDV), which is a defective RNA virus requiring surface antigen of hepatitis B virus; **hepatitis C virus** (HCV), a flavivirus; and **hepatitis E virus** (HEV), a probable calicivirus. The latter two viruses are the major cause of non-A, non-B hepatitis. Although various species of nonhuman primates are susceptible to experimental and natural infection, none of these agents is important as a cause of disease in domestic animals. Viruses very similar to hepatitis B virus, however, have been identified in woodchucks, ground squirrels, chimpanzees, and Peking ducks. These have been used to study the pathogenesis of the disease. The woodchuck virus has been used as a model for primary hepatocellular carcinoma, which is associated with the natural and experimental disease in woodchucks and is an important form of chronic HBV infection in humans.

References

Bradley DW. Hepatitis non-A, non-B viruses become identified as hepatitis C and E viruses. Prog Med Virol 1990;37:101–135.

Gust ID, et al. Taxonomic classification of hepatitis A virus. Intervirology 1983;20:1–7.

Gust ID, Burrell CJ, Coulepis AG, et al. Taxonomic classification of human hepatitis B virus. Intervirology 1986;25:14–29.

Montali RJ, Ramsay EC, Stephensen CB, et al. A new transmissible viral hepatitis of marmosets and tamarins. J Infect Dis 1989;160:759–765.

Popper H, et al. Woodchuck hepatitis and hepatocellular carcinoma: correlation of histologic with virologic observations. Hepatology 1981;1:91–98.

Roth L, King JM, Hornbuckle WE, et al. Chronic hepatitis and hepatocellular carcinoma associated with persistent woodchuck hepatitis virus infection. Vet Pathol 1985;22:338–343.

Shevtsova ZV, et al. Spontaneous and experimental hepatitis A in Old World monkeys. J Med Primatol 1988;17:177–194.

The A to F of viral hepatitis. Lancet 1990;336:1158–1160, 1990.

Tiollais P, Buendiam M-A. Hepatitis B virus. Sci Am 1991;264:116–123.

Zuckerman AJ. Woodchuck, squirrel and duck hepatitis viruses. Nature 1981;289:748–749.

TOROVIRIDAE

In 1972, a new virus was isolated in Berne, Switzerland, from a horse that died of enteritis and granulomatous and necrotizing hepatitis. Detailed descriptions of the agent, known as the **Berne virus,** were not published until 1983 (Weiss and others), at which time it was proposed that it did not belong to any existing family. In 1982, a related virus, termed **Breda virus** after the township of Breda, Iowa, was associated with neonatal calf diarrhea, and a similar agent was identified in cattle in France and named **Lyon 4 virus.** Since then, similar viruses have also been associated with diarrhea in cats, pigs, and humans. Serologic studies indicate that infection is widespread and common in horses and cattle. The Berne, Breda, Lyon-4, and other viruses are antigenically related. They may represent a distinct family *(Toroviridae)* or belong to a genus within *Coronaviridae.*

Morphologically, the virions are enveloped with a nucleocapsid of about 35 by 170 nm of variable shape. The nucleocapsid may appear as a rod or curved to the point of being kidney-shaped or as a disk. The genome is positive-sense, single-stranded RNA. Virions bud internally into the Golgi or through the rough endoplasmic reticulum.

The pathogenicity of these agents is still under study. Experimentally, infection of horses with Berne virus has not led to clinical disease, so despite its widespread occurrence, it would not appear to be a dangerous pathogen. Breda and related viruses, however, have been associated with natural epizootics of calf diarrhea and have been shown to cause diarrhea on experimental inoculation. Thus, it would appear that these agents are important to the pathogenesis of neonatal calf diarrhea along with coronaviruses, rotaviruses, and astroviruses.

Pathologically, Breda virus causes necrosis of intestinal epithelial cells from the mid-jejunum through and including the cecum and colon. In the small intestine, enterocytes of the villi and crypts are affected, and in the large intestine, crypt and dome villi (including both absorptive cells and M cells) are affected (Fig. 8-45F). Cell destruction leads to blunting and fusion of villi and accumulations of debris in dilated crypts. Neutrophils and mononuclear cells infiltrate an edematous lamina propria.

References

Beards GM, Green J, Hall C, et al. An enveloped virus in stools of children and adults with gastroenteritis that resembles the Breda virus of calves. Lancet 1984;1:1050–1052.

Fagerland JA, Pohlenz JFL, Woode GN. A morphological study of the replication of Breda virus (proposed family Toroviridae) in bovine intestinal cells. J Gen Virol 1986;67:1293–1304.

Horzinek MC, Flewett TH, Saif LJ, et al. A new family of vertebrate viruses: *Toroviridae.* Intervirology 1987;27:17–24.

Moussa A, Dannacher G, Fedida M. Nouveaux virus intervenant dans l'étiologie des entérites néonatales des bovins. Rec Méd Vét 1983;159:185–190.

Muir P, et al. A clinical and microbiological study of cats with protruding nictating membranes and diarrhoea: isolation of a novel virus. Vet Rec 1990;127:324–330.

Pohlenz JFL, Cheville NF, Woode GN, et al. Cellular lesions in intestinal mucosa of gnotobiotic calves experimentally infected with a new unclassified bovine virus (Breda virus). Vet Pathol 1984;21:407–417.

Weiss M, Horzinek MC. The proposed family Toroviridae: agents of enteric infections. Arch Virol 1987;92:1–15.

Weiss M, Horzinek MC. Morphogenesis of Berne virus (proposed family Toroviridae). J Gen Virol 1986;67:1305–1314.

Weiss M, Steck F, Horzinek MC. Purification and partial characterization of a new enveloped RNA virus (Berne virus). J Gen Virol 1983;64:1849–1858.

Woode GN. Breda and Breda-like viruses: diagnosis, pathology and epidemiology. Ciba Found Symp 1987;128:175–191.

Woode GN, Reed DE, Runnels PL, et al. Studies with an unclassified virus isolated from diarrhoeic calves. Vet Microbiol 1982;7:221–240.

Woode GN, Saif LJ, Quesada M, et al. Comparative studies on three isolates of Breda virus of calves. Am J Vet Res 1985;46:1003–1010.

ASTROVIRUS

The astroviruses are small nonenveloped viruses, whose shape is smooth or slightly concentrated with a solid star-shaped center, in contrast to caliciviruses, which have a hollow center. Astroviruses were first detected in association with diarrhea in human infants in 1975 and have since been identified in calves, lambs, puppies, kittens, piglets, and other species, both with and without diarrhea. Each appears to be antigenically distinct.

The pathogenic potential of astroviruses is not yet fully known; in most studies, although infection is established, clinical disease has not developed. Their pathogenicity is clearly enhanced in the presence of other viruses, such as rotavirus or Breda virus.

In calves, the virus invades epithelial cells of projecting villi, as well as those of dome villi, with a reduction of underlying lymphoid cells. There is blunting and fusion of villi and an infiltration of neutrophils and mononuclear cells in the lamina propria. In lambs, the distribution of infected cells is reportedly more analogous to rotavirus infection and is limited to enterocytes of villi (Fig. 8-45G).

An astrovirus is responsible for a severe hepatitis in ducks.

References

Appleton H, Higgins PG. Viruses and gastroenteritis in infants. Lancet 1975;1:1297.

Bridger JC. Detection by electron microscopy of caliciviruses, astroviruses and rotavirus-like particles in the faeces of piglets with diarrhoea. Vet Rec 1980;107:532–533.

Bridger JC, Hall GA, Brown JF. Characterization of a calici-like virus (Newbury agent) found in association with astrovirus in bovine diarrhea. Infect Immun 1984;43:133–138.

Gough RE, Collins MS, Borland E, et al. Astrovirus-like particles associated with hepatitis in ducklings. Vet Rec 1984;114:279.

Gough RE, Borland ED, Keymer LF, et al. An outbreak of duck hepatitis type II in commercial ducks. Avian Pathol 1985;14:227–236.

Gray EW, Angus KW, Snodgrass DR. Ultrastructure of the small intestine in astrovirus-infected lambs. J Gen Virol 1980;49:71–82.

Harbour DA, Ashley CR, Williams PD, et al. Natural and experimental astrovirus infection of cats. Vet Rec 1987;120:555–557.

Kurtz JB, Lee TW. Astroviruses: human and animal. Ciba Found Symp 1987;128:92–107.

Madeley CR, Cosgrove BP. Viruses in infantile gastroenteritis. Lancet 1975;2:124.

Snodgrass DR, Angus KW, Gray EW, et al. Pathogenesis of diarrhoea caused by astrovirus infections in lambs. Arch Virol 1979;60:217–226.

Woode GN, Pohlenz JF, Gourley NEK, et al. Astrovirus and Breda virus infections of dome cell epithelium of bovine ileum. J Clin Microbiol 1984;19:623–630.

FILOVIRIDAE

This newly proposed family contains two viruses, **Marburg virus,** first recognized in 1967, and **Ebola virus,** recognized in 1976. Neither agent nor any similar agent had been seen previously. The two are antigenically distinct, but morphologically identical, appearing as filaments or rods 80 nm wide and of variable length, usually around 800 nm, but up to 14,000 nm long. Virions develop in the cytoplasm of infected cells, where they accumulate and are visible by light microscopy as inclusion bodies. They acquire an envelope by budding. The genome is a negative-sense, single-stranded RNA. What are probably new members of the filovirus family have recently been found in cynomolgus monkeys imported from the Philippines.

Marburg virus disease

First described in 1967 in Marburg and Frankfurt, Germany, and Belgrade, Yugoslavia, Marburg virus disease is principally of importance as an infection of humans. The original episode occurred in laboratory workers in contact with tissues from African green monkeys (*Cercopithecus aethiops*) and in hospital workers caring for the patients. Of 31 cases reported in 1967, seven were fatal. Monkeys in the same shipment died of a disease similar to that seen in human patients. Since 1967, Marburg virus disease has been recognized in South Africa (1975), Kenya (1980), and Zimbabwe (1982). The infection is believed to be a zoonosis, but the reservoir host has not been identified. African green monkeys are not the reservoir, but are highly susceptible to the virus. The virus is also pathogenic for rhesus monkeys (*Macaca mulatta*), squirrel monkeys (*Saimiri sciureus*), guinea pigs, and hamsters.

Clinically, in humans and animals following an incubation period of 5 to 10 days, the disease is a severe hemorrhagic fever characterized by fever, prostration, vomiting, hematemesis, hemorrhagic diarrhea, and exanthematous rash. Pathologic findings are dominated by widespread focal necrosis, especially of the liver, lymphatic tissues, kidney, pancreas, adrenal glands, and skin. Nonsuppurative encephalitis with glial nodules and hemorrhage may also be present. Intracytoplasmic inclusion bodies composed of massed virions may be present, particularly in hepatocytes.

Ebola Virus Disease

This disease is caused by a virus antigenically distinct from Marburg virus, but the clinical and pathologic features are essentially identical. Episodes of Ebola disease were seen in Zaire and the Sudan in the 1970s. It is also thought to be a zoonosis with an unidentified reservoir. Closely related viruses have been recovered from cynomolgus monkeys (*Macaca fascicularis*) imported to the United States from the Philippines.

References

Baskerville A, Bowen ETW, Platt GS, et al. The pathology of experimental Ebola virus infection in monkeys. J Pathol 1978;125: 131–138.

Baskerville A, Fisher-Hoch SP, Neild GH, et al. Ultrastructural pathology of experimental Ebola haemorrhagic fever virus infection. J Pathol 1985;147:199–209.

Bechtelsheimer H, Jacob H, Solcher H. Zur Neuropathologie der Dursch Grune Meerkatzen (Cercopithecus aethiops) Ubertragenen Infektionskrankheiten in Marburg. Dtsche Med Wochenschr 1968;93:602–604.

Bechtelsheimer H, Jacob H, Solcher H. The neuropathology of an infectious disease transmitted by African green monkeys (Cercopithecus aethiops). Germ Med Mth 1969;14:10–12.

Bowen ETW, Platt GS, Lloyd G, et al. Viral haemorrhagic fever in Southern Sudan and Northern Zaire. Lancet 1977;i:571–573.

Centers for Disease Control. Ebola virus infection in imported primates - Virginia, 1989. MMWR 1989;38(48):831–2, 837–838.

Centers for Disease Control. [Updates on Filovirus infections among nonhuman primates.] MMWR 1990;39:22–24, 29–30, 221, 266–267, 273, 404–405.

Fisher-Hoch SP, Platt GS, Lloyd G, et al. Haematological and biochemical monitoring of Ebola infection in rhesus monkeys: implications for patient management. Lancet 1983;ii:1055–1058.

Fisher-Hoch SP, et al. Pathophysiology of shock and hemorrhage in a fulminating viral infection (Ebola). J Infect Dis 1985;152: 887–894.

Gear JSS, et al. Outbreak of Marburg virus disease in Johannesburg. Br Med J 1975;4:489–493.

Gedigk P, Bechtelsheimer H, Korb G. Die pathologische Anatomie der "Marburg-Virus"—Krankheit (sog. "Marburger Affenkrankheit"). Dtsch Med Wochenschr 1968;93:590–601.

Heymann DL, Weisfeld JS, Webb PA, et al. Ebola hemorrhagic fever: Tandala, Zaire, 1977–1978. J Infect Dis 1980;142:372–376.

Hofmann H, Kunz C. Ein mauspathogener Stature des "Marburg-Virus" (Rhabdovirus simiae). Arch Ges Virusforsch 1970;32: 244–248.

Jahrling PB, Geisbert TW, Dalgard DW, et al. Preliminary report: isolation of Ebola virus from monkeys imported to USA. Lancet 1990;335:502–505.

Johnson KM. Ebola virus and hemorrhagic fever: Andromeda strain or localized pathogen? Ann Intern Med 1979;91:117–119.

Johnson KM, Webb PA, Lange JV, et al. Isolation and partial characterization of a new virus causing acute haemorrhagic fever in Zaire. Lancet 1977;i:569–571.

Kiley MP, et al. Filoviridae: a taxonomic home for Marburg and Ebola viruses? Intervirology 1982;18:24–32.

Kiley MP, et al. Physicochemical properties of Marburg virus: evidence for three distinct virus strains and their relationship to Ebola virus. J Gen Virol 1988;69:1957–1967.

Kissling RE, Robinson RQ, Murphy FA, et al. Agent of disease contracted from green monkeys. Science 1968;160:888–890.

Korb G, Bechtelsheimer H, Gedigk P. Die Wichtigsten Histologischen Befunde Bei der Marburg Virus Krankheit. Jahrgang 1968;19: 1089–1096.

Maass G, Haas R, Oehlert W. Experimental infections of monkeys with the causative agent of the Frankfurt-Marburg syndrome (FMS). Lab Anim Handb 1969;4:155–165.

Pattyn S, Jacob W, van der Groen G, et al. Isolation of Marburg-like virus from a case of haemorrhagic fever in Zaire. Lancet 1977;i:573–574.

Siegert R, Shu HL, Slenczka W. Isolierung und Identifizierung des "Marburg-virus." Dtsch Med Wochenschr 1968;93:604–612.

Simpson DIH, Zlotnik I, Rutter DA. Vervet monkey disease. Experimental infection of guinea pigs and monkeys with the causative agent. Br J Exp Pathol 1968;49:458–464.

Simpson DIH. Marburg virus disease: experimental infection of monkeys. Lab Anim Handb 1969;4:149–154.

Smith DH, et al. Marburg-virus disease in Kenya. Lancet 1982;i: 816–820.

Zlotnik I, Simpson DIH, Howard DMR. Structure of the vervet-monkey disease agent. Lancet 1968;2:26–28.

Zlotnik I. Marburg agent disease: pathology. Trans R Soc Trop Med Hyg 1969;63:310–327.

Zlotnik I, Simpson DIH. The pathology of experimental vervet monkey disease in hamsters. Br J Exp Pathol 1969;50:393–399.

Borna disease

Borna disease is a progressive immune-mediated polio-encephalomyelitis of horses and sheep in Europe. It is caused by a single-stranded, negative-sense RNA virus, which has not yet been visualized and, therefore, remains unclassified. Recognized decades earlier, the disease derives its name from Borna in Saxony (Germany) where a severe outbreak was described in 1885. In Bavaria, the disease is known as **Kopfkrankheit.** Borna disease has also occurred in Romania, Libya, and Switzerland. It is not believed to occur in the Western Hemisphere, although antibodies against the virus have been detected in horses in the United States. Many species are experimentally susceptible to Borna disease virus, including chickens, rabbits, rats, guinea pigs, and monkeys. Borna disease virus-specific antibodies also have been identified in monkeys, humans, and birds. An encephalomyelitis leading to paralysis, which is caused by Borna disease virus or a closely related agent, has also been observed in ostriches in Israel. The virus has been suggested as a cause of encephalitis in cats ("staggering disease") and neuropsychiatric disorders in humans. This virus is also suspected to cause disease in cattle, goats, and other ruminants. An insect vector is not needed for transmission. The disease tends to predominate in spring and early summer. Transmission is via saliva and nasal secretions; possibly via colostrum and milk from infected horses with overt disease; or via individuals with a persistent infection, who serve as carriers of the virus. Rodents have been suspected as a potential source of infection.

The disease has been known to be infectious for decades and the agent can be grown in tissue culture, but specific infectious particles have not been identified. Particles of 100 nm in diameter surrounded by 20 nm granular zones have been described in the nucleus of infected cells, as have crystalline arrays and filaments, which are in the the cytoplasm as well, but their exact relationship to the virus has not been established. In tissue culture, the virus grows slowly as a persistent noncytopathic infection.

In contrast to other viral encephalitides, the incubation period is from 3 to 6 weeks and may extend for months or possibly years. Clinically, affected horses develop a slight fever followed by a course of 3 to 4 weeks of lethargy or restlessness, resulting in lethargy, ataxia, circling, paralysis, and death in most animals. Infection can occur without leading to clinical manifestations, but it does result in a carrier state. The virus replicates in neurons, astrocytes, and oligodendrocytes and has a predilection for grey matter of the cerebral hemispheres and brain stem. The most severe lesions are encountered in the olfactory bulbs, caudate nucleus, and hippocampus. The cerebellum is spared. The virus spreads via intra-axonal transport and may also spread centrifugally to peripheral nerves. Microscopically, the encephalitis is characterized by marked cuffing with lymphocytes, along with some macrophages and plasma cells, and gliosis. Neuronophagic nodules may be encountered, but neuronal necrosis is not a prominent feature. Acidophilic intranuclear inclusion bodies are present within neurons, particularly of the hippocampus. These were first described by Joest-Degen and termed **Joest bodies** or **Joest-Degen bodies.** They are considered specific for Borna disease.

The pathogenesis of the encephalitis is believed to be predominantly immune-mediated. The virus does not have direct cytopathic effects. Virally infected cells initiate a T-cell immune response, which leads to tissue destruction. Experimentally, the encephalitis can be modified by antibodies against CD8$^+$ cells and other immunosuppressive techniques.

DIAGNOSIS

Diagnosis is made histopathologically by the demonstration of Joest bodies. Specific diagnosis can be made with such techniques as *in situ* hybridization and polymerase chain reaction (PCR) viral amplification. Using these techniques, viral RNA has been demonstrated in neurons, astrocytes, Schwann cells, and ependymal cells.

References

Bilzer T, Stitz L. Immune-mediated brain atrophy. CD8$^+$ T cells contribute to tissue destruction during Borna disease. J Immunol 1994;153:818–823.

Blinzinger K, Anzil AP. Large granular nuclear bodies (karyosphaeridia) in experimental Borna virus infection. J Comp Pathol 1973;83:589–596.

Carbone KM, Duchala CS, Griffin JW, et al. Pathogenesis of Borna disease in rats: evidence that intra-axonal spread is the major route for virus dissemination and the determinant for disease incubation. J Virol 1987;61:3431–3440.

Carbone KM, Moench TR, Lipkin WI. Borna disease virus replicates in astrocytes, Schwann cells and ependymal cells in persistently infected rats: location of viral genomic and messenger RNAs by in situ hybridization. J Neuropathol Exp Neurol 1991;50:205–214.

Duchala CS, Carbone KM, Narayan O. Preliminary studies on the biology of Borna disease virus. J Gen Virol 1989;70:3507–3511.

Joest E, Degen K. Über eigentümliche kerneinschlüsse der ganglienzellen bei der enzootischen gehirn-rückenmarksentzundung der pferde. Z Infectionskr 1909;6:348–356.

Kao M, et al. Detection of antibodies against Borna disease virus in sera and cerebrospinal fluid of horses in the USA. Vet Rec 1993;132:241–244.

Koprowski H, Lipkin WI, ed. Borna disease. Curr Top Microbiol Immunol 1995;190:1–134.

Ludwig H, Bode L, Gosztonyi G. Borna disease: a persistent virus infection of the central nervous system. Prog Med Virol 1988;35:107–151.

Lundgren AL, Czech G, Bode L. Natural Borna disease in domestic animals other than horses and sheep. Zentralbl Veterinarmed [B] 1993;40:298–303.

Narayan O, Herzog S, Frese K, et al. Pathogenesis of Borna disease in rats: immune-mediated viral ophthalmoencephalopathy causing blindness and behavioral abnormalities. J Infect Dis 1983;148:305–315.

Nicolau S, Galloway IA. L-Encephalomyélite enzootique expérimentale (maladie de Borna). Ann Inst Pasteur 1930;44:457–523, 673–696.

Richt JA, et al. Borna disease virus: nature of the etiologic agent and significance of infection in humans. Arch Virol Suppl 1993;7:101–109.

Sasaki S, Ludwig H. In Borna disease virus infected rabbit neurons 100 nm particle structures accumulate at areas of Joest-Degen inclusion bodies. Zentralbl Veterinarmed [B] 1993;40:291–297.

Seifried O, Spatz H. Die ausbreitung der encephalitischen reaktion bei der Bornaschen krankheit der pferde und deren beziehungen zu die encephalitis epidemica, der Heine-medinschen krankheit und der Lyssa des menschen. Z Neurol Psychiat 1930;124:317–382.

Stitz L, Bilzer T, Richt JA, et al. Pathogenesis of Borna disease. Arch Virol Suppl 1993;7:135–151.

Waelchli RO, Ehrensperger F, Metzler A, et al. Borna disease in sheep. Vet Rec 1985;117:499–500.

Zimmerman W, Durrwald R, Ludwig H. Detection of Borna disease virus in naturally infected animals by a nested polymerase chain reaction. J Virol Methods 1994;46:133–143.

9

Diseases caused by mycoplasmatales, rickettsiales, and chlamydiales

The pathologist's approach to diagnosis of bacterial diseases is, in many ways, comparable to the approach used for diagnosis of viral diseases; both use tissue tropism and characteristics of the host reaction to narrow the possibilities. In addition, however, it is possible in many bacterial diseases to visualize the causative organism with light microscopy and determine certain attributes of the pathogen with special staining techniques.

Definitive identification and classification of bacteria requires an array of morphologic, physiologic, biochemical, and genetic measurements beyond the scope of this book. In general, we follow the classification and nomenclature of *Bergey's Manual of Systematic Bacteriology* (1984).

In this chapter, consideration is given to diseases caused by organisms that are distinct from viruses, yet have characteristics that set them apart from other bacteria. The mycoplasmas, in contrast to other bacteria, lack cell walls and are the smallest of bacteria. The rickettsias and chlamydias, in contrast to other bacteria, only multiply within cells. The classification of these organisms is depicted in Table 9-1.

DISEASES CAUSED BY MYCOPLASMATALES

Mycoplasmosis

The infectious agent involved in contagious bovine pleuropneumonia was first recognized by Nocard and Roux (1898), who were able to demonstrate the tiny organisms from infected bovine lungs by culturing them in celloidin bags implanted in the peritoneal cavity of rabbits. The organisms were seen undergoing brownian motion under the light microscope and were later proved to cause the disease in susceptible cattle. This organism is now called *Mycoplasma mycoides* (or *M.*

mycoides subsp *mycoides*), and it is the type species of the genus *Mycoplasma*.

Organisms of this genus are now considered to be the smallest free-living microbes that can be passed through bacteria-retaining filters. They grow on agar media without living cells, forming small, microscopically visible, disc-shaped colonies with a dark, thick center and lighter periphery. The electron microscope reveals the organisms to be pleomorphic, with no definite cell wall. This feature has caused the order Mycoplasmatales to be placed in a special category, i.e., class IV Mollicutes (meaning soft skin). Three genera in the order **Mycoplasmatales** are of medical interest: *Mycoplasma* and *Ureaplasma* (family **Mycoplasmataceae**) and *Acholeplasma* (family **Acholeplasmataceae**).

For many years the awkward name "pleuropneumonia-like organism," or "PPLO," was applied to all *Mycoplasma* organisms other than the causative agent of bovine pleuropneumonia. Fortunately, specific names are now available for most identifiable organisms in this genus. PPLO still remains in the older literature and may confound the newcomer.

A large number of distinct **Mycoplasma** species have been isolated from animals. Many of these are nonpathogenic commensals living on mucosal surfaces, especially of the respiratory and genital tracts. Some are of relatively low pathogenicity, producing only mild disease or becoming pathogenic only in conjunction with another insult, particularly viral and bacterial infections. There is no simple distinguishing feature differentiating pathogenic and nonpathogenic mycoplasmas. Certain respiratory pathogens (*M. mycoides* subsp *capri, Mycoplasma hyorhinis, Mycoplasma dispar*) have been shown to inhibit the activity of epithelial cilia, which is thought to aid in induction of disease. There are, however, mycoplasmas that are true pathogens, capable of

371

TABLE 9-1 **Classification of organisms**

Order:	Mycoplasmatales
Family:	Mycoplasmataceae
Genus:	*Mycoplasma*
	Ureaplasma
Family:	Acholeplasmataceae
Genus:	*Acholeplasma*
Order:	Rickettsiales
Family:	Rickettsiaceae
Tribe:	Ricketsieae
Genus:	*Rickettsia*
	Rrochalimaea
	Coxiella
Tribe:	Ehrlichieae
Genus:	*Ehrlichia*
	Cowdria
	Neorickettsia
Tribe:	Wolbachieae
Genus:	*Wolbachia*
	Rickettsiella
Family:	Bartonellaceae
Genus:	*Bartonella*
	Grahamella
Family:	Anaplasmataceae
Genus:	*Anaplasma*
	Aegyptianella
	Haemobartonella
	Eperythrozoon
Order:	Chlamydiales
Family:	Chlamydiaceae
Genus:	*Chlamydia*

producing both acute and chronic disease. Transmission may be aerosol, venereal, or *in utero*. Organisms may remain and be shed from animals after clinical signs have abated, providing a reservoir for spread of infection. Many mycoplasmas may remain viable in the environment for several days. In general, mycoplasmas are species-specific, although a few have been recovered from related species. Interestingly, most pathogenic mycoplasmas are associated with farm animals, particularly cattle, sheep, goats, swine, and poultry. To date, they are of lesser significance as causes of disease in horses, dogs, and cats.

Table 9-2 lists the important mycoplasmas of animals as well as many commensals of uncertain pathogenicity.

Ureaplasma species are differentiated from *Mycoplasma* species in that they hydrolyze urea with the production of ammonia. Two species, *Ureaplasma urealyticum* and *Ureaplasma diversum,* of several distinct species-specific serotypes, have been recovered from humans and animals, including cattle, sheep, goats, horses, swine, dogs, cats, monkeys, and birds. These organisms' pathogenicity is even less certain than many of the com-

TABLE 9-2 **Disease caused by Mycoplasmatales**

Organism	Disease
BOVINE MYCOPLASMAS	
M. mycoides subsp *mycoides* (SC type)	Contagious bovine pleuropneumonia
M. dispar	Respiratory commensal; subclinical or clinical pneumonia
M. alkalescens	Arthritis in calves; isolated from mastitis; genital commensal
M. bovigenitalium	Mastitis; chronic seminal vesiculitis; arthritis in calves; frequent commensal of vagina, seminal vesicles, and prepuce; endometritis, vulvovaginitis; suggested as a cause of infertility
M. bovirhinis	Mild mastitis; frequent respiratory commensal; often isolated from pneumonia
M. bovis	Severe mastitis; arthritis; associated with pneumonia; respiratory commensal
M. californicum	Acute mastitis
M. canadense	Mastitis; recovered from cases of calf arthritis; respiratory and genital commensal
M. bovoculi	Conjunctivitis; keratoconjunctivitis (usually in concert with another organism such as *Moraxella bovis*)
M. verecundum	Possible cause of conjunctivitis in calves
M. arginini	Respiratory, conjunctival, and genital commensal of cattle, sheep, and goats; recovered from dogs
M. alvi	Intestinal and genital commensal of cattle
OVINE AND CAPRINE MYCOPLASMAS	
M. mycoides subsp *capri* and strain F38	Contagious caprine pleuropneumonia
M. mycoides subsp. *mycoides* (LC type)	Pneumonia; arthritis; mastitis; septicemia
M. agalactiae	Contagious agalactia (mastitis); arthritis; pneumonia; keratoconjunctivitis; vulvovaginitis
M. capricolum	Polyarthritis with septicemia in goats; conjunctivitis; mastitis; vulvovaginitis; balanoposthitis; experimentally pathogenic to sheep, goats, and pigs; respiratory and genital commensal

(continued)

TABLE 9-2 (continued)

Organism	Disease
M. conjunctivae	Conjunctivitis and keratoconjunctivitis
M. ovipneumoniae	Chronic interstitial pneumonia; mastitis
M. putrefaciens	Mastitis in goats

MYCOPLASMAS OF SWINE

Organism	Disease
M. flocculare	Mild focal mononuclear pneumonia; respiratory and conjunctival commensal
M. hyopneumoniae	Enzootic pneumonia
M. hyorhinis	Arthritis and polyserositis; a common nasopharyngeal commensal; common isolate in conjunction with *M. hyopneumoniae*
M. hyosynoviae	Polyarthritis; persists indefinitely in oropharynx

OTHER MYCOPLASMAS

Organism	Disease
M. arthritidis	Polyarthritis in rats; associated with otitis media, conjunctivitis, and rhinitis; respiratory commensal; experimental arthritis in mice and rabbits
M. canis	Possibly not pathogenic; frequent respiratory, conjunctival, and genital commensal in dogs; associated with inflammatory disease of the urinary tract
M. caviae	Respiratory commensal of guinea pigs
M. cynos	Pneumonia in dogs
M. edwardii	Recovered from pneumonia in dogs; pathogenicity uncertain
M. equigenitalium	Frequent commensal of equine respiratory and genital tracts; pathogenicity unknown
M. equirhinis	Respiratory commensal of horses
M. fastidiosum	Recovered from equine nasopharynx; pathogenicity unknown
M. feliminutum	Has been recovered from respiratory tract of cat, dog, and horse; unknown pathogenicity
M. felis	Frequent respiratory and genital commensal of cats. Has been recovered from healthy horses and horses with respiratory disease
M. gateae	Frequent respiratory, conjunctival, and genital commensal of cats; periodically recovered from dogs and rarely, cattle
M. lipophilum	Recovered from throat of rhesus monkeys (also humans); unknown pathogenicity

Organism	Disease
M. maculosum	Common respiratory commensal of dogs; occasionally of conjunctivae and genital tract
M. moatsii	Respiratory and genital commensal of African green monkeys
M. molare	Infrequent respiratory commensal of dogs
M. neurolyticum	Common respiratory commensal of mice; associated with conjunctivitis; experimentally in mice and occasionally in rats, an exotoxin induces neurologic signs and sometimes lesions in the central nervous system ("rolling disease")
M. opalescens	Occasional respiratory and genital commensal of dogs
M. primatum	Oral and genital commensal of Old and New World monkeys
M. pulmonis	A frequent inhabitant of respiratory tract of mice and rats; highly pathogenic: chronic murine mycoplasmosis (rhinitis, pneumonia, otitis, oophoritis, salpingitis, endometritis, pyometra, urethritis, arthritis)
M. spumans	Common respiratory commensal of dogs; suggested association with granulomatous colitis in boxer dogs

MYCOPLASMAS OF HUMANS

Organism	Disease
M. buccale	Uncommon commensal of oropharynx
M. faucium	Uncommon commensal of oropharynx
M. fermentans	Uncommon commensal of urogenital tract
M. hominis	Urogenital disease
M. orale	Common commensal of oropharynx
M. pneumoniae	Primary atypical pneumonia
M. salivarium	Common commensal of oropharynx of humans and monkeys; has been recovered from horses
M. genitalium	Commensal of urogenital tract

UREAPLASMAS

Organism	Disease
U. diversum	Host specific strains recovered from many animal species, including cattle, horses, swine, dogs, cats; has been associated with pneumonia, conjunctivitis, mastitis, vulvovaginitis, and infertility
U. urealyticum	Genitourinary, oropharyngeal, and anal commensal of humans; associated with urethritis, endometritis, infertility

(continued)

TABLE 9-2 (continued)

Organism	Disease
ACHOLEPLASMAS	
A. laidlawii	Recovered from oral, respiratory, and genital mucosae of many species including humans, cattle, sheep, goats, swine, dogs, cats, monkeys, birds; also isolated from sewage and soil
A. granularum	Recovered from respiratory mucosae and conjunctivae of swine and horses
A. axanthum	Recovered from cattle (mucosae and serum) and rodents
A. modicum	Recovered from swine and cattle (tissues and semen)
A. oculi	Keratoconjunctivitis and pneumonia in goats; has been recovered from cases of infectious bovine keratoconjunctivitis and from nasal cavity of normal calves, horses, and swine
A. equifetale	Recovered from normal respiratory mucosae and aborted equine fetuses
A. hippikon	Recovered from aborted equine fetuses
A. morum	Recovered from bovine serum and calf kidney cultures

mensal *Mycoplasma* species, but they are associated with bovine mastitis, enzootic pneumonia, bovine abortion, and infertility in cattle and sheep.

Members of the genus *Acholeplasma* differ from *Mycoplasma* species and *Ureaplasma* species in that they do not need serum or cholesterol for growth. They can occur as saprophytes in soil and sewage, but some species are mucosal commensals of animals (swine, cattle, horses, and rodents) and have been detected in conjunction with keratoconjunctivitis, pneumonia, and abortion.

References

Freundt EA. Present status of the medical importance of mycoplasmas. Pathol Microbiol 1974;40:155–187.
Krieg NR and Holt JG, ed. Bergey's manual of systematic bacteriology. Vol. 1. Baltimore: Williams and Wilkins 1984.
Maramorosch K, ed. Mycoplasma and mycoplasma-like agents of human, animal, and plant diseases. Ann NY Acad Sci 1973;225:5–532.

Bovine pleuropneumonia

This infectious disease of cattle is caused by *Mycoplasma mycoides* subsp *mycoides*. It is the only mycoplasma divided into subspecies; *M. mycoides* subsp *capri* is the cause of caprine pleuropneumonia. Two groups or strains of *M. mycoides* subsp *mycoides* are recognized in culture: a small colony (SC) strain and a large colony (LC) strain. The SC strain causes contagious bovine pleuropneumonia. The LC strain resembles *M. mycoides* subsp *capri* and is associated with pneumonia, arthritis, mastitis, and septicemia in goats.

Contagious bovine pleuropneumonia has been known as a specific entity for more than 200 years. In the nineteenth century, it spread from Europe to many parts of the world, including the United States. The disease was eliminated from this country before 1892 by an intensive campaign involving slaughter and quarantine of infected and exposed animals, and fortunately, it has not reappeared. Around 1854, the disease was introduced from the Netherlands into South Africa, where it spread rapidly, causing the death of more than 100,000 cattle over 2 years. It has remained an important disease in Africa and Asia.

Animals with chronic infection or subclinical disease are important reservoirs of infection and make control of the disease difficult. Recovered animals with sequestered lesions containing viable organisms are also thought to be reservoirs, but evidence has been presented to the contrary (Windsor and Masiga, 1977).

SIGNS

Although the disease can be acute, leading to death within a week, the more usual course is two to several weeks after a prolonged incubation period. The affected individual exhibits signs of pneumonia, which clinically is indistinguishable from pneumonia of nonspecific cause. In the acute stage, a dry and painful cough, which later becomes moist, is followed by labored respiration with grunting, halting expiration. When the lungs are extensively involved, respiratory distress is exhibited by dyspnea so severe that the animal stands with its elbows turned out. In the later stages, mucopurulent discharge from the nose and sometimes edematous infiltration of the lower thorax may be seen. Weakness and emaciation usually become apparent, and swelling of the joints (polyarthritis) is sometimes seen in young calves. The organism may invade the placenta and fetus, resulting in abortion. Morbidity is high, although clinical signs may develop in only 50% or less of affected herds. Mortality rates range from 10% to 90%.

LESIONS

In the typical case of pleuropneumonia, the lesions of the lung are characteristic. They usually are limited to one lung, but occasionally are bilateral; however, they never symmetrically involve contralateral lungs. The pleural cavity over the affected lung usually contains an excess of pleural fluid, which may be blood-stained and include strands of fibrin; as a rule, the pleura adheres to the thoracic wall at some points. The parenchyma does not collapse when the thorax is opened, but remains firm and raised above the relatively normal adjacent lung tissue. The cut surface has a marbled appearance, with red and grayish areas of parenchyma separated by thick yellowish interlobular septa. The presence of unequally distended lymph spaces often imparts a "beaded" appearance to these septa. In cases of long standing, zones of necrosis within groups of lobules tend to become sequestrated from the adjacent lung and surrounded by a dense layer of connective tissue. Within these sequestra, which often are large, the original configuration of lung parenchyma may be retained for a time. Eventually abscesses may form in the encapsulated tissue, and their rupture may cause an acute exacerbation of the symptoms or the entire sequestrum may be converted to scar tissue.

The outstanding histologic characteristic of the lung is the separation of the lobules into distinct compartments by the heavily thickened interlobular septa, in which there is not only edema but organization as well. The lobules contain areas in which the alveoli are patent, although they are completely consolidated in many other locations. A particularly intense infiltration of round cells, chiefly lymphocytes and plasma cells, is seen around blood vessels and bronchi. Similar focal collections of leukocytes are found within the interlobular septa.

The lesions in other organs are not specific for this disease, but the liver may be infiltrated by round cells in the hepatic triads, with necrosis of individual liver cells near central veins. These necrotic liver cells are acidophilic, have dark pyknotic nuclei, and are believed by some to be the result of gradual anoxia. In the spleen, the germinal centers may be enlarged, mature lymphocytes decreased in number, plasma cells increased, and red blood cells and blood pigment present in excessive amounts.

DIAGNOSIS

The diagnosis may be established by the history, the clinical symptoms, the gross and microscopic lesions, and recovery of the organism. Immunoflourescent staining techniques are particularly useful, and results are often positive, even in the absence of positive culture. Serologic tests and a skin test can be used to identify chronically affected and recovered animals. A vaccine exists, but its effectiveness is limited to 2 years or less.

References

Boothby JT, Jasper DE, Zinkl JG, et al. Prevalence of mycoplasmas and immune responses to *Mycoplasma bovis* in feedlot calves. Am J Vet Res 1983;44:831–838.

Daubney R. Contagious bovine pleuropneumonia. Note on experimental reproduction and infection by contact. J Comp Pathol Ther 1935;48:83–96.

Howard CJ, Thomas LH. Inhibition by *Mycoplasma dispar* of ciliary activity in tracheal organ cultures. Infect Immun 1974;10:405–408.

Nocard E, Roux ER. Le Microbe de la péripneumonia. Ann Inst Pasteur (Paris) 1898;12:240–262.

Oghiso Y, et al. Pathological studies on bovine pneumonia in special references to isolation of mycoplasmas. Jpn J Vet Sci 1976;38:15–24.

Piercy DW. Synovitis induced by intra-articular inoculation of inactivated *Mycoplasma mycoides* in calves. J Comp Pathol 1970;80:549–558.

Piercy DWT, Bingley JB. Fibrinous synovitis in calves inoculated with killed *Mycoplasma mycoides*. Elevated plasma fibrinogen concentration and increased permeability of the synovium. J Comp Pathol 1972;82:279–290.

Piercy DWT. Reaction to killed *Mycoplasma mycoides* in joints in specifically sensitized calves. J Comp Pathol 1972;82:291–294.

Trichard CJV, Basson PA, Van Der Lugt JJ, et al. An outbreak of contagious bovine pleuropneumonia in the Owambo Mangetti area of South West Africa/Namibia: microbiological, immunofluorescent, pathological and serological findings. Onderstepoort J Vet Res 1989;56:277–284.

Watson GL, Slocombe RF. Mycoplasmosis in a Thomson's gazelle. Vet Pathol 1986;23:329–331.

Windsor RS, Masiga WN. Investigations into the role of carrier animals in the spread of contagious bovine pleuropneumonia. Res Vet Sci 1977;23:224–229.

Other bovine mycoplasmoses

Several other mycoplasmas of bovine origin can serve as primary pathogens or participate in concert with other infectious agents in several diseases, including: mastitis; urogenital infections; keratoconjunctivitis; enzootic pneumonia; and arthritis. These diseases are discussed in the following sections.

Bovine mastitis

Mycoplasma bovis (*Mycoplasma agalactiae* var *bovis, Mycoplasma bovimastiditis*) is the most important agent in primary mycoplasma mastitis in cows; the second is *Mycoplasma californicum*. Additionally, bovine mastitis may be caused by *Mycoplasma bovigenitalium, Mycoplasma alkalescens, Mycoplasma canadense,* and *Mycoplasma bovirhinis. Acholeplasma* species may also cause mastitis. *M. bovis* has also been recovered from calves with arthritis.

The disease caused by *M. bovis* occurs worldwide in an acute, highly contagious form. The organism can be carried as a respiratory mucosal commensal and can survive in the environment for long intervals, making meticulous sanitation a prerequisite for control. The disease is characterized by a sudden onset of agalactia with a swollen firm udder. All four quarters are affected. Morbidity rates within a herd are high. Systemic signs are usually absent, although the organism can cause arthritis and pneumonia in conjunction with mastitis. The milk contains large numbers of neutrophils, and although when first drawn it appears normal, on standing it rapidly separates into a flaky deposit and a clear supernatant. Apparent recovery usually occurs in 2 to 3 weeks with a marked decrease in size of the udder, but mycoplasmas are excreted for months.

LESIONS

The lesions involve mammary acini, interlobular ducts, and interstitial stroma. At the outset, all acini in the lobule become filled with purulent exudate. The interlobular ducts may also become filled with neutrophils, and the epithelium becomes hyperplastic. As the disease progresses, the ductal epithelium undergoes squamous metaplasia, and some ducts and acini are filled with lipogranulomatous exudate. The interstitial stroma is initially edematous and infiltrated by lymphocytes and plasma cells, but eventually undergoes fibrosis. Eosinophils are a common component of the exudate, both in natural and experimental infections.

Bovine genital infections

Several *Mycoplasma* species are normal commensals of the urogenital tract of cows and bulls and may cause disease. Although experimental data suggests that they can be primary pathogens, precipitating factors are probably necessary. *M. bovigenitalium,* which is also associated with **mastitis** and **arthritis,** is the *Mycoplasma* species most often recovered from animals with inflammatory disease of the urogenital tract and may be responsible for some cases of sterility or low fertility in bovines. Several species of *Mycoplasma* have been recovered from bovine fetuses and have been suggested to cause abortions.

LESIONS

The lesions in experimentally infected cows were not evident grossly and were limited to the uterus, oviducts, and related peritoneum. The endometrium was at first edematous, then infiltrated with lymphocytes and plasma cells. Neutrophils soon were evident in the lumen. The lymphocytic inflammation often extended to the serosal surface of the uterus and oviducts. In long-standing lesions, collections of lymphocytes and sometimes eosinophils were noted in the stroma surrounding uterine glands.

M. bovigenitalium and *Ureaplasma* species are also associated with **bovine granular venereal disease (granular vulvovaginitis)** and infertility. *M. bovigenitalium* has been recovered from animals with this disease and has caused the disease after being instilled into the vagina of normal cows. The gross lesions of bovine granular vulvovaginitis consist of mucopurulent discharge and the appearance of tiny granular elevations of the vulvar and vaginal epithelium. Microscopically, these elevated nodules consist of aggregations of lymphocytes that elevate and thin the overlying epithelium. The epithelium sometimes is necrotic, and the stroma is edematous and infiltrated by eosinophils.

Seminal vesiculitis and epididymitis in bulls may be the result of infection by *M. bovigenitalium.* Experimental infection has resulted in inflammatory disease in these and other parts of the genital tract of the bull.

Infectious bovine keratoconjunctivitis

This disease is caused by *Moraxella bovis* (Chapter 10); however, *Mycoplasma bovoculi* is also often recovered from cases (and outbreaks) of infectious bovine keratoconjunctivitis, and the organism appears to augment the severity of the disease. By itself, *Mycoplasma bovoculi* only causes a mild conjunctivitis. Ureaplasmas have also been recovered from animals with conjunctivitis and experimentally have been shown to cause more severe conjunctivitis than that induced experimentally by *M. bovoculi.* Other mycoplasmas, such as *Mycoplasma arginini* and *Mycoplasma verecundum,* are commensals on the conjunctiva and may or may not produce mild conjunctivitis. In some examples, *Acholeplasma oculi* has been isolated.

ENZOOTIC PNEUMONIA OF CALVES

Enzootic pneumonia (Chapter 20) is a term used for pneumonias occurring not only in calves but also lambs and young pigs housed in groups. Ordinarily, it is not a severe or fatal disease, although it is of considerable importance as a cause of subnormal growth. It is not a specific disease with a single cause but the result of the interaction of a combination of infectious agents, which include respiratory viruses, bacteria, acholeplasmas, mycoplasmas, and ureaplasmas.

Several bovine mycoplasmas are respiratory commensals (Table 9-2) and are often recovered in association with pneumonia, but *M. dispar* is recognized as a primary respiratory pathogen (in addition to *M. mycoides* subsp *mycoides* and *Mycoplasma bovis*).

LESIONS

The lesions are usually limited to a few lobules in apical or cardiac lobes and result in consolidation of small groups of lobules, sharply demarcated from adjacent ones. Microscopically, the lesions are centered around bronchioles, with purulent exudate and debris in the lumen, and nodules of lymphocytes distorting the bronchial wall. This is consistent with the fact that mycoplasmas grow on epithelial surfaces of the respiratory tract. This type of bronchiolitis is reminiscent of the lesions of murine chronic respiratory disease.

Bovine Mycoplasmal Arthritis

Polyarthritis in calves and cows can be caused by several of the bovine mycoplasmas. It can accompany bovine pleuropneumonia, occur after use of the vaccine for pleuropneumonia, or result from invasion of *Mycoplasma bovis* , *M. canadense,* or *M. alkalescens.*

Mycoplasmas, when they gain access to the blood stream of any species, tend, in general, to localize in synovial membranes and mesothelial surfaces. Affected joints become swollen and painful, leading to lameness. Pathologically, there is increased synovial fluid, which is cloudy and may contain fibrin. The synovial membrane is thickened as a result of villous hyperplasia and infiltrates of mononuclear cells, chiefly lymphocytes. Most animals probably recover without progression to serious chronic arthritis.

References

Al-Aubaidi JM, McEntee K, Lein DH, et al. Bovine seminal vesiculitis and epididymitis caused by *Mycoplasma bovigenitalium.* Cornell Vet 1972;62:581–596.

Afshar A. Genital diseases of cattle associated with mycoplasma. Vet Bull 1967;37:879–884.

Bennett RH, Jasper DE. Nasal prevalence of *Mycoplasma bovis* and IHA titers in young dairy animals. Cornell Vet 1973;67:361–373.

Blom J, Erno H, Birch-Andersen A. Mycoplasmosis: experimental seminal vesiculitis. Electron microscopy of infected tissue. Acta Pathol Microbiol Scand 1973;81B:176–178.

Boughton E. Mycoplasma bovis mastitis. Vet Bull 1979;49:377–387.

Boughton E, Hopper SA, Gayford PJR. *Mycoplasma canadense* from bovine fetuses. Vet Rec 1983;112:87.

Bushnell RB. *Mycoplasma* mastitis. Vet Clin North Am (Large Anim Pract) 1984;6:301–312.

Dellinger JD, Jasper DE, Ilic M. Characterization studies on mycoplasma isolates from bovine mastitis and the bovine respiratory tract. Cornell Vet 1977;67:351–360.

Edward DC, Hancock JL, Hignett SL. Isolation of a pleuropneumonia-like organism from the bovine genital tract. Vet Rec 1947;59:329–330.

Erno H, Blom E. Mycoplasmosis: experimental and spontaneous infections of the genital tract of bulls. Acta Vet Scand 1972;13:161–174.

Erno H, Blom E. Mycoplasmosis: experimental seminal vesiculitis. Demonstration of locally occurring antibody. Acta Vet Scand 1973;14:332–334.

Gourlay RN. Significance of mycoplasma infections in cattle. J Am Vet Med Assoc 1973;163:905–908.

Gourlay RN, Mackenzie A, Cooper JE. Studies of the microbiology and pathology of pneumonic lungs of calves. J Comp Pathol 1970;80:575–584.

Gourlay RN, Thomas LH. The experimental production of pneumonia in calves by the endobronchial inoculation of T-mycoplasmas. J Comp Pathol 1970;80:585–594.

Hale HH, Helmboldt CF, Plastridge WN, et al. Bovine mastitis caused by a *Mycoplasma* species. Cornell Vet 1962; 52:582–591.

Hartman HA, Tourtellotte ME, Nielsen SW, et al. Experimental bovine uterine mycoplasmosis. Res Vet Sci 1964;5:303–310.

Hirth RS, Nielsen SW. Experimental pathology of bovine salpingitis due to mycoplasma insemination. Lab Invest 1966;15:1132–1133.

Hirth RS, Nielsen SW, Tourtellotte ME. Characterization and comparative genital tract pathogenicity of bovine mycoplasmas. Infect Immun 1970;2:101–104.

Hjerpe CA, Knight HD. Polyarthritis and synovitis associated with *Mycoplasma bovimastitidis* in feedlot cattle. J Am Vet Med Assoc 1972;160:1414–1418.

Jasper DE. Mycoplasmas: their role in bovine disease. J Am Vet Med Assoc 1967;151:1650–1655.

Jasper DE. The role of *Mycoplasma* in bovine mastitis. J Am Vet Med Assoc 1982;181:158–162.

Jasper DE, Al-Aubaidi JM, Fabricant J. Epidemiologic observations on mycoplasma mastitis. Cornell Vet 1974;64:407–415.

Karbe E, Nielsen SW, Helmboldt CF. Pathology of experimental mycoplasma mastitis in the cow. Zentbl Vet Med 1967;14B:7–31.

Kehoe JM, Norcross NL, Carmichael LE, et al. Studies of bovine *Mycoplasma* mastitis. J Infect Dis 1967;117:171–179.

Kelly JI, Jones GE, Hunter AG. Isolation of *Mycoplasma bovoculi* and *Acholeplasma oculi* from outbreaks of infectious bovine keratoconjunctivitis. Vet Rec 1983;112:482.

Langford EV. Mycoplasma infections in the bovine genital tract. Can Vet J 1974;15:300–301.

Langford EV, Leach RH. Characterization of mycoplasma isolated from infectious bovine keratoconjunctivitis: *M. bovoculi* sp. nov. Can J Microbiol 1973;19:1435–1444.

Leach RH. Further studies on classification of bovine strains of Mycoplasmatales, with proposals for new species. *Acholeplasma modicum* and *Mycoplasma alkalescens.* J Gen Microbiol 1973;75:135–153.

Liberal MHT, Boughton E. Isolation of *Acholeplasma oculi* from calves. Vet Rec 1987;120:71.

Lopez A, Maxie MG, Ruhnke L, et al. Cellular inflammatory response in the lungs of calves exposed to bovine viral diarrhea virus, *Mycoplasma bovis,* and *Pasteurella haemolytica.* Am J Vet Res 1986;47:1283–1286.

Nicolet J, Buttiker W. Isolation of *M. bovoculi* from eye lesions of cattle in the Ivory Coast. Vet Rec 1974;95:442–443.

Panangala VS, Winter AJ, Wijesinha A, et al. Decreased motility of bull spermatozoa caused by *Mycoplasma bovigenitalium.* Am J Vet Res 1981;42:2090–2093.

Parsonson IM, Al-Aubaidi JM, McEntee K. *Mycoplasma bovigentalium:* experimental induction of genital disease in bulls. Cornell Vet 1974;64:240–264.

Pirie HM, Allan EM. Mycoplasmas and cuffing pneumonia in a group of calves. Vet Rec 1975;97:345–349.

Rosenbusch RF, Knudtson WU. Bovine mycoplasmal conjunctivitis: experimental reproduction and characterization of the disease. Cornell Vet 1980;70:307–320.

Ruhnke HL, Palmer NC, Doig PA, et al. Bovine abortion and neonatal death associated with *Ureaplasma diversum.* Theriogenology 1984;21:295–301.

Ryan MJ, Wyand DS, Hill DL, et al. Morphologic changes following intraarticular inoculation of *Mycoplasma bovis* in calves. Vet Pathol 1983;20:472–487.

Salih BA, Rosenbusch RF. Attachment of *Mycoplasma bovoculi* to bovine conjunctival epithelium and lung fibroblasts. Am J Vet Res 1988;49:1661–1664.

Shimizu T, Nosaka D, Nakamura N. An enzootic of calf pneumonia associated with *Mycoplasma bovirhinis.* Jpn J Vet Sci 1973;35:535–537.

Singh UM, Doig PA, Ruhnke HL. Mycoplasma arthritis in calves. Can Vet J 1973;12:183–185.

Stalheim OHV, Proctor SJ. Experimentally induced bovine abortion with *Mycoplasma agalactiae* subsp. *bovis.* Am J Vet Res 1976;37:879–884.

Thornber PM. Ureaplasma association with bovine infertility in southwest Scotland. Vet Rec 1982;111:591.

Contagious caprine pleuropneumonia

This respiratory disease of goats is very similar to bovine pleuropneumonia. The classic disease, which has occurred for centuries, is caused by *Mycoplasma mycoides* subsp *capri;* however, an essentially identical entity is caused by *Mycoplasma mycoides* subsp *mycoides* (LC type) and a mycoplasma known as strain F38. The disease occurs in Africa, Asia, the Middle East, and parts of Europe.

The incubation period of 7 to 10 days tends not to be protracted, as it is in bovine pleuropneumonia.

SIGNS

The signs usually seen include fever, nasal discharge, accelerated respiration, and depression. Incubation periods have been recorded as 8 to 28 days for the natural infection and 3 to 24 days for the experimentally induced disease. The mortality rate is high, often reaching 100% in an outbreak.

LESIONS

The pulmonary lesions resemble those of bovine pleuropneumonia, except that sequestration of lung tissue is less common. In the peracute form, the lungs are uniformly consolidated with fibrinopurulent exudate on the pleura. In the less fulminant form, the pulmonary lobules have a variegated appearance. Edema is extensive in the interlobular septa and under the pleura. There is fibrinous pleuritis and pericarditis. In addition to pneumonia, infection with *M. mycoides* subsp *mycoides* (LC type) may lead to arthritis or mastitis.

References

Barber TL, Yedloutschnig RJ. Mycoplasma infections of goats. Cornell Vet 1970;60:297–308.

Bölske G, Engvall A, Renström LHM, et al. Experimental infections of goats with *Mycoplasma mycoides* subspecies *mycoides,* LC type. Res Vet Sci 1989;46:247–252.

Brogden KA, Rose D, Cutlip RC, et al. Isolation and identification of mycoplasmas from the nasal cavity of sheep. Am J Vet Res 1988;49:1669–1672.

DaMassa AJ, Brooks DL, Adler HE. Caprine mycoplasmosis: widespread infection in goats with *Mycoplasma mycoides* subspecies *mycoides* (large-colony type). Am J Vet Res 1983;44:322–325.

DaMassa AJ, Brooks DL, Holmberg CA. Induction of mycoplasmosis in goat kids by oral inoculation with *Mycoplasma mycoides* subspecies *mycoides.* Am J Vet Res 1986;47:2084–2089.

DaMassa AJ, Brooks DL, Holmberg CA, et al. Caprine mycoplasmosis: an outbreak of mastitis and arthritis requiring the destruction of 700 goats. Vet Rec 1987;120:409–413.

Moulton WM: Contagious caprine pleuropneumonia in the United States? J Am Vet Med Assoc 1980;176:354–355.

Okoh AEJ, Ocholi RA. Disease associated with *Mycoplasma mycoides,* subspecies *mycoides* in sheep in Nigeria. Vet Rec 1986;118:212.

Rosendal S. Experimental infection of goats, sheep, and calves with the large colony type of *Mycoplasma mycoides* subsp. *mycoides.* Vet Pathol 1981;18:71–81.

Contagious agalactia of goats and sheep

This disease has been known for about a century in many countries where goats and sheep are important sources of milk and meat for human consumption. Contagious agalactia has been reported to occur in Romania, Yugoslavia, Switzerland, many Mediterranean countries, Sudan, Iran, the former Soviet Union, Pakistan, India, and South America. The disease causes considerable economic loss, principally from lowered milk production. Goats appear to be more susceptible in nature, but sheep are infected readily by experimental methods. The causative organism, *Mycoplasma agalactiae,* was first isolated by Bridré and Donatien (1923). *Mycoplasma putrefaciens* and *Mycoplasma ovipneumoniae* have also been identified as a cause of mastitis in goats in Europe and the United States, as well as *M. mycoides* subsp *mycoides* (LC type), which is discussed above.

Experimental infection with *M. agalactiae* results in bacteremia, followed by excretion of organisms in milk within 6 days (Watson and others, 1968). Mammary infection persists for months, and the organisms may be isolated from blood, milk, or joint fluid.

SIGNS

The signs appear first at lambing time as mastitis in the lactating females. The infection may be very acute, leading to septicemia and death in ewes and kids before overt mastitis is evident. The milk may become greenish-yellow, and the solids tend to sediment. Polyarthritis (particularly in males), pneumonia, and keratoconjunctivitis often appear.

Mycoplasma agalactiae has been associated with **granular vulvovaginitis** of goats in India (Singh, Rajya, and Mohanty, 1974). The lesions consist of multiple tiny nodules of lymphocytes and plasma cells in the lamina propria and muscularis of the vagina and vulva. These aggregations of lymphocytes are visible grossly as tiny translucent granules that elevate the mucosa. This appearance led to the descriptive term granular vulvovaginitis.

Ureaplasmas have also been associated with vulvovaginitis in sheep as well as mastitis in ewes.

References

Ball HJ, McCaughey WJ. Experimental production of vulvitis in ewes with a ureaplasma isolate. Vet Rec 1982;110:581.
Bridré J, Donatien A. Le Microbe de l'agalaxie contagieuse et sa culture in vitro. CR Acad Sci (Paris) 1923;177:841–843.
Kennedy S, Ball HJ. Pathology of experimental ureaplasma mastitis in ewes. Vet Pathol 1987;24:302–307.
Singh H, Rajya BS, Mohanty GC. Granular vulvovaginitis (GVV) in goats associated with *Mycoplasma agalactiae.* Cornell Vet 1974;64:435–442.
Singh N, Rajya BS, Mohanty GC. Pathology of *Mycoplasma agalactiae* induced granular vulvovaginitis (GVV) in goats. Cornell Vet 1975;65:363–373.
Turner AW. Pleuropneumonia group of diseases. In: Stableforth AW, Galloway LA, ed. Infectious diseases of animals. Vol. 2. London: Butterworth 1959;437–480.
Watson WA, Cottew GS, Erdag O, et al. The investigation of the pathogenicity of *Mycoplasma* organisms isolated from sheep and goats in Turkey. J Comp Pathol 1968;78:283–291.

Other mycoplasmoses in goats and sheep

Aside from *M. mycoides* var *capri* and *M. agalactiae,* which are important pathogens of goats and sheep in many parts of the world, several mycoplasmas have been isolated from diseased tissues in the United States. In some instances, evidence is convincing that the organisms recovered caused the disease. In others, it appears that mycoplasmas may be carried by essentially healthy sheep and goats.

Mycoplasma capricolum is a true pathogen for goats, causing, as with many mycoplasmas, diverse lesions ranging from acute septicemia to fibrinopurulent arthritis, conjunctivitis, mastitis, vulvovaginitis, and balanoposthitis. Sheep are experimentally susceptible. The disease occurs worldwide. Interstitial pneumonia of sheep and, probably, goats can result from *M. ovipneumoniae* infection. As described in Australia and the United States, the lesions are characterized by thickening of alveolar septae, proliferation of alveolar lining cells, hyperplasia of bronchiolar epithelium, and lymphocytic infiltrates. Keratoconjunctivitis (pink eye) in sheep and goats may be caused by any of those mycoplasmas already discussed, but *M. conjunctivae* is more often recovered in animals with this disorder and has been shown to reproduce the disease.

Ureaplasmas have been associated with granular vulvitis and infertility in sheep.

References

Adler HE, DaMassa AJ, Brooks DL. Caprine mycoplasmosis: *Mycoplasma putrefaciens,* a new cause of mastitis in goats. Am J Vet Res 1980;41:1677–1679.
Alley MR, Quinlan JR, Clarke JK. The prevalence of *Mycoplasma ovipneumoniae* and *Mycoplasma arginini* in the respiratory tract of sheep. NZ Vet J 1975;23:137–142.
Barile MF, Guidice RA Del, Tully JG. Isolation and characterization of *Mycoplasma conjunctivae* sp. n. from sheep and goats with keratoconjunctivitis. Infect Immun 1972;5:70–76.
Cordy DR, Adler HE, Yamamoto R. A pathogenic pleuropneumonia-like organism from goats. Cornell Vet 1955;45:50–68.
Cottew GS. Characterization of mycoplasmas isolated from sheep with pneumonia. Aust Vet J 1976;47:591–596.
Cottew GS, Lloyd LC. An outbreak of pleurisy and pneumonia in goats in Australia attributed to a mycoplasma species. J Comp Pathol 1965;75:368–374.
Goltz JP, Rosendal S, McCraw BM, et al. Experimental studies on the pathogenicity of *Mycoplasma ovipneumoniae* and *Mycoplasma arginini* for the respiratory tract of goats. Can J Vet Res 1986;50:59–67.
Greig A. Ovine keratoconjunctivitis. In Pract 1989;11:110,113.
Jones GE. Mycoplasmas of sheep and goats: a synopsis. Vet Rec 1983;113:619–620.
Jones GE. The pathogenicity of some ovine or caprine mycoplasmas in the lactating mammary gland of sheep and goats. J Comp Pathol 1985;95:305–318.
Langford EV. Mycoplasma and associated bacteria isolated from ovine pink-eye. Can J Comp Med 1971;35:18–21.
Livingston CW Jr, Gauer BB. Effect of venereal transmission of ovine ureaplasma on reproductive efficiency of ewes. Am J Vet Res 1982;43:1190–1193.
McCauley EH, Surman PG, Anderson DR. Isolation of Mycoplasma from goats during an epizootic of keratoconjunctivitis. Am J Vet Res 1971;32:861–870.
McGowan B, Moulton JE, Shultz G. Pneumonia in California lambs. J Am Vet Med Assoc 1957;131:318–323.

St. George TD, Sullivan ND, Love JA, et al. Experimental transmission of pneumonia in sheep with mycoplasma isolated from pneumonia sheep lung. Aust Vet J 1971;47:282–283.

St. George TD, Carmichael LE. Isolation of *Mycoplasma ovipneumoniae* from sheep with chronic pneumonia. Vet Rec 1975;97:205–206.

Murine chronic respiratory disease

This classification of disease includes chronic murine pneumonia, epizootic bronchiectasis of rats, infectious catarrh of rats, and rodent pulmonary mycoplasmosis.

For many years, chronic infection of the respiratory system of laboratory rats has been an important disease problem. Evidence now available indicates that *Mycoplasma pulmonis* is the cause of a specific syndrome that involves the nasal passages, nasal sinuses, middle ear, larynx, trachea, bronchi, and lungs. Rats are most commonly affected, but mice may be infected experimentally and by contact with infected rats.

M. pulmonis was first isolated by Kleineberger and Steabben (1937). The pathogenicity of the organism has been convincingly demonstrated by Kohn and Kirk (1969), Lindsey and associates (1971), and others. Concurrent infection with murine viruses, such as Sendai virus; exposure to excessive environmental (intracage) ammonia; and other stresses significantly enhance the severity of *M. pulmonis* infection (Shoeb and others, 1985; Shoeb and Lindsey, 1987).

SIGNS

Some rats may be severely affected but display few indications. Others may exhibit purulent rhinitis with nasal and ocular discharge, coughing, sneezing, and snuffling. Involvement of the inner ear often results in loss of equilibrium, twisting, and rotary movements. A rat held up by the tail characteristically undergoes rapid twisting or twirling motions. In the late stages, infected rats may exhibit polypnea, humped posture, inactivity, roughened hair coat, and loss of weight. Usually death occurs sporadically, and often, lesions are detected only by postmortem examination after sacrifice.

LESIONS

Purulent exudate in the nasal cavities and middle and internal ear may be recognized grossly, but in some instances, they can be detected only by aspiration of material with a capillary pipette. Similar exudate may be present in the trachea and bronchi. The subepithelial stroma of the entire upper respiratory tract is infiltrated by lymphocytes and plasma cells.

The lungs often have a gross gray color and characteristically have a cobblestone appearance on the surface caused by the dilated and thick-walled bronchi. In early lesions, the walls of bronchi are thick as a result of collections of lymphocytes and plasma cells. In long-standing cases, the bronchi become dilated and often contain pus. This bronchiectasis is often the dominant and characteristic feature. Squamous metaplasia of the bronchial epithelium is a common finding. Atelectasis often occurs, and some alveoli may be involved.

The electron microscope reveals large numbers of mycoplasma organisms on the surface of epithelial cells in intimate contact with the villi. Some organisms may be seen in membrane-bound vacuoles within these cells. Lymphocytes and plasma cells predominate in the tissue exudate involving the bronchial wall.

In addition to the respiratory and middle ear lesions, *M. pulmonis* also causes seropurulent polyarthritis (see discussion of *M. arthritidis*) and purulent and lymphocytic inflammatory disease of the entire female reproductive tract.

DIAGNOSIS

The microscopic lesions are characteristic and adequate for presumptive diagnosis of murine mycoplasmosis. Confirmation may be accomplished (1) by cultural isolation of *Mycoplasma pulmonis* from bronchial, tracheal, or nasal exudate; (2) by demonstration of mycoplasma antigens in tissue sections of lung, using immunofluorescence; (3) by transmission of the disease to germ-free rats or mice; or (4) by demonstration of mycoplasma in electronmicrographs of the lesions.

Murine mycoplasmosis must be differentiated from infection with the filamentous cilia-associated respiratory (CAR) bacillus, which often exists in conjunction with mycoplasmosis.

References

Cassell GH, Wilborn WH, Silvers SH, et al. Adherence and colonization of *Mycoplasma pulmonis* to genital epithelium and spermatozoa in rats. Isr J Med Sci 1981;17:593–598.

Davis JK, Cassell GH. Murine respiratory mycoplasmosis in LEW and F344 rats: strain differences in lesion severity. Vet Pathol 1982;19:280–293.

Ebbesen P. Chronic respiratory disease in BALB/c mice. I. Pathology and relation to other murine lung infections. Am J Pathol 1968;53:219–233.

Ebbesen P. Chronic respiratory disease in BALB/c mice. II. Characteristics of the disease. Am J Pathol 1968;53:235–243.

Ganaway JR, Allen AM, Moore TD, et al. Natural infection of germ-free rats with *Mycoplasma pulmonis*. J Infect Dis 1973;127:529–537.

Gay FW, Maguire ME, Baskerville A. Etiology of chronic pneumonia in rats and a study of the experimental disease in mice. Infect Immun 1972;6:83–91.

Giddens WE Jr, Whitehair CK, Carter GR. Morphologic and microbiologic features of trachea and lungs in germ-free, defined-flora, conventional, and chronic respiratory disease-affected rats. Am J Vet Res 1971;32:115–130.

Giddens WE Jr, Whitehair CK, Carter GR. Morphologic and microbiologic features of nasal cavity and middle ear in germ-free, defined-flora, conventional, and chronic respiratory disease-affected rats. Am J Vet Res 1971;32:99–114.

Halliwell WH, McClune EL, Olson LD. *Mycoplasma pulmonis*-induced otitis media in gnotobiotic mice. Lab Anim Sci 1974;24:57–61.

Jersey GC, Whitehair CK, Carter GR. *Mycoplasma pulmonis* as the primary cause of chronic respiratory disease in rats. J Am Vet Med Assoc 1973;163:599–604.

Kleineberger E, Steabben DB. On a pleuropneumonia-like organism in lung lesions of rats, with notes on the clinical and pathologic features of the underlying condition. J Hyg (Camb) 1937;37:143–153.

Kohn DF, Kirk BE. Pathogenicity of *Mycoplasma pulmonis* in laboratory rats. Lab Anim Care 1969;19:321–330.

Kohn DF. Sequential pathogenicity of *Mycoplasma pulmonis* in laboratory rats. Lab Anim Sci 1972;21:849–855.

Kohn DF. Bronchiectasis in rats infected with *Mycoplasma pulmonis*—an electron microscopy study. Lab Anim Sci 1972;21:856–861.

Lindsey JR, Baker HJ, Overcash RG, et al. Murine chronic respiratory disease. Significance as a research complication and experimental production with *Mycoplasma pulmonis*. Am J Pathol 1971;64: 675–717.

Lindsey JR, Davidson MK, Schoeb TR, et al. *Mycoplasma pulmonis*-host relationships in a breeding colony of Sprague-Dawley rats with enzootic murine respiratory mycoplasmosis. Lab Anim Sci 1985;35:597–608.

Schoeb TR, Lindsey JR. Exacerbation of murine respiratory mycoplasmosis by sialodacryoadenitis virus infection in gnotobiotic F344 rats. Vet Pathol 1987;24:392–399.

Schoeb TR, Kervin KC, Lindsey JR. Exacerbation of murine respiratory mycoplasmosis in gnotobiotic F344/N rats by Sendai virus infection. Vet Pathol 1985;22:272–282.

Whittlestone P, Lemcke RM, Olds RJ. Respiratory disease in a colony of rats. II. Isolation of *Mycoplasma pulmonis* from the natural disease, and the experimental disease induced with a cloned culture of this organism. J Hyg (Camb) 1972;70:387–407.

Murine mycoplasmal arthritis

Arthritis is a fairly common occurrence in laboratory rats and mice. In many instances, this disease is associated with the presence of *Mycoplasma arthritidis*, an almost ubiquitous organism, which has been recovered from infected joints, as well as from examples of otitis media and conjunctivitis. It is also pathogenic for mice, but most other laboratory animals are refractory to infection. The joints of limbs are most often involved. Usually only a single joint is involved, but occasionally two or more are affected. The joints are swollen, hot, tender, and fixed, as in acute arthritis in any species. After a time, proliferation of synovia and accumulation of fluid in the joint is accompanied by the appearance of purulent and lymphocytic inflammation in the adjacent tissues. Other organisms may also cause arthritis in these species; among them are *Corynebacterium kutscheri*, streptococci, and *Streptobacillus moniliformis*.

References

Findlay GM, Mackenzie RD, MacCallum FO, et al. The aetiology of polyarthritis in the rat. Lancet 1939;11:7–10.

Freundt EA. Arthritis caused by *Streptobacillus moniliformis* and pleuropneumonia-like organisms in small rodents. Lab Invest 1959;8: 1358–1375.

Hannan PCT, Hughes BO. Reproducible polyarthritis in rats caused by *Mycoplasma arthritidis*. Ann Rheum Dis 1971;30:316–321.

Harwick HJ, Kalmanson GM, Fox MA, et al. Mycoplasmal arthritis of the mouse: Development of cellular hypersensitivity to normal synovial tissue. Proc Soc Exp Biol Med 1971;144:561–563.

Hill A, Dagnall GJR. Experimental polyarthritis in rats produced by *Mycoplasma arthritidis*. J Comp Pathol 1975;85:45–52.

Sokoloff L. Osteoarthritis in laboratory animals. Lab Invest 1959;8: 1209–1217.

Stewart DD, Buck GE. The occurrence of *Mycoplasma arthritidis* in the throat and middle ear of rats with chronic respiratory disease. Lab Anim Sci 1975;5:769–773.

Mycoplasmal arthritis and polyserositis in swine

Two mycoplasmas are important causes of polyarthritis in young swine; *Mycoplasma hyosynoviae* and *M. hyorhinis*. Both organisms are common commensals of the nasopharynx, and young swine are infected by their mothers at an early age. Infection with *M. hyorhinis* also results in polyserositis.

Overt disease does not necessarily follow infection with either organism. Most often infection is subclinical. Stress of one sort or another appears to allow the mycoplasma to enter the bloodstream and localize in joints and, in the case of *M. hyorhinis*, serous surfaces.

LESIONS

The lesions of the experimental disease are described in detail by Roberts and colleagues (1963). The pericarditis, pleuritis, and peritonitis (collectively referred to as "polyserositis") is characteristic; each serous surface is affected in essentially the same way. Within 6 days of intraperitoneal instillation of organisms, fibrinopurulent exudate may be seen grossly on serous surfaces. This exudate becomes more extensive at 10 days after inoculation, but wanes by the thirtieth day. The peritoneum and pleura are severely involved, the pericardium much less so in the experimental disease. The full-blown lesion consists of fibrinopurulent exudate on the serous surface, with swelling and disorganization of the serosal lining cells. Underlying these cells are lymphocytes, macrophages, and plasma cells. Hyperemia and vascularization are features during this stage. As the disease runs its course over 15 to 30 days, the fibrinous exudate may organize, particularly over the pleural and peritoneal surfaces. This results in adhesions, which may persist for a long time. In an occasional case, severe exudation in the pericardial sac may lead to organizing epicarditis, which eventually interferes with cardiac function. The lymphocytic exudate sometimes extends into the subpleural alveoli and Glisson's capsule of the liver but otherwise does not affect parenchymatous organs. The tunica vaginalis may be affected by extension from the peritoneum. In some cases, lymphocytic leptomeningitis may be demonstrable.

The lesions of **arthritis** usually follow those of polyserositis. Both *M. hyorhinis* and *M. hyosynoviae* induce comparable lesions in the joints. One or more joints may become involved, with swelling, congestion, and pain resulting in lameness. In the least severely affected joints and early in the course of the disease, the joint capsule may be slightly hyperemic and the synovial fluid excessive in volume. In more severely affected joints, the synovial fluid becomes yellow or turbid and contains numerous neutrophils and, sometimes, strands of fibrin. The synovial membranes may become edematous, hyperemic, and yellowish in color. The membranes contain large numbers of lymphocytes and macrophages. The villi are edematous, redundant, and hyperemic. Nodules of lymphocytes sometimes form. In young swine, disorganization may be seen in the columns of cartilage in the epiphyseal plate. The cartilage columns lose their straight orderly arrangement and are distorted and irregular, with congested vascular spaces between them. Fibrous thickening of the joint capsule may result in partial or complete ankylosis of the affected joint.

DIAGNOSIS

The diagnosis of mycoplasma infections is made on the basis of the gross and microscopic lesions and the demonstration of the organisms by cultural methods, immunofluorescence, or electron microscopy.

The "fibrinous-serosa-joint inflammation" of young pigs, called Glässer's disease, is pathologically nearly identical to *M. hyorhinis* infection, but Hjärre and Wramby (1942) associated Glässer's disease with swine influenza and infection with *Hemophilus influenzae suis* (Figs. 9-1, 9-2). On the basis of recent evidence, it seems reasonably certain that *H. influenzae suis* and *M. hyorhinis* are distinct causes of polyserositis and arthritis in swine. Hjärre reserves the eponym Glässer's disease for the disease caused by *H. influenzae suis*, and distinguishes it from mycoplasmosis in that purulent meningitis is found in 80% of spontaneous cases of Glässer's disease, whereas purulent meningitis is not a feature of mycoplasmal infection. However, as noted previously, meningitis may develop in animals with *M. hyorhinis* infection. For accurate differentiation, attempts should be made to culture both organisms.

References

Barden JA, Decker JL. *Mycoplasma hyorhinis* swine arthritis. 1. Clinical and microbiologic features. Arthritis Rheum 1971;14:193–201.

Barden JA, Decker JL, Dalgard DW, et al. *Mycoplasma hyorhinis* swine arthritis. III. Modified disease in Piney Woods swine. Infect Immun 1973;8:887–890.

Barthel CH, Duncan JR, Ross RF. Histologic and histochemical characterization of synovial membrane from normal and *Mycoplasma hyorhinis*-infected swine. Am J Vet Res 1972;33:2501–2510.

Davenport PG, Shortridge EH, Voyle B. Polyserositis in pigs caused by infection with mycoplasma. NZ Vet J 1971;18:165–167.

Decker JL, Barden JA. *Mycoplasma hyorhinis* arthritis of swine: A model for rheumatoid arthritis. Rheumatology 1975;6:338–345.

Duncan JR, Ross RF. Fine structure of the synovial membrane in *Mycoplasma hyorhinis* arthritis in swine. Am J Pathol 1969;57:171–186.

Duncan JR, Ross RF. Experimentally induced *Mycoplasma hyorhinis* arthritis of swine: pathologic response to 26th post-inoculation week. Am J Vet Res 1973;34:363–366.

Ennis RS, et al. *Mycoplasma hyorhinis* swine arthritis. II. Morphologic features. Arthritis Rheum 1971;14:202–211.

Hjärre A. Enzootic virus pneumonia and Glässer's disease of swine. Adv Vet Sci 1958;4:235–263.

Hjärre A, Wramby G. On Fibrinös Serosaled inflammation (Glässer) Hos Svin. Skand vet-tidskr 1942;32:257–289.

King SJ. Porcine polyserositis and arthritis—with particular reference to mycoplasmosis and Glasser's disease. Aust Vet J 1968;44:227–230.

McNutt SH, Leith TS, Underbjerg GK. An active agent isolated from hogs affected with arthritis. Am J Vet Res 1945;6:247–251.

Moore RW, Redmond HE, Livingston CW Jr. Pathologic and serologic characteristics of a mycoplasma causing arthritis in swine. Am J Vet Res 1966;27:1649–1656.

Neil DH, et al. Glasser's disease of swine produced by the intratracheal inoculation of *Haemophilus suis*. Can J Comp Med 1969;33:187–193.

Potgieter LND, Ross RF. Demonstration of *Mycoplasma hyorhinis* and *Mycoplasma hyosynoviae* in lesions of experimentally infected swine by immunofluorescence. Am J Vet Res 1972;33:99–105.

Roberts DH, Johnson CT, Tew NC. The isolation of *Mycoplasma hyosynoviae* from an outbreak of porcine arthritis. Vet Rec 1972;90:307–309.

Roberts ED, Switzer WP, Ramsey FK. Pathology of the visceral organs of swine inoculated with *Mycoplasma hyorhinis*. Am J Vet Res 1963;24:9–18.

Roberts ED, Switzer WP, Ramsey FK. The pathology of *Mycoplasma hyorhinis* arthritis produced experimentally in swine. Am J Vet Res 1963;24:19–31.

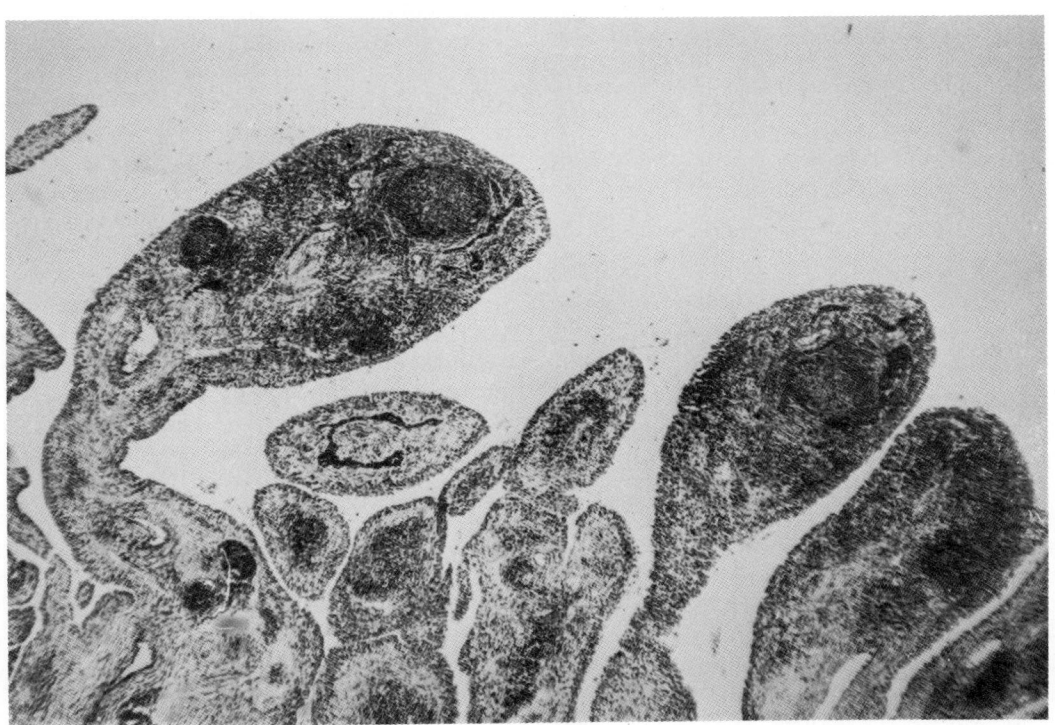

FIG. 9-1 *Mycoplasma hyorhinis* arthritis. Villous hypertrophy of synovial membrane in affected pig. Focal collections of lymphocytes are present within thickened villi. (Courtesy of Dr. J. R. Duncan and *American Journal of Veterinary Research*.)

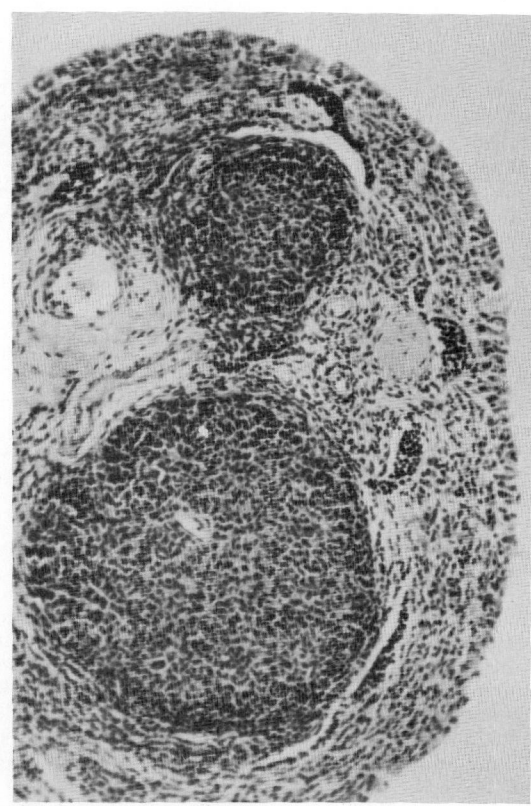

FIG. 9-2 *Mycoplasma hyorhinis* arthritis. Lymphocytic nodule in hypertrophic synovial villus. (Courtesy of Dr. J. R. Duncan and *American Journal of Veterinary Research.*)

Robinson FR, Moore RW, Bridges CH. Pathogenesis of Mycoplasma hyoarthrinosa infection in swine. Am J Vet Res 1967;28:483–496.

Ross RF, Dale SE, Duncan JR. Experimentally induced *Mycoplasma hyorhinis* arthritis of swine: immune response to 26th post-inoculation week. Am J Vet Res 1973;34:367–372.

Ross RF, Switzer WP, Duncan JR. Experimental production of *Mycoplasma hyosynoviae* arthritis in swine. Am J Vet Res 1971;32:1743–1750.

Ross RF, Spear ML. Role of the sow as a reservoir of infection for *Mycoplasma hyosynoviae.* Am J Vet Res 1973;34:373–378.

Enzootic mycoplasmal pneumonia of swine

The cause of this widespread pulmonary disease of young swine has been in question until recently, although the disease, "virus pig pneumonia" or "enzootic pneumonia of swine," has been recognized for many years. On the basis of experimental infection of young gnotobiotic pigs with pure cultures of *Mycoplasma* organisms, demonstration of the organisms in association with the lesions ultrastructurally and by immunofluorescence, and recovery of *Mycoplasma* organisms from affected lungs, it appears that these organisms are the principal, if not sole, cause of this pneumonia of swine. The organism *M. hyopneumoniae* (synonym for *M. suipneumoniae*) is the principal one involved, although in some cases *M. hyorhinis* or *M. flocculare* are recovered.

SIGNS

The clinical signs are limited to a prolonged course with subnormal weight gain, chronic cough, and high morbidity and low mortality rates.

LESIONS

The gross lesions are seen principally in the apical and cardiac lobes of the lung, with lobular consolidations and atelectasis, enlarged peribronchial lymph nodes, and sometimes serofibrinous pleuritis, peritonitis, and pericarditis. These latter findings are similar to those seen in mycoplasmal polyserositis and arthritis in swine.

The microscopic lesions include peribronchial and peribronchiolar accumulations of lymphocytes and plasma cells in large numbers, with some cellular and mucous exudate in the lumen. Mucous-secreting cells in the bronchiolar and bronchial epithelium are hyperplastic and produce excess mucus. Neutrophils, lymphocytes, and macrophages accumulate between alveoli and, in some instances, fill the alveoli. In some cases, lymphocytic encephalitis may be found.

ULTRASTRUCTURE

Ultrastructural studies (Livingston and associates, 1972; Baskerville and Wright, 1973) reveal that the mycoplasma are in the lumen of bronchi and bronchioles, applied to the surface of epithelial cells, and occasionally enclosed by invagination of the cell membrane near the ciliated border. Organisms are not usually found in alveoli, although purulent and lymphocytic exudate may be conspicuous at this site. Hyperplasia of type II pneumocytes is common (Baskerville, 1972). The pathogenic mechanisms are obscure, although it appears that excessive mucus secretion and partial bronchiolar occlusion may cause the exudate in alveoli. The organisms on the surface of the bronchial and bronchiolar epithelium may inhibit ciliary activity and stimulate secretion of mucus. The organisms are also thought to produce peroxide, which may affect cells lining airways and alveoli.

DIAGNOSIS

The diagnosis may be established by finding characteristic microscopic lesions and demonstrating mycoplasma on the bronchial or bronchiolar surface epithelium with electronmicroscopic preparations or by immunofluorescence (Potgieter and Ross, 1972).

References

Armstrong CH, Friis NF. Isolation of *Mycoplasma flocculare* from swine in the United States. Am J Vet Res 1981;42:1030–1032.

Baskerville A. Development of the early lesions in experimental enzootic pneumonia of pigs: an ultrastructural and histological study. Res Vet Sci 1972;13:570–578.

Baskerville A, Wright CL. Ultrastructural changes in experimental enzootic pneumonia of pigs. Res Vet Sci 1973;14:155–160.

Furlong SL, Turner AJ. Isolation of *Mycoplasma hyopneumoniae* and its association with pneumonia of pigs in Australia. Aust Vet J 1975;47:28–31.

Gois M, Pospisil Z, Cerny M, et al. Production of pneumonia after intranasal inoculation of gnotobiotic piglets with three strains of *Mycoplasma hyorhinis.* J Comp Pathol 1971;81:401–409.

Goodwin RFW, Pomeroy AP, Whittlestone P. Production of enzootic pneumonia in pigs with a mycoplasma. Vet Rec 1965;77:1247–1249.

Goodwin RFW. Experiments on the transmissibility of enzootic pneumonia of pigs. Res Vet Sci 1972;13:257–261.

Hjärre A. Enzootic virus pneumonia and Glasser's disease of swine. Adv Vet Sci 1958;4:235–263.

Huhn RG. Enzootic pneumonia of pigs: a review of the literature. Vet Bull 1970;40:249–257.

Jericho KWF. Pathogenesis of mycoplasma pneumonia of swine. Can J Vet Res 1986;50:136–137.

Livingston CW, Stari EL, Underdahl NR, et al. Pathogenesis of mycoplasmal pneumonia in swine. Am J Vet Res 1972;33:2249–2258.

Maré CJ, Switzer WP. Mycoplasma hyopneumoniae. A causative agent of virus pig pneumonia. Vet Med Small Anim Clin 1965;60:841–846.

Maré CJ, Switzer WP. Virus pneumonia of pigs: filtration and visualization of a causative agent. Am J Vet Res 1966;27:1677–1685.

Maré CJ, Switzer WP. Virus pneumonia of pigs: Propagation and characterization of a causative agent. Am J Vet Res 1966;27:1687–1693.

Marley J, Spradbrow PB, Watt DA. The isolation of mycoplasmas from porcine pneumonias. Aus Vet J 1971;47:375–378.

Piffer IA, Ross RF. Effect of age on susceptibility of pigs to *Mycoplasma hyopneumoniae* pneumonia. Am J Vet Res 1984;45:478–481.

Potgieter LND, Ross RF. Demonstration of *Mycoplasma hyorhinis* and *Mycoplasma hyosynoviae* in lesions of experimentally infected swine by immunofluorescence. Am J Vet Res 1972;33:99–106.

Roberts DH. Experimental infection of pigs with *Mycoplasma hyopneumoniae (suipneumoniae)*. Br Vet J 1974;130:68–74.

Switzer WP. Mycoplasmal pneumonia of swine. J Am Vet Med Assoc 1972;160:653–654.

Terpstar JE, Akkermans JPWM, Pomper W. A mycoplasma as a cause of enzootic pneumonia of a swine. Neth J Vet Sci. 2:5–11, 1969.

Young TF, Ross RF, Drisko J: Prevalence of antibodies to *Mycoplasma hyopneumoniae* in Iowa swine. Am J Vet Res **44**:1946–1948, 1983.

Mycoplasmosis in other species

HUMANS AND OTHER PRIMATES

Several species of *Mycoplasma* may be recovered from the oral, respiratory, and genital mucosae of humans and several other primate species. In only a few instances are these organisms clearly associated with any disease process. *Mycoplasma pneumoniae* (Eaton's agent) is clearly associated with many cases of primary atypical pneumonia. This respiratory disease is especially prevalent among young adults closely associated with one another (e.g., recruits in a military camp). The urogenital tract may be colonized by *M. hominis* or *Ureaplasma urealyticum* (T-mycoplasma) and is sometimes associated with "nongonococcal" urethritis. A causative role for *Mycoplasma* species in human rheumatoid arthritis has been suspected, but the evidence for such a role at this time is controversial. Other mycoplasmas of humans are cited in Table 9-2.

Marmosets are susceptible (Mutanda and Ufson, 1977) to experimental inoculation of *Mycoplasma pneumoniae*, but rhesus monkeys (*Macaca mulatta*) are somewhat resistant (Friedlaender and others, 1976). *Ureaplasma* (T-mycoplasma) species have been recovered from genital mucosae of chimpanzees and are thought to be related to infertility (Brown and others, 1976; Swenson and O'Leary, 1977). Similar organisms have been found in the oropharynx and genital tract of marmosets *(Callithix jacchus)* (Furr and others, 1976) and in the genital tract of Talapoin monkeys *(Miopithecus talapoin)* in association with reproductive failure (Kundsin and others, 1975).

It was suggested that arthritis in a rhesus monkey was caused by mycoplasma on the basis of complement-fixation tests, but organisms were not recovered (Obeck and others, 1976).

GUINEA PIGS

Organisms identified as *Mycoplasma caviae*, *Mycoplasma* species, and *Acholeplasma* species have been isolated from conventional and "specific pathogen-free" guinea pigs. These organisms maintain themselves in the nasal cavity and vagina, but no disease has been associated with them (Hill, 1971; Stalheim and Matthews, 1975).

DOGS

Mycoplasmas have been recovered repeatedly from conjunctiva, respiratory systems, and genital tracts of dogs. The organisms that are the most common inhabitants of dogs are *Mycoplasma spumans*, *M. canis*, *M. maculosum*, *M. opalescens*, *M. feliminutum*, *M. edwardii*, *M. cynos*, *M. molare*, and *M. gateae*. The last species is also often isolated from cats. *M. arginini* and *M. bovigenitalium* as well as *Acholeplasma laidlawii* and ureaplasmas have also been recovered from dogs. Some organisms have been recovered from lesions, such as those of pneumonic lungs, balanoposthitis, vaginitis, and urinary tract infections; the organisms may have a causative relationship to these diseases. Viruses (such as adenoviruses) and bacteria are often present as well, and attempts to reproduce the disease with *Mycoplasma* species often fails. The pathogenic significance of mycoplasma in dogs therefore remains equivocal at this time.

CATS

Several *Mycoplasma* species and one *Acholeplasma* species are quite often recovered from sick and normal cats. Tan and Miles (1974) recovered 407 strains from 236 sick cats in New Zealand. Table 9-3 shows some species isolated with the frequency indicated.

Although an association with severe conjunctivitis

TABLE 9-3 **Mycoplasmas recovered from 236 cats**

	Organisms recovered from		
Genus/species	**Sick cats %**	**Sick cats sacrificed %**	**Well cats %**
M. felis	29.7	38.0	4.4
M. arginini	16.5	9.2	6.7
M. gateae	46.2	43.1	62.2
A. laidlawii	0.5	0	22.2

appears to be established in many cases in which *Mycoplasma felis* was isolated, in many other instances a causative relationship has not been clearly established. *M. felis* has occasionally been associated with upper respiratory diseases in which viruses and chlamydias have also been recognized. Commensal or synergistic relationships have been suspected among these organisms, but not proven.

HORSES

No specific disease caused by a mycoplasma has been identified in horses. Several different mycoplasmas have been recovered from normal horses and a few have been associated with disease, most probably as opportunistic infectious agents. *M. felis* is one of the more frequently isolated mycoplasmas and has been associated with pleuritis.

References

Mycoplasmoses in Man and Other Primates

Barile MF. Mycoplasmal flora of simians. J Infect Dis 1973;127: S17–S20.

Brown WJ, Jacobs NF Jr, Arum ES, et al. T-strain mycoplasma in the chimpanzee. Lab Anim Sci 1976;26:81–83.

Friedlaender RP, et al. Experimental production of respiratory tract infection with *Mycoplasma pneumoniae* in Rhesus monkeys. J Infect Dis 1976;133:343–346.

Furr PM, Taylor-Robinson D, Hetherington CM. The occurrence of ureaplasmas in marmosets. Lab Anim 1976;10:393–398.

Furr PM, Hetherington CM, Taylor-Robinson D. Ureaplasmas in the marmoset *(Callithrix jacchus)*: transmission and elimination. J Med Primatol 1979;8:321–326.

Hill A. The isolation of mycoplasmas from nonhuman primates. Vet Rec 1977;101:117.

Hutchison VE, Pinkerton ME, Kalter SS. Incidence of mycoplasma in nonhuman primates. Lab Anim Care 1970;20:914–922.

Kundsin RB, et al. T-strain mycoplasmas and reproductive failure in monkeys. Lab Anim Sci 1975;25:221–224.

Madden DL, et al. The isolation and identification of mycoplasma from *Macaca mulatta*. Lab Anim Care 1970a;20:467–470.

Madden DL, et al. The isolation and identification of mycoplasma from *Cercopithecus aethiops*. Lab Anim Care 1970b;20:471–473.

Madden DL, et al. *Mycoplasma moatsii*, a new species isolated from recently imported grivet monkeys *(Cercopithecus aethiops)*. Intl J Syst Bact 1974;24:459–464.

Mutanda LN, Ufson MA. Experimental *Mycoplasma pneumoniae* infection of marmosets. Lab Anim Sci 1977;27:119.

Obeck DK, Toft JD II, Dupuy HJ. Severe polyarthritis in a rhesus monkey: suggested mycoplasma etiology. Lab Anim Sci 1976;26: 613–618.

Swensen CE, O'Leary WM. Genital ureaplasmas in nonhuman primates. J Med Primatol 1977;6:344–348.

Taylor-Robinson D, Barile MF, Furr PM, et al. Ureaplasmas and mycoplasmas in chimpanzees of various breeding capacities. J Reprod Fertil 1987;81:169–173.

Mycoplasmoses in Guinea Pigs

Hill A. *Mycoplasma caviae*, a new species. J Gen Microbiol 1971;65: 109–113.

Stalheim OHV, Matthews PJ. Mycoplasmosis in specific-pathogen-free and conventional guinea pigs. Lab Anim Sci 1975;25:70–73.

Mycoplasmoses in Dogs

Armstrong D, et al. Canine pneumonia associated with mycoplasma infection. Am J Vet Res 1972;33:1471–1478.

Binn LN, et al. Upper respiratory disease in military dogs: bacterial, mycoplasma, and viral studies. Am J Vet Res 1968;29: 1809–1815.

Jang SS, Ling GV, Yamamoto R, et al. Mycoplasma as a cause of canine urinary tract infection. J Am Vet Med Assoc 1984;185:45–47.

Kirchner BK, Port CD, Magoc TJ, et al. Spontaneous bronchopneumonia in laboratory dogs infected with untyped *Mycoplasma spp.* Lab Anim Sci 1990;40:625–628.

Rosendal S. Mycoplasmas as a possible cause of enzootic pneumonia in dogs. Acta Vet Scand 1972;13:137–139.

Rosendal S. *Mycoplasma molare*, a new canine mycoplasma species. Int J Syst Bact 1973a;23:49–54.

Rosendal S. Canine mycoplasmas. 1. Cultivation from conjunctivae, respiratory and genital tracts. Acta Pathol Microbiol Scand 1973b;81B:441–445.

Rosendal S. *Mycoplasma cynos*, a new canine *Mycoplasma* species. Int J Syst Bact 1974;23:125–130.

Rosendal S. Canine mycoplasmas. I. Cultural and biochemical studies of type and reference strains. II. Serological studies of type and reference strains, with a proposal for the new species, *Mycoplasma opalescens*. Acta Pathol Microbiol Scand 1975;83B:457–462, 463–470.

Rosendal S. Canine mycoplasmas: their ecologic niche and role in disease. J Am Vet Med Assoc 1982;180:1212–1214.

Mycoplasmoses in Cats

Campbell LH, Snyder SB, Reed C, et al. *Mycoplasma felis*-associated conjunctivitis in cats. J Am Vet Med Assoc 1973;163:991–995.

Tan RJS, Miles JAR. Characterization of mycoplasmas isolated from cats with conjunctivitis. NZ Vet J 1973;21:27–32.

Tan RJS, Miles JAR. Incidence and significance of mycoplasmas in sick cats. Res Vet Sci 1974;16:27–34.

Mycoplasmoses in Horses

Ogilvie TH, Rosendal S, Blackwell TE, et al. *Mycoplasma felis* as a cause of pleuritis in horses. J Am Vet Med Assoc 1982;182: 1374–1376.

Rosendal S, et al. Detection of antibodies to *Mycoplasma felis* in horses. J Am Vet Med Assoc 1986;188:292–294.

RICKETTSIAL DISEASES

Microorganisms classified in the family Rickettsiaceae (order Rickettsiales) include several agents that cause disease in humans and animals. The group is named after Howard Taylor Ricketts who beautifully characterized the ecology and biologic features of Rocky Mountain spotted fever in 1906 and 1907. The organisms are minute obligate parasites that are found in the cytoplasm of tissue cells but not in erythrocytes. The organisms are often transmitted from one vertebrate species to another by arthropod vectors in which transovarian transmission is common. Rodents can carry certain of the pathogens in this group and serve as reservoirs of infection. Six pathogenic genera are presently included in this family: *Rickettsia, Rochalimaea, Coxiella, Cowdria, Ehrlichia,* and *Neorickettsia* (Table 9-4). The several species comprising the genus *Rickettsia* are divided into three groups based on their effect on humans: the **typhus group** (*R. prowazekii, R. typhi*); the **spotted fever group** (*R. rickettsii, R. conorii, R. sibirica, R. akari*); and the **scrub typhus** group (*R. tsutsugamushi*) (Table 9-4). The organisms are transmitted by arthropods and, although a number of wild animals (mice, rats, squirrels, rabbits) are susceptible, the diseases are principally diseases of humans. Dogs are susceptible to *Rickettsia rickettsii*, but clinical signs of Rocky Mountain spotted fever are not usually seen. **In humans,** the diseases are characterized by fever, rash, and hemorrhage. The rash

TABLE 9-4 **Diseases caused by Rickettsiaceae**

Genus and species	Vectors	Hosts*	Disease
Typhus Group			
Rickettsia prowazekii	Louse (*Pediculus humanus*)	Humans (guinea pig)	Typhus fever (epidemic typhus)
	Louse (*Neohaematopinus scuiropteri*)	Southern flying squirrel	Flying squirrel typhus, Brill-Zinsser disease
R. typhi (R. mooseri)	Rat louse (*Polyplax spinulosus*)	Humans, rats, mice, (guinea pigs)	Murine typhus of humans
	Rat flea (*Xenopsylla cheopis*)		
	Human flea (*Pulex irritans*)		
	Human louse (*Pediculus humanus*)		
Spotted Fever Group			
R. rickettsii	Ticks (*Dermacentor andersoni, D. variabilis, Haemaphysalis leporis palustris, Amblyomma americanum, A. cajannense*)	Humans, squirrels, rabbits, mice, dogs (guinea pigs)	Rocky Mountain spotted fever
R. conorii	Dog ticks (*Rhipicephalus sanguineus*)	Humans, rodents, dogs, (guinea pigs)	Boutonneuse fever
R. sibirica	Ticks (*Dermacentor, Haemaphysalis,* and *Rhipicephalus* spp.	Humans, squirrels, mice, hares	North Asian tick typhus
R. australis	Ticks (*Ixodes holocyclus*)	Humans, marsupials, (newborn mice)	Queensland tick typhus
R. akari	Mites (*Allodermanyssus sangineus*)	Humans, mice, other rodents (guinea pigs)	Rickettsial pox
Scrub Typhus Group			
R. tsutsugamushi	Trombiculid mites (*Leptotrombidium diliense, L. akamushi,* etc.)	Humans, rhesus, gibbon, rodents (guinea pigs, hamster, moles, rats, gerbils, mice)	Tsutsugamushi fever (scrub typhus)
Rochalimaea quintana	Louse (*Pediculus humanus*)	Humans, (rhesus monkeys)	Trench fever
Neorickettsia helminthoeca	Fluke (*Nanophyetus salmincola*)	Dogs, foxes, bears	Salmon disease of dogs (neorickettsiosis)
Coxiella burnetii	Ticks (many species); aerosol transmission	Humans, cattle, sheep, goats, birds (rabbits, guinea pigs, hamsters, mice)	Q fever
Cowdria ruminantium	Ticks (*Amblyomma* sp.)	Cattle, sheep, goats	"Heartwater"
Ehrlichia phagocytophila	Ticks (*Ixodes ricinus*)	Cattle, sheep, goats, wild deer, bison	Tickborne fever

(continued)

TABLE 9-4 (continued)

Genus and species	Vectors	Hosts*	Disease
E. risticii	Unknown	Horses (cats, dogs)	Potomac horse fever
E. equi	Ticks suspected	Horses (sheep, goats, dogs, cats, monkeys)	Equine ehrlichiosis
E. bovis (Rickettsia bovis)	Ticks (Rhipicephalus and Hyalomma spp.)	Cattle, wild ruminants	Bovine ehrlichiosis ("mild disease of cattle")
E. ovina (Rickettsia ovis)	Ticks ((Rhipicephalus bursa, Hyalomma sp.)	Sheep	Ovine ehrlichiosis ("mild disease of sheep")
E. canis (Rickettsia canis)	Ticks (Rhipicephalus sanguineus)	Dogs	Canine ehrlichiosis
E. sennetsu (Rickettsia sennetsu)	Unknown	Humans	Sennetsu rickettsiosis (glandular fever)
E. platys	Ticks (?)	Dogs	Severe thrombocytopenia
Cytoecetes ondiri	Unknown	Cattle	Bovine petechial fever (Ondiri disease)
Colesiota conjunctivae	Unknown	Sheep, goats, cattle, swine	Keratoconjunctivitis

*Experimentally susceptible hosts in parentheses.

is centrifugal in the typhus group, centripedal in the spotted fever group, and mild to lacking in the scrub typhus group. *Rickettsia* species have a predilection for growth in endothelial cells, which accounts for most lesions.

Pathologically, the predominant lesion is a vasculitis of capillaries, arterioles, and venules with endothelial hypertrophy and hyperplasia and cuffing with leukocytes and thrombosis, which may lead to necrotic foci in the skin and, in typhus and spotted fever, in visceral organs as well. Necrosis of the vessel wall is common in spotted fever, because the organisms extend from endothelial cells and invade vascular smooth muscle. Severity of the diseases may vary widely. Interestingly, *R. prowazekii,* the cause of typhus, may occur as a reactivated infection years after initial exposure. Under these circumstances, the disease is milder and called Brill-Zinsser disease.

The other genera within *Rickettsiaceae* include *Rochalimaea quintana,* the cause of trench fever in humans, and several genera of interest as causes of disease in domestic animals. These include the following:

Neorickettsia contains the single species *N. helminthoeca,* the cause of salmon disease of dogs, which has a predilection for reticuloendothelial cells.
Coxiella contains a single species, *C. burnetii,* the cause of Q fever, which is primarily of importance as an infection of humans. It localizes in many tissues.
Cowdria also contains a single species, *C. ruminantium,* the cause of bovine heartwater. These organisms localize in endothelial cells.
Ehrlichia contains several species that affect animals, ordinarily causing a mild disease. These organisms localize in various leukocytes.
Colesiota and *Ricolesia* are other genera that are very poorly classified. Organisms termed *Colesiota* and *Ricolesia* have been associated with conjunctivitis and keratitis in ruminants and swine respectively.
Cytoecetes is a genus name that has been used for several organisms now bearing another designation. For example, *Ehrlichia phagocytophila* has been termed *Cytoecetes phagocytophila.* The exact position of *Cytoecetes* is uncertain, but it is applied to the causative organism of bovine petechial fever (*C. ondiri*).
The genera *Wolbachia* and *Rickettsiella* are not mammalian pathogens.

References

Heisey GB, Gan E, Shirai A, et al. Scrub typhus antibody in cynomolgus monkeys *(Macaca fascicularis)* in Malaysia. Lab Anim Sci 1981;31:289–291.

Ridgway RL, Oaks SC Jr, LaBarre DD. Laboratory animal models for human scrub typhus. Lab Anim Sci 1986;36:481–485.
Walker DH, Cain BG. The rickettsial plague. Evidence for direct cytopathic effect of *Rickettsia rickettsii*. Lab Invest 1980;43:388–396.

Rocky mountain spotted fever

Of the *Rickettsia* species that cause disease in humans (Table 9-4), only *Rickettsia rickettsii*, the cause of Rocky Mountain spotted fever, is of significance as a cause of disease in domestic animals. Dogs are naturally and experimentally susceptible to a disease that ranges in severity from inapparent to fatal. The disease is transmitted by ticks, chiefly the American dog tick (*Dermacentor variabilis*) in the eastern United States and the wood tick *(D. andersoni)* in the Rocky Mountain area. Other ticks, including the brown dog tick (*Rhipicephalus sanguineus*), are also capable of transmitting the disease. The prevalence of infection far exceeds overt clinical disease.

SIGNS

Signs in natural and experimental infection are variable. Experimental disease signs have been detailed by Keenan and associates (1977) and include fever, anorexia, and lethargy followed by mucocutaneous lesions and ocular and nasal discharge. There is hyperemia with petechiae and ecchymoses of the ocular, oral, and genital mucous membranes. Hyperemia is seen in the skin, particularly on the abdomen, muzzle and ears. Edema of the lips, scrotum, and sheath are common. In some male dogs, a macular rash with petechiae and ulceration develops on the scrotum. Lymph nodes are enlarged. Anterior uveitis may be found. Internal bleeding may be manifest by epistaxis and melena. Some dogs manifest signs of central nervous system dysfunction, such as ataxia, paresis, seizures, or coma. Leukocytosis (neutrophilia with lymphopenia, eosinopenia, and monocytosis) and thrombocytopenia develop in most dogs, and the erythrocyte sedimentation rate is markedly elevated. Bleeding time is prolonged.

The **gross findings** reflect the primary vascular lesion, with hyperemia and variably sized hemorrhages on mucous membranes, skin, gastrointestinal mucosa, serosa, and pleura. Lymph nodes are enlarged and hemorrhagic, and splenomegaly is apparent.

Microscopically, the underlying lesion is a generalized necrotizing vasculitis of venules and veins, reflecting the propensity rickettsial organisms have for vascular endothelium. *R. rickettsii* infection extends beyond the endothelium to a greater extent than other rickettsial disease and invades smooth muscle as well. Vessels are surrounded by accumulations of neutrophils and lymphocytes. Vasculitis is seen in almost all organs: skin, gastrointestinal tract, myocardium, lung, testicle, epididymis, kidney, lung, urinary bladder, pancreas, meninges, retina, and skeletal muscle.

DIAGNOSIS

Diagnosis is made on the basis of a history of tick bites and the characteristic signs and lesions and confirmed by detecting the causative rickettsia through intraperitoneal inoculation of guinea pigs with blood or by culture techniques. In recovered animals, a rise in serum antibodies can be measured by an indirect fluorescent antibody test or other serologic procedures.

References

Breitschwerdt EB, et al. Canine Rocky Mountain spotted fever: a kennel epizootic. Am J Vet Res 1985;46:2124–2128.
Breitschwerdt EB, et al. Antibodies to spotted fever-group rickettsiae in dogs in North Carolina. Am J Vet Res 1987;48:1436–1440.
Davidson MG, et al. Vascular permeability and coagulation during *Rickettsia rickettsii* infection in dogs. Am J Vet Res 1990;51:165–170.
Folds JD, Walker DH, Hegarty BC, et al. Rocky Mountain spotted fever vaccine in an animal model. J Clin Microbiol 1983;18:321–326.
Greene CE. Rocky Mountain spotted fever. J Am Vet Med Assoc 1987;191:666–671.
Greene CE, Burgdorfer W, Cavagnolo R, et al. Rocky Mountain spotted fever in dogs and its differentiation from canine ehrlichiosis. J Am Vet Med Assoc 1985;186:465–472.
Keenan KP, Buhles WC Jr, Huxsoll DL, et al. Studies on the pathogenesis of *Rickettsia rickettsii* in the dog: clinical and clinicopathologic changes of experimental infection. Am J Vet Res 1977;38:851–856.
Keenan KP, et al. Pathogenesis of infection with *Rickettsia rickettsii* in the dog: a disease model for Rocky Mountain spotted fever. J Infect Dis 1977;135:911–917.
Kelly DJ, Osterman JV, Stephenson EH. Rocky Mountain spotted fever in areas of high and low prevalence: survey for canine antibodies to spotted fever rickettsiae. Am J Vet Res 1982;43:1429–1431.
Magnarelli LA, Anderson JF, Philip RN, et al. Antibodies to spotted fever-group rickettsiae in dogs and prevalence of infected ticks in southern Connecticut. Am J Vet Res 1982;43:656–659.
Smith RC, Gordon JC, Gordon SW, et al. Rocky Mountain spotted fever in an urban canine population. J Am Vet Med Assoc 1983;183:1451–1453.

Q fever

A febrile disease of slaughterhouse workers was originally described in Queensland Australia by Derrick (1937), who named the disease "Q" fever (for query, i.e., of questionable or unknown cause). The disease occurs in widely scattered parts of the world, including the United States and Europe. The infectious agent, now classified with the rickettsial organisms and called *Coxiella burnetii (Rickettsia burnetii, R. diaporica)*, is harbored by cattle, sheep, goats, dogs, cats, and other species, but as a rule, the infection in animals is inapparent or mild. Although the organism can be transmitted by ticks (*Dermacentor andersoni, D. occidentalis, Rhipicephalus sanguineus, Otobius megnini*, and others) an intermediate vector is not required (in contrast to other *Ricketttsia* species). Human beings usually acquire the infection by contact with freshly slaughtered infected cattle or sheep or by consuming raw milk or butter in which the organisms are present. Particularly high concentrations of the organism are present at parturition, and the placenta may contain millions of organisms per gram. There have been several cases of Q fever in laboratories employing sheep as research subjects. The organisms can be passed through filters that retain most bacteria, but they are demonstrable in tissues stained by Giemsa or Macchiavello methods, where they appear as minute pleomorphic organisms in the form of lanceolate rods,

0.05 μ in width and 0.05 μ long; as bipolar forms about 1.0 μ in length; or as diplobacillary forms that attain a length of 1.5 μ. Clusters of these organisms appear in the cytoplasm of tissue cells and occasionally are seen extracellularly. *Coxiella burnetii* are poorly stained by ordinary bacterial methods, thus conforming to the characteristics of the rickettsiae.

LESIONS

Organisms have been recovered from cows that exhibited no signs of infection, and postmortem examination of such animals has disclosed few, if any, specific lesions. It is necessary to study the tissues of experimentally infected guinea pigs for information concerning the lesions of Q fever. According to Lillie (1942), the lesions in guinea pigs are characterized by focal perivascular exudation of lymphoid cells (less often by monocytes and fibroblasts) and "vascular endotheliosis," particularly in the myocardium, lungs, alveolar tissue generally, adrenals, renal cortex and medulla, and epididymis. In the lungs, small foci made up of collections of epithelioid cells are seen in alveoli, and some lymphocytes and other mononuclear cells are located in the interalveolar stroma. In later stages of the disease, small nodules of epithelioid cells are found in the spleen, liver, and vertebral marrow; less often in the heart, mediastinal and mesenteric fat, pancreas, kidney, adrenal, bladder mucosa, testicle, and brain. These small granulomas often contain large, multinucleated giant cells, which may replace the entire nodule. Serous exudate is common in alveolar tissues of the renal pelvis and rare in the epididymis.

In humans, the lesions in the natural infection are those of an interstitial pneumonia and disseminated epithelioid granulomas.

DIAGNOSIS

Recognition of infection in cattle depends on the isolation and identification of organisms, usually by inoculation of guinea pigs. Neutralization tests using convalescent serum to protect guinea pigs are of value in differential diagnosis. A complement-fixation test is also employed.

References

Biberstein EL, et al. A survey of Q fever *(Coxiella burnetii)* in California dairy cows. Am J Vet Res 1974;35:1577–1582.
Brooks DL, et al. Q fever vaccination of sheep: challenge of immunity in ewes. Am J Vet Res 1986;47:1235–1238.
Curet LB, Paust JC. Transmission of Q fever from experimental sheep to laboratory personnel. Am J Obstet Gynecol 1972;114:566–568.
Davis GE, Cox HR, Parker RR, et al. A filter-passing infectious agent isolated from ticks. I. Isolation from *Dermacentor andersoni*, reactions in animals and filtration experiments. II. Transmission by *Dermacentor andersoni*. III. Description of the organism and cultivation experiments. IV. Human infection. Pub Health Rep 1938;53:2259–2282.
Derrick EH. "Q" fever, a new fever entity: clinical features, diagnosis and laboratory investigation. Med J Aust. 1937;2:281–299.
Enright JB, et al. The behavior of Q fever rickettsiae isolated from wild animals in northern California. J Wildl Dis 1971;7:83–90.
Heggers JP, Billups LH, Hinrichs DJ, et al. Pathophysiologic features of Q fever-infected guinea pigs. Am J Vet Res 1975;36:1047–1052.
Hall WC, White JD, Kishimoto RA, et al. Aerosol Q fever infection of the nude mouse. Vet Pathol 1981;18:672–683.
Lillie RD. Pathologic histology in guinea pigs following intraperitoneal inoculation with the virus of "Q" fever. Pub Health Rep 1942;57:296–306.
Perrin TL, Bengston IA. The histopathology of experimental "Q" fever in mice. Pub Health Rep 1942;57:790–798.
Pinsky RL, Fishbein DB, Greene CR, et al. An outbreak of cat-associated Q fever in the United States. J Infect Dis 1991;164:202–204.
Singh SB, Lang CM. Q fever serologic surveillance program for sheep and goats at a research animal facility. Am J Vet Res 1985;46:321–325.
Spinelli JS. Managing the Q fever crisis. How UCSF made a bureaucracy work fast. Lab Anim 1981;10:29–38.
Spinelli JS, et al. Q fever crisis in San Francisco: controlling a sheep zoonosis in a lab animal facility. Lab Anim 1981;10:24–27.

Salmon disease of dogs and foxes ("salmon poisoning," canine neorickettsiosis)

A febrile, often fatal, disease of dogs and foxes has been known for some time to occur in conjunction with a diet that includes salmon, trout, and other fish.

Salmon disease, originally thought to be a poisoning, is caused by *Neorickettsia helminthoeca*, a rickettsial-like organism which is carried by a fluke. The fluke, *Troglotrema (Nanophyetus) salmincola*, parasitizes the small intestine of the family Canidae. Eggs, excreted in the feces, first develop in a snail, *Goniobasis plicifera* (*Oxytrema silicula* in the United States), with subsequent development of encysted metacercariae in fish of the family *Salmonidae* (salmon, trout). Adult flukes mature in the small intestine of canines consuming infested fish and allow *N. helminthoeca* to invade. The disease is limited to the Pacific Northwest in the United States.

SIGNS

The signs usually appear about 5 days after the ingestion of infected fish, starting with a fever, which continues for 4 to 8 days. Anorexia is a characteristic feature and is accompanied by depression, weakness, and weight loss. Vomiting and diarrhea, with scant, yellowish, watery, or occasionally bloody and mucoid feces, accompanied by tenesmus, are prominent manifestations. Occasionally, a serous nasal discharge is observed, and a tenacious conjunctival exudate may collect at the inner canthus of the eye.

LESIONS

According to Cordy and Gorham (1950), lymphoid tissues suffer particularly in this disease; the visceral nodes of the abdomen may be enlarged to six times normal size (Fig. 9-3), with the somatic lymph nodes somewhat less severely affected. These enlarged nodes are usually yellowish with prominent white follicles in their cortex. Some edema may surround them, and occasionally an opaque grayish fluid can be expressed from a nodule. The tonsils, which are enlarged and yellowish with prominent follicles and occasional petechiae, may be everted from the fossae. The spleen is often enlarged. The splenic follicles are prominent in

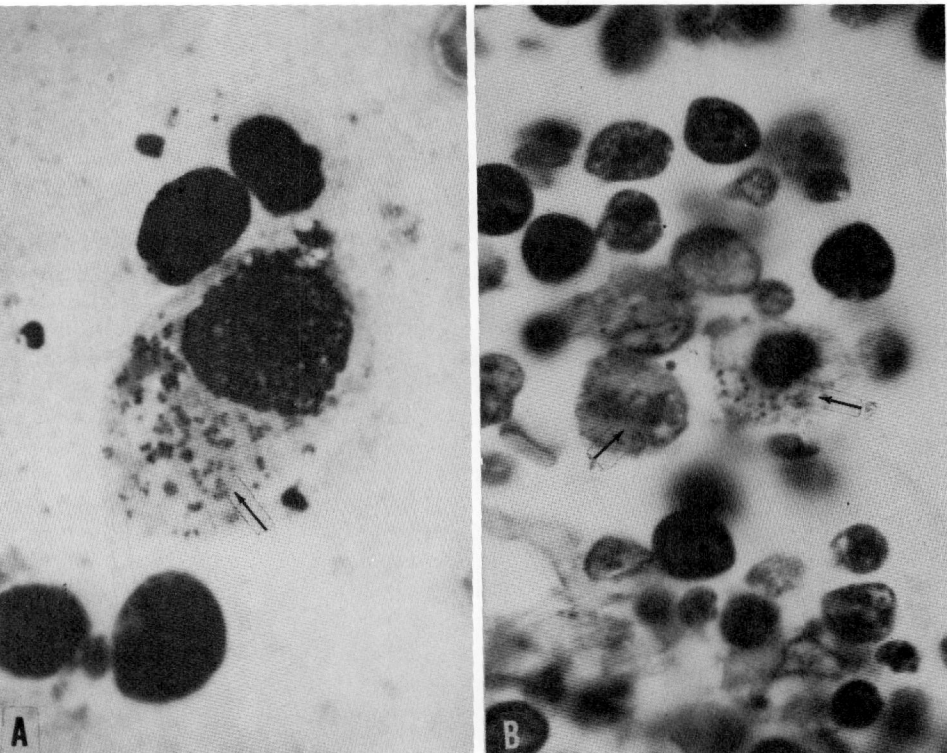

FIG. 9-3 "Salmon disease" in dog. **A.** Smear from a mesenteric lymph node (Giemsa stain, × 1500). **B.** Tissue section from another lymph node. (Giemsa stain, × 500.) Arrows indicate organism, *Neorickettsia helmintheca*. (Courtesy of Dr. Wm. J. Hadlow.)

foxes but unrecognizable in dogs. The lymphoid tissue of the intestinal tract is especially hyperplastic (Fig. 23-17). The intestinal contents may include free blood, especially in animals in which flukes have damaged the intestinal mucosa. Petechiae usually are seen in the intestinal mucosa, particularly over the enlarged lymphoid follicles. Bleeding from small ulcers may be noted in the pylorus. Intussusception of the small intestine is not uncommon. Although the liver often appears grossly normal, rupture is a possibility, with hemoperitoneum as the usual consequence. Hemorrhages have been observed in the gallbladder and the urinary bladder. The lungs usually are studded with many bright or dark red subpleural hemorrhagic puncta, 5 mm to 20 mm in diameter.

The microscopic findings, prominent in the lymph nodes, are dominated by hyperplasia of reticuloendothelial elements and depletion of small lymphocytes (Fig. 9-3). Foci of necrosis are common and many include hemorrhages. Elementary bodies of *Neorickettsia* organisms in reticuloendothelial cells, both in sinuses and parenchyma, are demonstrated by Giemsa or Macchiavello's stain. The thymus, in younger dogs, is the site of prominent changes, including depletion of small lymphocytes, proliferation of reticuloendothelial cells, increase in neutrophils, and the presence of small islands of necrosis throughout the gland. In the intestine, flukes may be demonstrated deep in the intestinal villi and occasionally in duodenal glands. There is surprisingly little tissue reaction to these flukes, aside from a few foci of neutrophils and a slight increase in lymphoid and plasma cells in the lamina propria. Small

hemorrhages in the intestinal mucosa or submucosa may be seen, although not necessarily in relation to the flukes.

According to Hadlow (1957), the brain contains microscopic lesions in 91% of fatal cases. These changes consist of: "*(a)* slight to moderate accumulation of mononuclear cells in the leptomeninges, most intense over the cerebellum; *(b)* cellular exudative and proliferative changes in sheaths of small and medium-sized intracerebral blood vessels; and *(c)* focal collections of glial, mesenchymal cells, or both." The intracerebral lesions, less intense than those of the meninges, occur in the cerebral cortex, brain stem, and cerebellum. Similar lesions may occur in the neurohypophysis. Aside from the hemorrhages, which are recognized grossly, microscopic changes in other viscera are minimal and believed to be nonspecific.

DIAGNOSIS

The presence of adult flukes in the small intestine or their eggs in the feces must be confirmed. The small intracytoplasmic "elementary" bodies in reticuloendothelial cells in lymphoid tissue and occasionally in large mononuclear cells of liver, lungs, and blood are of particular significance in the diagnosis of this disease. These bodies are coccoid or coccobacillary in shape and uniformly about 0.3 μ in diameter. With Giemsa's stain, these bodies are purple; with Macchiavello's stain, red or blue; with Levaditi's method, black or dark brown; with hematoxylin and eosin, pale bluish-violet. They are gram-negative. In some cells, they form nearly solid "plaques," filling the cytoplasm. In some smears, they are found free, apparently released from ruptured cells. They have not been observed in epithelium, endothelium, fibroblasts, or muscle cells.

The organisms have been propagated in tissue cultures and may be demonstrated by specific immunofluorescence (Brown and others, 1972; Kitao and others, 1973).

An unnamed rickettsial organism has been demonstrated in black bears (*Ursus americana*) infected with *Troglotrema salmincola*; this organism differs serologically and by immunofluorescence from *Neorickettsia helminthoeca*, and produces a slightly different disease in dogs. This disease has been called "Elokomin fluke fever" (after the Elokomin River in Washington) (Farrell and others, 1973; Sakawa and others, 1973; and Kitao and others, 1973). Another agent, *Rickettsia sennetsu*, is believed to be the cause of Hyuga or Kagami fever and was isolated from human patients in Kyushu, Japan. The human disease follows consumption of raw bora fish (*Mugil cephalus*), and it appears that an endoparasite of the fish may be the vector host (Kitao and others, 1973).

References

Acha PN, Szyfres B. Nanophyetiasis. In: Zoonoses and Communicable Diseases Common to Man and Animals. 2nd ed. Washington DC: PAHO, Sci Publ No. 503, 1987;673–675.

Brown JL, Huxsoll DL, Ristic M, et al. In vitro cultivation of *Neorickettsia helminthoeca*, the causative agent of salmon poisoning disease. Am J Vet Res 1972;33:1695–1706.

Cordy DR, Gorham JR. The pathology and etiology of salmon disease in the dog and fox. Am J Pathol 1950;26:617–637.

Farrell RK, Leader RW, Johnston SD. Differentiation of salmon poisoning disease and Elokomin fluke fever: studies with the black bear (*Ursus americanus*). Am J Vet Res 1973;34:919–922.

Foreyt WJ, Gorham JR, Green JS, et al. Salmon poisoning disease in juvenile coyotes: clinical evaluation and infectivity of metacercariae and rickettsiae. J Wildl Dis 1987;23:412–417.

Frank DW, McGuire TC, Gorham JR, et al.. Lymphoreticular lesions of canine neorickettsiosis. J Infect Dis 1974;129:163–171.

Hadlow WJ. Neuropathology of experimental salmon poisoning of dogs. Am J Vet Res 1957;18:898–908.

Karr SL, Wong MM. Experimental infection of monkeys with *Nanophyetus salmincola*. J Parasitol 1974;60:358.

Kitao T, Farrell RK, Fukuda T. Differentiation of salmon poisoning disease and Elokomin fluke fever: Fluorescent antibody studies with *Rickettsia sennetsu*. Am J Vet Res 1973;34:927–928.

Philip CB, Hadlow WJ, Hughes LE. *Neorickettsia helmintheca*, a new rickettsia-like disease agent of dogs in western United States transmitted by a helminth. Proc 6th Internat Cong Microbiol (Rome) 1953;4:70–82.

Sakawa H, Farrell RK, Mori M. Differentiation of salmon poisoning disease and Elokomin fluke fever: Complement fixation. Am J Vet Res 1973;34:923–926.

Weiseth PR, Farrell RK, Johnston SD. Prevalence of *Nanophyetus salmincola* in ocean-caught salmon. J Am Vet Med Assoc 1974;165:849–850.

"Heartwater" of cattle, sheep, and goats

This disease, which is significant in ruminant populations on the African continent, is named for its characteristic lesion: hydropericardium. The disease is also recognized in the Caribbean and, therefore, could easily enter the United States. The causative agent, *Cowdria* (formerly *Rickettsia*) *ruminantium*, is an intracellular parasite transmitted by ticks of the genus *Amblyomma*, chiefly the bont ticks *A. hebraeum* and *A. variegatum*. It

is currently differentiated from the rickettsia, which may be transmitted through the egg to succeeding generations of ticks. *C. ruminantium* may be carried through metamorphosis of larva to nymph or nymph to adult, but not through the egg. The organism is a tiny, rod-shaped, often diplococcoid organism, which can be demonstrated with Giemsa's stain in endothelial cells of the jugular vein, vena cava, renal glomerular capillaries, and cerebral gray matter as well as in reticuloendothelial cells and neutrophils.

The organisms seen with the electron microscope are quite pleomorphic, in coccoid, ovoid, filamentous, irregular, horseshoe, and polygonal shapes, measuring roughly 0.49 μ to 2.7 μ in diameter. Each organism is enclosed within a two-unit membrane and contains a structure made up of electron-dense granules ("cytoplasm") and less dense fibrillar material ("nucleoid"). The organisms are found in the cytoplasm of cells and, in the mature form at least, are bound by a cell membrane that separates them from cytoplasmic organelles. The organisms multiply by binary fission and apparently by multiple budding as well (du Plessis, 1970, 1975; Pienaar, 1970).

Cattle, sheep, goats, and wild ruminants are susceptible, but there is significant variation in susceptibility between breeds. Amongst cattle, Brahman and Jersey are particularly susceptible. The disease may be peracute and fatal or inapparent. More usually, there is fever followed by a course of 2 to 3 weeks, characterized by signs of central nervous system dysfunction, such as unsteady gait, twitching of muscles, circling, aggressive behavior, convulsions, and coma. The characteristic necropsy findings are hydropericardium, pulmonary edema, hydrothorax, ascites, and lymphadenopathy. Microscopically, tissues are edematous and there is generalized perivascular leukocytic infiltration. As indicated, the organisms invade vascular endothelium and are demonstrable there.

References

Bezuidenhout JD. Natural transmission of heartwater. Onderstepoort J Vet Res 1987;54:349–351.

Birnie EF, Burridge MJ, Camus E, et al. Heartwater in the Caribbean: isolation of *Cowdria ruminantium* from Antigua. Vet Rec 1985;116:121–123.

Brown CC, Skowronek AJ. Histologic and immunochemical study of the pathogenesis of heartwater (*Cowdria ruminantium* infection) in goats and mice. Am J Vet Res 1990;51:1476–1480.

Dardiri AH, Logan LL, Mebus CA. Susceptibility of white-tailed deer to experimental heartwater infections. J Wildl Dis 1987;23:215–219.

du Plessis JL. Pathogenesis of heartwater: I. *Cowdria ruminantium* in the lymph nodes of domestic ruminants. Onderstepoort J Vet Res 1970;37:89–95.

du Plessis JL. Electron microscopy of *Cowdria ruminantium* infected reticuloendothelial cells of the mammalian host. Onderstepoort J Vet Res 1975;42:1–13.

Kocan KM, Morzaria SP, Voigt WP, et al. Demonstration of colonies of *Cowdria ruminantium* in midgut epithelial cells of *Amblyomma variegatum*. Am J Vet Res 1987;48:356–360.

Mebus CA, Logan LL. Heartwater disease of domestic and wild ruminants. J Am Vet Med Assoc 1988;192:950–952.

Oberem PT, Bezuidenhout JD. Heartwater in hosts other than domestic ruminants. Onderstepoort J Vet Res 1987;54:271–275.

Pienaar JG, et al. Studies on the pathology of heartwater (Cowdria

Rickettsia) ruminantium Cowdry, 1926. I. Neuropathological changes. Onderstepoort J Vet Res 1966;33:115–138.

Pienaar JG. Electron microscopy of *Cowdria (Rickettsia) ruminantium* (Cowdry, 1926) in the endothelial cells of the vertebrate host. Onderstepoort J Vet Res 1970;37:67–78.

Uilenberg G. Experimental transmission of *Cowdria ruminantium* by the Gulf Coast tick *Amblyomma maculatum:* danger of introducing heartwater and benign African theileriasis onto the American mainland. Am J Vet Res 1982;43:1279–1282.

Uilenberg G. Heartwater (*Cowdria ruminantium* infection): current status. Adv Vet Sci Comp Med 1983;27:427–480.

Walker JB, Olwage A. The tick vectors of *Cowdria ruminantium* (Ixodoidea, Ixodidae, genus *Amblyomma*) and their distribution. Onderstepoort J Vet Res 1987;54:353–379.

Canine ehrlichiosis (canine rickettsiosis, tropical canine pancytopenia)

Caused by *Ehrlichia canis,* canine ehrlichiosis is principally of importance in Africa, Asia, and India, although it also exists in the United States, the Virgin Islands, and Puerto Rico. The disease is transmitted by the tick, *Rhipicephalus sanguineus.* The organism multiplies in reticuloendothelial cells, lymphocytes, and monocytes and may be visualized in stained smears of peripheral blood or tissue impressions, although visualization is often difficult. The life cycle of the parasite is not yet completely understood, but three intracellular forms can be recognized. Initial bodies are small (1 to 2 μ) spherical structures, which are believed to develop into larger bodies described as mulberry bodies, or morulae, composed of multiple subunits. The morula is thought to dissociate to small granules called elementary bodies. The disease is usually mild, except in young puppies or when complicated by another disease, such as infection with *Babesia canis.* In Asia, the disease has been called canine tropical pancytopenia. Most Canidae appear susceptible; German shepherds are reportedly more predisposed to serious infection than other breeds. Most infections in dogs are subclinical; reports indicate that from 11% to more than 50% of dogs have antibodies to *E. canis.* Human infection with *E. canis* has been reported. Dogs are also susceptible to *E. equi,* which is associated with a milder disease. Concurrent ehrlichiosis and babesiosis also occurs; the signs of babesiosis often overshadow those of ehrlichiosis.

SIGNS

Ewing (1965, 1969) describes the clinical signs as recurrent fever, serous nasal discharge, photophobia, vomiting, splenomegaly, and signs of central nervous system derangement. Epistaxis, emaciation, and edema of the limbs may also be observed (Hildebrandt and associates, 1973). Leukopenia, thrombocytopenia, anemia, and hypergammaglobulinemia, with increased levels of gamma globulin and glycoglobulin in the serum, are clinical features observed late in the disease. The clinical course runs from 4 weeks to several months. Subclinical chronic infection may last for years and may eventually result in severe chronic disease. Several authors have associated *E. canis* with polyarthritis, after having found ehrlichia morula in circulating neutrophils and neutrophils in synovial fluid.

LESIONS

The lesions encountered grossly consist of hemorrhages in the mucosae of the gastrointestinal and urogenital tracts and kidney, edematous or hemorrhagic enlargement of most lymph nodes, and edema of the limbs. Many animals are emaciated at the time of death, and epistaxis may be evident at this time. Rarely, icterus is observed (Hildebrandt and others, 1973).

The microscopic lesions consist of widespread perivascular accumulations of lymphoreticular and plasma cells, particularly in the meninges, kidneys, liver, and lymphopoietic tissues. The bone marrow is usually hypoplastic. Degeneration and acute necrosis is common in the center of lobules of the liver, presumably the result of anemia. There is also multifocal Kupffer's cell hyperplasia. In the spleen, there are crescent-shaped perifollicular hemorrhages. In the central nervous system, hemorrhages and plasma cell accumulations occur in the meninges, and occasionally lymphocytic and plasma cell infiltrations are present in the brain parenchyma.

Ehrlichia platys has also been identified recently as a cause of disease in dogs. Infection with this organism leads to severe but transient thrombocytopenia of uncertain pathogenesis. Parasitemia and thrombocytopenia occur in cycles of 10 to 14 days, giving rise to the term **infectious canine cyclic thrombocytopenia** for the disease.

DIAGNOSIS

The diagnosis may be confirmed by identifying the organisms in sections of tissues in fatal cases. Serologic identification of specific antibodies may be accomplished by an indirect immunofluorescence test. The organisms in tissues may also be identified by electron microscopy.

References

Anziani OS, Ewing SA, Barker RW. Experimental transmission of a granulocytic form of the tribe Ehrlichieae by *Dermacentor variabilis* and *Amblyomma americanum* to dogs. Am J Vet Res 1990;51:929–931.

Baker DC, Simpson M, Gaunt SD, et al. Acute *Ehrlichia platys* infection in the dog. Vet Pathol 1987;24:449–453.

Bellah JR, Shull RM, Shull Selcer EV. *Ehrlichia canis*-related polyarthritis in a dog. J Am Vet Med Assoc 1986;189:922–923.

Buhles WC Jr, Huxsoll DL, Ristic M. Tropical canine pancytopenia: Clinical, hematologic, and serologic response of dogs to *Ehrlichia canis* infection, tetracycline therapy, and challenge inoculation. J Infect Dis 1974;130:357–367.

Codner EC, Farris-Smith LL. Characterization of the subclinical phase of ehrlichiosis in dogs. J Am Vet Med Assoc 1986;189:47–50.

Codner EC, Roberts RE, Ainsworth AG. Atypical findings in 16 cases of canine ehrlichiosis. J Am Vet Med Assoc 1985;186:166–169.

Cowell RL, Tyler RD, Clinkenbeard KD, et al. Ehrlichiosis and polyarthritis in three dogs. J Am Vet Med Assoc 1988;192:1093–1094.

Du Plessis JL, Fourie N, Nel PW, et al. Concurrent ehrlichiosis and babesiosis in the dog: blood smear examination supplemented by the indirect fluorescent antibody test, using *Cowdria ruminantium* as antigen. Onderstepoort J Vet Res 1990;57:151–155.

Ewing SA. Canine ehrlichiosis. Adv Vet Sci 1969;13:331–353.

Ewing SA, Buckner RG. Manifestations of babesiosis, ehrlichiosis, and combined infections in the dog. Am J Vet Res 1965;26:815–828.

Groves MG, Dennis GL, Amyx HL, et al. Transmission of *Ehrlichia canis* to dogs by ticks (*Rhipicephalus sanguineus*). Am J Vet Res 1975;36:937–940.

Harvey JW, Simpson CF, Gaskin JM. Cyclic thrombocytopenia induced by a *Rickettsia*-like agent in dogs. J Infect Dis 1978;137:182–188.

Hildebrandt PK, et al. Pathology of canine ehrlichiosis (tropical canine pancytopenia). Am J Vet Res 1973;34:1309–1320.

Huxsoll DL, et al. *Ehrlichia canis*—the causative agent of a haemorrhagic disease of dogs. Vet Rec 1969;85:587.

Keefe TJ, Holland CJ, Salyer PE, et al. Distribution of *Ehrlichia canis* among military working dogs in the world and selected civilian dogs in the United States. J Am Vet Med Assoc 1982;181:236–238.

Kuehn NF, Gaunt SD. Clinical and hematologic findings in canine ehrlichiosis. J Am Vet Med Assoc 1985;186:355–358.

Leeflang P, Perie NM. A comparative study of the pathogenicities of Old and New World strains of *Ehrlichia canis*. Trop Anim Health Prod 1972;4:107–108.

Nims RM, et al. Epizootiology of tropical canine pancytopenia in Southeast Asia. J Am Vet Med Assoc 1971;158:53–63.

Madewell BR, Gribble DH. Infection in two dogs with an agent resembling *Ehrlichia equi*. J Am Vet Med Assoc 1982;180:512–514.

Maeda K, et al. Human infection with *Ehrlichia canis*, a leukocytic rickettsia. N Engl J Med 1987;316:853–856.

Nyindo M, et al. Cell-mediated and humoral immune responses of German Shepherd dogs and Beagles to experimental infection with *Ehrlichia canis*. Am J Vet Res 1980;41:250–254.

Pyle RL: Canine ehrlichiosis. J Am Vet Med Assoc 1980;177:1197–1199.

Reardon MJ, Pierce KR. Acute experimental canine ehrlichiosis. I. Sequential reaction of the hemic and lymphoreticular systems. II. Sequential reaction of the hemic and lymphoreticular system of selectively immunosuppressed dogs. Vet Pathol 1981;18:48–61, 384–395.

Seamer J, Snape T. *Ehrlichia canis* and tropical canine pancytopaenia. Res Vet Sci 1972;13:307–314.

Simpson CF. Structure of *Ehrlichia canis* in blood monocytes of a dog. Am J Vet Res 1972;33:2451–2454.

Walker JS, et al. Clinical and clinicopathologic findings in tropical canine pancytopenia. J Am Vet Med Assoc 1970;157:43–55.

Ziemer EL, Keenan DP, Madigan JE. *Ehrlichia equi* infection in a foal. J Am Vet Med Assoc 1987;190:199–200.

Ovine and bovine ehrlichiosis ("tick-borne fever," "mild disease of sheep")

Febrile disease of a mild, nonfatal nature, associated with tick infestation in both sheep and cattle, was first recognized in Scotland in 1932. The disease is caused by a rickettsial organism called *Ehrlichia phagocytophila* or *Cytoecetes phagocytophila* (*Rickettsia phagocytophila* or *Cytoecetes bovis*). It is transmitted by the tick *Ixodes ricinus*. Goats and other ruminants are also susceptible. The disease occurs in Great Britain, Ireland, Norway, the Netherlands, Finland, Austria, the Middle East, India, and South Africa.

The infections have not been well characterized. The principal clinical finding is fever of several days' duration. Lymphopenia followed by neutropenia and thrombocytopenia are consistent findings. The lymphopenia is principally the result of a decline in B lymphocytes with an accompanying suppression of humoral immune response. The infection often occurs in conjunction with other infectious diseases, which it also has been experimentally shown to exacerbate.

DIAGNOSIS

Diagnosis is made by identifying the organisms in circulating granulocytes and monocytes. They are visible in up to 50% of circulating cells and may remain visible for periods from several weeks to as long as 2 years. Giemsa or Wright-Leishman stains are best for identification. The disease is not fatal, and few pathologic features are associated with infection other than splenomegaly.

References

Buchanan RE, Gibbons NE. Bergey's Manual of Determinative Bacteriology. 8th ed. Baltimore: Williams & Wilkins 1974;894–895.

Foster WNM, Cameron AE. Thrombocytopenia in sheep associated with experimental tickborne fever infection. J Comp Pathol 1968;78:251–254.

Foster WNM, Foggie A, Hisbet DI. Haemorrhagic enteritis in sheep experimentally infected with tickborne fever. J Comp Pathol 1968;78:255–258.

Gordon WS, Brownlee A, Wilson DR, et al. Tickborne fever. J Comp Pathol 1932;45:301–312.

Hudson JR. The recognition of tickborne fever as a disease of cattle. Br Vet J 1950;106:3–17.

Woldehiwet Z. Tick-borne fever: a review. Vet Res Commun 1983;6:163–175.

Equine ehrlichiosis

This disease, caused by *Ehrlichia equi,* has been chiefly described as occurring in the foothills of northern California but has been sporadically reported elsewhere in the United States, including the East Coast. In California, the occurrence is seasonal, with the greatest incidence during late fall, winter, and spring. The disease can be transmitted via blood-containing organisms, and ticks are suspected but not yet proved to transmit the disease in nature. Sheep, goats, dogs, cats, and monkeys are experimentally susceptible, but they develop only a mild disease. Details of the infection in horses have been studied by Gribble (1969), Stannard and colleagues (1969), and Madigan and Gribble (1987).

SIGNS

The infection is more serious in horses over 3 years of age. The clinical features include fever, anorexia, depression, edema of the legs, and ataxia. Clinical laboratory findings include leukopenia, thrombocytopenia, elevated plasma icterus index, decreased packed cell volume, and lymphopenia. The organisms appear as granular bodies in the cytoplasm of neutrophils and eosinophils.

LESIONS

The experimentally induced lesions in horses and donkeys are seen grossly as petechiae, ecchymoses, and edema in muscles, fascia, and subcutis. Icterus and orchitis are common. The microscopic lesions consist of arteritis and phlebitis, particularly in muscles and fascia, but also in kidneys, heart, brain, and lungs. The blood vessels undergo necrosis as well as swelling of endothelium and smooth muscle cells. This is accompanied by accumulation of lymphocytes, plasma cells, and occasionally neutrophils.

DIAGNOSIS

The diagnosis is made on the basis of clinical findings and may be confirmed by the demonstration of organisms in neutrophils or eosinophils. They stain characteristically blue with Giemsa's or Wright-Leishman's stain and are gram-positive. The organisms are spherical, single or multiple, and vary in size from 200 mμ to 5 μ in diameter. The pleomorphic organisms, with two peripheral membranes, may be demonstrated with the electron microscope.

References

Gribble DH. Equine ehrlichiosis. J Am Vet Med Assoc 1969;155:462–469.

Lewis GE Jr, Huxsoll DL, Ristic M, et al. Experimentally induced infection of dogs, cats, and nonhuman primates with *Ehrlichia equi* etiologic agent of equine ehrlichiosis. Am J Vet Res 1975;36:85–88.

Madigan JE, Gribble D. Equine ehrlichiosis in northern California: 49 cases (1968–1981). J Am Vet Med Assoc 1987;190:445–448.

Madigan JE, Hietala S, Chalmers S, et al. Seroepidemiologic survey of antibodies to *Ehrlichia equi* in horses of northern California. J Am Vet Med Assoc 1990;196:1962–1964.

Sells DM, et al. Ultrastructural observations on *Ehrlichia equi* organisms in equine granulocytes. Infect Immun 1976; 13:273–280.

Stannard AA, Gribble DH, Smith RS. Equine ehrlichiosis: A disease with similarities to tick-borne fever and bovine petechiae fever. Vet Rec 1969;84:149–150.

Potomac Horse Fever (Equine Monocytic Ehrlichiosis, Equine Ehrlichial Colitis)

This disease, caused by *Ehrlichia risticii*, was first recognized near the Potomac River in 1979. Although most reports have emanated from Maryland and Virginia, the disease has been recognized across the United States to and including California, as well as abroad. The causative organism is antigenically related to *E. sennetsu*, the cause of human sennetsu rickettsiosis (ehrlichiosis; "infectious mononucleosis"; glandular fever; Hyuga fever; Kagami fever), a disease essentially limited to Western Japan. *E. risticii* is also related to *E. canis*. Potomac horse fever is seasonal, occurring in the summer months with most cases in July and August. This suggests an arthropod vector as with other *Ehrlichia* organisms, but an intermediate host has not yet been identified. Inoculation studies and serologic surveys indicate that cats and dogs are susceptible.

SIGNS

The signs in affected horses are initially characterized by fever, followed by anorexia, depression, colic, and diarrhea. The fever can be biphasic. There is leukopenia, with a decrease in neutrophils, lymphocytes, and eosinophils, and thrombocytopenia. A rebound leukocytosis may follow. The organisms are visible in circulating monocytes, but they are small, not numerous, and easily missed. There may also be anemia. Diarrhea can be explosive, leading to dehydration and shock. Laminitis may follow. Mortality rates are as high as 30%.

LESIONS

Pathologically, there are no diagnostic lesions. Most commonly, the cecum and colon are congested, hemorrhagic, and often eroded or ulcerated. The contents are watery. The stomach and small intestines are less severely affected. Organisms occur in the cytoplasm of colonic epithelium, and macrophages in the lamina propria. Mesenteric lymph nodes are enlarged and congested and may contain hemorrhage. The subcutaneous tissues of the thorax, abdomen, and often the legs are edematous. Lesions of laminitis are common.

DIAGNOSIS

The diagnosis is confirmed by demonstrating the organism in circulating monocytes or colonic epithelium. An indirect fluorescent antibody test has been developed but may not be positive during the acute phase of the disease. Recovered horses have positive results on the test. Other causes of acute gastrointestinal disease must be considered, such as salmonellosis and viral diseases. The **pathogenesis** of the lesions has yet to be defined.

References

Brewer BD, Harvey JW, Mayhew IG, et al. Ehrlichiosis in a Florida horse. J Am Vet Med Assoc 1984;185:446–447.

Cordes DO, Perry BD, Rikihisa Y, et al. Enterocolitis caused by *Ehrlichia* sp. in the horse (Potomac horse fever). Vet Pathol 1986;23:471–477.

Dawson JE, Abeygunawardena I, Holland CJ, et al. Susceptibility of cats to infection with *Ehrlichia risticii*, causative agent of equine monocytic ehrlichiosis. Am J Vet Res 1988;49:2096–2100.

Dutta SK, Penney BE, Myrup AC, et al. Disease features in horses with induced equine monocytic ehrlichiosis (Potomac horse fever). Am J Vet Res 1988;49:1747–1751.

Holland CJ, Ristic M, Cole AI, et al. Isolation, experimental transmission, and characterization of causative agent of Potomac horse fever. Science 1985;227:522–524.

Olchowy TWJ, Ames TR, Molitor TW. Serodiagnosis of equine monocytic ehrlichiosis in selected groups of horses in Minnesota. J Am Vet Med Assoc 1990;196:1967–1970.

Palmer JE, Whitlock RH, Benson CE. Equine ehrlichial colitis (Potomac horse fever): recognition of the disease in Pennsylvania, New Jersey, New York, Ohio, Idaho, and Connecticut. J Am Vet Med Assoc 1986;189:197–199.

Perry BD, et al. Epidemiology of Potomac horse fever: an investigation into the possible role of non-equine mammals. Vet Rec 1989;125:83–86.

Rikihisa Y, Reed SM, Sams RA, et al. Serosurvey of horses with evidence of equine monocytic ehrlichiosis. J Am Vet Med Assoc 1990;197:1327–1332.

Ristic M, Holland CJ, Dawson JE, et al. Diagnosis of equine monocytic ehrlichiosis (Potomac horse fever) by indirect immunofluorescence. J Am Vet Med Assoc 1986;189:39–46.

Ristic M, Dawson J, Holland CJ, et al. Susceptibility of dogs to infection with *Ehrlichia risticii*, causative agent of equine monocytic ehrlichiosis (Potomac horse fever). Am J Vet Res 1988;49:1497–1500.

Robl MG. Potomac horse fever: closing in on an unknown killer. Vet Med Small Anim Clin 1985;80(10):49–58,

Schmidtmann ET, Robl MG, Carroll JF. Attempted transmission of *Ehrlichia risticii* by field-captured *Dermacentor variabilis* (Acari: Ixodidae). Am J Vet Res 1986;47:2393–2395.

Steele KE, Rikihisa Y, Walton AM. Ehrlichia of Potomac horse fever identified with a silver stain. Vet Pathol 1986;23:531–533.

Ziemer EL, Whitlock RH, Palmer JE, et al. Clinical and hematologic variables in ponies with experimentally induced equine ehrlichial colitis (Potomac horse fever). Am J Vet Res 1987;48:63–67.

Bovine petechial fever (ondiri disease)

An infrequent disease confined to high altitudes of Kenya, bovine petechial fever resembles erlichiosis in clinical signs and gross lesions. The causative agent, named by Tyzzer in 1938, is *Cytoecetes ondiri,* a member of the family Rickettsiaceae, whose exact characterization and classification, however, is unclear. The infection is often confined to particular paddocks or woodlots, and the organism is suspected but not proven to be carried by an arthropod vector. Disease is usually mild, may be latent, and is only rarely fatal. There is fever, and petechiae may be visible on mucosal surfaces. Leukopenia, characterized by a drop in neutrophils, lymphocytes, and eosinophils and thrombocytopenia are present. In severe cases, extensive hemorrhage and enlargement of lymph nodes are more extensive than in milder cases. Organisms are demonstrable in circulating neutrophils and monocytes during infection and for 4 weeks or so after recovery.

References

Cooper JE. Attempted transmission of the Ondiri disease (bovine petechial fever) agent to laboratory rodents. Res Vet Sci 1973;15:130–133.

Danks WBC. (First description of bovine petechial fever). Annu Report Agri Dept, Kenya 1933;375.

Davies FG, Odegaard OA, Cooper JE. The morphology of the causal agent of bovine petechial fever (Ondiri disease). J Comp Pathol 1972;82:241–246.

Dawe PS, Ohder H, Wegener J, et al. Some observations on bovine petechial fever (Ondiri disease) passaged in sheep. Bull Epizoot Dis Afr 1970;18:361–368.

Jaffery MS, Mwangota AU. Hyperacute bovine petechial fever. Vet Rec 1974;95:212–213.

Snodgrass DR. Pathogenesis of bovine petechial fever. Latent infections, immunity, and tissue distribution of *Cytoecetes ondiri.* J Comp Pathol 1975;85:523–530.

Snodgrass DR, Karstad LH, Cooper JE. The role of wild ruminants in the epidemiology of bovine petechial fever. J Hyg 1975;4:245–250.

Walker AR, Cooper JE, Snodgrass DR. Investigations into the epidemiology of bovine petechial fever in Kenya and the potential of trombiculid mites as vectors. Trop Anim Health Prod 1974;6:193–198.

Colesiota Conjunctivitis

A rickettsial-like organism termed *Colesiota conjunctivae (Rickettsia conjunctivae; Ricolesia bovis; R. conjunctivae bovis)* has been found in association with conjunctivitis in sheep, goats, and cattle, principally in South Africa. The organism is so poorly classified that it is not possible to ascertain its taxonomic position nor whether multiple organisms are involved. Conjunctivitis and keratoconjunctivitis in chickens in South Africa is caused by another organism, *Colesiota conjunctivae-galli (Ricolesia conjunctivae). Ricolesia lestoquardii (Rickettsia conjunctivae-suis)* causes conjunctivitis and keratitis in swine. Organisms may be visualized in conjunctival epithelial cells.

DISEASES CAUSED BY BARTONELLACEAE

Diseases caused by organisms presently classified in the family Bartonellaceae are considered here (Table 9-5). These small, markedly pleomorphic organisms are found in erythrocytes of several species. The organisms take Giemsa's stain intensely, but are only lightly stained with aniline dyes. They are gram-negative and are distinguished from protozoa by the absence of recognizable cytoplasm around their nucleus.

Two genera currently make up this family: *Bartonella* and *Grahamella*; each of them contains parasitic species. *Bartonella bacilliformis,* the only species now recognized in this genus, is the cause of a disease syndrome of humans called Oroya fever, verruga peruviana, or Carrion's disease. This organism parasitizes the erythrocytes, reticuloendothelial system, and vascular endothelium, occurring in the form of tiny polymorphous cocci and rods. Human bartonellosis is of considerable importance in South America, particularly in Peru and Colombia, but also occurs in Central America. It is transmitted by several species of *Phlebotomus.*

The second genus, *Grahamella,* consists of rod-shaped to club-shaped organisms, 0.1 to 1.0 μ in size, which occur in the erythrocytes of several hosts. Two species, *Grahamella talpae,* a parasite of voles, and *Grahamella peromysci,* a parasite of deer mice, are currently recognized. These organisms stain light blue with Giemsa's stain; the club-shaped ends of the organism are usually a darker blue.

DISEASES CAUSED BY ANAPLASMATACEAE

In the present scheme of classification, the family Anaplasmataceae (order Rickettsiales) now contains organisms grouped in five genera (*Bergey's Manual of Systematic Bacteriology,* 1984). These genera are *Anaplasma,*

TABLE 9-5 **Diseases caused by Bartonellaceae**

Organism	Vectors	Hosts	Disease
Bartonella bacilliformis	*Phlebotomus sp.*	Humans	Human bartonellosis (Oroya fever, *Verruga peruviana*)
Grahamella talpae	Unknown	Moles (*Talpa sp.*)	Erythrocytes parasitized
G. peromysci	Unknown	Deer, mice (*Peromyscus leucopus novaboracensis*)	Erythrocytes parasitized

Paranaplasma, Aegyptianella, Haemobartonella, and *Eperythrozoon.* These organisms are obligate parasites, found on or within erythrocytes or free in the plasma of wild and domestic vertebrates. Stained with Giemsa's stain, the organisms appear rod-shaped, spherical, coccoid, or ring-shaped; reddish-violet; and 0.2 to 0.4 μm in diameter. Each organism is enclosed in a membrane with an internal structure that resembles rickettsiae (Fig. 9-4). The organisms may occur in short chains or irregular groups within erythrocytes or in plasma. They are gram-negative, are not acid-fast, multiply by binary fission, and are transmitted by arthropods. Anemia is the usual clinical feature manifested in infected animals.

Anaplasmosis

The organisms responsible for anaplasmosis are presently grouped into a single genus, *Anaplasma.* Three species are of pathogenic importance: *Anaplasma marginale, A. centrale,* and *A. ovis* (Table 9-6). With Romanowsky-type stains, such as Giemsa's, these organisms appear as dense, bluish-purple, homogeneous round structures within erythrocytes near the margin or in the center of the cell. With the electron microscope, these structures are separated from the cytoplasm of the erythrocyte by a membrane that encloses one to eight subunits, or initial bodies, which are the parasitic bacteria. The organisms are each 0.3 to 0.4 μm in diameter and enclose electron-lucid plasma, in which are embedded electron-dense aggregates of fine granular material (Fig. 9-5).

Within the genus **Paranaplasma** are two organisms,

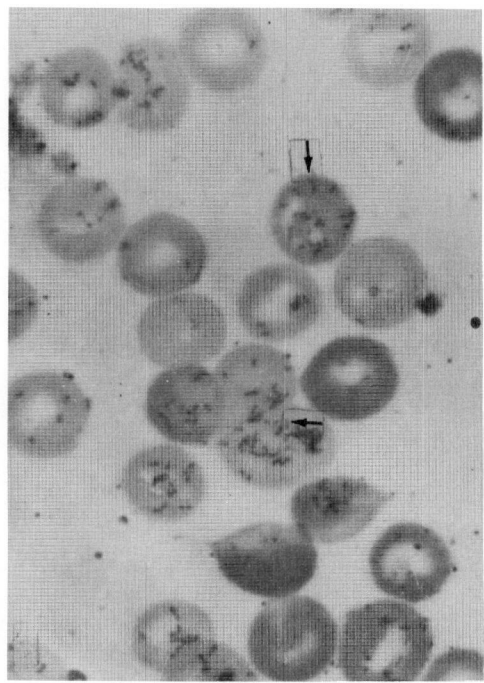

FIG. 9-4 *Bartonella* organisms *(arrows)* in human blood (× 1650).

P. caudatum (A. caudatum) and **P. discoides (A. discoides).** These are found in cattle infected with *Anaplasma marginale* (Kreier and Ristic, 1963) and may be distinguished by their predilection for infection of cattle over deer or sheep and by their distinctive morphology. By electron microscopy and fluorescent antibody stain, *P. caudatum* is seen to have a distinctive body and an appendage, which may resemble a tail, loop, or ring, connecting two organisms into a dumbbell shape. *Paranaplasma discoides* may be distinguished in waterlysed erythrocytes, using phase microscopy, as ovoid, disc-shaped structures with a dense mass at each pole. The pathogenic effect of these two organisms is not clearly established.

Anaplasma marginale, which parasitizes the red cells of cattle, causes an important disease of worldwide distribution. Deer and a number of other wild ruminants are susceptible. Sheep and goats can be infected but do not develop disease. In cattle, the disease is unusual in that infection results in overt disease only in adult animals (similar to babesiosis); most young calves undergo an inapparent infection unless splenectomized before exposure. Parasitemia, however, may remain in these animals (as well in recovered adults), and they can serve as a continuous source of infection for naive cattle.

The organism, *Anaplasma marginale,* is a tiny, spherical body, 0.3 to 0.8 μm in diameter, which is found within the cytoplasm of erythrocytes near the periphery of the cell. It is best demonstrated in blood smears with Giemsa's stain. Studies by Ristic and Watrach (1963) indicate that four developmental stages of *Anaplasma* species are recognizable in infected erythrocytes. These stages are *(a)* early stage, consisting of **initial bodies,** the infective form; *(b)* mixed population with marginal and initial bodies; *(c)* vigorous growth and transfer; and *(d)* massive multiplication with a predominance of marginal bodies. According to these investigators, the organisms reproduce by binary fission and pass through the four stages of development after penetration of the erythrocytic cell membrane by initial bodies, and then they are transferred to other mature erythrocytes by direct contact between cells. Simpson and co-workers (1967) described the initial body as spherical and surrounded by a double membrane. The marginal body contains up to six subunits (initial bodies) and is surrounded by a single membrane.

TRANSMISSION

The infection can be transmited to a normal animal by carrying over a minute amount of blood. This can occur by the use of improperly sterilized phlebotomy needles or by dehorning or castration without previous aseptic precautions, but usually in nature, it is spread by bites of ticks (*Boophilus annulatus, Dermacentor andersoni, D. occidentalis, D. variabilis,* and others), biting flies (*Tabanus* species), and less often by mosquitoes (*Psorophora* species). Ticks are the most important vectors, because they can carry the organisms for long periods of time. The transfer in utero between bovine

TABLE 9-6 **Diseases caused by Anaplasmataceae**

Organism	Vectors	Hosts	Disease
Anaplasma marginale	Ticks, horseflies	Cattle, zebu, water buffalo, bison, deer, elk, camel, blesbuck, and duiker	Severe anaplasmosis
A. centrale	Ticks, horseflies	Cattle	Mild anaplasmosis
A. ovis	Ticks, horseflies	Sheep and goats	Mild to severe anaplasmosis
Paranaplasma caudatum	Probably ticks and horseflies	Cattle	Mixed infection with *A. marginale*
P. discoides	Probably ticks and horseflies	Cattle	Mixed infection with *A. marginale*
Aegyptianella pullorum (*A. granulosa, A. granulosa penetrans, Babesia pullorum, Balouria anserina, B. gallinarum, Spirochaeta granulosa penetrans*)	Ticks (*Argas persicus*)	Chickens, geese, ducks, turkeys, guinea fowl, pigeons, quail, ostrich	Aegyptianellosis
Haemobartonella muris (*Bartonella muris*)	Rat louse (*Polyplax spinulosa*)	Albino mouse, albino rat, some wild mice, hamster	Anemia only following splenectomy
H. felis (*Eperythrozoon felis*)	Unknown	Domestic cat	Hemobartonellosis
H. canis (*Bartonella canis*)	Unknown	Domestic dog	Anemia only after splenectomy
Eperythrozoon coccoides (*Gyromorpha musculi*)	Mouse louse (*Polyplax serrata*)	Albino and wild mice, albino rats, rabbits, and hamsters	Eperythrozoonosis
E. ovis	Horsefly, other arthropods	Sheep, goats, deer	Anemia
E. suis	Unknown	Swine	"Icteroanemia"
E. parvum	Pig louse (*Haematopinus suis*)	Swine	Anemia after splenectomy
E. wenyonii (*Haemobartonella wenyonii*)	Unknown	Cattle	Anemia after splenectomy

mother and fetus has also been reported. The presence of carriers has long posed a problem in the control of disease. The detection of such carriers is rarely possible by examination of blood smears, but a complement-fixation test can be used to detect carriers.

SIGNS

Fever of short duration is manifest in adult cattle but may be undetected or overshadowed by the later findings. Anemia is the essential effect produced by the organism and is manifested by weakness, pallor of mucosae, accelerated respiration, jaundice, decreased red blood cell count, decreased hemoglobin level, and occasionally by muscular trembling, depression, anorexia, and excessive salivation. Anemia results from increased destruction of parasitized erythrocytes by the reticuloendothelial system and not by hemolysis; therefore, hemoglobinuria is not seen. Immune mechanisms are

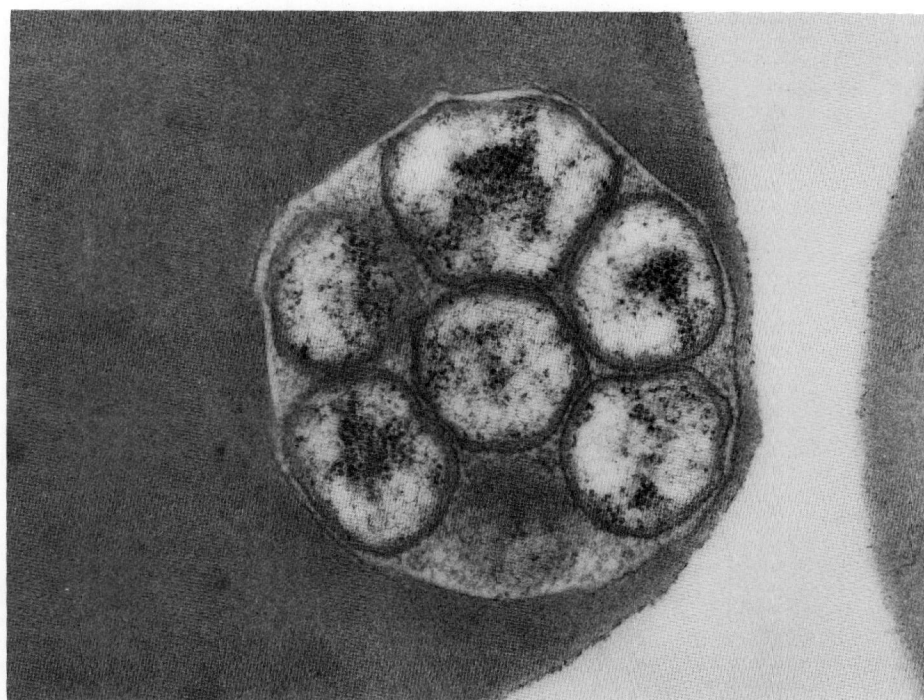

FIG. 9-5. *Anaplasma marginale.* An anaplasma body (marginal body) containing six subunits (initial bodies) (× 60,000). (Courtesy of Dr. C. T. Simpson and *American Journal of Veterinary Research.*)

most likely involved in phagocytosis and destruction of erythrocytes. Death occurs in many cases, but recovery is not infrequent; the recovered animals remain carriers of the infection for some time.

LESIONS

The gross postmortem findings in fatal cases are those of severe anemia, with pallor of the tissues and occasionally with icterus. The spleen is usually greatly enlarged, with reddish-brown pulp and enlarged splenic follicles. The liver is enlarged and has rounded edges, and it is yellowish in cases with icterus. The gallbladder is usually distended, with dark grumous bile. Petechiae may be encountered in the pericardium, and catarrhal inflammation may be evident in the gastrointestinal tract. The microscopic findings indicate severe demands on the hematopoietic system, with hyperplasia of the bone marrow and extramedullary hematopoiesis in the spleen and other organs. *Anaplasma* organisms can be demonstrated (with difficulty) in erythrocytes in tissue sections.

The number of organisms demonstrable in smears of peripheral blood is highly variable. Before the onset of anemia, the majority of erythrocytes may harbor organisms, but, with the sudden removal from the circulation, their numbers decrease. Immature erythrocytes (reticulocytes) that enter the circulation in response to the anemia are, for reasons poorly understood, resistant to the parasites.

Whether *Anaplasma centrale* warrants consideration as a separate species is doubtful; it may be a variant of *A. marginale.* It produces a mild infection in cattle, and has been employed to immunize cattle to *A. marginale.*

A. centrale usually localizes near the center of the red blood cell.

Anaplasma ovis is infectious for sheep and goats; cattle are not susceptible. The disease is mild, only rarely resulting in clinical signs of anemia.

DIAGNOSIS

The diagnosis is made on the basis of the clinical signs and demonstration of *Anaplasma* organisms in erythrocytes. The complement-fixation test can be used for the detection of clinically silent carriers.

References

Christensen JF, Howarth JA. Anaplasmosis transmission by *Dermacentor occidentalis* taken from cattle in Santa Barbara County, California. Am J Vet Res 1966;27:1473–1475.

Cox FR, Dimopoullos GT. Demonstration of an autoantibody associated with anaplasmosis. Am J Vet Res 1972;33:73–76.

Espana C, Espana EM, Gonzalez D. Anaplasma marginale. I. Studies with phase contrast and electron microscopy. Am J Vet Res 1959;20:795–805.

Fowler D, Swift BL. Abortion in cows inoculated with *Anaplasma marginale.* Theriogenology 1975;4:59–67.

Franklin TE, Redmond HE. Observations on the morphology of *Anaplasma marginale* with reference to projections or tails. Am J Vet Res 1958;19:252–253.

Jones EW, Kleiwer IO, Norman BB, et al. *Anaplasma marginale* infection in young and aged cattle. Am J Vet Res 1968;29:535–544.

Jones EW, Norman BB, Kliewer IO, et al. *Anaplasma marginale* infection in splenectomized calves. Am J Vet Res 1968;29:523–533.

Keeton KS, Jain NC. Scanning electron microscopic studies of *Paranaplasma* sp. in erythrocytes of a cow. J Parasitol 1973;59:331–336.

Kocan KM, Yellin TN, Ewing SA, et al. Morphology of colonies of *Anaplasma marginale* in nymphal *Dermacentor andersoni.* Am J Vet Res 1984;45:1434–1440.

Kreier JP, Ristic M, Schroeder W. Anaplasmosis. XVI. The pathogenesis of anemia produced by infection with anaplasma. Am J Vet Res 1964;25:343–352.

Kuttler KL. Clinical and hematologic comparison of *Anaplasma marginale* and *Anaplasma centrale* infections in cattle. Am J Vet Res 1966;27:941–946.

Lotze JC, Yiengst MJ. Mechanical transmission of bovine anaplasmosis by the horsefly, *Tabanus sulcifrons* (Macquart). Am J Vet Res 1941;2:323–326.

Lotze JC, Yiengst MJ. Studies on the nature of anaplasma. Am J Vet Res 1942;3:312–320.

Piercy PL. Transmission of anaplasmosis. Ann NY Acad Sci 1956;64:40–48.

Potgieter FT, Kocan KM, McNew RW, et al. Demonstration of colonies of *Anaplasma marginale* in the midgut of *Rhipicephalus simus*. Am J Vet Res 1983;44:2256–2261.

Ristic M, Watrach AM. Studies in anaplasmosis. II. Electron microscopy of *Anaplasma marginale* in deer. Am J Vet Res 1961;22:109–166.

Ristic M, Watrach AM. Anaplasmosis. VI. Studies and a hypothesis concerning the cycle of development of the causative agent. Am J Vet Res 1963;24:267–277.

Roby TO, et al. Immunity in bovine anaplasmosis after elimination of *Anaplasma marginale* infections with imidocarb. Am J Vet Res 1974;35:993–995.

Ryff JF, Weibel JL, Thomas GM. Relationship of ovine to bovine anaplasmosis. Cornell Vet 1964;54:407–414.

Schmidt H. Manifestations and diagnosis of anaplasmosis. Ann NY Acad Sci 1956;64:27–30.

Schroeder WF, Ristic M. Anaplasmosis. XVII. The relation of autoimmune processes to anemia. Am J Vet Res 1965;26:239–245.

Simpson CF, Kling JM, Love JN. Morphologic and histochemical nature of *Anaplasma marginale*. Am J Vet Res 1967;28:1055–1065.

Smith RD, Woolf A, Hungerford LL, et al. Serologic evidence of *Anaplasma marginale* infection in Illinois white-tailed deer. J Am Vet Med Assoc 1982;181:1254–1256.

Summers WA, Padgett F. Electron microscopy of negatively stained *Anaplasma marginale*. Theiler, 1910. Am J Vet Res 1970;31:1679–1686.

Trueblood MS, Swift BL, Bear PD. Bovine fetal response to *Anaplasma marginale*. Am J Vet Res 1971;32:1089–1090.

Young MF, Kuttler KL, Adams LG. Experimentally induced anaplasmosis in neonatal isohemolytic anemia-recovered calves. Am J Vet Res 1977;38:1745–1747.

Zaugg JL. Bovine anaplasmosis: transplacental transmission as it relates to stage of gestation. Am J Vet Res 1985;46:570–572.

Zaugg JL, Kuttler KL. *Anaplasma marginale* infections in American bison: experimental infection and serologic study. Am J Vet Res 1985;46:438–441.

Zaugg JL, Stiller D, Coan ME, et al. Transmission of *Anaplasma marginale* Theiler by males of *Dermacentor andersoni* Stiles fed on an Idaho field-infected, chronic carrier cow. Am J Vet Res 1986;47:2269–2271.

Haemobartonellosis

Organisms of the genus *Haemobartonella* are currently classified in the family Anaplasmataceae (Table 9-6). The organisms are obligate parasites, found within shallow or deep indentations of the cell wall of red blood cells. The organisms occur as cocci or chains of coccoid organisms, in pairs or in groups, in indentations of the surface of erythrocytes. They stain well with Giemsa's stain but poorly with many other aniline dyes. They are not acid-fast, are gram-negative, and have a limiting membrane but not a cell wall or nucleus (Fig. 9-6). Growth of *Haemobartonella* organisms is inhibited by arsenicals and tetracyclines but not by penicillin or streptomycin. They have not been cultivated outside the host.

Only three species have been accepted as valid (*Bergey's Manual of Systematic Bacteriology*, 1984). These are *Haemobartonella muris*, *H. felis*, and *H. canis*. Several other species have been identified in various hosts and await validation as distinctive species. These include: *H. peromyscii* var *maniculata*, from the gray-backed deer mouse; *H. microtii*, the vole; *H. tyzzeri*, the guinea pig; *H. bovis*, cattle; *H. sturmanii*, buffalo; *H. peromyscii*, the deer mouse; *H. blarinae*, the short-tailed shrew; and *H. sciuri*, the gray squirrel. *Haemobartonella* infections of erythrocytes have also been reported in an owl monkey (*Aotus* species), rhesus monkeys, and squirrel monkeys (*Saimiri sciureus*). In most species, with the exception of the cat, the disease is mild or without clinical signs until the host is splenectomized. Removal of the spleen is followed by anemia in most infected animals.

References

Adams MR, Lewis JC, Bullock BC. Hemobartonellosis in squirrel monkeys (*Saimiri sciureus*) in a domestic breeding colony: case report and preliminary study. Lab Anim Sci 1984;34:82–85.

Baker HJ, Cassell GH, Lindsey JR. Research complications due to *Haemobartonella* and *Eperythrozoon* infections in experimental animals. Am J Pathol 1971;64:625–652.

Benjamin MM, Lumb WV. *Haemobartonella canis* infection in a dog. J Am Vet Med Assoc 1959;135:388–390.

Carr DT, Essex HE. Bartonellosis: a cause of severe anemia in splenectomized dogs. Proc Soc Exp Biol Med 1944;57:44–45.

Handcock WJ. Clinical haemobartonellosis associated with the use of corticosteroid. Vet Rec 1989;125:585.

Harvey JW. *Haemobartonella canis* in the blood of dogs with parvovirus disease. [letter] J Small Anim Pract 1982;23:800–801.

Ingle RT. *Bartonella* infection in a dog. North Am Vet 1946;27:501–502.

Lotze JC, Bowman GW. The occurrence of *Bartonella* in cases of anaplasmosis and in apparently normal cattle. Proc Helminth Soc Washington, DC. 1942;9:71–72.

McKeen AE, Ziegler RF, Giles RC. Scanning and transmission electron microscopy of *Haemobartonella canis* and *Eperythrozoon ovis*. Am J Vet Res 1973;34:1196–1201.

Mulhern CR. A note on two blood parasites of cattle, (*Spirochaeta theileri* and *Bartonella bovis*), recorded for the first time in Australia. Aust Vet 1946;22:118–119.

Peters W, Molyneux DH, Howells RE. *Eperythrozoon* and *Haemobartonella* in monkeys. Ann Trop Med Parasitol 1974;68:47–50.

Pryor WH, Bradbury RP. *Haemobartonella canis* infection in research dogs. Lab Anim Sci 1975;25:566–569.

Simpson CF, Love JN. Fine structure of *Haemobartonella bovis* in blood and liver of splenectomized calves. Am J Vet Res 1970;31:225–231.

Small E, Ristic M. Morphologic features of *Haemobartonella felis*. Am J Vet Res 1967;28:845–851.

Tanaka H, et al. Fine structure of *Haemobartonella muris* as compared with *Eperythrozoon coccoides* and *Mycoplasma pulmonis*. J Bact 1965;90:1735–1749.

Tyzzer EE. "Interference" in mixed infections of *Bartonella* and *Eperythrozoon* in mice. Am J Pathol 1941;17:141–153.

Tyzzer EE. A comparative study of *Grahamellae*, *Haemobartonellae* and *Eperythrozoa* in small mammals. Proc Am Philos Soc 1942;85:359–398.

Venable JH, Equing SA. Fine structure of *Hemobartonella canis* (Rickettsiales: Bartonellacea) and its relation to the host erythrocyte. J Parasitol 1968;54:259–268.

Weinman D. On the cause of the anemia in *Bartonella* infection of rats. J Infect Dis 1938;63:1–9.

West HJ. Haemobartonellosis in the dog. J Small Anim Pract 1979;20:543–549.

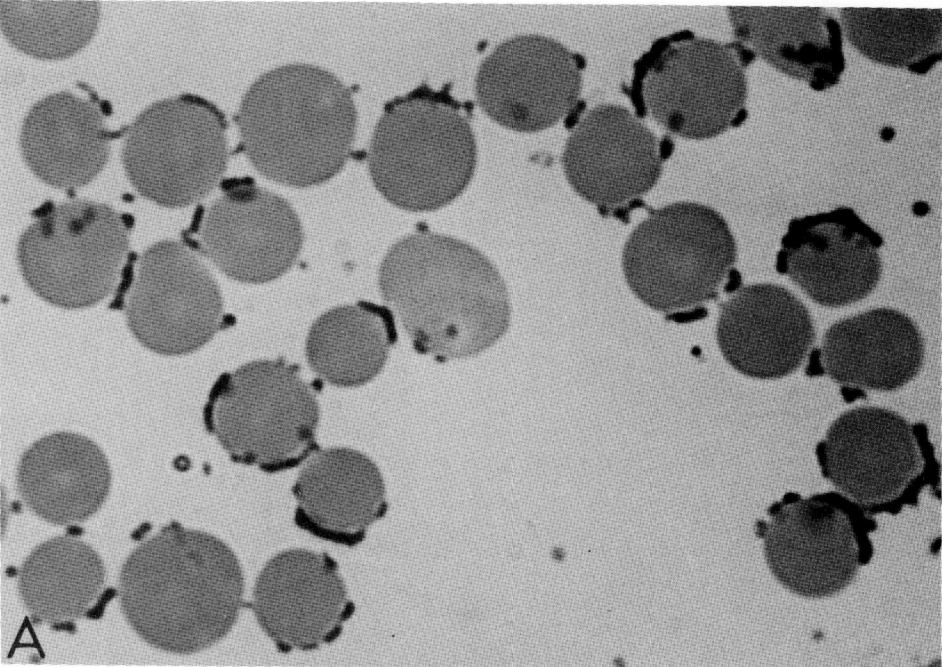

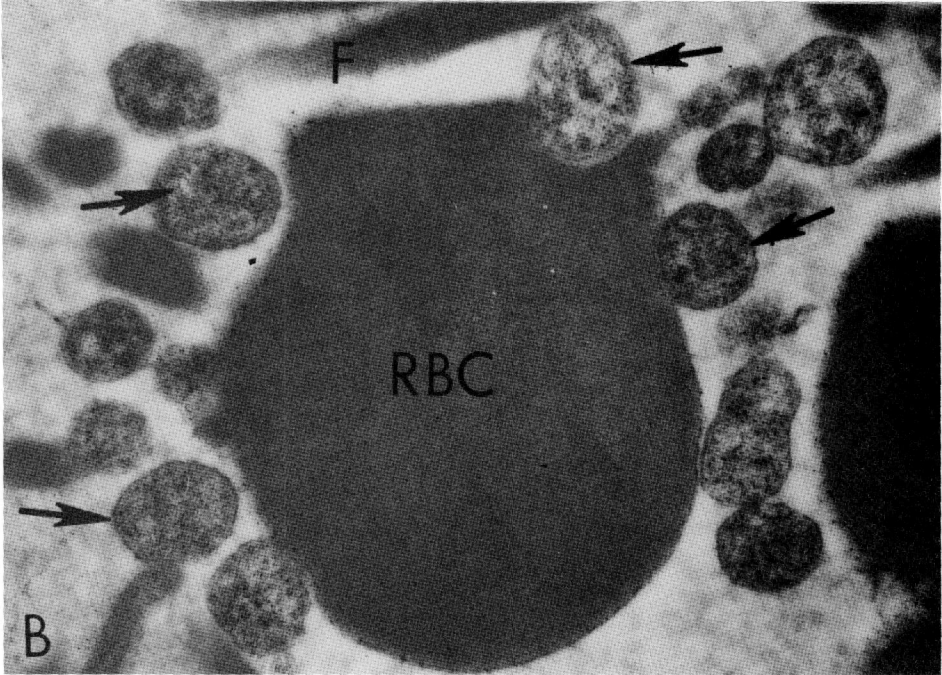

FIG. 9-6 *Haemobartonella bovis.* **A.** Organisms on periphery and surface of erythrocytes *(RBC)* from a splenectomized calf. **B.** Coccoid and rod-shaped organisms *(arrows)* on an erythrocyte (× 40,000). *F,* fibrin. (Courtesy of Dr. C. F. Simpson and *American Journal of Veterinary Research.*)

Feline infectious anemia (feline haemobartonellosis)

This disease of domestic and feral cats is caused by *Haemobartonella felis.* It is the only *Haemobartonella* infection of animals of importance as a cause of primary disease in its host. Even here, infection usually does not lead to disease in the absence of complicating factors, such as concurrent infection with feline leukemia virus or other insults that compromise the immune system.

Haemobartonella felis organisms are seen as small coccoid, ring-shaped, or rod-shaped bodies on erythrocytes of affected cats. These are best seen in blood smears stained with Giemsa's or Wright's stain (Fig. 9-7). The natural mode of transmission is not known; blood-sucking insects, such as fleas, are suspected. Experimentally, the injection of a small amount of blood containing parasitized erythrocytes can transmit the disease.

In its earliest stages, feline infectious anemia (haemobartonellosis) is manifested by fever, anorexia,

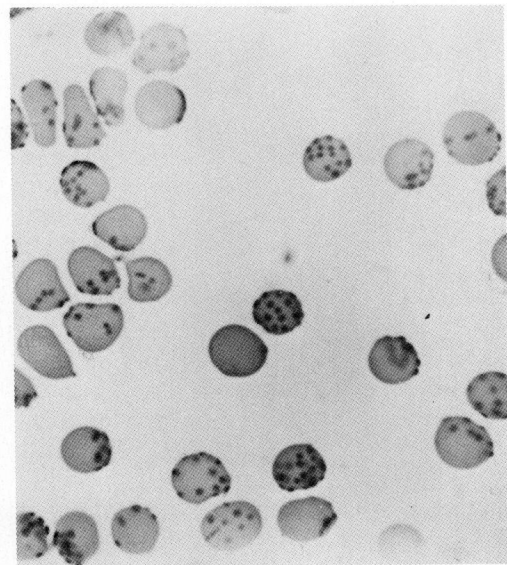

FIG. 9-7. *Haemobartonella felis* on the erythrocytes of cat with feline infectious anemia (Giemsa stain, × 1200). (Photograph by Dr. Rue Jensen; contributed by Dr. Jean C. Flint, Colorado State University.)

depression, and macrocytic, hemolytic anemia. The anemia is evidenced by pale, occasionally icteric, mucous membranes, weakness, and a characteristic blood picture, in which the hemoglobin and packed cell volumes are severely decreased. The hemoglobin levels usually decrease from a normal of 11 g/dL of blood to as low as 1.5 g/dL in severe cases. Levels of 6.0 g/dL of blood or lower are usually considered typical of this disease. Macrocytosis and anisocytosis are usually prominent features, and in early stages, nucleated erythrocytes are present in large numbers. Reticulocytes are also increased in number, and some of them may contain *Haemobartonella felis*. These organisms are not readily demonstrable in all stages of the disease, which complicates the diagnostic problem in many cases.

The leukocyte count in the acute stage is usually elevated, a point of diagnostic significance in eliminating panleukopenia, but as the disease progresses, the leukocyte count gradually falls. After a prolonged illness, leukopenia may be severe and abnormal "reticuloendothelial cells" may appear in the peripheral circulation.

Severely affected animals may die with evidence of a severe hemolytic anemia; others may recover, with or without treatment; and still others undergo relapses and eventually die after a prolonged illness.

LESIONS

The lesions are those of a hemolytic anemia. Icterus is a feature in some acute cases. The spleen is enlarged many times, and its cut surface is dark, firm, and bulges. Microscopically, this appearance is caused by congestion and extramedullary hematopoiesis. Hemo-

globin may stain the urine in the bladder, and hemorrhages may be present, particularly on serous surfaces. Fatty infiltration may be evident in the pale yellowish color of the liver, and central or paracentral necrosis may also be seen in microscopic sections of this organ. These changes are believed to be secondary to the anemia. The bone marrow is usually solidly red in the long bones and contains large numbers of hematopoietic cells in approximately normal proportions. The lymph nodes are usually grossly enlarged and moist in all parts of the body, and microscopic sections reveal that the enlargement is caused by reactive hyperplasia.

The lesions found at necropsy of animals that die after the prolonged illness are often subtle and are not clearly understood. The reactive hyperplasia of lymph nodes seen in the acutely fatal case is also a feature of the illness of longer duration, and the spleen may be large but not as hyperplastic. Icterus is rarely evident, and the bone marrow is hyperplastic. Ulceration of intestinal mucosae may be present, and sometimes hemorrhage may follow this ulceration. (Color plate II.)

References

Bobade PA, Nash AS, Rogerson P. Feline haemobartonellosis: clinical, haematological and pathological studies in natural infections and the relationship to infection with feline leukaemia virus. Vet Rec 1988;122:32–36.

Demaree RS Jr, Messmith WB. Ultrastructure of *Haemobartonella felis* from a naturally infected cat. Am J Vet Res 1972;33:1303–1308.

Flint JC, Moss LC. Infectious anemia in cats. J Am Vet Med Assoc 1953;122:45–48.

Flint JC, Roepke MH, Jensen R. Feline infectious anemia. I. Clinical aspects. Am J Vet Res 1958;19:165–168.

Flint JC, Roepke MH, Jensen R. Feline infectious anemia. II. Experimental cases. Am J Vet Res 1959;20:33–40.

Grindem CB, Corbett WT, Tomkins MT. Risk factors for *Haemobartonella felis* infection in cats. J Am Vet Med Assoc 1990;196:96–99.

Hatakka M. Haemobartonellosis in the domestic cat. Acta Vet Scand 1972;13:323–331.

Jain NC, Keeton KS. Scanning electron microscopic features of *Haemobartonella felis*. Am J Vet Res 1973;34:697–700.

Maede Y, Hata R. Studies on feline haemobartonellosis. II. The mechanism of anemia produced by infection with *Haemobartonella felis*. Jpn J Vet Sci 1975;37:49–54.

Maede Y, Sonoda M. Studies of the feline haemobartonellosis. III. Scanning electron microscopy of *Haemobartonella felis*. Jpn J Vet Sci 1975;37:209–211.

Small E, Ristic M. Morphologic features of *Haemobartonella felis*. Am J Vet Res 1967;28:845–851.

Eperythrozoonosis

The genus *Eperythrozoon* is presently grouped in the family Anaplasmataceae; the organisms are similar to *Haemobartonella* species and are often difficult to distinguish from them. The principal features differentiating *Haemobartonella* species from *Eperythrozoon* species are that eperythrozoa occur both in the erythrocytes of the host and in the plasma, whereas *Haemobartonella* organisms rarely are found free in the plasma and are seldom in ring forms, which are common in eperythrozoa. Five species of *Eperythrozoon* are currently accepted as valid (Table 9-6) (Kreier and Ristic, 1984). *E. coccoides* is a parasite of mice transmitted by the mouse louse (*Poly-*

plax serrata). It is widely distributed, but infection is generally subclinical. *E. suis* and *E. parvum* affect swine and are also widespread. *E. parvum* is not associated with disease, whereas *E. suis,* when parasitemia is high, results in clinical signs of anemia, a disease termed **icteroanemia.** Most infections are, however, subclinical. The mode of transmission is not established but probably involves insect vectors. Infection with *E. wenyonii,* a widespread parasite of cattle, can also cause mild anemia, but it is usually latent. In sheep, *E. ovis* infection is associated with hemolytic anemia. There are several reports of eperythrozoonosis in llamas.

Eperythrozoon organisms are seen in blood smears stained by Giemsa's method as tiny pleomorphic structures within the erythrocytes, lying on their surface or free in the plasma. The organisms are delicate pale purple to pinkish-purple and are predominantly ring-shaped, 0.5 to 1.0 μ in diameter or occasionally slightly larger. Triangular, ovoid, rod, dumbbell, and tennis-racket shapes may be seen. One to a dozen organisms may be present in a single red blood cell, and large numbers are uniformly distributed throughout the plasma. Organisms are much more numerous in blood smears taken at the height of infection.

The mode of transmission is not clearly established for all species of *Eperythrozoon,* but arthropods are generally suspected. *Eperythrozoon coccoides,* which infects mice, is transmitted by a louse, *Polyplax serrata.* Biting flies have been tentatively incriminated as vectors in other hosts. Experimental infection is greatly facilitated by the use of splenectomized animals.

SIGNS

Clinical disease caused by eperythrozoonosis is essentially restricted to sheep and swine; infection with the other eperythrozoa only causes anemia in splenectomized animals. In sheep and swine, evidence of infection may appear spontaneously, particularly in young animals exposed to other deleterious influences, such as helminthic parasitism, or may be brought forth by splenectomy of animals already harboring the infection. The natural disease in swine has been called "icteroanemia," and has similarities to anaplasmosis of herbivora. It is, of course, difficult to distinguish from anaplasmosis when sheep are involved. The symptoms start with fever (104°F to 107°F), which appears 6 to 10 days following exposure or splenectomy of animals with latent infection. This is accompanied by gradually increasing depression and weakness. The total red blood cell count drops precipitously to 1 to 2 million/mm^3, hemoglobin is decreased to 2 to 4 g/dL, and the packed red blood cell volume goes down to 4% to 7%. Hemoglobinuria has been noted in sheep, indicating the anemia is indeed hemolytic. The icteric index is elevated to 18 to 25, and the sedimentation rate is greatly accelerated, reaching 75 mm/min in some cases. The white blood cell count is usually not changed, although leukocytosis occurs in a few cases. Death may occur in an acute episode, as described, but animals recover more often and then are prone to have repeated recrudescences.

In cattle, the most usual sign of eperythrozoonosis is edema of the hind limbs and teats.

LESIONS

The gross lesions are compatible with the hemolytic anemia resulting from the effect of *Eperythrozoon* infection on the red blood cells. Icterus is a prominent feature; the blood is thin and watery; the liver is yellowish brown; and the gallbladder contains thick gelatinous bile. Hydropericardium and ascites are present in some cases, and the heart is pale and flabby. Petechiae may be seen in the mucosa of the urinary bladder. The bone marrow is predominantly red rather than fatty.

Microscopic changes are seen in the bone marrow, which is hyperplastic; the liver, which is rich in hemosiderin, shows some fatty change and central or paracentral necrosis of liver lobules. The latter is presumed to be an effect of anoxia. The organisms are difficult to demonstrate in tissue sections.

DIAGNOSIS

Eperythrozoonosis must be differentiated from anaplasmosis, haemobartonellosis, babesiosis, and other hemolytic anemias. The differentiation is most readily made by the precise identification of the causative organisms in the erythrocytes.

References

Adams EW, et al. Eperythrozoonosis in a herd of purebred Landrace pigs. J Am Vet Med Assoc 1959;135:226–228.

Daddow KN, Dunlop LB. The serological and microscopic monitoring of a natural outbreak of eperythrozoon infection in sheep. Queensland J Agric Anim Sci 1976;33:233–236. (Vet Bull 1978;48:4806.)

Keeton KS, Jain NC. *Eperythrozoon wenyoni:* a scanning electron microscope study. J Parasitol 1973;59:867–873.

Kreier JP, Ristic M. Morphologic, antigenic, and pathogenic characteristics of *Eperythrozoon ovis* and *Eperythrozoon wenyonii.* Am J Vet Res 1963;24:488–500.

Kreier JP, Ristic M. Genus IV. *Eperythrozoon* Schilling 1928, 1854. In: Krieg NR, Holt JG, ed. Bergey's Manual of Systematic Bacteriology. Vol. 1. Baltimore:Williams and Wilkins 1984;726–729.

Martin BJ, Chrisp CE, Averill DR Jr, et al. The identification of *Eperythrozoon ovis* in anemic sheep. Lab Anim Sci 1988;38:173–177.

McLaughlin BG, et al. An *Eperythrozoon*-like parasite in llamas. J Am Vet Med Assoc 1990;197:1170–1175.

Neitz WO. Eperythrozoonosis in sheep. Onderstepoort J Vet Sci Ind 1937;9:9–30.

Poole DBR, Cutler RS, Kelly WR, et al. *Eperythrozoon wenyoni* anaemia in cattle. Vet Rec 1976;99:481.

Purnell RE, Brocklesby DW, Young ER. *Eperythrozoon wenyoni,* a possible cause of anaemia in British cattle. Vet Rec 1976;98:411.

Reagan WJ, et al. The clinicopathologic, light, and scanning electron microscopic features of eperythrozoonosis in four naturally infected llamas. Vet Pathol 1990;27:426–431.

Smith JA, et al. *Eperythrozoon wenyonii* infection in dairy cattle. J Am Vet Med Assoc 1990;196:1244–1250.

Splitter EJ. *Eperythrozoon suis,* the etiologic agent of ictero-anemia or an anaplasmosis-like disease in swine. Am J Vet Res 1959;11:324–330.

Splitter EJ, Williamson RL. Eperythrozoonosis in swine. A preliminary report. J Am Vet Med Assoc 1950;116:360–364.

Sutton RH, Jolly RD. Experimental *Eperythrozoon ovis* infection of sheep. NZ Vet J 1973;21:160–166.

Zachary JF, Basgall EJ. Erythrocyte membrane alterations associated with the attachment and replication of *Eperythrozoon suis:* a light and electron microscopic study. Vet Pathol 1985;22:164–170.

Diseases caused by Chlamydiaceae

The organisms previously placed together as the psitta-cosis-lymphogranuloma-trachoma group are currently classified in a separate order, Chlamydiales; a single family, Chlamydiaceae, and one genus, *Chlamydia* (*Bergey's Manual of Systematic Bacteriology,* 1984). The name of this genus, *Chlamydia,* supplants several now considered obsolete: *Miyagawanella* (Brumpt, 1938); *Bedsonia* (Meyer, 1953); *Prowazekia* (Coles, 1953), and *Rakeia* (Levaditi and others, 1964). Two species are presently accepted as valid: *C. psittaci* and *C. trachomatis.*

Chlamydia organisms are minute (0.2 to 1.5 μm) bacteria that propagate only within host cells of vertebrates, including humans, other mammals, and birds. The organisms are nonmotile, spherical, and gram-negative, and they have a cell wall. The basic unit is termed an **elementary body,** which is a spherule measuring 0.2 to 0.4 μm in diameter; it contains an electron-dense nucleus and ribosomes surrounded by a trilaminar wall. This elementary body is the infectious form of the organism, which attaches to host cells, presumably through specific receptors, and enters the cell in a phagosome. Elementary bodies can also be taken up by phagocytes. The phagosomes do not fuse with lysosomes. Once inside the cell, the elementary body undergoes morphologic changes. It becomes larger (0.6 to 1.5 μm) and gains more ribosomes, and the nucleus becomes lacy or reticular and is termed a **reticulate body.** Reticulate bodies divide by binary fission and ultimately reorganize into elementary bodies, which are released from the cell. Release mechanisms are not understood, but the cell can simply burst, liberating its entire contents.

Transmission of *Chlamydia* infection is direct; however, in the case of psittacosis in humans, the transmission cycle usually involves birds, with human infection being accidental. *Chlamydia* organisms have been recovered from arthropods, particularly ticks, which under some conditions can mechanically transmit the organisms.

The intracellular organisms may be stained with Giemsa's, Machiavello's, Gimenez's, or Castañeda's methods. They may also be demonstrated in unstained preparations (wet mounts) of infected cells with a phase-contrast optical system. They have characteristic features under the electron microscope.

As stated previously, only two species of chlamydiae are recognized: *C. trachomatis* and *C. psittaci.* There are, however, multiple strains of each species, which are quite host-specific and associated with characteristic diseases. These are listed in Table 9-7.

Chlamydia trachomatis strains cause several syndromes in humans including trachoma and lymphogranuloma venereum. These strains are highly specific for humans. Another distinct strain causes *pneumonitis* in mice (not to be confused with "mouse pneumonitis virus"). This murine agent ordinarily establishes a latent infection, which does not lead to pneumonia. With serial passage of murine tissues (particularly lung), however, the agent causes interstitial pneumonia with mononuclear and polymorphonuclear infiltrates. The disease can be fatal. Peribronchial lymphocytic cuffing, as seen in murine mycoplasmosis, is not a feature.

Certain organisms have been so poorly characterized that it is not possible to ascertain whether they should be classified as *Chlamydia. Colesiota conjunctivae* (*Rickettsiae conjunctivae, Ricolesia bovis; R. conjunctivae bovis*) has been found in association with conjunctivitis of sheep, goats, and cattle in South Africa. Apparently

TABLE 9-7 **Disease caused by Chlamydiae**

Organism	Disease	Species affected
C. trachomatis	Trachoma	Humans
	Inclusion body conjunctivitis	
	Urogenital inflammatory disease	
	Lymphogranuloma venereum	
	Pneumonia	
	Murine pneumonitis	Mice
C. psittaci	Psittacosis (ornithosis)	Humans, birds
	Sporadic bovine encephalomyelitis	Cattle
	Polyarthritis	Cattle, sheep, horses
	Enzootic bovine abortion	Cattle
	Enzootic ovine abortion	Sheep
	Abortion	Horses, swine
	Feline pneumonitis and rhinitis	Cats
	Pneumonia	Cattle, sheep, goats, horses, dogs, rabbits
	Conjunctivitis	Sheep, cats, guinea pigs, hamsters
	Enteritis	Cattle, pigs, muskrats, snowshoe hares

this organism is not the cause of keratoconjunctivitis in cattle in the United States. Conjunctivitis and keratoconjunctivitis in chickens in South Africa is caused by another organism, *Colesiota conjunctivagalli (Ricolesia conjunctivae)*. *Ricolesia lestoquardii (Rickettsia conjunctivaesuis)* causes conjunctivitis and keratitis in swine.

References

Brumpt E. *Rickettsia intracellulaire stomacale (Rickettsia culicis* N. Sp.) de Culex fatigans. Ann Parasitol 1938;16:153–158.

Coles JDW. Classification of rickettsiae pathogenic to vertebrates. Ann NY Acad Sci 1953;56:457–483.

Hargis AM, Prieur DJ, Gaillard ET. Chlamydial infection of the gastric mucosa in twelve cats. Vet Pathol 1983;20:170–178.

Jones H, Rake G, Stearns B. Studies on lymphogranuloma venereum. III. The action of the sulfonamides on the agent of lymphogranuloma venereum. J Infect Dis 1945;76:55–69.

Levaditi JC, Roger F, Destombes P. Tentative de classification des Chlamydiaceae (Rake, 1955) tenante compte de leurs affinités tissulaires et du leur épidemiologie. Ann Inst Pasteur (Paris) 1964; 107:656–662.

Matsumoto A, Manire GP. Electron microscopic observations on the fine structure of cell walls of *Chlamydia psittaci.* J Bact 1970;104: 1332–1337.

McKercher DG, Wada EM, Ault SK, et al. Preliminary studies on transmission of *Chlamydia* to cattle by ticks (*Ornithodoros coriaceus*). Am J Vet Res 1980;41:922–924.

Meyer KF. Psittacosis group. Ann NY Acad Sci 1953;56:545–556.

Moulder JW. Order II. Chlamydiales Storz and Page 1971, 334. In: Krieg NR, Holt JG, ed. *Bergey's Manual of Systematic Bacteriology.* Vol. 1. Baltimore: Williams & Wilkins 1984;729–739.

Page LA. Revision of the family Chlamydiaceae Rake (Rickettsiales): Unification of the psittacosis-lymphogranuloma venereum-trachoma group of organisms in the genus Chlamydia Jones, Rake and Stearns, 1945. Int J Systemat Bacteriol 1966;16: 223–252.

Pienaar JG, Schutte AP. Occurrence and pathology of chlamydiosis in domestic and laboratory animals: a review. Onderstepoort J Vet Res 1975;42:77–89.

Pospischil A, Wood RL. Intestinal *Chlamydia* in pigs. Vet Pathol 1987;24:568–570.

Tamura A, Matsumoto A, Manire GP, et al. Electron microscopic observations on the structure of the envelopes of mature elementary bodies and developmental reticulate forms of *Chlamydia psittaci.* J Bact 1971;105:355–360.

Woollen N, Daniels EK, Yeary T, et al. Chlamydial infection and perinatal mortality in a swine herd. J Am Vet Med Assoc 1990; 197:600–601.

Psittacosis (ornithosis, parrot fever)

A febrile pulmonary disease of humans, believed since the latter half of the nineteenth century to be contracted from sick parrots ("parrot fever"), is caused by an infectious agent harbored not only by parrots, but also by a wide variety of other birds. The causative agent is *Chlamydia psittaci.* Its biologic and morphologic features are discussed in the preceding section. Psittacine birds (family Psittacidae), including parrots, parakeets, cockatoos, macaws, cockatiels, and masked love birds, were the first in which the infection was demonstrated, both in an inapparent form and with obvious signs of illness. Several birds, including finches, canaries, and rice birds, acquire the infection by contact with parrots and transport the disease to humans. Pigeons, ducks, fulmars, sea gulls, chickens, and turkeys are naturally infected and also serve as reservoirs for human infection. Thus, various species of birds are considered the primary hosts for these strains of *C. psittaci,* with infection of humans being incidental. Strains of *C. psittaci* that cause psittacosis and are spread directly from human to human without an avian host have been identified. These organisms, termed TWAR strains, are considered primary human pathogens. Those disorders of domestic animals listed in Table 9-7 as being caused by *C. psittaci* are not to be confused with psittacosis.

SIGNS

The disease in humans is manifested by sudden onset of a febrile illness with upper respiratory involvement, pneumonia, and severe debility. Although the disease is not usually fatal, deaths occur with alarming frequency in some outbreaks. Antibiotic therapy has reduced the death rate dramatically.

In birds, psittacosis may appear as a fulminant, highly fatal disease or as a smoldering, inapparent infection demonstrable only by laboratory study or the appearance of the disease in human contacts. Infection in birds does not produce characteristic clinical manifestations; hence, necropsy and laboratory examination are necessary for definitive diagnosis. Infected birds are sleepy, listless, and refuse to eat. Their wings droop and their feathers can be pulled out easily. There is usually a nasal and ocular discharge and greenish, occasionally blood-tinged diarrhea that stains the feathers around the cloaca. The mortality rate is likely to be higher in parrots than in parakeets, but losses, particularly among young birds, may be great in both species. Recovered birds may excrete the organism for long periods of time.

LESIONS

Psittacine birds that die of the disease or are sacrificed while they have definite symptoms are emaciated and have many maculae, 2 to 4 mm in diameter, on the skin over the body and legs. The nares may be plugged with mucopurulent exudate. Fibrinous or fibrinopurulent exudates are found over the pericardial sac, peritoneum, pleura, and air sacs. The liver is enlarged, its edges are rounded, and it is yellowish, with mottling or patchy discoloration in shades of green or brown. In some cases, the liver may be studded with petechiae and small yellowish foci of necrosis. The spleen is always enlarged, dark blood-red, and occasionally has yellowish necrotic foci on its surface. The kidneys may be swollen, pale, and friable. The lungs are affected only rarely, and the changes are limited to a few small areas of consolidation.

In parrots, parakeets, and other psittacine birds with latent infection, the spleen may be greatly enlarged, but no other gross lesions are apparent.

The microscopic changes in tissues in acute symptomatic psittacosis are associated with the presence of the organism in various tissue cells. The spleen is moderately to intensely infiltrated by mononuclear cells containing organisms, and its hemosiderin content is often increased. Hyperplasia of the reticuloendothelial cells is commonly observed. The liver often contains focal lesions involving isolated islands of parenchymal cells that undergo necrosis and replacement with a mass of hyaline amorphous material. Fibrin and lymphocytes may be noted on the liver capsule, and the portal areas are rich in lymphocytes and plasma cells. The epithelium of the kidney may be packed with large numbers of LCL bodies; these are minute, spherical basophilic bodies, discovered by Levinthal, Coles, and Lillie (hence the acronym). Destruction of this epithelium is followed by interstitial accumulation of epithelioid cells. In the lungs, a few alveoli may contain serous exudate, but frank pneumonic consolidation is rare. The superficial mucosa of the intestine is usually eroded, and the underlying lamina propria and submucosa are infiltrated with lymphocytes and plasma cells. The kidney may show destruction of tubular epithelium. Within macrophages and epithelial cells, cytoplasmic bodies, which represent the organism, may be visible, sometimes few and sometimes in very large numbers. They are best observed with Giemsa, Macchiavello, Casta Zeda, or immunofluorescent techniques.

DIAGNOSIS

The clinical manifestations and gross features at necropsy are generally insufficient for definitive diagnosis. Necropsies must be performed by aseptic methods with adequate protection for the prosector, and special care must be taken to prevent desiccation and subsequent scattering of any infective material. Histologic study of smears or sections of peritoneal or pericardial lesions and liver or spleen appropriately stained will disclose intracellular organisms in most acute cases. Intracranial or intraperitoneal injection of mice with tissue suspensions from birds that have the infection in an asymptomatic form usually causes death in 4 or 5 days, and organisms are demonstrable in the mouse tissues. In some instances, at least one blind passage is required to establish the agent in mice. The organism also grows well in embryonated eggs and tissue culture.

The complement-fixation test is of value in the detection of antibodies in birds that have latent infections or are convalescent.

References

Beasley JN, Watkins JR, Bridges CH. Experimental omithosis in calves. Am J Vet Res 1962;23:1192–1199.

Bland JCW, Canti RG. The growth and development of psittacosis virus in tissue cultures. J Pathol Bact 1935;40:231–241.

Buttery RB, Wreghitt TG. Outbreak of psittacosis associated with a cockatiel. Lancet 1987;ii:742–743.

Durfee PT, Pullen MM, Currier RW II, et al. Human psittacosis associated with commercial processing of turkeys. J Am Vet Med Assoc 1975;167:804–808.

Grayston JT, Kuo C-C, Wang S-P, et al. A new *Chlamydia psittaci* strain, TWAR, isolated in acute respiratory tract infections. N Engl J Med 1986;315:161–168.

Lillie RD. The pathology of psittacosis in animals and the distribution of *Rickettsia psittaci* in the tissues of humans and animals. Nat Inst Health Bull 1933;161:47–66.

Pierce KR, Moore RW, Carroll LH, et al. Experimental ornithosis in ewes. Am J Vet Res 1963;24:1176–1188.

Todd WJ, Storz J. Ultrastructural cytochemical evidence for the activation of lysosomes in the cytocidal effect of *Chlamydia psittaci*. Infect Immun 1975;12:638–646.

Tomlinson TH Jr. An outbreak of psittacosis at the National Zoological Park, Washington, DC. Pub Health Rep 1941;56:1073–1081.

Wachendorfer JG. Epidemiology and control of psittacosis. J Am Vet Med Assoc 1973;162:298–303.

Sporadic bovine encephalomyelitis

A disease of young calves and, less often, older cattle, described by McNutt in Iowa, has now been reported in several states, i.e., Idaho, South Dakota, California, Oklahoma, and Texas, as well as in Australia, Europe, and Japan. It probably is more widespread than published reports indicate. The disease is caused by an infectious agent currently designated as *Chlamydia psittaci* (*C. pecoris*).

Organisms identified as *Chlamydia psittaci* have been recovered from several different disease syndromes of cattle, including enteritis of calves, latent intestinal infection, pneumonia, polyarthritis, placental infection, and abortion. These syndromes are taken up on the following pages as they were described originally as distinct, separate diseases. As strains of the organisms are studied more extensively, it may become apparent that only one causative organism is involved, even though many different organ systems are affected. If this proves to be true, the disease should be identified as psittacosis or chlamydiosis, which may have varying clinical and pathologic manifestations.

SIGNS

The onset is sudden, with fever (105°F to 107°F), anorexia, depression, decreased activity, excessive salivation with drooling, and nasal discharge. Dyspnea with a cough is observed in about half the cases, but diarrhea, either mild or severe, is more common. Within a few days, calves have difficulty in walking, exhibiting stiffness and knuckling in the fetlock joints. They move aimlessly in circles, stagger, and fall with the head extended in opisthotonos. In the final stages, the limbs appear weak or paralyzed; death occurs in 5 to 7 days in most cases and is rarely delayed for as long as a month.

Although calves are most susceptible, the report of Menges and others (1953) indicates that adult cattle are also subject to the infection. These authors reported 21 herds totalling 1774 cattle of all ages, of which 269 (15%) exhibited symptoms and 75 (28% of those affected) died from the disease. Among 892 calves in these herds, however, 224 (25%) contracted the disease and 64 (29% of those affected) died. Outbreaks of sporadic bovine encephalomyelitis usually follow introduction of new animals into a herd.

LESIONS

The most constant gross lesion in fatal cases is serofibrinous peritonitis. Excessive amounts of clear yellow peritoneal fluid are present in early cases; in more prolonged cases, adhesive strands of fibrin form an exudate over the omentum, liver, and spleen. The spleen is sometimes enlarged. A similar fibrinous exudate lies over the pleura and pericardium in about one half of the fatal cases. A patchy lobular pneumonia may be seen in a few instances. The brain and spinal cord usually appear edematous and their vasculature is congested.

The microscopic lesions consist of fibrinous peritonitis, pleuritis, pericarditis, and perisplenitis, with addition of severe, diffuse meningoencephalomyelitis. The entire brain and spinal cord are involved in an intense inflammatory reaction; the meninges at the base of the brain are particularly affected. Proliferation of vascular endothelium and infiltration of the vessel walls with mononuclear and occasionally polymorphonuclear cells may be observed. Severe damage to neurons, both in brain and cord, has been described and is believed by some to be secondary to the severe vascular lesions. Minute elementary bodies are demonstrable in mononuclear cells in the serosal exudates and in the brain or spinal cord. These bodies occur singly or in small clusters in the cytoplasm of these cells. They vary in size, but usually are less than a micron in diameter. They stain pink-red with Macchiavello's stain.

In guinea pigs, a fatal disease may be experimentally induced with this agent; the organisms are demonstrable in the guinea pig tissues. Chick embryos are also susceptible; the embryos die 5 to 7 days after adaptation of the agent.

DIAGNOSIS

The gross and microscopic lesions are characteristic, although not diagnostic, of sporadic bovine encephalomyelitis. Demonstration of the typical elementary bodies is helpful. Transmission of this disease to the guinea pig with subsequent demonstration of the elementary bodies is confirmatory. All clinical and pathologic data must be carefully evaluated to eliminate rabies, "shipping fever," listeriosis, and malignant catarrhal fever.

References

Littlejohns IR, Harris ANA, Harding WB. Sporadic bovine encephalomyelitis. Aust Vet J 1961;37:53 (VB 3956–61).

McNutt SH. A preliminary report of an infectious encephalomyelitis of cattle. Vet Med 1940;35:228–231.

McNutt SH, Waller EF. Sporadic bovine encephalomyelitis (Buss disease). Cornell Vet 1940;30:437–448.

Menges RW, Harshfield GS, Wenner HA. Sporadic bovine encephalomyelitis. Studies on pathogenesis and etiology of the disease. J Am Vet Med Assoc 1953;122:294–299.

Omori T, Ishii S, Matumoto M. Miyagawanellosis of cattle in Japan. Am J Vet Res 1960;21:564–573.

Price DA, Hardy WT. Sporadic bovine encephalomyelitis—isolation and antibiotic susceptibility of a Texas strain. J Am Vet Med Assoc 1956;128:308–310.

Tustin RC, Maré J, van Heerden A. A disease of calves resembling sporadic bovine encephalomyelitis. J S Afr Vet Med Assoc 1961;32:117–123(VB 129–162).

Wenner HA, Harshfield GS, Chang TW, et al. Sporadic bovine encephalomyelitis. II. Studies on the etiology of the disease. Isolation of nine strains of an infectious agent from naturally infected cattle. Am J Hyg 1953;57:15–29.

Wenner HA, Menges RW, Carter J. Sporadic bovine encephalomyelitis. A serologic survey of cattle in the midwestern United States. Cornell Vet 1955;45:68–77.

Polyarthritis of calves

In circumstances essentially analogous to those of polyarthritis of sheep, a variety of infectious organisms are capable of inducing polyarthritis in calves. *Mycoplasma mycoides* infection and vaccination can cause polyarthritis, as can several other species of mycoplasma discussed earlier in this chapter. *Erysipelas insidiosa* and a variety of other bacteria (*Salmonella, Pasteurella,* diplococci, streptococci, staphylococci) are known to cause polyarthritis, often after umbilical infection. Studies by Storz and colleagues (1966) indicate that polyarthritis in calves can result from infection by *Chlamydia psittaci.* The organism has been isolated from field cases of polyarthritis and induced arthritis following experimental inoculation. The infection as described by Storz and colleagues principally affected calves 1 to 3 weeks of age and was characterized by involvement of practically all joints of the limbs, as well as vertebral and mandibular articulations. The joints were swollen and the synovial tissues edematous and thickened. The synovial fluid of the joints and tendon sheaths was increased in volume, turbid, yellow-gray, and contained numerous flakes of fibrin. Large plaques of fibrin often adhered to the synovial tissue and filled the pouches of the joint cavities. Cellular elements of the synovial fluid were increased in number and elementary bodies could be demonstrated in monocytic cells and synovial cells in smears stained with Giemsa.

Chlamydia organisms frequently inhabit the digestive tracts of bovine animals. Usually the infection remains inapparent in adult cattle, but in young calves, the organisms may cause **enteritis** and may reach the blood and be carried to the joints. Under experimental conditions, the organisms produce severe enteritis in newborn calves, but in adult cattle, the carrier state is more apt to result (Page and associates, 1973; Smith and colleagues, 1973; Doughri and others, 1973, 1974; Eugster and Storz, 1971).

References

Doughri AM, Altero KP, Storz J. Host cell range of chlamydial infection in the neonatal bovine gut. J Comp Pathol 1973;83:107–114.

Doughri AM, Altera KP, Storz J, et al. Ultrastructural changes in the *Chlamydia*-infected ileal mucosa of newborn calves. Vet Pathol 1973;10:114–123.

Doughri AM, Young S, Storz J. Pathologic changes in intestinal chlamydial infection of newborn calves. Am J Vet Res 1974;35:939–944.

Eugster AK, Joyce BK, Storz J. Immunofluorescence studies on the pathogenesis of intestinal chlamydial infections in calves. Infect Immun 1970;2:351–359.

Eugster AK, Storz J. Effect of colostral antibodies on the pathogenesis of intestinal chlamydial infections in calves. Am J Vet Res 1971;32:711–718.

Eugster AK, Storz J. Pathogenetic events in intestinal chlamydial infections leading to polyarthritis in calves. J Infect Dis 1971;123:41–50.

Hughes KL, Edwards MJ, Hartley WJ, et al. Polyarthritis in calves caused by *Mycoplasma* sp. Vet Rec 1966;78:276–281.

Moulton JE, Rhode ER, Wheat JD. Erysipelatous arthritis in calves. J Am Vet Med Assoc 1953;123:335–340.

Page LA, Matthews PJ, Smith PC. Natural intestinal infection with

Chlamydia psittaci in a closed bovine herd: serologic changes, incidence of shedding, antibiotic treatment of herd, and biologic characteristics of the chlamydiae. Am J Vet Res 1973;34:611–614.

Simmons GC, Johnston LAY. Arthritis in calves caused by *Mycoplasma* sp. Aust Vet J 1963;39:11–14.

Smith PC, Cutlip RC, Page LA. Pathogenicity of a strain of *Chlamydia psittaci* of bovine intestinal origin for neonatal calves. Am J Vet Res 1973;34:615–619.

Storz J, Smart RA, Marriott ME, et al. Polyarthritis of calves: isolation of psittacosis agents from affected joints. Am J Vet Res 1966;27:633–641.

Storz J, Shupe JL, Smart RA, et al. Polyarthritis of calves: experimental induction by a psittacosis agent. Am J Vet Res 1966;27:987–995.

Enzootic abortion of ewes

First reported in 1950 by Stamp in Scotland, enzootic abortion of ewes has since been recognized in Europe and the United States. The disease, which may also occur in goats, is caused by *Chlamydia psittaci*. The infection has been described as a zoonosis causing severe septicemia and abortion in pregnant women.

In sheep, abortion usually occurs in the last month of gestation but earlier abortion, stillbirth, and birth of weak lambs may occur. Fetal membranes are often retained, which results in clinical disease in the ewe; otherwise, specific signs of infection are not seen in the ewe. Placentitis is the major lesion. Cotyledons are gray to dark red and the periplacentome is thickened, opaque yellow-pink, and covered with a flaky, clay-colored exudate. The uterine surface of the chorion is of a tough, granular consistency, pink-yellow, and covered with a flaky, yellowish exudate. Microscopically there is focal necrosis, edema, vasculitis, and a mononuclear cell infiltration. Cytoplasmic elementary bodies can be demonstrated in tissue sections or smears stained by the Giemsa, Macchiavello, or Gimenez techniques. Lesions in the lamb are not striking.

DIAGNOSIS

Diagnosis is based on clinical and pathologic findings supported by demonstration of elementary bodies or isolation of the infectious agent.

References

Djurov A. Die pathohistologishen Veränderungen der Feten beim enzootischen Virusabort der Schafe. Zentralbl Veterinaermed [B]. 1972;19:578–587.

Gunson DE, Acland HM, Gillette DM, et al. Abortion and stillbirth associated with *Chlamydia psittaci* var *ovis* in dairy goats with high titers to *Toxoplasma gondii*. J Am Vet Med Assoc 1983;183:1447–1450.

Krauss H, Wandera JG, Lauerman LH Jr. Isolation and identification of *Chlamydia* in Kenya sheep and serologic survey. Am J Vet Res 1971;32:1433–1438.

Morgan KL, Wills JM, Howard P, et al. Isolation of *Chlamydia psittaci* from the genital tract of lambs: a possible link with enzootic abortion of ewes. Vet Rec 1988;123:399–400.

Novilla MN, Jensen R. Placental pathology of experimentally induced enzootic abortion in ewes. Am J Vet Res 1970;31:1983–2000.

Parker HD, Hawkins WW Jr, Brenner E. Epizootiologic studies of ovine virus abortion. Am J Vet Res 1966;27:869–877.

Parker HD. A virus of ovine abortion—isolation from sheep in the United States and characterization of the agent. Am J Vet Res 1960;21:243–250.

Pavlov N, Vesselivova A. Morphology of the natural infection in lambs with the virus of lamb abortion. Zentbl Vet Med 1965;12B:517–526.

Stamp JT, McEwen AD, Watt JAA, et al. Enzootic abortion in ewes. I. Transmission of the disease. Vet Rec 1950;62:251–254.

Storz J. Comparative studies on EBA and EAE, abortion diseases of cattle and sheep resulting from infection with psittacosis agent. In: Faulkner LC, ed. Abortion Diseases of Livestock. Springfield: Charles C Thomas, 1968.

Studdert MJ. Bedsonia abortion of sheep. II. Pathology and pathogenesis with observations on the normal ovine placenta. Res Vet Sci 1968;9:57–64.

Studdert MJ, McKercher DG. Bedsonia abortion of sheep. I. Aetiological studies. Res Vet Sci 1968;9:48–56.

Studdert MJ, Kennedy PC. Enzootic abortion of ewes. Nature (Lond) 1964;203:1088–1089.

Tunnicliff EA. Ovine virus abortion. J Am Vet Med Assoc 1960;136:132–134.

Chlamydial Abortion in Cattle

Chlamydia psittaci has been associated with spontaneous abortion in cattle in the United States and Europe, and experimental inoculation with *Chlamydia* organisms has been shown to lead to abortion in cattle. The extent and importance of chlamydiae as a cause of abortion, however, is not fully understood. Chlamydiae had been considered the cause of **epizootic bovine abortion**; however, it now appears that this is not the case and that this enzootic disease in California is caused by an as yet unidentified infectious agent (spirochetes, Chapter 10). One of the first associations of chlamydiae with bovine abortion was their recovery from aborted calves in California in association with epizootic bovine abortion. This makes interpretation of some of the earlier literature difficult, as it is not a simple task to determine which disease syndrome is being presented. It has also been suggested that some of the chlamydial isolates described may have represented contaminants, even though experimentally they may be capable of inducing abortion. Strains isolated from the gastrointestinal tract are antigenically similar to chlamydiae recovered from cases of abortion. Pregnant cattle are susceptible to the chlamydial agent of enzootic abortion of ewes and pregnant sheep are susceptible to experimental infection with the bovine agent; however, the exact relationship of the two agents and disease requires further study.

Experimental inoculation of pregnant cows with chlamydial agents recovered from aborted bovine fetuses causes only minimal clinical signs other than late abortion. The principal pathologic finding is placentitis comparable to that seen in chlamydial abortion of sheep (enzootic abortion of ewes). Elementary bodies can be demonstrated with appropriate staining techniques.

Chlamydiae have also been recovered from semen, epididymides, and seminal vesicles of bulls and has been suggested as a cause of seminal vesiculitis syndrome.

References

Bassan Y, Ayalon N. Abortion in dairy cows inoculated with epizootic bovine abortion agent (*Chlamydia*). Am J Vet Res 1971;32:703–710.

Boulanger P, Bannister GL. Abortion produced experimentally in cattle with an agent of the psittacosis-lymphogranuloma-venereum group of viruses. Can J Comp Med 1959;**23**:259–265. [Vet Bull 1960;30:1449]

Kwapien RP, Lincoln SD, Reed DE, et al. Pathologic changes of placentas from heifers with experimentally induced epizootic bovine abortion. Am J Vet Res 1970;31:999–1015.

Reed DE, Lincoln SD, Kwapian RP, et al. Comparison of antigenic structure and pathogenicity of bovine intestinal *Chlamydia* isolate with an agent of epizootic bovine abortion. Am J Vet Res 1975;36:1141–1143.

Storz J, McKercher DG. Etiological studies on epizootic bovine abortion. Zentralbl Veterinaermed 1962;9:411–427, 520–541. [Vet Bull 1963;33:153]

Storz J, Carroll EJ, Ball L, et al. Isolation of a psittacosis agent *(Chlamydia)* from semen and epididymis of bulls with seminal vesiculitis syndrome. Am J Vet Res 1968;29:549–555.

Storz J, Carroll EJ, Stephenson EH, et al. Urogenital infection and seminal excretion after inoculation of bulls and rams with Chlamydiae. Am J Vet Res 1976;37:517–520.

Storz J, McKercher DG, Howarth JA, et al. The isolation of a viral agent from epizootic bovine abortion. J Am Vet Med Assoc 1960;137:509–514.

Chlamydial pneumonia of cattle and sheep

Organisms of the genus *Chlamydia* have been isolated from naturally occurring cases of enzootic pneumonia of cattle, sheep, and goats. Cultures of these organisms on chicken yolk-sac preparations inoculated intratracheally in these species have also produced the disease. The relationship of these respiratory organisms to the chlamydiae that have been incriminated in sporadic bovine encephalomyelitis, polyarthritis of cattle or sheep, epizootic bovine abortion, enzootic abortion of ewes, follicular conjunctivitis of sheep, and other syndromes is not at all clear (Fig. 9-8). It appears that the organisms are all of the same species *(Chlamydia psittaci)*, but may differ in some minor antigens or in pathogenicity. As was mentioned in the discussion of sporadic bovine encephalomyelitis, each of the "syndromes" described in the literature may be differing clinical and pathologic aspects of the same etiologic complex. The answer lies in more thorough comparisons of the strains of chlamydiae involved.

Cattle have been experimentally susceptible to ovine pneumonia isolates, and sheep, to the bovine isolates. Enzootic pneumonia, which is principally but not exclusively of importance in young animals, is clinically nonspecific, characterized by fever, nasal discharge, cough, dyspnea, and depression.

LESIONS

Lesions, which are comparable in cattle and sheep, are most often restricted to the anterior lobes of the lung. Microscopically, the lesions are dominated by an extensive infiltration of lymphocytes, macrophages, and plasma cells, particularly in the bronchiolar mucosa and surrounding bronchioles and blood vessels but also within alveolar septae. The exudate often has a follicular arrangement and compresses bronchioles and alveoli. Bronchioles and alveoli contain macrophages and variable numbers of neutrophils, but purulent exudate is lacking unless secondary bacterial invaders initiate a more characteristic picture of bronchopneumonia, as is often the case. There is proliferation and epithelialization of alveolar lining cells, which contributes to alveolar consolidation.

DIAGNOSIS

As in other infections caused by *Chamydia psittaci*, elementary bodies are more easily demonstrated in tissue impressions than tissue sections. Positive diagnosis requires isolation of the causative organism. It is essential that this infection be distinguished from the "enzootic pneumonia" caused by *Mycoplasma* infection. The lymphocytic aggregations around the bronchial tree are characteristic of the microscopic lesions of myco-

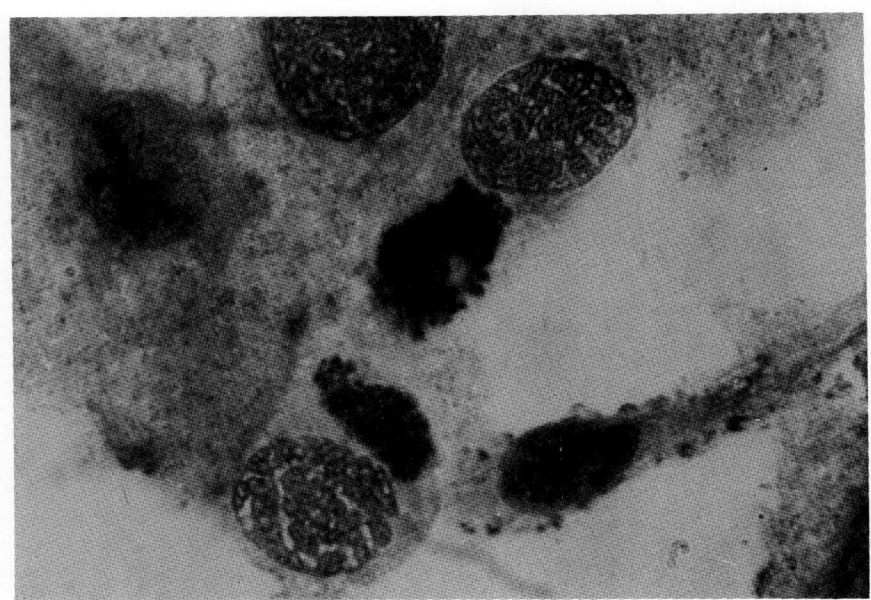

FIG. 9-8 Chlamydial inclusions 60 hours after infection in vitro with agent of ovine abortion. (Courtesy of Dr. J. Storz.)

plasmosis. The organisms also may be differentiated by their morphology and cultural characteristics.

References

Carter GR, Rowsell HC. Studies on pneumonia of cattle. II. An enzootic pneumonia of calves in Canada. J Am Vet Med Assoc 1958;132:187–190.

Dungworth DL, Cordy DR. The pathogenesis of ovine pneumonia. II. Isolation of virus from faeces: comparison of pneumonia caused by faecal, enzootic abortion and pneumonitis viruses. J Comp Pathol Ther 1962;72:71–79.

Dungworth DL, Cordy DR. The pathogenesis of ovine pneumonia. I. Isolation of a virus of the PL group. J Comp Pathol Ther 1962;72:49–70.

Ide PR. The etiology of enzootic pneumonia of calves. Can Vet J 1970;11:194–202.

Matumoto M, et al. Studies on the disease of cattle caused by a psittacosis-lymphogranuloma group virus (Miyagawanella). VI. Bovine pneumonia caused by this virus. Jpn J Exp Med 1955;25:23–34.

McKercher DG. A virus possibly related to the psittacosis-lymphogranuloma-pneumonitis group causing a pneumonia in sheep. Science 1952;115:543–544.

Omar AR. The aetiology and pathology of pneumonia in calves. Vet Bull 1966;36:259–273.

Palotay JL, Christensen MS. Bovine respiratory infections. I. Psittacosis-lymphogranuloma venereum group of viruses as etiological agents. J Am Vet Med Assoc 1959;134:222–230.

Phillip JIH, et al. Pathogenesis and pathology in calves of infection by Bedsonia alone and by Bedsonia and reovirus together. J Comp Pathol 1968;78:89–99.

Storz J. Psittacosis-lymphogranuloma agents in bovine pneumonia. J Am Vet Med Assoc 1968;152:814–819.

Polyarthritis of sheep

One form of so-called "stiff lamb disease" is not the result of lesions in the muscles, but in the joints. Various organisms have been incriminated from time to time, including *Erysipelothrix rhusiopathiae (insidiosa)* and *Mycoplasma* species. A specific and rather widespread cause of arthritis appears to be *Chlamydia psittaci* (Fig. 9-9), which can be isolated from joints, feces, cerebrospinal fluid, urine, blood, and viscera. Affected lambs are de-

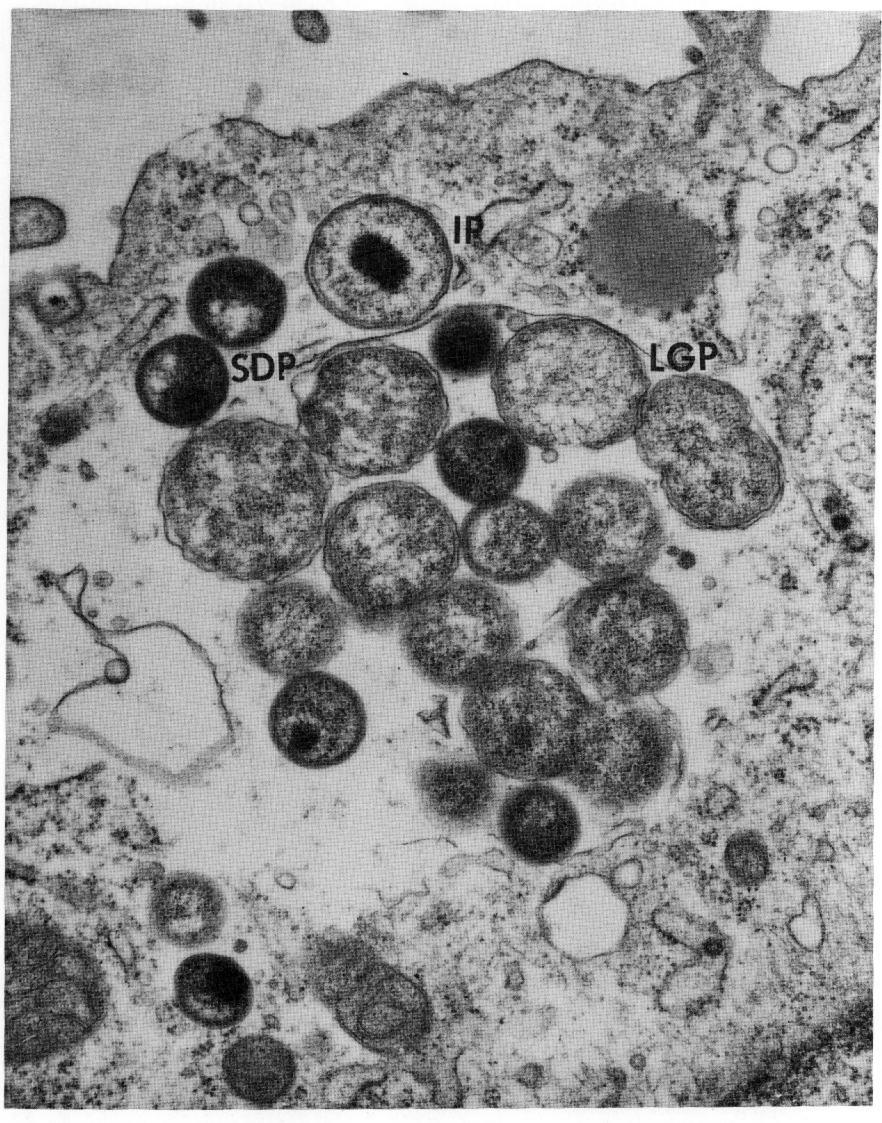

FIG. 9-9 Electron micrograph of a chlamydial inclusion of the agent of polyarthritis of lambs in tissue culture. Several stages of development are recognizable: small dense particles *(SDP)*, intermediate particles *(IP)*, and large granular particles *(LGP)*, some of which are dividing. (Courtesy of Dr. Randall C. Cutlip and *Infection and Immunity*.)

tected by a characteristic lameness involving one or more joints. Some lambs are depressed, with a high fever (106°F); others lose weight and are slow to recover. Some animals appear to recover completely, but others remain permanently lame.

LESIONS

The lesions in early stages consist mostly of serofibrinous or fibrinous synovitis, occasionally with edema around the affected joint and greenish-gray masses of material in the articular spaces. Microscopically, affected synovial membranes are edematous; lining cells are swollen, often disorganized, detached, and covered with fibropurulent debris. The subsynovial connective tissue contains granulomatous accumulations of mononuclear cells. In most examples, large numbers of elementary bodies can be demonstrated in smears or sections of synovia or joint fluid stained with Giemsa's or Macchiavello's stain; however, arthritis may persist in the absence of demonstrable organisms.

DIAGNOSIS

The diagnosis can be made by isolation of the infective agent in chick embryos, tissue culture, or guinea pigs and by demonstration of elementary bodies in association with characteristic lesions.

References

Cutlip RC. Electron microscopy of cell cultures infected with a chlamydial agent causing polyarthritis of lambs. Infect Immun 1970;1:499–502.

Cutlip RC, Ramsey FK. Ovine chlamydial polyarthritis: Sequential development of articular lesions in lambs after intraarticular exposure. Am J Vet Res 1973;34:71–76.

Hopkins JB, Stephenson EH, Storz J, et al. Conjunctivitis associated with chlamydial polyarthritis in lambs. J Am Vet Med Assoc 1973;163:1157–1160.

Mendlowski B, Segre D. Polyarthritis in sheep. I. Description of the disease and experimental transmission. Am J Vet Res 1960;21: 68–73.

Mendlowski B, Kraybill WH, Segre D. Polyarthritis in sheep. II. Characteristics of the causative virus. Am J Vet Res 1960;21:74–80.

Norton WL, Storz J. Observations on sheep with polyarthritis produced by an agent of the psittacosis-lymphogranuloma venereum trachoma group. Arthritis Rheum 1967;10:1–12.

Shupe JL, Storz J. Pathologic study of psittacosis-lymphogranuloma polyarthritis of lambs. Am J Vet Res 1964;25:943–951.

Stevenson RG, Robinson G. The pathology of pneumonia in young lambs inoculated with Bedsonia. Res Vet Sci 1970;11:469–474.

Storz J, et al. Polyarthritis of lambs induced experimentally by a psittacosis agent. J Infect Dis 1965;115:9–18.

Storz J, Shupe JL, James LF, et al. Polyarthritis of sheep in the Intermountain Region caused by a psittacosis-lymphogranuloma agent. Am J Vet Res 1963;24:1201–1206.

Feline pneumonitis

Feline pneumonitis, a chlamydial infection of domesticated cats, is a problem in catteries and in experimental laboratories where cats are congregated. The disease starts as an acute upper respiratory infection, with sneezing and catarrh; later symptoms are nasal and conjunctival mucous discharges, transitory fever, and some inappetence. The disease runs a course of about 2 weeks and terminates fatally in a small percentage of cases. Recovery followed by exacerbation of clinical signs is not unusual. The disease may be adapted to mice by serial passage of infected material inoculated intranasally. A feature of value in the recognition of the disease is the presence of elementary bodies of the organism, which can be demonstrated most readily in the lung tissues of experimentally infected mice and occasionally in feline tissues.

Chlamydial infection has also been associated with peritonitis, and organisms have been identified in and recovered from mucus-producing cells of the gastric mucosa of healthy cats. Experimentally, the latter have been shown to cause pulmonary disease resembling natural feline pneumonitis. It is thought that persistent infection in the gastrointestinal tract may provide a reservoir for chlamydial infection.

LESIONS

Aside from catarrhal inflammatory changes in the upper respiratory passages, the principal lesions are usually found in the lungs. Sharply demarcated patches of what appears to be consolidation may be seen in the various lobes. These patches are usually light reddish-brown to gray or even prune-colored, contrasting sharply with the light pink lung tissue.

Microscopic examination reveals that these affected areas are distributed around terminal bronchioles and consist principally of alveolar collapse rather than consolidation, although in some areas inflammatory cells, lymphoid and polymorphonuclear, fill the alveoli. Of diagnostic significance is the presence of elementary bodies, which usually appear in loose aggregates in the cytoplasm of epithelial and mononuclear cells. These bodies are tiny spherical structures, approximately .5 μ in diameter. In smears, they stain selectively with Macchiavello's stain, appearing brightly eosinophilic and usually coccoid. In some instances, the elementary bodies coalesce into a plaque, forming a solid eosinophilic body, which distends the cytoplasm of epithelial and occasionally of leukocytic cells. These organisms are currently considered to be a strain of *Chlamydia psittaci*. Older names include *Chlamydia felis* and *Miyagawanella felis*.

Schachter and colleagues (1969) have described a case of acute keratoconjunctivitis in humans caused by the feline pneumonitis agent.

References

Baker JA. A virus causing pneumonia in cats and producing elementary bodies. J Exp Med 1944;79:159–172.

Dickie CW, Sniff ES. Chlamydia infection associated with peritonitis in a cat. J Am Vet Med Assoc 1980;176:1256–1259.

Gaillard ET, Hargis AM, Prieur DJ, et al. Pathogenesis of feline gastric chlamydial infection. Am J Vet Res 1984;45:2314–2321.

Hargis AM, Prieur DJ, Gaillard ET. Chlamydial infection of the gastric mucosa in twelve cats. Vet Pathol 1983;20:170–178.

Hoover EA, Kahn DE, Langloss JM. Experimentally induced feline chlamydial infection (feline pneumonitis). Am J Vet Res 1978;39:541–547.

Mitzel JR, Strating A. Vaccination against feline pneumonitis. Am J Vet Res 1977;38:1361–1363.

Schachter J, Ostler HB, Meyer KR. Human infection with the agent of feline pneumonitis. Lancet 1969;31:1063–1065.

Other chlamydial infections

INCLUSION CONJUNCTIVITIS OF GUINEA PIGS

This natural disease was first described by Murray (1964) as a mild, self-limiting conjunctivitis of young guinea pigs. The inclusions in impressions of conjunctival epithelium are similar to those found in human inclusion blennorrhea (conjunctivitis). The causative organism in guinea pigs has the characteristics of *Chlamydia psittaci,* rather than those of *Chlamydia trachomatis,* the agent in the human disease. The genital tract of guinea pigs may be infected with organisms isolated from conjunctiva and cultivated on chick embryo yolk-sacs. This experimental disease resembles lymphogranuloma venereum and trachoma of the human patient to some extent (Mount and others, 1972, 1973; Howard and others, 1976; Reed and others, 1977; and Robinson, 1969).

ENZOOTIC PNEUMONIA IN RABBITS

This disease, not uncommon in young rabbits, is considered, with good reason, to be caused by *Pasteurella multocida.* In a few instances, Flatt and Dungworth (1971) were able to recover chlamydiae from occult lesions in lungs of apparently healthy young rabbits. The significance of this infection in pulmonary disease of rabbits appears yet to be established.

CHLAMYDIAL POLYARTHRITIS IN FOALS

In one case, described by McChesney and others (1974), chlamydiae were cultured from joint exudate from a young foal with spontaneous polyarthritis. This disease appears to be much less frequent in foals than in lambs or calves.

CHLAMYDIAL INFECTION IN DOGS

Although chlamydial antibody titers have been demonstrated in as many as 50% of dogs in some surveys, clinical disease is reported much less often in this species. Dogs are susceptible to experimental infection, however (Young and colleagues, 1972). A chlamydial agent recovered from a case of ovine polyarthritis produced disease in five of six dogs when inoculated intraperitoneally or intravenously. The principal lesions were focal necrosis of the liver, lymphocytic and reticuloendothelial hyperplasia in spleen and lymph nodes, acute leptomeningitis, and polyarthritis.

CHLAMYDIAL INFECTIONS IN MUSKRATS AND SNOWSHOE HARES

Strains of chlamydiae were isolated from dead muskrats *(Ondatra zibethicus)* and snowshoe hares *(Lepus americanus)* during an outbreak in Saskatchewan, Canada in 1961 (Spalatin and others, 1966). Experimental infection in these species was reproduced with these cultures of chlamydiae (Iversen and others, 1970).

FOLLICULAR CONJUNCTIVITIS OF SHEEP

A specific ocular disease of sheep is known in Australia as contagious conjunctivokeratitis, pink eye, snow blindness, or heather blindness. This has been compared to trachoma of humans by Cooper (1974). Chlamydiae isolated from affected sheep have been propagated in yolk-sac cultures and subsequently used to reproduce the disease in susceptible sheep (Cooper, 1974). Chlamydiae have also been isolated from the conjunctival sac of sheep suffering from a similar disease, follicular conjunctivitis, in the United States (Storz and others, 1967).

CHLAMYDIAL INFECTIONS OF NONHUMAN PRIMATES

Natural infection of two crab-eating macaques *(Macaca fascicularis)* with chlamydiae has been reported by Morita and associates (1971). Taiwan rock macaques *(Macaca cyclopis)* are susceptible to experimental infection with *Chlamydia trachomatis,* originally isolated from human trachoma. Owl monkeys *(Aotus* species) are even more susceptible to trachoma infection and have been used extensively in research on this disease (Fraser and Bell, 1971; Fraser and others, 1975; Fraser, 1976). *Chlamydia trachomatis,* isolated from a human patient with nongonococcal urethritis, produced urethritis and persistent infection after instillation into the urethra of male baboons (DiGiacomo and others, 1975).

References

Cooper BS. Transmission of chlamydia-like agent isolated from contagious conjunctivo-keratitis of sheep. NZ Vet J 1974;22:181–184.

DiGiacomo RF, Gale JL, Wang SP, et al. Chlamydial infection of male baboon urethra. Br J Vener Dis 1975;51:310–313.

Flatt RE, Dungworth DL. Enzootic pneumonia in rabbits: naturally occurring lesions in lungs of apparently healthy young rabbits. Am J Vet Res 1971;32:621–626.

Flatt RE, Dungworth DL. Enzootic pneumonia in rabbits: microbiology and comparison with lesions experimentally produced by *Pasteurella multocida* and a chlamydial organism. Am J Vet Res 1971;32:627–637.

Fraser CEO, Bell SD. Experimental trachoma in owl monkeys and Taiwan monkeys. In: Goldsmith EI, Moor-Jankowski.J, ed. Medical Primatology. Basel: S. Karg 1971;783–791.

Fraser CEO, McComb DE, Murray ES, et al. Immunity to chlamydial infections of eye. Arch Ophthamol 1975;94:518–521.

Fraser CEO. The owl monkey *(Aotus trivirgatus)* as an animal model in trachoma research. Lab Anim Sci 1976;26:1138–1141.

Howard LV, O'Leary MP, Nichols RL. Animal model studies of genital chlamydial infections. Immunity to re-infection with guinea pig inclusion conjunctivitis agent in the urethra and eye of male guinea pigs. Br J Vener Dis 1976;52:261–265.

Iversen JO, et al. The susceptibility of muskrats and snowshoe hares to experimental infection with a chlamydial agent. Can J Comp Med 1970;34:80–89.

McChesney AE, Becerra V, England JJ. Chlamydial polyarthritis in a foal. J Am Vet Med Assoc 1974;165:259–261.

Morita M, Yoshizawa S, Inaba Y. Spontaneous cases of a disease of cynomolgus monkeys *(Macaca irus)* probably caused by the psittacosis-lymphogranuloma-trachoma group *(Chlamydia).* Jpn J Vet Sci 1971;33:261–270.

Mount DT, Bigazzi PE, Barron AL. Infection of genital tract and transmission of ocular infection to newborns by the agent of guinea pig inclusion conjunctivitis. Infect Immun 1972;5:921–926.

Mount DT, Bigazzi PE, Barron AL. Experimental genital infection of male guinea pigs with the agent of guinea pig inclusion conjunctivitis and transmission to females. Infect Immun 1973;8:925–930.

Murray ES. Guinea pig inclusion conjunctivitis virus. I. Isolation and identification as a member of the psittacosis-lymphogranuloma-trachoma group. J Infect Dis 1964;114:1–12.

Reed C, Campbell LH, Soave OA. Limited survey of genital infection by guinea pig inclusion conjunctivitis agent. Am J Vet Res 1977;38:1383–1387.

Robinson GW. A naturally occurring latent bedsonia infection in guinea-pigs. Br Vet J 1969;125:23–25.

Spalatin J, et al. Agents of psittacosis-lymphogranuloma venereum group, isolated from muskrats and snowshoe hares in Saskatchewan. Can J Comp Med 1966;30:260–264.

Storz J, Pierson RE, Marriott ME, et al. Isolation of psittacosis agents from follicular conjunctivitis of sheep. Proc Soc Exp Biol Med 1967;125:857–860.

Young S, Storz J, Maierhofer CA. Pathologic features of experimentally induced chlamydial infection in dogs. Am J Vet Res 1972;33:377–383.

10

Diseases caused by bacteria

Under the heading Bacteria is a vast array of pathogenic organisms capable of causing a diversity of diseases. In contrast to viruses and the organisms considered in the previous chapter, most bacteria are extracellular pathogens or facultative intracellular pathogens, such as *Mycobacterium* and *Brucella* species. All bacteria contain both DNA and RNA, lack a nucleus, have few cytoplasmic organelles, and generally reproduce by binary fission. They are classified on the basis of a myriad of morphologic, cultural, biochemical, antigenic, and nucleic acid parameters, which are not specifically addressed in this book. Certain features discernible in tissue sections or stained smears and impressions of tissues are, however, very useful to the pathologist as aids to diagnosis. The many species are varied in morphology: round (micrococci); in chains of cocci (streptococci); rod-shaped (bacilli); or filamentous often with branching (actinomyces). Some bacteria have cilia or flagella; others produce spores. They can be divided into two broad groups by means of their staining reaction with Gram's stain: they are either gram-positive or gram-negative. Other staining techniques can further distinguish certain groups, such as acid-fast staining of mycobacteria.

The relative virulence or pathogenicity of various bacteria and the mechanisms whereby they cause disease are also diverse. Some organisms, such as certain species and types of staphylococci and streptococci, inhabit the nasopharynx and skin of normal animals and only produce disease if introduced by way of a wound or in compromised individuals. *Streptococcus pneumoniae* (pneumococcus) is a classic example of this type of host/organism relationship. Many normal adults carry pneumococci; it is a significant cause of pneumonia in humans during epidemics of influenza or in immunosuppressed individuals. Other strains of streptocci are not normal inhabitants, and if animals are exposed to them, they usually cause disease. These and organisms such as *Bacillus anthracis*, the cause of anthrax, or *Mycobacterium tuberculosis*, the cause of tuberculosis, are always pathogenic. Certain bacteria are highly invasive; they multiply and spread rapidly throughout the host, creating what is termed bacteremia or septicemia.

The cause of anthrax is an example. Others tend to be localized, either at the point of entry or at another site after an interval of systemic spread through bacteremia. *Clostridium tetani*, the cause of tetanus, is an example of an an organism that is not very invasive and remains at the site of entry, whereas mycobacteria may spread throughout the body and become established in localized lesions. Still other bacteria produce disease without ever invading a host. Botulism and staphylococcal food poisoning are examples of bacterial diseases resulting from the ingestion of toxins formed outside the body.

While data concerning the causative organisms are plentiful, the mechanisms whereby bacteria cause specific diseases are not always clear. Several different ways are, however, recognized. Many bacteria produce toxins; these can be divided into exotoxins, endotoxins, and other bacterial products. Exotoxins are deleterious substances, often enzymes, elaborated by bacteria, which interfere with host metabolism. Some are highly specific, such as the toxin elaborated by *Clostridium tetani* known as tetanospasmin, a potent neurotoxin that blocks inhibitory transmitter substance; or the toxin of *Clostridium botulinum*, which blocks cholinergic neurotransmitters and causes paralysis. The diseases caused by these organisms are entirely the result of these lethal exotoxins. The same is true for diptheria (*Corynebacterium diphtheriae*) and cholera (*Vibrio cholerae*) in humans. Both of the latter toxins lead to ribosomal dysfunction; the former curtails the assembly of polypeptides on ribosomes and the latter leads to the generation of excessive cyclic adenosine monophosphate (cAMP). One of the exotoxins of *Bacillus anthracis* (the cause of anthrax) and the enterotoxin of *Escherichia coli* also lead to ribosomal dysfunction, resulting in an increase in cAMP.

Endotoxins are complex lipopolysaccharides that are components of the cell wall of gram-negative bacteria and are released on their disintegration. These compounds have severe systemic effects, including fever, hypotension, hemorrhage, intravascular coagulation, and destruction of neutrophils with release of enzymes.

There are also sundry other products of bacteria;

413

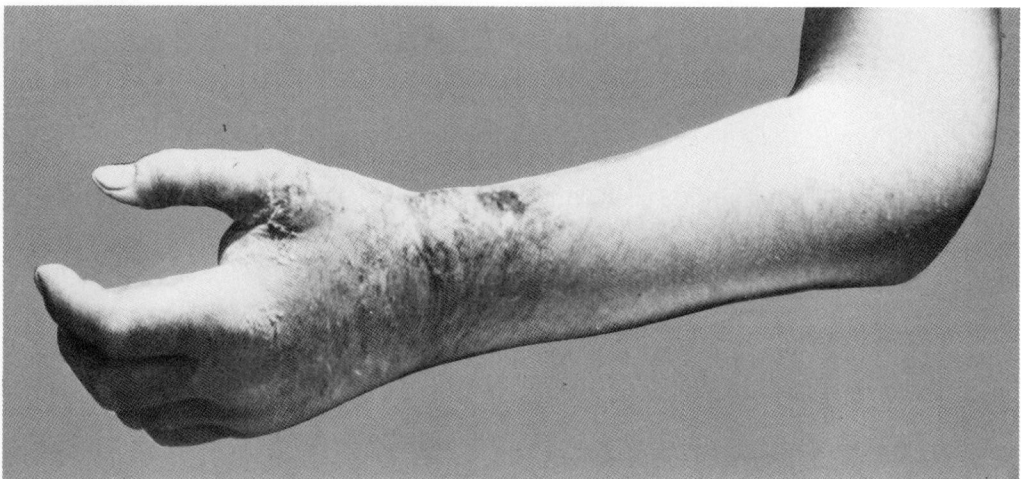

FIG. 10-1 Cutaneous anthrax in humans. This man and his wife skinned a cow that had recently died of anthrax. The carcass was fed to hogs, which soon exhibited "quinsey." *Bacillus anthracis* was isolated in pure culture from the lesion illustrated, from the swine, and the cow. The wife escaped infection. (Courtesy of Dr. Hubert Schmidt.)

they include hemolysins, fibrinolysins, coagulases, and other enzymes that are deleterious to the host. In cases of overwhelming septicemia, bacterial products and waste products are thought to interfere with host metabolism, often fatally. Host responses also contribute to the mechanisms whereby bacteria cause disease. Pyogenic bacteria, if not overcome by polymorphonuclear phagocytes and macrophages, cause the release of many chemical mediators responsible for fever and accompanying inflammation (see Chapter 5 on inflammation). Cellular immune mechanisms (hypersensitivity) contribute to the development of the lesions of tuberculosis. Immune-complex glomerulonephritis and immune-mediated arthritis may also be precipitated by bacterial infections.

This chapter is organized into three principal sections. The first includes diseases caused by various Gram-positice and Gram-negative cocci and rods. The second section includes members of the family Spirochaetales (spirochetes). The final section covers actinomycetes and mycobacteria.

Details concerning the classification of the many organisms covered in this chapter can be found in Bergey's Manual of Systematic Bacteriology (1984, 1986).

References

Holt JG, ed. Bergey's Manual of Systematic Bacteriology. Vol I & II. Baltimore: Williams & Wilkins, 1984, 1986.
Timoney JF, Gillespie JH, Scott FW, et al. Hagan and Bruner's Microbiology and Infectious Diseases of Domestic Animals. 8th ed. Ithaca: Comstock Publishing Associates, 1988.

THE GENUS BACILLUS

Bacillus anthracis has for many years been considered the only pathogenic member of the genus Bacillus (endospore-forming, gram-positive, aerobic or facultatively anaerobic, rod-shaped organisms). It appears, however, that other members of this large group of organisms are also pathogenic under certain conditions.

Anthrax

Anthrax is not only of current significance as an infection of animals and humans, but also of historical interest, for it was investigated intensively by the founders of bacteriology. Robert Koch, in 1876, was the first to isolate the causative organism in pure culture and to reproduce the disease with the culture. Pasteur, Rous, and Chamberland, in 1881, demonstrated active immunization with attenuated anthrax cultures in the famous experiment at Pouilly-le-Fort. Their dramatic demonstration of the immunizing properties of attenuated cultures of anthrax bacilli before a special French Commission has been hailed for years as a significant milestone in the history of bacteriology.

Anthrax is principally a disease of herbivorous animals, but it may affect a wide variety of species, including humans. Sheep and cattle are most susceptible; horses and mules are slightly more resistant to natural infection. Swine are even more resistant, as are dogs, cats, and other species, although anthrax does occur in these animals. In the more susceptible species (sheep, cattle, horses), the disease is usually seen as a fulminant septicemia. In the more resistant animals (swine), the disease may be localized and confined to the regional lymph nodes, particularly those of the cervical region. Humans usually acquire anthrax from contact with infected animals or animal products (hides, wool, shaving brushes made from infected hog bristles). The disease manifests as a localized, persistent cutaneous pustule, a malignant carbuncle, or a systemic, often fatal pulmonary disease, woolsorters' disease (Fig. 10-1).

Of the thirty-some species within the genus, *Bacillus anthracis* is the most important as a pathogen. *Bacillus anthracis* is a relatively large, encapsulated, rod-shaped bacillus, which produces spores. It grows well under aerobic conditions and is gram-positive. In smears from tissues, it often appears as short chains of square-ended rods, but spores are not formed until it has been exposed to air. Giemsa's stain should reveal red capsules on a minority of the organisms.

The organism can grow and sporulate in alkaline soil and organic material; highly resistant spores released from infected animals can cause contamination of the location in which infection has occurred, rendering it potentially hazardous for many years. Infected animal products also serve as an important source of virulent organisms. In addition to carcasses of animals dead of the disease, animal wastes and such products as bone meal, wool, bristles, and hides from abattoirs have been implicated in many infections. Anthrax occurs worldwide and throughout the United States, though it is particularly prevalent in the more tropical countries. Infection can follow ingestion or inhalation of spores or vegetative forms of the organism or entry of the organism through broken skin. On entry, spores germinate and, after localized multiplication, spread by means of lymphatics to lymph nodes and further to the bloodstream, leading to massive septicemia. There is little in the way of cellular reaction of the host to the organisms, whose capsules render them resistant to phagocytosis (as well as to neutralizing antibodies). The severity of the disease is the result of the elaboration of exotoxins, first described by Smith and colleagues (1955), which have been resolved into three components designated edema factor (EF), protective antigen (PA), and lethal factor (LF) or factors I, II, and III. EF has been shown to be an adenylate cyclase that causes an increase in cAMP, a feature shared by the enterotoxins of *Vibrio cholerae* and *Escherichia coli*.

SIGNS

The signs of anthrax in **cattle** and **sheep** are variable and may be overlooked in cases of short duration, in which death is the first indication of the presence of disease. In those instances in which symptoms have been observed, anthrax is recognized as a febrile disease with manifestations of depression, weakness, bloody discharges from body orifices, cyanosis, dyspnea, and occasional edematous subcutaneous swellings. Most animals so affected die within a few hours or a day.

Swine and dogs are usually infected by ingestion of infected meat from diseased sheep or cattle. Infection is usually localized to the pharynx, with enlargement of the cervical lymph nodes, or appears as an acute hemorrhagic gastroenteritis.

Pharyngeal or enteric disease is also the usual picture in horses. The cutaneous form, malignant carbuncle of humans, ordinarily is not recognized in animals.

LESIONS

The gross lesions in fatal cases of the disseminated form of anthrax include edematous and hemorrhagic changes in any part of the body, particularly in serous membranes. The spleen is greatly enlarged and engorged with dark, unclotted blood (Fig. 10-2). Lymph nodes are usually swollen, edematous, and occasionally hemorrhagic. Lesions in other organs are inconstant, although hemorrhages and swelling may occur in the intestinal tract, liver, and kidneys. In localized infections in swine, edema and hemorrhages are seen in the pharynx and cervical lymph nodes. In cases of longer standing, the lymph nodes become enlarged and solid, with yellowish foci surrounded by fibrous connective tissue.

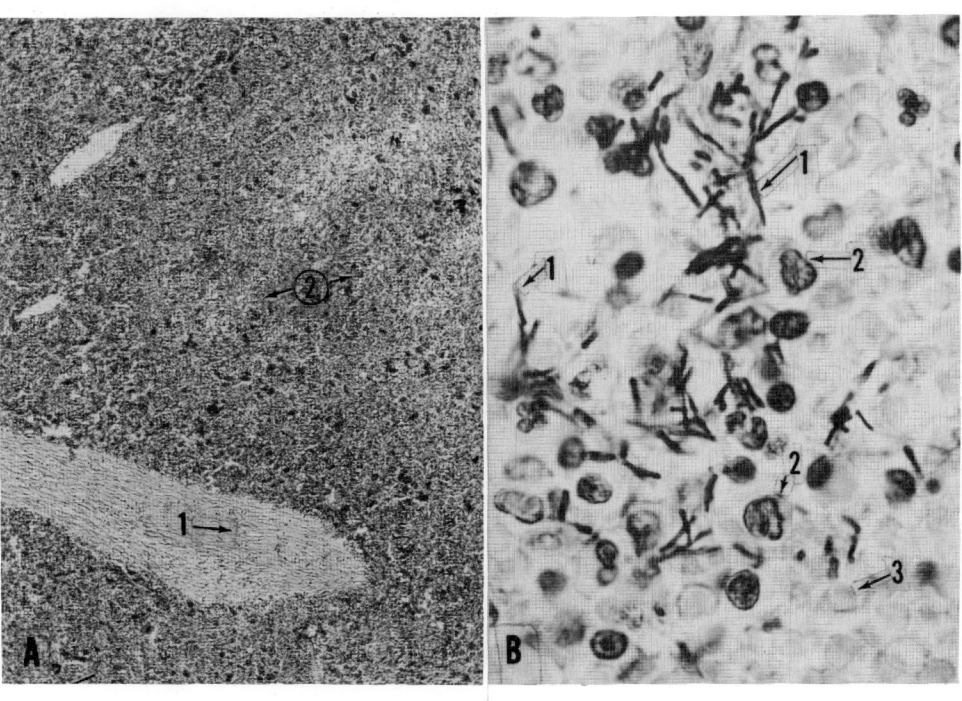

FIG. 10-2 Anthrax. **A.** Spleen in a fatal bovine case (hematoxylin and eosin [H & E], × 62). Lymphoid elements are obscured and trabeculae (1) are widely separated by the massive hemorrhage (2). **B.** Spleen of a guinea pig that was experimentally infected with anthrax from a bovine (× 1500). Gram's stain of a tissue section. Note gram-positive bacilli (1), lymphoid cells (2), and erythrocytes (3). (Courtesy of Dr. C. L. Davis, and Armed Forces Institute of Pathology.)

The microscopic findings in generalized cases are dominated by the presence of large numbers of anthrax bacilli in the blood and most other tissues. These large rod-shaped organisms can be demonstrated in smears or tissue sections, but they cannot be distinguished from saprophytic bacilli without culturing them and determining their pathogenicity in laboratory animals. In the spleen, the architecture is obscured by the presence of large numbers of erythrocytes. The lymphoid follicles are not discernible; only the trabeculae remain as tiny islands in a sea of red cells and nuclear debris, which floods the splenic sinuses and the cords of Bilroth. Bacilli are readily demonstrated in sections of the spleen with Gram's stain.

Localized infection in lymph nodes of swine result in foci of necrosis surrounded by a layer of granulation tissue. Giant cells usually are not present.

DIAGNOSIS

Presumptive diagnoses are made largely on the basis of the history (few premonitory symptoms, with sudden death of several animals in a herd) and the characteristic gross lesions found at necropsy. The diagnosis is confirmed by demonstration of *Bacillus anthracis* in large numbers in blood and tissues of animals dead of the disease. It is important that the organisms be identified and differentiated from saprophytes on the basis of pathogenicity as well as morphologic and cultural characterists. Inoculation of organisms, usually intraperitoneally, kills a mouse in 12 to 24 hours and a guinea pig in 24 to 36 hours. Organisms are readily seen in and cultured from the tissues of such inoculated animals.

Other organisms in the genus, such as *Bacillus cereus (B. anthracoides, B. pseudoanthracis)* and *B. thuringiensis,* both closely related to *B. anthracis* and *B. licheniformis,* have sometimes been associated with abortion and perinatal mortality, mastitis, and localized lesions in cattle and sheep. These and others have also been associated with food poisoning in humans. Other potential pathogens include *B. alvei, B. brevis, B. sphaericus, B. coagulans, B. pumilus,* and *B. subtilis.* None are clearly the sort of pathogen that *B. anthracis* is. Although associated with certain lesions, most have not been proven to be pathogenic. *B. cereus* has been shown to experimentally cause disease in cattle and sheep. *Bacillus piliformis,* the cause of Tyzzer's disease, is not a true member of the genus Bacillus.

References

Beall FA, Dalldorf FG. The pathogenesis of the lethal effect of anthrax toxin in the rat. J Infect Dis 1966;116:377–389.

Cartwright ME, McChesney AE, Jones RL. Vaccination-related anthrax in three llamas. J Am Vet Med Assoc 1987;191:715–716.

Dalldorf FG, et al. Transcellular permeability and thrombosis of capillaries in anthrax toxemia. Lab Invest 1969;21:42–51.

Dalldorf FG, Kaufmann AF, Brachman PS. Wool-sorters' disease. An experimental model. Arch Pathol 1971;92:418–426.

Fried BM. The infection of rabbits with the anthrax bacillus by way of the trachea. Arch Pathol 1930;10:213–223.

Fox MD, et al. Anthrax in Louisiana, 1971: epizootiologic study. J Am Vet Med Assoc 1973;163:446–451.

Fox MD, et al. An epizootiologic study of anthrax in Falls County, Texas. J Am Vet Med Assoc 1977;170:327–333.

Gleiser CA. Pathology of anthrax infection in animal hosts. Fed Proc 1967;26:1518–1521.

Holden C. What is Siberian ulcer doing in Sverdlovsk? Science 1980;208:37.

Kirkbride CA, Collins JE, Gates CE. Porcine abortion caused by Bacillus sp. J Am Vet Med Assoc 1986;188:1060–1061.

Leppla SH. Anthrax toxin edema factor: a bacterial adenylate cyclase that increases cyclic AMP concentrations in eukaryotic cells. Proc Natl Acad Sci USA 1982;79:3162–3166.

Plotkin SA, et al. An epidemic of inhalation anthrax, the first in the twentieth century. I. Clinical features. Am J Med 1960;29:992–999.

Ross JM. On the histopathology of experimental anthrax in the guinea pig. Br J Exp Pathol 1955;36:336–342.

Schuh J, Weinstock D. Bovine abortion caused by Bacillus cereus. J Am Vet Med Assoc 1985;187:1047–1048.

Smith H, Stoner HB. Anthrax toxic complex. Fed Proc 1967;26:1554–1558.

Smith ID, Frost AJ. The pathogenicity to pregnant ewes of an organism of the genus Bacillus. Aust Vet J 1968;44:17–19.

Smith ID. Ovine perinatal mortality associated with Bacillus cereus. Res Vet Sci 1972;13:499–501.

Van Ness GB. Ecology of anthrax. Science. 1971;172:1303–1307.

Wohlgemuth K, Bicknell EJ, Kirkbride CA. Abortion in cattle associated with Bacillus cereus. J Am Vet Med Assoc 1972;161:1688–1690.

Wohlgemuth K, Kirkbride CA, Bicknell EJ, et al.. Pathogenicity of Bacillus cereus for pregnant ewes and heifers. J Am Vet Med Assoc 1972;161:1691–1695.

Van Ness GB. Ecology of anthrax. Science 1971;172:1303–1307.

CLOSTRIDIAL INFECTIONS

Organisms of the genus Clostridium are sporulating, anaerobic bacteria of rather large size, usually about 0.8μ in width and 3 to 8μ in length, which occur singly, in pairs or in chains. Most members of the genus are nonpathogenic and are commonly found in soil and in the intestinal tract of humans and animals. Several members of the group are responsible for a number of diseases of humans and animals.

These organisms can be divided into two groups; those that produce disease through tissue invasion and those that owe their pathogenicity to the production of toxins. This division is, however, somewhat arbitrary, since all clostridia produce toxins that contribute to their pathogenicity.

Clostridium botulinum, the cause of botulism, is completely noninvasive; disease results from ingestion of toxins formed outside the body. *C. tetani,* the cause of tetanus, is not particularly invasive; disease results from circulating toxin produced by organisms, which, after entry into the body, remain localized within sites of tissue damage with low oxygen tension. The invasive clostridia, such as *C. chauvoie, C. novyi,* and *C. haemolyticum* cause diseases characterized by extensive tissue invasion and necrosis. Tissue invasion by these organisms, however, requires initial "priming" by means of tissue damage initiated through other mechanisms to produce an appropriate anaerobic environment. The pathogenesis of diseases caused by *C. perfringens* may involve invasive and noninvasive mechanisms. It may be a pathogen in cases of (1) food poisoning by toxins produced outside the body, (2) various enterotoxemias resulting from tox-

TABLE 10-1 **Pathogenic Clostridiae**

Species	Disease and principal animal species affected
C. chauvoei	Blackleg, cattle and sheep; wound infections (gangrene), many species
C. septicum	Malignant edema, many species; braxy, sheep
C. haemolyticum	Bovine bacillary hemoglobinuria
C. novyi	Black disease, sheep; wound infections (gangrene), many species
C. difficile	Pseudomembranous colitis (enterotoxemia), humans, hamsters, rabbits, guinea pigs
C. spiroforme	Enterotoxemia, rabbits
C. sordelli	Wound infections (gangrene), many species
C. carnis	Wound infections (gangrene), many species
C. histolyticum	Wound infections (gangrene), many species
C. villosum	Wound infections and pyothorax, cats
C. limosum	Rare isolate from cattle, dogs, guinea pigs
C. tetani	Tetanus, many species
C. perfringens, Types A–E	See Table 10-2
C. botulinum	Botulism; see Table 10-3

ins elaborated within the gastrointestinal tract, with or without significant tissue invasion, and (3) gas gangrene (also caused by other clostridia), resulting from initial proliferation in areas of tissue damage with low oxygen tension. Many of the clostridia (e.g., *C. septicum*) are normal inhabitants of the intestinal tract and, after death of the host, can widely invade and multiply. They are easily visualized or cultured under such circumstances, and caution must be exercised so as not to consider them as the cause of death.

The pathogenic clostridia and associated diseases are listed in Table 10-1.

Blackleg

The causative agent of blackleg is *C. chauvoie* (*C. feseri, Bacillus chauvoie*), an organism almost identical in culture and toxigenic characteristics to *C. septicum*, the cause of malignant edema (Fig.10-3). Each produces the same four toxins: alpha toxin, which is both necrotizing and hemolytic; beta toxin, which is a DNase; gamma toxin, a hyaluronidase; and delta toxin, a hemolysin. The most distinguishing feature between the two organisms is the nature of the diseases they cause.

Blackleg is an acute, highly fatal disease of cattle and occasionally of other species, such as sheep, goats, swine, mink, and, rarely, horses. The infection appears sporadically in certain areas where the organisms live in the soil. In some instances, the disease has appeared in cattle that have access to a newly excavated pond. It is postulated that disturbing the soil in some way exposes the bacteria or causes them to become pathogenic (Barnes and others, 1975).

C. chauvoie is also (along with other clostridia) a common secondary invader of traumatic or surgical wounds, resulting in gas gangrene or clostridial sepsis. This, however, is not the pathogenetic mechanism of blackleg. In blackleg, spores of *C. chauvoie* are ingested, the bacteria multiply in the intestine, and, in some manner, cross the intestinal mucosa and enter the general circulation, to be deposited in a variety of organs and tissues, including skeletal muscle. Here, spores remain dormant until damage to the muscle sets up an appropriate anaerobic environment for germination and proliferation. The mechanisms that lead to this appropriate environment are not clear; overt wounds are usually not apparent; and attempts to reproduce the syndrome usually fail. It is unknown why damage to other tissues where the latent spores may reside, such as the liver, doesn't initiate disease. Once the organisms begin to multiply, the release of toxins locally leads to myonecrosis and systemic spread of toxins via the bloodstream results in death.

SIGNS

The disease runs an acute, usually fatal course, and affected animals are often found dead before signs of illness have been observed. In some cases, there may be lameness or visible swelling of muscle groups. Any striated muscle may be affected, including the tongue, diaphragm, and myocardium, but the shoulder and pectoral muscles are most often involved. The disease is most common in young animals (6 months to 2 years of age) on a good plane of nutrition.

LESIONS

The lesions consist of crepitant swelling in the musculature, particularly of the extremities, which produces a stiff characteristic extension of the limbs a short time after death. Affected muscles incised at necropsy are dark brown or dark red, streaked with black. Some areas appear moist and, on pressure, yield dark, gas-filled exudate. Other groups of muscles are dry and sponge-like, with numerous gas bubbles. A peculiar sweetish odor may be noticed. The subcutaneous tissues overlying affected muscles are usually yellowish, gelatinous, blood-tinged, and contain gas bubbles. Similar lesions are often demonstrated in the heart but rarely in the tongue (could be confused with "woody

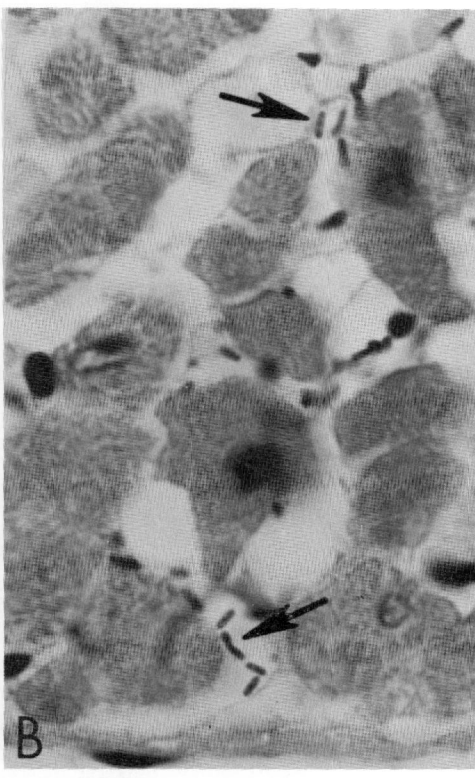

FIG. 10-3 Blackleg, bovine muscle. **A.** Fragmented myofibers are separated by edema, cellular infiltration, and gas bubbles. **B.** The large causative bacilli (arrows) demonstrated with Giemsa stain. (Courtesy of Dr. C. L. Davis.)

tongue"); diffuse hemorrhagic lesions in the lung may even occur.

Microscopically, the essential lesions are found in the skeletal musculature. Gas bubbles in the fixed tissues are indicated by spherical spaces separating muscle bundles and fascia. There are irregular areas of necrosis and collections of neutrophils and lymphocytes along the muscle septa. Edema is uncommon. Gram-positive organisms are demonstrable in sections, appearing singly or in small, irregular clumps.

DIAGNOSIS

A presumptive diagnosis can be made by the characteristic gross lesions and by demonstration of fairly numerous single or, possibly, paired bacilli with rounded ends and occasional spores near, but not at the end of, the cell. As is typical of clostridia, the spore is somewhat greater in diameter than the bacillus in which it forms. The lesions must be differentiated from other clostridial infections of muscle, particularly C. septicum; therefore, the diagnosis should be confirmed by culture or use of specific immunologic staining techniques.

Bovine bacillary hemoglobinuria

A disease apparently first described in California in 1916 by K. F. Meyer, bovine bacillary hemoglobinuria occurs principally in sharply delimited geographic areas in the western and southern United States but has also been reported in Wisconsin, Florida, New Zealand,

Mexico, South America, and Europe (Fig.10-4). The disease is caused by *Clostridium haemolyticum (C. haemolyticus bovis)*, which is very similar (identical in some respects) to *C. novyi* type B. The diseases caused by the two organisms are also very similar. Bergey's Manual of Systematic Bacteriology states that "*C. haemolyticum* cannot be distinguished from *C. novyi B* by any phenotypic or morphological test yet devised except by toxin neutralization in laboratory animals"; yet it continues ". . . antisera to one does not protect against infection with the other. . . ." Bovine bacillary hemoglobinuria is also

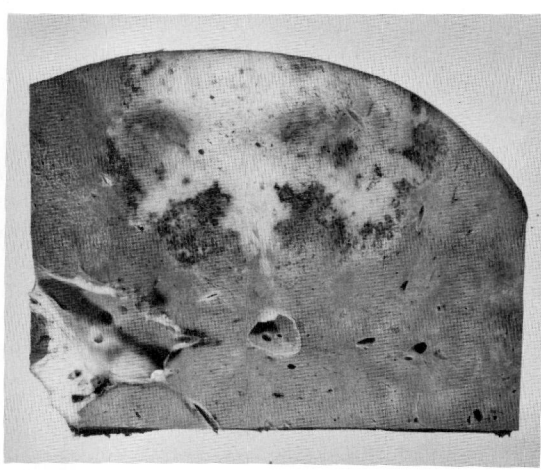

FIG. 10-4 Bovine bacillary hemoglobinuria. Necrotic lesion in liver of a 2-year-old Holstein heifer. (Courtesy of Dr. W. J. Hadlow.)

known as **red water disease** and **infectious icterohemoglobinuria.**

In a manner similar to certain other clostridia (*C. novyi, C. chauvoie*), organisms in the soil are ingested by the host, multiply in the intestinal tract, and somehow gain entry into the systemic circulation. *C. haemolyticum* then localizes in the liver and remains latent until an appropriate anaerobic environment allows its multiplication at this site. The migration of liver flukes is believed to represent the most effective mode of initiating hepatic damage, with resultant activation of the clostridia. Exotoxins then contribute to further hepatic damage, with the production of a characteristic "infarct," hemolysis, and death. The principal toxin is beta toxin (identical to that of *C. novyi*), a phospholipase C that hydrolyzes lecithin and sphingomyelin and hemolyzes red blood cells.

SIGNS

The disease, for which the mortality rate is high, is characterized by sudden onset of hemoglobinuria, fever, anemia, leukocytosis, collapse, and death within a day or two.

LESIONS

The typical lesion is a large area of necrosis, resembling an infarct, in the liver. It is almost always a solitary lesion, in contrast to black disease, where multiple areas of hepatic necrosis can occur. Microscopically, the necrotic tissue contains the gram-positive bacilli and is surrounded by a modest polymorphonuclear infiltrate. The kidneys are mottled as a result of hemoglobinuria, and any urine in the bladder is deep red.

DIAGNOSIS

Diagnosis is based on the pathologic findings (hepatic infarct, hemoglobinuria) and isolation of *C. haemolyticum*. The disease must be differentiated from many other bovine situations that are accompanied by hemoglobinuria.

Malignant edema

Originally isolated by Pasteur, who called it *"Vibrion septique," Clostridium septicum* is another ubiquitous organism that is found in soil and in the gastrointestinal tract of animals. It is similar in almost all characteristics to *C. chauvoie.* Malignant edema is seen as a sequel to wounds, such as those incurred in shearing or docking, or to parturition during which aseptic precautions were ignored. It is most common in horses, sheep, and cattle, but most animal species and humans are susceptible, although it is rare in dogs and cats.

The disease is essentially a form of gas gangrene, although in malignant edema gas production is minimal. *C. septicum* owes its pathogenicity to various toxins, as do the other clostridia. Of the several toxins elaborated by *C. septicum,* a hemolytic and necrotizing toxin referred to as alpha toxin is the most dangerous.

The disease is characterized by a febrile course of short duration with hot, painful swelling at sites of infection. These swollen areas later become even more edematous but less painful and cooler. At necropsy, the involved tissues are edematous and often hemorrhagic, and they contain some gas bubbles. Septicemia often occurs, with hemorrhages distributed throughout the body. The lungs are congested and edematous. Serous, blood-tinged effusion from the peritoneum may also be observed. *Clostridium septicum* is readily demonstrable in the affected tissues.

Braxy

Braxy (bradsot) is an acute infection of sheep caused by *Clostridium septicum* and characterized by hemorrhagic abomasitis. The disease is principally seen in Scotland and Scandinavia but also occurs in Iceland, Canada, and the northern United States. Its occurrence is associated with cold weather and the ingestion of frost-covered foods, but the pathogenesis is not understood. The infection mainly affects young sheep and usually occurs during the winter months. Death is sudden, with few or no clinical signs. The wall of the abomasum is thickened, edematous, and hemorrhagic. Similar lesions may be encountered in the small intestine. The large causative bacilli can be seen in tissue section and are readily isolated from the lesions.

Black disease

Also known as infectious necrotic hepatitis, black disease is an acute fatal infection of sheep and, rarely, cattle caused by *Clostridium novyi (C. oedematiens).* The organism is widely distributed in soil as three strains (A, B, and C) and is a common inhabitant of the intestinal tract of sheep. The strains are differentiated on the basis of toxin production. Type A produces alpha toxin, a necrotizing and lethal toxin; type B produces both alpha toxin and beta toxin, a necrotizing, hemolytic, and lethal toxin; and type C is nontoxigenic and nonpathogenic. *C. haemolyticum,* a very similar organism that only produces the beta toxin, is considered by some to be a toxigenic variant of *C. novyi.* The type B strain, which is nearly identical to *C. haemolyticum,* is the strain that causes black disease.

Black disease was first reported in Australia but subsequently has been recognized in New Zealand, the United States, the United Kingdom, Europe, Turkey, India, and the African nation of Mali (Bagadi, 1974). Similarities with the pathogenesis, etiology, and lesions of bovine bacillary hemoglobinuria are obvious. A similar disease has also been described in a horse (Dumaresq, 1939). In a high percentage of animals in enzootic areas, *C. novyi* pass through the intestinal wall and lodge in the liver, where they remain as a latent infection. An anaerobic environment produced by the migration of liver flukes (*Fasciola hepatica, Dicrocoelium dendriticum*) activates the bacteria, which release exotoxins, further contributing to hepatic necrosis and producing fatal toxemia. The principal toxin is necrotizing and called alpha toxin, or lethal toxin. A beta toxin is also produced, which is a necrotizing and hemolyzing lecithinase identical to the beta toxin of *C. haemolyticum*. Death of the host may result without premonitory signs. Pathologic changes include characteristic multiple foci of necrosis in the liver, petechiae on the epicardium and endocardium, and hydropericardium. Subcutaneous venous congestion causes a dark discoloration of the pelt, which is the reason for the name "black disease."

DIAGNOSIS

Diagnosis is made on the basis of pathologic findings and isolation of *C. novyi*. The organisms may be demonstrated with fluorescent antibody technique in smears or sections of the liver, but since the organisms are normal inhabitants at this site and proliferate rapidly after death from any cause, the clinical manifestations and gross and microscopic lesions must also be considered in establishing a diagnosis.

Gas gangrene (clostridial wound infections)

Type A *C. novyi* is a common contaminant of wounds and a cause of gas gangrene in several species,, including humans. In young rams, it may, as a consequence of head wounds sustained during fighting, result in a condition referred to as big head. The principle toxin of the type A strain is alpha toxin.

Gas gangrene is the term applied to clostridial infections of traumatic or surgical wounds. Most often it is applied to such infections in humans. Malignant edema, discussed above, is the term used for such a condition in animals, although in this disorder gas production is limited. Clostridia most often associated with gangrene include *C. perfringens, C. septicum, C. novyi, C. chauvoei, C. sordelli, C. histolyticum,* and *C. carnis. C. villosum* is often isolated from bite-wound abscesses in cats and also often recovered from cases of pyothorax in cats. Gas gangrene is initiated by proliferation of clostridial organisms in areas of tissue damage with low oxygen tension and is characterized by extensive necrosis of muscle with considerable edema and cellulitis. The affected areas are swollen, exude serosanguineous fluid, and have a putrid odor. Gas bubbles of varying size are interspersed with necrotic tissue. The lesion is the result of potent toxins, released from the offending bacteria, which may enter the circulation and lead to hemolytic anemia and necrotizing lesions at other sites.

Tetanus

Tetanus, or "lockjaw," occurs in humans and animals. It has become far less common than in the past because of more effective treatment of wounds and widespread use of tetanus toxoid. The causative organism, *Clostridium tetani*, is a normal inhabitant of the intestinal tract of herbivorous animals and is found in humus-rich soil. It is a gram-positive, sporulating, anaerobic, rod-shaped bacillus. Tetanus is usually a sequel of wounds, often insignificant ones, such as nail-pricks, or those pro-

duced by castration, docking, or shearing or those received during parturition. The anaerobic environment of certain wounds allows germination of the spores, multiplication of the organism, and release of a potent neurotoxin that prevents the function of inhibitory spinal interneurons by interfering with release of transmitter substance at the presynaptic terminals. Several biochemical events are initiated, but the most important is the interference with release of glycine, the inhibitory transmitter at this site. The toxin, called *tetanospasmin*, reaches the interspinal site by entering the bloodstream, attaching to peripheral nerve endings, and traveling along nerves to the central nervous system. *C. tetani* also releases two other toxins, **tetanolysin** (a hemolysin) and **"nonspasmogenic toxin."** The former may assist *C. tetani* to establish itself in wounds, and the latter may interfere with motor nerve function. It is tetanospasmin, however, which is responsible for the clinical picture of tetanus.

SIGNS

The disease is characterized by prolonged spasmodic contractions of muscles, with extension of limbs, stiffness, and immobilization. The muscles of mastication are often affected, immobilizing the jaws. The entire musculature is eventually involved, and death follows.

DIAGNOSIS

Diagnosis is based on clinical signs and a history of trauma; however, a wound is often not demonstrable, and if present, the bacilli are difficult to demonstrate. Specific lesions have not been described.

Enterotoxemia

A group of disorders, loosely gathered under the heading of enterotoxemia, are the result of the elaboration of toxins by *C. perfringens* in the gastrointestinal tract. Some of these disorders are true enterotoxemias (those caused by the type D organism), but others are characterized by a necrotizing enterocolitis more analogous to the disease associated with *C. difficile* described as pseudomembranous colitis. The latter do result, however, from elaboration of toxins and are reproducible with bacteria-free filtrates of intestinal contents.

There are five strains of *C. perfringens* (types A, B, C, D, and E), which owe their pathogenicity to the elaboration of one or more of four toxins, designated alpha, beta, epsilon, and iota. There are others, but these are the toxins of principal importance. The relative production of these four toxins by the five types of *C. perfringens* and the associated diseases are indicated in Table 10-2.

Alpha toxin, produced by all five types, is a phospholipase C that causes cell lysis (necrosis) and hemolysis: It is the toxin of importance in gas gangrene caused by *C. perfringens*.

Beta toxin, produced by types B and C, is not characterized, but is associated with increased vascular permeability and necrosis.

TABLE 10-2 *Clostridium perfringens* **types, toxins, and diseases**

Type	Toxins				Diseases
	Alpha	Beta	Epsilon	Iota	
A	+	−	−	−	Gas gangrene, food poisoning, infectious diarrhea in humans; enterotoxemia in lambs, cattle, goats, horses, dogs, mink; colitis X in horses; gastric dilation in primates
B	+	+	+	−	Lamb dysentery; enterotoxemia in calves, foals, guinea pigs
C	+	+	−	−	Enterotoxemia (necrotic enteritis) in lambs, goats, cattle, pigs; struck in adult sheep; darmand and pig-bel in humans
D	+	−	+	−	Enterotoxemia (overeating disease, pulpy kidney disease) in sheep, goats, cattle.
E	+	−	−	+	Enterotoxemia in calves, lambs, guinea pigs, rabbits

+, type contains this toxin; −, type does not contain this toxin.

Epsilon toxin, produced by types B and D, is first elaborated as a nontoxic compound, which is converted to a potent toxin by proteolytic enzymes such as trypsin: It causes increased vascular permeability and tissue necrosis.

Iota toxin, produced by type E, is also first elaborated as a protoxin and converted to its active form by proteolytic enzymes: It increases vascular permeability markedly and causes necrosis.

All five types of *C. perfringens* are extremely common in the gastrointestinal tract of animals. Types B and E are considered obligate parasites. Type A is additionally found in soil.

TYPE A

C. perfringens type A is the most common cause of gas gangrene in humans and animals and is a cause of some forms of food poisoning in humans. Type A enterotoxemia, often termed **yellow lamb disease,** has been described in lambs and calves in the western United States, but it is apparently a rare disease. It is an acute syndrome of short course and a high rate of mortality, characterized by intense icterus, hemolytic anemia, and hemoglobinuria. Lesions include icterus, anemia, excess pericardial fluid, dark kidneys, and an enlarged, friable liver. *C. perfringens* type A has also been associated with a syndrome in neonatal calves characterized by rumen tympany and abomasitis. A disease of horses termed colitis X has been associated with *C. perfringens* type A, but the exact causal relationship is not clearly established. Colitis X is characterized by foul-smelling, profuse diarrhea and dehydration. Aside from hemorrhage in various organs, lesions are restricted to the colon, where there is hemorrhage and necrosis of the mucosa. Type A organisms have also been associated with enteric disease in goats, dogs, and mink. In dogs, it often accompanies parvoviral enteritis.

TYPE B

C. perfringens type B is the cause of an enterotoxemia of lambs, calves, and foals in England, Scotland, Wales, South Africa, and the Middle East. It is a disease of the very young, affecting lambs less than 2 weeks of age, calves up to 10 days of age, and foals in the first 2 days of life, rarely after. The syndrome in lambs, known as **lamb dysentery,** is extremely acute. Death may occur without premonitory signs or lambs may be seen having watery, often bloody, diarrhea, lying down, refusing to suckle, and exhibiting signs of abdominal pain. The characteristic lesion is hemorrhagic enteritis, often with ulceration and occasionally with perforation and peritonitis. Lesions are usually restricted to the small intestine, but may also affect the colon. Petechiae and ecchymoses are common on serous membranes of the epicardium and endocardium, and the pericardial cavity contains excess fluid. The type B organism has also been associated with a wasting disease of older lambs in England referred to as "pine." Microscopically, the lesion is not pathognomonic and is characterized by focal areas of necrosis involving the entire thickness of the mucosa and extending into the muscularis. The lesions in calves and foals are also characterized by hemorrhagic enteritis and ulceration.

TYPE C

Two distinct forms of type C enterotoxemia have been described; one occurs in adult sheep and the other in neonatal lambs, calves, and piglets. The first form of type C enterotoxemia to be described was called struck, a disease of adult sheep in Britain. It occurs most commonly during the winter and early spring months. Clinical signs usually are not noted. The lesions are hemorrhagic enteritis with ulceration of the mucosa, particularly of the jejunum and duodenum. A striking feature is peritonitis with a large volume of clear yellow fluid in the peritoneal cavity. A very similar entity has been ascribed to *C. perfringens* type D in feedlot cattle.

In the United States, a form of type C enterotoxemia known as **enterotoxic hemorrhagic enteritis** occurs in calves, lambs, and foals in the first few days of life. Clinically, there is diarrhea, but, as with other forms of enterotoxemia, death often occurs in the absence of noted signs. The lesions are characterized by hemorrhagic enteritis with ulceration, particularly of the jejunum and ileum. Hemorrhages are common beneath the epicardium, in the thymus, and elsewhere.

Type C enterotoxemia also occurs in suckling piglets, usually during the first week of life. Most affected pigs die within 12 to 48 hours after onset of clinical signs, which include depression, dehydration and diarrhea that is often bloody. The pathologic changes, described in detail by Hogh (1969), are dominated by a hemorrhagic or necrotizing enteritis principally affecting the jejunum. There is hemorrhagic lymphadenitis of draining lymph nodes; serosanguineous fluid in the peritoneal, pleural, and pericardial cavities; and hemorrhage in the epicardium, endocardium, and kidneys.

TYPE D

C. perfringens type D is responsible for enterotoxemia of sheep, goats, and cattle. In sheep, the disease occurs in fatting lambs and, less regularly, in adult sheep and is known as **"pulpy kidney disease"** or **"overeating disease."** It occurs throughout the world and is often associated with diets high in concentrated grains. Decreasing the total amount of food or changing from a high concentration of grains with little roughage to a ration consisting almost entirely of hay or similar material appears to be an effective preventive measure. Lambs are usually found dead, but if observers are present, they may detect a period of one-half to a few hours during which opisthotonos progresses into premortal coma. In a few cases, convulsions take the place of coma, and death is more prompt. Occasionally, animals show a desire to push the forehead against a solid wall, which is the characteristic attitude of "blind staggers," as seen in many forms of indigestion in various species. Some investigators have found these acute symptoms to be preceded by a day or more of anorexia and diarrhea or mucus-covered feces, at least in some animals. There

is usually hyperglycemia and glycosuria. The disease in goats and calves is similar.

The pathologic findings are the result of absorption of epsilon toxin produced by *C. perfringens* within the intestinal lumen. Its injurious effect on vascular endothelium leads to hemorrhage, edema, and damage to parenchymal organs and the brain. There are petechial and ecchymotic hemorrhages beneath the epicardial and endocardial surfaces, the serous surfaces of the intestines, in abdominal muscles, in the diaphragm, and in the thymus. Hydropericardium is usually noted. In addition to distortion of other normal values in the blood chemistry, there is pronounced glycosuria. Also noted by some observers are distention of the rumen, reticulum, abomasum, and lower intestine by ingesta and gas. The intestinal mucosa is often hyperemic, and there may be microscopic evidence of superficial necrosis. The gallbladder is often distended. The kidneys are soft and friable, giving rise to the epithet "pulpy kidney disease"; often, this is entirely the result of postmortem autolysis, which proceeds rapidly. However, in some cases, particularly those with a longer clinical course, there is necrosis of the convoluted tubules.

Neurologic signs are explained by lesions in the central nervous system, which are the most specific and diagnostic for the disease. These consist of bilaterally symmetrical focal malacia of the basal ganglia, substantia nigra, and thalamus and bilaterally symmetrical demyelination in the internal capsule, subcortical white matter, and cerebellar peduncles. The harmful effect of the toxin on endothelium is particularly obvious in the brain. Damaged endothelial cells develop pyknotic nuclei, and the vessels become surrounded by a zone of edema. Ultrastructurally, the perivascular astrocyte endfeet are markedly swollen.

The ultrastructural changes in experimental disease (Morgan and Kelley, 1974) consist of periaxonal and intramyelinic edema in cerebellar white matter and swelling of axon terminals and dendrites in gray matter adjacent to lateral ventricles. Swelling of mitochondria is also an early feature. Occlusion of capillaries by aggregated platelets, accompanied by petechiae in relation to the malacia, suggests that changes in vascular endothelium may be the primary effect of the toxin. This concept is supported by evidence that the capillaries in affected parts of the brain leak conspicuously within 20 minutes after administration of *C. perfringens* type D toxin (Morgan and associates, 1975).

TYPE E

Type E *C. perfringens* has been found in calves and lambs, but the status of the disease with respect to frequency and importance is not known. Available data do not suggest that the disease is of significance.

Pseudomembranous Colitis (*C. difficile* and *C. spiroforme* Enterotoxemia)

Clostridium difficile (so named because of difficulty surrounding its isolation) has long been recognized as an inhabitant of the gastrointestinal tract of humans and animals, but it was not until 1977 that it was recognized as a cause of disease. Its usual association with disease results from the use of antibiotics to which *C. difficile* is resistant, allowing the organism to proliferate and secrete potent toxins. Under circumstances that are not understood, the organism has caused disease in the absence of antibiotic therapy in humans, nonhuman primates, and swine. Two toxins have been identified: toxin A or enterotoxin, which leads to marked fluid accumulation in the intestines by unknown mechanisms (not comparable to those of *Vibrio comma*); and toxin B, which is cytopathic. The toxins are similar to those produced by *C. sordelli*, an organism recovered from various infections. In fact, antibodies to *C. sordelli* toxins are used for identification of *C. difficile* toxin to confirm diagnosis.

The disease, which is characterized by severe colitis and often ileitis and cecitis, has been seen in hamsters, rabbits, guinea pigs, swine, foals, nonhuman primates, and humans. Pathologically, the lesions begin in the superficial mucosa as focal areas of necrosis, which progress to almost complete necrosis of the mucosa and its replacement by fibrin and debris. There is an intense neutrophilic inflammatory response and thrombosis of submucosal venules. The organisms are not invasive, but remain within the lumen. These lesions are very similar to those induced by *C. perfringens* enteritis (so-called enterotoxemia).

Clostridium spiroforme causes a similar disease in rabbits. Here the condition is also characterized by diarrhea and necrotizing colitis and typhlitis. It may occur spontaneously or in association with antimicrobial therapy. The disease has also been called iota-enterotoxemia, because the offending toxin is neutralized by antiserum to *C. perfringens* type E iota toxin.

Botulism

Clostridium botulinum is responsible for an extremely serious food intoxication, botulism. The bacterium was first named *Bacillus botulinus* by Emile Pierre Marie van Ermengem, who took the name from the Latin word botulus (sausage) because of the common association of the disease with ingestion of sausage. *C. butulinum* is divided into seven different toxigenic strains (A through G) based on antigenically distinguishable toxins released on dissolution of the organism.

On the basis of culture characteristics, these toxigenic strains are divided into four groups. Group I consists of proteolytic organisms, including all strains of type A and proteolytic strains of types B and F. Group II contains nonproteolytic strains of types B and F and all strains of type E. Group III contains types C and D, and Group IV consists of the type G strain, which has also been termed *C. argentinense*.

For the most part, each toxigenic strain produces a single toxin of the same designation; however, certain strains that produce more than one toxin or more than one variant of the same toxin have been identified. Two strains of type C organisms exist: type C-alpha and type C-beta. C-alpha mainly produces classical neurotoxin (designated C1). C-beta produces C2 toxin, which is not a neurotoxin; but it is cytotoxic through interference with adenosine diphosphate. The latter is not involved in the disease botulism.

Further complicating the situation is the fact that organisms distinct from *C. botulinum*, such as *C. barati* and *C. butyricum*, have been shown to produce botulinum toxin and have been implicated in cases of botulism. Type A strains of *C. novyi* also are very similar to Group III type C organisms. In general, all the botulinum neurotoxins behave in the same manner. Molecularly, they are very similar to tetanospasmin.

Botulism almost always results from the ingestion of preformed toxin in a food source. There are, however, two other pathogenetic mechanisms which have been termed toxicoinfectious. The first is **wound botulism,** first reported in 1951, in which *C. botulinum* contaminates wounds, grows in them, and produces toxin in them. This form of botulism has been associated only with proteolytic strains of type A and type B. It occurs in humans (types A and B) and horses (type B) but probably occurs in other species as well. Note that nonproteolytic strains do not grow and produce toxin at body temperature. The second mechanism in which toxin is not ingested results from colonization of the gastrointestinal tract with *C. botulinum* (types A and B), with subsequent production of toxin and absorption by the host. This is a true enterotoxemia, which in humans has been referred to as **infant botulism.** In humans, it is primarily seen in infants less than 6 months of age; all reported cases are less than 1 year of age, although the disease is suspected to occur in adults. The condition results from ingestion of foods containing spores of the organism, not the toxin. The most often implicated food in humans is honey. Enterotoxic botulism also occurs in pheasants, chickens, and probably other birds.

SIGNS

The signs of botulism follow a 1–day to 5–day "incubation period" and are characterized by a descending and symmetrical paralysis. After absorption into the bloodstream, the toxin enters peripheral nerves at their synaptic junctions, binds to nerve membranes, and prevents release of acetylcholine by synaptic vesicles. Only peripheral cholinergic nerves are affected: the toxin does not enter the central nervous system. Cranial nerves are first affected, but ultimately all muscles of the body may be affected. Almost all animal species, including birds and fishes, are susceptible.

In **humans,** most botulism results from the consumption of inadequately sterilized canned food that is neutral in acidity; the organisms produce their powerful neurotoxin in these foods. The food source varies in different parts of the world, but in the United States, canned vegetables and some fish products are the most common offenders.

In **cattle,** most botulism results from the ingestion of animal carcasses and their contaminated foodstuffs. Many small animals and birds carry type D organisms as part of their normal intestinal flora, and after death,

TABLE 10-3 **Botulism in animals and humans**

Type	Principal victims	Frequent vehicles	Greatest frequency
A	Humans, mink	Canned vegetables, fruits, meat, and fish	Western United States, Europe, Japan
B	Humans, horses, cattle, sheep	Meat, usually pork; silage and forage	Eastern United States, Europe
Cα	Cattle, sheep, horses, dogs, mink, birds, turtles	Fly larvae, rotting vegetation, silage, carrion	North and South America, South Africa, Australia
D	Cattle, horses, birds	Carrion	South Africa, Australia
E	Humans, mink, fish	Fish and marine animal foods	United States, Canada, Japan, Northern Europe, Russia
F	Humans	Liver paste	Denmark
G	Humans	Soil	Argentina, Switzerland

the carcass can become extremely toxic. Botulism often results from cattle with phosphorous deficiency chewing on bones (and remaining bits of decaying meat). This bone-chewing form of botulism is known as **lamsiekte** in South Africa, **bulbar paralysis** in Australia, and **loin disease** in the southwestern United States.

Forage poisoning is a form of botulism in cattle, which results from the ingestion of silage or hay that has become contaminated with a dead animal. Type C is most often implicated in this disease. Poultry litter containing type C or type D toxin has also been implicated in botulism in cattle. Type B toxin in grains and silage has proven an important source in the Netherlands. In Senegal, botulism (known as **Gnideo**) is common, resulting from drinking water contaminated with toxic animal carcasses.

Botulism in **sheep** is comparable to that in cattle. It is most common in South Africa and Australia and is associated with phosphorous deficiency and bone chewing.

In **horses,** botulism is seen sporadically worldwide. It is usually caused by ingestion of hay contaminated with a dead cat, an excellent source of type C toxin, to which cats themselves are highly resistant. Wound botulism resulting from type B toxin has been described in horses and foals ("shaker foal syndrome").

Swine are relatively resistant to botulism, apparently because the toxin is poorly absorbed. Type B toxicosis has, however, been described. In **dogs,** botulism resulting from type C toxin may occur, but it is not common.

Botulism is seen in most species of birds, except vultures, which are resistant. A peculiar form of torticollis is seen, resulting in the designation **limber neck.** Most

often, it results from type C toxin, but types D and E toxicoses have been reported. Toxicoinfectious or enterotoxemic botulism occurs in birds.

The various toxigenic types of *C. botulinum* are indicated in Table 10-3 along with the species usually affected. There is no specific histopathologic lesion.

References

Abbitt B, et al. Catastrophic death losses in a dairy herd attributed to type D botulism. J Am Vet Med Assoc 1984;185:798–801.

Allen JP, Wilson SS. A bibliography of references to avian botulism. US Fish and Wildlife Service Special Report No. 204. Washington, DC: US Department of the Interior 1977;1–6.

Allison MJ, Maloy SE, Matson RR. Inactivation of Clostridium botulinum toxin by ruminal microbes from cattle and sheep. Appl Environ Microbiol 1976;32:685–688.

Arnon SS, Midura TF, Clay SA, et al. Infant botulism: epidemiological, clinical, and laboratory aspects. JAMA 1977;237:1946–1951.

Bagadi HO. Infectious necrotic hepatitis (black disease) of sheep. Vet Bull 1974;44:385–388.

Barnes DM, Bergeland ME, Higbee JM. Selected blackleg outbreaks and their relation to soil excavation. Can Vet J 1975;16:257–259.

Barsanti JA, Walser M, Hatheway CL, et al. Type C botulism in American Foxhounds. J Am Vet Med Assoc 1978;172:809–813.

Bartlett JG, Onderdonk AB, Cisneros RL, et al. Clindamycin-associated colitis due to a toxin-producing species of Clostridium in hamsters. J Infect Dis 1977;136:701–705.

Bartlett JG, Chang TW, Gurwith M, et al. Antibiotic-associated pseudomembranous colitis due to toxin-producing clostridia. N Engl J Med 1978;298:531–534.

Beiers PR, Simmons GC. Botulism in pigs. Aust Vet J 1967;43:270–271.

Bennetts HW. Carrion poisoning in sheep (botulism). Aust Vet J 1928;4:105–106.

Bergeland ME. Pathogenesis and immunity of Clostridium perfringens type C enteritis in swine. J Am Vet Med Assoc 1972;160:568–571.

Bernard W, Divers TJ, Whitlock RH, et al. Botulism as a sequel to open castration in a horse. J Am Vet Med Assoc 1987;191:73–74.

Borriello SP, Carman RJ. Association of iota-like toxin and Clostridium spiroforme with both spontaneous and antibiotic-associated diarrhea and colitis in rabbits. J Clin Microbiol 1983;17:414–418.

Britton JW, Cameron HS. So-called enterotoxemia in lambs in California. Cornell Vet 1944;34:19–29.

Britton JW, Cameron HS. Experimental reproduction of so-called enterotoxemia. Cornell Vet 1945;35:1–8.

Bullen JJ. Enterotoxemia of sheep: Clostridium welchii, Type D, in the alimentary tract of normal animals. J Pathol Bact 1952;64:201–206.

Butler HC, Marsh H. Blackleg of the fetus in ewes. J Am Vet Med Assoc 1956;128:401–402.

Buxton D, Morgan KT. Studies of lesions produced in the brains of colostrum deprived lambs by Clostridium welchii (Cl. perfringens) type D toxin. J Comp Pathol 1976;86:435–447.

Buxton D, Linklater KA, Dyson DA. Pulpy kidney disease and its diagnosis by histological examination. Vet Rec 1978;102:241.

Carman RJ, Borriello SP. Infectious nature of Clostridium spiroforme-mediated rabbit enterotoxemia. Vet Microbiol 1984;9:497–502.

Carman RJ, Evans RH. Experimental and spontaneous clostridial enteropathies of laboratory and free living lagomorphs. Lab Anim Sci 1984;34:443–452.

Chang J, Rohwer RG. Clostridium difficile infection in adult hamsters. Lab Anim Sci 1991;41:548–552.

Clark DM, Harvey HJ, Roth L, et al. Clostridial peritonitis associated with a mast cell tumor in a dog. J Am Vet Med Assoc 1986;188:188–190.

Clay HA. A case of "blackquarter" in the pig. Vet Rec 1960;72:265–266.

Cohen A, Tamarin R. Investigations of two mass outbreaks of a botulism-like disease in cattle. IV. Bacteriological investigations. Refuah Vet 1978;35:109–115.

Crowe DT Jr, Kowalski JJ. Clostridial cellulitis with localized gas formation in a dog. J Am Vet Med Assoc 1976;169:1094–1096.

DiGiacomo RF, Missakian EA. Tetanus in a free-ranging colony of Macaca mulatta: a clinical and epizootiologic study. Lab Anim Sci 1972;22:378–383.

Divers TJ, Bartholomew RC, Messick JB, et al. Clostridium botulinum type B toxicosis in a herd of cattle and a group of mules. J Am Vet Med Assoc 1986;188:382–386.

Dodd S. The aetiology of black disease. J Comp Pathol 1921;34:1–26.

Dumaresq JA. A case of black disease in the horse. Aust Vet J 1939;15:53–57.

Edgar G. On the occurrence of black disease bacilli in the livers of normal sheep, with some observations on the causation of the disease. Aust Vet J 1928;4:133–141.

Eklund MW, Poysky FT, Peterson ME, et al. Type E botulism in salmonids and conditions contributing to outbreaks. Aquaculture 1984;41:293–310.

Farrow BRH, Murrell WG, Revington ML, et al. Type C botulism in young dogs. Aust Vet J 1983;60:374–377.

Finn CW Jr, et al. The structural gene for tetanus neurotoxin is on a plasmid. Science 1984;224:881–884.

Gardner DE. Pathology of Clostridium welchii type D enterotoxaemia. I. Biochemical and haematological alterations in lambs. J Comp Pathol 1973;83:499–507.

Gardner DE. Pathology of Clostridium welchii type D enterotoxaemia. II. Structural and ultrastructural alterations in the tissues of lambs and mice. J Comp Pathol 1973;83:509–524.

Gardner DE. Pathology of Clostridium welchii type D enterotoxaemia. III. Basis of the hyperglycaemic response. J Comp Pathol 1973;83:525–529.

Gitteo M. Botulism in mink: an outbreak caused by type-C toxin. Vet Rec 1959;71:868–871.

Goodwin WJ, Haines RJ, Bernal JC. Tetanus in baboons of a corral breeding colony. Lab Anim Sci 1987;37:231–232.

Griesemer RA, Krill WR. Enterotoxemia of beef calves—30 years' observation. J Am Vet Med Assoc 1962;140:154–158.

Griner LA, Bracken FK. Clostridium perfringens (type C) in acute hemorrhagic enteritis of calves. J Am Vet Med Assoc 1953;122:99–102.

Griner LA, Carlson WD. Enterotoxemia of sheep. I. Effects of Clostridium perfringens type D toxin on the brains of sheep and mice. II. Distribution of I131 radioiodinated serum albumin in brains of Clostridium perfringens type D intoxicated lambs. III. Clostridium perfringens type D antitoxin titers of normal, non-vaccinated lambs. Am J Vet Res 1961;22:429–442, 443–446, 447–448.

Griner LA, Johnson HW. Clostridium perfringens (type C) in hemorrhagic enterotoxemia of lambs. J Am Vet Med Assoc 1954;125:125–127.

Hagemoser WA, Hoffman LJ, Lundvall RL. Clostridium chauvoei infection in a horse. J Am Vet Med Assoc 1980;176:631–633.

Hartigan PJ. Botulism in horses. Irish Vet J 1985;39:194–197.

Hatheway CL. Toxigenic clostridia. Clin Microbiol Rev 1990;3:66–98.

Herd RP, Riches WR. An outbreak of tetanus in cattle. Aust Vet J 1964;40:356–357.

Hogh P. Necrotizing infectious enteritis in piglets, caused by Clostridium perfringens type C. I. Biochemical and toxigenic properties of the Clostridium. Acta Vet Scand 1967;8:26–38.

Hogh P. Necrotizing infectious enteritis in piglets, caused by Clostridium perfringens type C. II. Incidence and clinical features. Acta Vet Scand 1967;8:301–323.

Hogh P. Necrotizing infectious enteritis in piglets, caused by Clostridium perfringens type C. III. Pathologic changes. Acta Vet Scand 1969;10:57–83.

Holmes HT, Sonn RJ, Patton NM. Isolation of Clostridium spiroforme from rabbits. Lab Anim Sci 1988;38:167–168.

Jamieson S. Studies in black disease. 1. The occurrence of the disease in sheep in the north of Scotland. Vet Rec 1948;60:11–14.

Jamieson S. The identification of Clostridium oedematiens and an experimental investigation of its role in the pathogenesis of infectious necrotic hepatitis ("black disease") of sheep. J Pathol Bact 1949;61:389–402.

Jones MA, Hunter D. Isolation of pigs. Vet Rec 1983;112:253.

Jones RL, Adney WS, Alexander AF, et al. Hemorrhagic necrotizing enterocolitis associated with Clostridium difficile infection in four foals. J Am Vet Med Assoc 1988;193:76–79.

Jones RL, Shideler RK, Cockerell GL. Association of Clostridium difficile with foal diarrhea. Proc 5th Int Conf on Equine Infectious Diseases. Lexington, KY: University Press of Kentucky 1988.

Kao I, Drachman DB, Price DL. Botulinum toxin: mechanism of presynaptic blockade. Science 1976;193:1256–1258.

Kerry JB. A note on the occurrence of Clostridium chauvoei in the spleen and livers of normal cattle. Vet Rec 1964;76:396–397.

Langford EV. Feed-borne Clostridium chauvoei infection in mink. Can Vet J 1970;11:170–172.

Lewis GE Jr, Kulinski SS, Metzger PW, et al. Detection of Clostridium botulinum type G toxin by ELISA. Appl Environ Microbiol 1981;42:1018–1022.

Love DN, Jones RF, Bailey M. Clostridium villosum sp. nov. from subcutaneous abscesses in cats. Int J Syst Bacteriol 1979;29:241–244.

Love DN, Jones RF, Bailey M, et al. Isolation and characterisation of bacteria from pyothorax (empyaemia) in cats. Vet Microbiol 1982;7:455–461.

Lowe BR, Fox JG, Bartlett JG. Clostridium difficile-associated cecitis in guinea pigs exposed to penicillin. Am J Vet Res 1980;41:1277–1279.

Lund BM. Foodborne disease due to Bacillus and Clostridium species. Lancet 1990;335:982–986.

Macarie I, Cure C, Pop A. Histopathology of natural Clostridium perfringens type A infection in mink. Lucr Stiint Inst Agron "Nicolae Balcescu" C 1980;23:23–27.

MacKay RJ, Berkhoff GA. Type C toxicoinfectious botulism in a foal. J Am Vet Med Assoc 1982;180:163–164.

Mansfield PD, Wilt GR, Powers RD. Clostridial myositis associated with an intrathoracic abscess in a cat. J Am Vet Med Assoc 1984;184:1150–1151.

Marlow GR, Smart JL. Botulism in foxhounds. Vet Rec 1982;111:242.

Mason JH. Tetanus in the dog and cat. J S Afr Vet Med Assoc 1964;35:209–213.

McFarland LV, Mulligan ME, Kwok RYY, et al. Nosocomial acquisition of Clostridium difficile infection. N Engl J Med 1989;320:204–210.

McGowan B, Moulton JE, Rood SE. Lamb losses associated with Clostridium perfringens type A. J Am Vet Med Assoc 1958;133:219–221.

Moon HW, Bergeland ME. Clostridium perfringens type C enterotoxemia of the newborn pig. Can Vet J 1965;6:159–161.

Morgan KT, Kelly BG. Ultrastructural study of brain lesions produced in mice by the administration of Clostridium welchii type D toxin. J Comp Pathol 1974;84:181–191.

Morgan KT, Kelly BG, Buxton D. Vascular leakage produced in the brains of mice by Clostridium welchii type D toxin. J Comp Pathol 1975;85:461–466.

Nakamura S, Kimura I, Yamakawa K, et al. Taxonomic relationships among Clostridium novyi types A and B, Clostridium haemolyticum and Clostridium botulinum type C. J Gen Microbiol 1983;129:1473–1479.

Niilo L, Moffatt RE, Avery RJ. Bovine "enterotoxemia." II. Experimental reproduction of the disease. Can Vet J 1963;4:288–298.

Notermans S, Dufrenne J, Oosterom J. Persistence of Clostridium botulinum type B on a cattle farm after an outbreak of botulism. Appl Environ Microbiol 1981;41:179–183.

Notermans S, Hagenaars AM, Kozaki S. The enzyme-linked immunoabsorbent assay (ELISA) for the detection and determination of Clostridium botulinum toxins A, B, and E. Methods Enzymol 1982;84(Part D):223–239.

Olander HJ, Hughes JP, Biberstein EL. Bacillary haemoglobinuria: induction by liver biopsy in naturally and experimentally injected animals. Pathologia Vet 1966;3:421–450.

Osborne RH, Bradford HF. Tetanus toxin inhibits amino acid release from nerve endings in vitro. Nature New Biol 1973;244:157–158.

Pearson EG, Hedstrom OR, Sonn R, et al. Hemorrhagic enteritis caused by Clostridium perfringens type C in a foal. J Am Vet Med Assoc 1986;188:1309–1310.

Plaisier AJ. Enterotoxaemia in piglets caused by Clostridium perfringens type C. Tijdschr Diergeneeskd 1971;96:324–340.

Poonacha KB, Donahue JM, Nightengale JR. Clostridial myositis in a dog. J Am Vet Med Assoc 1989;194:69–70.

Popoff MR. Bacteriological examination in enterotoxaemia of sheep and lamb. Vet Rec 1984;114:324.

Quinlivan TD, Wedderburn JF. Bacillary haemoglobinuria in cattle in New Zealand. NZ Vet J 1959;7:113–115.

Ramsay WR. An outbreak of tetanus-like disease in cattle. Aust Vet J 1973;49:188–189.

Rastas VP, Myers GH, Lesar S. Bacillary hemoglobinuria in Wisconsin cattle. J Am Vet Med Assoc 1974;164:1203–1204.

Rebhun WC, Shin SJ, King JM, et al. Malignant edema in horses. J Am Vet Med Assoc 1985;187:732–736.

Rehg JE, Lu Y-S. Clostridium difficile colitis in a rabbit following antibiotic therapy for pasteurellosis. J Am Vet Med Assoc 1981;179:1296–1297.

Roeder BL, Chengappa MM, Nagaraja TG, et al. Experimental induction of abdominal tympany, abomasitis, and abomasal ulceration by intraruminal inoculation of Clostridium perfringens type A in neonatal calves. Am J Vet Res 1988;49:201–207.

Ryden EB, Lipman NS, Taylor NS, et al. Clostridium difficile typhlitis associated with cecal mucosal hyperplasia in Syrian hamsters. Lab Anim Sci 1991;41:553–558.

Schofield FW. Enterotoxemia (sudden death) in calves due to Clostridium welchii. J Am Vet Med Assoc 1955;126:192–194.

Scholtens RG, Coohon DR. Botulism in animals and humans, with special reference to type E, Clostridium botulinum. Sci Proc AVMA 1964;224–230.

Schwab ME, Suda K, Thoenen H. Selective retrograde transsynaptic transfer of a protein, tetanus toxin, subsequent to its retrograde axonal transport. J Cell Biol 1979;82:798–810.

Sinclair KB. Black disease—a review. Br Vet J 1956;112:196–200.

Smith LDS. Botulism: the organism, its toxins, the disease. Springfield, IL: Charles C Thomas 1977;113–141.

Smith LDS, Sugiyama H Botulism: the organism, its toxins, the disease. 2nd ed. Springfield, IL: Charles C Thomas 1988;1–171.

Sonnabend O, et al. Isolation of Clostridium botulinum type G and identification of type G botulinal toxin in humans: report of five sudden unexpected deaths. J Infect Dis 1981;143:22–27.

Sterne M, Edwards JB. Blackleg of pigs caused by Clostridium chauvoei. Vet Rec 1955;67:314–315.

Sugiyama H. Clostridium botulinum neurotoxin. Microbiol Rev 1980;44:419–448.

Swerczek TW. Toxicoinfectious botulism in foals and adult horses. J Am Vet Med Assoc 1980;176:217–220.

Swerczek TW. Experimentally induced toxicoinfectious botulism in horses and foals. Am J Vet Res 1980;41:348–350.

Tunnicliff EA. A strain of Clostridium welchii producing fatal dysentery in lambs. J Infect Dis 1933;52:407–412.

Turk J, et al. Enteric Clostridium perfringens infection associated with parvoviral enteritis in dogs: 74 cases (1987–1990). J Am Vet Med Assoc 1992;200:991–994.

Van Kampen KR, Kennedy PC. Experimental bacillary hemoglobinuria. II. Pathogenesis of the hepatic lesion in the rabbit. Pathologia Vet 1969;6:59–75, 1969.

Van Kampen KR, Kennedy PC. Experimental bacillary hemoglobinuria: intrahepatic detection of spores of Clostridium haemolyticum by immunofluorescence in the rabbit. Am J Vet Res 1968;29:2173–2177.

Van Ness GB, Erickson K. Ecology of bacillary hemoglobinuria. J Am Vet Med Assoc 1964;144:492–496.

STREPTOCOCCAL INFECTIONS

Certain of the gram-positive spherical organisms that grow in pairs or chains and are classified in the genus *Streptococcus* are pathogenic for humans and animals. The significance of these infections has decreased greatly during the past few years because of the widespread use of antibiotics. Several differing systems of streptococci classification have been proposed, but usually the various species are organized according to their Lancefield Group (a system based on antigens known as **group-specific antigens,** which are polysaccharides or teichoic acids) and the type of hemolysis induced in culture. This does not allow classification of all streptococci, but does allow differentiation of most of the important pathogens. These along with their associated diseases are listed in Table 10-4. In addition to these relatively specific diseases, streptococci are common invaders of wounds, leading to local purulent inflammation that, on occasion, can spread to distant organs. They are often recovered from purulent otitis media, arthritis, pneumonia, lymphadenitis, and other diseases.

Strangles (adenitis equorum)

Strangles is an upper respiratory infection accompanied by purulent lymphadenitis of horses caused by *Streptococcus equi*, an obligate parasite of horses that rarely affects other animals. The disease, most common in young horses living in crowded conditions, is usually introduced by carrier horses.

SIGNS

Following an incubation period of a few days, the signs are characteristic, although they vary strikingly in severity. There is fever, a mucopurulent nasal discharge, often conjunctivitis, and edematous swelling of the pharyngeal regions, which may produce inspiratory dyspnea, giving the impression that the animal is strangling. The submaxillary lymph nodes become enlarged and hot and soon form abscesses, which yield large quantities of creamy yellowish pus when they rupture spontaneously or are incised. In uncomplicated cases, recovery usually follows drainage of the abscess, but in

TABLE 10-4 **Streptococcal infections**

Organism	Lancefield group	Diseases
S. pyogenes	A	Scarlet fever in humans; pyogenic infections in monkeys; rarely affects animals
S. agalactiae	B	Bovine mastitis; mastitis in sheep and goats; pyogenic infections in humans
S. dysgalactiae	C	Bovine mastitis
S. equi	C	Equine strangles
S. equisimilis	C	Cervical abscesses in horses; various pyogenic infections in pigs, dogs
S. zooepidemicus	C	Pyogenic infections, including pneumonia, in horses; mastitis in cattle
S. bovis	D	GI commensal in cattle, sheep; rare cause of endocarditis in humans
S. equinus	D	GI commensal in horses
S. faecalis (genus Enterococcus)	D	Pyogenic infections in various animals
S. uberis	Mixed	Bovine mastitis
S. porcinus	E	Cervical abscesses in swine
S. canis	G	Genital infections in dogs and cats; abscesses in cats
S. suis	D	Septicemia, meningitis, arthritis in swine
S. pneumoniae	None	Lobar pneumonia in humans, monkeys; rare cause of disease in domestic animals

GI, gastrointestinal.

some horses, the infection spreads to other lymph nodes or reaches the general circulation. In such cases, abscesses may form in any organ but are most common in the lungs, kidneys, liver, and spleen and less common in the brain. A fatal outcome may be expected in overwhelming infections or in those instances in which abscesses form in a critical organ.

LESIONS

Organisms that penetrate the upper respiratory mucosa cause acute inflammation in the adjoining structures, particularly the lymph nodes, where abscesses form. In some cases, abscesses of microscopic size have been demonstrated in parapharyngeal lymph nodes by one of us (Jones) within 24 hours of the first evidence of fever. Such abscesses may become encapsulated or, more commonly, rupture into the oral or pharyngeal cavities or through the skin of the intermandibular region. There is catarrhal or purulent rhinitis and pharyngitis, often with small abscesses in the pharynx and on the soft palate. Metastatic abscesses occur in the lung (sometimes with cavitation), liver, kidney, spleen, and occasionally, the brain. Septicemia is sometimes observed, with few or absent abscesses. Abscesses in the retropharyngeal lymph nodes may drain into the guttural pouches, leading to empyema of these structures.

Purpura hemorrhagica may be a complication of strangles, and in such cases, large subcutaneous areas of edema and hemorrhage are associated with septic emboli in blood vessels of the tissues involved.

DIAGNOSIS

The clinical history, the presence of characteristic gross lesions, and the demonstration of S. equi in abscesses are sufficient to establish the diagnosis at necropsy. Demonstration and identification of the organisms in submaxillary or other abscesses confirms the clinical diagnosis in living animals.

Streptococcal mastitis

Streptococcus agalactiae, an obligate parasite of the bovine mammary gland, is the most important streptococcus as a cause of bovine mastitis. It represents a specific contagious disease of cattle that is transmitted from cow to cow by means of contaminated milking equipment or a milker's hands. The bacteria enter by way of the teat canal and colonize within ducts, ductules, and acini. The infection is thought to be permanent. Although the streptococci do not invade deep into the interstitium of the gland, the lining epithelium is disrupted and an intense polymorphonuclear inflammatory reaction follows. This gives way to replacement by macrophages, proliferative fibroblastic connective tissue, and nodules of lymphocytes. Ducts may become obstructed, resulting in cysts lined by villous epithelial projections, and on occasion, metaplastic squamous epithelium. Multiple foci of acute inflammation resulting in chronic inflammation and scarring ultimately culminate in a fibrotic gland, which is firm rather than soft to the touch. During the acute stages of the disease, the milk may contain fibrin and pus, but later the gland becomes dry.

Other streptococci that do not require the mammary gland for survival are also important as causes of mastitis, but the associated diseases are not solely dependent on the presence of the bacterium, as is the case with S. agalactiae. These include *Streptococcus uberis, Streptococcus dysgalactiae, Streptococcus fecalis, Streptococcus zooepidemicus,* and members of Lancefield groups G and L. In a few instances, streptococci of human origin (*Streptococcus pyogenes*) may be involved in outbreaks of bovine mastitis and contribute to concomitant epidemics of "septic sore throat" in persons who drink the milk from infected cows. With the exception of *S. uberis,* these other streptococci cause acute purulent mastitis. *S. uberis* is associated with less severe but more chronic disease. Bovine mastitis is described more fully in Chapter 25.

Urogenital infections

Streptococci are often associated with vaginitis, cervicitis, and endometritis. On occasion they are also responsible for placentitis and abortion. In horses, *S. zooepidemicus,* and in dogs, *Streptococcus canis* are the most common isolates. These infections do not represent a specific contagious disease but rather opportunistic entry of the organism into a susceptible host after parturition or coitus. Unrecognized low-grade inflammation with recovery is probably the most usual sequela. Streptococci also sometimes cause inflammatory lesions of the testes and male accessory sex glands, as well as urethritis and pyelonephritis. In none of these situations are the lesions distinctive; the predominant finding is purulent exudation.

Cervical lymphadenitis of swine

Abscesses (jowl abscess, swine strangles) are not uncommon in the cervical lymph nodes of swine. Streptococci of Lancefield group E are the most commonly isolated organisms. These have been termed *Streptococcus porcinus* along with related streptocci of Groups P, U, and V also recovered from such lesions. Other bacterial species, including group C streptococci, *Corynebacterium pyogenes,* *Pasteurella multocida,* and *Staphylococcus aureus* have also been recovered from abscesses of cervical lymph nodes.

The disease may be transmitted to susceptible swine by instilling virulent cultures into the nasal or oral cavities. Transmission to other swine by direct contact has been demonstrated, and some swine may recover from the disease but still harbor streptococci in the nasal or oral cavities and thus be a source of contagion. Hematogenous spread of the organisms occurs occasionally, causing abscesses in other parts of the body or streptococcal endocarditis or meningitis. Immunization is possible through use of a preparation made from a mutant, less virulent strain of group E streptococci.

Streptococcal meningitis and arthritis in swine

A specific streptococcal infection of young swine is caused by *S. suis,* an organism with several different serovars. Although *S. suis* reacts with Lancefield Group D antiserum, the organism also has antigens designated R, S, and RS. The bacterium may be carried in the oropharynx of swine, and transmission occurs through contact; the organism enters by way of the oral or respiratory routes. Newly established infections may be subclinical or result in pharyngitis and cervical lymphadenitis. In some young pigs, particularly during cold weather, septicemia may develop with localization of the organism in the meninges and joints, leading to fibrinopurulent meningitis and polyarthritis. Other manifestations may include purulent bronchopneumonia and endocarditis.

Streptococcal infections of guinea pigs

Streptococcal infections of Lancefield type C are frequently encountered in enzootic infections of guinea pigs. Abscesses occur in the lymph nodes of the head and neck and may lead to generalized dissemination of the organisms to pleura, lungs, peritoneum, pericardium, or lymph nodes generally. The organism most frequently isolated is usually designated *Streptococcus zooepidemicus, S. pyogenes animalis,* or simply serologic group C streptococci.

LESIONS

The lesions in the localized form are usually described as abscesses of lymph nodes, filled with cream-colored pus, sometimes reaching a large size. The reaction on pleural and peritoneal surfaces is usually fibrinopurulent, with thromboses and necrotic zones in infarcted lungs. The disease may be differentiated from pneumococcal infection by identification of the organisms.

Neonatal streptococcal infections

Streptococcal infections are a particular hazard for neonates in humans and most domestic animals, particularly foals, calves, lambs, and pigs. Infection is usually thought to gain entrance by way of the umbilicus, but there is little evidence to substantiate this portal of entry. The infection most often results in suppurative polyarthritis ("joint-ill") and meningitis, but localization in the valvular endocardium, kidneys, and choroid of the eye are not uncommon, especially in lambs. Despite the virulence of streptococci in neonates, the strains usually isolated from them are not pathogenic for adult animals. *S. equisimilis* and *S. zooepidemicus* are two of the most frequently recovered organisms.

Pneumococcal infections in animals

Streptococcus pneumoniae (formerly *Diplococcus pneumoniae*) is the most common cause of lobar pneumonia in humans. Infection in humans is endemic; a high percentage of normal adults carry the organism, providing a constant source of infection for susceptible individuals. Pneumococcal infection in humans may also lead to meningitis, pericarditis, arthritis, otitis media, and abscesses. *S. pneumoniae* may also be carried by several species of Old World primates and may cause pneumonia, meningitis, panophthalmitis, and septicemia. Pulmonary and extrapulmonary disease caused by S. pneumoniae have also been described in guinea pigs. Septicemia and mastitis have been seen in cattle, sheep, and goats.

References

Armstrong CH, Payne JB. Bacteria recovered from swine affected with cervical lymphadenitis (jowl abscess). Am J Vet Res 1969;30:1607–1612.

Armstrong CH, Boehm PN, Ellis RP. Experimental transmission of streptococcic lymphadenitis (jowl abscess) of swine. Am J Vet Res 1970;31:823–829.

Blakemore E, Elliott SD, Hart-Mercer J. Studies on suppurative polyarthritis (joint-ill) in lambs. J Pathol Bact 1941;52:57–82.

Collier JR, Noel J. Streptococcic lymphadenitis of swine: a contagious disease. Am J Vet Res 1971;32:1501–1506.

Collier JR, Noel J. Streptococcic lymphadenitis of swine: an immune carrier of Streptococcus suis. Am J Vet Res 1971;32:1507–1510.

Collier JR, Noel J. Streptococcal lymphadenitis of swine: prolonged carrier state and bacterial dynamics in the induction of disease. Am J Vet Res 1974;35:799–802.

Cutlip RC, Shuman RD. Susceptibility of rabbits to infection with Lancefield's group E streptococci. Cornell Vet 1971;61:607–616.

Doane RM, Oliver SP, Walker RD, et al. Experimental infection of lactating bovine mammary glands with Streptococcus uberis in quarters colonized by Corynebacterium bovis. Am J Vet Res 1987;48:749–754.

Elliot SD, Alexander TJL, Thomas JH. Streptococcal infection in young pigs. II. Epidemiology and experimental production of the disease. J Hyg Camb 1966;64:213–220.

Fallon MT, Reinhard MK, Gray BM, et al. Inapparent Streptococcus pneumoniae type 35 infections in commercial rats and mice. Lab Anim Sci 1988;38:129–132.

Field HI, Butain D, Done JT. Studies on piglet mortality. I. Streptococcal meningitis and arthritis. Vet Rec 1954;66:453–455.

Garnett NL, et al Hemorrhagic streptococcal pneumonia in newly procured research dogs. J Am Vet Med Assoc 1982;181:1371–1374.

Gibbons WJ. The histopathology of mastitis. Cornell Vet 1938;28:240–249.

Gilbert SG, Reuhl KR, Wong JH, et al. Fatal pneumococcal meningitis in a colony-born monkey (Macaca fascicularis). J Med Primatol 1987;16:333–338.

Goldman PM, Moore TD. Spontaneous Lancefield group G streptococcal infection in a random source cat colony. Lab Anim Sci 1973;23:565–566.

Gosser HS, Olson LD. Chronologic development of streptococcic lymphadenitis in swine. Am J Vet Res 1973;34:77–82.

Gunning OV. Joint-ill in foals (pyosepticemia). Vet J 1947;103:47–67, 104–111, 129–148.

Jones FS. The streptococci of equines. J Exp Med 1919;30:159–178.

Jones JET. The experimental production of streptococcal endocarditis in the pig. J Pathol 1969;99:307–318.

Knight AP, Voss JL, McChesney AE, et al. Experimentally induced Streptococcus equi infection in horses with resultant guttural pouch empyema. Vet Med Small Anim Clin 1975;70:1194–1195, 1198–1199.

Kunstyr I, Matthiesen T. Two forms of streptococcal infection (serologic group C) in guinea pigs. Versuchstierkd 1973;15:348–357.

McCrea CT. Pneumococcal septicaemia in calves. Vet Rec 1971;88:518–519.

McDonald JS, and Anderson AJ. [1] Experimental infection of bovine mammary glands with Streptococcus agalactiae during the nonlactating period. [2] Experimental infection of bovine mammary glands with Streptococcus uberis during the nonlactating period. Am J Vet Res 1981;42:462–464, 465–467.

McDonald TJ, McDonald JS. Streptococci isolated from bovine intramammary infections. Am J Vet Res 1976;37:377–381.

Miller RB, Olson LD. Frequency of jowl abscesses in feeder and market swine exposed to group E streptococci as nursing pigs. Am J Vet Res 1983;44:945–948.

Mitchell CA, Plummer PJG. Septic arthritis caused by Streptococcus equi. Can J Comp Med 1942;6:24–25.

Morrill CC. A histopathological study of the bovine udder. Cornell Vet 1938;28:196–210.

Parker GA, Russell RJ, De Paoli A. Extrapulmonary lesions of Streptococcus pneumoniae infection in guinea pigs. Vet Pathol 1977;14:332–337.

Prescott JF, Srivastava SK, deGannes R, et al. A mild form of strangles caused by an atypical Streptococcus equi. J Am Vet Med Assoc 1982;180:293–294.

Riley MGI, Morehouse LG, Olson LD. Distribution of group E streptococcus in head and neck regions of swine. Am J Vet Res 1973;34:1163–1166.

Riley MGI, Morehouse LG, Olson LD. Detection of tonsillar and nasal colonization of group E streptococcus in swine. Am J Vet Res 1973;34:1167–1170, 1973.

Sanford ES, Tilker AME. Streptococcus suis type II-associated diseases in swine. J Am Vet Med Assoc 1982;181:673–676.

Schueler RL, Morehouse LG, Olson LD. Intravenous exposure of swine to group E streptococci: clinical signs, hemic and lymphatic distribution of streptococci, and resistance to subsequent exposure. Am J Vet Res 1972;33:1797–1800.

Schueler RL, Morehouse LG, Olson LD. Intravenous exposure of swine to group E streptococci: Articular and cardiac lesions associated with experimentally induced septicemic infection of swine with group E streptococci. Am J Vet Res 1972;33:1801–1812.

Stallings B, Ling GV, Lagenaur LA, et al. Septicemia and septic arthritis caused by Streptococcus pneumoniae in a cat: possible transmission from a child. J Am Vet Med Assoc 1987;191:703–704.

Sweeney CR, Whitlock RH, Meirs DA, et al. Complications associated with Streptococcus equi infection on a horse farm. J Am Vet Med Assoc 1987;191:1446–1448.

Sweeney CR, et al. Description of an epizootic and persistence of Streptococcus equi infections in horses. J Am Vet Med Assoc 1989;194:1281–1286.

Swindle MM, Narayan O, Luzarraga M, et al. Contagious streptococcal lymphadenitis in cats. J Am Vet Med Assoc 1980;177:829–830.

Windsor RS, Elliott SD. Streptococcal infection in young pigs. IV. An outbreak of streptococcal meningitis in weaned pigs. J Hyg (Camb) 1975;75:69–78.

Wood RL, Cutlip RC, Shuman RD. Osteomyelitis and arthritis induced in swine by Lancefield's group A streptococci (Streptococcus pyogenes). Cornell Vet 1971;61:457–470.

STAPHYLOCOCCAL INFECTIONS

There are over two dozen distinct species of staphylococci, but only a few are pathogenic enough to be commonly associated with disease. These organisms excrete an assortment of toxins, including coagulases, fibrinolysins, hyaluronidase, hemolysins (alpha, beta, gamma, and delta), and enterotoxins, among others. Pyogenic infections of various organs and tissues, particularly of the skin, mammary glands, lungs, joints, and uterus, caused by staphylococci are seen on occasion in almost all species of animals (Fig. 10-5). The important pathogenic staphylocci include *S. aureus, S. epidermidis, S. intermedius,* and *S. hyicus.*

S. aureus is a hemolytic, coagulase-positive organism that can cause a variety of purulent inflammatory diseases. In humans, it is identified with septicemia, severely necrotizing and purulent pneumonia, endocarditis, upper respiratory infections, subcutaneous abscesses (furuncles and boils), cellulitis, enterocolitis, and toxic shock syndrome. *S. aureus* is also a cause of food poisoning, which results from the ingestion of preformed heat-stable enterotoxins elaborated by its growth in contaminated foods. In animals, *S. aureus* is associated with purulent lesions of the skin (**pyoderma, furunculosis, impetigo**), which on occasion may become dissemin-

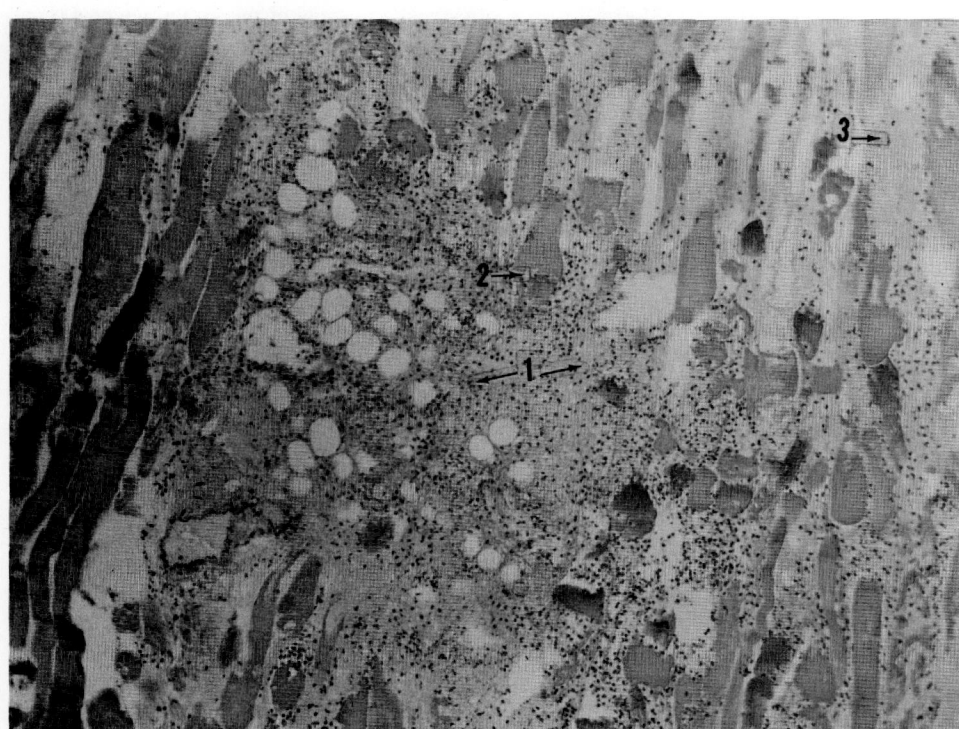

FIG. 10-5 Inflammatory edema in panniculus muscle of a horse with purpura hemorrhagica after respiratory infection with *Streptococcus pyogenes* (× 100). Septic emboli were found in adjacent tissues. Note cellular and albuminous exudate (1), fragmented muscle bundles (2), and loss of muscle fiber (3). (Courtesy of Army Veterinary Research Laboratory, and Armed Forces Institute of Pathology.)

ated. One such example is **"tick pyemia"** in sheep, a generalized staphylococcal infection introduced into young lambs by bites of the sheep tick, *Ixodes ricinus,* and characterized by multiple disseminated abscesses and polyarthritis. The pathogenesis of these types of disorders is not entirely understood; the virulence of the bacterium and the status of the host regarding trauma, nutritional status, concomitant diseases, and general hygiene all potentially influence the development of these disorders. The most interesting consequences of *S. aureus* infection in animals are **botryomycosis** and **staphylococcal bovine mastitis.**

Botryomycosis

This disease is a chronic pyogranulomatous inflammation caused by staphylococcus. More often than not, the specific causative species of staphylococcus has not been identified. Botryomycosis occurs in cattle, sheep, horses, dogs, cats, and pigs and probably in other species as well.

LESIONS

The lesions are most often in the subcutaneous tissues, but may occur in any organ. In cattle, the mammary gland may be affected (granulomatous staphylococcal mastitis) (Fig. 10-6), and in horses, the stub of the spermatic cord in geldings is a common site.

Grossly, the lesions are composed of multiple firm nodules with purulent cores containing white granules referred to as grains, which are comparable to the "sulfur granules" seen in some other bacterial and mycotic granulomas, although the grains are seldom suffi-

ciently firm to be felt with the fingers, as the granules usually are in actinomycosis. Microscopically, a core of neutrophils is surrounded by granulation tissue, containing epithelioid cells, some lymphocytes, plasma cells, and rarely multinucleated giant cells. This granulation tissue is, in turn, surrounded by considerable fibrous connective tissue. Within the core are brilliantly eosinophilic "rosettes" (**Splendore-Hoeppli** material) that closely resemble the rosettes of actinomycosis and actinobacillosis but which show less tendency to form "clubs" at the periphery. These are the grains seen grossly. Gram's stain shows these rosettes to surround colonies of cocci, although the organisms often have died out in the center, the oldest part of the colony.

Staphylococcal bovine mastitis

This may occur as a chronic infection that results in botryomycosis, as described above, as an acute gangrenous inflammation, or as an acute to clinically inapparent purulent lesion. Variations in the virulence of the infecting organisms, which gain entry via the teat, probably account for the differing severities of the infection. *S. aureus* also causes mastitis in sheep, goats, swine, and horses.

Exudative epidermitis of swine

Staphylococcus hyicus is a common inhabitant of the skin of pigs and sometimes cattle, in which it has been associated with mastitis. Porcine strains may cause polyarthritis and it is believed to be the primary cause of exu-

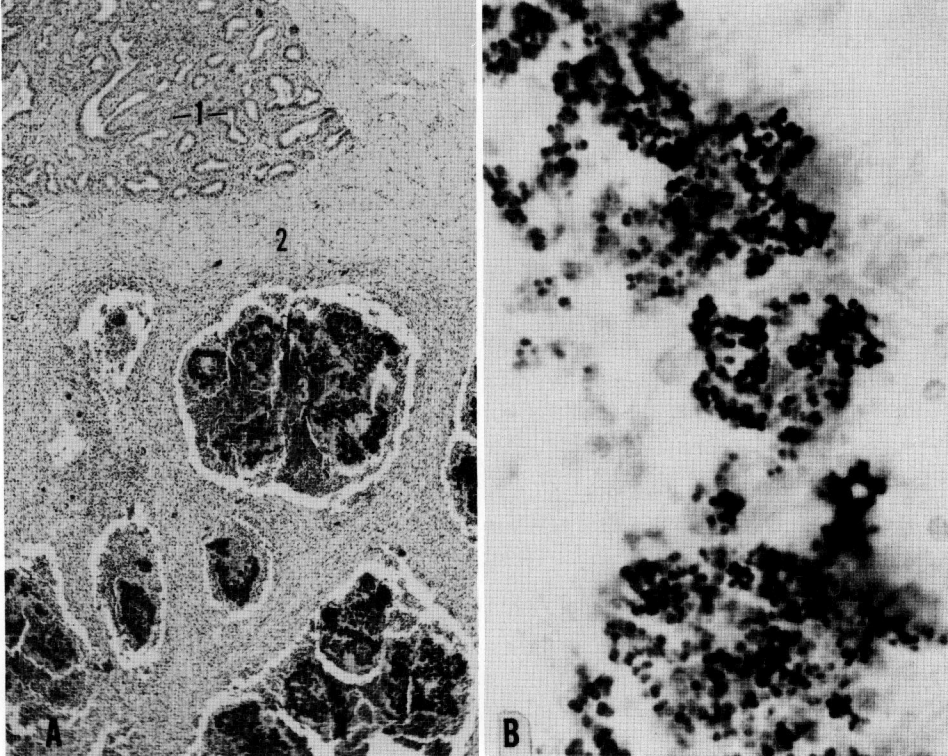

FIG. 10-6 Granulomatous staphylococcal mastitis, udder of a cow. **A.** Mammary lobules (1) are separated by dense bands of connective tissue (2) from the colonies of staphylococci (3), which are surrounded by a narrow zone of pus (× 48). **B.** Part of a bacterial colony stained by Gram's method (× 1000). Note spherical staphylococci. (Courtesy of Dr. E. A. Benbrook.)

dative epidermitis of swine. This condition is fully discussed in Chapter 18.

Other Staphylococcal infections

S. epidermidis is an opportunistic pathogen most often associated with abscesses and other purulent inflammmatory processes of wounds. *S. intermedius* is a common inhabitant of the skin and nasopharynx of carnivores. In dogs, it may cause pyoderma (multiple skin abscesses), otitis, conjunctivitis, and mastitis.

References

Anderson JC. Experimental staphylococcal mastitis in the mouse: the effect of inoculating different strains into separate glands of the same mouse. J Comp Pathol 1974;84:103–111.

Berg JN, Wendell DE, Vogelweid C, et al. Identification of the major coagulase-positive Staphylococcus sp of dogs as Staphylococcus intermedius. Am J Vet Res 1984;45:1307–1309.

Brown RW. Intramammary infections produced by various strains of Staphylococcus epidermidis and Micrococcus. Cornell Vet 1973;63:630–645.

Chandler RL. Ultrastructural pathology of mastitis in the mouse. A study of experimental staphylococcal and streptococcal infections. Br J Exp Pathol 1970;51:639–645.

Cohen JO. Staphylococcus. J Am Vet Med Assoc 1987;190:150–152.

Crandell RA, Huttenhauer GA, Casey HW. Staphylococcic dermatitis in mink. J Am Vet Med Assoc 1971;159:638–639.

Dennis SM. Perinatal staphylococcal infections of sheep. Vet Rec 1966;79:38–40.

Derbyshire JB. The pathology of experimental staphylococcal mastitis in the goat. J Comp Pathol Ther 1958;68:449–454.

Everitt JI, Fetter AW, Kenney RM, et al. Porcine necrotizing endometritis. Vet Pathol 1981;18:125–127.

Gudding R, McDonald JS, Cheville NF. Pathogenesis of Staphylococcus aureus mastitis: bacteriologic, histologic, and ultrastructural pathologic findings. Am J Vet Res 1984;45:2525–2531.

Lomax LG, Cole JR. Porcine epidermitis and dermatitis associated with Staphylococcus hyicus and Dermatophilus congolensis infections. J Am Vet Med Assoc 1983;183:1091–1092.

Markel MD, Wheat JD, Jang SS. Cellulitis associated with coagulase-positive staphylococci in racehorses: nine cases (1975–1984). J Am Vet Med Assoc 1986;189:1600–1603.

Morrill CC. A histopathological study of the bovine udder. Cornell Vet 1938;28:196–210.

Nickerson SC, Heald CW. Histopathologic response of the bovine mammary gland to experimentally induced Staphylococcus aureus infection. Am J Vet Res 1981;42:1351–1355.

Phillips WE Jr, King RE, Kloos WE. Isolation of Staphylococcus hyicus subsp hyicus from a pig with septic polyarthritis. Am J Vet Res 1980;41:274–276.

Poutrel B. Staphylococcus sciuri subsp lentus associated with goat mastitis. Am J Vet Res 1984;45:2084–2085.

Richardson JA, Morter RL, Rebar AH, et al. Lesions of porcine necrotic ear syndrome. Vet Pathol 1984;21:152–157.

Schalm OW, Lasmanis J, Jain NC. Conversion of chronic staphylococcal mastitis to acute gangrenous mastitis after neutropenia in blood and bone marrow produced by an equine antibovine leukocyte serum. Am J Vet Res 1976;37:885–890.

Seeger W, et al. Staphylococcal-toxin-induced vascular leakages in isolated perfused rabbit lungs. Lab Invest 1990;63:341–349.

Sheagren JN. Staphylococcus aureus: the persistent pathogen (Parts I and II). N Engl J Med 1984;310:1368–1373, 1437–1442.

Shults FS, Estes PC, Franklin JA, et al. Staphylococcal botryomycosis in a specific pathogen-free mouse colony. Lab Anim Sci 1973;23:36–42.

Spencer GR, McNutt SH. Pathogenesis of bovine mastitis. Am J Vet Res 1950;11:188–198.

Tessler J. Vesicular lesions produced in guinea pigs by a Staphylococcus aureus strain. Can J Comp Med 1973;37:323–324.

Thawley DG, Marshall RB, Cullinane L, et al. Atypical staphylococcal

mastitis in a dairy herd. J Am Vet Med Assoc 1977;171:425–428.
Tranter HS. Foodborne staphylococcal illness. Lancet 1990;336:1044–1046.

Campylobacter infections

The genus Campylobacter contains several pathogenic bacteria, which were formerly classified in the genus Vibrio. Campylobacter species are slender, spirally curved, motile, gram-negative rods that are associated with infections of the genital tract, resulting in abortion and infections of the gastrointestinal tract (Table 10-5). The organisms invade and proliferate within epithelial cells (chorionic epithelium or gastrointestinal tract epithelium), causing cell death or, by some unknown mechanism, proliferation. Organisms are visible with special staining techniques (such as Warthin-Starry, modified Koster's acid-fast, and immunofluorescence) and by electron microscopy, as slightly curved (comma-shaped) organisms within epithelial cells of affected tissues. Campylobacter also elaborate an enterotoxin similar in action to that of *Vibrio cholera*, which causes increased secretion and profuse diarrhea. A closely related organism, *Helicobacter pylori*, causes gastritis in humans.

TABLE 10-5 **Diseases associated with *Campylobacter* species**

Species	Hosts and diseases
C. fetus subsp *venerealis*	Endometritis, sterility, abortion in cattle
C. fetus subsp *fetus*	Abortion in sheep (occasionally in cattle); possible cause of enteritis in sheep, cattle, swine
C. jejuni (*C. fetus* subsp *jejuni*)	Abortion in sheep; enteritis in humans, nonhuman primates, cattle, foals, dogs, cats, and other species; proliferative (adenomatous) enteritis in many species
C. coli	Enteritis in humans, nonhuman primates, and other animals
C. sputorum subsp *bubulus*	Commensal of female genital tract of cattle and sheep
C. sputorum subsp. *mucosalis*	Associated with swine proliferative ileitis syndrome; adenomatosis in swine
C. upsaliensis	Probable cause of enteritis in dogs, cats, and humans
Helicobacter pylori (*C. pylori*)	Antral gastritis in children and nonhuman primates

Campylobacter fetus subsp *venerealis*

Previously known as *Vibrio fetus* var *venerealis*, this organism is the cause of a specific venereal disease of cattle. It is transmitted either by coitus or in the course of artificial insemination. Infection of bulls is not associated with any lesion or disease. In bulls, the infection may be eliminated spontaneously, but some bulls can carry the organism for protracted periods of time. Passive transfer of infection by the bull is considered unlikely because growth of organisms on the penis or within the prepuce is necessary for numbers to be adequate to cause infection in the cow. The infection in cows is principally characterized by temporary infertility and prolonged estrus cycles. The cow is infected during breeding and, although fertilization and implantation are normal, *C. fetus* subsp *venerealis*, which has a marked tropism for chorionic epithelium, soon kills the embryo and incites endometritis. Neither death of the embryo nor the endometritis are manifested by clinical signs. Endometritis may prevent conception at succeeding estrus periods, but most cattle conceive before resolution of the disease. Recovered cows are usually resistant to reinfection. *C. fetus* subsp *venerealis*, on occasion, may also cause observable abortions, usually between 4 and 7 months of gestation.

LESIONS

Lesions in cattle are usually subtle. In experimentally induced disease, Estes and coworkers (1966) described the lesions as a subacute, diffuse mucopurulent endometritis. Uterine glands contain neutrophils, lymphocytes, eosinophils, and sloughed epithelium. The uterine mucosa is infiltrated with lymphocytes, often in the form of small nodules. Similar infiltrates may be found in the cervix and vagina. When recognizable abortion occurs, the fetus and placenta are autolyzed as a result of intrauterine death. Placental necrosis may be evident along with neutrophilic and lymphocytic placentitis.

DIAGNOSIS

Diagnosis is often possible from the herd history, but the disease must be differentiated from trichomoniasis. *Campylobacter* species may be visible in tissue sections of the placenta and can be specifically identified with immunologic staining techniques. *C. sputorum* subsp *bubulus* is a common commensal of the male and female genital tract of cattle and must be differentiated from the pathogenic species.

Campylobacter fetus subsp *fetus*

Also known as *C. fetus* subsp *intestinalis* and *Vibrio fetus* var *intestinalis*, this organism infects sheep, but in contrast to the subspecies *venerealis* infection in cattle, it is not a venereal disease and is characterized by abortion. Infection is acquired by the oral route; the ram does not play a role in transmission. Birds have been identified as capable of carrying the organism, contributing to its spread. In ewes, the organism localizes in the pregnant uterus and, after a brief bacteremia, results in late abortion, stillbirth, or birth of weak lambs, which usually die soon after birth. Immunity follows abortion, but certain ewes may carry the organsim in the gastrointestinal tract.

Cattle are susceptible to *C. fetus* subsp *fetus* and late abortion may occur, but the incidence is far less than it is in sheep. Abortion has also been ascribed to *C. fetus* subsp *fetus* in horses, and the organism may also cause enteritis in cattle, sheep, pigs, and horses similar to that caused by *C. jejuni*. *Campylobacter jejuni* has also been shown to be a cause of abortion in sheep with lesions similar to those caused by *C. fetus* subsp fetus.

LESIONS

Lesions are found most often in the placenta but may also occur in the fetus; however, autolytic changes usually preclude adequate pathologic study. The bacteria first localize in the hilar zone of the placentomes, resulting in vascular damage and thrombosis of small vessels, causing separation of the chorion with formation of hematomas. Subsequent invasion of the chorion and chorionic capillaries leads to necrosis at this site and invasion of the fetus. Both hypoxia from placental damage and fetal invasion contribute to fetal death. The placenta, particularly the cotyledons, are edematous and infiltrated with neutrophils and mononuclear cells and contain foci of necrosis. The fetus is edematous and often macerated. In some, relatively specific lesions are present in the form of a focal diffuse necrotizing hepatitis observable grossly as multiple tan to gray foci, 1 mm to 2 mm in diameter. Diagnosis can be made by finding and identifying the organisms in the placenta or fetus.

Campylobacter jejuni

Also known as *C. fetus* subsp. *jejuni* or *Vibrio jejuni*, this organism is a normal inhabitant of the intestinal tract of cattle, sheep, goats, dogs, cats, rabbits, many species of birds, and probably many other animals. *C. jejuni* and some other campylobacters (*C. laridis, C. upsaliensis,* and others) have emerged in recent years as an important cause of enteritis and diarrhea in humans, dogs, cats, cattle, foals, rabbits, ferrets, hamsters, mink, and nonhuman primates, either as a primary pathogen or in concert with enteric viruses. In humans, the infection can be a zoonosis, acquired from dogs, cats, sheep, birds, and other infected animals.

LESIONS

In most examples, the lesions are not specific, consisting of stunting and fusion of villi, dilation of crypts and crypt abscesses, mild cellular infiltration of the mucosa, and occasionally ulceration and hemorrhage. In some examples, the mucosa is thickened as a result of hyperplasia of glandular epithelium. Lesions tend to be most severe in the proximal small intestine, but can af-

fect the entire small intestine and colon. With silver stains, the comma-shaped organisms can be seen on the surface of epithelial cells and within the lamina propria.

C. jejuni has been implicated in and considered by some to be the specific cause of peculiar diseases characterized by marked proliferation of intestinal and/or colonic epithelium. The mechanism whereby the bacteria initiate such lesions, however, remains to be elucidated. These diseases include proliferative ileitis of hamsters, proliferative colitis in ferrets, duodenal hyperplasia in guinea pigs, intestinal adenomatosis of foals, terminal ileitis of lambs, intestinal adenomatosis in blue fox, typhlitis in rabbits, and similar lesions in dogs, rats, and deer. Each of these disorders is characterized by multiple foci to diffuse proliferation of mucosal epithelium into the lumen and sometimes "invasion" into the wall of the intestine. Organisms are found within the apical cytoplasm of crypt and glandular epithelial cells of the proliferative zones but not elsewhere in the gut. The disorders are similar to the intestinal adenomatous complex of swine.

C. jejuni is a recognized cause of late abortion and stillbirths in sheep and goats, which must be differentiated from that caused by *C. fetus* subsp *fetus*. *C. jejuni* may also cause mastitis in cattle. A similar campylobacter has been recovered from aborted puppies.

Campylobacter sputorum subsp mucosalis and Campylobacter hyointestinalis

These organisms have been recovered from swine that have what has been termed the **"swine proliferative ileitis syndrome."** Included within the complex are porcine intestinal adenomatosis, proliferative ileitis, regional ileitis, terminal ileitis, necrotic enteritis, and hemorrhagic enteritis, all of which may be variations on the same theme. *Campylobacter* organisms can be found within the apical cytoplasm of crypt and glandular epithelial cells and isolated with regularity in this syndrome, and some attempts to reproduce the disorder have met with success. The proliferative lesions commense in and principally involve the epithelium of crypts and glands, where the cells become hypertrophied with larger than normal vesicular nuclei. Hyperplasia results in crowding of cells, development of a pseudostratified appearance, and elongated crypts and branching glands, which may extend into the submucosa. Individual glands may assume a dysplastic appearance. Villi overlying such areas become shortened (atrophic) and fused. Crypts contain neutrophils and mononuclear cells, and there is extensive mononuclear inflammation in the mucosa and submucosa. The terminal ileum is most severely affected. Necrotic enteritis and hemorrhagic enteritis are characterized by either extensive necrosis or necrosis accompanied by hemorrhage of an "adenomatous" mucosa. In either circumstance there is an extensive polymorphonuclear inflammatory response to the necrotic tissue in these conditions. Further descriptions are found in the chapter on the digestive system.

Campylobacter coli

This organism, on occasion, has been considered as a cause of enteritis in humans and animals, but it does not appear to be an important pathogen. It had once been considered the cause of winter dysentery (probably caused by coronavirus) in cattle and swine dysentery (caused by *Treponema hyodysenteriae*), but this is not the case.

Helicobacter pylori

This organism, originally named *Campylobacter pylori*, a gram-negative spiral bacterium, was first identified in 1982 in association with gastritis of humans in Australia. It is now recognized as a major cause of gastritis in humans, is important to the pathogenesis of peptic ulcer disease, and has a strong association with an increased risk for gastric carcinoma.

Vibrio species

Vibrio, the former classification of *Campylobactor*, remains a viable genus but does not contain pathogens for domestic animals. It does, however, contain pathogens of great importance to humans. The most significant species is *Vibrio cholerae*, the cause of cholera, a disease resulting from elaboration of an enterotoxin (an ADP-ribosyl transferase), leading to excess cAMP, which causes marked excess mucosal secretion and profuse diarrhea and, in turn, leads to dehydration and hypovolemic shock. Other pathogenic species are: *V. parahaemolyticus*, which also causes diarrhea; *V. alginolyticus* and *V. vulnificus*, which cause skin infections and septicemia.

Aeromonas

The genus *Aeromonas*, Family Vibrionaceae, contains anaerobic gram-negative organisms that are found in fresh water and sewage, which may be pathogens of fish, amphibians and reptiles. *Aeromonas hydrophila*, associated with colitis and diarrhea in humans, also has recently been observed to cause septicemia in nonhuman primates.

References

Al-Mashat RR, Taylor DJ. Production of diarrhoea and dysentery in experimental calves by feeding pure cultures of Campylobacter fetus subspecies jejuni. Vet Rec 1980;107:459–464.

Anderson KL, Hamoud MM, Urbance JW, et al. Isolation of Campylobacter jejuni from an aborted caprine fetus. J Am Vet Med Assoc 1983;183:90–92.

Ardrey WB, Armstrong P, Meinershagen WA, et al. Diagnosis of ovine vibriosis and enzootic abortion of ewes by immunofluorescence technique. Am J Vet Res 1972;33:2535–2538.

Atherton JG, Ricketts SW. Campylobacter infection from foals. Vet Rec 1980;107:264–265.

Boncyk LH, Brack M, Kalter SS. Hemorrhagic-necrotic enteritis in a baboon (Papio cynocephalus) due to Vibrio fetus. Lab Anim Sci 1972;22:734–738.

Broczyk A, Thompson S, Smith D, et al. Water-borne outbreak of Campylobacter laridis-associated gastroenteritis. Lancet 1987;i: 164–165.

Bronsdon MA, Goodwin CS, Sly LI, et al. Helicobacter nemestrinae sp. nov., a spiral bacterium found in the stomach of a pigtailed macaque (Macaca nemestrina). Int J Syst Bacteriol 1991;41:148–153.

Bryant JL, Stills HF, Lentsch RH, et al. Campylobacter jejuni isolated from patas monkeys with diarrhea. Lab Anim Sci 1983;33:303–305.

Bulgin MS, Ward ACS, Sriranganathan N, et al. Abortion in the dog due to Campylobacter species. Am J Vet Res 1984;45:555–556.

Burnens AP, Nicolet J. Detection of Campylobacter upsaliensis in diarrheic dogs and cats, using a selective medium with cefoperazone. Am J Vet Res 1992;53:48–51.

Chalifoux LV, Hajema EM, Lee-Parritz D. Aeromonas hydrophila peritonitis in a cotton-top tamarin (Saguinus oedipus), and retrospective study of infections in seven primate species. Lab Anim Sci 1993;43:355–358.

Chang K, Kurtz HJ, Ward GE, et al. Immunofluorescent demonstration of Campylobacter hyointestinalis and Campylobacter sputorum subsp mucosalis in swine intestines with lesions of proliferative enteritis. Am J Vet Res 1984;45:703–710.

Clark BL, Dufty JH, Monsborough MJ, et al. Studies on venereal transmission of Campylobacter fetus by immunized bulls. Aust Vet J 1975;51:531–532.

Corbeil LB, Corbeil RR, Winter AJ. Bovine venereal vibriosis: activity of inflammatory cells in protective immunity. Am J Vet Res 1975;36:403–406.

Corbeil LB, et al. Bovine venereal vibriosis: ultrastructure of endometrial inflammatory lesions. Lab Invest 1975;33:187–192.

Dobson AW, Bierschwal CJ Jr, McDougle HC. Induced estrus as an aid in detection of bovine genital vibriosis by means of the virgin heifer test. J Am Vet Med Assoc 1970;156:1584–1588.

Dooley CP, et al. Prevalence of Helicobacter pylori infection and histologic gastritis in asymptomatic persons. N Engl J Med 1989;321:1563–1566.

Dozsa L, Mitchell RG, Olson NO. Histologic changes of the uterine mucosa following the duration of Vibrio infection and the subsequent development of immunity. Am J Vet Res 1962;23:769–776.

Drumm B, Sherman P, Cutz E, et al. Association of Campylobacter pylori on the gastric mucosa with antral gastritis in children. N Engl J Med 1987;316:1557–1562.

Drumm B, Perez-Perez GI, Blaser MJ, et al. Intrafamilial clustering of Helicobacter pylori infection. N Engl J Med 1990;322:359–363.

Duhamel GE, Wheeldon EB. Intestinal adenomatosis in a foal. Vet Pathol 1982;19:447–450.

Eden AN. Perinatal mortality caused by Vibrio fetus. J Pediatr 1966;68:297–304.

Elwell MR, Chapman AL, Frenkel JK. Duodenal hyperplasia in a guinea pig. Vet Pathol 1981;18:136–139.

Estes PC, Bryner JH, O'Berry PA. Histopathology of bovine vibriosis and the effects of Vibrio fetus extracts on the female genital tract. Cornell Vet 1966;56:610–622.

Firehammer BD, Myers LL. Campylobacter fetus subsp jejuni: its possible significance in enteric disease of calves and lambs. Am J Vet Res 1981;42:918–922.

Fleming MP. Association of Campylobacter jejuni with enteritis in dogs and cats. Vet Rec 1983;113:372–374.

Fox JG. Campylobacteriosis - a "new" disease in laboratory animals. Lab Anim Sci 1982;32:625–637.

Fox JG, Claps M, Beaucage CM. Chronic diarrhea associated with Campylobacter jejuni infection in a cat. J Am Vet Med Assoc 1986;189:455–456.

Fox JG, Maxwell KO'N, Ackerman JI. Campylobacter jejuni associated diarrhea in commercially reared beagles. Lab Anim Sci 1984;34:151–155.

Fox JG, Moore R, Ackerman JI. [1] Canine and feline campylobacteriosis: epizootiology and clinical and public health features. [2] Campylobacter jejuni-associated diarrhea in dogs. J Am Vet Med Assoc 1983;183:1420–1424, 1430–1433.

Gebhart CJ, Ward GE, Chang K, et al. Campylobacter hyointestinalis (new species) isolated from swine with lesions of proliferative ileitis. Am J Vet Res 1983;44:361–367.

Hedstrom OR, et al. Pathology of Campylobacter jejuni abortion in sheep. Vet Pathol 1987;24:419–426.

Hong CB, Donahue JM. Campylobacteriosis in an aborted equine fetus. J Am Vet Med Assoc 1989;194:263–264.

Hosie BD, Nicolson TB, Henderson DB. Campylobacter infections in normal and diarrhoeic dogs. Vet Rec 1979;105:80.

Hunter DB, Prescott JF, Hoover DM, et al. Campylobacter colitis in ranch mink in Ontario. Can J Vet Res 1986;50:47–53.

Jensen R, Miller VA, Molello JA. Placental pathology of sheep with vibriosis. Am J Vet Res 1961;22:169–185.

Kazi JL, et al. Ultrastructural study of Helicobacter pylori-associated gastritis. J Pathol 1990;161:65–70.

Lander KP, Gill KPW. Campylobacter mastitis. Vet Rec 1979;105:333.

Lander KP, Gill KPW. Experimental infection of the bovine udder with Campylobacter coli/jejuni. J Hyg 1980;84:421–428.

Landsverk T. Intestinal adenomatosis in a blue fox (Alopex lagopus). Vet Pathol 1981;18:275–278.

La Regina M, Lonigro J. Isolation of Campylobacter fetus subspecies jejuni from hamsters with proliferative ileitis. Lab Anim Sci 1982;32:660–662.

Lawson GHK, Rowland AC. Intestinal adenomatosis in the pig: a bacteriological study. Res Vet Sci 1974;17:331–336.

Lawson GHK, Leaver JL, Pettigrew GW, et al. Some features of Campylobacter sputorum ssp. mucosalis new subspecies revised name and their taxonomic significance. Int J Syst Bacteriol 1981;31:385–391.

Lomax LG, Glock RD. Naturally occurring porcine proliferative enteritis: pathologic and bacteriologic findings. Am J Vet Res 1982;43:1608–1614.

Lomax LG, Glock RD, Hogan JE. Experimentally induced porcine proliferative enteritis in specific-pathogen-free pigs. Am J Vet Res 1982;43:1615–1621.

Lomax LG, Glock RD, Harris DL, et al. Porcine proliferative enteritis: experimentally induced disease in cesarean-derived colostrum-deprived pigs. Am J Vet Res 1982;43:1622–1630.

Lowrie DB, Pearce JH. The placental localization of Vibrio fetus. J Med Microbiol 1970;3:607–614.

McOrist S, Lawson GHK, Rowland AC, et al. Early lesions of proliferative enteritis in pigs and hamsters. Vet Pathol 1989;26:260–264.

Moon HW, Cutlip RC, Amtower WC, et al. Intraepithelial vibrio associated with acute typhlitis of young rabbits. Vet Pathol 1974;11:313–326.

Morgan G, Chadwick P, Lander KP, et al. Campylobacter jejuni mastitis in a cow: a zoonosis-related incident. Vet Rec 1985;116:111.

Nomura A, et al. Helicobacter pylori infection and gastric carcinoma among Japanese Americans in Hawaii. N Engl J Med 1991;325:1132–1136.

Olson P, Sandstedt K. Campylobacter in the dog: a clinical and experimental study. Vet Rec 1987;121:99–101.

Osborne JC. Pathologic responses in animals after Vibrio fetus toxin shock. Am J Vet Res 1965;26:1056–1067.

Osborne JC, Smibert RM. Vibrio fetus toxin. I. Hypersensitivity and abortifacient action. Cornell Vet 1964;54:561–572.

Osburn BI, Hoskins RK. Experimentally induced Vibrio fetus var. intestinalis infection in pregnant cows. Am J Vet Res 1970;31:1733–1741.

Osburn BI, Hoskins RK. Infection with Vibrio fetus in the immunologically immature fetal calf. J Infect Dis 1971;123:32–40.

Parsonnet J, et al. Helicobacter pylori infection and the risk of gastric carcinoma. N Engl J Med 1991;325:1127–1131.

Peterson WL. Helicobacter pylori and peptic ulcer disease. N Engl J Med 1991;324:1043–1048.

Prescott JF, Munroe DL. Campylobacter jejuni enteritis in man and domestic animals. J Am Vet Med Assoc 1982;181:1524–1530.

Redman DR, Trapp AL, Hamdy AH, et al. Ovine vibriosis in Ohio. J Am Vet Med Assoc 1963;143:1094–1095.

Reed KD, Berridge BR. Campylobacter-like organisms in the gastric mucosa of rhesus monkeys. Lab Anim Sci 1988;38:329–331.

Roberts L, Lawson GHK, Rowland AC. The experimental infection of neonatal pigs with Campylobacter sputorum subspecies mucosalis. Res Vet Sci 1980;28:145–147.

Rowland AC, Lawson GHK. Intestinal adenomatosis in the pig: immunofluorescent and electron microscopic studies. Res Vet Sci 1974;17:323–330.

Rowland AC, Lawson GHK. Porcine intestinal adenomatosis: a possible relationship with necrotic enteritis, regional ileitis and proliferative haemorrhagic enteropathy. Vet Rec 1975;97:178–180.

Russell RG, Krugner L, Tsai C-C, et al. Prevalence of Campylobacter in infant, juvenile and adult laboratory primates. Lab Anim Sci 1988;38:711–714.

Russell RG, et al. Epidemiology and etiology of diarrhea in colony-born Macaca nemestrina. Lab Anim Sci 1987;37:309–316.

Samuelson JD, Winter AJ. Bovine vibriosis: the nature of the carrier state in the bull. J Infect Dis 1966;116:581–592.

Schoeb TR, Fox JG. Enterocolitis associated with intraepithelial Campylobacter-like bacteria in rabbits (Oryctolagus cuniculus). Vet Pathol 1990;27:73–80.

Schutte AP, McConnell EE, Bosman PP. Vibrionic abortion in ewes in South Africa: preliminary report. J S Afr Vet Med Assoc 1971;42:223–226.

Svedhem A, Norkrans G. Campylobacter jejuni enteritis transmitted from cat to man. Lancet 1980;i:713–714.

Taylor NS, Ellenberger MA, Wu PY, et al. Diversity of serotypes of Campylobacter jejuni and Campylobacter coli isolated in laboratory animals. Lab Anim Sci 1989;39:219–221.

Wilkie BN, Winter AJ. Location of Vibrio fetus var. venerealis within the endometrium of the cow. Infect Immun 1971;3:854–856.

Wilkie BN, Winter AJ. Bovine vibriosis: the distribution and specificity of antibodies induced by vaccination and infection and the immunofluorescent localization of organisms in infected heifers. Can J Comp Med 1971;35:301–312.

Williams CE, et al. Ovine campylobacteriosis: preliminary studies of the efficacy of the in vitro serum bactericidal test as an assay for the potency of Campylobacter (Vibrio) fetus subsp intestinalis bacterins. Am J Vet Res 1976;37:409–415.

Wilson TM, et al. Porcine proliferative enteritis: serological, microbiological and pathological studies from three field epizootics. Can J Vet Res 1986;50:217–220.

THE GENUS *ERYSIPELOTHRIX*

This genus contains only one pathogenic member, *Erysipelothrix rhusiopathiae,* the cause of swine erysipelas.

Swine erysipelas

Swine erysipelas is an important disease in many parts of the world (Figs. 10-7 and 10-8). Not only does the causative organism produce infections in swine, but it also infects a wide variety of other species, including birds (turkeys, chickens, geese, ducks, pigeons, parrots, quail, and many other wild species), cattle, sheep, horses, dogs, fish, and porpoises. It causes **erysipeloid** of humans, particularly in persons who work in slaughterhouses and fish markets. The cutaneous lesions of erysipeloid are usually local but may explode into a fulminant disease, with widespread exanthematous or bullous lesions on the hands, face, or body. In humans, the term erysipelas is used to denote cutaneous infections with beta-hemolytic streptococci.

The causative organism, *Erysipelothrix rhusiopathiae (E. insidiosa),* is small, pleomorphic, and rod-shaped, either straight or curved. It is gram-positive and may have a beaded appearance. The organism forms tiny colonies on ordinary agar media. It survives for extremely long periods in alkaline soil, decaying flesh, and water; is resistant to such preservative processes as salting, smoking, and pickling; and many pigs carry the organism in their oropharynx. Thus, sources of infection are easily provided. Once infection is established, large

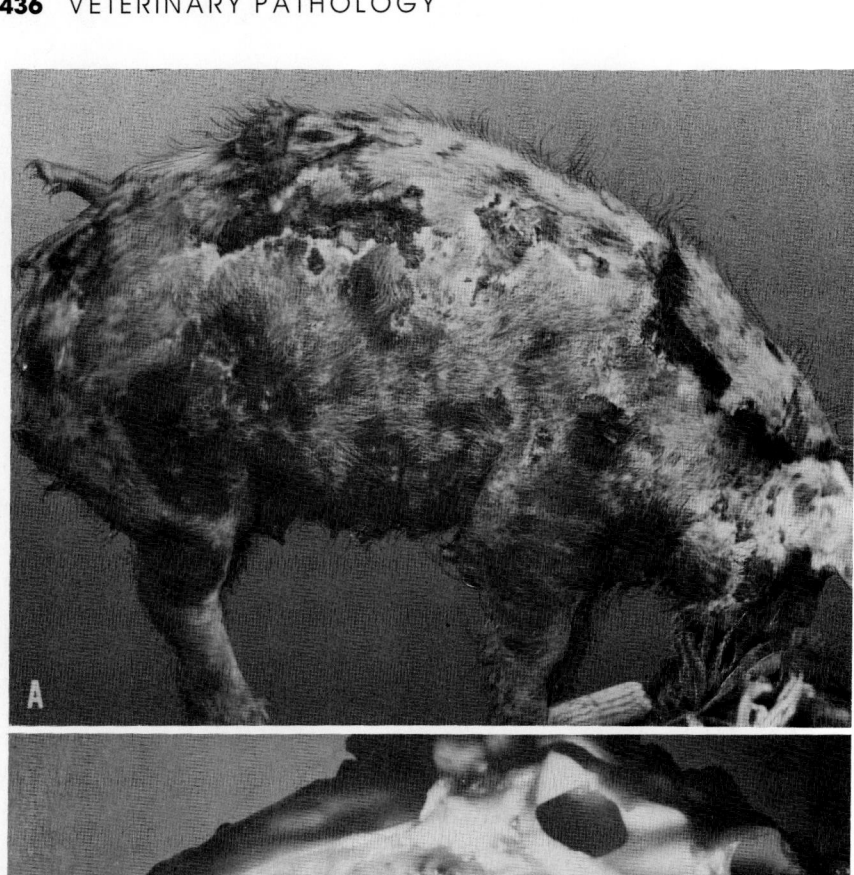

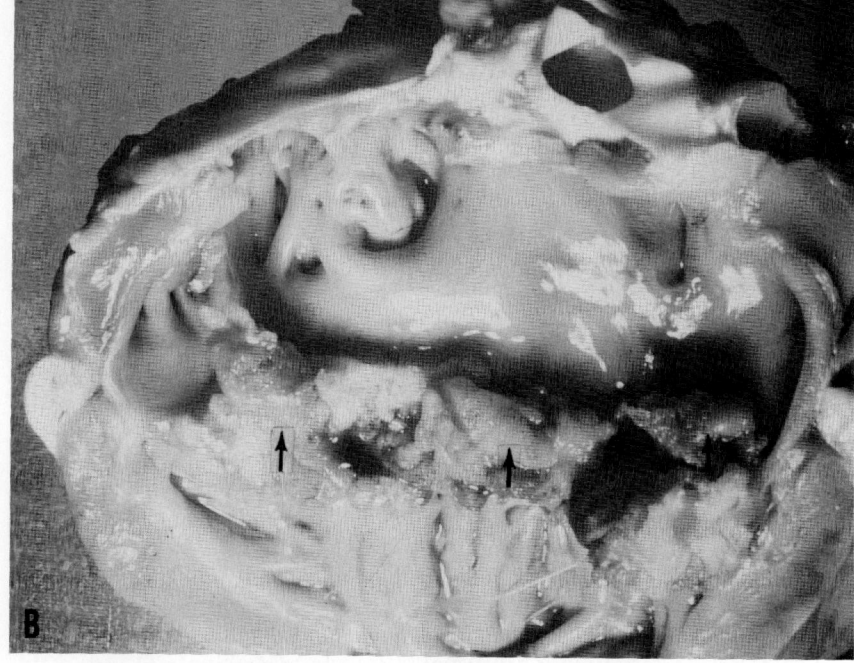

FIG. 10-7 Swine erysipelas. **A.** Sloughing of large areas of skin. **B.** Valvular endocarditis affecting the left atrioventricular (bicuspid or mitral) valve (arrows).

numbers of bacteria are excreted and furnish the principal basis for spread within a herd. Although infection can be initiated through broken skin, most often it is established through the oral route.

In swine, the disease presents as a peracute, acute, or chronic condition. The peracute form is a febrile disease with a high rate of mortality; death occurs before any specific lesions can be detected. The only outward sign may be discoloration of the skin. In less severe infections, appearance of rhomboid-shaped areas of intense erythema in the skin are characteristic, and therefore, the common name "diamond-skin disease" is

frequently applied to this entity. These erythematous lesions may progress to necrosis; large patches of epidermis slough as healing occurs. Chronic infection is chiefly characterized by localization of the organisms in the heart valves or joints, leading to vegetative endocarditis or arthritis. Arthritis in one or more joints is manifested by sudden onset of painful hot swelling, particularly of the carpal or tarsal articulations. Vegetative endocarditis is a common sequel and may result in sudden death. Hypersensitivity appears to play an important role in this disease, but evidence is still accumulating on this point. Lesions closely resembling the

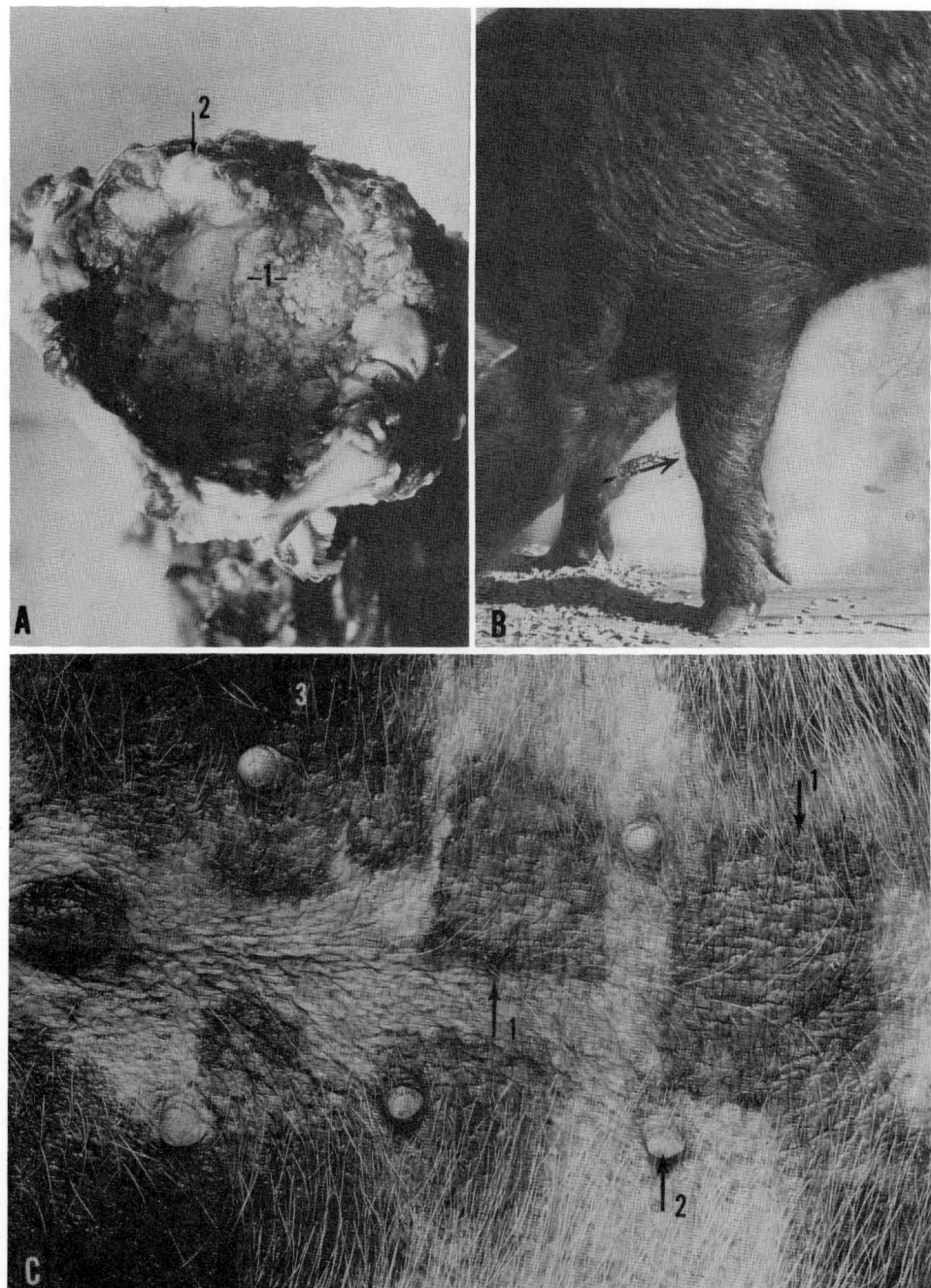

FIG. 10-8 Swine erysipelas. **A.** Arthritis, with roughened synovial surface (1) and thick joint capsule (2). **B.** Acute arthritis with enlargement of the joint (arrow). **C.** Rhomboid areas of congestion in the skin ("diamond skin disease"). Note sharp margin (1) of the lesion. Normal teat (2) and pigmented skin (3). (Courtesy of Bureau of Animal Industry, U.S. Department of Agriculture, and Armed Forces Institute of Pathology.)

arthritic disease have been produced in swine, lambs, and rabbits by direct instillation of cell-free materials from cultures of *E. rhusiopathiae* (Ajmal, 1971; Piercy, 1971; White and Puls, 1969).

LESIONS

In acute septicemic cases of swine erysipelas, non-specific lesions such as hemorrhages may occur in serous surfaces and elsewhere. Specific lesions of diagnostic significance develop as the disease progresses. The distinguishing lesions of the less florid disease are found in the skin, synovial membranes, and endocar-

dium. The cutaneous lesions, which are most common on the abdomen but may occur anywhere on the skin, vary in size but are almost always of diamond, rhomboid, or rectangular shape and are sharply demarcated from the adjacent normal skin. At first, they are bright red, but later they become purplish and, eventually, a dark blue. Necrosis in older lesions accounts for darkening of the skin; the overlying epidermis dries and eventually peels off. Forcible removal of scabs from an incompletely healed lesion uncovers a raw, bleeding surface. The reason for the shape of the skin lesions is not thoroughly understood, although the lesions themselves are believed to result from bacterially induced arteriolitis and thrombosis, which can be observed microscopically.

Microscopic evidence of synovitis may be seen in the subacute form of the disease, but in chronic erysipelas damage to affected joints may be recognized grossly. The joint capsule is obviously enlarged, thickened, and distended with excessive fluid, and the articular surfaces are roughened. Rugose thickening of the joint capsule is particularly evident at the margins of the articular surfaces. Microscopically, the joint capsule is seen to be infiltrated with lymphoid cells; occasional nests of neutrophils are present; and the synovial lining is prominent and often thrown up into folds. Cell detritus and leukocytes may be found free in the lumen of the joint capsule. Organisms may be identified in the synovial tissues early in the course of arthritis but generally cannot be found in chronic arthritis, which has led to the belief that the lesions result from immune mechanisms.

Lesions in the heart are usually the consequence of subacute bacterial endocarditis. Most prominent are the large, irregularly coarse masses on the leaves of the mitral (bicuspid) valve or, less often, on the pulmonary valves. These nodular masses project into the lumen of the left ventricle and, at times, almost occlude it. The material adheres rather tenaciously to the valve leaflets, but it can be broken loose. Hypertrophy of the affected ventricle occurs in chronic cases. Microscopically, the thickened valves are covered with fibrinous exudates made up of zones of organization, necrosis, leukocytes, and colonies of Erysipelothrix organisms.

In sheep, *E. rhusiopathiae* is an important cause of polyarthritis. It is most often seen in lambs; the organism gains entry after docking or castration. Affected lambs are lame, but usually lack signs and lesions of systemic disease. The joints are swollen and contain fibrin and pus. The lesions progress to degenerative osteoarthritis. Valvular endocarditis, septicemia, cutaneous lesions, or pneumonia may also develop in affected sheep.

DIAGNOSIS

Typical symptoms and lesions are usually sufficient for diagnosis, but recovery and identification of the organism is necessary in acute septicemic cases and advisable in others. The organisms can be readily demonstrated by Gram's stain of tissue.

References

Ajmal M. Experimental Erysipelothrix arthritis. Parts I. and II. Res Vet Sci 1971;12:403–411, 412–419.

Bratberg AM. Selective adherence of Erysipelothrix rhusiopathiae to heart valves of swine investigated in an in vitro test. Acta Vet Scand 1981;22:39–45. [Vet Bull 1981;51:5505]

Chineme CN, Slaughter LJ, Highley SW. Cardiovascular lesions associated with erysipelas in a sheep. J Am Vet Med Assoc 1973;162:278–279.

Drew RA. Erysipelothrix arthritis in pigs as a comparative model for rheumatoid arthritis. Proc R Soc Med 1972;65:994–998.

Dreyfuss DJ, Stephens PR. Erysipelothrix rhusiopathiae-induced septic arthritis in a calf. J Am Vet Med Assoc 1990;197:1361–1362.

Drommer W. Schulz L-Cl, Pohlenz J. Experimental infection of erysipelas in the pig. Disturbance of permeability and malacia in the central nervous system. Pathol Vet 1970;7:455–473.

Ehrlich JC. Erysipelothrix rhusiopathiae infection in man. Arch Int Med 1946;78:565–577.

Griffiths IB, Done SH, Readman S. Erysipelothrix pneumonia in sheep. Vet Rec 1991;128:382–383.

Hirsch DC, Boorman GA, Jang SS. Erysipelas in a black and red tamarin. J Am Vet Med Assoc 1975;167:646–647.

Klauder JV. Erysipelothrix rhusiopathiae infection in swine and in human beings. Arch Dermat Syph 1944;50:151–159.

Morita M, Nozaki C, Shibuga S, et al. Histopathology of muscle in experimental acute swine erysipelas. Jpn J Vet Sci 1973;35:261–267.

O'Brien JJ, Baskerville A, McCracken A. Chronic rheumatoid arthritis in pigs associated with Erysipelothrix infection. Ir Vet J 1973;27:21–25.

Piercy DWT. Synovitis induced by killed Erysipelothrix rhusiopathiae. Extended reaction in passively immunized lambs. J Comp Pathol 1971;81:557–562.

Rebhun WC. Erysipelothrix insidiosa septicemia in neonatal calves. Vet Med Small-Anim Clin 1976;71 684–686.

Sakuma S, Doi K, Okawa H, et al. Vascular and perivascular lesions in experimental Erysipelothrix insidiosa infection in rats. Natl Inst Anim Health Q (Tokyo) 1973;13:203–210.

Sakuma S, Doi K, Okawa H, et al. Articular lesions in experimental Erysipelothrix insidiosa infection in rats. Natl Inst Anim Health Q (Tokyo) 1975;15:86–93.

Seibold HR, Neal JE. Erysipelothrix septicemia in the porpoise. J Am Vet Med Assoc 1956;128:537–539.

Sikes D, Neher GM, Doyle LP. Studies on arthritis in swine. I. Experimental erysipelas and chronic arthritis in swine. Am J Vet Res 1955;16:349–366.

Sikes D, Neher GM, Doyle LP. Swine erysipelas I. A discussion of experimentally induced disease. J Am Vet Med Assoc 1956;128:277–281.

Shuman RD, Wood RL, Monlux WS. Sensitization by Erysipelothrix rhusiopathiae (insidiosa) with relation to arthritis in pigs. I, II, III, IV. Cornell Vet 1966;55:378–386, 387–396, 397–411, 444–453.

Simpson CF, Wood FG, Young F. Cutaneous lesions in a porpoise with erysipelas. J Am Vet Med Assoc 1958;133:558–560.

Wallach JD. Erysipelas in two captive Diana monkeys. J Am Vet Med Assoc 1977;171:979–980.

White TG, Puls JL. Induction of experimental chronic arthritis in rabbits by cell-free fragments of Erysipelothrix. J Bact 1969;98:403–406.

White TG, Puls JL, Mirikitani FK. Rabbit arthritis induced by cell-free extracts of Erysipelothrix. Infect Immun 1971;3:715–722.

Wood RL, Packer RA. Isolation of Erysipelothrix rhusiopathiae from soil and manure of swine-raising premises. Am J Vet Res 1972;33:1611–1620.

Wood RL. Survival of Erysipelothrix rhusiopathiae in soil under various environmental conditions. Cornell Vet 1973;63:390–410.

Wood RL. Isolation of pathogenic Erysipelothrix rhusiopathiae from feces of apparently healthy swine. Am J Vet Res 1974;35:41–43.

Wood RL. Swine erysipelas - a review of prevalence and research. J Am Vet Med Assoc 1984;184:944–949.

INFECTIONS CAUSED BY HAEMOPHILUS ORGANISMS

Haemophilus organisms are short, gram-negative bacteria that reside in the oropharynx or genital tract of humans and many species of animals. Most are either nonpathogenic or of very limited pathogenic potential. Certain of them, under appropriate (not always identified) conditions, are capable of causing specific and serious disease. These are listed in Table 10-6.

Glasser's disease

Haemophilus parasuis (H. suis), a normal resident of the oropharynx of swine, is the cause of Glasser's disease.

TABLE 10-6 **Principal diseases caused by *Haemophilus* species**

Species	Disease and species affected
H. pleuropneumoniae (*Actinobacillus pleuropneumoniae*)	Contagious pleuropneumonia, meningitis and arthritis in swine
H. parasuis	Polyserositis, meningitis, and arthritis (Glasser's disease) in swine; pneumonia in swine
H. somnus	Infectious thromboembolic meningoencephalitis, pneumonia and arthritis in cattle
H. agni	Meningitis, pneumonia, and arthritis in sheep
H. haemoglobinophilus	Genital commensal of dogs; recovered from balanoposthitis, vaginitis, and cystitis in ?
H. paragallinarum	Fowl coryza (infectious coryza)
H. influenzae	Upper respiratory tract infections and pneumonia in humans (several other *Haemophilus* species are associated with respiratory, endocardial, and brain infections in humans)
H. equigenitalis	Contagious equine metritis

The disease, seen in young swine after some form of stress, such as weaning or transport, is characterized by sudden onset of fever, lameness, respiratory distress, and neurologic signs. Affected swine become languid, and develop convulsions and paresis.

LESIONS

The lesions, designated as polyserositis, are characterized by serofibrinous inflammation of the meninges, pleura, pericardium, peritoneum, and synovia of joints. Meningitis is most severe in the basal meninges but may be more extensive and also involve the spinal meninges. Extensive deposits of fibrin cover the serosa of body cavities along with some fluid exudation. Joints are swollen, contain excessive cloudy fluid, and the lining is covered with accumulated fibrin. The limb joints and the atlanto-occipital joints are usually the most severely affected. Aside from fibrinous inflammation, microscopic features are not remarkable. The lesions resemble and must be differentiated from Mycoplasmal polyserositis of swine (Chapter 9). The latter condition is usually more protracted and microscopically characterized by a significant lymphocytic infiltrate.

Diagnosis of Glasser's disease can be confirmed by isolation of the organism.

H. parasuis is also a cause of pneumonia in swine, most often in conjunction with swine influenza virus.

Contagious pleuropneumonia of swine

Contagious pleuropneumonia of swine is caused by *Haemophilus pleuropneumoniae* (*H. parahaemolyticus*), a specific pathogen of swine which, in contrast to *H. parasuis*, is not carried by healthy animals. The exact taxonomic classification of *H. pleuropneumoniae* is uncertain; recent evidence suggests that it be renamed *Actinobacillus pleuropneumoniae*. Infection is spread via the respiratory route by infected animals and swine with subclinical disease. Young animals, up to 6 months of age, are most susceptible to infection, which is most prevalent in the winter months. Infection can be very acute and cause death in a day or two, but usually infection causes a pneumonia of several days duration. Mortality rates may be more than 50%. Signs include fever, respiratory distress, and nasal discharge, which is often tinged with blood.

LESIONS

The lesions are those of an acute fibrinopurulent pneumonia with extensive necrosis and hemorrhage. There is accompanying fibrinous pleuritis. Large zones may become sequestered and walled off by granulation tissue, only to be discovered as incidental findings in slaughtered swine. Meningitis and arthritis may accompany the pneumonia. Hani and colleagues (1973) and others point out that the early lesions resemble those of endotoxic shock, and indeed, Haemophilus endotoxins are believed to be primary contributors to the pathogenesis of the lesions. These include alveolar and interlobular edema, dilation of lymphatics, congestion, hemorrhage, and intravascular fibrinous thrombosis.

Diagnosis is confirmed by isolation of the organism from affected lung.

Infectious thromboembolic meningoencephalitis of cattle

First reported in Colorado by Griner and others (1956), infectious thromboembolic meningoencephalitis of cattle is now recognized throughout the United States as well as in Canada and Europe. The causative organism was recovered by Kennedy and associates (1960) from an outbreak in California and named *Haemophilus somnus*. Although the exact classification of the organism is uncertain, the disease has been experimentally reproduced by inoculation with cultures of the bacterium. *H. somnus* is carried in the nasal cavities, prepuce, and female genital tract of healthy cattle and is easily transmitted. On occasion, it has been associated with bovine abortion. The pathogenic potential is realized under conditions of stress, such as shipping and overcrowding in feedlots.

SIGNS

The course is rapid, and clinical signs may often go unnoticed. When observed, signs include fever, weakness, staggering, somnolence, ataxia, blindness, and paralysis. Signs of pneumonia (dyspnea) and arthritis are also common. Mortality rates are high.

LESIONS

Grossly, the most characteristic lesions are multiple foci of necrosis and hemorrhage in the brain. Any part of the brain may be affected. The meninges are opaque and roughened. Petechiae and ecchymoses may be present in any viscus; lymph nodes are often enlarged; and serofibrinous laryngitis, tracheitis, pleuritis, pneumonia, arthritis, pericarditis, and peritonitis are frequent findings. Microscopically, the basic and characteristic lesion is vasculitis with thrombosis and septic infarction. Vasculitis is most common in the brain but may be generalized. Necrotic foci contain bacterial colonies and become infiltrated with neutrophils. The thrombi are primarily fibrinous. Meningitis is characterized by a fibrinopurulent exudate. Lesions in other organs and in the respiratory tract, in addition to vasculitis and thrombosis, are characterized by fibrinopurulent inflammation.

Diagnosis is made on the basis of the lesions and recovery and identification of *H. somnus*.

Haemophilus somnus is also associated with diseases of other organ systems, in the absence of central nervous system lesions. These include polyarthritis, endometritis and abortion, orchitis, septicemia, and, especially, bronchopneumonia. *H. somnus* pneumonia is most prevalent in calves and is characterized by necrotizing bronchiolitis and fibrinopurulent bronchopneumonia and pleuritis.

Haemophilus septicemia of lambs

An acute septicemia of lambs caused by an organism of uncertain classification, termed *Haemophilus agni*, was described by Kennedy and others (1958).

SIGNS

Clinical signs include fever, depression, and reluctance to move, but since the course is usually less than 12 hours, affected animals are often found dead without premonitory signs.

LESIONS

Gross changes are dominated by multiple hemorrhages throughout the body, including skeletal muscle, where they are reported to be of diagnostic value. Focal necrosis of the liver and splenomegaly are almost constant findings. Fibrinopurulent arthritis, choroiditis, and basilar meningitis may develop in the rare lamb that survives 24 hours or longer. Microscopically identifiable generalized bacterial embolism and vasculitis account for the gross findings. All tissues may be involved, particularly the liver and skeletal muscle.

Definitive diagnosis requires isolation and identification of *H. agni*.

Contagious equine metritis

In horses, a condition known as contagious equine metritis is caused by an organism tentatively classified as *Haemophilus equigenitalis (Taylorella equigenitalis)*. This disease is described in Chapter 25.

References

Andrews JJ, Anderson TD, Slife LN, et al. Microscopic lesions associated with the isolation of Haemophilus somnus from pneumonic bovine lungs. Vet Pathol 1985;22:131–136.

Bailie WE, Anthony HD, Weide KD. Infectious thromboembolic meningoencephalitis (sleeper syndrome) in feedlot cattle. J Am Vet Med Assoc 1966;148:162–166.

Bendixon PH, Shewen PE, Rosendal S, et al. Toxicity of Haemophilus pleuropneumoniae for porcine lung macrophages, peripheral blood monocytes, and testicular cells. Infect Immun 1981;33:673–676.

Bertram TA. Quantitative morphology of peracute pulmonary lesions in swine induced by Haemophilus pleuropneumoniae. Vet Pathol 1985;22:598–609.

Bertram TA. Intravascular macrophages in lungs of pigs infected with Haemophilus pleuropneumoniae. Vet Pathol 1986;23:681–691.

Crandell RA, Smith AR, Kissil M. Colonization and transmission of Haemophilus somnus in cattle. Am J Vet Res 1977;38:1749–1751.

Davidson JN, King JM. An outbreak of Haemophilus parahaemolyticus pneumonia in growing pigs. Cornell Vet 1980;70:360–364.

Dawkins BG. Haemophilus influenzae septic pyarthrosis in a cynomolgus monkey. J Am Vet Med Assoc 1982;181:1430–1431.

Didier PJ, Perino L, Urbance J. Porcine Haemophilus pleuropneumoniae: microbiologic and pathologic findings. J Am Vet Med Assoc 1984;184:716–719.

Dukes TW. The ocular lesions in thromboembolic meningoencephalitis (TEME) of cattle. Can Vet J 1971;12:180–182.

Greenway JA. Haemophilus pneumonia in B.C. swine. [letter] Can Vet J 1981;22:20–21.

Griner LA, Jensen R, Brown WW. Infectious embolic meningoencephalitis in cattle. J Am Vet Med Assoc 1956;129:417–421.

Hani H, Konig H, Nicolet J, et al. Zur Haemophilus-Pleuropneumonie beim Schwein. V. Pathomorphologie. Schwiz Arch Tierheilkd 1973;115:191–203.

Hani H, Konig H, Nicolet J, et al. Zur Haemophilus-Pleuropneumonie beim Schwein. VI. Pathogenese. Schweitz Arch Tierheilkd 1972;115:205–212.

Humphrey JD, Stephens LR. "Haemophilus somnus": a review. Vet Bull 1983;53:987–1004.

Jackson JA, Andrews JJ, Hargis JW. Experimental Haemophilus somnus pneumonia in calves. Vet Pathol 1987;24:129–134.

Kennedy PC, Frazier LM, Theiler GH, et al. A septicemic disease of lambs caused by Hemophilus agni (new species). Am J Vet Res 1958;19:645–654.

Kennedy PC, et al. Infectious meningo-encephalitis in cattle, caused by a haemophilus-like organism. Am J Vet Res 1960;21:403–409.

Kume K, Nakai T, Sawata A. Isolation of Haemophilus pleuropneumoniae from the nasal cavities of healthy pigs. Jpn J Vet Sci 1984;46:641–647. [Vet Bull 1985;55:2591]

Little TWA. Haemophilus infection in pigs. Vet Rec 1970;87:399–402.

Metz AL, Haggard DL, Hakomaki MR. Chronic suppurative orchiepididymitis associated with Haemophilus somnus in a calf. J Am Vet Med Assoc 1984;184:1507–1508.

Miller RB, Barnum DA. Effects of Haemophilus somnus on the pregnant bovine reproductive tract and conceptus following cervical infusion. Vet Pathol 1983;20:584–589.

Miller RB, Barnum DA, McEntee KE. Haemophilus somnus in the reproductive tracts of slaughtered cows: location and frequency of isolation and lesions. Vet Pathol 1983;20:515–521.

Miller RB, Van Camp SD, Barnum DA. The effects of intra-amniotic inoculation of Haemophilus somnus on the bovine fetus and dam. Vet Pathol 1983;20:574–583.

Momotani E, Yabuki Y, Miho H, et al. Histopathological evaluation of disseminated intravascular coagulation in Haemophilus somnus infection in cattle. J Comp Pathol 1985;95:15–23.

Nielsen R, Mandrup M. Pleuropneumonia in swine caused by Haemophilus parahaemolyticus. A study of the epidemiology of the infection. Nord Vet Med 1977;29:465–473. [Vet Bull 1978;48:2103]

Panciera RJ, Dahlgren RR, Rinker HB. Observations on septicemia of cattle caused by a Haemophilus-like organism. Path Vet 1968;5:212–226.

Potgieter LND, et al. Experimental bovine respiratory tract disease with Haemophilus somnus. Vet Pathol 1988;25:124–130.

Saunders JR, Thiessen WA, Janzen ED. Haemophilus somnus infections. I. A ten year (1969–1978) retrospective study of losses in cattle herds in western Canada. Can Vet J 1980;21:119–123. [Vet Bull 1980;50:6298]

Schiefer B, Greenfield J. Porcine Hemophilus parahemolyticus pneumonia in Saskatchewan. II. Bacteriological and experimental studies. Can J Comp Med 1974;38:105–110.

Sebunya TNK, Saunders JR. Haemophilus pleuropneumoniae infection in swine: a review. J Am Vet Med Assoc 1983;182:1331–1337.

Stephens LR, Little PB. Ultrastructure of Haemophilus somnus, causative agent of bovine infectious thromboembolic meningoencephalitis. Am J Vet Res 1981;42:1638–1640.

Stephens LR, Little PB, Wilkie BN, et al. Humoral immunity in experimental thromboembolic meningoencephalitis in cattle caused by Haemophilus somnus. Am J Vet Res 1981;42:468–473.

Swaney LM, Breese SS Jr. Ultrastructure of Haemophilus equigenitalis, causative agent of contagious equine metritis. Am J Vet Res 1980;41:127–132.

Udeze FA, Latimer KS, Kadis S. Role of Haemophilus pleuropneumoniae lipopolysaccharide endotoxin in the pathogenesis of porcine Haemophilus pleuropneumonia. Am J Vet Res 1987;48:768–773.

Van Dreumel AA, Curtis RA, Ruhnke HL. Infectious thromboembolic meningoencephalitis in Ontario feedlot cattle. Can Vet J 1970;11:125–130.

Van Dreumel AA, Kierstead M. Abortion associated with Hemophilus somnus infection in a bovine fetus. Can Vet J 1975;16:367–370.

Walker RL, LeaMaster BR, Biberstein EL, et al. Serodiagnosis of Histophilus ovis-associated epididymitis in rams. Am J Vet Res 1988;49:208–212.

Ward GE, Nivard JR, Maheswaran SK. Morphologic features, structure, and adherence to bovine turbinate cells of three Haemophilus somnus variants. Am J Vet Res 1984;45:336–338.

Diseases Resulting from Escherichia Infection

The Escherichiae are members of the Family Enterobacteriaceae, a large group of gram-negative rods, which also includes the genera *Shigella, Salmonella, Citrobacter, Klebsiella, Enterobacter, Erwinia, Serratia, Proteus,* and *Yersinia.* The group contains many primary pathogens of importance to domestic animals and humans, most of which are associated with enteric disease. Others in the family are often opportunistic pathogens.

Colibacillosis

There are hundreds of serotypes of *Escherichia coli,* which are classified on the basis of various surface antigens referred to as O (somatic), K (capsular), H (flagellar), and F (fimbrial). Only a few *E. coli,* however, can be considered true pathogens. These are predominantly associated with enteric disease and are referred to as enteropathogenic (enterotoxic) *E. coli;* they are important causes of diarrhea in humans, swine, cattle, sheep, horses, and probably other species. *E. coli* is also the cause of edema disease of swine, which results from elaboration of a toxin that is absorbed into the bloodstream (enterotoxemic *E. coli*). Other strains are responsible for septicemia, especially in calves. *E. coli* are also often associated with septic infections, such as inflammation of the lower urinary tract, pyelonephritis, infected wounds, pneumonia, peritonitis, mastitis, and meningitis. In these conditions, *E. coli* is considered an opportunistic pathogen rather than a primary pathogen, although the degree of invasiveness varies between strains.

ENTERIC COLIBACILLOSIS

Three distinct pathogenetic mechanisms have been identified with the enteropathogenic *E. coli:* enterotoxic colibacillosis, enteroinvasive colibacillosis, and enteroadherent colibacillosis.

Enterotoxic colibacillosis The most common form of colibacillosis in domestic animals, this disease results from (1) colonization of *E. coli* on the surface of enterocytes, and (2) the elaboration of toxins. The ability to adhere to mucosal cells is a specific attribute of these pathogens and results from distinctive antigens on the surface of these *E. coli,* referred to as fimbrial antigens, which bind to ganglioside receptors on enterocytes.

Two classes of toxins are produced: heat labile enterotoxin (LT) and heat stable enterotoxin (ST). The heat labile enterotoxin acts in a manner similar to cholera toxin by activation of adenylate cyclase leading to an increase in intracellular cyclic-AMP, which causes a marked increase in cellular excretion, resulting in diarrhea. The action of LT is of relatively slow onset and long duration. ST specifically activates particulate guanylate cyclase, also inducing fluid loss and diarrhea. Two types of ST have been identified; STa and STb. The action of ST is more rapid and of shorter duration than that of LT. Although there may be villous atrophy, lesions in either form of enterotoxic colibacillosis are minimal to absent, an aid in differentiating the disease from the several enteric viral diseases, such as those caused by rotaviruses and coronaviruses. This form of colibacillosis is most common naturally in young piglets, calves, and lambs during the first week of life. A condition known as post-weaning enteritis (post-weaning diarrhea) of piglets also results from toxigenic *E. coli.* This entity is often seen in association with edema disease.

Enteroinvasive colibacillosis Primarily a disease of humans, there are a few examples of enteric colibacillosis in swine and cattle. This form of colibacillosis has been likened to shigellosis or salmonellosis. The organisms penetrate enterocytes, invade the lamina propria, and may extend to mesenteric lymph nodes and beyond. The responsible enteropathogenic *E. coli* are also believed to elaborate a toxin that inhibits protein synthesis, leading to necrosis of enterocytes, usually in the colon. The toxin has been called shigalike toxin, or SLT. In contrast to enterotoxic colibacillosis, microscopic lesions, consisting of blunting of villi, lengthening of crypts, focal ulceration, and an accompanying acute inflammatory response, are present in the enteroinvasive form.

Enteroadherent colibacillosis This is a more recently recognized form of colibacillosis that has been described in humans, calves, pigs, and rabbits. It is caused by recognized enteropathogenic serotypes that do not elaborate toxins. Rather, the organisms penetrate the glycocalyx, adhere closely to the mucosal cell surface, and destroy microvilli. They have been termed "attaching and effacing" *E. coli*. Histologically, there is blunting of villi, crypt hypertrophy, and inflammatory cell influx in the lamina propria. Ultrastructurally, organisms are seen adherent to enterocytes displacing microvilli. The colon is usually more severely affected than the small intestine.

EDEMA DISEASE OF SWINE (ENTEROTOXEMIC COLIBACILLOSIS)

First reported by Shanks in Ireland in 1938, this disease has been encountered with some frequency in most of the swine-producing areas of the world. It attacks previously healthy animals without warning, occurring most often following weaning or a change in diet. The course is short and characterized by incoordination and paralysis of the limbs, pain, coma, and often diarrhea, causing death within a number of hours or a day or two. It is not contagious, but herd morbidity rates may approach 35%. Mortality rates for sick animals may reach 100%.

The pathogenesis is not entirely clear, but the disease appears to result from the elaboration of a toxin by certain strains of *E. coli* that adhere to and colonize the intestinal mucosa. The mechanism whereby the organisms adhere is not established, but it is not dependent on fimbrial antigens, as in enterotoxic colibacillosis. The toxin, referred to as edema disease toxin (Shiga-like toxin II), is absorbed into the circulation and acts on small arteries and arterioles, where it causes a necrotizing arteritis, characterized by swelling and proliferation of endothelium and necrosis and hyalinization of the media, resulting in noninflammatory edema. Lesions can be detected as early as two days after experimental induction of the disease. Hypertension has also been demonstrated in affected swine, which would further contribute to the development of edema. Necrotizing arteritis can be found in almost all organs of the body, including the brain, where focal symmetrical encephalomalacia, particularly of the thalamus, basal ganglia, and nuclei of the brain stem, may be found.

The edema is typically, but not invariably, found in the wall of the stomach, where it may involve the cardiac region or the greater curvature, or the whole organ. The thickness of the gastric wall may be increased just perceptibly, or it may increase to 3 cm. The coiled portion of the colon, with its mesentery, is another common location of edema, but these regions are by no means the only sites that may be involved. The body cavities usually contain varying amounts of fluid; other parts of the intestinal tract sometimes are involved. The face and eyelids are edematous in a high proportion of cases, as can be observed during life. Less often, the tarsal and carpal regions and the ventral belly wall contain an excess of fluid. The parenchymatous organs of the abdomen usually appear normal, as do the brain and, usually, the lungs. Subepicardial hemorrhages sometimes occur, but inflammatory changes are typically absent from all organs.

What has been described as possibly a separate entity under the name swine cerebrospinal angiopathy has also been ascribed to enterotoxic *E. coli*. Necrotizing arteritis and arteriolitis with the occurrence of perivascular PAS-positive eosiniphilic droplets accompanied by malacia and demyelination, particularly of the medulla oblongata, pons, and mid-brain, characterize the syndrome. Other changes characteristic of edema disease are not pronounced, but may be present to some degree.

SEPTICEMIC COLIBACILLOSIS (COLISEPTICEMIC FORM)

In this form of the disease, the organisms invade the host (possibly through the oral cavity, respiratory system, pharynx, or umbilicus) and produce an endotoxin that apparently causes the lesions. Unless the enterotoxic form occurs simultaneously, the bacteria do not reach the small intestine. Thus diarrhea or intestinal lesions do not occur. This form is most dramatic and has been best described in young calves. Calves that are deficient in immunoglobulin (usually as a result of failure to receive colostrum) are most susceptible.

The signs and lesions are typical of bacterial arthritis, polyserositis, meningitis, ophthalmitis, and pyelonephritis, with bacterial emboli and necrotizing, purulent, or fibrinous exudation.

SUMMARY

Thus, different strains of *Escherichia coli* have the ability, under certain conditions of the host, to produce pathologic manifestations involving at least five pathogenetic mechanisms. It appears likely that new concepts will change or details will deepen with respect to this problem, since many investigators are currently conducting research on it.

References

Anderson JC, Burrows MR, Bramley AJ. Bacterial adherence in mastitis caused by Escherichia coli. Vet Pathol 1977;14:681–628.

Ansari MM, Renshaw HW, Gates NL. Colibacillosis in neonatal lambs: onset of diarrheal disease and isolation and characterization of enterotoxigenic Escherichia coli from enteric and septicemic forms of the disease. Am J Vet Res 1978;39:11–14.

Bertschinger HU, Pohlenz J. Bacterial colonization and morphology of the intestine in porcine Escherichia coli enterotoxemia (edema disease). Vet Pathol 1983;20:99–110.

Christie BR, Waxler GL. Experimental colibacillosis in gnotobiotic baby pigs. I. Microbiological and clinical aspects. II. Pathology. Can J Comp Med 1973;37:261–270, 271–280.

Clugston RE, Nielson NO, Smith DLT. Experimental edema disease of swine (E. coli enterotoxemia). III. Pathology and pathogenesis. Can J Comp Med 1974;38:34–43.

Cooke EM. Escherichia coli - an overview. J Hyg (Camb) 1985;95:523–530.

Cordy DR. Pathomorphology and pathogenesis of bacterial meningoventriculitis of neonatal ungulates. Vet Pathol 1984;21:587–591.

Dorn K, et al. Studies on pigs. V. Chemical studies on pigs with edema disease. Arch Exp Vet Med 1962;16:1187–1203.

Dreyfus LA, Robertson DC. Solubilization and partial characterization of the intestinal receptor for Escherichia coli heat-stable enterotoxin. Infect Immun 1984;46:537–543.

Du Pont HL, et al. Pathogenesis of Escherichia coli diarrhea. N Engl J Med 1971;285:1–9.

Fox MW, Haynes E. Neonatal colibacillosis in the dog. J Small Anim Pract 1966;7:599–603.

Gay CC. Escherichia coli and neonatal disease of calves. Bact Rev 1965;29:75–101.

Gill DM, Richardson SH. Adenosine diphosphate-ribosylation of adenylate cyclase catalyzed by heat-labile enterotoxin of Escherichia coli: comparaison with cholera toxin. J Infect Dis 1980;141:64–70.

Gitter M, Lloyd MK. Haemolytic Bact. coli in the bowel edema syndrome. II. Transmission and protection experiments. Br Vet J 1957;113:212–218.

Green SL, Smith LL. Meningitis in neonatal calves: 32 cases (1983–1990). J Am Vet Med Assoc 1992;201:125–128.

Guerrant RL, Hughes JM, Chang B, et al. Activation of intestinal guanylate cyclase by heat-stable enterotoxin of Escherichia coli: studies of tissue specificity, potential receptors, and intermediates. J Infect Dis 1980;142:220–228.

Guerrant RL, et al. Effect of Escherichia coli on fluid transport across canine small bowel: mechanism and time-course with enterotoxin and whole bacterial cells. J Clin Invest 1973;52:1707–1714.

Hall GA, et al. Dysentery caused by Escherichia coli (S102–9) in calves: natural and experimental disease. Vet Pathol 1985;22:156–163.

Harper M, Turvey A, Bramley AJ. Adhesion of fimbriate Escherichia coli to bovine mammary-gland epithelial cells in vitro. J Med Microbiol 1978;11:117–123.

Hornich M, et al. Enteric Escherichia coli infections. Morphological findings in the intestinal mucosa of healthy and diseased piglets. Vet Path 1973;10:484–500.

Johannsen U. Pathology and pathogenesis of spontaneous coli enterotoxaemia and the experimental coli endotoxin syndrome in pigs. VII. Pathology of the mesenteric nodes. Arch Exp Veterinaermed 1974;28:455–475.

Johnson WM, Lior H, Bezanson GS. Cytotoxic Escherichia coli 0157:H7 associated with haemorrhagic colitis in Canada. Lancet 1983;i:76.

Jones JET, Smith HW. Histological studies on weaned pigs suffering from diarrhea and oedema disease produced by oral inoculation of Escherichia coli. J Pathol 1969;97:168–172.

Jones TO. Escherichia coli mastitis in dairy cattle - a review of the literature. Vet Bull 1990;60:205–231.

Kennedy DJ, Akaike Y, Miyachi T, et al. Production of heat-stable enterotoxin component by Escherichia coli strains enteropathogenic for swine. Natl Inst Anim Health Q 1981;21:21–25.

Kennedy DJ, Greenberg RN, Dunn JA, et al. Effects of Escherichia coli heat-stable enterotoxin STb on intestines of mice, rats, rabbits and piglets. Infect Immun 1984;46:639–643.

Kernkamp HCH, et al. Epizootiology of edema disease of swine. J Am Vet Med Assoc 1965;146:353–357.

Kurtz HJ, et al. Pathologic changes in edema disease of swine. Am J Vet Res 1969;30:791–806.

Kurtz HJ, Short EC Jr. Pathogenesis of edema disease in swine: Pathologic effects of hemolysin, autolysate, and endotoxin of Escherichia coli (0141). Am J Vet Res 1976;37:15–24.

Luke D, Gordon WAM. Oedema of the bowel in pigs. Nature (Lond) 1950;165:286.

MacLeod DL, Gyles CL, Wilcock BP. Reproduction of edema disease of swine with purified Shiga-like toxin-II variant. Vet Pathol 1991;28:66–73.

Methiyapun S, Pohlenz JFL, Bertschinger HU. Ultrastructure of the intestinal mucosa in pigs experimentally inoculated with an edema disease-producing strain of Escherichia coli (0139:K12:H1). Vet Pathol 1984;21:516–520.

Meyer RC, Saxena SP, Rhoades HE. Polyserositis induced by Escherichia coli in gnotobiotic swine. Infect Immun 19713:41–44.

Moon HW, Nielsen NO, Kramer TT. Experimental enteric colibacillosis of the newborn pig: histopathology of the small intestine and changes in plasma electrolytes. Am J Vet Res 1970;31:103–112.

Moon HW. Pathogenesis of enteric diseases caused by Escherichia coli. Adv Vet Sci Comp Med 1974;18:179–211.

Moon HW, Isaacson RE, Pohlenz J. Mechanisms of association of enteropathogenic Escherichia coli with intestinal epithelium. Am J Clin Nutr 1979;32:119–127.

Moon HW, Whipp SC, Argenzio RA, et al. Attaching and effacing activities of rabbit and human enteropathogenic Escherichia coli in pig and rabbit intestines. Infect Immun 1983;41:1340–1351.

Morris DD, Cullor JS, Whitlock RH, et al. Endotoxemia in neonatal calves given antiserum to a mutant Escherichia coli (J-5). Am J Vet Res 1986;47:2554–2565.

Mushin R, Basset CR. Haemolytic Escherichia coli and other bacteria in oedema disease of swine. Aust Vet J 1964;40:315–320.

Nakamura K, et al. Swine cerebrospinal angiopathy with demyelination and malacia. Vet Pathol 1982;19:140–149.

O'Brien AD, Holmes RK. Shiga and Shiga-like toxins. Microbiol Rev 1987;51:206–220.

Olson P, Hedhammar Å, Wadström T. Enterotoxigenic Escherichia coli infection in two dogs with acute diarrhea. J Am Vet Med Assoc 1984;184:982–983.

Pearson GR, McNulty MS, Logan EF. Pathological changes in the small intestine of neonatal calves with enteric colibacillosis. Vet Pathol 1978;15:91–101.

Pearson GR, Logan EF. Ultrastructural changes in the small intestine of neonatal calves with enteric colibacillosis. Vet Pathol 1982;19:190–201.

Peeters JE, Charlier GJ, Raeymaekers R. Scanning and transmission electron microscopy of attaching effacing Escherichia coli in weanling rabbits. Vet Pathol 1985;22:54–59.

Philip JR, Shone DK. Some observations on oedema disease and a possibly related condition in pigs in Southern Rhodesia. J S Afr Vet Med Assoc 1960;31:427–434.

Priouzeau M. Gastrite oed,mateuse des bovid,s. Res Med Vet 1954;130:377–380.

Reynolds DJ, et al. Microbiology of calf diarrhoea in southern Britain. Vet Rec 1986;119:34–39.

Rose R, Whipp SC, Moon HW. Effects of Escherichia coli heat-stable enterotoxin b on small intestinal villi in pigs, rabbits, and lambs. Vet Pathol 1987;24:71–79.

Rothbaum R, McAdams AJ, Giannella R, et al. A clinocopathologic study of enterocyte-adherent Escherichia coli: a cause of protracted diarrhea in infants. Gastroenterology 1982;83:441–454.

Smith HW, Halls S. The production of oedema disease and diarrhea in weaned pigs by the oral administration of E. coli. Factors that influence the course of the experimental disease. J Med Microbiol 1968;1:45–59.

Snodgrass DR, et al. Aetiology of diarrhoea in young calves. Vet Rec 1986;119:31–34.

Staley TE, Jones EW, Corely LD. Attachment and penetration of Escherichia coli into intestinal epithelium of the ileum in newborn pigs. Am J Pathol 1969;56:371–392.

Staley TE, Jones EW, Corely LD, et al. Intestinal permeability to Escherichia coli in the foal. Am J Vet Res 1970;31:1481–1483.

Tennant B, Harrold D, Reina-Guerra M. Physiologic and metabolic factors in the pathogenesis of neonatal enteric infections in calves. J Am Vet Med Assoc 1972;161:993–1007.

Thomlinson JR, Buxton A. Anaphylaxis in pigs and its relationship to the pathogenesis of oedema disease and gastroenteritis associated with Escherichia coli. Immunology 1963;6:126–139.

Timoney JF. Experimental production of oedema disease of swine. Vet Rec 1949;61:710.

Timoney JF. Oedema disease of swine. Vet Rec 1950;62:748–756; 1956;68:849–851; 1957;69:1160–1175.

Todhunter DA, Smith KL, Hogan JS, et al. Gram-negative bacterial infections of the mammary gland in cows. Am J Vet Res 1991;52:184–188.

Ulshen MH, Rollo JL. Pathogenesis of Escherichia coli gastroenteritis in man—another mechanism. N Engl J Med 1980;302:99–101.

Underdahl NR, Stair EL, Young GA. Transmission and characterization of edema disease of swine. J Am Vet Med Assoc 1963;142:27–30.

Waxler GL, Britt AL. Polyserositis and arthritis due to Escherichia coli in gnotobiotic pigs. Can J Comp Med 1972;36:226–233.

Wilson RA, Keefe TJ, Davis MA, et al. Strains of Escherichia coli associated with urogenital disease in dogs and cats. Am J Vet Res 1988;49:743–746.

Wray C, Thomlinson JR. The effects of Escherichia coli endotoxin in calves. Res Vet Sci 1972;13:546–553.

Wray C, Thomlinson JR. Lesions and bacteriological findings in colibacillosis of calves. Br Vet J 1974;130:189–199.

INFECTIONS CAUSED BY KLEBSIELLA ORGANISMS

Klebsiella pneumoniae (Friedlander's bacillus) is the only member of this genus to have pathologic significance. It is a member of the Enterobacteriaceae and is a normal inhabitant of the gastrointestinal tract. Under conditions that are poorly understood, *K. pneumoniae* may be a causative factor in a variety of inflammatory processes. In humans and nonhuman primates, it is an important cause of severe pneumonia and upper respiratory and middle ear infections. Pneumonia caused by *K. pneumoniae* is only seen rarely in domestic animals. Other conditions associated with *K. pneumoniae* include meningitis in nonhuman primates, mastitis in cattle and swine, genitourinary infections in mares and bitches, and wound infections in many species.

Brief mention is made here of the genera *Serratia* and *Proteus*, other members of the Enterobacteriaceae. Members of these genera are opportunistic pathogens and have been associated with mastitis, diarrhea, and nosocomial infections. *Serratia marcescens* has been increasingly associated with disease in domestic animals, especially mastitis.

References

Armstrong PJ. Systemic Serratia marcescens infections in a dog and a cat. J Am Vet Med Assoc 1984;184:1154–1158.

Bowman GL, Hueston WD, Boner GJ, et al. Serratia liquefaciens mastitis in a dairy herd. J Am Vet Med Assoc 1986;189:913–915.

Braman SK, Eberhart RJ, Asbury MA, et al. Capsular types of Klebsiella pneumoniae associated with bovine mastitis. J Am Vet Med Assoc 1973;162:109–111.

Brown JE, Corstvet RE, Stratton LG. A study of Klebsiella pneumoniae infection in the uterus of the mare. Am J Vet Res 1979;40:1523–1530.

Colahan PT, Peyton LC, Connelly MR, et al. Serratia spp infection in 21 horses. J Am Vet Med Assoc 1984;185:209–211.

Done SH. Observations on an outbreak of Klebsiella mastitis in sows. Acta Vet Acad Sci Hung 1975;25:211–215.

Ewart S, Brown B, Derksen F, et al. Serratia marcescens endocarditis in a horse. J Am Vet Med Assoc 1992;200:961–963.

Fox JG, Rohovsky MW. Meningitis caused by Klebsiella spp in two rhesus monkeys. J Am Vet Med Assoc. 1975;167:634–636.

Fox JG, Rohovsky MW. Klebsiella in monkeys. J Am Vet Med Assoc 1976;168:276.

Giles RC Jr, Hildebrandt PK, Tate C. Klebsiella air sacculitis in the owl monkey (Aotus trivirgatus). Lab Anim Sci 1974;24:610–616.

Glickman LT. Veterinary nosocomial (hospital-acquired) Klebsiella infections. J Am Vet Med Assoc 1981;179:1389–1392.

Kageruka P, Mortelmans J, Vercruysse J. Klebsiella pneumoniae infections in monkeys. Acta Zool Pathol Antwerp 1971;52:83–88.

Ruegg PL, et al. Microbiologic investigation of an epizootic of mastitis caused by Serratia marcescens in a dairy herd. J Am Vet Med Assoc 1992;200:184–189.

Schmidt RE, Butler TM. Klebsiella-enterobacter infections in chimpanzees. Lab Anim Sci 1972;21:946–949.

Timoney PJ, McArdle JF, Bryne MJ. Abortion and meningitis in a Thoroughbred mare associated with Klebsiella pneumoniae, type 1. Equine Vet J 1983;15:64–65.

Wyand DS, Hayden DW. Klebseilla infection in muskrats. J Am Vet Med Assoc 1973;163:589–592.

BRUCELLOSIS

The discovery and identification of the bacteria now grouped in the genus *Brucella* were important steps in the development of knowledge concerning the complex disease of humans and animals now known as brucellosis. *Brucella melitensis*, the first genus to be recognized, was isolated in 1887 from the spleen of patients dead of "Mediterranean fever" or "gastric fever" (later called "Malta fever") by David Bruce, whose name identifies the organism and the disease (Fig. 10-9). In 1905, the infection was traced to the milk goat, which even today is the most common source of the organism, although it also has been isolated from the milk of infected cattle and from aborted fetuses of sheep.

A second step, in 1897, was the isolation and identification of *Brucella abortus* from aborted bovine fetuses and fetal membranes by the Danish veterinarian, Frederick Bang. The infection of cattle caused by that organism has since been known as "Bang's disease" or "Bang's abortion disease." Eventually it was proven that the causative organism was ubiquitous; natural infections occur not only in cattle, but also in humans, horses, fowl, sheep, dogs, deer, and bison. One important source of infection for humans is cow's milk, although contact with aborted bovine fetuses or slaughtered cattle has also produced the disease. The characteristic undulating or recurrent fever often observed in the human disease has given rise to the name "undulant fever."

The third organism to be included in the genus *Brucella* was originally identified by Traum in 1914 in aborted swine fetuses. This organism, *Brucella suis*, also infects humans and has been isolated from naturally infected horses, cattle, fowl, and dogs. The disease in humans, usually acquired from contact with swine, differs little from brucellosis caused by *B. abortus*, except that it tends to be more severe and persistent.

The three species of the genus *Brucella* (*melitensis*, *abortus*, and *suis*) are similar in morphologic and other characteristics but may be differentiated by bacteriologic methods. Some bacteriologists, however, contend that each of these is but a strain of the same species.

For our purposes, members of the genus Brucella may be described as small, gram-negative bacillary organisms, varying from 0.4 to 3.0 μ in length and 0.4 to 0.8 μ in width, with coccoid forms outnumbering rod forms under some culture conditions.

The remaining two pathogenic *Brucella* species were more recently identified: *Brucella ovis*, as the cause of epididymitis in rams in the 1950s; and *Brucella canis*, as the cause of abortion in dogs in the 1960s.

Pathogenesis and signs

After entry into the host, Brucella organisms first localize in regional lymph nodes, where they proliferate within reticuloendothelial cells. Most infections are acquired by ingestion of Brucella organisms, which have been shown by Ackerman and associates (1988) to enter and traverse intestinal epithelial cells overlying Peyer's patches through endocytosis. Subsequent entry into lymphatics and development of bacteremia allows localization of the bacteria in a variety of tissues; the bacteria

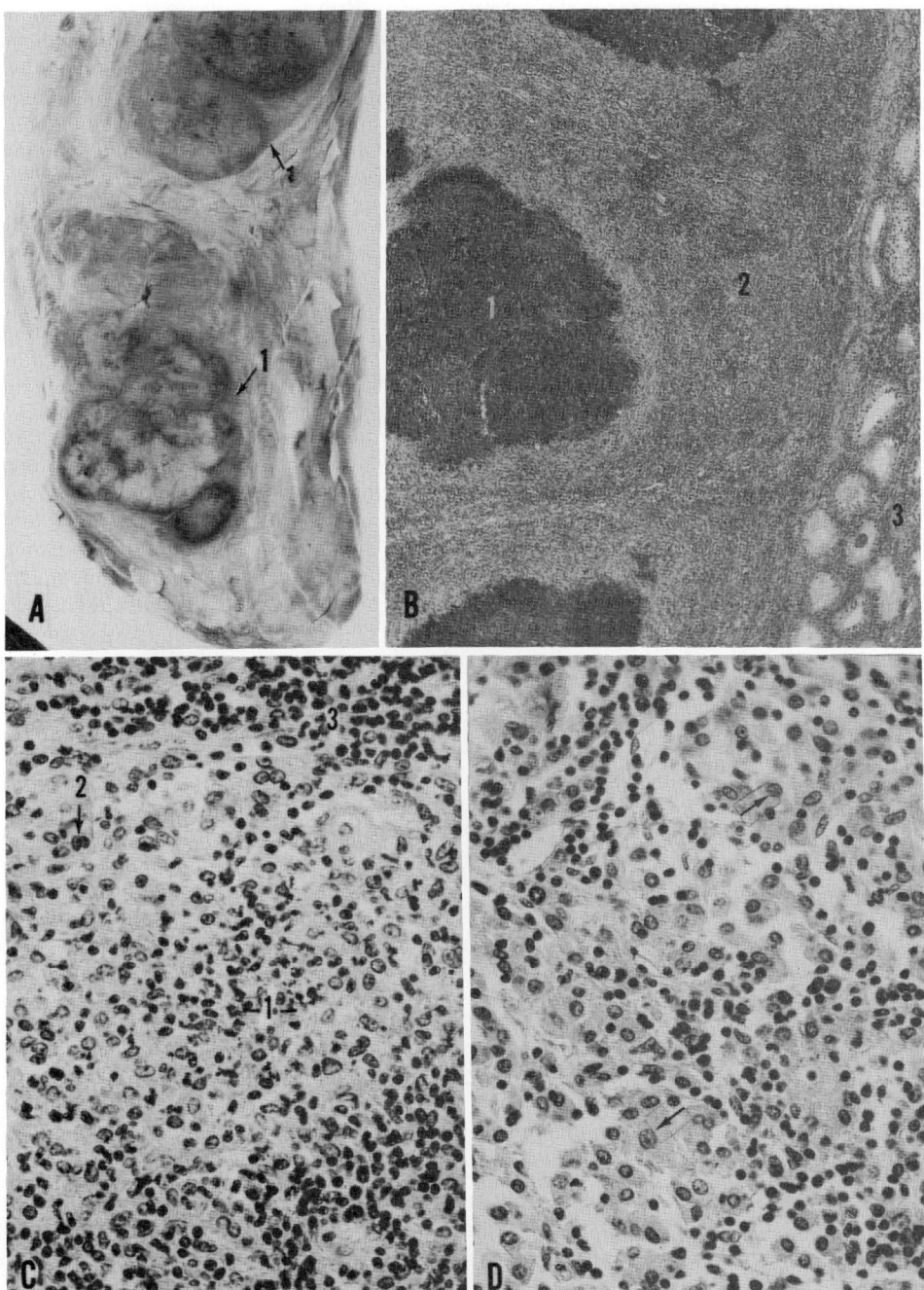

FIG. 10-9 Brucellosis. **A.** Granulomatous lesions (1) in the seminal vesicle of a bull. (Contributor: Bureau of Animal Industry, U.S. Department of Agriculture) **B.** Necrotic foci (1) surrounded by epithelioid granulation tissue (2), displacing seminiferous tubules (3) of swine testicle. (Contributor: Dr. H. C. H. Kernkamp.) **C.** Experimental brucellosis, lung of guinea pig (× 300). Necrotic center (1) surrounded by epithelioid cells (2) and lymphocytes (3). **D.** Another field of C (× 300). Epithelioid cells (arrows) mixed with lymphocytes. (Courtesy of Dr. J. Victor, and Armed Forces Institute of Pathology.)

have a particular affinity for male and female reproductive organs, placenta, fetus, and mammary glands. The organisms may, however, localize in other organs and tissues, such as lymph nodes, spleen, liver, joints, and bone, resulting in diverse clinical signs. At all sites Brucella organisms proliferate intracellularly. The affinity of the bacteria for the placenta and fetus, in particular for chorioallantoic trophoblasts, has been correlated with the presence of erythritol in these tissues. This sugar also promotes growth of Brucella species in vitro. It is the dramatic proliferation of Brucella organisms in trophoblasts that leads to placentitis, infection of the fetus, and abortion, which so often characterizes brucellosis in animals. Most often, infections with Brucella species are chronic or persistent, often without clinical signs.

Brucellosis in cattle is almost always caused by *B. abortus;* however, cattle can be infected with *B. melitensis* and *B. suis. B. abortus* may also infect sheep, dogs, horses, wild ruminants, and, of course, humans. The infection in cattle is of world-wide distribution and is usually spread by contact and ingestion of infective uterine discharge, aborted fetus, or placenta. The organism is also excreted in the milk. Coital transmission is rare; bulls are relatively resistant to infection. Prepubertal animals are susceptible to infection, but most eliminate the organism and only a few become persistently infected. In cows exposed after puberty, a persistent infection and disease is the usual outcome. The principal sign is abortion between the seventh and eighth months of gestation. Although brucellosis was once a major cause of abortion, control programs, including the use of vaccines, in the United States and many other countries have dramatically reduced its incidence.

Brucellosis in swine is usually caused by *B. suis*, although swine can be infected with *B. abortus* and *B. melitensis*. *B. suis* may also infect dogs, horses, reindeer, rodents, and humans. Transmission is typically coital. Infected sows abort between the second and third months of gestation. Orchitis occurs in infected boars. Localization in other tissues, particulary the skeleton, is much more common in swine than in other species.

Brucellosis in sheep and goats caused by *B. melitensis,* is characterized by late abortion and, on occasion, orchitis in billy goats. Transmission is as with *B. abortus* in cattle. Sheep and goats are also susceptible to *B. abortus* and *B. melitensis* can infect cattle, pigs, dogs, and humans. *B. ovis* is only recognized as a natural infection of sheep, though goats, cattle, deer, rodents, and other species can be experimentally infected. Infection of rams, which is highly contagious, leads to epididymitis in rams and abortion in ewes.

Canine brucellosis, caused by *B. canis,* is transmitted both by exposure to uterine discharges or aborted fetuses and by coitus. The infection in bitches leads to abortion, usually after 50 days of gestation, and in male dogs to orchitis and epididymitis. *B. abortus, B. melitensis,* and *B. suis* can infect dogs. Infection of humans with *B. canis* has been reported.

Brucellosis in horses, caused by *B. abortus* along with *Actinomyces bovis,* is associated with "poll-evil" and "fistulous withers", disorders initiated by *Onchocerca cervicalis.*

LESIONS

The lesions of brucellosis in animals are as protean as the clinical manifestations. As indicated above, after the onset of bacteremia, the organisms localize in a variety of tissues, differing somewhat according to animal species and species of Brucella. In the tissues, particularly the lymphoreticular system, the organisms attract macrophages and proliferate within them, leading to small granulomas. Macrophages may take on the morphologic appearance of epithelioid cells and become surrounded by lymphocytes. As the granuloma grows, caseous necrosis occurs in the center and large numbers of neutrophils enter the lesions. Fibrous connective tissue is ultimately laid down at the periphery. Multinucleated giant cells are usually not part of the lesion. These granulomas may be visible grossly or be microscopic in size. Although this process is the classic lesion of brucellosis, it is not always a feature of the disease, except with *B. suis* infection, where granulomas are the

rule in all tissues. Also, granuloma formation is usually not the lesion seen in the placenta associated with abortion (again, except for *B. suis*), which is the most serious outcome of brucellosis in most domestic animals.

In the bovine placenta, there is extensive proliferation of *B. abortus* in the chorionic epithelium and trophoblasts, leading to necrosis of cotyledons, which are dull and granular in appearance. The intercotyledonary chorion is edematous and becomes filled with an odorless, sticky, brownish exudate that resembles soft caramel candy. As the disease advances, yellowish granular necrotic areas are clearly visible in the cotyledons and the rest of the chorion is opaque and thickened, with a leathery consistency. Microscopically, many organisms can be demonstrated in the chorionic epithelial cells. There is necrosis and an inflammatory infiltrate, composed of both macrophages and neutrophils. Granulomas are not evident in the placenta, although small collections of epithelioid cells may be present in the endometrium. Comparable lesions are seen in sheep and goats affected with *B. melitensis,* and similar lesions may be caused by *B. ovis;* however, the latter organisms are most often associated with epididymitis. In contrast, the lesions caused by *B. suis* in swine (or other affected species) are typical granulomas. The aborted bovine fetus is edematous, with serosanguineous fluid in the body cavities. Fetal bronchopneumonia is the most characteristic lesion; the pneumonia, however, is predominantly characterized by a mononuclear infiltrate with a decreased number of neutrophils. Fetal lymph nodes are hyperplastic, and the thymus may be smaller than normal.

The bovine mammary gland and the supramammary lymph nodes are common sites of localization of *B. abortus,* and induration may be the result. Microscopically, diffuse inflammation has been demonstrated; lymphocytes and neutrophils predominate and collections of epithelioid cells and occasional Langhans' giant cells are present in some areas. As the disease progresses, there is atrophy of the glandular tissue and fibrosis. The epididymis and testicle of the bull occasionally exhibit lesions caused by localization of *B. abortus.* The scrotum becomes enlarged and indurated, a feature that can be detected in the living animal. The thickened tunica vaginalis usually surrounds large areas of thick fibrous connective tissue, which may compress or replace the testicle or epididymis. In rare instances, necrosis of the contents of the sac formed by the tunica may result in suppuration, rupture, and discharge of the contents. *B. abortus* can usually be recovered in pure culture from the affected scrotal contents.

In swine, *B. suis* most often produces lesions in the uterus, but the infection is also often generalized with localization in many organs, including bone, mammary glands, testicles, epididymis, seminal vesicles, lymph nodes, spleen, liver, kidneys, and brain. Grossly, the infected organs bear tiny white to yellowish nodules, usually under 5 mm in diameter. Microscopically, these are typical Brucella granulomas with caseous necrosis, containing some neutrophils in their centers. On occasion, the number of neutrophils approaches that of an abscess surrounded by macrophages and epithelioid cells.

In rams, *B. ovis* infection characteristically involves the tail of the epididymis. The lesions begin as perivascular edema and lymphocytic infiltration, with subsequent hyperplasia and degeneration of the tubular epithelium and intertubular fibrosis. Escape of spermatozoa from damaged tubules incites a granulomatous response, which accounts for the major alteration of the epididymis. Primary lesions do not occur in the testicle; however, stasis results in secondary testicular degeneration. The disease is closely mimicked clinically and pathologically by infection with *Actinobacillus seminis,* an infection principally seen in rams in Australia. Fetal lambs experimentally infected with *B. ovis* develop inflammatory changes in the lung, liver, lymph nodes, spleen, and kidneys. The nature of the lesions varies from reticuloendothelial hyperplasia to well-formed nodules of reticuloendothelial cells, lymphocytes, and plasma cells. Necrosis and a cellular infiltration occur in the placenta. The lesions associated with *B. melitensis* infection of sheep and goats resemble those described for *B. abortus* infection of cows.

B. canis infection in the bitch is accompanied by uterine and placental lesions analogous to bovine brucellosis. Bronchopneumonia is seen in aborted pups. Lesions described in a spontaneous outbreak in a laboratory colony of dogs included hyperplasia and plasmacytosis of lymph nodes, orchitis, epididymitis, prostatitis, and hyaline thickening of glomerular tufts (Gleiser and others, 1971). *B. canis* has also been associated with osteomyelitis in dogs, as has *B. suis* and *B. abortus.* Dogs have been suspected as sources of human infection with both *B. canis* and *B. suis.*

In horses, *B. bovis* has been isolated from persistent necrotizing and purulent lesions involving the ligamentum nuchae. These lesions may occur near the occipital attachment of the ligamentum nuchae; at this site, the age-old name "poll evil" indicates some of its clinical characteristics. In the region of the thoracic attachment of the ligamentum nuchae, similar necrotizing and purulent lesions have led to its being called "fistulous withers." Other organisms, such as *Spherophorus necrophorus,* have also been recovered from such lesions, but Brucella species appear to be the important pathogens.

B. abortus infection is occasionally reported in dogs. The lesions, attributed to infection, include arthritis, orchitis, epididymitis, and abortion.

Brucella neotomae, a species recovered from wood rats *(Neotoma lepida)* and ticks from them, appears to be rare and apparently of little significance to public or animal health (Meyer, 1974).

Diagnosis

The precise diagnosis of brucellosis is often difficult, in humans and animals. Isolation of the organism is the most reliable method. An agglutination test and complement fixation test can be used to detect antibodies. Immunologic staining or the use of molecular probes are precise techniques that can be used to detect the presence of organisms in tissues.

References

Ackermann MR, Cheville NF, Deyoe BL. Bovine ileal dome lymphoepithelial cells: endocytosis and transport of Brucella abortus strain 19. Vet Pathol 1988;25:28–35.

Anderson TD, Cheville NF, Meador VP. Pathogenesis of placentitis in the goat inoculated with Brucella abortus. II. Ultrastructural studies. Vet Pathol 1986;23:227–239.

Anderson TD, Meador VP, Cheville NF. Pathogenesis of placentitis in the goat inoculated with Brucella abortus. I. Gross and histologic lesions. Vet Pathol 1986;23:219–226.

Anderson WA, Davis CL. Nodular splenitis in swine associated with brucellosis. J Am Vet Med Assoc 1957;131:141–145.

Barr SC, Eilts BE, Roy AF, et al. Brucella suis biotype 1 infection in a dog. J Am Vet Med Assoc 1986;189:686–687.

Barron SJ, Kocan AA, Morton RJ, et al. Susceptibility of male white-tailed deer (Odocoileus virginianus) to Brucella ovis infection. Am J Vet Res 1985;46:1762–1764.

Biberstein EL, McGowan B, Olander H, et al. Epididymitis in rams. Study on pathogenesis. Cornell Vet 1964;54:27–41.

Bicknell SR, Bell RA, Richards PA. Brucella abortus in the bitch. Vet Rec 1976;99:85–86.

Brown IW, Forbus WD, Kerby GP. The reaction of the reticulo-endothelial system in experimental and naturally acquired brucellosis of swine. Am J Pathol 1945;21:205–232.

Bulgin MS. Brucella ovis epizootic in virgin ram lambs. J Am Vet Med Assoc 1990;196:1120–1122.

Carmichael LE. Canine abortion caused by Brucella canis. J Am Vet Med Assoc 1968;152:605–616.

Clegg FG, Rorrison JM. Brucella abortus infection in the dog: a case of polyarthritis. Res Vet Sci 1968;9:183–185.

Cohen ND, Carter GK, McMullan WC. Fistulous withers in horses: 24 cases (1984–1990). J Am Vet Med Assoc 1992;201:121–124.

Cuba-Caparo A, Myers DM. Pathogenesis of epididymitis caused by Brucella ovis in laboratory animals. Am J Vet Res 1973;34:1077–1086.

Dawkins BG, Machotka SV, Suchmann D, et al. Pyogranulomatous dermatitis associated with Brucella canis infection in a dog. J Am Vet Med Assoc 1982;181:1432–1433.

Denny HR. Brucellosis in the horse. Vet Rec 1972;90:86–91.

Deyoe BL. Histopathologic changes in male swine with experimental brucellosis. Am J Vet Res 1968;29:1215–1220.

Enright FM, Walker JV, Jeffers G, Deyoe BL. Cellular and humoral responses of Brucella abortus-infected bovine fetuses. Am J Vet Res 1984;45:424–431.

Feldman WH, Olson C. Spondylitis of swine associated with bacteria of the brucella group. Arch Pathol 1933;16:195–210.

Forbes LB. Brucella abortus infection in 14 farm dogs. J Am Vet Med Assoc 1990;196:911–916.

Gleiser CA, Sheldon WG, Van Hoosier GL, et al.. Pathologic changes in dogs infected with a brucella organism. Lab Anim Sci 1971;21:540–545.

Gordon JC, Pue HL, Rutgers HC. Canine brucellosis in a household. J Am Vet Med Assoc 1985;186:695–698.

Gorham SL, Enright FM, Snider TG III, et al. Morphologic lesions in Brucella abortus infected ovine fetuses. Vet Pathol 1986;23:331–332.

Henderson RA, Hoerlein BF, Kramer TT, et al. Discospondylitis in three dogs infected with Brucella canis. J Am Vet Med Assoc 1974;165:451–455.

Hofstad MS. The changes produced by Brucella abortus in the milk and udder of cows infected with Bang's disease. Cornell Vet 1942;32:289–294.

Hopper BR, Sanborn MR, Bantle JA. Detection of Brucella abortus in mammalian tissue, using biotinylated, whole genomic DNA as a molecular probe. Am J Vet Res 1989;50:2064–2068.

Kennedy PC, Frazier LM, McGowan B. Epididymitis in rams: pathology and bacteriology. Cornell Vet 1963;53:303–319.

Kernkamp HC, Roepke MH, Jasper DE. Orchitis in swine due to Brucella suis. J Am Vet Med Assoc 1946;108:215–221.

Libal MC, Kirkbride CA. Brucella ovis-induced abortion in ewes. J Am Vet Med Assoc 1983;183:553–554.

Luchsinger DW, Anderson RK. Longitudinal studies of naturally acquired Brucella abortus infection in sheep. Am J Vet Res 1979;40:1307–1312.

McCormick N, Hill WA, Van Hoosier GL Jr, et al. Enzootic abortion in a canine production colony. II. Characteristics of the associated organism, evidence for its classification as Brucella canis, and antibody studies on exposed humans. Lab Anim Care 1970;20:205–208.

Meador VP, Hagemoser WA, Deyoe BL. Histopathologic findings in Brucella abortus-infected pregnant goats. Am J Vet Res 1988;49:274–280.

Meador VP, Deyoe BL, Cheville NF. [1] Pathogenesis of Brucella abortus infection of the mammary gland and supramammary lymph node of the goat. [2] Effect of nursing on Brucella abortus infection of mammary glands of goats. Vet Pathol 1989;26: 357–368, 369–375.

Meinershagen WA, Frank FW, Waldhalm DG. Brucella ovis as a cause of abortion in ewes. Am J Vet Res 1974;35:723–724.

Meyer ME. Advances in research on brucellosis, 1957–1972. Adv Vet Sci Comp Med 1974;18:231–150.

Nicoletti P. The epidemiology of bovine brucellosis. Adv Vet Sci Comp Med 1980;24:69–98.

Osburn BI. The relation of fetal age to the character of lesions in fetal lambs infected with Brucella ovis. Path Vet 1968;5:395–406.

Osburn BI, Kennedy PC. Pathologic and immunologic responses of the fetal lamb to Brucella ovis. Path Vet 1966;3:110–136.

Prichard WD, Hagen KW, Gorham JR, et al. An epizootic of brucellosis in mink. J Am Vet Med Assoc 1971;159:635–637.

Ray WC, et al. Bovine brucellosis: an investigation of latency in progeny of culture-positive cows. J Am Vet Med Assoc 1988;192:182–186.

Smeak DD, Olmstead ML, Hohn RB. Brucella canis osteomyelitis in two dogs with total hip replacements. J Am Vet Med Assoc 1987;191:986–990.

Smith H, et al. Foetal erythritol: a cause of the localization of Brucella abortus in bovine contagious abortion. Nature 1962;193:47–49.

Swenson RM, Carmichael LE, Cundy KR. Human infection with Brucella canis. Ann Intern Med 1972;76:435–438.

INFECTIONS CAUSED BY BORDETELLA ORGANISMS

The genus Bordetella, which are gram-negative aerobic rods, contains three pathogenic species; *B. pertussis, B. parapertussis,* and *B. bronchiseptica. B. pertussis,* an obligate parasite of humans, is the cause of the respiratory infection known as "whooping cough." *B. parapertussis* is also an obligate parasite of humans that causes respiratory disease. It has recently been shown to be pathogenic for sheep, being associated with a condition called chronic nonprogressive pneumonia in New Zealand. *B. bronchiseptica* is also an obligate parasite, but with a broad host range (dogs, cats, swine, horses, guinea pigs, rabbits, rodents, raccoons, nonhuman primates, and occasionally, humans and other species) and, in contrast to *B. pertussis,* can be carried in the absence of disease. The organism is readily spread between individuals by contact and aerosols, establishing itself in the ciliated respiratory mucosa, where it proliferates among the cilia without invading beyond. A mucopurulent laryngotracheitis develops, which may progress to mucosal erosion. Certain strains are ciliostatic, which undoubtedly contributes to their pathogenicity. Upper respiratory disease caused by *B. bronchiseptica* has been seen in most of the species listed above, but the infection in dogs and swine has received the greatest attention. In dogs, *B. bronchiseptica* is considered an important bacterial pathogen in infectious tracheobronchitis ("kennel cough") and frequently contributes to the pneumonia in canine distemper. In swine, the organism is often found in cases of atrophic rhinitis and is considered by some to be the primary pathogen in this disease; however, its role remains controversial. Experimentally, it has induced a form of atrophic rhinitis in rats. *B. bronchiseptica* has also been recovered from and experimentally shown to cause chronic fibrosing pneumonia in swine.

References

Bayly WM, Reed SM, Foreman JH, et al. Equine bronchopneumonia due to Bordetella bronchiseptica. Equine Pract 1982;4:25–27, 30–32 [Vet Bull 1983;53:906]

Bemis DA, Kennedy JR. An improved method for studying the effect of Bordetella bronchiseptica on the ciliary activity of canine tracheal epithelial cells. J Infect Dis 1981;144:349–357.

Bemis DA, Greisen HA, Appel MJG. Pathogenesis of canine bordetellosis. J Infect Dis 1977;135:753–762.

Chen W, Alley MR, Manktelow BW, et al. Pneumonia in lambs inoculated with Bordetella parapertussis: bronchoalveolar lavage and ultrastructural studies. Vet Pathol 1988;25:297–303.

Drummond JG, Curtis SE, Meyer RC, et al. Effects of atmospheric ammonia on young pigs experimentally infected with Bordetella bronchiseptica. Am J Vet Res 1981;42:963–968.

Fisk SK, Soave OA. Bordetella bronchiseptica in laboratory cats from central California. Lab Anim Sci 1973;23:33–35.

Goodnow RA. Biology of Bordetella bronchiseptica. Microbiol Rev 1980;44:722–738.

Holt LB. The pathology and immunology of Bordetella pertussis infection. J Med Microbiol 1973;5:407–424.

Kimman TG, Kamp EM. Induced atrophic rhinitis in rats. Am J Vet Res 1986;47:2426–2430.

Meyer RC, Beamer PD. Bordetella bronchiseptica infections in germ-free swine: an experimental pneumonia. Vet Pathol 1973;10:550–556.

Saxegaard F, Teige J Jr, Fjellheim P. Equine bronchopneumonia caused by Bordetella bronchiseptica. A case report. Acta Vet Scand 1971;12:114–115.

Snyder SB, Fisk SK, Fox JG, et al. Respiratory tract disease associated with Bordetella bronchiseptica infection in cats. J Am Vet Med Assoc 1973;163:293–294.

Thompson H, McCandlish IAP, Wright NG. Experimental respiratory disease in dogs due to Bordetella bronchiseptica. Res Vet Sci 1976;20:16–23.

Underdahl NR, Socha TE, Doster AR. Long-term effect of Bordetella bronchiseptica infection in neonatal pigs. Am J Vet Res 1982;43:622–625.

INFECTIONS CAUSED BY FRANCISELLA ORGANISMS

The genus *Francisella* was established relatively recently to incorporate *Francisella tularensis,* the cause of tularemia (Figs. 10-10 and 10-11). There is a single report of another probable species, *F. novida,* which, although pathogenic for several species of laboratory animals, is apparently not a natural pathogen for domestic animals or humans.

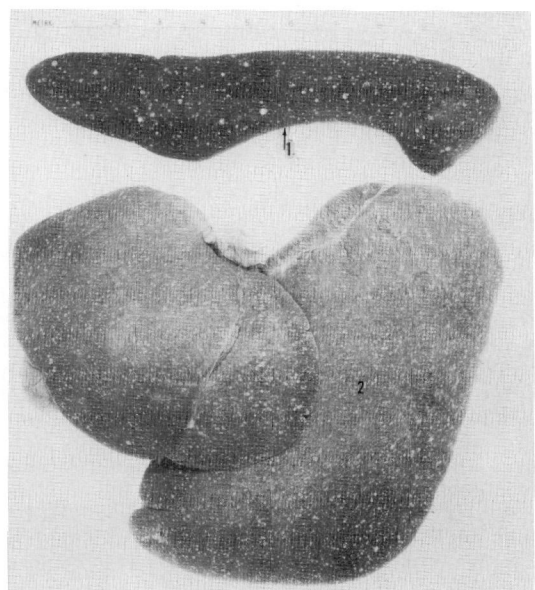

FIG. 10-10 Tularemia, spleen (1) and liver (2) of a ground hog *(Marmota flaviventer)*. Note uniform distribution of tiny white foci. (Courtesy of Dr. E. Francis, and Armed Forces Institute of Pathology.)

Tularemia

The history of tularemia begins in 1910, with the isolation of a bacterial organism from lesions of a "plague-like disease" of ground squirrels by McCoy. He named the organism *Bacterium tularense* after Tulare County, California, in which the first infected ground squirrels had been found. The organism was subsequently desig-

nated *Pasteurella tularensis* and more recently *Francisella tularensis.* Accidental infection of laboratory workers with this organism was soon to follow, and eventually the natural occurrence of the human disease was established. A human disease in Utah, for several years popularly known as "deer-fly fever," was later identified as tularemia. Localized cutaneous ulceration and lymphadenitis followed the bite of a blood-sucking fly, *Chrysops discalis,* which is probably responsible for spread of the disease among wild animals. A more important source of human infection was established by Francis (1925), who demonstrated tularemia organisms in the livers of wild rabbits collected from a market in Washington, DC (Fig. 10-11). "Rabbit fever," well known in the rabbit market, also proved to be tularemia, a form of the disease that still is the most common.

Two biovars of *F. tularensis* with differing virulence are recognized. Biovar *tularensis,* found only in North America, is the most virulent; has its reservoir in wildlife, particularly rabbits; and is transmitted by direct contact with infected animals or by bites of ticks or deer flies. Biovar *palaearctica,* which occurs in Europe, Asia, and the Americas, is less virulent and is maintained in wild rodents.

Tularemia is most important as a disease of humans and wild rabbits and rodents; however, it may occur in dogs, sheep, horses, nonhuman primates, and other species. Most mammals are undoubtedly susceptible. In the laboratory, the guinea pig is readily infected. The disease in humans is described as "ulceroglandular" when the site of entry and initial lesion is cutaneous; "oculoglandular" when initial entry is via the conjunctivae; or "glandular" when the site of entry is not explicit.

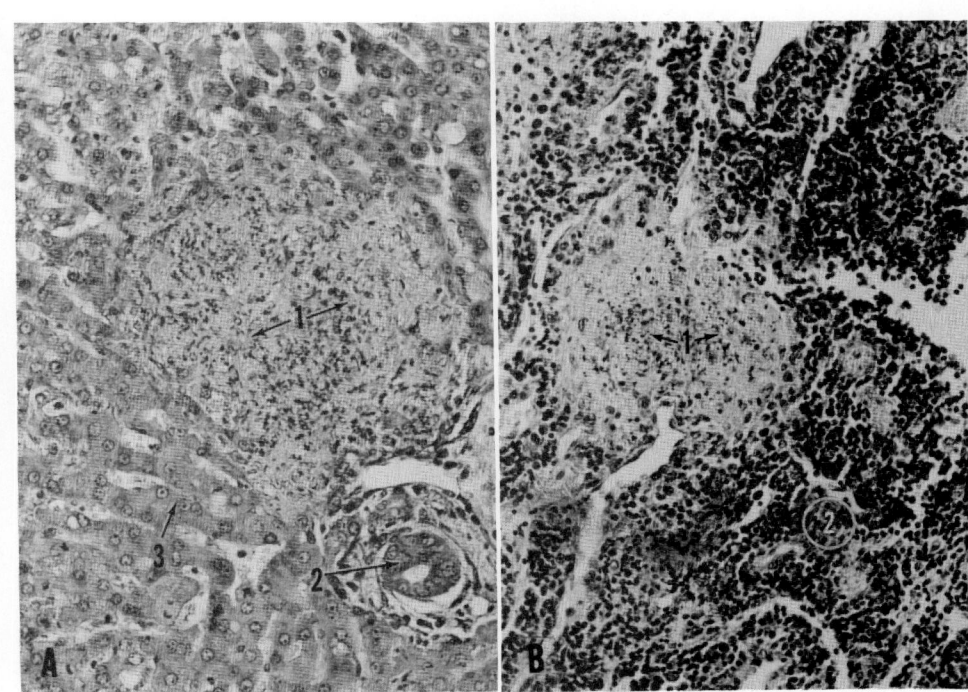

FIG. 10-11 Tularemia. **A.** Liver of a rabbit (× 120). Note necrotic focus (1) near portal area containing bile duct (2). Intact liver columns (3). **B.** Lymph node (× 210) of a rabbit. Necrotic lesions (1) displacing lymphoid cells (2). (Courtesy of Dr. W. J. Hadlow, and Armed Forces Institute of Pathology.)

LESIONS

In humans, the ulceroglandular form is the most common; the first sign is a small cutaneous indurated swelling at the site of an insect bite or on the fingers or hands after dressing wild rabbits. The lesion becomes hot and painful, eventually filling with pus and ulcerating. This is followed by extension to regional lymph nodes, which become enlarged and painful and may also ulcerate through the skin. Generalized lymphadenopathy follows with involvment of other viscera, such as the spleen, liver, lungs, heart, and bones. This widespread involvement generally results in death.

In rabbits and ground squirrels, the disease is usually recognized by the discovery of multiple chalky focal lesions scattered through the liver, spleen, and lymph nodes. These vary from pinpoint size to large, irregularly shaped foci several millimeters in diameter.

Microscopically, a central mass of caseous necrosis is surrounded by a zone of lymphocytes, mixed with a few neutrophils, macrophages, and occasionally multinucleated giant cells. Early lesions may have a purulent core, but it is soon replaced by necrotic tissue debris. Thrombosis of small blood vessels is common and areas of necrosis may coalesce. The causative organisms, being gram-negative, are difficult to demonstrate in tissue sections, but are present in large numbers, particularly in phagocytes at the margin of lesions.

DIAGNOSIS

The diagnosis can be made on the basis of the gross and microscopic lesions, isolation of the causative organisms, or specific identification with fluorescence antibody techniques. Increased agglutination-antibody ti-

ter is of diagnostic value in nonfatal human cases. Tularemia must be differentiated from other diseases that produce similar lesions in the liver. These include Tyzzer's disease, salmonellosis, listeriosis, toxoplasmosis, and mousepox.

References

Coffee WM, Miller J. Acute canine tularemia. J Am Vet Med Assoc 1943;102:210–212.
Francis E. Tularemia. J Am Med Assoc 1925;84:1243–1250.
Goodpasture EW, House SJ. The pathologic anatomy of tularemia in man. Am J Pathol 1928;4:213–226.
La Regina M, Lonigro J, Wallace M. Francisella tularensis infection in captive, wild caught prairie dogs. Lab Anim Sci 1986;36:178–180.
Moe JA et al. Pathogenesis of tularemia in immune and nonimmune rats. Am J Vet Res 1975;36:1505–1510.
Quin AH Jr. Tularemia, a disease transmissible from animal to man. North Am Vet 1925;6:36–38.
Rohrbach BW. Tularemia. J Am Vet Med Assoc 1988;193:428–432.
Schricker RL, Eigelsbach HT, Mitten JQ, et al. Pathogenesis of tularemia in monkeys aerogenically exposed to Francisella tularensis 425. Infect Immun 1972;5:734–744.

INFECTIONS CAUSED BY PSEUDOMONAS ORGANISMS

Of the numerous species of *Pseudomonas*, only three are responsible for diseases of animals: *P. mallei* (glanders), *P. pseudomallei* (melioidosis), and *P. aeruginosa* (purulent infections).

Glanders

An age-old respiratory disease of equines and humans, glanders is now rare in the United States but still com-

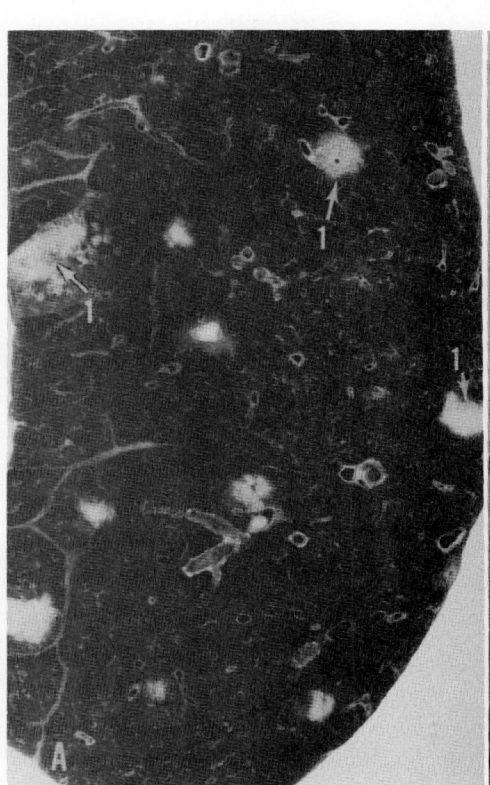 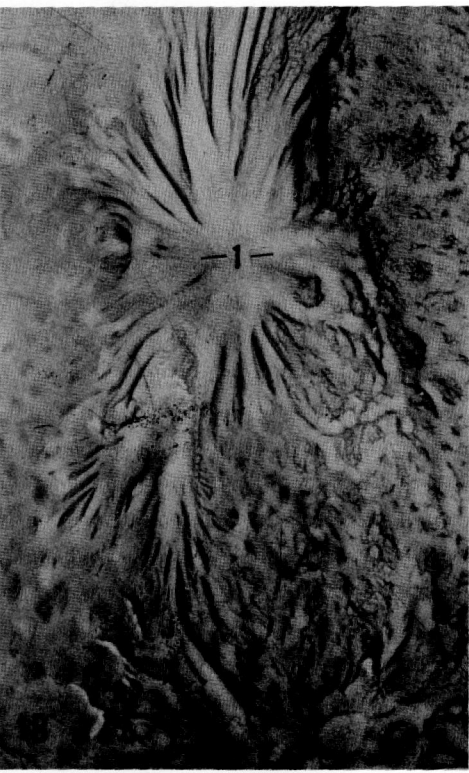

FIG. 10-12 Glanders. **A.** Sharply demarcated consolidated lesions (1) in the lung of a horse. (Courtesy of Capt. R. A. Kelser, and Armed Forces Institute of Pathology.) **B.** Scar (1) in the nasal mucous membrane of a horse. (Courtesy of School of Veterinary Medicine, Texas A&M University.)

mon in some parts of Asia (Fig. 10-12.). The respiratory mucosae and lungs are most commonly affected, but disseminated lesions may occur. Nasal involvement is indicated by a copious and persistent nasal discharge, which is first catarrhal, later purulent. Ulceration often occurs in the nasal mucosa, and chronic cough may indicate pulmonary infection. Cutaneous involvement ("farcy") produces indolent ulcers in the skin, with thickening of the superficial lymphatics, sometimes leading to abscesses in superficial lymph nodes.

The causative organism, *P. mallei (Malleomyces mallei, Loefferella mallei, Pfeiferella mallei, Bacillus mallei, Actinobacillus mallei)* is a short, rod-shaped organism with rounded ends. It is gram-negative, nonsporulating, aerobic, and an obligate parasite. Infection is passed from one animal to another through inhalation of nasal exudates or possibly by ingestion of contaminated food or water. Humans are susceptible, where the disease may occur as an acute, often fatal pyemia or a chronic granulomatous disease, as is usually seen in horses. Dogs and cats are also susceptible, acquiring the infection from ingestion of contaminated horse meat. The disease has been seen in large cats in zoos. Guinea pigs are readily infected. Intraperitoneal injection of infected material into male guinea pigs (Strauss test) results in acute purulent orchitis in 3 or 4 days, and the organisms can be isolated in pure culture from the testicular lesions.

LESIONS

The nasal lesions of glanders appear as erosive, deep ulcerations of the mucosa, particularly over the septum. After a prolonged course, the ulcers heal, leaving star-shaped scars (Fig. 10-12B). The pulmonary lesions are usually discrete granulomatous nodules resembling tubercles, but occasionally they coalesce. In a few cases, the disease is manifested as acute purulent bronchopneumonia. The granulomas usually have a caseous necrotic center surrounded by epithelioid cells, a few giant cells, and some lymphocytes. Granulomas occasionally occur in the liver, spleen, or other viscera.

The skin lesions, most common on the legs, appear as persistent ulcers connected by tortuous, indurated, thick-walled lymphatics. Superficial lymph nodes often become involved, suppurating and discharging thick tenacious pus. Healing occurs slowly with scarring, and the healed areas may break down, leaving persistent indolent ulcers.

DIAGNOSIS

Clinical diagnosis is usually confirmed by means of the intradermal mallein test, which has been an effective means for detecting asymptomatic infections and making control of the disease possible. Diagnosis at necropsy is based on the presence of typical lesions and the demonstration of *P. mallei* by culture methods or guinea pig inoculation.

References

Galati P, Puccini V, Contento F. An outbreak of glanders in lions. Histopathologic findings. [abstr] Vet Pathol 1974;11:445.

Mendelson RW. Glanders. US Armed Forces Med J 1950;1:781–784.
Verma RD. Glanders in India with special reference to incidence and epidemiology. Indian Vet J 1981;58:177–183. [Vet Bull 1982;52:523]

Melioidosis

Melioidosis is a disease resembling glanders (often called pseudoglanders) caused by *P. pseudomallei (Malleomyces pseudomallei, Loefferella mallei, Flavobacterium pseudomallei, Bacilli whitmori, Loefferella whitmori, Pfeiferella whitmori)*. Although infection may be latent, melioidosis is often a fatal disease of humans, nonhuman primates, rabbits, guinea pigs, goats, swine, dogs, horses, cattle, and wild rodents. Most mammals appear to be susceptible. Infection is acquired from other infected animals or from contaminated soil and water. It is most prevalent in Laos, Thailand, and Ceylon but has also been reported in Malaysia and Australia. The disease has come to recent attention in the United States after importation of infected nonhuman primates (stump-tailed macaque, *Macaca arctoides;* pig-tailed macaque, *M. nemestrina;* and chimpanzee, *Pan troglodytes*). Military dogs serving in the war in Vietnam were also occasionally reported to be infected.

LESIONS

According to Omar (1963), the lesions are characterized by the formation of granulomatous nodules with a caseous center, which in some cases become purulent. The solid, granulomatous nature of the nodules distinguishes them from frank abscesses. The organisms are found in colonies in the nodules' caseous center, surrounded by layers of granulation tissue, which give the gross appearance a laminated look. Giant cells are seldom seen, but purulent reactions, particularly in confluent nodules, is common.

In young swine, the lungs are most frequently affected by bronchopneumonia, and the intrathoracic lymph nodes are edematous or contain granulomas. In adult swine, nodules are more apt to be seen involving lungs, thoracic lymph nodes, liver, spleen, and less often, other lymph nodes.

Affected goats commonly are emaciated, have a head tilt, and terminally, are comatose. The lesions are usually more widely distributed than in swine, and the nodules are smaller. Ulcers may be found in the mucosa of the nasal septum and trachea; nodules and consolidated areas occur in the lungs; and multiple nodules are evident in the respiratory lymph nodes, spleen, and liver. A few nodules may be found in the heart, the wall of the cecum, the bladder wall, and the mesentery. Nodules, 2 to 3 mm in diameter, are also described in the lungs of affected horses; the nodules have a yellowish caseous center. The lungs may be edematous and consolidated; peritoneal effusion is evident; and occasionally purulent pyelitis may be associated with the presence of the organism.

DIAGNOSIS

The diagnosis is dependent on demonstration, isolation, and identification of the causative organism, *P.*

pseudomallei. Intraperitoneal inoculation of guinea pigs may lead to orchitis (Straus reaction), as with *Pseudomonas mallei.*

References

Butler TM, Schmidt RE, Wiley GL. Melioidosis in a chimpanzee. Am J Vet Res 1971;32:1109–1117.

Kaufmann AF, et al. Melioidosis in imported non-human primates. J Wildl Dis 1970;6:211–219.

Ketterer PJ, Donald B, Rogers RJ. Bovine melioidosis in south-eastern Queensland. Aust Vet J 1975;51:395–398.

Ladds PW, Thomas AD, Speare R, et al. Melioidosis in a koala. Aust Vet J 1990;67:304–305. [Vet Bull 1991;61:949]

Moe JB, Stedham MA, Jennings PB. Canine melioidosis. Clinical observation in three military dogs in Vietnam. Am J Trop Med Hyg 1972;21:351–355.

Omar AR, Cheah Kok Kheong, Mahendranathan T. Observations on porcine melioidosis in Malaya. Br Vet J 1962;118:421–429. [Vet Bull 1962;416–63]

Omar AR. Pathology of melioidosis in pigs, goats and a horse. J Comp Pathol 1963;73:359–372.

Rogers RJ, Andersen DJ. Intrauterine infection of a pig by Pseudomonas pseudomallei. Aust Vet J 1970;46:292.

Stedham MA. Melioidosis in dogs in Vietnam. J Am Vet Med Assoc 1971;158:1948–1950.

Strauss JM, et al. Melioidosis with spontaneous remission of osteomyelitis in a macaque (Macaca nemestrina). J Am Vet Med Assoc 1969;155:1169–1175.

Pseudomonas aeruginosa

P. aeruginosa (Bacterium aeruginosum, B. aerugineum, Micrococcus pyocyaneus, Bacillus aeruginosus, B. pyocyaneus, Pseudomonas pyocyanea, Bacterium pyocyaneum, or Pseudomonas polycolor) is associated with the production of blue-green pigments; is a normal inhabitant of skin and mucous membranes; and is associated with sporadic infections of plants, animals, and humans, often in association with other bacteria or fungi. Usually, infections in humans or animals are subsequent to some debilitating trauma or treatment, such as severe burns, extensive surgery, or a course of broad-spectrum antibiotics, corticosteroids, or antimetabolites. Nearly all domestic and laboratory animals have been reported to be sporadically infected, and in some (mink, chinchilla), severe epizootics have occurred.

The organism is a small, gram-negative, rod-shaped organism, 1.5 to 3.0 μ in length and 0.3 to 0.6 μ wide. It is actively motile, with one to three polar flagellae, and does not produce spores. It is not acid-fast, some strains may be encapsulated, and it may occur singly, in pairs, or in short chains. Most, but not all, strains produce characteristic blue-green pigment in tissues and in cultures. The pigments are complex and include pyocyanin and pyoverdin. Other substances with antibiotic and bacteriocidal properties have been recovered from the organisms. Their pathogenic properties appear to be a result of extracellular toxins, including protease and elastase, produced by the organisms.

LESIONS

The lesions are noncharacteristic, consisting of necrotizing, purulent, and hemorrhagic inflammatory reactions of affected tissues. The more common situations include pneumonia (which is very severe in mink and chinchilla), otitis media, traumatic reticulitis, mastitis, metritis, enteritis, dermatitis, and keratitis. In acute pneumonia, the lesions are described as vasculitis with infiltration by large numbers of bacteria in the walls, but not the lumen, of arteries and veins. More prolonged infection of any organ or tissue results in the formation of abscesses or granulomas with purulent cores, called "botryomycosis" (see staphylococcal infections).

References

Cross MR, Cooper JE, Needham JR. Observations on a post-operative septicaemia in experimental dogs with particular reference to *Pseudomonas aeruginosa.* J Comp Pathol 1975;85:445–451.

Dominguez J, Crasem D, Soave O. A case of pseudomonas osteomyelitis in a rabbit. Lab Anim Sci 1975;25:506.

Donovan GA, Gross TL. Cutaneous botryomycosis (bacterial granulomas) in dairy cows caused by *Pseudomonas aeruginosa.* J Am Vet Med Assoc 1984;184:197–199.

Ediger RD, Rabstein MM, Olson LD. Circling in mice caused by *Pseudomonas aeruginosa.* Lab Anim Sci 1972;21:845–848.

Kirk JH, Bartlett PC. Nonclinical *Pseudomonas aeruginosa* mastitis in a dairy herd. J Am Vet Med Assoc 1984;184:671–673.

Lausen NCG, Richter AG, Lage AL. *Pseudomonas aeruginosa* infection in squirrel monkeys. J Am Vet Med Assoc 1986;189:1216–1218.

Long GG, Gorham JR. Field studies: Pseudomonas pneumonia of mink. Am J Vet Res 1981;42:2129–2133.

Long GG, Gorham JR. Pseudomonas pneumonia of mink. J Am Vet Med Assoc 1982;181:1343–1344.

Olson LD, Ediger RD. Histopathologic study of the heads of circling mice infected with *Pseudomonas aeruginosa.* Lab Anim Sci 1972;22:522–527.

LEGIONELLACEAE

The family Legionellaceae contains six species of small gram-negative rods. At least four are human pathogens, collectively causing pneumonias grouped under the heading legionellosis. *Legionella pneumophila* is the cause of legionnaires' disease, an acute serious pneumonia, as well as a less severe nonpneumonic febrile disease called Pontiac fever. *L. micdadei* is the cause of a severe pneumonia called Pittsburgh pneumonia. *L. dumoffii* and *L. bozemanii* are two other species recovered from cases of human pneumonia. Although serologic evidence of infection in animals has been reported, there is no conclusive proof that *Legionella* organisms cause spontaneous disease in domestic animals.

References

Baskerville A, Fitzgeorge RB. Legionnaires' disease. Comp Pathol Bull 1989;21(1):3–4.

Cho S-N, Collins MT, Reif JS. Serologic evidence of Legionella infection in horses. Am J Vet Res 1984;45:2600–2602.

Collins MT, Cho S-N, Reif JS. Prevalence of antibodies to *Legionella pneumophila* in animal populations. J Clin Microbiol 1982;15:130–136.

Katz SM, Hashemi S. Electron microscopic examination of the inflammatory response to *Legionella pneumophila* in guinea pigs. Lab Invest 1982;46:24–32.

Myerowitz R. Legionnaires' disease: the problem of pathogenesis. Lab Invest 1982;47:507–509.

Winn WC Jr, Davis GS, Gump DW, et al. Legionnaires' pneumonia after intratracheal inoculation of guinea pigs and rats. Lab Invest 1982;47:568–578.

CHROMOBACTERIOSIS

Chromobacterium violaceum (Chromobacterium janthinum, C. manilae, C. laurentium) is a motile, rod-shaped, gram-negative bacterium which, in appropriate culture media, produces a violet-colored pigment, violacein. This identifying pigment is soluble in ethanol, but not in chloroform or water. The organism is a mesophilic facultative anaerobic bacterium that grows well in water and soil in tropical and subtropical climates and, on occasion, has infected humans and animals. Infections have been reported from the southern United States, Malaysia, the Philippines, and Thailand.

In addition to humans, infections have been reported in swine, cattle, buffalo, nonhuman primates, a Malaysian Sun bear, and a dog. The disease is usually manifested as an acute septicemia with few premonitory signs and death in a day or two. In swine, a few cases of prolonged duration have been observed.

Lesions

The lesions are large, circumscribed foci of necrosis in liver, spleen, lungs, kidneys, and adrenal glands. Organisms can usually be recovered from all of these organs and from the blood in fatal cases. The microscopic appearance of the lesions is usually one of sharply circumscribed foci of necrosis with little or no inflammatory reaction. In cases of prolonged duration, some encapsulation of the necrotic tissue may be evident.

DIAGNOSIS

The diagnosis may be suspected from the nature of the lesions and confirmed by recovery of the organisms in culture.

References

Groves MG, et al. Natural infections of gibbons with a bacterium producing violet pigment *(Chromobacterium violaceum).* J Infect Dis 1969;120:605–610.

Johnsen DO, Pulliam JD, Tanticharoenyos P. Chromobacterium septicemia in the gibbon. J Infect Dis 1970;122:563.

Johnson WM, DiSalvo AF, Steuer RR. Fatal *Chromobacterium violaceum* septicemia. Am J Clin Pathol 1971;56:400–406.

Joseph PG, et al. *Chromobacterium violaceum* infection in animals. Kajian Vet 1971;3:55–66.

Kornegay RW, Pirie G, Brown CC, Newton JC. Chromobacteriosis *(Chromobacterium violaceum)* in three colobus monkeys *(Colobus polykomos).* J Zoo Wildl Med 1991;22:476–484.

McClure HM, Chang J. *Chromobacterium violaceum* infection in a nonhuman primate *(Macaca assamensis).* Lab Anim Sci 1976;26:807–810.

Sipple WL, Medina G, Atwood MB. Outbreaks of disease in animals associated with *Chromobacterium violaceum.* I. The disease in swine. J Am Vet Med Assoc 1954;124:467–471.

SALMONELLOSIS

The genus *Salmonella,* named for the veterinary bacteriologist D.E. Salmon, contains hundreds of serovars (species), which are subdivided into five subgenera on the basis of biochemical characteristics; they are all members of the family Enterobacteriaceae. The pathogenic members, primarily belonging to subgenera I and III, are principally associated with enteric diseases. In humans, **typhoid fever** is the classic form of salmonellosis and remains today a major world health problem. In animals, the infections are often referred to as **paratyphoid.** Salmonella are rod-shaped, 0.7–1.5 μm wide by 2.0–5.0 μm in length, gram-negative, nonsporulating, and motile by peritrichous flagella. Certain of the Salmonella are host-specific, whereas others may infect a wide variety of animal species. *S. typhi,* the cause of typhoid fever in humans, and *S. choleraesuis* of swine are examples of host-specific Salmonella. In contrast, *S. typhimurium* produces gastroenteritis, occasionally leading to septicemia, in cattle, horses, rodents, swine, humans, and other species. The more important pathogenic members of the genus are listed in Table 10-7. Salmonellosis occurs in all animals but is most frequent in cattle *(S. dublin, S. typhimurium),* horses *(S. typhimurium),* and swine *(S. choleraesuis, S. typhimurium).* It is rare in dogs and cats. Birds are affected by their own species of salmonella as well as by *S. typhimurium.*

All of the events in the pathogenesis of Salmonella enteritis are not clear, but infection is acquired by ingestion of material contaminated with infected feces from either clinically ill animals or carrier animals. The carrier state is particularly important in the maintenance and transmission of the disease and exemplified by the classic story of "typhoid Mary." The bacteria ad-

TABLE 10-7 **Some of the more frequently isolated Salmonellae**

Host	*Organisms*
Horses	*S. typhimurium, S. newport, S. heidelberg, S. anatum, S. copenhagen, S. senftenberg, S. agona, S. abortus equi*
Cattle	*S. dublin, S. typhimurium, S. anatum, S. newport, S. montevideo*
Sheep and goats	*S. abortus ovis, S. montevideo, S. typhimurium, S. dublin, S. arizonae*
Swine	*S. choleraesuis, S. typhimurium, S. dublin, S. heidelberg*
Dogs and cats	*S. typhimurium, S. panama, S. anatum*
Poultry	*S. pullorum, S. gallinarum, S. typhimurium, S. agona, S. anatum*
Laboratory rodents	*S. enteritidis, S. typhimurium*
Humans	*S. typhi, S. paratyphi-A, S. typhimurium, S. enteritidis*

here to enterocytes by way of fimbriae or pili and colonize the small intestine. They then penetrate enterocytes, where further multiplication occurs before they cross to the lamina propria and continue to proliferate both free and within macrophages. Many Salmonella infections do not progress further; however, with some of the more pathogenic serovars, especially in young animals, the organisms are transported by macrophages to mesenteric lymph nodes. Further multiplication leads ultimately to **septicemia,** with localization of bacteria in many organs and tissues, including the spleen, liver, meninges, brain, and joints. Thus, the infection may range from a mild enteritis to serious and often fatal enteritis with septicemia. In humans, the mildest presentation of salmonellosis is food poisoning resulting from ingestion of contaminated foods, which often presents as an outbreak or epidemic. Fluid loss from diarrhea is important to the development of clinical signs and the outcome of the infection. The mechanism appears to involve both an enterotoxin that causes increased secretion by enterocytes (as in cholera and *E. coli* infections) and exsorption resulting from the inflammatory process. Abortion may occur during the acute enteritic or septicemic form of salmonellosis, especially in cattle and, on occasion, in the absence of obvious disease in the cow; in addition, however, certain of the Salmonella species cause abortion in the absence of overt enteritis. Such is the case with *S. abortus ovis* in sheep and *S. abortus equi* in horses.

Lesions

The lesions of salmonellosis or "paratyphoid fever" in animals are those of enterocolitis and septicemia. The stomach and proximal small intestine are usually spared, with enteritis commencing in the ileum and extending through the colon. The mucosa is hyperemic to frankly hemorrhagic, thickened, and often covered with a red, yellow, or gray exudate; it may contain distinct ulcers. Microscopically in the mucosa there is hemorrhage, edema, necrosis, and leukocytic infiltration, principally composed of macrophages. Lesions in other organs are less consistent. Although not pathognomonic, more specific lesions are found in the liver. These include small foci of necrosis and the so-called "paratyphoid nodules" ("typhoid" nodules in typhoid fever of humans). The latter consist of small aggregations of reticuloendothelial cells (histiocytes, macrophages), which may occur in association with or independent of hepatic necrosis. The Kupffer's cells become prominent, and the sinusoids may contain numerous leukocytes.

Reticuloendothelial hyperplasia is present in lymph nodes and the spleen, which may cause enlargement of these tissues. Hemorrhage and necrosis is common in mesenteric lymph nodes. In septicemic cases, petechiae or ecchymoses on the pleura, peritoneum, endocardium, kidney, and meninges invariably develop.

In the septicemic form, microscopic examination reveals fibrinoid necrosis of vessel walls and hyaline material deposited in glomerular capillaries and minor vessels of the dermis. This material is believed to be the result of thrombosis with fibrin and densely packed erythrocytes. This situation has been compared to the generalized Shwartzman reaction (Chapter 7) and has been reproduced in swine by the intravenous injection of killed *Salmonella cholerasuis,* which was repeated 24 and 48 hours later. This procedure resulted in disseminated vascular thromboses and bilateral cortical necrosis of the kidneys characteristic of the generalized Shwartzman reaction.

Rectal stricture in swine has been observed to follow prolonged ulcerative proctitis associated with infection caused by *Salmonella typhimurium.* The strictures result from annular fibrous thickening of the submucosa and muscularis at a point 2 to 5 cm anterior to the anus. Partial or complete obstruction of the rectum occurs with subsequent distention of the rectum, colon, and abdomen and with stunting of growth and emaciation. This syndrome has been reproduced experimentally by infecting pigs with *S. typhimurium.*

Abortion

S. abortus equi is a cause of abortion in mares but is no longer a common disease in the United States. *S. abortus ovis* and *S. montevideo* are causes of abortion in sheep in Great Britain, Europe, and the Middle East. Characteristically, either abortion occurs late in gestation or infected foals or lambs are born at term and die within a few days. There are no specific lesions in the placenta or fetus. The placenta is edematous and contains focal hemorrhage and necrosis. There is usually edema of the fetus.

Diagnosis

Salmonellosis can be suspected on the basis of gross and histopathologic findings; however, the lesions are not specific, and isolation or identification of the causative agent in association with lesions is necessary for confirmation.

References

Adamson PJW, Jang SS. Ulcerative keratitis associated with Salmonella arizonae infection in a horse. J Am Vet Med Assoc 1985; 186:1219–1220.

Arbuckle JBR. Villous atrophy in pigs infected with Salmonella cholerae-suis. Res Vet Sci 1975;18:322–324.

Baskerville A, Dow C. Pathology of experimental pneumonia in pigs produced by Salmonella cholerae suis. J Comp Pathol 1973;83:207–215.

Borland ED. Salmonella infection in dogs, cats, tortoises and terrapins. Vet Rec 1975;96:401–402.

Bruner DW, Morgan AB. Salmonella infection of domestic animals. Cornell Vet 1949;39:53–63.

Bulgin MS, Anderson BC. Salmonellosis in goats. J Am Vet Med Assoc 1981;178:720–723.

Calvert CA, Leifer CE. Salmonellosis in dogs with lymphosarcoma. J Am Vet Med Assoc 1982;180:56–58.

Carter JD, Hird DW, Farver TB, et al. Salmonellosis in hospitalized horses: seasonality and case fatality rates. J Am Vet Med Assoc 1986;188:163–167.

Casebolt DB, Schoeb TR. An outbreak in mice of salmonellosis caused by Salmonella enteritidis serotype enteritidis. Lab Anim Sci 1988;38:190–192.

Centers for Disease Control and Prevention. Typhoid fever - Skagit County, Washington. MMWR 1990;39(42):749–751.

Cordy DR, Davis RW. An outbreak of salmonellosis in horses and mules. J Am Vet Med Assoc 1946;108:20–24.

Donahue JM. Emergence of antibiotic-resistant Salmonella agona in horses in Kentucky. J Am Vet Med Assoc 1986;188:592–594.

Gianella RA, Gots RE, Charney AN, et al. Pathogenesis of Salmonella-mediated intestinal fluid secretion. Activation of adenylate cyclase and inhibition by indomethacin. Gastroenterology 1975;69:1238–1245.

Gorham JR, Cordy DR, Quortrup ER. Salmonella infections in mink and ferrets. Am J Vet Res 1949;10:183–192.

Harp JA, Myers LL, Rich JE, et al. Role of Salmonella arizonae and other infective agents in enteric disease of lambs. Am J Vet Res 1981;42:596–599.

Hinton MH. Salmonella dublin abortion in cattle. Vet Rec 1973;93:162.

Hook EW. Typhoid fever today. N Engl J Med 1984;310:116–118.

Innes JRM, Wilson C, Ross MA. Epizootic Salmonella enteritidis infection causing septic pulmonary phlebothrombosis in hamsters. J Infect Dis 1956;98:133–141.

Jack EJ. Salmonell abortus ovis: an atypical Salmonella. Vet Rec 1968;82:558–562.

Kent TH, Formal SB, Labrec EH. Salmonella gastroenteritis in rhesus monkeys. Arch Pathol 1966;82:272–279.

Keteran K, Brown J, Shotts EB Jr. Salmonella in the mesenteric lymph nodes of healthy sows and hogs. Am J Vet Res 1982;43:706–707.

Klumpp SA, Weaver DS, Jerome CP, et al. Salmonella osteomyelitis in a rhesus monkey. Vet Pathol 1986;23:190–197.

Meinershagen WA, Waldhalm DG, Frank FW. Salmonella dublin as a cause of diarrhea and abortion in ewes. Am J Vet Res 1970;31:1769–1771.

Morse EV, Duncan MA, Page EA, et al. Salmonellosis in Equidae: a study of 23 cases. Cornell Vet 1976;66:198–213.

Murray MJ. Salmonella: virulence factors and enteric salmonellosis. J Am Vet Med Assoc 1986;189:145–147.

Nakoneczna I, Hsu HS. The comparative histopathology of primary and secondary lesions in murine salmonellosis. Br J Exp Pathol 1980;61:76–84.

Nordstoga K. Porcine salmonellosis. I. Gross and microscopic changes in experimentally infected animals. Acta Vet Scand 1970;11:361–369.

Onyekaba CO. Salmonella ochiogu: [1] experimental infection of laboratory rabbits (Oryctolagus cuniculus). [2] experimental infection of laboratory rats (Rattus rattus). Lab Anim 1985;19:32–34, 148–151.

Palmer JE, Benson CE, Whitlock RH. Salmonella shed by horses with colic. J Am Vet Med Assoc 1985;187:256–257.

Palmer JE, et al. Comparison of rectal mucosal cultures and fecal cultures in detecting Salmonella infection in horses and cattle. Am J Vet Res 1985;46:697–698.

Peterson KJ, Coon RE. Salmonella typhimurium infection in dairy cows. J Am Vet Med Assoc 1967;151:344–350.

Reed WM, Olander HJ, Thacker HL. Studies on the pathogenesis of Salmonella heidelberg infection in weanling pigs. Am J Vet Res 1985;46:2300–2310.

Reed WM, Olander HJ, Thacker HL. Studies on the pathogenesis of Salmonella typhimurium and Salmonella choleraesuis var kunzendorf infection in weanling pigs. Am J Vet Res 1986;47:75–83.

Rout WR, Formal SB, Dammin GJ, et al. Pathophysiology of Salmonella diarrhea in the rhesus monkey: intestinal transport, morphological and bacteriological studies. Gastroenterology 1974;67:59–70.

Seghetti L. Observations regarding Salmonella choleraesuis (var. kunzendorf) septicemia in swine. J Am Vet Med Assoc 1946;109:134–137.

Seps SL, Cera LM, Terese SC Jr, et al. Investigations of the pathogenicity of Salmonella enteritidis serotype Amsterdam following a naturally occurring infection in rats. Lab Anim Sci 1987;37:326–330.

Smith BP, Reina-Guerra M, Hardy AJ, et al. Equine salmonellosis: experimental production of four syndromes. Am J Vet Res 1979;40:1072–1077.

Smith HW, Jones JET. Observations on experimental oral infection with Salmonella dublin in calves and Salmonella choleraesuis in pigs. J Pathol Bact 1967;93:141–156.

Timoney JF, Neibert HC, Scott FW. Feline salmonellosis: a nosocomial outbreak and experimental studies. Cornell Vet 1978;68:211–219.

Traub-Dargatz JL, Salman MD, Jones RL. Epidemiologic study of salmonellae shedding in the feces of horses and potential risk factors for development of the infection in hospitalized horses. J Am Vet Med Assoc 1990;196:1617–1622.

Tutt JB, Hoare DIB. Disease associated with S. typhimurium in cattle. Vet Rec 1974;95:334–337.

Wenkoff MS. Salmonella typhimurium septicemia in foals. Can Vet J 1973;14:284–287.

ACTINOBACILLOSIS

Five members of the genus Actinobacillus cause disease in animals. *A. equuli* and *A. suis* cause septicemia in foals and piglets respectively; *A. lignieresii* is the cause of woody tongue of cattle; a fourth organism of uncertain classification, but tentatively termed *A. seminis,* causes epididymitis and polyarthritis in sheep. There is a report of a fifth organism, classified as *A. capsulatus,* as a cause of arthritis in laboratory rabbits. Members of the genus *Actinobacillus* share features with *Pasteurella* and *Haemophilus.* Pleuropneumonia of swine caused by *Haemophilus pleuropneumoniae,* which may be more appropriately named *Actinobacillus pleuropneumoniae,* is discussed under Haemophilus infections.

Actinobacillus equuli

A specific infection of young foals is caused by *A. equuli (Shigella equuli, S. equirulis, S. viscosa).* The organism, a tiny rod-shaped bacterium that is gram-negative and nonsporulating, is often carried in the gastrointestinal tract of normal horses and has frequently been recovered from verminous aneurysms caused by *Strongylus vulgaris.* Foals are infected in utero or shortly after birth. Migrating strongyles may serve to infect the fetus. The organism has been recovered in numerous instances from newborn foals, the disease being contracted in utero, at parturition, or during the first days after birth. Most infected foals die within the first 3 days of life, sometimes within 18 hours, but others may survive for a month or longer. Occasionally, adult horses are affected. The organisms have been isolated from involved joints, fetal membranes, viscera (especially kidneys), umbilical cords, and heart blood and occasionally from infected verminous lesions in mesenteric arteries. *A. equuli* is the most common cause of pyosepticemia neonatorum, "joint-ill," "navel ill," "sleepy foal disease," and "septicemia of foals."

The disease must be suspected in newborn foals that are weak; are unable to stand to nurse; have swollen, hot, and painful joints; have fever and depression; or that die suddenly within a few days of birth.

LESIONS

Lesions may be difficult to discern in foals that die shortly after birth with a fulminant, septicemic infection, but if the foal survives a few days, gross lesions may

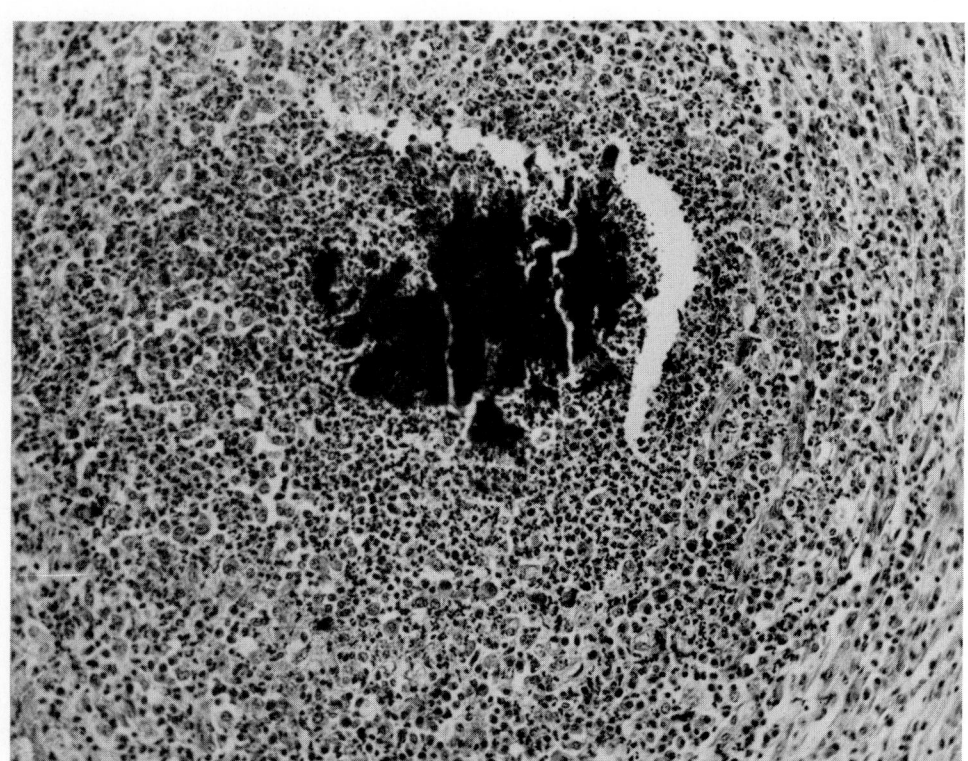

FIG. 10-13 Actinobacillosis, lung of a cow (× 160). Colony of *Actinobacillus lignieresi* in the center of a tiny abscess. (Courtesy of Dr. C. L. Davis, and Armed Forces Institute of Pathology.)

become recognizable. Infected joints are enlarged and contain excessive amounts of synovial fluid admixed with sanguineous or purulent exudate. The most characteristic gross changes are observed in the kidney, in which tiny gray foci, approximately equal in size, are uniformly distributed throughout the cortex. The renal medulla may contain hemorrhages, but it is remarkably free from the gray foci, which are demonstrable microscopically as tiny abscesses. These abscesses result from a shower of bacterial emboli that lodge in the capillaries, particularly in the glomerular tufts. Similar abscesses may occur in other organs, but much less frequently than in the kidney.

Actinobacillus equuli and another distinct organism, *Actinobacillus suis,* have been reported infrequently as causes of infection in swine. The infection, which resembles *A. equuli* in foals, is usually a septicemia of piglets, although pneumonia and arthritis have been described in older animals. Both organisms have been associated with vegetative endocarditis in piglets. *A. suis* has also been recovered from healthy horses and from equine abortuses. A single report (Moon and colleagues, 1969) has described *A. equuli* infection in New World monkeys.

DIAGNOSIS

Diagnosis can be confirmed by isolation of the organisms or by demonstration of typical gross and microscopic lesions in which the bacteria are present.

References

Baker JP. An outbreak of neonatal deaths in foals due to Actinobacillus equuli. Vet Rec 1972;90:630–632.

Dimock WW. Edwards PR, Bullard JF. Bacterium viscosum equi: a factor in joint-ill and septicemia in young foals. J Am Vet Med Assoc 1928;73:163–172.

Dimock WW, Edwards PR, Bruner DW. Infections of fetuses and foals. Ky Agric Exp Sta Bull 1947;509:1–40.

Edwards PR, Taylor EL. Shigella equirulis infection in a sow. Cornell Vet 1941;31:392–393.

Jang SS, Biberstein EL, Hirsh DC. Actinobacillus suis-like organisms in horses. Am J Vet Res 1987;48:1036–1038.

Kim BH, Phillips JE, Atherton JG. Actinobacillus suis in the horse. Vet Rec 1976;98:239.

Liven E, Larsen HJ, Lium B. Infection with Actinobacillus suis in pigs. Acta Vet Scand 1978;19:313–315.. [Vet Bull 1979;49:1142]

Mair NS, et al. Actinobacillus suis infection in pigs. A report of four outbreaks and two sporadic cases. J Comp Pathol 1974;84:113–119.

Moon HW, Barnes DM, Higbee JM. Septic embolic actinobacillosis: a report of 2 cases in New World monkeys. Pathol Vet 1969;6:481–486.

Webb RF, Cockram FA, Pryde L. The isolation of Actinobacillus equuli from equine abortion. Aust Vet J 1976;52:100–101.

Werdin RE, Hurtgen JP, Bates FY, et al. Porcine abortion caused by Actinobacillus equuli. J Am Vet Med Assoc 1976;169:704–706.

Windsor RS. Actinobacillus equuli infection in a litter of pigs and a review of previous reports on similar infections. Vet Rec 1973;92:178–180.

Actinobacillus lignieresii

A. lignieresii (named for J. Lignieres) is carried in the oral cavity of cattle and sheep. After a traumatic injury (or unknown mechanism), the organisms may invade adjacent tissues and, occasionally, spread systemically to produce lesions. The disease is most common in cattle and may produce signs and lesions that resemble those of actinomycosis, but differ in several respects. This organism may infect the jaw of cattle, but with far greater frequency it invades the tongue ("woody tongue"), lymph nodes of the head, neck, and thorax; it less often invades the lung (Fig. 10-13) and, rarely, other organs. This infection in cattle is therefore much more common in soft tissues than in bones: a point of differentiation from actinomycosis. In the rare instances in which actinobacillosis occurs in sheep, it most often affects the soft tissues and lymph nodes related to the mouth and pharynx. Lesions in internal organs are rare. Actinobacillosis does occur in other species, including dogs and humans, but examples are not common.

LESIONS

Microscopically, the lesions closely resemble actinomycosis, with discrete colonies of organisms surrounded by radiating clubs, suspended in pus, and encapsulated with rather dense connective tissue. The colonies tend to be much smaller, the radiating clubs longer and more slender, and the purulent exudate more abundant than in actinomycosis. Gram's stain of smears or sections reveals gram-negative, rod-shaped organisms in the center of the colonies, but they may be difficult to detect because of the acidophilic staining of the background.

In the tongue, where the abscesses are usually small, diffuse proliferation of connective tissue sometimes causes such great enlargement that the stiff, partially immobile tongue protrudes from the mouth. This is the so-called woody tongue of cattle. In lymph nodes, the usual change consists of the formation of an abscess, one to several centimeters in diameter, filled with thick, smooth, shiny pus that has marked cohesive but slight adhesive properties. In the lungs and other tissues, the abscesses are usually much smaller.

DIAGNOSIS

In tissue sections, gram-negative material in the center of the colonies suffices to distinguish actinobacillosis from actinomycosis, nocardiosis, and staphylococcal infections ("botryomycosis"). Demonstration of rosettes and the absence of gram-positive organisms in fresh preparations also establish the diagnosis in bovine material. Culture and identification of the organisms may be used to confirm the diagnosis.

References

Arseculeratne SN. A preliminary report on actinobacillosis as a natural infection in laboratory rabbits. Ceylon Vet J 1961;9:5–8. [Vet Bull 1962;32:82]

Arseculeratne SN. Actinobacillosis in joints of rabbits. J Comp Pathol 1962;72:33–39.

Campbell SG, Whitlock RW, Timoney JF, et al. An unusual epizootic of actinobacillosis in dairy heifers. J Am Vet Med Assoc 1975;166:604–606.

Chladek DW, Ruth GR. Isolation of *Actinobacillus lignieresi* from an

epidural abscess in a horse with progressive paralysis. J Am Vet Med Assoc 1976;168:64–66.

Cutlip RC, Amtower WC, Zinober MR. Septic embolic actinobacillosis of swine: a case report and laboratory reproduction of the disease. Am J Vet Res 1972;33:1621–1626.

Osbaldiston GW. Enteric actinobacillosis in calves. Cornell Vet 1972;62:364–371.

Actinobacillus seminis

First described as a cause of epididymitis in rams, the exact classification of *A. seminis* remains uncertain. Some isolates have been termed *Histophilus ovis*. Most reports of disease associated with *A. seminis* have come from Australia, New Zealand, and South Africa, where the organism is apparently widespread in sheep. Two reports have described the disease in the United States. The organism, which is present in semen, localizes in the epididymis and testis, producing a chronic pyogranulomatous inflammation comparable to that caused by *Brucella ovis*. The severity ranges from inapparent to gross distortion of the epididymis and testis with ulceration and draining abscesses. Systemic signs of fever and malaise are usually absent. *A. seminis* has also been associated with polyarthritis in sheep in Australia and has been suggested as a cause of abortion in sheep and goats in South Africa.

References

Baynes ID, Simmons GC. Ovine epididymitis caused by *Actinobacillus seminis*, n. sp. Aust Vet J 1960;36:454–459.

Livingston CW Jr, Hardy WT. Isolation of *Actinobacillus seminis* from ovine epididymitis. Am J Vet Res 1964;25:660–663.

Rahaley RS. Pathology of experimental *Histophilus ovis* infection in sheep. Vet Pathol 1978;15:631–637.

Sponenberg DP, et al. Suppurative epididymitis in a ram infected with *Actinobacillus seminis*. J Am Vet Med Assoc 1983;182:990–991.

van Tonder EM, Bolton TFW. The isolation of *Actinobacillus seminis* from bovine semen: a preliminary report. J S Afr Vet Med Assoc 1970;41:287–288. [Vet Bull 1971;41:2205]

van Tonder EM. *Actinobacillus seminis* infection in sheep in the Republic of South Africa. I. Identification of the problem. Onderstepoort J Vet Res 1979;46:129–133.

STREPTOBACILLUS INFECTIONS

Streptobacillus moniliformis, a gram-negative pleomorphic bacillus, is a normal inhabitant of the nasopharynx of rats. In humans, following a rat bite the organism may cause **rat-bite fever,** a disease characterized by rash, fever, and arthralgia. It has also followed ingestion of contaminated milk (termed **Haverhill fever**). The disease is usually self-limiting and not serious, but if left untreated, mortality rates are 10%. Complications include endocarditis, pneumonia, or brain abscesses. In laboratory mice, *S. moniliformis* infection may occur as an acute septicemia, but usually presents as purulent polyarthritis and tenosynovitis. Draining lymph nodes will often contain abscesses. In the septicemic form of infection, purulent and necrotizing lesions are found in the lungs, liver, spleen, and lymph nodes. The infection may be sporadic or occur as an epizootic. In guinea pigs, *S. moniliformis* causes abscess formation in submaxillary and cervical lymph nodes and, on occasion, abscesses in the lungs. Turkeys are also susceptible; purulent tenosynovitis and arthritis develop. Rat bites are believed to be the usual source of infection for turkeys. Rats tolerate the organism's presence, although it has been recovered from cases of pneumonia and other purulent lesions.

References

Acha PN, Szyfres B. Rat-bite fever. PAHO Sci Publ 1987;503:144–146.

Acha PN, Szyfres B. Bacterial zoonoses. PAHO Sci Publ 1987;503:205.

Aldred P, Hill AC, Young C. The isolation of *Streptobacillus moniliformis* from cervical abscesses of guinea-pigs. Lab Anim 1974;8:275–277.

Russell EG, Straube EF. Streptobacillary pleuritis in a koala *(Phascolarctos cinereus).* J Wildl Dis 1979;15:391–394.

Wullenweber M, Kaspareit-Rittinghausen J, Farouq M. *Streptobacillus moniliformis* epizootic in barrier-maintained C57BL/6J mice and susceptibility to infection of different strains of mice. Lab Anim Sci 1990;40:608–612.

Yamamoto R, Clark GT. *Streptobacillus moniliformis* infection in turkeys. Vet Rec 1966;79:95–100.

SHIGELLOSIS

Bacillary dysentery

Primates are the only hosts that are naturally susceptible to infection with dysentery bacilli. The disease is well known in humans and has been described in a variety of nonhuman primate species. It represents a disease of particular importance and frequency in Old World monkeys. *Shigella flexneri* is the most prevalent pathogen, but *S. sonnei* and *S. dysenteriae* also commonly occur. The strains of these shigellae species are infectious to humans, but they are not the strains that produce severe dysentery in humans, and fortunately, transmission from monkeys to humans is rare. The infection is readily transmissible among monkeys and often occurs as an epizootic. Control is hampered by infectious carriers that shed the bacilli in the absence of clinical disease.

Clinically, the dysentery varies from mild diarrhea to severe watery or mucoid diarrhea mixed with blood. Animals become dehydrated and rapidly lose condition. The pathologic changes are varied, nonspecific, and usually confined to the colon. The colonic mucosa is swollen and granular, with patchy or diffuse hemorrhage. Ulceration may or may not be present. The intestinal lumen contains varied quantities of mucus and blood. Other findings may include serosal petechiae, hyperemia of the mesentery, and enlarged and hemorrhagic mesenteric lymph nodes.

LESIONS

Microscopically, the colitis is characterized by hyperemia, edema, hemorrhage, necrosis, and desquamation of the mucosal epithelium. Large numbers of neutrophils and macrophages infiltrate the mucosa. The submucosa is usually edematous and hyperemic, but only rarely is there necrosis or cellular exudation. In electron micrographs, the organisms may be seen within the intestinal epithelial cells, either free in the cytoplasm or surrounded by a membrane. It is by means of this ability to penetrate epithelial cells that *Shigella* organisms exert their pathogenic effects.

DIAGNOSIS

Diagnosis requires isolation and identification of the causative organism.

References

Cooper JE, Needham JR. An outbreak of shigellosis in laboratory marmosets and tamarins (family: Callithricidae). J Hyg 1976;76:415–424.

Formal SB, Gemski P Jr, Giannella RA. Mechanisms of Shigella pathogenesis. Am J Clin Nutr 1972;25:1427–1432.

Levine MM, Dupont HL, Formal SB. Pathogenesis of Shigella dysenteriae 1 (Shiga) dysentery. J Infect Dis 1973;127:261–270.

Mulder JB. Shigellosis in nonhuman primates. A review. Lab Anim Sci 1971;21:734–738.

Ogawa H. Experimental approach in studies on pathogenesis of bacillary dysentery—with special references to the invasion of bacilli into intestinal mucosa. Acta Pathol Jpn 1970;20:261–277.

Rout WR, Formal SB, Giannella RA, et al. Pathophysiology of Shigella diarrhea in rhesus monkey: intestinal transport, morphological and bacteriological studies. Gastroenterology 1975;68:270–278.

Takasaka M, et al. Experimental infection with Shigella sonnei in cynomolgus monkeys (Macaca irus). Jpn J Med Sci Biol 1969;22:389–393.

Takasaka M, et al. Bacillary dysentery in cynomolgus monkeys following the administration with Shigella flexneri 2A by the anal route. Jpn J Med Sci Biol 1971;24:379–385.

Takeuchi A, FormaL SB, Sprinz H. Experimental acute colitis in the rhesus monkey following peroral infection with Shigella flexneri: an electron microscopic study. Am J Pathol 1968;52:503–529.

Takeuchi A, Sprinz H, La Brec EH, et al. Experimental bacillary dysentery—an electron microscopic study of the response of the intestinal mucosa to bacterial invasion. Am J Pathol 1965;47:1011–1044.

Takeuchi A, Jervis HR, Formal SB. Animal model of human disease: monkey shigellosis or dysentery. Am J Pathol 1975;81:251–254.

PASTEURELLOSIS

Among the gram-negative, facultatively anaerobic, rod-shaped bacteria is a group of organisms placed in the genus *Pasteurella* (after Louis Pasteur, who described the type species, *Pasteurella multocida,* and demonstrated it to be the cause of fowl cholera). At present, two groups of organisms have been removed from Pasteurella by the taxonomists and placed in two new genera, *Yersinia* and *Francisella.* Both of these contain pathogenic organisms that cause disease and are described in this chapter under their own headings.

Two species of Pasteurella, *P. multocida* and *P. haemolytica,* are important pathogens for cattle, sheep, and pigs. A third member, *P. pneumotropica,* is an occasional cause of pneumonia in laboratory animals, and a fourth member, *P. granulomatis,* a recently isolated organism, is associated with Lechiguana (panniculitis) of cattle in Brazil. Although both *P. multocida* and *P. haemolytica* are obligate parasites, they exist as normal commensals in the oropharynx of cattle, sheep, and other mammals. On the basis of capsular (most pathogenic strains produce capsules) and somatic antigens and other characteristics, there are multiple serotypes of each species, often with distinct geographic distributions, some of which are more highly pathogenic than others. Individual types are associated with specific disease manifestations. The events that allow these organisms to induce disease are not entirely clear, but during various stressful situations, such as inclement weather, shipping (hence "shipping fever"), or dipping, the most pathogenic strains outgrow others that are present. Initiation of disease by other organisms, such as viruses or mycoplasmas, also paves the way for Pasteurella species to become important secondary invaders in pneumonia. Several clinical entities, which are listed in Table 10-8, are associated with Pasteurella organisms.

Hemorrhagic septicemia is an acute infection of cattle, sheep, goats, and buffalo caused by *P. multocida* serotypes B and E. Except for its occurrence in bison in the United States, the disease is seen only in Asia and Africa. Occurring during the rainy season, the infection can spread rapidly among groups of animals, causing a mortality rate of almost 100%.

There are few clinical signs other than high fever and prostration. Widespread petechiae and ecchymoses on mucous and serous membranes are the principal pathogical findings. There may be edema of subcutaneous tissue, pericardium, lungs, and other tissues.

P. multocida is also an important cause of pneumonia in cattle, sheep, goats, and swine. Its occurrence is usually associated with inclement weather, stress of transport, or the occurrence of other infectious diseases, particulary pneumotropic viruses. *P. haemolytica*, however, is the more common cause of pneumonia in these species and is the usual pathogen in **"shipping fever"** of cattle. Serotype A is the most frequent offender. The pneumonia is a classic fibrinous or lobar pneumonia principally affecting the cranioventral portions of the lungs. Interlobular septae are thickened, the pleura is covered with fibrin, and alveoli are filled with neutrophils and mononuclear inflammatory cells. Numerous bacteria are present as are areas of necrosis.

A **septicemic disease** of sheep is caused by *P. haemolytica* biotype T. The condition principally affects lambs, but sheep of all ages are susceptible. Affected individuals die suddenly without any specific clinical signs. Pathologically, there are widespread hemorrhages on serosal surfaces, congestion and edema in lungs and lymph nodes and necrotizing pharyngitis. Microscopically, bacterial emboli are widespread throughout most organs, often not in association with any inflammatory lesion. *P. haemolytica* (biotype A) is also a cause of enzootic pneumonia of sheep and a form of mastitis, commonly referred to as "blue bag," characterized by extensive necrosis.

Both *P. multocida* and *P. haemolytica* are sporadic causes of various inflammatory disorders of most species of animals. These include mastitis, arthritis, otitis, sinusitis, meningitis, and encephalitis, among others. *P. multocida* type D along with *Bordetella bronchiseptica* are related to atrophic rhinitis (which is discussed in the chapter on the respiratory system).

In rabbits, *P. multocida* causes a common upper respiratory disease called **"snuffles."** Pleuritis and pneumonia may accompany the condition, which sometimes progresses to an acutely fatal septicemia.

P. pneumotropica occasionally causes enzootic pneumonia of mice, rabbits, and other laboratory animals. It may occur in the nasopharynx of humans and dogs. Occasionally, it is isolated from wound infections in human patients.

An apparently new organism, *P. granulomatis*, is believed responsible for a disease termed Lechiguana, which occurs in cattle in Brazil. This disorder is characterized by fibrogranulomatous panniculitis leading to large (up to 20 cm in diameter), hard subcutaneous swellings. The lesions are made up of dense fibrous connective tissue containing granulomas composed of macrophages, epithelioid cells, neutrophils, and large numbers of eosinophils. The centers of the granulomas contain necrotic debris and colonies of bacteria, which are often surrounded by eosinophilic clubs (Splendore-Hoeppli material). Similar granulomas may develop in draining lymph nodes. The pathogenesis of this disorder is not understood, but it has been suggested that infection with *Dermatobia hominis* may play a role in initiating infection.

TABLE 10-8 **Diseases associated with *Pasteurella* species**

Pasteurella multocida
  Hemorrhagic septicemia in cattle and buffalo in Asia and Africa
  Primary and secondary pneumonia in cattle, swine, and occasionally other animal species
  Snuffles, otitis media, pneumonia, and septicemia in rabbits
  Often associated with atrophic rhinitis in swine
  Assorted inflammatory lesions in any species
  Fowl cholera
Pasteurella haemolytica
  "Shipping fever" of cattle
  Primary and secondary pneumonia in cattle, sheep, and goats
  Septicemia in sheep
  Mastitis ("blue-bag") of sheep
  Assorted inflammatory lesions in any species
Pasteurella pneumotropica
  Secondary pneumonia in rats, mice, and rabbits
Pasteurella anatipestifer (Moraxella anatipestifer)
  Infectious serositis of ducks; new duck disease
Pasteurella granulomatis
  Lechiguana (fibrogranulomatous panniculitis) in cattle

References

Ackermann MR, Cheville NF, Gallagher JE. Colonization of the pharyngeal tonsil and respiratory tract of the gnotobiotic pig by a toxigenic strain of Pasteurella multocida type D. Vet Pathol 1991;28:267–274.
Bagadi HO, Razig SE. Caprine mastitis caused by Pasteurella mastitidis (P. haemolytica). Vet Rec 1976;99:13.

Benjamin SA, Lang CM. Acute pasteurellosis in owl monkeys (Aotus trivirgatus). Lab Anim Sci 1971;21:258–262.

Biberstein EL, Kennedy PC. Systemic pasteurellosis in lambs. Am J Vet Res 1959;20:94–101.

Carter GR. Pasteurella infections as sequelae to respiratory viral infections. J Am Vet Med Assoc 1973;163:863–864.

Carter GR. Pasteurellosis: Pasteurella multocida and Pasteurella hemolytica. Adv Vet Sci 1967;11:321–379.

DiGiacomo RF, Garlinghouse LE Jr, Van Hoosier GL Jr. Natural history of infection with Pasteurella multocida in rabbits. J Am Vet Med Assoc 1983;183:1172–1175.

DiGiacomo RF, Deeb BJ, Giddens WE Jr, et al. Atrophic rhinitis in New Zealand white rabbits infected with Pasteurella multocida. Am J Vet Res 1989;50:1460–1465.

Flatt RE, Dungworth DL. Enzootic pneumonia in rabbits: microbiology and comparison with lesions experimentally produced by Pasteurella multocida and a chlamydial organism. Am J Vet Res 1971;32:627–638.

Fox RR, Norberg RF, Meyers DD. The relationship of Pasteurella multocida to otitis media in the domestic rabbit (Oryctolagus cuniculus). Lab Anim Sci 1971;21:45–48.

Frank GH. Serotypes of Pasteurella haemolytica in sheep in the midwestern United States. Am J Vet Res 1982;43:2035–2037.

Gilmour NJL, Thompson DA, Fraser J. The recovery of Pasteurella haemolytica from the tonsils of adult sheep. Res Vet Sci 1974;17:413–414.

Hagen KW. Enzootic pasteurellosis in domestic rabbits. I. Pathology and bacteriology. J Am Vet Med Assoc 1958;133:77–80.

Haritani M, Narita M, Murata H, et al. Immunoperoxidase evaluation of pneumonic lesions induced by Pasteurella multocida in calves. Am J Vet Res 1989;50:2162–2167.

Harris G. An outbreak of pasteurellosis in lambs. Vet Rec 1974;94:84–85.

Johnson RB, Dawkins HJS, Spencer TL. Electrophoretic profiles of Pasteurella multocida isolates from animals with hemorrhagic septicemia. Am J Vet Res 1991;52:1644–1648.

Manning PJ. Serology of Pasteurella multocida in laboratory rabbits: a review. Lab Anim Sci 1982;32:666–671.

O'Sullivan BM, Bauer JJ, Stranger RS. Bovine mastitis caused by Pasteurella multocida. Aust Vet J 1971;47:576.

Panciera RJ, Corstvet RE. Bovine pneumonic pasteurellosis: model for Pasteurella haemolytica- and Pasteurella multocida-induced pneumonia in cattle. Am J Vet Res 1984;45:2532–2537.

Pass DA, Thomson RG. Wide distribution of Pasteurella haemolytica type 1 over the nasal mucosa of cattle. Can J Comp Med 1971;35:181–186.

Riet-Correa F, Mendez MC, Schild AL, et al. Bovine focal proliferative fibrogranulomatous panniculitis (Lechiguana) associated with Pasteurella granulomatis. Vet Pathol 1992;29:93–103.

Rogers RJ, Elder JK. Purulent leptomeningitis in a dog associated with an aerogenic Pasteurella multocida. Aust Vet J 1967;43:81–82.

Sawada T, Rimler RB, Rhoades KR. Hemorrhagic septicemia: naturally acquired antibodies against Pasteurella multocida types B and E in calves in the United States. Am J Vet Res 1985;46:1247–1250.

Slocombe RF, Derksen FJ, Robinson NE. Interactions of cold stress and Pasteurella haemolytica in the pathogenesis of pneumonic pasteurellosis in calves: changes in pulmonary function. Am J Vet Res 1984;45:1764–1770.

Stamp JT, Watt JAA, Tomlinson JR. Pasteurella hemolytica septicemia in lambs. J Comp Pathol 1955;65:183–196.

Suckow MA, Chrisp CE, and Foged NT: Heat-labile toxin-producing isolates of Pasteurella multocida from rabbits. Lab Anim Sci 1991;41:151–156.

Thomson RG, Benson ML, Savan M. Pneumonic pasteurellosis of cattle: Microbiology and immunology. Can J Comp Med 1969;33:194–206.

Vestweber JG, Klemm RD, Leipold HW, et al. Clinical and pathologic studies of experimentally induced Pasteurella haemolytica pneumonia in calves. Am J Vet Res 1990;51:1792–1798.

Vestweber JG, Klemm RD, Leipold HW, et al. Pneumonic pasteurellosis induced experimentally in gnotobiotic and conventional calves inoculated with Pasteurella haemolytica. Am J Vet Res 1990;51:1799–1805.

Watson WT, Goldsboro JA. Williams FP, et al. Experimental respiratory infection with Pasteurella multocida and Bordetella bronchiseptica in rabbits. Lab Anim Sci 1975;25:459–464.

YERSINIOSIS

Three important intracellular pathogens are contained in the genus *Yersinia;* these are *Y. pestis; Y. pseudotuberculosis;* and *Y. enterocolitica.* Three other species in the genus, *Y. intermedia, Y. kristensenii,* and *Y. frederiksenii* are probably not pathogens. *Y. ruckeri* is the cause of a disease of fish called red mouth disease.

Y. pestis is the cause of bubonic plague ("black death") in humans. It is principally an infection of rats, ground squirrels, and other rodents. It is transmitted between rodents and to humans by the rat flea, *Xenopsylla cheopis.* The bacteria infect the flea, causing esophageal obstruction and regurgitation of the deadly bacteria when they take their blood meal. The disease in humans is an extremely acute septicemia. Also in humans, septicemia caused by *Capnocytophaga canimorsus,* a normal inhabitant of the canine and feline mouth, has been confused with plague. Plague is not a disease of domestic animals, although there have been isolated reports, particularly in cats.

Y. pseudotuberculosis and *Y. enterocolitica* produce enteric and systemic diseases which are similar but not identical. Unfortunately, both diseases have been described as "pseudotuberculosis," largely because of the gross appearance of the visceral lesions. We suggest that the term "yersiniosis" be used for these two infections. This may reduce the confusion slightly (see Corynebacterium infections, p. 479).

Y. pseudotuberculosis infection principally causes disease in guinea pigs, rats, other rodents, and birds, but has been reported in many other species, including humans, rabbits, mice, deer, cats, swine, monkeys, sheep, goats, chinchillas, mink, horses, and many exotic mammals. The infection may occur as a fatal acute septicemia with few specific gross lesions or, more often, as a chronic infection that results in discrete white or gray nodules in the liver, spleen, lymph nodes, and lung.

Abortion has been described in cattle, sheep and goats, with typical lesions in the placenta and fetus.

Microscopic lesions of *Y. pseudotuberculosis* consist of a necrotic core of pus and bacteria surrounded by a zone of macrophages. Epithelioid cells may be present in lesions of prolonged duration, and a fibrous capsule may be formed. Giant cells are absent. In the intestine, especially the lower ileum, the necrotic lesions containing colonies of organisms often include the mucosa to the level of muscularis mucosa.

Y. enterocolitica, a similar organism, but distinguishable from *Y. pseudotuberculosis,* has a similar host range. It produces an enteric infection, usually limited to intestines and mesenteric lymph nodes, but it may become generalized in some instances and result in visceral lesions. Ulcers in Peyer's patches in the lower ileum have been described, as well as focal necrosis in liver, spleen, and lymph nodes. Colonies of organisms are seen under the light microscope in the necrotic zones, which in turn are surrounded by neutrophils and macrophages.

References

Acha PN, Szyfes B. Plague. PAHO Sci Publ 1987;503:131–140.

Baggs RB, Hunt RD, Garcia FG, et al. Pseudotuberculosis (Yersinia enterocolitica) in the owl monkey (Aotus trivirgatus). Lab Anim Sci 1976;26(Part II):1079–1083.

Bresnahan JF, Whitworth UG, Hayes Y, et al. Yersinia enterocolitica infection in breeding colonies of ruffed lemurs. J Am Vet Med Assoc 1984;185:1354–1356.

Bronson RT, May BD, Ruebner BH. An outbreak of infection by Yersinia pseudotuberculosis in nonhuman primates. Am J Pathol 1972;69:289–308.

Cappucci DT Jr, et al. Caprine mastitis associated with Yersinia pseudotuberculosis. J Am Vet Med Assoc 1978;173:1589–1590.

Centers for Disease Control and Prevention. Pneumonic plague - Arizona, 1992. MMWR 1992;41(40):737–739.

Centers for Disease Control and Prevention. Capnocytophaga canimorsus sepsis misdiagnosed as plague - New Mexico, 1992. 1993;42(4):72–73.

Chang J, Wagner JL, Kornegay RW. Fatal Yersinia pseudotuberculosis infection in captive bushbabies. J Am Vet Med Assoc 1980; 177:820–821.

Cover TL, Aber RC. Yersinia enterocolitica. N Engl J Med 1989;321:16–24.

Harper PAW, Hornitzky MAZ, Rayward DG. Enterocolitis in pigs associated with Yersinia pseudotuberculosis infection. Aust Vet J 1990;67:418–419. [Vet Bull 1991;61:3923]

Hubbert WT. Yersiniosis in mammals and birds in the U.S. Am J Trop Med Hyg 1972;21:458–463.

Jerrett IV, Slee KJ. Bovine abortion associated with Yersinia pseudotuberculosis infection. Vet Pathol 1989;26:181–183.

Karbe E, Erickson ED. Ovine abortion and stillbirth due to purulent placentitis caused by Yersinia pseudotuberculosis. Vet Pathol 1984;21:601–606.

Krogstad O. Yersinia enterocolitica infection in goats. A serological and bacteriological investigation. Acta Vet Scand 1974;15:597–608.

Lee LA, et al. Yersinia enterocolitica O:3 infections in infants and children associated with the household preparation of chitterlings. N Engl J Med 1990;322:984–987.

Mair NS, Ziffo GS. Isolation of Y. pseudotuberculosis from a foal. Vet Rec 1974;94:152–153.

Mair NS, et al. Pasteurella pseudotuberculosis infection in the cat: two cases. Vet Rec 1967;81:461–462.

McClure HM, Weaver RE, Kaufmann AF. Pseudotuberculosis in nonhuman primates: infection with organisms of the Yersinia enterocolitica group. Lab Anim Sci 1971;21:376–382.

McEvedy C. The bubonic plague. Sci Am 1988;258(2):118–123.

Obwolo MJ. A review of yersiniosis (Yersinia pseudotuberculosis infection). Vet Bull 1976;46:167–171.

Papageorges M, Higgins R, Gosselin Y. Yersinia enterocolitica enteritis in two dogs. J Am Vet Med Assoc 1983;182:618–619.

Raflo NL. Bubonic plague in a cat. J Am Vet Med Assoc 1986;188:534–535.

Robinson M. Pasteurella pseudotuberculosis infection in the cat Vet Rec 1972;91:676–677.

Rosenberg DP, Lerche NW, Henrickson RV. Yersinia pseudotuberculosis infection in a group of Macaca fascicularis. J Am Vet Med Assoc 1980;177:818–819.

Skavlen PA, Stills HF Jr, Steffan EK, et al. Naturally occurring Yersinia enterocolitica septicemia in patas monkeys (Erythrocebus patas). Lab Anim Sci 1985;35:488–490.

Slee KJ, Button C. [1] Enteritis in sheep, goats and pigs due to Yersinia pseudotuberculosis infection. [2] Enteritis in sheep and goats due to Yersinia enterocolitica infection. Aust Vet J 1990;67:320–322, 396–398. [Vet Bull 1991;61:990, 3922]

Spearman JG, Hunt P, Nayar PSG. Yersinia pseudotuberculosis infection in a cat. Can Vet J 1979;20:361–364.

Tsubokura M, Otsuki K, Itagaki K. Studies on Yersinia enterocolitica. I. Isolation from swine. Jpn J Vet Sci 1973;35:419–424.

Weber J, Finlayson NB, Mark JBD. Mesenteric lymphadenitis and terminal ileitis due to Yersinia pseudotuberculosis. N Engl J Med 1970;283:172–174.

Witte ST, Sponenberg DP, Collins TC. Abortion and early neonatal death of kids attributed to intrauterine Yersinia pseudotuberculosis infection. J Am Vet Med Assoc 1985;187:834.

Wooley RE, Shotts EB Jr, McConnell JW. Isolation of Yersinia enterocolitica from selected animal species. Am J Vet Res 1980;41:1668–1668.

LISTERIOSIS

A small, rod-shaped, gram-positive intracellular parasite, *Listeria* (formerly *Listerella*) *monocytogenes* causes disease in most species of animals and humans (Figs. 10-14 and 10-15). The organism gains its name from the occurrence of mononucleosis in the systemic form of the disease in rabbits and rodents. The organism is ubiquitous in nature and can be recovered from soil, vegetation, dairy products, animal feces, and sometimes the oropharynx and tissues of healthy animals. The circumstances necessary for the bacterium to invade and cause disease are not understood.

Listeriosis occurs as three distinct syndromes, which ordinarily do not occur together: **encephalitis** in humans, cattle, sheep, goats, and swine; **systemic infection** (septicemia) in humans, cattle, sheep, swine, dogs, cats, and rodents; and **abortion** in humans, cattle, and sheep. Less commonly, *L. monocytogenes* is a cause of endocarditis and purulent lesions in other organs and tissues.

Encephalitis

Involvement of the central nervous system, the most characteristic form of the disease in ruminants, is manifested by the animal's abnormal posturing of the head and neck, walking aimlessly in a circle ("circling disease"), nystagmus, blindness, and paralysis. The encephalitic form of listeriosis may also occur in horses, dogs, swine, rodents, and humans. The organism is thought to invade the central nervous system by way of as-

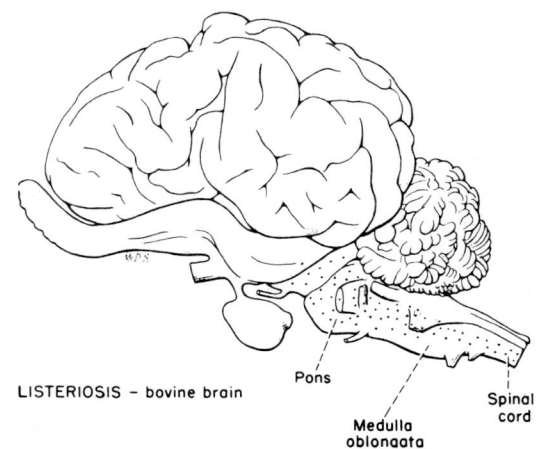

LISTERIOSIS – bovine brain

Pons

Medulla oblongata

Spinal cord

FIG. 10-14 Listeriosis, bovine brain. Localization of lesions indicated by dots in pons, medulla, and spinal cord. Compare with Figure 8-40.

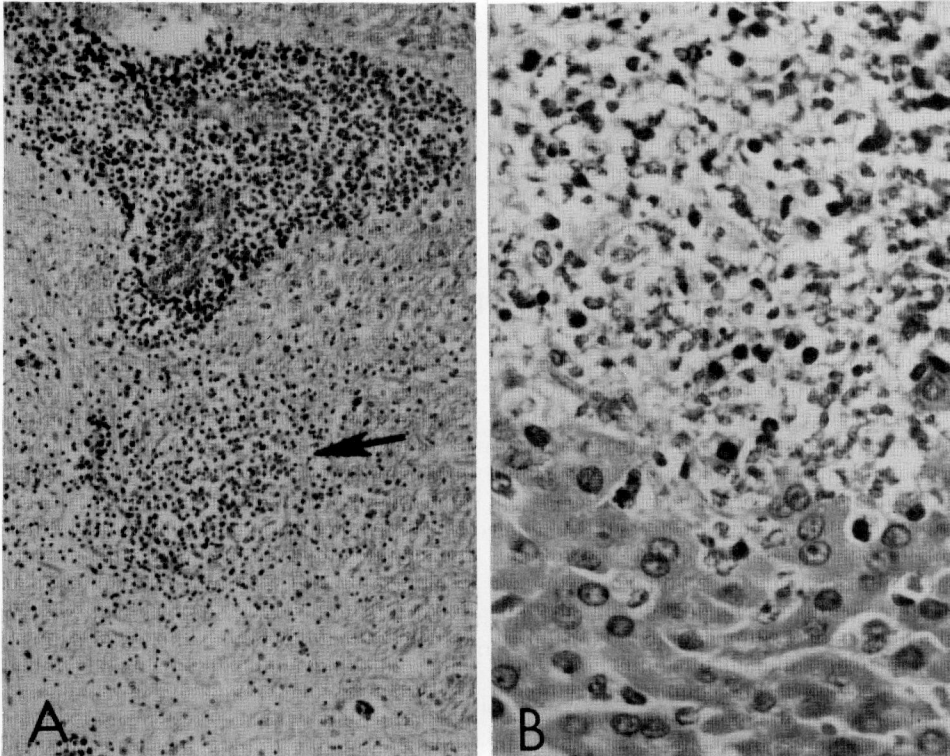

FIG. 10-15 Listeriosis. **A.** Brain of a cow. Note perivascular cuffing and a "microabscess" (arrow). (Courtesy of Dr. C. L. Davis.) **B.** Liver of a rat. There is focal necrosis with a moderate infiltration of neutrophils. (Courtesy of Animal Research Center, Harvard Medical School.)

cending peripheral nerves, particularly the trigeminal nerve.

The lesions in the central nervous system can be recognized only by microscopic examination and are confined to the brain stem, particularly the medulla oblongata and spinal cord. The primary lesion is a circumscribed collection of mononuclear cells, with or without neutrophils, in close proximity to blood vessels. Diffuse cellular infiltration and frank microabscesses may occur, but there is relatively little tissue necrosis. Nerve cells can be destroyed, but the lesions are not restricted to gray matter. In some cases, the gasserian ganglia are involved. The organisms, being gram-positive, can be demonstrated in tissue sections without difficulty with appropriate stains. They are found in the center of the lesions in the medulla oblongata or spinal cord. Intense meningeal infiltration of lymphoid cells is a characteristic accompaniment.

Visceral lesions similar to those described below in septicemic listeriosis may be encountered in both cattle and sheep with listeric encephalitis.

Septicemia

Generalized listeriosis is the more common form in monogastric animals and in human newborns and infants. The most characteristic lesion in this form is focal necrosis of the liver; less commonly, lesions occur in the spleen, lymph nodes, lungs, adrenal glands, myocardium, gastrointestinal tract, and brain. Microscopically, the lesions consist of focal areas of necrosis infiltrated with mononuclear cells and some neutrophils. The or-

ganisms are easily demonstrated with appropriately stained tissue sections.

ABORTION

Listeric abortion in animals is principally of importance in cattle and sheep. Abortion usually occurs in the last quarter of gestation without signs of infection in the dam. The fetus dies in utero and may be severely autolyzed when finally expelled. If not obscured by autolysis, focal hepatic necrosis containing stainable organisms in the fetal liver is the principal lesion of diagnostic value. An organism termed *Listeria ivanovii*, which is distinguishable from *L. monocytogenes*, is described as a cause of abortion in sheep.

PATHOGENESIS

Listeria have the ability to penetrate epithelial cells (in the conjunctiva, urinary bladder, and intestine), where they multiply, destroy the cells, and then are released to be phagocytized. Transport by macrophages is thought to result in a septicemic phase in some cases. Evidence points toward the centripetal movement of organisms within branches of the trigeminal nerve, eventually to reach the medulla oblongata. Bacteria appear to move along fiber tracts, but also within axons. In experimentally infected ewes in the latter half of gestation, Listeria organisms were believed to penetrate the placenta and reach the fetal liver. Here multiplication occurred, resulting in the death of the fetus. Listeria organisms can be carried and excreted in the feces of animals in the absence of disease.

DIAGNOSIS

The diagnosis of listeric encephalitis can be confirmed in suspicious cases by demonstration of the typical microscopic lesions, which include (1) microabscesses, diffuse purulent inflammation, or glial nodules; (2) perivascular accumulation of lymphocytes; and (3) lymphocytic leptomeningitis in combination with the gram-positive organisms associated with these lesions. Although the lesions in listeric septicemia and abortion are less specific than in listeric encephalitis, demonstration of the organisms within the necrotic lesions allows presumptive diagnosis. Confirmation can be made by isolation of the organisms in appropriate culture media inoculated with suspensions of tissue.

References

Attleberger MH, Seibold HR. Listeria infection of bovine mesenteric lymph nodes. J Am Vet Med Assoc 1956;128:202–204.

Barza M. Listeriosis and milk. N Engl J Med 1985;312:438–440.

Biester HE, Schwarte LH. Listerella infection in swine. J Am Vet Med Assoc 1940;96:339–342.

Borman G, Olson C, Segre D. The trigeminal and facial nerves as pathways for infection of sheep with Listeria monocytogenes. Am J Vet Res 1960;21:993–1000.

Briones V, et al. Biliary excretion as possible origin of Listeria monocytogenes in fecal carriers. Am J Vet Res 1992;53:191–193.

Busch RH, Barnes DM, Sautter JH. Pathogenesis and pathologic changes of experimentally induced listeriosis in newborn pigs. Am J Vet Res 1971;32:1313–1320.

Charlton KM, Garcia MM. Spontaneous listeric encephalitis and neuritis in sheep. Light microscopic studies. Vet Pathol 1977;14:297–313.

Charlton KM. Spontaneous listeric encephalitis in sheep. Electron microscopic studies. Vet Pathol 1977;14:429–434.

Cordy DR, Osebold JW. The neuropathogenesis of Listeria encephalomyelitis in sheep and mice. J Infect Dis 1959;104:164–173.

Courtieu AL. Latest news on listeriosis. Comp Immunol Microbiol Infect Dis 1991;14:1–7.

Decker RA, Roger JJ, Lesar S. Listeriosis in a young cat. J Am Vet Med Assoc 1976;168:1025.

De Heer E, Kersten MC, Van der Meer C, et al. Electron microscopic observations on the interaction of Listeria monocytogenes and peritoneal macrophages of normal mice. Lab Invest 1980;43:449–455.

Fleming DW, et al. Pasteurized milk as a vehicle of infection in an outbreak of listeriosis. N Engl J Med 1985;312:404–407.

Harcourt RA. Listeria monocytogenes in a piglet. Vet Rec 1966;78:735.

Jakob W. Further experiments on the pathogenesis of cerebral listeriosis in sheep. I. Pathological changes caused by freshly-isolated strains. Arch Exp Veterinaermed 1966;20:367–381.

Jones D. Foodborne listeriosis. Lancet 1990;336:1171–1174.

Kidd ARM, Terlecki S. Visceral and cerebral listeriosis in a lamb. Vet Rec 1966;78:453–454.

King LS. Primary encephalomyelitis in goats associated with listerella infection. Am J Pathol 1940;16:467–478.

Ladds PW, Dennis SM, Njoku CO. Pathology of listeric infection in domestic animals. Vet Bull 1974;44:67–74.

Linnan MJ, et al. Epidemic listeriosis associated with Mexican-style cheese. N Engl J Med 1988;319:823–828.

Macleod NSM, Watt JA, Harris JC. Listeria monocytogenes type 5 as a cause of abortion in sheep. Vet Rec 1974;95:365–367.

McClure HM, Strozier LM. Perinatal listeric septicemia in a Celebese black ape. J Am Vet Med Assoc 1975;167:637–638.

Miller JK, Burns J. Histopathology of Listeria monocytogenes after oral feeding to mice. Appl Microbiol 1970;19:772–775.

Njoku CO, Dennis SM, Cooper RF. Listeric abortion studies in sheep. I. Maternofetal changes. Cornell Vet 1972;62:608–627.

Njoku CO, Dennis SM. Listeric abortion studies in sheep. II. Fetoplacental changes. Cornell Vet 1973;63:171–172.

Njoku CO, Dennis SM. Listeric abortion studies in sheep. IV. Histopathologic comparison of natural and experimental infection. Cornell Vet 1973;63:211–219.

Njoku CO, Dennis SM, Noonday JL. Listeric abortion studies in sheep. III. Fetoplacental-myometrial interaction. Cornell Vet 1973;63:193–210.

Olafson P. Listerella encephalitis (circling disease) of sheep, cattle, and goats. Cornell Vet 1940;30:141–150.

Smith RE, Reynolds IM, Clark GW, et al. Experimental ovine listeriosis. IV. Pathogenesis of fetal infection. Cornell Vet 1970;60:450–462.

Smith RE, Reynolds IM, Bennett RA. Listeria monocytogenes and abortion in a cow. J Am Vet Med Assoc 1955;126:106–110.

Smith RE. Reynolds IM, Clark GW. Experimental ovine listeriosis. I. Inoculation of pregnant ewes. Cornell Vet 1968;58:169–179.

Watson GL, Evans MG: Listeriosis in a rabbit. Vet Pathol 1985;22:191–193.

Welsh RD. Equine abortion caused by Listeria monocytogenes serotype 4. J Am Vet Med Assoc 1983;182:291.

TYZZER'S DISEASE

Tyzzer's disease was originally described as an infection of mice caused by *Bacillus piliformis*, a gram-negative, curved rod 10 to 40 μ long and 0.5 μ or less wide (Tyzzer, 1917), and of no relation to the genus containing *Bacillus anthracis* (Fig. 10-16). The organism is an obligate intracellular parasite, which has only been cultivated in tissue culture. *B. piliformis* appears to live as a saprophyte in many mouse colonies, producing disease under adverse environmental conditions and other forms of stress. This organism is currently classified as *Clostridium piliforme* on the basis of 16S rRNA sequence analysis (Duncan, et al. 1993).

Tyzzer's disease has been demonstrated with increasing frequency in recent years as a disease of several animal species, including foals, dogs, cats, rats, gerbils, rabbits, guinea pigs, monkeys, muskrats, and hamsters. There is also a report of the disease in a calf. The disease in horses occurs as an acute, usually fatal disease in foals 4 weeks of age or younger.

Lesions

The gross lesions consist of circular gray-white foci, 1 to 2 mm in diameter, on the capsular and cut surfaces of the liver. Microscopically, these foci consist of areas of hepatic necrosis surrounded by a zone of neutrophils and a lesser number of lymphocytes and macrophages. Numerous organisms are present around the necrotic foci in the inflammatory zone and in intact hepatocytes. They usually cannot be seen in tissue sections stained with hematoxylin and eosin, but are clearly evident in sections stained by the Giemsa, Gomori's methenamine silver, and methylene blue techniques. Organisms are also found in intestinal epithelial cells, occasionally resulting in necrotizing enteritis. The mesenteric lymph nodes may contain small abscesses.

References

Allen AM, et al. Tyzzer's disease syndrome in laboratory rabbits. Am J Pathol 1965;46:859–882.

Boschert KR, Allison N, Allen TLC, et al. Bacillus piliformis infection in an adult dog. J Am Vet Med Assoc 1988;192:791–792.

Canfield PJ, Hartley WJ. Tyzzer's disease (Bacillus piliformis) in Australian marsupials. J Comp Pathol 1991;105:163–173.

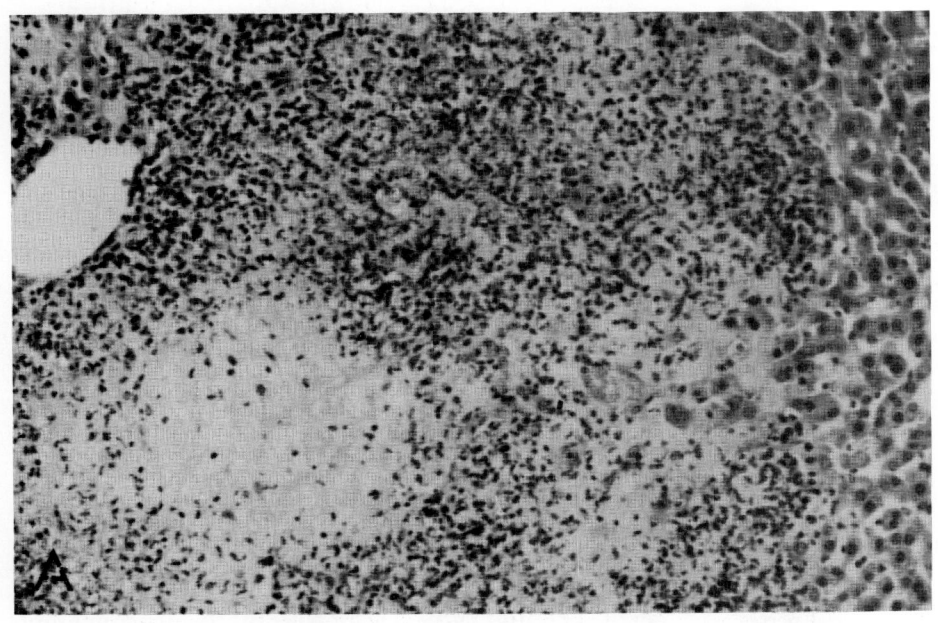

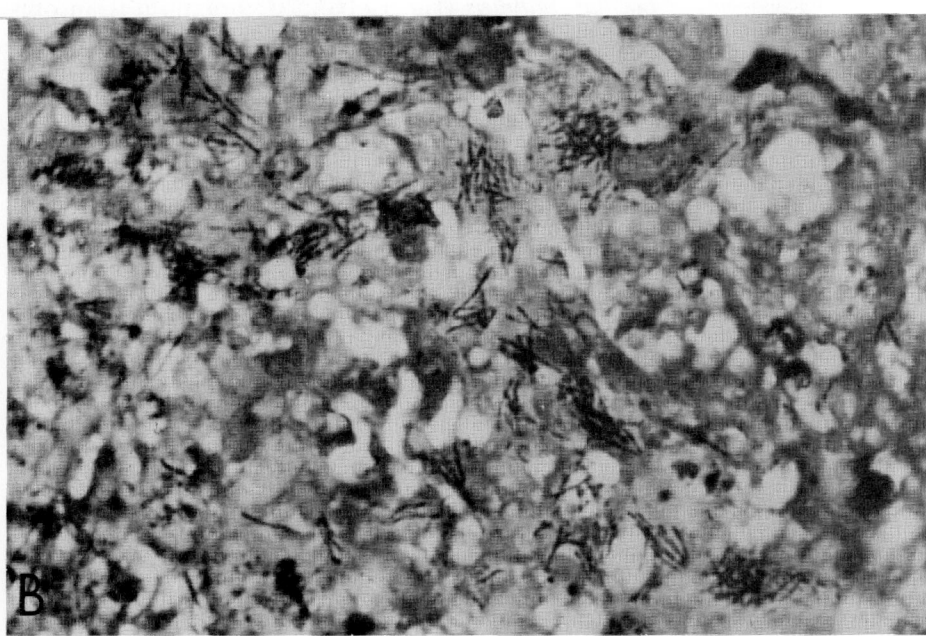

FIG. 10-16 Tyzzer's disease in a mouse. **A.** Focal hepatic necrosis surrounded by a zone of inflammatory cells. **B.** Filamentous Clostridium piliforme in the cytoplasm of hepatocytes (Gomori's methenamine silver stain). (Courtesy of Dr. C. L. Davis.)

Carter GR, Whitenack DL, Julius LA. Natural Tyzzer's disease in mongolian gerbils (Meriones unguiculatus). Lab Anim Care 1969;19:648, 651.

Cutlip RC, Amtower WC, Reall CW, et al. An epizootic of Tyzzer's disease in rabbits. Lab Anim Sci 1971;21:356–361.

Duncan AJ, Carmen RJ, Olsen GJ, Wilson KH. Assignment of the agent of Tyzzer's disease to *Clostridium piliforme* comb. nov. on the basis of 16S rRNA sequence analysis. Int J Syst Bacteriol 1993, 43: 314–318.

Ganaway JR. [1] Tyzzer's disease, liver, mouse, rat, hamster. [2] Tyzzer's disease, intestine, mouse, rat, hamster. In: Jones TC, Mohr U, Hunt RD, ed. Digestive system. New York: Springer-Verlag 1985;156–165, 330–333.

Hall WC, Van Kruiningen HJ. Tyzzer's disease in a horse. J Am Vet Med Assoc 1974;164:1187–1189.

Harrington DD. Naturally-occurring Tyzzer's disease (Bacillus piliformis infection) in horse foals. Vet Rec 1975;96:59–63.

Harrington DD. Bacillus piliformis infection (Tyzzer's disease) in two foals. J Am Vet Med Assoc 1976;168:58–59.

Kovatch RM, Zebarth G. Naturally occurring Tyzzer's disease in a cat. J Am Vet Med Assoc 1973;162:136–138.

Kubokawa K, et al. Two cases of feline Tyzzer's disease. Jpn J Exp Med 1973;43:413–421.

McLeod CG, Stookey JL, Harrington DG, et al. Intestinal Tyzzer's disease and spirochetosis in a guinea pig. Vet Pathol 1977;14:229–235.

Nold JB, Swanson T, Spraker TR. Bacillus piliformis infection (Tyzzer's disease) in a Colorado foal. J Am Vet Med Assoc 1984;185:306–307.

Port CD, Richter WR, Moize SM. An ultrastructural study of Tyzzer's disease in the Mongolian gerbil (Meriones unguiculatus). Lab Invest 1971;25:81–87.

Pulley LT, Shively JN. Tyzzer's disease in a foal. Light and electron-microscopic observations. Vet Pathol 1974;11:203–211.

Qureshi SR, Carlton WW, Olander HJ. Tyzzer's disease in a dog. J Am Vet Med Assoc 1976;168:602–604.

Riley LK, Franklin CL, Tyzzer's disease, rat, mouse and hamster. in: Jones TC, Popp & Mohr U (eds) Monograph on Pathology of Laboratory Animals, Digestive System. Springer V, Heideberg, Berlin. New York 2nd Edition 1997 *in press*

Takasaki Y, Oghiso Y, Sato K, et al. Tyzzer's disease in hamsters. Jpn J Exp Med 1974;44:267–270.

Tyzzer EE. A fatal disease of the Japanese waltzing mouse caused by spore-bearing bacillus (Bacillus piliformis, N. Sp.). J Med Res 1917;38:307–338.

Waggie KS, Ganaway JR, Wagner JE, et al. Experimentally induced Tyzzer's disease in Mongolian gerbils (Meriones unguiculatus). Lab Anim Sci 1984;34:53–57.

Waggie KS, Thornburg LP, Wagner JE. Experimentally induced Tyzzer's disease in the African white-tailed rat (Mastomys albicaudatus). Lab Anim Sci 1986;36:492–495.

Waggie KS, Wagner JE and Kelley ST. Naturally occurring Bacillus piliformis infection (Tyzzer's disease) in guinea pigs. Lab Anim Sci 1986;36:504–506.

Webb DM, Harrington DD, Boehm PN. Bacillus piliformis infection (Tyzzer's disease) in a calf. J Am Vet Med Assoc 1987;191:431–434.

Whitwell KE. Four cases of Tyzzer's disease in foals in England. Equine Vet J 1976;8:118–122.

Wilkie JSN, Barker IK. Colitis due to Bacillus piliformis in two kittens. Vet Pathol 1985;22:649–652.

FILAMENTOUS CILIA-ASSOCIATED RESPIRATORY (CAR) BACILLUS

Currently unclassified, the filamentous cilia-associated respiratory (CAR) bacillus (unrelated to the genus containing *Bacillus anthracis*) is a respiratory pathogen of rats and mice. Hamsters infected experimentally develop mild disease, whereas guinea pigs and rabbits, which also can be experimentally infected, do not develop any lesions. The CAR bacillus, only recently cultured on artificial media, has been suggested to be related to the so-called "gliding bacteria." Based on sequencing, it is most closely related to *Flavobacterium ferrugineum* and *Flexibacter sancti*. The bacilli are gram-negative, PAS-positive, and agyrophilic and stain particularly well with the Warthin-Starry and Grocott's methods. CAR bacilli often complicate murine mycoplasmosis and respiratory viral diseases of rats and mice.

CAR bacillus colonizes the respiratory epithelium, particularly the ciliated epithelium of bronchi and bronchioles. The filamentous character of the bacilli resembles cilia and, with preparations stained with hematoxylin and eosin, may be impossible to differentiate from cilia, although with heavy infestation bacilli appear more prominent than normal cilia.

The lesions resemble those seen in murine mycoplasmosis with a marked lymphocytic and plasmacytic infiltration extending from the respiratory tree lamina propria into the pulmonary parenchyma, giving rise to thick collars of inflammatory cells. These may be bronchiectasis and atelectasis and foci of purulent pneumonia. Bronchial epithelium is focally thickened and disorganized and there may be proliferation of type II epithelial cells. Bronchial and mediastinal lymph nodes are hyperplastic. The nasal cavity, eustachian tube, and middle ear may also be affected.

A morphologically similar and antigenically related organism has been found in cattle. The only associated pathologic change noted was a decrease in the number of cilia.

References

Brogden KA, Cutlip RC, Lehmkuhl HD. Cilia-associated respiratory bacillus in wild rats in central Iowa. J Wildl Dis 1993;29:123–126.

Shoji-Darkye Y, Itoh T, Kagiyama N. Pathogenesis of CAR bacillus in rabbits, guinea pigs, Syrian hamsters, and mice. Lab Anim Sci 1991;41:567–571.

Hastie AT, Evans LP, Allen AM. Two types of bacteria adherent to bovine respiratory tract ciliated epithelium. Vet Pathol 1993;30:12–19.

Kurisu K, Kyo S, Shiomoto Y, et al. Cilia-associated respiratory bacillus infection in rabbits. Lab Anim Sci 1990;40:413–415.

Matsushita S. Ultrastructure of respiratory tract epithelium of rats experimentally infected with the CAR bacillus. J Vet Med Sci 1991;53:361–363.

Matsushita S, Joshima H. Pathology of rats intranasally inoculated with the cilia-associated respiratory bacillus. Lab Anim 1989;23:89–95.

Matsushita S, Joshima H, Matsumoto T, et al. Transmission experiments of cilia-associated respiratory bacillus in mice, rabbits and guinea pigs. Lab Anim 1989;23:96–102.

Schoeb TR, Dybvig K, Davidson MK, et al. Cultivation of cilia-associated respiratory bacillus in artificial medium and determination of the 16S rRNA gene sequence. J Clin Microbiol 1993;31:2751–2757.

Shoji Y, Itoh T, Kagiyama N. Pathogenicities of two CAR bacillus strains in mice and rats. Jikken Dobutsu 1988;37:447–453.

INFECTIONS CAUSED BY MORAXELLA ORGANISMS

Gram-negative cocci and coccobacilli are currently grouped in the family Neisseriaceae, which contains four genera, three of which are of interest because of their pathogenicity (*Neisseria*, *Branhamella*, and *Moraxella*); organisms in the genus *Acinetobacter* are saprophytic.

Moraxella bovis is the cause of infectious bovine keratoconjunctivitis. The frequent recovery of *M. bovis* from healthy conjunctivae caused considerable confusion and debate as to the importance of this organism as a pathogen, but it is now recognized that differing strains exist and that only piliated strains are capable of adhering to corneal epithelial cells and are associated with the disease. Other environmental factors are, however, important to precipitating development of disease. These include exposure to sunlight, dust, insects, and other infections. The disease occurs worldwide. *M. bovis* can be carried by resistant or recovered animals in the ocular and nasal tissues, providing a constant source for new infections.

The clinical features of this bovine disease are summarized as: acute onset of photophobia, excessive lacrimation, purulent blepharitis, ulceration with peripheral vascularization of the cornea, and iridospasm. The lesions usually heal, though often with a corneal scar. In severe cases, the cornea may rupture, leading to loss of an eye.

Microscopically, the lesions are not specific, however, organisms can be found within and on the surface of corneal and conjunctival epithelial cells and within necrotic tissue overlying ulcers. There is necrosis of corneal epithelium and an infiltrate of neutrophils and mononuclear cells.

Generalized and localized infections of piglets with a Moraxella species have been described in Denmark (Larsen, Billie, and Nielsen, 1973). Other species of *Moraxella* and *Branhamella* (a subgenus) have been associated with keratoconjunctivitis in several animal species, but their exact role as pathogens has not been determined.

References

Gerber JD, Frank SK. Enhancement of *Moraxella* bovis-induced keratitis of mice by exposure of the eye to ultraviolet radiation and ragweed extract. Am J Vet Res 1983;44:1382–1384.

Gerhardt RR, Allen JW, Greene WH, et al. The role of face flies in an episode of infectious bovine keratoconjunctivitis. J Am Vet Med Assoc 1982;180:156–159.

Jayappa HG, Lehr C. Pathogenicity and immunogenicity of pilated and nonpilated phases of *Moraxella bovis* in calves. Am J Vet Res 1986;47:2217–2221.

Kopecky KE, Pugh GW Jr, McDonald TJ. Influence of outdoor winter environment on the course of infectious bovine keratoconjunctivitis. Am J Vet Res 1981;42:1990–1992.

Larsen JL, Billie N, Nielsen NC. Occurrence and possible role of Moraxella species in pigs. Acta Pathol Microbiol Scand 1973;81B:181–186.

Nayar PSG, Saunders JR. Infectious bovine keratoconjunctivitis. I. Experimental production. Can J Comp Med 1975;39:22–31.

Pedersen KB. *Moraxella bovis* isolated from cattle with infectious keratoconjunctivitis. Acta Pathol Microbiol Scand 1970;78B:429–434.

Pugh GW Jr, Hughes DE, McDonald TJ. Bovine infectious keratoconjunctivitis: serological aspects of *Moraxella bovis* infection. Can J Comp Med 1971;35:161–166.

Pugh GW Jr, Hughes DE, Schulz VD, et al. Experimentally induced infectious bovine keratoconjunctivitis: resistance of vaccinated cattle to homologous and heterologous strains of *Moraxella bovis*. Am J Vet Res 1976;37:57–60.

Rogers DG, Cheville NF, Pugh GW Jr. [1] Pathogenesis of corneal lesions caused by *Moraxella bovis* in gnotobiotic calves. [2] Conjunctival lesions caused by *Moraxella bovis* in gnotobiotic calves. Vet Pathol 1987;24:287–295, 554–559.

Schurig GG, Lightfoot DR, Troutt HF, et al. Genotypic, phenotypic, and biological characteristics of *Moraxella bovis*. Am J Vet Res 1984;54:35–39.

Vandergaast N, Rosenbusch RF. Infectious bovine keratoconjunctivitis epizootic associated with area-wide emergence of a new *Moraxella bovis* pilus type. Am J Vet Res 1989;50:1437–1441.

VandeWoude SJ, Luzarraga MB. The role of *Branhamella catarrhalis* in the "bloody-nose syndrome" of cynomolgus monkeys. Lab Anim Sci 1992;41:401–406.

INFECTIONS CAUSED BY NEISSERIA ORGANISMS

Gram-negative cocci, in the genus *Neisseria* (family Neisseriaceae) are principally human pathogens, but some cause infection in animals. *Neisseria gonorrhoeae* ("gonococcus") is the cause of the human venereal disease, gonorrhea. The chimpanzee is susceptible to experimental exposure to this organism. *Neisseria meningitidis* ("meningococcus") is the cause of some cases of meningitis in human patients.

Several other species of Neisseria recovered from humans and a variety of animal species (cats, sheep, guinea pigs, rabbits, dolphins, and iguanas), usually from the oral cavity, are not considered pathogens. *N.*

canis has been associated with cat-bite infections in humans. *Neisseria ovis,* tentatively classified in this genus, has been recovered from the conjunctival sac of sheep with keratoconjunctivitis or with clinically normal cornea and conjunctiva. Pure cultures of this organism, injected into the cornea, only rarely produce any significant disease in sheep. The role of this organism as a sole pathogen for sheep remains in question.

References

Brown WJ, Lucas CT, Kuhn USG. Gonorrhea in the chimpanzee: infection with laboratory-passed gonococci and by natural transmission. Br J Vener Dis 1972;48:177–179.

Guibourdenche M, Lambert T, Riou JY. Isolation of *Neisseria canis* in mixed culture from a patient after a cat bite. J Clin Microbiol 1989;27:1673–1674.

Hoke C, Vedros NA. Characterization of "atypical" aerobic Gram-negative cocci isolated from humans. J Clin Microbiol 1982;15:906–914.

Plowman CA, Montali RJ, Phillips LG Jr, et al. Septicemia and chronic abscesses in iguanas (*Cyclura cornuta* and *Iguana iguana*) associated with a Neisseria species. J Zoo Anim Med 1987;18(2/3):86–93.

Spradbrow P. Experimental infection of the ovine cornea with *Neisseria ovis*. Vet Rec 1971;88:615–616.

DISEASES CAUSED BY SPIROCHAETALES ORGANISMS

These bacterial organisms, commonly called spirochetes, are currently grouped in one order, Spirochaetales, containing two families; Spirochaetaceae and Leptospiraceae (Table 10-9). The family Spirochaetaceae contains four genera, three of which contain species pathogenic for animals and humans. The family Leptospiraceae contains two genera, only one of which contains pathogens. In general, the organisms are slender, helically coiled, single-celled bacteria measuring 5 to

---

TABLE 10-9 Classification of Spirochaetales

Family I. Spirochaetaceae
  Genus I. *Spirochaeta*
       Six or more species free-living in water, sewage; none are pathogenic
  Genus II. *Cristispira*
       Many organisms found in marine and fresh water species of univalve and bivalve molluscs; none known to be pathogenic
  Genus III. *Treponema*
       Four pathogenic and nine (or more) nonpathogenic species (see Table 10-11)
  Genus IV. *Borrelia*
       Many species of varying pathogenicity (see Table 10-12)

Family II. Leptospiraceae
  Genus I. *Leptospira*
       One pathogenic species (*L. interrogans*), subdivided into several serogroups containing numerous serovars, which cause leptospirosis in humans and animals (see Table 10-10)

---

250 microns in length. They are motile by means of periplasmic flagella (periplasmic fibrils, axial filaments, axial fibrils, endoflagella), which are encased within the outer sheath of the organisms. They multiply by binary fission and are best observed by phase-contrast or dark-field microscopy and silver staining techniques. Specific species are causes of important diseases of humans (syphilis, yaws, pinta, relapsing fever, Lyme disease, leptospirosis) and animals (spirochetosis, leptospirosis, and borreliosis).

Leptospirosis

The genus Leptospira is currently composed of two species; *L. biflexa,* which is nonpathogenic, and the pathogenic species *L. interrogans.* The pathogenic species is composed of almost 200 different, but related, organisms. On the basis of serologic relatedness as determined by cross-agglutination and agglutinin-absorption tests, these species are divided into several serogroups (serotypes), such as *canicola, icterohaemorrhagiae,* and *pomona* (Fig.10-17). Within each serogroup there are multiple antigenically distinct organisms, which are referred to as serovars. The pathogenic serogroups and serovars are not limited to a single host species. The various serovars cause leptospirosis, a disease of humans and animals with varying clinical and pathologic manifestations. In all species, after an interval of bacteremia, the organisms parasitize the kidney where they multiply in the lumen of the proximal convoluted tubule and are excreted in the urine, providing the principal mode of transmission as well as leading to acute or chronic nephritis. Leptospira can remain viable in moist areas

for extended periods. Certain serovars are well adapted to their hosts (reservoir hosts) and remain in the kidney for long periods, serving as a constant source of infection to other members of the same species or accidentally infecting a species in which the organism is less well adapted, but in which more serious disease may result. For example, rats infected with serovar icterohaemorrhagiae shed the organism in urine for life with little or no ill effect to the host. Ordinarily disease, if present in the reservoir host, is limited to chronic nephritis. When dogs (and other susceptible species) are exposed to infectious rat urine, the same organism can cause serious disease (Fig. 10-18). Infection in these "accidentally" infected hosts can vary from subclinical to peracute. The incidence of infection in most species far exceeds the occurrence of overt disease. Clinical signs and lesions, which may be quite acute and severe, may develop during the bacteremic phase of infection, before localization in the kidneys (Figs. 10-19 and 10-20). The signs and lesions vary somewhat, depending on the species affected and the serogroup of leptospira, but include extensive hemorrhage, hemolytic anemia, hepatocellular damage leading to icterus, and abortion. In addition to the kidney, Leptospira may localize for extended periods in other tissues, including the uterus, where reproductive disorders follow, and the aqueous humor, where they have been associated with chronic or recurrent iridocyclitis.

Organisms in the genus Leptospira conform to the general characteristics of the family Spirochaetaceae and have some specific features. The spiral organisms are single, flexuous, and helical, with bent, hooked, or curved ends. Their dimensions are 6 to 20 μm or more

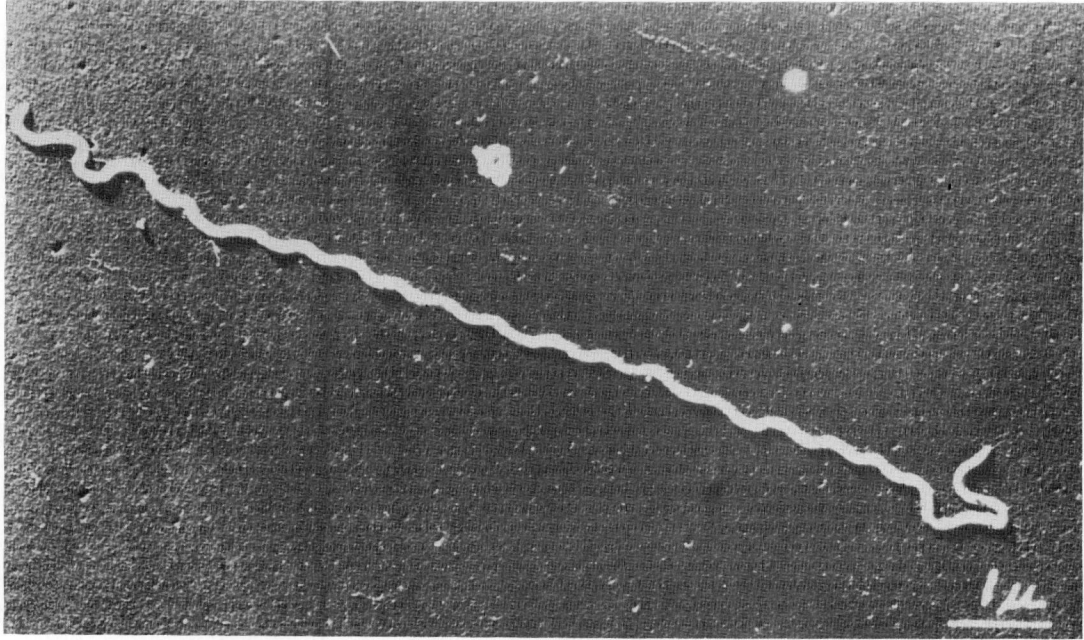

FIG. 10-17 Electron photomicrograph of Leptospira canicola. (Courtesy of Division of Veterinary Medicine, Walter Reed Army Institute of Research.)

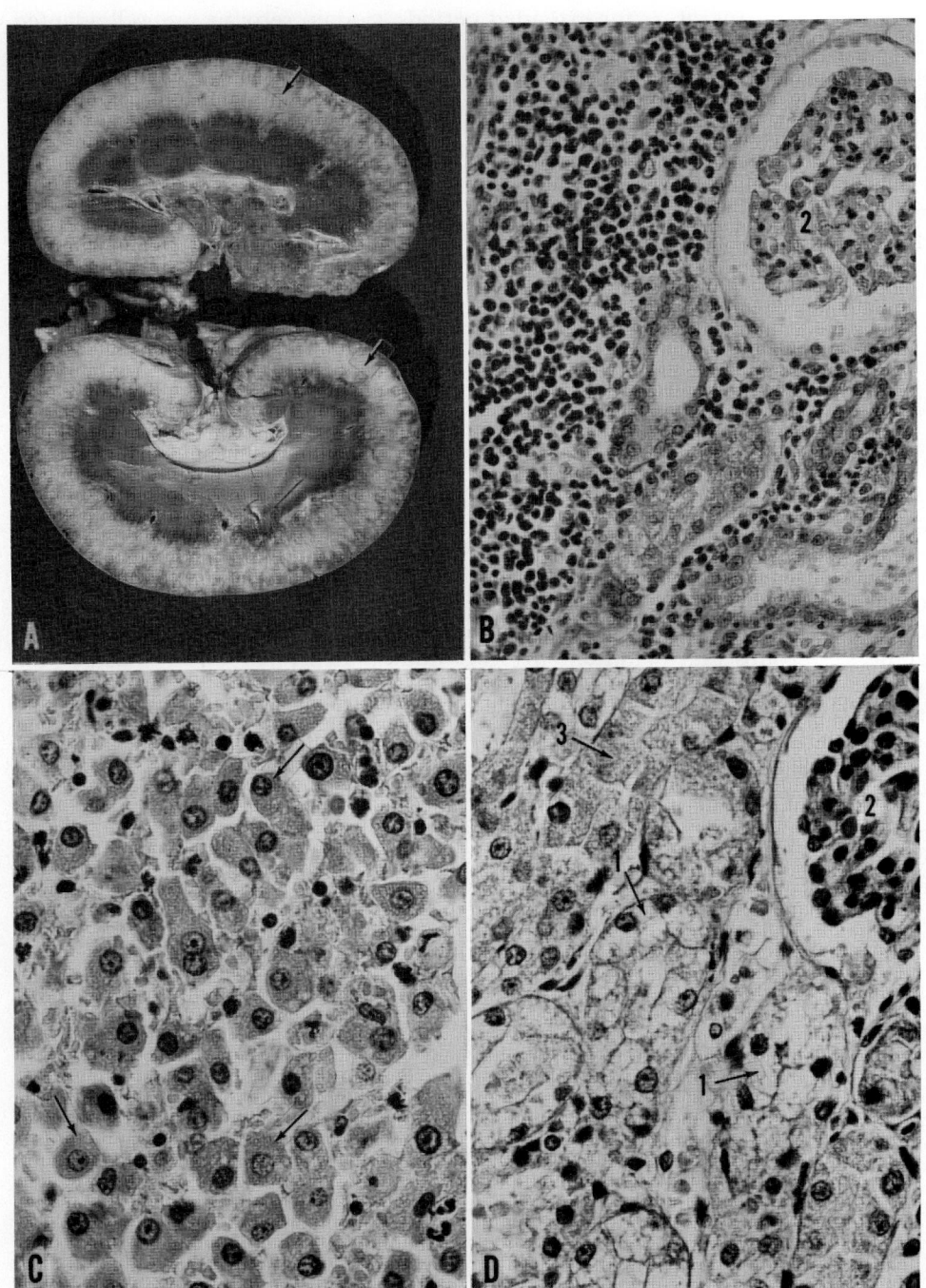

FIG. 10-18 Leptospirosis in the dog. **A.** Kidney of a dog with active infection following a subacute course. Note gray masses (arrows) replacing cortex. (Contributor: Dr. C. L. Davis.) **B.** Accumulation of lymphoid cells (1) in renal cortex in subacute case ($\times$ 260). Note glomerulus is spared. (Contributor: USAF Hospital, Lackland Air Force Base.) **C.** The liver in acute leptospirosis ($\times$ 490). Note dissociation of liver cells (arrows), which disrupts liver cell columns. **D.** The kidney in acute leptospirosis ($\times$ 490). Same dog as C. Note vacuoles in cytoplasm of some convoluted tubules (1). The glomerulus (2) and other convoluted tubules (3) are not affected. (Courtesy of Armed Forces Institute of Pathology.) Contributor: Division of Veterinary Medicine, Walter Reed Army Institute of Research.

in length by 0.1 μm in diameter. They are motile by means of periplasmic flagella (endoflagella, axial fibrils, or axial filaments), which are enclosed within an external sheath. They are best visualized by darkfield microscopy as well as the electron microscope. They may be stained with some silver-impregnation methods, but are not differently stained by aniline dyes.

The electron microscope reveals that the organisms consist of a cellular body wound on an axistyle with an external sheath surrounding both elements (Fig. 10-19). The cell body, approximately circular in transverse

section, contains nuclear material, cytoplasm, and a limiting cell membrane. The axistyle is a single structure, consisting of two filaments, each of which is inserted near one terminal end of the organism. The free ends are near the middle of the organism.

Leptospira are aerobic and may be cultivated on media containing inorganic salts, buffered with phosphates. Some media containing serum enhance the growth of certain serogroups.

Some of the more prevalent serogroups are listed in Table 10-10.

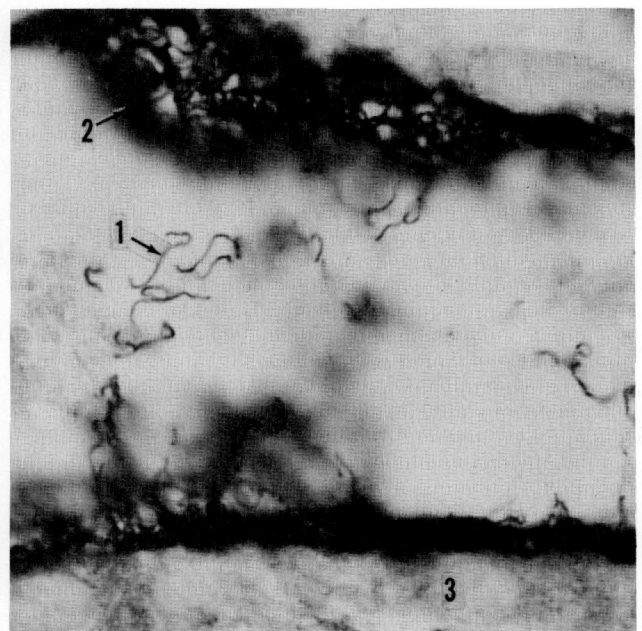

FIG. 10-19 Leptospirosis. Leptospira (× 1670) in the lumen (1) and in the epithelium (2 and 3) of a convoluted tubule, kidney of a dog with subacute infection. (Courtesy of Armed Forces Institute of Pathology.) Contributor: US Army Veterinary Research Laboratory.

References

Hanson LE: Leptospirosis in domestic animals: the public health perspective. J Am Vet Med Assoc 1982;181:1501–1509.

Johnson RC, Faine S. Genus I. Leptospira Noguchi 1917, 755. In: Krieg NR, Holt JG, ed. Bergey's Manual of Systematic Bacteriology. Vol. I. Baltimore: Williams & Wilkins 1984;62–67.

Songer JG, Thiermann AB. Leptospirosis. J Am Vet Med Assoc 1988;193:1250–1254.

Thiermann AB. Leptospirosis: current developments and trends. J Am Vet Med Assoc 1984;184:722–725.

CANINE LEPTOSPIROSIS

Leptospirosis in dogs can result from infection with several different serogroups of *Leptospira*. Serogroup *canicola* is the most common organism that infects dogs, the reservoir host for this serogroup, with transmission mainly occurring from dog to dog. Serogroup *icterohaemorrhagiae,* acquired from chronically infected rats, is also a frequent cause of leptospirosis in dogs, with members of other serogroups, such as *gryppotyphosa,* occurring sporadically. The incidence of infection, especially with serogroup *canicola,* far exceeds the incidence of clinical disease.

Leptospirosis in dogs may present, clinically and pathologically, as either an acute to peracute infection, with hemorrhage, hepatic dysfunction, and icterus as the predominant signs, or as a subacute nephritis. Usually the former is associated with serogroup *icterohaemorrhagiae,* and the latter with serogroup *canicola.* The two are, however, not distinct entities. Both organisms can be associated with either syndrome, and dogs recovering from the acute hepatic disease may succumb to uremia from nephritis. The acute disease is characterized by fever, hemorrhages, bloody diarrhea, vomiting, icterus, accelerated erythrocyte sedimentation rate, albuminuria, severe debilitation, and an often fatal outcome. The peracute form, with few signs other than hemorrhage, is most frequent in puppies. The nephritic form of the disease, known as **Stuttgart disease,** is characterized by typical signs of uremia and include "uremic" breath, ulcerative stomatitis, vomiting (often bloody), weight loss, dehydration, coma, and death.

Lesions For convenience, the lesions in these "acute" and "subacute" phases of the disease are described separately.

ACUTE PHASE LESIONS In dogs dying during the "acute" or septicemic stage of the disease, the lesions are dominated by severe dehydration and icterus, with many petechiae on the pleura, peritoneum, and nasal and oral mucosae. The liver usually exhibits characteristic microscopic changes, although few may be recognized grossly. The most striking lesion is in the liver cells, which shrink and become dissociated from one another, breaking up the normal columns of liver cells into individually discrete cells. This individualization of liver cells (Fig. 10-18) is not limited solely to leptospirosis, but is particularly striking in this disease. The affected liver cells often have coarsely granular, eosinophilic cytoplasm and small hyperchromic nuclei. Regeneration of liver parenchyma may at times be evidenced by binucleate cells, large hyperchromic nuclei, and mitotic figures. Foci of necrosis of liver parenchyma may be found. Bile retention is indicated by plugging of bile canaliculi, but larger bile ducts usually are empty. Kupffer cells contain large amounts of hemosiderin, and portal vessels are usually congested. Characteristic leptospirae may be demonstrated with appropriate silver impregnation technique. These organisms are seen in sinusoids and within liver cells as slender, tightly coiled, spiral organisms with hook-shaped ends (Fig. 10-19).

The changes in the kidney during this acute stage, except for grossly visible petechiae, may be somewhat subtle, but are definite and recognizable on careful microscopic examination. The glomeruli may show little change, but convoluted tubules are usually severely altered. The epithelial cells of the convoluted tubules in particular areas are swollen, coarsely granular, and deeply eosinophilic, or vacuolated and partially or completely desquamated into the lumen. In some tubules, only the bare basement membrane of the tubule is left. In others, the lumen is filled with eosinophilic epithelial cytoplasmic debris, in which are some nuclei and occasional erythrocytes. Some tubules may contain regenerating epithelium, as indicated by mitoses, hyperchromatic nuclei, and cells that coalesce to appear as multinucleated giant cells. Leptospirae are demonstrable singly or in small groups in affected tubules by use of silver impregnation techniques. Affected tubules are usually surrounded by lymphocytes, plasma cells, and occasional erythrocytes, which diffusely infiltrate the interstitial stroma.

Lymph nodes and spleen are usually grossly enlarged and may contain areas of edema and hemor-

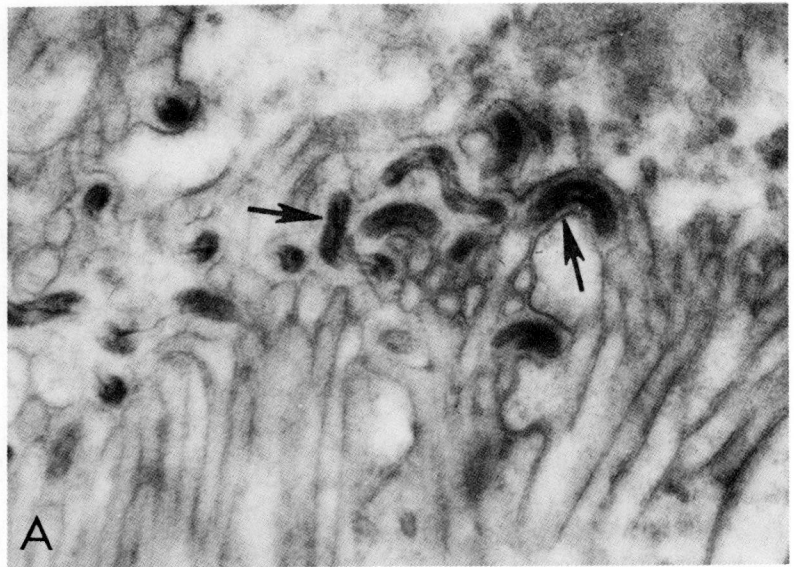

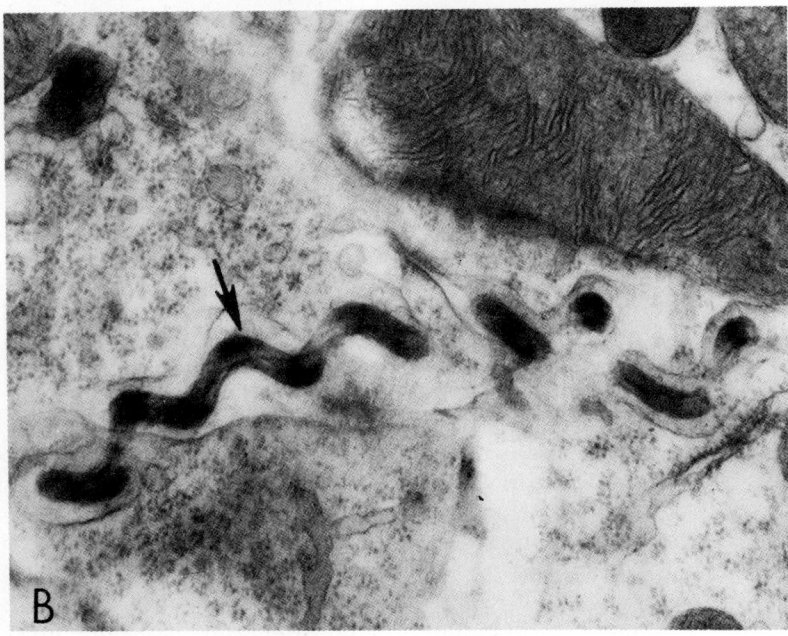

FIG. 10-20 Leptospirosis. **A.** *Leptospira pomona* closely associated with microvilli of a proximal convoluted tubule cell in the kidney of a hamster. **B.** *Leptospira pomona* within a proximal tubule cell in the kidney of a hamster. (Courtesy of Dr. N. G. Miller and American Journal of Veterinary Research.)

rhage. Microscopically, there is a paucity of mature lymphocytes and an apparent increase in reticular cells. Erythrocytes are often present in the medullary sinuses, either free or in macrophages. Diffuse hemorrhages are common in the fundic portion of the gastric mucosa, and may be associated with necrosis, neutrophilic infiltration, and desquamation of the mucosa. Hemorrhages also may be seen in the submucosa and less often in the muscularis. The intestine may contain small petechiae in the serosa and mucosa, but these are not so severe as those in the stomach, nor are the hemorrhages associated with necrosis.

Hemorrhages and areas of edema may be seen in other organs, such as myocardium, submucosa, and muscularis of the urinary bladder, adrenal gland, pancreas, gall bladder, and lung. In the lung, gross hemorrhages on the pleural surface may be particularly strik-

ing, the entire surface being covered with tiny spherical hemorrhages or larger ones a few millimeters in diameter.

SUBACUTE PHASE LESIONS Animals that live through or escape the "acute" septicemic form of the disease, only to die of uremia caused by renal involvement, may manifest a subacute course. At necropsy of such animals, dehydration, emaciation, and a strong "uremic" odor are observed, but icterus and hemorrhages are unusual. The renal lesions are most significant; those in other viscera are inconstant or related only to uremia. The kidneys are grossly enlarged, the surface usually is smooth, the capsule is tense and white or grayish, sometimes with hemorrhages showing through from the parenchyma. The renal parenchyma cuts with only slightly increased resistance, but the cut surface is moist and turgid, bulging away from the capsule. Petechiae may

TABLE 10-10 **Host/organism relationship for some of the Leptospira**

Serogroup	Serovar	Reservoir host	Other susceptible hosts
L. icterohaemorrhagiae	icterohaemorrhagiae	Rats, other wild mammals	Dogs, cattle, swine, humans
L. canicola	canicola	Dogs, wild mammals	Cattle, swine, humans
L. pomona	pomona	Swine, skunk	Cattle, sheep, horses, sea lions, humans
L. grippotyphosa	grippotyphosa	Raccoon, skunk	Cattle, swine, dogs
L. sejroe	hardjo balcanica	Cattle	Sheep, humans Cattle
L. australis	bratislava	Horses	
L. hebdomadis	szwajizak		Cattle

be seen anywhere on the cut surface, but the most striking changes usually are located at the corticomedullary junction. Here grayish masses of firm, turgid tissue replace the normal renal parenchyma. This gray tissue may form a wide band on the inner margin of the cortex or may obliterate most of the cortex. In animals sacrificed during recovery, these lesions may be focal in pattern.

The microscopic appearance of these lesions is characteristic. Convoluted tubules undergoing degenerative changes are surrounded or replaced by large dense masses of cells, including lymphocytes, plasma cells, macrophages, occasional neutrophils, and sometimes small nests of erythrocytes. Although convoluted tubules are severely affected, glomeruli are often spared or involved only secondarily. Except in cases treated with antibiotics, silver preparations demonstrate leptospirae in the lumen of tubules or in the cytoplasm of the tubular epithelium. The organisms occur singly or in tangled nests (Fig. 10-19).

Lesions resulting from uremia are found elsewhere in the body. They include severe gastric hemorrhages with microscopic deposits of calcium in the gastric mucosa and calcareous deposits in the walls of the aorta and large arteries (Chapter 21).

References

Bloom F. Histopathology of canine leptospirosis. Cornell Vet 1941;31:266–268.
Carlos ER, et al. Leptospirosis in the Philippines: canine studies. Am J Vet Res 1971;32:1451–1454.
Coffin DL, Maestrone G. Detection of leptospires by fluorescent antibody. Am J Vet Res 1962;23:159–164.
Jones TC, Roby TO, Davis CL, et al. Control of leptospirosis in war dogs. Am J Vet Res 1945;6:120–128.
Marler RJ, Cook JE, Kerr AI. Experimentally induced leptospirosis in coyotes (Canis latrans). Am J Vet Res 1979;40:1115–1119.
Meyer KF, Stewart-Anderson B, Eddie B. Canine leptospirosis in the United States. J Am Vet Med Assoc 1939;95:710–729.
Monlux WS. III. Clinical pathology of canine leptospirosis. Cornell Vet 1948;38:109–121.
Monlux WS. III. Pathology of canine leptospirosis. Cornell Vet 1948;38:199–208.
Morton HE, Anderson TF. Morphology of Leptospira icterohemorrhagiae and L. canicola as revealed by the electron microscope. J Bact 1943;45:143–146.
Moulton JE, Howarth JA. The demonstration of Leptospira canicola in hamster kidneys by means of fluorescent antibody. Cornell Vet 1957;57:523–532.
Thiermann AB. Canine leptospirosis in Detroit. Am J Vet Res 1980;41:1659–1661.

BOVINE LEPTOSPIROSIS

Leptospirosis in cattle is associated with a wide gamut of clinical signs and syndromes, which include hemolytic anemia, hemoglobinuria, icterus, mastitis, abortion, and nephritis. Several different serovars have been identified with disease in cattle: *hardjo,* for which cattle are the reservoir hosts; *pomona,* which is usually maintained by swine, but which is also well adapted to cattle; *icterohaemorrhagiae; grippotyphosa; canicola; szwajizak;* and *balcanica.*

Acute disease is most severe in calves and is principally characterized by hemolytic anemia. In animals that survive this phase or in which the bacteremic phase is subclinical, the leptospira localize in the kidneys, leading to interstitial nephritis. Abortion may occur during the acute or chronic phase of the infection and sometimes may occur in animals without any other signs of leptospirosis. Most often, abortion occurs in the latter half of pregnancy and is not associated with specific lesions in the placenta or fetus, although the fetus is usually autolyzed before being expelled. Mastitis is most often associated with serovar *hardjo*.

Lesions The disease in cattle in many respects parallels its counterpart in dogs. It may occur in an **acute septicemic form** or as a **chronic nephritic type** of disease. The latter is rarely fatal. The lesions in these two bovine types are similar to those observed in dogs.

In the acute case, icterus, a swollen yellowish liver, and petechiae are the principal gross findings, as in dogs. Hemolytic anemia, which is not a feature of the canine disease, accounts for hemoglobinuria and partially contributes to the icterus and hepatic lesions. Microscopic changes include portal hepatic lymphocytic infiltration, with splenic hemosiderosis in some outbreaks, and severe centrilobular necrosis of the liver caused by anemic anoxia in others. In certain outbreaks in Israel with organisms of the *grippotyphosa* serotype, leptospirosis took a protracted clinical course. The microscopic lesions included hepatic cell dissociation, cholangitis, and congestion and hemosiderosis of the spleen. In the kidneys, swelling and disorganization of convoluted tubular epithelium were associated with bile pigment and hemoglobin in the lumen.

Animals that survive the systemic disease have grayish to white focal lesions in the kidney parenchyma. These foci are usually discrete and scattered through the cortex, not concentrated at the corticomedullary junction, as is often the case in dogs. Microscopically, the principal lesions are based on changes in the tubular epithelium. The epithelial cells and affected tubules have granular, swollen, or vacuolated cytoplasm, sometimes associated with fragmentation of the cytoplasm and detachment of the cells. These affected tubules are surrounded by dense masses of leukocytes, chiefly lymphocytes and plasma cells. In some cases, syncytial giant cells of the Langhans' type have been described. Leptospirae are usually, but not constantly, demonstrable in sections impregnated with silver, located within affected tubular epithelium or in the lumen of the tubule.

References

Amatredo A. Bovine leptospirosis. Vet Bull 1975;43:875–891.

Baker JA, Little RB. Leptospirosis in cattle. J Exp Med 1948;88:295–307.

Burdin ML. Renal histopathology of *Leptospira grippotyphosa* in farm animals in Kenya. Res Vet Sci 1963;4:423–430.

Cordy DR, Jasper DE. The pathology of an acute hemolytic anemia of cattle in California associated with leptospira. J Am Vet Med Assoc 1952;120:175–178.

Ellis WA, Michna SW. Experimental leptospiral abortion in cattle. Vet Rec 1974;94:255.

Ellis WA, Thiermann AB. Isolation of leptospires from the genital tracts of Iowa cows. Am J Vet Res 1986;47:1694–1696.

Hadlow WJ, Stoenmer HG. Histopathologic findings in cows naturally infected with *Leptospira pomona*. Am J Vet Res 1955;16:45–56.

Imbabi SE, Sleight SD, Conner GH, et al. Experimental leptospirosis: *Leptospira canicola* infection in calves. Am J Vet Res 1967;28:413–419.

Langham RF, Morse EV, Morter RL. Pathology of experimental ovine leptospirosis. *Leptospira pomona* infections. J Infect Dis 1958;103:285–290.

Morsi HM, Shibley GP, Strother HL. Renal leptospirosis: challenge exposure of vaccinated and nonvaccinated cattle to *Leptospira ict-*

erohaemorrhagiae and *Leptospira canicola*. Am J Vet Res 1973;34:175–179.

Murphy JC, Jensen R. Experimental pathogenesis of leptospiral abortion in cattle. Am J Vet Res 1969;30:703–713.

Reinhard KR, Tierney WF, Roberts SJ. A study of two enzootic occurrences of bovine leptospirosis. Cornell Vet 1950;40:148–164.

Reinhard KR. A clinical pathologic study of experimental leptospirosis of calves. Am J Vet Res 1951;12:282–291.

Reinhard KR, Hadlow WJ. Experimental bovine leptospirosis—pathological, hematological, bacteriological and serological studies. Proc Am Vet Med Assoc 1954;205–216.

Thiermann AB, Handsaker AL. Experimental infection of calves with *Leptospira interrogans* serovar *hardjo:* conjunctival versus intravenous route of exposure. Am J Vet Res 1985;46:329–331.

PORCINE LEPTOSPIROSIS

Swine, as most other species, are susceptible to several serogroups of *Leptospira*. The most common pathogen is the serovar *pomona*, for which swine are the reservoir host. Most infections with this serovar are subclinical. Urinary excretion perpetuates the organism in swine and serves as a source of infection for other species, which are more severely affected, such as cattle and humans (in whom the disease has been termed swineherd's disease). Serovar *pomona* infection is primarily associated with chronic lymphocytic interstitial nephritis; this serovar along with others, such as *icterohaemorrhagiae* and *canicola,* are an important cause of abortion, stillbirths, and deaths of neonatal pigs. In young pigs, the latter two serovars can cause acute leptospirosis comparable to that seen in cattle, with hemolytic anemia, hemoglobinuria, hepatitis, and icterus.

Stillborn pigs and aborted fetuses, which are expelled mainly in the last third of gestation, are often macerated, precluding accurate examination. The most characteristic lesion in aborted fetuses and stillborns is focal necrosis of the liver, without significant cellular infiltration. Organisms can generally be isolated, but may be difficult to demonstrate in tissues.

References

Bolin CA, and Cassells JA. Isolation of *Leptospira interrogans* serovar *bratislava* from stillborn and weak pigs in Iowa. J Am Vet Med Assoc 1990;196:1601–1604.

Chaudhary RK, Fish NA, Barnum DA. Experimental infection with *L. pomona* in normal and immune piglets. Can Vet J 1966;7:106–112.

Cheville NF, Huhn R, Cutlip RC. Ultrastructure of renal lesions in pigs with acute leptospirosis caused by *Leptospira pomona*. Vet Pathol 1980;17:338–351.

Fennestead KL, Borg-Petersen C. Experimental leptospirosis in pregnant sows. J Infect Dis 1966;116:57–66.

Gochenour WS Jr, Johnson RV, Yager RH, et al. Porcine leptospirosis. Am J Vet Res 1952;13:158–160.

Hanson LE, Reynolds HA, Evans LV. Leptospirosis in swine caused by serotype *grippotyphosa*. Am J Vet Res 1971;32:855–860.

Langham RF, Morse EV, Morter RL. Experimental leptospirosis. V. *Leptospira pomona* infection in swine. Am J Vet Res 1958;19:395–400.

Michna SW, Campbell RSF. Leptospirosis in pigs: Epidemiology, microbiology and pathology. Vet Rec 1969;84:135–138.

Scanziani E, Sironi G, Mandelli G. Immunoperoxidase studies on leptospiral nephritis of swine. Vet Pathol 1989;26:442–444.

Sleight SD, Langham RF, Morter RL. Experimental leptospirosis: the early pathogenesis of *Leptospira pomona* infection in young swine. J Infect Dis 1960;106:262–269.

LEPTOSPIROSIS IN OTHER SPECIES

Serologic evidence indicates that leptospirosis is a relatively common infection in **horses,** but overt disease is rare. Serovars *icterohaemorrhagiae, pomona,* and *hardjo* have been associated with ill-defined febrile illnesses, abortion, periodic ophthalmia (Chapter 28), and rarely, icterus. Experimental inoculation with serovars *icterohaemorrhagiae* and *pomona* has been shown to result in a disease characterized by fever, hemolytic anemia, and icterus. In contrast to other genera, Leptospira do not establish themselves in the kidney with resultant excretion in urine, with the possible exception of serovar *bratislava,* for which horses may be the reservoir host.

Leptospirosis in **sheep and goats** resembles the disease in **cattle.** Acute hemolytic disease, abortion and interstitial nephritis have been the predominant conditions associated with leptospirosis in these species. Serovars *pomona* and *hardjo* have been the most frequently reported isolates.

Cats are susceptible to several leptospiral serovars, but infection has not been associated with clinical or pathologic changes.

New World and Old World **monkeys** are susceptible to leptospirosis, but reports of spontaneous disease are rare. Leptospirosis has also been reported in **great apes.** Acute hepatic disease, abortion and nephritis have been the principal findings.

Serovar *pomona* has been associated with illness, abortions, and stillbirths among **Californa sea lions.**

Most laboratory **rodents** are susceptible, but leptospirosis is not an important spontaneous disease. Wild rodents carrying Leptospira can serve as reservoirs of infection for many species of animals and humans.

References

Arean VM. The pathologic anatomy and pathogenesis of fatal human leptospirosis (Weil's disease). Am J Pathol 1962;40:393–423.

Bryans JT. Studies on equine leptospirosis. Cornell Vet 1955;45:16–50.

Carlos ER, et al. Leptospirosis in the Philippines: feline studies. Am J Vet Res 1971;32:1455–1456.

Davidson JN, Hirsh DC. Leptospirosis in lambs. J Am Vet Med Assoc 1980;176:124–125.

Ellis WA, O'Brien JJ, Cassells JA, et al. Leptospiral infection in horses in Northern Ireland: serological and microbiological findings. Equine Vet J 1983;15:317–320.

Famatiga EG. Leptospirosis in Philippine monkeys. Southeast Asian J Trop Med 1973;4:316–318.

Fear FA, et al. A leptospirosis outbreak in baboon (*Papio* sp.) colony. Lab Anim Care 1968;18:22–28.

Hartley WJ. Ovine leposirosis. Aust Vet J 1952;28:169–170.

Lucke VM, Crowther ST. The incidence of leptospiral agglutination titres in the domestic cat. Vet Rec 1965;77:647–648.

Marshall RB. Ultrastructural changes in renal tubules of sheep following experimental infection with *Leptospira interrogans* serotype *pomona.* J Med Microbiol 1974;7:505–508.

Michna SW, Campbell RSF. Leptospirosis in wild animals. J Comp Pathol 1970;80:101–106.

Minette HP. Leptospirosis in primates other than man. Am J Trop Med Hyg 1966;15:190–198.

Minette HP, Shaffer MF. Experimental leptospirosis in monkeys. Am J Trop Med Hyg 1968;17:202–212.

Roberts SJ. Sequelae of leptospirosis in horses on a small farm. J Am Vet Med Assoc 1958;133:189–194.

Roth EE. Leptospirosis in wildlife in the United States. Proc Am Vet Med Assoc 1964;211–218.

Shive RJ, et al. Leptospirosis in Barbary apes *(Macaca sylvana).* J Am Vet Med Assoc 1969;155:1176–1178.

Smith AW, Brown RJ, Skilling DE, et al. *Leptospira pomona* and reproductive failure in California sea lions. J Am Vet Med Assoc 1974;165:996–999.

Smith BP, Armstrong JM. Fatal hemolytic anemia attributed to leptospirosis in lambs. J Am Vet Med Assoc 1975;167:739–741.

Smith RE, Williams IA, Kingsbury ET. Serologic evidence of equine leptospirosis in the Northeast United States. Cornell Vet 1976;66:105–109.

Smith RE, Reynolds IM, Sakai T. Experimental leptospirosis in pregnant ewes. III. Pathologic features. Cornell Vet 1960;50:115–122.

Songer JG, Chilelli CJ, Reed RE, et al. Leptospirosis in rodents from an arid environment. Am J Vet Res 1983;44:1973–1976.

Tripathy DN, Hanson LE, Mansfield ME, et al. Experimental infection of lactating goats with *Leptospira interrogans* serovars *pomona* and *hardjo.* Am J Vet Res 1985;46:2512–2514.

Tripathy DN, Hanson LE, Bedoya M, et al. Experimental infection of pregnant and lactating goats with *Leptospira interrogans* serovars *hardjo* and *swajizak.* Am J Vet Res 1985;46:2515–2518.

Vedros NA, et al. Leptospirosis epizootic among California sea lions. Science 1971;172:1250–1251.

Verma BB, Biberstein EL, Meyer ME. Serologic survey of leptospiral antibodies in horses in California. Am J Vet Res 1977;38:1443–1444.

Watson ADJ, Wannan JS. The incidence of leptospiral agglutinins in domestic cats in Sydney. Aust Vet J 1973;49:545.

Yager RH, Gochenour WS Jr, Wetmore PW. Recurrent iridocyclitis (periodic ophthalmia) of horses. I. Agglutination and lysis of leptospiras by serums deriving from horses affected with recurrent iridocyclitis. J Am Vet Med Assoc 1950;117:207–209.

TREPONEMAL INFECTIONS

Treponema organisms are most significant as pathogens of humans; *T. pallidum,* the cause of syphilis, is the most important (Table 10-11). Two are of consequence as causes of disease in animals, *T. hyodysenteriae,* the cause of swine dysentery, and *T. paraluis-cuniculi,* the cause of venereal spirochaetosis of rabbits. There are several nonpathogenic species, which are commensals of humans and animals. The Treponema species are gram-negative, but are best visualized in tissue sections with silver impregnation staining methods. In wet smears or cultures, dark field illumination is best. They are helical in shape, 5 to 20 micrometers in length, motile by means of periplasmic flagella, and anaerobic.

References

Brandt AM. The syphilis epidemic and its relation to AIDS. Science 1988;239:375–380.

Kajdacsy-Balla A, Howeedy A, Bagasra O. Syphilis in the syrian hamster: a model of human venereal and congenital syphilis. Am J Pathol 1987;126:599–601.

Sell S, Baker-Zander S, Powell HC. Experimental orchitis in rabbits: ultrastructural appearance of *Treponema pallidum* during phagocytosis and dissolution by macrophages in vivo. Lab Invest 1982;46:355–364.

Swine dysentery (porcine ulcerative spirochaetosis)

Although swine dysentery was recognized as a clinical entity over 50 years ago, it was not until the 1970s that *T. hyodysenteriae* was established as the cause. The disease can be reproduced by administration of pure cul-

---

TABLE 10-11 **Diseases caused by *Treponema* organisms**

Organism	Disease and host
T. pallidum	Syphilis in humans; Syrian hamsters and rabbits susceptible to experimental exposure
T. pertenue	Yaws of humans; rabbits and hamsters susceptible; guinea pigs refractory
T. carateum	Pinta or Carate in humans; chimpanzees susceptible; rabbits, hamsters, and guinea pigs resistant
T. paraluis-cuniculi	Venereal spirochaetosis of rabbits (rabbit spirochaetosis); latent infection can be produced in mice, guinea pigs, and hamsters
T. hyodysenteriae	Swine dysentery
T. denticola	Nonpathogenic commensal of oral cavity of humans and chimpanzees
T. vincentii, scoliodontum	Nonpathogenic commensal of oral cavity of humans
T. refringens	Nonpathogenic commensal of genital tract of humans and animals
T. minutum	Nonpathogenic commensal of genital tract of humans
T. phagedenis	Nonpathogenic commensal of genital tract and anal areas of humans and chimpanzees
T. succinifaciens	Nonpathogenic commensal of colon of swine
T. bryantii	Nonpathogenic; isolated from bovine rumen
T. innocens	Nonpathogenic; isolated from intestinal tract of swine and dogs

tures of *T. hyodysenteriae,* but much remains to be learned of the pathogenetic mechanisms, because the disease cannot be reproduced in gnotobiotic pigs unless certain other "normal" colonic bacteria are also introduced. These include the enteric anaerobe *Bacteroides vulgatus* and another anaerobe, *Fusobacterium necrophorum.*

The disease is spread by recovered swine, which may carry the organism for several months after recovery, and by wild rodents, which can carry the organism without clinical disease. The organism is easily spread among rodents and, experimentally, can lead to typhlitis in mice. *T. hyodysenteriae* does not survive well in the environment. On ingestion, the organism establishes itself in colonic epithelium and goblet cells but does not invade deeper. Infection leads to diarrhea containing mucus and blood. Within a herd, morbidity rates of up to 90% with mortality rates of up to 50% result from dehydration and electrolyte imbalance. Piglets 8 to 14 weeks of age are the most susceptible.

LESIONS
The lesions are restricted to the colon, cecum, and rectum, but they are most constant and severe in the spiral colon. The affected mucosa is folded and rugose, covered with a fibrinous mucinous exudate with foci of hemorrhage and, eventually, ulcers. Microscopically, the mucosa is particularly involved; initially it is thickened, but then the superficial cells become necrotic and are sloughed. The fibrinous mucous exudate becomes conspicuous on the surface. Mucus lost from the goblet cells fills the crypts. The lamina propria becomes distended with leukocytes as epithelial cells are lost. Crypts and epithelial cells contain many spirochaetes. Other organisms, including *Vibrio coli* may exist in large numbers in the lumen of the crypts and among tissue debris in the lumen.

DIAGNOSIS
The diagnosis is established by the nature of the lesions and by demonstrating the spirochaetes in the colonic mucosa, using silver stains, immunofluorescent techniques, or electron microscopy.

References
Akkermans JPWM, Pomper W. Aetiology and diagnosis of swine dysentery. Tijdschr Diergeneeskd 1973;98:649–654.

Fisher LF, Olander HJ. Shedding of *Treponema hyodysenteriae,* transmission of disease, and agglutinin response of pigs convalescent from swine dysentery. Am J Vet Res 1981;42:450–455.

Hamdy AH, Glenn MW. Transmission of swine dysentery with *Treponema hyodysenteriae* and *Vibrio coli.* Am J Vet Res 1974;35:791–798.

Harcourt RA. Porcine ulcerative spirochaetosis. Vet Rec 1973;92:647–648.

Harris DL, Glock RD. Swine dysentery. J Am Vet Med Assoc 1972;160:561–565.

Harris DL, Glock RD, Christensen CR, Kinyon JM. Swine dysentery. I. Inoculation of pigs with *Treponema hyodysenteriae* (new species) and reproduction of the disease. Vet Med Small Anim Clin 1972;67:61–64.

Harris DL, et al. Swine dysentery: Studies of gnotobiotic pigs inoculated with *Treponema hyodysenteriae, Bacteroides vulgatus,* and *Fusobacterium necrophorum.* J Am Vet Med Assoc 1978;172:468–471.

Hughes R, Olander HJ, Gallina AM, et al. Swine dysentery. Induction and characterization in isolated colonic loops. Vet Pathol 1972;9:22–37.

Hughes R, Olander HJ, Williams CB. Swine dysentery: Pathogenicity of *Treponema hyodysenteriae.* Am J Vet Res 1975;36:971–978.

Hughes R, Olander HJ, Kanitz DL, et al. A study of swine dysentery by immunofluorescence and histology. Vet Pathol 1977;14:490–507.

Joens LA. Experimental transmission of *Treponema hyodysenteriae* from mice to pigs. Am J Vet Res 1980;41:1225–1226.

Kennedy GA, Strafuss AC. Scanning electron microscopy of the lesions of swine dysentery. Am J Vet Res 1976;37:395–401.

Meyer RC, Simon J, Byerly CS. The etiology of swine dysentery. I. Oral inoculation of germ-free swine with *Treponema hyodysenteriae* and *Vibrio coli.* Vet Pathol 1974;11:515–526.

Meyer RC, Simon J, Byerly CS. The etiology of swine dysentery. II.

Effect of known microbial flora, weaning and diet on disease production in gnotobiotic and conventional swine. Vet Pathol 1974;11:527–534.

Wilcock BP, Olander HJ. Studies on the pathogenesis of swine dysentery. I. Characterization of the lesions in colons and colonic segments inoculated with pure cultures or colonic contents containing *Treponema hyodysenteriae*. Vet Pathol 1979;16:450–465.

Venereal spirochaetosis of rabbits (treponematosis of rabbits, rabbit syphilis, cuniculosis, vent disease)

A natural disease of domesticated rabbits, caused by *Treponema paraluis-cuniculi (T. cuniculi),* should be distinguished from the infection produced experimentally in rabbits by injection of *Treponema pallidum* from lesions of human syphilis. The rabbit spirochaetosis is readily transmitted by coitus and may spread rapidly through a breeding colony of rabbits (Small and Newman, 1972).

LESIONS

Initial lesions develop on the vulva and preputial skin and may then extend throughout the perineum. Lesions may also appear on the skin of the face, nostrils, eyelids, and ears from either direct contact or spirochaetemia. Beginning as tiny, slightly raised, erythematous lesions, they progress to tiny vesicles followed by ulcers and, ultimately, raised areas of hyperkeratosis. The vesicles contain treponemes, which are demonstrable by dark-field examination. Lesions may not regress for months.

Microscopically, there is marked acanthosis and hyperkeratosis of the epidermis along with foci of necrosis, vesiculation, microabscesses, and ulceration. Underlying the dermis there is an infiltration of lymphocytes, macrophages, and heterophils. Lymph nodes may contain many nests of epithelioid cells, which replace much of the lymphocytic tissue. Orchitis can be induced experimentally.

DIAGNOSIS

The diagnosis may be established by the demonstration of treponemes in darkfield preparations. The organisms are difficult to demonstrate in tissue sections with silver stains. Serologic tests useful in detecting infection in a colony include the use of a fluorescent treponemal antigen and a rapid plasma reagin card.

References

Bayon H. A new species of Treponema found in the genital sores of rabbits. Br Med J 1913;2:1159.

Cunliffe-Beamer TL, Fox RR. Venereal spirochetosis of rabbits: [1] Description and diagnosis. [2] Epizootiology. [3] Eradication. Lab Anim Sci 1981;31:366–371, 372–378, 379–381.

DiGiacomo RF, Talburt CD, Lukehart SA, et al. *Treponema paraluis-cuniculi* infection in a commercial rabbitry: epidemiology and serodiagnosis. Lab Anim Sci 1983;33:562–566.

Hougen KH, Birch-Andersen A, Jensen HJS. Electron microscopy of *Treponema cuniculi*. Acta Pathol Microbiol Scand (B) 1973; 1:15–26.

Noguchi H. Venereal spirochaetosis in American rabbits. J Exp Med 1922;35:391–408.

Small JD, Newman B. Venereal spirochetosis of rabbits (rabbit syphilis) due to *Treponema cuniculi*: a clinical, serological, and histopathological study. Lab Anim Sci 1972;22:77–89.

Smith JL, Pesetsky BR. The current status of *Treponema cuniculi*: Review of the literature. Br J Vener Dis 1967;43:117–127.

Warthin AS, Buffington E, Wanstrom RC. A study of rabbit spirochaetosis. J Infect Dis 1923;32:315–332.

Borreliosis

Spirochaetal organisms of the genus *Borrelia* have been identified in epidemic and endemic relapsing fever in humans, Lyme disease, avian spirochaetosis, and many lice and ticks (Table 10-12). Several isolates, recovered from ticks in widely scattered parts of the world, have been assigned species names that future studies may prove to be unwarranted. Until these organisms can be compared, their taxonomic relationships remain unsettled.

RELAPSING FEVER (LOUSEBORNE AND TICKBORNE RELAPSING FEVER OF HUMANS)

Relapsing fever of humans occurs as **louse-borne relapsing fever,** caused by *Borrelia recurrentis,* and **tick-borne relapsing fever,** caused by several species of Borrelia (Table 10–12). The louseborne disease is the most serious. Both are characterized by periodic intervals of febrile disease with a rash, separated by an interval of about a week free of symptoms. The diseases resemble Rocky Mountain spotted fever (Chapter 9, *Rickettsia*) both clinically and pathologically. Louse-borne relapsing fever has been reproduced in African green monkeys (*Cercopithecus aethiops*), in which the organism causes a clinical course and pathologic lesions similar to those of the human disease.

Signs Initially, fever, inactivity, and leukocytosis are associated with spirochaetes circulating in the blood. After the initial infection, lasting 4 to 7 days, the signs subside, but relapses then follow after 4 to 6 days of remission. Convalescence may last up to 22 days; death may occur during the first episode, but it is more likely during the second or third remission. (Judge and others, 1974).

Lesions The lesions in Grivet monkeys are similar to those in humans, with severe purulent myocarditis, focal necrosis, and leukocytic infiltration in spleen and liver. Infarcts in the spleen are also frequent. Spirochaetal organisms may be seen in the lesions of each organ (Judge and others, 1974).

LYME DISEASE (LYME BORRELIOSIS)

Lyme disease was first reported as a clinical entity in humans in 1977 as a peculiar form of arthritis occurring in Lyme, Connecticut. The disease is now recognized to occur throughout the United States, Europe, Asia, and Australia. Further, retrospective inquiries indicate that the disease has existed for several decades in Europe and probably elsewhere. The disease is now recognized as a complicated multisystem syndrome caused by *Borrelia burgdorferi,* a spirochaetal organism first isolated and associated with the disease in 1982 by Burgdorfer and colleagues.

The spirochete is transmitted by *Ixodes* ticks: *I. dam-*

TABLE 10-12 **Diseases caused by *Borrelia* organisms**

Organism	Genus and species of vector	Geographic distribution	Disease(s)
B. anserina	Argus persicus, A. reflexus, A. miniatus, others	Worldwide	Avian borreliosis; borreliosis or spirochaetosis of birds
B. burgdorferi	Ixodes dammini, I. scapularis, I. pacificus	United States	Lyme disease
	I. ricinus	Europe	_____
	I. persulcatus	Asia	_____
B. recurrentis	Pediculus humanus (body louse)	Potentially cosmopolitan	Human epidemic relapsing fever (louse-borne fever)
B. hispanica	Ornithodorus erraticus	Middle East and Mediterranean areas	Human endemic relapsing fever (tick-borne fever)
B hermsii	O. hermsi	North America	Human endemic relapsing fever (tick-borne fever)
B. duttonii	O. moubata	Africa	Human endemic relapsing fever (tick-borne fever)
B. parkeri	O. parkeri	North America	Human endemic relapsing fever (tick-borne fever)
B. venezuelensis	O. rudis	South America	Human endemic relapsing fever (tick-borne fever)
B. mazzottii	O. talaje	Mexico and Guatemala	Human endemic relapsing fever (tick-borne fever)
B. persica	O. tholozani	Central Asia and Middle East	Human endemic relapsing fever (tick-borne fever)
B. turicatae	O. turicata	North and South America	Human endemic relapsing fever (tick-borne fever)
B. latyschewii	O. tartakovskyi	Central Asia	Human endemic relapsing fever (tick-borne fever)
B. caucasica	O. verrucosus	Caucasus	Human endemic relapsing fever (tick-borne fever)
B. braziliensis	O. braziliensis	Brazil	Human endemic relapsing fever (tick-borne fever)
B. dugesii	Ornithodoros dugesi	Mexico	Human endemic relapsing fever (tick-borne fever)
B. graingeri	O. graingeri	East Africa	Human endemic relapsing fever (tick-borne fever)
B. crocidurae	O. erraticus, sonrai	Africa, Near East, and Central Asia	Mildly pathogenic for humans
B. harveyi	Unknown	Africa	Mildly pathogenic for humans, monkeys, mice, rats
B. tillae	O. zumpti	South Africa	Borreliosis in rats, mice, monkeys
B. theileri	Rhipicephalus decoloratus, R. evertsi, Boophilus micropus	South Africa and Australia	Borreliosis of cattle and horses

mini in the northeastern and midwestern United States; *I. scapularis* in southeast United States; *I. pacificus* in western United States; *I. ricinis* in Europe; and *I. persulcatus* in Asia. Although the organisms have been identified in other insects, they have not been proven to be important as transmitters of the disease. The organism is maintained in the white-footed mouse, *Peromyscus leucopus,* which is the preferred host for the larvae and nymph stages of the tick. The mice serve as the reservoir hosts for *B. burgdorferi,* carrying the spirochete without developing any disease. Serologic studies have shown that a number of different wild rodents, deer, and other animals are susceptible to infection but probably do not participate in perpetuation of the disease. Ducks have been shown to be susceptible and capable of shedding the organism in their droppings. The adult ticks feed on white-tailed deer, which are important to the tick cycle but not as reservoir hosts for the spirochete. The ticks parasitize humans and domestic animals, although they are not the preferred hosts.

Lyme disease is most important in humans, where in many respects it resembles syphilis. Initial infection is characterized by an expanding pruritic skin rash referred to as **localized erythema migrans,** which usually resolves in 3 to 4 weeks but may last for several months and resolve only to recur. The initial signs are referred to as **Stage 1** or the **localized stage** of the disease. It may be accompanied by headache, musculoskeletal discomfort, and regional lymphadenopathy. This may be followed by **Stage 2** or a **disseminated stage,** which appears several days or weeks later. Disseminated infection is associated with a multiplicity of signs, which include: secondary dermatitis; myocarditis with arrhythmias (especially atrioventricular heart block); pericarditis; neurologic signs of meningitis, severe headache, Bell's palsy, radiculoneuritis, and ataxia; ophthalmitis; myalgia and arthralgia; hepatitis; orchitis; lymphadenopathy; and severe fatigue. This stage lasts weeks to months. **Late infection** or **Stage 3,** also referred to as **persistent infection,** occurs one or more years after the initial signs and is principally characterized by chronic arthritis, most commonly of one to a few large joints, particularly the knee. Chronic cardiac and central nervous system manifestations are also features of this stage.

Lesions The lesions have not yet been well characterized; however, at all stages the various affected tissues are infiltrated with lymphoblasts and plasma cells, and there is often an associated vasculitis. Polyclonal lymphoplasmacytic cells are found in the cerebrospinal fluid of patients with Lyme disease meningopolyneuritis. There may be necrosis (as well as cellular infiltration) in lymph nodes and the spleen. Arthritis is characterized by proliferative synovitis, fibrinaceous deposits, and aggregates of lymphoblasts, plasma cells, and mast cells. Late in its course, there are erosions of cartilage and bone.

Organisms are most demonstrable (using silver staining or immunologic staining methods) in the early skin lesions. In stage 2 or 3 lesions, it is unusual to locate or recover the spirochete, although, on occasion, they have been demonstrated. They are extracellular, often around or within blood vessels. The pathogenesis of the lesions is still to be elucidated, but immune mechanisms are thought to play an important role in both the initial and chronic lesions. The occurrence of chronic arthritis in Lyme disease has been associated with specific alleles of the major histocompatibility complex, indicating that it may result from immune responses in genetically susceptible people.

Serologic evidence of infection with *Borrelia burgdorferi* has been documented in several domestic animals (dogs, horses, and cattle). In some surveys, the incidence has exceeded 50%. None of the domestic species are considered reservoirs for Borrelia species. A variety of clinicopathologic findings have been suggested as caused by the spirochete in animals: arthritis (one of the most consistently associated lesions); encephalitis; uveitis; myocarditis; heart block; hepatitis; pneumonia; lymphadenopathy; lymphoblastic/plasmacytic infiltration of various tissues; and immune complex glomerulonephritis. This list is comparable to many of the manifestations of the disease found in humans. *B. burgdorferi* has been isolated or specifically demonstrated in conjunction with the lesions in several reported examples, but in many cases, the organism cannot be demonstrated or isolated. This is also comparable to the experience with human infection. Most attempts to experimentally reproduce disease in animals have established infection but have not resulted in lesions. Arthralgia, fever, and depression have followed experimental infection of dogs, and these results have been reproduced in rats and hamsters. The true significance of Lyme disease in domestic animals remains to be elucidated.

References

Anonymous. Lyme disease in Europe. Lancet 1987; 264–265.

Barthold SW, et al. Experimental Lyme arthritis in rats infected with *Borrelia burgdorferi.* J Infect Dis 1988;157:842–846.

Bernard WV, Cohen D, Bosler E, et al. Serologic survey for *Borrelia burgdorferi* antibody in horses referred to a mid-Atlantic veterinary teaching hospital. J Am Vet Med Assoc 1990;196:1255–1258.

Burgdorfer W, et al. Lyme disease—a tick-borne spirochetosis? Science 1982;216:1317–1319.

Burgdorfer W. Discovery of the Lyme disease spirochete and its relation to tick vectors. Yale J Biol Med 1984;57:515–520.

Burgess EC. Natural exposure of Wisconsin dogs to the Lyme disease spirochete *(Borrelia burgdorferi).* Lab Anim Sci 1986;36:288–290.

Burgess EC. *Borrelia burgdorferi* infection in Wisconsin horses and cows. Ann NY Acad Sci 1988;539:235–243.

Burgess EC, Mattison M. Encephalitis associated with *Borrelia burgdorferi* infection in a horse. J Am Vet Med Assoc 1987;191:1457–1458.

Burgess EC, Gendron-Fitzpatrick A, Wright WO. Arthritis and systemic disease caused by *Borrelia burgdorferi* infection in a cow. J Am Vet Med Assoc 1987;191:1468–1470.

Burgess EC, Gillette D, Pickett JP. Arthritis and panuveitis as manifestations of *Borrelia burdorferi* infection in a Wisconsin pony. J Am Vet Med Assoc 1986;189:1340–1342.

Cohen D, et al. Epidemiologic studies of Lyme disease in horses and their public health significance. Ann NY Acad Sci 1988;539:244–257.

Duray PH. Clinical pathologic correlations of Lyme disease. Rev Infect Dis 1989;11(Suppl 6):S1487–S1493.

Duray PH. Histopathology of clinical phases of human Lyme disease. Rheum Dis Clin North Am 1989;15:691–710.

Grauer GF, Burgess EC, Cooley AJ, et al. Renal lesions associated with

Borrelia burgdorferi infection in a dog. J Am Vet Med Assoc 1988;193:237–239.

Greene RT, et al. Clinical and serologic evaluations of induced *Borrelia burgdorferi* infection in dogs. Am J Vet Res 1988;49:752–757.

Hechemy PKE. Lyme disease: a review. Bull Soc Pathol Exot Filiales 1986;79:9–21.

Hejka A, Schmitz JL, England DM, et al. Histopathology of Lyme arthritis in LSH hamsters. Am J Pathol 1989;134:1113–1123.

Hulinska D, Jirous J, Valesova M, et al. Ultrastructure of *Borrelia burgdorferi* in tissues of patients with Lyme disease. J Basic Microbiol 1989;29(2):73–83.

Kornblatt AN, Urband PH, Steere AC. Arthritis caused by *Borrelia burgdorferi* in dogs. J Am Vet Med Assoc 1985;186:960–964.

Lastavica CC, Wilson ML, Berardi VP, et al. Rapid emergence of a focal epidemic of Lyme disease in coastal Massachusetts. N Engl J Med 1989;320:133–137.

Lissman BA, Bosler EM, Camay H, et al. Spirochete-associated arthritis (Lyme disease) in a dog. J Am Vet Med Assoc 1984;185:219–220.

Magnarelli LA, Anderson JF, Kaufmann AF, et al. Borreliosis in dogs from southern Connecticut. J Am Vet Med Assoc 1985;186:955–959.

Magnarelli LA, Anderson JF, Schreier AB, et al. Clinical and serologic studies of canine borreliosis. J Am Vet Med Assoc 1987;191:1089–1094.

Post JE, Shaw EE, Wright SD. Suspected borreliosis in cattle. Ann NY Acad Sci 1988;539:488. [Vet Bull 1990;60:1495]

Reotutar R. The ominous spread of *Borrelia burgdorferi* infection. J Am Vet Med Assoc 1989;194:1387–1391.

Roush JK, Manley PA, Dueland RT. Rheumatoid arthritis subsequent to Borrelia burgdorferi infection in two dogs. J Am Vet Med Assoc 1989;195:951–953.

Steere AC. Lyme disease. N Engl J Med 1989;321:586–596.

Steere AC, et al. Lyme athritis: an epidemic of oligoarticular arthritis in children and adults in three Connecticut communities. Arthritis Rheum 1977;20:7–17.

Wasmoen TL, et al. Examination of Koch's postulates for *Borrelia burgdorferi* as the causative agent of limb/joint dysfunction in dogs with borreliosis. J Am Vet Med Assoc 1992;201:412–418.

Wright SD, Nielsen SW. Experimental infection of the white-footed mouse with *Borrelia burgdorferi*. Am J Vet Res 1990;51:1980–1987.

BORRELIA THEILERI (BOVINE BORRELIOSIS)

Bovine borreliosis was first described by Theiler in South Africa in 1904. The causative organism, *Borrelia theileri*, which has been found in the blood of cattle in South Africa, Nigeria, Australia, Brazil, and Mexico, is transmitted by *Rhipicephalus evertsi, Margaropus decoloratus, Boophilus annulatus* and *Boophilus microplus*. *B. theileri* is relatively nonpathogenic, but it has been associated with fever, hemoglobinuria, and anemia. Sheep and horses are susceptible, and may develop very mild disease.

References

Callow LL. Observations on tick-transmitted spirochaetes of cattle in Australia and South Africa. Br Vet J 1967;123:492–496.

Smith RD, Miranpuri GS, Adams JH, et al. *Borrelia theileri*: isolation from ticks (*Boophilus microplus*) and tick-borne transmission between splenectomized calves. Am J Vet Res 1985;46:1396–1398.

Theiler A. Spirillosis of cattle. J Comp Pathol Ther 1904;17:47–55.

Trees AJ. The transmission of *Borrelia theileri* by *Boophilus annulatus* (Say, 1982). Trop Anim Health 1978;10:93–94.

OTHER SPIROCHAETAL INFECTIONS

Borrelia anserina is the cause of avian borreliosis, a disease of geese, chickens, ducks, and turkeys. The disease, which is transmitted by argasid ticks, occurs worldwide and carries a high mortality rate. Spirochaetal organisms have been seen in the large intestine of humans and nonhuman primates (Takeuchi and others, 1971; Takeuchi and Zeller, 1972) in close association with the microvilli of the brush border. The organisms are associated with loss of microvilli and are seen in contact with the plasma membrane but apparently do not result in any changes within the intestinal cell membrane. At present these organisms are difficult to study, and their pathogenic significance is not clear. Further study of these organisms and their effects on intestinal epithelial cells is needed.

References

Centers for Disease Control and Prevention. Common source outbreak of relapsing fever - California. MMWR 1990;39(34):579, 585–586.

Dzhankov I, Nikolov N, Kirev T. Recent findings in the pathogenesis of avian spirochaetosis (*Borrelia anserina* infection). Vet Med Nauki 1982;19:14–21. [Vet Bull 1983;53:1008]

Felsenfeld O. Borrelia. Meth Microbiol 1973;8:75–94.

Felsenfeld O, Wolf RJ. Immunology of borreliosis in nonhuman primates. Fed Proc 1975;34:1656–1660.

Judge DM, LaCroix JT, Perine PL. Experimental louse-borne relapsing fever in the grivet monkey, *Cercopithecus aethiops*. I. Clinical course. II. Pathology. III. Crisis following therapy. Am J Trop Med Hyg 1974;23:957–961, 962–968, 969–973.

Takeuchi A, Sprinz H, Sohn A. Intestinal spirochetosis in the monkey and man. Lab Invest 1971;24:450.

Takeuchi A, Zeller JA. Ultrastructural identification of spirochetes and flagellated microbes at brush border of large intestinal epithelium of the rhesus monkey. Infect Immun 1972;6:1008–1018.

Epizootic Bovine Abortion

First described in California in 1956 by Howarth and colleagues, epizootic bovine abortion represents an important cause of abortion in cattle in the foothill ranges of California. The disease, which occurs endemically (**not epizootically,** as its name suggests), is apparently limited in distribution to the range of the tick *Ornithodoros coriaceus,* believed to be the vector of an as yet unidentified infectious agent. The disease can be reproduced by allowing the tick to feed on pregnant cows. The tick also can be found on cattle in Nevada, Oregon, and northern Mexico. The disease had formerly been considered to be caused by *Chlamydia psittaci,* but this is no longer considered. A spirochete-like organism has been identified in bovine fetuses and in *O. coriaceus* and has been shown to be transmitted by the bite of the ticks. Inoculation of pregnant heifers with spirochetes recovered and concentrated from normal fetuses has not resulted in duplication of the disease but has resulted in the development of mild lesions in the fetus (Osebold and others, 1987). The exact classification of the organism has not been determined, but it has features of a Borrelia species. A virus, which is presently under study, has also been isolated from experimentally infected (by way of tick exposure) fetuses (Kimsey and colleagues, 1983).

Epizootic bovine abortion is principally a disease of the fetus, causing abortion, stillbirth, or birth of weak calves that die within a few days. No clinical evidence of disease is seen in the cow either before or after the abortion. Abortions usually occur between the seventh and ninth months of gestation, but earlier abortion may occur. The disease is described as a chronic fetal infection, as typical lesions are only observed in fetuses recovered 100 or more days after maternal tick exposure (Kennedy and others, 1983; Kimsey and others, 1983).

LESIONS

The pathologic features have been described in detail by Kennedy and colleagues (1960, 1983). Gross findings are dominated by generalized enlargement of lymph nodes, splenomegaly, and a small, edematous thymus that often contains petechiae. There may also be subcutaneous edema; pleural and peritoneal effusion; petechiae on the oral mucous membranes, larynx, trachea, and conjunctivae; small gray foci in the myocardium and kidneys; and a swollen, friable, coarsely nodular liver.

Microscopically, enlargement of lymph nodes and the spleen is caused by marked hyperplasia of lymphocytes and macrophages. The subcapsular sinuses of lymph nodes become filled with large macrophages, which also infiltrate perinodal tissues. In the cortical mantle of the thymus, there is replacement of small thymocytes with cells containing more vesicular nuclei, and there are many macrophages in the medulla. A granulomatous inflammatory process may involve any or all body organs, but in particular the liver, meninges, brain, kidney, heart, and skin. Individual lesions consist of focal necrosis and collections of macrophages, epithelioid cells, lymphocytes, and neutrophils. There is widespread vasculitis characterized by infiltration of the walls with inflammatory cells and hyperplasia of endothelium. Deposits of IgG and IgM have been detected in the vascular walls. The placenta is expelled normally and lacks any lesions of note.

DIAGNOSIS

The diagnosis of epizootic bovine abortion is dependent on finding the characteristic histopathologic lesions in the fetus.

References

Howarth JA, Moulton JE, Frazier LM. Epizootic bovine abortion characterized by fetal hepatopathy. J Am Vet Med Assoc 1956;128:441–449.

Kennedy PC, Olander HJ, Howarth JA. Pathology of epizootic bovine abortion. Cornell Vet 1960;50:417–429.

Kennedy PC, et al. Epizootic bovine abortion: histogenesis of the fetal lesions. Am J Vet Res 1983;44:1040–1048.

Kimsey PB, et al. Studies on the pathogenesis of epizootic bovine abortion. Am J Vet Res 1983;44:1266–1271.

Lane RS, Burgdorfer W, Hayes SF, et al. Isolation of a spirochete from the soft tick, Ornithodoros coriaceus: a possible agent of epizootic bovine abortion. Science 1985;230:85–87.

Osebold JW, Spezialetti R, Jennings MB, et al. Congenital spirochetosis in calves: association with epizootic bovine abortion. J Am Vet Med Assoc 1986;188:371–376.

Osebold JW, Osburn BI, Spezialetti R, et al. Histopathologic changes in bovine fetuses after repeated reintroduction of a spirochete-like agent into pregnant heifers: association with epizootic bovine abortion. Am J Vet Res 1987;48:627–633.

Schmidtmann ET, Bushnell RB, Loomis EC, et al. Experimental and epizootiologic evidence associating Ornithodoros coriaceus Koch (Acari: Argasidae) with the exposure of cattle to epizootic bovine abortion in California. J Med Entomol 1976;13:292–299. [Vet Bull 1977;47:3779]

The HIGHER BACTERIA ORDER ACTINOMYCETALES

The order Actinomycetales is composed of several families, some of which contain pathogenic organisms. These organisms, referred to as higher bacteria, often produce lesions that resemble those produced by fungi, discussed in Chapter 11. Some of the organisms themselves also have morphologic and biochemical characteristics that are shared by fungi. They are, however, bacteria lacking eukaryotic nuclei and mitochondria. The classification we have employed is oversimplified, but the important animal pathogens are in the following genera; *Actinomyces, Nocardia, Rhodococcus, Corynebacterium, Dermatophilus, Streptomyces,* and *Mycobacterium.*

Infections Caused by Corynebacterium Organisms

Bacterial organisms classified in the genus *Corynebacterium* are involved in a wide variety of lesions in many domestic and wild animals, as well as in humans. The best known organism in this genus is *Corynebacterium diphtheriae,* the causative agent of human diphtheria. Other members of this group are often referred to collectively as "diphtheroid bacteria." Many of these are of low pathogenicity, existing as commensals in otherwise normal animals. Predisposing factors, generally not identified, appear to be necessary for their induction of disease. The lesions produced by various species of Corynebacterium show much variety; the tissue reaction to some is predominantly necrotizing, to most it is suppurative, and to others granulomatous.

Corynebacteriae are gram-positive, not acid-fast, and occasionally "beaded" in stained tissue sections. They share features with *Mycobacteriae* and *Nocardia,* but are readily differentiated. The pathogenic Corynebacteriae are listed in Table 10-13.

Corynebacterium pyogenes, now termed *Actinomyces pyogenes,* is a common and important organism in pyogenic processes in cattle, swine, sheep, and goats. In cattle, the organisms are found in abscesses, many of which are heavily encapsulated, and in necrotic and suppurative pneumonias. They have also been isolated from the suppurative arthritis and umbilical infections in calves and from purulent metritis and mastitis in cows. In swine, the "diphtheroid" organisms produce diseases resembling those of cattle; infection often follows farrowing, and arthritis is a common manifestation. In sheep and goats, purulent pneumonias and abscesses in the upper respiratory tract have been described.

Corynebacterium renale is commonly associated with **"bacillary" pyelonephritis** of cattle, in which chronic purulent cystitis and urethritis accompany the inflammatory changes in the ureters and renal pelvis. Horses and sheep may become infected, but rarely dogs. In cattle, the disease is primarily confined to cows; it is rare in bulls. In affected herds, *C. renale* can be recovered from healthy individuals. The lesions can affect the entire urinary tract. The bladder, ureters, and renal pelvi

TABLE 10-13 **Pathogenic *Corynebacteriae***

Organism	Principal disease
Corynebacterium diphtheriae	Diptheria in humans
C. renale	Pyelonephritis, ureteritis, cystitis in cows
C. cystitidis	Hemorrhagic cystitis and pyelonephritis in cows
C. pilosum	Cystitis and pyelonephritis in cows
C. pseudotuberculosis	Caseous lymphadenitis in sheep and goats; ulcerative lymphangitis and pectoral abscesses in horses
C. bovis	Rare cause of mastitis in cattle
C. suis (Eubacterium suis)	Pyelonephritis and cystitis in swine
C. kutscheri	Pseudotuberculosis in rodents
C. pyogenes (Actinomyces pyogenes)	Suppurative infections in cattle, sheep, goats, and swine
C. ulcerans	Wound infections and abscesses in many species
C. equi (Rhodococcus equi)	Pneumonia in horses

are dilated with thickened walls and necrosis and hemorrhage of the mucosa, which becomes covered with a fibrinonecrotic membrane. Abscesses may be present throughout the kidneys.

Two other Corynebacteriae also cause cystitis and pyelonephritis in cows. *C. pilosum* causes a disease similar to that produced by *C. renale* and can also be recovered from the urogenital tract of healthy cows; however, in contrast to *C. renale,* it is not recovered from healthy cows. *C. cystitidis* is associated with a particularly severe hemorrhagic cystitis and often pyelonephritis in cows; however, also in contrast to *C. renale,* it is not recovered from healthy cows but is found as a commensal in the prepuce of bulls. In swine, an organism that has been called *C. suis,* but is now classified as *Eubacterium suis,* is a cause of cystitis, pyelonephritis, and metritis in sows. This organism is carried by boars, but not by sows.

Corynebacterium ulcerans is a strain that appears to be intermediate between *C. diphtheriae* and *C. pseudotuberculosis* and has been recovered from the nasopharynx of persons with upper respiratory infection. It appears to be the causative agent in infection of bite wounds and pulmonary abscesses in nonhuman primates (*Macaca mulatta, M. fascicularis,* and *Presbytis entellus*) (May, 1972). The organism has also been isolated from cases of mastitis in dairy cattle and a bonnet macaque (*Macaca radiata*).

Corynebacterium pseudotuberculosis (*C. ovis,* Preiz-Nocard bacillus) is the cause of caseous lymphadenitis or pseudotuberculosis of sheep and goats (Fig. 10-21). *C. pseudotuberculosis* also affects horses, causing ulcerative lymphangitis, pectoral abscesses, and folliculitis.

Corynebacterium kutscheri (*C. pseudotuberculosis murium*) is the cause of pseudotuberculosis in mice and

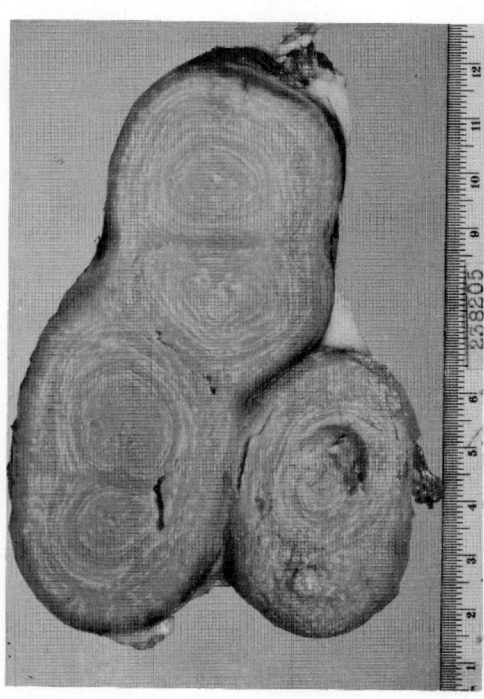 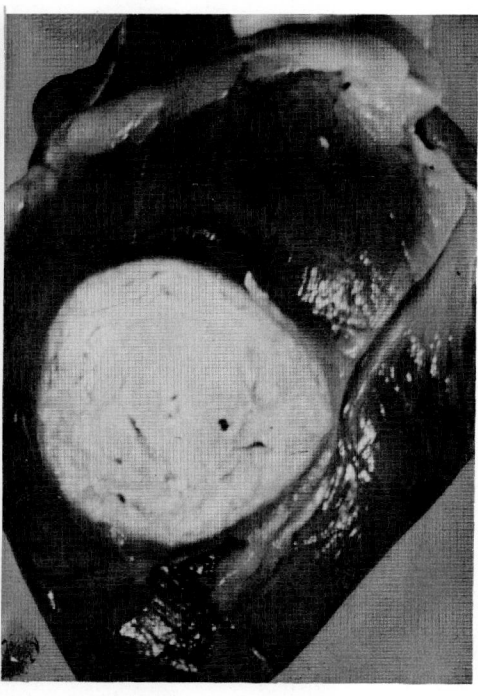

FIG. 10-21 Caseous lymphadenitis. **A.** Thoracic lymph nodes of a sheep. Note concentric laminations. (Courtesy of Dr. C. L. Davis, and Armed Forces Institute of Pathology.) **B.** A lesion in the myocardium of a sheep. (Courtesy of Dr. C. L. Davis.)

rats. The lesions consist of disseminated caseopurulent foci, particularly in the lungs, lymph nodes, liver, and kidneys (see also *Yersinia pseudotuberculosis*). Usually the infection is subclinical and only seen when animals are stressed with cortisone, irradiation, nutritional deficiency, or other challenges. The disease may run an acute or chronic course.

A bacterium that has been called *Corynebacterium equi*, but is more appropriately classified as *Rhodococcus equi*, is the cause of a specific pneumonia of foals and, occasionally, pneumonia in cattle, sheep, humans, and other species. This is discussed under Rhodococcus.

Corynebacterium bovis is the name given to an organism that is a frequent commensal of the bovine udder. Although resembling other member of this genus, the bacterium is not a true *Corynebacterium* and should be classified elsewhere. It has, on occasion, been associated with bovine mastitis. A *Corynebacterium* species has been associated with a multifocal dermatitis and wool loss (termed Bolo disease) in sheep in South America.

OVINE CASEOUS LYMPHADENITIS
(Pseudotuberculosis of Sheep And Goats)

Caseous lymphadenitis is a chronic disease of sheep and goats, which often occurs as an inapparent infection, being encountered only as an incidental finding in slaughtered animals. The causative organism is *Corynebacterium pseudotuberculosis (C. ovis)*, a gram-positive diphtheroid bacillus that produces an exotoxin (a phospholipase D) and bears toxic surface lipid, which allows the organism to survive within macrophages. The organism gains entry by way of abrasions in the skin or oral mucous membranes and, less commonly, through inhalation. Infection is rarely seen in cattle, although the disease was first described in 1888 from a case of bovine lymphangitis. The disease is characterized by abscesses of lymph nodes, usually the prescapular and prefemoral, but may become generalized with abscesses in many different lymph nodes as well as the lungs, liver, kidneys, and brain.

Lesions The lesions are usually restricted to lymph nodes, particularly the prescapular, prefemoral, and mediastinal nodes and, less often, the lungs, kidneys, and other viscera. Microscopic evidence indicates that the lesion starts as a small nidus of epithelioid cells but is soon overtaken by caseation necrosis, which becomes the predominant feature. The central caseous mass is soon surrounded by a thin layer of epithelioid cells admixed with lymphocytes, to which an external reinforcing layer of fibrous connective tissue is added. As the lesion grows, the epithelioid and fibrous reactive layers undergo necrosis; the epithelioid layer dies first. While the fibrous layer still remains visible, new reactive layers form outside it and successively become necrotic. The result is a spherical, onion-like, concentrically laminated mass, which may reach a diameter of several centimeters. Calcification may occur, but giant cells are not seen.

The gross appearance of lymph nodes is character-

istic; the entire node is greatly enlarged and almost replaced by a single globoid lesion. In cross section, it is concentrically laminated; layers of fibrous capsule alternate with caseous, friable material that may be greenish and occasionally gritty. In the lungs, the lesions may resemble an abscess, with a central, semifluid mass of yellowish or greenish pus.

Diagnosis The gross and microscopic features, if typical, are practically diagnostic. Identification of the causative organism depends on demonstrating its diphtheroid morphology and accepted culture characteristics. Pathogenicity tests are commonly unfruitful.

References

Ayers JL. Caseous lymphadenitis in goats and sheep: a review of diagnosis, pathogenesis, and immunity. J Am Vet Med Assoc 1977;171:1251–1254.
Biberstein EL, Knight HD, Jang S. Two biotypes of *Corynebacterium pseudotuberculosis*. Vet Rec 1972;89:691–692.
Brown CC, Olander HJ. Caseous lymphadenitis of goats and sheep: a review. Vet Bull 1987;57:1–12.
Brownstein DG, Barthold SW, Adams RL, et al. Experimental *Corynebacterium kutscheri* infection in rats: bacteriology and serology. Lab Anim Sci 1985;35:135–138.
Brumbaugh GW, Ekman TL. *Corynebacterium pseudotuberculosis* bacteremia in two horses. J Am Vet Med Assoc 1981; 178:300–301.
Cimprich RE, Rooney JR. *Corynebacterium equi* enteritis in foals. Vet Pathol 1977;14:95–102.
Colly PA, et al. Bolo disease: a specific, localised skin disease of woolled sheep. J S Afr Vet Assoc 1990;61:90–93.
Counter DE. Outbreak of bovine mastitis associated with *Corynebacterium bovis*. Vet Rec 1981;108:560–561.
Ellis JA. Immunophenotype of pulmonary cellular infiltrates in sheep with visceral caseous lymphadenitis. Vet Pathol 1988;25:362–368.
Feldman WH, Moses HE, Karlson AG. *Corynebacterium equi* as a possible cause of tuberculous-like lesions of swine. Cornell Vet 1940;30:465–481.
Foss JO. Identification of *Corynebacterium renalis* from the kidney and bladder of a horse. J Am Vet Med Assoc 1944;104:27.
Fox JG, Niemi SM, Ackerman J, et al. Comparison of methods to diagnose an epizootic of *Corynebacterium kutscheri* pneumonia in rats. Lab Anim Sci 1987;37:72–75.
Gezon HM, Bither HD, Hanson LA, et al. Epizootic of external and internal abscesses in a large goat herd over a 16–year period. J Am Vet Med Assoc 1991;198:257–263.
Giddens WE Jr, Keahey KK, Carter GR, et al. Pneumonia in rats due to infections with *Corynebacterium kutscheri*. Pathol Vet 1968;5:227–237.
Hayashi A, Yanagawa R, Kida H. Adhesion of *Corynebacterium renale* and *Corynebacterium pilosum* to epithelial cells of bovine vulva. Am J Vet Res 1985;46:409–411.
Heffner KA, White SD, Frevert CW, et al. Corynebacterium folliculitis in a horse. J Am Vet Med Assoc 1988;193:89–90.
Higgins RJ, Weaver CR. *Corynebacterium renale* pyelonephritis and cystitis in a sheep. Vet Rec 1981;109:256.
Hinton M. *Corynebacterium pyogenes* and bovine abortion. J Hyg (Camb) 1974;72:365–368.
Hughes JP, Biberstein EL. Chronic equine abscesses associated with *Corynebacterium pseudotuberculosis*. J Am Vet Med Assoc 1959;135:559–562.
Hughes JP, Biberstein EL, Richards WPC. Two cases of generalized *Corynebacterium pseudotuberculosis* infection in mares. Cornell Vet 1962;52:51–62.
Jones JET. Cystitis and pyelonephritis associated with *Corynebacterium suis* infection in sows. Vet Annu 1984;24:138–342.
Jones JET, Dagnall GJR. The carriage of *Corynebacterium suis* in male pigs. J Hyg 1984;93:381–388. [Vet Bull 1985;55:1356]
Marsh H. *Corynebacterium ovis* associated with arthritis in lambs. Am J Vet Res 1947;8:294–498.

May BD. *Corynebacterium ulcerans* infections in monkeys. Lab Anim Sci 1972;22:509–513.

Miers KC, Ley WB. *Corynebacterium pseudotuberculosis* infection in the horse: study of 117 clinical cases and consideration of etiopathogenesis. J Am Vet Med Assoc 1980;177:250–253.

Percy DH, Ruhnke HL, Soltys MA. A case of infectious cystitis and pyelonephritis of swine caused by *Corynebacterium suis*. Can Vet J 1966;7:291–292.

Pijoan C, Lastra A, Leman A. Isolation of *Corynebacterium suis* from the prepuce of boars. J Am Vet Med Assoc 1983;183:428–429.

Schiefer B, Pantekoek JFCA, Moffatt RE. The pathology of bovine abortion due to *Corynebacterium pyogenes*. Can Vet J 1974;15:322–326.

Smith RE, Reynolds IM, Clark GW, et al. Fetoplacental effects of *Corynebacterium pyogenes* in sheep. Cornell Vet 1971;61:573–590.

Soltys MA. *Corynebacterium suis* associated with a specific cystitis and pyelonephritis in pigs. J Path Bact 1961;81:441–446.

Stoops SG, Renshaw HW, Thilsted JP. Ovine caseous lymphadenitis: disease prevalence, lesion distribution, and thoracic manifestations in a population of mature culled sheep from western United States. Am J Vet Res 1984;45:557–561.

Suzuki E, Mochida K, Nakagawa M. Naturally occurring subclinical *Corynebacterium kutscheri* infection in laboratory rats: strain and age related antibody response. Lab Anim Sci 1988;38:42–45.

Van Pelt RW. Infectious arthritis in cattle caused by *Corynebacterium pyogenes*. J Am Vet Med Assoc 1970;156:457–465.

Van Tonder EM, et al. Bolo disease: a bacteriological survey. J S Afr Vet Assoc 1990;61:96–101.

Actinomycosis

Actinomycosis is the result of infection by organisms classified in the genus Actinomyces (Figs. 10-22 and 10-23). Although not fungi, the lesions produced by these bacteria closely mimic the true mycotic diseases. The currently recognized organisms, their hosts, and the diseases they cause are summarized in Table 10-14. Other species exist but are not known to be pathogenic. All of the Actinomyces are of low pathogenicity and, in general, are commensals in the oral cavity and intestinal tract, gaining entry into tissues through injuries. The classic disease, caused by *Actinomyces bovis,* occurs in cattle, but many species may be infected under natural conditions. The most frequent and obvious manifestation of actinomycosis in cattle is the hard, irregular enlargement that results from infection of the mandible or, less often, the maxilla and gives the disease its common name, "lumpy jaw." Similar infection of the mandible has been observed in wild ruminants, such as elk. In dogs, actinomycosis, most often caused by *A. hordeovulneris,* usually affects soft tissues and may become generalized. In humans, *A. israeli* is the usual infecting organism; the cheek, mouth, skin of the chest, appendix, and intestine are the usual sites of involvement. Actinomycotic infection of the porcine mammary glands, caused by *A. suis* (an organism of tentative classification), is not uncommon. *A. suis* and *A. naeslundii* also have been associated with abortion in swine, causing typical actinomycotic lesions in the uterus and the fetus, particularly in the lungs. Actinomycetes have also been identified in association with *Brucella abortus* in equine "fistulous withers."

LESIONS

The organisms grow in tenacious colonies of microscopic size, located in tiny purulent centers surrounded by dense granulation tissue, which displaces the nearby normal tissues. When the organisms penetrate bone, the bone becomes enlarged and honeycombed as a result of destructive rarefaction and regenerative proliferation. The cut surface of the lesion usually is white and glistening from the dense connective tissue in which the small abscesses are embedded. Occasional sinus tracts may be demonstrated, with drainage through the skin or into the oral cavity. Expression of the yellowish pus from the abscesses yields tiny, hard masses called "sulfur granules" because of their gross consistency and yellowish color. Microscopically, these masses may appear as rosettes, and although early investigators considered them the "ray fungus," they are now known to be merely separate colonies of actinomyces organisms growing in characteristic fashion. In sections stained with hematoxylin and eosin, a colony appears as a basophilic irregularly shaped mass, 20 microns or more in diameter, surrounded by a zone of radially arranged eosinophilic projections known as Splendore-Hoeppli material (Chapter 11).

The central part of the colony can be demonstrated by Gram's stain to be made up of a tangled mass of gram-positive, rod-shaped, or long filamentous organisms, which are often beaded and occasionally branched. Beyond the radiating clubs there is usually a zone of neutrophils, surrounded by an outer area of large mononuclear (epithelioid) cells with abundant, often foamy, cytoplasm. Giant cells of the Langhans' type and lymphocytes are occasionally found in this region. The dense, moderately vascular connective tissue that separates the many abscesses from one another usually encapsulates the entire lesion.

The colonies of actinomyces may become calcified in cases of long standing, in which event they assume a gritty texture as blue-staining granules of calcium salts replace the organisms. Actinomycosis of other tissues and in other species may have an identical histologic appearance. In some situations, however, as in actinomycotic pleuritis or peritonitis, one of the more frequent presentations in dogs, the lesions are a more diffuse purulent inflammation without distinct granuloma formation.

DIAGNOSIS

The characteristic lesions can be identified positively by using Gram's stain on sections of fixed tissue to differentiate the gram-positive organisms at the center of the colonies. Organisms can also be demonstrated in smears of fresh, unfixed material stained by Gram's method. The rosettes with the shiny, refractile, radiating clubs can be demonstrated in wet preparations of fresh pus compressed under a cover glass and examined under low illumination.

Differential diagnosis must include other granulomatous infections, but in particular actinobacillosis, nocardiosis, and staphylococcosis (botryomycosis). The morphology of the bacterial colonies and individual organisms and their staining reactions, which differ in each of these infections, allow ready differentiation.

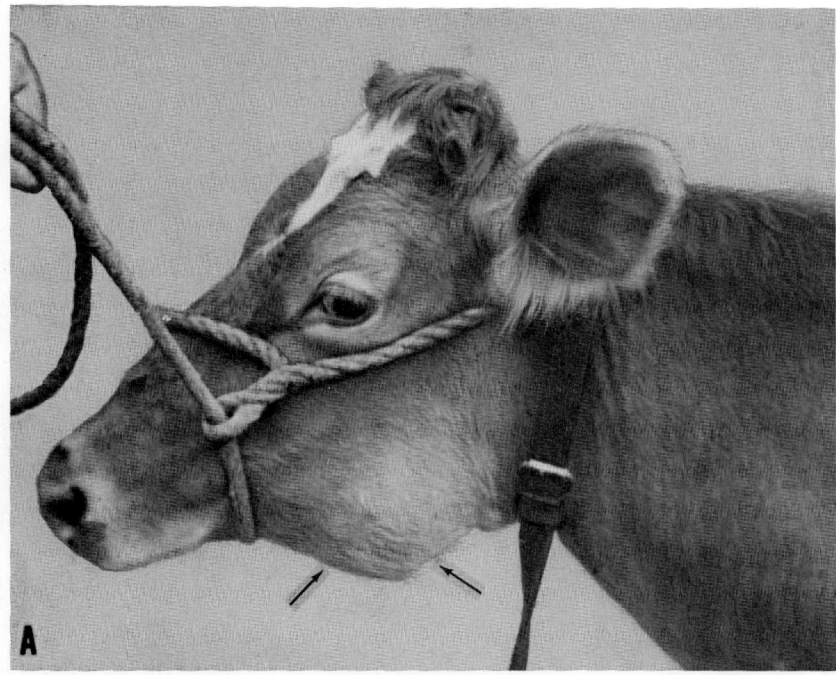

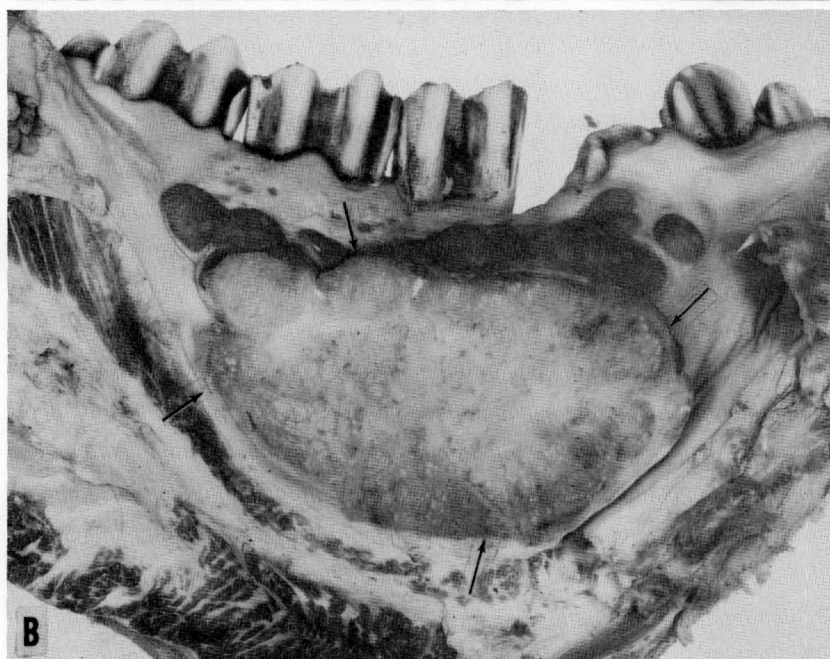

FIG. 10-22 Actinomycosis.   **A.** Lesions in mandible of a Guernsey cow. Case from clinic of College of Veterinary Medicine, Iowa State University.   **B.** Gross specimen from mandible of a similar case. (Courtesy of Major Lytle, V.C., and Armed Forces Institute of Pathology.)

References

Altman NH, Small JD. Actinomycosis in a primate confirmed by fluorescent antibody technics in formalin fixed tissues. Lab Anim Sci 1973;23:696–700.

Ayers KM, DePaoli A. Actinomycosis of the testes and spermatic cord in a dog. Vet Pathol 1977;14:287–288.

Bertone AL, Rebhun WC. Tracheal actinomycosis in a cow. J Am Vet Med Assoc 1984;185:221–222.

Bestetti G. Morphology of the "sulphur granules" (Drusen) in some actinomycotic infections. A light and electron microscopic study. Vet Pathol 1978;15:506–518.

Brown JR, von Lichtenberg F. Experimental actinomycosis in mice. Arch Pathol 1970;90:391–402.

Buchanan AM, Scott JL. *Actinomyces hordeovulneris*, a canine pathogen that produces L-phase variants spontaneously with coincident calcium deposition. Am J Vet Res 1984;45:2552–2560.

Chastain CB, et al. Actinomycotic peritonitis in a dog. J Am Vet Med Assoc 1976;168:499–501.

Coleman M, Georg LK. Comparative pathogenicity of *Actinomyces naeslundii* and *Actinomyces israelii*. Appl Microbiol 1969;18:427–432.

Davenport AA, Carter GR, Patterson MJ. Identification of *Actinomyces viscosus* from canine infections. J Clin Microbiol 1975;1:75–78.

Eustis SL, Kirkbride CA, Gates C,et al. Porcine abortion associated with fungi, *Actinomycetes*, and *Rhodococcus* sp. Vet Pathol 1981;18:608–613.

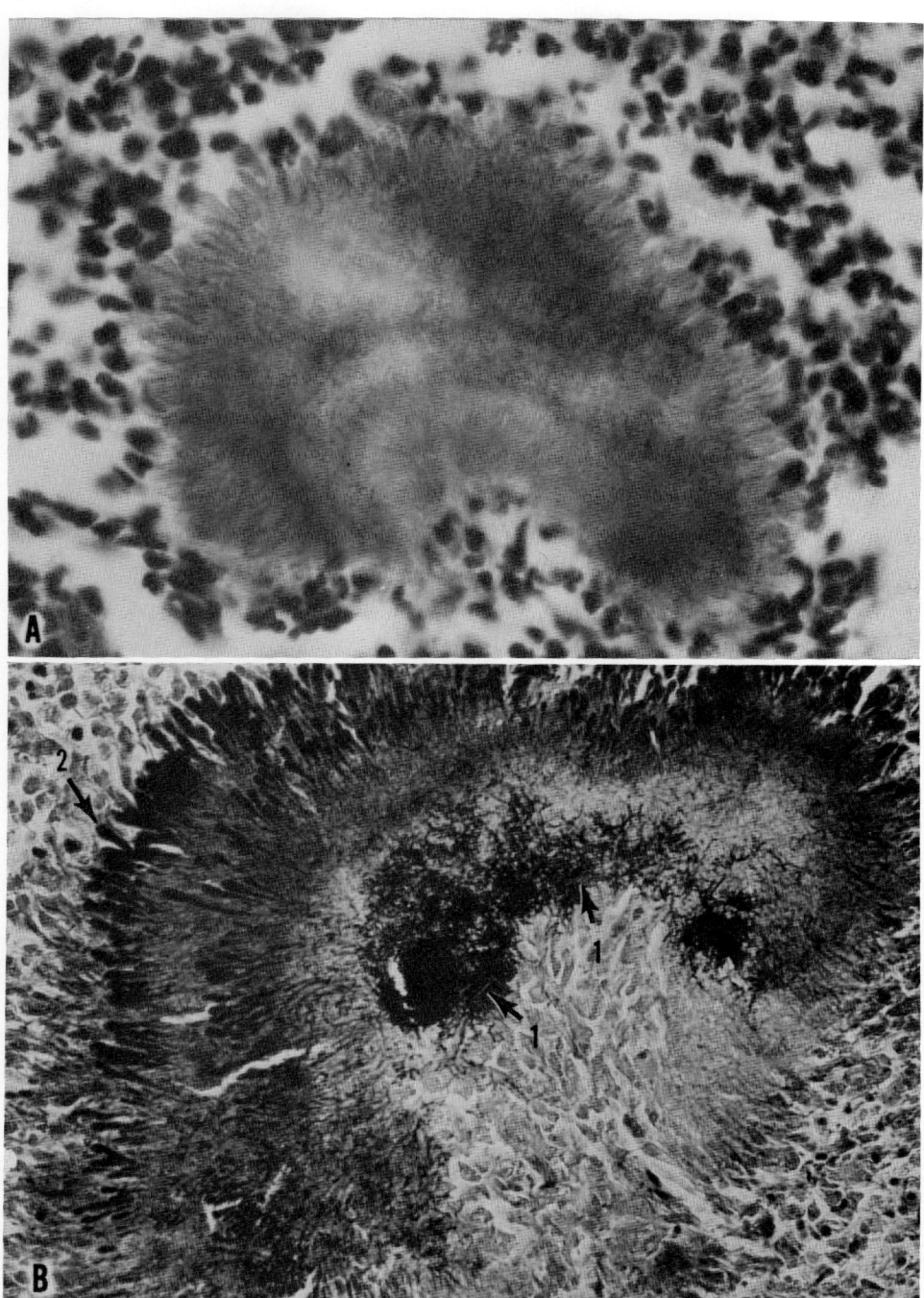

FIG. 10-23 Actinomycosis. **A.** Colony of *Actinomyces bovis* (× 500), in a tissue section stained with hematoxylin and eosin. (Contributor: Major Lytle, V.C.) **B.** A similar colony of Actinomyces bovis (× 500) in a tissue section stained by Gram's method. Note tangled, branching, gram-positive organisms in the center (1) surrounded by zones of radiating club-shaped structures (2). (Courtesy of Dr. H. R. Seibold, and Armed Forces Institute of Pathology.)

Georg LK, Brown JM, Baker HJ, et al. *Actinomyces viscosus* as an agent of actinomycosis in the dog. Am J Vet Res 1972;33:1457–1470.

Ginsberg A, Little ACW. Actinomycosis in dogs. J Path Bact 1948;60:563–572.

Menges RW, Larsh HW, Habermann RT. Canine actinomycosis. J Am Vet Med Assoc 1953;122:73–78.

Robboy SJ, Vickery AL. Tinctorial and morphologic properties distinguishing actinomycosis and nocardiosis. N Engl J Med 1970;282:593–596.

Ryff JF. Encephalitis in a deer due to *Actinomyces bovis*. J Am Vet Med Assoc 1953;122:78–80.

Shahan MS, Davis CL. The diagnosis of actinomycosis and actinobacillosis. Am J Vet Res 1942;3:321–328.

Swerczek TW, Schiefer B, Nielsen SW. Canine actinomycosis. Zentbl Vet Med 1968;15B:955–970.

Yamini B, Slocombe RF. Porcine abortion caused by *Actinomyces suis*. Vet Pathol 1988;25:323–324.

Nocardiosis

Nocardia are aerobic, gram-positive, filamentous (mycelial) organisms that, under some conditions, have "acid-fast" staining properties. These organisms infect humans and animals, particularly dogs and cattle, causing purulent, necrotizing, and at times, granulomatous dis-

TABLE 10-14 **Actinomycosis**

Organism	Host(s)	Anatomic systems affected
Actinomyces bovis	Cattle, swine, horses, elk	Mandible, maxilla, soft tissues, or generalized
A. israelii	Humans, cattle, swine	Soft tissues, may be generalized
A. meyeri	Humans	Soft tissues
A. naeslundii	Humans	Bony and soft tissues, eye
	Swine	Fetus (abortion)
A. odontolyticus	Humans	Periodontal disease, eye, subcutis, lungs
A. pyogenes	Humans, cattle, sheep, horses	Skin abscesses, mastitis, peritonitis, lymphadenitis
A. hordeovulneris	Dogs	Pleuritis, peritonitis, visceral abscesses, arthritis
A. suis	Swine	Mammary gland, fetus (abortion)
A. viscosus	Humans, swine, cats, dogs, hamsters	Bony and soft tissues, periodontal disease
A. denticolens	Cattle	Oral cavity commensal
A. howellii	Cattle	Oral cavity commensal
A. humiferus	Soil	Nonpathogenic

ease. The genus *Rhodococcus* has similar morphology and staining characteristics and is easily confused with *Nocardia*. Although *Actinomyces* species are not acid-fast (which is not a reliable differential feature), nocardiosis can also be confused with actinomycosis. Nocardiosis is most often caused by *Nocardia asteroides*, but *N. brasiliensis* and *N. caviae* are also pathogenic and occasionally identified. An organism termed *N. farcinica* was formerly considered to be the cause of a disease of cattle known as bovine farcy; however, the causative organism is now recognized as *Mycobacterium farcinogenes*.

LESIONS

In dogs, infection of the lungs and pleura or skin is most common, although systemic infection can occur, and the organisms may localize in peritoneal and pleural cavities, in the brain, or in any visceral organ. The lesions are seen microscopically as tangled, indistinct colonies of organisms surrounded by necrotic cellular debris, purulent exudate, and granulation tissue. Distinct granulomas are usually not a feature; however,

chronic lesions are characterized by a surrounding zone of macrophages, lymphocytes, plasma cells, and sometimes multinucleated giant cells along with a fibrovascular connective tissue. Ordinarily, eosinophilic clubs (Splendore-Hoeppli material) are not present surrounding the colonies of organisms, but they have been reported, making the differentiation from actinomycosis very difficult. The colonies are not surrounded by radiating clubs. The organisms can usually be demonstrated in the tissues as gram-positive, branching filaments, which are acid-fast when appropriately stained. Culture identification of the organism is necessary to establish the diagnosis, although presumptive diagnoses can be made from tissue sections.

Nocardiosis is less common in other species, but is a sporadic cause of mastitis or pneumonia in cattle and pneumonia in monkeys. The lesions in these or other species are similar to those described in the dog. The organism recovered from dogs and nonhuman primates has sometimes been identified as *Nocardia caviae*, a species closely related to *N. asteroides*.

Infection of the bovine fetus and placenta with resulting abortion has been associated with nocardiosis.

References

Bakerspigel A. An unusual strain of Nocardia isolated from an infected cat. Can J Microbiol 1973;19:1361–1365.

Beaman BL, Sugar AM. Nocardia in naturally acquired and experimental infections in animals. J Hyg (Camb) 1983;91:393–419.

Biberstein EL, Jang SS, Hirsh DC. *Nocardia asteroides* infection in horses: a review. J Am Vet Med Assoc 1985;186:273–277.

Bohl EH, et al. Nocardiosis in the dog. J Am Vet Med Assoc 1953;122:81–85.

Boncyk LH, McCullough B, Grotts DD, et al. Localized nocardiosis due to *Nocardia caviae* in a baboon (*Papio cynocephalus*). Lab Anim Sci 1975;25:88–91.

Cuttino JT, McCabe AM. Pure granulomatous nocardiosis: a new fungus disease distinguished by intracellular parasitism. Am J Pathol 1949;25:1–47.

Davenport DJ, Johnson GC. Cutaneous nocardiosis in a cat. J Am Vet Med Assoc 1986;188:728–729.

Deem DA, Harrington DD. *Nocardia brasiliensis* in a horse with pneumonia and pleuritis. Cornell Vet 1980;70:321–328.

Ginsberg A, Little ACW. Actinomycosis in dogs. J Pathol Bact 1948;60:563–572.

Jonas AM, Wyand DS. Pulmonary nocardiosis in the rhesus monkey. Importance of differentiation from tuberculosis. Pathol Vet 1966;3:588–600.

Kinch DA. A rapidly fatal infection caused by Nocardia caviae in a dog. J Pathol Bact 1968;95:540–546.

Liebenberg SP, Giddens WE Jr. Disseminated nocardiosis in three macaque monkeys. Lab Anim Sci 1985;35:162–166.

Mahajan VM, et al. Experimental pulmonary nocardiosis in monkeys. Sabouraudia 1977;15:47–50.

McClure HM, Chang J, Kaplan W, et al. Pulmonary nocardiosis in an orangutan. J Am Vet Med Assoc 1976;169:943–945.

Mitten RW. Vertebral oesteomyelitis in the dog due to Nocardia-like organisms. J Small Anim Pract 1974;15:563–570.

Pier AC, Gray DM, Fossatti MJ. *Nocardia asteroides*—a newly recognized pathogen of the mastitis complex. Am J Vet Res 1958;19:319–331.

Ridell M. Taxonomic study of *Nocardia farcinica* using serological and physiological characters. Int J Systematic Bacteriol 1975;25:124–132.

Sakakibara I, Sugimoto Y, Minato H, et al. Spontaneous nocardiosis with brain abscess caused by *Nocardia asteroides* in a cynomolgus monkey. J Med Primatol 1984;13:89–95.

Swerczek TW, Trutwein G, Nielsen SW. Canine nocardiosis. Zentralbl Veterinaermed 1968;15B:971–978.

Thordal-Christensen A, Clifford DH. Actinomycosis (nocardiosis) in a dog. Am J Vet Res 1953;14:298–306.

Tuttle PA, Chandler FW. Deep dermatophytosis in a cat. J Am Vet Med Assoc 1983;183:1106–1108.

Wohlgemuth K, Knudtson W, Bicknell EJ, et al. Bovine abortion associated with *Nocardia asteroides*. J Am Vet Med Assoc 1972;161:273–288.

Rhodococcus equi

Rhodococcus, a genus of bacteria that closely resembles *Nocardia,* are gram-positive, usually filamentous (mycelial), and partially acid-fast. Of the several species, only *Rhodococcus equi* is a significant pathogen for animals. This species, formerly classified as *Corynebacterium equi,* is a variably acid-fast coccobacillus that is an important cause of a specific granulomatous pneumonia of horses and occasionally of cattle, sheep, swine, and other species. *R. equi* has also been associated with pyogranulomatous submandibular and cervical lymph nodes of swine and arthritis in lambs; it has been reported as a cause of pneumonia and pleuritis in a monkey. It has also emerged as an important cause of pneumonia in immunosuppressed human patients, most often in individuals with a history of exposure to horses.

The organism, found in soil, is believed to enter via the respiratory route. The incidence of infection is highest in dry, dusty environments. Foals between 2 and 4 months of age are most susceptible; infection in horses over 6 months of age is rare unless they are immunocompromised. Morbidity rates can approach 20%, and mortality rates may be up to 80%. The pneumonia is a severe bronchopneumonia characterized by filling of alveoli with neutrophils, macrophages, and multinucleated giant cells. Enlarging foci of necrosis surrounded by this mixed cell infiltrate and fibrosis leads to multiple, often coalescing pyogranulomas. Microscopically, these pyogranulomas have a central region of caseous necrosis containing neutrophils surrounded by macrophages and multinucleated giant cells. The infection may be systemic with pyogranulomatous inflammation in many viscera and joints. Enteritis, metritis, abortion, and lymphangitis may result from *R. equi* infection in foals, independently of pneumonia. Purulent and mononuclear enterocolitis, often with ulcers and associated pyogranulomatous lymphadenitis, is the most frequent of these findings. In all forms of the infection, the organisms can be found within macrophages.

There is also a report (Edwards and Simpson, 1988) of the isolation of *R. rubropertinctus* from an equine abortus.

References

Barton MD, Hughes KL. *Corynebacterium equi:* a review. Vet Bull 1980;50:65–80.

Barton MD, Hughes KL. Ecology of *Rhodococcus equi*. Vet Microbiol 1984;9:65–76.

Edwards JF, Simpson RB. Nocardioform actinomycete *(Rhodococcus rubropertinctus)*-induced abortion in a mare. Vet Pathol 1988;25:529–530.

Etherington WG, Prescott JF. *Corynebacterium equi* cellulitis associated with Strongyloides penetration in a foal. J Am Vet Med Assoc 1980;177:1025–1027.

Falcon J, Smith BP, O'Brien TR, et al. Clinical and radiographic findings in *Corynebacterium equi* pneumonia of foals. J Am Vet Med Assoc 1985;186:593–599.

Hillidge CJ. Review of *Corynebacterium (Rhodococcus) equi* lung abscesses in foals: pathogenesis, diagnosis and treatment. Vet Rec 1986;119:261–264.

Johnson JA, Prescott JF, Markham RJF. The pathology of experimental *Corynebacterium equi* infection in foals following [1] intrabronchial [2] intragastric challenge. Vet Pathol 1983;20:440–449, 450–459.

Perdrizet JA, Scott DW. Cellulitis and subcutaneous abscesses caused by *Rhodococcus equi* infection in a foal. J Am Vet Med Assoc 1987;190:1559–1561.

Scott M, Tham K, Verrall R, et al. *Rhodococcus equi* - an increasingly recognized opportunistic pathogen [abstr 527]. Lab Invest 1991;64:90A.

Stein FJ, Stott G. *Corynebacterium equi* in the cottontop marmoset *(Saguinus oedipus):* a case report. Lab Anim Sci 1979;29:519–520.

Dermatophilus infection (cutaneous streptothricosis)

Infection by *Dermatophilus congolensis* has been termed mycotic dermatitis, cutaneous streptothricosis, lumpy wool, strawberry foot rot (sheep), cutaneous actinomycosis, and other terms that contain erroneous implications regarding the nature of the causal agent (Fig. 10-24). The disease is most common in tropical countries, but occurs worldwide. Dermatophilus infection (the preferred designation) has been described in cattle, sheep, goats, deer, horses, pigs, dogs, monkeys, cats, fowl, raccoons, lizards, cottontail rabbits, polar bears, and humans. Rabbits, mice, and guinea pigs have been experimentally infected. In each of these species, with the exception of humans, the gross and histopathologic changes are similar.

LESIONS

The infection is usually limited to the skin, producing raised, alopecic, and sometimes papillomatous lesions covered by thick keratinaceous incrustations. The lesions may be well-circumscribed or confluent and may affect the skin of any portion of the body. In some instances, the organisms may reach lymph nodes resulting in a granulomatous response.

The microscopic features are unique and best understood by explaining the pathogenesis of the infection. The organism invades and multiplies within the epidermis as branching filaments, which divide in a characteristic multidimensional fashion, giving rise to multiple rows of coccoid organisms. They do not invade the dermis, but induce an extensive purulent exudate beneath the epidermis, separating it from the dermis. The invaded epidermis cornifies and a new epidermis forms under the exudate, which in turn is invaded by hyphae at the periphery of the lesion. A second inflammatory exudate separates the new epidermis from the dermis, and a third epithelium is generated. The process is repeated, resulting in a thick scab composed of alternate strata of cornified epidermis and exudate. The organisms can usually be seen in tissue sections stained with hematoxylin and eosin and are clearly visi-

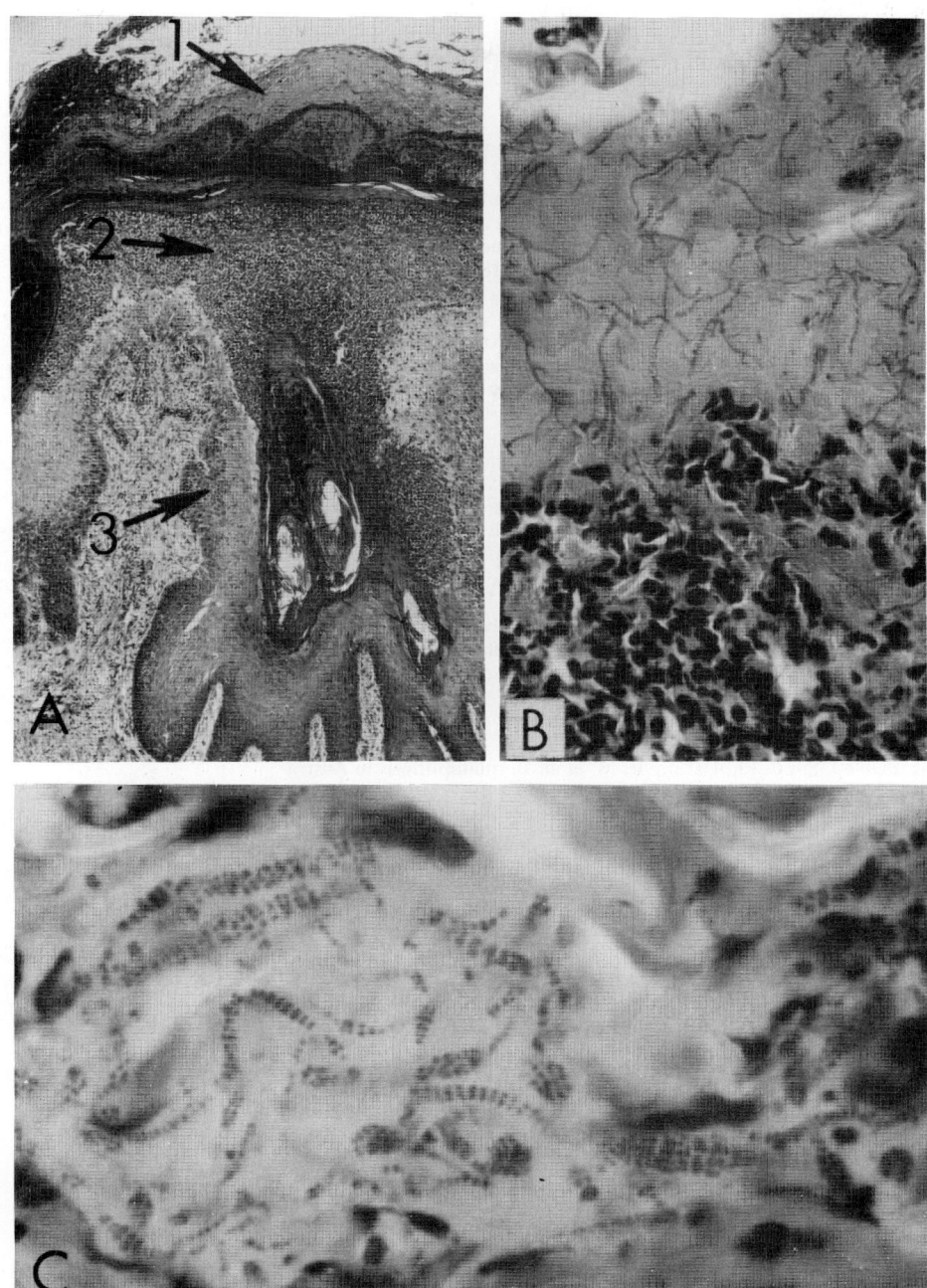

FIG. 10-24 Dermatophilus infection, skin, owl monkey *(Aotus trivirgatus)*. **A.** Characteristic lamination of cornified epithelium (1), purulent exudate (2), and regenerating epithelium (3). **B.** Mycelia in cornified epithelium. **C.** Characteristic multidimensional division of *Dermatophilus congolensis*. (Courtesy Dr. N. W. King, Jr.)

ble as gram-positive filaments or chains of cocci in sections stained with the Gram's technique.

The disease is transmitted by the coccoid forms, which result from the multidimensional division of the hyphae. This stage, known as a zoospore, is motile and released when the scabs are exposed to moisture. Transmission can be direct or indirect through contaminated water or grasses. Insect transmission, which has been demonstrated with flies and ticks, is believed to be a principal means of spreading zoospores.

Rarely, Dermatophilus infection affects tissues other than the skin. There have been reports of granulomatous lesions containing colonies of organisms in the subcutis, lymph nodes, tongue, tonsils, and urinary bladder in cats, cattle, sheep, goats, swine, humans, and a lizard. In one report of subcutaneous and lymph node granulomas in cattle (Gibson and others, 1983), colonies of *D. congolensis* were surrounded by radiating clubs (Splendore-Hoeppli material) resembling actinomycosis. The granulomas consisted of a central core of neutrophils containing the organisms, surrounded by a zone of macrophages, multinucleated giant cells, and fibrous connective tissue.

DIAGNOSIS

Diagnosis can usually be made from the morphology of the exudate and demonstration of the organisms. If necessary, the organism can be cultured.

References

Abu-Samra MT, Imbabi SE, Mahgoub S el. Experimental infection of domesticated animals and the fowl with *Dermatophilus congolensis*. J Comp Pathol 1976;86:157–172.

Bentinck-Smith J, Fox FH, Baker DW. Equine dermatitis (cutaneous streptothricosis) infection with dermatophilus in the U.S. Cornell Vet 1961;51:334–349.

Bridges CH, Romane WM. Cutaneous streptothricosis in cattle. J Am Vet Med Assoc 1961;138:153–157.

Carakostas MC, Miller RI, Woodward MG. Subcutaneous dermatophilosis in a cat. J Am Vet Med Assoc 1984;185:675–676.

Chastain CB, et al. Dermatophilosis in two dogs. J Am Vet Med Assoc 1976;169:1079–1080.

Fox JG, et al. Dermatophilosis (cutaneous streptothricosis) in owl monkeys. J Am Vet Med Assoc 1973;163:642–644.

Gibson JA, Thomas RJ, Domjahn RL. Subcutaneous and lymph node granulomas due to *Dermatophilus congolensis* in a steer. Vet Pathol 1983;20:120–122.

Jones RT. Subcutaneous infection with *Dermatophilus congolensis* in a cat. J Comp Pathol 1976;86:415–421.

Kaplan W. Dermatophilosis in primates. In: Lloyd DH, Sellers KC, ed. Dermatophilus infection in animals and man. New York: Academic Press 1976;128–140.

King NW, et al. Cutaneous streptothricosis (dermatophiliasis) in owl monkeys. Lab Anim Sci 1971;21:67–74.

Kistner TP, Shotts EB Jr, Greene EW. Naturally occurring cutaneous streptothricosis in a white tailed deer. Path Vet 1970;7:1–6.

LeRiche PD. The transmission of dermatophilosis (mycotic dermatitis) in sheep. Aust Vet J 1968;44:64–67.

Migaki G. Dermatophilosis in a titi monkey (Calicebus moloch). Am J Vet Res 1976;37:1225–1226.

Montali RJ, Smith EE, Davenport M, et al. Dermatophilosis in Australian bearded lizards. J Am Vet Med Assoc 1975;167:553–556.

Newman MS, Cook RW, Appelhof WK, et al. Dermatophilosis in two polar bears. J Am Vet Med Assoc 1975;167:561–564.

Oduye OO. Effects of various induced local environmental conditions and histopathological studies in experimental *Dermatophilus congolensis* infection on the bovine skin. Res Vet Sci 1975;19:245–252.

Richard JL, Pier AC, Cysewski SJ. Experimentally induced canine dermatophilosis. Am J Vet Res 1973;34:797–799.

Richard JL, Pier AC. Transmission of *Dermatophilus congolensis* by *Stomoxys calcitrans* and *Musca domestica*. Am J Vet Res 1966;27:419–423.

Roberts DS. Dermatophilus infection. Vet Bull 1967;37:513–521.

Roberts DS. The histopathology of epidermal infection with the actinomycete, *Dermatophilus congolensis*. J Pathol Bact 1965;90:213–216.

Salkin IF, Gordon MA, Stone WB. Dual infection of a white-tailed deer by *Dermatophilus congolensis* and *Alternaria alternata*. J Am Vet Med Assoc 1975;167:571–573.

Salkin IF, Gordon MA, Stone WB. Dermatophilosis among wild raccoons in New York State. J Am Vet Med Assoc 1976;169:949–951.

Schillhorn van Veen TW, Gregoricka MJ. Streptothricosis in a dairy herd. J Am Vet Med Assoc 1983;183:801.

Searcy GP, Hulland TJ. Dermatophilus dermatitis (streptothricosis) in Ontario. I. Clinical observations. II. Laboratory findings. Can Vet J 1968;9:7–21.

Shotts EB, Kistner TP. Naturally occurring cutaneous streptothricosis in a cottontail rabbit. J Am Vet Med Assoc 1970;157:667–670.

Smith CF, Cordes DO. Dermatitis caused by *Dermatophilus congolensis* infection in polar bears *(Thalacotos maritimus)*. Br Vet J 1972;128:336–371.

Stannard AA, Jang SS. Dermatophilosis in a lamb. J Am Vet Med Assoc 1973;163:1161–1164.

NECROBACILLOSIS

Necrobacillosis is a sweeping term applied to a number of lesions and disorders associated with *Fusobacterium necrophorum*. This organism (formerly called *Spherophorus necrophorus*), a filamentous, gram-negative strict anaerobe, is a commensal in the digestive tracts of animals and humans (Fig. 10-25). Although there is no doubt that *F. necrophorum* can be recovered from various lesions of animals, there is a question as to whether it is a primary pathogen. There is no question, however, that it does produce a variety of exotoxins and endotoxins that, once ensconced in necrotic tissue, allow it to cause considerably more progressive necrosis.

In horses, *F. necrophorum* (as well as other organisms) is associated with a necrotizing disease of the feet in animals that are forced to remain for long periods in deep, manure-soaked and urine-soaked mud. This "gangrenous dermatitis" usually starts at the heel or in the deep structures of the frog, and results in irregular ar-

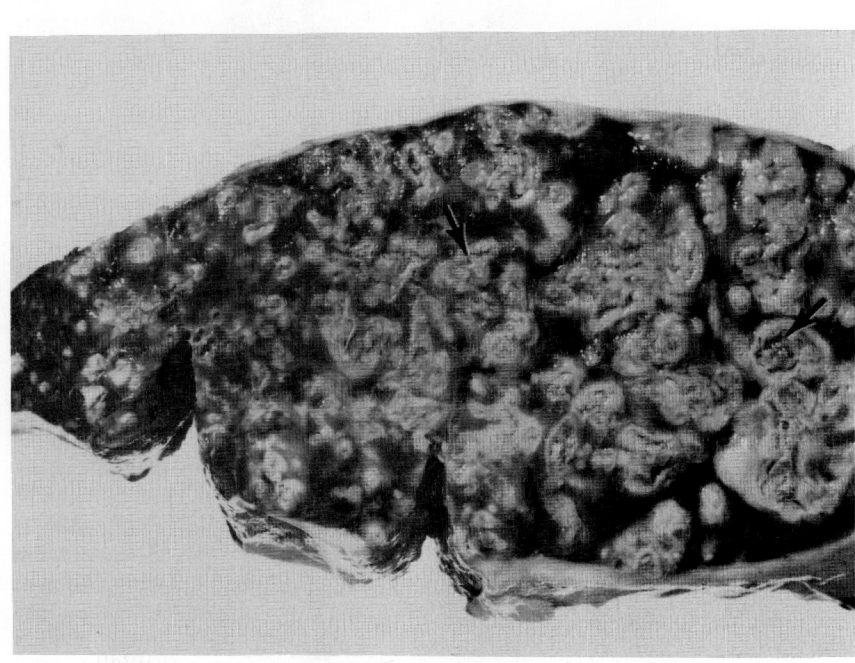

FIG. 10-25 Necrobacillosis. Irregularly shaped necrotic and encapsulated lesions (arrows) in a bovine spleen. (Courtesy of Dr. Wm. J. Hadlow.)

eas of sharply demarcated necrosis involving large amounts of tissue. It often produces serious disability.

In cattle, necrophorus organisms are found in the elevated, tenacious, necrotic plaques of the larynx, pharynx, and trachea, commonly referred to as "calf diphtheria." They also have been demonstrated in bovine cases that terminated fatally in pneumonia. Large, sharply delimited foci of necrosis also occur in the liver and spleen of adult cattle, particularly those which are heavily fed. The hepatic lesions are associated with ulcerations of the rumen and are discussed further in Chapter 23. In the Sudan, the disease in cattle has been reported to involve the subcutis, lymph vessels, and nodes, with occasional spread to internal organs, or in some cases, the internal organs are infected without apparent lesions in the subcutis ("bovine farcy").

Foot rot (infectious pododermatitis) in cattle and sheep is invariably associated with *F. necrophorum,* but the exact causes of the disease are not entirely understood. It appears that the disease only develops in the presence of the obligate anaerobe and obligate parasite of the hoof, *Bacteroides nodosus.* Progression of the disease is due to *B. nodosus,* not *F. necrophorum.* The disease can be induced by experimentally infecting the interdigital skin of normal animals with both organisms. *Actinomyces pyogenes* has also been recovered from bovine and ovine foot rot, and *Spirochaeta penortha* from ovine foot rot. Other species of *Bacteroides,* which are normal inhabitants of the gastrointestinal tract and found in feces, are occasionally recovered from various purulent inflammatory lesions. They are most likely not primary pathogens. Certain strains of *B. fragilis* produce an enterotoxin and have been demonstrated to cause severe enteritis in lambs, calves, piglets, foals, rabbits, and humans. The lesions are predominantly localized to the cecum and colon, where there is extensive exfoliation of enterocytes and crypt hyperplasia with a limited inflammatory cell infiltration.

Foot abscesses and "lip-and-leg ulceration" have been ascribed to necrophorous infection; however, it is doubtful that this organism is the cause of these diseases in sheep.

Ulcerative, necrotizing stomatitis and enteritis in swine have been questionably attributed to *Spherophorus necrophorus,* as has a disfiguring type of rhinitis ("bull-nose"). The similarity of the external appearance of the nose of affected swine is some evidence that this latter entity might have been confused in the past with atrophic rhinitis.

References

Benno Y, Mitsuoka T, Shirasaka S. Anaerobic bacteria isolated from abscesses in pigs. Jpn J Vet Sci 1982;44:309–315. [Vet Bull 1982;52:7130]

Berg JN, Loan RW. *Fusobacterium necrophorum* and *Bacteroides melaninogenicus* as etiologic agents of foot-rot in cattle. Am J Vet Res 1975;36:1115–1122.

Berg JN, Scanlan CM. Studies of *Fusobacterium necrophorum* from bovine hepatic abscesses: biotypes, quantitation, virulence, and antibiotic susceptibility. Am J Vet Res 1982;43:1580–1586.

Egerton JR, Roberts DS, Parsonson IM. The aetiology and pathogenesis of ovine foot-rot. I. A histological study of the bacterial invasion. J Comp Pathol 1969;79:207–215.

Glenn J, Carpenter TE, Hird DW: A field trial to assess the therapeutic and prophylactic effect of a foot rot vaccine in sheep. J Am Vet Med Assoc 1985;187:1009–1012.

Gradin JL, Sonn AE, Bearwood DE, et al. Electron microscopic study of *Bacteroides nodosus* pili and associated structures. Am J Vet Res 1991;52:206–211.

Holt SC, Ebersole J, Felton J, et al. Implantation of *Bacteroides gingivalis* in nonhuman primates initiates progression of periodontitis. Science 1988;239:55–57.

Jensen R, Flint JC, Griner LA. Experimental hepatic necrobacillosis in beef cattle. Am J Vet Res 1954;15:5–14.

Jensen R, et al. Laryngeal diphtheria and papillomatosis in feedlot cattle. Vet Pathol 1981;18:143–150.

Love DN, Jones RF, Calverley A. Asaccharolytic black-pigmented Bacteroides strains from soft-tissue infections in cats. Int J Syst Bacteriol 1984;34:300–303.

Mackey DR. Calf diphtheria. J Am Vet Med Assoc 1968;152:822–823.

Marsh H. Necrobacillosis of the rumen in young lambs. J Am Vet Med Assoc 1944;104:23–25.

Myers LL, Shoop DS. Association of enterotoxigenic *Bacteroides fragilis* with diarrheal disease in young pigs. Am J Vet Res 1987;48:774–775.

Myers LL, Shoop DS, Byars TD. Diarrhea associated with enterotoxigenic *Bacteroides fragilis* in foals. Am J Vet Res 1987;48:1565–1567.

Myers LL, Shoop DS, Collins JE. Rabbit model to evaluate enterovirulence of *Bacteroides fragilis.* J Clin Microbiol 1990;28:1658–1660.

Myers LL, Firehammer BD, Shoop DS, et al. *Bacteroides fragilis:* a possible cause of acute diarrheal disease in newborn lambs. Infect Immun 1984;44:241–244.

Myers LL, Shoop DS, Bradbury WC. Diarrheal disease caused by *Bacteroides* fragilis in infant rabbits. J Clin Microbiol 1989;27:2025–2030.

Myers LL, et al. Isolation of enterotoxigenic *Bacteroides fragilis* from humans with diarrhea. J Clin Microbiol 1987;25:2330–2333.

Roberts DS, Egerton JR. The aetiology and pathogenesis of ovine foot-rot. II. The pathogenic association of *Fusiformis nodosus* and *F. necrophorus.* J Comp Pathol 1969;79:217–227.

Scanlan CM, Hathcock TL. Bovine rumenitis-liver abscess complex: a bacteriological review. Cornell Vet 1983;73:288–297.

Simon PC, Stovell PL. Isolation of *Sphaerophorus necrophorus* from bovine hepatic abscesses in British Columbia. Can J Comp Med 1971;35:103–106.

Simon PC, Stovell PL. Diseases of animals associated with *Sphaerophorus necrophorus:* characteristics of the organism. Vet Bull 1969;39:311–315.

Walker RD, Richardson DC, Bryant MJ, et al. Anaerobic bacteria associated with osteomyelitis in domestic animals. J Am Vet Med Assoc 1983;182:814–816.

TUBERCULOSIS

Tuberculosis is the name applied to the disease caused by certain of the organisms within the genus *Mycobacterium,* which are curved or rod-shaped, sometimes filamentous, acid-fast bacteria. They are related to the genera *Nocardia, Corynebacterium,* and *Rhodococcus.* Many species of *Mycobacterium,* other than those causing tuberculosis, are pathogenic for humans and animals. These are listed in Table 10-15. Additionally, the genus contains saprophytes and members, which, although recovered from animals, are not known to be pathogenic. Other less well characterized mycobacteria have been recovered from granulomatous lesions in animals, and acid-fast organisms have been identified in "tuberculous" lesions, but have not been isolated. Such is the case with "tuberculous skin lesions" in cattle.

Aside from cattle, swine, nonhuman primates, and

TABLE 10-15 **Mycobacterial infections**

Organism	Host(s)	Disease
M. tuberculosis	Humans, nonhuman primates, dogs, rarely other domestic animals	Tuberculosis
M. bovis	Humans, cattle, nonhuman primates, dogs, cats, sheep, goats, swine, horses, parrots	Tuberculosis
M. avium	Domestic and wild fowl, swine, humans, nonhuman primates, rarely other domestic animals	Tuberculosis
M. microti	Voles	Tuberculosis
M. ulcerans	Humans	Indolent skin ulcers
M. intracellulare	Humans, nonhuman primates, cattle, swine	Pulmonary disease (tuberculosis)
M. kansasii	Humans, cattle	Pulmonary disease, lymphadenitis
M. africanum	Humans	Pulmonary disease (tuberculosis)
M. marinum	Humans, fish	"Swimming pool granuloma" of skin
M. scrofulaceum	Humans	Cervical lymphadenitis of children (scroful Tb)
M. chelonae	Humans	Ear and wound infections
M. farcinogenes and M. senegalense	Cattle	"Bovine farcy"
M. lepraemurium	Rats, possibly other animals	Nodular skin disease ("rat leprosy")
	Cats ?	Feline leprosy
M. paratuberculosis	Cattle, sheep	Paratuberculosis, Johne's disease
M. leprae	Humans, armadillo	Leprosy
M. fortuitum	Humans, dogs, cats, cattle, swine	Soft tissue infections
M. smegmatis	Cattle	Mastitis (usually a commensal)

domestic fowl, tuberculosis is not a common disease of animals (Figs. 10-26 thru 10-32). Throughout most of the world, the bovine disease is widespread, but in the United States, Great Britain, Europe, and Canada, and some other countries, its incidence has been greatly reduced by tuberculin testing and elimination of infected animals. In these countries, the control of bovine tuberculosis has dramatically reduced the prevalence of infection of the bovine type in both humans and animals. Four species of Mycobacterium cause tuberculosis.

Mycobacterium tuberculosis is the type species and

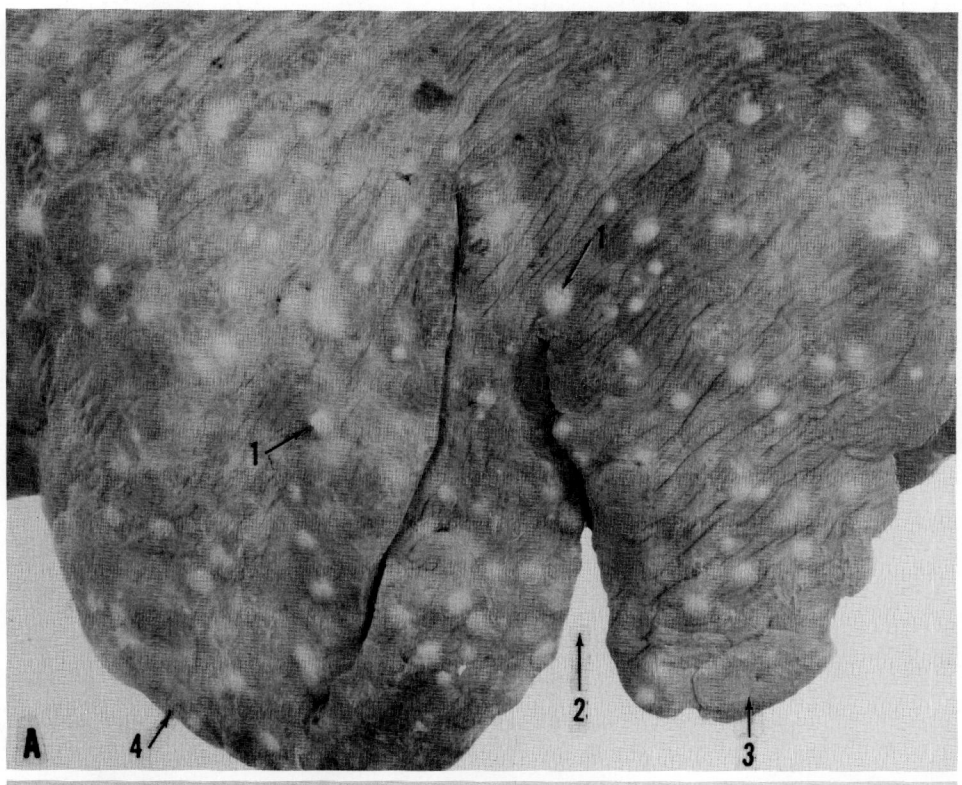

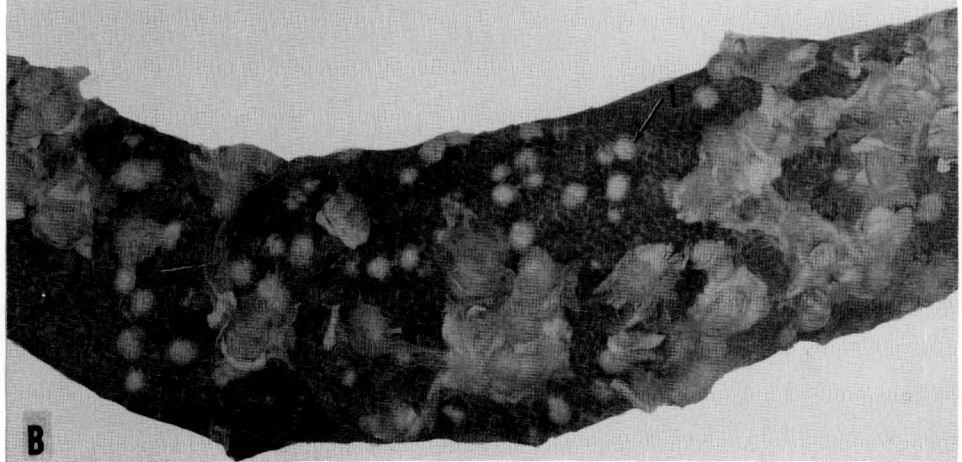

FIG. 10-26 Tuberculosis in swine. **A.** Lung. Sharply demarcated nodules (1) elevating the pleura. Cardiac notch (2), apical lobe (3), and inferior border (4) of the lung. **B.** Nodules in the spleen (1), adhesions of mesentery (2). (Courtesy of Dr. B. A. Walter, and Armed Forces Institute of Pathology.)

the principal cause of tuberculosis in humans and nonhuman primates. It is occasionally encountered as a cause of tuberculosis in dogs, but other domestic animals, such as cattle and cats, are relatively resistant. Among laboratory animals, guinea pigs and hamsters are highly susceptible, but rabbits and birds are resistant. Spread of infection is principally by aerosol from infected humans; the organism is rarely maintained in other species.

Mycobacterium bovis, which is closely related to *M. tuberculosis,* is the chief cause of tuberculosis in cattle, as well as in other domestic animals. Humans are also susceptible, usually acquiring the infection from ingestion of infected milk. It is also pathogenic for sheep, goats, dogs, cats, horses, swine, and some species of birds, such as parrots. Rabbits, guinea pigs, and nonhu-

man primates, are easily infected, whereas hamsters and mice are more resistant. The organism is only slightly pathogenic for rats. Domestic fowl are not susceptible. The organism is maintained in cattle and is spread in cattle principally by aerosol, but calves can be infected by ingestion of milk or in utero.

Mycobacterium avium is the main cause of tuberculosis in domestic fowl and wild birds. It is also an important pathogen for swine, but rarely a cause of tuberculosis in other animals, although it may infect dogs, cats, horses, sheep, goats, nonhuman primates, and humans. It is closely related to *Mycobacterium intracellulare,* and isolates are often dubbed *M. avium-intracellulare.* These are encountered on occasion as the cause of tuberculosis in animals as well as in humans, especially immunocompromised individuals. *M. avium* is not

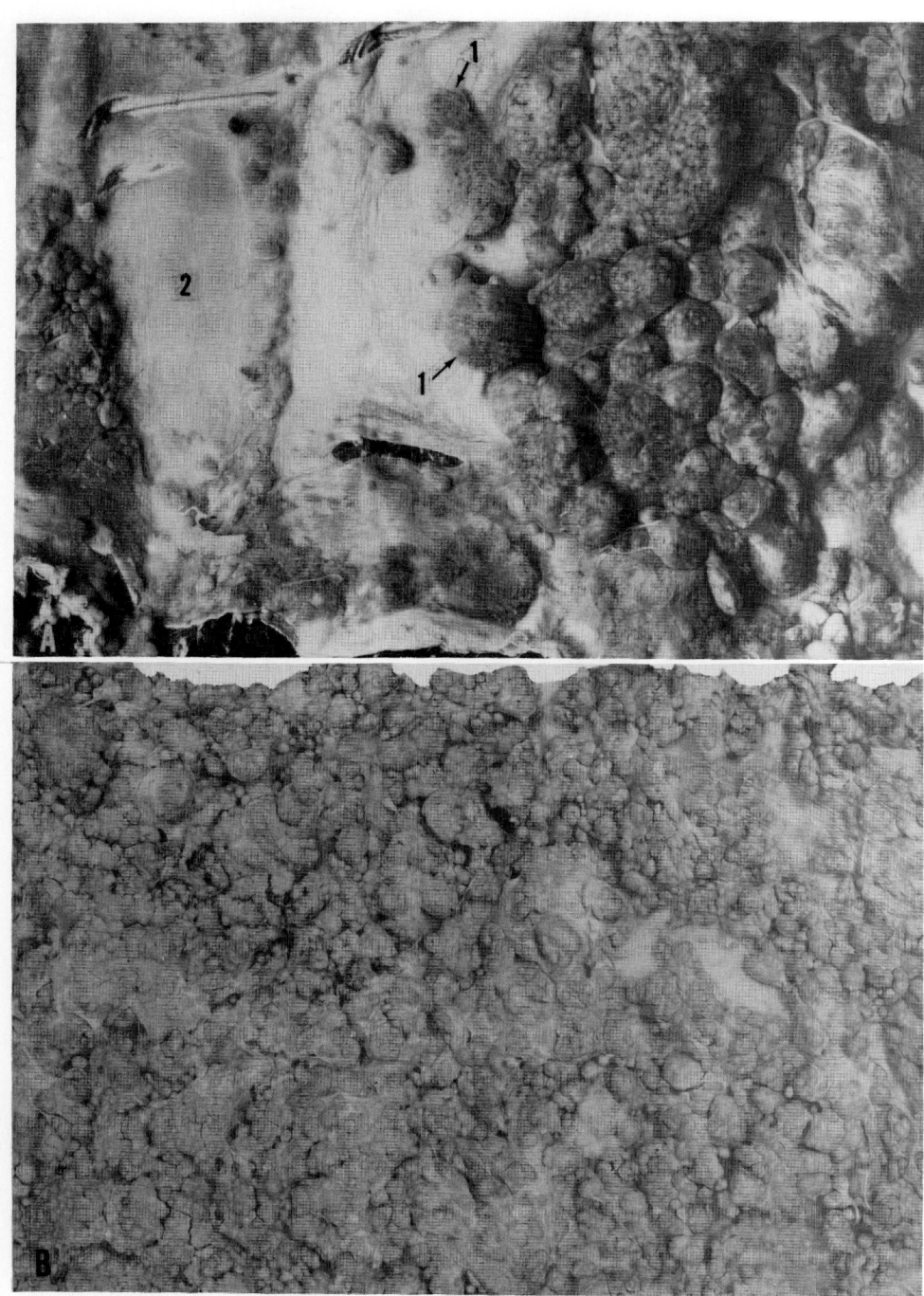

FIG. 10-27 Bovine tuberculosis. **A.** Involvement of pleura by coarse nodules (1). Inner surface of rib (2). (Contributor: Major Lytle, V.C., U.S. Army.) **B.** Tuberculous involvement of the omentum of a cow. (Courtesy of Station Veterinarian, U.S. Army, Fort Bayard, NM, and Armed Forces Institute of Pathology.)

pathogenic for guinea pigs or rats but will infect rabbits and mice. *M. avium* is maintained in birds and spread principally by ingestion. The source of infection in other species is not always related to contact with infected birds. In both swine and nonhuman primates, healthy animals may carry the organism in their digestive tracts, the most common site of lesions. Immunosuppression allows its presence to progress to disease in nonhuman primates, but this is not the case with swine, where lesions may be present in a high percentage of certain herds.

Mycobacterium microti is the cause of tuberculosis in voles and not of importance in domestic animals.

Lesions

The characteristic lesion of tuberculosis is the tubercle, a classic granuloma composed of a collection of epithelioid cells surrounded by a rim of fibroblasts with interspersed lymphocytes. Often the center of the granuloma is necrotic and calcified. Comparable with lesions of many other infectious diseases, the tubercle lesion is the

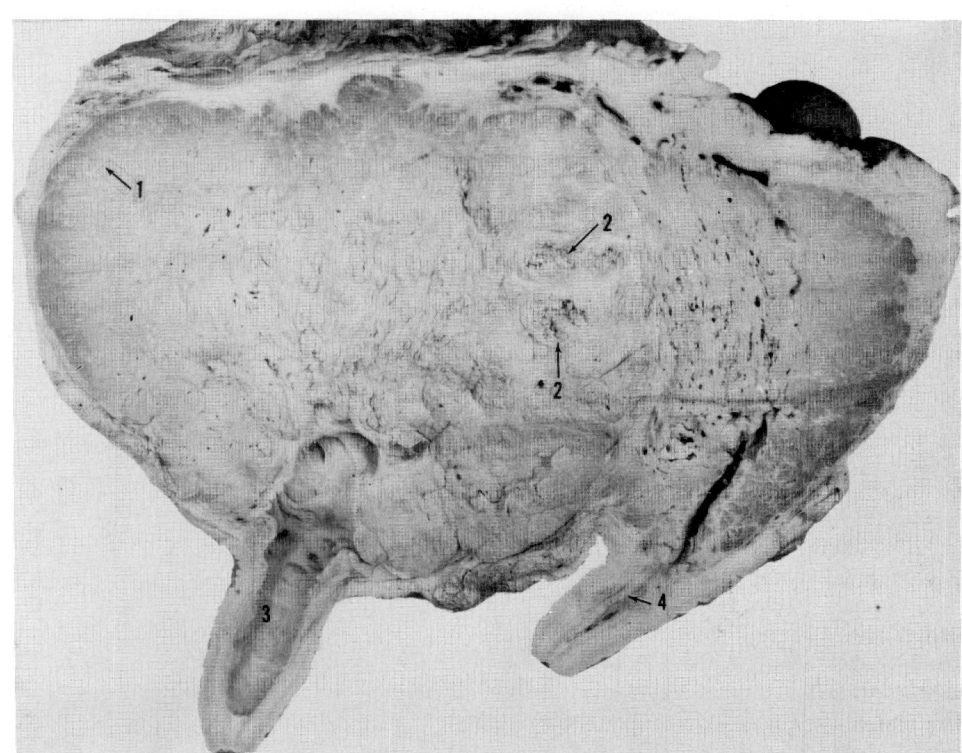

FIG. 10-28 Tuberculous mastitis, udder of a cow. Tiny discrete tubercles are seen at (1), confluent lesions with central necrosis at (2), normal teat canal (3), partially obstructed canal (4). (Courtesy of Major Lytle, V.C., U.S. Army, and Armed Forces Institute of Pathology.)

host's reaction to the invading organisms, and its pathogenesis is dependent on an immunologic response, usually referred to as hypersensitivity. The initial lesion consists of a cluster of neutrophils surrounding invading bacilli, which is replaced in a few hours by a whorl of macrophages. The mycobacteria are ingested, but multiply intracellularly, owing in part to mycobacterial glycolipids that prevent fusion of phagosomes with lysosomes. With unchecked intracellular multiplication, the organisms may gain entry into lymphatics to be carried to regional lymph nodes and distant sites.

With the onset of an immune response, the lesion develops the typical features of a granuloma. The whorl of macrophages takes on a different appearance; the cells become reminiscent of epithelial cells with abundant eosinophilic cytoplasm and are termed **epithelioid cells.** Although derived from circulating monocytes and phagocytes, epithelioid cells contain abundant endoplasmic reticulum suggestive of an adaptation to a secretory cell. Coalescence of epithelioid cells (less often by nuclear division) leads to the presence of multinucleated giant cells up to 50 microns in diameter. These are usually Langhans' giant cells, in which the nuclei are arranged in a wreath or crescent at the periphery of the cell. As the granuloma increases in size, the central cells undergo caseous necrosis. Calcification may occur in the caseous center of the tubercle, except in avian tuberculosis in birds, where it is practically unknown. Tubercle bacilli in varying numbers can be demonstrated with acid-fast stains in the cytoplasm of Langhans' giant cells, epithelioid cells, and in the case-

ous necrotic debris. Their number may be very few, and finding them may require a diligent search.

As the lesion ages, collagenous connective tissue surrounding the lesion increases in amount and maturity. If the bacteria in the lesion are eventually overcome, the tubercle is reduced to a small mass of fibrous or hyaline scar tissue. There is some evidence, however, that even with healing, the organisms may not be entirely eliminated but persist as a latent infection. If the immune responses are not effective, the lesions continue to grow in size, develop large cavitary centers, and continue to disseminate to other organs. Most tubercles are usually between 1 mm and 2 cm in diameter, but conglomerate tubercles may be formed by the growth and coalescence of one or more adjacent single tubercles.

Infection with tubercle bacilli does not always result in the formation of typical tubercles. This is particularly true of meningeal tuberculosis, a rapidly fatal infection, in which the pathologic changes consist of a scanty fibrinous or fibrinopurulent exudate on the surface of the pia mater and only a scattering of epithelioid cells in the meninges. Tissue reaction of a similar diffuse type may occur in overwhelming infections in sensitized animals.

The gross appearance of a tubercle, whether deep in soft tissue like liver and lungs, or bulging from a mucous or serous surface, is usually that of a firm or hard, white, gray, or yellow nodule. On cut section, its yellowish, caseous, necrotic center is dry and solid in contrast to the pus in an abscess. Calcification is common in

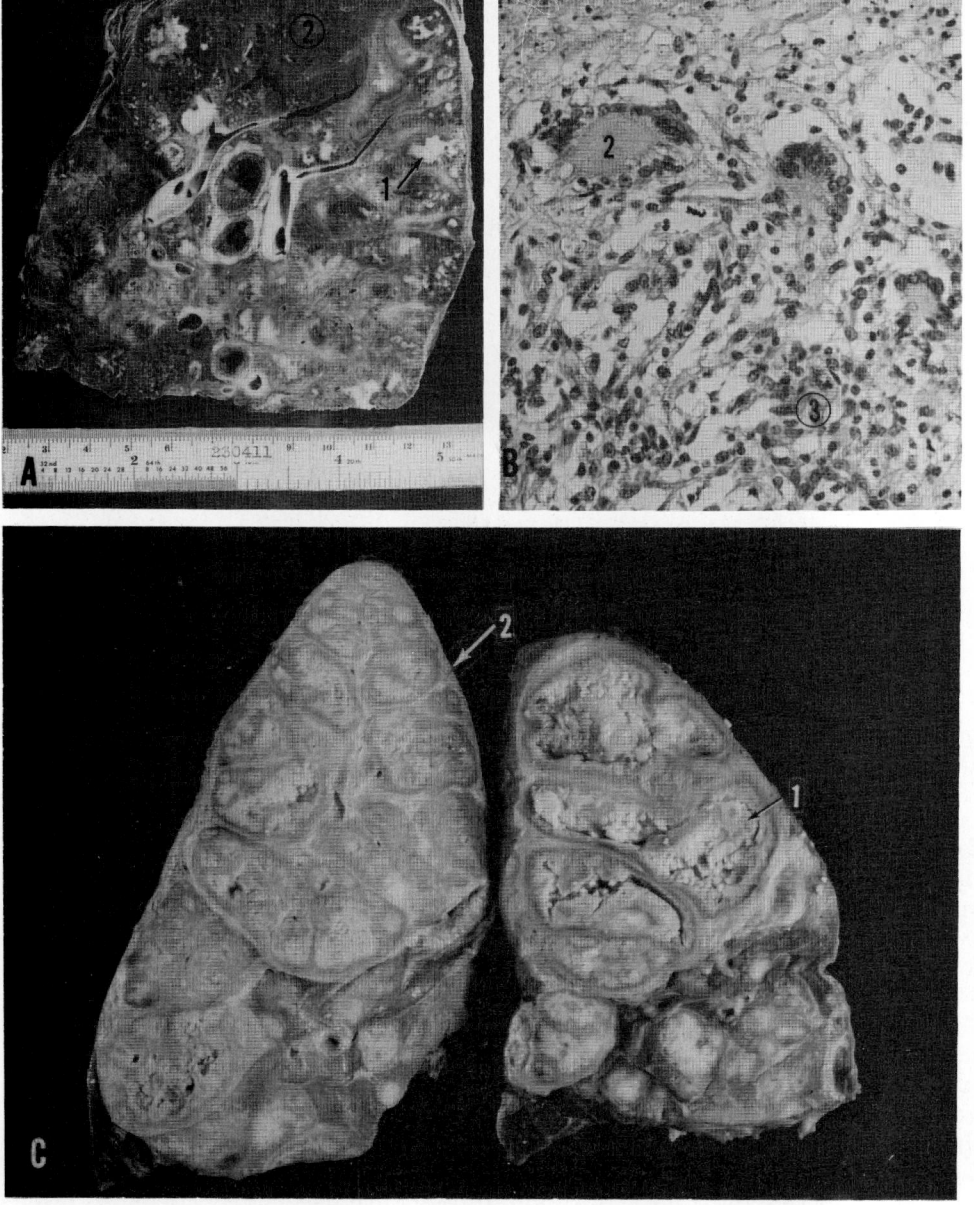

FIG. 10-29 Tuberculosis. **A.** Lobular pneumonia of tuberculosis, lung of a tapir. The white foci (1) represent pus in consolidated lobules, contrasting with less consolidated lung (2). (Contributor: National Zoological Park.) **B.** Margin of a tubercle in a bovine lung (× 260). Caseous necrosis (1), Langhans' giant cell (2), and epithelioid cells (3). **C.** Consolidated apical lobes of a bovine lung. Same animal as Case B. Note caseous areas (1) and thickening of pleura (2) and interlobular septa. (Courtesy of Dr. Wm. H. Feldman, and Armed Forces Institute of Pathology.)

many animals, and in sectioning a tubercle, a gritty sensation and grating sound indicate the presence of calcareous material.

Occasionally a tubercle breaks into a blood vessel, or by other means the blood is seeded with large numbers of tubercle bacilli, which lodge in capillaries of the parenchyma of visceral organs, where they give rise to myriad tubercles, 2 to 3 mm in diameter, all of the same age and size. Because these lesions suggested a sprinkling of millet seeds to early observers, they gave the name **miliary tuberculosis** to infection of this rapidly fatal type.

LESIONS IN DIFFERENT SPECIES

Although the general features of tuberculosis are evident in lesions from most species, certain differences in tissue reaction are more or less specific. In the **bovine,** calcification is often prominent, particularly in lymph nodes. Disseminated tubercles over the pleural and peritoneal surfaces are also fairly common. The appearance of these individual tubercles, usually from 0.5 to 1.0 cm in diameter, gives this manifestation a common descriptive name, pearl disease. Of particular interest are certain bovine skin lesions which, though histologically indistinguishable from those of typical

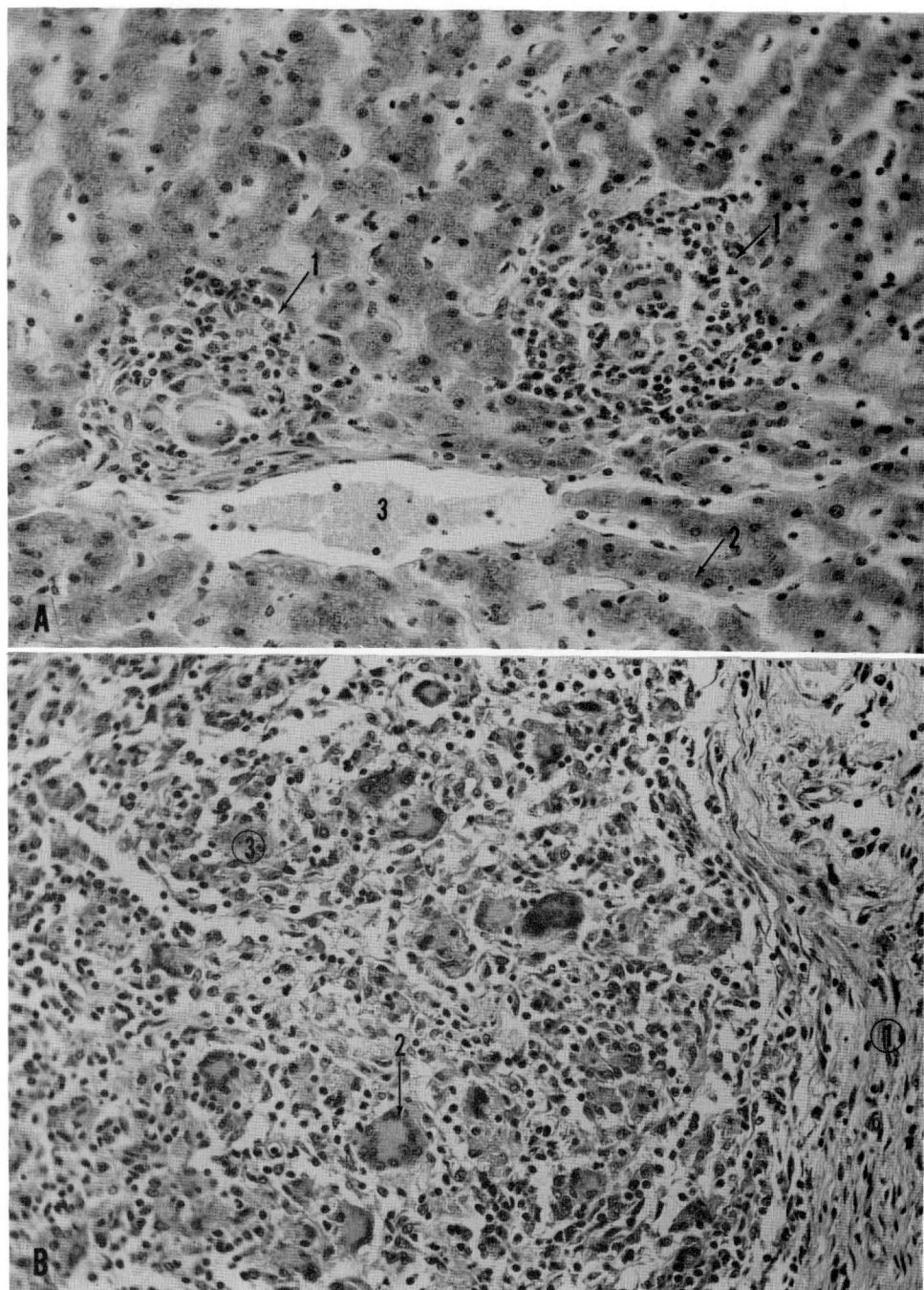

FIG. 10-30 Tuberculosis in a horse. **A.** Early tubercles in the liver (1) (× 260). Liver cell columns (2), central vein (3). **B.** Margin of a well-developed tubercle in the liver (× 260). The lesion is encapsulated (1) and contains many Langhans' giant cells (2) and epithelioid cells (3). (Courtesy of Dr. J. R. M. Innes, and Armed Forces Institute of Pathology.)

tuberculosis, are not caused by infection with tubercle bacilli. Acid-fast bacilli that apparently do not cause systemic disease produce these tuberculoid lesions. The organisms of particular interest cause certain bovine skin lesions that occur most frequently on the legs and are often associated with lymphangitis. This disease has been termed "skin tuberculosis," and, although the disease is histologically indistinguishable from those of typical tuberculosis, it is not caused by infection with tubercle bacilli. In most examples, organisms cannot be cultured; however, a species termed *M. vaccae* has been recovered from some lesions and from lacteal glands of

cattle. The disease produces sensitivity to bovine tuberculin, a point of considerable practical importance.

In the **horse,** the lesions of tuberculosis are usually of chronic, proliferative character and rarely exhibit caseation or calcification. Alimentary infection is the usual form, with possible extension elsewhere (Fig. 10-30). In **birds** also, calcification is seldom observed. In contrast, the lesions of tuberculosis of the avian type in **swine** appear as multiple caseocalcareous, encapsulated foci, most often affecting lymph nodes of the head and neck, mesenteric lymph nodes, and intestinal mucosa.

In **dogs** and **cats,** the lesions may be discrete granu-

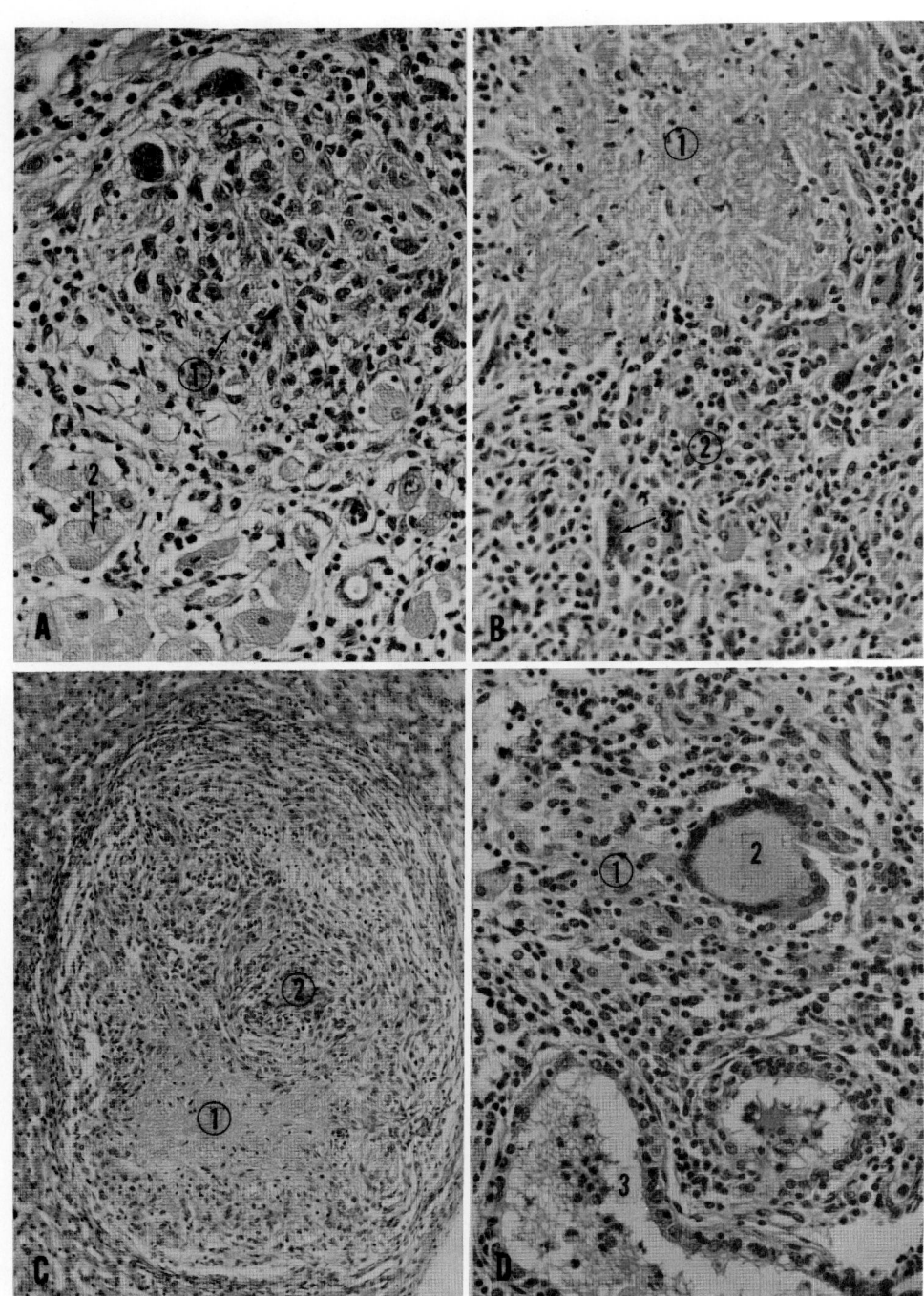

FIG. 10-31 Tuberculous lesions in different species. **A.** Tuberculous myocarditis in a pig (× 260). Note epithelioid cells (1) displacing myocardial fibers (2). (Contributor: Dr. C. L. Davis.) **B.** Tubercle in the spleen of a pig (× 260). Caseous necrosis (1), epithelioid cells (2), and giant cells (3). (Contributor: Dr. C. L. Davis.) **C.** Confluent tubercles in the liver of a dog (× 100). Note caseous necrosis (1) and epithelioid cells (2). Giant cells are absent. (Contributor: Dr. R. B. Oppenheimer.) **D.** Tuberculous mastitis in a cow (× 260). Note epithelioid cells (1), Langhans' giant cell (2), and mammary acinus (3). (Courtesy of Dr. Wm. H. Feldman, and Armed Forces Institute of Pathology.)

lomas with caseous centers, or they may be characterized by a more diffuse admixture of epithelioid cells, Langhans' giant cells, and connective tissue lacking organizational structure, caseation, and calcification.

In **nonhuman primates,** the disease is usually pulmonary and may run a fulminating course; miliary lesions are frequent, caseation is often prominent, and calcification is rare. Langhans' giant cells may be numerous or absent.

Infection by *Mycobacterium avium-intracellulare* often results in lesions of a very different nature from those already described. Although *M. avium* infection can

clearly lead to the formation of classic tubercles, there are a number of circumstances in which the lesions are characterized by infiltration of tissues by diffuse sheets of epithelioid cells containing a myriad of organisms. The numbers of organisms in any given cell can be so numerous that, with acid-fast stains, individual bacteria cannot be discerned nor cellular morphology recognized, everything being reduced to a red mass. Giant cells, necrosis, calcification, and fibroplasia are entirely absent. This pattern is seen in *M. avium-intracellulare* infection in nonhuman primates, where the lesion primarily affects the intestinal mucosa and mesenteric

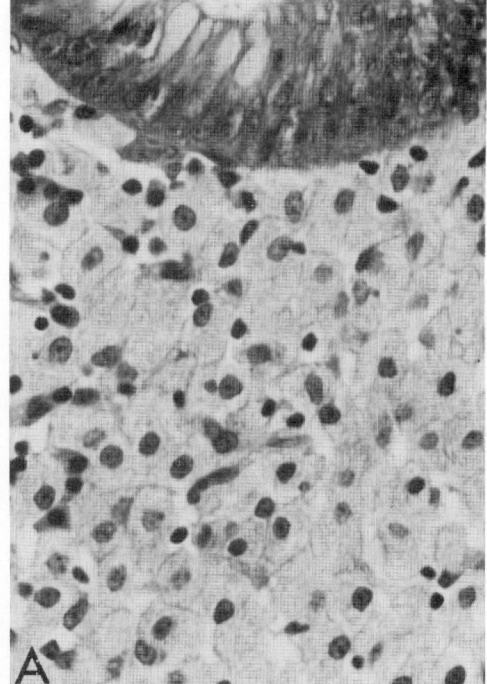

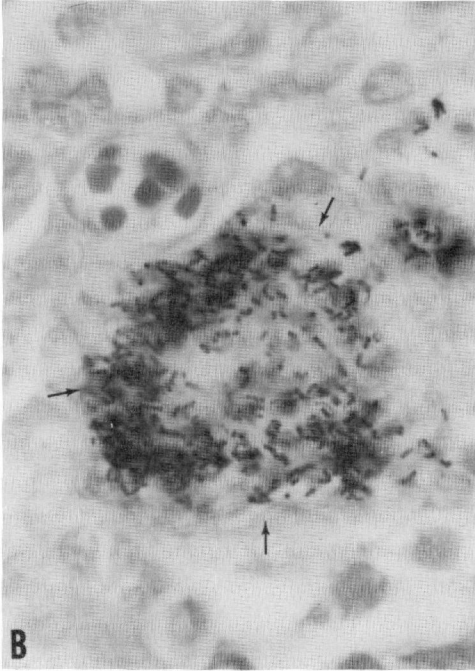

FIG. 10-32 Avian tuberculosis in a monkey. **A.** Large macrophages (epithelioid cells) in the lamina propria of the small intestine. **B.** A single macrophage (arrows) filled with tubercle bacilli (acid-fast stain). (Contributed by Dr. C. L. Davis.)

lymph nodes and resembles Johne's disease. Most often, this disorder of monkeys has been associated with immunosuppression induced by retroviruses. Similar lesions, but containing numerous Langhans' giant cells, have been seen in **horses.** There are also occasional reports in other species of infection characterized by epithelioid cells stuffed with organisms.

Diagnosis

The diagnosis of tuberculosis in the living animal may be based on roentgenographic findings, the tuberculin test, and demonstration of the organisms in exudates or excretions.

In tissues obtained surgically or at necropsy, demonstration of acid-fast organisms within typical tubercles is sufficient to establish the diagnosis, although bacteriologic isolation of the organism is necessary to establish its type. Acid-fast bacteria (mycobacteria) appear to infect many different species, hence it is important that in each instance organisms be recovered in culture for careful identification.

References

Barton MD, Acland HM. *Mycobacterium avium* serotype 2 infection in a sheep. Aust Vet J 1973;49:212–213.

Bellinger DA, Bullock BC. Cutaneous *Mycobacterium avium* infection in a cynomolgus monkey. Lab Anim Sci 1988;38:85–86.

Bone JF, Soave OA. Experimental tuberculosis in owl monkeys (Aotus trivirgatus). Lab Anim Care 1970;20:946–948.

Brooks OH. Observations on outbreaks of Battery type mycobacteriosis in pigs raised on deep litter. Aust Vet J 1971;47:424–427.

Capucci DT, Oshea JL, Smith GD. Epidemiologic account of tuberculosis transmitted from man to monkey. Am Rev Respir Dis 1972;106:819–823.

Carpenter JL, et al. Tuberculosis in five Basset hounds. J Am Vet Med Assoc 1988;192:1563–1568.

Cassidy DR, Morehouse LG, McDaniel HA. *Mycobacterium avium* infection in cattle: a case series. Am J Vet Res 1968;29:405–410.

Clarkson MJ, Smith MW. An outbreak of tuberculosis in experimental monkeys caused by the bovine organism. Trans R Soc Trop Med Hyg 1969;63:24.

Clifton-Hadley RS, Wilesmith JW. Tuberculosis in a deer: a review. Vet Rec 1991;129:5–12.

Cline JM, Schlafer DW, Callihan DR, et al. Abortion and granulomatous colitis due to *Mycobacterium avium* complex infection in a horse. Vet Pathol 1991;28:89–91.

Collins CH, Grange JM. A review. The bovine tubercle bacillus. J Appl Bacteriol 1983;55:13–29.

Dannenberg AM. Cellular hypersensitity and cellular immunity in the pathogenesis of tuberculosis: specificity, systemic and local nature, and associated macrophage enzymes. Bact Rev 1968;32:85–102.

Drolet R. Disseminated tuberculosis caused by *Mycobacterium avium* in a cat. J Am Vet Med Assoc 1986;189:1336–1337.

Duffield BJ, Young DA. Survival of *Mycobacterium bovis* in defined environmental conditions. Vet Microbiol 1985;10:193–197.

Ellsworth S, Kirkbride CA, Johnson DD. Excretion of *Mycobacterium avium* from lesions in the intestine and tonsils of infected swine. Am J Vet Res 1980;41:1526–1530.

Feldman WH. Histology of experimental tuberculosis in different species. Arch Pathol 1931;11:896–913.

Feldman WH, Fitch CP. Histologic features of the intradermic reactions to tuberculin in cattle. Arch Pathol 1936;22:495–509.

Ferber JA, Scherzo CS. Tuberculosis in a dog. J Am Vet Med Assoc 1983;183:117.

Fleischman RW, du Moulin GC, Esber HJ, et al. Nontuberculous mycobacterial infection attributable to *Mycobacterium intracellulare* serotype 10 in two rhesus monkeys. Am Vet Med Assoc 1982;181:1358–1362.

Flores JM, Canchez J, Castaño M. Avian tuberculosis dermatitis in a young horse. Vet Rec 1991;128:407–408.

Foster ES, Scavelli TD, Greenlee PG, et al. Cutaneous lesions caused by *Mycobacterium tuberculosis* in a dog. J Am Vet Med Assoc 1986;188:1188–1190.

Fox JG, et al. Tuberculosis spondylitis and Pott's paraplegia in a Rhesus monkey *(Macaca mulatta).* Lab Anim Sci 1974;24:335–339.

Francis J. Tuberculosis in animals and man. A study in comparative pathology. London: Cassell and Co. 1958.

Glassroth J, Robins AG, Snider DE Jr. Tuberculosis in the 1980s. N Engl J Med 1980;302:1441–1450.

Goodwin RT, Jerome CP, Bullock BC. Unusual lesion morphology and skin test reaction for *Mycobacterium avium complex* in macaques. Lab Anim Sci 1988;38:20–24.

Hix JA, Jones TC, Karlson AG. Avian tubercle bacillus infection in a cat. J Am Vet Med Assoc 1961;138:641–647.

Holmberg CA, et al. Immunologic abnormality in a group of *Macaca arctoides* with high mortality due to atypical mycobacterial and other disease processes. Am J Vet Res 1985;46:1192–1196.

Innes JRM. The pathology and pathogenesis of tuberculosis in domesticated animals compared with man. Br Vet J 1940;96:42–50, 96–105, 391–407.

Innes JRM. Tuberculosis in the horse. Br Vet J 1949;105:373–383.

Jang SS, Eckhaus MA, Saunders G. Pulmonary *Mycobacterium fortuitum* infection in a dog. J Am Vet Med Assoc 1984;184:96–98.

Janssen DL, Anderson MP, Abildgaard S, et al. Tuberculosis in newly imported macaques *(Macaca thibetans)*. J Zoo Wildl Med 1989;20:315–321.

Jarnagin JL, Himes EM, Richards WD, et al. Isolation of *Mycobacterium kansasii* from lymph nodes of cattle in the United States. Am J Vet Res 1983;44:1853–1855.

Jorgensen JB, Haarbo K, Dam A, et al. An enzootic of pulmonary tuberculosis in pigs caused by M. avium. I. Epidemiological and pathological studies. Acta Vet Scand 1972;13:56–67.

Karlson AG, Thoen CO. *Mycobacterium avium* in tuberculous adenitis of swine. Am J Vet Res 1971;32:1257–1261.

Kearns TJ, Russo PK. The control and eradication of tuberculosis. A summary report. N Engl J Med 1980;303:812–814.

Leathers CW, Hamm TE Jr. Naturally occurring tuberculosis in a Squirrel monkey and a Cebus monkey. J Am Vet Med Assoc 1976;169:909–911.

Lesslie IW, Davies DRT. Tuberculosis in a horse caused by the avian type tubercle bacillus. Vet Rec 1958;70:82–84.

Liu S-K, Weitzman I, Johnson GG. Canine tuberculosis. J Am Vet Med Assoc 1980;177:164–167.

Lowry PW, et al. *Mycobacterium chelonae* causing otitis media in an ear-nose-and-throat practice. N Engl J Med 1988;319:978–982.

Machotka SV, Chapple FE III, Stookey JL. Cerebral tuberculosis in a rhesus monkey. J Am Vet Med Assoc 1975;167:648–650.

Marks J. A new practical classification of the mycobacteria. J Med Microbiol 1976;9:253–261.

Matthews JA, Liggitt HD. Disseminated mycobacteriosis in a cat. J Am Vet Med Assoc 1983;183:701–702.

McGavin MD, Mallmann VH, Mallmann WL, et al. Pathological changes in calves injected intradermally with *Mycobacterium intracellulare* serotype Davis and M. avium serotype 2. Vet Pathol 1977;14:56–66.

Montali RJ, ed. Mycobacterial infections of zoo animals. Washington, DC: Smithsonian Institution Press 1978.

Moore TD, Allen AM, Ganaway JR, et al. A fatal infection in the opossum due to *Mycobacterium intracellulare*. J Infect Dis 1971;123:569–578.

Orr CM, Kelly DF, Lucke VM. Tuberculosis in cats. A report of two cases. J Small Anim Pract 1980;21:247–253.

Richardson A. The experimental production of mastitis in sheep by *Mycobacterium smegmatis* and *Mycobacterium fortuitum*. Cornell Vet 1971;61:640–646.

Safranek TJ, et al. *Mycobacterium chelonae* wound infections after plastic surgery employing contaminated gentian violet skin-marking solution. N Engl J Med 1987;317:197–201.

Sakula A. Robert Koch. the story of his discoveries in tuberculosis. Irish J Med Sci 1985;154(5, Suppl 1):3–9.

Sapolsky RM, Else JG. Bovine tuberculosis in a wild baboon population: epidemiological aspects. J Med Primatol 1987;16:229–235.

Saunders G. Pulmonary *Mycobacterium tuberculosis* infection in a circus elephant. J Am Vet Med Assoc 1983;183:1311–1312.

Schultze WD, Brasso WB. Characterization and identification of *Mycobacterium smegmatis* in bovine mastitis. Am J Vet Res 1987;48:739–742.

Sesline DH, et al. *Mycobacterium avium* infection in three rhesus monkeys. J Am Vet Med Assoc 1975;167:639–645.

Sills RC, Mullaney TP, Stickle RL, et al. Bilateral granulomatous guttural pouch infection due to *Mycobacterium avium* complex in a horse. Vet Pathol 1990;27:133–135.

Smith EK, et al. Avian tuberculosis in monkeys, a unique mycobacterial infection. Am Rev Respir Dis 1973;107:469–471.

Snider WR. Tuberculosis in canine and feline populations. Review of the literature. Am Rev Respir Dis 1971;104:877–887.

Snyder S, Peace T, Soave O, et al. Tuberculosis in an owl monkey *(Aotus trivirgatus)*. J Am Vet Med Assoc 1970;157:712–713.

Soave O, Jackson S, Ghumman JS. Atypical mycobacteria as the probable cause of positive tuberculin reactions in squirrel monkeys *(Saimiri sciureus)*. Lab Anim Sci 1981;31:295–296.

Stamp JT. Tuberculosis of the bovine udder. J Comp Pathol Ther 1943;53:220–230.

Tasler GRW, Hartley WJ. Foal abortion with Mycobacterium terrae infection. Vet Pathol 1981;18:122–125.

Thoen CO, et al. *Mycobacterium bovis* infection in baboons (Papio papio). Arch Pathol 1977;101:291–293.

Thoen CO, et al. Experimentally induced *Mycobacterium avium* serotype 8 infection in swine. Am J Vet Res 1976;37:177–182.

Thoen CO, Himes EM, Richards WD, et al. Bovine tuberculosis in the United States and Puerto Rico: a laboratory summary. Am J Vet Res 1979;40:118–120.

Turnwald GH, et al. Survival of a dog with pneumonia caused by *Mycobacterium fortuitum*. J Am Vet Med Assoc 1988;192:64–66.

Waggie JS, Wagner JE, Lentsch RH. [1] A naturally occurring outbreak of Mycobacterium avium-intracellulare infections in C57BL/6N mice. [2] Experimental murine infections with a *Mycobacterium avium-intracellulare* complex organism isolated from mice. Lab Anim Sci 1983;33:249–253, 254–257.

White SD, et al. Cutaneous atypical mycobacteriosis in cats. J Am Vet Med Assoc 1983;182:1218–1222.

Zumpe D, Silberman MS, Michael RP. Unusual outbreak of tuberculosis due to *Mycobacterium bovis* in a closed colony of rhesus monkeys *(Macaca mulatta)*. Lab Anim Sci 1980;30:237–240.

PARATUBERCULOSIS (JOHNE'S DISEASE)

Paratuberculosis is a specific infection with an acid-fast organism, *Mycobacterium paratuberculosis*, which is known to affect cattle, sheep, goats, and other ruminants (Figs. 10-33 and 10-34). Swine and horses can be infected, but lesions are minimal to absent. Most laboratory animals are generally resistant to infection; however, a model of the disease has been reproduced in athymic mice. An organism very similar to *M. paratuberculosis* has been recovered from humans with Crohn's disease and from stump-tailed macaques *(Macaca arctoides)* with a similar granulomatous ileocolitis. In cattle, it causes a wasting illness with a prolonged course, during which intractable diarrhea results in dehydration, emaciation, and eventually death. The disease is of worldwide distribution and constitutes an important economic problem in cattle; but it is less frequently encountered in other species.

Young calves are most susceptible to infection, which is usually acquired during the first year of life. Clinical signs are apparent only after several months. Infection in cattle and sheep does not always lead to clinical disease; even in the absence of recognizable infection, the organism is shed in the feces, providing a source of infection for young animals. Although lesions are usually restricted to the intestinal tract and lymph nodes, the organism can infect other tissues, including the uterus, which may lead to congenital infection and abortion.

Feces containing the organisms serve as the primary

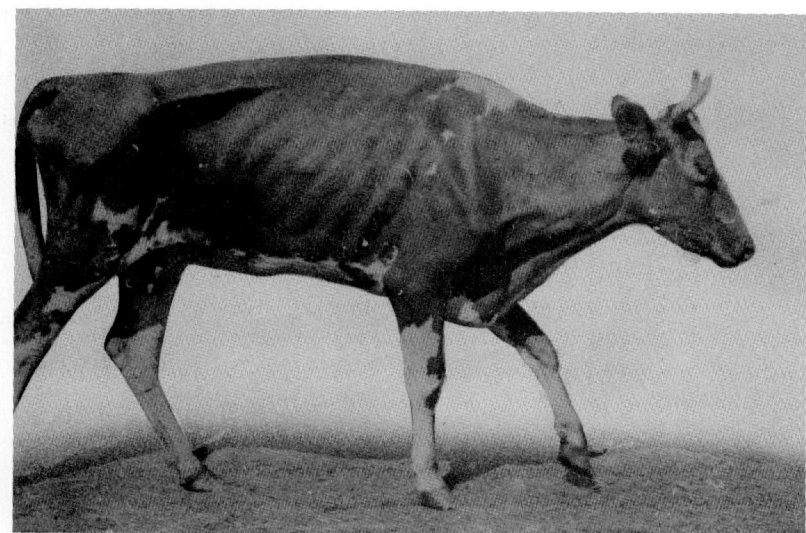

FIG. 10-33 Paratuberculosis. Emaciation and dehydration are significant features in this affected cow.

source of infection, which is acquired by ingestion. The organisms penetrate the intestinal mucosa and set up residence within macrophages, where they multiply intracellularly without killing the host cell and, like other mycobacteria, are resistant to cellular digestion. There is evidence to indicate that intestinal M cells play a key role in the transport of the bacteria across the mucosa, which would explain the primary localization of lesions to the terminal ileum.

Lesions

The terminal part of the ileum is the most common site of the specific lesions, which also occur in the remainder of the small and large intestines and the mesenteric lymph nodes. Microscopic sections reveal the lamina propria of the mucosa to be closely packed with large, discrete epithelioid cells that have abundant foamy cytoplasm and are often multinucleated. These cells also infiltrate and thicken the submucosa but leave the muscularis mucosae and the muscularis intact. Nests of these same epithelioid cells may be found in mesenteric lymph nodes, but seldom elsewhere. In impression smears or sections through these lesions, Ziehl-Neelsen's stain demonstrates quantities of acid-fast, rod-shaped organisms crowding the cytoplasm of the epithelioid cells where they multiply. As with the mycobacteria that cause tuberculosis, *M. paratuberculosis* is resistant to cellular digestion.

Secondary changes in the intestinal mucosa in paratuberculosis include edema, which results from local interference with circulation; nests of neutrophils; and increased numbers of eosinophils, the latter perhaps explainable on the basis of helminthic parasitism. Of importance is the absence of caseous necrosis, nodule formation, and calcification. In contrast to cattle, nod-

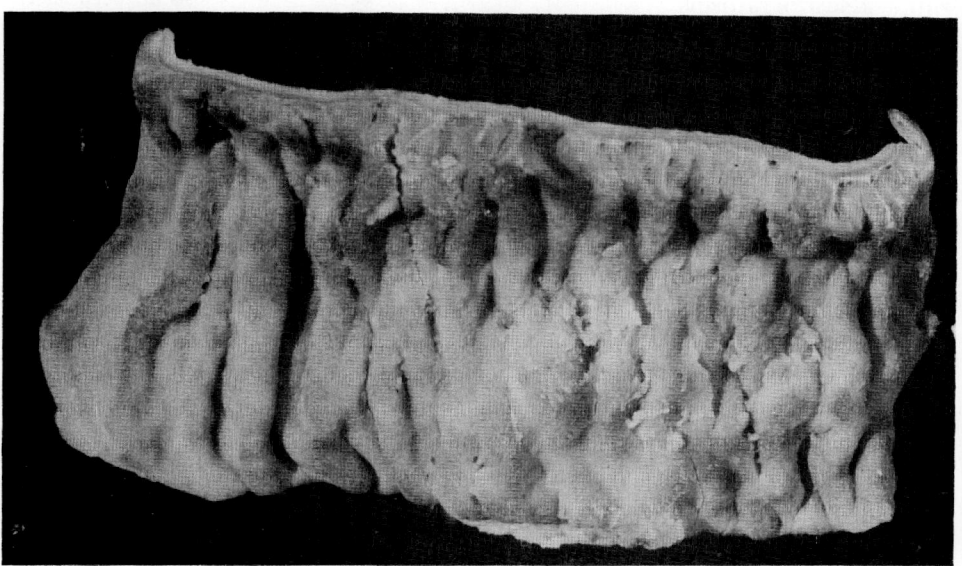

FIG. 10-34 Paratuberculosis (Johne's Disease), small intestine of a cow. Note thick, rugose mucosa. (Courtesy of Dr. Edward Records, and Armed Forces Institute of Pathology.)

ule formation with necrosis and calcification has been described in sheep, goats, and wild ruminants.

The gross appearance is directly related to the microscopic changes. The affected intestinal wall is thickened, sometimes edematous, and its mucosal surface bears many broad, closely placed, transverse folds, or rugae. These rugae result from thickening of villi and give the surface a corrugated appearance, which does not disappear when the intestinal wall is stretched (Fig. 10-34).

Although lesions are usually confined to the intestines and lymph nodes, generalized infection has been described in both naturally infected and experimentally infected cattle, sheep, and goats, with lesions occurring in the liver, spleen, lungs, kidneys, uterus, placenta, and nonmesenteric lymph nodes.

Diagnosis

The gross lesions in the intestine are highly suggestive, but confirmation of the diagnosis depends on the demonstration of epithelioid cells containing acid-fast bacilli in huge numbers in smears or sections of mucosa or submucosa. In about 60% of affected cattle, the lesions and organisms extend into the colon and rectum, which makes it possible to diagnose the disease in the living animal by microscopic examination of mucosal scrapings collected from the rectum.

The diffuse nature of the lesions, their confinement to the intestinal mucosa and mesenteric lymph nodes, and the presence of a myriad of acid-fast bacilli serve to differentiate paratuberculosis from tuberculosis, in which nodule formation, fibrosis, necrosis, calcification, and only few acid-fast bacilli are characteristic. In sheep and goats, lesions with caseation and calcification require greater caution in differentiating tuberculosis; however, the diffuse distribution of the lesions of paratuberculosis usually allows this distinction.

Avian tubercle bacilli produce similar lesions in nonhuman primates. Culture and identification of the organisms is essential in this and all other infections with acid-fast organisms.

If the disease cannot be confirmed by biopsy, various serologic tests and the intradermal johnin test can be employed, but neither approach is completely satisfactory.

References

Bendixen PH, Bloch B, Jorgensen JB. Lack of intracellular degradation of *Mycobacterium paratuberculosis* by bovine macrophages infected in vitro and in vivo: light microscopic and electron microscopic observations. Am J Vet Res 1981; 42:109–113.

Buergelt CD, Hall C, McEntee K, et,al. Pathological evaluation of paratuberculosis in naturally infected cattle. Vet Pathol 1978;15:196–207.

Chiodini RJ, Van Kruiningen HJ. Eastern white-tailed deer as a reservoir of ruminant paratuberculosis. J Am Vet Med Assoc 1983;183:168–169.

Chiodini RJ, Van Kruiningen HJ. Characterization of *Mycobacterium paratuberculosis* of bovine, caprine, and ovine origin by gas-liquid chromatographic analysis of fatty acids in whole-cell extracts. Am J Vet Res 1985;46:1980–1989.

Chiodini RJ, Van Kruiningen HJ, Merkal RS. Ruminant paratuberculosis (Johne's disease): the current status and future prospects. Cornell Vet 1984;74:218–262.

Dierckins MS, Sherman DM, Gendron-Fitzpatrick A. Probable paratuberculosis in a Sicilian ass. J Am Vet Med Assoc 1990;196:459–461.

Doyle TM. Foetal infection in Johne's disease. Vet Rec 1958;70:238.

Hallman ET, Witter JF. Some observations on the pathology of Johne's disease. J Am Vet Med Assoc 1933;83:159–187.

Hamilton HL, Cooley AJ, Adams JL, et al. *Mycobacterium paratuberculosis* monoassociated nude mice as a paratuberculosis model. Vet Pathol 1991;28:146–155.

Harding HP. Experimental infection with *Mycobacterium johnei*. 2. Histopathology of infection in experimental goats. J Comp Pathol 1957;67:37–52.

Harding HP. The histopathology of *Mycobacterium johnei* infection in small laboratory animals. J Pathol Bact 1959;78:157–169.

Hines SA, Buergelt CD, Wilson JH, et al. Disseminated *Mycobacterium paratuberculosis* infection in a cow. J Am Vet Med Assoc 1987;190:681–683.

Hole NH. Johne's disease. Adv Vet Sci 1958;4:341–387.

Howarth JA. Paratuberculous enteritis in sheep. Cornell Vet 1937;27:223–234.

Johne HA, Frothingham L. Ein eigenthumlicher Fall von Tuberculose beim Rind. Deutsch Zeit Thiermed verg Pathol 1895;21:438–454.

Kim JCS, Sanger VL, Whitenack DL. Ultrastructural studies of bovine paratuberculosis (Johne's disease). Vet Med Small Anim Clin 1976;71:78–83.

Kopecky KE, Larsen AB, Merkal RS. Uterine infection in bovine paratuberculosis. Am J Vet Res 1967;28:1043–1045.

Kluge JP, Monlux WS, Kopecky KE, et al. Experimental paratuberculosis in sheep after oral, intratracheal, or intravenous inoculation: lesions and demonstration of etiologic agent. Am J Vet Res 1968;29:953–962.

Larsen AB, Moon HW, Merkal RS. Susceptibility of swine to *Mycobacterium paratuberculosis*. Am J Vet Res 1971;32:589–595.

Larsen AB, Moon HW, Merkal RS. Susceptibility of horses to *Mycobacterium paratuberculosis*. Am J Vet Res 1972;33:2185–2189.

Larsen AB, Kopecky KE. *Mycobacterium paratuberculosis* in reproductive organs and semen of bulls. Am J Vet Res 1970;31:255–258.

Lominski I, Cameron J, Roberts GBS. Experimental Johne's disease in mice. J Pathol Bact 1956;71:211–221.

Majeed S, Goudswaard J. Aortic lesions in goats infected with *Mycobacterium johnei*. J Comp Pathol 1971;81:571–576.

McQueen DS, Russell EG. Culture of *Mycobacterium paratuberculosis* from bovine foetuses. [letter] Aust Vet J 1979;55:203–204.[Vet Bull 1980;50:553.]

Merkal RS. Paratuberculosis: advances in cultural, serologic, and vaccination methods. J Am Vet Med Assoc 1984;184:939–943.

Merkal RS, Kopecky KE, Monlux WS, et al. Experimental paratuberculosis in sheep after oral, intratracheal, or intravenous inoculation: serologic and intradermal tests. Am J Vet Res 1968;29:963–969.

Merkal RS, Kopecky KE, Larsen AB, et al. Immunologic mechanisms in bovine paratuberculosis. Am J Vet Res 1970;31:475–486.

Merkal RS, Whipple DL, Sacks JM, et al. Prevalence of *Mycobacterium paratuberculosis* in ileocecal lymph nodes of cattle culled in the United States. J Am Vet Med Assoc 1987;190:676–680.

M'Fadyean J. Histology of the lesions of Johne's disease. J Comp Pathol Ther 1918;31:73–87.

Momotani E, Whipple DL, Thiermann AB, et al. Role of M cells and macrophages in the entrance of *Mycobacterium paratuberculosis* into domes of ileal Peyer's patches in calves. Vet Pathol 1988;25:131–137.

Nakamatsu M, Fujimoto Y, Satoh H. The pathological study of paratuberculosis in goats, centered around the formation of remote lesions. Jpn J Vet Res 1969;16:103–120.

Pearson JKL, McClelland TG. Uterine infection and congenital Johne's disease in cattle. Vet Rec 1955;67:615–616.

Rajya BS, Singh CM. Studies on the pathology of Johne's disease in sheep. III. Pathologic changes in sheep with naturally occurring infections. Am J Vet Res 1961;22:189–203.

Sweeney RW, Whitlock RH, Rosenberger AE. *Mycobacterium paratuber-*

culosis isolated from fetuses of infected cows not manifesting signs of the disease. Am J Vet Res 1992;53:477–480.

Taylor AW. Experimental Johne's disease in cattle. J Comp Pathol 1953;63:355–367.

Thayer WR, Chiodini R, Van Kruiningen H, et al. Mycobacteria in inflammatory bowel disease. Falk Symp 1988;46:89–92.

Thoen CO, Baum KH. Current knowledge on paratuberculosis. J Am Vet Med Assoc 1988;192:1609–1611.

Williams ES, Snyder SP, Martin KL. Pathology of spontaneous and experimental infection of North American wild ruminants with *Mycobacterium paratuberculosis*. Vet Pathol 1983;20:274–290.

LEPROSY

Leprosy, also known as Hansen's disease, is caused by *Mycobacterium leprae* (Fig. 10-35). It is a slowly progressive infection of humans that principally affects the skin (especially of the face, hands, and feet), peripheral nerves, eyes, testes, and upper airways. Although not highly communicable, the disease remains an endemic infection in many tropical countries, with an estimated 10 to 12 million people afflicted.

The lesions of what is termed **lepromatous leprosy** are characterized by diffuse to nodular collections of vacuolated macrophages containing relatively large numbers of acid-fast bacilli. The macrophages are laden with lipid, taking on a distinctive appearance, and are termed **lepra cells.** As the disease progresses, similar lesions develop in the lymph nodes, liver, and spleen. In another expression of the disease in which there is a strong cell-mediated immune response, the lesions closely resemble those of tuberculosis. This form of the disease is termed **tuberculoid leprosy** and is characterized by very few stainable organisms within the lesions.

M. leprae has not been cultured and, until recently, was not thought to infect species other than humans.

Early in the 1970s, however, the nine-banded armadillo *(Dasypus novemcinctus)* was shown to be experimentally susceptible. Subsequently, naturally affected armadillos were identified in southern Louisiana and later in the Texas Gulf Coast where the disease is now recognized as endemic. The disease in armadillos is of the lepromatous type and more rapidly progressive than in humans, with extensive systemic lesions. Seven-banded *(Dasypus hybridus)* and eight-banded *(Dasypus sabanicola)* armadillos are also susceptible. More recently, naturally acquired leprosy has been observed in mangabey monkeys *(Cercocebus atys)* and a chimpanzee. The disease has been experimentally reproduced in mangabeys as well as in rhesus monkeys *(Macaca mulatta),* African green monkeys *(Cercopithecus aethiops),* and a chimpanzee.

References

Arnoldi J, et al. Species-specific assessment of *Mycobacterium leprae* in skin biopsies by in situ hybridization and polymerase chain reaction. Lab Invest 1992;66:618–623.

Balentine JD, Chang SC, Issar SL. Infection of armadillos with *Mycobacteriumn leprae.* Arch Pathol Lab Med 1976;100:175–181.

Baskin GB, et al. Experimental leprosy in the mangabey *(Cercocebus atys):* necropsy findings. Int J Lepr Other Mycobact Dis 1985;53:269–277.

Baskin GB, et al. Experimental leprosy in a rhesus monkey: necropsy findings. Int J Lepr Other Mycobact Dis 1987;55:109–115.

Convit J, Pinardi ME. Leprosy: confirmation in the armadillo. Science 1974;184:1191–1192.

Donham KJ, Leininger JR. Spontaneous leprosy-like disease in a chimpanzee. J Infect Dis 1977;136:132–136.

Gormus BJ, et al. A second sooty mangabey monkey with naturally acquired leprosy: first reported possible monkey-to-monkey transmission. Int J Lepr Other Mycobact Dis 1988;56:61–65.

Leininger JR, Donham KJ, Rubino MJ. Leprosy in a chimpanzee. Pathology of the disease and characterization of the organism. Vet Pathol 1978;15:339–346.

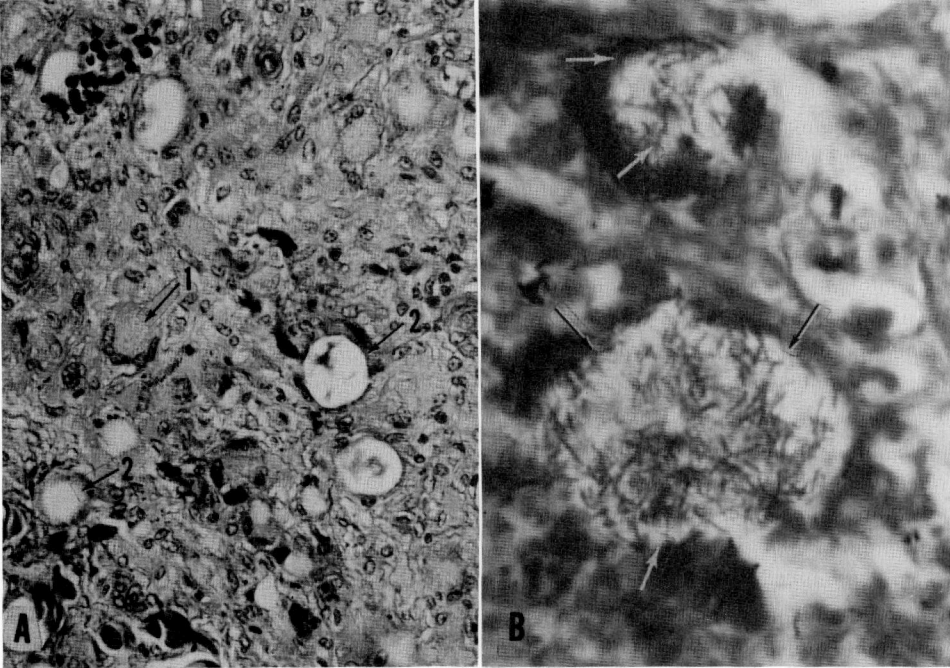

FIG. 10-35 Leprosy of buffaloes. **A.** A section of a dermal nodule (× 300). Giant cells (1) and large macrophages, many containing large "globules" (2). **B.** Higher magnification (× 1250) of a section stained for acid-fast bacilli. The "globules" (arrows) are filled with acid-fast organisms. (Courtesy of Dr. K. W. Wade, and Armed Forces Institute of Pathology.)

Malaty R, et al. Histopathological changes in the eyes of mangabey monkeys with lepromatous leprosy. Int J Lepr Other Mycobact Dis 1988;56:443–448.

Meier JL, Folse DS, Smith JH. Leprosy in wild armadillos *(Dasypus novemcinctus)* in the Texas Gulf Coast: ultrastructure of the liver and spleen. Lab Invest 1983;49:281–290.

Meyers WM, Gormus BJ, Walsh GP, et al. Naturally acquired and experimental leprosy in nonhuman primates. Am J Trop Med Hyg 1991;44(Suppl):24–27.

Meyers WM, et al. Comparative pathology of disseminated multibacillary leprosy. Comp Pathol Bull 1984;16(2):1,5–6.

Meyers WM, et al. Leprosy in a mangabey monkey — naturally acquired infection. Int J Lepr Other Mycobact Dis 1985;53:1–14.

Noordeen SK, Bravo LL. The world leprosy situation: the global situation. World Health Stat Q 1986;39:122–137.

Storrs EE. The nine-banded armadillo: A model for leprosy and other biomedical research. Int J Lepr 1971;39:702–703.

Storrs EE, Walsh GP, Burchfield HP, et al. Leprosy in the armadillo: new model for biomedical research. Science 1974;183:851–852.

Wolf RH, et al. Experimental leprosy in three species of monkeys. Science 1985;227:529–531.

Murine leprosy

Murine leprosy, a spontaneous disease of rats that closely resembles human leprosy, was first described in 1903 by Stefansky. The disease, which occurs endemically throughout the world in wild rats, is caused by *Mycobacterium lepraemurium*. Mice are susceptible and a limited, nonprogressive infection can be established in rabbits and monkeys. The same organism, or one that is very similar, causes feline leprosy.

LESIONS

The lesions in murine leprosy are the result of aggregations of cells packed with bacilli, diffusely infiltrating the dermis, subcutis, and all viscera except the kidney, or forming nodules in these tissues. These enlarged cells with foamy cytoplasm laden with acid-fast bacilli are called "lepra cells." They usually are derived from the reticuloendothelial system but occasionally from epithelial cells of the epidermis, testicular tubules, or epididymis. Some lepra cells contain such excessive numbers of bacilli and such quantities of lipid that they form vacuolated globi, identical with those that occur in human or bovine leprosy.

Granulomas resembling the nodular lesions of leprosy have been described in frogs, but their significance and relationship to leprosy have not been established.

References

Closs O, Haugen OA. Experimental murine leprosy. 3. Early local reaction to Mycobacterium lepraemurium in C311 and C57/BL mice. Acta Pathol Microbiol Scand A 1975;83:51–58.

Fite GL. Leprosy: The pathology of experimental rat leprosy. US Natl Health Bull. Washington, DC: US Pub Health Serv 1940;173:45–76.

Krakower C, Gonzales LM. Mouse leprosy. Arch Pathol 1940;30:308–329.

Lowe J. Rat leprosy, a critical review of the literature. Int J Lepr 1937;5:311–328, 463–482.

Machicao N, La Placa E. Lepra-like gramulomas in frogs. Lab Invest 1954;3:219–227.

Pinkerton H, Sellards AW. Histological and cytological studies of murine leprosy. Am J Pathol 1938;14:435–442.

Sellards AW, Pinkerton H. The behavior of murine and human leprosy in foreign hosts. Am J Pathol 1938;14:421–434.

Stefansky WK. Eine lepraähnliche Erkrankung der Haut und der Lymphdru ausen bei Wanderraten. Zentralbl Bakteriol Orig (pt. 1). 1903;33:481–487.

FELINE LEPROSY

Leprosy of the domestic cat *(Felis catus)* was first described in New Zealand (Brown and others, 1962) as a nontuberculous granulomatous disease involving the dermis and subcutis. The disease has at this writing been reported in Australia, Great Britain, the Netherlands, the western United States, and western Canada. The causative agent has not been specifically identified, but is very similar to *Mycobacterium lepraemurium*. The disease has been experimentally transmitted from cats to rats and mice and back to cats.

Lesions

The lesions usually appear as single or multiple nodules involving the skin and subcutis in almost any part of the body, but particularly the head and limbs. They may also develop in the oral and nasal cavities. The overlying epidermis or mucosa is occasionally ulcerated. Microscopically, the lesions resemble leprosy of humans, taking the form of either tuberculoid or lepromatous leprosy. In the former, the lesions resemble typical tubercles consisting of granulomas composed of epithelioid cells containing multinucleated giant cells and scattered lymphocytes and plasma cells with a caseous core. Calcification is not a feature, nor is there significant fibrosis. The lepromatous form consists of more diffuse granulomatous infiltrates of epithelioid cells lacking a defined structure, lacking caseous necrosis, and with fewer multinucleated cells and lymphocytes. Features of both forms may be present in a single individual. The cells are foamy, but less so when compared to leprosy in humans. Large numbers of acid-fast bacilli are present within the cytoplasm of the epithelioid cells. Involvement of peripheral nerves, as is typical of human leprosy, is also absent, however, there may be granulomatous lymphadenitis. In experimentally infected rats, the lesions become generalized, as seen in natural murine leprosy caused by *M. lepraemurium* in this species.

References

Brown LR, May CD, Williams SE. A non-tuberculous granuloma in cats. N Z Vet J 1962;10:7–9.

Lawrence WE, Wickham N. Cat leprosy: infection by a bacillus resembling *Mycobacterium lepraemurium*. Aust Vet J 1963;39:390–393.

Leiker DL, Poelma FG. On the etiology of cat leprosy. Int J Lepr 1974;42:312–315.

McIntosh DW. Feline leprosy: a review of forty-four cases from western Canada. Can Vet J 1982;23:291–295.

Robinson M. Skin granuloma of cats associated with acid-fast bacilli. J Small Anim Pract 1975;16:563–567.

Scheifer B, Gee BR, Ward GE. A disease resembling feline leprosy in Western Canada. J Am Vet Med Assoc 1974;165:1085–1087.

Schiefer HB, Middleton DM. Experimental transmission of a feline mycobacterial skin disease (feline leprosy). Vet Pathol 1983;20:460–471.

Thompson EJ, Little PB, Cordes DO. Observations of cat leprosy. NZ Vet J 1979;27:233–235.

Wilkinson GTA. A non-tuberculous granuloma of the cat associated with an acid-fast bacillus. Vet Rec 1964;76:777–778, 833–834.

LEPROSY OF BUFFALOES (LEPRA BUBALORUM)

A disease of water buffaloes (carabao) characterized by persistent cutaneous and subcutaneous nodules on the legs and lower parts of the abdomen and thorax occurs in Java and other East Indian countries. It is of particular interest because of the similarity of its histologic features to those of human leprosy. Apparently the disease is uncommon and ordinarily does not result in death or serious disability. The causative organism, although demonstrable in tissue, has not been cultured successfully. A similar but even less frequent disease *(Lepra bovinum)* has been described in cattle in the East Indies.

Lesions

The cutaneous nodules result from accumulation of large numbers of epithelioid cells in the dermis. Microscopically, these individually discrete cells are seen to have greatly distended, foamy, often vacuolated cytoplasm in which numerous acid-fast bacilli are demonstrable. The large vacuoles are believed to be the result of lipid production by the bacilli and are identical to those in the large "lepra cells" of human leprosy. Giant cells of Langhans' type may be seen, but caseation necrosis and calcification do not occur. The gross appearance of the lesion is not distinctive. A solid, uniform nodule, with a diameter as great as 4 to 5 cm, may be firmly attached to the dermis and elevate the epidermis.

Diagnosis

In countries where the disease occurs, the diagnosis can be made on the basis of the collections of "lepra cells" in the dermis, these cells being laden with acid-fast bacilli.

References

Lobel LWM. Lepra bubalorum. Int J Lepr 1936;4:79–96.

BOVINE FARCY

This disease, not known to occur in the United States, has been described in the Sudan, the Far East, and Latin America. Originally the causative organism was considered to be *Nocardia farcinica;* however, it is now believed to result from infection with *Mycobacterium farcinogenes* or *Mycobacterium senegalense.* The disease occurs as a chronic suppurative granulomatous inflammation of the skin, lymphatics and draining lymph nodes, usually confined to the limbs. Reportedly, the prescapular region is involved particularly often. In fatal infections, there is spread to the lungs, liver, spleen, and internal lymph nodes.

References

Awad FI, Karib AA. Studies on bovine farcy (nocardiosis) among cattle in the Sudan. Zentralbl Veterinarmed 1958;5:265–272.
Mostafa IE. Bovine nocardiosis (cattle farcy). A review. Vet Bull 1966;36:189–193.
Salih MAM, Sanousi SM el, Tag el Din HM. Predilection sites of bovine farcy lesions in Sudanese cattle. Bull Anim Health Prod Afr 1978;26:168–171.
Sanousi SM el, Tag el Din MH. On the aetiology of bovine farcy in the Sudan. J Gen Microbiol 1986;132:1673–1675

11

Diseases caused by fungi

The vast majority of fungi are saprophytes and do not cause disease in animals even when they gain entrance to the body through inhalation or other means. The only obligate parasites within the fungi are the dermatophytes, which live in keratin layers of the skin and cause ringworm. Theses are termed **superficial mycoses.** Dermatophytes do not live as saprophytes and transmission is direct; however, they are not invasive. All other disease-producing fungi live as saprophytes and only cause disease when the host is unable to restrict their growth in tissues. Most often, the organisms are destroyed after entry into the host and do not lead to disease.

A select group of organisms, however, are capable of establishing themselves in normal individuals. These fungi cause **systemic mycoses** and include histoplasmosis, coccidioidomycosis, blastomycosis, and sporotrichosis; they generally live as mycelial forms in soil or on plants and as yeast forms in tissue (dimorphic fungi). Even these organisms are usually checked after entering an animal host. Debilitated and immunocompromised animals are the most susceptible.

A third group of mycoses are the **subcutaneous mycoses** or **mycetomas.** Infection with these saprophytic fungi usually follows their entry into the skin through wounds where they grow in mycelial form, producing localized lesions that ordinarily do not disseminate.

A fourth group of fungi are capable of causing localized and disseminated disease, growing as mycelia in tissue. Included in this group are aspergillosis and the zygomycoses. These are most frequent in, but certainly not restricted to, debilitated animals.

The yeasts comprise a fifth group. Yeasts grow as single-celled fungi, although some form pseudomycelia. They are not highly pathogenic and rarely cause disease in the normal animal. Candidiasis is the most common yeast infection and is usually a superficial infection of mucous membranes, but may cause serious systemic disease. Cryptococcosis is the other yeast infection of significance in animals.

Many bacteria (so-called higher bacteria) induce disease that closely resembles the mycoses and are frequently included in discussions of diseases caused by fungi. They include *Actinomyces, Nocardia, Dermatophilus,* and *Mycobacteria.* These have been discussed in the preceding chapter on bacterial diseases.

LESIONS

In almost all cases the organisms can be easily seen in routine tissue sections stained with either hematoxylin and eosin or with special stains, such as Gomori methenamine silver (GMS), periodic acid-Schiff (PAS) reaction, or Gridley stain. A distinctive morphologic feature of certain of these diseases is the presence of a homogeneous, brightly eosinophilic material, known as **Splendore-Hoeppli material,** surrounding individual organisms or colonies of organisms. It exists as a variably-sized rim, frequently exceeding 100 microns, often with a serrated edge, or as a surrounding collar of radially arranged clubs or baseball bats. These clubs are usually coarse, 3–10 microns in diameter and 10–30 microns in length. Although their exact nature is not understood, it appears that they are a product of the host, most likely an antigen-antibody complex. Splendore-Hoeppli material is a relatively consistent feature of coccidioidomycosis and sporotrichosis, but may also be a feature of many other mycoses, as well as certain diseases caused by higher bacteria, such as actinomycosis.

The lesions produced by the tissue dwelling fungi are, in general, classic granulomas. A central core of necrotic debris exists, usually containing pus which, in turn, is surrounded by a zone of epithelioid cells, macrophages, and multinucleated giant cells. Variable numbers of lymphocytes, plasma cells, and on occasion eosinophils may be present. The entire lesion is surrounded by fibrovascular connective tissue of varying maturity. With coalescence, the characteristic spherical shape may be lost, but all distinctive elements are present.

The superficial mycoses (dermatophytoses) do not induce the formation of granulomas because the organisms are restricted to the superficial layers of the skin and are not invasive.

Excellent detailed descriptions of the pathology of diseases caused by fungi and many of the granuloma-forming bacteria, along with wonderful photomicrographs in color, can be found in the books by Chandler

505

and Watts (1987), Chandler et al., (1980) and Rippon (1988).

References

Baker RD, et al. (eds). International symposium on opportunistic fungus infections. Lab Invest 1962;11:1017–1241.

Chandler FW, Watts JC. Pathological diagnosis of fungal infections. Chicago: ASCP Press, 1987.

Chandler FW, Kaplan W, Ajello L. A colour atlas and textbook of the histology of mycotic diseases. London: Wolfe Med Publ, Ltd, 1980.

Connole MD, Johnston LAY. A review of animal mycoses in Australia. Vet Bull 1967;37:145–153.

Emmons CW, Binford CH, Utz JP, et al. Medical mycology, 3rd ed. Philadelphia: Lea & Febiger, 1977.

Kaplan W. Epidemiology of the principal systemic mycoses of man and lower animals and the ecology of their etiologic agents. J Am Vet Med Assoc 1973;163:1043–1047.

Kelley DC, Mosier JE. Public health aspects of mycotic diseases. J Am Vet Med Assoc 1977;171:1168–1170.

Purchase IFH, ed. Mycotoxins. New York: Elsevier Science Publishers, 1974.

Rippon JW. Medical mycology: the pathogenic fungi and pathogenic actinomycetes, 3rd ed. Philadelphia: WB Saunders, 1988.

Aspergillosis

Aspergillus spp. are saprophytic molds that are extremely common in nature, occurring on foodstuffs and plants as a white, fluffy, sporulating mold (Figs. 11-1 and 11-2). Ordinarily they are not pathogens, but rather opportunists; however, once established in a susceptible host, aspergillosis can be a serious disease. Circumstances allowing infection are usually not clear, although debilitated or immunocompromised animals and those on prolonged antibiotic therapy are at particular risk. Most infections are established by inhalation of spores leading to pneumonia. Hematogenous spread is common because of the faculty of *Aspergillus* to invade blood vessels and establish mycelial emboli. Certain *Aspergillus* spp. also produce toxins, known as aflatoxins, which cause mycotoxicosis (aflatoxicosis); mycotoxicosis is discussed later in this chapter. Of the over 100 species in the genus *Aspergillus*, *A. fumigatus*, *A. flavus*, *A. niger*, *A. nidulans*, and *A. terreus* are the most frequently associated with disease in animals.

Aspergillosis is most common and severe in poultry, especially young chicks and turkey poults, which become infected from contaminated bedding, usually while they are in the brooder stage of growth, hence the term "brooder pneumonia." The infection may occur as an epizootic with high mortality. Captive penguins, especially the king or emperor varieties in zoological gardens, are particularly susceptible to aspergillosis. In mammals, aspergillosis is seen in most species, but most often as an isolated event. The infection is not communicable. Superficial infections of the skin and cornea occur in most species as does pneumonia, sometimes with dissemination to other organs, such as the kidneys, gastrointestinal tract, liver, spleen, and central nervous system. In cattle, mastitis, placentitis and abortion, rumenitis, and gastritis may result from aspergillosis, often in concert with other fungi. Infection of the guttural pouch in horses results in a clinical syndrome manifested by recurrent epistaxis and visual and locomotor disturbances. The infectious granulomata may spread from the guttural pouch to the nasal cavity and, via the optic nerves, to the optic chiasma and cerebrum.

LESIONS

Acute or invasive aspergillosis is principally characterized by extensive necrosis and hemorrhage with a

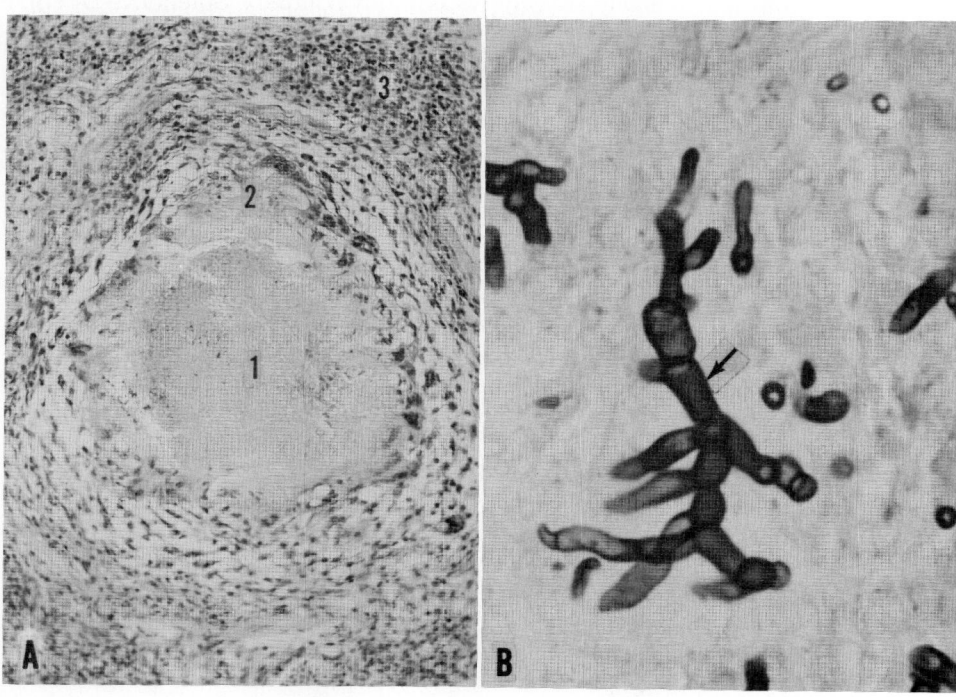

FIG. 11-1 Aspergillosis. **A.** Granuloma in lung of a chick (×185). Necrotic center (1) of the granuloma is surrounded by giant cells (2) and lymphocytes (3) in connective tissue. **B.** Gridley fungus stain of a section (×840) to demonstrate the septate, branching fungus. (Courtesy of Armed Forces Institute of Pathology and Dr. C.L. Davis.)

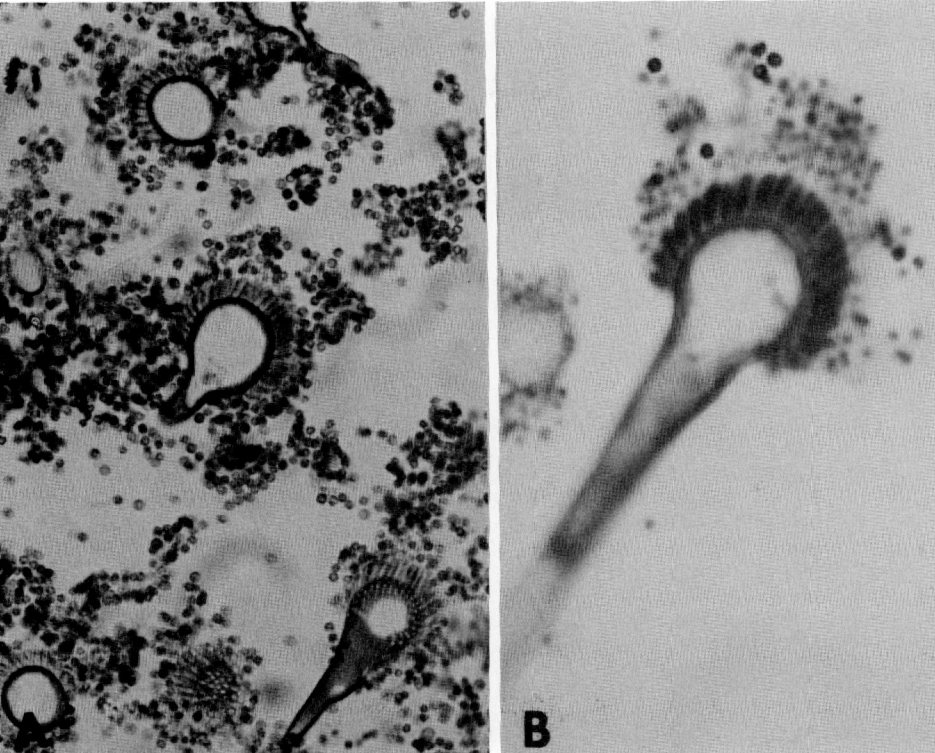

FIG. 11-2   Aspergillosis, lung of a chicken.   **A.** Conidiophores of *Aspergillus fumigatus*. These sporulating structures only form in the presence of high-oxygen tension. **B.** Higher magnification of a conidiophore.

purulent and mononuclear inflammatory response. Colonies of organisms are large and indiscriminately invade adjacent tissues. Invasion into the walls of arteries leads to thrombosis and infarction, further extending the necrotizing lesion. Lesions of longer standing take the form of granulomas with a central core of caseation necrosis in which the organisms are found surrounded by a wide zone of epithelioid cells. Multinucleated giant cells of the foreign body type may be present, as well as lymphocytes and a collar of fibroblasts in chronic lesions.

In tissue, the organisms may exist as large colonies of radiating hyphae, typical of the invasive disease, or as small colonies of irregularly dispersed hyphae, which is the more usual appearance within granulomas or superficial infections. The hyphae are slender, 3–6 microns wide, of uniform diameter, and of variable length. They are septate and branching. The branches form at acute angles and are of the same diameter as the parent hyphae. The hyphae are usually basophilic, but often do not stain well with hematoxylin and eosin. Stains for glycogen (PAS, Bauer, Gridley fungus) differentiate the mycelia by coloring the cell wall intensely. Spores are ordinarily not formed in tissues, but on surfaces exposed to air, such as those on air sacs and the lining of external orifices and trachea; the organism may produce long, aerial, mycelia-bearing conidiophores, which project into the lumen. The mycelial growth in these sites is like that in cultures on artificial media. On occasion, mycelia are surrounded by eosinophilic, radiating clubs (Splendore-Hoeppli material) similar to that seen in actinomycosis and certain other mycotic infections.

DIAGNOSIS

The diagnosis can be confirmed by demonstrating the characteristic organisms with their slender, dichotomously branching septate hyphae, in tissue sections or by recovering them in cultures from typical lesions.

References

Allo MD, Miller J, Townsend T, et al. Primary cutaneous aspergillosis associated with Hickman intravenous catheters. N Engl J Med 1987;317:1105–1108.

Cook WR, Campbell RSF, Dawson C. The pathology and aetiology of guttural pouch mycosis in the horse. Vet Rec 1968;83:422–428.

Griffin RM. Pulmonary aspergillosis in the calf. Vet Rec 1969;84:109–111.

Harvey CE. Nasal aspergillosis and penicilliosis in dogs: results of treatment with thiobendazole. J Am Vet Med Assoc 1984;184:48–50.

Hatziolos BC, Sass B, Albert TF, et al. Ocular changes in a horse with gutturomycosis. J Am Vet Med Assoc 1975;167:51–54.

Hill MWM, Whiteman CE, Benjamin M, et al. Pathogenesis of experimental bovine mycotic placentitis produced by *Aspergillus fumigatus*. Vet Pathol 1971;8:175–192.

Johnson JH, Merriam JG, Attleberger M. A case of guttural pouch mycosis caused by *Aspergillus nidulans*. Vet Med Small Anim Clin 1973;68:771–774.

Kabay MJ, Robinson WF, Huxtable CRR, et al. The pathology of disseminated *Aspergillus terreus* infection in dogs. Vet Pathol 1985;22:540–547.

Kahler JS, Leach MW, Jang S, et al. Disseminated aspergillosis attributable to *Aspergillus deflectus* in a Springer Spaniel. J Am Vet Med Assoc 1990;197:871–874.

Khoo TK, Sugai K, Leong TK. Disseminated aspergillosis. Case report and review of the world literature. Am J Clin Pathol 1966;45:697–703.

Lingard DR, Gosser HS, Monfort TN. Acute epistaxis associated with guttural pouch mycosis in two horses. J Am Vet Med Assoc 1974;164:1038–1041.

Mason RW. Porcine mycotic abortion caused by *Aspergillus fumigatus.* Aust Vet J 1971;47:18–19.

Matsui T, et al. Pulmonary aspergillosis in apparently healthy young rabbits. Vet Pathol 1985;22:200–205.

Merkow LP, et al. The pathogenesis of experimental pulmonary aspergillosis. An ultrastructural study of alveolar macrophages after phagocytosis of *A. flavous* spores *in vivo.* Am J Pathol 1971;62: 57–74.

Mullaney TP, Levin S, Indrieri RJ. Disseminated aspergillosis in a dog. J Am Vet Med Assoc 1983;182:516–518.

Patton NM. Cutaneous and pulmonary aspergillosis in rabbits. Lab Anim Sci 1975;25:347–350.

Pier AC, Cysewski SJ, Richard JL. Mycotic abortion in ewes produced by *Aspergillus fumigatus:* intravascular and intrauterine inoculation. Am J Vet Res 1972;33:349–356.

Prystowsky SD, et al. Invasive aspergillosis. N Engl J Med 1976;295: 655–658.

Qualls CW Jr, Chandler FW, Kaplan W, et al. Mycotic keratitis in a dog: concurrent *Aspergillus* sp and *Curvularia* sp infections. J Am Vet Med Assoc 1985;186:975–976.

Rehm S, Waalkes MP, Ward JE. *Aspergillus* rhinitis in Wistar (Crl:(WI)BR) rats. Lab Anim Sci 1988;38:162–166.

Samuelson DA, Andresen TL, Gwin RM. Conjunctival fungal flora in horses, cattle, dogs, and cats. J Am Vet Med Assoc 1984; 184:1240–1242.

Slocombe RF, Slauson DO. Invasive pulmonary aspergillosis of horses: an association with acute enteritis. Vet Pathol 1988;25:277–281.

Southard C. Bronchopulmonary aspergillosis in a dog. J Am Vet Med Assoc 1987;190:875–877.

Thurston JR, Peden WM, Driftmier KM, et al. Histopathologic and antibody responses of rabbits exposed to aerosols containing spores of *Aspergillus fumigatus:* comparison of single and multiple exposures. Am J Vet Res 1986;47:919–923.

Weber A, Rudolph R. Mycotic rhinitis in two dogs caused by *Aspergillus fumigatus.* Zentralbl Veterinaermed B 1972;19:503–510.

Whiteman CE, Benjamin MM, Ball L, et al. Bovine aspergillosis produced by the inoculation of conidiospores of *Aspergillus fumigatus* into a mesenteric or jugular vein. Vet Pathol 1972;9: 408–425.

Wood GL, et al. Disseminated aspergillosis in a dog. J Am Vet Med Assoc 1978;172:704–707.

BLASTOMYCOSIS (NORTH AMERICAN BLASTOMYCOSIS, GILCHRIST DISEASE)

Blastomycosis is an infectious disease of humans and animals caused by the thermal dimorphic (i.e., yeast form in tissue, mycelial in culture) *Blastomyces dermatitidis.* The infection occurs in North America, the Middle East, and Africa. In the United States, it is most frequent in the Mississippi and Ohio River basins, around the Great Lakes, and in the Southeast. Among animals, blastomycosis is most frequent in dogs, but has been reported in cats (particularly Siamese), horses (mammary gland), a Stellar sea lion, and an African lion. Why blastomycosis is not seen in other domestic animals is not known. Blastomycosis reportedly occurred in dogs and humans of the same household. The fungus has been recovered from soil and infection is acquired by inhalation; it is not a communicable disease.

In dogs and cats, pulmonary infection is most common, but dissemination of the organisms may result in involvement of any system. Lung, skin, bone, lymph node, testicle, and eye are the most frequently affected organs. In humans, the infection often presents as cutaneous blastomycosis, but the primary site of disease is the lung, with secondary spread to the skin.

LESIONS

Blastomycosis is characterized by a mixed cellular reaction. A purulent reaction is characteristic of early lesions, whereas a typical granulomatous reaction characterizes lesions of longer standing. The typical lesion in dogs consists of a central core of neutrophils and caseous necrosis surrounded by an intensive infiltration by epithelioid cells in which foci of neutrophils and diffusely distributed lymphocytes may be found. Multinucleated giant cells may be present. Little tendency toward encapsulation of the lesions exists.

In the human skin, intraepithelial abscesses with epithelioid reaction in the dermis and subcutis, ulceration, and slow healing of the epidermis are described. In the lungs of dogs, circumscribed gray nodules of solidification may be manifest in some cases, and diffuse consolidation of the lung with the cut surfaces yielding purulent exudate, in others. Microscopically, the pulmonary lesion is characterized by intensive infiltration by epithelioid cells, in which foci of neutrophils and diffusely distributed lymphocytes may be found. Caseation necrosis may occur, and although some fibroblasts are recognizable, little tendency toward encapsulation of the lesions exists. Multinucleated giant cells of the foreign body type may be seen, but Langhans giant cells are rare. Calcification is infrequent.

The causative organisms, which vary in number from a few to a myriad, are found in the lesions, free, or in macrophages, as spherical, yeast-like cells, 8–20 μ in diameter, with double-contoured walls. In hematoxylin- and eosin-stained sections, the organisms usually are seen as a central granular mass surrounded by a refractile, double-contoured, unstained zone which is bounded by a thin outer wall. An occasional cell may be seen extruding a daughter cell (budding). The buds are always single with a broad base, an important aid in differential diagnosis. Although not always clearly visible, each yeast cell contains several nuclei. Stains for bound glycogen (PAS, Bauer, Gomori methenamine silver, Gridley fungus) will stain the outer wall of the organism selectively, differentiating it more clearly from the surrounding tissue.

The lesions may be limited to the lungs, but dissemination with abscess formation has been described in the subcutis, spleen, kidneys, lymph nodes, liver, brain, bones, adrenal glands, eye, and intestines.

DIAGNOSIS

Microscopic examination of affected tissues is necessary to establish the diagnosis. The organisms can be demonstrated readily in typical lesions and can be stained differentially with glycogen stains (PAS, Bauer, Gridley fungus). They are larger than *Histoplasma capsulatum*, smaller than *Coccidioides immitis* (a fungus that contains endospores and does not reproduce by budding), and do not have the wide, mucicarmine-staining capsule of *Cryptococcus neoformans.* The tissue reactions in histoplasmosis and cryptococcosis are also unlike that of blastomycosis. Cultural identification of the organisms is of value, but it is more important that any fungus recovered in culture also be demonstrated in characteristic lesions.

South American blastomycosis contrasts with North American blastomycosis. The South American disease is caused by *Paracoccidioides braziliensis,* an organism that also affects humans and animals, but which can be differentiated in tissues by its manner of budding. This organism reproduces in tissues by multiple budding, in contrast to the single bud that grows out from the cell wall of each spherule of *Blastomyces dermatitidis* (Fig. 11-3).

References

Alden CL, Mohan R. Ocular blastomycosis in a cat. J Am Vet Med Assoc 1974;164:527–528.

Archer JR, Trainer DO, Schell RF. Epidemiologic study of canine blastomycosis in Wisconsin. J Am Vet Med Assoc 1987;190:1292–1295.

Benbrook EA, Bryant JB, Saunders LZ. Blastomycosis in the horse. J Am Vet Med Assoc 1948;112:475–478.

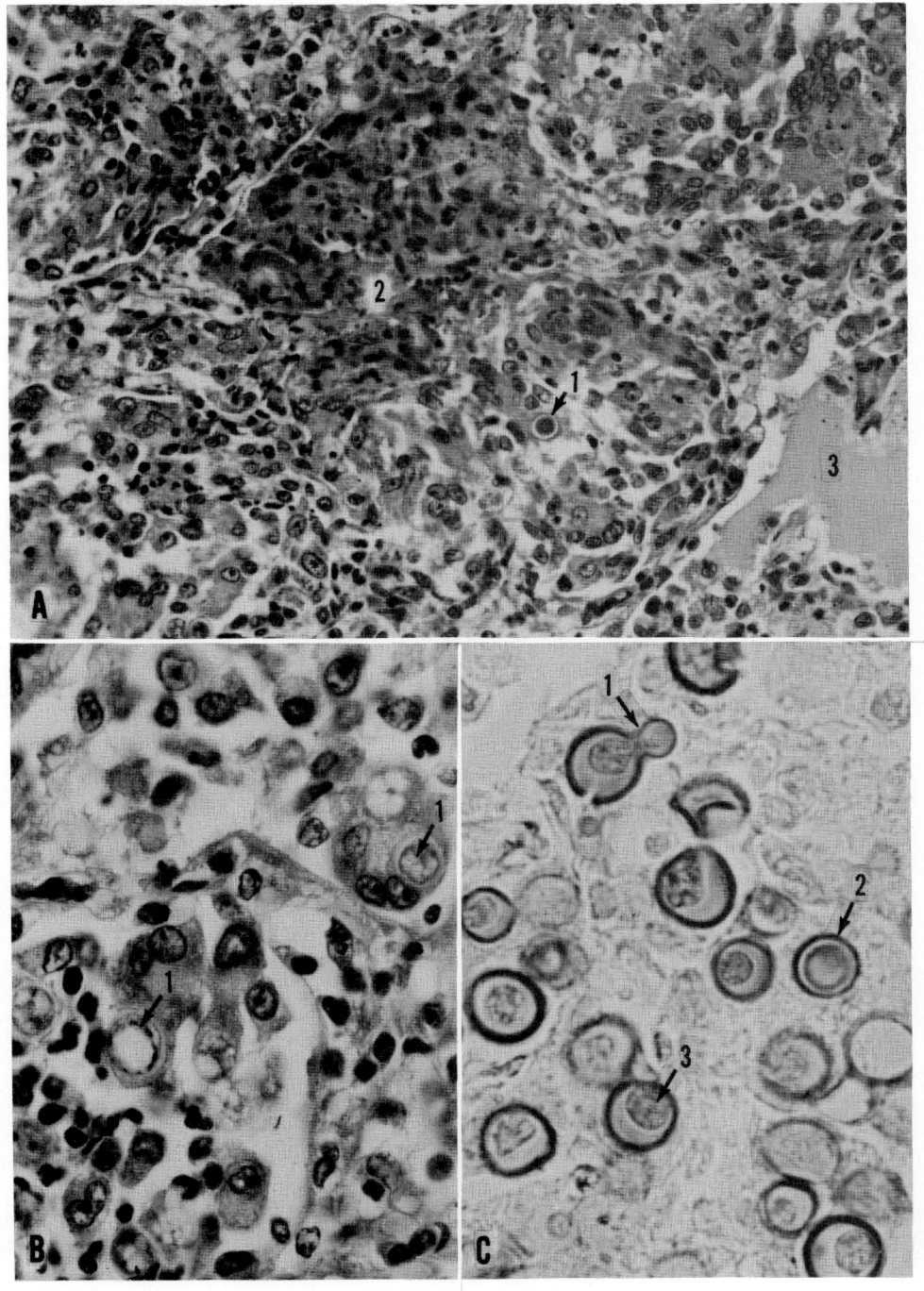

FIG. 11-3 Blastomycosis in canine lung. **A.** *Blastomyces dermatitidis* (1) surrounded by large masses of epithelioid cells, (2) alveolus, and (3) (×210). (Contributor: Dr. W.H. Riser.) **B.** Numerous organisms (1) in macrophages in alveoli in a fulminant case (×660). (Contributor: Dr. J.R. Rooney, II.) **C.** Higher magnification (×1050) of a section stained with Gridley fungus stain. Note (1) budding, (2) thick walls, and (3) the internal structure of the organisms. (Courtesy of Armed Forces Institute of Pathology and Dr. C.G. Loosli.)

Breider MA, Walker TL, Legendre AM, et al. Blastomycosis in cats: five cases (1979–1986). J Am Vet Med Assoc 1988;193:570–572.

Buyukmihci N. Ocular lesions of blastomycosis in the dog. J Am Vet Med Assoc 1982;180:426–431.

Easton KL. Cutaneous North American blastomycosis in a Siamese cat. Can Vet J 1961;2:350–351.

Furcolow ML, Smith CD, Turner C. Supportive evidence by field testing and laboratory experiment for a new hypothesis of the ecology and pathogenicity of canine blastomycosis. Sabouraudia 1974;12:22–32.

Johnson WD, Lang CM. Paracoccidioidomycosis (South American blastomycosis) in a squirrel monkey (*Saimiri sciureus*). Vet Pathol 1977;14:368–371.

Klein BS, et al. Isolation of *Blastomyces dermatitidis* in soil associated with a large outbreak of blastomycosis in Wisconsin. N Engl J Med 1986;314:529–534.

Kurtz HJ, Sharpnack S. *Blastomyces dermatitidis* meningoencephalitis in a dog. Pathol Vet 1969;6:375–377.

Lacroix LJ, Riser WH, Karlson AG. Blastomycosis in the dog. North Am Vet 1947;28:603–606.

Sarosi GA, Eckman MR, Davies SF, et al. Canine blastomycosis as a harbinger of human disease. Ann Intern Med 1979;197:733–735.

Saunders LZ. Cutaneous blastomycosis in the dog. North Am Vet 1948;29:650–652.

Seibold HR. Systemic blastomycosis in dogs. North Am Vet 1946;27:162–168.

Sheldon WG. Pulmonary blastomycosis in a cat. Lab Anim Care 1966;16:280–285.

Shull RM, Hayden DW, Johnston GR. Urogenital blastomycosis in a dog. J Am Vet Med Assoc 1977;171:730–735.

Soltys MA, Sumner-Smith G. Systemic mycoses in dogs and cats. Can Vet J 1971;12:191–199.

Trevino GS. Canine blastomycosis with ocular involvement. Pathol Vet 1966;3:652–658.

Wilson RW, Van Dreumel AA, Henry JNR. Urogenital and ocular lesions in canine blastomycosis. Vet Pathol 1973;10:1–11.

COCCIDIOIDOMYCOSIS (COCCIDIOIDAL GRANULOMA)

Coccidioidomycosis has been recognized as a human disease since 1892, when the first case was reported by Posada from Argentina. It is most prevalent in the arid regions of the southwestern United States, northern and central Mexico, and parts of South America. Coccidioidomycosis was first recognized as a spontaneous infection of animals by Giltner, who reported a bovine case in 1918. It is now known to occur in a wide variety of wild and domesticated animals, including wild deer, Bengal tigers, mice, pocket mice, grasshopper mice, kangaroo rats, pack rats, ground squirrels, gorillas, monkeys, dogs, sheep, cattle, and horses. In humans, the infection is usually subclinical or may present as an acute, febrile, respiratory infection with a short, favorable course (so-called San Jauquin Valley Fever). In a small percentage of humans, the infection progresses to an intractable disease with disseminated lesions and fatal outcome. In animals, the disease usually assumes the chronic progressive form with primary lesions in the lungs and dissemination initially to regional lymph nodes, then to most any viscus. Inapparent pulmonary infection has been recognized in cattle. Among domestic animals, disseminated coccidioidomycosis is most frequent in dogs.

The causative organism, *Coccidioides immitis (Oidium coccidioides)*, is a dimorphic fungus that lives in desert soil. Inhalation of spores (arthroconidia) produced by the mycelia causes the disease in either humans or animals. Direct transmission from one animal host to another apparently does not occur, although certain rodents have been suspected of being reservoirs of infection. The organisms grow well in cultures, producing aerial mycelia which form a small, fluffy-white, spherical colony. In tissues, however, mycelial structures are not observed, the fungus taking the form of spherules 5–50 μ in diameter with double-contoured walls. Reproduction in tissues is by endosporulation; hence, endospores may be found in some of the larger spherules.

Signs are absent in many cases, particularly in cattle, and the first indications of infection are lesions of the pulmonary lymph nodes found in apparently healthy animals at slaughter. Generalized infections run a slow course; the signs are nonspecific and may include emaciation, inappetence, low-grade fever, and occasional cough.

LESIONS

The gross lesions of coccidioidomycosis resemble those of tuberculosis in many respects. They may appear as discrete or confluent granulomas, with or without suppuration or calcification. In cattle, the lesions often are limited to small nodules in the lungs and, more frequently, to nodules or diffuse enlargements of bronchial or mediastinal lymph nodes. Large or small purulent foci may be surrounded by a wide band of granulation tissue and a fibrous capsule. Incision of an affected lymph node may permit the expression of thick, yellowish pus. In the disseminated form of the disease, as in the dog, grayish nodules of various sizes may be found in the lungs, lymph nodes, liver, spleen, meninges, eye, bone marrow, and other organs. The nodules are usually irregular in size and shape and may exude material when put under pressure. A close relationship to larger blood vessels may be demonstrated. In some species (dog, monkey), lesions may be disseminated throughout the skeletal system. Ocular involvement may also occur as the presenting lesion.

The microscopic appearance is characteristic, but varies to some extent in relationship to the developmental stage of the fungus which predominates in the lesion. The largest spherules, often filled with endospores, are usually surrounded by a wide zone of epithelioid cells, admixed with a few neutrophils and some lymphocytes. In cattle, these large spherules may be surrounded by a corona of radiating club-shaped structures (Splendore-Hoeppli material) (Fig. 11-4), somewhat resembling the "rosette" around a colony of *Actinomyces bovis*. When the wall of a large spherule ruptures, releasing its endospores, the tissue reaction becomes rich in neutrophils and lymphocytes, with fewer epithelioid cells. As these endospores mature, leukocytes and epithelioid cells tend to predominate in the inflammatory exudate. Because organisms in all stages may occur in a single lesion, mixed-tissue reactions are common. The organisms within the cytoplasm of Langhans giant cells are clearly seen in sections stained with hematoxy-

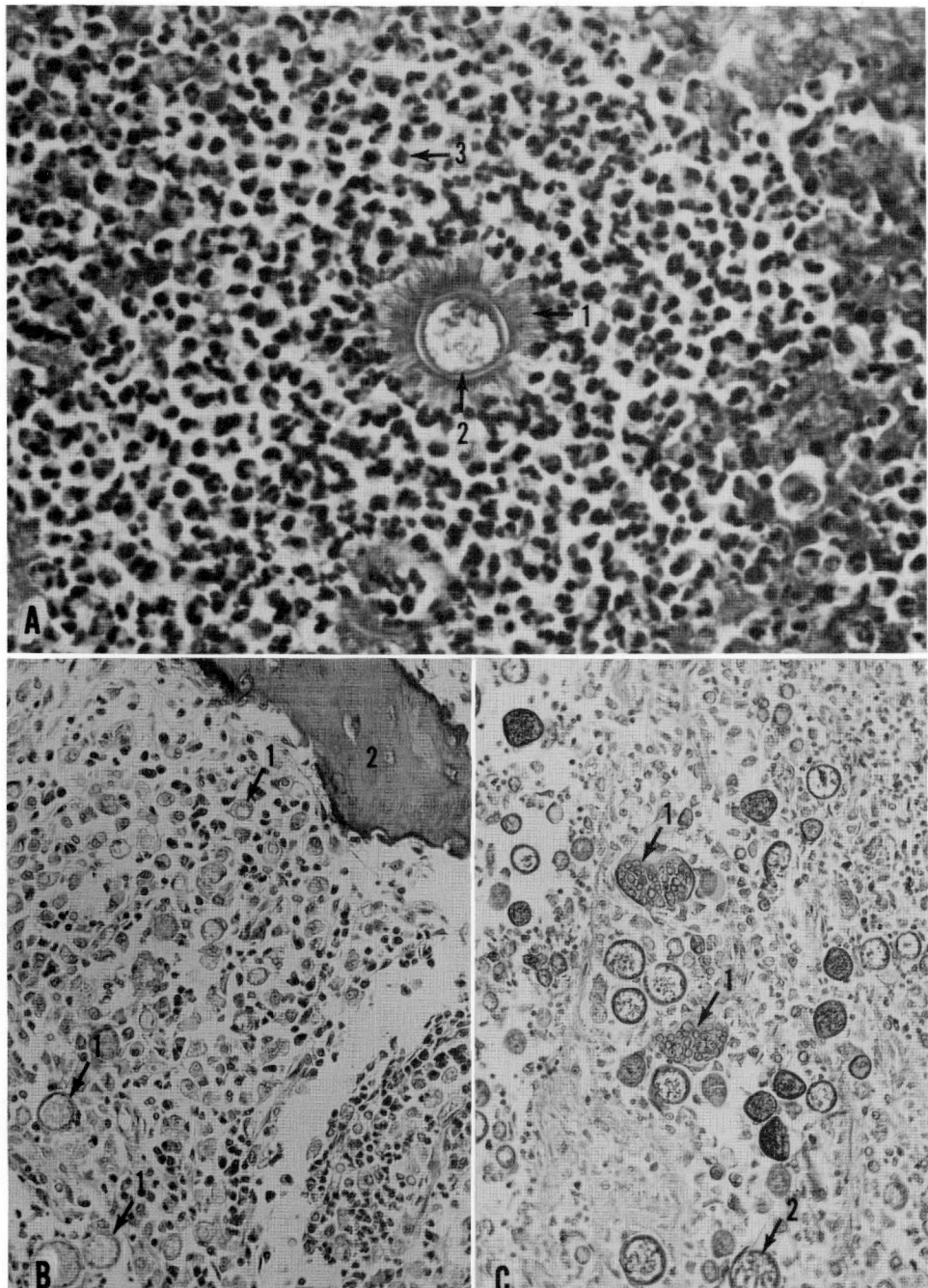

FIG. 11-4 Coccidioidomycosis. **A.** Lesions in a mediastinal lymph node of a cow (×100). Note (1) radiating club-shaped structures (2) around the thick-walled organism, (3) which lay in a pool of neutrophils. (Contributor: Dr. H.R. Seibold.) **B.** Lesion in bone marrow of a dog (×185). Organisms (1) of various sizes in macrophages which replace the normal marrow. Bone trabecula (2). **C.** Another section of *B* stained with Gridley fungus stain (×235). Large organisms (1) filled with endospores which are just starting to develop in smaller organisms (2). (Courtesy of Armed Forces Institute of Pathology and Dr. H.A. Smith.)

lin and eosin, but stains for bound glycogen (PAS, Gridley fungus, Bauer) will demonstrate the double-contoured wall selectively. In the liver, spleen, and lung, the lesions are usually spherical and sharply circumscribed and obviously are expanding to displace normal tissues; in lymph nodes and bone marrow, the feature of circumscription is usually lost. In the meninges, spherical nodules of microscopic size, containing one or two organisms in a mantle of epithelioid cells, may appear in the pia-arachnoid.

DIAGNOSIS

Microscopic demonstration of the organisms in characteristic lesions usually establishes the diagnosis. When organisms are few, special stains (PAS, Gridley fungus, Bauer) are helpful in revealing them. The size of the largest spherules ($50~\mu$), the presence of endospores, and absence of budding all serve to distinguish *Coccidioides immitis* from *Blastomyces dermatitidis* or *Cryptococcus neoformans*. The spherules of *Chrysosporium parvum* (adiaspiromycosis) may be similar in appearance and even larger in size, but they do not contain endo-spores. The spherules of *Rhinosporidium seeberi* are more similar to those of *Coccidioides*, but may be much larger, have a thicker wall, and contain larger endospores.

References

Angell JA, Merideth RE, Shively JN, et al. Ocular lesions associated with coccidioidomycosis in dogs: 35 cases (1980–1985). J Am Vet Med Assoc 1987;190:1319–1322.
Angell JA, Shively JN, Merideth RE, et al. Ocular coccidioidomycosis in a cat. J Am Vet Med Assoc 1985;187:167–169.
Ashburn LL, Emmons CW. Spontaneous coccidioidal granuloma in the lungs of wild rodents. Arch Pathol 1942;34:791–800.
Beaman L, Holmberg C, Henrickson R, et al. The incidence of coccidioidomycosis among nonhuman primates housed outdoors at the California Primate Research Center. J Med Primatol 1980;9:254–261.
Bellini S, Hubbard GB, Kaufman L. Spontaneous fatal coccidioidomycosis in a native-born hybrid baboon (*Papio cynocephalus anubis/Papio cynocephalus*). Lab Anim Sci 1991;41:509–511.
Burton M, Morton RJ, Ramsay E, et al. Coccidioidomycosis in a ring-tailed lemur. J Am Vet Med Assoc 1986;189:1209–1211.
Castleman WL, Anderson J, Holmberg CA. Posterior paralysis and spinal osteomyelitis in a rhesus monkey with coccidioidomycosis. J Am Vet Med Assoc 1980;177:933–934.
Cieplak W, Merbs CF. Coccidioidomycosis in an Arizona chimpanzee colony. Am J Phys Anthrop 1977;47:123.
Crane CS. Equine coccidioidomycosis. Vet Med 1962;57:1073–1074 VB 1503–1563.
Davis CL, Stiles GW Jr, McGregor AN. Pulmonary coccidioidal granuloma: a new site of infection in cattle. J Am Vet Med Assoc 1937;91:209–215.
Emmons CW. Coccidioidomycosis. Mycologia 1942;34:452–463.
Forbus WD, Bestebreurtje AM. Coccidioidomycosis: a study of 95 cases of the disseminated type with special reference to the pathogenesis of the disease. Mil Surgeon 1946;99:653–719.
Giltner LT. Occurrence of coccidioidal granuloma (oidiomycosis) in cattle. J Agric Res 1918;14:533–542.
Hugenholtz PG, et al. Experimental coccidioidomycosis in dogs. Am J Vet Res 1958;19:433–439.
Maddy KT. Disseminated coccidioidomycosis of the dog. J Am Vet Med Assoc 1958;132:483–489.
Pryor WH Jr, Huizenga CG, Splitter GA, et al. *Coccidioides immitis* encephalitis in two dogs. J Am Vet Med Assoc 1972;161:1108–1112.
Rapley WA, Long JR. Coccidioidomycosis in a baboon recently imported from California. Can Vet J 1974;15:39–41.
Reed RE, Hoge RS, Trautman RJ. Coccidioidomycosis in two cats. J Am Vet Med Assoc 1963;143:953–956.
Rehkemper JA. Coccidioidomycosis in the horse. A pathologic study. Cornell Vet 1959;49:198–211.
Rosenberg DP, Gleiser CA, Carey KD. Spinal coccidioidomycosis in a baboon. J Am Vet Med Assoc 1984;185:1379–1381.
Shively JN, Whiteman CE. Ocular lesions in disseminated coccidioidomycosis in 2 dogs. Pathol Vet 1970;7:1–6.
Smith HA. Coccidioidomycosis in animals. Am J Pathol 1948;24:223–233.
Stiles GW, Davis CL. Coccidioidal granuloma (coccidioidomycosis). Its incidence in man and animals and its diagnosis in animals. J Am Med Assoc 1942;119:765–769.
Zontine WJ. Coccidioidomycosis in the horse, a case report. J Am Vet Med Assoc 1958;132:490–492.

Adiaspiromycosis (Haplomycosis)

Adiaspiromycosis is a self-limiting disease resulting from the inhalation of nonreplicating spores of the fungi *Chrysosporium parvum* var. *parvum* or *Chrysosporium parvum* var. *crescens* (Fig. 11-5). The organism has been classified under several different names (*Emmonsia parva*, *Emmonsia crescens*, or *Haplosporangium parvum*). The name of the disease, originally proposed by Emmons (1948), stems from the offending spores known as adiaspores, which are spores that grow in size, but do not replicate. The "infection," thus, resembles a foreign-body inhalation pneumonia. The disease is obviously not contagious.

Adiaspiromycosis has been reported in a wide variety of wild animals, such as ground squirrels, pine squirrels, pocket mice, white-footed mice, kangaroo rats, wood rats, beavers, rock and cottontail rabbits, mink, martins, skunks, opossums, weasels, foxes, raccoons, wombats, wallabies, and armadillos. The organisms have also been found in the lungs of a dog and a goat and several reports of the disease in human beings have appeared since 1964. It is seen worldwide. In the United States, it is most frequent in the West.

LESIONS

Lesions of adiaspiromycosis are confined to the lung and may rarely include draining lymph nodes. The inhaled spores incite a granulomatous reaction consisting of epithelioid cells and multinucleated giant cells (Langhan's and foreign-body types) surrounded by fibrous connective tissue. The inflammatory cell reaction is usually rather thin. Mild lymphocytic infiltration may be present, but neutrophils are few. Some granulomas surround disintegrating organisms, which may be engulfed by giant cells. The organisms grow in size (but do not reproduce) from rather minute forms to extremely large spherical structures up to 400 microns in diameter. They have thick walls, 20–70 microns, which are doubly refractile. The outer third of the wall stains with eosin, with the inner two-thirds not staining. The organisms are clearly visible with hematoxylin and eosin, but when the usual stains for fungi are employed the entire wall is stained.

DIAGNOSIS

The spores of adiaspiromycosis are typical and not duplicated by other fungi. Those of *Coccidioides* and *Rhinosporidium* may bear a resemblance, but they are usually smaller, have thinner walls, and contain endospores.

References

Albassam MA, Bhatnager R, Lillie LE, et al. Adiaspiromycosis in striped skinks in Alberta, Canada. J Wildl Dis 1986;22:13–18.
Ashburn LL, Emmons CW. Experimental *Haplosporangium* infection. Arch Pathol 1945;39:3–8.
Cano RJ, Taylor JJ. Experimental adiaspiromycosis in rabbits: host response to *Chrysosporium parvum* and *C. parvum* var. *crescens* antigens. Sabouraudia 1974;12:54–63.
Ciferri R, Montemartini A. Taxonomy of *Haplosporangium parvum*. Mycopath Mycol Appl 1959;10:303–316.
Emmons CW. Coccidioidomycosis and haplomycosis. Proc. Fourth Internat. Cong Trop Med Malaria. Washington, DC. 1948;2:1278–1286.
Emmons CW, Jellison WL. *Emmonsia crescens sp: n.* and adiaspiromycosis (haplomycosis) in mammals. Ann NY Acad Sci 1960;89:91–101.
Koller LD, Patton NM, Whitsett DK. Adiaspiromycosis in the lungs of a dog. J Am Vet Med Assoc 1976;169:1316–1317.

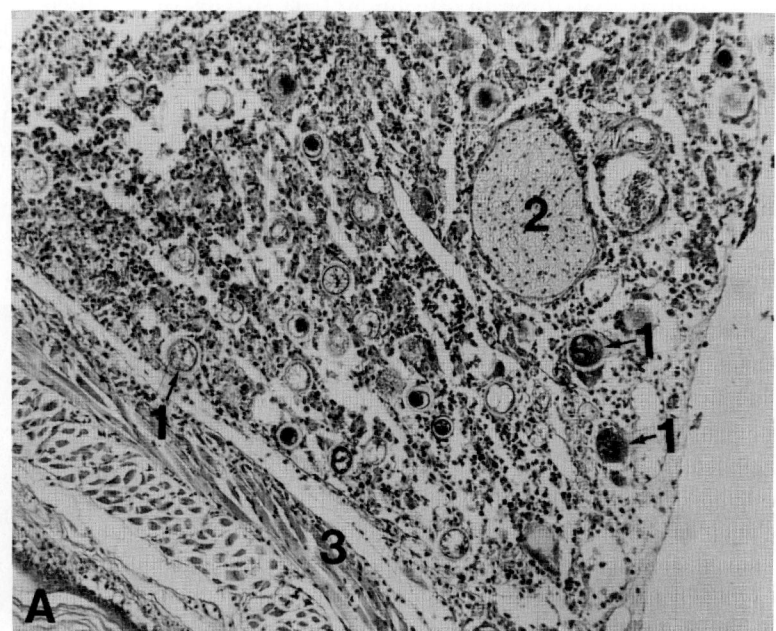

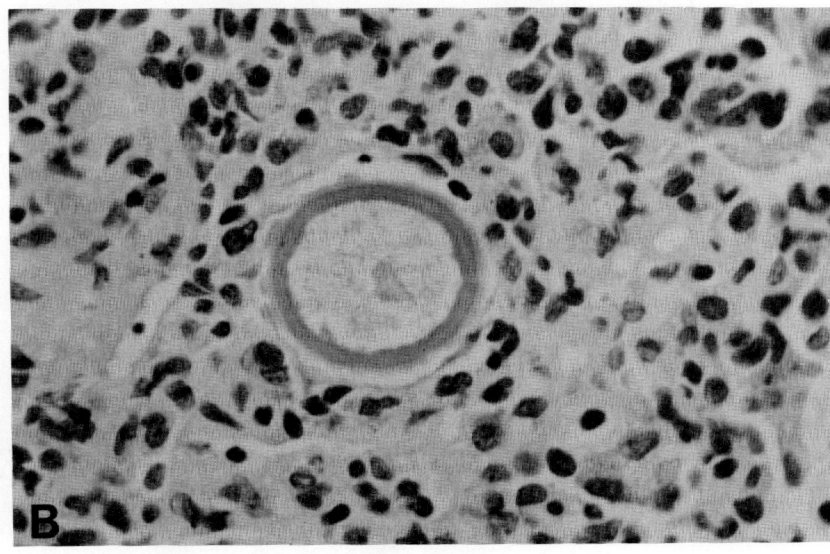

FIG. 11-5 Adiaspiromycosis. **A.** Organism (1) without endospores in mediastinum of a mouse. Nerve (2), esophagus (3). (Preparation courtesy of Dr. R. T. Haberman.) **B.** A single spherule in the lung of an armadillo. Note thick wall and absence of endospores. (Courtesy of Animal Research Center, Harvard Medical School).

Koller LD, Helfer DH. Adiaspiromycosis in the lungs of a goat. J Am Vet Med Assoc 1978;173:80–81.

Mason RW, Gauhwin M. Adiaspiromycosis in South Australian hairy-nosed wombats *(Lasiorhinus latifrons).* J Wildl Dis 1982;18:3–8.

Menges RW, Habermann RT. Isolation of *Haplosporangium parvum* from soil and results of experimental inoculations. Am J Hyg 1954;60:106–116.

Otcenasek M, Krivanec K, Slais J. *Emmonsia parva* as causal agent of adiaspiromycosis in a fox. Sabouraudia 1975;13:52–57.

Nasal Granuloma of Cattle

Polypoid or sessile masses are sometimes found in the nasal cavity of cattle. Most of these are apparently of allergic origin and are discussed in the chapter on the respiratory system. In certain parts of the country, most notably the west and south, true granulomatous lesions, in which fungi have been observed, are encountered in the nasal cavity; however, the etiology of such granulomas is not clearly established. It is probable that more than one causative agent may be involved. In India, a form of nasal granuloma, caused by the fluke, *Schistosoma nasalis* is seen in cattle.

Spherical organisms, undoubtedly fungal, were described in histologic sections of nasal granulomas, and cultures of *Helminthosporum* were recovered from these lesions by Davis and Shorten (1936), but the disease was not reproduced experimentally. Comparisons of the infection with haplomycosis and coccidioidomycosis have been made, but no conclusions reached.

Bridges reviewed the problem of bovine nasal granuloma, and published three cases from central Texas (1960). He was able to demonstrate both pigmented and nonpigmented hyphae and chlamydospores in the lesions, and by comparing their morphologic features, he determined that these organisms were a species of *Helminthosporum*. This organism has been isolated from cases of maduramycosis, suggesting that nasal granuloma is merely a form of this latter disease.

LESIONS

Lesions are confined to the external nares and appear as nodules that project from any part of the nasal mucosa into the nasal cavity (Fig. 11-6). The resulting partial obstruction may be accentuated by accumulation over the nodules of mucous and purulent exudates, which also stream from the external nostrils. The nodules have a glistening surface and are grayish yellow to red on cut section. Microscopically, the lesions underlying the elevated and often ulcerated nasal epithelium consist of granulomas, in which epithelioid and

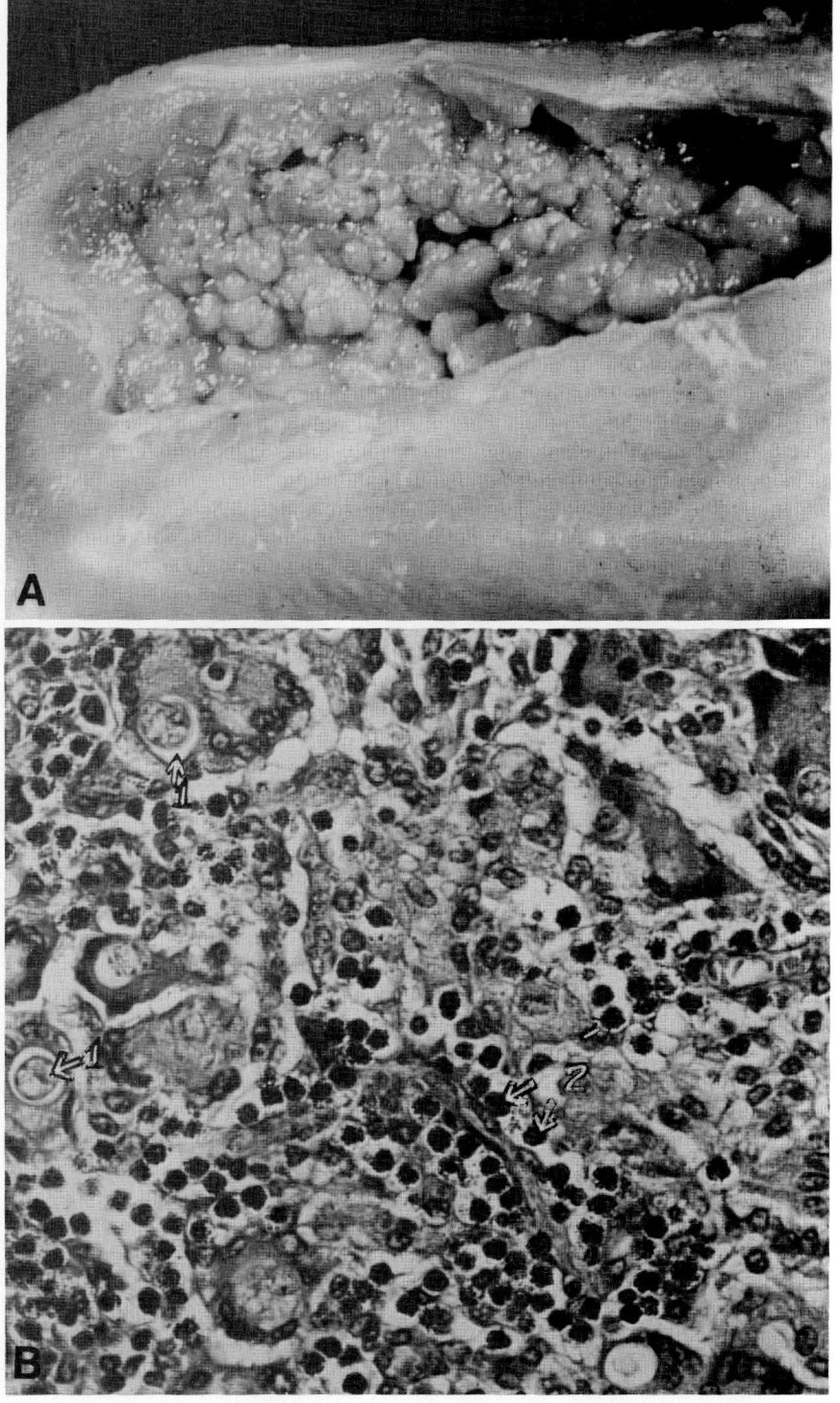

FIG. 11-6 Nasal granuloma of cattle. **A.** Polypoid masses on nasal septum. (Courtesy of Dr. C. L. Davis.) **B.** Section of a nasal granuloma (hematoxylin and eosin stain, ×400.) Note (1) fungal organisms and (2) eosinophils.

foreign-body giant cells predominate. Lymphocytes and eosinophils may make up a large part of some lesions. Spherical bodies, with thick walls and indistinct contents suggesting a fungus, are often seen within epithelioid and giant cells. In some reported cases, these organisms have not been found, although the possibility remains that they were present in parts of the lesion not examined microscopically.

References

Bridges CH. Maduramycosis of bovine nasal mucosa (nasal granuloma of cattle). Cornell Vet 1960;50:469–484.

Creech GT, Miller FW. Nasal granuloma in cattle. Vet Med 1933;28:279–284.

Davis CL, Shorten HL. Nasal swelling in a bovine. J Am Vet Med Assoc 1936;89:91–96.

Dikmans G. Nasal granuloma in cattle in Louisiana. North Am Vet 1934;15:20–24.

Roberts ED, McDaniel HA, Carbrey EA. Maduramycosis of the bovine nasal mucosa. J Am Vet Med Assoc 1963;142:42–68.

Robinson VB. Nasal granuloma. Am J Vet Res 1951;12:85–89.

MADURAMYCOSIS (MADURAMYCOTIC MYCETOMA, MADURA FOOT)

An age-old disease of barefooted people ("Madura foot") was originally named for an area in which the disease was first described (Madura, India). Many different organisms have been recovered from such cases and may well have etiologic significance. The clinical disease in human patients has been divided into: "eumycetomas," caused by *Eumycetes* or true fungi; "actinomycetomas," caused by organisms of the genera *Actinomyces, Nocardia, Actinomadura,* and *Streptomyces;* "botryomycosis," caused by *Staphylococcus sp., Actinobacillus lignieresi, Escherichia coli, Proteus sp., Pseudomonas aeruginosa,* and nonhemolytic streptococci. In this section, only those lesions in animals caused by true fungi are considered.

In tissues, the causative organisms currently grouped under this term form definite colonies or "grains" which are composed of cohesive masses of large, segmented mycelial filaments with well-defined walls, chlamydospores, or other spores and, in most cases, pigment (Fig. 11-7). Fungi that do not produce pigment are involved in "white-grained maduramycosis." Colonies that contain pigment are visible to the unaided eye as "black grains," suggesting tiny bits of coal.

A variety of different fungi have been identified in characteristic lesions of maduramycosis, most of which have undergone several name changes. Specific genera include: *Pseudoallescheria (Petriellidium, Allescheria); Curvularia; Madurella; Fusarium; Acremonium; Helminthosporium;* and *Brachycladium.* These, as well as the causative agents of actinomycetomas, are traumatically introduced into tissues. These same organisms may also be associated with superficial inflammatory lesions in the absence of an enlarging nodule. One, reported as *Petriellidium boydii (Allescheria boydii),* was described as a cause of placentitis and abortion in horses and cattle.

LESIONS

The lesions of maduramycosis are distinguished by the presence of discrete colonies of fungi, which appear grossly as tiny black, brown, or hyalin flecks ("grains") 1–3 mm wide, embedded in a large mass of granulation tissue. These colonies are tenaciously discrete and can be expressed by pressure from the narrow zone of pus that surrounds them. The lesions in animals are most frequent on the extremities, but may involve the nasal mucosa, peritoneum, or skin at any site. The coiled

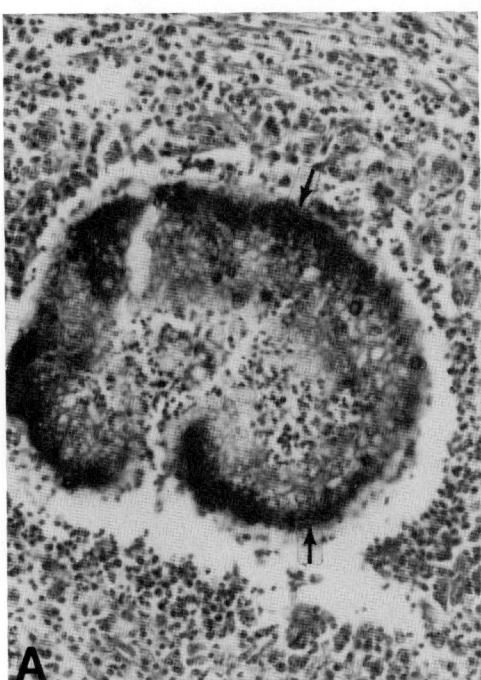
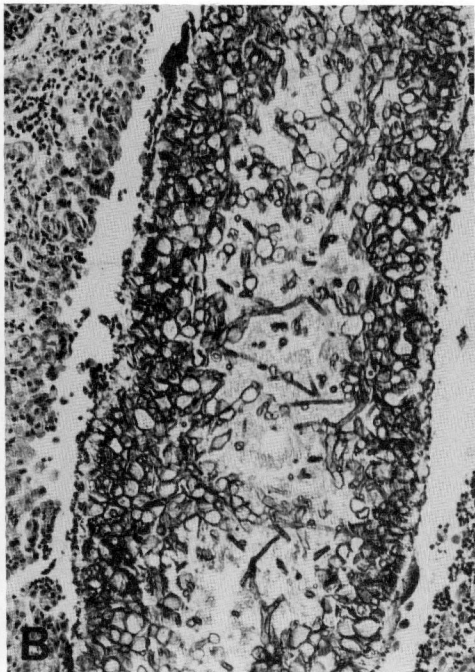

FIG. 11-7 Maduramycosis. **A.** Nasal granuloma in a horse (×224). Note pigment in tenacious colony. (Courtesy of Armed Forces Institute of Pathology and Dr. Leon Z. Saunders.) **B.** Granuloma of one year's duration in the foot of a dog (×130). *Curvularia geniculata* was isolated from the lesion. Note colony of organisms without pigment.

glands of the foot pad of dogs appear to be sites of predilection. These mycotic granulomas may become quite large and are generally resistant to any treatment short of surgical excision.

The microscopic appearance is distinctive. Colonies of the fungi are seen as brown, irregularly spherical bodies embedded within a pocket of neutrophils. These purulent centers are separated by abundant amounts of granulation tissue richly infiltrated with macrophages, plasma cells, and lymphocytes. The organisms in the fungal colony cling together tenaciously and form an outer coronal zone consisting of coarse, irregular, often swollen hyphae and thick-walled chlamydospores. The center of the colony is usually less dense and contains many branching, septate hyphae. The hyphae are of irregular length, but rarely more than 10 μ in width. The chlamydospores have thicker walls, are usually spherical, and may attain a diameter of 25 μ or more. The periodic-acid Schiff (PAS), Bauer, and Gridley fungus stains are particularly useful in demonstrating the morphology of the fungi in tissue sections (Fig. 11-7).

DIAGNOSIS

The diagnosis may be made by demonstration of typical fungal colonies in characteristic granulomas. Organisms should be cultured in order to establish the identity of the causative agent.

References

Baszler T, Chandler FW, Bertoy RW, et al. Disseminated pseudallescheriasis in a dog. Vet Pathol 1988;25:95–97.

Bridges CH. Maduromycotic mycetomas in animals. *Curvularia geniculata* as an etiological agent. Am J Pathol 1957;33:411–427.

Bridges CH, Beasley JN. Maduromycotic mycetomas in animals — *Brachycladium spiciferum,* Bainier as an etiologic agent. J Am Vet Med Assoc 1960;137:192–201.

Brodey RS, 1967. et al. Mycetoma in a dog. J Am Vet Med Assoc 1967,151:442–451.

Friedman DS, et al. *Pseudallescheria boydii* keratomycosis in a horse. J Am Vet Med Assoc 1989;195:616–618.

McEntee M. Eumycotic mycetoma: review and report of a cutaneous lesion caused by *Pseudallescheria boydii* in a horse. J Am Vet Med Assoc 1987;191:1459–1461.

Reinke SI, et al. Actinomycotic mycetoma in a cat. J Am Vet Med Assoc 1986;189:446–448.

Schauffler AF. Maduromycotic mycetoma in an aged mare. J Am Vet Med Assoc 1972;160:998–1000.

Seibold HR. Mycetoma in a dog. J Am Vet Med Assoc 1955;127:444–445.

Walker RL, Monticello TM, Ford RB, et al. Eumycotic mycetoma caused by *Pseudallescheria boydii* in the abdominal cavity of a dog. J Am Vet Med Assoc 1988;192:67–70.

CRYPTOCOCCOSIS (TORULOSIS, EUROPEAN BLASTOMYCOSIS)

Cryptococcosis, a disease of many animal species and humans, is distributed worldwide and is caused by the basidiomycetous yeastlike fungus *Cryptococcus neoformans* (*C. hominis* or *Torula histolytica*) (Fig. 11-8). Two varieties exist, *C. neoformans* var. *gratti* and *C. neoformans* var. *neoformans*. Most infections in animals, especially in the United States, are due to var. *neoformans*. In nature, *C. neoformans* var. *neoformans* is found in manure, especially that of birds, particularly pigeons. It is postulated that the natural host for the fungus is a common grass that birds (especially pigeons) eat, resulting in passage of encapsulated yeast cells through their gastrointestinal tract and subsequent wide dispersal. *C. neoformans* var. *gratti* is a parasite of flowering buds of the river red gum tree (*Eucalyptus camaldulensis*). In Australia, koalas may pass the yeast cells in their feces and cryptococcosis has been observed in koalas and Australian Aborigines who feed on or shelter under these trees, respectively (Ellis and Pfeiffer, 1990). This specific eucalyptus has been exported widely and the occurrence of infection with var. *gratti* corresponds with

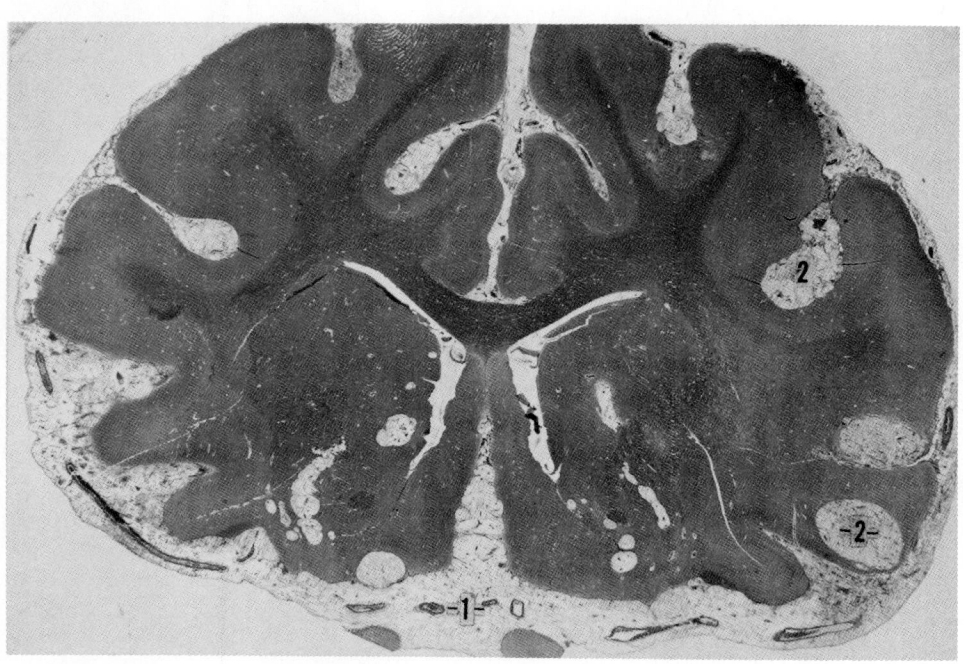

FIG. 11-8 Cryptococcosis, brain of a cat. Large masses of organisms in leptomeninges (1) give them an edematous appearance and result in distention of depths of sulci (2). (Courtesy of Armed Forces Institute of Pathology and Dr. John Mills.)

the distribution of the tree. Cryptococcosis is usually acquired by inhalation, is noncommunicable, and is generally an opportunistic infection in immunocompromised animals. The disease occurs in most domestic animals, laboratory animals, and a variety of wild species including: cattle; sheep; swine; horses; cats; dogs; rhesus (*Macaca mulatta*), Taiwan (*M. cyclopis*), and patas (*Erythrocebus patas*) monkeys; foxes; mink; ferrets; and guinea pigs. Most animal species are probably susceptible.

Cryptococcosis may involve many different organ systems, but most commonly affects the respiratory and central nervous systems. Any portion of the respiratory system may be invaded: from the external nares to the lungs. Lesions in the nasal cavity leading to obstruction are common. The organism has a strong affinity for the cerebrospinal meninges and brain, and may gain entry via hematogenous spread or by direct extension through the turbinates. Although disseminated cryptococcosis occurs, it is not a usual finding. Outbreaks of intractable mastitis have occurred in dairy cattle, with involvement of the supramammary lymph nodes, but ordinarily without further dissemination. Placentitis, fetal infection, and abortion have been described in horses.

LESIONS

Gross lesions are not diagnostic, but often unique. Although they may appear as nodules typical of other granulomatous diseases, more often the lesions consist of expanding masses of a mucinous or gelatinous translucent material. The tumorlike masses project from and displace the affected organ.

Microscopically, the findings are diagnostic, consisting of masses of organisms proliferating with little or no restriction.

The organisms occur in tissues as ovoid or spherical, thick-walled, yeast-like bodies that occasionally show single budding and are surrounded by a wide, gelatinous capsule (Fig. 11-9). The cell inside the capsule is usually 5–20 μ in diameter; the capsule increases the overall diameter to a maximum of 30 μ. In sections stained with hematoxylin and eosin, the cell wall and sometimes its contents are visible, but the capsule remains unstained. This capsule stains selectively by the mucicarmine technique and the PAS method for glycogen.

In most situations, the organisms grow and multiply rapidly, forming a cystic space occupied by myriads of organisms, whose mucoid capsules account for the glistening appearance and slimy consistency encountered grossly. This is a prominent feature in brain; the organisms grow in the pia mater over the surface and deep into the cerebral convolutions where they form cystic areas and displace brain parenchyma. Cystic lesions may occur in lungs, adrenal glands, lymph nodes, and mammary glands. In such sites, the tissue reaction of the host is difficult to detect, although occasional macrophages with engulfed organisms may be found. In some cases of cryptococcosis, the organisms are less numerous and the tissue reaction much more profound.

In lesions of this type, which may be adjacent to a cystic lesion, numerous epithelioid cells with an admixture of lymphocytes are partially or completely surrounded by connective tissue. This granulomatous reaction is particularly prominent in some cases of cryptococcal mastitis, but has also been observed in lesions in brain, lung, and other organs.

DIAGNOSIS

The diagnosis is readily made from characteristic microscopic lesions in which the organisms can be demonstrated and identified culturally or morphologically. The wide mucoid capsule, which selectively absorbs the mucicarmine stain, differentiates *Cryptococcus neoformans* in tissue from *Blastomyces dermatitidis*. The budding of *Cryptococcus neoformans*, as well as its smaller size and capsule, serves to distinguish it from *Coccidioides immitis*, which produces endospores and is not encapsulated.

References

Al-Doory Y. Bibliography of cryptococcosis. Mycopathol Mycol Appl 1971;45:1–60.

Barron CN. Cryptococcosis in animals. J Am Vet Med Assoc 1955; 127:125–132.

Cho D-Y, Pace LW, Beadle RE. Cerebral cryptococcosis in a horse. Vet Pathol 1986;23:207–209.

Chuck SL, Sande MA. Infections with *Cryptococcus neoformans* in the acquired immunodeficiency syndrome. N Engl J Med 1989;321: 794–799.

Dickson J, Meyer EP. Cryptococcosis in horses in Western Australia. Aust Vet J 1970;46:558.

Ellis DH, Pfeiffer TJ. Ecology, life cycle, and infectious propagule of *Cryptococcus neoformans*. Lancet 1990;336:923–925.

Frothingham L. A tumor-like lesion in the lung of a horse caused by a blastomyces (*Torula*). J Med Res 1902;8:31–42.

Hodgin EC, Corstvet RE, Blakewood BW. Cryptococcosis in a pup. J Am Vet Med Assoc 1987;191:697–700.

Holzworth J, Coffin DL. Cryptococcosis in the cat. Cornell Vet 1953;43:546–550.

Howell JM, Allan D. A case of cryptococcosis in the cat. J Comp Pathol 1964;74:415–418.

Innes JRM, Seibold HR, Arentzen WP. The pathology of bovine mastitis caused by *Cryptococcus neoformans*. Am J Vet Res 1952;13: 469–475.

Jergens AE, Wheeler CA, Collier LL. Cryptococcosis involving the eye and central nervous system of a dog. J Am Vet Med Assoc 1986;189:302–304.

Kavit AY. Cryptococcic arthritis in a Cocker Spaniel. J Am Vet Med Assoc 1958;133:386–389.

Krogh P, Basse A, Hesselholt M, et al. Equine cryptococcosis: a case of rhinitis caused by *Cryptococcus neoformans* serotype A. Sabouraudia. 1974;12:272–278.

Medleau L, Hall EJ, Goldschmidt MH, et al. Cutaneous cryptococcosis in three cats. J Am Vet Med Assoc 1985;187:169–170.

Olander HJ, Reed H, Pier AC. Feline cryptococcosis. J Am Vet Med Assoc 1963;142:138–143.

Panciera DL, Bevier D. Management of cryptococcosis and toxic epidermal necrolysis in a dog. J Am Vet Med Assoc 1987;191:1125–1127.

Roussilhon C, Postal J-M, Ravisse P. Spontaneous cryptococcosis of a squirrel monkey (*Saimiri sciureus*) in French Guyana. J Med Primatol 1987;16:39–47.

Rubin LF, Craig PH. Intraocular cryptococcosis in a dog. J Am Vet Med Assoc 1965;147:27–32.

Ryan MJ, Wyand DS. *Cryptococcus* as a cause of neonatal pneumonia and abortion in two horses. Vet Pathol 1981;18:270–272.

Scott EA, Duncan JR, McCormack JE. Cryptococcosis involving the

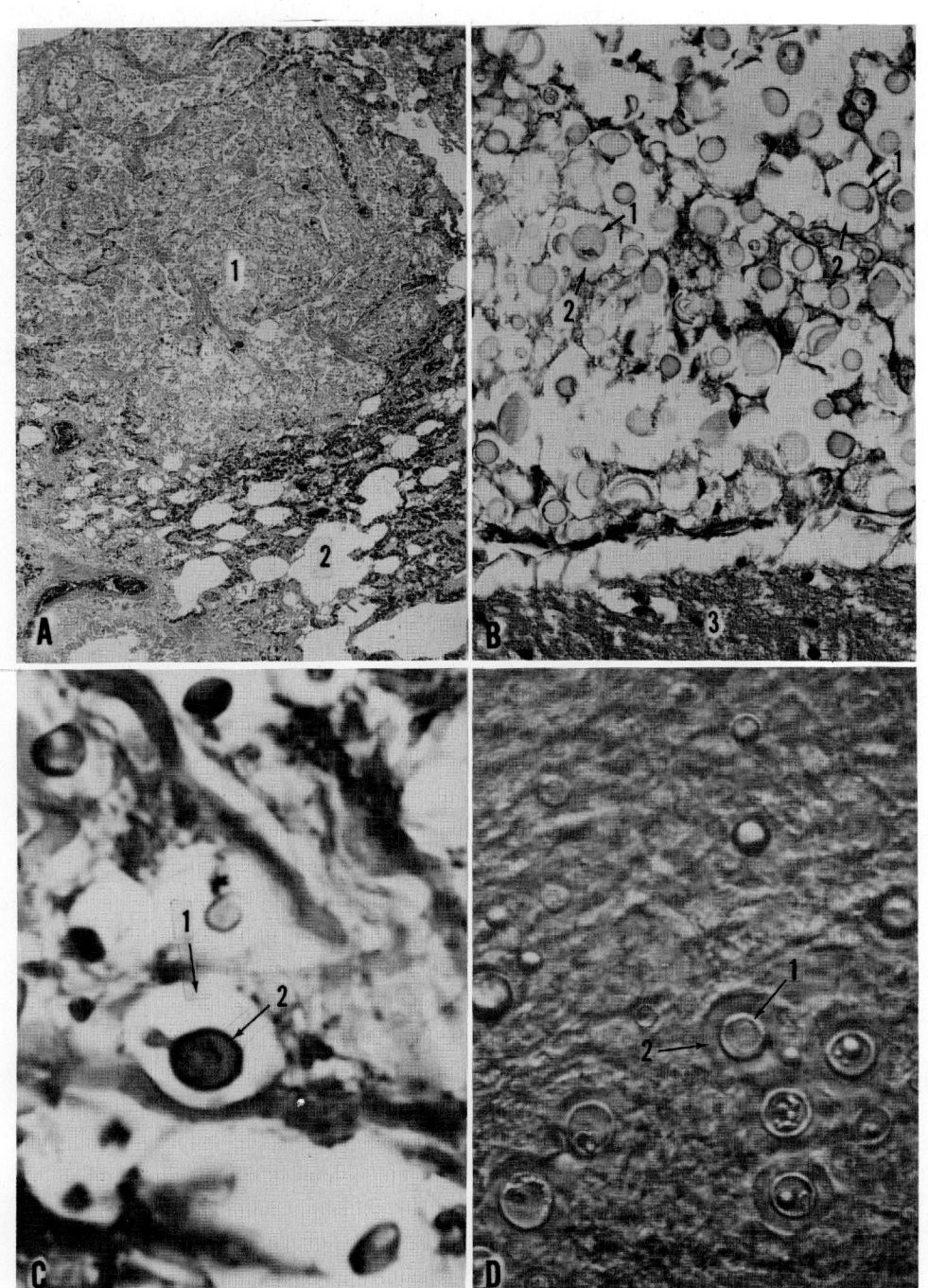

FIG. 11-9 Cryptococcosis. **A.** Lung of a cat (×48). Consolidated area (1) filling and compressing alveoli (2). **B.** Organisms in pia mater of a cat (×300). Note spherical organisms (1) surrounded by a wide, clear capsule (2). Cerebral cortex (3). (Contributor: Dr. John Mills.) **C.** Organisms in cat lung (×1045), same case as **A.** Note wide, unstained capsule (1) surrounding a budding organism (2). (Courtesy of Armed Forces Institute of Pathology and Dr. Jean Holzworth.) **D.** Unstained smear preparation viewed with phase contrast: (1) cell body and (2) capsule (×925).

postorbital area and frontal sinus in a horse. J Am Vet Med Assoc 1974;165:626–627.

Seibold HR, Roberts CS, Jordan EM. Cryptococcosis in a dog. J Am Vet Med Assoc 1953;122:213–215.

Shadomey HJ, Lurie HI. Histopathological observations in experimental cryptococcosis caused by a hypha-producing strain of *Cryptococcus neoformans* (Coward strain). Sabouraudia 1971;9:6–9.

Simon J, Nichols RE, Morse EV. An outbreak of bovine cryptococcosis. J Am Vet Med Assoc 1953;122:31–35.

Sly DL, London WT, Palmer AE, et al. Disseminated cryptococcosis in a Patas monkey (*Erythrocebus patas*). Lab Anim Sci 1977;27:694–699.

Smith DLT, Fisher JB, Barnum DA. Generalized *Cryptococcus neoformans* infection in a dog. Can Med Assoc J 1955;72:18–20.

Takos MJ, Elton NW. Spontaneous cryptococcosis of marmoset monkeys in Panama. Arch Pathol 1953;55:403–407.

Trautwein B, Nielsen SW. Cryptococcosis in 2 cats, a dog and a mink. J Am Vet Med Assoc 1962;140:437–442.

Weidman FD, Ratcliffe HJ. Cryptococcosis in a cheetah at the Philadelphia Zoo. Arch Pathol 1934;18:362–369.

Weitzman I, Bonaparte P, Guevin V, et al. Cryptococcosis in a field mouse. Sabouraudia 1973;11:77–79.

Wilkinson GT. Feline cryptococcosis: a review and seven case reports. J Small Anim Pract 1979;20:749–768.

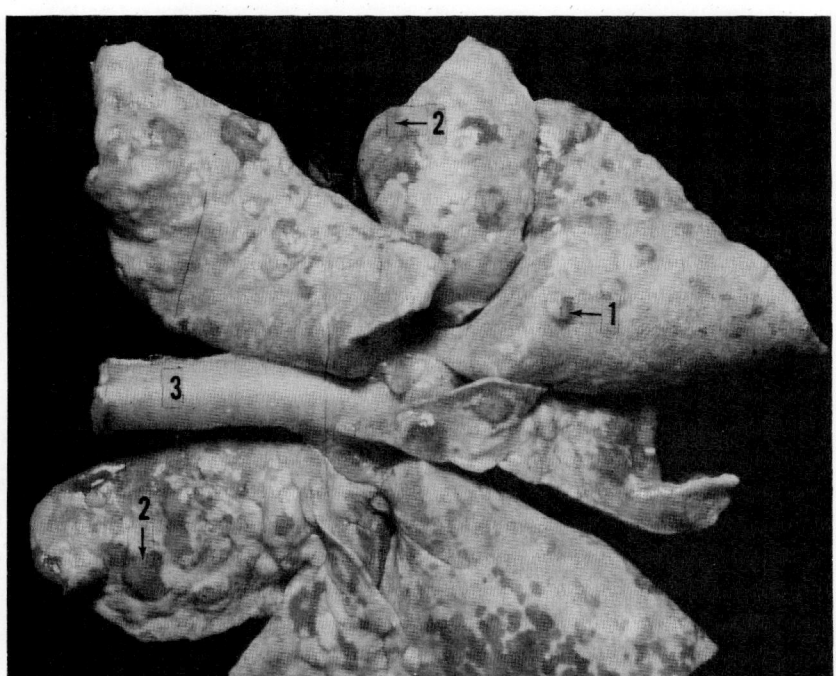

FIG. 11-10 Histoplasmosis. (1) Nodules in the lung of a dog. (2) Consolidated lobules. (3) Trachea. (Courtesy of Armed Forces Institute of Pathology and Dr. Karl S. Harmon.)

HISTOPLASMOSIS (*HISTOPLASMA CAPSULATUM*, CLASSIC HISTOPLASMOSIS)

Three species of *Histoplasma* are of medical significance (Figs. 11-10 and 11-11): *Histoplasma capsulatum,* the cause of classic histoplasmosis, the most common form of histoplasmosis in the world; *Histoplasma capsulatum* var. *duboisii,* the cause of African histoplasmosis; and *Histoplasma farciminosum,* the cause of epizootic lymphangitis of horses. *H. capsulatum* is a dimorphic fungus that grows readily in culture media and soil as a white-to-brown mold that bears spores of two types: spherical, minutely spiny microconidia, 3–4 μ in diameter, and spherical, or rarely clavate, macroconidia, 8–12 μ in diameter, with evenly spaced fingerlike projections over the surface. The parasitic phase in the mammalian host develops from either of these conidia into a yeast-like form.

Infection is acquired through inhalation of spores from infected soil. Its growth and spread in nature is aided by bird droppings. Initially, the infection is established in the lung where the yeast form of the fungus proliferates within macrophages and subsequently may be spread throughout the mononuclear phagocyte system. Although for many years the disease in humans was believed to occur only as a rare, consistently fatal, disseminated infection, it is now known that an acute, nonfatal form is much more prevalent both in humans and lower animals. The disease is not spread by direct contact between hosts, but it may appear in animals and humans sharing the same environment; therefore, so-called epidemics of histoplasmosis are related to an environmental source of infection rather than to spread of contagion from host to host. Both the benign inap-

parent and the fatal disseminated forms of the disease occur in a wide variety of animals. The disease is most frequent in dogs, but also occurs in cats, cattle, horses, guinea pigs, bats, rats, mice, woodchucks, skunks, opossums, foxes, raccoons, and monkeys.

It has been reported in many parts of the United States, South and Central America, and less frequently other parts of the world, but apparently histoplasmosis is most common in certain regions of the United States, specifically those bordering the Missouri, Ohio, and Mississippi Rivers.

The benign form of the disease in animals is seldom recognized unless pulmonary lesions are present or organisms are recovered at necropsy, although in some instances radiographic examination has revealed lesions in subjects with histoplasmin sensitivity. Benign histoplasmosis in humans may become apparent as an acute febrile pneumonitis with weight loss and adenopathy, or by radiographic evidence of dense, sometimes calcified "coin lesions" in the lungs, usually associated with histoplasmin sensitivity. The fatal disseminated form in animals, observed most frequently in dogs, usually runs a prolonged course with progressive weight loss, lymphadenopathy, diarrhea, weakness, anemia, hepatomegaly, and ascites. Although it is difficult to recognize in the living animal, histoplasmosis has been diagnosed from the signs and course and confirmed by demonstration of organisms in the circulating blood.

LESIONS

The dominant feature of tissue changes in histoplasmosis is the extensive proliferation of reticuloendothelial cells (macrophages, endothelioid, epitheli-

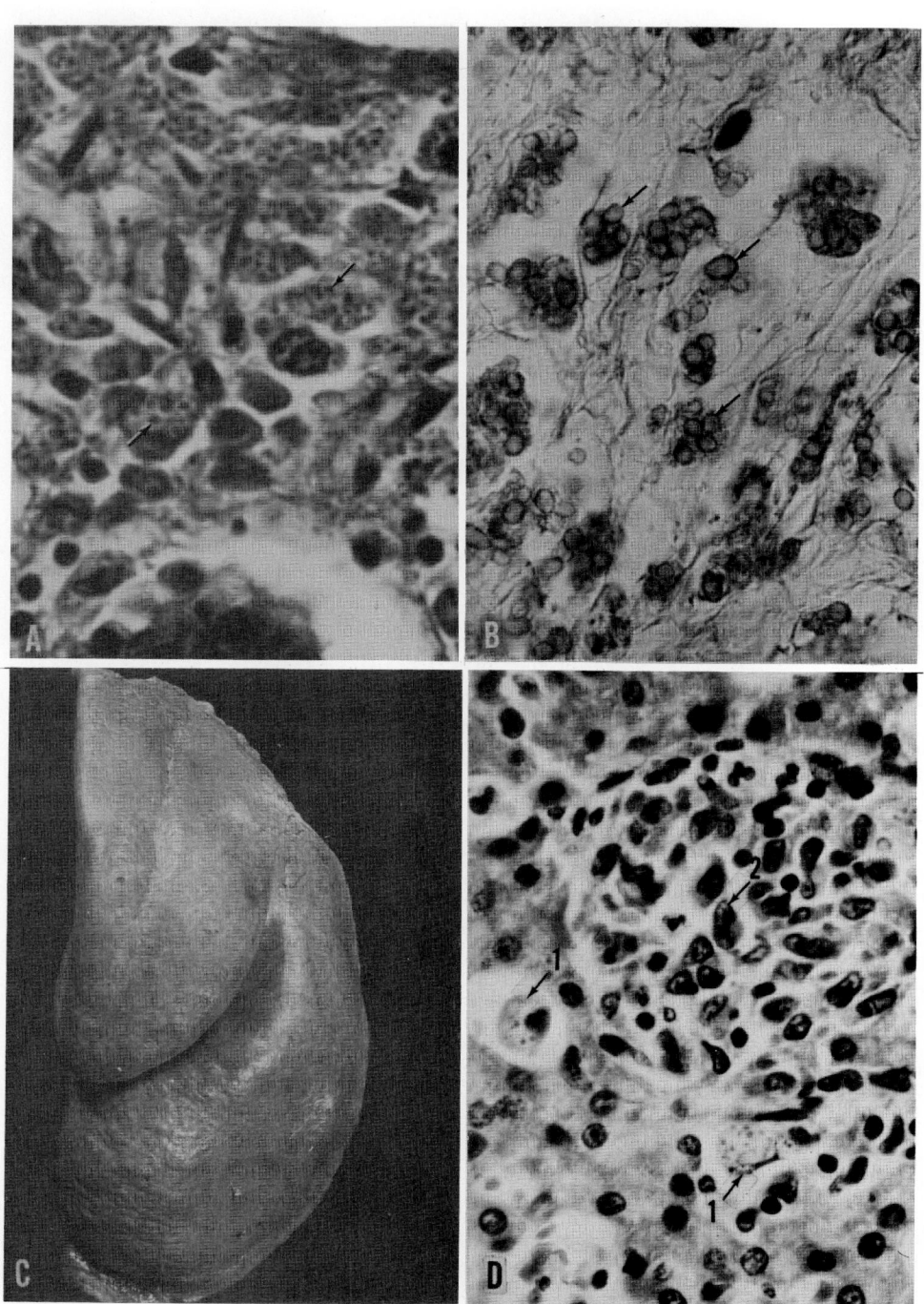

FIG. 11-11 Histoplasmosis. **A.** Macrophages (arrows) laden with *Histoplasma capsulatum* in submucosa of the ileum (×1000) of a dog. (Contributor: Dr. R. F. Birge.) **B.** Organisms (arrows) stained by Gridley fungus stain. The cell wall is stained red, causing the organisms to look larger than in A, although the magnification is the same (×1000). **C.** Enlarged gray liver of a dog. Same as Case B. (Contributor: Dr. Karl S. Harmon.) **D.** Lesion in the liver (×630) of a dog. Note macrophages laden with organisms (1) and reticuloendothelial cells (2). (Courtesy of Armed Forces Institute of Pathology and Dr. H.R. Seibold.)

oid cells), many of which contain yeast forms of the causative organism, either a few or so many that the cytoplasm is distended and tremendously enlarged. It is the proliferation of reticuloendothelial cells that causes displacement of normal tissues, interference with function, and gross enlargement of organs. The disease has been more adequately studied in the dog; hence, the following remarks on these lesions apply especially to the dog.

Primary disease in the lung may take the form of classic granulomas composed of epithelioid cells and multinucleated giant cells, which may contain demonstrable organisms, with or without central caseous cores. With recovery, these lesions regress to fibrocalcareous nodules that remain in the lung for years. Less frequently, this typical granulomatous reaction may also be found in other organs.

In the disseminated form, the alveoli and interstitial stroma may be flooded with lymphocytes, plasma cells, and epithelioid cells, many containing organisms. The yeastlike bodies, which are always located in the cytoplasm, are irregularly egg-shaped and measure from

2 by 3 μ to 3 by 4 μ. They reproduce with tiny buds connected by a narrow base. In sections stained with hematoxylin and eosin, a central, spherical, usually basophilic body is surrounded by an unstained zone which, in turn, is encircled by a thin cell wall. This may give the impression of a capsule around the central body, but the organism has no true capsule; the clear halo is actually within the cell wall. By PAS, Bauer, GMS, or Gridley fungus method, the wall is stained selectively, leaving its contents unstained; thus, the organism appears as an empty red or black ring. These stains are particularly useful in visualizing organisms when only a few are present and in differentiating them from other phagocytized particles, especially tissue debris.

The lymph nodes in the disseminated disease are tremendously enlarged by the proliferation of reticuloendothelial cells. Grossly, the nodes are firm and uniform in appearance, not unlike those of malignant lymphoma. The mononuclear phagocyte proliferation in severely affected nodes may obliterate the normal nodal architecture. Necrosis, purulent inflammation, calcification, and multinucleated giant cells are seldom observed. The predominant cell is mononuclear with tremendously expanded cytoplasm, often packed with organisms. Lymphocytes and plasma cells may be present in smaller numbers.

The spleen is enlarged to several times its normal size, light gray, and firm as the result of the reticuloendothelial proliferation, which masks much of the splenic architecture.

The liver is also enlarged, firm, and light gray because of the diffuse interlobular and intralobular proliferation of mononuclear phagocytes. These cells displace liver parenchyma and thus obviously interfere with liver function. As elsewhere, little tendency for lesion encapsulation exists in the disseminated form. Lymphocytes and plasma cells may be present in varying numbers.

The intestine, when involved, has a thickened rugose or nodular mucosal surface, and its wall is thickened by mononuclear phagocytes proliferation in the lamina propria and submucosa. Ulceration is unusual. The lymph nodules and adjacent lymph nodes are greatly enlarged, their architecture distorted by the characteristic large macrophages laden with organisms. The ileocecal junction and the adjacent lymph nodes are often severely affected.

The adrenal glands may be largely replaced by macrophages filled with organisms. This is particularly striking in fatal cases, but less so in affected animals sacrificed before the terminal stages of the disease.

Other organs, including skin, pancreas, heart, genitalia, kidneys, and eyes are usually less severely affected, but may be involved by the characteristic mononuclear phagocytes proliferation. Fatal infection leading to abortion has been described.

DIAGNOSIS

In the living animal, the diagnosis can be established by demonstration of typical mononuclear phagocyte proliferation and organisms in tissues at biopsy (tonsils, lymph node, liver). In some cases, monocytes,

neutrophils, or eosinophils containing *H. capsulatum* can be demonstrated in smears of circulating blood. Serologic tests are available, but are not reliable. A radioimmunoassay test for detection of *H. capsulatum* antigen in urine and serum has been shown to be useful in the diagnosis of histoplasmosis in humans (Wheat et al., 1986). Microscopic examination of tissue sections usually permits definitive diagnosis, but in some cases identification of the organisms in cultures is advisable. The organism of epizootic lymphangitis *(Histoplasma farciminosum)* cannot be differentiated in tissue sections (Fig. 11-12); hence, cultures are necessary to distinguish these two infections. However, the different geographic distribution and the anatomical location of the two diseases usually eliminate difficulty.

Differentiation from other mycotic and protozoan organisms may sometimes be difficult. Immunologic staining techniques allow accurate diagnosis; however, other staining and morphologic features are useful and often adequate. *Leishmania donovani* may appear to be like *Histoplasma*. The distinguishing feature is the bar-shaped kinetoplast seen in *Leishmania,* but this requires careful examination. *Toxoplasma gondii* may also resemble *Histoplasma,* but are smaller and lack the clear ring encircling each *Histoplasma* organism. On occasion, intracellular forms of *Cryptococcus neoformans* may resemble *Histoplasma*. The mucicarmine stain will usually, but not always, permit differentiation. Similarly, *Blastomyces dermatitidis* can be confused with *Histoplasma*. Ordinarily, these organisms are larger, and the bud has

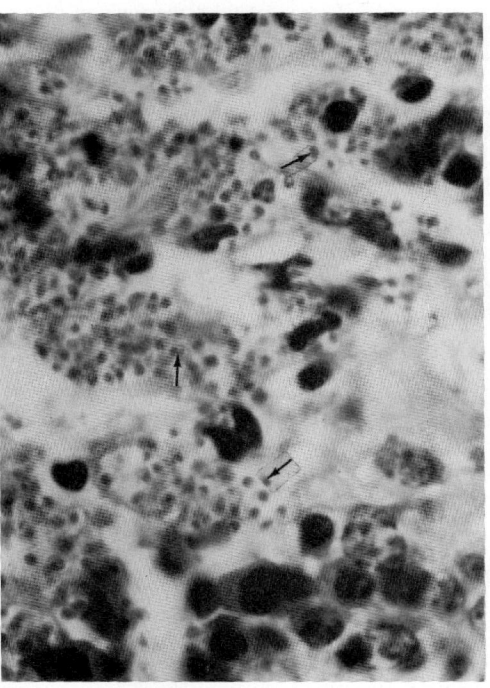

FIG. 11-12 Epizootic lymphangitis, skin of a mule ($\times$1200). Large number of *Histoplasma farciminosum (arrows)* are seen in macrophages. (Courtesy of Armed Forces Institute of Pathology and the Ninth Medical Service Detachment Laboratory, U.S. Army.)

a broad base compared to the narrow budding base of *Histoplasma*. The agent of sporotrichosis, *Sporothrix schenckii*, may not be easily distinguished, and the use of immunologic staining techniques may be necessary.

Some malignant neoplasms (malignant lymphoma, reticulum cell sarcoma), in which tissue necrosis and phagocytosis of cell debris have occurred, may have gross and microscopic features erroneously suggesting histoplasmosis, but can be distinguished by the absence of unequivocal organisms.

References

Bauman DS, Chick EW. Experimental histoplasmosis in rhesus monkeys. Infectious dose and extrapulmonary dissemination determination. Chest 1973;63:254–258.

Bauman DS, Chick EW. Acute cavitary histoplasmosis in rhesus monkeys: influence of immunological status. Infect Immun 1973;8:245–248.

Birge RF, Riser WH. Canine histoplasmosis. North Am Vet 1945;26: 281–287.

Clinkenbeard KD, Cowell RL, Tyler RD. Disseminated histoplasmosis in cats: 12 cases (1981–1986). J Am Vet Med Assoc 1987;190: 1445–1448.

Clinkenbeard KD, Cowell RL, Tyler RD. Identification of *Histoplasma* organisms in circulating eosinophils of a dog. J Am Vet Med Assoc 1988a;192:217–218.

Clinkenbeard KD, Cowell RL, Tyler RD. Disseminated histoplasmosis in dogs: 12 cases (1981–1986). J Am Vet Med Assoc 1988b;193:1443–1447.

Correa WM, Pacheco AC. Naturally occurring histoplasmosis in guinea pigs. Can J Comp Med Vet Sci 1967;31:203–206.

Del Favero JE, Farrell RL. Experimental histoplasmosis in gnotobiotic dogs. Am J Vet Res 1966;27:60–66.

De Monbreun WA. The dog as a natural host for *Histoplasma capsulatum*. Am J Trop Med 1939;19:565–588.

Dumont A, Robert A. Electron microscopic study of phagocytosis of *Histoplasma capsulatum* by hamster peritoneal macrophages. Lab Invest 1970;23:278–286.

Emmons CW. Histoplasmosis. Bull NY Acad Med 1955;31:627–638.

Emmons CW, Ashburn LL. Histoplasmosis in wild rats. Pub Health Rep 1948;63:1416–1422.

Farrell RL, Cole CR. Experimental canine histoplasmosis with acute fatal and chronic recovered courses. Am J Pathol 1968;53: 425–445.

Gwin RM, Makley TA Jr, Wyman M, et al. Multifocal ocular histoplasmosis in a dog and cat. J Am Vet Med Assoc 1980;176: 638–642.

Harmon KS. Histoplasmosis in dogs. J Am Vet Med Assoc 1948;108: 60–62.

Panciera RJ. Histoplasmic (*Histoplasma capsulatum*) infection in a horse. Cornell Vet 1969;59:306–312.

Percy DH. Feline histoplasmosis with ocular involvement. Vet Pathol 1981;18:163–169.

Rowley DA, Habermann RA, Emmons CW. Histoplasmosis: pathologic study of fifty cats and fifty dogs from Loudon County, Virginia. J Infect Dis 1954;95:98–108.

Saunders JR, Matthiesen RJ, Kaplan W. Abortion due to histoplasmosis in a mare. J Am Vet Med Assoc 1983;183:1097–1099.

Seibold HR. Histoplasmosis in a dog. J Am Vet Med Assoc 1946; 109:209–211.

Tomlinson WJ, Grocott RG. Canine histoplasmosis. A pathologic study of the three reported cases and the first case found in the Canal Zone. Am J Clin Pathol 1945;15:501–507.

VanSteenhouse JL, DeNovo RC. Atypical *Histoplasma capsulatum* infection in a dog. J Am Vet Med Assoc 1986;188:527–528.

Weller RE, Dagle GE, Malaga CA, et al. Hypercalcemia and disseminated histoplasmosis in an owl monkey. J Med Primatol 1990; 19:675–680.

Wheat LJ, Kohler RB, Tewari RP. Diagnosis of disseminated histoplasmosis by detection of *Histoplasma capsulatum* antigen in serum and urine specimens. N Engl J Med 1986;314:83–88.

AFRICAN HISTOPLASMOSIS (*HISTOPLASMA CAPSULATUM* VAR. *DUBOISII*)

African histoplasmosis is caused by *Histoplasma capsulatum* var. *duboisii*, a fungus that cannot be differentiated in culture from *H. capsulatum* var. *capsulatum*, the cause of classic histoplasmosis. In tissues, however, the two organisms are dissimilar. Var. *duboisii* looks like var. *capsulatum* with narrow-based buds and an intracellular location, but is larger, 8–15 microns in diameter. It is more likely to be confused with *Blastomyces dermatitidis*, but differs in that the latter buds with a broad base and contains multiple nuclei.

African histoplasmosis is essentially confined to Africa and Madagascar (with a few cases reported in Japan, Canada, and United States), or individuals coming from Africa, and has been described as affecting only humans and baboons. The lesions primarily affect the skin, lymph nodes, and bone, although its portal of entry is respiratory. Microscopically, in contrast to classic histoplasmosis, the lesions are characterized by granulomas composed of macrophages and numerous foreign-body and Langhans multinucleated giant cells containing yeast cells. The granulomas become surrounded by fibrous connective tissue.

References

Butler TM, Hubbard GB. An epizootic of histoplasmosis duboisii (African histoplasmosis) in an American baboon colony. Lab Anim Sci 1991;41:407–410.

Butler TM, Gleiser CA, Bernal JC, et al. Case of disseminated African histoplasmosis in a baboon. J Med Primatol 1988;17: 153–161.

Mariat F, Segretain G. Etude mycologique d'une histoplasmose spontanee du singe Africaine (*Cynocephalus babuin*). Ann Inst Pasteur 1956;19:874–891.

Walker J, Spooner ETC. Natural infection of the African baboon *Papio papio* with a large-cell form of *Histoplasma*. J Pathol Bacteriol 1960;80:436–438.

Williams AO, Lawson EA, Lucas AO. African histoplasmosis due to *Histoplasma duboisii*. Arch Pathol 1971;92:306–318.

EPIZOOTIC LYMPHANGITIS

Epizootic lymphangitis is a disease of the skin and superficial lymphatics of horses (and other equidae), but rarely humans, caused by a mycotic organism currently known as *Histoplasma farciminosum* (*Cryptococcus farciminosus, Blastomyces farciminosus, Saccharomyces farciminosus, Endomyces farciminosa, Saccharomyces equi,* or *Zygomonema farciminosum*). The organism is yeast shaped in tissue and cannot be differentiated from *Histoplasma capsulatum*. The disease does not occur in the Western Hemisphere and has been eradicated from Western Europe. It remains endemic in Africa (especially Egypt and Sudan), Eastern Europe, Russia, and Asia. The clinical features are those of chronic indurative ulceration of the skin, especially of the limbs, with thickening of the superficial lymphatics, enlargement of regional lymph nodes, formation of abscesses, and discharge of purulent material, followed by the development of new indolent ulcers. Less frequently, infection may occur as conjunctivitis or nasolacrimal infection, and rarely becomes generalized, involving internal viscera. The disease runs a chronic course over a period of months, but eventually resolves.

The mode of transmission is not established. Direct contact does not appear important unless infective material is conveyed to previously injured skin. Experimentally, flies *(Musca and Stomoxys)* have been shown capable of transmitting the infection.

With the exception of rabbits, most laboratory animals are refractory to infection.

LESIONS

Sections of the cutaneous lesions reveal granulomatous tissue reactions with a predominance of large macrophages and sometimes multinucleated giant cells. Their cytoplasm is distended with oval organisms, each about 2.0 by 3.0 μ, and enveloped by a thin, clear capsule. The central mass of the fungus is demonstrable in sections stained with hematoxylin and eosin; the peripheral capsule remains unstained. Stains for bound glycogen (PAS, Bauer, and Gridley) identify the capsule selectively, staining it red and leaving the central body unstained. Lymphocytes, plasma cells, and a scattering of neutrophils are present within the granulomatous tissue reaction. Secondary infection leads to the formation of abscesses which may drain to the surface.

DIAGNOSIS

The diagnosis of epizootic lymphangitis can be confirmed by the demonstration of typical organisms in characteristic lesions, tissue sections, cultures, or stained smears of exudate. The organisms cannot be differentiated from *H. capsulatum,* but the nature of the two diseases is different. *Sporothrix schenckii* (sporotrichosis) may closely resemble *H. farciminosum* and produce a similar disease and lesions. Usually *Sporothrix schenckii* is oval in shape.

References

Fawi MT. *Histoplasma farciminosum,* the aetiological agent of equine cryptococcal pneumonia. Sabouraudia 1971;9:123–125.

Fouad K, Saleh MS, Sokkar S, et al. Studies on lachrymal histoplasmosis in donkeys in Egypt. Zentralbl Veterinaermed B 1973;20:584–593.

Khater AR, Iskander M, Mostafa A. A histomorphological study of cutaneous lesions in equine histoplasmosis (epizootic lymphangitis). J Egypt Vet Med Assoc 1968;28:165–174.

Singh T. Studies on epizootic lymphangitis. I. Modes of infection and transmission of equine histoplasmosis (*Epizootic lymphangitis*). Indian J Vet Sci 1965;35:102–110.

Singh T, Varmani BML. Studies on epizootic lymphangitis. A note on pathogenicity of *Histoplasma farciminosum* (Rivolta) for laboratory animals. Indian J Vet Sci 1966;36:164–167.

Singh T, Varmani BML. Some observations on experimental infection with *Histoplasma farciminosum* (Rivolta) and the morphology of the organism. Indian J Vet Sci 1967;37:47–57.

ZYGOMYCOSIS (PHYCOMYCOSIS) AND PYTHIOSIS

The term, **zygomycosis** encompasses those disorders caused by fungi classified in the **Class Zygomycetes,** formerly classified as **Phycomycetes** and the diseases referred to as **phycomyces** (Table 11-1). The term, **mu-**

TABLE 11-1   **The Zygomycoses and Oomycoses (Pythiosis)**

Organism	*Disease*
Kingdom: Fungi	
Class: Zygomycetes	
Family: Mucoraceae	**Mucormycosis, Phycomycosis**
Absidia corymbifera	Seen in most animal species.
(*Mucor corymbifera,*	Common expressions include:
Lichthemia corymbifera)	cutaneous granulomas,
Mucor racemosus	rumenitis, gastritis,
Mucor ramosissimus	enteritis, placentitis,
Rhizopus microsporus	pneumonia, disseminated
(*Mucor speciosus*)	infections.
Rhizomucor spp	
Mortierella wolfii	
Cunninghamella spp	
Syncephalastrum spp	
Saksenaea spp	
Family: Entomophthoraceae	**Entomophthoromycosis**
Basidiobolus ranarum	Cutaneous and nasal
(*B. haptosporus*)	granulomas in horses
Conidiobolus coronatus	
(*Entomophthora coronatus*)	
Kingdom: Protista	
Class: Oomycetes	
Family: Pythiaceae	**Pythiosis (Oomycosis)**
Pythium spp	Cutaneous granulomas
(*Hyphomyces destruens*)	in horses ("leeches"),
	rarely cattle

cormycosis is often used to designate diseases caused by members of this group, as the **Order Mucorales** contains several of the more important potential pathogens, specifically the genera *Mucor, Absidia, Rhizopus, Rhizomucor, Mortierella, Cunninghamella, Syncephalastrum,* and *Saksenaea* (Fig. 11-13). Other **zygomycetes** associated with disease include members of the genera *Basidiobolus* and *Conidiobolus,* classified in the **Family Entomophthoraceae,** and their associated diseases termed **entomophthoromycoses.** A third group often included under the heading phycomycosis are the *Pythium* spp. These are not true fungi, but rather members of the **Kingdom Protista, Class Oomycetes** and therefore should probably be considered in a separate section; however, we include the discussion here because of the similarity of the lesions and their essentially identical appearance to the zygomycetes in tissue section. Infections with this latter group are termed **oomycosis** or **pythiosis.** These organisms have been associated principally with disease in horses, although infection has also been described in beef calves and cats. In nature, zygomycetes grow on decaying vegetation and are ordinarily not highly pathogenic; however, under appropriate conditions—such as intercurrent disease, long-term administration of antibiotics, or immunosuppression—they can cause serious disease. In tissue sections, none of the various fungi included in the zygomycetes can be differentiated from one another.

Many species, including humans as well as fish and arthropods, may be infected. Lesions commonly affect the skin or mucous membranes of the oral and nasal cavities; the diseases may be disseminated or restricted to a specific organ. The lungs, placenta, mammary glands, rumen, stomach, kidneys, and brain are frequent sites. No specific clinical syndrome exists; the clinical findings wholly depend on the tissues and organs affected. In cattle, placentitis, fetal infection, and abortion are the most frequent expressions of mucormycosis with *Absidia corymbifera, Mucor racemosus,* and *Mortierella wolfii* as frequent isolates. Abortion usually occurs in the last trimester, more often in the winter months. *Mucor* also has been shown to cause placentitis and abortion in horses. Infection of the rumen and abomasum by *Absidia, Mucor,* or *Rhizopus* is another common manifestation of mucormycosis in cattle. The digestive tract is the most frequent location of infection in dogs. In horses and rarely cattle, a dermal mycosis known as "leeches" or "kunkers," characterized by subcutaneous granulomatous inflammation, particularly of the legs (but may occur elsewhere), is caused by a *Pythium* sp. (formerly *Hyphomyces destruens*). This fungus is in the **Class Oomycetes** of the **Kingdom Protista** and the condition is termed **oomycosis** or **pythiosis.** Cutaneous granulomas in horses may also result from infection with *Basidiobolus haptosporus* (entomophthoromycosis). These three fungi cannot be easily differentiated on the basis of lesions or morphology in tissue section. *Conidiobolus (Entomophthora) coronata* produces similar granulomas in horses, usually localized to the nasal region.

LESIONS

In general, lesions induced by zygomycetes are diffuse and not in the form of discrete granulomas. The organisms are highly invasive, coursing through tissues,

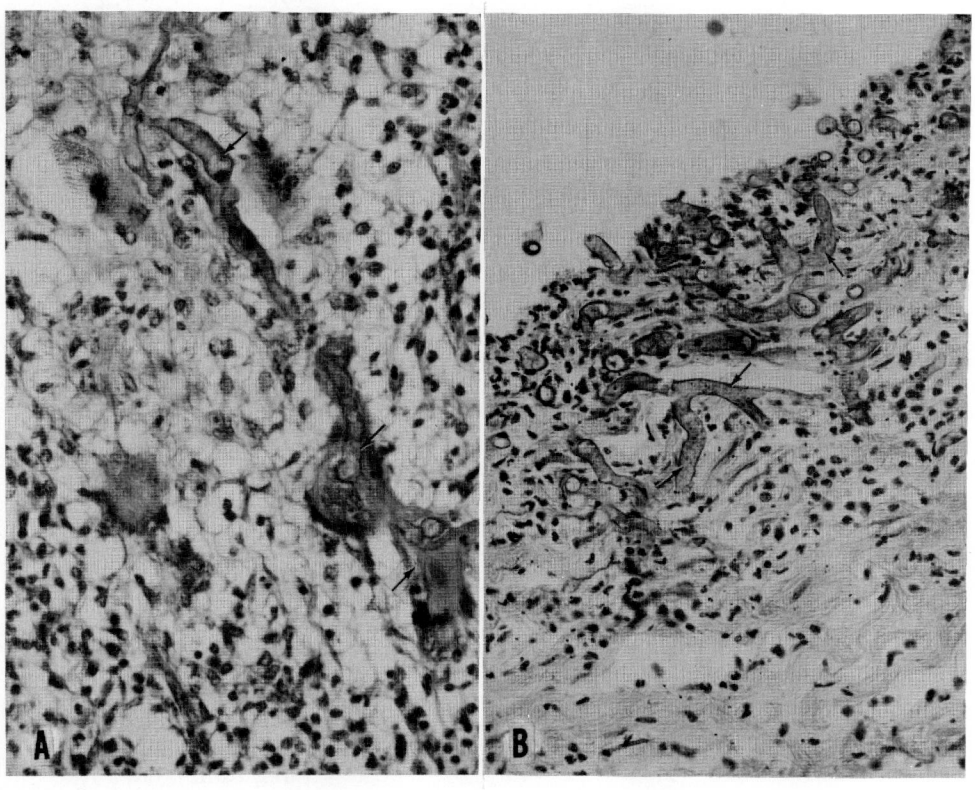

FIG. 11-13 Mucormycosis. **A.** Bovine mesenteric lymph node (×310). Note long mycelium (arrows) in a large giant cell. (Courtesy of Dr. C. L. Davis.) **B.** Organisms (arrows) in the depth of an ulcer in the stomach of a dog (×130). (Courtesy of Armed Forces Institute of Pathology and Dr. M.A. Troy.)

particularly into blood vessel walls, comparable to that seen in aspergillosis. This **angioinvasive** characteristic leads to thrombosis, hemorrhagic infarction, and dissemination of infection. The lesions are characterized by an influx of macrophages, often accompanied by multinucleated giant cells, necrosis, and variable numbers of neutrophils, giving a picture of diffuse pyogranulomatous inflammation with necrosis and pus.

As stated, all of the zygomycetes look alike in tissue section, appearing as pleomorphic, irregular, coarse, branching hyphae which are rarely septate. The hyphae range 3–25 microns in diameter with considerable variation along their courses, and often appear folded or distorted. Branching is often irregular and not dichotomous, with branches smaller than the parent hyphae and often at right angles. The hyphae usually stain basophilic with hematoxylin and eosin and are not any more clearly visualized with special staining techniques.

DIAGNOSIS

Specific diagnosis should be based on demonstration of characteristic organisms in granulomatous lesions. Isolation of organisms from the lesions is necessary for further identification, but histologic demonstration of the fungus within tissues that are obviously reacting to its presence is critical in establishing the causal relationship. Identification of the organism recovered in culture is not decisive because these fungi grow free in nature and can easily contaminate cultures taken under many circumstances.

The zygomycetes must be differentiated from *Aspergillus* spp. The latter have more uniform width, are regularly septate, and have a uniform, dichotomous branching pattern. *Aspergillus* spp. also do not stain as well with hematoxylin and eosin as do the zygomycetes.

References

Allison N, Gillis JP. Enteric pythiosis in a horse. J Am Vet Med Assoc 1990;196:462–464.

Angus KW, Renwick CC, Robinson GW. Segmental necrosis of the ileum in a lamb associated withphycomycete. Vet Rec 1971;88:654–656.

Austwick PKC, Copland JW. Swamp cancer. Nature 1974;250:84.

Baskin GB, Chandler FW, Watson EA. Cutaneous zygomycosis in rhesus monkeys *(Macaca mulatta)*. Vet Pathol 1984;21:125–128.

Bissonnette KW, et al. Nasal and retrobulbar mass in a cat caused by *Pythium insidiosum*. J Med Vet Mycol 1991;29:39–44.

Bridges CH, Emmons CW. A phycomycosis of horses caused by *Hyphomyces destruens*. J Am Vet Med Assoc 1961;138:579–589.

Bridges CH, Romane WM, Emmons CW. Phycomycosis of horses caused by *Entomophthora coronata*. J Am Vet Med Assoc 1962;140:673–677.

Brown CC, McClure JJ, Triche P, et al. Use of immunohistochemical methods for diagnosis of equine pythiosis. Am J Vet Res 1988;49:1866–1868.

Chauhan HVS, et al. A fatal cutaneous granuloma due to *Entomophthora coronata* in a mare. Vet Rec 1973;92:425–427.

Chihaya Y, Matsukawa K, Mizushima S, et al. Ruminant forestomach and abomasal mucormycosis under rumen acidosis. Vet Pathol 1988;25:119–123.

Connole MD. Equine phycomycosis. Aust Vet J 1973;49:214–215.

Cordes DO, Carter ME, di Menna ME. Mycotic pneumonia and placentitis caused by *Mortierella wolfii*. II. Pathology of experimental infection of cattle. Vet Pathol 1972;9:190–201.

Cordes DO, di Menna ME, Carter ME. Mycotic pneumonia and pla-

centitis caused by *Mortierella wolfii*. I. Experimental infections in cattle and sheep. Vet Pathol 1972;9:131–141.

Counter DE. An outbreak of mycotic abortion apparently due to mould-infected sugar beet pulp. Vet Rec 1973;93:425.

Cysewski SJ, Pier AC. Mycotic abortion in ewes produced by *Aspergillus fumigatus:* pathologic changes. Am J Vet Res 1968;29:1135–1151.

Davis CL, Anderson WA, McCrory BR. Mucormycosis in food-producing animals. J Am Vet Med Assoc 1955;126:261–267.

Dawson CO. Phycomycosis in animals in the tropics. Ann Soc Belg Med Trop 1972;52:357–364.

Fragner P, Vitovec J, Vladik P, et al. Liver disease in hog caused by *Rhizopus cohnii*. Mycopathologia 1973;49:249–254.

Gisler DB, Pitcock JA. Intestinal mucormycosis in the monkey (*Macaca mulatta*). Am J Vet Res 1962;23:365–366.

Gitter M, Austwick PKC. Mucormycosis and moniliasis in a litter of suckling pigs. Vet Rec 1959;71:6–11.

Gleiser CA. Mucormycosis in animals. J Am Vet Med Assoc 1953;123:441–445.

Goad MEP. Pulmonary pythiosis in a horse. Vet Pathol 1984;21:261–262.

Gregory JE, Golden A, Haymaker W. Mucormycosis of the central nervous system. Bull Johns Hopkins Hosp 1953;73:405–419.

Hessler JR, et al. Mucormycosis in a rhesus monkey. J Am Vet Med Assoc 1967;151:909–913.

Hillman RB. Bovine mycotic placentitis in New York State. Cornell Vet 1969;59:269–288.

Hillman RB, McEntee K. Experimental studies on bovine mycotic placentitis. Cornell Vet 1969;59:289–302.

Hutchins DR, Johnston KG. Phycomycosis in the horse. Aust Vet J 1972;48:269–278.

Jacobson ER, Calderwood MB, Clubb SL. Mucormycosis in hatchling Florida softshell turtles. J Am Vet Med Assoc 1980;177:835–837.

Johnson CT, Lupson GR, Lawrence KE. *Mortierella wolfii* abortion in British cows. Vet Rec 1990;127:363.

Knudtson WU, Bergeland ME, Kirkbride CA. Bovine fetal cerebral absidiomycosis. Sabouraudia 1975;13:299–302.

Lehrer RI, et al. Mucormycosis (UCLA Conf). Ann Intern Med 1980;93(Part 1):93–108.

Mahaffey LW, Adam NM. Abortions associated with mycotic lesions of the placenta in mares. J Am Vet Med Assoc 1964;144:24–32.

Martin JE, et al. Rhino-orbital phycomycosis in a rhesus monkey. J Am Vet Med Assoc 1969;155:1253–1257.

Migaki G, Toft JD II, Schmidt RE. Disseminated entomophthoromycosis in a mandrill (*Mandrillus sphinx*). Vet Pathol 1982;19:551–554.

Miller RI. Nomenclature of fungal diseases. Vet Pathol 1983;20:251–253.

Miller RI. Gastrointestinal phycomycosis in 63 dogs. J Am Vet Med Assoc 1985;186:473–478.

Miller RI, Campbell RSF. The comparative pathology of equine cutaneous phycomycosis. Vet Pathol 1984;21:325–332.

Miller RI, Turnwald GH. Disseminated basidiobolomycosis in a dog. Vet Pathol 1984;21:117–119.

Miller RI, Olcott BM, Archer M. Cutaneous pythiosis in beef calves. J Am Vet Med Assoc 1985;186:984–986.

Mitchell G, Esnouf D, Pritchard R. Mucormycosis in canaries (*Serinus canarius*) fed damp germinated seed. Vet Pathol 1986;23:625–627.

Murray DR, Ladds PW, Johnson RH, et al. Metastatic phycomycosis in a horse. J Am Vet Med Assoc 1978;172:834–836.

Owens WR, Miller RI, Haynes PF, et al. Phycomycosis caused by *Basidiobolus haptosporus* in two horses. J Am Vet Med Assoc 1985;186:703–705.

Pavletic MM, MacIntire D. Phycomycosis of the axilla and inner brachium in a dog: surgical excision and reconstruction with a thoracodorsal axial pattern flap. J Am Vet Med Assoc 1982;180:1197–1200.

Rapp JP, McGrath JT. Mycotic encephalitis in weanling rats. Lab Anim Sci 1975;25:477–480.

Reed WM, Hanika C, Mehdi NAQ, et al. Gastrointestinal zygomycosis in suckling pigs. J Am Vet Med Assoc 1987;191:549–550.

Roberts RJ. Ulcerative dermal necrosis (UDN) of salmon (*Salmo salar* L.). Symp Zool Soc Lond 1972;30:53–81.

Roy AD, Cameron HM. *Rhinophycomycosis entomophthorae* occurring in a chimpanzee in the wild in East Africa. Am J Trop Med Hyg 1972;21:234–237.

Sanford SE. Gastric zygomycosis (mucormycosis) in 4 suckling pigs. J Am Vet Med Assoc 1985;186:393–394.

Sanford SE, Josephson GKA, Waters EH. Submandibular and disseminated zygomycosis (mucormycosis) in feeder pigs. J Am Vet Med Assoc 1985;186:171–174.

White LO, Smith H. Placental localisation of *Aspergillus fumigatus* in bovine mycotic abortion: enhancement of spore germination in vitro by foetal tissue extracts. J Med Microbiol 1974;7:27–34.

Wohlgemuth K, Knudtson W. Bovine abortion associated with *Candida tropicalis*. J Am Vet Med Assoc 1973;162:460–461.

Rhinosporidiosis

Infection with *Rhinosporidium seeberi,* a fungus that has yet to be cultured in a cell-free medium, causes a polypoid granulomatous lesion, particularly of the nasal mucosa. It is known to infect humans, horses, cattle, dogs, and aquatic birds (ducks and geese) (Fig. 11-14). It is

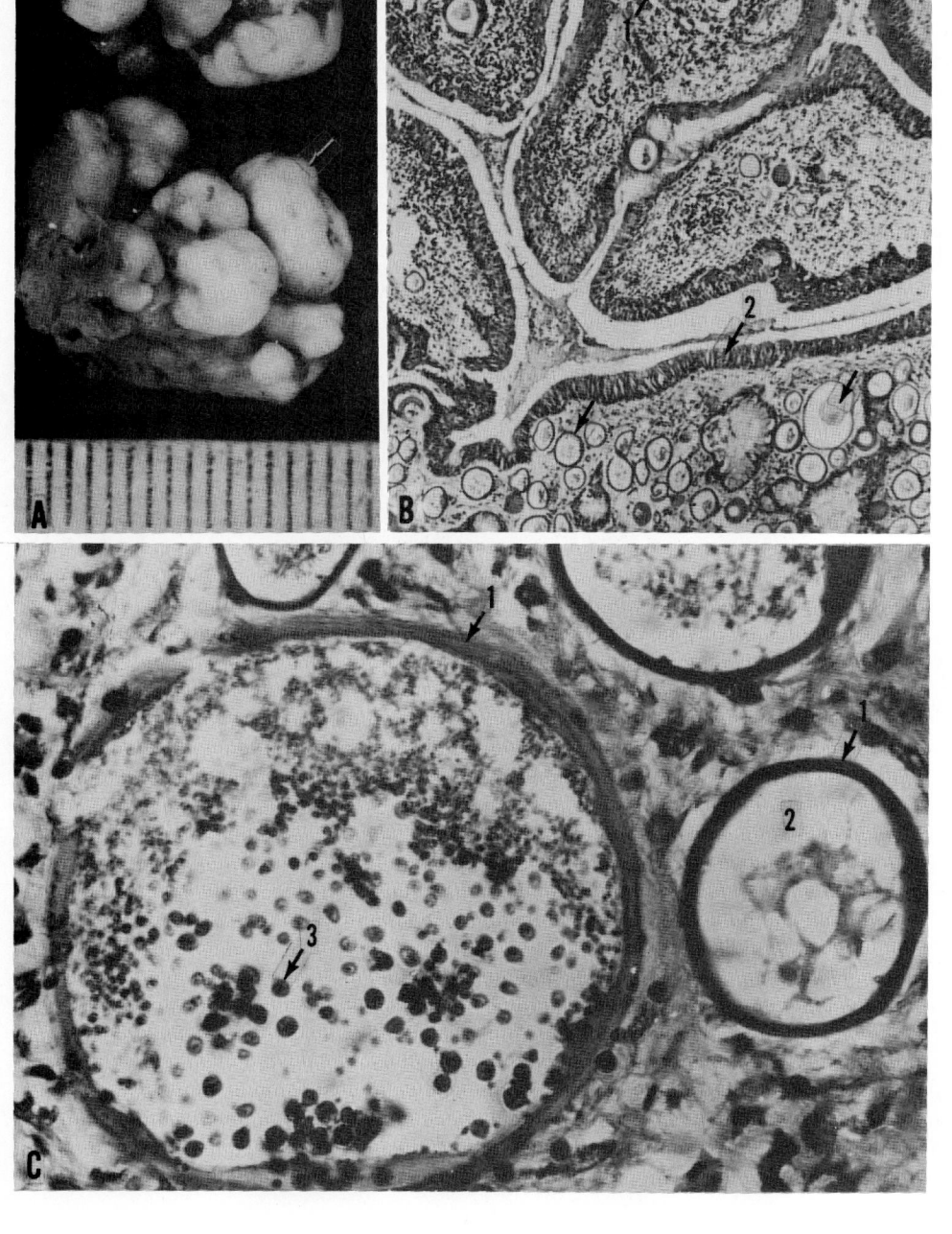

FIG. 11-14 Rhinosporidiosis. **A.** Polypoid masses from nasal mucosa of a horse. **B.** Section (×100) of one of the polyps. *Rhinosporidium seeberi* containing endospore (1) or as empty-cysts, elevating the mucous membrane (2). **C.** The organism (×600); note (1) thick wall, (2) empty organisms, and (3) others containing small and large endospores. (Courtesy of Armed Forces Institute of Pathology and Col. M.W. Hale.)

common in India, Sri Lanka, and Southeast Asia, and is reported infrequently in North and South America. The source of infection is not known, but the disease is associated with stagnant water.

In animals, as in humans, the organism invades the subepithelial stroma of the nasal mucosa and less frequently further within the respiratory tree or skin. It induces a chronic inflammation often leading to polyp formation. The polyps are single or multiple, irregular in size and shape, and may become large enough to occlude the nasal passages. In the horse in the Americas, nasal polyps are reportedly limited in extent, amenable to surgery, and probably self-limited in duration.

Microscopic examination of the polyps discloses a stroma filled with spherical organisms with a thick, double-contoured wall. Mature organisms (**sporangium**) measure up to 300 microns in diameter and are filled with endospores 2–10 microns in diameter. Endospores are larger and more uniformly round within the center of the sporangia and each contains several eosinophilic bodies. Smaller, often flattened, immature endospores lay at the periphery. Endospores are released by rupture of the cell wall at the so-called pore where it is thinnest and develop to **trophocytes,** which are up to 100 microns in diameter and contain a single nucleus with a prominent nucleolus. These are believed to, in turn, mature to sporangia containing endospores. The tissue reaction resembles that incited by *Coccidioides immitis,* which resembles *R. seeberi* in morphology. The sporangia are surrounded by an inflammatory infiltrate composed of epithelioid cells, multinucleated giant cells, lymphocytes, neutrophils, and fibrovascular connective tissue. Released endospores incite a more purulent response. Fragmented cell walls from mature organisms are found throughout the lesion.

Rhinosporidiosis must be differentiated from coccidioidomycosis. Distinguishing characteristics include: *Rhinosporidia* are larger; the sporangia contain endospores in varying stages of development which are larger than those of *C. immitis*; the endospores completely stain with fungal stains, such as PAS, whereas only the walls of *C. immitis* endospores stain; and the endospores of *R. seeberi* contain inner granules, but those of *C. immitis* do not. The spherules of adiaspiromycosis are also large, but have a much thicker wall and lack endospores.

References

Allison N, Willard MD, Bentinck-Smith J, et al. Nasal rhinosporidiosis in two dogs. J Am Vet Med Assoc 1986;188:869–871.

Davidson WR, Nettles VF. Rhinosporidiosis in a wood duck. J Am Vet Med Assoc 1978;171:989–990.

Easley JR, et al. Nasal rhinosporidiosis in the dog. Vet Pathol 1986;23:50–56.

Fain A, Herin V. Two cases of nasal rhinosporidiosis in a wild goose and a wild duck. Mycopathol Mycol Appl 1967;8:54–61.

Jimenez JF, Cornelius JB, Gloster ES. Canine rhinosporidiosis in Arkansas. Lab Anim Sci 1986;36:54–55.

Levy MG, Meuten DJ, Breitschwerdt EB. Cultivation of *Rhinosporidium seeberi* in vitro: interaction with epithelial cells. Science 1986;234:474–476.

Mosier DA, Creed JE. Rhinosporidiosis in a dog. J Am Vet Med Assoc 1984;185:1009–1010.

Myers DD, Simon J, Case MT. Rhinosporidiosis in a horse. J Am Vet Med Assoc 1964;145:345–347.

Smith HA, Frankson MC. Rhinosporidiosis in a Texas horse. Southwest Vet 1961;15:22–24.

Stuart BP, O'Malley N. Rhinosporidiosis in a dog. J Am Vet Med Assoc 1975;167:941–942.

Weller CV, Riker AD. *Rhinosporidium seeberi:* pathological histology and report of the third case from the United States. Am J Pathol 1930;6:721–732.

Zschokke E. Ein rhinosporidium beim Pferd. Schweitz Arch Tierheilkd 1913;55:641–650.

SPOROTRICHOSIS

Sporotrichosis is a granulomatous disease caused by the dimorphic fungus *Sporothrix schenckii* (*Sporotrichum schenkii*). It occurs in humans, dogs, cats, horses, mules, cattle, birds, and other animals. Among animals, it has been described most often in horses and cats. In nature, the fungus grows on plants (moss, hay, decaying vegetation), soil, and wood; infection is believed to be acquired by entry through abrasions. Sphagnum moss has been frequently incriminated as the source of infection. Ordinarily, like so many of the mycotic diseases, it has not been considered contagious; however, infected cats have been reported to be the source of infection for humans. In contrast to the disease in most species, the numbers of fungi within lesions in affected cats are high, which may account for their ability to serve as a source of infection. Chronic peritonitis and orchitis can be produced experimentally in male rats, mice, and hamsters by the intraperitoneal injection of material containing *S. schenckii.* In these experimentally induced lesions, the organisms are much more numerous and more easily seen and identified.

LESIONS

The lesions of sporotrichosis occur in the skin and cutaneous lymphatics, particularly over the legs, thorax, and abdomen. Spherical nodules, 1–4 cm in diameter, are formed in the dermis and subcutis along the course of cutaneous lymphatics, which are thickened and pursue a tortuous course between the nodules. Occasionally, the nodules ulcerate, yield small amounts of thick, creamy pus, and then heal slowly. Dissemination to other tissues, particularly bones and joints, occurs, but is rare. It has been more frequently reported in humans, cats, and dogs. Involvement of lungs, liver, spleen, kidneys, and internal lymph nodes can occur. Microscopic sections of the nodules reveal a purulent center surrounded by a wide band of epithelioid granulation tissue containing giant cells and lymphocytes. The lesion is usually surrounded by a dense connective-tissue capsule. The organisms, generally sparse, are not ordinarily visible in hematoxylin-and-eosin-stained tissue sections, except for infected cats where they are exceptionally numerous. When stained with GMS, PAS, and similar techniques, they appear as small, cigar-shaped (sometimes round) yeasts 4–6 microns (occasionally up to 12 microns) long, that have single and rarely multiple buds attached with a narrow base. They are located within the purulent core of the lesions and in the cytoplasm of macrophages and multinucleated giant cells.

The disease must be differentiated from epizootic lymphangitis in horses caused by *Histoplasma farciminosum*. The two yeasts may appear to be similar, requiring the use of animal inoculation, culture or immunologic staining techniques to distinguish between the two.

References

Barbee WC, Ewert A, Davidson EM. Animal model of human disease: sporotrichosis. Am J Pathol 1977;86:281–284.

Centers for Disease Control. Multistate outbreak of sporotrichosis in seedling handlers, 1988. MMWR 1988;37:652–653.

Davis HH, Worthington EW. Equine sporotrichosis. J Am Vet Med Assoc 1964;145:692–693.

Dunstan RW, Langham RF, Reimann KA, et al. Feline sporotrichosis: a report of five cases with transmission to humans. J Am Acad Dermatol 1986;15:37–45.

Dunstan RW, Reimann KA, Langham RF. Feline sporotrichosis. J Am Vet Med Assoc 1986;189:880–883.

Goad DL, Goad MEP. Osteoarticular sporotrichosis in a dog. J Am Vet Med Assoc 1986;189:1326–1328.

Jones TC, Maurer FD. Sporotrichosis in horses. Bull U. S. Army Med Dept 1944;74:63–73.

Kaplan W, Ochoa AG. Application of the fluorescent antibody technique to the rapid diagnosis of sporotrichosis. J Lab Clin Med 1963;62:835–841, 1251–1264.

Kier AB, Mann PC, Wagner JE. Disseminated sporotrichosis in a cat. J Am Vet Med Assoc 1979;175:202–204.

Scott EN, Kaufman L, Brown AC, et al. Serologic studies in the diagnosis and management of meningitis due to *Sporothrix schenckii*. N Engl J Med 1987;317:935–940.

Zamri-Saad M, Salmiyah TS, Jasni S, Cheng BY, et al. Feline sporotrichosis: an increasingly important zoonotic disease in Malaysia. Vet Rec 1990;127:480.

CANDIDIASIS (MONILIASIS, THRUSH)

Candidiasis, caused by species of the fungus *Candida* (most often *Candida albicans*), is principally a superficial mycosis of mucous membranes. It is encountered most frequently in avian species, affecting the mouth, esophagus, crop, and proventriculus. Superficial infection of oral mucous membranes is also the most common form of candidiasis in mammals, where it has been seen in humans, dogs, cats, cattle, swine, and nonhuman primates. Superficial infection of the skin is another manifestation. Systemic candidiasis is less frequent, but has been described in humans, calves, swine, and mice. In cattle, systemic disease may affect the gastrointestinal tract, lungs, liver, kidneys, or brain. Mastitis and abortion have also been ascribed to *Candida*. In swine, especially young piglets, infection of the stomach is the most frequent expression, usually along with oral and esophageal infection. In general, candidiasis is most common in young animals, debilitated patients, and as a complication of antibiotic therapy.

LESIONS

Gross lesions in the superficial form of candidiasis are characterized by a white pseudomembrane overlying the skin or mucous membranes. Microscopically, the membrane is composed of masses of entangled pseudohyphae, septate, hyphae, and budding yeastlike organisms 3–4 μ in diameter, which invade the epithelium, but rarely beyond the basal layer. The organisms can be difficult to discern in hematoxylin and eosin-stained tissue sections, but are clearly demonstrated with the periodic acid-Schiff, Gridley, and Gomori methenamine silver techniques. Pseudohyphae are chains of yeastlike cells, referred to as blastoconidia or blastospores, which have remained attached after division. They are distinguished from true hyphae by marked constrictions at the points of attachment of the individual yeasts. A leukocytic infiltration predominantly composed of neutrophils and lymphocytes accumulated beneath the epidermis. Lesions in systemic candidiasis, which may involve various internal organs but in particular the kidneys, are characterized by necrosis and suppuration. Rarely is a granulomatous reaction encountered.

DIAGNOSIS

Diagnosis depends upon demonstration of the organisms in characteristic lesions. The presence of blastoconidia and pseudohyphae is diagnostic. When only yeastlike forms are present, other mycoses, such as histoplasmosis or blastomycosis, must be considered. Certain *Candida* sp.—which cause disease in humans, most notably *Candida glabrata*—do not form hyphae and the yeastlike cells are small (2–3 microns), requiring immunologic staining techniques to differentiate them from *Histoplasma* sp.

References

Foley GL, Schlafer DH. Candida abortion in cattle. Vet Pathol 1987;24:532–536.

Goetz ME, Taylor DON. A naturally occurring outbreak of *Candida tropicalis* infection in a laboratory mouse colony. Am J Pathol 1967;50:361–369.

Goldstein E, et al. Studies on the pathogenesis of experimental *Candida guilliermondii* infection in mice. J Infect Dis 1965;115:293–302.

Kaufmann AF, Quist KD. Thrush in a rhesus monkey: report of a case. Lab Anim Care 1969;19:526–527.

Kitamura H, Anri A, Fuse K, et al. Chronic mastitis caused by *Candida maltosa* in a cow. Vet Pathol 1990;27:465–466.

Kral F, Uscavage JP. Cutaneous candidiasis in a dog. J Am Vet Med Assoc 1960;136:612–615.

McCullough B, Moore J, Kuntz RE. Multifocal candidiasis in a capuchin monkey (*Cebus apella*). J Med Primatol 1977;6:186–191.

Mills JHL, Hirth RS. Systemic candidiasis in calves on prolonged antibiotic therapy. J Am Vet Med 1967;150:862–870.

Patterson DR, et al. *Candida albicans* infections associated with antibiotic and corticosteroid therapy in spider monkeys. J Am Vet Med Assoc 1974;164:721–722.

Ray TL, Wuepper KD. Experimental cutaneous candidiasis in rodents. J Invest Dermatol 1976;66:29–33.

Reynolds IM, Miner PW, Smith RE. Cutaneous candidiasis in swine. J Am Vet Med Assoc 1968;152:182–186.

Richard JL, McDonald JS, Fichtner RE, et al. Identification of yeasts from infected bovine mammary glands and their experimental infectivity in cattle. Am J Vet Res 1980;41:1991–1994.

Schmidt RE, Butler TM. Esophageal candidiasis in a chimpanzee. J Am Vet Med Assoc 1970;157:722–723.

Wikse SE, Fox JG, Kovatch RM. Candidiasis in simian primates. Lab Anim Care 1970;20:957–963.

GEOTRICHOSIS

Geotrichosis is a rare, opportunistic mycosis of humans and animals caused by *Geotrichum candidum*, a fungus common on fruits, vegetables, and dairy products. It has been described as causing mastitis and abortion in cattle, lymphadenitis in swine, and systemic infection in dogs. In humans, geotrichosis has been described as chronic bronchitis, stomatitis, enteritis, conjunctivitis, dermatitis, and disseminated mycosis.

Cutaneous geotrichosis has been reported by Spanoghie et al. in aged red flamingoes (*Phoenicopterus ruber*) kept for 16 years in a zoo in Brussels, Belgium (1976). Lesions on the webs and legs of these birds contained organisms, demonstrated by culture and histologic sections. The infection was transmitted to chickens and mice. Pathogenesis was believed to be the result of aging and trauma to the feet of the flamingoes.

LESIONS

Lesions have been described as predominantly necrotizing and suppurative with variable numbers of macrophages and multinucleated giant cells, and as well-defined granulomas. The disseminated disease reported in dogs affected lung and kidney in two examples, and additionally lymph nodes, myocardium, liver, spleen, bone marrow, choroid plexus of the eye, and brain in a third example. The organisms in lesions appear as: round, yeastlike cells, 3–7 microns in diameter; chains of yeast cells forming pseudohyphae; and true septate hyphae with nonparallel contours and branching at acute angles.

DIAGNOSIS

Diagnosis requires demonstration of the organism in tissue section and differentiation from *Candida albicans*. Isolation of the organism is necessary for positive identification, but cannot be the sole means of diagnosis because of the ubiquitous presence of *Geotrichum spp.* in nature.

References

Lincoln SD, Adcock JL. Disseminated geotrichosis in a dog. Pathol Vet 1968;5:282–289.
Rhyan JC, Stackhouse LL, Davis EG. Disseminated geotrichosis in two dogs. J Am Vet Med Assoc 1990;197:358–360.
Spanoghie L, Devos A, Vianene N. Cutaneous geotrichosis in the red flamingo (*Phoenicopterus ruber*). Sabouraudia 1976;14:37–42.

LOBOMYCOSIS (LOBO DISEASE, KELOIDAL BLASTOMYCOSIS)

Lobo disease, or keloidal blastomycosis, is a chronic granulomatous infection of the human skin caused by a fungus, *Loboa loboi* (Fig.11-15). The disease is limited to Central and South America. Aside from humans, the infection has been recognized only in Atlantic bottle-nosed dolphins *(Tursiops truncatus)* in coastal waters of Florida. The disease has not been recognized in humans in the United States.

LESIONS

Lesions are localized to the dermis of the skin and rarely extend to the subcutis or beyond. They are characterized by dense collections of histiocytes and multinucleated giant cells with little proliferation of fibrous connective tissue. Small collections of neutrophils are usually present. The causative organisms are principally located within histiocytes and giant cells, appearing as round to oval yeastlike bodies 5–10 μ in diameter, containing a faintly basophilic central body 1–2 μ in diameter. They are often arranged in branching chains connected by short, thick tubes. The individual organisms may resemble *Paracoccidioides* or *Blastomyces,* but these rarely form chains through budding. They are best demonstrated with stains for carbohydrates (PAS, Gridley).

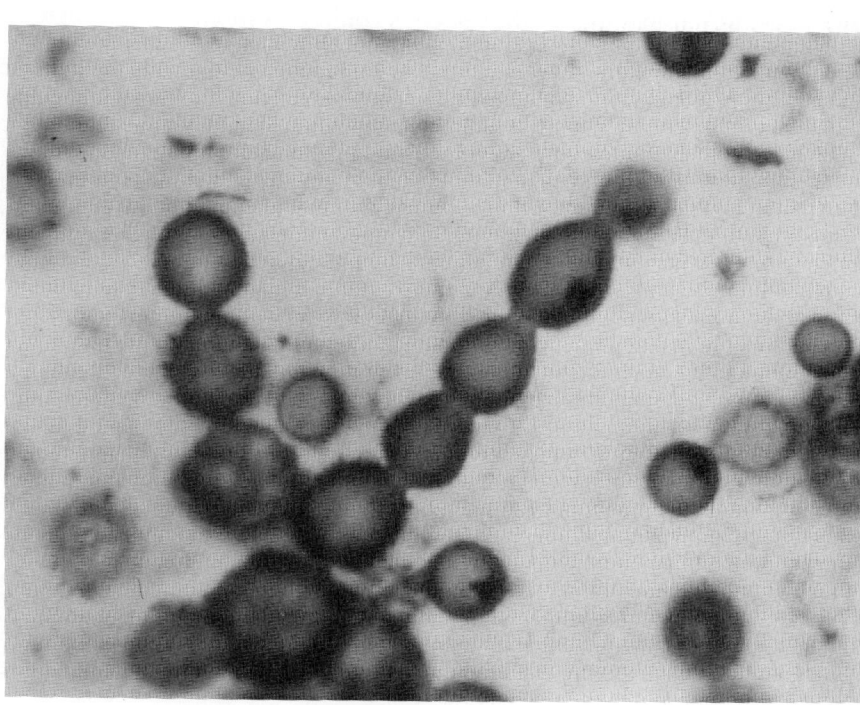

FIG. 11-15 Lobomycosis, Atlantic bottlenose dolphin. A branching chain of the fungus *Loboa loboi*. (Courtesy of Dr. G. Migaki.)

Diagnosis depends on demonstrating the characteristic organisms in tissue sections; the fungus has not been successfully cultured.

References

Bossart GD. Suspected acquired immunodeficiency in an Atlantic bottlenosed dolphin with chronic-active hepatitis and lobomycosis. J Am Vet Med Assoc 1984;185:1413–1414.

Caldwell DK, et al. Lobomycosis as a disease of the Atlantic bottlenosed dolphin (Tursiops truncatus) (Montagu, 1821). Am J Trop Med Hyg 1975;24:105–114.

Migaki G, Valerio MG, Irvine B, et al. Lobo's disease in an Atlantic bottlenose dolphin. J Am Vet Med Assoc 1971;159: 578–582.

Woodard JC. Electron microscopic study of lobomycosis (Loboa loboi). Lab Invest 1972;27:606–612.

PAECILOMYCOSIS

Although usually considered a nonpathogenic species and common laboratory contaminant, several species of *Paecilomyces* have been associated with disease in humans and animals; however, the reported examples are few. Aside from the disease in humans, disseminated infection has been reported in dogs, cats, a horse, and chameleons *(Chameleo lateralis)*, as well as pneumonia in green sea turtles *(Chelonia mydas)*, and one case in a rhesus monkey with subcutaneous and laryngeal lesions.

LESIONS

Lesions are usually granulomatous and may be localized or disseminated throughout the body, involving lungs, liver, bone, bone marrow, brain, and other tissues. Microscopically, the granulomas are composed of epithelioid cells, macrophages, and multinucleated giant cells, often with central cavitation or a collection of neutrophils. Lymphocytes, plasma cells, and eosinophils may be interspersed. The organisms appear as septate, variably branching mycelia with periodic bulbous swellings, which in some examples bear conidiophores. Yeast forms have also been described. Although the bulbous swellings along the hyphae are fairly unique, culture is required for identification.

References

Fleischman RW, McCracken D. Paecilomycosis in a nonhuman primate (*Macaca mulatta*). Vet Pathol 1977;14:387–391.

Elliott GS, Whitney MS, Reed WM, et al. Antemortem diagnosis of paecilomycosis in a cat. J Am Vet Med Assoc 1984;184:93–94.

Jang SS, Biberstein EL, Slauson DP, et al. Paecilomycosis in a dog. J Am Vet Med Assoc 1971;159:1775–1779.

Littman MP, Goldschmidt MH. Systemic paecilomycosis in a dog. J Am Vet Med Assoc 1987;191:445–447.

Patnaik AK, et al. Paecilomycosis in a dog. J Am Vet Med Assoc 1972;161:806–813.

Uys CJ, Don PA, Schrire W, et al. Endocarditis following cardiac surgery due to the fungus Paecilomyces. S Afr Med J 1963;37:1280–1296.

van den Hoven E, McKenzie RA. Suspected paecilomycosis in a dog. Aust Vet J 1974;50:368–369.

PHAEOHYPHOMYCOSIS (PHAEOMYCOTIC GRANULOMA)

This term is applied to a group of mycotic infections, subcutaneous or systemic, caused by fungi that grow in the hosts' tissues with dark-walled (dematiacious) septate mycelia. Many distinct fungi are included within this group, but they cannot be distinguished in histologic sections where most all appear as hyphae of varying length, 2–6 microns in width, with dark pigmented walls. Bulbous or vesicular swellings occur randomly along the length of the hyphae. Individual, yeastlike cells may also be seen as can chains of cells or pseudohyphae with marked constrictions where each cell is joined. Incriminated fungi include various species of the following genera: *Phialophora, Wangiella, Exophiala, Drechslera, Dactylaria, Cladosporium, Xylohypha, Moniliella,* and *Alternaria*. Most reported examples of phaeohyphomycosis have been in cats with some reports in dogs; however, it more than likely can be encountered in any species. The skin is the most usual site of involvement, followed by the central nervous system. *Dactylaria gallopava* is an important cause of cerebral phaeohyphomycosis in chickens and turkeys.

LESIONS

Most often, infections present as dermal and/or subcutaneous lesions, which are microscopically composed of multiple granulomas. The granulomas are characterized by a central cyst or core of neutrophils surrounded by epithelioid cells, multinucleated giant cells, and connective tissue. *Cladosporium* spp. have a predilection for brain, causing lesions characterized by large zones of necrosis and suppuration surrounded by epithelioid cells and multinucleated giant cells.

DIAGNOSIS

Diagnosis is made by finding the pigmented fungi within the lesions, but culture is necessary for identification of the specific fungus. Other pigmented fungi have distinct differentiating characteristics. The mycetomas are characterized by "grains" or entangled masses of pigmented hyphae, which are not seen in phaeohyphomycosis. The agents of chromoblastomycosis are also pigmented, but usually do not form hyphae in tissue and their division by septation is distinctive.

References

Dhein CR, Leathers CW, Padhye AA, et al. Phaeohyphomycosis caused by *Alternaria alternata* in a cat. J Am Vet Med Assoc 1988;193:1101–1103.

Dillehay DL, Ribas JL, Newton JC Jr, et al. Cerebral phaeohyphomycosis in two dogs and a cat. Vet Pathol 1987;24:192–194.

Hill JR, Migaki G, Phemister RD. Phaeomycotic granuloma in a cat. Vet Pathol 1978;15:559–561.

Kaplan W, et al. Equine phaeohyphomycosis caused by Drechslera spicifera. Can Vet J 1975;16:205–208.

McKenzie RA, Connole MD, McGinnis MR, et al. Subcutaneous phaeohyphomycosis caused by *Moniliella sauveolens* in two cats. Vet Pathol 1984;21:582–586.

Migaki G, Casey HW, Bayles WB. Cerebral phaeohyphomycosis in a dog. J Am Vet Med Assoc 1987;191:997–998.

Miller DM, Blue JL, Winston SM. Keratomycosis caused by *Cladosporium* sp in a cat. J Am Vet Med Assoc 1983;182:1121–1122.

Muller GH, Kaplan W, Ajello L, et al. Phaeohyphomycosis caused by Drechslera spicifera in a cat. J Am Vet Med Assoc 1975;166:150–154.

Rippon JW. Medical mycology: the pathogenic fungi and the pathogenic actinomycetes, 3rd ed. Philadelphia: WB Saunders Co., 1988.

Sisk DB, Chandler FW. Phaeohyphomycosis and cryptococcosis in a cat. Vet Pathol 1982;19:554–556.

Sousa CA, Ihrke PJ, Culbertson R. Subcutaneous phaeohyphomycosis (*Stemphylium* sp and *Cladosporium* sp infections) in a cat. J Am Vet Med Assoc 1984;185:673–675.

CHROMOBLASTOMYCOSIS

Rare reports have appeared describing chromoblastomycosis in dogs, cats, horses, and frogs. The condition, however, is principally a chronic fungal infection of the skin of humans chiefly seen in Latin America and Africa. It is caused by one of several different dematiaceous fungi, all of which have similar appearance in histologic sections. These include *Fonsecaea pedorosoi, F. compacta, Phialophora verrucosa, Cladosporium carrionii, Rhinocladiella (Acrotheca) aquaspersa,* and *R. cerophilum.* Other distinct species of *Phialophora* and *Cladosporum* are causes of phaeohyphomycosis.

The organisms incite a pyogranulomatous inflammatory reaction that is not distinctive, but the organisms are. They occur as chestnut-brown or light yellow-brown, thick-walled cells 5–15 um in diameter that are described as "muriform" and sclerotic. In contrast to other fungi, they divide by septation along one or two planes, generating two or four cells. Ordinarily the lesions, although often multiple, are restricted to the skin and subcutis. In humans, they rarely disseminate, but usually to the central nervous system.

References

Abid HN, Walter PA, Litchfield H. Chromomycosis in a horse. J Am Vet Med Assoc 1987;191:711–712.

McKeever PJ, Cywood DD, Perman V. Chromomycosis in a cat: successful medical therapy. J Am Anim Hosp Assoc 1983;19:533–536.

DERMATOMYCOSES (TRICHOPHYTOSIS, RINGWORM, FAVUS, TINEA, SUPERFICIAL MYCOSES, DERMATOPHYTOSIS)

Dermatomycoses are those infections of the skin and its adnexae caused by the dermatophytic fungi (dermatophytes) (Figs. 11-16 and 11-17). These fungi comprise many species that inhabit the skin of humans or animals and produce lesions under certain conditions. Forty-two species of dermatophytes are recognized (Babel and Rogers, 1983). The most important of these are listed in Table 11-2. Members of the genera *Microsporum* and *Trychophyton* infect animals and humans. Humans are also infected by a third genus, *Epidermophyton.* Infection is acquired by contact with infected individuals or contaminated fomites. Animals may serve as reservoirs for human infection and humans may transmit infection to animals. Those primarily infecting humans are called, **anthropophilic** while those primarily affecting animals are termed, **zoophilic.** A third group, **geophilic,** are primarily soil saprophytes and occasionally infect both humans and animals. The dermatomycoses are generally categorized as **ringworm** or, in human infections, **tinea** (from the Latin for gnawing worm).

In humans, these superficial mycoses are classified on the basis of the anatomical site of the lesion, as well as their clinical appearance. Included are: **tinea pedis,** "athletes' foot" or ringworm; **tinea cruris** (eczema marinatum), ringworm of the groin or "jock itch;" **tinea capitis,** ringworm of the scalp; **tinea favus,** a form of tinea capitis with a honeycomb appearance; **tinea unguium,** ringworm of the nails (onchomycosis); **tinea glabrosa,** also called **tinea circinata** or **tinea corporis** (**tinea imbricata** when particularly severe), ringworm of the gla-

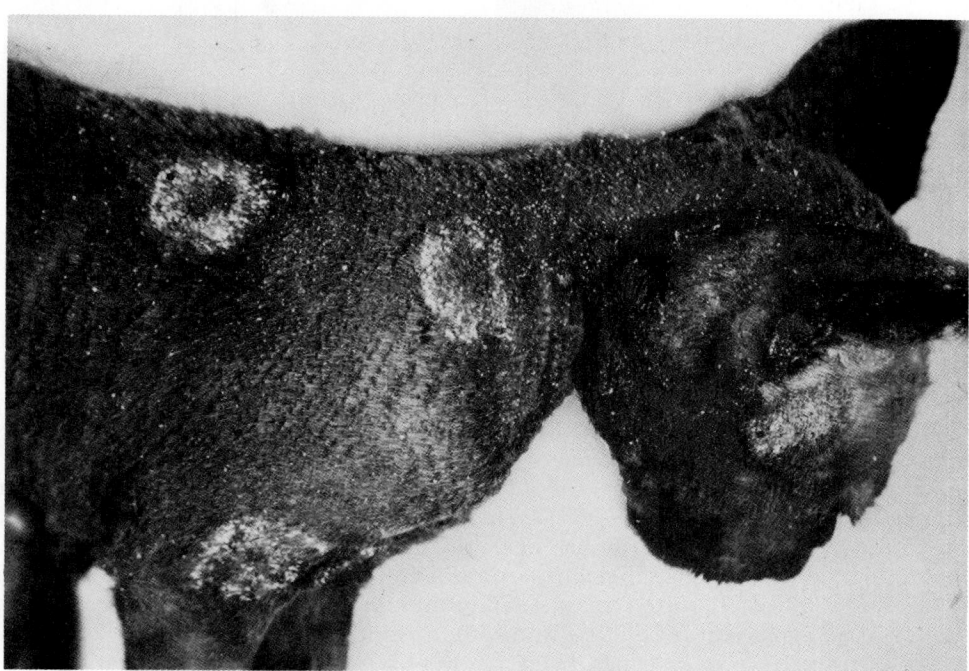

FIG. 11-16 Dermatomycosis ("ringworm") due to *Microsporum canis* in a kitten. (Courtesy of Angell Memorial Animal Hospital.)

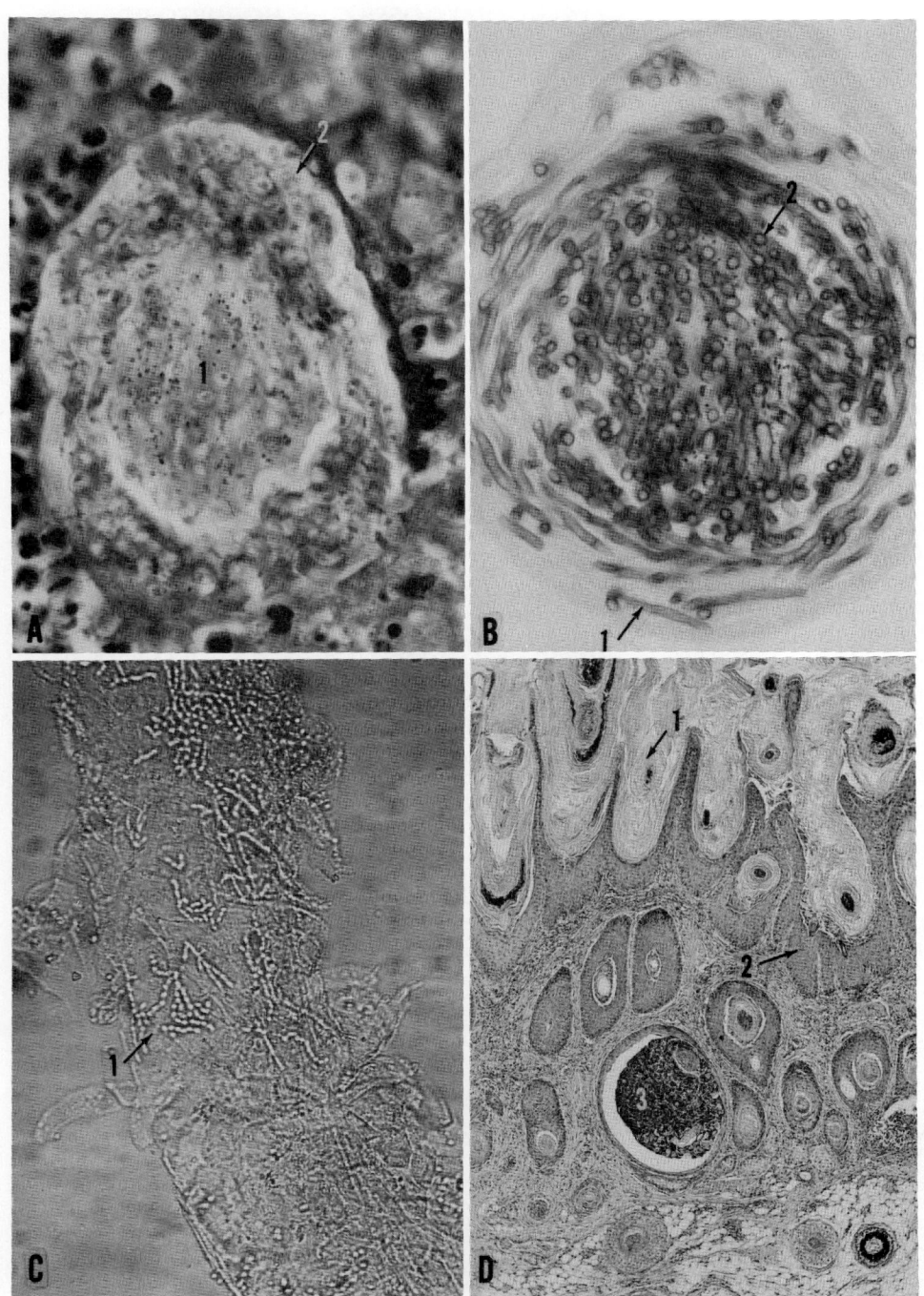

FIG. 11-17 Dermatomycosis. **A.** Hair follicle (×730) in the skin of a monkey: hematoxylin and eosin stain. Organisms are indistinctly seen in (1) hair and (2) surrounding it. **B.** Replicate section of **A,** (×730) stained with Gridley fungus stain. Note hyphae of fungi in (1) longitudinal and (2) cross section. **C.** A fresh preparation of hair, showing fungi on surface (1) of the hair. **D.** Skin of monkey (×35). Same case as **A** and **B**. Note (1) severe hyperkeratosis, (2) acanthosis, and (3) abscess in one hair follicle. (Courtesy of Armed Forces Institute of Pathology and Dr. Mervin G. Rhoades.)

brous skin; **tinea barbae,** "barber's itch," ringworm of the bearded area; and others. Other superficial mycoses of the skin of humans caused by distinct organisms include **tinea versicolor,** caused by *Malassezia furfur;* **tinea nigra,** caused by *Exophiala werneckii* or *Stenella araguata;* **black piedra,** caused by *Piedraia hortai;* and **white piedra,** caused by *Trichosporon beigelii (T. cutaneum).* Tinea versicolor, caused by *M. furfur,* has been described on the udders of milking goats. **Trichosporonosis** due to *T. beigelii* has also been reported as a dermal granuloma in one cat and as a cause of cystitis in another. Another trichosporon, *T. capitatum,* has been recovered from

cattle and humans, but rarely. *Trichosporon* has been reported to be more invasive in immunocompromised patients.

The dermatomycoses are characterized by growth of organisms upon or within the hairs, in the stratum corneum of the epidermis in the hair follicles, or the nails. The infection does not disseminate to deeper structures of the body. In these structures, the organisms appear as septate hyphae and individual or chains of arthrospores, derived from the mycelial form. *In vitro,* the fungi produce both micro- and macroconidia which are useful in identification, but are not produced

TABLE 11-2 **Principal causes of ringworm in man and animals**

Genus *Microsporum* *

M. canis (zoophilic)	Dogs, cats; sheep, calves, monkeys, apes also infected; tinea capitis in humans
M. audouinii (anthropophilic)	Epidemic urban tinea capitis, in humans, infects dogs, monkeys
M. gypseum (geophilic)	Sporadic ringworm of scalp (rare); also infects dogs, cats, horses, pigs
M. nanum (zoophilic)	Swine
M. distortum (zoophilic)	Dogs, cats, monkeys

Genus *Trichophyton* **

T. mentagrophytes (zoophilic)	Tinea capitis in humans (rare), (three varieties exist) tinea cruris, tinea barbae, tinea pedis; ringworm in dogs, cats, cattle, sheep, goats, horses, mice, rats, muskrats, foxes, chinchillas, rabbits, guinea pigs, monkeys, etc.
T. rubrum (anthropophilic)	Primary cause of tinea corporis, tinea pedis and tinea cruris in humans; tinea barbae; ringworm (rare) in dogs, foxes, monkeys, mice, squirrels, muskrats, etc.
T. tonsurans (anthropophilic)	Tinea capitis (currently most frequent form), and tinea corporis of man
T. schoenleinii (anthropophilic)	Cats, mice, rats, rabbits; tinea favosa (favus), man
T. concentricum (anthropophilic)	Tinea imbricata, man (rare)
T. violaceum (anthropophilic)	Tinea imbricata and tinea barbae of man
T. verrucosum (zoophilic)	Cattle; also horses, sheep, dogs; tinea favosa and tinea barbae of man
T. megninii (anthropophilic)	Tinea favosa of man
T. equinum (zoophilic)	Horses; also cattle; tinea barbae of man
T. gallinae (zoophilic)	Chickens, turkeys, man

Genus *Epidermophyton* (Sabouraud, 1910)

E. floccosum (anthropophilic)	Tinea cruris, tinea pedis, tinea unguium, tinea corporis of man

*Gruby, 1843
**(Malmsten, 1845)

in tissue. The organisms are often easiest to see in or on hair where two principal types of growth are seen: **ectothrix** dermatophytes, characterized by mycelial invasion within the hair with arthrospores on the outside of the hair shaft; and **endothrix** mycelia and arthrospores, found within the hair. All animal pathogens are of the ectothrix type.

LESIONS

The lesions of dermatomycosis are limited to the hairs, nails, epidermis, and dermis. The fungi grow within or upon the surface of the stratum corneum or the hairs. Growth of the fungi often binds hairs together or causes them to shed, depending upon the fungus and host. Dry, scaly, or powdery crusts may form, or the hair may be bound together in a scutulum, which leaves a red, sometimes raw and bleeding surface when it is removed. The lesions are often circumscribed and may involve any part of the skin surface. The name "ringworm" is suggested by the circinate lesions that sometimes result from the outward growth of the organisms from the healing areas in the center.

The microscopic appearance of the lesions is subtle and easily overlooked in routine sections. Thickening of the stratum corneum may be all that can be seen in sections stained with hematoxylin and eosin, but special methods, such as Bauer stain, PAS reaction, and Gridley fungus stain, often make it possible to recognize the fungi in tissue sections. Hypertrophy of the epidermis occurs in severe cases, accompanied by congestion and lymphocytic infiltration of the underlying dermis. In deeper infections in which hair follicles are involved, severe destruction of the follicle with much resulting inflammation in the dermis may be seen. Organisms also can be identified in hairs and skin scrapings cleared with a concentrated aqueous solution of sodium or potassium hydroxide and examined under the microscope, using decreased illumination.

DIAGNOSIS

The clinical recognition of some of the superficial mycoses is facilitated by the use of filtered ultraviolet light (Wood's light) to examine the lesions in a darkened room. Some species, particularly of *Microsporum*, exhibit fluoresence under ultraviolet light, making it possible to recognize mild infections. Ringworm is most frequently seen in dogs and cats with *M. canis* as the most frequent agent, and cattle, where *T. verrucosum* is the usual cause. Horses housed in groups are frequently affected with *T. equinum*. The disease in swine is now rare, and sheep are seldom affected.

References

Abu-Samra MT, Imbabi SE, Mähgoub ES. *Microsporum canis* infection in calves. Sabouraudia 1975;13:154–156.
Babel DE, Rogers AL. Dermatophytes: their contribution to infectious disease in North America. Clin Microbiol Newslett 1983;5:81–85.
Bagnall BG, Grunberg W. Generalized *Trichophyton mentagrophytes* ringworm in capuchin monkeys (*Cebus nigrivitatus*). Br J Dermatol 1972;87:565–570.
Baker HJ, Bradford LG, Montes LF. Dermatophytosis due to *Microsporum canis* in a rhesus monkey. J Am Vet Med Assoc 1971;159:1607–1611.

Banks KL, Clarkson TB. Naturally occurring dermatomycosis in the rabbit. J Am Vet Med Assoc 1967;151:926–929.

Bliss EL. Tinea versicolor dermatomycosis in the goat. J Am Vet Med Assoc 1984;184:1512–1513.

Cadigan C Jr, Chaicumpa V. Infections among Thai gibbons and humans caused by atypical *Microsporum canis.* Lab Anim Sci 1973;23:226–231.

Connole MD. A review of dermatomycoses of animals in Australia. Aust Vet J 1963;39:130–134.

Doster AR, Erickson ED, Chandler FW. Trichosporonosis in two cats. J Am Vet Med Assoc 1987;190:1184–1186.

Errington PL. Observations on a fungus skin disease of Iowa muskrats. Am J Vet Res 1942;3:195–201.

Fowle LP, Georg LK. Suppurative ringworm contracted from cattle. Arch Derm Syph 1947;56:780–793.

Fuentes CA, Bosch ZE, Boudet CC. Occurrence of *Trichophyton mentagrophytes* and *Microsporum gypseum* on hairs of healthy cats. J Invest Dermatol 1954;23:311–313.

Fuentes CA, Aboulafia R. *Trichophyton mentagrophytes* from apparently healthy guinea pigs. Arch Dermatol Syph 1955;71:478–480.

Georg LK, Kaplan W, Canap LB. Equine ringworm with special reference to Trichophyton equinum. Am J Vet Res 1957;18:798–810.

Ginther OJ. Clinical aspects of *Microsporum nanum* infection in swine. J Am Vet Med Assoc 1965;146:945–953.

Greene CE, Miller DM, Blue JL. *Trichosporon* infection in a cat. J Am Vet Med Assoc 1985;187:946–948.

Kaplan W, Hopping JL Jr, Georg LK. Ringworm in horses caused by the dermatophyte, Microsporum gypseum. J Am Vet Med Assoc 1957;131:329–332.

Korinek JK, Guarda LA, Bolivar R, et al. *Trichosporon* hepatitis. Gastroenterology 1983;85:732–734.

Kushida T, Watanabe S. Canine ringworm caused by *Trichophyton rubrum:* probable transmission from man to animal. Sabouraudia 1975;13:30–32.

Leeper AWD. Experimental bovine *Trichophyton verrucosum* infection. Preliminary clinical, immunological and histological observations in primarily infected and reinoculated cattle. Res Vet Sci 1972;13:105–115.

Mansfield PD, Stringfellow JS. Isolation of *Microsporum vanbreuseghemii* from the skin lesions of a dog. J Am Vet Med Assoc 1990; 197:875–876.

Menges RW, Georg LK. An epizootic of ringworm among guinea pigs caused by *Trichophyton mentagrophytes.* J Am Vet Med Assoc 1956;128:395–398.

Parrish HJ, Craddock S. A ringworm epizootic in mice. Br J Exp Pathol 1931;12:209–212.

Pascoe RR, Connole MD. Dermatomycosis due to *Microsporum gypseum* in horses. Aust Vet J 1974;50:380–383.

Vries GA de, Jitta CRJ. An epizootic in horses in the Netherlands caused by *Trichophyton equinum* var. *equinum.* Sabouraudia 1973;11:137–139.

PROTOTHECOSIS

Colorless algae of the genus *Prototheca,* though usually saprophytic, have been reported to cause disease in humans and animals (Fig. 11-18). *Prototheca* are considered achlorophyllous relatives of green algae of the genus *Chlorella;* however, their exact taxonomic position is uncertain. Two species have been associated with disease, *Prototheca wickerhamii* and *P. zopfii.* Although a rare disease, the number of reports in humans and animals has increased in recent years. In humans, infection is mostly limited to the skin, but in animals systemic or generalized infection with or without involvement of the skin is more usual. Protothecosis in animals was first described as a cause of mastitis in cattle and has since been reported in dogs, cats, deer, a beaver, and a fruit bat. In systemic infection of dogs, the organisms seem to have a predilection for brain and eyes with blindness or other neurologic abnormalities common clinical expressions. Disseminated lesions have also been described in the kidneys, heart, liver, gastrointestinal tract, lymph nodes, muscle, bone, and skin. In cattle, mastitis is the most frequent expression, with occasional extension to lymph nodes. The cutaneous form of the disease has been described in cats.

LESIONS

In tissue sections, *Prototheca* spp. appear as round, oval, or angular cells, 8–20 μm in diameter with a refractile wall and granular cytoplasm. Individual organisms contain a single nucleus; however, reproduction occurs by endosporulation, which produces 2–20 "endospores" or daughter cells within a single organism (morula). Each daughter cell contains cytoplasm and a cell wall in contrast to endospores of fungi. The morula eventually ruptures, releasing individual daughter cells.

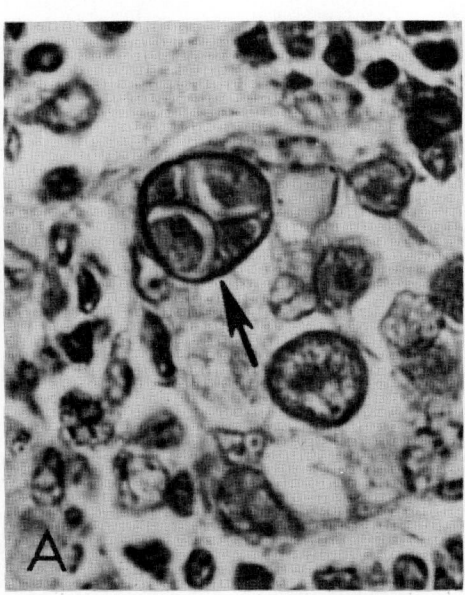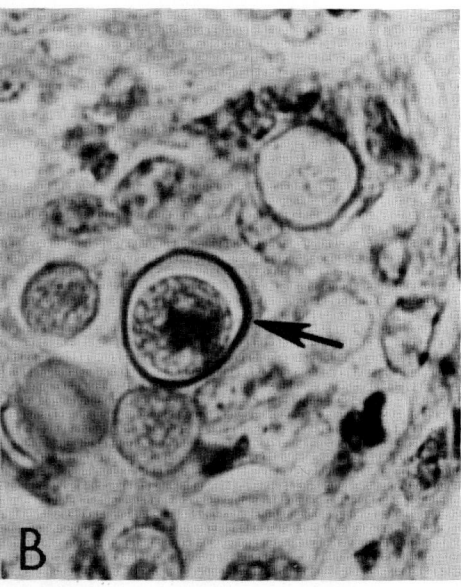

FIG. 11-18 Protothecosis, bovine lymph node. **A.** Several organisms, one composed of four daughter cells within a single-cell wall (arrow), Mayer mucicarmine stain. **B.** Single organisms have distinct cell walls (arrow) and one or more nuclei, Mayer mucicarmine stain. (Courtesy of Dr. G. Migaki and *Pathologia Veterinaria.*)

The endospores tend to fill the morula laying in juxtaposition to one another and are often angular in contrast to those seen in *Coccidioides* and similar fungi. The cell wall stains poorly in hematoxylin-and-eosin-stained tissue sections and the organisms, if few, can be easily missed; however, the wall is strongly positive to stains for carbohydrate (PAS, Gridley, Bauer, GMS). The numbers of organisms within lesions may be massive or sparse.

Tissue reaction is variable. In some cases little inflammatory response occurs, even to large numbers of organisms. Most commonly, diffuse pyogranulomatous reaction or typical granulomatous response with epithelioid cells and multinucleated giant cells transpires.

DIAGNOSIS

Diagnosis is based on finding the typical organisms in tissue section, but isolation is required for species identification. The organisms closely resemble *Chlorella* spp., but can be distinguished by finding PAS-positive starch granules in the cytoplasm of *Chlorella*, which are anisotropic in unstained tissue sections. In fresh smears of lesions containing *Chlorella*, the organisms are green due to chlorophyl.

References

Anderson KL, Walker RL. Sources of *Prototheca* spp in a dairy herd environment. J Am Vet Med Assoc 1988;193:553–556.

Buyukmihci N, Rubin LF, DePaoli A. Protothecosis with ocular involvement in a dog. J Am Vet Med Assoc 1975;167:158–161.

Carlton WW, Austin L. Ocular protothecosis in a dog. Vet Pathol 1973;10:274–280.

Cheville NF, McDonald J, Richard J. Ultrastructure of *Prototheca zopfii* in bovine granulomatous mastitis. Vet Pathol 1984;21:341–348.

Coloe PJ, Allison JF. Protothecosis in a cat. J Am Vet Med Assoc 1982;180:78–79.

Cook JR Jr, Tyler DE, Coulter DB, et al. Disseminated protothecosis causing acute blindness and deafness in a dog. J Am Vet Med Assoc 1984;184:1266–1272.

Dillberger JE, Homer B, Daubert D, et al. Protothecosis in two cats. J Am Vet Med Assoc 1988;192:1557–1559.

Font RL, Hook SR. Metastatic prototheccal retinitis in a dog. Electron microscopic observations. Vet Pathol 1984;21:61–66.

Frank N, Ferguson LC, Cross RF, et al. Prototheca, a cause of bovine mastitis. Am J Vet Res 1969;30:1785–1794.

Gaunt SD, McGrath RK, Cox HU. Disseminated protothecosis in a dog. J Am Vet Med Assoc 1984;185:906–907.

McDonald JS, Richard JL, Cheville NF. Natural and experimental bovine intramammary infection with *Prototheca zopfii*. Am J Vet Res 1984;45:592–595.

Migaki G, Garner FM, Imes GD Jr. Bovine protothecosis. A report of three cases. Pathol Vet 1969;6:444–453.

Migaki G, Font RL, Sauer RM, et al. Canine protothecosis: review of the literature and report of an additional case. J Am Vet Med Assoc 1982;181:794–797.

Moore FM, Schmidt GM, Desai D, et al. Unsuccessful treatment of disseminated protothecosis in a dog. J Am Vet Med Assoc 1985;186:705–708.

Povey RC, Austwick PKC, Pearson H, et al. A case of prothothecosis in a dog. Pathol Vet 1969;6:396–402.

Rakich PM, Latimer KS. Altered immune function in a dog with disseminated protothecosis. J Am Vet Med Assoc 1984;185:681–683.

Rogers RJ. Prototheccal lymphadenitis in an ox. Aust Vet J 1974;50:281–282.

Sudman MS. Protothecosis: a critical review. Am J Clin Pathol 1974;61:10–19.

Sudman MS, Majka JA, Kaplan W. Primary mucocutaneous protothecosis in a dog. J Am Vet Med Assoc 1973;163:1372–1374.

Tyler DE, Lorenz MD, Blue JL, et al. Disseminated protothecosis with central nervous system involvement in a dog. J Am Vet Med Assoc 1980;176:987–993.

van Kruiningen HJ. Prototheccal enterocolitis in a dog. J Am Vet Med Assoc 1970;157:56–63.

van Kruiningen HJ, Garner FN, Schiefer B. Protothecosis in a dog. Pathol Vet 1969;6:348–354.

CHLORELLOSIS

Chlorellosis is infection with green algae of the genus *Chlorella*. The organisms resemble those of *Prototheca* spp., but contain chlorophyl. The disease, which is even more infrequent than protothecosis, has been described in sheep, cattle, and a beaver *(Castor canadensis)*. In most examples, lesions have been restricted to lymph nodes, but lesions in the lungs, liver, and kidney have also been reported in sheep. The most distinctive feature is that grossly the lesions are green. The microscopic features have been described as ranging from primarily necrotizing with only a slight infiltration of neutrophils and macrophages to typical granulomas with epithelioid cells and multinucleated giant cells. The organisms occur singly and as morulae containing two or more daughter cells and superficially cannot be distinguished from *Prototheca* spp. The green pigmentation is lost in processing, but is evident in fresh smears. *Chlorella* are also distinguished by the presence of PAS-positive starch granules, which are anisotropic in unstained tissue sections.

References

Chandler FW, Kaplan W, Callaway CS. Differentiation between *Prototheca* and morphologically similar green algae in tissue. Arch Pathol Lab Med 1978;102:353–356.

Cordy DR. Chlorellosis in a lamb. Vet Pathol 1973;10:171–176.

Jones JW, McFadden HW, Chandler FW, et al. Green algal infection in a human. Am J Clin Pathol 1983;80:102–107.

Kaplan W. Protothecosis and infections caused by morphologically similar green algae. PAHO Sci Publ 1978;356:218–232.

Kaplan W, Chandler FW, Choudary C, et al. Disseminated unicellular green algal infection in two sheep in India. Am J Trop Med Hyg 1983;32:405–411.

Rogers RJ, et al. Lymphadenitis of cattle due to infection with green algae. J Comp Pathol 1980;90:1–9.

MYCOTOXICOSES (MOLDY FEEDS)

The diseases caused by fungi discussed up to this point have concerned disorders in which the organisms themselves invade tissue, no matter how superficially. Many of these are true pathogens or obligate parasites and many others represent opportunistic infections by fungi that are usually saprophytic or pathogens of plants. A large number of disorders remain, in which illness or death is attributable to the ingestion of molds or their products (toxins) produced by fungi (molds) in or on the animals' feed.

Collectively, these are grouped as mycotoxicoses. Diseases resulting from mycotoxins have been recognized for centuries, ergotism having been described in the Middle Ages and used medicinally for several hundred years. Other conditions were associated with molds earlier this century, such as stachybotryotoxicosis

TABLE 11-3 **Mycotoxicoses**

Disease	Fungus	Toxin	Species (exp.) *	Major pathologic features	Principal plant	Geographic location
Gangrenous ergotism	*Claviceps purpurea*	Ergotamine, other alkaloids (lysergic acid derivatives)	Cattle, horses, pigs, humans (all suscep.) Swine	Gangrene Agalactia	Grains, grasses	Worldwide
Convulsive or nervous ergotism	*Claviceps paspali*	Tremorigens (paspalitrems; paxilline, paspalanine)	Cattle, sheep, horses	Unknown	Dallis grass (*Paspalum* grasses)	Worldwide
Aflatoxicosis	*Aspergillus flavus*	Aflatoxins B_1, B_2, G_1, G_2	Poultry, dogs, swine, cattle, humans, trout	Toxic hepatitis, cirrhosis, hepatic adenomas and adenocarcinomas	Groundnut meal, corn, cottonseed, etc.	Worldwide
Facial eczema	*Pithomyces chartarum*	Sporodesmin	Sheep, cattle	Toxic hepatitis, cirrhosis, photosensitization	Pasture plants, esp. ryegrass	New Zealand, Australia, South Africa, Texas
Slobbers	*Rhizoctonia leguminicola*	Slaframine (converted to acetylcholinelike compound)	Cattle, sheep, horses	Salivation	Red clover	midwestern U.S.
Lupinosis	*Phomopsis leptostromiformis*	Phomopsin	Sheep, horses, cattle, swine	Toxic hepatitis, cirrhosis	Lupines	Europe, New Zealand, Australia, South Africa, Montana
Porcine vulvovaginitis	*Fusarium roseum*	Zearalenone (estrogenic)	Swine	Hyperplasia of uterus, vagina, mammary gland	Corn, barely, wheat, oats	Worldwide
Ill-defined (diarrhea, tremors, convulsions)	*Penicillium cyclopium*	Cyclopiazonic acid	Sheep, horses, cattle	Toxic hepatitis	Many foods	England
Ill-defined	*Penicillium rubrum*	Rubratoxins	Swine, cattle	Hepatic necrosis	Corn, other foods	United States (probably worldwide)
Tibial dyschondroplasia	*Fusarium roseum*	Unknown	Poultry	Tibial dyschondroplasia	Unknown	Worldwide
Stachybotryotoxicosis	*Stachybotrys alternans, S. chartarum*	Stachybotryotoxin (satratoxin)	Horses, humans	Hemorrhagic necrosis and ulceration of mouth, stomach, intestine; leukopenia	Hays	Russia, Eastern Europe
Alimentary toxic aleukia	*Fusarium poae, F. sporotrichioides*	Unknown	Humans	Dermatitis, stomatitis, leukopenia, lymphoid necrosis	Grains	Russia
Ulcerative stomatitis, gastroenteritis	*Fusarium, Cephalosporium, Myrothecium, Trichothecium, Trichodermia*	Trichothecenes	Cattle, swine, horses, humans	Dermatitis, gastroenteritis; hemorrhages, radiomimetic effect	Corn, barley, rice (many plants)	Worldwide

TABLE 11-3   (continued)

Disease	Fungus	Toxin	Species (exp.) *	Major pathologic features	Principal plant	Geographic location
Cardiac beriberi (Shoskin-Kakke)	*Penicillium citreoviride*	Citreoviridin	Humans (dogs, cats, mice, horses, sheep)	Cardiac distress, neurologic signs (Tremors, convulsions paralysis)	Rice	Japan
Hepatic necrosis	*Penicillium islandicum*	Luteoskyrin cyclochlorotine	Humans, chicks, mice, rabbits	Toxic hepatitis, cirrhosis, hepatocarcinoma	Rice	Japan
"Atypical interstitial pneumonia" of cattle	*Fusarium solani, F. frimbriata*	4-Ipomeanol	Cattle	Pulmonary edema, alveolar cell proliferation, hyaline membranes	Sweet potatoes	U.S.
Mold nephrosis of swine	*Aspergillus ochraceus, Penicillium viridicatum*	Ochratoxins, citrinin	Swine, poultry	Toxic nephrosis	Maize, wheat, barley, oats, alfalfa (others)	Denmark, Ireland, Wisconsin
Unknown	*Aspergillus versicolor*	Sterigmatocystin	Humans (rats, monkeys)	Hepatic and renal necrosis, cirrhosis hepatoma	Decaying animal and vegetable products	Worldwide
Moldy corn poisoning, equine encephalomalacia	Unknown (*Fusarium moniliforme?*)	Unknown	Horses	Encephalomalacia	Corn	Worldwide
Neurotoxicosis	*Penicillium patulum*	Patulin	Cattle	Convulsions, edema, hemorrhage	Malted barley, wheat	Europe, U.S., Japan
Kikuyu poisoning	*Myrothecium verrucaria, M. roridum*	Trichothecenes(?)	Cattle, sheep	Ulcerative rumenitis, reticulitis, omasitis	Kikuyu grass (*Pennisetum clandestinum*)	New Zealand
Fescue foot	*Balansia spp.?*	Probably a mycotoxicosis, but not proved (see Fescue grass, Chapter 16).				
Perrenial rye grass staggers	*Penicillium* spp.	Tremorigens	Cattle, sheep, horses	Tremors, ataxia, etc.	Perrenial ryegrass	Australia, New Zealand

*Experimentally susceptible species in parentheses.

of horses in the U.S.S.R. in the 1940s, and facial eczema in sheep in New Zealand in the 1950s. With the recognition of aflatoxicosis in the 1960s, interest in mycotoxins expanded rapidly, and many new and old diseases were recognized as being caused by toxic metabolites of molds. The search for other mycotoxins has resulted in the laboratory identification of additional mycotoxins, many of which have not yet been associated with naturally occurring disease, although such an association is to be expected.

No common clinical or pathologic features occur with mycotoxicoses. Many are hepatotoxic, but their effects are varied, ranging from neoplasia to neurologic

dysfunction. Some of the more important and better studied mycotoxicoses are listed in Table 11-3. Good reviews of mycotoxins can be found among the references that follow.

References

Austwick PKC. Mycotoxins. Br Med Bull 1975;31:222–229.
Berry CL. Review article. The pathology of mycotoxins. J Pathol 1988;154:301–311.
Cheeke PR, Shull LR. Natural toxicants in feeds & poisonous plants, In: Mycotoxins. Westport: AVI Publ Co, 1985;393–476.
Natl Res Council. Interactions of mycotoxins in animal production. Proc Symp July 13, 1978. Washington, DC: Natl Acad Sci, 1979.
Newberne PM. Mycotoxins: toxicity, carcinogenicity, and the influence

of various nutritional conditions. Environ Health Perspect 1974;9:1–32.

Pier AC. An overview of the mycotoxicoses of domestic animals. J Am Vet Med Assoc 1973;163:1259–1261.

Purchase IFH, ed. Mycotoxins. Amsterdam: Elsevier Scientific Publishing Company, 1974.

Shreeve BJ, Patterson DSP. Mycotoxicosis. Vet Rec 1975;97:279–280.

Smith JE, Henderson RS, eds. Mycotoxins and Animal Foods. Boca Raton: CRC Press Inc, 1991.

Stuart BP, Bedell DM. Mycotoxicosis in swine. Vet Clin North Am Large Anim Pract 1982;4:377–388.

Wilson BJ, Harbison RD. Rubratoxins. J Am Vet Med Assoc 1973;163:1274–1275.

Ergot

Most of the agricultural "small grains" and many different grasses are parasitized by the ascomycetic fungus, *Claviceps purpurea*. Each sclerotium (a compact collection of mycelia) of the fungus is a hard, black, elongated body that destroys and replaces a grain or seed of the maturing plant, being usually somewhat larger than the neighboring grains. These sclerotia constitute the substance called ergot (French for rooster's spur), the poisonous properties of which have long been familiar. Ergot contains a variety of toxic substances, including several alkaloids, the principal toxins responsible for the disease. These include derivatives of lysergic acid (ergotamine) and isolysergic acid (ergo-cristine). As late as the early nineteenth century, humans were not infrequently poisoned by contaminated flour. In animals, including birds, poisoning may occur through the feeding of contaminated grain, but in herbivora, it results more frequently from the use of hay or straw containing a considerable proportion of parasitized plants.

In general, the action of ergot is to stimulate smooth muscle by stimulating adrenergic nerves. This action upon the uterine musculature is responsible for its use as an oxytocic. Long-continued contraction of the vascular musculature is the principal basis for its poisonous effects. The usual manifestation of chronic poisoning by ergot, which is known as ergotism, consists of dry gangrene of the limbs, tail, and ears, so that after several weeks of ingestion of small amounts the most distal parts of the extremities may drop off. The early stages are characterized by lameness, irregular gait, and evidence of pain in the feet, the posterior extremities being chiefly affected. Palpation of the parts involved shows them to be cold and insensitive. These signs may begin as early as one week after the first consumption of contaminated material. Occasionally, gangrene has been moist instead of dry, at least in the feet and phalanges. As would be expected, a clear line of demarcation and an inflammatory zone just proximal to it usually exist. In birds, the comb, tongue, and beak become gangrenous. Less noticeable signs based upon involvement of the gastrointestinal musculature may precede or accompany those arising in the extremities. They include indigestion, colic, vomiting, and either diarrhea or constipation. Pregnant animals often abort. Decreased milk production (agalactia) occurs, which may be the only sign in swine.

The above-described signs mark the usual "gangrenous form." The rare "spasmodic form" (convulsive form, nervous form) causes tonic contractions of the flexors of the limbs, trembling of the muscles, opisthotonos, tetanic spasms of the whole body, convulsions, delirium, and death. This type of reaction is presumed to be related to failing blood supply in the central nervous system.

Postmortem lesions are obvious in the gangrenous cases. In addition, congestion and occasionally hemorrhage are described in the visceral organs.

Another related fungus, *Claviceps paspali*, produces different effects on animals and, therefore, is considered separately. Gangrenous ergotism is identical in appearance to fescue poisoning.

References

Anderson JF, Werdin RE. Ergotism manifested as agalactia and gangrene in sows. J Am Vet Med Assoc 1977;170:1089–1091.

Bacon CW, Porter JK, Robbins JD. Toxicity and occurrence of *Balansia* on grasses from toxic fescue poisoning. Appl Microbiol 1975;29:553–556.

Burfening PJ. Ergotism. J Am Vet Med Assoc 1973;163:1288–1290.

Dillon BE. Acute ergot poisoning in cattle. J Am Vet Med Assoc 1955;126:136.

Dollahite JW. Ergotism produced by feeding *Claviceps cinera* growing on Tobosagrass (*Hilaria mutica*) and Galletagrass (*Hilaria jamesii*). SW Vet 1963;16:295–296.

Greatorex JC, Mantle PG. Effect of rye ergot on the pregnant sheep. J Reprod Fertil 1974;37:33–41.

Lumb JW. Ergotism of cattle in Kansas. J Am Vet Med Assoc 1932;81:812–816.

Mantle PG, Gunner DE. Abortions associated with ergotised pastures. Vet Rec 1965;77:885–886.

Woods AJ, Jones JB, Mantle PG. An outbreak of gangrenous ergotism in cattle. Vet Res 1966;78:742–749.

Dallis Grass Poisoning (*Claviceps Paspali*)

Another fungus, *Claviceps paspali*, grows upon Dallis grass (*Paspalum dilatatum*), a pasture plant of the southern United States, and produces what is known as Dallis-grass poisoning (paspalum staggers) in cattle, sheep, and horses. This ergot (sclerotium), as the seed it replaces, is much smaller than that of *Claviceps purpurea* and often of a brownish color. Symptoms of Dallis grass poisoning appear after animals have had access to parasitized seedheads of the grass for a few or several days. The animals are essentially nervous in character and exhibit: (1) nervous hyperirritability, excitability, and even belligerency; and (2) muscular incoordination. The latter is worse when the cow or horse is excited and results in frequent falling and eventual inability to stand. Many animals recover with a change in feed. Gross lesions are minimal and microscopic studies appear to have been neglected. However, some have attributed certain forms of dermatitis to this fungus.

A symptomatically similar disease has occurred in certain years among cattle on the "bunch grass" ranges of the northern Rocky Mountain regions (Columbia basin of the state of Washington), and an ergot on the grass has been suspected. Neurologic sequelae have also been associated with Bermuda-grass and rye grass, but the cause or relationship to a mycotoxin has not been established. *Penicillium spp.* and *Aspergillus spp.* are also

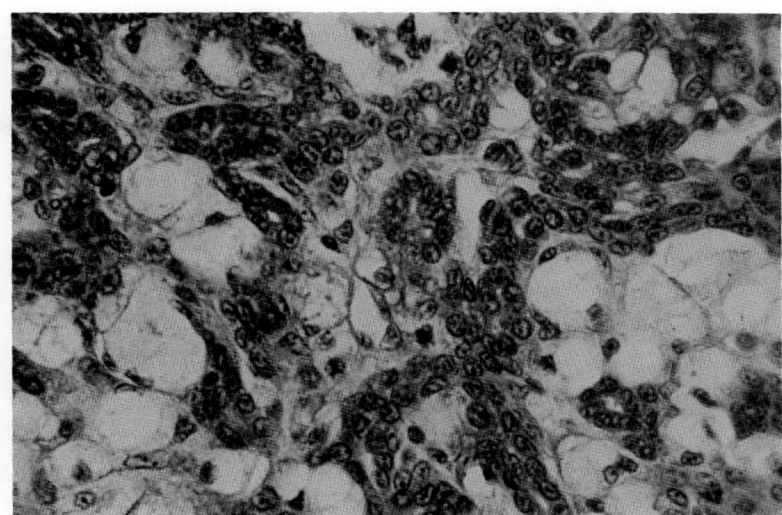

FIG. 11-19 Poisoning due to aflatoxin. Liver of rat, proliferation of bile ducts and vacuoles in hepatocytes. (Courtesy of Dr. Paul M. Newberne.)

known to produce neurotoxins that cause tremors and other neurologic signs in domestic and experimental animals. The term ergotism, as commonly understood, applies only to the disease caused by *C. purpurea; C. paspali* is not associated with gangrene.

References

Cysewski SJ. Paspalum staggers and Tremorgen intoxication in animals. J Am Vet Med Assoc 1973;163:1291–1292.
Perek M. *Claviceps paspali* in pasture as a cause of poisoning in cattle in Israel. Refuah Vet 1955;12:106–110.
Perek M. Ergot and ergot-like fungi as the cause of vesicular dermatitis (sod disease) in chickens. J Am Vet Med Assoc 1958;132:529–533.
Simms BT. Dallis grass poisoning. Auburn Veterinarian, Summer, 1945.

Tatrishvili PS. Pathology of experimental *Claviceps paspali* poisoning in livestock. Trud Vesesoyuz Inst Eksp Vet 1957;20:226–237. Abstr Vet Bull 1958;3383.

Aflatoxins (mycotoxin, aflatoxicosis, groundnut poisoning, toxin of aspergillus spp.)

Aflatoxins are highly toxic and carcinogenic metabolites produced by the fungi *Aspergillus flavus* and *A. parasiticus* when environmental conditions favor their growth on certain cereal grains, nuts, and seeds (Figs. 11-19 to 11-22). At least 17 different aflatoxins exist, all structurally related to coumarins. Those of greatest concern, designated aflatoxins B_1, B_2, G_1, G_2, and M_1, are

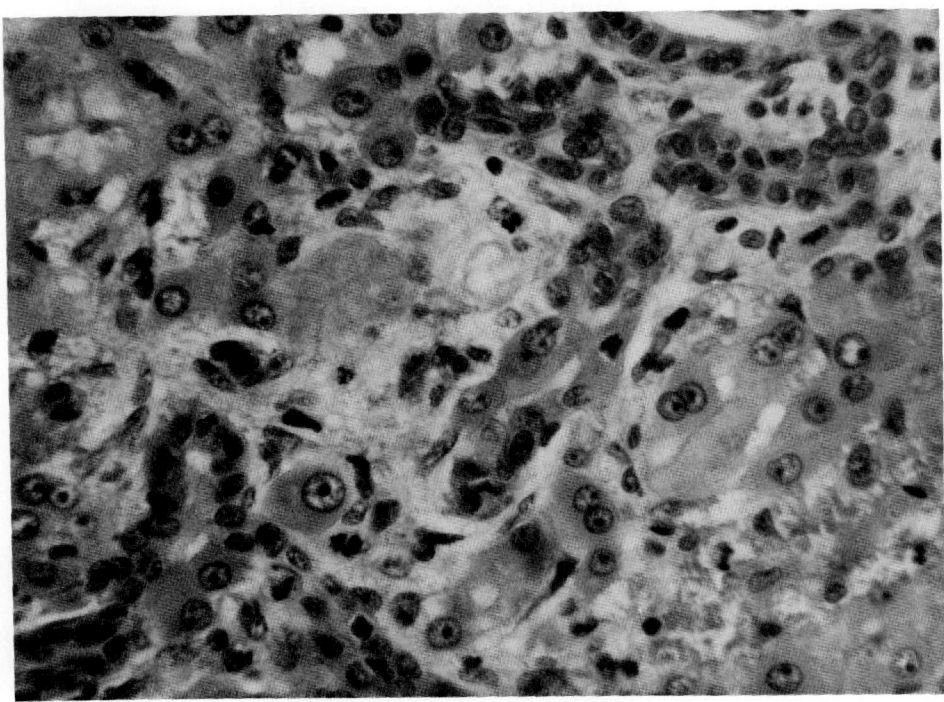

FIG. 11-20 Poisoning due to aflatoxin. Liver of dog. Proliferation of bile ducts, disorganization of hepatocytes. (Courtesy of Dr. Paul M. Newberne.)

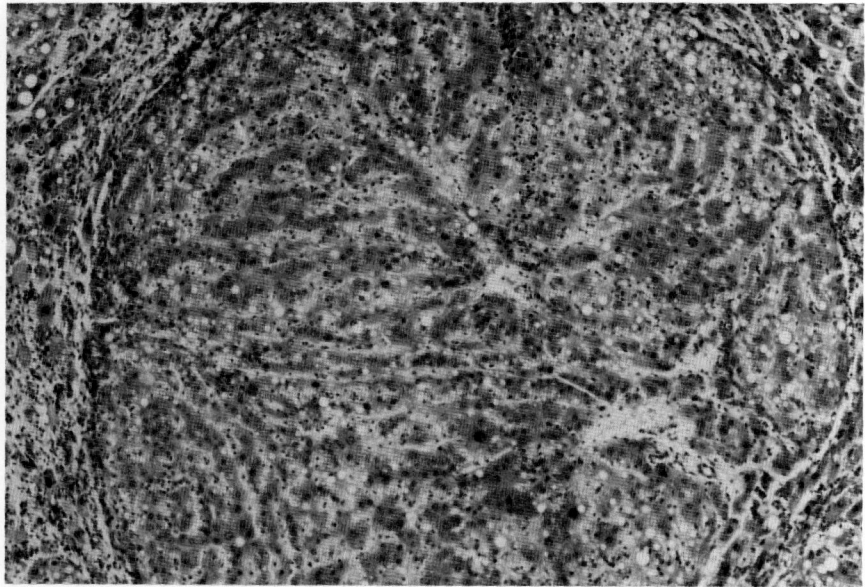

FIG. 11-21 Poisoning by aflatoxin. Hepatoma of rat. (Courtesy of Dr. Paul M. Newberne.)

the most widespread (the designations B and G refer to whether they flouresce blue or green in ultraviolet light). Of these, aflatoxin B_1 is the most prevalent and toxic. Aflatoxin M_1, a mammalian metabolite of B_1, is excreted in milk. In the United States, the most frequently contaminated foods are peanuts, corn, and cottonseed.

The first descriptions of what is now known to be aflatoxicosis appeared in 1952 when Seibold and Bailey described an epizootic toxic hepatitis ("hepatitis X") in dogs that was later demonstrated by Newberne et al. (1955) to be the result of feeding commercial dog foods that contained contaminated peanut meal. It was, however, investigations into a previously unrecognized disease of turkeys ("turkey X disease") in Great Britain

that killed over 100,000 turkeys, which first led to the identification of Brazilian groundnut meal as the common factor in the disorder and to the ultimate chemical isolation of aflatoxins. At about the same time, outbreaks of disease in pigs and calves were traced to Brazilian groundnut meal and the occurrence of hepatomas in hatchery-raised trout in the United States was traced to cottonseed meal contaminated with aflatoxins. A recent report describes an outbreak involving 30 Angora rabbit farms in India.

Based upon observations of natural poisonings and experimental data, it would appear that all animals, as well as fish, are susceptible to the hepatotoxicity of aflatoxins, and probably also to its carcinogenic attribute leading to primary liver cancer. Additionally, good evi-

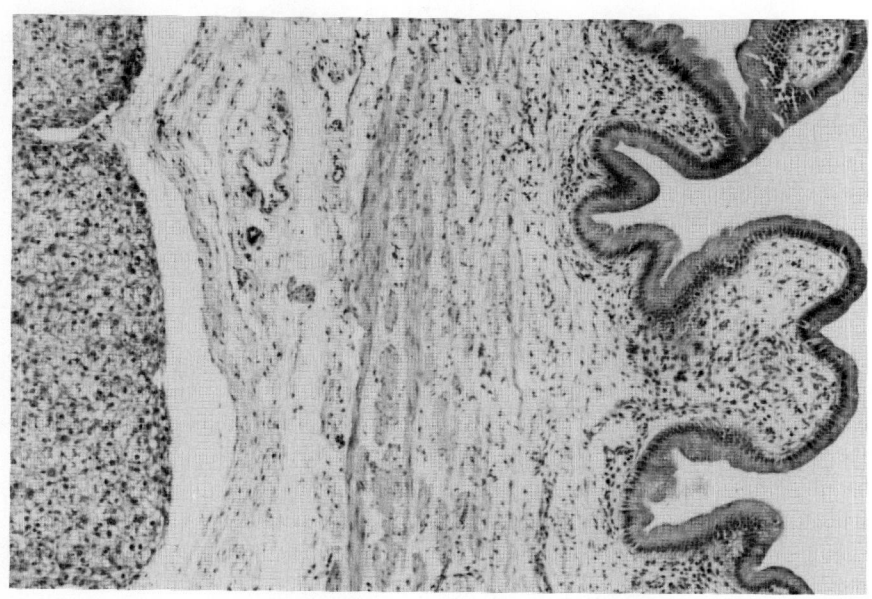

FIG. 11-22 Poisoning due to aflatoxin. Edema of the gallbladder of a dog. (Courtesy of Dr. Paul M. Newberne.)

dence suggests that humans are also susceptible and that serious outbreaks of acute poisoning have occurred in India and Africa. However, no obvious evidence that aflatoxins cause cancer in humans exists.

LESIONS

A variety of factors influence the effects of aflatoxins. Young animals are considerably more susceptible and males are more vulnerable than females. Poor nutritional status increases sensitivity. Considerable species variation also occurs. Young turkeys and ducklings are extremely more susceptible than chickens. Rats are more susceptible than mice, particularly to the carcinogenic effects of aflatoxins. Natural disease has been documented in dogs, pigs, and cattle, but has rarely been described in sheep and goats. Horses are relatively resistant. The dose of aflatoxin and the duration of exposure also influence the effects of its toxicity. Aflatoxins bind to nucleic acids and disrupt polyribosomes, leading to interference with both nucleic acid and protein synthesis. They also result in impaired T cell function.

Acute aflatoxicosis, resulting from ingestion of large quantities of aflatoxins, leads to severe hepatic necrosis within hours. Signs referable to liver damage develop rapidly and include icterus, widespread hemorrhage, and elevation of serum hepatic enzymes. Necrosis is primarily **periportal** in turkeys, ducklings, chickens, adult rats, and cats; **midzonal** in rabbits; and **centrilobular** in pigs, cattle, dogs, and guinea pigs. Diffuse necrosis is seen in neonatal rats and trout. Edema and hemorrhage in the gallbladder wall are consistent findings in pigs and dogs.

Chronic aflatoxicosis, the more usual form of the disease, results from exposure to a lower dosage of aflatoxins over a longer period of time. The effects develop over several days to months, but may be evident pathologically within one week. Signs include decreased growth rate, lowered productivity and, eventually, signs of liver disease. The most striking and consistent lesion in all species is marked proliferation of small bile ductules at the periphery of hepatic lobules, seen within days of exposure. Changes in hepatocytes include fatty change, swelling, and necrosis, although necrosis is not as extensive as in acute exposure. As the lesions progress, proliferation of fibrovascular connective tissue occurs, leading to periportal fibrosis or cirrhosis which dissects the liver. This is accompanied by nodular regeneration of hepatocytes: the occurrence of hepatocytes with marked variation in nuclear size and megalocytic hepatocytes.

The carcinogenic activity of aflatoxin is well established, although the precise conditions under which neoplasia develops are not completely understood. Hepatomas, hepatic cell carcinomas, and cholangiocarcinomas have been produced experimentally by feeding aflatoxin to ducklings, turkeys, rats, guinea pigs, trout, sheep, swine, and monkeys. Additionally in rats, aflatoxins induce carcinoma of the esophagus, glandular stomach, colon, and kidney. Among domestic animals, hepatic cell carcinomas have been observed only in swine poisoned by aflatoxins.

References

Aller WW Jr, Edds GT, Asquith RL. Effects of aflatoxins in young ponies. Am J Vet Res 1981;42:2162–2164.

Baker DC, Green RA. Coagulation defects of aflatoxin intoxicated rabbits. Vet Pathol 1987;24:62–70.

Blount WP. Turkey "X" disease. J Br Turkey Fed 1961;9:52.

Bortell R, Asquith RL, Edds GT, et al. Acute experimentally induced aflatoxicosis in the weanling pony. Am J Vet Res 1983;44:2110–2114.

Butler WH, Barnes JM. Carcinoma of the glandular stomach in rats given diets containing aflatoxin. Nature Lond 1966;209:90.

Carnaghan RBA, Lewis G, Patterson DSP, et al. Biochemical and pathological aspects of groundnut poisoning in chickens. Pathol Vet 1966;3:601–615.

Clark JD, Hatch RC, Miller DM, et al. Caprine aflatoxicosis: experimental disease and clinical pathologic changes. Am J Vet Res 1984;45:1132–1135.

Colvin BM, Harrison LR, Gosser HS, et al. Aflatoxicosis in feeder cattle. J Am Vet Med Assoc 1984;184:956–958.

Coppock RW, et al. Acute aflatoxicosis in feeder pigs, resulting from improper storage of corn. J Am Vet Med Assoc 1989;195:1380–1381.

Cysewski SJ, et al. Clinical pathologic features of acute aflatoxicosis in swine. Am J Vet Res 1968;29:1577–1590.

Davila JC, Edds GT, Osuna O, et al. Modification of the effects of aflatoxin B_1 and warfarin in young pigs given selenium. Am J Vet Res 1983;44:1877–1883.

DeJongh H, et al. Investigation of the factor in groundnut meal responsible for "turkey X disease." Biochem Biophys Acta 1962;65:548–551.

Ellis J, DiPaolo JA. Aflatoxin B_1 induction of malformations. Arch Pathol 1967;83:53–57.

Gagné WE, Dungworth DL, Moulton JE. Pathologic effects of aflatoxin in pigs. Pathol Vet 1968;5:370–384.

Harding JDJ, et al. Experimental groundnut poisoning in pigs. Res Vet Sci 1963;4:217–229.

Krishna L, Dawra RK, Vaid J. An outbreak of aflatoxicosis in Angora rabbits. Vet Hum Toxicol 1991;33:159–161.

Krishnamachari KAVR, Bhat RV, Nagarajan V, et al. Hepatitis due to aflatoxicosis. An outbreak in western India. Lancet 1975;1:1061–1063.

Madhavan TV, Tulpule PG, Gopalan C. Aflatoxin-induced hepatic fibrosis in rhesus monkeys. Pathological features. Arch Pathol 1965;79:466–469.

McGavin MD, Knake R. Hepatic midzonal necrosis in a pig fed aflatoxin and horse fed moldy hay. Vet Pathol 1977;14:182–187.

Miller DM, Crowell WA, Stuart BP. Acute aflatoxicosis in swine: clinical pathology, histopathology, and electron microscopy. Am J Vet Res 1982;43:273–277.

Miller DM, Clark JD, Hatch RC, et al. Caprine aflatoxicosis: serum electrophoresis and pathologic changes. Am J Vet Res 1984;45:1136–1141.

Newberne JW, Bailey WS, Seibold HR. Notes on a recent outbreak and experimental reproduction of hepatitis X in dogs. J Am Vet Med Assoc 1955;127:59–62.

Newberne PM, Carlton WW, Wogan GN. Hepatomas in rats and hepatorenal injury in ducklings fed peanut meal or *Aspergillus flavus* extract. Pathol Vet 1964;1:105–132.

Newberne PM, et al. Histopathologic lesions in ducklings caused by *Aspergillus flavus* cultures, culture extracts and crystalline aflatoxins. Toxic Appl Pharmacol 1964;6:542–556.

Newberne PM, Russo R, Wogan GN. Acute toxicity of aflatoxin B_1 in the dog. Pathol Vet 1966;3:331–340.

Newberne PM, Harrington DH, Wogan GN. Effects of cirrhosis and other liver insults on induction of liver tumors by aflatoxin in rats. Lab Invest 1966;15:962–969.

Newberne PM, Wogan GN. Sequential morphologic changes in aflatoxin B_1 carcinogenesis in the rat. Cancer Res 1968;28:770–781.

Newberne PM, Butler WH. Acute and chronic effects of aflatoxin on the liver of domestic and laboratory animals: a review. Cancer Res 1969;29:236–250.

Ray AC, et al. Bovine abortion and death associated with consumption of aflatoxin-contaminated peanuts. J Am Vet Med Assoc 1986;188:1187–1188.

Seibold HR, Bailey WS. Art epizootic of hepatitis in the dog. J Am Vet Med Assoc 1952;121:201–206.

Shotwell OL. Aflatoxins. Clin Microbiol Newslett 1983;5:101–103.

Sisk DB, Carlton WW, Curtin TM. Experimental aflatoxicosis in young swine. Am J Vet Res 1968;29:1591–1602.

Svoboda D, Grady HJ, Higginson J. Aflatoxin B_1 injury in rat and monkey liver. Am J Pathol 1966;49:1023–1051.

Lupinosis (phomopsis)

Lupinosis or European lupinosis was recognized as distinct from other forms of lupine poisoning in the nineteenth century. Early workers suggested that the plant poisoning (see Chapter on Poisons) characterized by neurologic signs was due to a specific alkaloid, but that lupinosis was the result of a hepatotoxic factor possibly related to a fungus. Despite these early observations, confusion between the two syndromes continued until well into the twentieth century. It is now recognized that lupinosis is caused by a mycotoxin (phomopsin) produced by the fungus *Phomopsis leptostromiformis* which may grow on sweet and bitter lupines. Lupinosis occurs in Europe, New Zealand, Australia, and South Africa.

Field outbreaks of lupinosis are restricted mainly to sheep, caused by greater use of lupines as a forage crop for sheep; however, the disease is reported in cattle, horses, and pigs. Experimentally, goats, dogs, rabbits, and mice are susceptible. Clinically, anorexia, icterus, and death occur within a few days to two weeks after exposure. Serum glutamic oxaloacetic transaminase, lactic dehydrogenase, alkaline phosphatase, and bilirubin are elevated in serum. Pathologically, pronounced icterus is manifest, and the liver is enlarged, yellow, and friable. Photosensitization may accompany lupinosis.

LESIONS

Hepatic lesions are initially characterized by focal necrosis, principally in the central and midzonal regions. The lesions progress to scarring, characterized by interlinking radiating bands of connective tissue connecting central and periportal regions, resulting in distortion of the normal lobular pattern. Hyperplasia of bile ductules and Kupffer cells occurs. Myopathy resembling white muscle disease has also been described in lupinosis.

References

Allen JG. The emergence of a lupinosis-associated myopathy in sheep in Western Australia. Aust Vet J 1978;54:548–549. [Vet Bull 1979; 49:3259.]

Allen JG. An evaluation of lupinosis in cattle in Western Australia. Aust Vet J 1981;57:212–215. [Vet Bull 1982;52:181.]

Gardiner MR. Lupinosis — an iron storage disease of sheep. Aust Vet J 1961;37:135–140.

Gardiner MR. Recent advances in lupinosis research — a progress report. J Dep Agric West Aust 1964;5:890–897.

Gardiner MR. The pathology of lupinosis of sheep, gross and histopathology. Pathol Vet 1965;2:417–445.

Gardiner MR. Fungus-induced toxicity in lupinosis. Br Vet J 1966;122: 508–516.

Gardiner MR. Lupinosis. Adv Vet Sci 1967;11:85–138.

Gardiner MR, Parr WH. Pathogenesis of acute lupinosis in sheep. J Comp Pathol 1967;77:51–62.

Gardiner MR, Petterson DS. Pathogenesis of mouse lupinosis induced by a fungus *(Cytospora spp.)* growing on dead lupins. J Comp Pathol 1972;82:5–13.

Jago MV, Peterson JE, Payne AL, et al. Lupinosis: response of sheep to different doses of phomopsin. Aust J Exp Biol Med Sci 1982;60:239–251. [Vet Bull 1982;52:7748.]

Papadimitriou JM, Bradshaw RD, Petterson DS, et al. Histological, histochemical and biochemical study of the effect of the toxin of lupinosis on murine liver. J Pathol 1974;112:45–53.

Papadimitriou JM, Walter MN-I, Petterson DS, et al. Hepatic ultrastructural changes in murine lupinosis. J Pathol 1973;111: 221–228.

Facial eczema (sporidesmin)

Facial eczema is one of the earlied-recognized diseases caused by a mycotoxin; it was first described in sheep in New Zealand. Cattle are also affected; it is also recognized in Australia and South Africa, and is suspected to occur in the United States. It results from the mycotoxin, sporidesmin produced by the fungus *Pithomyces chartarum*, which is a saprophyte on certain pastures. It is most often associated with ryegrass, and the disease is most frequent in the fall.

LESIONS

The toxin is principally a hepatotoxin, and the outstanding lesion from which the disease gets its name is the result of hepatotoxic photosensitization due to circulating phylloerythrin. In sheep, the face and ears are the most severely affected sites, whereas in cattle, the udder and teats are affected. Cholangiohepatitis—characterized by necrosis of biliary epithelium, fibrosis, and ductular hyperplasia—as the outstanding hepatic lesion. Focal hepatic necrosis and regenerative hyperplasia may be seen. Extrahepatic bile ducts are enlarged and edematous, as is the wall of the gallbladder. Hemorrhage in the wall of the gallbladder and urinary bladder are common.

A phototoxic syndrome, characterized by ophthalmitis and dermatitis, has been produced in mice by Budiarso et al. (1972) and McCracken et al. (1974), with *Penicillium viridicatum,* the mold associated with nephrosis in swine.

References

Budiarso IT, Carlton WW, Tuite JF. Phototoxic syndrome induced in mice by rice cultures of *Penicillium viridicatum* and exposure to sunlight. Pathol Vet 1970;7:531–546.

Dodd DC. The pathology of facial eczema. Symposium on Facial Eczema Research. Proc. New Zealand Soc. Anim. Prod., 19th Annual Conf., 1959;48–52.

McCracken MD, Carlton WW, Tuite J. *Penicillium viridicatum* mycotoxicosis in the rat: I. Ocular lesions. II. Scrotal lesions. III. Hepatic and gastric lesions. Food Cosmet Toxicol 1974;12:70–88, 89–98, 99–105.

Mortimer PH, Taylor A. The experimental intoxication of sheep with sporidesmin, a metabolic product of *Pithomyces chartarum.* I. Clinical observations and findings at postmortem examination. Res Vet Sci 1962;3:147–171.

Richard JL. Mycotoxin photosensitivity. J Am Vet Med Assoc 1973;163:1298–1300.

Synge RLM, White EP. Sporodesmin: a substance from *Sporodesmium bakeri* causing lesions characteristic of facial eczema. Chem Indust 1959;49:1546–1547.

Ochratoxicosis (mold nephropathy of swine, citrinin toxicity)

In 1928, Larson reported a peculiar nephropathy of swine in Denmark and associated it with ingesting moldy grains; however, it was not until several decades later that the offending mycotoxin(s) was identified. Several nephrotic mycotoxins, which are isocoumarin derivatives of phenylalanine, have been identified that are produced by species of *Penicillium* and *Aspergillus,* especially *P. viridicatum* and *A. ochraceus.* **Ochratoxin A** is believed to be the mycotoxin of principal importance in natural poisonings that have been reported in swine and poultry. Horses are suspected to suffer the same mycotoxicosis. Dogs are especially susceptible to ochratoxin A experimentally, but natural poisoning has not been described. The fungi can grow on a variety of animal feeds including corn, oats, wheat, and barley. The same fungi also produce another nephrotoxin, **citrinin,** which produces an essentially identical syndrome in swine and birds. Citrinin is a quinone methide that is believed to contribute to porcine and avian nephropathy in conjunction with ochratoxin, but does not represent a primary cause (Fig. 11-23).

The outstanding clinical signs of value are polydipsia, polyuria, and dehydration. Increased urinary excretion of leucine aminopeptides, glucose, and protein occurs; serum creatine and urea nitrogen are elevated. Growth rate is significantly retarded.

LESIONS

Pathologically, lesions are restricted to the kidney. Grossly, the kidneys are enlarged, gray-yellow, and firmer than normal. Ochratoxin in swine is specifically toxic to the proximal convoluted tubule (Fig. 11-24). Microscopi-cally, the epithelial cells lose their brush border and become shorter than usual, with enlarged vesicular nuclei. Later, pyknosis and necrosis of the cells occur, which may slough to the lumen. The tubular basement membranes become greatly thickened. Secondarily, peritubular fibrosis is manifest, which becomes progressively more extensive until most of the kidney, including the glomeruli, are sclerotic. These lesions have been reproduced in swine experimentally poisoned. The report of Szczech et al. also described necrotizing gastroenteritis as a feature of experimental ochratoxicosis in swine, similar to that seen in other species experimentally exposed (1973).

Experimentally, ochratoxin is also nephrotoxic in dogs, rats, chicks, and trout. The effect is principally on the proximal convoluted tubule, but degeneration of the distal tubule has also been described. In contrast to swine, lesions develop in other tissues in these species, including fatty change and focal necrosis of the liver; focal erosive and ulcerative enteritis and colitis; and proctitis and necrosis of lymphoid tissues. Carlton et al. experimentally induced a disease characterized by marked perirenal edema and renal necrosis by feeding swine a strain of *P. viridicatum* that did not produce citrinin or ochratoxin (1973). The significance of this finding was not understood.

Ochratoxin is suspected to be a cause of abortion in cattle fed moldy hay. Fetal death and resorption have been produced in rats. Ochratoxin is also suspected to cause fatal chronic nephropathy in humans in the Balkans (Krogh et al., 1977).

References

Albassam MA, Yong SI, Bhatnagar R, et al. Histopathologic and electron microscopic studies on the acute toxicity of ochratoxin A in rats. Vet Pathol 1987;24:427–435.

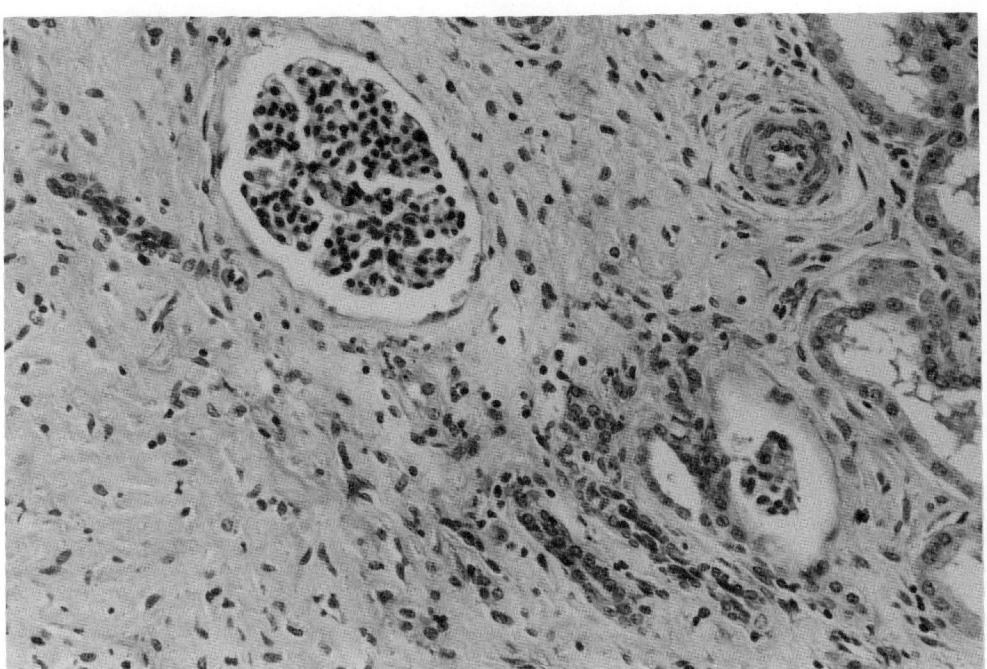

FIG. 11-23 Mycotoxic porcine nephropathy due to ochratoxin. Extensive cortical fibrosis represents the advanced stage of the disease. (Courtesy of Dr. P. Krogh.)

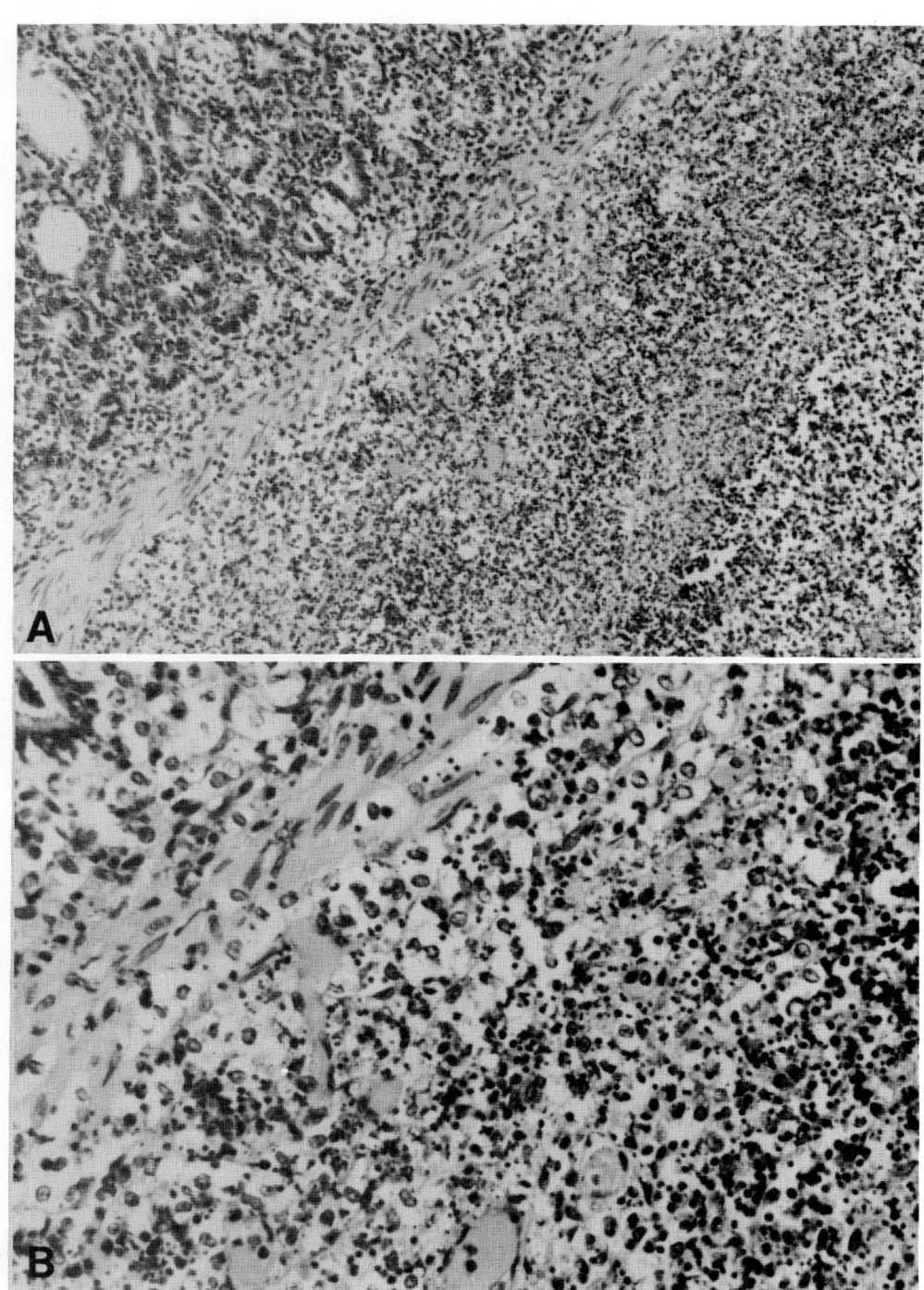

FIG. 11-24 Experimental ochratoxin A poisoning. **A.** Necrosis of submucosal lymphoid tissue in colon of a beagle dog. **B.** High magnification of submucosal lymphoid necrosis. (Courtesy of Drs. W.W. Carlton and G.M. Szczech.)

Applegate KL, Chipley JR. Ochratoxins. Adv Appl Microbiol 1973;16: 97–109.

Buckley HG. Fungal nephrotoxicity in swine. Irish Vet J 1971;25: 194–196.

Carlton WW, Tuite J. Nephropathy and edema syndrome induced in miniature swine by corn cultures of *Penicillium viridicatum.* Pathol Vet 1970;7:68–80.

Carlton WW, Tuite J, Caldwell R. *Penicillium viridicatum* toxins and mold nephrosis. J Am Vet Med Assoc 1973;163:1295–1297.

Cook WO, Osweiler GD, Anderson TD, et al. Ochratoxicosis in Iowa swine. J Am Vet Med Assoc 1986;188:1399–1402.

Elling F. Ochratoxin A-induced mycotoxic porcine nephropathy: alterations in enzyme activity in tubular cells. Acta Pathol Microbiol Scand 1979;87A:237–243. [Vet Bull 1980;50:152.]

Friis P, Hasselager E, Krogh P. Isolation of citrinin and oxalic acid from *Penicillium viridicatum* West and their nephrotoxicity in rats and pigs. Acta Pathol Microbiol Scand 1969;77:559–560.

Hanika C, Carlton WW, Hinsman EJ, et al. Citrinin mycotoxicosis in the rabbit: ultrastructural alterations. Vet Pathol 1986;23:245–253.

Harvey RB, Huff WE, Kubena LF, et al. Evaluation of diets cocontaminated with aflatoxin and ochratoxin fed to growing pigs. Am J Vet Res 1989;50:1400–1405.

Kitchen DN, Carlton WW, Hinsman EJ. Ochratoxin A and citrinin induced nephrosis in beagle dogs. III. Terminal renal ultrastructural alterations. Vet Pathol 1977;14:392–406.

Kitchen DN, Carlton WW, Tuite J. Ochratoxin A and citrinin induced nephrosis in beagle dogs. I. Clinical and clinicopathological features. Vet Pathol 1977;14:154–172.

Krogh P, Hald B, Plestina R, et al. Balkan (endemic) nephropathy and foodborne ochratoxin A: preliminary results of a survey of foodstuffs. Acta Pathol Microbiol Scand B1977;85:238–240.

Krogh P, et al. Experimental porcine nephropathy. Changes of renal function and structure induced by ochratoxin A-contaminated feed. Acta Pathol Microbiol Scand 1974;32(suppl 246):22.

Krogh P, et al. Porcine nephropathy induced by long-term ingestion of ochratoxin A. Vet Pathol 1979;16:466–475.

Larsen S. On chronic degeneration of the kidneys caused by mouldy rye (in Danish). Maanedsskr Dyrl 1928;40:259–284, 289, 300.

Mehdi NAQ, Carlton WW, Boon GD, et al. Studies on the sequential development and pathogenesis of citrinin mycotoxicosis in turkeys and ducklings. Vet Pathol 1984;21:216–223.

Szczech GM, Carlton WW, Hinsman EJ. Ochratoxicosis in Beagle dogs. III. Terminal renal ultrastructural alterations. Vet Pathol 1974;11:385–40.

Szczech GM, Carlton WW, Tuife J. Ochratoxicosis in beagle dogs. I. Clinical and clinicopathological features. Vet Pathol 1973;10:135–154.

Szczech GM, Carlton WW, Tuife J. Ochratoxicosis in beagle dogs. II. Pathology. Vet Pathol 1973;10:219–231.

Szczech GM, Carlton WW, Tuite J, et al. Ochratoxin A in swine. Vet Pathol 1973;10:347–364.

Estrogenic mycotoxicosis

Zearalenone, also known as F-2 toxin, is a mycotoxin with estrogenic activity produced by *Fusarium roseum* (*graminearum*) (*Gibberella zea*) and other species of *Fusarium*, which are fungal contaminants of corn, especially in the midwestern United States, but also of worldwide distribution. A disease of sows, recognized over 60 years ago and termed, vulvovaginitis, is now known to result from ingestion of this toxin. The toxicosis simulates estrus, resulting in enlarged vulvae, mammary glands, and nipples, and occasionally prolapse of the vagina. Sows are infertile and may demonstrate nymphomania or pseudopregnancy. The ovaries are atrophic, and the uterus and cervix are grossly enlarged. Ingestion early in pregnancy leads to embryonic death. In young male swine, feminization occurs with testicular atrophy and gynecomastia.

LESIONS

Microscopically, ovarian follicular atresia is manifest, as well as edema and cellular proliferation of all layers of the uterus and ductular proliferation in the mammary glands. Focal squamous metaplasia may be seen in the tubular reproductive organs and mammary ducts. Stillbirths, small litters, and neonatal mortality may also result. Miller et al. also described incoordination of the hindlimbs in pigs born to exposed sows (1973). In males, signs of feminization include testicular atrophy, swelling of the prepuce, and enlargement of the mammary gland.

Zearalenone toxicity is suspected to be responsible for similar occurrences and reduced fertility in cattle. Swine, rats, mice, guinea pigs, rabbits, and poultry are experimentally susceptible.

References

Bristol FM, Djurickovic S. Hyperestrogenism in female swine as the result of feeding mouldy corn. Can Vet J 1971;12:132–135.

Chang K, Kurtz HJ, Mirocha CJ. Effects of the mycotoxin zearalenone on swine reproduction. Am J Vet Res 1979;40:1260–1267.

Kurtz HJ, et al. Histologic changes in the genital tracts of swine fed estrogenic mycotoxin. Am J Vet Res 1969;30:551–556.

Long GG, Diekman MA. Characterization of effects of zearalenone in swine during early pregnancy. Am J Vet Res 1986;47:184–187.

Long GG, Diekman M, Tuite JF, et al. Effect of *Fusarium roseum* corn culture containing zearalenone on early pregnancy in swine. Am J Vet Res 1982;43:1599–1603.

McErlean BA. Vulvovaginitis of swine. Vet Rec 1952;64:539–540.

McNutt SH, Purevin P, Murray C. Vulvovaginitis in swine. J Am Vet Med Assoc 1929;73:484–492.

Miller JK, Hacking A, Harrison J, et al. Stillbirths, neonatal mortality and small litters in pigs associated with the ingestion of *Fusarium* toxin by pregnant sows. Vet Rec 1973;93:555–559.

Pier AC, Richard JL, Cysewski SJ. Implications of mycotoxins in animal disease. J Am Vet Med Assoc 1980;176:719–724.

Roine K, Korpinen EL, Kallela K. Mycotoxicosis as a probable cause of infertility in dairy cows. Nord Vet Med 1971;23:628–633.

TRICHOTHECENES

The trichothecenes are a group of highly toxic mycotoxins produced by several species of *Fusarium* and certain other fungi. These fungi affect grains in the field, but toxin production is accentuated by storage at cool temperatures; therefore, natural poisonings are most frequent in areas with cooler climates. At least two score of distinct trichothecenes have been identified, but only a few have received much attention as causes of naturally occurring disease. For the most part, no highly defined, naturally occurring clinical or pathologic syndromes are associated with specific trichothecenes. This results, in part, from the multiplicity of toxins, the fact that more than one toxin often exists in the same contaminated grain, and the difficulty of identifying incriminating toxins in a clinical setting. Those toxins best studied include **T-2 toxin, DAS** (diacetoxyscirpenol), **vomitoxin** (deoxynivalenol or DON), and **satratoxin. T-2 toxin** and **DAS** are highly toxic, causing necrosis of skin and mucous membranes (mouth, pharynx, esophagus, rumen, stomach) on contact, much like a caustic, and also extensive necrosis of a variety of internal tissues (described as radiomimetic). The consistent lesions in experimental poisonings include rapid necrosis of lymphoid and myeloid tissues and alimentary epithelium. These toxins are potent inhibitors of protein synthesis, which accounts for their cytotoxicity. T-2 toxin has also been shown to interfere with migration of neutrophils and with the phagocytic ability of macrophages. Ingestion of **vomitoxin** leads to anorexia and vomiting, especially in swine, but most species are susceptible to this effect. It apparently acts on central nervous system receptors without inducing morphologic lesions. Rapid recovery follows removal of the toxin from the diet.

Various syndromes have been ascribed to trichothecene toxicity, especially in cattle, swine, horses, and poultry. Clinical manifestations include oral ulceration, anorexia, vomiting, diarrhea, hemorrhage, leukopenia, icterus, depression, and incoordination. The most specific pathologic findings are necrosis of all lymphoid organs, bone marrow, and gastrointestinal epithelium. Necrosis in the liver, kidney, heart, and pancreas have also been described. In cattle, a condition recognized for years and referred to as **"mouldy corn poisoning"** is believed to result from T-2 toxin. This disorder is predominantly characterized by extensive hemorrhage, a feature not experimentally reproduced with T-2 toxin. Hemorrhage is, however, an expected result of thrombocytopenia due to the radiomimetic effects of this toxin and is a feature of stachybotryotoxicosis. Kikuyu is a condition of cattle and sheep in New Zealand resembling trichothecene toxicity with ulcerative rumenitis, reticulitis, and omasitis. It is associated with the fungi *Myrothecium verrucaria* and *M. roridum.* A condition in humans called alimentary toxic aleukia (ATA), which occurred as a serious outbreak in the Soviet Union, was believed to be due to T-2 toxin, and in Japan and Korea conditions called alkali toxicosis and scabby grain toxicosis have been suspected to result from trichothecenes.

Stachybotryotoxicosis, a disease first described in 1931, results from ingestion of a trichothecene known as **satratoxin** (stachybotryotoxin) produced by *Stachybotrys atra, S. alterans,* and possibly other fungi. It has occurred in horses, cattle, sheep, swine, poultry, and humans in the USSR, Hungary, Czechoslovakia, Romania, Finland, France, and South Africa following consumption of moldy straw or hay. The disease and lesions are comparable to those of T-2 toxin with ulceration of the oral mucous membranes, leukopenia, thrombocytopenia, widespread hemorrhage, and necrosis of the gastrointestinal mucosa. Signs of central nervous dysfunction may be evident.

References

Ciegler A. Trichothecenes: occurrence and toxicoses. J Food Protect 1978;41:399–403.
Corrier DE, Holt PS, Mollenhauer HH. Regulation of murine macrophage phagocytosis of sheep erythrocytes by T-2 toxin. Am J Vet Res 1987;48:1304–1307.
Côté LM, et al. Survey of vomitoxin-contaminated feed grains in midwestern United States, and associated health problems in swine. J Am Vet Med Assoc 1984;184:189–192.
Harvey RB, et al. Effects of treatment of growing swine with aflatoxin and T-2 toxin. Am J Vet Res 1990;51:1688–1693.
Hoerr FJ, Carlton WW, Yagen B. Mycotoxicosis caused by a single dose of T-2 toxin or diacetoxyscirpenol in broiler chickens. Vet Pathol 1981;18:652–664.
Hsu I-C, Smalley EB, Strong FM, et al. Identification of T-2 toxin in moldy corn associated with a lethal toxicosis in dairy cattle. Appl Microbiol 1972;24:684–690.
Lillehoj EB. Feed sources and conditions conducive to production of aflatoxin, ochratoxin, *Fusarium* toxins, and zearalenone. J Am Vet Med Assoc 1973;163:1281–1284.
Martinovich D, Smith B. Kikuyu poisoning of cattle. 1. Clinical and pathological findings. NZ Vet J 1973;21:55–63.
Martinovich D, Mortimer PH, di Menna ME. Similarities between so-called kikuyu poisoning of cattle and two experimental mycotoxicoses. NZ Vet J 1972;20:57–58.
Niyo KA, Richard JL, Niyo Y, et al. Pathologic, hematologic, and serologic changes in rabbits given T-2 mycotoxin orally and exposed to aerosols of *Aspergillus fumigatus* conidia. Am J Vet Res 1988;49:2151–2160.
Pang VF, Adams JH, Beasley VR, et al. Myocardial and pancreatic lesions induced by T-2 toxin, a trichothecene mycotoxin, in swine. Vet Pathol 1986;23:310–319.
Schneider DJ, Marasas WFO, Kuys JCD, et al. A field outbreak of suspected stachybotryotoxicosis in sheep. J S Afr Vet Assoc 1979;50:73–81.
Smalley EB. T-2 toxin. J Am Vet Med Assoc 1973;163:1278–1281.
Smith B, Martinovich D. Kikuyu poisoning of cattle. 2. Epizootiological aspects. NZ Vet J 1973;21:85–89.
Thurman JD, Creasia DA, Quance JL, et al. Adrenal cortical necrosis caused by T-2 mycotoxicosis in female, but not male, mice. Am J Vet Res 1986;47:1122–1124.
Thurman JD, Creasia DA, Trotter RW. Mycotoxicosis caused by aerosolized T-2 toxin administered to female mice. Am J Vet Res 1988;49:1928–1931.

Equine leukoencephalomalacia—moldy corn poisoning

As evident from Table 11-3, many different mycotoxin-producing molds may contaminate corn. Therefore, the term "moldy corn poisoning" may encompass a number of different syndromes; it is often used, however, to designate a specific disorder of horses and donkeys, which should more appropriately called **equine leukoencephalomalacia.** The syndrome has been associated with the feeding of moldy corn in the United States and other parts of the world since the nineteenth century. The experimental work of Schwarte et al. clearly established the causative status of moldy corn (1937). The syndrome has been experimentally reproduced by feeding cultures of *Fusarium moniliforme* to horses.

Affected horses are drowsy, tend to circle and stagger, and develop paralysis. The lesions, which are often grossly visible, consist of softening and liquefactive necrosis, chiefly of the white matter of the cerebrum. Edema and congestion occur, but with little cellular inflammatory reaction.

References

Lapcevic E, Pribicevic S, Kozic L. Poisoning in horses with the wheat rust fungus, *Puccinia graminis.* Vet Glasn 1953;7:268–271.
Schwarte LH, Biester HE, Murray C. A disease of horses caused by feeding moldy corn. J Am Vet Med Assoc 1937;90:76–85.
Wilson BJ, Maronpot RR. Causative fungus agent of leucoencephalomalacia in equine animals. Vet Rec 1971;88:484–486.

OTHER MYCOTOXINS

Rubratoxins, produced by *Penicillium rubrum* and *P. purpurogenum* and possibly species of *Aspergillus,* have been associated with moldy corn. Two have been identified: rubratoxin A and the more toxic rubratoxin B. These mycotoxins are absorbed slowly from the gastrointestinal tract and, therefore, are not highly toxic. They have, however, been suspected of poisoning swine and cattle. Their toxicity is also accentuated when fed in conjunction with other mycotoxins. They have been shown to cause necrosis of the liver, kidneys, and lymph organs, with clinical signs of icterus and hemorrhage.

Patulin is a mycotoxin produced by several different fungi, including species of *Aspergillus, Penicillium,* and

Byssochlamys, that has been suspected, but not proved, in natural poisonings of cattle and sheep. In foodstuffs, rotten apples seem to be a principal source of the toxin. Experimentally, toxicity is described as leading to extensive edema, congestion, and hemorrhage.

Cyclopiazonic acid is a toxin produced by *Penicillium cyclopium* as well as other species of *Penicillium* and *Aspergillus.* Its importance in natural poisonings is not known, but it is a frequent contaminant of stored corn and other grains. It is known to be toxic to swine, dogs, and laboratory animals, causing necrosis of the gastrointestinal tract, liver, kidney, pancreas, myocardium, skeletal muscle, and lymphoid organs.

References

Hayes AW, Neville JA, Hollingsworth EB. Acute toxicity of rubratoxin B in dogs. Toxicol Appl Pharmacol 1973;25:606–616.

Lomax LG, Cole RJ, Dorner JW. The toxicity of cyclopiazonic acid in weaned pigs. Vet Pathol 1984;21:418–424.

Nuehring LP, Rowland GN, Harrison LR, et al. Cyclopiazonic acid mycotoxicosis in the dog. Am J Vet Res 1985;46:1670–1676.

Purchase IFH. The acute toxicity of the mycotoxin cyclopiazonic acid to rats. Toxicol Appl Pharmacol 1971;18:114–123.

Richmond ML, Gray JI, Stine CM. The rubratoxins: causative agents in food/feedborne disease. J Food Protect 1980;43:579–586.

Wilson BJ, Harbison RD. Rubratoxins. J Am Vet Med Assoc 1973;163:1274–1276.

Wogan GN, Edwards GS, Newberne PM. Acute and chronic toxicity of rubratoxin B. Toxicol Pharmacol 1971;19:712–720.

12

Diseases due to protozoa

The subkingdom or phylum Protozoa (Kingdom Protista) is comprised of a diverse group of single-celled eukaryotic animals, the vast majority of which (as with most of the organisms discussed in previous chapters) are free-living and not pathogenic to either animals or humans. However, a number of important diseases are caused by protozoan parasites. As a disparate group of organisms, several different and complicated schemes of classification exist. A classification based upon *An Illustrated Guide to the Protozoa* (Lee et al., 1985), including only the pathogenic species, is presented in Table 12-1.

Mastigophora (a subphylum of the phylum Sarcomastigophora)includes those protozoa whose trophozoites have one or more flagella. These may occur as extracellular parasites as exemplified by *Giardia* in the digestive tract, *Trichomonas* in the digestive tract or tubular reproductive tract, or *Trypanosoma* spp. in the vascular system; or as intracellular parasites such as *Leishmania* and *Histomonas* (a parasite of turkeys). Their life cycles, which allow their transmission from host to host, may include: direct transmission with no extra-host stage; direct transmission with a resistant cyst stage outside their mammalian hosts *(Giardia);* indirect transmission with a parasitic stage in some bug or insect, which serves as an intermediate host *(Leishmania, Trypanosoma);* or, in the case of *Histomonas*, the trophozoites enter and reside in eggs of the roundworm *Heterakis gallinae*.

Sarcodina (a subphylum of the phylum Sarcomastigophora) includes those protozoa which utilize pseudopodia for locomotion. The parasitic species are extracellular parasites of the intestinal lumen which are capable of invading the intestinal wall and disseminating to other organs. Included are *Entamoeba, Acanthamoeba, Endolimax,* and *Iodamoeba.* Their life cycles are direct with a cyst stage outside of their hosts.

Apicomplexa (a phylum; formerly Sporozoa) includes several different families containing some of the most important pathogenic protozoa. These lack obvious means of locomotion (e.g., cilia, flagella or pseudopodia). Their life cycles may be: direct with an encysted extra-host form, as in the case of *Eimeria, Isospora, Klos-* *siella,* and *Cryptosporidium;* or indirect, with an intermediate host, as in the case of *Sarcocystis, Toxoplasma, Babesia, Plasmodium, Hepatocystis, Besnoitia, Neospora, Frenkelia,* and *Hammondia.* With a number of these parasites, it is the intermediate stage in various mammalian tissues that is of primary interest (although mammals also serve as the definitive hosts with sexual reproduction in intestinal epithelial cells). These include members of the family Sarcocystidae: *Sarcocystis, Toxoplasma, Frenkelia, Besnoitia, Neospora* and *Hammondia. Babesia, Plasmodium, Hepatocystis,* and *Theileria* which are all intracellular parasites.

Microspora (a phylum) contains a single parasite of significance, *Encephalitozoon cuniculi,* which is transmitted directly via spores in the urine and may also be transmitted *in utero.*

Ciliophora are dikaryotic protozoa with cilia, cirri or other compound ciliary structures for locomotion. The macronucleus is primarily concerned with cell metabolism and the micronucleus with genetics. Most are free-living or commensals. *Balantidium coli,* the only pathogen of concern, is transmitted directly via cysts.

In this chapter, the effects of protozoa upon various animal hosts are described and the life cycles of some of the parasitic protozoa are outlined, with emphasis on those features that influence pathogenesis. In some instances, the effects upon the host have been rather clearly demonstrated and the tissue changes are well known; in others, practically nothing is known. The poorly understood protozoan diseases of animals, therefore, present many challenges to the research-minded veterinary pathologist.

Many excellent photomicrographs in color and line drawings of life cycles can be found in *An Atlas of Protozoan Parasites in Animal Tissues* (Gardiner et al., 1988).

References

Gardiner CH, Fayer R, Dubey JP. An atlas of protozoan parasites in animal tissues. USDA, Agric. Res. Svc., Agric. Handbook No. 651. Washington, DC, 1988.

Kudo RR. Protozoology, 5th ed. Springfield: Charles C Thomas, 1966.

Lee JJ, Hutner SH, Bovec EC. An illustrated guide to the protozoa. Lawrence: Soc. Protozool., 1985.

TABLE 12-1 **Classification of Pathogenic Protozoa**

Subkingdom Protozoa
  Phylum Sarcomastigophora
    Subphylum Mastigophora
      Class Zoomastigophorae
        Order Kinetoplastida
          Family Trypanosomatidae
            Genus *Leishmania*
                  Trypanosoma
        Order Diplomonadida
          Family Hexamitidae
            Genus *Hexamita*
                  Giardia
        Order Trichomonadida
          Family Trichomonadidae
            Genus *Tritrichomonas*
                  Trichomonas
          Family Monocercomonadidae
            Genus *Histomonas*
    Subphylum Sarcodina
      Class Lobosea
        Order Amoebida
          Family Vahlkampfiidae
            Genus *Naegleria*
          Family Acanthamoebidae
            Genus *Acanthamoeba*
          Family Hartmannellidae
            Genus *Hartmannella*
          Family Entamoebidae
            Genus *Entamoeba*
                  Endolimax
                  Iodamoeba
  Phylum Apicomplexa
    Class Sporozoasida
      Order Eucoccidiorida
        Family Klossiellidae
          Genus *Klossiella*
        Family Haemogregarinidae
          Genus *Haemogregarina*
                Hepatozoon
        Family Eimeriidae
          Genus *Eimeria*
                Isospora
                Caryospora
        Family Cryptosporidiidae
          Genus *Cryptosporidium*
        Family Sarcocystidae
          Genus *Toxoplasma*
                Cystoisospora
                Besnoitia
                Hammondia
                Sarcocystis
                Frenkelia
                Neospora
        Family Calyptosporidae
          Genus *Calyptospora*
        Family Plasmodiidae
          Genus *Haemoproteus*
                Leucocytozoon
                Hepatocystis
                Plasmodium
        Family Babesiidae
          Genus *Babesia*
        Family Theileriidae
          Genus *Theileria*
                Cytauxzoon

TABLE 12-1 (continued)

    Phylum Microspora
      Class Microsporididae
        Order Pleistophoridida
          Family Pleistophoridae
            Genus *Encephalitozoon*
    Phylum Ciliophora
      Subphylum Rhabdophora
        Class Litostomatea
          Order Haptorida
            Family Balantidiidae
              Genus *Balantidium*
Unknown Classification
            Genus *Pneumocystis*

Levine ND. Protozoan parasites of domestic animals and man. Minneapolis: Burgess Pub. Co., 1961.

Levine ND, et al. A newly revised classification of the protozoa. The Committee on Systematics and Evolution of the Society of Protozoologists. J Protozool, 1980;27:37–58.

Soulsby EJL. Helminths, arthropods and protozoa of domesticated animals (Monnig), 6th ed. Philadelphia: Lea & Febiger, 1968.

Weinman D, Ristic M. Infectious blood diseases of man and animals: diseases caused by protista. Vol. II. The Pathogens, the Infections and the Consequences. Vol. 2. New York: Academic Press, 1968.

COCCIDIOSIS

Coccidiosis is the name applied to the disease produced by protozoa of genera of the order Eucoccidiorida.

Clinically, "*coccidiosis*" is applied to the diseases produced by the genera *Eimeria* and *Isospora,* in the family Eimeriidae, order Eucoccidiorida. The order Eucoccidiorida, however, includes many additional parasitic organisms referred to as coccidia, but the diseases associated with these are generally named after the appropriate genera, (e.g., toxoplasmosis, sarcosporidiosis). Most of the protozoa within the latter group were once thought to have only a tissue phase to their life cycles; however, it is now recognized that these also have an enteric cycle. Thus, the enteric phases of *Toxoplasma, Sarcosporidia, Besnoitia,* and other organisms would also be included under the disease classification of coccidiosis. Many coccidia affect animals and birds; the species and the tissues attacked depend upon the **obligate** preferences of each parasite. Coccidiosis is especially common in cattle, sheep, and poultry, and represents a disease of major economic importance. A few of the important coccidial parasites of animals are listed in Table 12-2.

Life Cycle

The life cycles of coccidia are similar and must be understood in order to visualize their effects upon the host. The oocysts are thick-walled, usually ovoid forms of the organism which resist drying and provide the means of transfer of infection from one host to an-

TABLE 12-2 *Eimeria* and *Isospora* of Animals

Cattle	Eimeria bovis E. quernii E. alabamensis E. auburnensis E. ellipsoidalis	Small intestine, cecum, colon
Sheep	Eimeria ovinoidalis E. ahsatta E. ovina E. parva	Intestine
Goats	Eimeria ninakohlyakimovae E. arloingi	Intestine
Swine	Eimeria debliecki E. porci E. scabra E. neodebliecki Isospora suis	Intestine
Dogs	Isospora canis I. ohioensis I. burrowsi I. neorivolta	Intestine
Cats	Isospora rivolta I. felis	Intestine
Rabbits	Eimeria stiedae E. perforans	Bile ducts Intestine
Mink	Eimeria heipei	Bile ducts
Man	Isospora belli (I. hominis) I. natalensis	Intestine
Nonhuman primates	Isospora spp.	Intestine

other. The oocysts of each species are distinctive morphologically, but have essentially similar features. Within the genus *Eimeria,* each fully-matured oocyst contains four sporocysts, each sporocyst bearing two sporozoites, with a total of eight sporozoites to each oocyst. Oocysts of *Isospora* contain two sporocysts, each with four sporozoites; thus the total number of sporozoites is also eight. *Isospora* oocysts are identical in appearance to those produced by the sexual, intestinal phase of *Toxoplasma, Sarcocystis, Besnoitia, Frenkelia,* and *Hammondia.* Each oocyst has at one pole a tiny pore, the **micropyle,** which is sealed by a substance which, like the rest of the wall, is resistant to drying as well as to many chemical substances. When oocysts are ingested and reach the small intestine, the trypsin-kinase of the pancreatic juice digests the seal of the micropyle, and through this opening the tiny sporozoites, now vigorously motile, escape from the oocyst.

Intestinal infection is believed to take place by direct invasion of the intestinal epithelium. Each sporozoite enters a single epithelial cell, where it undergoes asexual development known as **schizogony.** The sporozoite gradually increases in size and complexity, becoming first a trophozoite and finally a schizont, which liter-

ally fills the cytoplasm of the host cell, displacing the nucleus to one pole. Each mature schizont contains many elongated spores, similar morphologically to sporozoites, but known as **merozoites.** The schizont ruptures its own and the host's cell wall, liberating the merozoites, which infect other epithelial cells and continue this asexual life cycle.

At a certain stage, some of the merozoites enter into the sexual phase of the life cycle, known as **gametogenesis.** Each of these predestined merozoites develops within an individual host epithelial cell, into a female form, a macrogamete, or into its male counterpart, a microgametocyte. The microgametocyte eventually ruptures to release a large number of tiny motile microgametes. One of the microgametes unites with a single macrogamete, which, once thus fertilized, soon becomes an oocyst. Further development within the oocyst, known as **sporogony,** requires oxygen and certain other conditions which are met outside the body of the host. When the oocysts are taken in with food or water by a new host, the life cycle is repeated.

This cycle, which is usually enteric, is depicted in Figure 12-1; it is consistent for all species of *Eimeria* and for most of the common Isospora. The cycle of certain *Eimeria* spp. occurs in tissues other than the intestine. For example, in rabbits, *Eimeria stiedae* replicates in intrahepatic bile ducts, with the sporozoites reaching these ducts via portal veins or lymphatics and not by way of the common bile duct. Hepatic coccidiosis is a very common disease of rabbits. *E. hiepi* causes a similar intrahepatic coccidiosis in mink, and intrahepatic biliary coccidiosis with cholangiohepatitis has been reported in a dog (probably *Isospora*) and a calf. *Eimeria* spp. have also been found in the gallbladder and mesenteric lymph nodes of goats and sheep.

The life cycle is also consistent for most *Isospora* spp.; however, some spp. may utilize an intermediate or transport host. These are referred to as *Cystoisospora* and are included in the family Sarcocystidae. The intermediate host ingests the oocyst and the released sporozoites enter internal organs where they remain as a small cyst containing a single sporozoite (cystozoite). Upon ingestion by the definitive host, the released sporozoite enters intestinal epithelium to repeat the cycle as described. This scheme is depicted in panel 3 of Figure 12-3.

The other members of the order Eucoccidiorida, family Sarcocystidae also have an enteric asexual and sexual cycle in their definitive hosts that is nearly identical to the coccidia, and their oocysts are nearly identical to those of *Isospora.* These, however, also have an asexual tissue phase in an intermediate host (which can be the same as the definitive host) and are termed the tissue cyst-forming coccidia (i.e., Sarcocystidae). It is the tissue phase in the intermediate host that is of most interest. This tissue cycle has two stages: an acute infection characterized by cellular necrosis, and a chronic infection characterized by more or less dormant or latent collections of organisms. Following ingestion of oocysts and the release of sporozoites, individual organisms, termed **tachyzoites,** invade beyond the gastrointestinal tract and enter cells of other viscera. The

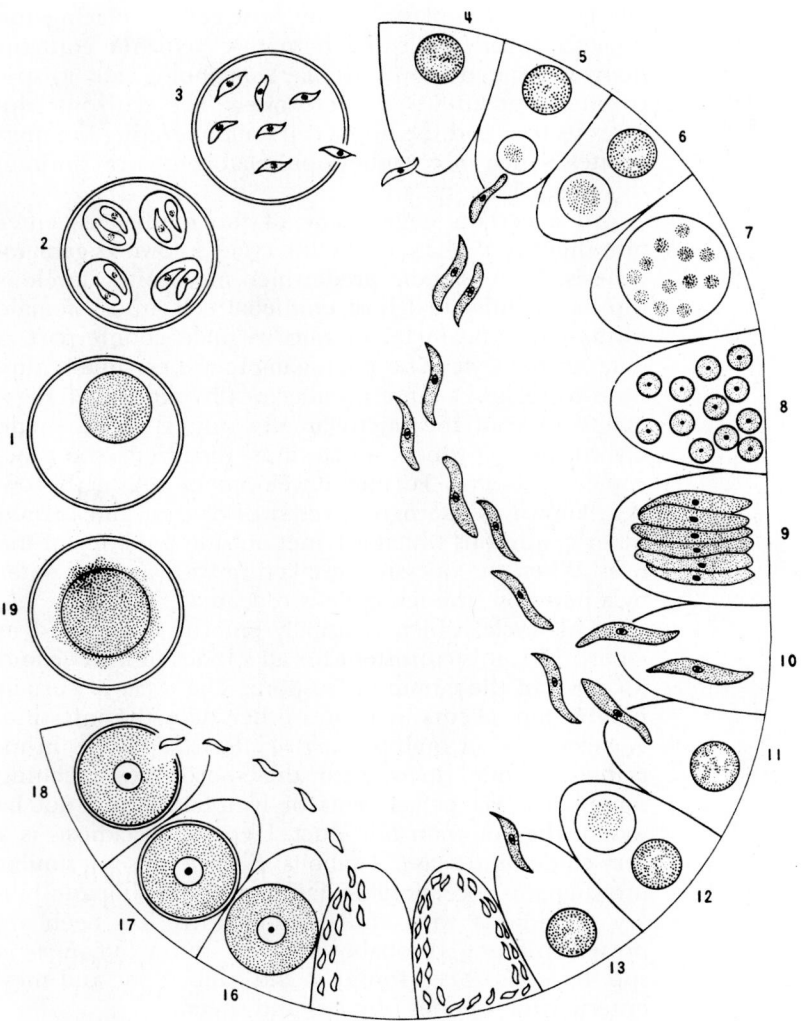

FIG. 12-1 Life cycle of *Eimeria* (diagrammatic). (1) Oocyst; (2) Sporulated oocyst; (3) Liberation of sporozoites; (4) Sporozoites entering epithelial cells; (5–11) Schizogony: formation of schizonts and merozoites; (12) Sporogony: formation of macrogametocyte; (13–15) Sporogony: formation of microgametocytes; (16–17) Development of macrogametocy; (18) Fertilization; and (19) Formation of oocyst.

tissue specificity varies with organism: *Toxoplasma* invade most cell types; *Hammondia,* lymphoid cells; *Sarcocystis,* hepatocytes; *Frenkelia,* hepatocytes and Kupffer cells. The organisms multiply by internal budding (endodyogeny) producing a group of tachyzoites (analogous to a schizont and erroneously called a pseudocyst) which eventually destroys the cell; the tachyzoites then infect another cell, repeating the cycle. This phase of acute infection may go unnoticed or be associated with extensive tissue necrosis, as in acute toxoplasmosis.

The chronic phase is characterized by formation of cysts containing individual organisms called **brady-zoites,** which slowly multiply by endodyogeny. The cysts localize in specific sites, again peculiar to each organism: *Sarcocystis* and *Hammondia* in skeletal and cardiac muscle; *Frenkelia* in brain and spinal cord, *Besnoitia* in fibroblasts; and *Toxoplasma* in many cell types.

Completion of the cycle depends on the carnivorous habits of the final hosts, in which the sexual cycle occurs in the intestinal epithelium (Fig. 12-2). This newer knowledge has resulted in multiple names for certain coccidia (formerly considered single organisms). For example, *Isospora bigemina* of dogs and cats is now recognized as the sexual stage for species of *Toxoplasma, Sarcosporidia, Hammondia,* and *Besnoitia.* Examples of these cycles are depicted in Figure 12-3.

Clinical manifestations

Coccidiosis affects the living host in many ways, depending upon the tissue preference of the particular parasite involved and the number of oocysts in the initial infection. Most of these parasites attack the mucosa of the intestinal tract; therefore symptoms are predominantly enteric. Sudden onset of bloody diarrhea with fever, followed by dehydration, emaciation, and occasionally death, are the expected manifestations, but more frequently, little or no evidence of infection is observed in the living animal. Hepatic coccidiosis in rabbits is rarely accompanied by diarrhea, and young animals may die suddenly without showing any obvious

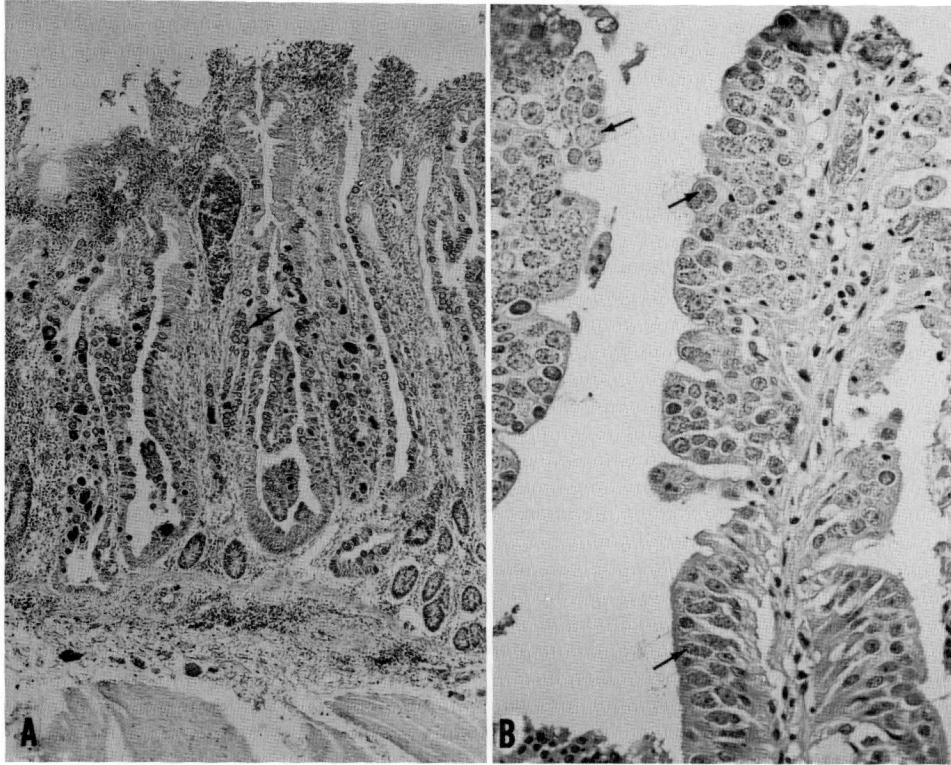

FIG. 12-2 Intestinal coccidiosis. **A.** Small intestine of a goat (×50). Note elongated crypts and villi lined with hyperplastic, tall columnar epithelial cells containing coccidia (arrow). (Contributor: Dr. L. Z. Saunders.) **B.** Small intestine of a mink (×260). Many coccidia (arrows) in epithelial cells. (Courtesy of Armed Forces Institute of Pathology; contributor: Dr. C. L. Davis.)

signs of disease, although jaundice and emaciation may be recognized in older animals.

Lesions

Coccidia are obligate intracellular parasites whose development within the cytoplasm of epithelial cells results in the death of each cell that is parasitized. The total effect on the host depends upon:

(1) The magnitude of the initial infecting dose of oocysts, which determines the number of cells invaded at the outset by sporozoites; and

(2) The spread of infection during schizogony, which is affected to a great extent by immunity acquired by the host.

As increasing numbers of organisms enter the sexual phase (gametogenesis), infection of new cells by merozoites diminishes and the disease gradually abates.

When many cells of the intestinal epithelium are parasitized at one time, the denuded mucosa may bleed freely, and intense inflammation involves the lamina propria and sometimes the submucosa. As large numbers of epithelial cells are destroyed, the remaining epithelium is stimulated to replace that which was lost. This eventually causes hyperplasia of the intestinal epithelium, which is cast into long papillary fronds as replacement of epithelial cells exceeds their loss. In lesions exhibiting this hyperplasia, coccidia in various stages of gametogenesis are most numerous. This is in contrast to the erosive, hemorrhagic stages, in which organisms in various stages of schizogony are most common.

Certain coccidia parasitize cells other than those of the intestinal tract. The most notable of these is hepatic coccidiosis in the rabbit, due to *Eimeria stiedae*, which affects the intrahepatic biliary epithelium in somewhat the same manner that other species of coccidia affect the intestinal epithelium. The destruction of biliary epithelium dominates the picture in early lesions, but in those animals in which the course is somewhat longer, proliferation of this epithelium becomes the predominant feature. The bile ducts become enormously enlarged by proliferation of epithelium, which is thrown up into papillary folds simulating adenomatous hyperplasia. These greatly enlarged segments of the bile ducts displace the adjacent liver parenchyma and appear grossly as irregularly shaped grayish areas, which are seen as depressions in the surface of the capsule (Fig. 12-2). A similar hepatic coccidiosis has also been reported in a dog, a calf, and in the gallbladder of a goat.

The gross lesions of intestinal coccidiosis may be envisaged from the foregoing account to appear as intensely congested, eroded, and bleeding areas of certain segments of the small intestine, sometimes alternating with, or replaced by, areas in which the mucosa is opaque and thickened.

Diagnosis

The clinical diagnosis is usually based upon the presence of oocysts in fecal specimens, associated with sudden onset of typical bloody diarrhea. The microscopic lesions at necropsy are characteristic and are confirmed by demonstrating the organisms in tissue sections.

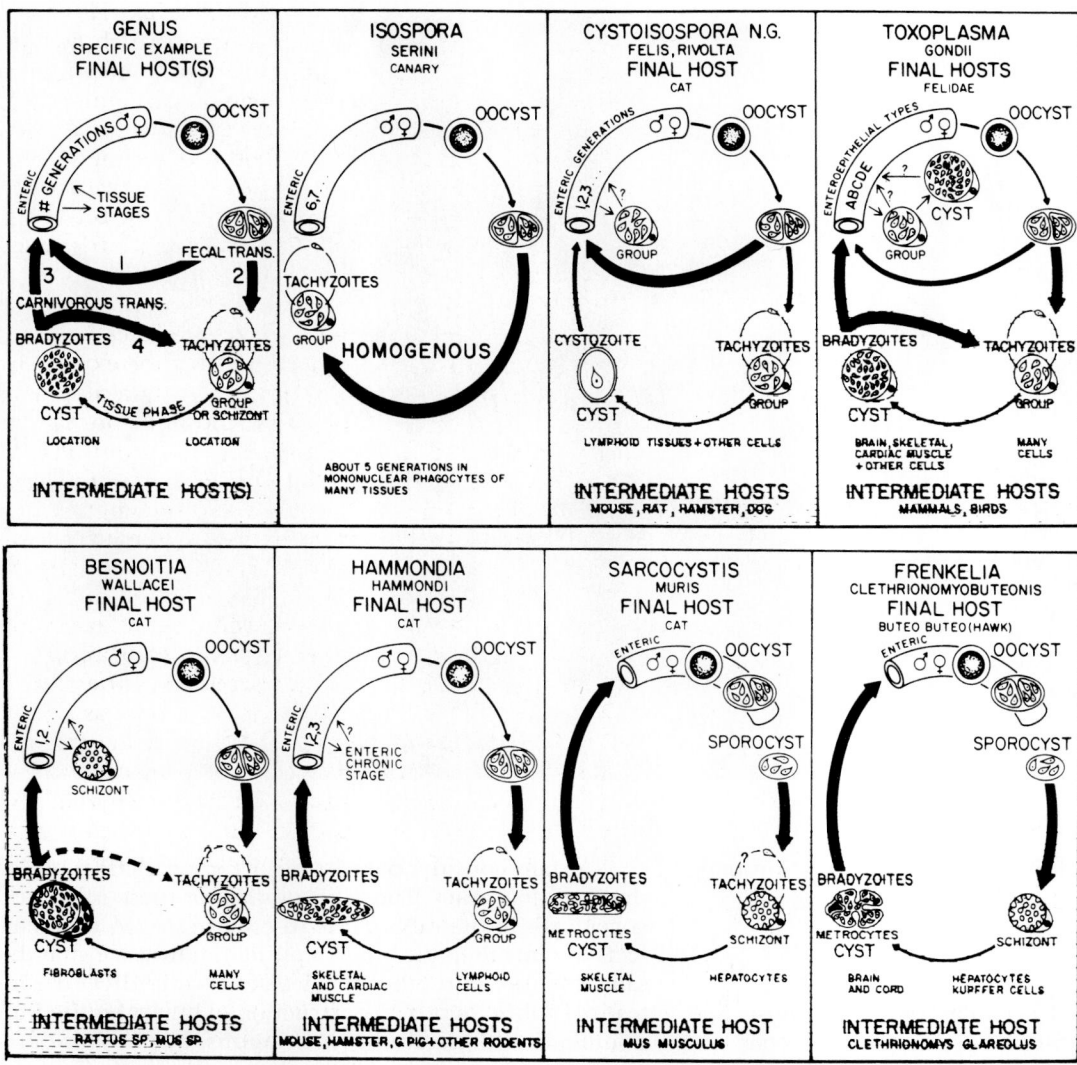

FIG. 12-3 The several types of cycles of *Isospora* and *Coccidia* other than *Eimeria*. The first panel depicts the several pathways by four arrows: 1. Oocyst to same host (homogenous, fecal); 2. Oocysts to intermediate host (heterogenous, fecal); 3. Cyst to final host (heterogenous, carnivorous); and 4. Cyst to intermediate host (homogenous, carnivorous). In the other panels, the heavy arrows indicate the most important route of transmission for the various parasites (Courtesy of Dr. J. K. Frenkel; J Parasitol 1977;63:611.)

References

Biester HE, Murray C. Studies in infectious enteritis of swine: VII. *Isospora suis* (N. Sp.) in swine. J Am Vet Med Assoc 1934;85:207–219.

Carpenter JW, Spraker TR, Novilla MN. Disseminated visceral coccidiosis in whooping cranes. J Am Vet Med Assoc 1980;177:845–848.

Collins JE, Dubey JP, and Rossow KD. Hepatic coccidiosis in a calf. Vet Pathol 1988;25:98–100.

Davis CL, Chow TL, Gorham JR. Hepatic coccidiosis in mink. Vet Med 1953;48:371–373.

Davis LR, Bowman GW. The endogenous development of *Eimeria zurnii*, a pathogenic coccidium of cattle. Am J Vet Res 1957;18:569–574.

Dubey JP. Experimental *Isospora canis* and *Isospora felis* infection in mice, cats, and dogs. J Protozool 1975; 22:416–417.

Dubey JP. Coccidiosis in the gallbladder of a goat. Proc Helminthol Soc Wash 1986;53:277–281.

Eustis SL, Nelson T. Lesions associated with coccidiosis in nursing piglets. Vet Pathol 1981;18:21–28.

Grafner G, Graubmann H-D, Dobbriner W. Hepatic coccidiosis in mink caused by a new species, *Eimeria hiepei*. Mh Vet Med 1968;22:696–700, Vet Bull 1968;2638:38.

Hammond DM, Davis LR, Bowman GW. Experimental infections with *Eimeria bovis* in calves. Am J Vet Res 1994;5:303–311.

Hitchcock DJ. The life of *Isospora felis* in the kitten. J Parasitol 1955;41:383–397.

Lee CD. The pathology of coccidiosis in the dog. J Am Vet Med Assoc 1934;85:760–781.

Levine ND, Ivens V. *Isospora* species in the dog. J Parasitol 1965;51:859–864.

Lipscomb TP, Dubey JP, Pletcher JM, et al. Intrahepatic biliary coccidiosis in a dog. Vet Pathol 1989;26:343–345.

Lotze JC. The pathogenicity of the coccidian parasite *Eimeria arloingiin* domestic sheep. Cornell Vet 1952;42:510.

Peeters JE, Geeroms R, Froyman R, et al. Coccidiosis in rabbits: a field study. Res Vet Sci 1981;30:328–334.

Pout DD. Review article: Coccidiosis of sheep. Vet Bull 1969;39:609–618.

Pout DD. Coccidiosis of lambs. III. The reaction of the small intestinal mucosa to experimental infections with *E. arloingi* "B" and *E. crandallis*. IV. The clinical response to infection of *E. arloingi* "B" and *E. crandallis* in laboratory-reared lambs. Br Vet J 1974; 130:45–53, 54–61.

Ruiz AV. On the natural history of coccidial infections in range and feeder cattle. Zentralbl Veterinaermed 1973;20B:594–602.

Sangster LT, Styer EL, and Hall GA. Coccidia associated with cutaneous nodules in a dog. Vet Pathol 1985;22:186–188.

Sharma Deorani VP. Histopathological studies in natural infection of goat coccidiosis. Indian Vet J 1966;43:122–127.

Sivadas CG, Rajan A, Nair MK. Studies on pathology of coccidiosis in goats. Indian Vet J 1965;42:474–479.

Smetana H. Coccidiosis of the liver in rabbits. I. Experimental study on the excystation of oocysts of *Eimeria stiedae*. Arch Pathol 1933;15:175–192.

Smetana H. Coccidiosis of the liver in rabbits. II. Experimental study on the mode of infection of the liver by sporozoites of *Eimeria stiedae*. Arch Pathol 1933;15:330–339.

Smetana H. Coccidiosis of the liver in rabbits. III. Experimental study of the histogenesis of coccidiosis of the liver. Arch Pathol 1933;15:516–536.

Spindler LA. Investigations on coccidia of sheep and goats. Am J Vet Res 1965;26:1068–1070.

Stockdale PHG, Niilo L. Production of bovine coccidiosis with *Eimeria zuernii*. Can Vet J 1976;17:35–37.

TOXOPLASMOSIS

Toxoplasma gondii, a small crescentic protozoan parasite, was first described in 1908 in material from a small rodent, the gondi, by Nicolle and Manceaux (1908); however, its widespread distribution in the animal kingdom was not generally recognized until more than 20 years later. The organisms were rediscovered by Sabin and Olitsky in 1935 in the brains of guinea pigs that were being used to propagate encephalitis viruses. Shortly thereafter the incrimination of *Toxoplasma* as the cause of a diffuse encephalitis and chorioretinitis in a 31-day old infant by Wolfe, Cowan, and Paige (1939) stimulated great interest in toxoplasmosis (Table 12-3).

The recent discovery of *Neospora* has complicated both the diagnosis and the interpretation of past reports of toxoplasmosis in all species. *Neospora* is nearly identical in appearance to *Toxoplasma* and induces similar lesions, especially in the central nervous system. It is discussed separately.

Life cycle

Studies by Work and Hutchinson (1969) demonstrated an inffective cyst in feces of cats experimentally infected with toxoplasma from mouse tissues. This cyst was identified by Frenkel et al. as an oocyst, typical of the genus *Isospora*, and associated with schizonts, micro-, and macrogametocytes in the intestinal epithelium (1969). These findings clarified a previously elusive life cycle and led the way to understanding the life cycle of other poorly understood organisms, such as sarcosporidia.

The sexual cycle of *Toxoplasma* (Fig. 12-3) occurs in the cat (and certain other felines), which is the definitive host and the most important source of infection for other animals in the perpetuation of toxoplasmosis. After consumption of infected meat or sporulated oocysts, the organism undergoes schizogeny in the cat's intestine with a typical coccidian cycle, leading to the production of oocysts. For one to two weeks after initial infection, cats shed millions of oocysts which are resistant to environmental influences and are infective after schizogeny. The sporulated oocysts, containing eight sporozoites, are capable of infecting a wide variety of intermediate hosts leading to either subclinical, acute or chronic infection, characterized respectively by formation of groups of tachyzoites or cysts of bradyzoites in a variety of tissues. Most mammals and birds, as well as cats, may serve as intermediate hosts. Infection of intermediate hosts and cats may follow exposure to cat feces or materials contaminated by cat feces (e.g., soil, sand boxes), or by the consumption of or exposure to infected tissues of intermediate hosts containing tachyzoites or bradyzoites. Congenital transmission may also occur in intermediate hosts during the acute phase by invasion of tachyzoites across the placenta. *Toxoplasma* have also been identified in milk and semen, which are also potential sources of infection. Released sporozoites, ingested tachyzoites, or bradyzoites first locally multiply intracellularly, usually in the intestine and lymph nodes. By endodyogeny they produce two tachyzoites per cell. These disseminate to other organs and tissues where they continue to reproduce and either lead to tissue damage and clinical disease or encyst as a collection of bradyzoites. The sexual stages in the intestinal tract have been observed so far only in cats, but the disease caused by the asexual parasites (tachyzoites and bradyzoites) is known to occur in humans and nearly all wild and domesticated mammals and birds.

Clinical manifestations

The intestinal infection in felines is not associated with clinical signs or pathologic lesions of any consequence; therefore, the disease, toxoplasmosis, usually refers to the results of the tissue phase in intermediate or final hosts.

Most infections with *Toxoplasma* go unrecognized. The incidence of infection approaches 75% in some populations of animals and humans. Clinical disease is most frequent in young animals or the aged. Animals that are immunocompromised for any reason are also more susceptible to developing signs of illness following infection. Inapparent infection or recovery from acute disease leads to immunity; however, tissue cysts containing viable bradyzoites remain for long intervals (over one year) and can serve as a source of recrudescence to active infection. Immune system infections and viral infections may serve to activate such cysts, but often the cause is unknown. In dogs, toxoplasmosis often accompanies canine distemper.

As the organisms can infect a variety of cell types, a wide diversity of manifestations have been attributed to toxoplasmosis, making it difficult to ascribe limits to the clinical signs. The organisms most often affect the brain, myocardium, lymph nodes, lungs, intestinal muscularis, pancreas, liver, uterus, placenta, and fetus; consequently, symptoms of toxoplasmosis may be referable to involvement of any one or more of these organs. In dogs, toxoplasmosis is most frequent in puppies and is

TABLE 12-3 **Characteristics of Tissue Cyst-Forming Coccidia**

Organism	Definitive host*	Intermediate host	Initial proliferative form	Cyst
Toxoplasma	Cats	All species	Tachyzoites: 　4–6 μm long 　4–6 rhoptries 　In parasitophorous 　　vacuole 　In multiple cell types	In multiple tissues 　10–100 μm diameter 　Thin-walled 0.5 μm
Neospora	Unknown	Dogs, cats, cattle, sheep, horses	Tachyzoites: 　4–7 μm long 　Numerous rhoptries 　No parasitophorous 　　vacuole 　In multiple cell types	Restricted to CNS 　Thick-walled 1–4 μm
Besnoitia	Cats & unknown	Bovines, equines, rodents, reptiles	Tachyzoites: 　5–9 μm long 　Contain enigmatic 　　bodies 　In parasitophorous 　　vacuole	Restricted to connective 　tissue 　Huge—(>11)mm in 　　size 　Contains host cell 　　nucleus in wall
Hammondia	Cats, dogs	Rodents	Tachyzoites: 　In lymphocytic cells 　Contain rhoptries 　In parasitophorous 　　vacuole	In skeletal and cardiac 　muscle 　300×95 μm 　Small cysts in CNS
Sarcocystis	Cats, dogs, humans, etc.	Principally herbi- vores, but seen in most species	Merozoites: 　In endothelial cells 　No rhoptries 　No parasitophorous 　　vacuole 　Often appear as 　　rosettes	In myofibers 　Septate 　In parasitophorous 　　vacuole 　Bradyzoites have 　　rhoptries
Frenkelia	Predator birds	Rodents, voles, muskrats	Merozoites: 　In liver	Multilobulated or 　septate 　Large—up to 1 mm 　In CNS
Cystoisospora (Levineia)	Cats, dogs & unknown	Mice, rats, dogs, chickens	Multiple tissues contain 　a single sporozoite	
Caryospora	Birds of prey, reptiles	Rodents, dogs	Gamogony in definitive 　and intermediate 　host	Sporulated oocysts and 　caryocysts containing 　a single sporozoite in 　tongue, skin, and 　other tissues

*Coccidial cycle in gastrointestinal tract

usually characterized by neurologic signs, gastrointestinal disease with diarrhea, or pneumonia, often in conjunction with canine distemper virus infection. The most common expressions in cats are pneumonia, encephalitis and pancreatitis. In sheep and goats, toxoplasmosis is an important cause of abortion, associated with necrosis and inflammation in the cotyledons of the placenta; it is also associated with infection of the fetus, especially of the central nervous system. Congenitally infected lambs and kids may be born with encephalitis. Disseminated infection is less frequent in sheep and goats. The manifestations in swine include pneumonia, encephalitis and abortion. Toxoplasmosis is apparently not common in cattle or horses. Many examples of protozoal abortion and congenital infection attributed to toxoplasmosis have been seen in cattle; however, it is now recognized that a large number of these are the result of infection with *Neospora* or a similar, but as yet unidentified, protozoan. Nonhuman primates are very susceptible to infection, usually developing disseminated disease. In humans, toxoplasmosis is recognized most frequently as a congenitally acquired infection of the newborn, manifested by encephalitis, chorioretinitis, microencephaly, macroencephaly, cerebral calcifications, convulsive disorders, and mental retardation. In adults, chorioretinitis, lymphadenopathy, myocarditis, pneumonia, and meningoencephalitis have been associated with *Toxoplasma*.

Characteristics of toxoplasma

Toxoplasma gondii is believed to be the single species of this parasite that infects all varieties of animals, as well as humans (Figs. 12-4, 12-5). The organism is readily maintained in the laboratory by cultivation in the peritoneal cavity of the mouse or in tissue cultures. In these situations, the organism is crescentic or arc-shaped, with one end rounded and the other pointed. It measures 2–4 μ in width and 4–7 μ in length. It has a nucleus, most clearly demonstrated with Giemsa stain, located near one pole of the cell. Its cytoplasm contains mitochondria, microtubules, endoplasmic reticulum, ribosomes, Golgi apparatus, and a number of organelles unique to protozoa. Among the latter are structures called rhoptries, which are osmiophilic, dense, vase-shaped, gland-like structures with their narrow portion at the pointed end of the organism and their broader base near the nucleus. Their function is unknown, but can be useful in differentiating various sarcocystidae. *Toxoplasma* have 4–6 rhoptries. At the narrow end of the organism, convoluted tubules of fibrils called toxonemes or micronemes are also present which may have some relationship to rhoptries. Toxoplasma lack a kinetoplast. The organisms are frequently found in parallel pairs (Fig. 12-6), indicating that reproduction occurs by longitudinal division (endodyogeny). These organisms, up to now considered as the only form of *Toxoplasma*, now appear to be tachyzoites, which have the ability to multiply in animal tissues and form collections of organisms. Under certain conditions (especially in brain), these collections of organisms may become encysted collections of bradyzoites.

In tissue sections, tachyzoites of *Toxoplasma* may be crescentic, but also occur in rounded and ovoid form. Presumably because of shrinkage in fixation, the organisms usually appear smaller in sections than in smears, about 2 μ wide and 4 μ long. They are most frequently found in the cytoplasm of cells, but may also be free. A large number of the organisms may be encountered in a single cell, or they may be contained by a thin, poorly defined membrane. Within the cell the tachyzoites are contained within a vacuole, termed a parasitophorous vacuole, which does not fuse with lysosomes. It is not visible in ordinary tissue sections, but can be discerned by electron microscopy. This characteristic is helpful in the differentiation from certain other members of the family Sarcocystidae such as *Neospora*, which is free in the cytoplasm. Chronic infection is characterized by larger cysts filled with bradyzoites, which represent a resting stage of the parasite; this is because they are often seen in the absence of reaction in the adjacent host tissues, and they are apparently more resistant to deleterious influences in this stage.

Electron photomicrographs and histochemical studies indicate that the cyst wall is actually formed by the organisms; thus, the term "pseudocyst" is not valid.

Lesions

Following initial replication, most usually in the intestine and associated lymph nodes, parasitemia disseminates the protozoa to various other tissues where *Toxoplasma* actively penetrate a variety of cell types. Most cell types are vulnerable. In all affected tissues, in addition to invasion of the principal parenchymal cell type, *Toxoplasma* can be found in macrophages, fibroblasts, and smooth muscle cells. Their continued intracellular replication leads to cell death. Thus, the characteristic lesion is distinguished by the presence of intracellular

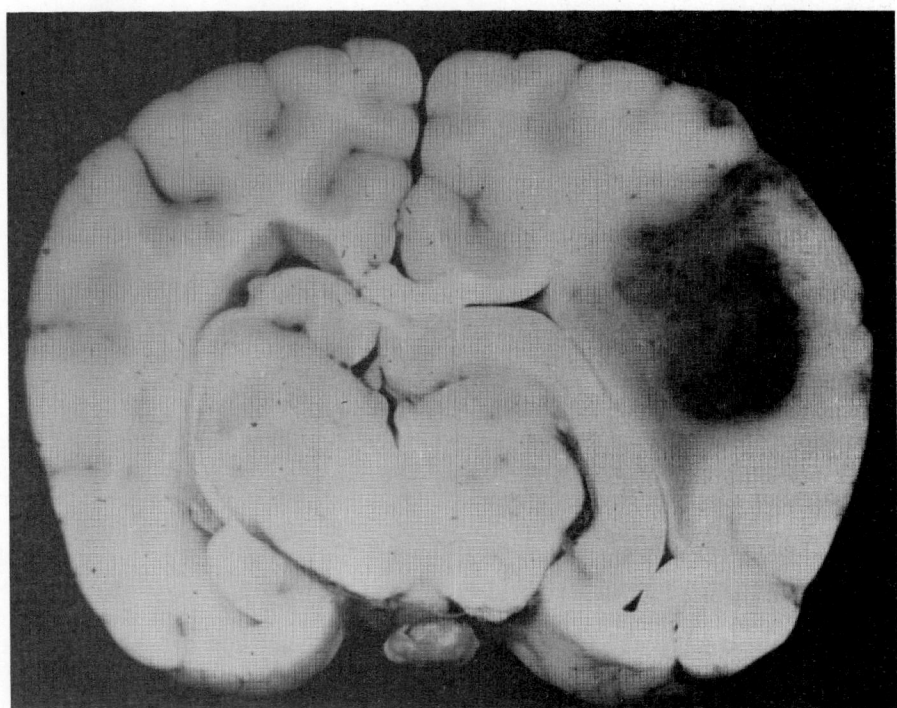

FIG. 12-4 Toxoplasmosis. Necrotic and hemorrhagic lesion in the left cerebral hemisphere of a four-year-old poodle. Myriads of *Toxoplasma gondii* were demonstrated in microscopic sections of this lesion. (Courtesy of Angell Memorial Animal Hospital.)

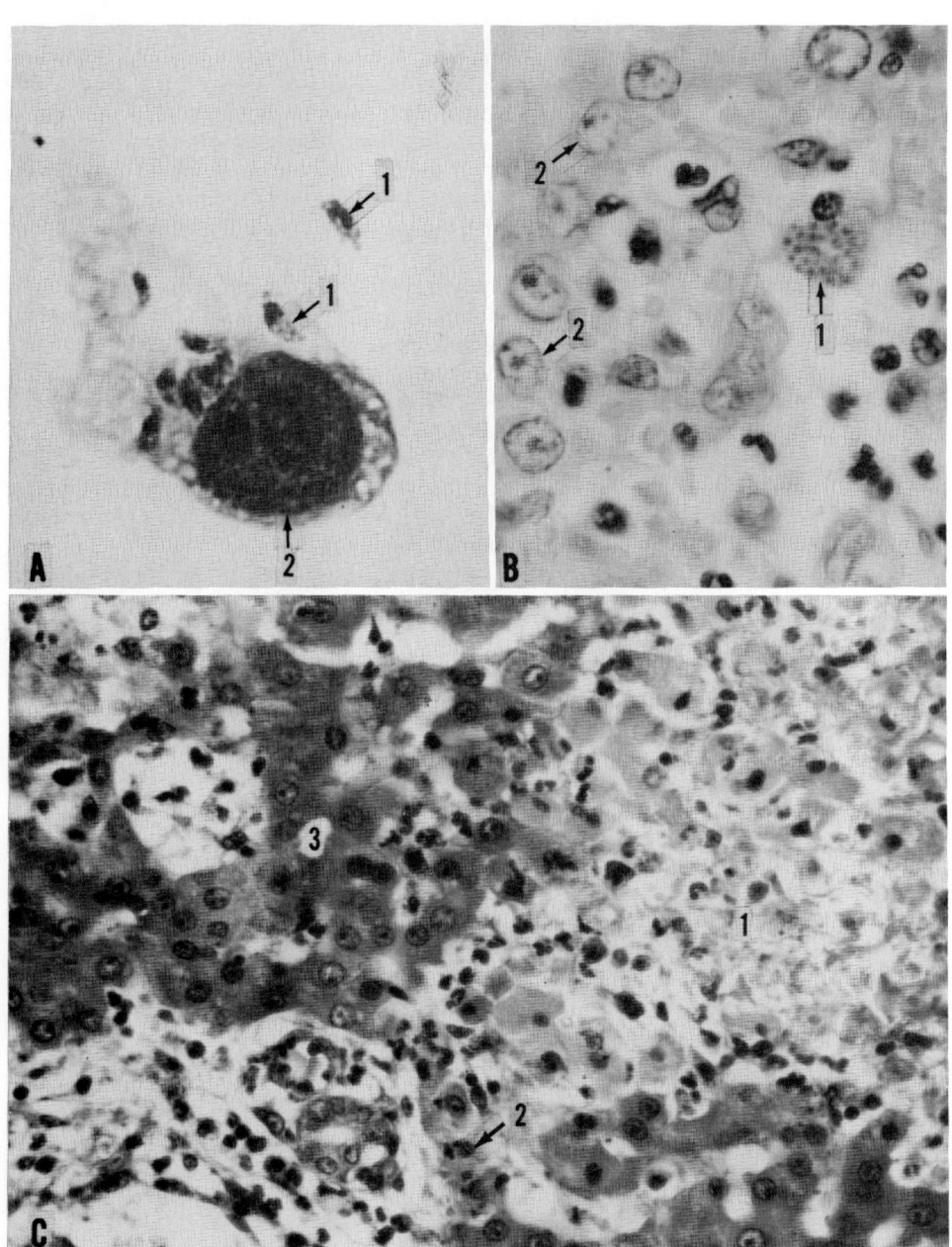

FIG. 12-5 Toxoplasmosis. **A.** (1) Tachyzoites of *Toxoplasma gondii;* and (2) In mouse peritoneum, most organisms in macrophage. (Contributor: Dr. W. B. Dublin.) **B.** Tachyzoites of *Toxoplasma gondii.* (1) In lung of a cat. Note proliferation and cuboidal shape; and (2) Of cells lining alveoli. (Contributor: Dr. M. Zimmerman.) **C.** Sharply demarcated necrotic lesion. (1) In liver of a dog (×500), (2) Necrotic, and (3) Viable liver cells are present. (Courtesy of Armed Forces Institute of Pathology; contributor: Angell Memorial Animal Hospital.)

tachyzoites, variably sized foci of necrosis, and an associated inflammatory reaction predominantly composed of mononuclear cells. As indicated, most infections are subclinical. In these cases, the organisms may form tissue cysts, especially in brain, but also in the liver, kidney and skeletal muscle, which may remain viable for years in the absence of any host reaction.

In brain, *Toxoplasma* chiefly invade neurons and astrocytes, leading to diffuse necrotizing and nonsuppurative infiltration of brain parenchyma, particularly adjacent to the meninges, which may be similarly infiltrated. Lymphocytic cells accumulate within the Robin-Virchow spaces and are scattered through the parenchyma. Vacuoles may occur in the white matter. *Toxoplasma* tachyzoites may be found scattered singly or in pairs through the pa-

renchyma, or in aggregations containing up to 50 organisms. Necrotizing lesions have been observed in the basilar arteries in the cat, but their relationship to toxoplasmosis is not clearly established.

The liver in frank toxoplasmosis contains large, sharply delimited, microscopic-sized areas of coagulation necrosis involving any part of the hepatic lobules. The necrotic areas, containing eosinophilic material and cell debris, are surrounded by apparently normal hepatic cells with little or no cellular reaction. Tachyzoites may be found within liver or Kupffer's cells, in cysts containing a large number of organisms, or singly or in pairs scattered sparsely in both the necrotic and viable tissues. Organisms may be few in number even when severe necrosis is present.

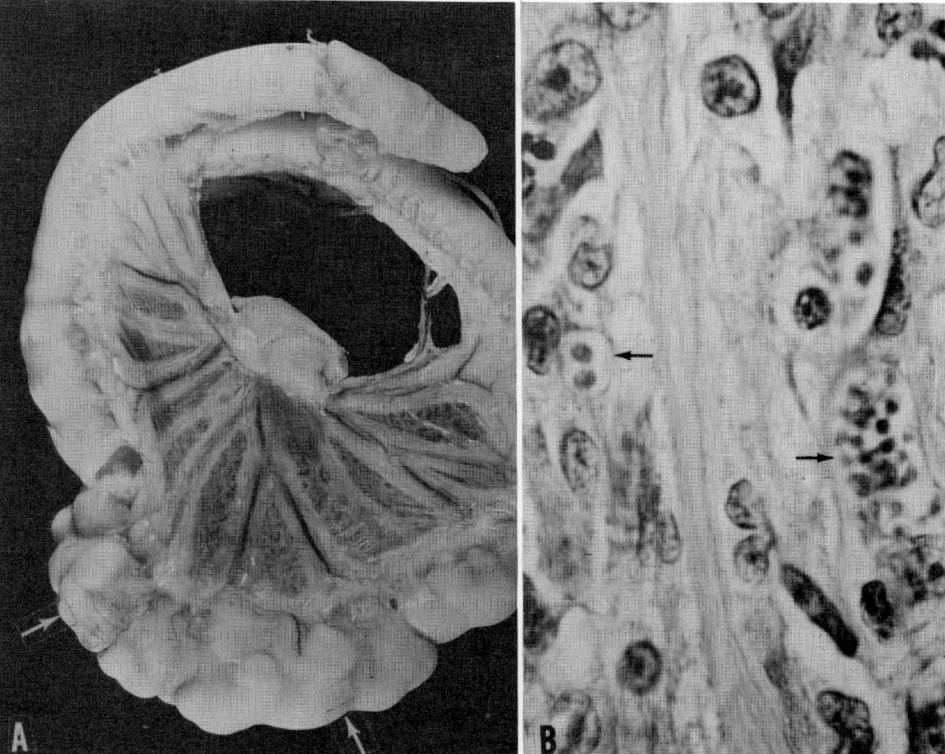

FIG. 12-6 Toxoplasmosis. **A.** Nodular granulomatous lesion in the intestinal muscularis of a cat. **B.** Involved muscularis of intestine (×1283). Tachyzoites of *Toxoplasma gondii* all and large groups within smooth muscle cells (arrows). (Courtesy of Armed Forces Institute of Pathology; contributor: Dr. Leo L. Lieberman.)

In the lung, *Toxoplasma* invade type I and II pneumocytes, and bronchiolar epithelial cells, as well as macrophages, fibroblasts, endothelial cells, and smooth muscle cells. This leads to foci of necrosis and a rather striking proliferative reaction, particularly in cats, although other species may develop similar lesions. The changes are particularly evident in the alveolar walls, whose lining becomes cuboidal or columnar and rich in cells, suggesting in this respect the appearance of fetal lung (so-called "fetalization" of lung). This feature also has superficial resemblances to pulmonary adenomatosis. The alveoli are filled with large mononuclear cells and leukocytes with aggregations of Toxoplasma in the cells lining the alveoli. These lesions have a nodular distribution throughout the lung, appearing grossly as small, gray, tumorlike masses scattered throughout one or all lobes. Foci of alveolar wall necrosis may accompany this change or may be the only lesion evident.

The lymph nodes, particularly those contiguous to affected parenchymal organs, are commonly involved in active cases. They are usually enlarged to several times their normal size, are firm in consistency and densely congested. Extensive coagulation necrosis is seen microscopically, usually in sharply demarcated but irregular zones with slight leukocytic infiltration around the margins. Tachyzoites may be found adjacent to these necrotic areas, particularly in endothelial cells of veins, but may be within the cytoplasm of monocytic cells or free in the tissues. Usually both lymphocytic and reticuloendothelial hyperplasia occurs.

Ulcers in the **intestine,** presumably resulting from necrosis of submucosal lymph nodules, have been described in toxoplasmosis. Upon occasion, *Toxoplasma* invade the muscularis of the intestine, where a chronic necrotizing lesion followed by production of granulation tissue results in large, grossly detectable granulomatous nodules, which may replace the wall and impinge upon the lumen. The organisms are clearly demonstrable in small and large groups in the muscularis and the granulation tissue.

The **pancreas** may be a site of localization in toxoplasmosis, and here the acute necrotizing lesions arouse intense lymphocytic infiltration, edema, and swelling.

The **eye** may be infected in human adults, and ocular infection has been reported in animals. The lesion is one of granulomatous chorioretinitis in which *Toxoplasma* are demonstrable.

The **myocardium** is frequently invaded by *Toxoplasma*, which may be present in large or small groups within the cytoplasm of cardiac muscle cells. In some instances, severe lymphocytic inflammation is evoked; in others, the organisms are present with little associated inflammation.

Placental invasion leads to focal necrosis (Fig. 12-7), often accompanied by calcification. Tachyzoites are found free and within trophoblasts. Abortion may follow with or without invasion of the fetus. This usually follows acute infection of the pregnant animal, but abortion may also follow reactivation of chronic infection. In the infected fetus, lesions are most common in brain. Placental transmission may also cause stillbirth and neonatal death.

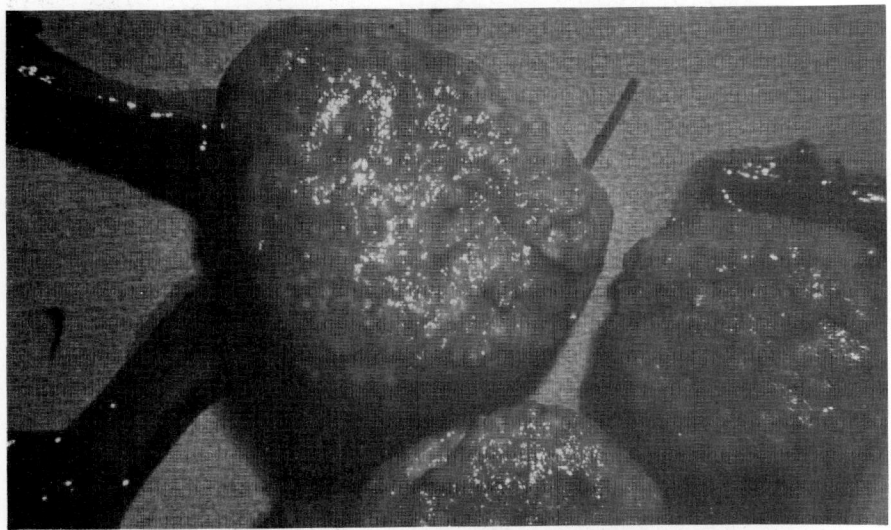

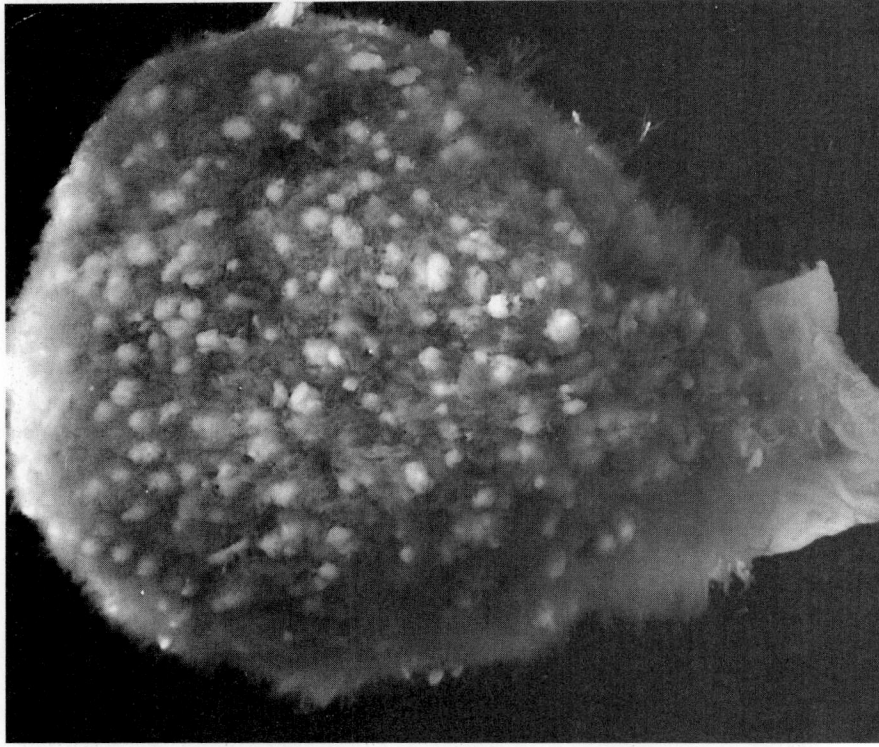

FIG. 12-7 Toxoplasmosis. Multiple foci of necrosis in the placental cotyledons in: **A.** A cow (Courtesy of Dr. W. A. Watson); and **B.** a sheep (Courtesy of Dr. J. P. Dubey, ARS, USDA, Beltsville, MD).

Diagnosis

The diagnosis of toxoplasmosis in the living animal is presently more of a problem than at necropsy. An array of assays (complement fixation, hemagglutination, Sabin-Feldman dye, latex agglutination, ELISA, indirect fluorescent antibody, direct and indirect carbon immunoassay) are valuable to detect antibodies, but due to the high percentage of serologic positivity, demonstration of antibody cannot distinguish between current and past infection. The combined testing for both IgM and IgG class antibody titers can help eliminate this problem as the IgM class antibody develops earlier and decreases more rapidly than do IgG class antibodies to

Toxoplasma. Detection of circulating antigen or isolation of organisms by mouse inoculation or other means permit recognition of active infection. At necropsy, the demonstration of *Toxoplasma* in tissue sections in characteristic lesions should be supported by isolation of the organisms or by use of immunologic staining techniques. In tissue sections, the microscopic appearance of other members of the family Sarcocystidae are similar, as are the leishmanial forms of *Trypanosoma cruzi.* *Neospora caninum* is the most similar in appearance and, until its discovery in 1988, has frequently been misdiagnosed as *Toxoplasma.* Distinguishing features are listed in Table 12-3. The intermediate hosts for several of these are shared (e.g., *Toxoplasma* and *Neospora*); however, for some (e.g., *Frenkelia, Hammondia*) it is restricted, often allowing their elimination from consideration. The leishmanial forms of *Trypanosoma cruzi* may be distinguished by their centrosome and kinetoplast, which can be seen in some organisms. *Besnoitia* may be distinguished by the giant nuclei in the well-developed wall of the cyst, in which the small organisms are found.

HAMMONDIA

Tissue stages of *Hammondia* are more difficult to differentiate, but the facts that intermediate hosts are limited to rodents, in which groups of tachyzoites are limited to lymphoid cells, and that cysts are limited to striated muscle are helpful. The application of the fluorescent antibody test to tissue sections or smears provides a useful method to more specifically identify *Toxoplasma*.

Hammondia hammondi is an organism which is similar to Toxoplasma and classified in the same family (Frenkel and Dubey, 1975). It has a two-host cycle, with sexual reproduction in the intestine of cats (*H. hammondi*) or dogs (*H. heydorni*). Various rodents serve as intermediate hosts where tachyzoites proliferate in lymphoid cells and cysts of bradyzoites are limited to skeletal and cardiac muscle. In contrast to *Toxoplasma*, *Hammondia* has an obligatory two-host life cycle; infection of cats is dependent upon ingestion of infected tissues of the intermediate host and the intermediate host is apparently only infected by ingestion of oocysts. Dogs have been shown to be experimentally susceptible intermediate hosts, but the role of *Hammondia* in clinical or pathologic disease has not been determined.

References

Al-Khalidi NW, Weisbrode SE, Dubey JP. Pathogenicity of *Toxoplasma gondii* oocysts to ponies. Am J Vet Res 1980;41:1549–1551.

Anderson DC and McClure HM. Acute disseminated fatal toxoplasmosis in a squirrel monkey. J Am Vet Med Assoc 1982;181:1363–1366.

Averill DR Jr, deLahunta A. Toxoplasmosis of the canine nervous system: clinicopathologic findings in four cases. J Am Vet Med Assoc 1971;159:1134–1141.

Beverley JKA, Watson WA, Payne JM. The pathology of the placenta in ovine abortion due to toxoplasmosis. Vet Rec 1971;88:124–128.

Beverley JKA, Watson WA, Spence JB. The pathology of the foetus in ovine abortion due to toxoplasmosis. Vet Rec 1971;88:174–178.

Bjerkås I. Neuropathology and host-parasite relationship of acute experimental toxoplasmosis of the blue fox (*Alopex lagopus*). Vet Pathol 1990;27:381–390.

Bjerkås I, Presthus J. The neuropathology in toxoplasmosis-like infection caused by a newly recognized cyst-forming sporozoan in dogs. Acta Pathol Microbiol Immunol Scand 1989;97:459–468.

Capen CC, Cole CR. Pulmonary lesions in dogs with experimental and naturally occurring toxoplasmosis. Path Vet 1966;3:40–63.

Dreesen DW. *Toxoplasma gondii* infections in wildlife. J Am Vet Med Assoc 1990;196:274–276.

Dubey JP. Experimental *Hammondia hammondi* infection in dogs. Br Vet J 1975; 131:741–743.

Dubey JP. Persistence of encysted *Toxoplasma gondii* in caprine livers and public health significance of toxoplasmosis in goats. J Am Vet Med Assoc 1980;177:1203–1207.

Dubey JP. Epizootic toxoplasmosis associated with abortion in dairy goats in Montana. J Am Vet Med Assoc 1981;178:661–670.

Dubey JP. Persistence of encysted *Toxoplasma gondii* in tissues of equids fed oocysts. Am J Vet Res 1985;46:1753–1754.

Dubey JP. Toxoplasmosis. J Am Vet Med Assoc 1986;189:166–170.

Dubey JP. *Toxoplasma gondii* cysts in placentas of experimentally infected sheep. Am J Vet Res 1987;48:352–353.

Dubey JP. [1] Lesions in transplacentally induced toxoplasmosis in goats. [2] Long-term persistence of *Toxoplasma gondii* in tissues of pigs inoculated with *T. gondii* oocysts and effect of freezing on viability of tissue cysts in pork. Am J Vet Res 1988;49:905–909, 910–913.

Dubey JP. Lesions in goats fed *Toxoplasma gondii* oocysts. Vet Parasitol 1989;32:133–144.

Dubey JP. [1] Status of toxoplasmosis in cattle in the United States. [2] Status of toxoplasmosis in sheep and goats in the United States. [3] Status of toxoplasmosis in pigs in the United States. J Am Vet Med Assoc 1990;196:257–259, 259–262, 270–274.

Dubey JP, Adams DS. Prevalence of *Toxoplasma gondii* antibodies in dairy goats from 1982 to 1984. J Am Vet Med Assoc 1990;196:295–296.

Dubey JP, Kirkbride CA. Toxoplasmosis and other causes of abortions in sheep from north central United States. J Am Vet Med Assoc 1990;196:287–290.

Dubey JP, Frenkel JK. Cyst-induced toxoplasmosis in cats. J Protozool 1972;19:155177.

Dubey JP, Sharma SP. Prolonged excretion of *Toxoplasma gondii* in semen of goats. Am J Vet Res 1980;41:794–795.

Dubey JP, Urban JF Jr. Diagnosis of transplacentally induced toxoplasmosis in pigs. Am J Vet Res 1990;51:1295–1299.

Dubey JP, Welcome FL. *Toxoplasma gondii*-induced abortion in sheep. J Am Vet Med Assoc 1988;193:697–700.

Dubey JP, Carpenter JL, Topper MJ, et al. Fatal toxoplasmosis in dogs. J Am Anim Hosp Assoc 1989;25:659–664.

Dubey JP, Gendron-Fitzpatrick AP, Lenhard AL, et al. Fatal toxoplasmosis and enteroepithelial stages of *Toxoplasma gondii* in a Pallis cat (*Felis manul*). J Protozool 1988;35:528–530.

Dubey JP, Miller NL, Frenkel JK. The *Toxoplasma* gondiioocyst from cat feces. J Exp Med 1970;132:636–662.

Dubey JP, Miller S, Powell EC, et al. Epizootiologic investigations on a sheep farm with *Toxoplasma gondii*-induced abortions. J Am Vet Med Assoc 1986;188:155–158.

Dubey JP, Miller S, Desmonts G, et al. *Toxoplasma gondii*-induced abortion in dairy goats. J Am Vet Med Assoc 1986;188:159–162.

Dubey JP, Schlafer DH, Urban JF Jr, et al. Lesions in fetal pigs with transplacentally-induced toxoplasmosis. Vet Pathol 1990;27:411–418.

Dubey JP, Sonn RJ, Hedstrom O, et al. Serologic and histologic diagnosis of toxoplasmic abortions in sheep in Oregon. J Am Vet Med Assoc 1990;196:291–294.

Dubey JP, Zajac A, Osofsky SA, et al. Acute primary toxoplasmic hepatitis in an adult cat shedding *Toxoplasma gondii* oocysts. J Am Vet Med Assoc 1990;197:1616–1618.

Dubey JP, et al. Caprine toxoplasmosis: abortion, clinical signs, and distribution of Toxoplasma in tissues of goats fed *Toxoplasma gondii* oocysts. Am J Vet Res 1980;41:1072–1076.

Frenkel JK. Ocular lesions in hamsters with chronic *Toxoplasma and Besnoitia* infection. Am J Ophthalmol 1955;39:203–225.

Frenkol JK. Host, strain and treatment variation as factors in pathogenesis of toxoplasmosis. Am J Trop Med Hyg 1953;2:390–415.

Frenkel JK. Toxoplasmosis: parasite life cycle, pathology and immunology. in: Hammond DM, Long PD, eds. The coccidia. Baltimore: University Park Press, 1973; 343–410.

Frenkel JK. [1] Pathology and pathogenesis of congenital toxoplasmosis. [2] Breaking the transmission chain of *Toxoplasma*: a program for the prevention of human toxoplasmosis. Bull NY Acad Med 1974;50:181–191, 228–235.

Frenkol JK. Transmission of toxoplasmosis and the role of immunity in limiting transmission and illness. [2] Toxoplasmosis in human beings. J Am Vet Med Assoc 1990;196:233–240, 240–248.

Frenkol JK, Dubey JP. Toxoplasmosis and its prevention in cats and man. J Infect Dis 1972;126:664–673.

Frenkol JK. *Hammondia hammondi*: a new coccidium of cats producing cysts in muscle of other mammals. Science 1975;189:222–224.

Frenkel JK, Dubey JP, Miller NL. *Toxoplasma gondii*: fecal forms separated from eggs of the nematode *Toxocara cati*. Science 1969;164: 432–433.

Frenkel JK. *Toxoplasma gondii* in cats: fecal stages identified as coccidian oocysts. Science 1970;167:893–896.

Frenkel JK, Ruiz A. Human toxoplasmosis and cat contact in Costa Rica. Am J Trop Med Hyg 1980;29:1167–1180.

Heidel JR, et al. Myelitis in a cat infected with *Toxoplasma gondii* and feline immunodeficiency virus. J Am Vet Med Assoc 1990;196:316–318.

Hartley WJ, Kater JC. The pathology of toxoplasma infection in the pregnant ewe. Res Vet Sci 1963;4:326–332, Vet Bull 2333:63.

Hubbard G, Witt W, Healy M, et al. An outbreak of toxoplasmosis in zoo birds. Vet Pathol 1986;23:639–641.

Hutchison WM, Dunachie JF, Siim J, Chr, et al. Coccidian-like nature of *Toxoplasma gondii*. Br Med J 1970;1:142–144.

Joiner KA, Fuhrman SA, Miettinen HM, et al. *Toxoplasma gondii*: fusion competence of parasitophorous vacuoles in Fc receptor-transfected fibroblasts. Science 1990;249:641–646.

Koestner A, Cole CR. Neuropathology of canine toxoplasmosis. Am J Vet Res 1960;21:813–830.

Koestner A, Cole CR. Neuropathology of porcine toxoplasmosis. Cornell Vet 1960;50:362–384.

Ladiges WC, DiGiacomo RF, Yamaguchi RA. Prevalence of *Toxoplasma gondii* antibodies and oocysts in pound-source cats. J Am Vet Med Assoc 1982;180:1334–1335.

Lappin MR, Greene CE, Prestwood AK, et al. Diagnosis of recent *Toxoplasma gondii* infection in cats by use of an enzyme-linked immunosorbent assay for immunoglobulin M. Am J Vet Res 1989;50:1580–1585.

Leighty JC. Strategies for control of toxoplasmosis. J Am Vet Med Assoc 1990;196:281–286.

Leland MM, Hubbard GB, Dubey JP. Clinical toxoplasmosis in domestic rabbits. Lab Anim Sci 1992;42:318–319.

Malik MA, Dreesen DW, de la Cruz A. Toxoplasmosis in sheep in northeastern United States. J Am Vet Med Assoc 1990;196:263–265.

McCabe R, Remington JS. Toxoplasmosis: the time has come. N Engl J Med 1988;318:313–315.

Meier H, Holzworth J, Griffiths RC. Toxoplasmosis in the cat, 14 cases. J Am Vet Med Assoc 1957;131:395414.

Miller NL, Frenkel JK, Dubey JP. Oral infections with *Toxoplasma* cysts and oocysts in felines, other mammals and birds. J Parasitol 1972;58:928–937.

Moller T, Nielsen SW. Toxoplasmosis in distemper-susceptible carnivora. Path Vet 1964;1:189–203.

Nichols BA, O'Connor GR. Penetration of mouse peritoneal macrophages by the protozoon *Toxoplasma gondii*: new evidence for active invasion and phagocytosis. Lab Invest 1981;44:324–335.

Nicolle C, Manceaux L. Sur une infection a corps de Leishman (ou organismes voisins) du gondi. Compt Rend Acad d Sc 1908;147:763–766.

Parker GA, Langloss JM, Dubey JP, et al. Pathogenesis of acute toxoplasmosis in specific-pathogen-free cats. Vet Pathol 1981;18:786–803.

Piper RC, Cole CR, Shadduck JA. Natural and experimental ocular toxoplasmosis in animals. Am J Ophthalmol 1970;69:662–668.

Rhyan JC, Dubey JP. Ovine abortion and neonatal death due to toxoplasmosis in Montana. J Am Vet Med Assoc 1984;184:661–664.

Ruiz A, Frenkel JK. [1] *Toxoplasma gondii* in Costa Rican cats. [2] Intermediate and transport hosts of *Toxoplasma gondii* in Costa Rica. Am J Trop Med Hyg 1980;29:1150–1160, 1161–1166.

Siim JC, Hutchison WM, Work K. Transmission of *Toxoplasma gondii*: further studies on the morphology of the cystic form in cat faeces. Acta Path Microbiol Scand 1969;77:756–757.

Smith C. Staining of *Toxoplasma* in histological sections. Br J Ophthalmol 1953;37:504–505.

Stalheim OHV, Fayer R, Hubbert WT. Update on bovine toxoplasmosis and sarcocystosis, with emphasis on their role in bovine abortions. J Am Vet Med Assoc 1980;176:299–302.

Tisseur H, et al. Histological diagnosis of toxoplasmosis in animals. Recl Med Vet 1966;142:15–23.

Uggla A, Sjöland L, Dubey JP. Immunohistochemical diagnosis of toxoplasmosis in fetuses and fetal membranes of sheep. Am J Vet Res 1987;48:348–351.

Wilson M, Ware DA, Juranek DD. Serologic aspects of toxoplasmosis. J Am Vet Med Assoc 1990;196:277–281.

Zimmerman JJ, Dreesen DW, Owen WJ, et al. Prevalence of toxoplasmosis in swine from Iowa. J Am Vet Med Assoc 1990;196:266–270.

NEOSPORA CANINUM

The existence of *Neospora caninum* was not recognized until 1988, when it was described by Dubey et al. in a review of specimens from dogs as far back as 1948, in which toxoplasmosis had been diagnosed. It has since been also identified as a parasite of cats, cattle, sheep, and horses. The life cycle has not been elucidated, but would presumably involve an enteric cycle in a definitive host comparable to other members of the cyst-forming coccidia in the family Sarcocystidae, phylum Apicomplexa. In tissues, *Neospora caninum* resembles *Toxoplasma gondii*, occurring as intracellular tachyzoites 4–7 μm long, which divide by endodyogeny, forming groups of variable numbers of organisms. Tissue cysts, which are found only in the central nervous system, have a thick wall (1–4 μm) and contain PAS-positive bradyzoites. Transplacental infection is the only means of transmission thus far identified; however, ingestion of unidentified oocysts or infected tissues, analogous to *T. gondii*, is also most likely to occur.

N. caninum can affect dogs of all ages, but appears to be most frequent in young animals, many of which may have acquired the infection in utero. The most frequent clinical expression relates to involvement of the central nervous system with variable degrees of ataxia, stiffness, incoordination, irregular movements, circling, and paresis, particularly of the hind limbs. Clinical signs may also include anorexia, listlessness, myalgia, and signs related to myocardial insufficiency or hepatic dysfunction. In cattle, *Neospora*, and protozoa described as *Neospora*-like, have been identified as an important cause of fetal infection leading to abortion. Experimentally, abortion and congenital infection have been produced in sheep.

Lesions

N. caninum can invade cells of most all tissues, but has a predilection for the central nervous system, myocardium, skeletal muscle, and endothelium, leading to encephalomyelitis and polymyositis as the principal pathologic findings. The liver, lung, pancreas, dermis, endothelium, retina and choroid, and smooth muscle cells of the gastrointestinal tract and vascular tree are other sites where the organism may proliferate. Intracellular multiplication of the tachyzoites leads to varying sized foci of necrosis, which is the predominant pathologic finding. An inflammatory cell reaction, most usually composed of various mononuclear cells, and an associated vasculitis surround and infiltrate the necrotizing lesions. Neutrophils may accompany the inflammation, but are rarely the predominant cell type. Proliferation of connective tissue may also develop adjacent to the lesions. Depending upon the most prominent feature, the lesions are those of necrotizing or granulomatous inflammation. In brain, the picture is of a nonsuppurative meningoencephalitis of both gray and white matter, with necrosis, gliosis and perivascular collections of mononuclear cells. Organisms are found intracellularly in all affected tissues as groups of tachyzoites. These collections of organisms lack any wall. In brain, in addition to proliferating collections of tachyzoites, thick-walled cysts containing bradyzoites may be present, often in areas without significant necrosis or inflammation. In aborted fetuses, the principal lesion is a multifocal, necrotizing and nonsuppurative encephalomyelitis, but disseminated disease may also be present as can placentitis. Fatal congenital infection has also been described in a one-week-old lamb with encephalitis and in an aborted equine fetus with proliferating organisms in the lung. In cats, experimental infection with *N. caninum* leads to myositis and encephalitis.

Diagnosis

The lesions and the light microscopic features of *N. caninum* closely resemble those of *Toxoplasma gondii* and the two diseases are easily confused. Retrospective studies demonstrated that previously recorded examples of toxoplasmosis were in fact infection with *N. caninum*. The diagnosis is best confirmed with the use of immunohistochemical staining techniques that have been developed. Distinguishing morphologic characteristics also exist, and are tabulated in Table 12-3.

The principal features distinguishing *N. caninum* from *T. gondii* are: *Neospora* tachyzoites lie in the host cell cytoplasm without a parasitophorous vacuole, whereas *Toxoplasma* are within a parasitophorous vacuole; *Neospora* organisms contain more numerous rhoptries than do *Toxoplasma*; the wall of the cyst stage of *Neospora* is thicker than that of *Toxoplasma*; and the cyst stage of *Neospora* has been identified only in the central nervous system. Congenital infection in cattle leading to abortion must be differentiated from sarcosporidiosis. In both infections in cattle, organisms may be located principally within endothelial cells. Those organisms described as *Neospora*-like in cattle resemble *N. caninum*, but do not totally cross-react, indicating an as yet unidentified but closely related protozoan.

References

Anderson ML, et al. Neospora-like protozoan infection as a major cause of abortion in California dairy cattle. J Am Vet Med Assoc 1991;198:241–244.

Barr BC, Anderson ML, Dubey JP, et al. *Neospora*-like protozoal infections associated with bovine abortions. Vet Pathol 1991;28:110–116.

Barr BC, Conrad PA, Dubey JP, et al. *Neospora*-like encephalomyelitis in a calf: pathology, ultrastructure, and immunoreactivity. J Vet Diagn Invest 1991;3:39–46.

Barr BC, et al. Bovine fetal encephalitis and myocarditis associated with protozoal infections. Vet Pathol 1990;27:354–361.

Dubey JP. *Neospora caninum*: a look at a new *Toxoplasma*-like parasite of dogs and other animals. Compend Contin Educ Pract Vet 1990;12:653–663.

Dubey JP, Lindsay DS. Transplacental *Neospora caninum* infection in cats. J Parasitol 1989;75:765–771.

Dubey JP, Lindsay DS. Transplacental *Neospora caninum* infection in dogs. Am J Vet Res 1989;50:1578–1579.

Dubey JP, Lindsay DS. *Neospora caninum* induced abortion in sheep. J Vet Diagn Invest 1990;2:230–233.

Dubey JP, Porterfield ML. *Neospora caninum* (Apicomplexa) in an aborted equine fetus. J Parasitol 1990;76:732–734.

Dubey JP, Hartley WJ, Lindsay DS. Congenital *Neospora caninum* infection in a calf with spinal cord anomaly. J Am Vet Med Assoc 1990;197:1043–1044.

Dubey JP, Koestner A, Piper RC. Repeated transplacental transmission of *Neospora caninum* in dogs. J Am Vet Med Assoc 1990;197:857–860.

Dubey JP, Leathers CW, Lindsay DS. *Neospora caninum*-like protozoon associated with fatal myelitis in newborn calves. J Parasitol 1989;75:146–148.

Dubey JP, Lindsay DS, Lipscomb TP. Neosporosis in cats. Vet Pathol 1990;27:335–339, 1990.

Dubey JP, Hartley WJ, Lindsay DS, et al. Fatal congenital *Neospora caninum* infection in a lamb. J Parasitol 1990;76:127–130.

Dubey JP, Hattel AL, Lindsay DS, et al. Neonatal *Neospora caninum* infection in dogs: isolation of the causative agent and experimental transmission. J Am Vet Med Assoc 1988;193:1259–1263.

Dubey JP, Higgins RJ, Smith JH, et al. *Neospora caninum* encephalomyelitis in a British dog. Vet Rec 1990;124:193–194.

Dubey JP, Miller S, Lindsay DS, et al. *Neospora caninum*-associated myocarditis and encephalitis in an aborted calf. J Vet Diagn Invest 1990;2:66–69.

Dubey JP, Schlafer DH, Urban JF Jr, et al. Lesions in fetal pigs with transplacentally-induced toxoplasmosis. Vet Pathol 1990;27:411–418.

Dubey JP, Carpenter JL, Speer CA, et al. Newly recognized fatal protozoan disease of dogs. J Am Vet Med Assoc 1988;192:1269–1285.

Dubey JP, Lindsay DS, Anderson ML, et al. Induced transplacental transmission of *Neospora caninum* in cattle. J Am Vet Med Assoc 1992;201:709–713.

Hay WH, Shell LG, Lindsay DS, et al. Diagnosis and treatment of *Neospora caninum* infection in a dog. J Am Vet Med Assoc 1990;197:87–89.

Hoskins JD, Bunge MM, Dubey JP, et al. Disseminated infection with *Neospora caninum* in a ten-year-old dog. Cornell Vet 1991;81:329–334.

Lindsay DS, Dubey JP. *Neospora caninum* (Protozoa: Apicomplexa) infections in mice. J Parasitol 1989;75:772–779.

Lindsay DS, Dubey JP. Immunohistochemical diagnosis of *Neospora caninum* in tissue sections. Am J Vet Res 1989;50:1981–1983.

Thilsted JP, Dubey JP. Neosporosis-like abortions in a herd of dairy cattle. J Vet Diagn Invest 1989;1:205–209.

CARYOSPORA

Caryospora are coccidia that are of little known importance to domestic animals; however, infection has been documented in dogs (Dubey et al., 1990). These coccidia have a complicated life cycle in which asexual and sexual cycles may occur in both the primary (definitive) and secondary (intermediate) hosts. The primary hosts are either reptiles or raptors in which a coccidian life cycle occurs in the intestinal tract leading to production of oocysts. Sporulated oocysts contain a single sporocyst with eight sporozoites. Ingestion of sporulated oocysts by the primary host results in repetition of the intestinal cycle. However, upon ingestion of sporulated oocysts by secondary hosts, which for most species of *Caryospora* are rodents, the sporozoites enter tissues and initiate schizogony as well as gametogony with production of oocysts that sporulate. Sporozoites released in tissue, in turn, develop into a stage termed a caryocyst, a form containing a single sporozoite. The most usual tissue site in the secondary host is the dermis or tongue. Upon ingestion of caryocyst-containing tissue by another secondary host this tissue cycle can be repeated or, when ingested by primary hosts, the intestinal cycle can be repeated. Thus, the tissue phase in secondary hosts can be perpetuated without the need of the definitive host, a situation analogous to what can occur in *Toxoplasma*. In the report of *Caryospora* infection in dogs, the disease was characterized by pyogranulomatous dermatitis and lymphadenitis with the presence of schizonts, macrogamonts and microgamonts, unsporu-

lated and sporulated oocysts, and numerous caryocysts. The occurrence of oocysts and the unique unicellular caryocysts allows differentiation from other tissue coccidia.

References

Dubey JP, et al. *Caryospora*-associated dermatitis in dogs. J Parasitol 1990;76:552–556.

Sundermann CA, Lindsay DS. Ultrastructure of in vivo-produced caryocysts containing the coccidian *Caryospora bigenetica* (Apicomplexa: Eimeriidae). J Protozool 1989;36:81–86.

Lindsay DS, Sundermann CA. Recent advances in the biology of the coccidian genus *Caryospora*. J Vet Parasitol 1989;3:1–5.

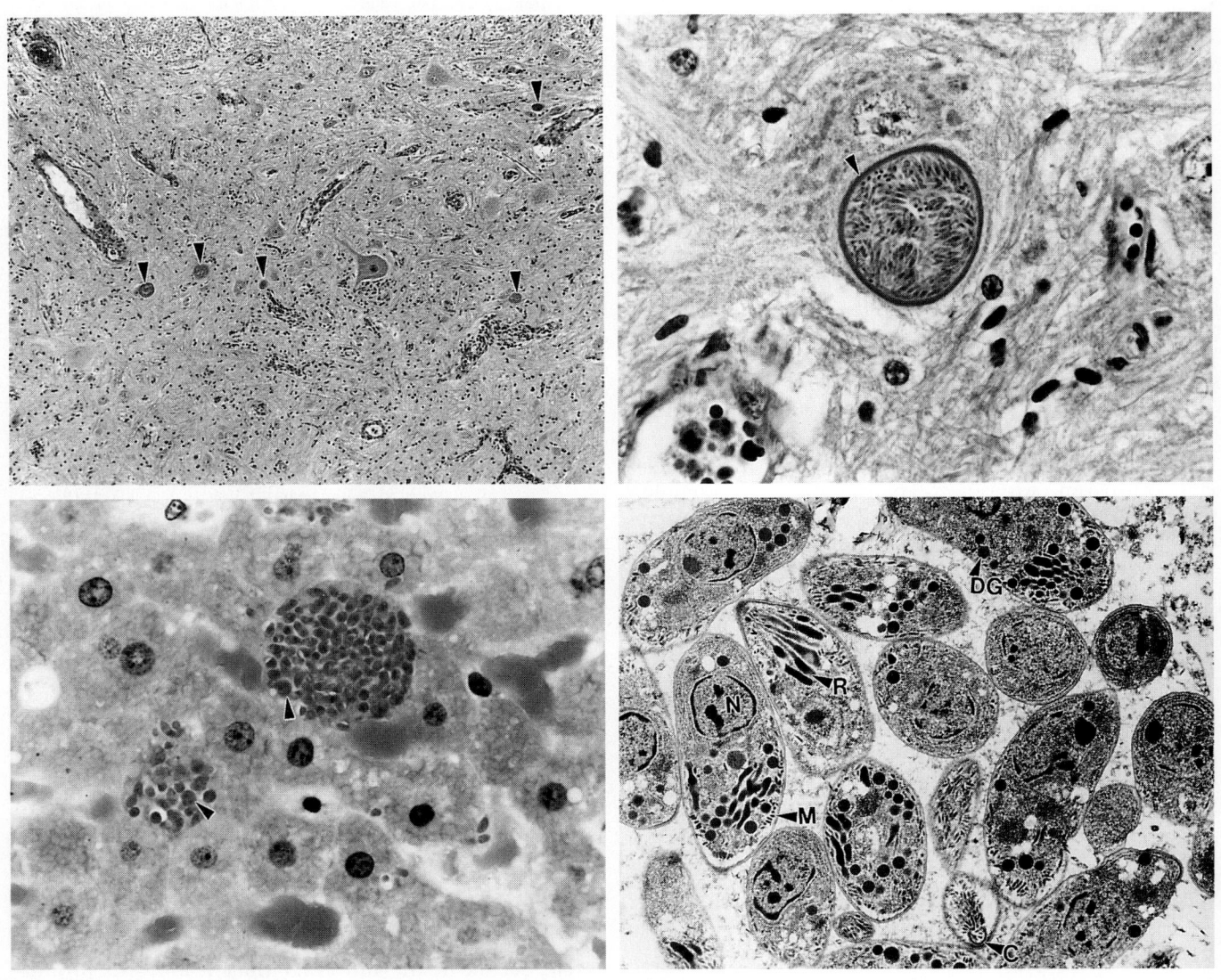

FIG. 12-8 *Neospora caninum.* **A.** Induced myelitis in spinal cord of a calf. Four tissue cysts (arrowheads) are present (hematoxylin and eosin stain, ×75). **B.** Tissue cyst in a neuron in the spinal cord of a naturally infected calf. Note the cyst wall (arrowhead) is thicker than the enclosed bradyzoites (hematoxylin and eosin stain, ×750). **C.** Numerous tachyzoites in hepatocytes of an experimentally infected rat. Note that numerous dividing tachyzoites (arrowheads) are larger than nondividing tachyzoites (hematoxylin and eosin stain, ×750). **D.** Transmission electron micrograph of a group of *Neospora caninum* tachyzoites in the spinal cord of a naturally infected dog. Although the host tissue is autolysed, parasite structures are preserved. Note several longitudinally cut tachyzoites with numerous rhoptries (R), micronames (M) located perpendicular to plasmalemma, a conoid (C), dense granules (DG), and the nucleus (N) (×13,000). (Courtesy of Dr. CP Dubey, Agricultural Research Service, USDA, Beltsville, MD)

SARCOSPORIDIOSIS

Tiny tubular cysts filled with crescentic bodies have been recognized for over a century as extremely common within skeletal and cardiac muscle fibers of aquatic birds and most mammals, particularly herbivora. *Sarcocystis* spp. were once considered of little pathologic significance; however, they are now recognized as important pathogens which may cause encephalitis, generalized disease, and abortion. They were first described by Miescher in 1843 in the musculature of a house mouse and were later called "Miescher's bodies, sacs, or tubules." Their classification, life cycle, source of infection, and significance were, however, a complete mystery until Rommel et al. (1972), Heydorn and Rommel (1972), Fayer and Johnson (1974), and Ruiz and Frenkel (1976) demonstrated that the parasitic cysts in muscle represent intermediate stages of intestinal coccidia, and that the life cycle is similar to that of Toxoplasma (Fig. 12-8). They are currently classified as Protozoa in the class Sporozoasida, family Sarcocystidae.

Only a few sarcosporidia have been studied in any detail and correlated with specific intestinal coccidia.

Over the years, numerous species names have been given to members of the genus *Sarcocystis*, and various classification systems have been proposed. For the most part, the proliferating or encysted organisms look identical, and techniques that allow differentiation in tissue section are not available, making species identification ordinarily not possible. Of special interest is another type found in the tongue, esophagus, and occasionally other muscles of sheep. This type, called *Balbiania gigantea*, forms quite large, grossly visible, multinucleated saccules containing a fibrillar network within which myriads of crescentic spores are found. A partial listing of those species affecting domestic animals is given in Table 12-4.

Quiescent sarcocysts are encountered in myofibers in many other species, usually as incidental findings. This is also true of dogs and cats, which ordinarily are definitive hosts for various species of *Sarcocystis*. Generalized infection with extensive proliferation of merozo-

TABLE 12-4 **Nomenclature of Some *Sarcocystis* Species**[a]

Species[b]	Host Intermediate	Host Definitive	Comments
S. hirsuta (S. bovifelis)	Bovine	Cat	Thick-walled cyst (6.0 μm) Low pathogenicity
S. cruzi (S. bovicanis)	Bovine	Canidae	Thin-walled cyst (0.5 μm) Highly pathogenic
S. hominis (S. bovihominis)	Bovine	Man, monkey	Thick-walled cyst (5.9 μm) Low pathogenicity
S. tenella (S. ovifelis)	Sheep	Cat	Thin-walled cyst Low pathogenicity
S. ovicanis	Sheep	Dog	Thick-walled cyst, radially striated Pathogenic
S. gigantea (Balbiani gigantea)	Sheep	Cat	Very large
S. bertrami (S. equicanis)	Horse	Dog	Thin-walled cyst
S. fayeri	Horse	Dog	Thin-walled cyst
S. canis	Dog	?	Disseminated disease in dogs
S. neurona	Horse	?	Associated with meningoencephalitis in horses
S. miescheriana (S. suicanis)	Pig	Dog	
S. porcifelis (S. suifelis)	Pig	Cat	Pathogenic
S. suihominis	Pig	Man	
S. orientalis	Goat	?	
S. capracanis	Goat	Dog	Can cause disseminated disease in goats
S. muris	Mouse	Cat	

[a] Based on Dubey, 1977.
[b] Former name in parenthesis.

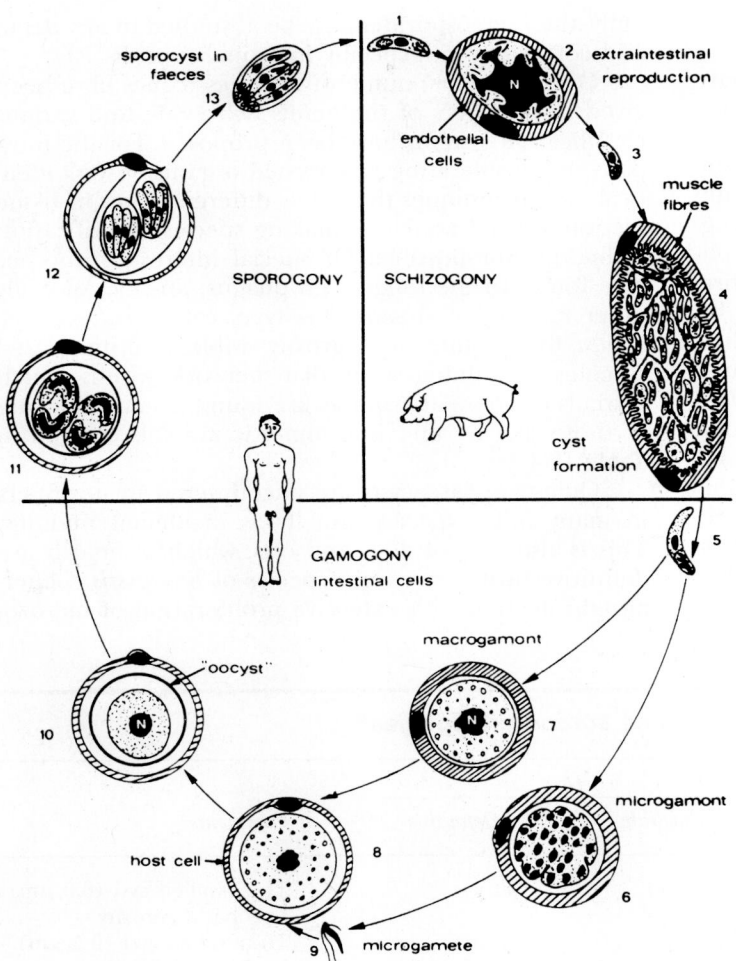

FIG. 12-9 Diagrammatic representation of the life cycle of *Sarcocystis suihominis*. (Courtesy of Dr. J. K. Frenkel and Zeitschrift for Parasitenkunde.)

ites leading to necrosis and inflammation in many different organs is recognized as an important form of sarcosporidiosis in animals.

Life cycle

Sarcocystis has an obligatory two-host life cycle as depicted in Figs. 12-3 and 12-9. Following ingestion of sporulated oocysts by an intermediate host, released sporozoites invade beyond the intestinal tract and first multiply by endopolygony in endothelial cells of arteries into groups of merozoites (first-generation meronts). The multiplication by endopolygony causes a rosette of merozoites, a distinguishing feature from other Sarcocystidae. Released merozoites undergo a second cycle in capillary endothelium in many tissues, forming second generation meronts whose released merozoites then parasitize circulating mononuclear cells, undergo endodyogeny (division in two) and are freed to enter type I and type II myofibers of skeletal muscle or heart, where the metrocytes divide into large numbers of bradyzoites forming the typical sarcocyst. The cycle is completed when the definitive host ingests muscle and released bradyzoites develop directly into micro- and

macrogamonts which, in turn, form oocysts to be released in the feces as infective sporulated oocysts. The sporulated oocysts of *Sarcocystis* are identical to those of *Isospora* with two sporocysts each containing four sporozoites. Variations in morphology, tissue distribution, and pathogenicity for certain *Sarcosporidia* spp. have been described.

The final hosts for many species of *Sarcocystis* have not been identified. Both cats and dogs have been identified as final hosts for bovine, ovine, porcine, and equine sarcosporidia. The intestinal stage in dogs and cats was formerly called *Isospora bigemina*. Humans are hosts for the sexual stages of sarcosporidia of bovines and swine. The intestinal stage in humans was previously called *Isospora hominis*. Based on the two hosts involved in the life cycles of sarcosporidia, new nomenclature has been proposed. Table 12-4 lists the nomenclature presented by Dubey (1977).

The sarcocysts within muscle fibers are variable in size but usually become slightly wider than a muscle fiber and several times longer than their width. The wall of the cyst appears clear or hyaline and may have a diagonally laminated structure. Often tiny strands or septae extend from the wall, which divide the cyst into tiny subcompartments in which the bradyzoites lay. The bradyzoites are strongly basophilic and elliptical or banana-shaped, each measuring about 4 by 8 μ. Often degeneration occurs in the centers of larger sarcocysts.

Lesions

In most examples, sarcocysts are encountered distorting myofibers of the heart or skeletal muscle without any inflammatory reaction. Purkinje fibers may also be affected, but whether this has any effect on the conduction system is not known. Smooth muscle is not affected. These mature sarcocysts, filled with their bradyzoites, represent the final stage in the life cycle, awaiting ingestion by the definitive host, and are more of an incidental finding than of pathologic significance. On occasion, rupture of a sarcocyst stimulates an inflammatory reaction which may be granulomatous in nature. More often than not, no clinical sign or lesion precedes their maturation.

Sarcosporidiosis can, however, lead to significantly more serious disease and clinical signs during the initial events of its cycle in the intermediate host. If infection is heavy, the multiplication of merozoites in endothelial cells as well as invasion and proliferation in parenchymal cells, including neurons and myocardial fibers, has been associated with fever, anemia, thrombosis, hemorrhage, and even death. This results from the extensive proliferation of merozoites leading to arteritis and capillary damage, tissue necrosis and inflammatory reactions. The organisms have a particular predilection for the vascular tree of the central nervous system where they may cause encephalitis, but pneumonia, hepatitis, dermatitis, polymyositis, and necrotizing and inflammatory lesions in other organs and tissues can be encountered (Figs. 12-10, 12-11).

Sarcocystis is also a recognized cause of abortion in cattle, sheep, goats, and pigs. Extensive multiplication of merozoites in endothelial cells throughout tissues of the fetus and within the placenta lead to fetal death and expulsion. The organisms are associated with vasculitis and necrosis of affected tissues which can include most organs, but especially the brain. The aborting cows may be otherwise normal.

Certain cases of eosinophilic myositis in the bovine have been attributed to sarcosporidiosis, but this interpretation is believed to be based upon insufficient evidence. Although Sarcocystis may be present in moderate numbers in muscles affected with eosinophilic myositis, it is rare that the lesions and parasites can be topographically related and no changes are evident in the organisms. The more valid conclusion is that eosinophilic myositis of unknown etiology may occur in skeletal muscle already affected with sarcosporidiosis.

Sarcocysts in tissue sections of skeletal or cardiac muscle are quite distinctive and usually do not pose a diagnostic problem. Distinguishing characteristics of these cysts are given in Table 12-4. Extensive proliferation of merozoites prior to their encystment in muscle, however, must be differentiated from diseases caused by other members of the family Sarcocystidae, particularly Toxoplasma, Neospora, and Caryospora. Key points include: multiplication of Sarcosporidia merozoites is restricted to endothelial cells; multiplication occurs by endopolygeny, giving rise to a rosette appearance; Sarcosporidia merozoites lack rhoptries and at this stage lay directly in the cytoplasm of the affected cell, not within a parasitophorous vacuole (Table 12-4). Immunologic staining techniques may be required for positive identification.

References

Barrows PL, Prestwood AK, Green CE. Experimental Sarcocystis suicanis infections: disease in growing pigs. Am J Vet Res 1982;43:1409–1412.

Colwell DD, Mahrt JL. Development of Sarcocystis alceslatrans in the small intestine of dogs. Am J Vet Res 1983;44:1813–1818.

Dubey JP. A review of sarcocystis of domestic animals and of other coccidia of cats and dogs. J Am Vet Med Assoc 1976;169:1061–1078.

Dubey JP. Toxoplasma, Hammondia, Besnoitia, Sarcocystis, and other tissue cyst-forming coccidia of man and animals. In: Kreier JP, ed. Parasitic protozoa. Vol. III. Gregarines, haemogregarines, coccidia, plasmodia, and haemoproteids. New York: Academic Press, 1977;101–237.

Dubey JP. [1] Coyote as a final host for Sarcocystis species of goats, sheep, cattle, elk, bison, and moose in Montana. [2] Sarcocystis species in moose (Alces alces), bison (Bison bison), and pronghorn (Antilocapra americana) in Montana. Am J Vet Res 1980;41:1227–1229, 2063–2065.

Dubey JP. Clinical sarcocystosis in calves fed Sarcocystis hirsuta sporocysts from cats. Vet Pathol 1983;20:90–98.

Dubey JP, Bergeron JA. Sarcocystis as a cause of placentitis and abortion in cattle. Vet Pathol 1982;19:315–318.

Dubey JP, Speer CA. Sarcocystis infections in mule deer (Odocoileus hemionus) in Montana and the descriptions of three new species. Am J Vet Res 1986;47:1052–1055.

Dubey JP, Speer CA. Sarcocystis canis n. sp. (Apicomplexa: Sarcocystidae), the etiologic agent of generalized coccidiosis in dogs. J Parasitol 1991;77:522–527.

Dubey JP, Hartley WJ, Badman RT. Fatal perinatal sarcocystosis in a lamb. J Parasitol 1989;75:980–982.

Dubey JP, Leek RG, Fayer R. Prevalence, transmission, and pathogenicity of Sarcocystis gigantea of sheep. J Am Vet Med Assoc 1986;188:151–154.

Dubey JP, Perry A, Kennedy MJ. Encephalitis caused by a Sarcocystis-like organism in a steer. J Am Vet Med Assoc 1987;191:231–232.

Dubey JP, Udtujan RM, Cannon L, et al. Condemnation of beef because of Sarcocystis hirsuta infection. J Am Vet Med Assoc 1990;196:1095–1096.

Dubey JP, Weisbrode SE, Speer CA, et al. Sarcocystosis in goats: clinical signs and pathologic and hematologic findings. J Am Vet Med Assoc 1981;178:683–699.

Dubey JP, et al. Sarcocystis neurona n. sp. (Protozoa: Apicomplexa), the etiologic agent of equine protozoal myeloencephalitis. J Parasitol 1991a;77:212–218.

Dubey JP, et al. Sarcocystosis-associated clinical encephalitis in a golden eagle (Aquila chrysaetos). J Zoo Wildl Med 1991b;22:233–236.

Edwards JF, Ficken MD, Luttgen PJ, et al. Disseminated sarcocystosis in a cat with lymphosarcoma. J Am Vet Med Assoc 1988;193:831–832.

Fayer R. Development of Sarcocystis fusiformis in the small intestine of a dog. J Parasitol 1974;60:660–665.

Fayer R, Johnson AJ. Development of Sarcocystis fusiformis in calves infected with sporocysts from dogs. J Parasitol 1973;59:1135–1137.

Fayer R, Johnson AJ. Sarcocystis fusiformis: development of cysts in calves infected with sporocysts from dogs. Proc Helminth Soc 1974;41:105–108.

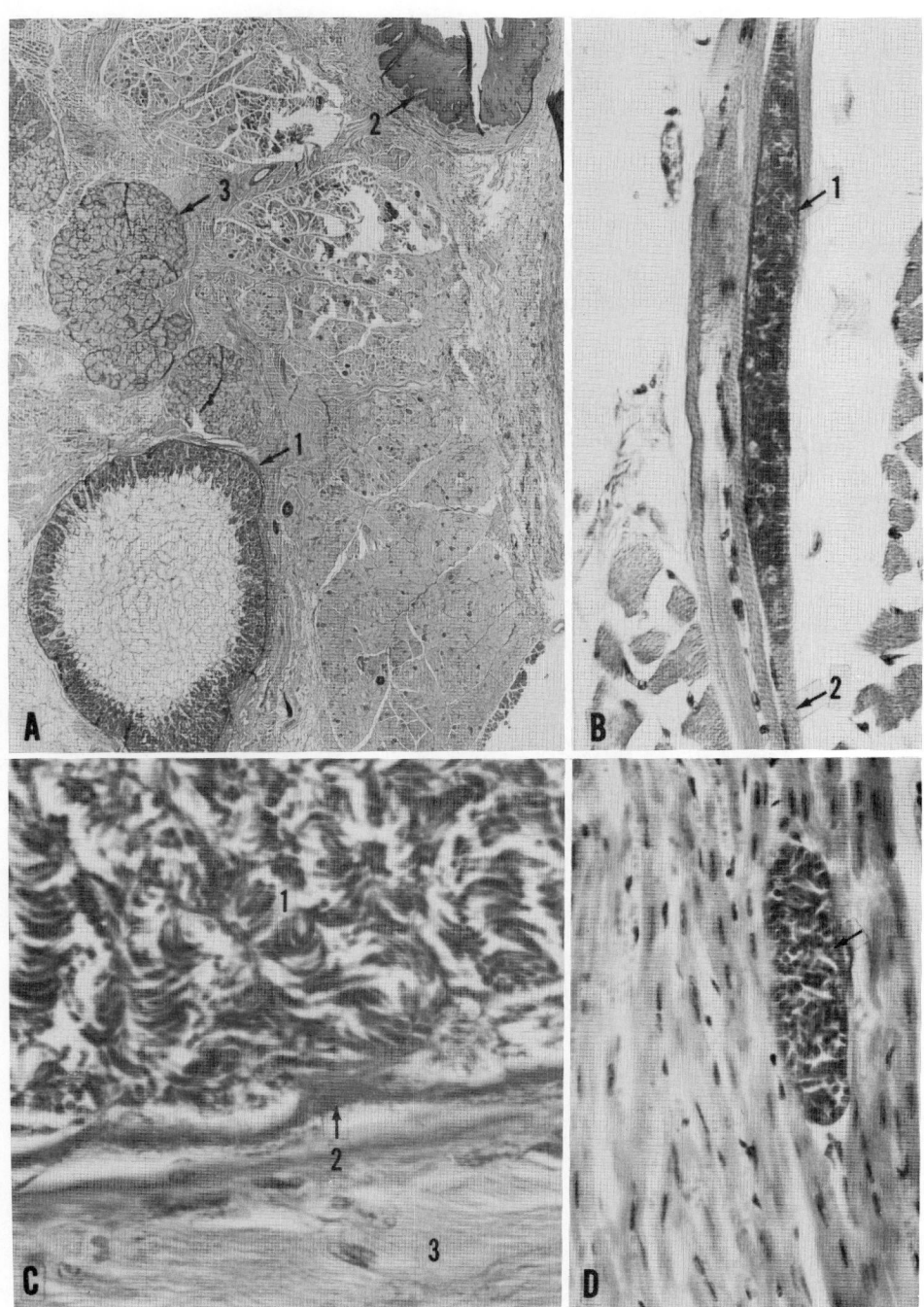

FIG. 12-10 Sarcosporidiosis. **A.** *Balbiania (sarcocystis) gigantea* (1) in the tongue of a sheep (×15); lingual epithelium (2), and lingual salivary glands (3). **B.** *Sarcocystis blanchardi:* (1) in the tongue of a cow (×330). (2) Note the muscle bundle contains the organism. **C.** Higher magnification of organisms in A (×650). Note (1) spores, (2) cyst wall, and (3) muscle fibers. (Courtesy of Armed Forces Institute of Pathology; contributor: Dr. C. L. Davis.) **D.** *Sarcocystis blanchardi* in the myocardium of a cow (×330).

Fayer R. Multiplication of *Sarcocystis bovicanis* in the bovine bloodstream. J Parasitol 1979;65:980–982.

Fayer R, Prasse KW. Hematology of experimental acute *Sarcocystis bovicanis* infection in calves: I. Cellular and serologic changes. Vet Pathol 1981;18:351–357.

Ford GE. Prey-predator transmission in the epizootiology of ovine sarcosporidiosis. Aust Vet J 1974;50:38–39.

Frelier PF, Lewis RM. Hematologic and coagulation abnormalities in acute bovine sarcocystosis. Am J Vet Res 1984;45:40–48.

Frelier P, Mayhew IG, Fayer R, et al. *Sarcocystosis:* a clinical outbreak in dairy calves. Science 1977;195:1341–1342.

Frenkel JK, Heydorn AO, Mehlhorn H, et al. Sarcocystinae: *Nomina dubia* and available names. Z Parasitenkd 1979;58:115–139.

Gasbarre LC, Suter P, Fayer R. Humoral and cellular immune responses in cattle and sheep inoculated with *Sarcocystis*. Am J Vet Res 1984;45:1592–1596.

Hong CB, Giles RC Jr, Newman LE, et al. Sarcocystosis in an aborted bovine fetus. J Am Vet Med Assoc 1982;181:585–588.

Jolley WR, Jensen R, Hancock HA, et al. Encephalitic sarcocystosis in a newborn calf. Am J Vet Res 1983;44:1908–1911.

Kimura T, Ito J, Suzuki M, et al. *Sarcocystis* found in the skeletal muscle of common squirrel monkeys. Primates 1987;28:247–255.

Kirkpatrick CE, Dubey JP, Goldschmidt MH, et al. *Sarcocystis* sp. in muscles of domestic cats. Vet Pathol 1986;23:88–90.

Markus MB, Killick-Kendrick R, Garnham PCC. The coccidial nature and life cycle of *Sarcocystis*. J Trop Med Hyg 1974;77:248–259.

Miescher F. Ueber Eigenthumliche Schlauche in den Muskeln einer Hausmaus. Ber ü d Verhandl Naturforsch Gesellsch Basel 1843;5:198–203.

Powell EC, Pezeshkpour G, Dubey JP, et al. Types of myofibers parasitized in experimentally induced infections with *Sarcocystis cruzi* and *Sarcocystis capracanis*. Am J Vet Res 1986;47:514–517.

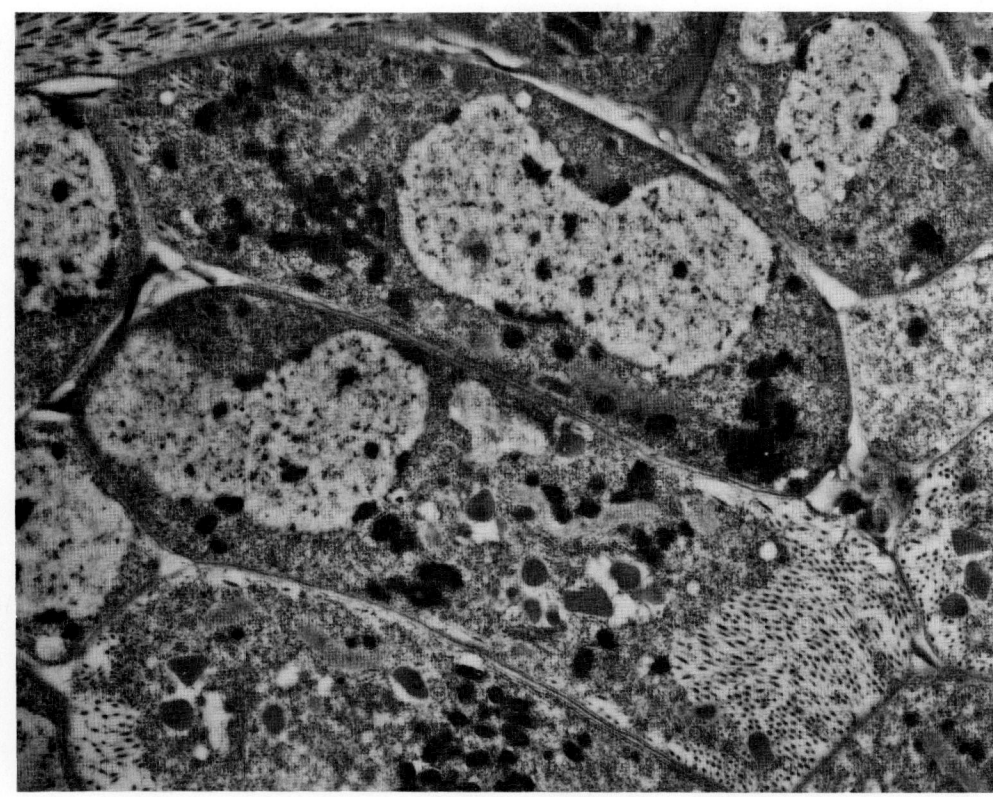

FIG. 12-11 *Sarcocystis fusiformis.* Electron micrograph (×18,000). (Courtesy of Dr. Charles F. Simpson and The Journal of Parasitology.)

Prasse KW, Fayer R. Hematology of experimental acute *Sarcocystis bovicanis* infection in calves. II. Serum biochemistry and hemostasis studies. Vet Pathol 1981;18:358–367.

Ruiz A, Frenkel JK. Recognition of cyclic transmission of *Sarcocystis muris* by cats. J Infect Dis 1976;133:409–418.

Schmitz JA, Wolf WW. Spontaneous fatal sarcocystosis in a calf. Vet Pathol 1977;14:527–531.

Simpson CF. Electron microscopy of *Sarcocystis fusiformis.* J Parasitol 1966;52:607–613.

FRENKELIA

Members of the genus *Frenkelia* are protozoa similar to sarcosporidia and classified in the same family. Sexual reproduction in the final host (various predatory birds) occurs in intestinal epithelium. Upon ingestion of sporulated oocysts (sporocyst) by intermediate hosts, the organisms undergo schizogony in hepatocytes and Kupffer's cells, and subsequently form extremely large, multilobulated cysts filled with bradyzoites in the central nervous system (Fig. 12-12). They were previously termed M-organisms or *Toxoplasma microti.* The cysts have been observed in voles, meadow mice (*Microtus* sp.), lemmings, muskrats, and rats. Usually there is no reaction to their presence, but granulomatous type inflammation is occasionally encountered, presumably after rupture of a cyst. Degeneration in the center of the cysts is not unusual.

References

Hayden DW, King NW, Murthy ASK. Spontaneous *Frenkelia* infection in a laboratory reared rat. Vet Pathol 1976;13:337–342.

Kennedy MJ, Frelier PF. *Frenkelia* sp. from the brain of a porcupine (*Erethizon dorsatum*) from Alberta, Canada. J Wildl Dis 1986; 22:112–114.

Lindsay DS, Blagburn BL. *Caryospora uptoni* and *Frenkelia* sp.-like coccidial infections in red-tailed hawks (*Buteo borealis*). J Wildl Dis 1989;25:407–409.

Lindsay DS, Ambrus SI, Blagburn BL. *Frenkelia* sp.-like infection in the small intestine of a red-tailed hawk. J Wildl Dis 1987;23: 677–679.

BESNOITIOSIS

A chronic debilitating and occasionally fatal disease with cutaneous and systemic manifestations in cattle has been described from South Africa and called besnoitiosis after the cyst-forming protozoa, *Besnoitia besnoiti.*

Earlier names for the organism, *Globidium besnoiti,* and the disease, "globidiosis," appear to have been based on erroneous data and therefore should be abandoned. *B. besnoiti* has also been found in the blue wildebeest (*Connochaetes taurinus*), impala (*Aepyceros melampus*), and a kudu (*Tragelaphus strepsiceros*) in the Transvaal of South Africa. Rabbits are susceptible to experimental infection, develop cutaneous lesions similar to those of cattle, and therefore serve as a good experimental model.

Besnoitia organisms found in a number of other animal species have been given specific names. These include: *B. bennetti,* horses and burros; *B. tarandi,* reindeer and caribou; *B. jellisoni,* white-footed mice in Idaho and kangaroo rats in Utah; and *B. darlingi,* lizards in Panama. Another species, *B. wallacei,* experimentally affects mice and rats. Similar organisms have

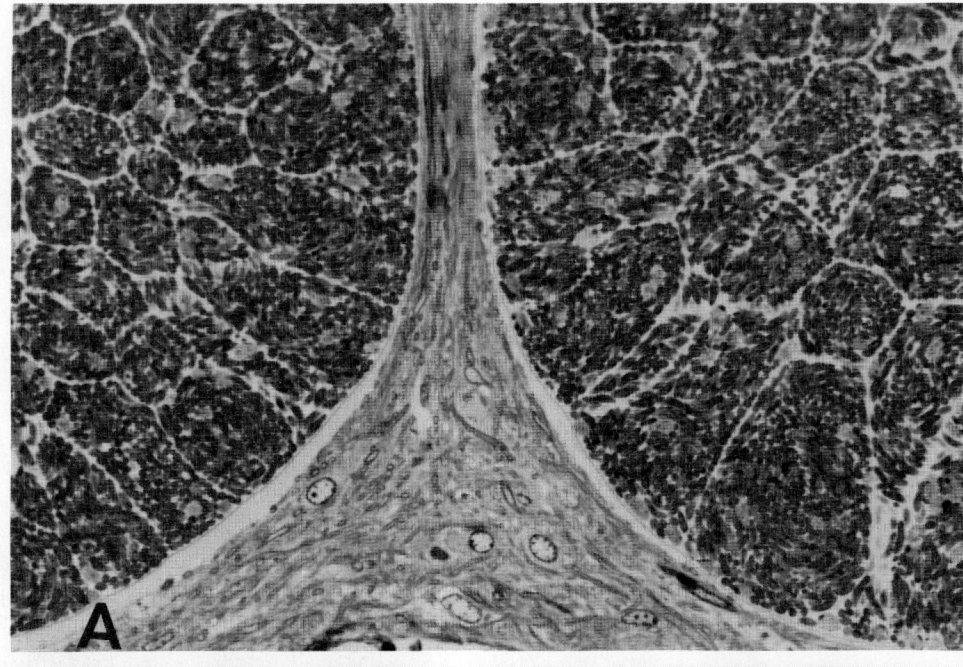

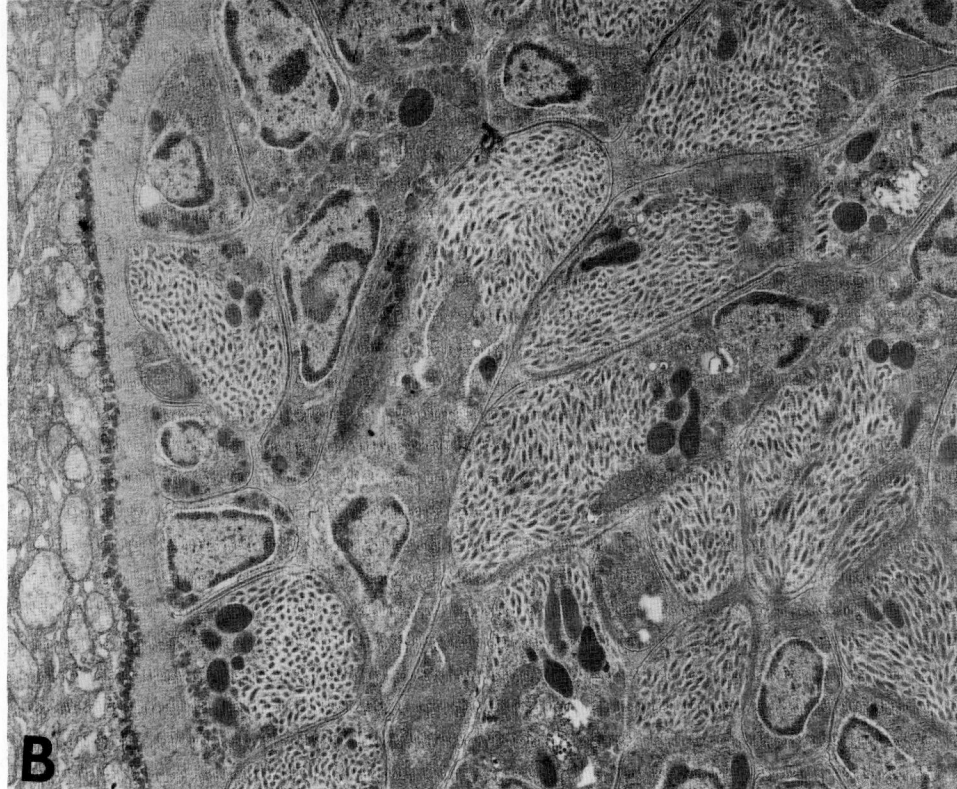

FIG. 12-12 *Frenkelia* sp. in brain of a rat. **A.** Metrocyst containing numerous crescent-shaped bradyzoites separated by fine, interlacing septae. (Courtesy of Dr. N. W. King. Jr. and Veterinary Pathology.) **B.** Ultrastructure of bradyzoites of *Frenkelia*. (Courtesy of Dr. N. W. King, Jr.)

been described in so-called "Bangkok hemorrhagic disease" of chickens. An organism resembling *Besnoitia*, and which is characterized by very large schizonts, is occasionally encountered in the mucosa of the abomasum and duodenum of sheep and goats. It has been termed *Globidium gilruthi* or *Eimeria gilruthi;* however, only the giant schizont stage has been recognized. Although minor differences have been detected in these

Besnoitia, it is not known whether they actually represent different species.

Life cycle

Besnoitia are classified in the family Sarcocystidae, as is the genus *Toxoplasma* and the genus *Hammondia*. It has a two-host life cycle (Fig. 12-13), with sexual reproduc-

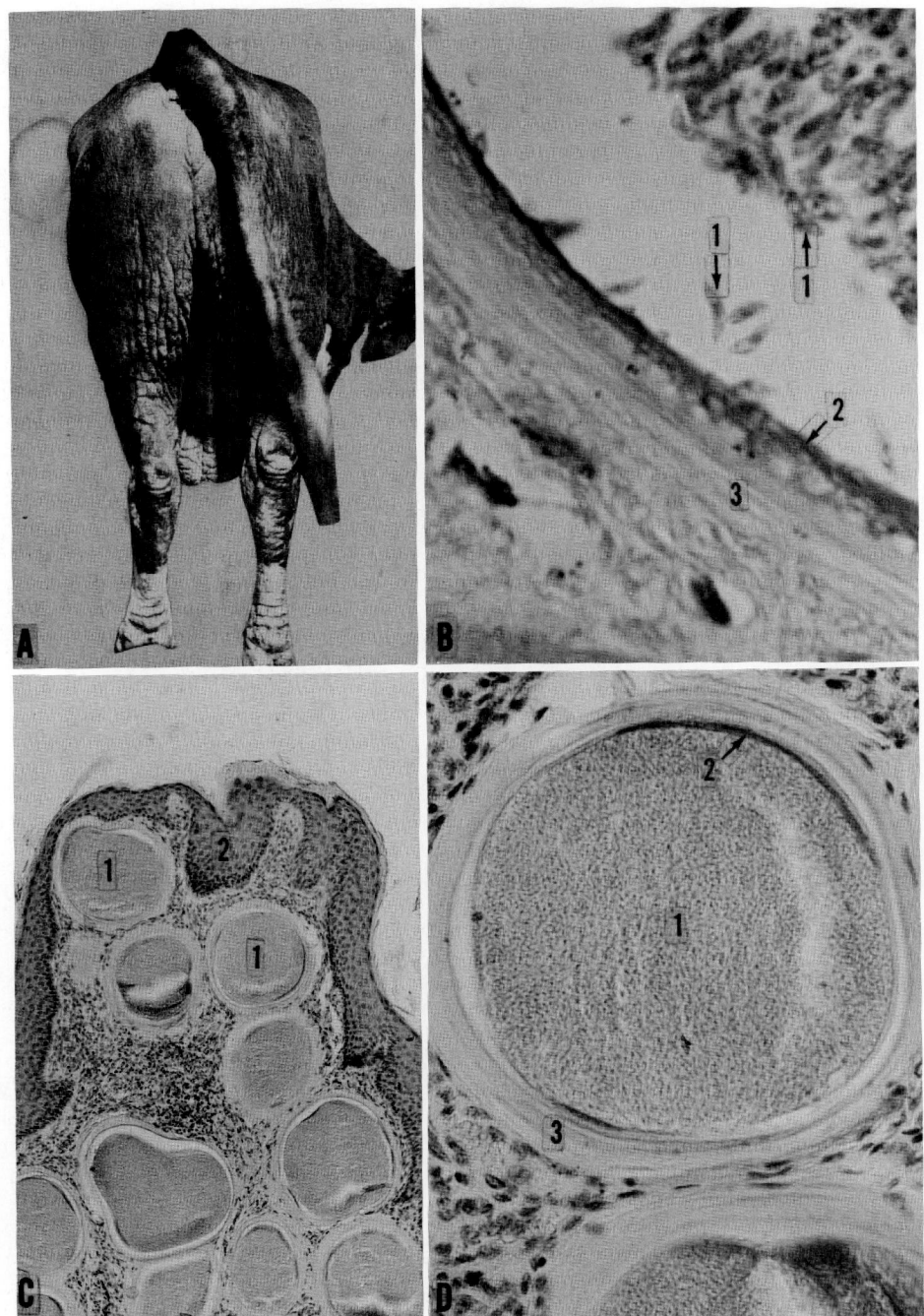

FIG.   12-13 Besnoitiosis. **A.**
Thickened rugose skin of thigh,
legs, and scrotum of Hereford bull
in South Africa. **B.** High magnification (×1300) of: (1) the wall of a
cyst containing spores, (2) acellular
wall, and (3) a dense, fibrous capsule. From the dermis of a burro.
(Contributor: Col. J. H. Rust, III.)
C. Section of skin of the bull shown
in A (×75). Note: (1) cysts in dermis, (2) covered by acanthotic epidermis. **D.** Higher magnification
(×330) of C: (1) Cyst filled with
spores, (2) large nucleus flattened
against cyst wall, and (3) fibrous
component of the wall. (Courtesy of
Armed Forces Institute of Pathology;
contributor: Dr. W. S. Monlux.)

tion occurring in the intestinal tract of the final host,
leading to production of oocysts. Cats serve as the definitive hosts for *Besnoitia besnoiti* and *B. wallacei.* The
definitive hosts for the other species are unknown.
Upon ingestion of oocysts by intermediate hosts, the
organisms invade many cell types, producing small
groups of tachyzoites indistinguishable from *Toxoplasma.* This acute infection can be severe and lead
to death, but it usually goes unrecognized. Tachyzoites
subsequently invade fibroblasts and produce large cysts
filled with bradyzoites, the infectious stage for the final
host. The cysts are large, often up to 2 mm in diameter,

and hence may be visible to the unaided eye (Fig. 12-
14).

The organisms in cattle, horses, and burros are encountered most frequently in the cyst form, at which
stage they have an unmistakable appearance. The cysts
are smoothly spherical in well-fixed tissues, 0.1–0.5 mm
in diameter, and are surrounded by a dense, uniformly
eosinophilic wall which is homogeneous or concentrically laminated, and which appears to come from host
tissue. Inside this wall are one or more giant ovoid nuclei which become compressed against the periphery by
the enlarging mass of spores within. These giant nuclei

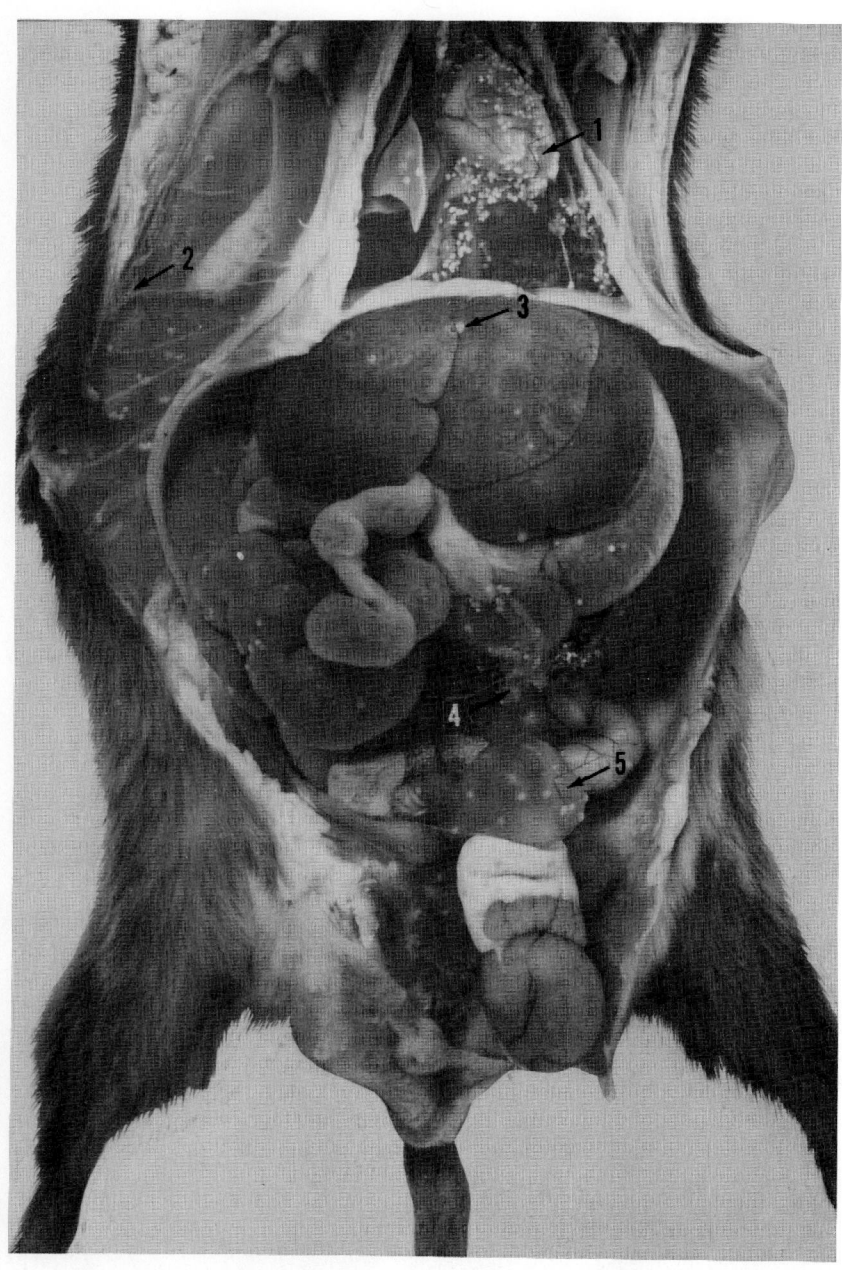

FIG. 12-14 *Besnoitia jellisoni* in: (1) pleura and pericardium, (2) subcutis, (3) serosa of the liver, (4) mesentery, and (5) urinary bladder of a deer mouse (*Peromyscus* sp.; photograph courtesy of Dr. W. J. Hadlow.)

are surrounded by a narrow band of cytoplasm which encircles the inner wall and sends one or more narrow dividing septa across the cyst. The inner contents are made up of many tiny crescentic spores, which in size and morphology are similar to *Toxoplasma.*

Lesions

The lesions in cattle and horses are closely related to the organisms, which may not only localize in the skin but may spread to all parts of the body. The cutaneous lesions are usually seen grossly as thickened, rugose, partially hairless areas of skin, particularly on legs, thighs, and scrotum. The microscopic picture is dominated by the large spherical cysts, which may occur in deeper areas and are frequently seen in the walls of small blood vessels. Invasion of the scrotum, epididymis, and testis, as well as upper gastrointestinal tract, is common and may be accompanied by a severe granulomatous tissue reaction, particularly when numerous spores are released into the tissue. In contrast, the mature cysts with their wide, hyaline wall are usually surrounded by little other inflammatory tissue reaction.

The lesions in antelopes appear to be limited to the presence of the cysts in the cardiovascular system. The intima of veins, such as the jugular and peripheral veins of limbs, is the site of predilection for the cysts, although some may be found in the muscularis or adventitia. In the impala, cysts are found especially in the walls of subcutaneous lymphatics. Some organisms may be found in the endocardium (McCully et al., 1966).

Diagnosis

The diagnosis is based upon demonstration of the organisms in tissue sections, which does not present a problem in the cyst stage. Extensive proliferation of tachyzoites prior to encystment, however, requires differentiation from other Sarcocystidae, especially *Toxoplasma*, *Neospora*, and *Sarcosporidia* (Table 12-3). Ultrastructurally, the tachyzoites of *Besnoitia* contain membrane-bound, spindle-shaped bodies with an electron-dense core, called enigmatic bodies, which are not present in other genera.

References

Bigalke RD, Naude TW. The diagnostic value of cysts in the scleral conjunctiva in bovine besnoitiosis. J S Afr Vet Med Assoc. 1962;33:2–27.

Bigalke RD, et al. The relationship between *Besnoitia* of antelopes and *Besnoitia besnoiti* (Marotel, 1912) of cattle. Bull Off Int Epizootol 1966;66:903–905.

Bigalke RD, et al. Studies on the relationship between *Besnoitia* of blue wildebeest and impala, and Besnoitia besnoiti of cattle. Onderstepoort J Vet Res 1967;34:7–28.

Binninger CE, McGuire TC. Atypical globidiosis in a lamb. J Am Vet Med Assoc 1967;151:606–608.

Bwangamoi O. *Besnoitiosis* and other skin diseases of cattle (*Bos indicus*) in Uganda. Am J Vet Res 1968;29:737743.

Campbell JG. Bangkok haemorrhagic disease of chickens: an unusual condition associated with an organism of uncertain taxonomy. J Pathol Bact 1954;68:423–429.

Fox MT, Higgins RJ, Brown ME, et al. A case of *Eimeria gilruthi* infection in a sheep in northern England. Vet Rec 1991;129:141–142.

Frenkel JK. Ocular lesions in hamsters with chronic *Toxoplasma* and *Besnoitia* infection. Am J Ophthalmol 1955;39:203–255.

Frenkel JK. Besnoitia wallacei of cats and rodents: with a reclassification of other cyst-forming isosporid coccidia. J Parasitol 1977;63:611–628.

Frenkel JK. Chronic besnoitiosis of golden hamsters (*Mesocricetus auratus*). Am J Pathol 1977;86:749–752.

Hadwen S. Cyst-forming protozoa in reindeer and caribou, and a sarcosporidian parasite of the seal (*Phoca richardi*). J Am Vet Med Assoc 1922;61:374–382.

Jellison WL. On the nomenclature of *Besnoitia besnoiti*, a protozoan parasite. Ann NY Acad Sci 1956;64:-270.

Jellison WL, Fullerton WJ, Parker H. Transmission of the protozoan *Besnoitia jellisoni* by ingestion. Ann NY Acad Sci 1956;64: 271–274.

Lane JG, Lucke VM, Wright AI. Parasitic laryngeal papillomatosis in a horse. Vet Rec 1986;119:591–593.

McCully RM, et al. Observations on besnoitia cysts in the cardiovascular system of some wild antelopes and domestic cattle. Onderstepoort J Vet Res 1966;33:245–275.

Neuman M. An outbreak of besnoitiosis in cattle. Refuah Vet 1962;19:106–110.

Pols JW. The artificial transmission of *Globidium besnoiti* Marotel, 1912, to cattle and rabbits. J S Afr Vet Med Assoc 1954;25:37–44.

Pols JW. Studies on bovine besnoitiosis with special reference to the aetiology. Onderstepoort J Vet Res 1960;28:265–356, Vet Bull 1426–61.

Pols JW. Preliminary notes on the behavior of *Globidium besnoiti* (Marotel, 1912) in the rabbit. J S Aft Vet Med Assoc 1954;25: 45–47.

Schulz KCA. A report on naturally acquired besnoitiosis in bovines with special reference to its pathology. J S Afr Vet Med Assoc 1960;31:21–35, Vet Bull 1427–61.

Terrell TG, Stookey JL. *Besnoitia bennetti* in two Mexican burros. Vet Pathol 1973;10:177–184.

Wallace GD, Frenkel JK. Besnoitia species (Protozoa, Sporozoa, Toxoplasmatidae): recognition of cyclic transmission by cats. Science 1975;188:369–371.

KLOSSIELLA

These coccidia localize in the convoluted tubules of the kidney. Among these parasites are: *Klossiella equi*, (Fig. 12-15) in horses, zebras, and asses (*Equidae*); *Eimeria truncata* in the goose; and *Klossiella cobayae* in the guinea pig. *Klossiella* has also been described in the kidneys of rats, bats, several South American and Australian marsupials, snakes, prosimians, and owls. Schizogony occurs in endothelial cells and epithelium of Bowman's capsule, releasing merozoites which infect tubular epithelial cells, where gametogenesis occurs. Oocytes are shed in the urine. Although these organisms destroy some renal epithelium, their total effect appears slight. Usually there are no clinical signs; the parasites are usually found incidentally at necropsy.

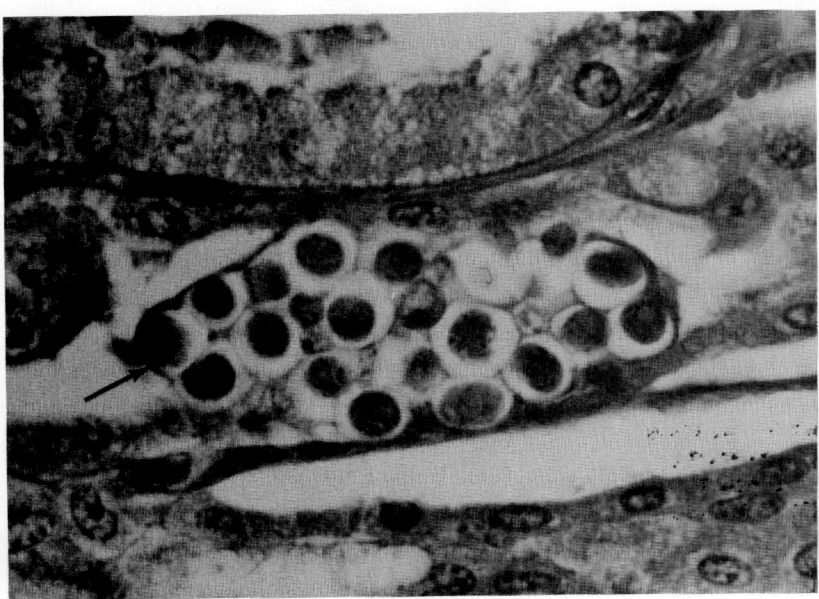

FIG. 12-15 *Klossiella equi* in convoluted renal tubules of a zebra. (Specimen courtesy of Dr. M. J. Eggert.)

References

Beemer AM, Kuttin ES, Birnbaum SC. Occurrence of *Klossiella* N. sp. in rats. Refuah Vet 1972;29:61–65.

Hartman HA. The protozoan parasite, *Klossiella* equi, in the Mexican burro. Am J Vet Res 1961;22:1126–1129.

Meshorer A. Interstitial nephritis in the spiny mouse *(Acomys cahirinus)* associated with *Klossiella* sp. infection. Lab Anim 1970;4: 227–232.

Mullin SW, Colley FC. *Eimeria* and *Klossia* spp. (Protozoa: Sporozoa) from wild mammals in Borneo. J Protozool 1972;19:406–408.

Pierce L. *Klossiella* infection of the guinea pig. J Exp Med 1916;23: 431–442.

Schoeb TR. *Klossiella* sp. infection in a galago. J Am Vet Med Assoc 1984;185:1381–1382.

Seibold HR, Thorsen RE. *Klossiella* equi, N. sp. (Protozoa-Klossielidae) from the kidney of an American jack. J Parasitol 1955;41: 285–288.

Seidelin H. *Klossiella* sp. in the kidney of a guinea pig. Ann Trop Med Parasitol 1941;8:553–564.

Smith T, Johnson HP. On a coccidium (*Klossiella muris,* gen. et. spec. Nov) parasitic in the renal epithelium of the mouse. J Exp Med 1902;6:303–316.

Vetterling JM, Thompson DE. *Klossiella* equi Baumann, 1946 (Sporozoa: Eucoccidia: Adeleina) from equids. J Parasitol 1972;58: 589–594.

Winter H, Watt D. *Klossiella hydromyos* n. sp. from the kidneys of an Australian water rat *(Hydromys chrysogaster).* Vet Pathol 1971;8: 222–231.

CRYPTOSPORIDIOSIS

Cryptosporidiosis, a disease of most domestic and wild animals, birds, fish, reptiles, and humans, is caused by members of the genus *Cryptosporidium*. First described as a parasitic protozoan of mice in 1907 by Tyzzer *(C. muris)*, cryptosporidia were not recognized as pathogens of any importance to humans or domestic animals until many decades later. *Cryptosporidia* are members of the phylum Apicomplexa, order Eucoccidiorida, and closely resemble the non-tissue cyst coccidia *Eimeria* and *Isospora*. In contrast to the coccidia, however, cryptosporidia are extremely small. Like coccidia, the organisms are located intracellularly, but are just beneath the cell membrane, giving the appearance that they are extracellular and attached to the microvillus border of parasitized cells. They have a typical coccidian life cycle of trophozoites, schizonts (or meronts) containing merozoites, macro- and microgametocytes, and oocysts, all of which are under 3 μm in diameter. Transmission is direct via sporulated oocysts that contain four sporozoites. In contrast to most coccidia, cryptosporidia also are not host-specific; however, some twenty different species have been described, most of which are named after the host from which they were recovered (e.g., *Cryptosporidium bovis* from cattle, *C. felis, C. muris*). Species identification, however, cannot be made from tissue section or simple examination of oocysts; therefore, most examples of disease due to *Cryptosporidium* are designated only as cryptosporidiosis (Fig. 12-16).

The majority of cryptosporidia of mammals parasitize intestinal epithelial cells, most usually of the distal small intestine, but also of the cecum and colon and occasionally bile ducts, trachea, and bronchi. Abomasal cryptosporidiosis has also been described in cattle. Various species of birds are susceptible to intestinal and gastric cryptosporidiosis, and to infection of the respira-

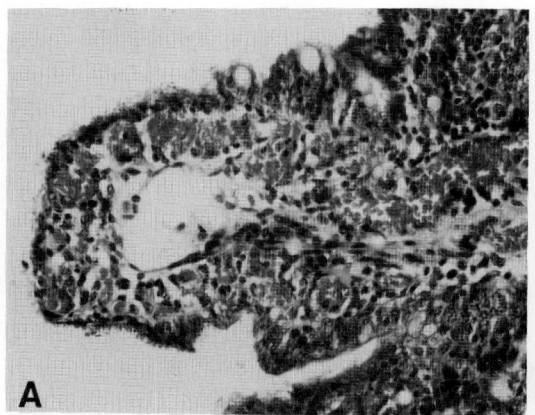
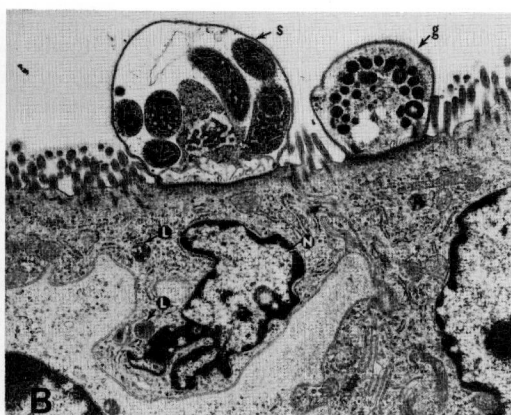
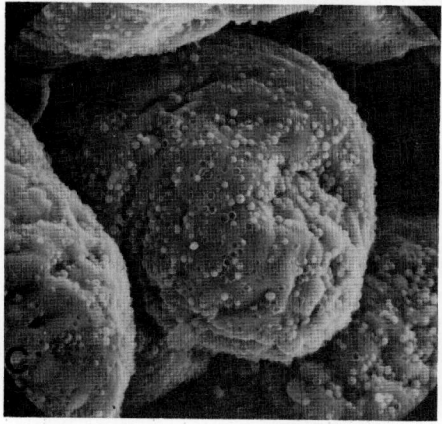

FIG. 12-16 Cryptosporidiosis in calves. **A.** Atrophic intestinal villus with numerous, barely discernible cryptosporidia adherent to the surface. **B.** Schizont (s) and gamete (g) in brush border of intestinal epithelium. **C.** Scanning electron micrograph of atrophic villus. Many cryptosporidia (white nodules) adherent to surface. Black circles are craters left when parasites leave surface or are rinsed off. (Courtesy of Dr. Harley W. Moon and Journal of the American Veterinary Medical Association.)

tory mucosa and the conjunctiva. In humans, the intestinal tract is also the most frequent site, but cryptosporidia have been identified in the respiratory tract as well. Cryptosporidiosis is often subclinical. Overt disease characterized by diarrhea is most frequent in young animals or in association with immunosuppressive disorders. The disease is of greatest importance in calves, lambs and laboratory animals.

Lesions

In tissue sections of small intestine or colon, the small, basophilic organisms are found embedded in microvilli of intestinal epithelial cells. Lesions may be minimal. Infected cells may be slightly more eosinophilic than normal, but extensive necrosis is not a feature of infection. There may be villous atrophy and fusion, dilatation of crypts and cellular infiltration of the lamina propria with lymphocytes and plasma cells and lesser numbers of neutrophils and eosinophils.

Diagnosis

Diagnosis in tissue section depends upon demonstration of the organism. The use of Giemsa stain and thin sections is helpful. Oocysts also are acid fast, a useful characteristic to aid identification in both tissue section and fecal flotation preparations. Phase-contrast microscopy also assists in identification of oocysts, which are brightly refractile in fecal flotations.

References

Anderson BC. Cryptosporidiosis: a review. J Am Vet Med Assoc 1982;180:1455–1457.

Anderson BC. Cryptosporidiosis in Idaho lambs: natural and experimental infections. J Am Vet Med Assoc 1982;181:151–152.

Anderson BC. Location of cryprosporidia: review of the literature and experimental infections in calves. Am J Vet Res 1984;45:1474–1477.

Anderson BC. Abomasal cryptosporidiosis in cattle. Vet Pathol 1987;24:235–238.

Angus KW. Cryptosporidiosis in domestic animals and humans. In Pract 1987;9:47–49.

Angus KW, Tzipori S, Gray EW. Intestinal lesions in specific-pathogen-free lambs associated with a *Cryptosporidium* from calves with diarrhea. Vet Pathol 1982;19:67–78.

Card CE, Perdrizet JA, Georgi ME, et al. Cryptosporidiosis associated with bacterial enteritis in a goat kid. J Am Vet Med Assoc 1987;191:69–70.

Carlson BL, Nielsen SW. Cryptosporidiosis in a raccoon. J Am Vet Med Assoc 1982;181:1405–1406.

Current WL, et al. Human cryptosporidiosis in immunocompetent and immunodeficient persons: studies of an outbreak and experimental transmission. N Engl J Med 1983;308:1252–1257.

Davis AJ, Jenkins SJ. Cryptosporidiosis and proliferative ileitis in a hamster. Vet Pathol 1986;23:632–633.

Dubey JP, Speer CA, Fayer R, eds. Cryptosporidiosis of Man and Animals. Boca Raton: CRC Press, 1990.

Fenwick BW. Cryprosporidiosis in a neonatal gazella. J Am Vet Med Assoc 1983;183:1331–1332.

Fukushima K, Helman RG. Cryptosporidiosis in a pup with distemper. Vet Pathol 1984;21:247–248.

Gibson SV, Wagner JE. Cryptosporidiosis in guinea pigs: a retrospective study. J Am Vet Med Assoc 1986;189:1033–1034.

Greene CE, Jacobs GJ, Prickett D. Intestinal malabsorption and cryptosporidiosis in an adult dog. J Am Vet Med Assoc 1990;197:365–367.

Hayes EB, et al. Large community outbreak of cryptosporidiosis due to contamination of a filtered public water supply. N Engl J Med 1989;320:1372–1376.

Klesius PH, Haynes TB, Malo LK. Infectivity of *Cryptosporidium* sp. isolated from wild mice for calves and mice. J Am Vet Med Assoc 1986;189:192–193.

Levine JF, Levy MG, Walker RL, et al. Cryptosporidiosis in veterinary students. J Am Vet Med Assoc 1988;193:1413–1414.

Lindsay DS, Blagburn BL, Hoerr FJ. Experimentally induced infections in turkeys with *Cryptosporidium baileyi* isolated from chickens. Am J Vet Res 1987;48:104–108.

Moon HW, Bemrick WJ. Fecal transmission of calf cryptosporidia between calves and pigs. Vet Pathol 1981;18:248–255.

Moon HW, Schwartz A, Welch MJ, et al. Experimental fecal transmission of human cryptosporidia to pigs, and attempted treatment with an ornithine decarboxylase inhibitor. Vet Pathol 1982;19:700–707.

Poonacha KB, Pippin C. Intestinal cryptosporidiosis in a cat. Vet Pathol 1982;19:708–710.

Rehg JE, Gigliotti F, Stokes DC. Cryptosporidiosis in ferrets. Lab Anim Sci 1988;38:155–158.

Sanford SE. Enteric cryptosporidial infection in pigs: 184 cases (1981–1985). J Am Vet Med Assoc 1987;190:695–698.

Sisk DB, Gosser HS, Styer EL, et al. Intestinal cryptosporidiosis in two pups. J Am Vet Med Assoc 1984;184:835–836.

Sundberg JP, Hill D, Ryan MJ. Cryprosporidiosis in a gray squirrel. J Am Vet Med Assoc 1982;181:1420–1422.

Turnwald GH, et al. Cryptosporidiosis associated with immunosuppression attributable to distemper in a pup. J Am Vet Med Assoc 1988;192:79–81.

Tzipori S, Angus KW, Gray EW, et al. Diarrhea in lambs experimentally infected with *Cryptosporidium* isolated from calves. Am J Vet Res 1981;42:1400–1404.

Wilson DW, Day PA, Brummer MEG. Diarrhea associated with *Cryptosporidium* spp. in juvenile macaques. Vet Pathol 1984;21:447–450.

Wilson RB, Holscher MA, Lyle SJ. Cryptosporidiosis in a pup. J Am Vet Med Assoc 1983;183:1005–1006.

Wolfson JS, et al. Cryptosporidiosis in immunocompetent patients. N Engl J Med 1985;312:1278–1282.

ENCEPHALITOZOONOSIS (NOSEMATOSIS)

Encephalitozoon cuniculi, a microsporidian protozoan best known as a cause of encephalitis and nephritis in rabbits, may also affect rats, mice, guinea pigs, monkeys, cats, dogs, wild carnivores, humans, and other species. Infection is most often subclinical, even in rabbits. At one time the organism was suggested to belong to the genus Nosema, a group of organisms which cause disease of bees, silkworms and other invertebrate species. The microsporidia are classified in a separate Phylum, Microspora. They are obligate intracellular parasites which lack mitochondria and have a coiled polar filament that is utilized to inject the parasite's sarcoplasm into the host's cells. *E. cuniculi* is the most important pathogen for animals; however, other species have recently emerged as meaningful opportunistic infections in humans, especially in immunocompromised individuals: *Enterocytozoon bieneusi* infects enterocytes leading to diarrhea; a *Pleistophora* sp. has been associated with myositis; and *Nosema corneum* is a cause of keratoconjunctivitis.

The infection is acquired by ingestion of spores excreted in urine. Ingestion of infected tissues containing spores is another potential source of infection. Transplacental infection of the fetus is also an important means of transmission. In dogs and blue foxes

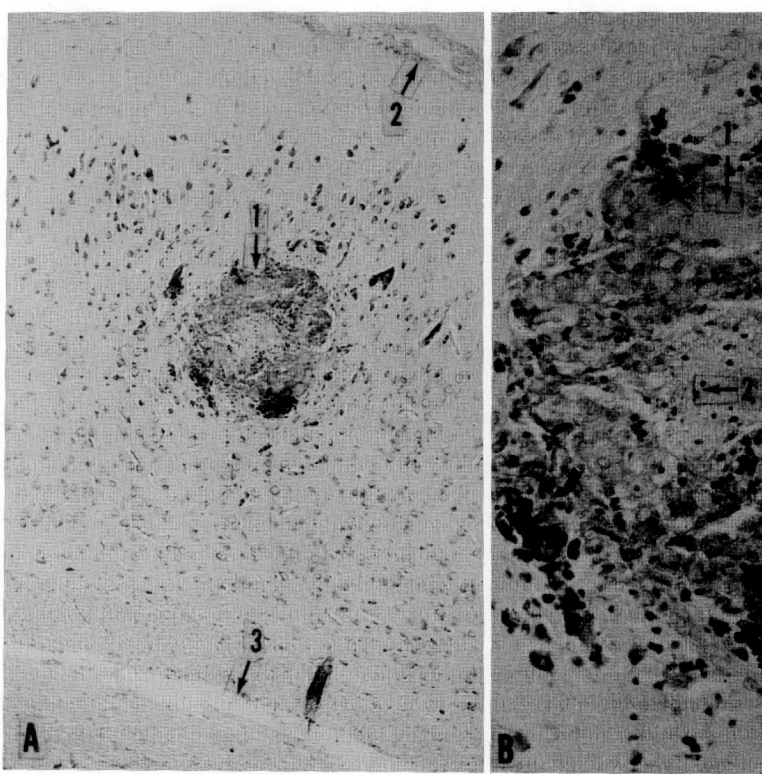

FIG. 12-17 Encephalitozoon infection in brain of a rabbit. **A.** Low power (×45) to show: (1) granuloma in the cerebral cortex. (2) Pia mater and (3) ependyma of lateral ventricle. **B.** Higher magnification of granuloma. Large, foamy macrophages (1) surrounding necrotic center containing organisms (i). (Courtesy of Armed Forces Institute of Pathology; contributor: U.S. Army Environmental Health Laboratory.)

(Alopex lagopus), severe disease may develop in neonates which acquired encephalitozoonosis in utero. In one outbreak in Norway, 1500 blue fox cubs died although the parent vixens remained healthy. *Encephalitozoon* invades a variety of cell types and proliferates within parasitophorous vacuoles in the host cell cytoplasm. Neurons, ependyma and choroid plexus epithelium, renal tubular epithelium, endothelium, and macrophages are the cell types in which the organisms are most often seen.

Clinical signs are usually not detected. Rabbits may develop a head tilt or other neurologic signs such as paralysis, but more often than not this is the result of middle ear infection or other causes.

Lesions

In rabbits the usual experience is to find the lesions and the organisms incidentally in histologic sections from rabbits which have shown no recognizable signs of infection. In brain, focal lesions are chiefly in the cerebral cortex, but may occur anywhere. Microscopic-sized granulomas (Fig. 12-17) made up of epithelioid cells surrounding a tiny necrotic center are the common finding in these occult infections. Larger areas of necrosis may be seen in fatal cases, and perivascular lymphocytic cuffing may be prominent. The organisms are demonstrable in the necrotic centers of the granulomas, usually appearing singly as short, plump, rod-shaped bodies with rounded ends, measuring about 1 by 2 μm. They are stained intensely by silver impregnation methods (Warthin-Starry), accept Giemsa stain, are acid-fast

and gram-positive, but are usually not visible in sections stained with hematoxylin and eosin.

Encephalitozoon cuniculi is also a cause of chronic nephritis in rabbits characterized by lymphocytic infiltration, granulomas (Fig. 12-18), and small focal scars. The organisms may be found in association with the lesions and in tubular epithelium (Fig. 12-19). Myocarditis and vasculitis are also features of encephalitozoonosis.

In blue foxes and dogs, granulomatous meningoencephalomyelitis and nephritis are the chief findings. In cases of longer standing, widespread polyarteritis characterized by endothelial hypertrophy and hyperplasia, splitting of the internal elastic membrane,

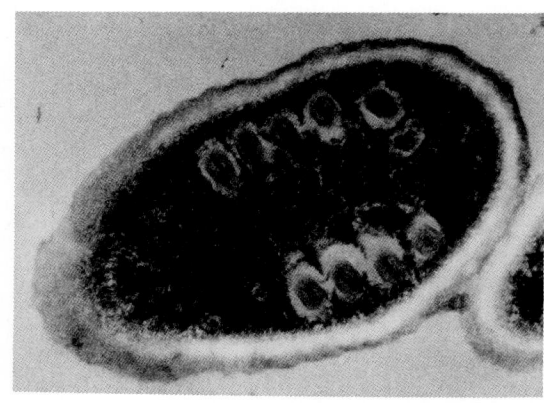

FIG. 12-18 *Encephalitozoon cuniculi* (×36,800). Note cross section of polar filament. (Courtesy of Dr. J. A. Shadduck, Ohio State University, and Science.)

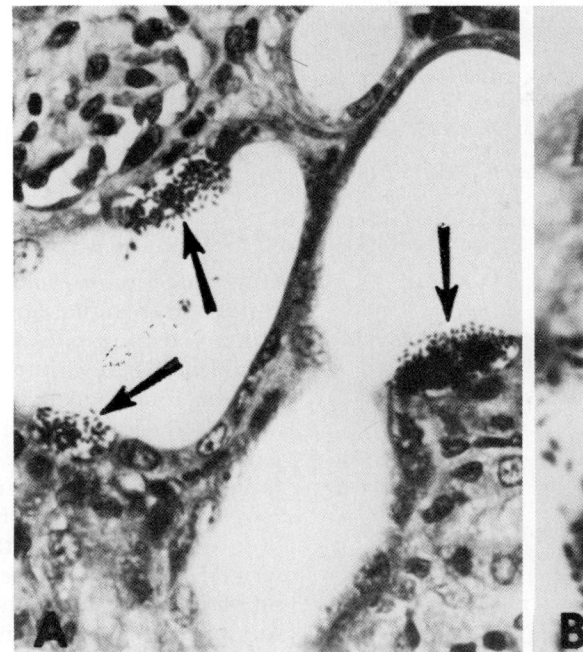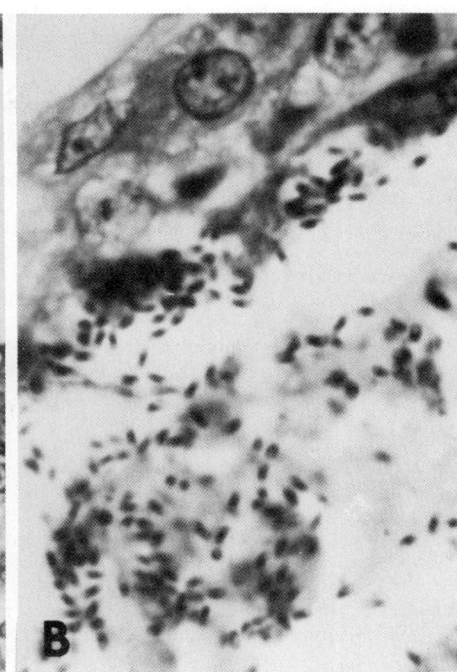

FIG. 12-19 Encephalitozoonosis, rabbit. **A.** *Encephalitozoon (Nosema) cuniculi* (arrows) within renal tubular epithelial cells. **B.** Organisms being extruded from epithelial cells and free within tubular lumen.

scarring of the media, and adventitial mononuclear infiltration have been described as prominent features. Such lesions in the coronary arteries have been associated with papillary epicardial mesotheliomas.

Diagnosis

Diagnosis depends upon demonstrating the organisms in tissue section, isolation in tissue culture, or mouse inoculation. The staining characteristics in tissue sections, particularly the fact that the spores are acid-fast and Gram-positive, help differentiate *E. cuniculi* from other small protozoan parasites. Another most helpful feature is that the spores of *E. cuniculi* (and other microsporidia) are birefringent (anisotropic). In the mouse peritoneum, the organism may be demonstrated to extrude its polar filament and be actively motile. Electron micrographs reveal that *E. cuniculi* is found within parasitophorous vacuoles and the distinctive polar filament is evident (Fig. 12-18). The spores are about 2 microns long and also contain a laminated structure known as the polaroplast. Serologic tests have also been developed.

References

Anver MR, King NW, Hunt RD. Congenital encephalitozoonosis in a squirrel monkey *(Saimiri sciureus)*. Vet Pathol 1972;9:475–480.

Beckwith C, Peterson N, Liu JJ, et al. Dot enzyme-linked immunosorbent assay (dot ELISA) for antibodies to *Encephalitozoon cuniculi*. Lab Anim Sci 1988;38:573–576.

Bjerkås I, Nesland JM. Brain and spinal cord lesions in encephalitozoonosis in the blue fox. Acta Vet Scand 1987;28:15–22.

Buyukmihci N, Bellhorn RW, Hunziker J, et al. *Encephalitozoon* (Nosema) infection of the cornea in a cat. J Am Vet Med Assoc 1977;171:355–357.

Canning EU, Hollister WS. *Enterocytozoon bieneusi* (Microspora): prevalence and pathogenicity in AIDS patients. Trans R Soc Trop Med HYG 1990;84:181–186.

Cole JR Jr, Sangster LT, Sulzer CR, et al. Infections with *Encephalitozoon cuniculi* and *Leptospira interrogans,* serovars *grippotyphosa* and *ballum,* in a kennel of Foxhounds. J Am Vet Med Assoc 1982;180:435–437.

Cutlip RC, Beall CW. Encephalitozoonosis in Arctic lemmings. Lab Anim Sci 1989;39:331–333.

Didier ES, et al. Isolation and characterization of a new human microsporidian, *Encephalitozoon hellem* (n. sp.), from three AIDS patients with keratoconjunctivitis. J Infect Dis 1991;163:617–621.

Flatt RE, Jackson SJ. Renal nosematosis in young rabbits. Pathol Vet 1970;7:492–497.

Hollister WS, Canning EU, Viney M. Prevalence of antibodies to *Encephalitozoon cuniculi* in stray dogs as determined by an ELISA. Vet Rec 1989;124:332–336.

Hunt RD, King NW Jr, Foster HL. Encephalitozoonosis: evidence for vertical transmission. J Infect Dis 1972;126:212–214.

Innes JRM, Zeman W, Frenkel JK, et al. Occult, endemic encephalitozoonosis of the central nervous system of mice. J Neuropathol Exp Neurol 1962;21:519–533.

Koller LD. Spontaneous *Nosema cuniculi* infection in laboratory rabbits. J Am Vet Med Assoc 1969;155:1108–1114.

Lainson R, Garnham PCC, Killick-Kendrick R, et al. Nosematosis, a microsporidial infection of rodents and other animals, including man. Br Med J 1964;2:470–472.

Liu JJ, Greeley EH, Shadduck JA. Murine encephalitozoonosis: the effect of age and mode of transmission on occurrence of infection. Lab Anim Sci 1988;38:675–679.

Lyngset A. A survey of serum antibodies to *Encephalitozoon cuniculi* in breeding rabbits and their young. Lab Anim Sci 1980;30:558–561.

Matsubayashi H, et al. A case of encephalitozoon-like body infection in man. Arch Pathol 1959;67:181–187.

Nordstoga K, Landsverk T. Papillary epicardial mesotheliomas associated with encephalitozoonosis in blue foxes. Vet Pathol 1981;18:564–566.

Nordstoga K, Westbye K. Polyarteritis nodosa associated with nosematosis in blue foxes. Acta Pathol Microbiol Scand 1976;84A:291–296.

Pakes SP, Shadduck JA, Cali A. Fine structure of *Encephalitozoon cuniculi* from rabbits, mice, and hamsters. J Protozool 1975;22:481–488.

Pang VF, Shadduck JA. Susceptibility of cats, sheep, and swine to a rabbit isolate of *Encephalitozoon cuniculi.* Am J Vet Res 1985;46:1071–1077.

Poonacha KB, Williams PD, Stamper RD. Encephalitozoonosis in a parrot. J Am Vet Med Assoc 1985;186:700–702.

Rensburg IBJ van, Plessis JL du. Nosematosis in a cat: a case report. J S Afr Vet Med Assoc1971;42:327–331.

Shadduck JA. *Nosema cuniculi:* in vitro isolation. Science 1969; 166:516–517.

Shadduck JA, Baskin G. Serologic evidence of *Encephalitozoon cuniculi* infection in a colony of squirrel monkeys *(Saimiri sciureus).* Lab Anim Sci 1989;39:328–330.

Szabo JR, Shadduck JA. Experimental encephalitozoonosis in neonatal dogs. Vet Pathol 1987;24:99–108.

Tiner JD. Birefringent spores differentiate *Encephalitozoon* and other microsporidia from coccidia. Vet Pathol 1988;25:227–230.

Van Heerden J, Bainbridge N, Burroughs REJ, et al. Distemper-like disease and encephalitozoonosis in wild dogs *(Lycaon pictus).* J Wildl Dis 1989;25:70–75.

Waller T, Bergquist NR. Rapid simultaneous diagnosis of toxoplasmosis and encephalitozoonosis in rabbits by carbon immunoassay. Lab Anim Sci 1982;32:515–517.

Weber R, et al. Improved light-microscopical detection of microsporidia spores in stool and duodenal aspirates. N Engl J Med 1992;326:161–166.

Zeman DH, Baskin GB. Encephalitozoonosis in squirrel monkeys *(Saimiri sciureus).* Vet Pathol 1985;22:24–31.

AMEBIASIS

Parasitic protozoa classified within the class Sarcodina—those with pseudopodia—are best known as pathogens of humans, but also of nonhuman primates and less frequently other animals. These organisms usually inhabit the intestinal tract and may be present in the absence of recognizable effects. However, under some circumstances, severe dysentery may result from their presence. The ameba may ulcerate and invade the intestinal wall, and possibly migrate to the liver or brain, resulting in "amebic" abscesses.

The diphthong (oe) is used in the names of some of these protozoa; however, in the United States, it is dropped when generally referring to the disease or organisms. Another point of possible confusion lies in the names of amebae of the genera *Entamoeba* and *Endamoeba*. At one time these organisms were considered in one genus; currently, they are separated. *Entamoeba* includes pathogens of humans and other mammals; *Endamoeba* are generally found in lower invertebrates.)

The most important pathogen in this group is *Entamoeba histolytica,* the cause of amebic dysentery in humans.

Most species of nonhuman primates are susceptible to E. histolytica and may develop amebic dysentery. *E. histolytica* can also infect many species of domestic animals (e.g., dogs, cats, pigs, cattle), but the presence of the organism only rarely results in disease (Fig. 12-20). Even in humans many asymptomatic carriers exist. The life cycle is direct. Following their proliferation in the intestinal tract, trophozoites then become cysts which are excreted into the environment. The organism may be transmitted between hosts by contamination of food or water by food handlers who are carriers, by means of cysts borne by flies or cockroaches, or by consumption of contaminated water, in which amebic cysts may survive for long periods.

Several other species of *Entamoeba* exist which are oral or gastrointestinal commensals of humans and animals that are not considered pathogenic. Members of the genera *Endolimax* and *Iodamoeba* are also commensals of humans, nonhuman primates and, rarely, other species.

Lesions

Once infection is established, reproduction is by binary fission, and under appropriate but unknown circumstances, trophozoites invade and undermine the mucosa, leading to variously sized ulcers. The trophozoites may be found deep in the wall of the colon, usually associated with a flask-shaped ulcer of the mucosa. The parasite is presumed to secrete a lytic enzyme under some as yet undetermined circumstances. The trophozoites may disseminate to other organs, particularly the liver and brain where they produce large lytic lesions, termed amebic abscesses, characterized by liquifaction necrosis of the parenchyma and, less frequently, frank suppuration. A distinctive feature of the necrotizing lesions in the colon and in other sites is the almost total lack of a cellular inflammatory response. This may result from the secretion of products that inhibit leukocyte chemotaxis.

The trophozoites of amebae are recognized in tissue sections as irregularly spherical organisms without cilia but often having pseudopodia. They have a distinct or indistinct nucleus, depending upon the species, and their abundant cytoplasm is often vacuolated and may contain phagocytized erythrocytes or tissue debris. Their overall size is variable, as they range from 10–60 μm in diameter. They may be seen in intestinal crypts, in necrotic foci in the submucosa, or at the margins of sharply demarcated ulcers.

Diagnosis

The diagnosis may be made tentatively by identifying trophozoites of E. histolytica in the feces in the presence of dysentery, and confirmed by demonstrating the organisms in ulcers or abscesses.

References

Brandt, H, and Tamayo RP. Pathology of human amebiasis. Hum Pathol 1970;1:351–385.

Burrows RB, Lillis WG. Intestinal protozoan infection in dogs. J Am Vet Med Assoc 1967;150:880–883.

Giménez-Scherer JA, et al. Ultrastructural changes associated with the inhibition of monocyte chemotaxis caused by products of axenically grown *Entamoeba histolytica.* Lab Invest 1987;57:45–51.

Haq A, Sharma A, Ahmad S, et al. Experimental infection of rhesus monkeys with *Entamoeba histolytica* mimics human infection. Lab Anim Sci 1985;35:484–484.

Jordan HE. Amebiasis *(Entamoeba histolytica)* in the dog. Vet Med Small Anim Clin 1967;62:61–64.

Loomis MR, Britt JO Jr, Gendron AP, et al. Hepatic and gastric amebiasis in black and white colobus monkeys. J Am Vet Med Assoc 1983;183:1188–1191.

McGowan K, et al. *Entamoeba histolytica* causes intestinal secretion: role of serotonin. Science 1983;221:762–764.

Miller MJ, Bray RS. *Entamoeba histolytica* infections in the chimpanzee (Pan satyrus). J Parasitol 1966;52:386–388.

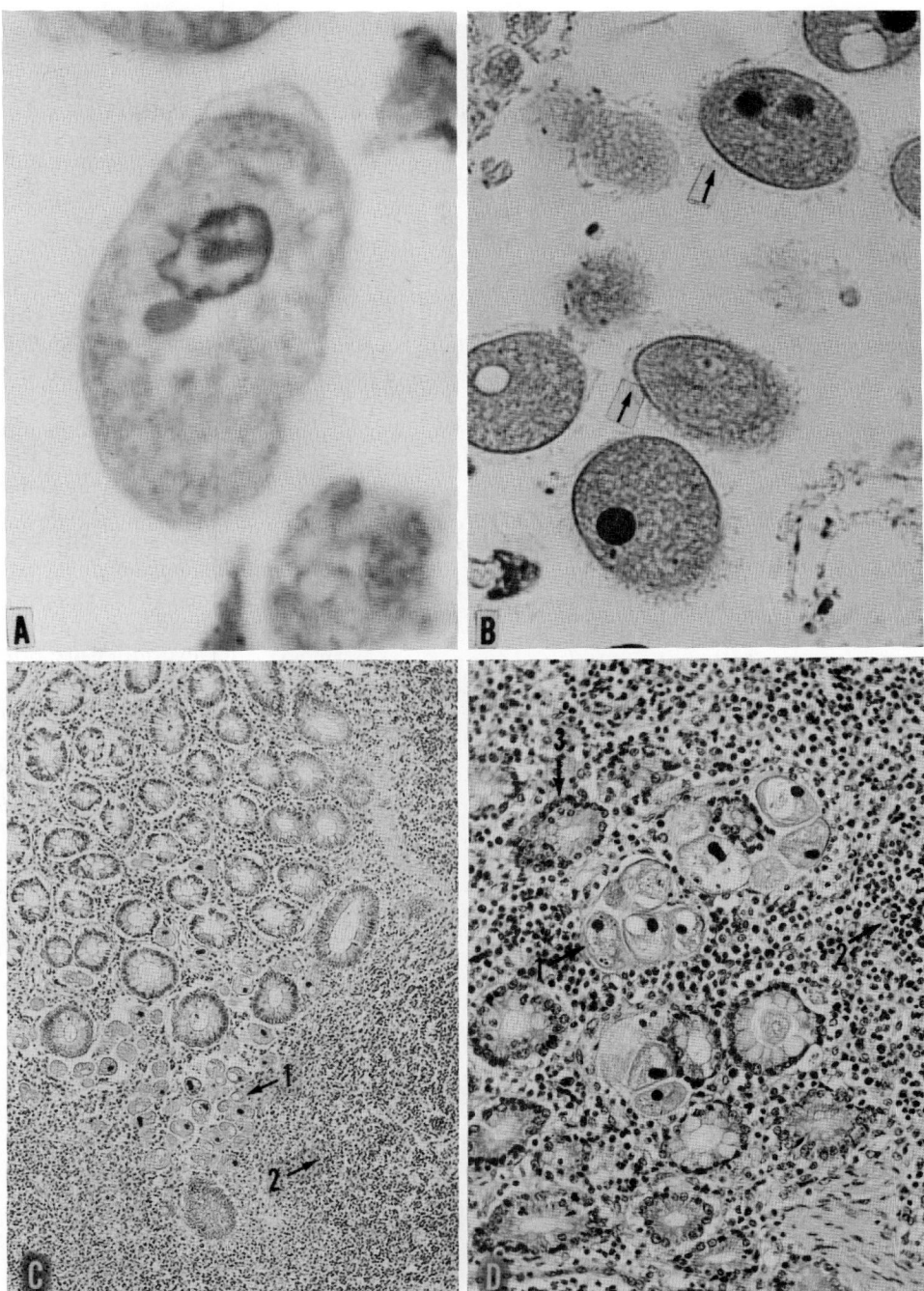

FIG. 12-20 **A.** *Entamoeba histolytica* (×1750) in experimental amebiasis in a kitten. (Contributor: Dr. H. E. Melleney.) **B.** *Balantidium coli* (×600) from colon of an orangutan. Note cilia (arrows). **C.** *Balantidium coli* (1) deep in the mucosa of the colon of an orangutan (×75). (2) Note lymphocytes. (Contributor: National Zoological Park.) **D.** *Balantidium coli* (×185) in: (1) mucosa of ileum of a pig, (2) lymphocytes, and (3) intestinal epithelium. (Courtesy of Armed Forces Institute of Pathology; contributor: Lt. Col. F. D. Maurer.)

Palmieri JR, Dalgard DW, Connor DH. Gastric amebiasis in a silvered leaf monkey. J Am Vet Med Assoc 1984;185:1374–1375.

Rees CW. Pathogenesis of intestinal amoebiasis in kittens. Arch Pathol 1929;7:1–26.

AMEBIC MENINGOENCEPHALITIS (NAEGLERIA; ACANTHAMOEBA; HARTMANNELLA)

Most of the numerous other members in the class Sarcodina, order Amoebidae are free-living and not pathogenic. A few, however, do on occasion invade tissue and result in disease. Most examples have involved humans, with only a few reports in animals. The circumstances fostering tissue invasion are not clear, but many examples of disease have occurred in immunosuppressed patients. In humans, *Naegleria fowleri* (the only *Naegleria* sp. which has been associated with disease) and certain species of *Acanthamoeba* can cause meningoencephalitis by invading through the cribriform plate. Several species of *Acanthamoeba* also have been identified as causing encephalitis in humans and are believed to reach the brain by hematogenous spread. *Acanthamoeba* is also a cause of keratitis in humans. Infection with these protozoa is often associated with swimming and diving in stagnant waters and unchlorinated pools. Disease has been reproduced experimentally in animals and there are isolated reports of its spontaneous occurrence in animals. An example of gangrenous bronchopneumonia in a bull caused by another free-living protozoan, *Hartmannella,* has been reported by McConnell et al. (1968).

Lesions

The lesions in the central nervous system caused by *Naegleria* in humans are those of a purulent, hemorrhagic and necrotizing meningoencephalitis, particularly of the cortical gray matter. *Acanthamoeba* cause a granulomatous encephalitis.

Diagnosis

Diagnosis depends on identifying the protozoa within lesions and/or their cultivation (Figs. 12-21, 12-22). In some examples, they may be present in large numbers, but in others they are extremely scarce. The trophozoites are 10–30 μm in diameter with a clear nucleus containing a distinct nucleolus. Encysted organisms are smaller, about 9 μm in diameter, and surrounded by a wall containing two or more pores (Fig. 12-21).

References

Ayers KM, Billups LH, Garner FM. Acanthamoebiasis in a dog. Vet Pathol 1972;9:221–226.

Butt CG. Primary amebic meningoencephalitis. N Engl J Med 1966; 274:1473–1476.

Culbertson CG, Smith JW, Cohen HK, et al. Experimental infection of mice and monkeys by *Acanthamoeba.* Am J Pathol 1959; 35:185–197.

Fuentealba IC, Wikse SE, Read WK, et al. Amebic meningoencephalitis in a sheep. J Am Vet Med Assoc 1992;200: 363–365.

Martinez AJ, Nelson EC, Duma RJ. Primary amebic meningoencephalitis, *Naegleria meningoencephalitis:* CNS protozoal infection. Am J Pathol 1973;73:545–548.

McConnell EE, Garner FM, Kirk JH. Hartmannellosis in a bull. Pathol Vet 1968;5:1–6.

Ziegler EE. Hematoxylin-eosin tissue stain, an improved and uniform technique. Arch Pathol 1944;37:68–69.

GIARDIASIS

Protozoa of the genus *Giardia* are pyriform in shape and bilaterally symmetrical. The anterior end is rounded and the posterior is elongated, nearly pointed. The convex ventral surface bears a large sucking disc. Each organism has four pair of flagella. These organisms are common inhabitants of the small intestine and colon of humans and animals without signs of disease.

Giardia can, however, be an important cause of diarrhea, best established in humans. In animals, giardiasis is seen most often in dogs, cats, rats, mice, guinea pigs, other small laboratory animals, and occasionally cattle. Distinct species of *Giardia* are associated with each animal (*G. canis, G. cati, G. muris, G. bovis,* etc.); however, they are not host-specific. The organisms localize in the small intestine on the surface of epithelial cells. Clinically the diarrhea tends to be chronic, often lasting for several weeks, and sometimes recurrent. The stools tend to be bulky, malodorous, and light colored. The prolonged course can lead to malabsorption syndrome with weight loss.

Lesions

Morphologic lesions in the intestinal tract may be minimal or stunting of villi and an inflammatory infiltrate in the lamina propria can occur. Organisms may be dif-

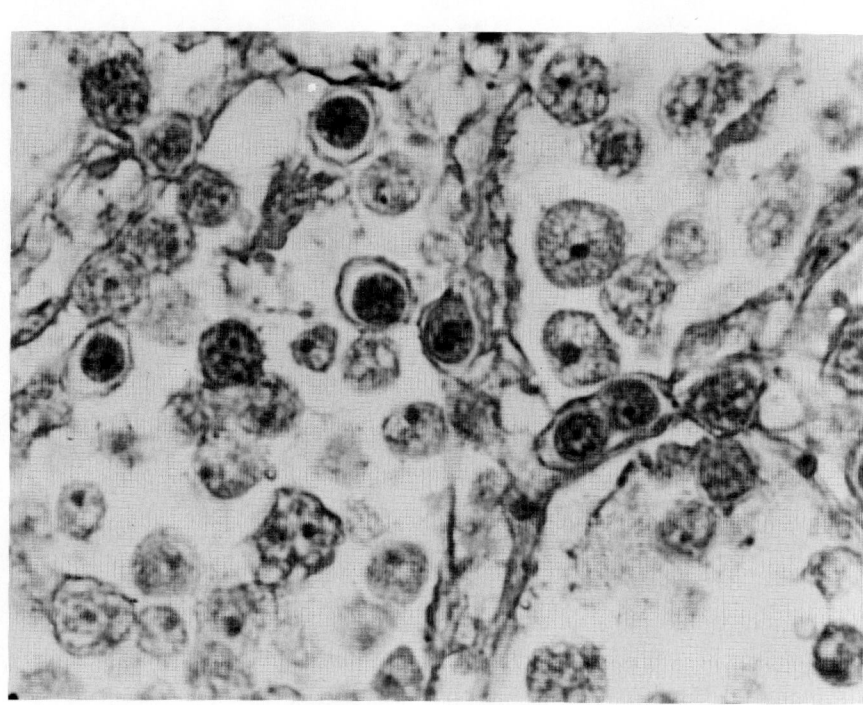

FIG. 12-21 *Hartmannella sp.* from a bovine lung (×900). Note trophozoite and cyst forms. (Courtesy of Col. F. N. Garner, V.C., Armed Forces Institute of Pathology.)

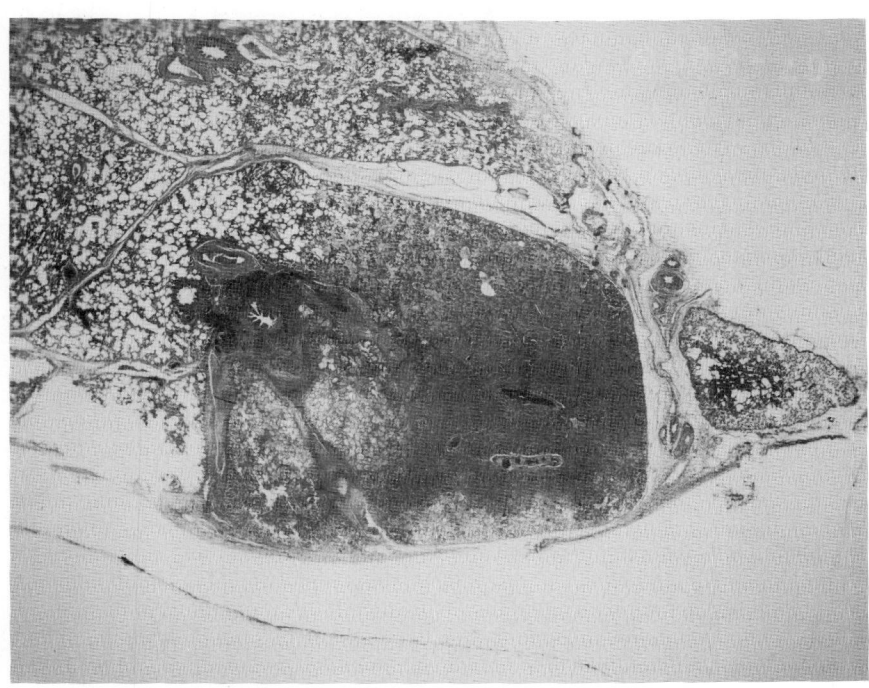

FIG. 12-22 Pneumonia, lung of a bull due to *Hartmannella* sp. (Courtesy of Col. F. N. Garner, V.C., Armed Forces Institute of Pathology.)

ficult to discern in tissue section and are better identified in fecal specimens where the typical trophozoites or cysts can be found.

Hexamita spp., morphologically similar to *Giardia*, can occur as free-living protozoa or commensals in the intestinal tract of various animals, birds, fish, and insects. They are not significant pathogens to domestic animals; however, they may cause diarrhea and enteritis in laboratory mice and can be opportunistic pathogens in immunocompromised individuals.

References

Barlough JE. Canine giardiasis: a review. J Small Anim Pract 1979;20:613–623.

Boorman GA, Van Hooft JIM, Van der Waaij D, et al. Synergistic role of intestinal flagellates and normal intestinal bacteria in a post-weaning mortality of mice. Lab Anim Sci 1973;23:187–193.

Burrows RB, Lillis WG. Intestinal protozoan infections in dogs. J Am Vet Med Assoc 1967;150:880–883.

Csiza CK, Abelseth MK. An epizootic of protozoan enteritis in a closed mouse colony. Lab Anim Sci 1973;23:858–861.

Dykes AC, et al. Municipal waterborne giardiasis: an epidemiologic investigation. Beavers implicated as a possible reservoir. Ann Intern Med 1980;92:165–170.

Flatt RE, Halvorsen JA, Kemp RL. Hexamitiasis in a laboratory mouse colony. Lab Anim Sci 1978;28:62–65.

Gillin FD, Reiner DS, Wang C-S. Human milk kills parasitic intestinal protozoa. Science 1983;221:1290–1292.

Hahn NE, Glaser CA, Hird DW, et al. Prevalence of *Giardia* in the feces of pups. J Am Vet Med Assoc 1988;192:1428–1429.

Kirkpatrick CE, Farrell JP. Feline giardiasis: observations on natural and induced infections. Am J Vet Res 1984;45:2182–2188.

Kirkpatrick CE, Laczak JP. Giardiasis in a cattery. J Am Vet Med Assoc 1985;187:161–162.

Kirkpatrick CE, Skand DL. Giardiasis in a horse. J Am Vet Med Assoc 1985;187:163–164.

Letvin NL, O'Connell MJ, Blake BJ, et al. Hematogenous hexamitiasis in a macaque monkey with an immunodeficiency syndrome. J Infect Dis 1984;149:828.

Osterholm MT, et al. An outbreak of foodborne giardiasis. N Engl J Med 1981;304:24–28.

Rogers KT, Hawkins JA, Vulgamott JC. Cystic and peritoneal giardiasis in a dog. J Am Vet Med Assoc 1984;185:669–670.

Van Kruiningen HJ, Knibbs DR, Burke CN. Hexamitiasis in laboratory mice. J Am Vet Med Assoc 1978;173:1202–1204.

Wagner JE, Doyle RE, Ronald NC, et al. Hexamitiasis in laboratory mice, hamsters, and rats. Lab Anim Sci 1974;24:349–354.

Watson ADJ. Giardiosis and colitis in a dog. Aust Vet J 1980;56:444–447, Vet Bull 1981;51:2400.

Wenrich DH. A species of *Hexamita* (Protozoa, Flagellata) from the intestine of a monkey (*Macacus rhesus*). J Parasitol 1933;19:225–229.

PNEUMOCYSTOSIS

A protozoan organism of uncertain taxonomic classification, *Pneumocystis carinii* (Fig. 12-23) is known to inhabit the pulmonary alveoli of humans and animals, and under certain conditions, causes severe disruption of respiratory function. *Pneumocystis* pneumonia has been recognized in humans, dogs, horses, swine, goats, rats, mice, and monkeys, and the organisms have been identified in the lungs of many additional species in the absence of clinical disease. The disease is seen in animals and humans suffering from immunodeficiency. *Pneumocystis* pneumonia is the most common opportunistic infection in patients with AIDS. Although the organisms in the various hosts are morphologically indistinguishable, some evidence indicates that each may be specific for the respective species. Failure to infect hamsters and rabbits with rat strains, and the absence of common complement-fixing antigens in human and rat strains, supports this concept of species specificity.

The organisms are located in alveoli closely adhered to type I and, on occasion, type II pneumocytes. Microscopically, there is little inflammatory reaction,

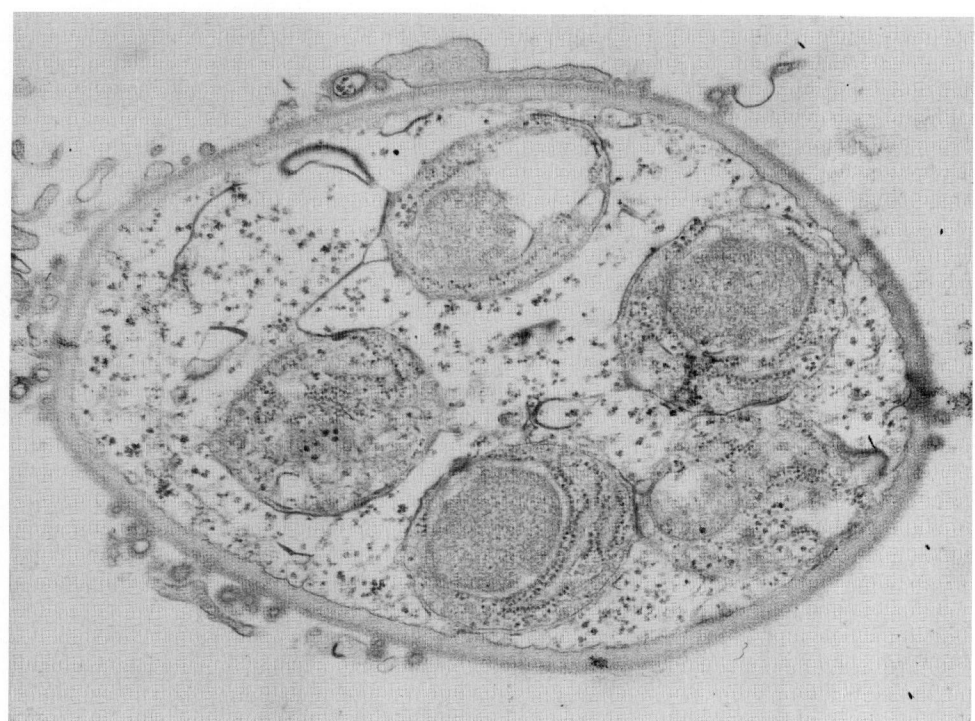

FIG. 12-23 *Pneumocystis carinii*, from the lung of a rat following treatment with cortisone acetate. Electron micrograph (×25,000) of thick-walled organism with five intracystic bodies. Courtesy of Drs. Earl G. Barton, Jr., Wallace G. Campbell, Jr. and The American Journal of Pathology.)

but type II alveolar lining cells may be enlarged. The alveoli appear filled with a pink frothy material which represents vast collections of organisms. *P. carinii* proliferates as trophozoites 1–4 μm in diameter, irregular in shape and containing a single nucleus. These in turn become cysts, which are larger (4–8 μm in diameter), round, slightly wrinkled, cup-shaped or crescentic, with a thick wall. Each cyst contains up to eight intracystic bodies or sporozoites. Neither form stains very well in hematoxylin-and-eosin-stained tissue sections. The trophozoites are best visualized with Giemsa stain, the nucleus staining red and the cytoplasm blue. The wall of the cyst stage stains well with *Gomori methenamine* silver stain or PAS. Immunoperoxidase and immunofluorescent staining techniques are the most specific methods for positive identification. If the infection were to resolve, however, it would not confer any immunity. A case of *P. carinii* induced osteomyelitis in a human with common variable immunodeficiency has been reported.

References

Barton EG, Campbell WG Jr. *Pneumocystis carinii* in lungs of rats treated with cortisone acetate. Ultrastructural observations relating to the life cycle. Am J Pathol 1969;54:209–236.

Chandler FW, McClure HM, Campbell WG Jr, et al. Pulmonary pneumocystosis in nonhuman primates. Arch Pathol Lab Med 1976;100:163–167.

Chandler FW Jr, Frenkel JK, Campbell WG Jr. *Pneumocystis carinii* pneumonia in the immunosuppressed rat. Am J Pathol 1979;95:571–574.

Copland JW. Canine pneumonia caused by *Pneumocystis carinii*. Aust Vet J 1974;50:515–518.

Cushion MT, Ruffolo JJ, Walzer PD. Analysis of the developmental stages of *Pneumocystis carinii*, in vitro. Lab Invest 1988;58:324–331.

Esolen LM, Fasano MB, Flynn J, et al. Pneumocystis carinii osteomyelitis in a patient with common variable immunodeficiency. N Engl J Med 1992;326:999–1001.

Farrow BRH, Watson ADJ, Hartley WJ, et al. Pneumocystis pneumonia in the dog. J Comp Pathol 1972;82:447–453.

Frenkel JK, Good JT, Shultz JA. Latent pneumocystis infections of rats, relapse, and chemotherapy. Lab Invest 1966;15:1559–1577 .

Long EG, Smith JS, Meier JL. Attachment of *Pneumocystis carinii* to rat pneumocytes. Lab Invest 1986;54:609–615.

Phair J, et al. The risk of *Pneumocystis carinii* pneumonia among men infected with human immunodeficiency virus type 1. N Engl J Med 1990;322:161–165.

Seibold HR, Munnell JF. *Pneumocystis carinii* in a pig. Vet Pathol 1977;14:89–91.

Shively JN, et al. *Pneumocystis carinii* pneumonia in two foals. J Am Vet Med Assoc 1973;162:648–652.

Shively JN, Moe KK, Dellers RW. Fine structure of spontaneous *Pneumocystis carinii* pulmonary infection in foals. Cornell Vet 1974;64:72–88.

Sundberg JP, Burnstein T, Shultz LD, et al. Identification of *Pneumocystis carinii* in immunodeficient mice. Lab Anim Sci 1989;39:213–218.

Weir EC, Brownstein DG, Barthold SW. Spontaneous wasting disease in nude mice associated with *Pneumocystis carinii* infection. Lab Anim Sci 1986; 36:140–144.

TRICHOMONIASIS

The family Trichomonadidae (subphylum Mastigophora) includes flagellated organisms which are subdivided in part on the number of anterior flagellae. Most are not pathogenic. Two genera are, however, of interest: *Tritrichomonas* (with three anterior flagellae); and *Trichomonas* (with four anterior flagellae).

Tritrichomonas foetus is the cause of bovine trichomoniasis, an important genital infection of cattle. The organism is transported by coitus. The infection in bulls generally goes unrecognized. Microscopically, there may be a mild mononuclear and neutrophilic inflammation in the penis and prepuce, but it is of little consequence. In cows, however, infection leads to vaginitis, endometritis, placentitis, fetal infection, early abortion, and pyometra. Following coitus with an infected bull, cows conceive normally, but the pregnancy terminates early in gestation. Most abortions occur in the first half of pregnancy or earlier and most often go unrecognized; however, trichomoniasis may cause abortion in the last trimester. The principal sign of trichomoniasis in a herd is infertility, which can affect a high percentage of animals and result in significant economic loss. Cows ordinarily eventually clear the infection.

Lesions in the female reproductive tract are usually not extensive, consisting of non-specific inflammation, unless pyometra develops, which is not the usual outcome. In the fetus, lesions may be absent, although in those aborted late in gestation there may be a pyogranulomatous bronchopneumonia with multinucleated giant cells.

The diagnosis is established by demonstrating *Tritrichomonas foetus* in vaginal, uterine, or preputial exudates in association with a herd history of decreased fertility, abortions, vaginitis, metritis, and balanitis. Direct microscopic examination may not be adequate if numbers of trichomonads are small, as is often the case in bulls. Culture of the organisms is more accurate. Test matings are also effective in diagnosing infected bulls.

T. suis is found in the digestive and upper respiratory tracts of swine, but its pathogenicity is not completely established. *T. gallinae* is the etiologic agent in avian trichomoniasis, a serious inflammation of the upper gastrointestinal tract of pigeons, turkeys, chickens, and wild birds. T. vaginalis is found in the vagina, urethra, and prostate of women and men. It may be carried without producing signs, especially in men, but also may result in vaginitis or urethritis. It is transmitted by coitus. *T. fecalis (T. equi)* is a common organism of the intestinal flora of normal horses. It has been blamed as a cause of gastroenteritis, but there is no good evidence in support of this supposition. Other species of trichomonads have been suspected in cases of gastrointestinal infection (Bennett and Franco, 1969) but it is difficult to prove that these organisms are pathogenic in the digestive tract where they may thrive in the absence of disease. *Tritrichomonas* and *Trichomonas* spp. are common inhabitants of the intestinal tract and have been associated with enteritis and diarrhea in a number of different animal species; however, only a few reports present convincing evidence to support their role as pathogens.

References

Bennett SP, Franco DA. Equine protozoan diarrhea (equine intestinal trichomoniasis) at Trinidad racetracks. J Am Vet Assoc 1969;154: 58–60.
BonDurant RH, et al. Prevalence of trichomoniasis among California beef herds. J Am Vet Med Assoc 1990;196:1590–1593.
Bunton TE, Lowenstine LJ, Leininger R. Invasive trichomoniasis in a *Callicebus moloch.* Vet Pathol 1983;20:491–494.
Damron GW. Gastrointestinal trichomonads in horses: occurrence and identification. Am J Vet Res 1976;37:25–28.
Goodger WJ, Skirrow SZ. Epidemiologic and economic analyses of an unusually long epizootic of trichomoniasis in a large California dairy herd. J Am Vet Med Assoc 1986;189:772–776.
Kimsey PB, Darien BJ, Kendrick JW, et al. Bovine trichomoniasis: diagnosis and treatment. J Am Vet Med Assoc 1980;177:616–619.
Rhyan JC, Stackhouse LL, Quinn WJ. Fetal and placental lesions in bovine abortion due to Tritrichomonas foetus. Vet Pathol 1988;25:350–355.
Scimeca JM, Culberson DE, Abee CR, et al. Intestinal trichomonads (*Tritrichomonas mobilensis*) in the natural host *Saimiri sciureus* and *Saimiri boliviensis*. Vet Pathol 1989;26: 144–147.
Skirrow SZ, BonDurant RH. Bovine trichomoniasis. Vet Bull 1988;58:591–603.

BALANTIDIASIS

The only member of the ciliated Protozoa, the Infusoria, which is of pathogenic significance (and this is questionable) is *Balantidium coli (B. suis)*. This comparatively large (50–200 μm), single-celled organism is a natural inhabitant of the digestive tract of swine, humans, nonhuman primates, and sometimes other vertebrates, usually living in the lumen or between the villi and causing no recognizable effect on the host. Under some imperfectly understood circumstances, *Balantidium coli* will invade the intestinal mucosa, penetrating into the submucosa, localizing particularly in lymphoid nodules. Occasionally, it may reach the genital tract. This tissue penetration results in varying degrees of acute inflammation in the vicinity and may result in some manifestations of enteric disease. Because its pathogenicity is questioned and most certainly limited, *Balantidium coli* is of interest to the pathologist as an organism that may be present with frank pathogens, but should not be mistakenly considered the cause of every disease with which it is associated (Fig. 12-20).

References

Hatziolos BC. Balantidium in bovine respiratory tract. Delt Hellen Kten Hetair 1973;24:8–18.
Savchenko VF, Karput IM. Pathology and histology of Balantidium infection in pigs. Uchen Zap Vitebsk Vet Inst 1970;22:22–26.

TRYPANOSOMIASIS

Trypanosomiasis is often thought of as an exotic disease that occurs only in tropical Africa, India, and other far-off places. It is true that this disease is most serious in humans and animals in certain regions of the world, but trypanosomes are distributed throughout all parts of the globe, often producing no recognizable disease in the host in which they reside. The disease trypanosomiasis is divided into two major forms: American trypanosomiasis caused by *Trypanosoma cruzi;* and African trypanosomiasis caused by the other pathogenic members of the genus. Additionally, several other trypanosomes are found in Africa and the New World which cause disease in domestic animals (Table 12-5). In humans, African trypanosomiasis, which has gone by many names, such as African sleeping sickness, tsetse fly disease, maladie du sommeil, Schlaffkrankheit, and doenca do sono, has influenced the course of history,

TABLE 12-5 **Important Trypanosomes of Man and Animals**

Species	Definitive host	Intermediate hosts (vectors)	Geographic distribution	Disease
T. lewisi	Rats	Fleas—several species	Cosmopolitan	None
T. theileri	Cattle	Tabanid flies	Cosmopolitan	None
T. melophagium	Sheep	Louse fly (Melophagus ovinus)	Temperate zones	None
T. theodori	Horses	Louse fly (Lipoptena caprina)	Palestine, Syria	None
T. cruzi	Man, armadillo, cat, opossum, dog	"Kissing bug" (Triatoma sp.)	S. America	Chagas' disease American trypanosomiasis
T. evansi	Horse, mule, ass, cattle, buffalo	Horse flies (Tabanidae and Stomoxys)	Africa, Asia, S. America, Far East	Surra
T. equiperdum	Horse, ass	Trans. by coitus	Cosmopolitan	Dourine
T. vivax (uniforme)	Cattle, sheep, horse, goat, camel	Tsetse fly (Glossina sp.)	Central and S. America, Martinique, Guadaloupe, Mauritius and Africa	Souma
T. caprae	Horse, sheep, cattle	Tsetse fly	Tanzania Nyasaland	Trypanosomiasis
T. congolense, dimorphon	Cattle, horse, goat, sheep, ass, pig, dog, camel	Tsetse fly	Tropical Africa	Trypanosomiasis
T. simiae	Monkey, pig, horse, sheep	Tsetse fly	East Africa	Trypanosomiasis
T. brucei	Man, domestic and wild mammals, except goats	Tsetse fly	Tropical Africa	Nagana
T. rhodesiense	Man, antelope	Tsetse fly	East Africa	Acute "sleeping sickness"
T. gambiense	Man, antelope	Tsetse fly	Tropical Africa	Chronic "sleeping sickness"

particularly in Africa, by denying people the use of certain lands and causing them to go to war over those areas relatively free of the disease. The disease in domesticated livestock has also played a similar historical role. Although urbanization and control measures have reduced the frequency of the disease, it still remains a serious problem in some areas of Africa and South America.

Life cycle

These protozoa are flagellated, motile parasites that frequent the blood of many vertebrate and invertebrate hosts and localize in tissues, sometimes in a nonflagellated form. Trypanosomes have certain common anatomic features such as: an ovoid or rounded body in the nonflagellate stage, and a slender elongate body when it becomes flagellated; a flagellum which arises from the dot-shaped blepharoplast and extends to or projects from the anterior pole of the organism; an un-dulating membrane that extends along the border of the organism, with the flagellum forming its margin; a spherical or rod-shaped structure, the parabasal body, which together with the blepharoplast makes up the kinetoplast. A relatively large round or ovoid nucleus containing a more deeply staining karyosome is usually located near the middle of the body. Trypanosomes usually can be identified by their morphologic features, such as size, shape, position, arrangement, and development of the organelles (Fig. 12-24), but no completely satisfactory classification scheme has yet been devised. Most species of trypanosomes do not produce serious effects upon their host, but a few are important pathogens (Table 12-5).

Most all trypanosomes are transmitted by arthropods, which act as biological vectors. An exception is *Trypanosoma equiperdum*, the cause of dourine, which is transmitted by coitus. Mechanical transmission of trypanosomes may be accomplished by certain biting flies (*Tabanus, Stomoxys*), but this is not an important means of

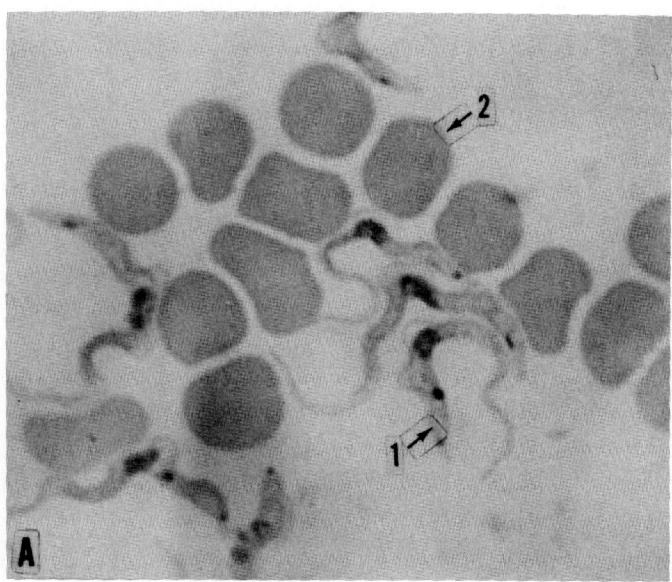

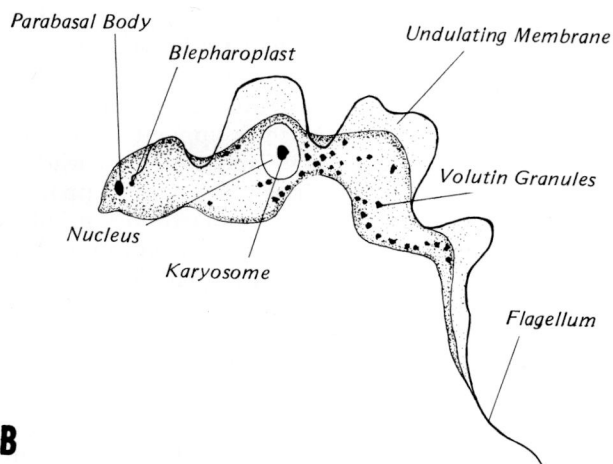

FIG. 12-24 Trypanosomiasis. **A.** *Trypanosoma equiperdum:* (1) in the blood of a rat. (2) Erythrocyte. (Courtesy of Armed Forces Institute of Pathology; contributor: Dr. Kent Davis.) **B.** Diagram of the morphology of a trypanosome.

transmission, except for *T. evansi,* the cause of surra in horses and dogs. Definite cyclic development occurs in the body of true invertebrate hosts. In these hosts, the trypanosomes multiply in various forms in the digestive tract, eventually migrate as infective forms to the salivary glands and are injected into the mammalian host with the vectors saliva at the time of the bite. *T. cruzi,* the cause of American trypanosomiasis, is an exception. Here the infectious stage is located in the hind gut and is excreted in the feces of the *Triatoma* bug, when the arthropod defecates at the time of its bite. When they are transmitted through vector saliva, trypanosomes are referred to as salivarian; when they are transmitted through arthropod feces, they are stercorarian.

Pathogenesis and general findings

The pathogenesis of trypanosomiasis in humans and animals is not thoroughly understood. The mechanisms that induce disease or cause death are essentially unknown with the exception of Chagas disease (American

trypanosomiasis) caused by *T. cruzi.* This organism invades cells, which partially explains the disease; however, the trypanosomes of African trypanosomiasis do not. Following introduction into the mammalian host, the trypanosomes of African trypanosomiasis (salivarian) rapidly multiply by binary fission as trypanomastigotes within the blood stream, leading to parasitemia. The parasitemia remains largely unabated by the hosts' immune response owing to the parasites unique ability to undergo almost endless antigenic variation through changes in surface glycoproteins. Because of their variability, these surface antigens are called varian surface glycoprotein, or VSG. Trypanosomes may enter the interstitial space as well, where multiplication also occurs. Continued stimulation of the immune system explains the reticuloendothelial, lymphocytic, and plasmacytic hyperplasia seen in the spleen and lymph nodes of many affected animals. Glomerulonephritis and vasculitis, which may also be features of chronic trypanosomiasis, may additionally result from the continuous immune response and the formation of antigen-antibody complexes. Anemia is a frequent finding and, although its pathogenesis is not settled, may also be immunologically mediated. It is at least in part hemolytic and in part due to erythrophagocytosis. Hypersensitivity to trypanosomal antigens may explain some acute deaths. The pathogenesis of inflammatory reactions in various tissues are hypothesized to be immune mediated. They are principally characterized by proliferation and activation of macrophages. Toxic products of the organisms may also play a role in the pathogenesis of tissue damage, which can include cellular necrosis. Usually leukocytosis, thrombocytopenia, and IgM hypergammaglobulinemia occur.

Specific infections

NAGANA (TSETSE FLY DISEASE)

Nagana is most commonly used as a collective term for African trypanosomiasis of domesticated animals, particularly those infections caused by *Trypanosoma brucei* (Bruce, 1894), *T. congolense* (Broden, 1904), and *T. vivax* (Ziemann, 1905). *T. vivax* and *T. congolense* are highly pathogenic for cattle. *T. brucei* is pathogenic for many domestic animals, particularly horses, dogs, and camels. Cattle, sheep, and goats are less susceptible and the disease in these species tends to be chronic. The local term "Souma" is sometimes applied to infection with *T. vivax*. A large number and variety of wild animals may serve as reservoirs of infection, apparently with impunity to themselves. Nagana occurs in all domesticated animals in tropical Africa, resulting in acute or chronic manifestations with irregular fever, anemia, emaciation, subcutaneous edema, weakness, conjunctivitis, photophobia, lacrimation, and neurologic signs of tremor, hyperexcitability, incoordination, paresis, dullness, and coma. Death may occur following an acute illness or after a prolonged course, during which gradual wasting is a dominant feature. Postmortem examination usually discloses severe emaciation with edematous changes in all fatty tissues. The lymph nodes are swollen, edematous, occasionally with hemorrhage in the medulla; the liver is enlarged and congested. The spleen is either enlarged, normal, or atrophic with prominent malpighian corpuscles. Hemorrhages are common, particularly in subendocardial and epicardial locations. Pericardial fluid may be excessive. Congestion and hemorrhage may be a prominent feature in the gastrointestinal tract. Trypanosomes are found in blood and other body fluids as well as free in tissues, where they incite an inflammatory reaction, predominantly mononuclear. Mononuclear inflammation may occur in virtually every body tissue, including skeletal muscle, myocardium, brain, spinal cord, and meninges, eye, liver, adrenal gland, uterus, and skin. Lymph nodes and spleen are hyperplastic. Erythrophagocytosis may be conspicuous throughout the reticuloendothelial system.

SURRA

The important trypanosomiasis of Asia occurs principally in Equidae, but dogs, elephants, and ruminants may be infected, and wild ruminants can act as reservoirs. Camels are also susceptible, and guinea pigs can be experimentally infected. The causative organism, *Trypanosoma evansi* (Evans, 1880), is transmitted mechanically by the bite of horse flies (*Tabanus, Stomoxys*). The disease is recognized most frequently in a severe form with the following characteristics: paroxysms of intermittent fever associated with trypanosomes in the blood; gradual emaciation in spite of good appetite; serous nasal discharge; patchy alopecia; petechiae and ecchymoses of visible mucosae; weakness and incoordination; edema of the limbs, lower abdomen, and thorax; icterus; progressive anemia; and fatal termination.

MAL DE CADERAS

This trypanosomiasis of tropical and subtropical South America, which affects Equidae in particular, is caused by *Trypanosoma equinum* (Voges, 1901). The disease is an acute infection similar to surra.

MURRINA DE CADERAS (DERRENGADERA DE CADERAS)

This occurs in Central America and is caused by *Trypanosoma hippicum*, first described by Darling in 1910. Horses and mules are particularly susceptible; cattle act as reservoirs of infection. The disease is essentially similar to surra, although a more prolonged course is described, with weakness, emaciation, anemia, ecchymoses, edema, splenomegaly, and paralysis being important features.

Trypanosomiasis in African swine, ascribed to *T. simiae*, a species originally recovered from monkeys, causes an acute fatal disease in pigs. In other domestic animals, the infection is transient.

DOURINE

A disease of Equidae, dourine has a cosmopolitan distribution but is now rare in the United States. In contrast to other trypanosomiases, the causative agent, *Trypanosoma equiperdum*, is transmitted by coitus, rarely by biting flies. The disease is manifest by edematous lesions in the genital tract and ventral body wall, persistent ulcerous plaques in the genitalia and skin, and occasionally by anemia, incoordination, and paralysis. The causative trypanosome is demonstrable in the lesions, particularly those of the genitalia. The lesions are those of a mononuclear or granulomatous inflammation. Rabbits and deer mice are experimentally susceptible.

CHAGAS DISEASE (AMERICAN TRYPANOSOMIASIS)

Trypanosoma cruzi was shown in 1909 by Chagas to be the cause of human trypanosomiasis in South America. The vectors were also proved by Chagas to be reduviid or "kissing" bugs (*Triatoma*). Dogs, cats, armadillos, monkeys, and small wild animals harbor the infection and are subject to a disease similar to the human infection. *T. cruzi*, in contrast to the other trypanosomes discussed, is of particular interest because it multiplies within the cytoplasm of cells in the mammalian hosts. After release of the infectious stage in the feces of the *Triatoma* bug, the organisms enter the blood stream as typical trypanosomes (trypanomastigotes), but do not multiply within the blood stream. Instead, they invade host cells, particularly cardiac and skeletal muscle, where they transform to amastigotes, a form closely resembling *Leishmania* and often referred to as the leishmanial form of *T. cruzi.* The amastigotes multiply within the cytoplasm of the infected cells, forming collections of organisms called pseudocysts. The amastigotes differentiate into trypanomastigotes, which are released upon rupture of the infected cells to the circulation where they are available to infect the intermediate host or invade another cell to repeat the cycle.

Lesions

The lesions result in part from the growth and activity of *T. cruzi* in the blood, but are most influenced by its intracellular activities, particularly in the myocardium. The initial lesion, seen in humans following the bite of a reduviid bug, is a hard, red, painful edematous mass occurring at the site of the bite. This soon subsides as the organisms spread. The lymph nodes may become enlarged, edematous, and show intense histiocytic proliferation, and occasionally may contain microabscesses. Giant cells may form and contain leishmanial forms of *T. cruzi.* The heart is particularly affected. Myocardial fibers are penetrated by the organism, which proliferates, filling and destroying muscle cells and resulting in severe myocarditis (Fig. 12-25). The heart becomes enlarged, the myocardium mottled with yellow, and the pericardial sac distended with fluid. Large cystic collections of leishmanial forms are demonstrable microscopically in cardiac muscle cells. The experimental disease in mice often results in myocarditis, particularly in the right ventricle. The right ventricle becomes distended and the ventricular wall thin. Passive congestion of liver and spleen is an expected result.

Skeletal and smooth muscle may also be invaded. In humans, megaesophagus and megacolon are frequent findings in patients with chronic infection. Although the pathogenesis is not entirely understood, it is believed to result from damage to the parasympathetic nervous system. This finding has not been reported in animals.

In brain, *T. cruzi* may produce edema and congestion, particularly in the meninges, with some perivascular lymphocytic infiltration. Nodules of mononuclear and glial cells may occur throughout the brain. Within these areas the leishmanial forms of the trypanosomes are found in the cytoplasm of cells and free in the tissue. Destruction of neurons may lead to chronic neurologic sequelae.

The testicle may be severely invaded by *T. cruzi;* the germinal cells become laden with organisms, and intense lymphocytic infiltration occurs in the interstitial stroma.

Diagnosis

The diagnosis depends upon demonstration of *T. cruzi* in blood or tissues of infected animals.

References

Anosa VO, Kaneko JJ. Pathogenesis of Trypanosoma brucei infection in deer mice *(Peromyscus maniculatus):* [1] hematologic, erythrocyte biochemical, and iron metabolic aspects; [2] light and electron microscopic studies on erythrocyte pathologic changes and phagocytosis. Am J Vet Res 1983a;44:639–644, 645–651.
Anosa VO, Kaneko JJ. Pathogenesis of *Trypanosoma brucei* infection in deer mice *(Peromyscus maniculatus):* V. Macrophage ultrastructure and function. Vet Pathol 1983b;20:617–631.
Anosa VO, Kaneko JJ. Pathogenesis of *Trypanosoma brucei* infection in deer mice *(Peromyscus maniculatus).* [1] Ultrastructural pathology of the spleen, liver, heart, and kidney. [2] Light and electron microscopic study of testicular lesions. Vet Pathol 1984;21:229–237, 238–246.
Anosa VO, Kaneko JJ. Ultrastructural pathology of hemopoietic organs in *Trypanosoma vivax* infection of goats. Vet Pathol 1989;26:78–83.
Barr S, Baker D, Markovits J. Trypanosomiasis and laryngeal paralysis in a dog. J Am Vet Med Assoc 1986;188:1307–1309.
Chagas C. Ueber eine neue Trypanosomiasis des Menschen. Mem Inst Oswaldo Cruz 1909;1:159–218.
Crane M St.J, Dvorak JA. Vertebrate cells express protozoan antigen after hybridization. Science 1980;208:194–196.
Esievo KAN, Saror DI. Immunochemistry and immunopathology of animal trypanosomiasis. Vet Bull 1991;61:765–777.
Fernandez DB, Rico F, Dumag PU. Observations on an outbreak of surra among cattle. Philipp J Anim Ind 1965;21:221–224, Vet Bull 1967;37:517.
Fiennes RNTW, Jones ER, Laws SG. The course and pathology of *Trypanosoma congolense* (Broden) disease of cattle. J Comp Pathol Ther 1946;56:1–27.
Fletcher KC, Hubbard GB. Fatal cardiomyopathy caused by *Trypanosoma cruzi* in an aardwolf. J Am Vet Med Assoc 1985;187:1263–1264.
Fox JC, Ewing SA, Buckner RG, et al. *Trypanosoma cruzi* infection in a dog from Oklahoma. J Am Vet Med Assoc 1986;189:1583–1584.
Gardiner PR, Pearson TW, Clarke MW, et al. Identification and isolation of a variant surface glycoprotein from *Trypanosoma vivax.* Science 1987;235:774–777.
Gleiser CA, Yeager RG, Ghidoni JJ. *Trypanosoma cruzi* infection in a colony-born baboon. J Am Vet Med Assoc 1986;189:1225–1226.
Ikede BO. Ocular lesions in sheep infected with *Trypanosoma brucei.* J Comp Pathol 1974;84:203–213.
Ikede BO, Losos GJ. Pathological changes in cattle infected with *Trypanosoma brucei.* Vet Pathol 1972;9:272–277.
Ikede BO, Losos GJ. Pathology of the disease in sheep produced experimentally by *Trypanosoma brucei.* Vet Pathol 1972;9:278–289.
Ikede BO, Losos GJ. Spontaneous canine trypanosomiasis caused by *T. brucei:* meningoenceophalomyelitis with extra-vascular localization by trypanosomes in the brain. Bull Epizoot Dis Afr 1972;20:221–228.
Ikede BO, Losos GJ. Pathogenesis of *Trypanosoma brucei* infection in sheep. I. Clinical signs. II. Cerebro-spinal fluid changes. III. Hypophysial and other endocrine lesions. J Comp Pathol 1975;85:23–31, 33–36, 37–44.
John DT, Hoppe KL. *Trypanosoma cruzi* from wild raccoons in Oklahoma. Am J Vet Res 1986;47:1056–1059.
Johnson CM. Cardiac changes in dogs experimentally infected with *Trypanosoma cruzi.* Am J Trop Med 1938;18:197–206.
Kaliner G. *Trypanosoma congolense.* II. Histopathologic findings in experimentally infected cattle. Exp Parasitol 1974;36:20–26.
Killick-Kendrick R. The diagnosis of trypanosomiasis of livestock: a review of current techniques. Vet Bull 1968;38:191–197.
Kobayashi A, Tizard IR, Woo PTK. Studies on the anemia in experimental African trypanosomiasis. II. The pathogenesis of the anemia in calves infected with *Trypanosoma congolense.* Am J Trop Med Hyg 1976;25:401–406.

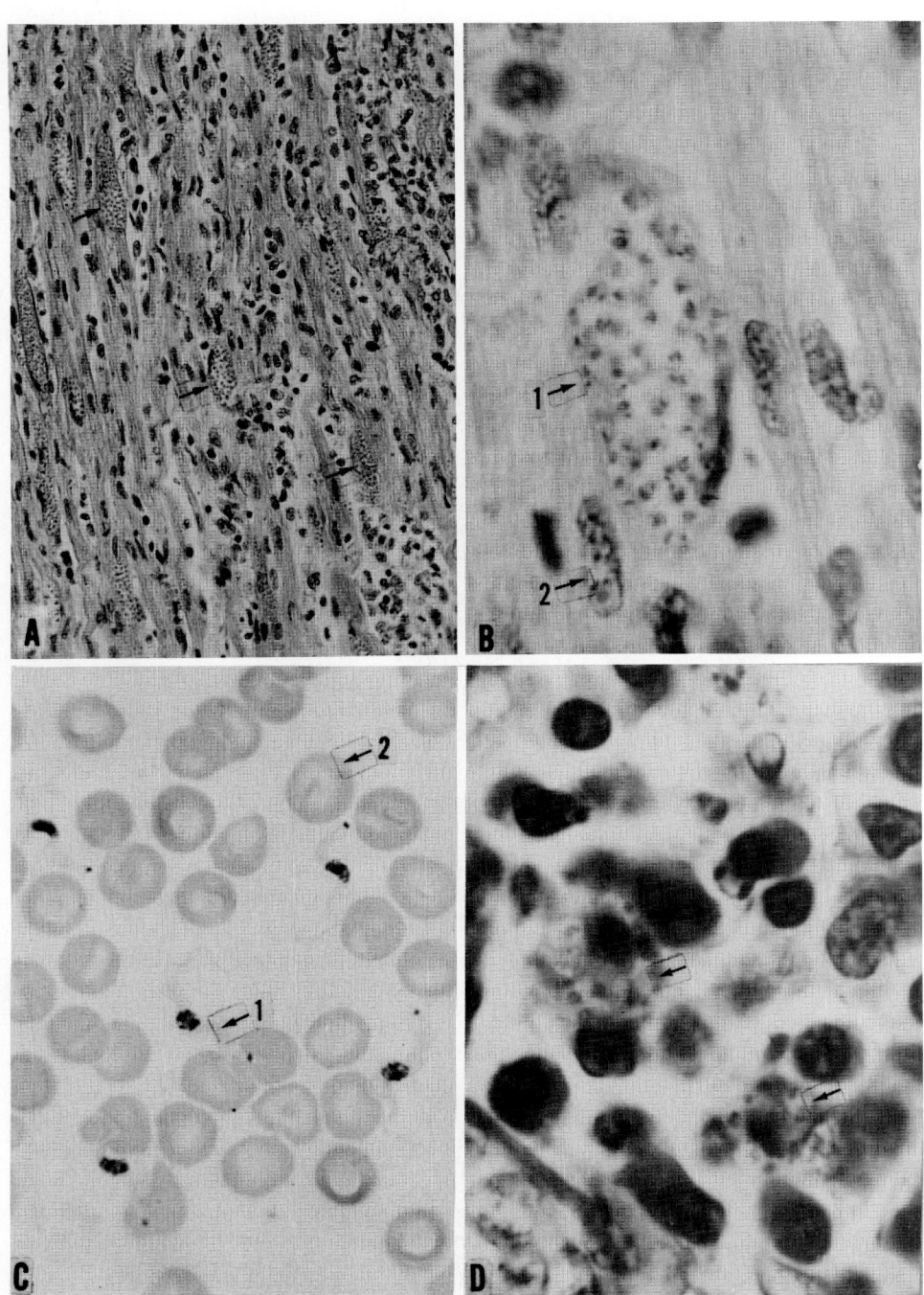

FIG. 12.25 **A.** *Trypanosoma cruzi* (arrows) (×240) in the myocardium of a dog. **B.** Higher magnification (×1240) showing leishmanial forms of Tr. cruzi in the cytoplasm (1) of a cardiac muscle bundle. (2) One nucleus of a cardiac muscle cell is indicated. (Contributor: Dr. Francisco Laranja.) **C.** Tr. cruzi (1) in the blood of a rat. (2) Erythrocytes. (Contributor: Lt. Col. F. D. Maurer.) **D.** Leishmaniasis, lymph node of dog (×1780); organisms (arrows) are in cytoplasm of macrophages. (Courtesy of Armed Forces Institute of Pathology; contributor: Dr. W. S. Bailey.)

Leach TM. African trypanosomiases. Adv Vet Sci Comp Med 1973;17:119–162.

Losos GJ, Ikede BO. Review of pathology of diseases in domestic and laboratory animals caused by *Trypanosoma congolense, T. vivax, T. brucei, T. rhodesiense* and *T. gambiense.* Vet Path 1972;9(Suppl).

McCully RM, Neitz WO. Clinicopathological study on experimental *Trypanosoma brucei* infections in horses. II. Histopathological findings in the nervous system and other organs of treated and untreated horses reacting to Nagana. Onderstepoort J Vet Res 1971;38:141–176.

Morrison WI, Murray M, Bovell DL. Response of the murine lymphoid system to chronic infection with *Trypanosoma congolense.* I. The spleen. Lab Invest 1981;45:547–557.

Mortelmans J, Neetens A. Ocular lesions in experimental *Trypanosoma brucei* infection in cats (and dogs). Acta Zool Path Antverp 1975;62:149–172.

Moulton JE. Relapse infection after chemotherapy in goats experimentally infected with *Trypanosoma brucei:* pathological changes in the central nervous system. Vet Pathol 1986;23:21–28.

Moulton JE, Coleman JL, Gee MK. Pathogenesis of *Trypanosoma equiperdum* in rabbits. Am J Vet Res 1975;36:357–366.

Moulton JE, Sollod AE. Clinical, serologic, and pathologic changes in calves with experimentally induced *Trypanosoma brucei* infection. Am J Vet Res 1976;37:791–802.

Nagle RB, Dong S, Janacek LL, et al. Glomerular accumulation of monocytes and macrophages in experimental glomerulonephritis associated with *Trypanosoma rhodesiense* infection. Lab Invest 1982;46:365–377.

Naylor DC. The haematology and histopathology of *Trypanosoma congolense* infection in cattle. I. Introduction and histopathology. Trop Anim Health Prod 1971;3:95–100.

Olson LC, Skinner SF, Palotay JL, et al. Encephalitis associated with *Trypanosoma cruzi* in a Celebes black macaque. Lab Anim Sci 1986;36: 667–670.

Ouaissi MA, Cornette J, Afchain D, et al. *Trypanosoma cruzi* infection inhibited by peptides modeled from a fibronectin cell attachment domain. Science 1986;234:603–607.

Packchanian A. Studies on *Trypanosoma gambiense* infection in various species of experimental animals. Tex Rep Biol Med 1964;22: 707–715.

Preston JM, Wellde BT, Kovatch RM. *Trypanosoma congolense:* calf erythrocyte survival. Exp Parasitol 1979;48:118–125, Vet Bull 1980; 50:674.

Seiler RJ, Omar S, Jackson ARB. Meningoencephalitis in naturally occurring *Trypanosoma evansi* infection (surra) of horses. Vet Pathol 1981;18:120–122.

Snider TG III, Yeager RG, Dellucky J. Myocarditis caused by *Trypanosoma cruzi* in a native Louisiana dog. J Am Vet Med Assoc 1980;177:247–249.

Tomlinson MJ, Chapman WL Jr, Hanson WL, et al. Occurrence of antibody to *Trypanosoma cruzi* in dogs in the southeastern United States. Am J Vet Res 1981;42:1444–1446.

LEISHMANIASIS

Infections in humans and animals with protozoan organisms of the genus *Leishmania* have various local names but can be grouped together on the basis of their common characteristics. Several pathogenic species and variously named subspecies of *Leishmania* are recognized; however, they cannot be differentiated from one another in tissue section. They have different geographic distributions and the diseases they induce are relatively distinct, although there may be overlap in clinical signs and lesions.

Leishmania occur in vertebrate hosts within parasitophorous vacuoles in macrophages and reticuloendothelial cells as amastigotes (leishmanial forms), which are small oval protozoans about 1–2 μm wide by 2–4 μm long, with neither flagellum nor undulating membrane. In Romanovsky-stained preparations, they have pale blue cytoplasm containing, near the posterior end, a reddish nucleus with a deeper staining central karyosome. Tangential and anterior to the nucleus is a deep violet, rod-shaped body, the kinetoplast, which contains the parabasal body and the dot-shaped blepharoplast. In its invertebrate host (sandflies) or in cultures, the organisms assume shapes varying from the leishmanial to the leptomonad form, the latter, being slender and spindle-shaped, from 14–20 μ in length and 1.5–4 μ in width. This form is motile by means of a flagellum that arises from the blepharoplast and projects from the anterior pole of the organism.

Life cycle

Leishmania reproduce in the vertebrate host by binary fission, but the complete life cycle and maintenance of virulence depend upon an intermediate host or vector. Many species of sandflies (*Phlebotomus*) are involved in the transmission of *Leishmania* and are necessary for their perpetuation, but certain flies, such as *Stomoxys calcitrans,* may mechanically transmit the infection.

Clinical forms of leishmaniasis

Classically, leishmaniasis is divided into three major forms, although there may be considerable variation. Each form is associated with specific species of *Leishmania*. The most notable difference between the forms is the generalized spread of organisms in visceral leishmaniasis and their localized confinement in the other forms.

Visceral leishmaniasis (Kala-azar, Dum dum fever) is principally caused by *L. donovani*. It occurs naturally in humans, dogs, cats, squirrels, cattle, horses, and sheep, but many laboratory animals, especially hamsters and dogs, are susceptible to experimental infection. It has a wide geographic distribution, but is most prevalent in countries bordering the Mediterranean, large areas of Africa, India, and China. In Central and South America a variant organism termed *L. donovani chagasi* is the main cause of visceral leishmaniasis. Most cases reported in the United States are in animals which contracted the infection in countries where the disease is endemic; however, endemic foci have been identified recently in Texas and Oklahoma.

Visceral leishmaniasis in animals usually is observed as a chronic debilitating disease with periods of fever, gradual weight loss, anemia, and leukopenia. Lymph nodes are enlarged and there is splenomegaly and hepatomegaly. A history of persistent cutaneous ulcer(s) that heals slowly may sometimes be obtained. Most often the infection slowly progresses to death.

The lesions of visceral leishmaniasis are characterized by massive infiltration of multiple organ systems with huge macrophages whose cytoplasm is filled with leishmaniae. The architecture of the lymph nodes and spleen, which are particularly affected, may be completely obscured by the phagocytic cells. Large numbers of plasma cells are usually also present. The liver, bone marrow, kidneys, lungs, gastrointestinal tract and, less often, other viscera and skin may be affected. Gross findings at necropsy consist of: severe emaciation; enlarged lymph nodes, spleen and liver; sometimes pallor of mucosae and serous surfaces; soft red bone marrow; and ulcers of the intestine. Some fibrosis may accompany the infiltrates, but this is not a remarkable feature, nor is necrosis. Immune complex glomerulonephritis may be present.

Cutaneous Leishmaniasis (Fig. 12-26) caused by *L. tropica* or *L. major* occurs principally in Southern European and Northern African countries bordering the Mediterranean. It is also known as Old World cutaneous leishmaniasis, Oriental sore, Delhi sore, Baghdad boil, or bouton de Crete. The reservoirs for human infection are various wild rodents, although dogs, mice, guinea pigs, and monkeys are susceptible to experimental infection. The infection is characterized by single or multiple very slowly developing nodules or ulcers of the skin that usually heal spontaneously, but only over a pe-

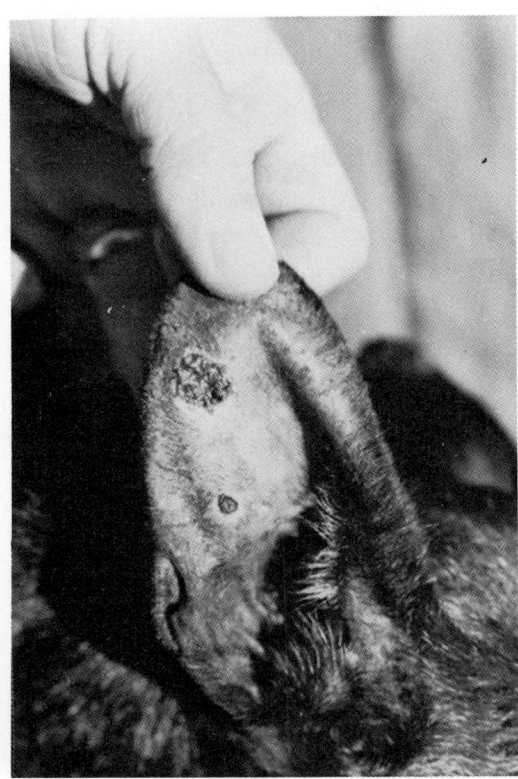

FIG. 12-26 Cutaneous leishmaniasis. Elevated ulcerated lesions in skin of the ear of a dog. (Courtesy of Dr. A. Herrer and American Journal of Tropical Medicine and Hygiene.)

riod of months. The lesions are characterized by dermal infiltration of macrophages accompanied by lymphocytes, plasma cells, and rarely eosinophils. Numerous parasites are present within the macrophages. Lesions of long-standing are circumscribed by fibroblastic connective tissue, giving them the appearance of a typical granuloma.

Mucocutaneous Leishmaniasis, also known as New World cutaneous leishmaniasis or American leishmaniasis, is caused by *L. braziliensis* or *L. mexicana*. It occurs in Mexico and Central and South America. Animals are not frequently found infected, although ground squirrels, dogs, cats, and monkeys are susceptible. The infection resembles Old World cutaneous leishmaniasis, but in addition to the skin, chronic ulcers often are localized at mucocutaneous junctions and may occur in oral and nasal cavities. The lesions are comparable to those of cutaneous leishmaniasis.

Diagnosis

Other diseases that also cause proliferation of reticuloendothelium present the most problems in differential diagnosis. These include histoplasmosis, toxoplasmosis (some cases), salmon disease, blastomycosis, and epizootic lymphangitis. Final determination must be based upon demonstration and identification of the causative organisms in tissue sections, smears or cultures. Identification of the kinetoplast and the small nucleus in *Leishmania*, which are not present in the organisms mentioned above, allows differentiation. The tissue phase of *Trypanosoma cruzi* (Chagas disease) does have a kinetoplast, but the distribution and character of the lesions are different. Tissues taken by biopsy are most useful to demonstrate the organisms in a living animal or human patient.

References

Anderson DC, Buckner RG, Glenn BL, et al. Endemic canine leishmaniasis. Vet Pathol 1980;17:94–96.

Broderson JR, Chapman WL Jr, Hanson WL. Experimental visceral leishmaniasis in the owl monkey. Vet Pathol 1986;23:293–302.

Chang K-P. Human cutaneous *Leishmania* in a mouse macrophage line: propagation and isolation of intracellular parasites. Science 1980;209:1240–1242.

Ferrer L, Fondevila D, Marco A, et al. Atypical nodular leishmaniasis in two dogs. Vet Rec 1990;126:90.

Ferrer L, Juanola B, Ramos JA, et al. Chronic colitis due to *Leishmania* infection in two dogs. Vet Pathol 1991;28:342–343.

Giannini SH, et al. Karyotype analysis of *Leishmania* species and its use in classification and clinical diagnosis. Science 1986;232:762–765.

Herrer A, Christensen HA. Natural cutaneous leishmaniasis among dogs in Panama. Am J Trop Med Hyg 1976;25:59–63.

Keenan CM, Hendricks LD, Lightner L, et al. Visceral leishmaniasis in the German shepherd dog. I. Infection, clinical disease, and clinical pathology. Vet Pathol 1984a;21:74–79.

Keenan CM, Hendricks LM, Lightner L, et al. Visceral leishmaniasis in the German shepherd dog. II. Pathology. Vet Pathol 1984b;21:80–86.

McConnell EE, Chafee EF, Cashell IG, et al. Visceral leishmaniasis with ocular involvement in a dog. J Am Vet Med Assoc 1970;156:197–203.

Ponce C, et al. *Leishmania donovani chagasi*: a new clinical variant of cutaneous leishmaniasis in Honduras. Lancet 1991;337:67–70.

Pung OJ, Kuhn RE. Experimental American leishmaniasis in the Brazilian squirrel monkey *(Saimiri sciureus)*: lesions, hematology, cellular, and humoral immune responses. J Med Primatol 1987;16:165–174.

Simpson CF, Harvey JW, French TW. Ultrastructure of amastigotes of *Leishmania donovani* in the bone marrow of a dog. Am J Vet Res 1982;43:1684–1686.

Swenson CL, et al. Visceral leishmaniasis in an English Foxhound from an Ohio research colony. J Am Vet Med Assoc 1988;193:1089–1092.

White MR, Chapman WL Jr, Hanson WL, et al. Experimental visceral leishmaniasis in the opossum. Vet Pathol 1989;26:314–321.

MALARIA

Malaria has been recognized as an important disease of humans for most of recorded history and is still one of the most important infectious diseases in spite of great strides toward its eradication. It is estimated that there are about 100 million clinical cases of malaria in humans annually with a new infection rate of over 4 million persons per year. The disease is most prevalent in tropical and subtropical regions, but is not unknown in temperate parts of the globe. It is especially deleterious to young children, often combining with hookworm, tuberculosis, and other diseases to debilitate and kill. The name of the malady, malaria, comes from the Italian words mala (bad) and aria (air), in reference to the "miasmic vapors" which were believed to come from swamps.

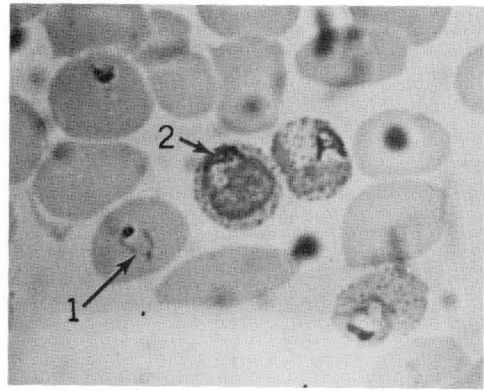

FIG. 12-27 Malaria in a cynomolgus monkey *(Macaca fascicularis)*. (1) Schizonts and (2) gametocytes of *Plasmodium cynomolgi* are present in erythrocytes. (Courtesy of New England Regional Primate Research Center, Harvard Medical School.)

One of the causative parasites was discovered by a French Army physician, Laveran, who in 1880 found what are now considered to be microgametocytes, probably of the organism now called *Plasmodium falciparum.* It was not until after the turn of the century that Sir Ronald Ross demonstrated mosquitoes to be the "miasmas" arising from swamps to spread the disease (1910). The causative protozoa, classified among the sporozoa, are currently all members of the genus *Plasmodium,* (Fig. 12-27) which includes many pathogenic species.

Malaria is most important as a disease of humans, but many species of animals are susceptible to their own specific species of *Plasmodium,* including birds, rodents, reptiles, and nonhuman primates. In general, however, malaria is not of veterinary importance except in experimental model systems. Those spontaneous infections encountered in animals, which includes infections in the United States, are not associated with significant clinical disease or pathological findings. The simian malarias are an occasional exception, but even here malaria in monkeys is usually an incidental finding. Nonhuman primate malarias are important models for human malaria (as are those of rodents and birds), but are also of interest as humans are susceptible to certain of the simian *Plasmodium* spp.

Life cycle

The life cycles of *Plasmodium,* as far as currently known, are quite similar. Two hosts are required: (1) vertebrates (humans, other mammals, birds, and reptiles), in which schizogony takes place in erythrocytes and other cells; and (2) invertebrate blood-sucking insects (mosquitoes). The cycle is started when a female mosquito penetrates the skin of the vertebrate host, introducing sporozoites into the peripheral circulation. After a few days of exoerythrocytic development in endothelial cells or hepatocytes as schizonts, merozoites are released and enter red blood cells where they reside within parasitophorous vacuoles. Here they initially appear as ring forms that enlarge to a stage called trophozoites which, in turn, divide into schizonts containing up to 24 or more merozoites. Merozoites released upon rupture of the infected erythrocyte reinfect other red blood cells. This repeated schizogony, progressing geometrically, results in the paroxysmal recurrence of the signs of fever and anemia. Some of the merozoites ultimately develop into gametocytes, and remain in the blood as macro- and microgametocytes until ingested by a mosquito or eliminated by phagocytosis as their life span is completed. The organisms incompletely catabolize hemoglobin, leaving a brownish pigment, hemozoin, easily visible on stained smears.

The macro- and microgametocytes ingested by female mosquitoes (the males do not ingest blood) undergo further development in the stomach of the mosquito; the macrogametocyte becomes one macrogamete and the microgametocyte becomes 4–8 microgametes. Fusion of gametes results in a motile zygote, called ookinete, which enters the gastric mucosa of the mosquito and becomes an oocyst, which then lies in the stroma adjacent to the gastric epithelium. Repeated nuclear divisions result in the formation of many sporozoites, which are set free by rupture into the hemolymph, permitting migration to the salivary glands of the mosquito. From this site, the sporozoites are available to infect a new vertebrate host when the female mosquito takes her blood meal.

Clinical manifestations

The signs in malaria are related to the numbers of parasites in the blood, and appear 5–14 or more days following infection; the incubation period depends to some extent upon the exoerythrocytic period of the parasites. Bouts of chills and fever appear at intervals roughly comparable to the periods of reproduction of the malaria parasite. The terms tertian (third) and quartan (fourth) apply to the usual interval between paroxysms. In tertian malaria, such as in *Plasmodium vivax* and *P. falciparum* infection, the signs reappear on the third day after a 48-hour cycle. In the case of quartan malaria, the cycle of the parasite *(P. malariae)* is about 76 hours, and the signs reappear each fourth day. Malaria due to *P. falciparum* may also have a cycle less than 48 hours (subtertian) due to presence of two broods of parasites. These features are covered in Table 12-6. Relapses often occur in human malaria, sometimes after long intervals, thus providing a carrier state. This state also appears to occur in other animals.

Lesions

The pathologic effects of malaria vary to some extent with the organism involved, but are similar in most vertebrate hosts. The destruction of parasitized erythrocytes results in hemolysis and anemia, to which most of the clinical and pathologic findings can be ascribed. Marked splenomegaly and hepatomegaly are manifest, resulting from congestion, hemorrhage, hyperplasia of

TABLE 12-6 **Malarias**

Organism	Vertebrate hosts	Disease	Geographic distribution
Plasmodium falciparum	Man	Malignant tertian, falciparum, or subtertian malaria	Widely distributed in tropics, some in subtropics
P. malariae	Man, chimpanzee	Quartan malaria	Philippine Islands, India
P. ovale	Man	Mild tertian malaria	Africa, Philippines and India
P. vivax	Man, chimpanzee (experimental)	Benign tertian or vivax malaria	Tropical, subtropical, some temperate regions, South and North America, England, Sweden, Argentina, Australia, Natal
P. knowlesi	*Macaca fascicularis* (crab-eater macaque) *M. cyclopis* (Taiwan macaque) *M. nemestrina* *Presbytis melalophus* Man	Simian malaria	Malaya, Philippines
P. gallinaceum	Domestic fowl (other birds suscept. exper.)	Avian malaria	India
P. relictum	Penguins, sparrows, many birds	Avian malaria	U.S.A. (zoos)
P. brazilianum	*Cebus apella* (capuchin), *Alouatta seniculus,* *A. fusca* (howler monkeys), *Cacajao calvus* (uakari), *Chiropotes chiropotes* (saki), *Ateles paniscus p.,* *A. paniscus chemek* (spider monkey), *Lagothrix lagotricha,* *L. cana* (woolly monkeys), *Brachyteles arachnoides* (woolly spider monkey), *Callicebus torquatus* (titi), *Saimiri sciureus* (squirrel monkey), man	Simian malaria (quartan type)	South and Central America
P. simium	*Alouatta fusca, Brachyteles arachnoides,* occasionally man	Simian malaria (benign-tertian type)	Brazil
P. cynomolgi	*Macaca fascicularis,* *M. nemestrina* (pig-tailed macaque), *M. cyclopis* (Taiwan macaque), *M. radiata* (bonnet monkey), *Cynopithecus niger, Presbytis sp.* Man	Simian malaria	Philippines, Taiwan, Malaya, Java, Ceylon, India, Cambodia, Pakistan
P. coatneyi	*Macaca fascicularis*	Simian malaria	Philippines, Malaya
P. inui	*Macaca fascicularis,* *M. mulatta* (rhesus), *M. radiata,* *M. nemestrina,* *M. cyclopis,* *Cynopithecus niger,* *Presbytis sp.* Man	Simian malaria	Indochina, Philippines, tropical Asia
P. fieldi	*M. nemestrina* *M. fascicularis*	Simian malaria	Malaya
P. fragile	*M. radiata, M. sinica*	Simian malaria	Ceylon

(continued)

TABLE 12-6 (continued)

Organism	Vertebrate hosts	Disease	Geographic distribution
P. simiovale	M. sinica	Simian malaria	Ceylon
P. pitheci	Pongo pigmaeus (orangutan)	Simian malaria	Borneo
P. youngi	Hylobates lar (gibbon)	Simian malaria	Malaya
P. jefferyi	Hylobates lar	Simian malaria	Malaya
P. eylesi	Hylobates lar	Simian malaria	Malaya
P. hylobates	Hylobates lar	Simian malaria	Java
P. gonderi	Cerocebus galeritus, C. aterrimus, C. atys, Mandrillus leucophaeus	Simian malaria	West Africa
P. reichenowi	Gorilla gorilla (gorilla), Pan troglodytes (chimpanzee)	Simian malaria	West and Central Africa
P. rhodhaini	Pan troglodytes	Simian malaria	West and Central Africa
P. schwetzi	Gorilla gorilla Pan troglodytes Man	Simian malaria	West and Central Africa
Hepatocystis (Plasmodium) kochi (Hepatocystis simiae)	Cercopithecus sp. Papio sp., etc.	Simian malaria Hepatocystis	Africa

reticuloendothelial cells, and an influx of macrophages, both of which cells contain phagocytized free parasites, parasitized erythrocytes and malaria pigment (hemozoin). Hemorrhages in brain may be associated with blood vessels occluded by parasitized red blood cells and thrombi. Immune complex glomerulonephritis may accompany acute and chronic infection.

Diagnosis

The diagnosis of malaria is usually established by demonstrating the organisms in erythrocytes in thin or thick smears stained with Giemsa's or Wright-Giemsa stain.

References

Abilgaard C, Harrison J, DeNardo S, et al. Simian *Plasmodium knowlesi* malaria: studies of coagulation and pathology. Am J Trop Med Hyg 1975;24:764–768.

Anonymous. World malaria situation. World Health Stat Q 1987;40:142–151.

Atkinson CT, Aikawa M. Ultrastructure of malaria-infected erythrocytes. Blood Cells 1990;16:351–368.

Coatney GR. Simian malarias in man: facts, implications, and predictions. Am J Trop Med Hyg 1968;17:147–155.

Collins WE. Primate malarias. Adv Vet Sci Comp Med 1974;18:1–23.

Conrad ME. Pathophysiology of malaria. Hematologic observations in human and animal studies. Ann Intern Med 1969;70:134–141.

Donovan JC, Stokes WS, Montrey RD, et al. Hematologic characterization of naturally occurring malaria (*Plasmodium inui*) in cynomolgus monkeys (Macaca fascicularis). Lab Anim Sci 1983;33:86–89.

Garnham PCC. Malaria in mammals excluding man. Adv Parasitol 1967;5:139–204.

Held JR. Primate malaria. Ann NY Acad Sci 1969;162:587–593.

Hutt MSR, Davies DR, Voller A. Malarial infections in *Aotus trivirgatus* with special reference to renal pathology. II. *P. falciparum* and mixed malaria infections. Br J Exp Pathol 1975;56:429–438.

Ross R. The Prevention of Malaria. London: Murray, 1910.

Schmidt LH. Infections with *Plasmodium falciparum* and *Plasmodium vivax* in the owl monkey: model systems for basic biological and chemotherapeutic studies. Trans R Soc Trop Med Hyg 1973;67:446–474.

Schmidt LH, Esslinger JH. Courses of infections with *Plasmodium falciparum* in owl monkeys displaying a microfilaremia. Am J Trop Med Hyg 1981;30:5–11.

Schofield LD, Bennett BT, Collins WE, et al. An outbreak of *Plasmodium inui* malaria in a colony of diabetic rhesus monkeys. Lab Anim Sci 1985;35:167–168.

Stokes WS, et al. Acute clinical malaria (*Plasmodium inui*) in a cynomolgus monkey (*Macaca fascicularis*). Lab Anim Sci 1983;33:81–85.

Voller A. Immunopathology of malaria. Bull WHO 1974;50:177–186.

Voller A, Davies DR, Hurt MSR. Quartan malarial infections in *Aotus trivirgatus* with special reference to renal pathology. Br J Exp Pathol 1973;54:457–468.

Young MD, Baerg DC, Rossan RN. Parasitological review: experimental monkey hosts for human plasmodia. Exp Parasitol 1975;38:136–152.

HEPATOCYSTIS

The genus *Hepatocystis,* classified in the same family as the genus *Plasmodium,* contains thirteen or more species of parasites which exist in tropical countries, particularly in Africa and Asia. They are recognized as affecting a variety of different monkeys as well as fruit bats, oriental squirrels, deer mice, and hippopotomi. The organisms have been found in primates of the genera *Ma-*

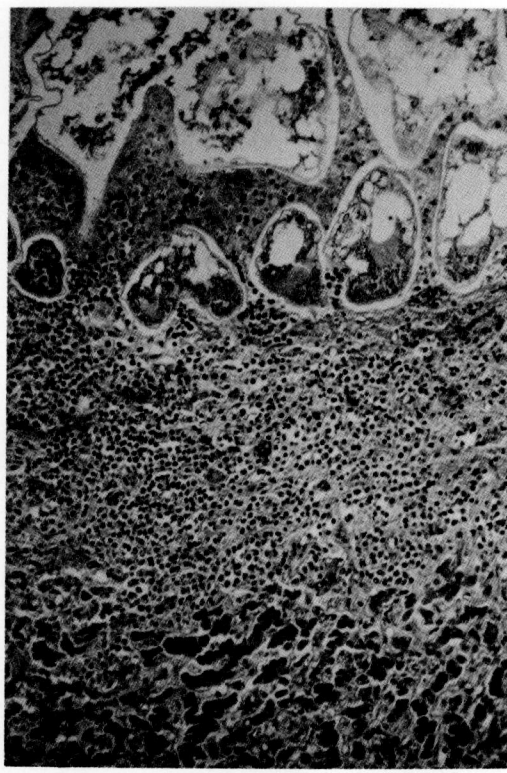

FIG. 12-28 *Hepatocystis kochi*, liver of a baboon. The section includes part of the cyst (too), a zone of reaction, and liver cells (bottom).

caca, Papio, Hylobates, and *Cercopithecus.* Species affecting nonhuman primates include *Hepatocystis kochi* (Fig. 12-28), *H. bouillezi, H. cercopitheci, H. simiae, H. semnopitheci,* and *H. taiwanensis.* The infection is apparently of little consequence to the health of the mammalian host; however, the parasites in erythrocytes can be confused with other protozoan diseases, such as malaria, and the schizonts in the liver can pose a diagnostic dilemma to the novice.

Life cycle

Culicoides species *(C. fulvithorax, C. adersi)* have been identified as intermediate hosts for nonhuman primate species of *Hepatocystis.* Sexual reproduction occurs in the insect, leading to the formation of sporozoites, which are the infectious stage for the mammalian host. Sporozoites invade hepatocytes and develop into schizonts which, over a period of one to two months, become large and are termed merocysts. One distinguishing feature of *Hepatocystis* is the size of the mature merocysts which are grossly visible, up to 2 mm in diameter with a central, fluid-filled space. Microscopically, the circumference of the merocyst is occupied by myriads of tiny merozoites; the central core consists of eosinophilic colloidal or granular material. Early schizonts and merocysts consist of irregular arrays of merozoites lacking the central acellular cyst. Released merozoites reinvade hepatocytes to repeat the process or parasitize

erythrocytes as ring forms, which then develop into gametocytes.

Lesions

Lesions in the liver consist of the large merocysts with or without a significant tissue reaction. The most frequent reaction is granulomatous with multinucleated giant cells admixed with macrophages, eosinophils, and lymphocytes (Fig. 12-28). Remnants of merocysts, lacking merozoites and surrounded by a granulomatous reaction, may be all that is seen in some cases. Ultimately, fibrous connective tissue replaces the cyst with a scar. The erythrocytic stage consists of ring form trophozoites, macrogametocytes and microgametocytes. As with *Plasmodium,* hemozoin pigment is present in the gametocytes.

References

Desowitz RS. Observations on *Hepatocystis* of white-cheeked gibbon *(Hylobates concolor).* J Parasitol 1970;56:444–446.
Fallis AM, Desser SS. On species of *Leucocytozoon, Haemoproteus,* and *Hepatocystis.* In: Kreier JP, ed. Parasitic Protozoa, Vol. III: Gregarines, haemogregarines, coccidia, plasmodia, and haemoproteids. New York: Academic Press, 1977;238–266.
Garnham PCC. Exoerythrocytic schizogony in *Plasmodium kochi,* Laveran: a preliminary note. Trans Roy Soc Trop Med Hyg 1947;40:719–722.
Garnham PCC. The developmental cycle of *Hepatocystes (Plasmodium) kochi* in the monkey host. Trans Roy Soc Trop Med Hyg 1948;41:601–616.
Manwell RD, Kuntz RE. Hepatocystis in Formosan mammals with a description of a new species. J Protozool 1966;13:670–672.
Shiroishi T, Davis J, Warren M. Hepatocystis in white-cheeked gibbon, *Hylobates concolor.* J Parasitol 1968;54:168.
Vickers JH. *Hepatocystis kochi* in Cercopithecus monkeys. J Am Vet Med Assoc 1966;149:906–908.
Warren McW, Shiroishi T, Davis J. A hepatocystis-like parasite of the gibbon. Trans Roy Soc Trop Med Hyg 1968;62:4.

HEPATOZOON INFECTIONS

Organisms of the genus *Hepatozoon* are placed in the class Sporozoa of the Protozoa and contain several pathogenic species. Schizogony occurs in endothelial cells of the liver; gametocytes may be found in either erythrocytes or leukocytes of the vertebrate host, depending upon the species of the protozoa. Sporogony occurs in blood-sucking arthropods.

Life cycle

Hepatozoon canis has been reported in dogs, cats, hyenas, jackals, and a number of wild felidae. For the most part, the infection is limited to the Middle East, North Africa, the Far East, and rarely Europe. In some locales the incidence of infection is high. It has been seen in the United States in a cat which had been to Hawaii, and has also been reported in two bobcats in California, indicating that the organism and therefore the disease can be encountered in the United States. The developmental cycle of the organism involves the brown dog tick, *Rhipicephalus sanguineus,* which, when infected, carries sporocysts in its body cavity. Ingestion of the infected vector tick by the vertebrate host results in release of sporozoites, which penetrate the intestinal wall to reach the spleen, liver, lungs, lymph nodes, myocardium, and bone marrow by way of the bloodstream. The parasites enter tissue cells to become schizonts, reproducing several generations in these cells. Eventually, merozoites are produced, which parasitize erythrocytes or leukocytes and become gametocytes, or gamonts. These gametocytes become differentiated into macro- and microgametocytes in the body of the vector tick, and sexual union results in a motile zygote, the ookinete. This ookinete migrates to the hemocoel of the tick, where it grows to a large oocyst, 100 μm in diameter, in which large numbers of sporozoites are formed within sporocysts. The sporozoites are released from the oocyst after the tick is ingested by the vertebrate host.

Clinical manifestations

Most frequently, the parasites are encountered as incidental findings in the absence of clinical signs or tissue reaction. However, infection may lead to signs of fever, anemia, splenomegaly, progressive emaciation, and sometimes paralysis. Death may occur four to eight weeks following outset of clinical signs.

Lesions

The lesions are those of anemia and focal necrotizing granulomas in affected tissues.

Diagnosis

The diagnosis is based on demonstration of the organisms: gametocytes in leukocytes in blood smears, or schizonts in biopsy or necropsy specimens of liver, spleen, bone marrow, or other tissue. Intercurrent disease apparently accentuates the pathogenicity of hepatozoon (McCully et al., 1975).

Several other organisms of this genus are known to infect vertebrates; some of them are: *Hepatozoon cuniculi* (host: rabbit in Europe); *H. muris* (brown rat, *Rattus norvegicus*, or black rat, *Rattus rattus*; the vector is the rat mite, *Echinolaelaps echidminus*); *H. procyonis* (raccoon); *Hepatozoon* sp. (impala in South Africa); *H. musculi* (white mouse in England).

References

Basson PA, et al. Observations on a *Hepatozoon*-like parasite in the impala. J S Afr Vet Med Assoc 1967;38:12–14, Vet Bull 1967; 37:4651.

Gaunt PS, Gaunt SD, Craig TM. Extreme neutrophilic leukocytosis in a dog with hepatozoonosis. J Am Vet Med Assoc 1983;182: 409–410.

Klopfer U, Nobel TA, Neumann F. *Hepatozoon*-like parasite (schizonts) in the myocardium of the domestic cat. Vet Pathol 1973;10: 185–190.

Lane JR, Kocan AA. *Hepatozoon* sp infection in bobcats. J Am Vet Med Assoc 1983;183:1323–1324.

McCully RM, et al. Observations on naturally acquired hepatozoonosis of wild carnivores and dogs in the Republic of South Africa. Onderstepoort J Vet Res 1975;42:117–133.

Schneider CR. *Hepatozoon procyonis* Richards, 1961, in a Panamanian raccoon, *Procyon cancrivorus panamensis* (Goldman). Rev Biol Trop 1968;15:123–135.

Soulsby EJL. Helminths, arthropods and protozoa of domesticated animals (Monnig), 6th ed. Philadelphia: Lea & Febiger, 1968.

Babesiosis (piroplasmosis, tick fever, "red water")

Organisms of the genus *Babesia*, Protozoa of the order Sporozoa, parasitize the erythrocytes of a wide variety of vertebrate hosts, multiplying in the erythrocytes by means of binary fission and giving rise to two or four daughter individuals. Ticks act as intermediate host-vectors in which the parasites reproduce, sometimes penetrating the egg to infect the young tick. *Babesia*, first described in 1888 by Babes in Roumania, were not recognized as important pathogens until Smith and Kilborne (1893) reported them as the cause of Texas cattle fever. Their work demonstrated for the first time that an infection of any kind could be transmitted by an arthropod vector, a major scientific achievement and a milestone in the conquest of disease.

Several score of *Babesia* spp. (Table 12-7) have been identified, all of which are pathogenic, but there is considerable variation in the severity of disease caused by the different species and strains of organisms. In cattle, severity of infection is also determined by breed. *Bos indicus* breeds are relatively resistant. Infection in young animals is usually mild (due to the effects of colostrum) and affords future protection. Recovery from infection in adults confers relatively good immunity. The infection is more severe following splenectomy. Of the 71 species in the genus *Babesia*, only a few affect domestic animals. *Babesia* spp. have been considered to be relatively host-specific; recently, however, cross-species infections have been recognized. Dogs, cattle, horses, sheep, swine, humans, and nonhuman primates are susceptible to one or more separate species of *Babesia*, but the general features of the disease are similar in all hosts.

The organisms occur in circulating erythrocytes as pyriform or ovoid bodies, usually in pairs or multiples thereof. They can be divided into two groups based on their size: the larger (*Babesia bigemina*, *B. major*, *B. caballi*, *B. motasi*, *B. canis*, *B. trautmanni*) measuring 4–5 μm long by 2–3 μm wide; and the smaller (*B. bovis*, *B. argentina*, *B. ovis*, *B. gibsoni*, *B. felis*, *B. divergens*, *B. equi*) measuring 1–2 μm long by about 0.5 μm wide. They are readily distinguished from *Plasmodium* spp. by the absence of hemoglobin-derived pigment. *Babesia* spp. completely catabolize hemoglobin, whereas the *Plasmodia* retain the brownish pigment (hemozoin). *Babesia* are particularly well demonstrated by Romanovsky-type stains.

Clinical signs

Clinical Signs are variable, but include fever, malaise, listlessness, anorexia, anemia, icterus, hemoglobinuria, and ascites. Coma may appear prior to death.

TABLE 12-7 **_Babesia_ Infections**

Organism	Animals affected	Geographic distribution	Tick vectors
B. bigemina	Cattle, zebu, water buffalo, deer	Central and South America, Africa, Australia, Southern Europe	_Boophilus annulatus, B. microplus, B. australis, B. calcaratus, B. decoloratus, Rhipicephalus evertsi, Rh. bursa, Rh. appendiculatus, Haemaphysalis punctata_
B. bovis	Cattle, roe deer, stag	Southern Europe, Africa, Asia	_Ixodes ricinus, I. persulcatus, Boophilus calcaratus, Rhipicephalus bursa_
B. argentina	Cattle	Central and South America, Australia	_Boophilus miroplus_
B. divergens	Cattle	Northern Europe	_Ixodes ricinus, Dermacentor reticulatus_
B. major	Cattle	Europe, Africa	_Haemophysalis punctata_
B. canis	Dog, wolf, jackal	Asia, Africa, Southern Europe, United States, Central and South America, Soviet Union	_Rhipicephalus sanguineus, Dermacentor reticulatus, D. marginatus, Haemophysalis leachi, Hyalomma plumbeum_
B. gibsoni	Dog, wolf, fox, jackal	India, Ceylon, China, Turkestan, North Africa, United States	_Haemaphysalis bispinosa, Rhipicephalus sanguineus_
B. equi	Horse, mule, donkey, zebra	Asia, Africa, United States, Europe, South America, Soviet Union	_Dermacentor reticulatus, D. marginatus, Rhipicephalus bursa, Rh. sanguineus, Rh. evertsi, Hyalomma excavatum, Hy. plumbeum, Hy. dromedarii_
B. caballi	Horse, donkey, mule	Southern Europe, Asia, Soviet Union, Africa, Panama, United States	_Dermacentor marginatus, D. silvarum, D. nitens, Hyalomma excavatum, Hy. dromedarii, Hy. scupense, Hy. truncatum Rhipicephalus bursa, Rh. sanguineus, Dermacentor reticulatus_
B. motasi	Sheep, goats	Southern Europe, Middle East, Soviet Union, Asia, Africa	_D. silvarum, Haemaphysalis punctata, Rhipicephalus bursa_
B. ovis	Sheep, goats	Tropics, Southern Europe, Soviet Union	_Rh. bursa_
B. trautmanni	Pig, wart hog, bush pig	Southern Europe, Soviet Union, Congo, Tanzania	_Rh. turanicus, Rh. sanguineus, Boophilus decoloratus, Dermacentor reticulatus_
B. felis	Domestic cat, wildcat, lion, leopard, puma, American lynx	Sudan, South Africa, U.S. (Zoos)	Unknown

Lesions

Necropsy of the emaciated carcasses of animals dead of the disease discloses the blood to be thin and watery and the plasma is red-tinged. The subcutaneous, subserous, and intramuscular connective tissue is edematous and yellow, and the fat is similarly affected. Icteric discoloration is clearly recognizable in all viscera. The spleen is constantly enlarged four to five times normal size, and its parenchyma is soft and dark red. The splenic corpuscles are usually prominent. Lymph nodes are often enlarged. The liver is enlarged and yellow-brown, with the gallbladder distended with dark green bile. The lungs are slightly edematous and the urinary bladder usually contains red-colored urine.

The microscopic findings are characteristic of severe hemolytic anemia. Hemoglobinuric nephrosis, centrilobular and paracentral necrosis of the liver, edema, excessive fluid in the peritoneal, pericardial and pleural cavities, and serosal hemorrhages are usual findings. *Babesia* may be demonstrable in large numbers in capillaries in brain, and in the optic choroid, even though they cannot be found elsewhere. The organisms in these sites are described as being both free in the lumen and in packed erythrocytes. The organisms may be associated with small thrombi, foci of hemorrhage and necrosis.

Bovine babesiosis (Texas Fever, Tick Fever, Piroplasmosis). This disease of cattle is of historical interest because it has now been virtually eliminated from the southern United States where it was once prevalent. Its eradication was accomplished by elimination of the tick vector *Boophilus annulatus*. Babesiosis, however, is still present in many other parts of the world. Of the several species that affect cattle, *B. bigemina* and *B. bovis* are the most prevalent and important.

Equine babesiosis is caused by either *B. equi* or *B. caballi*, which occur worldwide. *B. caballi* is reportedly less pathogenic than *B. equi*.

Canine babesiosis is the result of infection with either *B. canis*, which occurs in the Western Hemisphere, Africa, Europe, parts of Asia and the Soviet Union, or *B. gibsoni*, which principally occurs in India, Sri Lanka, China, Turkestan, and North Africa. *B. gibsoni* has recently been identified in the United States.

In humans, babesiosis was first reported in 1957 (Skrabalo and Deanovic) in a patient in Yugoslavia affected with *B. bovis*. Additional reports have followed from various parts of the globe. Most examples have occurred on Nantucket and Martha's Vineyard Islands in Massachusetts and are ascribed to infection with *B. microti*, a *Babesia* of mice and rodents. *B. divergens* has also been identified in a human patient. Babesiosis has been recognized in nonhuman primates as well, as has infection with a closely related parasite, *Entopolypoides macaci*.

Diagnosis

The diagnosis is confirmed by identification of *Babesia* in blood smears; however, all clinical manifestations must be judiciously weighed, because of their variety and the occurrence of non-pathogenic *Babesia* in animals which may be ill from other causes. The organisms may be identified by their morphology and their stimulation of specific antibodies in the serum of infected animals. These antibodies may be detected by hemagglutination, complement fixation, fluorescent antibody, and agglutination tests.

References

Allen PC, Frerichs WM, Holbrook AA. Experimental acute *Babesia caballi* infection. I. Red blood cell dynamics. Exp Parasitol 1975;37:67–77.

Anderson JF, et al. Canine *Babesia* new to North America. Science 1979;204:1431–1432.

Anderson JF, Magnarelli LA, Sulzer AJ. Canine babesiosis: indirect fluorescent antibody test for a North American isolate of *Babesia gibsoni*. Am J Vet Res 1980;41:2102–2105.

Basson PA, Pienaar JG. Canine babesiosis: a report on the pathology of three cases with special reference to the "cerebral" form. J S Afr Vet Med Assoc 1965;36:333–341.

Blouin EF, De Waal DT. The fine structure of developmental stages of *Babesia caballi* in the salivary glands of *Hyalomma truncata*. Onderstepoort J Vet Res 1989;56:189–195.

Breitschwerdt EB, et al. Babesiosis in the Greyhound. J Am Vet Med Assoc 1983;182:978–982.

Brocklesby DW, Sellwood SA, Harradine DL, et al. *Babesia major* in Britain: blood-induced infections in splenectomized and intact calves. Int J Parasitol 1973;3:671–680.

Brown JMM, cited by Malherbe WD. The manifestations and diagnosis of *Babesia* infections. Ann NY Acad Sci 1956;64:128–146.

Callow LL, Johnston LAY. *Babesia* spp. in the brains of clinically normal cattle and their detection by a brain smear technique. Aust Vet J 1963;39:25–31.

Cullen JM, Levine JF. Pathology of experimental *Babesia microti* infection in the Syrian hamster. Lab Anim Sci 1987;37:640–643.

Cullen JM, Levine JK. Babesiosis. Comp Pathol Bull 1989;21:3–4.

Dorner JL. A hematologic study of babesiosis of the dog. Am J Vet Clin Pathol 1967;1:67–75.

Emerson CL, Tsai C-C, Holland CJ, et al. Recrudescence of *Entopolypoides macaci* Mayer, 1933 (Babesiidae) infection secondary to stress in long-tailed macaques *(Macaca fascicularis)*. Lab Anim Sci 1990;40:169–171.

Everitt JI, Shadduck JA, Steinkamp C, et al. Experimental *Babesia bovis* infection in Holstein calves. Vet Pathol 1986;23:556–562.

Farwell GE, LeGrand EK, Cobb CC. Clinical observations on *Babesia gibsoni* and *Babesia canis* infections in dogs. J Am Vet Med Assoc 1982;180:507–511.

Fitzpatrick JEP, et al. Human case of piroplasmosis (babesiosis). Nature 1968;217:861–862.

Harvey JW, Taboada J, Lewis JC. Babesiosis in a litter of pups. J Am Vet Med Assoc 1988;192:1751–1752.

Healy GR. Babesiosis. Clin Microbiol Newslett 1982;4:33–35.

Hirsh DC, et al. An epizootic of babesiosis in dogs used for medical research. Lab Anim Care 1969;19:205–208.

Kuttler KL, Gipson CA, Goff WL, et al. Experimental *Babesia equi* infection in mature horses. Am J Vet Res 1986;47:1668–1670.

Malherbe WD. The manifestations and diagnosis of *Babesia* infections. Ann NY Acad Sci 1956;64:128–146.

Malherbe WD. Clinico-pathological studies of *Babesia canis* infection in dogs. I. The influence of the infection on Bromsulphalein retention in the blood. J S Afr Vet Med Assoc 1965;36:25–30.

Malherbe WD. Clinico-pathological studies of *Babesia canis* infection in dogs. II. The influence of the infection on plasma transaminase activity. III. The influence of the infection on plasma alkaline phosphatase activity. J S Afr Vet Med Assoc 1965;36:173–178, 179–182.

Malherbe WD. Clinico-pathological studies of *Babesia canis* infection in dogs. V. The influence of the infection on kidney function. J S Afr Vet Med Assoc 1966;37:261–264.

Maurer FD. Equine piroplasmosis—another emerging disease. J Am Vet Med Assoc 1962;141:699–702.

Rogers RJ. Observations on the pathology of *Babesia argentina* infections in cattle. Aust Vet J 1971;47:242–247.

TABLE 12-8 **Theileriases**

Organism	Animals affected	Geographic distribution	Tick vector
Theileria parva	Cattle, African buffalo, Indian water buffalo	Africa	Rhipicephalus appendiculatus
Th. annulata	Cattle, zebu, water buffalo	North Africa, Middle & Far East, Southern Europe, Soviet Union	Hyalomma detritum, H. dromedarii, H. excavatum, H. turanicum, H. savignyi, H. plumbeum, H. scupense
Th. mutans (th. sergenti)	Cattle, deer	Africa, Asia, Australia, Soviet Union, United States, England	Rhipicephalus appendiculatus, Rh. evertsi, Haemaphysalis bispinosa, H. punctata
Th. hirci	Sheep, goats	North & East Africa, Iraq, Turkey, Soviet Union, Greece	Rhipicephalus bursa (?)
Th. ovis	Sheep, goats	Africa, Asia, India, Soviet Union, Europe	Rhipicephalus bursa, Rh. evertsi, Dermacentor sylvarum, Haemaphysalis sulcata, Ornithodorous lahorensis
Th. lawrencei	Cattle, buffalo	Africa	Rhipicephalus appendiculatus
Th. cervi	White tailed deer	United States	Unknown

Roher DP, Anderson JF, Nielsen SW. Experimental babesiosis in coyotes and coydogs. Am J Vet Res 1985;46:256–262.

Ruebush TK II, et al. Human babesiosis on Nantucket Island, Clinical features. Ann Intern Med 1977;86:6–9.

Scholtens RG, Braff EK, Healy GR, et al. A case of babesiosis in man in the United States. Am J Trop Med Hyg 1968;17:810–813.

Schroeder WF, Cox HW, Ristic M. Anaemia, parasitaemia, erythrophagocytosis, and haemagglutinins in Babesia rodhaini infection. Ann Trop Med Parasitol 1966;60:31–38.

Seneviratna P. The pathology of Babesia gibsoni (Patton, 1910) infection in the dog. Ceylon Vet J 1965;13:107–110.

Seneviratna P. Studies of Babesia gibsoni infections of dogs in Ceylon. Ceylon Vet J 1965;13:1–6.

Simpson CF, Kirkham WW, Kling JM. Comparative morphologic features of Babesia caballi and Babesia equi. Am J Vet Res 1967;28:1693–1697.

Sippel WL, et al. Equine piroplasmosis in the United States. J Am Vet Med Assoc 1962;141:694–698.

Skrabalo Z, Deanovic A. Piroplasmosis in man: report on a case. Doc Med Geogr Trop 1957;9:11–16.

Smith T, Kilborne FL. Investigations into the nature, causation and prevention of Texas or Southern cattle fever. US Dept Agric Bur Anim Ind Bull no. 1, 1893.

Smith RD, et al. Bovine babesiosis: pathology and heterologous species immunity of tick-borne Babesia bovis and B. bigemina infections. Am J Vet Res 1980;41:1957–1965.

Western KA, et al. Babesiosis in a Massachusetts resident. N Engl J Med 1970;283:854–856.

Wright IG. An electron microscopic study of intravascular agglutination in the cerebral cortex due to Babesia argentina infection. Int J Parasitol 1972;2:209–215.

THEILERIASIS

Protozoan parasites of the genus *Theileria*, like *Babesia*, are found in the erythrocytes but reproduce by schizogony in lymphocytes or histiocytes, and are classified in the family Theileriidae. Two related genera are *Gonderi*, whose members reproduce by schizogony in lymphocytes and by fission in erythrocytes, and *Cytauxzoon*, which multiply by schizogony in histiocytic cells and by fission in erythrocytes. Table 12-8 indicates the important pathogenic *Theileria*.

Theileria parva, the cause of East Coast fever, a disease of cattle of much importance in Africa, is transmitted by several species of ticks the most important of which is *Rhipicephalus appendiculatus*. The life cycle in the mammalian hosts is not totally clear; however, following introduction into the host by saliva of the tick, *Theileria* invade lymphocytes and histiocytes, first in the regional lymph nodes, but then throughout all lymph nodes, spleen, liver, and other organs, as well as circulating cells. Here they develop in the cytoplasm of affected cells into macroschizonts, which are up to 16 μm in diameter and contain 8 or more nuclei of 1 μm in diameter. These large bodies, termed Koch's bodies after their discoverer, are considered characteristic and diagnostic of the disease. After about 10 days, forms termed micrischizonts appear in lymphocytes and particularly histiocytes. These are characterized by considerably more nuclei (up to 100 or more). It is not clear if microschizonts form following release of merozoites from macroschizonts or through another mechanism. Released "micromerozoites" (destroying the cell in the process) parasitize erythrocytes as tiny rod-, comma- or ring-shaped bodies somewhat smaller than *Babesia*, which do not undergo further division. Their pleomorphism distinguishes them from *Babesia*.

Clinical manifestations

The clinical manifestations start with fever, which appears about 15 days following exposure by the bite of infected ticks. Several days after *Theileria* becomes demonstrable in the blood, the appetite is gradually lost, rumination ceases, and milk secretion decreases. The superficial lymph nodes become noticeably enlarged, the muzzle dry, the hair coat rough, and salivation as well as lacrimation becomes excessive. Respiratory distress may follow pulmonary edema, and death may result from asphyxia. As the disease progresses, severe leukopenia of all white blood cell types develops and enlarged lymph nodes may regress to less than normal size. Anemia, which has been postulated to be of immune origin, may also be present. In some cases, death follows gradual emaciation, delirium, and coma. When signs relevant to central nervous system are present, the disease has been termed "turning disease." Mortality is high, approaching 100%.

Lesions

The most constant lesion found at necropsy is generalized enlargement of lymph nodes, although in some cases hyperplastic lymph nodes may have regressed to smaller than normal. Lymph nodes are edematous and may contain hemorrhage. The spleen may appear normal, large, or small. Usually the following occurs: pulmonary edema and emphysema, subcutaneous and intramuscular edema, and excessive pericardial and pleural fluid. The liver is generally enlarged, yellowish, and frequently mottled. White foci of various sizes may be seen in the renal cortex. The meninges may be congested and focal hemorrhage present in brain.

The principal microscopic finding is proliferation of lymphocytic cells in lymph nodes, spleen, Peyer's patches, liver, kidneys, and elsewhere. Blood vessels, including cerebral vessels, may be filled with parasitized lymphocytes, which apparently impede blood flow, leading to focal infarction. Koch's bodies may be found in tissue sections of many organs. In cases where lymph nodes have regressed in size, there is marked depletion of lymphocytes, edema and hemorrhage.

Theileria annulata, the cause of tropical theileriasis in cattle, is similar to East Coat Fever, but less severe. *Th. lawrencei* affects cattle and buffalo causing what is called Buffalo disease or Corridor disease, which if severe resembles East Coast Fever. *Th. mutans* also affects cattle, but is of little pathogenic importance. *Th. sergenti* is relatively nonpathogenic to cattle. Sheep are affected by *Th. hirci,* which can cause a disease resembling East Coast Fever, and *Th. ovis* which rarely causes clinical disease. Other species of *Theileria* which have been identified appear to be of no pathogenic significance, as have species of a closely related genus, *Haematoxenus,* which affects cattle and sheep.

Gonderia bovis is an organism similar to *Theileria;* in fact, Gonderia was once synonymous with Theileria. Infection, when severe, is similar to theileriasis.

Diagnosis

The diagnosis of theileriasis depends upon demonstration of the organisms in erythrocytes and in lymphocytes (Koch's bodies). Babesiosis is the most important disease from which it must be differentiated. Various tests for circulating antibodies have also been used with success.

References

Hooshmand-Rad P. The pathogenesis of anaemia in *Theileria annulata* infection. Res Vet Sci 1976;20:324–329.
Hooshmand-Rad P, Hawa NJ. Malignant theileriosis of sheep and goats. Trop Anim Health Prod 1973;5:97–102.
Jarett WFH, Brocklesby DW. Preliminary electron microscopic studies on East Coat fever. Parasitol 1965;55:13.
Jarett WFH, Brocklesby DW. A preliminary electron microscopic study of East Coast fever (*Theileria parva* infection). J Protozool 1966;13:301–310.
Krier JP, Ristic M, Watrach AM. *Theileria* sp. in a deer in the United States. Am J Vet Res 1962;23:657–663.
Matson BA. Theileriosis due to *Theileria parva, T. lawrencei* and *T. mutans.* Bibliography 1897–1966. Weybridge: Commonwealth Bureau of Animal Health, 1967;44.
Rensburg IBJ van. Bovine cerebral theileriosis: a report of five cases with splenic infarction. JS Afr Vet Assoc 1976;47:137–141.
Splitter EJ. *Theileria mutans* associated with bovine anaplasmosis. J Am Vet Med Assoc 1950;117:134–135.
Steck W. Histologic studies on East Coast fever. 13th & 14th Reports. South Africa: Onderstepoort, 1928; Part 1:243–282.
Wilde JKH. East Coast fever. Adv Vet Sci 1967;11:207–259.

CYTAUXZOONOSIS

Cytauxzoonosis, caused by species of *Cytauxzoon* within the family Theileriidae, is an infection thought to have been limited to various wild ungulates in Africa. However, a disease pathologically similar is now recognized to occur sporadically in domestic and wild cats in the United States (Fig. 12-29). Cytauxzoonosis in cats has been seen in Missouri, Arkansas, Mississippi, Georgia, Texas, Oklahoma, Florida, and Louisiana. The life cycle is not known, but presumably the organism is transmitted by ticks, comparable to that known for *Theileria* spp. Schizogony occurs in endothelial-associated macrophages with a piroplasma form in erythrocytes. Domestic cats are not believed to represent the usual host, as the disease is invariably fatal. A less severe infection has been recognized in bobcats, which may represent the natural host for the organism and the reservoir for infection in cats.

Clinically, the disease in cats is characterized by fever, depression, dehydration, dyspnea, anorexia, enlargement of lymph nodes, anemia, pale mucous membranes, and icterus, leading to death in three to six days. Gross findings include pallor or icterus of mucous membranes, with petechiae and ecchymoses in and on the lung, heart, lymph nodes, and mucous membranes. Lymph nodes and spleen are enlarged. Excessive fluid is present in the pericardial sac in most cases. The distinctive microscopic feature is the presence of numerous large schizonts (Fig. 12-30) within the cytoplasm of endothelial-associated macrophages. Each schizont contains numerous small merozoites (cytomeres). They lack a parasitophorous vacuole and the individual merozoites contain rhoptries. The affected macrophages are huge (up to 75 μm in diameter) and may occlude the

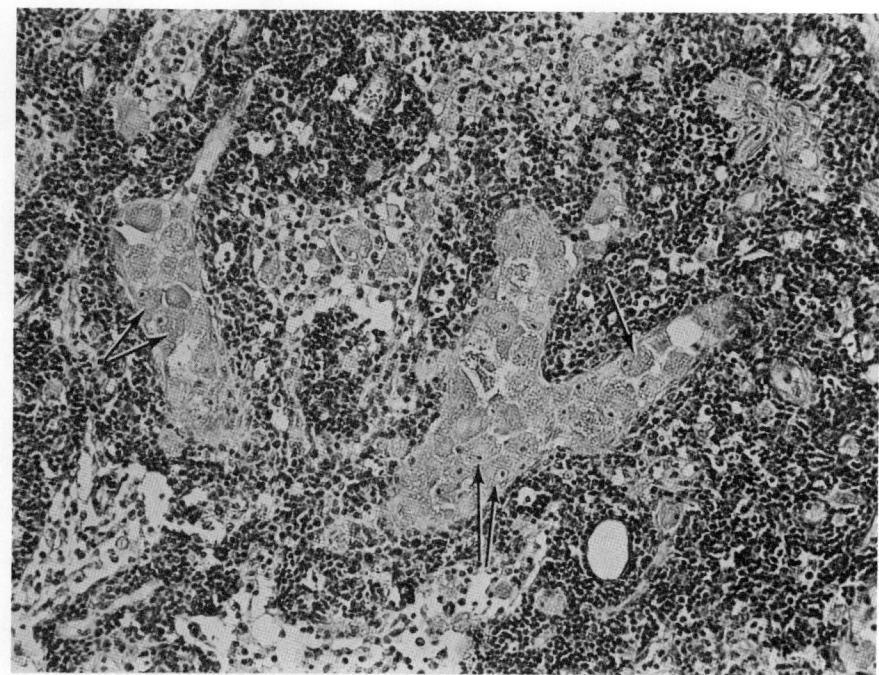

FIG. 12-29 Feline *Cytauxzoon*-infected cells (arrows) in veins and sinuses of a mesenteric lymph node of a cat. Typically, nuclei of infected cells are not distinct and the cytoplasm appears foamy. (Courtesy of Dr. Ann Kier.)

lumen. Such cells may be found in almost any tissue including the lung, myocardium, lymph nodes, spleen, liver, kidneys, brain, and bone marrow. Merozoites, released from schizonts without killing the macrophage, are believed to enter erythrocytes to form the intraerythrocytic stage, which is variable in appearance and best seen on smears of peripheral blood or tissue impressions. They occur as round, oval or signet ring shaped bodies 1–5 μm in diameter, with a small peripherally placed basophilic nucleus. More than one organism may parasitize a single erythrocyte. Up to 25% of erythrocytes may be affected.

References

Glenn BL, Stair EL. Cytauxzoonosis in domestic cats: report of two cases in Oklahoma, with a review and discussion of the disease. J Am Vet Med Assoc 1984;184:822–825.

Glenn BL, Kocan AA, Blouin EF. Cytauxzoonosis in bobcats. J Am Vet Med Assoc 1983;183:1155–1158.

Hauck WN, Snider TG III, Lawrence JE. Cytauxzoonosis in a native Louisiana cat. J Am Vet Med Assoc 1982;180:1472–1474.

Kier AB, Wagner JE, Morehouse LG. Experimental transmission of *Cytauxzoon felis* from bobcats (*Lynx rufus*) to domestic cats (*Felis domesticus*). Am J Vet Res 1982;43:97–101.

Kier AB, Wightman SR, Wagner JE. Interspecies transmission of *Cytauxzoon felis*. Am J Vet Res 1982;43:102–105.

McCully RM, Keep ME, Basson PA. Cytauxzoonosis in a giraffe (*Giraffa camelopardalis* [Linnaeus, 1758]) in Zululand. Onderstepoort J Vet Res 1970;37:7–9, Vet Bull 1971;41:5294.

Simpson CF, Harvey JW, Carlisle JW. Ultrastructure of the intraerythrocytic stage of Cytauxzoon felis. Am J Vet Res 1985;46:1178–1180.

Simpson CF, et al. Ultrastructure of schizonts in the liver of cats with experimentally induced cytauxzoonosis. Am J Vet Res 1985;46:384–390.

Wagner JE. A fatal cytauxzoonosis-like disease in cats. J Am Vet Res Assoc 1976;168:585–588.

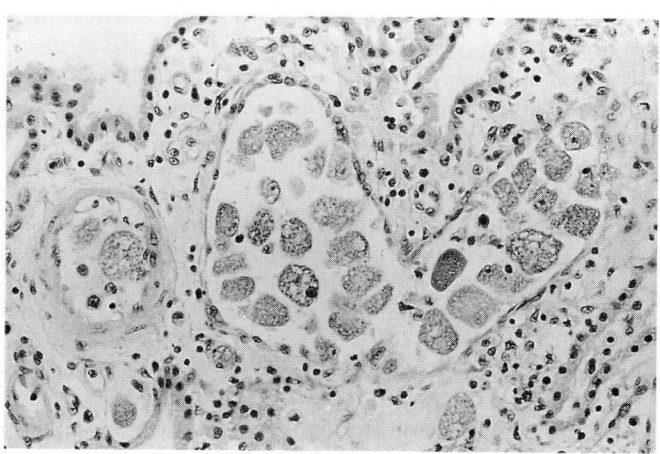

FIG. 12-30 Cytauxzoonosis in a cat. Large schizonts within the vasculature of the choroid plexus. (Specimen courtesy of Kansas State University College of Veterinary Medicine, Department of Pathology, Manhattan, KS.)

13

Diseases caused by parasitic helminths and arthropods

Metazoan parasites comprise a large and diverse group of organisms of considerable importance to veterinary medicine throughout the world.

Literally thousands of parasitic helminths and arthropods can affect animals. Because many have restricted geographic distributions, affect only wild animals, or are rare, we will not attempt to cover them all here. For a relatively complete commentary on parasites of animals, refer to Soulsby's text (1982, reprinted 1986). In the United States, many parasitisms of animals have been well controlled, and most of those affecting humans have been reduced to a minimum. In many countries, however, metazoan parasites remain among the most frequent and significant causes of disease: for example, schistosomiasis in humans. In addition to being primary causes of disease, metazoan parasites may also serve as vectors for other infectious organisms. This is especially true of arthropods, which serve as vectors for many viruses, as well as protozoan parasites.

Many parasites have indirect life cycles involving one or more intermediate hosts. Both the adult parasites and their intermediate stages have a pathologic effect on their respective hosts. Both stages may affect animals discussed in this text, or they may involve an insect, fish, or some other species not covered here. Depending upon the particular parasite, the stage of interest to the veterinary pathologist may be either the adult parasite in the definitive stage or the intermediate stages.

PARASITIC HELMINTHS

Parasitic helminths, or worms, are important causes of disease in all species of animals. Although in many cases they produce little serious damage to the host, these parasites are never beneficial; in some cases they can produce severe and even fatal disease. The effect of various helminths upon animal hosts is given chief consideration in this chapter. Life cycles, host range, immunity, and infectivity are also briefly discussed. The reader is referred to standard texts and the selected references at the ends of these topics for more detailed information on the many other important aspects of helminthic parasitism (**helminthiasis**).

The parasitic helminths to be considered in this chapter are classified by the International Code of Zoological Nomenclature in three phyla, as follows:

Phylum Platyhelminthes, including the **trematodes** or **flukes,** and the **cestodes** or **tapeworms**;

Phylum Nemathelminthes, including the **nematodes** or **roundworms,** which infect a wide variety of hosts including animals, humans, and plants; and **Phylum Acanthocephala,** including the **thorny-headed worms,** a few of which are important parasites of animals.

Effects of Helminthic Parasites upon the Host

Helminthic parasites produce harmful effects upon their hosts in a wide variety of ways. These can be outlined as follows:

1. Mechanically interfere with function
   a. Obstruct blood or lymph channels
      (1) Right ventricle and pulmonary artery—*Dirofilaria immitis* (dog)
      (2) Carotid arteries—*Elaeophora schneideri* (sheep)
      (3) Lymphatic channels—*Dracunculus insignis* (dogs)
      (4) Mesenteric arteries—*Strongylus vulgaris* (horses)
      (5) Aorta—*Spirocerca lupi* (dogs); *Strongylus vulgaris* (horses)
      (6) Vena cava—*Schistosoma bovis, S. hematobium*
   b. Obstruct ducts or tracts
      (1) Bile duct—liver flukes, ascarids, fringed tapeworms
      (2) Esophagus—*Spirocerca lupi* (dogs)
      (3) Intestinal lumen—ascarids, tapeworms

601

(4) Respiratory tract—*Filaroides osleri, Metastrongylus apri*

(5) Urinary tract—*Dioctophyma renale*

c. Attach to or use functional tissue
(1) Stomach mucosa—*Trichostrongylus axei* (sheep, cattle), *Draschia megastoma* (horses)
(2) Small intestine—hookworms
(3) Cecum and large intestine—strongyles (horses), cecal worms (turkeys, dogs)

d. Act as foreign bodies, with resultant tissue reactions displacing normal structures
(1) Schistosome ova (flukes)
(2) Dead larvae of many nematodes—*Toxocara canis, Dirofilaria immitis*

2. Invade and displace cells and tissues, producing necrosis, loss of function and hypersensitivity reactions
a. Skin—hookworm larvae, *Habronema* larvae, *Rhabditis* sp., *Onchocerca* larvae, *Elaeophora schneideri* larvae, *Stephanofilaria stilesi*
b. Liver—giant liver flukes, kidney worm larvae, cysticercus, echinococcus and coenurus cysts, ascarid larvae, *Capillaria hepatica* (rats, humans)
c. Intestinal wall—nodular worms (*Oesophagostomum* sp.), larvae of strongyles (horses)
d. Brain and spinal cord—coenurus, echinococcus, filaria, other helminth larvae
e. Lung—lungworms, ascarid larvae, hookworms
f. Musculature—trichinae, cysticerci

3. Devour blood and thereby cause anemia
a. Hookworms (dogs, cattle)
b. Stomach worms (cattle and sheep)

4. Use food needed by the host:
a. Tapeworms
b. Ascarids

5. Induce or predispose to neoplasia:
a. Esophagus—*Spirocerca lupi* (dogs)
b. Liver—*Cysticercus fasciolaris* (rats)
c. Urinary bladder—*Schistosoma hematobium* (humans)

6. Introduce bacterial or other infection into tissues of the host
a. Lungs—lungworms, ascarid larvae
b. Intestinal wall—hookworms, nodule worms, salmon flukes (dogs)
c. Cecum—cecal worms (histomonads of turkeys)
d. Perirenal tissues—*Stephanurus dentatus*

7. Devour tissues of host
a. Ascarids
b. Stomach worms

8. Secrete toxic products (hemolysins, histolysins, anticoagulants)
a. Hookworms, nodule worms
b. Stomach worms
c. Strongyles

Identification of helminths in tissues

The discovery of one or more fragments of a helminth in histologic sections of tissue presents a challenge to pathologists. In order to effectively evaluate the significance of such a finding, they must know the potentialities of the parasite: its origin; where it was going when trapped by the fixative; and what its total effect upon the host might be. The identification of the parasite is therefore critical. Whenever possible, it is necessary to secure complete, well-preserved specimens for referral to a parasitologist whenever possible. However, presumptive identification of the parasite can often be made from fragments of the organism in tissues; or, it may be possible to tease parasites in recognizable form from fixed gross tissues. Although far from complete, the information concerning the appearance of helminths in tissue sections is now sufficient to permit the recognition of many species.

In determining the identity of a parasite in tissues, several factors may be used to narrow the field of consideration: the host and its usual parasites; the anatomic location of the parasite; the nature of the tissue reaction; and, most important, the morphologic features of the parasite itself. Helminths must also be differentiated from arthropods and pentastomids, which may be encountered in tissue sections. (These organisms are discussed at the end of this chapter.) Identification of these major groups of parasitic metazoa by morphologic features is aided by the following key, based on Chitwood and Lichtenfels, 1972.

1.
A. Internal organs embedded in parenchymatous matrix; body usually flattened dorsoventrally..Platyhelmintha 2
B. Internal organs suspended or free in body cavity; body usually not flattened 3

2.
A. Segmented; attached by scolex; contain calcareous corpuscles; lack digestive tract; muscle layers separated..Cestoda
B. Leaf-shaped; attached by suckers; lack calcareous corpuscles; have digestive tract .... Trematoda

3.
A. Somatic musculature not striated (smooth); attached to body wall throughout length...........4
B. Somatic musculature striated; attached to body wall only at ends 6

4.
A. Hypodermis thicker than muscular layer; contains lacunar channels; digestive system absent.. Acanthocephala
B. Hypodermis thinner than muscular layer, with no lacunar channels; digestive system present, but may be rudimentary.....................................5

5.
A. Cuticle usually with areoles; lateral hypodermal chords absent; ventral nerve chord usually prominent; digestive system rudimentary..Nematomorpha
B. Cuticle may be smooth, striated, or annulated, but areoles absent; hypodermal chords present; digestive system well developed...........Nematoda

6.
   A. Chitinous exoskeleton may be segmented, with jointed appendages.............................Arthropoda
   B. Pseudosegmented, when present; pseudopodia not jointed.......................................Pentastomida

Nematodes have an external cuticle supported by a thin membrane, the hypodermis, within which is a muscular wall surrounding the body cavity. They have an alimentary canal and the sexes are separate. All of these features can be detected in cross sections of the adults and, in some cases, of the larvae. The midsomatic muscular wall of the nematodes has some distinguishing features: the muscle cells are arranged longitudinally in a single layer just within the hypodermis; in cross section of most species, muscle cells are visibly divided into four groups by cords of cells (chords) of the hypodermis; and, these chords project toward the center. Thus, one dorsal, one ventral, and two lateral chords are formed by the hypodermis. These cells in many species vary distinctively in size and number. When numerous long slender muscle cells, running lengthwise along the body wall, protrude into the body cavity and are divided into four longitudinal units (by dorsal, ventral, and lateral chords made up of a single row of cells), nematodes are said to have a **polymyarian** somatic musculature (*Ascaris, Filaria,* and *Dracunculus*) (Fig. 13-6). Those nematodes with closely packed, somewhat flattened muscle cells in units containing three or four cells are classified as **meromyarian,** and include such genera as *Enterobius, Ancylostoma,* and *Necator.* In a third group of nematodes, the muscle cells, although closely packed, are not divided by chords, and the body cavity is completely surrounded by longitudinally running muscle cells. This group is classified as **holomyarian** and includes the genus **Trichuris.**

The eggs or larvae can serve as a guide in the identification of some adult parasites in tissues. Sections are often made through the ovary or uterus of adult worms, in which numerous ova or larvae are present. The size, shape, and shell of many ova are distinctive for the species; for example, the ovoid egg with double-contoured shell of *Strongylus,* the single polar eminence of ova of *Oxyuris,* and the double polar eminence of ova of *Capillaria* (Fig. 13-21). Nematodes in which the ova embryonates and hatches in the uterus, with the larvae escaping as free forms, are termed **viviparous** (*Dirofilaria*); others are ovoviviparous, in that they produce ova which are embryonated, but the larvae are still within the egg shell when they are expelled from the parasite (*Spirocerca*).

Trematodes and cestodes generally can be differentiated from nematodes in tissue sections. They are flat dorsoventrally and they do not have a body cavity, although some of the larval forms may be suspended in a bladder (see cysticerci). Most of them are hermaphroditic; hence, male and female sex organs can often be seen in tissue sections of a single parasite. The anatomic site in which cestodes and trematodes are found,

the nature of the tissue reaction they evoke, and their structural form are often guides to the tentative identification of these parasites in tissues. Familiarity with their life cycle, host range, and morphology is thus an asset to the pathologist.

The cestodes possess a specialized structure, the scolex, which can often be detected in larval forms as well as in adult in tissue sections. The scolex may bear two or more elongated suctorial grooves, or they may have cup-shaped sucking discs and a proboscis. In some species, the proboscis is armed with characteristic hooklets (Fig. 13-29). An external cuticle surrounding a germinal layer from which scolices, or brood capsules containing scolices, may arise also serves to identify cestodes in tissue sections. The body of cestodes is almost always segmented. The outer longitudinal muscles are separated from the inner circular muscles by parenchyma, within which are suspended calcareous corpuscles. Cestodes lack a digestive tract.

In contrast to cestodes, trematodes are leaf-shaped and nonsegmented. They contain a digestive tract, lack calcareous corpuscles, and have longitudinal and circular muscle layers that are close to one another. Their cuticle is usually thinner than that of cestodes. The eggs of trematodes are also distinctive. They are usually pigmented, operculated, and birefringent (anisotropic). The presence of some trematodes in the body may be determined by the identification of the ova of the parasite, even though the adult is not found. This is of particular value in schistosomiasis, in which many ova are carried by the blood stream to various organs, where they become embedded in small granulomas. Some of the filarid worms are seldom seen in adult form in the tissues, but their larval forms are sufficient for diagnosis.

Host response to parasites

Parasites are extremely adept at evading the host's immune system, a feature that allows their development and persistence. Most infections with helminths are chronic. Those parasites that reside in the lumen of the intestinal tract or in airways, such as adult ascarids or *Paragonimus,* are removed from direct contact with humoral and cellular immune mechanisms and their escape from immune attack is not surprising. However, even intravascular parasites, which should be the most vulnerable, may escape immune destruction. Adult *Dirofilaria immitis* may remain viable within pulmonary arteries for long periods of time. Those parasites that reside in tissue, or spend part of their life cycles migrating through tissue, often do so with impunity from immune attack. Several mechanisms exist that allow parasites to dodge rejection. Comparable to certain protozoa (e.g., trypanosomes), developing helminths disguise themselves through antigenic variation, presenting a camouflage to humoral and cellular immune responses, thus allowing them to complete their maturation. This allows migrating larvae to proceed unabated on first encounter, producing tissue damage primarily due to mechanical insult. However, on repeated exposure this mechanism begins to fail and fewer larvae reach their final destination as adults. Parasites may also acquire surface antigens that are remarkably similar to those of their hosts, which help them escape immune destruction. Exposure to helminths in utero also imparts a degree of unresponsiveness on the part of the host's immune system. Certain parasites also have been demonstrated to secrete substances that suppress immune function and the inflammatory response. Thus, helminths may migrate through tissues or reside as adults with a minimal tissue reaction.

This is not to say that an immune response does not exist nor that it is not important. Helminths contain a wide spectrum of antigens that do elicit both humoral and cellular immunity. It is this response which provides some degree of immunity to challenge in previously exposed individuals; these antigens also encourage expulsion of adult worms from the intestinal tract, and the formation of the inflammatory lesions that have been seen surrounding helminth eggs, larvae, and adults in tissue section. The severity of the response is dependent upon the parasite, its site, and whether or not there has been previous exposure. The type of inflammatory response to parasitisms is also highly variable and includes all the diverse forms of inflammatory reaction, from purulent to granulomatous. A unique feature of many parasitisms is the occurrence of eosinophils in both the inflammatory/immune response and the circulation. Eosinophils seem to be particularly important to the host's defense against helminthic parasites, releasing their cytotoxic granules on the parasite's surface. Their occurrence and effectiveness are, however, highly variable. The Inflammation chapter discusses why eosinophils are more prominent in diseases caused by helminths, and the factors that cause them to release.

References

Behnke JM, ed. Parasites: immunity and pathology. The consequences of parasitic infection in mammals. London: Taylor & Francis, Ltd., 1990.

Benbrook EA. Outline of parasites reported for domesticated animals in north america. 6th ed. Ames: Iowa State Univ Press, 1963.

Chitwood M, Lichtenfels JR. Identification of parasitic metazoa in tissue sections. Exp Parasitol 1972;32:407–519.

Flynn RJ. Parasites of laboratory animals. Ames: Iowa State Univ Press, 1973.

Foreyt WJ. Diagnostic parasitology. Vet Clin North Am Small Anim Pract 1989;19:979.

Georgi JR. Parasitology for veterinarians. 3rd ed. Philadelphia: WB Saunders, 1980.

Griffiths HJ. A handbook of veterinary parasitology: domestic animals of North America. Minneapolis: Univ of Minnesota Press, 1978.

Hsu C-K. Parasitic diseases: how to monitor them and their effects on research. Lab Anim 1980;9:48–53.

Kelly JD. Mechanisms of immunity to intestinal helminths. Aust Vet J 1973;49:91–97.

Lapage G. Veterinary parasitology. 2nd ed. Springfield: Charles C Thomas, 1968.

Larsh JE Jr, Weatherly NF. Cell-mediated immunity in certain parasitic infections. Curr Top Microbiol Immunol 1974;67:113–137.

Larsh JE Jr, Weatherly NF. Cell-mediated immunity against certain parasitic worms. Adv Parasitol 1975;13:183–222.

Michel JF. The epidemiology and control of some nematode infections in grazing animals. Adv Parasitol 1976;14:355–397.

Noble ER, Noble GA. Parasitology: the biology of animal parasites. 5th ed. Philadelphia: Lea & Febiger, 1982.

Poynter D. Some tissue reactions to the nematode parasites of animals. Adv Parasitol 1966;4:321–383.

Sloss MW, Kemp RL. Veterinary clinical parasitology. 5th ed. Ames: Iowa State Univ Press, 1978.

Soulsby EJL. Helminths, arthropods and protozoa of domesticated animals. 7th ed. London: Baillière Tindall, 1982.

Whitlock JH. Diagnosis of veterinary parasitisms. Philadelphia: Lea & Febiger, 1960.

Ascariasis (common roundworm infection, ascarid worm infection)

Ascarids (phylum: Nemathelminthes; family: Ascaridae) are extremely common roundworms whose adult forms are found in abundance in the gastrointestinal tracts of birds and mammals throughout the world (Fig. 13-1). Ascarids occur not only in great numbers but in many varieties. Most of them are host-specific. Larval migration may, however, occur in other than the true host, which are referred to as **paratenic hosts.** The principal ascarids are listed in Table 13-1.

The adults are usually large robust worms found in the small intestine, the cecal worms of chickens being an exception (Fig. 13-1). The eggs are thick-shelled and unsegmented when laid, and a period of incubation and two molts within the shell are required before the embryo becomes infective. The eggs are resistant to desiccation, low temperatures, and many chemical agents. Young animals are particularly susceptible to infection with ascarids; many adults lose their ascarid parasites spontaneously.

Ascarids are among the most common intestinal parasites of animals, and are especially significant to dogs, cats, swine, and horses (Fig. 13-2). Cattle are less frequently infected, and infection in sheep and goats is rare to nonexistent. A few representative species listed by their currently preferred names are presented in Table 13-1.

The **life cycles** of all ascarids are direct; however, several variations in the migratory patterns of larvae are possible. In the typical life cycle, using *Ascaris suum* as the prototype, embryonated eggs containing second-stage larvae are ingested and hatch in the stomach wall; they then enter the portal veins and invade the hepatic parenchyma, where they may molt to third-stage larvae and wander for a period of time before entering the general circulation to be carried to the lungs (Fig. 13-2). Here, the third-stage larvae break through to the alveoli and ascend the bronchi and trachea to be swallowed. In the intestine, two additional molts occur before maturation to adult worms. This **tracheal migration** occurs for *Toxocara canis, T. cati, T. vitulorum, Parascaris equorum,* and *Ascaris suum.* The principal variation is that the molt to third-stage larvae occurs in the pulmonary alveoli for *T. canis, T. cati,* and *P. equorum.*

Of the important ascarids of domestic animals, only *Toxocaris leonina* varies from this general migratory pattern. The second-stage larvae of *T. leonina* penetrate the

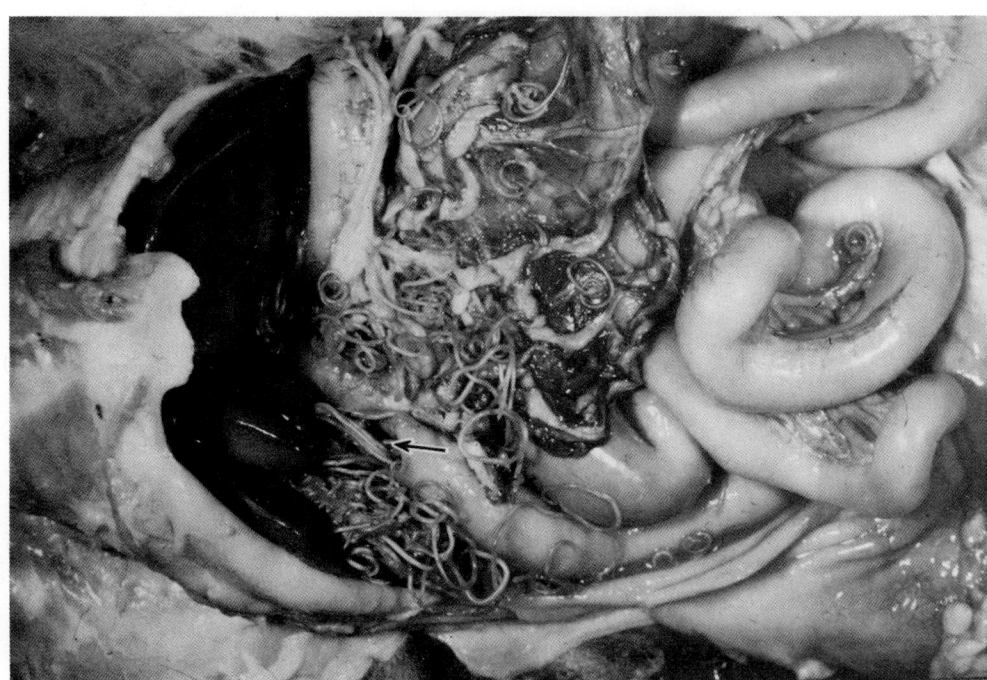

FIG. 13-1 Ascariasis. Unusually severe infection of a seven-week-old Collie puppy with *Toxocara canis* resulted in rupture of duodenum (arrow) and death. (Courtesy of Angell Memorial Animal Hospital.)

intestinal wall and do not migrate further. They undergo their molts here and reenter the lumen as fourth-stage larvae, which mature to adults.

Larvae of *T. canis, T. cati,* and *T. vitulorum* may, in addition to entering pulmonary alveoli, remain in the circulation to be widely distributed throughout the body. This pattern is termed **somatic migration** of larvae. The second-stage larvae lodged in various tissues do not undergo further development, but remain alive for months or years. Others die at these sites, instigating small granulomas. Localization of such migrating larvae in the brain or retina, which are not uncommon sites, leads to serious sequelae. An important feature of somatic migration in dogs is that, during the latter third of pregnancy, these larvae can migrate from their tissue location to the uterus, cross the placenta, and infect pups in utero. Prenatal infection does not occur with *T. cati* or *T. vitulorum;* however, larvae of these species and *T. canis* can enter the mammary glands and

milk to infect pups, kittens, and calves as neonates. Somatic migration, rather than tracheal migration, is much more likely to occur in older dogs. In cats, tracheal migration is the more usual route, regardless of age.

Yet another variation in the life cycles of *T. canis* and *T. cati* involves infection of paratenic hosts. A number of different species, including rodents and even humans, can support initial development of these parasites. Tracheal migration leads to the larvae's demise as further development in the gastrointestinal tract does not occur; however, systemic migration in the paratenic host may lead to viable second-stage larvae embedded in tissues, where they incite an inflammatory reaction. This is known as visceral larval migrans, and is especially important in young children where the larvae may locate in the brain. *Toxocara canis* is the most important cause of **visceral larval migrans** in humans; however, other animal parasites (e.g., *Ascaris suum, Capillaria hepatica* and *Dirofilaria immitis*) may also lead to this condition. When the tissues of a paratenic host are ingested by a dog or cat, the second-stage larvae may develop to mature worms in the alimentary tract. Third and fourth-stage larvae develop in the wall of the stomach and reenter the lumen without the need of tracheal migration.

Thus, the means by which dogs can become infected with adult *T. canis* include: (1) ingestion of eggs; (2) in utero; (3) via milk; or (4) ingestion of paratenic hosts. *T. cati* may use each of these routes except in utero infection.

It is readily apparent that ascarid larvae can penetrate various tissues of the host, where they may remain

TABLE 13-1 **Representative species of Ascaridae**

Species of Ascarid	Definitive hosts
Ascaris lumbricoides (suum)	Humans, swine (var. suis)
Toxocara canis	Dog
Toxocara cati	Cat, wildcat, lion, leopard
Toxascaris leonina	Dog, cat, lion, tiger, fox
Toxocara vitulorum	Cattle
Parascaris equorum	Horse
Ascaridia galli	Chickens, turkeys

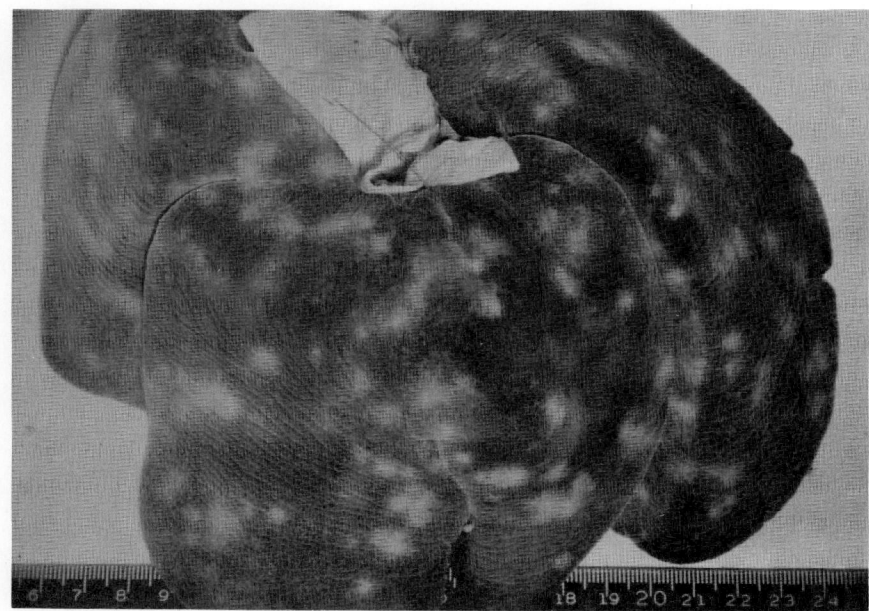

FIG. 13-2 Ascariasis. Liver of a young pig. Gray, fibrous areas are caused by migration of ascaris larvae.

for some time and produce tissue damage. While the intestinal wall, the liver, and the lungs are the common routes for larval migration, any tissue of the body can be invaded. The interval between ingestion of infective forms and the appearance of eggs in the feces of the final host is called the **prepatent period.** This is a period during which the host can sustain serious damage from the migration and development of larvae in the tissues. The prepatent period for different species of worms var-

ies; it may be relatively long, for example, 60 or more days for *A. lumbricoides* (Fig. 13-3).

LESIONS

Adult ascarids ordinarily live free in the lumen of the small intestine. They feed on the intestinal contents, occasionally abrade the mucosa and, by a swimming movement, maintain their position in the tract in spite of peristaltic action. Several factors may enhance

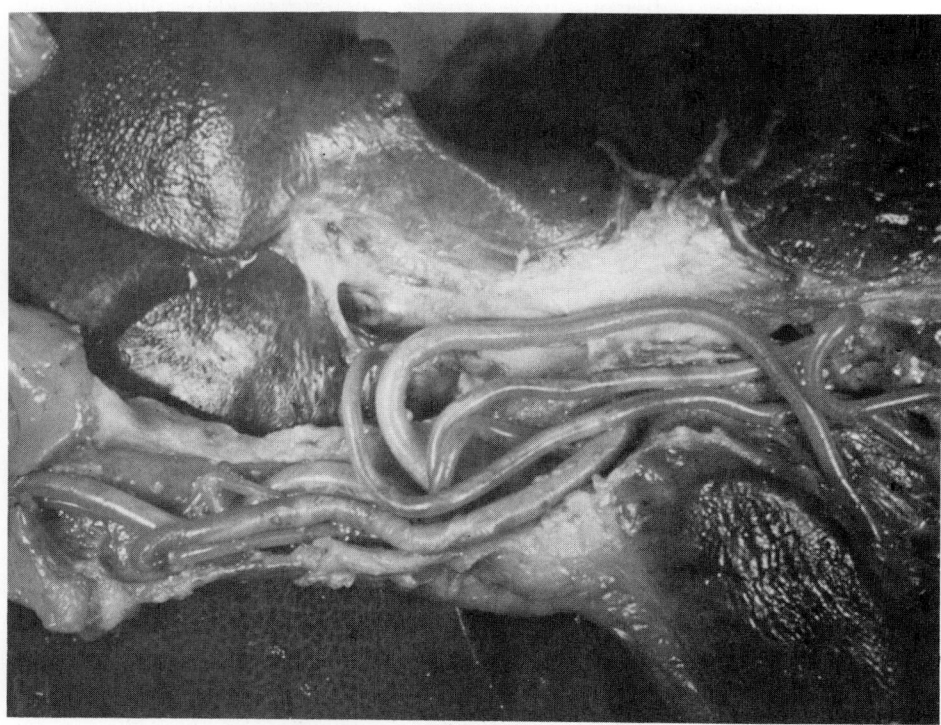

FIG. 13-3 *Ascaris lumbricoides,* var. *suis* in bile ducts of a pig. (Courtesy of Dr. C. L. Davis.)

their motility, among which are increased temperature (fever in the host) and starvation. On the other hand, they may be unable to maintain their position against the exaggerated peristalsis that occurs in diarrhea or after purging, and thus be swept out of the intestine. When their motility increases, it is not uncommon for ascarids to move into the stomach or the hepatic or pancreatic ducts. They may produce obstruction in the bile ducts, resulting in icterus. Jaundice of this origin is a fairly common reason for condemnation of hog carcasses inspected in abattoirs. Adult ascarids that remain in their usual location may become so numerous that they cause obstruction of the intestinal lumen; this may be fatal, particularly in young animals. On occasion, penetration of the intestinal wall has produced peritonitis in the host. Inanition in the host and retardation of growth of the young animal are the most common effects produced by ascarids, for they deprive the host of food and interfere with its digestive processes.

The lesions produced by the infective larvae during their migration and development in the tissues of the host range from minimal to severe. As the larvae migrate, tissues along the route are damaged and reparative processes become part of the pathologic picture. Larvae that penetrate the intestinal mucosa may carry bacteria into the tissues. In the liver, heavy infection with larvae often produces intense inflammation, with edema, neutrophils, eosinophils, and lymphocytes as components of the inflammatory reaction. It is possible to identify larvae in a central mass of characteristic caseous necrosis surrounded by epithelioid cells, eosinophils, lymphocytes, and neutrophils. The portal areas are most severely involved, but subsequent fibrosis may obliterate entire lobules. However, in the average case seen at necropsy, tissue changes are negligible. In swine, a diffuse, subcapsular fibrosis is believed to mark the sites of previous larval invasion of the liver. Larval migration through the lungs sets up an inflammatory reaction that may result in mild to severe respiratory involvement, and which usually heals with few residual lesions. Hemorrhages occur as the larvae break out of the pulmonary capillaries to enter the alveoli, and in heavy infection loss of bronchiolar epithelium and infiltration of leukocytes may occur.

Ascarid larvae may wander throughout the body and produce granulomatous nodules in many sites. They are most commonly encountered in the kidney, but may localize in any tissue, including the liver, lung, myocardium, brain, eye, and lymph nodes.

DIAGNOSIS

Clinical diagnosis of ascariasis is based upon demonstration of ova or adults in the feces and the correlation of these findings with the clinical signs. During the prepatent period, ova will not be found in the feces, although immature forms may be present in the tissues or intestinal lumen. Ascarid larvae may be identified in tissue sections and their relationship to lesions clearly demonstrated. Serologic tests are useful to diagnose visceral larval migrans, which may mimic many granulomatoses and occasionally neoplastic diseases. Eosinophilia usually accompany larval migrans. Occlusion of hepatic ducts by adult ascarids may occur, and is usually recognized at necropsy.

References

Barron CN, Saunders LZ. Visceral larva migrans in the dog. Pathol Vet 1966;3:315–330.

Clayton HM, Duncan JL, Dargie JD. Pathophysiological changes associated with *Parascaris equorum* infection in the foal. Equine Vet J 1980;12:23–25.

Dubey JP. *Toxocara cati* and other intestinal parasites of cats. Vet Rec 1966;79:506–508.

Fitzgerald PR, Mansfield ME. Visceral larva migrans (*Toxocara canis*) in calves. Am J Vet Res 1970;31:561–566.

Glickman LT, Summers BA. Experimental *Toxocara canis* infection in cynomolgus macaques (*Macaca fascicularis*). Am J Vet Res 1983; 44:2347–2354.

Glickman LT, Schantz PM, Cypess RH. Canine and human toxocariasis: review of transmission, pathogenesis, and clinical disease. J Am Vet Med Assoc 1979;175:1265–1269.

Glickman LT, Grieve RB, DeGregory KT, et al. Toxocara antigen and mitogen-induced lymphocyte blastogenesis for diagnosis of visceral larva migrans: clinical and experimental findings in macaques and human beings. Am J Vet Res 1984;45:1235–1237.

Greve JH. Age resistance to *Toxocara canis* in ascarid-free dogs. Am J Vet Res 1971;32:1185–1192.

Hayden DW, Van Kruiningen HJ. Experimentally induced canine toxocariasis: laboratory examinations and pathologic changes, with emphasis on the gastrointestinal tract. Am J Vet Res 1975; 36:1605–1614.

Hughes PL, Dubielzig RR, Kazacos KR. Multifocal retinitis in New Zealand sheep dogs. Vet Pathol 1987;24:22–27.

Koutz FR, Groves HF, Scothorn MW. The prenatal migration of *Toxocara canis* larvae and their relationship to infection in pregnant bitches and in pups. Am J Vet Res 1966;27:789–795.

Matoff K, Komandarey S. Comparative studies on the migration of the larvae of *Toxascaris leonina* and *Toxascaris transfuga*. Z Parasitenkd 1965;25:538–555.

Moncol DJ, Batte EF. Peripheral blood eosinophilia in porcine ascariasis. Cornell Vet 1967;57:96–107.

Morrow DA. Pneumonia in cattle due to migrating *Ascaris lumbricoides* larvae. J Am Vet Med Assoc 1968;153:184–189.

Mossalam I, Hosney Z, Atallah OA. Larva migrans of *Toxocara cati* in visceral organs of experimental animals. Acta Vet Acad Sci Hung 1971;21:405–412.

Nicholls JM, Clayton HM, Pirie HM, et al. A pathological study of the lungs of foals infected experimentally with *Parascaris equorum*. J Comp Pathol 1988;88:261–274.

Randall EL. Visceral larva migrans. Clin Microbiol Newslett 1982;4 (6):39–41.

Rubin LF, Saunders LZ. Intraocular larva migrans in dogs. Pathol Vet 1965;2:566–573.

Schantz PM, Glickman LT. Canine and human toxocariasis: the public health problem and the veterinarian's role in prevention. J Am Vet Med Assoc 1979;175:1270–1273.

Schantz PM, Stehr-Green JK. Toxocaral larva migrans. J Am Vet Med Assoc 1988;192:28–32.

Schwartz B. Experimental infection of pigs with *Ascaris suum*. Am J Vet Res 1959;20:7–13.

Scothorn MW, Koutz FR, Groves HF. Prenatal *Toxocara canis* infection in pups. J Am Vet Med Assoc 1965;146:45–48.

Swerczek TW, Nielsen SW, Helmboldt CF. Transmammary passage of *Toxocara cati* in the cat. Am J Vet Res 1971;32:89–92.

Tomimura T, Yokota M, Takiguchi H. Experimental visceral larva migrans in monkeys. I. Clinical, hematological, biochemical and gross pathological observations of monkeys inoculated with embryonated eggs of the dog ascarid, *Toxocara canis*. Jpn J Vet Sci 1976;38:533–538.

Ueckert B. Larva migrans, a review. Southwestern Vet 1962;15: 223–230.

Wilder HC. Nematode endophthalmitis. Tr Amer Acad Ophthalmol 1950;99–108.

Wiseman RA. Toxocariasis in man and animals. Vet Rec 1969;84: 214–216.

Ancylostomiasis (hookworm disease)

Hookworms (family: Ancylostomidae) are important parasites of mammals, and in some parts of the world they produce widespread disease in humans. These parasites are cosmopolitan in distribution, although limited to certain areas by environmental conditions such as moisture and temperature. One or more species of hookworm occurs in every domestic mammal, with the exception of the horse. A few important hookworms are listed in Table 13-2.

The life cycle of each of the hookworms has not been totally worked out, but several different migratory patterns have been identified. The adult worms of *Ancylostoma caninum*, for example, inhabit the small intestine, where they attach to the mucosa with well-developed buccal cavities containing hooklike structures. Eggs are passed in the feces and, under favorable conditions of a moist warm environment, rapidly hatch and develop into rhabditiform larvae. Hatching may actually occur within the gut. Following two molts, the larvae become nonfeeding filariform larvae and may infect another host by penetration of the skin or through ingestion. When ingested, the larvae migrate briefly in the mucosa and then develop directly to adults in the small intestine. After penetrating the skin, the larvae migrate systemically to reach the lungs where they penetrate to alveoli, are coughed up and are swallowed to develop into adults in the small intestine. Some species (e.g,. *Ancylostoma caninum*) may enter the systemic circulation to be deposited in muscle as arrested third-stage larvae. These can become reactivated and enter the milk of bitches, infecting neonatal pups; they may, rarely, penetrate the pregnant uterus and infect the fetus. Hookworms are host specific; however, larvae can penetrate the epidermis of aberrant hosts, producing a specific dermatitis called creeping eruption. These larvae do not go on to an adult stage.

LESIONS

The dominant effect of hookworms results from the parasite's ingestion of blood, leading to anemia and hypoproteinemia. The anemia in acute overwhelming infection, as may be seen in neonates infected by way of the milk, is normocytic and normochromic; however, because it is microcytic and hypochromic, in more chronic disease it usually presents as an iron deficiency anemia. Even a small number of A. caninum can lead to severe anemia, although a small to moderate burden of other species of hookworms may not lead to anemia. Infection with particular parasites, such as A. braziliense and U. stenocephala in dogs, is usually not associated with anemia, although hypoproteinemia may occur. Extensive edema, hydrothorax, and ascites may accompany the anemia and hypoproteinemia.

Changes in the intestinal mucosa may be minimal, although diarrhea is a common clinical finding. Hookworms attach to the mucosa and often change positions, leaving small denuded areas in the epithelium that continue to bleed and appear as small punctate hemorrhages at autopsy. There may be blunting and fusion of intestinal villi, and inflammation and fibrosis of the lamina propria, which heightens the disease by causing malabsorption.

Larval migration often occurs without associated clinical signs or lesions; however, severe infestation may lead to pulmonary hemorrhage, and even pneumonia. Entry through the skin leads to dermatitis in the natural host ("ground itch", or "water itch" in humans) and in aberrant hosts where it is known as creeping eruption. The dermatitis is most severe in previously sensitized animals and is characterized by irregular reddish patches; these may take the form of linear serpiginous

TABLE 13-2 **Important hookworms**

Hookworm	Host(s)	Comment
Agriostomum vryburgi	Cattle	In India and Sumatra
Ancylostoma duodenale	Humans	Rare infections in swine
A. caninum	Dog, fox, wolf	Mainly in tropical countries Most pathogenic of canine hookworms
A. braziliense	Dog, cat, fox	Infection usually not characterized by anemia
A. ceylanicum	Dog, cat	Limited to Asia. Rare infections in humans
A. tubaeforme	Cat	Widely distributed
Bunostomum phlebotomum	Cattle	Important pathogen
B. trigonocephalum	Sheep, goats, deer	
Gaigeria pachyscelis	Sheep, goats	In Southeast Asia and Africa
Globocephalus urusubulatus	Swine	In North and South America, Europe, and Asia
G. longemucronatus	Swine	In Europe, Africa and Asia
Necator americanus	Humans, monkeys	Rare infections in dogs
Uncinaria lucasi	Fur seal	Important pathogen of seals
U. stenocephala	Dog, cat, fox	Usually no anemia

tunnels 1–2 mm in diameter, which extend for a few centimeters.

Microscopically, the tissue reaction is limited to the vicinity of the migratory path of the larvae and features an infiltration of eosinophils, lymphocytes, and macrophages.

References

Baker KP, Grimes TD. Cutaneous lesions in dogs associated with hookworm infestation. Vet Rec 1970;87:376–379.

Buelke DL. Hookworm dermatitis. J Am Vet Med Assoc 1971;158: 735–739.

Lee KT, Little MD, Beaver PC. Intracellular (muscle-fiber) habitat of *Ancylostoma caninum* in some mammalian hosts. J Parasitol 1975;61:589–598.

Migasena S, Gilles HM, Maegraith BG. Studies in *Ancylostoma caninum* infection in dogs. I. Absorption from the small intestine of amino-acids, carbohydrates and fat. Ann Trop Med Parasitol 1972;66:107–128.

Migasena S, Gilles HM, Maegraith BG. Studies in *Ancylostoma caninum* infection in dogs. II. Anatomical changes in the gastrointestinal tract. Ann Trop Med Parasitol 1972;66:203–207.

Miller TA. Blood loss during hookworm infection, determined by erythrocyte labeling with radioactive chromium. I. Infection of dogs with normal and with x-irradiated *Ancylostoma caninum*. J Parasitol 1966;52:844–855.

Miller TA. Blood loss during hookworm infection, determined by erythrocyte labeling with radioactive [51] chromium. II. Pathogenesis of *Ancylostoma braziliense* infection in dogs and cats. J Parasitol 1966;52:856–865.

Orihel TC. *Necator americanus* infection in primates. J Parasitol 1971;57:117–121.

Soulsby EJL, Venn JAJ, Green KN. Hookworm disease in British cattle. Vet Rec 1955;67:1124–1125.

Spellman GG Jr, Nossel HL. Anticoagulant activity of dog hookworm. Am J Physiol 1971;220:922–927.

Stone WM, Girardeau M. Transmammary passage of *Ancylostoma caninum* larvae in dogs. J Parasitol 1968;54:426–429.

Trichostrongylosis

The superfamily Trichostrongyloidea is comprised of several families, including Trichostrongylidae, which in turn includes several genera that parasitize the gastrointestinal tracts of a variety of animal species. Some of the more important and common representatives are listed in Table 13-3. The genera of greatest significance are those which inhabit the abomasum of sheep and cattle, particularly members of the genera *Ostertagia* and *Haemonchus*. The superfamily Trichostrongyloidea contains a number of additional gastrointestinal parasites of animals. Many of these are not important in the United States, and others are parasites of rabbits, birds, and wild mammals. Other significant families included are Dictyocaulidae, Metastrongylidae, and Filaroididae, which contain many important lungworms discussed later in this chapter.

Helminths of the superfamily Trichostrongyloidea are small, slender worms in which the buccal cavity is absent or rudimentary, without leaf crowns, and usually toothless; their spicules are usually long and filiform, or short and stout with protuberances. Their life cycles are direct; ellipsoidal ova pass to the ground in the feces of the host, hatch into filariform larvae, develop through larval stages in the soil, and produce infection in a new host when they are ingested with fresh grass. The larvae burrow between and beneath epithelial cells of the abomasum, stomach, or small intestine (but generally remain above the basement membrane), where they undergo further development to adult worms. They do not systemically migrate. The consequences of infection vary among the trichostrongyles.

Heamonchosis

Haemonchus contortus, which parasitizes sheep and goats, and *H. placei* of cattle are extremely important parasites of the abomasum, and frequently associated with disease. They are commonly known as "barber-pole worms," "twisted stomach worms," or "common stomach worms," and are the largest of the trichostrongyles, with female worms measuring up to 30 mm in length. The common names are derived from the appearance of the female worms in which the ovaries are spirally wrapped around the blood filled intestine. Optimal larval development requires a warm and moist environment; consequently, most serious infections are seen from late spring to late summer, depending upon the geographic location. Larvae do not survive cold winters nor hot dry summers; however, the parasites have adapted to unfavorable environmental conditions through arrested larval development (hypobiosis) within their hosts, which allows their perpetuation. Infective third-stage larvae, after they are ingested, reach the abomasum; there they penetrate between epithelial cells and molt to the fourth stage, when they attach to the mucosa. Sexual maturity is reached in about two weeks for *H. contortus* and about four weeks for *H. placei*. Both the fourth-stage larvae and adults suck blood, attaching to the mucosa with their lancets (buccal teeth). Not only do they rob the host of large quantities of blood, but they leave lacerations on the mucosa which predispose the host to gastritis.

Anemia and hypoproteinemia (due to blood loss) are the principal manifestations of haemonchosis. In severe infection with large numbers of worms, death may occur in the absence of clinical signs. More often, the disease is protracted with signs of weakness, loss of weight, and edema of dependent parts, especially under the jaw and along the abdomen.

LESIONS

Lesions depend upon the duration of infection, but always are characterized by multifocal hemorrhages on the mucosa of the abomasum, with attached and free nematodes readily visible. The abomasal contents are reddish brown. Mucous membranes are pale and edema may be widespread. Hydropericardium, hydrothorax, and ascites may be present. The body fat undergoes mucoid degeneration and becomes highly edematous. The liver is light brown and often friable, with areas of fatty change. In Southeast Asia and Central America, the trichostrongyle *Mecistocirrus digitatus*, an important pathogen of ruminants, has similar manifestations to haemonchosis. It is similar in appearance, but larger; it also has a buccal lancet and sucks blood. Swine are also susceptible.

Trichostrongylosis

Many species of the genus *Trichostrongylus* affect animals. The most important are: *Trichostrongylus axei*, which parsitizes the abomasum of cattle, sheep, and goats and the stomach of horses; *T. colubriformis*, which parasitizes the the small intestine of cattle, sheep, and goats; *T. vitrinus*, *T. capricola*, and *T. probolurus* of the sheep and goat small intestine; and *T. longispicularis* of

the small intestine of cattle, sheep, and goats. Representative species and their usual location are listed in Table 13-3. The life cycle is direct. Following ingestion of infective third-stage larvae, they exsheath and penetrate beneath the abomasal or intestinal epithelium, but above the basement membrane; or, in the case of horses, deep into dilated gastric glands. The larvae pass through two more stages to become sexually mature in about 20 days. These adults remain partially embedded in the superficial mucosa. Larvae of *Trichostrongylus* spp are much more resistant to drying and winter temperatures than are *Haemonchus* spp. Their development is,

TABLE 13-3 **Representative species of Trichostrongyloidea**

Parasite	Location of adult	Host(s)
Family Trichostrongylidae		
Trichostrongylus axei	Abomasum, stomach	Sheep, goat, cattle, pig, horse, donkey, humans
T. colubriformis	Abomasum, anterior small intestine	Sheep, goat, cattle, pig, rabbit, dog, humans
T. vitrinus	Small intestine	Sheep, goat, pig, deer, rabbit, dog, humans
T. capricola	Small intestine	Sheep, goat
T. longispicularis	Small intestine	Sheep, cattle
T. retortaeformis	Small intestine, stomach (rare)	Rabbit, hare, goat
T. affinus	Small intestine	Rabbit, sheep, other ruminants
T. tenuis	Small intestine, cecum	Ducks, geese, fowl, guinea fowl, pheasant, partridge
Haemonchus contortus	Abomasum	Sheep, goat, cattle, other ruminants
H. placei	Abomasum	Cattle
H. similis	Abomasum	Cattle, deer
Ostertagia ostertagi	Abomasum	Sheep, goat, cattle, horse
O. circumcincta	Abomasum	Sheep, goat
O. trifurcata	Abomasum	Sheep, goat, cattle
Cooperia punctata	Small intestine, abomasum (rare)	Cattle, sheep (rare)
C. pectinata	Small intestine, abomasum (rare)	Cattle, sheep (rare)
C. oncophora	Small intestine, abomasum (rare)	Cattle, sheep, horse (rare)
C. curticei	Small intestine, abomasum (rare)	Sheep, goat, cattle (rare)
C. spatulata	Small intestine, abomasum (rare)	Sheep, cattle
Nematodirus filicollis	Small intestine	Sheep, goat, cattle, deer
N. spathiger	Small intestine	Sheep, cattle, other ruminants
N. battus	Small intestine	Sheep, cattle, other ruminants
Mecistocirrus digitatus	Abomasum, stomach	Sheep, goat, cattle, pig, buffalo, human (rare)
Marshallagia sp.	Abomasum, duodenum (rare)	Sheep, goat, wild ruminants
Hyostrongylus rubidus	Stomach	Swine
Graphidium strigosum	Stomach, small intestine	Rabbit, hare
Obeliscoides cuniculi	Stomach	Rabbit
Ornithostrongylus quadriradiatus	Crop, proventriculus, small intestine	Pigeon
Family Ollulanidae		
Ollulanus tricuspis	Stomach	Cat, fox, wild *Felidae*, swine

however, optimal during the warm moist seasons. Comparable to *Haemonchus* spp, larvae may remain in arrested development to allow their survival of adverse environmental conditions; however, they generally rely on persistence of adults for their perpetuation.

Trichostrongylus spp are not nearly as important pathogens as *Haemonchus* spp, and their presence may not be associated with clinical disease. More typically they are found along with other nematodes, including *Ostertagia* spp, which are more important parasites. Trichostrongylosis can, however, be characterized by wasting, diarrhea, and hypoproteinemia. Pathologically, abomasitis, gastritis, or enteritis may occur. The mucosa of the abomasum or stomach is usually covered with a layer of mucous and, microscopically, epithelial hyperplasia and mucous metaplasia is evident. This leads to achlorhydria. Small erosions may be present, and the lamina propria is infiltrated with eosinophils, neutrophils, lymphocytes, and plasma cells. Villous atrophy with an increased number of goblet cells is the principal finding when the small intestine is parasitized.

Ostertagiosis

Ostertagia spp. are important parasites of cattle and sheep. *O. ostertagi* is the most significant species in cattle and *O. circumcincta* the most important to sheep and goats. Other species of *Ostertagia* which parasitize cattle and sheep are listed in Table 13-3. Species of the genus *Marshallagia*, which resemble *Ostertagia*, parasitize sheep and wild ruminants. *Ostertagia* spp. resemble abomasal *Trichostrongylus* spp., but are much more important as pathogens, especially to cattle. The life cycle is direct and the parasites are more resistant to drying and cold temperatures than *Trichostrongylus* spp. Even so, hypobiosis is common. After ingestion, the larvae penetrate the mucosa, where they undergo further development. Mature worms may remain partially embedded in the mucosa or be found free. Diarrhea results, which may be severe and wasting; hypoproteinemia may be evident, as well as edema of dependent parts. Grossly, the abomasum is thickened and covered with multiple nodules, giving rise to the descriptive term "morocco leather" appearance. The nodules, which may coalesce, contain larvae and often a projecting adult worm. Microscopically, the nodules can be seen to result from dilation of glands along with marked epithelial hyperplasia and mucous metaplasia. Differentiated cells are replaced with a more flattened epithelium. A definite loss of parietal cells results, as well as achlorhydria. The lamina propria is infiltrated with eosinophils, neutrophils, lymphocytes, and plasma cells. Areas of mucosal necrosis also exist in severe infections.

Cooperia and nematodirus

Cooperia and *Nematodirus* spp. are trichostrongyles that parasitize the upper small intestine of cattle, sheep, and other ruminants, including lambs, goats, and deer. The species of most significance include: *Cooperia punctata*, *C. pectinata*, and *C. oncophora* of cattle; *C. curticei* of sheep and goats; *Nematodirus spathiger* and *N. filicollis* of sheep, cattle, goats, and other ruminants, including deer; *N. battus* of sheep; and *N. helvetianus* of cattle and sheep. Their life cycles are direct, with ingested larvae penetrating the intestinal mucosa, which can lead to extensive destruction. Clinically, affected animals develop diarrhea, hypoproteinemia, and wasting. Microscopically, the mucosa is atrophic with villous atrophy, and with dilated glands contain the parasites. There may be erosions and an associated inflammatory infiltrate in the lamina propria.

Hyostrongylus rubidus

Hyostrongylus rubidus is a trichostrongylid gastric parasite that is common in swine, but ordinarily of little significance. It has a direct life cycle, with ingested third-stage larvae burrowing deeply into gastric glands. When mature adults, some return to the gastric lumen, but others remain deep in the gastric glands, where they cause grossly visible nodules comparable to those caused by *Ostertagia* spp. in ruminants. These lesions are characterized by dilation of glands with epithelial hyperplasia and mucous metaplasia. An admixture of inflammatory cells infiltrates the lamina propria, and neutrophils may be found in the dilated glands. Occasionally, *Hyostrongylus* produces ulcerations or diphtheric gastritis in which the mucosa is covered with a yellowish membrane or tenacious mucous exudate. The mucosa in such examples is thickened, hyperemic, and infiltrated with large numbers of lymphocytes. In areas of erosion or ulceration, neutrophils, eosinophils, and fibrin are part of the exudate. Other gastric nematodes of swine—excluding trichostrongyles—include *Ascarops strongylina*, *Physocephalus sexalatus* and *P. cristatus*, *Simondsia paradoxa*, and *Gongylonema pulchrum*. Gongylonemiasis is discussed later in this chapter.

Ollulanus tricuspis

Ollulanus tricuspis is a small trichostrongyle (family Ollulanus) that parasitizes the stomach of cats, other felidae, and sometimes swine. The parasite is vivaparous, with third-stage larvae developing in the uterus. The infection is spread via vomit. Ordinarily, the infection goes unnoticed and is of little consequence. The parasites do, however, burrow into gastric glands and cause gastritis characterized by hyperplasia, erosions, and an infiltration of inflammatory cells, particularly lymphocytes, into the lamina propria. Species of *Physaloptera* and *Gnathostoma* are spirurids (discussed elsewhere), and also stomach parasites of felines and other carnivores.

References

Baker NF, Fisk RA. Seasonal occurrence of infective nematode larvae in California Sierra foothill pastures grazed by cattle. Am J Vet Res 1986;47:1680–1685.

Barker IK. Intestinal pathology associated with *Trichostrongylus colubriformis* infection in sheep: histology. Parasitology 1975;70: 165–171.

Barker IK. A study of the pathogenesis of *Trichostrongylus colubriformis* infection in lambs with observations on the contribution of gastrointestinal plasma loss. Int J Parasitol 1973;3:743–757.

Barker IK. Scanning electron microscopy of the duodenal mucosa of lambs infected with *Trichostrongylus colubriformis*. Parasitology 1973;67:307–314.

Barker IK. Relationship of abnormal mucosal microtopography with distribution of *Trichostrongylus colubriformis* in the small intestines of lambs. Int J Parasitol 1974;4:153–163.

Barker IK. Location and distribution of *Trichostrongylus colubriformis* in the small intestine of sheep during the prepatent period, and the development of villus atrophy. J Comp Pathol 1975;85:417–426.

Baskerville A, Ross JG. Observations on experimental and field infections of pigs with *Hyostrongylus rubidus*. Br Vet J 1970;126:538–542.

Becklund WW, Walker ML. Nematodirus of domestic sheep, *Ovis aries,* in the United States with a key to the species. J Parasitol 1967;53:777–781.

Blanchard JL, Gallina AM, Wescott RB. Pathologic changes in lambs with *Ostertagia circumcincta* infections associated with decreased infectivity of *Haemonchus contortus*. Am J Vet Res 1986;47:309–314.

Coop RL, Angus KW, Mapes CJ. The effect of large doses of *Nematodirus battus* on the histology and biochemistry of the small intestine of lambs. Int J Parasitol 1973;3:349–361.

Dodd DC. Hyostrongylosis and gastric ulceration in the pig. NZ Vet J 1960;8:100–103.

Durham PJK, Elliott DC. Experimental *Ostertagia* infection of sheep: pathology following a single high dose of larvae. NZ Vet J 1975;23:193–196.

Hargis AM, Prieur DJ, Blanchard JL. Prevalence, lesions, and differential diagnosis of *Ollulanus tricuspis* infection in cats. Vet Pathol 1983;20:71–79.

Hargis AM, Prieur DJ, Blanchard JL, et al. Chronic fibrosing gastritis associated with Ollulanus tricuspis in a cat. Vet Pathol 1982;19:320–323.

Hotson IK. Ostertagiosis in cattle. Aust Vet J 1967;43:383–388.

Jennings FW, et al. Experimental *Ostertagia ostertagi* infections in calves: studies with abomasal cannulas. Am J Vet Res 1966;27:1249–1257.

Kates KC, Turner JH. Observations on the life cycle of *Nematodirus spathiger*, a nematode parasitic in the intestine of sheep and other ruminants. Am J Vet Res 1955;16:105–115.

Kendall SB, Thurley DC, Peirce MA. The biology of *Hyostrongylus rubidus*. I. Primary infection in young pigs. J Comp Pathol 1969;79:87–95.

Nicholson TB, Gordon JG. An outbreak of helminthiasis associated with *Hyostrongylus rubidus*. Vet Rec 1959;71:133.

Osborne JC, Batte EG, Bell RR. The pathology following single infections of *Ostertagia ostertagi* in calves. Cornell Vet 1960;50:223–224.

Ritchie JDS, et al. Experimental *Ostertagia ostertagi* infections in calves: parasitology and pathogenesis of a single infection. Am J Vet Res 1966;27:659–667.

Ross JG, Dow C. The course and development of the abomasal lesion in calves experimentally infected with the nematode parasite *Ostertagia ostertagi*. Br Vet J 1965;121:228–233.

Ross JG, Purcell A, Dow C, et al. Experimental infections of calves with *Trichostrongylus axei*: observations on lethal infections. Res Vet Sci 1968;9:314–318.

Rowlands DapT, Probert AJ. Some pathological changes in young lambs experimentally infected with *Nematodirus battus*. Res Vet Sci 1972;13:323–329.

Snider TG III, Williams JC, Karns PA, et al. High concentration of serum gastrin immunoreactivity and abomasal mucosal hyperplasia in calves infected with *Ostertagia ostertagi* and/or *Trichostrongylus axei*. Am J Vet Res 1988;49:2101–2104.

Stockdale PHG. The pathogenesis of *Hyostrongylus rubidus* in growing pigs. Br Vet J 1974;130:366–373.

Stockdale PHG, Ashton GK, Howes MA, et al. Hyostrongylosis in Ontario. Can Vet J 1973;14:265–268.

Taylor SM, Pearson FR. *Trichostrongylus vitrinus* in sheep. I. The location of nematodes during parasitic development and associated pathological changes in the small intestine. II. The location of nematodes and associated pathological in the small intestine during clinical infection. J Comp Pathol 1979;89:397–403, 405–412.

Wiggin CJ and Gibbs HC. Pathogenesis of simulated natural infections with *Ostertagia ostertagi* in calves. Am J Vet Res 1987;48:274–280.

Oesophagostomiasis (nodule worm disease)

An important parasitic disease is produced in cattle, sheep, and goats in many parts of the world by nodule worms. The more significant species, which are members of the family Strongylidae, are: *Oesophagostomum columbianus* in sheep; *O. radiatum* in cattle; and *O. dentatum* in swine. Several other species of *Oesophagostomum* may infect these animals, but they are less pathogenic. *Oesophagostomum* spp. may also infect nonhuman primates, particularly Old World species. The parasite is a small, slender nematode that has a direct life cycle. Adults in the large intestinal lumen produce ova that pass out in the feces, and after a period outside the host, develop into infective larvae. These larvae, when ingested by another host, penetrate the intestinal mucosa, become encysted, molt in the submucosa, and eventually return to the lumen, where they reach maturity. Percutaneous infection has been demonstrated experimentally, but is not considered important to natural transmission.

CLINICAL MANIFESTATIONS

Signs are most often observed in young animals. Profuse diarrhea is the most constant sign, and apparently is more intense when the larvae are returning from the submucosa to the intestinal lumen. Heavy, long-standing infections usually result in chronic diarrhea, anemia, emaciation, cachexia, prostration, and death. Even though signs are mild, lesions may be found at postmortem inspection.

LESIONS

Mucus and inflammatory cells exuding from the intestinal mucosa of the host is believed to be the result of irritation caused by substances secreted by the adult parasite, perhaps from its cephalic or esophageal glands. It is believed that this exudate is the chief source of food for the worms, for they are not blood suckers, and neither do they attach themselves to the mucosa or cause obstruction of the lumen. Although the mechanism is not understood, the adult parasites do cause intestinal hemorrhage, which may lead to anemia.

The larvae, on the other hand, produce severe and striking lesions (Fig. 13-4). They penetrate the mucosa at any point from the pylorus to the anus in order to reach the deeper parts of the submucosa, where they encyst and undergo a molt. Some may encyst in the lamina propria on the superficial face of the muscularis mucosae, but most of them are found in the submucosa on the deeper side of the muscularis mucosae. Larvae are capable of migrating into the peritoneal cavity and

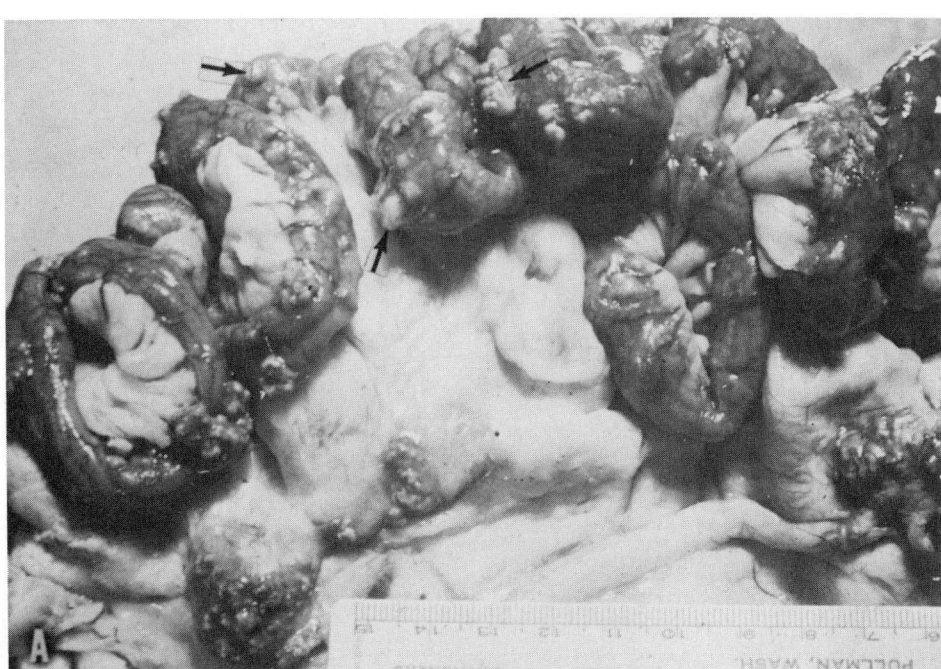

FIG. 13-4 Oesophagostomiasis in small intestine of a sheep. Subserosal nodules are indicated by arrows. (Courtesy of Dr. C. L. Davis.)

encysting in walled-off granulomas on the surface of various abdominal viscera. In initial infections, the larvae shed a striated skin and return to the intestinal lumen as fourth-stage larvae in five or six days, having produced only transitory inflammation in the mucosa and submucosa; however, their ecdysis leads to small ulcers and intestinal bleeding. Some fourth-stage larvae of *O. columbianum* have been demonstrated to undergo a second intestinal invasion, where further development is usually arrested. In contrast, local tissue sensitivity develops in animals repeatedly exposed to these parasites, and the subsequent entry of larvae into the submucosa evokes an intense tissue reaction. Large numbers of eosinophils, lymphocytes, macrophages, and foreign body giant cells surround the larvae and infiltrate the adjacent submucosa and mucosa. The center of these lesions becomes caseated, often calcified, and is surrounded by a dense capsule, which preserves the nodular character of the lesions. A few larvae survive and escape by wandering through the muscularis, but most of them die without finding their way back to the lumen.

The nodules may become infected and enlarged, and displace the muscularis to serve as a nidus for local or generalized peritonitis, but usually they remain as calcified, encapsulated nodules. These lesions give the intestine a nodular appearance as they thicken the wall and project from the serosal surface. When present in large numbers, these nodules sometimes interfere with peristalsis and intestinal absorption.

DIAGNOSIS
Clinical diagnosis may be made by finding eggs or fourth-stage larvae in fecal specimens. At necropsy, the lesions are recognized by their characteristic gross and microscopic features, for which the popular term, nodule disease, is an especially graphic summation.

Chabertia

Another member of the family Strongylidae that closely resembles equine strongyles, as well as *Oesophagostomum* spp., is *Chabertia ovina,* an inhabitant of the colon of sheep, goats, cattle, and wild ruminants. The male species measure up to 14 mm long, and females as much as 20 mm. A large buccal capsule on the anterior end is used to attach to the mucosa. The parasites draw in a piece of the mucosal epithelium, digest it with their esophageal secretions and may ingest blood. Hemorrhage and loss of blood may lead to anemia and death of the host. The life cycle is comparable to *Oesophagostomum* spp., with a histotropic phase in the small intestine, but *Chabertia* does not cause nodules. Marked diarrhea with blood and mucus may be present in severely affected animals. A harmful effect upon the growth of wool has also been ascribed to this parasite.

References
Andrews JS, Maldonado JF. Intestinal pathology in experimental bovine esophagostomiasis. Am J Vet Res 1942;3:17–27.

Berger H, Ribelin WE. Pathology of the swine nodular worm, *Oesophagostomum dentatum* in rabbits. J Parasitol 1969;55:1099–1101.

Bremner KC, Fridemanis R. *Oesophagostomum radiatum* in calves: intestinal hemorrhage associated with larval emergence. Exp Parasitol 1974;36:424–429.

Bremner KC, Keith RK. *Oesophagostomum radiatum:* adult nematodes and intestinal hemorrhage. Exp Parasitol 1970;28:416–419.

Dash KM. The life cycle of *Oesophagostomum columbianum* (Curtice, 1890) in sheep. Int J Parasitol 1973;3:843–851.

Dobson C. Globule leucocytes, mucin and mucin cells in relation to *Oesophagostomum columbianum* infections in sheep. Aust J Sci 1966;28:434.

Dobson C. Pathological changes associated with *Oesophagostomum columbianum* infestations in sheep: haematological observations on control worm-free and experimentally infected sheep. Aust J Agric Res 1967;18:523–538.

Elek P, Durie PH. The histopathology of the reactions of calves to experimental infection with the nodular worm, *Oesophagostomum radiatum* (Rudolphi, 1803). II. Reaction of the susceptible host to infection with a single dose of larvae. Aust J Agric Res 1967;18:549–559.

Gerber HM. Percutaneous infestation of calves and lambs with *Oesophagostomum* spp. J S Afr Vet Assoc 1975;46:273–275.

Hass DK, Brown LJ, Young R Jr. Infectivity of *Oesophagostomum dentatum* larvae in swine. Am J Vet Res 1972;33:2527–2534.

Herd RP. The parasitic life cycle of *Chabertia ovina* (Fabricius, 1788) in sheep. Int J Parasitol 1971;1:189–199.

Herd RP, Arundel JH. Life cycle, pathogenicity and immunogenicity of *Chabertia ovina*. Vet Rec 1969;84:487–488.

McCracken RM, Ross JG. The histopathology of *Oesophagostomum dentatum* infections in pigs. J Comp Pathol 1970;80:619–623.

Skelton GC, Griffiths HJ. *Oesophagostomum columbianum:* experimental infection in lambs: effects of different types of exposure in the intestinal lesions. Pathol Vet 1967;4:413–434.

Soulsby EJL. Helminths, arthropods, and protozoa of domestic animals. 7th ed. London: Baillière Tindall, 1982;185–186.

Dirofilariasis (canine filariasis, heart worm disease)

Animals and humans are subject to infection with a number of filarial (Filarioidea) parasites. A selected list is presented in Table 13-4. The "heart worm," *Dirofilaria immitis*, is one of the more important filarial parasites (Fig. 13-5), and is not uncommon, particularly in the southern and eastern coastal regions of the United

TABLE 13-4 **Filarial parasites of animals**

Filarial parasite	Definitive host	Adult location	Intermediate host
Dirofilaria immitis	Canidae, Felidae	Right ventricle	Mosquitos
D. repens	Canidae, Felidae	Subcutis	Mosquitos
D. corynodes	Canidae, Felidae	Subcutis	Mosquitos
D. conjunctivae	Humans	Subcutis of head	Mosquitos
D. roemeri	Kangaroo, wallaby	Subcutis	Flies
D. tenuis	Procyonidae, humans	Subcutis	Mosquitos
Suifilaria suis	Swine	Subcutis	Unknown
Brugia malayi	Humans, monkey, dog, cat	Lymphatics	Mosquitos
B. pahangi	Cat, dog, monkey	Lymphatics	Mosquitos
Wucheria bancrofti	Humans	Lymphatics	Mosquitos
Loa loa	Humans	Eye, skin	*Chrysops* spp.
Parafilaria multipapillosa	Equidae	Skin	*Haematobia atripalpis*
P. bovicola	Bovidae	Skin	*Musca* spp.
Elaeophora schneideri	Sheep, deer, elk	Arteries	Horseflies
E. poeli	Cattle, buffalo	Aorta	Unknown
Wehrdikmansia cervipedis	Cervidae	Subcutis	Simuliidae
Setaria equina	Equidae	Peritoneal cavity	Mosquitos
S. digitata	Bovidae	Peritoneal cavity	Mosquitos
S. cervi	Cervidae	Peritoneal cavity	Mosquitos
S. yehi	Cervidae	Peritoneal cavity	Mosquitos
S. labiato-papillosa	Cattle, deer	Peritoneal cavity	Mosquitos
Dipetalonema reconditum	Canidae	Subcutis	Fleas, ticks
D. perstans	Humans, apes	Peritoneal and pleural cavity	*Culicoides* spp.
D. dracunculoides	Canidae	Peritoneal cavity	*Hippobosca longipennis*
D. grassi	Dogs	Subcutis	*Rhipicephalus sanguineus*
D. evansi	Camels	Arteries	Mosquitos
Stephanofilaria stilesi	Cattle	Subcutis	*Lyperosia titillans, Haematobia irritans*
S. assamensis	Cattle	Subcutis	*Musca conducens*
S. dedoesi	Cattle	Subcutis	Flies
S. okinawaensis	Cattle	Subcutis	Flies
Onchocerca cervicalis	Equidae	Ligamentum nuchae	*Culicoides* spp.
O. reticulata	Equidae	Tendons of leg	*Culicoides* spp.
O. gutturosa	Cattle	Ligamentum nuchae	Simuliidae
O. lienalis	Cattle	Gastrosplenic ligament	Simuliidae
O. gibsoni	Cattle	Subcutis	*Culicoides* spp.
O. armillata	Cattle, sheep, goats	Aorta	unknown
Dracunculus medinensis	Humans, dog, horse	Subcutis	*Cyclops* spp.
D. insignis	Canidae	Subcutis	*Cyclops* spp.

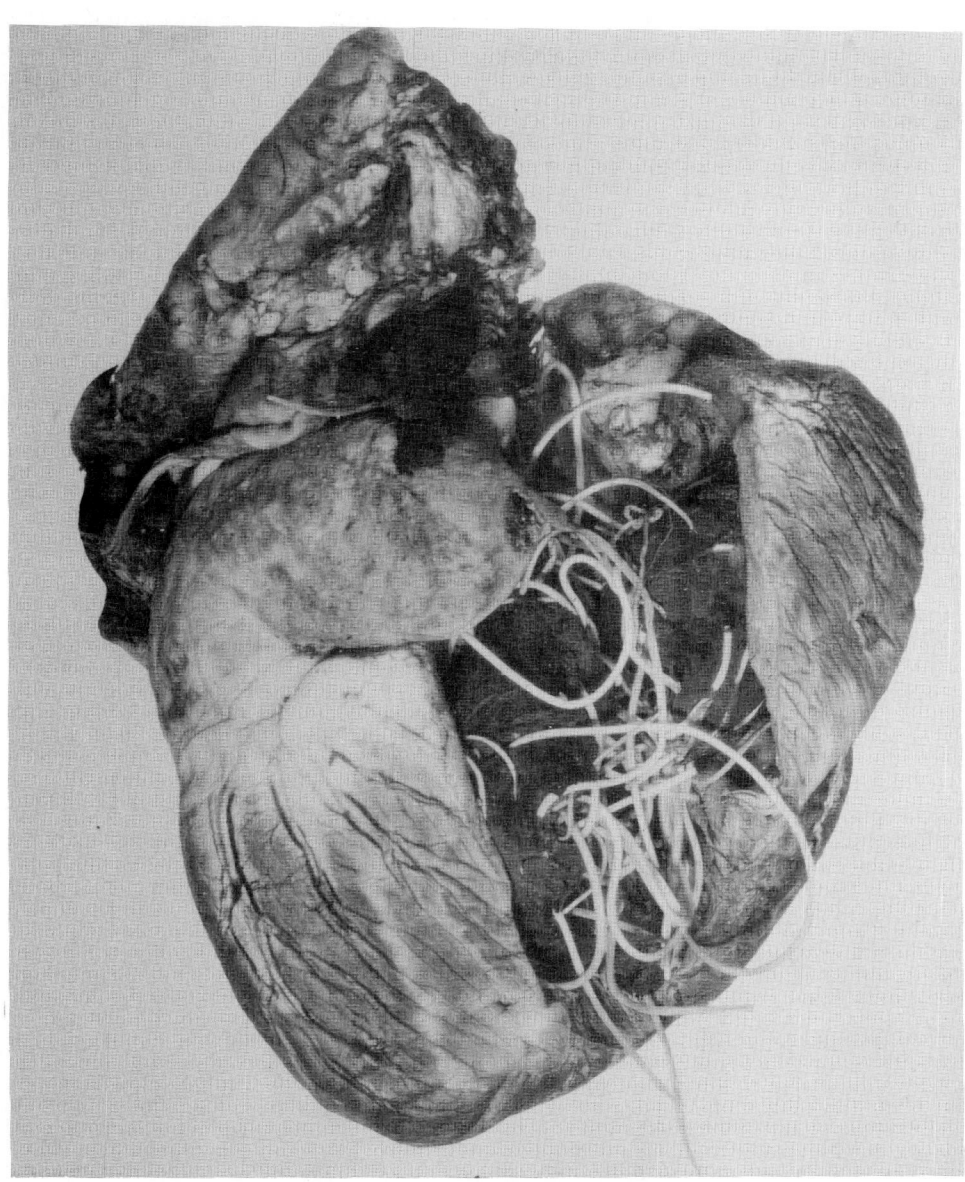

FIG. 13-5 Dirofilariasis. Many adult *Dirofilaria immitis* in right ventricle (opened) of a dog. (Courtesy of Armed Forces Institute of Pathology; contributor: Col. Wm. P. Hill, V.C.)

States. Dogs, cats, foxes, wolves, muskrats, and rarely other species, such as horses, sea lions, and humans, have been reported to be infected. *Dirofilaria repens* is a subcutaneous parasite of dogs, cats, and rarely humans in Europe and the Far East. Adult worms of a closely related species, *Dirofilaria tenuis,* have been reported in the subcutis of raccoons (*Procyon lotor*) in Florida and Louisiana (Orihel and Beaver, 1965). This species has also been found in the subcutis of humans, as has *Dirofilaria conjunctivae* (which may be the same as *D. tenuis*). *Angiostrongylus vasorum* is another parasite that resides in the right heart of dogs. This parasite and other species of *Angiostrongylus* are discussed under Pulmonary Nematodiasis.

The adult worms are slender, almost threadlike, filarial parasites. Males, 12–30 cm long, and females 25–31 cm long, are found in the right ventricle of the heart, and less often in the right auricle pulmonary artery and vena cava. The males and females copulate in these sites; the viviparous female releases highly motile microfilariae, which circulate with the blood. These microfilariae are taken up from the cutaneous circulation by certain biting insects (mosquitoes), in whose bodies they undergo stages of development. The infective filariae then gain access to the tissues of a new host through the bite of the intermediate host. These filarial larvae undergo further development in muscles, subcutaneous, and adipose tissues of the new host. When they reach a length of about 5 cm, they enter veins and are carried to the right heart. The cycle is complete when adult filariae start reproduction in the right ventricle of the host. Transplacental infection of fetal pups with microfilariae may occur, but these do not develop into adults, and disappear after two months.

CLINICAL MANIFESTATIONS

The disease in its earliest stages may give rise to few signs, but severely affected animals will exhibit shortness of breath, weakness, cardiac enlargement, hepatomegaly, ascites, occasionally hypertrophic pulmonary osteoarthropathy and may die with failure of the right heart. In a few instances, fatal outcome may be the result of pulmonary embolism by adult *Dirofilaria*, which die and are swept into the smaller branches of the pulmonary artery. In one case, we have observed dead worms lodged in the pulmonary artery, resulting in a thrombus and aneurysm in the branch of this artery supplying the diaphragmatic lobe. Subsequent rupture of the aneurysm into the adjacent bronchus resulted in severe hemoptysis and exsanguination in a few minutes.

LESIONS

The principal effects of *Dirofilaria immitis* are produced by the adult worms, which interfere with circulation through the right heart (Fig. 13-6). Mechanical interference applied over long periods produces compensatory hypertrophy and enlargement of the right ventricle; insufficiency of the right heart results in passive congestion of the lungs, liver, and spleen, as well as ascites. Occasional adults die and are transported through the pulmonary artery to the lungs where they produce pulmonary embolisms, sometimes leading to infarction. This complication is relatively infrequent, except in dogs treated with certain filaricidal drugs.

Changes in the pulmonary arterial system regularly develop over a period of months. Lesions first develop in the smaller branches of the pulmonary arteries, but progress over time to ultimately involve the extrapulmonary segments. The initial damage is to the endothelial cells, which become swollen and disoriented with disruption of cell junctions. Platelets and leukocytes adhere to the damaged endothelium and an endarteritis ensues with an intimal infiltration of eosinophils. The internal elastic lamina becomes discontinuous; hypertrophy and hyperplasia of medial smooth muscle cells extend into the intima and project into the lumen. The release of platelet-derived growth factor (PDGF) is believed to trigger the marked proliferation of smooth muscle. This leads to the formation of longitudinally arranged rows of villous projections into the lumen (Figs. 13-7A, 13-7B). Grossly, the intima of the arterial tree is uneven, rough or shaggy, an effect considered pathognomonic of dirofilariasis. The proliferative lesion may almost occlude the lumen of the smaller pulmonary arteries, leading to pulmonary hypertension. The presence of adult worms and the damaged endothelium often leads to thrombosis and thromboembolism to the lungs, which can bring on infarction. Fragments of dead Dirofilariae may also lodge in the lungs, stimulating a granulomatous imflammatory reaction. Often, pulmonary hemosiderosis results, and diffuse pulmonary fibrosis with hyperplasia of alveolar epithelium resembling interstitial pneumonia.

In heavy infestations, *D. immitis* may occupy the vena cava, resulting in phlebosclerosis of the vena cava and hepatic veins. Rarely, adult parasites are found in the left side of the heart, aorta, or peripheral arteries, and occasionally outside the vascular tree in such locations as the peritoneal cavity, eye, or ventricles of the brain.

The microfilariae (Fig. 13-7) that circulate freely

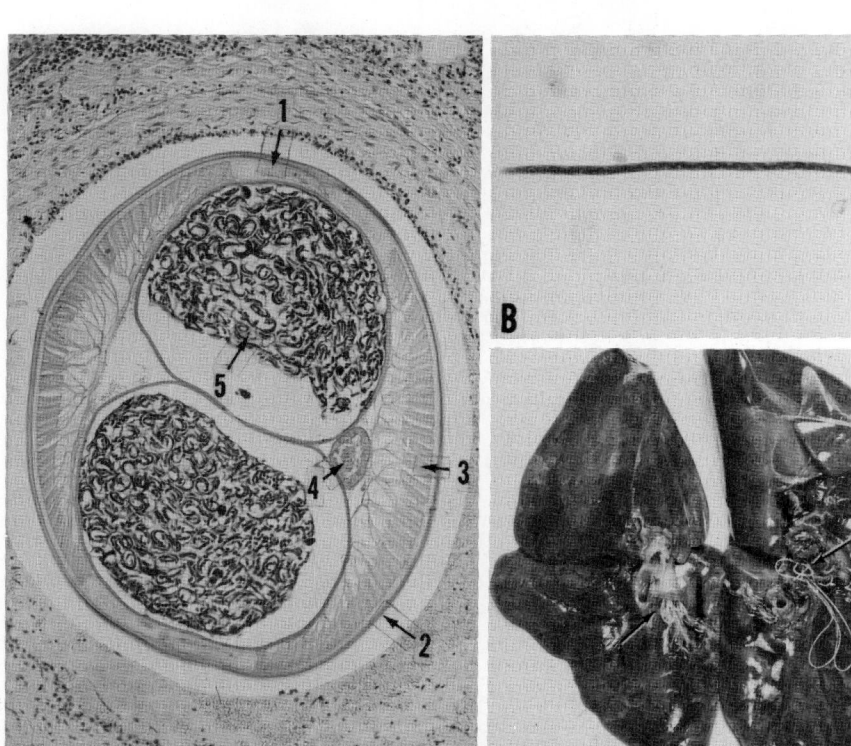

FIG. 13-6 Dirofilariasis. **A.** Adult female *Dirofilaria immitis* in a branch of the pulmonary artery of a dog. (1) Note lateral chord cells; (2) Continuous with the hypodermis, which lay just under the cuticula; (3) The musculature of the worm; (4) Its digestive tube; and (5) Uterus filled with microfilariae. (Courtesy of Armed Forces Institute of Pathology; contributor: Army Veterinary Research Laboratory.) **B.** A single microfilaria of *Dirofilaria immitis* in a fixed specimen from peripheral blood. **C.** *Divofilaria immitis* filling the pulmonary arteries (arrows).

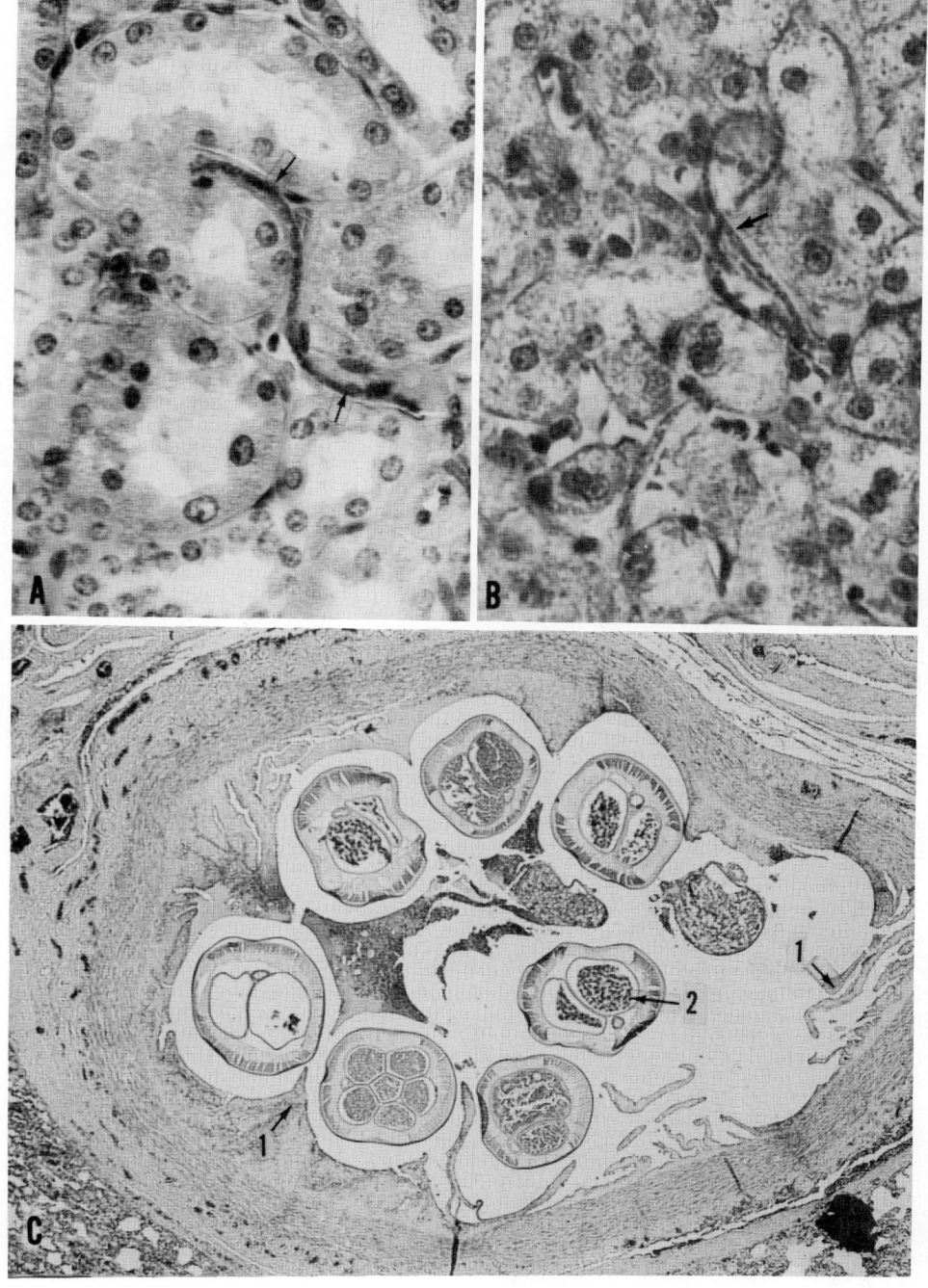

FIG. 13-7 Dirofilariasis. **A.** Microfilaria (arrows) in a capillary in the renal cortex (×300). **B.** Microfilaria (arrow) in sinusoid of liver (×515). **C.** Adult *Dirofilaria immitis* in the pulmonary artery (×30). (1) Note villous proliferation of intima; and (2) Microfilaria in uterus of a female worm. (Courtesy of Armed Forces Institute of Pathology; contributor: Army Veterinary Research Laboratory.)

with the blood appear to produce little tissue damage, for they are frequently found in tissue sections, usually in the absence of a demonstrable inflammatory or other tissue reaction. Some microfilariae die, however, and a small granuloma usually forms around them. Such tiny granulomas have been seen in the interstitial stroma of the kidney in infected dogs. Immune complex glomerulonephritis is another complication of dirofilariasis. Interstitial nephritis and cystitis have been observed in dogs infected with *Dirofilaria*, but the causal relationship of the parasite to these lesions has not been established.

DIAGNOSIS

Presumptive clinical diagnosis can be based upon the symptoms. Adult worms can be visualized as radiolucencies using angiocardiography, a technique used to assess the extent of damage and effect of treatment. Diagnosis is confirmed by demonstration of microfilariae in peripheral blood; however, absence of circulating microfilariae does not preclude infection.

Up to 20% of cases may be occult, without detectable circulating microfilariae. Several different tests are available for the detection of microfilariae; however, once detected, it is necessary to distinguish *Dirofilaria*

TABLE 13-5 **Comparison of *Dirofilaria immitis* and *Dipetalonema reconditum***

Dirofilaria immitis	*Dipetalonema reconditum*
Microfilaria: Length: 307–322 μm width: 6.7–7.1 μm Tails: mostly straight Develop in mosquitos (*Anopheles quadri- maculatus*)	*Microfilaria:* Length: 269–283 μm width: 4.3–4.8 μm Tails: curved, "button-hook" Develop in fleas (*Ctenocepha- lus canis*)
Adults: Found in right ventri- cle and pulmonary artery	*Adults:* Found in subcutis

immitis from other filariae, particularly *Dipetalonema reconditum. D. reconditum,* a fairly common parasite of dogs in the United States, is a relatively innocuous parasite whose adult forms are found in the subcutis, and which is transmitted by fleas and ticks. Several distinguishing features are listed in Table 13-5.

The simplest method of identification, in fresh blood smears, is adequate when the number of microfilariae is large. The microfilariae of *D. immitis* are actively motile, undulating more or less in place, while those of *D. reconditum* tend to migrate across the slide. The odds of finding microfilariae is greatly improved by employing various concentration techniques. The standard method is the Knott technique (Newton and Wright, 1956), in which 1 ml of whole blood is mixed with 9 ml of 1–2% formalin, shaken, centrifuged, and the supernatant decanted. A few drops of 1:1000 methylene blue is added to the sediment, which is then placed on a slide with a coverslip. Cresyl blue is also a satisfactory stain. The morphologic characteristics of the microfilariae are then determined. The most distinguishing features between *D. immitis* and *D. reconditum* are that microfilariae of *D. immitis* are longer, wider, and have a straight tail in contrast to the shorter, narrower *D. reconditum* with its "button-hook" tail. Other concentration techniques are available, including the use of membrane filters; however, these do not preserve the morphologic features as well. Staining for the localization of acid phosphatase (Fig. 13-8), as described by Chalifoux and Hunt (1971), provides an accurate method to distinguish the species. In microfilariae of *D. immitis*, acid phosphatase activity is limited to narrow bands at the excretory and anal pores, whereas in those of *D. reconditum* the enzyme activity is uniformly distributed throughout the parasite (Fig. 13-8). The acid phosphatase technique also has been used to differentiate *Brugia malayi* from *Brugia pahangi*, two filarial parasites of humans. Serologic methods also can be employed to diagnose heartworm infection. Enzyme-linked immunosorbent assay (ELISA) and indirect immunofluorescent assays for adult or microfilarial antigens are both sensitive.

Differentiation among microfilariae of various species of *Dirofilaria* may not be obvious, but due to the geographic restriction of many species, not always of great concern. Cloned specific DNA probes provide a highly specific method to differentiate microfilariae of various filarid parasites, but are not in general use. Adult worms can also be similar in appearance and, because their location is not always restricted to a single site, appearance cannot be the sole criterion for differentiation. Scanning electron microscopy studies of several species of *Dirofilariae* provide a means of distinguishing *D. immitis* from others, as its cuticle lacks the longitudinal ridges present in *D. repens, D. tenuis,* and others (Wong and Brummer, 1978).

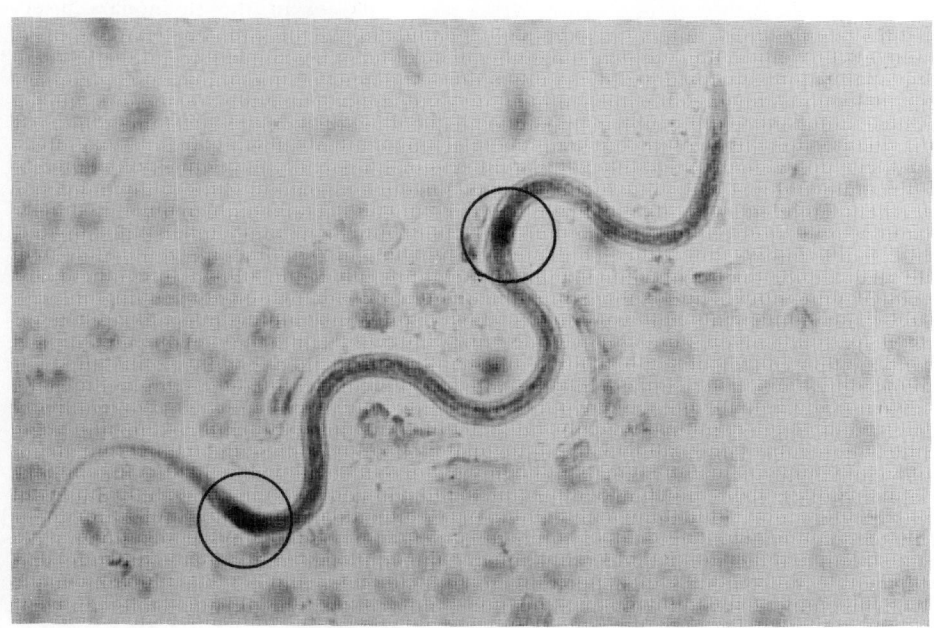

FIG. 13-8 Microfilaria of *Dirofilaria immitis* stained for the demonstration of acid phosphatase activity. Two distinct bands of activity at the excretory and anal pores (circles) allow accurate differentiation from microfilariae of *Dipetalonema reconditum* in which acid phosphatase activity is uniformly distributed. The background is stained with methyl green. (Courtesy of New England Regional Primate Research Center, Harvard Medical School.)

Several other species of *Dipetalonema* affect humans and animals, two of which parasitize dogs: *D. dracunculoides*, whose adults live in the peritoneal cavity and which occurs in Africa and Asia; and *D. grassi*, which is a subcutaneous parasite of dogs in southern Europe and Africa.

References

Abbott PK. Feline dirofilariasis in Papua. Aust Vet J 1966;42:247–249.

Adcock JL. Pulmonary arterial lesions in canine dirofilariasis. Am J Vet Res 1961;22:655–662.

Baskin GB, Eberhard ML. *Dirofilaria immitis* infection in a rhesus monkey (*Macaca mulatta*). Lab Anim Sci 1982;32:401–402.

Bech-Nielsen S, Sjogren U, Lundquist H. *Parafilaria bovicola* (Tubangui 1934) in cattle: epizootiology—disease occurrence. Am J Vet Res 1982;43:945–947.

Bech-Nielsen S, et al. *Parafilaria bovicola* (Tubangui 1934) in cattle: epizootiology—vector studies and experimental transmission of *Parafilaria bovicola* to cattle. Am J Vet Res 1982;43:948–954.

Brunner CJ, Hendrix CM, Blagburn BL, et al. Comparison of serologic tests for detection of antigen in canine heartworm infections. J Am Vet Med Assoc 1988;192:1423–1427.

Calvert CA, Mandell CP. Diagnosis and management of feline heartworm disease. J Am Vet Med Assoc 1982;180:550–552.

Campbell JR, et al. The silvered leaf monkey (Presbytis cristata) as a model for human Bancroftian filariasis. Lab Anim Sci 1987;37:502–504.

Castleman WL, Wong MM. Light and electron microscopic lesions associated with retained microfilariae in canine occult dirofilariasis. Vet Pathol 1982;19:355–364.

Chalifoux L, Hunt RD. Histochemical differentiation of *Dirofilaria immitis* and *Dipetalonema reconditum*. J Am Vet Med Assoc 1971;158:601–605.

Chapleau MW, Fish RE, Levitzky MG. Regional hypoxic pulmonary vasoconstriction in dogs with asymptomatic dirofilariasis. Am J Vet Res 1985;46:1341–1345.

Cooley AJ, Clemmons RM, Gross TL. Heartworm disease manifested by encephalomyelitis and myositis in a dog. J Am Vet Med Assoc 1987;190:431–432.

Courtney CH, Cornell JA. Evaluation of heartworm immunodiagnostic tests. J Am Vet Med Assoc 1990;197:724–729.

Dillon AR, Braund KG. Distal polyneuropathy after canine heartworm disease therapy complicated by disseminated intravascular coagulation. J Am Vet Med Assoc 1982;181:239–242.

Dillon R, Sakas PS, Buxton BA, et al. Indirect immunofluorescence testing for diagnosis of occult *Dirofilaria immitis* infection in three cats. J Am Vet Med Assoc 1982;180:80–82.

Ferenc SA, Copeman DB, Turk SR, et al. *Onchocerca gutturosa* and *Onchocerca lienalis* in cattle: effect of age, sex, and origin on prevalence of onchocerciasis in subtropical and temperate regions of Florida and Georgia. Am J Vet Res 1986;47:2266–2268.

Forrester DJ, Jackson RF, Miller JF, et al. Heartworms in captive California sea lions. J Am Vet Med Assoc 1973;163:568–570.

Fukushima K, Hutsell D, Patton S, et al. Aberrant dirofilariasis in a cat. J Am Vet Med Assoc 1984;184:199–201.

Gardiner CH, Oberdorfer CE, Reyes JE, et al. Infection of man by *Dirofilaria repens*. Am J Trop Med Hyg 1978;27:1279–1281.

Grieve RB, et al. Canine *Dirofilaria immitis* infection in a hyperenzootic area: examination by parasitologic findings at necropsy and by two serodiagnostic methods. Am J Vet Res 1986;47:329–332.

Griffiths HJ, Schlotthauer JC, Gehrman FW. Feline dirofilariasis. J Am Vet Med Assoc 1962;140:61.

Gulber DJ. A comparative study of the distribution, incidence and periodicity of the canine filarial worms *Dirofilaria immitis* (Leidy) and *Dipetalonema reconditum* (Grassi) in Hawaii. J Med Entomol 1966;3:159–167.

Hendrix CM, Bemrick WJ, Schlotthauer JC. Natural transmission of *Dirofilaria immitis* by Aedes vexans. Am J Vet Res 1980;41:1253–1255.

Jackson RF, von Lichtenberg F, Otto GF. Occurrence of adult heartworms in the venae cavae of dogs. J Am Vet Med Assoc 1962;141:117–121.

Kamalu BP. Canine filariasis caused by *Dirofilaria repens* in southeastern Nigeria. Vet Parasitol 1991;40:335–338.

Klein JB, Stoddard ED. *Dirofilaria immitis* recovered from a horse. J Am Vet Med Assoc 1977;171:354–355.

Knight DH. Heartworm infection. Vet Clin North Am Small Anim Pract 1987;17:1463–1518.

Kotani T, Powers KG. Developmental stages of *Dirofilaria immitis* in the dog. Am J Vet Res 1982;43:2199–2206.

Kotani T, et al. Pathological studies on the ectopic migration of *Dirofilaria immitis* in the brain of dogs. Jpn J Vet Sci 1975;37:141–154.

Krakowka S. Transplacentally acquired microbial and parasitic diseases of dogs. J Am Vet Med Assoc 1977;171:750–753.

Lavers DW, Spratt DM, Thomas C. *Dirofilaria immitis* from the eye of a dog. Aust Vet J 1969;45:284–286.

Lindsey JR. Identification of canine microfilariae. J Am Vet Med Assoc 1965;146:1106–1114.

Lok JB, Cupp EW, Bernardo MJ. *Simulium jenningsi* Malloch (Diptera: Simuliidae): a vector of *Onchocerca lienalis* Stiles (Nematoda: Filarioidea) in New York. Am J Vet Res 1983;44:2355–2358.

Luttgen PJ, Crawley RR. Posterior paralysis caused by epidural dirofilariasis in a dog. J Am Anim Hosp Assoc 1981;17:57–59.

MacLean JD, Beaver PC, Michalek H. Subcutaneous dirofilariasis in Okinawa, Japan. Am J Trop Med Hyg 1979;28:45–48.

Mantovani A, Jackson RF. Transplacental transmission of microfilariae of *Dirofilaria immitis* in the dog. J Parasitol 1966;52:116.

Matherne CM, Green SP, Corwin RM, et al. Detection of circulating *Dirofilaria immitis* antigens in random source laboratory dogs: evaluation of two commercial serodiagnostic tests. Lab Anim Sci 1988;38:584–587.

McCall JW. Heartworm infections: diagnosis and control. Pract Vet 1978;49:32–34.

Moreland AF, Battles AH, Nease JH. Dirofilariasis in a ferret. J Am Vet Med Assoc 1986;188:864.

Narama I, Miura K, Tsuruta M, et al. Microfilarial granulomas in the spleens of wild-caught cynomolgus monkeys (*Macaca fascicularis*). Vet Pathol 1985;22:355–362.

Newton WL, Wright WH. The occurrence of a dog filariid other than *Dirofilaria immitis* in the United States. J Parasitol 1956;42:246–258.

Orihel TC, Beaver PC. Morphology and relationship of *Dirofilaria tenuis* and *Dirofilaria conjunctivae*. Am J Trop Med Hyg 1965;14:1030–1043.

Pampiglione S, Rivasi F, Trotti GC. Human pulmonary dirofilariasis in Italy. Lancet 1984;i:333.

Parrott TY, Greiner EC, Parrott JD. *Dirofilaria immitis* infection in three ferrets. J Am Vet Med Assoc 1984;184:582–583.

Patton S, Faulkner CT. Prevalence of *Dirofilaria immitis* and *Dipetalonema reconditum* infection in dogs: 805 cases (1980–1989). J Am Vet Med Assoc 1992;200:1533–1534.

Rawlings CA. Cardiopulmonary function in the dog with *Dirofilaria immitis* infection: during infection and after treatment. Am J Vet Res 1980;41:319–325.

Rawlings CA, Keith JC Jr, Schaub RG. Development and resolution of pulmonary disease in heartworm infection: illustrated review. J Am Anim Hosp Assoc 1981;17:711–720.

Rawlings CA, Dawe DL, McCall JW, et al. Four types of occult *Dirofilaria immitis* infection in dogs. J Am Vet Med Assoc 1982;180:1323–1326.

Rothstein H, Brown ML. Vital staining and differentiation of microfilaria. [*D. immitis* and *Dipetalonema*.] Am J Vet Res 1960;21:1090–1094.

Schnelle GB, Roby TO, Young RM, et al. Canine filariasis. North Am Vet 1945;26:155–164.

Schnelle GB, Jones TC. *Dirofilaria immitis* in the eye and in an interdigital cyst. J Am Vet Med Assoc 1945;107:14–15.

Scholtens RG, Patton S. Evaluation of an enzyme-linked immunosorbent assay for occult dirofilariasis in a population of naturally exposed dogs. Am J Vet Res 1983;44:861–864.

Scott DW. Nodular skin disease associated with *Dirofilaria immitis* infection in the dog. Cornell Vet 1979;69:233–240.

Shires PK, Turnwald GH, Qualls CW, et al. Epidural dirofilariasis causing paraparesis in a dog. J Am Vet Med Assoc 1982;180:1340–1343.

Sim BKL, et al. Identification of *Brugia malayi* in vectors with a species-specific DNA probe. Am J Trop Med Hyg 1986;35:559–564.

Stackhouse LL, Clough E. Clinical report: five cases of feline dirofilariasis. Vet Med Small Anim Clin 1972;67:1309–1310.

Sutton RH, Atwell RB. Lesions of pulmonary pleura associated with canine heartworm disease. Vet Pathol 1985;22:637–639.

Taguchi M, Takehara B, Uriu I. Aberrant *Dirofilaria immitis* in the lateral ventricle of the brain in a dog. J Jpn Vet Med Assoc 1959;12:430–432, (Engl summary) Vet Bull 1960;30:1499.

Tankersley WG, Richter CB, Batson JS. Therapy of filariasis in tamarins. Lab Anim Sci 1979;29:107–110.

Thilsted JP, et al. Comparison of four serotests for the detection of *Dirofilaria immitis* infection in dogs. Am J Vet Res 1987;48:837–841.

Tolbert RH, Johnson WE Jr. Potential vectors of *Dirofilaria immitis* in Macon County, Alabama. Am J Vet Res 1982;43:2054–2056.

Winter H. The pathology of canine dirofilariasis. Am J Vet Res 1959;20:366–371.

Wong MM. Experimental dirofilariasis in macaques. II. Susceptibility and host responses to *Dirofilaria repens* of dogs and cats. Am J Trop Med Hyg 1976;25:88–93.

Wong MM, Brummer MEG. Cuticular morphology of five species of Dirofilaria: a scanning electron microscope study. J Parasitol 1978;64:108–114.

References

Benbrook EA. The occurrence of the guinea worm, *Dracunculus medinensis*, in a dog and a mink with a review of this parasitism. J Am Vet Med Assoc 1940;96:260–263.

Chandler AC. The guinea-worm, *Dracunculus insignis* (Leidy, 1858): a common parasite of raccoons in east Texas. Am J Trop Med 1942;22:153–157.

Cheatum EL, Cook AH. On the occurrence of the North American guinea-worm in mink, otter, raccoon, and skunk in New York State. Cornell Vet 1948;38:421–423.

Crichton VFJ, Beverley-Burton M. Observations on the seasonal prevalence, pathology and transmission of *Dracunculus insignis* (Nematoda: Dracunculoidea) in the raccoon (*Procyon lotor* (L)) in Ontario J Wldlf Dis 1977;13:273–280.

Elder C. Dracunculiasis in a Missouri dog. J Am Vet Med Assoc 1954;124:390–391.

Johnson GC. *Dracunculus insignis* in a dog. J Am Vet Med Assoc 1974;165:533.

Panciera DL, Stockham SL. *Dracunculus insignis* infection in a dog. J Am Vet Med Assoc 1988;192:76–78.

Schwabe CW, Meier H, Bent CF. A case of dracontiasis in a New England dog. J Parasitol 1956;42:651.

Tirgari M, Radhakrishnan CV. A case of *Dracunculus i* in a dog. Vet Rec 1975;96:43–44.

Turk RD. Guinea-worm (*Dracunculus insignis;* Leidy, 1858) infection in a dog. J Am Vet Med Assoc 1950;117:215–216.

Dracunculosis

Two species of *Dracunculus* or "guinea-worms" can infect animals, but only one is common in the Americas. Both have an indirect life cycle utilizing *Cyclops* as the intermediate host. The classic guinea-worm, *Dracunculus medinensis* ("serpent-worm", "dragon-worm," or "medinaworm") is principally a parasite of humans in tropical and subtropical countries, particularly the Middle East, Asia, and Africa. It may also affect dogs and rarely cats, horses, and cattle. In North America, *D. insignis* parasitizes dogs and wild carnivores, and is common in racoons, skunks, mink, and otters.

The adult parasites, the females of which may reach up to 400 cm in length, reside in the subcutis, particularly of the limbs. Less often, adults may locate in other connective tissue, a body cavity, the heart, or the eye. In the subcutis, the parasites cause painful inflammatory swellings that tend to ulcerate, and which are subject to secondary bacterial infection. The head of the worm may protrude from the ulcer, and the uterus, when in contact with water, prolapses and releases larvae. Larval development to the infective stage requires the intermediate host, *Cyclops*. The definitive host becomes infected after drinking water in which the crustaceans live. The *Cyclops* in the intestine release infective larvae, which migrate through tissues for several months to reach the subcutis; there, lesions become evident some 10–12 months after initial infection.

Diagnosis depends on identification of the adult parasites in the lesions. When in unusual sites, they must be differentiated from *Dirofilaria immitis*. On occasion, *Dracunculus* larvae have demonstrated in circulating blood and must be distinguished from other filarial parasites with microfilaremia. Affected animals may exhibit eosinophilia.

Equine strongylidosis

The family Strongylidae contains well over 50 species of worms that parasitize the cecum and colon of horses and other equidae, causing disease (conveniently designated as **strongylidosis**) with protean manifestations. All have direct life cycles. The **larger strongyles** of the genus *Strongylus,* slender worms about 1–2 inches in length, are the most important as pathogens. Three species, *Strongylus vulgaris, S. equinus* and *S. edentatus,* cause disease through blood sucking by the adult worms and extensive tissue damage due to larval migration. Three other genera of large strongyles, *Triodontophorus, Craterostomum,* and *Oesophagodontus,* are of little significance. The **small strongyles,** classified in the subfamily Cyathostominae (or family Trichonematidae), include about 40 species within six or more genera (*Cyathostomum, Cylicocyclus, Cylicodontophorus, Cylicostephanus, Posteriostomum,* and *Gyalocephalus*) all formerly classified as *Trichonema* spp. These parasites are less injurious to the host, since they neither attach themselves to the intestinal mucosa nor ingest blood; also, they do not undergo extensive tissue migration as larvae, as do the important larger varieties.

CLINICAL MANIFESTATIONS

Clinical signs are varied and depend upon the severity of the infection caused by the adult worms and the anatomic localization of the larval forms. General debility, weakness, emaciation, diarrhea, and anemia can result from the presence of numerous large strongyles in the cecum and colon. The larvae of *Strongylus vulgaris* often give rise to lesions in the mesenteric arteries; this results in intestinal infarction that manifest as severe abdominal pain (colic). The larvae may also produce thrombi in the aorta or iliac arteries, which may partially occlude these vessels, causing serious weakness in one or both rear limbs; this symptom is accentuated by exercise. Migration of *S. equinus* and *S. edentatus* through the liver and peritoneal cavity can lead to peritonitis, colic and, in severe infections in foals, even death.

Specific strongyles

Strongylus vulgaris, the common or double-toothed strongyle, is found in the cecum, usually attached to the mucosa. The males are about 16 mm in length, the females approximately 24 mm, and as a rule, the worms are red from ingested blood. The life cycle is direct; eggs pass in the feces and first-stage larvae hatch out, eventually developing to second-stage and finally to third-stage infective larvae. Following ingestion, third-stage larvae penetrate the wall of the intestine, molt in the submucosa, and penetrate terminal branches of intestinal arteries. This migration results in small hemorrhages throughout the wall of the intestine and an infiltration of lymphocytes, neutrophils, and eosinophils. Submucosal arteries present similar inflammation and thrombosis, and contain fourth-stage larvae. The fourth-stage larvae migrate up the lumen of mesenteric arteries, in the intima, to reach the anterior mesenteric artery at one of its major branches by two to three weeks after infection, where they remain for three or more months. Here they are responsible for striking arterial lesions, particularly in the anterior mesenteric artery, and less frequently in the aorta, iliac, renal, and other arteries. The fourth-stage larvae then return by way of arteries to the wall of the cecum and colon, where they again induce local hemorrhage and inflammation. They then enter the lumen and mature to adults.

Larvae burrowed in arteries evoke proliferation of intima and endothelium, sometimes associated with hemorrhage and necrosis. Fibrin and cellular debris accumulate over the roughened intimal areas, extend out into the lumen, and occasionally cause occlusion. In long-standing cases, the wall of the artery becomes greatly thickened by the proliferation of both intimal and adventitial fibrous tissue. Collections of lymphocytes often gather in the thickened wall of the artery. This is the most common lesion and is appropriately regarded as **verminous arteritis.** In a less common lesion, the arterial wall becomes both thickened and sacculated, forming a dilated segment with a relatively smooth lining. This is properly considered a **verminous aneurysm.** Rupture of such aneurysms is almost unknown, although in some encountered at necropsy, the wall is extremely thin at certain points.

The worms are found in the lumen of the affected artery, firmly attached to the intima, and associated with varying degrees of inflammation. In some cases, only a few parasites are seen in an arterial lesion; in others, as many as 50 may be found. The worms may also be found at times in emboli or thrombi that arise from those arterial lesions. Fifth-stage larvae have been found in association with lesions in the spinal cord of a pony, and similar spinal lesions, without the parasite, have been reported in the horse (Pohlenz, et al., 1965). When mature young adults, parasites return to the intestine by way of lumens of arteries, again inducing local hemorrhage and inflammation.

Strongylus equinus, the triple-toothed strongyle, sclerostome, or bloodworm, is found in its adult form in the cecum and rarely in the colon of equines (Fig. 13-9). It is usually attached to the mucosa and engorged with blood. The male is about 35 mm long; the females, up to 55 mm. Ingested third-stage larvae penetrate the

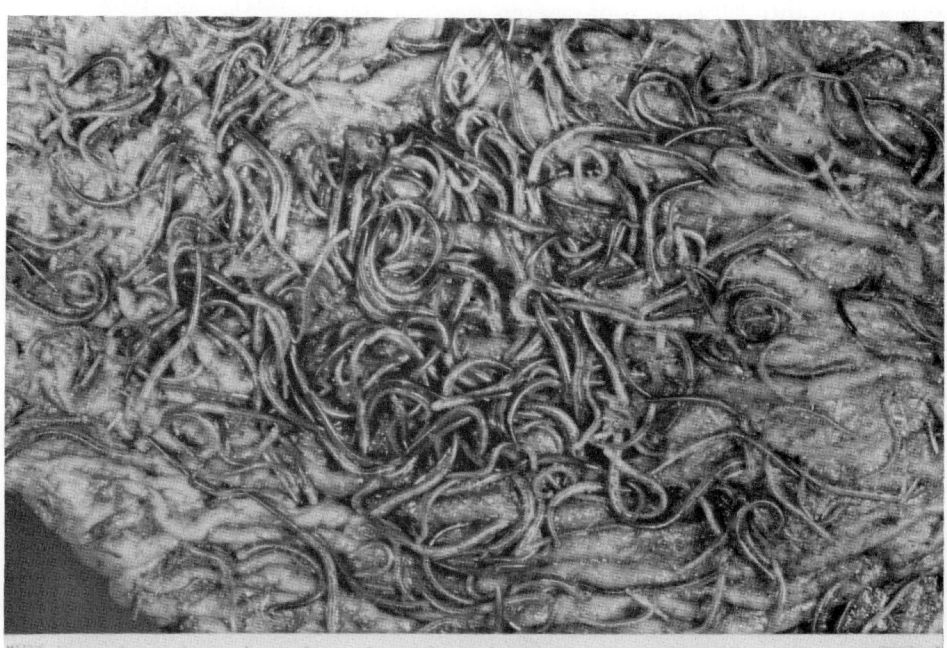

FIG. 13-9 Equine strongylidosis. Adult *Strongylus equinus* in the cecum of a two-year-old gelding. (Courtesy of Dr. C. R. Cole, Ohio State University.)

wall of the cecum or colon, causing small hemorrhages and inflammatory nodules before migrating into the peritoneal cavity and entering the liver, where they wander for six to seven weeks. Their migration leads to paths of hepatic necrosis and eosinophilic inflammation. Larvae leave the liver by way of the hepatic ligament, enter the pancreas and then the peritoneal cavity, where they molt to the fifth stage and presumably migrate directly to the intestinal lumen.

Strongylus edentatus, the toothless strongyle, occurs in adult form in the cecum and colon of equines, usually attached to the mucosa. The males are about 28 mm long; the females as much as 44 mm. The life cycle is direct; infective third-stage larvae penetrate the wall of the intestine and reach the liver by way of portal veins. The larvae develop to fourth-stage larvae, which migrate within the liver, producing necrosis and inflammation. Larvae are believed to leave the liver within hepatic ligaments, and make their way to the retroperitoneal tissue of the right flank, where they remain as fourth-stage and early fifth-stage larvae for about three months, and cause small hemorrhages and inflammatory nodules. They then migrate through the mesentery to the wall of the cecum and colon, again causing nodules before reentering the lumen to become adults.

S. edentatus infection is associated with striking nodules in the small and large intestines, which have been termed *haemonomelasma ilei* by Cohrs (1954) (Fig. 13-20B). The subserous masses are about 3 mm high, 5 mm wide, and one to several centimeters long. These lesions, when fresh, are bright red from recent hemorrhage; later, they turn to shades of yellow and brown as the blood cells disintegrate to release blood pigment, which remains as hematoidin or hemosiderin.

Microscopically, these subserosal lesions are made up of edema, connective tissue, free red blood cells, leukocytes, macrophages, blood pigment, and in some sections, a central fragment of caseous necrotic debris. It is difficult to find larvae in the subserosal lesions, but occasionally a tract can be followed through the muscularis into the submucosa. Occasionally, the offending larvae may be cut in cross section in histologic preparations. These lesions, in spite of their florid appearance, seem to have little effect upon the host; consequently, their proper evaluation is important.

Larvae of any of the migrating strongyles may occasionally be encountered in aberrant locations, such as the lung or brain. The small strongyles also have direct life cycles and are believed to develop in small nodules in the wall of the large intestine similar to *Oesophagostomum* species.

The small strongyles are relatively nonpathogenic, even though they may occur in great numbers. They may, however, cause lesions that can lead to clinical signs of enteritis, including diarrhea and colic. After ingestion, infective larvae penetrate the mucosa of the colon, where they remain for variable periods and cause inflammatory nodules, which can be numerous. They then return to the lumen, where they mature to adults 0.5–2 cm in length. Their migration leads to hemorrhage and eosinophilic enteritis.

DIAGNOSIS

Quantitative determination of the strongyle ova in the feces are used to estimate the parasitic burden in the living animal. This is necessary because these parasites are so common that a few ova in a fecal specimen have no diagnostic significance. The diagnosis of equine strongylidosis must be based upon mature evaluation of all symptoms and ova counts. Verminous arteritis and lesions due to migration of the parasite are usually recognized at necropsy.

References

Blackwell NJ. Colitis in equines associated with strongyle larvae. Vet Rec 1973;93:401–402.
Craig TM, Bowen JM, Ludwig KG. Transmission of equine cyathostomes (Strongylidae) in central Texas. Am J Vet Res 1983;44:1867–1869.
Cohrs P. Lehrbuch der Speziellen Pathologischen Anatomie der
Drudge JH, Lyons ET. Equine parasites, problems and control. Pract Vet 1978;49:5–7, 9.
Duncan JL, Pirie HM. The life cycle of *Strongylus vulgaris* in the horse. Res Vet Sci 1972;13:374–379.
Duncan JL, Pirie HM. The pathogenesis of single experimental infections with *Strongylus vulgaris* in foals. Res Vet Sci 1975;18:82–93.
Foster AO, Clark HC. Verminous aneurysm in equines of Panama. Am J Trop Med 1937;17:85–99.
Jasko DJ, Roth L. Granulomatous colitis associated with small strongyle larvae in a horse. J Am Vet Med Assoc 1984;185:553–554.
Klei TR, Torbert BJ, Ochoa R, et al. Morphologic and clinicopathologic changes following *Strongylus vulgaris* infections of immune and nonimmune ponies. Am J Vet Res 1982;43:1300–1307.
Little PB, Lwin US, Fretz P. Verminous encephalitis of horses: experimental induction with *Strongylus vulgaris* larvae. Am J Vet Res 1974;35:1501–1510.
Little PB, Lwin US, Fretz P. *Strongylus vulgaris* in the horse: a review. Can Vet J 1976;17:150–157.
McCraw BM, Slocombe JOD. *Strongylus edentatus:* development and lesions from ten weeks postinfection to patency. Can J Comp Med 1978;42:340–356.
Ogbourne CP. Studies of the epidemiology of *Strongylus vulgaris* infection of the horse. Int J Parasitol 1975;5:423–426.
Pohlenz J, Schulze D, Eckert J. (Spinal infection with *Strongylus vulgaris* in a pony.) Dtsch Tieaerztl Wochenschr 1965;72:510–511, Vet Bull 1966;36:1472.
Segal M. "Mal seco," enfermedad de equidos, contribucion al conocimiento de su etiopatogenia, observaciones y experiencia en Junin de los Andes (Nequen). Buenos Aires: Rev Vet Milit 1959;7:3–10, 66–68, 70–74, 106, 108–116, Vet Bull 1960;30:752.
Turk MAM, Klei TR. Effect of ivermectin treatment on eosinophilic pneumonia and other extravascular lesions of late *Strongylus vulgaris* larval migration in foals. Vet Pathol 1984;21:87–92.

Spirocercosis

Infection with the spiruroid worm, *Spirocerca lupi* (*Spirocerca sanguinolenta, Spiroptera sanguinolenta, Filaria sanguinolenta,* esophageal worm) is particularly common in southern parts of the United States, but it has also been reported from many parts of the world. The adult worms, which are usually bright red, have been found coiled in nodules in the wall of the esophagus, aorta, stomach and other organs of the dog, fox, wolf, and cat. The males measure 30–54 mm long; the females,

54–80 mm. The eggs are thick-walled, about 37 by 15 μ in maximum dimensions, and contain larvae when deposited.

LIFE CYCLE

The life cycle of this helminth is complex. The embryonated eggs are passed in the feces and do not hatch until ingested by certain coprophagous beetles. In these intermediate hosts, the larvae develop into the infective (third) stage, then encyst. When eaten by an abnormal host (paratenic host), such as a frog, snake, lizard, or any one of many birds and mammals, the larvae burrow into the mesentery, where they remain in a viable state for some time. When infected beetles or other transport hosts are eaten by one of the final hosts (dog, fox, wolf, cat), the larvae penetrate the stomach wall; then, by following the course of the arteries and migrating through adventitia and media, they reach the wall of the aorta and localize in the adventitia, usually of the upper thoracic portion. The parasites reach the aorta one to two weeks after ingestion and develop there for about 90 days, when they migrate to the adjacent esophagus and burrow into its wall; there, they develop to adults in cystic nodules. Patent infection is established 50–70 days later, with the eggs reaching the esophageal lumen through a small opening in the nodule. Rarely, the adults localize in an abnormal location, such as the wall of the stomach or lungs.

CLINICAL MANIFESTATIONS

Clinical signs may be absent in mild infections; or, persistent dysphagia and vomiting may be caused by esophageal obstruction. Sudden death from hemorrhage from aortic lesions has been reported.

LESIONS

The principal lesions in this disease are produced by the adult worms as a result of their localizing in the adventitia of the aorta and the submucosa of the esophagus. The worms become the center of a tumorlike nodule in the aortic wall; this may initiate the formation of aneurysm, with possible rupture and fatal hemorrhage. In microscopic sections of active lesions in the aorta, worms may be found in areas of the adventitia and media where normal tissue is destroyed and replaced by leukocytes and debris. Sometimes the worms are seen burrowing into the media, with necrotic tracts leading to the intima. The intimal stroma undergoes considerable proliferation, and mineralization and ossification may occur in the intima and media. In most instances, however, the worm eventually departs from the aortic media or adventitia for the esophagus, leaving a lesion in the wall in the aorta. In an animal that presents previous localization of the aorta, it is not uncommon to observe well-developed worm-containing nodules in the esophagus. On the intimal surface, these lesions appear as roughened, slightly elevated plaques of various sizes, or as depressed aneurysmal scars.

The esophageal lesions are most common near its terminus, usually a few centimeters from the cardia of the stomach. Grossly, one or several nodules are seen on the luminal surface, elevating the epithelium a centimeter or more. One or several worms may be embedded in each nodule, with parts of the worms protruding from a small orifice. Cross section of one of the nodules usually reveals a thick fibrous wall partially covered by epithelium, enclosing a cavity containing worms and yellowish pus. Microscopically, the worms form the center for a mass of neutrophils, surrounded by a thick wall of connective tissue infiltrated with macrophages, lymphocytes, and plasma cells. Strangely, eosinophils are usually absent. The adult worms have a thick cuticle surrounding a meromyarian muscle wall, interrupted by a double row of very large specialized muscle cells arranged along each side of the body cavity. Ova within the gravid uterus are flattened and ovoid, and are embryonated before they are discharged through the genital pore.

Some affected dogs develop vertebral spondylosis or "deformative ossifying spondylitis" of the thoracic vertebrae, which is believed to be related to the migration and encystment of Spirocerca lupi. This lesion (Figs. 13-10, 13-11) is characterized by irregular coarse exostoses of the ventral surfaces of the bodies of certain thoracic vertebrae.

Malignant neoplasms may develop within the wall of *Spirocerca lupi* granulomas. These are either fibrosarcomas or osteosarcomas that may metastasize to the lung. Their pathogenesis is not known, but their close association with the parasite suggests it is the cause. Hypertrophic pulmonary osteoarthropy is a frequent finding in dogs with large esophageal malignancies.

DIAGNOSIS

Infection with *Spirocerca lupi* in the living animal is confirmed by the identification of embryonated ova in the feces. Postmortem diagnosis is easily made by demonstration of characteristic lesions in the aorta, esophagus, or ventral face of thoracic vertebrae in association with the adult parasites.

References

Anantaraman M, Se K. Experimental spirocercosis in dogs with larvae from a paratenic host, *Calotes versicolor,* the common garden lizard in Madras. J Parasitol 1966;52:911–912.

Anantaraman M, Se K. Parasites and cancer: sarcoma in dogs associated with *Spirocerca lupi.* Ann NY Acad Sci 1963;108:890–923.

Bailey WS. *Spirocerca lupi:* a continuing inquiry. J Parasitol 1972;58: 3–22.

Bwangamoi O. Spirocercosis in Uganda and its association with fibrosarcoma in a dog. J Small Anim Pract 1967;8:395–398.

Chhabra RC, Singh KS. Life history of *Spirocerca lupi:* route of migration of histotropic juveniles in dog. Indian J Anim Sci 1972;42: 540–547.

Dixon KG, McCue JF. Further observations on the epidemiology of *Spirocerca lupi* in the southern United States. J Parasitol 1967; 53:1074–1075.

Murray M. Incidence and pathology of *Spirocerca lupi* in Kenya. J Comp Pathol 1968;78:401–405.

Rajan A, Mohiyuddeen S. Incidence of spirocercosis in some uncommon sites. Kerala J Vet Sci 1974;5:139–142.

Ribelin WE, Bailey WS. Esophageal sarcomas associated with *Spirocerca lupi* infection in the dog. Cancer 1958;2:1242–1246.

Seibold HR, et al. Observations on the possible relation of malignant

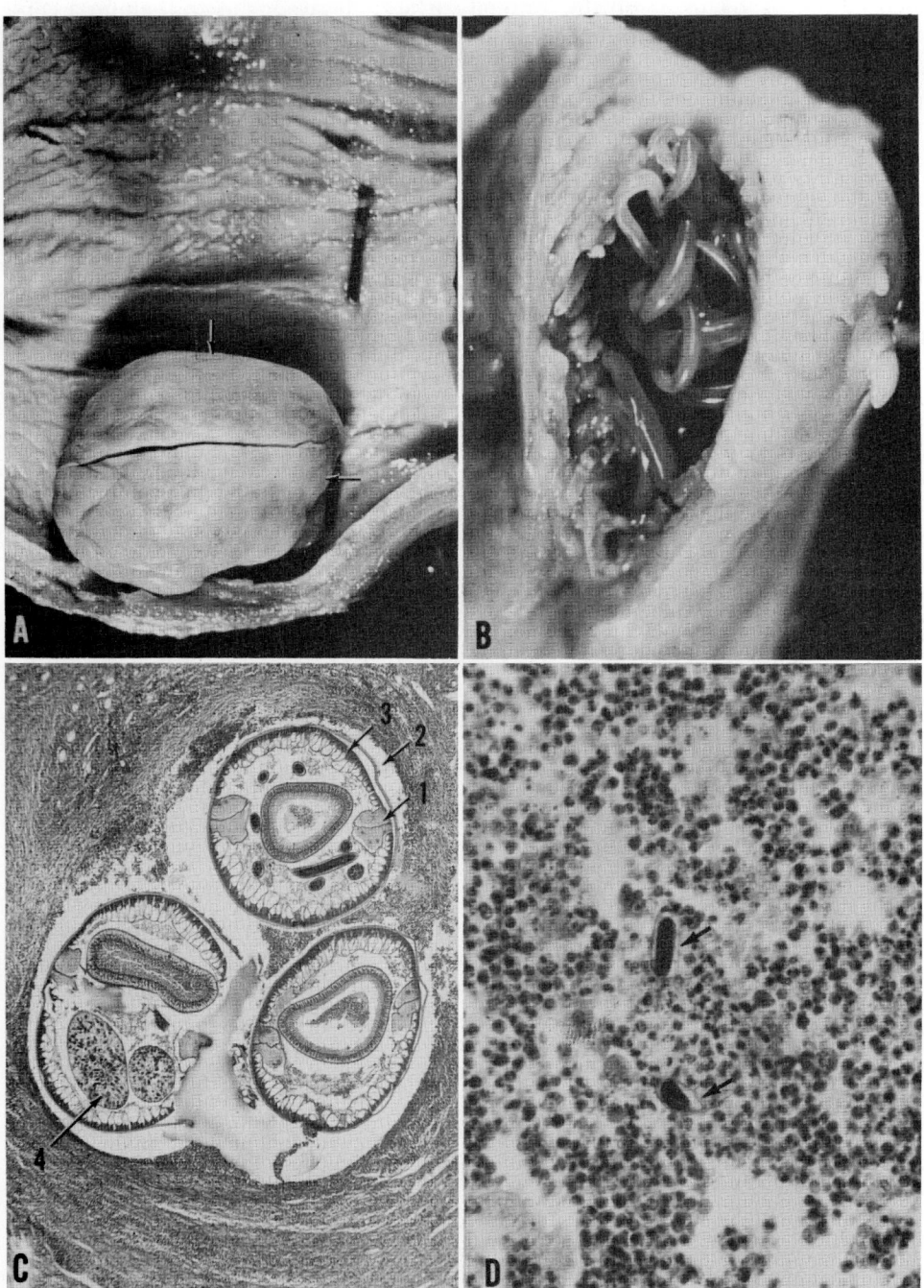

FIG. 13-10 Spirocercosis. **A.** Nodule (arrows) in thoracic esophagus of a dog. **B.** A nodule opened to show the coiled nematodes within. (Courtesy of Major C. N. Barron.) **C.** Section through a nodule (×48) containing adult worms. (1) Note lateral chord cells; (2) Cuticula; (3) Muscle cells; and (4) Uterus filled with ova (Contributor: Major C. N. Barron.) **D.** Ova of *Spirocerca lupi* (×300) surrounded by pus in an esophageal nodule. (Courtesy of Armed Forces Institute of Pathology; contributor: Major C. N. Barron.)

esophageal tumors and *Spirocerca lupi* lesions in the dog. Am J Vet Res 1955;16:5–14.

Stephens LC, Gleiser CA, Jardine JH. Primary pulmonary fibrosarcoma associated with *Spirocerca lupi* infection in a dog with hypertrophic pulmonary osteoarthropy. J Am Vet Med Assoc 1983;182:496–498.

PHYSALOPTERA

Several species of Physaloptera (order Spirurida, family Physalopteridae) parasitize the stomach and duodenum of cats, dogs, rodents, monkeys, and other animals. These are listed in Table 13-6. Infection follows ingestion of an intermediate host, which includes cockroaches, crickets and beetles. The adults attach to the mucosa and suck blood, leaving small erosions and ulcers when they change positions. Hyperplasia of the gastric mucosa may lead to nodular projections resembling tumors, especially in monkeys infected with *P. tumefasciens*. As a rule, *Physaloptera* infections do not lead to clinical disease.

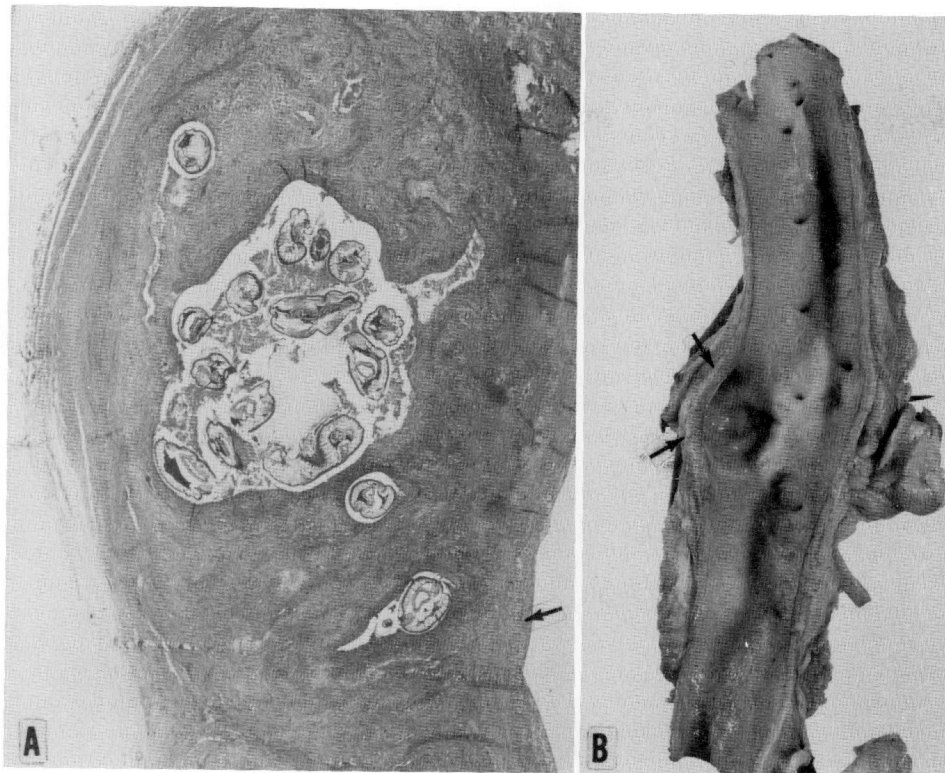

FIG. 13-11 Spirocercosis. **A.** Section of aorta (×12) with a large worm-filled nodule in the adventitia. The intima is indicated by an arrow. (Contributor: Dr. H. R. Seibold.) **B.** A large sacculate lesion (arrows) in the aorta resulting from spirocercosis. (Courtesy of Armed Forces Institute of Pathology; contributor: Major C. N. Barron.)

TABLE 13-6 **Selected species of *Physaloptera* and animals affected**

Physaloptera rara	Dogs, wild Canidae, and Felidae
P. praeputialis	Cats
P. pseudopraeputialis	Cats, coyotes
P. canis	Dogs, cats
P. felidis	Cats
P. tumefaciens	Macaque monkeys
P. dilitata	New World monkeys
P. (Abbreviata) caucasia	Old World monkeys
P. (A.) poicilometra	Old World monkeys
P. maxillaris	Raccoons, skunks, badgers, weasels

References

Slaughter LJ, Bostrom RE. Physalopterid (*Abbreviata poicilometra*) infection in a sooty mangabey monkey. Lab Anim Care 1969; 19:235–236.

Windle DW, Reigel DH, Heckman MG. *Physaloptera tumefaciens* in the stump-tailed macaque (*Macaca arctoides*). Lab Anim Care 1970;20:763–767.

Gnathostoma

Gnathostoma spinigerum (order Spirurida, family Gnathostomatidae) is a parasite of the stomach of cats, dogs and wild carnivores. Two intermediate hosts are required, a *Cyclops* and a fresh water fish, frog, or reptile. Infective third-stage larvae may also encyst in a variety of mammals, including mice, rats, dogs, and primates. Encysted larvae are released after ingestion and migrate through the liver and other viscera, where extensive damage may occur. Ultimately, the adult worms reach the wall of the stomach where they dwell in large cavities within the submucosa. Several worms inhabit a single thick-walled cyst filled with serosanguinous fluid. Eggs escape through a small opening leading to the lumen of the stomach.

References

Kirkpatrick CE, Lok JB, Goldschmidt MH, et al. Gastric gnathostomiasis in a cat. J Am Vet Med Assoc 1987;190:1437–1439.

Trichospirura

Trichospirura leptostoma is a small spirurid nematode (family Thelaziidae) whose adults inhabit the pancreatic ducts of various species of tamarins and marmosets. The parasites may be encountered with little associated reaction, but often their presence leads to periductal fibrosis, chronic pancreatitis with parenchymal necrosis and atrophy, and ductular proliferation. Embryonated eggs pass through the pancreatic ducts to reach the feces which, when expelled, is then ingested by intermediate host cockroaches (*Blatella germanica* or *Supella longipalpa*). Monkeys become infected by eating the cockroaches.

References

Beglinger R, Illgen B, Pfister R, et al. The parasite *Trichospirura leptostoma* is associated with wasting disease in a colony of common marmosets, *Callithrix jacchus*. Folia Primatol 1988;51:45–51.

Cosgrove GE, Humason G, Lushbaugh CC. *Trichospirura leptostoma*, a nematode of the pancreatic ducts of marmosets (*Saguinus* spp.). J Am Vet Med Assoc 1970;157:696–698.

Illgen-Wilcke B, Beglinger R, Pfister R, et al. Studies on the developmental cycle of *Trichospirura leptostoma* (Nematoda: Thelaziidae): experimental infection of the intermediate hosts *Blatella germanica* and *Supella longipalpa* and the definitive host *Callithrix jacchus* and development in the intermediate hosts. Parasitol Res 1992;78:509–512.

Cerebrospinal nematodiasis (neurofilariasis, setariasis)

Certain nematodes have selective affinity for the central nervous system, and several may accidentally wander into the brain or spinal cord (Fig. 13-12), especially in an aberrant host. The migration of larval parasites to sites other than customary for their life cycles is not unusual; however, their localization to tissues outside the central nervous system usually does not lead to clinical disease. Such migration into the nervous system may also be encountered only as incidental findings, but on occasion it leads to clinical signs typically characterized by paralysis.

Setaria digitata

Setaria are filarid worms whose adults parasitize the peritoneal cavity of a variety of herbivores. Ordinarily neither the adults nor the circulating microfilariae

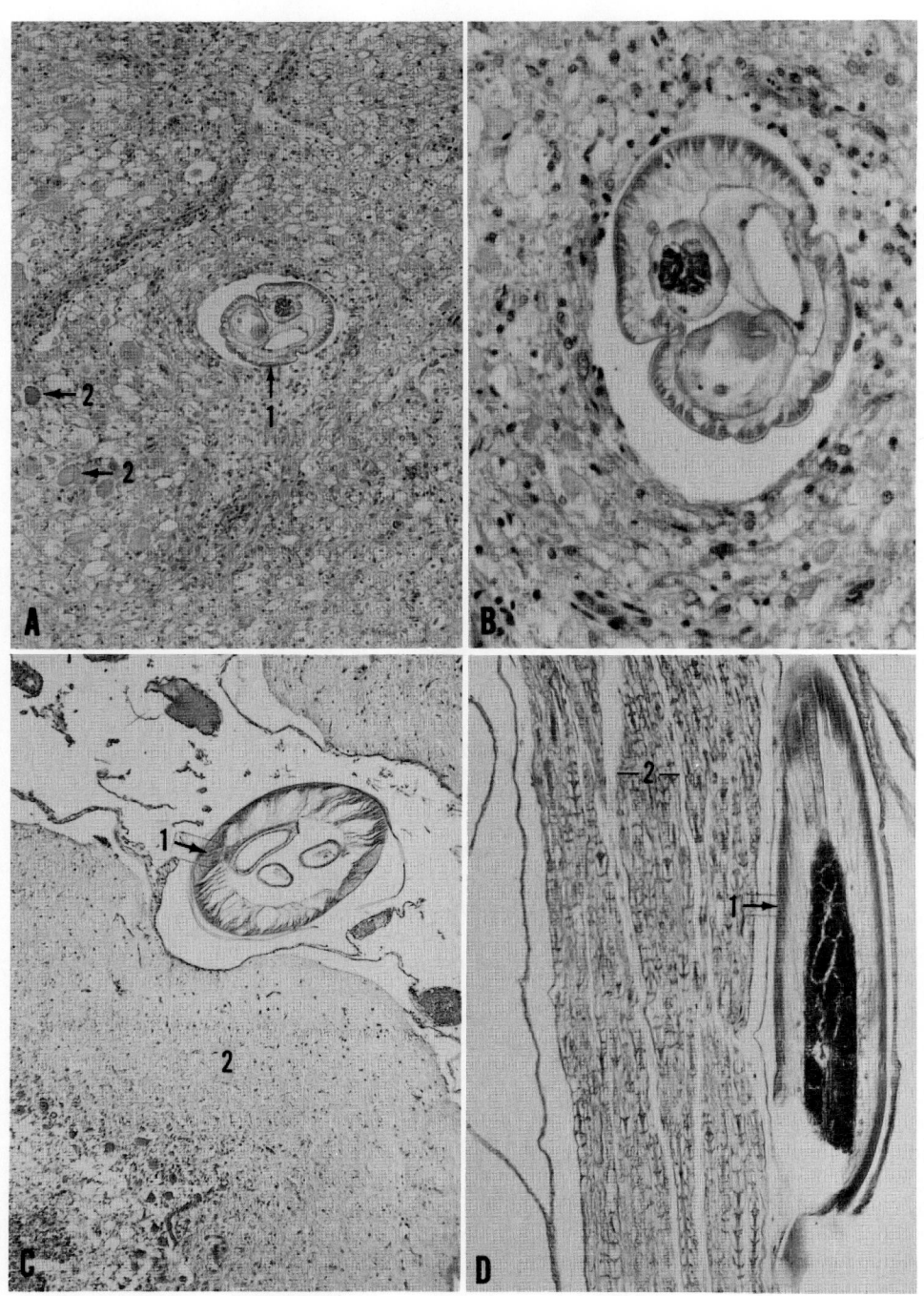

FIG. 13-12 Cerebrospinal nematodiasis. **A.** Nematode. (1) In the spinal cord (×77) of a sheep; (2) Note swollen axones. B. Higher magnification (×215) shows the parasite in greater detail. (Contributor: Dr. Peter Olafson.) **C.** Nematode. (1) In the pia mater (×53) of a horse; (2) Cerebellar cortex. **D.** Another larva. (1) In the longitudinal section (×100) in a spinal nerve; (2) From the same horse as C. (Courtesy of Armed Forces Institute of Pathology; contributor: 406th Medical General Laboratory.)

cause serious disease. Occasionally, the parasites locate in other sites, such as the pleural cavity or eye. Selected species are listed in Table 13-4. *Setaria digitata,* a parasite of the peritoneal cavity of cattle in the Far East and Asia, is a cause of cerebrospinal nematodiasis when it affects aberrant hosts such as sheep, goats, and horses. Immature worms wander randomly throughout the brain, leaving necrotic paths. Gitter cells and a slight to moderate infiltration of eosinophils and neutrophils surround the tracts. Clinical signs include incoordination, weakness, and paralysis, which in sheep and goats has been termed "lumbar paralysis" and in horses, "kumri".

Pneumostrongylus tenuis

Pneumostrongylus tenuis (Parelaphostrongylus, Odocoileostronglus, Elaphostrongylus, Neurofilaria cornelliensis) is a parasite of white-tailed deer *(Odocoileus virginianus)* whose adults inhabit the subdural space and venous sinuses. The parasitism is of little consequence in white-tailed deer; however, in other species such as moose, elk, caribou, black-tailed deer, red deer, llamas, sheep, and goats, the parasites cause considerable damage. The parasite has an indirect life cycle with larval development in various species of snails and slugs. After ingestion of the intermediate hosts, larvae first migrate to the dorsal column of the spinal cord, enter the subdural space, then migrate to the subdural space of the brain and enter venous sinuses. Eggs travel by way of the venous system to the lung, where they hatch, pass up the bronchial tree to be swallowed, and exit via the feces. The destructive lesions in aberrant hosts are primarily caused by wandering parasites. Several species of the related genus *Elaphostrongylus* also have been associated with neurologic signs and lesions in deer.

Angiostrongylus cantonensis

Angiostrongylus cantonensis, a lungworm of rats, normally migrates through the brain as part of its life cycle in rats, and has been recognized as a cause of eosinophilic meningoencephalitis in humans and dogs. Its life cycle is similar to *Pneumostrongylus,* utilizing gastropods as intermediate hosts, and crabs and frogs as paratenic hosts. Other species of *Angiostrongylus* infect the lungs of mink (*A. [Perostrongylus] pridhami*) and pulmonary arteries of dogs and foxes (*A. vasorum*). *Angiostrongylus costaricensis* is a parasite of subserosal arteries of wild rats in Central and South America, which may also affect humans and nonhuman primates. It does not affect the brain or lung. Infection with *Gurltia paralysans,* a filarid that resides in the spinal veins of cats and wild *Felidae* of South America, may lead to paralysis.

Halicephalobus (Micronema) deletrix

Halicephalobus (Micronema) deletrix, which is apparently a saprophytic filarid nematode, has been recognized as a cause of encephalitis and nasal granulomas in horses in the United States and Egypt. Migrating larvae of **Stron-** **gylus vulgaris** are another of the more important causes of verminous encephalitis in horses in the United States; also, the horse stomach worm, **Draschia megastoma,** has also been reported as a cause of cerebrospinal nematodiasis in horses.

Various species of ascarids are occasionally encountered in the brain. The common ascarids of raccoons and skunks, **Baylisascaris (Ascaris) procyonis** and **B. (A.) columnaris** respectively, are important causes of cerebrospinal nematodiasis in many different species, having been observed in dogs, foxes, rabbits, squirrels, woodchucks, prairie dogs, and mice, as well as a variety of birds. **Toxocara canis** is an important cause of cerebrospinal nematodiasis in children (visceral larval migrans), and also is encountered in the true host, the dog. **Meningonema peruzzi** and **Dipetalonema perstans** have been found in the brain of monkeys. The latter species, as well as **Wuchereria bancrofti** and **Loa loa,** may invade the brain of humans.

In addition to nematodes, other metazoan parasites, discussed later in this chapter, parasitize the central nervous system. These include *Coenurus cerebralis,* various *Cysticerci, Echinococcus, Troglotrema, Oestrus ovis,* and *Hypoderma bovis,* and *H. lineatum.*

CLINICAL MANIFESTATIONS

Manifestations of cerebrospinal nematodiasis are extremely varied. Mildly affected animals may show only motor weakness, incoordination, or slight loss of balance. Animals with severe lesions may exhibit paresis of one or all limbs, the hind legs being most frequently and severely affected. The onset may be dramatically sudden in some cases, more insidious in others; death may intervene within a few days; or, recovery may follow, with or without residual nervous manifestations, such as drooping of eyelid or ear, weakness, or impaired gait.

LESIONS

Grossly visible lesions are unusual, except in those infrequent instances in which hemorrhage occurs in the primary malacic focus caused by the migration of the parasites. Meticulous microscopic study of the brain and spinal cord is usually necessary to uncover the affected areas. The primary foci may be single or multiple, and may occur in any part of the central nervous system, although the spinal cord and thalamus appear to be favored sites. The lesions are usually asymmetric, each appearing as a solitary, raggedly bound focus of cavitation, rarely containing hemorrhage. Under low magnification, these foci appear as cracks, crevices, or spongy areas; in some, tracts leading from the nearby meninges can be detected. Under higher magnification, nervous tissue appears partially or completely lost in the center of the affected zone. Around this, axis cylinders in cross section are visibly large, irregularly shaped, rounded bodies; they are stained darkly eosinophilic in hematoxylin and eosin preparations, and are heavily impregnated when the Bodian method is employed. Longitudinal sections of these axis cylinders show that they are irregularly enlarged, tortuous, and fragmented.

Axons similarly affected are seen in ascending and descending tracts extending above and below the primary malacic locus. Axonal damage is associated with swelling and distortion of myelin sheaths; in long-standing cases, it is associated with glial proliferation. The secondary (wallerian) degeneration is no different from the degeneration that results from injuries to the central nervous system. The degenerative lesion in nerve-fiber tracts may lead to the primary lesion, when sufficient numbers of serial sections are prepared and examined.

Cellular infiltration composed of lymphocytes, neutrophils, or occasionally eosinophils is frequently observed in the pia mater near the primary malacic foci. These cells may also be seen in irregular nests in the pia arachnoid, in subdural and epidural locations, and sometimes extending along the spinal nerve roots. Perivascular lymphocytic cuffing may be prominent adjacent to primary malacic foci.

The offending helminths will be seen in tissue sections only fortuitously, unless a diligent search of serial sections through characteristic lesions is made. It is assumed that migratory larvae not only can invade nervous tissue, but can also wander out again. In some cases it is possible to demonstrate the parasites only by filtration of the spinal fluid, although evidence of their invasion of nervous tissue may be readily found.

DIAGNOSIS

Definitive diagnosis can be made only after meticulous microscopic examination of the central nervous system. Typical lesions must be found, and some should contain the causative nematodes. Clinical diagnosis is made in geographic regions in which the disease is enzootic, but at present can be based only upon presumptive evidence.

References

Alden C, Woodson F, Mohan R, et al. Cerebrospinal nematodiasis in sheep. J Am Vet Med Assoc 1975;166:784–786.

Anderson RC. Neurological disease in moose infected experimentally with *Pneumonstrongylus tenuis* from white-tailed deer. Pathol Vet 1964;1:289–322.

Anderson RC. The development of *Pneumonstrongylus tenuis* in the central nervous system of white-tailed deer. Pathol Vet 1965;2:360–379.

Anderson RC. The pathogenesis and transmission of neurotropic and accidental nematode parasites of the central nervous system of mammals and birds. Helminth Abstr 1968;37:191–210.

Anderson RC, et al. Further experimental studies of *Pneumonstrongylus tenuis* in cervids. Can J Zool 1966;44:851–861.

Anderson RC, et al. Experimental cerebrospinal nematodiasis (*Pneumonstrongylus tenuis*) in sheep. Can J Zool 1966;44:889–894.

Anderson RC, et al. The penetration of *Pneumonstrongylus tenuis* into the tissues of white-tailed deer. Can J Zool 1967;45:285–289.

Anderson RC, et al. The effect of *Pneumonstrongylus tenuis* (Nematoda: Metastrongyloidea) on kids. Can J Comp Med 1969;33:280–286.

Beautyman W, Woolf AL. An ascaris larva in the brain in association with acute anterior poliomyelitis. J Pathol Bact 1951;63:635–647.

Cho DY, Hubbard RM, McCoy DJ, et al. *Micronema* granuloma in the gingiva of a horse. J Am Vet Med Assoc 1985;187:505–507.

Dade AW, Williams JF, Whitenack DL, et al. An epizootic of cerebral nematodiasis in rabbits due to *Ascaris columnaris*. Lab Anim. Sci 1975;25:65–69.

Dixon D, Reinhard GR, Kazacos KR, et al. Cerebrospinal nematodiasis in prairie dogs from a research facility. J Am Vet Med Assoc 1988;193:251–253.

Dubey JP: *Baylisascaris procyonis* and eimerian infections in raccoons. J Am Vet Med Assoc 1982;181:1292–1294.

Ferris DH, Levine ND, Beamer PD. *Micronema deletrix* in equine brain. Am J Vet Res 1972;33:33–38.

Frauenfelder HC, Kazacos KR, Lichtenfels JR. Cerebrospinal nematodiasis caused by a filariid in a horse. J Am Vet Med Assoc 1980;177:359–362.

Innes JRM, Shoho C. Cerebrospinal nematodiasis: focal encephalomyelomalacia of animals caused by nematodes (*Setaria digitata*), a disease which may occur in man. Arch Neurol Psychiat 1953;70:325–349.

Innes JRM, Pillai CP. Kumri—so-called lumbar paralysis—of horses in Ceylon (India and Burma), and its identification with cerebrospinal nematodiasis. Br Vet J 1955;111:223–235.

Jortner BS, Troutt HF, Collins T, et al. Lesions of spinal cord parelaphostrongylus in sheep: sequential changes following intramedullary larval migration. Vet Pathol 1985;22:137–140.

Kazacos KR, Kazacos EA. Experimental infection of domestic swine with *Baylisascaris procyonis* from raccoons. Am J Vet Res 1984;45:1114–1121.

Kazacos KR, Reed WM, Kazacos EA, et al. Fatal cerebrospinal disease caused by *Baylisascaris procyonis* in domestic rabbits. J Am Vet Med Assoc 1983;183:967–971.

Kelly WR, Innes JRM. Cerebrospinal nematodiasis with focal encephalomalacia as a cause of paralysis of beavers (*Castor canadensis*) in the Dublin Zoological Gardens. Br Vet J 1966;122:285–287.

Kennedy PC, Whitlock JH, Roberts SJ. Neurofilariosis, a paralytic disease of sheep. I. Introduction, symptomatology, pathology. Cornell Vet 1952;42:118–124.

Krogdahl DW, Thilsted JP, Olsen SK. Ataxia and hypermetria caused by *Parelaphostrongylus tenuis* infection in llamas. J Am Vet Med Assoc 1987;190:191–193.

Kurtz HJ, Loken K, Schlotthauer JC. Histopathologic studies on cerebrospinal nematodiasis of moose in Minnesota naturally infected with *Pneumonstrongylus tenuis*. Am J Vet Res 1966;27:548–557.

Larson DJ, Greve JH. Encephalitis caused by *Baylisascaris* migration in a silver fox. J Am Vet Med Assoc 1983;183:1274–1275.

Little PB. Cerebrospinal nematodiasis of Equidae. J Am Vet Med Assoc 1972;160:1407–1413.

Mayhew IG, Lichtenfels JR, Greiner EC, et al. Migration of a spiruroid nematode through the brain of a horse. J Am Vet Med Assoc 1982;180:1306–1311.

Myers RK, Monroe WE, Greve JH. Cerebrospinal nematodiasis in a cockatiel. J Am Vet Med Assoc 1983;183:1089–1090.

Nettles VF, Davidson WR, Fisk SK, et al. An epizootic of cerebrospinal nematodiasis in cottontail rabbits. J Am Vet Med Assoc 1975;167:600–602.

Nichols DK, Montali RJ, Phillips LG, et al. *Parelaphostrongylus tenuis* in a captive reindeer and sable antelope. J Am Vet Med Assoc 1986;188:619–621.

Orihel TC, Esslinger JH. *Meningonema peruzzii* gen. et sp. n. (Nematoda: Filarioidea) from the central nervous system of African monkeys. J Parasitol 1973;59:437–441.

Pletcher JM, Howerth E. *Micronema deletrix* infection in the horse. J Am Vet Med Assoc 1980;177:1090.

Richter CB, Kradel DC. Cerebrospinal nematodosis in Pennsylvania groundhogs (Marmota monax). Am J Vet Res 196425:1230–1235.

Roth L, Georgi ME, King JM, et al. Parasitic encephalitis due to *Baylisascaris* sp. in wild and captive woodchucks (Marmota monax). Vet Pathol 1982;19:658–662.

Rubin HL, Woodard JC. Equine infection with *Micronema deletrix*. J Am Vet Med Assoc 1974;165:256–258.

Schueler RL. Cerebral nematodiasis in a red squirrel. J Wldlf Dis 1973;9:58–60.

Smith HJ, Archibald RMcG. Moose infected with the common cervine parasite, *Elaphostrongylus tenuis*. Can Vet J 1967;8:173–177.

Spalding MG, Greiner EC, Green SL. *Halicephalobus* (*Micronema*) *deletrix* infection in two half-sibling foals. J Am Vet Med Assoc 1990;196:1127–1129.

Sprent JFA. On the invasion of the central nervous system by nematodes. I. The incidence and pathological significance of nematodes in the central nervous system. Parasitology 1955;45:31–40.

Sprent JFA. On the invasion of the central nervous system by nematodes. II. Invasion of the nervous system by ascariasis. Parasitology 1955;45:41–55.

Thomas JS. Encephalomyelitis in a dog caused by *Baylisascaris* infection. Vet Pathol 1988;25:94–95.

Tiner JD. The migration, distribution in the brain and growth of ascarid larvae in rodents. J Infect Dis 1953;92:105–113.

Trichinosis (trichiniasis, trichinelliasis)

Although they are seldom seriously affected by trichinosis, animals are the source of infection for humans, in whom the disease may be debilitating or fatal. The causative agent is a tiny, slender nematode that spends its adult life in the mucosa of the small intestine of a wide variety of animals, including humans, domestic and wild swine, rats, bears, dogs, and cats. The female is 3–4 mm in length, and the male about half as long. The females are viviparous. They larvae they produce are the principal excitants of symptoms and lesions because they burrow through tissues and encyst in striated muscles. The causative parasite, *Trichinella spiralis*, is classified among the Nematoda under the family Trichinellidae, and is the chief pathogen in this family. Based on cross-breeding experiments, it has recently been demonstrated that several other species of *Trichinella* exist; however, the parasites are morphologically identical.

LIFE CYCLE

Completion of the life cycle of *Trichinella spiralis* depends upon consumption by the host of raw or undercooked flesh containing encysted larvae. Pork products provide the principal source of infections for humans. The action of digestive juices releases the infective larvae from the ingested muscle; then, in rapid succession, they undergo four molts and mature into adults. After copulation the male dies, but the female burrows into the lamina propria of the intestinal villi and deposits large numbers of larvae in the lymphatic spaces. Some larvae may escape into the intestinal lumen, but most of them are carried to the blood stream and reach the musculature. The larvae invade the muscle bundles (Fig. 13-13), where they encyst and remain throughout the life of the host. Further development of the parasite follows upon ingestion of the infected muscle by another host. The fetuses of rats, mice, and rabbits may become infected in utero under experimental conditions (Hartmannova and Chroust, 1969).

CLINICAL MANIFESTATIONS

The symptoms and signs of trichinosis, rarely observed in animals, are varied and often nonspecific in humans. Even in humans, small numbers of trichina larvae undoubtedly can reach the muscle without provoking detectable symptoms, but in large numbers they produce muscular pain, nausea, vomiting, diarrhea, fever, edema of the face, increased respiratory rate, and urticarial skin manifestations. Invasion of cardiac muscle by the larvae may result in feeble or dicrotic pulse, muffled heart sounds, systolic murmur, or palpitation. When larvae invade the central nervous system, a plethora of signs may appear, including disorientation, apathy, stupor, delirium, paralysis, and coma. The most significant clinical laboratory evidence of the infection is in the blood cell count. Leukocytosis with eosinophilia, which in extreme cases may reach 90%, is characteristic. Although fluctuating within wide limits, the circulating eosinophilia may persist for months, or even years. Identification of adult trichinae in the stools, or demonstration of larvae in biopsy specimens of muscle, is decisive in confirming the clinical diagnosis of trichinosis.

LESIONS

Except for transitory catarrhal enteritis provoked by the activities of the adults, the lesions of trichinosis are confined to the skeletal and, to a much smaller extent, the cardiac musculature, and are the result of invasion and encystment of the larvae. In humans, the muscles most frequently and heavily parasitized are the diaphragmatic, intercostal, masseteric, laryngeal, lingual, and ocular. The heart muscle may be invaded by young larvae during the time that they are being liberated in the intestinal villi, but encysted larvae are rarely found in cardiac muscle. The larvae penetrate the skeletal muscle bundles, most frequently near the tendinous portion, eliciting some inflammatory reaction in the adjacent stroma. This inflammation, manifested by edema, neutrophils, lymphocytes, and eosinophils, soon subsides as each larva becomes encased in a muscle bundle. The sarcoplasm is replaced at the site of invasion by the encapsulated worm, and adjacent parts of the muscle bundle may undergo some degenerative changes. The parasite distorts the sarcolemma; the nuclei increase in size and number; and the sarcoplasm may become granular and lose its cross striations. Droplets of fatty material collect in the sarcolemma near the poles of the cyst containing the parasite. After some time, calcium salts may be deposited; first in the thick hyaline capsule around the parasite, now dead or dying; and later, in the parasite itself. Fully calcified lesions, appearing as short chalk-colored streaks in skeletal muscle, are sometimes visible to the naked eye.

DIAGNOSIS

Histologic demonstration of the trichina larvae in the muscles of animals is sufficient to establish the nature of the parasitism, but not enough to prove that the larvae were the cause of any clinical symptoms. This is a somewhat academic problem in animals, although it is more important in humans. Trichina larvae can be demonstrated by digestion of muscle and collection of the parasites in the Baermann apparatus.

A European meat inspection practice uses bits of fresh skeletal muscle (usually the diaphragm), which are compressed between two heavy glass plates and examined under low magnification; this practice was originally advocated by Virchow, and has been practiced since 1866. Larvae are readily recognized in these preparations, but in mild infections this method may not disclose any larvae. Routine histologic sections will also

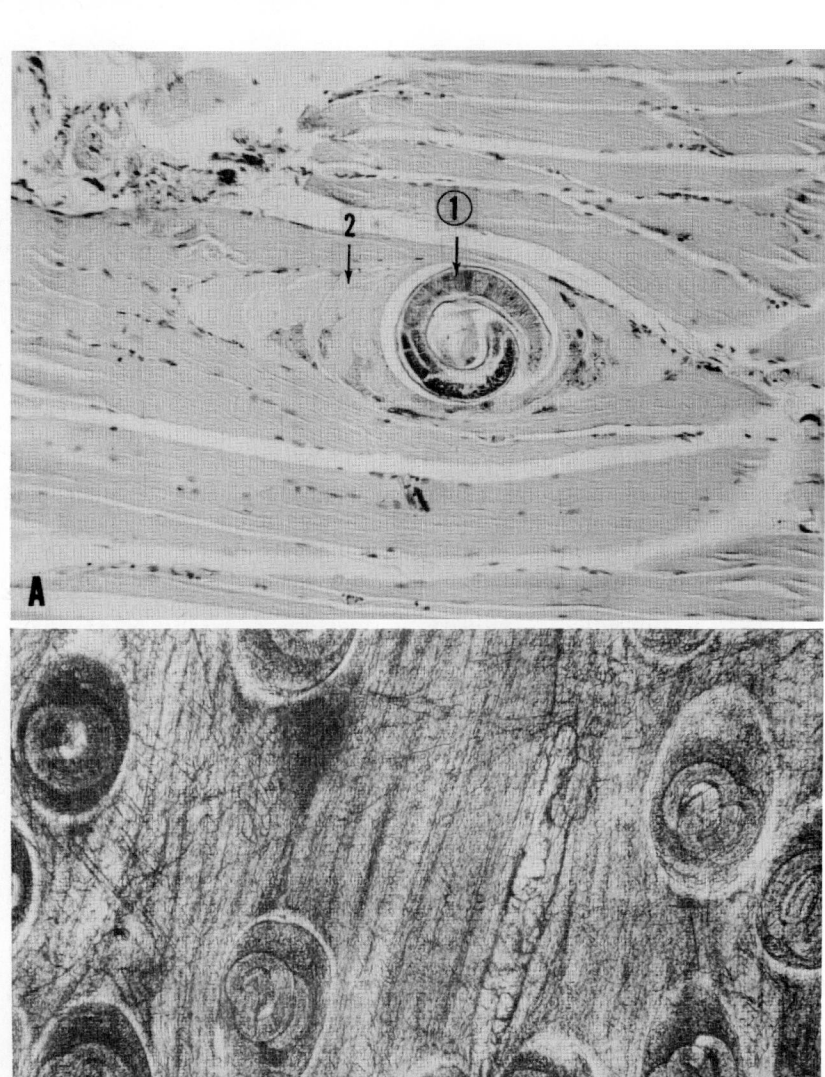

FIG. 13-13 Trichinosis. **A.** *Trichinella spiralis* larva. (1) Encysted in a skeletal muscle bundle of a rat; (2) Note capsule around nematode (×80). (Courtesy of Armed Forces Institute of Pathology; contributor: Dr. J. C. Swartz.) **B.** Crush preparation of skeletal muscle containing *Trichinella spiralis* larvae.

reveal the encysted larvae coiled within a hyaline membrane inside a muscle bundle (Fig. 13-13).

References

Cypess RH, Lubiniecki A, DeSeau V, et al. Observations on trichinosis in the Rhesus monkey. J Med Primatol 1977;6:23–32.

Geller EH, Zaiman H. Incidence of infection with *Trichinella spiralis* in dogs. J Am Vet Med Assoc 1965;147:253–254.

Hanbury RD, Doby PB, Miller HO, et al. Trichinosis in a herd of swine: cannibalism as a major mode of transmission. J Am Vet Med Assoc 1986;188:1155–1159.

Holzworth J, Georgi JR. Trichinosis in a cat. J Am Vet Med Assoc 1974;165:186–191.

Horning B. Short report concerning *Trichinella* in Switzerland (1975–1976). Wiadom Parazytol 1978;24:123–124.

Hugh-Jones ME, et al. Prevalence of trichinosis in southern Louisiana swine. Am J Vet Res 1985;46:463–465.

Hunt GR. *Trichinella spiralis* in dogs and cats. Parasitology 1967;53:659.

Lin T-M, Olson LJ. Pathophysiology of reinfection with *Trichinella spiralis* in guinea pigs during the intestinal phase. J Parasitol 1970;56:529–539.

McCracken RO, Taylor DD. Mebendazole therapy of parenteral trichinosis. Science 1980;207:1220–1222.

Pullen MM, Seymour MR, Zimmermann WJ. Trichinosis in sows slaughtered at a Kentucky abattoir. J Am Vet Med Assoc 1977;171:1171–1172.

Rice L, Frongillo MK, Randolph JF. Trichinosis in a dog. J Am Vet Med Assoc 1990;197:480–482.

Schad GA, Leiby DA, Duffy CH, et al. Swine trichinosis in New England slaughterhouses. Am J Vet Res 1985;46:2008–2010.

Shaikenov B, Tazieva ZCh, Horning B. The etiology of sylvatic trichinellosis in Switzerland. Acta Tropica 1977;34:327–330.

Steele JH, Arambulo PV III. Trichinosis. A world problem with extensive sylvatic reservoirs. Int J Zoon 1975;2:55–75.

Strafuss AC, Zimmermann WJ. Hematologic changes and clinical signs of trichinosis in pigs. Am J Vet Res 1967;28:833–838.

Worley DE, Seesee FM, Espinosa RH, et al. Survival of sylvatic *Trichinella spiralis* isolates in frozen tissue and processed meat products. J Am Vet Med Assoc 1986;189:1047–1049.

Pulmonary nematodiasis (lungworm disease, dictyocauliasis, dictyocaulosis, metastrongylidosis, verminous pneumonia)

The adults of a number of different genera of nematodes, each containing several species, reside in the lung, producing pulmonary nematodiasis or lungworm disease (Fig. 13-14). Larval migration of other nematodes may also cause lung damage, but these are not considered here. Other parasites of the lungs include: flukes (*Paragonimus, Schistosoma, Troglotrema,* and *Fasciola*) sp.; intermediate stages of cestodes (hydatid cysts); and arthropods *Pneumonyssus* sp., *Linguatula serrata*). Those that inhabit the upper respiratory passages include: *Linguatula serrata* (nasal passages of dogs); species of *Mammomonogamus,* related to the gapeworm *Syngamus,* (nasal passages of cats and cattle in Asia and the West Indies); and the flukes *Schistosoma nasalis* and *Troglotrema acutum.* The lungworms, listed in Table 13-7, often produce disease that leads to death, but they may live in the lungs with little apparent effect on the host. Serious disease is most likely to be encountered in young animals.

Dictyocaulus

Dictyocaulus species, which are among the most important nematodes that parasitize the lung, include: *D. viviparus* of cattle, deer, buffalo, and camels; *D. filaria* of sheep and goats; and *D. arnfieldi* of horses and donkeys. These have a direct life cycle. Adults reside in the bronchi, where eggs are deposited, some of which may

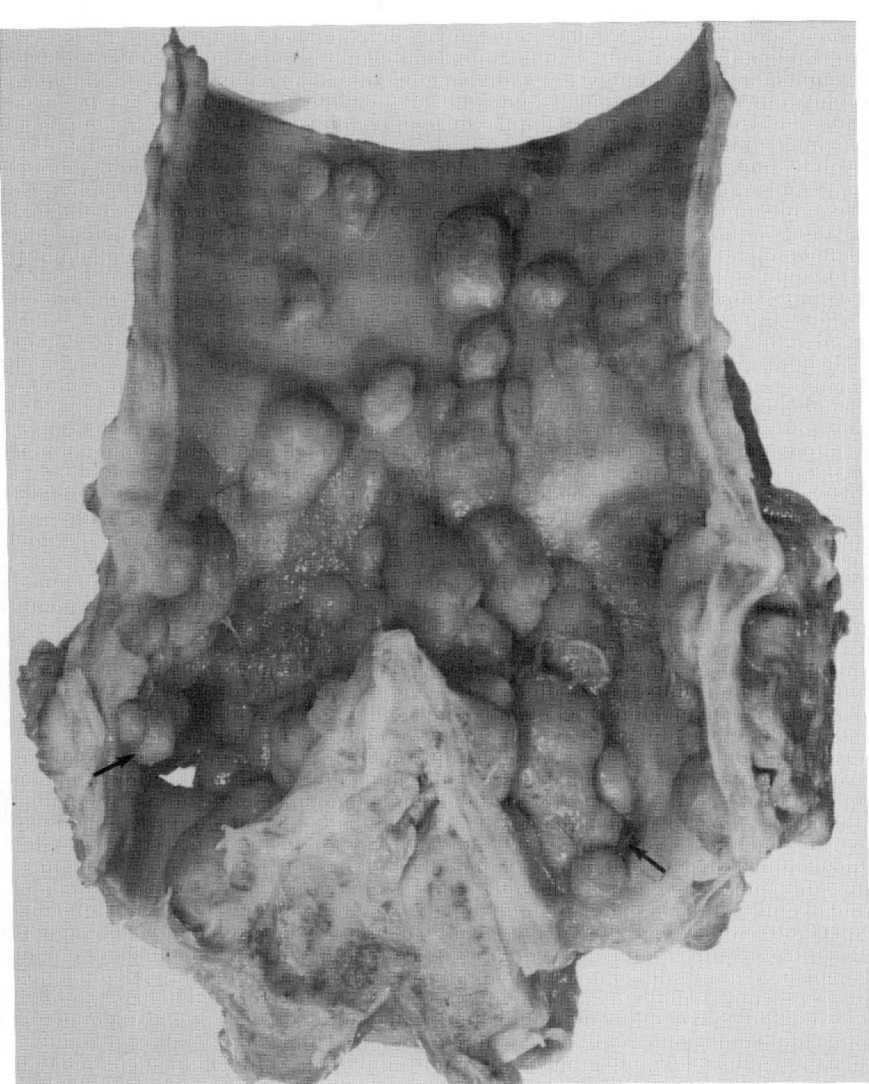

FIG. 13-14 Pulmonary nematodiasis. Nodules containing adult *Filaroides osleri* in the tracheal mucosa near the bifurcation. Note that the nodules produce partial stenosis of the lumen of the bronchi (arrows). (Courtesy of Armed Forces Institute of Pathology; contributor: Dr. F. D. Gentry.)

TABLE 13-7 **Common lungworms**

Parasite	Principal hosts	Site of adult parasite
Dictyocaulus filaria	Sheep, goats	Bronchi, bronchioles
D. viviparus	Cattle	Bronchi, bronchioles
D. arnfieldi	Horses, donkeys	Bronchi, bronchioles
Metastrongylus salmi, M. apri (elongatus), M. pudentectus	Swine	Bronchi, bronchioles
Protostrongylus rufescens, P. skjabini	Sheep, goats	Bronchioles
P. rushi, P. stilesi	Sheep, goats, bighorn sheep	Bronchioles
P. boughtoni	Rabbits (wild)	Bronchi, bronchioles
Muellerius capillaris	Sheep, goats	Alveoli
Cystocaulus ocreatus (nigrescens)	Sheep, goats	Alveoli
Crenosoma vulpis	Fox, dog, raccoon	Trachea, bronchi, bronchioles
C. striatus	Hedgehogs	Trachea, bronchi, bronchioles
Capillaria aerophila	Foxes, dogs, cats	Trachea, bronchi
C. goblei	Raccoons	Trachea, bronchi, bronchioles
C. didelphis	Opossum	Bronchi
Aelurostrongylus abstrusus	Cats	Bronchioles, alveolar ducts
A. pridhami	Mink	Bronchioles
Troglostrongylus subcrenatus	Cats	Alveolar ducts
Filaroides osleri	Dogs	Trachea, bronchi
F. milksi, F. hirthi	Dogs	Bronchi, bronchioles, alveoli
F. rostratus	Cats	Bronchi
F. martis	Mink	Adventitia of pulmonary arteries
F. cebus	New World monkey	Bronchioles, alveoli
Angiostrongylus vasorum	Dogs, foxes	Pulmonary arteries
A. cantonensis	Rats	Pulmonary arteries and capillaries
Perostrongylus pridhami	Mink	Bronchioles, alveolar ducts
P. falciformis	Badgers	Bronchioles, alveolar ducts

hatch in the airways. Eggs and/or larvae are coughed up, swallowed, and passed in the feces; they then develop to infective third-stage larvae in moist, cool soil. Ingested larvae penetrate the intestinal mucosa and migrate via lymphatics to mesenteric lymph nodes, where they develop to fourth-stage larvae. These reach the lungs by way of lymphatics and pulmonary arteries. They enter the pulmonary alveoli and, ultimately, bronchioles and bronchi, where they reach sexual maturity.

CLINICAL MANIFESTATIONS

Clinical signs of infection with *Dictyocaulus sp.* in sheep, goats, and cattle may be barely recognizable, or so severe that death results. Severe infection is limited almost exclusively to young animals. The presence of a few lungworms usually causes only a hacking cough. Heavy infestation, however, may result in labored respiration, anorexia, diarrhea, and stunted growth. Occasionally, death may follow pulmonary consolidation caused by secondary bacterial infection of occluded bronchioles and alveoli. Infection with *D. arnfieldi* is usually mild.

LESIONS

As the larvae break through the capillary and alveolar walls, they cause hemorrhage and necrosis. They also incite an inflammatory cellular infiltrate chiefly composed of eosinophils, which fill the alveoli, alveolar septae, and terminal bronchioles. Occasional larvae (and later, adults and eggs) die and may be surrounded by a granulomatous reaction, with multinucleated giant cells. When the number of larvae is large, this initial phase of the infection can lead to grossly visible foci of consolidation randomly distributed throughout the lungs. Heavy infestation is also often associated with extensive pulmonary edema and interstitial emphysema, which is believed to result from a hyperimmune response. With maturation to adults in bronchioles and bronchi, the alveolar lesions begin to resolve and are overshadowed by lesions in the bronchi. While the larvae induce lesions throughout the lungs, lesions associated with the adults tend to concentrate in the dorsocaudal lung. The bronchial epithelium becomes hyperplastic, and eosinophils and lymphocytes infiltrate the wall and peribronchial tissues. Eosinophils and mucous plug the bronchial lumens, which, when occluded,

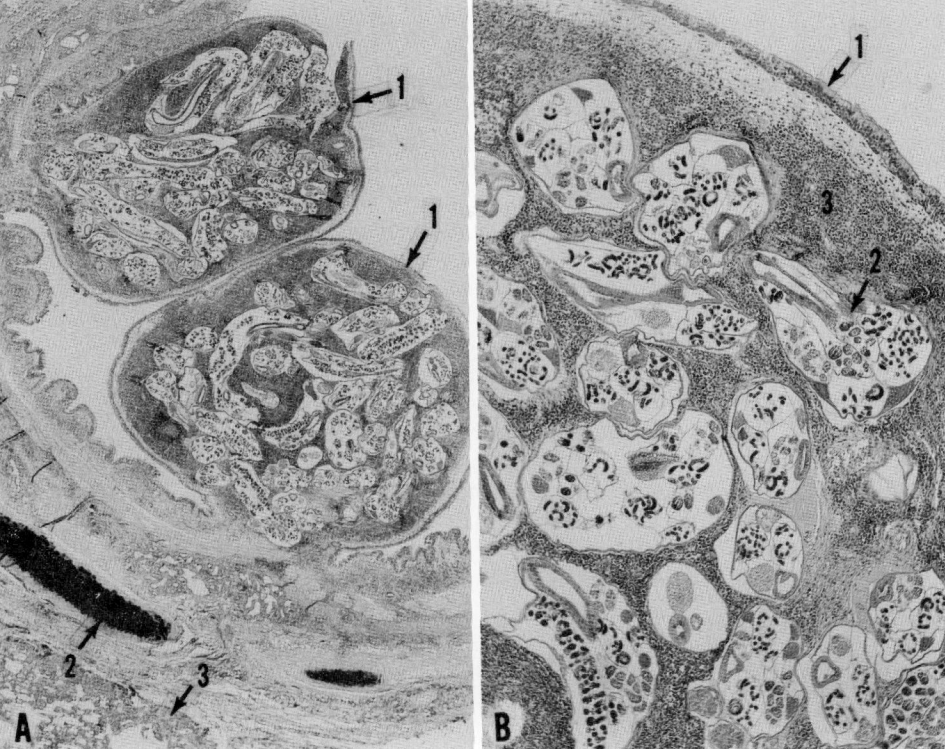

FIG. 13-15 Pulmonary nematodiasis. **A.** Two nodules filled with adult *Filaroides osleri* in the bronchial mucosa of a dog (×13). (1) The epithelium is elevated; (2) Bronchial cartilage; and (3) Lung parenchyma. **B.** Enlarged view (×50) of one of the nodules in A. (1) Bronchial epithelium; (2) Adult worms containing larvae; (3) Lymphocytic inflammatory reaction. (Courtesy of Armed Forces Institute of Pathology; contributor: Dr. F. D. Gentry.)

lead to atelectasis or consolidation of the related alveoli. The adults, feeding head down on mucus and cellular detritus, deposit ova; these are coughed up as embryonating eggs or hatched larvae, or they may lodge in alveoli, initiating a foreign body reaction.

Metastrongylus

Three species of *Metastrongylus* parasitize the bronchi and bronchioles of swine: *Metastrongylus apri (M. elongatus), M. pudendotectus,* and *M. salmi.* The life cycle is in-

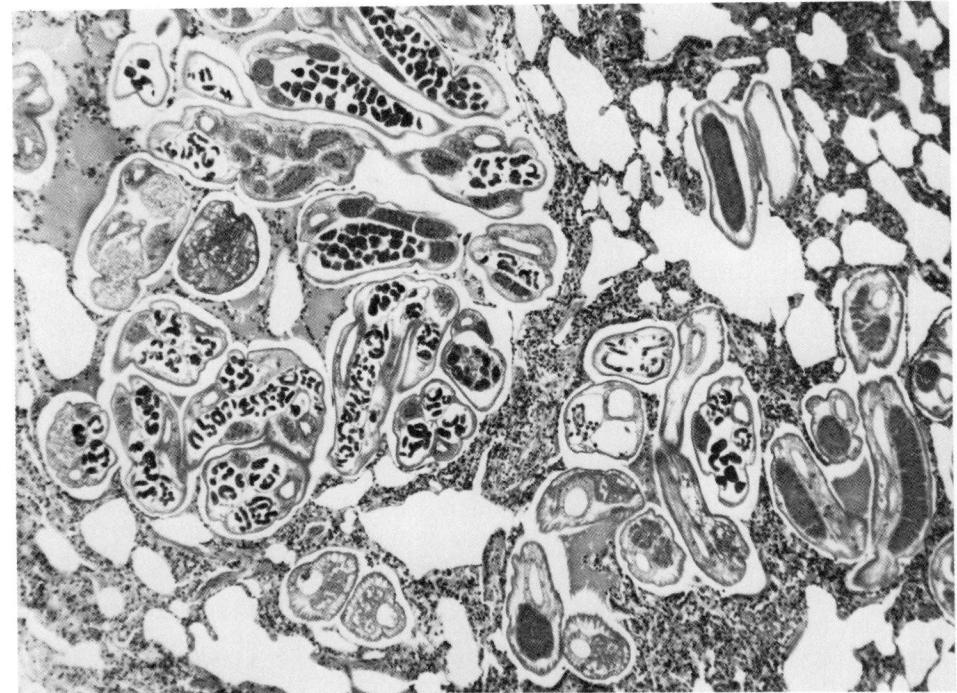

FIG. 13-16 Pulmonary nematodiasis. *Filaroides cebus* within pulmonary alveoli of a squirrel monkey.

direct. Eggs laid in the bronchial tree are coughed up, swallowed, and passed in the feces; there, they (or larvae that hatch in the soil) must be ingested by an appropriate species of earthworm, in which further development occurs. Earthworms may harbor a large number of larvae for extended intervals without any ill effects, allowing the parasite to overwinter. Swine are infected when they ingest infected earthworms, or larvae that earthworms released when they died of other causes. Larvae subsequently penetrate the intestinal mucosa and migrate to mesenteric lymph nodes, where they undergo a molt. They then proceed to the lungs. The lesions are comparable to those induced by *Dictyocaulus* sp. in ruminants, but not nearly as severe (Fig. 13-19). Ordinarily, lesions are not grossly visible and clinical signs are more related to poor performance rather than respiratory signs. In addition to alveolitis and bronchitis, the lungs of affected swine often contain grossly visible granulomas incited by dead parasites and their eggs.

Protostrongylus

Protostrongylus rufescens is a nematode that parasitizes small bronchioles of sheep, goats, and deer. It has an indirect life cycle, with eggs hatching in the lungs and then passed as larvae in the feces. Further development requires that they be ingested by a snail. After ingestion of the snail by the animal, larvae penetrate the intestinal mucosa, pass to mesenteric lymph nodes, molt, and then move on to the lungs. The infection is not severe, but the parasites incite an inflammatory response in the wall of the affected bronchiole, and cause consolidation of the related alveoli. Several other species of *Protostrongylus* (*P. stilesi, P. rushi, P. hobmaieri, P. brevispiculum*) also affect sheep, goats, and bighorn sheep.

Muellerius

Muellerius capillaris is a common lungworm of sheep and goats, but infestation rarely leads to clinical disease. The life cycle is indirect and similar to *Protostrongylus*, with first-stage larvae passed in the feces and a snail or slug required for further development. After ingestion of the snail by sheep or goats, the fourth-stage larvae reach the lung, presumably through the lymphatics. The larvae enter alveoli, mature to adults, and deposit eggs; the eggs then hatch to first-stage larvae, and eventually pass up the bronchial tree. The adults, eggs, and newly hatched larvae all inhabit alveoli, where they incite an inflammatory reaction leading to grossly visible nodules. For reasons unknown, most of the parasites are located immediately beneath the pleura. The inflammatory response varies with the age of the lesion and previous exposure. Early lesions are characterized by an infiltration of lymphocytes in the alveolar septae and some alveolar hemorrhage. Later, and in previously exposed animals, the infiltrate contains numerous eosinophils, macrophages (and often multinucleated giant cells); these distend the septae and fill the alveoli surrounding the parasites. Alveolar walls also become fibrotic. The lesions may progress to an inflammatory

nodule or granuloma with a core of parasites; necrotic material (often calcified) is surrounded by macrophages and giant cells, which in turn are surrounded by fibrous connective tissue. Bronchioles contain mucus and inflammatory cells, and their lining may be hyperplastic; however, bronchiolitis is not a usual feature.

Another parasite, *Cystocaulus ocreatus (nigrescens)*, also affects the lungs of sheep and goats, residing in alveoli and resulting in subpleural nodules. Its life cycle also requires a snail. This parasite occurs in Europe, the Middle East, and Russia.

Filaroides

Several species of the genus *Filaroides parasitize* the respiratory tract of dogs and cats. *Filaroides osleri* (Fig. 13-15A) affects the trachea and bronchi of dogs; it resides in the mucosa, where it produces nodules about one centimeter in diameter. The life cycle is direct. Mature worms deposit eggs containing larvae, which leave the nodules through small pores. These pass through the feces, with pups usually acquiring the infection from their dam. The nodules are predominantly composed of parasites, which are themselves surrounded by a connective tissue capsule containing a few inflammatory cells. Dead worms incite a stronger reaction. The presence of nodules may cause a chronic cough, but generally does not affect the overall health of the dog. Although *F. osleri* occurs throughout the world, it is not common. *F. milksi* and *F. hirthi*, which also have direct life cycles, inhabit alveoli and small bronchioles of dogs. Reaction may be minimal, or granulomatous, with the presence of eosinophils that cause small nodules somewhat similar to those induced by *Muellerius*. Hyperinfection with *F. hirthi* can occur in immunosuppressed dogs; larvae reenter the host through the intestinal tract, and return to the lung or a variety of other organ. *F. martis*, which has an indirect life cycle, is a common parasite of mink in North America. *F. (Anafilaroides) rostratus*, a parasite of cats that resides in the mucosa of bronchi, has only been reported from Sri Lanka.

Crenosoma

Crenosoma species are common parasites of the trachea, bronchi, and bronchioles of wild carnivores and insectivores. The best studied is *Crenosoma vulpis*, a parasite of foxes and occasionally dogs. Its life cycle requires a snail which, after ingested, releases larvae that make their way to the lung via lymphatics. The parasites induce bronchitis, bronchiolitis, and tracheitis, principally characterized by an infiltration of eosinophils. Focal areas of alveolar consolidation may also develop. Other species of *Crenosoma* include *C. goblei* of raccoons, *C. mephiditis* of skunks, and *C. striatum* of hedgehogs.

Capillaria

Capillaria species affect a wide variety of animals and reside in many different tissues, including the small intestine, urinary bladder, skin, and liver. *Capillaria aero-*

phila localizes in the trachea and bronchi of dogs, foxes, various wild mammals, and occasionally cats. Its life cycle is direct, with infective larvae developing in operculated eggs. Larvae released in the intestine make their way to the respiratory tract, where the adults develop and cause mild tracheitis and bronchitis.

Aelurostrongylus

Aelurostrongylus abstrussus, which has an indirect life cycle, is a common lungworm of cats (Fig. 13-17); the adult parasites (Fig. 13-18) live in terminal bronchioles and alveolar ducts. Larvae that are passed in the feces must be ingested by various snails or slugs for further development. These in turn may be ingested by trans-

port hosts, which include rodents, frogs, lizards, and birds, in which the larvae remain infective. Cats become infected by eating the intermediate or transport hosts. Larvae released in the gastrointestinal tract move to the lung via the blood stream to ultimately lie in the bronchial tree. Eggs, which hatch to larvae, form small, nodular collections within alveoli. These tend to be located at the periphery of the lung and can be seen grossly as 1–10 mm pale projections. Microscopically (Fig. 13-19), the lesions consist of: alveoli packed with eggs and larvae; disrupted alveolar septae; and an infiltration of eosinophils, lymphocytes, macrophages, and often multinucleated giant cells. The adult worms initiate a mild peribronchiolar inflammation containing eosinophils and mononuclear cells. *Aelurostrongylus* is believed to be

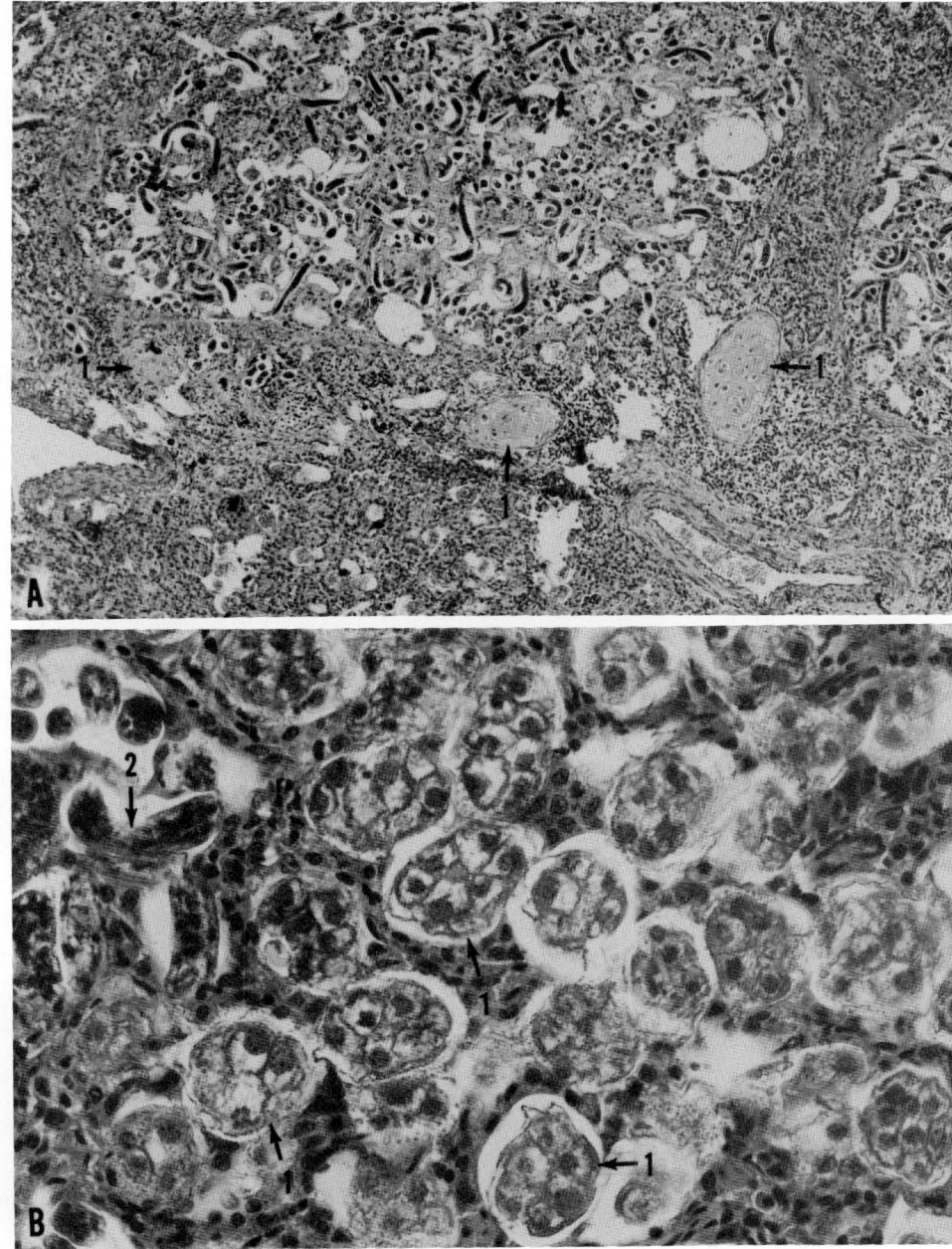

FIG. 13-17 Pulmonary nematodiasis. *Aelurostrongylus abstrusus* in the lung of a cat. **A.** Larvae filling a small bronchus outlined by its cartilage. (1) (×83). **B.** Another area in the same lung with embryonating ova. (1) In alveoli; and (2) Larvae in alveolar duct (×385). (Courtesy of Armed Forces Institute of Pathology; contributor: Dr. W. S. Bailey.)

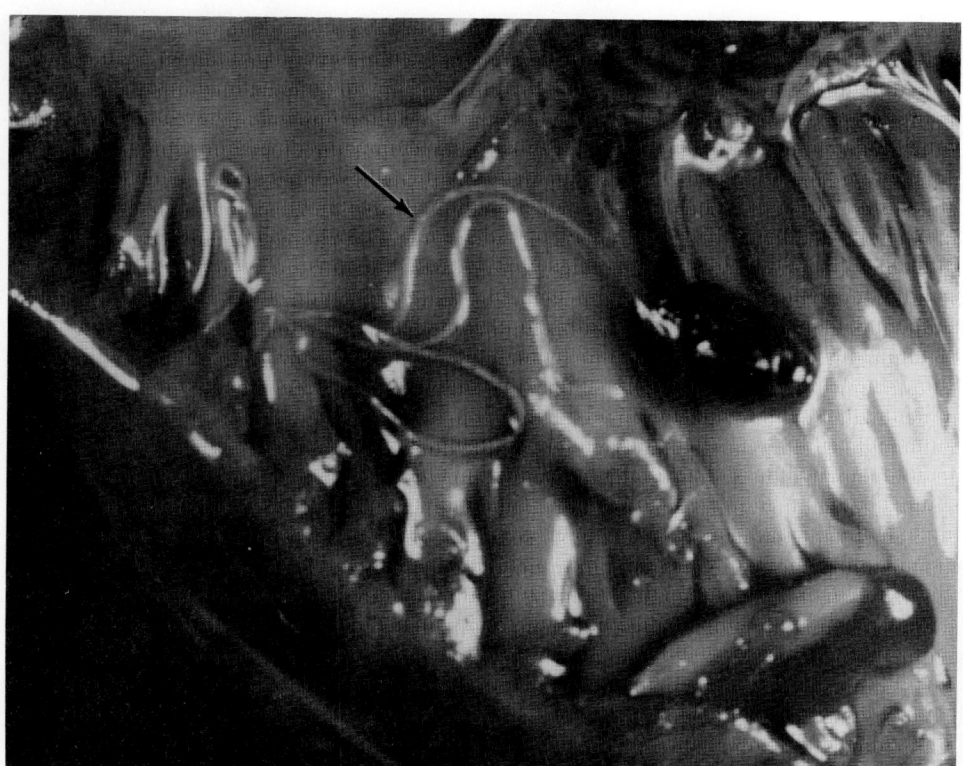

FIG. 13-18 *Aelurostrongylus abstrusus* (adults) in right ventricle of a four-year-old male tabby and white cat. (Courtesy of Angell Memorial Animal Hospital.)

the chief cause of medial hyperplasia and hypertrophy of the smooth muscle of pulmonary arteries, which is so frequently encountered in cats. Troglostrongylus subcrenatus, a worm resembling *A. abstrussus,* also affects the cat lung, causing similar nodules.

Angiostrongulus

Several species of *Angiostrongylus* parasitize the lung and pulmonary arteries. The adults of *Angiostrongylus vasorum,* which reside in the pulmonary arteries and right ventricle of dogs and foxes, incite a proliferative endarteritis comparable to that induced by *Dirofilaria immitis.* Eggs pass as far as the pulmonary capillaries, where they lodge and hatch. Released larvae penetrate into the alveolar spaces, are coughed up, swallowed, and passed in the feces; they may then be ingested by snails and slugs, which serve as intermediate hosts. In the lungs, the eggs and larvae damage capillaries and small arterioles, leading to thrombosis and occlusion, accompanied by a granulomatous reaction surrounding the parasites. Several infections may lead to pulmonary hypertension, as well as right heart hypertrophy and failure. A. cantonensis, a common parasite of the lungs of rats in Australia and the Pacific islands, has also been identified in rats in the southern United States. It spends part of its life cycle in brain before eggs lodge in pulmonary capillaries. It is most important as a cause of cerebrospinal nematodiasis (discussed previously). A. pridhami parasitizes the lungs of mink. A. costaricensis is not a lung worm, but a parasite of intestinal subserosal arteries

and the anterior mesenteric artery of cotton rats in South and Central America. It may affect humans, leading to **abdominal angiostrongylosis,** which is characterized by eosinophilic granulomas in the wall of the intestine. Examples of this condition, acquired by children in the United States, have recently been reported.

DIAGNOSIS

The diagnosis of lungworm disease can be suspected from the signs and confirmed by identifying lungworm eggs or larvae in the feces of the living animal. Demonstration of adult lungworms in the bronchi or bronchioles and ova and larvae in the lung parenchyma at necropsy is often necessary to establish the nature of a herd infection. Careful examination with the naked eye and use of the hand lens are advisable, especially when searching for the smaller lungworms, and histopathologic examination is recommended.

References

Alicata JE. Present status of *Angiostrongylus cantonensis* infection in man and animals in the tropics. J Trop Med Hyg 1969;72:53–63,.

August JR, Powers RD, Bailey WS, et al. *Filaroides hirthi* in a dog: fatal hyperinfection suggestive of autoinfection. J Am Vet Med Assoc 1980;176:331–334.

Beresford-Jones WP. Observations on *Muellerius capillaris* (Muller, 1889) (Cameron, 1927). II. Experimental infection of mice, guinea-pigs, and rabbits with third-stage larvae. Res Vet Sci 1966;7:287–291.

Burrows CF, O'Brien JA, Biery DN. Pneumothorax due to *Filaroides osleri* infestation in the dog. J. Small Anim Pract 1972;13:613–618.

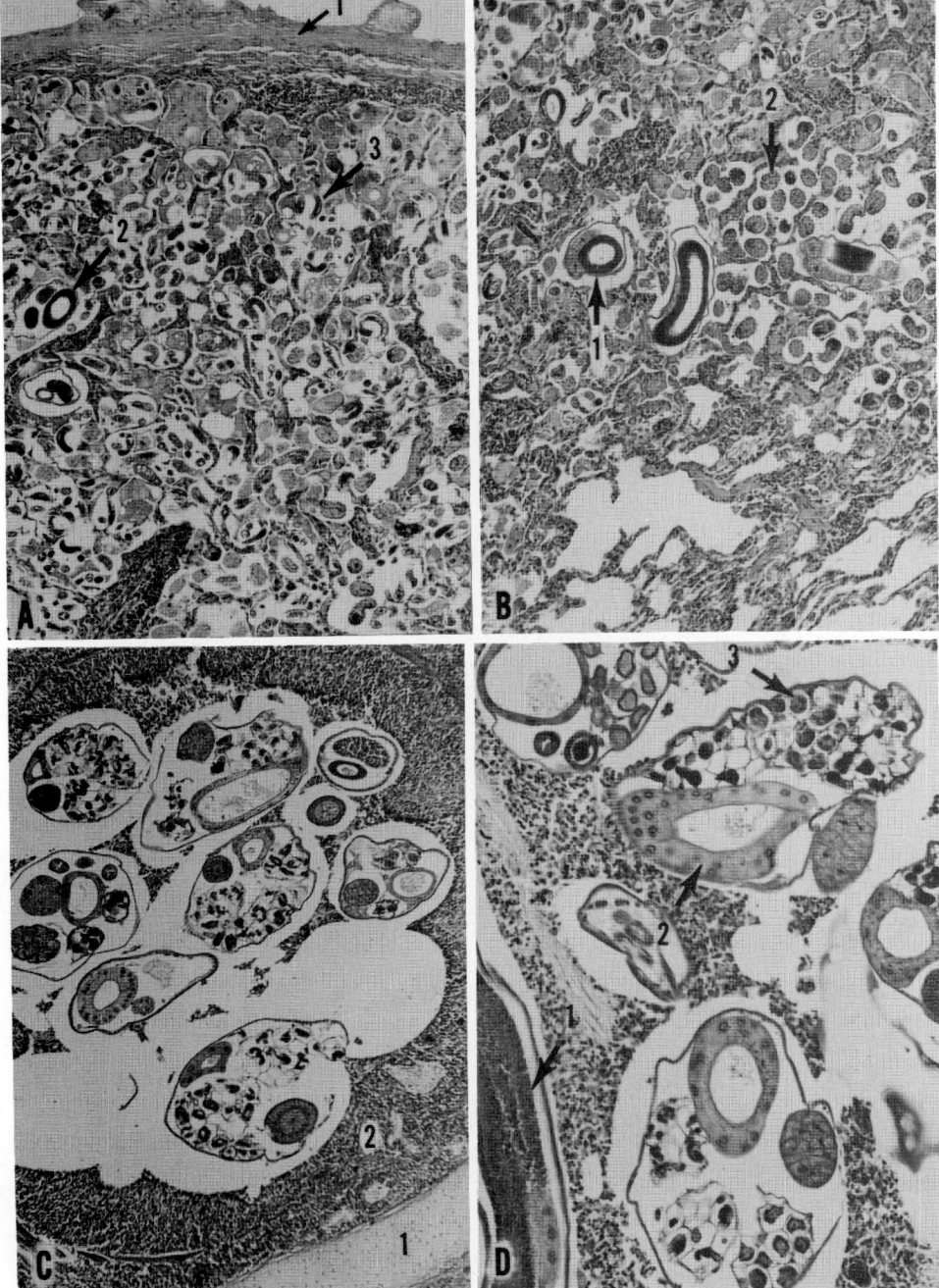

FIG. 13-19 Pulmonary nematodiasis. **A**. *Muellerius minutissimus* in the lung (×45) of a bighorn sheep *(Ovis canadensis)*. (1) Note the pleura; (2) Young adult worms; and (3) Larvae. **B**. Higher magnification of A (×70). (1) Young adult larvae and (2) Embryonating ova. Most alveoli are consolidated. (Contributor: Dr. C. L. Davis.) **C**. *Metastrongylus apri* in a bronchus of a pig (×62). (1) Bronchial cartilage; and (2) Inflammatory exudate in the mucosa. **D**. Slightly higher magnification (×75) of C. (1) Adult worms in longitudinal and cross section; (2) The intestinal tube; and (3) Ovary. (Contributor: Dr. R. J. Byrne.) (A, D, Courtesy of Armed Forces Institute of Pathology.

Cameron TWM. Observations on the life history of *Aelurostrongylus abstrusus* (Railliet) the lungworm of the cat. J Helminthol 1927;15:55–66.

Cuadrado R, Maldonado-Moll JF, Segarra J. Gapeworm infection of domestic cats in Puerto Rico. J Am Vet Med Assoc 1980;176:996–997.

Dodd K. *Angiostrongylus vasorum* (Baillet, 1866) infestation in a Greyhound kennel. Vet Rec 1973;92:195–197.

Dorrington JE. Preliminary report on the transmission of *Filaroides osleri* (Cobbold, 1879) in dogs. J S Afr Vet Med. Assoc 1965;36:389, Vet Bull 1966;36:3563.

Dorrington JE. *Filaroides osleri* (Cobbold, 1879): infestation in the dog. J S Afr Vet Med Assoc 1967;38:91, Vet Bull 1968;38:1942.

Dorrington JE. Studies on *Filaroides osleri* infestation in dogs. Onderstepoort J Vet Res 1968;35:225–285, Vet Bull 1969;39:1684.

Dubey JP, Beverley JKA, Crane WAJ. Lung changes and *Aelurostrongylus abstrusus* infestation in English cats. Vet Rec 1968;83:191–194.

Forrester DJ, Porter JH, Belden RC, et al. Lungworms of feral swine in Florida. J Am Vet Med Assoc 1982;181:1278–1280.

Genta RM, Schad GA. *Filaroides hirthi:* hyperinfective lungworm infection in immunosuppressed dogs. Vet Pathol 1984;21:349–354.

Georgi JR, Georgi ME, Fahnestock GR, et al. Transmission and control of *Filaroides hirthi* lungworm infection in dogs. Am I Vet Res 1979;40:829–831.

Hamilton JM. Parenteral infection of the cat by larvae of *Aelurostrongylus abstrusus*. J Helminthol 1969;43:31–34.

Hamilton JM. Experimental lungworm disease of the cat: association of the condition with lesions of the pulmonary arteries. J Comp Pathol 1966;76:147–157.

Heyneman D, Lim B-L. *Angiostrongylus cantonensis:* proof of direct transmission with its epidemiological implications. Science 1967; 158:1057–1058.

Hirth RS, Hottendorf GH. Lesions produced by a new lungworm in Beagle dogs. Vet Pathol 1973;10:385–407.

Hobmaier M. Newer aspects of the lungworm (Crenosoma) in foxes. Am J Vet Res 1941;2:352–354.

Jindrak K. The pathology of radicular involvement in angiostrongylosis as observed in experimentally infected calves and pigs. Virchows Arch Path Anat 1968;345:228–237.

Jindrak K, Alicata JE. Comparative pathology in experimental infection of pigs and calves with larvae of Angiostrongylus cantonensis. J Comp Pathol 1968;78:371–382.

Jindrak K, Alicata JE. Experimentally induced Angiostrongylus cantonensis infection in dogs. Am J Vet Res 1970;31:449–456.

Jonas AM, Swerczek TW, Downing SE. Vaso-occlusive pulmonary hypertension a feline model system. Lab Invest 1970;22:502.

Jubb KV. The lesions caused by Filaroides milksi in a dog. Cornell Vet 1960;50:319–325.

Lyons ET, Tolliver SC, Drudge JH, et al. Lungworms (Dictyocaulus arnfieldi): prevalence in live equids in Kentucky. Am J Vet Res 1985;46:921–923.

Mahaffey MB, Losonsky JM, Prestwood AK, et al. Experimental canine angiostrongylosis: II. Radiographic manifestations. J Am Anim Hosp Assoc 1981;17:499–502,.

Michel JF, MacKenzie A. Duration of the acquired resistance of calves to infection with Dictyocaulus viviparus. Res Vet Sci 1965;6:344–395.

Mills JHL, Nielsen SW. Canine Filaroides osleri and Filaroides milksi infection. J Am Vet Med Assoc 1966;149:56–63.

Pinckney RD, Studer AD, Genta RM. Filaroides hirthi infection in two related dogs. J Am Vet Med Assoc 1988;193:1287–1288.

Poynter D, Selway S. Diseases caused by lungworms. Vet Bull 1966;36:539–554.

Prestwood AK, Greene CE, Mahaffey EA, et al. Experimental canine angiostrongylosis: I. Pathologic manifestations. J Am Anim Hosp Assoc 1981;17:491–497.

Rose JH. Lungworms of the domestic pig and sheep. Adv Parasitol 1973;11:559–599.

Rosen L, Ash LR, Wallace GD. Life history of the canine lungworm Angiostrongylus vasorum (Baillet). Am J Vet Res 1970;31:131–143.

Schelling CG, Greene CE, Prestwood AK, et al. Coagulation abnormalities associated with acute Angiostrongylus vasorum infection in dogs. Am J Vet Res 1986;47:2669–2673.

Simpson CF, et al. Pathological changes associated with Dictyocaulus viviparus (Block) infection in calves. Am J Res 1957;18:747–755.

Stockdale PHG. Pulmonary lesions in mink with a mixed infection of Filaroides martis and Perostrongylus pridhami. Can J Zool 1970;48:757–759.

Stockdale PHG. The pathogenesis of the lesions elicited by Aelurostrongylus abstrusus during its prepatent period. Pathol Vet 1970;7:102–115.

Stockdale PHG, Hulland TJ. The pathogenesis, route of migration, and development of Crenosoma vulpis in the dog. Pathol Vet 1970;7:28–42.

Subramaniam T, D'Souza BA, Victor DA. Broncho-pneumonia in baby pigs due to Metastrongylus apri. Indian Vet J 1967;44:121–127.

Taffs LF. Lungworm infection in swine. Vet Rec 1967;80:554.

Willard MD, Roberts RE, Allison N, et al. Diagnosis of Aelurostrongylus abstrusus and Dirofilaria immitis infections in cats from a humane shelter. J Am Vet Med Assoc 1988;192:913–916.

Williams JF, Lindemann B, Padgett GA, et al. Angiostrongylosis in a Greyhound. J Am Vet Med Assoc 1985;186:1101–1103,.

Wilson GI. Investigations on the pathogenicity and immunology of Dictyocaulus filaria in sheep and goats. Diss Abstr 1966;26:5612–5613, Vet Bull 1967;37:619.

Renal dioctophymosis

The giant kidney worm *Dioctophyma* renale is an uncommon parasite of a wide variety of species that includes dogs, cats, mink, foxes, horses, cattle, pigs, and humans, to name a few. In domestic animals it is most common in dogs, which are considered an abnormal host. Mink, the most commonly affected animals, are believed to be the normal definitive host. The adult worms are the largest of the nematodes and reside in the pelvic kidney, although they may also be encountered in the peritoneal cavity. Eggs laid by adult worms pass in the urine and undergo a prolonged development of one to several months in water; they are then ingested by the intermediate host, a free-living annelid, *Lumbriculus variegatus*. Here they hatch, undergo further development, and encyst. Frogs and fish may serve as paratenic hosts. Dogs, mink, and other susceptible species become infected by ingesting the intermediate, or paratenic, hosts. Larvae released in the intestinal tract penetrate the wall, enter the peritoneal cavity, and subsequently penetrate the kidney to reside in the pelvis. This entire process requires a minimum of about three months, but may take several years.

In dogs, the right kidney is more frequently affected than the left, but because dogs are not a usual host the parasite is more often found restricted to the peritoneal cavity, where it obviously cannot complete its life cycle. The presence of the worms in the renal pelvis leads to slow destruction of the renal parenchyma, ultimately leading to a fluid-filled sac. In the peritoneal cavity, the worms and their eggs incite a chronic peritonitis with adhesions. They often are in close proximity to the liver where they may cause strangulation of a lobe.

CLINICAL MANIFESTATIONS

Clinical signs may be absent. Compensatory hypertrophy of the unaffected kidney precludes renal failure; however, bilateral involvement leads to death from uremia.

Diagnosis

Diagnosis can be made by finding eggs in the urine.

References

Cooperrider DE, Robinson VB, Staton LB. Dioctophyma renale in a dog. J Am Vet Med Assoc 1954;124:381–383.

Eubanks JW, Pick JR. Dioctophyma renale infection in a dog. J Am Vet Med Assoc 1963;143:164–169.

Hallberg CW. Dioctophyma renale (Goetze, 1782): a study of the migration routes to the kidneys of mammals and resultant pathology. Am Microscop Soc 1953;72:351–363.

Karmanova EM: The life cycle of the nematode Dioctophyma renale (Goeze, 1782). Dokl Akad Nauk SSSR 1960;127:700–702.

McLeod JA. Dioctophyma renale infections in Manitoba. Can J Zool 1967;45:505–508.

McNeil CW. Pathologic changes in the kidney of mink due to infection with Dioctophyma renale (Goetze, 1782), the giant kidney worm of mammals. Am Microscop Soc 1948;67:257–261.

Osborne CA, et al. Dioctophyma renale in the dog. J Am Vet Med Assoc 1969;155:605–620.

Woodhead AE. Life history cycle of the giant kidney worm, Dioctophyma renale (Nematoda), of man and many other mammals. Am Microscop Soc 1950;69:21–46.

Habronemiasis

The stomach worms of horses are of three species: *Habronema muscae*, *H. majus* (*H. microstoma*), and *Draschia megastoma* (*Habronema megastoma*). The adults of *H. muscae* and *H. majus* reside on the surface of the gastric mucosa, whereas *D. megastoma* penetrates through the mucosa, leading to grossly visible large nodules. *H. muscae* and *H. majus* may cause mild catarrhal gastritis and small erosions and ulcers; rarely do they lead to significant lesions or clinical disease. Although the size of the nodules or tumors induced by *D. megastoma* may lead to mechanical interference, these also rarely lead to clinical disease. The nodules, with a small opening to the gastric lumen, are characterized by a granulomatous inflammatory reaction containing numerous eosinophils, with the center containing the parasites and necrotic debris. All three parasites have an indirect life cycle. Eggs passed in the feces are ingested by larvae (maggots) of the housefly *(Musca domestica)*, in the cases of *H. muscae* and *H. majus,* and of the stable fly *(Stomoxys calcitrans),* in the case of *D. megastoma.* The larvae undergo further development in the pupae of the fly, then migrate, as infective larvae, into the proboscis of the adult flies. The infective larvae are believed to be deposited on the lips of horses and eventually swallowed, to develop into adults in the stomach.

Cutaneous habronemiasis

Cutaneous habronemiasis (summer sores), a persistent disease of the skin of equines, results from the activity of larvae of stomach worms, especially *Draschia megastoma.* The larvae are deposited on the skin by flies, which are attracted to a pre-existing ulceration or wound in the skin. Lesions are particularly common in the skin of the pectoral region, between the forelegs. The larvae penetrate deeply into the dermis and elicit granulomatous tissue in which eosinophils are conspicuous. The skin loses its hair and becomes encrusted by serous exudate, which oozes from the surface. This le-

sion is not uncommon in horses during the summer months, but its true nature is often not suspected until larvae expressed from the lesion are identified by microscopic examination.

Habronema larvae may be deposited in the eye, leading to granulomatous conjunctivitis. They have been observed in granulomas in the lung, although the portal of entry is not understood. There also is a recent report of cutaneous habronemiasis in a dog.

References

de Jesus Z. Observations on habronemiasis in horses. Philipp J Vet Med 1963;2:133–152, Vet Bull 1965;35:3901.

Dikmans G. Skin lesions of domestic animals in the United States due to nematode infestation. Cornell Vet 1948;38:3–23.

Lewis JC, Seddon HR. Habronemic conjunctivitis. J Comp Pathol Ther 1918;31:87–94.

Sanderson TP, Niyo Y. Cutaneous habronemiasis in a dog. Vet Pathol 1990;27:208 209.

Strongyloidiasis

Several species of Strongyloides (not to be confused with *Stronglus,* p. 20) affect animals. Those of most importance include: *S. papillosus* of cattle, sheep, and goats; *S. westeri* of horses, swine, and zebras; *S. ransomi* of swine; *S. cati* and *S. tumefaciens* of cats; *S. stercoralis* of humans, monkeys, foxes, dogs, and cats; *S. ratti* and *S. venezuelensis* of rats; and *S. fuelleborni* of monkeys (Figs. 13-20, 13-22D).

LIFE CYCLE

Strongyloides are unusual parasites in that they may occur as either parasites of the intestinal tract, or as free-living nonparasitic worms. Only the female worm, which is trisomic and reproduces parthenogenetically,

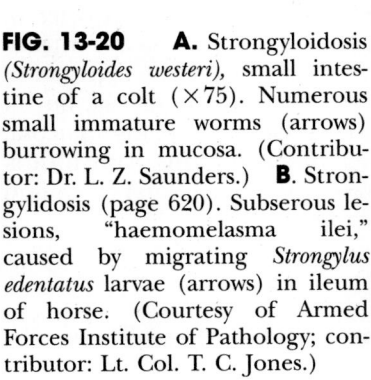

FIG. 13-20 **A.** Strongyloidosis *(Strongyloides westeri),* small intestine of a colt (×75). Numerous small immature worms (arrows) burrowing in mucosa. (Contributor: Dr. L. Z. Saunders.) **B.** Strongylidosis (page 620). Subserous lesions, "haemomelasma ilei," caused by migrating *Strongylus edentatus* larvae (arrows) in ileum of horse. (Courtesy of Armed Forces Institute of Pathology; contributor: Lt. Col. T. C. Jones.)

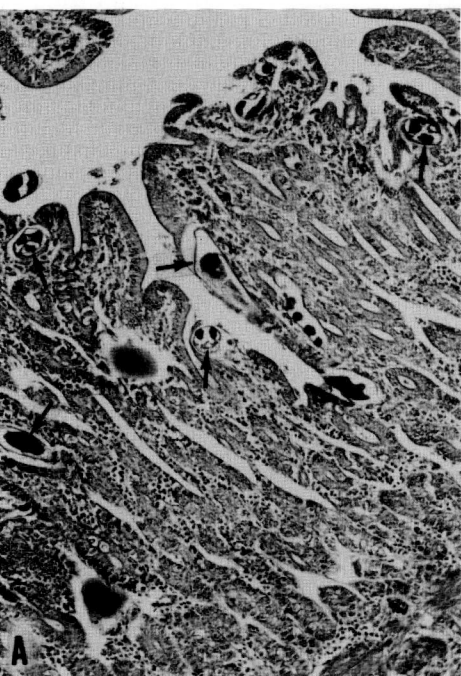
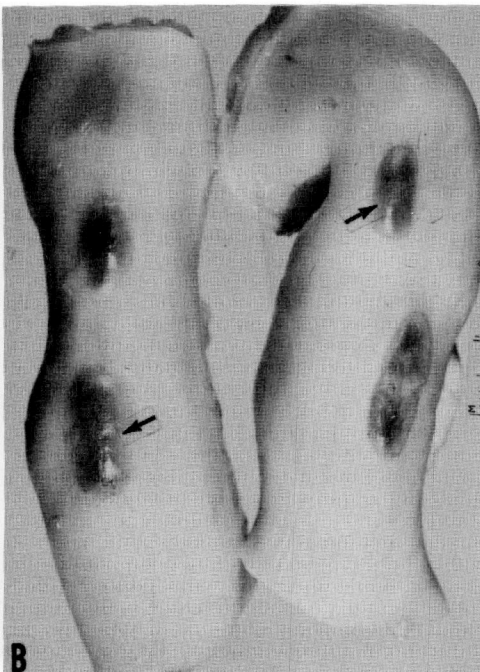

is parasitic. The worms range from 1–6 mm in length, depending on the species, and reside deep in the crypts of of the small intestine. Embryonated eggs may hatch in the lumen of the small intestine or be passed in the feces. They are of three types: diploid, haploid, and triploid. In the soil, triploid eggs give rise to infective third-stage larvae; diploid eggs hatch to free-living female adults; and haploid eggs hatch to free-living male adults. These free-living worms may produce either additional free-living forms, or parasitic third-stage female triploid larvae. Larvae gain access to a host primarily by penetrating the skin and entering the venous circulation, although infection per os can also occur.

The larvae are then carried to the lungs, where they break into the alveoli; they are coughed up, swallowed, and ultimately reach the intestine, where they develop into adults. Transmammary and prenatal infection may occur for some species of *Strongyloides* in the absence of intestinal parasitism, a situation similar to that of some species of ascarids. These routes are believed to be of major importance in swine infected with *S. ransomi*. Another unique feature of *Strongyloides* is that hyperinfection may occur, with completion of the reproductive cycle occurring within the host. In this situation, the larvae hatch in the lower intestine, penetrate the intestinal wall, and cycle through the lungs. This is most frequent in humans.

LESIONS

Upon entry, the larvae cause minimal mechanical damage to the skin and lungs; however, in previously exposed (hypersensitive) animals, this migration may lead to allergic dermatitis and pneumonia, although usually transient. The adult parasites lie deeply burrowed in the crypts of the anterior small intestine. When their numbers are small, clinical signs and significant lesions may not exist; an occasional parasite may be encountered as an incidental finding in routine histologic sections. The presence of larger numbers, however, leads to diarrhea and often serious disease, which may lead to death. The mucosa of the small intestine is edematous and infiltrated with neutrophils, lymphocytes, eosinophils; occasionally, epithelioid cells form small granulomas. Small erosions and hemorrhages may occur. Villi become blunted. The associated diarrhea is believed to result from malabsorption. In severe infections, especially in hyperinfection as described above, numerous migrating filariform larvae are present throughout the wall of the intestine and in many distant organs, including the liver, lungs, and brain. Often, bacteria brought along with the larvae leads to sepsis. This is not common in domestic animals, but is not unusual in humans and nonhuman primates, especially the great apes. *S. tumefaciens* infection of cats is associated with nodular (tumorlike) proliferative lesions in the colon.

DIAGNOSIS

Diagnosis of strongyloidiasis is made by demonstrating the eggs or larvae in the feces. Histopathologically, the lesions are characteristic.

References

Genta RM, Schad GA. Strongyloidiasis. Comp Pathol Bull 1986; 18:2, 4.

Greer GJ, Bello TR, Amborski GF. Experimental infection of *Strongyloides westeri* in parasite-free ponies. J Parasitol 1974;60:466–472.

Lyons ET, Drudge JH, Tolliver SC. On the life cycle of *Strongyloides westeri* in the equine. J Parasitol 1973;59:780–787.

Malone JB, Breitschwerdt EB, Little MD, et al. *Strongyloides stercoralis*-like infection in a dog. J Am Vet Med Assoc 1980;176:130–133.

Moncol DJ. Supplement to the life history of *Strongyloides ransomi* (Schwartz and Alicata, 1930) (Nematoda: Strongyloididae) of pigs. Proc Helminthol Soc Wash 1975;42:86–92.

Moncol DJ, Batte EG. Transcolostral infection of newborn pigs with *Strongyloides ransomi*. Vet Med Small Anim Clin 1966;61:583–586.

Pfeiffer H, Supperer R. Studies on the genus *Strongyloides*. VII. Prenatal infection in pigs. Wien Tieraerztl Mschr 1966;53:90–94, Vet Bull 1966;36:3144.

Stewart TB, Stone WM, Marti OG. *Strongyloides ransomi*: prenatal and transmammary infection of pigs of sequential litters from dams experimentally exposed as weanlings. Am J Vet Res 1976;37:541–544.

Stone WM, Simpson CF. Larval distribution and histopathology of experimental *Strongyloides ransomi* infection in young swine. Can J Comp Med 1967;31:197–202, Vet Bull 1968;38:1483.

Turner JH, Shalkop WT. Larval migration and accompanying pathological changes in experimental ovine strongyloidiasis. J Parasitol 1958;44:28–38.

Uemura E, Houser WD, Cupp CJ. Strongyloidiasis in an infant orangutan (*Pongo pygmaeus*). J Med Primatol 1979;8:282–288.

Pinworms

Several members of the family Oxyuridae are parasitic in animals and humans. These include *Enterobius vermicularis* (humans), *E. anthropopitheci* (apes and monkeys), *Oxyuris equi* (equines), *Skrjabinema ovis* (sheep and goats), *Passalurus ambigus* (rabbits), *Syphacia obvelata* (rodents), and *Aspicularis tetraptera* (mice).

LIFE CYCLE

The life cycle is direct. Fertilized adult females lay singly operculated eggs in clusters in the perianal region. The eggs reach the infectious stage within a few hours, and are either licked off by a new host, or fall off and are subsequently ingested. The larvae are released in the intestine and mature to adults, which reside in the cecum or colon. Fertilized females migrate to the lower rectum and anus to deposit their eggs.

LESIONS

Pinworms are relatively innocuous parasites and are rarely associated with serious disease. The activities of the female worm result in pruritus, and heavy infestation is believed to cause ulcerative colitis. The adult worms do not attach themselves to the mucosa, but in ulcerative colitis they may migrate into the mucosa, along with larvae Whether the association with ulcerative colitis and tissue invasion is coincidental or caused by other factors is not established.

DIAGNOSIS

Diagnosis of pinworm infestation is usually made by either recognizing adult worms at the anus, or eggs recovered from the perianal area. Cellophane or similar clear, sticky tape is useful to recover the eggs.

Probstmayria vivipara, another parasite of the colon of horses, is in the same superfamily, but a different family (Kathlaniidae) than the pinworms. It is much smaller than *Oxyuris equi,* is not associated with lesions and, as its name implies, it is viviparous.

References

Drudge JH, Lyons ET. Equine parasites, problems and control. Pract Vet 1978;49:5–7, 9.

Holmes DD, Kosanke SD, White GL, et al. Fatal enterobiasis in a chimpanzee. J Am Vet Med Assoc 1980;177:911–913.

Kellogg HS, Wagner JE. Experimental transmission of *Syphacia obvelata* among mice, rats, hamsters, and gerbils. Lab Anim Sci 1982;32:500–501.

Lichtenfels JR. Helminths of domestic equids. Proc Helminthol Soc Wash 1975;42:1–92.

Moore G, Myers BJ. Parasites of non-human primates. Washington, D.C.: Am Assoc Zoo Vet (Annual Proceedings) 1974;79–86.

Ross CR, Wagner JE, Wightman SR, et al. Experimental transmission of Syphacia muris among rats, mice, hamsters, and gerbils. Lab Anim Sci 1980;30:35–37.

Schmidt RE, Prine JR. Severe enterobiasis in a chimpanzee. Pathol Vet 1970;7:56–59.

Slocombe JOD, McCraw BM. Gastrointestinal nematodes in horses in Ontario. Can Vet J 1973;14:101–105.

CAPILLARIA, TRICHOSOMOIDES AND ANATRICHOSOMA

The genus *Capillaria* parasitizes a large number of species of mammals, birds, and fish, but only a few are of concern as pathogens of animals.

Capillaria hepatica (Hepaticola hepatica)

Capillaria hepatica (Hepaticola hepatica) is primarily a parasite of rats and mice, but may also infect dogs, cats, rabbits, beavers, muskrats, squirrels, peccaries, horses, monkeys, humans, and other species. The adult worm is a slender nematode related to whipworms (*Trichuris* sp.), but without the broader posterior extremity. The adults live in the liver parenchyma, where ova and excreta accumulate, causing tissue destruction leading to fibrosis. The life cycle is continued only when the infected liver is eaten by a new (intercalary host), in which the ova are released but do not hatch. Ova with bipolar plugs (typical of the genus) are passed with the feces of this second host and embryonate on the ground to reach the infectious stage. Ova ingested by a third host contain larvae that penetrate the intestinal wall, eventually reaching the liver (Fig. 13-21). The disease is not uncommon in wild rodents, but is rarely encountered in laboratory animals.

Capillaria feliscati and C. plica

These slender worms are about 30–60 mm long, and are found in the urinary bladder and occasionally the ureters and renal pelvis. *C. feliscati* has been reported in cats and *C. plica* in dogs, cats and foxes. It is possible that these helminths are identical. In some kennels, the incidence of infection has been observed to exceed 75%. *C. mucronata* affects the urinary bladder of mink. Ordinarily, these worms produce little effect on the urinary tract; however, the parasites do invade the mucosa, which can lead to hematuria. Their presence may be detected by microscopic demonstration of bipolar ova in the urine.

Capillaria aerophila, a related species that infects the lung, was discussed under Pulmonary Nematodiasis. *Capillaria putorii* is a rarely reported parasite of the stomach and upper small intestine in cats, pigs, and a number of wild species such as bears, raccoons and bobcats.

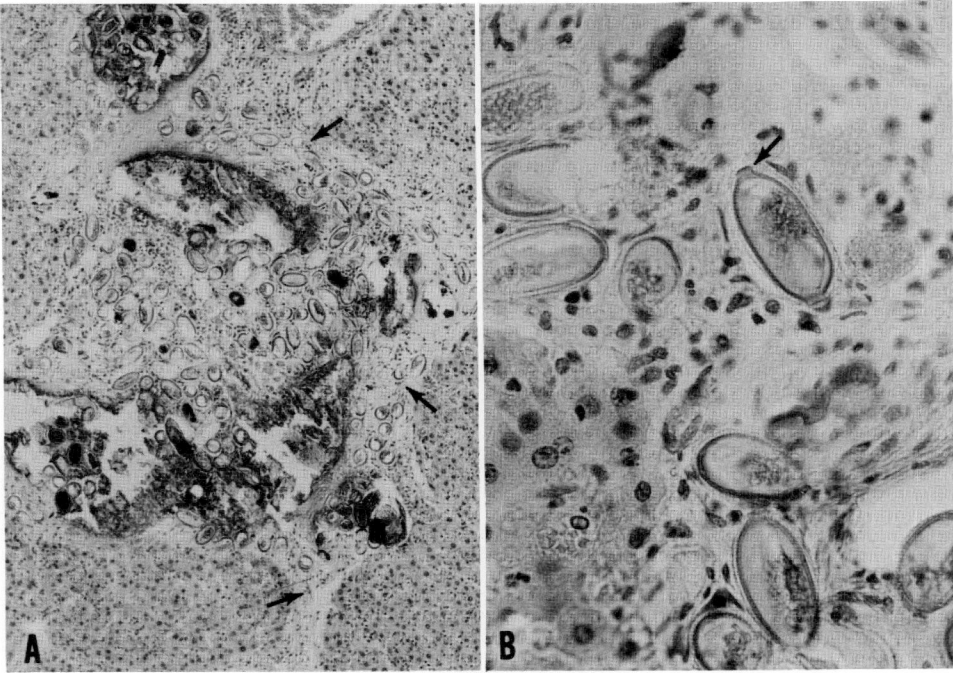

FIG. 13-21 *Capillaria hepatica* infection in the liver of a rat. **A.** Accumulation of ova in portal areas (arrows) with resultant fibrosis (×76). **B.** Higher magnification (×440). Note ova with polar eminence (arrow) at each end, characteristic of the genus.

In rats, a parasite within this same family, *Trichosomoides crassicauda*, inhabits the urinary bladder with no apparent ill effects, although it has been considered a cause of neoplasia of the bladder.

Anatrichosoma cutaneum

Anatrichosoma cutaneum is a nematode that resides in the nasal mucosa and, less frequently, the skin around the nares, lips, and eyes of Old World monkeys and apes. Most often they are incidental findings, but they may lead to small nodules in the skin and nasal passages. Microscopically, the coiled worms and bipolar eggs are found in the submucosa or dermis, surrounded by a mixed inflammatory cell infiltrate predominantly composed of lymphocytes, plasma cells, and eosinophils. The mucosa or epidermis is hyperplastic and hyperparakeratotic or hyperkeratotic.

References

Allen AM. Occurrence of the nematode, *Anatrichosoma cutaneum*, in the nasal mucosa of *Macaca mulatta* monkeys. Am J Vet Res 1960;21:389–392.

Breznock AW, Pulley LT. *Anatrichosoma* infection in two white-handed gibbons. J Am Vet Med Assoc 1975;167:631–633.

Greve JH, Kung FY. *Capillaria putorii* in domestic cats in Iowa. J Am Vet Med Assoc 1983;182:511–513.

Karr SL Jr, Henrickson RV, Else JG. A survey for *Anatrichosoma* (Nematoda: Trichinellida) in wild-caught *Macaca mulatta*. Lab Anim Sci 1979;29:789–790.

Senior DF, Solomon GB, Goldschmidt MH, et al. *Capillaria plica* infection in dogs. J Am Vet Med Assoc 1980;176:901–905.

Schmidt RE, Prine JR. Severe enterobiasis in a Chimpanzee. Pathol Vet 1970;7:56–59.

Waddell AH. *Capillaria feliscati* in the bladder of cats in Australia. Aust Vet J 1967;43:297.

Waddell AH. Further observations on *Capillaria feliscati* infections in the cat. Aust Vet J 1968;44:33–34.

Weisbroth SH. Diagnosis of *Trichosomoides crassicauda* in laboratory rats. BLU:LETTER (Blue Spruce Farms, Inc., Altamont, NY), 1970;2:2–3.

Weisbroth SH, Scher S. *Trichosomoides crassicauda* infection of a commercial rat breeding colony. I. Observations on the life cycle and propagation. Lab Anim Sci 1971;21:54–61.

Trichuriasis

The so-called **whipworms** include members of the Trichuridae, which were so-named because one part of their body is thick and the rest is thin, resembling the shape of a whip. Interestingly, the name *Trichuris* means "hair-tail" and resulted from failure to observe that the posterior portion of the worm is thickest. "Hair-head" (*Trichocephalus*) is presumably more correct, but *Trichuris* has priority. Several species are of interest: *Trichuris ovis* is found in the cecum of cattle, sheep, goats, and many wild ruminants; *T. discolor* in the cecum and colon of cattle, sheep, and goats; *T. suis* inhabits the cecum of the domestic and wild pig and wild boar, and is similar if not identical morphologically to *T. trichiura*, a parasitic in humans and other primates; *T. vulpis*, which infects dogs and foxes; *T. campanula* and *T. serrata* of cats; and *T. globulosa* of sheep, goats, cattle, and camels.

The parasites are oviparous (Fig. 13-22). Infective bipolar eggs are ingested and hatch in the intestine, liberating larvae that penetrate the mucosa of the cecum and colon. After a period of about two weeks, the posterior portion protrudes into the intestinal lumen, while the filamentous head remains embedded in the mucosa.

Although light to moderate infections produce little detectable effects, heavy parasitic loads may lead to catarrhal, hemorrhagic, or necrotizing typhlitis and colitis. Clinical and pathologic findings are most frequent in swine. During periods of drought (Farleigh, 1966a), whipworms apparently increase and may be found in large numbers in the cecum and colon of sheep. Death may result under these conditions.

References

Beer RJ, Rutter JM. Spirochaetal invasion of the colonic mucosa in a syndrome resembling swine dysentery following experimental *Trichuris suis* infection in weaned pigs. Res Vet Sci 1972;13:593–595.

Beer RJS. Experimental infection of man with pig whipworm. Br Med J 1971;2:44.

Beer RJS. Studies on the biology of the life-cycle of *Trichuris suis* (Schrank, 1788). Parasitology 1973;67:253–262.

Beer RJS, Lean IJ. *Clinical trichuriasis* produced experimentally in growing pigs. I. Pathology of infection. Vet Rec 1973;93:189–195.

Farleigh EA. Observations on the pathogenic effects of *Trichuris ovis* in sheep under drought conditions. Aust Vet J 1966a ;42:462–463.

Farleigh EA. Whip worm (*Trichuris ovis*) of sheep. Vet Insp NSW 1966;30:70–71.

Hall GA, Rutter JM, Beer RJS. A comparative study of the histopathology of the large intestine of conventionally reared, specific pathogen-free and gnotobiotic pigs infected with Trichuris suis. J Comp Pathol 1976;86:285–292.

Loomis MR, Wright JF. Gastric trichuriasis in a black and white colobus monkey. J Am Vet Med Assoc 1986;189:1214–1215.

Perdrizet JA, King JM. Whipworm (*Trichuris discolor*) infection in dairy replacement heifers. J Am Vet Med Assoc 1986;188:1063–1064.

Onchocerciasis

Onchocerca are large parasites whose adults usually reside in connective tissues, especially of the subcutis, tendons, and fascia. Most incite a chronic inflammatory response leading to the formation of dense fibrous nodules. Each produces microfilariae, many of which locate in the skin where they are available to various insects, the obligatory intermediate hosts. Several species of interest exist. *Onchocerca volvulus*, which is transmitted by blackflies (*Simulium sp.*), is the cause of serious disease of humans in Africa and Central America. The adults reside in the subcutaneous tissues, where they produce fibrous nodules; a more serious consequence is that, microfilariae may localize in the chambers of the eye and cause blindness.

O. gibsoni, transmitted by *Culicoides* sp., parasitizes cattle, most frequently locating in the subcutaneous tissue of the brisket and the hind limbs. It is restricted to Asia, Australia, and southern Africa. O. gutturosa also parasitizes cattle, most often localizing in connective tissue adjacent to the nuchal ligament or fascia adjacent to major bones of the limbs. Its microfilariae concen-

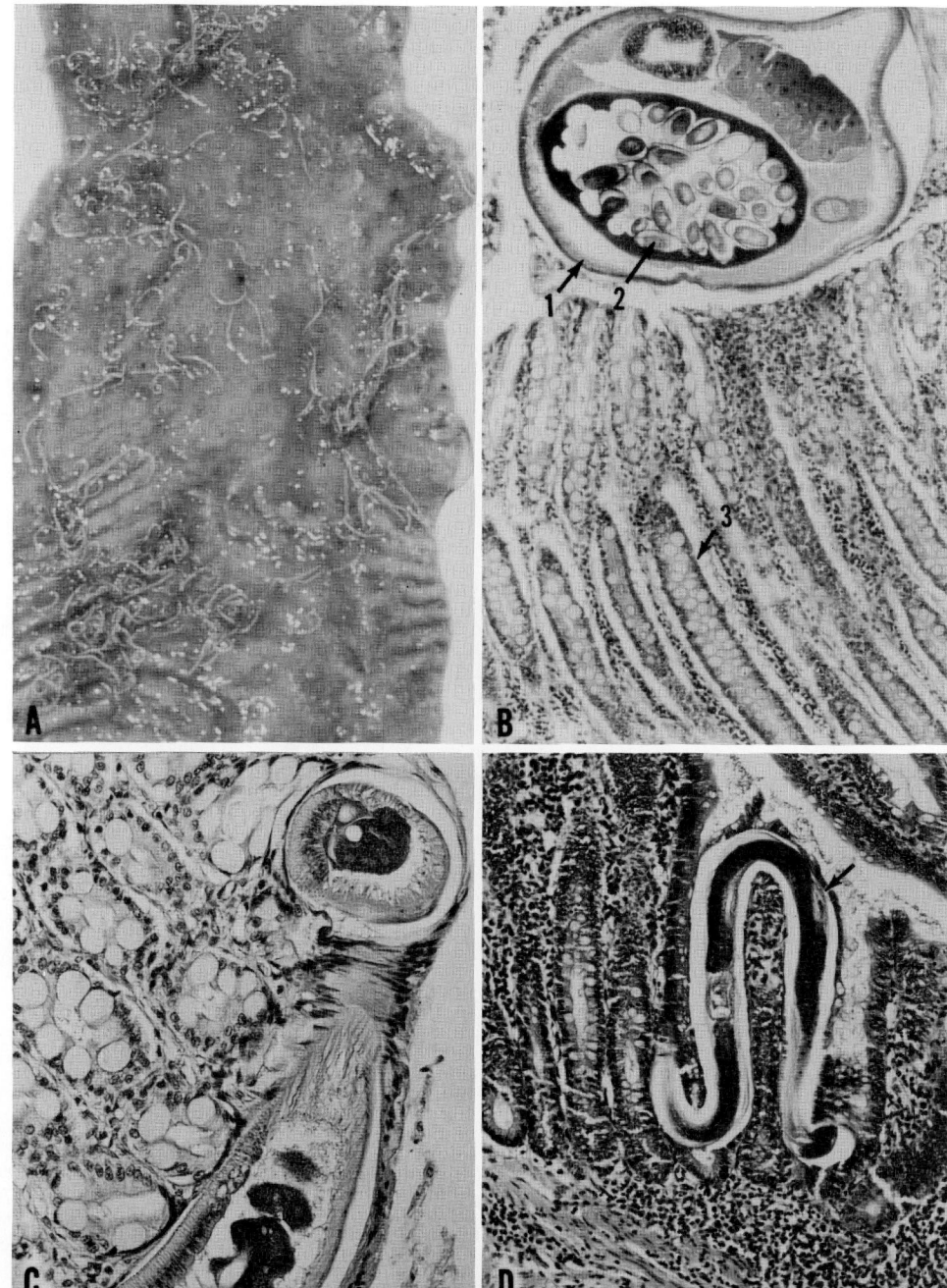

FIG. 13-22 A. Trichuriasis. Colon of a dog. (Contributor: Army Veterinary School.) **B.** *Trichuris vulpis* in the mucosa of the colon of a dog (×100). (1) Note muscular layer in wall; and (2) Ova in uterus of the worm; (3) Lymphocytic infiltration of the lamina propria separates the epithelial components. **C.** Another segment of *Tr. vulpis* (×200) embedded in the mucosa of the colon. (Contributor: Army Veterinary School.) **D.** Strongyloidosis. Small intestine of a spider monkey. Note the worm (arrow) buried in the mucosa. (Contributor: Dr. C. N. Woolsey.) (A, B, D, Courtesy of Armed Forces Institute of Pathology.)

trate in the skin at sites frequented by the most prominent intermediate host in the particular geographic locale. It is transmitted by *Simulium* sp. and occurs throughout most of the world. Neither the microfilariae nor the adults elicit any significant pathologic change. Another species that affects cattle in the United States and Australia is *O. lienalis*, which localizes in the gastrosplenic ligament. *O. armillata* (Fig. 13-23) occurs in cattle, sheep, and goats in Africa and Asia, and is particularly frequent in Ghana. The adults of this parasite form tunnels, nodules, and cysts in the aortic wall, with microfilariae concentrating in the skin.

In the horse, the adults of *O. cervicalis* are slender, filariform worms ranging from 27–75 mm in length; they are found in the ligamentum nuchae and occasionally in nodular cutaneous lesions. The microfilariae concentrate in the skin of the abdomen adjacent to the umbilicus, the flank, or in the eyelids and other ocular tissues. *O. cervicalis* is common in horses, and the worms are believed to have some etiologic relationship to "poll evil," "fistulous withers," periodic ophthalmia, and remittent dermatitis; however, no sound evidence exists to attribute these maladies to onchocerciasis. *O. reticulata* inhabits the suspensory ligaments of the fore-

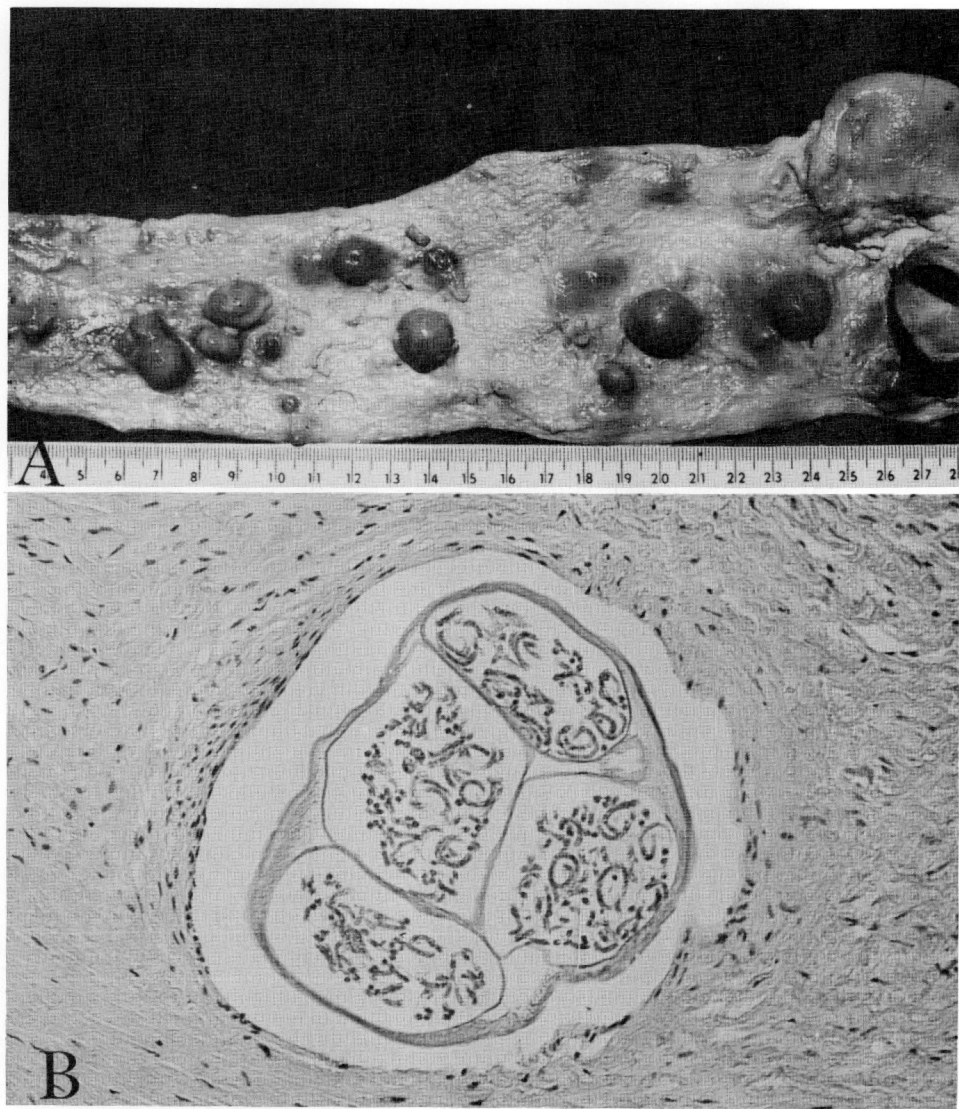

FIG. 13-23 Bovine onchocerciasis. **A.** Nodules in the adventitia of the aorta produced by *Onchocerca armillata*. **B.** Cross section of *O. armillata* in the media of the aorta. (Courtesy of Dr. A. H. Cheema and Veterinary Pathology.)

limbs of horses. The incidence of infection is high, ranging from 10% in young horses to 90% in horses over 16 years of age. The lesions are also more apparent in older horses and are described as mineralization and granuloma formation around adult worms in the nuchal ligaments. *O. reticulata* inhabits the suspensory ligaments of the forelimbs of horses. Both of these equine parasites are transmitted by *Culicoides* sp.

References

Chadnik KS. Histopathology of the aortic lesions in cattle infected with *Onchocerca armillata*. Ann Trop Med Parasitol 1958; 52:145–148.

Cummings E, James ER. Prevalence of equine onchocerciasis in southeastern and midwestern United States. J Am Vet Med Assoc 1985;186:1202–1203.

Dikmans G. Skin lesions of domestic animals in the United States due to nematode infestation. Cornell Vet 1948;38:3–23.

Eichler DA, Nelson GS. Studies on *Onchocerca gutturosa* (Neumann, 1910) and its development in *Simulium ornatum* (Meigen, 1818). I. Observations on *O. gutturosa* in cattle in Southeast England. J Helminthol 1971;45:245–258.

ElBihari S, Hussein HS. Location of the microfilariae of *Onchocerca armillata*. J Parasitol 1975;61:656.

Gunders AE, Neumann E. Parasitology and diagnosis of onchocerciasis with special reference to the outer eye. Isr J Med Sci 1972;8:1139–1142.

Harty TM, Ferenc SA, Copeman DB, et al. *Onchocerca gutturosa* and *Onchocerca lienalis* in cattle: variation in length of microfilariae by site of recovery. Am J Vet Res 1989;50:169–172.

Hilmy N, Khamis MY, Selim MK. The role of *Onchocerca reticulata* as the cause of fistulous withers and ulcerative wounds of the back in solipeds, and its treatment. Vet Med J Giza 1967;14:149–164, Vet Bull 1969;39:2979.

Ivanov IV. Histological changes in the skin of cattle with onchocerciasis. Trudy vses Inst Gel'mint 1964;11:59–61, Vet Bull 1966; 36:1477.

Klei TR, Torbert B, Chapman MR, et al. Prevalence of *Onchocerca cervicalis* in equids in the Gulf Coast region. Am J Vet Res 1984;45:1646–1647.

Marolt J, Zukovic M, Molan M. Onchocerciasis in horses. Dtsch Tierarztl Wochenschr 1966;73:130–134, Vet Bull 1966;36:3555.

Mellor PS. Studies on *Onchocerca cervicalis* (Railliet and Henry, 1910). II. Pathology in the horse. J Helminthol 1973;47:111–118.

Rabalais FC, Eberhard ML, Ashley DC, et al. Survey for equine onchocerciasis in the midwestern United States. Am J Vet Res 1974;35:125–126.

Rabalais FC, Votava CL. Cutaneous distribution of microfilariae of *Onchocerca cervicalis* in horses. Am J Vet Res 1974;35:1369–1370.

Schmidt GM, Krehbiel JD, Coley SC, et al. Equine onchocerciasis: lesions in the nuchal ligament of midwestern US horses. Vet Pathol 1982a;19:16–22.

Schmidt GM, Krehbiel JD, Coley SC, et al. Equine ocular onchocerciasis: histopathologic study. Am J Vet Res 1982b;43:1371–1375.

Stannard AA, Cello RM. *Onchocerca cervicalis* infection in horses from the western United States. Am J Vet Res 1975;36:1029–1031.

Elaeophoriasis (filarial dermatosis of sheep)

Three species of *Elaeophora* affect animals, but only one, *Elaeophora schneideri*, is of concern in the United States. This "arterial worm" is a filarial parasite common in western and southwestern U.S. in sheep, elk, and deer. Deer (white-tailed and mule) suffer few consequences from the parasitism and are considered the normal or reservoir hosts. In sheep, the parasitism results in "filarial dermatosis" and in elk, arterial lesions leads to infarction. Its life cycle is indirect, utilizing horse flies (*Hybomitra* and *Tabanus*) as intermediate hosts.

LESIONS

In **sheep,** the adult worms are found most frequently in the carotid arteries, but the mesenteric, iliac, and other arteries may also be parasitized. The adults are 6–12 cm in length, slender, threadlike, and glossy white. Microfilariae measuring 18 by 270 μm localize in the dermis of specific sites and lead, in most cases, to circumscribed dermatitis over the head, poll, and face. The skin of the abdomen and hind feet may be involved, as well as the cornea and oral and nasal mucosae. The lesion is accompanied by considerable pruritis, vesicles, and small pustules; epilation and crust formation follow. Proliferation of the horns in normally hornless rams sometimes occurs. The microscopic changes in the skin in this disease have been studied by Davis and Kemper (1951) and Jensen and Seghetti (1955). The affected epithelium is covered with a thick hyperkeratotic or parakeratotic layer variously infiltrated with cell debris and exudative fluid, and shows severe localized acanthosis with clubbing of the rete pegs. Areas of ulceration are associated with hemorrhagic and serous exudation. Superficial vesicles or bullae in the epithelium are common, and some are filled with serum or an admixture of serum, red blood cells, and eosinophils. The dermis is severely involved in an inflammatory process of granulomatous nature, centering around microfilariae in vascular channels or enclosed in the inflammatory exudate. In some foci of inflammation, histiocytes and giant cells predominate, with some lymphocytes and plasma cells in the surrounding tissue; in others, eosinophils are predominant. These changes are undoubtedly influenced by the age of the lesion, death of larvae, and sensitization of the host. The dermis is often completely involved to the level of the musculature. Localization of the larvae in skin (Fig. 13-24) and mucous membranes exposed to the external environment suggests a tropism for such localities. The adult worms may cause thrombosis of the arteries in which they are found.

In elk, the adult worms most frequently locate in common brachiocephalic and leptomeningeal arteries, and in those arteries supplying the eye. The arterial lesions, in contrast to sheep, are more pronounced and lead to serious sequelae. The parasites incite marked intimal proliferation, granulomatous inflammation, and fibrosis that may occlude affected arteries. Thrombosis is common and leads to infarction in brain, and in the optic nerve, retina, and skin about the head; this, then, leads to neurologic signs and blindness. Necrotizing lesions in the skin are most frequent about the muzzle, nostrils, and ear tips, and are often associated with malformed antlers.

Two other species of *Elaeophora* affect animals, but neither occurs in the United States, nor do they lead to clinical disease. **Elaeophora poeli** is a parasite of the aorta of cattle and buffalo in Asia and Africa. The males reside entirely within fibrotic nodules while the females are partially embedded in the nodule, with their posterior portion hanging free in the lumen. **Elaeophora böhmi** is a parasite seen in horses in Austria. The adults reside within the media of arteries and veins of the distal extremities. Their presence leads to the formation of nodules and narrowing of the lumen.

DIAGNOSIS

Diagnosis can be made by finding characteristic microfilariae in microscopic sections of affected skin or in smears of skin scrapings. The adult worms are found only at necropsy.

References

Adcock JL, Hibler CP. Vascular and neuro-ophthalmic pathology of elaeophorosis in elk. Pathol Ve 1969;6:185–213.

Bindernagel JA. *Elaeophora poeli* (Nematoda: Filaroidea) in African buffalo in Uganda, East Africa. J Wldlf Dis 1971;7:296–298.

Clark GG, Hibler CP. Horse flies and *Elaeophora schneideri* in the Gila National Forest, New Mexico. J Wldlf Dis 1973;9:21–25.

Davis CL, Kemper HE. The histopathologic diagnosis of filarial dermatosis in sheep. J Am Vet Med Assoc 1951;118:103–106.

Douglas JR, Cordy DR, Spurlock GM. *Elaeophora schneideri,* (Wehr and Dikmans, 1935) (Nematoda, filarioidea) in California sheep. Cornell Vet 1954;44:252–258.

Foreyt WJ, Foreyt KM. *Elaeophora schneideri* in a White-Tailed deer from Texas. J Wldlf Dis 1979;15:55–56.

Hibler CP, Gates GH, Donaldson BR. Experimental infection of immature mule deer with *Elaeophora schneideri*. J Wldlf Dis 1974;10:44–46.

Hibler CP, Gates GH, White R, et al. Observations on horseflies infected with larvae of *Elaeophora schneideri*. J Wldlf Dis 1971;7:43–45.

Hibler CP, Metzger CJ. Morphology of the larval stages of *Elaeophora schneideri* in the intermediate and definitive hosts with some observations on their pathogenesis in abnormal definitive hosts. J Wldlf Dis 1974;10:361–369.

Jensen R, Seghetti L. Elaeophoriasis in sheep. J Am Vet Med Assoc 1955;127:499–505.

Kemper HE. Filarial dermatosis of sheep. North Am Vet 1938;19:36–41.

Robinson RM, Jones LP, Galvin TJ, et al. Elaeophorosis in Sika deer in Texas. J Wldlf Dis 1978;14:137–141.

Titche AR, Prestwood AK, Hibler CP. Experimental infection of white-tailed deer with *Elaeophora schneideri*. J Wldlf Dis 1979;15:273–280.

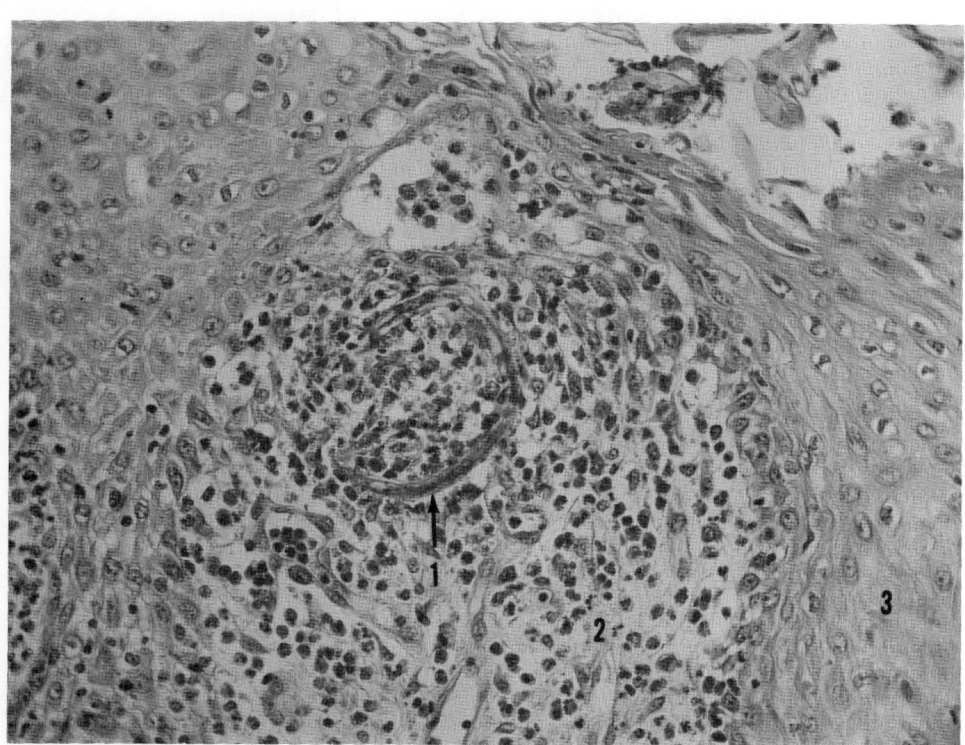

FIG. 13-24 Elaeophoriasis. Skin of sheep (×260). (1) Larva of *Elaeophora schneideri;* (2) In dermal papilla, which is congested and infiltrated with lymphocytes and eosinophils; (3) The epidermis is acanthotic. (Courtesy of Armed Forces Institute of Pathology; contributor: Bureau of Animal Industry, U.S. Department of Agriculture.)

Worley DE. Observations on epizootiology and distribution of *Elaeophora schneideri* in Montana ruminants. J Wldlf Dis 1975;11:486–488.

Rhabditis dermatitis (Pelodera dermatitis)

The family Rhabditidae contains many free-living nematodes that reside in moist decaying organic matter. Ordinarily these are not pathogenic. On occasion, however, some are associated with dermatitis or other superficial lesions. In dogs, cattle, and rarely horses, *Pelodera strongyloides (Rhabditis strongyloides)* can be found within localized areas of dermatitis characterized by erythema, pustules, and hyperkeratosis, especially on the ventral abdomen and limbs. The nematodes are not believed to be capable of penetrating intact skin, but instead invade skin previously damaged from other causes. Microscopically, the nematodes are most conspicuous within hair follicles, but may also be found within the dermis. They do not invade beyond the skin. They can be identified in tissue section by their rhabditiform esophagus (anterior wide portion, narrow midsection, and terminal bulbous portion). *Rhabditis bovis* is a free-living nematode that has been seen in association with otitis media in cattle of East Africa.

References

Chitwood BG. The association of *Rhabditis strongyloides* with dermatitis in dogs. North Am Vet 1932;13:35–40.

Chitwood M, Lichtenfels JR. Parasitological review: identification of parasitic metazoa in tissue sections. Exp Parasitol 1972;32:407–519.

Georgi JR. Parasitology for Veterinarians. 2nd ed. Philadelphia: WB Saunders, 1974.

Jibbo JMC. Bovine parasitic otitis. Bull Epizoot Dis Afr 1966;14:59–63.

Rhode EA, et al. The occurrence of *Rhabditis* in cattle. North Am Vet 1953;34:634–637.

Schlotthauer CF, Zollman PE. The occurrence of *Rhabditis strongyloides* in association with dermatitis in a dog. J Am Vet Med Assoc 1955;127:510–511.

Stephanofilariasis

Nematode dermatitis occurring in cattle in widely scattered parts of the world is caused by several related filarial worms. *Stephanofilaria stilesi*, originally recognized by Stiles and described by Dikmans (1948), has been reported in skin lesions of cattle in most of the western and midwestern states, as well as Louisiana. This filarid causes a circumscribed dermatitis usually located on the abdomen near the midline. *S. dedoesi* has been reported from Java, Sumatra, Celebes, and Indonesia; it produces lesions on the sides of the neck, withers, dewlap, shoulders, and around the eyes. *S. assamensis*, occurring in Assam and other parts of India, causes a chronic dermatitis in Zebu cattle, known as "hump sore." In Malaya, *S. kaeli* is reported to produce "filarial sores" on the lower legs of cattle. *S. zaheeri* is associated with dermatitis of the ears of buffalo in India. In Japan, a sixth species, *S. okinawaensis*, causes dermatitis of the muzzle and teats of cattle.

Each has an indirect life cycle, with various species of flies ingesting microfilariae as they feed on the lesions. Infective larvae, which are found in the proboscis, develop in the fly after an interval of about 10 days.

Horn flies, *Haematobia (Lyperosia) irritans*, and *H. (L.) titillans*, are the principal intermediate hosts for *S. stilesi*. *Musca conducens* has been identified as the intermediate host for *S. kaeli*, *S. assamensis*, and *S. okinawaensis*.

LESIONS

The adult forms of *Stephanofilaria stilesi* are found either in small cysts with epithelial linings in the base of hair follicles or in the dermis near the epidermis (Fig. 13-25). In either site, the worms are surrounded by a zone of inflammation containing eosinophils, lymphocytes, some neutrophils, and histiocytes, and often a layer of connective tissue. The microfilariae are found a short distance from the adults in spaces in the dermal papillae. The adults and microfilariae can often be seen in the same field when the low power of the microscope is used (Fig. 13-25). Hyperkeratosis and parakeratosis may be noted in the epidermis of parasitized areas, and crusts of exuded serum and detritus may collect on the surface. Death of the parasites and sensitization of the host result in a severe dermatitis.

Studies on *S. assamensis* in zebu cattle with "humpsore," in Bangladesh, have revealed that the microfilariae reside within eggs whose shells do not stain with H & E, but can be visualized with Gram stain.

DIAGNOSIS

The diagnosis may be established by the demonstration of adults and microfilariae in biopsy, or necropsy specimens of affected skin. The parasites can also be collected by deep scrapings of skin and identified by microscopic examination.

References

Dewan ML, Rahman MM. Isolation of microorganisms from stephanofilariasis (humpsore) and their roles in the initiation of the disease. Bangladesh Vet J 1970;4:25–30, Vet Bull 1972;42:6983.

Dewan ML. Histopathology of stephanofilariasis (humpsore) at different stages of its development. Bangladesh J Agric Sci 1975;2: 51–58.

Dikmans G. Skin lesions of domestic animals in the United States due to nematode infestation. Cornell Vet 1948;38:3–23.

Hibler CP. Development of *Stephanofilaria stilesi* in the horn fly. J Parasitol 1966;52:890–898.

Kono I, Fukuyoshi S. Leucoderma of the muzzle of cattle induced by a new species of *Stephanofilaria*. II. Jpn J Vet Sci 1967;29:301–313, Vet Bull 1968;38:4627.

Levine ND, Morrill CC. Bovine stephanofilarial dermatitis in Illinois. J Am Vet Med Assoc 1955;127:528–530.

Loke YW, Ramachandran CP. Histopathology of *Stephanofilaria kaeli* lesions in cattle. Med J Malaya 1966;20:348–353, Vet Bull 1967;37:931.

Oduye OO. Stephanofilarial dermatitis of cattle in Nigeria. J Comp Pathol 1971;81:581–583.

Pal AK, Sinha PK. *Stephanofilaria assamensis* as the cause of common chronic ulcerated growth at the base of the dewclaws in cattle in West Bengal. Ind Vet J 1971;48:190–193.

Ramachandran CP, Loke YW, Nagendram C. Studies on *Stephanofilaria kaeli* in cattle. Med J Malaya 1966;20:344–347.

Sharma Deorani VP. Studies on the pathology of *Stephanofilariasis assamensis* in cattle. Curr Sci 1965;34:410–411.

Thelaziasis

Thelazia ("eye worms") are parasites that reside in the conjunctival sac and lacrimal duct of many animal species. *Thelazia californiensis* occurs in the United States in sheep, dogs, deer, and rarely cats and humans. *T. lacrymalis* affects horses worldwide. *T. gulosa* and *T. skrjabini* are parasites of cattle, and are also distributed world-

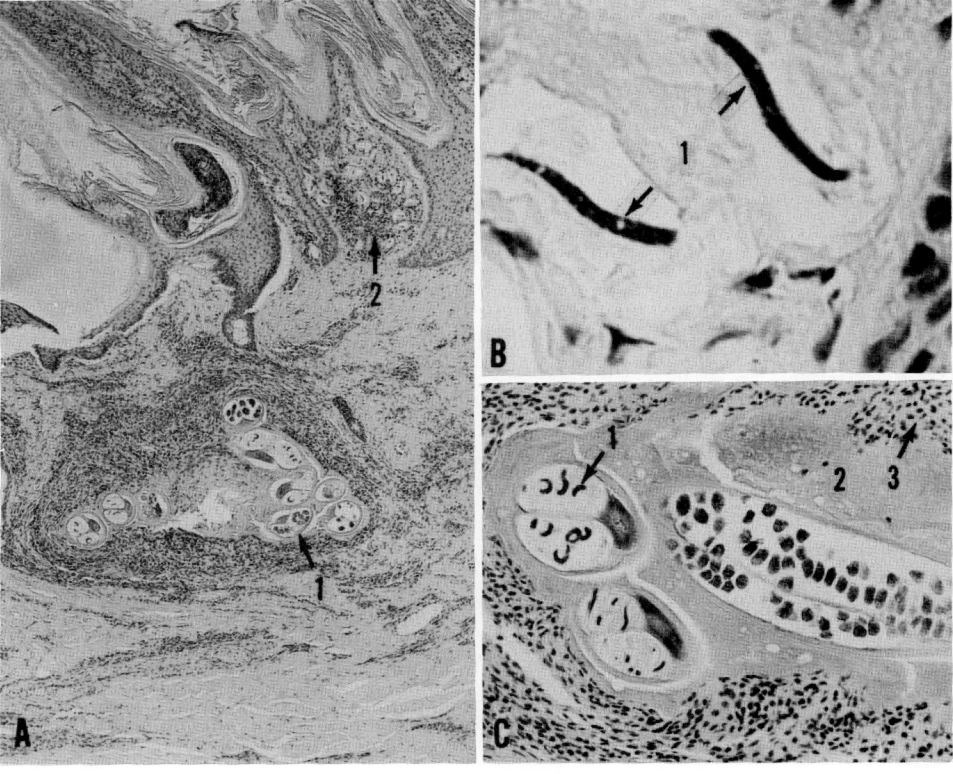

FIG. 13-25 Stephanofilariasis. Bovine skin. **A.** Section of skin (×75) containing coiled adult *Stephanofilaria stilesi*. (1) Deep in a hair follicle; and (2) Larvae in the dermal papillae. Note acanthosis and hyperkeratosis. **B.** Larvae (×900). (1) In papilla. **C.** Adult (×150) worm. (1) Larvae in uterus; (2) Hyaline material surrounding it; and (3) Zone of inflammation. (Courtesy of Armed Forces Institute of Pathology and Dr. C. L. Davis.)

wide. *T. alfortensis*, which may be the same as *T. gulosa*, affects cattle in Europe. *T. callipaeda* occurs in Asia in dogs, and less frequently in rabbits and humans. *T. rhodesii* has been reported from Asia, Africa, and Europe in cattle, sheep, goats, and buffaloes.

The life cycles (Soulsby, 1968) of these spiruroid worms depend upon various species of *Musca* or, in the case of *T. californiensis*, species of Fannia as intermediate hosts and vectors. The larvae move from the gut to develop first in the ovary of the fly, where they penetrate and develop in ovarian follicles. They spend their second and third stages in the ovary; then, as third-stage infective larvae, they migrate to the mouth parts of the fly, ready to be transferred to the conjunctivae of cattle.

Their presence in the conjunctival sac results in considerable photophobia and excessive lacrimation; if not removed, they are reported to cause blindness, presumably through production of corneal opacity. The diagnosis is made by finding and identifying the parasites in the conjunctiva.

References

Barker IK. *Thelazia lacrymalis* from the eyes of an Ontario horse. Can Vet J 1970;11:186–189.

Fitzsimmons WM. Verminous ophthalmia in a cow in Berkshire: a review of *Thelazia* infections as a veterinary problem. Vet Rec 1963;75:1024–1027.

Geden CJ, Stoffolano JG Jr: Bovine thelaziasis in Massachusetts. Cornell Vet 1980;70:344–359.

Lyons ET, Drudge JH. Two eyeworms, *Thelazia gulosa* and *Thelazia skrjabini*, in cattle in Kentucky. J Parasitol 1975;61:1119–1122.

Lyons ET, Drudge JH. *Thelazia lacrymalis* in horses in Kentucky and observations on the face fly (*Musca autumnalis*) as a probable intermediate host. J Parasitol 1976;62:877–880.

Lyons ET, Drudge JH, Tolliver SC. Age distribution of horses in Kentucky infected with the eye worm *Thelazia lacrymalis*. J Am Vet Med Assoc 1980;176:221–223.

Lyons ET, Tolliver SC, Drudge JH, et al. Eyeworms (Thelazia lacrymalis) in one- to four-year-old Thoroughbreds at necropsy in Kentucky (1984–1985). Am J Vet Res 1986;47:315–316.

Weinmann CJ, Anderson JR, Rubtzoff PI, et al. Eyeworms and face flies in California. Calif Agric 1974;28:4–5.

Stephanuriasis (kidney worm disease)

The swine kidney worm, *Stephanurus dentatus,* is a stout parasitic nematode, 20–40 mm in length, found principally in the perirenal fat and adjacent tissues. It is especially common in the southern United States. These worms form cystic cavities that communicate with the lumen of the ureter and permit the discharge of ova with the urine. The larvae hatch only in moist, shaded soil, and remain infective for some time unless exposed to direct sunlight and desiccation. The infective larvae may be ingested by the host or penetrate the mudcaked skin. Earthworms may serve as transport hosts. The larvae lose their sheaths to reach the fourth stage in one of two sites, depending upon the route of entry. Orally ingested worms molt in the wall of the stomach, while those that penetrate the skin undergo this change in the abdominal muscles. The fourth-stage larvae soon migrate to the liver either via the portal veins when in-

gested or, following penetration of the skin, through the lungs and systemic circulation. They remain in the liver for two or three months, their movements exciting severe tissue reaction. Eventually the larvae break out of the liver into the peritoneal cavity and wander extensively, most of them eventually reaching the perirenal fat. Here the successful adults copulate and the female lays her eggs in a cyst, which then empties into the ureter. This life cycle requires about six months. Infected swine are commonly emaciated in spite of a good appetite, and ascites is frequent as a result of liver damage. Death may occur following secondary infection, extensive tissue destruction, or urinary obstruction. The condemnation of livers and carcasses of infected animals slaughtered for food makes the disease an important economic problem.

LESIONS

Both the larvae and the adult forms of this nematode produce severe effects upon the host. Nodules and edema in the subcutis and transitory enlargement of superficial lymph nodes are produced by the passage of larvae, but their most serious effect is upon the liver. Not only do these worms burrow into the liver, but during their relatively long stay they move about aggressively. This restive sojourn in the liver eventually results in extensive portal fibrosis, which may spread to obliterate many liver lobules. The fibrotic change is accompanied by intense tissue eosinophilia, foci of coagulation necrosis, and infiltration by other leukocytes. The lesions are often so severe that they render the liver totally unfit for human food.

This parasite, to a greater extent than most others, wanders through the host's tissue producing widespread damage. Although the successful worms find their way to the vicinity of the ureters, many wander to other sites, where they excite a local purulent tissue reaction. *S. dentatus* has been found in the kidney, lumbar muscles, myocardium, lungs, pleural cavity, spleen, and even the spinal canal. Paralysis may result from destruction of the lumbar spinal cord by the migrations of these worms.

DIAGNOSIS

The diagnosis may be made by demonstrating the ova in the urine, or by finding the worms at necropsy. Leukocytic infiltration and fibrosis in the liver are usually much more intense and extensive than the changes in this organ caused by other larvae (e.g., ascarids), a point that may be used in histologic differentiation.

References

Ashizawa H, Nosaka D, Tateyama S, et al. Pathological findings in stephanuriasis in pigs. I. Route of penetration of worms into the urinary passages. II. Pathological changes in the kidneys, ureters, and adjacent tissues. Bull Fac Agricul Miyazaki 1972;19:155–165, 167–178.

Ashizawa H, Nosaka D, Tateyama S, et al. Pathological findings in stephanuriasis in pigs. III. Pathological changes in the liver and lungs. Bull Fac Agricul Miyazaki, 1972;19:179–192.

Batte EG, Moncol DJ, Barber CW. Prenatal infection with the swine kidney worm *(Stephanurus dentatus)* and associated lesions. J Am Vet Med Assoc 1966;149:758–765.

Peneyra RS, Naui VC. Observations on the incidence and pathology of kidney-worm infection in swine (slaughterhouse material). Philipp J Vet Med 1967;4:129–140.

Gongylonemiasis

The adults of these tiny worms lie within the stratified squamous epithelium of the esophagus, the rumen, and stomach. They are often encountered in histologic sections of these organs, coiled in the epithelium (Fig. 13-26), apparently inciting little or no host reaction. The life cycle is indirect, using various coprophagous beetles as intermediate hosts. *Gongylonema pulchrum* occurs in sheep, cattle, goats, pigs, buffalo, and occasionally the horse, camel, wild boar, and donkey. It has been reported in humans. *G. verrucosum* inhabits the rumen of sheep, goats, cattle, deer, and zebu. It is known in the United States, India, and South Africa. *G. monnigi* infects sheep and goats in South Africa. Other species infect the rat *(G. neoplasticum)* nonhuman primates (Fig. 13-26), and birds.

References

Chitwood M, Lichtenfels JR. Parasitological review: identification of parasitic metazoa in tissue sections. Exp Parasitol 1972;32:407–519.

Georgi JR. Parasitology for Veterinarians. 2nd ed. Philadelphia: WB Saunders, 1974.

Lichtenfels JR. Morphological variation in the gullet nematode, *Gongylonema pulchrum* (Molin, 1857), from eight species of definitive hosts with a consideration of gongylonema from *Macaca* spp. J Parasitol 1971;57:348–355.

Soulsby EJL. Helminths, arthropods and protozoa of domesticated animals. 6th ed. Philadelphia: Lea & Febiger, 1968.

Zinter DE, Migaki G. *Gongylonema pulchrum* in tongues of slaughtered pigs. J Am Vet Med Assoc 1970;157:301–303.

Acanthocephalan infections

The Acanthocephalan, or thorny-headed, worms are classified in a separate phylum *(Acanthocephala)* from the nematodes. The worms are characterized by a spiny proboscis that attaches and burrows into the intestinal wall this may lead to perforation, but usually the worms are well-tolerated. They parasitize many species of mammals, birds, and fish; however, except for swine, they are not important to most species of domestic animals. They all have indirect life cycles. *Macrocanthorhynchus hirudinaceus (Echinorhynchus gigas)*, which infects domestic swine, uses various beetles as intermediate hosts. These parasites attach to the wall of the small intestine, often moving from site to site, where they penetrate the mucosa and muscularis and induce small ulcers surrounded by neutrophils and granulation tissue. Rarely, the parasites penetrate the wall, leading to peritonitis.

In dogs and wild carnivores, the thorny-headed worm Oncicola canis, a small worm that embeds its spiny proboscis in the wall of the small intestine, induces lesions comparable to those of M. hirudinaceus. *Prosthenorchis elegans* (Figs. 13-27, 13-28) is a common parasite of South American monkeys that uses cockroaches as one of its intermediate hosts. The numbers of parasites can be so numerous they almost occlude the lumen, but they are well tolerated and rarely lead to clinical disease.

References

Arambulo PV III, Blanea MR. The occurrence of *Macracanthorhynchus hirudinaceus* in swine in the Philippines with a note on its zoonotic implications. Kajian Veterinaire Malaysia-Singapore, 1972;4:5–8.

Dunn FL. Acanthocephalans and cestodes of South American monkeys and marmosets. J Parasitol 1963;49:717–722.

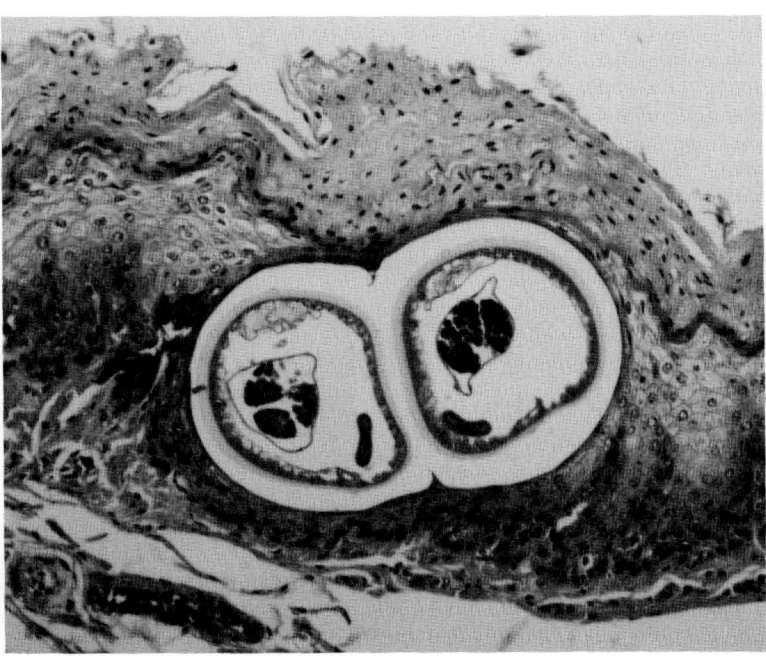

FIG. 13-26 *Gongylonema* sp. Cross sections of a parasite embedded in the epithelium of the tongue of a rhesus monkey *(Macaca mulatta).* (Courtesy New England Regional Primate Research Center, Harvard Medical School.)

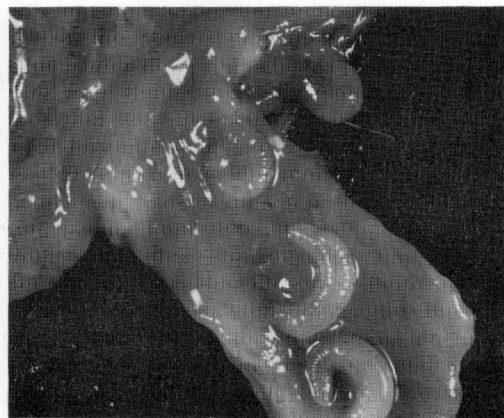

FIG. 13-27 *Prosthenorchis elegans* in a marmoset *(Saguinus oedipus)*. These acanthocephalids characteristically embed their thorny heads in the mucosa of the terminal ileum. (Courtesy New England Regional Primate Research Center, Harvard Medical School.)

Moore JG. Epizootic of acanthocephaliasis among primates. J Am Vet Med Assoc 1970;157:699–705.

Richart R, Benirschke K. Causes of death in a colony of marmoset monkeys. J Pathol Baet 1963;86:221–223.

Takos MJ, Thomas LJ. The pathology and pathogenesis of fetal infections due to an acanthocephalid parasite of marmoset monkeys. Am J Trop Med Hyg 1958;7:90–94.

Van Cleave HJ. Acanthocephala of *North American mammals. Ill Biol Monograph* 1953;23:(1–2):1–179.

Cestodiasis (tapeworm disease, taeniasis)

Cestodes, or tapeworms (phylum: Platyhelminthes, class: Cestoda), are common parasites of all vertebrate animals, including humans. An exception occurs in the United States, where the pig seems to be singularly free of tapeworms. The adult forms in the intestinal tract of the definitive host are flat worms made up of a chain of independent, hermaphroditic segments (proglottides); they are fastened together and usually attach to the intestinal mucosa by a specialized segment (scolex) at the anterior end. Each proglottid contains male and female genitalia and is complete in other respects; consequently, the tapeworm is in reality a colony of individuals attached to one another in a tapelike chain. As proglottides of most tapeworms mature, those at the caudal end are shed and expelled from the body with the feces, to release their innumerable ova.

All tapeworms have one or more larval stages (Fig. 13-29) through which they pass in various intermediate hosts, including insects and mammals; some tapeworms require more than one intermediate host. Only one tapeworm, *Hymenolepis nana*, a parasite of rodents, has a direct life cycle; here, the definitive host serves also for the stages of development usually completed within the intermediate host. These larval forms invade animal tissues, and by replacing vital cells can produce serious effects upon the host. Certain tapeworm larvae were recognized for a long time before their connection with the adult form was appreciated. For this reason, the lar-

val form may have a separate, well-established name; for example, *Cysticercus cellulosae* (Fig. 13-30), the bladderworm of "measly pork," is the larval form of *Taenia solium,* a tapeworm of humans.

The class Cestoda is usually divided into eleven orders, nine of which include parasites of fishes, annelids, reptiles, or amphibia, and two, Pseudophyllidea and Cyclophyllidea, in which are classified all tapeworms parasitic for humans and other mammals. The Pseudophyllidea are largely parasites of fish; the adult of only one species, *Diphyllobothrium latum,* is parasitic in mammals. Species of this order have a scolex that has no hooks and narrow, deep grooves, and **bothria,** instead of suckers. The eggs are usually operculated, resembling those of trematodes. All of the rest of the species of tapeworms parasitic for mammals are classified in the order Cyclophyllidea.

LIFE CYCLES

The adult tapeworms apparently produce little serious effect upon the host except in heavy infections, in which they interfere with digestion or cause partial obstruction. The adults all reside in the intestine, with the exception of a few species, such as: *Thysanosoma actinoides* (the fringed tapeworm); *Stilesia hepatica* (limited to Africa), which inhabit bile ducts in ruminants; and *Hymenolepis microstoma,* in bile ducts of rodents.

The parasites in their intermediate stages produce more important effects upon the host. The pathologist may encounter these intermediate stages of tapeworms in animal tissues; therefore, the identifying features of the different types are of diagnostic significance. The larvae usually develop in one of two possible ways, to become solid larvae and bladder larvae. In the first (solid) type, the ovoid, operculate ovum is passed out of the uterus to hatch into a ciliated motile embryo—the **coracidium,** which escapes through the operculum and becomes free-living. The coracidium is ingested by a freshwater crustacean, in whose tissues it develops into an elongated form, the **procercoid** larva. Development of this larva continues after the arthropod is swallowed by a second intermediate host (often a fish), until it becomes an elongated solid larva **(plerocercoid; sparganum),** with a head resembling that of the mature tapeworm. The broad fish tapeworm (*Diphyllobothrium latum*) provides an example of larval development of this type. "Spargana" is a term applied to certain plerocercoid larvae of other pseudophyllidae and the larvae of *Mesocestoides* spp., intermediate cestodes between pseudophyllidae and cyclophyllidae. The second (bladder) type of larvae, however, are most commonly termed **tetrathridia.**

In development of the second type, the larvae arise from eggs that are usually round or nearly square; the proglottid releases the larvae from the uterus when it disintegrates, or by discharge through one or more uterine pores by those species that have them. These eggs are fully developed when they escape from the uterus, in that they contain a larva, the **onchosphere** or **hexacanth** embryo, surrounded by a dense membrane. In the intestine of the intermediate host, the oncho-

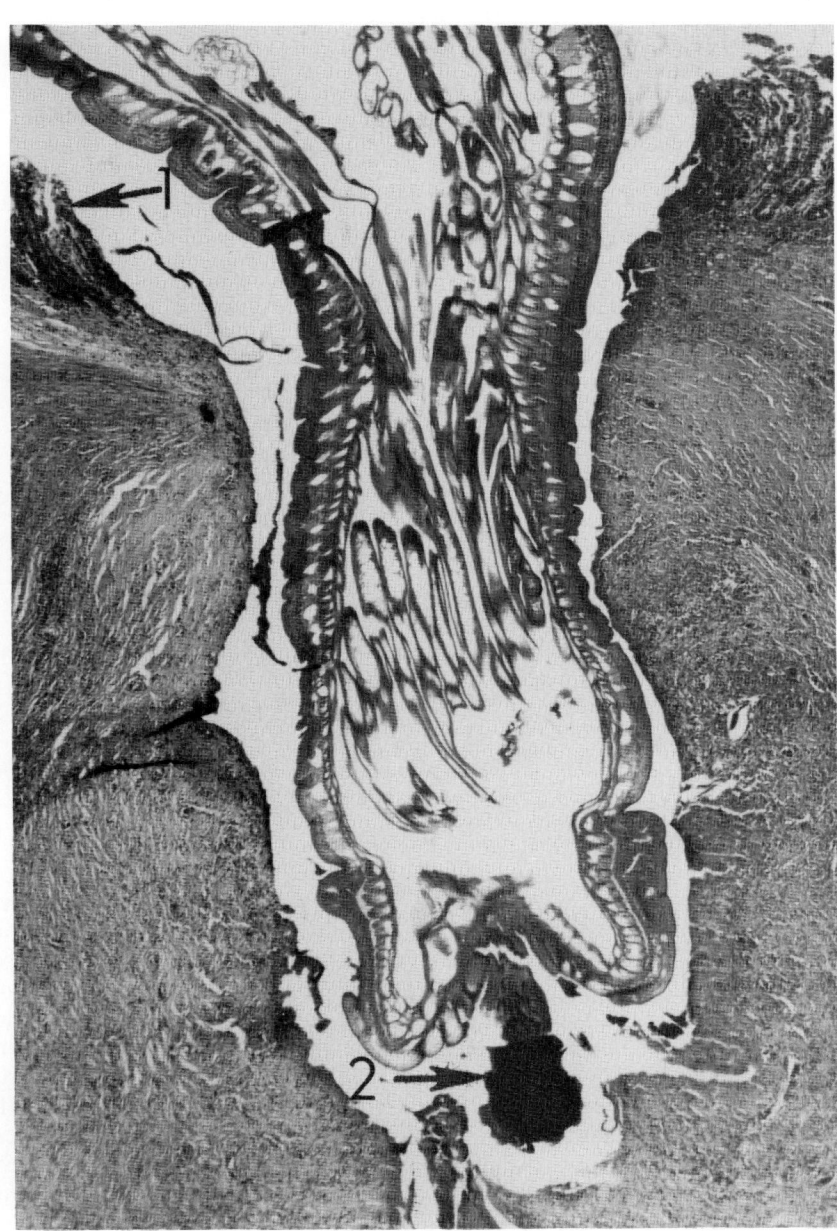

FIG. 13-28 Acanthocephalid in a marmoset *(Saguinus oedipus). Prosthenorchis elegans.* (1) Penetrated through the mucosa of the ileum; (2) Assisted by its thorny proboscis. (Courtesy New England Regional Primate Research Center, Harvard Medical School.)

sphere is released to migrate through the intestinal mucosa and enter the lymph or blood; it circulates to other tissues, where it becomes transformed into a bladder-shaped structure with one or more inverted scolices in an invaginated portion of the wall. When the larva has a solid caudal portion and a bladderlike proximal portion, it is called a **cysticercus.** Modifications of the cysticercus include: the **strobilocercus,** with an invaginated scolex attached to a small bladder by a segmented portion; the coenurus or **multiceps,** with a germinal layer capable of producing multiple scolices beneath the bladder wall; and the **echinococcus** or **hydatid cyst,** with a germinal layer that produces brood capsules within which scolices develop. **Cysticercoid,** a form usually found in invertebrates, consists of a small vesicle with a tiny cavity and one scolex. The scolices in all of these larval stages possess suckers and (in armed species)

hooklets identical to those of the adult stage. When ingested by the definitive host, the scolex evaginates and attaches itself to the intestinal mucosa; growth of the tapeworm then proceeds by proliferation of segments at the posterior extremity.

Some of the features of important tapeworms of domestic animals are outlined in Table 13-8.

Cysticercosis

The presence of larvae of certain tapeworms in the tissues of humans or animals results in a disease known as **cysticercosis** (beef or pork "measles," bladderworm disease). The effect upon the host depends largely on the organs involved and the degree of parasitism. In some sites, such as peritoneum and subcutis, the cysticerci are tolerated with little reaction, but those species

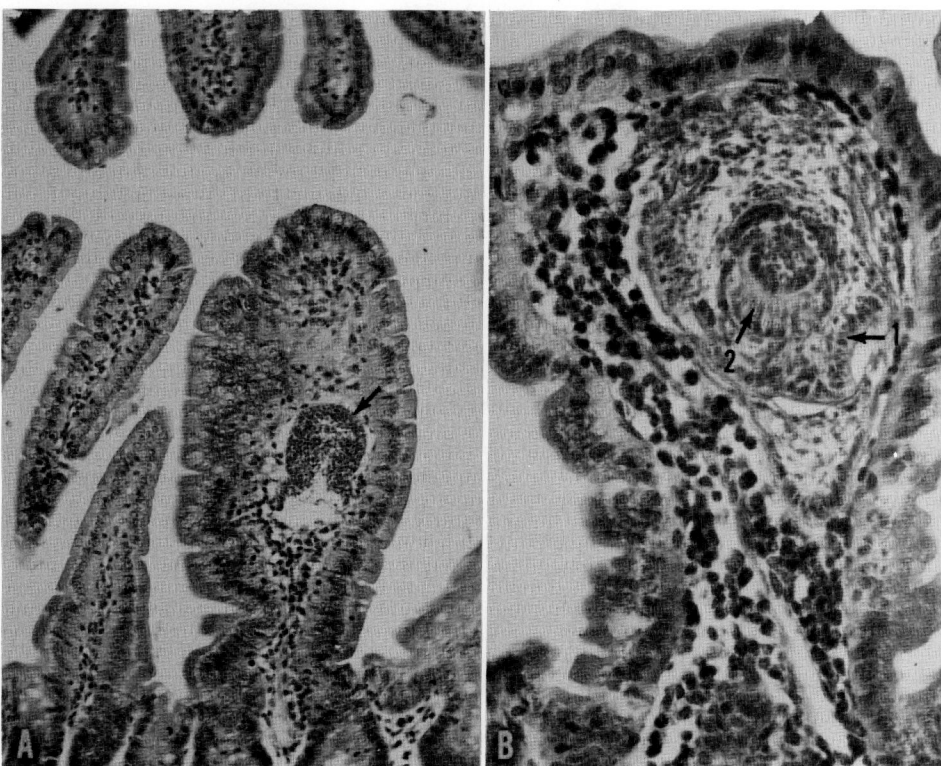

FIG. 13-29 Cestodiasis. **A.** Cysticercoid larva (arrow) of *Hymenolepis nana* (×45) in intestinal villus of a mouse. **B.** Later stage in larval development (×395). (1) Note sucker; and (2) Hooklets of the larva encysted in the lamina propria of the intestinal villus. (Courtesy of Armed Forces Institute of Pathology; contributor: Dr. W. S. Bailey.)

that invade and displace tissue in critical organs (liver, heart, brain) may produce grave signs or death.

Cysticercus bovis (larva of *Taenia saginata,* beef bladderworm), which may be found in muscle, liver, heart, lungs, diaphragm, lymph nodes, and other parts of the body of cattle, is important because the bovine parasite is the intermediate stage of a human tapeworm. Few symptoms are produced in cattle, but in some cases of massive infection death may occur following a febrile course. The cysticerci are usually found on postmortem inspection as small cysts, up to 9 mm in diameter; they occur in musculature or, in the heart, partly embedded and partly projecting from the surface. The cysts are white or gray; a small yellowish spot representing the scolex is unarmed (without hooklets). As a rule, the principal tissue change is displacement of normal cells, with little inflammatory reaction surrounding the viable bladderworm. In long-standing cases, however, death of the parasite is followed by dense encapsulation, which eventually forms a scar. Microscopic sections through the lesion may disclose the thin bladder wall and the invaginated scolex of the cysticercus bearing hooklets. The adult *T. saginata* has four suckers, but lacks a rostellum and has no hooks.

Cysticercus cellulosae (the pork bladderworm, or worm of "pork measles"), is the intermediate stage of *Taenia solium,* the adult that occurs in the small intestine of humans. In some instances this bladderworm has been found in cattle, sheep, deer, and humans. The cysticerci resemble *C. bovis* and are most frequent in striated muscles, particularly of the neck, cheek, shoul-

der, and tongue; however, the heart, abdominal wall, liver, lungs, brain, and eye may be involved. This bladderworm strongly resembles *Cysticercus bovis,* except that the scolex bears a double row of hooklets. This tapeworm is serious in humans because of the possibility of autoinfection, with cysticerci developing in the tissues. Diagnosis in humans is often possible by radiography because of the frequent calcification of mature cysts.

Cysticercus ovis, the intermediate stage of *Taenia ovis,* a tapeworm of dogs, foxes, wolves, coyotes, and other carnivores, is the cause of sheep "measles," or ovine cysticercosis. The bladderworms are found in the connective tissue of the heart, voluntary muscles, diaphragm, esophagus, and rarely, the lungs of sheep and goats. The effect of this parasite on its intermediate host is similar to that of the other cysticerci that invade the same tissues. Experimental feeding of large numbers of gravid proglottides of *Taenia ovis* has caused death in sheep. Heavy infections are also the cause of condemnation of animals slaughtered for food.

Coenurus cerebralis, the larval stage of a dog tapeworm, *Taenia (Multiceps) multiceps,* is the causative agent of an uncommon disease of the central nervous system of sheep known as "gid" or "sturdy." It may also infect other herbivorous animals and, rarely, carnivores, monkeys, and humans. Symptoms indicating central nervous involvement depend upon localization of the bladderworms in the brain or spinal cord, and vary from incoordination to paralysis. The larvae wander through the body before localizing in nervous tissue in the form of cysts, which reach a diameter of 50 mm or more.

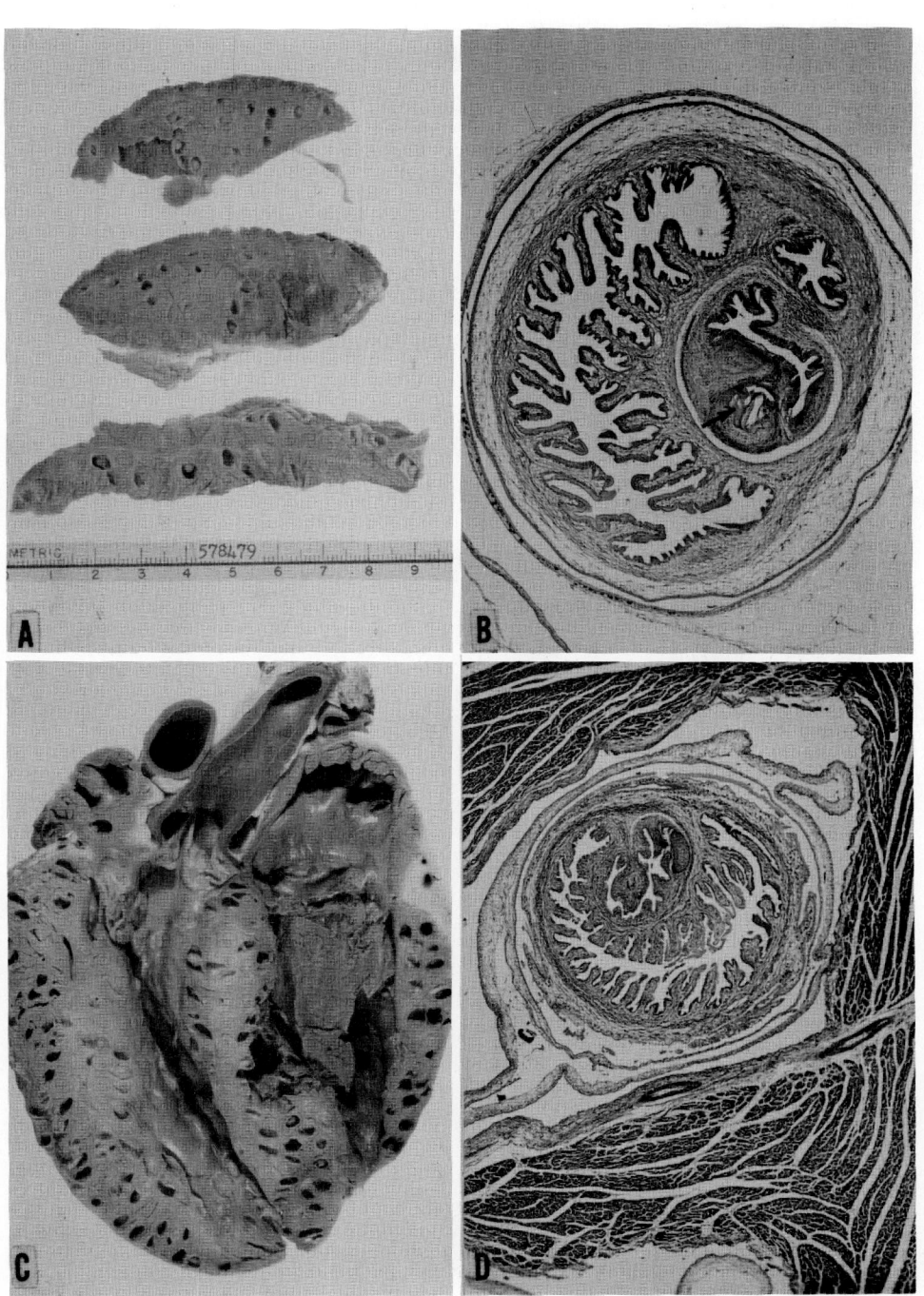

FIG. 13-30 Cestodiasis. An unusual bovine infection with the pork tapeworm *Cysticercus cellulosae (Taenia solium)*. **A.** Skeletal muscles containing cysticerci. **B.** A single inverted scolex (×38). Note hooklets (arrow) which distinguish this larva from that of the more common beef tapeworm, *Cysticercus bovis (Taenia saginata)*. **C.** Cysticerci in the myocardium. **D.** A single cysticercus (×21) in the heart muscle. (Courtesy of Armed Forces Institute of Pathology; contributor: Major C. N. Barron.)

Each cyst is filled with clear fluid and contains as many as 500 scolices, visible through the thin walls of the cyst as small white foci. The **coenurus** is a modified cysticercus with a germinal layer and the ability to produce many scolices. The disease has not been recognized in sheep in the United States for several decades. A relatively recent report described a coenurus in the brain of a cat in New York (Georgi et al., 1969).

Cysticercus tenuicollis, the intermediate stage of a tapeworm of dogs and other carnivores, *Taenia hydatigena*, is found chiefly in the liver, mesentery, and omentum of squirrels, cattle, wild ruminants, sheep, and swine. The cysticerci may be large, often attaining a diameter of 80 mm, but they contain only a single scolex armed with a double row of hooklets. The effect upon the intermediate host may not be obvious; the cysticerci may merely be noted during postmortem examination. The migration of the larvae through the liver results in necrotic tracts similar to those caused by *Fasciola hepatica*.

Other cysticerci that may be encountered by the veterinary pathologist include *Cysticercus pisiformis*, which occurs on the peritoneum and liver capsule of rabbits, squirrels, and other small rodents. The adult

TABLE 13-8 **Features of some important tapeworms**

Name of tapeworm	Adult host	Intermediate stage		
		Anatomic site	Type of larva	Intermediate hosts
Taenia saginata	Humans	Heart, skeletal muscle	Cysticercus (bovis)	Cattle
T. solium	Humans	Muscle, heart, viscera	Cysticercus (cellulosae)	Swine
Echinococcus granulosus	Humans, dog, fox, wolf, jackal	Liver, lungs, other viscera	Echinococcus (granulosus)	Humans, cattle, swine, sheep, deer, horse, moose, etc.
E. multilocularis	Humans, dog, fox, wolf, jackal	Liver, lungs, other viscera	Echinococcus (multilocularis)	Humans, cattle, swine, sheep, deer, horse, moose, etc.
Taenia hydatigena	Dog	Peritoneal cavity	Cysticercus (tenuicollis)	Squirrels, cattle, wild ruminants, sheep, goats, swine
T. ovis	Dog, fox, wolf, coyote	Muscles	Cysticercus (ovis)	Sheep, goats
T. pisiformis	Dog, cat, fox, wolf	Liver capsule, peritoneum	Cysticercus (pisiformis)	Rabbit, squirrel, other small rodents
T. taeniaeformis (syn.: *T. crassicollis*)	Cat, dog, fox	Liver	Cysticercus (fasciolaris)	Rats, mice, rabbits
T. (Multiceps) multiceps	Dog	Brain, spinal cord	Coenurus (cerebralis)	Sheep, goats
T. serialis	Dog, other carnivores	Subcutis	Coenurus (serialis)	Rabbit
Diphyllobothrium latum	Humans, bear, dog, cat, pig, fox	Muscles	Procercoid and plerocercoid	Microcrustacea, freshwater fish
Spirometra (Diphyllobothrium) mansonoides	Dog, cat	Peritoneal cavity	Procercoid and plerocercoid (sparganum)	Snakes, humans, monkeys, dog
Mesocestoides corti, M. lineatus	Dog, cat, wild carnivore, humans	Peritoneal and pleural cavities, liver, lung, other organs	Tetrathridium	Mites and wild rodents, dogs, cat, other mammals, reptiles
Dipylidium caninum	Dog, cat		Cysticercoid	Dog flea, biting lice
Moniezia expansa	Sheep, goats, cattle	—	Cysticercoid	Mites: *Galumna, Scheloribates, Scutovertex minutus*
M. benedeni	Sheep, goats, cattle	—	Cysticercoid	*Scutovertex minutus*
Anoplocephala magna	Equines	—	Cysticercoid	Mites of family *Oribatidae*
A. perfoliata	Equines	Intestinal tract	Cysticercoid	*Oribatidae*
Paranoplocephala mammillana	Equines	—	Cysticercoid	*Oribatidae*
Thysanosoma actinioides	Sheep, cattle, goats, deer	—	Cysticercoid	*Oribatidae*
Spirometra mansonoides	Cat	Connective tissue	Sparganum	Snakes, rodents

stage of this parasite *(Taenia pisiformis)* is attained in the small intestine of the dog, cat, fox, wolf, and other carnivores. A similar parasite, *Cysticercus fasciolaris* (or crassicollis), is found embedded in the liver of rats, mice, and other rodents; the adult form *(Taenia taeniaeformis)* is a tapeworm of the cat, less often of the dog, fox, and other carnivores. *Cysticercus fasciolaris* is of particular interest because of the undifferentiated sarcoma that often develops in the rat liver adjacent to the parasites. A bladderworm found in the subcutis of rabbits is known

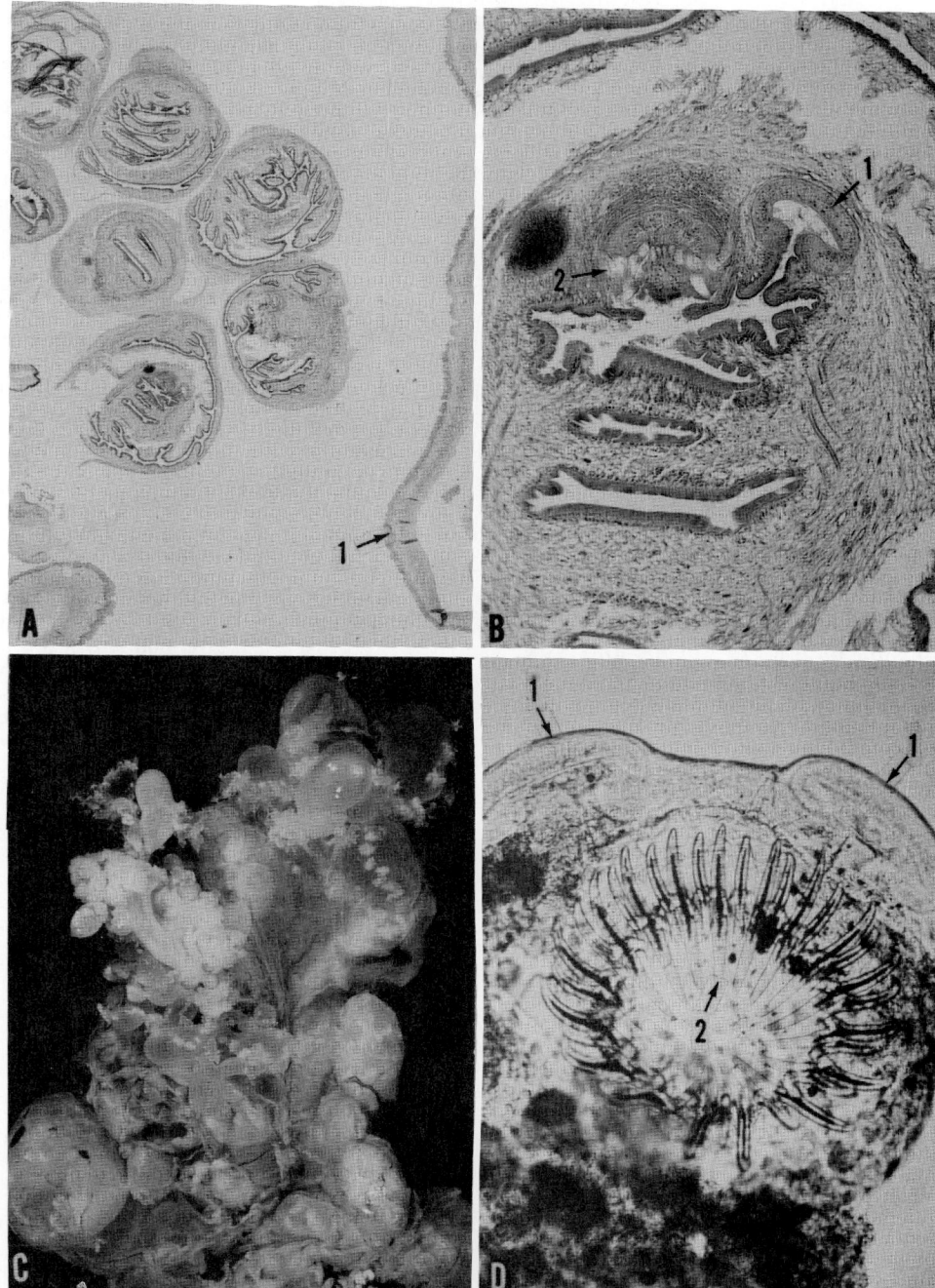

FIG. 13-31 Cestodiasis. A. Coenurus of *Multiceps serialis* (×12) in muscle of a rabbit. (1) Note several scolices and wall of cyst. B. A single inverted scolex of *M. serialis* (×50). (1) Note sucker; and (2) Hooklets. (Contributor: Capt. Morris Schneider, V.C.) C. *Multiceps serialis*. Larvae from the subcutis of a monkey. (Contributor: National Zoological Park.) D. Everted scolex (×150) of *Taenia pisiformis*. Larva from the peritoneum of a deer. (1) Note suckers; and (2) Hooklets. (Courtesy of Armed Forces Institute of Pathology; contributor: Capt. James R. Prine.)

as *Coenurus serialis* and is the intermediate stage of *Taenia (Multiceps) serialis* (Fig. 13-31), a tapeworm of the dog and closely related carnivores.

Sparganosis

Sparganosis is a term used to designate infection with the larva (**sparganum**) of certain Pseudophyllidea; the adults occur in mammals. The sparganum is an elongated, solid larva (**plerocercoid**) that may increase in number by transverse division. The first intermediate hosts are species of **Cyclopidae**, and the second are frogs, snakes, and mammals. In some, the sparganum is

recognized, but the adult form has not been identified. *Sparganum proliferum* occurs in the muscles and connective tissues of humans in Taiwan and Japan. The adult stage is believed to be *Spirometra ranarum* and parasitic in frogs. *Spirometra mansoni,* found in dogs and cats in Asia, produces spargana that are found in the connective tissues of snakes and rodents. *Sparganum mansoni* may infect the eye of humans through the practice of applying the flesh of frogs to treat eye disease, or by the consumption of infected *Cyclops* sp., frogs or snakes.

Spirometra mansonoides parasitizes the cat, bobcat, and dog in North America. Larvae (procercoids) infect various *Cyclops* species (*C. leukarti, C. bicuspidatus,* and

C. viridis), and the second intermediate hosts are wild mice, rats, and snakes. Experimental infection of humans has been demonstrated.

Spirometra erinacei has been found in the intestine of foxes and cats in Asia and Australia.

Infected wild pigs that have been found in the same habitat are believed to have acquired spargana from infected crustaceans or frogs. The precise association and identification of the larvae and adult forms of these parasites are not clearly established.

Tetrathridiosis is an infection with the intermediate stages of *Mesocestoides* spp. These stages resemble spargana and are often referred to as such. The adult tapeworms, which are of little consequence, parasitize dogs, cats, humans, and other mammals. Although imperfectly understood, the life cycle uses two intermediate hosts: a mite, followed by dogs, cats, wild mammals, or reptiles. In the second intermediate host, tetrathridia develop in the peritoneal and pleural cavities, lung, liver, and other organs, where they may incite an intense purulent and necrotizing inflammatory response; this may ultimately progress to a granulomatous reaction. *M. corti* occurs in North and Central America, and *M. lineatus*, in Europe and Asia.

References

Banerjee D, Singh KS. Studies on *Cysticercus fasciolaris*. III. Histopathology and histochemistry of rat liver in cysticerciasis. Indian J Anim Sci 1969;39:242–249.

Barclay WP, Phillips TN, Foerner JJ. Intussusception associated with *Anoplocephala perfoliata* infection in five horses. J Am Vet Med Assoc 1982;180:752–753.

Cárdenas-Ramírez L, Celis-Salgado P, Hernández-Jauregui P. Ocular and orbital cysticercosis in hogs. Vet Pathol 1984;21:164–167.

Clark JD. Coenurosis in a Gelada baboon (*Theropithecus gelada*). J Am Vet Med Assoc 1969;155:1258–1263.

Corkum KC. Sparganosis in some vertebrates of Louisiana and observations on human infection. J Parasitol 1966;52:444–448.

Davis JA, Donkaewbua S, Wagner JE, et al. *Cysticercus fasciolaris* infection in a breeding colony of mice. Lab Anim Sci 1989;39:250–252.

Dinnik JA, Sachs R. Cysticercosis, echinococcosis, and sparganosis in wild herbivores in East Africa. Vet Med Rev 1969;2:104–114.

Fertig DL, Dorn CR. *Taenia saginata* cysticercosis in an Ohio cattle feeding operation. J Am Vet Med Assoc 1985;186:1281–1285.

Gemmell MA. Hydatidosis and cysticercosis. 2. Distribution of *Cysticercus ovis* in sheep. Aust Vet J 1970;46:22–24.

Georgi JR, DeLahunta A, Percy DH. Cerebral coenurosis in a cat: report of a case. Cornell Vet 1969;59:127–134.

Greve JH, Tyler DE. *Cysticercus pisiformis* (Cestoda: Taenidae) in the liver of a dog. J Parasitol 1964;50:712–716.

Hayunga EG, Sumner MP, Rhoads ML, et al. Development of a serologic assay for cysticercosis, using an antigen isolated from *Taenia* spp cyst fluid. Am J Vet Res 1991;52:462–470.

Hernandez-Jauregui PA, Márquez-Monter H, Sastre-Ortiz S. Cysticercosis of the central nervous system in hogs. Am J Vet Res 1973;34:451–453.

Irfan M, Hatch C. The pathology of *Taenia hydatigena* infection in Irish lambs. Irish Vet J 1969;23:62–66.

Ivens V, Conroy JD, Levine ND. *Taenia pisiformis* cysticerci in a dog in Illinois. Am J Vet Res 1969;30:2017–2020.

Jones ND, Brooks DR, Harris RL. *Macaca mulatta*: a new host for *Choanotaenia* cestodes. Lab Anim Sci 1980;39:575–577.

Kassai T, Mahunka S. Vectors of *Moniezia*. Magy Allatorv Lap 1964;19:531–538, Vet Bull 1965;35:4282.

Larsh JE Jr, Race GJ, Esch GW. A histopathologic study of mice infected with the larval stage of *Multiceps serialis*. J Parasitol 1965;51:45–52.

Lloyds TS. Hepatitis cysticercosa causing sudden death in a pig. Vet Rec 1964;76:1080.

Lyons ET, Drudge JH, Tolliver SC, et al. Prevalence of *Anoplocephala perfoliata* and lesions of *Draschia megastoma* in Thoroughbreds in Kentucky at necropsy. Am J Vet Res 1984;45:996–999.

McIntosh A, Miller D. Bovine cysticercosis, with special reference to the early developmental stages of *Taenia saginata*. Am J Vet Res 1960;21:169–177.

Migaki G, Zinter DE. Hepatic lesions caused by *Cysticercus tenuicollis* in sheep. J Am Vet Med Assoc 1974;164:618–619.

Pawlowski Z, Schultz MG. Taeniasis and cysticercosis (*Taenia saginata*). Adv Parasitol 1972;10:269–343.

Pearson GR, Davies LW, White AL, et al. Pathological lesions associated with *Anoplocephala perfoliata* at the ileo-caecal junction of horses. Vet Rec 1993;132:179–182.

Silverman PH, Hulland TJ. Histological observations on bovine cysticercosis. Res Vet Sci 1961;2:248–252, Vet Bull 1961;61:4022.

Smith MC, Bailey CS, Baker N, et al. Cerebral coenurosis in a cat. J Am Vet Med Assoc 1988;192:82–84.

Sulaiman S, Williams JF, Wu D. Natural infections of vervet monkeys (*Cercopithecus aethiops*) and African red monkeys (*Erythrocebus patas*) in Sudan with taeniid cysticerci. J Wildl Dis 1986;22:586–587.

Tazieva AK. Histological differences between cysticerci of small ruminants. Parazity sel'skokhoz zhivotnykh Kazakhstan 1964;3:7–29, Vet Bull 1965;35:975.

Thompson JE. Some observations on the European broad fish tapeworm *Diphyllobothrium latum*. J Am Vet Med Assoc 1936;89:77–86.

Todd KS Jr, Simon J, DiPietro JA. Pathological changes in mice infected with tetrathyridia of *Mesocestoides corti*. Lab Anim 1978;12:51–53.

Vickers JH, Penner LR. Cysticercosis in four rhesus brains. J Am Vet Med Assoc 1968;153:868–871.

Voge M, Berntzen AK. Asexual multiplication of larval tapeworms as the cause of fatal parasitic ascites in dogs. J Parasitol 1963;49:983–988.

Williams JF, Shearer AM. Longevity and productivity of *Taenia taeniaeformis* in cats. Am J Vet Res 1981;42:2182–2183.

Williams JF, Lindsay M, Engelkirk P. Peritoneal cestodiasis in a dog. J Am Vet Med Assoc 1985;186:1103–1105.

Echinococcosis

The larval or intermediate stages of tapeworms in the genus *Echinococcus* are known as hydatid cysts, and the disease they induce is called **echinococcosis** or **hydatid disease.** The adult tapeworms are of little concern; however, the larval forms, which localize in the liver, lungs, and other vital organs, induce serious disease. Four species of *Echinococcus* exist. Dogs and wild carnivores serve as the principle definitive hosts for *E. granulosus,* whose larvae are most commonly encountered in sheep, but can also infect cattle, horses, deer, moose, swine, monkeys, rodents, and humans and other species. It is distributed worldwide. Several strains exist with affinity for a particular intermediate host. Foxes serve as the principal definitive hosts for the adults of *E. multilocularis,* but dogs, cats, and coyotes can also serve that function. Larval forms occur in various rodents, chiefly voles, field mice, shrews, and ground squirrels, although humans can be infected. This species occurs in the Northern Hemisphere, particularly Canada and northern Europe. *E. oligarthus* is a parasite of various wild felids in Central and South America. Agoutis serve as intermediate hosts. *E. vogeli* occurs in central and northern South America as a parasite of dogs, with the intermediate stages in pacas and other rodents, and on occasion, humans.

Eggs ingested by the appropriate intermediate host hatch in the small intestine; the released onchospheres invade a venule or lymphatic, pass to the liver or lungs, where they may lodge; or, they pass into the general circulation and are disseminated elsewhere to develop into a hydatid that slowly grows. The hydatid of *E. granulosus* is unilocular, consisting of a thick concentrically laminated outer membrane encasing a germinal membrane, from which numerous spheric brood capsules arise. These may be attached by a short stalk, or be free in the cyst where they are termed "hydatid sand". Each brood capsule contains germinal epithelium from which as many as 40 scolices (Fig. 13-32) arise. Each scolex is ovoid and bears a crown of 32–40 hooklets, 21–29 μm in length. Daughter cysts may form within the parent cyst and, when the outer membrane ruptures, external to the parent cyst. The hydatids of *E. multilocularis* regularly produce multilocular hydatids with external daughter cysts. *E. oligarthus* and *E. vogeli* are polycystic. Hydatids may be sterile, lacking scolices.

The effect on the host depends upon the organ parasitized and the size attained by the hydatid cyst, which may measure up to several inches. The hydatids are usually surrounded by mononuclear cells, eosinophils, multinucleated giant cells, and fibrous connective tissue. The inflammatory reaction becomes severe when the cyst ruptures. In humans, rupture of the cyst can lead to anaphylactic shock or other severe allergic reactions. Adjacent tissues undergo compression atrophy. Hydatids may degenerate spontaneously, in which case they undergo calcification.

DIAGNOSIS

The presence of the adult worm in the intestinal tract can be verified by the demonstration of segments and ova in the feces, but the intermediate stage presents more difficulties. The hydatid cysts may be identified by pathologic examination of tissue removed at exploratory laparotomy or at necropsy. Complement fixation test, delayed hypersensitivity tests, hemagglutination tests, fluorescent antibody test, and other immunologic procedures have been used with varying results.

References

Binhazim AA, Harmon BG, Roberson EL, et al. Hydatid disease in a horse. J Am Vet Med Assoc 1992;200:958–960.

Crellin JR, Marchiondo AA, Andersen FL. Comparison of suitability of dogs and cats as hosts of *Echinococcus multilocularis*. Am J Vet Res 1981;42:1980–1981.

Crosby WM, Ivey MH, Shaffer WL, et al. *Echinococcus cysts* in the Savannah baboon. Lab Anim Care 1968;18:395–397.

Dent CHR. Cerebral hydatids in a cow. Aust Vet J 1966;42:28–30.

Foley GL, Georgi M. Hydatidosis in a horse. Vet Pathol 1986;23:646–647.

Gelberg HB, Todd KS, Duckett WM, et al. Hydatid disease in a horse. J Am Vet Med Assoc 1984;184:342–343.

Goldberg GP, Fortman JD, Beluhan FZ, et al. Pulmonary *Echinococcus granulosus* in a baboon (*Papio anubis*). Lab Anim Sci 1991;41:177–180.

Hatch C. Hydatidosis in Irish horses. Irish Vet J 1972;26:74–77.

Healy GR, Hayes NR. Hydatid disease in rhesus monkeys. J Parasitol 1963;49:837.

Hutchison WF. Studies on *Echinococcus granulosus*. III. The rhesus monkey (*Macaca mulatta*) as a laboratory host for the larval stage. J Parasitol 1966;52:416.

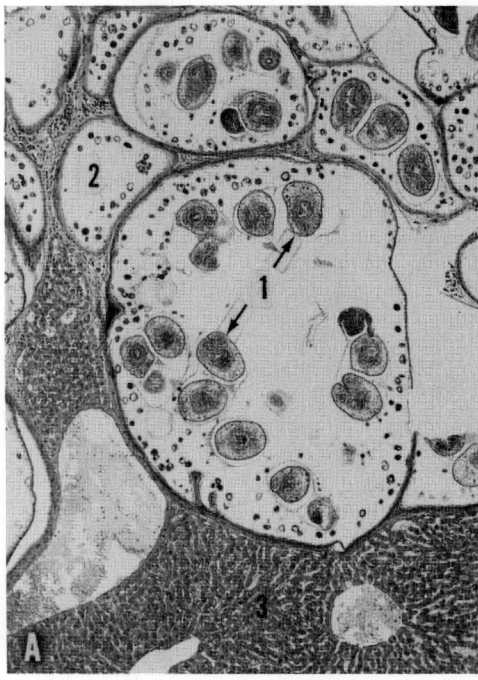 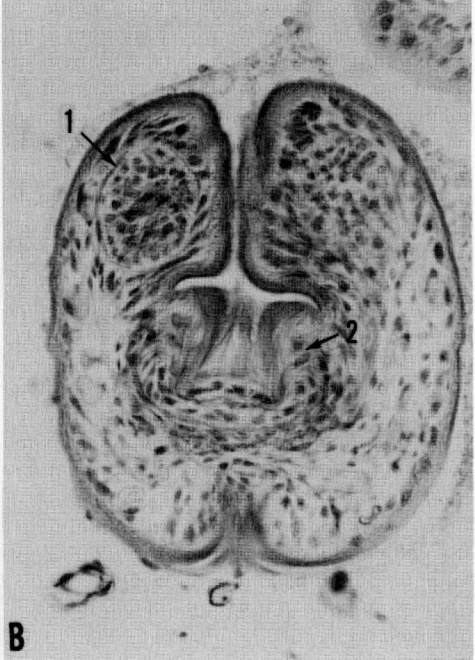

FIG. 13-32 Echinococcosis. **A.** *Echinococcus multilocularis* (×50) in the liver of a vole. (1) Note many inverted scolices, some surrounded by a thin, brood capsule; (2) Some daughter cysts do not yet contain fully developed scolices; (3) Liver parenchyma is displaced by the cysts. **B.** A single scolex (×525). (1) Note part of inverted sucker; and (2) Hooklets. (Courtesy of Armed Forces Institute of Pathology; contributor: Dr. Robert Rausch.)

Islam AWMS. *Echinococcus granulosus* in dogs in Bangladesh. Am J Vet Res 1980;41:415–416.

Kamiya M, Sato H. Complete life cycle of the canid tapeworm *Echinococcus multilocularis,* in laboratory rodents. FASEB J 1990;4:3334–3339.

Leiby PD. Cestode in North Dakota: echinococcus in field mice. Science 1965;150:763.

Leiby PD, Kritsky DC. *Echinococcus multilocularis:* a possible domestic life cycle in central North America and its public health implications. J Parasitol 1972;58:1213–1215.

Leiby PD, Olsen OW. The cestode *Echinococcus multilocularis* in foxes in North Dakota. Science 1964;145:1066.

Matoff K, Yanchev Y. The fox as definitive host of *Echinococcus granulosus.* Acta Vet Hung 1965;15:155–160, Vet Bull 1966;36:640.

Myers BJ, Kuntz RE, Vice TE. Hydatid disease in captive primates *(Colobus* and *Papio).* J Parasitol 1965;51:22.

Powers RD, Price RA, Houk RP, et al. Echinococcosis in a drill baboon. J Am Vet Med Assoc 1966;149:902–905.

Rausch R. Studies on the helminth fauna of Alaska. XX. The histogenesis of alveolar larvae of *Echinococcus* species. J Infect Dis 1954;94:178–186.

Verster AJM. Review of echinococcus species in South Africa. Onderstepoort J Vet Res 1965;32:7–118.

Ward JW. Additional records of *Echinococcus granulosus* from dogs in the lower Mississippi region. J Parasitol 1965;51:552–553.

Trematodiasis (distomiasis)

Trematodes are flat worms in the same family (Platyhelminthes) as the cestodes. Most are leaflike in shape and have one or two suckers. The term **distoma,** which was the former name of a specific genus, has come to be synonymous with trematode. There exist three subclasses of trematodes, but all that are parasitic in domestic animals lie within the subclass Digenea. Each has an indirect **life cycle.** In the typical life cycle, the hermaphroditic parasites deposit ova which, for most of the parasitic flukes, exit through the feces. Fluke eggs are usually operculated, yellow-brown, and anisotropic; these are features that aid in their identification in tissue sections. Each ovum, under warm moist conditions, produces a free-living ciliated larva **(miracidium),** which either bores into the body or is ingested by one of several varieties of snails. Here, they encyst to become a **sporocyst,** which reproduces asexually to produce daughter sporocysts or several generations of **rediae** that begin to take on the appearance of an adult fluke. The final stages in the snail are motile **cercariae,** which leave the intermediate host and usually encyst on plants to become the infective stage **(metacercariae).** Many flukes require a second intermediate host (e.g., *Dicrocoelium dendriticum*) in which the metacercariae are formed. Infection in the final host is established by ingestion of the metacercariae. Those flukes that inhabit the liver (Figs. 13-33, 13-34) are the most important to animals. Flukes may also reside in the intestinal tract, pancreatic ducts, lungs, and veins (Schistosoma). Tables 13-9 and 13-10 list many of the parasitic trematodes of animals.

Hepatic distomiasis (liver fluke disease, fascioliasis, fascioloidiasis, dicrocoeliasis)

Liver flukes are significant pathogens in domestic animals, particularly sheep and cattle. The most important species are *Fasciola hepatica* (common liver fluke), *Fasciola gigantica* (large African liver fluke), *Fascioloides magna* (large liver fluke), and *Dicrocoelium dendriticum*

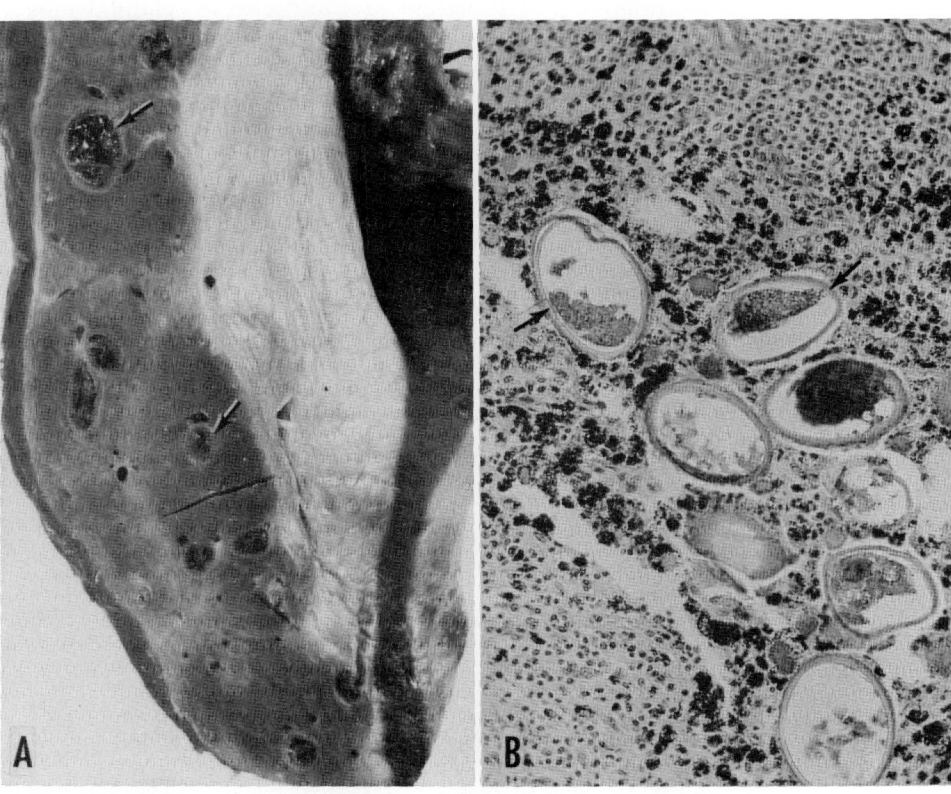

FIG. 13-33 Distomiasis. **A.** Liver of a sheep with distended, thick-walled bile ducts (arrows) containing *Dicrocoelium dendriticum.* (Contributor: Dr. G. Dikmans.) **B.** Ova of *Fascioloides magna* (arrows) in a bovine liver (×150). Note black granular pigment interspersed among the ova. (Courtesy of Armed Forces Institute of Pathology; contributor: Dr. Henry J. Griffiths.)

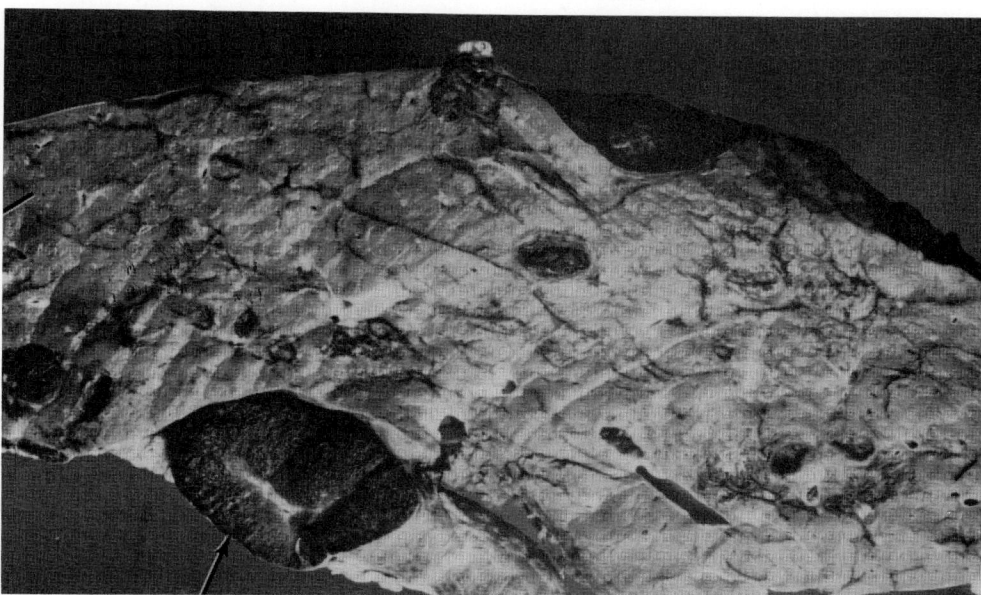

FIG. 13-34 Circumscribed zones of black pigment in the liver of a deer infected with *Fascioloides magna,* the large liver fluke. The adjacent lymph nodes contained similar pigment.

(lancet fluke). Many other species also infect the liver of various animals (Table 13-9), some of which are briefly discussed at the end of this section.

Fasciola hepatica

Fasciola hepatica in its adult form is found in the liver, bile ducts, and gallbladder of cattle and sheep, but it may also parasitize the horse (rarely), goat, dog, cat, rabbit, guinea pig, squirrel, deer, beaver, pig, and humans. The adult fluke is 20–30 mm long and about 13 mm wide; it is flattened and leaflike, and usually reddish-brown. It is hermaphroditic and reproduces by depositing ova in the biliary passages, through which they reach the intestine and are expelled with the feces. The life cycle, which typically follows that described above, uses several species of amphibious snails of the genus *Lymnaea.* Following ingestion, infective metacercariae encyst in the duodenum, penetrate the wall, and migrate through the abdominal cavity to the liver. The immature flukes migrate in the liver for about six weeks and start to reach the bile ducts, where they become adults during the seventh week.

LESIONS

The lesions produced by the common liver fluke are most constant and important in the liver, although occasional parasites may wander into the lungs or other tissues. The lesions in the liver can be divided into those caused by migrating larvae, and those induced by the adults; however, the effects of both may be present simultaneously. After initial penetration of the liver parenchyma by the flukes, hepatic cells are destroyed as the larvae migrate and cause tracts of blood, fibrin, and cellular debris. These tracts soon become filled with neutrophils, eosinophils, and lymphocytes. Macrophages, epithelioid cells, and multinucleated giant cells become increasingly numerous in older lesions, particularly around dead larvae. The lesions ultimately heal by ingrowth of granulation tissue, causing random scarring. If exposed to large numbers of metacercariae, this early migration results in extensive damage to the liver, causing an acute syndrome characterized by anemia, eosinophilia, peritonitis (due to initial migration), and sudden death. This acute syndrome is more frequent in sheep than in cattle.

Flukes that reach the bile ducts start producing eggs by the tenth week following oral infection. Their presence in the biliary passages excites considerable tissue reaction, leading to cholangiohepatitis. The biliary epithelium is stimulated to papillary and glandular hyperplasia, in some places, and is eroded in others. The walls of the ducts become infiltrated with eosinophils, lymphocytes, and macrophages, and eventually become significantly thickened from fibrous proliferation. Partial or complete occlusion of the bile ducts is a frequent effect. The extensive fibrosis and calcification of bile ducts, most frequent in cattle, gives rise to the descriptive term "pipe-stem liver." Small granulomas may form around eggs that become lodged in small bile ducts.

Extensive infection interferes with liver function, causing weight loss or failure to gain normally. Elevated serum hepatic enzymes, eosinophilia, hypoproteinemia, and progressive anemia are usual findings. Low serum albumin due to plasma leakage through bile ducts causes the hypoproteinemia. Anemia results from both hemorrhage into the migrating larval tracts, as well as blood-sucking by the adults and hemorrhage into the bile ducts. The anemia may be normocytic, normochromic, macrocytic, or have the characteristics of iron deficiency anemia.

Fasciola gigantica

Fasciola gigantica resembles *Fasciola hepatica,* but is larger, the adults measuring up to 75 mm in length and about 12 mm wide. These flukes are common parasites

TABLE 13-9 **Representative species of trematodes (flukes)**

Parasite	Hosts	Site of adult	Intermediate host(s)
Family: Diplostomidae			
Alaria spp.	Dog, cat, fox, mink	Small intestine	Snail and tadpole, frogs
Family: Dicrocoeliidae			
Dicrocoelium dendriticum	Sheep, goat, deer, pig, dog	Bile ducts	Snail and ant
Platynosomum fastosum	Cats	Liver, bile ducts	Snail and lizard, crustaceans
Athesmia foxi	New World monkeys	Bile ducts	Molluscs, possibly others
Eurytrema pancreaticum	Sheep, goat, cattle	Pancreatic and bile ducts, duodenum	Snail and grasshopper, crickets
Concinnum procyonis	Raccoon, fox, cat	Pancreatic and bile ducts	Snail, possibly others
Family: Heterophyidae			
Heterophyes heterophyes	Dog, cat, fox, humans	Small intestine	Snail and fish
Mentagonimus yokogawai	Dog, cat, pig, humans	Small intestine	Snail and fish
Euryhelmis squamula E. monorchis	Mink, fox	Small intestine	Snail and frogs
Apophallus donicum	Dog, cat, fox, humans	Small intestine	Snail and fish
Cryptocotyle spp	Dog, cat, fox, mink	Small intestine	Snail and fish
Family: Opisthorchiidae			
Opisthorchis tenuicollis	Dog, cat, fox, pig	Pancreatic and bile ducts	Snail and fish
Chlonorchis sinensis (*Opisthorchis sinensis*)	Dog, cat, pig, humans	Bile ducts, duodenum	Snail and fish
Pseudamphistomum truncatum	Dog, cat, fox	Bile ducts	Snail and fish
Metorchis albidus	Dog, cat, fox	Bile ducts	Snail and fish
M. conjunctus	Dog, cat, fox, mink	Bile ducts	Snail and fish
Family: Nanophyetidae			
Nanophyetus salmincola	Dog, cat, fox, mink, raccoon, skunk	Small intestine	Snail and fish
Family: Fasciolidae			
Fasciola hepatica	Cattle, sheep, goat, dog, cat, horse, humans	Bile ducts	Snail
Fasciola gigantica	Cattle, sheep	Bile ducts	Snail
Fascioloides magna	Cattle, sheep, horse, pig	Liver	Snail
Fascioloides buski	Pig, humans	Small intestine	Snail
Family: Echinostomatidae			
Echinochasmus perfoliatus	Dog, cat, fox, pig	Small intestine	Snail, fish
Isthmiophora melis	Cat, fox, mink	Small intestine	Snail
Family: Hasstilesiidae			
Skrjabinotrema ovis	Sheep	Colon	Snail
Family: Troglotrematidae			
Troglotrema acutum	Fox, mink	Frontal and ethmoid sinuses	Snail

(continued)

TABLE 13-9 (continued)

Parasite	Hosts	Site of adult	Intermediate host(s)
Family: Paragonimidae			
Paragonimus westermani	Dog, cat, pig	Lungs	Snail and crawfish
P. kellicotti	Dog, cat, pig, mink	Lungs	Snail and crawfish
Family: Paramphistomatidae			
Paramphistomum cervi and other spp.	Cattle, sheep, goat	Rumen	Snail
Cotylophoron cotykophorum			
Calicophoron calicophorum			
Ceylonocotyle streptocoelium			
Fishoederius spp.			
Gastrothylax crumenifer			
Carmyerius spp.			
Gastrodiscus aegyptiacus	Horse, pig	Small intestine	Snail
Pseudodiscus collinsi	Horse	Colon	Snail
Gigantocotyle explanatum	Cattle, buffalo	Bile ducts	Snail
Family: Schistosomatidae*			

*See Table 13-10.

---

of cattle and sheep in Africa, Taiwan, Hawaii, and the Philippines. *F. gigantica* also occurs in Europe and the southern United States. The intermediate hosts are also species of Lymnaea. The effects of this trematode are similar to those caused by *Fasciola hepatica.*

Fascioloides magna, the large liver fluke, occurs in the liver of cattle, deer (Fig. 13-34), sheep, moose, horse, wapiti, yak, bison and rarely swine, and has also been reported in the lungs of some of these hosts. Rabbits and guinea pigs are susceptible to experimental infection. This fluke is similar in appearance to the common liver fluke, except that it is larger, 30 by 80 mm in greatest dimension, and has more rounded ends. It is hermaphroditic and its life cycle is similar to that of *Fasciola hepatica;* snails are required as intermediate hosts. The infective forms penetrate the intestinal wall and wander around in the peritoneal cavity before invading the liver. Within the liver parenchyma, the migrations of this fluke produce severe damage in some hosts, and less in others. In the "true" hosts (deer, wapiti, moose), the parasite is well-tolerated. Although it soon becomes encysted, the cyst wall is thin and its lumen communicates with bile ducts. Thus, ova of the fluke escape with its excreta into the intestinal lumen of the host, a factor that favors the completion of the life cycle of the parasite.

In Bovidae (cattle, bison, yak), however, the flukes wander briefly through the liver parenchyma, destroying tissue and eliciting a reaction of the host, which encapsulates the parasites. A cyst soon forms, but its lumen rarely communicates with the bile ducts; consequently, excreta and ova accumulate around the fluke. Black granular pigment collects in the cyst and is phagocytized by the macrophages of the host. This distinctive pigment is believed to be part of the excrement of the fluke, because similar material can be found within its alimentary tract. The black, sooty pigment is often grossly visible in affected liver. The failure of the fluke to establish and maintain continuity with the bile ducts in these hosts prevents the ova from escaping. For this reason, cattle and bison are unfavorable hosts for the propagation of the parasite.

In sheep, the migration of this large liver fluke through the liver is almost entirely unchecked; hence, severe tissue destruction and marked clinical disease result. A severe neutrophilic and eosinophilic tissue reaction, with little attempt at encapsulation, is the rule in the liver of infected sheep. Even a few flukes may, by their wanderings through the liver, produce severe symptoms and death in sheep. They also wander in and out of the hepatic vascular system, causing phlebitis, arteritis, and thrombosis, which further accentuates hepatic damage. The death of this host brings to a halt the life cycle of the parasite; therefore, the sheep is not considered a true host for *Fascioloides magna.*

Dicrocoelium dendriticum

Dicrocoelium dendriticum, the Old World, or lancet, fluke, is capable of infecting cattle, sheep, goats, horses, camels, deer, elk, pigs, dogs, rabbits, and humans. This parasite, smaller than the other flukes, is 5–12 mm long and about 1 mm wide. It is slender, flat, and lancet-shaped, with pointed ends.

The life cycle of the lancet fluke has been elucidated by the work of Krull and Mapes (1953), who found that this parasite requires not only a snail as intermediate host, but also an ant *(Formica fusca)* as a second intermediate host. A fascinating bit of biologic knowledge lies in the report of Anokhin (1966), who

TABLE 13-10 **Schistosomiasis**

Species	Natural definitive hosts	Anatomic site of adult fluke	Geographic distribution
Schistosoma japonicum	Humans, dog, cat, rat, cattle, sheep, water buffalo, goat, horse, swine	Mesenteric and portal veins, hemorrhoidal plexus	China, Japan, Taiwan, Celebes, Philippines
S. hematobium	Humans, monkey	Pelvic veins, esp. vesical and mesenteric, vesicoprostatic, pubic, and uterine plexus	Africa, Western Asia, Southern Europe, Australia
S. mansoni	Humans, monkey	Mesenteric and portal veins, hemorrhoidal plexus	Africa, South America, West Indies
S. bovis	Cattle, sheep, goat, horse, mule, antelope, baboon	Portal and mesenteric veins	Africa, Southern Asia, Sardinia
S. spindale	Cattle, sheep, goat, antelope, water buffalo, dogs	Mesenteric and portal veins	India, Sumatra, Africa
S. hippopotami	Hippopotamus	Cardiovascular system generally	South Africa
S. incognitum	Dog, pig	Mesenteric and portal veins	India
S. nasalis	Cattle, goats, horses	Nasal veins	India
S. indicum	Cattle, sheep, goats, horse, camels	Mesenteric, portal, and pelvic veins	India
S. intercalatum	Humans, horses, cattle, sheep	Mesenteric and portal veins	Africa
S. mattheei	Cattle, sheep, goats, horses, and rarely humans	Mesenteric and portal veins	Africa
Schistosomatium douthitti	Meadow mouse, vole, hare, muskrat	Mesenteric veins	North America
Trichobilharzia ocellata	Wild and domesticated ducks	Mesenteric veins	Europe and North America
T. stagnicolae	Canaries, possibly other birds	Mesenteric veins	North America
T. physellae	Ducks, teal	Mesenteric veins	North America
Heterobilharzia americana	Dog, raccoon, bobcat, rabbit, nutria	Mesenteric veins	North America
Ornithobilharzia bomfordi	Zebu, cattle	Mesenteric veins	India
O. turkestanicum	Cattle, sheep, goats, horses, camels, cats	Mesenteric veins	Eurasia

confirmed Hohorst's observation that encysted metacercariae in the brains of ants (Formica nigricans) cause the ants to remain on herbage after normal ants return to their nest. This presumably increases the possibility that infected ants will be ingested by a grazing cow or sheep. The final hosts are infected by the ingestion of ants containing encysted metacercariae. When released in the small intestine, the metacercariae migrate to the liver by way of the common bile duct. The adult flukes are found in the bile ducts of the definitive host. The infection is less severe than that or Fasciola hepatica; also, because they are smaller, they may be found in smaller bile ducts. Hyperplasia of bile duct epithelium occurs; also, although superficial erosions are present, plasma or blood loss is not extensive. The walls of the bile ducts become thickened, and general periportal fibrosis may be produced by the parasite. Liver parenchyma rarely tends to be destroyed.

DIAGNOSIS
Distomiasis can be recognized in the living host by the identification of characteristic ova (Fig. 13-33) in the feces. At necropsy or biopsy of the liver, the lesions in the liver are typical and the parasite can usually be found in the liver parenchyma or affected biliary system.

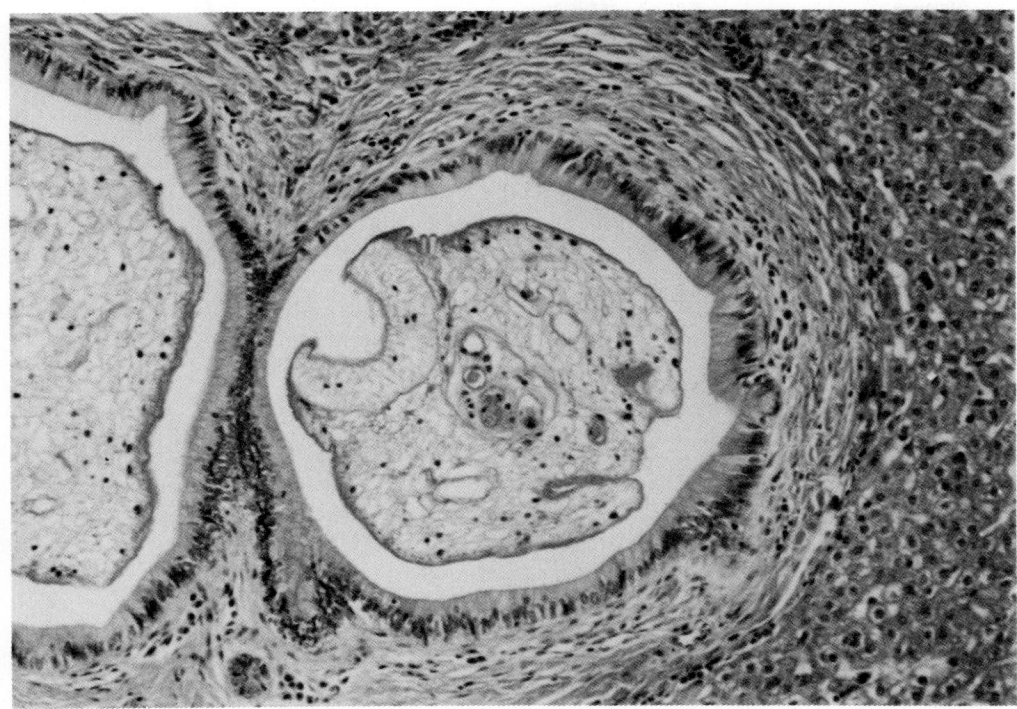

FIG. 13-35 A typical trematode *(Athesmia foxi)* within a bile duct of a *Cebus albifrons* monkey. The infestation is accompanied by slight periductal fibrosis.

Hepatic distomiasis in dogs and cats

Hepatic distomiasis in dogs and cats is caused by several different flukes. *Metorchis conjunctis,* the most common, resides in bile ducts causing cholangiohepatitis characterized by biliary necrosis, hyperplasia, eosinophilic, and mononuclear infiltration and fibrosis. Hepatic function may be impaired and there may be an associated eosinophilia. It requires two intermediate hosts: a snail *(Amnicola limosa porosa)* and the suckerfish *(Castostomus commersonii).* Other species that affect the bile ducts include: *Platynosomum fastosum* in cats in the Far East, Latin America, the Caribbean, and southern United States; *Metorchis albidis* of dogs in Alaska; *Clonorchis sinensis* of dogs, cats, swine, and humans in the Orient; *Opisthorchis tenuicollis* of dogs, cats, foxes, and swine, which may also reside in pancreatic ducts; *Pseudamphistomum truncatum* of dogs, cats, foxes, and humans in Europe, Russia and India; and *Concinnum procyonis* of cats, foxes, and raccoons in the United States.

Infestation with any of these flukes may lead to hyperplastic cholangiohepatitis, and some have a strong association with **cholangiosarcoma,** particularly *Clonorchis sinensis* infection in humans.

References

Anokhin IA. The diumal rhythm of ants invaded by *Dicrocoelium lanceatum* metacercariae. Dokl Akad Nauk SSSR 1966;166:757–759.
Ashizawa H. Pathological studies on fascioliasis. I. The liver of goats. II. The liver of sheep. III. The liver of cattle. IV. The liver of experimentally infected goats, rabbits and guinea pigs. Bull Fac Agric Univ Miyazaki 1963/65;9:1–44, 143–191; 10:1–40, 189–221, Vet Bull 1965;35:3886.
Ashizawa H. Pathological studies on fascioliasis. V. Parasitic bronchiectasis in cattle caused by *Fasciola* sp. Bull Fac Agric Univ Miyazaki 1966;12:1–57, Vet Bull 1967;37:4779.
Baker DW, Nelson SK. *Dicrocoelium dendriticum* infections in New York State cattle. Cornell Vet 1943;33:250–256.
Bengtsson E, et al. Infestation with *Dicrocoelium dendriticum*—the small liver fluke—in animals and human individuals in Sweden. Acta Path Microbiol Scand 1968;74:85–92.
Beresford OD. A case of fascioliasis in man. Vet Rec 1976;98:15.
Cheema AH. Adenomatous cholecystis in cattle with chronic fascioliasis. Vet Pathol 1974;11:407–416.
Conboy GA, Hayden DW, Stromberg BE. Hepatic and pulmonary pathology of experimental *Fascioloides magna* infection in guinea pigs. J Comp Pathol 1991;105:213–223.
Dawes B, Hughes DL. Fascioliasis: the invasive stages in mammals. Adv Parasitol 1970;8:259–274.
Dow C, Ross JG, Todd JR. The pathology of experimental fascioliasis in calves. J Comp Pathol 1967;77:377–385.
Dow C, Ross JG, Todd JR. The histopathology of *Fasciola hepatica* infections in sheep. Parasitology 1968;58:129–135.
Foreyt WJ, Hunter RL. Clinical *Fascioloides magna* infection in sheep in Oregon on pasture shared by Columbian white-tailed deer. Am J Vet Res 1980;41:1531–1532.
Foreyt WJ, Leathers CW. Experimental infection of domestic goats with Fascioloides magna. Am J Vet Res 1980;41:883–884.
Fox JN, Mosley JG, Vogler GA, et al. Pancreatic function in domestic cats with pancreatic fluke infection. J Am Vet Med Assoc 1981;178:58–60.
Hjerpe CA, Tennant BC, Crenshaw GL, et al. Ovine fascioliasis in California. J Am Vet Med Assoc 1971;159:1266–1271.
Hoover RC, Lincoln SD, Hall RF, et al. Seasonal transmission of *Fasciola hepatica* to cattle in northwestern United States. J Am Vet Res Assoc 1984;184:695–698.
Huffman JE, Fried B, Roscoe DE, et al. Comparative pathologic features and development of *Sphaeridiotrema globulus* (Trematoda) infections in the mute swan and domestic chicken and chicken chorioallantois. Am J Vet Res 1984;45:387–391.

Kendall SB, Parfitt JW. The life-history of some vectors of *Fasciola gigantica* under laboratory conditions. Ann Trop Med Parasitol 1965;59:10–16.

Krull WH, Mapes CR. Studies on the biology of *Dicrocoelium dendriticum* (Rudolphi, 1819) (Looss, 1899)—including its relation to the intermediate host, *Cionella lubrica* (Muller). III. Observations on the slimeballs of *Dicrocoelium dendriticum*. Cornell Vet 1952;42:253–276.

Krull WH, Mapes CR. Studies on the biology of *Dicrocoelium dendriticum* (Rudolphi, 1819) (Looss, 1899)—including its relation to the intermediate host, *Cionella lubrica* (Muller). IV. Infection experiments involving definitive hosts. Cornell Vet 1952;42:277–285.

Krull WH, Mapes CR. Studies on the biology of *Dicrocoelium dendriticum* (Rudolphi, 1819) (Looss, 1899)—including its relation to the intermediate host *Cionella lubrica*. IX. Notes on the cyst, metacercaria, and infection in the ant, Formica fusca. Cornell Vet 1953;43:389–410.

Migaki G, Zinter DE, Garner FM. *Fascioloides magna* in the pig: three cases. Am J Vet Res 1971;32:1417–1421.

Nansen P, Andersen S, Hesselholt M. Experimental infection of the horse with *Fasciola hepatica*. Exp Parasitol 1975;37:15–19.

Pullan NB, Sewell MMH, Hammond JA. Studies on the pathogenicity of massive infections of *Fasciola hepatica* in lambs. Br Vet J 1970;126:543–558.

Rahko T. The pathology of natural *Fasciola hepatica* infection in cattle. Pathol Vet 1969;6:244–256.

Robinson VB, Ehrenford FA. Hepatic lesions associated with liver fluke *(Platynosomum fastosum)* infection in a cat. Am J Vet Res 1962;23:1300–1303.

Ross JG, Dow C, Todd JR. A study of *Fasciola hepatica* infections in sheep. Vet Rec 1967;80:543–546.

Ross JG, Dow C, Todd JR. The pathology of *Fasciola hepatica* infection in pigs: a comparison of the infection in pigs and other hosts. Br Vet J 1967;123:317–322.

Schillhorn van Veen TW. Prevalence of *Fascioloides magna* in cattle and deer in Michigan. J Am Vet Med Assoc 1987;191:547–548.

Stromberg BE, Conboy GA, Hayden DW, et al. Pathophysiologic effects of experimentally induced *Fascioloides magna* infection in sheep. Am J Vet Res 1985;46:1637–1641.

Simesen MG, et al. Chronic fascioliasis in sheep. I. Clinical, clinical-pathological and histological studies. Nord Vet Med 1968; 20:638–650, Vet Bull 1969;39:2100.

Stemmermann GN. Human infestation with *Fasciola gigantica*. Am J Pathol 1953;29:731–753.

Swales WE. The life cycle of *Fascioloides magna* (Bassi, 1875): the large liver fluke of ruminants in Canada. Can J Res 1935;12: 177–215.

Swales WE. Further studies on *Fascioloides magna* (Bassi, 1875) (Ward, 1917), as a parasite of ruminants. Can J Res 1936;14:83–95.

Symons LEA, Boray JC. The anaemia of acute and chronic ovine fascioliasis. Z Tropenmed Parasitol 1968;19:451–472, Vet Bull 1969; 39:1648.

Thorpe E, Ford EJH. Serum enzyme and hepatic changes in sheep infested with *Fasciola hepatica*. J Pathol 1969;97:619–629.

Watson TG, Croll NA. Clinical changes caused by the liver fluke *Metorchis conjunctus* in cats. Vet Pathol 1981;18:778–785.

Wiedosari E, Graydon R, Copeman DB. Comparative pathological stude of hepatic changes induced by *Fasciola gigantica* and *Gigantocotyle explanatum* in Javanese thin-tailed sheep. J Comp Pathol 1991;105:146–155.

Intestinal trematodiasis

A number of flukes inhabit the gastrointestinal tract of animals; however, most are of little consequence. In dogs and cats, species of *Alaria*, *Heterophyes*, *Anophallus*, *Cryptocotyle*, *Echinochasmus*, and *Isthmiophora* are encountered in various parts of the world, but only in heavy infestations do they lead to enteritis. *Nanophyetus salmincola* by itself is also of little significance to dogs and cats;

however, this fluke carries the *reckettsia*, which causes salmon poisoning and Elokomin fluke fever.

In cattle and sheep, several genera of flukes in the family Paramphistomatidae (Table 13-9) inhabit the forestomachs, where they are essentially harmless. The metacercariae, however, excyst in the duodenum and heavy infestation with the immature flukes may lead to severe hemorrhagic duodenitis, which can be fatal. After maturing, the flukes migrate forward to the rumen.

Those species listed in Table 13-9 as affecting the intestinal tract of horses and swine are generally of little concern.

Schistosomiasis

Studies of ancient Egyptian records and mummies indicate that since the pre-Christian era the people of the Middle East have been subject to a disease in which hematuria, dysentery, and cirrhosis were prominent features. It was not until 1851 that Bilharz observed adult flukes in the veins of an Egyptian, and even later before he demonstrated the relation of the organisms to this prevalent and historic disease. Many more years elapsed before Leiper (1918) demonstrated experimentally that two separate parasites were responsible for the human disease, and that snails were necessary intermediate hosts for the blood flukes.

The schistosomes, or blood flukes, affect hundreds of millions of people and animals, causing serious disease worldwide. In the United States, however, except for some infections of wild birds and *Heterobilharzia americana* infection of wild mammals and occasionally dogs, schistosomiasis is not prevalent. The adults of most schistosomes live in portal and mesenteric veins, others reside in pelvic veins and *S. nasalis* resides in veins of the nasal cavity.

These worms are small trematodes that live in the blood vessels of their hosts; their ova, which circulate as emboli and lodge in tissue as foreign bodies, produce the principal pathologic changes in the host. The females are slender round worms, 1.4–2.0 cm in length; the distinctive feature of the slightly shorter male is a long gynecophoric canal, a canoe-shaped structure in which the female is held during coitus. The blood flukes are classified as Trematoda within the suborder Strigeata, with the parasites of birds and mammals grouped in the family Schistosomatidae. Table 13-10 summarizes certain characteristics of important blood flukes of humans and animals.

LIFE CYCLE

All blood flukes have similar life cycles. The adult female, after copulation with the male within the lumen of a vein, moves against the venous blood stream into small venules, where she deposits the ova. Schistosomes that live in the mesenteric veins (*S. bovis*, *S. japonicum* (Fig. 13-36), *Heterobilharzia americana*, and *S. mansoni*) deposit their ova in venules of the intestine; those that dwell in the vesical and other pelvic veins (*S. hematobium* and occasionally *S. mansoni*) use venules of the urinary

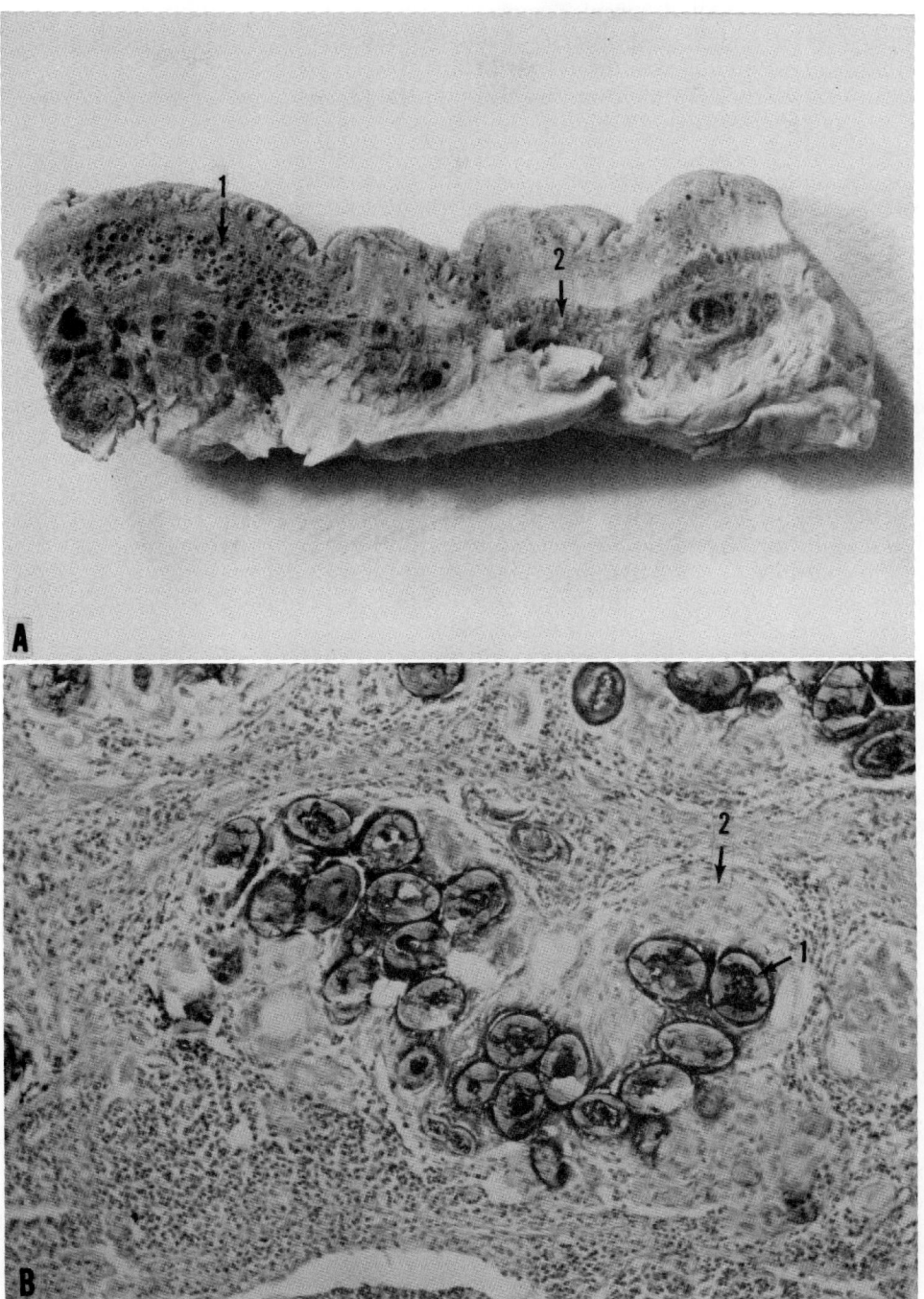

FIG. 13-36 Schistosomiasis. **A.** Small intestine of a dog. (1) Thickened submucosa and muscularis; (2) The inner part of the muscularis is marked. **B.** Ova of *Schistosoma japonicum* in a lymph node (×135) of a dog. (1) The ova; (2) Surrounded by epithelioid cells and fibrous stroma. (Courtesy of Armed Forces Institute of Pathology; contributor: 36th Evacuation Hospital.)

bladder. The deposited ova secrete cytolytic fluid through pores of the egg shell, which, assisted by the movement of the host's tissues, permits them to rupture the capillary walls and move through the tissues toward the lumen of the intestine or the urinary bladder. The successful ova leave the body of the host with the feces (*S. japonicum, S. bovis, H. americana,* and *S. mansoni*) or the urine (*S. hematobium, S. mansoni*). Unsuccessful ova may remain in any tissue through which they are unable to pass, or they may be transported via the blood stream to other organs, where they produce lesions. Fertile ova will not hatch in the tissues of the host; how-

ever, upon reaching a favorable external environment, a single, ovoid ciliated organism, a **miracidium,** quickly escapes from the ovum. The miracidium swims about in water until it finds a suitable intermediate host, a snail, whose body it penetrates by a head-on boring action with the aid of proteolytic enzymes secreted by its cephalic glands.

Each schistosome has an affinity for one or more species of snail, which it uses as an intermediate host. The availability of suitable gastropod hosts thus influences the geographic distribution of schistosomiasis.

Within the body of the snail, the miracidium soon

becomes a thin-walled saccular sporocyst that reproduces several daughter sporocysts. Each of these secondary sporocysts releases thousands of tiny fork-tailed organisms, **cercariae,** which wander through the tissues of the snail, occasionally killing it, and finally emerge into the surrounding water. These cercariae must find a suitable definitive host in order to carry their life cycle further. Upon meeting with such a host, the cercariae penetrate the skin, where they undergo structural changes to become immature flukes, termed **schistosomula.** These are carried by the venous circulation to the lungs, and then through the arterial system to the liver. Within the intrahepatic portal system the flukes grow in size, then eventually migrate to the portal, mesenteric, or pelvic veins, depending upon the species, where they attain their adult form and continue the reproductive cycle.

LESIONS

It is obvious from the life cycles of parasites of this group that injury to the definitive host can result from the presence of adults in the veins, ova in veins or tissues, or cercariae as they penetrate the skin.

The adult blood flukes living within the veins may produce some phlebitis, with intimal proliferation and occasionally venous thrombosis. Vascular lesions are most likely to be severe when the adult worms die or are trapped in unusual sites. The adult schistosomes also consume erythrocytes and discharge blood pigment, which is engulfed by macrophages and may be found in reticuloendothelial tissues in the liver and spleen. This pigment appears in the cytoplasm of macrophages as black granules, not unlike that seen in association with certain liver flukes.

The ova of the blood flukes are the most important factors in the production of lesions. The ova deposited in the venules reach venous capillaries, adhere to and become embedded within the endothelium, rupture the basement membrane by means of enzymes secreted through the pores of the egg shell by the miracidium within, and escape into the tissues to make their way to the lumen of the intestine or urinary bladder. This migration leads to small hemorrhagic ulcers, which in extensive infestations may lead to overt hemorrhage, anemia, and hypoproteinemia.

This ideal escape of ova, however, is overshadowed by the fact that most eggs do not escape to the outside; instead, they become embedded in tissues and elicit an extreme immunologic response to antigens released by the eggs. This hypersensitivity reaction leads to the formation of granulomas composed of neutrophils, lymphocytes, macrophages, and multinucleated giant cells. These granulomas or "pseudotubercles" are a characteristic feature of schistosomiasis and may be widespread, leading to extensive tissue damage. They become especially prominent in the wall of the intestine and throughout the liver as ova move up the portal veins into the hepatic parenchyma. Cirrhosis follows extensive hepatic involvement. Other ova gain access to the general circulation to be distributed widely throughout the body. These ova also incite granulomas that may be found in the spleen, lungs, brain, or any other organ of the body. With time, the eggs die and the host response abates, leading to healing, which may leave a small spheric scar. Within each granuloma lies an ovoid, schistosome egg, with a thick, hyaline, unstained, or yellow wall. Sometimes a single spine may be seen protruding from this wall. The spine is located along the lateral surface in ova of *S. mansoni* and at one terminal pole in *S. hematobium, S. bovis, S. indicum, S. intercalatum, S. nasalis,* and *S. spindale;* it is lateral, small, and inconspicuous on the ova of *S. japonicum.* The nature and location of the spine can be used to identify the type of infection in some cases. Microscopic sections of ova may contain recognizable parts of the miracidium, but in older lesions only the egg shell may be left. It is often ruptured in such situations, and only a fragment may be present; however, the tissue reaction and microscopic appearance of the egg shell are characteristic. The Ziehl-Neelsen stain is useful in differentiating some schistosome eggs. Eggs of *S. mansoni, S. nasalis,* and *S. intercalatum* are acid-fast, whereas *S. spindale, S. indicum, S. hematobium, S. mattheei, S. japonicum,* and *S. bovis* are negative.

Cutaneous lesions develop in humans and animals as a result of penetration of the skin by the cercariae of schistosomes. The intensity of the tissue reaction depends to some extent upon the sensitivity and resistance of the host to the parasite. As the cercariae reach the dermis, a leukocytic reaction of varying intensity results, including neutrophils, lymphocytes, and eosinophils. This is accompanied by urticaria, itching, and the formation of tiny nodules that elevate the epidermis. In sensitized animals or humans, a severe tissue reaction occurs, and death of the parasite in the dermis may set up a prolonged local tissue reaction. Cercariae have the ability to penetrate the epidermis of hosts in which complete development of the fluke does not occur; in this case, the cercariae die in the dermis. This is the basis of **cercarial dermatitis** ("swimmer's itch," "collector's itch," "swamp itch"), a problem to individuals exposed to infested waters (e.g., agricultural workers, swimmers). Numerous schistosomes of birds and mammals have demonstrated to cause cercarial dermatitis, but the most important appear to be *Trichobilharzia stagnicolae,* a blood fluke of canaries; *Trichobilharzia ocellata,* a parasite of ducks; *Trichobilharzia physellae* (wild ducks and teal), *Schistosomatium douthitti* (meadow mouse, muskrat) and *Schistosoma spindale* (cattle, sheep, goat, horse, antelope, and water buffalo).

A schistosome of some importance in parts of southern United States is *Heterobilharzia americana.* This parasite, reported for the first time by Malek et al. (1961) to be a parasite of the dog, usually has other definitive hosts: bobcat (*Lynx rufus*), rabbit (*Sylvilagus aquaticus*), raccoon (*Procyon lotor*), opossum (*Didelphis marsupialis*), white-tailed deer (*Odocoileus virginiana*), and the nutria (*Myocastor coypus*). The life cycle of this schistosome is essentially the same as others described previously. An ovum releases the free-swimming miracidium to penetrate a snail (*Lymnaea cubensis* or *Pseudosuccinea columella*), in whose digestive gland it undergoes development to a mature cercaria which, in turn, penetrates the skin of its mammalian host. After periods of maturation in the lung and liver, the adults move to the mesenteric veins and undergo copulation. Ova reach the intestine, liver, and other viscera, and incite the tissue reaction described previously for *S. japonicum* and *S. mansoni*. Ova appear in the feces about 68 days after cercariae penetrate the skin (the prepatent period). *Schistosomatium douthitti* is the only other schistosome that infests mammals in the United States.

In humans, carcinoma of the urinary bladder is a frequent complication of vesicular schistosomiasis. The carcinomas are often squamous cell types arising in metaplastic epithelium. The exact causal relationship has not been established. Experimentally, neoplasms have developed in nonhuman primates infected with *S. hematobium* and *S. intercalatum;* however, these have been composed of transitional epithelium and not squamous. *S. japonica* infection of humans has also been associated with hepatocellular carcinoma, but the association is not nearly as strong as that of cholangiocarcinoma and infection with *Clonorchis sinensis*. Abe et al. reported a case of hepatocellular carcinoma in a chimpanzee infected with *S. mansoni* (1993). Glomerulonephritis is also frequently associated with schistosomiasis in humans, and has been induced experimentally in chimpanzees (Cavallo et al., 1974). Evidence suggests an immune complex origin, but this has not been firmly established.

DIAGNOSIS

The clinical diagnosis of schistosomiasis can be confirmed by demonstration of schistosome ova in the feces, or by histologic examination of biopsy specimens of rectal mucosa, liver, or other affected organs. The adult parasite may be found in veins at necropsy, and the typical ova in granulomas are demonstrable by histologic examination of specimens collected at necropsy or biopsy.

References

Abe K, Kagei N, Teramura Y, et al. Hepatocellular carcinoma associated with chronic Schistosoma mansoni infection in a chimpanzee. J Med Primatol 1993;22:237–239.

Anonymous. Immunopathology of schistosomiasis. Lancet 1987; ii:194–195.

Barbosa FS, Barbosa I, Malgalhães-Filho A. Natural infection of cattle with Schistosoma mansoni. Proc 1st Int Congr Parasit Roma 1964;2:703–710, Vet Bull 1967;37:2698.

Bartsch RC, Ward BC. Visceral lesions in raccoons naturally infected with Heterobilharzia americana. Vet Pathol 1976;13:241–249.

Brackett S. Pathology of schistosome dermatitis. Arch Dermat Syph 1940;42:410–418.

Capron A, Dessaint JP, Capron M, et al. Immunity to schistosomes: progress toward vaccine. Science 1987;238:1065–1072.

Cheever AW, et al. Animal model of human disease: carcinoma of the urinary bladder in Schistosoma haematobium infection. Proliferative urothelial lesions in nonhuman primates infected with Schistosoma haematobium. Am J Pathol 1976;84:673–676.

Cheever AW, Kuntz RE, Moore JA, et al. Proliferative epithelial lesions of urinary bladder in cynomolgus monkeys (Macaca fascicularis) infected with Schistosoma intercalatum. Cancer Res 1976;36: 2928–2931.

El-Cheikh MC, Dutra HS, Borojevic R. Eosinophil granulocyte proliferation and differentiation in schistosomal granulomas are controlled by two cytokines. Lab Invest 1991;64:93–97.

Goff WL, Ronald NC. Miracidia hatching technique for diagnosis of canine schistosomiasis. J Am Vet Med Assoc 1980;177:699–700.

Goff WL, Ronald NC. Certain aspects of the biology and life cycle of Heterobilharzia americana in east central Texas. Am J Vet Res 1981;42:1775–1777.

Goff WL, Ronald NC. Indirect hemagglutination for the diagnosis of Heterobilharzia americana infections in dogs. Am J Vet Res 1982;43:2038–2041.

Hsu HF, Davis JR, Hsu SYL. Histopathological lesions of rhesus monkeys and chimpanzees infected with Schistosoma japonicum. Z Tropenmed Parasitol 1969;20:184–205.

Hsu SYL, Hsu HF, Lust GL, et al. Organized epithelioid cell granulomata elicited by schistosome eggs in experimental animals. J Reticuloendothel Soc 1972;12:418–435.

Hussein MF. The pathology of experimental schistosomiasis in calves. Res Vet Sci 1971;12:246–252.

Kuntz RE, Cheever AW, Myers BJ. Proliferative epithelial lesions of the urinary bladder of non-human primates infected with Schistosoma haematobium. J Natl Cancer Inst 1972;48:223–235,.

MacHattie C, Chadwick CR. Schistosoma bovis and S. mattheei in Iraq with notes on development of eggs of S. haematobium pattern. Tr Roy Soc Trop Med Hyg 1932;26:147–156.

Malek EA, Ash LR, Lee HF, et al. Heterobilharzia infection in the dog and other mammals in Louisiana. J Parasitol 1961;47:619–623.

Muller RL, Taylor MG. On the use of the Ziehl-Neelsen technique for specific identification of schistosome eggs. J Helminthol 1972;46:139–142.

Olivier L, Weinstein PP. Experimental schistosome dermatitis in rabbits. J Parasitol 1953;39:280–291.

Penner LR. Possibilities of systemic infection with dermatitis-producing schistosomes. Science 1941;93:327–328.

Pierce KR. Heterobilharzia americana infection in a dog. J Am Vet Med Assoc 1963;143:496–499.

Price HF. Life history of Schistosomatium douthitti (Cort). Am J Hyg 1931;13:685–727.

Saeed AA, Nelson GS, Hussein MF. Experimental infections of calves with schistosomes. Trans R Soc Trop Med Hyg 1969;63:15.

Sharma DN, Dwivedi JN. Pulmonary schistosomiasis in sheep and goats due to Schistosoma indicum in India. J Comp Pathol 1976;86:449–454.

Sturrock RF. A review of the use of primates in studying human schistosomiasis. J Med Primatol 1986;15:267–279.

Thrasher JP. Canine schistosomiasis. J Am Vet Med Assoc 1964; 144:1119–1126.

Vercruysse J, Fransen J, Southgate VR, et al. The pathology of experimental Schistosoma curassoni infections in mice and hamsters. Vet Pathol 1986;23:668–672.

Von Lichtenberg F, Erickson DG, Sadun EH. Comparative histopathology of schistosome granulomas in the hamster. Am J Pathol 1973;72:149–178.

Warren KS. The pathology of schistosome infections. Helminthol Abs 1973;42A:591–633.

Warren KS. The pathology, pathophysiology and pathogenesis of schistosomiasis. Nature 1978;273:609–612.

Warren KS. The relevance of schistosomiasis. N Engl J Med 1980;303:203–206.

Wu K. Cattle as reservoir hosts of Schistosoma japonicum in China Am J Hyg 1938;27:290–297.

Paragonimiasis

Small reddish-brown, egg-shaped flukes of the genus Paragonimus are important parasites of humans and animals. These flukes are 8–12 mm long, 4–6 mm in diameter; they are hermaphroditic and have a spiny cuticle. Two species are of particular interest: *Paragonimus westermani*, which occurs in the Far East in a variety of animal species, including humans; and *P. kellicotti,* which occurs in North America in cats, dogs, pigs, and mink, all viewed as the natural hosts. The adults of *P. kellicotti* usually are found in pairs in lung cysts, and may or may not communicate with bronchi. The cysts often are lined with bronchial epithelium and surrounded by granulomatous inflammation. Released eggs lodge in the pulmonary parenchyma and incite an eosinophilic granulomatous response. Eggs can also enter the circulation and lodge in a variety of organs inciting granulomas. Rarely, adult flukes will locate in other tissues, such as the brain.

LIFE CYCLE

The life cycle involves two intermediate hosts (Table 13-9). Eggs that reach the bronchi are coughed up, swallowed, and expelled with the feces. The eggs are thick-walled, operculated, anisotropic, yellowish-brown, and measure 80–118 μ in length and 48–60 μ wide. Under most conditions, miracidia develop slowly in these ova, hatch into water, and then burrow into one of several species of freshwater snails. Cercariae that escape the snail then penetrate crayfish of the genus Cambarus, which live in small sluggish streams. Other species of crayfish and crabs serve as the second intermediate host for *P. westermani.* Metacercariae released from ingested crayfish excyst in the duodenum; immature flukes bore through the duodenal wall and reach the lungs through wandering in the peritoneal and pleural cavities. This journey can lead to peritonitis and pleuritis.

References

Ameel DJ. Paragonimiasis, its life history and distribution in North America and its taxonomy. Am J Hyg 1934;19:279–317.

Comfort CF, Axelson RD. Two reports of unusual parasites diagnosed in dogs. Can Vet J 1962;3:22–24.

Greve JH, et al. Paragonimiasis in Iowa. Iowa State Univ Vet 1963/64;26:21–28.

Herman LH, Helland DR. Paragonimiasis in a cat. J Am Vet Med Assoc 1966;149:753–757.

LaRue GR, Ameel DJ. The distribution of Paragonimus. J Parasitol 1937;23:382–388.

Nielson SW. Canine paragonimiasis. North Am Vet 1955;36:657–662.

Rendano VT Jr. Paragonimiasis in the cat: a review of five cases. J Small Anim Pract 1974;15:637–644.

Seed JR, Sogandares-Bernal F, Mills RR. Studies on American paragonimiasis. II. Serological observations of infected cats. J Parasitol 1966;52:358–362,.

Eurytrema pancreaticum

Eurytrema pancreaticum is a small red fluke that resides in the pancreatic duct of sheep, goats, cattle, and buffalo in Eastern Asia and Brazil. It may also parasitize humans. The flukes are slightly over 1 cm long. When present in large numbers, they may also cause fibrosis of the duct and the acinar tissue. Erosion of the mucosa may allow eggs to enter tissue, where they incite granulomas (Fig. 13-37). In the United States, the pancreatic fluke *Concinnum (Eurytrema) procyonis* affects cats, raccoons, and foxes and may cause chronic pancreatitis. In New World monkeys, the presence of the nematode *Trichospirura leptosoma,* which resides in the pancreatic ducts, may lead to pancreatitis. *Troglotrema acutum* re-

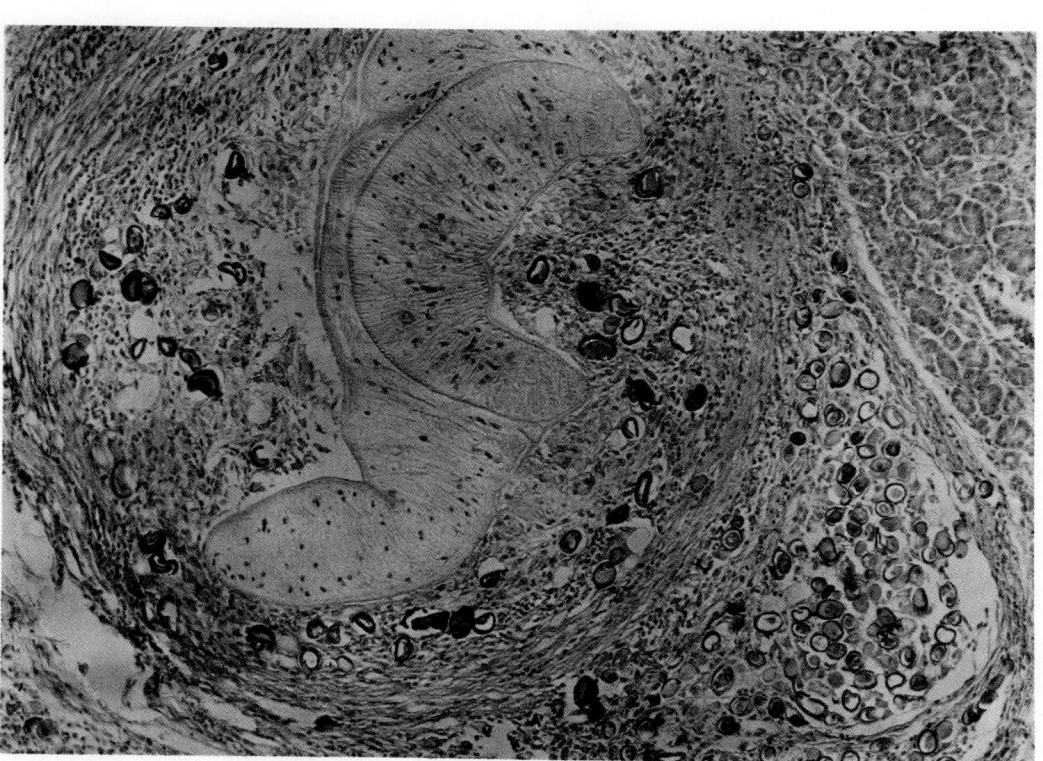

FIG. 13-37 A fluke, *Eurytrema pancreaticum,* in the pancreatic duct of a Brazilian cow. Note the large numbers of ova and the inflammation in the duct. (Contributor: Dr. A. V. Machado, University of Munas Gervais.)

sides in the frontal and ethmoid sinuses of foxes and mink in Europe. In foxes, these flukes attach to the mucosa; in mink, however, the parasites invade the mucosa, leading to granulomatous sinusitis and osteomyelitis.

References

Basch PF. Completion of the life cycle of Eurytrema pancreaticum (Trematoda: Dicrocoeliidae). J Parasitol 1965;51:350–355.

Nosaka D, Ashizawa H, Nagata Y. Pathological studies on Eurytrema infection in cattle. III. Behaviour of Eurytrema eggs in the wall and surrounding tissue of bovine pancreatic ducts infected with Eurytrema species. Bull Fac Agric Miyazaki 1970;17:104–132.

PARASITIC ARTHROPODS

The phylum Arthropoda is in general made up of organisms characterized by bilateral symmetry, metameric segmentation, jointed appendages, and a hardened exoskeleton. It is divided into five classes as follows:

Crustacea: crabs, crayfish, shrimp, copepods
Myriapoda: centipedes and millipedes
Insecta: six-legged insects (mosquitoes, flies)
Arachnida: spiders, scorpions, ticks, mites
Pentastomida: tongue worms (of uncertain classification)

The classes **Insecta** and **Arachnida** contain most of the parasitic species and the vectors of disease-producing viruses, protozoa, nematodes, rickettsia, and spirochetes. Each of these vectors is considered briefly in the part of this text devoted to the disease which it transmits. Many orders exist in the class **Insecta,** some of which contain species that are parasitic to animals; however, Diptera (flies, mosquitos, gnats), Hemiptera (bugs), Siphonaptera (fleas), Mallophaga (biting lice), and Anoplura (Siphunculata; sucking lice) are most significant. The class **Arachnida** (arachnids) also contains many orders that parasitize animals to varying degrees, the most important of which is Acarina. This order contains several suborders and families that include the hard and soft ticks and numerous mites, which cause various forms of mange. Other orders contain species of less interest that may act as vectors of disease, but these will not be discussed here. Fleas, lice, and bugs, although vexing and sometimes injurious parasites, do not often have a serious portent from the pathologist's viewpoint; hence, they will not be considered further. Flies, however, do incite specific and severe pathologic changes, and so they are pathogens in their own right.

Biting and blood sucking insects

Many species in both the class Insecta and Arachnida are parasites that bite animals or suck their blood. Horseflies, stable flies, tsetse flies, horn flies, gnats or black flies, sheep keds, midges, mosquitos, kissing bugs, bees, wasps, hornets, biting and sucking lice, fleas, and others are among the numerous organisms included here. Many are merely annoying or cause only tempo-

rary discomfort; however, their irritation can lead to traumatic dermatitis from the animals rubbing or biting the irritated skin. Others, such as fleas or lice, can be present in sufficient numbers to cause blood loss anemia. These and several of the other superficial insects and arachnids may also incite hypersensitivity skin diseases (Chapter 18).

Myiasis

Myiasis results from the invasion of the living tissues of animals by the larval stage of flies of the order Diptera. The sites of invasion of these larvae provide a basis for their clinical classification:

(1) Cutaneous—the larvae live in or under the skin (e.g., ox warble);
(2) Intestinal—in the stomach or intestines (e.g., horse "bots");
(3) Atrial—in the oral, nasal, ocular, sinusal, vaginal, and urethral cavities (e.g., *Oestrus ovis*);
(4) Wound-invading ("screw-worm larvae"); and
(5) External (bloodsucking larvae).

Some fly larvae occupy more than one of these sites during the course of development in the host. Many fly larvae are specific parasites of a certain host; others are accidental or nonspecific parasites in that they are deposited in or near diseased or wounded tissues in which they find a favorable environment.

BOTFLIES

The genus Gasterophilus contains three species whose larvae are parasitic for equines in the United States. *Gasterophilus intestinalis* (syn. *G. equi*; DeGeer, 1776), the most common botfly in the United States, is a brown fly that deposits its eggs on the hair of horse's fetlocks or forelegs, and sometimes in the scapular region. The female fly darts in quickly and attaches her pale yellow eggs to the hair with a tenacious material. These eggs are ready to hatch in five to ten days, but actual hatching requires licking or rubbing by the horse. This action also helps the larvae reach the animal's mouth, where they penetrate the mucosa of the tongue. The developing larvae remain in the tongue for 21–28 days, then migrate to the stomach; then, with their mouth parts, they attach to the cardiac portion of the mucosa. The bot larvae at this stage have a reddish color and are selective in their location; only rarely are they found attached to the fundic or pyloric portion of the stomach. Each larva causes a small, unbilicated ulcer at its site of attachment. Large numbers of bots obviously interfere with function in the affected part of the stomach, but only occasionally do they produce general debility in the host. Surprisingly, often the host tolerates them without recognizable effect. The larvae remain attached to the mucosa, living on blood and tissue, for 10–12 months. After this period, they loosen their hold and pass out with the feces; the larvae pupate in soil for three to five weeks, and then emerge as adults.

Gasterophilus hemorrhoidalis, (Linne, 1761), the

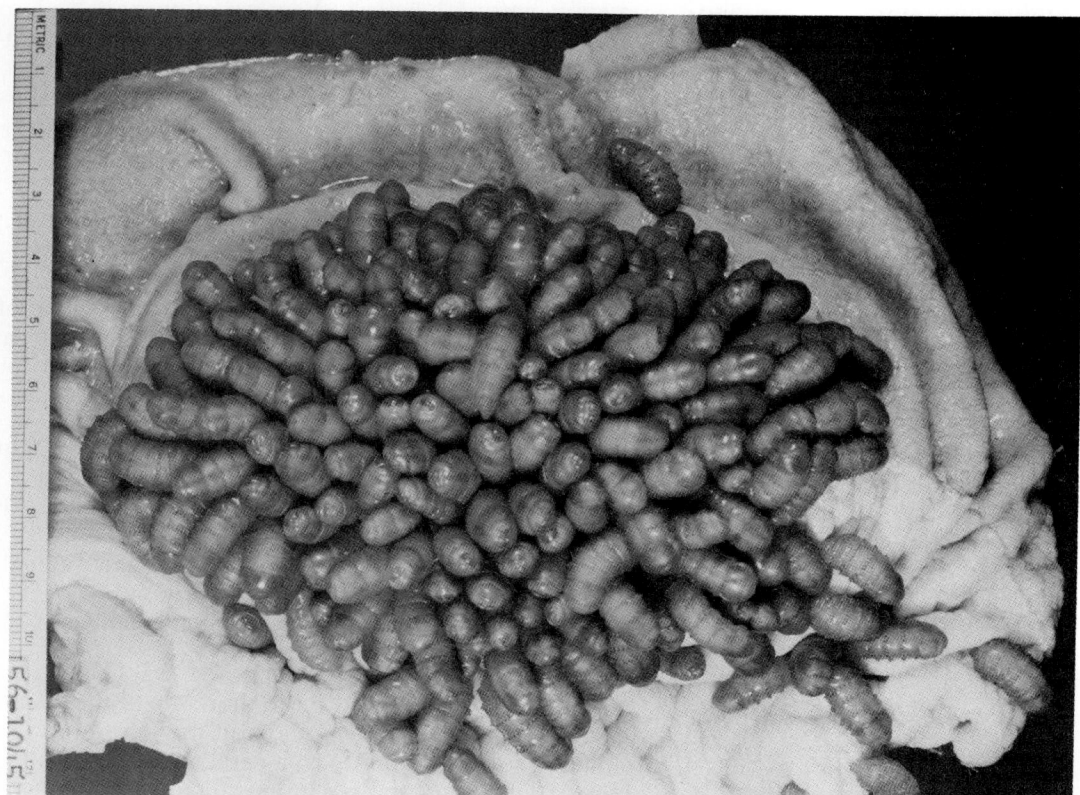

FIG. 13-38 Larvae of *Gasterophilus intestinalis*, "bots," attached to the stomach of a two-year-old gelding. (Courtesy of Dr. C. R. Cole, Ohio State University.)

"nose botfly," is a small red-tailed fly that lays its eggs on hairs around the mouth, nose, and cheeks of horses. The eggs of this species are dark brown or black and elongated; they are pointed at one end and have an operculum at the other. The larvae hatch from these eggs, then pierce the skin of the face and wander into the mouth. The young red-colored larvae are sometimes found in the pharynx, but eventually they become attached at the cardia of the stomach. Here they have a similar effect to that of *G. intestinalis*, (Fig. 13-38) and remain for 10–12 months at this site before passing to the rectum; there, they again attach for a few days before passing out with the feces. The rest of their life cycles are similar to that of *G. intestinalis*.

Gasterophilus nasalis, (Clark, 1897), (also known as *G. veterinus;* Linne, 1761), the "chin" or "throat" fly, lays it eggs on hairs in the intermandibular region of horses. The larvae are pale yellow and migrate to attach to the mucosa of the pylorus and duodenum. Otherwise, their life cycles and effects upon the host are similar to that of *G. intestinalis*.

Gasterophilus pecorum (Fabricus, 1794), is a botfly found in Europe but not in the United States. The female fly deposits her eggs on the hoofs of horses, and on inanimate objects such as food and other materials. The eggs are dark-colored and must be rubbed or licked by the host before the larvae can emerge. The larvae penetrate the mucosa of the cheeks and soon assume a blood-red color. The third-stage larvae attach to the stomach mucosa and, before leaving the host in the spring, attach to the rectal mucosa for a few days.

Gasterophilus inermis (Braurer, 1858), is principally a botfly of Europe, but has also been observed in North America. The adult fly deposits her eggs on hairs around the mouth and cheeks. The larvae may penetrate the skin and leave tracks as they wander toward the mucosa. The third-stage larvae attach to the mucosa of the rectum. Otherwise the life history is similar to that of *G. intestinalis*. Other species of *Gasterophilus* include *G. nigricornis* in Asia and parts of southern Europe, and *G. meridionalis* and *G. ternicinctus*, both of which affect zebra in Africa.

Oestrus ovis, the botfly or "head grub" of sheep, deposits its larvae in the nose of sheep; the larvae migrate into the nasal cavity and nasal sinuses, where they attach and undergo further development. Growth and migration of these larvae in these sites result in serious damage to the tissue and may cause death. The successful larvae eventually drop to the ground, where they pupate and later emerge as adult flies. The larvae of several other flies in the genera *Rhinoestrus, Cephalopsis,* and *Pharyngobolus* (in the same family) inhabit the nasal sinuses or pharynx of horses, camels, and elephants in Europe, Asia, and Africa.

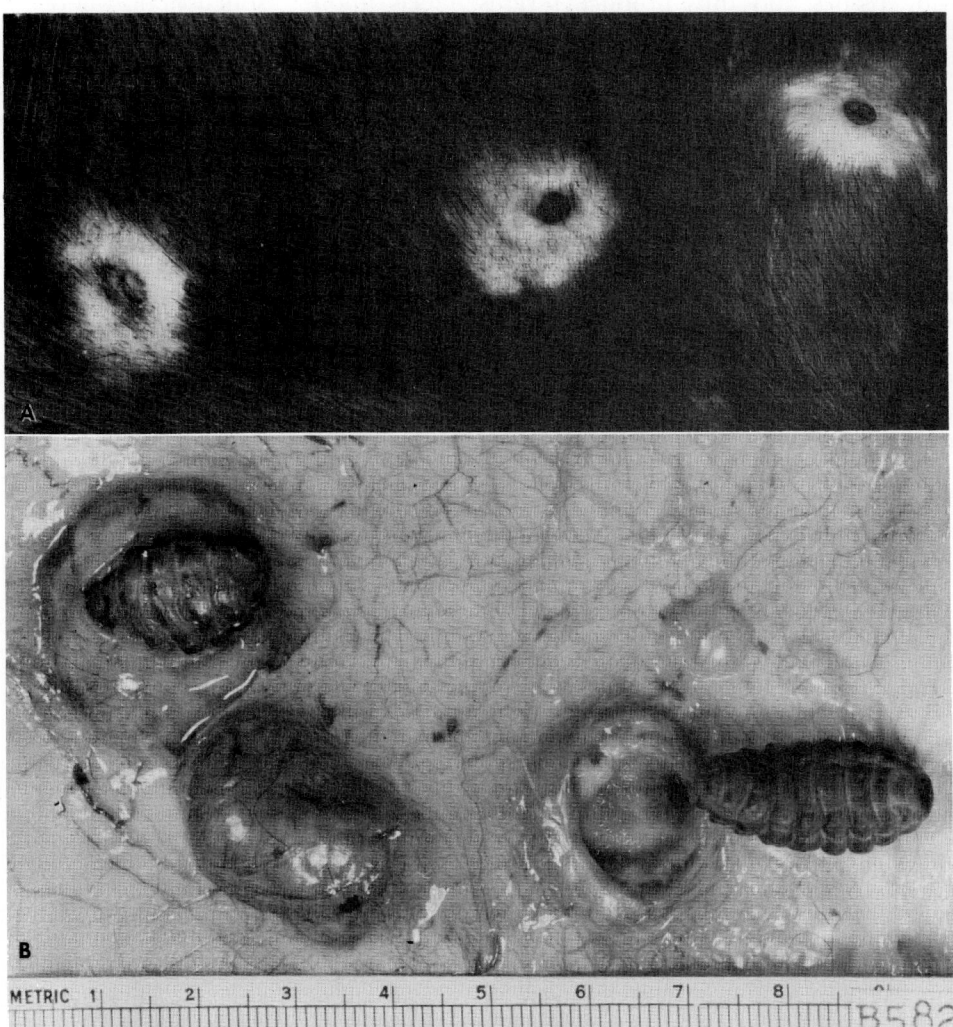

FIG. 13-39 *Hypoderma bovis,* "ox warble," in the bovine skin. **A.** Three holes viewed from the external surface of the skin. The larvae lie under these holes, which eventually enlarge to permit escape of the larvae. **B.** *H. bovis* larvae from the deep surface of the bovine skin. (Courtesy of Dr. C. R. Cole, Ohio State University.)

WARBLES, HEEL FLIES (HYPODERMA)

The genus Hypoderma, in the same family (Oestridae) as *O. ovis,* contains two important species in the United States; *Hypoderma bovis* (Fig. 13-39) and *H. lineatum,* the hairy yellow and black "warble" or heel flies of cattle, which occasionally attack horses and, rarely, humans. Several other species infect deer, sheep, and goats in Europe and Mediterranean countries, with analogous effects. Similar flies *(Oedemagena tarandi)* affect deer in Africa, and voles and muskrats in Europe *(Estromyia leporina).*

The female fly deposits her eggs on the hair of the legs (hence, heel flies), flanks, or dewlap of cattle, which produces irritation and excitement in their victims. The larvae hatch from these eggs and penetrate the skin to begin wandering throughout the body. *H. lineatum* eventually reaches the wall of the esophagus, and *H. bovis* reaches the epidural tissues of the spinal cord, where they reside for weeks during the winter months. In late winter or early spring the larvae migrate to the subcutaneous tissue of the back, where they remain in an encapsulated nodule. They gradually produce holes in the epidermis, through which the group of larvae eventually emerge. After reaching the ground, the larvae pupate and emerge as adult flies 40–50 days later. Surprisingly, the migration pathway of these larvae is usually sterile, even though considerable tissue destruction occurs along the way. Heavy infestation leaves the skin with many holes that make the hide unfit for use. Larvae may migrate to abnormal sites, such as brain, and cause death. Mechanical rupture of a cyst-containing larvae in the skin can also lead to serious hypersensitivity reactions, including anaphylaxis.

SCREW-WORM FLY

The "screwworm" flies *Callitroga hominivorax (Cochliomyia americana)* and *C. macellaria* are parasitic flies which are obligate parasites, their larvae only developing in wounds of animals and man leading to myiasis. Through extensive erradication programs screwworm myiasis has been erradicated in the United States. These and other species however, remain as important pathogens in other countries. The pathogenic effects of this fly are produced by the larvae, which feed upon living tissues and thus produce serious effects upon their host. In humans, harmful effects have been produced by maggots invading the nasopharynx (nasopharyngeal myiasis). In animals, the larvae attack any wounds by which they can gain entrance. In sheep and lambs, "needle" grass may produce the wounds that allow maggots to invade, although cuts in the skin made by shearing can also be troublesome. In cattle, the screw-worm larvae may invade the umbilicus of the newborn calf, or the vagina of its mother. Dehorning and castration may also provide wounds that invite the assault of this parasite.

The adult fly has a dark greenish-blue metallic abdomen; its face is orange or reddish, and three stripes cross the surface of the thorax. The female deposits her eggs in large numbers near wounds; after 11–21 hours, the larvae emerge to feed voraciously for three to five days. A prepupal stage lasts for a few hours to 3 days, and the pupal stage about 7 days. The entire cycle from egg to adult is completed in about 11 days.

DERMATOBIA AND CUTEREBRA
CUTANEOUS MYIASIS

Cutaneous myiasis may also be caused by larvae of flies of the family Cuterebridae. Two genera are of particular interest: Dermatobia and Cuterebra. *Dermatobia hominis* may infect humans, cattle, dogs, sheep, cats, rabbits, and other animals, particularly in tropical America. The adults do not feed, but survive on food stores obtained during the larval period. The adult female is about 12 mm long; her thorax is dark blue, and her short, broad abdomen is a brilliant blue. She glues her ova to the abdomen of a mosquito or blood-sucking fly. The larvae hatch on this transport host and penetrate the skin of a warm-blooded host, upon which the transport host feeds. The larvae of *D. hominis* develop in the subcutis, producing a painful enlargement that opens to the surface through a pore. The larvae require up to ten weeks to mature to about 25 mm in length, with rows of strong spines on their surface. They escape from the skin to the ground, where they pupate to become the mature flies.

The genus Cuterebra is made up of large flies with beelike bodies, 20 mm or more in length. The adult flies oviposit near the mouths of burrows of rodents and rabbits. Larvae hatch and penetrate the skin of the host; they mature in about a month, and produce large, subcutaneous lesions. The larvae pupate on the ground and also are covered with bands of characteristic spines. *Cuterebra buccata, C. americana,* and *C. lepivora* are usually parasitic in rabbits, but these and other species may also infect dogs, cats, and humans. Another species, *C. emasculator,* usually parasitizes mice and chipmunks, but may involve other species. Larvae may invade brain, scrotum, or other tissues, as well as the subcutis.

BLOWFLIES (CALLIPHORINE MYIASIS, STRIKE)

In contrast to the other causes of myiasis, the blowflies are not obligate parasites; the larvae are capable of complete development in dead tissues of carcasses. The eggs, however, can also be deposited in wounds or soiled wool, where they can initiate, or exacerbate existing, lesions. Although such invasion can occur in any species, it is most frequent in sheep and referred to as "strike". The primary blowflies include species of Lucilia, Calliphora, Phormia, and Chrysomyia. Species of these genera are capable of establishing a dermatitis that rapidly becomes secondarily infected. It is commonly about the soiled skin of the perineum. Certain species of Chrysomyia and Microcalliphora may deposit eggs in existing blowfly lesions without initiating the disease. These are referred to as secondary blowflies and exacerbate the lesions. Less invasive flies such as the common house fly *(Musca domestica),* not usually associated with living tissue, may also invade such lesions. These are called tertiary flies. *Calliphorine myiasis* is a particularly important disease of sheep in Australia.

References

Beesley WN. Recent work on the ox warble flies (Hypoderma). Vet Bull 1965;35:1–6.
Beesley WN. Further observations on the development of Hypoderma lineatum de Villiers and Hypoderma bovis, Degeer (Diptera, Oestridae) in the bovine host. Br Vet J 1966;122:91–98.
Cowell AK, Cowell RL, Tyler RD, et al. Severe systemic reactions to Hymenoptera stings in three dogs. J Am Vet Med Assoc 1991;198:1014–1017.
Cunningham DG, Zanga, JR. Myiasis of the external auditory meatus. J Pediatr 1974;84:857–858.
Davis CL, Leadbetter WA. Fatal brain hemorrhage in the bull caused by the cattle grub (Hypoderma bovis). North Am Vet 1952;33:703–705.
Eyre P, Boulard C, Deline T. Local and systemic reactions in cattle to Hypoderma lineatum larval toxin: protection by phenylbutazone. Am J Vet Res 1981;42:25–28.
Gardiner CH, James VS, Valentine BA. Visceral myiasis caused by Musca domestica in a cat. J Am Vet Med Assoc 1983;182:68–69.
Greve JH, Cassidy DR. Aberrant Hypoderma bovis infection in a cow. J Am Vet Med Assoc 1967;150:627–628.
Hatziolos BC. Cuterebra larva in the brain of a cat. J Am Vet Med Assoc 1966;148:787–793.
Hatziolos BC. Cuterebra larva causing paralysis in a dog. Cornell Vet 1967;57:129–145.
Johnson BW, Helper LC, Szajerski ME. Intraocular Cuterebra in a cat. J Am Vet Med Assoc 1988;193:829–830.
Olander HJ. The migration of Hypoderma lineatum in the brain of a horse: a case report and review. Pathol Vet 1967;4:477–483.
Roberts IH, Colbenson HP. Larvae of Oestrus ovis in the ears of sheep. Am J Vet Res 1963;24:628–630.
Sartin EA, Hendrix CM, Dillehay DL, et al. Cerebral cuterebrosis in a dog. J Am Vet Med Assoc 1986;189:1338–1339.
Simmons SW. Some histopathological changes caused by Hypoderma larvae in the esophagus of cattle. J Parasitol 1937;23:376–381.
Zumpt F. Myiasis in man and animals. London: Butterworth, 1965.

Acariasis

Within the class Arachnida, the order Acarina includes the ticks and mites, both of which are at times parasitic in their relation to animals (Table 13-11). These and other exoparasites, such as fleas and lice, usually are not associated with serious disease, except when present in large numbers. All of these parasites cause variable degrees of inflammation at the site of attachment or bite, which results from mechanical irritation, immediate hypersensitivity reactions (localized anaphylaxis or arthus-type reaction), delayed hypersensitivity reaction

TABLE 13-11 **Acarid (mite) animal parasites**

Name	Anatomic site	Disease	Hosts
Demodex folliculorum, D. phylloides, D. cati, D. canis, D. bovis, D. equi, D. ovis	Hair follicles, sebaceous glands	Demodectic mange	Humans, swine, dog, cat, cattle, horse, sheep
Sarcoptes scabiei var. suis, bovis, etc.	Epidermis, general	Scabies, sarcoptic mange	Dog, cat, cattle, sheep, swine, horse, humans
Notoedres cati, N. muris	Epidermis, esp. ears, face, neck	Notoedric mange	Cat, mouse
Psoroptes ovis	Epidermis, general	Psoroptic mange, sheep scab	Sheep, cattle
P. equi	Epidermis, general	Psoroptic mange	Horse
P. cuniculi	Ears	Psoroptic mange	Rabbit, sheep, goat, horse
Chorioptes equi, C. bovis, C. ovis	Epidermis, legs, base of tail	Chorioptic mange	Horse, cattle, sheep
Otodectes cynotis	Ears	Otodectic mange	Dog, cat
Psorergates ovis	Epidermal cysts, skin	Psorergatic mange	Sheep
P. simplex	Epidermal cysts, skin	Mouse mange	Mice
Cheyletiella parasitivorax	Epidermis, general	Mange	Dog, cat, rabbit
C. yasguri	Epidermis, general	Mange	Dog
Myobia musculi	Epidermis, general	Mange	Mice
Pneumonyssus caninum	Paranasal sinuses	Mite infection	Dog
P. simicola	Bronchioles, alveoli	Pulmonary acariasis	Old World monkeys
Linguatula serrata	Nasal and respiratory passages	Pentastomiasis or linguatuliasis	Dog, fox, wolf, horse, goat, sheep, humans
Trixacarus caviae	Epidermis, general	Mange	Guinea pigs
T. diversus	Epidermis, general	Mange	Rats
Trombicula autumnalis and related species	Epidermis, general	Chiggers	All species

(contact dermatitis), or the introduction of secondary bacteria.

Ticks are particularly important as vectors of disease-producing agents, but except when present in large numbers or in particular sites, as in the ears, do not produce any immediate or serious effect upon the host. An important exception is **tick paralysis,** a dramatic paralytic disease observed in humans, sheep, dogs, cats, and other species. Twenty-two species of ticks have been associated with paralysis in various parts of the world. In the United States, *Dermacentor andersoni* (wood tick) is the most important, and in Australia, *Ixodes holocyclus.* The paralysis ensues within about one week after one or more ticks are attached to the skin; it may disappear dramatically when the offending ticks are removed, or slowly abate in several days. Young and small animals are more susceptible to the condition, with fewer ticks required to induce paralysis. Death occurs in animals and humans when the ticks are not detected and removed in time. The paralysis is believed to result from a neuroparalytic toxin secreted by the tick, but its mode of action has not been elucidated, although it is believed to interfere with release of acetylcholine. A short-lived immunity follows exposure, and immune serum can be made from hyperimmunized animals.

The tissue-burrowing habits of mites cause them to produce more obvious lesions in animals than do ticks.

Common mites that are pathogenic for animals are listed in Table 13-11. These mites can be appropriately considered in groups according to the body system which they attack, i.e., pulmonary, cutaneous, intestinal, and urinary.

PULMONARY ACARIASIS

The frequent occurrence of pulmonary lesions in monkeys, caused by a lung mite *Pneumonyssus simicola,* (Fig. 13-40) and related species, is important to the experimental use of these animals. Nearly all imported rhesus monkeys are infected with lung mites, whose presence in the bronchiolar system incites characteristic lesions. Clinical manifestations are not usually observed. The life cycle is not understood, but the occurrence of pulmonary acariasis in monkeys born in captivity (United States) suggests direct transmission.

These acarids, barely large enough to be seen with the unaided eye, are found in the bronchi and bronchioles. Apparently, they move down the bronchial tree until the lumen becomes small enough to impede their progress. Their presence results in accumulation of mucus, localized bronchiolitis, peribronchiolitis, and occasional bronchiectasis. The mites can often be found in a pool of mucus and cellular debris, surrounded by the thickened remnants of the bronchiolar wall, which is largely replaced by lymphoid cells. The nodule thus formed can be recognized grossly. A characteristic crys-

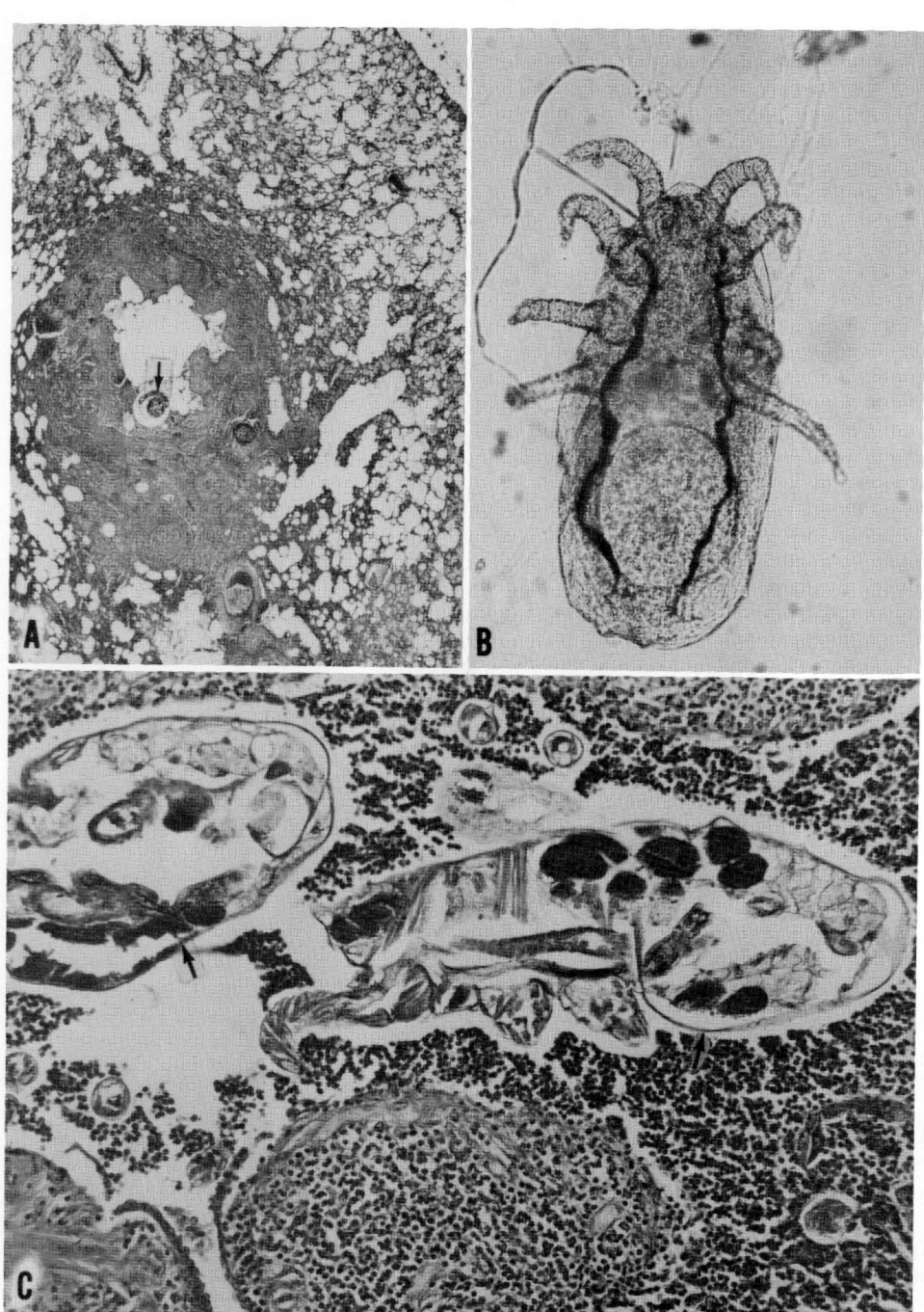

FIG. 13-40 Pulmonary acariasis. **A.** *Pneumonyssus simicola* (arrow) in a dilated bronchiole with thickened wall, in lung of a rhesus monkey *(Macaca mulatta)*. **B.** A female, egg-bearing mite teased from a lesion. **C.** Section of two mites in a bronchiole. (Courtesy of Dr. J. R. M. Innes.)

talline pigment that is microscopically demonstrable accumulates in affected lungs, sometimes at points distant from the parasite. In lymphatic spaces, this pigment occurs as golden brown, coarsely granular or needlelike anisotropic crystals; the crystals may also be refractile and anisotropic, light-brown, phagocytized or free, and finely granular. The pigment is difficult to analyze, but it contains iron and lipofuscin, and probably derives from the excreta of the mites.

A related mite, *Pneumonyssus caninum,* is encountered occasionally in the paranasal sinuses and upper respiratory tracts of dogs. The presence of these mites may result in purulent sinusitis, but this is rarely recognized in the living animal. Mites of another genus, *Cytoleichus,* are found in the air sacs of birds.

PENTASTOMIASIS

Organisms related to the mites and grouped in the class Pentastomida include several genera that are parasitic in mammals. All have indirect life cycles. *Linguatula serrata (Pentastomum taenioides)* is a tongue-shaped, wormlike arthropod that inhabits the respiratory passages of the fox, dog, wolf, horse, goat, sheep, and human. The adults are slightly convex dorsally and

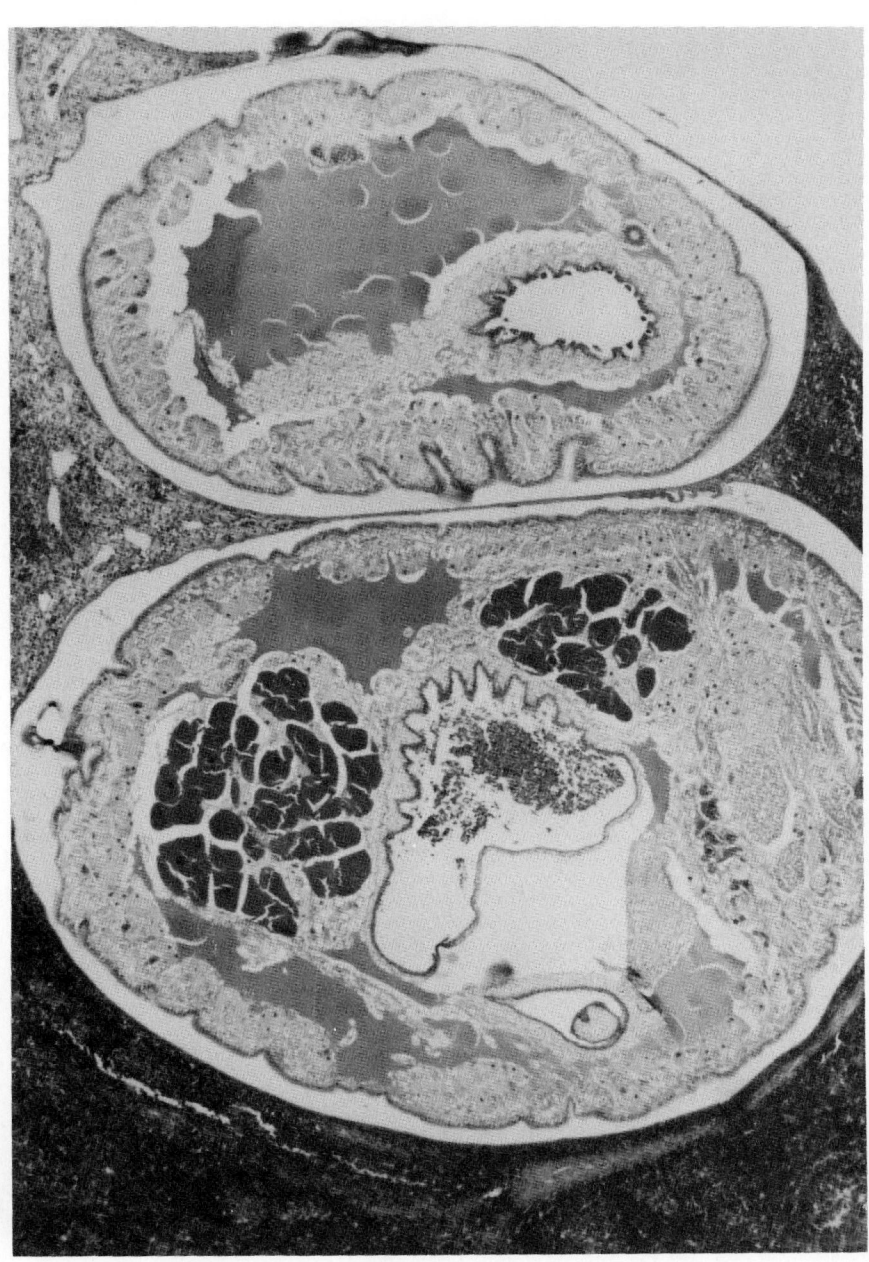

FIG. 13-41 Pentastomiasis. In a rhesus monkey *(Macaca mulatta).* Pentastome nymphs *(Armillifera armillatus)* embedded in the spleen. (Courtesy of New England Regional Primate Research Center, Harvard Medical School.)

flattened ventrally; males measure up to 2 cm and females up to 13 cm in length. The cuticle is transversely striated. Eggs expelled from the nostrils are ingested by suitable intermediate hosts; these are usually sheep or cattle, but swine, horses, rabbits, and other species can be infected. The eggs hatch in the digestive tract, penetrate the intestinal wall, and localize in mesenteric lymph nodes or other tissues. There, the larvae grow to the infective stage. Dogs are believed to become infected by eating tissues containing larvae.

The larvae of a related species, Armillifer armillatus (Fig. 13-41), have been reported to infect viscera of cattle, monkeys, swine, and humans (du Toit and Sutherland, 1968; Challier et al., 1967). The larvae of another species, *Porocephalus clavatus,* are particularly common in various species of nonhuman primates. The larvae of these species are most frequently found in the lungs and liver, but may occur in most any viscus and brain. The adults reside in the respiratory tract of snakes.

CUTANEOUS ACARIASIS (MANGE, SCABIES, SCAB, MITE INFESTATION) (Figs. 13-42 to 13-46).

A wide variety of mites parasitize the skin of animals (Fig. 13-44), and many of them produce serious lesions. In general, each species of mite has its preferred host and will not flourish on any other. Collectively, parasitism with mites is called mange.

Demodectic mange (follicular mange, red mange)
Mites of the genus *Demodex,* which are small and cigar-shaped, are parasites of hair follicles and sebaceous glands of most all animals, including humans. Small numbers of parasites may go unnoticed, but when they

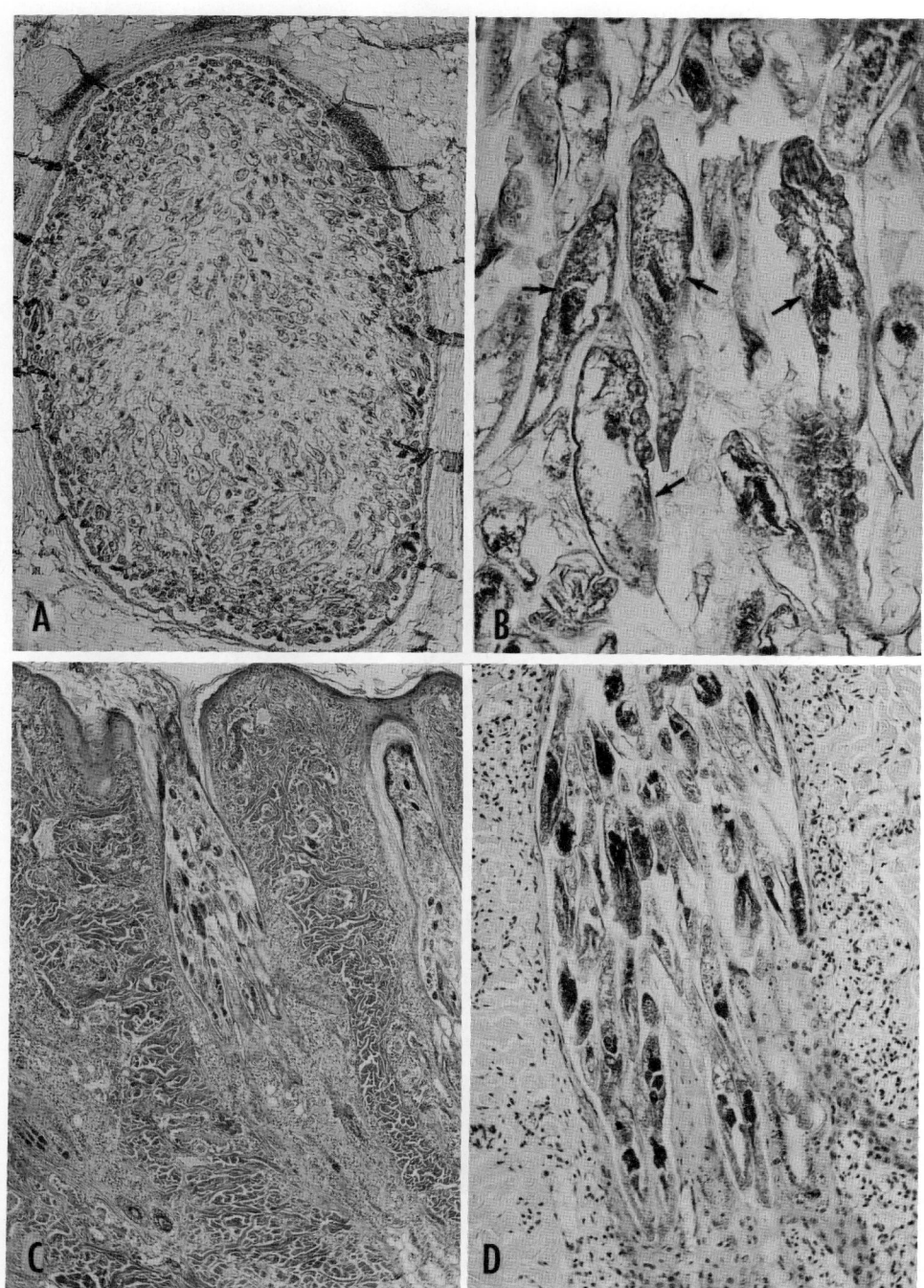

FIG. 13-42 Cutaneous acariasis. **A.** Demodectic mange in the skin of a pig (×35). Large dilated hair follicle filled with *Demodex phylloides*. **B.** Higher magnification (×210) of A shows detail of sections of mites (arrows). (Contributor: Dr. C. L. Davis.) **C.** Demodectic mange in skin of a dog (×35). Note the acanthosis and prominent, distended hair follicles. **D.** A single follicle (×115) from C containing many *Demodex folliculorum*. (Courtesy of Armed Forces Institute of Pathology; contributor: Dr. R. D. Turk.)

are present in large numbers they lead to severe lesions of the skin (Figs. 13-42, 43). It is not clear what allows the mites to proliferate unchecked in some individuals. Although few exist among mites recovered from different species, each recognizable difference is given a specific name. These include *Demodex canis, D. cati, D. bovis, D. ovis, D. equi, D. phylloides* (swine), and *D. folliculorum* (humans). *Demodex spp.* are obligate parasites in which no stage of their cycles occurs outside the skin. Transmission is by direct contact. Clinical disease is most frequent and common in dogs, cattle, and swine. These

mites burrow into the hair follicles of the skin (Fig. 13-43), which produces intense itching accompanied by alopecia and scaling of the epidermis. The itching causes the animal to rub the affected part, which accentuates the symptoms and promotes exudation of serum and scab formation on the denuded surface. The mites may burrow into sebaceous or sweat glands, or to the depths of hair follicles, which causes proliferation and then necrosis of the epithelium, followed by intense inflammation of the underlying dermis; this takes the form of small abscesses, granulomas with giant cells, and diffuse

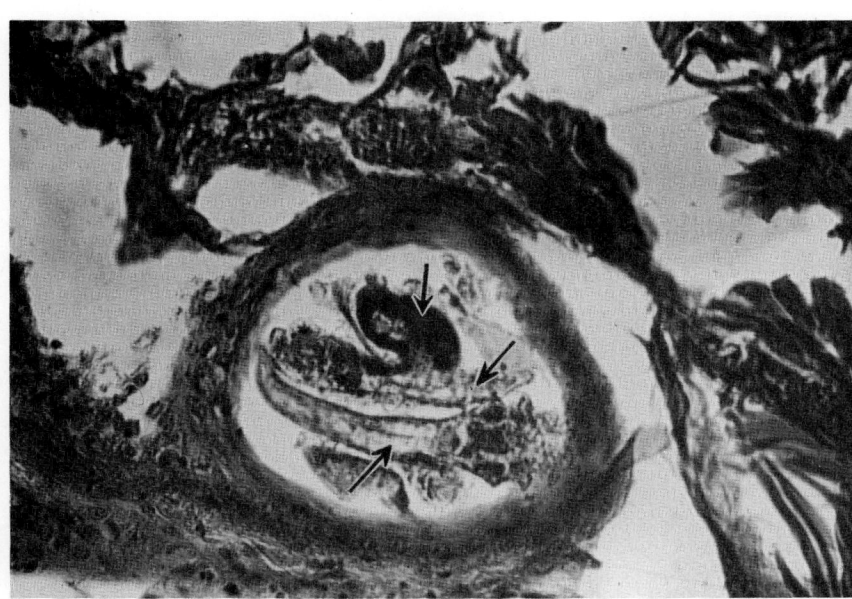

FIG. 13-43 *Demodex folliculorum,* acarid mites (arrows) in a hair follicle cut in cross section. Skin of a dog. (H & E ×250.)

infiltration of lymphocytes. In some cases, the mites migrate even deeper and reach lymph nodes. Secondary pyogenic infections can result in death. Deep folliculitis and dermatitis is recognizable in tissue sections, in which the parasites are easily demonstrated. Deep scrapings of affected skin may also be examined microscopically for the mites.

Sarcoptic mange (Fig. 13-44A) is caused by a specific mite, *Sarcoptes scabiei* (sarcoptic mange mite), which may attack many species, including cattle, sheep, dogs, swine, horses, and humans. Morphologically indistinguishable varieties of *S. scabiei* (such as *bovis* and *suis*) are found in each host species, each variety of mite having its definite host preference; cross-infection of heterologous species rarely occurs. The sarcoptic mange mite burrows in the deeper parts of the stratum corneum, or the superficial layers of the stratum malpighii of the skin, and rarely goes deeper. It completes its entire life cycle at this level. Even in this superficial position, however, the mites cause severe itching, hyperkeratosis, and acanthosis, and loss of hair or wool results. The intense pruritus causes rubbing of the skin, which in turn causes loss of epithelium and secondary infection of the dermis. In dogs, the pruritus is much more intense in sarcoptic than in demodectic mange.

Notoedric mange, which resembles sarcoptic mange, is principally a disease of cats caused by *Notoedres cati.* The lesions predominate around the ears, face, and neck, but may extend and become generalized. *N. muris* affects the ears of rats.

Psoroptic mange occurs in several species of animals, but in domestic animals it is most important in sheep (sheep scab) and cattle, where it is caused by *Psoroptes ovis. P. cuniculi* (Fig. 13-46) is important to laboratory rabbits, where the mites live in the external auditory meatus and produce severe lesions that may lead to middle or inner ear infection, and death. Psoroptes

spp. do not burrow into the epidermis, but remain on the surface.

Chorioptic mange (Fig. 13-45), caused by species of *Chorioptes,* is most frequent in horses *(C. equi),* cattle *(C. bovis)* (Fig. 13-45), and sheep *(C. ovis).* In horses, the mites tend to localize on the legs, which leads to foot mange or leg itch.

Otodectic mange, common in dogs, cats, and wild carnivores, is caused by *Otodectes cynotis,* which resides in the ear canal and rarely elsewhere. The mites live on the surface but incite intense itching, which leads to head-shaking and scratching. This commonly results in hematomas of the pinna. It may also lead to otitis media or interna, and even encephalitis.

Psorergatic mange (Fig. 13-44B, C) is principally a disease of sheep caused by *Psorergates ovis,* which lives on the skin surface and causes pruritis and dermatitis.

Other mites that affect the skin include: *Cheyletiella parasitivorax* and other *Cheyletiella* spp. of rabbits, dogs and cats; *Myobia musculi* of laboratory mice; and *Trombicula autumnalis* and related spp., which are free-living mites whose larvae parasitize humans and most species of animals and birds, causing irritation and dermatitis.

References

Anderson RK. Norwegian scabies in a dog: a case report. J Am Anim Hosp Assoc 1981;17:101–104.

Arlian LG, Kaiser S, Estes SA, et al. Infestivity of Psoroptes cuniculi in rabbits. Am J Vet Res 1981;42:1782–1784.

Baker EW. Ectopic ear mite infestation in the dog. J Am Vet Med Assoc 1974;164:1125–1126.

Baker DW, Nutting WB. Demodectic mange in New York State sheep. Cornell Vet 1940;40:140–142.

Baker KP. The histopathology and pathogenesis of demodecosis of the dog. J Comp Pathol 1969;79:321–327.

Baker KP. Infestation of domestic animals with the mite Cheyletiella parasitivorax. Vet Rec 1969;84:561.

Beresford-Jones WP. Occurrence of the mite *Psorergates simplex* in mice. Aust Vet J 1965;41:289–290.

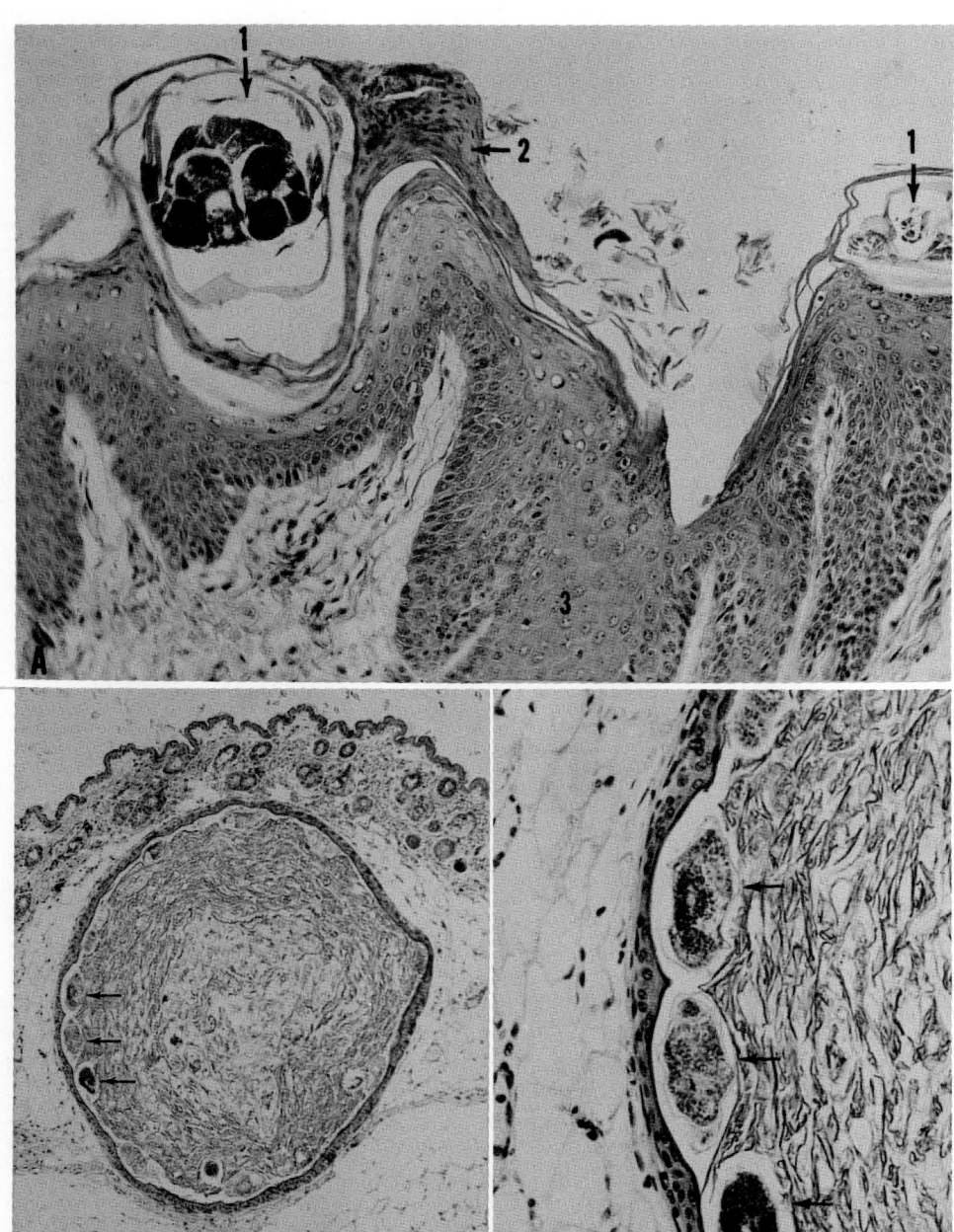

FIG. 13-44 Cutaneous acariasis. **A.** Sarcoptic mange. (1) The mites are in the superficial epidermis; (2) Parakeratosis; and (3) Acanthosis. (Contributor: Col. J. H. Rust, V. C.) **B.** Acariasis in the skin of a mouse (×70). The mites (*Psorergates simplex*) (arrows) cause the formation of epidermal inclusion cyst. **C.** The mites (arrows) in the cyst (×250). (Courtesy of Armed Forces Institute of Pathology; contributor: Dr. Robert J. Flynn.)

Carter HB. A skin disease of sheep due to an ectoparasitic mite, *Psorergates ovis* (Womersley 1941). Aust Vet J 1941;17:193–201.

Challier A, Gidel R, Traore S. Porocephalosis caused by *Armillifer (Nettorhynchus) armillatus* (Wyman 1847) in a bull and pig. Revue Elev Med Vet Pays Trop 1967;20:255–259.

Danilov I. Lethal infestation of goats with juvenile forms of *Linguatula serrata*. Vet Sbir 56:24–25, Vet Bull 1959;3513–3559.

Dawson DV, Whitmore SP, Bresnahan JF. Genetic control of susceptibility to mite-associated ulcerative dermatitis. Lab Anim Sci 1986;36:262–267.

Desch C, Nutting WB. *Demodex cati* Hirst 1919: a redescription. Cornell Vet 1979;69:280–285.

Dodd K. *Cheyletiella yasguri*: widespread infestation in a breeding kennel. Vet Rec 1970;86:346–347.

Doube BM. Cattle and the paralysis tick *Ixodes holocyclus*. Aust Vet J 1975;51:511–515.

Doube BM, Kemp DH. Paralysis of cattle by *Ixodes holocyclus* Neumann. Aust J Agric Res 1975;26:635–640.

Du Toit R, Sutherland KJ. *Armillifer armillatus* (Wyman) (Order: Pentastomida) from slaughter stock. J S Afr Vet Med Assoc 1968;39:77–79.

Durden LA, DeBruyn EJ. Louse infestations of tree shrews (*Tupaia glis*). Lab Anim Sci 1984;34:188–190.

Ewing SA, Mosier JE, Foxx TS. Occurrence of *Cheyletiella* spp. on dogs with skin lesions. J Am Vet Med Assoc 1967;151:64–67.

Flatt RE, Patton NM. A mite infestation in squirrel monkeys (*Saimiri sciureus*). J Am Vet Med Assoc 1967;155:1233–1235.

Flynn RJ, Jaroslow BN. Nidification of a mite (*Psorergates simplex* (Tyr-

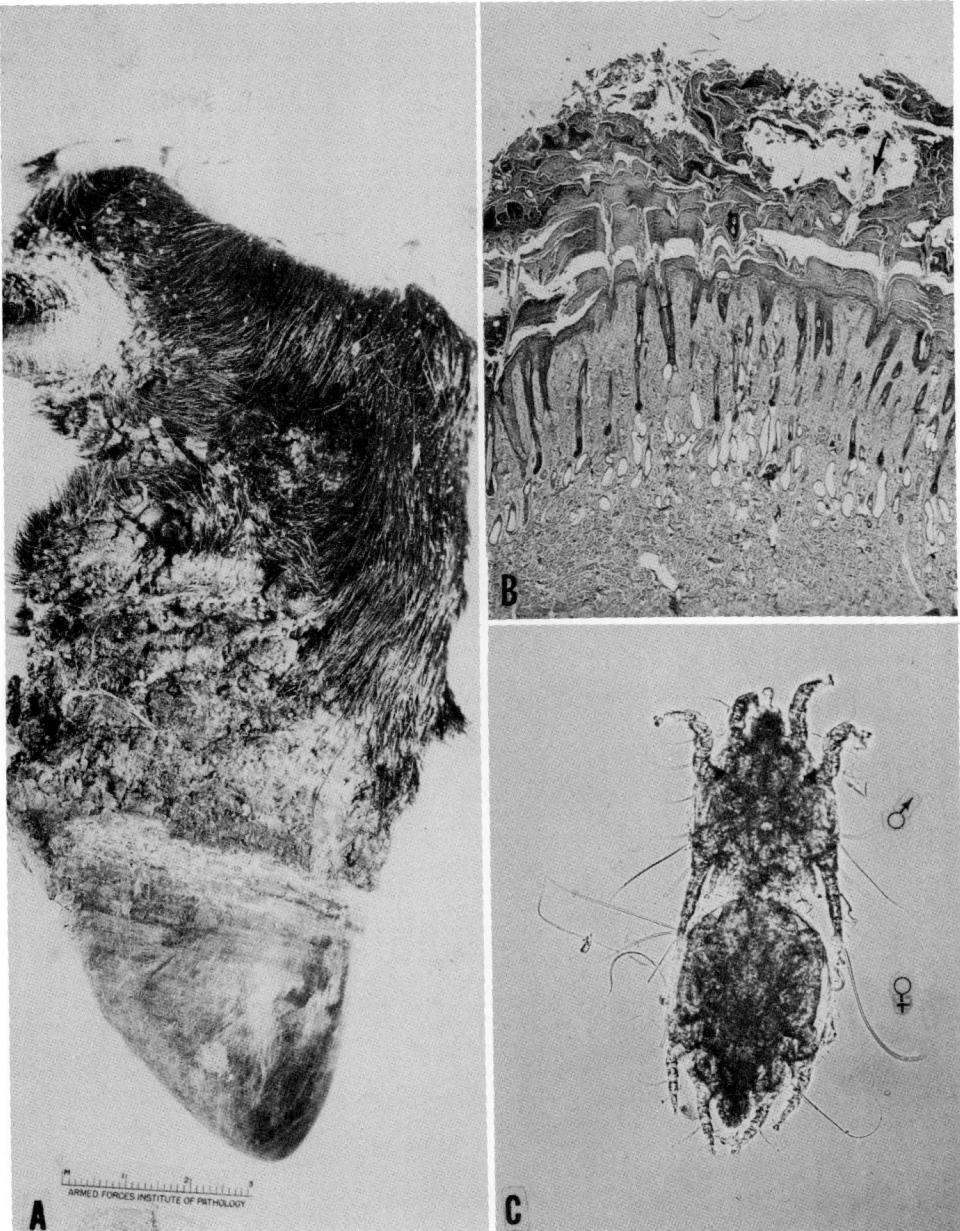

FIG. 13-45 Chorioptic mange in fetlock region of an Angus steer. **A.** Tenacious, thick scales adhering to hairs. **B.** Section (×10) of the affected skin. Note thick exudate adhering to epidermis. Arrow points to the mites. **C.** Pair of mites in coitus, teased from the fixed specimen and cleared in phenol (×75). (Courtesy of Armed Forces Institute of Pathology; contributor: Dr. E. R. Derflinger.)

rell, 1883) (Myobiidae) in the skin of mice. J Parasitol 1956;42:49–52.

Foxx TS, Ewing SA. Morphologic features, behavior, and life history of *Cheyletiella yasguri.* Am J Vet Res 1969;30:269–285.

Frederickson RG, Haines DE, Hall JE. Pentastomid nymph from the brain of a squirrel monkey *(Saimiri sciureus).* II. Morphology of the host response. J Med Primatol 1985;14:209–223.

French FE. *Demodex canis* in canine tissues. Cornell Vet 1964;54:271–290.

Friedman S, Weisbroth SH. The parasitic ecology of the rodent mite *Myobia musculi.* II. Genetic factors. Lab Anim Sci 1975;25:440–445.

Gething MA. Cheyletiella infestation in small animals. Vet Bull 1973;43:63–69.

Greene RT, Scheidt VJ, Moncol DJ. Trombiculiasis in a cat. J Am Vet Med Assoc 1986;188:1054–1055.

Gresham ACJ. Porcine infestation with *Parasitus consanguineus.* Vet Rec 1990;127:525.

Griffin CA, Dean DJ. Demodectic mange in goats. Cornell Vet 1944;34:308–311.

Grono LR. Studies of the ear mite, *Otodectes cynotis.* Vet Rec 1969;85:6–8.

Hall JE, Haines DE, Frederickson RG. Pentastomid nymph from the brain of a squirrel monkey *(Saimiri sciureus).* I. Morphology of the nymph. J Med Primatol 1985;14:195–208.

Harvey RG. Dermatitis in a cat associated with *Spilopsyllus cuniculi.* Vet Rec 1990;126:89–90.

Hawkins JA, McDonald RK, Woody BJ. *Sarcoptes scabiei* infestation in a cat. J Am Vet Med Assoc 1987;190:1572–1573.

Hickey TE, Kelly WA, Sitzman JE. Demodectic mange in a tamarin *(Saguinus geoffroyi).* Lab Anim Sci 1983;33:192–193.

Innes JRM, Colton MW, Yevich PP, et al. Pulmonary acariasis as an enzootic disease caused by *Pneumonyssus simicola* in imported monkeys. Am J Pathol 1954;30:813–835.

Khalil GM, Schacher JF. *Linguatula serrata* in relation to halzoun and the Marrara syndrome. Am J Trop Med Hyg 1965;14:736–746.

Kim CS, Bang BG. Nasal mites parasitic in nasal and upper skull tissues in the baboon (Papio sp.). Science 1970;169:372–373.

Kirkwood A, Kendall SB. Demodectic mange in cattle. Vet Rec 1966;78:33–34.

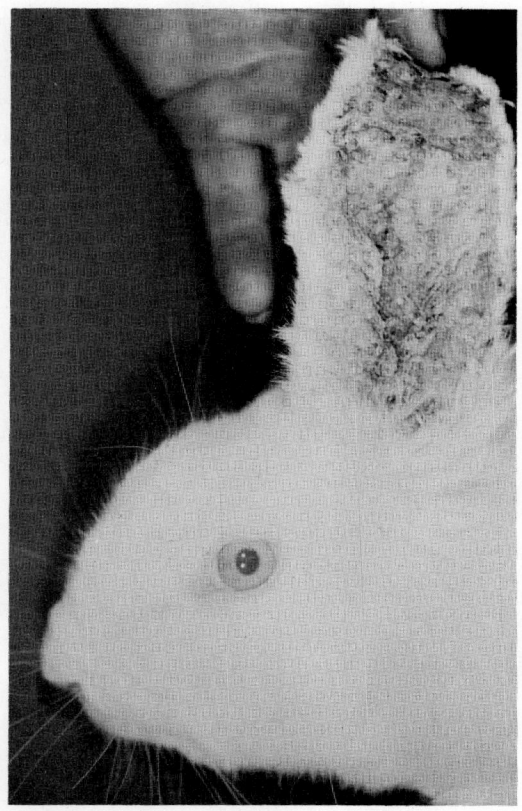

FIG. 13-46 Lesions of ear mites *(Psoroptes communis v. cunuliculi)* in the ear of a New Zealand white rabbit.

Kummel BA, Estes SA, Arlian LG. *Trixacarus caviae* infestation of guinea pigs. J Am Vet Med Assoc 1980;177:903–908.

Kunkle GA, Greiner EC. Dermatitis in a horse caused by the straw itch mite. J Am Vet Med Assoc 1982;181:467–469.

Leerhoy J, Jensen HS. Sarcoptic mange in a shipment of cynomolgus monkeys. Nord Vet Med 1967;19:128–130.

Lindquist WD, Cash WC. Sarcoptic mange in a cat. J Am Vet Med Assoc 1973;162:639–640.

Lok JB, Kirkpatrick CE. Pentastomiasis in captive monkeys. Lab Anim Sci 1987;37:494–496.

Martin HM, Deubler MJ. Acariasis *(Pneumonyssus* sp.) of the upper respiratory tract of the dog. Univ of Pa Bull 1943;43:21–27.

McConnell EE, Basson PA, de Vos V. Laryngeal acariasis in the chacma baboon. J Am Vet Med Assoc 1972;161:678–682.

McDonald SE, Lavoipierre MMJ. *Trixacarus caviae* infestation in two guinea pigs. Lab Anim Sci 1980;30:67–70.

McKeever PJ, Allen SK. Dermatitis associated with *Cheyletiella* infestation in cats. J Am Vet Med Assoc 1979;174:718–720.

McLennan H, Oikawa I. Changes in function of the neuromuscular junction occurring in tick paralysis. Can J Phys Pharmacol 1972;50:53–58.

Miller JK, Tompkins VN, Sieracki JC. Pathology of Colorado tick fever in experimental animals. Arch Pathol 1961;72:149–157.

Morgan K. Aural haematomata, cauliflower ears, and *Psoroptes ovis* in sheep. Vet Rec 1991;128:459–460.

Nelson WA, Bainborough AR. Development in sheep of resistance to the ked, *Melophagus ovinus.* III. Histopathology of sheep skin as a clue to the nature of resistance. Exp Parasitol 1963;13:118–127, Vet Bull;63:3570.

Powell MB, Weisbroth SH, Roth L, et al. Reaginic hypersensitivity in *Otodectes cynotis* infestation of cats and mode of mite feeding. Am J Vet Res 1980;41:877–882.

Prathap K, Lau KS, Bolton JM. Pentastomiasis: a common finding at autopsy among Malaysian aborigines. Am J Trop Med Hyg 1969;18:20–27.

Schaffer MH, Baker NF, Kennedy PC. Parasitism by *Cheyletiella parasitivorax.* A case report of the infestation in a female dog and its litter. Cornell Vet 1958;48:440–447.

Schnelle GB, Jones TC. Occurrence of the cereal mite in war dogs. J Am Vet Med Assoc 1944;104:213–214.

Sharma Deorani VP, Chaudhuri RP. On histopathology of the skin lesion of goats affected by sarcoptic mange. Indian J Vet Sci 1965;35:150–156.

Sheahan BJ. Pathology of *Sarcoptes scabiei* infection in pigs. I. Naturally occurring and experimentally induced lesion. II. Histological, histochemical and ultrastructural changes at skin test sites. J Comp Pathol 1975;85:87–95, 97–110.

Sloan CA. Mortality in sheep due to *Ixodes* species. Aust Vet J 1968;44:527–528.

Smith EB, Claypoole TF. Canine scabies in dogs and in humans. J Am Med Assoc 1967;199:59–64.

Walder EJ, Howard EB. Persistent insect bite granuloma in a dog. Vet Pathol 1981;18:839–841.

Whitney RA, Kruckenberg SM. Pentastomid infection associated with peritonitis in Mangabey monkeys. J Am Vet Med Assoc 1967;151:907–908.

Wimsatt JH, Houston RS, Maul DH. An infestation of sucking lice in a juvenile rhesus macaque. Lab Anim Sci 1988;38:203–204.

Yasgur I. Parasitism of kennel puppies with the mite *Cheyletiella parasitivorax.* Cornell Vet 1964;54:406–407.

Zajac A, Williams JF, Williams CSF. Mange caused by *Trixacarus caviae* in guinea pigs. J Am Vet Med Assoc 1980;177:900–903.

14

Pathologic effects of ionizing radiations

An understanding of the pathologic effects of radiation has increased in importance over the past several years, and its significance will continue to grow with the expanding development of nuclear energy. The explosion of a nuclear bomb produces huge quantities of radioactive substances that may be scattered widely by blast and wind with possible hazard to humans and animals. The use of nuclear energy as a controlled source of power in nuclear reactor and atomic "piles" presents the potential hazard of accidental exposure.

Release of radioactivity into the atmosphere, as the result of accidents involving nuclear power plants, has become a matter of public concern. It is sometimes difficult to learn of the facts involving an actual or potential nuclear accident amid the outcries of proponents and opponents of nuclear power. The potential hazards to animal and human life are real and must be evaluated dispassionately if they are to be understood and dealt with effectively.

To the veterinarian, ionizing radiation should be seen as one of the causes of injury to animals and must be distinguished from all other causes of disease or injury. To do this, it is essential that the types of radiation and their effects on animal tissues be known, as well as the doses of radiation. The detection of exposure requires specialized instruments and knowledge.

Hopefully, these two sources of radiation will remain controlled.

Radiation will continue to increase in importance in the diagnosis and treatment of disease and, in its many forms, will be a valuable tool to animal research. It is important, therefore, to study the biologic effects of radiation from whatever source.

Radiation of the types to be considered, which exists in both electromagnetic and particulate form, gives up energy and, in general, produces effects upon cells and tissues by ionization. This property, the ionization of matter, also provides the usual means for detection of radiation of this type; thus, the term, ionizing radiation is appropriate and useful to differentiate it from radiation of other types that are nonionizing (visible light, infrared, microwaves, and radio waves). Ionization is the production of ions (atoms or molecules that possess an electrical charge) by a sequence of atomic events leading to displacement of electrons and transfer of energy.

Details of atomic physics lay outside the scope of this book, but some of the nomenclature must be used in studying the lesions produced by ionizing radiation. Therefore, a few terms will be discussed prior to considering the biologic effects of ionizing radiation.

References

Anon. Radiation quantities and units. International Commission on Radiation Units and Measurements. Washington, D.C.: Report 33, 1980.

Anon. The accident at the Chernobyl nuclear power plant and its consequences. USSR state committee on the utilization of atomic energy. Report to an expert meeting in Vienna, 25–29 August, 1986.

Goldman M. Chernobyl: a radiobiological perspective. Science 1987;238:622–623.

Lindell B. Radiation and health. Bull WHO 1987;65:139–143.

TYPES OF IONIZING RADIATION

As indicated previously, ionizing radiation may be either electromagnetic or particulate.

Electromagnetic radiation

Electromagnetic radiation includes a broad spectrum of energy waves: radio waves, infrared waves, ultraviolet waves, visible light, gamma (γ) rays, x-rays (roentgen rays), and cosmic rays. All have their specific wavelengths and frequencies and travel at the speed of light. Those with short wavelengths and high frequencies are ionizing radiations, and include γ, x-, and cosmic rays. Ionization results from the ejection of electrons from target molecules.

γ Rays are electromagnetic radiations of short wavelengths emitted from the nucleus of radioisotopes. They are essentially similar to x-rays but usually of higher energy, and generally come from different sources. γ Rays have long range and deep penetration in tissues, but low ionization per unit of matter penetrated. These rays may penetrate deep into the body and produce an effect upon the entire body (total body effect).

X-rays or roentgen rays are penetrating electromagnetic radiation having wavelengths less than those of visible light. Although similar to γ rays, x-rays usually are of much lower energy and are produced by the bombardment of a metallic target by fast-moving electrons in a high vacuum. Their biologic effects are similar to those of γ rays.

Cosmic rays are complex radiation phenomena that originate in outer space and are largely absorbed by the earth's atmosphere. Some constituents of cosmic rays are capable of extremely deep penetration, even in dense matter, such as rock.

Particulate radiation

A variety of discrete particles, which may be released from radioisotopes or accelerated artificially, comprise particulate radiation. As particles, they all have lesser penetrability into tissues than electromagnetic radiation, but possess greater capacity for ionization.

The alpha (α) particle is a helium nucleus consisting of two protons and two neutrons with a double-positive charge and having a definite mass. A stream of α particles (so-called α ray) has high ionizing but very low penetrating properties and a short range; a thin sheet of paper, the keratin layer of the skin, or other material of comparable thickness will prevent its passage. It has little biologic effect except when α-emitting isotopes (such as radium) are deposited in tissues where prolonged effects are produced.

The beta (β) particle is a charged particle (negative or positive) emitted from the nucleus of an atom; its mass and charge are equal in magnitude to those of the electron. A positive electron is called a positron (β+). Depending on its energy, a β particle has a longer range and deeper penetration than an α particle, but causes only a medium degree of ionization. Radioactive isotopes that emit β particles ("β emitters") may produce lesions in the skin upon continued contact and may be particularly dangerous when concentrated in bone (as in radioactive isotopes deposited in bone; i.e., "bone seekers").

Neutrons (n) are elementary nuclear particles that bear no electrical charge and have a mass approximately the same as that of hydrogen atoms. Neutrons have very long range, deep penetration, and may induce radioactivity. They may be artificially accelerated in the form of a beam, which provides a useful means of tissue analysis by induction of radioactivity (neutron activation analysis).

Protons are also constituents of atomic nuclei with the same mass as a neutron but bearing a positive charge equal and opposite to that of an electron. They have high ionizing capacity and may induce radioactiv-ity. Proton beams can also be artificially created and used to induce radioactivity for tissue analysis (proton activation analysis). Proton beams are more definable in outline than the more diffuse neutron beams.

MEASUREMENT OF RADIATION

The roentgen (r) is a unit of x- or γ radiation used in measuring dosage. It is defined as that quantity of x- or γ radiation which is of such magnitude that its associated corpuscular emission per 0.001293 g of air produces in-air ions carrying one electrostatic unit of electricity of either sign. The intensity of the roentgen is measured in air; hence, it is not an accurate indication of radioactivity absorbed by tissue. In order to overcome this discrepancy, a unit of measurement of absorbed dosage of radiation, the rad, was adopted by the International Commission on Radiologic Units at the Seventh International Congress of Radiology, Copenhagen, in 1953. The rad is a measure of the energy (100 ergs/g) imparted to matter by ionizing particles per unit mass of unit material at the place of interest. Another unit, the Gray (Gy), is an absorbed dose 100 times greater than one rad. In biologic systems, the matter irradiated is usually stated as a specific tissue.

The curie (Ci) is that quantity of radioactive material having associated with it 3.7×10^{10} disintegrations per second. It is therefore a measure of radioactivity and is most commonly used in biology as millicurie (mc) or microcurie (μc) units.

The specific activity of radioactive material is the activity of a sample per unit mass.

The half-life of a radioactive substance is the length of time (in seconds, hours, days, or years) required for the substance to lose 50% of its radioactivity by decay. The biologic half-life of a substance is the time required for the body to eliminate one-half of an administered dose of the substance by the usual process of elimination. The lethal dose (LD) of radiation is usually stated as the amount required to kill a given number of animals within a specified period of time. Thus, LD 50/30 is the dosage of radiation required to kill 50% of a group of animals in 30 days.

An electron volt (eV) is a unit of energy equivalent to the amount of energy gained by an electron passing through a potential difference of 1 volt. Large multiples of this unit are commonly used, viz., kev (thousand electron volts), mev (million electron volts), and bev (billion electron volts).

Linear energy transfer (LET) is a term used to express the quality of radiation. It concerns the spatial distributions of energy transfers that occur along and within the tracks of particles as they penetrate matter. These energy transfers influence the effectiveness of irradiation in producing physical, chemical, or biologic changes, and are independent of other physical factors, such as total energy dissipated, absorbed dose, absorbed dose rate, and absorbed dose fractionation. Relative biologic effectiveness (RBE) is used to compare the absorbed dose of two forms of radiation to produce the same biologic effect. The precise, technical definition of these terms may be found in the report of the International Commission on Radiation Units and Measurements (1980).

RADIOISOTOPES

An isotope of an element is one of several nuclides of that element having the same number of protons in their nuclei—hence the same atomic number—but differing in the number of neutrons and consequently in mass number. Isotopes of a particular element have almost identical chemical properties, and may be stable or unstable. Unstable isotopes undergo radioactive decay, and are therefore called radioactive isotopes or radioisotopes. Only a few radioisotopes occur in nature and generally these do not constitute a large source of radioactivity. The fission reaction in the atomic bomb or the neutron bombardment of stable isotopes in a nuclear reactor can produce large quantities of artificial radioisotopes that have wide use in science, industry, and medicine. Isotopes are usually designated by their chemical symbol and mass number: thus, radium-223 (^{223}Ra), potassium-40 (^{40}K), and uranium-238 (^{238}U) are naturally occurring radioisotopes; iodine-131 (^{131}I) and phosphorus-32 (^{32}P) are artificially produced radioisotopes; while potassium-39 (^{39}K), carbon-13 (^{13}C), and oxygen-16 (^{16}O) are stable isotopes. These symbols may be written with left (^{32}P) or right (P^{32}) superscripts. The convention using the left superscript for the mass number and a left subscript for the atomic number of the element may also be encountered (i.e., $^{1}_{1}$H for hydrogen; $^{2}_{1}$H for heavy hydrogen: deuterium). The student is referred to the texts listed in the references for further information.

References

Anon. The international system of units (SI). National Bureau of Standards Special Publication 330, U.S. Government Printing Office, Washington D.C., 1977.

Lapp RE, Andrews HL. Nuclear radiation physics, 2nd ed. New York: Prentice-Hall, 1954.

National Council on Radiation Protection and Measurements. Radiation protection in veterinary medicine. NCRP Report No. 36, 15, Washington, D.C., August 1970.

Upton AC. Radiation injury. Chicago: Univ. Chicago Press, 1969.

EFFECTS OF RADIATION ON BIOLOGIC SYSTEMS

Direct effects

Direct effects of radiation may be explained on the basis of the target theory, particularly in relationship to viruses, genes, and chromosomes. The target is visualized as one of relatively large molecular dimensions, and the effect is attributed to a single ionization, or a small number of ionizations anywhere within the structure. It is presumed that a chemical change is produced in a molecule when ionization occurs directly within it. A larger molecule is more likely to be hit than a smaller one, thus the dose required to change a quantity of a substance by radiation will be inversely proportional to its molecular weight. A method based upon this principle has been used to determine the molecular weight of some proteins.

Quantitation of direct effects depends upon the target size, type of radiation, and intensity of radiation dosage.

Indirect effects

Indirect action of radiation is particularly applicable in aqueous solution and depends upon ionization, which produces free radicals, and then, in turn, may react chemically. These free radicals (for example, hydroxyl [OH-] and perhydroxyl [HO$_2$] radicals) are highly reactive and may become responsible for chemical changes in other molecules in the solution. This indirect effect upon molecules would depend upon the number of free radicals released and not upon molecular size or concentration. If a single substance in solution were radiated, changes in that solute would increase linearly with the dose of radiation. If two or more substances were present in the irradiated solution, one may elicit a protective effect by competing for the free radicals.

Enzymes and enzyme systems

The inactivation of vital enzymes or enzyme systems in cells has been postulated as one of the possible means by which radiant energy could injure cells. Purified enzymes, such as ribonuclease, in the solid state may be partially inactivated by x-radiation when very large doses are used (i.e., 20×10^6 rads). This appears to be due to a direct effect of the radiation. In dilute aqueous solution, a purified enzyme is inactivated more readily, but increased concentrations appear to be protective, suggesting an indirect effect of the radiation. Many compounds, particularly those such as cysteine and glutathione which have an affinity for reaction with oxidizing radicals, exert a protective effect upon enzymes radiated in solution. Oxidative phosphorylation in biologic systems results in the generation of adenosine triphosphate (ATP) from adenosine diphosphate (ADP) or monophosphate (AMP). This generation of ATP in cells is accomplished principally in the mitochondria. Radiation of isolated mitochondria, in vitro, has little effect on their phosphorylation potential unless very high doses are used (10,000 rads). Conversely, mitochondria from spleen or thymus of irradiated rats (700 rads), have decreased phosphorylating capacity. Isolated calf thymic nuclei, in vitro, have phosphorylating activity that can be inactivated by radiation. Phosphorylation of nuclear histone is also depressed by γ irradiation. Synthesis of deoxyribonucleic acid (DNA) is also inhibited in plant cells following irradiation, particularly when done prior to the onset of mitosis.

Viruses

The direct effect of radiation on viruses appears to be most significant in purified, dry, or concentrated solution, or in the presence of protective substances. The mean lethal dose may be correlated with the size of some plant and phage viruses. However, with the larger vaccinia virus, the target volume appears to be smaller than the virus itself, perhaps indicating a more radiosensitive component of the virus complex.

Bacteria

The survival of bacteria has been studied following ionizing radiation in the dry state or suspended in water or nutrient media. Curves prepared of the logarithmic numbers of surviving bacteria usually indicate an exponential relationship to dose, but in some instances an increasing percentage of bacteria is killed by each increment of radiation dosage before this exponential relationship is reached. In some conditions, bacteria are protected from the lethal effects of radiant energy by freezing or by the presence of reducing agents in the solution.

Mammalian cells

The radiosensitivity of cells, in vitro, has been demonstrated for many types of neoplastic and normal animal cells. Many neoplastic murine cells (lymphoma, Ehrlich ascites, sarcoma, mammary carcinoma, and squamous cell carcinoma) have been exposed, in vitro, to x-rays or γ rays under varying experimental conditions. Of interest is the observation that most of these tumor cells are much more radiosensitive in the oxygenated as compared to the anoxic state. The sensitivity of these cells also varies widely in relationship to the stage of mitotic cycle in which they are irradiated. All cells are most radiosensitive during mitosis, then are resistant for a period, until the start of DNA synthesis. After completion of DNA synthesis, these cells remain radioresistant until mitosis resumes.

Some heritable changes occurred in cultures of irradiated mammalian cells. The nucleus of most cells is clearly more sensitive to radiation than is the cytoplasm. Although most cells irreparably injured by radiation are unable to reproduce subsequently, many functions of the cell are not impaired until the cell actually undergoes necrosis. A few cells, particularly oocytes and lymphocytes, are quite sensitive in interphase, undergoing necrosis shortly after receiving a small dose.

Nonlethal doses of radiant energy may produce lesions in chromosomes which are of particular interest. γ Irradiation is of greatest significance in whole-body irradiation, but when radioisotopes are introduced into tissue, α-emitters are 15–20 times more damaging to chromosomes than either γ- or β-emitters. Modern cytogenetic techniques make it possible to examine chromosomes in metaphase and to detect anomalies in number and morphology. These effects have been observed in human patients who were irradiated for treatment of one of various disorders and in radiation workers whose circulating lymphocytes were subsequently studied by cytogenetic methods. These abnormalities have also been seen in many animal karyotypes. Certain lesions in chromosomes are considered unstable in that they are usually lost as the cell undergoes mitosis. These include: chromatid breaks (fracture of one arm of the chromosome), acentric fragments (bits of chromosome with no centromere, resulting from fracture), dicentric chromosomes (with two centromeres, resulting from fracture and rejoining at centromere), tricentric chromosomes (three centromeres), and aneuploidy (more or less than the normal diploid number). Stable or permanent lesions include: reciprocal translocations (exchange transfer of parts of chromatids between two chromosomes), ring chromosomes (breaks with fusion of telomeric ends of chromosomes), and aneuploidy (trisomy especially, may also be unstable).

Lesions in chromosomes occur in increased numbers in lymphocytes of patients and experimental animals following x-ray treatment. Similar breaks occur in unirradiated patients, but usually in 1% of cells examined. Following irradiation, these may constitute as much as 37% of the cells karyotyped. These defects undoubtedly change the metabolism of the affected cells, but have not been shown to affect germ cells and thus influence the genetic makeup of offspring.

Genes

The rearrangement, loss, or addition of parts of a chromosome doubtlessly has an effect upon the metabolism and progeny of the affected cell. It is also possible for radiant energy to cause chemical alteration in the DNA of cells, resulting in mutation. The mutagenic effect of ionizing radiation has been clearly demonstrated in such organisms as the bread mold, Neurospora, and fruit fly, Drosophila. The evidence for such mutagenic effects in mammals, such as mice, is not as convincing. It is possible that mutagenic effects do occur in mammalian germ cells, but resulting gametes are less viable, resulting in fewer zygotes carrying the mutant gene.

Carcinogenesis

Several obvious examples exist to indicate that some forms of neoplasia appear with increased frequency in animals and humans following exposure to ionizing radiation (See Neoplasia). The possible interaction of certain oncogenic viruses in some neoplasms is yet to be explained. Leukemia in Japanese people who were exposed to irradiation at Hiroshima or Nagasaki clearly became more frequent than in those who were unirradiated. Irradiated mice also have significant increased frequency of lymphoma (so-called leukemia). The appearance of squamous cell carcinomas on the hands of radiologists and veterinarians following x-ray injury also is acceptable evidence. Clearly, ionizing radiation may be an antecedent event in certain types of malignant disease, although the precise etiologic relationship and pathogenetic mechanisms are not yet established.

Environmental pollution

Some forms of radioactivity, particularly resulting from atomic explosions, may become concentrated by biologic processes and therefore represent a special kind of pollutant. Radioiodine is one example, the ^{131}I is concentrated in the thyroid of animals after consumption of contaminated forage. Radiostrontium is more important in this respect because it is metabolized as a chemical analogue of calcium and is concentrated by aquatic plants and animals. Here it becomes part of the food chain of animals and humans and, therefore, a hazard. Radiostrontium (^{90}Sr) is stored in bones of animals and excreted in milk. However, specific biologic discrimination by the cow (i.e., intestinal absorption of only part of the ^{90}Sr, deposit of some of it in bone and subsequent urinary excretion with calcium) makes milk one of the safest sources of calcium in an area contaminated by radioactive fallout. In other words, foods directly contaminated would provide relatively more ^{90}Sr to be absorbed and metabolized as calcium.

References

Anon. Ionizing radiation: sources and biological effects. United Nations Scientific Committee on the Effects of Atomic Radiation. Report to the General Assembly. New York: United Nations, 1982.

Comar CL. Radioisotopes in biology and agriculture. New York: McGraw-Hill, 1955.

Moore W Jr, Gillespie LJ. Persistence of chromosomal damage following in utero irradiation of the dog. Am J Vet Res 1967;28:890–891.

Russell WL. The effect of radiation dose rate and fractionation on mutation in mice. In: Sobels FH, ed. Repair from genetic radiation damage. Oxford: Pergamon Press, 1963;205–217.

Sasser LB, Bell MC, Cross FH. Hematologic response of sheep and cattle to whole-body gamma irradiation and gastrointestinal and skin beta irradiation. Am J Vet Res 1973;34:1555–1560.

Spalding JF, Brooks MR, Archuleta RF. Genetic effects of x-irradiation of 10, 15 and 20 generations of male mice. Health Phys 1964;10:293–296.

RADIOSENSITIVITY OF TISSUES

The susceptibility of tissues to radiation varies widely even in the same species. In general, those tissues undergoing the most rapid growth are most susceptible to the injurious effects of ionizing radiation; conversely, cells that have a slower rate of reproduction are most resistant. Tissues with the least degree of differentiation also are more sensitive than those that are highly differentiated. Thus, cells may be listed in order of their susceptibility to radiation:

Extreme Radiosensitivity

Lymphocytes
Immature hematopoietic cells
Intestinal epithelium
Germinal cells

High Radiosensitivity

Endothelium
Urinary bladder epithelium
Gastric epithelium
Epithelium of the skin
Epithelium of mouth, pharynx, and esophagus

Intermediate Radiosensitivity

Connective tissue cells
Cartilage and growing bone cells
Renal epithelium

Hepatic epithelium
Pancreatic epithelium
Thyroid epithelium
Adrenal epithelium
Pulmonary epithelium

Low Radiosensitivity

Skeletal muscle cells
Mature bone cells
Mature connective tissue
Neurons
Mature hematopoietic cells

SUSCEPTIBILITY OF DIFFERENT SPECIES

The susceptibility of various animal species to ionizing radiation differs within wide limits. In large animals, the LD 50/30 is also influenced by the source of the radiation and the dosage rate. The following list indicates the approximate LD (50/30) of x- or γ-radiation given in one dose over the total body:

Species	rad
Sheep	200–300
Swine	200–300
Dog	240–320
Goat	250–300
Burro	250–300
Guinea pig	400–500
Rhesus monkey	500–600
Mouse	525–775
Rabbit	700–800
Rat	700–820

Simpler forms of life are, in general, much more resistant to the lethal effects of radiation. For example, 750,000 r are required to kill all bacteria in milk: sporulating bacteria may require as much as 500,000 r to kill all spores; tobacco mosaic virus is killed by 1,800,000 r; and although some enzyme systems show measurable effects after this large amount of radiation, many times this dose is required to destroy all enzyme systems in tissues.

References

Gleiser CA. The determination of the lethal dose 50/30 of total body x-radiation for dogs. Am J Vet Res 1953;14:284–286.

Rust JH, et al. The lethal dose of whole-body tantalum 182 gamma irradiation for the burro (Equus asinus asinus). Radiology 1953;60:579–582.

Rust JH, Trum BF, Kuhn USG III. Physiological aberrations following total body irradiation of domestic animals with large doses of gamma rays. Vet Med 1954;49:318.

WHOLE-BODY RADIATION

In contrast to radiation delivered to a specific part of the body (as in radium or x-ray therapy), whole-body radiation is the exposure of the entire surface of the body so as to give a uniform dose of ionizing radiation to all parts of the body. This type of radiation injury may be produced experimentally by x- and γ rays and may occur following the detonation of an atomic bomb. If dosages were sufficiently high, several systems of the body would be affected, resulting in radiation sickness.

Clinical manifestations

The clinicopathologic changes in animals exposed to whole-body radiation include immediate and severe lymphopenia with a slow recovery in surviving animals. Within a few days, the polymorphonuclear cells in the circulating blood decrease. Thrombocytes in blood are progressively reduced and return slowly to the circulation. This thrombocytopenia undoubtedly underlies the hemorrhagic phenomena that follow. Anemia slowly becomes evident, probably due to the reduction of the red cell precursors; blood clot retraction is delayed and blood levels of alkaline phosphatase are reduced. The iodine uptake by the thyroid may be decreased, the respiratory quotient is reduced, and urea excretion is slightly increased.

The signs observed in animals exposed to lethal doses of ionizing radiation depend, to some extent, upon the dose, as well as the dose rate. A few dogs, which receive twice the 100% LD (2 × LD 100/30) of total body radiation, may die suddenly within 72 hours without manifesting significant signs. Diarrhea may develop in some animals, and after a time the stools may become tarry or bloody. Other animals receiving similar doses may not show any effects for seven to nine days following radiation. Hemorrhages then may be observed in visible mucosae; septicemia follows the severe agranulocytosis and death soon supervenes. Animals exposed to very high doses may suddenly exhibit severe disturbances of locomotion and die within 72 hours. Symptoms, therefore, are nonspecific and easily could be mistakenly attributed to several causes. Infection and septicemia are common following high or lethal doses of radiation and are often responsible for death. The killing of leukocyte stem cells is of primary importance, but high doses also impair chemotaxis and phagocytosis of fully differentiated neutrophils.

Gross lesions

The most prominent gross change in animals dying after lethal doses of whole-body radiation is hemorrhage, which may occur anywhere in the body, but most frequently involves the heart, and gastrointestinal and genitourinary systems (Figs. 14-1, 14-2). In early stages, congestion of small blood vessels of heart, brain, lungs, mesentery, intestine, and subcutis may be the only findings. Later, however, scattered petechiae also may be found in these organs. The hemorrhages observed in severely affected animals vary from small petechiae to extensive extravasations with occasional hematomas. In goats and pigs, petechiae have been described in the renal cortices and pelves, with large blood clots in the pelves.

Hemorrhages may be seen in the musculature of the back, abdomen, legs, thorax, and diaphragm. This is particularly common in guinea pigs, rare in rats, and occasionally seen in goats and pigs. The lymph nodes and tonsils are characteristically hemorrhagic, edematous, enlarged, and dark red; on cut surfaces, hemolytic areas are interspersed with gray, moist-appearing lymphoid tissue. Hemorrhages and ulcerations are the predominant lesions in the gastrointestinal tract. Ulcers are most common in the large intestine and are superficial. Fibrinous membranes, stained with feces, may be removed from the mucosal surface with difficulty, leaving raw, eroded areas in the underlying mucosa. The bone marrow usually loses its deep-red color and appears pale and often gelatinous with a yellowish tint.

Microscopic lesions

The microscopic findings in lethal whole-body radiation generally can be correlated with the gross as well as the clinical manifestations. The degree of injury to

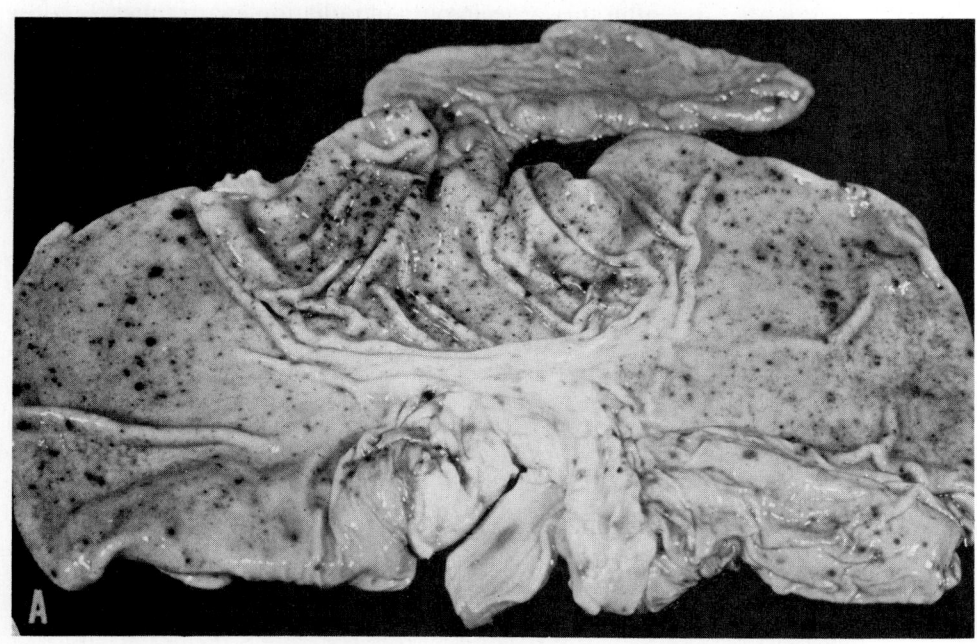

FIG. 14-1 Whole-body radiation: hemorrhage in the stomach of a pig. Contributor: Medical Section, Joint Task Force No. 1, Operation Crossroads. (Courtesy of Armed Forces Institute of Pathology.)

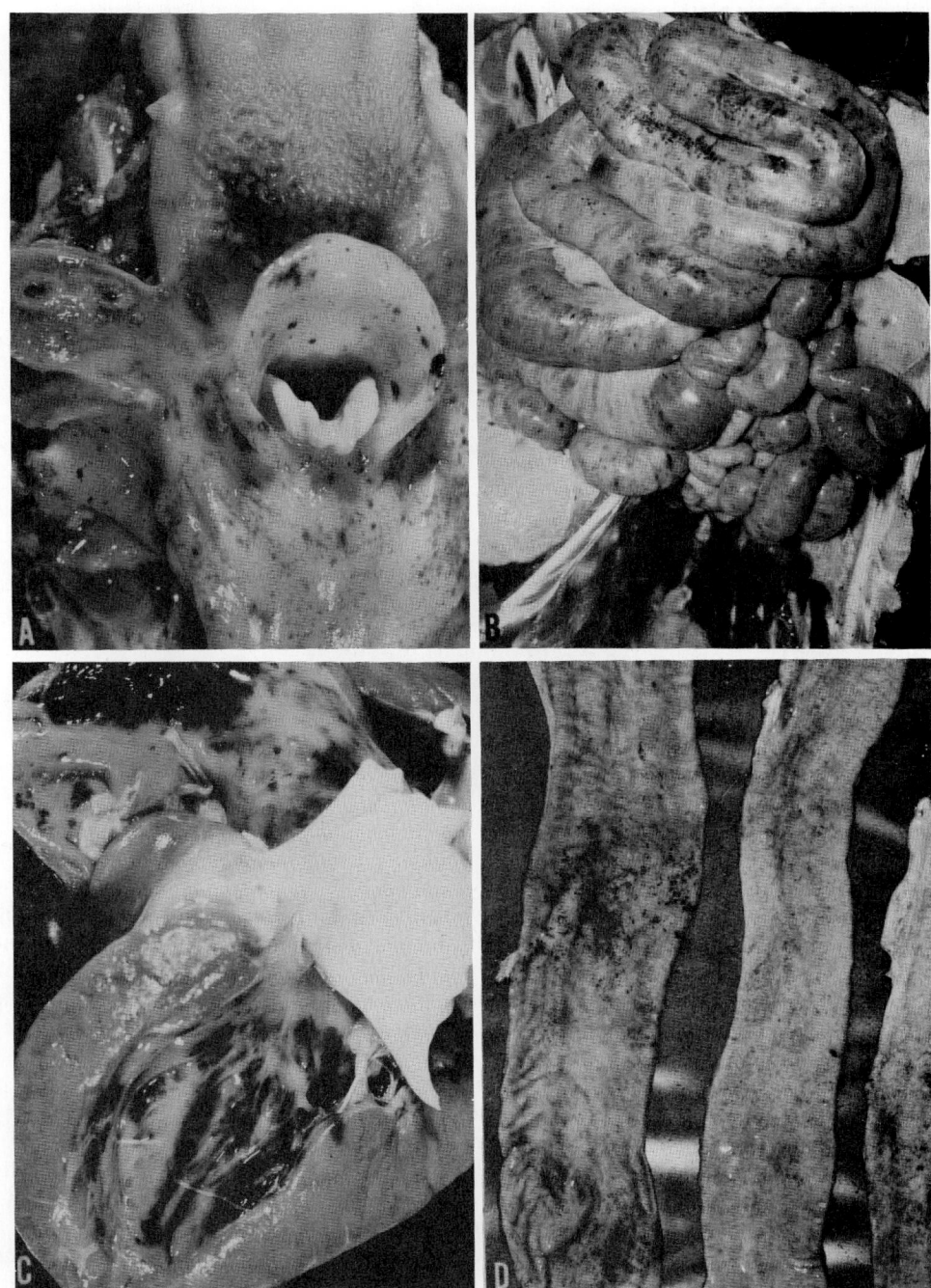

FIG. 14-2 Whole-body radiation. **A,** Hemorrhage in the mucosa of the pharynx and epiglottis of a pig. **B,** Hemorrhage in the intestinal serosa of a pig. **C,** Subendocardial hemorrhage in the heart of a pig. **D,** Hemorrhage in the intestinal wall of a pig. Contributor: Medical Section, Joint Task Force No. 1, Operation Crossroads. (Courtesy of Armed Forces Institute of Pathology.)

tissues depends somewhat upon dosage, but to a greater extent upon the radiosensitivity of tissue. Lymphoid cells, being most susceptible, will manifest the most severe changes, while mature bone will be least affected.

In general, lesions resulting from radiation at the level of the cell or the body as a whole are not unique. This is exemplified by the reference to effects of certain drugs and even viruses as radiomimetic. Following irradiation, cells may undergo degenerative changes and necrosis similar to those described in Chapter 2. Nuclear chromatin becomes clumped and the nucleus may swell or become pyknotic and fragment (karyorrhexis).

The entire cell becomes swollen and vacuolated, as do individual cytoplasmic organelles (Fig. 14-3). These events and cell death may not occur until after mitosis or until after several divisions, indicative of chromosomal damage. The loss of cells or necrosis leads to the varying consequences of necrosis caused by other injurious agents (e.g., impairment of function, atrophy, regeneration, repair, fibrosis). Thus, a spectrum of chronic histopathologic lesions may be seen even years subsequent to the initial injury.

Changes in the reproductive capacity of a cell is another effect of radiation on cells. Although it may appear morphologically normal, an irradiated cell may

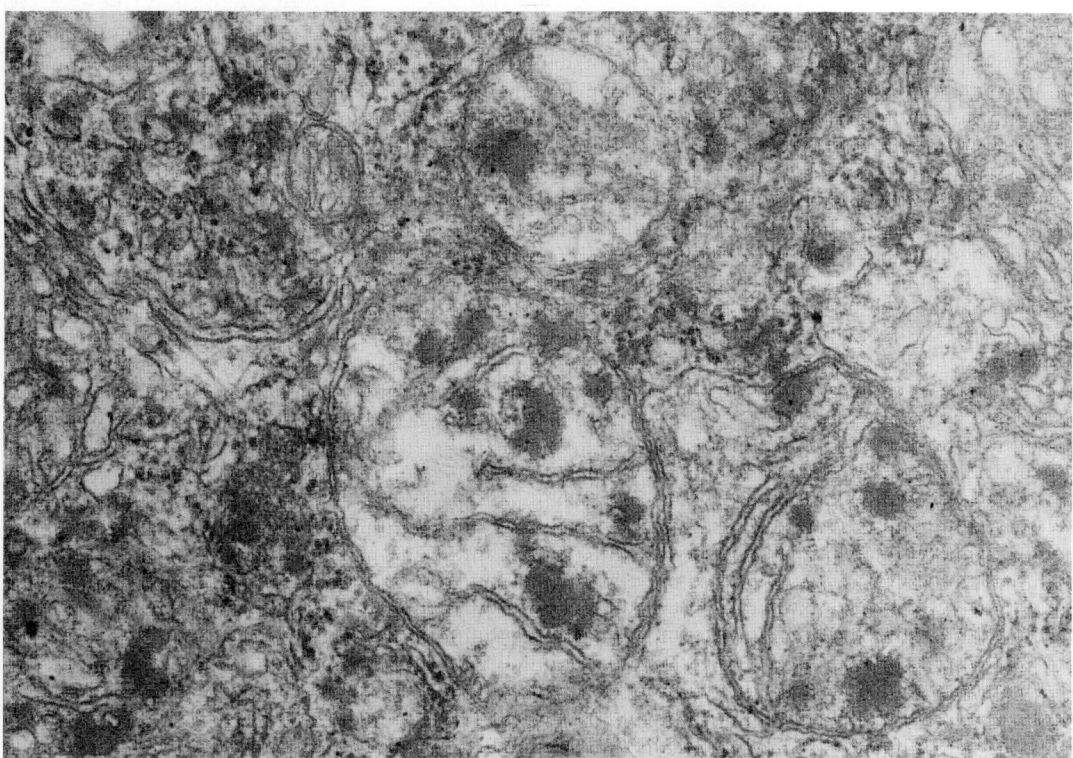

FIG. 14-3 Mitochondrial swelling and disruption of cristae in the kidney of a mouse following 2.01×10^6 rads of x-ray exposure. These changes developed within two minutes after exposure. (Courtesy of Scott W. Jordan, M.D.)

lose its ability to divide or may replicate without cellular division, leading to the formation of multinucleated giant cells. Multinucleated giant cells, particularly in fibroblasts, are a clue to radiation damage. Other causes, such as certain viral infections, must be excluded.

Damage to blood vessels account for some of the acute effects of irradiation and is responsible for a number of chronic sequelae. Initially, vascular dilation leads to hyperemia, which is believed to result from release of various chemicals, as in inflammation. Subsequently, endothelial cells become swollen and vacuolated, leading to increased permeability and egress of plasma and cells. Over a period of months, the walls of arteries and arterioles become sclerotic and hyalinized, and the number of lining endothelial cells increases. Resultant reduction of blood flow leads to further functional impairment and fibrosis of affected organs.

LYMPHOID TISSUE

Lymphoid tissues, such as lymph nodes, spleen, thymus, and tonsils, are affected promptly, and this is reflected in the microscopic alterations. Necrosis of lymphocytes, as evidenced by pyknosis, karyorrhexis, and karyolysis of nuclei, is the earliest and most significant finding. As a result, the germinal centers soon appear "washed out," leaving only the reticuloendothelial cells. The sinuses are dilated and filled with macrophages,

some of which have engulfed erythrocytes as well as tissue debris. Recent hemorrhage may be evident; in cases of longer duration, collections of blood pigment may appear. Secondary changes due to abscesses, ulcers, hemorrhages, or other lesions in organs drained by a particular lymph node may occur in animals with prolonged survival time.

BONE MARROW

Microscopically, detectable lesions occur in the bone marrow within a few hours after heavy doses of radiation. Necrosis of hematopoietic cells, particularly the most immature, occurs early. Myelocytes appear to be most susceptible, megakaryocytes and erythrocytes less so, and reticular cells quite resistant. The sinuses become dilated with plasma or red blood cells. Within one to two weeks, most radiosensitive elements disappear from the bone marrow, leaving aplastic, acellular marrow that contains only fat cells, reticular cells, edema, and hemorrhage. Secondary infection may be the means by which colonies of fungi or bacteria are transplanted in the marrow, where they grow, usually without apparent inflammatory reaction to their presence. Bloom described a change in irradiated small animals in which the bony trabeculae on the diaphyseal side of the epiphyseal cartilage disappear and are replaced by fibrillar stroma (1948). The resulting separation of the epiphyseal cartilage from the spongy bone on the diaphyseal side has been referred to as "severance" of the epiphyseal plate.

DIGESTIVE SYSTEM

Shallow ulcers with little or no underlying leukocytic infiltration are common in the oral and pharyngeal mucous membranes, especially along the margins of the tongue and adjacent to the tonsillar crypts. These shallow ulcers have a necrotic base; leukocytes appear only when the animal begins to recover from agranulocytosis. The mucous membrane of the digestive tract from the esophagus to the anus is severely affected by whole-body radiation. Edema of the submucosa and subserosa is common throughout the tract, and is usually associated with necrosis of the mucosal epithelium and frequent hemorrhages in all parts of the wall. The necrosis of the epithelium rarely extends deeper than the submucosa, and perforation seldom occurs. Blood vessels of the lamina propria and submucosa adjacent to ulcers may be dilated and contain fibrin thrombi. Individual epithelial cells may be seen to have undergone several changes; namely, vacuolization of cytoplasm or nuclei, and distortion in size and shape. Hyaline changes in the submucosal stroma may occur late in association with formation of bizarre fibroblasts and fibrocytes. Strictures may result from fibrosis, causing intestinal obstruction.

GENITAL SYSTEM

The germinal cells of the testis and ovary are among the most radiosensitive cells of the animal body; hence, they are readily destroyed by radiation. In the acute stage, hemorrhage and edema may be seen, but the most specific effect is the destruction of spermatogonia as well as spermatocytes, with little effect upon spermatozoa. Whole-body radiation in sufficient dosage to destroy germinal cells would be enough to kill the animal; therefore, sterility would be an academic problem. If the same dosage were applied only to the gonads, the whole-body effect would be nil, but sterility of temporary or permanent duration would result.

SKIN

Radiation injury to the skin is frequent after radiation therapy of tumors and is one of the principal tissues affected by radioactive fallout. Lesions are discussed in detail in the next section.

RESPIRATORY SYSTEM

Respiratory epithelium is relatively resistant to radiation damage. High doses will lead to swelling and desquamation of alveolar lining cells and epithelium of the bronchial tree. Most of the acute and chronic effects result from vascular damage, causing pulmonary edema in the acute stage and alveolar fibrosis and consolidation as chronic manifestations. Pulmonary edema may account for the immediate cause of death following whole-body irradiation. A hyaline material free in alveoli and within alveolar macrophages and proliferation of granular pneumocytes have been described in humans and dogs.

URINARY SYSTEM

Therapeutic doses of X and γ radiation in humans have been followed by renal lesions termed, radiation nephropathy. Similar lesions have been observed in animals following experimental irradiation, which indicates that endothelial cells in glomeruli and around the convoluted tubules are most sensitive to irradiation. The earliest morphologic manifestation of radiation injury appears to be the attachment of neutrophils to the glomerular capillary endothelium. This is followed by transudation and enigration of plasma components, leukocytes, erythrocytes, and platelets into pericapillary and mesangial tissue. Pericapillary edema with reduction in the capillary lumen follows.

The molecular events that lead to these anatomical changes are not completely understood but appear to begin with the release of toxic oxygen species by the effect of radiation. Radiation releases a chemotactic factor for neutrophils, possibly a lipid product of the lipoxygenase pathway, which causes the attachment of leukocytes to the glomerular capillary endothelium. This, in turn, may also affect increased leukocytic adhesive molecules via cytokine-activated endothelial attraction with increased levels of intracellular adhesion molecule.

Platelet thrombi appear in the glomerular and peritubular capillaries and mesangial proliferation becomes extensive. Periglomerular and interstitial fibrosis become evident as the effects progress. These changes eventually interfere seriously with renal function.

The transitional epithelium of the urinary bladder is also radiosensitive, and in contrast to the kidney, the lesions are acute. The epithelial cells become necrotic and slough, leading to ulcers. Infection is a frequent complication. Fibrosis from healing may result in distortion of the bladder.

BONE AND CARTILAGE

Mature osteocytes and chondrocytes are radioresistant, and lesions in these tissues are of little consequence in adults. Proliferating osteoblasts and chondroblasts, however, are more radiosensitive. In growing animals, damage to these cells will result in retarded or distorted growth.

HEART

Although the myocardium has been generally considered relatively radioresistant, radiation-induced heart disease has been reported in a number of human patients following radiation therapy and has been experimentally produced in animals. It is characterized by fibrous pericarditis, interstitial fibrosis of the myocardium, and perivascular accumulations of mononuclear cells. In monkeys, the extent of myocardial fibrosis suggests healed infarcts. All of these lesions probably result from ischemia caused by vascular damage.

OTHER TISSUES AND LESIONS

Chronic vascular lesions may result in impaired circulation to many tissues, with the resultant lesions of anoxia. Therefore, chronic effects may be encountered even in radioresistant tissues, such as the nervous system. During embryogenesis, when all tissues are less differentiated and rapidly dividing, irradiation may cause a variety of congenital abnormalities. Cataract formation is not infrequent following irradiation of the lens. Carcinogenesis is one of the most serious of the chronic sequelae following irradiation; a variety of different neoplasms has been associated with radiation (Chapter 4).

References

Crosson JT, Keane WF, Anderson WR. Radiation nephropathy. In: Tishner CG, Brenner BM, eds. Renal pathology. Philadelphia: Lippincott, 1989;866–876.

Faulkner CS II, Connolly KS. The ultrastructure of ^{60}Co radiation pneumonitis in rats. Lab Invest 1973;28:545–553.

Gillett NA, Stegelmeier BL, Kelly G, et al. Expression of epidermal growth factor receptor in plutonium-239–induced lung neoplasms in dogs. Vet Pathol 1992;29:46–52.

Glatstein E, Fajardo LF, Brown JF. Radiation injury in the mouse kidney. I. Sequential light microscopic study. Int J Radiat Oncol Biol Phys 1977;2:933–943.

Jaenke RS, Robbins MEC, Baywaters T, et al. Capillary endothelium: target site of renal radiation injury. Lab Invest 1993;68:396–405.

Kunkler PB, Farr RF, Luxton RW. Limits of renal tolerance to X-rays. Br J Radiol 1952;25:190–201.

Mewissen DJ, Comar CL, Trum BF, et al. A formula for chronic radiation dosage versus shortening of life span: application to a large mammal. Radiat Res 1957;6:450–459.

Nelson AC, Shah-Yukich A, Babayan R. Radiation damage in rat kidney microvasculature. Scanning Electron Microsc 1984;3:1273–1277.

Phillips SJ, Macken DL, Rugh R. Pathologic sequelae of acute cardiac irradiation in monkeys. Am Heart J 1971;81:528–542.

Raulston GL, Gray KN, Gleiser CA, et al. A comparison of the effects of 50 MeV D-BE neutron and cobalt-60 irradiation on the kidneys of rhesus monkeys. Radiology 1978;128:245–249.

Reinhold HS, Hopewell JW, Calvo W, et al. Vasculoconnective tissue. In: Scherer E, Streffer CH, Trott KR, eds. Radiopathology of organs and tissues. Berlin: Springer Verlag, 1991;243–268.

Robbins MEC, Soper M, Gunn Y. Techniques for the measurement of individual kidney function in the pig. Int Appl Radiat Isot 1984;35:853–858.

Robbins MEC, Campling D, Rezvani M, et al. Radiation nephropathy in mature pigs following the irradiation of both kidneys. Int J Radiat Biol 1989;56:83–98.

Robbins MEC, Woodridge MJA, Jaenke RS, et al. A morphological study of radiation in the pig. Radiat Res 1991;126:317–327.

Rust JH, Folmar GD Jr, Lane JJ, et al. The lethal dose of total body cobalt-60 gamma radiation for the rabbit. Am J Roentgen 1955;74:135–138.

Rust JH, et al. Effect of 200 roentgens fractional whole body irradiation in the burro. Proc Soc Exp Biol Med 1954;85:258–261.

Rust JH, et al. Effects of 50 roentgens and 25 roentgens fractional daily total-body r-irradiation in the burro. Radiat Res 1955;2:475–482.

Rust JH, et al. Lethal dose studies with burros and swine exposed to whole body cobalt-60 irradiation. Radiology 1954;62:569–574.

Slauson DO, et al. Inflammatory sequences in acute pulmonary radiation injury. Am J Pathol 1976;82:549–572.

Snider RS, Raper JR. Histopathological effects of single doses of total-surface beta radiation of mice. In: Zirkle RE, ed. Effects of external beta radiation. New York: McGraw-Hill, 1951;152–178.

Trum BF, et al. Effect of 400 fractional whole body gamma irradiation in the burro (Equus asinus asinus). Am J Physiol 1953;174:57–60.

Trum BF, et al.. The histopathology of radiation lesions. Physiol Rev 1944;24:225–238.

Wise D, Turbyfill CL. The acute mortality response of the miniature pig to pulsed mixed gamma-neutron radiations. Radiat Res 1970;41:507–515.

RADIOACTIVE FALLOUT

The explosion of a thermonuclear weapon releases not only vast quantities of energy in the form of heat, light, and blast, but also great amounts of radioactivity. Part of this radioactivity is released instantaneously in the form of neutrons and γ rays, which can produce radiation effects within their range. This range—or distance through which this radiation travels and thus produces biologic effects—depends upon the energy of the explosion, but is not great, even in the most powerful explosions. However, fast-moving neutrons can penetrate deeply into matter and induce radioactivity in otherwise stable substances. This induced or secondary radioactivity, under certain circumstances, can be an important source of ionizing radiation.

Of far greater significance in an explosive fission reaction is the release of radioactive substances in particulate form. These particles consist of radioactive fission products, matter (sea water, air, soil) in which radioactivity has been induced, and perhaps, remnants of the original fissionable material. The explosive power of the bomb may send great quantities of these radioactive materials high into the earth's atmosphere, wind currents move them as clouds over great distances, and then rain or other atmospheric conditions cause the particulate matter to fall back to earth. This fallout may constitute a serious hazard to humans, plants, and animals in areas downwind from the point of detonation (Fig. 14-4). The areas of serious radioactivity would vary in size according to such factors as yield and height of burst, the nature of the surface over which the burst occurs, and the meteorologic conditions. The radioactive material may lodge on the skin of the backs of animals which are out in the open, or may fall on pasture or animal feed, where it may be ingested and cause internal radiation, a condition that is discussed later.

The fallout of radioactive materials may occur as a shower of dry, flaky material or as minute, invisible particles, perhaps accompanied by rain. The fact that radioactivity is associated with particles has an important influence upon skin lesions resulting from contact with this material. The chemical nature of material in radioactive fallout depends upon the composition of the bomb, as well as the medium in which it was exploded (air, sea, underground). Most radioisotopes of importance in such radioactive clouds decay by emission of β particles and γ rays. α Particle emitters are a possibility, but because of their low penetrability would have little effect upon the skin.

The effect of radioisotopes on the skin depends upon the following:

(1) Their energy and type of emission,
(2) Duration of contact with skin,

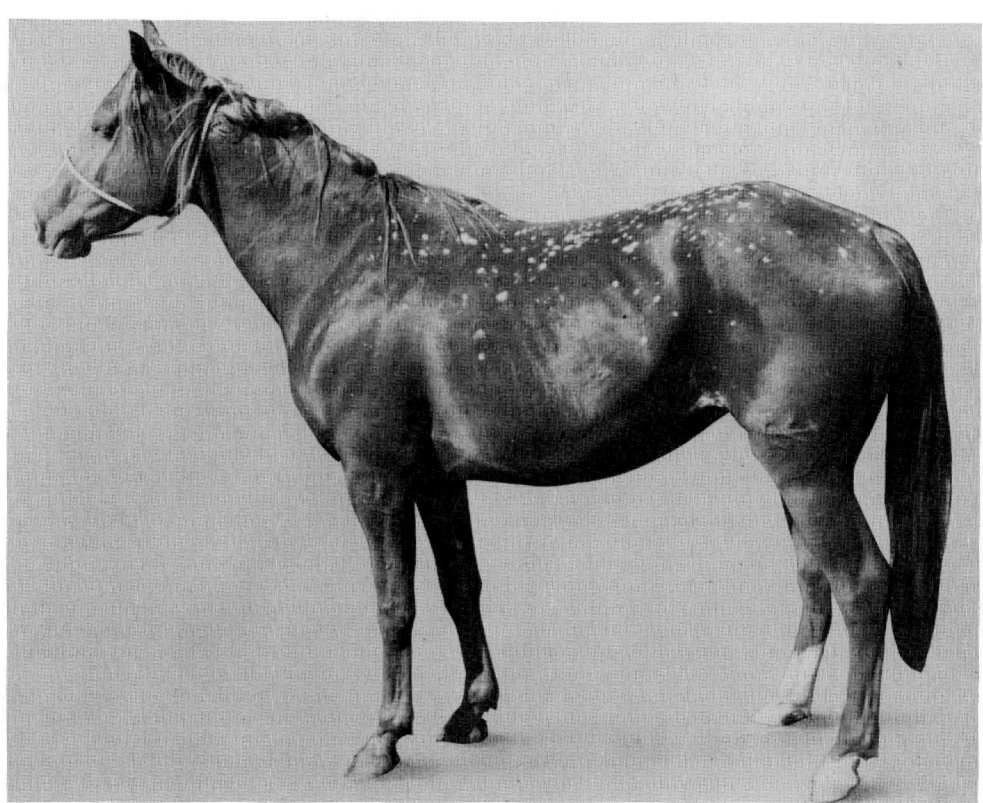

FIG. 14-4 Effect of radioactive fallout. The lesions are discrete and located on the dorsal portions of the body of this horse. (Courtesy of Lt. Col. B. F. Trum, V.C.)

(3) Radioactive half-life, and
(4) Any irritating effect due to their chemical nature.

Lesions

Lesions will develop in the skin of animals exposed to radioactive fallout, provided the material is in contact with the skin for a sufficient length of time (Fig. 14-5). As indicated previously, α particles do not penetrate the keratin layer; hence, they produce no effect upon the skin. γ Rays penetrate deeply but have low-specific ionization in the superficial layers; therefore, they produce little direct effect upon the skin. β Particles, conversely, penetrate most layers of skin, have high-specific ionization, and produce severe effects. Skin lesions caused by β particles have been called "beta burns," but they are not strictly burns because no heat is involved.

The sequence of changes resulting from contact with β-emitting radioisotopes has been studied by Moritz and Henriques (1952), who placed β-emitting plaques in contact with the skin of swine. These authors used radioisotopes of different energies—sulfur-35 (0.17 MeV), cobalt-60 (0.31 MeV), cesium-137 (0.55 MeV), yttrium-91 (1.53 MeV), and strontium-yttrium-90 (0.61 and 2.2 MeV)—to demonstrate the relationships between the energy of the isotope and the surface, or transepidermal, dose to the resultant radiation injury. These studies provide information on the development of changes following radiation of this type; some of these changes have been observed in "field" cases of injury due to radioactive fallout. The remarks that follow are based on the reports of Moritz and Henriques.

The first observable change in swine skin following exposure to these radioactive isotopes is erythema, which may appear within 24 hours. When it persists 72 hours or longer, erythema is indicative of injury severe enough to result in chronic radiation dermatitis. Edema of dermal papillae, when recognizable within 48 hours following irradiation, will be followed by transepidermal necrosis. Death of cells in the basal and deeper malpighian layers of the epidermis, demonstrated by increase in staining intensity of their nuclei, occurs within 24 hours following high dosage, but with lower dosage may not appear for 10–14 days.

Epidermal atrophy, one of the least severe changes, is recognized in microscopic sections only and is seen one to two weeks following radiation. This change is evidenced by thinning of the rete, presumably as a result of depression of cell division in the basal layer plus continued desquamation of surface layers. It persists for two to four weeks and appears to be completely reversible because no residua occur. Exfoliation and crust formation follow more severe injury, begin during the second week, and may be precursors of chronic radiation dermatitis. A scaling brown crust is shed for weeks or months, apparently because of accelerated maturation of malpighian cells without loss of their nuclei, which results in parakeratosis. Death of individual cells in the deeper parts of the epidermis may continue for many weeks after irradiation.

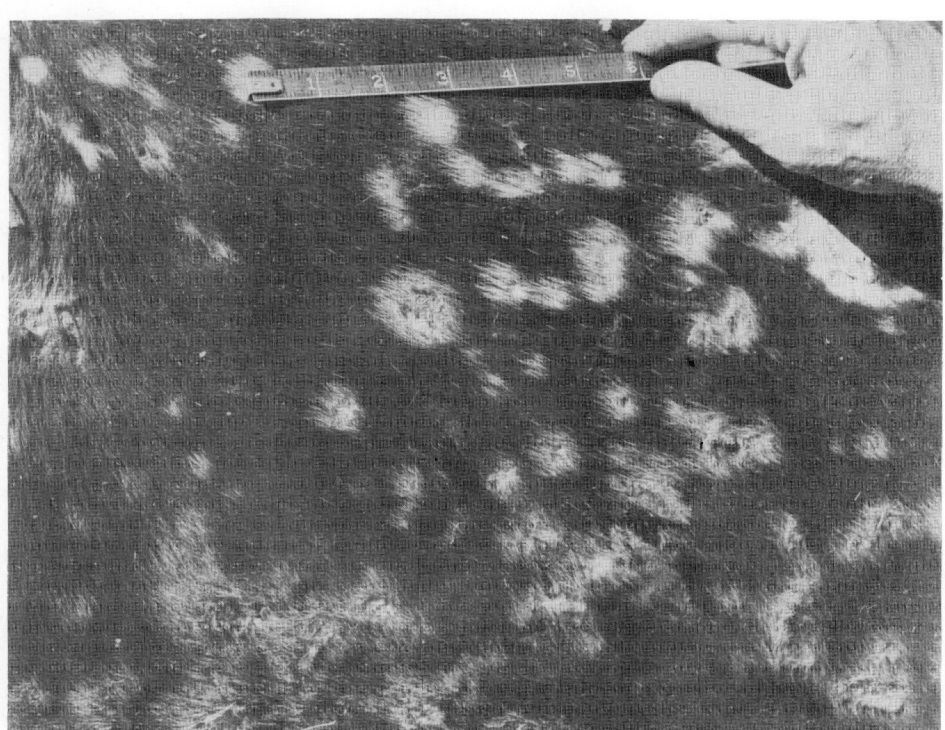

FIG. 14-5 Radioactive fallout. Lesions in the skin of the back of a horse. Depigmentation of hair in sharply circumscribed areas with alopecia and ulceration in the center of some. (Courtesy of Lt. Col. B. F. Trum, V.C.)

Epidermal necrosis and exfoliation follow higher dosages of radiation. The first indication of probable irreversible injury is swelling and vacuolation of cytoplasm of epidermal cells, which may appear ragged or coagulated into round, acidophilic hyaline masses. Disorganization of the basal and malpighian layers occurs, with vesicles appearing at the dermal-epidermal interface. Transepidermal necrosis, with ulceration of the entire target area, follows still higher dosage, and may be complete within 48 hours. With lower dosage, several weeks may elapse before necrosis of the epidermis is complete. Radiation of lower energy (sulfur-35, 0.17 MeV) produces shallow ulcers with little damage to the dermis, while higher energy β radiation—from strontium-yttrium-90 (0.61 and 2.2 MeV), cobalt-60 (0.31 MeV), and cesium-137 (0.55 MeV)—results in deep injury to the dermis and is followed by chronic radiation dermatitis.

Changes in the dermis and subcutis are observed only when the epidermis is damaged. The earliest lesion is hyperemia of the capillaries in the dermal papillae, followed by edema, asteroid swelling of fibrocytes, and exudation of lymphocytes and neutrophils in relationship to the ulceration of epidermis. Edema, capillary ectasia, and degenerative changes in arterioles may persist after regeneration of epithelium, but the dermis in this state apparently cannot support the growth of epithelium; therefore, ulceration recurs.

Epilation takes place when the dosage of higher energy β particles is sufficient to produce recognizable injury in the epidermis; lower energy β radiation from sulfur-35, however, does not produce epilation. When they receive sufficient radiation to cause hair loss, dermal papillae become atrophic and contracted, particularly in length. Atrophy occurs in epithelial cells of the hair matrix, including the inner root sheath, and may be associated with swelling and squamous metaplasia. Sometimes columns of cells from hair follicles may persist, but they undergo central dissolution, producing epithelial-lined cysts, which may communicate with the surface. In severe injury, hair follicles are permanently destroyed.

Other skin adnexa, sebaceous, and sweat glands may disappear completely after high-energy β radiation in sufficient dosage to destroy the epidermis. These structures are not replaced. Less severely affected tubular glands may become atrophic and be surrounded by a dense hyaline membrane.

In chronic radiation dermatitis, characterized clinically by persistent exfoliation with crust formation of one- to three-months' duration, the microscopic findings (Fig. 14-6) include parakeratosis with atrophy (or less often, hyperplasia) of the epidermis associated with chronic inflammation in the dermis. In some instances, proliferation and downward growth of the epithelium occur, with pleomorphism, loss of polarity, and increased numbers of mitotic figures. This change suggests a trend toward neoplasia.

The skin of cattle studied several years after exposure to severe doses of radiation from fallout presented with irregular areas of scarring, surrounded by zones of epilation and white hair. The scarred areas were partially covered by dense layers of tough, horny material several centimeters in thickness. Microscopically, these scarred areas were covered by thick, stratified squamous epithelium with an overlying dense layer of keratin. The rete pegs, hair follicles, sebaceous, and sweat glands were absent under the affected epithelium, but occasionally were present, although atrophic, at the edges of lesions (Fig. 14-6).

In horses exposed to radioactive fallout, focal areas of ulceration surrounded by a wide zone of white hair (Fig. 14-5) have been reported. Because radioactivity emitted from particulate fallout usually arises from a point source and radiates nearly equally in all directions, the volume of skin affected will be roughly hemispherical in depth, while the surface lesion will be round.

Solar radiation results in similar, but less rapidly progressive, precancerous lesions in the skin.

References

Archambeau JO, Fairchild RG, Commerford SL. Response of skin of swine to increasing exposures of 250 KVP x-ray. In: Bustad LK, McClellan RO, eds. Swine in biomedical research. Richland: Battelle Memorial Institute, 1966;463–489.

Ballard RV, et al. Iodine 129 in thyroids of grazing animals. Health Phys 1976;30:345–350.

Bogen DC, et al. "Fallout tritium" distribution in the environment. Health Phys 1976;30:203–208.

Brown DG, Reynolds RA, Johnson DF. Late effects in cattle exposed to radioactive fallout. Am J Vet Res 1966;27:1509–1514.

Dagle GE, Phemister RD, Legel JL, et al. Plutonium-induced popliteal lymphadenitis in beagles. Radiation Res 1975;61:239–250.

George LA, Bustad LK. Comparative effects of beta irradiation of swine, sheep and rabbit skin. In: Bustad LK, McClellan RO, eds. Swine in biomedical research. Richland: Battelle Memorial Institute, 1966;491–500.

Shively JN, Phemister RD, Epling GP, et al. Pathogenesis of radiation-induced retinal dysplasia. Invest Ophthalmol 1970;9:888–900.

Shively JN, Phemister RD, Epling GP, et al. Dose relationships of pathologic alterations in the developing retina of irradiated dogs. Am Vet Res 1972;33:2121–2134.

Tessmer CF. Radioactive fallout effects on skin. I. Effects of radioactive

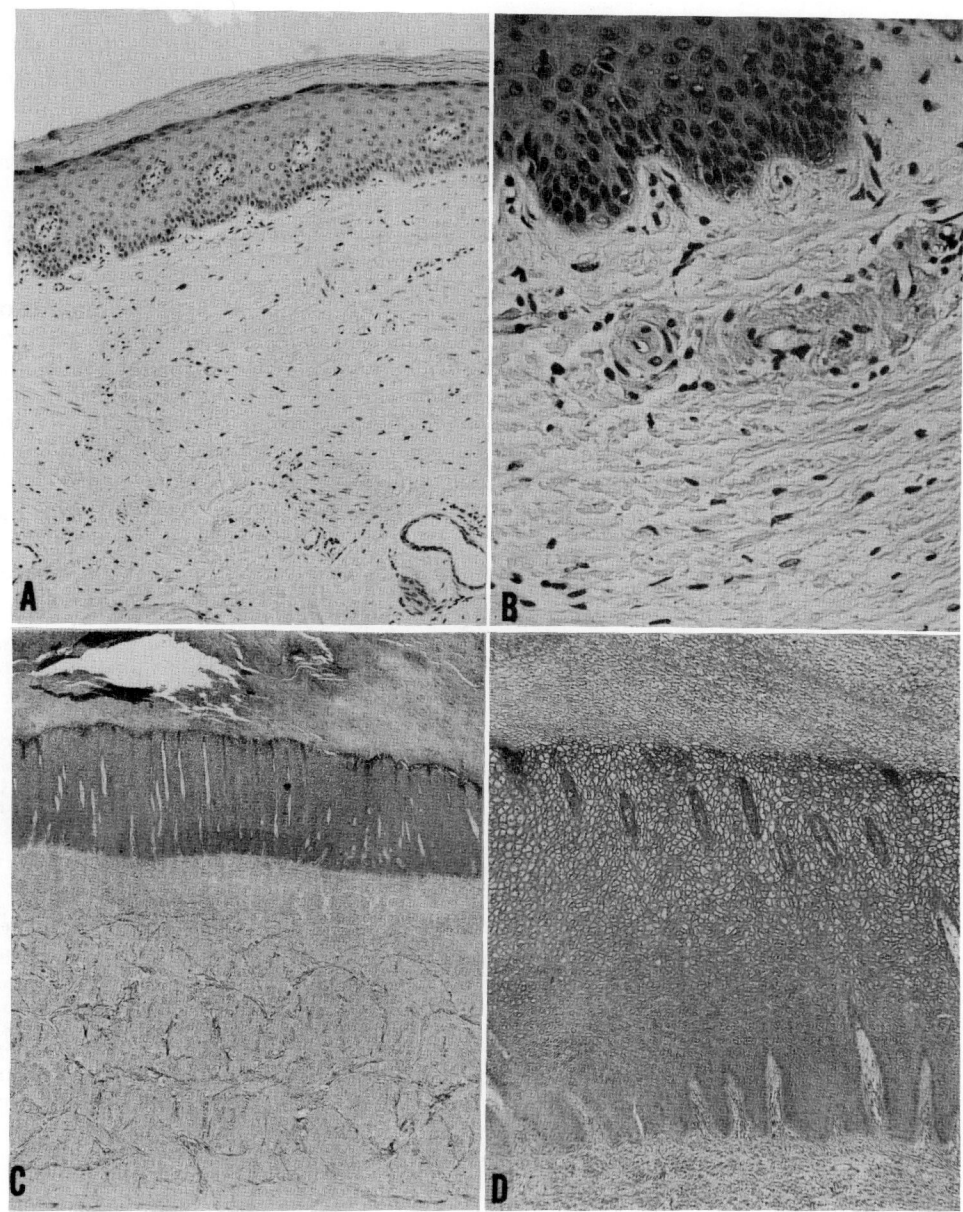

FIG. 14-6 A, Radioactive fallout in bovine skin (×75). Note absence of sebaceous glands and remnant of sweat gland in dermis. **B,** Radioactive fallout in bovine skin (×250). Thickened hyaline wall in capillary of dermis. Specimen taken several years after exposure.   **C,** Radioactive fallout in bovine skin (×11). Several years after exposure. Severe hyperkeratosis, acanthosis, and loss of adnexa.   **D,** Higher magnification of area depicted in Figure C (×48), illustrating acanthosis and part of the layer of hyperkeratosis. (Courtesy of Armed Forces Institute of Pathology. Contributor: Dr. Cyril Comar.)

FIG. 14-7 Positive print of an autoradiograph of the femur of a dog which had received strontium-90. (Courtesy of Dr. Arthur Lindenbaum, Argonne National Laboratory.)

fallout on skin of Almagordo cattle. Arch Pathol 1961;72: 175–190.

Tessmer CF, Brown DG. Carcinoma of skin and bovine exposed to radioactive fallout. J Am Med Assoc 1962;179:210–214.

Tullis JL, Warren S. Gross autopsy observation in the animals exposed at Bikini: preliminary report. J Am Med Assoc 1947;134:1155–1158.

Tullis JL, Lawson BC, Madden SC. Pathology of swine exposed to total body gamma radiation from an atomic bomb source. Am J Pathol 1955;31:41–51.

INTERNAL RADIATION

Radioactive isotopes may gain access to the human or animal body by inhalation, ingestion, parenteral injection, or absorption through wounds in skin. The effect produced by these isotopes depends upon many factors, the most important of which are the following: the quantity, specific ionization, and energy of radioactivity taken into the body; its deposition in critical or radiosensitive tissues; the biologic half-life of the isotope; and the size and importance to life of the organ in which the isotope is deposited. Except in the immediate region of an explosion and close-in areas of fallout, internal radiation is a much greater hazard than is external radiation because the isotope is in contact with animal tissue for longer periods, and even when of low energy, may be deposited in critical tissues (bone, thyroid) in intimate enough contact to cause serious damage. Sources of radioactivity that possibly could become internal radiation hazards to animals include fallout following explosions of atomic weapons, with contamination of animal water or pastures, and contamination of feed or water by inadequate disposal of radioactive wastes from atomic "piles," power reactors, or industrial and medical facilities in which radioisotopes are used.

Radioactive isotopes are metabolized in the body in exactly the same manner as are nonradioactive isotopes of the same element. Therefore, radioiodine (^{131}I) is rapidly concentrated in the thyroid exactly as is stable iodine (^{127}I). Radiocalcium (^{45}Ca) is deposited in bone as are its nonradioactive isotopes (e.g., ^{40,42}Ca), and is eliminated not only in feces and urine but in milk. Radiosodium (^{24}Na) is distributed more widely through the tissues and is eliminated rapidly; hence, it is not as great a hazard as ^{131}I or ^{45}Ca.

Many radioisotopes are not ordinarily metabolized by the body, but are deposited in tissue in much the same way as are similar chemical elements. The most important of these include the "bone seekers," which include strontium-90, radium-226, uranium, radioactive rare earths, and plutonium. Bone-seeking radioisotopes are deposited in growing bone, at first most heavily concentrated in the metaphysis, particularly adjacent to the epiphyseal line, where they remain in greatest concentration. After a time, radioactivity can be demonstrated also in the diaphyses of the long bones by radioautographs (Fig. 14-7), prepared by placing slabs of affected bone in contact with photographic film for a period of time, then developing the film. Radioactive components darken the film, indicating their site of deposition in tissue.

The deposition of radioactivity in bone may destroy the hematopoietic elements, thus producing aplastic anemia, and may adversely affect the growing bone, predisposing the human or animal to osteogenic sarcoma. Aside from these effects upon the individual, radioactive bones in meat-producing animals could become a food hazard to humans or other animals.

Radioiodine (^{131}I) in sufficient dosage can cause enough destruction of thyroid tissue to interfere seriously with the function of the gland. Internal radiation from these isotopes has especially deleterious effects on young animals.

References

Casey HW, Cordy DR, Goldman M, et al. Influence of chronic acceleration on the effects of whole-body irradiation in rats. Aerosp Med 1967;38:451–457.

Cockerham LG, Doyle TF, Trumbo RB, et al. Acute post-irradiation canine intestinal blood flow. Int J Radiat Biol 1984;45:65–72.

Dungworth DL, Goldman M, Switzer J, et al. Development of a myeloproliferative disorder in beagles continuously exposed to 90Sr. Blood 1969;34:610–632.

Moulton JE, Rosenblatt LS, Goldman M. Mammary tumors in a colony of beagle dogs. Vet Pathol 1986;23:741–749.

Nold JB, Miller GK, Benjamin SA. Parnatal and neonatal irradiation in dogs: hematologic and hematopoietic responses. Radiat Res 1987;112:490–499.

Pool RR, Williams RJ, Goldman M. Induction of tumors involving bone in beagles fed toxic levels of strontium 90. Am J Roentgenol Radium Ther Nucl Med 1973;118:900–908.

Raabe OG, Book SA, Parks NJ, et al. Lifetime studies of 226Ra and 90Sr toxicity in beagles—a status report. Radiat Res 1981;86: 515–528.

15

Diseases due to extraneous poisons

Poisonous substances in the environment, called xenobiotics, are numerous and have toxic and carcinogenic properties that are often hazardous to people and animals.

The public has become increasingly aware of the hazards, from nature and from industrial production or waste products, resulting in demands on the government to control or eliminate all such threats to public health. The United States Congress and state legislatures have responded by acts and appropriations that mount huge efforts to identify all such hazards and eliminate them. Industrial, academic, and governmental agencies have expanded their scientific capabilities to meet these needs.

The discipline of pathology, in all its aspects, has proved necessary to identify the effects of xenobiotics on laboratory animals as a step toward assessing the potential hazards to human health. As a result, the specialty of "toxicologic pathology" has expanded greatly in resources and personnel to produce a large and expanding body of knowledge. Veterinary parhologists have found their background in biologic sciences and pathology useful and many have sought the specialized knowledge and skills to qualify as toxicologic pathologists.

Toxicologic pathology has grown at such a rate that it is not possible to include much of its specialized information in a text such as this one. However, toxic substances are hazards to animal populations and veterinarians are required to recognize the hazards and do what is necessary to control or eliminate them. It is toward the beginning of the training of new veterinarians that this chapter is aimed. It is also hoped that the information here will prove useful as a reference.

Despite the length of this chapter, it is by no means a complete list of poisonous substances. We have purposely avoided including many poisonous plants not found in the Americas, and the scores of plants identified as toxic by isolated reports concerning one or two animals. The rapid expansion of industrial chemicals also precludes complete coverage of these compounds.

Only those associated with natural poisonings are discussed. Finally, hardly any drug exists (both pharmaceutical and biologic) that will not, under some circumstances, produce an adverse reaction. Although some drugs are included here, a more detailed treatment is addressed by pharmacology.

Considerable effort may be necessary for the reader to keep clearly in mind the characteristic signs and lesions that accompany each of the poisonings described in this chapter. To facilitate this process, the various poisons have been grouped in accordance with some outstanding lesion which, upon being encountered, may afford a clue to the diagnosis. To effect such a grouping is by no means easy, not only because the manifestations of a given poisoning vary in different individuals, but more so because many poisons attack by several mechanisms and produce a number of lesions, no one of which is salient among the others. It, thus, becomes most difficult to decide to which pathologic family a particular poison belongs. An exception to this approach occurs with respect to mycotoxins. These are discussed as a group at the conclusion of Chapter 11.

Whenever it is possible to use pathologic and clinical features to decrease the number of suspected etiologic agents, further investigation is simplified. Chemical identification of the poison or clear demonstration of its ingestion or contact should always be attempted when the situation permits. In only a few poisonings are lesions characteristic enough to permit definitive diagnosis. As with infectious diseases, it is important to demonstrate the etiologic agent in association with the lesions that it is expected to cause.

Many poisonous plants are referred to in this chapter by their common and scientific names. No further effort is made to identify the plants. This identification is admirably accomplished by John M. Kingsbury in the book, *Poisonous Plants of the United States and Canada* (Prentice-Hall, 1964).

Extraneous poisons will be addressed in the sequence as illustrated in Table 15-1.

TABLE 15-1 **Extraneous poisons**

Group	Pathologic features	Poisons		
A	Local injury	Venoms Phenol	Lewisite Mustard gas	
B	Gastroenteritis	Arsenic Salt Petroleum Sodium fluoroacetate Ground glass Dynamite Urea Nicotine Nightshades	Castor beans Locust tree Tung oil tree Flourensia cernua Oaks Oleander Milkweeds Red squill Blister beetle	
C	Hepatotoxicity; often nephrotoxicity	Phosphorus Phosphates Copper Carbon tetrachloride Tetrachloroethylene Phenothiazine Phenanthridinium Clay pigeons (pitch) Hydrogen sulfide Gossypol Cocklebur Senecios	Crotalaria Heliotrope Tarweed Lantana Sacahuiste Drymaria Lechuguilla Phyllanthus Mushrooms Lupines Vetch Algae Hepatotoxic mycotoxins	
D	Nephrotoxicity	Turpentine Sulfonamides Oxalates ethylene glycol Broomweed	Chloroform Chinese tallow tree Bitterweed Nephrotoxic mycotoxins	
E	Cardiac insufficiency	Selenium Death camas Aconite	Baileya Jimson weed Pimelea	
F	Extensive hemorrhage	Dicoumarin Bracken fern	Aspirin	
G	Anemia	Molybdenum Naphthalene	Onions	
H	Methemoglobinemia	Nitrates Nitrites	Chlorates	
I	Carboxyhemoglobinemia	Carbon monoxide	Cyanides	
J	Edema	Naphthyl thiourea (ANTU)		
K	Pulmonary dysfunction	Rape Kale	Stinkwood Paraquat	
L	Lesions of bone and teeth	Fluorine		
M	Hypercalcemia	*Solanum malacoxylon*	*Cestrum diurnum*	
N	Loss of hair or wool	Thallium	Jumbay tree	

(continued)

TABLE 15-1 (continued)

Group	Pathologic features	Poisons	
O	Epithelial hyperplasia	Chlorinated dibenzodi-oxins Chlorinated naphthalenes	Polychlorinated biphenyls Polybrominated biphenyls
P	Nervous malfunction	Strychnine Loco Vetchlike Astragali Atropine Equisetum Hemlocks Phalaris grass Lathyrus Larkspur Yellow Star Thistle 3-nitro-4-hydroxy phenyl-arsonic acid	Anguina Carbon disulfide Ortho-tricresyl phosphate Lead Mercury Chlorinated hydrocarbons Organic phosphates Cycada Arsanilic acid
Q	Degeneration of cardiac and skeletal muscles	Coffee senna Coyotillo	Hairy vetch
R	Teratogenic effects on embryo or fetus	Veratrum californicum Thalidomide Pine needles	Lupin Selenium Lathyrus
S	Miscellaneous or unclassified	Small head sneeze weed Box Grasstree Pokeweed Yew Sorghum Sesbania Djenkol bean Estrogen Nitrogen dioxide	Cobalt Chloroquine Zinc Zinc phosphide Cadmium Gidyea tree Wild everlasting Chinaberry tree Aspirin Benzoic acid Carpet weed Fish (shellfish)

GROUP A: LOCAL INJURY

Poisons that produce local injury (necrosis and inflammation) to the tissues with which they come in contact are included in this group. An appropriate degree of concentration is essential to produce this effect. Strong acids and alkalies are categorized in this group, but are not discussed here.

Venoms of snakes and other creatures

Snake bites, at least those of North American rattlesnakes, copperheads, and moccasins, promptly cause an extremely rapid though weakening heart beat, but their most spectacular effect is tremendous local swelling, which is well under way within minutes after the bite is inflicted. The swelling is the result of inflammatory edema, or more precisely, of serous inflammatory exudation. Within three or four hours the maximum is reached, and when the bite is on the nose, as it usually is in horses and may be in the case of dogs and cattle, suffocation may ensue from closing of the nostrils or glottis. If the animal were to survive, the swelling would subside in four to seven days, but the toxic injury would be sometimes so severe that necrosis and sloughing of a large mass of tissue may supervene. Hemolysis is another effect of the venom, perhaps to the extent that hemoglobinuria and hemolytic icterus may be noticeable. Interference with clotting of the blood also occurs. Certain venoms are also strongly neurotoxic, leading to restlessness, irritability, and trembling followed by paralysis. Postmortem findings include the foregoing changes plus extreme passive congestion of all organs and hemorrhages in the region of the bite. Local gas gangrene or tetanus occasionally supervenes, initiated by the bacterial contamination of the serpent's mouth.

Many species of **toads** (*Bufo* sp.) throughout the world produce toxins (venoms) in their parotid glands that are responsible for poisoning animals, especially dogs and occasionally cats and humans. Poisoning usually follows when a dog plays with the toad and absorbs the toxin through the buccal and gastric mucosa. The toxins are digitalis-like, leading to irregularities in cardiac function, which may result in death.

The **stings of bees** and various other insects are similar to snake bites in causing an extreme degree of serous exudation. This fluid in either type of poisoning exerts a valuable protective effect by diluting the poison and causing so much local pressure that circulation of the blood and the consequent dissemination of the poison are inhibited. The severity of the reaction to the stings of bees and scorpions and the bites of ants varies greatly in different individuals of any species, apparently on an allergic basis. Even horses have died from multiple bee stings, methemoglobinemia and bilirubinemia being noted.

The **black widow spider** (*Latrodectus mactans*), requires careful consideration in the diagnosis of sudden canine illnesses in practically all parts of the United States and many other countries. Although some dogs appear to be immune (possibly from previous exposure), the bite of this black spider with the red "hour-glass" spot on its abdomen may well be fatal to a dog or, presumably, to a cat. The period of illness may terminate fatally in two hours or it may continue for two or three days with recovery or death. Early symptoms commence with pain at the site of the bite, which may be severe. Edema (serous inflammatory exudate) also develops around the bite. The whole integument becomes painful and hypersensitive to slight pressure; the abdominal wall becomes rigid through reflex contraction of the muscles. In some cases, hyperesthesia, which appears to reside in the articular surfaces, causes fleeting but pronounced pain which, in a matter of minutes, may shift from one limb to another. If intoxication were to persist, gradually increasing paralysis may appear on the second or third day; meanwhile, the pain may subside, but paralysis may become so extensive as to produce death. Postmortem examination reveals little but venous congestion.

References

Baerg WJ. The black widow: its life history and the effects of the poison. Scient Monthly 1923;17:535–547.
Bedford PGC. Toad venom toxicity and its clinical occurrence in small animals in the United Kingdom. Vet Rec 1974;94:613–614.
Comstock JH. The spider book. Ithaca: Comstock Pub. Co., Inc., 1948.
Crimmins ML. Facts about Texas snakes and their poisons. J Am Vet Med Assoc 1927;71:704–712.
Ditmars RL. Snake bites among domestic animals. J Am Vet Med Assoc 1939;94:383–388.
Fitzgerald WE. Snakebite in the horse. Aust Vet J 1975;51:37–39.
McNellis R. Rattlesnake bite. J Am Vet Med Assoc 1949;114:145–146.
Nighbert EM. Effects of bites of poisonous snakes on dogs. North Am Vet 1943;24:363–364.
Palumbo NE, Perri S, Read G. Experimental induction and treatment of toad poisoning in the dog. J Am Vet Med Assoc 1975;167:1000–1005.
Parrish HM, Scatterday JE, Pollard CB. The clinical management of snake venom poisoning in domestic animals. J Am Vet Med Assoc 1957;130:548–551.
Perry BD, Bracegirdle JR. Toad poisoning in small animals. Vet Rec 1973;92:589–590.
Pritchard CW. Black widow spider and snake venom in small animals. J Am Vet Med Assoc 1940;96:356–358.
Schöll, G. Todlicher Kreuzotterbiss bei einem Dackel. (Necropsy findings in a dachshund bitten by a common viper.) Die Kleintierpraxis 1968;13:113–115.
Wirth D. Bienenstichvergiftung beim Pferd. (Bee sting poisoning in horses.) Wien Tierärztl Monatschr 1943;30:129–134.

Phenol

Phenol, or carbolic acid, is used in medicine much less than formerly, but poisoning through accidental ingestion or by absorption through the skin is still occasionally seen. In general, symptoms are those of nervous shock and nervous depression, paralysis, and coma. The salient lesion results from the action of all but high dilutions of phenol as a potent tissue fixative. Mucous membranes (mouth, stomach) with which it comes in contact promptly become firm and white, a state of coagulative necrosis. Microscopically, the white, coagulated tissue is found to be perfectly preserved, while adjoining areas may show postmortem autolysis in keeping with the time between death and preservation of tissue.

References

Angus KW, Smith PH. Ultrastructural features of lung lesions in sheep dipped in a carbolic dip. J Comp Pathol 1983;93:33–42.
Carlisle CH. Toxicity of flufenamic acid in the cat. J Small Anim Pract 1983;24:653–658.

Lewisite

This gas, chlorovinyldichloroarsine or a mixture of closely related compounds, is vesicant and necrotizing on the skin or other tissues with which it comes in contact. The eyes and air passages suffer severely when the gas is inhaled: the mouth and whole gastrointestinal tract when ingested. Absorption of the material also occurs, with the result that the blood-borne poison produces the usual changes of acute toxic hepatitis and less severe toxic nephrosis. The epithelium of the bile ducts and gallbladder may suffer necrosis as the result of elimination of some of the poison in the bile. Shock, comparable to that which results from ordinary burns, may develop after a few days, with fatal termination.

Reference

Cameron GR, Carlton HM, Short RHD. Pathological changes induced by lewisite and allied compounds. J Pathol Bact 1946;58:411–422.

Mustard gas

Animals have been poisoned by eating forage or pasturage contaminated with this deadly war gas, which chemically is B, B_1-dichloroethyl sulfide. Clinical signs include profuse salivation, lacrimation and conjunctivitis, mucous rhinitis, refusal to eat, pain in the mouth and pharynx, nausea, and rapid pulse and respiration. Lesions are chiefly due to the local irritant and necrotizing action upon the mucous membranes of the mouth, esophagus, and stomach. These could lead to confusion with "mucosal disease" or in sheep, with contagious ecthyma or possibly with other viral infections. Hemorrhages and focal prenecrotic degeneration are reported in the myocardium. Burns, of course, can occur on the skin when the poisonous liquid or vapor comes in contact with it. Coagulative necrosis is the fundamental change, with ulceration supervening. In fatal cases, death after several days is partly attributable to secondary infection of the ulcerated surfaces.

References

Koschnick H. Gelbkreuz-(Lost-) vergiftungen bei Pferden Z Veterinärk. 1943;55:57–63.

Pullinger BD. Some characters of coagulation necrosis due to mustard gas. J Pathol Bact 1947;59:255–259.

Watson JF. Mustard gas poisoning in the horse. Vet Rec 1943;55:338.

Young L. Effects of mustard gas on the rat. Can J Res Sect E 1947;25:141–151.

GROUP B: GASTROENTERITIS

Poisons in group B have **gastroenteritis** as the prominent pathologic feature. However, lesions in other organs are present in most of these poisonings and clinical signs may be diverse.

Arsenic

Animals frequently acquire arsenic in poisonous quantities through the accidental ingestion of such compounds as lead arsenate and Paris green, which are kept on farms for use as insecticidal sprays, and lead arsenite, which is used as a cutaneous parasiticide (dips) for ticks and mites (Fig. 15-1). Another frequent accident consists of animals eating plants and weeds that have been sprayed with arsenicals intentionally, to kill the plants, or inadvertently, while the spray was being applied to fruit trees. Poisoning occurs readily through cutaneous absorption when animals are dipped in a solution that is too concentrated. Occasional poisoning results from excessive administration of arsenic medicaments, such as Fowler's solution or neoarsphenamine. Chronic poisoning also occurs in animals grazing on land subject to precipitated fumes from smelters and blast furnaces using arsenic-containing ores. Arsenous acid, in the experience of one of the authors (Jones), has accidentally contaminated commercial dog food, with numerous fatalities. Arsanilic acid (an organic arsenic) is used in poultry and swine feeds as a stimulant to growth. It is also occasionally used to control dysentery in swine. These practices have added to the possibility of causing arsenic poisoning by error in compounding feed or by contamination of feeds intended for other species.

The outstanding lesion of acute arsenic poisoning is severe gastritis or gastroenteritis, often hemorrhagic. The usual signs of severe abdominal pain, vomiting (dogs, pigs), purgation, and tenesmus obviously depend upon this lesion; the same may be true of the acceleration of pulse and respiration and general collapse. Gastroenteritis is said to occur regardless of the route by which the poison enters the body. Dehydration of the tissues occurs with abundant fluid in the bowels (diluting the irritant).

In less acute poisonings, diarrhea usually marks the presence of moderately severe gastroenteritis. In these cases, stupor, incoordination, convulsions, and subnormal temperature are manifest. Such cases in cows have been mistaken for milk fever.

The chronic form is more rare now than previously, when arsenicals were often used in treatment of several obscure diseases. The principal lesions include:

(1) Toxic hepatitis (hydropic degeneration, fatty change, and necrosis);
(2) Chronic dermatitis with excessive pigmentation (in white skins) and extreme hyperkeratosis;
(3) "Neuritis" causing atrophy of the optic nerve and blindness. Peripheral motor nerves and their neu-

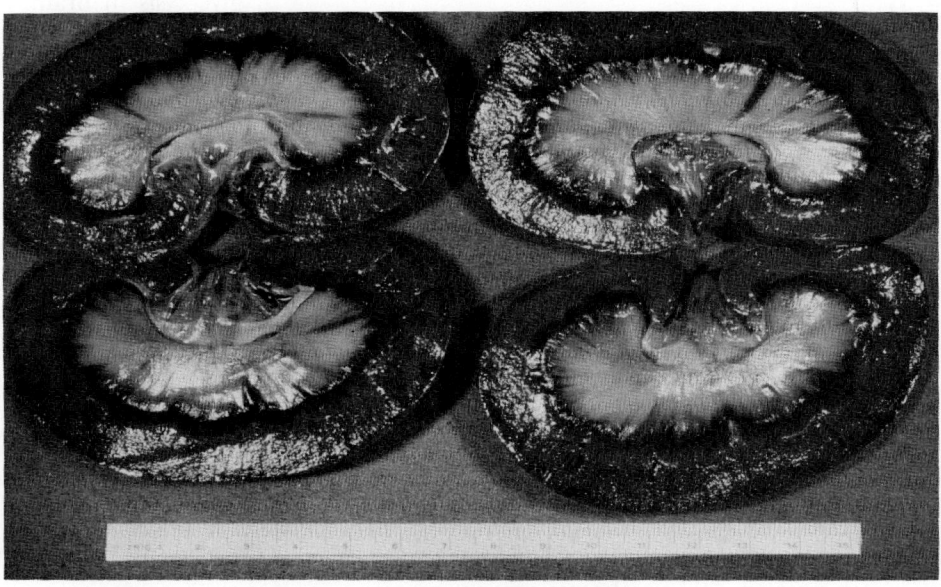

FIG. 15-1 Arsenic poisoning, kidneys of a four-year-old male foxhound. Note dark, congested corticomedullary junction and blanched medulla. (Courtesy of Angell Memorial Animal Hospital.)

rons in the cord may also be destroyed, leading to paraplegia and dysphagia; and,

(4) In cattle, an unexplained periarticular fibrosis sometimes occurs, producing stiffness and asymmetric enlargements of hocks or other joints of the limbs.

Arsenic is chemically rather indestructible, and can be detected in the liver and other tissues years after death and burial. The element is also detectable in the urine.

Arsanilic acid (p-aminophenylarsonic acid) and 3-nitro-4-hydroxyphenylarsonic acid are each organic arsenical compounds which are used in pig feed to promote growth and control enteric infections. Under certain conditions, these chemicals may cause toxic effects in the nervous system. These effects are discussed under Group Q toxins in this chapter.

References

Byron WR, et al. Pathological changes in rats and dogs from two-year feeding of arsenite and sodium arsenate. Toxicol Appl Pharmacol 1967;10:132–147.

Harding JDJ, Lewis G, Done JT. Experimental arsanilic acid poisoning in pigs. Vet Rec 1968;83:560–564.

Lindgren A, Danielsson BRG, Nightenhelser LK. Embrotoxicity of arsenate: distribution in pregnant mice and monkeys and effects on embryonic cells in vitro. Acta Pharmacol Toxicol 1984; 54:311–320.

McCulloch EC, St John JL. Lead arsenate poisoning of sheep and cattle. J Am Vet Med Assoc 1940;96:321–326.

Moxham JW, Coup MR. Arsenic poisoning of cattle and other domestic animals. NZ Vet J 1968;16:161–165.

Peoples SA. Arsenic toxicity in cattle. Ann NY Acad Sci 1964;111:644–649.

Thatcher CD, Meldrum JB, Wikse SE, et al. Arsenic toxicosis and suspected chromium toxicosis in a herd of cattle. J Am Vet Med Assoc 1985;187:179–182.

Tsukamoto H, Parker HR, Gribble DH, et al. Nephrotoxicity of sodium arsenate in dogs. Am J Vet Res 1983;44:2324–2330.

Tsukamoto H, Parker HR, Peoples SA. Metabolism and renal handling of sodium arsenate in dogs. Am J Vet Res 1983;44:2331–2335.

Salt

Swine and poultry are sometimes poisoned by sodium chloride when the salty (60%) brines used for the preservation of meats on farms are discarded in such a manner that animals have access to them. Other animals are occasionally poisoned by consuming too much when the usual free supply of salt, with or without other minerals, has been unavailable for some time and then is abruptly replenished. Other forms of accidental ingestion of excessive amounts have been reported.

Chickens and other farm birds are most susceptible, by far, to poisoning by sodium chloride. Swine are next most susceptible. For baby chicks, physiologic salt solution (0.9% NaCl) as the exclusive source of drinking water is regularly fatal in a few days. A concentration of 0.5% administered in the same way may also kill them, but 0.25% does not. Adult hens are able to consume appreciably more, especially if the salt were administered dry, mixed with the food. In the latter form of administration, 30% in the ration was sometimes fatal, but 20% evoked no unfavorable signs. In young

pigs, salt amounting to 2.5% of the ration and mixed with the feed caused severe nervous symptoms but no fatalities, unless the supply of water was restricted. Cattle are sometimes poisoned, as mentioned previously; conversely, they have been unharmed by the prolonged consumption of two pounds (900 g) of salt per day as long as the large consumption of water that resulted remained unrestricted. It can be said with respect to all species that it is not easy to produce poisoning as long as animals are allowed all the water they wish to drink.

The signs include nervous derangement and hyperirritability. Blindness, stumbling, walking backward or in circles, and convulsive seizures are most frequently mentioned. In experimental cases the following have been reported: deranged consciousness, blindness, epileptiform seizures beginning with twitching of the nose and progressing clonus of the neck muscles, circling or running movements, retropulsion, pleurothotonos, opisthotonos, and sialorrhea. As the effects become more severe, signs of abdominal pain become paramount. Thirst is always excessive.

Lesions following the sudden ingestion of excessive amounts of salt, especially when unlimited water has not been available, consist of severe, acute inflammation of the gastric and upper intestinal linings. Sometimes crystals of undissolved salt adhere to the inflamed mucosa. In cases of continued consumption of moderately excessive amounts of salt over a period of days, usually experimental, the principal lesion is edema of both tissues and body cavities. A microscopic lesion that appears to be pathognomonic in swine, but not necessarily in poultry, has been called eosinophilic meningoencephalitis. It is characterized by a startlingly, extensive infiltration of eosinophils into the perivascular (Virchow-Robin) spaces of brain, along with edema and sometimes encephalomalacia. Experimental work indicates that sodium becomes concentrated in brain tissue, its high osmotic pressure then being responsible for edema. Sodium is also a strong inhibitor of anaerobic glycolysis in brain. Sodium and chloride of the blood are elevated.

In poultry, salt poisoning causes a form of nephritis which is believed by many to be the same as a disease known by such names as nephrosclerosis of poultry or pullet disease.

References

Blaxland JD. Toxicity of sodium chloride for fowls. Vet J 1946;102:157–173.

Franson JC, Sileo L, Fleming WJ. Iatrogenic salt poisoning in captive sandhill cranes. J Am Vet Med Assoc 1981;179:1211–1213.

Sautter JH, Sorenson DK, Clark JJ. Symposium on salt poisoning: salt poisoning in swine. J Am Vet Med Assoc 1957;130:12–22.

Scarratt WK, Collins TJ, Sponenberg DP. Water deprivation-sodium chloride intoxication in a group of feeder lambs. J Am Vet Med Assoc 1985;186:977–978.

Schlifferli C, Savio R. Eosinophilic meningoencephalitis in swine-salt poisoning. Arch Med Vet Chile 1981;13:44–47. [Vet Bull 1982;52:2621.]

Smith DLT. Poisoning by sodium salt. A cause of eosinophilic meningoencephalitis in swine. Am J Vet Res 1957;18:825–850.

Swayne DE, Shlosberg A, Davis RB. Salt poisoning in turkey poults. Avian Dis 1986;30:847–852.

Petroleum

When one observes the lack of gustatory discrimination shown by most bovine animals, one is not too greatly astonished to see cattle drinking crude petroleum that has escaped from an oil tank or pipeline and is standing in a pool on the ground or floating on the surface of a pond or stream. Just how toxic a given specimen of crude oil is remains unknown. Well-purified petroleum oil constitutes the liquid petrolatum of the Pharmacopeia and is practically inert in the digestive tract. Conversely, the volatile fractions of petroleum are irritating and definitely poisonous. It can be said with certainty that fresh oil is consequently more toxic than that which has been out of the ground long enough for much of the volatile material to have evaporated. One specimen of crude oil used as tractor fuel was found to be lethal at the rate of 1 gallon (3800 ml) for a bovine weighing 450 pounds (200 kg). Although other species are not immune, their different habits usually protect them.

Signs have usually included fetid and hemorrhagic diarrhea, although constipation has been noted, probably as an initial change. Oil is usually detectable in feces and it may be regurgitated. Bloating commonly occurs. The temperature is somewhat elevated; respiration and heart beat are accelerated. Terminally, dilated pupils and muscular incoordination occur. Some animals recover in a few days.

Postmortem lesions include acute enteritis with marked enteric edema, renal hyperemia, perhaps with hemorrhages, and acute cystitis. Pulmonary congestion and edema are prominent when the oil contained much volatile material.

Kerosene is occasionally administered accidentally and more often is given by the laity for some supposed medicinal effect. Not all of the victims die, but in those who do, pneumonia is usually an outstanding lesion, presumably because of inhalation of irritant fumes. Central nervous system dysfunction, which is a well-recognized sequela to kerosene poisoning in humans, is believed to result from hypoxia. It is sometimes applied externally (e.g., for lice) and has caused loss of hair in the horse. In cattle, severe dermatitis and hematuria have been reported.

References
Barber DML, Cousin DAH, Seawright D. An episode of kerosene poisoning in dairy heifers. Vet Rec 1987;120:462–463.
Kerr LA, Edwards WC. Chromate poisoning in livestock from oil field wastes. Vet Hum Toxicol 1981;23:402–402.
Leighton FA. Morphological lesions in red blood cells from Herring gulls and Atlantic puffins ingesting Prudhoe Bay crude oil. Vet Pathol 1986;23:254–263.
Toofanian F, Aliakbari S, Ivoghli B. Acute diesel fuel poisoning in goats. Trop Anim Health Prod 1979;11:98–101. [Vet Bull 1979;49:7554.]

Sodium fluoroacetate

This compound of fluorine, sometimes sold as "Formula 1080," inhibits the citric acid cycle. It is used as a poison for destroying rats. It is sometimes accidentally eaten by dogs when it is placed in meat as bait and by cattle which may ingest contaminated forage or grain. Signs include increasing weakness and rapidity of the heart beat; the heart eventually becomes exhausted. Signs of severe abdominal pain and nausea are prominent in dogs and swine (experimentally). Nervous disturbances terminate in opisthotonos and convulsions, with death in a few or several hours after ingestion of the poison. It is said that the prognosis is hopeless once symptoms have appeared. Lesions are few, but ordinarily severe inflammation of the small intestine occurs. As a result of cardiac failure and anoxia, the blood is dark and subepicardial and subendocardial petechiae are evident. Studies of the nervous tissues have not been reported.

References
Jensen R, Tobiska JW, Ward JC. Sodium fluoroacetate poisoning in sheep. Am J Vet Res 1948;9:370–372.
Murphy SD. Pesticides. In: Doull J, Klaasen CD, Amdur MO, eds. Toxicology: the basic science of poisons. New York: Macmillan, 1980;395–396.
Nichols HC, et al. Poisoning of two dogs with 1080 rat poison (sodium fluoroacetate). J Am Vet Med Assoc 1949;115:355–356.
Schnautz JO. Sodium fluoroacetate poisoning in cattle. J Am Vet Med Assoc 1949;114:435.
Schwarte LH. Toxicity of sodium monofluoroacetate for swine and chickens. J Am Vet Med Assoc 1947;111:301–303.

Ground Glass

More or less finely shattered glass is administered from time to time to humans or animals with felonious intent. In a majority of cases, no effects are noticed. In some instances, transient abdominal discomfort, diarrhea, and mild gastroenteritis ensue.

References
Mayo NS. Effect of "ground glass" on the gastrointestinal tract of dogs. J Am Med Assoc 1919;55:202–203.
Simmons JS, Von Glahn WC. Effect of "ground glass" on the gastrointestinal tract of dogs. J Am Med Assoc 1918;71:2127.

Dynamite

Cattle are sometimes poisoned by eating dynamite or its wrappings. One suspects that the native bovine curiosity, which is sometimes manifested in most incongruous ways, has more to do with the animal's eating a substance of this kind than has the actual appetite. Nitroglycerine, of course, is available as a drug, and would have the same effect as dynamite when ingested in excessive amounts.

Signs are polyuria and polydipsia, nausea, colic, and perhaps coma. In fatal cases, death occurs in 24–36 hours. Postmortem lesions are acute gastroenteritis, acute toxic tubular nephritis, dark or chocolate-colored blood due to the formation of methemoglobin, and often petechiae due to terminal anoxia.

References
Buffington RM. Nitroglycerine (dynamite) poisoning in cattle. Vet Bull 1928;21:197–198.
Holm LW, et al. Experimental poisoning of cattle and sheep with dynamite. Cornell Vet 1952;42:91–96.
Kinnell GN. Dynamite poisoning. Am Vet Rev 1894;17:554–556.

Urea (ammonia)

Because the practice of feeding cattle and other ruminants artificially concocted feeds containing urea as a substitute for protein nitrogen has developed, deaths attributed to poisoning by this substance have ceased to be rare. It appears that 2–3% of the total ration (dry-weight basis) can safely be urea, but that larger amounts are likely to produce poisoning. Urea is much better tolerated when mixed with plentiful amounts of other feeds than when, for any reason, it enters the digestive tract less well diluted; hence, the occurrence of poisoning is erratic. Poisoning is due to the local and generalized effects of ammonia released by hydrolysis of the urea by urease. Ammonium salts are also used in feeds, and their use in fertilizer provides another source of exposure. The effects of urea and ammonium salts are comparable.

Signs arise suddenly and may lead to death in one to two hours or less. However, illness does not necessarily develop at the first ingestion of the urea-containing feed, but apparently occurs whenever—through intestinal inactivity or other functional irregularity—a sufficient amount of ammonia is released at one time and, judging from experimental administration via the stomach tube, in the same region of the digestive canal. Signs are attributable to the effect of ammonia on the nerve centers, and include twitching of eyelids, lips, and tail, ataxia in locomotion, and convulsions. Salivation may be prominent, with frothing at the mouth. Pulse and respirations become progressively slower and death follows. The resemblance to strychnine poisoning is often marked. Blood-urea nitrogen, as well as ammonia-nitrogen in the rumen, are elevated. The pH of the blood and urine are abnormally high.

Postmortem lesions are not extensive. Usually severe, acute catarrhal or, at times, hemorrhagic enteritis is manifest. In the experience of some, the inflammation has been found in the stomach (abomasum); in the experience of Hilton Smith, severe inflammation always occurs in the last third of the small intestine. Mild toxic hepatitis and toxic tubular nephrosis accompany enteric injury. In the lungs, hemorrhages may be evident, either peribronchial or intra-alveolar, as well as mild, acute catarrhal bronchitis. The central nervous lesions, consisting of neuronal degenerations, pial hemorrhages, and congestion, are probably attributable to the direct effects of ammonia.

References

Salam AA, Chooi KF, Osman A, et al. Accidental urea poisoning in beef cattle. Vet Rec 1986;119:407–408.

Zarnke RL, Taylor WP Jr. Urea poisoning in free-ranging Alaskan bison. J Am Vet Med Assoc 1982;181:1417.

Nicotine

"Nicotine has been consumed in the form of tobacco and other plants for many hundreds of years. The compulsive use of tobacco has been observed in nearly every culture into which tobacco has been introduced. Nearly 30 percent of adult Americans smoke despite, in most cases, a desire to quit and despite common knowledge of the health hazards. Their failure to quit smoking is attributed in large part to the addictive properties of nicotine." (Benowitz, 1988).

Poisoning by nicotine occurs in animals almost exclusively from the improper use of insecticidal solutions on the skin or nicotine sulfate as an anthelmintic internally. One of the most deadly poisons known, nicotine is promptly absorbed from mucous membrane or skin and acts rapidly, producing at first nervous stimulation and then depression. When swallowed, local pain in the throat and stomach is experienced. Muscular tremors and weakness cause the animal to fall. Convulsions are followed in a matter of minutes by loss of voluntary movement, so that the patient lies quietly. Concurrently with vomiting and purging, the pulse and respiration become weaker and slower, with death from respiratory failure and collapse, all within two to three hours. A case of a dog being poisoned by eating cigarette stubs (equivalent of 15–20 cigarettes per day) is on record. Depression and polyuria were followed by vomition and then by diarrhea lasting four days. Another reported fatality, in a three-month-old puppy, resulted from eating a pack of cigarettes.

As would be expected from the rapidity of the poisonous action, lesions are minimal. Acute inflammation of the stomach (abomasum) and intestines is likely to be pronounced, even when the mode of entry is by cutaneous absorption. Mesenteric vessels are severely hyperemic, the blood being bright red.

References

Benowitz NL. Pharmacologic aspects of cigarette smoking and nicotine addiction. N Engl J Med 1988;319:1318–1330.

Boissière. Intoxication du chien par le tabac. Rec mé vét. 1938;114:35.

Crawshaw HA. Nicotine poisoning in lambs. Vet Rec 1944;56:276–277.

Fincher MG. Blackleaf 40 poisoning. Cornell Vet 1934;24:86.

Kaplan B. Acute nicotine poisoning in a dog. Vet Med Small Anim Clin 1968;63:1033–1034.

Nightshades (genus solanum)

Plants of the genus *Solanum* are globally distributed and include a large number of species that are useful as feed for animals or food for humans, sometimes are ornamental and often poisonous. Some of these species are listed in Table 15-2. Their toxic properties, in general, are the result of the production of one or more glycoalkaloids.

The signs and lesions that follow consumption of these plants are varied depending on the active principle and quantity involved. Some produce gastrointestinal effects with vomiting, tympanitis, and diarrhea, some result in nervous signs and lesions, others lead to calcinosis which is particularly intense in the cardiovascular system, and some are teratogenic.

Deadly nightshade (belladonna) is described on page 755; *S. malacoxylon* and other calcinosis-producing plants are described on page 744.

TABLE 15-2 *Solanum* **(Nightshades)**

Species	Common name	Toxin effect	Region
Dimidiatum	Potato weed	Solanine, choconine neuropathy, cattle	Texas
Kwebense		Purkinje cell neuropathy, cattle	South Africa
Fastigiatum		Purkinje cell neuropathy, cattle	Brazil
Bonariensis		Purkinje cell neuropathy	Uruguay
Malacoxylon Syn:glaucum		Vit D3, analogue calcinosis	Americas, Hawaii
Torvum		Vit D3, analogue calcinosis	New Guinea
Glaucophyllium		Vit D3, analogue calcinosis	Europe
Verbacifolium		Vit D3, analogue calcinosis	Europe
Aviculare		"Diosgenin"	Australia and New Zealand, Eastern Europe
Incanum	Bitter apple	Dimethylnitrosamine carcinogen	Africa
Eleangnifolium	White horse nettle	Spirosolane (solasodine) teratogen	Americas
Tuberosum	Common potato sprouts and green skin	a-solanine, a-chaconine teratogen (hamsters)	Global
Dulcamera	Poinsettia	Spirosolane (solasodin) soladulein, teratogen	Europe, Americas

References

James LF, Keeler RF, Bailey EM Jr, et al. Poisonous plants: Proc 3rd Int Symp. Ames: Iowa State Univ Press, 1992.

Keeler RF, Tu AT, eds. Handbook of natural toxins. Vol I. Plant and fungal toxins. New York: Marcel Dekker, 1983.

Kellerman TS. Plant poisoning and mycotoxicosis in livestock in Southern Africa. Capetown: Oxford Univ Press, 1988.

Koslowski B. Dermatitis in unweaned pigs from feeding green potatoes to the sows. Méd vét Varsovie 1953;9:505. [Vet Bull 1954;3290.]

Sever JL. Potatoes and birth defects: summary. Teratology 1973;8:319–320.

Simic WJ. Solanine poisoning in swine. Vet Med 1943;38:353–354.

CASTOR BEANS (RICINUS COMMUNIS)

The meal remaining after the extraction of oil from castor beans contains ricin, an extremely potent poison that is water-soluble; hence, it is not found in the castor oil. Ricin resembles bacterial exotoxins in that an animal can be hyperimmunized to it so that the serum has high-antitoxic properties. As in the case of bacterial toxins, heat (about 56°C) destroys a toxic fraction (toxophore) and leaves an immunizing fraction (haptophore). Boiling the meal or whole seeds renders them nonpoisonous.

Signs appear a few hours after ingestion of small amounts of meal or the whole seeds. They consist chiefly of vomiting violent diarrhea, signs of severe abdominal pain (grinding of teeth, humping of back), tumultuous heart action, slightly elevated temperature, and collapse. Horses show profuse sweating, and tetanic spasms have occurred. Lesions include severe, acute gastritis (abomasitis in ruminants), with reddening and edema continuing into the upper small intestine, where they are accompanied by petechiae. Free blood may be found in the bowel. Microscopically, the epithelium of the affected gastrointestinal areas is necrotic, although sometimes still present. Hepatocytes undergo hydropic degeneration, fatty change, and areas of necrosis (acute toxic hepatitis). The renal epithelium displays a less severe fatty degeneration and necrosis (acute toxic nephritis). Striking destruction of lymphocytes occurs in the lymphoid organs (possibly simulating that seen in rinderpest and in irradiation). Necrosis has been demonstrated in brain. In horses, severe edema is reported in the lungs, with a less severe degree in bronchial, mesenteric, and hepatic nodes, as well as elsewhere. Much fluid pools in the inflamed digestive tract. Treatment is symptomatic unless serum from a previously hyperimmunized animal is available.

References

Clarke EGC. Poisoning by castor seed. Vet J 1947;103:273–278.

Geary T. Castor bean poisoning. Vet Rec 1950;62:472–473.

McCunn J, Andrew H, Clough GW. Castor-bean poisoning in horses. Vet J 1945;101:136–138.

Locust tree

The seeds, leaves, bark, and roots of the black locust tree (*Robinia pseudoacacia*) have long been known to be poisonous, several different alkaloidal or glycosidal poisonous principles having been described. The clammy locust (*Robinia viscosa*) is also known to be poisonous, and presumably the same is true of other locusts. Horses and also humans have been poisoned by chewing the bark of young trees: chickens, by eating leaves and young sprouts.

Signs appear several hours after the poisonous material is ingested and include extreme muscular weakness, mental depression, and maximum dilatation of the pupils. Serious cardiac depression occurs; the beat may be weak, but in the terminal stages it is frequently reported to be characterized by a loud thump, audible for some distance. Signs of abdominal pain may be evident, and humans report nausea, but rarely, if ever, followed by purgation. Salivation and bleeding from the mouth have been described in the horse. Many humans and animals afflicted recover after a few days and gradually regain strength.

Necropsy of those that die reveals mucous inflammation of the gastrointestinal tract and occasionally more severe gastroenteritis. Venous congestion occurs, and some have described a yellowish discoloration of the mucous membranes (icterus).

Some experimental evidence indicates that the toxicity is seasonal (early and midsummer), or at least that locust trees are not constantly poisonous.

References

Barnes MF. Black locust poisoning of chickens. J Am Vet Med Assoc 1921;59:370–372.
Gardiner WW. Locust-tree bark poisoning. Am Vet Rev 1903;27:599–600.
Pammel LH. The toxicity of black locust. North Am Vet 1927;8:41–43.
Waldron CA. Poisoning from locust bark. Am Vet Rev 1908;33:456–459.

Tung oil tree

The tung tree (*Aleurites fordi*) is cultivated in warm countries for its oil, which is valuable in paints and varnishes. Poisoning of farm animals, including chickens, has resulted from attempts to feed the meal that remains after extraction of the oil from the tung nuts. It also can occur from ingestion of foliage—not from the tree directly—but in the form of cut leaves and branches, which have considerable palatability to cattle.

Profuse watery or bloody diarrhea occurs after an interval of a few days and is the chief sign. Illness lasts from one to three weeks before terminating fatally. Lesions include severe hemorrhagic gastroenteritis, severe congestion of the splanchnic organs, and early toxic changes in the liver.

References

Davis GK, et al. Tung meal in rations for growing chicks. Poult Sci 1946;25:74–79.
Emmel MW, et al. Toxicity of foliage of *Aleurites fordi* for cattle. J Am Vet Med Assoc 1942;101:136–137.
Hurst E. The poison plants of New South Wales. Sydney: Univ. of Sydney and N.S.W. Dept. Agric., 1942.

Fluorensia cernua

Known popularly as **blackbush** or **tarbush,** this plant is indigenous to the arid areas of the southwestern United States and Mexico. Poisoning occurs almost exclusively in sheep and goats, which eat the berrylike fruit, sometimes merely in the course of being driven through an infested area.

Signs include salivation, grinding of teeth, and severe abdominal pain, evident from groaning and arching of the back. Muscular twitchings are not infrequent. If the animal were to live for some time, mucous rhinitis would likely be manifest. Death frequently occurs in 24–48 hours; animals that survive five days usually recover. Lesions include severe inflammation of the abomasum and duodenum. In cases of some standing, the inflammatory infiltration of fluid and leukocytes extends into the muscularis.

Reference

Mathews EP. Toxicity of the ripe fruit of blackbrush, tarbush (*Fluorensia cernua*). Exp Sta Bull 644, College Station: Texas A. & M. College, 1944.

Oaks

Several hundred species of oak trees or shrubs are known, and poisoning by members of this genus (*Quercus*) has been recognized for a long time, but is not fully understood. The principle toxins of oaks are tannins (*gallotannins*), which are broken down into gallic acid and pyrogallol, both of which are toxic.

The usual form of oak poisoning occurs when the young leafbuds and flowers appear annually during springtime, and accordingly is often called "oak-bud poisoning." The usual outbreaks of the disease result from the ingestion of buds and young leaves of certain, small shrublike species known as shin-oak or shinnery oak, *Quercus havardi,* indigenous to the southwestern United States, and it may well be that this species is more poisonous than others. However, typical oak-bud poisoning has occurred when budding branches of large oak trees have been made accessible to cattle or sheep in the course of lumbering operations. It is unknown to what extent some or all oaks are more poisonous during the budding and early leafing stage, and to what extent the occurrence of poisoning at that time may be related to the contemporary shortage of other green feed and an appetite for the oaks. Oak poisoning may also result from consuming acorns in large quantity. In contrast to oak-bud poisoning, acorn poisoning occurs in the fall. Green acorns are more toxic than mature acorns.

Signs of oak-bud poisoning are chiefly alimentary and urinary in nature. Although a few animals have diarrhea from the outset, the great majority have severe constipation with tenesmus. The frequent efforts at defecation produce small, hard balls of mucus-covered feces, to which blood is sometimes adherent. After several days, the constipation commonly gives way to a fetid and hemorrhagic diarrhea. Blood-stained nasal exudate is a frequent sign. Ventral edema of renal origin is also characteristic, especially in sheep. The severe injury to the kidneys, which appears always to be a part of the syndrome, is evidenced by polydipsia and polyuria, clear urine of low specific gravity voided at frequent intervals. The illness may terminate fatally in 24 hours, after several days, or may yield to slow recovery in two or three weeks. New cases may appear for approximately one week after the herd or flock has been removed from access to budding oaks.

The lesions are those that would be predicted from the signs. Mucous enteritis involves the last half of the digestive canal and becomes partly or eventually almost entirely hemorrhagic. The mesenteric lymph nodes are edematous. In addition to the subcutaneous edema already mentioned, usually hydropericardium and hydroperitoneum occur. The liver is congested and shows a moderate degree of acute toxic hepatitis. The gallbladder is distended with viscid, brownish bile. The kidneys are of the large, pale type, but rather uniformly sprinkled with petechiae 2–3 mm in diameter. The medulla is congested. The microscopic renal picture is almost pathognomonic. Numerous proximal convoluted tubules contain dense casts of albumin, their pink color being stained with brown, doubtless from bile pigment and possibly also from hemoglobin. The necrotic epithelial lining cells are usually so intimately mixed with the proteinaceous contents of the lumen that the whole forms a dense, homogeneous mass limited by the basement membrane and interstitial tissue. Adjacent to such a tubule are others that appear quite uninjured. The glomeruli undergo little change, and the medulla remains nearly normal in appearance except for congestion.

The **pathogenesis** of oak poisoning has been subject to several hypotheses. One of the most recent is based upon the following: After cattle eat oak leaves or buds (rarely acorns), oak tannins of high-molecular weight are released into the rumen, but are not absorbed directly. Products of degradation of tannins include phenolic compounds of low-molecular weight that are absorbed into the circulation and produce toxic effects on the kidneys and other organs.

References

Basden KW, Dalvi RR. Determination of total phenolics in acorns from different species of oak trees in conjunction with acorn poisoning in cattle. Vet Hum Toxicol 1987;29:305–306.

Sandusky GE, Fosnaugh CJ, Smith JB, et al. Oak poisoning of cattle in Ohio. J Am Vet Med Assoc 1977;171:627–629.

Shi Z. Research on the pathogenesis of oak leaf poisoning in cattle. In: James LF, Keeler RF, Bailey EM JR, Cheeke PR, Hegarty MP, eds. Poisonous plants: Proc 3rd Int Symp. Ames: Iowa State Univ Press, 1992;503–516.

Smith HA. The diagnosis of oak poisoning. Southwest Vet 1959;13:343–349.

Spier SJ, Smith BP, Seawright AA, et al. Oak toxicosis in cattle in northern California: clinical and pathologic findings. J Am Vet Med Assoc 1987;191:958–964.

Zimmer MA. An investigation of the pathogenesis and pathomorphology of blackjack oak (*Quercus marilandica*) leaf toxicity. Diss Abstr Int B 1986;46:4192.

Oleander

The oleander (*Nerium oleander*), native to most of the warmer parts of the world and grown as an ornamental plant in the southern United States, has been known for its extreme toxicity since ancient times. Humans have been fatally poisoned not only by eating a few leaves, but even when oleander twigs were used as skewers in meat. Horses, cattle, and sheep usually do not eat it; most cases of poisoning occur when cuttings from a garden are thoughtlessly thrown into a dry lot, especially where animals are accustomed to having hay placed before them. Although the presenting signs and lesions focus on the gastrointestinal tract, death occurs from heart failure. The toxic principles of oleander are cardiac glycosides (oleandrin, neriine), similar in action to digitalis.

Signs include abdominal pain, nausea, vomiting, diarrhea, and tenesmus, plus a digitalis-like stimulation of the heart and constriction of vessels. As a result, extremities are cold, while the general body temperature is raised. Respirations are augmented both in rate and depth. Bradycardia or tachycardia may be associated with various arrhythmias. Tremors and tetanic stiffness give way to paralysis and death, usually without convulsions. The duration of symptoms is usually less than 24 hours.

Lesions are chiefly those of severe catarrhal or hemorrhagic gastroenteritis, the irritation even beginning in the pharynx in some cases. Terminal petechial and ecchymotic hemorrhages are common on the heart, and serous and mucous membranes, including the gallbladder and meninges. Blood-stained or clear fluid is frequent in the serous cavities. In an equine case studied by Hilton A. Smith, petechiae in the renal cortex were accompanied by hematuria. Early toxic hepatitis and toxic tubular nephrosis were evident in this animal. The cortical tubules were largely in a state of coagulative necrosis and contained casts of hemoglobin-stained protein.

References

Oehme FW. The hazard of plant toxicities to the human population. In: Keeler RF, Van Kampen KR, James LF, eds. Effects of poisonous plants on livestock. New York: Academic Press, 1978;67–80.

Panisset L. Noxiousness of rhododendron (oleander). North Am Vet 1923;4:255–256.

Ratigan WJ. Oleander poisoning in a bear. J Am Vet Med Assoc 1921;60:96–98.

Schwartz WL, et al. Toxicity of *Nerium oleander* in the monkey (*Cebus apella*). Vet Pathol 1974;11:259–277.

Steyn DG. The toxicology of plants in South Africa. Johannesburg: Central News Agency, Ltd., 1934.

Milkweeds

The plants known as milkweeds, at least in North America, belong to the genus *Asclepias* named for the Greek god of medicine. The common broad-leafed milkweeds, *A. eriocarpa* and *A. latiformis* have caused fatalities, and *A. speciosa*, a similar species, is considered moderately poisonous. The whorled milkweed, *A. subverticillata* (syn. *A. galioides*) and, and the dwarf *A. pumila* are much more common causes of poisoning. These latter plants have slender leaves and an appearance different from that of the common broad-leafed milkweeds. *A. crispa*, *A. fruticosa*, and *A. physocarpa* are narrow-leafed species that have been reported as poisoning animals in South Africa.

The milkweeds are readily recognized by the milky fluid that exudes from a broken stem, leaf, or root. Range livestock do not ordinarily eat these plants, but will do so when nothing else is available. Of biologic interest is the accumulation of active toxins in the bodies of insects, especially monarch butterflies (*Danaus Plesippus*), whose larvae feed exclusively on milkweeds. The chemical accumulation protects the insect from its potential predators, such as birds, that soon learn of its emetic potency and thereafter avoid this distinctively marked butterfly. Another interesting aside is the previous use of a related milkweed, *Calotropis procera*, to treat the tips of poisonous arrows in Africa.

Many biologically active toxins have been isolated from milkweeds. Most of them are classified as cardiac glycosides, or cardenolides, and have been given names based upon their source as well as chemical nature. These include: labriformin and uscaridin (from *Asclepias labriformis* and *A. eriocarpa*); calotropin and calactin (isolated from A. curassavica). Other medically useful cardenolides from different sources and with slightly different chemical structure are ouabain, digitoxin, and digoxin.

The effects of these toxic cardenolides seem to be much the same in all species. Signs are related to the cardiac, nervous, and gastrointestinal systems.

Depression and apathy, great weakness, loss of mucular control, falling, dilated pupils, and respiratory paralysis represent the former group; intestinal stasis and fermentation, foul odors from the mouth, and occasionally a terminal fetid diarrhea belong to the latter. All species of farm animals, including chickens, are susceptible. Depending on the degree of toxicity and the amount eaten, signs commence in 2–14 hours after ingestion of the plants and continue for one or two to several hours. Lesions include acute catarrhal gastroenteritis and congestion of the lungs. The kidneys may also be severely congested. Terminal dilation of the ventricles of the heart is frequent.

References

Benson JM, Seiber JN, Keeler RF, et al. Studies on the toxic principle of Asclepias eriocarpa and Asclepias labriformis. In: Keeler RF, Van Kampen KR, James LF, eds. Effects of poisonous plants on livestock. New York: Academic Press, 1978;273–284.

Seiber JN, Lee SM, Benson JM. Cardiac glycosides (cardenolides) in species of Asclepias (Asclepiadaceae). In: Keeler RF, Tu AT, eds. Handbook of natural toxins. Vol I. Plant and fungal toxins. New York: Marcel Dekker, 1983;43–83.

Red squill

Also known as the sea onion, *Urginea maritima*, red squill is notably emetic, as well as nauseating, for many species. The red variety is used to poison rats, which like it and do not vomit. Most other animals do not eat it, but dogs have been known to do so. Swine have eaten red squill when it was accidentally mixed with their feed. Dogs usually vomit promptly, and hence are not likely to be killed by it. Cats dislike it but have been poisoned by it.

The signs are vomition in the dog, usually not in other species, depression, collapse, incoordination, twitching, and convulsions in severe cases. Death may ensue in two to three days. Lesions include hyperemia and inflammation of gastric and intestinal mucosae, often with terminal bronchopneumonia. In most cases, toxic changes in the liver and kidney occur, but large experimental doses killed swine before these changes had become pronounced.

References

Gwatkin R, Plummer PJG. Toxicity of red squill for swine and rats. Can J Comp Med 1943;7:244–249.

Nagle AC. Red squill poisoning in a dog. J Am Vet Med Assoc 1948;112:139.

Rietz JH, Moore EN. Red squill poisoning in swine. J Am Vet Med Assoc 1943;102:120–121.

Blister beetle

The source of the name for the striped blister beetles of the genus **Epicauta** is from the action of **cantharidin,** a substance in their hemolymph which, when applied topically, causes acantholysis leading to formation of intraepidermal vesicles. The beetles feed on alfalfa, and dead beetles may be incorporated into alfalfa hay which, when consumed by horses, leads to acute poisoning. Although the geographic range of the beetles is wide, reports of poisoning in horses have been limited to Tennessee, Texas, and Oklahoma. The clinical and pathologic features of natural poisoning in horses have been reviewed and the disease experimentally reproduced. The most consistent clinical signs include abdominal pain, fever, depression, frequent urination, and increased pulse and respiration rates. Laboratory findings indicate hemoconcentration, and a slight increase in blood urea nitrogen occurs, as well as a decrease in serum calcium and hematuria. The tissue changes (Fig. 15-2) appear to result from local action of the toxin on the gastrointestinal tract, as well as on systemic effects following absorption, but the biochemical action of cantharidin is unknown.

Erosion and ulceration of the mucosa of the distal esophagus and esophageal part of the stomach are frequent, which results from separation of epithelial cells and their necrosis. Little inflammatory reaction is manifest at these sites, but the glandular stomach, small intestine, and colon are hyperemic and edematous. The contents are watery. Mild, toxic tubular nephritis is evident, but rarely is there extensive necrosis. Grossly, the urinary bladder is hyperemic and contains petechiae or larger hemorrhages. Microscopically, focal necrosis of transitional epithelium, erosion, and ulceration are evident. Discrete gray-red or pale yellow patches of necrosis up to 5 cm in greatest dimension in the ventricular myocardium are visible on the epicardial, endocardial, and cut surfaces. Histologically, the muscle fibers are swollen, have increased eosinophilia, and lose their striations. The lungs are hyperemic and edematous, and centrilobular congestion of the liver occurs. These lesions apparently result from myocardial failure.

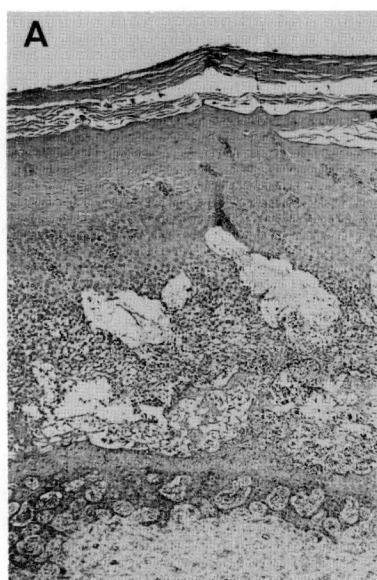

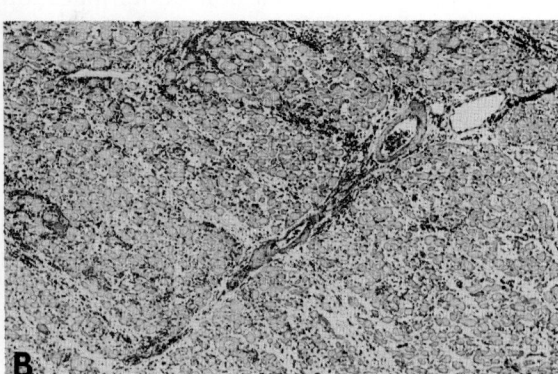

FIG. 15-2 Blister beetle poisoning in a horse. **A.** Acantholysis of the squamous gastric mucosa. **B.** Necrosis, edema, and hemorrhage of the myocardium. (Courtesy of Dr. T. R. Schoeb.)

None of these lesions is pathognomonic, but this combination of findings should suggest blister beetle poisoning, and the beetles should be sought in hay.

References

Ray AC, Post LO, Hurst JM, et al. Evaluation of an analytical method for the diagnosis of cantharidin toxicosis due to ingestion of blister beetles (Epicauta lemniscata) by horses and sheep. Am J Vet Res 1980;41:932–933.

Schoeb TR, Panciera RJ. Blister beetle poisoning in horses. J Am Vet Med Assoc 1978;173:75–77.

Schoeb TR, Panciera RJ. Pathology of blister beetle (Epicauta) poisoning in horses. Vet Pathol 1979;16:18–31.

GROUP C—HEPATOTOXICITY: OFTEN NEPHROTOXICITY

Poisons in Group C are primarily **hepatotoxic,** resulting in fatty change, necrosis, and acute or chronic hepatitis. Many hepatotoxins are also nephrotoxic and clinical signs may reflect damage to both organ systems. Signs of central nervous system derangement, such as depression, hyperirritability, and convulsions, in the absence of morphologic changes in brain, are frequent.

Phosphorus

Because of changes in manufacturing methods and popular customs, traditional poisoning by phosphorus matches has all but disappeared, and that due to the accidental ingestion of fireworks is not far behind. Animals (dogs, pigs) are poisoned most often by eating preparations intended for the consumption of rats, ants, or other pests. Phosphorus poisoning has also occurred in herbivorous animals pastured on former battlefields where certain weapons have been used.

Although a peracute poisoning marked by coma, convulsions, and fatal central nervous depression has been described, the usual case is characterized by ab-

dominal signs, which appear some hours after ingestion. Nausea, vomiting, and abdominal pain then appear, and are succeeded by fever, polydipsia, and polyuria. The appearance of jaundice is followed by delirium, convulsion, and coma, the whole illness lasting usually from two to five days.

At autopsy, mild inflammation of parts of the gastrointestinal tract may be evident, but the principal lesions consist of degenerative changes in the liver and kidneys. Icterus is prominent and is said to be due in many cases to obstructive swelling of the bile duct. However, the outstanding lesion is fatty change, for which phosphorus poisoning is one of the classic causes. In the liver, the majority of the cells are filled with fat droplets, and centrilobular necrosis would supervene if the patient were to live for a while. Fatty change of the kidney and heart is pronounced, and smaller amounts of fat can be demonstrated in other tissues. In the kidney of a dog, at least, most of the fat appears in the epithelium of the ascending loops of Henle in the medullary rays. The distal convoluted tubules contain the second largest amount of fat; other structures of the kidney may have slight amounts. The accumulation of lipids is due to interference with lipoprotein synthesis and excretion. Hydropic degeneration is marked in the proximal convoluted tubules. The spleen is regularly small and atrophic. Hydrothorax and more or less generalized edema occur in some cases, doubtless because of gradual failure of the degenerating heart muscle. One author noted severe hemorrhagic enteritis, cholecystitis, and urinary cystitis in an experimental dog (unpublished data). Ecchymotic hemorrhages sometimes occur in the heart and elsewhere.

Phosphates

Cattle are poisoned rarely by eating commercial fertilizers, which are usually mixtures of phosphates, nitrates, potassium, and ammonium. It appears, however, that these poisonings are chiefly attributable to nitrates or potassium rather than to phosphates. Ammonium nitrate is surprisingly harmless. Chickens and other birds have been poisoned by zinc phosphate, which is used as a treatment for seed-wheat. Characteristic features include dullness, anorexia, thirst, and terminal nervous effects, ending fatally a few hours after ingestion. A garliclike odor of $Zn_3 (PO_4)_2$ was noted in the contents of the crop. (See also organic phosphates, Group Q.)

References

O'Hara PJ, Cordes DO. Superphosphate poisoning of sheep: a study of natural outbreaks. NZ Vet J 1982;30:153–155.

O'Hara PJ, Fraser AJ, James MP. Superphosphate poisoning of sheep: the role of fluoride. NZ Vet J 1982;30:199–201.

Swan JB, McIntosh IG. Toxicity of North African phosphate and superphosphate to milking cows. Proc NZ Soc Anim Prod 1952;12:83–88.

Copper

Copper poisoning in humans and animals appears in two general forms: an acute form following ingestion of toxic quantities of copper salts and a chronic form which results from gradual accumulation of copper in the liver and other tissues. A sudden release of copper in the chronic form, for reasons not understood, causes severe effects resembling those of the acute form.

SIGNS

Signs in the acute form of toxicosis result from sudden onset of severe gastroenteritis with weakness, exhaustion (trembling), arching of the back, icterus, hemoglobinuria, and hemolytic anemia. Liver enzymes, such as alanine transaminase and alkaline phosphatase, are usually elevated in blood. The signs in fatal cases endure for 24–48 hours before death intervenes. The toxic amounts of copper may come from many sources, such as herbage grown on copper-rich or contaminated soil, wet pastures treated with copper sulfate to control snails, misuse of medications containing copper, feeding salt to which copper salts are added, runoff from mines or smelters, or even chicken litter used as fertilizer from flocks fed diets to which copper sulfate or oxide was added.

LESIONS

Lesions found at necropsy following the acute form consist of icterus, friable and yellow colored liver, swollen spleen with dark colored parenchyma, and swollen yellowish or dark-stained kidneys. Microscopic changes in the liver consist of centrilobular necrosis and fatty change with diffuse infiltration of inflammatory cells. Toxic nephrosis is evident in the kidneys plus tubular casts of erythrocytes or hemoglobin.

CHRONIC FORM

In the chronic form of copper poisoning, copper is conjugated to a protein (copperthionein) and accumulated in lysosomes, especially in liver cells, followed by fibrosis and nodular regeneration (cirrhosis). Cop-

per can be identified specifically by use of rhodanine stain on biopsy specimens from the liver. Eventually these events, possibly abetted by other insults to the liver, lead to liver failure, necrosis of liver cells, and release of large amounts of copper into the circulation. This has the effect of precipitating signs and lesions which resemble the acute form of copper toxicity. Most striking is the appearance of a hemolytic crisis, with intravascular hemolysis, hemoglobinuria, icterus, and methemoglobinuria. The combined effects on the liver, kidneys, and hemopoietic system are usually fatal. This syndrome is more frequent in sheep and has been referred to as enzootic icterus or icterohemoglobinuria.

A hereditary defect in the excretion of copper is known in humans and some breeds of dogs. Hereditary copper toxicosis has been described in Bedlington terriers and a possibly less severe form in West Highland white terriers. Inheritance of a recessive autosomal gene which affects the enzyme necessary for the release of copper from a hepatic lysosomes is the underlying cause. A similar syndrome occurs in humans as Wilson disease, hepatolenticular, or hepatocerebral degeneration.

References

Bath GF. Enzootic icterus—a form of chronic copper poisoning. J S Afr Vet Assoc 1979;50:3–14.

Gooneratne SR, Howell JM, Aughey E. An ultrastructural study of the kidney of normal, copper poisoned and thiomolybdate-treated sheep. J Comp Pathol 1986;96:593–612.

Hoogenraad TU, Rothuizen J. Compliance in Wilson's disease and in copper toxicosis of Bedlington Terriers. Lancet 1986;ii:170.

Hultgren BD, Stevens JB, Hardy RM. Inherited, chronic, progressive hepatic degeneration in Bedlington terriers with increased liver copper concentrations: clinical and pathologic observations and comparison with other copper-associated liver diseases. Am J Vet Res 1986;47:365–377.

Johnson GF, Sternlieb I, Twedt DC, et al. Inheritance of copper toxicosis in Bedlington terriers. Am J Vet Res 1980;41:1865–1866.

Johnson GF, Gilbertson SR, Goldfischer S, et al. Cytochemical detection of inherited copper toxicosis of Bedlington terriers. Vet Pathol 1984;21:57–60.

Ludwig J, Owen CA Jr, Barham SS, et al. The liver in the inherited copper disease of Bedlington terriers. Lab Invest 1980;43:82–87.

Thornburg LP, et al. Hereditary copper toxicosis in West Highland white terriers. Vet Pathol 1986;23:148–154.

Thornburg LP, Rottinghaus G, McGowan M, et al. Hepatic copper concentrations in purebred and mixed-breed dogs. Vet Pathol 1990;27:81–88.

Carbon tetrachloride and tetrachloroethylene

Humans become poisoned by carbon tetrachloride through inhalation of its vapor, as in the clothes-cleaning industry. In animals, poisoning is not altogether infrequent as the result of the use of this substance as an anthelmintic. Such poisoning is ordinarily acute. Signs include loss of appetite, gastrointestinal pain, diarrhea (after a few hours), and blood-stained feces. Icterus is often but not always present. Collapse and death ensue in about 24 hours.

Lesions consist of acute catarrhal or hemorrhagic gastritis and enteritis, and acute toxic changes in the liver and kidneys. The hepatic changes are those usually found in acute toxic hepatitis, namely hydropic degeneration, fatty change, and necrosis with cellular infiltrations, when the animal lives long enough develop these signs. Often little evidence, except necrosis, is manifest at death. Necrosis tends to be central, but often becomes massive, involving whole groups of lobules in their entirety. In the kidney, the changes are often less pronounced, but consist principally of fatty change and necrosis of the epithelium of the tubules. Nevertheless, in some cases, death must be attributed to renal failure. Petechiae, said to be due to thrombocytopenia, may be present in various organs and tissues. In chronic cases, which are unusual, acute toxic hepatitis becomes chronic toxic hepatitis: in other words, cirrhosis.

The injurious effects of halomethanes (including carbon tetrachloride and tetrachloroethylene) have been the subject of extensive laboratory studies directed toward the mechanisms of toxicity. New information and new theories abound and are currently being accepted or rejected by the scientific community. These factors cause this subject to be mostly outside the scope of this text. However, some information seems to have a solid foundation, is useful to the understanding of toxic effects of these chemicals, and is therefore presented here. Continued research will likely either modify, confirm, or make these concepts obsolete.

The toxic properties of carbon tetrachloride (CCL_4) do not appear to be innate properties of the stable form of the chemical, but are the result of its conversion to active metabolites in the smooth endoplasmic reticulum of hepatocytes or other cells. This conversion to active forms is controlled by the cytochrome P450-mixed oxidase enzyme system. Inhibition of this system reduces the toxicity of the chemical.

Necrotizing effects of the immediate metabolites on the liver cell are believed to be the result of two actions:

1. Covalent binding of the metabolite, or immediate products, to the protein or lipid targets within the cell; and,
2. Peroxidation of membrane lipids initiated by the same metabolic products.

Tetrachloroethylene is considerably less toxic than carbon tetrachloride; hence, it is more desirable as an anthelmintic, but both have similar actions. A preventive effect in nicotinic acid or tryptophane has been demonstrated. These substances are precursors of the respiratory cofactors, pyridine nucleotides.

Poisonings have been reported in several unique situations. One of the most interesting is the high sensitivity of male mice of certain inbred strains. A minute amount of carbon tetrachloride, released into an animal room, may cause the death of many adult male mice. Male mice of the inbred strains Balb/c, A/He, C_3H, and Swiss are susceptible in that order. Inbred strains C58, DBA/2, SJL, AKR, and RF are apparently quite as resistant as all females and young. This sensitivity in mice is similar to that observed with chloroform.

Exposure of dogs, monkeys, rats, and mice to carbon tetrachloride vapor under varying simulated altitudes, led to the conclusion that higher altitudes (with 100% oxygen) had an additive effect upon the toxicity of carbon tetrachloride on these species.

References

Ahmed EA, Kubic VL, Stevens JL, et al. Carbon tetrachloride: metabolism and toxicity. Fed Proc 1980;35:3150–3155.

Cagen SZ, Klassen CD. Carbon tetrachloride-induced hepatotoxicity: studies in developing rats and protection by zinc. Fed Proc 1980;39:3124–3128.

Martinez-Hernandez A. The hepatic extracellular matrix. II. Electron immunohistochemical studies in rats with CCl4–induced cirrhosis. Lab Invest 1985;53:166–186.

Sáez JC, Bennett MVL, Spray DC. Carbon tetrachloride at hepatotoxic levels blocks reversibly gap junctions between rat hepatocytes. Science 1987;236:967–969.

Phenothiazine

This important anthelmintic drug produces highly variable toxic effects, principally in horses. Two important factors appear to determine whether poisoning will result from a given dose. The first and most crucial is the diet and nutritional state of the affected animal. As is the case with many hepatotoxic drugs, a well-nourished animal on a high-protein diet with ample stores of glycogen in the liver is much less apt to suffer ill effects than an animal in the opposite condition. The second factor is the degree of refinement of the phenothiazine and the presence or absence of diphenylamine, which is a contaminant of the crude drug. Poisoned animals show more or less severe anemia, which reaches its height a few days after the drug is ingested. This is hemolytic anemia, and it is occasionally rapid enough to cause hemoglobinuria. Acute toxic hepatitis and nephrosis of varying degrees of severity also occur. Hepatic injury is of such a nature that photosensitization occasionally arises. Symptoms include depression, dullness, weakness, and coma, in addition to the derangements directly traceable to the pathologic changes. Many animals recover from the signs of depression after some hours, and from the anemia and hepatorenal symptoms after several days.

Phenothiazine is also a cause of primary photosensitizational dermatitis, which is described in Chapter 3.

References

Baird JD, Hutchins DR, Lepherd EE. Phenothiazine poisoning in a thoroughbred horse. Aust Vet J 1970;46:496–499.

Biswal G, Patnaik B. Photosensitized keratitis in calves and kids following administration of phenothiazine. Indian Vet J 1961;38:400–403.

Britton JW. Phenothiazine poisoning in pigs. Cornell Vet 1943;33:368–369.

Hebden SP, Setchell BP. Phenothiazine toxicosis. Aust Vet J 1962;38:399.

McSherry BJ, Roe CK, Milne FJ. The hematology of phenothiazine poisoning in horses. Can Vet J 1966;7:3–12.

Woolf FP, Simms BT. Studies of the toxicology of phenothiazine in horses and mules. North Am Vet 1943;24:595–599.

Phenanthridinium and other trypanocidal drugs

Certain compounds of phenanthridinium—especially 2:7-diamino-9-phenyl-10 methyl phenanthridinium bromide, commonly called dimidium bromide, and ethidium bromide, which is identical except that it has an ethyl group instead of the methyl radical—are currently used parenterally to treat animals with trypanosomal infections. Quinapyramine sulfate and chloride, usually in a mixture bearing the common name of antrycide, have the same therapeutic use. Of these, dimidium bromide is toxic and poisoning may occur when the amount administered is too great or too frequently repeated. The effects of a single or repeated dose are commonly delayed for five to seven weeks, during which the animal, usually a bovine, loses weight severely. The van den Bergh reaction and other tests show impaired hepatic function. The principal lesion is acute toxic hepatitis, beginning with hydropic or vacuolar degeneration of the hepatic cells at the periphery of the lobule. This is followed by fatty change, which spreads toward the center of the lobule. Photosensitization follows in some individuals, especially when the dose is later repeated. In the case of antrycide, toxic tubular nephritis is more severe than the hepatitis and is accompanied by anemia. Many animals recover from the toxicity of either drug.

References

Burdin ML, Plowright W. Toxic effects of four trypanocidal substances for East African type of zebu cattle. Vet Rec 1952;64:635–639.

Ford EJH, Boyd JW. Cellular damage and changes in biliary excretion in a liver lesion of cattle. J Pathol Bacteriol 1962;83:39–48.

Gretillat EH. Observations sur les accidents toxiques survenus a la suite du traitement de la trypanosomiase bovine par le bromure de la trypanosomiase bovine par le bromure de dimidium dans quelques troupeaux du Kwango. Bull Agric Congo Belge 1953;44:787–812.

Plowright W, Burdin ML, Thorold PW. Delayed toxicity due to dimidium bromide. J Comp Pathol Ther 1952;62:136–140, 178–195.

"Clay-pigeon" poisoning—coal-tar pitch

Trap shooters may rent farmland for shooting contests and then the land may be used by farmers. The "clay pigeons" that are used as targets to be shattered in the air by the marksman are constructed of an amalgam held together by a kind of pitch derived from coal tar, a heterogeneous and variable mixture in which a number of poisonous chemical compounds have been identified. The fragments remain in the soil and are tasty to pigs, which may be pastured on the contaminated ground. At least a few days are required for illness to develop, depending on the amount of the material consumed. Usually only a few hours of nonspecific symptoms occur.

The principal postmortem lesion consists of severe centrilobular necrosis of the liver with blood replacing the lost cells and filling the center of the lobule. The supporting reticular tissue of the lobule appears to remain intact. Because involvement of the liver tends to be patchy, the organ is grossly spotted with reddish and yellowish areas. Limited fibrinous or adhesive perihepatitis may develop. Other lesions include well-marked anemia, with erythrocyte counts and hemoglobin often approximating half the normal, jaundice, edema of lymph nodes, and ascites. Blood glucose is also reduced prior to death, and thymol turbidity, serum chloride, and phosphorus are increased. White cell counts, sedimentation rate, serum protein, calcium, and creatinine are not changed.

References

Davis JW, Libke KG. Hematologic studies in pigs fed clay pigeon targets. J Am Vet Med Assoc 1968;152:382–384.

Graham R, Hester HR, Henderson JA. Coal-tar pitch poisoning in pigs. J Am Vet Med Assoc 1940;96:135–140.

Giffee JW. Clay pigeon poisoning in swine. Vet Med 1945;40:97.

Rummler HJ. Pigsty flooring materials containing tar and bitumen. Mh Vet Med 1962;17:482–487.

Hydrogen sulfide

Animals have been poisoned by the inhalation of H_2S in the atmosphere of stables so constructed that the gases from manure pits could enter them. (In some cold countries, the excreta are collected and stored in underground pits, where decomposition processes reduce it to a semi-liquid mass, useful as fertilizer.) A concentration of as much as 0.03% H_2S in the air is dangerous. Although harmless in medicinal amounts, the accidental feeding of a large quantity of sulfur has resulted in a similar type of poisoning, H_2S being formed as a decomposition product.

Signs, which may last for a few hours, include dyspnea, cyanosis, mucous exudate from the upper respiratory passages, depression, and apathy, or in some species, convulsions. Lesions include severe pulmonary edema, hyperemia, and catarrhal inflammation of the air passages, acute toxic hepatitis and nephrosis, and subendocardial and other hemorrhages. Tissues of the gastrointestinal tract and brain are edematous but not congested. Blood is dark brown due to formation of sulfhemoglobin.

Experimental exposure of Fischer-344 rats to hydrogen sulfide gas at a concentration of 560 mg of H_2S per cubic meter for four hours results in necrosis and exfoliation of respiratory and olfactory, but not squamous, epithelial cells in the nasal mucosa. Injured olfactory cells continue to exfoliate for up to 44 hours, but respiratory mucosal cells are quickly replaced. A single four-hour exposure of Fischer-344 rats to an atmosphere containing 615 mg per cubic meter results in pulmonary edema and fibrinocellular alveolitis in proximal regions of the lung. Ultrastructural evidence indicates necrosis of only bronchiolar epithelial cells which are rapidly replaced.

References

Dahme E, Bilzer T, Dirksen G. Neuropathology of manure gas (hydrogen dulfide) poisoning in cattle. Dtsch Tierarztl Wochenschr 1983;90:316–320.

Lorenz A, Prior M, Lillie LE, et al. Histologic and ultrastructural alterations in lungs of rats exposed to sublethal concentrations of hydrogen sulfide. Vet Pathol 1988;25:376–384.

Lopez A, Prior M, Yong S, et al. Nasal lesions in rats exposed to hydrogen sulfide for four hours. Am J Vet Res 1988;49:1107–1111.

Gossypol

A byproduct of the cotton industry, cottonseed meal is a valuable protein concentrate for cattle and other farm animals. A small amount of a poisonous substance, gossypol, remains in the meal which is made from the seeds after cottonseed oil has been extracted from them. The processor endeavors to keep the gossypol at a level approximating 0.02–0.04%, but because of variations in temperature with the hydraulic-press process and to undesirable solvents in other processes, this amount may be greatly exceeded.

Swine are much more susceptible to poisoning than other species, and it is usually recommended that cottonseed meal not exceed 9% of the total ration of these animals. Signs commonly develop after pigs have been fed one to three months on rations containing excessive amounts of gossypol. They consist principally of dyspnea, panting, weakness, and anorexia, and last commonly for several, rarely for many, days before death occurs.

Lesions account readily for the signs. Most conspicuous are hydrothorax, hydropericardium, hydroperitoneum, and edema of the lungs, many or all lymph nodes, and often the subcutaneous tissues. Edema of the wall and attachments of the gallbladder is conspicuous in half the cases. Passive congestion is prominent in the lungs, liver, and kidneys. All this is readily explained as cardiac edema and congestive heart failure when the heart is examined. Dilatation of the ventricles is readily demonstrable in nearly all cases, with well-marked hypertrophy in the more prolonged ones. "White muscles," a definite paleness of various skeletal muscles, exist in two-thirds of affected individuals. Icterus is noticeable in a minority of cases. The liver is most often redder than normally, because of the congestion, but some, containing less blood, show the paleness indicative of necrosis and other changes (Fig. 15-3). In either case, the lobular architecture is more distinct even than that which is normal for the pig, so that the experienced prosector has little doubt grossly of the existence of some form of toxic hepatitis.

Microscopic changes are in accord with what is seen grossly, those in the liver and heart requiring special mention. The fundamental hepatic lesion is centrilobular necrosis. The space left by the lost parenchymal cells is filled with blood, the scanty reticulum of Kupffer's cells remaining, at least for a time. In 80% of the livers, necrosis in practically all lobules is so extensive that hepatic cells remain in only a narrow peripheral zone, perhaps only three or four cells wide; the rest of the lobule is filled with blood. This condition is obviously responsible for the red color of these livers grossly. In a minority of livers, a limited zone of cells in a state of fatty degeneration exists between the peripheral living zone and the blood-filled central area. It is unknown whether the centrilobular necrosis should be attributed to direct toxic injury by the gossypol or to anoxia resulting from cardiac insufficiency. Both conditions are

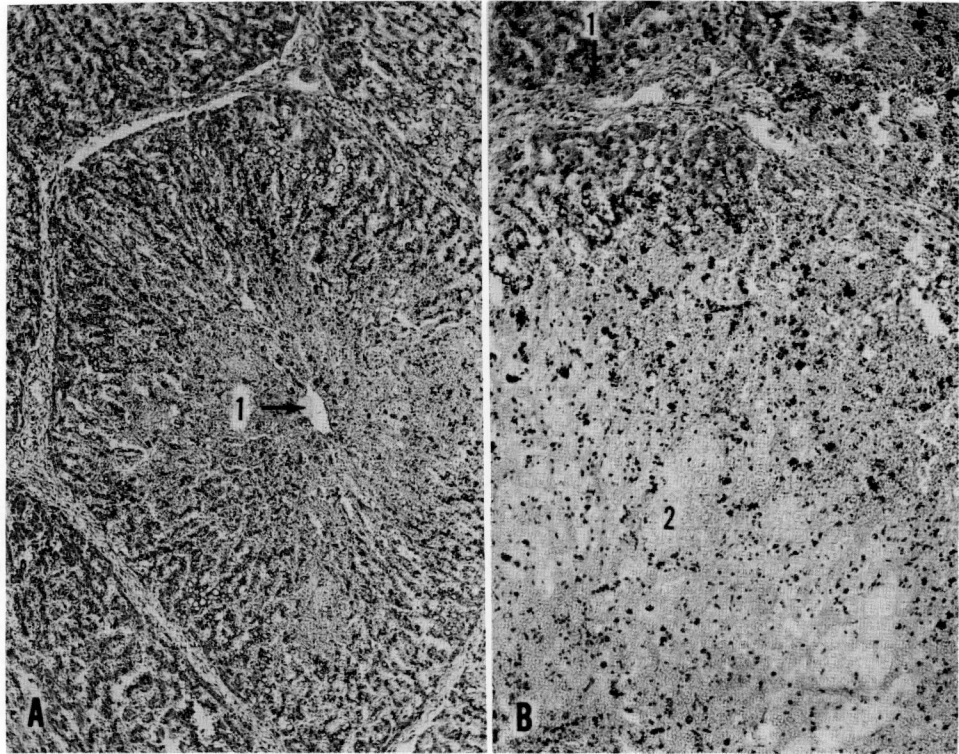

FIG. 15-3 Liver of a pig poisoned by gossypol. **A.** Necrosis of hepatic cells around central vein (1) (×60). **B.** Same liver (×100). Portal area (1) is relatively unaffected, but necrosis and hemorrhage are extensive in the center of the lobule (2).

present, but the extent of necrosis is greater than that which usually results from cardiac disease alone. Microscopic examination of the heart reveals: necrosis or degeneration of numerous myocardial fibers; some fibers are without the normal number of nuclei; some have large and poorly outlined vacuoles in the cytoplasmic areas; and some are greatly atrophied. Except in the hearts of pigs that die early, fibers showing compensatory hypertrophy mingle with those that have degenerated. Hypertrophy is evidenced by a limited increase in the size of the fiber, but more especially by a marked increase in both the size and the number of nuclei in the hypertrophic fiber.

Diagnosis can be made with considerable assurance on the basis of the combination of cardiac changes, marked edema, and hepatic changes. When available, the clinical history is important; however, it is usually inconclusive as to the amount of gossypol consumed. Poisoning by coal-tar pitch occurs in swine and produces comparable hepatic changes, but no cardiac injury. In hepatosis diaetetica, hepatic necrosis is not uniform.

References

Eisele GR. A perspective on gossypol ingestion in swine. Vet Hum Toxicol 1986;28:118–122.

Holmberg CA, Weaver LD, Guterbock WM, et al. Pathological and toxicological studies of calves fed a high concentration cotton seed meal diet. Vet Pathol 1988;25:147–153.

Montamat EE, et al. Inhibitory action of gossypol on enzymes and growth of Trypanosoma cruzi. Science 1982;281:288–289.

Morgan S, Stair EL, Martin T, et al. Clinical, clinicopathologic, pathologic, and toxicologic alterations associated with gossypol toxicosis in feeder lambs. Am J Vet Res 1988;49:493–499.

Patton CS, Legendre AM, Gompf RE, et al. Heart failure caused by gossypol poisoning in two dogs. J Am Vet Med Assoc 1985;187:625–627.

Shandilya LN, Clarkson TB. Hypolipidemic effects of gossypol in cynomolgus monkeys (Macaca fascicularis). Lipids 1982;17:285–290.

Smith HA. Pathology of gossypol. Am J Pathol 1957;33:353–365.

Stephens DT, Critchlow LM, Hoskins DD. Mechanisms of inhibition by gossypol of glycolysis and motility of monkey spermatozoa in vitro. J Reprod Fertil 1983;69:447–452.

Cocklebur

Cockleburs *(Xanthium strumarium)* are most poisonous, as well as more palatable, at or shortly after the two-leaf seedling stage. Pigs are more often poisoned than other species, but cattle and sheep have also suffered. Signs appear several hours after ingestion of the plants and are those of gastrointestinal pain and irritation and of cardiac and muscular weakness. Opisthotonos and convulsions also occur. The failing heart, with weak and rapid pulse, is responsible for death after an illness of a few hours.

Lesions include subepicardial and other subserous hemorrhages, and a moderate degree of gastritis and enteritis, but toxic injury to the liver, kidneys, and heart is more important. The liver undergoes the usual changes of acute toxic hepatitis, with fatty change predominant in some individuals, necrosis in others. Necrosis is preceded by acute cellular swelling and narrowing of the hepatic cords; it is centrilobular at first, but may extend throughout all but the most peripheral parts of the lobule. Fatty change, of patchy distribution and demonstrable only by fat stains, is present in various parts of the myocardium. In the kidney, fat is prominent in the ascending loops of Henle, and incipient necrosis of the proximal convoluted tubules is usually present. The lower tubules often contain albuminous casts. Changes in the central nervous system appear not to have been investigated.

The toxic principle has been demonstrated to be carboxyatractyloside, a compound extracted by aqueous solution of *Xanthium strumaruium,* and produces typical effects in the pure chemical form when administered to swine.

Xanthium pungens, the Noogoora bur, causes a similar form of poisoning in Australia.

References

Forrest GP. Cocklebur poisoning. J Am Vet Med Assoc 1938;93:42–43.

Kenny GC, Everist SL, Sutherland AK. Noogoora bur poisoning of cattle. Queensland Agric J 1950;70:172–177.

Martin T, Stair EL, Dawson L. Cocklebur poisoning in cattle. J Am Vet Med Assoc 1986;189:562–563.

Stuart BP, Cole RJ, Gosser HS. Cocklebur (Xanthium strumarium L. var. strumarium) intoxication in swine: review and redefinition of the toxic principle. Vet Pathol 1981;18:368–383.

Pyrrolizidine alkaloids

The toxicity of several, unrelated plants results from their content of pyrrolizidine alkaloids, which are esters of the amino-alcohols derived from the heterocyclic pyrrolizidine nucleus.

More than 250 pyrrolizidine alkoloids are known, about half are toxic to animals, and several have been demonstrated to be carcinogenic to rats. These pyrrolizidine alkaloids include monocrotaline, retronecine, dehydroretronecine, heliotrine, lasiocarpine, symphytine, monocrotaline pyrrole, retrorsine, isatidine, petasitenine, senkirkine, hydroxysenkirkine, and clivorine. Others also have specific effects on animal cells or tissues, thus are of intense interest in biology.

Pyrrolizidine alkaloids are produced by a large number of plants with worldwide distribution and are classified in seven families containing many genera. These plant families, with representative poisonous genera, include the following: Apocynaceae (Parsonsia); Boraginaceae (Heliotropium, Amsinckia); Celastraceae (Bhesa); Compositae (Conoclinium, Eupatorium, Senecio); Leguminosae (Crotalaria); Rannunculaceae (Caltha); and Scrophulariacae (Castilleja). Poisoning of animals associated with some of these plant species (Senecio, Crotalaria, Heliotropium, and Amsinckia) are described in more detail in following paragraphs.

Although variance occurs in the alkaloids between the plants and in the conditions of poisoning of humans and domestic animals, the lesions produced by these alkaloids are remarkably similar. They are all hepatotoxic, causing varying degrees of hepatocellular necrosis, megalocytosis, fibrosis, and bile ductule proliferation. Many of the alkaloids also cause occlusive lesions of veins, especially in the liver, leading to a syndrome referred to as Budd-Chiari syndrome in humans, and in the lung leading to cor pulmonale or right heart failure. Megalocytosis of renal tubular epithelium and glomerulosclerosis resulting from endothelial damage are also frequent findings.

Reference

Peterson JE, Culvenor CCJ. Hepatotoxic pyrrolizidine alkaloids. In: Keeler RF, Tu AT, eds. Handbook of natural toxins. Vol 1. Plant and fungal toxins. New York: Marcel Dekker, 1983;637–671.

Senecios

Plants of the genus Senecio are woody herbs with terminal clusters of yellow flowers, bushy, and commonly reaching a height of 20–50 cm. Like most poisonous plants, they are eaten only when more palatable pasturage is not available. Certain species are popularly known in many localities as ragworts or groundsels. In Europe, South Africa, New Zealand, or the plains region of the United States and Canada, at least the following species are known to be poisonous: *S. aquaticus, burchelli, ilicifolius, integerrimus, jacobaea, longilobus, plattensis, riddellii,* and *scleratus.* Chemically, it has been shown that pyrrolizidine alkaloids, retrorsine, and seneciophylline are responsible for toxicity.

Poisoning involves horses and cattle chiefly, sheep being much less susceptible. In earlier times what is now known to be poisoning by senecios was described as several different diseases before the true nature was recognized. Of these, the principal ones included Molteno disease of cattle in Cape Colony (Africa), Winton disease of horses and cattle in New Zealand, Pictou disease of cattle in Canada, and Van Es walking disease of horses in Nebraska. Zd'ar disease of horses in Bohemia and probably Schweinsberger disease in Bavaria have also been added to this list.

Signs appear after the animal has consumed varying amounts of the plant for a number of days or as long as three weeks. A disturbance of consciousness causes the animal to walk aimlessly but stubbornly, and to press the head continually against an object with which it collides. In the later stages of the illness, which usually lasts a few days, mania may ensue. Semidomesticated cattle of the western ranges, especially, may become dangerously belligerent, with a behavior suggestive of rabies but without the terminal paralysis that characterizes the latter disease. In addition, jaundice and severe intestinal irritation occur, which result in frequent watery defecations with marked tenesmus and even eversion of the rectum.

Senecios can be classified with the strong hepatotoxic poisons. Postmortem lesions (Fig. 15-4) are those of chronic toxic hepatitis, with actively acute inflammation usually still in progress, as well as jaundice and abdominal edema. Hepatic changes vary from megalocytosis and necrosis of the hepatic cells to full-fledged portal cirrhosis, depending on the duration of the disease, its severity, and rapidity of progress. Fibrous tissue tends to spread into the lobule in an irregular fashion, differing in this respect from the typical portal, or atrophic, cirrhosis. Proliferation of new bile ducts is prominent in many areas, perhaps somewhat more so than in the usual examples of portal cirrhosis. With necrosis of hepatic parenchymatous cells, conspicuous attempts at regeneration frequently occur. Such areas are recognized by the unusually large size of the cells and their nuclei and the relative frequency of cells with more than one nucleus. As a result of the architectural derangement, bile canaliculi are occluded in various areas. Such areas show considerable deposits of bile pigment microscopically; grossly, greenish-brown discoloration of icteric liver tissue is evident. Because considerable congestion also manifests in the less fibrotic areas, the typical liver has totally irregular mottling grossly, and is unduly hard in proportion to the amount of cirrhosis. The hepatic lymph nodes may be enlarged due to reticuloendothelial proliferation. The lumens of hepatic veins, especially the central veins, become constricted as a result of reticulum and collagenous tissue proliferation, edema, and endothelial hypertrophy. It is believed that endothelial cells become metaplastic and contribute to the reticulum and collagen fiber deposition. Passive congestion results from cirrhosis and veno-occlusive disease.

Generalized toxic jaundice is usually of conspicuous severity and is stated to be invariably present. Abdominal edema is widely diffused in the subserosa of the intestines and often of the stomach. The mesenteries are often markedly thickened with fluid. The gallbladder not only has a highly edematous wall, but also is distended with unused bile, sometimes to enormous proportions. The bile is stated to be of normal quality; hence, the condition is presumed to represent a combination of edema based upon intrahepatic obstruction and the usual accumulation of bile that occurs in the absence of cholecystikinetic stimuli from the intestine. Considerable edema commonly occurs in the mucosa and submucosa of the stomach and intestine. Because this is not proportional to the subserosal edema, and because a certain degree of catarrhal enteritis is demonstrable on the basis of hyperemia and other changes, the submucous fluid should doubtless be considered inflammatory. Although the toxic action of senecio plants mainly affects the liver, a noticeable degree of toxic tubular nephrosis with megalocytosis occurs, as seen in the liver. Petechiae and ecchymoses are prominent on the heart, mesentery, and omentum, and are attributable to toxic injury of capillaries.

Pulmonary lesions have been produced in experimental poisoning in rats. They are not well described in natural poisonings, but probably are a consistent finding. They are discussed in more detail under crotalaria poisoning.

No extensive studies of brain appear to address whether the manic symptoms are based upon cerebral lesions or merely upon the tendency for nervous hyperirritability, which frequently accompanies hepatic diseases. The violent behavior has been reported chiefly

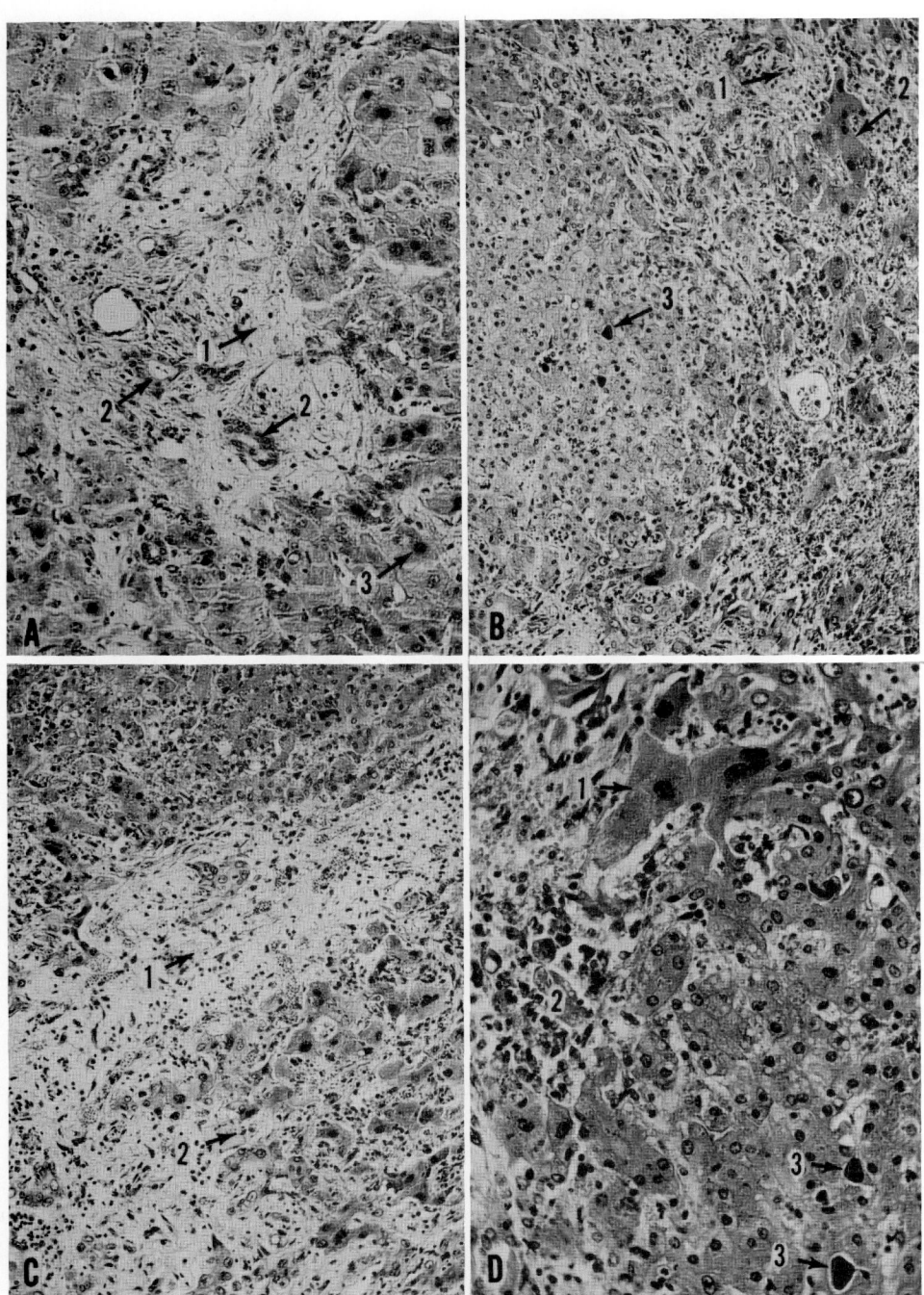

FIG. 15-4 A. Bovine liver (×150) in Senecio poisoning. Periportal fibrosis (1), hyperplasia of bile ducts (2), and hyperchromatism in hepatic nuclei (3). (Photograph courtesy of Dr. C. L. Davis.) **B.** Equine liver in crotalaria poisoning (×100). Periportal fibrosis (1), regenerating liver cells (2), and distended bile canaliculi (3). **C.** Another field, equine liver in B (×100). Note portal fibrosis (1), which extends into the lobule (2). **D.** Equine liver (same as B and C; × 210). Regenerating liver cells (1), leukocytes in portal region area (2), and distended bile canaliculi (3). (Courtesy of Dr. H. R. Seibold.)

by Mathews and to those familiar with the untamed range cattle with which he worked; their belligerency is understandable merely as an expression of the bodily discomfort which they undoubtedly felt. Even these cattle, Mathews reported, commonly showed no bellicose symptoms when, during the course of experimental studies, they were fed the plants while confined in a small pen.

Hepatic tumors were reported in experimentally poisoned rats.

Diagnosis must be based upon a combination of presence of the plant, symptoms, and lesions. No specific tests exist; few other equally hepatotoxic substances are likely to be encountered under circumstances where senecio plants would be ingested.

References

Burns J. The heart and pulmonary arteries in rats fed on Senecio jacobaea. J Pathol 1972;106:187–194.

Chase WH. The Molteno cattle disease. Agric J Cape Good Hope 1904;25:675–678.

Goeger DE, Cheeke PR, Ramsdell HS, et al. Comparison of the toxicities of Senecio jacobaea, Senecio vulgaris and Senecio glabellus in rats. Toxicol Lett 1983;15:19–23.

Johnson AE, Smart RA. Effects on cattle and their calves of tansy rag-wort (Senecio jacobaea) fed in early gestation. Am J Vet Res 1983;44:1215–1219.

Kinghorn AD. Carcinogenic and cocarcinogenic toxins from plants. In: Keeler RF, Tu AT, eds. Handbook of natural toxins. Vol 1. Plant and fungal toxins. New York: Marcel Dekker, 1983;239–298.

Kirkland PD, Moore RE, Walker KH, et al. Deaths in cattle associated with Senecio lautus consumption. Aust Vet J 1984;59:64.

Mathews FP. Poisoning of cattle by species of groundsel. Exp Sta Bull, 481. College Station: Texas A. & M. College, 1933.

Mendel VE, et al. Pyrrolizidine alkaloid-induced liver disease in horses: an early diagnosis. Am J Vet Res 1988;49:572–578.

Miranda CL, Henderson MC, Buhler DR. Dietary copper enhances the hepatotoxicity of Senecio jacobaea in rats. Toxicol Appl Pharmacol 1981;60:418–423.

Pethick WH. Special report on Pictou cattle disease. Canadian Dept. Agriculture, No. 8, (Cited by Mathews.), 1906.

Van der Watt JJ, Purchase IFH, Tustin RC. Chronic toxicity of ret-rorsine, a pyrrolizidine alkaloid, in vervet monkeys. J Pathol 1972;107:279–287.

Vanek J. Poisoning with Senecio erraticus as the cause of Zd'ár disease of horses. Schweiz Z Allg Pathol 1958;21:821–848. Vet Bull 1959;3724.

Van Es L, Cantwell LR, Martin HM, et al. Nature and cause of the "walking disease" of northwestern Nebraska. Exp Sta Bull No 43. Lincoln: Univ. of Nebraska, 1929.

White RD, Swick RA, Cheeke PR. Effects of dietary copper and molyb-denum on tansy ragwort (Senecio jacobaea) toxicity in sheep. Am J Vet Res 1984;45:159–161.

Crotalaria

The Crotalaria genus includes several leguminous plants that are used as soil-building cover crops or, in some cases, to provide hay or forage of rather questionable value. Some species are weeds in other parts of the world, particularly South Africa and Australia (Table 15-3). *Crotalaria spectabilis* (Figs. 15-5 to 15-7) is probably the most poisonous species. With certain other, less toxic species, it grows extensively in the southeastern United States. Humans and all species of farm animals are susceptible, including chickens and turkeys.

In general, acute and chronic forms of poisoning occur. In the former, the period of illness is at most a few days, although the poison has usually been accumulating as the result of repeated ingestion over weeks or months. Signs include gastrointestinal disturbance accompanied by salivation, weakness, and relatively nonviolent nervous malfunction, such as staggering, incoordination, and ultimately inability to stand. Diarrhea with severe tenesmus and partial eversion of the rectum have been prominent in bovines. In more chronic cases, the illness persists for a few weeks or several months, with signs of anorexia, inactivity, and terminal emaciation. Horses may press against solid objects, the so-called "blind staggers." Icterus is especially noticeable in chronic cases. Emphysema—initially pulmonary and subsequently subcutaneous—is characteristic.

In North America, the outstanding postmortem lesion is hemorrhage, which appears in the form of petechiae or large ecchymoses. These hemorrhages, characterized by as yet unexplained bright red color, involve serous and mucous surfaces.

All organs are congested; many are edematous, especially the abomasum, omasum, and gallbladder. Severely congested liver in acute cases may progress to cirrhosis if the poisoning were prolonged. The lesions resemble those of Senecio poisoning. In the lungs, emphysema alternates with atelectasis and hemorrhages.

TABLE 15-3 **Crotalaria poisoning**

Pyrrolizidine alkaloid	Plant species	Disease	Species affected	Organ systems	Region
Fulvine	fulva	Infantile cirrhosis	Human	Hepatic	India, Jamaica
Fulvine, crispatine, monocrotaline	crispata	Crotalariosis	Bovine	Hepatic	Southern Africa
Monocrotaline	retusa	"Walkabout," "Kimberly horse disease"	Equine	Nervous	Australia
Monocrotaline	spectabilis	Crotalariosis	Bovine, swine. equine	Hepatic, respiratory, renal	United States
Monocrotaline	spectabilis	Experimental	Macaca mulatta	Hepatic	United States
Monocrotaline	spectabilis	Experimental crotalariosis	Guinea pig	Hepatic	United States
Dicrotaline	dura globifera juncea	Crotalariosis equorum, "equine jaagsiekta"	Equine	Respiratory, hepatic	Southern Africa
Unknown	spartioides	Crotalariosis	Bovine	Respiratory, hepatic	Southern Africa
Unknown	burkeana	"Stiff sickness"	Bovine, caprine, equine, ovine	Cutaneous	Southern Africa

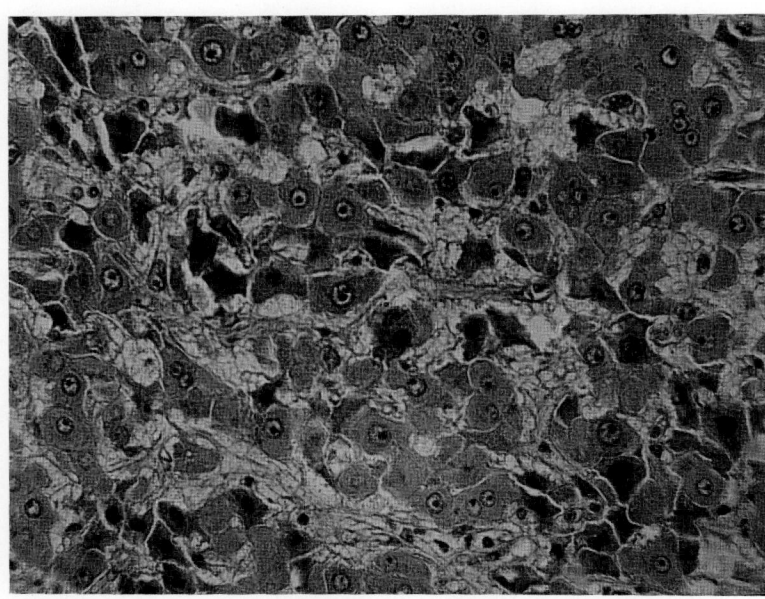

FIG. 15-5 Poisoning due to *Crotalaria spectabilis* seed. Liver of rhesus monkey *(Macaca mulatta).* Individualization of hepatocytes, variation in cell size, staining of nuclei, and distortion of nuclei. (Courtesy of Dr. J. R. Allen and American Journal of Veterinary Research.)

In South Africa, *Crotalaria dura* and *C. globifera,* both known as wild lucerne, cause chronic poisoning having many of the features just outlined, but also affect horses and sheep with repeated febrile episodes of pulmonary disease and eventually fatal termination. Early in the course of the disease, pulmonary emphysema—alveolar and interstitial—is the salient feature. Spreading from the lungs via the hilus, air appears in the mediastinal tissues and ultimately in the subcutaneous tissues of the neck. Terminally, the lungs undergo a chronic proliferative process involving all parts. The proliferated cells are largely epithelioid, probably originating from the alveolar walls. Glandlike proliferations of the bronchial epithelium also occur and resemble "jaagsiekte;" they are sometimes called by that name. Partial to complete occlusion of pulmonary capillaries

and arterioles, apparently on the same basis as in veno-occlusive disease in the liver, may be seen in natural poisoning and has been reproduced in experimental animals. This leads to pulmonary hypertension and cardiac hypertrophy.

In South Africa, *Crotalaria burkeana,* the "rattle bush," also causes bovine "stiff-sickness," in which the animal suffers at first from generalized stiffness and then from laminitis in all four feet. The latter condition is prolonged; the hoofs become greatly elongated and horizontally wrinkled (compared with selenium poisoning, p. 729), and a layer of granulation tissue fills the space between the separated sensitive and insensitive laminae. Experimentally, the laminitis has appeared in as little as six days after consuming the toxic plant. Its pathogenesis is probably related to an inflammatory en-

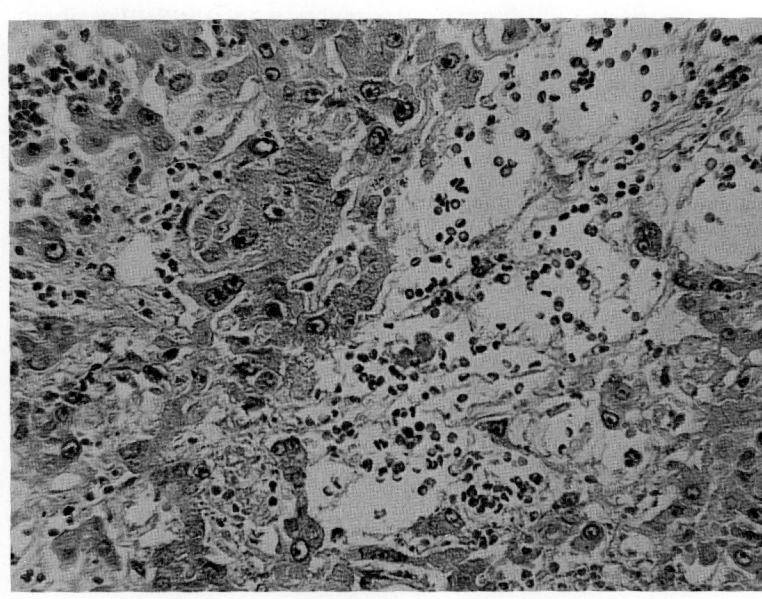

FIG. 15-6 Poisoning due to *Crotalaria spectabilis* seed. Liver of *Macaca mulatta.* Focal necrosis with loss of hepatocytes. (Courtesy of Dr. J. R. Allen and American Journal of Veterinary Research.)

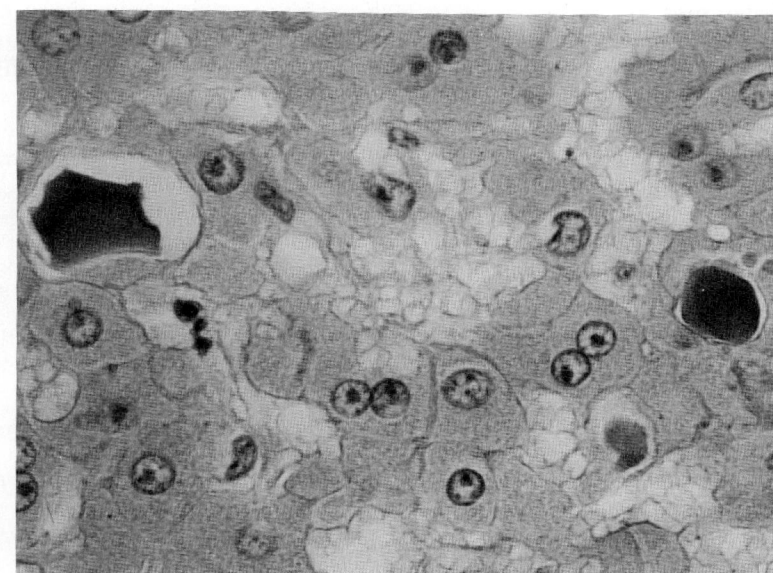

FIG. 15-7 Poisoning due to *Crotalaria spectabilis.* Liver of *Macaca mulatta.* Vacuoles in hepatocytes and bile stasis. (Courtesy of Dr. J. R. Allen and American Journal of Veterinary Research.)

teric disorder, as is believed to be true of laminitis under other circumstances.

In Northern Australia, *Crotalaria retusa* and *C. crispata* have been incriminated as the cause of "walkabout" or "Kimberly horse disease." This disease is characteristic of crotalaria poisoning, although cases due to *C. crispata* usually are more acute.

Swine poisoned by *Crotolaria spectabilis* develop typical hepatic lesions and extensive nephrosis characterized by glomerulosclerosis resulting from endothelial cell damage. Megalocytosis of tubular epithelium, as seen in many species, is also a feature.

In children, infantile cirrhosis, in which occlusion of intrahepatic veins is a significant feature, has been described in Jamaica, and is associated with ingestion of "bush-tea" made from *Crotalaria fulva* or other plants. The similarity of the lesions in fatal cases in children and animals suggested the possibility of Crotalaria poisoning. Pulmonary lesions have not been reported in humans. Simian primates *(Macaca mulatta)* are susceptible to acute poisoning, with lesions essentially similar to those observed in other species. *Crotalaria spectabilis* seeds, finely ground and added to the diet of *M. mulatta* at the level of 0.25–1%, result in ascites, hydrothorax, subcutaneous edema, leukopenia, decrease in serum albumin, acute toxic hepatitis, pulmonary edema, and occasional leukocytic infiltration of the adventitia of pulmonary arteries.

In guinea pigs, a naturally-occurring disease due to contamination of feed with seeds of Crotalaria has been recognized and reproduced experimentally. Seeds of *Crotalaria spectabilis* added to the guinea pig diet at the level of 5% resulted in disease typical of crotalaria poisoning.

Monocrotaline, one of the pyrrolizidine alkaloids produced by plants of the genus Crotalaria, has been shown by experimental studies to induce in rats increased thickness of the media of branches of the pul-

monary artery, right ventricular hypertrophy, and pulmonary hypertension. These effects can be produced by feeding ground *Crotalaria spectabilis* plants or by injecting monocrotaline pyrrole intraperitoneally. The thickening of the wall of the pulmonary artery branches is the result of extension of muscle into media of these arteries. This hypertrophy of the media of arteries and hypertrophy of the right ventricle are similar to the lesions demonstrated in humans with pulmonary hypertension. This combination of lesions has also been observed in several poisonings of animals by plants in the genus Crotalaria.

Among the three alkaloids from Crotalaria, fulvine appears to be most toxic to rabbits; monocrotaline and crispatine, in order, are slightly less toxic. Each of these produces slightly different lesions when fed in pure form to rabbits (Gardiner et al., 1965). Monocrotaline poisoning in rabbits results in enlargement of most hepatic cells, with much variation in size and shape of nuclei. Abnormal mitotic figures are frequent in hepatocytes, and marginated or depleted chromatin is common. Proliferation of small cholangioles and bile ductules with portal fibrosis is also conspicuous. Frank necrosis is infrequent. The lungs are not affected.

Crispatine in rabbits produces lesions essentially similar to those caused by monocrotaline, but subcutaneous injection is often followed by tonic and clonic convulsions, lasting 15–20 minutes. Lesions of centrilobular fibrosis suggesting veno-occlusive disease are seen infrequently.

Fulvine administered subcutaneously to rabbits produces centrilobular necrosis and fibrosis of the liver. Hypertrophy of liver cells and proliferation of bile ducts are much less conspicuous. At lower doses, changes in the lung with thickened fibrotic alveolar walls, proliferation and desquamation of alveolar phagocytes and fibroblasts are conspicuous features.

References

Kellerman TS, Coetzer JAW, Naude TW. Plant poisoning and myco-toxicoses of livestock in Southern Africa. Capetown: Oxford Univ Press, 1988.

Meyrick B, Reid L. Development of pulmonary arterial changes in rats fed Crotalaria spectabilis. Am J Pathol 1979;94:37–50.

Meyrick B, Gamble W, Reid L. Development of Crotalaria pulmonary hypertension: hemodynamic and structural study. Am J Physiol 1980;239(Heart Circ Physiol 8):H692–H702.

Peterson JE, Culvenor CCJ. Hepatotoxic pyrrolizidine alkaloids. In: Keeler RF, Tu AT, eds. Handbook of natural toxins. Vol 1. Plant and fungal toxins. New York: Marcel Dekker, 1983;637–671.

Todrovitch-Hunter L, Johnson DJ, Ranger P, Keeley FW, Rabinovitch M. Altered elastin and collagen synthesis associated with progressive pulmonary hypertension induced by monocrotaline: a biochemical and ultrastructural study. Lab Invest 1988;58:184–195.

Heliotrope

Wild heliotrope *(Heliotropium europaeum)* is eaten by sheep and is poisonous by virtue of a slowly progressive toxic hepatitis, symptoms of illness appearing perhaps months after access to the plant has ceased. Jaundice is the salient feature. The usual fatty and other changes of acute toxic hepatitis progress to cirrhosis and a shrunken, "hob-nailed" liver. The effect of this plant is due to pyrrolizidine alkaloids (lasiocarpine, heliotrine), and is thus similar to that of the senecios and a number of other plants (Table 15-3). It is especially important in Australia. Intestinal atrophy has been induced in sheep, rats, and mice injected with lasiocarpine or heliotrine.

References

Anonymous: Plant toxicology. Proceedings of the Australia-US poisonous plant symposium. Brisbane, Australia, May 14–18, 1984. Plant Toxicol 1985:3–611.

Jones RT, Drummond GR, Chatham RO. Heliotropium europaeum poisoning of pigs. Aust Vet J 1981;57:396.

Klopfer U, et al. First cases in Israel of chronic poisoning in calves caused by ingestion of Heliotropium europaeum. 2. Prognostic evaluation of liver lesions. Refuah Vet 1981;38:88–94.

Tarweed

Tarweed, *Amsinckia intermedia,* is a weed that often seriously contaminates the wheat fields of the Pacific region of the United States and occasionally other areas. The rather small seeds are harvested with the crop and are separated from the wheat at the flour mill, going into the cull portion known as "screenings." The latter are commonly returned to the farm to be used as feed for animals, chiefly swine. After a few or many weeks on a diet containing considerable amounts of the seeds, icterus and other signs of toxic hepatitis appear. As evidence of alimentary irritation and disturbance, small ulcers often appear in the mouth. Mild ataxia and the central nervous disturbances characteristic of many hepatic disorders appear in the later stages. The behavior of horses is comparable to that seen in Van Es walking disease, in other words, senecio poisoning. As in Senecio and Crotalaria, the toxic principles are pyrrolizidine alkaloids. Swine often reach marketable age with no

more conspicuous disturbance than general unthriftiness, and at slaughter are determined to have "hard-liver disease;" the lesions are those of acute or chronic toxic hepatitis or, most often, both.

References

McCulloch EC. Hepatic cirrhosis of horses, swine and cattle due to ingestion of seeds of the tarweed, Amsinckia intermedia. J Am Vet Med Assoc 1940;96:5–17.

McCulloch EC. Use of grain containing tarweed seed as poultry feed. J Am Vet Med Assoc 1942;101:481–483.

Woolsey JH, Jasper DE, Cordy DR, et al. Two outbreaks of hepatic cirrhosis in swine in California, with evidence incriminating tarweed. Vet Med 1952;47:55–58.

Lantana

Lantana camara includes a complex array of many closely related, but poorly classified, taxa. All of them are shrubs with coarse, woody stems that are roughly square in cross section, have a pithy center and small prickles along the angles. Several of these plants have been reported to be poisonous to cattle in the southern United States, Australia, Mexico, and Africa. Certain other related species have little toxicity; all of them are unpalatable.

The known biologically active compounds found in *Lantana camara* include pentacyclic triterpene acids; the first two are lantadene A and lantadene B.

The toxicity is principally manifest by hepatotoxic photosensitivity, icterus, and varying degrees of gastrointestinal irritation. The lips and muzzle are particularly affected by photosensitivity dermatitis. The mildest form of poisoning to be noticed is the "pink nose" of Australian cattle. In this condition, the hairless parts of the muzzle are merely inflamed and red. In many of the more severe cases, the visible lesions are almost exclusively those of photosensitization. The skin of the muzzle and surrounding regions becomes inflamed, thickened, and cracked, and tends to peel, leaving severely inflamed, ulcerated areas. The same condition affects the mouth, producing ulcerative stomatitis, with drooling of saliva and, of course, refusal to eat. Mild dermatitis is manifest with itching over various other areas of the integument. Such cases recover after several weeks.

The most severe forms are acute, often being fatal after three or four days of illness. Clinically, symptoms of gastrointestinal disturbances arise, with bloody feces, icterus, and marked weakness. At necropsy, the principal lesions include acute hemorrhagic gastroenteritis with blood clots and pseudomembranes in the gut. Icterus is marked. Subcutaneous edema and subepicardial hemorrhages also occur. The usual changes of acute toxic hepatitis, varying from barely discernible to extensive necrosis, are seen in the liver. Photosensitization is present in those animals that live a few days. No doubt some injury to hepatic cells always occurs and accounts for photosensitization.

The lesions in sheep and cattle may be produced by the ingestion of predetermined amounts of powdered leaves of *Lantana camara*. Icterus, photosensitization, swollen, ochre-colored livers, distended gallbladders, dry feces in the colon anterior to the ansa spiralis, and excessive mucus in the remainder of the large intestine, ascites, and pulmonary edema were the principal findings at necropsy. Microscopic lesions in the liver in the less severely affected sheep were limited to vacuolization of hepatic cells in the portal region of the lobules, with proliferation of bile ductules. Hepatocytes in the center of the lobules were apparently unaffected. In severely affected sheep, necrosis involved most of the liver cells, with disorganization of lobular architecture, proliferation of bile ductules, and regeneration of liver cells. In the kidney, necrosis of proximal convoluted tubules was the essential feature, which resulted in proteinuria, bilirubinuria, and in some cases, uremia. Some necrosis of isolated cardiac muscle fibers suggested a possible direct effect of Lantana on the heart muscle.

Ultrastructural changes in hepatocytes from sheep poisoned with *Lantana camara* have also been described to start with distention of the bile canaliculi and proliferation of the villi into the canaliculi (Figure 15-8). A space containing new microvilli forms between plasma membranes of adjacent hepatocytes at points where the plasma membranes are normally contiguous and parallel. Only at the terminal bars do the plasma membranes remain in contact. Characteristic blebs often form as modification of the wall of the canaliculus. These changes are believed by Seawright to be characteristics of lantana poisoning. In severely damaged hepatocytes, the endoplasmic reticulum is often fragmented and dispersed. The nuclear membrane many disintegrate or lose its definition. The mitochondria remain intact. In some severely affected cells, rounded masses formed from the plasma membranes may be seen in the newly formed intercellular spaces. Deposits of bile may surround the distended endoplasmic reticulum. Invagination of nuclear membrane containing cytoplasmic organelles was sometimes seen. Large pinocytic vesicles, deposits of bile, and distended or fragmented endoplasmic reticulum occupied the cytoplasm of severely affected hepatocytes.

Seawright proposed that hepatocytes at the periphery of the lobules are so damaged by lantana poisoning to permit the bile to regurgitate from the canaliculi to the sinusoids. This would account for the biliary retention and accumulation of bile in the peripheral blood without microscopic evidence of bile stasis in the hepatocytes or bile ducts.

Reference

Seawright AA, Everist SL, Hrdlicka J. Comparative features of lantana, myoporum and pimelea toxicities in livestock. In: Keeler RF, Tu AT, eds. Handbook of natural toxins. Vol 1. Plant and fungal toxins. New York: Marcel Dekker, 1983;511–541.

Sacahuiste

Sacahuiste, sacahuista, or beargrass *(Nolina texana)* is a perennial plant that grows in the moderately arid parts of the southwestern United States, principally in central and western Texas. Because of its extremely long, bladelike leaves (60–160 cm long, 2–5 mm wide), which rise to a height of 50–75 cm, then bend and droop on all sides, the plant resembles a large tuft of grass. In early spring, it sends up flowering stems, which bear panicles of fine flowers of inconspicuous grayish color. Only the flowering panicles and buds are poisonous, according to the experimental work of Mathews (1940). Sheep and goats more frequently eat poisonous amounts than do cattle.

This is a photosensitizing plant; if the animal were to eat adequate amounts of chlorophyll-containing material and concurrently were exposed to sunlight, the usual edema and necrosis of the unpigmented skin would result. These changes are most prominent in the face and ears. The ears of sheep may swell to a thickness of 2–3 cm, drooping because of the added weight. Dermatitis is frequently characterized by severe pruritus. Necrosis of areas of skin may supervene, depending on the severity of this phase of the disease. Other outstanding signs of poisoning by sacahuiste include icterus, which appears within one to two days after the first loss of appetite, a discharge of tenacious, yellow exudate from the nostrils, and copious conjunctival exudate, which is serous at first and later purulent. The urine is dark yellow or sometimes reddish. The latter discoloration appears to be due to hemoglobin; at least no hematuria occurs. A band of purplish discoloration encircling the hoof just below the coronary band is believed by Mathews to represent an aspect of photosensitization. Poisoned animals usually live a week or more after the appearance of symptoms, meanwhile seeking water and shade; a few recover.

The lesions are those of acute toxic hepatitis, so that grossly the liver has a greenish paleness and greasy feeling. Upon incision, greenish casts of inspissated bile can be expressed from the severed ducts. Microscopically, the hepatic changes are disorganization of the hepatic cords, fatty change, chiefly centrilobular, biliary casts containing cholesterol clefts, and a minimal amount of necrosis. The other principal changes include: toxic tubular nephrosis; large, pale kidney grossly; hydropic degeneration; and fatty change most prominent microscopically. As in the liver, actual necrosis is minimal. Albuminous casts are numerous and may extend into Bowman's capsules. Bile pigment tends to produce a greenish-brown discoloration macroscopically, which is carried over into the microscopic sections to temper the usual staining reactions of the cells.

In diagnosis, the absence of marked changes in the gallbladder and the frequent presence of photosensitization help to differentiate this poisoning from that caused by senecios and possibly from those due to some other plants having the same geographical habitat. It is doubtful that any of the chemical poisons produce precisely this combination of changes.

Reference

Mathews FP. Poisoning in sheep and goats by sacahuiste (Nolina texana) buds and blooms. Exp Sta Bull 585. College Station: Texas A. & M. College, 1940.

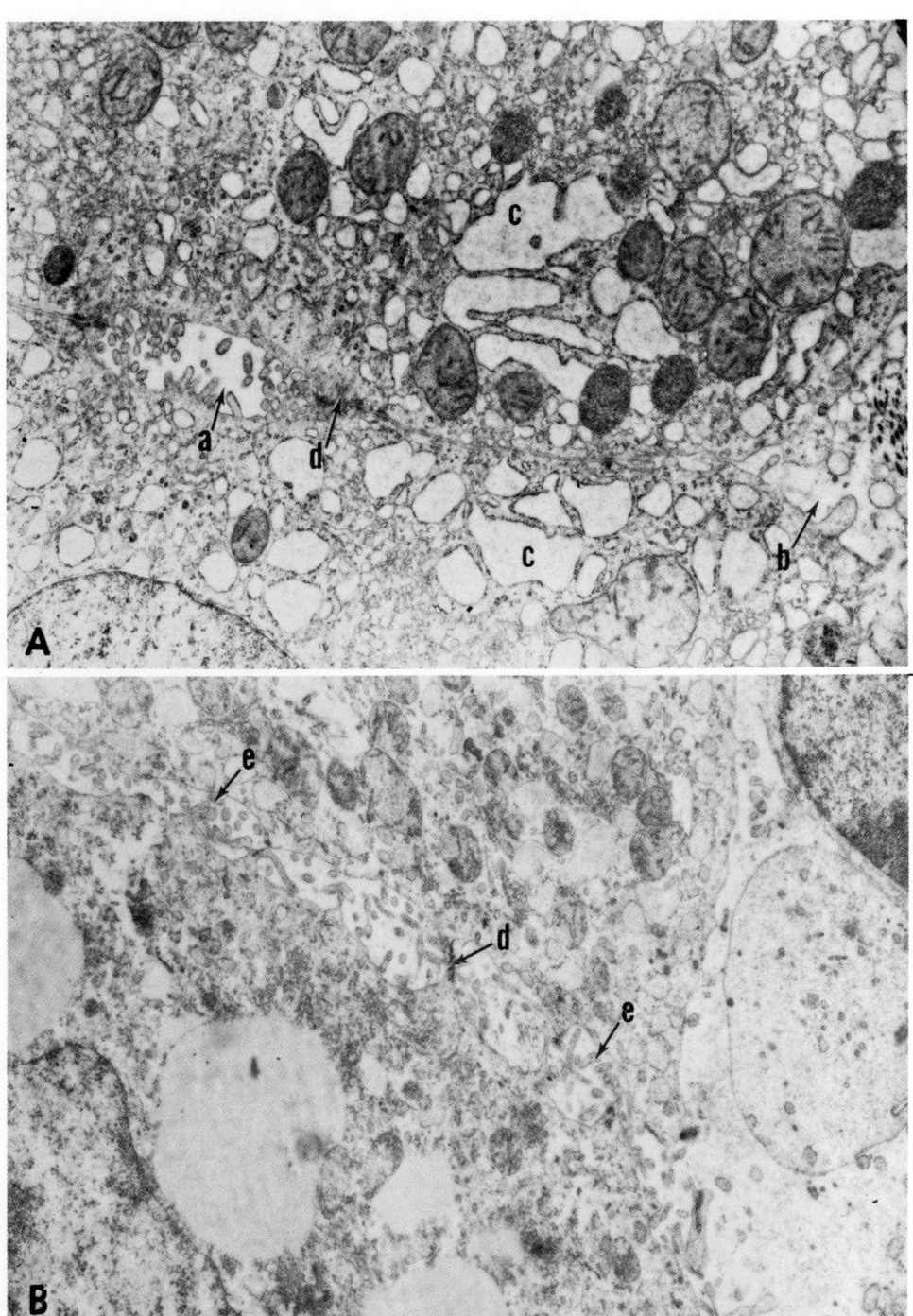

FIG. 15-8 Lantana poisoning, sheep. **A.** Electron micrograph of liver cells of normal, fasted sheep. Note the intercellular membrane between hepatocytes, extending from the bile canaliculus (a) to the space of Disse (b). The endoplasmic reticulum (c) is distended and the terminal bar (d) is intact. **B.** Electron micrograph of liver cells of sheep poisoned by Lantana. Note intercellular space (e) formed by microvilliform changes in the plasma membranes of contiguous hepatocytes. The terminal bar (d) indicates the location of the modified plasma membranes. (Courtesy of Dr. A. A. Seawright and Pathologia Veterinaria.)

Drymaria pachyphylla

This plant, found on the arid ranges of the southwestern United States, has been shown by Mathews (1933) to be highly poisonous to sheep and somewhat less so to cattle and goats. A member of the "chickenweed" group, the plant grows flat on the ground, reaching a width of as much as 40 cm. Its rather sparse, trailing branches bear ovate leaves about 1 cm in length, which are thick and juicy. (Pachyphylla means thick-leaved.) Its fruits and seeds are tiny and are borne where the short leaf-stalks extend from the branches.

Signs appear in a little less than 24 hours after ingestion of the plant (experimentally) and may be followed by death in two hours or possibly by recovery in about two days. They consist of diarrhea and evidence of mild abdominal pain. Lethargy, coma, and death tend to follow rapidly, depending on the severity of the poisoning. Pulse and respiration remain practically normal.

Lesions include hemorrhagic inflammation, at least of the ileum, and at times of higher portions of the intestine. This is accompanied by severe serous and often hemorrhagic cholecystitis, with edematous pericholecystitis and pericholangitis. Ecchymotic hemorrhages are described as numerous in the diaphragm, epicardium, and outer myocardium. The liver and spleen are congested. The liver also undergoes centrilobular necrosis, usually coagulative, with acidophilic staining of the cytoplasm. Fatty change occurs more peripherally. Toxic changes in the kidneys are much more limited and without casts.

Diagnosis is not likely to be possible on the basis of lesions alone, but should become reasonably certain when the availability of the plant and the unavailability of normal and palatable forage are known to exist. The poison may be classified as enteritis-producing and hepatotoxic.

Reference

Mathews FP. The toxicity of Drymaria pachyphylla for cattle, sheep and goats. J Am Vet Med Assoc 1933;83:255–260.

Lechuguilla

Agave lechuguilla is a plant of the arid southwestern United States, Mexico, and similar regions; it is eaten, upon necessity, by sheep and goats. In addition to the usual signs of general illness, such as weakness and emaciation, symptoms include a yellow, tenacious mucous exudate from the eyes and nose, icterus, and high blood urea nitrogen or nonprotein nitrogen. The latter change can be detected by examination as early as the eighth day after ingestion of the plant begins. If the animal were exposed to bright summer sunlight, photosensitization manifests by edematous swelling ("bighead") of the ears and face, the overlying skin sometimes becoming necrotic. Leukocytosis then occurs in addition to hematologic abnormalities. A short period of coma usually precedes death.

Postmortem lesions include those that would be expected from the symptoms: acute toxic hepatitis and acute toxic tubular nephrosis. Fatty change of the liver is marked and is principally responsible for the pale or yellow color grossly. Centrilobular necrosis is of moderate degree. Lymphocytic infiltrations in or around the islands of Glisson (portal spaces) are usually noticeable. Considerable retention and inspissation of bile occur, which form precipitated masses in some intrahepatic bile ducts. In the kidneys, dilation of the tubules is pronounced. This distention is probably due to obstruction by large albuminous casts in the case of some nephrons, but hypertrophic dilation and regeneration of epithelium also are evident. Fatty change occurs in the ascending loops of Henle. In addition to frequent, obstructing casts, a precipitate of albumin is manifest in most of the proximal convoluted tubules. Edema, cutaneous necrosis, and subsequent inflammatory exudation are typical in those that develop photosensitization.

Reference

Mathews FP. Lechuguilla poisoning in sheep and goats. J Am Vet Med Assoc 1938;93:168–175.

Phyllanthus

A plant popularly classed as a spurge, *Phyllanthus abnormis* or *P. drumondii*, has poisoned cattle in the southern and western parts of Texas. It produces a slowly progressive intoxication, characterized by depression, inappetence, and cachexia, with diarrhea and slight icterus. Postmortem lesions show this to be another example of hepatotoxic and nephrotoxic poisoning. In chronic cases, the usual changes of acute toxic hepatitis progress to cirrhosis. Renal damage occurs in the necrosis and degenerative epithelial changes characteristic of acute toxic tubular nephrosis, together with albuminous material in the tubules, which is perhaps more in the nature of proteinaceous debris from disintegrating cells than of albuminous excretion.

Reference

Mathews FP. Toxicity of a spurge (Phyllanthus abnormis) for cattle, sheep and goats. Cornell Vet 1945;35:336–346.

Mushrooms

Certain species of mushrooms, especially *Amanita phalloides, A. pantherina,* and *A. verna* (popularly called "destroying angel"), are well known to be poisonous, human fatalities being only too frequent. Cattle may develop a notable liking for these mushrooms when they are numerous in the pasture because of optimal growing conditions (warm, humid climates); cases of fatal poisoning have been reported.

Signs include vomiting, painful defecation, sometimes with eversion and ulceration of the rectal mucosa, muscular spasms, drowsiness, and death. In humans, hallucinations occur. Illness begins several hours after ingestion of the mushrooms and is likely to last for several days. Principal lesions include acute catarrhal gastroenteritis throughout the tract, and hemorrhages on the heart, liver, and other organs. Gross appearances indicate a considerable degree of acute toxic hepatitis and toxic tubular nephrosis. In humans poisoned by *Amanita phalloides*, hepatic and renal toxic changes are the principal lesions, with marked fatty change of these organs and the heart. Complete microscopic studies appear not to have been made in animals.

References

Burton HA. Mushroom poisoning in cattle. Vet Med 1944;39:290.

Piercy PL, Hargis G, Brown CA. Mushroom poisoning in cattle. J Am Vet Med Assoc 1944;105:206–208.

Ridgway RL. Mushroom (Amanita pantherina) poisoning. J Am Vet Med Assoc 1978;172:681–682.

Lupines

Lupines are leguminous plants of the pea family, native to most of the temperate regions of the world. Most of the 100 or more species of the genus Lupinus are native to the western United States, but have also been traced to the poisoning of livestock in Australia, South Africa, and Central and Western Europe. In Europe, the plants were introduced as a means of providing nitrogenous forage and improving poor soil. The Greeks and Romans used the seeds of certain lupines for making flour after first loosening the hulls by cooking, and then soaking out the bitter, poisonous principles in running water.

Several species have been identified with losses of livestock. In the western United States, these include: *L. sericeus, L. leucophyllus, L. argenteus, L. caudatus, L. perennis, L. pusillus, L. laxifloris,* and *L. onustus.* In South Africa, *L. angustifolius,* widely used as a cover crop and feed for sheep, has occasionally caused severe losses in sheep, cattle, and sometimes swine. In Australia, *L. digitatus* is the commonest variety, widely cultivated and naturalized after its introduction during the late nineteenth century. This blue lupine is usually involved in livestock losses from lupines in Australia.

Certain alkaloids found in lupines have been identified as the cause of illness in animals; development of new genetic strains ("sweet lupines"), which do not contain these alkaloids, has eliminated losses due to this cause. The following alkaloids have been isolated from lupine species: lupinine, lupinidine or l-sparteine, d-lupanine, hydroxy-(oxy) lupanine, and spathulatine. The toxic effects of these lupine alkaloids have been grouped under the terms lupine poisoning, American lupinosis, alkaloidal poisoning, or lupine madness. Gardiner proposed that the term, lupine poisoning be used for lupine alkaloid poisoning, to differentiate it from another syndrome associated with lupines but unrelated to toxic alkaloids (1967). This latter syndrome Gardiner termed lupinosis or European lupinosis, and is due to a mycotoxin produced by the fungus *Phomopsis leptostomiformis,* which may grow on sweet and bitter lupines. This is discussed elsewhere with other mycotoxicoses.

Lupine poisoning, due to the effects of one or more of the lupine alkaloids, is manifest by severe effects on nerve centers, especially respiratory and vasomotor centers, which are first stimulated, then paralyzed. This effect results in decrease of blood pressure, slow heart rate, dilation of pupils, and death by asphyxia associated with convulsions. All mammals are susceptible, but natural poisonings have been observed in sheep, horses, cattle, goats, swine, and deer. Signs of poisoning may appear a few hours after ingesting poisonous lupines. In sheep, nervous manifestations predominate, with erratic behavior, confused running, dyspnea, excessive frothy salivation, convulsions, stupor, or coma leading to death. Gross and microscopic lesions in this type of poisoning due to lupine alkaloids apparently are not distinctive.

A distinctive congenital syndrome, crooked calf disease, occurs in range cattle in certain western states and Alaska and has been shown to be caused by the teratogenic effect of lupines consumed by cows on days 40–70 of pregnancy. The disease is seen in newborn calves from cows that have access to lupines on the range, and has been reproduced by feeding pregnant cows dried lupine plants, especially Lupinus sericeus. The cows exhibit lethargy, nervousness, incoordination, muscular twitching, and dry, rough hair coat as a result of feeding on lupines months before delivery of the deformed calves.

Affected calves are born with any or all of several anomalies (Fig. 15-9), including arthrogryposis, scoliosis, torticollis, and cleft palate. Most calves are viable and may survive to become adults, but some abortions are recorded among affected cattle. This disease, known by ranchers for many years in certain regions, was originally believed to be hereditary, but genetic evidence was not convincing and experimental data now clearly point toward lupines as the cause.

Evidence currently points to a quinolizidine alkaloid, anagyrine, as the putative, active principle involved in the teratogenic effects of some lupines. Anagyrine is produced by many plants of the genus Lupinus, especially L. laxiflora, sericeus, and caudatus. Conversely, the active teratogen in Lupinus formosus is reported to be another quinolizidine alkaloid, named ammodendrine.

Other plants, such as deadly hemlock plants, have been demonstrated to cause similar teratogenic effects

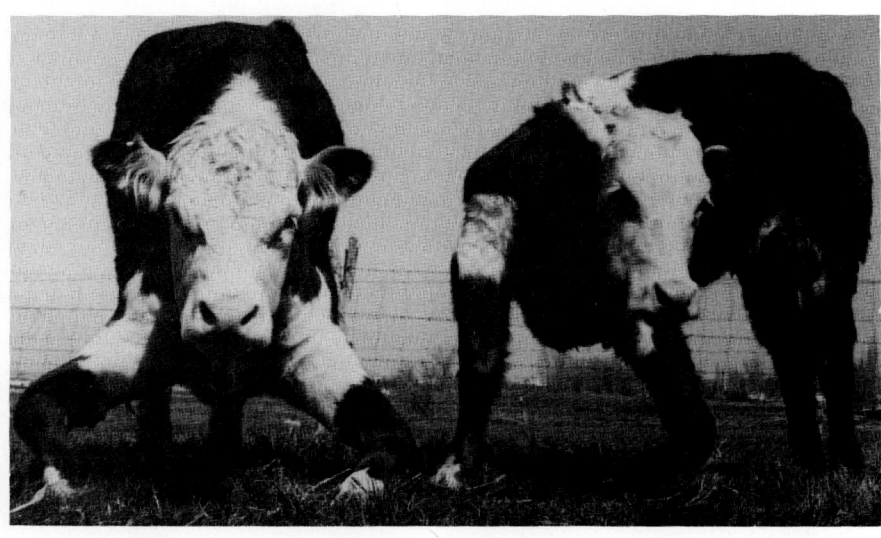

FIG. 15-9 Arthrogryposis and scoliosis of calves following lupine poisoning. (Courtesy of Dr. J. L. Shupe and Journal of the American Veterinary Medical Association.)

(arthrogryposis, torticollis, and scoliosis) in cattle, swine, and Syrian hamsters. *Conium maculatum* contains a piperidine alkaloid, coniine, which is reported to be teratogenic to cattle. The stalks of tobacco plants, *Nicotiana tabacum,* are under some conditions palatable to swine. Pregnant sows, after consuming these plants during the early stages of pregnancy, may deliver piglets with skeletal anomalies. The active principle in the tobacco plants is probably not nicotine. The active teratogen in *Nicotiana glauca* appears to be a piperidine alkaloid named anabasine.

Pregnant hamsters, after consuming many of the suspected plants on days 7 or 8 after conception, produce deformed young with congenital skeletal anomalies. These animals provide a useful model for screening plants for suspected teratogens.

References

Allen JG. Recent advances with cultivated lupins with emphasis on toxicological aspects. In: James LF, Keeler RF, Bailey EM Jr, Cheeke PR, Hegarty MP, eds. Poisonous plants: Proc 3rd Int Symp. Ames: Iowa State Univ Press, 1992;229–233.
Crowe MW. Tobacco—a cause of congenital arthrogryposis. In: Keeler RF, Van Kampen KR, James LF, eds. Effects of poisonous plants on livestock. New York: Academic Press, 1978;419–427.
Gardiner MR. Lupinosis. Adv Vet Sci 1967;11:85–138.
Keeler RF, Panter KE. Induction of crooked calf disease by the piperidine alkaloid-containing plant Lupinus formosus. In: James LF, Keeler RF, Bailey EM Jr, Cheeke PR, Hegarty MP, eds. Poisonous Plants: Proc 3rd Int Symp. Ames: Iowa State Univ Press, 1992;239–244.
Shupe JL, et al. Lupine, a cause of crooked calf disease. J Am Vet Med Assoc 1967;151:198–203.
Shupe JL, James LF, Binns W. Observations on crooked calf disease. J Am Vet Med Assoc 1967;151:191–197.

Vetch

Vetches *(Vicia spp.)* are leguminous plants related to the lupines genetically and also in their toxicology. Several species, especially *Vicia sativa,* the "common vetch," are raised, like certain lupines, as proteinaceous forage or as nitrogen-fixing soil-builders. The seeds of this and some other species contain poisonous amounts of prussic acid, especially before maturity. However, in most cases, toxic effects of vetches in hay or forage are different. The illness, which usually extends over several days or longer, is characterized especially by vague digestive disturbances and icterus. In more acute forms, muscular twitchings and definite signs of gastroenteritis are manifest. In the case of *Vicia faba,* the "broad bean" or "horse bean," hemolytic anemia and hemoglobinuria are also signs. Lesions include those of acute toxic hepatitis with or without gastroenteritis.

Panciera et al. associated a syndrome in cattle with feeding upon pastures containing hairy vetch (*Vicia villosa;* 1966). This disease differs in several ways from that usually associated with other vetch poisoning. The disease was observed in 13 herds, in which dermatitis, conjunctivitis, and diarrhea were the principal signs of illness. Approximately 800 cattle were observed, about 7% of them were sick, and about half of these sick cattle died. The affected skin became thickened, folded, and

in places, denuded of hair. Lesions occurred in pigmented, as well as nonpigmented, areas of the skin. A few pregnant cows aborted.

Lesions in fatal cases were distributed through the myocardium, kidney, adrenal, lymph nodes, and thyroid, and appeared grossly as focal or confluent grayish infiltrations, usually moderately firm and sharply demarcated from the adjacent tissue. Microscopically, these focal lesions were formed by necrosis of parenchyma and infiltration by macrophages, multinucleated giant cells, eosinophils, and lymphocytes. Myocardial fibers were necrotic, sometimes mineralized, and the sarcoplasma was often absent, leaving sarcolemmal nuclei and many giant cells. Necrosis of renal tubules was also observed in this syndrome, accompanied by replication of tubular epithelial cells, intense infiltration by leukocytes, principally lymphocytes, and peculiar membranous thickening of the glomerular tufts.

A specific hemolytic anemia, favism, in certain human patients depends upon a genetic factor and the ingestion of the broad bean, *Vicia faba.* The inherited defect in susceptible human patients results in a deficiency of the enzyme glucose-6–phosphate dehydrogenase (G-6–PD). Deficiency of this enzyme is reflected in reduced glutathione in red blood cells. Extracts of *Vicia faba* beans have had a destructive effect upon the erythrocytes of susceptible individuals in vitro; therefore, it is believed that the beans may act similarly on susceptible red blood cells in vivo, resulting in hemolytic anemia.

References

Bowman JE, Walker DG. Action of Vicia faba on erythrocytes: possible relation to favism. Nature 1961;189:555–556.
Kerr LA, Edwards WC. Hairy vetch poisoning of cattle. Vet Med Small Anim Clin 1982;77:257–258.
Panciera RJ. Hairy vetch (Vicia villosa Roth) poisoning in cattle. In: Keeler RF, Van Kampen KR, James LF, eds. Effects of poisonous plants on livestock. New York: Academic Press, 1978;555–563.
Panciera RJ, Johnson L, Osbum BI. A disease of cattle grazing hairy vetch pasture. J Am Vet Med Assoc 1966;148:804–808.
Steyn DG. Toxicology of plants in South Africa. Johannesburg: Central News Agency, 1934.

Algae

Green or blue-green algae ("water bloom," "cyanobacterial bloom") of several species have been associated with poisoning of domestic or wild animals in several parts of the world. These algae grow on or beneath the surface of lakes, ponds, or streams and at some times are concentrated by wind or other factors to become extremely poisonous to all animals that drink the water. Poisoning incidents have been reported involving cattle, sheep, swine, dogs, and bats.

Several species of algae have been identified and demonstrated experimentally to contain toxin. Identified organisms include the following: *Anabaena spiroides, A. circinalis, Nodularis spumigena, Microcystis aeruginosa,* and *Anabaena flos-aquae.* In some instances an irreversible anticholesterase effect has been demonstrated with contents of these organisms.

Death occurs suddenly within approximately one to two hours after drinking the water. Symptoms include acute prostration followed by convulsions, or else rapidly developing general paralysis. Postmortem lesions are usually absent, except possibly the presence of hydroperitoneum. Conversely, subacute and chronic cases are reported in South Africa. In the former, acute toxic hepatitis occurs with icterus, the liver being yellow and friable. Bloody or yellowish fluid in the serous cavities, acute swelling of the spleen, and sometimes hemorrhagic enteritis develop. In a few chronic cases, the liver is described as hard, presumably cirrhotic. In cattle which have recovered, severe cutaneous lesions characteristic of photosensitization have developed. Water toxicity can be demonstrated in experimental animals orally or parenterally, but toxic conditions in lakes may change quickly, with the "water-bloom" being blown elsewhere, or by other means.

References

Beasley VR, et al. Apparent blue-green algae poisoning in swine subsequent to ingestion of a bloom dominated by Anabaena spiroides. J Am Vet Med Assoc 1983;182:413–313.

Galey FD, et al. Blue-green algae (Microcystis aeruginosa) hepatotoxicosis in dairy cows. Am J Vet Res 1987;48:1415–1420.

Jackson ARB, McInnes A, Falconer IR, et al. Clinical and pathological changes in sheep experimentally poisoned by the blue-green algae Microcystis aeruginosa. Vet Pathol 1984;21:102–113.

Kerr LA, McCoy CP, Eaves D. Blue-green algae toxicosis in five dairy cows. J Am Vet Med Assoc 1987;191:829–832.

Mahmood NA, Carmichael WW, Pfahler D. Anticholinesterase poisonings in dogs from a cyanobacterial (blue-green algae) bloom dominated by Anabaena flos-aquae. Am J Vet Res 1988;49:500–503.

Pybus MJ, Hobson DP, Onderka DK. Mass mortality of bats due to probable blue-green algal toxicity. J Wildl Dis 1986;22:449–450.

GROUP D: NEPHROTOXICITY

Poisons in Group D are primarily nephrotoxic. Some of these poisonings may also affect other organ systems, but in general, less so than with the hepatotoxins discussed in the previous section.

Turpentine

Turpentine is a local and diffusible irritant. Skin is readily blistered within one to two hours after a single topical application. Ingested without adequate dilution, turpentine causes severe gastroenteritis, in addition to stomatitis and esophagitis. When it is inhaled, the result is bronchopneumonia. A considerable amount, however, is tolerated in the digestive tract when properly diluted. Fatalities result from acute toxic tubular nephrosis, which develops within a few days. Most cases of poisoning result from attempts to use the substance for therapeutic purposes. An unusual case of fatal nephritic poisoning occurred when a dog walked upon a freshly painted floor and the owner used turpentine to wash the animal's feet (unpublished data). Giffee reported sudden, fatal poisoning when turpentine was applied to castration wounds in little pigs (1939). Symptoms of acute peritonitis appeared within minutes and death of several occurred within one to two hours.

Reference

Giffee JW. Turpentine poisoning in pigs. J Am Vet Med Assoc 1939;95:509.

Sulfonamides

The usual toxic effects of sulfonamide drugs, as seen in domestic animals, depend upon obstruction of renal tubules by precipitated crystals of sulfonamide (Fig. 15-10). With the unaided eye, masses of the yellowish crystals can often be seen in the renal papillae and pelvis, or even forming pale radial lines, which mark distended medullary tubules. It is said that their amount is sometimes so great as to act as obstructive calculi in the ureter. Microscopically, the crystals in the papillae lay within the ducts of Bellini and collecting tubules, which they commonly obstruct; the lining of the tubules and ducts are mechanically irritated by the sharp points of the crystals. Fatalities appear to be possible from these effects alone but, in some instances, the obstructive changes may be accompanied by the formation of albuminous casts, suggesting more subtle renal injury. This is accompanied by mild, degenerative changes in the cells of the proximal convoluted tubules.

In humans, the kidneys often contain foci of necrosis, in and around which the heavy accumulation of reticuloendothelial and other inflammatory cells amounts to a granulomatous reaction. This is the so-called nephrotoxic reaction; it is considered an allergic process, supposedly depending on previous sensitization. The rarity or nonexistence of this phenomenon in animals may be attributable to the infrequency with which an animal has more than one illness treated by sulfonamides. However, when one considers the alacrity and nonchalance with which ranchers administered sulfonamide drugs (until antibiotics replaced them) for illnesses of all sorts, such an explanation seems doubtful.

Other disorders that have resulted from the administration of sulfonamides include temporary nervous dysfunctions, such as blindness, failure of optical adaptation and accommodation, hyperesthesia, incoordination, ataxia, and convulsions. These usually follow a single, excessive dose of the drug. Demyelinization of nerves has also resulted, and serious or fatal results have followed the application of sulfonamide medications where they came into contact with central or peripheral nervous tissue.

The therapeutic administration of sulfonamides occasionally leads to detectable porphyrinuria in humans. No reports of accompanying photosensitization exist, but the situation may well be different in the case of a farm animal, normally exposed to much sunlight, which suffered provocative hepatic damage. Experimentally, in rats, sulfonamides administered to the pregnant mother have inhibited ossification of the bones of the fetus. In young chickens, as little as 0.06% of sodium sulfaquinoxaline in the drinking water for four days

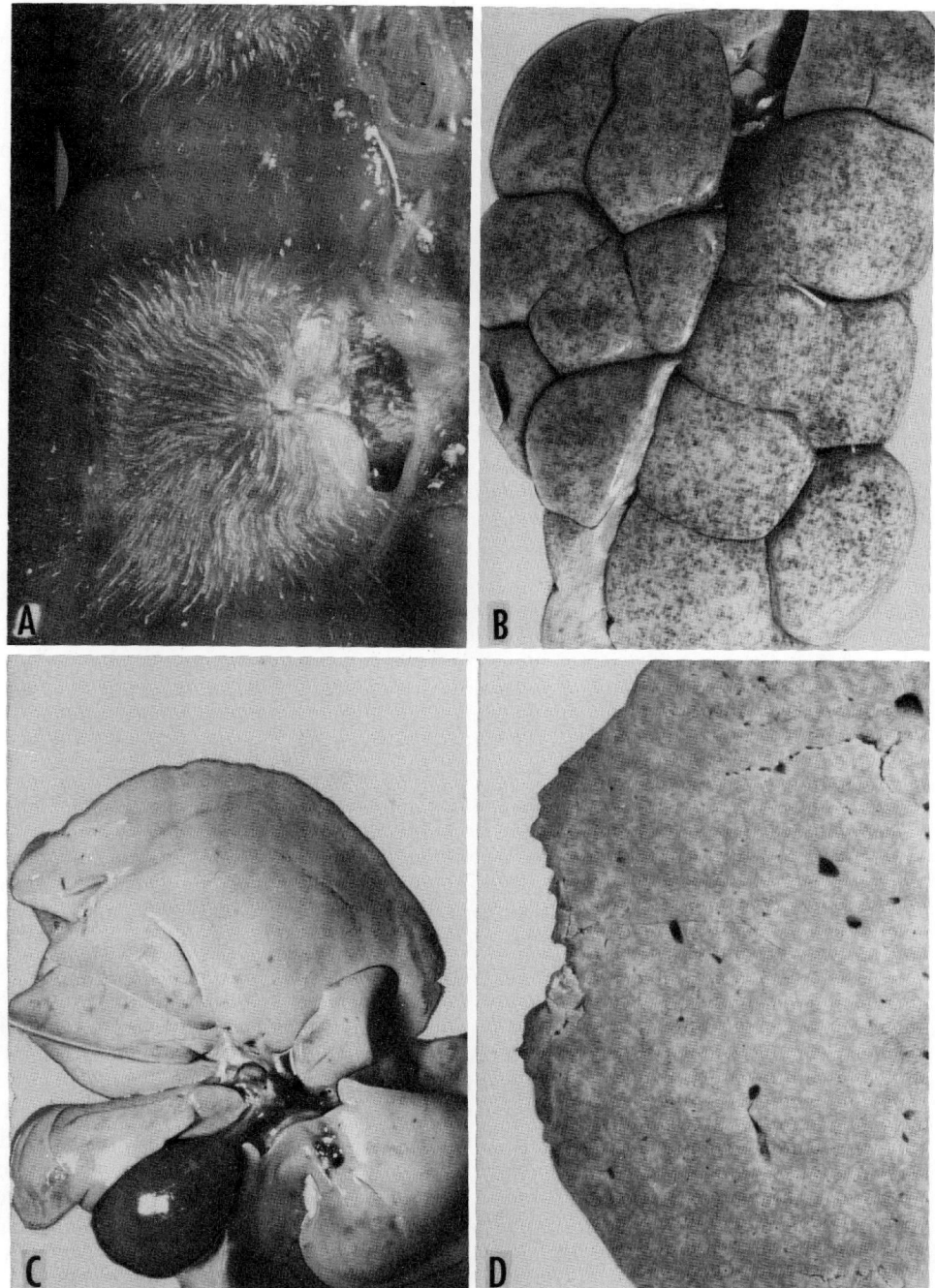

FIG. 15-10 A. Poisoning by sulfathiazole, kidney of a three-week-old calf. Crystals fill collecting tubules. (Case at Texas Sch. Vet. Med.) **B.** Kidney of a Brahman heifer poisoned by eating oak buds. (Case at Texas Sch. Vet. Med.) **C.** Liver of a dog which survived three days after being poisoned by phosphorus. The liver was pale yellowish in color. (Case at Iowa Sch. Vet. Med.) **D.** Liver of a horse with toxic hepatitis, probably due to crotalaria poisoning.

has produced a hemorrhagic syndrome of serious import.

In spite of the several dangerous possibilities, however, sulfonamides remain highly useful therapeutic agents. Crystallization in the renal tubules as the glomerular filtrate is concentrated into urine, the most likely catastrophe, is rendered improbable by promoting alkalinity in those species having acidic urine, and even more by copious intake of water.

References

Blackwell TE, Werdin RE, Eisenmenger MC, FitzSimmons MA. Goitrogenic effects in offspring of swine fed sulfadimethoxine and ormetoprim in late gestation. J Am Vet Med Assoc 1989;194:519–523.

Reece RL, Barr DA, Gould JA. Poisoning in a chicken flock caused by sulphachloropyrazine. Vet Rec 1986;119:324–325.

Oxalate-bearing plants and ethylene glycol

Oxalate poisoning may result from ingestion of:

1. Plants that contain toxic levels of oxalate;
2. Ethylene glycol;
3. Oxalate salts; or,
4. Plants infected with fungi that produce oxalates.

Ordinary garden rhubarb *(Rheum rhaponticum)* is one of the oxalate-containing plants, but of more significance in causing losses of livestock are halogeton *(Halogeton glomeratus)* and greasewood *(Sarcobatus vermiculatus),* both of which grow in the Rocky Mountain region of the United States. In dry weather, halogeton has been known to contain oxalates, largely sodium and potassium oxalate, equivalent to 19% of anhydrous oxalic acid. Soursob *(Oxalis cernua),* indigenous to South Australia, is another plant that owes its poisonous qualities to oxalates, as is also the common sorrel, *Rumex acetosa* and other members of the genus Rumex.

Another plant demonstrated by analysis to contain high levels of oxalate is *Amaranthus retroflexus,* pigweed, redroot, or careless weed (Marshall et al., 1967). The leaves of this plant may contain as much as 30% of total oxalate on a dried weight basis. Oxalate poisoning from ingestion of these plants is primarily a disease of sheep. Cattle and horses are relatively resistant.

The poisonous effects of calcium oxalates are also produced in some species (humans, dogs, cats) by the ingestion of toxic amounts of ethylene glycol. This colorless, odorless, slightly viscous, dihydric alcohol has a sweetish taste and is widely used as a solvent in manufacturing. Its common use as a nonvolatile antifreeze makes it available in many households, and its taste appeals to some people, cats, and dogs. Ethylene glycol is metabolized in the liver by alcohol dehydrogenase, which results in the formation of oxalates. This enzyme is also necessary for the degradation of ethyl alcohol. The simultaneous administration of ethyl alcohol competes for this enzyme in the liver and decreases the formation of oxalate. This fact is utilized in the treatment of ethylene glycol poisoning (Wacker et al., 1965). Intravenously administered 4–methylpyrazole, an inhibitor of alcohol dehydrogenase, is also effective in treating ethylene glycol toxicosis in humans.

The initial effect of oxalate poisoning is hypocalcemia, resulting from the formation of insoluble calcium oxalate. Serum calcium levels may decrease to less than half of normal. Signs of acute poisoning are observed within two to four hours. In sheep, these include depression, anorexia, slight to moderate bloating, weakness, restlessness, frequent attempts to urinate, occasional reddish-brown urine and brownish-black feces, blood-tinged nasal exudate, and coma, followed by death. Ethylene glycol poisoning in dogs results in the rapid development of ataxia, polydipsia, depression, miosis, tachycardia, tachypnea, hyperpnea, bradycardia, and coma. Convulsions and vomiting are frequent. In most cases, death follows the administration of 6.6 ml/kg of body weight or more.

The neurologic signs are believed to be the result of hypocalcemia. Precipitation of calcium oxalate in cerebral blood vessels, however, may contribute in some manner.

Calcium oxalate is precipitated (Fig. 15-11) in the renal tubules during the process of elimination, and a fatal outcome may occur from renal insufficiency and uremia after the earlier symptoms have abated. Conversely, recovery is possible, with blood urea levels slowly subsiding after about one month. Cystitis and urethritis may be a part of this syndrome.

Postmortem diagnosis can usually be made in these cases by the presence of numerous, nearly transparent crystals in the renal tubules. Visible when light is sharply reduced or polarized, these crystals may be single, irregularly rhomboidal, and 30–40 μ long. Often, however, the crystals lay closely packed in a radial arrangement, the whole rosettelike structure more than filling the lumen of the tubule and occupying space at the expense of the epithelial cells (Fig. 15-11). The latter eventually become necrotic, although the extent of cellular damage depends upon whether death occurred early or late. Severe congestion of all parts of the kidney also occurs, as well as moderate increase in cellularity of the glomeruli, and marked albuminous precipitate in the tubules. Those epithelial cells not directly affected by the crystals show little toxic injury. Oxalate nephrosis has been reported in fetal kidneys of sheep exposed to oxalic acid during pregnancy.

Widespread hemorrhage and edema found at postmortem, particularly in the rumen of sheep poisoned by halogeton, are associated with deposits of calcium oxalate in the walls of blood vessels. The presence of oxalate at these sites appears to damage the blood vessel wall, but the interference with clotting due to hypocalcemia is probably of greater significance.

Diagnosis The diagnosis is usually established postmortem by the demonstration of characteristic birefringent crystals in renal tubules and cerebral blood vessels (Fig. 15-11). Nonfatal doses do not appear to produce permanent damage to renal tubules.

Studies of the toxicity of ethylene glycol administered to three species of Old World monkeys *(Macaca mulatta, M. fascicularis,* and *M. radiata)* revealed lesions similar to those described in other species. The toxic dose in these species is believed to be similar to that in humans: 1.6 ml/kg of body weight.

PERIRENAL EDEMA DISEASE

Perirenal edema disease has been observed in swine given access to pastures bearing heavy growth of common piglot weeds, such as *Amaranthus retroflexus,* or the weed called lambs' quarters *(Chenopodium album).* Other weeds, such as black nightshade *(Solanum nigrum),* buffalo burr *(Solanum rostratum),* and Jimson weed *(Datura stramonium),* have also been suspected as causative.

The signs in perirenal edema syndrome include trembling, weakness, incoordination, sternal recumbency, and coma, followed by death. The characteristic postmortem lesion is the presence of a large amount of edema surrounding the kidney between the renal capsule and the perirenal peritoneum. Sometimes this edema fluid is tinged with blood, but the affected kidneys are usually pale and normal in size. Edema in the wall of the abdomen, around the rectum, and in the wall of the stomach may also be present. Clear, transparent, or straw-colored fluid may distend the peritoneal and pleural cavities. The renal capsule usually is not affected, although edema may extend into the renal parenchyma. Micro-

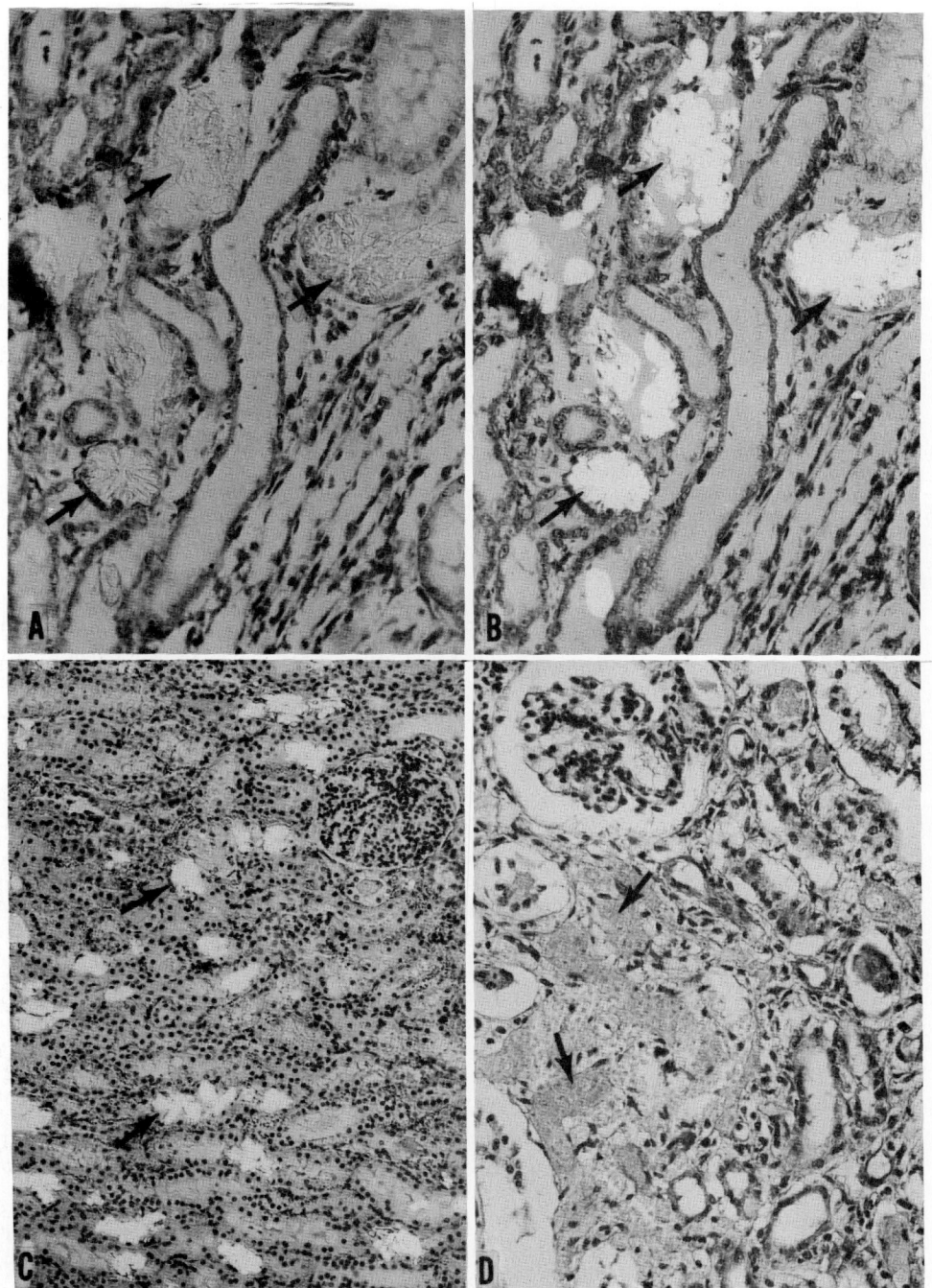

FIG. 15-11 **A.** Kidney of a kitten poisoned by ethylene glycol (antifreeze) (×210). Note oxalate crystals (arrows) in tubules. **B.** Same section as A photographed under polarized light. Note brilliance of oxalate crystals (arrows). (Courtesy of Dr. Wm. J. Hadlow.) **C.** Kidney of a sheep poisoned by eating Halogeton plants (×125). Note oxalate crystals (arrows), photographed under polarized light. (Courtesy of Dr. Wayne C. Anderson.) **D.** Kidney of a steer poisoned by eating buds of an oak tree (×210). Necrosis (arrows) of certain convoluted tubules.

scopic evidence of toxic tubular nephrosis with interstitial edema in the renal cortex has been described. The pathogenesis of the syndrome has not been elucidated. A similar syndrome is described in cattle, also associated with Amaranthus poisoning (Stuart et al., 1975).

Lesions are not typical of oxalate poisoning: oxalate crystals are not readily identifiable in tissue section; hence, the precise pathogenetic mechanisms are not known. It is possible that nitrate is an etiologic factor because *A. retroflexus* may contain elevated levels of nitrate. Feeding this plant to swine appears to have produced this syndrome.

References

Andrews EJ. Oxalate nephropathy in a horse. J Am Vet Med Assoc 1971;159:49–52.

Baud FJ, et al. Treatment of ethylene glycol poisoning with intravenous 4–methylpyrazole. N Engl J Med 1988;319:97–100.

Boermans HJ, Ruegg PL, Leach M. Ethylene glycol toxicosis in a pigmy goat. J Am Vet Med Assoc 1988;193:694–696.

Dickie CW, Hamann MH, Carroll WD, et al. Oxalate (Rumex venosus) poisoning in cattle. J Am Vet Med Assoc 1978;173:73–74.

Hadlow WJ. Acute ethylene glycol poisoning in a cat. J Am Vet Med Assoc 1957;130:296–297.

James LF. Serum electrolyte, acid-base balance, and enzyme changes in acute halogeton glomeratus poisoning in sheep. Can J Comp Med 1968;32:539–543.

Lincoln SD, Black B. Halogeton poisoning in range cattle. J Am Vet Med Assoc 1988;176:717–718.

Littledike ET, James L, Cook H. Oxalate (halogeton) poisoning of sheep: certain physiopathologic changes. Am J Vet Res 1976;37:661–666.

Marshall VL, Buck WB, Bell GL. Pigweed (Amaranthusretroflexus): an oxalate-containing plant. Am J Vet Res 1967;28:888–889.

Peterson CD, Collins AJ, Himes JM, et al. Ethylene glycol poisoning. Pharmacokinetics during therapy with ethanol and hemodialysis. N Engl J Med 1981;304:21–23.

Roberts JA, Seibold HR. Ethylene glycol toxicity in the monkey. Toxicol Appl Pharmacol 1969;15:624–631.

Shupe JL, James LF. Additional physiopathologic changes in Halogeton glomeratus (oxalate) poisoning in sheep. Cornell Vet 1969;59:41–55.

Stuart BP, Nicholson SS, Smith JB. Perirenal edema and toxic nephrosis in cattle, associated with ingestion of pigweed. J Am Vet Med Assoc 1975;167:949–950.

Thrall MA, Grauer GF, Mero KN. Clinicopathologic findings in dogs and cats with ethylene glycol intoxication. J Am Vet Med Assoc 1984;184:37–41.

Wacker WEC, et al. Treatment of ethylene glycol poisoning with ethyl alcohol. JAMA 1965;194:1231–1233.

Broomweed

The broomweeds or broom snakeweeds, particularly *Gutierrezia sarothrae* and *G. microcephala,* are plants that grow over large areas of arid ranges of the western United States. These plants may be eaten by cattle and sheep and are commonly, but not always, poisonous.

The plant is a somewhat herbaceous perennial which makes a bushy growth to a height of about 1 foot (30 cm). It has fine foliage, covered with a sticky exudate, and large numbers of tiny yellow flowers.

Signs appear after an animal has been eating appreciable amounts of the plant for at least a few days, and begin with anorexia, listlessness, arched back, and drooping head. A noticeable degree of icterus is present. Appropriate tests reveal uremia; in severe, acute cases, hematuria also is evident. Abortion often occurs in pregnant sheep or cattle.

The lesions can be summarized as those of acute toxic tubular nephrosis and a rather unusual form of toxic hepatitis. The proximal and distal convoluted tubules and the ascending loops of Henle are affected by hydropic degeneration and disintegration of the cytoplasm of their epithelial cells, with ultimate necrosis if the animal were to live long enough. In the more acute cases, hemorrhage occurs into Bowman's capsules and tubules, as well as into intertubular tissue, while in animals with more prolonged courses (one to two weeks), a considerable degree of lymphocytic infiltration is manifest. The hepatic changes consist of hydropic degeneration and necrosis, diffusely distributed without regard to any particular zone in the lobule. Although many diseases are characterized by toxic nephrosis and hepatitis, it would seem that hemorrhage into the nephron and hydropic degeneration of the liver cells would serve to distinguish broomweed poisoning from many other nephrotoxic and hepatotoxic poisonings.

Broom snakeweeds accumulate selenium when grown on soil containing excessive selenium, but this does not appear to account for all of their toxic properties. The basic toxic principle in a related species, Xan-

thocephalum, appears to be saponin, which produces the clinical signs, including abortion, when administered to pregnant rabbits, cows, and goats.

References

Dollahite JW, Anthony WV. Poisoning of cattle with Gutierrezia microcephala, a perennial broomweed. J Am Vet Med Assoc 1957;130:525–530.

Dollahite JW, Shaver T, Camp BJ. Injected saponins as abortifacients. Am J Vet Res 1962;23:1261–1263.

Mathews FP. Toxicity of broomweed (Gutierrezia microcephala) for sheep, cattle and goats. J Am Vet Med Assoc 1936;88:55–61.

Shaver TN, Camp BJ, Dollahite JW. The chemistry of a toxic constituent of Xanthocephalum species. Ann NY Acad Sci 1964; 111:737–743.

Chloroform

Chloroform toxicity serves to emphasize specific sexual dimorphisms and genetically determined sensitivity in certain inbred strains of laboratory mice. Experience has taught laboratory workers to avoid opening a bottle of chloroform in a room in which inbred mice are kept. Even a slight exposure to chloroform vapor will cause the death of male mice. The following inbred strains are particularly susceptible: CBA-p, DBA, C_3H,A, and HR. Immature males, adult females, and castrated males are relatively insusceptible. Castrated males become sensitive after administration of testosterone.

Inhalation of chloroform vapor by these susceptible mice results in necrosis of liver cells, glomeruli, and proximal convoluted tubules. Animals that survive sublethal doses may later be demonstrated to have many calcified deposits in glomeruli and tubules in the renal cortex (Dunn, 1965).

References

Brown DM, Langley PF, Smith D, et al. Metabolism of chloroform. The metabolism of (14C) chloroform by different species. Xenobiotica 1974;4:151–163.

Christensen LR, et al. Accidental chloroform poisoning of Balb/cAn-NIcr mice. Z Versuchstierkd 1963;2:135–140.

Deringer MK, Dunn TB, Heston WE. Results of exposure of strain C_3H mice to chloroform. Proc Soc Exp Biol Med 1953;83:474–479.

Dunn TB. Spontaneous lesions of mice. In: Ribelin WE, McCoy JR, eds. The pathology of laboratory animals. Springfield: Charles C Thomas, 1965;303–329.

Eschenbrenner AB, Miller E. Induction of hepatomas in mice by repeated oral administration of chloroform, with observations on sex differences. J Nat Cancer Inst 1945;5:251–255.

Eschenbrenner AB, Miller E. Sex difference in kidney morphology and chloroform necrosis. Science 1945;102:302–303.

Hewitt HB. Renal necrosis in mice after accidental exposure to chloroform. Br J Exp Pathol 1956;37:32–39.

Chinese tallow tree

The Chinese tallow tree (*Sapium sebiferum, Croton sebiferum,* or *Stillingia sebifera*), originally imported from China, is grown in the United States as an ornamental plant. It is abundant along the Atlantic coast from South Carolina to Florida and along the Gulf Coast west to Texas and Oklahoma; it is suspected to cause poisoning in cattle. Leaves and fruit from these trees have been shown experimentally to be toxic to cattle, but less so for sheep and goats (Russell et al., 1969). Administration of material from this tree to cattle was followed by severe diarrhea, weakness, and dehydration within 12 hours. Usual hematologic values (packed cell volume, hemoglobin) were not affected. Total serum protein or serum glutamic oxaloacetic transaminase levels were not changed. Blood urea nitrogen and serum creatine phosphokinase levels were elevated in some animals.

Gross lesions were found in the intestines, which were thickened and irregularly hyperemic. The kidneys were slightly swollen, and one liver had a yellow, oily appearance. The principal lesion appeared to be toxic tubular nephrosis.

The Chinese tallow tree does appear to have a potential for poisoning cattle, although differing conditions of growth may affect the tree's toxic properties.

Reference

Russell LH, Schwartz WL, Dollahite JW. Toxicity of Chinese tallow tree (Sapium sebiferum) for ruminants. Am J Vet Res 1969;30:1233–1238.

Bitterweed

Hymenoxys odorata, also known as western bitterweed, pingue, or bitter rubberweed, is a weed native to southwestern United States which has caused considerable losses among sheep. *H. richardsonii* (Colorado rubberweed or Pingue) is also poisonous. The manifestations of bitterweed poisoning were studied by Witzel et al. (1977), who dosed young sheep with 1 g of dried H. odorata per kilogram body weight per day. Signs, which developed within four to five days, included anorexia, depression, mucoid nasal discharge, and weakness. Most animals died within two weeks.

The principal gross lesions were gaseous and liquid distention of the gastrointestinal tract, edema and congestion of the gastrointestinal tract, ascites, hydropericardium, and hemorrhage in the mucosa of the gallbladder.

Erosions have been reported in the epithelium of the rumen, reticulum, and abomasum. The lesions in the kidneys, detected by histologic examination, are distinctive and include increased cellularity, scattered pyknotic nuclei, and swelling of the glomerular tufts, causing them to fill Bowman's spaces. The epithelial cells of the convoluted tubules are necrotic in small foci and occasionally evidence regeneration. The lumena of the proximal tubules are filled with protein and the lower part of the mephron may contain granular or hyalin casts. In the liver, microscopic changes incude scattered small foci of vacuolated or necrotic hepatic cells and some small collections of leukocytes. Biliary stasis may be evident and occasional bile duct epithelial cells are swollen and occlude the lumen.

These plants may contain several toxic compounds. One group consists of sesquiterpene lactones, one of which has been isolated from *Hymenoxys odorata,* hymenoxon. Another compound of this group was named hymenovin and may be the same as hymenoxon.

References

Bowers DE, Jones DH, Sampson HW, et al. Acute exposure to hymenoxon: electron microscopic study of the mouse liver. Am J Vet Res 1984;45:383–386.
Ivie GW, et al. Hymenovin. Major toxic constituent of western bitterweed (Hymenoxys odorata DC). J Agric Food Chem 1975;23:841–845.
Kim HL, Anderson AC, Herrig BW, et al. Protective effects of antioxidants on bitterweed (Hymenoxys odorata DC) toxicity in sheep. Am J Vet Res 1982;43:1945–1950.
Witzel DA, Jones LP, Ivie GW. Pathology of subacute bitterweed (Hymenoxys odorata) poisoning in sheep. Vet Pathol 1977;14:73–78.
Witzel DA, Rowe LD, Clark DE. Physiopathologic studies on acute Hymenoxys odorata (bitterweed) poisoning in sheep. Am J Vet Res 1974;35:931–934.

GROUP E: CARDIAC INSUFFICIENCY

Poisons of Group E have cardiac insufficiency as their prominent clinical sign. The pathogenesis may include direct injury to the myocardium with conspicuous lesions, but more usually it is alkaloids that interfere with cardiac action without causing morphologically demonstrable myocardial lesions (see also Group P).

Selenium

The rare element, selenium exists in appreciable concentrations in the soil of certain areas in the arid western part of North America and in similar situations in other parts of the world. All plants able to grow in such soils tend to incorporate the element in their tissues. This amounts to 20–30 ppm in the case of most of the common cereal and forage plants, but certain uncultivated plants which thrive in selenium areas commonly harbor as much as 5000–15,000 ppm. In the latter group are species of the genus Astragalus, including the common loco weed and milk vetch (A. bisulcatus), as well as the woody aster (Aster parryi) and saltbush (Atriplex nuttallii); however, this does not imply that loco poisoning is due to selenium. Appreciable amounts of selenium in plants can be detected by a sulfurous odor when the plants are crushed in the hand.

Acute selenium poisoning occurs in herbivorous animals as the result of eating one or several meals of some of the strongly seleniferous weeds, such as those mentioned. Another source of acute poisoning is the administration of overdoses of selenium in the therapeutic or preventative treatment of animals suspected of being deficient in selenium. As little as 10 mg of sodium selenite given orally to young lambs has resulted in fatalities. Differences in susceptibility between species may be considerable, and many other factors, such as nature of the diet, chemical form of the selenium, and rate of administration, have been shown to modify the toxic effects. In cattle and horses, this form of poisoning is largely an acute congestive and enteric disease, with gastrointestinal symptoms and collapse from respiratory and myocardial failure in a few hours or one to two days. Postmortem lesions include hemorrhagic enteritis and proctitis, passive congestion of the lungs and abdominal viscera, early toxic changes in the liver and kidneys (acute toxic hepatitis and toxic tubular nephrosis), and terminal anoxic hemorrhages in the epicardium and elsewhere. Mucosae of both the bladder and gallbladder, as well as that of the folds of the omasum, are commonly inflamed, probably because the poisonous substance is eliminated through them.

Sheep are reported to be poisoned by grazing on plants which accumulate selenium, thus the term "phytogenic selenium poisoning." In one reported incident, large numbers of sheep died after grazing on plants that included stinking milkvetch (Astragalus praelongus), analyzed as containing 2,144 ppm of selenium, and fourwing saltbush (Artemisia canescens), which contained 80 ppm of selenium. Dried plants of both of these species caused death when fed to sheep (James et al., 1982).

Although sheep may graze on selenium-bearing plants for some time without apparent effect, sudden death may occur, presumably as highly toxic doses are reached. The sheep die without apparent struggle and are found on their sternums with blood-tinged froth about their nostrils. Gross lesions consist of severe edema and congestion of the lungs.

In swine, selenium poisoning may be manifest by sudden onset of paralysis followed by characteristic hemorrhage and congestion along the coronary band of the hoofs, leading to grooves in the hoof and separation from the underlying tissue.

Paralysis of front, hind, or all four limbs is consistently associated with lesions in the cervical and lumbar intumescences of the spinal cord. The lesions are symmetric, involve the ventral horns, and appear grossly as light yellow, brown-tinged foci or as pale depressed areas. Necrosis with loss of neurons, gliosis, cavitation, and congestion of the ventral horns, displace the normal tissues and are often surrounded by a cystic zone. Similar but smaller lesions may be seen in the intermediolateral gray zones, particularly in the lumbar cord. Similar foci of malacia may be found in the medulla oblongata, involving the nucleus of the facial nerve. The lesions are limited to the locations described.

These clinical signs and lesions have been associated with feed containing 19–24 ppm of selenium. Feeding the contaminated feed to pigs under controlled conditions resulted in replication of the spontaneous clinical disease (Harrison et al., 1983).

Chronic selenium poisoning has been described under two rather distinct syndromes, "blind staggers" and "alkali disease."

A rather violent termination of slow, cumulative poisoning is picturesquely, though inaccurately, designated by the name, blind staggers. This is a reversion to the layman's terminology of a century ago, when mad staggers meant violently painful spasmodic colic, blind staggers, any of the toxic or infectious nervous disturbances characterized by a desire to press forward; staggers, in general, suggested the antics of a horse in severe abdominal pain. This form of selenium poisoning, however, has been seen most commonly in cattle. Somewhat as in Van Es "walking disease" of horses, which is simply toxic hepatitis caused by senecio poisoning, the animal is impelled to seek relief from constant abdominal discomfort by continuous walking; as the condition worsens, nervous impairment of vision occurs, as well as other functions. Animals try to walk through obstacles that they would normally avoid. They frequently stand pressing their foreheads against some solid object, possibly gaining some relief. Great weakness and paralysis supervene, being most severe in the forelimbs; dyspnea, cyanosis, and death follow as the result of respiratory failure.

The form of chronic selenium poisoning known as alkali disease was once attributed to excessive ingestion of soil alkali (e.g., sodium carbonate, sulfate), which is commonly plentiful in the same arid areas where selenium is concentrated. It is now known to result from consumption of mildly seleniferous plants over a period of weeks or months. It is characterized by shedding hair, especially of the mane and tail (bob-tail disease), and a related malnutrition of the hoofs. The latter develop deep encircling grooves parallel to the coronary band that are more pronounced than those of laminitis. In more severe cases, the groove may become a painful crack that causes partial separation of the hoof. Occasionally, one or more hoofs become detached from the sensitive laminae and slough. More often, the distorted hoof remains attached and, with the amount of wear reduced by painful locomotion, the toe grows to an inordinate length, which deforms it with an anterior concavity. This applies to the hooves of either cattle or horses. Eroded joints also make walking difficult, and the animal may die from inability to obtain food and water. Erosions of the articular surfaces of the long bones, especially of the distal end of the tibia and the proximal end of the metatarsus, are common.

The lesions are basically similar in the two clinical syndromes of chronic selenium poisoning. Myocardial insufficiency accounts for chronic, passive congestion of the lungs and splanchnic viscera, and is itself based upon focal necroses in the heart muscle and a reaction that has been described as serofibrinous and spreading into the muscle from the endocardium. Lymphocytic infiltrations accompany these changes in advanced cases. Edema of the pericardial, thoracic, and peritoneal cavities, and of the lungs, brain, and lymph nodes, is traceable to a cardiac origin as well.

Petechiae and ecchymoses on the external and internal cardiac surfaces and in various other organs are apparently attributable to a direct toxic origin, as are the comparatively mild toxic changes in the liver and kidneys. In the liver, these are described as hydropic degeneration, fatty change and necrosis with eventual fibrous scarring. In sheep, hepatic damage may attain the status of acute yellow atrophy; in the slowly developing alkali disease of cattle, some livers become truly cirrhotic. In the kidney, swelling of the renal epithelium occurs, and hyaline changes and hyaline casts appear in the convoluted tubules.

Widespread hyaline degeneration and fibrinoid necrosis of arterioles, which were believed to be the basis for edema, hemorrhages, and visceral degenerative changes, have been described in experimental selenium poisoning in swine. In affected swine, edema and necrosis of the cerebral and cerebellar cortices and gray matter of the spinal cord also were manifest.

The gastrointestinal mucosa suffers from mild inflammatory changes in the omasum and upper intestine, which become less conspicuous in proportion to the duration of illness. Apparently due to a depressant action on smooth muscle, impaction of a dilated rumen and even of the omasum nearly always occurs. Hemorrhage and necrosis of the pancreas has been reported in swine. The accumulation of hemosiderin in the spleen in the most chronic (alkali disease) cases probably rests entirely upon chronic, passive congestion, although the possibility of a hemolytic action seems not to have been fully investigated. Hemolytic anemia has been induced in rats fed sodium selenite.

The fetus shares in the deposition of selenium and malformations are common (another example of nongenetic developmental anomalies). Eggs from selenium-fed hens show a constant and severe impairment of hatchability directly proportional to the amount of selenium ingested. Chicks that do hatch have little vitality.

References

Casteel SW, Osweiler GD, Cook WO, et al. Selenium toxicosis in swine. J Am Vet Med Assoc 1985;186:1084–1085.

Harrison LH, et al. Paralysis in swine due to focal symmetrical poliomalacia: possible selenium toxicosis. Vet Pathol 1983;20:265–273.

James LF, Smart RA, Shupe JL, et al. Suspected phytogenic selenium poisoning in sheep. J Am Vet Med Assoc 1982;180:1478–1481.

Kyle R, Allen WM. Accidental selenium poisoning of a flock of sheep. Vet Rec 1990;126:601.

Mensink CG, Koeman JP, Veling J, et al. Haemorrhagic claw lesions in newborn piglets due to selenium toxicosis during pregnancy. Vet Rec 1990;126:620–622.

Death camas

Zygadenus gramineus, Z. nuttallii, and other closely related species are known by the name of death camas or by the descriptive synonym of wild onion. These are among the most poisonous plants, toxic to all species but eaten most often by sheep. The signs usually do not appear for several hours after the plant is eaten. They consist of nausea and salivation, failing heart and respiration, and great weakness and nervous depression. Terminal coma may be several hours in duration. Postmortem lesions are usually limited to the congestions of anoxic heart failure and to early changes of acute toxic hepatitis and tubular nephrosis, demonstrable microscopically.

References

Marsh CD, Clawson AB, Marsh H. Zygadenus, or death camas. U. S. Dept Agric Bull 1915;125.

Morris MD. Nuttall death camas poisoning in horses. Vet Med 1944;39:462.

Nieman KW. Death camas poisoning in fowls. J Am Vet Med Assoc 1928;73:627–631.

Panter KE, Ralphs MH, Smart RA, et al. Death camas poisoning in sheep: a case report. Vet Hum Toxicol 1987;29:45–48.

Aconite

Aconitum columbianum, a flowering and ornamental plant known either as monkshood or aconite, is similar to, and often confused with, larkspur. Animals are occasionally poisoned by it, either on the ranges or through contact with garden plants. Therapeutically, the drug is used to slow the heart. In poisonous doses, it not only slows but weakens cardiac action. Signs include restlessness and anxiety, nausea, salivation, abdominal pain, increasing weakness and prostration, weakening and terminally rapid heart rate, and final asphyxia. Of special diagnostic significance are continual swallowing movements, due to a peculiar irritation of the throat, and pronounced risus sardonicus, the lips being maximally retracted and displaying the foam-covered teeth as the horse or other animal lies helpless on the ground. Cats and rabbits jump vertically into the air, topple over backwards and experience convulsions. Death is seldom delayed more than one to two hours; therefore, few lesions can be expected beyond hemorrhage and congestion incident to asphyxia.

Baileya multiradiata

This is a plant (also called "Desert Baileya") of the arid Southwest, from Texas to California, which sheep eat reluctantly with poisonous results. Its many slender stalks reach a height of 50–60 cm, bear elongated, tongue-shaped leaves on their lower parts, and terminate each in a single, yellow flower-head at the top. This is one of the large number of plants that produce chemicals classified as sesquiterpene lactones, which include "hymenovin," believed to be the most important toxin of *Baileya multiradiata.*

Signs include the usual arched back, loss of weight, and disinclination to move. Excessive salivation appears early. If the animal were forced to exercise, cardiac embarrassment—which is the fundamental disturbance—would be revealed by rapid, pounding heart action audible at a distance of several feet.

The lesions are those of congestive heart failure, including venous congestion of the liver, spleen, kidneys, and other abdominal viscera. Zenker's necrosis and preliminary degenerative changes proceed in the myocardium, commonly involving sporadic, individual muscle cells. Pursuant to the congestive and anoxemic state, parenchymatous cells of the liver and renal cortical tubules undergo hydropic degeneration and fatty change. If the illness were to continue for several days, acute dilatation of the damaged ventricles would develop. Conversely, if cardiac failure were to cause sudden anoxic death, widespread hemorrhage over the epicardium, diaphragm, and other areas would result, as is usually observed in terminal anoxia.

A considerable proportion of animals slowly recover after several days, during which all food is refused.

References

Ivie GW, Witzel DA. Sesquiterpene lactones: structure, biological action and toxicological significance. In: Keeler RF, Tu AT, eds. Handbook of natural toxins. Vol 1. Plant and fungal toxins. New York: Marcel Dekker, 1983;571.

Mathews FP. Toxicity of Bailey a multiradiata for sheep and goats. J Am Vet Med Assoc 1933;83:673–679.

Jimson weed, thornapple

Datura stramonium and a few other closely related species, known as Jimson weed, thornapple, mad apple, stinkweed, stinkwort, Jamestown lily, and some others, are of worldwide distribution. Although ordinarily unpalatable, the ingested plant has considerable toxicity, which is due to the powerful alkaloids, atropine and hyoscyamine. The domesticated herbivora, birds, and humans are sometimes poisoned.

Signs include chiefly nervousness with excitement, which may deepen into insane delirium somewhat suggestive of rabies, and which is usually followed by incoordination, coma, and death. Dilated pupils are of considerable diagnostic significance. Inhibition of salivary and related secretions leads to extreme thirst with consequent polyuria. The heart beat, no longer restrained by the paralyzed vagus, becomes rapid and weak, and death occurs from anoxia. Signs appear within minutes or after only a few hours. Recovery, if it were to occur, would require several days. Lesions include marked congestion and edema of the lungs, hydrothorax, congestion of the meninges, and dilation of the ventricles. Hemorrhages characteristic of asphyxia occur, as well as petechiae in brain, stomach, and upper intestine. Recognizable fragments of the large leaves or of the "thornapples" may be found in the stomach or forestomachs.

Jimson weed has been associated with congenital arthrogryposis in swine, but the causal relationship has not been firmly established.

References

El-Dirdiri NI, Wasfi IA, Adam SEI, et al. Toxicity of Datura stramonium to sheep and goats. Vet Hum Toxicol 1981;23:241–246.

Hightower CE. Jimsonweed. Vet Hum Toxicol 1979;21:360.

Nelson PD, Mercer HD, Essig HW, et al. Jimson weed seed toxicity in cattle. Vet Hum Toxicol 1982;24:321–325.

Pimelea

An obscure disease of cattle in Australia termed St. George disease has been recognized for several decades, but the cause of the syndrome has remained unknown. Outbreaks of the disease have been associated with the presence of *Pimelea simplex* (desertrice flower), a small perennial herb native to Queensland.

The Pimelea genus contains more than eighty species, but the plants demonstrated to be toxic include Pimelea simplex, continua, trichostachya, and elongatus. The active principles include several classes of chemicals, such as diterpene esters based on tigliane derivatives prostratin, "factor P%" and "subtoxin B." Others are found among the diaphnane esters, includ-ing the prototype, resiniferonol. The prototype orthoester irritant in Pimelea is simplexin. Other similar substances have been isolated from these plants. The diaphnane esters are of further interest for their tumor-promoting characteristics demonstrable in the two-stage carcinogenic model in mouse skin.

Feeding trials with the plant have reproduced most of the clinical and pathologic features of field cases of St. George disease. Although principally a disease of cattle, losses of horses have also been attributed to Pimelea, and experimentally the plant has been demonstrated to be toxic to horses.

Signs include diarrhea (often tinged with blood), weakness, anemia, and evidence of circulatory failure. This may include a jugular pulse and pronounced subcutaneous edema (anasarca), especially in the submaxillary and pharyngeal regions extending to the brisket, ventral abdomen and, to a lesser degree, the limbs. At necropsy, the most striking finding is extensive edema and congestion of all organs and tissues, especially the subcutis, thorax, and gastrointestinal tract.

Under light microscope, villous atropy, small ulcers, and hemorrhages may be present in the intestine, but the changes do not fully reflect the severity of diarrhea.

The resemblance of the signs and lesions of this disease to those of "high altitude disease" (page 722) is worth noting.

The heart is dilated without hypertrophy and small foci of myocardial necrosis are present. The liver is enlarged and dark purple. Hepatic sinusoids are dilated and hepatocytes are atrophic. Anemia, which is a consistent finding, may be characterized by hemoglobin levels as low as 5.5 g/100 mL. Pathogenesis is obscure: the bone marrow is neither suppressed nor hyperplastic, and hemorrhage rarely is extensive. It is postulated that it is primarily the result of hemodilution.

References

Seawright AA, Everist SL, Hrdlicka J. Comparative features of lantana, myosporum, and pimelea toxicities in livestock. In: Keeler RF, Tu AT, eds. Handbook of natural toxins. Vol 1. Plant and fungal toxins. New York: Marcel Dekker, 1983;511–541.

Seawright AA. Phlebectatic peliosis hepatis in Australian cattle. Vet Hum Toxicol 1984;26:208–213.

GROUP F: EXTENSIVE HEMORRHAGE
Dicoumarin

Sweet clover hay (not pasturage) contains a substance called coumarin, which not infrequently undergoes change into a related compound, known as dicoumarin or dicumarol. This substance is such a potent anticoagulant that it has been adopted as a drug for use when reduced coagulability of blood is desired, and has been utilized as a rat poison in the commercial product called warfarin. The anticoagulant action, although not completely understood, results primarily from depressing the synthesis of prothrombin and factors VII, IX, and X, all of which require vitamin K for formation. Vitamin K inhibits the anticoagulant effect, but apparently is not a complete antidote for poisoning. Interference with the synthesis of clotting factors results from the accumulation of a natural metabolite inhibitory to vitamin K (naphthoquinone [Vitamin K]-2, 3–epoxide). Normally, this epoxide is reduced to vitamin K, but in the presence of warfarin, the reductase is inhibited. Apparently capillary permeability is also affected by warfarin independently from anticoagulant activity. Loss of endothelial ground substances and organelles and degeneration of smooth muscle and elastic fibers have been described. Horses are not affected by this hay. Rabbits are susceptible and may be used to test the safety of a given supply of hay because they die from hemorrhage in a much shorter time than do cattle (6–12 days). Warfarin is poisonous to dogs (Fig. 15-12) and doubtless to all species.

Historically, the development of dicoumarin as an important anticoagulant drug started with the studies of Schofield on a new disease of cattle (1924). Schofield described this disease as manifest by large hemorrhages that occurred in animals recently fed hay made from sweet clover. He aptly named the disease sweet clover poisoning and correctly ascribed the signs and lesions to the anticoagulant effect of something in the sweet clover. Roderick demonstrated that this substance was water-soluble and easily extracted from sweet clover hay (1929,1931). Campbell and Link eventually isolated, crystallized, and identified the active ingredient as dicoumarin (1941).

Signs arise after cattle have consumed the poisonous hay for about one month, and consist of uncontrollable hemorrhage from accidental or operative wounds and slow internal hemorrhages as the result of bruises and minor injuries. Postmortem lesions take the form of "hematomas" in the subcutis, between the muscles, or beneath the capsules of organs. Ecchymoses occur in many places, commonly beneath the endocardium. The liver lobule is likely to contain petechiae and may undergo fatty change or hydropic degeneration. Necrosis and hyaline-droplet degeneration involve the renal tubules; scattered small foci of necrosis may be found in the heart.

Newborn calves may be affected because dicoumarin crosses the placenta, even though their dams do not manifest clinical signs at the time of parturition. This apparently results from a transient hypoprothrombinemia in calves, which is intensified by the transplacental passage of dicoumarin. Cows that produce such calves may be shown to be feeding on sweet clover hay, and the clotting time of their blood is prolonged.

References

Alstad AD, Casper HH, Johnson LJ. Vitamin K treatment of sweet clover poisoning in calves. J Am Vet Med Assoc 1985;187:729–731.

Bellah JR, Weigel JP. Hemarthrosis secondary to suspected warfarin toxicosis in a dog. J Am Vet Med Assoc 1983;182:1126–1127.

Benson ME, Casper HH, Johnson LJ. Occurrence and range of dicoumarol concentrations in sweet clover. Am J Vet Res 1981;42:2014–2015.

Campbell HA, Link KP. Studies on the hemorrhagic sweet clover disease. IV. The isolation and crystallization of the hemorrhagic agent. J Biol Chem 1941;138:21–33.

Cohen AJ. Critical review of the toxicology of coumarin with special reference to interspecies differences in metabolism and hepatotoxic response and their significance to man. Food Cosmet Toxicol 1979;17:277–289.

Osuna O, Edds GT. Toxicology of aflatoxin B1, warfarin, and cadmium in young pigs: [1] Performance and hematology. [2] Clinical chemistry and blood coagulation. [3] Metal residues and pathology. Am J Vet Res 1982;43:1380–1386, 1387–1394, 1395–1400.

Pritchard DG, Markson LM, Brush PJ, et al. Haemorrhagic syndrome of cattle associated with the feeding of sweet vernal (Anthoxan-

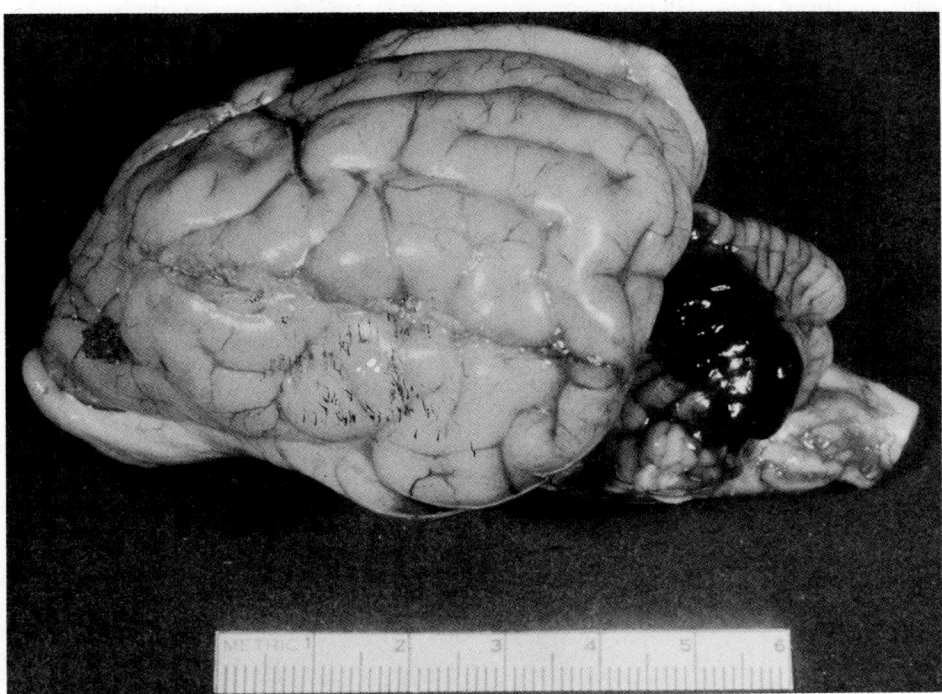

FIG. 15-12 Hemorrhage in the leptomeninges due to warfarin (dicoumarin) poisoning in a 15–year-old male mongrel collie. (Courtesy of Angell Memorial Animal Hospital.)

thum odoratum) hay containing dicoumarol. Vet Rec 1983;113:78–84.

Roderick LM. The pathology of sweet clover disease in cattle. J Am Vet Med Assoc 1929;74:314–324.

Roderick LM. A problem in the coagulation of the blood. "Sweet clover disease in cattle." Am J Physiol 1931;96:413.

Stahmann MA, Huebner CF, Link KP. Studies on the sweet clover disease. V. Identification and synthesis of the hemorrhagic agent. J Biol Chem 1941;138:513–527.

Schofield FW. Damaged sweet clover: the cause of a new disease in cattle simulating hemorrhagic septicemia and blackleg. J Am Vet Med Assoc 1924;64:553–575.

Bracken fern

Fern plants grow in most humid parts of the world and poisoning of cattle by them has been reported from the eastern and far northwestern United States, Central Europe, Great Britain, Central and South America, the Middle East, Southern India, Java, the Philippines, Australia, and New Zealand. The predominant fern species in the United States is *Pteridium aquilinum* (syn. *Pteris aquilina*). In New Zealand, only one species is recognized, *Pteridium esculantum,* but in Australia the important species is *Cheilanthus sieberi.* Each of these plant species contains varying amounts of ptaquiloside, a norsesquiterpenoid glycoside, which is capable of inducing toxic and carcinogenic effects of fresh or dried bracken fern. Illness appears after the plant has been consumed for several months. The manifestations of braken fern poisoning in ruminants (sheep, cattle) differ from those seen in monogastric animals (horse, rat, mouse).

In cattle and sheep, bracken fern causes severe hypoplasia or aplasia of the hematopoietic tissue, to which most signs and lesions can be ascribed. The illness may start suddenly with high fever, hemorrhage from any and often several body openings, delayed clotting time, thrombocytopenia, neutropenia, anemia, and death in one to three days. Diarrhea or upper respiratory inflammation may be noted. Hemorrhage results from thrombocytopenia, as well as increased levels of anticoagulant substances in blood. Secondary infection follows neutropenia, resulting in high fever. Under experimental conditions, as long as 15 months may be required before signs of toxicity ensue. The acute, and usually terminal, episode may occur weeks after removal from access to the plant. The active principle responsible for the depression of bone marrow has not been identified.

Experimental evidence supports the idea that bovine enzootic hematuria is a part of the syndrome resulting from poisoning by bracken fern. Prolonged feeding of bracken fern to cattle is followed by lesions in the bladder and generalized hemorrhagic syndrome.

Autopsy lesions include widespread petechiae and ecchymoses, especially on the heart and other serous surfaces, on mucous membranes, and in muscles and subcutaneous tissues. Abomasal ecchymoses in cattle may lead to ulceration. The large bowel often contains clotted blood. Necrotic areas in liver have been described by some. Thrombocytopenia is marked and is the cause of hemorrhages. Neutropenia and terminal anemia accompany thrombocytopenia and are due to destruction of early myeloid cells. Megakaryocytes disappear.

Lesions in the urinary system most often involve the bladder, but may also occur in the ureters or renal pelvis, and appear to represent a chronic but violently hyperplastic and hemorrhagic inflammation that leads to frank neoplasia. The transitional epithelium undergoes localized proliferation with metaplasia to mucinous columnar or stratified squamous types or a mixture of the two (Fig. 15-13). In many cases, the hyperplastic epithelium acquires neoplastic properties, developing into a squamous cell or adenocarcinoma, which is locally invasive and may metastasize to the regional lymph nodes and lungs. Capillaries of the inflammatory lesion also participate in hyperplasia, sometimes to the extent of forming hemangiomas in the stroma or projecting from the mucosal surface. These hemangiomas may be the source of much of the hemorrhage into the urine, and are capable of developing malignant qualities.

The carcinogenic properties of bracken fern have been demonstrated experimentally in cattle as well as laboratory animals, in which a variety of neoplasms have resulted, including intestinal adenocarcinomas in rats and quail, malignant lymphoma and pulmonary adenomas in mice, and bladder tumors in guinea pigs.

In Great Britain, bracken fern has been associated with a form of retinal atrophy in sheep known as bright blindness. The condition, which has been experimentally reproduced, develops in the absence of the changes just described. It is characterized by loss of rods and cones and reduction in the width of the outer nuclear layer. Lesions are most extensive in the tapetal region, and when advanced, the layer of rods and cones and outer nuclear layer are destroyed. The factor responsible has not been identified.

In differential diagnosis, hemorrhage in sweet clover poisoning is large, with hematomas often forming in the tissues, but with no accompanying fever. Blood transfusions are promptly curative in sweet clover poisoning. In crotalaria poisoning, hemorrhages may have no differential features, but the liver usually undergoes considerable fibrosis, the gallbladder is distended, and edema of the abomasal and duodenal tissues often occurs. In poisoning by trichloroethylene-extracted soybean meal, hemorrhage and anemia are the principal lesions, and differentiation may depend on the history. Anaplasmosis must be considered, but can usually be distinguished by the large spleen and by finding the causative organism in the erythrocytes. Leptospirosis causes fever and hemorrhage, but the latter is much less extensive. Icterus is present with both of these infections. Demonstration of a high serologic titer or of the leptospirae in the kidney or liver by silver techniques is decisive. In none of the above conditions, except at one stage of leptospirosis, is neutropenia comparable to that of bracken poisoning.

In horses and experimental rats, the usual bracken poisoning is cured by administration of thiamine, but this is not effective in cattle. Thiaminase appears to be one of the active toxic principles. Presumably cattle syn-

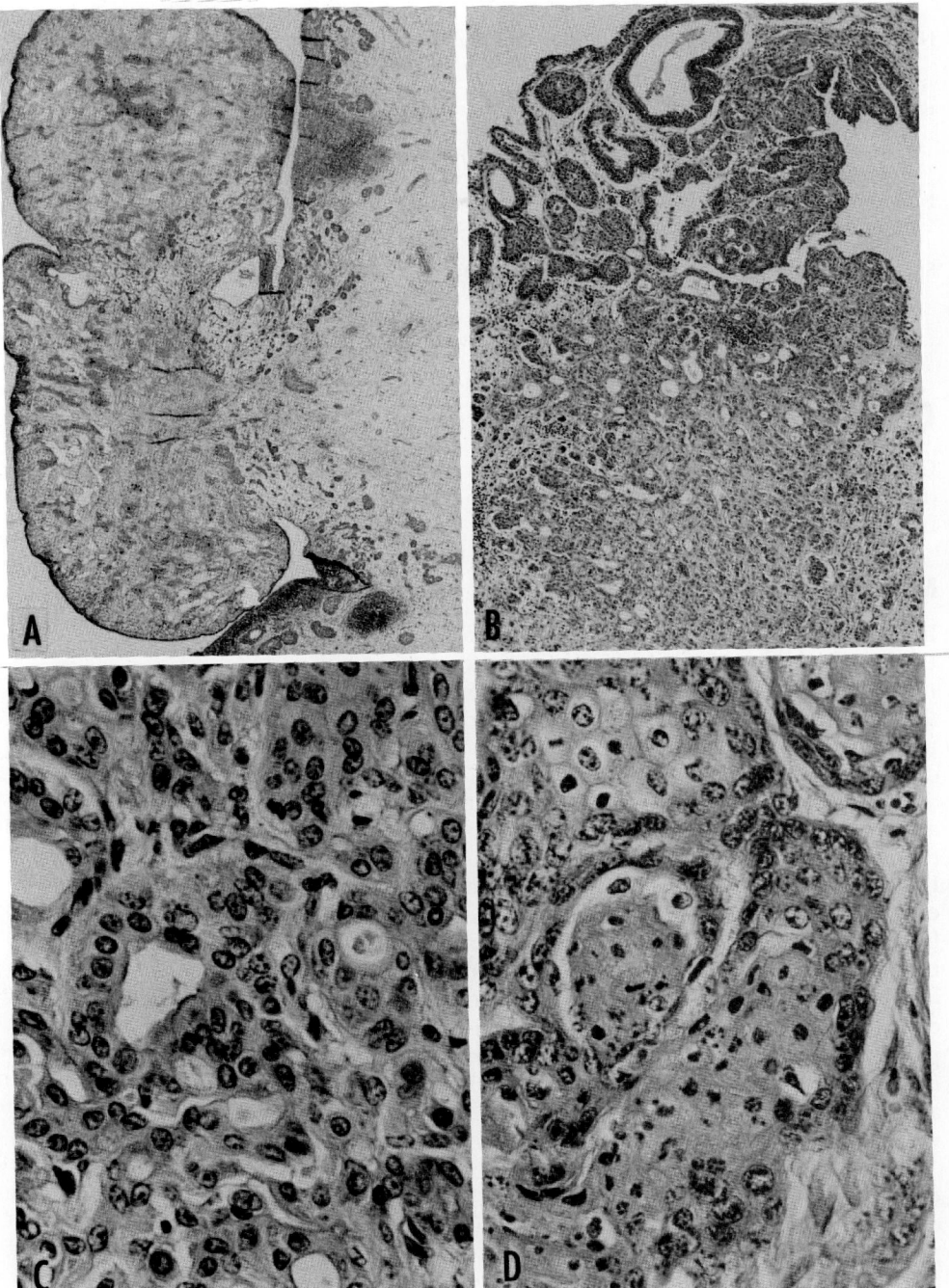

FIG. 15-13 Bovine enzootic hematuria. **A.** Papillomatous hemangioma in the urinary bladder (×24). **B.** Neoplastic transformation in the urinary bladder (×50) with transitional cell carcinoma and adenocarcinoma in juxtaposition. **C.** Adenocarcinoma (×350), higher magnification of B. **D.** Squamous cell carcinoma (×350) in bovine urinary bladder. (A, C, and D courtesy of Armed Forces Institute of Pathology; contributor: Dr. Sati Baran.)

thesize adequate thiamine and other B-vitamins, and the toxicity of the bracken fern is based upon other actions. In horses, therefore, bracken poisoning is similar to poisoning by equisetum and the lesions are those of thiamine deficiency. Affected horses become incoordinated and ataxic, develop tremors, may fall, and ultimately are recumbent. Although thrombocytopenia and depression of other hematopoietic elements are evident, neuropathologic sequelae overshadow these lesions. Presumably the hematopoietic changes are based

upon the same toxic principles as in cattle, but their relationship to thiamine deficiency is not resolved. In swine, focal myocardial necrosis, comparable to that caused by thiamine deficiency in this and other species, has been described in experimentally poisoned animals.

References

Chick BF, Carroll SN, Kennedy C, et al. Some biochemical features of an outbreak of polioencephalomalacia in sheep. Aust Vet J 1981;57:251–252.

Hirono I, et al. Separation of carcinogenic fraction of bracken fern. Cancer Lett 1984;21:239.

Hirono I, et al. Reproduction of acute bracken poisoning in a calf with ptaquiloside, a bracken constituent. Vet Rec 1984;115:375–378.

Kinghorn AD. Carcinogenic and cocarcinogenic toxins from plants. In: Keeler RF, Tu AT, eds. Handbook of natural toxins. Vol 1. Plant and fungal toxins. New York: Marcel Dekker, 1983;239–298.

Pamukcu AM, Milli U, Bryan GT. Protective effect of nicotinamide on bracken fern induced carcinogenicity in rats. Nutr Cancer 1981;3:86–93.

Smith BL, Embling PP, Lauren DR, et al. Carcinogenicity of Pteridium esculentum and Cheilanthes sieberi in Australia and New Zealand. In: James LF, Keeler RF, Bailey EM Jr, Cheeke PR, Hegarty MP, eds. Poisonous plants: Proc 3rd Int Symp. Ames: Iowa State Univ Press, 1992.

GROUP G: ANEMIA

Clearly, most poisonings characterized by hemorrhage, discussed in the preceding group, are also characterized by anemia.

Molybdenum

In Florida, California, and other areas of the western United States and England, certain muck or shale soils ("teart" soils in England) contain enough molybdenum that green pasture plants, but not cured hay, contain toxic amounts of the element. Ruminants are almost exclusively affected, principally cattle.

Signs include unthriftiness or emaciation, a faded and rough hair coat, apathy, anemia, foul and gaseous diarrhea, sterility, and evidence of painful locomotion. Lesions include hypochromic, microcytic anemia, and emaciation. Enlargement of the epiphyses of the long bones and of the costochondral articulations, comparable to those of ordinary rickets, may occur in the young; in older animals, rarefaction of bone occurs with susceptibility to fractures. Aspermatogenesis, likely to be permanent, occurs in bulls; in cows, reversible cessation of ovarian function is present. Among the progeny of affected animals, an unusually high percentage of developmental anomalies occurs.

Chemically, molybdenum appears to facilitate the excretion of phosphorus, which may be the mechanism of the disorders of bone, although the levels of blood phosphorus and calcium are usually normal. Molybdenum poisoning usually occurs in animals whose intake of copper is low, and for reasons unknown, increasing copper in the diet (copper sulfate, 1–2 g daily) prevents the deleterious effects of a surprising amount of molybdenum. Copper deficiency has also been noticed to have a more pronounced effect in the presence of molybdenum in the bovine diet. It is possible that the anemia given as a characteristic of molybdenum poisoning is due to lack of utilizable copper.

References

Britton JW, Goss H. Chronic molybdenum poisoning in cattle. J Am Vet Med Assoc 1947;108:176–178.

Cook GA, et al. Interrelationship of molybdenum and certain factors to the development of the molybdenum toxicity syndrome. J Anim Sci 1966;25:96–101.

Gardner AW, Hall-Patch PK. An outbreak of industrial molybdenosis. Vet Rec 1962;74:113–116.

Muir WR. The teart pastures of Somerset. Vet J 1941;97:387–400.

Naphthalene

Poisoning by naphthalene (naphthol, not naphtha) has occurred in humans from the accidental ingestion of mothballs, and in dogs experimentally. Although symptoms include anorexia and nausea, the principal effect is the destruction within a few days of a majority of erythrocytes with hemoglobinuria and hemolytic jaundice. The liver and kidneys develop toxic degenerative changes. The contrast with the pathologic effects of chlorinated naphthalenes is interesting.

References

Abelson SM, Henderson AT. Moth ball poisoning. U.S. Armed Forces Med J 1951;2:491–493.

Zuelzer WW, Apt L. Acute hemolytic anemia due to naphthalene poisoning. J Am Med Assoc 1949;141:185–190.

Onions

In onion-growing districts, it is not unusual for cattle and sheep to be given cull or unsalable onions (*Allium cepa*) as a major part of their diet. Even when somewhat decomposed, onions appear to be palatable and commonly harmless. Nevertheless, poisoning, often fatal, does occur unexpectedly in these animals and in horses and experimentally in dogs. Wild onions (*A. canadense, A. validum*) are also toxic and occasionally poison horses, cattle, and sheep grazing on pastures containing these plants. The toxic principle (hemolysin) of onions is n-propyl disulfide, which alters glucose-6-phosphatase, resulting in denaturation and precipitation of hemoglobin.

Both symptoms and lesions can be summarized as hemolytic anemia, hemolytic icterus, and hemoglobinuria. Signs may arise within a few days of consuming the onions; anemia, as estimated by hemoglobin determinations, may be extreme, but clinical recovery occurs in a few days when the animal, not yet moribund, is given a change in diet. The breath, urine, and tissues have a strong odor of onions, making diagnosis easy. Several species of wild onions exist and have the same propensities, but animals are not likely to get sufficient quantities to do more than flavor the milk, in the case of dairy cows. Experimental feeding of one species of wild onion (*Allium validum*) to pregnant ewes resulted in loss of appetite and weight, plus depression of erythropoietic tissues, but had no effect on fetal development.

References

Gill FA, Sergeant ESG. Onion poisoning in a bull. Aust Vet J 1981;57:484.

Harvey JW, Rackear D. Experimental onion-induced hemolytic anemia in dogs. Vet Pathol 1985;22:387–392.

Kirk JH, Bulgin MS. Effects of feeding cull domestic onions (Allium cepa) to sheep. Am J Vet Res 1979;40:397–399.

GROUP H: METHEMOGLOBINEMIA

Poisons in Group H are characterized by production of methemoglobin with chocolate-colored blood and the associated inability of hemoglobin to function as a carrier of oxygen.

Nitrates and nitrites

Humans, as well as animals, have been poisoned by drinking or ingesting with the food, water containing nitrates in solution. Such water always comes from shallow, surface wells (or possibly from ponds or pools). Water causing poisoning usually contains 1000–3000 ppm of nitrate; however, because the presence of nitrates indicates organic pollution, water containing any amount of nitrate is undesirable even if within the limits of chemical safety. Another possible source of poisoning is the swallowing of lubricating oil to which nitrites have been added by the manufacturer. This has happened in a human. The release of nitric oxide and nitrogen dioxide from automobile exhausts and other combustion sources provides another means of exposure. Herbivorous animals will also lick or eat commercial fertilizers left on their food supply and are poisoned by nitrates contained therein. Sheep are especially prone to eat such salty-tasting compounds, even when adequately supplied with sodium chloride. "Salting the range" was the spreading of salt-petre (potassium nitrate) in places where sheep would eat it, a practice which pioneers are said to have used in an effort to drive sheep-raisers and their flocks from an area of free range in the public domain of the then unsettled western United States.

The usual source of nitrate and nitrite poisoning in veterinary practice is from plants, growing or cured, which have derived large amounts of nitrate, chiefly KNO_3, from soil excessively rich in that substance. Among plants that have been found occasionally to contain poisonous amounts of nitrates are oats, either green, as hay, straw or stubble, barley, wheat, millets, flax, cornstalks (maize), sorghums, sugar-beet leaves, and a number of weeds, including pigweed (*Amaranthus retroflexus*) and variegated (or "bull") thistle (*Silybum marianum*). Some species of Astragalus that synthesize aliphatic nitro compounds may also cause nitrite poisoning. Astragalus species are also the cause of locoweed poisoning and selenium poisoning. The application of weed killers such as "2, 4–D," 2, 4–dichlorophenoxyacetic acid, sometimes causes a marked increase in the nitrate content of some plants, such as sugar beets, the harvested leaves of which are a standard feed for ruminants. The sorghums, of course, are noted for the development of hydrocyanic acid, but occasionally appear to have been poisonous through an excessive content of nitrate. To what extent the frequent "corn-stalk poisoning" has been poisoning by nitrates is a difficult question, but evidence indicates that some of the outbreaks may be linked to them.

Nitrates are irritants to the kidneys and urinary tract; potassium nitrate was at one time used as a diuretic. Poisoning by ingestion of excessive amounts of this chemical results in severe hemolytic anemia despite active hematopoiesis, as well as toxic injury to the renal parenchyma. Localized gastroenteritis occurs, and probably because of sensations originating in the gastrointestinal disorder, dogs show mental disturbances and depression. Decomposition of nitrate into nitrite is insignificant, and consequently methemoglobinemia is minimal or absent.

Quite the opposite is true of nitrates contained in tissues of plants. In the presence of moisture and possibly with the aid of bacteria, phytogenous nitrates are easily reduced to nitrites (and eventually to ammonia). This occurs either in the stomach, and especially the rumen, or externally, as in stacks of hay that have become wet from rain or snow. In certain experiments, the process (in oat hay) reaches a maximum in 20 hours after the application of moisture. Poisoning from excessive nitrates in the various plants, hay, and straw, then, is poisoning by nitrites, the principal effect of which is the formation of methemoglobin, sometimes from more than half of the total hemoglobin. The process involves transformation of the Fe atom from the ferrous to the ferric state, and hemoglobin so deranged has no oxygen-carrying capacity. Nitrites also markedly dilate the arterioles, thereby lowering blood pressure and accelerating the pulse.

Lethality of ingested nitrates is influenced by the manner and rate of administration. The LD_{50} for nitrate fed to cattle with forage is about 45 g/100 pounds of body weight. About one-third of this amount would produce lethality when administered in a drench.

Signs of nitrite poisoning that have attracted most attention include cyanosis, dyspnea, extremely rapid pulse (150/minute), great weakness and recumbency, diarrhea, and voiding of colorless urine every few minutes. Some mention terminal convulsions, but coma seems to be more usual.

The outstanding lesion is the dark, brownish color of the blood, the effect of methemoglobin. It is commonly described as chocolate-colored, but this must not be taken too literally. Clotting remains approximately normal. The mucous membranes are cyanotic, except those of the stomach and intestines, which is seen more or less hyperemia and inflammation. A few petechiae may appear, as in most anoxemias. Blood-stained pericardial fluid is a frequent finding. Discoloration of blood should be diagnostic, but tests for methemoglobin can be performed, remembering that small amounts are demonstrable in healthy cattle.

References

Burrows GE. Nitrate intoxication. J Am Vet Med Assoc 1980;177:82–83.

McFarland PJ, McRory FJ, Bell N, et al. Nitrite poisoning in pigs. Vet Rec 1980;106:201–202.

Nicholls TJ, Miles EJ. Nitrate/nitrite poisoning of cattle on ryegrass pasture. Aust Vet J 1980;56:95–96.

Troxler J. Intoxication mortelle de 19 gáenisses par la moutard jaune (Sinapis alba L.). [Fatal poisoning of 19 heifers fed fresh white mustard (Sinapis alba L.).] Schweiz Arch Tierheilkd 1981;123:495–497 [Vet Bull 1982;52:1315].

Williams MC, James LF. Effects of herbicides on the concentration of poisonous compounds in plants: a review. Am J Vet Res 1983;44:2420–2422.

Wood PA. The molecular pathology of chronic nitrate intoxication in domestic animals: a hypothesis. Vet Hum Toxicol 1980;22:26–27.

Chlorates

Sodium chlorate, a strong oxidizing agent, is used to kill noxious weeds, being sprayed on the foliage and on the ground in a concentration amounting to 4 pounds/ sq. rod (72 g/M^2). Trials indicate that animals are neither poisoned by eating any ordinary amount of sprayed foliage, especially when a few days have elapsed since the spraying, nor from the soil. Poisoning has occurred when animals accidentally gained access to supplies of the chemical, which is palatable because of its salty taste. The minimum lethal dose for sheep and probably for other farm mammals approximates 2–3 g/ kg of body weight, death ensuing in 6–48 hours.

Signs include somnolence and dyspnea, the temperature being normal. When small, sublethal amounts are ingested over a period of time, icterus and a dark or brownish discoloration of the conjunctivae can be expected. Postmortem lesions include methemoglobinemia. The musculature is dark or almost black, cut surfaces becoming somewhat lighter on exposure to air. Blood is dark or blackish, but clots readily. The liver is almost black; the lungs have the color of normal liver. The heart is flabby and dark. The spleen is dark but not enlarged. The abomasum contains ulcerated areas that are black; all other parts of the alimentary tract were without lesions. In addition to these changes, hemolytic anemia has been described in dogs. Concentrations of the chemical in ingesta or blood are too slight to respond to ordinary chemical tests.

References

McCulloch EC, Murer HK. Sodium chlorate poisoning. J Am Vet Med Assoc 1939;95:675–682.

Moore GR. Sodium chlorate poisoning in cattle. J Am Vet Med Assoc 1941;99:50–52.

Sheahan BJ, Pugh DM, Winstanley EW. Experimental sodium chlorate poisoning in dogs. Res Vet Sci 1971;12:387–389.

GROUP I: CARBOXYHEMOGLOBINEMIA

These poisons produce carboxyhemoglobin and inability of blood to transport oxygen.

Carbon monoxide

An important form of poisoning in humans, carbon monoxide (CO) poisoning, in veterinary practice, is ordinarily limited to pet animals which may chance to be confined in houses or basements where defective heating equipment may permit accidental accumulation of the gas.

Signs include incoordination and ataxia, vomiting, involuntary urination and defecation, and unconsciousness. In humans, fatal drowsiness often overcomes victims so stealthily that they are unaware of the danger. The one salient and usually diagnostic lesion is the bright cherry-red color of blood and tissues. This color is due to the formation of carboxyhemoglobin. The CO radical replaces the O of hemoglobin, which has greater affinity for CO. Inability of blood to transport oxygen leads to fatal asphyxia. When death occurs quickly, few or no lesions of significance are encountered aside from petechiae on serosal surfaces and white matter of the cerebral hemispheres. In patients surviving several days, bilateral necrosis of cerebral white matter, basal ganglia, and cortical gray matter (laminar necrosis) occurs, which may be visible grossly. In humans, focal subendocardial myocardial necrosis has also been described. Leuko- and polioencephalopathy are believed to result primarily from hypoxia, but acidosis may also play a role in pathogenesis. Lesions are not pathognomonic and may be encountered in other conditions characterized by hypoxia. Diagnosis should be based upon analysis for carboxyhemoglobin.

Reference

Dominick MA, Carson TL. Effects of carbon monoxide exposure on pregnant sows and their fetuses. Am J Vet Res 1983;44:35–40.

Cyanides

Although accidents with chemical preparations of cyanides are possible, the usual cause of cyanide poisoning in animals is ingestion of cyanogenic plants, such as sorghums of all kinds, Sudan, Johnson, arrow, and velvet grasses, African or giant star grass (*Cynodon plectostachyum*), a plant of Australia and certain southern parts of Africa, flax, suckleya (*Suckleya suckleyana*), reed sweetgrass (*Poa aquatica*), hydrangea, wild or domesticated members of the cherry family (including cherry pits eaten by chickens), and a number of others.

Many plants (about 2000 species) have been demonstrated to produce biological precursors of hydrogen cyanide, mostly in the form of cyanogenic glycosides that liberate cyanide when the plant is mascerated. In the single plant family Sapindaceae, cyanogenic lipids also occur. When the cyanogenic plant is macerated, specific β-glucosidase enzymes, normally in separate compartments of the plant, come in contact with the cyanogenic glycosides and accelerate the release of hydrogen cyanide. Known cyanogenic glycosides currently number 29. Their identification and synthesis is an interesting and continuing saga in chemistry.

Death may be instantaneous, but usually effects last for some minutes or an hour. The animal falls, with convulsions, frothing at the mouth, unconsciousness, and infrequent gasping respirations. Pupils are dilated and involuntary defecation and micturition occur. Respiration ceases while the heart still beats. Acute cases are without lesions in the organs, but a bright red, arterial color of the venous blood is a diagnostic change. It is seen best by putting a small amount of blood over a dark background; the bright red persists for several hours despite drying. The proverbial odor of almonds or cherry pits is seldom detectable. Seldom any erosion or inflammation of the alimentary mucosa is evident. In animals surviving longer or repeatedly exposed to cyanide, focal necrosis of gray and white matter in brain may be seen. Lesions are similar to those of carbon monoxide poisoning and are believed to result from hypoxia.

Poison acts by preventing the intracellular oxidative process, although blood does not lack for oxygen. This action is the reason for the bright red blood, which is prevented from losing its oxygen to the tissues.

Ruminants may convert cyanide to the less toxic thiocyanate, which is goitrogenic.

References

Egekeze JO, Oeme FW. Cyanides and their toxicity: a literature review. Vet Q 1980;2:104–114.

Majak W, McDiarmid RE, Hall JW. The cyanide potential of Saskatoon serviceberry (Amelanchier alnifolia) and chokecherry (Prunus virginiana). Can J Anim Sci 1981;61:681–686.

Shaw JM. Suspected cyanide poisoning in two goats caused by the ingestion of crab apple leaves and fruits. Vet Rec 1986;119:242–243.

Telles I, Johnson D, Nagel RL, et al. Neurotoxicity of sodium cyanate: new pathological and ultrastructural observations in Macaca nemestrina. Acta Neuropathol (Berl) 1979;47:75–79.

Vennesland B, et al. Cyanide metabolism. Fed Proc 1982;41:2639–2648.

Webber JJ, Roycroft CR, Callinan JD. Cyanide poisoning in goats from sugar gums (Eucalyptus cladocalyx). Aust Vet J 1985;62:28.

GROUP J: EDEMA

Poisons in Group J cause marked and conspicuous edema.

α-Naphthyl thiourea

α-Naphthyl thiourea (ANTU) is popular for killing rats; it is usually mixed with meat or grain for that purpose. It was originally heralded as not dangerous to dogs because it was believed they would rid themselves of the substance by vomiting. Experience has proved otherwise, in spite of the fact that vomition does occur. Symptoms include cardiac and respiratory embarrassment, with imperceptible but rapid pulse and rapid, shallow respiration. Vomitus is frothy and may become bloody. Diarrhea is severe, becoming bloody. Weak and comatose, the dog commonly lies in the sternal recumbent position, fluid from the lungs often running out from the mouth. The temperature becomes markedly subnormal before death. As a rule, all this transpires and death occurs in one to four hours after the ANTU is eaten.

Postmortem lesions of poisoning by ANTU are practically diagnostic. Hydrothorax is present in nearly all cases. When the thorax is opened carefully and without contaminating hemorrhage from the vessels, it is found to be full to overflowing with clear, watery fluid. Extremely severe edema of the lungs occurs almost without exception, fluid often running out the trachea when the thoracic organs are raised posteriorly. The lungs also undergo severe congestion, with diapedesis of erythrocytes into numerous alveoli. In the stomach, the fundic mucosa is severely inflamed and reddened

in more than half the cases, moderately so in most of the remainder. Microscopically, the stomach has considerable mucous exudate, as well as hyperemia. The surface epithelium is intact, but the chief cells are inconspicuous in appearance and numbers as compared to the parietal cells. This catarrhal inflammation continues into the small intestine and subsides gradually in the large bowel. Considerable amounts of bile collect in the upper intestine, although the gallbladder is not completely emptied. The kidneys are severely congested, often deep red. In the cortex and some of the medullary rays, fatty change of the epithelial cells is demonstrable. In the liver, the light color of vacuolization and central necrosis alternates in spots with the red of acute congestion. Fatty change, however, is absent. The spleen is small and empty of blood.

Poisoning by ANTU has also occurred in horses through the accidental ingestion of poison bait.

References

Hesse FE, Loosli CG. The lining of the alveoli in mice, rats, dogs, and frogs following acute pulmonary edema produced by ANTU poisoning. Anat Rec 1949;105:299–324.

Jones LM, Smith DA, Smith HA. Alphanaphthyl (ANTU) thiourea poisoning in dogs. Am J Vet Res 1949;10:160–167.

Michel RR, Hakim TS, Smith TT, Poulsen RS. Quantitative morphology of permeability lung edema in dogs induced by alpha-naphthylthiourea. Lab Invest 1983;49:412–419.

GROUP K: PULMONARY DYSFUNCTION

Pulmonary dysfunction is the principal feature of rape, kale, stinkwood, and paraquat poisoning, and are included in this group.

Rape, kale, and other plants of genus brassica

The disease recognized as rape poisoning commonly appears in a herd 7–10 days after the cattle or sheep have been placed in a pasture of this kind. Luxuriant growth, wet weather, and possibly, frosting, appear to increase the danger.

This disease has many features of a syndrome of unknown etiology associated with moving cattle from sparse to lush pasture which may be made up of one or many plant species. This syndrome has been called by many names, including "fog fever," "atypical intestinal pneumonia," and "acute bovine respiratory edema and emphysema." The eventual development of anemia, icterus, hemoglobinemia, or hemoglobinuria may serve to distinguish poisoning caused by eating members of the Brassica genus. These plants include *Brassica napa* (rape), *B. rapsus* (turnip), and *B. oleracea* (varieties include cabbage, kale, Brussel sprouts, cauliflower). Some of these plants, or their seeds under particular conditions, contain glucosinolate and are goitrogenic.

Signs include the following:

1. More or less digestive disturbance, usually absence of peristalsis and constipation, occasionally the reverse with fetid diarrhea;

2. Respiratory difficulties including dyspnea with open mouth and a thumping sound at each respiration; and,

3. Gradually increasing anemia, usually with hemoglobinuria and mild icterus.

It is unknown whether the icterus is hemolytic or toxic. Anemia has been described as hyperchromic and macrocytic. Weakness, ataxia, and nervous abnormalities, as well as blindness, are also described. When the cow is recently postparturient, the condition has been found to be indistinguishable from the poorly understood disorder called puerperal hemoglobinuria.

Of the lesions, severe and destructive pulmonary emphysema, accompanied by congestion and edema and involving all parts of both lungs, is the most spectacular. Microscopically, rupture of the pulmonary alveoli is uniformly widespread, and both emphysema and edema also involve the interlobular septa. Emphysema of the mediastinal and even subcutaneous tissues also develops in some cases when pulmonary emphysema has existed for a few days. Hemorrhage may occur in the trachea and bronchi. Moderately acute toxic hepatitis is evident, shown chiefly by centrilobular necrosis. The gallbladder is regularly distended with viscid bile which is characteristic of alimentary inactivity.

The pathogenetic mechanisms have been the subject of considerable speculation and study. Some suspect that the condition has an allergic basis. Schofield has found in a number of instances a heavy invasion of the contents of the alimentary canal by *Clostridium perfringens,* with evidence of toxin similar to that of enterotoxemia that develops under other circumstances and is associated with other species of clostridia. The concept of a specific poisonous substance is supported, not only by the variety of lesions produced, but to some extent, by the fact that rape seed has been found poisonous to fowls. Wild cabbage *(Brassica oleracea)* has been reported as poisoning cattle when in the seed stage only. Rape-seed cake has a locally irritant action with the production of vesicles. (See also the pulmonary emphysema-adenomatosis syndrome.)

Experimentally feeding kale to cattle, sheep, and goats has regularly induced anemia.

References

Carlson JR, Breeze RG. Cause and prevention of acute pulmonary edema and emphysema in cattle. In: Keeler RF, Tu AT, eds. Handbook of natural toxins. Vol 1. Plant and fungal toxins. New York: Marcel Dekker, 1983;85–115.
Clegg FG, Evans RK. Haemoglobinemia of cattle associated with the feeding of Brassica species. Vet Rec 1962;74:1169–1176.
Cote FT. Rape poisoning in cattle. Can J Comp Med 1944;8:38–41.
Crawshaw HA. Rape blindness. Vet Rec 65:254 and Dalton PJ. Ibid. p. 298, 1953.
Evans ETR. Kale and rape poisoning in cattle. Vet Rec 1951;63:348–349.
Grant CA, et al. Kale anaemia in ruminants. II. Observations on kale fed sheep. Acta Vet Scand 1968;9:141–150.
Greenhalgh JFD, Sharman GAM, Aitken JN. Kale anaemia. I. The toxicity to various species of animal of three types of kale. Res Vet Sci 1969;10:64–72.
Greenhalgh JFD, Sharman GAM, Aitken JN. Kale anaemia. II. Further

factors concerned in the occurrence of the disease under experimental conditions. Res Vet Sci 1970;11:232–238.
Kellermaan TS, Coetzer JAW, Naude TW. Plant poisonings and mycotoxicosis of livestock in southern Africa. Cape Town: Oxford Univ Press, 1988.
Penny RHC, David JSE, Wright AI. Observations on the blood picture of cattle, sheep, and rabbits fed on kale. Vet Rec 1964;76:1053–1059.
Schofield FW. Acute pulmonary emphysema of cattle. J Am Vet Med Assoc 1948;112:254–259.
Stamp JT, Stewart J. Haemolytic anemia with jaundice in sheep. J Comp Pathol Ther 1953;63:48–52.
Tucker EM. The onset of anaemia and the production of haemoglobin C in sheep fed on kale. Br Vet J 1969;125:472–479.
VanEtten CH, Tookey HL. Glucosinolates in cruciferous plants. In: Keeler RF, Van Kampen KR, James LF, eds. Effects of poisonous plants on livestock. New York: 1978;507–520.

STINKWOOD

This is another Australian poisonous shrub *(Zieria arborescens)* that may cause death in cattle. The principal signs and lesions are related to massive pulmonary edema. The disease has been experimentally reproduced in rabbits.

References

Mundy BL: *Zieria arborescens* (stinkwood) intoxication in cattle. Aust Vet J 44:501–502, 1968.
Mundy BL, Cummings R, Wilson BJ: Experimental *Zieria arborescens* (stinkwood) poisoning in rabbits. Res Vet Sci 17:270–272, 1974.

Paraquat

Paraquat (1,1–dimethyl-4, 4–dipyridylium dichloride) is a broad-spectrum herbicide responsible for poisonings in humans and domestic animals. The lung is the principal site of injury. Following a single large dose, regardless of route, pulmonary edema and hemorrhage develop within hours and may lead to death. In animals that recover from a single exposure or experience repeated smaller exposures, paraquat induces fatal progressive interstitial inflammation and fibrosis of the lung. Based on experimental poisoning in rats, type I alveolar epithelial cells are target cells in acute and chronic poisoning. Type II cells are less affected, and proliferate to replace defects left by necrosis of type I cells. Endothelial cell damage contributes to acute edema and hemorrhage. The mechanism leading to progressive fibrosis is not understood. Alveoli contain numerous macrophages, of which many contain hemosiderin.

The clinical signs focus on pulmonary distress, but signs resulting from local contact toxicity to the oral cavity and gastrointestinal tract may be the first to be encountered. Oral and gastrointestinal tract ulcers may be present following acute toxicity. Signs related to renal and hepatic failure have been reported, and focal hepatic and renal necrosis have been described in some but not all experimental studies. Rabbits are relatively resistant to the pulmonary effects of paraquat.

References

Johnson RP, Huxtable CR. Paraquat poisoning in a dog and cat. Vet Rec 1976;98:189–191.

Murray RE, Gibson JE. A comparative study of paraquat intoxication in rats, guinea pigs and monkeys. Exp Mol Pathol 1972;17:317–325.

Webb DB. The pathophysiology of paraquat nephrotoxicity in the sheep. Clin Toxicol 1983;19:911–929.

GROUP L: BONES AND TEETH

Fluorine is the single poison included in this group and is characterized by lesions in bones and teeth.

Fluorine

Fluorosis may occur in chronic or acute forms.

CHRONIC FLUORINE POISONING

Chronic fluorosis occurs in animals receiving more than a minute amount of fluorine in the diet over a long period of time. The minimum amount of fluorine in the form of soluble fluorides required to produce evidence of injury in cattle and other farm animals is 1–2 mg/kg of body weight per day, or 12–27 ppm of the diet. As a partially soluble contaminant of rock phosphate, a somewhat larger amount may possibly be harmless. In humans, the amount tolerated without lesions (in the teeth) is said to be much less. Chronic poisoning of this nature occurs in animals eating pasturage or forage contaminated by air-borne residues from aluminum manufacturers, phosphate refineries, and similar industrial installations, or drinking well-water containing soluble fluorides to the extent of 10 ppm or more. In Iceland, fluorosis has been noted to follow volcanic eruptions. Following the Hekla eruption of May 5, 1970, volcanic ash was demonstrated to have up to 2000 ppm fluoride, and grass up to 4300 ppm fluoride. The concentration rapidly decreased, but remained at toxic levels for several weeks. When, as is commonly the case, both water and forage contain considerable amounts of fluorine, the safe level for water alone is less than the figure given.

CLINICAL MANIFESTATIONS

The clinical signs of chronic fluorine poisoning in cattle according to Shupe et al. (1964) include:

1. Mottling and abrasion of teeth;
2. Intermittent lameness;
3. Periosteal hyperostosis, demonstrable radiographically; and,
4. Demonstration of > 6 ppm of fluorine in urine.

In fluorosis, as much as 30 ppm of fluorine may be present in urine, depending upon the age of the animal, specific gravity of the urine and length of time the animal has ingested fluorine.

LESIONS

The pathognomonic lesions of chronic fluorine poisoning involve the teeth, bones, and possibly kidneys (Figs. 15-14 to 15-17). The principal changes in the teeth include "chalky" areas, "mottling," excessive attrition, and hypoplastic pitting of the enamel. The chalky areas have received this description because the enamel

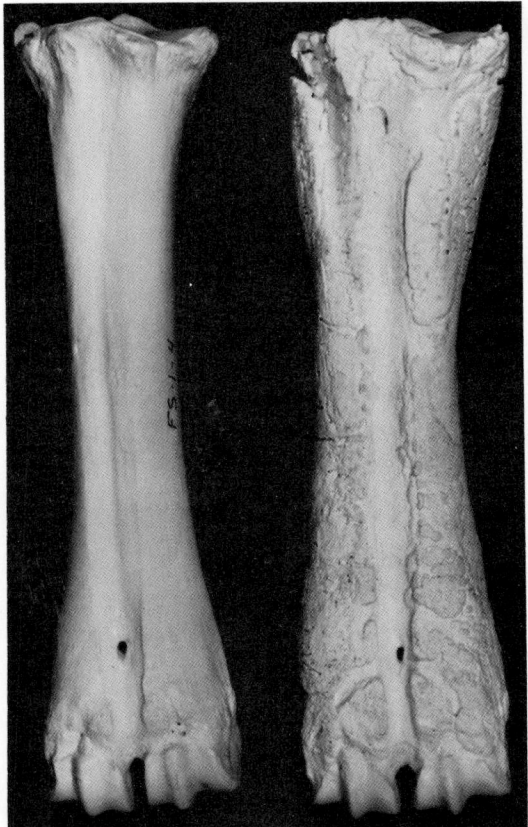

FIG. 15-14 Chronic bovine fluorosis. Left: normal metatarsal bone of a dairy cow after ingesting 12 ppm fluorine in the diet for about seven years. Right: hyperostosis and roughened periosteum of metatarsal bone of a dairy cow after consuming 93 ppm fluorine for approximately seven years. (Courtesy of Dr. J. L. Shupe and American Journal of Veterinary Research.)

has lost its shiny, translucent appearance and has assumed the dull, white opacity characteristic of chalk. Slight degrees of this condition are best detected by placing a light behind the tooth. The mottling consists of spots of yellow, brown, or greenish black. The pigmentation is in the enamel and cannot be removed, but may tend to be accentuated at the site of hypoplastic defects.

Excessive attrition results from abnormal softness of enamel and perhaps also of the dentine (Figs. 15-16, 15-17). Affected teeth are short because of rapid wear, which may reduce them to the level of the gums in the worst cases. The pitting consists of punctate or linear depressions on the side of the tooth due to deficient deposition of enamel at those places. The distribution of the hypoplastic "pits" may follow a horizontal pattern, considered to represent a chronologic period in the development of the tooth. Note that these dental lesions develop only when the fluorosis is present and active when the tooth is being formed. Once the tooth is fully formed, it is not affected by fluorosis. For this reason, the deciduous teeth do not develop lesions, and the permanent teeth which are formed earliest in life

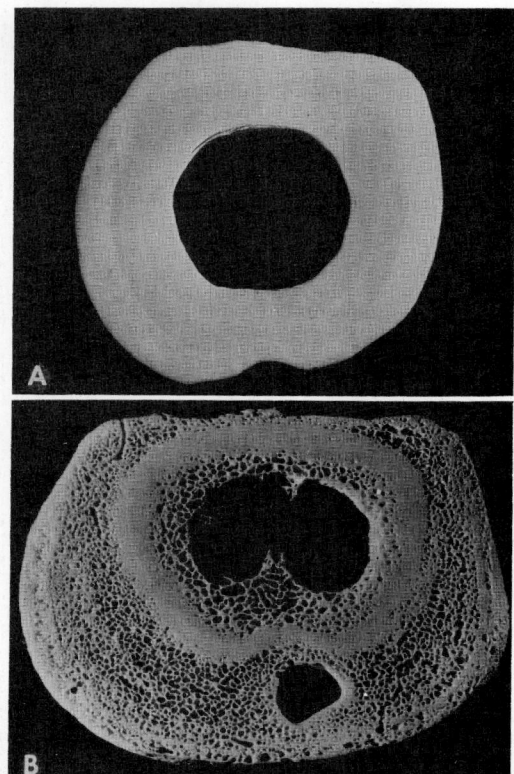

FIG. 15-15 Chronic bovine fluorosis, ground cross sections of metatarsus. **A.** Osteosclerosis in a cow which received slightly elevated levels of fluorine for several years. **B.** Osteoporosis with periosteal hyperostosis and endosteal resorption, in a cow which received high levels of fluorine in its diet for several years. (Courtesy of Dr. J. L. Shupe and Annals of New York Academy of Sciences.)

show the least damage. The more lateral incisors, as well as the later arriving molars and premolars, having been subjected to the fluorine over a longer period in most naturally occurring cases, are more worn and discolored than the older teeth, a situation contrary to the wear pattern of normal teeth.

Bony changes (Figs. 15-14, 15-15) are most pronounced in the metacarpals, metatarsals, and mandible, although all bones, like the teeth, store considerable amounts of fluoride and suffer from it. Bones become thicker and heavier than normal, the marrow cavity often being diminished in size, and the periosteal layer, in severe cases, is thickened. Microscopically, the bony trabeculae are thickened at the expense of the intertrabecular marrow spaces. The trabeculae have a dense appearance, with sharp, heavy outlines. However, it has been claimed that osteopetrotic changes, such as these, are due to calcium fluoride, but that sodium fluoride causes the opposite condition of osteoporosis. Another view concluded that osteosclerosis occurs in animals receiving low doses of fluorine over a long time (Shupe et al., 1964). Osteoporosis, with endosteal resorption and periosteal hyperostosis, conversely, is believed to result in animals receiving high doses of fluorine over a similarly prolonged period. The periosteal proliferation may result in microscopically demonstrable subperios-

teal thickening and often, in the more severely affected individuals, is accompanied by the formation of sessile exostoses, seldom more than 0.5 cm in length. These may be detectable clinically but, in company with the general periosteal disturbance, result in stiffness and lameness. Chemically bones of appreciably poisoned animals contain fluorine to the extent of 4000–15,000 ppm (1.5%). The concentration has been developed slowly over a period of years and could conceivably represent absorption of fluorine from environmental sources no longer present; the same, of course, is true of dental changes.

In the kidneys of experimental rats, degeneration and disintegration of the tubular epithelium, slight glomerular changes, thickened arterioles and terminal fibrosis are described. The fibrotic areas are radially arranged and are devoid of alkaline phosphatase. Polydipsia, polyuria, and poorly concentrated urine are concomitant signs.

The general health of the animal is not necessarily affected when mild dental changes are the only sign of fluorosis, but in more severe cases, signs appear, including lameness, anorexia, loss of weight, decreased production of milk, general unthriftiness, and perhaps intermittent diarrhea. Fluorine passes through the placenta and may accumulate in the bones of the fetus, but no significant direct effect upon fertility has been demonstrated.

The precise mechanisms involved in chronic fluorosis are unknown. One hypothesis is that fluoride ions replace hydroxyl radicals in the apatite crystal and that this results in abnormal osteoid. This, in turn, is believed to be responsible for the poor bony matrix, which is defective and irregularly mineralized. It is evident that osteoblastic activity is abnormal, as judged by the defective new bone and dentine.

Chronic fluorosis in the guinea pig has been identified as the underlying factor in a syndrome referred to in Australia as "slobbers." This descriptive name comes from the characteristic excessive salivation that results from abnormal teeth. The teeth grow irregularly, become elongated or wear excessively, and the enamel is eroded and often encrusted with tartar. The irregularly shaped teeth are believed to interfere with swallowing, resulting in drooling. Affected animals eventually die unless the diet is corrected. At necropsy, lesions in the teeth are most significant. Elevated levels of fluorine in bones of naturally and experimentally affected animals corroborate the diagnosis. Levels of up to 6700 ppm in naturally affected guinea pigs and over 5700 ppm in experimentally poisoned animals have been recorded, in contrast to levels of not greater than 160 ppm of fluorine in normal animals.

One source of fluorine in guinea pig feed appears to have been rock phosphate of high content used as a component of pelleted feed.

ACUTE FLUORINE POISONING

This type of poisoning results from accidents or the improper use of sodium fluoride, which is employed as a vermifuge in swine and externally for lice in poultry. It also occurs in dogs that eat dead rats poisoned by the

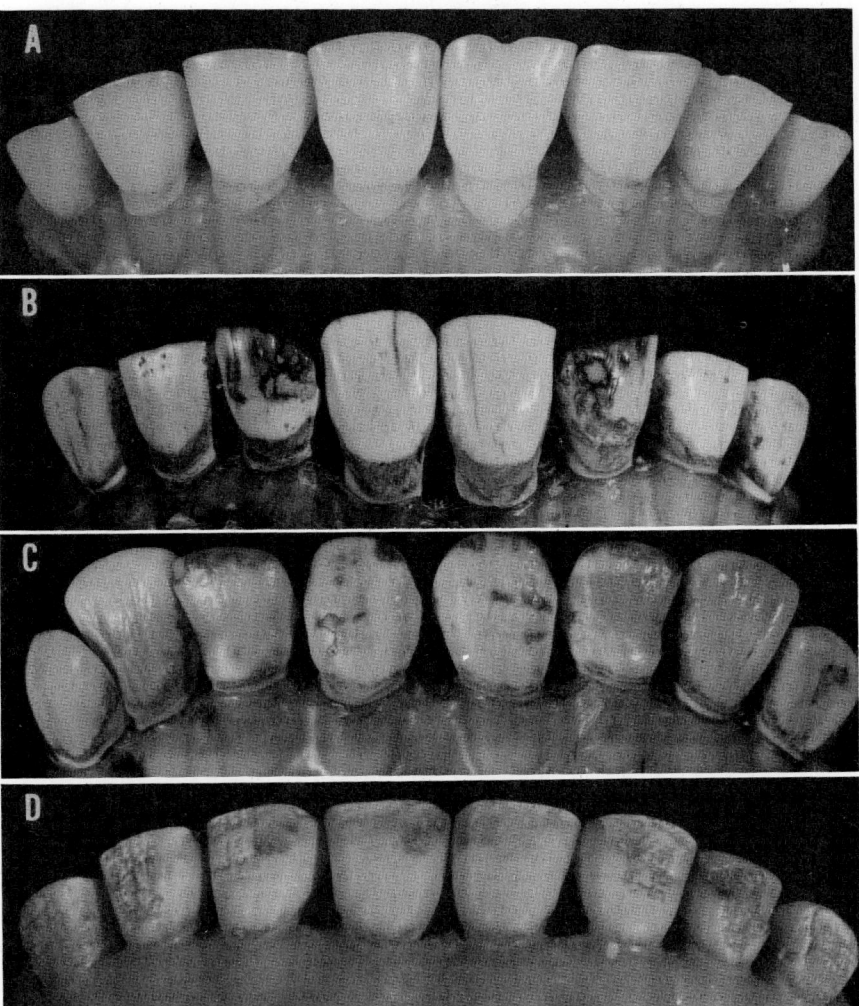

FIG. 15-16 Teeth in chronic bovine fluorosis. **A.** Normal incisors. **B-D.** Varying degrees of mottling of enamel of incisor teeth. (Courtesy of Dr. J. L. Shupe.)

rodenticide, sodium monofluoroacetate ("compounded 1080"), or when a domestic animal eats the bait directly. Lasting a few hours or a day or two, signs include extreme abdominal pain, convulsions, and frenzy alternating with weakness and lethargy. Diarrhea develops shortly. Collapse is followed by death from respiratory and myocardial arrest. Postmortem lesions include acute gastroenteritis.

The anesthetic agent methoxyflurane is recognized as nephrotoxic in humans and experimental animals. Prolonged exposure may lead to severe mitochondrial swelling and necrosis of proximal convoluted tubules mediated through inorganic fluoride released by metabolism of the anesthetic. Halothane, which is also a fluorinated anesthetic agent, is also recognized as nephrotoxic, but to a much lesser degree. In humans, repeated exposure to halothane may, in a small number of patients, result in acute hepatic necrosis. This is believed to result from an "allergic" basis and is not related to fluoride poisoning. Fluorinated hydrocarbons used in aerosol propellants (freons) have generally been considered to be inert. Recently, cardiac irregularities that may lead to death have been associated with these agents. The mechanism of action is not known.

References

Atkinson FF, Hard GC. Chronic fluorosis in the guinea-pig. Nature 1966;211:429–430.

Bond AM, Murray MM. Kidney functions and structure in chronic fluorosis. Br J Exp Pathol 1952;33:168–176.

Egyed MN, Shupe JL. Experimental acute fluoroacetamide poisoning in sheep and dogs. I. Symptomatology and pathology. Fluoride 1971;4:129–136.

Krook L, Maylin GA. Industrial fluoride pollution. Chronic fluoride poisoning in Cornwall Island cattle. Cornell Vet 1979;69(Suppl 8):1–70.

Maylin GA, Eckerlin RH, Krook L. Fluoride intoxication in dairy calves. Cornell Vet 1987;77:84–98.

Milhaud GE, Borbe MA, Krishnaswamy S. Effect of fluoride ingestion on dental fluorosis in sheep. Am J Vet Res 1987;48:873–879.

Schultz RA, Coetzer JAW, Kellerman TS, et al. Observations on the clinical cardiac and histopathologic effects of fluoroacetate in sheep. Onderstepoort J Vet Res 1982;49:237–245.

Shore D, et al. Aluminum-fluoride complexes: preclinical studies. J Environ Pathol Toxicol Oncol 1985;6:9–13.

Shupe JL, Eanes ED, Leone NC. Effects of excessive exposure to sodium fluoride on composition and crystallinity of equine bone tumors. Am J Vet Res 1981;42:1040–1042.

Shupe JL, et al. Relative effects of feeding hay atmospherically contaminated by fluoride residue, normal hay plus calcium fluoride, and normal hay plus sodium fluoride to dairy heifers. Am J Vet Res 1962;23:777–787.

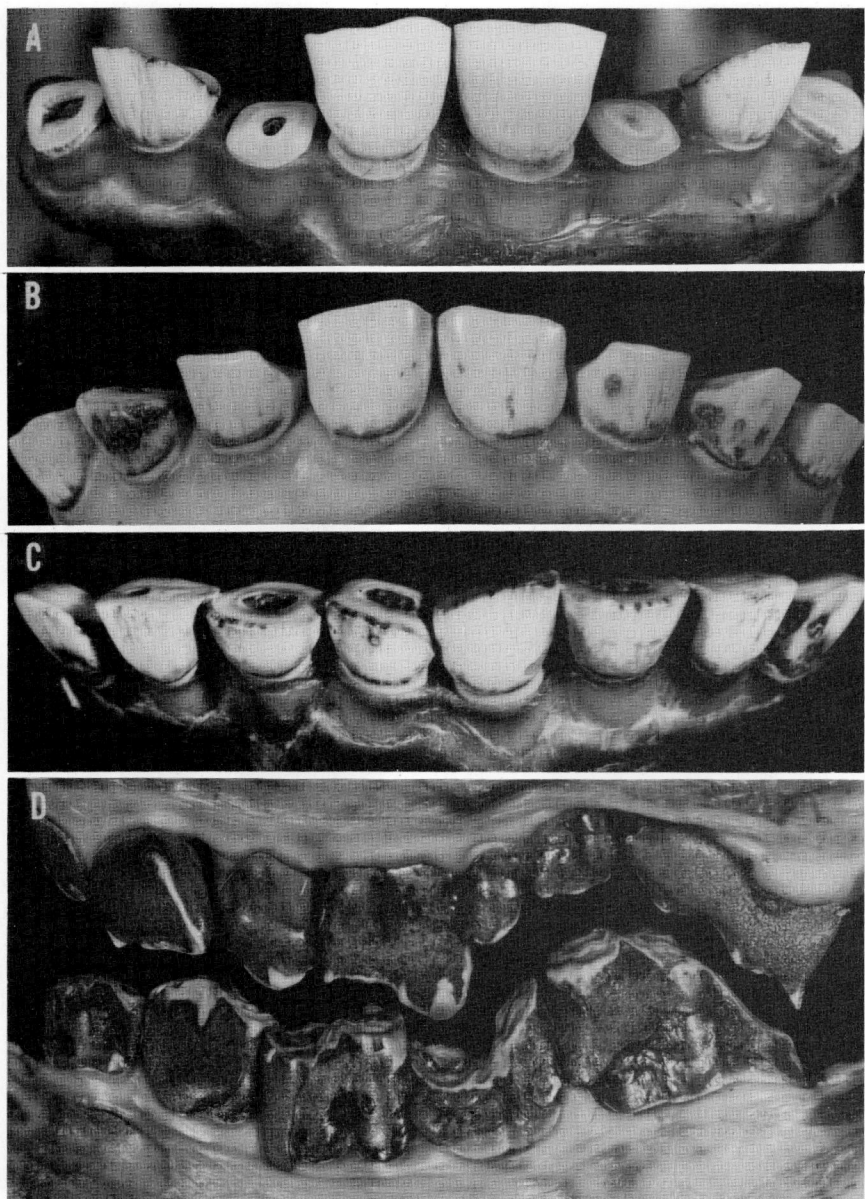

FIG. 15-17 Teeth in chronic bovine fluorosis. **A.** Irregular wear of incisors. **B.** Irregular mottling of incisors. **C.** Excessive wear of incisors. **D.** Irregular wear and stained enamel of molar teeth. (Courtesy of Dr. J. L. Shupe.)

Shupe JL, et al. The effect of fluorine on dairy cattle. V. Fluorine in the urine as an estimator of fluorine intake. Am J Vet Res 1963;24:300–306.

Shupe JL, et al. The effect of fluorine on dairy cattle. II. Clinical and pathologic effects. Am J Vet Res 1963;24:964–979.

Shupe JL, Miner ML, Greenwood DA. Clinical and pathological aspects of fluorine toxicosis in cattle. Ann NY Acad Sci 1964;111:618–637.

Shupe JL, Olson AE, Peterson HB, et al. Fluoride toxicosis in wild ungulates. J Am Vet Med Assoc 1984;185:1295–1300.

Whitford GM. The metabolism and toxicology of fluoride. In: Myers HM, ed. Monographs in oral science. Vol 13. Basel: Karger, 1989;160.

GROUP M: HYPERCALCEMIA

Group M contains poisonous plants that induce hypercalcemia, mimicking hypervitaminosis D_3.

Solanum malacoxylon

Severe, generalized calcifying arteriosclerotic disease ("enzootic calcinosis," hypercalcemia) of cattle and sheep has been recognized from certain tropical areas, particularly Jamaica, British West Indies, Argentina, and Hawaii. Its colloquial names in these places include "Manchester wasting disease," "enteque seco," and "Naalehu disease," respectively. This latter term comes from the name of the district in Hawaii meaning "covered with gray ashes." Only recently has each of these diseases been considered to represent the same syndrome and to be caused by the consumption of leaves and stems of the plant *Solanum malacoxylon* (syn: *S. glaucum* Dun.). The plant contains a molecule similar or identical to 1,25-dihydroxy vitamin D_3 combined with one or more carbohydrate moieties. Glycoside is believed to be cleaved in vivo to release the active form of vitamin D_3. Thus, the toxicity of *S. malacoxylon* is analogous to vitamin D_3 toxicity. The disease occurs naturally in cattle and sheep, but experimentally other domestic animals and laboratory animals are susceptible. Calves are less susceptible than are adult cows.

Other plants that have been demonstrated to contain this vitamin D3 analogue include: *Solanum verbascifolium, S. glaucophylium, S. torvum* (New Guinea), *Trisetum flavescens,* and *Cestrum diurnum* (United States).

The disease is manifest by progressive emaciation, stiffness of joints, and weakness. The clinicopathologic findings are those of vitamin D toxicity. Serum calcium is greatly elevated and serum phosphorus moderately increased. Extensive calcification of the media and intima of the aorta and all major and minor blood vessels occurs, as well as in the kidney, heart, lung, and other tissues. Bones may be thickened due to hyperostosis. A dark basophilic band separates new bone growth from preexisting bone. Its composition is not known, but presumably it is a mucopolysaccharide.

Poisoning by other species of Solanum is discussed on page 702.

References

Camberos HR, Davis GK, Djafar JI, et al. Soft tissue calcification in guinea pigs fed the poisonous plant Solanum malacoxylon. Am J Vet Res 1970;31:685–696,.
Done SH, Tokarnia CH, Dämmrich K, et al. Solanum malacoxylon poisoning in pigs. Res Vet Sci 1976;20:217–219.
Lynd FT, et al. Bovine arteriosclerosis in Hawaii. Am J Vet Res 1965;26:1344–1349.
Morris KML, Simonite JP, Pullen L, et al. Solanum torvum as a causative agent of enzootic calcinosis in Papua, New Guinea. Res Vet Sci 1979;27:264–266.
Peterlik M, et al. Further evidence for the 1,25–dihydroxyvitamin D-like activity of Solanum malacoxylon. Biochem Biophys Res Commun 1976;70:797–804.
Procsal DA, Henry HL, Hendrickson T, et al. 1, alpha, 25–dihydroxyvitamin D3–like component present in the plant Solanum glaucophyllum. Endocrinology 1976;99:437–444.
Rambeck WA, Zucker H. Vitamin D-artige Aktivitäten in calcinogen Pflanzen. [Vitamin D-like activity in calcinogenic plants.] Zentralbl Veterinarmed A 1982;29:289–296 [Vet Bull 1983;53:602].

Cestrum diurnum

This plant, also known as day-blooming jessamine, wild jasmine, day cestrum, or Chinese inkberry, is a member of the nightshade family (Solonaceae), but in contrast to most toxic plants in this group, *Cestrum diurnum* owes its toxicity to 1,25-dihydroxyvitamin D_3-glycoside. Its effect, therefore, resembles *Solanum malacoxylon* poisoning. The plant, introduced from the West Indies, is grown as an ornamental in warmer parts of the United States, including Florida, Texas, and California, as well as in India and Hawaii. It is especially abundant in southern Florida, where poisoning in horses and cattle have been described.

The disease was first recognized in 1970 in horses, in which most examples of poisoning have been observed. Affected horses lose weight over a period of months, become stiff and reluctant to move, and develop a short,

choppy gait. Flexor tendons and suspensory ligament are sensitive to palpation. The animals become progressively debilitated and are ultimately destroyed. Serum calcium is elevated (11.4–16.7 mg/100 mL), but serum phosphorus is normal. Pathologic soft-tissue calcification resulting from hypervitaminosis D is widespread in arteries, tendons, and ligaments. Calcification of the kidneys and lungs is not a feature of the disease. Generalized osteopetrosis (hyperostosis) has been described as resulting from retarded osteocytic osteolysis.

References

Harrington DD. Acute vitamin D2 (ergocalciferol) toxicosis in horses: case report and experimental studies. J Am Vet Med Assoc 1982;180:867–873.
Krook L, et al. Cestrum diurnum poisoning in Florida cattle. Cornell Vet 1975;65:557–575.
Krook L. Hypercalcemia and calcinosis in Florida horses: implication of the shrub, Cestrum diurnum, as the causative agent. Cornell Vet 1975;65:26–56.
Sarkar K, Narbaitz R, Pokrupa R, et al. The ultrastructure of nephrocalcinosis induced in chicks by Cestrum diurnum leaves. Vet Pathol 1981;18:62–70.
Wasserman RH, Corradino RA, Krook L. Cestrum diurnum: a domestic plant with 1,25–dihydroxycholecalciferol-like activity. Biochem Biophys Res Commun 1975;62:85–91.

GROUP N: LOSS OF HAIR OR WOOL
Thallium

Because it is a heavy metal with toxic effects and atomic weight similar to lead and mercury, thallium may be involved in poisonings of humans and animals. The thallous form, particularly thallous sulfate, is most active pharmacologically and is odorless, colorless, and tasteless; each of these characteristics favors its use as a pesticide. Although banned by federal law from sale to the general public for household use, accidental poisonings of children, dogs, and cats still occur. Cattle and sheep have also been reported to have eaten poisoned bait. Poisonings from industrial wastes and use of thallium as a depilatory seem to be decreasing.

The clinical signs reflect involvement of several body systems and depend, to some extent, on the amount of thallium ingested. Dogs exhibit these signs in order of frequency: vomiting, cutaneous alterations, depression, anorexia, nervous signs, diarrhea, respiratory distress, conjunctivitis, dehydration, and esophageal paralysis. Cutaneous lesions first appear as localized areas of erythema from the third to seventh day after poisoning. Serum oozes from these lesions, and in a few days they become covered with thick, crusty material. Hair may be plucked easily in early stages, later it may fall readily from large areas of skin. Necrosis and sloughing of skin may eventually occur.

Clinical laboratory findings in dogs, in order of frequency, include: lymphopenia, neutrophilia, eosinopenia, left shift of neutrophils, hemoconcentration, and circulating immature red blood cells. Blood urea nitrogen often is elevated. Serum glutamic pyruvic transaminase may be elevated, and serum glutamic oxaloacetic transaminase is usually elevated. Proteinuria and bilirubinuria may be present. Elevated specific gravity is characteristic of urine, presumably due to dehydration. Glycosuria may be evident, and granular casts, erythrocytes, leukocytes, and epithelial cells are usually excessive in urine sediment.

Microscopic lesions of thallotoxicosis are found in most systems of the body. Changes in the skin are striking and characteristic (Fig. 15-18A), consisting of severe acanthosis and parakeratosis involving epidermis and hair follicles, occasional intraepithelial and hair follicles, occasional intraepithelial abscesses, and congestion of epidermal capillaries. Necrosis of isolated renal convoluted tubules is also typical (Fig. 15-18B), with proteinaceous material in some Bowman's spaces. In later stages, some leukocytic infiltration may occur, completing the picture of toxic tubular nephrosis. Edema of the lungs is usual, and purulent bronchopneumonia may be found in about one-third of cases. Disseminated focal necroses of skeletal and cardiac muscle fibers are constant, with the expected leukocytic infiltration at the sites of necrosis. Spleens and lymph nodes are often edematous and enlarged with hyperpla-

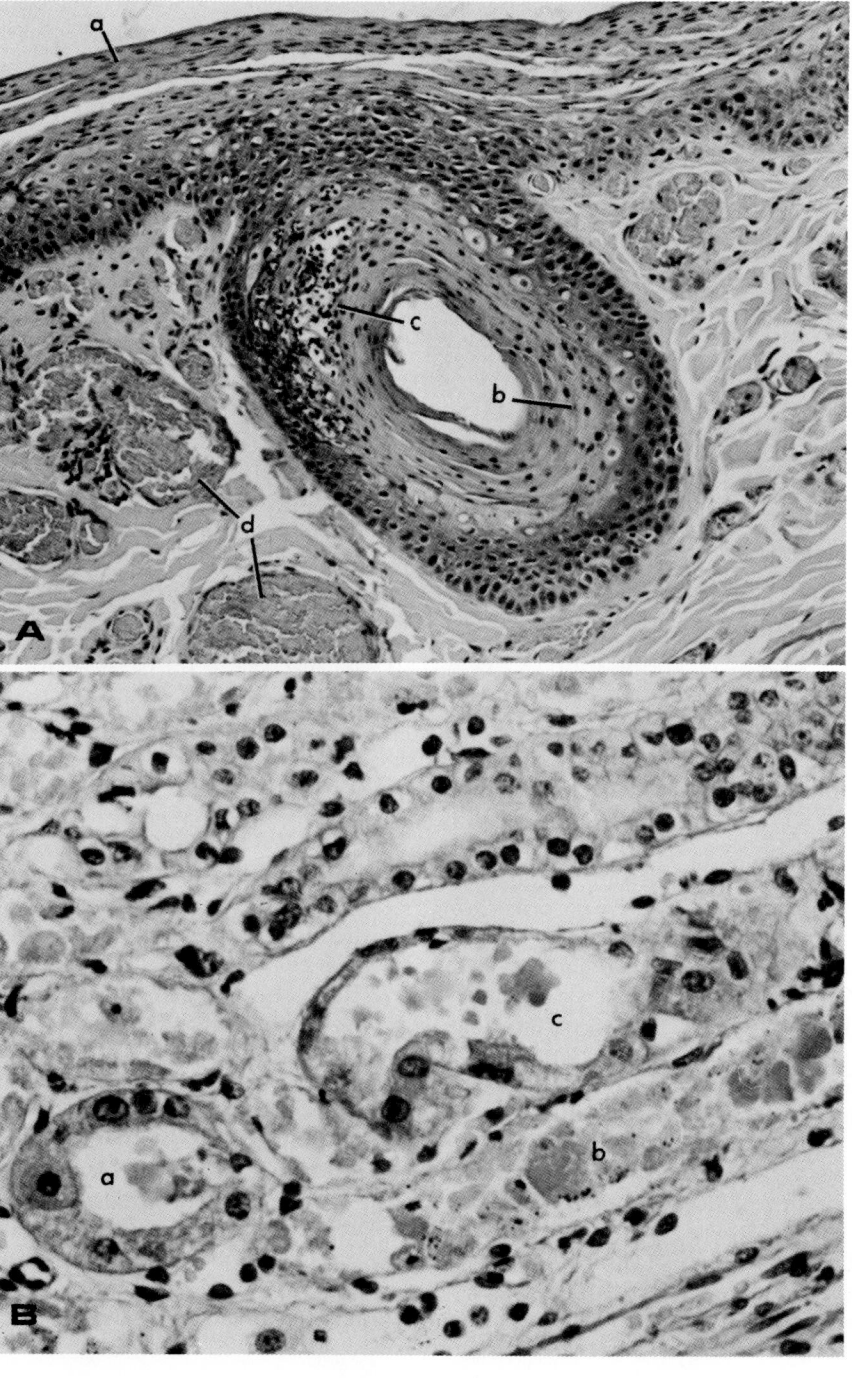

FIG. 15-18 Thallium poisoning. **A.** Thallium poisoning in a one-year-old male Scottish terrier. Note: (a) parakeratosis and acanthosis in the epidermis and the hair follicle (b); intraepithelial abscess (c), and congestion of capillaries (d). **B.** Kidney of a two-year-old, castrated male collie which died of thallium poisoning. Note: (a) renal tubule with slightly affected cells (cytoplasm swollen, cells partially individualized); tubule with completely necrotic epithelium (b), and part of tubule with some necrotic cells (c). (Courtesy of Angell Memorial Animal Hospital.)

sia of reticuloendothelial elements. Some myelinated nerves may have some degenerated axons with enlarged, empty myelin sheaths. Aspermatogenesis with formation of multinucleated masses of spermatids is evident in the testes. Ulceration of the esophagus, with focal necrosis in nearby muscle fibers, is a constant finding. Hepatic lesions are usually limited to early toxic hepatitis, with necrosis and distention of sinusoids near central veins. In brain, lesions may be found in animals in which neurologic involvement is indicated by clinical signs. These consist of disseminated early necrotic lesions (with chromatolysis and neuronophagia), and edema throughout the cerebellum and cerebrum.

Gross lesions, as may be judged from the clinical signs and microscopic findings, consist of the following: patchy or diffuse areas of cutaneous erythema, alopecia, or dermatitis; cardiac hypertrophy; subendocardial hemorrhages; severe congestion of the kidneys; edema and consolidations of the lungs; edema and enlargement of lymph nodes; enlargement of the spleen; and dilation, erosion, or ulceration of the esophagus.

The pathologic diagnosis is established by the microscopic lesions, particularly those in the skin, and by the chemical demonstration of thallium in urine or tissues.

References

Newsom IE, Loftus JB, Ward JC. The toxicity of thallium sulphate for sheep. J Am Vet Med Assoc 1930;76:826–832.

Pile CH. Thallium poisoning in domestic felines. Aust Vet J 1956;32:18–20.

Ruhe LP, Andries JK. Thallium intoxication in a dog. J Am Vet Med Assoc 1985;186:498–499.

Schwartzman RM, Kirschbaum JO. The cutaneous histopathology of thallium poisoning. J Invest Dermatol 1962;39:169–173.

Skelley JF, Gabriel KL. Thallium intoxication in the dog. Ann NY Acad Sci 1964;111:612–617.

Zook BC, Gilmore CE. Thallium poisoning in dogs. J Am Vet Med Assoc 1967;151:206–217.

Zook BC, Holzworth J, Thornton GW. Thallium poisoning in cats. J Am Vet Med Assoc 1968;153:285–299.

Jumbay tree (leucaena glauca)

Chronic poisoning of horses reported in the Bahamian Islands is due to the consumption for several weeks of the leaves and twigs of a small leguminous tree, *Leucaena glauca*, commonly known as the jumbay. *Leucaena glauca* is known as "ipil-ipil" in the Philippines, as "lamtoro" in Indonesia, and "cow bush" in Australia. In Hawaii, where it is cultivated extensively, it is called "kao haole," "ekoa," or "white popinac." It is able to grow in the worst kinds of soil and with little water, has good value as forage, may contain up to 30% protein (dry weight), and twice as much carotene as alfalfa.

The substance responsible for this toxicity is found in plants of the family Mimosaceae that includes *Leucaena glauca, L. leucocephala,* and other legumes, including *Mimosa spp.* It is a toxic amino acid, mimosine, [β-N-(3–hydroxyl-4–pyridone)-α-aminopropropionic acid]. Certain bacteria inhabiting the rumen of some cattle and sheep are believed to degrade a toxic intermediate product of mimosine, 3–hydroxy-4–(1H)pyridone, making it possi-

ble for these animals to consume Leucaena with impunity in amounts as much as 30%.

Horses and pigs are most frequently affected; ruminants are less susceptible than monogastric animals. The most striking symptom is partial to complete loss of the long hair of the mane, tail, and forelock; when the case is severe, patchy loss above and below the knees and hocks and in the flanks and neck occurs. Experimental feeding of high levels has produced severe stomatitis, hemorrhagic enteritis, proctitis, edema of the hind legs and genitals, and chronic laminitis with rings in the hoof. Recovery occurs after feeding is discontinued and possibly some tolerance develops.

The feeding of Leucaena to swine and rats reportedly causes fetal death and resorption, and polypodia of the forelimbs.

References

Keeler RF. Naturally occurring teratogens from plants. In: Keeler RF, Tu AT, eds. Handbook of natural toxins. Vol 1. Plant and fungal toxins. New York: Marcel Dekker, 1983;161–199.

Mullenax CH. A dietary cause of hair loss in Bahamian livestock. J Am Vet Med Assoc 1957;131:302.

Mullenax CH. Observations on Leucaena glauca. Aust Vet J 1963;39:88–91.

Wayman O, Iwanaga II, Hugh WI. Fetal resorption in swine caused by Leucaena leucocephala (Lam.) de Wit. in the diet. J Anim Sci 1970;30:583–588.

GROUP O: EPITHELIAL HYPERPLASIA

Group O contains several chlorinated compounds which have epithelial hyperplasia as their most prominent pathologic feature.

Chlorinated dibenzodioxins (TCDD, dioxin, toxic fat)

Several chlorinated dibenzodioxins are known to be toxic, with 2, 3, 7, 8–tetrachlorodioxin (TCDD), commonly referred to as dioxin, being one of the most toxic compounds known. Dioxins originate from various chlorophenol compounds, especially when treated with alkali, and therefore may contaminate products containing or derived from chlorophenols. Chlorophenols are widely used as antiseptics, disinfectants, fungicides, herbicides, hide preservatives, and wood preservatives. Dioxin has also been found as a contaminant of polychlorinated biphenyls.

Poisoning by dioxin in humans and a variety of animals has been well documented and may account for many mysterious illnesses. Dioxin may also be the active principle in chlorinated naphthalene poisoning, discussed following this section.

The first identification of dioxin as an important toxin took place in 1962 when it was shown to be the responsible cause of a mysterious disease of chickens first recognized in 1957. The disease in poultry was first named "edema disease," "water belly," and "ascitic disease" by poultry farmers and veterinarians, indicating the common postmortem findings. Following the recognition of a toxic factor in the unsaponifiable fraction of certain fats, it was labeled toxic fat poisoning. After five years of research, dioxin or TCDD was shown to be the cause. The source was shown to be fleshing grease from hides that had been treated with commercial pentachlorophenol. Millions of broilers died in the 1957 "outbreak." A subsequent outbreak occurred in 1969, which was traced to contaminated vegetable oil by-product fatty acids used in the feed. The vegetable oil refinery also formulated antimicrobial products that contained chlorophenols.

Subsequent to recognition of "edema disease" in poultry, poisoning by dioxin has been confirmed in other animal species and humans exposed to chemicals containing dioxin as a contaminant. Industrial accidents have occurred in Ludwigshafen, West Germany, the Netherlands, Derbyshire, England, and Seveso, Italy, and exposure of workers at a chemical plant in the United States have all been associated with human illness. The use of waste oil to control dust in riding arenas has also resulted in human and animal poisoning by dioxin. Currently, considerable attention has focused on the use of the herbicide, 2–4,5 trichlorophenoxyacetic acid (2–4,5–T or agent orange), which was widely sprayed in Vietnam, as well as in other countries, such as Colombia, and which contains dioxin as a contaminant.

Chloracne, a persistent and disfiguring form of acne, is the principal outward sign of toxicity in humans, and comparable lesions of the skin occur in animals experimentally or naturally exposed. These lesions closely resemble those described in greater detail in the following sections on chlorinated naphthalene and PCB poisonings.

Lesions of the skin, however, are by no means the only effect of dioxin toxicity. Other lesions include necrosis of the liver, edema, thrombocytopenia, and prothrombin deficiency leading to bleeding, conjunctivitis, abortion, congenital malformations, chromosomal aberrations, and carcinoma of the liver. The mortality rate may be low or high, but death occurs remarkably late after exposure, ranging from one month to one year.

The mechanism of toxicity of dioxin is not known, but it is speculated to be related to the fact that it is a potent inducer of aryl hydrocarbon hydroxysynthetase.

References

Bumb RR, et al. Trace chemistries of fire: a source of chlorinated dioxins. Science 1980;210:385–390.
McNulty WP. Toxicity and fetotoxicity of TCDD, TCDF, and PCB isomers in rhesus macaques (Macaca mulatta). Environ Health Perspect 1985;60:77–78.
Pellegrini S, Fabiani O, Lanfranchi A, et al. Ultrastructural studies on the liver and kidney of animals naturally or experimentally contaminated with dioxin (TCDD). Atti Soc Ital Sci Vet 1982;36:531–533.
Safe SH. Comparative toxicology and mechanism of action of polychlorinated dibenzo-p-dioxins and dibenzofurans. Annu Rev Pharmacol Toxicol 1986;26:371–399.
Tschirley FH. Dioxin. Sci Am 1986;254:29–35.

Chlorinated naphthalenes

A disease entity, known as hyperkeratosis previous to the discovery of its etiology, has been traced to the presence of highly chlorinated naphthalenes (probably ≥ 5

Cl ions; Figs. 15-19, 15-20), which gain access to the animal metabolism either through ingestion or cutaneous absorption. Although the disease was first described in connection with a wood preservative used on stables in which cattle were kept, a more common source of naphthalene compounds has been lubricating oils. Such compounds have been found to improve the lubricating properties of the oil, but minute amounts from the bearings of machines used in the process have contaminated commercially produced feeds, especially those made into pellets. Animals have also absorbed the poison through contact with farm machinery so lubricated. Cattle are ordinarily involved, although sheep have been poisoned experimentally.

Signs include lacrimation, which may develop within one week after the first contact with the poison, often salivation, afebrile depression, anorexia, emaciation, terminal diarrhea, and death after several weeks.

Lesions can be summarized as an overgrowth of epithelium. This includes an increase of the cornified layer (hyperkeratosis) on those surfaces where the epithelium is already stratified squamous, and squamous metaplasia in many places where it is normally of the columnar type. This results in marked thickening of the skin, especially over the neck and withers, with coarse, deep wrinkling, scaliness, and loss of hair. Microscopically (Fig. 15-20), some degree of acanthosis occurs with deepening of the rete pegs, but most of the increased thickness is in the cornified layer. The keratohyaline of this layer extends deep into the hair follicles, compressing the surrounding zone of cellular epithelium. The corium commonly shows a noticeable infiltration with lymphocytes.

On the mucosa of the mouth and lips and especially on the tongue, raised "plaques" of thickened, hyperkeratotic epithelium are likely to be manifest. These average 1 cm or more in diameter. Judging from early experimental cases, these plaques apparently are preceded by shallow ulcers. Similar, but smaller, nodular proliferations are likely to be found in the esophagus. The same tendency toward nodular increase of epithelium extends through the digestive tract where thickened spots or areas occasionally develop through hyperplasia of the columnar epithelium, forming cysts filled with mucus and cell debris. This general tendency is more likely to be seen in the gallbladder and in extrahepatic and intrahepatic bile ducts. The latter often develop thickenings characterized by irregular epithelial-lined cysts, which vary from microscopic in size to a diameter of 1 cm. Within the liver (Fig. 15-19), such ducts are encircled by increased fibrous tissue. In a few instances, the changes approach those of biliary cirrhosis. The ducts of the salivary glands and pancreas sometimes undergo metaplastic changes similar to those in the bile ducts.

In the kidneys, the same tendency toward epithelial hyperplasia reveals itself in enlargement and dilatation of tubules, chiefly the collecting tubules of the medullary rays. The epithelium of these tubules is not compressed but hyperplastic, even to the extent that small

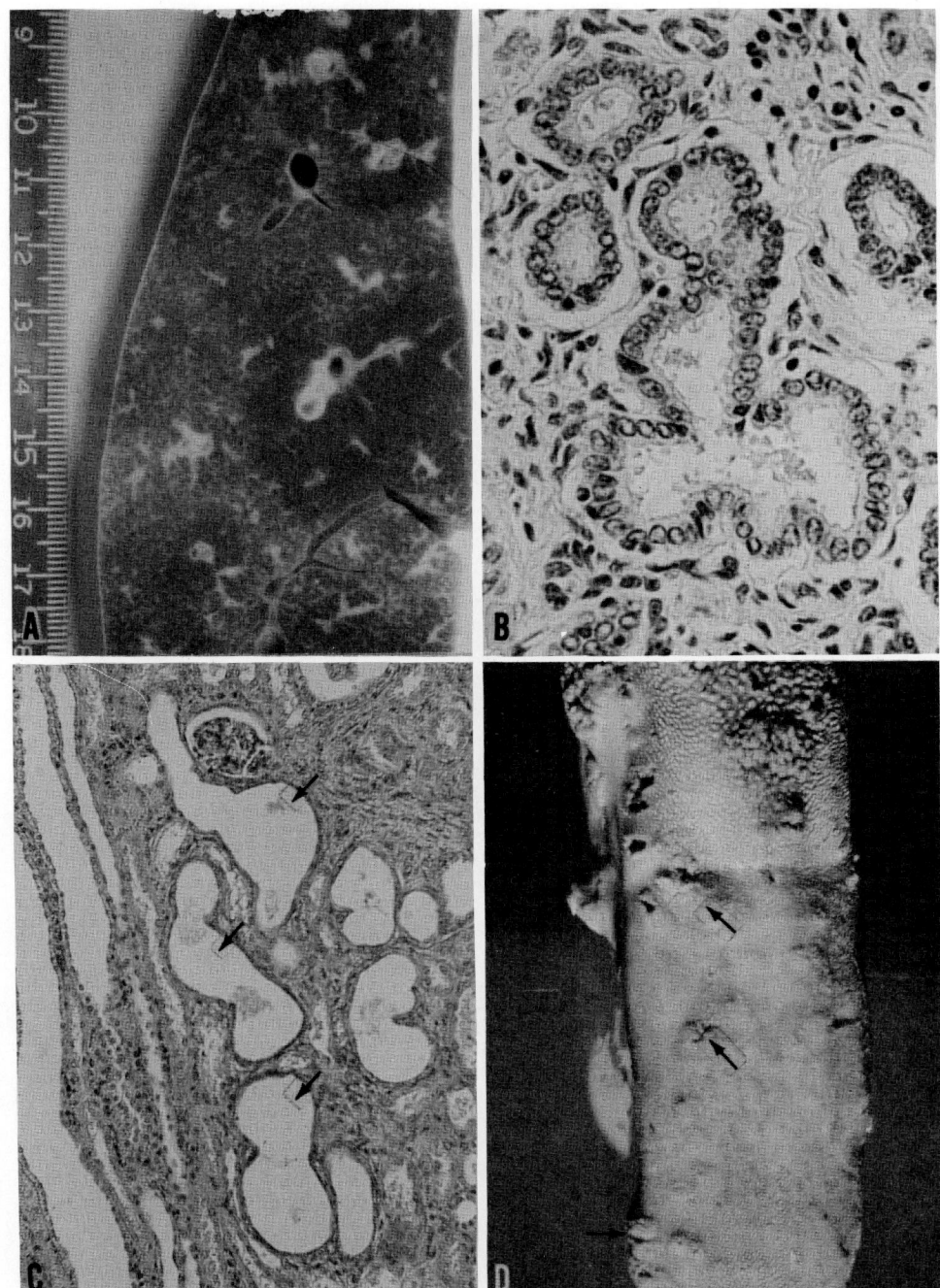

FIG. 15-19 Poisoning caused by chlorinated naphthalene (bovine hyperkeratosis). **A.** Bovine liver with prominent biliary system. **B.** Hyperplasia of bile ducts (×485) in portal region. (Contributor: Dr. J. F. Ryff.) **C.** Hyperplasia and dilatation of renal tubules (arrows) in a bovine kidney (×100). (Courtesy of Armed Forces Institute of Pathology; contributors: Drs. Kenneth McEntee and Peter Olafson.) **D.** Tongue of an affected cow. Note elevated lesions in epithelium (arrows). (Case at Iowa Sch. Vet. Med.)

papillary projections extend into the lumen. A certain amount of fibrosis accompanies these tubular changes when they are severe.

Squamous metaplasia and cornification are likely to be found in the tubular and glandular organs of the male genitalia, especially in the seminal vesicles.

In sheep, similar squamous metaplasia has been found in the endometrial lining and glands. The epithelium of the cervix may be hyperplastic in both cattle and sheep.

It is not to be expected that all of the above lesions will be found in the same animal. Usually any of them,

when unequivocally developed, are sufficient for a diagnosis.

A milder degree of epithelial hyperplasia and hyperkeratosis is characteristic of avitaminosis-A. Investigations have shown that in poisoning by chlorinated naphthalenes the amount of vitamin A in the blood declines sharply within five days after the first ingestion of the poison. It falls as low as 25 μg/100 ml, but does not reach zero as it almost does in experimental deprivation of the vitamin. This antivitamin-A effect persists for at least one month after ingestion of the poison has ceased. Feeding five times the normal requirement of

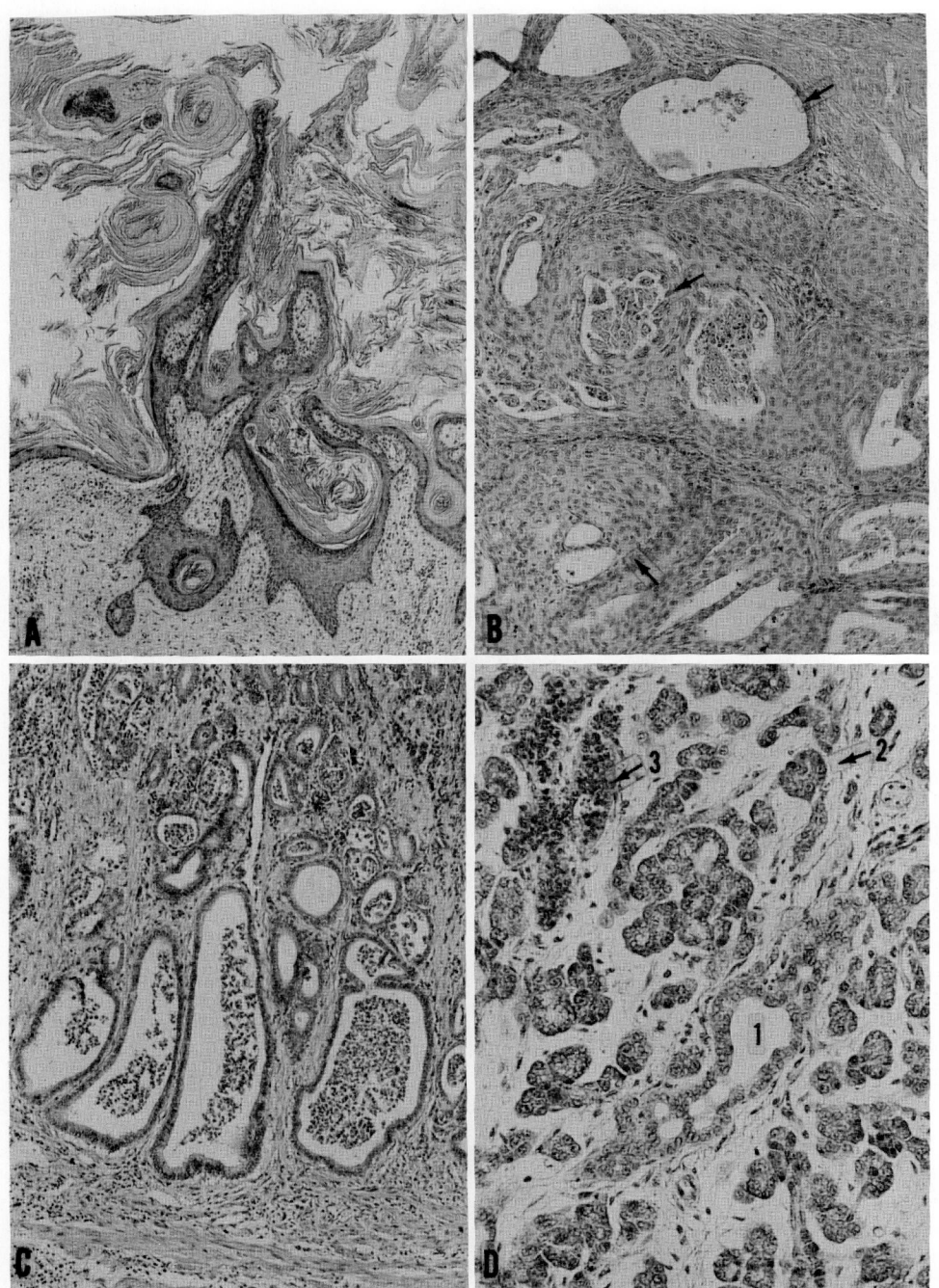

FIG. 15-20 Poisoning from chlorinated naphthalene (bovine hyperkeratosis). **A.** Severe hyperkeratosis in bovine skin (×56). (Contributor: Dr. J. F. Ryff.) **B.** Squamous metaplasia of tubular epithelium (arrows) of epididymis (×100). (Contributors: Drs. Kenneth McEntee and Peter Olafson.) **C.** Hyperplasia and cystic dilatation of epithelium in crypts of small intestine (×70). (Contributor: Dr. J. F. Ryff.) **D.** Hyperplasia of ductal epithelium, bovine pancreas (×195). Duct (1), stroma (2), and island of Langerhans (3). This is more severe than usual. (Courtesy of Armed Forces Institute of Pathology; contributor: Dr. J. F. Ryff.)

vitamin A (5 × 5000 IU vitamin A per 100 pounds of body weight per day) maintains a satisfactory amount of the vitamin in both blood and liver against a limited amount of the toxic feed, but this effect is transient. It does not appear that larger amounts of the vitamin are able to keep pace with increases of the poison. When administration of the vitamin is continued adequately beyond the period of poison ingestion, some animals recover. The question of just how the chlorinated naphthalene neutralizes the effect of vitamin A has baffled investigators. Evidence suggests that it interferes with conversion of carotene to vitamin A, doubtless through

impairment of the liver, but this is by no means the only toxic action; it is not possible to duplicate the lesions by vitamin deprivation, no matter how complete. The similarity of the lesions to dioxin poisoning raises the possibility that chlorinated naphthalenes are contaminated with dioxins.

Because the epithelial hyperplasia of this disease sometimes reaches such proportions to suggest neoplasia, the question arises as to whether chlorinated naphthalenes could possibly have carcinogenic actions. The answer, to date, is no; this is supported by extensive experimentation. To the question of whether any other substances can have the same effects as chlorinated naphthalenes, the answer is possibly less certain, but apparently is also negative.

References

Hansel W, McEntee K, Olafson P. The effects of two causative agents of experimental hyperkeratosis on vitamin-A metabolism. Cornell Vet 1951;41:367–376.

Hoekstra WG, Hall RE, Phillips PH. Relationship of vitamin-A to the development of hyperkeratosis (X disease) in calves. Am J Vet Res 1954;15:41–46.

Knocke KW. Hyperakeratose in einem Rinderbestand 13 Jahre nach Anwendung eines Holzschutmittels. Dtsche Tierärztl. 1961;68:701–703.

Olafson P. Hyperkeratosis (X disease) of cattle. Cornell Vet 1947;37:279–291.

Pallaske G. Zur pathologischen Anatomie der Chlornaphthalinvergiftung der Rinder. Monatsheft Veterinärmed 1956;11:677–678.

Sikes D, Bridges ME. Experimental production of hyperkeratosis ("X disease") of cattle with a chlorinated naphthalene. Science 1952;116:506–507.

Teuscher R. Ein seltener klinischer Fall von zweimaliger Vergiftung eines Rinderbestandes durch chloriente naphthaline. Monatsheft Veterinärmed 1956;11:675–677.

Wagener K. Hyperkeratosis of cattle in Germany. J Am Vet Med Assoc 1951;119:133–137.

Polychlorinated biphenyls and polybrominated biphenyls

Polychlorinated biphenyls (PCB), polychlorinated triphenyls (PTB), and polybrominated biphenyls (PBB) are relatively chemically inert compounds that resist high temperatures and are used in the manufacture of plastics, lubricants, wood coatings, and other products in which heat resistance is desired. The toxicity of PCB was first recognized in humans in Japan, where contaminated cooking oil caused an acneiform dermatitis termed "Yusko." Isolated reports of poisoning in animals have appeared in the past decade, and probably many poisonings have gone unrecognized. The most re-

cent experience occurred in Michigan in 1973, in which a PBB fire retardant ("Firemaster") was inadvertently used in the preparation of cattle feeds. Nearly 30,000 cattle and thousands of other farm animals were destroyed or quarantined, causing estimated losses of $75–100 million.

The most consistent outward signs included swelling of the eyelids, which become encrusted with exudate, loss of hair, particularly about the face and neck, but also on the back and thorax, and thickened and wrinkled skin. In cattle, abnormal growth of the hoofs may occur, causing them to grow long and curl upward and inward. Weight loss, subcutaneous edema, diarrhea, shrinking of the udder, decrease in milk production, embryonic resorption, and prolonged gestation are other reported signs.

Pathologically, the predominant finding is epithelial hypertrophy, hyperplasia, and metaplasia, especially of the skin (Fig. 15-21) and gastrointestinal tract. The epidermis is thickened and hyperkeratotic. Hair follicles become distorted into large, keratin-filled cysts. Squamous metaplasia of sebaceous glands and Meibomian glands leads to their enlargement, ultimately to large, keratin-filled cysts. The gastric mucosa undergoes hyperplasia and mucous metaplasia. Large cysts develop in the mucosa, and the epithelium invades extensively through the muscularis mucosa into the submucosa. Hyperplasia of the mucosa of the gallbladder and bile ductule proliferation and fibrosis may be prominent. Focal hepatic necrosis and renal tubular necrosis are often present, especially in the more acute stages. Hepatocellular hypertrophy may lead to gross enlargement of the liver.

The mechanism by which PCB and PBB bring about these changes is unknown. As with chlorinated naphthalenes, reduction in vitamin A levels has been noted, but it is doubtful that the lesions are solely related to this effect. Dioxin is a contaminant of PCB and may, in part, explain its toxicity.

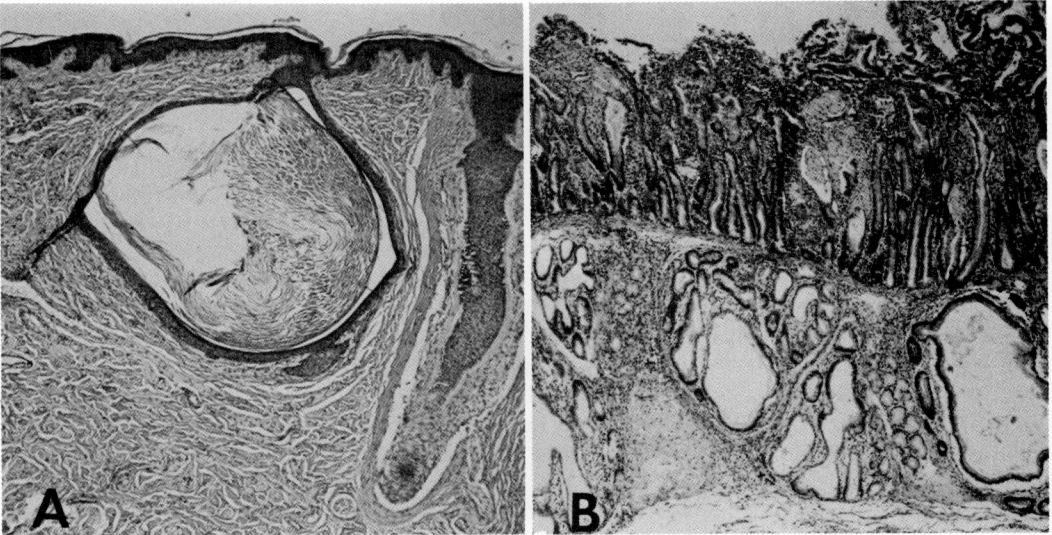

FIG. 15-21 Polychlorinated biphenyl intoxication (*Macaca mulatta*). **A.** Keratin-filled cyst in skin. **B.** Adenomatous hyperplasia of gastric mucosa. (Courtesy of Dr. J. R. Allen.)

References

Altman NH, New AE, McConnell EE, et al. A spontaneous outbreak of polychlorinated biphenyl (PCB) toxicity in rhesus monkeys (Macaca mulatta): clinical observations. Lab Anim Sci 1979;29:661–665.

Bailey J, Knauf V, Mueller W, et al. Transfer of hexachlorobenzene and polychlorinated biphenyls to nursing infant monkeys: enhanced toxicity. Environ Res 1980;21:190–196.

Collins WT, Capen CC. Biliary excretion of 125I-thyroxine and fine structural alterations in the thyroid glands of Gunn rats fed polychlorinated biphenyls (PCB). Lab Invest 1980;43:158–164.

Hori S, et al. Effect of polychlorinated biphenyls in cynomolgus monkey (Macaca fascicularis). Toxicology 1982;24:123–139.

Masuda Y, Yoshimura H. Chemical analysis and toxicity of polychlorinated biphenyls and dibenzofurans in relation to Yusho. J Toxicol Sci 1982;7:161–175.

Robens J, Anthony HD. Polychlorinated biphenyl contamination of feeder cattle. J Am Vet Med Assoc 1980;177:613–615.

Polybrominated biphenyls (PBB)

Dunckel AE. An updating on the polybrominated biphenyl disaster in Michigan. J Am Vet Med Assoc 1975;167:838–841.

Patterson DG, et al. Hyperkeratosis induced by sunlight degradation products of the major polybrominated biphenyl in firemaster. Science 1981;213:901–902.

Werner PR, Sleight SD. Toxicosis in sows and their pigs caused by feeding rations containing polybrominated biphenyls to sows during pregnancy and lactation. Am J Vet Res 1981;42:183–188.

GROUP P: NERVOUS MALFUNCTION

These poisons cause nervous malfunction with or without demonstrable lesions in the tissues. Note that many poisons in other groups (e.g., hepatotoxins) may also be characterized by nervous malfunction.

Strychnine

Intermittent tonic spasms, initiated by noises or other external stimuli, provide a well-known symptom that is practically diagnostic. Strychnine binds to synaptic membranes and antagonizes the hyperpolarizing action of glycine (a major inhibitory neurotransmitter), resulting in hyperirritability and lack of normal inhibitory restraint in the spinal part of the reflex arc. No postmortem lesions are manifest, except possibly petechiae resulting from the anoxia incident to arrest of respiration during spasms. The absence of lesions often has diagnostic significance when associated with typical symptoms. The drug can be identified by chemical procedures or by microscopic identification of typical crystals, but both methods are complicated. An infusion of suspected ingesta or urine can be inoculated either into the dorsal lymph space or the peritoneum of frogs or into the peritoneum of mice, with the result that the test animals show the characteristic tonic spasms when irritated by touch. This should occur within 20 minutes. The test is regarded as highly sensitive; the urine of any dog fatally poisoned is stated to contain sufficient strychnine at death for a positive test. In addition to malicious poisoning, accidents in the use of strychnine-containing rodent and grasshopper poisons afford instances of poisoning.

References

Blakley BR. Epidemiologic and diagnostic considerations of strychnine poisoning in the dog. J Am Vet Med Assoc 1984;184:46–47.

McConnell EE, van Rensburg IBJ, Minne JA. A rapid test for the diagnosis of strychnine poisoning. J S Afr Vet Med Assoc 1971;42:81–84.

Young AB, Snyder SH. Strychnine binding associated with glycine receptors of the central nervous system. Proc Natl Acad Sci USA 1973;70:2832–2836.

Loco

Locoweed poisoning is a nervous disorder (loco, Spanish for madness) related to consumption of certain plants (loco weeds). It was first recognized in the horses of De Soto and other Spanish conquistadors during their explorations of the New World. The offending plants grow particularly in the western United States and consist of a large number of species classified in two genera, Astragalus and Oxytropis. The toxic principle has been identified in the following species in North America: *Astragalus earlei*, *A. mollissimus* (purple woolly loco), *A. pubentissimus* (green river milkvetch), *A. lentigenosis* (spotted locoweed), *A. wootoni* (garbancillo), *A. nothoxys* (beaked milkvetch), *A. tophrodes* (ashen milkvetch), *A. humistratus* (ground cover milkvetch), *Oxytropis sericea* (white point locoweed), *O. campestris* (Canada), and *O. lambertii* (Lambert locoweed). In Australia, similar toxicoses are associated with consumption of plants in the genus *Swainsona*: *S. luteola*, *S. greyana*, and *S. galegifolia*. In sheep this Australian disease has been referred to as "pea struck."

Cattle, sheep, and horses are most frequently reported to be affected, but the disease has also been seen in wild ruminants.

SIGNS

Signs of the disease develop slowly in cattle and require consumption of plants over a period of 60 days in an amount equal to 90% of body weight. Ninety-eight days and consumption of 2.3 times the animal's weight are the minimum likely to cause death. In the horse, however, consumption equivalent to 30% of the animal's weight during a 49–day experimental period has been fatal. As a cumulative poison, signs may not develop until after ingestion has ceased.

In the horse, hyperexcitability, fright, and violent reactions to slight stimuli are the early signs of loco poisoning. Much of this reaction, however, may be due to inability to see clearly. The same impaired vision and disordered judgment cause a cow to perform all the movements of drinking while the mouth is six inches above the water. Sensory and motor derangements increase until the animal is unable to obtain food. Slowly increasing ataxia of the limbs becomes ascending paralysis; death results from a combination of nervous failure and starvation. Sheep are depressed from the start; goats suffer from posterior paresis and ascending paralysis in the initial stages and opisthotonos at the last. In all species, the terminal events are similar.

LESIONS.

Microscopic lesions (Figure 15-22), described in sheep experimentally poisoned with *Oxytropis sericea*, *Astragalus lentiginosus* or *A. pubentissimus*, tend to explain the clinical signs. Nearly identical vacuolar lesions

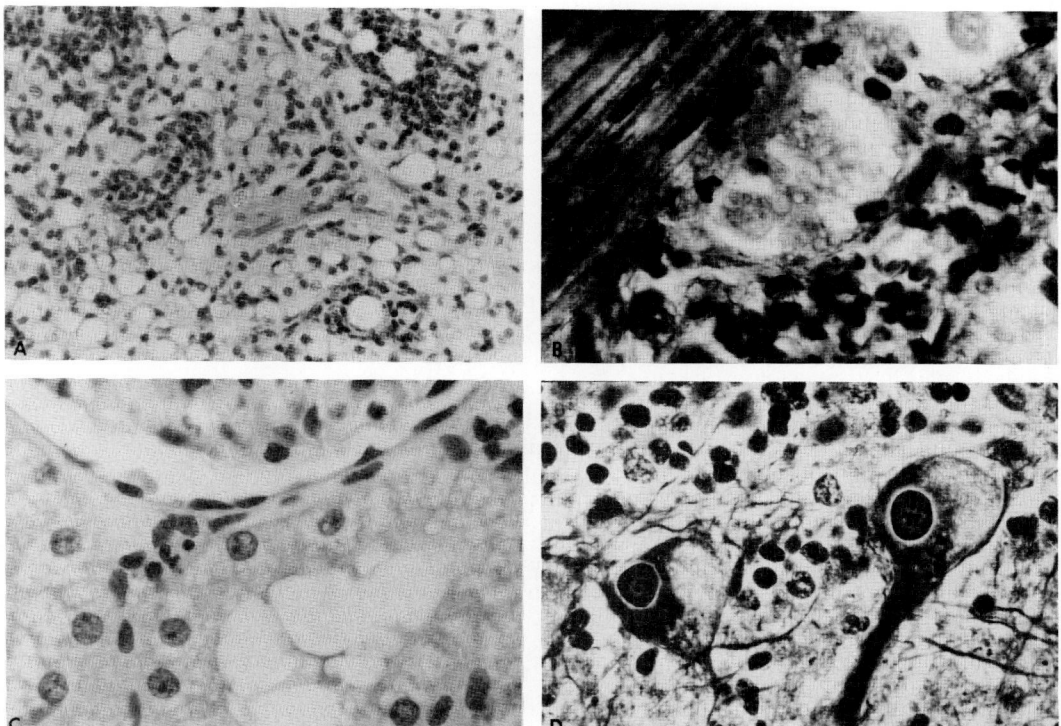

FIG. 15-22 Locoweed poisoning in sheep. **A.** Vacuolated cells in lymph node. **B.** Vacuolated neurons in Auerbach's plexus. **C.** Vacuoles in cells of convoluted tubule, kidney. **D.** Cytoplasmic vacuolation in Purkinje cells. (Courtesy of Dr. Kent R. Van Kampen and Pathologia Veterinaria.)

in neurons and renal epithelium have been encountered in sheep in Australia poisoned naturally and experimentally by eating plants, such as *Swainsona luteola* and *S. galegifolia*. The toxic effects on pregnant ewes of *Swainsona galegifolia, Astragalus pubentissimus,* and *A. lentiginosus* are quite similar, leading to the original idea that the active principle in all of these plants is the same.

The vacuolated appearance of the cytoplasm of neurons and other cells is not the result of accumulation of lipid or glycoprotein, as indicated by negative reactions to oil-red-O and PAS reactions. The vacuoles, visualized as membrane-bound in electron micrographs, are believed to have been lysosomes that are distended by incompletely catabolized α-manosyl residues, as explained in an earlier paragraph.

PATHOGENESIS

The most important active principle involved in locoweed poisoning is swainsonine, an indolizidine alkaloid, which acts as an inhibitor of α-mannosidase, an enzyme found in lysosomes. Decreased α-mannosidase activity interferes with the catabolism of α-mannosyl residues which accumulate in lysosomes of cells, especially those of the nervous system. This accumulation gives cells the vacuolated appearance seen in histologic sections.

This vacuolated feature in swainsonine poisoning is essentially similar to that of inherited mannosidosis that occurs in Angus cattle, Persian cats and humans, but the defective enzyme, α-mannosidase, results from a de-

fective mutant gene. In both of these conditions, swainsonine toxicosis and inherited mannosidosis, the lesion is the result of accumulation of α-mannosyl residues (constituents of many N-linked glycoproteins) in lysosomes, due to defective catabolism.

Locoweeds also may be poisonous through two other mechanisms:

1. Some plants concentrate selenium from the soil and cause selenium poisoning; and,
2. Others synthesize alphatic nitro compounds, which result in nitrite poisoning (page 737).

Damage to neurons is most significant and may be found in any part of the central or peripheral nervous systems, including the Meissner's and Auerbach's plexuses in the gastrointestinal tract. In late stages, karyolysis, karyorrhexis, or cytolysis leads to loss of neurons or mineralization of the necrotic remnants. Axonal degeneration may be found, but myelin is not significantly altered. Gliosis and neuronophagic nodules are not conspicuous. Perivascular edema is usually evident throughout the central nervous system. Spheroids (swollen axons) develop following neuronal necrosis.

Accumulation of material in lysosomes, similar to that noted in neurons, has been described in many other organs and tissues, including the follicular epithelium of the thyroid, chief cells of parathyroid, adrenal cortical cells, serous cells of salivary glands, hepatocytes, reticuloendothelial cells of lymph nodes and spleen, transitional epithelium of the urinary tract, spermatogonia, and chorionic epithelium. Widespread cytoplasmic vacuolation is also seen in fetuses of ewes that have consumed locoweed. In ewes experimentally fed *A. lentiginosus,* vacuoles have appeared within four hours in renal tubular epithelium and by eight days in neurons. Neuronolysis was evident by the sixteenth day.

GROSS LESIONS

Gross lesions are not diagnostic, but the enlargement of thyroids, emaciation, golden color of liver and renal cortex, generalized edema, and focal erosions of the abomasal mucosa near the pyloris have been described. In pregnant cows, severe edema may resemble hydrops amnii.

Teratogenic effects have been observed in nature and reproduced experimentally in sheep. Feeding of *Astragalus pubentissimus* to pregnant sheep results in the frequent occurrence of congenital anomalies in the offspring. The type of anomaly appears to depend upon the stage of pregnancy during which the locoweed is eaten. If locoweed were consumed by ewes during days 25–49 of pregnancy, aplasia of the lower jaw is the dominant congenital anomaly in the lambs. Ingestion during days 40–60 of pregnancy often results in hypermobility of the hock and stifle joints in affected lambs. Offspring with flexures of carpal joints result from feeding the plant during days 60–90 of pregnancy. Lambs born of ewes that ingested locoweed on days 100–125 of pregnancy are apt to have relaxed pastern joints. Abortions are common and some ewes die from this plant poisoning.

Oxytropis sericea also has been fed to ewes during days 82–102 of gestation, resulting in contracted flexor tendons (or muscles) in the offspring. A few cases of frank arthrogryposis in sheep poisoned in utero with locoweed have been seen (lupines, page 721).

Poisoning by locoweed (*Oxytropis sericea*) in cattle has been demonstrated to increase the severity and frequency of "high-altitude disease," with particularly severe hypertrophy of the right side of the heart and cardiac failure (page 752).

References

Alroy J, Orgad U, Ucci AA, et al. Swainsonine toxicosis mimics lectin histochemistry of mannosidosis. Vet Pathol 1985;22:311–316.

Hartley WJ, James LF. Microscopic lesions in fetuses of ewes ingesting locoweed (Astragalus lentiginosus). Am J Vet Res 1973;34:209–212.

James LF, Elbein AD, Molyneux RJ, et al. Swainsonine and related glycoside inhibitors. Ames: Iowa State Univ Press, 1989.

James LF, Hartley WF, Van Kampen KR, et al. Relationship between ingestion of the locoweed Oxytropis sericea and congestive right-sided heart failure in cattle. Am J Vet Res 1983;44:254–259.

James LF, Hartley WJ, Nielsen D, et al. Locoweed (Oxytropis sericea) poisoning and congestive heart failure in cattle. J Am Vet Med Assoc 1986;189:1549–1556.

James LF, Keeler RF, Bailey EM Jr, et al, eds. Poisonous plants: Proc 3rd Int Symp. Ames: Iowa State Univ Press, 1992.

James LF, Keeler RF, Binns W. Sequence in the abortive and teratogenic effects of locoweed fed to sheep. Am J Vet Res 1969;30:377–380.

James LF, Van Kampen KR, Hartley WJ. Comparative pathology of Astragalus (locoweed) and Swainsona poisoning in sheep. Pathol Vet 1970;7:116–125.

Laws L, Anson RB. Neuronopathy in sheep fed Swainsona luteola and S. galegifolia. Aust Vet J 1968;44:447–452.

Van Kampen KR, James LF. Pathology of locoweed poisoning in sheep. Pathol Vet 1969;6:413–423.

Van Kampen KR, James LF. Ophthalmic lesions in locoweed poisoning of cattle, sheep, and horses. Am J Vet Res 1971;32:1293–1295.

Van Kampen KR, James LF. Ovarian and placental lesions in sheep from ingesting locoweed (Astragalus lentiginosus). Vet Pathol 1971;8:193–199.

Van Kampen KR, James LF. Pathology of locoweed (Astragalus lentiginosus) poisoning in sheep. Sequential development of cytoplasmic vacuolation in tissues. Pathol Vet 1970;7:503–508.

Wolfe GJ, Lance WR. Locoweed poisoning in a northern New Mexico elk herd. J Range Manag 1984;37:59–63.

Vetchlike astragali

A number of small leguminous plants that resemble the true vetches and sometimes receive that designation produce poisoning on the ranges of the Rocky Mountain region of the United States. They are classified, however, in the genus Astragalus, which is notable because of locoweeds, which are also included in it. The form of poisoning produced, like loco, involves the nervous system principally, and does not resemble the hepatotoxic effects of the true vetches.

Under the name of timber milkvetch, *Astragalus decumbens, A. convallarius, A. hylophilus,* and *A. campestris* may be included, which are similar or identical species. The red-stemmed peavine, *A. emoryanus,* is a similar plant; it grows in the more southern regions, whereas the timber milkvetch reaches north into Canada.

Another classification of these plants places several varieties in a single genus, *Astragalus miser* (Williams et al., 1969). These include: *A. miser var oblongifolius, serotinus, hylophilus, miser, tenuifolius, praeteritus, decumbens,* and *crispatus.* The first three have been incriminated in poisoning of livestock. Cattle appear to be most susceptible, sheep much less so; rabbits and chickens may be poisoned experimentally. The basic sign is nervous weakness and incoordination involving the hindlimbs. When mild, this may be shown only by a momentary sinking of the hindquarters at the start of a forward movement. Later, distinct incoordination ensues, such as crossing of the legs and weakness, shown by "knuckling over" of the fetlock joints. Ultimately, the animal falls frequently and rises with difficulty. In cattle poisoned by milkvetch, the metatarsal and phalangeal joints are abnormally relaxed and poorly controlled, so that in walking the dewclaws (first metatarsal rudiments) strike the hoofs with a flapping sound. This has resulted in the nickname of "cracker-heel" for the disease. In sheep, another prominent, and at times primary, symptom is dyspnea accompanied by a loud rasping noise at inspiration and a cough frequently at expiration. The morphologic basis for this seems not to have been determined. It may be presumed the complete microscopic studies of the nervous system would reveal degenerative changes that would account for the posterior weakness. Conversely, the fact that a considerable number of victims die suddenly from acute dilatation of the heart, while the usual difficulties are yet at an early stage, raises the suspicion of interference with the metabolic processes of muscle. It should be noted that, although posterior weakness and paraplegia are much like the corresponding effects of the closely related locoweeds (*Astragalus mollissimus et spp.*), no disturbances of sensation or of the sensorium occur in the presently considered poisonings.

One toxic agent has been identified as miserotoxin, the β-glucoside of 3-nitro-1-propanol. This toxin is catabolized in vivo to two toxic fractions, inorganic nitrite and a 3-carbon nitro side chain. Nitrite (NO_2) produces methemoglobinemia, particularly in rabbits.

References

Mathews FP. Toxicity of red-stemmed peavine for cattle, sheep, and goats. J Am Vet Med Assoc 1940;97:125–134.

Newsom IE, et al. Timber milk vetch as a poisonous plant. Exper Sta Bull 425. Fort Collins: Colorado State College, 1936.

Panciera RJ. Hairy vetch (Vicia villosa Roth) poisoning in cattle. In: Keeler RF, Van Kampen KR, James LF, eds. Effects of poisonous plants on livestock. New York: Academic Press, 1978;555–563.

Williams MC, Van Kampen KR, Norris FA. Timber milkvetch poisoning in chickens, rabbits, and cattle. Am J Vet Res 1969;30:2185–2190.

Atropine (deadly nightshade, belladonna)

The foliage and unripe berries of the belladonna plant (*Atropa belladonna*) poison swine and rarely other animals by virtue of atropine (and other alkaloids). Other plant sources of tropane alkaloids (atropine, hyoscyamus) include *Datura stramonium* (jimsonweed, page 732) and *Hyoscyamus niger*.

Signs mostly include loss of nervous control with incoordination, shortly followed by convulsions and death, usually within 12 hours after the plant is eaten. Typically mydriasis, decreasing temperature, and failing heart are manifest. Postmortem lesions are not diagnostic, but may include subserous serofibrinous exudations, perhaps tinged with blood, especially around the kidneys and gallbladder. Of prime importance in diagnosis is the mydriatic action of belladonna. Not only are the patient's pupils dilated, but instillation of a small amount of the patient's urine into the conjunctival sac of a small experimental animal, particularly a cat, dog, or rabbit, should dilate the pupil within a few minutes.

References

Keeler RF. Naturally occurring teratogens from plants. In: Keeler RF, Tu AT, eds. Handbook of natural toxins. Vol 1. Plant and fungal toxins. New York: Marcel Dekker, 1983;178.

Smith HC, Taussig RA, Peterson PC. Deadly nightshade poisoning in swine. J Am Vet Med Assoc 1956;129:116–117.

Equisetum

Known by such names as horsetail, mare's tail and jointed rush, several species, of which *Equisetum arvense* is the most common, are poisonous, chiefly to horses. Signs include a nervous disorder and muscular weakness, the latter probably related to faulty innervation. Incoordination gradually increases until staggering, reeling, and ultimately inability to stand are manifest. Progressive muscular rigidity reaches the point where the animal can only lie on its side with the four limbs stiffly outstretched. Constipation and tenesmus are marked. Large amounts of watery urine are voided. The pupils are dilated; the animal's expression and actions reveal a state of apprehension, which deepens in to fright as the result of noises or other stimuli. In a recumbent state, the horse continues to live for several days, maintaining a good appetite until too weak to eat.

Lesions found postmortem include a pale and flabby state of the skeletal musculature, frequently hydroperitoneum, and congestion and inflammatory edema (serous exudate) of the cerebellar and spinal meninges. Microscopic studies are needed, especially of the nervous tissues and the kidneys, which from the polyuria appear to be damaged.

Poisoning by equisetum is prevented and usually cured by the administration of large amounts of thiamine (vitamin-B_1), but not by other components of the B-complex. From this it is inferred that equisetum owes its toxicity to a powerful opponent of thiamine; an extract of the plant has been shown to neutralize thiamine in vitro. Biochemical studies showed that carbohydrate metabolism was impaired in equisetum poisoning in the same way that it is in thiamine deficiency. Glycolysis by the blood in vitro was diminished. Glucose tolerance in the living animal was depressed, as were the amounts of glycogen in liver and muscle. Pyruvic acid in the blood rose to 1.52 mg/100 mL, with oxalic acid behaving similarly; phosphates reached levels of 13 mg, and potassium 50 mg. Levels of alkaline phosphatase and cholesterinase also increased (thiaminase, p. 734, and polioencephalomalacia, Chap. 27).

Lesions in the central nervous system should be comparable to those of thiamine deficiency or bracken fern poisoning.

References

Forenbacher S. Equisetum poisoning of horses and the vitamin B Complex. Vet Arch 1950;20:405–471, 1951;21:497–547. (English summary.) Abstr Vet Bull 1953;2671, also in Schweiz Arch Tierheilkd 1952;94:153–171.

Henderson JA, et al. The antithiamine action of equisetum. J Am Vet Med Assoc 1952;120:375–378.

Lott DG. The use of thiamin in mare's tail poisoning of horses. Can J Comp Med 1951;15:274–276.

Rich FA. Equisetum poisoning. Am Vet Rev 1903;26:944–954.

Hemlocks

Poisoning by deadly hemlock, *Conium maculatum*, has been recognized since the dawn of history. Ancient Greeks compelled condemned prisoners (Socrates the most famous) to drink an infusion of this plant, causing a relatively painless death. Herbivorous animals, including swine, occasionally eat the plant in spite of unpalatability and an offensive odor which it releases when bruised. After mild and transient stimulation, the plant acts as a nerve depressant, and it is upon this nervous depression that the signs are based. Although varying somewhat in different species, signs involve loss of muscular strength and gradual loss of the power of locomotion, the hindlimbs—as is usual in nervous and paralytic disorders—being most severely affected. In some cases, tremors and rarely generalized trembling occur, but more often the animal's activities quietly subside into a sort of coma, in which consciousness appears to be greatly depressed but not disordered. Death may come in about one hour, but many animals remain comatose for one or several hours and then quietly recover. In cattle, lacrimation, salivation, dyspnea, and fetid or bloody diarrhea have been described. Signs usually commence within one to two hours after the plants are eaten and last for several hours or one to two days.

Postmortem lesions are based upon the cardiac depressant action of the poison. As a consequence of the slow cardiac failure, widespread passive congestion is manifest, most noticeably in the lungs and liver and vessels that nourish the heart muscle. It would appear from descriptions of "watery blood" that probably hemolysis or decreased clotting power, or both occur, but opportunities for systematic studies have seldom arisen. Severe, localized catarrhal or hemorrhagic enteritis have been described in cattle. Recognizable fragments of leaves or stems may be found in the forestomachs of ruminants and true stomachs of other species, constituting a valuable aid in diagnosis.

Five piperidine alkaloids have been identified from *Conium maculatum*. Two, coniine (2–propylpiperidine) and γ coniceine (δ 1–2 propylpiperidine), are the most significantly toxic and teratogenic to animals, including cattle and swine. *Conium maculatum* fed to cows during the susceptible days of pregnancy (days 40–70), resulted in arthrogryposis in their newborn offspring. Feeding the seeds or plants to sows at various periods during pregnancy result in the following lesions in newborn piglets: cleft palate (days 30–45) and congenital arthrogryposis (days 43–53) in many of the newborn piglets. Less severe lesions followed feeding seeds or plants during days 51–61 of pregnancy.

Transient congenital limb deformities have been seen in newborn lambs from ewes fed the toxic plant during days 30–60 of pregnancy.

A similar plant, *Cicuta douglasii* grows in wet places in the Rocky Mountain region of the United States, and is known as hemlock, water hemlock, or poison hemlock. Its large, chambered primary stem and the adjoining roots are especially poisonous. It differs from *Conium maculatum* in causing convulsions of the greatest violence, which are almost always fatal.

Poisonous quails of North America, which in both biblical and modern times have poisoned people who ate their flesh, should also be mentioned here. Evidence indicates that the meat of the quails contained the poisonous principle of hemlock plants which the birds had eaten. The much greater resistance of birds to many poisons than that possessed by mammals is a well-known phenomenon.

References

Gunn A. Cattle poisoned by hemlock. Vet J Ann Comp Pathol 1881;13:233–235.
Hannam DAR. Hemlock (Conium maculatum) poisoning in the pig. Vet Rec 1985;116:322.
MacDonald H. Hemlock poisoning in horses. Vet Rec 1937;49:1211–1212.
Panter KE, Keeler RF, Buck WB. Induction of cleft palate in newborn pigs by maternal ingestion of poison hemlock (Conium maculatum). Am J Vet Res 1985;46:1368–1371.
Panter KE, Keeler RF, Buck WB. Congenital skeletal malformations induced by maternal ingestion of Conium maculatum (poison hemlock) in newborn pigs. Am J Vet Res 1985;46:2064–2066.
Panter KE, Bunch TD, Keeler RF. Maternal and fetal toxicity of poison hemlock (Conium maculatum) in sheep. Am J Vet Res 1988;49:281–283.

PHALARIS GRASS

This pasture plant (*Phalaris tuberosa*, "canary grass"), has been incriminated in poisoning of sheep and cattle in Australia, New Zealand, South Africa, California, and South America. In New Zealand, a related species, *Phalaris arundinacea*, appears to be involved. Sheep are the principal animals affected, but cattle have been poisoned in Australia by this plant.

SIGNS

Signs in sheep have been described as peracute, resulting in sudden death, acute, with transient neurologic signs, and chronic, or "phalaris staggers," manifested by progressive, usually fatal, neurologic disease.

The peracute and acute forms of the disease are believed to be caused by tryptamine alkaloids which, on occasion, accumulate in these plants.

In the chronic form, "phalaris staggers," the cause is not clearly established. The initial signs include incoordination, stilted gait, staggering, muscle tremors, and hyperexcitability. Some animals may move about on their knees, apparently unable to straighten their forelimbs. Eventually the affliction leads to lateral recumbency, convulsions, and death. Mortality rates vary in different outbreaks 5–50%.

Gross lesions are quite distinctive, with the presence of a gray-green to blue pigment in nervous tissues and, to a lesser extent, in the renal medulla and liver. Focal symmetric pigmentation is evident in the brainstem, ventral horns of the spinal cord, and in dorsal root ganglia.

This pigment is seen microscopically in neurons of particular nuclei in the brainstem, spinal cord, and ganglia. The pigment is yellow-brown and does not stain with the periodic acid Schiff reaction or luxol-fast-blue stain. Accumulation of the pigment eventually destroys the neurons. Wallerian degeneration of white matter of the spinal cord is sometimes evident.

Ultrastructural studies indicate that the pigment is somewhat amorphous and is first seen in mitochondria. Pigment in lysosomes is believed to have been picked up after release from the mitochondria.

References

East NE, Higgins RJ. Canary grass (Phalaris sp.) toxicosis in sheep in California. J Am Vet Med Assoc 1988;192:667–669.

Hartley WJ. Chronic phalaris poisoning or phalaris staggers. In: Keeler RF, Van Kampen KR, James LF, eds. Effects of poisonous plants on livestock. New York: Academic Press, 1978;390–393.

Lathyrus (lathyrism)

Although several other closely related toxic species exist, the principal one is *Lathyrus sativus*. Several common names are in use, including Indian pea, dogtooth pea, flat pea, and Singletary pea. *Lathyrus odoratus* is the common sweet pea grown in flower gardens for its fragrance. *L. sativus* is also known in some English-speaking countries as "chickling vetch," but it is not to be confused with the usual vetches, which belong to a different genus, although they are leguminous plants of generally similar appearance. *Lathyrus sativus*, frequently in mixture with the closely related *L. cicera* and *L. clymenum,* are grown as forage plants especially in Mediterranean countries and India, and the seeds are a frequent article of human food. Under the name of "lathyrism," poisoning from excessive consumption of the seeds is well known in humans and domestic animals, especially horses. Because, in limited amounts, it is a nutritious legume rich in protein, and because of its hardiness, it has been introduced into the agricultural regions of Africa, Canada, and the mountainous ranges of the United States.

Poisoning only occurs when large amounts of seeds are eaten over a period of at least a few weeks, more often months. In humans and animals, the one outstanding effect is gradually increasing paralysis of the posterior (inferior) limbs. This is said to depend upon degeneration and disappearance of neurons in the spinal cord accompanied by gliosis and ultimate atrophy of the cord. Because many well-established cases recover, humans and animals, it is difficult to believe that irreversible changes occur until the late stages of illness. Some refer to the changes in the cord as inflammatory rather than degenerative. Paralysis of the recurrent laryngeal nerve with the production of "roaring" has been noted several times in horses. In cattle, blindness, torticollis, and anesthesia of the skin are additional symptoms. In any species, the pulse becomes rapid and weak because of incipient vagal paralysis. Constipation and mild digestive disturbances occur occasionally. Death ensues from respiratory paralysis.

In addition to the lesions of the spinal cord, mild, chronic enteritis is manifest, perhaps with cecal or other impactions, terminal subepicardial hemorrhages (asphyxiative), and pulmonary congestion. A neurotoxin, β-N-oxalyl-L-α, β-diaminopropionic acid (ODAP), has been isolated from seeds of *L. sativus*. The mode of action is suggested to be due to interference with ammonia metabolism in brain, leading to chronic ammonia toxicity.

Ground sweet pea seeds (*Lathyrus odoratus*) fed to growing rats result in striking skeletal deformities and changes in other mesodermal tissues. Periosteal new bone formation, kyphoscoliosis, and dissecting aneurysms of the aorta occurred, presumably as a result of severe disturbance of the growth of cartilage, bone, or elastic tissues. Paralysis in these rats appeared to result either from pressure upon segments of the spinal cord, as a consequence of the severe scoliosis, or from specific destruction of neurons in the cord. The effect upon bone, cartilage, and tendons is considered to be the result of cross-linkage impairment of elastin and collagen molecules. The active principles are often referred to as osteolathyrogens or neurolathyrogens, depending upon their effects. Some evidence has accrued that some of these compounds may affect both bone and nervous tissue. The principal lathyrogenic compounds now known include: aminoacetonitrile, a,r-diaminobutyric acid, β-aminopropionitrile, β-cyanoalanine, β-N-oxalyl-L-2,3 diaminopropionic acid, r-glutamyl-β-cyanoalanine, and r-glutamyl-β-aminopropionitrile.

Poisoning of pregnant animals, particularly sheep, has been shown to result in abortions, intrauterine death, contracted tendons, and aplasia of the lower jaw in the offspring. Thus, this group of plant toxins has a teratogenic potential.

In turkeys, lathyrism is associated with dissecting aneurysms of the aorta.

References

Hegarty MP. Toxic amino acids of plant origin. In: Keeler RF, Van Kampen KR, James LF, eds. Effects of poisonous plants on livestock. New York: Academic Press, 1978;575–586.

Keeler RF. Naturally occurring teratogens from plants. In: Keeler RF, Tu AT, eds. Handbook of natural toxins. Vol 1. Plant and fungal toxins. New York: Marcel Dekker, 1983;161–200.

Levene CI, Gross J. Alterations in state of molecular aggregation of collagen induced in chick embryos by β-aminopropionitrile (lathyrus factor). J Exp Med 1959;110:771–789.

Mennin S, Thomas DW. Comparative effects of an osteolathyrogen and a neurolathyrogen on brain and connective tissues. Proc Soc Exp Biol Med 1970;134:489–491.

Rasmussen MA, Foster JG, Allison MJ. Lathyrus sylvestris (flatpea) toxicity in sheep and rumenal metabolism of flatpea neurolathyrogens. In: James LF, Keeler RF, Bailey EM Jr, Cheeke PR, Hegarty MP, eds. Poisonous plants: Proc 3rd Int Symp. Ames: Iowa State Univ Press, 1992;377–381.

Larkspur (delphinium sp.)

The genus of decorative plants, Delphinium, consists of many species, but only a few have been demonstrated to be poisonous to livestock. These include *Delphinium barbeyi* (tall larkspur), *D. nuttallianum* (low larkspur), *D. glaucescens,* and *D. occidentale* (probably the least toxic). *Delphinium barbeyi* thrives over large areas of western grazing land in the United States and is an important cause of death in cattle. In British Columbia of western Canada, a low-growing variety, *Delphinium nuttallianum,* has been incriminated as a leading toxic plant that is readily consumed by cattle.

At least 27 alkaloids have been identified from Delphinium plants, but evidence points toward methyllycaconitine and its congeners as the most likely cause of toxicity in cattle. Horses also are susceptible, but sheep are reported to graze on these plants, ususally with little adverse effect. Rats are susceptible to ground up whole plants and extracts from them.

SIGNS

Signs of poisoning by these plants usually start with uneasiness, stiff gait, characteristic "straddle stance" (hing legs placed far apart), and sudden collapse (usually first by the forelegs). Some animals may regain the ability to stand, but are weak and muscles involuntarily twitch. Nausea, abdominal pain, and vomition may occur and death may follow aspiration of vomitus. Constipation is nearly always observed. Death often appears to result from repiratory failure.

Postmortem lesions include acute catarrhal gastroenteritis (hyperemia chiefly) and widespread venous congestion typical of gradual cardiac failure. Congestion is especially prominent in the kidneys, as well as in the vena cava and large veins.

References

Bai Y, Benn MH, Majak W. The alkaloids of Delphinium nuttallianum: the cattle-poisoning low larkspur of interior British Columbia. In: James LF, Keeler RF, Bailey EM Jr, Cheeke PR, Hegarty MP, eds. Poisonous plants: Proc 3rd Int Symp. Ames: Iowa State Univ Press, 1992;304–308.

Cronin EH, Nielsen DB. Tall larkspur and cattle on high mountain ranges. In: Keeler RF, Van Kampen KR, James LF, eds. Effects of poisonous plants on livestock. New York: Academic Press, 1978;521–534.

Olson JD. Larkspur toxicosis: a review of current research. In: Keeler RF, Van Kampen KR, James LF, eds. Effects of poisonous plants on livestock. New York: Academic Press, 1978;535–543.

Yellow star thistle

A plant that grows abundantly in dry, weedy pastures in the northern valleys of California, *Centaurea solsitialis,* popularly known as yellow star thistle, is credited, on the basis of clinical and experimental studies, with causing an equine central nervous disorder called "chewing disease" by ranchers and nigropallidal encephalomalacia by pathologists.

A similar disease with essentially the same lesions has been seen in Colorado, and has been produced in horses by feeding dried Russian knapweed *(Centaurea repens).* They also described necrosis in the nucleus of the inferior colliculus, the mesencephalic nucleus of the trigeminal nerve, and the dentate nucleus.

Signs appear suddenly after the animal has been eating the plant for one to three months and has consumed several hundred pounds of it. They consist essentially of hypertonicity of the muscles of the face, lips, and tongue due to hyperirritability of the nervous mechanism controlling them, the whole being dependent upon loss of central control from the higher centers. Local reflexes and sensation remain intact. The horse performs involuntary chewing movements, but is unable effectively to obtain food or swallow it. The lips are rigid and the skin is puckered, although the angles of the mouth are not necessarily retracted as in the risus sardonicus of some other nervous disorders. The mouth may be held half open with the tongue protruding, although the animal is able to withdraw the latter and no (flaccid) paralysis occurs. A mild degree of som-

nolence usually prevails with some disturbance of gait, but death eventually results from starvation or thirst in horses so severely affected that they are unable to drink.

Postmortem, the dorsum of the tongue is regularly coated with dried salivary and other material that accumulates with cessation of swallowing; often a tendency toward local edema and buccal ulceration is evident, perhaps from injury in efforts to eat. Some cases develop enterocolitis, which may be due directly to the poison. The fundamental lesion was found to consist in localized encephalomalacia (necrosis) involving the anterior portions of the globus pallidus and substantia nigra. The necrotic areas were sharply demarcated, roundly elongated, and as much as 10–15 mm in greatest dimension. Slightly yellowish or buff in color, the areas were gelatinous and bulging in the early stages, distinctly soft at one or two weeks of age, and cavities filled with semifluid debris at three weeks. The lesions were usually bilaterally symmetric; when they were unilateral, the peripheral disturbances were contralateral. Microscopically, the early lesions (two to five days) showed pyknosis and karyolysis of neuroglial nuclei and gradual disappearance of neurons, with limited glial proliferation and slight accumulation of scavenger cells (gitterzellen). With time, proliferated neuroglia increased (gliosis), as well as the number of scavenger cells; at three to six weeks, a definite glial capsule had formed and some of the scavenger cells had developed into bizarre forms and giant cells. Although minute hemorrhages occurred in necrotic areas, hyperemia was not a feature. Cordy summarized the changes under the name of nigropallidal encephalomalacia.

The precise and consistent location of the lesions, naturally occurring or experimentally induced, in the nigrostriatal tract in the globus pallidus and substantia nigra in the equine brain suggests a specific toxic effect involving a single pathway. Similar induced lesions affecting the nigrostriatal pathway of rats result in signs and lesions analogous to those seen in horses. One possible explanation states that the initial signs are the result of massive release of dopamine (stored neurotransmitter). Similar effects have been demonstrated in macaque monkeys.

Identification of the exact toxin or toxins appears to be necessary to remove the principal obstacle to further understanding of the pathogenesis of this disease.

References

Cordy DR. Centaurea species and equine nigropallidal encephalomalacia. In: Keeler RF, Van Kampen KR, James LF, eds. Effects of poisonous plants on livestock. New York: Academic Press, 1978;327–336.

Cordy DR. Nigropallidal encephalomalacia in horses, associated with ingestion of yellow star thistle. J Neuropathol Exp Neurol 1954;13:330–342.

Denny-Brown D. The basal ganglia and their relation to disorders of movement. London: Oxford Univ Press, 1962.

Riopelle RJ, Boegman RJ, Little PB, et al. Neurotoxicity of sesquiterpene lactones. In: James LF, Keeler RF, Bailey EM Jr, Cheeke PR, Hegarty MP, eds. Poisonous plants: Proc 3rd Int Symp. Ames: Iowa State Univ Press, 1992;298–303.

Young S, Brown WW, Klinger B. Nigropallidal encephalomalacia in horses fed Russian knapweed Centaurea repens. L Am J Vet Res 1970;31:1393–1404.

Young S, Brown WW, Klinger B. Nigropallidal encephalomalacia in horses caused by ingestion of weeds of the genus Centaurea. J Am Vet Med Assoc 1970;157:1602–1605.

Anguina (rye grass poisoning, rye grass staggers)

Anguina agrostis is one of the many species of minute nematodes that infest plants. In the case of this species, microscopic larvae invade the seeds of certain grasses, causing the seed to become an enlarged, reactive mass known as a gall. The multitudinous larvae remain dormant in the gall until it is softened by moisture, when they escape and reproduce. Among the species of grass liable to be infested by this parasite are Chewings fescue, creeping red fescue, various kinds of bent grass, orchard grass, buffalo grass, red top, creeping timothy, sweet vernal grass, velvet grass, annual blue grass, and Kentucky blue grass. *Anguina lolii* has been identified as a parasite on Wimmera rye grass *(Lolium rigidum)* in Australia. This parasite acts as a vector for a *Corynebacterium sp.*, which grows as a yellow slime on the plants and in the galls. It is believed that the source of the toxicity is from the *Corynebacterium sp.*

As has been shown by Galloway, working on the irrigated grass fields of arid central Oregon, horses and cattle, as well as experimental rats and chickens, are poisoned when they consume sufficient amounts of infested grass seeds, either mixed with hay or in "screenings," the discarded imperfect seeds separated from harvested grass seed. The grass in which this occurred in Galloway's experience was Chewings fescue grass *(Festuca rubra v. commutata).*

Formerly viewed as manifestations of forage poisoning, the signs indicate that the toxic substance, which can be extracted with boiling alcohol, is a nerve poison. Prominent among these symptoms are staggering, knuckling of the feet, tucking the head between the forelegs, falling, and clonic spasms. The illness may arise when the toxic material has been consumed for about two weeks. Death may ensue in a matter of hours or the nervous symptoms may continue for a week or more. Gross lesions are not discernible; microscopic changes apparently have not been studied. Diagnosis is made by soaking the suspected seeds and galls and demonstrating the microscopic larvae, which are numerous.

References

Berry PH, Richards RB, Howell J McC, et al. Hepatic damage in sheep fed annual ryegrass, Lolium rigidum, parasitized by Anguina agrostis and Corynebacterium rathayi. Res Vet Sci 1982;32:148–156.

Fletcher LR, Harvey IC. An association of a Lolium endophyte with ryegrass staggers. NZ Vet J 1981;29:185–186.

Gallagher RT, White EP, Mortimer PH. Ryegrass staggers: isolation of potent neurotoxins lolitrem A and lolitrem B from staggers-producing pastures. NZ Vet J 1981;29:189–190.

Gallagher RT, et al. Ryegrass staggers: the presence of lolitrem neurotoxins in perennial ryegrass seed. NZ Vet J 1982;30:183–184.

Galloway JH. Grass seed nematode poisoning in livestock. J Am Vet Med Assoc 1961;139:1212–1214.

Haag JR. Toxicity of nematode infested Chewings fescue seed. Science 1945;102:406–407.

Lanigan GW, Payne AL, Frahn JL. Origin of toxicity in parasitized annual ryegrass (Lolium rigidum). Aust Vet J 1976;52:244–246.

Latch GCM, Falloon RE, Christensen MJ. Fungi and ryegrass staggers. NZ J Agric Res 1976;19:233–242.

Carbon disulfide

This highly volatile liquid has a number of industrial and laboratory uses, but domestic animals come in contact with it when it is administered as a treatment against gastric or intestinal parasites, chiefly in horses and swine. Serious excesses in dosage have been rare, but a more frequent accident has been the breaking of a capsule in the animal's pharynx. Violent spasm of the regional musculature is the result, and fatal arrest of respiration is a possibility. Signs of poisoning include transient local pain and inflammation, but are largely related to its nerve-depressant action, dullness and lethargy being followed by lower neuron paralysis and coma. Lesions, other than localized gastritis and enteritis in areas of contact, are neurologic. Nerve cells are destroyed sporadically in brain and spinal cord, and fiber tracts and peripheral nerves suffer demyelination.

Reference

Comporti M. Lipid peroxidation and cellular damage in toxic liver injury. Lab Invest 1985;53:599–623.

Orthotricresyl phosphate

Orthotricresyl phosphate, contained in a type of synthetic rubber used for shoe soles, scraps of which were eaten by chickens, was shown clinically and experimentally to be highly fatal. Signs in chickens were inappetence, fetid diarrhea, and progressive paralysis of the legs. Sensation, at least of pain, was not lost. The poisoning was invariably fatal in three to four weeks. Lesions consisted principally of enteritis with atrophy of the unused gastrointestinal tract and a full gallbladder. Wallerian degeneration of the myelin sheaths of peripheral nerves occurred, principally the sciatic and lumbosacrals, which resembled histologically the lesion of thiamine deficiency.

Reference

Hartwigk H. Lähmungen bei Hühnern durch Weichigelit. Monatsh Veternirm 1950;5:53–55.

Lead

Animals are sometimes poisoned by lead salts through licking painted surfaces, which is a habit of calves especially, or through the ingestion of discarded paint or putty. Puppies are most often poisoned by chewing or eating objects painted with lead-base paints, old paint chipped from surfaces to be repainted, linoleum containing lead, and less frequently, broken wet cell batteries, plumber's lead compounds, or lead-containing roofing material. Children may be poisoned from these same sources or possibly from lead-glazed cooking ware.

Waterfowl have been poisoned by metallic lead shot ingested from the sludge of lake bottoms, in which the discharges from guns of many hunters had accumulated. Fumes from burning storage batteries, cutaneous absorption from gasoline-containing tetra-ethyl lead, and other mechanisms have been rarely incriminated. Habitual exposure to fumes from lead smelters has poisoned horses working in or near them. The lead in wind-borne contamination of pastures in the vicinity of such smelters may reach 130 mg/kg of dry forage, and accumulations of lead in the soil to levels reaching 1000 ppm have been associated with poisoning of cattle and horses. Orchard sprays frequently contain lead arsenate, but the arsenical ion is the one of principal importance. In calves and sheep, a single dose of 200–400 mg/kg of body weight is regularly fatal, but a daily intake of about 6 mg/kg of body weight is necessary to produce cumulative poisoning in an adult cow. Horses appear to be somewhat more susceptible. The minimum lethal dose of lead in waterfowl has been found to approximate 8 mg/kg of body weight. Lead poisoning rarely occurs in swine, which seem to be more tolerant than other domestic species.

SIGNS AND LESIONS

Signs and lesions of lead poisoning in general focus on its effects on red blood cells (Fig. 15-23), the nervous system, kidney, and bone (Fig. 15-24); however, great variation exists in the extent of lesions in these tissues from one example of lead poisoning to another, as well as between species. The explanation for these variations is not clear, but in part, is related to the duration of exposure. Young animals and children appear to be more susceptible. Increased environmental temperature and vitamin D accentuate the poisoning. Un-

doubtedly, many more factors influence toxicity and development of lesions.

RED BLOOD CELLS

Anemia develops in almost all species. In dogs, anemia is usually slight, but regularly large numbers of nucleated red blood cells in peripheral circulation are manifest, often up to 100 or more per 100 white blood cells. Basophilic stippling occurs in almost all examples. The appearance of immature red blood cells with little anemia is a strong indication of lead poisoning in the dog. Lead inhibits two enzymes involved in hemoglobin synthesis: d-aminolevulinic acid dehydratase and ferrochelatase. Inability to synthesize hemoglobin is, in part, the basis of anemia. This also leads to increased urinary excretion of porphyrins and d-aminolevulinic acid, two measurements that can be useful as diagnostic aids. Erythrocytes accumulate protoporphyrin IX, which causes them to fluoresce red when exposed to 320–400 nm ultraviolet light. Inhibition of nucleotidase is believed to result in basophilic stippling, as well as in the increased fragility of red cells. The resultant shortened erythrocyte lifespan also contributes to anemia. Bone marrow, as to be expected, is hyperplastic.

NERVOUS SYSTEM

The neuropathologic effects of lead poisoning are of the greatest concern and have received the greatest attention, but are still not clearly understood. Signs in most species include restlessness, head pressing, hyperesthesia, colic, tremors, ataxia, convulsions, and blindness. Horses most often exhibit gradual paralysis. Laryngeal paralysis is quite characteristic, resulting in noisy respiration (roaring).

Lesions may be minimal or absent even in the pres-

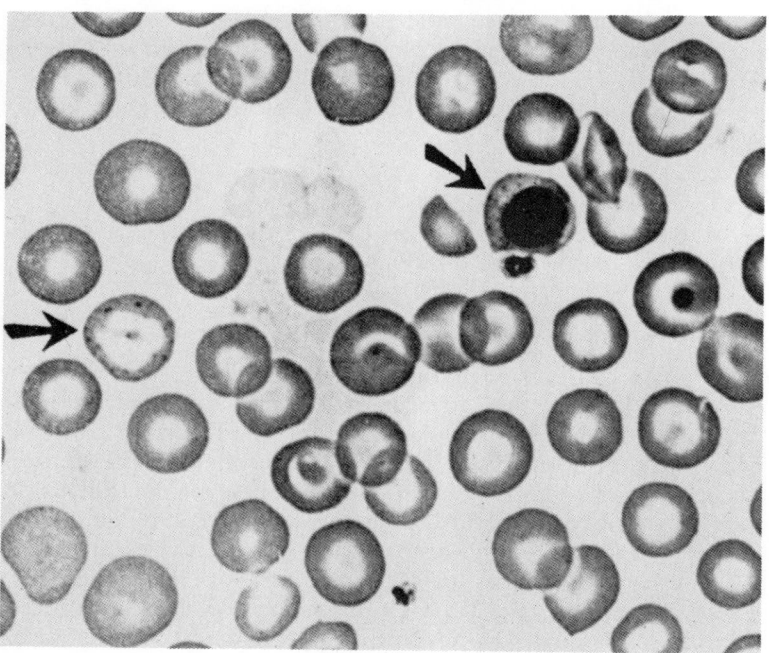

FIG. 15-23 Lead poisoning of a dog. Punctate-basophilic stippling in nucleated and nonnucleated erythrocytes (arrows) in a smear of peripheral blood stained with Wright-Giemsa stain. Note anisocytosis, poikilocytosis, hypochromia, "target" cells, and polychromatophilia involving red blood cells. (Courtesy of Dr. B. C. Zook and Journal of the American Veterinary Medical Association.)

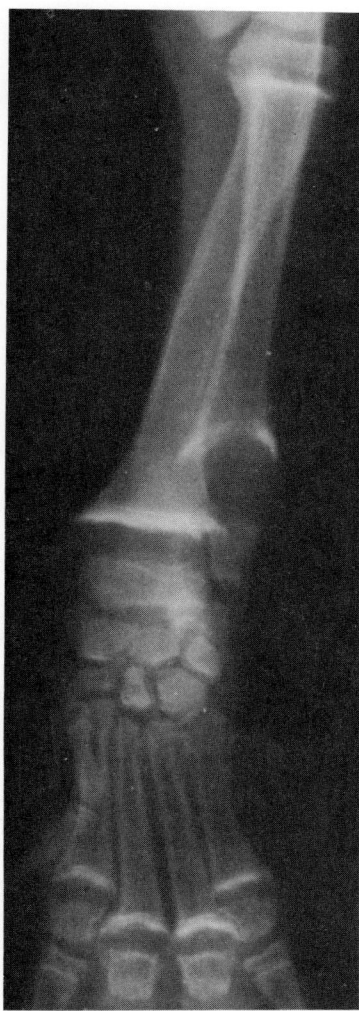

FIG. 15-24 Lead poisoning of a young dog. Radiograph of a foreleg. Radiographically dense bands in the distal metaphysis of radius, ulna, and metacarpal bones and proximal metaphysis of the radius. (Courtesy of Dr. B. C. Zook and Journal of the American Veterinary Medical Association.)

one of the common manifestations of lead poisoning in humans, and may account for the paralysis seen in horses. The peripheral nerves have not been studied extensively in animals, but the lesion in humans is wallerian degeneration of nerve roots. Segmental degeneration of axons and myelin have been reproduced in laboratory rats and guinea pigs.

KIDNEY

One of the most well-known lesions of lead poisoning is the occurrence of intranuclear inclusion bodies (Figs. 15-25, 15-26) in tubular epithelial cells of the kidney. Similar inclusion bodies develop in hepatocytes and osteoclasts. These inclusions are recognized by light microscopy by their acid-fast character when stained with carbol-fuchsin, and their failure to stain for DNA by the Feulgen reaction. In electron micrographs, the inclusion is a distinctive discrete body with a dense central core surrounded by a zone of fibrillar structures (Fig. 15-26). Inclusions isolated from cells after digestion with trypsin are seen as a dense homogeneous core surrounded by a membrane. Chemical analysis of isolated inclusions reveals them to contain lead and protein in relatively constant ratios. Although the presence of these inclusion bodies is considered pathognomonic for exposure to lead, caution should be used in assessing their usefulness to diagnose lead poisoning. They develop within hours of exposure and may be present in the absence of any clinical signs or other lesions of lead poisoning. Moreover, they are not invariably present in lead poisoning. Cytoplasmic inclusion bodies may also be present.

Renal tubular dysfunction, as indicated by proteinuria or aminoaciduria, has been noted in humans, dogs, and experimentally poisoned rats; however, tubular lesions have been described in almost all species. Acute lesions are principally restricted to the proximal convoluted tubule, whose epithelial cells have enlarged nuclei, become swollen, and may undergo necrosis and slough. Chronic nephropathy is described as an outcome of lead poisoning in humans and has been reproduced in rats and rabbits. It is characterized by tubular dilatation and fibrosis. The precise causal relationship to lead poisoning, however, deserves further study.

BONE

The lead line, a linear metaphyseal density seen on radiographs (Fig. 15-24), is another well-recognized lesion of lead poisoning in growing animals. Microscopically, this band is composed of trabeculae of calcified cartilage covered by a thin layer of bone. The bars of mineralized cartilage, which results from impaired resorption by osteoclasts, are wider than normal and project further into the metaphyseal marrow cavity than normal. Although they surround these spicules, numerous, multinucleated giant cells are apparently incapable of digesting the mineralized matrix. Many such cells bear acid-fast intranuclear inclusion bodies. Bone formation appears to be depressed, which is consistent with reports of osteoporosis resulting from lead poisoning. Lameness is a frequent clinical sign, and may result from the metaphyseal lesion.

ence of neurologic signs. Microscopically, the most consistent findings include cerebral edema and marked distention of many arterioles, venules, and capillaries. Endothelial cells are swollen and hyperplastic and occasionally pyknotic. In dogs, arteriolar walls may be hyalinized or contain hyalin thrombi. Laminar necrosis in the deeper cortical gray matter is often a feature that is believed to develop independently of vascular lesions. It is accompanied by astrocytosis. Astrocytosis may also be evident diffusely throughout both gray and white matter. Focal necrosis of basal nuclei and brainstem nuclei may also be encountered. Demyelinating encephalopathy has been associated with lead poisoning in nonhuman primates, but this is not consistent with the findings in other species, in which necrosis is principally confined to gray matter; the lesion has not been seen in experimentally poisoned monkeys.

Peripheral neuropathy leading to motor weakness is

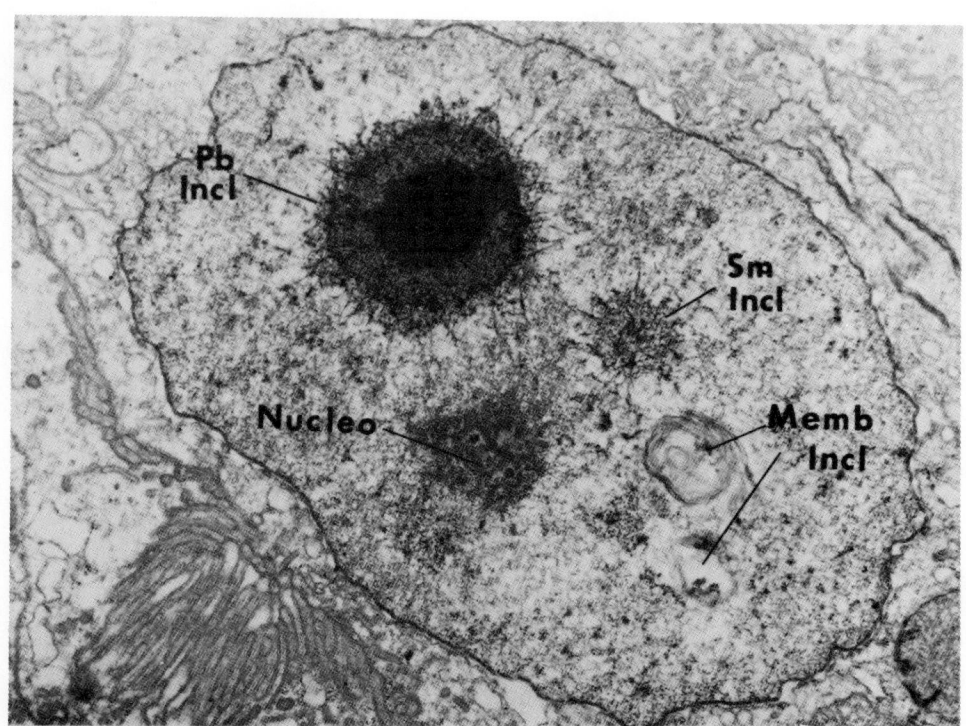

FIG. 15-25 Lead poisoning of a rat. Electron micrograph of nucleus of a proximal renal tubular epithelial cell. Inclusion body (Pb incl); nucleolus (nucleo); small, possibly incipient inclusion body (sm incl), and nonspecific invaginations of cytoplasmic fragments (memb incl). (Courtesy of Dr. Robert A. Goyer and Laboratory Investigation.)

OTHER TISSUES

A variety of changes has been reported in other tissues, but the lesions are less consistent and their relationship to lead poisoning not clear. These include pancreatic fibrosis, interstitial pneumonia, retarded embryonic development, oligospermia, focal myocardial necrosis, hepatic fatty change, and toxic hepatitis. Night blindness has been reported in experimentally poisoned monkeys, and a degenerative retinopathy in rabbits.

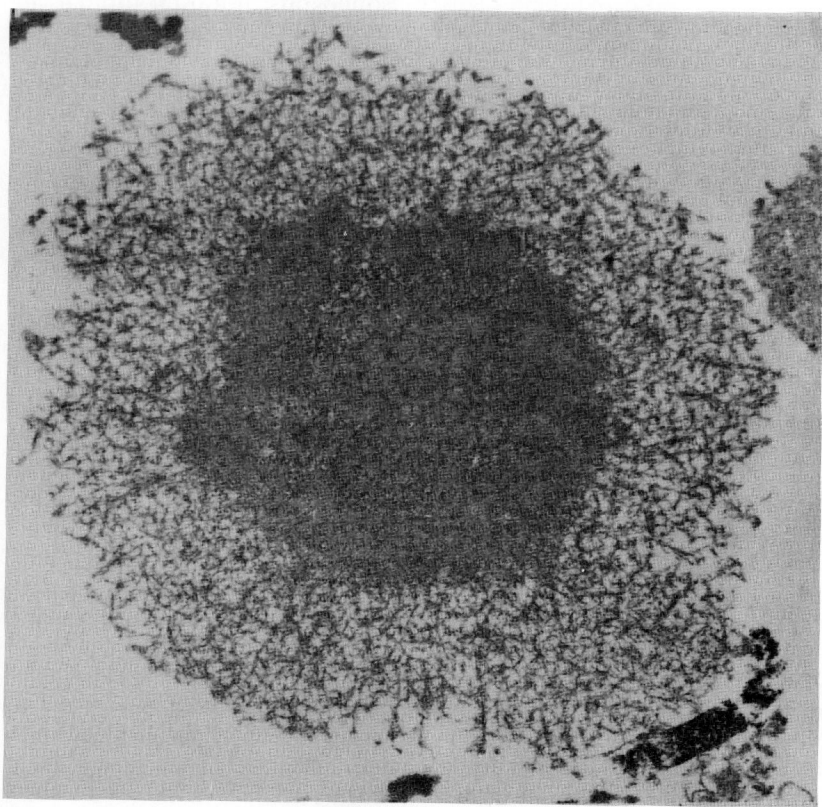

FIG. 15-26 Lead poisoning. Electron micrograph (×30,000) of an isolated inclusion body from renal tubular epithelium of a rat. Note fibrillar outer zone with attached granules. (Courtesy of Dr. Robert A. Goyer and Laboratory Investigation.)

DIAGNOSIS

It is frequently difficult to diagnose lead poisoning with certainty. The demonstration of lead in fluids and tissue is of value, but extreme variations are encountered. Zook et al. considered the following levels significant (1972): blood lead 35 μg or more/100 ml; urine lead 75 μg or more/L; urine lead 24 hours after starting chelation therapy, 821 μg or more/L; hair lead, 88 μg or more/g; liver lead (wet weight), and 3.6 μg or more/g. Reference has already been made to the usefulness of urinary excretion of porphyrins, d-aminolevulinic acid, and erythrocyte fluorescence. The occurrence of nucleated and other immature red blood cells in peripheral circulation, out of proportion to anemia, is one of the best diagnostic clues, especially in the presence of neurologic signs.

Pathologically, the lesions in the central nervous system, kidney, and bone are of greatest consistency. Lead-containing foreign bodies (e.g., paint, linoleum) may sometimes be demonstrated radiographically in the gastrointestinal tract. The classic "lead line," a dark bluish discoloration of the gingival mucosa adjacent to the teeth, is less useful and frequent in animals than, reportedly, it is in humans. This lead line is the result of precipitation of lead sulfide following interaction with blood-borne lead and hydrogen sulfide arising from decaying particles of food. In young dogs, increased radiographic density may be demonstrated at the epiphysis of long bones (Fig. 15-24).

References

DeVries CR, et al. Acute toxicity of lead particulates on pulmonary alveolar macrophages. Lab Invest 1983;48:35–44.

Goyer RA, Krall R. Ultrastructural transformation in mitochondria isolated from kidneys of normal and lead-intoxicated rats. J Cell Biol 1969;41:393–400.

Goyer RA, Rhyne BC. Pathological effects of lead. Int Rev Exp Pathol 1973;12:1–77.

Goyer RA, et al. Lead and protein content of isolated intranuclear inclusion bodies from kidneys of lead-poisoned rats. Lab Invest 1970;22:245–251.

Hamir AN. Review of lead poisoning in dogs. Vet Bull 1986;56:1059–1070.

Sass B, Banfield WG, Saffiotti U. Detection and cellular localization of lead by electron probe analysis in the diagnosis of suspected lead poisoning in rhesus monkeys. Toxicol Pathol 1991;19:30–34.

Zook BC, Carpenter JA, Leeds EH. Lead poisoning in dogs. J Am Vet Med Assoc 1969;155:1329–1342.

Zook BC, et al. Lead poisoning in dogs: analysis of blood, urine, hair, and liver for lead. Am J Vet Res 1972;33:903–909.

Zook BC, et al. Experimental lead poisoning in nonhuman primates. II. Clinical pathologic findings and behavioral effects. J Med Primatol 1980;9:286–303.

Zook BC. Lead poisoning in nonhuman primates. In: Jones TC, Mohr U, Hunt RD, eds. ILSI monographs on pathology of laboratory animals, nonhuman primates I. Heidelberg: Springer-Verlag, 1993;163–169.

Mercury

Acute mercurial poisoning may result from the accidental ingestion of mercury compounds (Fig. 15-27), chiefly the extremely poisonous mercuric chloride (bichloride of mercury) or the organic mercurial fungi-

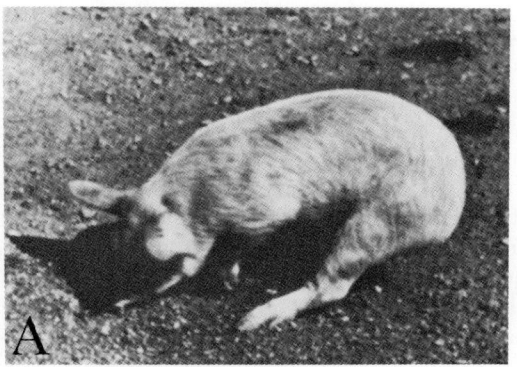
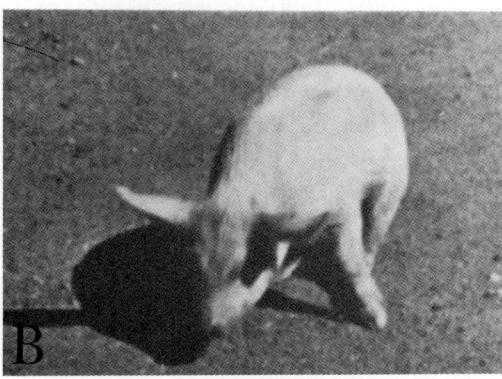
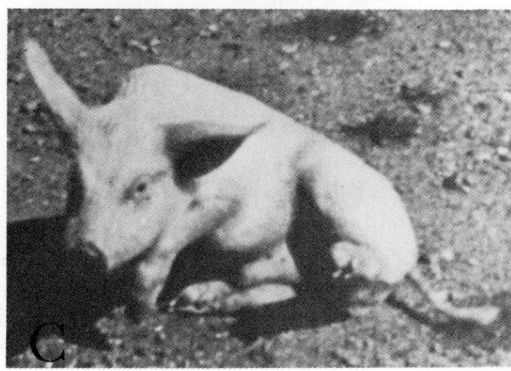

FIG. 15-27 Organo-mercurial poisoning. This affected pig demonstrates paresis, manifest by **A.** knuckling of fetlocks, and **B.** and **C.** falling backwards. (Courtesy of Dr. L. Tryphonas.)

cides. It may also occur as the result of excessive absorption from bichloride antiseptic solution, or possibly from mercuric iodide (red biniodide of mercury) used as a counterirritant or due to inhalation of mercury vapor from metallic mercury. In such cases, symptoms, arising within a period of some hours, include severe colicky pain, vomiting, and diarrhea. The chief lesion is severe and perhaps hemorrhagic gastroenteritis. The gastric mucosa undergoes coagulative necrosis, a change comparable to what happens to tissues subjected to mercurial fixatives in the pathology laboratory.

If the patient were to live a few days, severe and stubborn ulcerative colitis would develop because absorbed mercury is extensively eliminated through the colonic mucous membrane. About this time, anuria and uremia also develop because of destruction of the renal tubules. The proximal convoluted tubules and, to a lesser degree, the other tubules undergo hydropic degeneration and necrosis of the epithelium, the necrotic cytoplasm being desquamated and sometimes congealed to form albuminous casts in the lumen. If the patient were to survive, a new epithelial lining, at first low and flat, would be regenerated after about 10 days.

The use of mercurial drugs by ingestion or in ointment, douches, or other preparations, or exposure to metallic mercury—when continued for a time—produces a slower type of poisoning; soreness, swelling, bleeding, and ultimately, ulceration of the gums, tongue, and buccal mucosa occur. Necrosis may extend to the jaw bones; anemia, edema (renal origin), cachexia, and terminal infections lead to death. Nervous disorders based upon injury essentially similar to nervous changes accompany this form of poisoning, the whole syndrome sometimes being known as mercurialism. Local poisoning, characterized by paralysis of the hand and forearm involved, was reported in a man who rubbed an ointment containing mercuric iodide into the skin of cattle.

At present, the usual mercurial poisoning encountered in domestic animals results from using as feed for animals (chiefly swine), grains (e.g., wheat, oats, barley, rice) that had been set aside for seed and treated with an organic mercurial, such as methylmercury, arylmercury, ethylmercury phosphate, and mercury p-toluene sulfonanilide; these were used to control fungous diseases in germinating plants. The use of such seed grains for feed is not always accidental because of the temptation to avoid seed waste by using these chemicals. Industrial plants that discharge mercurial waste products into streams or rivers present a potent hazard to humans and animals.

At least one report concerned mercury poisoning of an 8-year-old girl, her 13-year-old brother, and 20-year-old sister. All were ill with similar signs of decreased vision, ataxia, and depression leading to coma. Toxic amounts of mercury were demonstrated in the urine of each patient. Each of these children, and four other members of the family, had eaten pork from swine slaughtered on their farm. Fourteen of seventeen swine on the farm had been ill with blindness and disturbance of gait. Twelve of the fourteen swine died. The swine had been fed seed grain treated with mercury dicyandiamide; mercury was demonstrated chemically in the pork and seed grain. This report appears to establish mercury poisoning of swine as a potential hazard to public health.

The signs and lesions of this form of mercurial poisoning are related almost entirely to the nervous system (Fig. 15-28). After 15–50 days on a diet of the treated grain, pigs become blind without ocular lesions, lose their appetites, become weak and incoordinated, and shortly can no longer stand. The usual experience with experimental pigs receiving minimal toxic amounts of treated seed has been that the animals then become increasingly comatose. They often live several days, lying on one side, with the head drawn backward but with the back arched and forelegs drawn rigidly backward against the sternum. They perform convulsive running movements periodically or when irritated, but ultimately lie still with slower and slower respirations and little evidence of life. In clinical cases, death usually ensues after an illness considerably shorter than the period of a week or more which was characteristic of the experimental poisonings.

Few gross lesions appear. Microscopically, the glandular organs (e.g., salivary glands, pancreas) show more conspicuous hydropic degeneration than does the liver. The renal tubules show hydropic degeneration or early necrosis. The lumens of the proximal convoluted tubules are commonly obliterated by swelling. Albuminous precipitate is seen in some of the tubules still patent. Commonly a well-marked increase of reticuloendothelial tissue in the spleen and lymph nodes is evident.

The nervous system is most severely affected. Throughout the brain, many nerve-cell bodies have the usual changes of degeneration and necrosis; a diffuse increase of microglia, including rod-shaped nuclei, occurs. Demyelinization of nerve tracts extends into the cord, and occasionally encephalomalacia and myelomalacia are seen. Neuronal necrosis is usually most extensive in the cerebral cortex, but may also develop in the cerebellar cortex or any other gray matter. Dorsal root ganglia are also affected, and wallerian degeneration of peripheral sensory nerves is a frequent finding. Often many peripheral nerve fibers are reduced to hollow cylinders containing only irregular globules of red-stained (hematoxylin and eosin stain) necrotic material. Perivascular cuffing with lymphocytes may be extensive in brain. In some species (notably cattle, swine, and rats), varying degrees of fibrinoid necrosis of the leptomeningeal artery media (Fig. 15-29) is a nearly consistent finding, and has been suggested to contribute to cortical necrosis through ischemia. This vascular lesion, however, does not accompany the neuropathologic sequelae of experimental organomercurial poisoning in most species.

Hyaline degeneration of Purkinje fibers and cardiac muscle fibers occurs in cattle. Zenker necrosis of skeletal muscle has been described in experimentally poisoned animals, but this may not be a primary lesion. In chronic organomercurial poisoning, hair concentrates the greatest amount of mercury, followed by the liver, gallbladder, and kidney. Other tissues, including brain, contain considerably less. Clearly, tissue sensitivity to the toxic effects of mercury is more important than concentration of the metal in some tissues.

Mercury remains in tissues for a considerable period of time. Following a single oral dose of methylmercury, about 35% (23% excluding hair) remains after 156 days. The concentration of methylmercury in brain resulting in neurologic signs is about 10 ppm.

Certain organomercurials, such as arylmercury, are metabolized more rapidly than others, and that poisoning by such compounds more closely resembles mercuric chloride poisoning, with colitis and renal tubular necrosis as the principal lesions without injury to the central nervous system.

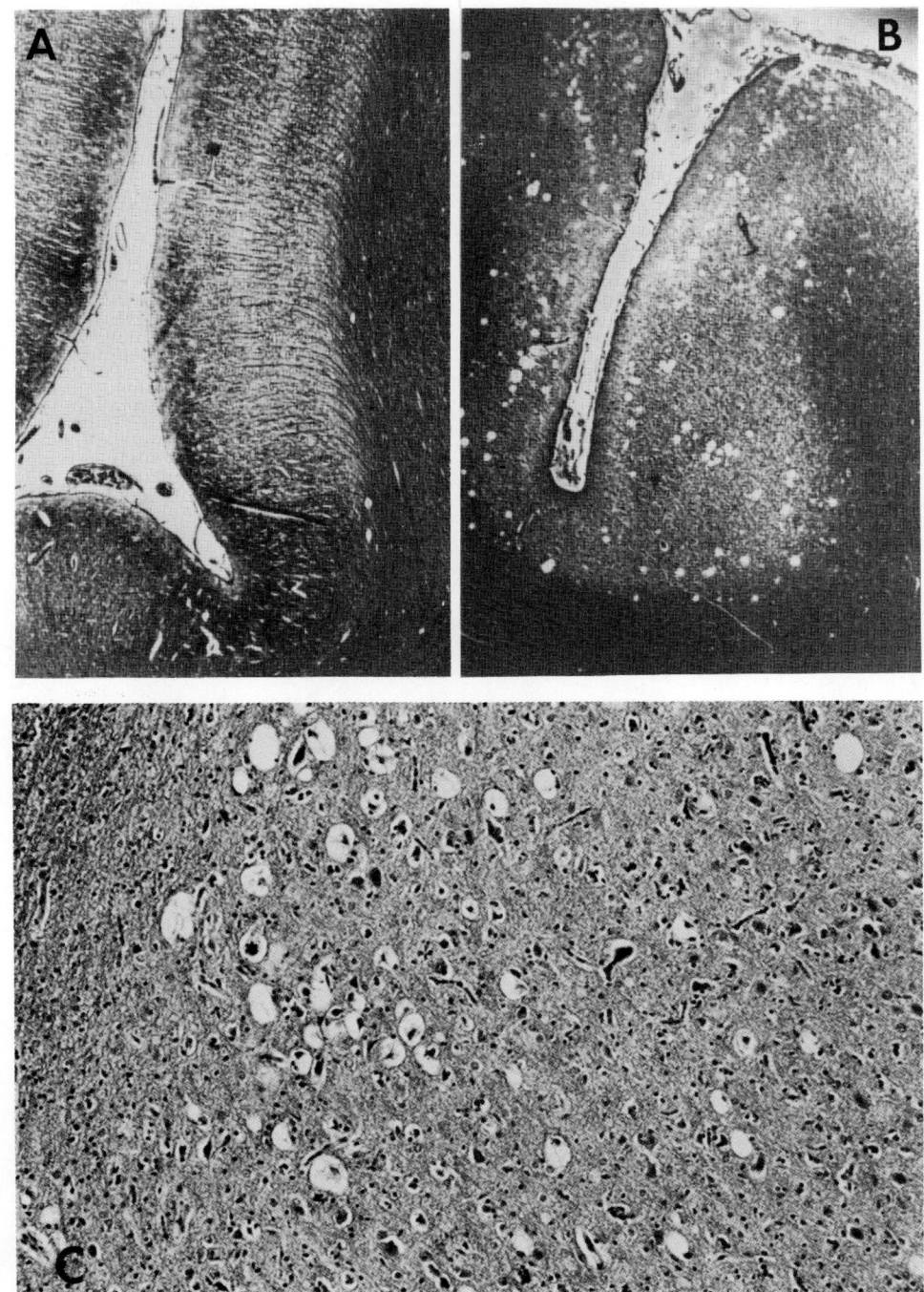

FIG.   15-28 Organomercurial poisoning, swine. **A.** and **B.** Necrosis of the occipital cerebral cortex. Bielchowsky stain. (Courtesy of Dr. L. Tryphonas.) **C.** Cerebrocortical neuronal necrosis in experimental swine methylmercury poisoning. (Courtesy of Dr. T. S. Davies and Dr. S. W. Nielsen.)

References

Burbacher TM, Monnett C, Grant KS, et al. Methylmercury exposure and reproductive dysfunction in the nonhuman primate. Toxicol Appl Pharmacol 1984;75:18–24.

Chen W-J, Body RL, Mottet NK. Biochemical and morphological studies of monkeys chronically exposed to methylmercury. J Toxicol Environ Health 1983;12:407–416.

Daoust R-Y, Wobeser G, Newstead JD. Acute pathological effects of inorganic mercury and copper in gills of rainbow trout. Vet Pathol 1984;21:93–101.

Hinglais N, Druet P, Grossetete J, et al. Ultrastructural study of nephritis induced in Brown Norway rats by mercuric chloride. Lab Invest 1979;41:150–159.

Merigan WH, Maurissen JPJ, Weiss S, et al. Neurotoxic actions of methylmercury on the primate visual system. Neurobehav Toxicol Teratol 1983;5:649–658.

Rice DC. Central nervous effects of perinatal exposure to lead or methylmercury in the monkey. In: Clarkson TW, Nordberg GF, Sager PR, eds. Reproduction and developmental toxicity of metals. New York: Plenum, 1983;517–539.

Insecticides of the chlorinated hydrocarbon group

The original and still important member of the chlorinated hydrocarbon group is dichloro, diphenyl trichloroethane (DDT). The discovery of this substance and

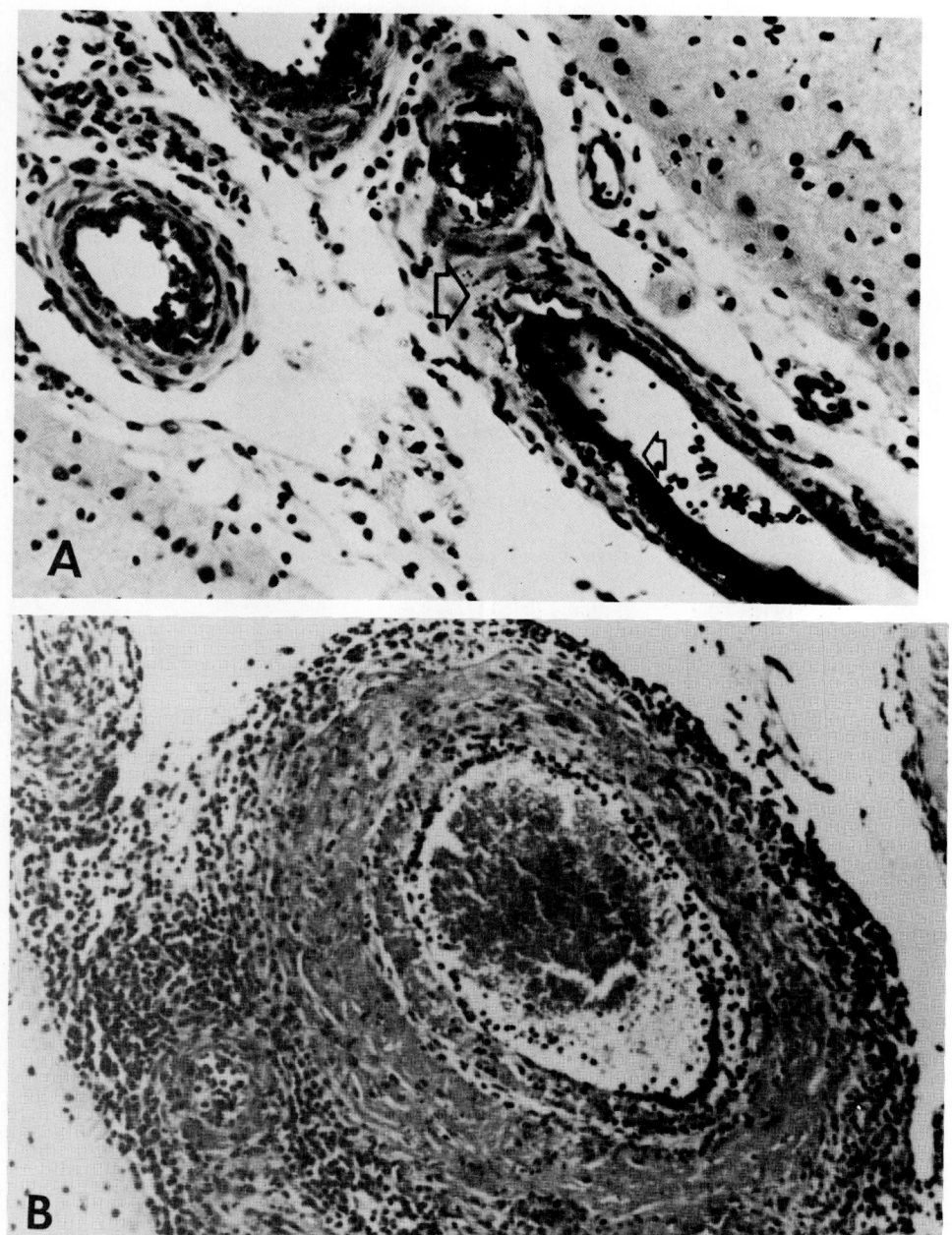

FIG. 15-29 Organomercurial poisoning in swine. **A.** Arterial fibrinoid necrosis in experimental swine methylmercury poisoning. Note fibrinoid deposits (small arrow) and medial necrosis (large arrow). (Courtesy of Dr. T. S. Davies and Dr. S. W. Nielsen.) **B.** Necrosis and vasculitis of a small cerebral artery. (Courtesy of Dr. L. Tryphonas.)

its insecticidal powers marked the advent of a series of insecticidal substances, which is still growing, and whose value to humans is beyond estimation. Other prominent members of the group include chlordane, lindane (which is the gamma isomer of benzene hexachloride), toxaphene, strobane, endrin, heptachlor (epoxide), methoxychlor, TDE, aldrin, and dieldrin. All of these chemicals have closely related hydrocarbons to which several chlorine atoms have been joined. Only the first four of the 11 compounds listed are commonly used on the skin of animals; all may be used against plant pests that prey upon farm crops and pastures. The limits of safety in the employment of these insecticides have been well established by extensive research, and as long as they are used as intended, either upon parasitized animals, feed crops, or buildings, poisoning is unlikely. However, errors in mixing or application, and accidents are all too numerous. The latter term, which is perhaps too mild, includes such incidents as one in which a farmer mixed DDT spray in the bucket used for calf feed, then unknowingly mixed calf feed with what remained of the spraying solution and fed it to the calves with fatal results. Another example includes a stockman who dipped a large herd of cattle in the proper dilution of a hydrocarbon insecticide, as he believed, to treat them for ticks. All died within a few hours. He complained to the manufacturer, but when it was demonstrated that his dipping fluid contained arsenic, he discovered that he had filled the vat with an arsenical intended for the cotton field. Baffling diagnostic problems are obviously presented in such cases, and unfortunately, they cannot be solved entirely by the observable aspects of the animals' illnesses.

A serious objection to the use of these insecticides is that they are not degraded by natural biologic processes, and therefore become a permanent part of the environment. They make their way into the water supply, are taken up by aquatic animals, and become part of the food chain because they are accumulated and concentrated, usually in fat, by many such animals. Deleterious effects on wildlife, especially birds, are reported. These effects include soft eggshells and loss of hatchability, which probably result from the known estrogenic actions of DDT. Decreased reproductive performance has also been noted in mammals.

The signs of these poisonings are more informative from the diagnostic standpoint than from the lesions. The earlier signs, which may appear within minutes and almost always within a few hours, are those of nervous hyperirritability and stimulation. Spasmodic twitching and quivering of various muscle groups, including those of the eyelids, increase in extent and frequency until almost the whole body is trembling. Apprehensiveness or occasionally belligerency deepens into frenzy; incoordination and various abnormal stances are replaced by convulsions. The animal may press its head against solid objects (blind staggers), may plunge headlong into an obstacle of any sort, or without warning, jump as if stung by the sudden lash of a whip and then fall in a convulsion. As in tetanus or strychnine poisoning, these symptoms are initiated or augmented by slight external stimuli, such as a sharp noise. A minority of animals become depressed, drowsy, and eventually comatose. Occasionally an animal licks continually at a certain spot of the body surface, simulating Aujeszky disease. Many of these animals die; others recover suddenly and completely after nervous seizures lasting a few minutes or hours. Simultaneously with the appearance of convulsions, the body temperature soars to unbelievable heights, perhaps 115°F. This rise is more than can be attributed to muscular activity and must depend on derangement of the heat-regulating center. Dyspnea and cyanosis accompany the convulsive seizures. Groaning, grunting, and grinding of teeth may occur; some have interpreted these as signs of severe pain, but to others they have appeared to stem from nervous derangement.

Lesions at necropsy include petechiae and ecchymoses on and in the heart and in many other places. These occur especially in association with convulsions and are explainable on the basis of dyspneic anoxia. Pulmonary congestion and edema, diffuse or localized, exist. The heart usually stops in systole. In spite of the startling symptoms of central nervous disorder, few changes in the central nervous cells and tissues are manifest. This, of course, is in conformity with the rapid and complete recovery that may follow some of the most violent symptoms. Some have reported Nissl degeneration and necrosis of neurons, especially in the ganglia of the medulla, cerebellum, and brainstem; others have found no central nervous lesions beyond congestion and increased cerebrospinal fluid. In the few cases in which symptoms have been prolonged for one to two days, the usual changes of acute toxic hepatitis and acute toxic tubular nephrosis have been noted, centrilobular necrosis being especially prominent. Focal necroses have been noted in skeletal muscle. Enteritis is noticeable only when the poison has been eaten. Dehydration and rapid depletion of depot fat are usual in these cases. The biochemist can demonstrate accumulation of chlorinated compounds in the body tissues, chiefly the stored fat.

References
Grisedale IM. Dieldrin poisoning in cats. Vet Rec 1984;114:363.
Mount ME, Traffas V, Milleret RJ, et al. An unusual occurrence of toxaphene poisoning in swine. J Am Vet Med Assoc 1980; 177: 445–447.
Saint Omer VV. Chronic and acute toxicity of the chlorinated hydrocarbon insecticides in mammals and birds. Can Vet J 1970; 11: 215–226.

Organic phosphates

Under the group name of organic phosphates are included certain "nerve gases" devised for use in warfare and a number of valuable insecticides, anthelmintics, and defoliants. Tetra-ethyl pyrophosphate (TEPP) is one belonging to both categories. Insecticides and antihelmintics are usually best known by specific trade names, the more important of which are currently parathion, o,o-diethyl p-nitrophenyl thiophosphate, and malathion, o,o-diethyl dithiophosphate. Others in this group include carbaryl (Sevin®), carbophenothion (Trithion®), ciodrin, coumaphos (Co-rad®), demetron, diazinon, dichlorvos (DDVP), trichlorfon, phosalone, dioxathion, disyston, endosulfan, ENP, ethion, guthion, methyl parathion, mevinphos (Phosdrin®), naled (Dibrom®), phorate (Thiomet®), ronnel, and trichlorophon (Dipterex®). Others, such as triaryl phosphate, have industrial use in lubricants.

Other organophosphate compounds that have been involved in accidental or inadvertent poisonings in humans or animals include the following: chlorpyrifos, chlorpyrifos-diazinon, crufomate, dimethoate, fenchlorphos, fonofos, haloxon, and posmet. A large number of similar compounds have been synthesized and many have been manufactured in large quantities; therefore, poisoning by accident or design remains a threat.

Known as anticholinesterases, these organic phosphates have essentially similar effects, which depend upon the ability to prevent or inhibit the action of cholinesterase. This leaves acetylcholine of the sympathetic and parasympathetic nerve endings free to act continuously and without release of effectors at the end of each stimulus. The oral lethal dose of parathion for dogs is estimated at 25–35 mg/kg body weight: for cats, 15 mg/kg; and for rabbits, 40 mg/kg.

Signs include excessive salivation, the saliva being copious but watery. Respiratory difficulty occurs, with labored and exaggerated respiratory movements, the mouth often being held partially open. Before death, loud pulmonary rales and soft grunts are evident. Twitching and fasciculation of muscles and ataxia occur, but convulsions only exceptionally. Asphyxia is the main cause of death. Signs commonly arise within one to two hours after a single contact with the poison, which may occur by inhalation or cutaneous absorption more often than by ingestion. Somewhat exceptionally, death ensues within five minutes of tetra-ethyl pyrophosphate being sprayed on the skin of cattle. Nonfatal cases recover within 48 hours. Susceptibility varies greatly among individuals of any species, and can be increased by frequently repeated mild exposure. The greater susceptibility appears to be due to exhaustion of the body's store of cholinesterase.

Postmortem lesions are minor. Hemorrhages appear in various locations, especially the heart, lungs, and gastrointestinal tube. Pulmonary congestion with edema is a prominent, but not necessarily constant, finding. The most specific lesion is axonal degeneration (Fig. 15-30), characterized by marked swelling up to 20 times normal. Pathogenesis of the lesion is ascribed to inhibition of esterases necessary to transport nutrients from the nerve cell body to more distal portions of the axon. The longest axons are affected first. Ultrastructurally, mitochondrial swelling, vacuolation of axoplasm, and separation of myelin lamellae occur.

Parenchymatous degeneration of the liver and kidneys has been reported but is probably exceptional.

Berger and Bayliss described a histochemical method for the detection of cholinesterase at motor end plates in teased preparations of skeletal muscles, which should be useful in detecting fatal accumulations of anticholinesterase (1952).

Decrease in the level of cholinesterase in circulating red blood cells is considered to be evidence of toxicity by organic phosphates.

Flea collars treated with the organic phosphate, dichlorvos, are also associated with allergic dermatitis.

References

Abdelsalam EB. Factors affecting the toxicity of organophosphorus compounds in animals. Vet Bull 1987;57:441–448.

Berger AD, Bayliss MW. Histochemical detection of fatal anticholinesterase poisoning. US Armed Forces Med J 1952;3:1637–1644.

Brack M, Rothe H. Organophosphate poisoning in marmosets. Lab Anim 1982;16:186–188.

Dalgaard-Mikkelson SV, Poulsen E. Toxicology of herbicides. Pharmacol Rev 1962;14:225–250.

Kurtz DA, Hutchinson L. Fonofos toxicosis in dairy cows: an accidental poisoning. Am J Vet Res 1982;43:1672–1674.

Leighton T, Marks E, Leighton F. Pesticides: insecticides and fungicides are chitin synthesis inhibitors. Science 1981;213:905–907.

Murphy SD. Pesticides. In: Doull J, Klaassen CD, Amdur MO, eds. Casarett and Doull's toxicology: the basic science of poisons. 2nd ed. New York: Macmillan, 1980;357–408.

Quick MF. Pesticide poisoning of livestock: a review of cases investigated. Vet Rec 1982;111:5–7.

Santon HC, Albert JR, Mersmann HJ. Studies on the pharmacology and safety of dichlorvos in pigs and pregnant sows. Am J Vet Res 1979;40:315–320.

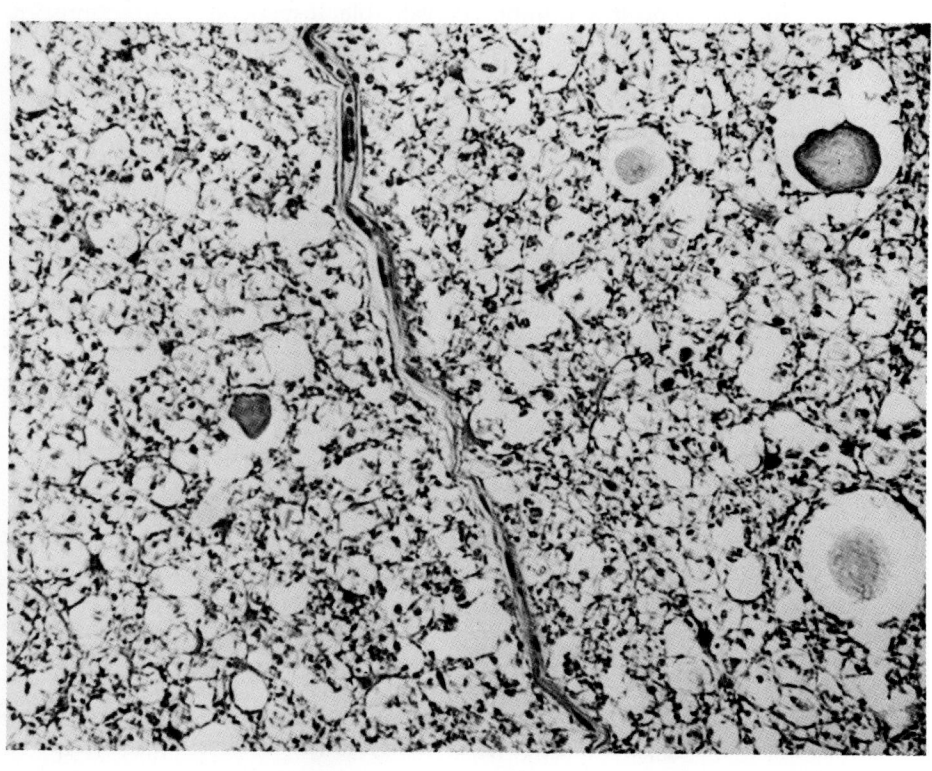

FIG. 15-30 Triaryl phosphate poisoning. Axonal degeneration in the spinal cord of a poisoned cow. Note swollen axons or spheroids. (Courtesy of Dr. B. E. Beck and Veterinary Pathology.)

Scheidt AB, Long GG, Knox K, et al. Toxicosis in newborn pigs associated with cutaneous application of an aerosol spray containing chlorpyrifos. J Am Vet Med Assoc 1987;191:1410–1412.

Cycada

Plants of the order Cycadales, particularly *Zamia integrifolia, Z. portoricoensis, Z. latafoleatus, Cycas circinalis, C. media, Bowenia serrulata, Macrozamia lucida,* and *M. reidlei,* are coarse, woody, fernlike, and grow in Australia, New Guinea, Puerto Rico, Dominican Republic, and Florida. The fruit and nuts have been used as a source of feed for humans and animals and the leaves are consumed by grazing stock. Both contain two toxins: a neurotoxin, which is resistant to drying, and hepatotoxin, which is readily destroyed by drying. Cattle and sheep are susceptible. In cattle, neurologic sequelae are the usual outcome, whereas in sheep, acute or chronic liver disease is more frequent. Although the plants grow in Florida, no poisonings of this type have been reported in the United States.

Poisoning of cattle, associated with these plants, results in nervous signs which have prompted such colloquial names as: "wobbles," "rickets," "zamia paralysis," cycad ataxia, derriengue (Dominican Republic), and ranilla (Puerto Rico). Clinical signs are chiefly neurologic, with ataxia involving the hindquarters initially. A peculiar involvement of the hind legs results in swaying, flexion of the hock and fetlock joints, wobbling, and malpositioning of the legs. Lesions are concentrated in the spinal cord (Fig. 15-31). Degeneration of myelin is evident in nerve fibers of all funiculi of the cord throughout its length. The Marchi and Guillery silver-staining methods are particularly useful in demonstrating these lesions (Hall and McGavin, 1968). Swollen axons, appearing as large, eosinophilic spheroids 10–50 μ in diameter, are present within the spinal tracts and medulla oblongata.

Hepatic necrosis in sheep has most often followed

consumption of *Macrozamia reidlei.* Acute poisoning is characterized by jaundice, ascites, hydrothorax, serosal hemorrhages, and extensive centrilobular hemorrhagic necrosis of the liver. Hepatic fibrosis is the predominant finding in chronic poisoning in sheep. The hepatotoxin is methylazoxymethanol, a compound similar in structure to dimethylnitrosamine, which inhibits hepatic protein synthesis. This active principle, a β-glycoside, needs to undergo hydrolysis by intestinal bacteria in order to be toxic or carcinogenic. It has been demonstrated to be a carcinogen in rats, mice, hamsters, and nonhuman primates.

References

De Luca P, Moretti A, Sabato S, et al. The ubiquity of cycasin in cycads. Phytochemistry 1980;19:2230–2231.

Gabbedy BJ, Meyer EP, Dickson J. Zamia palm (Macrozamia reidlei) poisoning of sheep. Aust Vet J 1975;51:303–305.

Gardiner MR. Chronic ovine hepatosis following feeding of Macrozamia reidlei nuts. Aust J Agric Res 1970;21:519–526.

Hall WTK, McGavin MD. Clinical and neuropathological changes in cattle eating the leaves of Macrozamia lucida or Bowenia serrulata (family Zamiaceae). Pathol Vet 1968;5:26–34.

Hirono I. Carcinogenicity and neurotoxicity of cycasin with special reference to species differences. Fed Proc 1972;31:1493–1497.

Hooper PT, Best SM, Campbell A. Azonal dystrophy in the spinal cords of cattle consuming the cycad palm, Cycas media. Aust Vet J 1974;50:146–149.

Mason MM, Whiting MG. Caudal motor weakness and ataxia in cattle in the Caribbean area following ingestion of cycads. Cornell Vet 1968;58:541–554.

Politis MJ, Schaumberg HH, Spencer PS. Neurotoxicity of selected chemicals. In: Spenser PS, Schaumberg HH, eds. Experimental and clinical neurotoxicology. Baltimore: Williams and Wilkins, 1980;613–630.

Rogers AE. Naturally occurring carcinogens in higher plants. In: Sontag JM, ed. Carcinogens in industry and the environment. New York: Marcel Dekker, 1981;519–534.

Senior DF, et al. Cycad intoxication in the dog. J Am Anim Hosp Assoc 1985;21:103–109.

Sieber SM, Correa P, Dalgard DW, et al. Carcinogenicity and hepatotoxicity of cycasin and its aglycone methylazoxymethanol acetate in nonhuman primates. JNCI 1980;65:177–189.

Arsanilic acid

Arsanilic acid (p-aminophenyl-arsonic acid) poisoning in swine is not characterized by gastroenteritis as is arsenic (Group B), but rather almost entirely by neurologic signs and lesions. Experimentally-induced poisoning in pigs has been produced by adding arsanilic acid to the feed at the rate of 611, 1000, or 2000 g to each (English) ton of feed; the usual recommended dose as a growth stimulant is 100 g/ton, or for treatment of dysentery, 250 g/ton. At all dose levels, signs of intoxication were produced. Clinical signs appeared earlier in pigs receiving higher dosages. Tremors, incoordination, progressively developing blindness, and eventual inability to stand were the principal signs. Poisoned animals remained alert with good appetites in spite of these severe signs. The principal lesions were microscopic and consisted of wallerian degeneration of optic nerves, optic tracts, and peripheral nerves. Ledet et al. described similar signs and lesions in pigs fed 1000 ppm arsanilic acid in their ration (1973). Neuropathologic changes

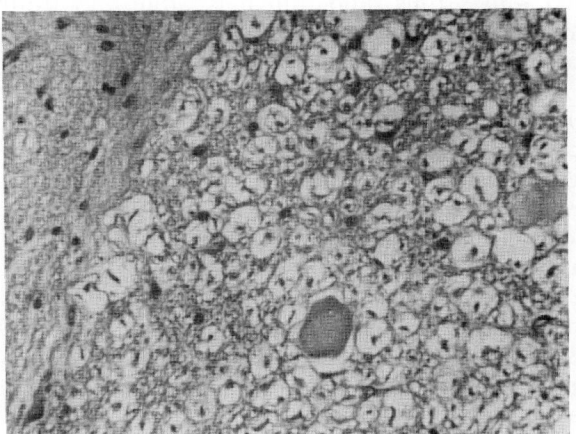

FIG. 15-31 Cycad palm poisoning. Spheroids and demyelination in the dorsolateral white matter of the cervical spinal cord in a steer poisoned by *Cycas armstrongii* (C. media). (Courtesy of Dr. P. T. Hooper and Australian Veterinary Journal.)

were limited to the same three sites and were characterized by necrosis of myelin-supporting cells and degeneration of myelin sheaths and axons. Cutaneous hyperemia and hyperesthesia were described as the earliest signs, appearing within five days. More severe neurologic signs appeared in almost two weeks.

References

Harding JDJ, Lewis G, Done JT. Experimental arsanilic acid poisoning in pigs. Vet Rec 1968;83:560–564.

Ledet AE, Duncan JR, Buck WB, et al. Clinical, toxicological, and pathological aspects of arsanilic acid poisoning in swine. Clin Toxicol 1973;6:439–457.

Oliver WT, Roe CK. Arsanilic acid poisoning in swine. J Am Vet Med Assoc 1957;130:177–178.

3-NITRO-4-HYDROXYPHENYLARSONIC ACID

This compound, 3-nitro-4-hydroxyphenylarsonic acid (3-nitro), is chemically related to arsanilic acid and both are used to promote growth and combat enteric disease in young swine. Under some conditions, they both are toxic to the nervous system. Signs resulting from 3-nitro toxicity consist of clonic episodes of convulsions, which are induced by exercise. Blindness and tremors are less conspicuous than in arsanilic acid toxicosis.

The microscopic lesions are similar with each neurotoxin, with destruction of axons and myelin, but their distribution is somewhat different. The 3-nitro compound produces lesions in the cervical, thoracic, and lumbar regions of the spinal cord with fewer and less extensive lesions in peripheral and optic nerves. The vagus nerve and dorsal root ganglia are not affected.

References

Kennedy S, Rice DA, Cush PF. Neuropathology of experimental 3-nitro-4-hydroxyphenylarsonic acid toxicosis in pigs. Vet Pathol 1986;23:454–461.

Prier RF, Nees PO, Derse PH. The toxicity of an organic arsenical, 3-nitro-4-hydroxyphenylarsonic acid. II. Chronic toxicity. Toxicol Appl Pharmacol 1963;5:526–529.

Rice DA, Kennedy S, McMurray CH, et al. Experimental 3-nitro-4-hydroxyphenylarsonic acid toxicosis in pigs. Res Vet Sci 1985;39: 47–52.

GROUP Q: DEGENERATION OF CARDIAC AND SKELETAL MUSCLE

Poisons in Group Q produce necrosis of cardiac and skeletal muscles as their principal lesions. Similar lesions may also be found in some other poisonings, such as selenium (Group E) and gossypol (Group C).

Coffee senna

Coffee senna (*Cassia occidentalis*, L.) received its common name because of the use of the bean as a substitute for coffee. The plant is an annual shrub that grows natively in the southeastern United States, as well as in many other parts of the world. The plant has drab green leaves and bright, golden yellow flowers. The seed pods are green with brown transverse bars when immature, and become brown when mature. Other sen-

nas are known to have cathartic properties and some may be toxic to animals (Kingsbury, 1964). Among these plants are: *Cassia fistula* (senna of commerce), *C. lindheimeriana*, *C. fasciculata* (partridge pea) and *C. tora* (sicklepod). Reported as poisonous to livestock first in 1911, episodes of toxicity in horses, cattle, and sheep have been recorded over the years. Experimental poisoning has also been recorded in cattle, rabbits, sheep, and goats.

Two similar plants, *Cassia roemeriana* (twin-leaf senna) and *Cassia obtusifolia* have different geographic distributions in the United States, but have been incriminated as causing similar toxicity in cattle and goats. The active compound in this problem has not been identified.

Calves given daily oral doses of ground beans of *Cassia occidentalis* at the dose rate of 0.5% or more of body weight survive at a rate inversely proportional to the dosage. Signs of poisoning include anorexia and diarrhea, followed by hyperpnea, tachycardia, and progressive muscular incapacitation, with stumbling and ataxic gait. Elevated levels of serum glutamic oxalacetic transaminase and phosphocreatine kinase are constant, and hemoglobin appears in the urine of about half of these cases. After a period of prostration and recumbency, death follows in a few hours due to heart failure.

Gross lesions consist of focal or diffuse pallor of skeletal muscles, generally distinguishable from the chalky whiteness and granular consistency observed in white-muscle disease. Stippling of pale muscles may be seen in calves. The myocardium is usually mottled or streaked (Fig. 15-32) with pale or yellow zones. These areas may be diffusely distributed or concentrated adjacent to the endocardium. Subepicardial hemorrhages may be seen, particularly along the course of the coronary arteries. Effusion into the pericardial sac sometimes occurs. The lungs are usually diffusely dark red, partially airless and heavy. The interlobular septa are thickened by edema. Trachea and bronchi are filled with serous fluid, which is white and frothy in part. Blood flows freely from the cut surface of the lung.

The earliest lesions seen with the light microscope in cardiac muscle consist of numerous, small, indistinct vacuoles among the myofibrils, in some cases giving them a distinctly fenestrated appearance. These vacuoles are demonstrated with electron microscopy to be due to swelling of the mitochondria, with loss of their matrix and fragmentation and disorganization of cristae. Electron-dense, spherical inclusions sometimes appear in these dilated mitochondria (Fig. 15-32). With loss of mitochondrial energy production, cellular swelling ensues, with loss of glycogen and degeneration of the sarcotubular system.

Lesions of skeletal muscles seen by light microscopy are compatible with classic Zenker necrosis of muscle. Affected muscle fibers are swollen, eosinophilic (amorphous), and sometimes fragmented. Occasional nuclei are necrotic and some proliferation of sarcolemmal nuclei is evident. Calcification is not reported.

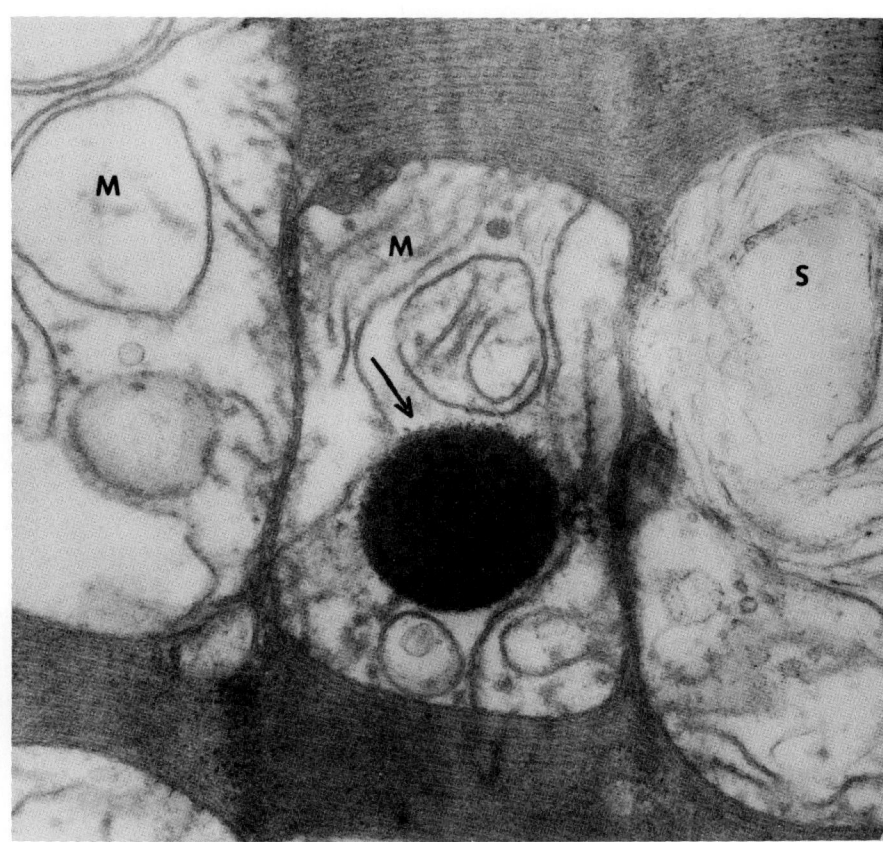

FIG. 15-32 Poisoning due to coffee senna. Electron micrograph of myocardium of a calf poisoned with *Cassia occidentalis* (×43,200). Note electron dense spherule (arrow) in swollen mitochrondrion of myocardial muscle cell. Note disorganized cristae and spheromembranous structure(s) in mitochondrion. (Courtesy of Dr. W. Kay Read and Laboratory Investigation.)

References

Brocq-Rousseau, Bruere P. Accidents mortels sur des cheveaux due a la graine de Cassia occidentalis. L Compt Rend Soc Biol 1925;92:555–557.

Colvin BM, Harrison LR, Sangster LT, et al. Cassia occidentalis toxicosis in growing pigs. J Am Vet Med Assoc 1986;189:423–426.

Dollahite JW, Henson JB. Toxic plants as the etiologic agent of myopathies in animals. Am J Vet Res 1965;26:749–752.

Graziano MJ, Flory W, Seger CL, et al. Effects of a Cassia occidentalis extract in the domestic chicken (Gallus domesticus). Am J Vet Res 1983;44:1238–1244.

Henson JB, et al. Myodegeneration in cattle grazing Cassia species. J Am Vet Med Assoc 1965;147:142–145.

Kingsbury JM. Poisonous plants of the United States and Canada. Englewood Cliffs: Prentice-Hall, 1964.

Martin BW, Terry MK, Bridges CH, et al. Toxicity of Cassia occidentalis in the horse. Vet Hum Toxicol 1981;23:416–417.

O'Hara PJ, Pierce KR, Read WK. Degenerative myopathy associated with ingestion of Cassia occidentalis L.: clinical and pathologic features of the experimentally induced disease. Am J Vet Res 1969;30:2173–2180.

Read WK, Pierce KR, O'Hara PJ. Ultrastructural lesions of an acute toxic cardiomyopathy of cattle. Lab Invest 1968;18:227–231.

Rowe LD, Corrier DE, Reagor JC, et al. Experimentally-induced Cassia roemeriana poisoning in cattle and goats. Am J Vet Res 1987;48:992–997.

Sullivan HB, Shommein AM. Toxic effect of the roasted and unroasted beans of Cassia occidentalis in goats. Vet Hum Toxicol 1986;28:6–11.

Coyotillo

The coyotillo plant *(Karwinskia humboldtiana)* is a spineless shrub with pinnately-veined leaves, small, greenish flowers, and ovoid, brown-black fruit. In sheep and goats, the fruit has been shown to cause a toxicosis called limberleg, which is manifest by progressive weakness of legs, muscular incoordination, recumbency, and death. In 1789, Indian children reportedly lost the use of their limbs, and some died after eating the fruit of the coyotillo.

This shrub is native to southwest Texas and Mexico, and in some regions it grows profusely.

Lesions of this toxicosis are found in cardiac and skeletal muscle, peripheral nerves, and liver. In the myocardium, disseminated focal lesions of coagulation necrosis involve a few muscle fibers in each location. A few fibers lose their sarcoplasma. In skeletal muscle, any or all muscles may be involved, and microscopic lesions are typical of Zenker necrosis. Isolated muscle fibers are swollen, eosinophilic, often fragmented, and occasionally associated with infiltration of lymphocytes and macrophages and proliferation of sarcolemmal cells. Toxic hepatitis is also a feature, with focal necroses of small numbers of hepatic cells, usually at the center of the lobules, plus some mild fatty change. Peripheral neuropathy with swollen Schwann cells, segmental demyelination, and wallerian degeneration has been found in goats.

Associated with these lesions are severe increases in the serum concentration of glutamic oxaloacetic transaminase and moderate increases in glutamic pyruvic transaminase. Serum alkaline phosphatase may be slightly decreased.

References

Charlton KM, Pierce KR. Peripheral neuropathy in experimental coyotillo poisoning in goats. Texas Rpts Biol Med 1969;27:389–399.

Charlton KM, Pierce KR. A neuropathy in goats caused by experimental coyotillo (Karwinskia humboldtiana) poisoning. II. Lesions in the peripheral nervous system—teased fiber and acid phosphatase studies. Pathol Vet 1970;7:385–407.

Charlton KM, Pierce KR. A neuropathy in goats caused by experimental coyotillo (Karwinskia humboldtiana) poisoning. III. Distribution of lesions in peripheral nerves. Pathol Vet 1970;7:408–419.

Charlton KM, Pierce KR. A neuropathy in goats caused by experimental coyotillo (Karwinskia humboltiana) poisoning. IV. Light and electron microscopic lesion in peripheral nerves. Pathol Vet 1970;7:420–434.

Charlton KM, et al. A neuropathy in goats caused by experimental coyotillo (Karwinskia humboldtiana) poisoning. V. Lesions in the central nervous system. Pathol Vet 1970;7:435–447.

Dewan ML, et al. Toxic myodegeneration in goats produced by feeding mature fruits from coyotillo plant (Karwinskia humboldtiana). Am J Pathol 1965;46:215–226.

Dollahite JW, Henson JB. Toxic plants as the etiologic agent of myopathies in animals. Am J Vet Res 1965;26:749–752.

GROUP R: TERATOGENS

These poisons cause teratogenic or other effects on the embryo or fetus. Other poisons are also teratogenic but are described elsewhere in this volume. These poisonous plants that are also teratogenic, are classified as species in the following genera: Lupinus (p. 721), Conium (p. 755), Nicotiana (p. 702), and Solanum (p. 702).

Veratrum californicum

This impressive perennial plant grows profusely in 11 western states, reaching three to eight feet in height. Its common names include: skunk cabbage, western helibore, false helibore, and wild corn. It is included in the lily family (Lileacea), in which seven other species in this genus are classified and are indigenous to North America. *Veratrum veride,* which grows in the eastern United States, and *V. album,* a European species, are the source of several alkaloids, some of which are used medicinally. Among these specific alkaloids are: veratridine, protoveratrine, veratrine, cevadine, and jirvine.

A striking and grotesque congenital malformation of lambs was first described by Binns et al. as occurring in sheep pastured on mountain ranges in southern Idaho, located at altitudes to 10,000 feet (1969; Fig. 15-33). The deformed lambs were usually born alive singly

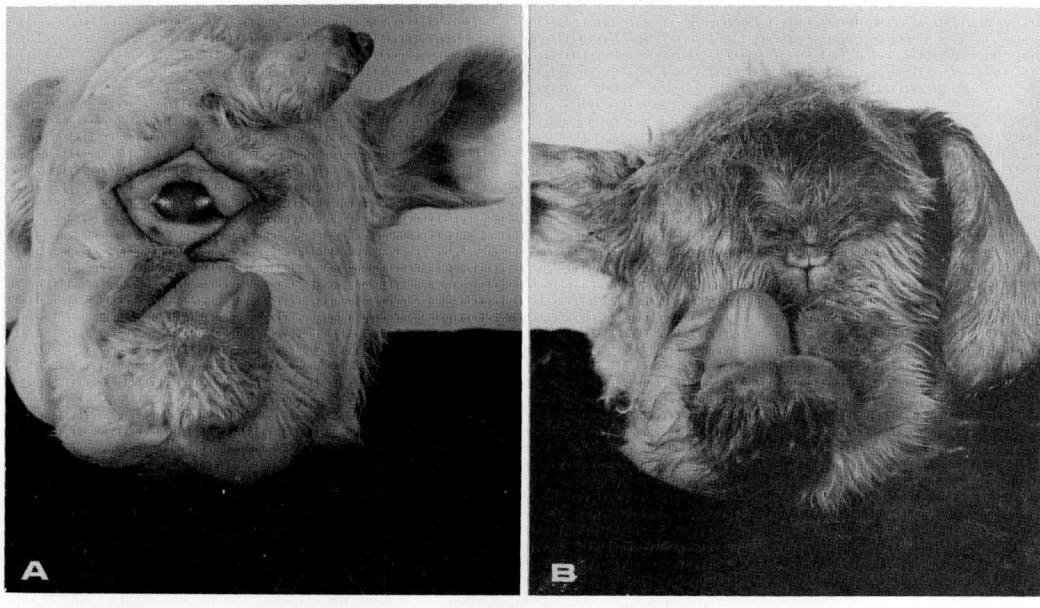

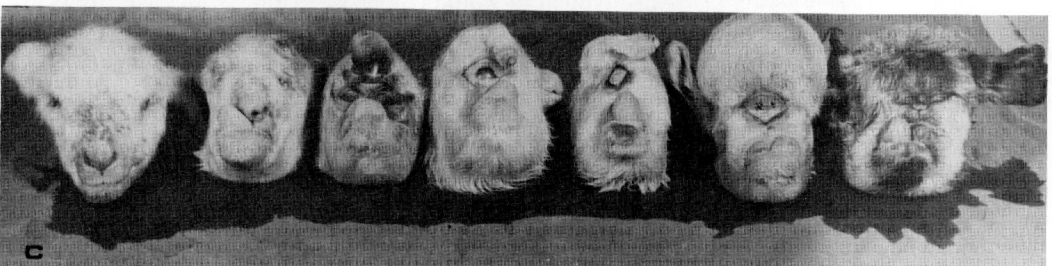

FIG. 15-33 Congenital malformations in newborn lambs resulting from feeding their mothers a plant, *Veratrum californicum* (false helibore) on day 14 of gestation. **A.** A lamb's head with cyclopia and other anomalies. **B.** A lamb with anophthalmia and other defects. **C.** Several lambs' heads with varying congenital deformities. Normal lamb at left. (Courtesy of Dr. Wayne Binns, United States Department of Agriculture.)

or with a living or dead twin which may have been affected. The malformations are limited to the head and represent several defects, the commonest being partial or complete cyclopia. A single eye or two fused eyes usually occupy a single orbit. The two fused eyes give the startling appearance that caused the sheepmen to call them "monkey-faced lambs." The upper jaw may be slightly distorted with a cleft palate or almost totally absent. The nose is distorted in varying degrees, and the lower jaw usually protrudes drastically. A large median cutaneous protuberance often occurs over the single eye. The cerebral hemispheres are frequently fused, and hydrocephalus involves the lateral ventricles. The optic nerves may be fused.

In many cases the pituitary of the fetus is absent, and this is associated with prolonged gestation and a large fetus, which is not delivered except by hysterotomy.

In a series of carefully conducted experiments, Binns et al. clearly established that this congenital malformation results from the consumption of the fresh or dried plant *Veratrum californicum,* or extracts thereof, by the ewe during days 13–15 of pregnancy. Several steroidal alkaloids (cyclopamine, veratramine, veratrosine, muldamine) have been isolated from *V. californicum* and have been demonstrated to cause the teratogenic effects just described, as well as other malformations. When the plant or certain alkaloids are fed to sheep on days 13 and 14 of pregnancy, the cyclopian deformity results. Exposure on days 17 and 18 results in motor nerve paralysis, whereas a multiplicity of abnormalities followed exposure from days 12 through 30, including cleft palate, hare-lip, brachygnathia, syndactylism, decrease in length and diameter of all bones, or shortening only of metacarpals and metatarsals and a decrease in number of coccygeal vertebrae. Exposure after day 30 only resulted in hypoplasia of the metacarpal and metatarsal growth plates. Some of the malformations have also been experimentally produced in cattle, goats, rabbits, rats, mice, hamsters, and chickens.

References

Binns W, et al. A congenital cyclopian-type malformation in lambs. J Am Vet Med Assoc 1969;134:180–183.

Binns W, et al. A congenital cyclopian-type malformation in lambs induced by maternal ingestion of a range plant, Veratrum californicum. Am J Vet Res 1963;24:1164–1175.

Binns W, et al. Toxicosis of Veratrum californicum in ewes and its relationship to congenital deformity in lambs. Ann NY Acad Sci 1964;111:571–576.

Brown D. Structure-activity relation of steroidal amine teratogens. In: Keeler RF, Van Kampen KR, James LF, eds. Effects of poisonous plants on livestock. New York: Academic Press, 1978;409–418.

Bryden MM, Perry C, Keeler RF. Effects of alkaloids of Veratrum californicum on chick embryos. Teratology 1973;8:19–28.

Crowe MW. Tobacco—a cause of congenital arthrogryposis. In: Keeler RF, Van Kampen KR, James LF, eds. Effects of poisonous plants on livestock. New York: Academic Press, 1978;419–427.

Keeler RF. Alkaloid teratogens from Lupinus, Conium, Veratrum, and related genera. In: Keeler RF, Van Kampen KR, James LF, eds. Effects of poisonous plants on livestock. New York: Academic Press, 1978;397–408.

Keeler RF. Naturally occurring teratogens from plants. In: Keeler RF, Tu AT, eds. Handbook of natural toxins. Vol 1. Plant and fungal toxins. New York: Marcel Dekker, 1983;174–175.

Keeler RF. Teratogenic compounds in Veratrum californicum (Durand). IX. Structure-activity relation. X. Cyclopia in rabbits produced by cyclopamine. Teratology 1970;3:169–174,175–180.

Keeler RF, Binns W. Chemical compounds of Veratrum californicum related to congenital ovine cyclopian malformations: extraction of active material. Proc Soc Exp Biol Med 1964;116:123–127.

Keeler RF, Binns W. Possible teratogenic effects of veratramine. Proc Soc Exp Biol Med 1966;123:921–923.

Van Kampen KR, Ellis LC. Prolonged gestation in ewes ingesting Veratrum californicum: morphological changes and steroid biosynthesis in the endocrine organs of cyclopic lambs. J Endocrinol 1972;52:549–560.

Thalidomide

This tranquilizing drug, introduced in Germany in the late 1950s, was eventually associated with a large number of congenitally malformed babies whose mothers had taken the drug during early pregnancy (days 21–36 postconception). The most striking malformations in these infants were absence of limbs (amelia) or shortening of the arms or legs to the point at which they resembled a seal's flippers (phocomelia, phoke = seal, melos = extremity). Other anomalies also were described in these children (Toms, 1962).

Although not a naturally-occurring teratogen for animals, thalidomide has been shown to produce congenital anomalies comparable to those seen in children in several species. Nonhuman primates develop the same anomalies as described in humans. The susceptible period is also comparable to humans, ranging from 22 through 30 days of gestation at dose levels of 5–50 mg/kg/day. Administration of 50–200 mg thalidomide daily to female rhesus monkeys *(Macaca mulatta)* started after mating appeared to kill the embryo or prevent implantation, because no young were born. Administration of the drug to rabbits (150 mg/kg body weight daily) from days 8–16 of pregnancy resulted in stillbirths and deformed offspring. Rats apparently reabsorbed fetuses in utero, but produced no deformed offspring when placed on a similar regimen. Congenital abnormalities in tail vertebrae, sternebrae, and extremities also occur in puppies whose mothers are given thalidomide during pregnancy.

Thalidomide also may produce phocomelia in the armadillo *(Dasypus novemcinctus mexicanus),* and a choriocarcinoma of the uterus with metastases has been associated. (Marin-Padilla and Benirschke, 1963). Injury to the myocardium of armadillo embryos has also been demonstrated (Marin-Padilla and Benirschke, 1965).

References

Hendrickx AG, Axelrod LR, Clayborn LD. "Thalidomide" syndrome in baboons. Nature 1966;210:958–959.

Lucey JF, Behrman RE. Thalidomide: effect on pregnancy in the rhesus monkey. Science 1963;139:1295–1296.

Marin-Padilla M, Benirschke K. Thalidomide-induced alterations in the blastocyst and placenta of the armadillo, Dasypus novemcinctus mexicanus, including a choriocarcinoma. Am J Pathol 1963;43:999–1016.

Marin-Padilla M, Benirschke K. Thalidomide injury to the myocardium of armadillo embryos. J Embryol Exp Morphol 1965;13:235–241.

Somers GF. Thalidomide and congenital malformations. Lancet 1:912–913, 1962.

Toms DA. Thalidomide and congenital malformations. Lancet 1962;2:400.

Vickers TH. The thalidomide embryopathy in hybrid rabbits. Br J Exp Pathol 1967;48:107–117.

Weidman WH, Young HH, Zollman PE. The effect of thalidomide on the unborn puppy. Staff Meeting Mayo Clin 1963;38:518–522.

Wilson JG. An animal model of human disease: thalidomide embryopathy in primates. Comp Pathol Bull 1973;5:3–4.

Pine needles

The consumption of the needles of yellow ponderosa pine *(Pinus ponderosa)* may lead to birth of weak calves or abortion in cattle. It is principally a problem of range cattle in western United States and Canada, the habitat of the ponderosa pine. Sheep appear to be resistant. In cattle, pine needle abortion most often occurs in late fall, winter, or early spring during the last trimester of pregnancy. Prior to abortion, cattle become depressed, and rapid edema of the vulva and udder occurs. Retention of the placenta is common following abortion. Histopathologic studies are limited, but necrosis of proximal convoluted tubules of the kidney of aborted fetuses has been reported.

The site of action may be the placentome (fetal/placental unit) where increased numbers of binucleated trophoblastic cells are reported in poisoned pregnant cows. Increased necrosis and phagocytosis of luteal cells in the corpus luteum of affected cows also occurs. Reduced levels of circulating progesterone may also be associated with toxic effects. The toxic principle has not been identified and the pathogenesis of the abortion is not clearly established.

References

Jensen R, et al. Evaluation of histopathologic and physiologic changes in cows having premature births after consuming ponderosa pine needles. Am J Vet Res 1989;50:285–289.

Panter KE, James LF, Molyneux RJ, et al. Ponderosa pine-induced premature bovine parturition. In: James LF, Keeler RF, Bailey EM Jr, Cheeke PR, Hegarty MP, eds. Poisonous plants: Proc 3rd Int Symp. Ames: Iowa State Univ Press, 1992;387–391.

Short RE, James LF, Staigmiller RB, et al. Pine needle abortion in cattle: associated changes in serum cortisol, estradiol and progesterone. Cornell Vet 1989;79:53–60.

Stuart LD, James LF, Panter KE, et al. Pine needle abortion in cattle: pathological observations. Cornell Vet 1989;79:61–69.

Wiedmeier RD, Pfister JA, Adams DC, et al. Effects of ponderosa pine needle consumption on ruminal microflora in cattle. In: James LF, Keeler RF, Bailey EM Jr, Cheeke PR, Hegarty MP, eds. Poisonous plants: Proc 3rd Int Symp. Ames: Iowa State Univ Press, 1992;382–386.

GROUP S: MISCELLANEOUS POISONS

Within the group of miscellaneous poisons are included a variety of poisonous plants and inorganic and organic chemicals which, for the most part, are not encountered frequently. This chapter will not address the single most conspicuous lesion or clinical sign in these poisons, in order to keep the number of poisons in each group to a minimum.

Small head sneeze weed

Small head sneeze weed *(Helenium microcephalum),* with such intriguing and descriptive common and scientific names, grows in Texas and Mexico. Many losses of cattle, sheep, and goats have been attributed to eating this plant. Toxicity has been demonstrated by feeding studies with calves, goats, rabbits, and sheep. The flowering plants were more toxic than those in earlier stages of growth. Experimentally-poisoned animals exhibit signs of excess salivation, nasal discharge, bloating, and severe abdominal pain within one hour, and die within 24 hours after eating these plants. Accelerated pulse and respiratory rates, vomiting, and diarrhea are often exhibited. Gross lesions consist of pulmonary edema, hydrothorax, ascites, hyperemia, and edema in the submucosa of the rumen and reticulum. Microscopically, edema of nervous tissue, lung, submucosa of rumen, and reticulum is conspicuous. Mild toxic tubular nephritis is seen occasionally, plus some fatty change in cardiac muscle.

The toxic principle has been identified as helenalin, one of the large group of sesquiterpene lactones which have been identified also in *Helenium autumnale* and *tenuifolium*. Other plants that produce large amounts of sesquiterpene lactones include: *Hymenoxys odorata, Hymenoxys richardsonii,* and *Dugaldia hoopesii*.

References

Dollahite JW, Hardy WT, Hanson JB. Toxicity of Helenium microcephalum (small head sneeze weed). J Am Vet Med Assoc 1964;145:694–696.

Herz W. Sesquiterpene lactones from livestock poisons. In: Keeler RF, Van Kampen KR, James LF, eds. Effects of poisonous plants on livestock. New York: Academic Press, 1978;487–497.

Witzel DA, Ivie GW, Dollahite JW. Mammalian toxicity of Helenium microcephalum (small head sneeze weed). Am J Vet Res 1976;37:859–861.

Box

The common box, boxwood, or boxtree *(Buxus sempervirens)* is native to Europe and Asia and is widely grown in the warmer climates of the United States as an ornamental or hedge. Losses of sheep, horses, pigs, cattle, and camels have been reported as a result of eating the leaves and stems of this plant. Severe gastroenteritis, sometimes with bloody diarrhea, are reported, and death occurs in a short time. Several alkaloids have been extracted from the plant, including boxine—a severe emetic or purgative.

References

Couch JF. The chemistry of stock-poisoning plants. J Chem Educ 1937;14:16–24.

Kingsbury JM. Poisonous plants of the United States and Canada. Englewood Cliffs: Prentice-Hall, 1964.

Van Soest H, Gottink WM, van den Vooren IJ. Poisoning in pigs and cows by boxtree leaves (Buxus sempervirens). Tijdschr Diergeneeskd 1965;90:387–389.

GRASSTREE

This plant *(Xanthorrhoea resinosa, X. hastile)* has been reported to cause poisoning of cattle only in Australia. The animals apparently eat this plant only when other feed is not available. The principal signs are "lurching to one side" and dribbling urine. In some animals, signs appear or are exacerbated two to three weeks after they have stopped eating the plant.

References

Hall WTK. Grasstree poisoning of cattle. Queensland Agric J 1965;91:504–506.
Kingsbury JM. Poisonous plants of the United States and Canada. Englewood Cliffs: Prentice-Hall, 1964.

POKEWEED (PHYTOLACCA)

Pokeweed poisoning has been recorded in swine from eating the roots of this plant *(Phytolacca americana)* and in cattle from eating the tops of its fruit (pokeberries). Signs of poisoning have appeared overnight after feeding green plants cut with corn silage. Signs included severe diarrhea and purgation, subnormal temperature, severe decrease in milk flow, convulsions, and paralysis, which may lead to death from respiratory failure.

Reference

Kingsbury JM, Hillman RB. Pokeweed (Phytolacca) posioning in a dairy herd. Cornell Vet 1965;55:534–538.

YEW

These ornamental shrubs *(Taxus cuspidata, T. baccata, T. canadensis)* are rarely eaten by animals, but severe toxicity has been ascribed to them. The European variety, *Taxus baccata,* is a more frequently reported cause of poisoning on that continent, principally affecting cattle. The Japanese yew, *Taxus cuspidata,* a popular ornamental shrub in the United States, has been incriminated in deaths of horses, deer, reindeer, and burros. Cattle have been reported to die after eating *Taxus canadensis,* but the toxicity of *Taxus brevifolia* has been imputed but not confirmed.

Signs of poisoning may be missed; animals may simply be found with the offending plant in mouth and stomach. Nervous manifestations, such as trembling, dyspnea, and collapse, may be evident during a short course. Lesions have not been recognized.

References

Alden CL, Fosnaugh CJ, Smith JB, et al. Japanese yew poisoning of large domestic animals in the midwest. J Am Vet Med Assoc 1977;170:314–316.
Kingsbury JM. Poisonous plants of the United States and Canada. Englewood Cliffs: Prentice-Hall, 1964.
Lowe JE, et al. Taxus cuspidata (Japanese yew) poisoning in horses. Cornell Vet 1970;60:36–39.

SORGHUM

Horses grazed in pastures rich in sudan grass *(Sorghum sudanese)* have been observed to develop chronic cystitis and occasionally ataxia. The urinary bladder in prolonged cases becomes thickened due to fibrosis, the epithelium is ulcerated, and abscesses may occur in the wall. The vagina may also be ulcerated and presumably infected, and abortion may occur. In one case, *Streptococcus zooepidemicus* was recovered. The basis for ataxia in some cases has not been explained.

In one report, eight pregnant heifers were grazed on a pasture made up principally of a regrowth of a hybrid sudan grass *(Sorghum sudanese x Sorghum bicolor cv. Sudax.* Subsequently, six of the eight cows with *dystocia* delivered calves affected with arthrogryposis. The last two were bred four months later, and were kept on the same pasture; they delivered normal calves. A teratogen was suspected to be in the sudan grass pasturage.

References

Knight PR. Equine cystitis and ataxia associated with grazing of pastures dominated by sorghum species. Aut Vet J 1968;44:257.
Romane WM, et al. Equine cystitis associated with grazing of sudan grass. J Am Vet Med Assoc 1966;149:1171.
Seaman JT, Smeal MG, Wright JC. The possible association of a sorghum (Sorghum sudanese) hybrid as a cause of developmental defects in calves. Aust Vet J 1981;57:351–352.

Sesbania

This South African shrub or small tree *(Sesbania punicea,* purple sesbane, purple rattlebox) has been reported to be toxic to most domestic animals and poultry.

The whole plant is poisonous; the seeds, flowers, and leaves each contain the toxic element. The poisoning is manifest by irritation of the gastrointestinal tract and cardiac failure. Terminal renal failure has been noted in some cases. Several North American species are also known to be poisonous. These are known under various scientific and common names. *Sesbania vesicaria,* bagpod, bladderpod, or coffeebean, is a vigorous annual that grows especially in damp soils in the coastal plain from North Carolina and Florida to Texas.

Sesbania drummondii, coffeebean, rattlebush or rattlebox, is a perennial shrub or small tree with a distribution similar to *S. vesicaria.* Sheep and goats have been poisoned under natural conditions and cattle, experimentally. *S. punicea* has been described as growing in Florida to Louisiana after its introduction as an ornamental from Mexico. The toxic principle in these plants is suspected to be saponin, but has not been clearly identified.

References

Flory W, Hebert CD. Determination of the oral toxicity of Sesbania drummondi seeds in chickens. Am J Vet Res 1984;45:955–958.
Terblanche M, et al. A toxicological study of the plant Sesbania punicea, Benth. J S Afr Vet Med Assoc 1966;37:191–197.

Estrogens

These hormones have been known to cause poisoning under two generally different conditions. Synthetic estrogen, diethylstilbestrol, is used in feed for cattle to stimulate economical growth and usually causes no overt ill effects in these animals. On occasion, however, the "premix" containing the synthetic estrogen has been erroneously mixed with feed under preparation for laboratory mice. Certain inbred strains of mice are sensitive to estrogens, and the effect upon a breeding colony is dramatic. In one incident in such a breeding colony of white mice, the number of pregnancies declined rapidly from 1000 a week to 20 per week. Litter size was reduced and many young were stillborn. About 90% of the adult males suddenly exhibited scrotal hernias, and sections of testes revealed complete azoospermia. After removal of the offending adulterated feed, reproduction gradually resumed in the mouse colony (Figure 15-34).

Experimental administration of diethylstilbestrol to mice has also been shown to produce lesions in the rete testis, including adenocarcinoma.

A second source of estrogens is in natural plants, such as subterranean clover (*Trifolium subterraneum*). This clover poisoning is a major problem to sheep in certain parts of Australia. Different strains of clover vary in estrogen content and toxicity. The effects include stillbirths, neonatal deaths, dystocia, prolapse of uterus, and infertility in ewes. Virgin ewes may undergo precocious mammary development and lactation. Castrated males (wethers) may also lactate. White clover (*T. repens*) has also been shown to have estrogenic effects.

In two herds of cattle in Mississippi, severe reduction in pregnancy rates, from 70% in the fall to 10% in the spring, have been attributed to grazing on pastures consisting largely of *Trifolium subterraneum* L. var *Mt. Barker*. Shortened estrous cycles and loss of pregnancy up to 60 days following conception were noted. Necropsy of 15 affected cows revealed lesions, such as mucometria (2), cystic endometrial hypoplasia (8), cystic Graafian follicles (4), and epithelial cysts in the fimbria of the oviducts (1).

Estrogenic mycotoxins are another source of exogenous estrogenic compounds; these are discussed in chapter 12.

References

Donaldson LE. Clover disease in two Mississippi cattle herds. J Am Vet Med Assoc 1983;182:412–413.
Hadlow WJ, Grimes EF. Influence of stilbestrol-contaminated feed on reproduction in a colony of mice. Proc Anim Care Panel 1955;6:19–25.
Hadlow WJ. Stilbestrol poisoning in mice. J Am Vet Med Assoc 1957;130:300–303.
Kelley RW, Hay RJM, Shackell GH. Formononectin content of grasslands Pawera red clover and its oestrogenic activity in sheep. NZ J Exp Agric 1979;7:131–134.
Lightfoot RJ, Adams NR. Changes in cervical histology in ewes following prolonged grazing on oestrogenic subterranean clover. J Comp Pathol 1979;89:367–373.
Newbold RR, Bullock BC, McLachlan JA. Adenocarcinoma of the rete testis: diethylstilbestrol-induced lesions of the mouse rete testis. Am J Pathol 1986;125:625–628.
Southey IN, Davis HL, Maller R. Oestrus cycles in ewes grazing different cultivars of subterranean clover. Aust Vet J 1976;52:297–298.

Nitrogen dioxide

This gas has been incriminated as a cause of "silo-fillers disease" in humans and pulmonary adenomatosis in cattle. Intratracheal instillation of nitrogen dioxide gas in controlled doses into cattle results in severe respiratory distress, methemoglobinemia, and death. Animals that survive 11–14 days following this exposure exhibit severe pulmonary consolidation and emphysema of the lungs. The respiratory epithelium undergoes squamous metaplasia in the trachea and proliferation in the rest of the bronchial tree. The alveolar epithelium proliferates and fills alveoli in some lobules; in others, fibrin precipitates in alveoli to form a hyaline membrane. The bronchiolar epithelium becomes redundant, and subepithelial fibrosis is conspicuous. Invasion by leukocytes into affected lungs may be extensive.

References

Cutlip RC. Experimental nitrogen dioxide poisoning in cattle. Pathol Vet 1966;3:474–485.
Lowry T, Schuman LM. Silo-filler's disease—a syndrome caused by nitrogen dioxide. J Am Vet Med Assoc 1956;162:153–160.
Seaton VA. Pulmonary adenomatosis in Iowa cattle. Am J Vet Res 1958;19:600–609.

Cobalt

Cobalt is necessary for bacterial synthesis of vitamin B_{12} in the rumen, and some soils are deficient in this element. This has led to application of cobalt sulfate to the soil, and sometimes to injudicious dosing of ruminants with this salt. Overdoses have led to death of cattle within a few hours. The principal findings at necropsy indicate severe congestion of the abomasal mucosa and microscopic evidence of toxic nephrosis. Cobalt may be demonstrated by spectrographic analysis to be present in liver and kidney.

In humans, endemic cardiomyopathy in heavy beer drinkers has been ascribed to cobalt (a beer additive). Necrotizing cardiomyopathy has been reproduced in rats given cobalt sulfate. Protein deficiency augmented the lesion. Many rats also developed vegetative endocarditis. Experimental canine cardiomyopathy, produced by administration of cobalt, has been proposed as a model for the study of heart failure.

References

McLaren APC, Johnston WG, Voss RC. Cobalt poisoning in cattle. Vet Rec 1964;76:1148–1149.
Rona F. Experimental aspects of cobalt cardiomyopathy. Br Health J 1971;33(Suppl 1):171–174.
Unverforth DV, et al. Canine cobalt cardiomyopathy: a model for the study of heart failure. Am J Vet Res 1983;44:989–995.

Chloroquine

Chloroquine has been used for the suppression or treatment of malaria in humans, as well as for treatment of systemic or discoid lupus erythematosus and rheumatoid arthritis. Tests of this drug in swine have revealed interesting toxicologic effects. Daily oral doses of 25

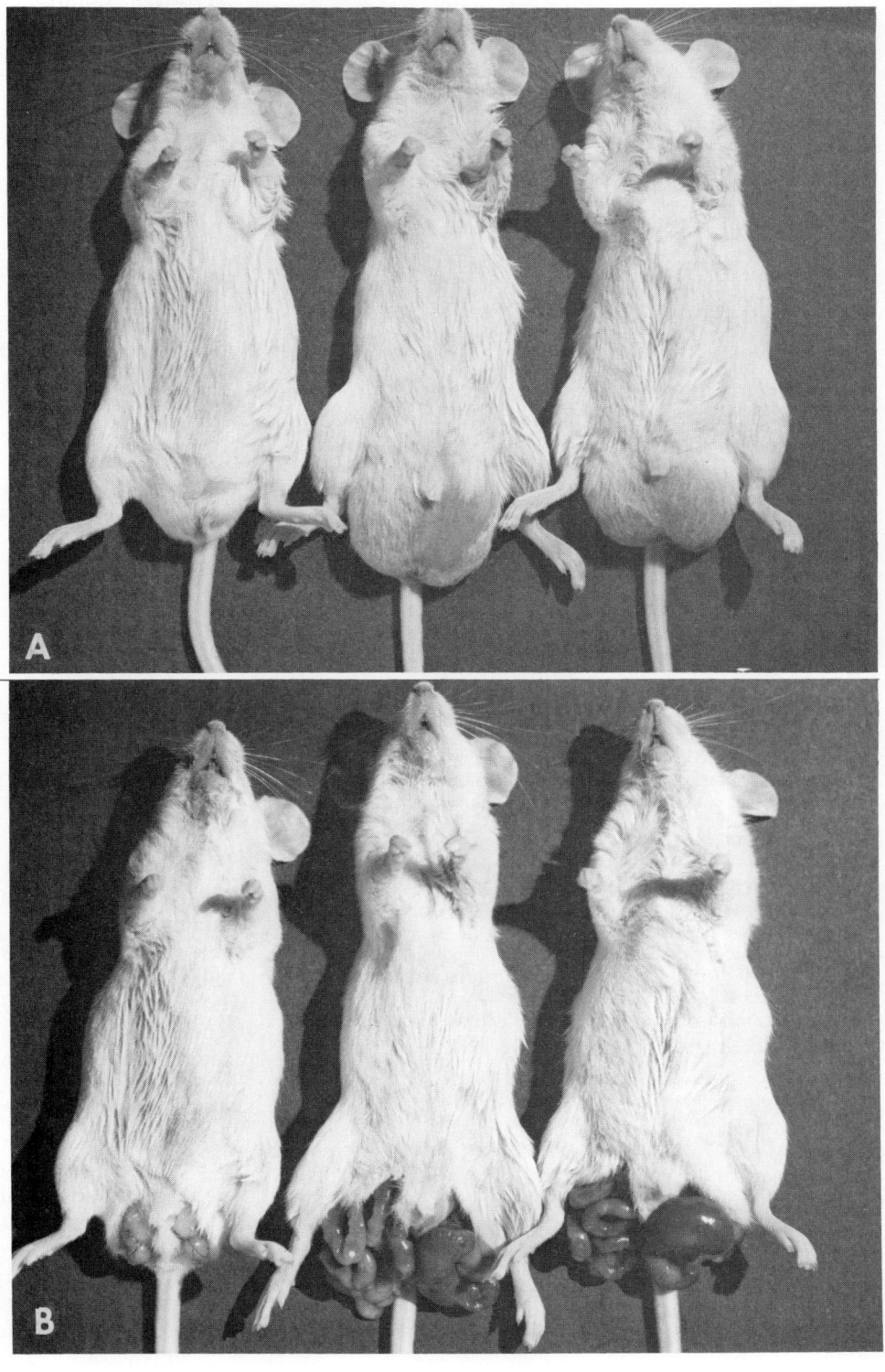

FIG. 15-34 Poisoning by diethylstilbestrol. Scrotal hernias in adult male mice. Normal mouse on the left. **A.** Intact mice. **B.** Scrotum incised to reveal intestinal content in two affected mice. (Courtesy of Dr. W. J. Hadlow and Proceedings of The Animal Care Panel.)

mg/kg body weight were not lethal, but pigs were killed by doses of 50–100 mg/kg/day. The significant pathologic lesions included diffuse myopathy of skeletal muscles, degenerative changes in neurons of the central nervous system and retina, necrosis of lymphocytes, and edema of the retina. Changes in skeletal muscles resembled Zenker necrosis. By light microscopy, the changes in neurons appeared as swollen, foamy cytoplasm with displacement of nuclei. Electron micrographs disclosed this foamy cytoplasm to contain numerous lamellated, membranous bodies.

References

Gleiser CA, et al. Study of chloroquine toxicity and a drug-induced cerebrospinal lipodystrophy in swine. Am J Pathol 1968;53:27–45.

Zinc

Deficiency of this element associated with parakeratosis of swine and its necessity in metabolism are discussed elsewhere (p. 808). It seems inevitable that poisoning with zinc will occur as a result of overzealous administration of zinc compounds. Experimentally, toxicity has been demonstrated in sheep and cattle. Depressed or depraved appetites result in cattle that have been fed zinc oxide in the diet at the rate of 0.9 g or more per kilogram of feed. Zinc accumulates in the blood, liver, pancreas, kidney, and bone, and in lesser amounts in hair, spleen, lung, and heart. After prolonged periods, hemoglobin and packed cell volumes in the blood are decreased.

Signs and lesions of osteochondrosis, osteoporosis, and nephrocalcinosis have been observed in a group of horses, especially foals, kept in a farm near a zinc smelter. Zinc and cadmium levels were severly increased in the pancreas, liver, and kidney of these animals. Osteochondrosis was considered characteristic of the lesions seen in horses fed experimental diets containing hing levels of zinc. Osteoporosis and mephrocalcinosis were consistent with lesions resulting from experimental cadmium poisoning in horses.

References

Fitzgerald PR, Peterson J, Lue-Hing C. Heavy metals in tissues of cattle exposed to sludge-treated pastures for eight years. Am J Vet Res 1985;46:703–707.

Gunson DE, Kowalczyk DF, Shoop R, et al. Environmental zinc and cadmium pollution associated with generalized osteochondrosis, osteoporosis, and nephrocalcinosis in horses. J Am Vet Med Assoc 1982;180:295–299.

Ott EA, et al. Zinc toxicity in ruminants. I. Effect of high levels of dietary zinc on gains, feed consumption and feed efficiency of lambs. II. Effect of high levels of dietary zinc on gains, feed consumption and feed efficiency of beef cattle. J Anim Sci 1966;25:414–418,419–423.

Ott EA, et al. Zinc toxicity in ruminants. III. Physiological changes in tissues and alterations in rumen metabolism in lambs. J Anim Sci 1966;25:424–431.

Ott EA, et al. Zinc toxicity in ruminants. IV. Physiological changes in tissues of beef cattle. J Anim Sci 1966;25:432–438.

Zinc phosphide

A gray-black powder, used as a rodenticide, which releases phosphine (PH_3) when mixed with water has caused poisoning in a variety of animal species in Europe, but only recently has poisoning been described in the United States. The histopathologic changes have not been well described, but clinically poisoning is characterized by vomiting, abdominal pain, lethargy, and convulsions.

Reference

Stowe CM, et al. Zinc phosphide poisoning in dogs. J Am Vet Med Assoc 1978;173:270.

Cadmium

A single subcutaneous dose of cadmium chloride ($CaCl_2$) into Wistar rats has been demonstrated to result in acute vascular lesions in the testes with ischemic necrosis in seminiferous tubules. These changes, after resolution of necrosis, may be followed by intratubular fibrosis and mineralization also involving the rete testis. After a prolonged period, interstitial (Leydig) cell tumors develop in some of these testes. In some, Sertoli-Leydig cell tumors have also been found, as well as adenocarcinoma, involving the rete testis. The addition of zinc to the feed potentiates this effect.

Cadmium has been shown to accumulate in the pancreas, liver, and kidney of horses grazed on pastures in the vicinity of a zinc smelter, and has been associated with severe osteoporosis and nephrocalcinosis. Accumulation of cadmium has also been noted in the kidneys of cattle kept for up to eight years on pastures fertilized by aerobically digested sludge, but no signs or lesions were associated with its presence.

References

Elinder C-G, Jonsson L, Piscator M, et al. Histopathological changes in relation to cadmium concentration in horse kidneys. Environ Res 1981;26:1–21.

Fitzgerald PR, Peterson J, Lue-Hing C. Heavy metals in tissues of cattle exposed to sludge-treated pastures for eight years. Am J Vet Res 1985;46:703–707.

Gunson DE, Kowalczyk DF, Shoop R, et al. Environmental zinc and cadmium pollution associated with generalized osteochondrosis, osteoporosis, and nephrocalcinosis in horses. J Am Vet Med Assoc 1982;180:295–299.

Rehm S, Waalkes MP. Mixed Sertoli-Leydig cell tumor and rete testis adenocarcinoma with cadmium chloride. Vet Pathol 1988;25:163–166.

Singhal RK, Anderson ME, Meister A. Glutathione, a first line of defense against cadmium toxicity. FASEB J 1987;1:220–223.

Gidyea tree

The leaves and pods of the gidyea tree (Acacia georginae) contain a poisonous principle that may be lethal to sheep and cattle. This poisoning is reported from the Georgina River basin in eastern Northern Territory and western Queensland of Australia, where it is known as Georgina River poisoning. The active poison is fluoroacetate ion. It is possible that this tree may concentrate fluoroacetate in its leaves and pods, under specific conditions, from soils rich in fluorine. Monofluoroacetic acid in significant quantities has been isolated from the "gifblaar" plant (Dichapetalum cymosum) in South Africa where severe losses of livestock have been associated with eating this plant. See also sodium monofluoroacetate poisoning, page 701.

The most significant lesion is reported to occur in the myocardium. Focal necroses of myocardial fibers, usually followed by leukocytic infiltration and in some cases fibrosis, are seen microscopically. These are associated with gross petechiae and ecchymoses under the endocardium and epicardium, and occasional focal scars in the myocardium.

References

Fowler ME. Plant poisoning in camelids. In: James LF, Keeler RF, Bailey EM Jr, Cheeke PR, Hegarty MP, eds. Poisonous plants: Proc 3rd Int Symp. Ames: Iowa State Univ Press, 1992;335–339.

Whittem JH, Murray LR. The chemistry and pathology of Georgina River poisoning. Aust Vet J 1963;39:168–173.

Helichrysum argyrosphaerum

This plant—also known as "Wild Everlasting," "Proprosie," "Sewejarrtjie"), native to Africa, long suspected as toxic—has been shown to cause a disease characterized by blindness and paralysis in sheep and cattle. Most field cases occur in sheep. The lesions, which have been reproduced experimentally are characterized by marked demyelination and necrosis of white matter in brain, optic nerves and chiasm, spinal cord, and peripheral nerves. Degeneration of the retina also occurs, commencing in the layer of rods and cones and extending to the inner nuclear layer. Cataracts characterized by necrosis of lens epithelium and lens cortex have been associated with natural outbreaks, but have not been reproduced.

Reference

Basson PA, et al. Blindness and encephalopathy caused by Helichrysum argyrosphaerum DC (Compositae) in sheep and cattle. Onderstepoort J Vet Res 1975;42:135–145.

Melia azedarch

Poisoning of livestock, principally sheep and swine, have been reported in Africa, Australia, and India from consumption of the fruits of the *Melia azedarch* (chinaberry tree, white cedar). Although the tree is naturalized in southern United States, examples of poisoning are rare. Signs of poisoning include gastroenteritis (principally diarrhea) and nervous dysfunction (trembling, depression, paralysis). Lesions have not been described in detail. Hemorrhagic gastroenteritis, focal necrosis of the liver, kidney, myocardium, lymph nodes, and spleen, meningeal congestion, cerebral hemorrhage, and perivascular cuffing have been recorded.

Reference

Kwatra MS, Singh B, Hothi DS, et al. Poisoning by Melia azedarch in pigs. Vet Rec 1974;95:421.

Aspirin

Aspirin (acetylsalicylic acid) is one of the most widely used drugs in human medicine, as an analgesic, antiphlogistic, and anticoagulant. In most species, an extremely wide margin of safety exists, but intolerance reflected as hypersensitivity reactions (atopy, anaphylaxis) are reported; its anticoagulant properties may lead to hemorrhage when used in high doses for prolonged periods. Cats are extremely intolerant of aspirin. Toxicity leads to hemorrhagic and ulcerative gastritis and toxic hepatitis with centrilobular necrosis. The principal effect of aspirin lies with its interference with the modulating role of prostaglandins on platelet aggregation and release of their contents. Aspirin, which inhibits cyclooxygenase, an enzyme necessary for prostaglandin production, leads to defective platelet aggregation and release. Other nonsteroid, antiinflammatory drugs have similar actions. Acetaminophen (metabolic product of phenacetin), another analgesic, is also toxic to cats and reported to induce hemolytic anemia and methemglobinemia.

References

Allen DG, Johnstone IB, Crane S. Effects of aspirin and propranolol alone and in combination on hemostatic determinants in the healthy cat. Am J Vet Res 1985;46:660–663.
Judson DC, Barton M. Effect of aspirin on haemostasis in the horse. Res Vet Sci 1981;30:241–242.
Schubert TA. Salicylate-induced seizures in a dog. J Am Vet Med Assoc 1984;185:1000–1001.
Whiting J, Salata K, Bailey JM. Aspirin: an unexpected side effect on prostacyclin synthesis in cultured smooth muscle cells. Science 1980;210:663–665.

Benzoic acid

Benzoic acid is commonly used as a preservative in some dog and cat foods. Poisoning has been suspected in cats, which appear to be more sensitive to its effects than dogs. Experimental poisoning of cats has been reported with meat containing 0.5–1.0% benzoic acid. The syndrome is characterized by aggression, hyperesthesia, convulsions, and death. The pathogenesis of these signs is unknown.

Benzyl alcohol has been used as a preservative in parenteral solutions, such as lactated Ringer's solution. Normally, in most species, benzyl alcohol is rapidly oxidized in the body to benzoic and hippuric acid and benzyl glucuronide. In the cat, only hippuric acid is formed due to inadequate capacity to conjugate benzyl glucuronide. This is believed to result in the accumulation of hippuric acid, which is toxic to the cat. Neonatal humans and other animals, also sensitive to benzoic acid toxicity, may have similar underdeveloped capacities in these metabolic pathways.

References

Bedford PGC, Clarke EGC. Experimental benzoic acid poisoning in the cat. Vet Rec 1972;99:53–58.
Cullison RF, Menard PD, Buck WB. Toxicosis in cats from the use of benzyl alcohol in lactated Ringer's solution. J Am Vet Med Assoc 1983;182:61.

Kallstroemia

Poisoning by carpet weed or hairy caltrop (*Kallstroemia hirsutissima*) has been documented in cattle and sheep, respectively. The plants are native to western United States. Poisoning is characterized by a peculiar knuckling over of the hind legs at the fetlock joints, which progresses to posterior paralysis and death. The forelimbs are unaffected. The basis for these unusual signs or death is not known. Severe gastroenteritis is reported in sheep.

References

Mathews FP. The toxicity of Kallstroemia hirsutisima (carpetweed) for cattle, sheep, and goats. J Am Vet Med Assoc 1944;95:152–155.
Dollahite JW. Toxicity of Kallstroemia parviflora (warty caltrop) to sheep, goats and rabbits. Southwest Vet 1975;28:135–139.

Fish poisoning

Poisoning from consumption of certain fishes and shellfish under appropriate conditions is well recognized in humans. Although most mammals are believed to be susceptible, few reported cases exist; similar poisonings in animals probably go unrecognized. Many different types of fish poison humans. Ciguatera and scombroid poisoning are the most common.

Ciguatera (from Spanish, poisonous snail) is most often associated with barracuda, red snapper, amberjack, and grouper. The heat-stable toxin is referred to as ciguatoxin, which is believed to enter fish through the food chain. It is a cholinesterase inhibitor, but its action is believed to be more complex. Signs of poisoning, which develop within a few minutes to 30 hours after ingestion, include abdominal cramps, nausea, vomiting, diarrhea, and paresthesia, particularly of the lips, tongue, and throat.

Scombroid fish poisoning is associated with tuna, mackerel, bonito, and shipjack, and the nonscombroid fish, mahi-mahi. The toxin, formed by bacteria on fish flesh, is called scombrotoxin, and is believed to consist of histamine and other heat-stable substances.

Symptoms begin within a few minutes to a few hours after ingestion, and include flushing, headache, dizziness, burning of the mouth and throat, abdominal cramps, nausea, vomiting, diarrhea, urticaria, and pruritus.

Shellfish poisoning results from ingestion of bivalve mollusks contaminated with neurotoxins of the dinoflagellates *Gonyaulax catenalla* or *Go. tamarensis*, which results in a paralytic disease commencing within 30 minutes, or *Gymnodinium breve*, which is associated with neurologic signs, such as ataxia, but not with paralysis. In both forms, nausea, vomiting, and diarrhea also occur. The toxins are heat-stable. Mussels, clams, oysters, and scallops are the main vehicles. When in abundance, these and other toxic dinoflagellates, as well as nontoxic dinoflagellates, impart a reddish brown color to the water, usually called a red tide.

References

Hughes JM, Merson MH. Fish and shellfish poisoning. N Engl J Med 1976;295:1117–1120.
Shimizu Y, Yoshioka M. Transformation of paralytic shellfish toxins as demonstrated in scallop homogenates. Science 1981;212:547–549.

16

Nutritional deficiencies

Deficiency of nutrients required to maintain homeostasis can lead to a vast array of pathologic conditions, affecting all organ systems. Deficiency of a single nutrient is rare as a natural disease, although a number of examples can be cited: iodine deficiency leading to goiter; iron deficiency leading to anemia; ingestion of thiaminase leading to thiamine deficiency; and molybdenum toxicosis leading to copper deficiency. In general, nutritional deficiencies occur multiply, and lead to complex disease states that are more difficult to analyze; these complex states also are difficult to compare with the single nutrient deficiencies produced in the laboratory. Nutritional deficiency can arise from several different mechanisms, including the following.

1. Simple dietary deficiency of one or more nutrients. This can arise from a diet of generally poor quality (starvation), a lack of specific ingredients in commercially prepared diets, or a diet specifically lacking in one or more essential nutrients.
2. Interference with intake. This has the same effect as inadequate supply, which may arise from causes, such as anorexia, mechanical obstruction, dental disease, and parasitism.
3. Interference with absorption of nutrients. This may be caused by: lack of digestive secretions caused by hepatic or pancreatic disease; enteritis; hypermotility of the intestinal tract; parasitism; or the formation of insoluble complexes, such as between calcium and phytate.
4. Interference with storage or utilization. For example, in thyroiditis, insufficient normal tissue may be available for the proper utilization of iodine.
5. Increased excretion or retention of nutrients. For example, diarrhea may result in loss of potassium, and hyperparathyroidism may cause a loss of calcium. Retention of phosphorus in renal disease leads to lowered levels of serum calcium.
6. Increased requirements. Pregnancy, lactation, or hyperthyroidism may cause deficiency states when the diet is not adjusted. Neonatal and young animals also have increased dietary requirements; therefore, this age group is more susceptible to deficiency.

7. Inhibition of nutrients. Certain inhibitors or analogs of nutrients may exist in the diet, and lead to deficiency. Analogs are known for several of the B vitamins. Imbalance of nutrients is also included in this categoty; for example, a diet that is excessively high in phosphorous results in lowered levels of serum calcium.
8. Inherited metabolic defects. These interfere with absorption, utilization, or other aspects of nutrient metabolism. A number of essential nutrients can also be toxic when fed in large amounts. This is true of vitamins A and D, as well as many minerals: for example, copper and selenium. These are also discussed in this chapter as well as in the chapter on poisons (Chapter 15).

References

Brown ML, ed. Present Knowledge in Nutrition. 6th ed. Washington, DC: Int Life Sci Inst, Nutr Foundation, 1990.
Combs GF Jr. The vitamins: fundamental aspects in nutrition and health. New York: Academic Press, 1992.
Follis RH Jr. Deficiency disease. Springfield: CC Thomas, 1958.
McDowell LR. Minerals in Animal and Human Nutrition. New York: Academic Press, 1992.
Schneider HA, Anderson CE, Coursin DB, eds. Nutritional support of medical practice. 2nd ed. Philadelphia: Harper and Row, 1983.

FAT SOLUBLE VITAMINS

Vitamin A

Vitamin A designates a large group of compounds, known as retinoids, that have similar qualitative biologic activity. The prototype or parent compound, **all-*trans*-retinol**, only exists in foods of animal origin, primarily as retinyl ester. Herbivores rely on a group of yellow pigmented compounds of plant origin, known as carotenoids; many carotenoids have provitamin A activity as their source of vitamin A. β-Carotene is the most important of these, and also occurs in animal products. Absorption of vitamin A and carotenoids requires bile and pancreatic enzymes. Rentinyl ester is absorbed in the small intestine after it is hydrolyzed to retinol (vitamin A alcohol). β-Carotene can be absorbed directly from the intestine to the bloodstream; or, it can be enzymatically converted into two molecules of retinal (vitamin A aldehyde) in the intestinal mucosa. Retinal is then converted to retinol. Absorbed carotene can also be converted to retinal, and then to retinol in the liver and other tissues. The absorption and cleavage process of β-carotene varies greatly among species, and even among breeds. Herbivores are most efficient in the process; omnivores are less so, and cats entirely lack the ability. Retinol from either source is reesterified in the intestinal mucosa, released, and then transported to the liver—primarily through the lymphatics—where it is stored. When mobilized from liver, retinyl esters are converted to retinol and transported in the blood, bound to **retinol-binding protein.** Retinal and retinoic acid also circulate in the blood, bound to their own specific proteins. At the level of target cells, specific surface receptors for the transport protein (not retinol) are required for its transport across the cell membrane. It is then bound to **cellular retinol-binding protein.**

Retinol is the most active of the vitamin A metabolites. In humans, it takes almost twice the amount of β-carotene to match the dietary requirement of vitamin A provided by retinol. Dietary retinoic acid can meet many of the vitamin A requirements (e.g., maintenance of epithelia), but it cannot be converted to retinol, retinal, or retinyl esters; therefore, it cannot meet the requirements for vision. Most retinoic acid is catabolized and excreted. This is a brief overview of the complex metabolism of the retinoids.

FUNCTIONS

The primary functions of vitamin A are to maintain vision and to differentiate epithelial cells. The first signs of deficiency are related to these roles. Hypovitaminosis A is also characterized by a number of other changes, including: skeletal and dental malformation; increased cerebrospinal pressure; reproduction failure; immunosuppression; developmental anomalies; and cancer. However, the mechanisms of these changes are less well understood.

DEFICIENCY

Vitamin A deficiency (Fig. 16-1) is not common, and is encountered only when inadequate diets are consumed for prolonged periods. The liver stores an amount adequate for a considerable period, during which total dietary deprivation produces no effect. This period is usually five or six months in cattle and horses, and two or three months in sheep and goats. **Zinc deficiency** has been shown to reduce the synthesis of retinol-binding protein and, therefore, to interfere with vitamin A transport. Zinc is also believed to be necessary for conversion of retinol to retinal, which is necessary for vision.

VISION

The earliest sign of deficiency of vitamin A is **night blindness** (nyctalopia); however, vitamin A is required for the function and integrity of both rods and cones.

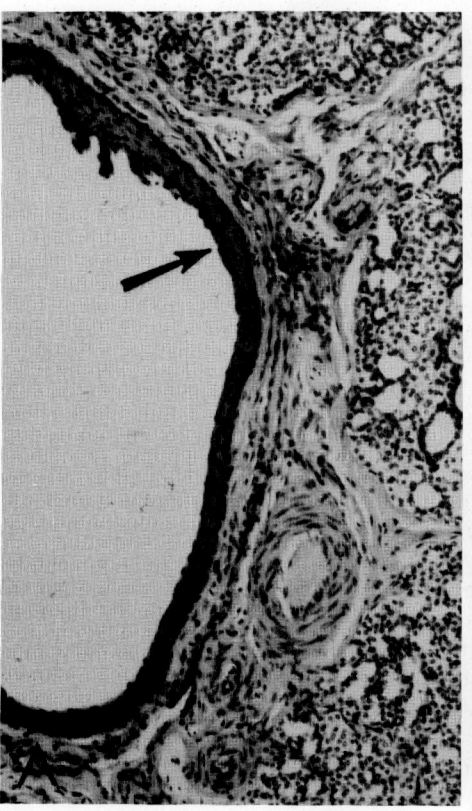 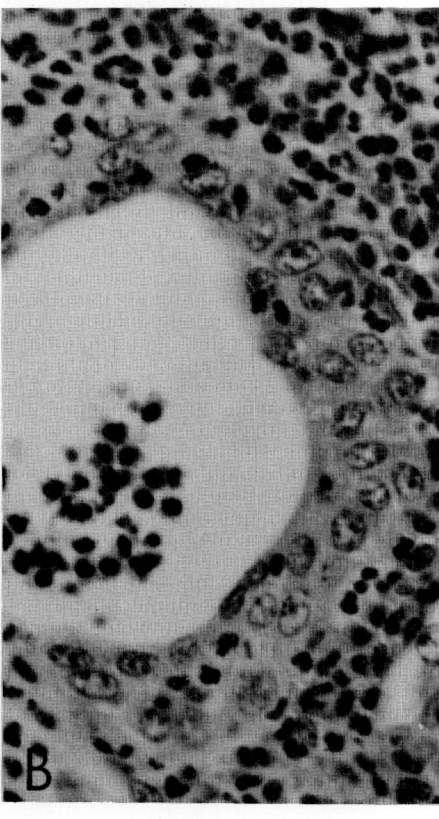

FIG. 16-1 Vitamin A deficiency. **A.** Squamous metaplasia of a major duct in the salivary gland of a calf. **B.** Squamous metaplasia of a collecting tubule in the kidney of a mink. Also note purulent exudate in the lumen of the tubule and interstitium.

Rods and cones contain proteins known as opsins which, when combined with 11–*cys*-retinal, become the photosensitive pigments of these cells: **rhodopsin** in rod cells, and three different **iodopsins** in cone cells. 11–*cys*-retinal is derived from circulating rentinol that is first oxidized to all-*trans*-retinal, and then isomerized to 11–*cys*-retinal. When exposed to light, a series of events occurs in which rhodopsin is reduced to all-*trans*-retinal and opsin; a nervous signal is then sent through the visual pathways. During dark adaptation most of the all-*trans*-retinal is reduced to retinol, some of which is reutilized; much of the retinol is lost, however, requiring a continuous source of circulating retinol. Rhodopsin is the most light-sensitive of the visual pigments, and is therefore important to vision in reduced light.

Histologically, atrophy of the retina occurs; atrophy is first evident in the rod segments; it subsequently affects all the photoreceptor cells and, ultimately, the entire thickness of the retina. Aberrant development of the optic foramina may occur during development of the fetus in deficient mothers; this is due to increased cerebrospinal pressure, and may also cause retinal changes. These are described below.

EPITHELIAL DIFFERENTIATION

The second most frequent sign of vitamin A deficiency is **xerophthalmia,** or dryness of the eyes. This is not a singular expression of vitamin A deficiency, but one of many changes in epithelia related to the role vitamin A plays in cellular differentiation. In vitamin A deficiency, normal cuboidal and columnar epithelial surfaces are replaced by keratinizing, stratified, squamous epithelium. This **squamous metaplasia** is particularly prominent on mucus-secreting surfaces; however, it is widespread throughout many systems, and is first evident in the conjunctiva. Squamous metaplasia of the ducts of lacrimal glands leads to deficiency of lacrimal secretion; this aggravates the conjunctival lesion, causing conjunctivitis, keratitis, and blindness. Squamous metaplasia is prominent in the mucosa of the respiratory, gastrointestinal, and genitourinary tracts; it also occurs in the ducts of glands, such as the pancreas. Desquamated keratin in the urinary tract leads to **urolithiasis.** Hyperplasia and hyperkeratosis of the skin and hair follicles are also features of hypovitaminosis A, and may result in dermatitis. All forms of vitamin A, including retinoic acid, effectively prevent these epithelial changes. Evidence exists for two mechanisms in which vitamin A is necessary for cellular differentiation. One suggests that vitamin A functions like a steroid hormone, acting through the nucleus to signal necessary transcriptional proteins for cell differentiation. The other proposes that the requirement for vitamin A to synthesize glycoproteins leads to their deficiency, which affects intercellular interactions important to differentiation.

Reproduction Loss of reproductive efficiency occurs in vitamin A deficiency, characterized by death and resorption of the fetus, and decreased spermatogenesis. Squamous metaplasia of the endometrial mucosa may

be partly responsible, because retinoic acid cannot correct or prevent the problem.

Bone and tooth growth Vitamin A is required for the effective function of osteoclasts, whose number declines in deficiency; this leads to an imbalance between bone formation (by osteoblasts) and bone resorption. This effect is most often encountered in young animals and in infants born to deficient mothers, where the imbalance is pronounced in the cranial bones; a disparity exists, then, between growth of the nervous system and its bony enclosure. The most noticeable effect of this disparity is a failure of the optic foramina to grow in sufficient diameter; this leads to constriction and degeneration of the optic nerves. Other nerves (e.g., spinal and acoustic) may also be affected, resulting in loss of hearing or other functions. In rats and guinea pigs, vitamin A deficiency also leads to loss of differentiation and function of odontoblasts and ameloblasts, resulting in defective formation of both dentin and enamel.

Cerebrospinal Fluid Increased cerebrospinal fluid pressure results, in part, from a reduction in size of the cranial vault; however, impaired absorption of cerebrospinal fluid via arachnoid villi is more important. This results from thickening of the dura matter, particularly of the tentorium cerebelli, which may become ossified. This is associated with optic nerve papilledema and signs of nervous dysfunction.

Immune function Hypovitaminosis A also impairs immune function. Deficiency in animals is associated with increased susceptibility to infection; in part, this is due to altered mucosal surfaces; however, retinoids also appear to be important to the differentiation of lymphocytes and macrophages.

Developmental Effects Developmental anomalies in addition to those described above are also encountered in animals born to deficient mothers. These include microphthalmia, corneal dermoids, anasarca, polydactyly, and cardiac anomalies, among others. They have been most frequently described in swine.

Cancer Studies with laboratory animals have found that, with certain model systems, vitamin A deficiency leads to increased susceptibility to cancer, and that increased doses of vitamin A are protective. Carotenoids may be equally or more important to these effects.

HYPERVITAMINOSIS A

Excessive intake of the retinoids in most any form is toxic (Fig. 16-2). This does not include the carotenoids, which are not known to be toxic, even when ingested in large amounts. Excessive consumption of carotenoid does, however, lead to a yellow/orange discoloration of adipose tissue that may be visible through the skin. As vitamin A is stored in the liver, signs of toxicity are apparent only after vitamin A levels exceed its storage capacity. Hypervitaminosis A may follow a single large dose or, more usually, prolonged excessive intake. The source is usually dietary supplementation; however, excessive consumption of liver may also be toxic, and is the usual cause of toxicity in cats. In animals, the le-

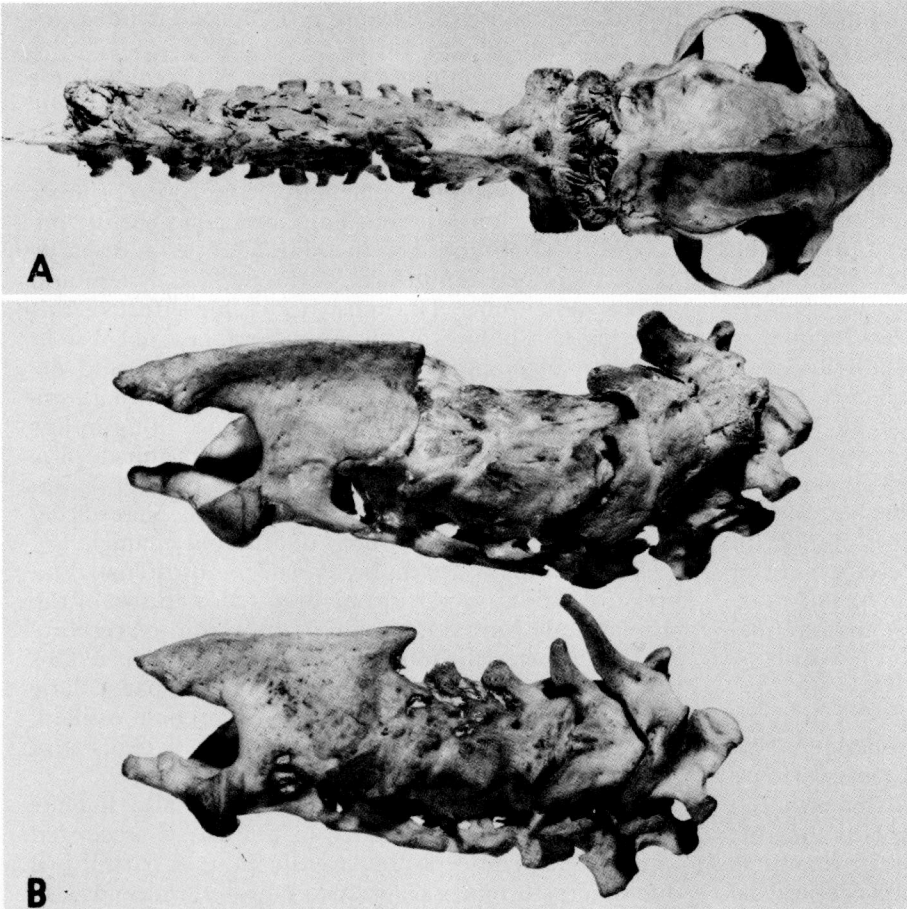

FIG. 16-2 Hypervitaminosis A, feline. **A.** Dorsal aspect of vertebral column and cranium in a natural case of the disease. Exostoses have resulted in fusion of vertebrae and fusion of the atlas to the occipital bone. **B.** Fusion of vertebrae in an experimentally induced case. (Courtesy of Dr. A. A. Seawright.)

sions, which focus on skeletal changes, take weeks to develop following either acute or chronic toxicity. In humans, an acute syndrome characterized by headache, vomiting, papilledema, and mental lethargy may follow a single large dose of vitamin A, but a comparable condition has not been described in animals.

The skeletal changes in animals can be divided into two classes: destruction of **cartilaginous growth plates** and **osteoporosis,** which is the outstanding lesion in young pigs, calves, and kittens; and a syndrome described as **deforming cervical spondylosis,** which develops in adult cats. In the former, the growth plates become thin and undergo premature, irregular degeneration. This leaves a plate that is in part continuing to grow and in part closed, which deforms and shortens the bones, leading to dwarfism. Metaphyseal flaring occurs; the tibial tuberosities, greater trochanters of the femur, and humoral tuberosities become elongated. There may also be rotation of the epiphyses. Decreased bone formation is also evident in the cranial bones, which may become thin; their sutures may prematurely close, resulting in increased cranial pressure. Exostoses may develop, but are not the hallmark of this form of hypervitaminosis A.

In adult cats, deforming cervical spondylosis is characterized by multiple exostoses that principally develop on the cervical and thoracic vertebrae, forelimbs, and ribs. Histologically, the exostoses are initially composed of irregular masses of cartilage, as well as new subperiosteal bone that, over time, matures to compact bone. The growths ultimately lead to ankylosis, and may also impinge nerves. Retarded growth and loss of teeth, along with gingivitis and osteoporosis of the jaw bones, is another feature of hypervitaminosis A in cats.

In contrast to hypovitaminosis A, excess vitamin A may lead to a drop in cerebrospinal fluid pressure, which is believed to result from a decreased formation of cerebrospinal fluid. Toxic levels of vitamin A administered by parenteral routes also induce calcification of arteries, heart, and kidney, comparable to the changes seen in hypervitaminosis D. Toxicity and lesions of hypervitaminosis D can be ameliorated, in part, by the administration of relatively large amounts of vitamin A.

In humans, severe and often fatal liver disease may follow vitamin A overdosage. This is characterized by perisinusoidal fibrosis and portal hypertension. Excessive vitamin A is also **teratogenic,** leading to such abnormalities as cleft palate, micro- or anopia, defective bone development, heart defects, pulmonary hypoplasia, and hydrocephalus.

References

Bendich A, Olson JA. Biological actions of carotenoids. FASEB J 1989;3:1927–1932.
Blomhoff R, Green MH, Berg T, et al. Transport and storage of vitamin A. Science 1990;250:399–404.

Butera ST, Krakowka S. Assessment of lymphocyte function during vitamin A deficiency. Am J Vet Res 1986;47:850–855.

Calhoun MC, Rousseau JE Jr, Hall JJ. Cisternal cerebrospinal fluid pressure during development of chronic bovine hypervitaminosis. Am J Dairy Sci 1965;48:729–732.

Cho DY, Frey RA, Guffy MM, et al. Hypervitaminosis A in the dog. Am J Vet Res 1975;36:1597–1603.

Clark I, Smith MR. Effects of hypervitaminosis A and D on skeletal metabolism. J Biol Chem 1964;239:1266–1271.

Clark L, Seawright AA. Skeletal abnormalities in the hind limbs of young cats as a result of hypervitaminosis A. Nature 1968;217:1174–1176.

Clark L, Seawright AA, Hrdlicka J. Exostoses in hypervitaminotic A cats with optimal calcium-phosphorus intakes. J Small Anim Pract 1970;11:555–561.

Davis TE, Krook L, Warner RG. Bone resorption in hypovitaminosis A. Cornell Vet 1970;60:90–119.

Divers TJ, Blackmon DM, Martin CL, et al. Blindness and convulsions associated with vitamin A deficiency in feedlot steers. J Am Vet Med Assoc 1986;189:1579–1582.

Doige CE, Schoonderwoerd M. Dwarfism in a swineherd: suspected vitamin A toxicosis. J Am Vet Med Assoc 1988;193:691–693.

Dreizen S, Levy BM, Bernick S. Studies on biology of periodontium of marmosets. II. Histopathologic manifestations of spontaneous and induced vitamin-A deficiency in oral structures of adult marmosets. J Dent Res 1973;52:803–809.

Dutt B. Effect of vitamin A deficiency on the testes of rams. Br Vet J 1959;115:236–238.

Dutt B, Vasudevan B. Clinical syndromes and histopathological changes in vitamin "A" deficiency in cow calves. Indian Vet J 1962;39:584–587.

Eaton HD. Chronic bovine hypo- and hypervitaminosis A and cerebrospinal fluid pressure. Am J Clin Nutr 1969;22:1070–1080.

Frier HI, et al. Rates of formation and absorption of cerebrospinal fluid in mild chronic bovine hypervitaminosis. J Dairy Sci 1970;53:1051–1057.

Frier HI, et al. Formation and absorption of cerebrospinal fluid in adult goats with hypo- and hypervitaminosis A. Am J Vet Res 1974;35:45–55.

Gallina AM, et al. Bone growth in the hypovitaminotic A calf. J Nutr 1970;100:129–142.

Gallina AM, et al. Bone lesions in mild chronic bovine hypervitaminosis A. Arch Exp Veterinaermed 1970;24:1091–1100.

Goodman DS. Vitamin A metabolism. Fed Proc 1980;39:2716–2722.

Goodman DS. Vitamin A and retinoids in health and disease. N Engl J Med 1984;310:1023–1031.

Gorgacz EJ, et al. Morphologic alterations associated with decreased spinal fluid pressure in chronic bovine hypervitaminosis A. Am J Vet Res 1985;36:171–180.

Grey RM, et al. Pathology of skull, radius and rib in hypervitaminosis A in young calves. Pathol Vet 1965;2:446–467.

Hayes KC, Nielsen SW, Eaton HD. Pathogenesis of the optic nerve lesion in vitamin A-deficient calves. Arch Ophthalmol 1968;80:777–787.

Ihrke PJ, Goldschmidt MH. Vitamin A-responsive dermatosis in the dog. J Am Vet Med Assoc 1983;182:687–690.

Lammer EJ, et al. Retinoic acid embryopathy. N Engl J Med 1985;313:837–841.

Lucke VM, et al. Deforming cervical spondylosis in the cat associated with hypervitaminosis A. Vet Rec 1968;82:141–142.

Marchok AC, Cone MV, Nettesheim P. Induction of squamous metaplasia (vitamin A deficiency) and hypersecretory activity in organ cultures. Lab Invest 1965;33:451–460.

Mills JHL, et al. Experimental pathology of dairy calves ingesting one-third the daily requirement of carotene. Acta Vet Scand 1967;8:324–346.

Nielsen SW, et al. Parotid duct metaplasia in marginal bovine vitamin A deficiency. Am J Vet Res 1966;27:223–233.

Noell WK, Delmelle MC, Albrecht R. Vitamin A deficiency effect on retina: dependence on light. Science 1971;172:72–75.

Olson JA, Bridges CDB, Packer L, et al. The function of vitamin A. Fed Proc 1983;42:2740–2746.

O'Toole BA, et al. Vitamin A deficiency and reproduction in rhesus monkeys. J Nutr 1974;104:1513–1524.

Palludan B. The teratogenic effect of vitamin A deficiency in pigs. Acta Vet Scand 1961;2:32–59.

Schmidt H. Vitamin A deficiencies in ruminants. Am J Vet Res 1941;2:373–389.

Seawright AA, English PB. Cervical spondylosis: cats. J Pathol Bacteriol 1964;88:503–509.

Seawright AA, Hrdlicka J. Pathogenetic factors in tooth loss in young cats on a high daily oral intake of vitamin A. Aust Vet J 1974;50:133–141.

Seawright AA, Hrdlicka J. Severe retardation of growth with retention and displacement of incisors in young cats fed a diet of raw sheep liver high in vitamin A. Aust Vet J 1974;50:306–315.

Seawright AA, English PB, Gartner RJW. Hypervitaminosis A and hyperostosis of the cat. Nature 1965;206:1171–1172.

Seawright AA, English PB, Gartner RJW. Hypervitaminosis A and deforming cervical spondylosis of the cat. J Comp Pathol 1967;77:29–39.

Sorsby A, Reading HW, Bunyan J. Effect of vitamin A deficiency on the retina of the experimental rabbit. Nature 1966;210:1011–1015.

Spratling FR, et al. Experimental hypovitaminosis-A in calves. Clinical and gross post-mortem findings. Vet Rec 1965;77:1532–1542.

Werler MM, Lammer EJ, Rosenberg L, et al. Maternal vitamin A supplementation in relation to selected birth defects. Teratology 1990;42:497–503.

Willett WC, MacMahon B. Diet and cancer: an overview (Parts I and II). N Engl J Med 1984;310:633–638, 697–703.

Wolke RE, Nielsen SW, Rousseau JE Jr. Bone lesions of hypervitaminosis A in the pig. Am J Vet Res 1968;29:1009–1024.

Wolke RE, et al. Qualitative and quantitative osteoblastic activity in chronic porcine hypervitaminosis. Am J Pathol 1969;97:677–686.

Vitamin D

The active metabolite of vitamin D functions as a hormone, differently from most vitamins. Also in contrast to other vitamins, with adequate exposure to sunlight their is no dietary requirement. Dietary sources of vitamin D can, however, fully meet all requirements. Vitamin D is formed from steroid precursors, or provitamins, of which two have been found in nature: ergosterol (provitamin D2), which is found in plants; and 7–dehydrocholesterol (provitamin D3), which is found in animal tissues. To be effective, the provitamins, either in the skin or in food, must be exposed to the radiant action of ultraviolet light; this is ordinarily sunlight, which converts ergosterol to vitamin D2 ergocalciferol, and 7–dehydrocholesterol to vitamin D3 cholecalciferol. It has been shown in light-skinned humans that relatively brief periods of exposure to sunlight are adequate to produce sufficient vitamin D3 to prevent deficiency. In fact, prolonged exposure to sunlight causes isomerization of vitamin D3 cholecalciferol to inactive lumisterol and tachysterol. With the exception of New World nonhuman primates and some birds that require vitamin D3, it appears that, for most animals, either source of vitamin D is effective in preventing deficiency. This does not, however, indicate that they are equally active. For many species, vitamin D3 is more active. This is of importance to the induction of hypervitaminosis D (described below). An exception to this distinction in source for vitamin D2 and D3 is the presence of vitamin D3 metabolites in certain plants. These include *Solanum malacoxylon, S. glaucophyllum, Cestrum diurnum,* and *Trisetum flavescens;* these contain several metabolites of vitamin D3, including its most active form (1,25(OH)2–vitamin D) which, when consumed, can lead to hypervitaminosis D.

After it is ingested or formed in the skin, vitamin D is transported to the liver by means of an a-globulin; there, it is converted to 25–hydroxycholecalciferol (25–OH-D3 or calcidiol), which is the major form of vitamin D in circulation. This in turn is further hydroxylated in the kidney to 1,25–dihydroxycholecalciferol [1,25–(OH)2D3 or calcitriol], the most active form of vitamin D. The formation of calcitriol in the kidney is controlled by several factors. In a classic hormone feedback loop, production of calcitriol decreases as its plasma level increases; and, conversely, its production increases as plasma levels of calcitriol decrease. Parathyroid hormone directly stimulates formation of calcitriol. Hypocalcemia stimulates this formation via increased secretion of parathyroid hormone; hypophosphatemia, however, acts directly to stimulate the formation. Conversely, hypercalcemia and hyperphosphatemia depress the formation of calcitriol. Both calcitonin and prolactin stimulate its formation. When production of calcitriol is depressed, 25–OH-D is converted to other metabolites that include 24,25–(OH)2D and 25,26–(OH)2D. These are functionally much less active than calcitriol. It is not known whether they—or several other metabolites of vitamin D that have been identified—serve another purpose.

FUNCTIONS

The primary function of vitamin D is to maintain serum calcium at optimal levels. This is achieved through several mechanisms that increase: (1) intestinal absorption of calcium (and phosphorus); (2) parathyroid-dependent renal tubular resorption of calcium (and phosphorus); and (3) parathyroid hormone-dependent mobilization of calcium from bone. Vitamin D is also required for mineralizing osteoid to bone. At the cellular level, vitamin D first binds to specific cellular receptors, to ultimately enter the nucleus; there, it binds to nuclear chromatin, and stimulates transcription of mRNAs; this allows synthesis of specific proteins responsible for these effects. At the level of bone, the mobilization of calcium is believed to be accomplished through stimulation of osteoclastic resorption of bone. Although vitamin D is required for this resorption, in vitamin D deficiency one may actually find a significant increase in bone resorption. This may seem paradoxic, along with the fact that vitamin D is also necessary for mineralizing osteoid and epiphyseal cartilage. Thus, deficiency increases resorption of bone and causes a failure to mineralize the growing epiphyseal cartilage and its unrestricted growth. The deposition of new osteoid also fails to mineralize and is resistant to resorption. Whether vitamin D is required for the deposition of new osteoid is not clear. In some examples of deficiency, marked osteoblastic activity occurs, with excessive production of osteoid; in other cases, little new osteoid formation results. These varying pictures and paradoxes probably reflect several variables, including: the relative severity of vitamin D deficiency; the amount of calcium in the diet; the possible activities of other

metabolites, such as 24,25–(OH)2D; and age. As stated, comparable to other hormones, the active form of vitamin D binds to specific receptors on the target organs. In addition to osteoblasts and intestinal and renal epithelial cells, receptors have been identified on many other cell types, including cells in brain, pancreas, mammary gland, smooth muscle, pituitary, and other tissues. This suggests that Vitamin D may have functions beyond calcium homeostasis.

DEFICIENCY

Deficiency of vitamin D may result from any combination of: (1) lack of exposure to sunlight; (2) inadequate dietary intake; (3) gastrointestinal diseases that impair absorption of fats; or (4) interference with synthesis of its active form, which can occur in chronic renal disease. Two conditions occur in humans, termed vitamin D-dependent rickets, types I and II. In type I, there occurs a genetic lack of the enzyme necessary to convert 25–OH-D to 1,25–(OH)2D; in type II, a defect is manifest in the cellular receptors for vitamin D. The outcome of vitamin D deficiency is rickets in growing animals, and osteomalacia in adults. Although vitamin D deficiency is the classic cause of rickets and osteomalacia, it is important to recognize that deficiency in dietary calcium and phosphorus can also lead to these disorders. Rickets (Fig. 16-3) is characterized by failure of the cartilage in growth plates to undergo provisional calcification and disintegration. This leads to marked and irregular extension of the growth plate into the diaphysis. Osteoid is deposited over the viable cartilage and may accumulate to a marked degree. This osteoid, and newly formed osteoid deposited elsewhere, fails to mineralize. Osteomalacia is characterized by failure to mineralize osteoid, resulting in an increased thickness of osteoid seams; this accumlation can lead to an overall increased thickness of the bone. Chapter 19 further discusses these diseases.

HYPERVITAMINOSIS D

Hypervitaminosis D is ordinarily the result of overzealous or accidental dietary supplementation. Vitamin D3 is generally more toxic than vitamin D2. The deleterious effects are due to hypercalcemia (Figs. 16-4, 16-5), resulting from increased intestinal absorption, increased mobilization from the skeleton, and decreased urinary excretion of calcium. The principal tissue change is metastatic calcification, predominantly as phosphate salts. Tissues most frequently affected are: the intima and media of arteries (where the lesions resemble Mönckeberg arteriosclerosis); endocardium; myocardium; gastric mucosa; lung; and kidney. Damage to the kidney may lead to renal failure. In the skeleton, two changes are seen. Osteoclastic activity is stimulated, leading to rarefication. The second change, which is pathognomonic of vitamin D toxicity, is osteoblastic production of a fibrillary, highly basophilic matrix that irregularly coats the surface of trabeculae, the endosteum, and the periosteal cortex. This material may extend into the fibrous periosteum itself; it may also be

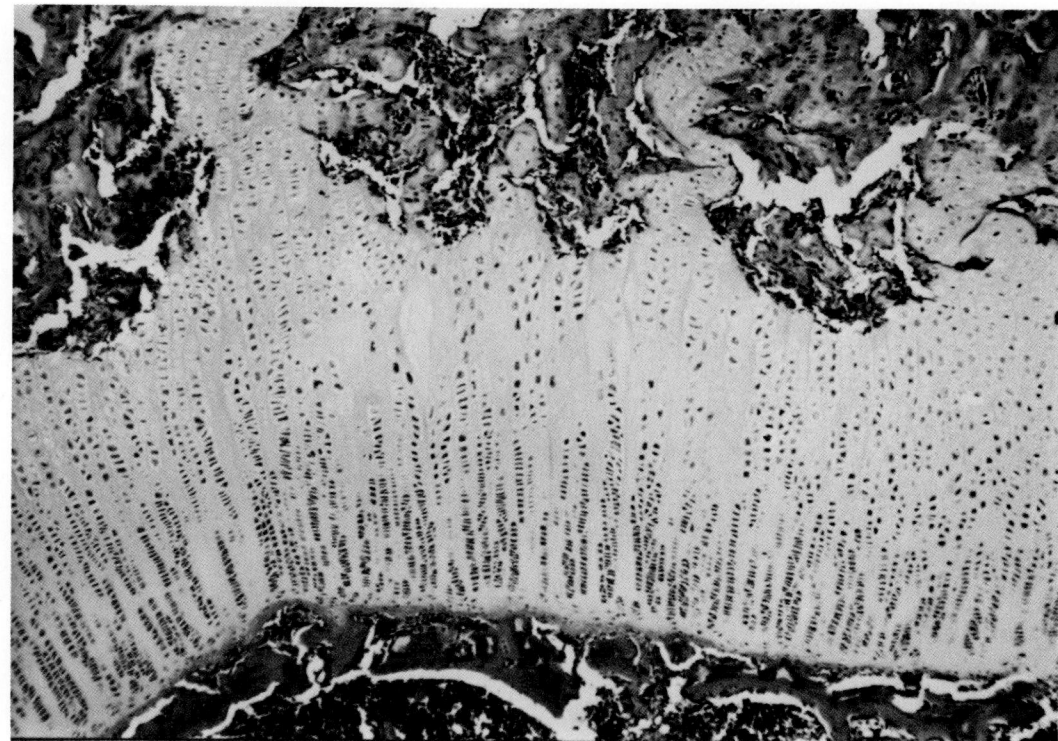

FIG. 16-3 Rickets. The cartilaginous growth plate is disorganized and extends irregularly into the metaphysis. The cartilage does not mineralize or die. No defect occurs in osteoid formation.

seen in the Haversian canals and canalicules. Periodic increased doses of vitamin D results in bones characterized by alternating layers of this basophilic matrix and normal bone.

References

Boyce RW, Weisbrode SE. Effect of dietary calcium on the response of bone to 1,25(OH)2D3. Lab Invest 1983;48:683–689.

Briggs MH, Briggs M. Vitamin D hormones: Part I. Med J Aust 1974;1:838–843.

Bronner F. Symposium: Vitamin D and membrane structure and function. Fed Proc 1982;41:60–87.

Burgisser H, Jacquier C, Leuenberber M. Hypervitaminosis D in pigs. Schweiz Arch Tierheilkd 1964;106:714–718.

Capen CC, Young DM. Fine structural alterations in thyroid parafollicular cells of cows in response to experimental hypercalcemia induced by vitamin D. Am J Pathol 1969;57:365–382.

Capen CC, Cole CR, Hibbs JW. The pathology of hyperviraminosis D in cattle. Pathol Vet 1966;3:350–378.

Clegg FG, Hollands JG. Cervical scoliosis and kidney lesions in sheep following dosage with vitamin D. Vet Rec 1946;98:144–146.

DeLuca HF. The kidney as an endocrine organ for the production of 1,25–dihydroxyvitamin D3, a calcium-mobilizing hormone. N Engl J Med 1973;289:359–365.

DeLuca HF. The kidney as an endocrine organ involved in the function of vitamin D. Am J Med 1975;58:39–47.

Fraser DR, Kodicek E. Unique biosynthesis by kidney of a biologically active vitamin D metabolite. Nature 1970;228:764–766.

Gill BS, Singh M, Chopra AK. Enzootic calcinosis in sheep: clinical signs and pathology. Am J Vet Res 1976;37:545–552.

Harrington DD. Acute vitamin D2 (ergocalciferol) toxicosis in horses: case report and experimental studies. J Am Vet Med Assoc 1982;180:867–873.

Harrington DD, Page EH. Acute vitamin D3 toxicosis in horses: case reports and experimental studies of the comparative toxicity of vitamins D2 and D3. J Am Vet Med Assoc 1983;182:1358–1369.

Haussler MR, McCain TA. Basic and clinical concepts related to vitamin D metabolism and action (Parts I and II). N Engl J Med 1977;297:974–983, 1041–1050.

Holick MF, et al. Synthesis of (6–3H)-1a-hydroxyvitamin D3 and its metabolism in vivo to (3H)-1a,25–dihydroxyvitamin D3. Science 1975;190:576–578.

Hunt RD, Garcia FG, Hegsted DM. Hypervitaminosis D in New World monkeys. Am J Clin Nutr 1969;22:358–366.

Lam HY-P, Schnoes HK, DeLuca HF. 1a-Hydroxyvitamin D2: a potent synthetic analog of vitamin D2. Science 1974;186:1038–1040.

Lee SW, Russell J, Avioli LV.: 25–Hydroxycholecalciferol to 1,25–dihydroxycholecalciferol: conversion impaired by systemic metabolic acidosis. Science 1977;195:994–996.

Long GG.: Acute toxicosis in swine associated with excessive dietary intake of vitamin D. J Am Vet Med Assoc 1984;184:164–170.

Minghetti PP, Norman AW. 1,25(OH)2–Vitamin D3 receptors: gene regulation and genetic circuitry. FASEB J 1988;2:3043–4053.

Norman AW. Evidence for a new kidney-produced hormone, 1,25–dihydroxy-cholecalciferol, the proposed biologically active form of vitamin D. Am J Clin Nutr 1971;24:1346–1351.

Norman AW, Mitra MN, Okamura WH, et al. Vitamin D: 3–deoxy-1a-hydroxyvitamin D3, biologically active analog of 1a,25–dihydroxyvitamin D3. Science 1975;188:1013–1015.

Penn GB. Calciphylactic syndrome in pigs. Vet Rec 1970;86:718–721.

Reichel H, Koeffler HP, Norman AW. The role of the vitamin D endocrine system in health and disease. N Engl J Med 1989;320:980–991.

Roe DA. Symposium: Nutritional implications of photochemical reactions. Fed Proc 1987;46:1875–1905.

Schnoes HK, DeLuca HF. Recent progress in vitamin D metabolism and the chemistry of vitamin D metabolites. Fed Proc 1980;39:2723–2729.

Wasserman RH. Calcium absorption and calcium-binding protein synthesis: Solanum malacoxylon reverses strontium inhibition. Science 1974;183:1092–1094.

Wong GL, Luben RA, Cohn DV. 1,25–dihydroxycholecalciferol and parathormone: effects on isolated osteoclast-like and osteoblast-like cells. Science 1977;197:663–665.

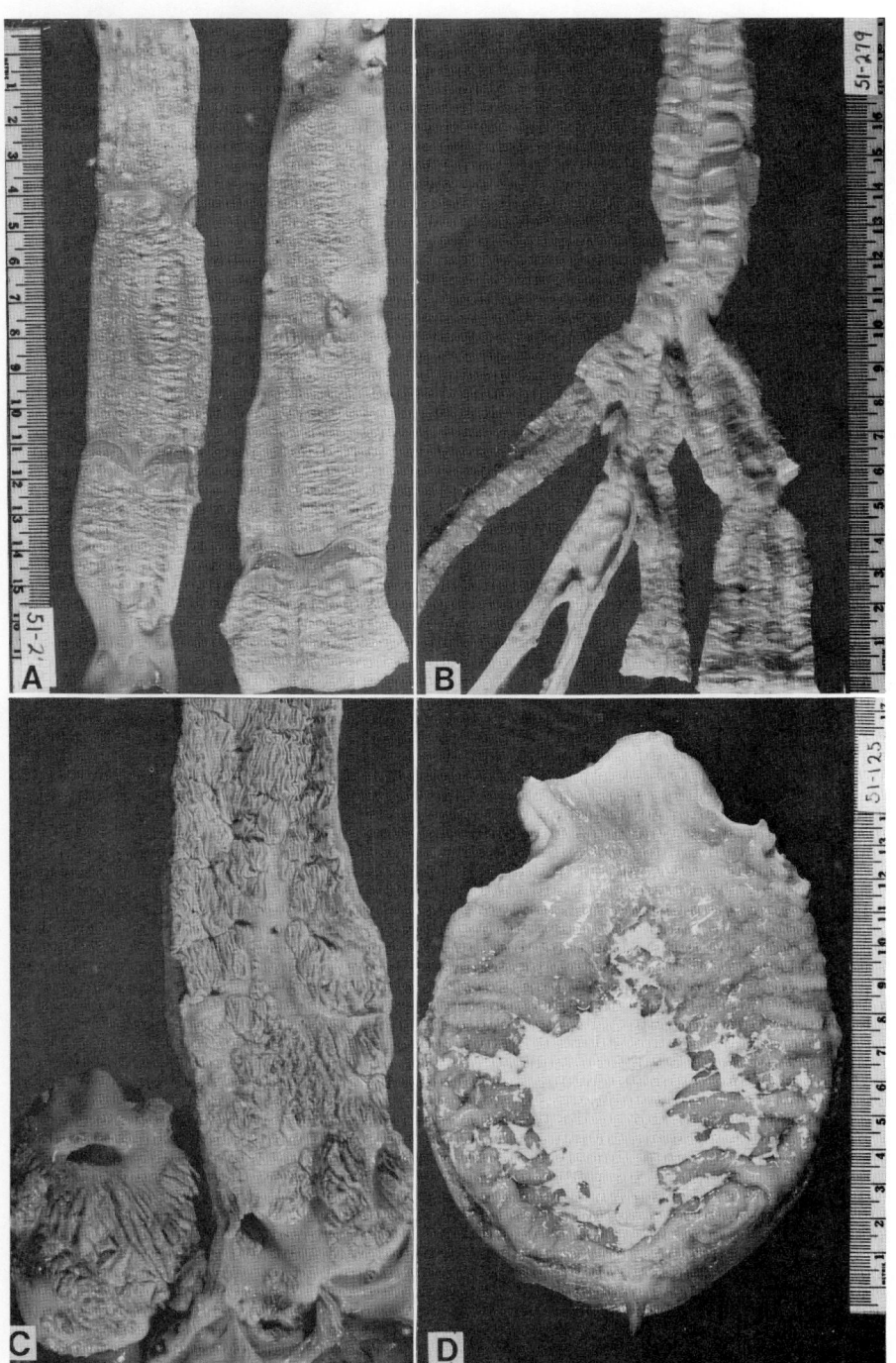

FIG. 16-4 Hypervitaminosis D. Lesions in a pregnant Jersey cow, (six years old), that was given 30 million IU of vitamin D (viosterol) for 20 days preceding parturition, and killed one day later. **A.** Jugular vein with transverse corrugations in roughened intima. **B.** Terminal aorta and its branches, with mineralization of media, resulting in loss of contractility and elasticity and irregular plaques (visible from the intimal surface). **C.** Aortic valves and aortic arch. Raised, rugose plaques of calcareous material are conspicuous from the intimal surface. **D.** Urinary bladder, containing white granular material. (Courtesy of Dr. C. R. Cole, Ohio State University.)

Vitamin E

Vitamin E is the term used to encompass the fat soluble tocopherols and tocotrienols. Four tocopherols have been identified: α-, β-, δ-, and lambda-tocopherol. α-Tocopherol is the most active biologically, and is found within chloroplasts of plants. In animal tissues vitamin E is located in cell membranes and within adipose tissue.

Vitamin E is an antioxidant that serves as a scavenger of free radicals. Without a mechanism to prevent their generation and capture, these radicals lead to chain reac-

tions, with further generation of highly reactive oxidizing radicals and the peroxidation of lipids. The polyunsaturated fatty acids of cell membranes are particularly susceptible to such reactions which, without the protective effects of vitamin E, would be completely oxidized to hydroperoxides. The bulk of vitamin E resides within cell membranes. In addition to vitamin E, other antioxidant mechanisms exist to reduce highly reactive oxygen radicals to water. These include the metalloenzymes, superoxide dismutases (which contain copper, zinc and manganese), catalase, and glutathione peroxidase. Selenium is

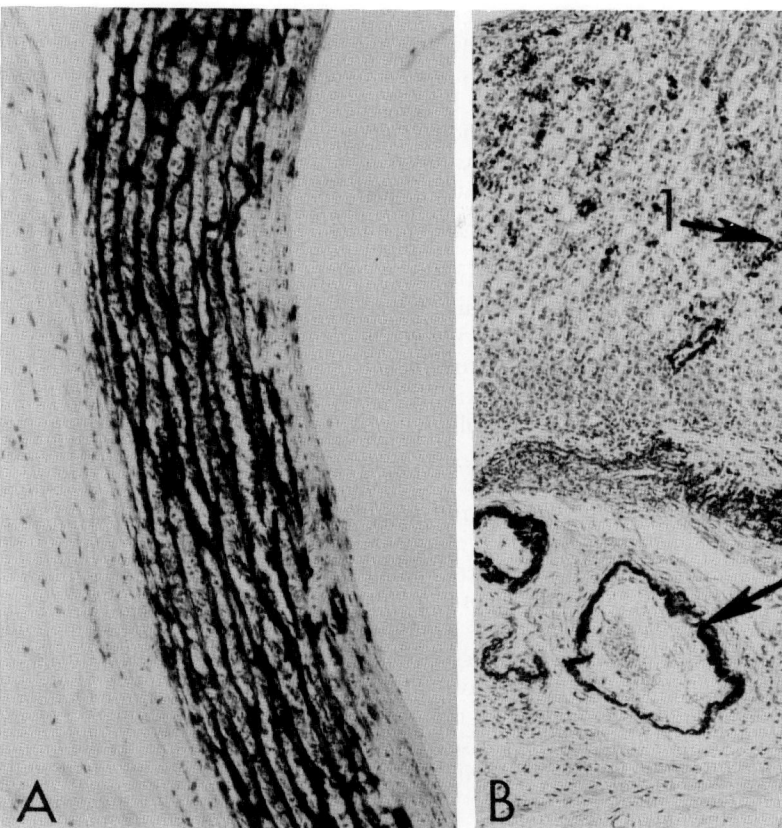

FIG. 16-5 Hypervitaminosis D, cebus monkey. **A.** Metastatic calcification of the aorta. **B.** Metastatic calcification of the gastric mucosa. (1) Muscularis mucosa; (2) Arteries; (3) In the muscularis. (Courtesy of New England Regional Primate Research Center, Harvard Medical School.)

an essential constituent of glutathione peroxidase. Diets high in selenium reduce the requirement of vitamin E, and diets low in selenium increase vitamin E requirement. Certain sulfur-containing amino acids also influence the vitamin E requirement. Cysteine—which can be synthesized from methionine—is essential for the synthesis of glutathione and, therefore, glutathione peroxidase. Measurement of glutathione peroxidase in red blood cells or other tissues is useful as an index of selenium status. The availability of selenium has been shown to be influenced by the amounts of other trace minerals in the diet, such as silver, copper, zinc, and cadmium. Diets high in polyunsaturated fatty acids increase the requirements for all of these antioxidants.

DEFICIENCY

Deficiency of vitamin E is so closely linked with deficiency of selenium that it is appropriate to refer to clinical deficiency as vitamin E-selenium deficiency. A range of syndromes has been associated with deficiency; however, what accounts for the varying expressions of deficiency is not clear. In swine, the use of iron complexes to treat iron deficiency anemia may augment the various maladies associated with vitamin E-selenium deficiency. Based upon experimentally induced deficiency and clinical observations, those conditions that have been described are listed in Table 16-1.

Myopathy Nutritional myopathy occurs in many species, but is most frequently encountered in cattle, sheep, pigs, and horses. It can result from deficiency of

vitamin E, selenium, or both. It is primarily a disease of young animals, often occurring in the first few days of life and even in utero; however, it may occur at any age. The disease, which has been known as white muscle disease, stiff-lamb disease and, in swine, Herztod, affects

---

TABLE 16-1 **Vitamin E-selenium deficiency: conditions and species affected**

Skeletal cardiac muscle necrosis (nutritional myopathy; white muscle disease): Most animal species, including cattle, sheep, goats, horses, pigs, dogs, mink, rats, mice rabbits, guinea pigs, nonhuman primates, and humans (Keshan disease in China)
Mulberry heart disease: pigs
Hepatic necrosis (hepatosis dietetica): pigs, rats, mice
Steatitis (yellow fat disease): cats, horses, swine rabbits
Intestinal lipofuscinosis: dogs
Encephalomalacia, neuronal necrosis, and axonal degeneration: chickens, dogs, rats, monkeys, humans
Testicular degeneration and aspermatogenesis: rats, guinea pigs
Fetal resorption: rats
Hemolytic or destructive anemia: swine, cattle, nonhuman primates, humans
Pigmentary retinal degeneration: dogs, nonhuman primates, humans
Cataracts: rabbits
Exudative diathesis: poultry, swine

both the myocardium and skeletal muscle. Although any skeletal muscle may be affected, it is the larger limb muscles that are most often involved. Lesions also are frequent in the neck muscles, and may be found in the tongue, and even the esophagus. Signs include irregular gait, stiffness, and weakness; paralysis may occur. When the myocardium and intercostal muscles are affected, dyspnea is a prominent sign. Grossly, the affected muscles are pale (white), opaque and may be gritty due to extensive calcification. When the heart is severely affected, gross lesions of heart failure, pulmonary edema, and hydrothorax may be evident. Microscopically, (Figs. 16-6, 16-7) myofibers undergo fragmentation, hyalinization, and calcification. Marked influx of macrophages, satellite cell proliferation, attempted myoregeneration, and repair by fibrovascular connective tissue occurs, which can give the lesion a cellular appearance. Usually, the microscopic feature is an admixture of continued necrosis and repair.

Mulberry heart disease Mulberry heart disease (dietetic microangiopathy) is a complex disorder of young swine that is one of several manifestations of vitamin E-selenium deficiency in this species. The circumstances that lead to the varying major manifestations of vitamin E-selenium deficiency in young swine are not clear, but obviously complicated. Mulberry heart disease is not a characteristic finding in experimental vitamin E-sele-

nium deficiency in swine, although myocardial and skeletal muscle necrosis is. Vitamin E-selenium supplementation neither prevents its occurrence, nor increases the levels of vitamin E in tissue, which are decreased in mulberry heart disease. Dietary increase in polyunsaturated fatty acids, however, does increase the incidence of the disease. It is suggested that the condition results from either a metabolic disorder in vitamin E metabolism, or from an increased requirement. Mulberry heart disease is characterized by extensive edema, myocardial hemorrhage, myocardial degeneration, cerebral leukoencephalomalacia, and arteriolar necrosis. The disease occurs abruptly in previously healthy swine. Signs may be few or absent. Subcutaneous edema occurs, along with hydropericardium, hydrothorax, and ascites. The fluid is rich in fibrin, which may be evident as fibrin tags or clotting of the fluid at necropsy. Myocardial hemorrhage affecting the epicardium, endocardium, and myocardium may be extensive, and provides the basis for the term mulberry heart disease. Microscopic evidence of myodegeneration in the heart is present in animals that survive for 12 hours or more. Cerebral lesions also are only found in animals that have not died acutely. These are characterized by edema and necrosis of white matter, especially of the cerebral cortex, but may also involve deeper structures and the cerebellum. The arteriolar lesions are generalized to include brain, and are characterized by medial necrosis—described as fibrinoid necrosis—and hyalin thrombi. Arteriolar lesions are not a feature of vitamin E-selenium deficiency in other domestic species, nor is leukoencephalomalacia, except in chickens.

Hepatic necrosis Hepatic necrosis (hepatosis dietetica) is a vitamin E-selenium deficiency disorder of rapidly growing young swine which, like mulberry heart disease, has an acute onset. It is characterized by extensive hepatic necrosis and hemorrhage. It may be seen in association with skeletal and cardiac necrosis, arteriolar lesions, or yellow fat disease. Hepatic necrosis is not a feature of vitamin E-selenium deficiency in other species, but has been experimentally produced in rats and mice.

Steatitis Steatitis, or yellow fat disease (Fig. 16-8), is yet another manifestation of vitamin E deficiency that can develop in most species of animals, but apparently not in ruminants. It is most common in cats, mink, and swine. In each of these species it is associated with a diet of fish meal, fish offal, or other products of like origin that are increased in unsaturated fatty acids and decreased in vitamin E. Affected animals may have a fishy odor to their carcass. In swine, it is usually discovered as an incidental finding without clinical signs. Cats with yellow fat disease, however, develop a fever and a general malaise. Severe pain results when the cutaneous region is disturbed, either by manipulation or by the patient's own movements. Palpation reveals an abnormal denseness and lumpiness of the subcutaneous fat. Pronounced neutrophilia is manifest, as well as a shift to the left, and often eosinophilia. Without treatment the disease may terminate fatally. The yellow color, giving the disease its name, is due to the accumulation of a yellow to brown pigment

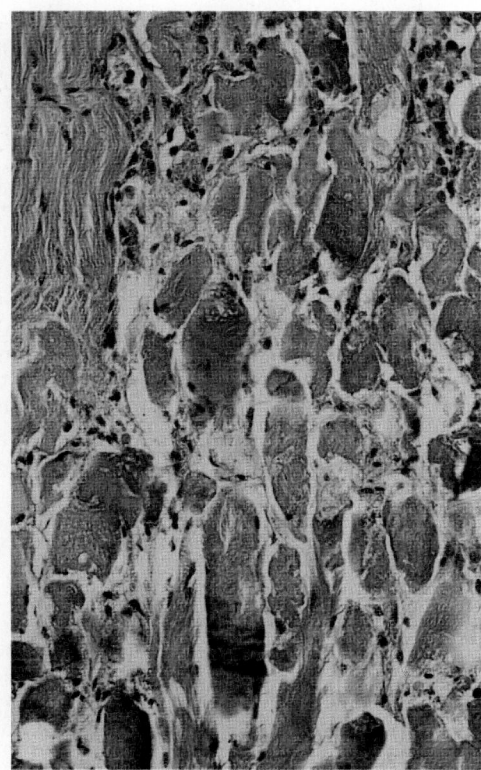

FIG. 16-6 Nutritional myopathy, white-muscle disease, skeletal muscle of a cow (×195). Fragmentation of muscle fibers with swelling and early calcification. (Courtesy of Armed Forces Institute of Pathology; contributor: Dr. J. F. Ryff.)

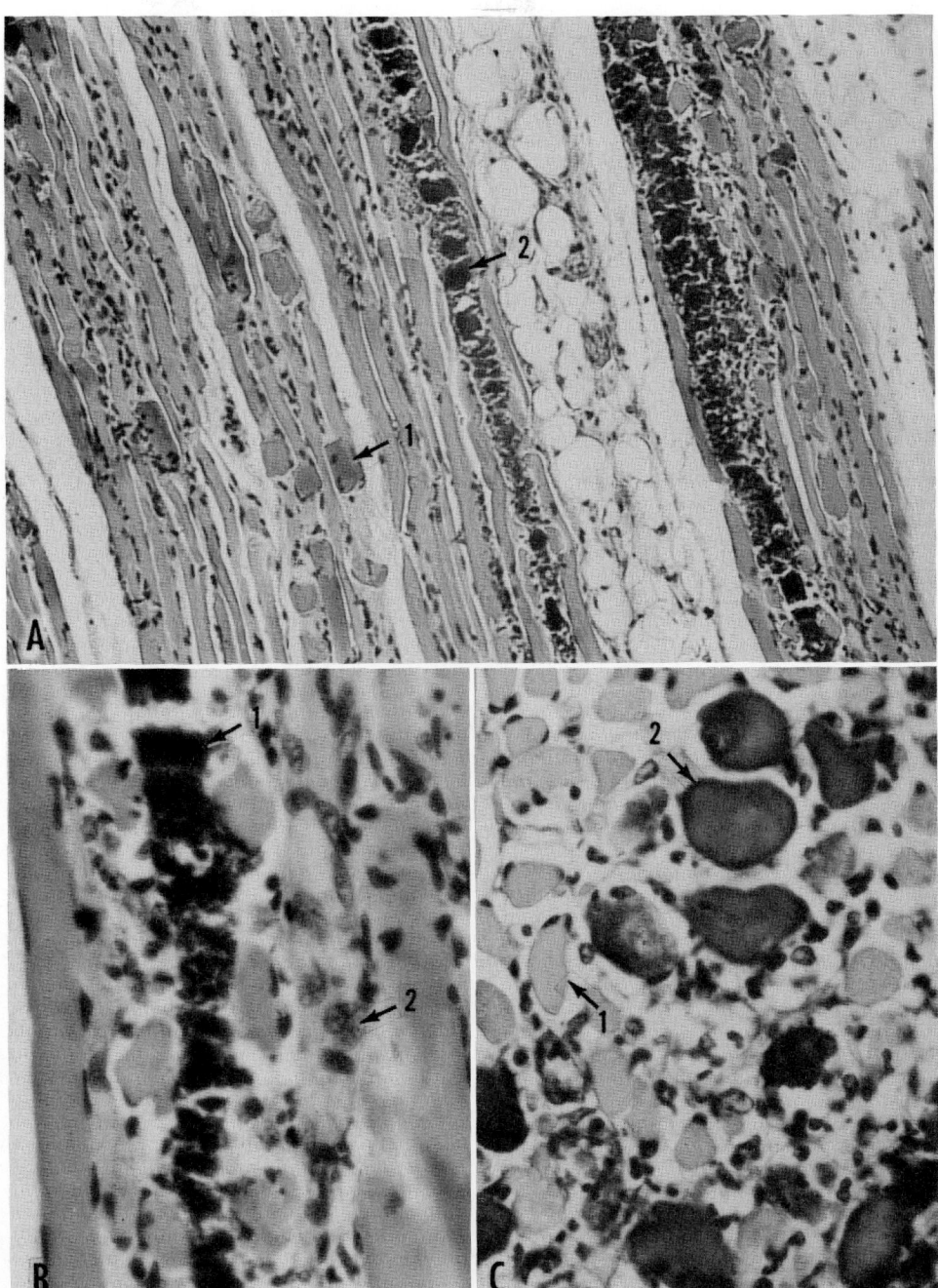

FIG. 16-7 Nutritional myopathy, white-muscle disease, in the tongue of a newborn foal. **A.** (1) Low power to show fragmentation of muscle bundles (×150); and (2) Calcification. **B.** Longitudinal section of muscle bundles (×500). (1) Calcification within muscle bundles; (2) Proliferation of sarcolemmal nuclei. **C.** Cross section of muscle fibers (×500). (1) Note normal muscle bundles; and (2) Calcified muscle bundles. (Courtesy of Armed Forces Institute of Pathology; contributor: Dr. W. O. Reed.)

at the interstices of adipose cells. Because of its waxy nature, it has received the name of ceroid. It is insoluble in fat solvents and is acid-fast. Adipose tissue becomes infiltrated with macrophages, and occasionally multinucleated giant cells, in which ceroid is also found. Pigment-laden macrophages may be found in regional lymph nodes. Yellow fat disease may also occur in foals deficient in vitamin E, in association with myodegeneration. It has been seen also in rabbits. Although yellow fat disease does not occur in dogs, a condition has been described termed

intestinal lipofuscinosis, characterized by a histologically and histochemically identical pigment in smooth muscle cells, particularly of the small intestine and spleen. It may be so extensive that it imparts a grossly visible brown color to the small intestine, and has been called "brown dog gut." The pigment has also been termed "leiomyometoplasts."

Encephalomalacia Encephalomalacia, resulting from vitamin E-selenium deficiency, is seen in swine with mulberry heart disease and in chickens. Axonal degener-

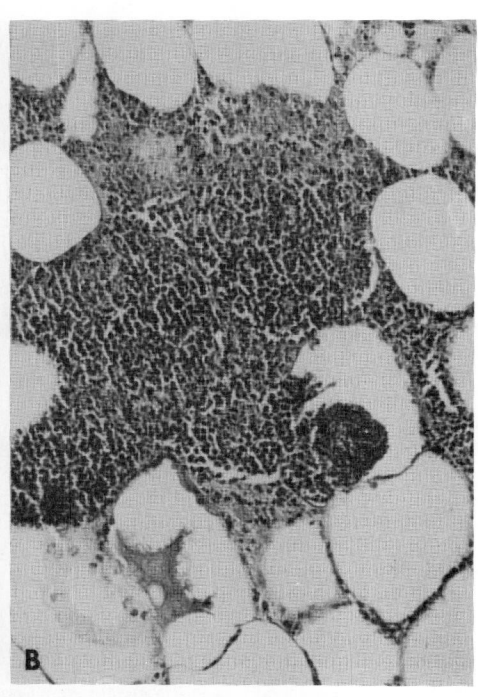

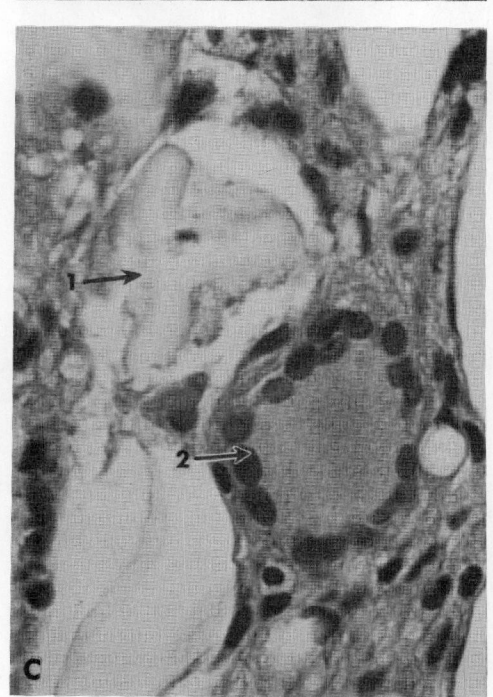

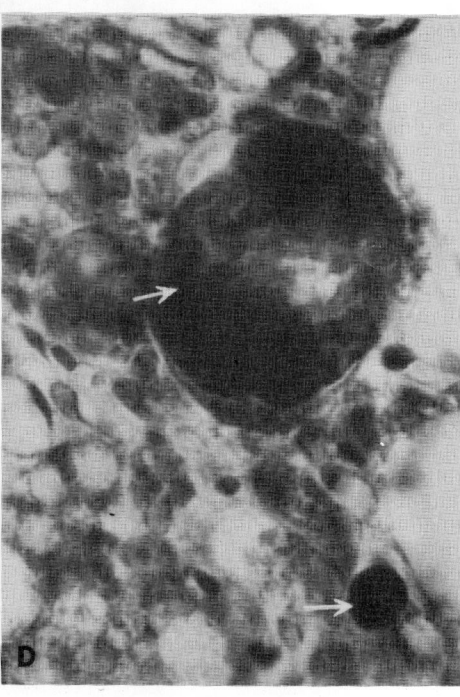

FIG. 16-8 Steatitis in the cat. **A.** Mesenteric fat of a 1 ½-year-old castrated male cat. The dark spots were bright yellow color, the rest of the abundant mesenteric fat was yellowish tan. **B.** Neutrophils in adipose tissue, in young obese cat that exhibited fever and severe neutrophilic leukocytosis (hematoxylin and eosin stain, ×110). **C.** Adipose tissue of a cat in a late stage of the disease. (1) Altered fat; and (2) Langhans' type giant cell (hematoxylin and eosin stain, ×540). **D.** A section of adipose tissue from the same cat as C, with globules of acid-fast ceroid pigment (arrows) (Ziehl-Neelsen acid-fast stain; ×540). (Courtesy of Angell Memorial Hospital and Journal of the American Veterinary Medical Association.)

ation—principally in the brainstem and spinal cord—may follow vitamin E deficiency in dogs, rats, and monkeys, and is also frequently encountered in clinically normal dogs. This suggests that vitamin E deficiency may be more frequent in dogs than usually suspected. The degenerating axons form eosinophilic, spheric bodies up to 150 m in diameter. Myelopathy attributed to vitamin E deficiency has also been described in Mongolian wild horses. Certain forms of axonal degeneration in humans are also attributed to vitamin E deficiency.

Testicular lesions Testicular degeneration and aspermatogenesis occurs in vitamin E-deficient rats. The lesions, which are irreversible, lead to necrosis of spermatogonia and the fusion of spermatogonia with the formation of multinucleated giant cells. Similar lesions have been described in guinea pigs, but they apparently do not occur in mice. In rats, hepatic and muscular necrosis may be seen in conjunction with the testicular lesions.

Reproduction Fetal resorption is a feature of experimental vitamin E deficiency in mice and rats as well as swine. The basis for fetal loss is not clear, but this effect on reproduction is reversible.

Retinal function Pigmentary retinal degeneration has been produced in dogs and monkeys fed vitamin E-deficient diets for prolonged periods, and is reportedly an effect of vitamin E deficiency in humans. The experimentally induced disease in dogs closely resembles naturally occurring pigment epithelial dystrophy (central progressive retinal atrophy). It is characterized by the accumulation of lipofuscin-like pigment in the pigmentary retinal epithelium. The epithelium undergoes hypertrophy and hyperplasia, thickening and forming irregular clumps described as dystrophic. The overlying photoreceptor degenerates, as do the outer nuclear and outer plexiform layers.

TOXICITY

Toxicity from vitamin E has not been recognized as occurring in animals. Extremely high levels can, however, interfere with vitamin A and vitamin K metabolism.

References

Anonymous. Vitamin E deficiency. Lancet 1986;i:423–424.

Ausman LM, Hayes KC. Vitamin E deficiency anemia in Old and New World monkeys. J Clin Nutr 1974;27:1141–1151.

Baustad B, Nafstad I. Haematological response to vitamin E in piglets. Br J Nutr 1972;28:183–190.

Cheville NF. The pathology of vitamin E deficiency in the chick. Pathol Vet 1966;3:208–225.

Danse LHJC, Steenbergen-Botterweg WA. Enzyme histochemical studies of adipose tissue in porcine yellow fat disease. Vet Pathol 1974;11:465–476.

Danse LHJC, Verschuren PM. Fish oil-induced yellow fat disease in rats. I. Histological changes. III. Lipolysis in affected adipose tissue. Vet Pathol 1978;15:114–124, 544–548.

Danse LHJC, Steenbergen-Botterweg WA. Fish oil-induced yellow fat disease in rats. II. Enzyme histochemistry of adipose tissue. Vet Pathol 1978;15:125–132.

Davis CL, Gorham JR. The pathology of experimental and natural cases of "yellow fat" disease in swine. Am J Vet Res 1954;15:55–59.

Dodd C, et al. Muscle degeneration and yellow-fat disease in foals. NZ Vet J 1960;8:45–50.

Droneman J, Wensvoort P. Muscular dystrophy and yellow fat disease in Shetland pony foals. Neth J Vet Sci 1968;1:42–48.

Endicott KM. Similarity of the acid-fast pigment ceroid and oxidized unsaturated fat. Arch Pathol 1944;37:49–53.

Ewan RC, Wastell ME, Bicknell EJ, et al. Performance and deficiency symptoms of young pigs fed diets low in vitamin E and selenium. J Anim Sci 1969;29:912–915.

Ewan RC, Wastell ME. Effect of vitamin E and selenium on blood composition of the young pig. J Anim Sci 1970;31:343–350.

Foreman JH, Potter KA, Bayly WM, et al. Generalized steatitis associated with selenium deficiency and normal vitamin E status in a foal. J Am Vet Med Assoc 1986;189:83–86.

Gershoff SN, Norkin SA. Vitamin E deficiency in cats. J Nutr 1962;77:303–308.

Gorham JR, Boe N, Baker GA. Experimental "yellow-fat" disease in pigs. Cornell Vet 1951;41:332–338.

Hayes KC, Nielsen SW, Rousseau JE Jr. Vitamin E deficiency and fat stress in the dog. J Nutr 1969;99:196–209.

Hayes KC, Rousseau JE Jr, Hegsted DM. Plasma tocopherol concentrations and vitamin E deficiency in dogs. J Am Vet Med Assoc 1970;157:64–71.

Hayes KC. Animal model of human disease: hemolytic anemia of premature infants associated with vitamin E deficiency. Am J Pathol 1974;77:123–126.

Hayes KC. Pathophysiology of vitamin E deficiency in monkeys. Am J Clin Nutr 1974;27:1130–1140.

Hidiroglou M, Jenkins KJ, Lessard JR, et al. Metabolism of vitamin E in sheep. Br J Nutr 1970;24:917–928.

Hoekstra WG. Biochemical function of selenium and its relation to vitamin E. Fed Proc 1975;34:2083–2089.

Langweiler M, Schultz RD, Sheffy BE. Effect of vitamin E deficiency on the proliferative response of canine lymphocytes. Am J Vet Res 1981;42:1681–1685.

Leach RM Jr. Biochemical function of selenium and its inter-relationship with other trace elements and vitamin E. Fed Proc 1975;34:2082.

Liu S-K, Dolensek EP, Adams CR, et al. Myelopathy and vitamin E deficiency in six Mongolian wild horses. J Am Vet Med Assoc 1983;183:1266–1268.

Liu S-k, Dolensek EP, Tappe JP, et al. Cardiomyopathy associated with vitamin E deficiency in seven gelada baboons. J Am Vet Med Assoc 1984;185:1347–1350.

Lohr JE, Mclaren RD. Yellow fat disease (pansteatitis) in wild hares in New Zealand. NZ Vet J 1971;19:266–269.

Maas J, Bulgin MS, Anderson BC, et al. Nutritional myodegeneration associated with vitamin E deficiency and normal selenium status in lambs. J Am Vet Med Assoc 1984;184:201–204.

Michel RL, Whitehair CK, Keahey KK. Dietary hepatic necrosis associated with selenium-vitamin E deficiency in swine. J Am Vet Med Assoc 1969;155:50–59.

Munson TO, et al. Steatitis ("yellow fat") in cats fed canned red tuna. J Am Vet Med Assoc 1958;133:563–568.

Nafstad I. Studies of hematology and bone marrow morphology in vitamin E-deficient pigs. Pathol Vet 1965;2:277–287.

Nafstad I. The vitamin-E deficiency syndrome in pigs. III. Light and electron microscopic studies on myocardial vascular injury. Vet Pathol 1971;8:239–255.

Nafstad I, Nafstad HJ. An electron microscopic study of blood and bone marrow in vitamin E deficient pigs. Pathol Vet 1968;5:520–537.

Nafstad I, Tollersrud S. The vitamin-E deficiency syndrome in pigs. I. Pathological changes. Acta Vet Scand 1970;11:452–480.

Nair PP, Kayden HJ, eds. Vitamin E and its role in cellular metabolism. Ann NY Acad Sci 1972;203:1–247.

Newberne PM, Hare WV. Axon dystrophy in clinically normal dogs. Am J Vet Res 1962;23:403–411.

Platt H, Whitwell KE. Clinical and pathological observations on generalized steatitis in foals. J Comp Pathol 1971;81:499–506.

Raychaudhuri C, Desai ID. Ceroid pigment formation and irreversible sterility in vitamin E deficiency. Science 1971;173:1028–1029.

Rice DA, Kennedy S. Vitamin E, selenium, and polyunsaturated fatty acid concentrations and glutathione peroxidase activity in tissues from pigs with dietetic microangiopathy (mulberry heart disease). Am J Vet Res 1989;50:2101–2104.

Riis RC, Sheffy BE, Loew E, et al. Vitamin E deficiency retinopathy in dogs. Am J Vet Res 1981;42:74–86.

Ringler DH, Abrams GD. Nutritional muscular dystrophy and neonatal mortality in a rabbit breeding colony. J Am Vet MEd Assoc 1970;157:1928–1934.

Ruth GR, Van Vleet JR. Experimentally induced selenium-vitamin E deficiency in growing swine: selective destruction of type I skeletal muscle fibers. Am J Vet Res 1974;35:237–244.

Scott ML. Advances in our understanding of vitamin E. Fed Proc 1980;39:2736–2739.

Sharp BA, Young LG, van Dreumel AA. Dietary induction of mulberry heart disease and hepatosis in pigs. 1. Nutritional aspects. Can J Comp Med 1972;36:371–376.

Stevens JB, Olson WG, Kraemer R, et al. Serum selenium concentrations and glutathione peroxidase activities in cattle grazing forage of various selenium concentrations. Am J Vet Res 1985;46:1556–1560.

Stowe HD, Whitehair CK. Gross and microscopic pathology of tocopherol-deficient mink. J Nutr 1963;81:287–300.

Sweeny PR, Brown RG. Ultrastructural changes in muscular dystrophy. I. Cardiac tissue of piglets deprived of vitamin E and selenium. Am J Pathol 1972;68:479–492.

Trapp AL, Keahey KK, Whitenack DL, et al. Vitamin E-selenium deficiency in swine: differential diagnosis and nature of field problem. J Sm Vet Med Assoc 1970;157:289–300.

Van Vleet JF. Experimentally induced vitamin E-selenium deficiency in the growing dog. J Am Vet Med Assoc 1975;166:769–774.

Van Vleet JF, Ferrans VJ. Comparative pathology of selenium and vitamin E deficiency and excess. Comp Pathol Bull 1985;17:1,4.

Van Vleet JF, Boon GD, Ferrans VJ. Induction of lesions of selenium-vitamin E deficiency in weanling swine fed silver, cobalt, tellurium, zinc, cadmium, and vanadium. Am J Vet Res 1981;42:789–799.

Van Vleet JF, Ferrans VJ, Ruth GR. Ultrastructural alterations in nutritional cardiomyopathy of selenium-vitamin E deficient swine. I. Fiber lesions. II. Vascular lesions. Lab Invest 1977;37:188–200, 201–211.

Van Vleet JF, Meyer KB, Olander HJ. Control of selenium-vitamin E deficiency in growing swine by parenteral administration of selenium-vitamin E preparations to baby pigs or to pregnant sows and their baby pigs. J Am Vet Med Assoc 1973;163:452–456.

Van Vleet JF, Ruth G, Ferrans VJ. Ultrastructural alterations in skeletal muscle of pigs with selenium-vitamin E deficiency. Am J Vet Res 1976;37:911–922.

Wilson TM, et al. Myodegeneration and suspected selenium-vitamin E deficiency in horses. J Am Vet Med Assoc 1976;169:213–216.

Hypovitaminosis K

Adequate dietary vitamin K is present in most animal food sources and it is freely synthesized by intestinal bacteria. The principal forms of Vitamin K are phylloquinones in plants and the menaquinones synthesized by bacteria. Menadione is a common synthetic form, usually used as a menadione sodium bisulfite complex. Deficiency of vitamin K is rare. It can occur in conjunction with disorders that interfere with lipid absorption: biliary stasis; prolonged use of antibiotics, which interfere with microbial synthesis; or by the presence of toxins, such as the coumarins (sweet clover poisoning, warfarin poisoning), which interfere with its metabolism. Vitmamin K is essential for the synthesis of prothrombin and clotting factors VII, IX and X. Deficiency is characterized by extensive hemorrhage. Vitamin K is also required for synthesis of other proteins and certain enzymes.

The phylloquinones are generally not considered toxic; however, menadione can precipitate several tissue changes. Renal tubular necrosis has been observed in horses receiving parenteral vitamin K as menadione sodium bisulfite. Increased doses of parenteral menadione in humans have been associated with hemolytic anemia in infants. This has also been induced in laboratory rats, along with necrotizing hepatitis and nephritis. The mechanism of toxicity appears to be related to the formation of menadione-glutathione conjugates and the generation of superoxide radicals.

References

Caldwell PT, Ren P, Bell RG. Warfarin and metabolism of vitamin K. Biochem Pharmacol 1974;23:3353–3362.

Rebhun WC, Tennant BC, Dill SG, et al. Vitamin K3–induced toxicosis in the horse. J Am Vet Med Assoc 1984;184:1237–1239.

Suttie JW. Control of clotting factor biosynthesis by vitamin K. Fed Proc 1969;28:1696–1701.

Suttie JW. Vitamin K—introduction to symposium. Fed Proc 1978; 37:2598.

Suttie JW. The metabolic role of vitamin K. Fed Proc 1980;39:2730–2735.

WATER-SOLUBLE VITAMINS

Thiamin (Vitamin B1)

Thiamin (vitamin B1) is an essential metabolite that exists in animals as thiamin pyrophosphate (TPP), also known as cocarboxylase. TPP serves as a cofactor for several enzymatic conversions, especially in carbohydrate metabolism; it is required for oxidative decarboxylation of α-keto acids by α-ketoacid dehydrogenases, and for the activity of transketolase in the pentose phosphate pathway. In deficient states, serum levels of pyruvate and lactate increase. Animals derive thiamin from animal tissues, where it occurs as TPP, or from plants, where it exists as free thiamin.

DEFICIENCY

Deficiency may result from: (1) simple dietary deficiency, which is not common; (2) the vitamin may be destroyed by dietary additives, such as sulfites or sulfur dioxide used as a preservative; (3) the diet may contain thiamin antagonists; or (4) the vitamin may be destroyed by the action of thiaminases in the diet. Thiaminases may be found in bracken fern (*Pteridium aquilinum),* horse tail (*Equisetum aroena),* the flesh of certain fish, coffee, tea, and some berries; or, it may be produced by certain organisms growing in the gastrointestinal tract (*Bacillus thiaminolyticus, B. aneurinolyticus, Clostridium thiaminolyticum, C. sporogenese).* The precipitating situation varies in different species. In cats, dogs, mink, and foxes—where the condition is most frequently encountered—deficiency usually results from eating raw fish containing thiaminase. Adult ruminants do not require thiamin in the diet, because the vitamin is produced by bacteria in their forestomachs. Calves and lambs, however, have no such activity early in life and are therefore susceptible to dietary deficiency. Adult ruminants may become deficient by consuming plants containing thiaminase, or by the activity of thiaminase-producing bacteria. Horses, on rare occasion, may also exhibit the deficiency after eating plants bearing thiaminase.

In humans, thiamin deficiency leads to **beriberi** or **Wernicke-Korsakoff syndrome** (Wernicke encephalopathy). Beriberi occurs as either "wet" beriberi, which is primarily characterized by myocardial failure and edema, or "dry" beriberi, in which peripheral neuropathy is the dominant manifestation. Wernicke-Korsakoff syndrome is characterized by focal symmetric malacia of the paraventricular gray matter.

Each of these forms can be encountered in animals. Involvement of the central nervous system, comparable to Wernicke-Korsakoff syndrome, is the most frequent expression of deficiency. It was originally described as **Chastek paralysis** when it was first encountered in cats, dogs, mink, and foxes. In ruminants, deficiency may lead to polioencephalomalacia or cerebrocortical necrosis. Peripheral neuropathy is the more usual finding in chickens and other birds. Thiamin deficiency also results in focal myocardial necrosis, which is encountered in most species. This may lead to heart failure, but it is usually not the prominent feature of deficiency.

Chastek paralysis is most frequent in cats, mink, and foxes consuming raw fish. Signs include ataxia, incoordination, opisthotonos, ascending paralysis, torticollis, and mydriasis. The lesions are usually limited to bilaterally symmetric zones of malacia involving the gray matter of brain. Although necrosis of the cortex may occur, it is the paraventricular nuclei that are most selectively destroyed. Any and all of the paraventricular nuclei may be affected, where necrosis of neurons may occur, as well as hyperemia, edema, and hemorrhage. In a recent study of experimental deficiency in dogs, the lesions were reported as most consistent in the caudal colliculi, followed by suprasplenial gyri of the occipital and parietal cortex, claustra, medial vestibular nuclei, and cerebellar noduli.

Polioencephalomalacia Polioencephalomalacia or cerebrocortical necrosis of ruminants—first described in Colorado—is a disease of sheep, cattle, and goats. The circumstances surrounding its occurrence are not clear, but it has been induced with thiamin deficiency; the administration of thiamin can lead to recovery. It is not clear, however, that it represents a single entity. It is probably etiologically nonspecific. This disease is more fully described in Chapter 27.

TOXICITY
The use of extremely high doses of thiamine has led to headache, irritability, insomnia, and rapid pulse in humans, but no specific disorder has been identified in animals.

References

Baggs RB, deLahunta A, Averill DR. Thiamine deficiency encephalopathy in a specific-pathogen-free cat colony. Lab Anim Sci 1978;28:323–326.

Draper HH, Johnson BC. Thiamine deficiency in the lamb and calf. J Nutr 1951;43:413–422.

Evans WC, et al. Induction of thiamine deficiency in sheep, with lesions similar to those of cerebrocortical necrosis. J Comp Pathol 1975;85:253–268.

Innes JRM, Saunders LZ, eds. Comparative neuropathology. XX. Deficiency diseases: thiamin deficiency in cats. New York: Academic Press, 1962:680.

Jubb KU, Saunders LZ, Costas HV. Thiamine deficiency encephalopathy in cats. J Comp Pathol 1956;66:217–227.

Loew FM, et al. Naturally occurring and experimental thiamin deficiency in cats receiving commercial cat food. Can Vet J 1970;11:109–113.

Markson LM, Terlecki S. The aetiology of cerebrocortical necrosis. Br Vet J 1968;124:309–315.

Markson LM, Edwin EE, Lewis G, et al. The production of cerebrocortical necrosis in ruminant calves by the intraruminal administration of amprolium. Br Vet J 1974;130:9–16.

Okada HM, Chihaya Y, Matsukawa K. Thiamine deficiency encephalopathy in foxes and mink. Vet Pathol 1987;24:180–182.

Pill AH. Evidence of thiamine deficiency in calves affected with cerebrocortical necrosis. Vet Rec 1967;81:178–181.

Read DH, Harrington DD. Experimentally induced thiamine deficiency in beagle dogs: clinical observations. Am J Vet Res 1981;42:984–991.

Read DH, Harrington DD. Experimentally induced thiamine deficiency in beagle dogs: clinicopathologic findings. Am J Vet Res 1982;43:1258–1267.

Read DH, Harrington DD. Experimentally induced thiamine deficiency in beagle dogs: pathologic changes of the central nervous system. Am J Vet Res 1986;47:2281–2289.

Sager RL, Hamar DW, Gould DH. Clinical and biochemical alterations in calves with nutritionally induced polioencephalomalacia. Am J Vet Res 1990;51:1969–1974.

Shreeve JE, Edwin EE. Thiaminase-producing strains of Clostridium sporogenes associated with outbreaks of cerebrocortical necrosis. Vet Rec 1974;94:330.

Studdert VP, Labuc RH. Thiamin deficiency in cats and dogs associated with feeding meat preserved with sulphur dioxide. Aust Vet J 1991;68:54–57.

Riboflavin (Vitamin B2)

Riboflavin, or vitamin B2, is key to the function of numerous enzymes that are essential for the metabolism of carbohydrates, amino acids, and lipids.

DEFICIENCY
Deficiency, which has been well-studied experimentally, can lead to a host of different signs and lesions. Spontaneous deficiency under natural conditions is, however, rarely reported in animals. Adult ruminants synthesize the vitamin in their forestomachs and do not require a dietary source. The most characteristic lesions include conjunctivitis and vascularization of the cornea leading to corneal opacity. Dermatoses characterized by scaling, dryness, alopecia, ulceration, and dermatitis have been described in many animal species. Deficiency also leads to a normocytic hypochromic anemia. In humans and under experimental conditions in animals, cheilosis, stomatitis, and glossitis are regular findings. Deficiency in chicks leads to myelin degeneration, especially the sciatic nerve; this results in a syndrome termed "curled-toe paralysis." Humans may also suffer neuralgia.

TOXICOSIS
Riboflavin is essentially nontoxic. Increased doses can lead to a darker yellow color to urine.

References

Heywood R, Partington H. Ocular lesions induced by vitamin B2 deficiency. Vet Rec 1971;88:251–252.

Johnson WD, Storts RW. Peripheral neuropathy associated with dietary riboflavin deficiency in the chicken. I. Light microscopic study. Vet Pathol 1988;25:9–16.

Jones TC. Riboflavin and the control of equine periodic ophthalmia. J Am Vet Med Assoc 1949;64:326–329.

Jones TC, Roby TO, Maurer FD. The relation of riboflavin to equine periodic ophthalmia. Am J Vet Res 1946;7:403–416.

Tandler B, Erlandson RA, Wynder EL. Riboflavin and mouse hepatic cell structure and function. I. Ultrastructural alterations in simple deficiency. Am J Pathol 1968;52:69–95.

Niacin

Niacin is essential for the pyridine nucleotides—nicotinamide adenine dinucleotide (NAD) and nicotinamide adenine dinucleotide phosphate (NADP)—on which many dehydrogenases and reductases are dependent. Niacin is, therefore, key to the metabolism of carbohydrates, fatty acids, and amino acids. In animal tissues, it occurs as NAD and NADP, and in plants as protein-bound nicotinic acid which, in many plants such as corn, is bound to complexes that are not digested and absorbed. NAD and NADP can be synthesized by animals and humans from the essential amino acid tryptophan; however, this conversion is not efficient and some foods such as corn are low in tryptophan. Pyridoxine (vitamin B6) is required for this conversion. Excess intake of the amino acid leucine, which is high in millet, also reduces this conversion.

DEFICIENCY

Deficiency of niacin is usually a combination inadequacy with other B vitamins, particularly pyridoxine, and tryptophan. The classic disorder in humans is pellagra. This is characterized by dermatitis, diarrhea, and dementia. Deficiency in animals has been described in pigs as "pig pellagra," and in dogs it has been termed "blacktongue." In swine, it is usually associated with a corn diet and is characterized by dermatitis, diarrhea, and anemia. Nervous disorders are also described. In dogs, blacktongue is characterized by necrotizing lesions of the tongue and buccal membranes, and diarrhea, which can be severe. The histopathologic changes have not been well described. In the skin, hyperemia occurs, as well as edema, fibrosis of the dermis, hyperkeratosis, and alopecia. The oral mucosa also develops hyperemia, edema, thinning, and necrosis. Atrophy of the gastrointestinal mucosa results, with shortened villi and enlarged crypts. The mucosa becomes hyperemic and may contain hemorrhages. In humans, degenerative changes are described in neurons. In birds, niacin deficiency leads to perosis of the hock joint similar to that caused by manganese or choline deficiency.

Niacin toxicity is not described in domestic animals, but the use of increased doses in humans leads to flushing—due to release of histamine—cardiac arrhythmias, hyperkeratosis, and hepatic necrosis.

References

Alhadeff L, Gualtieri CT, Lipton M. Toxic effects of water-soluble vitamins. Nutr Rev 1984;42:33–40.
Chittenden RH, Underhill FP. The production in dogs of a pathological condition which closely resembles human pellagra. Am J Physiol 1917;44:13–17.
Denton J. A study of the tissue changes in experimental blacktongue of dogs compared with similar changes in pellagra. Am J Pathol 1928;4:341–347.
Dreizen S, Levy BM, Bernick S. Studies on the biology of the periodontium of marmosets. XIII. Histopathology of niacin deficiency stomatitis in the marmoset. J Periodontol 1977;48:452–455.
Goldberger J, Wheeler GA. Experimental blacktongue of dogs and its relation to pellagra. Publ Health Rep 1928;43:172–177.
Gopalan C, Narasinga Rao BS. Experimental niacin deficiency. Methods Achiev Exp Pathol 1972;6:49–80.
Victoria CR, Meneghelli UG. (Morphometry and kinetics of jejunal epithelium in rats with niacin deficiency.) Morfometria e cinetica do epitelio jejunal em ratos com deficiencia de niacina. Arq Gastroenterol 1989;26:111–115.

Pyridoxine (Vitamin B6)

Pyridoxine, or vitamin B6, is present in meats, grains, and vegetables; however, like niacin, much of what is of plant origin is bound to complexes that render it unavailable. Vitamin B6 in animals is largely in the form of pyridoxal phosphate, and serves as a coenzyme necessary for transaminases, decarboxylases, racemases, and phosphorylases in amino acid and protein metabolism. Included is the conversion of tryptophan to niacin. Some drugs, such as isoniazid, inactivate the vitamin.

DEFICIENCY

Deficiency of pyridoxine as a single nutrient is not common. Experimentally, a variety of changes have been described in animals. In most species, a microcytic hypochromic anemia develops. Dermatitis is also a consistent feature, characterized by acanthosis, hyperkeratosis, hyperemia, and a leukocytic infiltrate in the dermis. Ataxia and convulsions are described in puppies, calves, swine, and rats. The basis for these signs is not well-described, but in swine, demyelination of peripheral nerves occurs. In kittens, necrosis of renal tubular epithelium develops, along with deposition of oxalate crystals and calcification.

TOXICITY

Pyridoxine toxicity in humans following large doses leads to a peripheral sensory and motor neuropathy.

References

Anonymous. Vitamin B6 toxicity: a new megavitamin syndrome. Nutr Rev 1984;42:44–46.
Anonymous. Sensory neuropathy from megadoses of pyroxidine. Nutr Rev 1984;42:49–51.
Blanchard PC, Bai SC, Rogers QR, et al. Pathology associated with vitamin B-6 deficiency in growing kittens. J Nutr 1991;121:S77–S78.
Johnson BC, Pinkos JA, Burke KA. Pyridoxine deficiency in the calf. J Nutr 1949;40:309–322.
Miller ER, Schmidt DA, Hoeffer JA, et al. The pyridoxine requirement of the baby pig. J Nutr 1957;62:407–419.
Schaumburg H, et al. Sensory neuropathy from pyridoxine abuse: a new megavitamin syndrome. N Engl J Med 1983;309:445–448.

Pantothenic acid

Pantothenic acid is a component of Coenzyme A (CoA), which is key to many metabolic functions, including the entrance of acetic acid into the tricarboxylic acid cycle ("Krebs cycle").

DEFICIENCY

Deficiency is rare, but has been recognized in growing swine under field conditions. The deficiency usually appears when corn (maize) is a significant part of the diet. The clinical signs are gradual loss of flesh, dirty scaly skin, and fluid feces, followed by stiffness in the rear legs and apparent weakness in the loin muscles. The muscular weakness progresses, and eventually the animals rest their weight on their hocks. Later the pigs assume a sitting position, with the hind-legs extended forward and to the side. The pigs eventually drag themselves about with their forelegs. Supplementation with pantothenic acid in the diet stops the appearance of new cases.

Experimental deficiency of pantothenic acid in swine results in mucous, hemorrhagic, and necrotizing colitis with consequent diarrhea. An ataxic gait and terminal recumbency are caused by necrosis of neurons in the dorsal spinal ganglia, degeneration of myelin, and axons in brachial and sciatic nerves. Experimental deficiency can also be produced in dogs, monkeys, rats, chicks, and other animals. Lesions in rats include dermatitis, achromotrichia, increased protoporphyrin secretion by the Harderian gland, and adrenal cortical necrosis. Naturally occurring deficiencies are rare because of the many sources of this vitamin.

Reference

Oakley GA. Pantothenic acid deficiency in a commercial herd of pigs. Vet Rec, 1970;86:252–253.

Vitamin B12 (cobalamin)

Vitamin B12 is a compound composed of a corrin ring (similar to porphyrin ring) containing cobalt. It is produced only by bacteria, either in the intestine or in fermented foods.

DEFICIENCY

Deficiency is rare, except in humans and nonhuman primates because animals obtain the vitamin from their diet of animal products, or it is synthesized in the intestinal tract and either absorbed or excreted, and obtained by coprophagy. Bacterial synthesis requires the presence of cobalt. Absorption of Vitamin B12 requires it to be bound to a protein, termed intrinsic factor, which is secreted by gastric parietal cells. This factor binds to specific receptors in the ileum. Vitamin B12 is required for the function of methylmalonyl CoA mutase, leucine mutase, and methionine synthetase. It is required for the conversion of 5–methyl-tetrahydrofolic acid (5–methyl-FH4) to tetrahydrofolic acid (FH4), the active form of folic acid. Thus, vitamin B12 deficiency leads to folic acid deficiency. In humans, several inherited defects of vitamin B12 metabolism have been identified.

DEFICIENCY

Deficiency in humans and monkeys is characterized by megaloblastic anemia and demyelinizing lesions. The neuropathy first develops in peripheral nerves, but progresses to the spinal cord with prolonged deficiency. Cobalt deficiency, which occurs in ruminants who synthesize their vitamin B12 in the rumen, is essentially a vitamin B12 deficiency and is discussed later in this chapter.

References

Agamanolis DP, et al. Neuropathology of experimental vitamin B12 deficiency in monkeys. Neurology 1976;26:905–914.

Goodman A, Harris JW, Hines JD. Biochemical megaloblastosis in B-12 deficient monkeys. Clin Res 1978;26:347A.

Hogan KG, Lorentz PP, Gibb FM. The diagnosis and treatment of vitamin B12 deficiency in young lambs. NZ Vet J 197321:234–237.

Kark JA, et al. Nutritional vitamin B12 deficiency in rhesus monkeys. Am J Clin Nutr 1974;27:470–478.

Marston HR. The requirement of sheep for cobalt or for vitamin B12. Br J Nutr 1970;24:615–633.

Oxnard CE. Some variations in the amount of vitamin B12 in the serum of the rhesus monkey. Nature 1964;201:1188–1191.

Oxnard CE, Smith WT. Neurological degeneration and reduced serum vitamin B12 levels in captive monkeys. Nature 1966;210:507–509.

Scherer HJ. Degeneration of the papillomacular bundles in apes and its significance in human neuropathology. J Neurol Neurosurg Psychiatry 1940;3:37–48.

Schuh S, et al. Homocystinuria and megaloblastic anemia responsive to vitamin B12 therapy: an inborn error of metabolism due to a defect in cobalamin metabolism. N Engl J Med 1984;310:686–690.

Van Bogaert L, Innes JRM. Neurologic diseases of apes and monkeys. In: Innes JRM, Saunders LZ, eds. Comparative neuropathology. New York: Academic Press, 1962:5:55–146.

Folic acid (pteroylglutamic acid)

Folic acid is widely distributed in animal products and plants. Its active form is tetrahydrofolic acid (FH4). FH4 is important in the metabolism of amino acids, and in purine nucleotide and pyrimidine nucleotide synthesis. It is, thus required for all cell proliferation, and the hematopoietic system is particularly sensitive. Signs of folic acid deficiency in humans and other animals therefore include leukopenia, macrocytic anemia, and megaloblastic cytologic changes in the bone marrow. The cat and cebus monkey are susceptible to experimental deprivation. Anemia due to folic acid deficiency is confirmed by adding folic acid to the diet, resulting in correction of the anemia.

References

Rasmussen KM, Hayes KC, Thenen SW. Folic acid deficiency in cebus monkey. 1977; 36:1121.

Thenen SW, Rasmussen KM. Megaloblastic erythropoiesis and tissue depletion of folic acid in the cat. Am J Vet Res, 1978;39:1205–1207.

Biotin

Biotin is widely distributed in foods of plant and animal origin, and deficiency is almost nonexistent. It is important in the function of carboxylase enzymes and, thus, the metabolism of fats, glucose and amino acids. Deficiency can be induced experimentally and has occurred by excessive consumption of raw egg whites, which contain a substance secreted by the oviducts termed avidin. Avidin forms an indigestible complex with biotin. Signs of deficiency include hyperkeratosis, dermatitis, alopecia and achromotrichia.

Vitamin C (ascorbic acid)

Vitamin C is synthesized by the liver in almost all mammals and most species of birds and, thus, is not a dietary requirement. Deficiency states are therefore limited.

DEFICIENCY

Among mammals, humans, nonhuman primates, guinea pigs, Indian fruit bats, and Indian pipistrels cannot synthesize vitamin C. These species lack the enzyme L-gulonolactone oxidase required for synthesis. Insects, invertebrates, and fish also generally do not synthesize vitamin C. Many functions are ascribed to vitamin C, but its role in the synthesis of collagen proteins is responsible for the classic form of deficiency known as

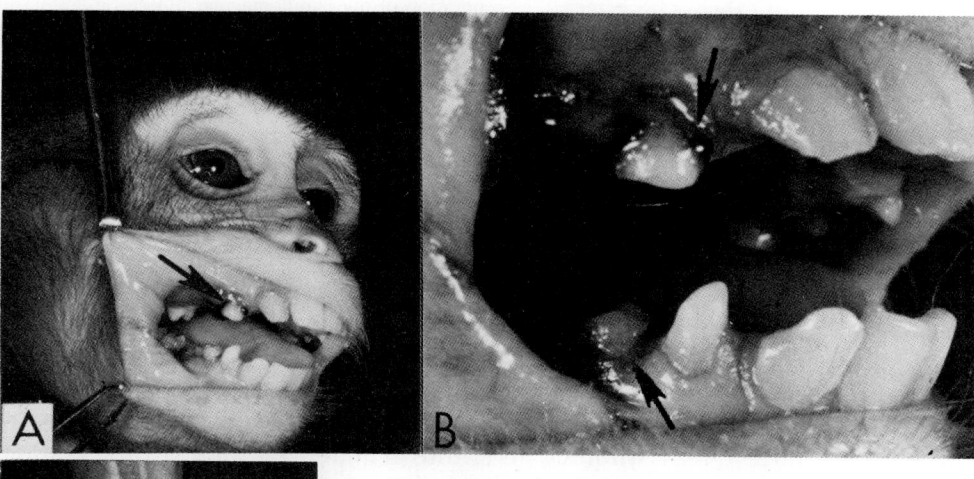

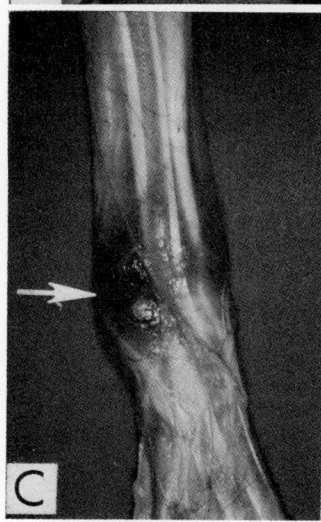

FIG. 16-9 Scurvy, in rhesus monkey *(Macaca mulatta)*. **A.** and **B.** Loosening of teeth and gingival hemorrhage (arrows). **C.** Subperiosteal hemorrhage at distal tibia (arrow). (Courtesy of New England Regional Primate Research Center, Harvard Medical School.)

scurvy. Vitamin C is required for the formation of hydroxyproline and hydroxylysine, which give collagen its helic structure, its rigidity and structural strength. Vitamin C is also required for the optimal function of a number of other enzymes, including those involved in the synthesis of carnitine.

Scurvy Scurvy, or scorbutus, in humans was known to be prevented in the eighteenth century by eating fresh fruit or green vegetables. Lime juice was required in the daily ration of sailors on British ships-of-war; hence came the nickname "Limeys." The signs of scurvy include gingivitis and bleeding gums, failure of wounds to heal, inappetence, dermatitis, loss of weight, and sudden death (Figs. 16-9, 16-10, 16-11). Guinea pigs succumb within three to four weeks after ascorbic acid is withdrawn from their diet; longer intervals usually are required in Old and New World monkeys and humans.

LESIONS The lesions consist chiefly of subperiosteal hemorrhages, abnormal ossification of long bones, and gingivitis. The fundamental disturbance is the inability of fibroblasts to form collagen or osteoid. This accounts for the failure of wounds to heal and for the pathologic changes in bones. The epiphysis is usually widened, due to a zone of calcified but unossified cartilage at the site of endochondral bone formation. The cartilaginous

side of the epiphyseal junction is convex and bulges into the disordered osseous side (Fig 16-11B). Focal necroses in the myocardium sometimes occur, accounting for sudden death.

DIAGNOSIS The diagnosis is arrived at from the clinical signs and lesions, and may be confirmed in living animals by the prompt response to the addition of ascorbic acid to the diet.

References

Baker EM, et al. Metabolism of ascorbic acid and ascorbic-2-sulfate in man and subhuman primate. Ann NY Acad Sci 1975;258:72–80.

Chatterjee IB, Majumder AK, Nandi BK, et al. Synthesis and some major functions of vitamin C in animals. Ann NY Acad Sci 1975;258:24–47.

Demaray SY, Altman NH, Ferrell TL. Suspected ascorbic acid deficiency in a colony of squirrel monkeys (Saimiri sciurius). Lab Anim Sci 1978;28:457–460.

DiFilippo NM, Blumenthal HJ. Cholelithiasis in the scorbutic guinea pig. J Am Osteopath Assoc 1972;72:284–287.

Gillespie DS. L-gulonolactone oxidase: the missing link in the biosynthesis of vitamin C. Lab Anim 1981;10:5155.

Hsu C-K. Vitamin C and immune response in rhesus monkeys. Fed Proc 1977;36:1177.

Jukes TH. Further comments on the ascorbic acid requirement. Proc Natl Acad Sci USA 1975;72:4151–4152.

Lehner NDM, Bullock BC, Clarkson TB. Ascorbic acid deficiency in the squirrel monkey. Proc Soc Exp Biol Med 1968;128:512–514.

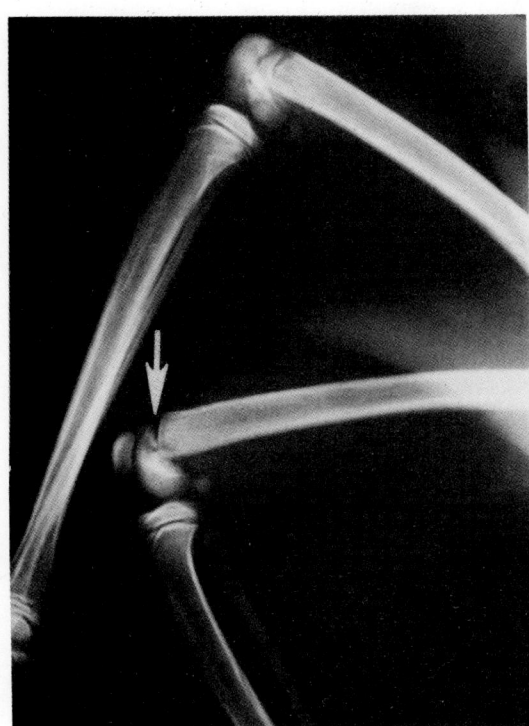

FIG. 16-10 Scurvy, in rhesus monkey *(Macaca mulatta)*. Epiphyseal fracture (arrow) of the distal femur. (Courtesy of New England Regional Primate Research Center, Harvard Medical School.)

Levine M. New concepts in the biology and biochemistry of ascorbic acid. N Engl J Med 1986;314:892–902.

MacKenzie IC, Kolar G, Kashani H, et al. Periodontal changes in ascorbic acid deficient monkeys. J Dent Res 1977;56:B111.

Ratterree MS, Didier PJ, Blanchard JL, et al. Vitamin C deficiency in captive nonhuman primates fed commercial primate diet. Lab Anim Sci 1990;40:165–168.

Sulkin NM, Sulkin DF. Tissue changes induced by marginal vitamin C deficiency. Ann NY Acad Sci 1975;258:317–328.

Tucker BW, Halver JE. Vitamin C metabolism in rainbow trout. Comp Pathol Bull 1986;18:1,6.

MINERALS

Calcium

About 99% of the body's calcium is in bones and teeth, with the remainder in extracellular fluid and cell membranes. In serum, 50% of the calcium occurs as the biologically active ionized form, with most of the remainder bound to globulin or albumin, which serves as a reserve, and a small portion in a variety of organic complexes. Optimal serum calcium levels are precisely maintained by the interaction of parathyroid hormone, thyrocalcitonin, and the active form of vitamin D, all of which are discussed under vitamin D earlier in this chapter and in Chapter 26, The Endocrine System. Because of the large skeletal reserve of calcium, these homeostatic mechanisms prevent a dietary deficiency of calcium from leading to hypocalcemia. Instead, deficiency of calcium leads to rickets, osteomalacia, or os-

teodystrophia fibrosa, also discussed under vitamin D and in the Skeletal System chapter (18).

DEFICIENCY

Deficiency of calcium can result from several different mechanisms:

1. Because cereal grains are low in calcium, and meat is also low in calcium and high in phosphorus, the diet may simply not contain adequate calcium;
2. Vitamin D deficiency, among other things, precludes adequate absorption of calcium;
3. Diets high in phosphorus relative to calcium interfere with absorption of calcium. A dietary ratio of 1:1 or 2:1 is desirable.
4. Dietary calcium may be complexed with other compounds preventing its absorption. Phytic acid, for example, hinders absorption of calcium, phosphorus, iron, manganese, and zinc. Oxalates also interfere with calcium absorption. An acid environment is also required for proper calcium absorption.
5. Interference with the normal flow of bile, coupled with a diet rich in fats, may produce steatorrhea and the formation of calcium soaps, preventing calcium absorption and leading to what has been termed celiac rickets; and,
6. Chronic renal disease can lead to hyperphosphatemia—and to an associated hypocalcemia and secondary parathyroidism—which then results in renal rickets; chronic renal disease can also reduce the effectiveproduction of adequate biologically active vitamin D.

Hypocalcemia In each of the above circumstances, serum calcium is maintained at or near normal levels. Hypocalcemia, a life threatening disorder, arises from other mechanisms. These include: hypoparathyroidism; parturient paresis or milk fever; eclampsia in bitches; and acute pancreatitis, where calcium is fixed as insoluble calcium soaps that release fatty acids during fat necrosis; this is believed to cause a rapid depletion of calcium in extracellular fluids. Hypocalcemia leads to interference with normal neuromuscular transmission. In most species, hypocalcemia is characterized by tetany; however, in cattle, parturient paresis, as its name implies, is characterized by paralysis.

Parturient paresis Parturient Paresis (milk fever, parturient hypocalcemia) is a disorder of dairy cows, and sometimes sheep; it occurs at or shortly after parturition, resulting from an acute hypocalcemia. The homeostatic mechanisms that maintain serum calcium are unable to meet the sudden demand for calcium required for lactation, and serum calcium levels fall to 50% of normal. The disease was first recognized with the development of heavily producing dairy breeds; the earliest references to it (according to Hutyra et al., 1938) are those of Eberhardt (1793), Price (1806), Jorg (1808), and Fabe (1837). It is seen more often in cows maintained on high-calcium diets, and is less frequent in cows on low-calcium diets. Older cows are the most vulnerable.

The affected cow is found lying on its sternum with the head characteristically turned toward the flank. The

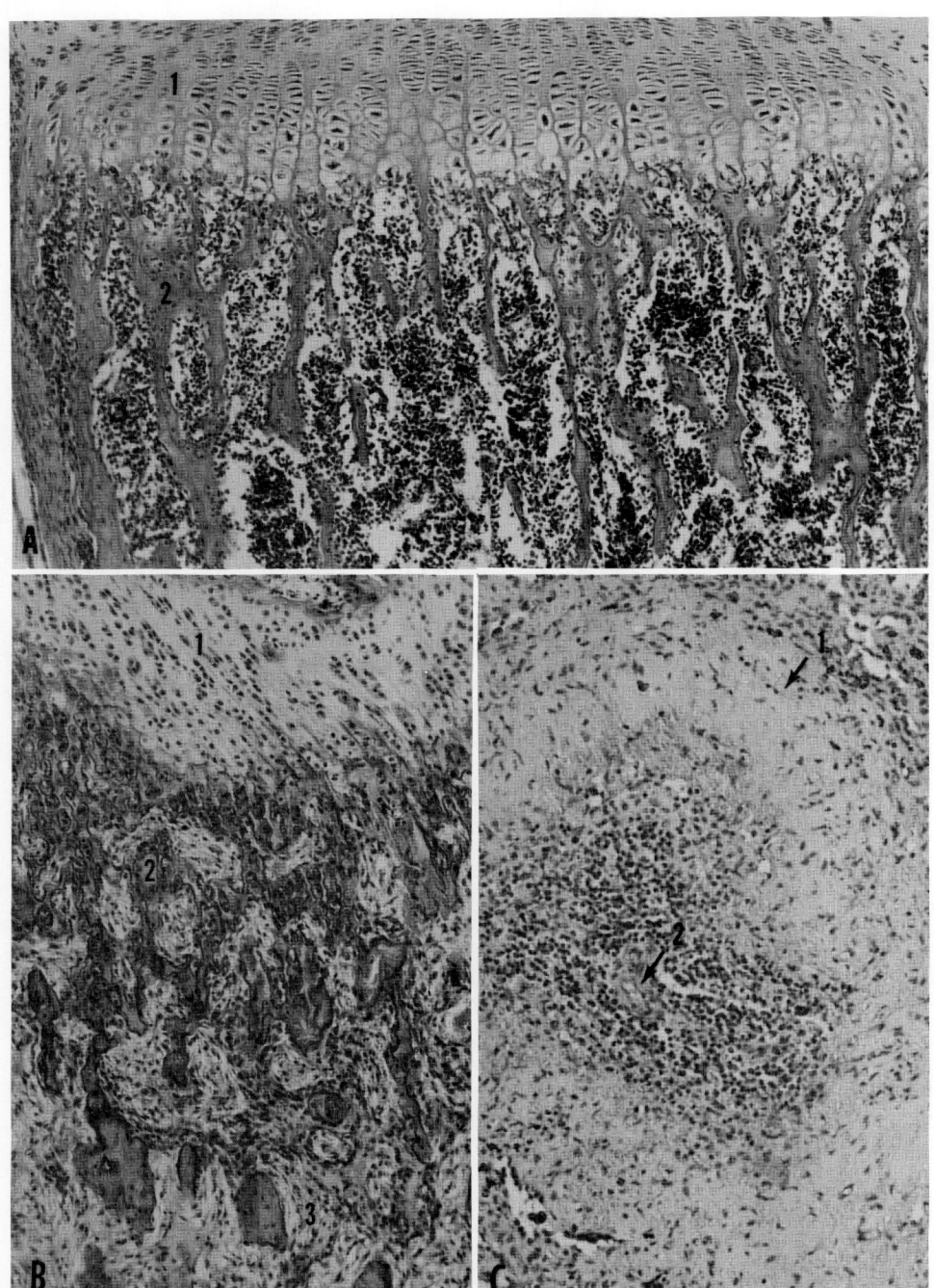

FIG. 16-11 Scurvy, in guinea pig. **A.** Femur of normal-guinea pig (×90). (1) Epiphyseal cartilage; (2) New-formed bone; and (3) Hematopoietic marrow. **B.** Femur of scorbutic guinea pig (×100). (1) Distorted epiphyseal cartilage; (2) Disrupted spicules of new bone; and (3) Fibrous marrow. **C.** Amyloidosis of spleen of scorbutic guinea pig (×150). (1) Amyloid surrounds and displaces lymphocytes of the splenic corpuscle; (2) Central artery. (Courtesy of Armed Forces Institute of Pathology; contributor: Army Medical Nutrition Laboratory.)

cow is unable to get to her feet and may die in a day or so when not treated. In ewes, an interval of hyperexcitability and tremors may precede paresis. No specific pathologic findings occur. Ultrastructural studies by Capen and Young (1967) and Capen (1971) show that the chief cells of the parathyroid are active and lack storage granules; this suggests that the cows are unable to handle the demand for parathormone. These studies also showed degranulation of parafollicular cells, the origin of thyrocalcitonin.

Eclampsia (puerperal tetany) Eclampsia in bitches and, less often, cats is a hypocalcemia that occurs 1–3 weeks after parturition. A comparable condition is sometimes seen in mares (lactation tetany). Clinically, the disorders are characterized by hyperexcitability, tremors, and tetany. These are also clinical expressions of hypocalcemia in humans. Why cows become paretic is not clear, but it has been suggested that cattle have a fundamental physiological difference in neuromuscular transmission.

HYPERCALCEMIA

Hypercalcemia is seen in hypervitaminosis D and hyperparathyroidism. It leads to calcification of a variety of tissues, especially the vasculature, kidneys, and gastric mucosa. Diets high in calcium do not lead to these changes, but can result in increased levels of serum calcitonin (due to C cell hyperplasia) and decreased levels of parathormone. A short interval of high dietary calcium does not lead to pathologic changes; however, when consumed for prolonged periods, the hypercalcitonemia leads to osteopetrosis, which is characterized by an increased thickness of bones due to retarded osteoclastic resorption. Osteophytes may also develop. Additionally, the physeal and articular cartilaginous growth plates fail to mature and become widened and disorganized with irregular protrusions into the metaphysis or subchondral bone. These cartilaginous changes could resemble rickets, but an absence of osteomalacia exists, and no apparent increase in osteoblastic activity.

Diets high in calcium increase the requirement for zinc and can lead to parakeratosis in swine. High dietary calcium also aggravates manganese deficiency.

References

Black HE, Capen CC, Yarrington JT, et al. Effect of a high calcium prepartal diet on calcium homeostatic mechanisms in thyroid glands, bone, and intestine of cows. Lab Invest 1973;29:437–448.

Blum JW, Ramberg CF Jr, Johnson KG, et al. Calcium (ionized and total), magnesium, phosphorus, and glucose in plasma from parturient cows. Am J Vet Res 1972;33:51–56.

Blum JW, Mayer GP, Potts JT Jr. Parathyroid hormone responses during spontaneous hypocalcemia and induced hypercalcemia in cows. Endocrinology 1974;95:84–92.

Bowen JM, Blackmon DM, Heavner JE. Neuromuscular transmission and hypocalcemic paresis in the cow. Am J Vet Res 1970;31:831–839.

Capen CC. Fine structural alterations of parathyroid glands in response to experimental and spontaneous changes of calcium in extracellular fluids. Am J Med 1971;59:598–611.

Capen CC, Young DM. The ultrastructure of the parathyroid glands and thyroid parafollicular cells of cows with parturient paresis and hypocalcemia. Lab Invest 1967;17:717–737.

Capen CC, Young DM. Thyrocalcitonin: evidence for release in a spontaneous hypocalcemic disorder. Science 1967;157:205–206.

Chisari FV, Hochstein HD, Kirschstein RL, et al. Parathyroid necrosis and hypocalcemic tetany induced in rabbits by L-asparaginase. Am J Pathol 1972;68:461–468.

Dryerre H, Greig R. Further studies on etiology of milk fever. Vet Rec 1928;8:721–728.

Fish PA. Physiology of milk fever: blood phosphates and calcium. Cornell Vet 1929;19:147–160.

Goedegebuure SA, Hazewinkel HAW. Morphological findings in young dogs chronically fed a diet containing excess calcium. Vet Pathol 1986;23:594–601.

Greig JR. Calcium gluconate as a specific in milk fever. Vet Rec 1930;10:115–120, 301–305.

Hutyra F, Marek J, Manninger R. Special pathology and therapeutics of the diseases of domestic animals. Vol III. Chicago: Alex Eger, 1938:454.

Kirk GR, Breazile JE, Kenny AD. Pathogenesis of hypocalcemia tetany in the thyroparathyroidectomized dog. Am J Vet Res 1974;35:407–408.

Kronfeld DS. Parturient hypocalcemia in dairy cows. Adv Vet Sci Comp Med 1971;15:133–135.

Krook L, Lutwak L, McEntee K. Dietary calcium ultimobranchial tumors and osteopetrosis in the bull. Am J Clin Nutr 1969;22:115–118.

Krook L, Lutwak L, McEntee K, et al. Nutritional hypercalcitoninism in bulls. Cornell Vet 1971; 61:625–639.

Little WL, Wright NC. The aetiology of milk fever in cattle. Vet Rec 1925;5:631–633.

Littledike ET, Whipp SC, Schroeder L. Studies on parturient paresis. J Am Vet Med Assoc 1969;155:1955–1962.

Posner AS. Problems in calcium metabolism. Bone mineral on the molecular level. Fed Proc 1973;32:1933–1937.

Reddy BS. Calcium and magnesium absorption: role of intestinal microflora. Fed Proc 1971;30:1815–1821.

Reitz RE, Mayer GP, Deftos LJ, et al. Endogenous parathyroid hormone response to thyrocalcitonin-induced hypocalcemia in the cow. Endocrinology 1971;89:932–935.

Resnick S. Hypocalcemia and tetany in the dog. Vet Med Small Anim Clin 1972;67:637–641.

Schryver HF, Hintz HF, Craig PH. Calcium metabolism in ponies fed a high phosphorus diet. J Nutr 1971;101:259–264.

Swartzman JA, Hintz HF, Schryver HF. Inhibition of calcium absorption in ponies fed diets containing oxalic acid. Am J Vet Res 1978;39:1621–1623.

Phosphorus

Like calcium, most (about 80%) of the body's phosphorus is in bones and teeth, and disorders in phosphorus metabolism are reflected in skeletal disease comparable to calcium or vitamin D deficiency. Nonskeletal phosphorus is widely dispersed, and is involved in most aspects of metabolism; this includes its role in energy metabolism (ATP), nucleoproteins, and regulation of acid base balance.

DEFICIENCY

Dietary deficiency of phosphorus may be the most common mineral deficiency of ruminants, especially in tropical countries where plants are low in this element. It is rare in other species. In ruminants, phosphorus deficiency is characterized by general weakness and weight loss (possibly related to its role in energy metabolism); however, the most striking and characteristic sign is a marked pica for phosphorus. Animals have a tendency to chew or lick bones of animals dead on the range. The consumption of clinging shreds of decaying musculature predisposes these animals to botulism, and in South Africa the disorder has been designated lamsiekte. Osteomalacia is the predominant pathologic finding. Serum phosphorus is usually maintained at normal levels.

Hypophosphatemia Hypophosphatemia is seen in primary hyperparathyroidism, prolonged diarrhea or vomiting, hyperadrenocorticism and renal disease, or prolonged use of diuretics. The effects of hypophosphatemia depend in part on its duration. Severe hypophosphatemia leads to myocardial and skeletal muscle dysfunction and necrosis, which is probably related to the role of phosphorus in energy metabolism. There also may be neurologic signs of irritability, seizures, coma, and a hemolytic anemia. When prolonged, hypophosphatemia will obviously result in osteomalacia.

HYPERPHOSPHATEMIA

Hyperphosphatemia—or a tendency in that direction—resulting from diets high in phosphorus and low in calcium, leads to secondary hyperparathyroidism and associated skeletal disease. The so-called "big head" of horses results from a diet high in wheat bran; in dogs and cats, a similar disorder can follow prolonged meat diets. Each of these sources are high in phosphorus and low in calcium.

References

Eicher EM, Southard JL, Scriver CR, et al. Hypophosphatemia: mouse model for human familial hypophosphatemic vitamin D-resistant rickets. Proc Natl Acad Sci USA 1976; 73:4667–4671.

Forrester SD, Moreland KJ. Hypophosphatemia: causes and clinical consequences. J Vet Intern Med 1989;3:149–159.

Morrow DA. Phosphorus deficiency and infertility in dairy heifers. J Am Vet Med Assoc 1969;154:761–768.

Symonds HW. The effect of thyroidectomy and thyroparathyroidectomy upon phosphorus homeostasis in the goat: a hypothesis for the cause of hypophosphataemia. Res Vet Sci 1970;11:260–269.

Magnesium

About 70% of the body's magnesium is present, along with calcium and phosphorus, in bone. In soft tissues, magnesium is the most abundant intracellular bivalent cation. It is known to be the activator of many enzyme systems, including alkaline phosphatase, as well as of most enzymes that utilize adenosine triphosphatase (ATP) or catalyze transfer of phosphate. Magnesium is therefore involved in many biologic activities, including: membrane transport; the activation of animo acid, acetate, or succinate; the synthesis of protein, nucleic acid, fat, or coenzymes; the generation and transmission of nerve impulses; and the contraction of muscle and oxidative phosphorylation.

Magnesium ions are present in the blood at the approximate level of 2.0 mg/100 ml. Dietary deficiency is believed to be the principal cause of lowered levels in the blood. Levels below 0.7 mg/100 ml cause nervous hyperirritability. Excessively increased levels cause depression, coma, and death. This occurs when euthenasia is accomplished by intravenous injection of a solution of magnesium sulfate.

DEFICIENCY

Dietary deficiency, or disturbances of magnesium metabolism, are rare, with the exception of grass tetany and milk tetany.

Grass tetany (grass staggers), milk tetany, (wheat poisoning), and winter tetany These disorders, characterized by hypomagnesemia, are seen in cattle, sheep, and rarely horses. Milk tetany and winter tetany represent dietary deficiency of magnesium in animals fed a magnesium-deficient diet for prolonged periods—either milk or poor hay. Grass tetany (grass staggers) results when animals have been pastured exclusively on lush and succulent grasses of various kinds or wheat and cereal crop pastures. The basis for hypomagnesemia is more complicated than a simple dietary deficiency. The increased protein and potassium contents of such pastures reduce the absorption of magnesium. Serum calcium is also frequently depressed in affected animals. It is most frequent in females of beef breeds,

especially lactating animals. The onset is acute, with serum magnesium falling from a normal of about 2.0 mg/dL to less than 1.0 mg/dL. Animals may be found dead or develop signs that include hyperirritability, apprehensiveness, and/or incoordination followed by sudden convulsive seizures. Signs are intermittent and initiated by excitement or exercise. The convulsions repeat at intervals and ultimately lead to death. No specific lesions occur: however, agonal hemorrhages and congestion may result.

References

Ashton DG, Jones DM, Gilmour JS. Grain-sickness in two nondomestic equines. Vet Rec 1977;100:406–407.

Blaxter JL, Rook JF. The magnesium requirements of calves. J Comp Pathol Ther 1954;64:176–186.

Christian KR, Williams VJ. Attempts to produce hypomagnesaemia in dry nonpregnant sheep. NZ J Agric Res 1960;3:389–398.

Flink EB, Jones JE, eds. The pathogenesis and clinical significance of magnesium deficiency. Ann NY Acad Sci 1969;162:705–984.

Fontenot JB, Wise MB, Webb KE Jr. Interrelationships of potassium, nitrogen and magnesium in ruminants. Fed Proc 1973;32:1925–1928.

Haggard DL, Whitehair CK, Langham RF. Tetany associated with magnesium deficiency in suckling beef calves. J Am Vet Med Assoc 1978;172:495–497.

Hall RF, Reynolds RA. Concentrations of magnesium and calcium in plasma of Hereford cows during and after hypomagnesemic tetany. Am J Vet Res 1972;33:1711–1714.

Harrington DD. Pathologic features of magnesium deficiency in young horses fed purified rations. Am J Vet Res 1974;35:503–513.

Heggtveit HA, Herman L, Mishra RK. Cardiac necrosis and calcification in experimental magnesium deficiency: a light and electron microscopic study. Am J Pathol 1964;45:757–782.

Herd RP. Grass tetany in sheep. Aust Vet J 1966;42:160–164.

Herd RP, Peebles RM. Hypomagnesaemia and grass tetany in sheep. Aust Vet J 1962;38:455–456.

Hughes JP, Cornelius CE. An outbreak of grass tetany in lactating beef cattle. Cornell Vet 1960;50:26–33.

Kemp A, et al. Hypomagnesemia in milking cows: intake and utilization of magnesium from herbage by lactating cows. Neth J Agric Sci 1961;9:134–149.

Marshak RR. Some metabolic derangements associated with magnesium metabolism in cattle. J Am Vet Med Assoc 1958;133:539–542.

Mayo RH, Plumlee MP, Beeson WM. Magnesium requirement of the pig. J Anim Sci 1959;18:264–274.

Mershon MM. Tetany in cattle on winter rations. J Am Vet Med Assoc 1959;135:435–439.

Moore LA, Hallman ET, Sholl LB. Cardiovascular and other lesions in calves fed diets low in magnesium. Arch Pathol 1938;26:820–838.

Owen JB, Sinclair KB. The development of hypomagnesaemia in lactating ewes. Vet Rec 1961;73:1423–1424.

Patterson R, Crichton C. Grass staggers in large scale dairying on grass. J Br Grass Soc 1960;15:100–105.

Rook JAF. Spontaneous and induced magnesium deficiency in ruminants. Ann NY Acad Sci 1969;162:727–731.

Rook JAF. Rapid development of hypomagnesaemia in lactating cows when given artificial rations low in magnesium. Nature 1961;191:1019.

Todd JR, Horvath DJ. Magnesium and neuromuscular irritability in calves, with particular reference to hypomagnesaemic tetany. Br Vet J 1970;126:333–346.

Udall RH. Low blood magnesium and associated tetany occurring in cattle in the winter. Cornell Vet 1947;37:314–324.

Wilcox GB, Hoff JE. Grass tetany: an hypothesis concerning its relationship with ammonium nutrition of spring grass. J Dairy Sci 1974;57:1085–1089.

Potassium

Potassium is the most abundant intracellular cation and plays a key role in regulation of acid-base balance, osmolality, activation of several enzymes, and in neurotransmission.

DEFICIENCY

Deficiency is rarely recorded, but may develop in patients with severe dehydration, chronic diarrhea, hyperadrenalism, medication with corticosteroids, or prolonged use of diuretics. Rarely is a dietary deficiency identified. Milk contains an increased level of potassium, which increases the dietary requirement in lactating animals. Signs of deficiency include loss of appetite, weight loss, rough hair coat, and muscular weakness. In grave deficiency, weakness and paralysis may develop due to defective neuromuscular transmission and rhabdomyolysis. Experimental deficiency in rats leads to focal necrosis of the myocardium, similar to the cardiac changes seen in thiamin deficiency.

HYPERKALEMIA

Hyperkalemia can result from supplementation of diets with excessive potassium, but not from most usual diets. Excessive dietary potassium does interfere with the metabolism of magnesium and predisposes to grass tetany. Hyperkalemia also occurs in acidosis resulting from chronic renal disease.

References

Belman AS, Schwartz WB. The nephropathy of potassium depletion. N Engl J Med 1956;255:195.

Dow SW, LeCouteur RA, Fettman MJ, et al. Potassium depletion in cats: hypokalemic polymyopathy. J Am Vet Med Assoc 1987;191:1563–1568.

Sodium and chlorine

Sodium and chlorine are the principal extracellular cations and anions; among other functions, they are both critical for the maintenance of acid-base balance and osmolality. Both ions are indispensable, but neither is the basis of a separate clinical deficiency. Practically speaking, the metabolism of these two elements is the metabolism of sodium chloride. Carnivorous animals obtain sufficient sodium chloride from the animal tissues that they eat. The need for salt on the part of humans (and domestic and wild herbivora) is such that access to the substance has been the basis of taxation, has occasioned wars, and has governed the strategy of generals and of hunters.

Inadequate dietary salt is most frequently encountered in cattle in tropical countries where forages are decreased in sodium. In cattle, and to a lesser degree other species, sodium deficiency leads to a marked craving for salt that becomes manifest within weeks. Deficient animals lick almost any object, including the sweat of other animals. More prolonged deficiency is further characterized by weakness, loss of appetite, weight loss or reduced growth rate, rough hair coat, general unthriftiness, and incoordination. Increased sweating associated with hot weather and hard work increases the need for dietary sodium, as does lactation.

Diets specifically low in chloride are rare; however, excessive vomiting can lead to deficiency. Experimental deficiency in calves leads to lethargy, loss of weight, and dehydration. Lesions include necrosis of renal tubular epithelium at the corticomedullary junction and medullary nephrocalcinosis.

TOXICOSIS

Sudden heavy excesses of salt in the absence of adequate water leads to salt poisoning in swine, cattle, sheep, and chickens. With ample water, however, a cow, for example, can consume as much as 2 pounds of sodium chloride daily over an indefinite period without ill effects. Salt poisoning is discussed in Chapter 15.

References

Blackmon DM, et al. Clinical aspects of experimentally induced chloride deficiency in Holstein calves. Am J Vet Res 1984;45:1638–1640.

McDougall JG, Coghlan JP, Scoggins BA, et al. Effect of sodium depletion on bone sodium and total exchangeable sodium in sheep. Am J Vet Res 1974;35:923–930.

Turpeinen O. The effects of deprivation of sodium on young puppies. Am J Hyg 1938;18:104–109.

Whitlock RH, Kessler MJ, Tasker JB. Salt (sodium) deficiency in dairy cattle: polyuria and polydipsia as prominent clinical features. Cornell Vet 1975;65:512–526.

Fluorine

There is no evidence to indicate that fluorine deficiency occurs in domestic animals. In fact, only marginal evidence exists that fluorine deficiency can be experimentally produced in mice and rats, and here the reports are conflicting. Some studies have reported reduced growth rate, anemia, and reduced fertility in rats and mice. No such examples exist for other animals. The strongest evidence for a beneficial effect or requirement for fluorine is its effect in reducing dental caries in humans when added to the water supply at levels of 1–2 ppm.

TOXICITY

Fluorine is highly toxic, leading to fluorosis. Toxic levels vary among species and due to other factors, but amounts as low as 40 ppm in feed can be toxic. Fluorosis is discussed in Chapter 15.

Reference

Messer HH, Armstrong WD, Singer L. Fertility impairment in mice on a low fluoride intake. Science 1972;177:893–894.

Sulfur

Dietary deficiency of sulfur does not occur in monogastric animals, although they do have a dietary dependency on methionine, a sulfur-containing amino acid.

Cystine and cysteine are also metabolically required, sulfur-containing amino acids, but these can be synthesized from methionine.

Ruminants depend upon bacterial synthesis of methionine in the rumen, and therefore require a dietary source of sulfur. Ordinarily, most diets will contain adequate sulfur for this purpose. It has been shown, however, that when the diet contains increased levels of non-protein nitrogen—such as urea—the requirement for sulfur is higher and supplementation is necessary. Signs of deficiency are nonspecific and include loss of appetite, poor growth, reduced lactation, poor quality of wool, and weakness.

Sulfur rickets is known, sulfur being able to replace phosphorus in the mineral of bones. This has happened when animals have been fed large amounts of sulfur: for example, when sulfur is used as an anticoccidial drug in chickens.

Selenium

Selenium is an essential nutrient that is also highly toxic. It is discussed as a poison in Chapter 15. Selenium is a component of the enzyme glutathione peroxidase, which serves to capture peroxides and prevent them from damaging cell membranes. Vitamin E in cell membranes serves a similar function, but both are required. Selenium deficiency and vitamin E deficiency are so interrelated that it is usual to refer to the diverse group of disorders ascribed to their deficiencies as vitamin E-selenium deficiency (refer to section on Vitamin E).

The dietary requirements of selenium for most species is 0.1–0.3 ppm of diet (mg/kg). Toxic levels range from 2–10 ppm, and greater amounts are rapidly lethal. Toxic levels may be exceeded in some situations by parenteral use of commercial selenium-vitamin E prepartaions (Van Fleet et al., 1974).

References

Ammerman CB, Miller SM. Selenium in ruminant nutrition: a review. J Dairy Sci 1975;58:1561–1577.

Hidiroglou M, Jenkins KJ, Wauthy JM, et al. A note on the prevention of muscular dystrophy by winter silage feeding of the cow or selenium implantation of the calf. Anim Prod 1972;14:115–118.

Jenkins KJ, Hidiroglou M, Mackey RR, et al. Influence of selenium and linoleic acid on the development of nutritional muscular dystrophy in beef calves, lambs, and rabbits. Can J Anim Sci 1970;50:137–146.

National Academy of Sciences. Selenium in Nutrition. Washington DC: 1971.

Rotruck JT, et al. Selenium: biochemical role as a component of glutathione peroxidase. Science 1973;179:588–590.

Scott ML. The selenium dilemma. J Nutr 1973;103:803–810.

Van Vleet JF, Carlton W, Olander HJ. Hepatosis dietetica and mulberry heart disease associated with selenium deficiency in Indiana swine. J Am Vet Med Assoc 1970;157:1208–1219.

Van Vleet JF, Meyer KB, Olander HJ. Acute selenium toxicosis induced in baby pigs by parenteral administration of selenium-vitamin E preparations. J Am Vet Med Assoc 1974;165:543–547.

Van Vleet JF, Ruth G, Ferrans VJ. Ultrastructural alterations in skeletal muscle of pigs with selenium-vitamin E deficiency. Am J Vet Res 1976;37:911–922.

Van Vleet JF, Ruth GR. Efficacy of supplements in prevention of sele-nium-vitamin E deficiency in swine. Am J Vet Res 1977;38:1299–1305.

Iron

Iron is an essential component of hemoglobin, myoglobin, and the cytochromes; it is also a part of, or required for, the function of several other enzymes. Iron deficiency can arise from: a lack of iron in the diet; certain gastrointestinal disorders, such as steatorrhea, long-tanding diarrhea, and achlorhydria; and chronic blood loss. Although nutritional iron deficiency has been recognized for centuries, it is not frequent, except in humans and young pigs. Most foods contain adequate iron to meet needs; however, milk is low in iron, and piglets raised without access to soil or pasture will develop deficiency within 2–4 weeks of birth. When left untreated, it may lead to death. Piglets that survive for several weeks will recover when they supplement their diet with the sow's food. The classic feature of iron deficiency is a hypochromic, microcytic anemia. Affected piglets are unthrifty, have labored breathing, and may be edematous. At necropsy, mucous membranes are pale and the lungs are edematous; also, fluid exists in the pericardial sac, thorax, and abdomen. Deficiency of copper, which is necessary for the availability of iron for hemoglobin synthesis, will augment iron deficiency; conversely, diets increased in copper can interfere with iron absorption. Iron deficiency associated with milk diets is also sometimes seen in cattle, horses, and other species, but is much less common.

A hereditary, sex-linked gene in mice (gene symbol sla) results in hypochromic anemia that resembles anemia caused by dietary deficiency of iron. The gene-controlled defect leads to failure to transfer iron from the intestinal mucosal cell to the plasma. Ferritin, therefore, accumulates in the absorptive cell and in vacuoles, as well as free in the cytoplasm. Accumulation of this ferritin is associated with a decrease in the rough endoplasmic reticulum, and with an increase in the smooth endoplasmic reticulum (Bedard et al., 1971).

Tremendously excessive amounts of iron are stored in various tissues in hemochromatosis.

In humans, hemochromatosis can occur as a genetic defect termed idiopathic or primary hemochromatosis; it may also occur as secondary hemochromatosis arising from frequent transfusions, or possibly from prolonged consumption of excessive iron. In primary hemochromatosis, iron is deposited in a wide variety of tissues and somehow interferes with cellular function. In secondary hemochromatosis, the hemosiderin is largely restricted to macrophages and hepatocytes. In animals, hemochromatosis is rare. Excessive storage of iron is seen in animals with diseases characterized by frequent bouts of hemolytic anemia; on occasion, the excess iron may result from excessive iron consumption. The iron is deposited as hemosiderin in macrophages, hepatocytes, and renal epithelium. It may be associated with cirrhosis, but usually not.

Like sulfer, iron is able to enter the calcium phosphate compound of the bone and cause rickets (osteomalacia). The compound thus formed is $Fe_3(PO_4)^2$. The disorder has occurred in poultry. A similar displacement is also theoretically possible when aluminum, magnesium, or beryllium are in excess.

References

Bedard YC, Pinkerton PH, Simon GT. Ultrastructure of the duodenal mucosa of mice with a hereditary defect in iron absorption. J Pathol 1971;104:45–51.

Cook JD. Absorption of food iron. Fed Proc 1977;36:2028–2032.

Cusak RP, Brown WD. Achromotricia in iron-deficient rats. Nature 1964;204:582–583.

Finch CA, Huebers H. Perspectives in iron metabolism. N Engl J Med 1982;306:1520–1528.

Jacobs A. Serum ferritin and iron stores. Fed Proc 1977;36:2024–2027.

Linder MC, Munro HN. The mechanism of iron absorption and its regulation. Fed Proc 1977;36:2017–2023.

Lindvall S, Moberg G, Nordblom B. Studies of sudden fatalities among piglets following parenteral iron therapy. Acta Vet Scand 1972;13:206–217.

Moore RW, Redmond HE, Livingston CW Jr. Iron deficiency anemia as a cause of stillbirths in swine. J Am Vet Med Assoc 1965;147:746–748.

Munro HN. Iron absorption and nutrition. Fed Proc 1977;36:2015–2016.

Nath I, Sood SK, Nayak NC. Experimental siderosis and liver injury in the rhesus monkey. J Pathol 1972;106:103–112.

Scrimshaw NS. Iron deficiency. Sci Am 1991;265:46–52.

Copper

Deficiency of copper is seen in animals throughout the world. Simple dietary deficiency can be seen in any animal species fed milk—which is low in copper—for prolonged periods. In adult animals, especially cattle and sheep, copper deficiency may occur in animals raised on copper-deficient pastures. Copper deficiency in ruminants is usually more complex than a simple dietary deficiency. In these species the availability of copper is influenced by the level of both molybdenum and sulfur in the diet. In the rumen, sulfur is reduced to sulfide that, with molybdenum, forms thiomolybdate that in turn reacts with copper, forming an insoluble complex reducing copper absorption. Absorbed thiomolybdate also binds copper in plasma making it unavailable. Increased levels of sulfur, in the absence of significant molybdenum, can also lead to the formation of insoluble copper sulfide. Conversely, decreased levels of dietary molybdenum and sulfur increase availability of copper, and predispose to copper poisoning. Increased dietary copper will reduce tissue molybdenum. Increased levels of zinc in the diet of any species reduces the absorption of copper.

Copper is an essential component of many enzymes (metalloenzymes) that have a diversity of functions; hence, copper deficiency leads to effects on multiple organ systems. Copper-containing enzymes include cytochrome c oxidase, superoxide dismutase, dopamine-β-hydroxylase, lysyl oxidase, tyrosinase, ceruloplasmin, and thiol oxidase. The more important effects of copper deficiency include anemia, osteoporosis (and other defects in collagen and elastin), enzootic ataxia (or swayback), and achromotrichia.

ANEMIA

Copper is part of ceruloplasmin, which is synthesized in the liver from stored copper; it is also the plasma carrier of copper from the liver to other tissues. Ceruloplasmin is also required for the oxidation of ferrous iron to ferric iron; it is therefore required for the incorporation of iron into hemoglobin or myoglobin, because only ferric iron can serve this purpose. Copper deficiency thus leads to a microcytic, hypochromic anemia. Copper is also part of superoxide dismutase, a copper-zinc enzyme that serves to prevent damage to cell membranes by superoxide molecules. It is not clear, however, whether copper deficiency leads to increased destruction of red cells from deficiency of superoxide dismutase.

SKELETAL SYSTEM

Copper is an essential component of the enzyme, lysyl oxidase which is necessary for the cross-linking and maturation of collagen and elastin. In copper deficiency, failure of bone matrix formation results, leading to osteoporosis. The cartilaginous growth plate proliferates and calcifies normally, or may be slightly thickened; but osteoblastic activity stops or markedly declines, along with the reduced formation of osteoid. Affected bones are fragile and break easily. The lesions bear a remarkable resemblance to those of scurvy, and are in direct opposition to the changes of rickets. Copper deficiency is believed to be important to the pathogenesis of osteochondrosis in suckling foals.

The failure to form cross-linking in elastin leads to defective arterial walls that rupture or form aneurysms, especially of the aorta. Myocardial necrosis and rupture have also been reported in copper deficiency.

ENZOOTIC ATAXIA OR SWAYBACK

Disorders of the central nervous system arise in lambs, kids, and piglets born to copper-deficient dams. The disease may be evident at birth, or it may develop over a period of weeks or months after birth. In either case, signs in affected animals include incoordination and weakness of the posterior limbs, spastic paralysis, and sometimes blindness. A swaying of the hind quarters gives the disorder one of its names. The lesions are most pronounced in newborn lambs, and consist of demyelinization, extensive malacia or necrosis, and disappearance of much of the white matter in the central portions of the cerebral hemispheres and spinal cord. In the severest cases, little is left of the hemispheres except the cortical shell of grey matter. Milder forms involve only areas of symmetric demyelinization, with gitter cells, central chromatolysis, and karyorrhexis of neurons. Demyelinization and necrosis may also be found in the cerebellum and peripheral nerves, especially in kids.

The pathogenesis of this disorder is not understood. It is speculated that the lesions could arise from altered cellular respiration and reduced synthesis of phospholipid and therefore myelin, both stemming from a deficiency of cytochrome oxidase or failure of superoxide dismutase to capture free radicals. Copper deficiency also causes reduced dopamine-β-hydroxylase, which then results in decreased synthesis of noradrenaline and increased dopamine in tissues.

ACHROMOTRICHIA

Achromotrichia, or lack of pigmentation of hair, develops in all animals (including feathers of birds) that are deficient in copper owing to a deficiency of tyrosinase, which is required to convert tyrosine to melanin. A deficiency of thiol oxidase leads to defective keratinization; this is most evident in hair and wool. The enzymatic defect reduces disulfide and manifests as straight wool, termed steely wool.

Other abnormalities caused by copper deficiency include weight loss, diarrhea, fetal resorption, and depressed humoral and cellular immunity. In cattle, a disease termed falling disease is characterized by sudden death with multifocal myocardial necrosis and fibrosis, and has been attributed to copper deficiency.

WILSON DISEASE

Wilson disease (hepatolenticular degeneration) in humans is an autosomal-recessive disorder of copper metabolism, in which copper is not transported from the liver into the circulation as ceruloplasmin or excreted into bile (usual route of excretion). Serum ceruloplasmin is decreased and stores of lysosomal hepatic copper are increased; circulating nonceruloplasmin copper that is loosely bound to albumin increases, along with urinary excretion of copper. The precise defect is not known, but it is postulated that the decreased ceruloplasmin synthesis by hepatocytes is not the primary defect; instead, it results from hepatotoxicity of excessive cellular copper which, for some reason, is not released from lysosomes and excreted in the bile. Signs and lesions of the disease usually do not become apparent until patients are five years of age or older. The hepatic changes are characterized by fatty change, necrosis, and cirrhosis. The increased nonceruloplasmin copper leads to increased tissue copper concentrations in many different organs, with associated tissue damage. Of particular concern is progressive cerebral damage, particularly of the basal ganglia. Another feature is the development of Kayser-Fleischer rings in the cornea, which represent deposits of copper in Descemet's membrane at the limbus. Bedlington terriers suffer a similar disorder that is also inherited as an autosomal recessive trait; however, it is estimated that fully two-thirds of all Bedlington terriers are affected. In contrast to Wilson's disease, circulating levels of ceruloplasmin are elevated. Hepatic copper levels are increased, and in older dogs chronic hepatitis and cirrhosis develop. Specific lesions in brain have not been described; how-

ever, increased aggressiveness has been described in dogs.

MENKES DISEASE

Menkes disease is an X-linked recessive disorder of humans, in which defective intestinal absorption of copper occurs, leading to copper deficiency. The disease is also known as kinky hair disease because the hair becomes like steel wool. Similar inherited disorders exist in mice; a condition has also been described in which inbred Alaskan Malamutes appear to suffer a similar autosomal recessive trait, causing a defect in copper absorption. The presenting sign in these dogs focuses on the effect of copper deficiency on the skeleton; affected dogs develop a chondrodysplasia, which leads to dwarfism (see also zinc).

The toxicosis of excess copper is discussed in Chapter 15.

References

Barlow RM, Field AC, Ganson NC. Measurement of nerve cell damage in the spinal cord of lambs affected with swayback. J Comp Pathol 1964;74:530–541.
Brewer NR. Comparative metabolism of copper. J Am Vet Med Assoc 1987;190:654–658.
Bridges CH, Womack JE, Harris ED, et al. Considerations of copper metabolism in osteochondrosis of suckling foals. J Am Vet Med Assoc 1984;185:173–178.
Bull LB, et al. Ataxia in young lambs. Bull Council Sci Indust Res Aust 1938;113:72.
Cancilla PA, Barlow RM. Structural changes of the central nervous system in swayback (enzootic ataxia) of lambs. II. Electron microscopy of the lower motor neuron. III. Electron microscopy of the cerebral lesions. Acta Neuropathol 1966;6:251–259, 260–265.
Cancilla PA, Barlow RM. Experimental copper deficiency in miniature swine: biochemistry, histochemistry, and pathology of the central nervous system. J Comp Pathol 1966;80:315–319.
Chalmers GA. Swayback (enzootic ataxia) en Alberta lambs. Can J Comp Med 1974;38:111–117.
Cordy DR, Knight HD. California goats with a disease resembling enzootic ataxia or swayback. Vet Pathol 1978;15:179–185.
Coulson WF, et al. Cardiovascular system in naturally occurring copper deficiency and swayback in sheep. Am J Vet Res 1967;27:815–818.
Goodrich RD, Tilman AD. Copper, sulfate, and molybdenum interrelationships in sheep. J Nutr 1966;90:76–80.
Gumbrell RC. Suspected copper deficiency in a group of full sib Samoyed dogs. NZ Vet J 1972;20:238–240.
Hoag GN, Brown RG, Smart ME, et al. Alaskan Malamute chondrodysplasia. VI. Copper absorption studies. Can Vet J 1977;18:349–351.
Howell J, Davison AN, Oxberry J. Observations on the lesions in the white matter of the spinal cord of swayback sheep. Acta Neuropathol 1969;12:33–41.
Huisungh J, Gomez GG, Matrone G. Interactions of copper, molybdenum, and sulfate in ruminant nutrition. Fed Proc 1973;32:1921–1924.
Innes JRM, Shearer GD. "Swayback", a semyelinating disease of lambs with affinities to Schilder's encephalitis in man. J Comp Pathol Ther 1940;53:1–41.
Irwin MR, Poulos PW Jr, Smith BP, et al. Radiology and histopathol-

ogy of lameness in young cattle with secondary copper deficiency. J Comp Pathol 1974;84:611–621.

Keen CL, Hurley LS. Copper supplementation in quaking mice: reduced tremors and increased brain copper. Science 1976;193:244–245.

Kincaid SA, Carlton WW. Experimental copper deficiency in laboratory mice. Lab Anim Sci 1982;32:491–494.

Leigh LC. Changes in the ultrastructure of cardiac muscle in steers deprived of copper. Res Vet Sci 1975;18:282–287.

Lewis G, Terlecki S, Allcroft R. The occurrence of swayback in the lambs of ewes fed a semi-purified diet of low copper content. Vet Rec 1967;81:415–416.

Lewis G, Terlecki S, Parker BNJ. Observations on the pathogenesis of delayed swayback. Vet Rec 1974;95:313–316.

McGavin MD, Ranby PD, Tammimagi L. Demyelination associated with low liver copper levels in pigs. Aust Vet J 1962;38:8–14.

Owen EC, et al. Pathological and biochemical studies of an outbreak of swayback in goats. J Comp Pathol 1965;75:241–251.

Rucker RB, Parker HE, Rogler JC. Effect of copper deficiency on chick bone collagen and selected bone enzymes. J Nutr 1969;98:57–63.

Shields GS, Coulson WF, Kimball DA, et al. Studies on copper metabolism. XXXII. Cardiovascular lesions in copper-deficient swine. Am J Pathol 1962;41:603–621.

Simpson CF, Harms RH. Pathology of the aorta of chicks fed a copper-deficient diet. Exp Molec Pathol 1964;3:390–400.

Su L-E, Owen CA Jr, Zollman PE, et al. A defect of biliary excretion of copper in copper-laden Bedlington terriers. Am J Physiol 1982;243:G231–G236.

Su L-E, Ravanshad S, Owen CA Jr, et al. A comparison of copper-loading disease in Bedlington terriers and Wilson's disease in humans. Am J Physiol 1982;243:G226–G230.

Suttle NF, Field AC, Barlow RM. Experimental copper deficiency in sheep. J Comp Pathol 1970;80:151–162.

Thornburg LP, Rottinghaus G, McGowan M, et al. Hepatic copper concentrations in purebred and mixed-breed dogs. Vet Pathol 1990;27:81–88.

Waisman J, Carnes WH. Cardiovascular studies on copper-deficient swine. X. The fine structure of the defective elastic membranes. Am J Pathol 1967;51:117–135.

Waisman J, Carnes WH, Weissman N. Some properties of the microfibrils of vascular elastic membranes in normal and copper-deficient swine. Am J Pathol 1969;54:107–119.

Weiner G. Genetic and other factors in the occurrence of swayback in sheep. J Comp Pathol 1966;76:435–447.

Cobalt

Cobalt is required for the synthesis of vitamin B12 (discussed earlier in this chapter), and therefore is only a dietary requirement for those species which synthesize their vitamin B12 in the gastrointestinal tract. These include the ruminants, horses, rabbits, and most herbivores. Those species that require a dietary source of vitamin B12, such as dogs, cats and swine, do not have a requirement for cobalt. Deficiency of cobalt in ruminants is primarily restricted to grazing animals, and has no characteristic features. It is essentially a wasting disease accompanied by an anemia. Rather than a megaloblastic anemia, as seen in humans, the anemia is normocytic and normochromic. Various disorders—such as "Grand Traverse disease" of the American Great Lakes region; "pine" in England; "hill sickness" in New Zealand; "coast disease," "wasting disease," and "enzootic marasmus" in Australia; and "Nakuruitis" in Kenya—are examples of cachectic syndromes in cattle and

sheep due to cobalt deficiency. They are characterized by poor appetite, weakness, and general wasting. Without supplementation the animals will ultimately die. Specific lesions are not present, although hemosiderosis occurs in the liver, spleen, and kidneys; this condition represents a storage of iron that should, but cannot, be utilized. Fatty change of the liver is prominent, especially in sheep. In the latter, what is believed to be cobalt deficiency has been termed "ovine white-liver disease". Demyelination of peripheral nerves is also described. Although horses and most other herbivores require dietary cobalt, their efficiency in producing vitamin B12 appears to preclude cobalt deficiency, unless the diet is entirely void of this element.

Cobalt has been described in one report as effective in prevention of cerbrocortical necrosis in sheep. This effect is believed to work through stimulation of rumenal bacteria; these bacteria produce thiamine or inhibit production of thiaminase.

References

Andres ED, Hart LI, Stephenson BJ. Vitamin B12 and cobalt concentrations in livers from healthy and cobalt-deficient lambs. Nature 1958;182:869–870.

Decker DE, Smith LE. The metabolism of cobalt in lambs. J Nutr 1951;43:87–100.

Filmer JF. Enzootic marasmus of cattle and sheep. Aust Vet J 1933;9:163–179.

Filmer JF, Underwood EJ. Enzootic marasmus: treatment with limonite fractions. Aust Vet J 1934;10:83–87.

Ibbotson RN, Allen SH, Gurney CW. An abnormality of the bone marrow of sheep fed cobalt-deficient hay chaff. Aust J Exp Biol Med Sci 1970;48:161–169.

Keener HA, Percival GP, Morrow KS. Cobalt deficiency in New Hampshire with sheep. J Anim Sci 1948;7:16–25.

MacPherson A, Moon FE, Voss RC. Biochemical aspects of cobalt deficiency in sheep with special reference to vitamin status and a possible involvement in the aetiology of cerebrocortical necrosis. Br Vet J 1976;132:294–308.

Tokarnia CH, et al. Cobalt deficiency in cattle in the state of Ceara, Brazil (TT). Arq Inst Biol Anim Rio de J 1963;4:195–202.

Underwood EJ. Cobalt. Nutr Rev 1975;33:65–69.

Wessels CC. Cobalt in relation to ruminant nutrition in South Africa. J S Afr Vet Med Assoc 1961;32:289–312.

Manganese

Manganese is a component of arginase, pyruvate carboxylase, and manganese-superoxide dismutase, and is an activator of several hydrolases, decarboxylases, and transferases. Experimentally, manganese deficiency has been induced in a number of animal species. Although it has been described in grazing cattle and poultry, deficiency is not common in domestic animals under normal conditions.

A variety of different lesions develops. One of the most striking and characteristic is abnormal bone growth; this has been described both experimentally in laboratory animals, swine, and cattle, and in natural deficiency in cattle, poultry, and possibly swine. Reduced activity of glycosyl-transferases interferes with synthesis of proteoglycan and cartilage. This leads to a form of chondrodystrophy, in which bones are shortened and grossly deformed; they may be twisted and weakened, and the joints may be enlarged. Osteoblastic and osteoclastic activity are also reportedly impaired. In chickens, this is one of the forms of perosis (slippage of the Achilles tendon), which can also be caused by deficiency of choline, biotin, or niacin. A unique feature of impaired cartilaginous matrix formation is seen in offspring of animals born manganese-deficient. Defective formation of the otoliths leads to impaired function of the inner ear, which manifests as irreversible ataxia and incoordination.

In guinea pigs, hypoplasia of the pancreas occurs, and in rats impaired synthesis of insulin results. Lipoprotein metabolism is also altered, and disruption of cellular membranes has been ascribed to either altered lipid content or deficiency of manganese-superoxide dismutase. Other more general features include weight loss, muscular weakness, small birth weights, and irregular estrus cycles.

References

Amdur MO, Norris LC, Heuser GF. The need for manganese in bone development by the rat. Proc Soc Exp Biol Med 1945;59:254–255.

Barnes LL, Sperling G, Maynard LA. Bone development in the albino rat on a low manganese diet. Proc Soc Exp Biol Med 1941;46:562–565.

Miller RC, et al. Manganese as a possible factor influencing the occurrence of lameness in pigs. Proc Soc Exp Biol Med 1940;45:50–51.

Neher GM, et al. Radiographic and histopathological findings in the bones of swine deficient in manganese. Am J Vet Res 1956;17:121–128.

Oliver JW. Interrelationships between athyreotic and manganese-deficient states in rats. Am J Vet Res 1976;37:597–600.

Rojas MA, Dyer IA, Cassatt WA. Manganese deficiency in the bovine. J Anim Sci 1965;24:664–667.

Zinc

Deficiency of zinc affects many different enzyme systems, including those that concern the synthesis of DNA, RNA, and protein; carbonic dehydrogenase, alkaline phosphatase, alcohol dehydrogenase, and scores of others. Deficiency then is expressed in a variety of disturbances of growth and repair; however, the pathogenesis of the various findings is not clear. Zinc is a component of the enzyme superoxide dismutase (which also contains copper and manganese), and failure to scavenge free radicals may in part explain some of the lesions. Zinc is also involved in vitamin A metabolism; deficient animals may exhibit night blindness and

photophobia. The mechanism is two fold: zinc is necessary for the formation of retinal binding protein; and it is part of the alcohol dehydrogenase necessary for conversion of vitamin A alcohol (retinol) to vitamin A aldehyde (retinal). In experimental deficiency in pregnant rats, the rate of fetal resorption is increased, and pups are born with microphthalmia or anophthalmia. The predominant clinical and pathologic expression in animals, however, is parakeratosis and thymic and lymphoid atrophy. Deficiency is most common in swine, but is also recognized in dogs, cats, cattle, sheep, and goats. Diets high in phytate significantly reduce the availability of zinc.

PARAKERATOSIS

Parakeratosis of swine, first described by Kernkamp and Ferrin (1953), is now accepted as the result of zinc deficiency. Although the exact circumstances that bring about zinc deficiency in swine are not entirely understood, it has been shown that excess dietary calcium interferes with zinc absorption. The addition of zinc to the ration, as well as adjusting calcium intake, dramatically cures or prevents parakeratosis. Available evidence suggests that calcium, in conjunction with either phytate or phosphate, forms a complex with zinc, making it unavailable for absorption.

Parakeratosis usually appears in young swine 10–20 weeks of age and is manifest by circumscribed erythematous areas, 3–5 cm in diameter; these occur particularly in the skin of the abdomen, medial surfaces of the thighs over joints of the lower limbs, the ears, around the mouth, and on the tail. These affected areas soon become elevated and scaly, and the lesions become widespread, with a symmetric distribution. The surface layer of keratin becomes increasingly thick, rough, horny, and fissured. The hairs are not lost, but are often entangled and matted in the superficial horny material. The appetite may be impaired and the rate of gain somewhat reduced, but often signs are inconstant and not specific.

The microscopic appearance of the affected skin is dominated by parakeratosis and acanthosis, with elongation and congestion of dermal papillae and disappearance of the stratum granulosum. In the thick, horny parakeratotic layer, retained nuclei are usually seen in undulating, irregular rows; sometimes the nuclei are mixed with cellular debris. In some areas, the stratum germinativum is thinner than normal, but acanthosis appears to be the rule. Hyperplasia also occurs, as well as an increase in the thickness of the parakeratotic layers of the oral mucosa and esophagus.

In cattle, sheep and goats, dietary zinc deficiency is shown to lead to parakeratosis, as well as to abnormal growth of horn and hoof in sheep. The lesions of the skin have a distribution comparable to those in swine, with greatest severity around the eyes and mouth, on the neck, inside the legs, and over the lower leg joints. Parakeratosis and hyperkeratosis occurs throughout the fore-stomachs. Joints are enlarged and the animals assume a peculiar bow-legged stance and an arched back. Anorexia and failure to gain proper weight results. Testicular hypoplasia or atrophy is also reported; this tendency has been seen in experimental zinc deficiency in laboratory rodents. Microscopically, failure of maturation of spermatogonia is apparent. Facial eczema, a disease of cattle described in New Zealand, manifests as eczema on the face and other parts of the body, weight loss, and occasionally death. Eczema responds favorably to dietary supplementation with zinc. Infectious pododermatitis of cattle is also reported to respond to oral zinc.

In cattle, an autosomal-recessive disorder occurs called **hereditary thymic hypoplasia,** or lethal trait A-46, in which the absorption of zinc is impaired. The disorder was first described in black pied Danish cattle of Friesian descent; it has since been described in Friesian cattle in Great Britain and Europe, and in shorthorn calves in the United States. Signs first appear in calves between two and eight weeks after birth, and will progress to death within six months when not treated. The condition is characterized by cutaneous exanthema, gastroenteritis, and thymic hypoplasia; it is analogous to a disease in humans termed **acrodermatitis enteropathica,** which is also inherited as an autosomal recessive lethal disease. Although absorption of zinc is impaired, it is not absolute, and providing oral supplementation can prevent or reverse the disorder in cattle and humans. In the disease in humans, it has been shown that zinc in cows milk is less available for absorption than zinc in human milk. In addition to parakeratotic skin lesions comparable to those described above, marked hypoplasia of the thymus, spleen, and lymph nodes results. The associated immunodeficiency leads to the occurrence of secondary infections, such as bronchopneumonia. The pathogenesis of the thymic and lymphoid hypoplasia is not understood; however, it is also a feature of experimental dietary zinc deficiency in several species. In bull terriers, a disorder exists termed lethal acrodermatitis, which is similar to lethal trait A46 in cattle or acrodermatitis enteropathica in humans. It is inherited as an autosomal-recessive trait, and is also characterized by parakeratosis and hypoplasia of the thymus and lymphoid tissues. Although plasma zinc levels are decreased, the disease does not respond to oral zinc supplementation.

There are a number of reports of zinc-responsive dermatosis in dogs. These cases fall into two broad groups that have been interpreted as two different syndromes; however, it is not known yet whether they truly are different.. The first group occurs in rapidly growing puppies of any breed raised on zinc-deficient diets, or on diets containing excessive calcium or phytates (which interfere with zinc absorption). In the second group, lesions do not develop until puberty or later, and are predominantly confined to Siberian huskies, Alaskan malamutes, Great Danes, and Doberman pinschers. In both circumstances, the disease is characterized by parakeratosis, especially of the head and limbs. Both respond to zinc supplementation, but when the disorder occurs in adult dogs, relapse may occur when supplementation is not continued.

Another disorder of Alaskan malamutes has a zinc connection. Hereditary autosomal-recessive chondrodysplasia leads to dwarfism in this species which is due to a defect in copper absorption. One feature of the disorder is delayed sexual maturity. This is associated with acrosomal defects in spermatozoa , an effect that is reversed with oral zinc supplementation. These animals do not have parakeratosis.

References

Andresen E, Flagstad T, Basse A, et al. Evidence of a lethal trait, A 46, in black pied Danish cattle of Friesian descent. Nord Vet Med 1970;22:473–485.

Blackmon DM, Miller WJ, Morton JD. Zinc deficiency in ruminants: occurrence, effects, diagnosis, treatments. Vet Med 1967;62:265–270.

Brown RG, Hoag GN, Smart ME, et al. Alaskan Malamute chondrodysplasia. V. Decreased gut zinc absorption. Growth 1978;42:1–6.

Brummerstedt E, Flagstad T, Basse A, et al. The effect of zinc on calves with hereditary thymus hypoplasia. Acta Pathol Microbiol Scand 1971;79A:686–687.

Degryse A-D, Fransen J, Van Cutsem J, et al. Recurrent zinc-responsive dermatosis in a Siberian Husky. J Small Anim Pract 1987;28:721–726.

Demertzis PN, Mills CF. Oral zinc therapy in the control of infectious pododermatitis in young bulls. Vet Rec 1973;93:219–222.

Fadok VA. Zinc responsive dermatosis in a Great Dane: a case report. J Am Anim Assoc 1982;18:409–414.

Flagstad T. Lethal trait A 46 in cattle: intestinal zinc absorption. Nord Vet Med 1976;28:160–169.

Jezyk PF, Haskins ME, McKay-Smith WE, et al. Lethal acrodermatitis in Bull Terriers. J Am Vet Med Assoc 1986;188:833– 839.

Kane E, Morris JG, Rogers QR, et al. Zinc deficiency in the cat. J Nutr 1981;111:488–495.

Kernkamp HCH, Ferrin EF. Parakeratosis in swine. J Am Vet Med Assoc 1953;123:217–220.

Kroneman J, van der Mey GJM, Helder A. Hereditary zinc deficiency in Dutch Friesian cattle. Zentralbl Veterinaermed 1975;22A:201–208.

Macapinlaf MP, et al. Production of zinc deficiency in the squirrel monkey (Saimiri sciureus). J Nutr 1967;93:499–510.

Miller JK, Miller WJ. Experimental zinc deficiency and recovery of calves. J Nutr 1962;76:47–474.

Miller WJ. Dynamics of absorption rates, endogenous excretion, tissue turnover, and homeostatic control mechanisms of zinc, cadmium, manganese, and nickel in ruminants. Fed Proc 1973;32:1915–1920.

Miller WJ, Pitts WJ, Clifton CM, et al. Experimentally produced zinc deficiency in the goat. J Dairy Sci 1964;47:556–559.

Mills CF, et al. The production and signs of zinc deficiency in the sheep. Proc Nutr Soc 1965;24:21–22.

Mills CF, Dalgarno AC, Williams RB, et al. Zinc deficiency and the zinc requirements of calves and lambs. Br J Nutr 1967;21:751–768.

Nelson DR, Wolff WA, Blodgett DJ, et al. Zinc deficiency in sheep and goats: three field cases. J Am Vet Med Assoc 1984;184:1480–1485.

Norrdin RW, Krook L, Pond WG, et al. Experimental zinc deficiency in weanling pigs on high and low calcium diets. Cornell Vet 1973;63:264–290.

Oberleas D, Muhrer ME, O'Dell BL. Effects of phytic acid on zinc availability and parakeratosis in swine. J Anim Sci 1962;21:57–61.

O'Dell BL. Symposium: History and status of zinc in nutrition. Fed Proc 1984;43:2821–2839.

Ohlen B, Scott DW. Zinc-responsive dermatitis in puppies. Canine Pract 1986;13:6–10.

Perryman LE, et al. Lymphocyte alterations in zinc-deficient calves with lethal trait A46. Vet Immunol Immunopathol 1989;21:239–248.

Pierson RE. Zinc deficiency in young lambs. J Am Vet Med Assoc 1966;149:1279–1282.

Price J, Wood DA. Zinc responsive parakeratosis and ill-thrift in a Friesian calf. Vet Rec 1982;110:478.

Reuter R, Bowden M, Besier B, et al. Zinc responsive alopecia and hyperkeratosis in Angora goats. Aust Vet J 1967;64:351–352.

Rickard BF. Facial eczema: zinc responsiveness in dairy cattle. NZ Vet J 1975;23:41–42.

Robertson BT, Burns MJ. Zinc metabolism and the zinc-deficiency syndrome in the dog. Am J Vet Res 1963;24:997–1002.

Russell RM, Cox ME, Solomons N. Zinc and the special senses. Ann Intern Med 1983;99:227–239.

Sanecki RK, Corbin JE, Forbes RM. Tissue changes in dogs fed a zinc-deficient ration. Am J Vet Res 1982;43:1642–1646.

Sanecki RK, Corbin JE, Forbes RM. Extracutaneous histologic changes accompanying zinc deficiency in pups. Am J Vet Res 1985;46:2120–2123.

Smith JC Jr. The vitamin A-zinc connection: a review. Ann NY Acad Sci 1980;355:62–75.

Sousa CA, Stannard AA, Ihrke PJ, et al. Dermatosis associated with feeding generic dog food: 13 cases (1981–1982). J Am Vet Med Assoc 1988;192:676–680.

Suliman HB, Abdelrahim AI, Zakia AM, et al. Zinc deficiency in sheep: field cases. Trop Anim Health Prod 1988;20:47–51.

Tucker HF, Salmon WD. Parakeratosis or zinc deficiency in the pig. Proc Soc Exp Biol Med 1955;88:613–616.

Vallee BL. Biochemistry, physiology, and pathology of zinc. Physiol Rev 1959;39:443–490.

van Adrichem PWM, van Leeuwen JM, van Kluijve JJ. Parakeratosis of the skin in calves. Neth J Vet Sci 1971;4:57–63.

van den Broek AHM, Stafford WL. Diagnostic value of zinc concentrations in serum, leucocytes and hair of dogs with zinc-responsive dermatosis. Res Vet Sci 1988;44:41–44.

van den Broek AHM, Thoday KL. Skin disease in dogs associated with zinc deficiency: a report of five cases. J Small Anim Pract 1986;27:313–323.

Vogt DW, Carlton CG, Miller RB. Hereditary parakeratosis in Shorthorn beef calves. Am J Vet Res 1988;49:120–121.

Weisman K, Flagstad T. Hereditary zinc deficiency (adema disease) in cattle, an animal parallel to acrodermatitis enteropathica. Acta Derm Venereol 1976;56:151–154.

Molybdenum

Molybdenum is a component of several enzymes, including: aldehyde oxidase, which concerns the detoxification of pyrimidines, purines, and pteridines; xanthine oxidase, which converts hypoxanthine to xanthine and xanthine to uric acid; and sulfite oxidase, which concerns the transformation of sulfite to sulfate. Specific molybdenum deficiency states do not occur naturally in domestic animals, with the possible exception of chickens. Experimental deficiency has been induced in several different species, with a variety of nonspecific findings. Tungsten is an antagonist of molybedenum and has been used to aggravate experimental deficiency.

Iodine

The halogen iodine is an indispensable nutrient that is an essential component of the thyroid hormones. It has no other function. Largely ingested as iodides, iodine is rapidly transported to the thyroid gland, where it is oxidized by thyroid peroxidase to iodine, and combined with tyrosine to form monoiodotyrosine, diiodotyrosine, triiodothyronine (T3), and tetraiodothyroxine (T4; thyroxine). Thyroglobulin, or colloid, is the storage form of these hormones.

Iodine deficiency occurs worldwide. Certain areas where the soil and water are especially low in iodine are known as endemic goitrogenic regions. These include the Great Lakes region and Pacific Northwest in the United States, the Swiss Alps, and parts of the Andes. In addition to simple deficiency, a number of dietary substances exist, referred to as goitrogens, which interfere with various steps in iodine metabolism and thyroxine synthesis and release. The effect of goitrogens, which is analogous to iodine deficiency, can be mediated through (1) interference with the uptake of iodine by the thyroid, (2) interference with oxidation of iodate to iodine by thyroid peroxidase and its subsequent organification, (3) interference with hormone secretion, (4) increased metabolism of thyroid hormone, and (5) interference with monodeiodinase, which converts T4 to T3. A partial list of goitrogens is presented in Table 16-2.

GOITER

Deficiency of iodine causes goiter, a compensatory hypertrophy and hyperplasia of the thyroid, which may be accompanied by other signs and lesions. The histopathologic features of the thyroid are presented in Chapter 26 (The Endocrine System). For signs other than enlargement of the thyroid to appear in adult animals, a deficiency of iodine must exist for months to over a year. Even then, signs may be minimal. They include anorexia, lethargy, dry scaly skin, rough and reduced hair or wool, and myxedema. Iodine deficiency is much more pronounced in the young and newborn. The deficiency also may be recognized as reproductive failure, characterized by fetal resorption, abortion, stillbirth, or birth of weak young. The thyroid of the dam is often enlarged and the goiters in the newborn are usually of conspicuous size. Newborns may have little hair and, if they survive, develop poorly and die prematurely.

A significant excess of absorbed iodine produces the condition known as iodism. This occurs when iodine or its compounds are administered internally or externally in maximal dosages over a period of time. It is characterized by depression, anorexia, poor development, lacrimation, and dry scaly skin with exfoliation of a dandruff-like material. In part, iodism is the result of hypothyroidism caused by the decreased release of thyroid hormones brought about by increased circulating levels of iodides.

TABLE 16-2 **Goitrogens and their mechanism of action and sources**

Interfere with uptake of iodine by the thyroid

Thiocyanate, isothiocyanate	Cassava, millet, cabbage, turnip
Thiooxazolidone	Brassica seed, sweet potatoes

Interfere with iodide oxidation by thyroid peroxidase and organification of iodine

Sulfonamides	
Disulfides	Onion, garlic
Thiourea, cyanogenic glycosides	
Flavonoids	Millet, sorghum, beans, groundnut
Pyridines	Mimosine in *Leucaena leucocephala*
Resorcinol, phenolics, dihydroxybenzoic acid	

Interfere with hormone secretion

Iodide, lithium

Increase metabolism of thyroid hormone

Phenobarbitol, benzodiazepines, calcium channel blockers, chlorinated hydrocarbons, polyhalogenated biphenyls

Interfere with monodeionase

FD&C Red No. 3, amiodarone, iopannic acid

References

Andrews FN, et al. Iodine deficiency in new-born sheep and swine. J Anim Sci 1948;7:298–310.

Capen CC. Pathophysiology of chemical injury to the thyroid gland. Toxicol Lett 1992;64/65:381–388.

Evvard JM. Iodine deficiency symptoms and their significance in animal nutrition and pathology. Endocrinology 1928;12:539–590.

Gaitan E. Goitrogens in food and water. Annu Rev Nutr 1990;10:21–39.

Amino Acids

Monogastric animals require a dietary source of protein to provide the essential (indispensable) amino acids (Table 16-3). These amino acids, along with the nonessential (dispensable) amino acids, are required for protein synthesis and a diversity of other functions. The division into essential and nonessential amino acids is traditional and demonstrable experimentally; however, diseases which disrupt metabolism may compromise the synthesis of certain nonessential amino acids in animals. Newborns may require a dietary source above that required by adults. This has led to the introduction of such terms as "conditionally indispensable" or "semi-indispensable." There also are species variations—for example, cats—which are unable to synthesize adequate taurine.

Deficiency

Deficiency of single amino acids is rare; however, several common farm feeds are moderately deficient in certain essential amino acids and may cause problems when fed alone. Indian corn (maize) is especially deficient in lysine and trytophan; other grains, linseed meal, and cotton-seed meal are less so in descending order. Peanuts are deficient in methionine, and soybeans less so. The principal signs of deficiency of amino acids in general are hypoproteinemia, anemia, poor growth, and delayed healing of wounds.

FELINE TAURINE DEFICIENCY

Taurine (β-aminoethanesulfonic acid) is an amino acid that most species synthesize from methionine and cysteine. In cats, this process is inadequate to meet the metabolic requirements; this is due to decreased activity of cysteine sulfinate decarboxylase, one of the enzymes required for conversion of cysteine to taurine. Cats also rely exclusively on taurine to conjugate bile acids. Ordinarily, meat contains ample taurine to meet requirements; however, certain commercial rations based largely on cereals are deficient. Taurine is absent from the plant kingdom. It is present in most animal cells, with increased concentrations in brain and muscle. Milk is low in taurine. The identification of taurine deficiency was first observed in cats fed a semipurified diet with casein as the protein source. The function of taurine is not fully understood, but it is believed to play a role in membrane transport of calcium, stabilizing membranes, and as an inhibitory neurotransmitter. It is important for the conjugation of bile acids, and is the only amino acid that conjugates bile acids in cats. Taurine is an amino acid that is not incorporated into protein.

Taurine deficiency in cats is characterized by multiple defects. The two principal conditions are **feline central retinal degeneration** and **dilated cardiomyopathy.** Feline central retinal degeneration is characterized by photoreceptor cell degeneration which, when not corrected early, leads to irreversible blindness. Cone cells are the first to be affected, but ultimately the rod cells also degenerate. The lesion begins in the central retina and, with time, extends peripherally. Another feature is loss of the membranes surrounding the intracytoplasmic inclusions in the tapetum.

TABLE 16-3 **Essential amino acids**

Histidine (during growth)
Isoleucine
Methionine
  Cystine can partially replace methionine
Phenylalanine
  Tyrosine can partially replace phenylalanine
Threonine
Tryptophan
Valine
Taurine (cats)
Carnitine
  Synthesized from methionine and lysine, but may be inadequate in dogs
Arginine (cats and dogs)

Dilated cardiomyopathy or taurine deficiency cardiomyopathy is another outcome of feline taurine deficiency, but requires longer to develop than the retinal degeneration. Cardiomyopathy results from a failure of contractility, with an associated decreased cardiac output and congestive heart failure. It is suggested that it is a consequence of an abnormal calcium ion balance in the myofibers. The affected heart has thin flabby walls with dilated chambers. Fibrosis of the myocardium may occur, but often no demonstrable microscopic finding exists.

Taurine deficiency also leads to fetal death and birth of weak kittens that fail to grow. In addition, fetal malformations may develop, including dysplasia of the cerebellar granular layer, which causes a spastic posterior paresis. Immune function may also be impaired. Cats are subject to an increased incidence of purulent inflammatory processes.

CARNITINE DEFICIENCY

Carnitine is an amino acid that ordinarily is synthesized from methionine and lysine; it is questionable whether most species require a dietary source. In humans and dogs, however, it appears that under some circumstances biosynthesis is not adequate to meet metabolic requirements. Carnitine functions in the transport of long-chain fatty acids into mitochondria, enabling them to enter the pathway of β-oxidation and ketone synthesis. Long-chain fatty acids, after activation to acyl-coenzyme A (CoA) esters at the outer mitochondrial membrane, must be transesterified by carnitine palmitoyl-transferase type 1 to form long-chain fatty acylcarnitine at the inner mitochondrial membrane. They are then transported into the mitochondria by carnitine acylcarnitine translocase. The enzyme carnitine palmitoyl-transferase type 2 then releases carnitine, and converts acylcarnitine back to acyl-CoA to enter the β-oxidation pathway. Deficiency of carnitine thus results in the failure of energy production, the accumulation of triglycerides in cells, and the intracellular accumulation of toxic acyl-CoA compounds. Most body carnitine lies within skeletal and cardiac muscle, both of which depend on long-chain fatty acids as a source of energy. Deficiency has been identified in humans and dogs. In humans, several genetic or familial disorders occur that affect carnitine metabolism, but not its biosynthesis. These include primary carnitine deficiency syndromes in which a defect occurs in the plasma membrane transporter of carnitine; this defect leads to failure of carnitine to enter into cells, failure of intestinal absorption, or failure of renal tubular reabsorption. Primary carnitine deficiency occurs in (1) myopathic form, characterized by skeletal muscular weakness, and (2) systemic form, characterized primarily by cardiomyopathy. Both are responsive to carnitine therapy. Secondary carnitine deficiency syndromes have also been identified, in which metabolic defects result, which lead to either increased utilization and loss of carnitine, or deficiencies of carnitine palmitoyl-transferase types 1 and 2 and carnitine acylcarnitine translocase. Secondary carnitine

deficiency is less responsive to carnitine supplementation. In both situations, fasting aggravates the disorder. Carnitine deficiency is characterized by cardiomyopathy, myopathy, and hepatic encephalopathy caused by fasting hypoketotic hypoglycemia. Depending on the syndrome, these lesions may appear singly or in combination.

Cardiomyopathy In dogs, a cardiomyopathy has been described in boxers. This condition appears to be a hereditary disorder that affects carnitine metabolism; it is believed to interfere with the transport of carnitine into the myocardium. Cardiomyopathy resembles primary systemic carnitine deficiency in humans. A similar disorder may exist in Doberman pinschers. Various forms of hypertrophic and dilated cardiomyopathies also occur in other breeds—especially the large breed dogs—but it is not known if these are related to carnitine deficiency. The disease of boxers is characterized by myocardial degeneration, which begins as fatty change and progresses to necrosis of myofibers, and their replacement by fibrous connective tissue and fatty infiltration. A mild mononuclear infiltrate occurs. The lesions are most severe in the right ventricular wall, but all portions of the heart are affected. Changes in skeletal muscle and neurologic signs, as seen in humans, have not been described.

ARGININE

Arginine is one of the semi-indispensable amino acids; growing animals require a dietary source of arginine, and adults are capable of its biosynthesis. Cats and, to a lesser extent, dogs appear to require arginine as adults. Experimentally, arginine-deficient diets lead to hyperammonemia, a variety of neurologic signs, and death. Experimental deficiency of **tryptophan,** a precursor of niacin, results in alopecia, cataracts, corneal vascularization, necrosis of skeletal muscle, and fatty change in the liver. **Methionine** deficiency also results in fatty change of the liver; this is believed to result from its role in choline synthesis. **Lysine** deficiency in rats causes achromotrichia.

Protein

More usual than an amino acid deficiency is simply a lack of adequate total dietary protein; this is ordinarily the result of inadequate food: in other words, starvation. It may also follow any disorder that leads to anorexia, or which interferes with food consumption by other means. Obviously, the effects are most pronounced in young growing animals. In humans, the most important manifestations of protein malnutrition are **nutritional marasmus** and **kwashiorkor.** The deficiency syndrome is not simple, because it is complicated by concomitant micronutrient deficiency. Lesions are not specific. The major pathologic changes include failure to grow, cessation of cell proliferation of epiphyseal cartilages, reduced osteoblastic activity, failure of collagen formation, atrophy of endocrine glands (including testicle and ovary, atrophy of thymus and lymphoid tissues, fatty liver, anemia, hypoproteinemia, and edema. It is further complicated by the superimposition of infections.

References

Angelini C, Vergani L, Martinuzzi A. Clinical and biochemical aspects of carnitine deficiency and insufficiency: transport defects and inborn errors of β-oxidation. Crit Rev Clin Lab Sci 1992;29:217–242.

Anonymous. Taurine requirements in long-term parenteral nutrition. Nutr Rev 1988;46:15–16.

Bhuyan UN, Ramalingaswami V. Lymphopoiesis in protein deficiency: stathmokinetic and tritiated thymidine uptake os the mesenteric lymph node of the guinea pig. Am J Pathol 1974;75:315–328.

Bieber LL. Carnitine. Annu Rev Biochem 1988;57:261–283.

Breningstall GN. Carnitine deficiency syndromes. Pediatr Neurol 1990;6:75–81.

Duran M, Loof NE, Dorland L. Secondary carnitine deficiency. J Clin Chem Clin Biochem 1990;28:359–363.

Feller AG, Rudman D. Role of carnitine in human nutrition. J Nutr 1988;118:541–547.

Felsenfeld O, Gyr K, Wolf RH. Malnutrition and susceptibility to infection with Vibrio cholerae in vervet monkeys (Cercopithecus aethiops). I. Induction of protein, B-vitamin complex, and calorie malnutrition. J Med Primatol 1976;5:186–194.

Fleagle JG, Samonds KW, Hegsted DM. Physical growth of cebus monkeys (Cebus albifrons) during protein or calorie deficiency. Am J Clin Nutr 1975;28:246–253.

Geist CR, Zimmermann RR, Smith OW, et al. Emergence of a kwashiorkor-like syndrome associated with protein-calorie malnutrition in the developing rhesus monkey (Macaca mulatta). Psychol Rep 1977;40:1330–1344.

Harpster NK. Boxer cardiomyopathy: a review of the long-term benefits of antiarrhythmic therapy. Vet Clin North Am Small Anim Pract 1991;21:989–1004.

Hayes KC. Taurine requirement in primates. Nutr Rev 1985;43:65–70.

Hayes KC. Taurine nutrition. Nutr Res Rev 1988;1:99–113.

Hayes KC, Trautwein EA. Taurine deficiency syndrome in cats. Vet Clin North Am Small Anim Pract 1989;19:403–413.

Hayes KC, Carey RE, Schmidt SY. Retinal degeneration associated with taurine deficiency in the cat. Nutr Rev 1985;43:84–86.

Jacobson HN. Protein deficiency in primates. J Clin Nutr 1975;28:801–802.

Keene BW. L-carnitine supplementation in the therapy of canine dilated cardiomyopathy. Vet Clin North Am Small Anim Pract 1991;21:1005–1009.

Lombardi B, Oler A. Choline deficiency fatty liver. Protein synthesis and release. Lab Invest 1967;17:308–321.

Manocha SL, Olkowski ZL. Experimental protein malnutrition in primates: cytochemistry of the nervous system. Am J Phys Anthropol 1973;38:439–445.

Pion PD, Kittleson MD, Rogers QR, et al. Myocardial failure in cats associated with low plasma taurine: a reversible cardiomyopathy. Science 1987;237:764–768.

Platt BS, Stewart RJC. Experimental protein-calorie deficiency: histopathological changes in the endocrine glands of pigs. J Endocrinol 1967;38:121–143.

Rebouche CJ. Carnitine function and requirements during the life cycle. FASEB J 1992;6:3379–3386.

Riopelle AJ, et al. Protein deficiency in primates. IV. Pregnant rhesus monkeys. Am J Clin Nutr 1975;28:20–28.

Roberts ED, Gallo JT, Maner JH. Protein deficiency in swine and use of opaque-2 corn to prevent changes in bone: light, fluorescence, and electron microscopy study. Am J Vet Res 1972;33:1985–1994.

Scholte HR, Periera RR, de Jonge PC, et al. Primary carnitine deficiency. J Clin Chem Clin Biochem 1990;28:351–357.

Stanley CA. Plasma and mitochondrial membrane carnitine transport defects. Prog Clin Biol Res 1992;375:289–300.

Stanley CA, Hale DE, Berry GT, et al. A deficiency of carnitine-acylcarnitine translocase in the inner mitochondrial membrane. N Engl J Med 1992;327:19–23.

Vinton NE, Geggel HS, Ament ME, et al. Taurine deficiency in a child on total parenteral nutrition. Nutr Rev 1985;43:81–83.

Lipids and carbohydrates

LIPIDS

Fat is an important dietary component because it supplies essential fatty acids, serves as a carrier for fat-soluble vitamins, has increased caloric value, and adds palatability to food. The three essential fatty acids are linoleic, linolenic, and arachidonic acids; their requirements, however, vary among species. Linoleic acid is essential for all species; most evidence supports linolenic as also essential for all species. Arachidonic acid can be synthesized by most species, with the exception of the cat.

DEFICIENCY

Deficiency of fat probably does not exist in domestic animals. Deficiency of essential fatty acids has been produced and studied in experimental animals, and is often suggested as a cause of ill-defined dermatoses in animals. Dietary deficiency of essential fatty acids is, however, rare. Deficiency can occur when absorption of fat is impaired in biliary or pancreatic disease. Dietary supplementation with fats occasionally results in improvement of certain skin disorders, but virtually no sound study has shown fatty acids to be specific for the "cure." Experimental fatty acid deficiency requires months to years to affect the skin of dogs and cats. The earliest change is dryness, followed by erythema, alopecia, scaling, ulceration, and failure of wounds to heal properly.

Microscopically, the epidermis is thickened, due to an increase in cells and hyperkeratosis. Hair follicles become hypercellular and plugged with keratin, and sebaceous glands increase in size. The dermis becomes edematous and infiltrated with mononuclear cells.

In cats, fatty change of the liver and kidneys may develop, as well as mineralization of the adrenal, and degeneration of testicular germinal epithelium; changes have also been seen in experimental fatty acid deficiency in rats.

Carbohydrates

Carbohydrates—or, in the case of ruminants, roughage—provide a major dietary source of energy; however, no specific carbohydrate deficiency state occurs. Dogs and cats do not even require a dietary source. Certain carbodydrate sources can lead to enteropathy. This is well known with gluten (wheat) enteropathy in humans. Gluten enteropathy has also been identified in Irish setters, and is characterized by villus atrophy and intraepithelial lymphocytic infiltration.

Reduction in available carbohydrates is a precipitating factor of ketosis in cattle, and of pregnancy toxemia in sheep and cattle.

References

Brady RO. The abnormal biochemistry of inherited disorders of lipid metabolism. Fed Proc 1973;6:1660–1667.

Crawford MA, Rivers JPW, Hassam AG. Comparative studies on the metabolic equivalence of linoleic and arachidonic acids. Nutr Metab 1977;21:189–190.

Dietschy JM, Wilson JD. Regulation of cholesterol metabolism (Parts I, II,and III). N Engl J Med 1970;282:1128–1138, 1179–1184, 1241–1250.

Hansen AE, Wiese HF. Fat in the diet in relation to nutrition of the dog. I. Characteristic appearance and gross changes of animals fed diets with and without fats. Texas Rep Biol Med 1951;9:491–515.

Hansen AE, Holmes SG, Wiese HF, Fat in the diet in relation to nutrition of the dog. IV. Histologic features of skin from animals fed diets with or without fat. Texas Rep Biol Med 1951;9:555–570.

Hansen AE, Sinclair JG, Wiese HF. Sequence of histologic changes in skin of dogs in relation to dietary fat. J Nutr 1954;52:541–554.

Hanson LJ, Sorensen DK, Kernkamp HCH. Essential fatty acid deficiency: its role in parakeratosis. Am J Vet Res 1958;19:921–930.

Hoilund LJ, et al. Essential fatty acid deficiency in the rat. I. Clinical syndrome, histopathology, and hematopathology. Lab Invest 1970;23:58–70.

MacDonald ML, Anderson BC, Rogers QR, et al. Essential fatty acid requirements of cats: pathology of essential fatty acid deficiency. Am J Vet Res 1984;45:1310–1317.

Rivers JPW, Sinclair AJ, Crawford MA: Inability of the cat to desaturate essential fatty acids. Nature 1975;258:171–173.

Rivers JPW, Hassam AG, Crawford MA. The comparative nutrition of essential fatty acid metabolism. Nutr Metab 1976;20:193.

Sinclair AJ, et al. Linolenic acid deprivation in capuchin monkeys. Proc Nutr Soc 1974;33:A49–A50.

Ketosis and hypoglycemia

Ketosis is the term used to describe the accumulation of excessive quantities of "ketone bodies" in the blood (ketonemia). The ketone bodies are β-hydroxybutyric acid, acetoacetic acid, and acetone. Ketosis follows excessive breakdown of adipose tissue as a source of energy when the availability of glucose is limited for any reason. The oxidation of free fatty acids through acetyl-CoA, however, depends on a continuous source of oxaloacetate; this allows its incorporation into the tricarboxylic acid cycle. In the face of active gluconeogenesis, which accompanies increased demands for glucose, inadequate oxaloacetate results, and acetyl-CoA is directed to ketogenesis. Normally, small amounts of ketone bodies are continuously generated and oxidized in the tissues. When produced in amounts that exceed tissue utilization, ketones are excreted in the urine (ketonuria); when produced in amounts which exceed the renal capacity for excretion, they accumulate in the blood and lead to ketosis. Ketosis can develop through (1) starvation, because of an increased demand for gluconeogenesis, (2) diabetes mellitus, because of an inability to utilize glucose, and (3) pregnancy and lactation, which place an increased demand for glucose. Diabetes is obviously characterized by hyperglycemia, whereas the other disorders associated with ketosis are usually associated with hypoglycemia. This is clearly an oversimplification for ketosis, but it is beyond the scope of this text to include a comprehensive review of the intermediary metabolism of carbohydrates and lipids.

BOVINE KETOSIS

Bovine ketosis can develop through starvation, or from diets containing excessive butyric acid; however, the usual form is a spontaneous ketosis, seen in lactating dairy cows on an increased plane of nutrition. It is believed that the immense demand of the mammary gland to synthesize lactose exceeds the available glucose; this leads to hypoglycemia. The disease is characterized by anorexia and depression, or sometimes excitability, incoordination, and terminal coma. Pregnancy toxemia of ewes ("pregnant ewe paralysis") is a disease that develops late in pregnancy, usually in ewes carrying twins or triplets; the ewes have, for some reason, become stressed or deprived of adequate food. This, coupled with the increased demand for glucose by the fetuses, leads to ketosis. It is characterized by depression, somnolence, and coma, but not true paralysis. The outstanding lesion of bovine ketosis and pregnancy toxemia of ewes is sever fatty change in the liver.

References

Ganaway JR, Allen AM. Obesity predisposes to pregnancy toxemia (ketosis) of guinea pigs. Lab Anim Sci 1971;21:40–44.

Jasper DE. Acute and prolonged insulin hypoglycemia in cows. Am J Vet Res 1953;14:184–191.

Jasper DE. Prolonged insulin hypoglycemia in sheep. Am J Vet Res 1953;14:209–213.

Krebs HA. Bovine ketosis. Vet Rec 1966;78:187–192.

Kronfeld DS. The hypoglycemia of bovine ketosis: its metabolic origin and clinical effects. Hanover: Proc 17th World Vet Congr, 1963;2:1315–1317.

Pehrson B. Studies on ketosis in dairy cows. Acta Vet Scand Suppl 1966;15:1–59.

Procos J. Ovine ketosis. I. The normal ketone body values. Onderstepoort J Vet Res 1961;28:557–567.

Reid IM. An ultrastructural and morphometric study of the liver of the lactating cow in starvation ketosis. Exp Mol Pathol 1973;18:316–330.

Reid RL. The physiopathology of undernourishment in pregnant sheep, with particular reference to pregnancy toxemia. Adv Vet Sci 1968;12:163–238.

Roderick LM, Harshfield GS, Hawn MC. The pathogenesis of ketosis: pregnancy disease of sheep. J Am Vet Med Assoc 1937;90:41–50.

Saba N, et al. Some biochemical and hormonal aspects of experimental ovine pregnancy toxaemia. J Agric Sci Camb 1966l67:129–138.

Sampson J. The significance of hypoglycemia. J Am Vet Med Assoc 1948;112:350–352.

Seibold HE. Ketosis in subhuman primates. Lab Anim Care 1969;19:826–830.

WATER

Water, which is the most abundant component of the animal body, is a dietary requirement, although not a nutrient in itself. A number of factors influence the daily need of water, including: environmental temperature and humidity; composition of the diet (especially with respect to the amount of sodium); and physical activity. Other conditions which can lead to an increased requirement for water are (1) fever, (2) diarrhea, (3) vomiting, (4) hemorrhage, and (5) polyuria from diabetes insipidus or diabetes mellitus. When healthy animals have access to water, deficiency is unlikely. Deprivation of water or inadequate replacement in ill animals are the likely causes of water deficiency; both of these conditions are more common in animals than published literature indicates. Animals may be herded into a lot without water and overlooked for days. The attendant may fail to give water to animals kept in enclosed quarters. The automatic drinking device or water bottle may become occluded for some reason and deprive laboratory animals of water. Freezing of water is always a hazard to livestock. Even though it is common knowledge that all animals require water from some source, still it happens that animals may be unwittingly deprived of essential water.

Pathologic findings in water loss or dehydration are minimal. Little or no fluid will be evident in the pericardial, pleural, and peritoneal cavities, and the serosal membranes are dry, sticky, and lack their usual glistening character. Polycythemia occurs. The skin is wrinkled and may seem too big for the body. Flanks and abdomen appear gaunt.

References

Lindley WH. Water deprivation in cattle. J Am Vet Med Assoc 1977;171:439–440.

Shimamura T, Trojanowski S. Effects of repeated deprivation of drinking water on the structure of renal medulla of rats. Am J Pathol 1976;84:87–92.

Sinha RP, Ganapathy MS. Studies on experimental dehydration in canines with particular reference to clinical picture, haemoglobin concentration, hematocrit, specific gravity of the plasma, and plasma sodium concentration. Indian Vet J 1967;44:127–136.

17

The skin and its appendages

The skin, or integument, is the single largest organ of the body. Representing the physical barrier between the environment and the organism, the skin performs many important functions, many of which have been known for decades. The skin prevents fluid loss, and keeps opportunistic organisms from invading the more vulnerable, underlying soft tissues. It functions in temperature regulation through neurologic communications between the hypothalamus and cutaneous vasculature. Moreover, the skin can reflect a wide variety of systemic disorders, most notably certain metabolic, viral, inflammatory, and endocrine diseases. Therefore, examination of the skin constitutes a key component of any thorough physical examination. However, the complexity of interactions between the normal components of the skin and other organ systems, particularly the immune system, has implicated the skin in many more functions than just those of a protective barrier. During the last two to three decades, there has been an explosion of new information regarding the numerous molecular, physiologic, and cellular functions that occur in the skin. For example, we now know that the skin has a number of unique cellular components of the immune system which selectively target to and reside within specific environments of the skin. We also know that keratinocytes, in addition to being the building blocks of the epidermis, conduct important paracrine communication functions through the secretion of important cytokines. Furthermore, the epidermis contains all of the components necessary for the initiation of an immune response against externally as well as internally-derived antigens. Thus, the skin serves important functions in the overall immune surveillance system of the body.

The discovery of these cutaneous functions has not only broadened our understanding of cellular interactions in general but has greatly enhanced our knowledge of the physiologic and histopathologic processes that occur in the skin. The following pages attempt to describe veterinary skin diseases in terms of morphologic patterns and mechanisms. For ease of reference

for the diagnostic pathologist, certain skin diseases have been grouped according to histomorphologic pattern, although with some dermatoses—particularly ones of a chronic nature—it should be remembered that significant overlap can be found between groups. In addition, some skin disorders of known cause have been better addressed in other chapters of this text; where applicable, one is instructed to read pertinent sections elsewhere.

NORMAL STRUCTURE AND FUNCTION

The skin of animals presents particular problems to the pathologist, not only because of the complexity of its components in various parts of the body, but because of the many differences between species. Knowledge of normal structure and function is therefore particularly important to the interpretation of lesions of the skin.

The skin has three principal layers: the epidermis, dermis, and subcutis (or hypodermis).

Epidermis

The epidermis is the most superficial layer of the skin and is composed of **stratified squamous epithelium** composed primarily of **keratinocytes** with smaller numbers of scattered **dendritic Langerhans cells, melanocytes, Merkel cells,** and migrating lymphocytes. The keratinocytes differentiate as they progress from the deeper portions of the epidermis to the surface, where they die leaving their cytoplasmic keratin protein as the cornified layer. In some parts of the skin, the epidermis projects into the dermis by way of elongate protrusions called **rete ridges.** Under normal conditions, the epidermis can be further subdivided into four layers based on this differentiation process and morphological appearance of the resident keratinocytes (Fig. 17-1).

The **stratum basale,** or basal layer, consists of a row of distinctive cuboidal cells with hyperchromatic nuclei

817

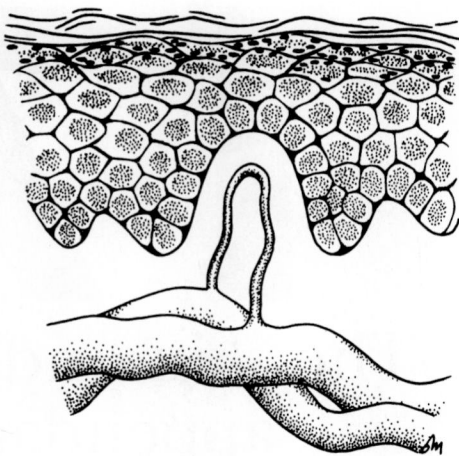

FIG. 17-1 Schematic illustration of the four layers of the epidermis (from bottom to top: the stratum basale, stratum spinosum, stratum granulosum and stratum corneum) and the superficial vasculature of the dermis consisting of an arteriole, a postcapillary venule and a dermal papillary capillary loop. (Courtesy of Dr. George F. Murphy, University of Pennsylvania School of Medicine).

lying just on the epidermal side of the basement membrane, which defines the dermal-epidermal junction. Indeed, the keratinocytes in this layer manufacture and secrete the extracellular matrix proteins comprising the basement membrane. This layer is responsible for keratinocyte replenishment; thus, mitotic figures are common. The basilar keratinocytes are firmly attached to the basement membrane by specialized anchoring structures called **hemidesmosomes.**

Just above the stratum basale lies the **stratum spinosum.** It is composed of polyhedreal cells, and these cells assume a more flattened morphology as they progress to the surface. Its name derives from the presence of numerous intercellular junctions between keratinocytes, called **desmosomes,** which because of artificial shrinkage during slide preparation sometimes give the microscopic appearance that they have "spines." These spines actually consist of fine cytoplasmic filaments (tonofibrils), which end at desmosomes attaching adjacent cell surfaces, giving the false impression of continuity between cells. These structures provide mechanical attachment between cells of the epithelium. The stratum spinosum and stratum basale together are sometimes referred to as the Malpighian layer.

Progressing next towards the surface is the **stratum granulosum,** or granular layer. It is made up of rows of two to five epithelial cells in depth, in which the cells are rhomboid shaped and flat. The nuclei are pale or shrunken, and the cytoplasm is filled with dark-staining basophilic keratohyalin granules. Keratohyalin consists of a mixture of proteins, RNA, lipids, and polysaccharides. A cationic protein called **filaggrin** has been isolated from keratohyalin which accumulates among keratin filaments and in the interstices of the keratinocytes as they flatten and become cornified cells.

The **stratum corneum** is the most superficial layer. It consists predominantly of the skeletons of dead keratinocytes, that is, keratin filaments. Keratohyalin granule-derived filaggrin comprises a large portion of the matrix surrounding the keratin filaments, and it is believed that it functions as the glue that holds the keratin filaments together. Thus, this layer is anucleate and consists principally of keratin filaments embedded in a filaggrin-rich matrix. The thickness and density of the stratum corneum varies considerably with location on the body. On hairless regions, it is relatively thin and sometimes appears in a "basketweave" pattern. In contrast, in regions subject to considerable abrasive forces, such as the foot pad, it is extremely thick and dense, sometimes normally up to 20 times the thickness of the other epidermal strata combined.

In hairless regions in some domestic animals, such as the bovine teat or canine foot pad, or in the thick skin of the human palms and soles, some histologists have defined a fifth epidermal layer, the **stratum lucidum.** Arguably representing modified stratum corneum, this layer lies between the stratum granulosum and the most superficial layer. It is composed of flattened, anucleate keratinocytes, and as its name implies, has a somewhat translucent appearance compared to the most superficial keratin in routine histologic sections. Other than keratinocytes, the epidermis is populated with scattered cells of multiple types and functions. **Melanocytes** are dendritic cells within the epidermis that make melanin, the pigment of the skin. These cells are formed embryologically from the neural crest and migrate to the epidermis during fetal development. There they tend to populate the basilar regions of the epidermis, but their dendrites extend for significant distances between keratinocytes throughout the stratum basale and stratum spinosum. Melanocytes are territorial, tending to separate themselves from one another, and thus are usually found singly, except in certain neoplastic processes. Melanin is produced by a tyrosine-dependent pathway; thus, melanocytes synthesize tyrosinase (a useful marker) and package melanin in specialized cytoplasmic organelles called melanosomes. Skin color is imparted by the transfer of these melanosomes from melanocytes to keratinocytes. Thus, it is these pigment-containing keratinocytes that absorb and disperse damaging energy from ultraviolet light. Tanning is accomplished by the increased production and transfer of melanin from melanocytes to keratinocytes and by increased production of resident epidermal melanocytes.

Like melanocytes, **Merkel cells** are found sporadically throughout the epidermis. They have been identified in a broad spectrum of species, including fish, amphibians, reptiles, birds, and mammals. Unlike normal melanocytes, Merkel cells can sometimes be found in clusters in the epidermis. Occasional solitary Merkel cells are found in the dermis. In humans, they are more abundant in areas typically involved with sensory perception, such as the face or hands. In routine histologic sections, epidermal Merkel cells are difficult to identify.

Artifactual shrinkage of these cells during processing is suggestive of their identity in tissue sections, but this criterion can be applied to other non-keratinocyte epidermal cells as well and thus cannot be used to definitively identify them. The presence of cytoplasmic neuroendocrine granules is their unique feature for identification, which can be seen ultrastructurally or demonstrated immunohistochemically. Clusters and solitary Merkel cells are frequently in intimate association with myelinated nerve fibers. The presence of neuropeptides, such as vasoactive intestinal polypeptide (VIP), and metenkephalin-like proteins, has been localized to these granules, which along with their close association with nerve terminals, has prompted investigators to propose that they either have a role in signal transduction for mechanoreceptors, subserve a neuromodulator function by influencing action potential thresholds of the adjacent sensory nerve terminal, or perhaps provide trophic navigational signals to developing neuronal axons.

Langerhans cells (LC) (Fig. 17-2) are suprabasilar bone marrow derived dendritic cells found in all squamous epithelia, including the follicular epithelium of skin. They constitute 2% to 8% of the epidermal cells and share a number of properties with cells of the mononuclear phagocyte system. These include high level of ATPase and nonspecific esterase activity, membrane expression of major histocompatibility complex (MHC) class II molecules, and receptors for the Fc portion of IgG and C3b component of complement.

Ultrastructurally, LCs can be identified in humans, monkeys, cattle and mice by the presence of a unique trilaminar "tennis racket"-shaped cytoplasmic organelle, the Birbeck granule (Fig. 17-2). The function of this structure is not known. In dog and cat skin, dendritic cells comparable to LCs do not contain Birbeck granules, but have many other features in common with human LCs. These cells lack cytoplasmic tonofilaments,

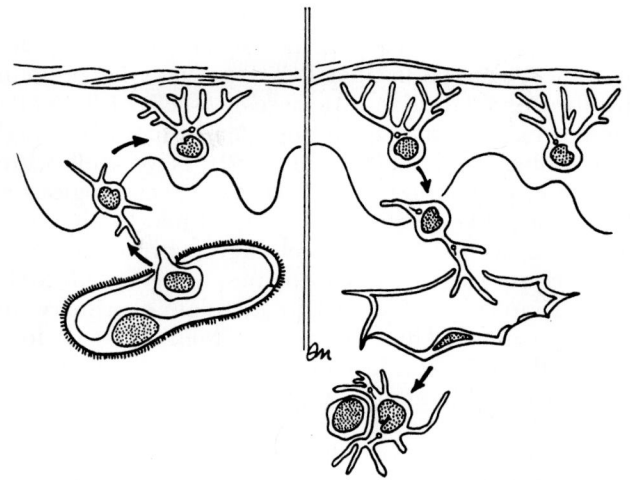

FIG. 17-3 Schematic illustration of the migration of a monocytic precursor from a dermal blood vessel to give rise to a Langerhans cells (left of midline), and exodus of a mature, antigenically-stimulated Langerhans cell from the epidermis into a dermal lymphatic (right of midline). The Langerhans cell-lymphocyte association depicted at the bottom most likely occurs in a regional lymph node but could conceivably also occur in the dermis. (Courtesy of Dr. George F. Murphy, University of Pennsylvania School of Medicine).

have large reniform nuclei, and abundant homogeneous cytoplasm. In the dog, as in humans, these cells express a number of surface molecules including MHC class II antigens, a spectrum of leukocyte antigens characteristic of dendritic cell differentiation including CD1a, CD1b, CD1c, preferentially express individual β_2 integrins CD11/CD18 and the leukocyte common antigen, CD45. Like macrophages and other dendritic cells, LCs represent a type of **antigen presenting cell** (APC) or **accessory cell,** responsible for the elicitation of immune reactions against foreign or tumor-associated antigens. A more complete discussion of antigen presentation is discussed in chapters 5 and 7. Langerhans cells, thus, represent a group of bone marrow-derived immune cells with potent antigen processing and immune stimulatory activities. Within squamous epithelia, LCs are able to entrap antigen, internalize it, degrade it into smaller antigenic peptides, and incorporate it in context with MHC Class II molecules for presentation on their cell surface membranes. Subsequently, antigen-expressing LCs traverse the dermal-epidermal basement membrane and do one of two things (Fig. 17-3). They can present the processed antigen to CD4+ memory T lymphocytes, found sparsely around superficial dermal vessels. In so doing, antigen-dependent T cell activation and proliferation occurs which ultimately results in a classic delayed hypersensitivity inflammatory reaction. Alternatively, if the host is native to the antigen and thus no memory cells reside in the dermis, the antigen-bearing LC can migrate to dermal lymphatics and be carried to a regional lymph node as a **veiled cell.** In the lymph node, the human LC loses its Birbeck granules

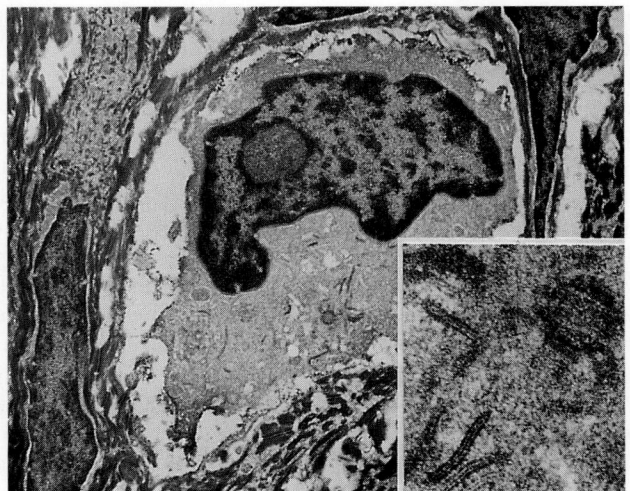

FIG. 17-2 Low-magnification electron micrograph of a Langerhans cell of the epidermis of a rhesus monkey. **Inset:** Characteristic trilaminar Birbeck granules.

and is believed to differentiate into a more efficient dendritic accessory cell. In fact, it has been suggested by some investigators that LCs represent the progenitors for the potent dendritic accessory cells of the nodal paracortex, the interdigitating dendritic cell (Stingl, 1990; Silberberg-Sinakin et al, 1980). Nevertheless, the migrating LC localizes to paracortical T cell regions of the lymph node, where it can present new foreign antigens to unprimed CD4+ T cells and provide the necessary accessory signals (i.e. cytokines, antigen with MHC Class II molecules) needed to stimulate a primary immune response. Thus, because of their strategic location in the skin, the fact that they have dendritic processes which extend to the surface of the epidermis, their ability to migrate to draining lymph nodes, and their potent accessory cell function, Langerhans cells are exquisitely adapted to provide protective immune surveillance activity for the host. Thus, the skin should not be thought of simply as a passive, protective barrier of the body but, instead, as an active and integral component of the host immune system. Thus, Streilein (1985) and colleagues have suggested that LCs represent the afferent component of "skin-associated lymphoid tissue ("SALT") comparable to gut and respiratory-associated lymphoid tissue.

In mouse skin, there is another dendritic cell within the epidermis which does not contain Birbeck granules and instead expresses the murine T cell membrane marker Thy-l. It has been referred to as the **Thy-1+ dendritic cell** or **dendritic epidermal T cell.** The function of these cells is not known, but they are believed to play a role in the control of cutaneous immune responses through antigen-specific immune suppressor circuits. An analogous cell in other mammals, including humans, has not been definitively identified. Lastly, there is a Langerhans-like cell in mammalian epidermis that is devoid of Birbeck granules but similar in other respects to LCs, including the expression of MHC Class II antigens. These **indeterminate cells** are likely either immature LCs or cells analagous to the murine Thy-l+ dendritic cells.

Dermis

Beneath the epidermis, separated by the basement membrane, lies the dermis. The dermis is the largest component of the skin and owing to abundant collagen, provides the tensile strength inherent in normal integument. Collagen is the most abundant material found in the dermis, and approximately 80% of dermal collagen is composed of Type I fibers; most of the remaining collagen is Type III. Type IV collagen is only found in the basement membrane. Elastic fibers and extracellular matrix consisting of fibronectin, glycosoaminoglycans, and filamentous glycoproteins are found in the interstices of collagen fibers and provide resilience and substrates important for cell migration and attachment.

The dermis is organized into two zones: the **papillary** and **reticular** dermis. The papillary region lies immediately adjacent to the epidermis and follows its contour, including around adnexa, such as hair follicles and sweat glands, and between rete ridges in the **dermal papillae.** In contrast to the reticular dermis, it is predominantly comprised of Type III collagen, the fibers of which have a smaller diameter. However, the reticular dermis makes up the bulk of the dermis. Its major component, Type I collagen fibers, are relatively thick in comparison to those within the papillary dermis. Approximately at the border between the papillary and reticular dermis, cutaneous arterioles ramify into the **superficial vascular plexus** (Fig. 17-1). These vascular channels give rise to capillary loops which extend into the papillary dermis, providing the nutritional support to the overlying epidermis. The post-capillary venules of the plexus are important to pathologists and dermatologists, because these vessels are the predominant site for inflammatory vascular alterations. Other than providing adequate blood supply to the skin and being the focus of cutaneous inflammatory disease, the cutaneous vasculature also plays an important role in thermoregulation.

The dermis is endowed with a number of different cell types, including fibroblasts, macrophages, endothelium, myocytes, mast cells, and lymphocytes. Fibroblasts are interspersed between collagen bundles, where they synthesize the collagen, elastin, and extracellular components. Macrophages are scattered throughout the dermis and can assist Langerhans cells in antigen processing and presentation while providing protective phagocytic functions. Dermal mast cells (Fig. 5-2) are found commonly around dermal vessels, where they act as "gatekeepers of the microvasculature" (Klein et al., 1989); they can directly modulate the activation state of endothelium by the local release of their cytoplasmic granular constituents. Mast cell degranulation is directly involved in type I hypersensitivity reactions and is likely involved in other inflammatory dermatoses of an acute and chronic nature. The integral nature of mast cells in the evolution of so many cutaneous inflammatory conditions is explained by the nature of vascular responses after exposure to the vasoactive substances found in mast cell granules. These compounds, including heparin, histamine, and possibly tumor necrosis factor-α, can directly influence both vascular dilatation and permeability (which accounts for redness, heat, and swelling) as well as the endothelial expression of adhesion molecules specific for leukocytes. These endothelial adhesion proteins, such as E-selectin (formerly ELAM-1) and VCAM-l, mediate attachment of circulating leukocytes to endothelium and thereby permit leukocytes to estravasate from the vasculature into the surrounding tissues. Thus, mast cells are likely instrumental in the initiation and propagation of many cutaneous inflammatory responses. For a more thorough discussion of inflammatory cells and the mechanisms related to inflammation, the reader is directed to pertinent sections of Chapter 5.

The skin is innervated by sensory and autonomic nerve fibers within the dermis. Sympathetic motor fibers innervate dermal sweat glands, arrector pili muscles, and vascular smooth muscle. The skin's sense of touch is accomplished predominantly by a network of free sensory nerve endings, which vary in density between anatomic locations. They richly supply the papillary dermis by extending their terminal portions into dermal papillae as well as the orifices of hair follicles. They represent the most widespread sensory receptors of the body. Dermal sensory nerves, however, can also be associated with either clusters of Merkel cells or specialized mechanoreceptors, such as Meissner's corpuscles of dermal papillae or Pacinian corpuscles of the deep dermis or hypodermis.

The adnexa include the specialized structures that arise from the epidermis. They are for the most part contained in the dermis but may extend into the subcutis in some situations. The adnexa include:

1. Sudoriferous or sweat glands ("merocrine" glands),
2. Apocrine glands,
3. Specialized tubular glands, such as lacrimal and mammary glands,
4. Sebaceous glands and modified sebaceous glands, e.g., circumanal (perianal) glands,
5. Hair follicles of two types, i.e. common "guard" hairs and tactile hairs.

Tactile follicles are distinguished in tissue sections by the large surrounding vascular spaces and the sensory nerve, which can usually be seen.

Subcutis

The subcutis, or hypodermis, is composed predominantly of lobules of adipose tissue. Near the border between the deep reticular dermis and the subcutis, lies the second vascular plexus of the skin, the **deep vascular plexus.** It is usually found within the deep reticular dermis, but vascular channels and tributaries can sometimes be found in the subcutis. It is similar to the superficial vascular plexus except that there are smaller numbers of capillaries originating from it. In most mammals, below the subcuticular adipose tissue, lies the panniculus carnosus, a thin layer of skeletal muscle responsible for skin movement in response to external stimuli; it has become vestigial in humans.

References

Bressler RS, Bressler CH. Functional anatomy of the skin. Clin Podiatr Med Surg 1989;6:229–246.
Compton CC, Gill JM, Bradford D, et al. Skin regenerated from cultured epithelial autografts on full-thickness burn wounds from 6 days to 5 years after grafting: A light, electron microscopic and immunohistochemical study. Lab Invest 1989;60:600–612.
Creed RFS. Histology of mammalian skin, with special reference to the dog and cat. Vet Rec 1958;70:1–7.
Cruz PD, Bergstresser PR. Antigen processing and presentation by epidermal Langerhans cells: Induction of immunity or unresponsiveness. Dermatol Clin 1990;8:633–647.
Gould VE, Moll R, Moll I, et al. Neuroendocrine (Merkel) cells of the skin: Hyperplasias, dysplasias, and neoplasms. Lab Invest 1985;52:334–353.
Klein LM, Lavker RM, Matis WL, et al. Degranulation of human mast cells induces an endothelial antigen central to leukocyte adhesion. Proc Natl Acad Sci USA 1989;86:8972–8976.
Lovell JE, Getty R: The hair follicles, epidermis, dermis and skin glands of the dog. Am J Vet Res 1957;18:873–885.
Maruyama T, Tanaka S, Bozoky B, et al. New monoclonal antibody that specifically recognizes murine interdigitating and Langerhans cells. Lab Invest 1989;61:98–106.
Montagna W. Cutaneous comparative biology. Arch Dermatol 1971;104:577–591.
Murphy GF. Cell membrane glycoprotein and Langerhans cells. Hum Pathol 1985;16:103–112.
Nordlund JJ. The lives of pigment cells. Dermatol Clin 1986;4:407–418.
Ringler DJ, Hancock WW, King NW, et al. Characterization of nonhuman primate epidermal and dermal dendritic Langerhans cells and indeterminate cells in the rhesus monkey. Lab Invest 1987;56:313–320.
Shimada S, Katz SI. The skin as an immunologic organ. Arch Pathol Lab Med 1988;112:231–234.
Silberberg-Sinakin I, Gigli I, Baer RL, et al. Langerhans cells: role in contact hypersensitivity and relationship to lymphoid dendritic cells and to macrophages. Immunol Rev 1980;53:203–232.
Sontheimer RD. Perivascular dendritic macrophages as immunobiological constituents of the human dermal microvascular unit. J Invest Dermatol 1989;93:96S-101S.
Sprecher E, Becker Y. Role of epidermal Langerhans cells in viral infections. Arch Virol 1988;103:1–14, 1988.
Stingl G: Dendritic cells of the skin. Dermatologic Clinics 1990;8:673–679.
Stingl G, Steiner G. Immunological host defense of the skin. Curr Probl Dermatol 1989;18:22–30.
Streilein JW: Circuits and signals of the skin-associated lymphoid tissue (SALT). J Invest Dermatol 1985;85:10S–13S.
Streilein JW, Grammer SF, Yoshikawa T, et al. Functional dichotomy between Langerhans cells that present antigen to naive and to memory/effector T lymphocytes. Immunol Rev 117:159–183, 1990.
Sullivan S, Bergstresser PR, Tigelaar RE, et al. Induction and regulation of contact hypersensitivity by resident, bone marrow-derived, dendritic epidermal cells: Langerhans cells and Thy-1+ epidermal cells. J Immunol 1986;137:2460–2467.
Toews TB, Bergstresser PR, Streilein JW: Langerhans cells: Sentinels of skin associated lymphoid tissue. J Invest Dermatol 1980;75:78–82.

RESPONSE TO INJURY

As with other tissues, the skin has limited means by which it can respond to injury. Dermatitides manifest all the hallmarks of inflammation seen in other tissues, namely vascular dilatation, edema, and leukocyte infiltration. Additionally, the mechanisms of inflammation in the skin are the same as described in previous chapters. However, because the skin represents the physical barrier between the host and the environment, in addition to influences from within, the skin is affected by a multitude of damaging agents and sensitizing antigens from the outside. Thus, how the skin responds to injury depends upon where the inciting injury occurs, the type and nature of the insult, and the duration, location to specific skin structures, and severity of the inciting agent. Although there are basic patterns of morphological changes in skin in response to different types of insults, remarkably, there are a number of changes which are common to many of the different types of cutaneous injury. In this section, some of these cutaneous reactive patterns will be reviewed. The more specific changes in skin in response to injury will be addressed individually in subsequent sections of this chapter.

Epidermis

As the most external layer of the skin, the epidermis bears the brunt of the collective insults from the external environment. Thus, most externally-derived injurious agents produce direct damage to cells of the epidermis. However, the epidermis can also be damaged from insults from below, specifically, cellular and humoral components of the immune system and foreign bloodborne agents. For many years, the epidermis was thought of as only a passive participant in these injurious reactions. However, it is now recognized that the epidermis is instead a dynamic, active participant in these reactions. Keratinocytes are able to generate powerful messenger (cytokine) stimuli on cells in the dermis as well as on adjacent cells within the epidermis, including themselves. Many of these actions of keratinocytes will be outlined below.

The epidermis is dynamic; there is continual movement and differentiation of cells from the deep stratum basale to the superficial stratum corneum. There is proliferation of keratinocytes in the stratum basale, differentiation of these cells as they move toward the skin surface, and similarly, corneocytes (largely keratin) are desquamated at the surface. In normal skin, the rates of mitosis, differentiation, and desquamation are in equilibrium. If the relative rates of each become unequal due to a variety of influences, then the thickness and character of the epidermis will change. Thus, the thickness of the epidermis is determined by the relative rate of all three processes.

If the proliferative rate of keratinocytes is increased (hyperplasia) without relative increases in differentiation and desquamation, then the thickness of the epidermis, particularly the stratum basale and stratum spinosum, increases. The presence of a thickened epidermis is defined as **acanthosis** (Fig.17-4). This change is particularly common in inflammatory skin diseases and is caused by epidermal cell injury and/or proliferative signals from the dermis. Often as the proliferative activity of the epidermis increases, subsequent increases in the number of basal keratinocytes at the basement membrane zone causes the overall length of the basal region to lengthen, causing undulations and elongations in the rete ridges.

Increased production of keratinocytes with decreased desquamation from the surface ultimately leads to **hyperkeratosis,** a term denoting a thickened stratum corneum. Although acanthosis is often seen in association with hyperkeratosis, it can occur alone in some specimens. There are two types of hyperkeratosis: **orthokeratotic** hyperkeratosis resembles normal but thickened stratum corneum while **parakeratotic** hyperkeratosis is characterized by a stratum corneum containing pyknotic nuclei of keratinocytes, usually with diminution or absence of the stratum granulosum. In theory, parakeratosis can result either from a failure to fully differentiate or cornify, or from sustained, accelerated differentiation with reduced transit time which does not permit complete cornification. However, in practice, it can occur much more quickly than these mechanisms would imply based on epidermal transit time. In fact, parakeratosis can be visualized in as little as a few hours in response to either direct focal epidermal injury or signals generated in the superficial dermis during an inflammatory reaction.

While parakeratosis represents incomplete cornification at the level of the stratrum corneum, **dyskeratosis** represents premature cornification, usually of individual keratinocytes scattered throughout the thickness of the epidermis. Dyskeratotic keratinocytes can be recognized in tissue sections by increased eosinophilia of their cytoplasm and the presence of small, hyperchromatic nuclei. On routine histology, it can be difficult to distinguish dyskeratotic keratinocytes from necrotic cells since the morphologic changes are basically identical. However, from a physiologic standpoint, the two processes are decidedly different. The eosinophilic cytoplasm in a dyskeratotic cell is the result of

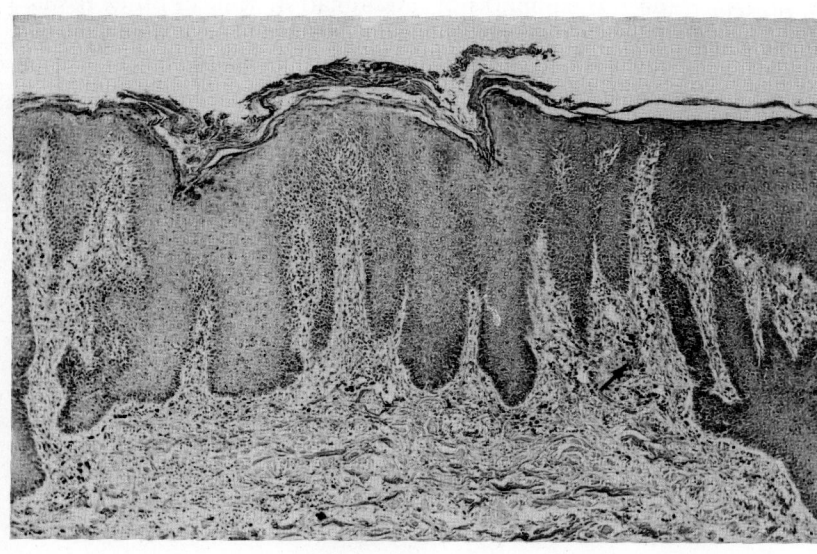

FIG. 17-4 Acanthosis nigricans, skin of a dog. Thick epidermis (×50) with elongated rete ridges. Melanin is increased in the epidermis and dermis (arrows). (Courtesy Armed Forces Institute of Pathology.) Contributor: Dr. M. A. Troy.

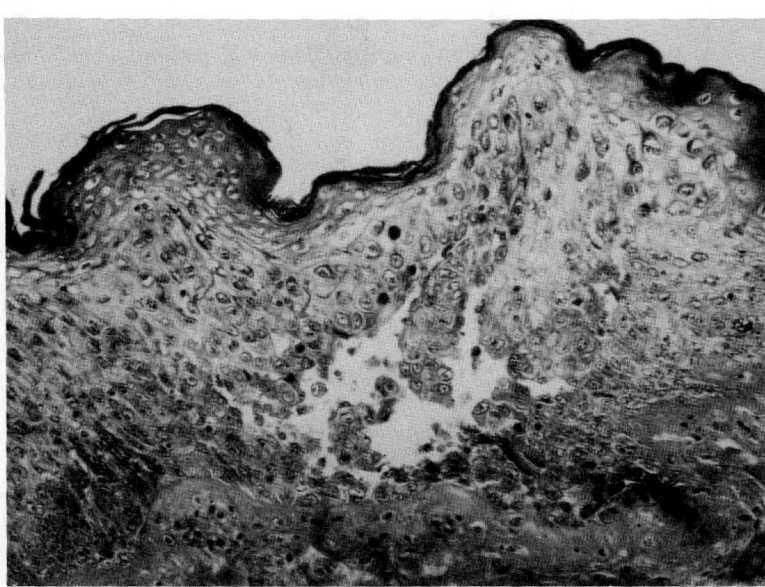

FIG. 17-5 Epithelial viral vesicle in the skin of a patas monkey *(Erythrocebus patas)* affected with herpes virus. (Courtesy of Dr. H. R. Seibold.)

abundant keratin filaments, while the same increased eosinophilia in a necrotic cell is secondary to increased eosin staining of denatured cytoplasmic proteins as well as degradation of cytoplasmic RNA, which when present, normally imparts a slight basophilic hue to the cytoplasm. Because the morphologic changes in an individual cell do not readily permit one to distinguish between dyskeratosis and necrosis, the entire epithelium must be assessed to arrive at a judgement as to whether a cell is dead or prematurely cornified. Electron microscopy can be used for further documentation of the process. Inflammatory, neoplastic, and some human genetic diseases, such as Darier's disease, induce dyskeratosis.

There are numerous epidermal changes that ultimately result in loss of epidermal integrity. Most of these changes are the result of damage or loss of intercellular adhesion, represented by strong desmosomal attachments and weaker intercellular attractive forces between keratinocytes. Damage or loss of adhesion between keratinocytes, in effect, creates potential spaces between cells, which subsequently fill with fluid because of the normal small but continuous net movement of fluid from the dermal vasculature to the interstitial space.

The first noticeable change associated with fluid exudation from the dermis into the intercellular spaces of the epidermis is termed **spongiosis.** This mild form of intercellular edema of the epidermis usually separates keratinocytes so that they only remain attached to each other by a few desmosomes. Spongiosis should be differentiated from intracellular **hydropic change,** or **ballooning degeneration,** which instead of involving loss of intercellular adhesion, represents the early consequence of direct cellular injury. Thus, ballooning degeneration, as its name implies, represents an early degenerative change resulting from impairment of the cell's ability to maintain intracellular fluid and

ion balance. If damage to intercellular attachments is prolonged and severe, then keratinocytes will ultimately die. When this results in focal loss of keratinocytes, spongiosis can progress to **vesicle ("blister")** formation with the development of a fluid-filled space within the epidermis (Fig.17-5). Both vesicle formation and spongiosis typically occur with inflammatory conditions associated with a marked influx of leukocytes, particularly polymorphonuclear cells, into the epidermis. It is critical that a vesicle be differentiated from **acantholysis,** a process associated with a number of disorders involving severe destruction of all intercellular adhesive forces. In these cases, unlike in a vesicle, the keratinocytes are completely viable, but round up into spheres, and float within the fluid-filled cavity. The presence of **acantholytic cells** in the fluid of epidermal vesicles or pustules is a useful diagnostic finding for a number of autoimmune diseases of the skin characterized by disruption of keratinocyte adhesion, specifically the pemphigus group. If acantholysis or vesiculation becomes so severe that the full-thickness of the epidermis is lost, an **ulcer** results. These are not the only mechanisms that lead to cutaneous ulceration, mechanical trauma is probably the most common cause. Not only are keratinocytes attached to each other through desmosomes, but basal keratinocytes are firmly attached to the underlying dermis by **hemidesmosomes,** specialized attachments that anchor these cells to the basement membrane. The basement membrane, in turn, is attached to the collagen fibers of the dermis by way of filaments and microfibrils. Any process which damages these anchoring structures will result in separation of the dermis from the epidermis, creating a vesicle if the epidermis remains intact. These vesicles can arise from damage and loss of basal keratinocytes, particularly in inflammatory skin diseases like lupus erythematosus, where the basal cells and basement membrane are the focus of the reaction. They can also be formed by direct destruction or damage of the basement membrane, as occurs in bullous pemphigoid, where autoantibodies are directed against components of the lamaina lucida of the basement membrane. Lastly, severe destructive inflammatory reactions in the papillary dermis can destroy the anchoring fibrils between dermal collagen fibers and basement membrane with subsequent cleft formation between the epidermis and dermis.

Dermis

It is virtually impossible to separate the response to injury in dermal and epidermal compartments, because injury to one results in changes in the other and vice versa. In particular, because the epidermis is avascular, all the components in an inflammatory response (e.g. edema fluid, increased vascular flow, leukocyte extravasation and infiltration, etc.) must arise from the vessels in the dermis. Indeed, the dermis is richly endowed with an elaborate network of vascular channels. Adjacent to these vessels lie a relatively rich supply of mast cells, which upon release of their preformed granules containing vasoactive amines, can mediate significant inflammatory vascular changes. Thus, the skin, like other environmental barriers such as mucosal surfaces, has the capacity to respond to injury rapidly and aggressively and, yet like other vascularized tissue of the body, this response is still stereotyped, with typical inflammatory sequelae that have been described in previous chapters. The main difference between the skin and parenchymal tissues in particular, is that in the skin, inflammatory changes in the dermis generally induce secondary disturbances in the epidermis, particularly affecting the rate of epidermal mitosis and differentiation. Although not fully understood, it was once thought that the signals needed to induce these changes in epidermal growth and differentiation originate from growth factors elaborated by either cells residing in the dermis (such as mast cells) or inflammatory cells brought to the dermis or epidermis. However, recently it has been recognized that the epidermis is not just an innocent bystander in this process. When injured or appropriately stimulated, the epidermis can produce proinflammatory molecules which have profound effects on the underlying dermal vasculature. Much of this work has been pioneered by Nickoloff and his colleagues at the University of Michigan (Barker et al., 1991; Nickoloff, 1988; Nickoloff and Griffiths, 1990). For example, urushiol, the agent responsible for poison ivy dermatitis, retinoic acid, or ultraviolet light can induce keratinocytes to secrete the cytokines TNF-α, IL-8, and IL-l in vitro (Fig.17-6). In addition, these agents are able to induce keratinocyte expression of E-selectin, the ligand for which is leukocyte function-associated-1 (LFA-l) molecule (Chapters 5 and 7). As Nickoloff (1991) has proposed, these keratinocyte-derived cytokines and ICAM-l can then begin to orchestrate the cellular inflammatory response. First, keratinocyte-derived IL-l and TNF-α can induce the nearby dermal vasculature to express the adhesion molecules, E-Selectin, VCAM-l, and ICAM-l. As described in previous chapters, these endothelial adhesion molecules interact with their respective leukocyte receptor, thereby causing leukocyte margination and subsequent migration from the vasculature. Second, once brought to the site, these extravasated leukocytes may do one of two things. They can remain in the dermis, where they can amplify the stimulatory signals to the epidermis (Fig. 17-6). Alternatively, they can migrate along IL-8-directed chemotactic gradients to the epidermis, where LFA-l-expressing leukocytes will adhere to ICAM-l-expressing keratinocytes. There, they can either provide growth or stimulatory signals to keratinocytes, or damage them by cell type-specific cytotoxic mechanisms. Thus, although these mechanisms of cutaneous inflammation are only just recently being elucidated and surely more will come, it is clear that cells residing in the epidermis and dermis interact in concert with one another to manifest pathologic changes in the skin. Unfortunately, most of the inflammatory dermatoses of humans or animals have not yet been examined in this detail. However, it is clear from in vitro experiments that keratinocytes have potential functional capabilities that far surpass those necessary to simply provide a protective barrier. Furthermore, without doubt that there are many more agents or environmental stimuli which have the capacity to induce keratinocyte elaboration or expression of inflammatory cytokines or important adhesion molecules.

Gross cutaneous lesions

There are a number of clinical descriptive terms used in dermatology, some of which are useful to the dermatopathologist when making a diagnosis. Unfortunately, in the literature, there is variation and nonuniformity in definitions of some of these clinical terms. In this chapter, the clinical terms we have chosen to describe primary skin lesions in animals are defined below.

Skin lesions that are flat, but of a different color than the adjacent skin, are either **macules** (< 1.0 cm in diameter) or **patches** (<1.0 cm in diameter) and can be the result of a number of different processes. Variations in the quantity of melanin pigment can result in either hyperpigmented or hypopigmented macules or patches. Many flat lesions are attributed to variations in the amount of blood flow to the area, such as in inflamed erythematous skin lesions. In these lesions, the erythrocytes, for the most part, remain in the dilated vessels so that the skin blanches when pressure is applied to it. When red blood cells have extravasated from the vessels and are free in the dermal collagen, the redness imparted to the skin does not blanche, and the lesions are usually dark red to purple. These **purpuric** lesions are referred to either as **petechiae** when they are pinpoint in size and **ecchymoses** when they are greater than 1 cm in diameter. Petechiae should always be differentiated from telangiectasis, which is a

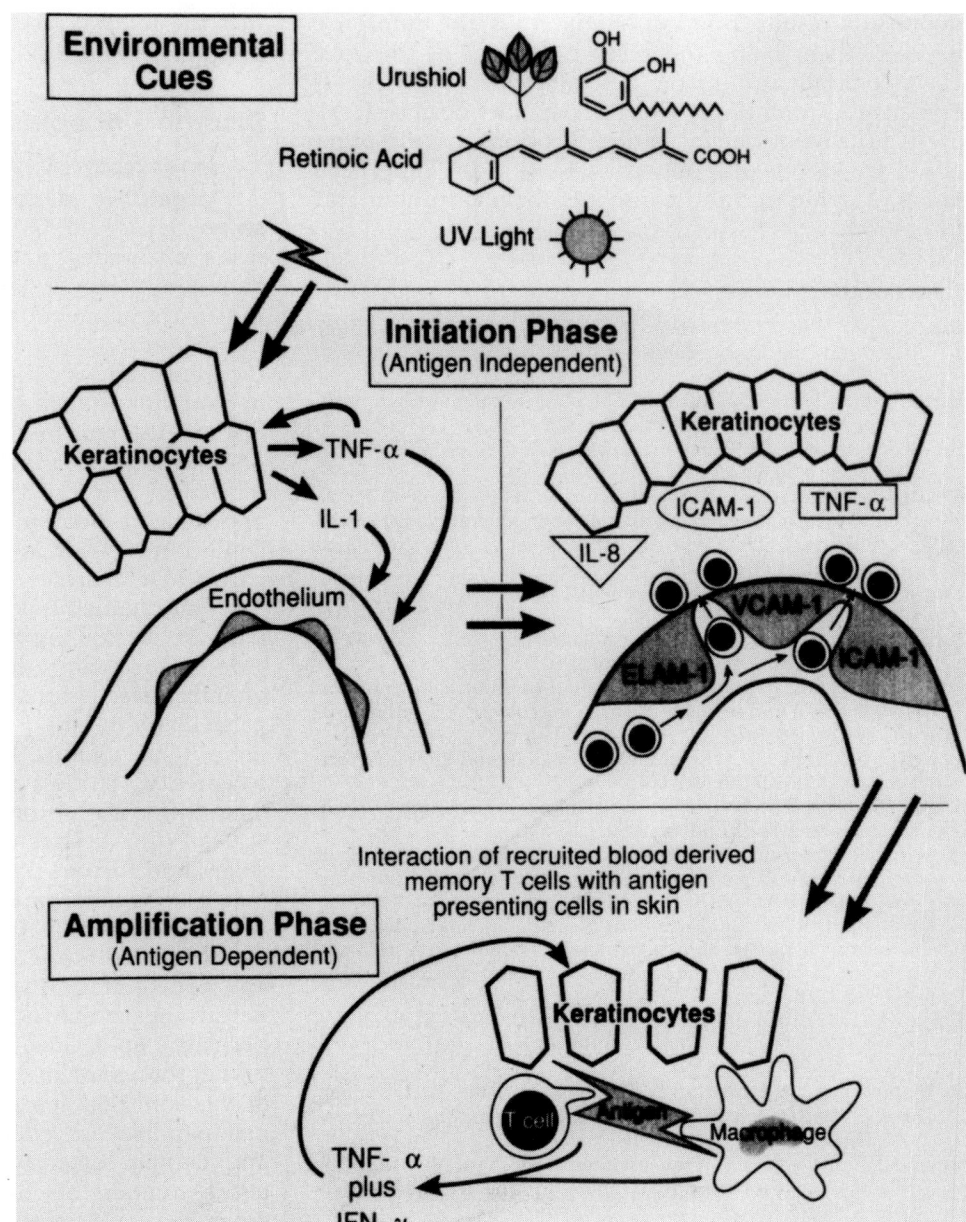

FIG. 17-6 Schematic illustration of how keratinocytes function as environmental signal transducers converting exogenous stimuli into the production of pro-inflammatory cytokines. (Barker JNWN, Mitra RS, Griffiths CEM, et al. Keratinocytes as initiators of inflammation. Lancet 1991;337:211–214, with permission of Dr. BJ Nickoloff and Lancet, Ltd.).

permanent dilatation of a single or multiple dermal capillaries. As the erythrocytes remain in the telangiectatic vessels, these lesions will blanche upon pressure.

A skin lesion that is raised, regardless if it is of a different color than the surrounding skin, is called a **papule** if it is less than 1.0 cm in diameter or a **plaque** if it is larger. Papules and plaques can result from either cellular infiltrates, metabolic deposits, or hyperplasia of specific components of the skin. They can be soft and often difficult or impossible to detect by palpation; visual examination with oblique light for the presence of shadows from these lesions is sometimes helpful in their detection. A **nodule,** on the other hand, is a solid, circumscribed elevation of any size that is readily palpable.

It usually results from massive infiltration of cells into the dermis and/or subcutis. A specific type of papule or plaque is a **wheal,** a rounded or flat-topped elevated lesion resulting from the accumulation of edema fluid within the dermis. These lesions, also called **urticarial eruptions,** are typically allergic responses (like type I hypersensitivity reactions) that disappear in a few hours. They can be many sizes and shapes and are usually pale red to white. Other raised lesions include **vesicles,** which are circumscribed, elevated lesions that contain fluid (Fig. 17-5), and **bullae,** which are vesicles <1.0 cm in diameter. Pustules are vesicles containing neutrophils and/or eosinophils exudate. Vesicles and bullae can be intraepidermal or subepidermal.

Depressed lesions include **ulcers** and **erosions.** The

depression results from loss of epidermis, the difference between them being the relative amount of this loss. Ulcers typically result from destruction of full-thickness epidermis as well as parts of the papillary dermis. Healing is usually by scar formation. Erosions, on the other hand, are lesions with only partial loss of the superficial layers of epidermis and consequently heal without scar formation.

References

Baadsgard O, Fisher G, Voorhees JJ, et al. The role of the immune system in the pathogenesis of psoriasis. J Invest Dermatol 1990;95:32S–34S.

Barker JNWN, Mitra RS, Griffiths CEM, et al. Keratinocytes as initiators of inflammation. Lancet 1991;337:211–214.

Bressler S, Bressler CH. Functional anatomy of the skin. Clin Podiatr Med Surg 1989;6:229–246.

Fitzpatrick TB, Bernhard JD. The structure of skin lesions and fundamentals of diagnosis. In: Dermatology in general medicine. 3rd ed. Fitzpatrick TB, Eisen AZ, Wolff K, et al., eds. New York: McGraw-Hill, 1987;4:20–49.

Krueger GG, Jorgensen CM. Experimental models for psoriasis. J Invest Dermatol 1990;95:56S–58S.

Krueger GG, Stingl G. Immunology/inflammation of the skin—a 50 year perspective. J Invest Dermatol 1989;92:32S–51S.

Lavker RM, Zheng P, Dong G. Aged skin: a study by light, transmission electron, and scanning electron microscopy. J Invest Dermatol 1987;88:44S–51S.

McKenzie RC, Sauder DN. Keratinocyte cytokines and growth factors. Dermatol Clin 1990;8:649–661.

Muller GH, Kirk RW, Scott DW. Small animal dermatology. 4th ed. Philadelphia: WB Saunders, 1989.

Nickoloff BJ. Role of interferon-gamma in cutaneous trafficking of lymphocytes with emphasis on molecular and cellular adhesion events. Arch Dermatol 1988;124:1835–1843.

Nickoloff BJ, Griffiths CEM. Abnormal cutaneous topobiology: the molecular basis for dermatopathologic mononuclear cell patterns in inflammatory skin disease. J Invest Dermatol 1990; 95:128S–131S.

Singer KH, Le PT, Denning SM, et al. The role of adhesion molecules in epithelial- T-cell interactions in thymus and skin. J Invest Dermatol 1990;94:85S–89S.

Siu G, Springer EA, Hedrick SM. The biology of the T-cell antigen receptor and its role in the skin immune system. J Invest Dermatol 1990;94:91S–100S.

Streilein JW. Speculations on the immunopathogenesis of psoriasis: T-cell violation of a keratinocyte sphere of influence. J Invest Dermatol 1990;95:20S–21S.

Van Damme J, Opdenakker G. Interaction of interferons with skin reactive cytokines: from Interleukin-1 to Interleukin-8. J Invest Dermatol 1990;95:93S–97S.

Wantzin GL, Ralfkiaer E, Lisby S, et al. The role of intercellular adhesion molecules in inflammatory skin reactions. Br J Dermatol 1988;119:141–145.

Wolff K, Kibbi A-G, Mihm MC. Basic pathologic reactions of the skin. In: Dermatology in general medicine. 3rd ed. Fitzpatrick TB, Eisen AZ, Wolff K, et al., eds. New York: McGraw-Hill, 1987;5:49–68.

DISORDERS OF THE EPIDERMIS

As previously discussed, it is often impossible to separate the response of injury to the epidermis from that of the dermis, since injury of one affects the other and vice versa. However, there are specific disease entities of the skin in animals where the predominant change is located in one of the cutaneous compartments. In an attempt to simplify microscopic diagnosis using organization of diseases by reaction patterns, we have classified the following skin diseases according to predominant lesion and location within the skin.

Disorders of epidermal maturation

HYPERKERATOSIS/PARAKERATOSIS/ACANTHOSIS

Vegetative dermatosis (dermatosis vegetans) in swine Hjarre (1953) described a syndrome in young swine in Sweden that involved a proliferative and inflammatory reaction of the skin and hoof associated with a granulomatous alveolar and interstitial pneumonia. The disease is genetically inherited as an autosomal recessive trait, as originally reported by Larrson (1953) in Sweden and confirmed by Percy and Hulland (1967) in Canada; thus, heterozygotic parents and siblings are phenotypically normal. The gene has only been described in swine of the Landrace breed, and common ancestors in Sweden appear to be responsible for the condition in swine in Norway, England, Canada, Australia, and Denmark.

The cutaneous lesions usually appear in newborn animals, as swelling and erythema of the coronary region of the main and accessory digits of all feet. Frequently, these lesions spread to other parts of the body, particularly the inner aspects of the legs and the abdomen. The cutaneous lesions progress to elevated, roughened, hairless plaques, which may become covered with yellow-brown, greasy scale. In addition, the wall of the hooves become thickened and develop ridges and furrows parallel to the coronary band which may lead to deformities.

Microscopically, the early cutaneous lesions consist mainly of acanthosis and hyperkeratosis (orthokeratotic and parakeratotic), with elongation of the rete ridges. Keratin pearls may occasionally be found within the hyperplastic epidermis. This marked epidermal proliferation accounts for the uneven appearance of the surface of the skin. Between the elongated rete ridges, the dermal papillae are edematous, have dilated capillaries, and contain extensive infiltrates of neutrophils and lesser numbers of eosinophils, sometimes forming microabscesses. Microabscesses may also be found within the acanthotic epidermis. Older lesions consist of severe acanthosis involving extensive areas of the epidermis, often associated with moderate to severe hyperkeratosis. In some cases, the dermis is thrown up into papillary folds. The sweat glands may be cystic due to occlusion of their ducts by the accumulation of excessive keratin.

Evensen and Bratberg (1990) in a longitudinal study of the lung lesions demonstrated that animals are born with normal lungs, but that a mononuclear interstitial and alveolar pneumonia with multinucleated giant cells develops by seven days of age (Fig. 17-7). These inflammatory cellular infiltrates are accompanied by hyperplasia of alveolar pneumocytes. Bronchi and bronchioles are not affected. The inflammation within the alveoli and interstitium increases progressively to a widespread granulomatous pulmonary infiltrate by the second month of life, after which, the inflammatory changes progressively subside. If the ani-

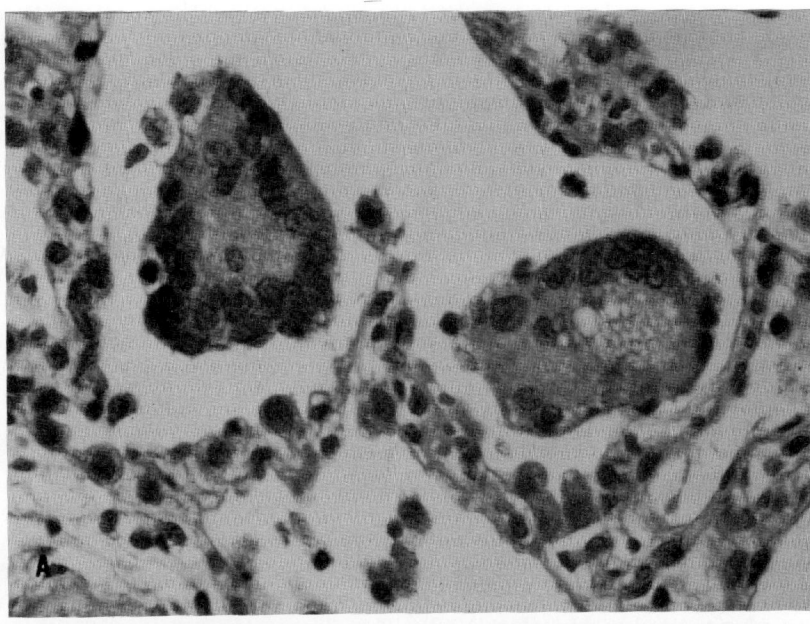

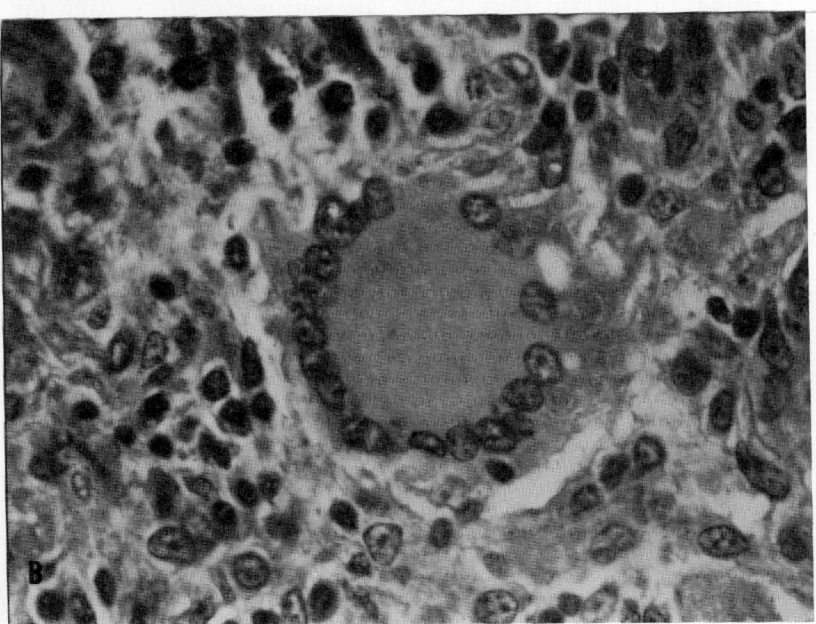

FIG. 17-7 Vegetative dermatosis of swine. **A.** Multinucleated giant cells with vacuolated cytoplasm in alveoli of lung. **B.** Langhan's type of multinucleated giant cell in bronchial lymph node. (Courtesy of Drs. Dean H. Percy, Thomas J. Hulland, and *Pathologia Veterinaria.*)

mal survives to one year of age, the lungs may contain moderate interstitial fibrosis, smaller and fewer granulomas, and moderate mononuclear interstitial inflammation.

The role of the defective gene product in the pathogenesis of the disorder has not been determined.

References

Done JT, Loosemore RM, Saunders CM. Dermatosis vegetans in pigs. Vet Rec 1967;80:292–298.

Evensen O, Bratberg B. Pulmonary multinucleate giant cells in dermatosis vegetans in swine: light microscopic and immunohistochemical investigations. Acta Vet Scand 1987;28:429–433.

Evensen O, Bratberg B. A sequential light microscopic study of the pulmonary lesions in porcine dermatosis vegetans. Res Vet Sci 1990;49:50–55.

Garrett KC, Richerson HB, Hunninghake GW. Pathogenesis of the granulomatous lung diseases. Am Rev Respir Dis 1984;130:476–496.

Hjarre A. Vegetierende Dermatosen mit Riesenzellem-pneumonien bei Schwein. Dtsch Tierarztl Wochenscher 1953;60:105–110.

Jericho KWF. Dermatosis vegetans—giant cell pneumonitis in pigs: further observations and interpretations. Res Vet Sci 1974;16:176–181.

Larsson EL. Klumpfotgrisar. Svenska Svinavelsfer Tidskr 1953;1:1– 15.

Percy DH, Hulland TJ. Dermatosis vegetans (vegetative dermatosis) in Canadian swine. Can Vet J 1967;8:3–9.

Percy DH, Hulland TJ. Evolution of multinucleate giant cells in dermatosis vegetans in swine. Pathol Vet 1967;5:419–428.

Percy DH, Hulland TJ. The histopathological changes in the skin of pigs with dermatosis vegetans. Can J Comp Med 1969;33:48–54.

Webb RF, Bourke CA. Dermatosis vegetans in pigs. Aust Vet J 1987;64:287–288.

Ichthyosis A rare disease of humans, cattle, dogs, swine, chickens, mice, and llamas (for which there has been a single report), ichthyosis is, in fact, a heterogeneous group of dermatoses characterized by excessive cutaneous scale formation causing the skin to resemble that of a fish. In most cases, the condition is present at birth, however, acquired examples of ichthyosis have been described in human patients with hyperparathyroidism, certain malignancies, and hypothyroidism, and in human beings and mice administered certain drugs that interfere with cholesterol metabolism (Elias et al., 1983).

In the veterinary literature, most cases have been in calves, with rare descriptions in the dog. In cattle, there is variation in the severity of the condition. The most severe form, termed ichthyosis fetalis (Harlequin fetus, from the grotesque garb of Harlequin clown), was first described in humans more than a century and a half ago. The harlequin calf has been described in Norwegian Red Poll and Swiss breeds. Affected calves are born hairless, or nearly so, and are covered with thick, scaly, horny skin, which is divided into plates by deep fissures. These fissures are often wide, with a red, raw-appearing base, and follow a pattern that corresponds to the cleavage planes of the skin (Fig. 17-8). The skin is everted around the lips, eyes, and other body orifices, giving the impression that it is too small for the body. The affected animals do not survive for more than a few hours, or at the most, a few days. Microscopic sections reveal the epidermis to be covered by an extremely thick, dense, and tightly adherent layer of keratin. Hyperkeratosis also involves the infundibulae of hair follicles. The rete ridges are elongated; the dermis is moderately thickened and contains congested capillaries, particularly in areas underlying the fissures.

Less severe forms of the disease have been described in Holstein calves (Julian, 1960). The condition is usually present at birth but varies in severity. Males appear to be affected more often than females, and the disease affects specific families of cattle. This form of the diseaese has been referred to as icthyosis congenita. The affected calves are born with thick, hard skin that folds along the neck, abdomen, and joints, with variable but sparse short hair. Cracks and fissures develop around the muzzle and ears.

Histologically, the surface of the skin is thrown into wrinkles and folds, and the stratum corneum is considerably thickened. The hyperkeratosis extends into the hair follicles. As parents are almost always phenotypically normal, this form of the disease is believed to be inherited as a single recessive trait.

More recently, rare reports of a similar disease in dogs have been described. Affected dogs have most if not all of their skin covered by dry, gray, tightly adherent scales (Fig. 17-9). Occasionally, the adherent scales will appear as feathered keratinaceous projections. Patches of dry scale are more prominent in the flexural creases and intertriginous areas. In two cases (Muller, 1976), the digital and carpal foot pads were involved and were reported to be thick and painful. Microscopically, the skin is marked by orthokeratotic hyperkeratosis and follicular plugging. The stratum granulosum is prominent, due to an increase in the number of keratohyaline granules. Ballooning change (hydropic swelling) of keratinocytes in the statum granulosum is sometimes present. The epidermis may or may not be acanthotic. Canine ichthyosis is thought to be inherited as an autosomal recessive trait.

In human beings, ichthyosis has been classified based on differences in clinical appearance, family history and mode of inheritance, histopathological changes in the skin, and most recently, quantitative enzyme assays from patient cells and lipid biochemical analyses of cutaneous scales. The two most common types of ichthyosis in humans are ichthyosis vulgaris,

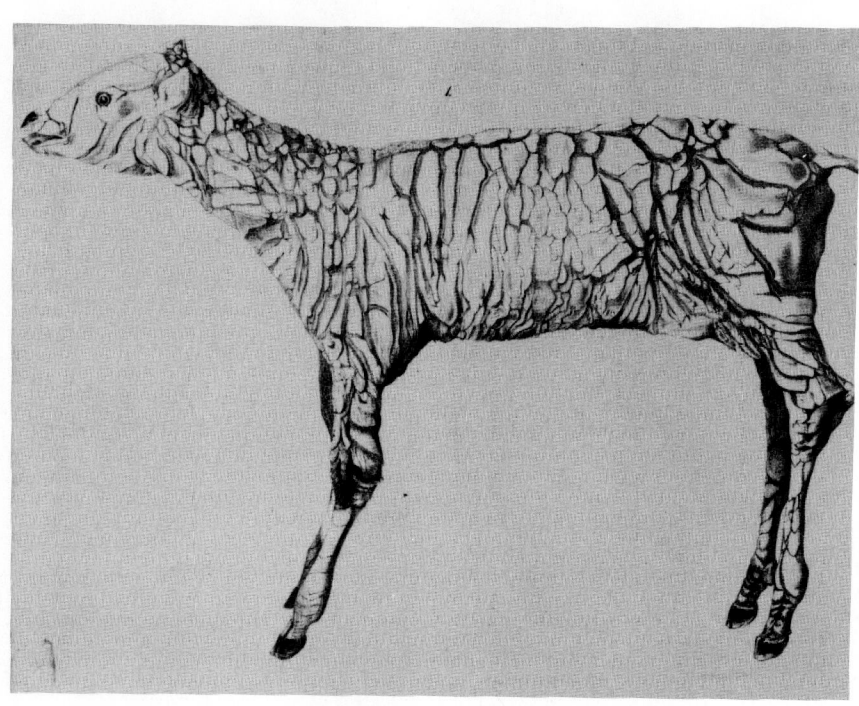

FIG. 17-8 Congenital ichthyosis, skin of a newborn calf. (Courtesy of Armed Forces Institute of Pathology.)

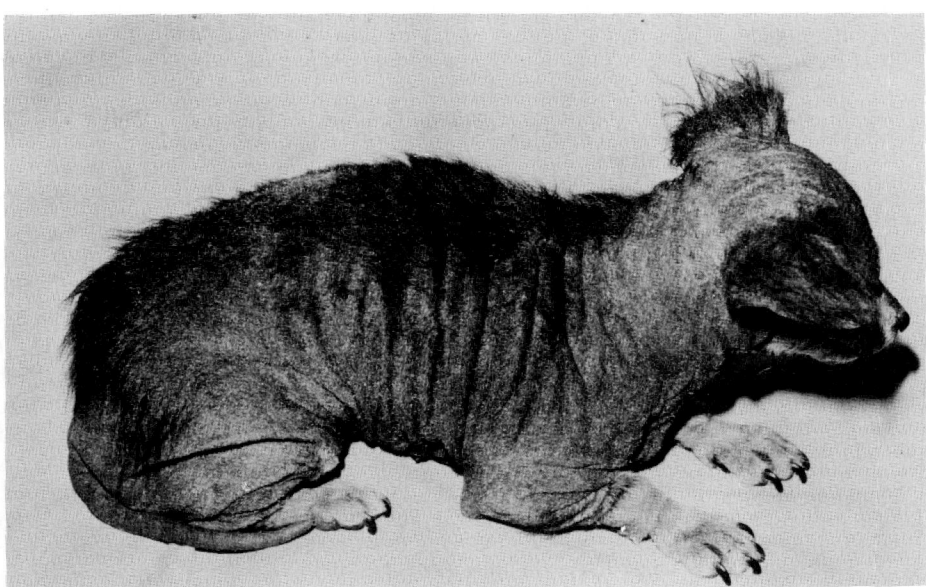

FIG. 17-9 Canine ichthyosis. There is little body hair, the skin is thickened and covered with keratin scales. (Courtesy of Dr. G. H. Muller and *Journal of the American Veterinary Medical Association*.)

which varies considerably in clinical severity and is inherited in an autosomal dominant fashion, and the recessive X-linked ichthyosis, which is associated with a deficiency in steroid sulphatase. This enzyme is important in the metabolism of estrogen and cholesterol sulphate. Affected males have relatively severe scaling, while heterozygous females have relatively minor clinical signs. Other types of ichthyosis include the congenital varieties: 1) lamellar ichthyosis (also referred to as nonbullous congenital ichthyosiform erythroderma), which has two subclasses, one inherited in an autosomal recessive fashion, the other as an autosomal dominant type, 2) the previously described lethal Harlequin ichthyosis, or ichthyosis fetalis, and 3) epidermolytic hyperkeratosis, or bullous congenital ichthyosiform erythroderma, which is inherited as an autosomal dominant trait. This type of ichthyosis has, in addition to the common orthokeratotic hyperkeratosis, vacuolization and ballooning change of the suprabasilar keratinocytes, often with clinically-visible bullae.

As mentioned in the introduction to this chapter, excessive scale can be the result of overproduction of stratum corneum and/or the excessive retention of keratin. In most forms of ichthyosis in humans, it is believed that abnormal retention of keratin is the mechanism for excessive scale formation. As the stratum corneum represents corneocytes embedded in a lipid-rich matrix glue, problems with epidermal lipid metabolism may interfere with normal corneocyte cohesion and disassociation and thus the normal rate of keratin desquamation from the surface. In that regard, there is compelling evidence that ichthyosiform dermatoses are associated with abnormal lipid metabolism: 1) the human X-linked variety is linked to an absence of steroid sulfatase activity, which results in the accumulation of cholesterol sulfate in skin and other tissues, 2) lipid

profiles of stratum corneum derived from patients with ichthyosiform dermatoses are often abnormal compared to those from normal patients, 3) in some varieties of ichthyosis, particularly lamellar ichthyosis, increased numbers of lipid inclusions can be found in the stratum corneum, and 4) humans and mice develop ichthyosiform changes when administered hypocholesterolemic drugs. Because of the rarity of the condition in animals, the possibility of classification into different types, perhaps with different pathophysiologic mechanisms, remains to be determined.

References

Arnold ML, Anton-Lamprecht I., Melz-Rothfuss B, et al. Ichthyosis congenita type III: clinical and ultrastructural characteristics and distinction within the heterogeneous ichthyosis congenita group. Arch Dermatol Res 1988;280:268–278.

August JR, Chickering WR, Rikihisa Y. Congenital ichthyosis in a dog: comparison with the human ichthyosiform dermatoses. Comp Cont Ed 1988;10:40–45.

Ballabio A, Sebastio G, Carozzo R, et al. Deletions of the steroid sulphatase gene in "classical" X-linked ichthyosis and in X-linked ichthyosis associated with Kallmann syndrome. Hum Genet 1987;77:338–341.

Baker JR, Ward WR. Ichthyosis in domestic animals: a review of the literature and a case report. Br Vet J 1985;141:1–8.

Belknap EB, Dunstan RW. Congenital ichthyosis in a llama. J Am Vet Med. Assoc 1990;197:764–767.

Bousema M, van Diggelen O, van Joost T, et al. Ichthyosis. Reliability of clinical signs in the differentiation between autosomal dominant and sex-linked forms.. Int J Dermatol 28:240–242, 1989.

Brown BE, Williams ML, Elia. PM. Stratum corneum lipid abnormalities in ichthyosis. Arch Dermatol 1984;120:204–209.

Edmonds HW, Dolan WD: Icthyosis congenita fetalis, severe type(harlequin fetus). Bull Internat Assoc Med Mus 1951;32:1–21.

Elias PM, Lampe MA, Chung J-C, et al. Diazacholesterol-induced ichthyosis in the hairless mouse. Lab Invest 1983;48:565–577.

Epstein EH, Williams ML, Elias PM. Biochemical abnormalities in the ichthyoses. Curr Prob Dermatol 1987;17:32–44.

Fleck RM, Barnadas M, Schulz WW, et al. Harlequin ichthyosis: an ultrastructural study. J Am Acad Dermatol 1989;21:999–1006.

Hutt FB. Inherited lethal characters in domestic animals. Cornell Vet 1934;24:1–25.

Jensen JE, Esterly NB. The ichthyosis mouse: histologic, histochemical, ultrastructural and autoradiographic studies of interfollicular epidermis. J Invest Dermatol 1977;68:23–31.

Julian RJ. Ichthyosis congenita in cattle. Vet Med 1960;55:35–41.

London RD, Lebwohl M. Acquired ichthyosis and hyperparathyroidism. J Am Acad Dermatol 1989;21:801–802.

McGrae JD, Jr. Keratitis, ichthyosis, and deafness (KID) syndrome. Int J Dermatol 1990;29:89–93.

Melnik B, Kuster W, Hollmann J, et al. Autosomal dominant lamellar ichthyosis exhibits an abnormal scale lipid pattern. Clin Genet 1989;35:252–256.

Muller GH. Ichthyosis in two dogs. J Am Vet Med Assoc 1976;169:1313–1316.

Piccirillo A, Auricchio L, Fabbrocini G, et al. Ocular findings and skin histology in a group of patients with X-linked ichthyosis. Br J Dermatol 1990;119:185–188.

Piraud M, Maire I, Zabot M. X-linked recessive echthyosis. Enzyme 1989;41:227–234.

Selmanowitz FJ. Ichthyosis. In: Andrews EJ, Ward BC, Altman NH, eds. Spontaneous animal models of human diseases. Vol. II. New York: Academic Press, 1979;145:4–5.

Steijlen PM, Perret CM, Schuunnans Stekhoven JH, et al. Ichthyosis bullosa of siemens: further delineation of the phenotype. Arch Dermatol Res 1990;282:1–5.

Primary idiopathic seborrhea A chronic skin condition of unknown cause, primary idiopathic seborrhea is a persistent disease more common in certain breeds of dogs, particularly the cocker spaniel, springer spaniel, bassett hound, Irish setter, Doberman pinscher, German shepherd, West Highland white terrier, dachshund, shar pei, Labrador retriever, and poodle. There appears to be a genetic predisposition for its development. There is no cure, so affected animals have the condition for life, but topical treatments can ameliorate some of the clinical signs.

The disease is characterized by the appearance of alopecia, scaling, and crusting on the face, extremities, and ventral trunk, which can appear as dry, flaky scale (seborrhea sicca) or oily adherent brown to yellow clumped scale (seborrhea oleosa). By definition, seborrhea means increased sebum production; while increased cutaneous lipid production with the oleosa variety is easy to appreciate clinically, it may not be as apparent in the sicca type. In fact, measurement of actual sebum production in dogs with seborrhea, to the authors' knowledge, has not been done. Kwochka and Rademakers (1989) have demonstrated that the sebaceous glands from Cocker Spaniels with idopathic seborrhea are hyperproliferative, which by inference in a holocrine type gland suggests that they have an increased secretory rate. Other gross manifestations of idiopathic seborrhea include comedones, alopecia, odor, keratinaceous plaques, and ceruminous otitis. Idiopathic seborrhea can sometimes be associated with inflammation, in which case it is referred to as **seborrheic dermatitis.** In seborrheic dermatitis erythema can be added to the clinical signs. Seborrheic dermatitis has also been recognized in other species, most commonly humans, where it occurs in babies and adults and involves the scalp, face, and trunk.

Histologically, seborrheic skin is acanthotic, has keratin plugging of the follicular infundibulae, and vari-

able amounts of parakeratosis, particularly around the shoulders of follicular ostia. Spongiosis may or may not be present. Inflammation, if present, consists of a mild perivascular, mononuclear infiltrate in the superficial dermis. Variable numbers of neutrophils may also be present in the dermis, and keratin scale near the follicular ostia may contain collections of neutrophils as well.

As these changes are not specific for primary idiopathic seborrhea, this disorder can only be diagnosed on the basis of excluding other causes of epidermal and follicular scale. Identical changes occur with **secondary seborrhea,** which occurs secondarily to either: 1) inflammatory conditions, such as ectoparasites, autoimmune diseases, hypersensitivity reactions, bacterial or fungal infections, or 2) those of a metabolic nature, such as endocrinopathies including hypothyroidism (Fig. 17-10), hyperadrenalcorticism, gonadal hormone abberations, diabetes mellitus and nutrional deficiencies, including protein, fat, vitamins A and E, and zinc. Secondary seborrhea stemming from nutritional deficiencies can be the result of dietary inadequacies, malabsorption, maldigestion, or intestinal parasitism. As a rule, primary idiopathic seborrhea does not respond favorably to dietary supplementation with vitamins, minerals, protein, or fat. Thus, the diagnosis of primary idiopathic seborrhea can only be made after an exhaustive search for associated causes of secondary seborrhea.

Although the etiology of primary idiopathic seborrhea is not known, some aspects of its pathogenesis have been characterized. First, cell kinetic studies have shown that compared to normal dogs, affected dogs have accelerated cellular proliferation of the interfollicular epidermis, upper follicular external root sheath, and sebaceous glands (Baker and Maibach, 1987; Kwochka and Rademakers, 1989; Kwochka, 1990). In these studies, it was found that the cell renewal time of epidermis from affected dogs is approximately 7 days, while that from normal dogs is approximately 22 days. Thus, in affected dogs, there is more rapid epidermal proliferation, which without concomitant keratin loss from the surface, leads to the formation of adherent scale. Most investigators attribute, at least in part, the hyperkeratosis associated with this condition to this epithelial hyperproliferation, but as suggested by Kwochka and Rademakers (1989), retention of the keratinized scale may also play a role, particularly if the lipid content of the epidermis is also altered. Although, to our knowledge, quantitative sebum analyses have not been reported on canine seborrheic skin, there are relative increases of free fatty acids and decreases of diester waxes compared to normal dogs (Ihrke, 1979). These observations have led investigators to speculate that primary idiopathic seborrhea represents abnormalities of epidermal maturation/keratinization and perhaps sebum production. However, as mentioned at the beginning of this chapter, dermal constituents can have profound influences on the epidermis and vice versa. Thus, as investigations continue into the nature of the signals and pathways activated in the skin that influence the

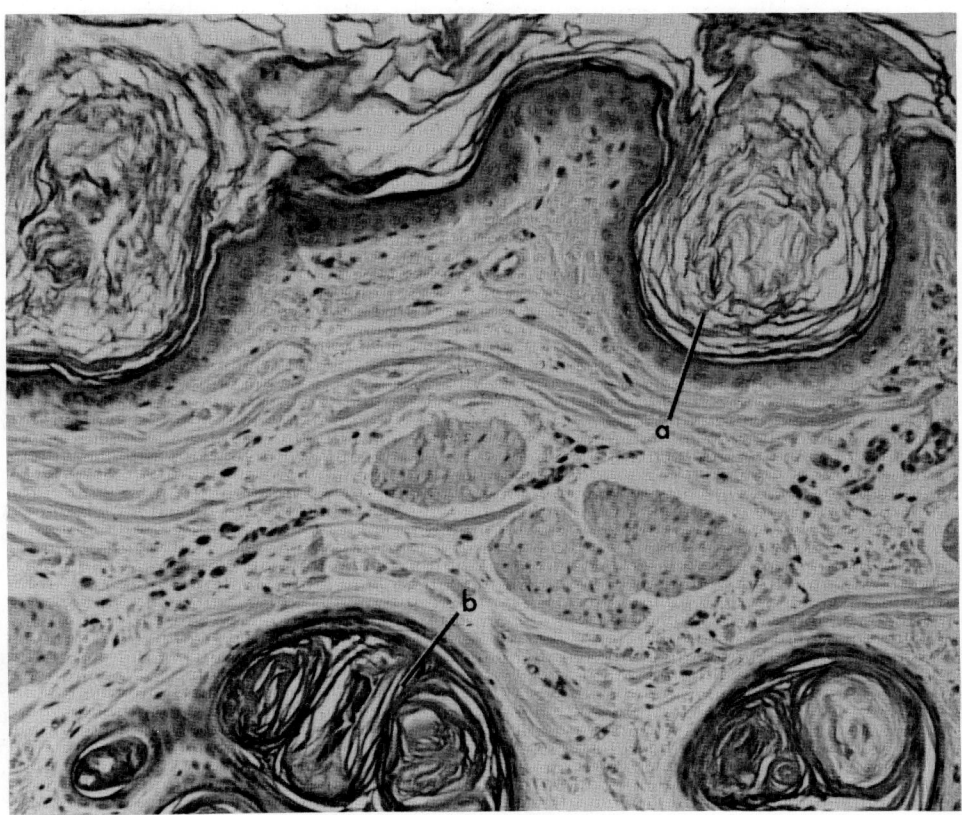

FIG. 17-10 The skin in canine hypothyroidism. A seven-year-old female Chihuahua with characteristic clinical signs. Note hyperkeratosis involving epidermis (*a*) and the hair follicles (*b*). (Courtesy of Angell Memorial Animal Hospital.)

function of other components of the skin, it is possible that the altered epidermal turnover and sebum production in canine idiopathic seborrhea may, in fact, be related to each other via a common pathway.

References

Baker BB, Maibach HI. Epidermal cell renewal in seborrheic skin of dogs. Am J Vet Res 1987;48:726–728.

Brenner S, Horwitz C. Possible nutrient mediators in psoriasis and seborrheic dermatitis: I. Prevalence, etiology, symptomatology, histological and biochemical features. World Rev Nutr Diet 1988;55:153–164.

Brenner S, Horwitz C. Possible nutrient mediators in psoriasis and seborrheic dermatitis: II. Nutrient mediators: essential fatty acids; vitamins A, E and D; vitamins Bl, B2, B6, niacin and biotin; vitamin C, selenium; zinc; iron. World Rev Nutr Diet 1988;55:165–182.

Halliwell RE. Seborrhea in the dog. Comp Cont Ed 1979;1:227–236.

Hoger H, Gialamas J, Adamiker D. Inherited seborrheic dermatitis— a new mutant in mice. Laboratory Animals 1987;21:299–305.

Ihrke PJ. Canine seborrheic disease complex. Vet Clin North Am 1979;9:93–106.

Kwochka KW. Cell proliferation kinetics in the hair root matrix of dogs with healthy skin and dogs with idiopathic seborrhea. Am J Vet Res 1990;51:1570–1573.

Kwochka KW, Rademakers AM. Cell proliferation kinetics of epidermis, hair follicles, and sebaceous glands of cocker spaniels with idiopathic seborrhea. Am J Vet Res 1989;50:1918–1922.

Muller GH, Kirk RW, Scott DW. Chapter 14 Keratinization defects. In: Small animal dermatology. 4th ed.. Philadelphia: WB Saunders, 1989;14:715–726.

Newcomer CE, Fox FG, Taylor RM, et al. Seborrheic dermatitis in a rhesus monkey (*Macaca mulatta*). Lab Anim Sci 1984;34:185–187.

Plewig G: Seborrheic dermatitis. In:Fitzpatrick TB ,Eisen AZ, Wolff K, et al., eds. Dermatology in general medicine. 3rd ed.New York: McGraw-Hill, 1987;84:978–981.

Vitamin A-responsive dermatosis of dogs A chronic exfoliative skin disease affecting primarily cocker spaniels, vitamin A-responsive dermatosis clinically resembles primary idiopathic and secondary seborrhea. The skin has varying degrees of generalized to focal crusting, scaling, and alopecia. There is marked follicular plugging with comedo-like horny plugs and hyperkeratotic plaques. These plaques often have frond-like projections of keratin protruding from their surface. These plaques can be found anywhere on the body but are especially prominent on the ventral and lateral chest and abdomen.

Histologically, the plaques are characterized by striking dilatation of the follicular infundibulae, with extreme follicular orthokeratotic hyperkeratosis. There is only mild epidermal orthokeratotic hyperkeratosis with little or no parakeratosis. The epidermis is either normal in thickness or only mildly acanthotic. In the dermis, there may or may not be an inflammatory infiltrate. If present, it consists mainly of mononuclear inflammatory cells located around the superficial dermal vessels. Diagnosis is made by clinical findings, microscopic changes in the skin, and positive response to large doses of orally-administered vitamin A. Although hyperkeratosis of the follicular ostia also occurs in seborrhea, it is not as consistent or as strikingly severe as it is in vitamin A-responsive dermatosis.

The lesions are very similar to the cutaneous changes seen in humans and animals with vitamin A deficiency. In this deficiency, marked follicular keratosis, dry skin, scaling, and pruritus have been described. However, in animals with vitamin A-responsive dermatosis, there is no history of, or other clinical signs of hypovitaminosis A. Thus, the pathogenesis of this disorder is unknown, and the influences on follicular keratinization by exogenously-administered vitamin A, in amounts exceeding recommended canine dietary requirements, is also not understood.

References

Boyd AS. An overview of the retinoids. Am J Med 1989;86:568–574.

Cohen PR, Prystowsky JH. Pityriasis rubra pilaris: a review of diagnosis and treatment. J Am Acad Dermatol 1989;20:801–807.

Ihrke PJ, Goldschmidt MH. Vitamin A-responsive dermatosis in the dog. J Am Vet Med Assoc 1983;182:687–690.

Miller WH. Nutritional considerations in small animal dermatology. Vet Clin North Am Small Anim Pract 1989;19:497–511.

Muller GH, Kirk RW, Scott DW. Chapter 14 Keratinization defects. In: Small animal dermatology. 4th ed. Philadelphia: WB Saunders, 1989;14:726–727.

Scott DW. Vitamin A-responsive dermatosis in the cocker spaniel. J Am Anim Hosp Assoc 1986;22:125–129.

Zinc-responsive dermatoses Zinc is an essential trace element for hundreds of metalloenzymes important for normal nucleic acid, protein, and membrane metabolism. As such, deficiencies result in a multitude of clinical effects, ranging from marked growth retardation, thymic atrophy, lymphoid depletion with defects in cellular immunity, chronic diarrhea, skin changes, and hypogonadism, to more subtle abnormalities such as alterations in taste acuity. As skin changes are often one of the first clinical signs of zinc deficiency in a number of animal species, including dogs, swine, rats, sheep, cattle, goats, cats, ducks, chickens, and humans, and because they resemble other hyperkeratotic skin disorders, we will describe these skin alterations in this section of the book. For a more thorough discussion of the other systemic signs of zinc deficiency, the reader is encouraged to see Chapter 17.

A biologic deficiency of zinc can occur in a variety of ways. True dietary deficiencies of zinc in domestic animals fed commercially-prepared food are extremely uncommon. However, the effective absorption of zinc from the gut is influenced by a number of other nutrients. Calcium, phytate (organic phosphorus found in plant proteins), copper, or cadmium, when present in sufficient quantities in the diet, can interfere with the absorption of zinc from the gut. A relative zinc deficiency can ensue when these compounds are in relative high amounts in the diet combined with marginal or normal levels of dietary zinc. For example, in **parakeratosis of swine,** first described by Kernkampp and Ferriin (1953), it has been established that excess dietary calcium interferes with zinc absorption and predisposes young swine to the disease. Addition of zinc to the ration and adjusting calcium intake dramatically cures or prevents parakeratosis. Likewise, in rapidly-growing puppies fed diets oversupplemented with minerals (e.g. calcium), or in dogs fed generic foods based on corn and wheat (e.g. high phytate), an exfoliative dermatosis resembling experimental zinc deficiency results (Sousa et al., 1988; Miller, 1989). Moreover, genetic defects of

zinc absorption from the intestine have been described in humans and animals, resulting in reduced zinc bioavailability, deficiency, and exfoliative skin disease. In humans, Black Pied Danish cattle, and the bull terrier, **acrodermatitis enteropathica** is a lethal, autosomal recessive trait. In humans and cattle, zinc supplementation results in complete cure; in the bull terrier, serum zinc levels are reduced, but supplementation of dietary zinc does not ameliorate the clinical signs or prevent death (Jezyk et al., 1986). In Alaskan malamutes and Siberian huskies, there is a **zinc-responsive dermatosis,** that at least for malamutes, appears to be the result of reduced absorption of intestinal zinc. As its name implies, dietary zinc therapy is usually rapidly successful. Other causes of functional zinc deficiency include steatorrhea, inflammatory bowel disease, renal disease, thermal injuries, and the therapeutic use of chelating agents for other medical reasons.

As all of the above conditions are effectively the result of reduced bioavailability of zinc, the skin lesions are similar and thus represent a recognizable functional consequence of zinc deficiency. There is partial alopecia and tightly adherent scaling and crusting of the distal portions of the extremities, face, mucocutaneous junctions, and pressure points, often in a bilaterally symmetrical pattern. A zone of erythema often demarcates the lesions. Erosions, ulcerations, papules, pustules, and sometimes exudative lesions may be observed in more advanced lesions, occasionally with regional lymphadenopathy. In dogs, the foot pads frequently have fissures, cracks, and focal erosions.

Histologically, the lesions are characterized by marked parakeratosis, with moderate acanthosis and mild orthokeratotic hyperkeratosis. Parakeratotic hyperkeratosis is particularly prominent near and within follicular ostia. Occasionally, neutrophil exocytosis into the epidermis and follicular epithelium is seen. Ballooning change in epidermal cells may or may not be present. In dogs fed generic food or puppies receiving nutritional supplementation, dyskeratotic keratinocytes have been described (Sousa et al., 1988). In the dermis, there is a mild to moderate perivascular mixed inflammatory cell infiltrate.

References

Fadok VA. Zinc responsive dermatosis in a Great Dane: a case report. J Am Ani Hosp Assoc 1982;18:409–414.

Jezyk PF, Haskins ME, MacKay-SmithWE, et al. Lethal acrodermatitis in bull terriers. J Am Vet Med Assoc 188:833–839, 1986.

Kernkamp HCH, Ferrin ER. Parakeratosis in swine. J Am Vet Med Assoc 1953;123:217–220.

Kunkle GA. Zinc-responsive dermatoses in dogs. In: Kirk RW, ed. Current veterinary therapy VII: small animal practice. . Philadelphia: WB Saunders, 1980;472–476.

McClain CJ, Kasarskis EJ, Jr., Allen JJ. Functional consequences of zinc deficiency. Prog Food Nutr Sci 1985;9:185–226.

Miller WH, Jr. Nutritional considerations in small animal dermatology. Vet Clin North Am Small Anim Pract 1989:19:497–511.

Muller GH, Kirk RW, Scott DW. Chapter 14. Keratinization defects. In: Small animal dermatology. 4th ed. Philadelphia: WB Saunders, 1989;17:801–806.

Ohlen B, Scott DW. Zinc responsive dermatitis in puppies. Canine Pract 1986;13:6–10.

Prasad AS. Clinical, endocrinological and biochemical effects of zinc deficiency. Clin Endocrinol. Metab 1985;14:567–589.

Robertson BT, Burns MJ. Zinc metabolism and the zinc-deficiency syndrome in the dog. Am J Vet Res 196324:997–1002.

Sanecki RK, Corbin JE, Forbes RM. Tissue changes in dogs fed a zinc-deficient ration. Am J Vet Res 1982;43:1642–1646.

Sousa CA, Stannard AA, Ihrke PJ,et al. Dermatosis associated with feeding generic dog food: 13 cases (1981–1982). J Am Vet Med Assoc 1988;192:676–680.

Van Den Broek AHM. Diagnostic value of zinc concentrations in serum, leucocytes and hair of dogs with zinc-responsive dermatosis. Res Vet Sci 1988;44:41–44.

Van Den Broek AHM, Thoday KL. Skin disease in dogs associated with zinc deficiency: a report of 5 cases. J Small Anim Pract 1986;27:313–323.

Wright RP: Identification of zinc-responsive dermatoses. Vet Med. 1985;80:37–40.

Dermatophilosis (cutaneous streptothricosis) Dermatophilosis is an extremely hyperkeratotic and pyogenic disease of the skin that affects a wide variety of species including horses, cattle, sheep, goats, wild ruminants, and rarely cats, dogs, nonhuman primates and humans. It is caused by the gram-positive actinomycete, *Dermatophilus congolensis,* an organism that usually does not invade the normal epidermis. Although it occurs sporadically in most parts of the world; it occurs most commonly in warm tropical and subtropical geographic regions having a long rainy season. Under these conditions, prolonged exposure of the skin to heavy rainfall interferes with the protective function of the stratum corneum and sebaceous secretions of the skin. Lesions commonly occur on the back, but any area of the skin may be affected. Grossly, the lesions appear as raised, thick, yellow-brown discrete or confluent crusts containing matted hair on the surface of the skin. These crusts, when peeled from the skin, may leave areas of erosion. This prolonged dampness of the skin, coupled with trauma from biting insects, such as ticks, flies and mosquitoes, all of which can serve as mechanical vectors of *D. congolensis,* or wounds incurred during shearing or simply grazing in areas of coarse grasses, allows dormant zoospores of the organism to germinate and colonize the damaged epidermis. These zoospores are highly resistant to drying and extreme environmental temperatures and persist in dried exudates for many months even in recovered animals. Once the zoospores germinate in the damaged stratum corneum they become mobile and invade deeper portions of the epidermis down to the basement membrane. During this process they form branching filaments within which the organism undergoes a characteristic multidimensional division producing both longitudinal and transverse separation. The presence of such filaments is diagnostic of dermatophilosis. Early in infection, *D. congolensis* undergoes marked proliferation in the epithelium of the outer root sheath of hair follicles causing premature keratinization of these cells. At the same time, it provokes edema of the superficial dermis and neutrophil infiltration in the affected areas of epidermis with formation of microabscesses. As a consequence of the premature keratinization, epidermal cells beneath these areas respond by undergoing a reactive hyperplasia, which produces new cells that in turn are also invaded by the motile zoospores and the cycle is repeated. This results in the accumulation of a thick, elevated crust composed of alternating layers of parakeratotic and orthokeratotic hyperkeratosis with intervening zones of degenerating neutrophils. The underlying dermis typically is edematous and contains a mixture of acute and chronic inflammatory cells. Although rare, *D. congolensis,* has been reported to invade the dermis of cats, where it causes a pyogranulomatous dermatitis.

References

Bida SA, Dennis SM. Sequential pathological changes in natural and experimental dermatophilosis in Bunaji cattle. Res Vet Sci 1977;22:18–22.

Caracostas MC, Miller RI, Woodward MG. Subcutaneous dermatophilosis in a cat. J Am Vet Med Assoc 1984;185:675–676.

Hyslop NS. Dermatophilosis (streptothricosis) in animals and man. Comp Immunol Microbiol Infect Dis 1980;2:389–404.

Lloyd DH, Jenkinson DM. The effect of climate on experimental infection of bovine skin with *Dermatophilus congolensis.* Br Vet J 1980;136:122–134.

Roberts DS: The histopathology of epidermal infection with the actinomycete *Dermatophilus congolensis.* J Pathol Bacteriol 1965;90:213–216.

Lichenoid-psoriasiform dermatosis of springer spaniels A rare disorder of young (less than two years of age) Springer Spaniels, lichenoid-psoriasiform dermatosis, as its name implies, is characterized by the simultaneous appearance of two histologic changes in the same sample of skin. Lichenoid skin reactions refer to a "band-like" infiltrate of inflammatory cells in the upper dermis, often obscuring the dermal-epidermal junction. In human medicine, the prototypic disease of lichenoid skin reactions is lichen planus. **Psoriasiform skin reactions** refer to a type of epidermal hyperplasia (acanthosis) characterized by elongated rete ridges, a thin suprapapillary plate above the dermal papillae, variable amounts of othokeratotic and parakeratotic hyperkeratosis, hypogranulosis above the dermal papillae with hypergranulosis intervening elsewhere. Psoriasiform skin reactions occur in a number of human and animal skin diseases, but psoriasis of human beings is the disorder most often cited as displaying this type of reaction. The dermatosis of springer spaniels described in this section has features which are both lichenoid and psoriasiform. The lesions begin as erythematous papules and plaques on the medial aspect of the pinnae and caudoventral portion of the abdomen, with involvement of the prepuce in males. In more advanced cases, scaly, erythematous papules and plaques can also be found around the eyes, anus, mouth, nose, and extremities.

Histologically, psoriasiform hyperplasia of the epidermis is diffuse, and orthokeratotic hyperkeratosis is mild to moderate and associated with underlying hypergranulosis. Parakeratotic hyperkeratosis is present multifocally, often in mounds containing dense collections of neutrophils (Munro microabscesses). Hypogranulosis, if present, can be found beneath the parakeratotic mounds. Within the thickened epidermis are pustules containing neutrophils. Spongiosis and exocytosis of neutrophils and lymphocytes are seen within the deeper epidermis.

Within the dermis, there is a lichenoid infiltrate of

plasma cells, lymphocytes, and macrophages, often obscuring the dermal-epidermal junction. Marginated neutrophils can sometimes be seen in superficial dermal vessels. Mild basilar cell damage associated with this lichenoid infiltrate is variable.

Limited immunofluorescent studies have demonstrated granular deposits of C3 at dermoepidermal junction. Antibiotics and corticosteroids are palliative only and not curative. As Gross et al. (1986) and Mason et al. (1986) discuss, this disorder may be a clinical variation of canine seborrhea. However, the lichenoid infiltrate and the discrete papules and proliferative plaques suggest a separate entity, the etiology and pathogenesis of which are not known.

References

Gross TL, Halliwell RE, McDougal BJ, et al. Psoriasiform lichenoid dermatitis in the springer spaniel. Vet Pathol 1986;23:76–78.
Mason KV, Halliwell REW, McDougal BJ. Characterizaton of lichenoid- psoriasiform dermatosis of springer spaniels. J Am Vet Med Assoc 1986;189:897–901.

Solar dermatitis (actinic dermatosis). Solar energy is a form of nonionizing radiation that can induce an exfoliative dermatitis in human beings and animals. The radiation reaching the earth is in the range from ultraviolet (UV), high energy light (290–400 nm) to lower energy, infrared light (>760 nm). Visible light is in the range of 400 to 760 nm in wavelength. The most damaging solar radiation occurs to nonpigmented, hairless skin by radiation in the UV range, and more specifically in the UVB spectrum (290–320 nm). Although UVA (320–400 nm) radiation is able to penetrate deeper into the skin, its damaging effects are not nearly as noticeable as those produced by UVB radiation. UVB radiation is able to induce cutaneous injury by directly stimulating light absorbing molecules in the skin named **chromophores.** Sole cutaneous chromophores include keratin proteins, hemoglobins, porphyrins, carotene, nucleic acids, melanin, lipoprotein, peptide bonds, and some aromatic amino acids. These skin chromophores absorb specific wavelengths of light, during the course of which the energy in the light photoexcites the molecule by moving an electron to a different orbital (singlet state), and/or with a different spin (triplet state), or the electron is removed altogether (free radical). As discussed in the inflammation chapter (Chapter 5), free radicals are extremely reactive and damaging to surrounding tissue structures. Chromophore singlet or triplet states remain photoexcited only very briefly, in nanoseconds, and discharge their energy to surrounding molecules in the form of light, heat, or energy that induces a chemical reaction to form photoproducts. Thus, the process of dissipating solar energy through excitation and subsequent decay of skin chromophores can alter a number of important cell components Specifically, solar damage results in important changes to purines and pyrimidines of DNA, enzymes, and the hydrogen and disulfide bonds of proteins.

There are three major ways in which solar radiation can damage the skin. First, it can induce damage directly, without the aid of endogenous or exogenous photoactive chemicals or compounds in the skin. This **primary phototoxicity** is the typical sunburn reaction known to all of us. UVB radiation is the predominant type of solar energy responsible for this response. In contrast, **photoallergic responses** result from exposure of a cutaneously-applied chemical and UVA radiation. Following a refractory "sensitizing" period in days, subsequent exposures of the chemical and UVA radiation result in an inflammatory dermatosis resembling a delayed-type hypersensitivity reaction. In humans, chemicals in deodorant soaps and cosmetics are usually the offending agents. To our knowledge, this type of solar damage to the skin has not been documented in animals. Thirdly, and probably most important in domestic animals, is **photosensitization.** Photosensitization occurs when either exogenously-administered or endogenously-produced photodynamic chemicals or compounds circulate via the blood to the skin where they absorb solar radiation, predominantly of the UVA type, to induce tissue damage. Common sensitizing compounds include porphyrins, phyloerythrin (a degradation product of chlorophyll), certain other plant pigments, and drugs such as phenothiazine, sulfonamides, thiazine diuretics, and griseofulvin. Photosensitization is addressed in greater detail in Chapter 3 under Pigments.

Acute primary phototoxicity can be seen in exposed, nonpigmented, hairless skin of almost any domestic animal and is recognized grossly by erythema, peaking in intensity approximately 24 hours after sunlight exposure in mild and moderate reactions. In severe cases, progressive erythema peaks days after the initial solar insult, and alopecia, scaling, and crusting, rarely with sloughing, of skin can be seen. In severe cases, the astute clinician should consider photosensitizing agents as underlying causes of the solar reaction. Histologically, acute primary phototoxicity results in epidermal injury, characterized by so-called "sunburn cells" which are dyskeratotic keratinocytes. In addition, spongiosis and slight vacuolization of keratinocytes may be present. Lesions examined days after the initial insult will have acanthosis and orthokeratotic and parakeratotic hyperkeratosis. The dermal vasculature is dilated, and dermal edema, extravasated erythrocytes, and a scant perivascular mononuclear and purulent inflammatory infiltrate is present.

Chronic exposure to sunlight results in a chronic premalignant lesion, termed **actinic keratosis,** in unprotected skin. The association of sunlight, chronic dermatitis, and neoplasia is well recognized in human beings, where it is most frequent in middle-aged individuals with fair complexions. The incidence is highest in the southwestern United States and other sunny geographic locations throughout the world. The lesions resemble those induced in the skin by other forms of irradiation. Typically, the nose and ears of white cats, udders of goats, but essentially any nonpigmented, hairless region of any species can be involved. Grossly, these are rough, slightly raised papules or plaques, often erythematous with adherent scale or crusts and comedones. They vary in the amount of pigmentation, some even being black. The microscopic alterations include changes within the epidermis and dermis. The epidermis is acanthotic with predominantly parakeratotic hyperkeratosis, although orthokeratosis can also be present. Hyperkeratosis can be so pronounced in some lesions as to produce a **cutaneous horn,** a projectile mass of keratin. There is hypogranulosis, and the keratinocytes of the stratum basale and stratum spinosum are atypical or dysplastic, characterized by disorderly stratification. Instead of the typical transition from cuboidal basilar cells to flattened keratinocytes of the outer strata, cells of varying morphological appearances and differentiation stage inhabit all epidermal strata. Degenerative changes in the dermis, termed **dermal elastosis,** can be present. The dermal collagen is partly replaced by elastic fibers, and there is slight basophilic degeneration and homogenization of dermal collagen fibers. Lymphocytes and plasma cells tend to localize around telangiectatic dermal vessels. In human beings, actinic keratosis is associated with squamous cell carcinoma, basal cell carcinoma, and malignant melanoma. Similarly, in animals, solar keratosis preceded cutaneous squamous cell carcinoma in a population of beagle dogs (Hargis et al., 1977), and solar-induced injury is involved in the pathogenesis of squamous cell carcinoma arising in and around the eyes of white faced Hereford cattle and the skin of the pinnae of white cats (also see Chapter 14).

References

Griffi CE. Nasal dermatitis. Dermatol Rep 1983;2:1.

Hargis AM, Thomassen RW, Phemister RD. Chronic dermatosis and cutaneous squamous cell carcinoma in the beagle dog. Vet Pathol 1977;14:218–228.

Ihrke PJ. Nasal solar dermatitis. In: Kirk, RW, ed. Current veterinary therapy VII. Philadelphia: WB Saunders, 1981;440.

Irving RA, Day RS, Eales L. Porphyrin values and treatment of feline solar dermatitis. Am J Vet Res 1982;43:2067–2069.

Lim HW, Buchness MR, Ashinoff R, et al. Chronic actinic dermatitis. Arch Dermatol 1990;126:317–323.

Muller GH, Kirk RW, Scott DW. Neoplastic diseases. Chapter 20 In: Small animal dermatology. 4th ed. Philadelphia: WB Saunders, 1989; pp. 941.

Norris PG, Hawk JLM: Chronic actinic dermatitis: a unifying concept. Arch Dermatol 1990;126:376–378.

Schwartz RA, Stoll HL. Epithelial precancerous lesions. In: Fitzpatrick TB, Eisen AZ, Wolff K, et al., eds. Dermatology in general medicine. 3rd ed. Volume 1. New York: McGraw-Hill, 1987;74:733–746.

Willis I: Photosensitivity and Phototherapy. In: Dermatology, second edition, edited by SL Moschella, HJ Hurley. Philadelphia , W.B Saunders Co., 1985 Chapter 6, volume 1, pp. 389–424.

Yager JA, Scott DW. The Skin and appendages. In: Jubb KVF, Kennedy PC, Palmer N, eds. Pathology of domestic animals. 3rd ed. Volume 1. New York: Academic Press, 1985;407–549.

CONGENITAL HYPOPLASIA OF THE EPIDERMIS
Epitheliogenesis imperfecta. A congenital defect characterized by discontinuity of squamous epithelium is recognized in humans and many species of animals, including several breeds of cattle, swine, horses, dogs, and cats. It is most common in cattle, where it is inherited as an autosomal recessive trait. Affected calves may be aborted or succumb to infection shortly after birth. The epithelial defects most often affect the feet and claws, but may exist anywhere, including the oral mucosa. Microscopically, the normal epithelium terminates abruptly at the affected site.

Crowell WA, Stephenson C, Cosser HS. *Epitheliogenesis imperfecta* in a foal. J Am Vet Med Assoc 1976;168:56–58.

Gupta BN. *Epitheliogenesis imperfecta* in a dog. Am J Vet Res 1973; 34:443–444.

Leipold HW, Mills JHL, Huston K: *Epitheliogenesis imperfecta* in Holstein-Friesian calves. Can Vet J 1973;14:114–118.

Munday BL: *Epitheliogenesis imperfecta* in lambs and kittens. Br Vet J 1970;126:47.

ATROPHY OF THE EPIDERMIS
Atrophy or obvious thinning and loss of rete ridges of a previously normal epidermis may occur with, but is not necessarily diagnostic of, a number of systemic endocrine abnormalities, including hypothyroidism, hyperadrenalcorticism, gonadal hormone abnormalities, diabetes mellitus, etc. Depending upon its cause, epidermal atrophy may be associated with a variety of other histologic changes of the epidermis and dermis, including superficial and follicular hyperkeratotic hyperkeratosis, secondary seborrhea, pyoderma, epidermal hypermelanosis, atrophy of sebaceous glands and hair follicles, hypertrophy and vacuolization of arrector pili muscles, dermal mucinosis (myxedema), and calcinosis cutis. Typically, skin changes resulting from endocrine imbalances have a bilaterally symmetric pattern, but this is not always the case. Bilateral alopecia with or without epidermal thinning or thickening (lichenification) and hyperpigmentation are often the most striking clinical findings. These may be accompanied by dry or greasy seborrhea, a dull, brittle, easily epilated haircoat that grows back slowly, if at all,, and varying degrees of erythema depending upon the presence of secondary bacterial infection. Typically, non-infected endocrine associated alopecias are non-pruritic; but may become so if secondary bacterial infection intervenes.

SPONGIOTIC DISEASES OF THE EPIDERMIS
Allergic contact dermatitis This is a relatively uncommon skin disorder in dogs and cats caused by a type IV, delayed hypersensitivity reaction to an environmental allergen to which the affected animal has direct contact. Sensitization occurs through direct contact between the offending allergen and relatively hairless portions of the body (interdigital skin, groin, axillae, genitalia, muzzle, ears and perineum); heavily haired portions of the body are more protected. Grossly, the exposed areas develop erythema, papules, vesicles which rupture and result in crust formation. Chronic exposure may lead to alopecia, hyperpigmentation and lichenification. The lesions are variably pruritic. Microscopically, the early lesions of allergic contact dermatitis begin as areas of spongiosis (intercellular edema) that progress to vesiculation and infiltration of the affected epidermis by lymphocytes and lesser numbers of neutrophils. In chronic cases, there may be acanthosis, erosions, and secondary bacterial infection of affected areas due to self-inflicted trauma from licking, biting or scratching. The dermis beneath these areas have vari-

able degrees of superficial, perivascular infiltrates with lymphocytes, histiocytes and small numbers of eosinophils. This lesion has to be differentiated from irritant contact dermatitis.

References

Grant DI, Thoday KL. Canine allergic contact dermatitis: a clinical review. J Small Anim Pract 1980;21:127–37.

Gross TL, Ihrke PJ, Walder EJ. Spongiotic diseases of the epidermis. In: Veterinary dermatopathology. Mosby Year Book: St. Louis, 1992;4:51–57.

Krawiec DR, Gaafar SM. A comparative study of allergic and primary irritant contact dermatitis with DNCB in dogs. J Invest Dermatol 1975;65:248–251.

Muller GH, Kirk RW, Scott DW. Contact hypersensitivity. In: Small animal dermatology. 4th ed. Philadelphia: WB Saunders, 1989;464–470.

Reedy LM, Miller WHJ: Allergic skin diseases of dogs and cats. Philadelphia: WB Saunders, 1989, 159–169.

Irritant contact dermatitis. Although the gross and microsocpic lesions of this form of dermatitis can bear a striking resemblance to those of allergic contact dermatitis, the pathogenesis is different. This form of dermatitis is due to exposure of the skin to irritating chemical substances that directly damage epidermal cells, rather than being mediated by an allergic reaction. It differs from allergic contact dermatitis in that lesions occur after the initial exposure to the irritating substance, and thus no period of sensitization is required. In this form of dermatitis, the offending chemical may be much more easily identified than a suspected environmental allergen. Also, the lesions tend to be more painful than pruritic. The lesions begin with spongiosis that progresses to vesiculation, ballooning change (intracellular edema), vesicle formation and epidermal necrosis. Neutrophils tend to be more prominent in this form of dermatitis than in allergic contact dermatitis.

References

Gross TL, Ihrke PJ, Walder EJ. Spongiotic diseases of the epidermis. In: Veterinary Dermatopathology. St. Louis: Mosby Year Book, 1992;4:51–57.

Krawiec DR, Gaafar SM. A comparative study of allergic and primary irritant contact dermatitis with DNCB in dogs. J Invest Dermatol 1975;65:248–251.

VESICULAR-PUSTULAR DISEASES OF THE EPIDERMIS

Impetigo Impetigo, or puppy pyoderma, is a superficial pustular, bacterial epidermitis seen in sexually immature dogs of either sex and any breed. It is caused by *Staphylococcus intermedius*. Grossly, the affected areas of skin are marked by the presence of interfollicular crusty and/or erythematous papules and fragile, yellow-white pustules that rupture easily. The interfollicular location of the lesions differentiates this disease from the various forms of folliculitis in which a hair usually protruded from the pustule. Microscopically, the epidermis contains multiple discrete pustules located between hair follicles and just beneath the thin stratum corneum. The pustules are usually slightly elevated above the adjacent non-affected areas of epidermis and are filled with large numbers of neutrophils. There may be mild spon-

giosis of keratinocytes immediately adjacent to the pustule as well as mild acanthosis. Gram stains reveal gram-positive cocci in the exudate of intact pustules. The dermis beneath the pustules may be variably edematous and contains moderate numbers of neutrophils and fewer mononuclear inflammatory cells. This condition differs from pemphigus by the absence of acantholytic cells in the pustules.

References

Ihrke PJ. The management of canine pyoderma. In: Kirk RW, ed. Current veterinary therapy VIII.. Philadelphia: WB Saunders, 1983;505–517.

Gross TL, Ihrke PJ, Walder EJ. Spongiotic diseases of the epidermis. In: Veterinary dermatopathology. St. Louis: Mosby Year Book, 1992;4:51–57.

Superficial spreading folliculitis. This is a very common superficial bacterial infection of the skin of dogs that extends only into the upper portion of hair follicles. It affects glabrous skin more often than heavily haired areas and predisposing factors are thought to include frictional trauma such as that which occurs at the axillae and from scratching in the groin region. Poor hygiene and grooming practices probably contribute to its occurrence. As with impetigo in puppies, *Staphylococcus intermedius* is the most frequent cause, but other staphylococci and bacteria may be involved. The lesion tends to be variably pruritic.

Grossly, the affected areas of skin develop multiple pustules centered within the infundibulae of hair follicles; there is often a hair protruding from the pustule. Erythematous macules may spread concentrically from the central pustule causing elevation and peeling of the keratin at the periphery of the macules. This central area of erythema surrounded by a collar of elevated and peeling keratin is referred to clinically as an "epidermal collarette".

Microscopically, the lesions of superficial spreading pyoderma can be quite variable during the course of the infection. Typical lesions consist of small, areas of spongiosis that rapidly progress to ill-defined superficial epidermal pustules that become superficial crusts. Although early pustules usually arise from within the infundibulae of hair follicles, this may not be obvious in advanced cases. Gram positive cocci consistent with staphylococci can usually be found in the superficial keratin layer mixed with granular basophilic cellular debris and inflammatory cells. At the advancing margins of well-preserved lesions, the stratum corneum may be elevated corresponding to the crusty margin of a collarete. The dermis beneath the epidermal pustules generally contains superficial, perivascular infiltrates of neutrophils. Superficial spreading pyoderma differs from impetigo in that the pustules tend to be less discrete.

Pemphigus foliaceus This is one of four uncommon but related autoimmune diseases of the skin and, in some cases mucous membranes, that comprise the so-called **pemphigus complex.** The pemphigus complex occurs in humans, dogs and cats, and rarely in other species. These disorders have in common the development of autoantibodies, typically IgG, against components of desmosomes and glycoprotein surface molecules of keratinocytes of the skin and, in some instances, oral and genital mucous membranes. When these antibodies bind to the intercellular antigens, the epidermal cells internalize the antigen-antibody complex which causes the affected keratinocytes to synthesize and secrete the extracellular protease, plasminogen activator. This enzyme converts the plasma proenzyme plasminogen to plasmin which catalyzes the hydrolysis of peptide bonds of proteins. This activity leads to the destruction of attachments between cells causing the cells to become detached from one another, round up and float free in an epidermal vesicle or pustule. This process is referred to as **acantholysis,** which, literally interpreted, means lysis of spines, in this case, the desmosomes of the stratum spinosum. The cytoplasm of the rounded-up keratinocytes typically become more eosinophilic than that of normal keratinocytes, but their nuclear morphology remains unaltered indicating that they are still viable. These free-floating cells are known as **acantholytic keratinocytes** and are the microscopic hallmark of the pemphigus complex of skin diseases.

The four conditions comprising the pemphigus complex differ from one another in their clinical severity, anatomic distribution of the gross lesions, where within the epithelium the autoantibodies are deposited (subcorneal versus suprabasal) and the nature of the microscopic lesions produced, namely vesicles versus pustules.

Pemphigus folicaceus, the most common form of the pemphigus complex in animals, has been described predominantly in middle-aged dogs and cats and rarely in horses. In dogs, the bearded collie, Akita, chow chow, Newfoundland, schipperke and Doberman pinscher are reportedly most susceptible. Lesions often display bilateral symmetry and occur most often on the dorsal aspect of the muzzle, planum nasale, pinnae, periorbital skin, and footpads. Affected footpads frequently are thickened, hardened and may contain painful open cracks and fissures. The margins of the pads may be ulcerated. Other areas of the skin may occasionally be involved. Mucocutaneous junctions and mucosal surfaces are rarely affected. The lesions generally occur in waves of multiple vesicles and pustules that rapidly become covered with crusts that readily exfoliate. In this form of pemphigus, autoantibodies consistsing of IgG or rarely IgM and complement (C3) are typically deposited in intercellular areas of the superficial granular layer of the epidermis where they cause the formation of broad, discrete, **subcorneal** or **intragranular pustules** that may span multiple hair follicles and involve their infundibula. The pustules contain large numbers of neutrophils, variable numbers of eosinophils and scattered, free floating acantholytic keratinocytes. The presence of intact pustules distinguishes this disorder from pemphigus vulgaris where suprabasal clefts and intraepidermal vesicles lacking inflammatory cells are the hallmark. Early lesions of spongiosis, active acantholysis and vesicles may also be present adjacent to the more advanced pustules.

References

Gross TL, Ihrke PJ, Walder EJ. Veterinary dermatopathology. St. Louis: Mosby Year Book, 1992;16–18.
Halliwell REW, Goldschmidt MH. Pemphigus foliaceus in the canine: a case report and discussion. J Amer Animal Hosp Assoc 1977;13:431–436.
Ihrke PJ, Stannard AA, Ardans AA, et al. Pemphigus foliaceus in dogs: a review of 37 cases. J Am Vet Med Assoc 1985;186:59–66.
Ihrke PJ, Stannard AA, Ardans AA, et al. Pemphigus foliaceus of the footpads in three dogs. J Am Vet Med Assoc 1985;186:67–69.
Manning TO, Scott DW, Smith CA et al. Pemphigus diseases in the feline: seven case reports and discussion. J Amer Anim Hosp Assoc 1982;18:433–443.
Messer NT, Knight AP. Pemphigus foliaceus in a horse. J Am Vet Med Assoc 1982;180:938–940.
Muller GH, Kirk RW, Scott DW. Small animal dermatology. 4th ed. Philadelphia: WB Saunders, 1989;498–513.
Johnson ME, Scott DW, Smith VA, et al. Pemphigus foliaceus in the horse. J Equine Pract 1981;3:40–45.

Pemphigus erythematosus This form of the pemphigus complex is thought to be either a rare, milder variant of pemphigus folicaceus, or possibly a disorder somewhere between pemphigus and lupus erythematosus (LE). It differs from the other forms of pemphigus in that affected animals tend to be **antinuclear antibody (ANA) positive,** a feature of systemic but not discoid LE. It has been described in dogs and cats. In this disorder the vesicles, pustules and crusting is confined to the face where they also exhibit a bilaterally symmetrical distribution. As with both forms of LE, there may be depigmentation of the muzzle and planum nasale with resultant photosensitivity.

References

Scott DW, Walton DK, Slater MR, et al.: Immune-mediated dermatoses in domestic animals: ten years after—part I, Comp Cont Educ 1987;9:425–435.
Scott DW, Walton DK, Smith CA et al. Unusual findings in canine pemphigus erythematosus and discoid lupus erythematosus. J Amer Anim Hosp Assoc 1984;20:579–584.

Subcorneal pustular dermatosis This is an extremely rare and controversial idiopathic, superficial pustular dermatosis of dogs that is primarily diagnosed after exclusion of other better characterized pustular skin disorders. Affected animals develop transient, multifocal to generalized yellow-green, non-follicular, thin-walled pustules that rapidly become superficial crusts. Erythema, alopecia and epidermal collarettes may also be evident in the affected areas. Microscopically, this disease is characterized by the presence of prominent subcorneal pustules in which there are no acantholytic keratinocytes, no colonies of bacteria and no evidence of autoantibody or complement deposition in the affected skin. The exudate within the pustules consists primarily of neutrophils. Hair follicles generally are not affected.

References

McKeever PJ, Dahl MV. A disease of dogs resembling human subcorneal pustular dermatosis. J Am Vet Med Assoc 170:704–708;1977.
Muller GH, Kirk RW, Scott DW: Small animal dermatology. 4th ed. Philadelphia: WB Saunders, 1989;828–831.

VESICULAR AND BULLOUS ("BLISTERING") DISEASES OF THE EPIDERMIS

Pemphigus vulgaris This is the most common form of the pemphigus complex in humans, but the second most common form in animals. This rare, but severe, autoimmune disease affects the skin, particularly mucocutaneous junctions, and stratified squamous epithelium of mucosae of the oral cavity, esophagus, and genital tracts of people, dogs and cats.

There are isolated reports of its occurrence in nonhuman primates. The pathogenesis of pemphigus vulgaris is similar to that described above for pemphigus foliaceus. Autoantibodies bind to antigenic components of the glycoproteins of the surfaces of keratinocytes ultimately leading to plasmin-induced lysis of intercellular junctions and the formation of vesicles and bullae containing acantholytic keratinocytes. In this disorder, desmosomes of keratinocytes are destroyed, but the hemidesmosomes that attach basal cells to the underlying basement membrane are spared. This leads to the formation of **suprabasal clefts** (Fig. 17-11) that rapidly progress to fluid-filled vesicles and bullae containing acantholytic keratinocytes. The superficial portions of hair follicles may also be affected in this disease. The base of these fluid-filled sacs is lined by a single layer of intact basal cells; the top is covered by a thin layer of corneocytes. These vesicles and bullae are fragile and transient in nature because the thin layer of corneocytes is readily dislodged resulting in erosions and ulcerations. Once ruptured, the denuded surface may become secondarily infected by bacteria leading to purulent inflammation and crust on the surface. Un-

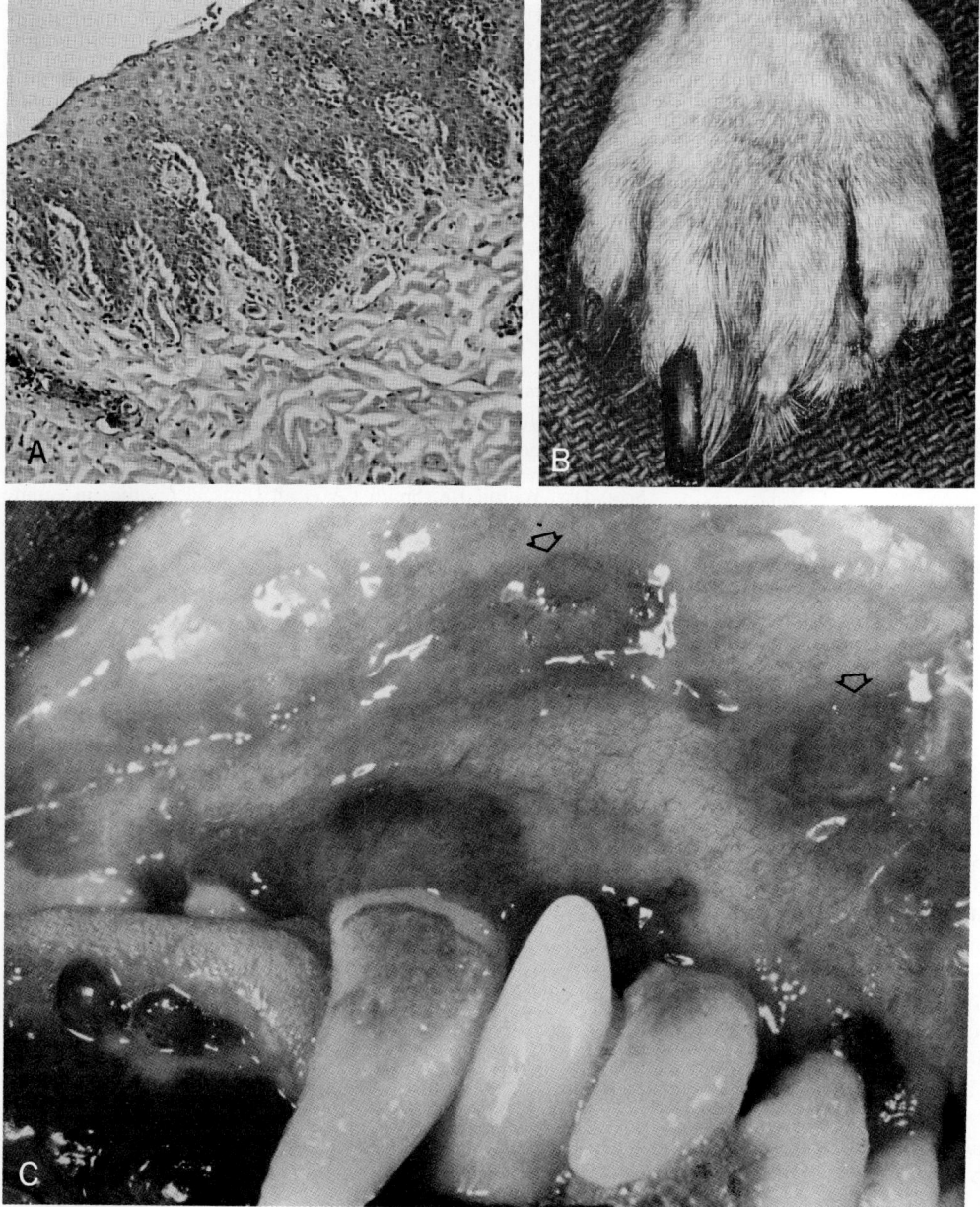

FIG. 17-11 Canine pemphigus vulgaris. **A.** Supra-basal acantholysis. **B.** Loss of claws and exposure of ungual processes. **C.** Erosions of oral mucous membrane (arrows). (Courtesy of Dr. A. I. Hurwitz and *Journal of the American Veterinary Medical Association*.)

like, pemphigus folicaceus, the intact vesicles and bullae that characterize pemphigus vulgaris do not contain inflammatory cells. By immunohistochemistry, immunofluorescence or immunoelectron microscopy, IgG deposits can be demonstated in the intercellular spaces and on the surfaces of affected keratinocytes. C3 may also occasionally be present. The dermis or lamina propria beneath affected areas may contain superficial infiltrates of lymphocytes, plasma cells and neutrophils.

References

Hurvitz AI, Feldman E. A disease in dogs resembling human pemphigus vulgaris; case reports. J Am Vet Med Assoc 1975;166:585–590.

Scott DW, Wolfe MJ, Smith CA, et al. The comparative pathology of non-viral bullous skin diseases in domestic animals. Vet Pathol 17:257–281, 1980.

Stannard AA, Gribble DH, Baker BB. A mucocutaneous disease in the dog resembling pemphigus vulgaris in man. J Am Vet Med Assoc 1975;166:575–582.

Suter MJ, Wilkinson JE, Dougherty EP, et al. Ultrastructural localization of pemphigus vulgaris antigen on canine keratinocytes in vivo and in vitro. Am J Vet Res 1990;51:507–511.

Pemphigus vegetans This is the least common form of the pemphigus complex. It has been reported in both the dog and cat where there apparently is no breed, age or sex predilection. It is generally regarded as a less severe form of pemphigus vulgaris in which the affected host is able to mount some unidentified form of resistance to the disease. Pemphigus vegetans is characterized as vesiculopustular dermatosis that progresses to a verrucous and papillomatous proliferation of the epidermis and the superficial follicular epithelium that ooze and are marked by pustules. Grossly, the lesions appear as erythematous plaques, and papillomatous areas with associated pustules. Microscopically, the epidermis contains areas of suprabasal acantholysis similar to pemphigus vulgaris but also contains suprabasal pustules that may extend through the entire thickness of the epidermis or follicular epithelium. These pustules contain eosinophils, lesser numbers of neutrophils and scattered acantholytic keratinocytes. The epidermis in the affected areas is markedly hyperplastic, thrown up into verrucous or papillary projections and is variably hyperkeratotic. These changes are useful in distinguishing this form of pemphigus from the others.

Reference

Scott DW. Pemphigus vegetans in a dog. Cornell Vet 1977;67:374–384.

Discoid lupus erythematosus (DLE) DLE is an autoimmune dermatosis of humans and dogs that is thought to be a mild variant of the more severe condition known as systemic lupus erythematosus (SLE). It differs from SLE in that lesions are confined to the non-haired portions of the skin and affected patients exhibit no signs of systemic illness. In dogs, the Shetland sheepdog, German shepherd, collie and Siberian husky breeds are at increased risk for discoid lupus. Solar radiation aggravates the condition and may play some role in its induction. In the past, the conditions referred to as **"Collie nose"** and **nasal solar dermatitis** were probably this immune-mediated dermatosis. DLE is recog-

nized most often in middle aged dogs (4 to 8 years) and occurs somewhat more often in females than males.

Affected animals initially develop areas of depigmentation, erythema, scaling, erosions, crusting and occasionally vesicles and bullae on non-haired or lightly haired portions of the body exposed to sunlight. These sites include the planum nasale, nostrils, dorsal muzzle, lips and less often the skin of the periorbital areas, pinnae and feet. Oral erosions or ulcers may be present in some cases. Chronic lesions are characterized by scarring, alopecia and hypopigmentation. The pathogenesis of DLE possibly involves solar radiation-induced alterations in the antigenic properties of basal cells of the epidermis such that the host develops autoantibodies against components of these cells. When these antibodies bind to the altered cell antigens, the resultant immune complex binds complement (C1) and initiates the classical complement pathway with the generation of C5a, which is highly chemotactic for neutrophils and the membrane attack complex which causes necrosis of basal cells.

Microscopically, the epidermal changes of DLE are rather characteristic and consist of moderate to severe vacuolar change and necrosis of basal cells. The necrotic basal cells round up, shrink and develop intensely eosinophilic cytoplasm and generally lose their nuclei. These necrotic cell remnants are commonly referred to as **Civatte or colloid bodies.** The basement membrane in affected areas is often thicker than normal. The dermis just beneath the altered epidermis contains a prominent, linear band-like (lichenoid) infiltrate of lymphocytes, macrophages and plasma cells that directly abut the dermal-epidermal junction. The lymphocytes in these infiltrates consist predominantly of CD4+ (helper) T lymphocytes. Also present are variable numbers of melanin-containing macrophages (melanophages) that have ingested pigment released by degenerating basal cells. This finding is often colorfully referred to as **pigmentary incontinence.** Direct immunofluorescent or immunohistochemical tests of cutaneous lesions reveals granular, rather than linear, deposits of host immunoglobulins (IgG, IgM or IgA) and C3 at the dermal-epidermal junction of lesional skin but not unaffected skin. This is in contrast to SLE where immunoglobulins and complement can be demonstrated at the dermal-epidermal junction even in unaffected skin after exposure to sunlight.

References

Griffith CE, et al. Canine discoid lupus erythematosus. Vet Immunol Immunopathol 1979;1:79–87.

Scott DW, Walton DK, Slater MR, et al. Immune-mediated dematoses in domestic animals: ten years after. Part II. Comp Cont Educ 1987;9:539–553.

Walton DK, Scott DW, Smith CA et al.: Canine discoid lupus erythematosus, J Am Anim Hosp Assoc 1981;17:851.

Systemic lupus erythematosus (SLE) This is a relatively rare autoimmune disorder that affects multiple organ systems, including the skin, of people, dogs, cats and certain strains of laboratory mice, particularly New

Zealand Black (NZB)-New Zealand White (NZW) hybrids. Individuals with SLE develop autoantibodies to a variety of antigens specific for certain cells or tissues (erythrocytes, platelets, granulocytes, lymphocytes, thyroglobulin etc.) as well as antigens that are common to many tissues or organs (nucleic acids, nucleoproteins, cellular organelles and phospholipids). A high percentage of affected animals will be ANA positive and LE cell positive. The development of such a wide array of autoantibodies is thought to result from a fundamental defect in immunoregulation, possibly involving an imbalance between helper and suppressor T lymphocyte function. Such a hypothetical defect would result in increased B lymphocyte function, the overproduction of circulating immunoglobulins, some of which are directed towards various self-antigens. The clinical and pathological features of SLE are due to hypersensitivity reactions resulting from the formation, circulation and deposition of immune complexes that damage cells and tissues. The clinical signs of SLE can be quite diverse depending upon what organ systems are affected. These include: symmetric nonerosive polyarthritis causing shifting leg lameness, skin lesions, glomerulonephritis, peripheral lymphadenopathey, hemolytic anemia, thrombocytopenic purpura, neurologic disorders, myositis, myocarditis and thyroiditis. Of these, only the cutaneous manifestations of SLE will be described here.

Clinically, the cutaneous signs of SLE are highly variable. Erythema, crusting, scaling, depigmentation and hair loss may be seen. Bullae that progress to ulcers may occur on the skin, mucocutaneous junctions and oral mucous membranes. Generalized exfoliative dermatitis, footpad ulcerations, and panniculitis may occur. The face, pinnae and distal limbs are frequent sites of involvement. Facial lesions in particular may exhibit some degree of symmetry. Exposure to sunlight often aggravates the lesions. Breeds that appears to be predisposed to SLE include the spitz, collie, Shetland sheepdog, German shepherd and poodle, whereas in cats the Siamese and other purebred breeds appear more at risk. In addition, one should be aware of the fact that cats receiving propylthiouracil therapy for hyperthyroidism may develop many of the clinical signs of SLE.

Microscopically, the lesions bear a remarkable resemblance to those described under discoid lupus erythematosus. In SLE basal cell vacuolization, necrosis and Civatte body formation may be more severe leading to vesicle formation and ulceration. The epithelium of the superficial portions of hair follicles may also be affected. As with DLE, the basement membrane may be thickened. The interface or lichenoid dermal infiltrates in SLE may not be as extensive or severe as in DLE. Direct immunofluorescence tests reveal granular deposits of immunoglobulins and complement at the basement membrane and dermal-epidermal interface of lesions. If there is an immune-complex vasculitis in the dermis of the affected skin, then these same antigen antibody complexes will also be present. Features that assist in differentiating SLE from DLE are the presence of clinical signs of other systemic disorders, i.e. lameness, anemia, renal dysfunction.

References
Lewis RM, Picut KA: Veterinary clinical immunology. From classroom to clinics. Philadelphia: Lea & Febiger, 1989;167–182.
Lewis RM, Schwartz R, Henry WB, Jr. Canine systemic lupus erythematosus. Blood 1965;25:143–147.
Muller GH, Kirk RW, Scott DW. Miscellaneous diseases Chapter 19. In: Small animal dermatology, 4th ed. Philadelphia: WB Saunders, 1989;828–831.

Hereditary lupoid dermatosis of German shorthair pointers This inherited, breed-specific dermatosis has none of the immunological characteristics of discoid or systemic lupus erythematosus, but microscopically the epidermal changes are quite similar. The disease usually becomes manifest between 5 and 7 months of age and is characterized by the development of prominent exfoliative scale and crusts beginning on the head and back and eventually becoming generalized. The affected skin may also be thicker than normal. Epidermal erosions and ulcerations are extremely rare in this disease and mucosal involvement has not been described. Microscopically, the epidermis is variably acanthotic, parakeratotic and hyperkeratotic and covered with crusts. There may be mild spongiosis and intra-epidermal neutrophils and lymphocytes. The most prominent microscopic feature and one that resembles lupus is severe vacuolar degeneration of basal cell layer of the epidermis and superficial follicular epithelium and necrosis of individual basal cells. These changes may be associated with mild separation of the dermal-epidermal junction. Macrophages containing phagocytized melanin from degenerate basal cells may also be present in the superficial dermis. Finally, the dermis contains mild to moderate perivascular and subepidermal infiltrates of lymphocytes, macrophages, mast cells, neutrophils and plasma cells. Direct immunofluorescent tests are negative for immunoglobulins and complement. Although its pathogenesis is not known, the disease could conceivably result from some inherited defect in basal cell survivability.

Reference
Gross TL, Ihrke PJ, Walder EJ. Veterinary dermatopathology. St. Louis: Mosby Year Book, 1992;26–28.

Bullous pemphigoid This is a rare autoimmune skin disease of humans and dogs. The Doberman pincher, collie and dachshund breeds are most often affected. Affected individuals develop autoantibodies against an antigen, known as the bullous pemphigoid antigen, that is synthesized by keratinocytes and is a normal component of the dermal-epidermal junction. When these antibodies bind to this antigen it causes cleavage of the lamina lucida of the basement membrane and the formation of large, fluid-filled bullae which, because of their subepidermal location, tend to remain intact longer than those that occur with the pemphigus complex. These bullae are found commonly in the oral mucosa mucocutaneous junctions of the mouth, anus, vulva and prepuce, and periorbital regions, but may occur anywhere on the skin but especially in the axillae, groin, skin around the nails and on the inner surface of the pinnae. These lesions eventually rupture leading to discrete, non-coalescent ulcers at the affected sites. Severely affected dogs may exhibit signs of systemic illness.

Microscopically, bullous pemphigoid is characterized by **subepidermal or subepithelial vesicles** and **bullae** that may contain small numbers of neutrophils, eosinophils, erythrocytes and fibrin. Dermal or lamina proprial changes are highly variable and consist of mild to marked perivascular infiltrates of neutrophils, eosinophils, lymphocytes and plasma cells. Direct immunofluorescent or immunohistochemical techniques reveals the presence of homogeneous linear deposits of IgG or IgM and C3 along the basement membrane of affected epithelia. Microscopically, the lesions of bullous pemphigoid may be indistinguishable from those of epidermolysis bullosa; however, in the latter there are no immunoglobulin deposits.

References

Kunkle G, Goldschmidt MJH, Halliwell REW: Bullous pemphigoid in a dog: A case report with immunofluorescent findings. J Am Anim Hosp Assoc 1978;14:52–57.

Scott DW, Manning TO, Smith CA, et al. Observations on the immunopathology and therapy of canine pemphigus and pemphigoid. J Am Vet Med Assoc 1982;180:48–52.

Epidermolysis bullosa. This is an extremely rare mechanobullous skin disease of humans, dogs and sheep. In humans, epidermolysis bullosa is hereditary and encompasses at least three types of disorders all of which are characterized by the formation of **subepidermal** or **subepithelial blisters** at sites of pressure, friction or trauma beginning shortly after birth. The various types differ in the sites of cleavage of the epidermis from the dermis along the basement membrane, whether it occurs due to degeneration of basal cells, structural fragility of the stratum lucidum of the basement membrane or defects in anchoring fibers or collagen that binds the dermis to the lamina densa of the basement membrane. In all forms, there is weakness of the dermal-epidermal junction. The one reported case in a cesarean section-delivered toy poodle had vesicles and bullae on the footpads, oral mucosa and tongue within 24 hours of birth. It was euthanatized at 3 days of age and was found to have cleavage of the lamina lucida zone of the basement membrane similar to the junctional form of epidermolysis bullosa of humans. The other cases involving the collie and Shetland sheepdog breeds reported in the literature are now regarded as probable mild forms of canine familial dermatomyositis. In sheep, epidermolysis bullosa has been reported in the Suffolk and South Dorset Down breeds. Affected lambs were either born with blisters and ulcerations of the skin and mucous membranes at the sites of frictional tauma (legs, bony prominences, joints, lips and oral cavity) or developed them during the first 2 weeks of life. In these ovine cases, the sites of cleavage was between the dermis and the lamina densa of the basement membrane.

Reference

Bruckner-Tuderman L, Guscetti F, Ehrensperger F. Animal model for dermolytic mechanobullous disease: Sheep with recessive dystrophic epidermolysis bullosa lack collagen VII. J Invest Dermatol 1991;96:452–458.

Dunstan RW, et al. A disease resembling junctional epidermolysis bullosa in a toy poodle. Am J Dermatopathol 1988;10:442–447.

Canine Familial Dermatomyositis. This is an autosomal dominant inherited disorder with "variable expressivity" that is characterized by inflammatory lesions of the skin and skeletal muscle of Shetland sheepdogs, collies and related crossbreeds. There is a similar disease of children. The precise pathogenesis of the canine disorder is not known, but autoimmunity and viral infection are suspected, based upon the fact that the severity of the disease waxes and wanes in direct relationship to the levels of circulating immune complexes in the peripheral blood.

The skin lesions first become apparent between 7 and 14 weeks of age when pups develop multifocal dermatitis of the face, pinnae, tip of the tail, distal portions of the extremities and over skeletal pressure points. Mucous membranes are not affected. The skin lesions begin as transient papules, vesicles and pustules that progress to erosions and crusts with loss of hair and hypo- or hyperpigmentation. Clinical signs of muscular involvement are not always apparent in dogs with this disorder, but when they do appear it is always after the appearance of the cutaneous lesions, generally between 12 and 20 weeks of age. Signs of muscular involvement include: facial palsy, diminished jaw tone, stiff gait, generalized muscular weakness, megaesophagus, dysphagia and atrophy of temporal and masseter muscles. Affected dogs are ANA negative but typically have elevated levels of circulating immune complexes, that fluctuate with the severity and duration of skin lesions.

Microscopically, the dermis and epidermis both contain significant lesions. In the epidermis and follicular epithelium scattered individual basal cells are either vacuolated or shrunken and intensely eosinophilic (Civatte bodies); these changes may be accompanied by vesicle formation at the dermal-epidermal junction. When present the vesicles often contain small numbers of erythrocytes. Vesicles may rupture leading to ulceration or superficial crusts. The epidermal changes bear a similarity to those seen in systemic lupus erythematosis; however, in canine familial dermatomyositis direct immunofluorescence tests for detection of immunoglobulins in the epidermis are negative. Characteristic dermal lesions consist of perifollicular, lymphocytic and histiocytic infiltrates, follicular atrophy, and superficial perivasculitis. Atrophy of adnexal structures may be found in chronic cases. Affected skeletal muscles, particularly those around the eyes and temporal and masseter muscles may contain mixed inflammatory infiltrates consisting of lymphocytes, macrophages, plasma cells and scattered neutrophils most evident in the peripheral portions of muscle bundles. These inflammatory changes are associated with degeneration, atrophy and fibrosis of myofibers.

Vasculitis of venules and arterioles may be found in affected skin and muscle. It is characterized by fibrinoid change in vessel walls, necrosis of intimal cells and neutrophilic infiltrates. These changes most likely are associated with deposition of immune complexes from the circulation.

A similar condition termed **ulcerative dermatosis of Shetland sheepdogs and collies** has been recognized only in adult dogs of these breeds. It may represent a late onset variant of canine familial dermatomyositis. It differs from the latter in that the degenerative changes in epidermal basal cells is more severe with numerous Civatte bodies being present. Degenerative changes may also involve keratinocytes of the stratum spinosum.

References

Gross TL, Kunkel GA: The cutaneous histology of dermatomyositis in collie dogs. Vet Pathol 1987;24:11–15.

Hargis AM, Haupt KH, Prieur DJ, et al. A skin disorder in three Shetland sheepdogs. Comparison with familial canine dermatomyositis of collies. Comp Cont Educ 1985;7:306–315.

Hargis AM, Haupt KH, Hegreberg GA, et al. Familial canine dermatomyositis. Initial characterization of the cutaneous and muscular lesions. Am J Pathol 1984;116:234–244.

NECROTIZING LESIONS OF THE EPIDERMIS

Thermal and chemical burns. In any species, direct exposure of the skin or mucous membranes to extremely hot solids or liquids or to caustic chemicals will cause immediate tissue damage referred to as a **burn.** The severity of the injury will vary depending upon the temperature of the object or liquid or concentration of the chemical, and with the duration of exposure. In veterinary practice burns are usually classified as partial-thickness if only the superficial layers of the skin are involved or full-thickness if the injury destroys adnexal structures, blood vessels and nerves of the dermis. In many cases burns can be differentiated from other forms of cutaneous injury by the history of exposure, characteristic pattern of the injury (Fig. 17-12), or the presence of residual quantities of the caustic chemical on the injured site. Burns are more easily recognized and often are more severe on relatively hairless portions of the body than on thickly haired sites. In the latter areas they may go unrecognized until the skin is actually lost from the site. Grossly, burns appear as well-circumscribed areas of erythema that progress to erosions or ulcerations depending upon the depth of the injury. The lesions may appear hard and dry or if the necrotic skin has sloughed there may be a large area of ulceration with varying amounts of serum and purulent exudate over a raw oozing surface.

Microscopically, in relatively mild partial-thickness lesions there will be coagulative necrosis of the epidermis with varying degrees of spongiosis and subepidermal vesicle ("blister") formation. These frequently ulcerate and become covered by scabs consisting of dried serum containing neutrophils. In more severe burns the coagulative changes involve the collagen of the dermis as well as adnexal glands, hair follicles and blood vessels, and in some cases even the subcutaneous adipose tissue (panniculus) Affected blood vessels may be thrombosed. These latter lesions heal by extensive scar formation (Fig. 17-12).

Reference

Gross TL, Ihrke PJ, Walder EJ: Veterinary dermatopathology. St Louis: Mosby Year Book, 1992;48–50.

Superficial necrolytic dermatitis (hepatocutaneous syndrome) This uncommon necrotizing skin disorder seen primarily in older dogs, has a number of synonymns, including diabetic dermatopathy and hepatocutaneous syndrome. Affected dogs usually have systemic metabolic disorders including diabetes mellitus or glucagon-secreting tumors of the pancreatic islet cells that may be associated with vacuolar changes in the liver. Mild to moderate increases in plasma glucagon

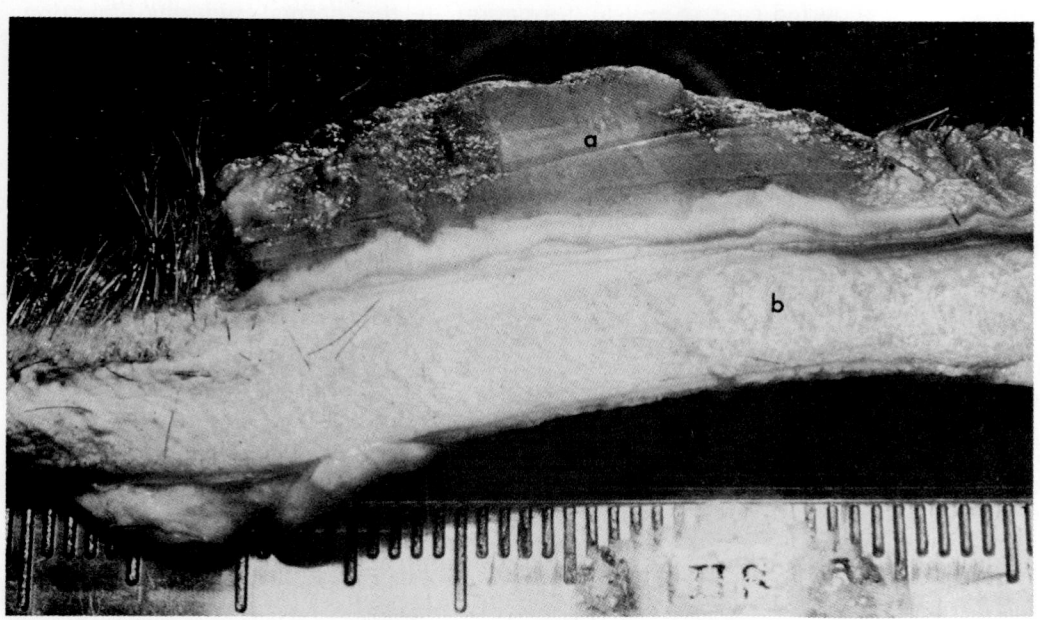

FIG. 17-12 "Brand papilloma" in the skin of a six-year-old male Hereford. Note the thick keratin layer *(a)* at the site of the scar caused by a hot-iron brand; dermis *(b)*.

have been demonstrated in dogs with this dermatosis even in animals without demonstrable endocrine tumors of the pancreas. The skin lesions are thought to be due to the marked decrease in plasma amino acid levels that have been documented in these cases.

Grossly, the skin lesions are characterized by bilaterally symmetrical erosions, ulcerations, alopecia, exudation and the presence of thick, adherent crusts on the footpads and mucocutaneous junctions of the lips, eyelids, anus, vulva. Lesions may also be seen on the pinnae, over various pressure points and on the scrotum. These lesions commonly become secondarily infected by opportunistic bacteria, dermatophytes and yeasts.

Histologically, the characteristic feature of this disease is the red (pink), white and blue laminated appearance of the epidermis. The red or pink outer zone consists of a layer of eosinophilic parakeratotic keratin. The middle pale white zone consists of an area of edema and lysis of keratinocytes. Finally, the inner basophilic zone consists of hyperplastic basal cells. Pustules and opportunistic microorganisms may be present in the outermost layer. The epidermis may separate at the middle zone creating intra-epidermal clefts which may become erosions or ulcerations. The superficial dermis contains variable numbers of perivascular neutrophils and lesser numbers of macrophages, lymphocytes and plasma cells. The concomitant association between skin lesions, liver abnormalities and diabetes mellitus or endocrine secreting pancreatic tumors differentiates this necrotizing dermatosis from others.

References

Gross TL, O'Brien TD, Davies AP, et al. Glucagon-producing pancreatic endocrine tumors in two dogs with superficial necrolytic dermatitis. J Am Vet Med Assoc 1990;197:1619–1622.
Miller WH, Scott DW, Buerger RG et al. Necrolytic migratory erythema in dogs. A hepatocutaneous syndrome. J Am Anim Hosp Assoc 1990;26:573–581.

Toxic epidermal necrolysis. This severe, life-threatening ulcerative disease of the skin and oral mucous membranes has been reported in dogs and cats. It is usually associated with a hypersensitivity reaction to some medication, or rarely with a visceral neoplasm or systemic infection. The epithelial injury is thought to be immunologically mediated. Clinically, the disease is seen initially as patchy areas of erythema that progress to confluency. The epidermis soon becomes necrotic and sheds in thin, broad sheets. It can also be displaced manually by simply rubbing the affected areas, a positive **Nikolsky's sign.** The skin of the face, mucocutaneous junctions and footpads are commonly affected, but any part of the body may be involved. The mucosa of the oral cavity, esophagus and tracheobronchial tree, as well as the gastrointestinal tract, may also contain lesions.

Microscopically, toxic epidermal necrolysis is characterized by acute coagulative necrosis and ballooning degeneration of keratinocytes of the epidermis. The necrotic epidermis eventually separates from the dermis to form large bullae that rupture leaving areas of ulceration. Inflammatory cells only appear in the dermis after the necrotic epidermis has desquamated. These changes are similar to what has been described in burns; hence it is important to determine if the affected animal is on any medication or has any evidence of a neoplasm in order to differentiate between these two conditions.

References

Muller GH, Kirk RW, Scott DW. Small animal dermatology. 4th ed. Philadelphia: WB Saunders, 1989;539–540.
Scott DW, et al. Toxic epidermal necrolysis in two dogs and a cat. J Am Anim Hosp Assoc 1979;15:271–279.

FOLLICULITIS AND FURUNCULOSIS

The term **folliculitis** denotes inflammation confined to a hair follicle, whereas **furunculosis** refers to an inflamed hair follicle that has ruptured, spilling inflammatory exudate and the causative agent into the surrounding dermis. There are many causes of folliculitis and furunculosis, including bacteria (especially *Staphylococcus intermedius* and others), fungi *(Microsporum spp.* and *Trichophyton spp.)* and certain ectoparasites *(Demodex spp.)* Folliculitis caused by bacteria and *Demodex spp.* tend to be pruritic, whereas mycotic folliculitis generally is not. With the exception of bacterial folliculitis, the causative agent (fungus or mite) can usually be found in biopsies of affected areas of skin.

Bacterial folliculitis Grossly, the lesions of bacterial folliculitis appear as pustules centered within hair follicles. An intact hair may protrude from affected follicles unless it has been lost. Because these pustules are fragile and rupture easily, crusted papules are seen with greater frequency. Erythema, swelling and alopecia of affected areas are variable. If these inflamed follicles rupture and form furuncles, the gross lesions are larger, firm papules or nodules. Crusty collarettes of desquamated keratin may surround individual pustules. Microscopically, affected follicles contain neutrophils, and in some cases eosinophils, and their periphery may be surrounded by similar cells that are migrating into the follicle. If the follicle is damaged to such an extent that it ruptures, the inflammatory exudate and necrotic cellular debris, including keratin, will be present in the surrounding dermis. If the condition persists, rather than resolves, increased numbers of macrophages, lymphocytes and plasma cells will be present in the dermis. There may also be some degree of perifollicular fibrosis.

Mycotic folliculitis. Grossly, the lesions of mycotic folliculitis are variable. They range from irregular areas of patchy alopecia to expanding circular areas of alopecia ("ringworm") with erythematous borders. The hair in these circular areas is often broken and appears as short, thick, stubble that protrudes just above the surface. In some cases, pustules can be found in the affected areas. Microscopically, the epidermis is acanthotic, often hyperkeratotic and there may be crusts composed of dried serum and neutrophils around broken hairs. The hair follicles are usually surrounded by lymphocytes and macrophages, and variable numbers of neutrophils. Hair shafts contain variable numbers of refractile to faintly basophilic fungal spores and hyphae. Occasionally an infected hair follicle will rupture giving rise to a pyogranulomatous dermatitis containing remnants of hairshafts, fungal spores and hyphae. This condition is referred to as a **kerion.** (See also Chapter 12).

Demodectic folliculitis (demodicosis) Mites of the genus *Demodex* are part of the normal flora of hair follicles of many species of healthy animals, but under states of putative immunosuppression these acarids undergo excessive proliferation and cause clinical disease, either localized or generalized. Demodicosis occurs in two forms, juvenile-onset and adult-onset. In the juvenile-onset form there is a breed and familial association, whereas cases of adult-onset demodicosis are frequently associated with immunosuppressive disorders such as hyperadrenalcorticism, various forms of neoplasia or subsequent to various forms of immunosuppressive therapy. Clinically, most cases of demodicosis begin as patchy, somewhat circumscribed, alopecic macules in which there may be erythema and superficial crusting. Early lesions occur most often around the eyes, commissures of the lips and forelimbs. Rarely, early lesions present as dermal nodules. When the disease becomes generalized it usually spreads from localized lesions. As the condition spreads and lesions progress, they become macular and alopecic. The feet are often most severely affected. Longstanding lesions may exhibit lichenification and hyperpigmentation and secondary bacterial folliculitis. Pruritis, pain and lymphadenopathy may accompany the disease.

Skin biopsies from lesions of demodicosis have acanthosis, hyperkeratosis, superficial seropurulent crusts and variable degrees of ulceration. Follicular changes vary from areas of no inflammatory infiltrates to follicles exhibiting extensive purulent folliculitis and furunculosis. Secondary bacterial infection of affected follicles is common. The surrounding dermis often contains plasma cells, macrophages, lymphocytes and neutrophils. Variable numbers of cigar-shaped mites are often present in affected follicles. In some instances, inflamed follicles rupture, spilling the mites and associated inflammatory cells into the surrounding dermis where they provoke discrete pyogranulomas in the surrounding dermis. Occasionally pyogranulomas occur within sebaceous glands of affected follicles. Mites may be present in the center of the pyogranulomas. Although rare, feline demodicosis is generally associated with milder, primarily lymphocytic and histiocytic inflammatory infiltrates surrounding, rather than infiltrating the affected hair follicles (also see Chapter 13).

References

Foil CS. Dermatophytosis. In: Greene CE, editor: Infectious diseases of the dog and cat. Philadelphia, 1990, WB Saunders, pp 659–668.

Gross TL, Ihrke PJ, Walder EJ. Veterinary dermatopathology. St. Louis, Mosby Year Book, Inc. 1992, pp. 252–260.

Healey MC, Gaafar SM. Immunodeficiency in canine demodectic mange. I. Experimental production of lesions using antilymphocyte serum. II. Skin reactions to phytohemagglutinin and conconavalin A. Vet Parasitol 1977; 3:121–131.

Krick SA, Scott DW. Bacterial folliculitis, furunculosis and cellulitis in the German Shepherd Dog: a retrospective analysis of 17 cases. J Am Anim Hosp Assoc 1989;25:23–30.

Kwochka, KW. Canine demod cosis. In: Kirk RW, editor: Current veterinary therapy X, Philadelphia, WB Saunders, 1986; pp 531–537.

Muller GH, Kirk RW, Scott DW. Small animal dermatology, 4th edition, Philadelphia, WB Saunders, 1989; pp 244–285.

Wilkie BN, Markham RJF, Hazlett C. Deficient cutaneous response to PHA-P in healthy puppies from a kennel with a high prevalence of demodicosis. Can J Comp Med 1979;43:415–419.

Wisselink MA, Willemse A, Koeman JP. Deep pyoderma in the German Shepherd Dog, J Am Anim Hosp Assoc 1985;21:773–776.

DISEASES OF THE DERMIS

Many of the skin disorders presented under disorders of the epidermis are associated with prominent inflammatory cellular infiltrates in various parts of the dermis; these will not be recounted under this heading. Instead, only those conditions where the primary inflammatory response appears to be centered in the dermis will be discussed. It should be emphasized that the pathologist cannot view inflammatory changes in the dermis in a vacuum, but must also determine what, if any, changes co-exist in the overlying epidermis before a meaningful interpretation and diagnosis can be made. It should be recalled from the discussion of epidermal injury at the earlier part of this chapter that the dermis and epidermis are intricately linked in terms of normal function and responses to injury. The epidermis is capable of responding in various ways to a wide variety of signals that it receives from normal cells of the dermis, as well as from cells that infiltrate the dermis in response to various inflammatory stimuli.

Hypersensitivity reactions involving the dermis

A number of localized cutaneous as well as systemic hypersensitivity reactions are characterized by inflammatory cellular infiltrates in the dermis, often in a perivenular location. The composition of these inflammatory infiltrates, as well as their location within the dermis, are important elements in any assessment of their cause.

Atopy or **atopic dermatitis** is a form of hypersensitivity reaction seen with some frequency in dogs and cats. Patients with this disorder have an inherited tendency to develop type I hypersensitivity reactions to environmental allergens, such as pollen. Breeds most susceptible to atopic dermatitis are West Highland white terrier, wirehaired fox terrier, cairn terrier, Scottish terrier, golden retriever, dalmatian, boxer, pug, Irish setter, English setter, miniature schnauzer, Lhasa apso and Chinese shar-pei. The allergen responsible for the skin lesions that occur in this disorder may be inhaled or absorbed directly through the skin. Upon initial exposure to the allergen, atopy-susceptible individuals develop reaginic antibodies of the IgE and IgGd subclasses to the specific allergen which bind to cutaneous mast cells. Upon re-exposure to the same allergen, these mast cell-bound antibodies bind the antigen, causing mast cells in the skin and other tissues to degranulate, releasing histamine. The histamine causes prurititis, vasodilatation, vascular leakage, edema and erythema. Repeated scratching or licking at affected sites, especially the face, dorsal aspect of the feet, ears, axilla and groin results in self-inflicted excoriations, alopecia, lichenification and hyperpigmentation. Erosions and ulcerations that result may become secondarily infected by bacteria. Microscopically, the dermis contains mild, superficial perivascular infiltrates of lymphocytes and macrophages, and variable numbers of mast cells. Eosinophils are not a prominent feature of atopic dermatitis. Neutrophils, when present, are usually the consequence of bacterial infection of self-inflicted erosions.

Food allergy is a less common cause of hypersensitivity dermatitis in dogs and cats that has to be differentiated from atopic dermatitis. The immunologic basis for the cutaneous and gastrointestinal signs of food allergy has not been characterized in dogs and cats, but in people it mainly involves a type I hypersensitivity reaction, and only occasionally types III and IV. In dogs, the miniature schnauzer, golden retriever, West Highland white terrier, and Chinese shar-pei are at increased risk for development of food allergy. Clinically, the cutaneous lesions of food allergy are extremely variable. They vary from erythematous papules, wheals, pustules and crusts to erosions, ulceration and excoriations resulting from persistent licking, biting and scratching. The cutaneous lesions of food allergy tend to be extremely pruritic, especially in cats. The skin lesions may be generalized or confined to the face, ears and feet. The head and neck are commonly affected in cats, where food allergy can be one of several causes of so-called "allergic miliary dermatitis."

Microscopically, in canine food allergy the dermis contains superficial and deep perivascular infiltrates of lymphocytes, plasma cells, eosinophils and mast cells that may become diffuse and extend down to and surround adnexal structures. There may be variable amounts of dermal edema. If the epidermis is severely traumatized, neutrophils may be present due to secondary bacterial infection. In cats, mast cell infiltrates may be extensive and extend into the superficial layers of the panniculus. Eosinophils are also present in significant numbers throughout the dermis. Involvement of the deep dermis and the presence of eosinophils are useful features that distinguish food allergy from atopy. However, food allergy has to be differentiated from other forms of allergic dermatitis characterized by dermal infiltrates of eosinophils, including canine flea allergy dermatitis, feline allergic miliary dermatitis, canine sarcoptic acariasis, feline notoedric acariasis, cheyletiellosis and cutaneous dirofilariasis.

Flea allergy dermatitis

Flea allergy dermatitis is the most common form of cutaneous hypersensitivity of dogs and cats. Affected animals become sensitized to the saliva of the common cat flea, *Ctenocephalides felis,* or the less prevalent dog flea, *C. canis* and develop IgE antibodies and sensitized T lymphocytes specific for it. The antibodies mediate a type I (immediate) and the sensitized T cells a type IV (delayed) hypersensitivity reactions in the skin. Atopic animals are probably more predisposed to flea allergy dermatitis than non-atopic individuals. Very few fleas or even a transient infestation will evoke an intense allergic dermatitis in hypersensitized dogs. There is also seasonal variation in the occurrence of this disorder, it being more common in the summer and fall when fleas are most active.

Clinically, flea allergy dermatitis is distinctive in terms of its distribution which corresponds to the favored feeding sites of the flea. These include the dorsal lumbosacral region, base of the tail, perineum and caudomedial aspect of the thighs. In cats, the head and neck are frequently affected. In longstanding cases the lesions may become generalized. The intense pruritis associated with this disorder provokes considerable self-inflicted trauma from persistent biting, scratching and licking at affected sites. The very early lesions appear as erythematous papules and wheals which rapidly progress to pustules, crusts, moist erosions and varying degrees of alopecia due to self-trauma. Chronic lesions are characterized by alopceia, crusting, lichenification and hyperpigmentation.

Histologically, the lesions of flea allergy dermatitis are characterized by superficial perivascular to diffuse infiltrates of eosinophils, mast cells, lymphocytes and macrophages. Affected areas exhibit varying degrees of edema. Depending upon the degree of self-trauma and secondary bacterial infection, neutrophils may also be present in the infiltrates. The lesions can generally be differentiated from atopy due to the presence of eosinophils, but may be extremely difficut to distinguish from food allergy. In such cases, the distribution of the lesions can be helpful in the differential diagnosis.

Mite-induced allergic dermatitis (mange)

Numerous species of mites that characteristically inhabit the superficial layers of the epidermis cause allergic reactions in the underlying dermis of the skin of domestic animals. These include different species-specific variants of *Sarcoptes scabei* (humans, swine, dogs, cattle and goats, rarely in horses, cats and sheep); *Notoedres cati* (cats, rabbits); several species of *Cheyletiella,* i.e. *C. yasguri* (dogs), *C. blakei* (cats), and *C. parasitovorax* (rabbits) and several species of *Psoroptes,* i.e. *P. ovis* (sheep, cattle); *P. cuniculi* (rabbits, horses, goats and sheep); *P. natalensis* (cattle) and *P. equi* (horses). Clinically, these different forms of mange are characterized by marked thickening of the skin, lichenification, crusting, scaling and areas of superficial erosions and ulcerations due to self-inflicted trauma. The lesions, as in flea allergy dermatitis, tend to be intensely pruritic. The distribution of the mite-induced lesions tends to be somewhat characteristic for each species. In swine, favorite sites of infestation include the inner aspect of the pinnae, rump, flank and abdomen; in dogs, the elbows, hocks, pinnae and ventral thorax; and in cattle, goats, horses and cats the head, neck and pinnae are favored sites. In all of these species, chronic infestations may become generalized, particularly in debilitated or immunosuppressed individuals.

Microscopically, the epidermis of the infected skin is variably acanthotic, parakeratotic, hyperkeratotic, and contains the characteristic mites in the stratum corneum beneath the thickened layer of superficial keratin. The presence of the mites is diagnostic in these cases, but these may be few in number and difficult to find. The dermal lesions consist of superficial vasodilatation, edema, and extensive infiltration by eosinophils, macrophages, mast cells, and lymphocytes, typically those cells seen in types I and IV hypersensitivity reactions. Neutrophils may also be present if there are self-inflicted epidermal erosions (also see Chapter 13).

Other parasites that affect the skin

Numerous other parasites can infest and cause lesions in the skin of domestic animals. These are listed in Table 17-1 by host species, parasite name and preferred sites of localization within the skin. They are discussed in greater detail in Chapter 13.

Vascular lesions of the dermis

Two types of vasculitides occur in the dermis: immune-mediated and septic. Both forms of vasculitis are rare. Immune-mediated vasculitis results from the deposition of circulating immune complexes in the wall of vessels within the dermis. This condition may be associated with vasculitis of visceral organs as well. Septic vasculitis, when it involves dermal vessels, usually results from direct extension of a bacterial infection involving hair follicles or surrounding tissues in the region of affected vessels. Clinically, dermal vasculitis is manifest by swelling of the skin at the affected site, erythema, purpura, hemorrhage, bullae and ulceration. The loss of blood supply is often associated with infarction of the overlying skin leading to cutaneous ulceration. Tissues most susceptible to vasculitis-associated cutaneous lesions are those with poor collateral circulation. These include the pinnae, paws, tip of the tail, lips, oral mucosa, and antecubital regions. Vessels in the subcutaneous adipose tissue are also occasionally affected. Animals with cutaneous vasculitis may show signs of systemic illness, including fever, malaise and anorexia related to vasculitis in other organs.

Microscopically, affected vessels in both forms of vasculitis contain neutrophil infiltrates within and surrounding the vessel wall. In immune complex vasculitis the neutrophils may be extensively fragmented, a feature often referred to as **leukocytoclastic vasculitis.** In septic vasculitis, the neutrophilic infiltrate may be more intense and bacterial emboli can be but are rarely present. In both types of vasculitis the vessel wall contains degenerative changes and thrombi are often present in the lumen. In other less common forms of immune-mediated vasculitis lymphocytes and histiocytes comprise the cellular infiltrate.

Pyogranulomatous and granulomatous diseases of the dermis and subcutis

A large number of infectious agents cause pyogranulomatous or granulomatous dermatitis in domestic animals. Many of these are described in those chapters of this text dealing with specific etiologic agents. Some of these lesions result from infections or parasitic infestations that spill from ruptured, inflamed hair follicles; others result from primary infections of the dermis that are initially introduced into the dermis at sites of prior inflammation or trauma, and still others are idiopathic. **Pyogranulomas** of the dermis, as in other tissues, have purulent centers composed of collections of neutrophils surrounded by variable numbers of histiocytes, macrophages, lymphocytes, plasma cells and an outer zone of fibroblasts. **Granulomas,** on the other hand, are composed almost exclusively of discrete or confluent masses of histiocytes (epithelioid cells) which may be associated with variable numbers of lymphocytes, plasma cells, multinucleated giant cells and fibroblasts.

As mentioned above, hair follicles inflamed as the result of infestation by *Demodex spp.* often rupture spilling the inflammatory exudate and mites into the surrounding dermis. The presence of mites free in the dermis provokes a pyogranulomatous dermatitis. In such cases the characteristic cigar-shaped mites can be found within the center of the pyogranulomas and in neighboring hair follicles.

Sporothrix schenckii, the causative agent of **sporotrichosis,** is a saprophytic fungus found commonly in soil and decaying vegetable matter. This organism when introduced into the dermis as a wound contaminant causes a multifocal to diffuse pyogranulomatous dermatitis and panniculitis. Infection occurs in people and in various laboratory and domestic animals. It is reported most often in cats and dogs, and cats have been known to transmit the disease to people. In tissues sections, the organism is cigar-shaped and varies from 4–9 μm in length by 1–2 μm in width. In cats, the lesions contain numerous organisms that are readily visible in hematoxylin and eosin stained tissue sections; whereas in dogs the organisms are usually few in number and difficult to find. Periodic acid-Schiff or Gomori's methenamine silver stains enhance one's ability to identify the organisms in canine lesions.

Mycobacterial infections of the skin occurs with some frequency in cats but are rare in dogs, except in the Basset breed. Agents involved in such infections include: *Mycobacterium lepraemurium*—the cause of feline leprosy, *M. fortuitum*, *M. chelonei*, *M smegmatis*, *M. avium-intracellulare* and others. These opportunistic, acid-fast organisms are generally introduced into the skin at sites of trauma. They generally cause solitary or multiple, slow-growing alopecic nodules in the skin and subcutis of the face, forelegs and thorax. Older lesions may eventually ulcerate. Microscopically, the dermis and subcutis contain diffuse nodular infiltrates of large, pale, foamy macrophages that may contain large vacuoles. Giant cells are not usually a feature of these forms of cutaneous mycobacteriosis. Ziehl-Neelsen or other

TABLE 17-1 **Parasitic diseases of the skin**

Hosts	Parasite	Location of lesion
Cattle, sheep, dog, man, swine, horse	*Sarcoptes scabiei*, var. *bovis, ovis, canis, suis*, etc.	Epidermis generally (scabies or sarcoptic mange)
Dog, cat, man, swine, sheep, cattle	*Demodex folliculorum*	Hair follicles, sebaceous glands, dermis, lymph nodes (demodectic mange)
Sheep, cattle, horses, rabbits	*Psoroptes communis*, var. *ovis, bovis, equi*, and *cuniculi*	Epidermis of ears and elsewhere
Cattle, sheep, horses, goats	*Chorioptes bovis*	Epidermis of feet and base of tail
Swine	*Demodex phylloides*	Hair follicles and sebaceous glands
Dogs, cats, sheep, deer, rarely man	*Thelazia californiensis*	Conjunctiva, membrana nictitans
Dogs, cattle	larvae of *Rhabditis strongyloides*	Dermis and hair follicles
Cat	*Notoedres cati*	Epidermis, esp. of neck (notoedric mange)
Cattle	larvae of *Hypoderma bovis* and *lineatum* (ox warble)	Subcutis and dermis of back
Cattle	*Thelazia rhodesi*	Conjunctiva, membrana nictitans
Cattle	*Onchocerca gutturosa*	Dermis and subcutis
Cattle	*Onchocerca gibsoni*	Subcutis
Cattle (U.S.)	*Stephanofilaria stilesi*	Hair follicles and dermis, usually of abdomen
Cattle (Indonesia)	*Stephanofilaria dedoesi*	Hair follicles and dermis of shoulders, eyelids, neck, withers, dewlap
Cattle (India)	*Stephanofilaria assamensis*	Dermis of shoulders and elsewhere
Cattle (Malaya)	*Stephanofilaria kaeli*	Dermis and epidermis of lower parts of legs
Cattle	*Parafilaria bovicola*	Subcutis
Sheep, deer	microfilaria of *Elaeophora schneideri*	Dermis of head, face, poll
Sheep	*Psorergates ovis*	Epidermis generally
Horses	microfilaria of *Onchocerca cervicalis*	Dermis of abdomen and pectoral region
Horses	larvae of *Habronema majus*	Dermis, pectoral region
Horses	larvae of *Draschia megastoma*	Dermis, pectoral region
Horses	larvae of *Habronema muscae*	Dermis, pectoral region
Horses, asses, mules	*Parafilaria multipapillosa*	Nodules, subcutis
Horses, asses, mules	*Onchocerca reticulata*	Subcutis, dermis
Man	larvae of *Schistosomes* of birds and mammals	Dermis ("swimmer's itch")
Man	larvae of *Ancylostoma*	Dermis ("creeping eruption")
Mice	*Psorergates simplex*	Epidermis generally
Poultry	*Dermanyssus gallinae*	Epidermis generally
Chicken	*Cnemidocoptes mutans*	Scales of legs
Chicken	*Cnemidocoptes gallinae*	Feather follicles
Dog, rabbit, cat	*Cheyletiella parasitivorax*	Epidermis generally
Dog, mink, otter, raccoon	*Dracunculus insignis*	Subcutis of limbs

acid-fast stains reveal massive numbers of acid-fast bacilli within the foamy macrophages with *M. lepraemurium* and *M. avium-intracellulare* infections, but organisms may be present in small numbers and difficult to
identify with the other mycobacterial agents. Some Bassett hounds have been shown to be genetically predisposed to *M. avium-intracellular* infection. Although not
documented, these dogs would appear to have some
dysfunction of T lymphocytes that renders them susceptible.

Cryptococcus neoformans causes systemic as well as cutaneous infection of cats, and rarely dogs. The cutaneous lesions tend to be located in the subcutis of the
head, neck and ears and consist of well-circumscribed,
clustered, firm to fluctuant nodules which rupture and
exude large amounts of mucinous exudate. Histologically, the dermis and subcutis contain large numbers of
5 to 20 μm, oval to spherical yeast forms surrounded
by a clear space consisting of a mucinous capsule. The
capsules impart a "soap bubble" appearance to the lesion. Capsules are best demonstrated by the mucicarmine stain which stains the clear space a bright red because of its mucin content. The organism also exhibits
narrow-based budding. Culture can also be used to
identify this agent. The inflammatory reaction in such
lesions is highly variable. It may be scant or consist of
large numbers of macrophages containing phagocytized
organsims. Neutrophils and lymphocytes may also be
scattered throught the affected tissues.

Other mycotic dermatitides include *Microsporum canis*
which causes dermatophytic mycetoma, particularly in
Persian cats, *Histoplasma capsulatum, Blastomyces dermatitidis,* and *Coccidioides immitis,* each of which can cause a
pyogranulomatous or granulomatous dermatitis in
many animal species, and *Pythium sp.* a plant pathogen
that has rarely been associated with pyogranulomatous
dermatitis in dogs (also see Chapter 11).

Feline eosinophilic granuloma complex

This complex of idiopathic skin lesions of cats includes:
eosinophilic plaque, linear granuloma and **eosinophilic
ulcer.**

Eosinophlic plaque is a common, severely pruritic lesion of the skin of cats, suspected but not proven to
represent a form of localized or systemic hypersensitivity. The lesions appear as single or multiple, sharply demarcated, erythematous round to ovoid, ulcerated
plaques that ooze serum. They occur most often on the
abdomen and inner aspect of the thighs. Microscopically, the epidermis adjacent to areas of ulceration are
acanthotic, spongiotic and may contain exocytosis of
eosinophils. The dermis also contains diffuse infiltrates
of eosinophils that may extend from the superficial dermis into the subcutaneous adipose tissue. These epidermal and dermal changes bear some resemblance to flea
allergy dermatitis, atopic dermatitis and food allergy
dermatitis all of which have been considered at one
time or another as possible etiologies of this disorder.

Linear granuloma occurs characteristically as a linear,
well-demarcated, pinkish-yellow, elevated firm lesion on
the caudal thighs. Histologically similar lesions have
also been reported on the forelimbs, pinnae, neck and
thorax, lip, chin, and footpads. Microscopically, linear
granuloma is characterized by epidermal acanthosis,
erosions, ulceration and serum exudation. The dermis
is diffusely infiltrated with large numbers of eosinophils
that are often arranged around variable sized foci of
brightly eosinophilic, degenerate dermal collagen. This
collagenolysis is mediated by major basic protein, a

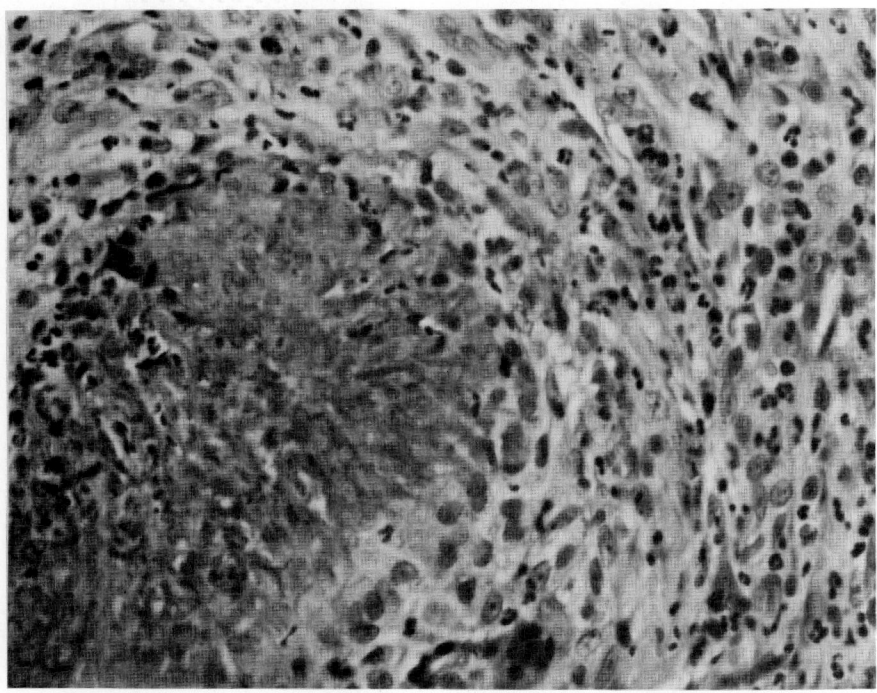

FIG. 17-13 Eosinophilic granuloma,
tongue of a cat. A central core of brightly
eosinophilic degenerate collagen is surrounded by macrophages, epithelioid
cells, and eosinophils. (Courtesy of Dr.
N. W. King, Jr.)

product of eosinophils granules. Macrophages and foreign body giant cells may also surround the degenerate collagen. The intervening areas of dermal connective tissue contains variable numbers of macrophages, mast cells and lymphocytes.

Eosinophilic ulcer is a disorder similar to linear granuloma, except that it involves tissues of the oral cavity, especially the tongue, frenulum, or soft palate. The lesions at these sites are histologically similar to linear granular in that there typically are areas of collagen degeneration surrounded by degranulating eosinophils with an admixture of histiocytes, foreign body type giant cells and lymphocyes (Fig.17-13). Interestingly, naked hairshafts are found with some frequency in these oral lesions. Their role, if any, in the causation of this condition has not been established.

Calcinosis circumscripta

This is an uncommon lesion in dogs and is exceedingly rare in cats. It is a poorly understood form of dystrophic calcification that affects the dermal connective of the skin over pressure points or at sites of trauma. It also occurs on rare occasions in the tongue. The condition occurs most often in large breeds of dogs, especially the German Shepherd, and in brachiocephalic breeds. Common sites for its occurrence include the feet and the margins of pinnae that have been surgically cropped. The pathogenesis of calcinosis circumscripta is not resolved; some have concluded that it represents deposition of calcium phosphate on areas of altered collagen, others feel that it arises within the lumens of cystic apocrine glands.

Clinically, the lesion usually appears as a single raised, nodular, firm to fluctuant mass located in the dermis and subcutis. The epidermis overlying larger masses may be ulcerated. On cut-section, the nodule is composed of one or more circumscribed masses of homogeneous, white, putty-like or gritty material surrounded by bands of connective tissue (Fig.17-14). The entire mass may also be somewhat encapsulated. At the sites of ear cropping the lesions may be small and multiple.

Microscopically, the deep dermis and subcutis contain one to several isolated or confluent masses of pale to intensely basophilic acellular material surrounded by zones of histiocytes, giant cells and bands of fibroblastic connective tissue containing variable numbers of lymphocytes and neutrophils (Fig.17-15). In rare cases, the mineralized material is surrounded by what appear to be epithelial, or perhaps epithelioid, cells giving the impression that the deposits arose within the lumens of glands, possibly apocrine glands. This remains an issue of controversy.

Cutaneous amyloidosis

The various forms of amyloidosis and the physico-chemical properties of the various types of amyloid are described in detail in Chapter 2. Cutaneous amyloidosis is a form of primary amyloidosis in which deposits of AL (im-

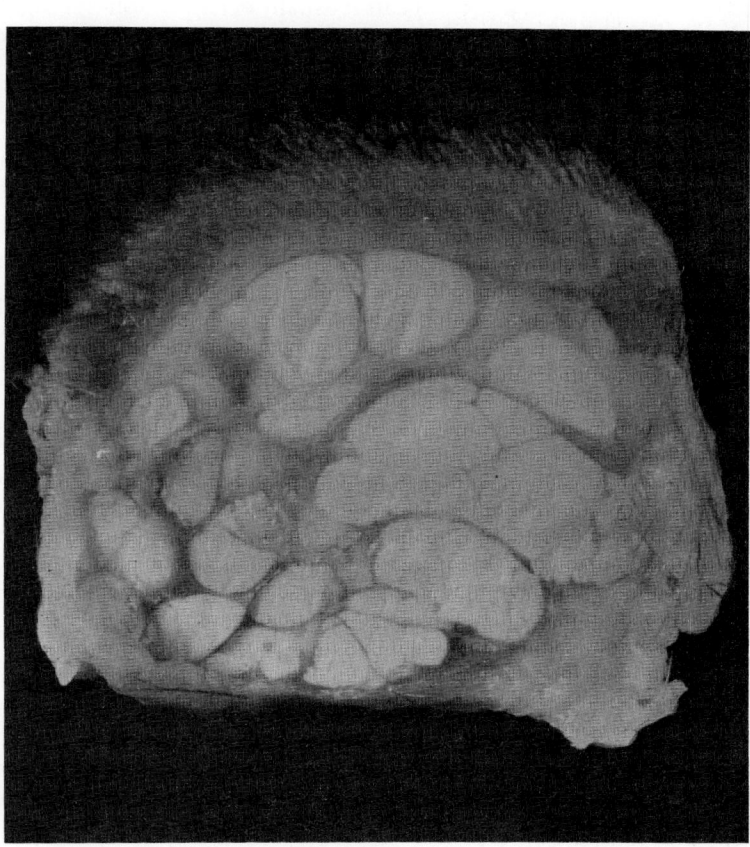

FIG. 17-14 Calcinosis circumscripta, skin of a male, three-year-old dachshund. Freshly cut specimen. (Courtesy of Angell Memorial Animal Hospital.)

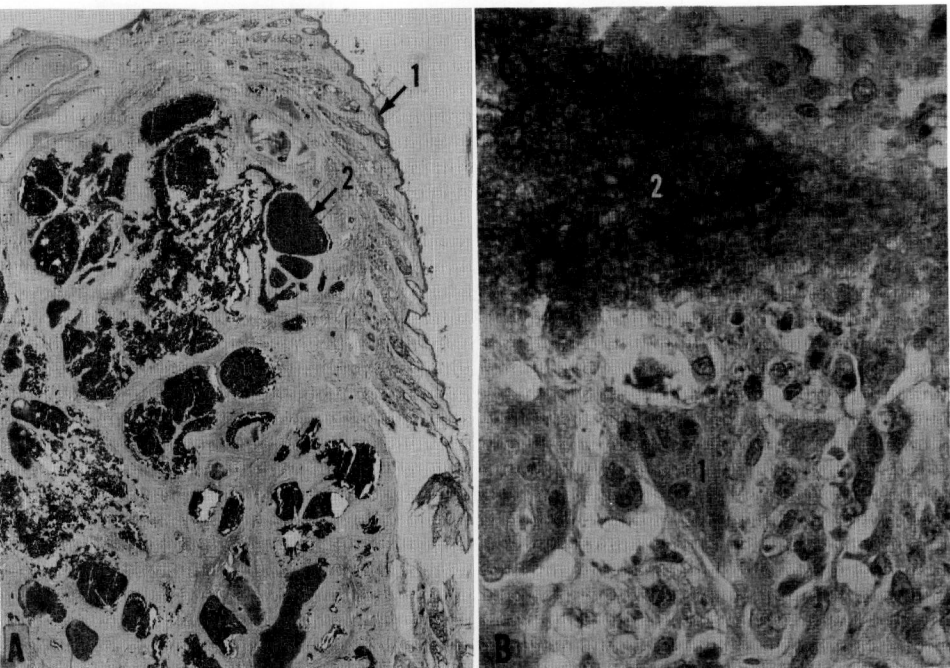

FIG. **17-15** Calcinosis circumscripta, skin of a dog. **A.** Low magnification (×7). Epidermis (1), circumscribed deposits (2) of calcium salts in the dermis. **B.** Same specimen as A (×440). Epithelioid cells (1) surrounding calcium salts (2). (Courtesy of Armed Forces Institute of Pathology and Dr. S. W. Stiles.

munoglobulin light chain) amyloid occur in the dermis. It occurs in humans, dogs and cats and probably other species in association with various forms of plasma cell dyscrasia, including multiple myeloma, cutaneous (extramedullary) plasmacytoma and in sites of localized plasma cell proliferation. In dogs and cats it usually occurs as solitary or multiple firm nodules in the dermis and subcutis, especially of the ear, but also at other sites. The acellular, eosinophilic deposits of amyloid occur in the dermal connective tissue intimately associated with the benign neoplastic plasma cells of a cutaneous plasmacytoma, a relatively common skin tumor of dogs. The deposits may be surrounded by histiocytes, lymphocytes and rare foreign body type giant cells.

Cutaneous dermal asthenia

This condition encompasses a number of different inherited defects of dermal collagen that lead to increased extensibility and decreased tensile strength of the skin, and hyperextensibility of joints. It has been described in people where it encompasses a number of disorders included in the **Ehlers-Danlos syndrome**; in dogs, cats, and mink, where it has been termed **cutaneous asthenia**; and in cattle and sheep where it is referred to as **dermatosparaxis**. In dogs, cats and mink, it is inherited as an autosomal dominant trait, whereas in cattle and sheep it is an autosomal recessive disorder. In dogs, the condition has been described in several breeds including the boxer, dachshund, English springer spaniel, greyhound, beagle, and in mixed breeds. Clinically, affected dogs and cats have extreme fragility of the skin leading to large gaping wounds as the result of minimal trauma. Microscopically, the epidermis and dermal collagen may appear normal, or in some cases there may be variability in the size of the

bundles of dermal collagen. Electron microscopy or biochemical analysis of the collagen is generally needed to confirm the diagnosis. Ultrastructurally, the collagen fibrils are inadequately packed and fail to form orderly, uniform cylindrical fibers that characterized normal collagen. The collagen generally persist as flattened, twisted ribbons (Fig.17-16).

NEOPLASMS

Neoplasms of the skin are of particular interest in veterinary medicine for they are common and readily accessible for surgical excision or other forms of treatment. The biologic characteristics and morphologic features of neoplasms are discussed in Chapter 4. Included here are primary neoplasms of the epidermis and the adnexae, and the neoplasms of the dermis that are most frequent in the skin or restricted to this location. Neoplasms that arise in specialized epidermal structures (e.g., mammary gland, ceruminous gland) are discussed elsewhere, as are neoplasms of supporting structures covered in other systems (e.g., hemangioma, neurofibroma). Table 17-2 lists cutaneous neoplasms by site of origin and indicates which are discussed in other sections of this book. The relative frequency of neoplasms of the skin in dogs and cats is listed in Table 17-3. The skin is the most common site for neoplasia in dogs, and second only to malignant lymphomas in cats.

Neoplasms of epidermis

PAPILLOMA

A papilloma or "wart", as it is commonly referred to, is a benign neoplasm of stratified squamous epithelium. Grossly, papillomas appear as single, or more of-

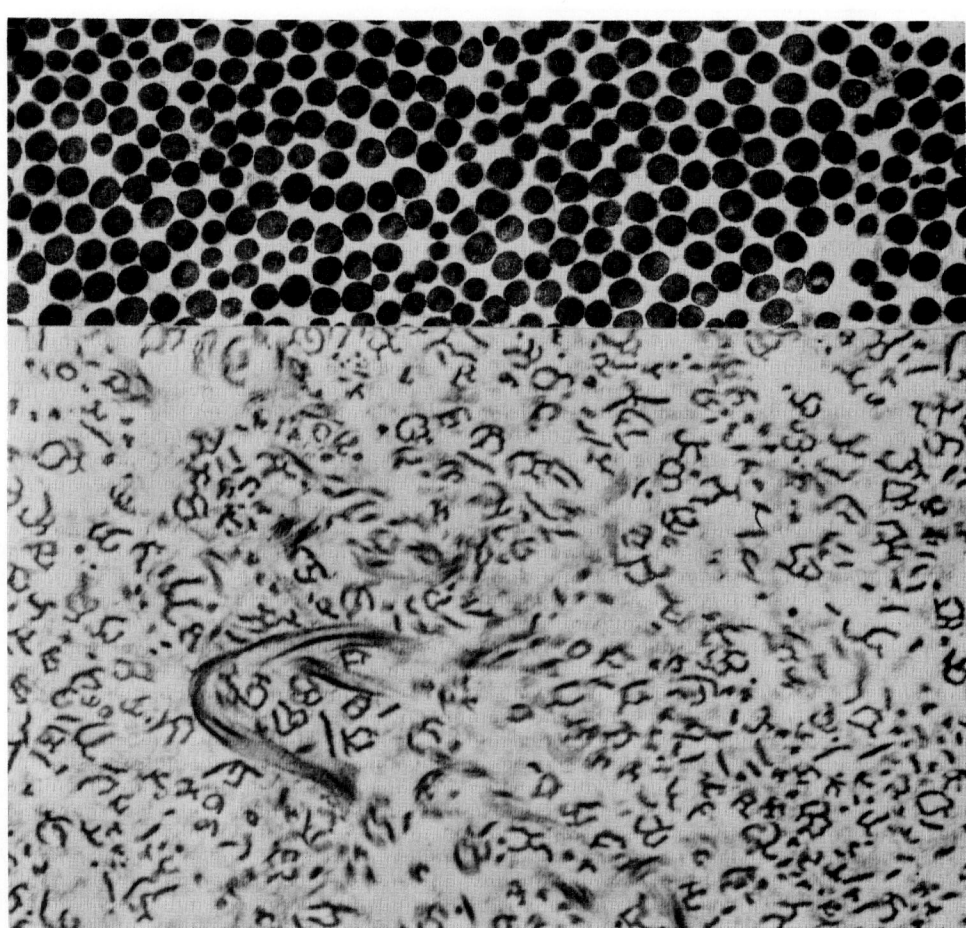

FIG. 17-16 Bovine dermal collagen (×49,400). *Top,* Normal collagen fibers in cross section. *Bottom,* Collagen of calf affected with dermatosparaxis. (Courtesy of Dr. W. Kay Read and *Laboratory Investigation.*)

ten multiple, raised, flat or cauliflower-like growths with either a smooth or more often an irregular surface. Papillomas are illustrated in Chapter 8. The face, neck, and oral mucosa are the most common sites, but they can arise anywhere including the esophagus, rumen and external genital tract. Transitional cell papillomas also occur in the urinary bladder.

Microscopically, a papilloma consists of an elevated mass composed of multiple papillary projections of fibrovascular connective tissue covered by a well-differentiated layer of heavily keratinized or cornified stratified squamous epithelium. Papillomas do not contain cutaneous adnexal structures or rete ridges. As with most tumors, the fibrovascular stroma is not neoplastic but is an extension of the normal dermis or lamina propria, depending upon the tissue affected, that is induced to proliferate by the neoplasm to maintain its blood supply. Most spontaneously occurring papillomas of humans and animals are induced by DNA-containing papillomaviruses; however, the etiology of some is not known. As described in Chapter 4, viral induced papillomas begin with extensive proliferation of the basal cells of the epidermis or mucosa without replication of the infectious virus. As the proliferating basal cells become more differentiated, they become permissive for viral replication and one can then find amphoteric in-

tranuclear inclusion bodies in the cells corresponding to the stratum spinosum and stratum granulosum of the normal epidermis. By electron microscopy these inclusion bodies are composed of masses of papillomavirus virions. With the progression of viral replication, infected cells undergo degenerative changes and die, releasing infectious viruses into the environment for dissemination to other susceptible individuals via insect vectors, fomites or direct contact. This cytolytic effect of the virus coupled with a cell-mediated immune response by the host generally leads to spontaneous regression of papillomas. Rarely, a papilloma will undergo malignant transformation resulting in a squamous cell carcinoma. This has been documented in experimental studies in animals and with genital warts and squamous cell carcinoma of the cervix of women.

For the most part, papillomaviruses are relatively species specific, but cross-species infections do occur occasionally as in the case of equine sarcoid which is thought to be caused by bovine papillomavirus. In addition, papillomas arising from different sites tend to be virus type specific. Oral papillomas, for example, are caused by a different papillomavirus than cutaneous papillomas. The molecular basis for papillomavirus-induced neoplastic transformation is described in Chapter 4.

TABLE 17-2 **Neoplasms of the skin**

Neoplasm	Chap.
Epidermis	
Papilloma	
Squamous cell carcinoma	
Keratoacanthoma	
Basal cell carcinoma	
Malignant melanoma	
Adnexa	
Adenoma and adenocarcinoma of sweat and apocrine glands	
Adenoma and adenocarcinoma of sebaceous glands	
Adenoma and adenocarcinoma of perianal gland	
Hair matrix tumor (benign calcifying epithelioma)	
Trichoepithelioma	
Adenoma and adenocarcinoma of ceruminous glands	28
Mammary gland neoplasms	25
Dermis and Subcutis	
Fibroma and fibrosarcoma	
Equine sarcoid	
Mast cell tumor	
Canine cutaneous histiocytoma	
Venereal tumor	25
Hemangioma, hemangiosarcoma	21
Lymphangioma, lymphangiosarcoma	21
Hemangiopericytoma	
Neurofibroma, neurofibrosarcoma	27
Lipoma, liposarcoma	
Tumor of brown fat (hibernoma)	
Xanthoma	
Myxoma, myxosarcoma	

In cattle, particularly white-faced cattle, smaller but similar appearing papillomas occur near the corneoscleral junction and constitute an early stage of squamous cell carcinoma. Whether malignant transformation of such papillomas is due to the original solar radiation induced mutation or a different mutational event is not known, but one should be reminded that carcinogenesis is generally a multi-mutational phenomenon.

Another, relatively uncommon form of papilloma is the **inverted papilloma.** It has been described in dogs where it occurs on the skin of the abdomen and inguinal areas. This neoplasm has many of the features of the exophytic form of papilloma, except that it is endophytic and rather than projecting from the surface of the skin, grows downward into the dermis. Grossly, the inverted papilloma appears as a slightly raised, 1–2 cm, firm dermal nodule that has a pore opening to the surface of the skin. Microscopically, the tumor is composed of numerous long papillary projections of hyperplastic stratified squamous epithelium supported by thin cores of fibrovascular connective tissue. The tumor is invaginated into the dermis where it grows by expansion com-

pressing the adjacent dermal connective tissue. The epithelial component has an orderly sequence of maturation with layers of keratin surrounding the papillary projections and filling the lumen. Cells of the stratum granulosum contain numerous basophilic keratohyalin granules and the nuclei of some of the cells contain ill-defined, eosinophilic viral inclusion bodies surrounded by a halo. By electron microscopy the inclusion bodies contained numerous papillomavirus virions.

SQUAMOUS CELL CARCINOMA

This, the commonest form of carcinoma of the skin, is derived from stratified squamous epithelium. The neoplastic epithelium may or may not cornify depending upon the nature of the epithelium from which it arises. Pigmentation and papillation (formation of rete ridges), however, are not features of this type of neoplasm. In a reasonably well-differentiated squamous cell carcinoma, the usual sequence of keratinocyte maturation may be somewhat preserved from the underlying connective-tissue stroma, the dark, basal stra-

TABLE 17-3 **Relative frequency (%) of neoplasms of skin, subcutis, and adnexa in dogs and cats***

	Dog	*Cat*
1. Mast cell tumor	18.2	15.6
2. Hemangiopericytoma	9.1	0
3. Lipoma	8.3	3.9
4. Adenoma, perianal gland	8.3	0
5. Canine cutaneous histiocytoma	8.2	0
6. Adenoma of sebaceous gland	6.8	2.6
7. Hair matrix tumor	6.5	1.3
8. Malignant melanoma	5.3	3.9
9. Keratoacanthoma	3.8	1.3
10. Hemangioma	3.4	0
11. Papillomatosis	3.4	0
12. Basal cell tumor	2.9	23.4
13. Adenocarcinoma of sebaceous gland	2.3	2.6
14. Adenocarcinoma of perianal gland	2.0	0
15. Fibrosarcoma	2.0	5.2
16. Adenoma of sweat gland	1.7	3.9
17. Adenocarcinoma of sweat gland	1.5	5.2
18. Hemangioendothelioma	1.5	7.8
19. Melanoma, benign	1.2	0
20. Tumor, unclassified	1.1	6.5
21. Squamous cell carcinoma	1.0	6.5
22. Ganglioneuroma	0.6	3.9
23. Fibroma	0.5	3.9
24. Neurofibroma	0.3	2.6
25. Liposarcoma	0.1	0
26. Tumor of brown fat	0.1	0
27. Mixed tumor of sweat gland	0.1	0
Total %	100	100
Total (No.)	(1370)	(77)

*Modified from Jones, 1971.

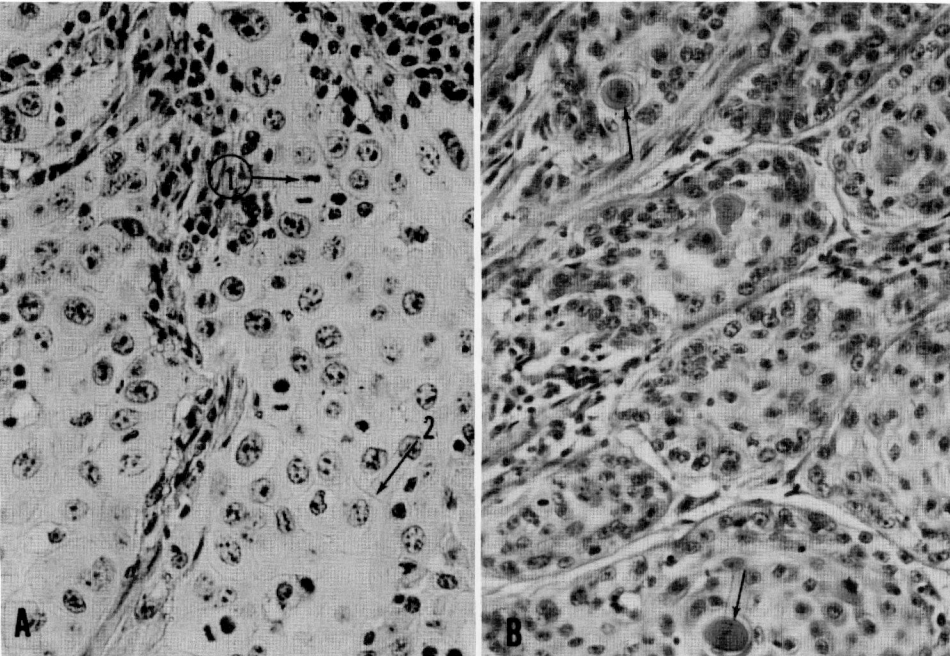

FIG. 17-17 Squamous cell carcinoma. **A.** From the corneal epithelium of a four-year-old Hereford cow. Mitotic figures *(1)* are frequent and cell borders *(2)* are prominent (×335). Contributor: Drs. C. N. Barron and G. T. Easley. **B.** Primary tumor in the vulva of a six-year-old Hereford cow. (×224). Keratinized centers of epithelial "pearls" are indicated by arrows. Contributor: Dr. C. L. Davis and the Armed Forces Institute of Pathology.

tum germinativum, the larger and paler cells of the stratum spinosum, gradually flattening to become the stratum corneum or cornified (keratinized) layer. However, the neoplastic squamous cells are not restricted to the outer surface of the neoplasm, as is the case in a papilloma. Instead, irregular masses and elongate cords of tumor cells extend haphazardly throughout the neoplasm. Cross sections of these cords appear as islands of neoplastic epithelium surrounded by stroma. The basal layer of epithelial cells is often situated at the periphery of such an island, with what would normally be the most differentiated, superficial epidermal cells occupying the center of the mass. In the case of a cornifying tumor, the red-staining keratin of the stratum corneum is produced at the center of the epithelial mass, becomes quite compact from the pressure of proliferating cells, and forms a round, concentrically laminated structure known as a **keratin pearl** (Fig. 17-17). The presence of intercellular bridges between adjacent cells (prickle cells) is a useful feature for identifying the cell of origin of the tumor. Keratin pearls and intercellular bridges, however, may be lacking in poorly differentiated squamous cell carcinomas.

The term **epidermal carcinoma** is sometimes used as a synonymn for these tumors, in as much as they are derived from the epidermis. The tongue, esophagus, rumen, ocular surfaces, and vagina are also sites of occurrence of squamous cell carcinomas.

The more anaplastic squamous cell carcinomas lack differentiation into distinct layers, and the epithelial masses consist of cells that are all more nearly uniform, with hyperchromatic nuclei, sometimes in the process of mitosis. Occasionally, the epithelial cells of a highly anaplastic carcinoma (squamous-cell or adenocarcinoma) assume a fusiform or spindle shape, so that it becomes difficult even to determine if the tumor is a

carcinoma or sarcoma. In such cases immunohistochemical staining for specific epithelial (cytokeratin), mesenchymal (desmin, vimentin) and endothelial (Factor 8–related antigen) cell markers and/or electron microscopy can be extremely useful in such differentiation.

Squamous cell carcinomas arise from the epidermis of the skin and the stratified squamous epithelium of various mucosal surfaces. They occur with some frequency in all domestic species. These, like other carcinomas, are especially prone to metastasize to the regional lymph nodes and from there to visceral organs. As with most neoplasms, the precise cause is not known, but there is a relationship to solar irradiation with the occurrence of squamous cell carcinoma of the eyelid (and corneoscleral junction) in cattle, the skin of the pinnae of white cats. In women, greater than 90 percent of squamous cell carcinomas of the cervix contain integrated copies of human papillomavirus type 16 or 18 in the DNA of neoplastic cells.

An unusual form of squamous cell carcinoma called **carcinoma of the horn or horn cancer** occurs at the junction of the skin and the horn. It is seen in Zebu cattle in India and Sumatra, where it is most common in castrated bulls, rare in cows, and nonexistent in intact bulls.

Pseudoepitheliomatous hyperplasia, as the name implies, must be differentiated from squamous cell carcinoma. The squamous cells in the former are hyperplastic, non-invasive and confined by a basement membrane. It represents a benign, proliferative response often adjacent to an area of ulceration and inflammation. The morphology of squamous cell carcinomas is frequently complicated by secondary inflammatory reactions arising from ulcerated surfaces, and the presence of cornified cells and keratin free in the dermis.

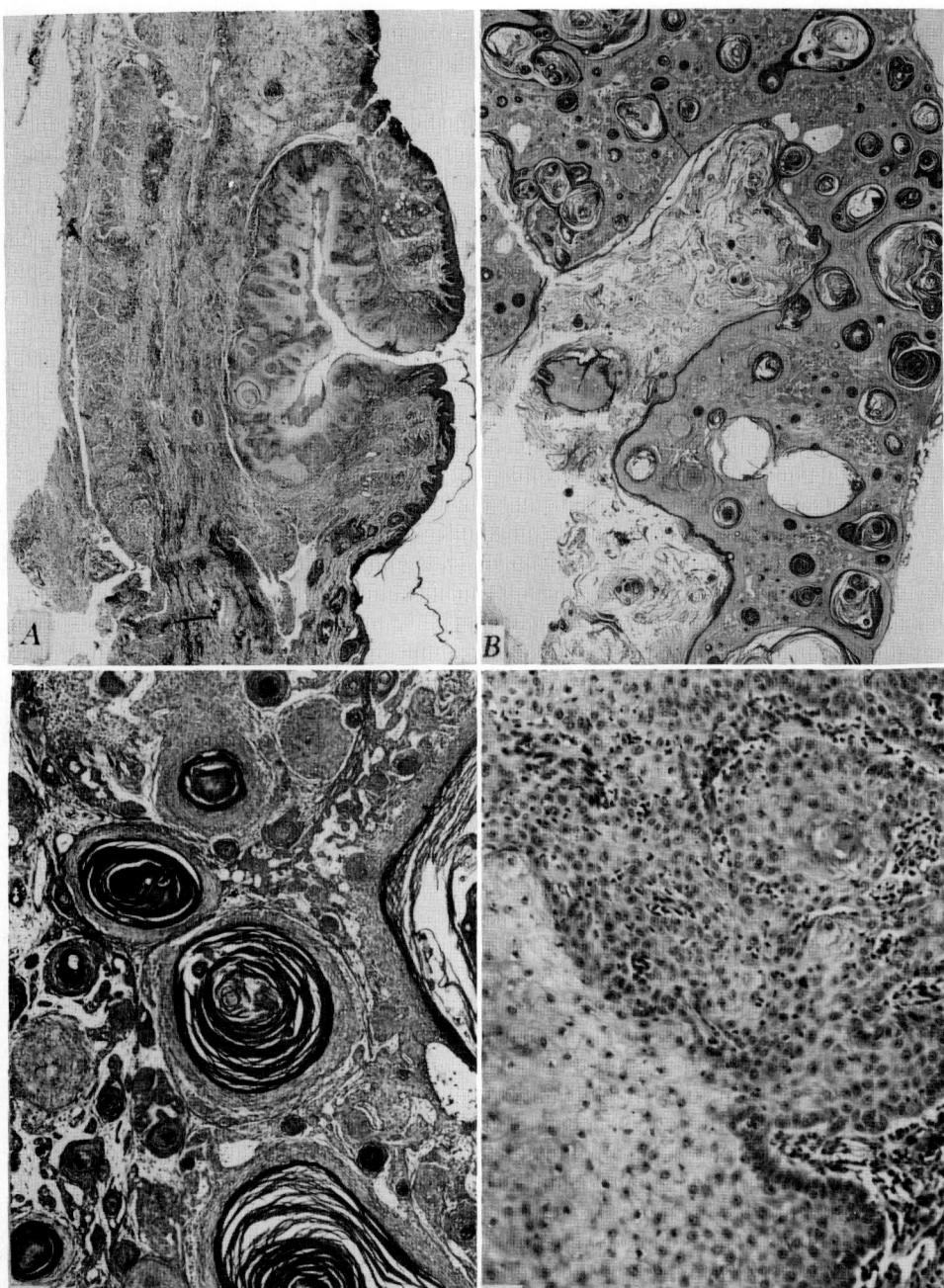

FIG. 17-18 Keratoacanthoma (canine). **A.** Early lesion (×9) arising from epidermis which is thickened and forced downward into the dermis. **B.** A more fully developed lesion (×9) with multiple keratin nests and a cystic center. **C.** Another lesion, with many epithelial nests filled with keratin and cords of cells between them (×50). **D.** Solid zones of epithelium in the early development of the lesion. (H & E, × 150.) (Courtesy of Angell Memorial Animal Hospital.)

INFUNDIBULAR KERATINIZING ACANTHOMA (KERATOACANTHOMA, INTRACUTANEOUS CORNIFYING EPITHELIOMA)

This benign, cystic neoplasm is thought to arise from the keratinized stratified squamous epithelium of the infundibular portion of hair follicles. The thickened, downward-growing epidermis forms a crypt, which eventually becomes a single or multiloculated cyst filled with entrapped keratin. These tumors have a pore that connects the keratin-filled cyst with the surface of the skin, similar to inverted papillomas. As the tumor cells grow down into the dermis, continued folding of the epithelium produces few or many concentri-

cally laminated masses of keratin (keratin pearls) surrounded by a uniform layer of squamous epithelium, the cells of which maintain the usual polarity and orderly arrangement. As the epithelial mass continues to expand, the central masses of keratin may become conspicuous and can at times be expressed from the pore on its surface (Fig.17-18). In most, but not all cases, columns of cuboidal cells grow out from the basal surface of the epithelium into the surrounding dermis and sometimes join one another to form interlacing cords or columns. This feature has been interpreted as an abortive attempt to form adnexal structures, but this has by no means been confirmed. Inflammation may become a prominent feature in the surrounding dermis, especially if the cyst ruptures, spilling keratin into the dermis.

All available evidence indicates that this is a self-limiting disease in the dog, as in humans, although multiple tumors and recurrent lesions are common. Stannard and Pulley (1975) observed up to 40 such growths on one dog, and suggested that Norwegian Elkhounds were more prone to this generalized form of the disease. Infundibular keratinizing acanthomas appear to be more frequent in males and occur in a younger population than most other cutaneous tumors.

BASAL CELL TUMOR

The term **basal cell tumor** is a categorical term that encompasses a number of morphologically distinct cutaneous neoplasms all of which are believed to be derived from basal cells of the epidermis and hair follicle but differ in their pattern of growth and differentiation. The traditional name for these tumors in human medicine is "basal cell carcinoma," but in animals their proclivity to remain localized makes this name inappropriate with respect to their usual biologic behavior. In humans these tumors tend to occur on those portions of the skin most exposed to solar radiation, i.e. the face, head and neck. In animals the following distinctive types of basal cell tumors are recognized:

Basal cell tumor and basal cell carcinoma. Tumors referred to by these names occur in both dogs and cats. The vast majority of these tumors behave in a benign clinical manner in that they tend to be remain localized, are non-invasive, and rarely recur following attempts at excision. In dogs, as in humans, the head, neck, shoulders, and thorax are common sites for its occurrence but a clear association with exposure to sunlight has not been established since they can occur in heavily haired portions of the body. Grossly, basal cell tumors appear as a well-circumscribed solitary, solid or cystic, sometime pigmented mass confined to the dermis and subcutis. They can vary considerably in size, especially in the dog. In cats they can be cystic and pigmented. The histologic distinction between benign and malignant basal cell tumors can be difficult and in most instances is based upon the degree of microscopic invasiveness of the latter. With few exceptions, excision is generally curative and metatasis is extraordinarily rare. A somewhat distinctive form of basal cell carcinoma is termed the **basosquamous cell carcinoma.** This particular variant has features of both basal cell tumor and squamous cell carcinoma in that some of the basal cells differentiate into keratinocytes that become cornified and keratinized. It tends to be more locally invasive and less circumscribed than simple basal cell tumors, but is not as aggressive as pure squamous cell carcinoma.

Microscopically, neoplasms referred simply as basal cell tumors are composed of solid or cystic masses of small round to fusiform shaped cells with an ovoid, deeply basophilic nucleus containing a single nucleolus and scant eosinophilic cytoplasm (Fig.17-19). Except for the **basosquamous carcinoma** type which contains areas

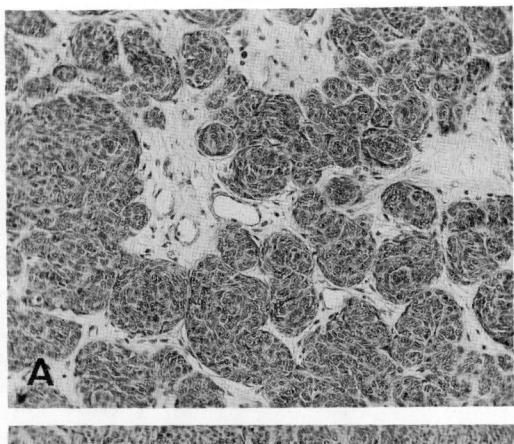
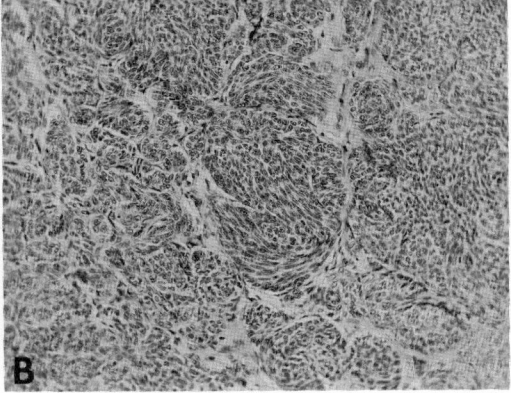

FIG. 17-19 Basal-cell tumor, skin of a cat. **A.** Discrete interconnecting islands of oval cells in a connective tissue stroma. **B.** From another area of the same neoplasm, the cells are more fusiform in shape. (Courtesy of Armed Forces Institute of Pathology.)

of cornified or keratinizing squamous cells, the common basal cell tumor contains no intercellular bridges, a feature that distinguishes them from keratinocytes. The neoplastic cells are arranged in multiple, focal and confluent, solid, nodular masses that displace bundles of dermal collagen and adnexal structures, or in multiple layers around varying sized, single or multiloculated cysts containing eosinophilic debris that may represent areas of cystic degeneration of tumor cells that were originally in a solid nodule. There is usually a variable amount of dense collagenous connective tissue surrounding the solid and cystic structures that tends to keep it localized. In some instances, particularly in cats, some of the tumor cells may contain melanin pigment in their cytoplasm.

Ribbon-type basal cell tumor (trichoblastoma) This very common histologic variant of basal cell tumor, also referred to as a **ribbon-type trichoblastoma,** has a distinctive pattern of growth that differs from the solid and cystic types. However, one occasionally encounters a neoplasm with features of both (Fig. 17-20). The term trichoblastoma refers to its origin from the trichoblastic epithelium of the hair bulb of a hair follicle, hence it is arguable as to whether this should be included as a neoplasm of the epidermis or adnexal structures. It is common in dogs, but rare in cats.

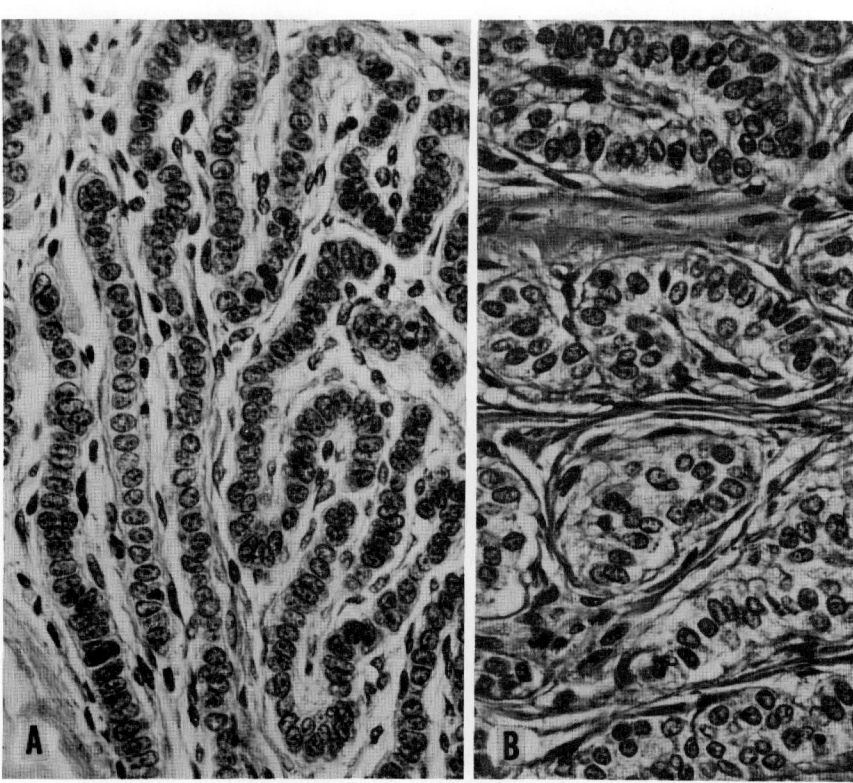

FIG. 17-20 Basal-cell tumor, skin of nose of a four-year-old male, mongrel dog. **A.** Characteristic long, tortuous cord of cells with elongated nuclei perpendicular to length of cord. (×400). **B.** Another area in same tumor (×400), with tumor cells forming nests. (Courtesy of Armed Forces Institute of Pathology.) Contributor: Dr. W. H. Cowan.

Histologically, the tumor cells are made up of undifferentiated basal type cells that are arranged in long, branching, serpentine ribbons or cords generally two cells thick (Fig. 17-20). These radiating ribbons often emanate from a central nidus, giving rise to the term "Medusa- head" pattern of growth. Within these ribbons the tumor cells are oriented such that their ovoid nuclei are perpendicular to the long axis of the ribbon. Typically, these ribbon-like structures are surrounded by a collagenous connective tissue stroma. A **trabecular variant of basal cell tumor,** also termed **trabecular trichoblastoma,** is seen in cats but rare in dogs. In this neoplasm the tumor cells proliferate in lobules made up of broad trabeculae of basal cells. These trabeculae are characterized by the presence of small basal cells containing very little cytoplasm, arranged in a palisading pattern at the periphery of the trabeculae, with somewhat larger basal cells containing moderate amounts of eosinophilic cytoplasm in the central portions of the trabeculae.

MELANOCYTOMA AND MELANOMA.

Recently, the term **melanocytoma** has been used to refer to all benign neoplasms of melanocytes. It replaces the older and somewhat confusing term **nevus** which has been ingrained in the human pathology literature for many years. The term **melanoma,** with or without the adjective malignant is used to refer to all malignant tumors of melanin-producing cells.

Cells that produce melanin (melanoblasts) arise embryologically in the neural crest, a derivative of the neuroectoderm. Early in embryonic life, these cells migrate to other positions in the body, particularly the skin, where they eventually produce melanin. This pigment enters into other tissue cells (e.g., dermis, epidermis, choroid, retina, ciliary processes, meninges) adjacent to the melanoblast. It is not surprising, therefore, that tumors of melanin-producing cells are most common in the skin but may originate elsewhere. Their nature and chemistry have been discussed in connection with melanin.

Melanocytomas and melanomas of the skin are common tumors in most species, including fish. Their pathogenesis has been the subject of much speculation and study. In humans, many cutaneous melanomas arise in the small raised, brown spots present in almost everyone's skin known as **pigmented nevi,** or more recently **melanocytomas.** Fortunately, most lesions of this type do not undergo malignant transformation. In human dermatopathology, nevi (melanocytomas) have been classified into three morphologic types, **junctional, intradermal and compound.** A lesion analogous to **junctional nevus** of humans has not been recognized in dogs but is recognized in swine. The lesion is composed of small, somewhat spherical clusters of variably pigmented round to polygonal cells confined to the basal and prickle cell layer of the epidermis and or follicular epithelium. The cells are often separated from one another due to acantholysis. If the cells are anaplastic, the lesion is believed to be the precursor of malignant melanoma. A histologically similar finding is seen in the epidermis overlying malignant melanomas in humans as well as animals. This finding is referred to as a **junctional change** and essentially is diagnostic of malignant melanomas in animals.

A **compound melanocytoma,** analagous to com-

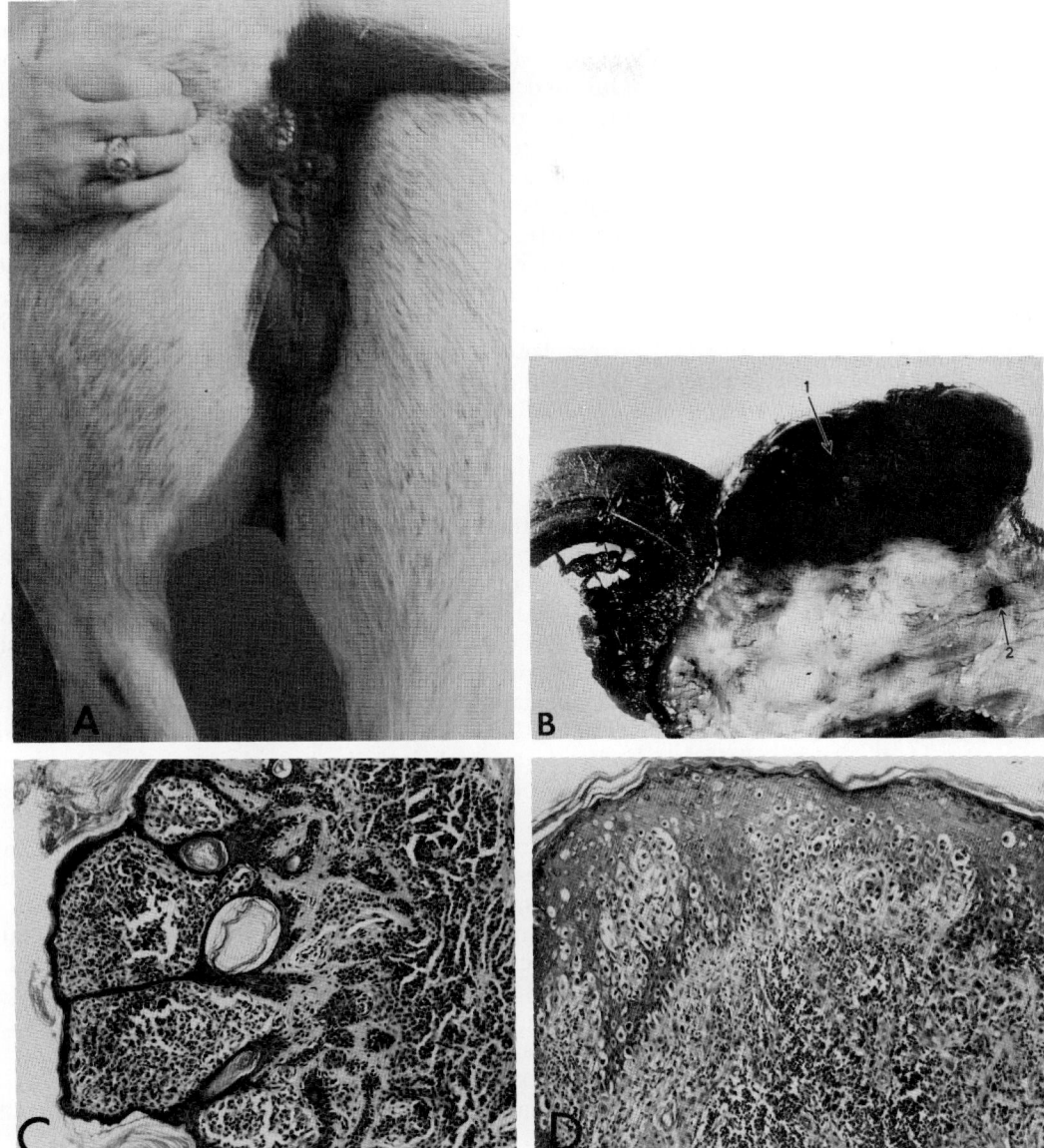

FIG. 17-21 **A.** Melanoma in the perineum of an aged mule. (Courtesy of Dr. Thomas Hardy.) **B.** Malignant melanoma arising at base of toe nail of a 16-year-old male dachshund-collie cross-bred dog. The tumor mass *(1)* is not encapsulated and a small mass is separated from it *(2)*. (Courtesy of Angell Memorial Animal Hospital.) **C.** Compound nevus in the skin of a human being. Although not infrequent in man, such lesions are rare to nonexistent in animals. **D.** Junctional change of the epidermis overlying a malignant melanoma. Epithelial cells of the basal and prickle cell layer are separated from one another, swollen, and disorganized.

pound nevus of humans (Fig. 17-21) occurs with some frequency in dogs. It is composed of a well-circumscribed, unencapsulated nodule of small spindle to large polygonal, variably pigmented melanocytes arranged in solid nests, sheets and whorls. The tumor cells are present in the epidermis and penetrate the basement membrane to occupy a portion of the superficial dermis. Mitotic figures are generally rare. Melanin-laden macrophages and mononuclear inflammatory cells may be present around the dermal portion of the tumor.

Dermal melanocytomas, analogous to dermal nevus of humans, is also recognized in dogs. These tumors are confined to the superficial dermis and may be separated from the epidermis by a thin zone of normal dermal collagen, or what is termed a Grenz zone. The tumor is composed of plump fusiform cells arranged in whorls or sheets similar to what one sees in tumors of nerve sheath origin. There is usually no stromal collagen between the closely packed, moderately pigmented tumor cells. The neoplastic cells have ovoid, vesicular nuclei with prominent nucleoli. Mitotic activity is generally low. Melanophages may be present in the immediate vicinity of the tumor. In some cases, the tumor cells are more epithelioid or dendritic in appearance and contain large melanin granules. In these cases, collagen may separate individual tumor cells.

Melanomas, or what are often termed **malignant melanomas,** are the malignant counterpart of melanocytoma. They occur with varying frequency in most animal species. The hallmark of melanomas is the great pleomorphism and variation in the patterns of growth and degree of pigmentation of the neoplastic cells. The cells may be so filled with the dark brown melanin that nuclei and cytoplasmic morphology are obscured, or at the other extreme, the neoplastic cells may contain no melanin at all in what is termed an **amelanotic melanoma.** The shape of the cells varies within the same and different tumors, from round or polygonal forms resembling epithelial cells to elongated, fusiform to stellate cells resembling mesenchymal cells. This feature of pleomorphism has led to the old dictum "if a tumor has areas that resemble a carcinoma and others that resemble sarcoma, always consider the possibility of melanoma". Typically the somewhat spindle-shaped cells dominate and fit together somewhat like the segments of an orange, within small compartments clearly or vaguely demarcated by thin fibrous trabeculae. The cytoplasm tends to be basophilic, and typically, when stained with the milder hematoxylin preparations (Mayer's), the nuclei have a distinctive violet hue which is not seen in other than melanoma cells. The nucleoli are large and prominent. In most cases, the large amounts of melanin in the cytoplasm of the tumor cells, as well as that phagocytized by melanophages in the vicinity, leave no doubt regarding the diagnosis, but some melanomas are so amelanotic that the diagnosis must be made on the morphologic features of the cells alone. A particularly useful, if not pathognomonic, feature is the occurrence of a junctional change in the epidermis overlying a dermal melanoma. This change is similar in appearance to a junctional nevus as described previously, but the islands of separated epidermal cells are more anaplastic and usually contain melanin. The basement membrane is lost and the altered epithelium blends with the dermal neoplasm and extends upward into the epidermis. Some rete ridges may be entirely replaced by junctional change. Other features that can be useful in distinguishing melanomas from melanocytomas include the presence of large, hyperchromatic nuclei, bizarre forms, and high mitotic activity. Obviously, invasion of lymphatics or small blood vessels is absolute evidence of malignancy.

Grossly, the melanoma is ordinarily recognized by its deep black color (Fig.17–21) and by the inky pigment that may diffuse from it into any aqueous medium with which the cut surface comes in contact. The true nature of an amelanotic melanoma may only be discerned by microscopic examination.

Melanomas occur in so many forms and locations that generalization is difficult. Quiescent or actively malignant melanomas are especially frequent in old gray horses, although they also occur in horses of other colors. They are particularly common in the perianal and perineal regions (Fig. 17-21), from where they spread to perirectal and other pelvic lymph nodes. In some equine cases, death results from metastasis to the spleen, lungs, or other internal organs without the primary lesion having been found.

The association of graying or loss of pigmentation, termed **vitiligo,** with melanoma has been recognized in humans and in Sinclair swine. In humans, vitiligo occurs in patients with melanoma 10 to 20 times more frequently than in the general population. This is thought to result from destruction of normal melanocytes through an immune mechanism stimulated by a melanoma. In Sinclair swine, which reportedly have a 20% incidence of multiple melanomas, there is depigmentation of normal skin as well as of the tumors, most of which ultimately regress. In horses, graying appears to precede development of melanoma, but this warrants further investigation.

In cattle, melanomas arise in the skin at various locations. In swine, cutaneous melanomas varying in diameter from a few millimeters to several centimeters, and usually somewhat elevated, are common. The smaller ones usually remain until the pig is slaughtered; larger ones may be successfully removed surgically. They are most frequent on the posterior half of the body. In the meat-producing animals, there is little opportunity to observe the ultimate outcome of these tumors. In the dog, cutaneous melanomas arise in various parts of the body and are one of the more common neoplasms of the lip and oral cavity in breeds having pigmented oral mucosa. In dogs, oral melanomas have a much more aggressive clinical course than those arising in the skin. Local recurrence and metastasis following attempts at surgical incision are common (Fig.17-22).

As indicated, most melanomas arise in the skin; those arising in the meninges and eyes are discussed in Chapters 27 and 28, respectively.

Neoplasms of adnexa

ADENOMAS AND ADENOCARCINOMAS OF SWEAT AND APOCRINE GLANDS.

The benign neoplasms resemble normal apocrine glands, but have more variation in size or papillary projections into the lumens. They are usually surrounded by abundant dense collagenous connective tissue. Adenocarcinomas have the usual features of malignancy, and the cells may form solid masses with little or no attempt at gland formation, in which case their histologic origin is difficult to ascertain. Adenocarcinomas of the apocrine glands that line the bilateral anal sacs of dogs are highly invasive and are almost always associated with a hypercalcemia due to secretion of a parathormone-like substance. Rarely, tumors of apocrine glands, especially of the skin, may contain myoepithelial cells and cartilage and resemble mixed tumors of the canine mammary gland . They are referred to as **mixed tumors of apocrine glands** (Fig. 17-23).

ADENOMAS AND ADENOCARCINOMAS OF SEBACEOUS GLANDS.

These are common neoplasms of the skin of dogs where they may be single or multiple. The head is a common site for their occurrence. Grossly they appear as yellow-white, raised, dome-shaped, or sometime pa-

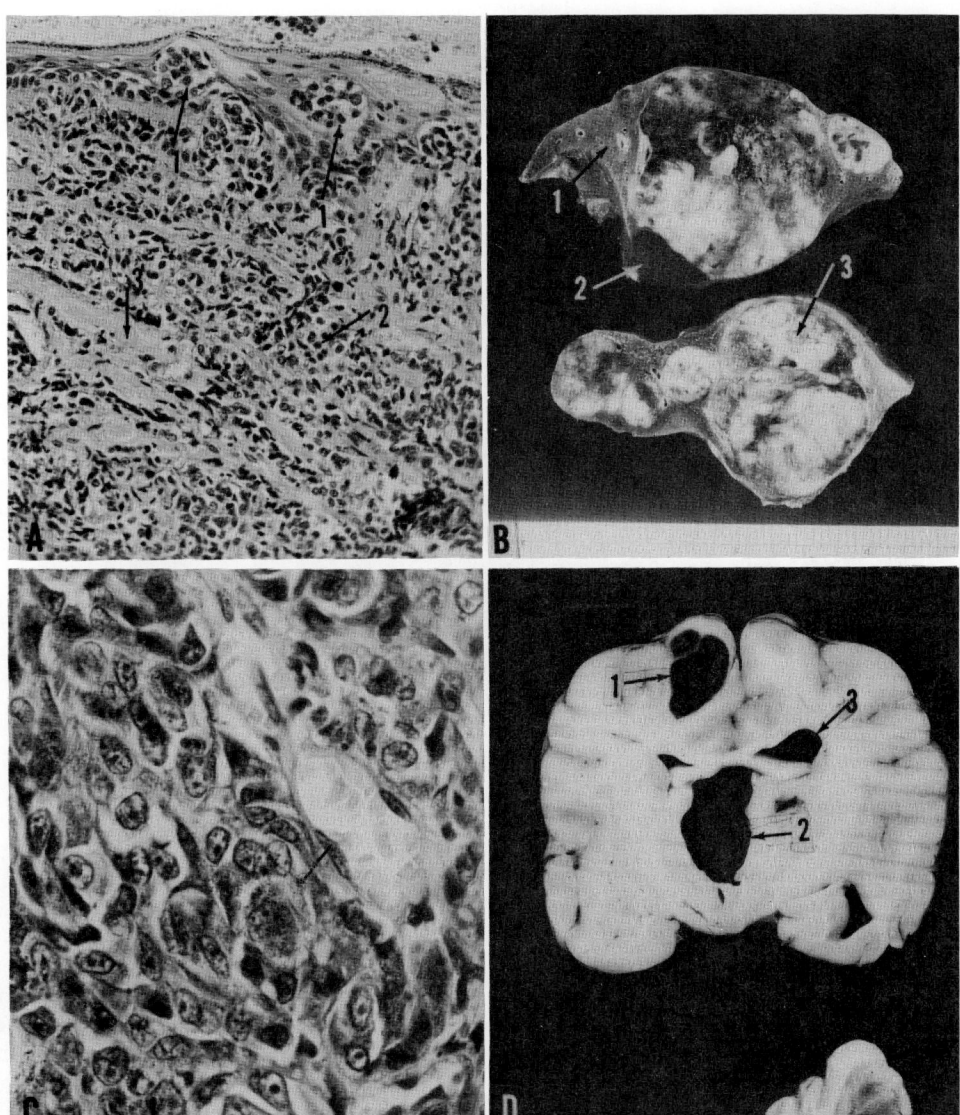

FIG. 17-22 Malignant melanoma. **A.** Primary lesion in tongue of a dog (×160). Note neoplastic cells in epidermis *(1)* and dermis *(2)*, displacing collagen fibers *(3)*. **B.** Metastatic malignant melanoma in lung *(1)* of a dog. Note melanotic *(2)* and amelanotic *(3)* areas. Contributor: Dr. M. L. Povar. **C.** High magnification (×574) of tumor in *A.* Large cells laden with melanin (arrow). Contributor: Dr. Leo L. Lieberman. **D.** Metastatic malignant melanoma *(1)* and *(2)* in brain of a dog. Note slight internal hydrocephalus *(3)*. (Courtesy of Armed Forces Institute of Pathology.) Contributor: Dr. C. L. Davis.

pillated, alopecic nodules often misinterpreted clinically as a "sebaceous cyst." Microscopically, the tumor cells simulate the normal sebaceous gland and ductal structures. Often there is little more than size to distinguish it from the normal or hyperplastic glands. The adenomas tend to be unencapsulated, sharply demarcated, expansile nodules that displace and compress the bundles of dermal collagen. Virtually identical tumors arise from the tarsal or meibomian glands of the eyelids of dogs and occasionally other species. Hyperplasia of sebaceous glands is more often a diffuse process, with many enlarged, hypercellular sebaceous glands scattered over a larger area of the dermis. An important element in differentiation of adenoma from hyperplasia is the fact that hyperplastic sebaceous glands maintain their normal positional relationship to hair follicles, whereas adenomas and adenocarcinomas do not.

Adenocarcinomas of sebaceous glands occur in dogs and histologically are much more anaplastic than adenomas. Many of the tumor cells are undifferentiated

and lack obvious lipid droplets in their cytoplasm; only a few cells will have vacuolated cytoplasm resembling normal sebaceous cells. They often extend randomly into the dermis as irregular nodules or nests with no orderly pattern of growth. Lymphatic invasion and metastasis also occur. In dogs, tumors of sebaceous glands are most frequent in the skin of the hindquarters, abdomen, and thorax.

ADENOMAS AND ADENOCARCINOMAS OF CIRCUMANAL (PERIANAL) GLANDS.

The circumanal or perianal glands of the skin of dogs are androgen-responsive, modified sebaceous glands. They extend from the tip of the tail to the lumbosacral region dorsally and to the preputial orifice ventrally in male dogs. Tumors can arise anywhere between these anatomic sites, but most often in the perianal region.

Adenomas of circumanal (perianal) glands are common, particularly in intact male dogs, and are usually sharply circumscribed, thinly encapsulated, spheri-

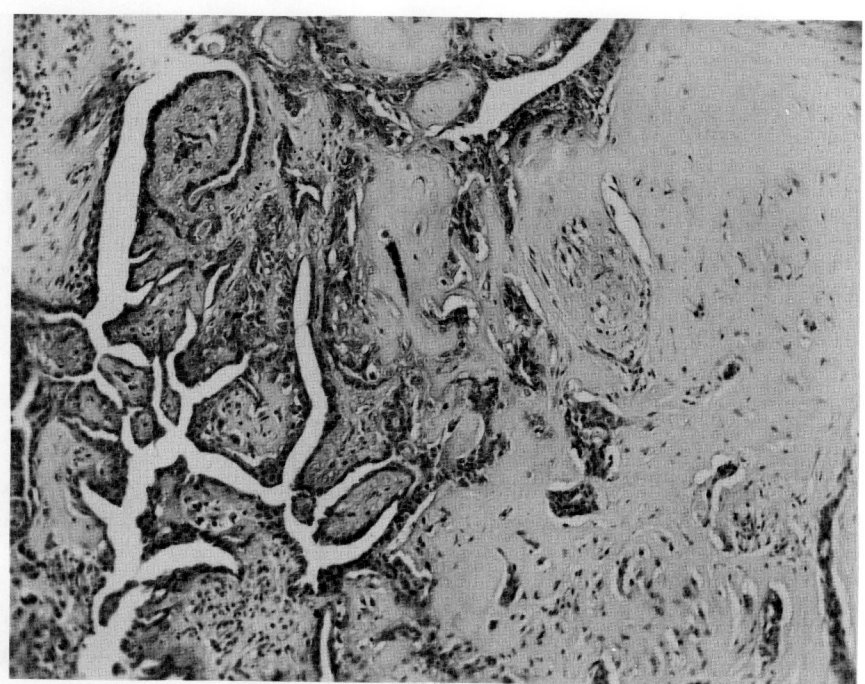

FIG. 17-23 Mixed tumor of apocrine gland. The neoplasm contains cartilage and glandular epithelium. (Courtesy of Armed Forces Institute of Pathology.)

cal masses of varying size (Fig. 17-24). Their cut surface is usually orange-tinted and greasy in texture, sometimes marked by areas of hemorrhage and ulceration of the overlying skin. Histologically, the adenoma closely resembles the normal gland, except that the glands are usually larger, more closely packed and form an expansile mass that displaces the surrounding tissues. The tumor cells are large, polygonal with abundant eosinophilic cytoplasm and a centrally placed round nucleus. They have been referred to as "hepatoid" cells because of their resemblance to hepatocytes. These cells are arranged in elongate solid lobules with smaller reserve cells situated at the periphery of the lobules. A thin connective tissue stroma separates the lobules from

each other within the main mass. There may be scattered ducts lined by flattened squamous epithelium present in the neoplasm. Ulceration and hemorrhage due to external trauma are frequent. The modified sebaceous cells cling together and usually have an orderly relationship to their scant stroma (Fig. 17-24).

Adenocarcinomas are much less frequent, but surprisingly, may arise in aged spayed females, in which the benign form is rare. This malignant form may metastasize to the iliac lymph nodes (Fig. 17-25) and thence to sublumbar and other intra-abdominal lymph nodes, and eventually reach the general circulation. The identifying feature of this adenocarcinoma is the presence of scattered individual and small nests of invasive neoplastic

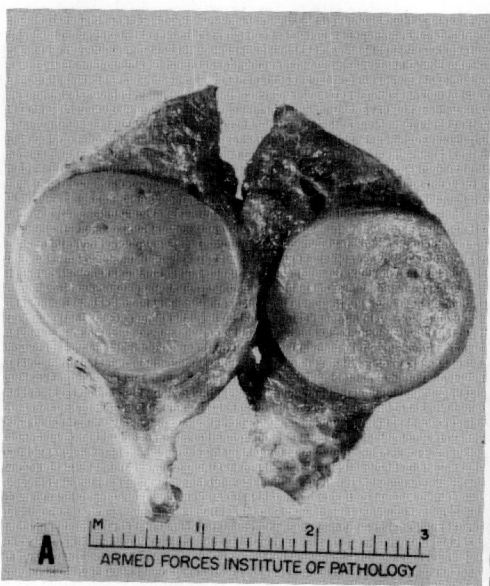
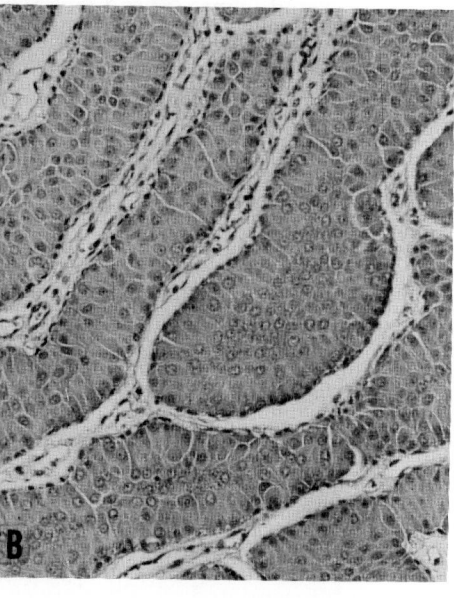

FIG. 17-24 Adenoma of perianal gland of a six-year-old male beagle. **A.** Gross specimen with its spherical outline and orange-tinted, greasy cut surface. **B.** Photomicrograph ($\times 150$) of the new growth. Irregular columns of large polyhedral cells supported by delicate stroma. (Courtesy of Armed Forces Institute of Pathology and Major C. N. Barron.)

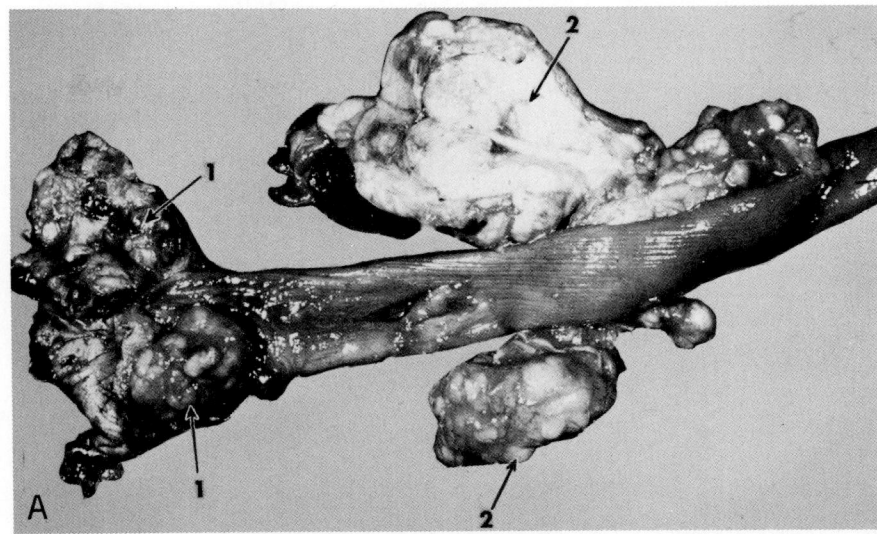

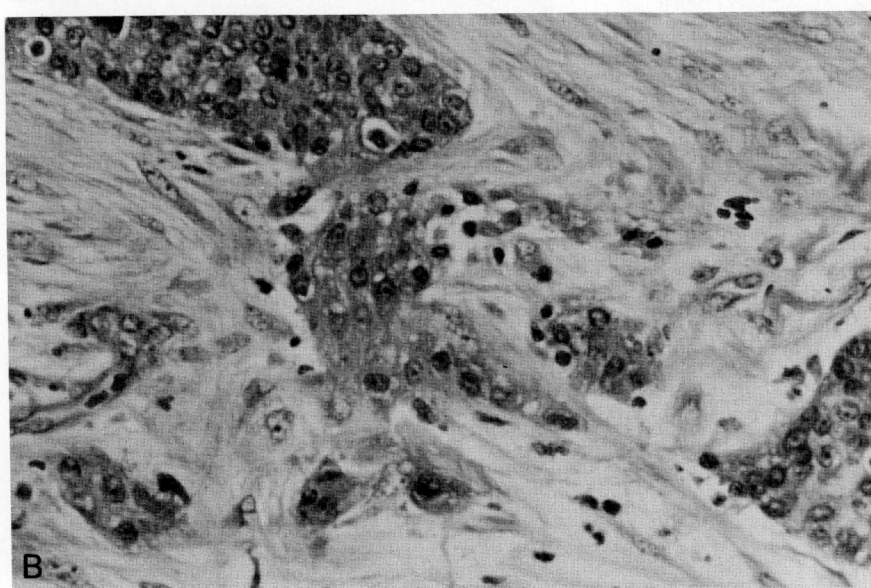

FIG. 17-25 Adenocarcinoma of perianal gland of a ten-year-old spayed female Cocker Spaniel. **A.** Two tumor masses *(1)* near anus, and metastatic tumors in iliac lymph nodes *(2)* adherent to the rectum. (Courtesy of Angell Memorial Animal Hospital.) **B.** Microscopic appearance of malignant cells of adenocarcinoma of perianal gland. Note irregular bizarre shape of the cells and their isolation into small groups in the cellular stroma.

cells in the dermal connective tissue surrounding the tumor (Fig. 17-25). This is the only reliable histologic criterion for malignancy in this tumor. To the uninitiated who has not studied and followed the biologic behavior of the neoplasm, many adenomas may appear to be malignant from their histologic appearance.

PILOMATRICOMA (HAIR MATRIX TUMOR, BENIGN CALCIFYING EPITHELIOMA)

This neoplasm is referred to by different names, largely based upon the personal preference of the pathologist involved. It is a benign, usually cystic neoplasm thought to be derived from the germinative cells of the follicular matrix or hair bulb. The tumor occurs commonly in dogs but is exceedingly rare in cats. It is composed of multiple solid masses or cystic spaces lined by an outer rim of cells that resemble the hair matrix (Fig. 17-26). The interior of these lobules is usually made up of masses of cells resem-

bling those at the periphery, but which fail to take the usual hematoxylin stain. The outlines of these necrotic cells, nevertheless, can be seen, leading to the term "ghost cells"—an apt description. These tumors are therefore cystic. In contrast to an **epidermal inclusion cyst** which is lined by a layer of well-differentiated keratinizing stratified squamous epithelium that surrounds a central mass of keratin (Fig.17-27), the cyst wall of a hair matrix tumor is lined by deeply basophilic, basaloid cells resembling the matrix cells of the hair bulb with an abrupt junction with the ghost cells. Calcification often starts in the center of the tumor lobules and may involve much of the necrotic tumor. These tumors are benign, often multicystic and may ulcerate to the overlying skin. If through rupture their necrotic content spills into the dermis, it incites a pyogranulomatous dermatitis. Malignant tumors of this type are extremely rare.

This tumor also differs from an epidermoid (der-

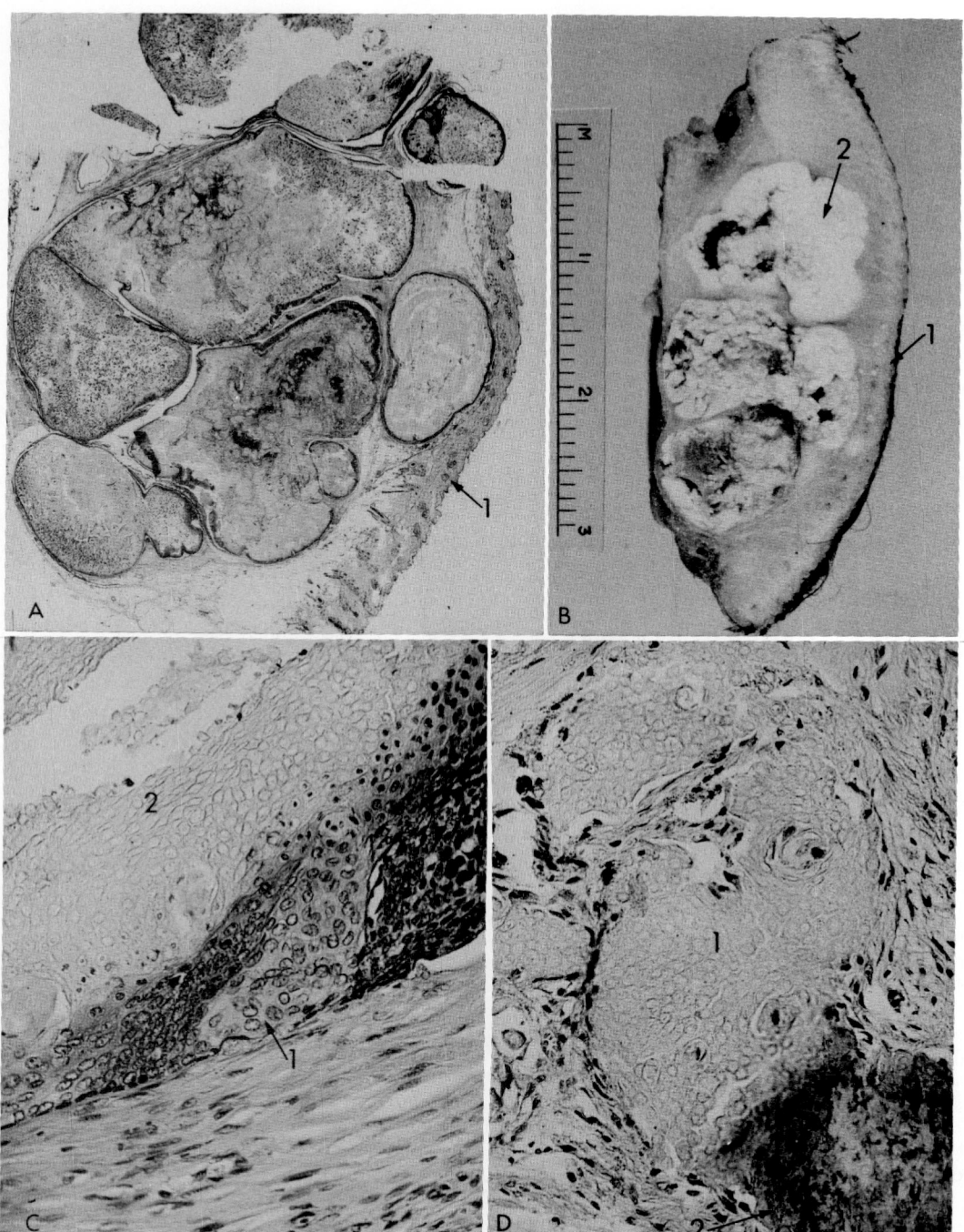

FIG. 17-26 Hair matrix tumor (benign calcifying epithelioma). **A.** Tumor (×4) in dermis and subcutis of right prescapular region of a three-year-old female French Poodle. Note the lobulated nature of the new growth. Epidermis *(1)*. **B.** Gross appearance of the same tumor. Epidermis *(1)* chalky, granular, and lobulated tumor *(2)*. Contributor: Dr. M. G. Rhoades. **C.** A similar tumor from the dermis of a two-year-old Kerry Blue Terrier (×250). Epithelial cells *(1)* simulating hair matrix, and cells *(2)* in center of lesion, which stain poorly but maintain their outline ("shadow" or "ghost" cells). **D.** Another area of same tumor as C (×200). Outlines of cells *(1)* in center of lesion; calcification is present *(2)*. Courtesy of Armed Forces Institute of Pathology and Dr. G. A. Goode.)

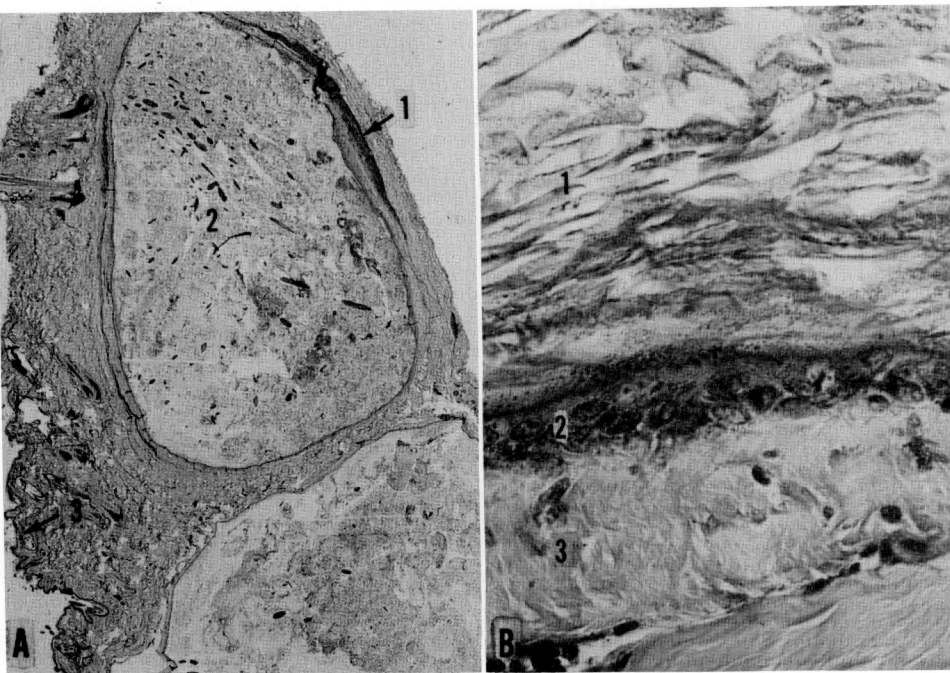

FIG. 17-27 Epidermal inclusion cysts in the skin of a dog. **A.** Cyst (×9) in dermis, with squamous wall *(1)*, keratinous contents *(2)*. Epidermis *(3)*. **B.** Same lesion as A (×490). Squames of keratin *(1)* in the center of the cyst, stratified squamous epithelium *(2)*, and dense collagen *(3)* in the cyst wall. (Courtesy of Armed Forces Institute of Pathology and Dr. Edward Baker.)

moid) cyst which, like an epidermal inclusion cyst is lined by keratinizing stratified squamous epithelium, but which also has hair follicles and sebaceous glands surrounding it that communicate with the cyst cavity. These lesions result from bits of ectoderm that become entrapped in the dermis during embryonic development. They contain mature hair and foul-smelling sebaceous secretion (Fig. 17-28).

TRICHOEPITHELIOMA

This tumor, like the trichoblastoma described above, is also thought to arise from hair follicles. It consists of multiple, varying sized cysts lined by basaloid cells that surround masses of either hair matrix type

ghost cells or laminated squames of keratin. In the latter type the basaloid cells differentiate into squamous cells near the center of the rudimentary hair follicle-like structures. Hair is not formed by these neoplastic cells. It is usual that both types of structures are found in individual tumors.

TRICHOLEMMOMA

This neoplasm is derived from the epithelium of the outer root sheath of hair follicles. The neoplasm generally occurs in older dogs and the Afghan hound is thought to be predisposed to this type of cutaneous neoplasm. This neoplasm is composed of numerous closely packed lobular masses of small polygonal cells

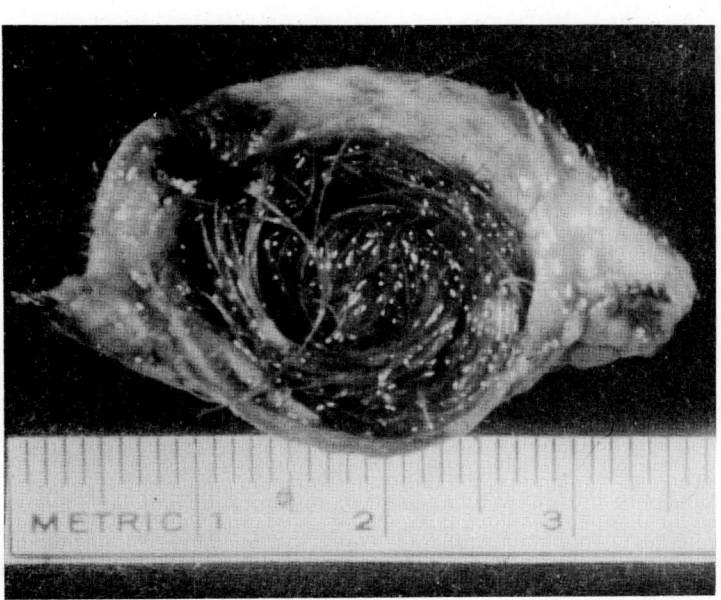

FIG. 17-28 Epidermoid cyst in the skin of the tail of a seven-year-old castrated male bloodhound. Note hair in cyst. (Courtesy of Angell Memorial Animal Hospital.)

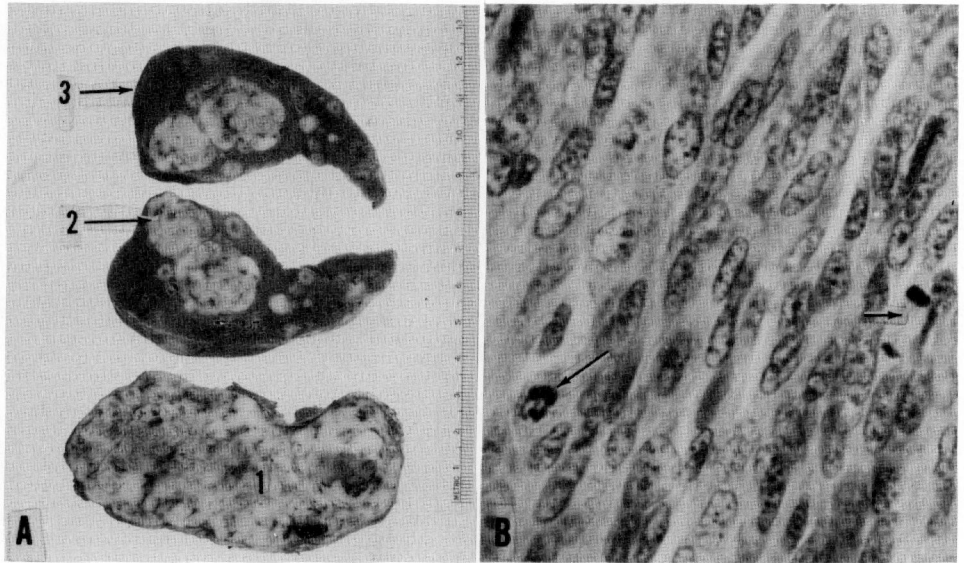

FIG. 17-29 A. Fibrosarcoma, primary *(1)*, in cheek of a 12-year-old male Scottish terrier, with metastases *(2)*, to lung *(3)*. **B.** Photomicrograph of same tumor (×700). Note spindle-shaped cells with ovoid nuclei and mitotic figures (arrows). (Courtesy of Armed Forces Institute of Pathology and Dr. John E. Craige.)

cuffed by a thick, hyaline basement membrane resembling the vitreous sheath of normal hair follicles. The majority of the cells have clear cytoplasm and palisade around the periphery of the masses. The cells in the center of the masses have eosinophilic cytoplasm and exhibit small focal areas of keratinization.

Neoplasms of the dermis and subcutis

FIBROMA; FIBROSARCOMA

In the skin, fibromas and fibrosarcomas are the most frequent mesenchymal tumors in most species, except the dog, in which the histiocytoma and mast cell tumors are more common. In general, fibrosarcomas occur with a somewhat higher frequency than fibromas. The tumors arise from fibrous connective tissue in its ubiquitous locations and resemble it in appearance. The cells with their collagenous fibrils proliferate in a variety of patterns. Long interlacing bundles of tumor cells is a frequent pattern (Fig. 17-29), and is useful in distinguishing the fibrosarcoma from nerve sheath tumors and hemangiopericytoma, tumors in which this is not a feature. In fibromas, the tumor cells generally make significant amounts of collagen that separates individual tumor cells from each other. The margins of fibromas also tend to be well-delineated even though the tumor is not encapsulated. Mitotic activity is extremely low in fibromas in contrast to fibrosarcoma. As mentioned in Chapter 4, fibromas in some species are caused by papillomaviruses. In contrast, fibrosarcomas are usually more cellular than fibromas, make less collagen, have a moderate to high mitotic index, and generally invade tissues rather than compress them. Other criteria of malignancy include cellular and nuclear pleomorphism and hyerchromasia and the presence of tumor giant cells. Fibrosarcomas of the skin of cats have been associated with feline sarcoma virus and adverse tissue reactions to several types of viral vaccines (see Chapter 4).

EQUINE SARCOID

A cutaneous growth peculiar to equines was first recognized by Jackson (1936), who named it equine sarcoid because, despite contrary clinical behavior, its histologic appearance is certainly that of a sarcoma of moderate malignancy. The lesion, often multiple, is most frequently found on the lower legs, head, and prepuce. It occurs perhaps even more frequently in mules and donkeys than in the horse. The growths may reach the size of a softball, have a variable sized base, and bulge from under the skin. The overlying skin is gener-

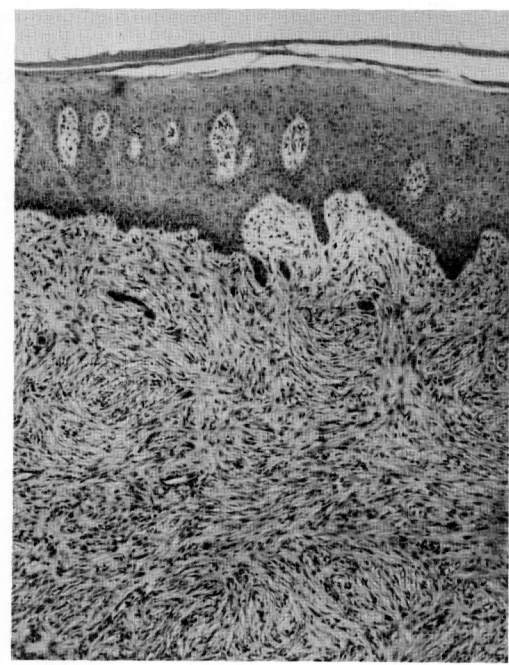

FIG. 17-30 Equine sarcoid, skin of a horse. Hyperplastic epithelium covers the mass within the dermis. The neoplasm resembles a neurofibrosarcoma.

ally thickened and rough (acanthotic), and sooner or later becomes ulcerated and infected. The expanding mass may extend into the subcutis, especially in lesions that recur after incomplete removal. The underlying skeletal muscle is usually not invaded.

Microscopically, the new growth is made up principally of interlacing bundles of spindle-shaped cells which may form whorls and bundles suggestive of a neurofibroma (Fig.17-30). It is not surprising that many pathologists, confronted with the lesion for the first time, consider it a neurofibroma, neurofibrosarcoma, fibroma or fibrosarcoma. The proportion of collagen fibrils to nuclei varies, but it is not so high that the sarcoid is likely to be mistaken for a keloid. Inflammatory infiltration is, of course, present near an ulcerated surface; a few lymphocytes and eosinophils may appear anywhere among the fibroblastic cells, but these are so few that there is no likelihood of mistaking the lesion for inflammatory granulation tissue. Neither is the number of capillaries great enough to favor such an interpretation. The real difficulty is in distinguishing the sarcoid from a sarcoma. Usually there is less anaplasia of nuclei and fewer mitoses than in a sarcoma, but in borderline cases differentiation may not be possible on histologic grounds alone. Indeed, someday it may be found that there is no real distinction. The overlying epidermis often sends long fronds deep into the mass, a feature which Jackson thought more or less confirmed his opinion that the epithelium participated in the neoplastic process. However, this bizarre epithelial proliferation is not unusual in any epidermis which is attempting to cover an expanding mass of any kind.

Anything less than complete removal is followed by a recurrent growth that tends to be more highly cellular, the spindle-shaped cells being increased in size, with large, hyperchromatic nuclei and more frequent mitotic figures. Metastasis, however, does not occur, the situation being reminiscent of the diagnosis of "sarcoma of local malignancy only." The association of this neoplastic growth with bovine papillomavirus is discussed under oncogenic viruses tumor-forming (Chapters 4 and 8).

LIPOMA; LIPOSARCOMA.

Lipomas, often multiple, occur in a great variety of locations as masses of adipose tissue of various sizes and shapes. They are most frequently encountered in the subcutis. The fat may be yellowish. These benign tumors are distinguished grossly from the excessive fat of obesity, which they frequently accompany, by the fact that they form discrete lumps or masses in contrast to the diffuse distribution of ordinary adipose tissue. Microscopically, close comparison shows a greater variation in the size and shape of the fat cells than occurs in normal adipose tissue. The liposarcoma, which is rare, is characterized by areas of anaplastic fibrous tissue in company with adipose tissue and an intermediate tissue in which only rudimentary fat cells with small vacuoles exist. A particular type of fatty tumor occurs in the subcutis in the midline of the back over the thorax or in the axilla. This is called a **"tumor of brown fat"** or **"hib-**

ernoma." It forms solid masses of cells which resemble those of the "brown fat" or "hibernating gland" of many animals. This fat is brownish grossly and the lipid in the cytoplasm is in the form of tiny droplets uniformly distributed throughout the rather dark brownish cytoplasm. These fat cells contain much more potential energy (they contain numerous mitochondria) than do ordinary fat cells. The tumors may reach large sizes but are usually benign. Dogs, rats, and wild animals have been found with these tumors.

MYXOMA; MYXOSARCOMA

These tumors are composed of connective tissue that forms mucin; in other words, connective tissue of embryonal type. The nuclei tend to be round or stellate; the intercellular fibrils are bluish (hematoxylin and eosin) and show little parallelism. These tumors are always more or less malignant, but the term myxoma is generally used in spite of that fact. They are encountered with some frequency in veterinary medicine. Some effort must be made to distinguish this neoplasm from a fibrosarcoma with myxomatous degeneration.

MAST CELL TUMOR

The mast cell tumor is the most frequent cutaneous neoplasm of the dog, where they arise in the dermis. They also occur in the skin of cats where they are less common, and occur rarely in swine and cattle. They have also been reported in laboratory animals, including monkeys.

The term "mastocytoma" often appears in the literature in reference to tumors derived from cutaneous mast cells. The prefix "mast" in this context comes from the German, meaning fattened or stuffed, and "cyte" comes from the Greek, *kytos,* meaning a hollow cell. The combining form "mast" from the Greek *mastos* (breast) has quite a different meaning. In deference to the sensitivities of our classical scholarly colleagues, the authors have chosen not to use this incorrect combination of two languages.

In dogs, mast cell tumors occur most often on the posterior part of the animal's body; the flank and scrotum are common sites. It appears as a bulging cutaneous mass 2 to 5 cm in diameter and a height of 1 to 3 cm. (Fig.17-31) Pruritis, erythema, bruising, edema and ulceration are common in skin containing a mast cell tumor because of the release of histamine from the neoplastic cells. Because these tumors tend to be diffusely infiltrative, they can pose problems for the surgeon in identifying their margins. For this reason, wide excision is imperative with this tumor, otherwise local recurrence can be a common problem. Metastasis also can occur.

In dogs, mast cell tumors are seldom a diagnostic challenge histologically. Typically, the neoplastic cells form diffuse sheets or densely packed cords of round to somewhat polygonal cells with a round, centrally placed nucleus and moderate amounts of coarsely granular basophilic cytoplasm (Fig.17-31). The cords of cells are often separated by bundles of dermal collagen. Scattered throughout the neoplastic infiltrates are variable num-

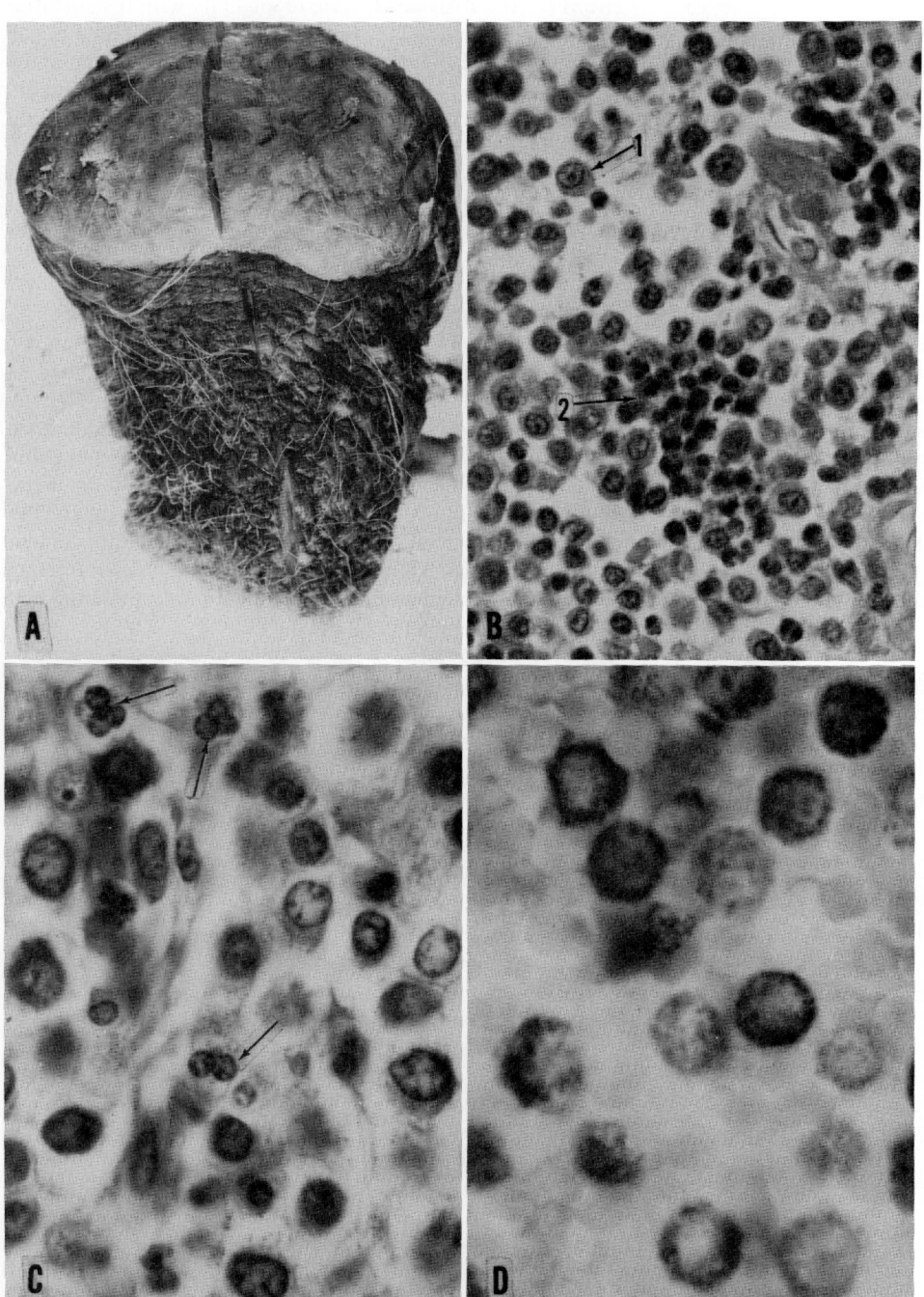

FIG. 17-31 Mast-cell tumor. **A.** Ulcerated tumor involving the skin of the scrotum of a thirteen-year-old male Spitz dog. Contributor: Dr. S. W. Stiles. **B.** Photomicrograph (×545) of a mast-cell tumor from the cheek of a ten-year-old male Cocker Spaniel. Mast cells *(1)* and nests of eosinophils *(2)* are present. (H & E.) Contributor: Dr. W. H. Riser. **C.** Higher magnification of a mast-cell tumor from the skin of the leg of a 12-year-old male Boston terrier. (H & E, ×650.) A few mast cells contain cytoplasmic granules. Eosinophils (arrows) are common. (Contributor: Army Veterinary School.) **D.** Section with Giemsa stain (×1200) to demonstrate metachromatic granules in the cytoplasm of the neoplastic mast cells. (Courtesy of Armed Forces Institute of Pathology.) Contributor: Dr. C. L. Davis.

bers of reactive eosinophils, no doubt in response to eosinophil chemotactic factor, a normal product of mast cell granules. Another feature found with some frequency in mast cell tumors, particularly those containing large numbers of reactive eosinophils, are scattered foci of highly eosinophilic, degenerate collagen. This is probably a collagenolytic change induced by products of eosinophil granules. Similar collagenolytic changes are also found in feline eosinophilic granuloma and linear granuloma. The neoplastic cells exhibit varying degrees of differentiation based upon the presence and prominence of their cytoplasmic granules

in hematoxylin and eosin-stained tissue sections. This feature, along with degree of pleomorphism and mitotic index of the cells, has been used subjectively to classify these tumors for prognostic purposes into three grades. In grade I, the most differentiated form with the best prognosis, the tumor cells are uniform in size and shape, have very prominent basophilic granules in their cytoplasm and a central round nucleus containing a single, small nucleolus. Mitotic figures are exceedingly rare. In grade III, the least differentiated type having the worst prognosis, the tumor cells have very few or no basophilic granules in their cytoplasm, have a large nuclear to cytoplasmic ratio, have nuclei that vary in size and shape and may contain binucleated tumor cells. The few granules that may be present in grade III mast cell tumors may require staining of the tissue section with a metachromatic stains such as Giemsa or toluidine blue to find them. Grade II mast cell tumors have features intermediate between grades I and III.

In the cat, mast cell tumors occur in two separate forms: a **primary cutaneous mast cell tumor** and a **visceral mast-cell tumor.** The cutaneous form appears as one or more small nodular dermal masses that seldom exceed 2 cm in diameter. The head and neck are favored sites in cats. Microscopically, cutaneous mast cell tumor of cats are composed of solid nodular masses of extremely uniform round to polygonal cells with round centrally placed, somewhat hyperchromatic nuclei. The cytoplasm of feline mast cells is not basophilic but instead clear to faintly eosinophilic. Granules are not a conspicuous feature of feline mast cells stained with hematoxylin and eosin, but can be demonstrated by metachromatic staining or electron microscopy. Eosinophils may be present but in smaller numbers than in many canine mast cell tumors.

Visceral mast cell tumors in cats often affect the spleen and, less often, lymph nodes, liver, bone marrow, lungs, kidneys, and skin. The spleen is usually markedly enlarged and has a characteristic deep mahogany color and fleshy consistency. Mast cells may be found in small numbers in the peripheral circulation in such cases, and the term mast cell leukemia has been used by some authors. These circulating cells are morphologically identical to tissue mast cells rather than basophils. An interesting concomitant feature is the presence of small, sharply demarcated ulcers in the mucosa of the pylorus or duodenum. These ulcers are probably due to hyperhistaminemia produced by the neoplastic mast cells.

An apparently third form of mast-cell tumor occurs in the intestine of cats. Intestinal mast cell tumors arise in the small intestine, less often in the colon, resulting in a segmental thickening of the wall not sharply demarcated from adjacent tissue. The bulk of the mass is confined to the muscularis, although it may extend into the mucosa. Metastasis is frequent. The cells have finely granular or vacuolated cytoplasm, but usually are more clear than other forms of mast cell tumors. These neoplasms were once thought to arise from enterochromaffin cells and likened to carcinoid tumors of humans. The studies of Alroy et al. (1975), however, have demonstrated that they are in fact mast cell tumors. Interestingly, intestinal ulcers do not occur in association with these tumors.

In horses, Altera and Clark (1970) described a rare condition termed **equine cutaneous mastocytosis,** which closely resembles mast cell tumors of dogs. Diffuse or sharply defined collections of mast cells associated with mature eosinophils and collagen degeneration with calcification were described in the skin from varied sites. It has been suggested (Cheville et al., 1972) that the cells are basophils and not mast cells and that the condition resembles urticaria pigmentosa of human beings. It does not appear to be a true neoplasm.

CANINE CUTANEOUS HISTIOCYTOMA

This is the most common cutaneous neoplasm of dogs less than 3 years of age, but it occurs in dogs of all ages. The face, pinnae, neck and distal extremities and scrotum are common sites for histiocytoma, but other sites can be involved. Grossly, the neoplasm appears as a rapidly growing, usually solitary but occasionally multiple, raised, 1.0 to 3.0 cm alopecic plaque or dome-shaped mass, often with superficial ulceration. Because of this appearance it is often referred to clinically as a "button tumor". These tumors, if left alone, will eventually undergo spontaneous regression after several weeks or, in some instances, months. Microscopically, histiocytomas are composed of nodular, non-encapsulated infiltrates of round to polygonal cells arranged in cords and solid sheets. The infiltrate generally destroys most adnexal structures at the affected site but an occasional hair follicle may persist. In the superficial dermis the neoplastic cells are arranged in rows or columns arranged perpendicular to the dermal-epidermal junction. Occasionally, small nests of cells will be present within the epidermis, resembling Pautrier's abscesses seen in the epidermotropic lymphoma known as mycosis fungoides. In deeper portions of the tumor, the neoplastic cells form solid sheets that separate bundles of dermal collagen and extend into the superficial portion of the subcutaneous adipose tissue (Fig. 17-32). Older tumors will contain infiltrates of lymphocytes along their deepest margin and will have areas of coagulative necrosis associated with spontaneous regression. The regression of this lesion is mediated by CD8+ $\alpha\beta$ T lymphocytes that infiltrate its deepest margins. Neutrophils may be present, particularly if the lesion is ulcerated and secondarily infected. The tumor cells present in the superficial cords are discrete and have distinct cell borders. They have small to moderate amounts of somewhat eosinophilic cytoplasm that may be vacuolated. Their nuclei vary from round to ovoid to reniform and mitotic activity is generally high until evidence of regression appears. The tumor cells arranged in sheets at the base of the tumor tend to have somewhat more cytoplasm but rather indistinct cell outlines because of their closely packed nature. Earlier histochemical and ultrastructural studies revealed that the tumor cells have many features in common with histiocytes. Until very recently the precise source of the neoplastic cells was not known. Using a wide range of monoclonal antibodies to canine leukocyte antigens, Moore et al. (1996) have demonstrated that the tumor cells express a variety of leukocyte antigens characteristic of activated canine Langerhan's cells. These, it will be recalled, are the antigen-presenting cells of the epidermis. These authors characterize this so-called "tumor" as a **localized form of self-limiting Langerhans cell histiocytosis.** Hence this lesion may not be a neoplasm at all, but instead a localized reactive proliferation of Langerhans cells due to some unknown cause. There is a disease of humans termed Langerhans cell histiocytosis that has some features in common with the canine disorder.

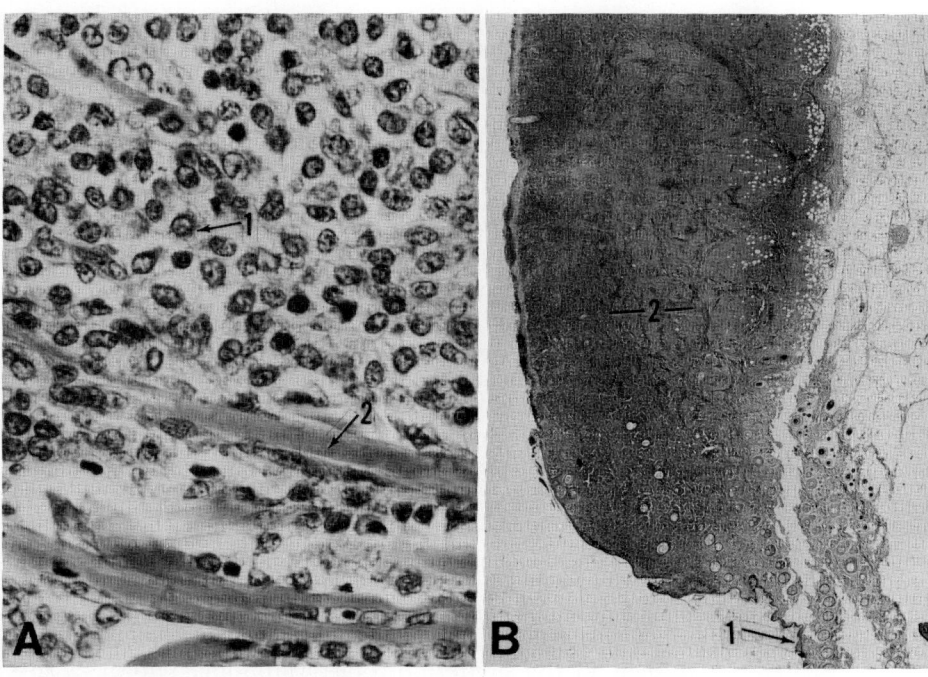

FIG. 17-32 Canine cutaneous histiocytoma. **A.** Cells of the new growth *(1)* infiltrating collagen bundles *(2)* of the dermis (×440). **B.** Low power view of the cutaneous nodule (×8). The epidermis *(1)* is elevated by the mass *(2)*, which also infiltrates the subcutis. (Courtesy of Armed Forces Institute of Pathology.) Contributor: Dr. Elihu Bond.

BENIGN CUTANEOUS AND SYSTEMIC HISTIOCYTOSIS

Three forms of histiocytosis have been described in dogs, two of these involve the skin. These differ from the common cutaneous histiocytoma just described.

The first, termed **benign cutaneous histiocytosis,** is characterized by the development of multiple non-pruritic, erythematous plaques and nodules in the panniculus of the face, neck, back and trunk. Mucous membrane involvement of the nares occurs in some cases. Multiple breeds are affected and the age of affected dogs has ranged from 2 to 13 years, with most animals being under 6 years of age. Lesions occasionally become ulcerated. The disease varies in severity between individual animals being severe and recurrent in some and mild and intermittent in others. This feature and its multicentric nature differentiate this condition from canine cutaneous histiocytoma. Histologically, this disorder is characterized by infiltrates of the dermis and panniculus with large histiocytic cells admixed with other inflammatory cells. Recent immunophenotyping studies have shown that the proliferating histiocytic cells in this disorder, as in canine cutaneous histiocytoma, are activated epidermal Langerhans cells.

The second, known as **systemic histiocytosis,** is a disorder that has thus far only been described in male Bernese Mountain dogs, 2–5 years of age. It is a familial disease characterized by the development of perivascular infiltrates of large, reactive, non-neoplastic histiocytes in the subcutis of the skin and in peripheral lymph nodes with variable involvement of visceral organs, conjunctiva and bone marrow. The disease typically has periods of remission and exacerbations. Microscopically, nodular accumulations of large, bland appearing histiocytes occur both within and surrounding the wall of dermal and subcutaneous blood

vessels. There may be infiltrates of lymphocytes and occasional neutrophils as well as fibrosis around affected sites. The cause of this disease is unknown. This disorder also appears to be a form of canine Langerhans cell proliferation.

A third lethal form of histiocytosis, termed **malignant histiocytosis** has also been recognized in the same family lines of Bernese Mountain dogs with systemic histiocytosis. In this disorder, the skin is apparently spared, lesions occurring most often in the lungs and tracheobronchial and less often in other visceral lymph nodes, liver, spleen and central nervous system. In this disorder the proliferating histiocytes are extremely pleomorphic, often forming multinucleated giant cells having pronounced cytological atypia and bizarre mitotic figures.

FIBROUS HISTIOCYTOMA, MALIGNANT FIBROUS HISTIOCYTOMA

These are rare tumors of the skin of dogs and cats characterized by a mixture of neoplastic cells having features of fibroblasts and histiocytes. The benign variety appears as a solitary, sometimes multiple, partially alopecic nodule usually less that 1 cm in diameter. They occur most often on the scrotum and legs, and less often at other sites. Microscopically it consists of a well-demarcated but unencapsulated dermal mass composed primarily of histiocytic cells arranged in solid sheets. There are lesser numbers of fibroblast cells admixed with the histiocytes but they make very little collagen. An occasional multinucleated giant cell may be present. These nodular infiltrates may extend to the dermal-epidermal junction and reportedly spares hair follicles.

Malignant fibrous histiocytomas are uncommon neoplasms of the skin of cats. They are rare in dogs. They appear as large, solitary, firm, poorly-circumscribed lobulated subcutaneous masses that may be alopecic and ulcerated. They are clinically aggressive and tend to recur following attempts at removal, however, metastasis has not been reported. Histologically, these tumors are composed of a mixture of two cell types, a histiocytic type and a fibroblastic type.The fibroblastic type is often arranged in a storiform or herring-bone type pattern. Multinucleated tumor giant cells may be found in malignant fibrous histiocytomas.

CUTANEOUS (EXTRAMEDULLARY) PLASMACYTOMA

These are benign neoplasms of plasma cells that affect the skin of the digits, lips, pinnae and ear canals of middle-aged dogs of both sexes. They appear as a solitary, sessile-based, spherical or dome-shaped, alopecic nodules which occasionally are pedunculatd. They generally do not exceed 2 cm in diameter. On cut surfaces they are pale tan to amber, or dark red from hemorrhage. Microscopically, the neoplastic cells range from those that are uniform in size and and bear remarkable resemblance to normal plasma cells, to those that are poorly differentiated with pleomorphic nuclei and marked variation in size of the cells. Binucleate and multinucleate tumor cells can be found in most tumors regardless of their degree of differentiation.The pattern of arrangement within the tumor varies from a prominent trabecular pattern to those that simply form broad sheets or nest. The neoplastic cells are confined to the dermis and superficial panniculus and never invade the epidermis. Most such tumors do not recur following excision, but there is some evidence that an extremely small percentage may progress to multiple myeloma.

CUTANEOUS LYMPHOMAS.

Lymphomas of the skin are of two basic types: non-epitheliotropic and epitheliotropic, the latter is often termed **mycosis fungoides.** The non-epitheliotropic forms are of B lymphocyte origin, the epitheliotropic are derived from T lymphocytes. Although visceral lymphomas occur with some frequency in most domestic animal species, cutaneous lymphoma is relatively rare. It is reported most often in cattle, dogs and cats. Unlike visceral lymphoma in cattle and cats, cutaneous lymphomas in these species are not associated with leukemia viruses.

Non-epitheliotropic cutaneous lymphomas appear as nodular to diffuse infiltrations of the dermis and subcutis by neoplastic lymphocytes. In this form of lymphoma, the epidermis generally is not invaded by tumor cells. Adnexal structures may be destroyed by the neoplastic infiltrates. The morphology of the neoplastic cells is highly variable depending upon the degree of differentiation. The cells may have features of lymphocytes, lymphoblasts, immunoblasts or even appear histiocytic. It is impossible to distinguish neoplastic B lymphocytes from neoplastic T lymphocytes based upon hematoxylin and eosin stained sections. Immunophenotyping studies using monoclonal antibodies to specific B and T lymphocyte markers are required to make this determination.

Epitheliotropic cutaneous lymphomas (mycosis fungoides and Sezary syndrome) are of T lymphocyte lineage and have an affinity for certain cells of the epidermis. In animals the mycosis fungoides type predominates, there being few cases of the Sezary phenotype. Grossly, the cutaneous lesions resemble those described for the non-epitheliotropic lymphoma, but microscopically there are characteristic differences. The most notable difference is the progressive accumulation of the neoplastic T lymphocytes around sites occupied by Langerhans cells to which these tumor cells are attracted. Similar infiltrates occur within the epithelium of hair follicles. At both sites, these small clusters of intraepidermal lymphocytes are termed Pautrier's abscesses, even though they contain no neutrophils. This type of cutaneous lymphoma also obliterates dermal adnexal structures and extends into the panniculus. Many of the mycosis fungoides cells have somewhat convoluted, pale nuclei and small amounts of relatively clear cytoplasm.

HEMANGIOPERICYTOMA.

The hemangiopericytoma is a relatively common subcutaneous neoplasm of dogs that is thought to originate from the pericytes that surround small blood vessels. It is rare in other species. The tumor cells, however, have never been unequivocally proven to be pericytes by histochemical and electron microscopic examination. Some feel that it may have a neural origin. Grossly, these tumors appear as solitary, multilobulated firm to fluctuant masses located mainly in the subcutis, but occasionally involving the deep dermis. They can become quite large and be difficult to separate from surrounding tissues (Fig. 17-33). Because of this they are prone to local recurrence because of incomplete excision. The neoplasm is composed of spindle-shaped cells with ovoid or elongated nuclei and considerable cytoplasm, which frequently becomes fibrillar. The distinctive feature of this neoplasm, however, is the presence of numerous small capillaries, open or collapsed, which are lined by endothelium but closely encircled by loosely arranged concentric rings of pleomorphic "spindle" cells with features of pericytes (Fig. 17-33). In some specimens, the encircling cells are flattened and extended in a circumferential direction; in others, their relationship to the vessel wall is less obvious, but the cells tend to form whorls or clusters around a capillary space. By reticulum stains, large and numerous reticular fibers can be demonstrated in the concentric layers around the vessels. The tumor is always subcutaneous. It has a tendency to recur locally after many months, or in some cases years. Metastasis is extremely rare. The term **perithelioma** has been applied to this tumor.

XANTHOMA.

This term refers to tiny yellowish nodules that form on the skin of the eyelids and on tendons and tendon sheaths in humans. They consist of collections of large, pale "foam cells," doubtless of reticuloendothelial origin, whose extensive cytoplasm is made granular by many minute droplets of cholesterol and other lipids.

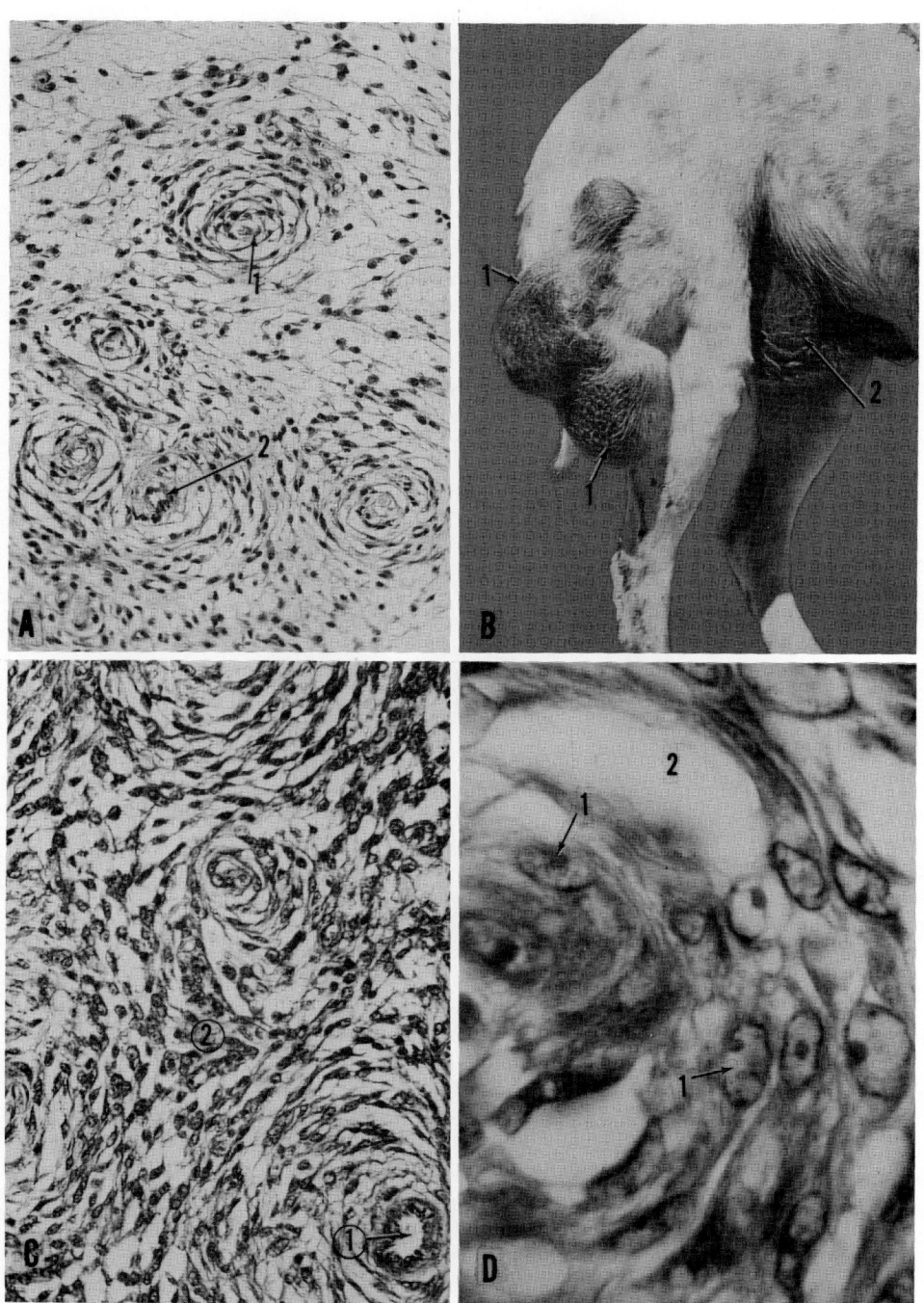

FIG. 17-33 Hemangiopericytoma of the subcutis of the dog. **A.** Photomicrograph (×160) with whorl arrangement of tumor cells around occult (1) and overt capillaries (2). Contributor: Dr. S. W. Stiles. **B.** Large subcutaneous hemangiopericytoma (1) in a 15-year-old terrior dog. Note metastasis to inguinal region (2). Contributor: Dr. W. J. Zontine. **C.** Section (×210) in a densely cellular area with capillaries (1) and spindle-shaped cells (2) concentrically arranged around them. Contributor: Dr. W. H. Riser. **D.** High magnification (×1080) of another tumor. Note ovoid nuclei (1), which are often vesicular and contain a single nucleolus. Clear, empty spaces (2) are common. (Courtesy of Armed Forces Institute of Pathology.) Contributor: Phillips Veterinary Hospital.

With them are fibroblasts and other phagocytes. This is not truly a neoplasm, but a reactive lesion. It possibly bears some significant relation to cholesterol metabolism.

Rather wide-based, sessile proliferations called xanthomas have been encountered subcutaneously in chickens. They consist mostly of connective tissue and "foamy," cholesterol-containing phagocytes similar to those in human xanthomas. The proliferations are quite irregular in contour but do not grow to extensive heights. They are not true neoplasms. A typical xanthoma also occurs with some frequency in subcutis of the shell parakeet (budgerigar) (Petrak and Gilmore, 1969).

References

Alroy J, Leav I, DeLellis RA, et al. Distinctive intestinal mast cell neoplasms of domestic cats. Lab. Invest 1975;33:159–167.

Altera K, Clark L. Equine cutaneous mastocytosis. Pathol Vet 1970;7:43–55.

Anderson LJ, Sandison AT. Tumours of connective tissues in cattle, sheep, and pigs. J Pathol 1969;98:253–263.

Baer KE, Patnaik AK, Gilbertson SR, et al. Cutaneous plasmacytomas in dogs: a morphologic and immunohistochemical study. Vet Pathol 1989;26:216–221.

Baker JR, Leyland A. Histological survey of tumours of the horse, with particular reference to those of the skin. Vet Rec 1975;96:419–422.

Bevier DF, Goldschmidt MH. Skin tumors in the dogs. I. Epithelial tumors and tumor-like lesions. Comp Cont Educ 1981;3:389–398.

Bolon B, Calderwood Mays MB, Hall BJ. Characterization of canine melanomas and comparison of histology and DNA ploidy to their biologic behavior. Vet Pathol 1990;27:96–102,.

Borland R., Webber AJ An electron microscope study of squamous cell carcinoma in Merino sheep associated with keratin-filled cysts of the skin. Cancer Res 1966;26:172–182,.

Bostock DE. The prognosis following surgical removal of mastocytomas in dogs. J Small Anim Pract 1973;14:27–40.

Bostock DE. Prognosis after surgical excision of canine melanomas. Vet Pathol 1979;16:32–40.

Calderwood Mays MB, Bergeron JA: Cutaneous histiocytosis in dogs. J Am Vet Med Assoc 1986;188:377–381.

Campbell KL, Sundberg JP, Goldschmidt CK, et al. Cutaneous inverted papillomas in dogs. Vet Pathol 1988;25:67–71

Carothers MA, Johnson GC, DiBartola SP, et al. Extramedullary plasmacytoma and immunoglobulin-associated amyloidosis in a cat. J Am Vet Med Assoc 1990;195:1593–1597.

Carpenter JL, Andrews LK, Holzworth J. Tumors and tumor-like lesions. In: Holzworth J, ed. Diseases of the cat. Philadelphia: WB Saunders, 1987;407–410.

Cheville NF, Prasse K, van der Maaten M, et al. Generalized equine cutaneous mastocytosis. Vet Pathol 9:394–407, 1972.

Diters RW, Goldschmidt MH. Hair follicle tumors resembling tricholemmomas in six dogs. Vet Pathol 1983;20:123–125.

Diters RW, Walsh JNL. Feline basal cell tumors: a review of 124 cases. Vet Pathol 1984;21:51–56.

Flatt RE, Middleton CC, Tumbleson ME, et al. Pathogenesis of benign cutaneous melanomas in miniature swine. J Am Vet Med Assoc 1968;153:936–941.

Fujimoto Y, Olson C. The fine structure of the bovine wart. Pathol Vet 1966;3:659–664.

Garner FM, Lingeman CH: Mast-cell neoplasms of the domestic cat. Pathol Vet 1970;7:517–530.

Goldschmidt MH, Bevier DE. Skin tumors in the dog. III. Lymphohistiocytic and melanocytic tumors. Comp Cont Educ 1981;3:588–594.

Goto N, Osasa M, Takahashi R, et al. Pathological observations of feline mast cell tumor. Jpn J Vet Sci 1974;36:483–494.

Greve JH, Moses HE. Histopathologic changes in xanthomatosis in chickens. J AmVet Med Assoc 1961;139:1106–1110.

Graves G, Bjorling DE, Mahaffey E. Canine hemangiopericytoma: 23 cases (1967–1984). J Am Vet Med Assoc 1988;192:99–102.

Hargis AM., Thomassen RW, Phemister RD. Chronic dermatosis and cutaneous squamous cell carcinoma in the beagle dog. Vet Pathol 1977;14:218–228.

Headington JT: Tumors of the hair follicle. Am J Pathol 1976;85:480–514.

Holzinger EA: Feline cutaneous mastocytomas. Cornell Vet 1973;63:87–93.

Hottendorf GH, Nielsen SW. Collagen necrosis in canine mastocytomas. Am J Pathol 1966;49:501–513.

Hottendorf GH, Nielsen SW. Pathologic report of 29 necropsies on dogs with mastocytoma. Pathol Vet 1968;5:102–121.

Howard EB, Sawa TR, Nielsen SW, et al.: Mastocytoma and gastroduodenal ulceration. Gastric and duodenal ulcers in dogs with mastocytoma. Pathol Vet 1969;6:146–158.

Johnson RM, Sanger VL. Lipids in avian xanthomatous lesions. Am J Vet Res 1963;24:1280–1282.

Jones TC. Comparative pathology of skin. Int Acad Pathol Monogr 1971;10:597–605.

Kelly DF. Canine cutaneous histiocytoma. A light and electron microscopic study. Pathol Vet 1970;7:12–27.

Lerner AB, Cage GW. Melanomas in horses. Yale J Biol Med 1973;46:646–649.

Lester SJ, Mesfin GM: A solitary plasmacytoma in a dog with progression the disseminated myeloma >AQ: Title doesn't make sense. Missing words?<. Can Vet J 1980;20:284–286,.

Lucke VM Primary cutaneous plasmacytomas in the dog and cat. J Small Anim Pract 1987;28:49–55.

Millikan LE, Boylon JL, Hook RR, et al. Melanoma in Sinclair swine: a new animal model. J Invest Dermatol 1974;62:20–30.

Millikan LE, Hook RR, Manning PJ. Immunobiology of melanoma. Gross and ultrastructural studies in a new melanoma model: the Sinclair swine. Yale J Biol Med 1973;46:631-640.

Mills JHL, Nielsen SW. Canine haemangiopericytomas—a survey of 200 tumours. J Small Anim Pract 1967;8:599–604.

Moore PF, Rosin A. Malignant histiocytosis of Bernese Mountain dogs. Vet Pathol 1986;23:1–10.

Moore PF, Schrenzel MD, Affolter VK, et al. Canine cutaneous histiocytoma is an epidermotropic Langerhans cell histiocytosis that expresses CD1 and specific β_2-integrin molecules. Am J Pathol 1966;148:1699–1708.

Morton LD, Barton CL, Elissalde GS, et al. Oral extramedullary plasmacytomas in two dogs. Vet Pathol 1986;23:637–639.

Mulligan RM. Neoplastic diseases of dogs: mast cell sarcoma, lymphosarcoma, histiocytoma. Arch Pathol 1948;46:477–492.

Mulligan RM. Hemangiopericytoma in the dog. Am J Pathol 1955;31:773–789.

Naik SN, Randelia HP, Dabholkar RD. Carcinoma of the horn in a cryptorchid bull. Pathol Vet 1970;7:265–269.

Nielsen SW, Aftosmis J. Canine perianal gland tumors. J AmVet Med Assoc 1964;144:127–135.

Nielsen SW, Cole CR. Canine mastocytoma—a report of one hundred cases. Am J Vet Res 1958;19:417 432.

Olson C, Jr. Equine sarcoid, a cutaneous neoplasm. Am J Vet Res 1948;9:333–341.

Olson C, Jr., Cook RH. Cutaneous sarcoma-like lesions of the horse caused by the agent of bovine papilloma. Proc Soc Exp Biol Med 1951;77:281–284.

Patnaik AK, Liu S-K, Hurvitz AI, et al. Nonhematopoietic neoplasms in cats. J Natl Cancer Inst 1975;54:855–860.

Peckham MC. Xanthomatosis in chickens. Am J Vet Res 1955;16:580–583.

Petrak ML., Gilmore CE. Neoplasms. In: Diseases of cage and aviary birds. Petrak ML, ed. Philadelphia, Lea & Febiger, 1969;459–489.

Pulley LT, Stannard AA. Tumors of the skin and soft tissues. In: Moulton J, editor. Tumors in domestic animals. 3rd ed. Berkely, CA: University of California Press, 1990.

Ragland WL, Keown GH, Gorham IR. An epizootic of equine sarcoid. Nature 1966;210:1399.

Rowland PH, et al. Cutaneous plasmacytomas with amyloid in six dogs. Vet Pathol 1991;28:125–130.

Sells DM, Conroy JD. Malignant epithelial neoplasia with hair follicle differentiation in dogs. J Comp Pathol 1976;86:121–129.

Shadduck JA, Reedy L, Lawton G, et al. Cutaneous lymphoproliferative disease resembling mycosis fungoides in man. Vet Pathol 1978;15:716–724.

Stannard AA, Pulley LT. Intracutaneous cornifying epithelioma (keratoacanthoma) in the dog: a retrospective study of 25 cases. J Am Vet Med Assoc 1975;167:385–388.

Strafuss AC. Basal cell tumors in dogs. J Am Vet Med Assoc 1976;169:322–324.

Thrall MA, Macy DW, Snyder SP, et al. Cutaneous lymphosarcoma and leukemia in a dog resembling Sezary syndrome in man. Vet Pathol 1984;21:182–186.

Walder EJ, Gross T. Neoplastic diseases of the skin. In: Gross TL, Ihrke PJ, Walder EJ, eds. Veterinary dermatopathology. St. Louis: Mosby Year Book, 1992;327–484.

Ward JM, Hurvitz AI. Ultrastructure of normal and neoplastic mast cells of the cat. Vet Pathol 1972;9:202–211.

Yost DH, Jones TC. Hemangiopericytoma in the dog. Am J Vet Res 1958;19:159–163.

Xu FN. Ultrastructure of canine hemangiopericytoma. Vet Pathol 1986;23:643–645.

18

Skeletal muscle

John F. Van Vleet

INTRODUCTION

Skeletal muscle primarily functions to allow support and movement of the body. It accounts for 40–50% of body weight. Skeletal muscles are composed of fibers, each representing a syncytium formed during myogenesis by fusion of hundreds to thousands of individual myoblasts. The fibers are specialized, with approximately 80% of their cell volume occupied by contractile elements. Normal function of these fibers depends upon a normal nervous system to provide the appropriate stimuli to initiate contraction; normal function also involves intricate control mechanisms that direct movement of calcium ions in and out of the sarcoplasmic reticulum during the contraction-relaxation cycle. Muscle fibers have increased energy requirements that are often needed on short notice; this is a metabolic feature that may predispose these cells to injury from certain chemical and drug toxicities. Use of histochemical staining procedures allows recognition of several fiber types, each with unique metabolic and functional features that may render a specific population of fibers to be susceptible to certain injurious insults. Critical nutrients needed to maintain the structural integrity of muscle fibers include adequate dietary intake of selenium, vitamin E, and protein.

The methods that the pathologist most often uses to study diseases of skeletal muscle encompass the gross, microscopic, and ultrastructural morphology, as well as histochemical features. Careful dissection of the muscles and detailed inspection of their surfaces, attachments, and cut sections are necessary to adequately distinguish gross features. Careful fixation and inclusion of both cross and longitudinal sections are vital to avoid distracting artifacts in histologic sections.

References

Bradley R, McKerrell RE, Barnard EA. Neuromuscular disease in animals. In: Walton J, ed. Disorders of voluntary muscle. 5th ed. New York: Churchill Livingstone, 1988;910–980.

Carpenter S, Karpati G. Pathology of skeletal muscle. New York: Churchill Livingston, 1984;740.

Hadlow WJ. Diseases of skeletal muscle. In: Innes JRM, Saunders LZ, eds. Comparative neuropathology. New York: Academic Press, 1962;147–243.

Kakulas BA. Experimental muscle diseases. In: Walton J, ed. Disorders of voluntary muscle. 5th ed. New York: Churchill Livingstone, 1988;427–454.

Kakulas BA, Adams RD. Diseases of muscle. 4th ed. New York: Harper and Row, 1985;1–830.

Mastaglia FL, Walton J. Skeletal muscle pathology. New York: Churchill Livingstone, 1982;1–630.

Schmalbruch H. Skeletal muscle. New York: Springer-Verlag, 1985;1–384.

Walton J, ed. Disorders of voluntary muscle. 5th ed. New York: Churchill Livingstone, 1988; 1–1166.

Embryogenesis

Skeletal muscle arises from mesodermal somites in the embryo during the first trimester of gestation. The somites give rise to myotomes—sites where embryonic muscle cells or myoblasts aggregate—that roughly correspond to the segments of the vertebral column; each somite receives a spinal nerve. Skeletal muscles of the adult will often contain muscle fibers of several myotomes following migration and fusion of embryonic myoblasts; thus, the muscles will also receive nerve supply from several myotomes. **Myoblasts,** the primitive mononuclear precursor cells of skeletal muscle fibers, elongate and fuse with each other to form myotubes. These cells rapidly form the early cytoplasmic components of mature muscle cells by producing thin (actin) and thick (myosin) myofilaments and Z band material that aggregate into sarcomeres; the sarcotubular membrane systems also form at this stage. Myotubes subsequently fuse with each other, and sarcomerogenesis continues as nuclei migrate to the subsarcolemmal positions. Finally, innervation occurs and fibers become organized for contractile function. Further growth of these fibers in width and length occurs during fetal life. Increased numbers of muscle fibers are produced by waves of growth in late gestation; these instances of growth are presumed to be the result of proliferation and activation of satellite cells that recapitulate the events of mus-

873

cle fiber development and maturation as described above.

Microscopic appearance

Muscle fibers or cells generally extend from tendon to tendon in a muscle, and do not branch or form syncytia. In the adult animal, muscle fibers in cross-sections have a polygonal or multifaceted shape. Many factors—such as species, breed, age, weight, sex, level of nutrition, position and function of the muscle, and exercise—influence the diameter of muscle fibers. Measurements of fibers in individual muscles will show variability in fiber size that will be reflected as a bell-shaped curve on a histogram. Differences in fiber size in various species are not directly related to body weight (pig<horse, cow, rabbit<sheep). Fiber size is greater in males than in females, and tends to increase with age to maturity.

The cellular features of skeletal muscle fibers are best appreciated in longitudinal sections. The fibers are bounded by the plasma membrane, or sarcolemma, that is covered by an external lamina (stained by periodic acid-Schiff reaction). The thin elongated nuclei are generally positioned beneath the sarcolemma in a spiral pattern spaced 10–50 μm apart. At myotendinous junctions, muscle fibers have numerous centrally located nuclei. Nuclei of satellite cells are positioned between the sarcolemma and the external lamina. Fibers contain hundreds of longitudinally aligned myofibrils; these are composed of repeating sarcomeres. The characteristic transverse striation of skeletal muscle fibers results from parallel alignment of the bands in adjacent myofibrils. The largest bands, termed according to their appearance in polarized light, are **A bands** (anisotropic or birefringent, appear bright) and **I bands** (isotropic, appear dark). The I bands, composed of thin myofilaments, are bisected by 2 lines (disks, bands) that form the end of each sarcomere; the A bands, composed of thick filaments, are bisected by the less birefringent **H bands.** The banding pattern, named for the appearance in polarized light, is reversed when studied by either light microscopy—with phase contrast optics or conventional optics on sections stained with the usual cationic dyes—or transmission electron microscopy.

Application of histochemical stains (such as ATPase or NADH-TR) to frozen sections of skeletal muscle allows demonstration of various fiber type populations that cannot be distinguished in paraffin-embedded sections stained with the usual stains (such as hematoxylin and eosin); however, differing fiber types are recognized by ultrastructural study. The histochemical uniqueness of these fiber types correlates with differences in their physiologic features: for example, contraction speed and fatigability, biochemical and metabolic activities, gross color, and structure (as revealed ultrastructurally). Table 18-1 summarizes these features.

Most muscles will have a mixture of all fiber types; this produces the so-called "checkerboard" pattern of differential histochemical staining. Fibers innervated by the same nerves will have the same fiber type, and reinnervated fibers may show reversal of fiber types. Some muscles will have a preponderance of one fiber type, such as the soleus in birds (red muscle high in type I fibers and capable of sustained action or weight-bearing) and the pectorals in birds (white muscle high in type II fibers and capable of sudden action and purposeful motion). The proportions of the various fiber types may vary with species, breed, age, exercise, and in certain muscular diseases.

SATELLITE CELLS

Satellite cells are thin cells with a nucleus and a scant amount of sarcoplasm interposed between the sarcolemma of muscle fibers and the external lamina. They are abundant in newborn animals; in muscle of mature animals, 3–5% of nuclei in muscle fibers belong to satellite cells. The cells serve an important role in normal development of fibers and in regeneration of damaged fibers by serving as stem cells that can be activated to undergo mitosis in adult life; subsequently, they differentiate to myoblasts, myotubes, and later to mature myofibers.

MOTOR END PLATES

Motor end plates (neuromuscular junctions)—generally recognized only by use of special techniques, such as metallic impregnation, intravital dyes, histochemical procedures, or electron microscopy—represent a complex and intimate attachment site of the motor nerve fiber on the surface of the skeletal muscle fiber. The end of the nerve fiber is unmyelinated and branches into axon terminals that invaginate into a thickened zone of subsarcolemmal sarcoplasm with numerous nuclei as synaptic clefts. The axon terminal has abundant synaptic vesicles that contain the neurotransmitter acetylcholine.

MUSCLE SPINDLES

Muscle spindles are fusiform structures of 0.5–3.0 mm length, found longitudinally at the edge of muscle fasciculi. The spindle has a thick surrounding fibrous capsule and contains multiple small variably-sized intrafusal fibers, nerve fibers, specialized nerve endings, and blood vessels. Muscle spindles have sensory function and serve to maintain muscle tone by responding to stretch.

The interstitial connective tissue of muscle is subdivided into the **epimysium** (surrounds the entire muscle), **perimysium** (surrounds large angular fascicles divided into primary fascicles of 10 to 100 fibers), and **endomysium** (surrounds individual muscle fibers). The endomysium contains capillaries, nerve fibers, fibroblasts, and collagen fibrils. Larger amounts of collagen fibrils and large blood vessels and nerves are in the perimysium.

Physiologic features

The unique structural differentiation of skeletal muscle fibers is closely integrated with their well-developed and specialized contractile function; this function allows for locomotion and maintenance of posture by conversion

TABLE 18-1 **Characteristics of major mammalian skeletal muscle**

| | *Fiber types* | | |
	Type 1	*Type 2A*	*Type 2B*
General characteristics			
Natural appearance	Dark	Dark	Pale
Surrounding capillary density	High	High	Low
Relative cytochemical activity			
Myofibrillar ATPase pH 9.4	Weak	Strong	Strong
Myofibrillar ATPase pH 4.6	Strong	Weak	Strong
Myofibrillar ATPase pH 4.3	Strong	Weak	Weak
NADH-tetrazolium reductase	Strong	Strong	Weak
Succinic dehydrogenase	Strong	Strong	Weak
Amylophosphorylase	Weak	Strong	Strong
Glycogen content	Low	High	High
Myoglobin content	High	High	Low
Lipid globules	Numerous	Numerous	Few
Electron microscopy			
Mitochondria	Many, small	Many, large	Few, small
Z disc	Intermediate	Wide	Narrow
Physiologic features			
Twitch speed	Slow twitch	Fast twitch	Fast twitch
Fatiguability	Resistant	Resistant	Susceptible
Other designations			
Stein and Padykula (1962)	B	C	A
Padykula and Gauthier (1967)	Intermediate	Red	White
Yellin and Guth (1970)	Beta	Alpha-beta	Alpha
Burke et al. (1971)	S	FR	FF
Peter (1973)	SO	FOG	FG

Abbreviations: FR—Fast, resistant: FF—Fast, fatigable: S—Slow: FOG—Fast, oxidative glycolytic: FG—Fast glycolytic: SO—Slow oxidative

of chemical energy into mechanical energy. Further specialization in form and function is provided by the differentiation of myofibers into various fiber types, each of which is specifically suited for certain physiologic applications.

The functional unit of the neuromuscular system is the motor unit consisting of (1) nerve cell bodies in the ventral horns or brainstem, (2) the axon of these neurons that course to the muscle and terminate as a motor end plate, and (3) the group of specific histochemical type of muscle fibers that are innervated by the neuron. The number of muscle fibers supplied by a neuron of a motor unit may vary widely, depending on the degree of refined movement needed by the muscle (e.g., 10 fibers per neuron, in extrinsic eye muscles, to 2000 fibers per nerve, in large limb muscles).

Contraction of muscle is the result of sarcomeres shortening with interdigitation of thin and thick myofilaments. According to the sliding filament hypothesis of contraction, the force of contraction is generated by the movement of cross-bridges that project from myosin

molecules along actin molecules. The chemical energy for contraction is supplied by high-energy phosphate compounds; these compounds are largely generated in type 1 fibers by mitochondrial oxidative phosphorylation via the electron transport system; this generation follows the oxidation of fatty acids and glucose via the Krebs cycle, and in type 2 fibers, by sarcoplasmic anaerobic glycolysis and glycogenolysis. Consequently, the metabolic differences of the various fiber types are associated with differences in their functional features, such as speed of contraction and resistance to fatigue.

CLINICAL PATHOLOGIC ALTERATIONS OF MUSCLE DISEASE

Degeneration and necrosis of skeletal muscle, when acute and extensive, results in elevation of certain serum enzymes; this elevation occurs in the development of myoglobinemia and myoglobinuria, and in creatinuria. The enzymes creatine kinase, aldolase, aspartate aminotransferase, and lactic dehydrogenase may all be elevated in the serum of animals after damage to skeletal muscle. Two enzymes are of special importance—muscle aldolase and MM creatine kinase (CK)—because they are regarded as specific for striated muscle. Aspartate aminotransferase (glutamic oxaloacetic transaminase, GOT) activity increases during training and exercise of horses. This enzyme is not as sensitive to muscle damage as CK. However, when elevated, GOT does have a much longer clearance rate than other enzymes, especially CK. The latter enzyme returns to normal within a few days (3–5) after cessation of active muscle damage, or within 24 hours after an elevation of activity due to exercise.

Postmortem alterations

Following somatic death, skeletal muscle will generally remain in relaxation for two to four hours until muscle glycogen stores are metabolized and sufficient energy to maintain the relaxed state is no longer present. **Rigor mortis** (stiffness of the muscles and immobility of the joints) then ensues for at least 24–48 hours. Subsequently, rigor will gradually dissipate as autolysis occurs, muscle proteins are denatured, and muscle fibers lose the ability to contract. The onset of rigor mortis will be rapid when the muscle has conditions of decreased pH and increased temperatures. Abundant muscular glycogen stores at the time of death will lead to delayed onset of rigor. Debilitated animals tend to have weak rigor.

Pallor develops in muscles following death—as also seen in necrotic muscle—and this is believed to be due to leaching of myoglobin by accumulated lactic acid. Following the death of debilitated animals with depleted glycogen stores, muscles may appear unusually dark.

References

Anderson PH, Barrett S, Patterson DS. The significance of elevated plasma creatine phosphokinase activity in muscle disease of cattle. J Comp Pathol 1976;86:531–538.

Bradley R. Skeletal muscle biopsy techniques in animals for histochemical and ultrastructural examination and especially for the diagnosis of myodegeneration in cattle. Br Vet J 1978;134: 434–444.

Cardinet GH III. Skeletal muscle function. In: Kaneko JJ, ed. Clinical biochemistry of domestic animals. 4th ed. New York: Academic Press, 1989;462–495.

Cardinet GH, Holliday TA. Neuromuscular diseases of domestic animals: a summary of muscle biopsies from 159 cases. Ann NY Acad Sci 1979;317:290–313.

Cullen MJ, Hudgson P, Mastaglia FL. Ultrastructural studies of diseased muscle. In: Walton J, ed. Disorders of voluntary muscle. 5th ed. New York: Churchill Livingstone, 1988;284–344.

Gauthier GF. The muscular tissue. In: Weiss L, ed. Cell and tissue biology. 6th ed. Baltimore: Urban and Schwartzenberg, 1988;255–276.

McGavin MD. Muscle biopsy in veterinary practice. Vet Clin North Am Small Anim Pract 1983;13:135–144.

Shelton GD, Cardinet GH III. Pathophysiologic basis of canine muscle disorders. J Vet Intern Med 1987;1:36–44.

DEVELOPMENTAL DISORDERS OF MUSCLE

A growing number of developmental disorders of muscle are becoming known in animals. We have chosen to present a summary of current knowledge by means of tabulation (Table 18-2). The diseases in different species often have similar lesions and clinical manifestations.

Muscular dystrophy

The muscular dystrophies represent a group of hereditary primary muscle disorders with an, as yet, unknown biochemical or metabolic aberration of the muscle fibers; this aberration leads to the delayed onset of a progressive syndrome of generalized muscular weakness. In dystrophy, the muscles have normal nervous system structure and function, in contrast to the denervation atrophies; however, many microscopic alterations are common to these two groups of disorders. Dystrophy is characterized by lack of effective regeneration of damaged fibers following degeneration and atrophy. Loss of fibers is accompanied by replacement with adipose tissue and collagenous connective tissue.

Inherited diseases of differentiated muscle cells have been described in humans, mice, Syrian hamsters, New Hampshire chickens, turkeys, Merino sheep, mink, and dogs. Probable muscular dystrophy has been described in cattle and cats, although the disease in these cases has not been completely established as inherited. The pattern of inheritance for dystrophic disease in mice, hamsters, chickens, turkeys, sheep, mink, and dogs is autosomal recessive.

X-linked muscular dystrophy is also described in humans, mice, dogs, and, apparently, domestic cats. This is the most common form of muscular dystrophy in humans, and is termed **Duchenne muscular dystrophy**. The X-linked muscular dystrophies are characterized by a deficiency of dystrophin, a cytoskeletal protein that is similar to A-actinin and spectrin.

References

Ashmore CR, Robinson DW. Hereditary muscular hypertrophy in the bovine. I. Histological and biochemical characterization. Proc Soc Exp Biol Med 1969;132:548–554.

Banker BQ. A pathological study of muscular dystrophy in the Bar Harbor 129 house mouse with particular reference to the ultrastructural features. In: Locke S, ed. Modern neurology. Boston: Little Brown, 1969;241–259.

Bourne GH, Golarz MN. Muscular dystrophy in man and animals. New York: Hafner Publishing, 1963;1–514.

Bradley R, Terlecki S. Muscle lesions in hereditary "daft" lamb disease of Border Leicester sheep. J Pathol 1977;123:225–236.

Bradley R, Wells GAH. Developmental muscle disorders in the pig. Vet Annu 1978;18:144–157.

Bradley R, McKerrell RE, Barnard EA. Neuromuscular disease in animals. In: Walton J, ed. Disorders of voluntary muscle. 5th ed. New York: Churchill Livingstone, 1988;910–980.

Carpenter JL, et al. Feline muscular dystrophy with dystrophin deficiency. Am J Pathol 1989;135:909–919.

Ducatelle R, Maenhout D, Coussement W, Hoorens JK. Spontaneous and experimental myofibrillar hypoplasia and its relation to splayleg in newborn pigs. J Comp Pathol 1986;96:433–445.

Goedegebaar SA, Hartman W, Hoebe HP. Dystrophy of the diaphragmatic muscles in adult Meuse-Rhine-Yssel cattle: electromyographical and histological findings. Vet Pathol 1983;20:32–48.

Hadlow WJ. Diseases of skeletal muscle. In: Innes JRM, Saunders LZ, eds. Comparative neuropathology. New York: Academic Press, 1962;147–243.

Hegreberg GA, Norton SL, Gorham JR. Muscular dystrophy of mink. Am J Pathol 1976;85:233–236.

TABLE 18-2 **Developmental disorders of skeletal muscle**

Species	Name of disease	Mode of inheritance	Features of disease	References
Dog	Progressive muscular dystrophy	S,R	Recognized in Irish terriers and golden retrievers by stiff gait and difficulty in swallowing; high muscle tone; decreased stamina. Progresses with gross atrophy of muscles. Histology: normal and abnormal fibers are mixed; Zenker degeneration often; phagocytosis of some fibers; nuclei often fall into rows. Dystrophin deficiency and cardiomyopathy in golden retriever.	Kornegay et al., 1988
Dog	Hereditary myopathy	A,R	Seen in Labrador retrievers. Onset at less than 6 months of age. Features include abnormal head and neck posture; stiff, hopping gait; loss of muscle mass: myotonia indicated by electromyotonic studies. Some relief with diazepam. Lesions: progressive loss of myofibrils, especially red type; usual destruction and partial repair similar to other muscle dystrophies.	Kramer et al., 1976, McKerrel and Braund, 1986
Cat	Muscular dystrophy with systrophin deficiency	S,R	Affected male DSH cats show "bunny hopping" gait, myotonia and muscular hypertrophy (diaphragm especially). Histology: variation in fiber size, degeneration, necrosis and fibrosis, accompanying myocardial necrosis.	Carpenter et al., 1989
Cow	Muscular dystrophy of diaphragm	?	Observed in adult meuse-Rhine-Yssel cattle in the Netherlands. Show anorexia and bloat.	Goedegebaar et al., 1983
Cow	Limber leg	A,R	Affected Jersey cattle have abnormal flexure and extension of joints.	Lamb et al., 1972
Sheep	Progressive ovine muscular dystrophy	A,R	In Merino sheep in Australia, recognized as early as one month of age by reduced flexion of femorotibial and tibial-tarsal joints and stiff gait. Bilaterally symmetric lesions occur, particularly in vastus intermedius muscles. Progressive loss of muscle fibers with irregular size, central rows of nuclei, replacement over years by adipose cells.	McGavin and Baynes, 1969
Sheep	Daft lamb disease	A,R	Affected Border Leicester sheep have progressive myopathy. Variation in fiber size.	Bradley and Terlecki, 1977

(continued)

TABLE 18-2 (continued)

Species	Name of disease	Mode of inheritance	Features of disease	References
Hamster	Cardiomyopathy; muscular dystrophy; myopathy	A,R	Disease appears at about 30 days of age in skeletal and cardiac muscle. Histology: progressive necrosis and some repair of muscle cells; nuclei become centrally placed in fibers and fall into long chains; coagulation necrosis of muscle fibers; focal fibrosis in myocardium.	Gertz, 1973
Mink	Muscular dystrophy	A,R	Manifest as early as two months of age by locomotor dysfunction; dysphasia and atrophy especially of muscles of head, pectoral, and pelvic girdles. Histology: striking variation in size of muscle fibers; hyaline degenerative changes; nuclei centralized; often regenerating multinucleated nuclei; increase of connective tissue. Serum enzymes elevated include: creatine phosphokinase, aldolase, glutamic-oxaloacetic transaminase.	Hegreberg et al., 1976
Mouse	Muscular dystrophy	dy/dy A,R LG IV	Weakness and atrophy of muscles begin to show at about three weeks of age; most die before 10th week. Histology: decrease in size of muscle fibers; increase in connective tissue and fat; some coagulation necrosis of muscle fibers; nuclei fall into closely-packed chains. Ultrastructure: loss of myofibrils, mitochondria often enlarged; endoplasmic reticulum swollen and lost.	Banker, 1969, Hadlow, 1962, Jones, 1978
Chicken	Muscular dystrophy	A,R	Mild, progressive disease; first sign is failure of fowl to right itself when placed on its back. Lesions, variation in muscle size, vacuolation of fibers, loss of fibers and replacement by adipose tissue.	Ashmore, 1968, Julian, 1973, Cardinet et al., 1972
Turkey	Muscular dystrophy	A,R	Seen in broad-breasted Bronze breed; atrophy of pectoral and wing muscles is evident first at 8–16 weeks of age; other muscles not affected. As in chickens, first sign is inability of fowl to right itself when placed on its back. Lesions: variation in size of myofibrils, necrosis of individual fibers, mild deposition of fat cells.	Harper and Parker, 1967

(continued)

TABLE 18-2 (continued)

Species	Name of disease	Mode of inheritance	Features of disease	References
Mouse, turkey	Muscular dysgenesis	mdg/mdg A,R	Homozygote born dead; lesions limited to skeletal muscle; myoblasts differentiate into myotubules and cross striations appear, then development ceases; necrosis of muscle cells eventually with pyknotic and karyorrhectic nuclei and dissolution of cytoplasm; macrophages engulf degenerated cell detritus. Also described in New Hampshire chicken ("crooked neck dwarfism").	Platzer and Gluecksohn-Waelsch, 1972
Mouse	Muscular dystonia	dt/dt LG XIII A,R	Atrophy of muscles secondary to degeneration of peripheral nerves, dorsal root ganglia, and gray matter of spinal cord.	Duchen and Strich, 1964
Swine	Hereditary metabolic myopathy; malignant hyperthermia	A,D (?) polygenic (?)	Inherited susceptibility to halothane, etc., which triggers severe muscular rigidity, high fever, elevated electrolytes and muscle enzymes in serum.	Chapter 6
Cattle, sheep	Congenital hyperplasia ("double muscles;" hereditary muscular hypertrophy)	A,R	Calves are born with muscles in shoulders and rump much larger than normal; may cause dystocia; fat deposits are reduced by about 60% from normal.	Ashmore and Robinson, 1969, Holmes and Robinson, 1970
Calves	Hereditary myopathy associated with hydrocephalus	A,R	Newborn Hereford calves are alive but unable to stand; limbs mobile and joints normal; hydrocephalus accompanied also by microphthalmia and cerebellar hypoplasia; muscles are atrophied, pale, soft, sometimes spongy. Histology: thin muscles with myofibers scattered in connective tissue; some hyalinization and necrosis of myofibrils, little regeneration, and few fat cells.	Hadlow, 1962, Green et al. 1974
Mouse	Hereditary motor endplate disease (MED); myopathy; hereditary myopathy	A,R	Considered a new form of hereditary myopathy; appears 11–14 days after birth, increased muscle weakness especially in hind legs, to almost complete loss of movement; no atrophic or dystrophic changes in motor endplates. In muscle: focal myofibrillar disorganization, enlarged mitochondria, autophagic vacuoles, engulfing sarcoplasm; increased acid phosphatase in membranes; possible diminished protein synthesis.	Duchen, 1970

(continued)

TABLE 18-2 (continued)

Species	Name of disease	Mode of inheritance	Features of disease	References
Dog	"Scottie cramp," muscular hypertonicity	A,R	Scottish terrier breed affected. Episodes of muscular hypertonicity result in arching of back, then forelimbs and neck causing head to lower; sometimes somersaults. No functional defect in peripheral axon myoneural junction, myomembrane, or contractile proteins. No morphologic lesion in muscle, nervous tissue, or parenchyma. Believed to originate in central nervous system.	Meyers, Padgett and Dickson, 1970
Calves, lambs, pigs, foals	Myopathy associated with congenital articular rigidity (arthrogryposis)	A,R in swine and Charolais cattle	Fixed joint(s) with muscular atrophy; multifactorial etiology may include maternal exposure to *Lupinus* spp. or akabane virus in cattle; *Astragalus* spp. or akabane virus in sheep; vitamin A and manganese deficiency or ingestion of tobacco (*Nicotiana tabacum*), thorn apple (*Datura stramonium*), hemlock (*Conium maculatum*), black cherry (*Prunus serontina*) in swine.	Bradley and Wells, 1978 Swatland, 1974
Swine	Myofibrillar hypoplasia ("splayleg," "spraddleleg")		Newborn piglets show muscular weakness and limb abduction ("splaying"). Multifactorial etiology. Histology: small, immature muscle fibers with myofibrils.	Ward, 1978, Thurley et al., 1967
Swine	"Creeper" syndrome	A,R	Occurs in Pietrain breed. Onset at two to four weeks of age of creeping gait. Histology: variation in fiber diameter and degenerative alterations in fibers.	Bradley and Wells, 1978 Done et al. 1975
Goat, dog, horse, sheep, mouse	Myotonia	?	Startled animals have continued muscle contraction, affected dogs have "bunny hopping" gait (Rhodesian Ridgeback, Staffordshire terrier, Fox terrier, West Highland terrier, Chow chow, German shepherd). Histology: muscle fiber hypertrophy and degeneration, some cases have no alterations.	Reed et al., 1988
Cattle, sheep, dog, cat, Japanese quail	Glycogenosis	A,R (cattle)	Muscular weakness. Histology: glycogen accumulation in fibers.	Edward and Richards, 1979, Manktelow and Hartley, 1975, Matsui et al., 1983, Ceh et al., 1976, Harvey et al., 1990
Cattle, sheep, swine	Steatosis	?	No clinical signs. Histology: replacement of muscle fibers by fat cells.	Hadlow, 1962

(continued)

TABLE 18-2 (continued)

Species	Name of disease	Mode of inheritance	Features of disease	References
Cattle	Xanthosis	?	No clinical signs in affected Ayrshires. Histology: lipofuscin accumulation in fibers.	Bradley and Duffell, 1982
Swine	Myositis ossificans	?	Histology: heterotopic bone formation.	Seibold and Davis, 1967
Dog, cat	Myasthenia gravis	A,R (dog)	Muscular weakness. Megaesophagus, dysphagia. Histology: no alterations.	Oda et al., 1984
Dog	Familial canine dermatomyositis	A, D	Affected collies and Shetland sheepdogs have cutaneous lesions and muscular atrophy. Histology: vasculitis and mixed inflammatory cell infiltration of muscle, fiber degeneration and fibrosis.	Hargis et al., 1984, Hargis et al., 1986

S = sex-linked; R = recessive; A = autosomal; ? = unknown; *dy* = gene symbol; LG = linkage groups; D = dominant.

Holmes JHG, Robinson DW. Hereditary muscular hypertrophy in the bovine: metabolic response to nutritional stress. J Anim Sci 1970;31:776–780.

Kornegay JN, Tuler SM, Miller DS, Levesque DC. Muscular dystrophy in a litter of Golden retriever dogs. Muscle Nerve 1988;11:1056–1064.

Kramer JW, Hegreberg GA, Bryan GM, Meyers K, Ott RL. A muscle disorder of Labrador retrievers characterized by deficiency of type II muscle fibers. J Am Vet Med Assoc 1976;169:817–820.

McGavin MD, Baynes ID. A congenital progressive ovine muscular dystrophy. Pathol Vet 1969;6:513–524.

McKerrell RE, Braund KG. Hereditary myopathy in Labrador retrievers: a morphologic study. Vet Pathol 1986;23:411–417.

Meyers KM, Padgett GA, Dickson WM. The genetic basis of a kinetic disorder of Scottish terrier dogs. J Hered 1970;61:189–192.

Reed SM, et al. Progressive myotonia in foals resembling human dystrophia myotonia. Muscle Nerve 1988;11:291–296.

Seibold HR, Davis CL. Generalized myositis ossificans (familial) in pigs. Pathol Vet 1967;4:79–88.

Swatland HJ. Developmental disorders of skeletal muscle in cattle, pigs, and sheep. Vet Bull 1974;44:179–202.

Szabo KT. Muscular system. In: congenital malformations in laboratory and farm animals. New York: Academic Press, 1989;184–191.

Telford IR. Experimental muscular dystrophies in animals: a comparative study. Springfield IL: Charles C Thomas, 1971;1–234.

Thurley DC, Gilbert FR, Done JT. Congenital splayleg of piglets: myofibrillar hypoplasia. Vet Rec 1967;80:302–304.

Valentine BA, Cooper BJ, de Lahunta A, O'Quinn R, Blue JT. Canine X-linked muscular dystrophy. An animal model of Duchenne muscular dystophy: clinical studies. J Neurol Sci 1988;88:69–81.

Ward PS. The splayleg syndrome in newborn pigs: a review. Parts I and II. Vet Bull 1978;48:279–295, 381–399.

Muscular hypoplasia and hyperplasia

A condition in newborn piglets termed myofibrillar hypoplasia ("splayleg" or "spraddleleg") represents a delayed maturation of muscle fibers. Affected piglets have small muscle fibers that contain few myofibrils surrounded by granular masses of sarcoplasm. Spontaneous resolution of the disease usually occurs by several weeks of age, when fibers mature adequately.

With muscular hyperplasia (also termed "**double-muscling**" and *Doppellander*), increased muscle mass may occur in cattle and sheep. Microscopically, the numbers of muscle fibers are increased, but the size of individual fibers is normal.

References

Ashmore CR, Robinson DW. Hereditary muscular hypertrophy in the bovine. I. Histological and biochemical characterization. Proc Soc Exp Biol Med 1969;132:548–554.

Ducatelle R, Maenhout D, Coussement W, Hoorens JK. Spontaneous and experimental myofibrillar hypoplasia and its relation to splayleg in newborn pigs. J Comp Pathol 1986;96:433–445.

Holmes JHG, Robinson DW. Hereditary muscular hypertrophy in the bovine: metabolic response to nutritional stress. J Anim Sci 1970;31:776–780.

Thurley DC, Gilbert FR, Done JT. Congenital splayleg of piglets: myofibrillar hypoplasia. Vet Rec 1967;80:302–304.

Ward PS. The splayleg syndrome in newborn pigs: a review. Parts I and II. Vet Bull 1978;48:279–295, 381–399.

Muscle glycogenosis

In animals, glycogenosis (glycogen storage disease) has been documented in a variety of species including cattle, sheep, dogs, cats, mice, rats, and quail. In some reports, intrasarcoplasmic and lysosomal accumulations of glycogen in skeletal muscle are described. Storage diseases are discussed in Chapter 2.

References

Ceh L, Hauge JG, Svenkerud R, Strande A. Glycogenosis III in the dog. Acta Vet Scand 1976;17:210–222.

Edwards JR, Richards RB. Bovine generalized glycogenosis type II: a clinicopathological study. Br Vet J 1979;135:338–348.

Harvey JW, Calderwood-Mays MB, Gropp KE, Denaro FJ. Polysaccharide storage myopathy in canine phosphofructokinase deficiency (type VII glycogen storage disease). Vet Pathol 1990;27:1–8.

Manketelow BW, Hartley WJ. Generalized glycogen storage disease in sheep. J Comp Pathol 1975;85:139–145.

Matsui T, Kuroda S, Mizutani M, Kiuchi Y, Suzuki K, Ono T. Generalized glycogen storage disease in Japanese quail (*Coturnix coturnix japonica*). Vet Pathol 1983;20:312–321.

Ossification of muscle

Ossifications of muscle represent heterotopic bone formations in muscle, and may follow trauma; this condition is termed **myositis ossificans.** A generalized form of myositis ossificans of suspected heritability has been described by Seibold and Davis in pigs (1967).

Reference

Seibold HR, Davis CL. Generalized myositis ossificans (familial) in pigs. Pathol Vet 1967;4:79–88.

Steatosis

The term steatosis has been used to designate a variant condition in the musculature of beef cattle, sheep, and swine. It is usually recognized at slaughter as an extensive increase in intramuscular fat, particularly in the muscles of the loin and back. This gross change is the result of replacement of many muscle fibers by adipose tissue cells (Figure 18-1). In this respect it resembles a lesion of muscular dystrophy ("pseudohypertrophy") in which the end stage is replacement of muscle fibers by adipose cells; such replacement results in grossly apparent enlargement of the muscle. The cause is unknown, but it may be under genetic control.

Reference

Hadlow WJ. Diseases of skeletal muscle. In: Innes JRM, Saunders LZ, eds. Comparative neuropathology. New York: Academic Press, 1962;147–243.

DISTURBANCES OF GROWTH

Atrophy

Atrophy is a common reaction of skeletal muscle fibers in response to influences such as denervation, disuse, emaciation, cachexia, senility, and compression by local lesions (Figure 18-2). Affected fibers are recognized by their decrease in cross-sectional area; this decrease is associated with regression in cell volume and a negative growth phase. Ultrastructural study of atrophic muscle fibers reveals a number of morphologic alterations that are common to this pathologic process, regardless of the primary initiating event. The contractile elements of affected fibers are altered, with thin myofibrils that eventually show malalignment and disruption in the late stages of atrophy. The plasma membrane shrinks to fit the smaller diameter of the fiber and pulls away from the external lamina. The external lamina appears convoluted and may have redundant layers. Sarcoplasmic membrane systems have increased prominence, including the sarcoplasmic reticulum, T-tubules, Golgi appara-

tus, and rough endoplasmic reticulum. Increased numbers of autophagic vacuoles, lipofuscin granules, and polysomes are often present. Satellite cells appear to increase in denervated atrophic fibers.

The biochemical mechanisms involved in muscle fiber atrophy are largely unknown. In principle, loss of the contractile elements in atrophy could result from either enhancement of protein degradation, decrease in protein synthesis, or a combination of both processes. The turnover rates of individual myofibrillar proteins show considerable heterogeneity. Selective loss of one type of filament in certain diseases may be associated with these differences. The role of muscle fiber proteases is still unclear in myofibrillar degradation and subsequent fiber atrophy. Muscle fibers contain several enzymes capable of degrading myofibrillar proteins, including calcium-activated protease, cathepsin B and cathepsin D. The role of endogenous inhibitors of these enzymes, which are known to exist in muscle fibers, is not established. Ultrastructural evidence of increased lysosomal activity in atrophic fibers is not impressive, and intralysosomal accumulation of myofibrillar debris is rarely observed. It has been suggested that initial degradation of myofibrillar proteins is extralysosomal and is mediated by calcium-activated protease; subsequent breakdown of resulting monomers and dimers of actin and myosin occur within lysosomes, under the influences of cathepsins B and D (Dayton et al., 1976).

Traditionally, muscular atrophy is classified according to cause: (1) **denervation atrophy** (also termed neurogenic atrophy); (2) **disuse atrophy**; (3) **atrophy of cachexia and emaciation**; (4) **senile atrophy**; and (5) **compression atrophy.** The most striking microscopic alterations tend to be observed in denervation atrophy. In animals, the most frequent primary lesions of the nervous system with denervation atrophy are seen in either (1) the spinal cord and nerve rootlets in conditions, such as intervertebral disc disease, trauma, neoplastic proliferation, or localized inflammation, or (2) peripheral nerve injury, such as traumatic damage to the radial or brachial nerve, or idiopathic damage to the recurrent laryngeal nerve. When denervation to the affected muscle is complete, then all fibers may be uniformly affected. However, generally denervation is incomplete and selective atrophy occurs in those fibers innervated by a damaged nerve fiber; adjacent fibers supplied by an intact nerve supply remain unaffected. Consequently, a typical pattern is observed with 3–15 atrophic fibers surrounded by 3–15 fibers of normal or increased (due to compensatory hypertrophy) size. Atrophic fibers assume an angulated shape. Endomysial connective tissue and adipose tissue appear prominent. In the late stages of atrophy, fibers may undergo degeneration and sarcoplasmic debris will be phagocytized by invading macrophages.

Disuse atrophy results from primary lesions, such as severed tendons, immobilization of limbs with fractures, ankylosis, and other painful disorders that inhibit limb movement; atrophy will also accompany the paralysis that occurs in denervating lesions. The atrophic process in disuse, as well as in cachexia and senility, tends to be

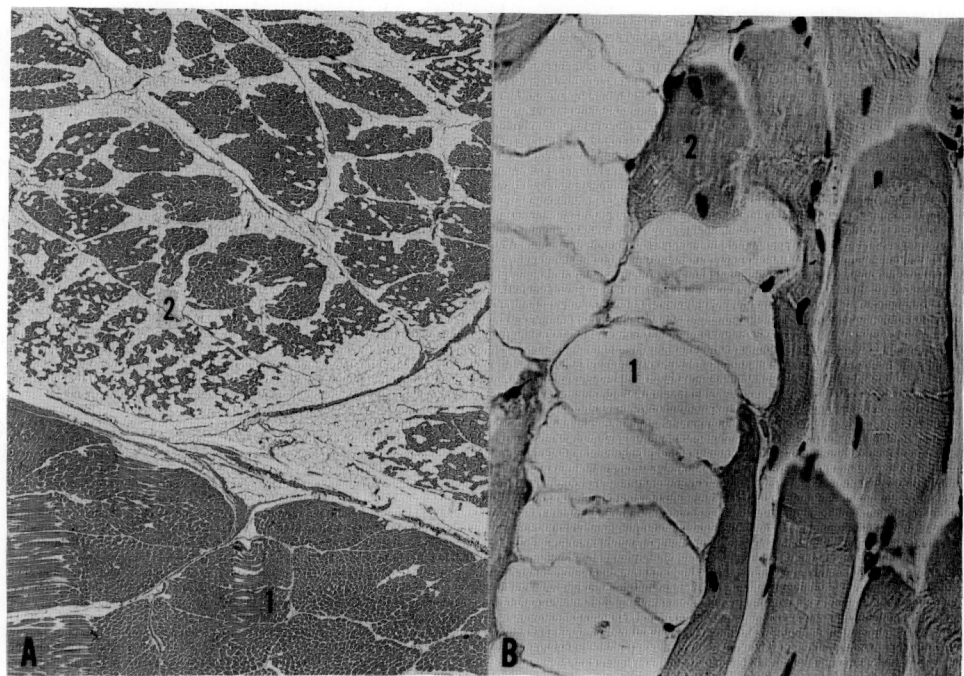

FIG. 18-1 A. Steatosis, psoas muscle (×10) of a steer. (1) Normal muscle; (2) Infiltrated and replaced by fat. **B.** The same muscle as A (×330). (1) Note fat cells; (2) Replacing muscle bundles. (Courtesy of Armed Forces Institute of Pathology; contributor: Colonel Russell McNellis, V.C.)

more widespread in the musculature and to develop more slowly than in denervation atrophy. Type 2 fibers are selectively affected in malnutrition atrophy (Hulland, 1993).

Atrophy of muscle fibers may be reversible when the causative factors are removed early in the course of the process. Even denervated muscle fibers may be restored to normal size and activity when reinnervation occurs; this is seen in some cases in which the nerve sheaths are preserved and allow slow regrowth of nerve fibers to reestablish contact with muscle fibers.

Hypertrophy

Increased size of muscle fibers, or hypertrophy, may occur physiologically as a response to increased workload, or it may be a compensatory alteration in certain muscular diseases. Athletic animals in training may show

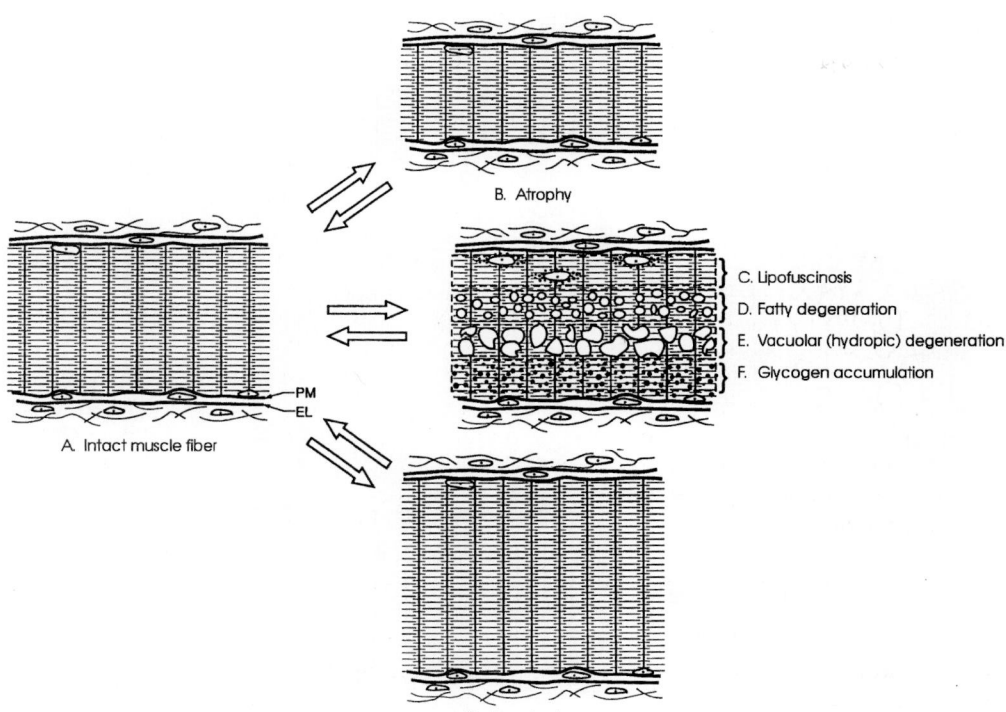

FIG. 18-2 Growth disturbances and degenerations of skeletal muscle fibers. (EL - external lamina, PM - plasma membrane).

muscular hypertrophy. Compensatory hypertrophy may develop in muscles with extensive fiber loss or atrophy, such as in chronic denervation atrophy and congenital neuromuscular disorders. Muscle fibers undergoing hypertrophy have increased numbers of myofibrils that are believed to arise from longitudinal splitting of existing myofibrils.

Physical injuries

Traumatic injury of muscles in animals by bruising is common, but only rarely results in apparent clinical signs. External trauma may result from attacks by other animals, striking immovable objects in the environment, and moving vehicles. Also, injuries may occur from violent exercise, overstretching of limbs from falling, penetration of foreign bodies, intramuscular injections of irritant compounds, and surgical incisions. Muscular damage from trauma may be complicated by secondary injury of soft tissue by sharp bone fragments from fractures. Sudden compression of the abdominal muscles in small animals struck by a moving vehicle may result in rupture of the diaphragm from elevated intra-abdominal pressure. In horses, a condition termed fibrotic or ossifying myopathy may develop following traumatic rupture of the posterior thigh muscles.

Muscle lesions following physical injury include edema, hemorrhage, and physical disruption. Healing is generally accompanied by scar tissue formation (Figure 18-3).

References

Dayton WR, Reville WJ, Goll DE, Stromer MH. A Ca2+-activated protease possibly involved in myofibrillar protein turnover: partial characterization of the purified enzyme. Biochemistry 1976;15:2159–2167.

Hulland TJ. Muscles and tendons. In: Jubb KVF, Kennedy PC, Palmer N, eds. Pathology of domestic animals, 4th ed. Vol 1.New York: Academic Press, 1993;183–265.

Turner AS, Trotter GW. Fibrotic myopathy in the horse. J Am Vet Med Assoc 1984;184:335–338.

Degeneration and necrosis

Unlike in most tissues, the difference between the reversible sublethal alterations of degeneration and the irreversible lethal change of necrosis is difficult to detect by microscopic study. Skeletal muscle fibers are large, long, multinucleated cells; often, it is not possible to view the entire length of the fiber in the plane of a tissue section to determine whether the sarcoplasmic damage involves the entire fiber or only a segment of the fiber. It seems likely that segmental degeneration occurs frequently, but necrosis of entire fibers is uncommon. In any event, the causes of both degeneration and necrosis are similar.

Specific morphologic types of degeneration have been described. The most common type is so-called **hyaline** or **waxy degeneration.** Affected muscles may be detected grossly by diffuse pallor or scattered pale streaks, especially when secondary calcification has occurred in damaged fibers. Microscopically, affected fibers appear swollen and hypereosinophilic, with loss of cross-striations. The altered contractile material frequently becomes fragmented into large blocks or discs scattered along the "tube" of persisting external lamina of the muscle fiber. Within 24 hours, the affected areas will be invaded by an occasional polymorphonuclear leukocyte and numerous macrophages. Macrophages are observed in the interstitium and also within injured muscle fibers. Ultrastructurally, the affected fibers show masses of disrupted contractile material tangled with damaged membranes of mitochondria, sarcoplasmic re-

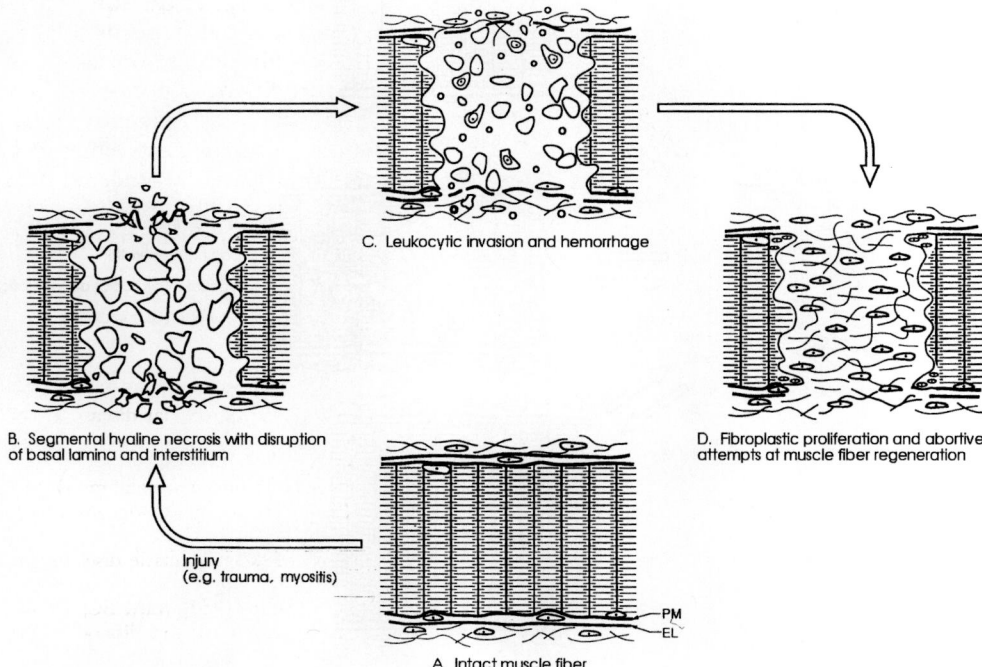

C. Leukocytic invasion and hemorrhage

B. Segmental hyaline necrosis with disruption of basal lamina and interstitium

D. Fibroplastic proliferation and abortive attempts at muscle fiber regeneration

Injury (e.g. trauma, myositis)

A. Intact muscle fiber

FIG. 18-3 Sequential events of skeletal muscle disruption and repair by fibrosis. (EL - external lamina, PM - plasma membrane).

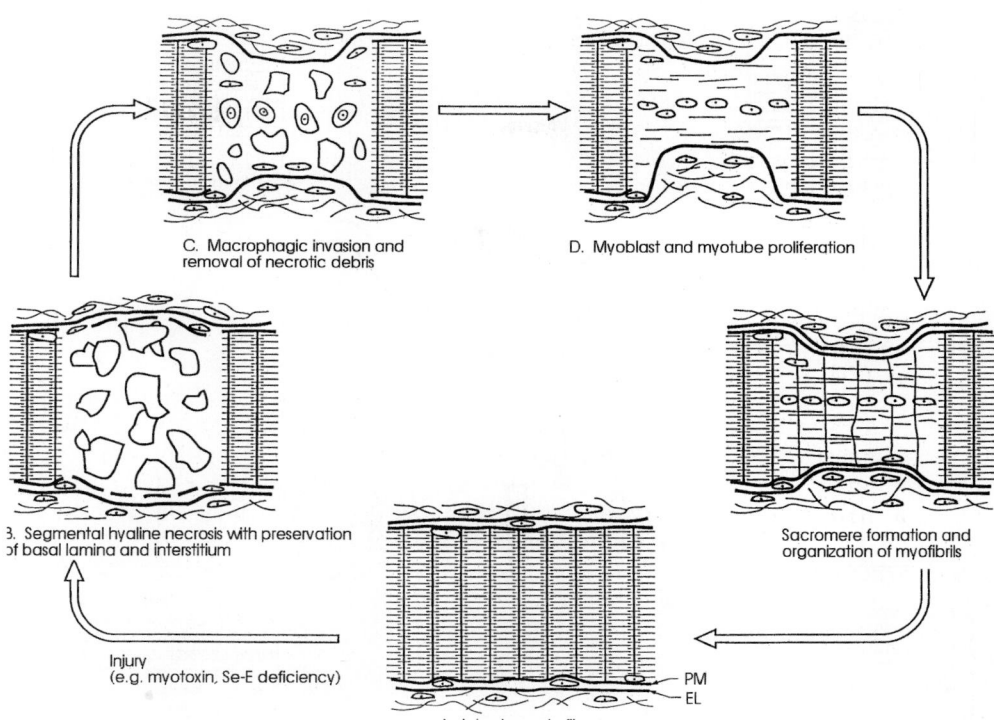

C. Macrophagic invasion and removal of necrotic debris

D. Myoblast and myotube proliferation

B. Segmental hyaline necrosis with preservation of basal lamina and interstitium

Sacromere formation and organization of myofibrils

Injury (e.g. myotoxin, Se-E deficiency)

A. Intact muscle fiber

PM
EL

FIG. 18-4 Sequential events of skeletal muscle degeneration/necrosis in skeletal muscle. (EL - external lamina, PM - plasma membrane).

ticulum, and plasmalemma. The "tube" of external lamina persists to guide regenerative events, and it may be focally disrupted to allow entry of macrophages (Figure 18-4).

Another type of degeneration described in skeletal muscle is **granular degeneration.** The microscopic appearance differs from hyaline degeneration in that the damaged contractile material appears as small basophilic granules that fill the "tube" of external lamina. The causes of granular and hyaline degeneration are similar; included are nutritional deficiencies, such as selenium/vitamin E, various myotoxic drugs and plants, and metabolic disorders, such as azoturia and capture myopathy (Van Vleet and Ferrans, 1986).

The spatial distribution and temporal pattern of lesions of degeneration and necrosis in skeletal muscle have been utilized to classify reactions: (1) **monophasic monofocal,** (2) **monophasic polyfocal,** (3) **polyphasic monofocal,** and (4) **polyphasic polyfocal** (Kakulas, 1988; Figure 18-5). Monophasic monofocal reactions result from an isolated single mechanical injury, such as external trauma or needle insertion. In monophasic polyfocal reactions, a single insult—such as exposure to various myotoxic drugs or chemicals or various metabolic disorders—may initiate widespread muscle lesions, but all the alterations are in the same phase of injury. Polyphasic monofocal reactions would be the result of repeated localized mechanical injury. Polyphasic polyfocal reactions are frequent in muscular diseases of animals, and result from continued insults applied over a prolonged time, such as from nutritional deficiencies and genetic disorders (as in muscular dystrophies). The lesions are widespread in the musculature and various pathological reactions—including necrosis, leukocytic

invasion during resolution, and regeneration—will occur concurrently.

Other less common types of degeneration in skeletal muscle fibers include **vacuolar** or **hydropic degeneration, fatty degeneration,** and **lipofuscinosis** (xanthomatosis). Vacuolar or hydropic type degeneration occurs with cortisol excess and with the inherited glycogenoses. The affected fibers have vacuolated lace-like areas in the sarcoplasm. Fatty degeneration is uncommon. It is seen as a non-specific response to injury, and it results in abundant small spherical lipid vacuoles scattered among myofibrils. Lipid deposits appear similar to vacuoles, but are less abundant, and are normally present in type I muscle fibers. Lipofuscinosis—also termed xanthomatosis when involvement is severe—occurs with cachexia, may accompany aging and chronic vitamin E deficiency in rats and mice, and is an inherited disease of Ayrshire cattle. Distinctive yellowish-brown perinuclear granules indicate the condition.

References

Bradley R, Duffell SJ. The pathology of the skeletal and cardiac muscles of cattle with xanthosis. J Comp Pathol 1982;92:85–97.

Bradley R, McKerrell RE, Barnard EA. Neuromuscular disease in animals. In: Walton J, ed. Disorders of voluntary muscle. 5th ed. New York: Churchill Livingstone, 1988;910–980.

Cullen MJ, Mastaglia FL. Pathological reactions of skeletal muscle. In: Mastaglia FL, Walton J, eds. Skeletal muscle pathology. New York: Churchill Livingstone, 1982;88–139.

DeGiorolami U, Smith TW. Pathology of skeletal muscle diseases. Am J Pathol 1982;107:235–276.

Hegreberg GA. Muscular system. In: Andrews EJ, Ward BC, Altman NH, eds. Spontaneous animal models of human disease. Vol II. New York: Academic Press, 1979;85–106.

Kakulas BA. Experimental muscle disease. In: Walton J, ed. Disorders

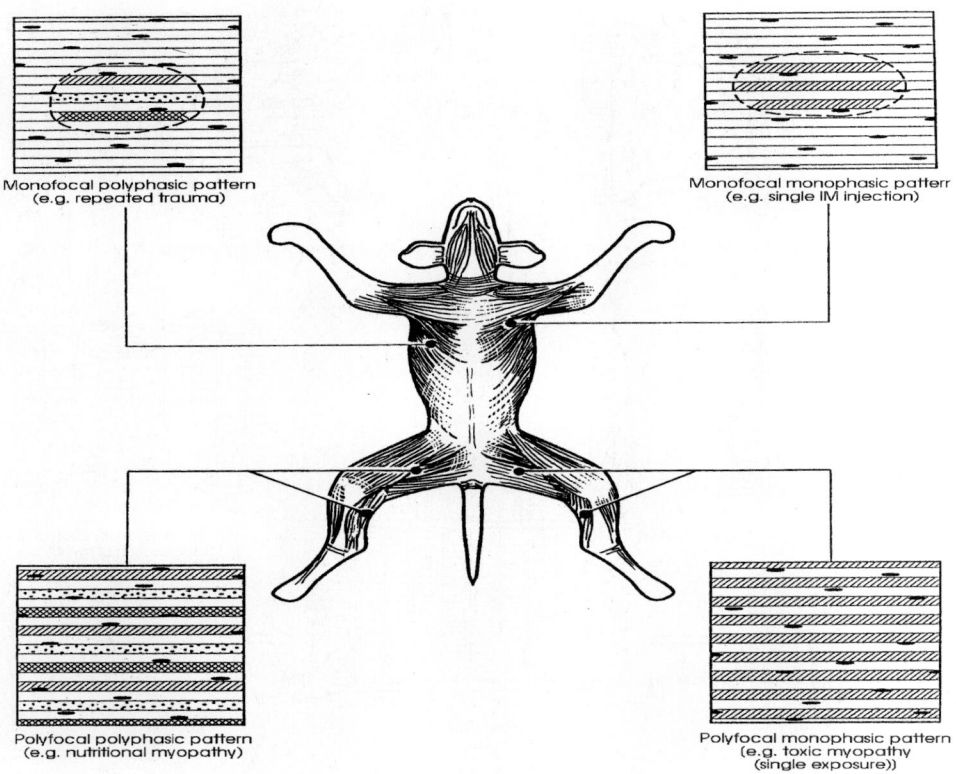

Monofocal polyphasic pattern
(e.g. repeated trauma)

Monofocal monophasic pattern
(e.g. single IM injection)

Polyfocal polyphasic pattern
(e.g. nutritional myopathy)

Polyfocal monophasic pattern
(e.g. toxic myopathy
(single exposure))

FIG. 18-5 Distribution and temporal pattern of the degenerative/necrosis in skeletal muscle.

of voluntary muscle. 5th ed. New York: Churchill Livingtone, 1988;427–454.

Scott-Moncrieff JCS, Hawkins EC, Cook JR Jr. Canine muscle disorders. Compend Contin Educ Pract Vet 1990;12:31–39.

Trump BF, et al. The role of calcium in cell injury: a review. Scan Electron Microsc 1980;2:437–462.

Van Vleet JF, Ferrans VJ. Myocardial diseases of animals. Am J Pathol 1986;124:98–178.

Wrogemann K, Pena SDJ. Mitochondrial calcium overload: a general mechanism for cell necrosis in muscle diseases. Lancet 1976;1:672–674.

Regeneration and repair

Many injuries of skeletal muscle heal by regeneration. This is especially true for the common monophasic or polyphasic polyfocal myopathies, such as those associated with nutritional deficiencies, metabolic disorders, and myotoxicities. In these diseases, extensive muscle fiber necrosis may occur; however, the scaffolding of external lamina of the muscle fiber and the innervation and blood supply to the damaged muscle are preserved; this permits regeneration, which is often virtually complete. Regeneration is further promoted in these conditions by the transient nature of the insult responsible for the muscle injury; this is in contrast to the prolonged expression of other types of insults, such as denervation or genetic derangements in those muscular diseases with limited effectiveness of regeneration. In severe muscle diseases, trauma, hemorrhage, or infection may cause extensive disruption of endomysial connective tissues and the "tubes" of external laminae of damaged myofibers; the outcome of healing will involve limited regeneration, and will be accompanied by extensive fibrosis and scarring.

The cellular events of regeneration are well-characterized, and center around the proliferation of mononucleated myogenic stem cells, termed myoblasts. Myoblasts arise from satellite cells; these are a population of resting and differentiated cells that persist in mature skeletal muscle and appear morphologically as very thin cells that lie between the plasma membrane and the external lamina of myofibers. For unknown reasons, satellite cells tend to be resistant to many insults that destroy mature myofibers. Following selective destruction of skeletal muscle fibers, the sarcoplasmic debris is removed rapidly by invasion of macrophages and phagocytic lysis. The persisting sarcolemmal "tubes" of external lamina rapidly become populated by elongated myoblasts. These myoblasts have large vesicular nuclei and prominent basophilic sarcoplasm that reflect the numerous polysomes present and the intense synthesis of cellular proteins in these cells. Myoblasts fuse to form multinucleated cells, termed sarcoblasts, which further elongate to form myotubes; these myotubes rapidly bridge the gap of disrupted sarcoplasm in damaged myofibers. Myotubes have rows of centrally located nuclei and peripheral masses of forming contractile myofilaments that soon become oriented into sarcomeres and myofibrils with restoration of cross-striations in the immature myofibers. Subsequently, the central nuclei will migrate to their normal subsarcolemmal location—as seen in mature fibers—and the regenerated muscle fibers may then be indistinguishable from adjacent fibers that have not suffered injury.

References

Kakulas BA. Experimental muscle diseases. In: Walton J, ed. Disorders of voluntary muscle. 5th ed. New York: Churchill Livingstone, 1988;389–416.

Reznik M. Current concepts of skeletal muscle regeneration. In: Pearson EM, Mostofi FK, eds. The striated muscle., Baltimore: Williams and Wilkins, 1973;185–225.

Schmalbrunch H. The morphology of regeneration of skeletal muscles in the rat. Tissue Cell 1976;8:673–692.

Snow MH. Origin of regenerating myoblasts in mammalian skeletal muscle. In: Mauro A, et al., eds. Muscle regeneration. New York: Raven Press, 1979;91–100.

Van Vleet JF. Pathological reactions of skeletal muscle to injury. In: Jones TC, Mohr U, Hunt RD, eds. ILSI monographs on pathology of laboratory animals: cardiovascular and musculoskeletal systems. New York: Springer Verlag, 1991;109–126.

Nutritional myopathy (white muscle disease)

The most susceptible species to nutritional myopathy are sheep, cattle, and pigs. Horses and goats are moderately susceptible. The disease also occurs in a wide variety of avian and laboratory animals, as well as in wild and fur-bearing animals, such as mink. Rapidly growing animals appear to be more susceptible. Nutritional myopathy typically occurs throughout the livestock-producing areas of the world, in late winter or early spring. The severity of muscle lesions may vary within a species and according to strain, a finding reported in the mouse.

The disease is due to a deficiency of vitamin E and/or selenium, and a variety of environmental and nutritional variables interact to either initiate or modify the disease process. Diets high in polyunsaturated fatty acids enhance the severity of the disease because they destroy or increase the dietary requirement for vitamin E. Low intake of sulfur-containing amino acids also makes animals more susceptible. Certain elements—silver, mercury, copper, cobalt, and cadmium—are antagonistic to selenium bioavailability and increase the dietary need for selenium. Exposure to pro-oxidants—such as ozone and iron—predisposes the animal to a deficiency of vitamin E and the development of muscle disease.

The enzyme glutathione peroxidase requires the element selenium and has decreased activity in the deficiency state. This enzyme, together with vitamin E found in the lipid component of cellular membranes, functions to protect membranes from peroxidation and free radical injury. These interactions are discussed further in Chapter 16.

In **cattle**, nutritional myopathy is most often observed in young beef calves 4–6 weeks of age, in dairy and beef calves 6–12 months of age, and in pregnant heifers. Calves may have the disease *in utero*. Outbreaks are associated with diets of poor quality hays and roughages for prolonged periods, and are often apparently precipitated by some unaccustomed physical activity. The incidence is increased in the spring, when calves are first placed in pasture; this involves a sudden increase in their exercise, often during inclement weather. The disease occurs predominantly in young animals. The incidence has increased in cattle, due to the replacement of proteins with urea; low dietary intakes of vitamin E, caused by reduced content in grains after treatment of moist grains with propionic acid, also result in increased disease. Affected calves have a stiff, shuffling gait; some become recumbent with signs of difficult respiration, and some die with signs of respiratory failure. Some calves have myoglobinuria; in these cases, the activity of creatine kinase is increased in the serum of affected cattle in proportion to the severity of the muscle lesions. Pregnant heifers with nutritional myopathy may also have increased incidence of abortion, stillbirths, and recumbency after parturition. Cardiac lesions in calves can result in increased mortality.

Gross lesions are observed when calcification is extensive; the lesions consist of white opaque flecks, patches, and streaks within skeletal muscle and the myocardium, especially of the left ventricle (Figure 18-6). Lesions are often extensive in the large muscles of the thigh and shoulder, but they are also found in the tongue and muscles of the neck.

Histopathologic alterations are described as polyphasic and polyfocal; they include hypercontracted myofibers that are larger than adjacent fibers; they are also rounded, hyaline, and intensely eosinophilic, with loss of striations. Myofibers undergo necrosis, with fragmentation of sarcoplasm and loss of sarcoplasm. Necrotic sarcoplasm undergoes calcification. Macrophages invade necrotic fibers and remove sarcoplasmic debris. Satellite-cell proliferation—with myotube formation—is extensive, and repair may be complete. Type I myofibers are preferentially affected, but not exclusively. Normal myofibers occur adjacent to necrotic muscle cells.

In **sheep**, nutritional myopathy is common in many regions of the world, affecting lambs at 2–4 weeks of age and 4–8 months of age, often in association with changes in diet. Precipitating factors for development of nutritional myopathy include: changes in weather; changes in diet, such as feeds low in selenium or vitamin E; and forced, increased, and unaccustomed activity.

Nutritional myopathy occurs in **pigs** as a result of selenium-vitamin E deficiency; however, other lesions of selenium-vitamin E deficiency are more common in pigs, such as **hepatosis dietetica** (more likely to be due to selenium deficiency) and **mulberry-heart disease.** Pigs of a wide age range may have skeletal muscle lesions; however, usually recently weaned pigs are affected. The injection of iron compounds to prevent anemia can result in an acute fatal myopathy in pigs only a few days old. These neonatal pigs are more susceptible because of their low vitamin E status, and because of the marked pro-oxidant activity of the injected iron. The iron-catalyzed lipid peroxidation causes membrane damage because peroxides are doubled in injected muscle.

With vitamin E-selenium deficiency, gross lesions are few in skeletal muscle; usually lesions are present in the liver and heart. Microscopic lesions are present and consist of myofiber degeneration and necrosis, macrophage invasion, phagocytosis, and regeneration. Regen-

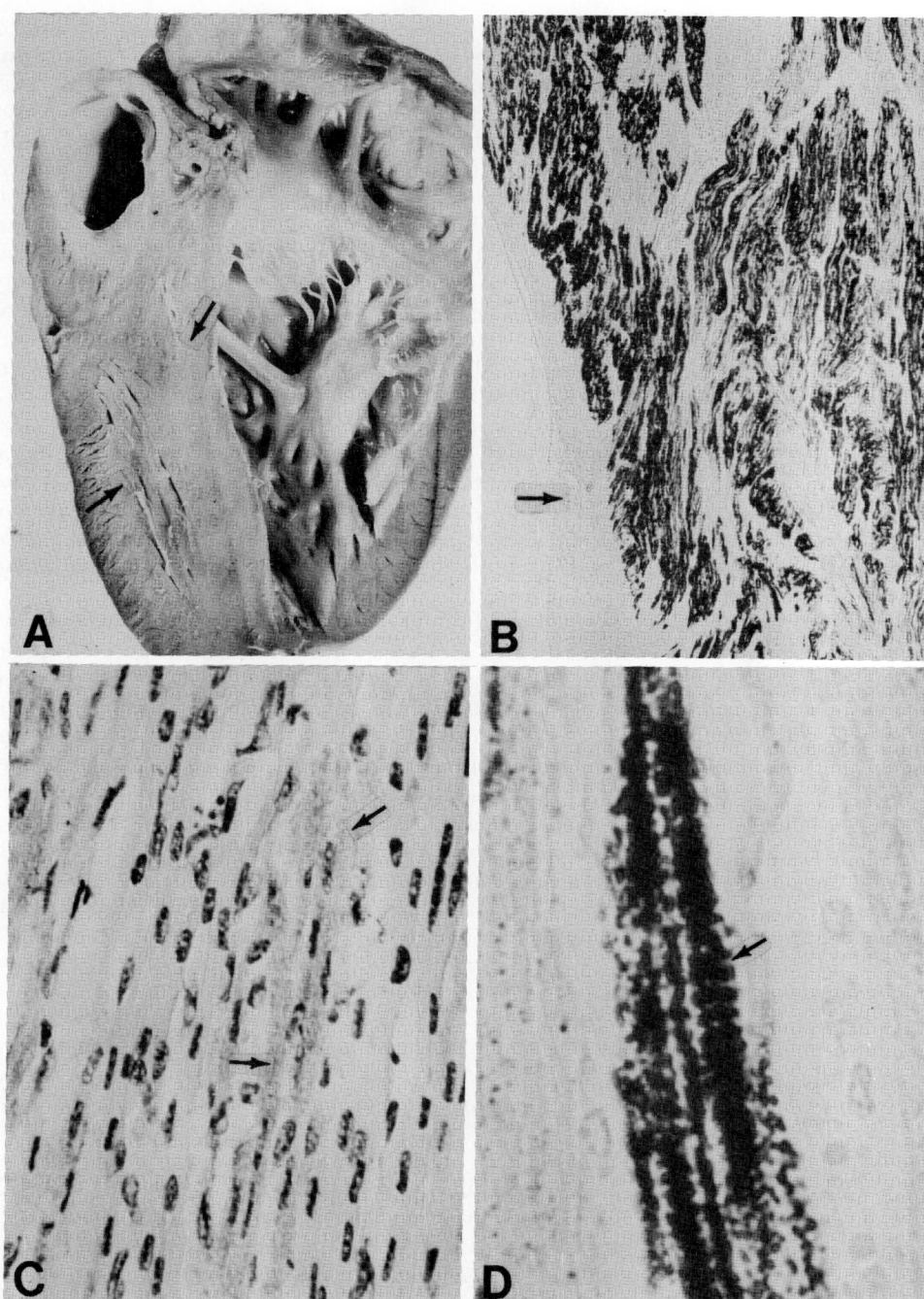

FIG. 18-6 Nutritional muscular degeneration in the heart of a newborn lamb. **A.** Gray areas in the myocardium (arrows). **B.** Section of myocardium (×45) stained with von Kossa method to demonstrate salts of calcium (black). Arrow indicates the endocardium. **C.** Another section (×515) stained with hematoxylin and eosin. Note dark granules (arrows) in fibers of cardiac muscle. **D.** Another section (×600) stained with von Kossa method. Note calcium salts (arrow), which outline the cross-striations. (Courtesy of Armed Forces Institute of Pathology; contributor: Dr. O. H. Muth.)

eration is rapid and may be complete in surviving pigs. Type I myofibers are principally involved in the degenerative process. The pattern of the distribution of necrotic myofibers is determined by the distribution of type I myofibers, which may be grouped in certain regions of certain muscles.

Foals have a myopathic disease much like vitamin E-selenium deficiency in cattle, sheep, and swine. The disease has also been described in adult horses.

Affected foals have lesions in the muscles of the shoulder, neck, and thigh; these lesions may be bilateral and locally extensive. Grossly, the lesions are opaque chalk-like flecks and streaks within muscles. The gross lesions represent calcification of necrotic myofibers. Some foals also have degeneration, necrosis, and calcification of the myocardium and necrotizing steatitis.

Nutritional myopathy is a rare disease in **dogs**; however, it and has been produced experimentally and has been observed in dogs with biliary fistula. In dogs, vitamin E-selenium deficiency is manifested by acute myocardial necrosis, as well as in skeletal muscle degeneration.

Nutritional myopathy due to deficiency of vitamin E-selenium is now a rare disease in **cats, mink,** and

foxes. In these species, hypovitaminosis E produces steatitis (pansteatitis), and is associated with diets increased in rancid unsaturated fats.

STEATITIS

Steatitis (yellow fat disease) is an inflammatory disease of adipose tissue. In cats, it is associated with diets with an increased concentration of fish, particularly red tuna. Affected cats have such signs as anorexia, fever, and leukocytosis; pain may occur on palpation of regions with deposits of adipose tissue, such as the abdomen and dorsal lumbar area. Microscopically, cellular infiltrates are present in the affected adipose tissue; also present may be deposits of ceroid, an acid-fast waxy yellow-brown pigment. Fat necrosis accompanies the neutrophilic infiltrates. In some foci the inflammatory reaction is granulomatous, with numerous epithelioid cells and Langhans-type giant cells.

Guinea pigs and rabbits are suitable species for the experimental production of myodegeneration of selenium-vitamin E deficiency. However, mice and rats are relatively resistant to the induction of nutritional myopathy. Naturally occurring nutritional myopathy is rare in laboratory animals, but has been observed in guinea pigs and rabbits.

References

Goedegebuure SA. Spontaneous primary myopathies in domestic mammals: a review. Vet Q 1987;9:155–171.

Kennedy S, Rice DA, Davidson WB. Experimental myopathy in vitamin E and selenium-depleted calves with and without dietary polyunsaturated fatty acids as a model for nutritional degeneration myopathy in ruminant cattle. Res Vet Sci 1987;43:384–394.

Kroneman J, Wensvoort P. Muscular dystrophy and yellow fat disease in Shetland pony foals. Neth J Vet Sci 1968;1:42.

Lannek N, Lindberg P. Vitamin E and selenium deficiencies (VESD) of domestic animals. Adv Vet Sci Comp Med 1976;19:127–164.

Nafstad I, Tollersrud S. The vitamin E-deficiency syndrome in pigs. I. Pathological changes. Acta Vet Scand 1970;11:452–480.

Nelson JS. Pathology of vitamin E deficiency. In: Machlin LJ, ed. Vitamin E: a comprehensive treatise. New York: Marcel Decker, 1980;397–428.

Ruth GR, Van Vleet JF. Experimentally induced selenium-vitamin E deficiency in growing swine: selective destructive of type I skeletal muscle fibers. Am J Vet Res 1974;35:237–244.

Van Vleet JF. Experimentally induced vitamin E-selenium deficiency in the growing dog. J Am Vet Med Assoc 1975;166:769–774.

Van Vleet JF. Amounts of 12 elements required to induce selenium-vitamin E deficiency in ducklings. Am J Vet Res 1982;43:851–857.

Exertion-induced myopathies

Exertional disease syndromes include equine exertional rhabdomyolysis, azoturia, porcine stress syndrome, and capture myopathy. **Equine exertional rhabdomyolysis,** (also known as "tying up"), and **azoturia** (also termed "paralytic myoglobinuria" or "Monday morning disease") are similar disorders; however, the former is generally mild, whereas the latter is often fatal. Both disorders occur in working horses following a few days of rest while on full rations. The diseases have similar clinical and pathologic features, consisting of variably severe gait abnormalities after periods of intense exercise. Horses have such signs as trembling, profuse sweating, and recumbency. Serum activities of creatine kinase, aldolase, and aspartate aminotransferase are increased in most circumstances; the increase in activities roughly correlate with the severity of clinical signs and skeletal muscle lesions.

Gross and microscopic lesions may vary in severity, depending on the time of examination after the period of exercise (Figure 18-7). Grossly, muscles have foci of

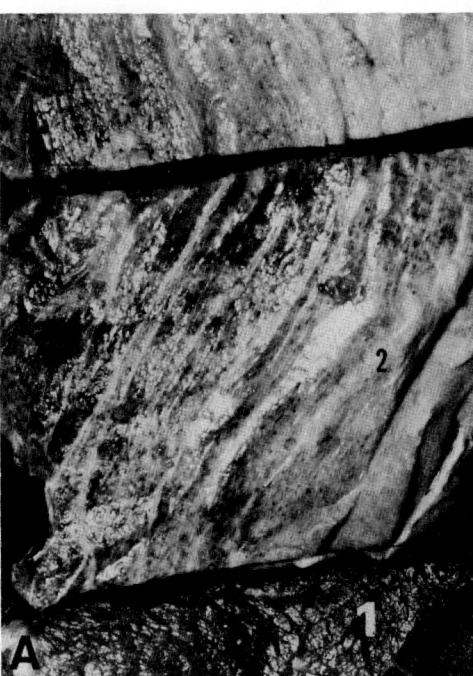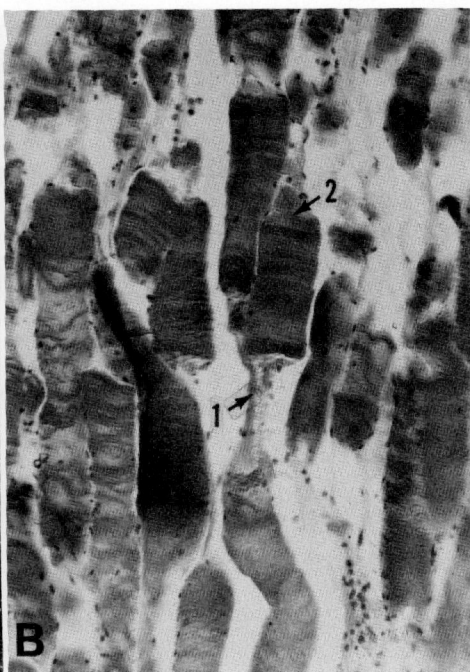

FIG. 18-7 Equine rhabdomyolysis. **A.** Muscle of a year-old colt tangled in halter rope (lived three days). (1) Normal dark red muscle; (2) Compare with white and degenerating muscle. (Courtesy College of Vet. Med., Iowa State University). **B.** Microscopic view of muscle fibers (×180). (1) Note atrophy; and (2) Enlargement. The latter appeared dark red and shiny in the section stained with hematoxylin and eosin. (Courtesy College of Vet. Med, Iowa State University).

discoloration and hemorrhages; the kidneys may be swollen and congested; and the urinary bladder may contain brown urine (myoglobinuria). Microscopically, myofiber degeneration and necrosis is characterized by swollen eosinophilic, hyaline, fragmented myofibers, with loss of striations in acute cases. In time, macrophages infiltrate areas of necrosis; phagocytosis is followed by regeneration in muscles of surviving animals. Renal tubular necrosis with myoglobin casts may be observed in cases of exertional rhabdomyolysis.

HERTZTOD

"Porcine stress syndrome," "malignant hyperthermia," and "back muscle necrosis" have also been termed hertztod and appear to represent a single syndrome. This syndrome is characterized by marked hyperthermia, and by severe acidosis associated with necrosis of skeletal muscle, particularly of the back muscles. Other muscles and the myocardium may also be affected. The stress of handling or transportation may cause the disorder in susceptible swine; they may die before lesions of myodegeneration are apparent. The susceptible genotype is probably an autosomal dominant trait that leads to abnormal regulation of muscle cell calcium; the release of increased levels of calcium into the myoplasm stimulates oxidative phosphorylation and glycolysis. Halothane anesthesia may also precipitate the disease in genetically predisposed swine, dogs, cats, horses, and humans. Lesions are characterized by muscular edema, hypercontraction, fragmentation, and granular degeneration.

CAPTURE MYOPATHY IN WILD ANIMALS

Conservation efforts involving capture and transport of large wild mammals has led to the recognition of an important disease termed capture myopathy ("exertional rhabdomyolysis," "overstraining disease," and "white muscle disease"). The condition becomes evident following the severe physical exertion associated with capture; the musculature is obviously involved, and myoglobinuria often occurs. The signs vary: some animals undergo severe depression, others have fever and muscular fibrillation; the animal may be reluctant to move, or may continually shift its weight from one leg to another. Convulsions, torticollis, or opisthotonos may be followed by paralysis and death in two to four days. Less severely affected animals may survive for two weeks to a month, and then succumb. In some species (zebras), severe acidosis has been recognized immediately following capture.

Grossly, the lesions observed in the muscles consist of sharply demarcated zones of hemorrhage; pale muscle is also apparent, and may be soft and gelatinous. The lesions are usually bilateral, but rarely symmetric. The kidneys are swollen and dark brown, and myoglobin may be demonstrated in the urinary bladder. Hemorrhages are evident in all layers of the adrenal cortex.

Levels of creatine kinase, glutamic oxaloacetic transaminase, and lactic dehydrogenase in the serum are all elevated. Blood pH may be decreased (6.5–6.45). The microscopic lesions in the skeletal muscles, with

calcification, are characteristic of Zenker necrosis. The renal lesions consist of tubular necrosis, acute glomerular degeneration, and necrosis.

The features of this syndrome in wild animals clearly resemble those of exertional rhabdomyolysis of equines and humans, as well as porcine stress syndrome. Further research may clarify whether the precise causal mechanisms of capture myopathy are the same as those of these other conditions.

References

Arighi M, Baird JD, Hulland TJ. Equine exertional rhabdomyolysis. Compend Contin Educ Pract Vet 1984;6:726–730.

Bartsch RC, McConnell EE, Imes GD, Schmidt JM. A review of exertional rhabdomyolysis in wild and domestic animals and man. Vet Pathol 1977;14:314–324.

Chalmers GA, Barrett MW. Capture myopathy. In: Huff GL, Davis JW, eds. Noninfectious diseases of wildlife. Ames: Iowa State Univ Press, 1982;84–94.

Christian LL, Lundstrom K. Porcine stress syndrome. In: Leman AD, et al., eds. Diseases of swine. 7th ed. Ames: Iowa State Univ Press, 1992;763–771.

Dodman NH, William R, Court MH, Norman WM. Postanesthetic hind limb adductor myopathy in five horses. J Am Vet Med Assoc 1988;193:83–86.

Done JT, Allen WM, Bailey J, DeGrunchy PH, Curran MK. Asymmetric hindquarter syndrome (AA-QS) in the pig. Vet Rec 1975;96:482–488.

Friend SCE. Postanesthetic myonecrosis in horses. Can Vet J 1981; 22:367–371.

Grandy JL, Steffey EP, Hodgson DS, Woliner MJ. Arterial hypotension and the development of postanesthetic myopathy in halothane-anesthetized horses. Am J Vet Res 1987;48:192–197.

Gronert GA. Malignant hyperthermia. Anesthesiology 1980;53:395–423.

Harthoorn AM, Young E. A relationship between acid-base balance and capture myopathy in zebra (Equus burchelli) and an apparent therapy. Vet Rec 1974;95:337–342.

Lindholm A, Johansson AE, Kjaersgaard P. Acute rhabdomyolysis (tying up) in standardbred horses. Acta Vet Scand 1974;15:325–339.

Lopez JR, Allen, PD, Alamo L, Jones D, Sreter FA. Myoplasmic free (Ca2+) during a malignant hyperthermia episode in swine. Muscle Nerve 1988;11:82–88.

McEwen SA, Hulland TJ. Histochemical and morphometric evaluation of skeletal muscle from horses with exertional rhabdomyolysis (tying up). Vet Pathol 1986;23:400–410.

Mugera GM, Wanders JG. Degenerative polymyopathies in East Africa domestic and wild animals. Vet Rec 1967;80:410–413.

Nelson TE. Malignant hyperthermia in dogs. J Am Vet Med Assoc 1994;198:989–994.

Owen R. Dystrophic myodegeneration in adult horses. J Am Vet Med Assoc 1977;171:343–349,.

Wallace RS, Bush M, Montali RJ. Deaths from exertional myopathy at the National Zoological Park from 1975 to 1985. J Wildl Dis 1987;23:454–462.

Myopathy of endocrinopathies

Myopathic changes have been described in some dogs with hypothyroidism, and in dogs with hyperadrenocorticism. Symmetric hair loss, thyroid damage, and atrophy of the skin may occur in obese hypothyroid dogs; variation in myofiber diameter may also occur, due to atrophy and hypertrophy. The atrophic fibers are predominantly type II.

Dogs with hyperadrenocorticism have clinical signs

of polydipsia, polyuria, alopecia, and pendulous abdomen. Muscular weakness, hindlimb spasticity, and generalized muscle atrophy are seen in affected dogs. Myopathic alterations include: variation in myofiber diameter; focal or multifocal internal nuclei; splitting myofibers; myofiber necrosis; phagocytosis; and focal perimysial and endomysial fibrosis.

References

Afifi AK, Bergman RA. Steroid myopathy—a study of the evolution of the muscle lesion in rabbits. Johns Hopkins Med J 1969;124:66–86.

Braund KG, Dillon AR, August JR, Ganjam UK. Hypothyroid myopathy in two dogs. Vet Pathol 1981;18:589–598.

Braund KG, Dillon AR, Mikeal RL, August JR. Subclinical myopathy associated with hyperadrenocorticism in the dog. Vet Pathol 1980;17:134–148.

Greene CE, et al. Myopathy associated with hyperadrenocorticism in the dog. J Am Vet Med Assoc 1979;174:1310–1315.

Toxic myopathy

The normal structure and function of skeletal muscle can be altered by a variety of chemicals and drugs (Table 18-3). Toxic myopathy of animals has occurred from exposure to ionophores that have been used as growth promotants and coccidiostats. Horses are uniquely susceptible to ionophore toxicity; ruminants are moderately susceptible, and birds are resistant. Myotoxicity may also be caused by exposure to gossypol (in cottonseed oil meal) or to certain plants (*Cassia spp., Karwinskia sp., Thermopsis sp., Eupatorium sp.*). Sensitivity to toxic agents may be enhanced because these substances tend to bind to skeletal muscle. Skeletal muscle dysfunction or damage has been induced by both indirect and direct mechanisms. Muscular atrophy can develop when interruptions occur in peripheral motor nerve function. No significant morphologic changes appear during neuromuscular blockade, and the blockade is usually reversed when the causative substance is removed. In some instances, toxicants have induced muscle necrosis by dramatically increasing motor nerve activity, or by allowing significant amounts of acetylcholine to accumulate at the myoneural junction.

A toxicant may also induce toxicity indirectly by provoking immunologic reactions that lead to generalized muscle weakness. Some toxicants may exert localized toxicity when injected into or near the muscle. Focal damage has occurred following intramuscular injection of narcotic analgesics and oxytetracycline. Agents such as pentazocine and meperidine cause a severe fibrotic reaction. Other toxicants can produce diffuse muscle damage when given systemically. The cell membrane represents an important cellular component that is usually exposed to the highest concentration of a substance. A change in electrical properties can occur when a substance alters the cell membrane.

Dioxocholesterol interferes with the biosynthesis of cholesterol; as a result, an accumulation of excessive amounts of desmosterol occurs in the cell membrane, leading to excessive chloride permeability and myoto-

nia. Myotonia also occurs, following exposure to the herbicidal compound 2, dichlorophenoxyacetic acid (2,4–D). Monensin, an Na + -selective carboxylic acid ionophore, consistently causes both skeletal and cardiac muscle necrosis in a variety of animals. Evidence suggests that these effects are due to calcium overloading. Injection of type A *Clostridium perfringens* toxin induces a unique myopathy. This toxin initially causes alterations in the muscle cell membrane.

Toxicants have been found to produce alterations in the sarcoplasmic reticulum. Intraperitoneal injections of doxorubicin have caused damage to the diaphragm muscle; this effect is associated with cytoplasmic vacuolization, due to dilation of the sarcoplasmic reticulum. Similarities exist in the myotoxic effects of colchicine and vincristine, both of which are known to interfere with the function of microtubules. Myofilamentous degeneration occurs following treatment with plasmocid. The agent causes selective loss of Z and I bands in the rat diaphragm and in cardiac muscle.

Certain amphiphilic cationic agents with diverse pharmacologic actions cause a myopathy that includes lysosomal phospholipid accumulation; this effect takes the form of large masses of concentric lamellae with peculiar structures known as curvilinear bodies. The antimalarial chloroquine is associated with this type of myopathy, as are aminodarone and perhexiline (Chapter 2).

A potentially serious drug-induced condition—characterized by muscular rigidity and myoglobinuria, hypermetabolism, and metabolic acidosis—occurs in genetically susceptible people undergoing routine surgery. Malignant hyperthermia is commonly precipitated in these individuals by exposure to halothane and succinylcholine. Other halogenated anesthetic agents, nitrous oxide, muscle relaxants, and certain local anesthetic agents may also induce this reaction. A condition similar to the human syndrome has been described in certain strains of pigs. Susceptible pigs are sensitive to stress and develop muscle rigidity, acidosis, and hyperkalemia. Death ensues due to heart failure when these pigs are subjected to stress. These sensitive pigs also react to halothane and depolarizing neuromuscular blocking agents. The malignant hyperthermic reaction appears due to an alteration in muscular control of intracellular calcium levels. Acute increases in this cation cause contracture of muscle fibers, decreased ATP levels, increased metabolism and temperature, and secondary changes in a variety of cellular components.

Prolonged corticosteroid therapy is known to cause a skeletal muscle myopathy. Those steroids—which are fluorinated in the 9 position (triamcinolone, dexamethasone, and betamethasone)—are most likely to be myotoxic; however, continuous treatment with any of the corticosteroids will also lead to a myopathy.

Prenatal exposure of rats to 6–mercaptopurine has led, after a latent period, to a continuous and progressive atrophic degeneration of muscle cells. These myotoxic effects are not seen when 6–mercaptopurine is administered during the postnatal period.

TABLE 18-3 Toxicants affecting skeletal muscle

Agents that induce necrosis and degeneration of muscle cells

Ionophores (e.g., monensin, lasalocid, narasin)
Oxytetracycline, others (intramuscular injection sites)
Corticosteroids
Antimalarials (e.g., choloroquine, plasmocid)
Others (e.g., iron dextran, selenium, dimethylsulfoxide, colchicine, 2, 4-D)
Toxic plants (*Cassia occidentalis, C. obtusifolia, Karwinskia humboltiana, Eupatorium rugosum, Trigonella foenumgraecum, Petiveria alliacea*)
Plant product [gossypol—*Gossypium* spp. (cottonseed oil meal)]
Animal toxins (snake venoms)
Bacterial toxins (*Clostridium chauvoei, C. septicum, C. novyi, C. perfringens*)
Mycotoxins (cyclopiazonic acid, tremorgans)

Agents that precipitate malignant hyperthermia episodes

Halothane, succinylcholine, other halogenated anesthetics, nitrous oxide, local anesthetics

Agents that alter protein synthesis

Corticosteroids (triamcinolone, dexamethasone, betamethasone)

Agents that cause immunologic modulations

D-penicillamine, procainamide

Agents that induce physical injury at intramuscular injection sites

Oxytetracycline, meperidine

Agents that induce cell membrane alterations in muscle fibers

Dioxocholesterol, 2,4-D, ionophores, type A *Clostridium perfringens* toxin, clofibrate

Agents that induce sarcoplasmic reticular alterations in muscle fibers

Doxorubicin

Agents that induce microtubular alterations in muscle fibers

Colchicine, vincristine

Agents that induce myofilament alterations in muscle fibers

Plasmocid, emetine

Agents that induce lysosomal alterations in muscle fibers

Amiodarone, chloroquine, perhexiline

Agents that alter neurogenic function

Neuromuscular blockage—aminoglycoside antibiotics
Increased motor nerve activity—heroin, amphetamine
Acetylcholine accumulation—cholinesterase inhibitors (paraoxon)
Denervation atrophy—antimicrobial agents (isoniazid, nitrofurantoin, sulfonamides, clioquinol, metronidazole, amphotericin B), antineoplastic agents (vincristine, procarbazine, nitrofurazone, cytosine arabinoside podophyllir, chlorambucil, antirheumatic drugs (gold, colchicine, chloroquine, indomethacin, phenylbutazone), hypnotics and psychotropics (thalidomide, methoqualone, glutethimide), cardiovascular drugs (perhexiline, amiodarone, hydralazine, disopyramide, clofibrate,

TABLE 18-3 (continued)

digitalis), and other drugs (phenytoin, disulfiram, dapsone, ergotamine, methimazole, propylthiouracil, methylthiouracil).

Agents that alter muscle cell differentiation

6-Mercaptopurine

Agents that produce neuromuscular blockage but no morphologic alterations

Aminoglycoside antibiotics (neomycin, kanamycin, streptomycin, gentamycin), polypeptide antibiotics (polymyxin B, colistins), other antibiotics (oxytetracycline, rolitetracycline, lincomycin, clindamycin), antirheumatic drugs (D-penicillamine, chloroquine), cardiovascular drugs (oxprenolol, practolol, quinidine, procainamide, propranolol, anticonvulsants (trimethadione, phenytoin) psychotropic drugs (lithium, chlorpromazine, promazine, phenelzine), anesthetics (diazepam, ketamine, propenidid, ether), and other drugs (busulfan, oral contraceptives, methoxyflurane, ACTH, corticosteroids, thyroid hormones, anticholinesterases, oxytocin, aprotinin, procaine, lidocaine).

Agents that produce myotonia but no morphologic alterations

20, 25-Diazacholesterol, propranolol, suxamethonium

References

Amend JF, Mallon FM, Wren WB, Ramos AS. Equine monensin toxicosis: some experimental clinicopathologic observations. Compend Contin Educ Pract Vet 1980;2:S173–S183.

Argov Z, Mastaglia FL. Drug-induced neuromuscular disorders in man. In: Walton J, ed. Disorders of voluntary muscle. 5th ed. New York: Churchill Livingstone, 1988;981–1014.

Baker DC, Keeler RF. Thermopsis montana-induced myopathy in calves. J Am Vet Med Assoc 1989;194:1269–1272.

Janzen ED, Radostits OM, Orr JP. Possible monensin poisoning in a group of bulls. Can Vet J 1981;22:92–94.

Kakulas BA. Skeletal muscle. In: Riddell RH, ed. Pathology of drug-induced and toxic diseases. New York: Churchill Livingstone, 1982;49–69.

Lane RJM, Mastaglia FL. Drug-induced myopathies in man. Lancet 1978;2:562–566.

Mastaglia FL. Adverse effects of drugs on muscle. Drugs 1982;24:304–321.

Mastaglia FL, Argov Z. Drug-induced myopathies and disorders of neuromuscular transmission. In: Manzo L, et al., eds. Advances in neurotoxicology. Oxford: Pergamon, 1981;319–328.

Nation PN, Crowe SP, Harries WN. Clinical signs and pathology of accidental monensin poisoning in sheep. Can Vet J 1982;23:323–326.

Umemura T, Kawaminami A, Goryo M, Itakara C. Enhanced myotoxicity and involvement of both type I and II fibers in monensin-tiamulin toxicosis in pigs. Vet Pathol 1985;22:409–414.

Van Vleet JF, Ferrans MA. Ultrastructural alterations in skeletal muscle of pigs with acute monensin myotoxicosis. Am J Pathol 1984;114:461–471.

Van Vleet JF, Amstutz HE, Weirich WE, Rebar AH, Ferrans VJ. [1] Acute monensin toxicosis in swine: effect of graded doses of monensin and protection of swine by pretreatment with selenium-vitamin E. [2] Clinical, clinicopathologic, and pathologic alterations of monensin toxicsis in swine. [3] Clinical, clinicopathologic, and pathologic alterations in acute monensin toxicosis of cattle. Am J Vet Res 1983;44:1460–1468, 1469–1475, 2133–2144.

Van Vleet JF, Ferrans VJ, Herman E. Cardiovascular and skeletal muscular systems. In: Haschek-Hock W, Rosseaux C, eds. Fundamentals of toxicologic pathology. New York: Academic Press, 1991;539–624.

Wilson JS. Toxic myopathy in a dog associated with the presence of monensin in dry food. Can Vet J 1980;21:30–31.

CIRCULATORY DISORDERS

Hemorrhage

In hemorrhage, the interstitial tissues are distended by extravasated erythrocytes. Causes include physical trauma, hemorrhagic diathesis, and conditions with extensive vascular damage, such as hemorrhagic myositis and septicemia.

Ischemia

Factors which operate to prevent ischemic injury of skeletal muscle include the rich vascular supply to this tissue and the presence of collateral arterial circulation. However, occasional instances occur in animals where ischemic necrosis develops. Arterial thrombosis of major vessels—as in aorto-iliac thrombosis of cats or horses—may result in ischemic necrosis of hindlimb muscles, unless collateral blood flow is adequate. Increases in intramuscular pressure may result in ischemic injury, as seen in the conditions termed: compartment syndrome, downer syndrome, muscle-crush syndrome, and postanesthesia myopathy in horses; and deep pectoral myopathy of turkeys and chickens. When ischemia is of short duration, the muscular lesions may be partially or even completely repaired by regeneration. However, prolonged ischemic damage will heal with extensive fibroblastic proliferation and scarring of the damaged muscle.

DEEP PECTORAL MYOPATHY

This myopathy has been described in turkeys and chickens; it involves the deep pectoral muscles, and is caused by ischemia following variable periods of muscular contraction. The supracoracoid muscle is enclosed in an inelastic osteofascial compartment, and this compartment prevents the free expansion of the muscle during exercise, resulting in vascular occlusion with development of ischemic necrosis. Grossly, focal or diffuse greenish discoloration is apparent in either one or both of the deep pectoral muscles, especially the middle portion; the muscle may consist of a green brittle core of necrotic tissue. Acutely affected muscles are swollen, edematous, and pale; the muscle may have a parboiled appearance. In older lesions, the middle and posterior thirds may be dry, necrotic, encapsulated, pink, or green; or, they may be reduced to a band of fibrous and adipose tissue. Microscopically, heterophil infiltrates and hemorrhages are present at the periphery of necrotic muscle, along with some macrophages and multinucleated muscle giant cells.

References

Siller WG, Wight PAL. The pathology of deep pectoral myopathy of turkeys. Avian Pathol 1978;7:583–617.

Siller WG, Wight PAL, Martindale L. Exercise-induced deep pectoral myopathy in broiler fowls and turkeys. Vet Sci Commun 1979;2:331–336.

Wight PAL, Siller WG, Martindale L. The sequence of pathological events in deep pectoral myopathy of broilers. Avian Pathol 1981;10:57–76.

INFLAMMATION—MYOSITIS

In myositis, the central focus of the tissue reaction involves the interstitial tissue components; this contrasts with common degenerative myopathies, where the foci center on alterations within the muscle fibers. The interstitial reaction in myositis is characterized by: influx of inflammatory cells and serous fluid; vascular congestion; and proliferation of interstitial connective tissue cells, as seen in any organ during inflammation. However, overlap occurs in the microscopic alterations of myositis and myopathy; myositis may have accompanying secondary damage to muscle fibers; primary degenerative myopathies with segmental necrosis of fibers also will elicit an influx of inflammatory cells into the area of damage. Thus, there may be some instances where it is difficult to determine whether the primary event in the altered muscle is inflammatory or degenerative in origin.

The types of inflammation observed in muscle are generally either hemorrhagic, necrotizing, suppurative, eosinophilic, or granulomatous. The duration of the reaction may be acute, subacute, or chronic. Most frequently, myositis in animals is associated with infections by various bacterial, viral, protozoal, or helminthic agents; some cases, however, are immunologically-mediated or, as yet, idiopathic.

Clostridial myositis

Clostridial infections of the skeletal muscle of domestic animals include malignant edema and blackleg (cattle and sheep) and gangrenous dermatomyositis (chickens and turkeys). The gram-positive, anaerobic, spore-forming clostridial bacilli produce rapidly progressive and fatal infections in animals; certain species of bacilli attack skeletal muscle, causing edema, hemorrhages, gas formation, and myofiber degeneration and necrosis.

MALIGNANT EDEMA

Malignant edema is a wound infection described in several animal species, principally cattle and sheep; this infection is associated with several clostridial species (Cl. septicum, Cl. sordelli, Cl. perfringens). Malignant edema is more often a cellulitis than a myositis, but it may have extensive necrosis and lysis of muscle fibers as well as extensive serosanguinous exudate. The edema fluid is poor in protein; it separates muscle fibers and extends into the perimysium. Necrotic myofibers are intensely eosinophilic and undergo lysis. Little or no cellular reaction is present, because histiocytes do not accumulate, and the few neutrophils are rapidly immobilized and killed by spreading toxins.

BLACKLEG

Blackleg, primarily a disease of young cattle caused by Cl. chauvoei, follows activation of latent infections in skeletal muscles. Clinically, circumscribed crepitant swellings are present over the thigh muscles, rump, back, and shoulders. Lesions are found in other locations, such as the tongue, diaphragm, and heart. Yellow gelatinous exudate, blood, and gas bubbles are present in subcutaneous and intermuscular connective tissues. Muscles are swollen and dark red to black; they are typically porous, spongy, and dry with a sweetish butyric acid odor. Microscopically, muscle necrosis is extensive and associated with gas bubbles, hemorrhages, lysed erythrocytes, small collections of inflammatory cells, and gram-positive bacilli (see also Chapter 10).

Viral myositides

Viral diseases with lesions in skeletal muscle include: ovine bluetongue and Ibaraki disease (cattle); epizootic hemorrhagic disease (deer); and Marek disease (birds). The lesions of bluetongue are the results of vascular damage; they include muscle necrosis and hemorrhages, and vascular necrosis and thrombosis (see also Chapter 8).

PARASITIC MYOSITIDES

Parasitic infections of skeletal muscle: include trichinosis, cysticercosis, toxoplasmosis, sarcocystosis, and numerous other parasites. Trichinosis (*Trichinella spiralis*) is characterized by the presence of larval forms within modified myofibers, called nurse cells. Skeletal muscle invasion is accompanied by leukocytosis with eosinophilia. The parasites in severe infections appear as small gray streaks or specks of calcification. Cellular response is slight to absent.

A variety of infections by larval tapeworms (cysticercosis, coenuriasis, hydatid disease) affect skeletal muscle and the heart. The severity of disease produced by the larval tapeworms depends upon the location (usually in the heart and masticatory muscles) and number of bladderworms. The cysts displace tissue, but rarely produce an inflammatory reaction; a few lymphocytes and eosinophils, however, may occur about some cysticerci.

Myositis may occur as one of the components of the variety of lesions in cases of toxoplasmosis, but toxoplasmal myositis is not considered common in either animals or humans. Polymyositis has been observed in dogs infected with *Toxoplasma gondii;* the multifocal inflammatory necrotizing lesions consist of myofiber degeneration and necrosis, with infiltrates of neutrophils, histiocytes, plasma cells, and lymphocytes. Toxoplasmal organisms are present within affected regions of the muscles (see also Chapter 12).

Cysts of *Sarcocystis sp.* in skeletal muscle and heart, without any inflammatory reaction, is a common finding in most domestic animals, and in rodents and rabbits. Sarcocystosis is apparently not common in nonhuman primates. Most infections are inapparent, but large doses of sporocysts of *S. ovicanis* in sheep produced clinical disease of anemia, anorexia, fever, and weight loss; gross lesions of hemorrhages were also produced, in skeletal muscles and visceral organs. Myositis of mild to moderate severity developed during both the meront and cyst-form-

ing stages; the inflammatory exudate were composed mostly of histiocytes and plasma cells. Chronic eosinophilic myositis was observed in a rhesus monkey infected with *Sarcocystis sp.* (see also Chapter 12).

IMMUNOLOGIC MYOSITIDES

Eosinophilic masticatory myositis of young dogs is a localized myopathic disease with a probable immune-mediated pathogenesis. An immunologic basis is suspected because: the cellular infiltrates contain eosinophils, lymphocytes, and plasma cells; serum globulins may be elevated; and the lesions are responsive to administration of corticosteroids. The masticatory muscles also are composed principally of type IIC myofibers; these myofibers have unique native myosin isozymes, myosin light chains, and myosin heavy chains by electrophoretic separation. Because they differ from type IIC myofibers of limb muscles, these myofibers have been designated as type IIM. Such data are significant in the pathogenesis of canine eosinophilic myositis because dogs with masticatory myositis have immune complexes limited to type IIM myofibers; their antibodies also are directed against type IIM myofibers.

Clinically, affected dogs have swollen, firm masticatory muscles (such as the masseter, temporalis, and pterygoid). The swelling and pain result in restricted movement of the jaws; pressure on the retrobulbar fat forces the globe forward and causes exophthalmos. The attacks last for 2–3 weeks; they recur at monthly intervals, and the recurrent episodes may extend over a period of years.

The lesions are bilateral and usually symmetric; they vary with the stage of the disease. Acutely, the muscles are swollen and edematous; later, they are dark red and doughy or firm in consistency. Scattered red foci of hemorrhages are present, as well as yellow to yellow-white streaks. The microscopic lesions also vary with the stage of the disease. The acute early lesions are multifocal collections of mainly eosinophils, with edema and hemorrhage. With time, the cellular composition changes to mainly plasma cells, lymphocytes, and histiocytes. Muscle fiber degeneration and necrosis, myofiber atrophy and loss, and myofiber regeneration are features of the subacute to chronic lesion. Atrophy of muscles and myofibers with fibrosis are found after several attacks (see also Chapter 7).

Polymyositis—believed to be immune-mediated—occurs in the dog. The inflammatory lesions are multifocal, and lymphocytes and plasma cells predominate.

Familial canine dermatomyositis Familial canine dermatomyositis is a newly recognized immune-mediated disease of juvenile collies and Shetland sheepdogs (Shelties); the disease has both cutaneous and muscle lesions. In the collie, genetic analysis suggests that the disease has an autosomal-dominant component of inheritance. In collies, the disease varies in severity from dog to dog; cutaneous lesions develop between 7–11 weeks of age, most often on the skin of the face, lips, pinna, tip of the tail, and skin over bony prominences. During the active disease phase, the cutaneous lesions include erythema, alopecia, scales, ulcers, crusts, and vesiculation.

Bilaterally symmetric, generalized muscular atrophy develops between 13–19 weeks of age, and coincides regionally with the cutaneous lesions. The lesions are more severe in the muscles of the head and distal extremities. Gross foci of pale tan, soft muscles contain cellular infiltrates. These infiltrates occur in the perimysium and endomysium, and about the blood vessels; they are composed of: lymphocytes, plasma cells, eosinophils, macrophages, neutrophils, and fibroblasts. Blood vessels often have alterations of vasculitis. Muscular lesions include myofiber degeneration, atrophy, and regeneration; the muscle lesions are multifocal and include fragmentation of myofibers with loss of cross striations, vacuolar change, and variation of myofiber diameter with internal nuclei especially in basophilic fibers with vesicular nuclei that have prominent nucleoli. Older lesions are characterized by perimysial and endomysial fibrosis. Both types I and II myofibers are smaller in areas of myositis. Dogs with progressive disease develop pyoderma, septicemia, megaesophagus, and secondary aspiration pneumonia. Sera of some collies have large amounts of circulating immune complexes and proportionally increased total IgG. The onset and severity of dermatitis and myositis correlate with content of circulating immune complexes, in which the immunoglobulin component consists principally of IgG.

IDIOPATHIC MYOSITIDES

Eosinophilic myositis is an uncommon lesion in cattle, sheep, and swine, without clinical signs associated with the muscle lesions. Diagnosis is made at slaughter by meat inspection. Grossly, well-demarcated green patches varying in size are seen when the affected muscles are first incised. Muscles of the back and thighs are most often affected, but lesions also occur in the tongue, diaphragm, and myocardium. Microscopically, muscle fasciculi and myofibers are separated by perimysial and endomysial edema, and by dense aggregates of eosinophils (Figure 18-8). Hyaline and vacuolar changes are present in some myofibers. More chronic lesions have macrophages, fibrosis, and calcified necrotic myofibers. Some lesions contain granulomas, and *Sarcocystis spp.* cysts are present in some of these lesions.

References

Despommier D. Adaptive changes in muscle fibers infected with Trichinella spiralis. Am J Pathol 1975;78:477–484.
Hamilton JM, McCance CM. Eosinophilic myositis in cattle. Vet Rec 1968;83:471–472.
Harcourt RA, Bradley R. Eosinophilic myositis in sheep. Vet Rec 1973;92:233–234.
Harding HP, Owen LN. Eosinophilic myositis in the dog. J Comp Pathol 1956;66:109–122.
Hargis AM, Haupt KH, Hegreberg GA, Prieur DJ, Moore MP. Familial canine dermatomyositis: initial characterization of the cutaneous and muscular lesions. Am J Pathol 1984;116:234–244.
Hargis AM, Prieur DJ, Haupt KH, Collier LL, Evermann JF, Ladiges WC. Postmortem findings in four litters of dogs with familial canine dermatomyositis. Am J Pathol 1986;123:480–496.
Jensen R, et al. Eosinophilic myositis and muscular sarcocystosis in the carcasses of slaughtered cattle and lambs. Am J Vet Res 1986;47:587–593.
Johnson AJ, Hildebrandt PK, Fayer R. Experimentally-induced sarcocystis in calves: pathology. Am J Vet Res 1975;36:995–999.
Juranek DD, Forbes LS, Keller Z. Taenia saginata cysticerci in muscles of beef cattle. Am J Vet Res 1976;37:785–789.
Karstad L, Winter A, Trainor DO. Pathology of epizootic hemorrhagic disease of deer. Am J Vet Res 1961;22:227–235.
Kornegay JN, et al. Polymyositis in dogs. J Am Vet Med Assoc 1980;176:431–438.

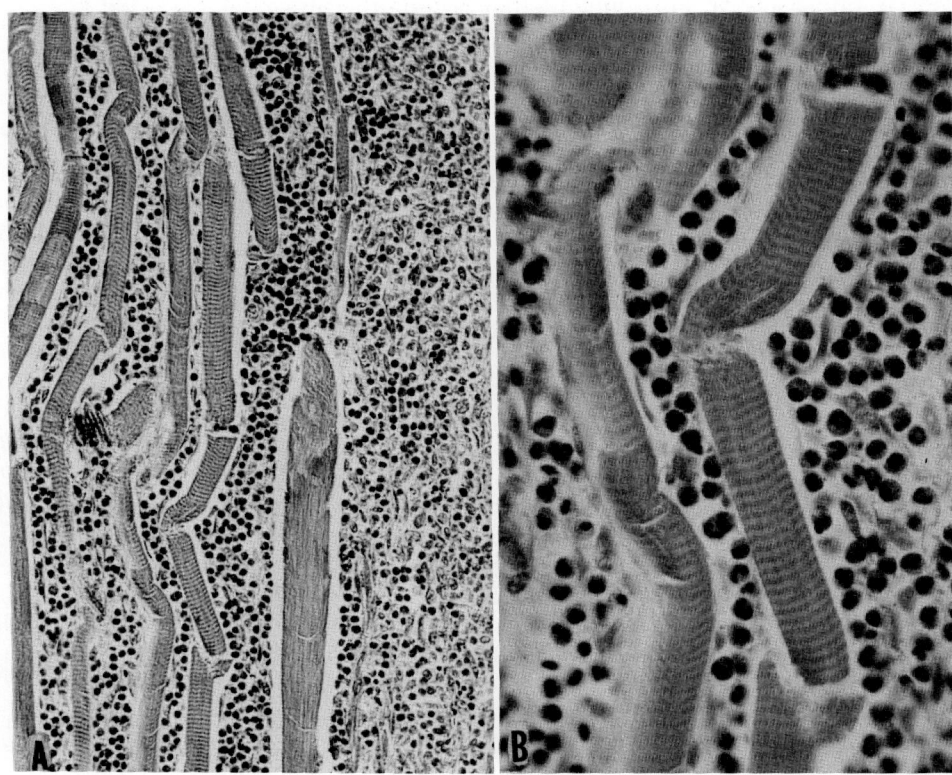

FIG. 18-8 Eosinophilic myositis, psoas muscle of a cow. **A.** Eosinophilic leukocytes isolating and replacing muscle bundles (×195). **B.** Details of A (×460). Distention and rupture of muscle bundles and replacement by eosinophils. (Courtesy of Armed Forces Institute of Pathology; contributor: Dr. C. L. Davis.)

Leek RG, Fayer R, Johnson AJ. Sheep experimentally infected with Sarcocystis from dogs. I. Disease in young lambs. J Parasitol 1977;63:642–650.

Moulton JE. Pathology of bluetongue of sheep. J Am Vet Med Assoc 1961;138:493–498.

Orvis JS, Cardinet GH. Canine muscle fiber types and susceptibility of masticatory muscles to myositis. Muscle Nerve 1981;4:354–359.

Rimiala-Parnanen E, Nikander S. Generalized eosinophilic myositis with sarcosporidiosis in a Finnish cow. Nord Vet Med 1980;32:96–99.

Samuels BS, Rietschel RL. Polymyositis and toxoplasmosis. JAMA 1976;235:60–61.

Shelton GD, Cardinet GH, Baudman E, Cudden P. Fiber type specific autoantibodies in a dog with eosinophilic myositis. Muscle Nerve 1985;8:783–790.

Shelton GD, Cardinet GH, Baudman E. Canine masticatory muscle disorders: a study of 29 cases. Muscle Nerve 1987;10:753–766.

Smith LDS. Clostridial diseases of animals. Adv Vet Sci 1957;3:463–524.

Stewart GL, Giannini SH. Sarcocystis, Trypanosoma, Toxoplasma, Brugia, Ancylostoma, and Trichinellaspp: a review of the intracellular parasites of striated muscle. Exp Parasitol 1982;53:406–447.

Neoplasia

In general, neither primary nor secondary neoplastic disease occurs frequently in skeletal muscle. Primary tumors, either benign or malignant, may arise from mature muscle fibers or precursor cells; they may occur in various connective tissues cells, or in vascular or neural tissues of muscle. Secondary tumors may arise by either hematogenous metastasis, or by local invasion of the primary neoplasm. The most frequently observed secondary neoplasms of muscle in animals are lymphoma, malignant melanoma, and hemangiosarcoma. However, even these neoplasms are infrequent in muscle, compared to their frequency in other metastatic sites (such as lungs and liver). It has been suggested that skeletal muscle offers a local environment that is unfavorable for the survival and proliferation of embolic tumor cells.

Rhabdomyoma

Rhabdomyoma or rhabdomyosarcoma are names given respectively to benign or malignant neoplasms arising from striated muscle, skeletal, or cardiac. Although known in many animals species, they are infrequent. The benign variety is essentially unknown in animals. Rhabdomyosarcoma has been reported to arise from skeletal muscle of the tongue, pharynx, and panniculus, and from the myocardium and urinary bladder. They have been reported most often in dogs; they are locally invasive and tend to metastasize early.

The microscopic features of rhabdomyosarcoma are varied and often difficult to identify with certainty (Figure 18-9). More differentiated tumors may have histologic features that clearly resemble those of immature striated muscle; incompletely or completely developed muscle fibers occur, with identifiable myofibrils and cross-striations. These are more easily identified. Others may be highly undifferentiated, containing pleomorphic cells with often bizarre, giant, and multiple nuclei. The cytoplasm may be abundant, but amorphous.

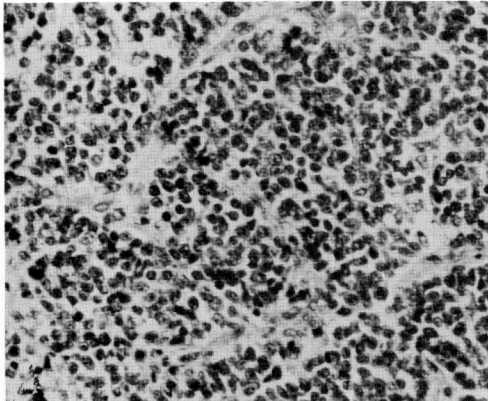
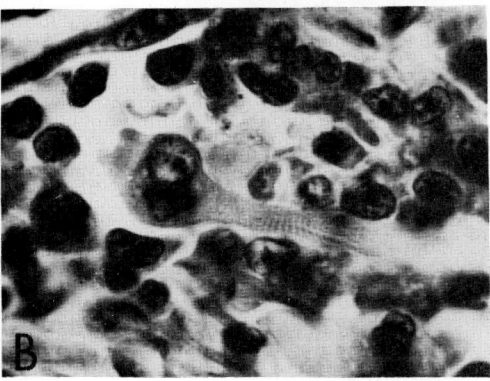

FIG. 18-9 Juvenile rhabdomyosarcoma in a dog. **A.** Undifferentiated region of tumor. **B.** Multinucleated "racquet" cell with cross-striations. (Courtesy of Dr. H.R. Seibold and Vet Path 1974;11:558–560.)

Sometimes, small amounts of eosinophilic cytoplasm are visible. Special stains, such as phosphotungstic acid hematoxylin, may be required to demonstrate the cross-striations that provide definitive identification.

Granular cell myoblastoma

Granular cell myoblastoma is a microscopically startling growth. It consists principally of large—even huge—polyhedral and spheric cells of epithelioid appearance; they have a comparatively small central nucleus, and an extensive, pale, granular cytoplasm. Collagen-bearing stroma may be apparent. In the human tongue, these cells appear related to and derived from striated muscle; this effect is responsible for the name applied to the tumor. One school of thought places the origin of the peculiar cells in nervous tissue; another considers them as altered fibroblasts. Cases have been reported in the horse, mouse, and tongue of a dog.

References

Hulland TJ. Tumors of the muscle. In: Moulton JE. Tumors in domestic animals. 3rd ed. Los Angeles: Univ Calif Press, 1989;88–101.

Kelly DF. Rhabdomyosarcoma of the urinary bladder in dogs. Vet Pathol 1973;10:375–384.

Ladds PW, Webster DR. Pharyngeal rhabdomyosarcoma in a dog. Vet Pathol 1971;8:256–259.

Misdorp W, Nauta-van Gelder HL. "Granular cell myoblastoma" in the horse: a report of 4 cases. Pathol Vet 1968;5:385–394.

Osborne CA, Low DG, Perman V, Barnes DM. Neoplasms of the canine and feline urinary bladder: incidence, etiologic factors, occurrence and pathologic features. Am J Vet Res 1968;29:2041–2055.

Peter CP, Kluge JP. An ultrastructural study of a canine rhabdomyosarcoma. Cancer 1970;26:1280–1288.

Seibold HR. Juvenile alveolar rhabdomyosarcoma in a dog. Vet Pathol 1974;11:558–560.

Wyand DS, Wolke RE. Granular cell myoblastoma of the canine tongue: case reports. Am J Vet Res 1968;29:1309–1313.

19

Skeletal system

James Carroll Woodard

BONE

Bone is primarily composed of mineral in the form of calcium hydroxyapatite and type I collagen in a ground substance of glycosaminoglycans. The collagenous matrix is known as **osteoid;** it is produced by the principal cell type of bone, the **osteoblast,** a cell that lines bone-forming surfaces. These cells later become entrapped within the matrix and are termed **osteocytes.** Osteoblasts contain alkaline phosphatase and have receptors for parathyroid hormone. **Osteoclasts,** which are multinucleated cells, are concerned with bone resorption and are found along bone surfaces; osteoclasts are associated with small resorption cavities, termed **Howship lacunae.** These cells are rich in acid phosphatase and lack receptors for parathyroid hormone. The noncollagenous proteins—also produced by osteoblasts—include: phosphoproteins, osteonectin, osteopontin, osteocalcin (bone glaprotein), bone proteoglycan, bone morphogenic protein, bone sialoprotein, and bone proteolipid.

Following the deposition of osteoid by osteoblasts, calcium salts are not deposited for five to ten days (mineralization lag time), depending upon the species. This leaves an unmineralized layer of osteoid—termed an **osteoid seam**—of 5–15 mm in thickness, depending upon the rate of bone formation. This may be visualized as an eosinophilic zone separated by a basophilic line (mineralization front) from the more basophilic mineralized osteoid. This distinction may not be apparent in decalcified tissue sections, and is best judged in undecalcified tissue sections. With the exception of the metaphysis of a growing bone, less than 20% of cancellous bone surfaces are covered with osteoid, and less than 2% of the bone volume is composed of osteoid. The collagen fibers of bone are arranged in an orderly parallel fashion. This is termed **lamellar bone.** In the fetus, the collagen fibers are deposited in an irregular fashion (woven or basket weave pattern), termed **woven bone.** This is replaced through remodeling. Woven bone is also seen in pathologic states when formation of osteoid and neoplasms of bone are rapid.

Normal development of bone

Bone is formed under two different situations by differing processes. One is known as **intramembranous bone formation,** in which fibroblastic-appearing cells of the inner or "cambium" layer of the periosteum gradually differentiate into osteoblasts—or bone-forming cells—and osteocytes, which are completely differentiated bone cells, each locked in its particular lacuna. This type of bone formation is responsible for the formation of the flat bones of the head and pelvis; such formation also occurs along the periosteal surfaces of the shafts (diaphyses) of the long bones as these grow in width.

Increase in length of long bones occurs by **endochondral bone formation,** principally at the cartilaginous growth plate that divides the epiphysis and metaphysis. After the animal has grown, endochondral bone formation occurs only on one side of the growth-plate cartilage (**physis**), the side toward the diaphysis. On the other (articular) side, growth cartilage abruptly joins the cancellous bone that is part of the developing secondary ossification center of the epiphysis. The epiphyseal secondary ossification center increases in size by inconspicuous endochondral ossification and transition from growth cartilage to bone along the base of the articular cartilage.

Endochondral bone development on the diaphyseal side of the growth-plate cartilage is characterized by a series of consecutive changes in this region, termed the metaphysis. Proceeding from the inactive cartilage of the growth plate (**resting cartilage zone**) we encounter a region of columnar cartilage. The first cells in the column undergo mitotic division (**proliferating cartilage zone**), and are responsible for interstitial growth within the cartilaginous growth plate. These cells in their lacunae are close together and stain darkly when hematoxylin-and-eosin stain is used. As the cells in the column differentiate to form the **maturing cartilage zone,** they synthesize cartilage matrix; this process further expands the interstitium. The last zone is com-

899

posed of degenerate, swollen cells with extensive, nearly colorless cytoplasm, called the **hypertrophic cartilage zone.** As the hypertrophic cartilage cells imbibe fluid from the matrix, the matrix proteoglycans become more concentrated; the intercellular matrix becomes more metachromatic with toluidine blue, and stains a deep blue or purple with hematoxylin. Degeneration of cartilage cells, formation of matrix vesicles, and synthesis of specialized matrix components lead to mineralization of the longitudinal cartilage septa (**calcified cartilage zone**). Mineralization allows cartilage to be invaded by mesenchymal tissue and capillaries reaching from the adjacent marrow spaces and carrying cells with lytic capacities. Multinucleated cells (chondroclasts/osteoclasts) reduce the mineralized cartilage to minute longitudinal trabeculae with scalloped edges. **Osteoprogenitor cells** surrounding the vessels proliferate and differentiate into osteoblasts. The osteoblasts deposit pink-staining osteoid onto the surfaces of the remaining cartilage cores, and the osteoid subsequently mineralizes. During the process of depositing osteoid on trabecular surfaces, some osteoblasts bury themselves within lacunae and become included in the primary bone trabeculae, the **primary spongiosa.** Osteoclasts, formed from mononuclear precursor cells arriving in blood, erode the trabecular surfaces of the primary spongiosa, causing most of the calcified cartilage to disappear as secondary and tertiary trabeculae form. Primary trabeculae of cancellous bone or initial plexiform bone of the cortex are composed of woven bone; lamellar bone ultimately replaces this immature bone type.

During growth, the bone changes shape and structure by the processes of bone modeling and remodeling. **Bone modeling** (Fig. 19-1) is a result of the architectural changes that occur during growth; these include changes in gross contour, spatial orientation, and size. During modeling, osteoblasts and osteoclasts function on different surfaces and can alter the bone's shape much like an artist would model clay. A good example of modeling is the maintenance of the funnel shape of the metaphyseal contour by osteoclastic resorption on the metaphyseal surface at the cut back or funnel zone. Other modeling activities include: the expansion of the medullary cavity by osteoclastic resorption, at the marrow-cancellous bone interface or at the cortical endosteum; and the increase in the bone's width by periosteal bone formation. When bone growth stops, modeling activity slows greatly and peak bone mass is reached. **Bone remodeling** is the process by which microscopic packages, called the **basic multicellular units** (BMU) (Fig. 19-2), remove old bone and replace it with new bone without altering the bone's gross structure. **Bone remodeling** of the metaphyseal trabeculae (Fig. 19-3) occurs as a sequence of events. Osteoclastic resorption followed by osteoblastic refilling at the same bone site creates a new lamellar bone packet that is delimited by a basophilic-staining, scalloped cement line called a **reversal line.** In cortical bone, (Fig. 19-2) remodeling occurs as resorption by osteoclast cuts

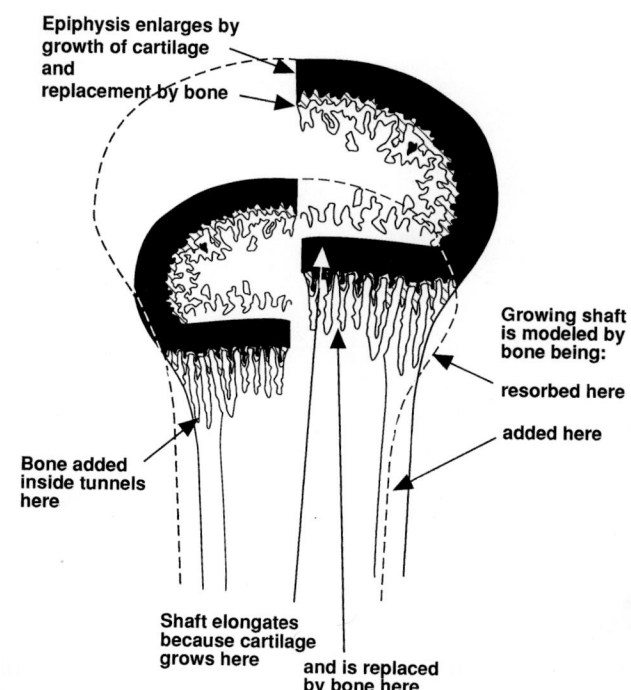

FIG. 19-1 Diagram of reshaping of a long bone (bone modeling) during longitudinal bone growth. The younger bone profile is on the left and the older is shown on the right. The outline of the earlier bone shape is shown as a superimposed dotted line on the right side of the figure. The bone has grown in length by endochondral ossification at the growth region beneath articular cartilage and at the physis. The general shape of the bone is retained by bone modeling; bone resorption occurs on some surfaces while bone deposition occurs on different surfaces, as indicated in the diagram. (Redrawn from Ham AW. J Bone Joint Surg 1952;34A:711.)

through primary bone, forming tunnels or "cutting cones;" these cones are then filled in centripetally by osteoblasts, forming successive layers of bone that constitute the haversian system or secondary osteons. No change in the bone balance occurs when bone resorption equals bone formation. Remodeling of both cancellous and cortical bone continues throughout life, producing successive generations of basic multicellular units seen as lamellar bone packets or secondary osteons. Preexisting lamellar bone or preexisting osteons lie between adjacent osteons, forming the interstitial lamellae.

In the metaphyseal region of a long bone, no outer wall of compact bone exists; even the marrow spaces are connected directly with the fibrous periosteum. Continual reshaping and modeling of the bone takes place here (Fig. 19-1); this process is necessary because continued growth causes bone elements that were in the metaphysis to take a diaphyseal position. A smooth transition between the wider epiphysis and the narrower diaphysis occurs at the **cut back** or **funnel** zone. Osteoclasts remove bone from the outside metaphyseal surface next to the growth plate; osteoblasts add bone

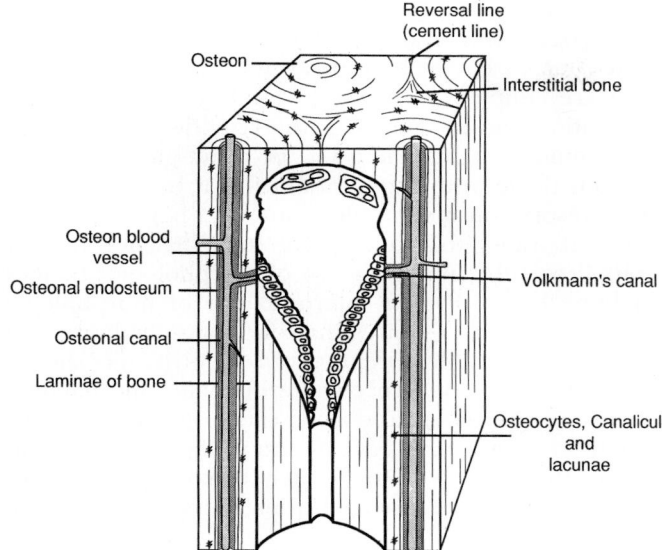

Reversal line
(cement line)

Osteon

Interstitial bone

Osteon blood
vessel

Osteonal endosteum

Osteonal canal

Laminae of bone

Volkmann's canal

Osteocytes, Canaliculi
and
lacunae

FIG. 19-2 Diagram of compact bone of the diaphysis illustrates the basic multicellular unit (BMU) and sequential events in remodeling of cortical bone. The leading end of the BMU is the cutting cone, and it moves through the bone cortex removing bone longitudinally and centrifugally. Gradual refilling with new bone results in the formation of a new osteon. The reversal cement line is formed at the peripheral limit of the osteon, and its location is determined by the centrifugal extent of osteoclastic resorption. The reversal line represents the point at which cell function reverses from osteoclastic resorption to formation of bone by osteoblasts. The temporal relationships and cellular events are similar to those illustrated for cancellous bone (Figure 19-3).

to the interior near the diaphysis, and fill in between the trabeculae (a process called **compaction**) that were formed by endochondral ossification. The marrow in this region is at first fibrous, but soon develops the usual myeloid and fatty pattern. As the trabeculae are moved from a position adjacent to the growth plate toward the diaphysis, the process of bone remodeling

increases the marrow space and leads to a reduction in the number of trabeculae and amount of cancellous bone. As the bone grows in length and as the diameter of the growth plate expands, the cortical diameter of the diaphysis increases by subperiosteal addition of new bone. The microstructural morphology of the developing bone cortex differs among animal species and has a relationship to the rate of body growth. Primary **lamellar bone** is the type formed when the process is slow, and it is arranged in circular rings around the periosteal circumference (circumferential lamellae). **Primary osteons** form when lamellae are arranged in concentric rings around individual vascular channels; osteons are found within well-organized primary lamellar bone. **Secondary osteons** differ from primary osteons because they do not have cement lines (reversal lines) as they are not produced by the remodeling process. **Plexiform bone** is formed in rapidly growing animals and is the most common type seen in the cortices of large domestic animals. This bone forms around intertwining vascular plexuses, and thickens by surface bone apposition to become dense cortical bone.

Mechanical usage, effects on bone

Although much of a bone's shape is genetically determined, mechanical usage affects the bone's shape and size. This is illustrated by the anatomical differences between bones from a normal active animal and those from an individual that has been paralyzed and inactive since birth. During growth, increased mechanical usage increases bone modeling and decreases bone remodeling. The amount of compacta increases, and the expansion of the marrow cavity is retarded (modeling). The rate of disappearance of spongiosa from the metaphysis decreases (remodeling). This leads to an increased external diameter of the bone, an increase in the cortical bone's cross section, and a dense metaphyseal spongiosa. In the adult, since bone modeling is no longer adding bone to the skeleton, increased mechanical usage

FIG. 19-3 Sequential events in remodelling of cancellous bone. Time sequence: *0,* old basic multicellular unit (BMU) with trabecular lamellae; *1,* early bone resorption with osteoclasts (OCL) the dominant cell type; *2,* late bone resorption with mononuclear (MON) cells the dominant cell type; *3,* preosteoblast (POB) cell phase; *4,* early matrix formation before the start of mineralization, OB Osteoblasts; *5,* late part of bone formation with osteoid seam and mineralized bone filling the resorptive cavity; *6,* completed new trabecular BMU. (Redrawn from Eriksen EF. Endocr Rev 1986;7:379–408.)

Trabecular
Remodeling Sequence

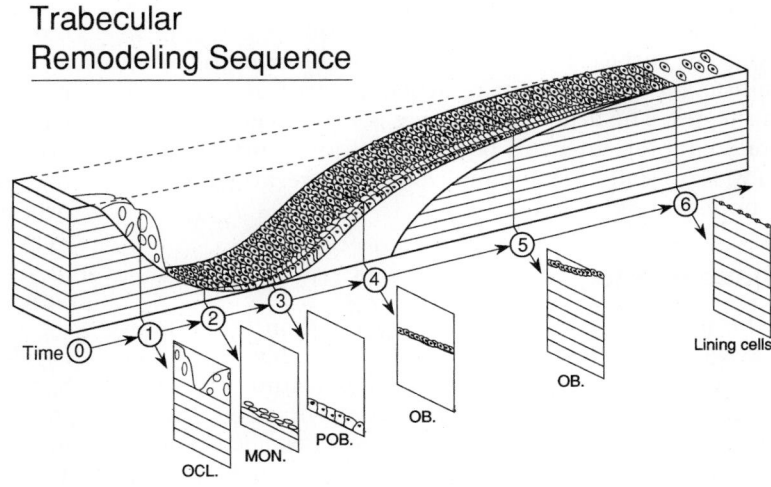

Time

OCL.

MON.

POB.

OB.

OB.

OB.

Lining cells

can only conserve the amount of bone that is already present by decreasing remodeling. The age-related expansion of the marrow cavity at the corticoendostium is retarded. Acute disuse releases the inhibition on bone remodeling, and remodeling activity increases (osteoporosis). In the growing animal with decreased mechanical usage, bone modeling is depressed. Retardation in the accumulation of compacta results, as well as an increased loss in the amount of spongiosa, and expansion of the marrow cavity diameter. The outside diameter of the bone decreases, along with the bone cross-sectional area. The compacta decreases and the marrow cavity enlarges.

Examination of skeleton

The required detail of the skeletal system examination depends upon the objectives of the necropsy procedure. At a minimum, the rib bones should be isolated and examined grossly for breaking strength and irregularities of the costochondral junction. The rib is easily handled; it represents cortical bone with high turnover and is easily trimmed to examine the growth region. Five major joints—in addition to those opened in the course of the necropsy procedure—should receive open inspection, and longitudinal saw cuts should be made through the middle of at least two long bones; bone marrow can also be obtained at this time. The examination of the limb bones is best accomplished by removing the muscular attachments surrounding the joint. The joint can then be opened using a pair of serrated shears or scissors, using caution not to let the tips touch articular cartilage; a knife or scalpel used in dissection may cause minor alterations in the articular cartilage surface. It is necessary to completely expose the joint so that the articular margins and bone grooves—through which ligaments pass—can be inspected closely. The formation of small osteophytic excrescences at locations where muscle tension pulls on ligamentous insertions may indicate joint disease before visual inspection of the joint cartilage surface reveals significant alterations. Visual inspection of the articular surface alone is insufficient to recognize many cartilaginous lesions. For example, the early changes of osteochondrosis can be visualized on bone sagittal sections prior to the appearance of surface lesions. The use of radiographs as an aid to the examination of articular cartilage offers advantages. The articular cartilage is radiolucent, and the radiographic interface between two joint surfaces actually represents the mineralized cartilage and the subchondral bone of each surface.

Bone histology

The proper recognition and interpretation of the morphologic changes in the skeleton, more than any other tissue, is highly dependent upon understanding normal organ anatomy, histology, and biologic function. Knowledge of recent advances in the field of skeletal biology is required to fully understand the pathogenesis of skeletal disease. It is an old idea that bone resorption and

formation are controlled by different hormones and are characteristic of different disease processes; the current concept is that bone resorption and bone formation are coupled processes. It is the balance between resorption and formation in the remodeling cycle that determines whether there will be a net gain or loss of osseous tissue of the basic multicellular unit. Because a bone resorption site may develop into a bone formation site with time, this concept of **bone balance** further complicates the interpretation of morphologic changes in bone tissue. Proper interpretation of morphologic changes in bone requires that one consider bone as a dynamic system. Measurement of bone dynamics should be made when the process altering the bone has had sufficient time to act, and when the remodeling process has reached a steady state. It should be recognized in this context that bone tissue may behave differently in disease than it does under normal physiologic circumstances.

Although quantitative bone histomorphometry is more useful as a research tool than it is as a diagnostic aid, the use of tetracycline bone labeling and undecalcified bone sections is a valued part of the histologic examination. Tetracycline labels sites of active mineralization and is deposited directly at the calcification front. Undecalcified bone sections allow the differentiation between mineralized and unmineralized bone or cartilage matrix; they also permit the examination of bone surfaces and cells with relatively little contraction artifact. Mononuclear and multinuclear osteoclasts can be identified on bone surfaces; the number of cells and extent of eroded bone surface are valid indices of the resorptive activity. The limit of each osteoclastic resorptive wave is marked by a narrow line of basophilic matrix, termed the **reversal line.** Variations in the rate of bone turnover cause a variation in the reversal line pattern. An exceptionally large number of lines gives rise to the description of bone having a "mosaic" pattern. Osteoblasts become larger and more numerous when making osteoid, and they appear as a prominent row of contiguous cells. Indices of bone formation are: estimates of the number of osteoblasts, quantitation of osteoid area, proportion of osteoid with active osteoblasts, and proportion of osteoid with calcification front. Osteoid thickness usually does not exceed 15 μm, and only a small percent of the osteoid surface is covered by plump osteoblasts. Except for the initial bone that is laid down during bone modeling, woven bone is not normally seen in tissue sections. **Woven bone** is the initial bone that is laid down in the fetus or in pathologic processes; it can be identified by the woven or basket-weave pattern of its collagen. Bone volume is a useful index for estimating osteopenia and osteosclerosis seen with certain metabolic bone diseases.

Certain bone diseases appear to affect one **bone envelope** (periosteal, haversian, endocortical, or trabecular) more than another (Fig. 19-4). In general, the trabecular bone envelope is more reactive and responsive than the haversian envelope because of its greater surface and higher turnover. Age also affects the responsiveness of the skeletal system. Fractures heal

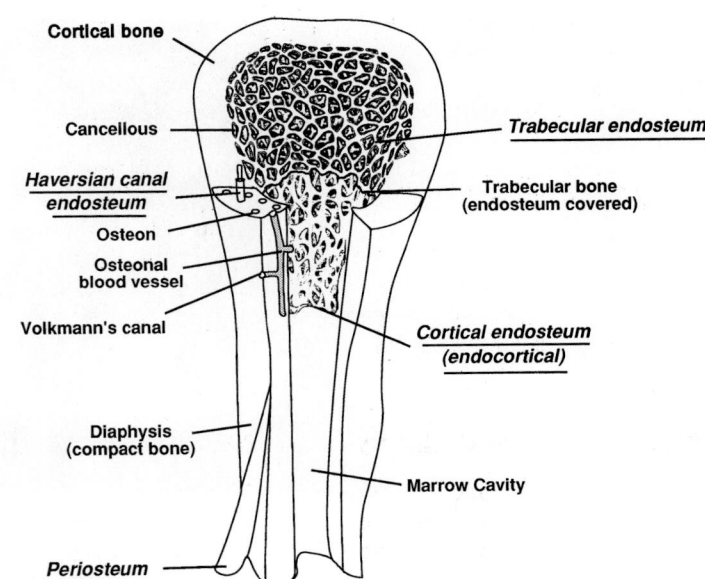

Cortical bone

Cancellous

Haversian canal endosteum

Osteon

Osteonal blood vessel

Volkmann's canal

Diaphysis (compact bone)

Periosteum

Trabecular endosteum

Trabecular bone (endosteum covered)

Cortical endosteum (endocortical)

Marrow Cavity

FIG. 19-4 Bone segment demonstrates the four bone envelopes: periosteal, haversian canal endosteal, cortical bone endosteal, and trabecular endosteal. (Redrawn from Banks WJ. Applied veterinary histology. Baltimore: Williams & Wilkins, 1981;117.)

less vigorously in older animals, compared to younger ones. Pathologic effects are more serious or proceed more rapidly in young animals; this is because the modeling and remodeling processes beneath the growth plates of growing animals are more active than what has been observed in cortical or cancellous bone of older animals. Conditions that cause bone resorption cause bone formation at a later time, and little change in bone mass may occur. When activation of new remodeling units increases—therefore increasing bone turnover by parathyroid or thyroid hormones—the initial bone resorption enlarges the **remodeling space;** consequently, temporary nonprogressive bone loss occurs. Conversely, depressed activation by calcitonin, estrogens, or increased dietary calcium reduces resorption first, then leads to small, nonprogressive net gains in the amount of bone. Some diseases—such as hyperparathyroidism or Cushing disease—affect several or all of the sequential bone remodeling stages, whereas others act on only one particular stage. The skeletal response to hormones and pharmacologic agents diminishes with time, particularly when the agent is administered continuously.

References

Baron R, Tross R, Bignery A. Evidence of sequential remodeling in rat trabecular bone: morphology, dynamic histomorphometry, and changes during skeletal maturation. Anat Rec 1984;45:137–145.

Brighton CT. Structure and function of the growth plate. Clin Orthop 1978;136:22–32.

Enlow DH. Principles of bone remodeling. Springfield: CC Thomas, 1963.

Frost HM. Intermediary organization of the skeleton. Boca Raton: CRC Press, 1986.

Parfitt AM. The cellular basis of bone remodeling: the quantum concept re-examined in light of recent advances in the cell biology of bone. Calcif Tissue Int 1984;36:S37–S45.

Recker RR. Bone histomorphometry: techniques and interpretation. Boca Raton: CRC Press, 1983.

FRACTURE OF BONES

Fracture types

A clean break separating a bone into two parts is called a **simple fracture** (Fig. 19-5). When many parts exist, it is a **comminuted fracture.** When, as rarely happens, one piece of bone is forcibly driven into another, the lesion is an **impacted fracture.** A fracture that causes incomplete bone separation without displacement is termed an infraction. When, in addition to the break in the bone, there exists an opening in the overlying skin, the lesion is a **compound fracture.** The latter is much more dangerous because infection is able to enter. A fracture in which the periosteum remains intact and holds the ends of bone in place is a **greenstick fracture.** When bone is under repeated stress, remodeling activity—which is possibly directed at microdamage repair—increases. When the stress continues, periosteal and endosteal calluses develop and help strengthen the bone while active remodeling takes place. A **stress fracture** develops as a last event. This chain of events is often repeated when young Thoroughbreds enter training and is termed "sore or bucked shins". The term **pathologic fracture,** is used to designate one that occurs, not as the result of any unusual trauma, but because the bone was previously weakened by some other disease (such as fibrous osteodystrophy or bone tumor).

Fracture repair

Following a fracture, a set of events with discrete steps lead to bone healing (Fig. 19-7). Tissue disruption leads to hemorrhage; necrosis of cortical bone extends a variable distance from the fracture site. Next, the injured region becomes a special sphere of influence, where normal physiologic processes are accelerated. This reaction has been termed a general metabolic shift or **re-**

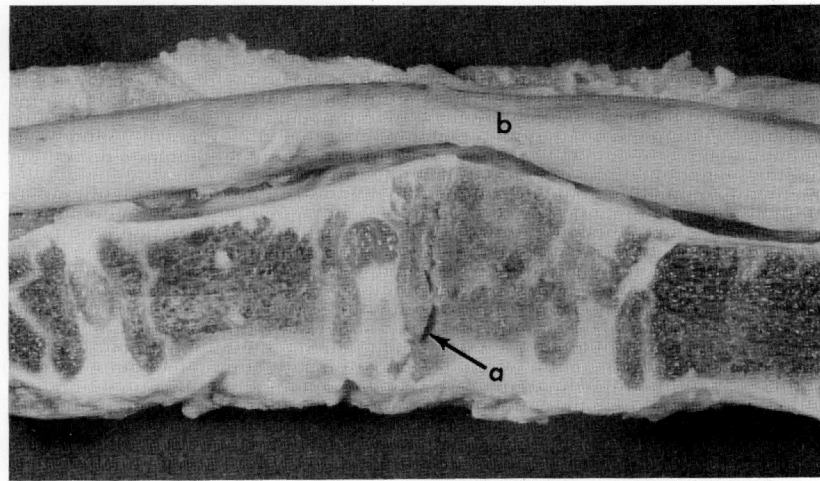

FIG. 19-5 Fracture of a vertebra; a nine-month-old female German shepherd was hit by a car. **A.** Fracture through the epiphysis, and **B.** resulting in compression of the spinal cord. (Photograph courtesy of Angell Memorial Animal Hospital.)

gional acceleratory phenomenon. Acute inflammation occurs with organization of the initial hematoma and formation of granulation tissue occur. This effect may progress to fibrosis in the case of a nonunion; eventually, pseudoarthrosis may develop when excessive mobility exists at the fracture site. Stability of the site allows a **fracture callus** to form (Fig. 19-6), a process that recapitulates bone growth during fetal development. On the periosteal and endosteal surfaces, cell proliferation results; mesenchymal cells differentiate into fibrous tissue and hyaline cartilage of the external and internal callus; later, there is endochondral ossification. Next, bone remodeling replaces the injured and necrotic original

cortical bone, and the newly produced woven bone of the callus, with lamellar bone. The remodeling process is based on the basic multicellular unit. The last phase consists of modeling, a process that is of much greater intensity in children than adults, where resorption and formation drifts tend to straighten crooked bones.

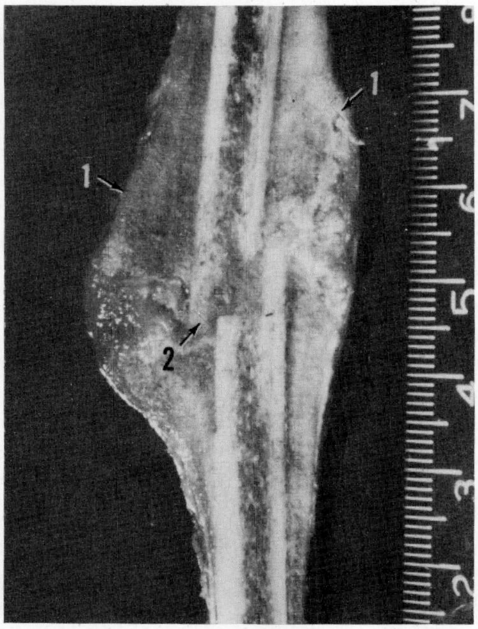

References

Frost HM. The biology of fracture healing: an overview for clinicians (Parts I and II). Clin Orthop 1989;248:283–309.
Rhinelander FW, Barogry RA. Microangiography of bone healing: undisplaced closed fractures. J Bone Am V 1962;44A:1273–1298.

REACTION TO INJURY

Bone responds to injurious agents a limited number of ways, and the responses that occur in bone during various diseases are exemplified by the reactions that occur during fracture healing. The bone reactions are listed below, with examples of selected diseases that illustrate the different reactions.

Bone necrosis

Bone necrosis is most commonly seen following fracture, or in association with bone inflammation or bone neoplasms. Zones of necrotic bone occur in which there is very little response in the surrounding tissue. Epiphyseal necrosis—most often of the head of the femur or humerus—is occasionally encountered in domestic animals and laboratory rats and mice. This necrosis regularly results from a fracture of the femoral neck that interferes with the vascular supply to the epiphysis, but it is also encountered without a clearly defined pathogenesis; vascular interference, however, is usually the underlying cause. Idiopathic osteocyte necrosis has been observed in normal bone in rhesus monkeys and mice.

Aseptic necrosis of the femoral head is seen as part of **Legg-Perthes disease** in immature, small-breed dogs before growth-plate closure. The disease develops in adolescent dogs; initial signs of lameness appear at 4–11

FIG. 19-6 Fracture of a rib of a year-old Guernsey calf. (1) Note bony callus; (2) Surrounding the fracture. (Courtesy of College of Veterinary Medicine, Iowa State University.)

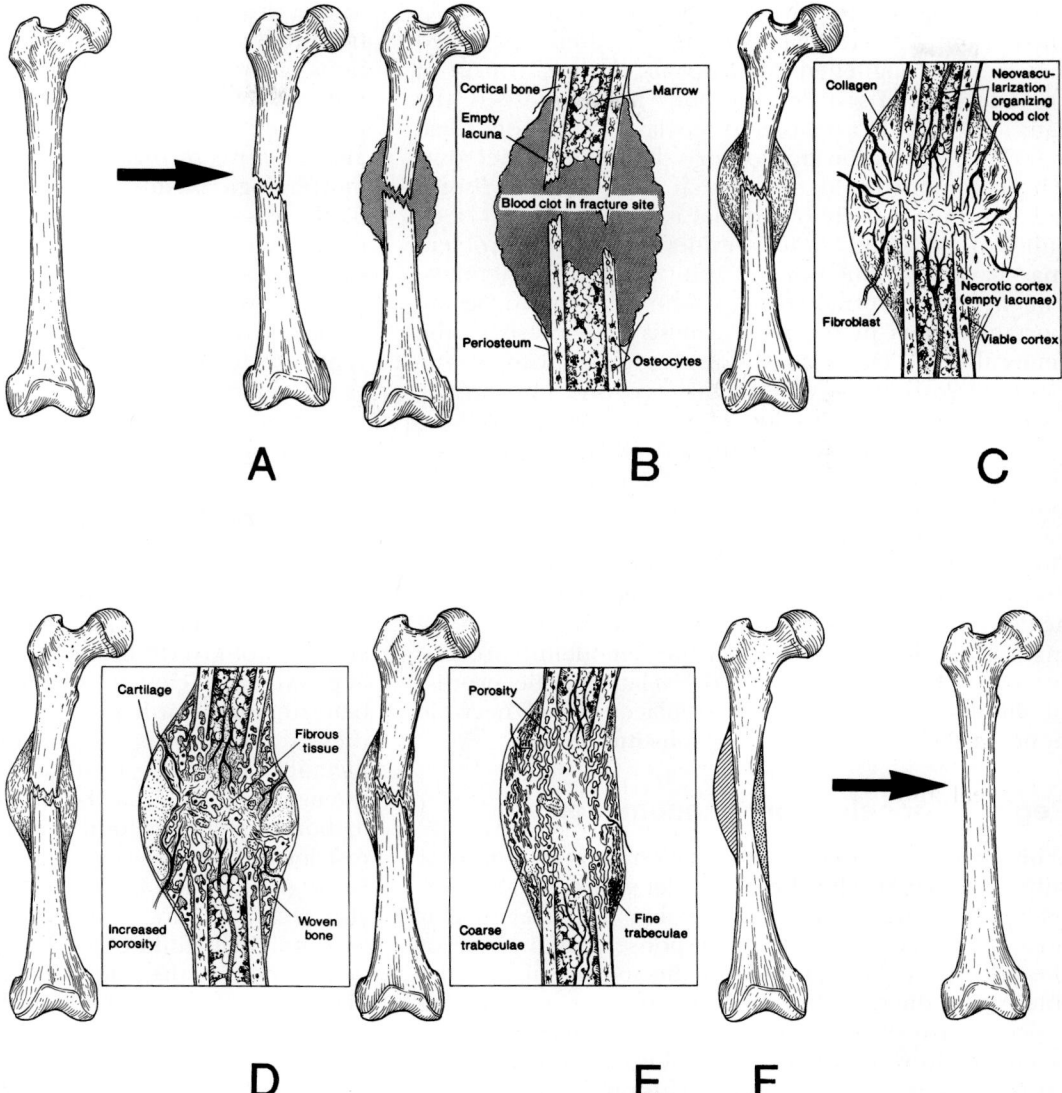

FIG. 19-7   Reaction to injury, fracture healing.   **A.** Injury. Break in continuity of the bone and periosteum. The moment a fracture occurs, the stage is set for repair, and all physiologic processes—including bone remodeling—are accelerated (regional acceleratory phenomenon, RAP.)   **B.** Hematoma phase. The degree of soft-tissue injury, the amount of the hemorrhage, and the amount of cortical bone necrosis depend upon the severity of the injury.   **C.** Inflammatory phase. Vascular dilatation and exudation of fluid and leukocytes are followed by organization of the blood clot by neovascularization and formation of granulation tissue.   **D.** Reparative phase. Pluripotential mesenchymal cells from the soft tissue, periosteum, and bone marrow form a callus composed of fibrous tissue, cartilage, and bone. The callus becomes consolidated, and continuity between fragments is restored by fusion of osteogenic layers on either side of the callus.   **E.** Remodeling phase. The size of the callus is reduced as newly formed woven bone is gradually converted to lamellar bone. The necrotic cortex is removed by accelerated remodeling (RAP) as cutting cones remove necrotic bone and give the cortex a trabecular appearance.   **F.** Modeling phase. In young animals, a malunion up to 30 degrees will straighten completely by a process of disproportionate osteoclastic resorption (hatched) and bone formation (stippled). (Modified from Woodard JC, Jee WSS. Skeletal system. In: Toxicologic pathology. Haschek, Rosusseaux, eds. San Diego: Academic Press, 1991;508.)

months. In young dogs, femoral head necrosis must be differentiated from the beginning lesions of hip dysplasia. Femoral head necrosis is seen in dogs weighing under 10 kilograms, whereas hip dysplasia usually occurs in dogs weighing over 25 kilograms. Initial radiographic changes in Legg-Perthes disease are widening of the

joint space and the presence of single or multiple foci of decreased density in the femoral head. As the disease progresses, the radiolucency increases and the head of the femur develops an irregular contour, indicating collapse of the articular cartilage. Gross lesions—which are best observed after midsagittal sectioning—vary from subtle changes in the shape of the femoral head to fragmentation; the articular cartilage is often discolored brown and roughened. Microscopic changes consist of osteonecrosis of subchondral bone and necrosis of the fatty marrow. Fibroplasia, osteoclasis, and additional new bone formation may occur subsequent to necrosis. The commonly held theory that Legg-Perthes disease can be caused solely by arterial ischemia has not been substantiated, and there is evidence that the problem may have a venous origin. Disturbed venous drainage and increased intraosseous pressure appear to be important factors in the pathogenesis of necrosis of the femoral head. Other conditions associated with aseptic bone necrosis are severe anemia, occlusive vascular disease, thrombosis, and pancreatic release of lipolytic enzymes. Necrotic bone is characterized histologically by disappearance of osteocytes from their lacunae. Usually, bone vascular channels are also empty. One must be careful not to confuse as a lesion the artifactual lack of tissue basophilia and nuclear staining that occurs when bone tissues have received prolonged treatment with acid in the demineralization process. Necrotic bone may be removed completely by the remodeling process, or it may become sequestered (isolated). The process of simultaneous removal and replacement of necrotic bone has been called **creeping substitution.**

Regional acceleratory phenomenon

When bone is injured or receives a noxious stimulus of sufficient magnitude, there is acceleration of the normal physiologic defense and healing processes in that area. The magnitude of the response and the size of the affected region varies with the individual and the intensity of the stimulus. When the defense and healing processes are evoked, most vital tissue processes are accelerated above their normal value. The accelerated processes include bone tissue perfusion, modeling, and remodeling. Accelerated modeling and remodeling can be seen with bone scintigraphy as areas of biphosphonate accumulation (hot-spots), and they can be detected with fluorochrome bone markers as regions of increased bone turnover. The regional acceleratory phenomenon can be observed in association with numerous diseases, trauma, denervation, burns, bone infections, and neoplasms. This phenomenon is responsible for the multiple cement lines or mosaic pattern that characterize certain disease states. A regional acceleratory phenomenon can often accelerate longitudinal bone growth following fracture, denervation, tumor, or a surgical procedure (such as periosteal stripping). Because the remodeling process may remain accelerated for more than a year following bone injury, serial biopsies from the same bone cannot be used with bone labeling to make comparisons of disease progress.

Inflammation and repair

Injury to bone can cause reactions that occur in all organs (refer to bone infections): acute inflammation, formation of granulation tissue, and fibrous repair.

These processes do not differ in the skeletal system from that seen in other systems. One of the major functions of the skeleton is biomechanical support. Disease may weaken or reduce skeletal strength, causing a pathologic fracture; therefore, inflammation, repair, and adaptive reconstruction often predominate in the morphologic picture, and may obscure the true nature of the disease. It is frequently necessary to study the progression of a particular condition and to examine early states of disease in order to fully understand the pathogenesis of the disease. Fibrous tissue is sometimes deposited as a substitute for bone when disease prevents normal ossification. The fibrous tissue formed in association with hyperparathyroidism, or seen in myelofibrosis of anemia, probably differs from simple reparative fibrosis.

Growth and mineralization

Many diseases result from interference with the normal bone growth process. Inanition or negative nitrogen balance can reduce longitudinal bone growth. When cessation of growth becomes severe, there is an attempt at growth-plate closure; a lateral plate of bone is formed beneath the growth plate. When growth is reinitiated, these transverse bone plates will be left behind in the metaphysis as the growth cartilage moves away from them. Bone plates may be visualized radiographically or in bone specimens, and are termed **Harris growth arrest lines.** With time, the line is eventually remodeled. Focal growth-plate closure or abnormal bone growth is also seen following trauma, certain mineral deficiencies, and toxic conditions. **Longitudinal bone growth** is determined by: the rate of cell division in the proliferating zone, enlargement caused by cell hypertrophy, and production of interstitial matrix within the maturing cartilage zone. Enlargement in metaphyseal diameter is accomplished by cell division and apposition at the perichondrial ring. Normally, longitudinal and transverse growth are coupled, but different factors affect growth at these two sites. Growth hormone governs growth rate at both locations indirectly; a deficiency (**dwarfism**) or excess (**gigantism**) causes a proportionate change in the bone width and length. When longitudinal growth is inhibited more than transverse appositional growth, then the bones will be short; they will, however, have a normal diameter. Such is the case with the osteochondrodysplasias. When transverse growth is inhibited more than longitudinal growth, the bones will be long and thin. Under pathologic conditions, bone may be produced with the deposition of woven bone, as it was during fetal growth or following bone fracture. This can occur on the periosteal, endocortical, or trabecular surfaces, and may be focal or generalized; examples include: **osteophytes, exostosis, and enostosis.** Whenever bone is injured, it may react with the formation of an osteophyte. Osteophytes (enthesiophytes) form at tendinous insertions following injury to Sharpey fibers; osteophytes also form when there is local hemorrhage. **Microscopically,** an exostosis is seen to consist of compact or woven bone that is not arranged into haversian systems. The outer limit of original normal bone is usually visible as a slender line; the new bone appears as an added layer. In some cases, the extreme tip of an exostosis is formed of hyaline cartilage. Adjacent soft tissue may undergo inflammatory changes. **Juxtaposed bone** is the deposition of woven bone—which may be unusually basophilic—on pre-existing viable or necrotic bone; this deposition may be seen in a number of conditions. A classic example is creeping substitution of dead bone; however, juxtaposed bone may be seen in toxic osteopathies, such as fluorosis. This type of bone formation indicates a sudden disruption of normal surface bone remodeling processes by an overpowering insult or inciting agent. Neoplasia can be considered to be cell growth where there is proliferation without adequate control. Conditions that affect calcium/phosphorus homeostasis interfere with cartilage or bone matrix mineralization and cause abnormal endochondral ossification. Abnormal mineral homeostasis in the adult leads to an increased mineralization lag time; wide osteoid seams are seen at remodeling sites. In some cases, osteoid is not mineralized properly because the matrix is abnormal. This is best visualized in microradiographs; hypomineralization of osteons or trabeculae can be seen in diseases such as fluorosis and *Solanum malacoxylon* toxicity, or in injury due to internal irradiation. **Pathologic** (heterotopic or ectopic) **ossification** is the development of bony structures in normally soft tissues. In veterinary medicine, it is commonly seen in the lung and skin; it also occurs in association with myositis ossificans and fibrodysplasia ossificans, and with hip masses in Doberman pinschers with von Willebrand disease.

Modeling and remodeling

Bone modeling as a process occurs principally during growth, but it continues to a lesser extent throughout life. Bone **modeling-dependent reactions** affect compact bone and lead to insufficient or excess accumulations of bone of mechanically inappropriate architecture. An example of abnormal modeling activity is seen in angular limb deformities in foals with congenital hypothyroidism caused by the maternal ingestion of excessive iodine. Another bone modeling abnormality occurs in acromegaly, when growth hormone reactivates growth-plate endochondral ossification and articular cartilage chondrocyte proliferation. Modeling drifts can be reactivated in adult animals, and the formation of marginal osteophytes can occur in association with degenerative joint disease. The production of woven bone in the adult and the resorption of bone in association with metastatic tumor can be considered modeling activities. Osteoclast-mediated bone resorption may occur because T lymphocytes secrete a lymphokine-, interleukin 1-, or osteoclast-activating factor in response to products of sensitized macrophages.

    Bone remodeling is a continuous ongoing process that is under the influence of many different factors, both systemic and local: it is a common pathway by which diverse influences can affect bone structure; it

is the process that repairs microdamage induced by mechanical activity; and it is responsible for maintaining mineral homeostasis when the capacity of the bone surface-canalicular system is over extended. Remodeling-dependent reactions to injury occur in growing animals (as the spongiosa is remodeled) and in the adult (after modeling has slowed). These reactions include: losses or gains in the amount of bone, improper distribution, and bone of abnormal quality. Metabolic bone diseases have their major effect on the remodeling sequence.

References

Enlow DH. Osteocyte necrosis in normal bone. J Dent Res 1966;45:213.

Liu SL, Ho TC. The role of venous hypertension in the pathogenesis of Legg-Perthes disease: a clinical and experimental study. J Bone Joint Surg 1991;73:194–200.

Riser WH, Brodey RS, Biery DN. Bone infarctions associated with malignant bone tumors in dogs. J Am Vet Med Assoc 1972;160:414–421.

Sokoloff L, Habermann RT. Idiopathic necrosis of bone in small laboratory animals. Arch Pathol 1958;65:323–330.

ABNORMALITIES OF BONE GROWTH AND DEVELOPMENT

Genetic abnormalities, biomechanics, environment (toxins), hormones, and nutrition all influence bone growth and maturation. Selection has been used to maintain unusual skeletal characteristics in certain breeds or strains of animals, and this selected genetic constitution predisposes the animals to develop certain osseous defects (such as in the Manx cat). Many examples of genetically controlled skeletal disorders have been recognized in animals, especially laboratory animals. These have been summarized by Jones (1978) and Woodard (1978). It is thought that environmental factors act in a complementary way with the genotype of the embryo to produce congenital malformations. **Malformations** are structural defects that occur during the embryonic period because of a localized error of development. **Deformities** occur as alterations in the size, shape, or structure of bone that was previously normal; deformities usually arise late in embryonic life or after birth. Malformations resulting from the administration of a teratogen represent a continuous spectrum from minor variations of normalcy to gross abnormality incompatible with life. Hormones and nutrition influence bone growth, as indicated in the section on growth and mineralization. Nutritional deficiencies or excesses can alter bone strength and structure, and lead to biomechanical effects. The stress of ambulation causes strain within the weakened bone, causing a secondary adaptation. Nutritional deficiencies of calcium and phosphorus, or trace minerals and excess iodine cause angular limb deformities (bone modeling).

    Growth-plate injuries may be caused by traumatic events or by nutritional deficiencies and excesses. Severe injuries may cause focal growth-plate closure. When lesions are of sufficient size, they cause the bone to develop an abnormal shape. Deviations in the forelimb growth are common in dogs, and are associated with conditions that cause premature closure of the growth plates. **Retained endochondral hypertrophied cartilage** in the metaphysis is considered one of the most probable causes of retarded ulnar growth in the giant-breed dogs. The occurrence of lesions in dogs are increased by overnutrition, where protein, energy, or calcium is increased. When growth of the ulna is retarded and the ulna becomes shorter than the radius, the animal may develop a characteristic abducted foot. The development of **valgus** (outward bowing) or varus (inward bowing) have been associated with disproportionate growth of parallel limb bones, or with slowing of endochondral ossification on the lateral sides of a single growth plate. Vertebral deformities (kyphosis, scoliosis) may also be associated with mechanical alterations (spastic paralysis or bony defect) or collagen abnormalities (Ehlers-Danlos syndrome, Marfan syndrome).

References

Anonymous. Nomenclature des maladies osseses constitutionelles. [International nomenclature of constitutional diseases of bone]. Ann Radiol 1983;26:456–462.

Jones TC. Hereditary disease. In: Benirschke K, Garner FM, Jones TC, eds. Pathology of laboratory animals. Vol II. New York: Springer Verlag, 1978;1981–2064.

Woodard JC. The musculoskeletal system. In: Benirschke K, Garner FM, Jones TC, eds. Pathology of laboratory animals. Vol I. New York: Springer Verlag, 1978;663–888.

SKELETAL DYSPLASIAS

The skeletal dysplasias are a heterogeneous group of inheritable connective-tissue disorders that lead to abnormalities in the size and shape of the limbs, trunk, and skull. **(Osteo)chondrodysplasia** (Figure 19-8) frequently results in disproportionate short stature. Interstitial expansion of cartilage contributes to growth-plate thickness; cartilage apposition increases growth-plate width. Combined morphologic and biochemical studies have provided valuable insight into the variety of pathogenetic mechanisms producing the dysplastic conditions. The skeletal dysplasias can be interpreted as disorders of normal bone growth or modeling, and they are frequently classified by the potential site of the anatomic defect in the skeleton (epiphysis, metaphysis, or diaphysis). Thus, epiphyseal and metaphyseal dysplasias exist; each can be further differentiated, depending on whether the cranium or spine is also involved (cranio- or spondylo-epiphyseal dysplasias, spondylometaphyseal dysplasias). The short-limbed or disproportionate dwarfisms can be divided into those disorders in which: the major area of shortening is in the proximal segments of the limbs **(rhizomelic)**; the major shortening involves the middle segments of the limbs **(mesomelic)**; and the shortening primarily affects the digits **(acromelic)**. This basic classification serves as the beginning of the differential diagnosis; each of these classes can further be divided into several distinct disorders based on a variety of other clinicopathologic differences. **Dwarfism** is frequently manifest at birth; animals may

be born dead, or they may live only for a short period. On occasion, chondrodysplasia may appear later in life; the syndrome of elbow and retinal dysplasia in Labrador retrievers is an example of this type of chondrodysplasia. Osteogenesis imperfecta, osteopetrosis, and cortical hyperostosis are constitutional diseases of bone that have an incompletely known pathogenesis. They are classified as bone dysplasias with abnormal bone density. Fibrous dysplasia and multiple cartilaginous exostoses are developmental disorders of fibrous and cartilaginous components of the skeleton.

Chondrodysplasia

Skeletal dysplasias that develop on the basis of defective cartilage development constitute the chondrodysplasias. Various forms of chondrodysplasia have been recognized in most species of laboratory and domestic animals. Those of domestic animals are summarized in Table 19-1. As is the case with other conditions that cause disproportionate dwarfism, the chondrodysplasias represent a heterogeneous group of conditions. The cause is frequently related to an abnormality in the cartilage matrix (non-collagenous proteins, abnormal organization of type-II collagen, structural alteration of the type-II collagen molecule, abnormal proteoglycan metabolism). Two different histologic types can be distinguished.

HYPOCHONDROPLASIA

Hypochondroplasia represents those diseases in which the growth plate appears well-organized and regular endochondral ossification occurs. Snorter dwarfism in cattle is an example of hypochondroplasia, where the growth-plate histology appears essentially normal but longitudinal bone growth is very slow. Similar changes occur in the human disease termed achondroplasia.

DYSCHONDROPLASIA

Dyschondroplasia represents those diseases characterized by differing forms of disorganization of endochondral ossification. Most diseases in domestic and laboratory animals fall under this classification; specific disease processes tend to recur in the same species, breed, or strain.

MULTIPLE CARTILAGENOUS EXOSTOSES

Multiple protuberances of bone and cartilage—predominantly arising from bones at or near epiphyseal cartilage—have been described in humans, horses, dogs, and cats. Inheritance in humans and horses is clearly due to a single, dominant gene.

FIBROUS DYSPLASIA

Fibrous dysplasia is a rare condition. Polyostotic fibrous dysplasia is described as a familial disease in Doberman pinschers. The lesion may be visualized radiographically by enlargements and by multicompartmental lucencies in distal metaphyses that become displaced as the bone grows. The inherited nature of the

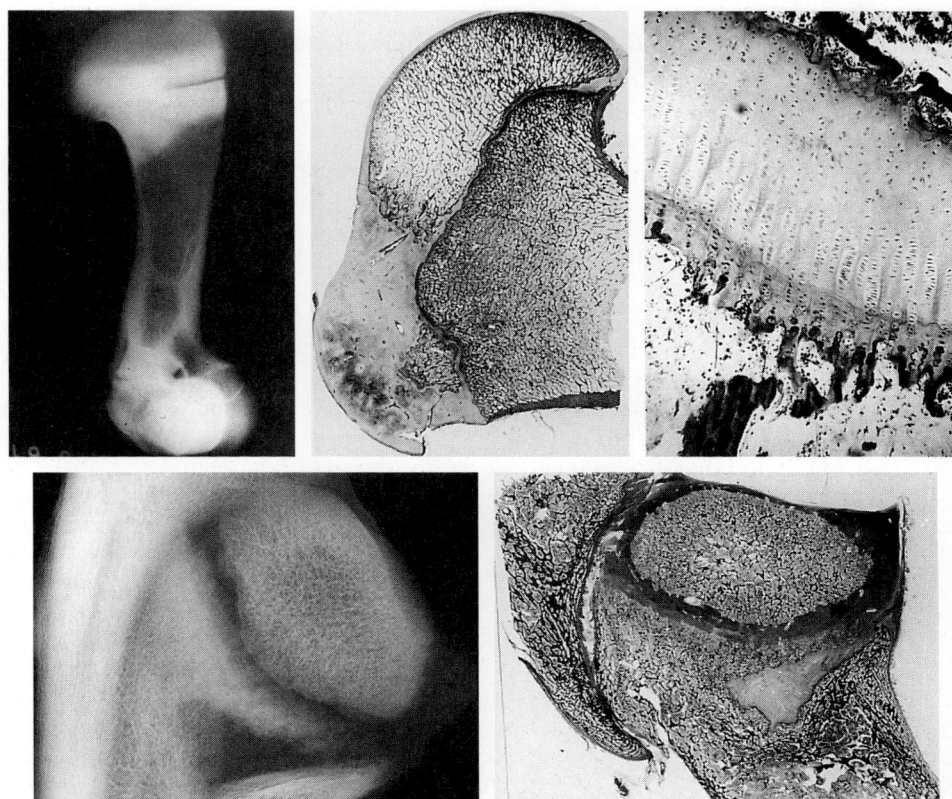

FIG. 19-8 Histologic types of osteochondrodysplasia. **A, B,** and **C:** hypochondroplasia, "snorter" dwarf calf. **A.** Radiograph of humerus; the bone is shorter than normal, and it has a dumbbell shape because the width is not reduced proportionally. **B.** Section of head of humerus illustrates narrow growth plate and incomplete development of the secondary ossification center. **C.** High magnification of the growth plate (hematoxylin-and-eosin stain); nearly normal morphology with some cartilage cells lined up in columns; reduced longitudinal growth is indicated by the narrow zone of hypertrophied cartilage cells, poor invasion by marrow capillaries, and apposition of osseous tissue adjacent to the metaphyseal surface of the growth plate. (Courtesy of A. Lorincz and W. Ennecking, and the University of Florida.) **D.** and **E.** Dyschondroplasia, equine neonate. **D.** Radiograph of a sagittal section of proximal radius; the growth plate is wide with flocculent radiodensity and a triangular radiolucent zone beneath. **E.** Histology of **D** (hematoxylin-and-eosin stain); growth plate is wide and disorganized; incomplete mineralization of hypertrophic cartilage occurs, as well as necrosis of hypertrophic chondrocytes and failure of endochondral ossification.

disease has not been established. Lesions of a similar nature are reported as monostotic lesions in horses, dogs, cats, pigs, and monkeys. Histologic appearance is that of fibrous replacement of bone containing woven-bone trabeculae that are formed by direct conversion of fibro-osseous tissue to bone (osseous metaplasia). The characteristic shapes of the trabeculae are curled configurations. Notably absent are mature plump osteoblasts; these form lamellar bone, and normally occur in rows lining trabeculae. Sometimes, fibrous dysplasia appears more primitive, with mitosis of mesenchymal cells, maturation of stroma toward osteoblasts, and distinct intramembranous formation of basophilic woven-bone trabeculae. The condition must be distinguished from other conditions, such as: metabolic bone disease that leads to fibrous osteodystrophy; bone tumors; and other conditions that cause bone cysts, including osteosarcoma.

OSTEOGENESIS IMPERFECTA

In humans, osteogenesis imperfecta occurs more frequently than does osteopetrosis; in animals, however, the converse is true. Osteogenesis imperfecta is a heterogenous group of diseases in which collagen abnormalities are considered the biochemical basis for the disease process. The condition is characterized by increased bone fragility. Histologically, poor collagen formation occurs in the bone trabeculae; or, the bone is hypercellular and composed of woven bone. Several structural defects in type I procollagen have been identified, but in many cases structural defects in type I collagen are less evident. Animals notably have increased bone fragility, and the conversion of fetal bone into an adult type is inhibited. The condition is recognized sporadically in dogs and cats, but is best-defined in cattle. Two different varieties of osteogenesis imperfecta are recognized as autosomal-dominant conditions in Holstein calves.

TABLE 19-1 **Osteochondrodysplastic dwarfism in domestic animals**[1]

Species	Disease name	Breed	Morphology	Inheritance	References
Canine[2]	Chondrodysplasia	Alaskan malamute	Spondylometaphyseal dysplasia	Recessive	Fletch (1971, 1972, 1973) Sande (1982) Bingel (1985) Smart (1971) Subden (1972)
	Chondrodysplasia	Scottish deerhound	Spondyloepimetaphyseal dysplasia	Recessive	Breur (1989)
	Pseudoachondroplastic dwarfism (Multiple epiphyseal dysplasia)	Beagle, miniature poodle	Spondyloepiphyseal dysplasia	Recessive	Rasmussen (1971, 1973) Cotchin (1956) Lodge (1966) Gardner (1959) Riser (1980)
	Chondrodysplasia	Norwegian elkhound	Spondylometaphyseal dysplasia, intracytoplasmic chondrocyte inclusions	Recessive	Bingel (1982)
	Chondrodysplasia	Great pyrenees	Spondylometaphyseal dysplasia micromelic	Recessive	Sande (1982)
	Ocular-skeletal dysplasia	Labrador retriever, samoyed	Multiple bone abnormalities	Unknown	Carrig (1977, 1988) Meyers (1983)
Bovine[2]	Dexter bull-dog, Telemark lethal, long-headed, short-headed	Numerous breeds of cattle from different countries	In general, micromelic animals with variation in grades of severity	Incompletely dominant or recessive[3]	Gregory (1967)
	Snorter dwarf	Angus, Hereford	Hypochondrodysplasia	Recessive	Jones (1982)
Ovine	Spider lambs	Suffolk, Hampshire	Epiphyseal dysplasia	Recessive	Rook (1988)
	Ancon type	Ancon, Otter, Cheviot	Rhizomelic	Recessive	Landauer (1949)
Equine	Rhizomelic	Mixed	Metaphyseal dysplasia	Unknown	Woodard (1990)

[1] Adapted from Sande and Bingel, 1982.
[2] Several breeds, English pointer, cocker spaniel, Scottish terrier, shorthorn and Aberdeen-angus, have been reported without data on pathology.

[3] Experiments suggest that all bovine chondrodystrophy genes are interrelated and components of the same genetic complex with the major conditioning-gene are recessive.

Overmodification of type I collagen has been demonstrated in calves and the two clinically identical bovine diseases can be distinguished easily by the osteonectin content of the bone matrix. Osteonectin is a noncollagenous bone matrix macromolecule. The Australian variety has a normal complement of osteonectin, whereas the Texas type has severely depleted osteonectin in bones. Similar changes in osteonectin have been noted in humans. Charolais cattle and sheep have also been reported to have the condition. Fragilitas ossium (fro)—an autosomal-recessive mutation in the mouse—is reported to have abnormalities similar to those found in the severe form of osteogenesis imperfecta.

References

Beachley MC, Graham FH Jr. Hypochondroplastic dwarfism (enchondral chondrodystrophy) in a dog. J Am Vet Med Assoc 1973; 163:283–284.
Bingel SA, Sande RD. Chondrodysplasia in the Norwegian elkhound. Am J Pathol 1982;107:219–229.
Bingel SA, Sande RD, Wight TN. Chondrodysplasia in the Alaskan malamute: characteristics of proteoglycans dissociatively extracted from dwarf growth plates. Lab Invest 1985;53:479–485.
Breur GJ, Zerbe CA, Slocombe RF, et al. Clinical, radiographic, pathologic, and genetic features of osteochondrodysplasia in Scottish deerhounds. J Am Vet Med Assoc 1989;195:606–612.
Carrig CB, Seawright AA. A familial canine polyostotic fibrous dyspla-

sia with subperiosteal cortical defects. J Small Anim Pract 1969;10:397–405.

Carrig CB, MacMillan A, Brundage S, et al. Retinal dysplasia associated with skeletal abnormalities in Labrador retrievers. J Am Vet Med Assoc 1977;170:49–57.

Carrig CB, Sponenberg DP, Schmidt GM, et al. Inheritance of associated ocular and skeletal dysplasia in Labrador retrievers. J Am Vet Med Assoc 1988;193:1269–1272.

Cotchin E, Dyce KM. A case of epiphyseal dysplasia in a dog. Vet Rec 1956;68:427–428.

Denholm LJ, Cole WG. Heritable bone fragility, joint laxity, and dysplastic dentin in Friesian calves: a bovine syndrome of osteogenesis imperfecta. Aust Vet J 1983;60:9–17.

Fletch SM, Smart ME, Pennock PW, et al. Clinical and laboratory features of an inherited skeletal defect in purebred Alaskan malamutes. J Am Vet Med Assoc 1971;158:1863.

Fletch SM, Pinkerton PH. An inherited anaemia associated with hereditary chondrodysplasia in the Alaskan malamute. Can Vet J 1972;13:270–271.

Fletch SM, Smart ME, Pennock PW, et al. Clinical and pathologic features of chondrodysplasia (dwarfism) in the Alaskan malamute. J Am Vet Med Assoc 1973;162:357–361.

Gardner DL. Familial canine chondrodystrophia foetalis (achondroplasia). J Pathol Bacteriol 1959;77:243–247.

Gardner EJ, Shupe LL, Leone NC, et al. Hereditary multiple exostosis: a comparative genetic evaluation in man and horses. J Hered 1975;66:318–326.

Gee BR, Doige CE. Multiple cartilagenous exostoses in a litter of dogs. J Am Vet Med Assoc 1970;156:53–59.

Gregory PW, Julian LM, Tyler WS. Bovine achondroplasia: possible reconstitution of the Telemark lethal. J Hered 1967;58:220–224.

Hare WCD, Wilkinson JS, McFeely RA, et al. Bone chondroplasia and a chromosome abnormality in the same dog. Am J Vet Res 1967;28:583–587.

Holmean JR, Baker JR, Davies ET. Osteogenesis imperfecta in lambs. Vet Rec 1964;76:980–984.

Jones JM, Jolly RD. Dwarfism in Hereford cattle: a genetic, morphological, and biochemical study. NZ Vet J 1982;30:185–189, Vet Bull 1983;53:4037.

Landauer W, Chang TK. The Ancon and Otter sheep: history and genetics. J Hered 1949;40:105–112.

Lodge D. Two cases of epiphyseal dysplasia. Vet Rec 1966;79:136–138.

Maroteaux P, Lamy M. Achondroplasia in man and animals. Clin Orthop 1964;33:91–103.

Mather GW. Achondroplasia in a litter of pups. J Am Vet Med Assoc 1956;128:327–328.

McKusick VA, Scott CI. A nomenclature for constitutional disorders of bone. J Bone Joint Surg 1971;53:978–986.

Meyers VN, Jezyk PF, Aguirre GD, et al. Short-limbed dwarfism and ocular defects in the Samoyed dog. J Am Vet Med Assoc 1983;183:975–979.

Pool RR, Carrig CB. Multiple cartilaginous exostoses in a cat. Vet Pathol 1972;9:350–359.

Pool RR. Tumors of bone and cartilage. In: Moulton JE, ed. Tumors in domestic animals. 3rd ed. Berkeley: Univ Calif Press, 1978;157–230.

Rasmussen PG. Multiple epiphyseal dysplasia in a litter of beagle puppies. J Small Anim Pract 1971;12:91–97.

Rasmussen PG, Reimann I. Multiple epiphyseal dysplasia with special reference to histologic findings. Acta Pathol Microbiol Scand 1973;81:381–389.

Riser WH, Haskins ME, Jezyk PF, et al. Pseudoachondroplastic dysplasia in Miniature poodles: clinical, radiologic, and pathologic features. J Am Vet Med Assoc 1980;176:335–341.

Rook JS, Trapp AL, Krehbiel J, et al. Diagnosis of hereditary chondrodysplasia (spider lamb syndrome) in sheep. J Am Vet Med Assoc 1988;193:713–718.

Sande RD, Bingel SA. Animal models of dwarfism. Vet Clin North Am Small Anim Pract 1982;13:71–89.

Sande RD, Alexander JE, Spencer GR, et al. Dwarfism in Alaskan malamutes: a disease resembling metaphyseal dysplasia in human beings. Am J Pathol 1982;106:224–236.

Smart ME, Fletch S. A hereditary skeletal growth defect in purebred Alaskan malamutes. Can Vet J 1971;12:31–32.

Subden RE, Fletch SM, Smart MA, et al. Genetics of the Alaskan malamute chondrodysplasia syndrome. J Hered 1972;63:149–152.

Woodard JC. Personal observations, 1990.

OSTEOPETROSIS

Congenital osteopetrosis in domestic animals rarely occurs. In those examples in animals which have been adequately studied, it has autosomal-recessive transmission. The disease has been recognized in most animal species; it represents a diverse group of conditions (Fig. 19-9) characterized by either abnormal osteoclast differentiation or function. In most cases, the disease is evident at birth and is lethal. Alterations in bone are associated with failure of osteoclastic resorption of cartilage as the primary spongiosa is formed; also, the woven bone initially laid down on the primary trabeculae fails to be resorbed. Consequently, the bone diaphysis becomes filled with cancellous bone. The bone frequently has an abnormal shape at the cut-back zone because of failure of the osteoclasts to function on the metaphyseal bone surface. Even though the metaphyseal bone diameter may be increased and the diaphysis is dense, bones are subject to pathologic fracture; this is because the medullary cavity contains woven bone, and no remodeling occurs to permit adaptation to biomechanical stress or to repair microdamage. The bone may contain few osteoclasts, or numerous osteoclasts may fail to function properly. In some examples of osteopetrosis, bone marrow transplantation may cure the condition by furnishing osteoclast precursor cells. In the case of a mutant strain of mice (OP), marked reduction and abnormal differentiation of osteoclasts have been associated with a failure to produce a functional macrophage colony-stimulating factor. A wide spectrum of morphologic changes may be observed (Table 19-2); for example, alterations in metaphyseal radiographic density in cattle indicate that osteoclasts operate appropriately at certain times. The juvenile form of osteopetrosis in dogs is often presented with spontaneous bone fracture or anemia. The external shape of the bone appears normal in this type of canine osteopetrosis, but the marrow cavity is filled with cancellous bone. Therefore, the osteoclasts function appropriately at the cut-back zone on the metaphyseal surface, but not within the marrow cavity. It seems that osteopetrosis is caused by failure of osteoclastic resorption; however, the pathogenesis that leads to failure of formation of mature osteoclasts or to proper function differs in each animal mutant.

References

Leipold HW, Cook JE. Osteopetrosis in Angus and Hereford calves. Am J Pathol 1977;86:745–748.

Marks SC Jr. Congenital osteopetrotic mutations as probes of the origin, structure, and function of osteoclasts. Clin Orthop 1984;189:239–263.

Nation PN, Klavano GG. Osteopetrosis in two foals. Can Vet J 1986;27:74–77.

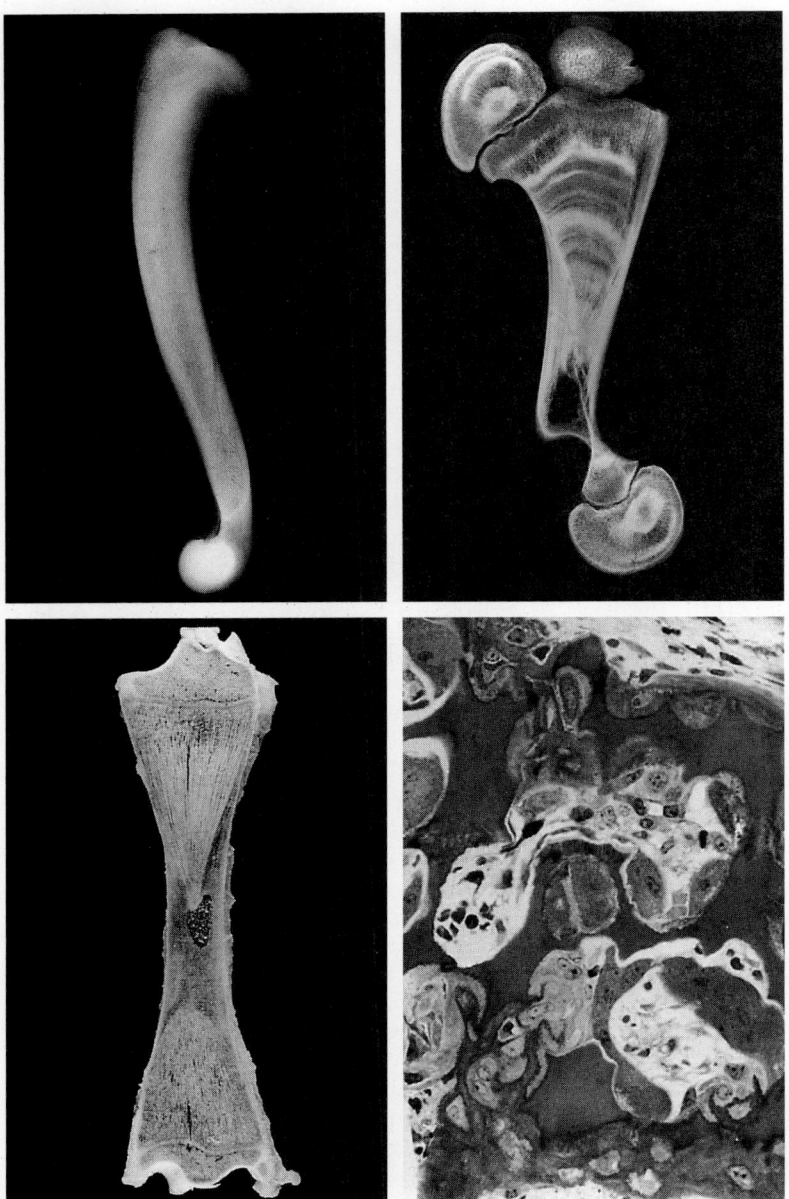

FIG. 19-9 Osteopetrosis. **A.** Canine juvenile form of osteopetrosis (osteopetrosis tarda). Radiograph of osteosclerotic humerus demonstrates small medullary cavity but a normal external bone contour. **B.** Congenital osteopetrosis, angus calf. Radiograph illustrates radiodense bands that correspond to retention of calcified cartilage caused by a temporal decrease in osteoclast function (Courtesy of David Young.) **C.** Equine neonatal osteopetrosis, tibia, Peruvian Paso foal. Triangular zones of metaphyseal bone—derived from the growth plate during bone elongation—are retained within the marrow cavity. In addition, diminished bone resorption of the external metaphyseal surface makes this region wider than normal, and the bone does not have its normal hour-glass appearance. **D.** Section from **C** illustrates the primary spongiosa. The darker mineralized cartilage is covered by lighter appearing osteoid. Howship lacunae are lined by numerous abnormally shaped osteoclasts. The retention of cartilage within the metaphysis indicates that resorption by individual osteoclasts is not proceeding at a normal rate.

Walker DG. Congenital osteopetrosis in mice cured by parabiotic union with normal siblings. Endocrinology 1972;91:916–920.

CORTICAL HYPEROSTOSIS

Cortical hyperostosis occurs as a familial disease in infant children, rhesus monkeys (Caffey disease), and newborn pigs **(congenital hyperostosis).** The condition in pigs is uncommon and is considered to follow an autosomal-recessive mode of inheritance. Pigs are born dead or die soon after birth. Limb involvement may be variable, but one or more of the forelimbs are always involved. Lesions are found in the long bones; the femur, scapula, and metacarpals are often normal. Muscle atrophy and subcutaneous edema is prominent in the affected limb. Bone lesions are limited to regions of periosteal modeling, where a subperiosteal layer of woven bone radiates perpendicular from the developing concentric lamellae of more normal cortex. Trabeculae

within the marrow cavity and the inner cortex appear normal. The excessive bone is deposited on the periosteal surface prior to birth; longitudinal bone growth and osteoblastic matrix calcification stop soon after the animal is born. The condition is rare in primates, but closely compares to the familial form of infantile cortical hyperostosis of children. The disease in the nonhuman primate has been noted to regress after the first year, as does the condition in infants. Lesions in the primate may be found in the long bones and mandible, and are usually bilaterally symmetric. The periosteum is markedly and diffusely thickened; significant proliferation of subperiosteal new bone manifests in the diaphyses, and preexisting marrow cavities appear normal. The original diaphyseal cortical bone appears to be multifocally replaced in an irregular fashion with cancellous bone trabeculae. Distinguishing bone dysplasia from inflammation is important in the differential diag-

TABLE 19-2 **Osteopetrosis in animals**

Species (gene symbol)	Osteoclast number (ruffled border)	Successful bone marrow transplant	Transmission
Mouse			
Gray-lethal (gl/gl)	Decreased	Yes	Recessive
Microphthalmic (mi/mi)	Normal	Yes	Recessive
Osteosclerotic (oc/oc)	Increased (abnormal)	No	Recessive
Osteopetrotic (op/op)	Greatly decreased	No	Recessive
Rat			
Incisors-absent (ia/ia)	Greatly increased (abnormal)	Yes	Recessive
Osteopetrotic (op/op)	Greatly decreased	Yes	Recessive
Toothless (tl/tl)	Greatly decreased	No	Recessive
Rabbit			
Osteosclerotic (os/os)	Decreased	Unknown	Recessive
Dog			
Newborn lethal	Unknown	Unknown	Recessive
Juvenile	Decreased	Unknown	Unknown
Cow			
Newborn lethal	Slightly increased	Unknown	Recessive
Equine			
Newborn lethal	Increased (abnormal)	Unknown	Recessive
Human			
Adult, benign form	Unknown	Unknown	Dominant
Juvenile malignant form	Decrease/increase	Yes/no	Recessive
Juvenile mild form	Unknown	Unknown	Recessive
Carbonic anhydrase II def.	Unknown	Unknown	Recessive
Infantile lethal	Unknown	Unknown	Recessive

*Modified from Marks SC. Congenital osteopetrotic mutations as probes of the origin, structure, and function of osteoclasts. Clin Orthop 1984; *189*:239–257.

nosis of cortical hyperostosis. Significant neutrophilic inflammation is not part of the conditions in pigs or rhesus, and growth plates and epiphyses appear normal.

References

Doize B, Martineau G-P. Congenital hyperostosis in piglets: a consequence of a disorganization of the perichondrial ossification groove of Ranvier. Can J Comp Med 1984;48:414–419.

Snook SS, King NW Jr. Familial infantile cortical hyperostosis (Caffey's disease) in rhesus monkeys (Macaca mulatta). Vet Pathol 1989; 26:274–277.

CRANIOMANDIBULAR OSTEOPATHY

Craniomandibular osteopathy ("lion jaw"), a hereditary bone disease of unknown pathogenesis of young dogs, is characterized by multiple bilateral exostoses of the mandible and tympanic bullae of the temporal bone (Figure 19-10). Less regularly, exostoses occur on the occipital, frontal, lacrimal, and maxillary bones; in some instances, bones of the limbs are involved. The disease is most frequent in Scottish terriers, West Highland White terriers, and Cairn terriers; however, it has been seen in other breeds as well. Exostoses of the mandibular processes and tympanic bullae mechanically obstruct the motion of the jaw; this causes difficulty in eating, which is usually the first sign of the disease. Distortion of the mandible is rarely the first recorded observation, owing to the long shaggy hair around the head of the breeds usually affected. As the lesions advance, the mouth may not be able to open more than 1 or 2 cm, and the mandible may approach twice the normal thickness. The exostoses are tender to the touch, and intermittent fever may occur (up to 40°C); however, aside from pain and the inability to eat, the condition does not cause other systemic signs. The disease is usually first seen in dogs three to seven months of age; it runs a course of intermittent progression and regression of the exostosis until 11–13 months of age, when the disease ceases to progress and may recede completely. Disappearance of the condition corresponds with closure of the growth plates.

The **gross lesions** involve the maxilla, tympanic bullae, long bones, and occasionally the parietal and frontal bones. The long bones may have exostoses extending outward from the preexisting cortex; or, fingerlike projections may extend from the metaphysis, surrounded by dense collagenous tissue. The mandible is thickened through its width and length, usually from the middle mental foramen caudally. The greatest change appears in the region of the angular process. The lesions are, in general, bilaterally symmetric. The tympanic bullae are enlarged three to four times their

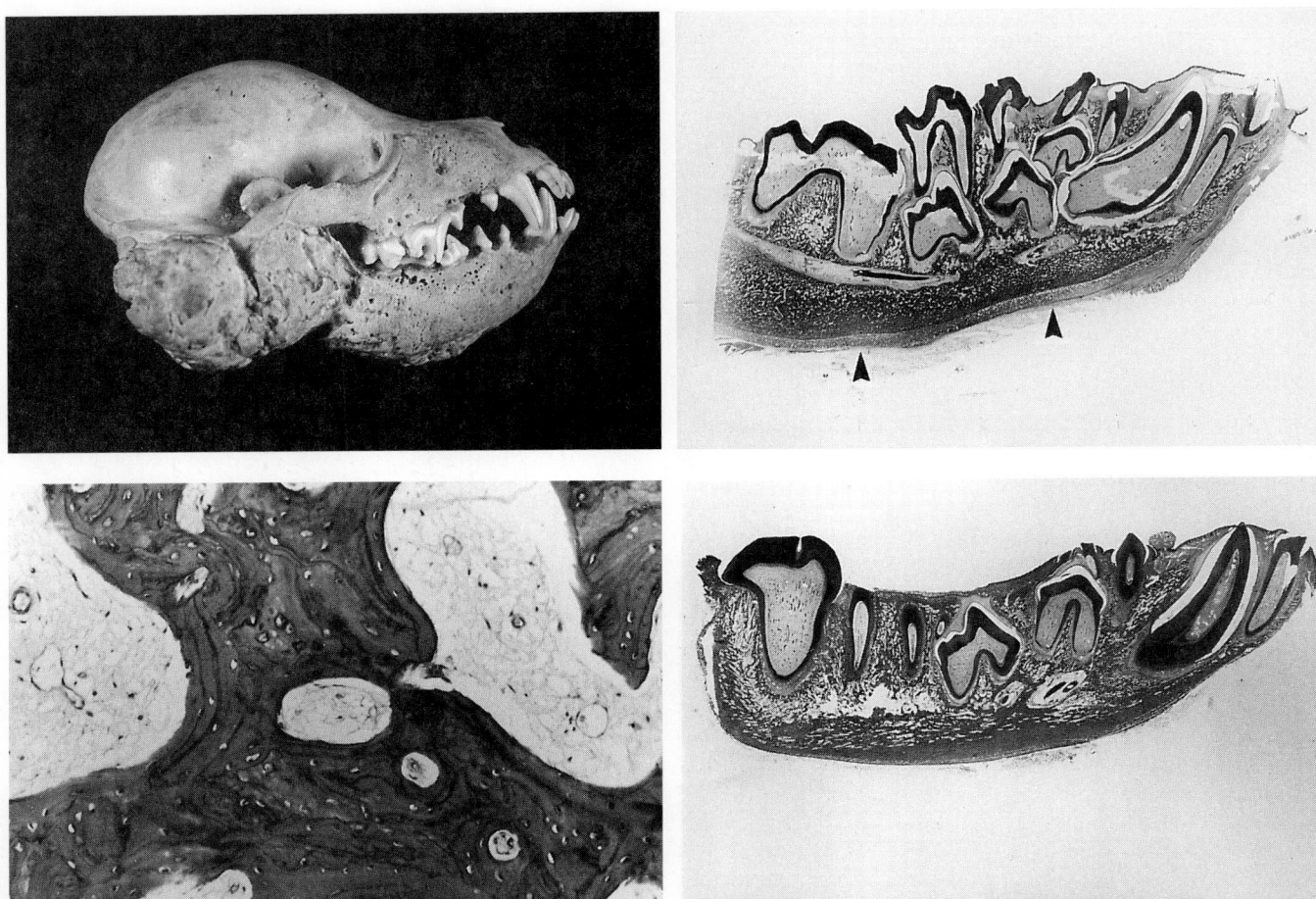

FIG. 19-10 Craniomandibular osteopathy. **A.** In this macerated specimen, portions of the mandible, maxilla, temporal, and occipital bones are thickened and fused by extraosseous bone. **B.** Mandible from affected dog. There has been subperiosteal proliferation of woven bone (arrowheads), and the cortex is less compact. Active bone resorption increases cortical porosity and produces a trabecular bone pattern. **C.** High magnification of porous area of affected mandible demonstrates trabecular bone pattern and prominent cement lines that separates underlying woven bone from overlying lamellar bone. **D.** Mandible from normal dog can be compared with affected animal in **B.** (Courtesy of Dr. Wayne H. Riser.)

normal diameter, and are filled with new bone. Each bulla is usually fused with the adjacent angular process of the mandible. This fusion obviously interferes with the movement of the mandible.

Microscopic lesions in the mandible consist of bony proliferation on the periosteal surface and internal replacement of cortical bone with osseous trabeculae. In some instances, osseous proliferation is not accompanied by inflammation; however, active areas of ossification or bone remodeling are often associated with suppurative foci. In other regions, trabeculae are separated by highly vascular fibrous stroma that contains a mixed inflammatory cell population of macrophages, neutrophils, lymphocytes, and plasma cells. Characteristic of the newly produced trabeculae is a mosaic pattern of irregular cement lines (reversal lines). The prominent cement-line pattern in trabeculae of the enlarged bone is evidence that intense remodeling activity occurred previously. Necrotic bone is observed in some trabeculae.

Although the condition in West Highland White

terriers has been shown to be an autosomal-recessive disorder, its pathogenesis has not been thoroughly investigated. It is basically an osseous proliferation disorder that resolves with time. It is unclear why some lesions are characterized by acute inflammation. In the differential diagnosis one must consider an infectious process; dissecting periostitis can lead to facial enlargement. Bone inflammation is one cause of the regional acceleratory phenomenon (refer to *bone reactions to injury*); accelerated remodeling can produce the cement-line mosaic pattern that also characterizes craniomandibular osteopathy. The inflammation of dissecting periostitis is much more intense than that characteristically seen in terriers with craniomandibular osteopathy. These lesions and the clinical features of the canine disease have some similarities to cortical hyperostosis.

References

Burk RL, Broadhurst JJ. Craniomandibular osteopathy in a Great Dane. J Am Vet Med Assoc 1976;169:635–636.
Padgett GA, Mostosky UV. The mode of inheritance of craniomandib-

ular osteopathy in West Highland White terrier dogs. Am J Med Genet 1986;25:9–13.

Riser WH, Parkes LJ, Shirer JR. Canine craniomandibular osteopathy. J Am Vet Radiol Soc 1967;8:23–31.

Watson AD, Huxtable CR, Farrow BR. Craniomandibular osteopathy in Doberman pinschers. J Small Anim Pract 1975;16:11–19.

METABOLIC BONE DISEASE

In the young, metabolic bone diseases interfere with normal bone growth and development; in adult animals, they interfere with normal bone remodeling. Rickets, osteomalacia, fibrous osteodystrophy, and osteoporosis are diseases that can be defined by a precise set of morphologic lesions that describe each disease. However, the lesions in one of the above conditions can overlap with the lesions of another, causing more complex metabolic disturbances in bone. Therefore, the lesions in an individual animal may not allow easy classification into one of these specific disease categories. Since many of the metabolic bone diseases are characterized by defective bone formation, they can also be classified as a type of osteodystrophy: for example, renal osteodystrophy and nutritional osteodystrophy. This nomenclature is convenient when the morphology of the metabolic processes overlaps, as occurs in conditions caused by secondary hyperparathyroidism. Understanding metabolic bone disease is difficult because the same disease name may have a different meaning when used by individuals in other disciplines. For example, biochemists frequently refer to any bone disease associated with vitamin D deficiency in a young animal as rickets, whereas the bone histology of that condition may not necessarily fit the disease rickets. Terms used to describe pathologic lesions may have a different connotation to clinicians. Radiologists use the term osteopenia when they are unable to distinguish between loss of bone with normal mineralization (osteoporosis) and decreased density due to incomplete mineralization of osteoid (osteomalacia). Another confusing factor is that the same terms are used to name a specific disease and to designate a morphologic lesion (diagnosis) that might characterize more than one disease. In order to clarify descriptions as much as possible, the following terms and their definitions should be used as morphologic diagnoses, regardless of disease designation:

(1) **Osteomalacia**—defective mineralization of bone matrix;
(2) **Fibrous osteodystrophy**—increased osteoclastic resorption of bone with fibrosis;
(3) **Osteosclerosis**—too much mineralized trabecular bone;
(4) **Osteopenia**—reduction in bone mass; and,
(5) **Osteoporosis**—reduction in the amount of bone that appears normally mineralized below what is normal for the animal's age, sex, and species.

Rickets and osteomalacia

Rickets (rachitis) is a disease characterized by abnormal endochondral ossification caused by failure to deposit

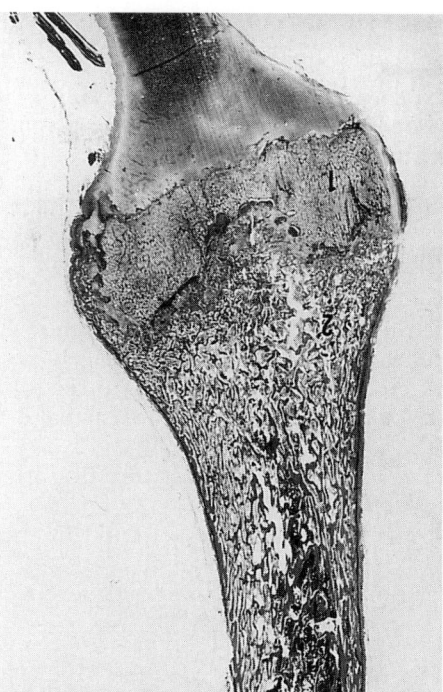

FIG. 19-11 Rickets: dog rib. (1) Failure to mineralize hypertrophic cartilage causes characteristic increased thickness of growth-plate cartilage and retention of cells in the hypertrophic cartilage zone. (2) The metaphysis adjacent to the growth plate demonstrates the affects that respiratory movement has on weakened bone structure. (Courtesy of Dr. Wayne H. Riser.)

adequate quantities of mineral in the bones of growing animals (Fig. 19-11) and children. The circumstances that cause rickets in young animals often lead to soft bones and the accumulation of excessive osteoid in adults. The disease in adults is termed osteomalacia.

GROSS APPEARANCE

The ends of the long bones are enlarged, as are the costochondral articulations. The former are observable during life; in severe cases the bones of the limbs become permanently bent under the weight of the animal's body, producing valgus ("bow legs") and other skeletal deformities. Due to the weakening of the muscles and tendons, the abdomen is pendulous. At necropsy the same changes are seen; the enlarged costochondral articulations—viewed collectively from the inner side—have been likened to a string of beads, the "rachitic rosary." This condition persists even after healing; the enlarged articulations become permanently calcified without regressing. Even the intestine may appear relaxed and dilated. When a long bone is sawed longitudinally, the growth cartilage is seen to be abnormally thick due to unimpaired proliferation of the cartilage. The bones are abnormally soft and can often be cut with a knife. In birds, a crooked sternum with deviation to one side frequently occurs and reflects a mild degree of rickets in early life.

MICROSCOPIC APPEARANCE

The principal microscopic changes include:

(1) An increase in thickness of the zone of hypertrophic cartilage cells adjacent to the primary spongiosa of the metaphysis;

(2) Disorderly arrangement of hypertrophic cartilage, as well as a crookedness and irregularity of this zone or line as it stretches from one side of the bone to the other. Normally, the cartilage cells form regular rows running lengthwise of the bone; in rickets no such rows exist. Because the whole bone is widened at this point, the cartilage is correspondingly increased in the transverse direction also;

(3) Disorderly penetration of the cartilage by blood vessels;

(4) Defective calcification and failure of normal degeneration of the cartilage;

(5) Great excess of uncalcified osteoid in the metaphysis;

(6) Marrow tends to be fibrosed with a corresponding reduction of myeloid cells.

Evidence of increased resorption is usually not a feature of rickets; in fact, osteoclasts are fewer in number than one might expect. However, when secondary hyperparathyroidism (in response to hypocalcemia) is severe, bone resorption and fibrous replacement become features of rickets, and the microscopic appearance, especially in the diaphysis, tends toward that of fibrous osteodystrophy. Often, rachitic animals are given dietary supplements before a bone specimen is taken for diagnostic purposes; the pathologist, therefore, is required to make a diagnosis when the lesion is in the initial reparative stage.

CAUSES AND PATHOGENESIS OF RICKETS AND OSTEOMALACIA

(1) Vitamin D deficiency is the classic cause of rickets in children or young animals. However, it is not possible to produce vitamin-D-deficiency rickets in a puppy when the dam had an adequate vitamin source. Apparently, the mother transfers sufficient vitamin D to the liver of her young to protect against disease. The microscopic lesions described above can develop as a result of an inadequate availability of calcium, or in any disorder favoring hypocalcemia;

(2) Dietary lack of calcium is a fundamental cause, but in actual practice this seldom occurs, probably because longitudinal bone growth declines in calcium deficiency;

(3) Continued escape of calcium from the intestinal tract in combination with fatty acids from unassimilated fat (celiac rickets) is theoretically important;

(4) Formation of other insoluble complexes between calcium and oxalate or phytate can prevent calcium absorption;

(5) Deficiency of phosphorus is able to cause rickets, since this element is essential in forming calcium phosphate. Phosphorus deficiency is common in herbivorous animals in certain parts of the world (Gulf Coast of the United States, and in South Africa) where the soil is deficient in this element. However, other signs resulting from chewing clostridial-infected bones usually direct attention to the deficiency before the impaired condition of the bones becomes apparent. In addition to simple dietary lack, phosphorus deficiency can arise from steatorrhea, formation of insoluble complexes, and changes in the pH of intestinal contents;

(6) A severely unbalanced calcium-phosphorus ratio in the diet is capable of causing rickets; such cases are encountered especially where inexperienced caregivers supply mineral mixtures to livestock. When the diet contains an excessive amount of phosphorus—for example, when animals are fed too much wheat bran or bone meal—such an imbalance develops; either Ca ion or PO4 ion tends to be excreted with the feces in combination with its counterpart, as $Ca_3 (PO_4)_2$;

(7) Strontium rickets is a special type of rickets, usually induced experimentally. Strontium interferes with the conversion—by the kidneys—of 25-hydroxycholecalciferol to 1,25-dihydroxycholecalciferol (the most active form of vitamin D);

(8) Drugs or disease may interfere with liver vitamin D metabolism. The metabolism of vitamin D is discussed further in Chapter 16;

(9) Certain drugs, such as biphosphonates, can interfere with cartilage matrix mineralization; and,

(10) Rickets may be an inherited disease. Vitamin-D-resistant rickets is caused by failure of renal absorption of phosphorus, or by renal tubular acidosis. Persistent hypophosphatemia is apparent; however, bone lesions can be partially prevented with pharmacologic doses of vitamin D. Vitamin-D-dependent rickets is caused by a deficiency of the 1-α hydroxylase enzyme in renal tubules; or, it is caused by a failure of the end organ to respond to normal levels of vitamin D hormone; both conditions can be treated with $1,25 (OH)_2 D_3$.

The lesions of rickets develop because of inadequate mineralization of growth-plate cartilage. When cartilage does not mineralize, metaphyseal blood vessels fail to penetrate the maturing cartilage zone; a lack of chondroclastic resorption results. Therefore, the unmineralized hypertrophic cartilage cells persist. In addition, the osteoid forming on the primary trabeculae fails to mineralize. Biomechanical stress causes creep of the pliable cartilage and microfractures. A reparative response leads to fibrous tissue deposition, more cartilage, and accumulation of additional osteoid. Finally, low serum calcium levels stimulate the parathyroid glands and produce secondary hyperparathyroidism. Oddly, rickets is rarely seen in animals in the United States, and it may be difficult to produce experimentally in certain species. It occurs more commonly in northern latitudes when animals are fed inadequate diets. Several possible explanations exist for the infrequent occurrence of rickets. First, animals may be born with a significant supply of vitamin D when the dams have been exposed to sunlight or fed a nutritionally adequate diet. Animals with little skin pigment—such as albino rats—can synthesize vitamin D when exposed to fluorescent room lights. When the diet contains adequate levels of calcium and phosphorus, the requirement for vitamin D is significantly reduced. The classic lesion of rickets is abnormal endochondral ossification.

SIGNIFICANCE AND EFFECT

Supporting weight on the poorly calcified bones is painful, and results in lameness or disinclination to move. Pathologic fractures, even of the vertebral column, are not infrequent. When the cause is corrected, normal ossification promptly begins. The strength and hardness of the bone become normal, although the deformities tend to persist for life.

Although the serum calcium level of blood in rickets may decrease slightly (10%), parathyroids maintain blood calcium at the proper level, even at the expense of bone. Only rarely is there severe hypocalcemia in rickets. In these cases, tetany may occur. Serum alkaline phosphatase levels and serum levels of bone gamma-carboxyglutamic acid protein (osteocalcin or bone gla protein) are elevated. As indicated earlier, in longstanding rickets the parathyroids undergo hypertrophy to two or three times their normal size. In cases of hyperparathyroidism (for example, when caused by a parathyroid tumor) the bones lose calcium; however, the effect is different from that of rickets, and is known as fibrous osteodystrophy.

In some species, the changes in bone that are characteristic of rickets need to be distinguished from those of avitaminosis C (refer to chapter 16 on *vitamin C*).

Osteomalacia Osteomalacia occurs in the bones of adults through the same mechanisms as rickets in the young; it is often called **adult rickets.** Osteoclasts remove bone during the normal activation of the remodeling cycle; osteoid replaces the bone and mineralizes through the formative action of osteoblasts. In osteomalacia, the calcification rate decreases and the time between osteoid deposition and the onset of mineralization (mineralization lag time) increases, which leads to an increase in the width of unmineralized osteoid and an increase in bone surfaces covered with osteoid **(hyperosteoidosis).** In tissues that have not been subjected to prolonged decalcification, excessive pink-staining osteoid is apparent; this staining usually occurs in the form of wide borders around a basophilic rim and the central portion that marks the zone of mineralization in each bony trabecula. These osteoid borders lined by prominent osteoblasts are the so-called "osteoid seams" upon which the histopathologic diagnosis of osteomalacia is based. Because osteoid cannot always be clearly distinguished in decalcified sections, critical measurements should be made with sections prepared from undecalcified bone. As in rickets, osteoid is resistant to osteoclastic resorption; this allows its continual buildup. Osteoclasis of calcified bone may be apparent, but it is seldom a striking finding unless secondary hyperparathyroidism ensues. In the latter event, resorption and

fibrous replacement of bone become paramount, and the pathologic picture progresses to that of fibrous osteodystrophy. In hypophosphatemic osteomalacia—seen with phosphorus deficiency and renal tubular defects in phosphorus resorption—the lesions are similar to vitamin-D deficiency, except that no evidence of hyperparathyroidism exists and the activation frequency of new remodeling sites remains normal.

Irregular, diffuse thickening of the bones occurs all along the diaphysis; however, the bone is soft, easily cut or sawed, and may become permanently deformed. Because growth is no longer in progress, the epiphyseal changes are absent or minimal. Still, enlargement at the carpal and tarsal regions occurs (at least in horses). The flat bones of the head and pelvis experience thickening and distortion. Due to the stresses of bearing weight, marked deformity of the pelvis often develops.

Causes have been given under rickets. Significance and effect are also similar.

References

Bullock BC, Bowen JA. Rickets and osteomalacia in squirrel monkeys (Saimiri sciureus). Fed Proc 1966;25:533.
Collins DH. Rickets, osteomalacia, scurvy, and other effects of vitamins. In: Collins DH, ed. Pathology of bone. London: Butterworths, 1966;4:87–109.
Gershoff SN, Legg MA, O'Connor FJ, et al. The effect of vitamin D-deficient diets containing various Ca:P ratios on cats. J Nutr 1957;63:79–93.
Huffer WE, Lacey DL. Studies on the pathogenesis of avian rickets. II. Necrosis of perforating epiphyseal vessels during recovery from rickets in chicks caused by vitamin D3 deficiency. Am J Pathol 1982;109:302–309.
Suda T, Takahashi N, Shinki T, et al. The common marmoset as an animal model for vitamin D-dependent rickets, type II. Adv Exp Med Biol 1986;196:423–435.

Fibrous osteodystrophy

Also known by the Latin names **osteitis fibrosa cystica** and **osteodystrophia fibrosa,** fibrous osteodystrophy (Fig. 19-12) is characterized by marked bone resorption, fibrous replacement, and the formation of cysts; often, accelerated osteoid formation does not become mineralized (osteomalacia). Osteodystrophy is the direct result of the continuous and excessive action of parathyroid hormone on bone. In humans, the disease has also been called **von Recklinghausen disease.** Bones—especially ones with higher turnover, such as the mandible and maxilla—gradually soften and become flexible and deformed; often, they become considerably enlarged. At the same time, they are easily fractured and are painful when bearing weight. Radiologic examination shows widespread areas of rarefaction, sometimes with cystic spaces in them.

GROSS AND MICROSCOPIC APPEARANCES

Gross and microscopic examinations of severely affected bones indicate a marked disappearance of mature bone; this disappearance results because activation of remodeling leads to bone resorption and an increase in the number of resorption cavities. Numerous osteoclasts may occupy Howship lacunae; reticulin stains

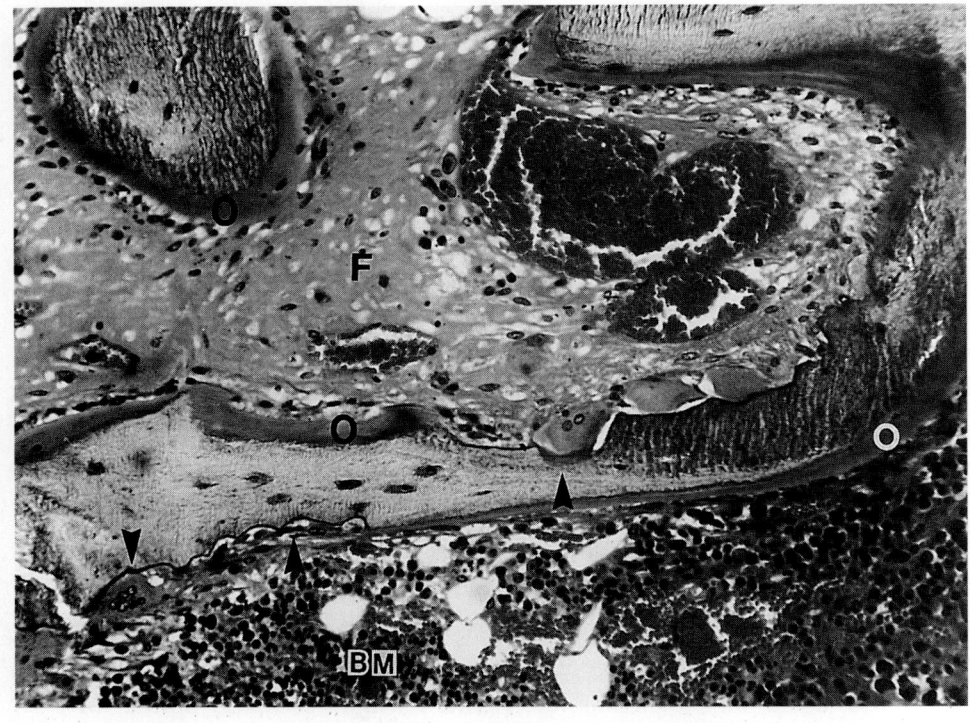

FIG. 19-12 Equine fibrous osteo-dystrophy. **A.** Section of mandible (×50) with replacement of marrow and cortex with irregular spicules of poorly calcified bone supported by a fibrous stroma. **B.** Mandible of an affected horse. Note great thickness of mandible, which was soft and easily cut with a knife. **C.** Section of mandible illustrates increased bone resorption by osteoclasts (arrowheads) and wide osteoid seams *(O)*. Normal bone marrow *(BM)* and fibrotic marrow *(F)*. Note that osteoclasts are not present on osteoid covered surfaces. Multiple stain of undecalcified methyl methacrylate section. (**A** and **B** Courtesy of Armed Forces Institute of Pathology; contributor: Colonels John J. Kintner and Rufus L. Holt.)

identify marrow fibrosis closely applied to the bone, initially in regions of resorption. As the condition progresses, dissection osteoclasia becomes a pathognomonic feature. Groups of osteoclasts visibly appear to bore into the center of bone trabeculae. In more severe cases, cortical bone is characterized by enlarged haversian canals, leading to a loss of bone substance. The remodeling space formerly occupied by calcified bone is filled by fibrous connective tissue; osteoclasts and osteoclastic giant cells line receding bone in some places,

and smaller osteoblasts attempt to replace the lost bone in others. The number of osteoblasts and the amount of osteoid deposition is variable and often extensive; these effects, coupled with large amounts of collagenous connective tissue, greatly increase the size of bones. As the disease becomes chronic, large portions of cortical bone are replaced by woven-bone trabeculae, many of which remain unmineralized (Fig. 19-13). A distinctive feature is the irregular pattern of osteoid mineralization. The degree of defective mineralization

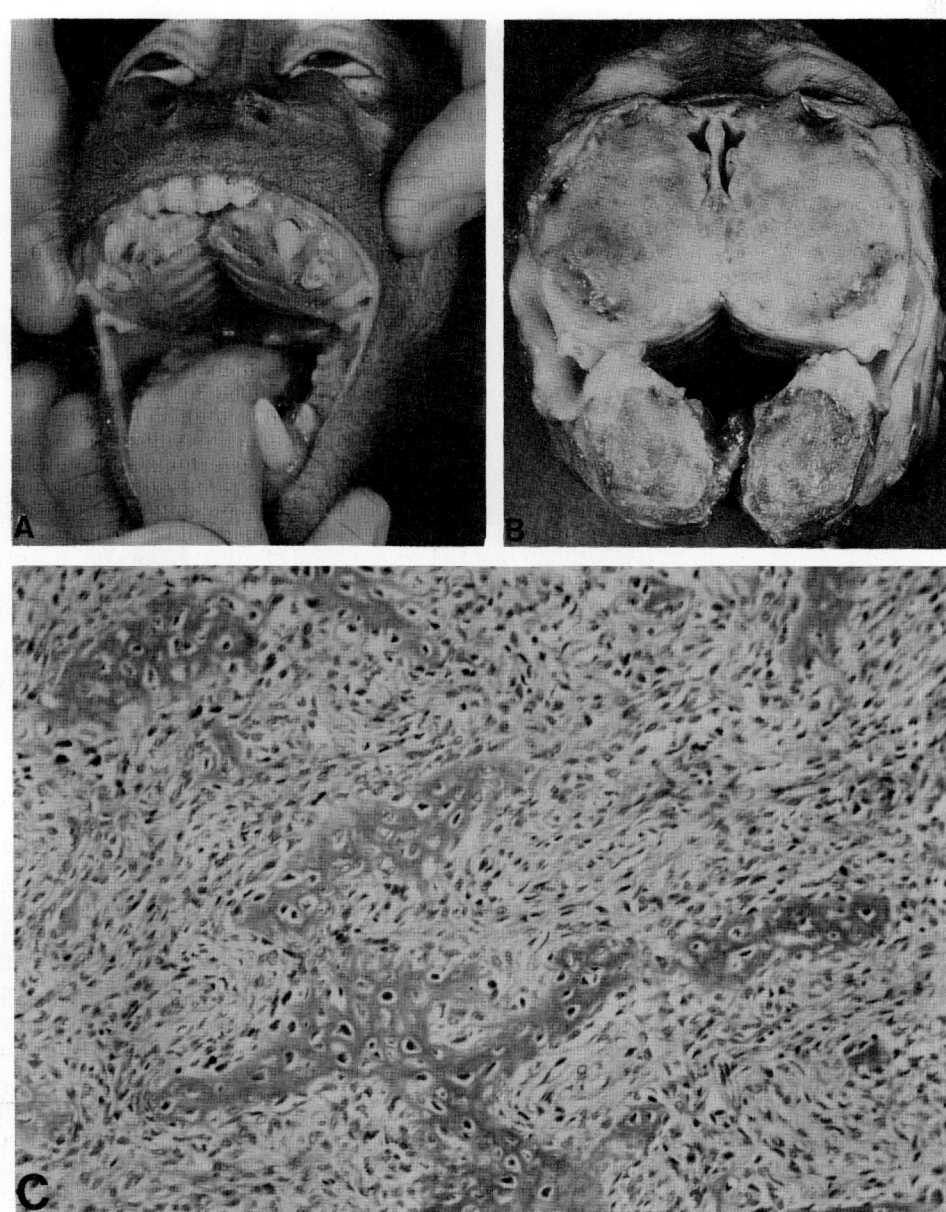

FIG. 19-13 Fibrous osteodystrophy in a 1 1/2-year-old male spider monkey. **A.** Thickened maxilla and deeply-embedded teeth in the living animal. **B.** Mandibles and maxillae, softened and thickened and encroaching on the nasal cavity; **C.** section of the maxilla with zones of unmineralized woven bone interspersed in fibrous marrow. (Hematoxylin-and eosin-stain, ×150.) (Courtesy of Angell Memorial Animal Hospital.)

differs depending upon the pathogenesis. The fibrous tissue may undergo cystic degeneration in places, probably because of insufficient blood supply. The bones, in addition to being deformed, may be so soft that they can be cut with a knife.

As indicated, the cause and pathogenesis of this startling disorder result from hyperparathyroidism, which can arise for several different reasons.

Primary hyperparathyroidism Primary hyperparathyroidism is usually the result of a functioning parathyroid adenoma, which is rare in animals. Parathyroid adenomas have been reported in horses, cattle, and dogs. In primary hyperparathyroidism, hypercalcemia occurs, as well as hypophosphatemia (renal loss) and marked elevation of serum alkaline phosphatase. Metastatic calcification of soft tissues is a consistent finding, and re-

nal mineralization can lead to an increase in serum phosphorus in animals with endstage kidneys.

Secondary hyperparathyroidism Secondary hyperparathyroidism is without question the most common cause of fibrous osteodystrophy (Fig. 19-14) in animals. Hypocalcemia, regardless of cause, is the stimulus for the increased activity of the parathyroid glands. In animals, secondary hyperparathyroidism occurs in nutritional deficiencies (nutritional secondary hyperparathyroidism) and in chronic renal disease. The lesions are similar to primary hyperparathyroidism, with added features of osteomalacia.

Renal secondary hyperparathyroidism Renal secondary hyperparathyroidism is most common in dogs, in which the disorder has been termed **renal rickets** or "rubber-jaw" (Fig. 19-15). Inability to excrete phos-

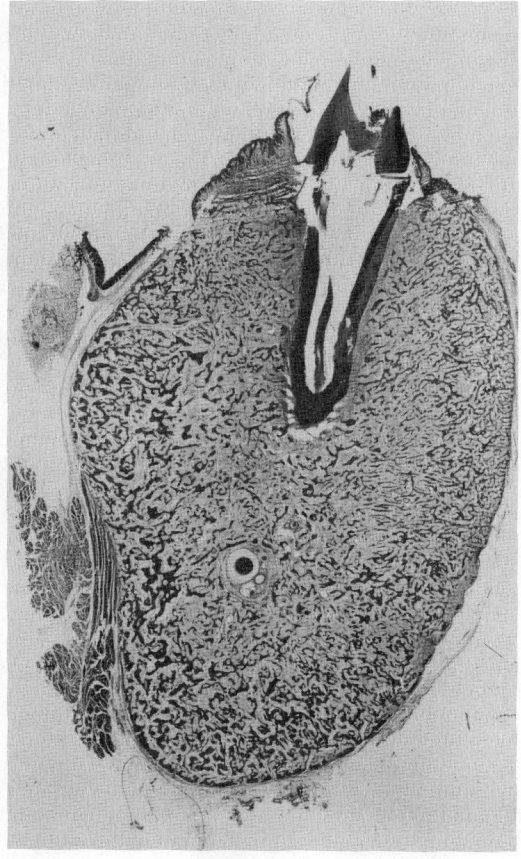

FIG. 19-14 Fibrous osteodystrophy, woolly monkey. The cortex, lamina dura and medullary cavity of the mandible have been entirely replaced with trabeculae of cancellous bone in a loose fibrous stroma. (Courtesy of New England Regional Primate Research Center, Harvard Medical School.)

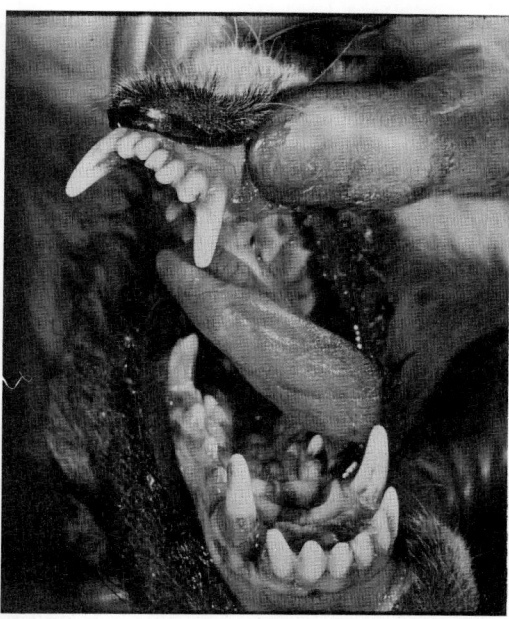

FIG. 19-15 The flexible "rubber jaws" of a 5 1/2-year-old male terrier with chronic interstitial nephritis. Normal jaws cannot be distorted in this manner. (Courtesy of Angell Memorial Animal Hospital.)

phates causes these ions to accumulate in the blood and leads to lowering of the serum calcium concentration. The damaged kidney and the inhibitory effects of increased phosphate decrease production of the active metabolite of vitamin D; the intestinal absorption of calcium subsequently decreases. Hyperparathyroidism in response to hypocalcemia causes marked resorption of bone, and hypocalcemia contributes to defective mineralization of osteoid (osteomalacia). Hyperphosphatemia is present throughout the course of the disease; serum alkaline phosphatase is also elevated. Unlike primary hyperparathyroidism—where serum calcium is elevated—serum calcium is usually low in renal secondary hyperparathyroidism. In dogs, the bones of the head undergo pronounced softening, enlargement, and radiographically detectable rarefaction; the jaws become "rubbery." **Microscopically,** the lesions are those of fibrous osteodystrophy and osteomalacia; resorption of bone occurs by osteoclastic resorption and fibrous replacement; and woven-bone trabeculae that fail to mineralize properly are excessively produced. Since osteoid retards osteoclastic activity, osteoclasts are found selectively on mineralized surfaces, and unmineralized bone tends to accumulate. All bones are affected to varying degrees, but the lesions are most striking in the facial bones and mandible. Metastatic calcification of soft tissues is a regular feature. All of the parathyroids are grossly enlarged. Tests for renal function are indicative of severe renal insufficiency.

Nutritional secondary hyperparathyroidism Nutritional secondary hyperparathyroidism has been described in most domestic animals as well as many exotic species. The usual nutritional imbalances associated with the development of fibrous osteodystrophy are deficiency of calcium or vitamin D, or excess of phosphorus. As indicated under rickets and osteomalacia, secondary parathyroid hyperplasia may develop, causing these diseases to progress to fibrous osteodystrophy.

Fibrous osteodystrophy Fibrous osteodystrophy, also described under the name **Bran disease,** occurred when horses—owned by flour-millers to whom bran was a cheap by-product—were fed bran almost exclusively. Similar changes can be seen when grain-fed animals are supplemented with hay of poor nutritional value, rather than alfalfa that is high in calcium. Changes in the head and facial outlines are commonly the first signs of the disease; it has therefore been described under the expressive designation of **"big head."** The sharp features of the head—especially in the region of the zygomatic arch and upper and lower jaws—become rounded and indefinite, giving the appearance of more swelling than really exists. Dissection shows a uniform thickening and rounding due to diffuse proliferation of imperfect bone in the subperiosteal region. The teeth may loosen and fall out. Lameness also occurs, and general tenderness of the joints. **Microscopically,** classic lesions of fibrous osteodystrophy (Fig. 19-16) with osteo-

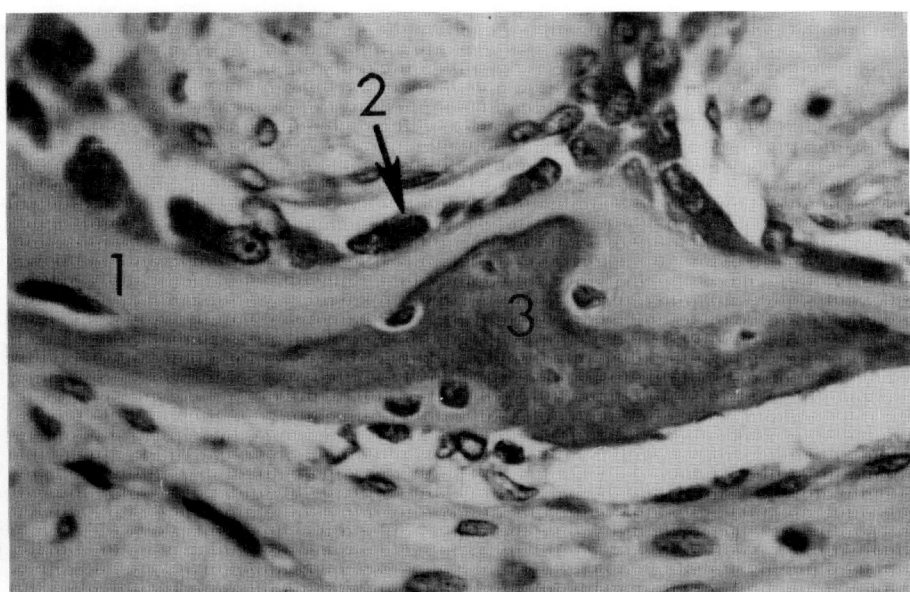

FIG. 19-16 Bone trabecula, fibrous osteodystrophy, in monkey. (1) The light staining osteoid; (2) Immediately beneath a layer of osteoblasts; (3) Overlays a mature spicula of bone; wide osteoid seams are the hallmark of osteomalacia.

malacia are most obvious in the facial bones and mandible; however, the lesions are generalized throughout the skeleton. The disorder is the result of diets low in calcium and high in phosphorus. Clinicopathologic findings may reveal hyperphosphatemia and hypocalcemia, but compensation may occur through the action of parathyroid hormone on bone and the kidneys. Serum alkaline phosphatase is elevated.

Young animals fed all-meat diets—particularly young cats fed a diet consisting almost exclusively of beef hearts (low in calcium and vitamins A and D, high in phosphorus)—get a severe osteopenic bone disease, causing pathologic fractures. Although the disease has features of fibrous osteodystrophy, the fact that the disease occurs during an active growth phase of the animal causes other lesions (refer to **osteoporosis**). Rather than appearing rachitic, the growth plate minimally thickens, and the zone of maturing cartilage cells appears almost normal. The tissue spaces in the region of the primary spongiosa are fibrous and may be almost devoid of trabeculae; or, a sparse number of thin cartilaginous trabeculae may be covered with inadequate amounts of bone matrix. It may be difficult to determine in decalcified sections whether bone matrix is adequately mineralized. The bone cortex is composed of plexiform bone in which maturation by perivascular filling is delayed; rather than being composed of compact bone, the diaphysis has the appearance of joining trabeculae lined by osteoblasts and separated by fibrous connective tissue. Although osteoblasts actively form osteoid, no marked increase in osteoid is seen as in the other forms of fibrous osteodystrophy. The bones are thin, not thickened. Pronounced subperiosteal osteoclastic activity may occur, and wide zones of osteoclasts may be seen adjacent to the growth plate or articular cartilage. The disease is caused by nutritional imbalance of calcium and phosphorus; this imbalance results in hypocalcemia and secondary hyperparathyroidism.

Unless compensated, hyperphosphatemia occurs with elevated serum alkaline phosphatase. The **signs** of the disease are nervousness and hyperirritability, reluctance to move, abnormal stance and gait, and spontaneous fractures.

Fibrous osteodystrophy used to be a frequent disorder of laboratory primates, and is still common in pet monkeys. The disease is almost exclusively encountered in New World monkeys (such as those from Central and South America); it has been the recipient of numerous inappropriate and misleading terms, such as goundou, Paget disease, simian bone disease, and cage paralysis. In monkeys, the disease is characterized by facial deformity, reluctance to move, bending of long bones, and multiple fractures leading to distortion of the limbs. **Microscopically,** the lesions are classic for fibrous osteodystrophy, with marked production of new bone causing gross enlargement of the skeleton, especially of the skull bones. The cause is not clear in each example, but in most cases it is the result of vitamin D deficiency. In New World monkeys, it has been demonstrated that vitamin D_2 is ineffective in promoting intestinal absorption of calcium; these species require vitamin D_3 in their diet or access to ultraviolet radiation or sunshine. The higher requirement of New World primates for vitamin D stems from the fact that they possess a distinctive receptor system for steroid hormones, including $1\alpha,25 \ (OH)_2 \ D_3$. The substitution of vitamin D_3 for vitamin D_2 in commercial primate diets has greatly reduced the incidence of fibrous osteodystrophy in laboratory monkeys. In pet monkeys, lack of vitamin D is important to the development of the disease, but the condition is also aggravated by unusual diets—such as baby foods made of cereal grains and bananas—which are often high in phosphorus and low in calcium.

In addition to the specific examples cited, fibrous osteodystrophy of nutritional origin has been described in cattle, goats, dogs, birds, and reptiles. Both renal and nutritional osteodystrophy are common in rats and hamsters. As a rule, in all species with nutritional or renal fibrous osteodystrophy, the parathyroid glands are grossly enlarged. **Microscopically,** the enlargement results from an increase in size and number of light chief cells. Many chief cells become vacuolated, and the number of water clear cells increase.

It has been emphasized here that rickets and osteomalacia may progress to fibrous osteodystrophy when severe hyperparathyroidism develops in the course of the disease. This progression is easy to understand; however, the presence in young animals of fibrous osteodystrophy without rickets (in some species, a frequent finding) may appear confusing. In nutritional secondary hyperparathyroidism, serum electrolyte values may remain normal because calcium is removed from the bone. Under these circumstances, endochondral ossification remains normal, and rickets does not develop. Fairly rapid longitudinal bone growth is necessary in order to get the typical morphologic lesions of rickets; when bone growth decreases, the requirement for mineral decreases and the thickness of the diseased growth plate declines. In addition, severe nutritional deficiencies frequently cause severe inanition and can lead to osteopenia (refer to *osteoporosis*).

References

Bienfet V, et al. A primary parathyroid disorder. Osteofibrosis caused by parathyroid adenoma in a Shetland pony: recovery after surgical removal. Ann Med Vet 1964;108:252–265.

Hunt RD, Garcia FG, Hegsted DM. A comparison of vitamin D2 and D3 in New World primates. I. Production and regression of osteodystrophia fibrosa. Lab Anim Care 1967;17:222–234.

Jowsey J, Gershon-Cohen J. Effect of dietary calcium levels on production and reversal of experimental osteoporosis in cats. Proc Soc Exp Biol Med 1964;116:437–441.

Nielsen SW, McSherry BJ. Renal hyperparathyroidism (rubber-jaw syndrome) in a dog. J Am Vet Med Assoc 1954;124:270–274.

Rowland GN, Capen CC, Nagode LA. Experimental hyperparathyroidism in young cats. Pathol Vet 1968;5:504–519.

Osteoporosis

Osteoporosis defines a group of skeletal disorders that are characterized by a diminution of bone mass (**osteopenia),** with the remaining bone appearing normal. The bones are therefore thin, brittle, and subject to fractures. It is an extremely common disorder in humans, especially post-menopausal women. It is far less frequent in animals. Histologically, the bone cortices are thinned and porous and the trabeculae are reduced in number, size, and connectivity. However, the bone morphology in fully developed cases gives little evidence as to how it became osteopenic.

GROSS AND MICROSCOPIC LESIONS

The cortical bone is reduced in thickness, and the porosity is increased. The medullary cavity may be increased in diameter. The amount of cancellous bone is also reduced and the bony spicules become thin, less numerous, and more widely separated. Abnormally bent bones, with thin cortices and increased bone diameter, may indicate that osteoporosis occurred as an aftermath of previous nutritional osteodystrophy. Usually, the histology of bone surfaces appears quiescent, indicating that the events that led to bone loss occurred previously or operated slowly. In some cases, biopsy may show active remodeling sites. In all cases, the trabeculae appear adequately mineralized.

Bone surfaces, or envelopes, tend to react differently in various disease conditions, including in osteoporosis. Osteoporosis mainly affects the endosteal envelope. The three bone envelopes are (1) the **periosteal** (which covers bone surfaces), (2) the **endosteal** (which is divided between the corticoendosteal and trabecular surfaces), and (3) the **haversian** and **Volkmann canal** surfaces. Normally, the turnover sites on the endosteal envelope and haversian systems on the inner third (paramedullary) of the cortex are in negative balance. **Negative balance** means that the depth of osteoclastic erosion is greater than the thickness of lamellar bone deposited during formation. The sites on the periosteal surfaces are slightly positive; the outside dimension of bones continues to expand slightly, even in old animals. The balance is neutral in the haversian systems of the external two thirds of the diaphyseal compacta. As animals age, the negative bone balance accounts for the continuous erosion and trabeculation of the cortices from within, as well as the thinning and losses of trabeculae in the center of the medullary cavity. This process is accelerated in osteoporosis (Figure 19-17).

PATHOGENESIS

Osteoporosis results from bone resorption exceeding bone formation. Two groups of pathogenic mechanisms can cause osteopenia; one occurs in young animals and the other in adults. The first is a **growth modeling-dependent** reaction. Longitudinal and transverse growth is ultimately responsible for the final amount of bone present in adults. During growth, bone modeling expands the outside and inside diameters of the bone at different rates. Too rapid expansion of the marrow cavity can lead to thin bone cortices. The amount of spongiosa that is retained is dependent upon its turnover and the degree of imbalance between the resorptive and formation process. In the adult, after growth has ceased and modeling is slow, osteopenias arise as a **remodeling-dependent** process. Rapid bone loss can occur because excessive depth of osteoclastic resorption leads to perforation and discontinuity of bone trabeculae. Osteoporosis may be the final morphologic effect in animals that have had previous episodes of osteomalacia or fibrous osteodystrophy. With severe mineral deficiency, the inner third of the subendosteal region of the bone cortex may be converted into trabecular structures (Fig. 19-18) that experience perforation. Slow bone loss results following formation of resorption cavities of normal or reduced size, but these cavities are incompletely filled by osteoblasts. **Reversible (high-turnover) osteopenia** arises when the remodeling space is increased due to activated osteoclastic resorption or a prolonged remodeling period. In

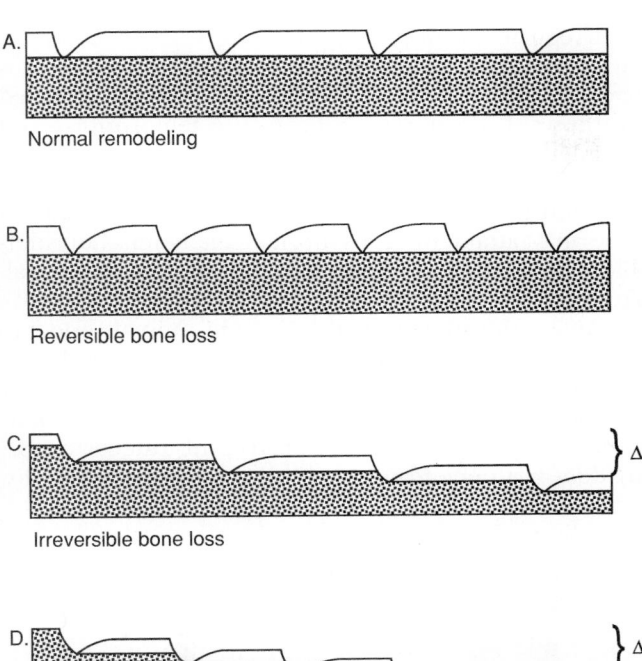

FIG. 19-17 Osteoporosis, relation between bone turnover, bone balance and bone loss. **A.** Normal remodelling sequence (Cf. Figure 19-3) with no imbalance between resorption and formation results in preservation of bone mass. **B.** Increased rate of formation of new remodelling sites (increased activation frequency) results in expansion of the remodelling space and reversible bone loss. **C.** Bone remodeling characterized by resorption exceeding formation results in a net irreversible loss of bone per remodeling cycle (delta B). **D.** Net irreversible bone loss, per remodeling cycle in combination with increased activation frequency, results in accelerated irreversible bone loss. (Redrawn from Eriksen EF. Endocr Rev 1986;7:379–408.)

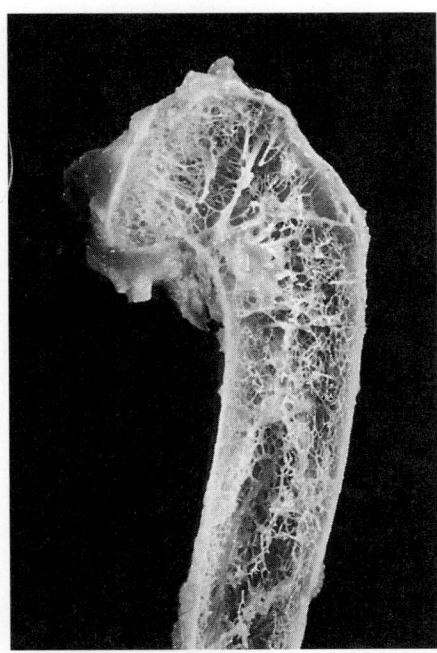

FIG. 19-18 Osteoporosis in New World primate. Humerus illustrates severe osteopenia of both cortical and cancellous bone.

the osteopenia of thyrotoxicosis or hyperparathyroidism, increased activation results. Drugs that depress activation can prevent reversible osteopenia. **Irreversible (low-turnover) osteopenia** is the result of absolute bone-volume deficits that usually arise on the trabecular and endocortical surfaces. During aging, the amount of bone removed during remodeling declines, but the amount of bone that refills the resorption bay declines even more; therefore, accelerated bone loss occurs, despite decreased bone resorption. Conditions that enhance the deficit cause an irreversible osteopenia.

Causes A number of recognized causes of osteoporosis exist. **Disuse osteoporosis** is caused by lack of physical exercise, reduction in weight bearing, and immobilization of limbs. In aging animals, a reduction in bone mass (**osteoporosis of senility**)—which is so frequent as to be considered normal—may be due in part to reduced physical activity. Other causes of osteoporosis include: **malnutrition** and chronic **metabolic acidosis;** imbalances of many hormones; **hyperadrenocorticism,** prolonged use of corticosteroids, and

thyrotoxicosis; and **hyperparathyroidism** (under appropriate but poorly defined circumstances). Hyperparathyroidism—possibly related to calcium and vitamin D intake—coupled with estrogen deficiency are thought to play the key roles in the development of osteoporosis in post-menopausal women. The osteopenia of scurvy, copper deficiency, osteogenesis imperfecta, and lathyrism occurs largely because of effects on bone matrical proteins.

Osteoporosis that is uncomplicated by fibrous osteodystrophy is rare, but not unknown in animals. The major causes of osteoporosis in veterinary medicine include disuse syndromes and improper nutrition. Many examples that have been designated osteoporosis have usually proved to arise from inadequate calcium deposition, and are thus more appropriately termed osteomalacia. When inadequate bone mineralization is microscopically evident, the disease should not be termed osteoporosis.

References

Detenbeck LC, Jowsey J. Normal aging in the bone of the adult dog. Clin Orthop 1969;65:76–80.

Doige CE. Pathological findings associated with locomotory disturbances in lactating and recently weaned sows. Can J Comp Med 1982;46:1–6.

Jaworski ZFG, Uhthoff HK. Disuse osteoporosis: current status and problems. In: Uhthoff HK, Stahl E, eds. Current concepts of bone fragility. New York: Springer Verlag, 1986;181–191.

Nordin BEC. The pathogenesis of osteoporosis. Lancet 1961;i:1011–1015.

Parfitt AM. Age-related structural changes in trabecular and cortical bone: cellular mechanisms and biomechanical consequences. Calcif Tissue Int 1984;36:S123–S128.

Scott PO, McKuseck VA, McKuseck AB. The nature of osteogenesis imperfecta in cats: evidence that the disorder is primarily nutritional, not genetic, and therefore not analog. J Bone Joint Surg 1963;45A:125–134.

Bone disease of unknown cause

HYPERTROPHIC (PULMONARY) OSTEOARTHROPATHY

Also known as **Marie disease** for its discoverer (in humans, 1890), this rare disease is reported in dogs, sheep, deer, cats, gibbons, horses, and lions. Often preceded a few months earlier by a cough, dyspnea, or other pulmonary disturbances, the characteristic lesions are chronic proliferation of new bone, producing marked thickening and deformity of the limbs. New bone is formed just beneath the periosteum, which is pushed outward (Fig. 19-19). The osteophytic growths are irregular because of intervening vascular channels and adventitial spaces; in some locations the bone is made extremely rough. The bones usually affected are those of all four limbs from the femorotibial and shoulder joints to the phalanges. The joint surfaces are not involved, although there periarticular proliferation and enlargement are apparent. Occasionally, a bone may attain twice its normal diameter. Considerable pain results on movement and, ultimately, on palpation.

Antedating the skeletal lesions in animals and humans are important and extensive lesions in the lungs, most often a space-occupying pulmonary abscess or neoplasm, such as lymphoma or metastatic osteosarcoma. The occurrence of hypertrophic osteoarthropathy does not depend so much on the nature of the dis-

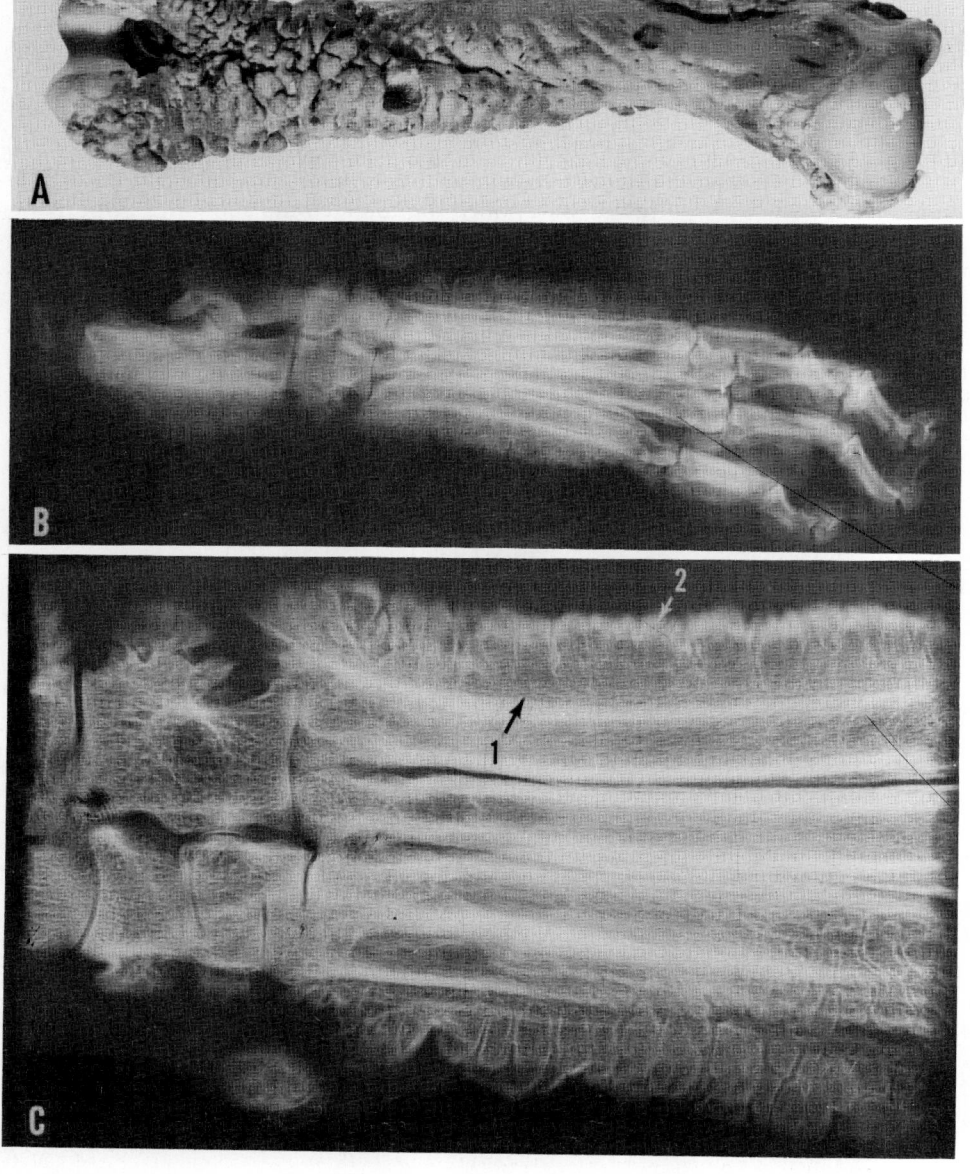

FIG. 19-19 Hypertrophic pulmonary osteoarthropathy. **A.** Humerus of a dog with severe exostosis. Note knoblike projections of bone from the cortex. **B.** Roentgenograph of the forelimb of a dog. Note severe exostoses on external surfaces of metacarpal bones, phalanges, and carpus. **C.** Roentgenograph of the specimen collected at necropsy from **B.** (1) The cortex of the bone is sharply demarcated; and (2) New bone growth; (3) Exterior to the cortex. (Courtesy of Armed Forces Institute of Pathology; contributor: Dr. H.R. Seibold.)

ease causing the lesion as it does on its location and duration. In some countries, advanced pulmonary tuberculosis is frequently present; chronic bronchiectatic, purulent process are occasionally found. Occasionally, cases without lung lesions are seen; the causative lesions are said to follow the distribution of the vagus and glossopharyngeal nerves. Urinary bladder or esophageal neoplasms are sometimes the cause; the occurrence of esophageal tumor is responsible for the relationship between infection with the canine esophageal worm, *Spirocerca lupi,* and hypertrophic osteoarthropathy. In humans, chronic heart diseases and insufficiencies have been concomitant with osteoarthropathy. In other human cases, osteoarthropathy is associated with a number of other lesions outside the thorax, including liver disease, colitis, and gastrointestinal tumors. The condition has been reported in single bones following infection of vascular grafts.

In view of the above circumstances, the cause is believed to be longstanding hypoxia. Accordingly, an experimental anastomosis shunting a part of the blood past the lungs is stated to have produced osteoarthropathy. Others suggest that hypertrophic osteoarthropathy (Fig. 19-20) develops because the lung fails to inactivate a vasodilator and bone-remodeling substance normally present in the systemic venous circulation. It is speculated that this substance may be platelet-derived growth factor; the lung may normally remove megakaryocytes or megakaryocyte fragments from the circulation and prevent them from reaching blood vessels of the limbs. It has been demonstrated that severing the vagus nerve quickly cures osteoarthropathy that has been caused by pulmonary neoplasia; the fundamental mechanism is still under study. Vagotomy results in a prompt decrease in blood flow to the limbs; this decrease of flow supports the hypothesis that increased peripheral blood flow is responsible for the bony growths. It has been hypothesized that inappropriate stimulation of the vagus or glossopharyngeal nerve leads to excess fluid and dilated vessels in all four limbs; these are secondary effects that are possibly mediated by a cerebral sodium homeostatic mechanism. It may be that more than one pathogenetic mechanism exists which causes excessive periosteal bony proliferation.

References

Carroll KB, Doyle L. A common factor in hypertrophic osteoarthropathy. Thorax 1974;100:262–264.
Dickinson CJ, Martin JF. Megakaryocytes and platelet clumps as the cause of finger clubbing. Lancet 1987;ii:1434–1435.
Doyle L. Pathogenesis of secondary hypertrophic osteoarthropathy: a hypothesis. Eur Respir J 1989;2:105–106.
Flavell G. Reversal of pulmonary hypertrophic osteoarthropathy by vagotomy. Lancet 1956;i:260–262.
Gerbode F, Birnstingl M, Braimbridge M. Experimental hypertrophic osteoarthropathy. Surgery 1966;60:1030–1035.
Martinez-Lavin M. Digital clubbing and hypertrophic osteoarthropathy: a unifying hypothesis. J Rheumatol 1987;14:6–8.
Shneerson JM. Digital clubbing and hypertrophic osteoarthropathy: the underlying mechanisms. Br J Dis Chest 1981;75:113–131.

PANOSTEITIS

This uncommon canine inflammatory bone disease, also called **eosinophilic panosteitis** or **enostosis,** is a self-limiting condition of unknown cause (Fig. 19-21). It is considered an inflammatory lesion because vascular congestion, intratrabecular fibrinous exudate, and moderate increases in inflammatory cells are seen in the initial stages, where enostosis begins around vessels at the intervertebral foramen. It may be associated with eosinophilia of the peripheral blood in 20% of cases. The disease is seen more frequently in females (ratio,

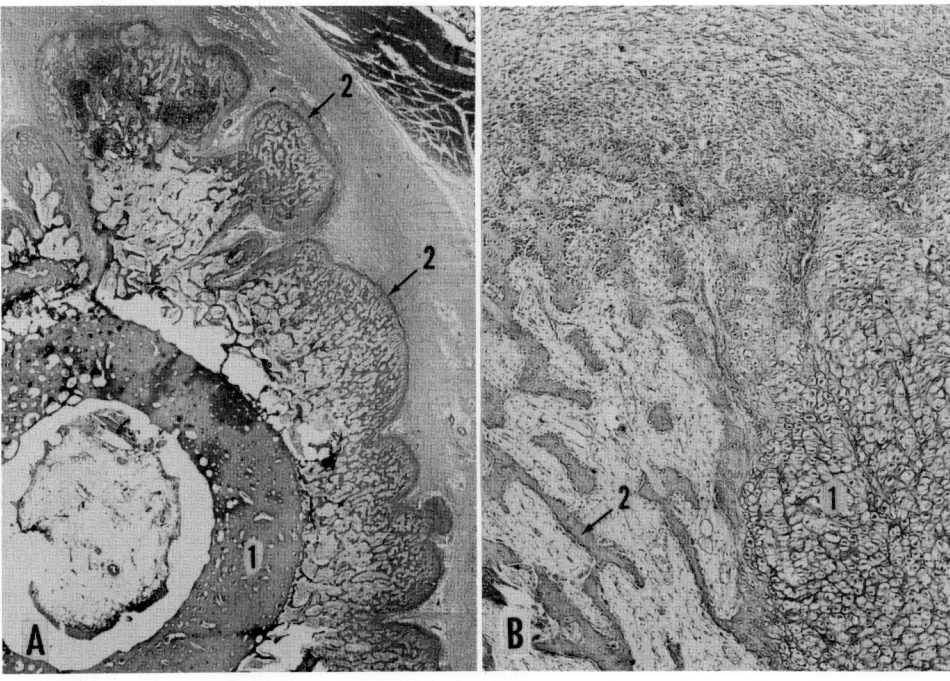

FIG. 19-20 Hypertrophic pulmonary osteoarthropathy. **A.** Cross section of tibia of a dog (×3 3/4). (1) Note porous bone cortex; and (2) Bulbous new bone; (3) Its exterior surface. **B.** Higher magnification (×40). (1) Cartilaginous; and (2) Osseous components. Courtesy of Armed Forces Institute of Pathology; contributor: Dr. H.R. Seibold.)

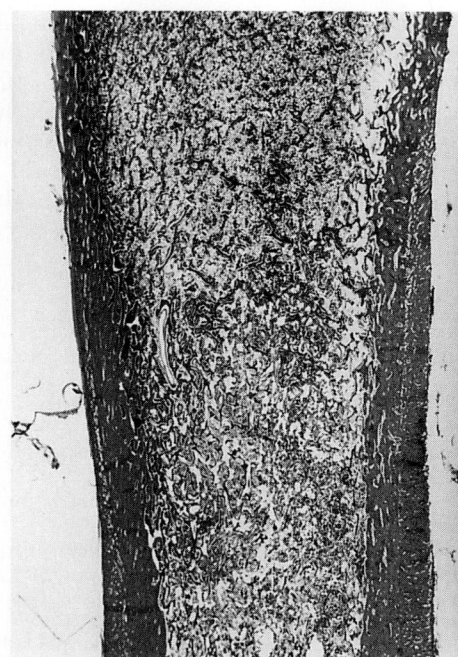

FIG. 19-21 Panosteitis in German shepherd. Medullary cavity is filled with trabeculae of woven bone, and increased porosity of the cortex is apparent.

4:1), and is more commonly observed in large-breed dogs, predominately German shepherd dogs. The condition primarily affects long bones of young growing animals and is seen clinically as an obscure, intermittent lameness affecting one or both forelimbs. The condition usually affects one bone at a time. Pain can be elicited by deep palpation, but no swelling or heat is apparent at the site. During the initial stages, some animals have fever; however, few other signs of systemic illness occur. Lameness may subside and reappear in the same or another limb, and spontaneous recovery invariably follows a course of two to nine months. The ulnae and radii are most commonly affected. The disease appears to cycle back and forth between the forelegs and the hindlegs. When the pain is severest, little radiographic evidence of bone abnormality is apparent; however, increased radiographic density occurs within 10 days in the region of the nutrient foramen. As the condition progresses, the patchy density of the medullary cavity greatly increases; the endosteal outline is accentuated and a well-defined periosteal new bone reaction may occur. Histologically, the first lesion is seen in the region of the nutrient foramen where there occurs proliferation of the adventitial cells accompanying the small medullary vessels. Increased vascularity and edema are observed; a small central area is formed, composed of woven-bone trabeculae. After formation of the initial nidus, satellites develop along the vascular system. The newly formed osseous trabeculae spread centrifugally within the marrow cavity, eventually stopping at the metaphysis. From the periphery to the center of the more fully developed lesion, bone maturity is increased. When a trabecular network fills most of the

marrow, subperiosteal osteophyte formation exists. As the lesion begins to resolve, the more mature central bone disappears first.

References

Herron MR. Eosinophilic panosteitis diagnosis and therapy. S West Vet 1970;23:103–105.

Van Sickle DC. Selected orthopedic problems in the growing dog. Am Anim Hosp Assoc 1975.

HYPERTROPHIC OSTEODYSTROPHY

Canine hypertrophic osteodystrophy (metaphyseal osteopathy) is an inflammatory bone disease of unknown cause that affects young dogs, usually of the larger breeds (Fig. 19-22). The spontaneous condition is characterized by clinical signs of pain, lameness, and pyrexia, and by swelling and hyperthermia of the metaphysis of the long bones; lesions are bilaterally symmetric. Radiographically, new bone formation may be seen in the periosteal region of the long bones; frequently, lipping of the metaphysis of long bones is apparent, and a transverse line of increased density is observed next to the growth plate (with an adjacent metaphyseal radiolucent zone). The costochondral junctions are enlarged, with increased radiodensity. The gross appearance depends upon the disease stage; however, in earlier stages, sawed sections of long bones have a 1–5 mm wide pale-yellow zone, with a soft, crumbly consistency on the metaphyseal side of the growth cartilage. In more chronic lesions, the ends of affected bones are markedly thickened by an enlarged periosteum, and by deposition of extraperiosteal bone and cartilage. Dogs may recover from the disease. In some instances, bone metaphyses remain malformed and animals appear dwarfed.

Early microscopic lesions are those of acute inflammation in which the intertrabecular tissue of the primary spongiosa is infiltrated with large numbers of

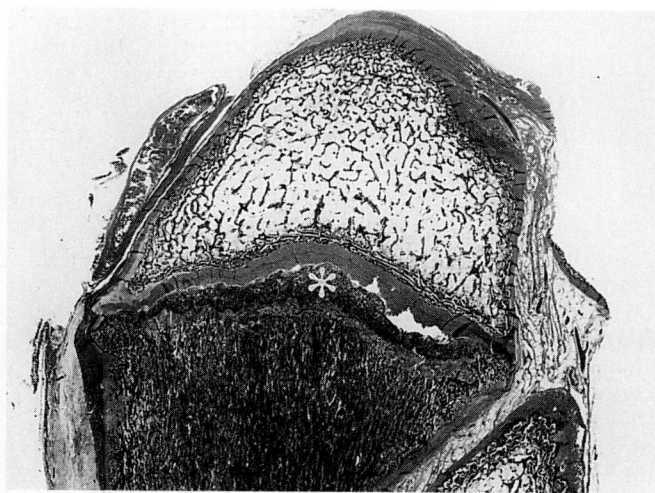

FIG. 19-22 Hypertrophic osteodystrophy. Distal radius from a 4-month-old Great Dane with recurrent disease. Suppurative exudate and detritus from trabecular fractures is present beneath growth plate within infraction region (*).

neutrophils. Inflammation results in necrosis of mesenchymal components of the primary spongiosa; necrosis of osteoblasts leads to failure of ossifications of cartilaginous trabeculae in this region. The thin, elongated mineralized cartilaginous trabeculae may fracture and cause infraction beneath the growth plate. Interruption in the metaphyseal vessels prevents normal growth-plate cartilage resorption and leads to elongation of the zone thickness of mineralized hypertrophic cartilage. Inflammation of osteochondral junctions (osteochondritis) is evident in many locations where no gross or radiographic lesions are apparent. Osteomyelitis may be evident in the mandible, particularly in the dental sac, and the incisor and molar teeth may have a gray-brown color. Soft-tissue lesions may include calcinosis in various organs, including skin, heart, spleen, kidneys, and stomach. These lesions are sometimes associated with suppurative foci. Hemorrhages are probably related to delayed blood clotting.

References

Alexander JW. Hypertrophic osteodystrophy. Canine Pract 1978;5:48–52.

Watson ADJ, Blair RC, Farrow BRH, et al. Hypertrophic osteodystrophy in the dog. Aust Vet J 197349:433–439.

Woodard JC. Canine hypertrophic osteodystrophy: a study of the spontaneous disease in littermates. Vet Pathol 1982;19:337–354.

OSTEOCHONDROSIS

Osteochondrosis occurs as a focal area of disordered endochondral ossification—including both chondrogenesis and osteogenesis—that occurs in a bone growth area that was previously normal (Figure 19-23). When lesions classified as osteochondrosis are limited by this definition, systemic diseases—such as metabolic bone disease and osteochondrodysplasia—are excluded from consideration under this heading. Osteochondrosis is an idiopathic condition, and it is possible that the lesion develops by several different pathogenetic mechanisms. Theories concerning the cause of osteochondrosis are ischemia, trauma, and a constitutional disease. The causes are not necessarily mutually exclusive, and all may play a pathogenetic role in individual cases. The finding of multiple bone involvement and bilateral symmetry is strong circumstantial evidence of a constitutional component. It is likely that biomechanical forces represent a fundamental cause, and physical stress initiates subsequent changes. Differences in the vascularity of growth cartilage at different ages of maturity between large- and small-breed animals may also play a pathogenetic role. When the articular cartilage or subchondral bone are abnormal, or when the animal is young enough that the osteochondral interface has not fully matured, then normal physical activity may induce injury. Osteochondrosis occurs in most domestic species, particularly in larger animals. For example, it is a common condition in giant-breed dogs, but uncommon in small dogs. It is rarely seen in wild animals.

Lesions of osteochondrosis represent three fundamental areas of abnormal endochondral ossification: (1) nonarticular epiphysis; (2) articular cartilage of the epiphysis; and (3) **growth plate.** Although the lesions appear similar in each location, a different mechanism exists, which leads to failure of proper endochondral ossification of cartilage.

In the nonarticular (apophysis) epiphyseal osteochondroses, the lesions occur principally at sites of attachment of tendons and ligaments. Excessive traction at tendon or ligamentous insertions can cause fracture or avulsion of cartilage at the point of attachment: for example, tuberosity of the tibia in Osgood Schlatter disease, and anconeal process in large dogs.

Early osteochondrotic lesions of the subarticular cartilage in swine are characterized by chondrocyte necrosis; later, dissection of cartilage occurs, as well as formation of a cartilage flap and development of free-joint bodies. The latter condition has been termed **osteochondritis dissecans,** although little inflammation occurs. Osteochondrosis of the humoral head in young Great Danes occurs in a region where the cartilage is thick and less mature. It is not known whether cartilage thickness is a predisposing factor or whether increased thickness represents an early stage in the pathogenesis. In young swine, small areas of cartilage necrosis develop in the cartilage growth region below definitive articular cartilage. Lesions are associated with cartilage-canal vessels with endothelial injury, and are not perfused. It is not known whether the vascular changes are the cause or result of the condition. These necrotic cartilage zones fail to mineralize or to undergo endochondral ossification; they leave tongues of degenerate cartilage behind as the bone-cartilage interface expands during growth. Multiple, small subarticular cartilage lesions develop in most pigs of modern swine breeds; unless lesions are large, cause cartilage dissection, or lead to osteoarthritis, they have little disease consequence. When osteochondrosis breaches the cartilage surface, a myxomatous reaction occurs in the subchondral marrow; an attempt to form fibrocartilage results. Reorganization of the subchondral trabeculae and myxomatous degeneration of the intertrabecular tissue leads to formation of a subchondral **pseudocyst.**

The pathogenesis of early growth-plate lesions in swine differs from that observed in articular cartilage. No evidence exists of cartilage necrosis, but a focal failure occurs in mineralizing hypertrophic cartilage cells. This mineralization failure leads to a focal rachitic lesion, with persistence of hypertrophic cartilage cells. **Eosinophilic streaks** are linear zones of acidophilic cartilage matrix and represent areas where the matrix is altered. They occur normally, and some represent regions of cartilage-canal chondrification or matrix degeneration. They are more prominent in osteochondrosis. Other alterations that could be the result of trauma or excess biomechanical stress are seen in the region. It is hard to know if these lesions are related to the cause, or if they are the result of osteochondrosis. Lesions include: metaphyseal trabecular fractures, abrupt displacement lines in the growth plate, cartilage-matrix degeneration, disorientation—similar to that observed following cartilage creep—of cartilage cells, and disorganization of the cartilage-growth pattern. Cartilage

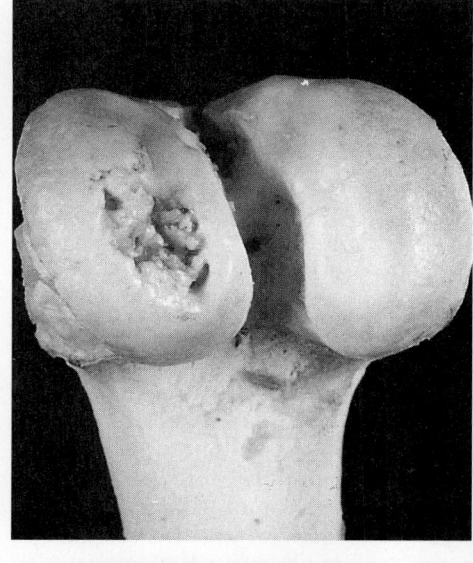
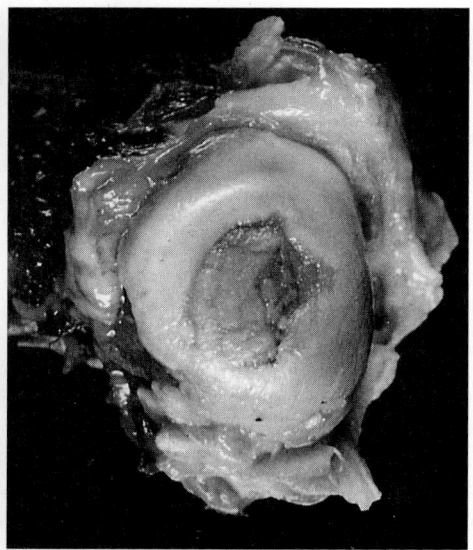
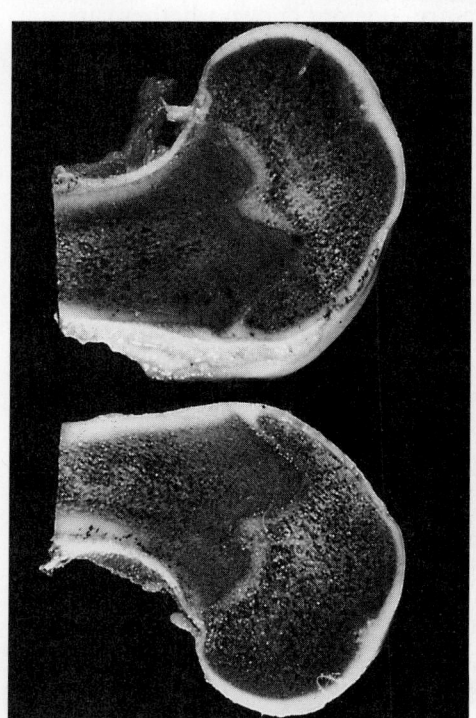
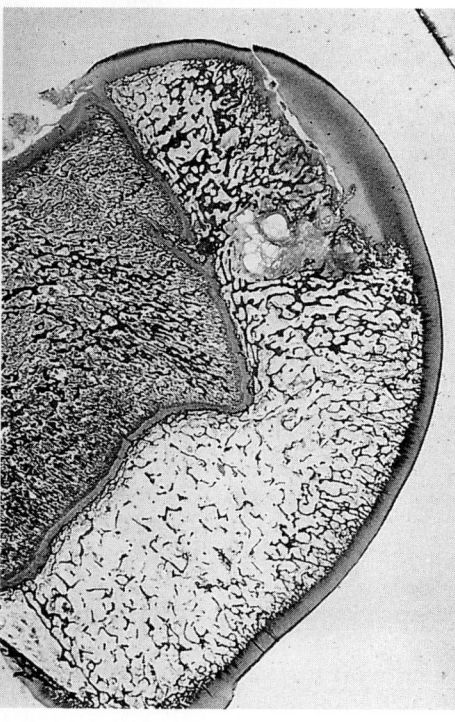

FIG. 19-23 Osteochondrosis. **A.** Distal humerus in pig. Macerated specimen illustrates that lesion extends into subchondral bone. **B.** Proximal humerus in Great Dane. Chronicity of lesion is indicated by proliferation of fibrocartilage that fills the lesion site, production of osteophytes along the articular rim of humoral head, and thickening of the articular capsula. **C.** Distal humerus in pig. Although lesions could not be identified on the articular surfaces, on the cut surface one can see focal early changes as areas of cartilage protruding into subchondral bone. **D.** Proximal humerus in dog. Cartilage flap is caused by a transverse cartilage fracture that propagates along the tidemark. Note also pseudocyst in subchondral bone and the small growthplate fracture beneath the articular lesion. (Courtesy of Dr. Wayne H. Riser.)

creep is the slow change in shape that may occur following plastic deformation. Focal failure of endochondral ossification can also be associated with bone inflammation or disruption of metaphyseal vessels; however, these conditions should not be classified as osteochondrosis.

Epiphysiolysis is separation of the epiphysis from the metaphyseal bone, probably due to trauma. Some consider osteochondrosis to predispose the growth plate to failure following trauma.

References

Birkeland R. Osteochondritis dissecans in the humeral head of the dog. Nord Vet Med 1967;19:294–305.

Bouchaert A, Matheews D. Avascular necrosis of the head of the femur in dogs: radiographic aspects of 50 cases. Vlaams Diergeneeskd Tijdschr 1973;43:125–133.

Bridges CH, Harris ED. Experimentally induced cartilaginous fractures (osteochondritis dissecans) in foals fed low-copper diets. J Am Vet Med Assoc 1988;193:215–221.

Bridges CH, Womack JE, Harris ED, et al. Considerations of copper metabolism in osteochondrosis of suckling foals. J Am Vet Med Assoc 1984;185:173–178.

Woodard JC, Becker HN, Poulos PW. Articular cartilage blood vessels in swine osteochondrosis. Vet Pathol 1987;24:118–123.

Infections of bone

Inflammation of bone **(osteitis)** is confined to the connective tissue spaces surrounding cortical bone **(osteoperiostitis),** or to the marrow spaces **(osteomyelitis)** in contact with the endosteum or cancellous bone. Osteomyelitis is generally infectious in origin. Infections most frequently follow penetrating wounds or compound bone fractures, but they also may be of hematogenous origin. Trauma and the use of orthopedic implant materials increase the likelihood of bone infection. Rarely, inflammation of the vertebrae (**spondylitis**) occurs following infection of the abdominal viscera, through retrograde spread of infection via the vertebral venous plexus. **Discospondylitis** is contiguous involvement of the vertebral body and intervertebral disk. Staphylococci and streptococci are the most frequent aerobic bacteria causing hematogenous infections; however, less pathogenic organisms—such as *E. coli* or *Fusobacterium necrophorum*—can be opportunists and cause acute osteomyelitis. *Corynebacterium pyogenes (Actinomyces pyogenes)* is a frequent isolate from cattle, sheep, and swine, and *Salmonella* are commonly isolated from foals. Anaerobic bacteria, or mixed aerobic and anaerobic infections, also are common causes of acute osteomyelitis.

Acute osteomyelitis of hematogenous origin is seen most often in young animals. The absence of epiphyseal fusion influences the localization of infection to either the epiphysis adjacent to the articular-cartilage growth zone or to the metaphysis adjacent to the growth plate. Here, arterioles form a loop at the growth cartilage-bone junction; they then drain into the cancellous bone marrow space without forming a capillary bed. During endochondral ossification, vascular sprouts form blind-ended vessels that are lined with an attenuated endothelium with no underlying basement membrane. Bacteria lodge in this region and attach to trabecular bone or cartilage-matrix surfaces, but not to adjacent vascular linings or erythrocytes.

Certain bacteria—such as *S. aureus* and *P. aeruginosa*—contain fibronectin-binding surface proteins with the ability to interact with collagen; or, bacteria may contain binding sites that attach to bone sialoprotein. Adherence stimulates the organisms to exude a glycocalyx, which becomes progressively more dense. This biofilm buries the organism and serves as a barrier against antibiotics and host defense mechanisms. Liberated bacterial toxins and ischemia lead to bone necrosis. The necrotic zones may coalesce into an avascular zone, permitting further bacterial proliferation. In the case of infection of foals with *Salmonella sp.*, a sequestrum may form. A **sequestrum** is a piece of dead bone that has become isolated during the process of necrosis. An **involucrum** is a sheath of pyogenic fibrous tissue or reactive bone that forms around the sequestrum. **Brodie abscess** is a suppurative metaphyseal focus surrounded by a sclerotic margin. The abscess occurs when the bacterial infection and inflammatory reaction become localized and chronic. After the inflammation is contained, continuation of longitudinal bone growth increases the distance between the metaphyseal inflammatory focus and the growth plate. **Puriform softening** of bone results from liberation of lysosomal enzymes from polymorphonuclear leukocytes and macrophages; however, in inflammation, a regional accelerator phenomenon also occurs, with activation of remodeling by osteoclasts. Tissue destruction within the metaphysis may be so ex-

tensive that the vascular supply to the growth plate is interrupted. Focal rachitic lesions with thickening of the physis develop because local inflammatory lesions prevent normal vascular invasion of the mineralized hypertrophic cartilage. Suppurative exudate may escape from the bone's interior at the periosteal-surface junction of the growth plate and cortical bone. Suppurative exudate, once outside of the bone, may invade the joint, leading to a secondary suppurative arthritis. Exudate also may flow between the periosteum and the cortex and isolate bone from its blood supply by shearing off the perforating arteries and devitalizing the cortex. When it is isolated from its dual blood supply by periosteal and marrow exudate, the cortical bone may undergo complete necrosis. As the suppurative exudate dissects between the bone cortex and the periosteum, it causes reactive bone to be formed. Thus, an involucrum may be formed around sequestrated cortical bone fragments. The purulent exudate may make a hole in the periosteum and skin, and form a draining sinus.

Chronic osteomyelitis is characteristic of certain infections that have a propensity to affect bone; these include brucellosis, tuberculosis, actinomycosis, and coccidioidomycosis. Chronic osteomyelitis—with lesions typically seen with each fungal disease—are sometimes found with aspergillosis, blastomycosis, histoplasmosis, cryptococcosis, and mycetoma. Brucellosis ordinarily forms an intra-osseous caseous abscess; the abscess is encapsulated by fibrous tissue with a mixture of leukocytes (including many eosinophils). In swine and calves, a frequent location is within one or two adjoining vertebrae. Actinomycosis and mycetoma are pyogranulomatous processes, whereas the lesions in cryptococcosis may be more histiocytic. Each of the other diseases produces a more typical granulomatous lesion. The inflammatory response is able to grow and proliferate by destroying the bony tissue around it. The bone tissue reacts with a reparative proliferation at the same time that adjoining areas are being resorbed. The result is a pronounced local enlargement that proves to be honeycombed when the soft tissues are removed by maceration. Because it involves the jaw bones of cattle ("lumpy jaw"), this type of lesion is especially conspicuous in actinomycosis. In the case of tuberculosis, the bone lesion is usually part of a generalized process; the same is usually the case with most of the mycotic diseases. In actinomycosis and brucellosis, the bone lesion is usually the only manifestation.

References

Buxton TB, Horner J, Hinton A, et al. In vivo glycocalyx expression by *Staphylococcus aureus* phage type 52/52A/80 in *S. aureus* osteomyelitis. J Infect Dis 1987;156:942–946.

Costerton JW. The etiology and persistence of cryptic bacterial infections: a hypothesis. Rev Infect Dis 1984;6:S608–S616.

Gristina AG, Costerton JW. Bacterial adherence and the glycocalyx and their role in musculoskeletal infection. Orthop Clin North Am 1991;15:517–535.

Morrissy RT, Haynes DW. Acute hematogenous osteomyelitis: a model with trauma as an etiology. J Pediatr Orthop 1989;9:447–456.

Speers DJ, Nade SM. Ultrastructural studies of adherence of *Staphylococcus aureus* in experimental acute hematogenous osteomyelitis. Infect Immun 1985;49:443–446.

JOINT DISEASE

Types of joints and their examination

Several different types of joints exist; they may join one or more bones. Most of the freely movable articulations are **synovial joints,** termed **diarthroses.** A synovial joint consists of a joint cavity surrounded by a synovial membrane and fibrous capsule joining two bones. Often, synovial joints are reinforced with ligaments. Other joints lack joint cavities; instead, they consist of **fibrous joints,** or **synarthroses** (which are seen in sutures), and **fibrocartilaginous** joints, or **amphiarthroses** (which include the intervertebral connections). The fibrous joints and fibrocartilagenous connections have much more limited motion than the synovial joints. Synovial joints are formed early in the process of limb-bud differentiation; the joints are vulnerable to various teratogens and other insults during this period.

The gross appearance of synovial fluid, the synovial membrane, and articular cartilage can be altered by local congestion and autolysis. Hemolysis of blood can cause synovial fluid and articular cartilage to be stained red. Normally, the synovial fluid is viscid and appears clear to yellow. **Grossly,** normal articular cartilage appears white, milky, and opaque in the thicker areas. In thin areas that overlie bone marrow, the cartilage may be translucent and slightly blue. On cut section, the thickness of the articular cartilage is variable, not only from joint to joint within an individual, but also from region to region within a given joint. A range of articular cartilage thickness exists between animal species. Synovial fossae are normal anatomical structures that appear as nonarticulating depressions in the joint surface. They are absent at birth, and the time of appearance, size, shape, and persistence of any given fossa varies. It is important to recognize synovial fossae and linear grooves as normal anatomical structures, and to distinguish them from areas of articular collapse or from lesions of osteoarthritis (Fig. 19-24). The gross color and transparency of menisci and articular discs also are regionally variable and reflect the thickness and composition of the structure. Thin portions of menisci and discs are translucent. With increasing thickness, opacity also increases; the color changes gradually from blue-gray to white. **Grossly,** most ligaments appear white and have a fibrous texture; however, ligaments that contain a significant amount of elastic tissue—such as the ligamentum nuchae—are yellow. The synovial lining of the joint capsule is pink, glistening, and usually smooth. Synovial villi are particularly prominent in certain places, such as a joint out-pouching or cul-de-sac. The villi are larger and more regularly spaced in animals than in humans, and they are more prominent in large domestic animals, such as horses.

Abnormalities of joint development

Joint laxity may lead to subluxation or luxation of the joint. **Atlantoaxial subluxation and luxation** occur in several species, but are most common in toy-breed dogs.

It is usually encountered in dogs less that one year of age and leads to compression of the spinal cord by dorsal displacement of the axis. The following cause rupture of the transverse ligament of the atlas: luxation of an intact dens, luxation due to congenital malformation of the dens, and dens fracture. Compression of the spinal cord causes cervical pain, which may progress to tetraplegia. Defective synthesis of type I collagen can cause hypermotility of the joint; another cause of hypermotility is a delay in motor-nerve development, which may be transitory. "Contracted foals" have congenital contraction of the axial or appendicular skeleton. The contracted condition arises during early pregnancy. Congenital joint dysplasia in association with hypoplasia of epiphyses (epiphyseal dysplasia, Table 19-1) can lead to deformations of the limbs or abnormal curvature of the spine. Other conditions—such as abnormal neuromuscular function—can also cause abnormal spinal curvature. **Scoliosis** is abnormal curvature of the spine, with lateral displacement. When the curvature is displaced ventrally, it is termed **lordosis.** With **kyphosis,** the curvature has a dorsal prominence.

Congenital **arthrogryposis**—the persistent flexure or contracture of a joint—is actually a disorder of the nervous system and skeletal muscles. Although the failure of joint-space development results in persistent fixation of the joint, arthrogryposis usually develops due to failure of proper muscle development (or atrophy) caused by fetal neurologic disturbances. The muscles are reduced to fibrous connective tissue, which precludes fetal movement and ultimately leads to fixation of the joints. Arthrogryposis can result from the ingestion of alkaloids from such plants as wild tree tobacco (*Nicotiana*), lupines (*Lupinus*), and poison hemlock (*Conium*). It is also seen in cattle and sheep following intrauterine infections with akabane or blue-tongue viruses.

JOINT DYSPLASIA

Abnormal development of the joint leads to joint incongruity, resulting in secondary osteoarthritis and lameness (Fig. 19-25). Elbow dysplasia is caused by several different conditions that lead to joint incongruity: for example, ununited anconeal process, fragmented coronoid process, patella cubiti (ectopic sesamoid bone of the elbow), osteochondrosis of the medial condyle, and ununited medial epicondyle. Hip dysplasia occurs most frequently in large-breed dogs; it is occasionally observed in cats, and rarely seen in farm animals. Conditions that induce pathologic changes during the intrauterine (fetal) period, the neonatal period (shortly after or during birth), or later during the animal's growth, may result in joint dysplasia. Gradual postnatal deformation of the joint results in **Canine hip dysplasia** (Fig. 19-26). Subluxation of the femoral head—perhaps due to inadequate muscle strength—allows a sequence of events that results in acetabular dysplasia and degenerative joint disease. The primary structural alterations probably occur during the neonatal period, when the animal's growth is most pronounced. Gentle mechanical forces, when persistently applied, may lead to gradual progressive deformation of normal bone structure.

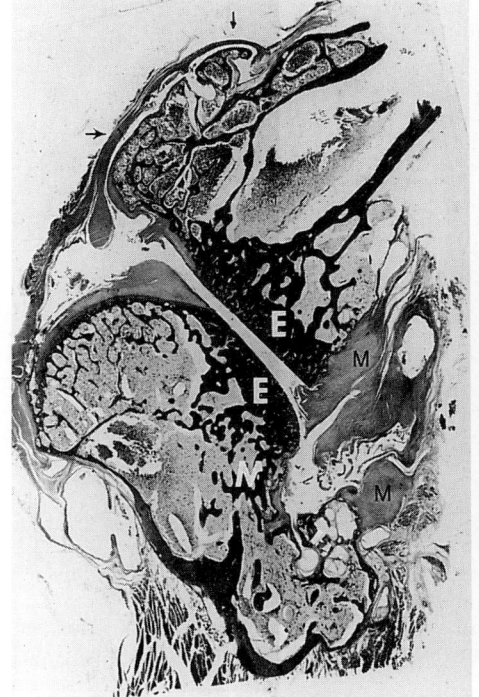

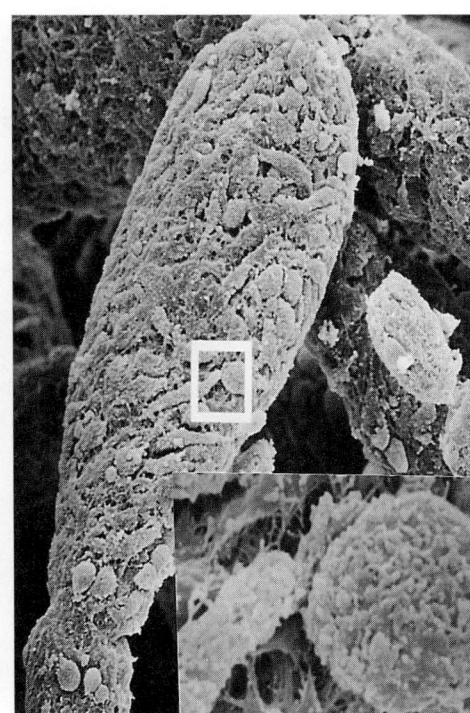

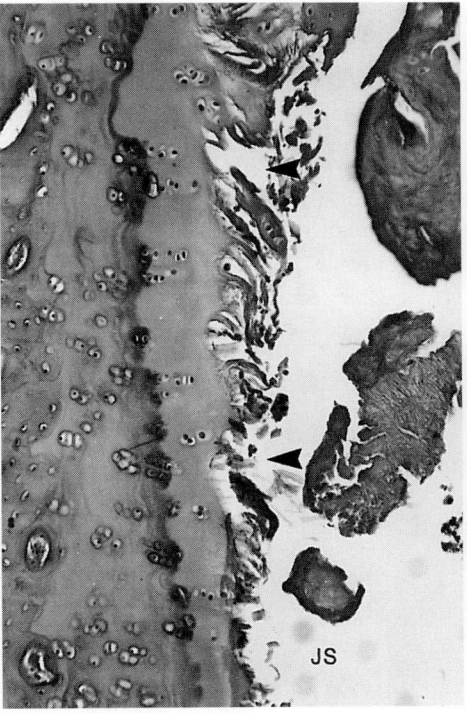

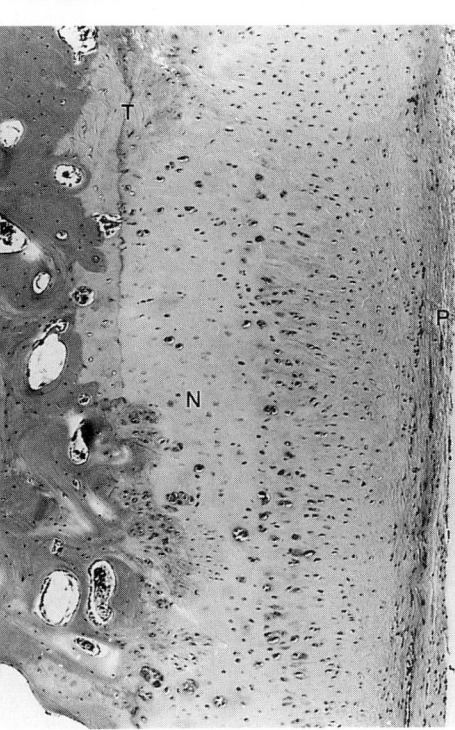

FIG. 19-24 Reaction of joint to injury. **A.** Osteoarthritis of scapulohumeral joint, in rabbit. Mature osteophyte (arrowheads) on the rim of the scapula, eburnation *(E)* of the articular surface, and cartilaginous metaplasia *(M)* of the synovium. **B.** Scanning electron micrograph of synovial villi, caprine-arthritis-encephalitis-virus arthritis. Hypertrophic synovial cells have numerous surface filopodia (inset). **C.** Fibrillated articular cartilage in osteoarthritis. Degenerative change in articular cartilage characterized by loss of cartilage matrix and development of clefts *(arrowheads)* between groups of cartilage cells. Joint space (JS). **D.** Chondromalacia in polyarthritis of greyhounds. Chondrocyte necrosis, empty lacunae (N), superficial to the tidemark (T) and within calcified cartilage. There is a thin pannus (P) veil of fibrovascular tissue on the articular surface.

Such deformation occurs much more readily during periods of excessively rapid growth. The largest loads placed on the hips are due to muscular forces, and abnormal muscle activity patterns influence the cartilage modeling process of the acetabulum. The mechanical forces that hold the femoral head firmly into the acetabular joint are a resultant force caused by muscles that pull vertically or medially on the hip. It has been shown that when the rear limb is held in extension or adduction, the hip tends to dislocate. Alterations causing hip dysplasia tend to concentrate the mechanical hip loads on the craniodorsal aspect of the acetabular rim; this excessive force retards cartilage modeling and causes the bone to become abnormally shaped. These structural changes lead to subluxation of the femoral head (Fig. 19-27). Early changes seen in dogs with hip dysplasia involve retarded development of the craniodorsal acetabular rim and lag in ossification, as well as

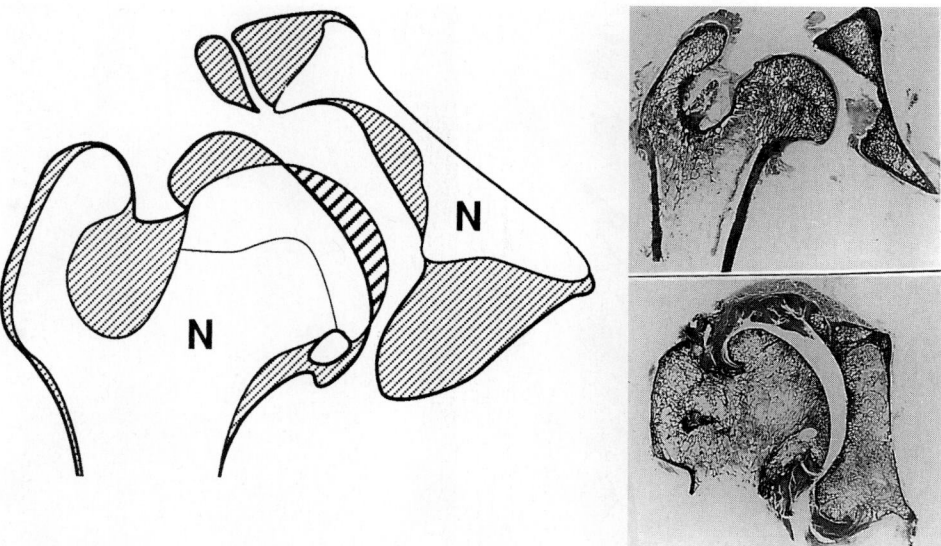

FIG. 19-25 Bone restructuring in hip dysplasia. The normal hip *(N)* (diagram and upper photograph), is overlaid with the dysplastic joint (lower photograph). In hip dysplasia, eburnation causes loss of articular cartilage and subchondral bone from the joint surface (heavily striped). Osteophytes fill the acetabular fossa and broadened the articulating surface (lightly striped).

the tearing of fibers in teres ligament and stretching of the joint capsule. Subluxation and bending of the greater trochanter occur later. Joint incongruity leads to secondary osteoarthritis. Progressive reconstruction of the femoral head, marginal osteophytes, osseous filling of the acetabular fossa, and changes in the contour of the acetabular rim all cause radiographic changes to become more noticeable after six months of age. The

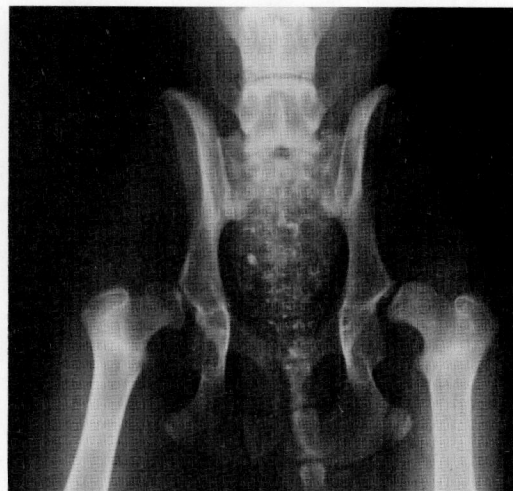

FIG. 19-26 Hip dysplasia. Radiograph of severe dysplasia (grade IV) in a six-month-old male German shepherd dog. Note that the acetabula appear shallow because of bone production and filling of the acetabular fossa; the femoral heads are not within the acetabulum on either side. The articular surface of the femoral head on the right is flattened. (Courtesy of Dr. G. B. Schnelle, Angell Memorial Animal Hospital.)

causes of hip dysplasia may be intrinsic to bone structure or to the strength of the supporting connective tissue that prevent joint laxity; however, the condition develops after birth and is more likely to be due to disproportionate muscle tone of the muscular groups that pull medially on the hip relative to those that pull vertically. Such differences could be neuromuscular function, or related to muscle strength.

References

Corley EA, Sutherland TM, Carlson WD. Genetic aspects of canine elbow dysplasia. J Am Vet Med Assoc 1968;153:543–547.

Lust G, Geary JC, Sheffy BE. Development of hip dysplasia in dogs. Am J Vet Res 1973;34:87–91.

Priester WA, Mulvihill JJ. Canine hip dysplasia: relative risk by sex, size, and breed, and comparative aspects. J Am Vet Med Assoc 1973;160:735–739.

Riser WH. The dog as a model for the study of hip dysplasia: growth, form, and development of the normal and dysplastic hip joint. Vet Pathol 1975;12:234–334.

Stevens DR, Sande RD. An elbow dysplasia syndrome in the dog. J Am Vet Med Assoc 1974;165:1065–1069.

Crystal deposition disease

Crystal deposition disease occurs when certain types of crystals are deposited in periarticular tissues, joints, bursae, or tendon sheaths. This causes pain when an inflammatory processes is induced. The deposition of monosodium urate crystals causes **gout** (Chapter 3), and appears as white foci (**tophi**) of granulomatous inflammation. Gout is not seen in domestic animals; this is because they have the enzyme uricase, which oxidizes uric acid to allantoin. Articular gout occurs in people that normally do not have uricase, and also in birds or reptiles that synthesize uric acid as their principal end-

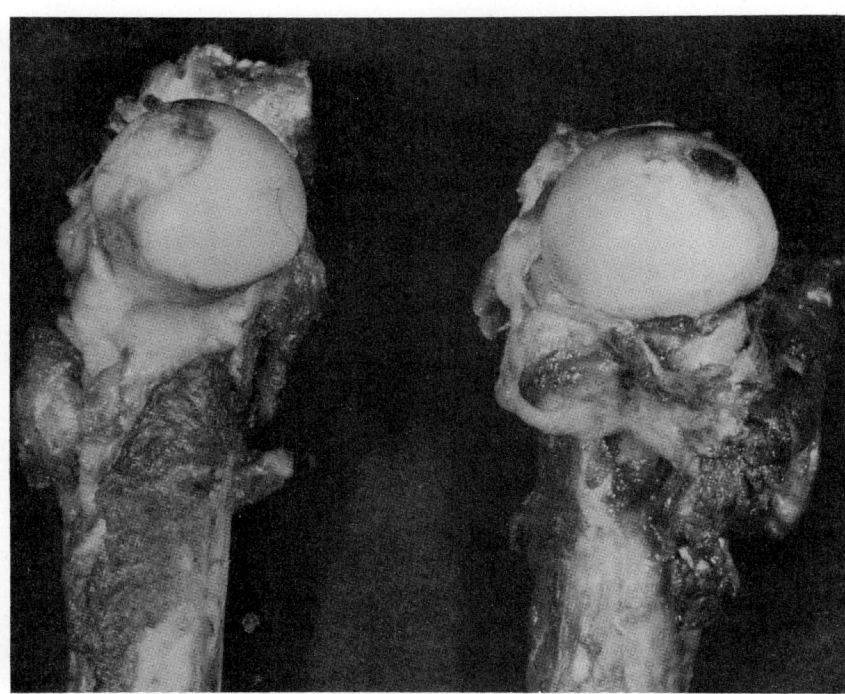

FIG. 19-27 Osteoarthritis of the femoral heads subsequent to hip dysplasia in a 10-year-old male German shepherd dog. The femoral heads are flattened and the articular surfaces eroded. (Courtesy of Angell Memorial Animal Hospital.)

product of nitrogen metabolism (uricotelic). Various forms of calcium phosphate may also be deposited in articular tissue and cause arthritis. Articular calcification is separable from other types of metastatic mineralization because the viscera are not involved. A variety of names have been applied (calcium gout, pseudogout, calcinosis); the name of the crystal type (apatite, calcium hydrogen phosphate dihydrate, calcium pyrophosphate dihydrate) has been used as a scheme to classify calcium phosphate crystal deposition. Pseudogout is the name generally applied when calcium pyrophosphate dihydrate is deposited (CCPD deposition disease). This classification system is not entirely satisfactory, because changes in the organic matrix possibly antedate and predispose to mineral deposition. Also, more than one crystal type is found within some deposits. Calcium phosphate deposition may affect single joints, or may be inherited and manifest as metabolic disease. In the latter case, serum levels of phosphorus or vitamin D metabolites may be abnormal; the disease may affect multiple joints. The inherited condition is autosomal-recessive and has been described in Great Danes and mice (ank/ank). It is also seen in clutches of newly hatched turtles. Periarticular calcification may also occur as localized masses (**tumoral calcinosis**). **Chondrocalcinosis** is the abnormal deposition of calcium salts in the hyaline or fibrocartilage of the joints; this term is generally used when cartilage calcification is nonspecific and crystal identification is lacking. It may be seen in the intervertebral disk, meniscus, or articular cartilage of the larger diarthrodial joints. Articular chondrocalcinosis is reported in dogs, primates, and rabbits. It occurs as isolated mineralized foci within articular cartilage and may not necessarily be associated with obvious osteochondrosis or osteoarthritis. When the deposited

mineral is dislodged from the articular surface, it leaves a small pinpoint crater. Although calcification of periarticular structures and tendons may be seen with degenerative joint disease, calcific tendonitis also occurs in the absence of degeneration.

References

Gibson JP, Roenigk WJ. Pseudogout in a dog. J Am Vet Med Assoc 161:912–915, 1972.

Heimann M, Carpenter JL, Halverson PB. Calcium pyrophosphate deposition (chondrocalcinosis) in a dog. Vet Pathol 1990;27:122–124.

Roberts ED, Baskin GB, Watson E, et al. Calcium pyrophosphate deposition in nonhuman primates. Vet Pathol 1984;21:592–596.

Woodard JC, Shields RP, Aldrich HC, et al. Calcium phosphate deposition disease in Great Danes. Vet Pathol 1982;19:464–485.

Reaction of joints to injury

The synovial membrane is a thin vascular lining that covers the inner surfaces of the articular capsule and the intraarticular ligaments and tendons. Synovial villi project into the joint at specialized regions, such as niches between the large fat folds. The synovial lining cells react to injurious agents by hypertrophy and hyperplasia (Fig. 19-24). The plump lining cells increase; these contain abundant quantities of rough endoplasmic reticulum. Inflammatory reactions that cause synovial cells to increase phagocytic activity increase synthesis of hydrolase enzymes and lysosome production. The synovial membrane has a tremendous capacity to undergo villous proliferation caused by low-grade inflammation. The stimulation of the synovial membrane in inflammation causes the proliferation of synovial vessels, producing a fibrovascular membrane (**pannus**) that extends to the articular surface; this membrane may penetrate defective cartilage. Secondary responses within the synovium include: deposition of hemosiderin, fibrosis and articular capsular hypertrophy, and mineralization within the synovial wall or joint capsule. In rare instances, the synovium may undergo metaplasia to form osteochondral nodules in association with chronic inflammation.

Too much pressure or a lack of sufficient contact on the bone end leads to alteration in articular cartilage. With too much pressure, cells in the superficial cartilage zone become necrotic, resulting in loss of matrix staining. Too little load results in decreased synthesis of proteoglycans and chondromalacia (soft cartilage). Next, where the normal collagen fibrils within the cartilage matrix become more apparent, cartilage **fibrillation** appears; cracks and crevices develop, which fragment the remaining cartilage into longitudinal clefts. With or because of synovial inflammation, destruction of the articular cartilage occurs. **Joint mice** are fragments of cartilage that break off from the joint surface. They may survive, grow, and ossify while being bathed by synovial fluid from which they derive nourishment. Whenever cartilage cell necrosis or loss of the superficial cartilage layers occurs, remaining cartilage cells undergo cell division; this produces daughter cells, cell clones, or chondrones. However, the ability of articular cartilage to replace itself following injury is limited. The response of articular cartilage to trauma depends largely upon the depth of the injury. Superficial lacerations evoke only a short-lived metabolic and enzymatic response, which fails to provide sufficient numbers of cells or matrix to repair the smallest injury. However, when the injury penetrates bone, a typical granulation tissue response occurs within the region. This phase is similar to that described under fracture repair, except that the cartilage wound edges are united only with fibrous tissue. The marrow space becomes filled with granulation tissue, and some cartilage—usually fibrocartilage—and reactive bone may be produced. The chondrification of mesenchymal tissue filling the marrow may be deficient and more characteristic of myxomatous tissue. When articular cartilage is breached— as occurs in chronic stages of degenerative arthritis or osteochondrosis—the synovial fluid pressure causes myxomatous degeneration of marrow tissue. Selective resorption of bone may occur; the surrounding trabeculae may become thick and produce a zone of sclerosis around the myxomatous tissue, forming a **pseudocyst.**

The underlying biochemical mechanisms involved in immune-mediated and nonimmune articular diseases are similar in that the production of local factors can lead to chondromalacia or degradation of articular cartilage. Heat-killed bacteria can induce arthritis when injected into experimental animals, and arthritogenicity is directly associated with the content of cell-wall peptidoglycans. Systemic administration of small molecular-weight peptidoglycans can induce acute polyarthritis by a nonimmune-mediated process. This initial inflammatory response is probably mediated by mast cell degranulation. The development of immune-mediated arthritis with peptidoglycans or other antigens is dependent upon the antigenic material being deposited in the joint and the development of delayed hypersensitivity. Nonimmunoglobin, T-cell-derived molecules (lymphokines) that bind specifically to the antigen are effector molecules. Immune complexes trapped in joint collagenous tissue provoke an inflammatory response, and the pathologic role of sequestered antigen in maintenance of the chronic inflammatory response lies in long-lasting leakage of antigen into surrounding tissue. Immune complexes can be absorbed by macrophages or synovial cells with the production of interleukin-I. Alternatively, complement is activated by immune complexes with the production of C3a and C5a components; these are known to induce interleukin-I secretion. Degradative changes in articular cartilage, leading to subchondral bone erosion, are features of both inflammatory and degenerative joint diseases. Prostaglandin E_2 inhibits cartilage proteoglycan synthesis and may mediate the loss of articular cartilage, due to normal matrix degradation exceeding synthesis. Lysosomal enzymes (collagenase, cathepsins, elastase, and arylsulfatase) are present in inflammatory, synovial, bone, and cartilage cells; these enzymes may cause degradation of proteoglycan (as in papain-induced or hypervitaminosis-A conditions). Enzymatically generated superoxide or peroxide can depolymerize polysaccharides and degrade synovial fluid and cartilage. Synovial lining cells can be induced to generate hydrogen peroxide constitutively following an inflammatory response. Neutral proteases act on collagen and proteoglycans and are produced by synoviocytes and chondrocytes. Their secretion is induced by a peptide released from cells of the immune system. Among these factors, interleukin-I plays an important role. Because interleukin-I is produced by synovial cells, an inflammatory condition does not seem necessary for it to be secreted.

References

Burkhardt H, Schwingel M, Menninger H, et al. Oxygen radicals as effectors of cartilage destruction: direct degradative effect on matrix components and indirect action via activation of latent collagenase from polymorphonuclear leukocytes. Arth Rheum 1986;29:379–387.

Kohashi O, Kohashi Y, Shigematsu N, et al. Acute and chronic polyarthritis induced by an aqueous form of 6-0-acyl and N-acyl derivatives of N-acetylmuramyl-L-alanyl-D-isoglutamine in euthymic rats and athymic nude rats. Lab Invest 1986;55:337–346.

McCord JM. Free radicals and inflammation: protection of synovial fluid by superoxide dismutase. Science 1974;185:529–531.

Spitznagel JK, Goodrum KJ, Warejcka DJ. Rat arthritis due to whole group B streptococci: clinical and histopathologic features compared with groups A and D. Am J Pathol 1983;112:37–47.

Stein H, Yarom R, Levin S, et al. Chronic self-perpetuating arthritis induced in rabbits by a cell-free extract of group A streptococci (37479). Proc Soc Exp Biol Med 1973;143:1106–1112.

Stuart JM, Watson WC, Kang AH. Collagen autoimmunity and arthritis. FASEB J 1988;22:2950–2956.

Tomoda K, Kitaoka M, Iyama K, et al. Endosteal new bone formation in the long bones of adjuvant treated rats. Pathol Res Pract 1986;181:331–338.

Van den Broek MF, van den Berg WB, van de Putte LBA, et al. Streptococcal cell wall-induced arthritis and flare-up reaction in mice induced by homologous or heterologous cell walls. Am J Pathol 1988;133:139–149.

DEGENERATIVE JOINT DISEASE

Osteoarthritis

Osteoarthritis (osteoarthropathy, hypertrophic arthritis, degenerative arthropathy) is the name generally applied in the United States to the most common form of articular disease that affects diarthrodial joints. Although inflammation may not be an outstanding feature or the primary cause of the condition, the name osteoarthritis emphasizes the role inflammation plays in the early stage of the disease processes. When the initial lesion is caused by an intrinsic alteration in the articular cartilage, **primary osteoarthritis** results. **Secondary osteoarthritis** is a consequence of some other joint disturbance, such as traumatic injury, joint dysplasia, or osteochondrosis. Osteoarthritis may be recognized in its early stages by the articular cartilage losing its normal hyaline appearance and becoming dull-white or light-yellow. Pits, depressions, and linear grooves appear in the articular surface, portions of which may break free to produce loose bodies (joint mice). Another lesion is the early development of marginal **osteophytes;** this lesion may be seen at the articular rim or as **enthesiophytes** at sites of muscular insertions. In advanced cases, constant friction results in eburnation, polishing, and grooving of the subchondral bone in contact areas. Eburnation and continued formation of perichondral cartilage and osteophytes alter the articular contour and produce the irregular margins (lipping) seen radiographically. In the late stages, subchondral pseudocysts—similar to those described in osteochondrosis—are produced; cystic changes can also be produced in the bone end by osteophytes surrounding synovial structures.

The initial microscopic lesion may be visualized with special stains as a loss of cartilage glycosaminoglycans. The articular cartilage appears less hyalin, and the fibrillary substratum of the cartilage becomes more apparent microscopically. The articular surface becomes fibrillated by developing deep clefts that separate strands of matrix. The remaining chondrocytes divide, develop clones or daughter cells (chondrones), and appear as clusters of chondrocytes arranged in rows. The articular cartilage is lost or worn away in some locations, which results in a progressive increase in the cartilage thickness at other sites. Endochondral ossification of the thickened cartilage adds bone to the surface. The synovial membrane may produce synovial cell hyperplasia, resulting in a mild lymphocyte infiltrate. Villous formation of the synovial membrane is occasionally observed, as well as chondroplasia and osseous metaplasia of synovial connective tissue or tendons.

Equines with osteoarthritis—probably biomechanically related—are excessively subject to exostoses of the limbs. A **ringbone** is an exostosis or group of exostoses arising on the second or—less commonly—first phalanx. It causes serious and painful **periarthritis. Splints** occur when inflammation along the interosseous ligament produces exostoses of the shaft and at the ends of the second and fourth metacarpal (rarely metatarsal) bones. Because of their less sensitive surroundings, they usually do not cause lameness. Exostoses frequently form on the medial portions of the distal bones of the tarsus. Such a lesion is called a (bone) **spavin.** Though small, it is a serious and stubborn cause of lameness.

NAVICULAR DISEASE

Navicular disease is a degenerative disease involving the equine distal sesamoid (navicular) bone and resulting in an associated inflammation of the podotrochlear bursa. The condition occurs almost exclusively in the forefeet. Gross lesions are not always apparent in clinically lame animals. Important pathologic changes include: degenerative changes and adhesions involving the fibrocartilaginous surface of the navicular bone and the deep flexor tendon, osteophyte formation, focal subchondral osteolysis (subchondral cysts), and mild villous hypertrophy of the bursal synovium. Manifestations of osteoarthritis (which appear to be age-related) include: degenerative changes in the fibrocartilaginous surfaces, development of osteophytes, and development of pseudocysts. The occurrence of osteoarthritis may not be associated with clinical signs, but extensive degenerative changes in navicular cartilaginous surfaces, together with subchondral bone cavitation (cysts) and adhesions, are consistent findings in horses with histories of navicular disease.

DEGENERATION OF THE INTERVERTEBRAL DISK

Age-related alterations occur in the structure of the intervertebral disk, and the disk becomes progressively more fibrous. In addition to aging fibrosis, certain breeds of dogs have an accelerated degeneration of the intervertebral disk. The chondrodystrophoid dog breeds—such as the dachshunds (Fig. 19-28), Pekingese, and French bulldogs—develop chondroid metaplasia of the nucleus pulposus at an early age. In other dog breeds—such as beagles and cocker spaniels—their chondrodystrophoid nature is less established, but they develop similar disk disease. The notocord cells of the nucleus pulposus are replaced by cartilage cells. Cartilaginous transformation begins in the periphery of the nucleus and progresses from the inner to the outer lamellae of the annulus fibrosus. Degeneration of the nucleus pulposus predisposes the disk to displacement through the annulus fibrosus. The direction of the prolapse varies and depends upon the surrounding anatomy of the vertebral column and the species of animal involved. Because of the relative immobility of the thoracic spine and the presence of the conjugal ligament that reinforces the dorsal annulus fibrosus, dorsal herniation of disks in the thoracic region is uncommon. Protrusion of the intervertebral disk into the spinal canal may cause injury to the spinal cord and paralysis. An initial inflammatory reaction to the liberated, degenerated disk material may involve the periosteum, longitudinal ligament, and dura matter. The inflammatory reaction becomes chronic, with marked fibroplasia. The degenerated disk material may calcify and cause a granulomatous reaction, leading to osseous metaplasia.

SPONDYLOSIS DEFORMANS

Spondylosis deformans is a degenerative arthropathy of vertebral amphiarthroses (intervertebral discs); it is characterized by osteophytes that grow toward each

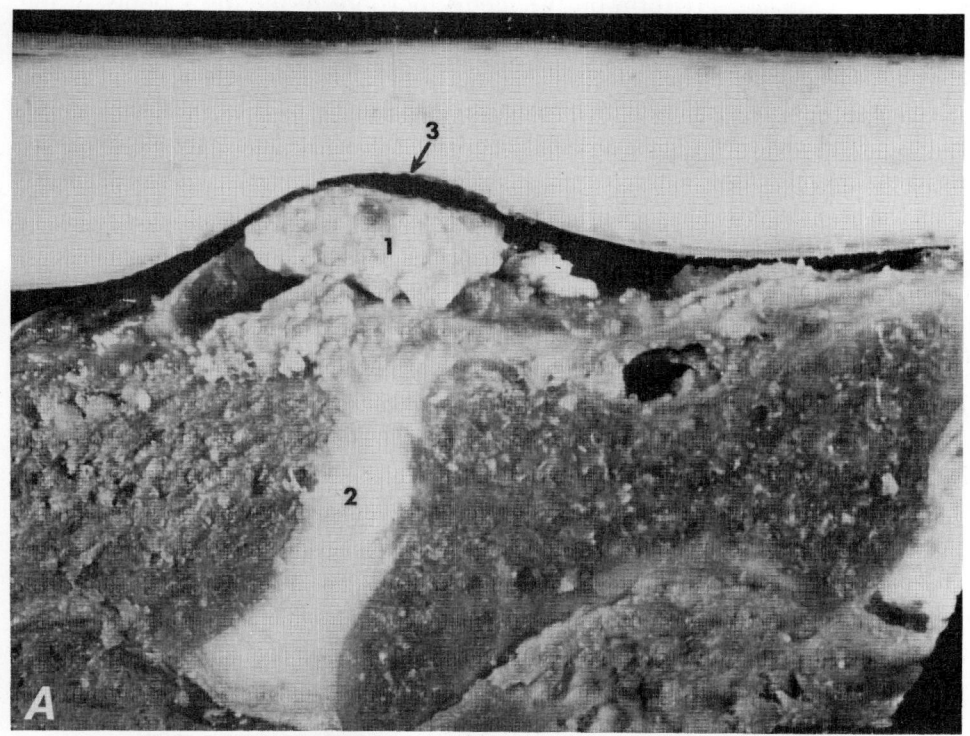

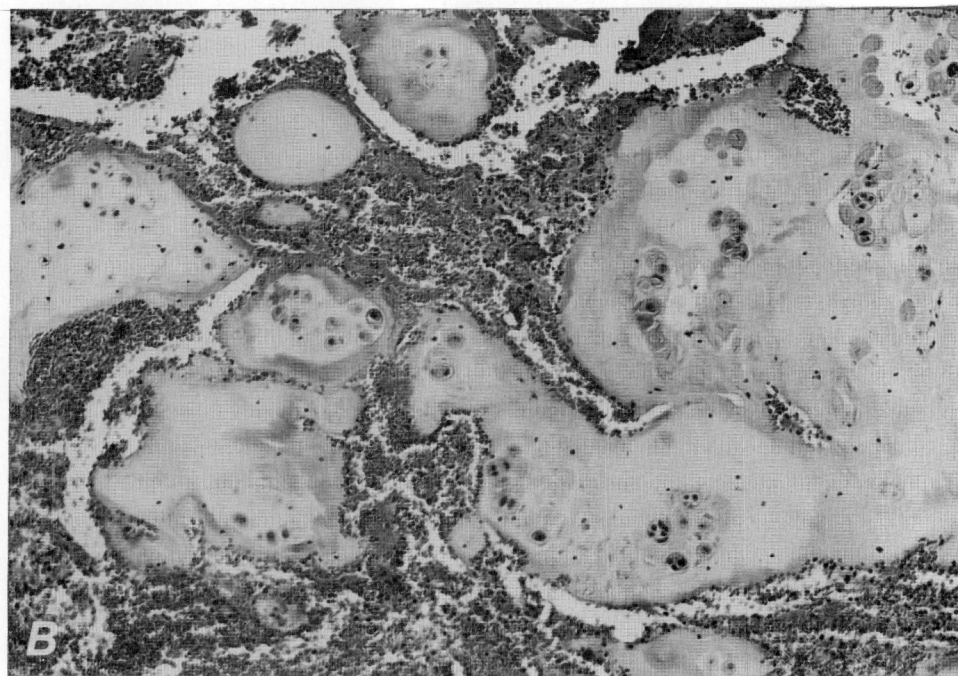

FIG. 19-28 A. Protrusion of intervertebral disc in a five-year-old male dachshund. (1) The protruded material; (2) From cervical disc 5-6; (3) Has compressed the spinal cord. The vertebral column and spinal cord were fixed in formalin and then cut sagittally. **B.** Chondroid material, hemorrhage, and debris from the nucleus pulposus, which has undergone chondroid metaplasia and has been expelled into the vertebral canal through a diseased annulus fibrosus. (Hematoxylin-and-eosin stain, ×150.) (Courtesy of Angell Memorial Animal Hospital.)

other and often bridge the ventral intervertebral space (Fig. 19-29). Protrusion of the intervertebral disk leads to spondylosis deformans when it is accompanied by avulsion of the fibers of the annulus fibrosus from its attachment site at the margin of the vertebral body. The development of osteophytes—at the attachment of the ventral longitudinal ligament to the vertebral body—is similar to the development of an enthesiophyte in osteoarthritis. Intervertebral disc degeneration may grad-

ually lead to protrusion of disc material. The outer fibers of the annulus are fused with the ventral longitudinal ligament. Rupture of the fibers of the annulus fibrosus produces traction on the ventral longitudinal ligament and provokes subperiosteal new bone production. Formation of an exostosis progresses; well-developed buttresses of bone from opposing vertebrae grow toward each other and may eventually fuse. A fibrocartilaginous separation usually occurs. Spondylosis

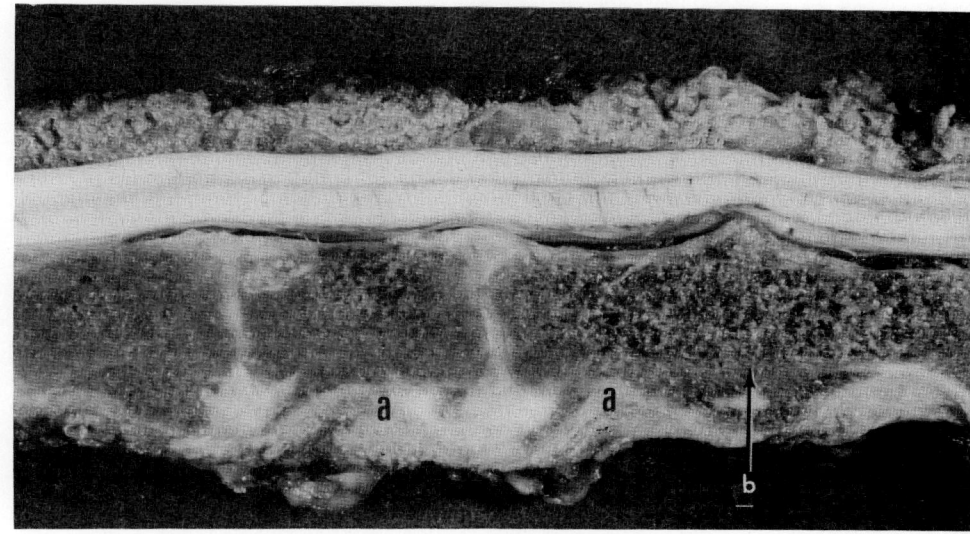

FIG. 19-29 Ankylosing spondylosis fusing lumbar vertebrae in a 15-year-old cross-breed terrier. **A.** Note buttresses of bone expand across narrowed intervertebral spaces, and **B.** loss of intervertebral disc. (Courtesy of Angell Memorial Animal Hospital.)

is associated with vertebral diseases other than protrusion of the intervertebral disk. It commonly occurs in cats, cattle, and swine. It is relatively rare in other domestic animals; it has been described as an occupational hazard of stud bulls, but the cause and pathogenesis has not been established. Severe spondylosis of cervical vertebrae in cats is usually due to hypervitaminosis A.

References

Doige CE, Hoffer MA. Pathological changes in the navicular bone and associated structures of the horse. Can J Comp Med 1983;47:387–395.

Ghosh P, Taylor TKF, Braund KG, Larsen LH. A comparative chemical and histochemical study of the chondrodystrophoid and non-chondrodystrophoid canine intervertebral disc. Vet Pathol 1976;13:414–427.

Goggin JE, Li AS, Franti CE. Canine intervertebral disk disease: characterization by age, sex, breed, and anatomic site of involvement. Am J Vet Res 1970;31:1687–1692.

Griffiths IR. Spinal cord infarction due to emboli arising from the intervertebral disc in the dog. J Comp Pathol 1973;83:225–232.

Hansen HJ. Comparative views on the pathology of disc degeneration in animals. Lab Invest 1959;8:1242–1265.

Johnson LC. Joint remodeling as the basis for osteoarthritis. J Am Vet Med Assoc 1962;141:1237–1241.

Lust G, Pronsky W, Sherman DM. Biochemical and ultrastructural observations in normal and degenerative canine articular cartilage. Am J Vet Res 1972;33:2429–2440.

Morgan JP, Pool RR, Miyabayashi T. Primary degenerative joint disease of the shoulder in a colony of beagles. J Am Vet Med Assoc 1987;190:531–540.

Riser WH. Canine hip dysplasia: cause and control. J Am Vet Med Assoc 1974;165:360–362.

Seawright AA, English PB. Cervical spondylosis: cat. J Pathol Bacteriol 1964;88:503–509.

Inflammatory joint disease

INFECTIOUS ARTHRITIS

Acute inflammation of a joint is commonly serous, fibrinous, or purulent. Synovial fluid is a dialysate of blood plasma into which hyaluronate is secreted by synovial cells. Serous inflammation is equivalent to an excessive formation of synovia, which distends the joint capsule and forms a "puffy" swelling. The articular and synovial surfaces show nothing more than a slight hyperemic redness. This type of arthritis is usually due to mild, often repeated trauma. When infection is present, the intracapsular exudate is fibrinous; or, in the presence of pyogenic organisms, it is purulent. In such cases, the articular surfaces may be eroded (Figure 19-30), and extreme pain results. The periarticular tissues are edematous.

Acute suppurative or acute fibrinous arthritides (which may progress to chronic arthritis) may be due to wounds that open the joint cavity to infective microorganisms. However, they are more frequently due to articular localization of generalized septicemic or pyemic infections. Pyogenic arthritis also is one of the most common complications of pyogenic osteomyelitis, and is seen more frequently in young animals than adults. Spread of infection from the carpal or tarsal bones to the joint is common in equines. Suppurative osteomyelitis commonly manifests in the articular ends of long tubular bone. Prior to growth-plate closure, infection may spread from the affected bone to the neighboring joint. The growth plate is a barrier to the spread of infection from the metaphysis to the joint. In the large diarthrodial joints, such as the stifle, infection often spreads from the bone interior to the periosteum and then into the joint at the site of attachment of the joint capsule.

Pyogenic arthritis may be a consequence of bacteremia and direct infection of the synovial membrane. The most common condition is pyosepticemia of the newborn (pyosepticemia neonatorum, "joint-ill") resulting from infection of the umbilicus at birth. A variety of microorganisms may be associated with infectious arthritis in both newborn and adult animals. In foals, *Actinobacillus equuli* (previously named *Shigella equirulis*) is the most common organism recovered, but other organisms such as *Streptococcus sp.*, *Salmonella sp.*, and *Escherichia coli* are also frequently recovered. *Erysipelothrix*

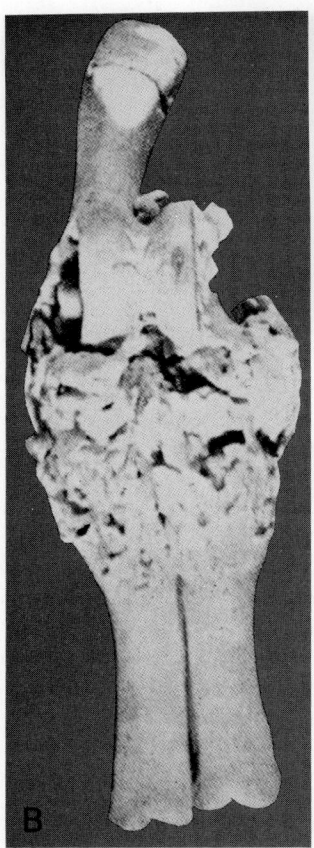

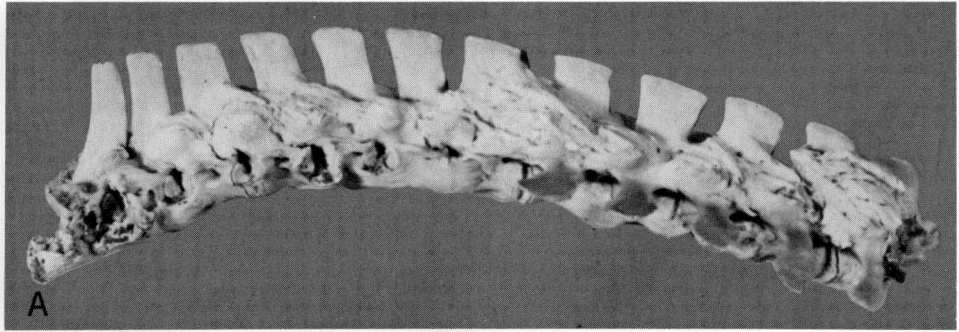

FIG. 19-30 Thoracic and lumbar spondylitis in a pig that, at the age of three months, was inoculated with a pure culture of *Erysipelothrix rhusiopathiae.* **A.** Most of the joints developed a proliferative and ankylosing inflammation that was continuously progressive until euthanasia at three years of age. **B.** Tarasometatarsal arthritis in same animal as **A.** (Courtesy of Dr. Dennis Sikes.)

rhusiopathiae is notable for causing a chronic low-grade arthritis and periarthritis in swine, lambs, and turkeys. *Corynebacterium ovis, Escherichia coli,* and *Streptococcus sp.* are also frequent causes of arthritis in sheep. *Mycoplasma sp.* are important causes of arthritis in swine, sheep, goats, and cattle. *Chlamydia psittaci* type 2 is a cause of sporadic or endemic arthritis in lambs and calves. *Hemophilus suis* produces polyserositis with arthritis in swine. *Brucella sp.* and *Streptococcus sp.* also frequently cause a suppurative arthritis in swine. In rats Mycoplasma, *Streptobacillus moniliformis, Diplococcus pneumoniae,* and *Corynebacterium kutcheri* are frequent causes of arthritis. It should be clear from this list that arthritis is an important manifestation of many infectious diseases, but noticeably absent are generalized infections of dogs and cats. Aside from reports of **Lyme arthritis** and other occasional joint infections such as cryptococcosis, little information exists about infectious joint disease in these species. Most examples of infectious arthritis in dogs and cats are the result of penetration wounds, in which case ordinary pyogenic bacteria are responsible.

Chronic arthritis Chronic arthritis may follow trauma or an acute infection, such as swine erysipelas. This type of arthritis may have am immune-mediated component that augments and prolongs the inflammatory processes. Antibodies may be formed in response to matrix constituents liberated from degenerating articular cartilage; or, antibodies may be complex with antigens derived from infecting organisms. *Borrelia burgdorferi*—the spirochete that causes Lyme disease—is known to infect wild animals and has been reported to cause arthritis in dogs, cats, and a cow. A small number of spirochetes are the antigenic stimulus for chronic synovial inflammation. Villous hyperplasia, lymphoplasmocytic cellular infiltrates, and fibrin deposition are nonspecific changes. Obliterative microvascular and fibrinoid lesions are more agent specific. **Granulomatous arthritis** is a special type of immune-mediated inflammation associated with delayed hypersensitivity. It is seen with mycotic infections, and also in tuberculous arthritis; arthritis may develop in any species and often localizes in the vertebral column.

Caprine arthritis-encephalitis infection Goats infected with the caprine arthritis-encephalitis retrovirus frequently develop a disease in which chronic arthritis is sometimes the principal manifestation. Up to 30% of the herd may show clinical signs. In addition to lameness, animals may have carpal hygromas; a dramatic reduction in milk production may also result. The joint capsules thicken in the atlantooccipital, carpal, stifle, and hock joints. The synovium contains a heavy inflammatory cell infiltrate composed principally of lymphocytes and plasma cells; the joint capsule is sometimes mineralized. The distended synovium is hypertrophic and has a villous surface. Fibrin may be attached to the synovial surface and appear as blood clots; or, serosanguinous joint fluid may contain small hard white grains of inspissated fibrin (so-called **rice grains**). Fibrillation and erosion of cartilage is seen in severe cases, as well as cartilage destruction by pannus, which rarely leads to joint fusion. Lesions are also found in brain, lung, and mammary gland.

References

Adams DS, Crawford TB, Klevjer-Anderson P. A pathogenetic study of the early connective tissue lesions of viral caprine arthritis-encephalitis. Am J Pathol 1980;99:257–278.
Cole BC, Washburn LR, Taylor-Robinson D. Mycoplasma-induced arthritis. In: Razin S, Barile MF, eds. The mycoplasmas. Vol IV. New York: Academic Press, 1985;107–160.
Johnston YE, et al. Lyme arthritis: spirochetes found in synovial microangiopathic lesions. Am J Pathol 1985;118:26–34.
Lowbeer L. Skeletal and articular involvement in brucellosis of animals. Lab Invest 1959;8:1448–1453.
Maierhofer CA, Storz J. Clinical and serologic responses in dogs inoculated with the chlamydial (psittacosis) agent. Am J Vet Res 1969;30:1961–1966.
Watt DA, Bamford V, Nairn ME. Actinobacillus seminis as a cause of polyarthritis and posthitis in sheep. Aust Vet J 1970;46:515.
Woodard JC, Gaskin JM, Poulos PW, et al. Caprine arthritis-encephalitis: clinicopathologic study. Am J Vet Res 1982;43:2085–2096.

NONINFECTIOUS ARTHRITIS

Canine rheumatoid arthritis Canine rheumatoid arthritis differs from the counterpart disease in humans by lacking systemic features; also, rheumatoid nodules do not usually develop in the dog. The canine disease is more severe in its early stages and progresses rapidly. Otherwise, the articular pathology and clinical signs are similar to the human condition, although rheumatoid factor is present in comparatively low titer and in only 25% of affected dogs. The canine disease is manifested by severe polyarthritis with swollen, painful joints, fever, and neutrophilia (in initial stages). The condition is rare and is seen more commonly in small- or toy-breed dogs. The joints associated with the small bones of the appendicular skeleton are more commonly affected, but other joints may be involved as well. Changes in synovial fluid indicate synovitis, with elevated total cell-count and a high population of neutrophils; mucin may variably decrease. Neutrophils are rarely seen in synovial biopsy specimens, and only in the early disease phase. Marked synovial hyperplasia occurs, with villous formation; the synovium is infiltrated with lymphocytes, plasma cells, and macrophages. Erosion of the articular cartilage is present at the cartilage margins. Granulation tissue from the inflamed synovium may extend across the articular surface as a pannus. A distinctive lesion is the undermining of cartilage and erosion of subchondral bone by pannus arising from the synovium.

Polyarthritis in greyhounds This disease of unknown cause occurs in young greyhounds and has been described in Australia, Europe, England, and the United States. **Grossly,** significant lesions are primarily limited to the affected joints and are most prominent in the stifle, elbow, carpal, and tibiotarsal joints. Fibrinous strands may bridge onto joint surfaces, and the articular surfaces contain irregular erosions. In other areas, the cartilage appears thin, grooved, and disrupted. The synovium is yellow-brown, appears slightly raised, and contains velvet textured plaques. Marginal osteophytes may be observed. **Microscopically,** full-thickness necrosis of articular cartilage has been reported and may be a distinguishing feature. Surface cartilage is sloughed, and erosions sometimes extend to the subchondral bone. A prominent feature is the necrosis of the deeper hyaline cartilage zones with relative sparing of the surface regions. The synovium has marked villus hypertrophy and is infiltrated with aggregate-forming lymphocytes. In addition to lymphocytes, plasma cells, and macrophages, occasional collections of neutrophils contribute to the inflammatory cell infiltrate. Hemosiderosis may be prominent, with iron pigment occurring in fibroblasts and synovial cells.

Progressive feline polyarthritis This is a specific entity affecting young adult male cats. Although the pathogenesis and precise cause is unknown, it is thought to be related to infections with feline-syncytia-forming-virus (FeSFV) and feline-leukemia-virus (FeLV). All affected animals have antibodies to FeSFV, and 70% have antibodies to FeLV. The disease has not been reproduced experimentally, and arthritis is thought to be an uncommon manifestation of retrovirus infection in genetically predisposed individuals. The arthritis appears in two forms. An erosive and deforming arthritis is the less common variant, in which the gross and microscopic features are similar to canine rheumatoid arthritis. Erosions are seen at the articular margins and central parts of the subchondral bone. The more common periosteal proliferative form is associated with extensive new bone formation surrounding the joint. Periarticular erosion results, with collapse of the joint space and fibrous ankylosis; however, bone deformity does not occur with this variant.

Nonerosive immune-mediated polyarthritis Nonerosive immune-mediated polyarthritis is an etiologically diverse condition that is probably mediated by similar immunopathologic mechanisms. It is seen in systemic lupus erythematosus; it also occurs secondarily in various infectious diseases (refer to *chronic inflammation* above) and has been reported following inflammatory bowel disease. Clinical signs include cyclic fever, malaise, anorexia, lameness, and generalized stiffness. When it occurs as part of systemic lupus erythematosus, the simultaneous occurrence of other systemic manifestations aid in making the diagnosis: for example, polymyositis, glomerulonephritis, thrombocytopenia, and hemolytic anemia. Otherwise, serologic abnormalities—such as the presence of antinuclear antibodies—may be the only finding that permits making a diagnosis of lupus. The arthralgia may be cyclic in nature, and the radiographic alterations are minimal. A predisposition exists for the condition to affect small distal limb joints, particularly the carpus and tarsus. A single, few, or many joints may be involved. Biopsy reveals a sparse mononuclear cell infiltrate with a moderate to severe superficial inflammation characterized by polymorphonuclear leukocyte infiltration and fibrin exudation. At necropsy, the gross lesions are not striking. The synovial membrane may be congested and edematous, and the amount of synovial fluid may be increased. Articular cartilage usually has a normal appearance. The condition is distinguished from other types of noninfectious arthritis because villous hypertrophy, marginal erosions of articular cartilage, and pannus formation are not prominent.

References

Halliwell RE, Lavelle RB, Butt KM. Canine rheumatoid arthritis: a review and a case report. J Small Anim Pract 1972;13:239–248.

Huxtable CR, Davis PE. The pathology of polyarthritis in young greyhounds. J Comp Pathol 1976;86:11–21.

Kendrick JW, Sittmann K. Inherited osteoarthritis of dairy cattle. J Am Vet Med Assoc 1966;149:17–24.

Krum SH, Cardinet GH III, Anderson BC, et al. Polymyositis and polyarthritis associated with systemic lupus erythematosus in a dog. J Am Vet Med Assoc 1977;170:61–64.

Lewis RM. Canine systemic lupus erythematosus. Am J Pathol 1972;69:537–540.

Lewis RM, Borel Y. Canine rheumatoid arthritis: a case report. Arth Rheum 1971;14:67–74.

Pedersen NC, Pool RR, O'Brien T. Feline chronic progressive polyarthritis. Am J Vet Res 1980;41:522–535.

Neoplasms of bone and joints

Osteosarcoma is the most frequent bone neoplasm, and in different studies is reported to represent between 65–85% of the primary bone neoplasms of the dog. Chondrosarcomas are the next most common primary bone tumor (15%) with fibrosarcomas and hemangiosarcomas occurring about equally. Osteosarcoma and fibrosarcomas are occasionally found in bones of small-breed dogs that have infarcts of multiple bones. Some primary bone tumors—such as liposarcoma, hemangioma, malignant mesenchymoma, and leiomyosarcomas—occur infrequently. Other primary bone tumors—such as schwannomas—are extremely rare. Osteoblastoma is reported in the radius of a horse, and a related tumor—osteoid osteoma—is reported in the vertebrae of a cat. Chordomas—rare malignant tumors of bone and soft tissue—arise along the axial skeleton and are reported most frequently in the lumbosacral or coccygeal region of ferrets, ranch mink, and rats. One must be careful to distinguish neoplasms from tumorlike lesions that are infrequently associated with bone and joints. Some examples of tumorlike lesions that may cause confusion are: simple or unicameral bone cysts, aneurysmal bone cysts, fibrous dysplasia, central giant cell granuloma, pigmented villonodular synovitis, nodular tenosynovitis, or ganglion. Epidermal inclusion cysts and epidermoid cysts may be found deep in vertebrae at the midline of Rhodesian Ridgeback dogs; or, epidermal inclusion cysts may be found in the nailbed involving the third phalanx.

Osteoma Osteoma is an uncommon tumor occurring most frequently in the head. The tumor grows slowly and progressively by intramembranous bone formation. It is attached to the bone surface by a broad base; when mature, it is difficult to distinguish from an osteophyte. It is composed of cancellous bone with fibrous connective tissue or fat-filled marrow spaces. The matrix may have a mucoid appearance. The periosteum is well-differentiated and composed of fibrous and osteogenic layers. Peripheral trabeculae are made up of woven bone bordered by typical osteoblasts. Lamellae are thickened by apposition and, in the center of the lesion, trabeculae may have borders of lamellar bone.

Ossifying fibroma Ossifying fibroma is a rare fibroosseous tumor of the jaw of horses and cattle. It is a sharply demarcated lesion; its expansive mass distorts the normal bone contour. Normal bone is replaced by a fibroosseous stroma composed of irregular trabeculae of osteoid and woven bone rimmed by osteoblasts. The lesion can be differentiated from osteoma because the intervening connective tissue is more cellular and contains more collagen fibers than does osteoma. Also, no truly recognizable periosteal membrane exists.

Osteosarcoma (osteogenic sarcoma, periosteal sarcoma, parosteal or juxtacortical sarcoma) Malignant neoplasms, identified as osteosarcomas (Fig. 19-31), are known in most species; however, they are more frequent in dogs, especially in the giant breeds. These tumors originate most often in the metaphysis of long bones where bone turnover is the greatest; they may, however, arise from any site, including the sesamoids. About 20% of osteosarcomas occur in the dog's axial skeleton. Osteosarcoma of the head is more frequent in the bovine and equine species. In dogs, osteosarcoma of the skull—including paranasal sinuses or calvarium—generally has a longer clinical survival than osteosarcoma of the limbs. **Periosteal osteosarcomas** arise from the surface of the diaphysis more frequently than from the metaphysis and are neoplasms of intermediated differentiation. **Parosteal** or **juxtacortical osteosarcomas** are tumors that arise on the surface of the bone and do not involve the medullary cavity. They are composed typically of well-differentiated but malignant fibroosseous tissue. Parosteal osteosarcomas are not prone to metastasis, but recur locally after incomplete removal. **Extraskeletal osteosarcomas** are uncommon tumors that most often arise, in dogs, in visceral organs (Fig. 19-32).

The diagnosis of osteosarcoma is dependent upon recognizing the production of osteoid and woven bone by unequivocally anaplastic stromal cells. Several morphologic variants of the tumor have different histologic characteristics; most, however, have a similar clinical behavior. In the most common variety, the characteristic feature of osteosarcoma is the presence of neoplastic osteoblasts that are seen histologically as short, spindle- or triangular-shaped cells with plump ovoid nuclei, usually closely packed together. They are oriented to point in various directions, and do not lay parallel to one another in bundles. The critical identifying characteristic of these cells is their ability to produce **osteoid,** the col-

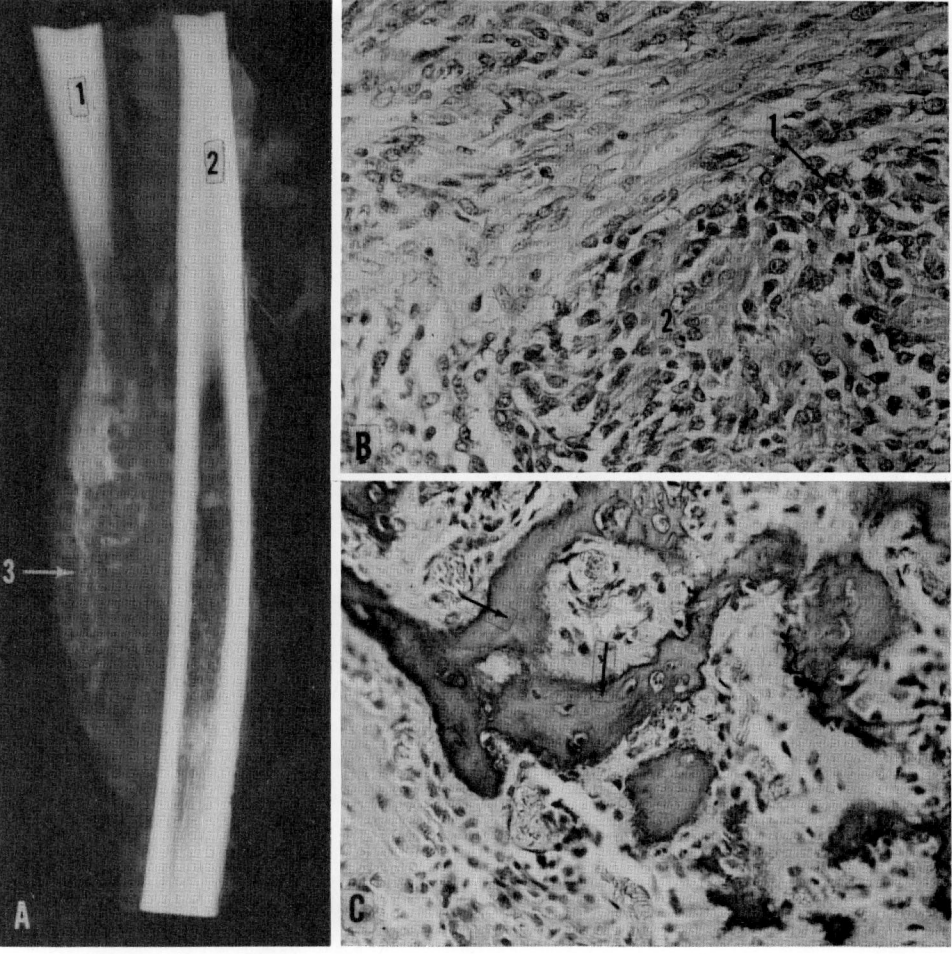

FIG. 19-31 Osteosarcoma of the ulna of a 10-year-old female golden retriever. **A.** Radiograph of the neoplasm (3) in (1) the distal third of the ulna. The radius (2) is not directly involved. **B.** Photomicrograph (×250) in an area of the neoplasm consisting of (1) densely-packed cells (2) that form osteoid. **C.** Photomicrograph (×250) of the same tumor from an area with irregular spicules of new bone (arrows). (Courtesy of Armed Forces Institute of Pathology; contributor: Fourth Medical Field Laboratory, U.S. Army.)

lagenous matrix that may become mineralized to form bone. Newly-formed osteoid is extracellular, dense, darkly eosinophilic staining material that may be fibrillar. Osteocytes may be trapped within it (Fig. 19-31), a feature also of normal bone. Multinucleated cells may also be present, and both osteoclasts and tumor giant cells can be identified. The recognition of newly formed osseous tissue as being an osteosarcoma is dependent upon identification of anaplastic characteristics of osteoblasts. Rarely, anaplastic characteristics of tumor cells may not be obvious. In these cases, helpful diagnostic features include: the identification of growth characteristics of tumor filling the intertrabecular spaces, the recognition of osteoid production as streamers and globules of unmineralized matrix, the appreciation of neoplastic cartilage, and the finding of global bone resorption in radiographs. Histopathologic variations include patterns with various predominating features. These patterns include sclerotic, cartilage, spindle-cell, large-cell, giant-cell, small- or round-cell, and vascular or cystlike (**telangiectatic osteosarcoma**) predominating characteristics. These patterns can be seen in all tumors in varying proportions; these varied histologic faces make diagnosis of osteosarcoma a most challenging exercise. Osteosarcomas metastasize to the lung very early, and the lung lesions may cause hypertrophic

pulmonary osteoarthropathy, a confounding factor in biopsy diagnosis. Approximately 10% of osteosarcomas metastasize to other locations in bone.

Chondroma Benign forms of cartilaginous tumor are reported but not frequent; they are distinguished from chondrosarcoma by their lack of local invasiveness, more orderly arrangement of the cartilage cells, and closer resemblance to normal mature cartilage. Primary chondromas are reported as benign lesions occurring in various bone or cartilage sites. They should be distinguished from lesions occurring in mixed tumors, multilobular tumor, synovial or bursal chondromatosis, osteochondroma, and enchondroma.

Osteochondroma Osteochondroma (**multiple cartilaginous exostoses, chondrodysplasia, diaphyseal aclasis, hereditary deforming chondrodysplasia**) are cartilage-capped, exophytic osseous lesions that usually occur in the metaphysis of young animals and cease to grow when the animal becomes mature. When they are removed from their primary location, the lesion cannot be distinguished from marginal osteophytes occurring secondarily in osteoarthritis. The condition is more common in dogs, cats, and horses, and may be monostotic (solitary) or polyostotic (osteochondromatosis). Osteochondromas are thought to arise from ectopic growth-plate cartilage. Histologically, the lesion points

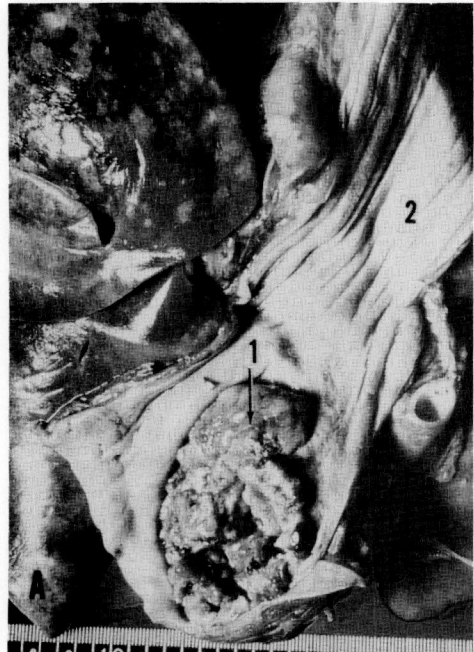
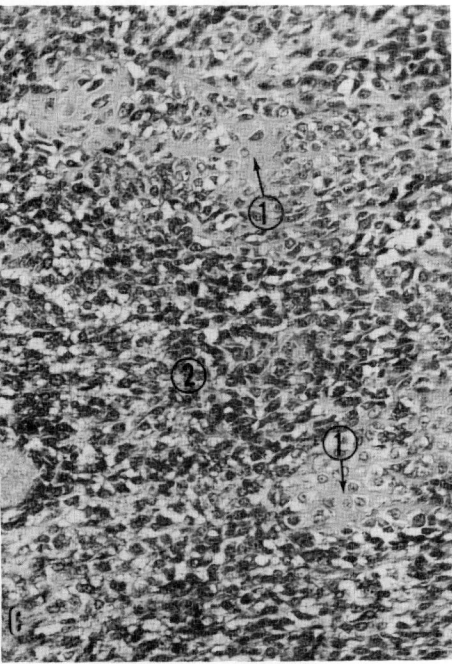

FIG. 19-32 Osteosarcoma, primary in the esophagus of a seven-year-old male hound. The neoplasm was associated with long-standing infection of the esophagus by *Spirocerca lupi.* **A.** (1) The tumor involves (2) the terminal esophagus. (3) The lung containing metastases. **C.** An area of the tumor (×150). (1) Osteoid surrounded by hyperchromatic, densely-packed osteoblasts. (Courtesy of Armed Forces Institute of Pathology; contributor: Dr. H.R. Seibold.)

away from the joint, and the cortex and spongiosa of the osteochondroma blend imperceptibly with the cortex and spongiosa of the host bone. Cartilaginous growth seems to be the initial factor, followed by ossification. Cartilage usually persists around the periphery of the masses, and the center becomes ossified. Malignant transformation to chondrosarcoma has been reported in three dogs. Senescent osteochondromas may have the cartilage cap completely replaced by bone. Multiple osteochondromas (hereditary multiple exostoses) occur as an autosomal-dominant inherited disorder in dogs and horses. Feline osteochondromatosis differs from the inherited disease and may be associated with intralesional retrovirus. The lesions in cats undergo progressive growth, even after maturity. Tumors may arise in flat bone and the sternum, as well as long bones. The histology of feline osteochondromas differs from the inherited type because the hyperplastic periosteum may directly form bone, and the cartilage lesions are more disorganized.

Enchondroma Enchondroma is a rare, benign cartilage tumor composed entirely of hyaline or fibrocartilaginous tissue arising in the bone medulla. It may be a mono- or polyostotic (enchondromatosis) lesion. It is a radiolucent, usually well-demarcated, expansive mass covered by a thin shell of bone. Histologically, islands of cartilage are surrounded by plates of lamellar to woven bone.

Multilobular tumor Multilobular tumor (**multilobular osteoma** or *chondroma, chondroma rodens, cartilage analogue of fibromatosis, juvenile aponeurotic fibroma*) consists of multiple small compact osteocartilaginous lobules, usually arising in the canine skull; however, it occurs in other bones and has been seen in cats and a horse. It is a distinct tumor type that has unique morphologic

features. Radiographic study reveals diffuse nodular or stippled densities in soft tissues around the skull. These are accompanied by rarefaction of the underlying cranial bones. Microscopic examination reveals small islands of chondroid, osseous, or osteocartilaginous tissue surrounded by spindle-shaped cells in connective tissue. Foci of calcification may be seen in the fibroblastic cells. This lesion is potentially aggressive, and its features suggest malignancy; it produces increased numbers of mitotic figures, has less distinct lobulation, and one of the mesenchymal components may overgrow the other. Multilobular sarcomas should be differentiated from the standard variety of chondrosarcoma or osteosarcoma. The disease causes progressive local tissue destruction, and the tumor has a high metastatic rate. Local lesions can recur when not completely removed, and sarcomas may metastasize to the lung.

Chondrosarcoma Chondrosarcoma tumor is made up of irregular, disorderly masses of immature cartilage that invade tissue and metastasize through the lymphatic and blood circulation. Tumor may infiltrate between host-bone trabeculae before the trabeculae are resorbed or altered by remodeling. The cartilage cells in lacunae of cartilaginous matrix vary in size and do not maintain any orderly polarity (Fig. 19-33). Because of the tendency of normal cartilage cells to become hypertrophic during the process of endochondral ossification, it is inadvisable to use cell or nuclear sizes as the main criteria of malignancy for cartilage tumors. In addition to nuclei becoming enlarged, they become hyperchromatic and develop other diagnostic features of malignancy: for example, having double nuclei per cell, large eosinophilic nucleoli, and multiple enlarged nucleoli. Perhaps one of the most helpful features is cel-

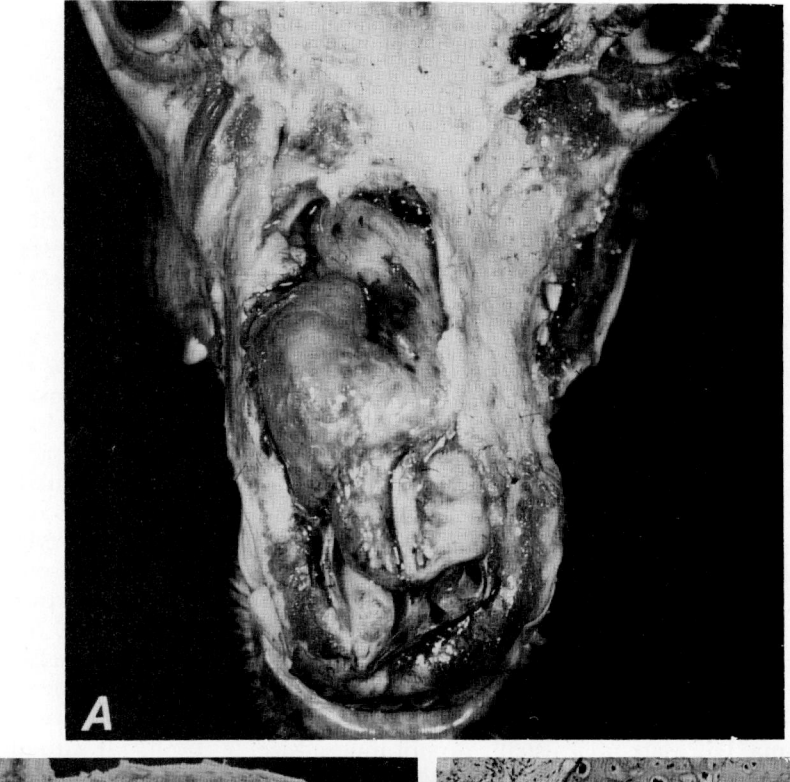

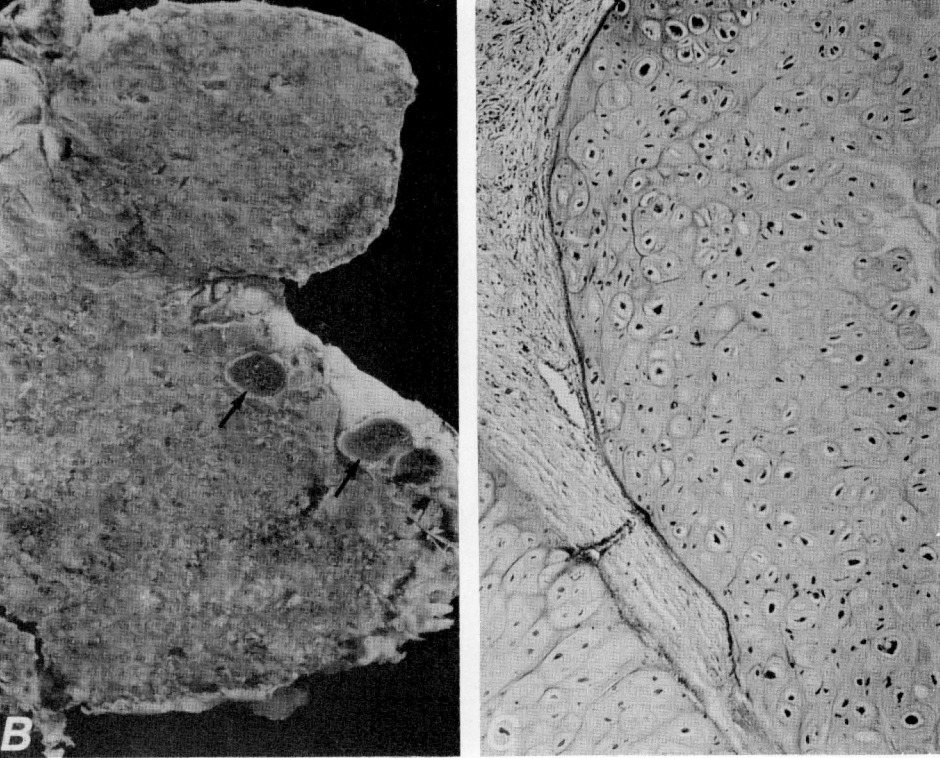

FIG. 19-33 A. Chondrosarcoma of nasal septum of a seven-year-old male pointer. (Courtesy of Angell Memorial Animal Hospital.) **B.** Chondrosarcoma of the ribs of a five-year-old ewe. The tumor metastasized to the lung. (Contributor: Dr. C.L. Davis.) **C.** Chondrosarcoma of the ribs of an aged ewe (×120). Note cells with irregular polarity and variable size in cartilaginous matrix. Metastasis to the lungs also occurred in this case. (Courtesy of Armed Forces Institute of Pathology; contributor: Dr. C.L. Davis.)

lular disorganization. Malignant cartilage lobules are often separated by bands of fibrous tissue. Malignancy is also evident by tumor invasiveness and metastases to the lungs and elsewhere. Types of chondrosarcoma include those composed of hyaline cartilage, and a fibromyxoid variety composed of myxoid fibrillary material. **Mesenchymal chondrosarcomas** are highly malignant tumors in which a large proportion of the tumor is composed of primitive spindly to ovoid mesenchymal stromal cells. Chondrosarcomas can contain regions of osseous metaplasia (chondroid bone), and neoplastic cartilage is commonly found in osteosarcomas. In order to distinguish chondrosarcoma from osteosarcoma, one should determine that the osteoid is not produced directly by malignant stromal cells, and that it goes through a cartilage phase first. Chondrosarcoma tends to arise from sites where normal cartilage exists, such as near rib cartilage, scapular cartilage, pelvis, and the nasal turbinates and septum (Figure 19-33).

Dogs are most often affected with bone tumors, and chondrosarcomas are second in frequency to osteosarcomas. They also tend to be malignant and recur (when excised). However, slightly more success following surgical removal is experienced with chondrosarcoma when compared to osteosarcoma.

Fibroma These tumors are extremely infrequent primary tumors of bone. They are circumscribed, usually encapsulated, and made up of more mature collagenous connective tissue. Their course is benign, although they may be locally disfiguring.

Fibrosarcoma This tumor may arise from connective tissue anywhere in the body; occasionally, it is primary in bone. Commonly, an extraskeletal fibrosarcoma invades bone. The cells are pleomorphic and vary from high undifferentiated, roughly spindle-shaped cells with round to ovoid nuclei, often in mitosis, to elongated cells interlacing bundles resembling immature connective tissue. This tendency for groups of cells to be parallel to one another is a valuable feature in identifying fibrosarcoma. Fibrosarcomas usually do not metastasize, even after several months; however, they may be associated with bone lysis and local extension. Canine maxillary fibrosarcomas are tumors of low-grade malignancy that arise on the outer bone surface and must be differentiated from invasive amelanotic melanomas.

Hemangiosarcoma A tumor arising from endothelium, the hemangiosarcoma (malignant hemangioen-dothelioma) may be primary in almost any tissue; in most species, however, it more frequently originates in spleen, liver, heart muscle (atrium), and bone. The histologic features include neoplastic cells with large hyperchromatic nuclei and scant cytoplasm. Cells often tend to form large vascular spaces, which may be distended with blood. The blood vessels are clearly formed by tumor cells and are not part of the supporting stroma. Mitoses are common, multiple sites may occur, and metastases can be expected. These tumors destroy bone locally—as do osteosarcomas and chondrosarcomas—and they metastasize just as readily.

Giant-cell tumor of bone Giant-cell tumor of bone (osteoclastoma) is rarely encountered in animals, but when seen most often involves dogs and cats. It occurs as an eccentric epiphyseal lesion of long bones and usually is confined within bone, being covered by a thin rim of osseous tissue. Histologically, the tumor is composed of ovoid or short spindly stromal cells, with masses of prominent osteoclastic giant cells that stain for tartrate-resistant acid phosphatase (a reaction characteristic of osteoclasts). Nuclei in the mononuclear and giant cells appear similar, are ovoid to reniform, contain small nucleoli, and have a finely stippled chromatin pattern. Some mesenchymal stromal cells react positively with antigens found to be present in mononuclear phagocytes, including leukocyte common antigen. Both benign and malignant tumors are reported. This tumor must be differentiated from other lesions containing giant cells, such as a simple bone cyst, aneurysmal bone cyst, hyperparathyroidism, fibrous dysplasia, giant cell variants of osteosarcoma, and reparative granuloma.

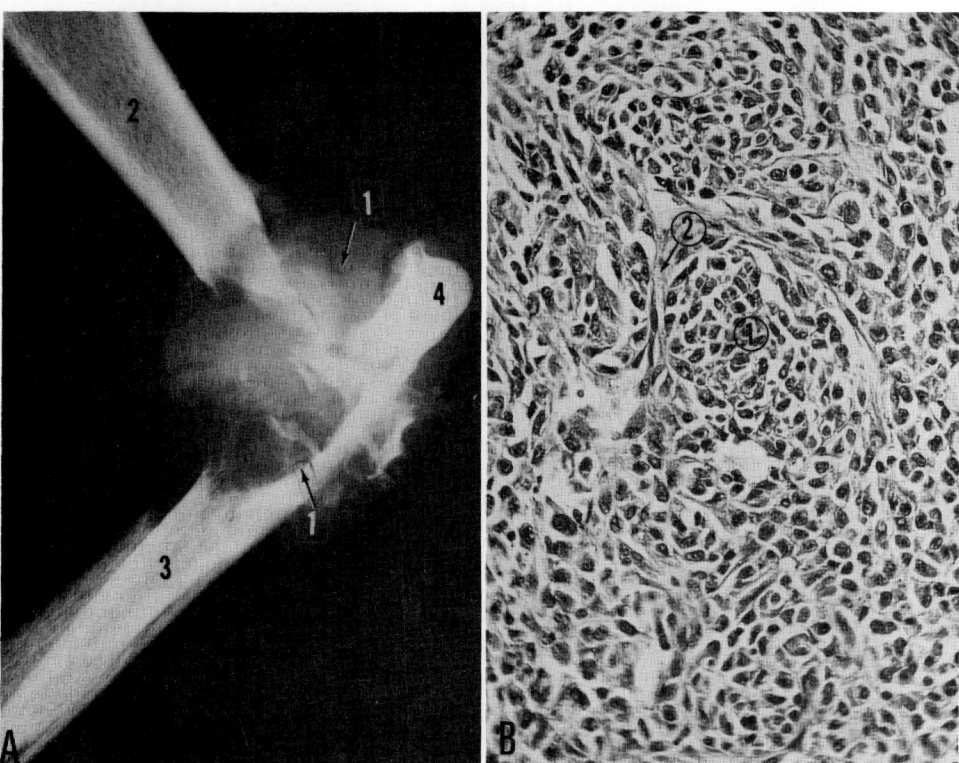

FIG. 19-34 Synovial sarcoma involving elbow joint, humerus, radius, and ulna of an 11-year-old female spitz dog. **A.** (1) Radiograph of the tumor, which replaces the joint and destroys (2) the distal part of the humerus, (3) proximal part of the radius, and (not shown) ulna. (4) The olecranon is partially invaded. **B.** Photomicrograph (×330) of (1) the highly cellular neoplasm with (2) indistinct stroma. (Courtesy of Armed Forces Institute of Pathology; contributor: Dr. Leo L. Lieberman.)

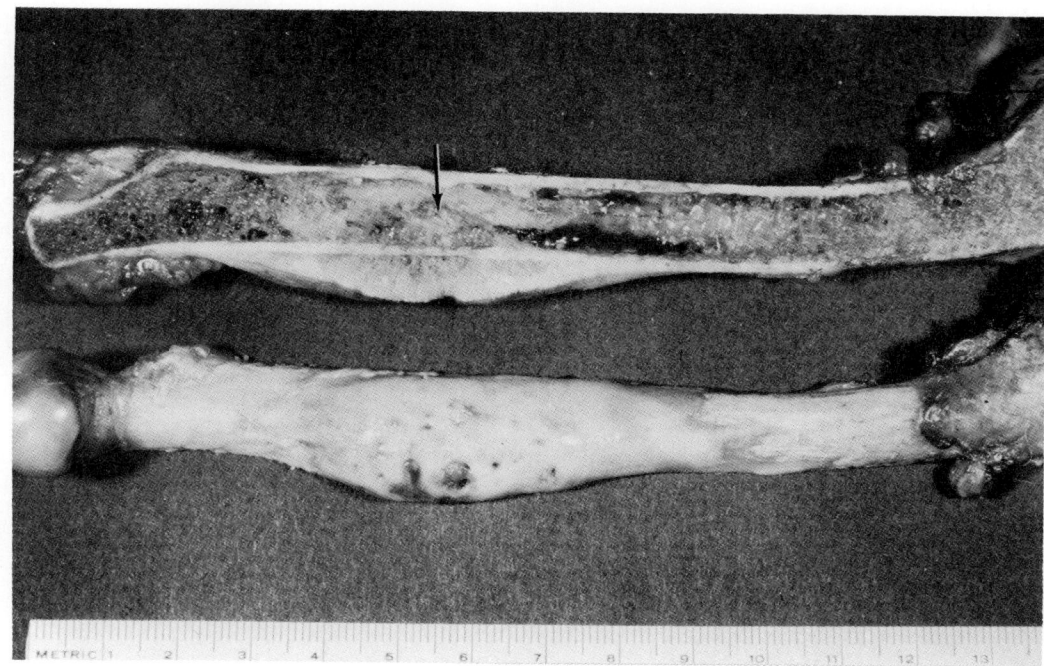

FIG. 19-35 Secondary, metastatic neoplasm in femur of a 12-year-old spayed female kerry blue terrier. The primary was a bronchiolar/alveolar cell carcinoma of the lung. (Courtesy of Angell Memorial Animal Hospital.)

Fibrous histiocytoma A dual histiocytic-fibrocytic tumor is rare; however, when seen it is a multilobular mass that encircles and invades bone and surrounding soft tissue. The tumor consists of pleomorphic polygonal mononuclear and pleomorphic spindle cells in various amounts of collagenous stroma. Tumors are often intermixed with bizarre giant cells, and frequently have a storiform pattern. Currently, some confusion still exists concerning differentiation of this lesion from true giant-cell tumor (osteoclastoma) of bone. Cloning of tumor cells establishes a cell line that resembles dermal fibroblasts and produces type I collagen; however, in contrast with true giant-cell tumors, the cloned cells do not react positively with antibodies to leukocyte common antigen. Inoculation of the cloned tumor cells produce tumors with the histology of fibrous histiocytoma and induce prominent macrophage infiltration.

Synovial sarcoma Locally destructive and metastasizing tumors infrequently arise from the synovial membrane of a joint (Fig. 19-34), and less commonly from tendons or synovial sheaths. Synovial sarcomas are rare in dogs and cats, and occur less frequently in cattle and horses. Tumors cause lameness, and a painless palpable mass is found on a major weight-bearing joint. The tumor growth may be slow at first and then accelerate; metastasis is rare. A radiolucent mass usually invades and replaces bone on both sides of an articulation. Actually, when the tumor encroaches on the bone end, it causes no direct damage to the articular cartilage; it erodes the articular margin, infiltrates at the joint cartilage infiltration line, or enters the epiphysis via the connective tissue of the epiphyseal vessels. The tumor is made up of a biphasic population of cells composed of varying proportions of two intermingled cellular elements of epithelioid and fibroblastic populations. Using immunohistochemical techniques, cells within synovial cell sarcomas again show a biphasic pattern, with spindle cells containing vimentin-positive, intermediate filaments and cytokeratin or desmoplakin staining of epithelial-type cells. Although these characteristics are considered typical diagnostic features, areas with clefts and tubular spaces lined by epithelioid cells are rare in most canine synovial sarcomas. More typical are solid masses of cells with round to ovoid nuclei and irregularly stellate cytoplasm. Giant cells may be a variable component.

Secondary tumors of bone Malignant neoplasms may metastasize to bone from primary sites in mammary gland, lung, oral mucosa, skin, subcutis, thyroid, and bone (Fig. 19-35). The clinical manifestations of secondary tumors in bone include lameness, pain, swelling, and less frequently, paraplegia. The radiographic appearance is often indistinguishable from a primary tumor. For example, secondary (metastatic) tumors may localize near the epiphysis, expand extensively, and be radiolucent. Sometimes they may contain spicules of bone. Definitive diagnosis is based upon identification of the tissue in histologic sections.

Some neoplasms, arising adjacent to bone, may either invade the bone or alter it by compression. Squamous cell carcinomas arising in the oral or pharyngeal mucosa may invade the mandible or maxilla, although their usual route is to the lymph nodes and then to lungs. Rhabdomyosarcoma and malignant fibrous histiocytoma are also reported to invade bone. Neoplasms of hemopoietic cells may originate in and displace the bone marrow. Lymphosarcoma and reticulum cell sarcoma (histiocytic lymphoma) tend to replace bone marrow and may cause bone infarction. Plasma cell tumors may occur as a solitary lesion with expansion of the medullary cavity, destruction of the cortex, and extension of the neoplasm into adjacent tissue. Alternatively, plasma-cell tumors may take the form of multiple myeloma, forming multicentric lytic lesions that have a characteristic radiographic appearance of a "punched-out" lesion without a sclerotic margin.

References

Brodey RS, Reid CF, Sauer RM. Metastatic bone neoplasms in the dog. J Am Vet Med Assoc 1966;148:29–43.

Liu SK, Dorfman HD, Patnaik AK. Primary and secondary bone tumors in the cat. J Small Anim Pract 1974;15:141–156.

Sullivan DJ. Cartilaginous tumors (chondroma and chondrosarcoma) in animals. Am J Vet Res 1960;21:531–535.

20

The respiratory system

The principal function of this system is the intake of oxygen and the elimination of carbon dioxide and other gases in the process of respiration. Some other functions are closely related: the olfactory system is closely housed and accompanies the inhalation of air. In some species, exchange of air is important in body cooling; some noxious gases are partially neutralized by the upper respiratory tract and some dusts are cleansed from inspired air. The specialized functions of the respiratory tract are made possible by the presence of specific types of cells which line that tract. The tissues made up of these specialized cells also have characteristic influences on the type of pathologic changes that occur in the respiratory tract.

Respiratory failure is serious—if not reversed promptly, it soon leads to death. Several conditions that have significant effects on the respiratory system are discussed in earlier chapters of this text. These include disturbances of circulation (Chapter 6), viral infections (Chapter 8), mycoplasmal and similar infections (Chapter 9), bacterial infections (Chapter 10), fungal infections (Chapter 11), protozoal diseases (Chapter 12), parasitic helminths and arthropods (Chapter 13), and extraneous poisons (Chapter 15).

Pathogenetic mechanisms will be discussed in those situations in which they are reasonably well-established; lesions and diagnostic criteria will be described in as succinct a manner as possible. Anatomic and species differences will be referred to in those conditions in which they are significant factors.

Upper Air Passages

The mucous membrane of the nares, paranasal sinuses, pharynx, larynx, trachea, and bronchi is subject to injury by chemical and infectious agents brought to it in the inspired air. Chemical injury is infrequent, being due to accidental inhalation of such gases as ammonia and chlorine, as well as war gases; injury by infectious microorganisms, including viruses, is frequent and often severe. As might be expected, the more external of the respiratory passages are more accessible to such injurious agents; the deeper structures, such as the bronchi, are less often attacked, but the effects of infections

here are most severe and more ominous than in the upper part of the respiratory tract. It is possible, however, for these mucous membranes to be attacked via the hematogenous route by infections or toxins which have an affinity for them. For instance, when material containing the virus of bovine malignant catarrhal fever is injected subcutaneously, the respiratory mucous membranes become the principal seat of disease just as if the infection had gained primary access to them.

The mucous membranes which line the upper nasal passages are made up of several types of epithelium: squamous at and near the external nares, then transitional, and respiratory in type. Olfactory epithelium is found particularly in the ethmoid region. Specialized epithelium makes up the vomeronasal organ. The epithelium covers extensive surface areas due to the tortuous projections of the turbinates into the nasal cavity. The anatomic and histologic features of the upper air passages vary greatly, depending on the species involved. Study of the pathologic responses of the system requires careful analysis of the anatomic and histologic features in the animal species involved. This is especially true in situations involving the experimental effects of toxicologic or infectious agents on the respiratory system.

References

Harkema JR, Morgan KT. Normal morphology of the nasal passages in laboratory rodents. In: Jones TC, Dungworth DL, Mohr U, eds. Monographs on pathology of laboratory animals, respiratory system. 2nd ed. New York: Springer Berlin Heidelberg, 1995;3–17.
Renne RA, Miller RA. Microscopic anatomy of toxicologically important regions of the larynx of the rat, mouse, and hamster. In: Jones TC, Dungworth DL, Mohr U, eds. Monograph on pathology of laboratory animals, respiratory system. 2nd ed. New York: Springer Berlin Heidelberg 1995;43–50.

Inflammations

Rhinitis (inflammation of the nasal mucosa), **sinusitis, pharyngitis, laryngitis, tracheitis,** and **bronchitis** usually commence as acute mucous (catarrhal) inflammations of the respective mucous membranes. They somewhat later tend to become purulent or fibrinous, depending on the nature of the agent, and fulfill the descriptions

TABLE 20-1 **Some causes of rhinitis**

Organisms	Affected Species	Reference
Viruses		
Canine Distemper virus	canine	Chapter 8
Equine herpes virus 1	equine	Chapter 8
Infectious bovine rhino-tracheitis virus	bovine	Chapter 8
Feline viral rhinotracheitis	feline	Chapter 8
Bovine malignant catarrh	bovine	Chapter 8
Inclusion body rhiniits	swine	Chapter 8
Bacteria		
Streptococcus equi	eqine	Chapter 10
Brucella bronchiseptica	canine	Chapter 10
Pasteurella multocida	rabbit	Chapter 10
Fungi		
Cryptococcus neoformans	feline	Chapter 11
Helminths and arthropods		
Oestrus ovis	ovine	Chapter 13

already given in the general study of inflammation. In most cases the infectious process, like the human "cold," starts as a rhinitis, and the extent to which it spreads into the lower air passages depends upon its virulence and the susceptibility of the patient. Some of them reach the lung parenchyma itself, causing pneumonia. Some of the causative factors of rhinitis are listed in Table 20-1.

Frontal sinusitis occurs in cattle from infection of the wound produced by dehorning. Extension of infection to the cranial cavity is similarly possible. Maxillary sinusitis, especially in the horse, results from disease of the molar teeth and the walls of the dental alveoli, which are surprisingly thin.

Infectious inflammations of the nasopharynx occasionally spread up the mucosa of one or both eustachian tubes in humans, more or less completely closing the lumen by the swelling produced, and in some cases spreading into the middle ear to produce **otitis media.** Called eustachitis, the condition may occur in domestic animals but, since the symptoms are chiefly subjective (interference with hearing, etc.), it is seldom diagnosed in veterinary practice.

In the horse, **catarrh of the guttural pouches** occurs as a continuation of a similar eustachitis. The pouches are filled and often distended with exudate, which is most often mucopurulent and tenacious. Since swelling of the tube, as well as its position, interferes with drainage, the catarrh is likely to become chronic, and the desiccated exudate may develop into caseous or even more solid concrements. **Tympanites of the guttural pouches** occurs as a bulging pneumatic swelling, usually bilateral, apparently related to the head being held downward, as in grazing. The more or less swollen tube

appears to have a valve-like action permitting air to be pumped in but not expelled as the animal chews. This is comparable to the development of subcutaneous emphysema from a wound in the axillary region. A similar meteorism of the guttural pouches is said to exist as the result of their distension by gases derived from putrefaction of the exudate in chronic catarrh, mentioned previously.

Arthropod and helminthic parasites

In sheep, the larvae of the **bot-fly,** *Oestrus ovis,* some 2 cm long when fully grown, migrate up the nares, usually into the frontal sinus, sometimes into the recesses of the turbinate bones. They cause the formation of a tenacious mucopurulent exudate, in which they are more or less buried. Naturally such a sinusitis is the cause of much suffering and interference with the general health. It is occasionally fatal by extension to the cranial cavity via the ethmoid. *Linguatula serrata* is a parasite which infects the nasal passages of dogs and, rarely, other species. Also in dogs, the paranasal sinuses and nasal passages may be infested with the mite *Pneumonyssus caninum.*

The nasal passages of Old World nonhuman primates as well as humans are occasionally infested with the nematodes *Anatrichosoma cutaneum* and *A. cynomolgi.* Two new species of *Anatrichosoma, A. rhina* and *A. nacepobi,* have been described from the nasal mucosa of Rhesus monkeys *(Macaca mulatta)* (Conrad and Wong, 1973). The anatrichosomes are somewhat rare and incompletely understood trichuroid worms, which are found in nasal passages of many Asian and African monkeys. The adult, egg-laying females inhabit the upper nasal passages and burrow into the squamous epithelium, which becomes hyperplastic. Their eggs reach the surface of the epithelium through tunnels and can be demonstrated by swab collection and microscopic examination. Mites identified as *Rhinophagus papionis* have been identified in the nasal fossae of the baboon *(Papio spp.).*

Leeches are distributed worldwide and may become parasitic on humans, domestic animals, or nonhuman primates that come in contact with them in their water habitat. They are most common in Sri Lanka, Thailand, Taiwan, India, Burma, and China. *Dinobdella ferox* is reported from nasal cavities of domestic cattle, buffalo, yak, deer, dogs, and monkeys *(Macaca mulatta* and *M. cyclopis).* This leech has a dorso-ventrally flattened body, blackish-brown in color, and varies in length from 35 to 60 mm. An anterior sucker is somewhat smaller than the posterior sucker. Their life cycle is direct, but apparently they do not reproduce during their sojourn in the nasal cavity. They can induce inflammation and impede breathing, as well as suck blood from their hosts.

Amyloidosis

Nodular amyloidosis of the nasal mucosa is occasionally seen in horses, albeit rarely. The amyloid is deposited surrounding blood vessels and glands and within the connective tissue. The cause is not known, but it is not associated with generalized amyloidosis.

Air sacs

Air sacs are mucosa-lined diverticula from the larynx or trachea occurring in several species of nonhuman primates including orangutan *(Pongo pygmaeus),* howler monkey *(Alouatta),* baboon *(Papio),* macaques *(Macaca),* and gibbons *(Hylobates),* as well as others. These air sacs may become infected, usually with several species of bacteria and lead to septicemia or aspiration pneumonia.

Nasal polyps

Nasal polyps (polypi) are inflammatory new growths which resemble true neoplasms. They are often pedunculated or elongated so that a single polypus fills most of the nasal lumen in which it lies. They are smoothly covered with mucous membrane. The inner tissue is fibrous and myxomatous with a generous infiltration of leukocytes, chiefly neutrophilic granulocytes and lymphocytes, the presence of which does not depend on any ulceration of the surface. These, together with numerous capillaries, suffice to indicate an inflammatory pathogenesis which puts polypi in the same category as the granulation tissue of wound healing, although the exact etiology is often not discernible. They have to be differentiated from nasal granuloma of bovines, rhinosporidiosis, granulomatous growths caused by the blood fluke, *Schistosoma nasalis* (at least in India), and by the larvae of the equine stomach worm, *Habronema sp.,* and probably by other occasional parasites, as well as true neoplasms, which are encountered rarely. In horses, nasal inflammatory polyps may be a source of hemorrhage. Feline nasal polyps are occasionally attached to similar inflammatory polyps which extend into the external auditory meatus (Fig. 20-1).

Epistaxis

Epistaxis, or **nosebleed,** occurs infrequently in domestic animals. If not caused by some trauma such as a heavy blow or the passing of a stomach tube, it is likely to be an indication of an ulcerative infection or neoplasm, a hemangioma (rare), or possibly a fractured bone which has lacerated a blood vessel in the region.

A study of epistaxis in horses indicates that the site of the hemorrhage depends to some extent upon the occupation of the horse. About 28% of 174 cases were bilateral and occurred in racehorses following competitive exercise, and the source was considered to be the lungs. Spontaneous hemorrhage appearing while the horse was at rest was usually unilateral and originated in the nasal cavity (10%) following viral infection or in the paranasal sinuses and labyrinth of the ethmoid (27%) due to hematoma (which may be bilateral) in the ethmoid region. Auditory tube diverticulum was the site of 34% of the hemorrhages, which were usually unilateral and due to erosion of blood vessels.

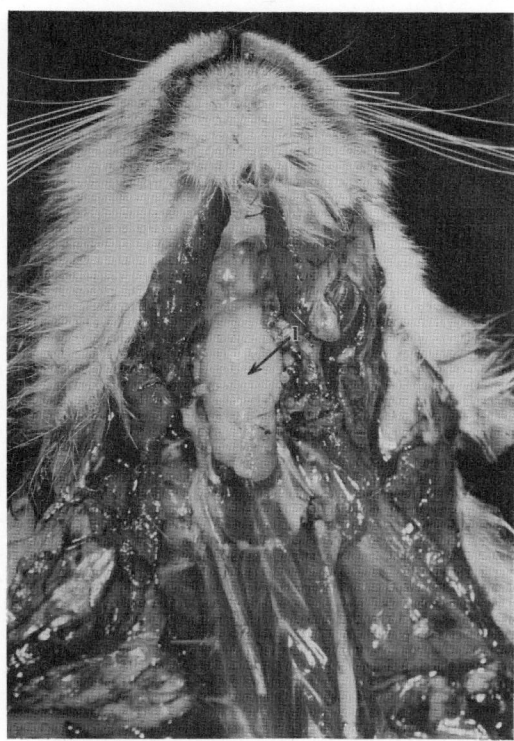

FIG. 20-1 A nasal polyp *(1)* extending from the nasopharynx of a nine-year-old female cat. A similar fibrinous, inflammatory mass extended through the eustachian tube and connected with another in the external auditory canal. (Courtesy of Angell Memorial Animal Hospital.)

"Exercise-induced pulmonary hemorrhage" in horses has been demonstrated to occur as an entity in thoroughbred and standardbred horses as well as in mixed breed animals used in polo or other competitive athletic events. The hemorrhage clearly comes from the lung, as detected by the use of a flexible fiberoptic endoscope, and is a frequent event following exercise. The precise cause of the hemorrhage at this writing is unknown.

References
Cook WR. Epistaxis in the racehorse. Equine Vet J 1974;6:45–48.
Pascoe JR, Ferraro GL, Cannon JH, et al. Exercise-induced pulmonary hemorrhage in racing thoroughbreds: A preliminary study. Am J Vet Res 1981;42:703–707.
Voynick BT, Sweeney CR. Exercise-induced pulmonary hemorrhage in polo and racing horses. J Am Vet Med Assoc 1986;188:301–302.

Laryngeal hemiplegia

Normally at each inspiration the arytenoid cartilages of the larynx are drawn outward by their muscles, as two double doors might be swung open, to admit air. In this disease of the horse there is a paralysis, usually partial, of one of the muscles of arytenoid cartilages which leaves it vapid in the rushing air currents. Commonly, the muscles have enough strength to hold it open during ordinary breathing, but not during the more violent respiration which goes with vigorous exercise, when the air current draws the flap of tissue into midstream. The result is that at each inspiration this fluttering obstruction not only limits the amount of air which can reach the lungs, but also sets up a considerable sound, which is responsible for the disease being called roaring.

The affected crico-arytenoideus muscle undergoes atrophy of many of its fibers, which progresses until they disappear completely, with replacement by fibrous tissue. Grossly the degenerated muscle is said to look like fish flesh. Successive stages of demyelinization and wallerian degeneration may be seen in the recurrent laryngeal nerve supplying the muscle.

It is almost always the left arytenoid cartilage, crico-arytenoideus muscle, and recurrent laryngeal nerve which are involved in this disorder. This is believed to be because of the unique course of the left nerve around the arch of the aorta and along the deep face of that vessel. Causes of certain infrequent cases which may be on either side include pressure by enlarged granulomatous lymph nodes, tumors, abscesses, aneurysms, and esophageal swelling. Congenital defects have been suspected. Many cases follow pneumonia.

References

Mason BJE. Laryngeal hemiplegia: a further look at Haslam's anomaly of the left recurrent nerve. Equine Vet J 1973;5:150–155.

Neumann-Kleinpaul K, Tabbert B. Zur aetiologie und pathologie der recurrenslahmung des pferdes. Arch Tierheilk. 1936;70:413–416.

Rooney JR, Delaney FM. An hypothesis on the causation of laryngeal hemiplegia in horses. Equine Vet J 1970;2:35–39.

Pharyngeal diverticulitis

In the pig, the diverticulum pharyngeum lies just dorsal to the origin of the esophagus. It is rather frequently the site of lodgement of capsules incorrectly administered for the treatment of intestinal helminthiasis or other diseases. Depending on the nature of the contained medicaments, severe inflammation or fatal gangrene may result from release of the drug in the diverticulum. Prosectors must not overlook a lesion of this kind.

Porcine atrophic rhinitis

This insidious disease of swine was first recognized in North America about 1940, although what was probably the same disease attracted attention in Northern Europe early in the nineteenth century. Commencing in young pigs with slight catarrh, nasal irritation, and sneezing, the disease progresses slowly over many months, with increasing dyspnea and anorexia and eventual death from inanition (Fig. 20-2).

The earliest lesions usually described are small, depressed, and congested foci on the mucosa of the turbinate bones. Erosion and disappearance of the mucous membrane follow and are accompanied by a heavy infiltration of inflammatory cells, chiefly lymphocytes and monocytes. Areas of the turbinate bones begin to soften, grossly. Microscopically, this appears first as a rarefaction and fading of the bony tissue. As destruction of the bone continues, large numbers of fibroblastic cells proliferate in the periosteal region. These are interpreted as osteoblasts, but no new bone is formed. Osteoblasts are never numerous. Bone resorption is believed to result from osteolysis. The turbinate bones disappear in 2 to 4 weeks following apparent experimental inoculation, leaving only a dense, fibrous band to mark their place of attachment. A tenacious mucopurulent exudate clings in the recesses of the turbinates as long as they remain, and in the cells of the ethmoid. Late in the course of the disease, the nasal septum likewise disappears, a process requiring some months. Growth of the snout is retarded so that its dorsal aspect becomes short and concave. Often the interference with growth is greater on one side than on the other, so that the snout curves slightly toward the most severely affected side. In the nasal passages of some advanced cases, little remains but the inflamed walls of the passages, bearing perhaps a coating of dried and clotted blood. In other cases, the nares are more or less plugged by solidified and inspissated exudate and dead tissue. In spite of the slow progress and rather low virulence of the disease, it does not appear that recovery ever occurs.

ETIOLOGY

The evidence for several years has indicated that a causative organism is *Bordetella bronchiseptica*. It now appears that another bacterium, *Pasteurella multocida*, may also inhabit the porcine nasal passages where it produces a dermonecrotic toxin. Presence of the organism or its toxin is associated with the lesions of Atrophic Rhinitis. Both organisms appear to produce a similar toxin and together cause the most severe disease. This toxin, when injected intramuscularly, has a deleterious effect upon the osteoblasts of turbinate bone.

References

Dominick MA, Rimler RB. Turbinate osteoporosis in pigs following intranasal innoculation of purified *Pasteurella* toxin: Histomorphometric and ultrastructural studies. Vet Pathol 1988;25:17–27.

Elling F, Pedersen KB. The pathogenesis of persistent turbinate atrophy induced by toxigenic *Pasteurella multocida* in pigs. Vet Pathol 1985;22:469–474.

Gois M, Barnes HJ, Ross RF. Potentiation of turbinate atrophy in pigs by long-term nasal colonization with *Pasteurella multocida*. Am J Vet Res 1983;44:372–378.

Kamp EM, Kimman TG. Induction of nasal turbinate atrophy in germ-free pigs, using *Pasteurella multocida* as well as bacterium-free crude and purified dermonecrotic toxin of *P. multocida*. Am J Vet Res 1988;49:1844–1849.

Nakai T, Sawata A, Kume K. Intracellular locations of dermonecrotic toxins in *Pasteurella multocida* and in *Bordetella bronchiseptica*. Am J Vet Res 1985;46:870–874.

Bovine nasal granuloma

Granulomatous inflammation in the mucosa of the bovine nasal cavity is not infrequent and appears to be due to at least four causes. In the United States, a form due to **mycotic** infection has been described. The iden-

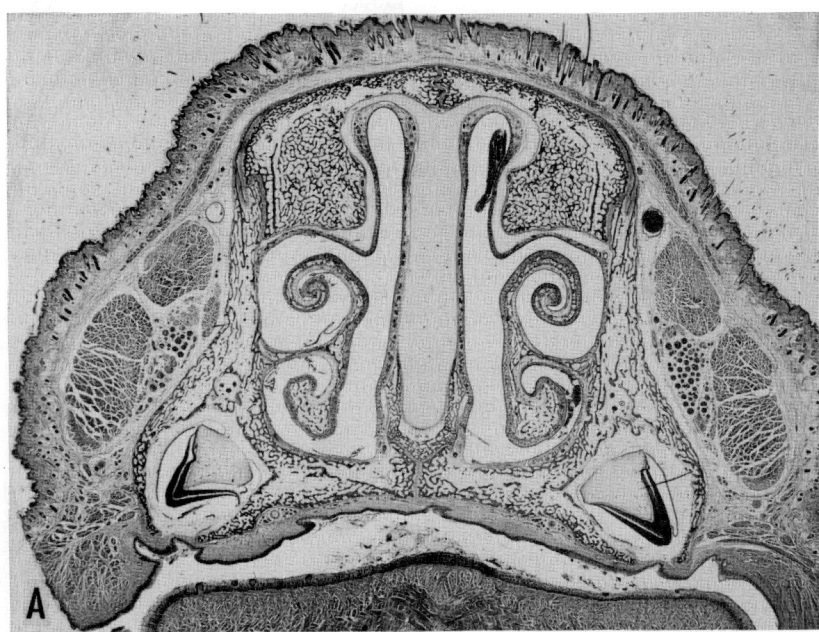

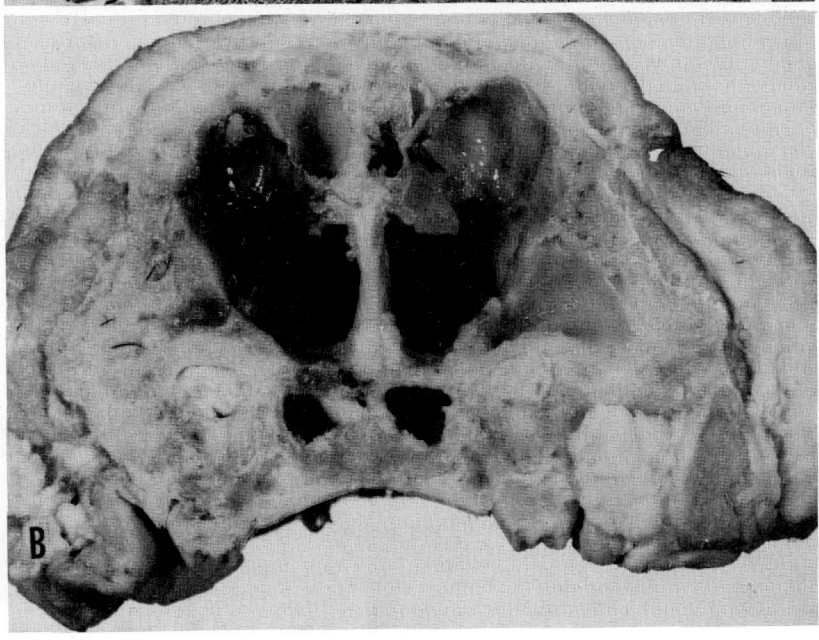

FIG. 20-2 Porcine atrophic rhinitis. **A.** Stained section through nose of a normal pig (×4). (Courtesy of Armed Forces Institute of Pathology.) Contributor: Lt. Col. T.C. Jones. **B.** Transverse section (gross specimen) through the nose of a pig with atrophic rhinitis. Except for part of the ethmoids, all the turbinates have been destroyed. (Courtesy of Armed Forces Institute of Pathology.) Contributor: Dr. C.L. Davis.

tity of the fungus seen in tissue sections has not been established.

In India, a type of granulomatous reaction in the nasal mucosa has been ascribed to a blood fluke, *Schistosoma nasalis.*

Actinobacillosis may also occur in the bovine nasal cavity, tiny abscesses in the nasal mucosa simulating some of the clinical features and gross lesions.

A fourth type of nasal granuloma (also called atopic or allergic rhinitis or chronic granular rhinitis) has been described in Australia, New Zealand, and, more recently, in the United States. The usual course starts with gradual onset over a period of weeks with a nasal discharge, at first mucous, then mucopurulent. Nasal pruritis is evident from the earliest stages. Exacerbation of

the signs is observed in the summer months, remission in the winter. The anterior third of the nasal mucosa becomes elevated by tiny nodules which give it a roughened "cobblestone" appearance.

The histologic features of the involved nasal mucosa are characteristic. The mucosa is altered by many closely-packed tiny polyps covered by acanthotic squamous epithelium projecting into the lumen. The underlying lamina propria is edematous, filled with capillaries, fibroblasts, eosinophils, mast cells, "globule cells", and plasma cells. The necks of the ducts of mucous glands are also made up of metaplastic pseudostratified columnar epithelium, and goblet cells are conspicuous, but deeper structures are not affected. Epithelioid macrophages of typical granulomas are not a feature of this lesion.

The evidence points toward this disease being caused by episodic type I hypersensitivity reaction to unidentified antigens. The granulation tissue is identifiable with type III hypersensitivity. Specific allergens responsible for this disease have not, at this time, been identified but affected cows are definitely hypersensitive to many antigens. These include a large number of plant pollens, tree pollens, fungi, and miscellaneous items such as mites. In one experiment, nasal lesions have been associated with induced hypersensitivity to hen egg albumin.

References

Carbonell PL. Bovine nasal granuloma. Gross and microscopic lesions. Vet Pathol 1979;16:60–73.

Krahwinkel DJ, Schmeitzel LP, Fadok VA, et al. Familial allergic rhinitis in cattle. J Am Vet Med Assoc 1979;192:1593–1596.

Congenital anomalies

Congenital malformations that involve the respiratory system are usually secondary. For example, malformations of the head and face (cyclopia, anencephalia, campylognathia, cebocephalus, among others) result in anomalies of the upper respiratory tract. Lesions in the thorax such as diaphragmatic hernia, occurring during gestation, lead to hypoplasia or atelectasis of the lung. Intrauterine poisoning of lambs due to *Veratrum californicum* is one of the serious causes of congenital malformations of the respiratory tract. In most instances, however, the cause is unknown, although hereditary factors have been identified in some types of malformations.

References

Dennis SM. Congenital respiratory tract defects in lambs. Aust Vet J 1975;51:347–350.

Heider L, et al. Nasolacrimal duct anomaly in calves. J Am Vet Med Assoc 1975;167:145–147.

Huston R, Saperstein G, Schoneweis D, et al. Congenital defects in pigs. Vet Bull 1978;48:645–675.

Thomson FG. Congenital bronchial hypoplasia of calves. Pathol Vet, 1966;3:89–109.

NEOPLASMS

Nasal passages and paranasal sinuses

Neoplasms of the upper respiratory tract are not frequent in animals but, if one considers all species of mammals and the literature, it appears that essentially every tissue type in these structures can give rise to a neoplasm. As newer methods are applied, the cell of origin of each neoplasm may be identified. This development makes the nomenclature even more complex and sometimes confusing, as new terminology may be applied prematurely before all the variables have been adequately studied. The authors prefer to name neoplasms according to the tissue or cell type of origin and degree of malignancy.

Adenocarcinoma is the most frequent neoplasm recognized as arising from the nasal or sinus epithelium. It is made up of columnar or cuboidal cells with the usual haphazard arrangement, zones of necrosis and hemorrhage and invasion of adjacent tissues. Acinar and papillary arrangements of the tumor cells may be recognized. Mitoses are usually numerous.

Neoplasms arising from olfactory epithelial cells usually are located in the dorsal nasal cavity and tend to invade the cribiform plate and the anterior lobes of the cerebrum. Many names have been applied to the tumors, the most common is **Neuroepithelial carcinoma of olfactory epithelium.** The tumor cells are pleomorphic but resemble the olfactory epithelium, with haphazard arrangement but often forming sheets of columnar cells and rosettes. The cells may resemble the basal cells of olfactory epithelium, adenosquamous sustentacular cells, or neuroblasts. These neoplasms may be encountered in the course of toxicologic studies with laboratory rats, particularly when nasal carcinogens are used.

In sheep and cattle a neoplastic disease arises in the olfactory mucosa and, from epizootiologic evidence, it is believed to be infectious. The lesion has been called **adinopapilloma, adenocarcinoma, ethmoid carcinoma** and other names. Viral particles have been seen with the electron microscope in tumor tissues and some evidence indicates that a retrovirus, such as the one involved in maedi/visna, might be the causative factor.

Squamous cell carcinoma is one of the more frequent neoplasms of the upper respiratory tract. It is most apt to arise in the nasal tract near to the external nares. An almost indistinguishable tumor may originate from oral mucosa around a tooth and invade the nasal structures, presenting a diagnostic problem involving its origin. In either case, the soft and bony tissues of the head may be extensively invaded and metastases to the regional lymphnodes should be expected.

Of interest is the spontaneous occurrence of hyperplasias and tumors of **neuroendocrine** cells in the larynx and trachea of the Syrian hamster (*Mesocricetus auratus*). These lesions are found in or beneath the epithelium lining the trachea or larynx. The frank tumors have been identified by various names: **carcinoid, clear cell carcinoma, carcinoid tumor, tumorlet, and neuroendocrine carcinoma.** The tumors start as small nests of cells with clear cytoplasm and spherical, hyperchromic nuclei, that grow and expand until much of the tracheal lumen is occluded. These cells may be further identified by their intense immunoreactivity for calcitonin, calcitonin gene-related peptide (CGRP), serotonin, neuron-specific enolase and synaptophysin.

Chondrosarcoma may arise from the nasal septum and is made up of solid masses of undifferentiated cartilage cells which produce immature cartilage.

Mucoepidermoid carcinoma, consisting of squamous cell elements and glandular cells with mucous secretion, are occasionally encountered. Other tumors (fibrosarcoma, adenoma, mast cell tumor, fibropapilloma, lymphosarcoma, hemangioma, sarcoma, and osteosarcoma) are much less frequent and are described in the chapters concerned with the system from which they most often arise.

THE TRACHEA AND BRONCHI

Lining cells of trachea, bronchi and bronchioles

The nasal epithelium nearest the nares is lined by stratified squamous epithelium, which toward the pharynx becomes typical pseudostratified respiratory epithelium. This type of epithelium extends to the origin of the bronchiole, where it becomes simple columnar. Nine types of epithelial cells have been identified in the tracheobronchial epithelium: ciliated, goblet, epithelial serous, brush, basal, intermediate, Kultschitzky-like (K type), special type, and Clara cells. One important function of the tracheobronchial epithelium is the production of mucus. This is accomplished by the epithelial serous cells, goblet cells, and mucous glands in the lamina propria, which are lined by serous and mucous cells and communicate with the lumen.

References

Plopper CG, Pinkerton KE. Overview of diversity in the respiratory system of mammals. In: Parent RA, ed. Comparative biology of the normal lung. Boca Raton, FL: CRC Press, 1992;3–5.
Parent RA. ed. Comparative biology of the normal lung. Boca Raton, FL: CRC Press, 1992;1–830

Bronchiectasis

This is a dilation of one or more bronchi. During violent or forced respiration, the bronchi and bronchioles dilate to full capacity and become round in cross section, but at other times all but the largest bronchi are contracted by their encircling musculature so that the mucosa is thrown into folds. In cross sections, these folds give the smaller and medium bronchi a star-like appearance. In bronchiectasis, they are dilated and the folds are stretched out to a full circle, a position which persists after death. This inelasticity and failure to return to the normal contracted state are due to small amounts of fibrous tissue in and around the bronchial wall, which has proliferated as the result of chronic inflammation. Commonly, a number of leukocytes and reticulo-endothelial cells are still visible in the peribronchial zone. The scar tissue also acts to keep the lumen distended by fixing the wall to surrounding structures. Bronchiectasis is thus an indication of a present or previous inflammation. The peribronchial tissue commonly shares in the inelasticity, so that the ability of the lung to collapse is impaired, and its functional efficiency diminished. Continued irritation results from these structural derangements, as is generally evidenced by catarrhal exudation and cough. This exudative state may be enhanced by continuing or recurrent infections of low virulence. Owing to chronic irritation, squamous metaplasia of the bronchial epithelium is a frequent finding. A striking example of bronchiectasis is a consistent feature of chronic murine (mycoplasmal) pneumonia. A specific type of bronchiectasis has been described in yearling feedlot cattle. This lesion is limited to single lobules, but involves all of the bronchial branches in the lobule. This lesion was encountered in 32 (1.6%) of 1988 necropsies of yearling cattle. Many bacterial organisms (*Pasteurella haemolytica, P. multocida, Corynebacterium pyogenes, Escherichia coli, Salmonella anatum, Staphylococcus spp.*) and one mycoplasma (*Mycoplasma arginini*) were isolated from these bronchi. The pathogenetic mechanisms remain obscure.

Bronchitis

Bronchitis has been mentioned in common with the upper respiratory diseases. It is most often an extension of one of these infections, but may rarely represent an extension of a pneumonic process which originated in the pulmonary parenchyma. The mild or early forms are characterized by catarrhal inflammation; later the exudate usually becomes fibrinous or purulent. The virulence and the importance of an upper respiratory infection can usually be gauged by how far it extends from the nares toward the lungs, bronchitis being the most formidable of the subpneumonic infections.

Canine tracheobronchitis or "kennel cough" is a clinical designation for a disease characterized by intermittent coughing. Although clinically the disease may appear as a single entity, there is little reason to consider it a specific disease with a single cause, anymore so than the human cold. Various viruses, including adenoviruses, influenza viruses, and herpes viruses have been reported to induce tracheobronchitis in dogs, but their respective roles in the natural disease are not established. There are few reports describing the gross or histopathologic features as the disease is not fatal. Inclusion bodies in tracheal and bronchial epithelium, similar to those produced by adenoviruses and herpes viruses, are occasionally encountered in dogs with a history of coughing.

Chronic bronchitis has been described in dogs, particularly from Great Britain, manifested particularly by a cough which persists for months to years. The findings at postmortem examination consist of mucous plugs in the tracheobronchial tree, thickened and hyperemic bronchial mucosae, occasional polypoid lesions in mucosa, and often moderately extensive subpleural emphysema. Microscopically, mucous exudate may be seen in the lumen of bronchioles, goblet cells are increased in number, and the lamina propria is infiltrated with inflammatory cells (lymphocytes and plasma cells). At severely affected sites, epithelial cells may lose cilia, undergo excessive proliferation or may be sloughed, leaving an ulcerated zone. Some degree of pneumonia may be associated with the bronchitis. The principal bacterial inhabitant appears to be *Bordetella bronchiseptica*.

A similar chronic bronchitis has been reproduced in Beagles by prolonged exposure to sulfur dioxide gas in closed chambers.

References

Adams LE, et al. An epizootic of respiratory tract disease in Sprague-Dawley rats. J Am Vet Med Assoc 1972;161:656–660.

Amis TC. Tracheal collapse in the dog. Aust Vet J 1974;50:285–289.

Bienenstock J, Johnston N, Perey DYE. Bronchial lymphoid tissue. I. Morphologic characteristics. Lab Invest 1973;28:686–692.

Bienenstock J, Johnston N, Perey DYE. Bronchial lymphoid tissue. II. Functional characteristics. Lab Invest 1973;28:693–698.

Booth BH, Talbot CH, Patterson R. Bronchial secretions in dogs with IgE mediated respiratory responses. Arch Allergy Appl Immunol 1971;40:639–642.

Breeze RG, Wheeldon EB, Pirie HM. Cell structure and function in the mammalian lung: the trachea, bronchi, and bronchioles. Vet Bull, 1976;46:319–337.

Chakrin LW, Saunders LZ. Experimental chronic bronchitis: pathology in the dog. Lab Invest, 1974;30:145–154.

Dill GS, Jr., Stookey JL, Whitney GD. Nodular amyloidosis in the trachea of a dog. Vet Pathol 1972;9:238–242.

Jensen R, et al. Bronchiectasis in yearling feedlot cattle. J Am Vet Med Assoc 1976;169:511–514.

Splitter GA, Butcher WI, Stevens MD. Tracheal basement membrane thickening in Rhesus monkeys. Vet Pathol 1974;11:278–288.

Wheeldon EB, Pirie HM, Fisher EW, et al. Chronic bronchitis in the dog. Vet Rec 1974;94:466–471.

Immotile cilia syndrome

This syndrome, first described in humans, more recently in dogs, involves chronic rhinitis and sinusitis, bronchiectasis and associated *situs inversus* of thoracic and abdominal viscera. It is also referred to as Kartagener's Triad or Syndrome in humans, a species in which immotile spermatozoa have also been described. The syndrome occurs infrequently in both sexes of several breeds of dogs and appears to be hereditary although the evidence for its inheritance is incomplete.

The basic lesion underlying the functional defect is demonstrable by electron microscopy in affected cilia and sperm tails. It has been postulated that ciliary immotility in the embryo affects embryo rotation to randomly result in *situs inversus* (transposition of abdominal and thoracic viscera from right to left). Electron microscopy reveals a transverse section of a single cilium to be circular, with an exterior wall surrounding several precisely arranged (doublet) tubules. A pair of single tubules is in the center of the cilium, nine of these microtubular doublets are arranged in a circle under the limiting membrane. Each of these doublets is connected to the adjacent ones by a pair of dynein arms. Lines drawn through the long axis of the central couplets in a large field of cilia will be parallel. Nexin links connect adjacent microtubules and radial spokes anchor the peripheral doublet pairs to a central sheath that surrounds the central doublet pair.

Studies of the ultrastructure of cilia of affected dogs reveal that not all cilia have detectable defects. Affected cilia may have varying numbers of peripheral doublets, dynein arms may be absent or reduced, or the configuration may be other than the 9 + 2 arrangement. Some cilia may have one or no central microtubles and some may be completely disorganized. Basal bodies (part of cilium below level of the cell membrane) may be unevenly spaced, and others contain a central plug of amorphous material, vesicles, or electron-dense material. The effect of this syndrome is to interfere with mucociliary clearance in the respiratory tract and lungs.

References

Afzelius BA, Carlsten J, Karlsson S. Clinical, pathologic, and ultrastructural features of *situs inversus* and immotile-cilia syndrome in a dog. J Am Vet Med Assoc 1984;184:560–563

Dhein CR, Prieur DJ, Riggs MW, et al. Suspected ciliary dysfunction in Chinese Shar Pei pups with pneumonia. Am J Vet Res 1990;51:439–446.

Edwards DF, Patton CS, Bemis DA, et al. Immotile ciliary syndrome in three dogs from a litter. J Am Vet Med Assoc 1983;183:667–672.

Morrison WB, Frank DE, Roth JA, et al. Assessment of neutrophil function in dogs with primary ciliary dyskinesia. J Am Vet Med Assoc 1987;191:425–430.

THE LUNG

The lung in all mammals has similar functions, but some differences in anatomy among various species affect the nature of pathologic lesions. The respiratory function, involving exchange of gases (particularly oxygen and carbon dioxide) between the bloodstream and the ambient air is preeminent, but the lung has other, nonrespiratory functions. These functions include self-cleansing mechanisms that deal with inadvertent intake of contaminated air, a water-drainage system that prevents flooding of the gas-exchanging surfaces, elaboration of essential biological products, such as surfactant, and other metabolic activities that keep the lungs continuously viable. The functions are influenced by autacoids (prostaglandins), catecholamines, and steroids.

The distribution and nature of pathologic lesions in the lung are influenced to some extent by anatomic features. A brief outline of some of the different infections among species is given in Table 20-1.

The alveolus

The terminal air saccule of the lung is shaped by a skeleton of connective tissue which contains a network of capillaries and is lined by an uninterrupted layer of cells, in turn covered by a film (surfactant) which separates them from the air. Three kinds of epithelial lining cells have been described.

The **type I pneumocyte** covers most of the alveolar surface. Its shape resembles that of a fried egg: the yolk corresponds to the nucleus and the peripheral egg white to the cytoplasm of the cell which extends around the alveolus into contact with other lining cells. Ribosomes are concentrated around the nucleus, but few organized structures occupy the thin part of the cell. The cell has sparse endoplasmic reticulum and a Golgi complex. Many vesicles occupy this type I cell, some contained entirely within the cell, others appearing to open to the surface. These vesicles serve to carry macromolecules across the epithelium between alveolar and interstitial spaces.

The **type II cell (granular pneumocyte or giant alveolar cell)** is interspersed among the type I cells and is apt to be located near the points where adjacent alveoli intersect. This cell is roughly cuboidal, is known to undergo rapid proliferation under some conditions, and is thought to be the progenitor of the type I cell. The cytoplasm contains numerous organelles, including cytosomes, mitochondria, and peroxisomes. The cytosomes are the most distinctive organelles, consisting of osmiophilic lamellae arranged in layers or whorls 0.2 to 1.0 μm in diameter. These lamellar bodies are the sites of storage and elaboration of surfactant.

Secretory activity is indicated by the presence of numerous mitochondria, a well-developed Golgi apparatus, and many multivesicular bodies. Histochemistry and cytochemistry studies have demonstrated the presence of many different enzymes, including hydrolases, esterases, catalase, and phosphatases. This is the cell that proliferates to give the alveolar lining its cuboidal appearance under many circumstances, a feature called by many names: "fetalization," "epithelialization," "adenomatosis," etc.

SURFACTANT

The surface of the alveoli of the lungs becomes covered in postnatal life by surface-active material generally referred to as surfactant. This material forms an insoluble film at the air-liquid interface of the alveolus, modifies surface tension depending on the alveolar surface area, and prevents atelectasis. As indicated, the source of this material is the type II pneumocyte. The cytoplasm of these cells contains membrane-bound inclusions which are ultrastructurally visible as laminated osmiophilic bodies. In fortuitous sections, these bodies may be seen open to the exterior and contributing their contents to the overlying surfactant layer.

The chemical content of surfactant at this writing is believed to consist of several fractions. The first consists of phosphatidylcholine, which contributes the unusual surface properties that lower the surface tension. A second component is phosphatidylglycerol, which is believed to give surfactant increased molecular mobility and increase its rate of adsorption to the alveolar interface. Other components consist of surfactant-associated apoproteins which are closely bound to the lipids.

Type II pneumocytes become able to produce and extrude surfactant at a critical time in late prenatal life. In the rabbit this time occurs within a 24-hour period at about the 29th day of pregnancy. The respiratory distress experienced by premature infants is believed to be for the most part due to the absence or incompetence of surfactant.

A **type III pneumocyte,** the "alveolar brush cell," has been described in rat lung, but at this writing its functions have not been uncovered.

ALVEOLAR MACROPHAGES

These cells, important to the defense functions of the lung, are derived from monocytes from the bone marrow that migrate through the alveolar wall to reach the lumen of the alveolus. They are active phagocytes and contain hydrolases, such as lysozyme, acid phosphatase, and cathepsin, which enable them to digest bacteria and neutralize other material. Lymphocytes and plasma cells are also present in small numbers in the alveolar wall and can increase greatly in numbers when the circumstances warrant.

MAST CELLS

The distribution of these important cells varies between species. Their functional components are contained in large metachromatic granules which contain heparin, lipids (slow-reacting substances of anaphylaxis), prostaglandins, amines (histamine and, in rat and mouse, serotonin), polypeptides (bradykinin and eosinophil leukocyte chemotactic factor of anaphylaxis), proteins (kallikrein), and other substances.

References

Adamson IYR, Bowden DM. Derivation of Type I epithelium from Type II cells in the developing rat lung. Lab Invest 1979;32:736–745.

Evans MJ, Cabral-Anderson LJ, Freeman G. Role of the Clara cell in renewal of the bronchiolar epithelium. Lab Invest 1978;38:648–655.

Kikkawa Y, Smith F. Cellular and biochemical aspects of pulmonary surfactant in health and disease. Lab Invest 1983;49:122–139.

Meyrick B, Reid L: The alveolar brush cell in rat lung—a third pneumonocyte. J Ultrastruct Res 1968;23:71–80.

Plopper CG. Structure and function of the lung. In: Jones TC, Dungworth DL, Mohr U, eds. Monograph on pathology of laboratory animals, respiratory system. Heidelberg, Springer Verlag 1995;135–150.

Robertson B, Enhorning G. The alveolar lining of the premature newborn rabbit after pharyngeal deposition of surfactant. Lab Invest 1974;31:54–59.

Rooney SA. Phospholipid composition, biosynthesis, and secretion. In: Parent RA, ed. Comparative biology of the normal lung. Boca Raton, FL: CRC Press, 1992;511–544.

Tyler WS, Julian MD. Gross and subgross anatomy of lungs, pleura, connective tissue septa,distal airways, and page 2 vp1220a structural units. In: Parent RA, ed. Comparative biology of the normal lung. Boca Raton, FL: CRC Press1992;37–48

Pneumonia, pneumonitis

Pneumonitis can properly refer to any inflammatory disease of the lungs, but its use usually is restricted to new infectious diseases of the lung, such as immunologically mediated pneumonitis and a more or less chronic reaction in which a prominent part is taken by fibroblasts of the interstitial tissue and the lining cells of the alveoli. The term pneumonia is usually reserved to apply to one of the acute infectious inflammations with copious exudate filling the alveoli.

Pneumonia

Acute inflammation of the lung, which is pneumonia, occurs in all species, but from a variety of causes. In many instances the gross and microscopic lesions are (to the diagnostician) disconcertingly similar regardless of what particular bacterium or virus is the cause (Fig. 20-3).

While pneumonia itself is a reaction taking place in the alveoli and their walls, the interlobular septa and other connective tissue structures are also distended

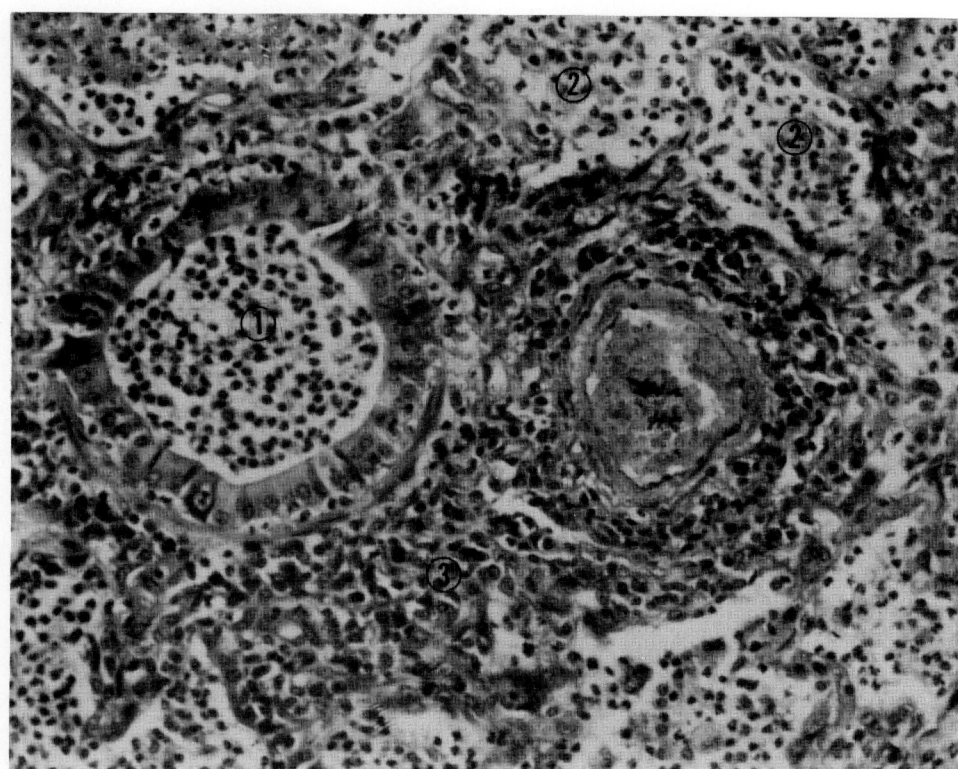

FIG. 20-3 Pneumonia associated with equine rhinopneumonitis. Lung of a young horse (×280). Mononuclear and polymorphonuclear cells fill the bronchioles *(1)*, alveoli *(2)*, and interstitial stroma *(3)*. (Courtesy of Armed Forces Institute of Pathology.) Contributor: Army Veterinary Research Laboratory.

with exudate, especially with the serous fluid. There is usually, but not always, a discernible bronchitis in the pneumonic area. This is recognized by desquamation and disappearance of the epithelial lining cells, by an infiltration of lymphocytes and other leukocytes in the wall of the bronchus or bronchiole, and an accumulation of exudate, usually polymorphonuclear, in the lumen. However, if a bronchial lumen contains pus or other exudate while the epithelium and wall still appear normal, it may be concluded that the exudate came from some other area, the bronchus merely serving as a drainage way.

The pleura over the pneumonic area may or may not share in the inflammatory process. If pleuritis (see below) is present, the exudate is usually fibrinous or fibrinopurulent on its surface and the causative organism or secondary invaders can be isolated there.

In some pneumonias, it is only in the immediate vicinity of the bronchi and bronchioles that the inflammatory changes and consolidation are in evidence, the infection having entered by the bronchial route. Such a form is known as **peribronchial** pneumonia, or even as peribronchitis and peribronchiolitis.

In the vicinity of the pneumonic changes, there are almost sure to be areas of atelectasis and areas of emphysema. The former are due to plugging of the bronchioles which served them by masses of exudate. The emphysema involves alveoli which expand unduly because of decreased space occupied by neighboring alveoli which are either atelectatic or consolidated.

Unfortunately, the prompt and complete resolution described above does not always occur and complica-

tions develop. One of these is the spreading of the pneumonic process to new areas of lung tissue. These must then proceed through the same series of stages, recovery of the patient being delayed by the time required for these stages. This is characteristic of lobular pneumonia (see below) in debilitated individuals. Also of considerable import is the fact that areas of lung adjoining the pneumonic parts usually suffer from marked inflammatory edema, which possibly represents spread of the pneumonia but which, at any rate, interferes seriously with pulmonary function.

With delayed resolution in a given area, certain changes may develop. The type II alveolar lining cells may undergo hyperplasia and resemble cuboidal epithelium. Their nuclei are very dark and the cells are conspicuous, sometimes being known as **cells of Tripier.** The condition has also been called **pulmonary adenomatosis** or **fetalization** of the lining cells, since they resemble those of the fetal lung. In Marsh's ovine chronic progressive pneumonia, this change becomes extreme, so that the area of lung may strikingly resemble an adenoma.

If a fibrinous or partially fibrinous exudate remains long (2 to 3 weeks) in the alveoli, the same thing happens that occurs when fibrin persists in a thrombus or in a fibrinous exudate elsewhere: the fibrin is organized by fibroblasts which build into it from surrounding tissues. Such an area is then converted permanently into fibrous tissue, a process known as **carnification** (*caro, carn,* flesh). Similarly, if the offending organism destroys pulmonary parenchyma (necrosis), healing is by scarring.

LESIONS

The distribution and extent of lesions deserve attention. From statements in the preceding description, it will be inferred that the areas of pneumonic consolidation do not necessarily involve a major portion of the pulmonary tissue, and this is true. It is unusual for more than a third of the total of the two lungs to be hepatized, and frequently the process is much more limited. In the great majority of pneumonias, which are bronchogenous in origin, the anterior and ventral portions of the lungs are first and most extensively affected. These are the apical and cardiac lobes in those species whose lungs are divided into lobes. Evidence indicates that this is because infective particles, when inhaled, fall most readily into the bronchial system of these lobes. The pneumonic process commonly progresses centrally in these lobes and may eventually involve the anterior part of the diaphragmatic lobes, not to mention the intermediate lobe in species which have it. The disease may be localized in one lung but more frequently it attacks both.

There are two routes by which pathogenic organisms may enter the lungs: via the bronchi (the **bronchogenous** route), and via the blood stream (the **hematogenous** route). The former is the more frequent. Coming down the arborization of the bronchial system, it is obvious that infected particles may drop into certain bronchioles and not into others. Around each infected bronchiole, a pneumonic area forms and extends to the limits of the histologic lobule supplied by the bronchiole in question. Other lobules become infected in the same way, with the result that the affected portion of the lung is spotted with hepatized and relatively normal lobules in an irregular pattern. This form constitutes **lobular pneumonia.** Since its origin is by way of the bronchial passages, it is also known as **bronchial pneumonia** or bronchopneumonia. While in some instances, infected particles fall or are sucked through a normal bronchial passageway, in other cases, the infection and the inflammation spread along the lining of the bronchus, infecting it bit by bit. In this case, the bronchopneumonia is accompanied by bronchitis and bronchiolitis.

Hematogenous pneumonia arises when the blood carries pathogenic organisms to produce, at least temporarily, a condition of septicemia. This happens in the case of certain viral infections, like psittacosis. It also occurs with bacterial septicemias. Pasteurellosis, while often bronchogenous, may reach the lungs in this way as is proven by the fact that the causative organisms often invade the pericardial space, which can be reached in no other way than by the blood. Pneumonia of hematogenous origin may be lobular or it may be lobar, meaning that it involves not a lobule here and lobule there, but that it affects all lobules in a considerable area, even a whole lobe. The term **fibrinous pneumonia** is often used synonymously with lobar pneumonia, but fibrinous describes the character of the exudate rather than the anatomical distribution, and should not be considered as a substitute for the term lobar. The virulence of the invading pathogen is of greater importance than the route by which the pathogen reaches the lung in determining if the resultant pneumonia is lobular or lobar. Many pneumonias arising by the bronchogenous route are lobar in distribution, if the offending organism is highly virulent or the host lacks resistance; in fact, many examples of lobar pneumonia in animals are aerogenous in origin.

The distinction between lobar and lobular pneumonia is less important in veterinary than in human medicine, where lobar pneumonia is a specific disease with a specific cause, the *Diplococcus pneumoniae*, a fibrinous reaction, and a specific course and treatment. Most pneumonias in animals are lobular (Fig. 20-4).

CAUSES

The causes of pneumonia are infections: bacterial, viral, and, exceptionally, fungal. Chemical irritants, such as gases like chlorine, sulfur dioxide, mustard gas, and ether vapor used as an anesthetic, and various irritating medicinal substances accidentally introduced via the trachea when intended for the esophagus, should be added to the list of causes conditionally. They are frequent inciting causes, but usually they merely produce an area of injury or necrosis with a distinctly limited inflammatory reaction. Inhaled bacteria, finding a fertile field of growth in the injured and debilitated area, then continue the irritation and are responsible for most of the pneumonic process. Chemicals do not reproduce themselves; bacteria multiply indefinitely. Likewise, metazoan parasites produce an initial injury, the injured area then becoming infected with inhaled bacteria which would not be able to colonize the healthy tissue.

An outline of the types of infectious agents that have been identified in pneumonic lungs is included in Table 20-2. This table undoubtedly does not include all such agents but may give a perspective to the complex susceptibility of the lung to infection.

It would be a matter of great diagnostic convenience if a characteristic type of pneumonic reaction could be attributed to each individual causative agent but only a few generalities are possible. In foals, a distinctly suppurative exudate with neutrophil polymorphs filling the alveoli is likely to be due to *Corynebacterium equi*. In other hosts a strongly suppurative reaction may be seen at times but can hardly be used to identify the offending pathogen. A reaction that is strongly fibrinous is suggestive of *Pasteurella sp.,* although not all *Pasteurella* pneumonias are fibrinous by any means. Streptococcal pneumonias are likely to be fibrinous (Fig. 20-5).

It is possible to make the general statement that pneumonia having a virus as its cause is usually characterized by a serous and mononuclear reaction, whereas most pneumonias of bacterial causation produce an exudate in which both the granulocytes and fibrin predominate. A number of viruses, mycoplasma, and members of the psittacosis-lymphogranuloma group of agents, either cause pneumonia independently or predispose to one or more of the bacterial invaders so that pneumonia becomes a feature of the typical syndrome

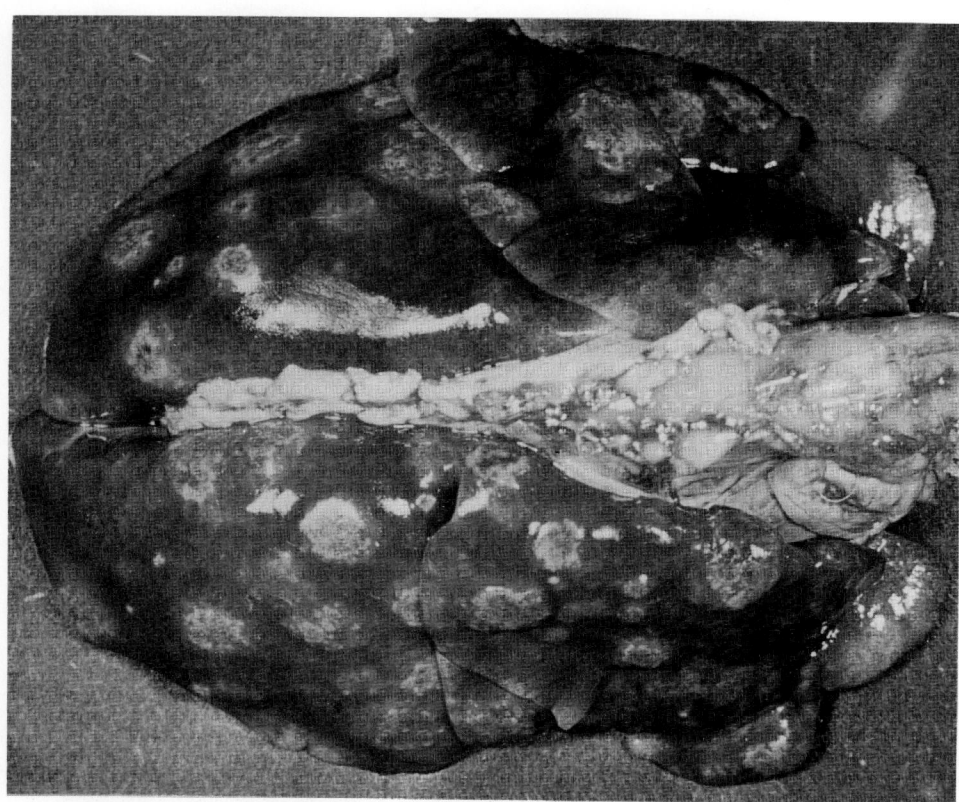

FIG. 20-4 Purulent pneumonia in the lungs of a one-year-old female tortoiseshell cat. (Courtesy of Angeli Memorial Animal Hospital.)

produced by them. These include the agents of equine rhinopneumonitis, bovine contagious pleuropneumonia, canine distemper, feline pneumonitis, a contagious mycoplasma pleuropneumonia of pigs, and contagious pleuropneumonia of goats. For the most part, pneumonias produced by these agents, in the absence of secondary bacterial invaders (and excluding bovine and caprine pleuropneumonia), are not comparable to the exudative lobular and lobar pneumonias described above. Instead the inflammatory reaction is predominantly interstitial, and appropriately the lesion is termed interstitial pneumonia, which is characterized by exudation within the interalveolar septa. The septa become greatly thickened by infiltrating lymphocytes, macrophages, and plasma cells, the accumulation of serum or fibrin, and by an increase in connective tissue fibers. Hyperplasia of alveolar lining cells is a frequent finding. Exudation of neutrophils into the alveoli is not a usual feature, however, free-lining cells and macrophages may occupy the alveoli. These features are also characteristic of **hypersensitivity pneumonitis.** In some infections, such as canine distemper, measles, and parainflueza-3 in calves, multinucleated giant cells are a component of the exudate in the septa and the alveolar lumens. Focal accumulation of lymphocytes often producing distinct nodules with germinal centers is a feature of many interstitial pneumonias, such as those in swine, calves, sheep, and rats caused by mycoplasmas and chlamydiae (Fig. 20-6).

Chilling of the body or a part of it lowers resistance and predisposes to pneumonia as it does to other respiratory infections. Extreme fatigue and severe hunger lower resistance to most infections, respiratory as well as others.

EFFECTS

Many cases of pneumonia are fatal. The pneumonia may be accompanied by morbid changes in other organs, as, for instance, in pasteurellosis. When the pulmonary disease alone is responsible for death, it may occur because too many of the alveoli are filled and unable to do their part in aerating the blood. This happens especially if non-hepatized areas are in a state of congestion and edema, conditions which also prevent the erythrocytes from getting and purveying oxygen. However, pneumonia is often fatal with very considerable portions of the lung tissue still functional. In such cases, death is attributed to toxic effects from the microorganisms and their products.

Bronchiectasis and carnification have been mentioned as unfavorable sequelae. In a few cases in which the invading organisms belong to the pyogenic group and are of high virulence, **abscesses** may form in the hepatized tissue. More frequently, however, pulmonary abscesses are of embolic origin in an otherwise healthy lung. In a few other pneumonias from non-pyogenic pathogens of high virulence, areas of tissue are killed by the toxins produced and gangrene results, but pulmonary gangrene usually has other causes.

References

Bowden DH. Unraveling pulmonary fibrosis: The bleomycin model. Lab Invest 1984;50:487–488.

Buergelt CD, Hines SA, Cantor G, et al. A retrospective study of pro-

TABLE 20-2 Putative infectious causes of pneumonia (organisms identified in pneumonic lungs)

Bacteria: (see Chapter 10)	Principal hosts:
Pasteurella multocida	many species
Pasteurella hemolytica	ruminants
Streptococcus spp.	several species
Corynebacterium pyogenes	ruminants, several species
Corynebacterium equi	horses
Bordetella bronchiseptica	dogs, swine, nonhumans primates
Hemophilus suis	swine
Hemophilus influenzae	nonhuman primates
Klebsiella pneumoniae	nonhuman primates, dogs
Staphylococcus spp.	dogs
Pseudomonas aeruginosa	cats, rabbits, several others
Diplococcus pneumoniae	nonhuman primates, rats
Corynebacterium pseudotuberculosis	sheep, rabbits
Mycobacterium tuberculosis	primates, all other species
Acytinobacillus lignieresi	cattle

Viruses: (see Chapter 8)	Principal hosts:
Equine influenza A	horses, mules, donkeys
Equine herpesvirus, 1-4	horses, mules, donkeys
Equine rhinovirus	horses, mules, donkeys
Equine parainfluenza-3	horses, mules, donkeys
Equine adenovirus	horses
Equine viral arteritis	horses
Equine horse-sickness	horses
Canine distemper	dogs, mink, ferrets
Canine herpesvirus	dogs
Canine adenovirus 1, 2	dogs, foxes
Parainfluenza, SV5	dogs
Canine reovirus-1	dogs
Infectious bovine rhinotracheitis	cattle
Bovine parainfluenza-3	cattle
Bovine respiratory syncytial	cattle
Bovine mucosal disease	cattle, sheep
Bovine reovirus	cattle
Feline herpesvirus	cats

Mycoplasma: (Chapter 9)	Principal hosts:
Mycoplasma dispar	ruminants
Ureaplasma	ruminants
Mycoplasma bovirhinis	ruminants
Mycoplasma mycoides	ruminants
Mycoplasma spp.	ruminants, swine
Mycoplasma pulmonis	rats
Mycoplasma hyopneumonia	swine

Chlamydia: (Chapter 9)	Principal hosts:
Chlamydia spp.	cattle
Chlamydia spp.	cats
Chlamydia psittaci	parrots and other birds, man

Fungi: (Chapter 11)	Principal hosts:
Aspergillus fumigatus, flavus, niger, nidulans	birds, mammals

TABLE 20-2 (continued)

Fungi: (Chapter 11)	Principal hosts:
Coccidioides immitis	many mammals
Blastomyces dermatidis	dogs, man
Histoplasma capsulatum	man, dogs
Cryptococcus neoformans	cats, man
Haplosporangium parvum	rodents, armadillo
Actinomyces bovis	cattle, swine
Nocardia spp.	several species
Sphaeropherus necrophorus	swine, cattle
Geotrichum candidum	dog

liferative interstitial lung disease of horses in Florida. Vet Pathol 1986;23:750–756.

Lay JC, Slauson DO. The bovine pulmonary inflammatory response: Adjuvant pneumonitis in calves. Vet Pathol 198219:506–520.

Turk JR, Brown CM, Johnson GC. Diffuse alveolar damage with fibrosing alveolitis in a horse. Vet Pathol 1981;18:560–562.

Winder NC, Gruenig G, Hermann M, et al. Fibrin/fibrinogen in lungs and respiratory secretions of horses with chronic pulmonary disease. Am J Vet Res 1990;51:945–949.

Special types of pneumonia

A number of types of pneumonia commonly receive special recognition because of peculiar characteristics.

PNEUMONIA DUE TO PARAINFLUENZA VIRUS 1

The first virus identified and later classified in the group of parainfluenza viruses (see Chapter 8) and currently placed in the genus *Paramyxovirus*, is also called the Sendai virus, after a city in Japan where it was first isolated from a laboratory mouse. This virus is an important pathogen in several species and its effects have been intensively studied, providing the basis for comparison with many other viral infections of the lung.

Sendai virus is transmitted by aerosol and contact, and a single infected mouse can infect up to 70% of susceptible mice by 24 hours of contact. Infection does depend on the immune state of exposed animals, athymic nude (immunodeficient) mice may become persistently infected. The virus replicates only in the respiratory tract although transient viremia may occur. The initial infection occurs in the ciliated and Clara cells of the terminal bronchioles. Its strict pneumotropism is believed to be, at least in part, due to the virus's dependence upon one or more respiratory serine endoproteases, such as Tryptase clara, which specifically cleaves the inactive viral nascent fusion glycoprotein at residue arginine-116 to the active form.

The microscopic lesions start in bronchial and bronchiolar epithelium, then extend to the pneumocytes II and to a lesser degree to pneumocytes type I. The earliest changes are segmental, the infected bronchiolar epithelial cells are enlarged, with eosinophilic, granular, foamy, or homogenous cytoplasm. Their nuclei are poorly polarized, and often fused, producing epithelial syncytia (See Fig. 20-7). Cellular infiltrate,

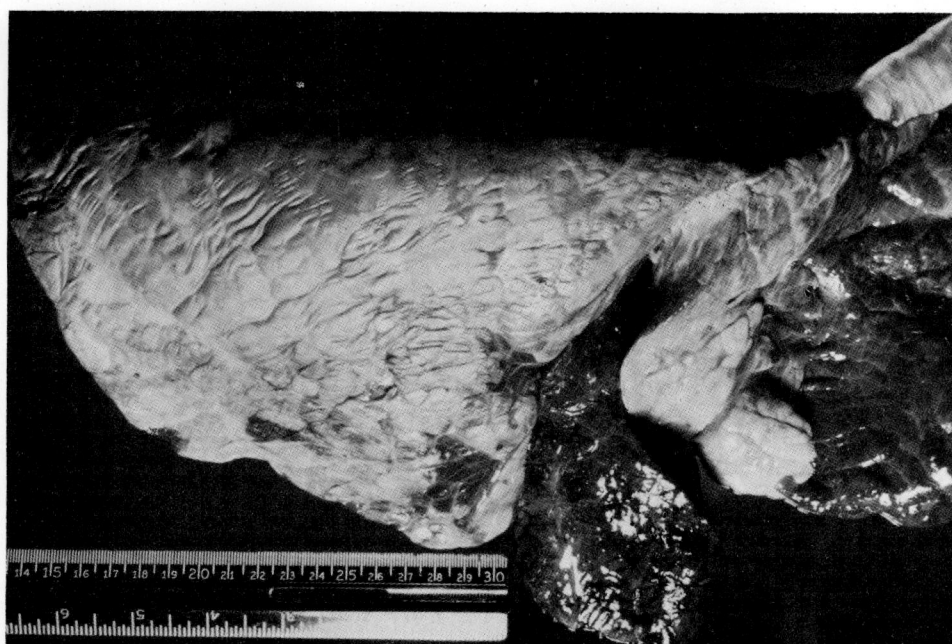

FIG. 20-5 Pneumonia involving apical and cardial lobes of the right lung of a male calf, four months of age. *Pasteurella spp.* was isolated from the affected lobes.

edema, and dilated lymphatics expand the lamina propria and adventitia. The inflammatory cells consist initially of polymorphonuclear leukocytes and lymphoid cells often with expanded and tinctorially altered cytoplasm. The peribronchiolar arterioles and venules are dilated with increased intimal cellularity and accumulations of lyphoid cells in the intima. These changes persist for 5 to 12 days which has been defined as the *acute phase*. Viral inclusions may be seen as homogeneous irregular or spherical cytoplasmic bodies surrounded by a halo, but they are frequently lost due to sloughing of the infected cells.

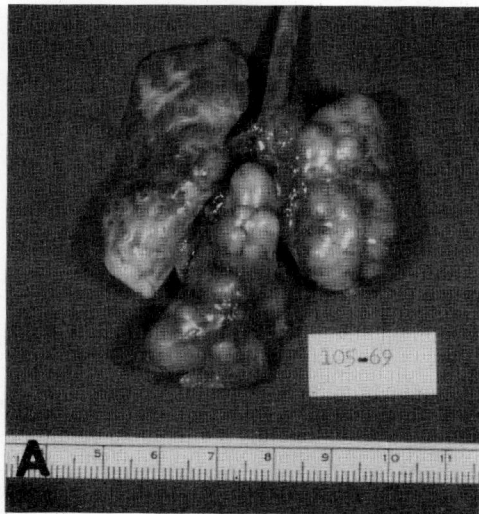

FIG. 20-6 Chronic murine pneumonia, rat, Bronchiectatic nodules. (Courtesy of Animal Research Center, Harvard Medical School.)

As the *acute phase* ends, infected epithelial cells are sloughed into bronchiolar lumens along with inflammatory exudate. Lymphoid aggregates accumulate in the lamina propria, causing the epithelium to bulge into the lumen. Some bronchioles may be devoid of epithelium, others nearby are lined by hypertrophied epithelial cells. Alveoli adjacent to affected bronchioles are filled with inflammatory exudate, consisting of neutrophils, macrophages, lymphocytes and desquamated pneumocytes (see Fig. 20-8). Alveolar septa become distended with edema, congested capillaries, and hypertrophied type II pneumocytes. Alveoli may fill with fibrin or blood, the fibrin accumulating along alveolar surfaces or filling alveolar spaces. Alveolar septa are thickened by mononuclear cells and some foci of emphysema may be present. In severe cases, the focal inflammation may become confluent, leading to lobar pneumonia.

The beginning of the *reparative phase* is indicated by the appearance of regenerating epithelium. This is usually clearly evident by the 8th to 12th day, although some few regenerating cells may be seen earlier. Initially, partially denuded bronchioles are newly covered with low cuboidal, polygonal or squamous cells, and as the lining is completed, the cells become columnar and assume their mucociliary appearance. Some terminal bronchioles become lined by stratified, nonkeratinizing, squamous epithelium. The adventitia and lamina propria becomes less edematous as repair proceeds, and are densely infiltrated by lymphocytes and plasma cells. As the reparative phase progresses, the inflammation shifts from the alveoli to the interstitium. In one form of repair, the septa are lined by cuboidal epithelium (alveolar epithelialization, adenomatous hyperplasia, alveolar bronchiolization). Initially undifferenti-

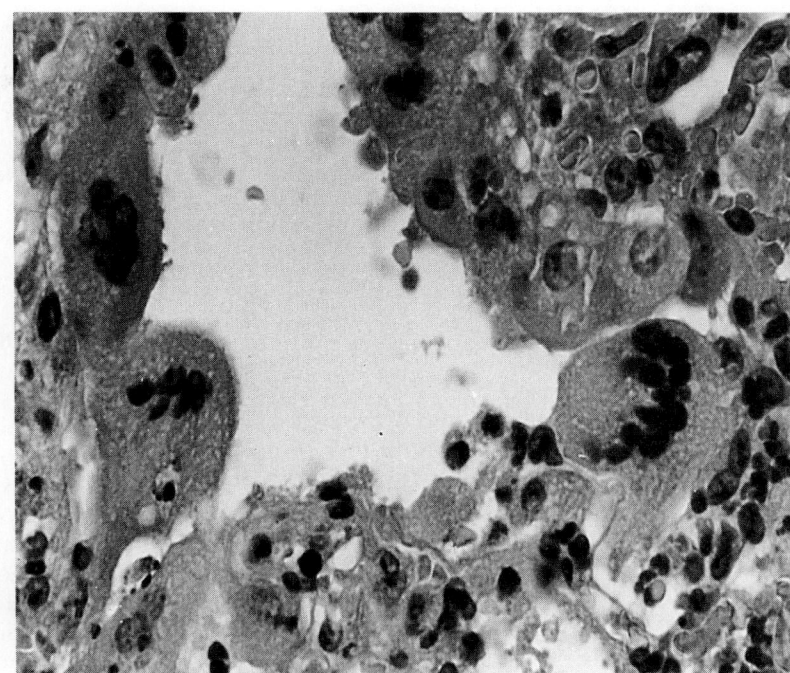

FIG. 20-7 Sendai virus infection, acute phase, lung, mouse. Bronchiolar epithelium is hypertrophied with loss of nuclear polarity and formation of syncytia. The adventitia is edematous and infiltrated with lymphocytes. (H & E, ×791.) (Courtesy of Dr. David G. Brownstein and Springer Verlag.)

ated, these cells soon differentiate into pneumocytes, mucous, ciliated, or Clara cells. In a second form of repair, partial or total atelectasis results from filling of alveolar spaces by metaplastic squamous epithelium. This results in partial or total atelectasis of the affected alveoli. If fibrin has been deposited, it undergoes lysis by macrophages which surround or infiltrate fibrin deposits, or it becomes organized as evidenced by the presence of large, plump fibroblasts and eventually by the identification of collagen.

The *resolution phase* may be short, with few identifiable residual lesions, but in some cases, perhaps for the

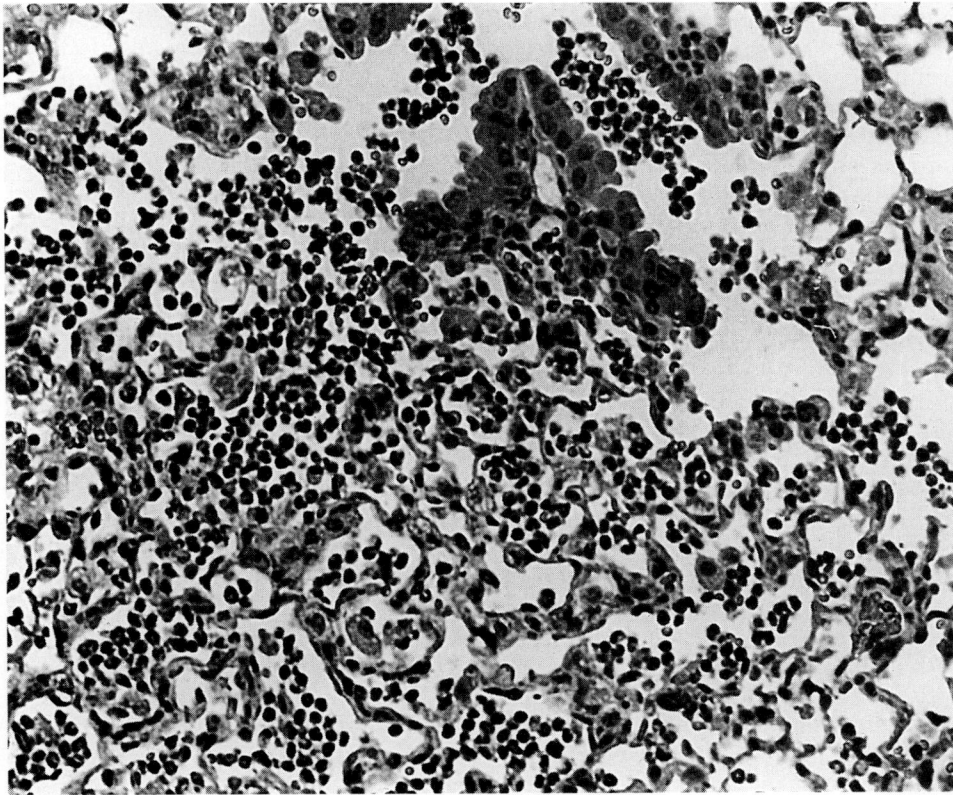

FIG. 20-8 Sendai virus infection, acute phase, lung, mouse. Alveoli adjacent to an infected bronchiole contain lymphocytes, macrophages and few polymorphonuclear leukocytes. Alveolar septa are edematous and infiltrated with mononuclear cells. (H & E, ×345.) (Courtesy of Dr. David G. Brownstein and Springer Verlag.)

life of the animal, an organizing alveolitis remains, with or without a fibrous obliterating bronchiolitis.

References

Brownstein DG, Smith AL, Johnson EA. Sendai virus infection in genetically resistant and susceptible mice. Am J Pathol 1981;105:156–163.

Brownstein DG. Sendai virus infection, lung, mouse, rat. In: Jones TC, Dungworth DL, Mohr U, eds. Monographs on pathology of laboratory animals, respiratory system, 2nd ed. Heidelberg, Springer Verlag, 1996;308–316

EMBOLIC PNEUMONIA

This is characterized by numerous pneumonic foci which are rather evenly scattered through all lobes of both lungs, the greatest number of foci being near the pleural surface until they become confluent and their site of origin becomes obscured. The sub-pleural location is attributable to the fact that this area contains the largest proportion of small arteries and arterioles in which an embolus may be lodged. In contrast, the hematogenous pneumonia which accompanies septicemic diseases is diffuse. However, it is more frequent that lodged emboli produce individualized abscesses (rarely other types of reaction, such as specific granulomas) rather than areas of hepatization. Microscopically, embolic pneumonia can be seen in its earlier stages to differ from bronchopneumonia in that the foci spread out from blood vessels and not from bronchi.

VERMINOUS PNEUMONIA

Verminous pneumonia is another form in which there is departure from the usual anteroventral distribution of lesions. In verminous pneumonia, the diaphragmatic lobes have their full share of pneumonic areas because these depend upon the localization of the worms. The larvae of ascarid worms pass through the lungs, especially in swine, but in non-immune animals, leave only negligible lesions. The inflamed areas in verminous pneumonia are usually small, scattered, and in different chronological stages, a fact of diagnostic value. The adult nematodes are usually found in the bronchi and bronchioles, where they incite a mucopurulent bronchitis. However, the exact site of localization of the adult nematodes varies among lungworms. Their embryonated ova or larvae are conspicuous in the bronchial exudate, by which they leave the lungs for the extraneous part of their existence. True pneumonic lesions develop when the tissue which the worms have injured is attacked by inspired pathogens from the throat region. Each individual inflammatory focus, small, large, or perhaps confluent, thus has the usual characteristics of bronchopneumonia, some of the usual organisms being demonstrable. However, there is considerable tendency to chronicity, not only through the consecutive development of different foci, but also within the individual lesions. These heal with difficulty or not at all until the worm lives its life span and disappears (several weeks), and there is often considerable reaction of the foreign-body type and fibrous encapsula-

tion. In the meantime, an extensive and fatal bacterial pneumonia may or may not develop. The immunologic aspects of repeated infections by lungworms are referred to in Chapter 7.

References

Kornegay RW, Giddens WE, Morton WR, et al. Verminous vasculitis, pneumonia and pulmonary infarction in a cynomologous monkey after treatment with Invermectin. Lab Anim Sci 1986;36:45–47.

GANGRENOUS PNEUMONIA

Gangrenous pneumonia is in veterinary medicine almost synonymous with what is variously called **aspiration pneumonia, foreign-body pneumonia, medication pneumonia, lipid pneumonia** and others of similar import. As previously stated, it is possible for some pneumonia-producing pathogens of high virulence to kill tissue outright, which then becomes subject to invasion by putrefactive saprophytes, thus fulfilling the specifications of **gangrene,** but such cases are rare. Pulmonary embolism and infarction with saprophytic invasion of the dead infarct are also possible but rare.

The usual cause of gangrenous pneumonia is the introduction into the lungs of medicines intended for the esophagus. Henceforth, what happens is largely dependent on the nature and quantity of the material introduced. Many drugs are highly irritant and entirely capable of producing necrosis of the pulmonary tissue, which is much less resistant than the mucus-protected lining of the stomach. Oily drugs are especially harmful, not because of their immediately irritating properties, but because the oil, especially mineral oil, is not capable of being absorbed and cannot be eliminated. In any case, these medicines are not sterile, nor is the pharyngeal mucosa over which they pass. We thus have an irritant chemical substance and a rather massive concentration of various kinds of bacteria in the same place. The result is very often, but not invariably, necrosis of the area followed by gangrene. In animals whose cough reflexes are impaired by anesthesia, paralysis, or coma, there is always the possibility of aspiration of drops of exudate, particles of food or vomitus. Indeed whole grains, heads of wheat, or parts of ears of corn are occasionally found in the lungs of the herbivorous animals (see Fig. 20-9). These usually carry high concentrations of bacteria of many kinds. Gangrene of the area involved is a common result, preceded by a very intense inflammation.

The definitive lesion of gangrenous pneumonia is death of tissue. It is accompanied by intense hyperemia and exudative and even hemorrhagic inflammation in the surrounding living tissue. The dead tissue soon liquefies (liquefaction necrosis) so that it can almost be said that the characteristic lesion is cavitation. Like other necrotic tissue, the remaining dead tissue may be white or black depending on the amount of blood in it. As putrefying bacteria multiply, foul odors appear. The liquefied material may be of pasty consistency at one stage, but ultimately becomes entirely fluid. These changes are commonly well established in a course of 2 or 3 days, although death may come earlier. Numerous foreign bodies have been reported to cause focal or diffuse pneumonic lesions. These include foreign feed or plant material inhaled by cats or swine; hair fragment emboli reaching the lungs of rats via the vasculature from the skin—introduced by a needle through the skin into a vein; and inhaled vegetable products that often reach the lung of brachiocephalic dogs (see Fig. 20-9).

HYALINE-MEMBRANE DISEASE

This designation has been applied to a fatal respiratory distress syndrome of premature infants in which one of the features is the presence, at postmortem, of hyaline membranes within alveoli. These membranes are probably the result of fibrinous and other debris in alveoli. This syndrome is associated with surfactant deficiency due to prematurity, disturbance of the fibrinolytic system, atelectasis, and pulmonary hypoperfusion, possibly induced by perinatal asphyxia. The exact cause is unknown.

Homologues of the human disease have been produced experimentally in premature lambs and nonhuman primates. A few natural cases have been reported in animals. These may or may not involve the same mechanisms seen in the human disease.

PNEUMONIA OF "SHIPPING FEVER"

This respiratory disease syndrome in young cattle is usually associated in time by transport from one place to another—often from the farm to a feedlot. The signs may be overlooked, but usually involve upper respiratory disease, which ends in recovery or fatal pneumonia. In a study of 1988 necropsies of cattle in feedlots, Jensen et al. (1976), found that 64% had lesions of the respiratory tract. "Shipping fever pneumonia" was identified in 75% of the necropsies involving respiratory disease. The lesions tended to be localized in the lower parts of the cardiac and intermediate lobes. The pneumonic areas were associated with bronchitis, accumulation of fibrinous exudate, lymphatic clots, intravascular clots, thrombosis, and focal necrosis. *Pasteurella spp., Mycoplasma,* and infectious bovine rhinotracheitis virus were isolated most frequently.

Hypothetical pathogenic processes, proposed by Jensen et al. (1976), are initiated by viral, *Pasteurella,* or other microbial growth in the upper respiratory system, which has a deleterious effect on the ciliated cells and mucous coating of the trachea, bronchi, and bronchioles. Pathogenic *Pasteurella* and other microorganisms from the nasopharynx reach the ventral bronchi and alveoli by gravitational drainage along the tracheal floor. *Pasteurella* endotoxin, produced by growth of the organisms in infected lobules, causes thrombosis of veins, capillaries, and lymphatics. This causes ischemic necrosis. Fibrinous exudate predominates in the alveoli but leukocytes and bacteria are also present. It is useful to have a hypothesis concerning pathogenetic mechanisms; such a theory often forms the basis for future study.

HYPOSTATIC PNEUMONIA

Hypostatic congestion has been described. The porous nature of pulmonary tissue is especially conducive to hypostatic congestion, as a result of which edema of the area is likely to develop. Tissue devitalized by these two circulatory disorders may well fall prey to inhaled upper respiratory pathogens which would be promptly destroyed in a healthy lung. Pneumonia thus develops, in recumbent patients, in the lower parts of the lower lung as a feature, all too frequently terminal, of many diseases.

GRANULOMATOUS PNEUMONIA

A group of infectious organisms often localize in the lung and do not induce pneumonia comparable to the acute exudative pneumonias or interstitial pneumonitis already described. These include many of the higher bacteria and fungi. Although tuberculous pneumonia occurs rarely as an acute febrile pulmonary inflammation which is clinically and pathologically much like the pneumonia already described, the usual tuberculous involvement of the lung is a very different matter, having a much slower course and being characterized by granulomatous rather than exudative lesions. This latter is well termed tuberculous pneumonia.

In the same group are other granulomatous infections that involve the lungs: actinomycosis, actinobacillosis, coccidioidomycosis, histoplasmosis, glanders, chronic aspergillosis, the usual chronic form of blastomycosis, and rarely mucormycosis and others. *Blastomyces dermatitidis* occasionally causes diffuse pneumonia in the dog, although granulomatous lesions are more usual.

PNEUMOCONIOSIS

Chronic inflammatory reaction to several inhaled mineral contaminants results in forms of granulomatous pneumonia. Such substances include various dusts from mines, quarries, grinding, sand-blasting, and other industries, the most formidable being silica (SiO_2), beryllium, and asbestos. Bauxite (impure Al_2O_3), graphite, and carbon are less important. Large quantities inhaled over a period of time are usually necessary to cause important disease, but eventual fatalities are not uncommon. The reaction to silicon dioxide is typically in the form of dense fibrous nodules, the condition being known as **silicosis. Asbestosis** is characterized by a more cellular and a more diffuse reaction and by **"asbestos bodies"** which can be found microscopically in the lesions. These are brownish, club-shaped filaments bearing some resemblance in size and shape to the broken mycelial filaments seen in mucormycosis. The "beryllium granuloma" resembles a non-caseating tubercle, even including Langhans' giant cells. Asteroid inclusion bodies of unique appearance are occasionally seen in the giant cells. The pneumoconioses are largely limited to humans and experimental animals for the reason that domestic animals are seldom exposed to the dusts which cause them. Horses and mules used in quarries and mines are subject to the same atmospheric contamination as the men and develop the same lesions, but such use of draft animals is largely past. The dust pneumonia of pigs belongs with the acute pneumonias. Anthracosis is frequent in dogs required to sleep in coal bins. Pneumonia due to *Pneumocystis carinii* has been described in Chapter 12. Chronic murine pneumonia is considered as a mycoplasmosis in Chapter 9, as is enzootic pneumonia of swine, sheep and calves.

References

Brody AR, Roe MW, Evans JN, et al. Deposition and translocation of inhaled silica in rats. Lab Invest 1982;47:533–542.

Farber JL. How do mineral dusts cause lung injury? Lab Invest 1983;49:379–380.

Haley PJ, Finch GL, Mewhinney JA, et al. A canine model of beryllium-induced granulomatous lung disease. Lab Invest 1989;61:219–227.

Hubbard AK. Role for T lymphocytes in silica-induced pulmonary inflammation. Lab Invest 1989;61:46–52.

Macdonald JL, Kane AB. Identification of asbestos fibers within single cells. Lab Invest 1986;55:177–185.

Mossman BT, Gee JBL. Asbestos-related diseases. N Engl J Med 1989;320:1721–1730.

Saltini C, Winestock K, Kirby M, et al. Maintenance of alveolitis in patients with chronic beryllium disease by beryllium-specific helper T cells. N Engl J Med 1989;320:1103–1109.

Wick G, Mark H, von der Dietrich H, et al. Globular domain of basement membrane collagen induces autoimmune pulmonary lesions in mice resembling human Goodpasture disease. Lab Invest 1986;55:308–317.

Pneumonitis

There is considerable diversity in the use of this term, which literally means an inflammation of the lungs. In general, it has been used for inflammatory conditions of the lung to which one hesitates to apply the term pneumonia. The latter we have already described in the classic way as an acute exudative filling of the lung alveoli, with a rather typical febrile clinical course. Many consider the term pneumonitis synonymous with interstitial pneumonia. Several special types of pneumonitis are now recognized in animals and it appears most useful to consider them in connection with their etiology.

HYPERSENSITIVITY PNEUMONITIS (ALLERGIC ALVEOLITIS)

Exposure to specific antigens, particularly products of mold growth, results in a hypersensitive immune state which is precipitated by reexposure into a severe tissue reaction. If the lung is the target organ, the tissue reactions and clinical signs are grouped under this term, hypersensitivity pneumonitis. This phenomenon has been demonstrated repeatedly in animals under experimental conditions and is also recognized in humans and animals as a disease phenomenon in nature.

A large number of antigens have been found to produce hypersensitivity upon inhalation by humans or animals. These antigens have been identified particularly in vegetable, animal, insect, bacterial, or viral products, particularly if contaminated by molds. The disease conditions have been long identified with the affected worker's occupation: "farmer's lung," "mushroom-worker's disease," "malt-worker's lung," "paprika-slicer's lung," "thatched-roof disease," "pigeon-breeder's disease," "miller's lung," etc. Some of the specific antigens have been identified. "Farmer's lung' was initially associated with farmers who had been working with moldy hay. The antigens are now associated with certain thermophilic actinomycetes, particularly *Micropolyspora faeni* and *Thermoactinomyces vulgaris*. Many other sensitizing organisms have been tentatively identified.

EQUINE PULMONARY EMPHYSEMA (CHRONIC DIFFUSE ALVEOLAR EMPHYSEMA, HEAVES, BROKEN WIND)

An equine disease long associated with moldy, dusty hay, and compared with chronic allergic bronchitis—asthma in humans—as early as 1887, its cause is not completely known. Sensitization to products of some common contaminants of a horse's environment has been demonstrated. *Aspergillus spp., Alternaria spp.,* and *Hormodendrum spp.* have been used as antigens to demonstrate sensitivity in affected horses by direct skin tests and passive cutaneous anaphylactic skin tests. Affected horses have also been shown to be sensitized to chickens.

Horses with pulmonary emphysema have a characteristic sign which consists of two successive expiratory movements, with the second forcibly expelling the last portion of tidal air. The lesions include diffuse and rather evenly distributed alveolar emphysema, which is identified by gross inspection of the lung. The emphysema appears to be secondary to chronic bronchiolitis, which may be associated with bronchiospasms that occlude the alveolar ducts. Hyperplasia of the bronchiolar musculature and peribronchiolar leukocytic infiltration has been noted in association with mucous and purulent exudate in bronchiolar lumens.

BOVINE ALLERGIC ALVEOLITIS (BOVINE-FARMER'S LUNG, BOVINE HYPERSENSITIVITY PNEUMONITIS)

If a farmer, while feeding moldy hay to his cows, becomes hypersensitive to the molds, it should be no surprise that the cows also become sensitized to the same molds, which is exactly what does happen. Typically, the bovine disease occurs during the winter months when the adult cows are housed indoors and fed last year's crop of hay. Affected cows cough frequently, have an increased rate of respiration, and a decrease in milk yield, weight, and appetite. The number of affected animals increases and severity of signs intensifies as the winter progresses. After some months, chronically affected animals may die.

Using double-diffusion tests, precipitating antibodies may be detected in antigen prepared from cultures of *Micropolyspora faeni*. Skin tests are also of value in detecting the antigen of *M. faeni* in affected cows. Induration of the skin at the site of antigenic inoculation may be present 2 to 4 hours after injection. Exposure of sensitized animals to aerosol suspensions of mold by way of the respiratory tract will accentuate the clinical signs.

Lesions The gross lesions in chronic cases are concentrated in the lungs. Lobules in all lobes may contain small gray foci, and peripheral alveoli are grossly distended. Excessive yellow mucus may be found in some bronchi. Microscopically, the bronchioles are particularly affected. Some are obliterated by protrusion of inflammatory exudate into the lumen, carrying the epithelium with it. The interstitial exudate contains macrophages, monocytes, lymphocytes, plasma cells, and occasional fibroblasts; a few multinucleated giant cells may be present. The affected bronchioles are surrounded by lymphocytes, plasma cells, globule cells, and occasionally eosinophils. These cells are numerous in the alveolar septa and may form small, discrete granulomas. In many areas, this interstitial exudate is accompanied by hyperplasia of cuboidal, sometimes ciliated cells, lining the alveoli.

EQUINE ALLERGIC PNEUMONITIS

A syndrome with many similarities to bovine and human "farmer's lung" has been described in horses. This disease is manifested by attacks of dyspnea and coughing associated with eosinophilia of peripheral blood and nasal secretions. Intracutaneous response was demonstrated to allergenic mixtures of dust from food and bedding. Precipitins develop for *Micropolyspora faeni* and *Aspergillus fumigatus*.

The lesions began as acute interstitial pneumonitis with interalveolar edema, intravascular fibrin masses, fibrillar hyaline membranes in alveoli, and extensive infiltration of interstitium and alveoli with monocytes and macrophages. Hyperplasia of the alveolar epithelium and fibrosis of interstitial tissues were seen in late stages.

BRONCHIAL ASTHMA

This disease is characterized by attacks lasting from one to many hours of very difficult, wheezing respiration, especially expiration, due to spasmodic contraction of the encircling musculature of the bronchioles and smaller bronchi, as well as to the production of large amounts of viscid mucous exudate which is strongly inclined to adhere to the bronchial walls. While some cases are secondary to a bronchial infection, the majority are allergic reactions to a great variety of inhaled organic substances to which the individual has become hypersensitive. That contraction of smooth muscle is an outstanding manifestation of the anaphylactic state has been demonstrated many times by suitable laboratory experiments.

Lesions The principal lesions in fatal cases include extensive infiltration of the bronchial and bronchiolar walls with lymphocytes, monocytes and usually large numbers of eosinophils, accumulation of dense mucous exudate in the lumens, as well as in the epithelial cells which produce it, and frequently an astonishing hyaline thickening of the bronchial basement membranes. The mucus sometimes condenses in peculiar spiral strings called Curschmann's spirals. There is marked secondary emphysema.

Causes Asthma is chiefly a human disease, but it has possibly occurred in cattle and certainly, though rarely, in cats and dogs. In the latter, it has been pro-

duced artificially in experimental work. The similarities in etiology and lesions causes us to consider asthma in relation to hypersensitivity pneumonitis. The antigens which affect animals have not yet been adequately studied. Hypersensitivity to pollens in the dog results from exposure through the respiratory tract, but the effects are manifest principally in the skin (atopy, atopic skin disease). Susceptibility appears to be inherited.

HYPERSENSITIVITY IN LUNGWORM INFECTION

Reinfection of previously infected cattle with the lungworm, *Dictyocaulus viviparous*, has been considered to produce acute respiratory distress. This situation can be differentiated from acute interstitial emphysema or "fog fever" on the basis of the clinical and pathologic features. It is known that initial infections with lungworms produce almost no tissue reaction in the lung until immune reactions have had sufficient time to appear. Animals (cattle or sheep especially) which were infected with lungworms one season and then reinfected at the beginning of the second season may exhibit signs of severe respiratory distress, and death may occur. Severe tissue reaction to the parasites is a constant feature of the pulmonary lesions. It appears that immunologic factors are important in this disease and require further study. See chapter 7.

Pleuritis

Inflammation of the pleura is known as pleuritis or by the older name of pleurisy. The ordinary forms of pleuritis belong to the acute exudative inflammations, usually being either serous, fibrinous, or purulent. If the pleuritis accompanies pneumonia, the pleuritic area overlies the hepatized portions of lung parenchyma, the condition is called **pleuropneumonia.** But there are many cases of pneumonia without pleuritis, and it is entirely possible for pleuritis to exist without pneumonia. The pulmonary pleura is first involved, as a rule, but the infection and the inflammatory reaction promptly spread to the contiguous areas of parietal pleura.

The usual attack of pleurisy begins with acute hyperemia and swelling of the thin covering membrane. During this stage, the friction of the visceral and parietal surfaces at each respiratory movement is very painful, causing a typical kind of breathing. After about 2 days a serous exudate appears, which lubricates and separates the two surfaces, and the pain is assuaged. The exudate may remain serous, filling the pleural cavity and compressing the lungs, or it may become fibrinous or purulent. Often all forms coexist, resulting in a sero-fibrino-purulent pleuritis. Microscopically, the pleural layer is infiltrated with lymphocytes and other inflammatory cells. Its thickness is increased several fold by edema fluid which fills the intercellular spaces and distends the numerous but previously unseen lymph vessels. Capillaries are numerous and greatly dilated. The surface layer of mesothelial cells is largely destroyed, and the surface is covered with a thin or thick layer of fibrin or with adherent dead neutrophils and other elements characteristic of a purulent exudate.

With the lapse of a few days the amount of seropurulent exudate collecting in the pleural cavity may become so great as to interfere seriously with expansion of the lungs, requiring drainage by thoracocentesis. In such cases, the exudate is very likely to become fibrinous, depending largely on the kind of organism that is causing it. The layers of fibrin on each of the two apposing surfaces tend to become organized by immigrating fibroblasts, and the two surfaces often become tied together by strands of fibrous connective tissue. These are known as **adhesions;** the inflammatory process is then called **adhesive pleuritis.** It is not unusual to find large areas of lung surface inseparably joined to the chest wall. Most animals so affected die while the process is still active. Some survive the causative

infection with adhesions of limited extent. These adhesions cause pain with respiratory movement, but this diminishes as the anatomical structures adjust themselves. There is no permanent disability in most cases.

Causes The causes of pleuritis are usually infectious, and, in general, they are the same kinds of organisms which cause pneumonia. Infection of the pleura may result by direct extension from the lung, but many cases of pleuritis arise by the hematogenous route without involvement of the lungs, especially in septicemic diseases of young animals. An important variant is seen in those bovines in which a swallowed metallic foreign body penetrates from the reticulum into the pleural cavity, carrying infection with it. A majority of these,

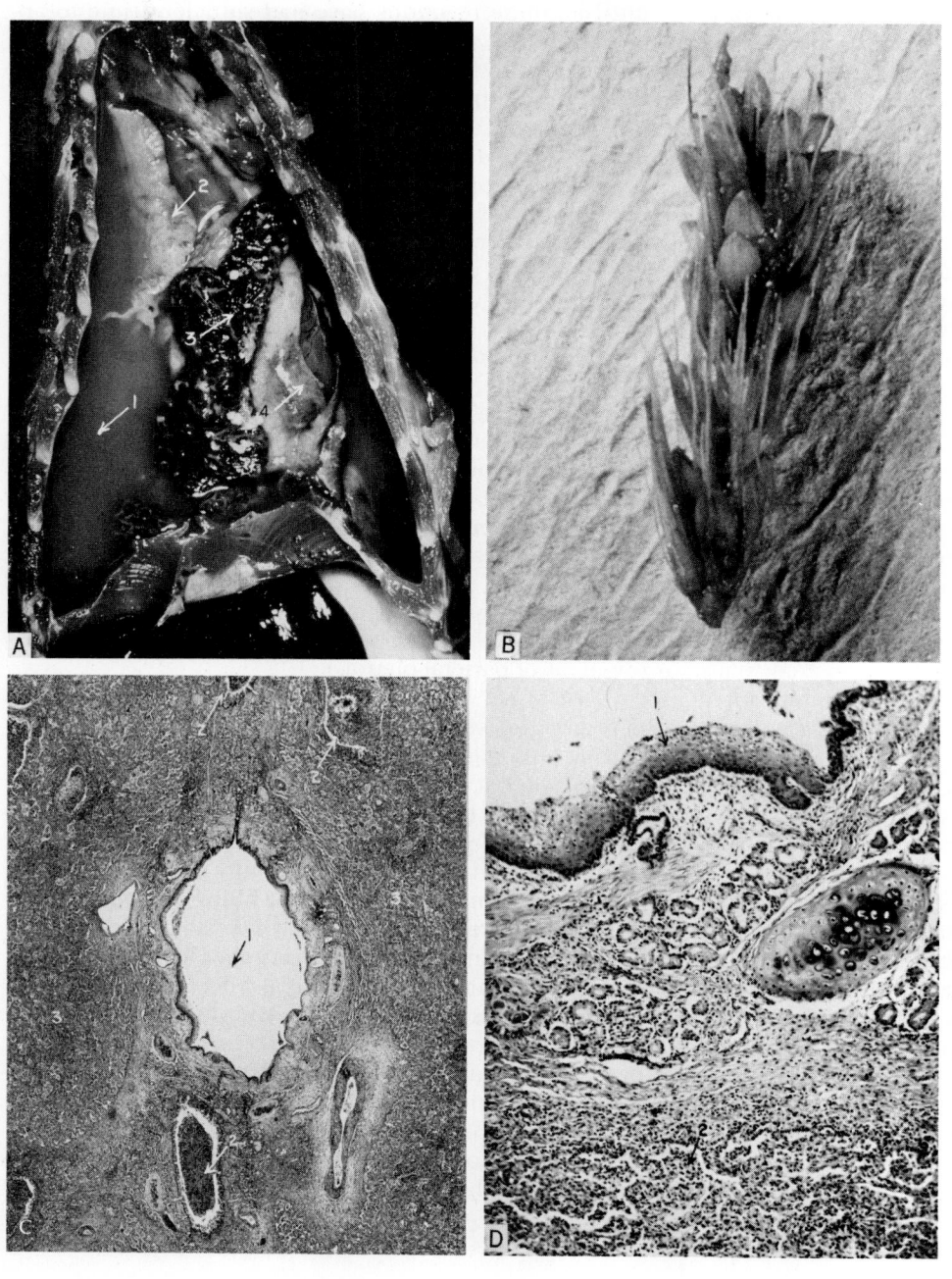

FIG. 20-9 Pyothorax and pneumonia secondary to aspiration of a grass awn by a male cat, age 1 1/2 years. **A.** the thorax at necropsy, containing purulent fluid (1), cardiac lobe of lung (2), fibrinous exudate in mediastinum (3), and fibrinous exudate on pericardium (4). **B.** Grass awn found in major bronchus at necropsy. **C.** Bronchus (1) in which the grass awn was found, secondary bronchi (2) and alveoli (3) are filled with purulent exudate. **D.** Higher magnification of **C.** Squamous metaplasia of bronchial epithelium (1) and consolidation (2) of alveoli. (H & E, ×125.) (Courtesy of Angell Memorial Animal Hospital.)

however, penetrate the pericardium and produce "traumatic pericarditis" rather than pleuritis. Tuberculous pleuritis is a fairly common accompaniment of tuberculosis of other parts. It manifests itself as "pearly disease," in which pleural surfaces, especially those of the thoracic wall, become studded with protruding, irregularly spherical tubercles, dense, white and shiny and thus reminiscent of pearls. They commonly have a diameter of 3 to 10 mm. Tuberculous infection may be hematogenous or it may be a direct extension from a tuberculous lung or possibly from a thoracic lymph node. In swine, pleuritis is part of a generalized serositis in two infections, Glasser's disease, caused by *Hemophilus suis,* and a serositis, caused by mycoplasma.

A considerable accumulation of purulent exudate (pus) in the pleural cavity is known as empyema. Hydrothorax denotes accumulation of (non-inflammatory) edema fluid in the pleural cavity. The watery fluid has the low specific gravity (1.017 or less) and the low protein content (4% or less) characteristic of a transudate. Hydrothorax is one of the manifestations of generalized edema, usually cardiac or renal. **Chylothorax** denotes the presence of chyle in the pleural cavity. This rare condition results from rupture or erosion of the thoracic duct. The chyle has a milky appearance. However, it is possible for edema fluid or serous exudate to appear milky from a high content of emulsified fat or albumin. Exudates may also accompany intrathoracic neoplasms. Pneumothorax is a rare condition in which air gains access to the pleural cavity. This may occur through a rupture of the chest wall, or through rupture of an emphysematous "bulla" or of some other air-containing lesion of the lung. If large amounts of air enter the pleural sac, the lung on the affected side collapses; pain and dyspnea result. In the horse, such an accident is likely to be fatal, for the right and left pleural cavities usually communicate, and the pneumothorax becomes bilateral. Cases are on record, nevertheless, of recovery from penetrating thoracic wounds.

References

Deem DA, Harrington DD. *Nocardia braziliensis* in a horse with pneumonia and pleuritis. Cornell Vet 1980;70:321–328.

Hultgren BD, Pearson EG, Lassen ED, et al. Pleuritis and pneumonia attributed to a conifer twig in a bronchus of a horse. J Am Vet Med Assoc 1986;189:797–798.

Kramek BA, Caywood DD, O'Brian TD. Bullus emphysema and recurrent pneumothorax in the dog. J Am Vet Med Assoc 1985; 186:971–974.

Fossum TW, Birchard SJ, Jacobs RM. Chylothorax in 34 dogs. J Am Vet Med Assoc 1986;188:1315–1318.

NON-INFLAMMATORY DISORDERS

Among the non-inflammatory disorders which may involve the lung, congestion, edema, infarction, thrombosis, and embolism have been treated at the appropriate places in the section on General Pathology.

Hemorrhages, usually recent, but sometimes old, with clotted fibrin occur in the lungs not only from septicemias and the other causes listed in the discussion of hemorrhage, but also as a result of uremia, presumably because of toxic injury to capillary walls. This may be an important explanation of the hemorrhages of leptospirosis.

While the lungs share in any generalized **passive congestion,** usually acute and terminal due to a failing heart muscle, it will be remembered that the usual chronic passive congestion is a result of interference with the prompt passage of blood through the left side of the heart. The resulting brown induration with its "heart-failure cells" due to phagocytized hemosiderin has been described. The possibility of hypostatic pneumonia supervening was mentioned under that heading.

In those cases in which recent and relatively acute pulmonary congestion and edema are prominent at autopsy, there is always the question whether one is dealing with active hyperemia and inflammatory edema which would have developed into full-fledged pneumonia if the patient had lived a few hours longer. The relative scarcity of pathogenic organisms when such lungs are submitted to bacterial culture suggests that most of these cases are the result of a failing heart rather than pneumonia. The tendency for the accumulation of fluid to be greatest in the more dependent portions of the lungs and the presence of congested vessels elsewhere in the body tend to confirm this interpretation. Acute hypersensitivity reactions may account for pulmonary edema, but in these examples there is diffuse involvement in all lobes. Anaphylaxis is a classic example, but hypersensitivity also plays a role in hypersensitivity pneumonitis of cattle.

The gross differentiation of the lung that is congested and edematous from one that is pneumonic may confuse the inexperienced. The former is voluminous with little or no tendency to collapse, well rounded and grayish pink, especially in the dorsal parts of the diaphragmatic lobes. It is doughy and "pits on pressure," but it does yield to pressure of the finger, while the hepatized lung is incompressible save for a slight "give" which lets the finger descend just a bit before it comes to an abrupt standstill. From the cut surface, a watery fluid, clear or blood stained, runs out either freely or upon the application of pressure, depending on the degree of severity. The microscopic differentiation is obvious from the nature of the processes involved.

Fibrin **emboli** lodge in the lungs if they are released into the circulation elsewhere but, on the whole, this is not frequent in animals. Fatty emboli are even more rarely recognized. Thrombi form in the vessels of the lungs during the course of severe pneumonias.

As has already been explained, infarction of the lung is unlikely to occur when the pulmonary and bronchial circulations are of normal force. Large infarcted areas tend to become gangrenous upon the advent of saprophytic bacteria, which are sure to be inhaled from time to time.

Atelectasis

This term means failure of the alveoli to open or to remain open; in other words, the empty alveoli are collapsed and do not contain air. The usual atelectasis involves one or more relatively small areas of lung. Such an area is slightly depressed and shrunken as compared to the surrounding tissue, and is sharply demarcated from it. The atelectatic area is dull red in color and has the feeling and consistency that one would expect, for instance, in liver. However, the hepatized tissue of pneumonia is swollen and not shrunken. Atelectatic, as well as hepatized, tissue sinks in water, or almost sinks if it still contains a bit of air. No fluid can be squeezed from its cut surface. Microscopically, the alveoli are compressed into scarcely recognizable slits, all lying parallel in a direction determined by adjacent pressures. Careful inspection will reveal that the cells are those which normally compose lung tissue. While well-filled capillaries may be seen, the total content of blood is less than the same tissue would have contained normally. The bronchioles are collapsed as far as their structure permits.

CAUSE

The cause of the usual atelectatic area is occlusion of the bronchus or bronchiole which supplies it. This results most often from a plug of mucous or purulent exudate. The air contained at the time the bronchus is closed is absorbed in a short time as is regularly the case with entrapped gases. The airless alveoli then collapse under surrounding pressures.

A lung collapsed because of pneumothorax is also obviously atelectatic, but the usual reference is merely to a portion of lung so affected. The collapse of the alveoli is scarcely so complete when it is the result of pneumothorax since the external pressure does not exceed that within the still patent bronchi. The same is true of areas of atelectasis resulting when pleural fluid occupies some of the space belonging to the lungs. Atelectasis also accompanies space-occupying lesions in the thoracic cavity and the accumulation of transudates and exudates when their volume is great.

Atelectasis neonatorum describes the non-aerated condition of the lungs of a newly born animal which has never breathed. The appearances are not remarkably different from those of atelectasis under other circumstances. The whole lung sinks in water. Determination of this condition may have legal import in settling controversies over breeding fees which are contingent upon the birth of living young. However, caution must be exercised in relying solely on whether the lung sinks in water, for such is occasionally the case in animals born alive, but dying in the perinatal period.

Emphysema

With a literal meaning of inflation, emphysema designates a condition in which there is air in the tissues. This may be, for instance, subcutaneous as the result of a cutaneous wound in such a location that movements exert a sucking or pumping action. It should not be confused with postmortem gas formation, which sometimes causes much gas to accumulate in the tissues as the result of bacterial action. Many times more frequent is pulmonary emphysema. Pulmonary emphysema is of two kinds, alveolar and interstitial (Fig. 20-10).

ALVEOLAR PULMONARY EMPHYSEMA

Without qualifying adjectives, it is alveolar pulmonary emphysema that is meant when reference is made to emphysema. In this ordinary emphysema, certain areas of lung are unduly distended with air. They are thereby distorted so that they project somewhat beyond the surrounding tissue, pale or almost white in color, dry, easily compressed by the finger, but not very resilient. This is because the compressing finger forces air out of the area through narrow openings and devious passageways; its movement can sometimes be recognized by the sensation in the finger. Then, upon removal of the finger the air returns slowly by the same route.

Microscopically, many alveoli are too large and many have wide openings into each other or into a common space due to rupture of alveolar walls. This situation is thus the exact opposite of atelectasis. The blunt ends of alveolar walls which have been broken often persist and become thickened and hyperplastic rounded knobs. Some of the walls are slightly thickened—hence, inelastic—but others are stretched and very thin. Blood-filled capillaries are scarce. The smooth muscle of the alveolar ducts is often hyperplastic.

Cause Frequently emphysematous areas of lung are seen near, or alternating with, areas of atelectasis. Such examples of emphysema represent areas of lung which have expanded unduly, under the pressure of inhaled air, to occupy the space left vacant by the collapsed, atelectatic portions. In doing this, some alveoli have been stretched beyond their capacity and have burst.

In other cases where there is difficult and forced respiration, a plug of mucus may have seriously but not completely impeded the passage of air in a given bronchus. At inspiration, the area connected with this bronchus slowly fills with air; then, by the forcible expiration which accompanies some acute respiratory diseases, the area in question is put under considerable pressure. The air cannot pass out through the bronchus as fast as this is accomplished in certain neighboring areas; the general pressure tends to force the full alveoli into space being vacated by neighboring emptying alveoli, and the full one is ruptured. The healing of ruptured alveoli involves enough light fibrosis to interfere with their elasticity, although it usually fails to restore the continuity of their walls.

INTERSTITIAL PULMONARY EMPHYSEMA

This is a condition in which air collects in the interlobular septa, beneath the pleura and wherever there is interstitial tissue in the lungs. Probably because of anatomical peculiarities, the condition is most often seen in necropsies on cattle. In these animals, various interlobular septa as much as 0.5 cm in thickness are seen in criss-crossing straight lines, usually at wider intervals than would be the case if every lobular wall were so thickened. The septum is shiny, well outlined, usually filled with large and small bubbles, and obviously distended with air. Microscopically, the increased width of

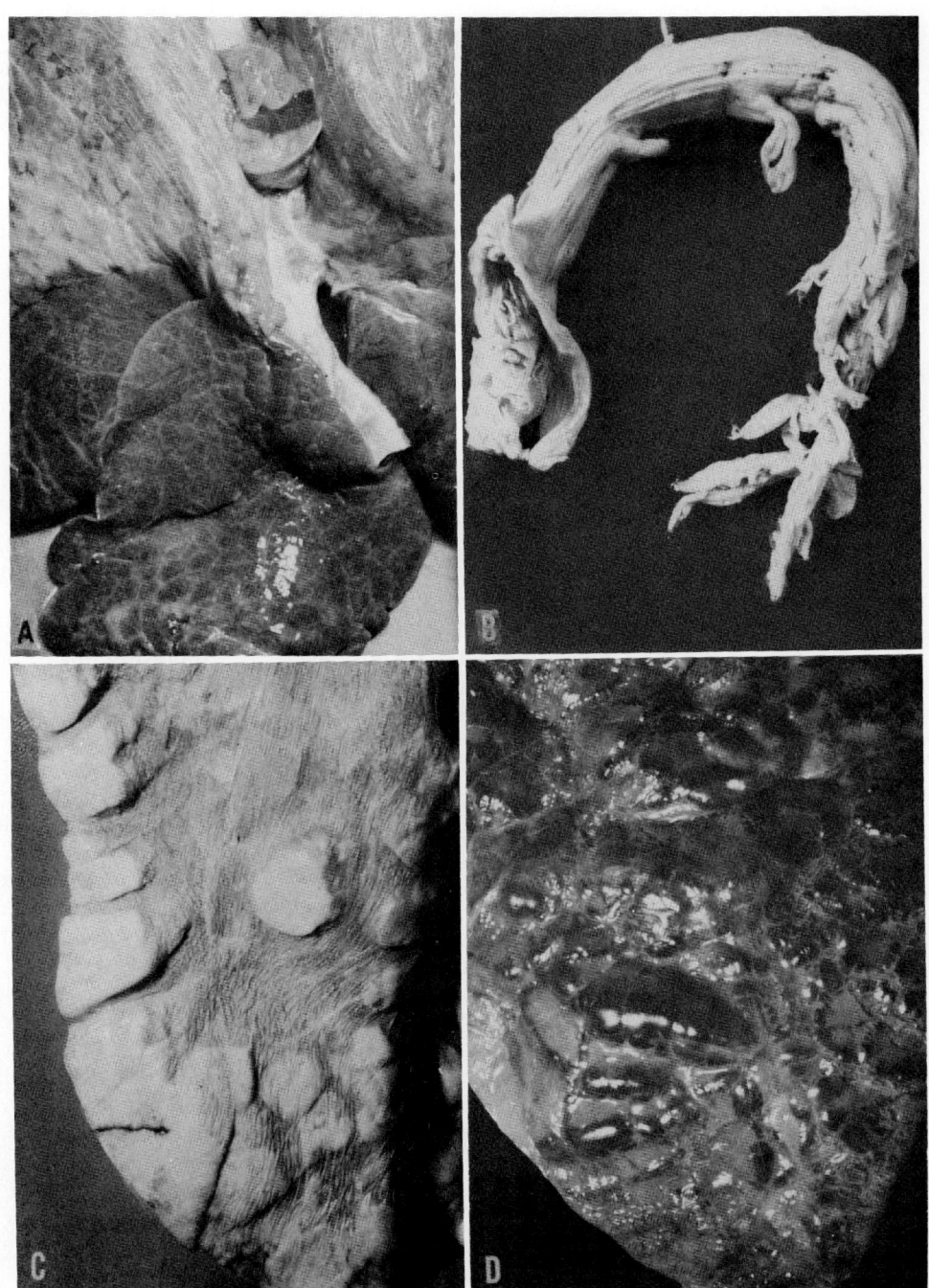

FIG. 20-10 A. Early red hepatization in the lung of a calf. **B.** A fibrinous cast from a bronchus and its branches. This was coughed up by a calf whose owner had noticed no sign of illness. **C.** Alveolar emphysema (raised pale areas) in the lung of a swine which died of swine erysipelas. **D.** Interstitial emphysema in the lung of a cow. Death was the result of pyelonephritis.

the septum is seen to be due to separation and distention of the fibers without any increase of tissue elements. It is reported that air from these emphysematous tissues sometimes finds its way into the mediastinal structures and even into the dorsal part of the neck.

Cause The air gains access to the interstitial tissues from alveoli which have ruptured during violent respiratory efforts. For this reason, this type of emphysema is most often seen as a terminal phenomenon when death from some other cause has been accompanied by violent efforts to compensate for growing anoxia. One of the most familiar situations of this sort is

death from loss of blood. This type of emphysema is clearly associated with severe respiratory efforts which appear to be caused by some impediment to the exchange of gases in the alveoli.

References

Goldring IP, et al. Histopathology and mechanical properties of the lung in experimental emphysema. Pathol Microbiol, 19703;5:176–180.

Kuhn C III, Tavassoli F. The scanning electron microscopy of elastase-induced emphysema: a comparison with emphysema in man. Lab Invest, 1976;34:2–9.

Kuhn C, et al. The induction of emphysema with elastase. II. Changes in connective tissue. Lab Invest, 1976;34:372–380.

McLauthlin RR, Jr., Edwards DW. Naturally occurring emphysema, the fine, gross and histopathologic counterpart of human emphysema. Am Rev Resp Dis, 1966;93:22–29.

Pushpakorn R, et al. Experimental papain-induced emphysema in dogs. Am Rev Respir Dis, 1970;102:778.

Strawbridge, HTG. Chronic pulmonary emphysema—an experimental study. Am J Pathol 1960;37:391–412.

BOVINE ACUTE PULMONARY EMPHYSEMA (ACUTE PULMONARY EDEMA AND EMPHYSEMA, "FOG FEVER," "ATYPICAL INTERSTITIAL PNEUMONIA")

This syndrome, described in many parts of the world, has often been confused with acute respiratory distress due to other diseases. Although diverse causes have been demonstrated, it appears that this syndrome has some fundamental features which merit considering it one disease, at least for the present. This disease appears abruptly, usually in adult cattle 2 to 10 days after they have been moved from dry, sparse grazing to lush, nutritious pasture. In Great Britain, beef-type adult cattle are usually affected during the fall months (August-November), after they have been moved to pasturage consisting of new growth which followed a recent cutting of hay. This grass that has regrown from an earlier cut for hay, is known by the ancient words "aftermath" or "foggage." Thus the name "fog fever" comes from "foggage" and has nothing to do with the event of nature that activates foghorns and sometimes closes airports.

The clinical onset is typically sudden in its severest form, with severe dyspnea, frothing at the mouth, mouth breathing, tachypnea and a loud expiratory grunt. Auscultation usually reveals inspiratory and expiratory sounds, occasionally with rales, and sometimes with the crackling sounds of emphysema. Death occurs within 2 days in about one third of the severely affected animals. The herd usually includes less severely affected animals that survive.

Gross lesions The gross lesions are essentially limited to the lungs, although severe congestion and hemorrhages are usually seen in tracheal and bronchial mucosa. The lumens of trachea and bronchi are filled with white frothy edema fluid. This fluid in terminal bronchi may be tinged with blood. Edema and emphysema are the most conspicuous lesions in the lungs. In severe cases, gas bubbles are seen in interlobular fascia in most lobes (most severe in diaphragmatic) of the lungs and form sub-pleural bullae up to 15 cm in diameter. The air also may extend into the mediastinum, mediastinal lymph nodes, and subcutis of the shoulders and back. Edema fluid often accompanies the gas bubbles. The lung is uniformly dark, congested and edematous, but not collapsed. The cut surface is smooth, homogeneous and exudes much edematous fluid.

Microscopic The microscopic features of the lesions include edema and hyaline membranes in most alveoli and alveolar ducts. The alveolar septae are edematous and congested. Alveolar epithelial cells are often conspicuous and type II pneumocytes are increased in number, usually lying in short rows. In non-fatal cases, killed several days after onset, proliferation of alveolar lining cells (type II pneumocytes) and accumulation of large monocytes in the alveoli are conspicuous features. This gives the lung an "edematous" or "fetalized" appearance. Monocytes and macrophages are numerous in the thickened, edematous septae, and some may be seen in alveoli. Emphysematous bullae may be seen under the pleura. The mediastinal lymph nodes are characteristically enlarged, congested, edematous, and filled with gas bullae.

Etiology At present writing, the etiology appears to consist of many factors, all perhaps acting through a common mechanism. The disease has been associated with lush pastures and specific types of plants including rape, turnips, *Brassica*, spoiled sweet potatoes, and other plants such as *Perilla frutescens* and stinkwood, (*Zieria arbonescens*). Of particular interest is the experimental production of the signs and lesions of this syndrome with several substances.

The amino acid DL tryptophan has been shown to produce this disease following oral administration. One ruminal fermentation product of tryptophan, 3-methylindole (skatole), has been shown to be even more active following intravenous or oral administration to cattle. Sheep and goats have also been reported to be susceptible to this experimental disease. A natural disease of sheep with many similarities to the bovine disease has been described. Demonstration of increased levels of tryptophan or 3-methylindole in the forage of naturally affected cattle has not been accomplished at this writing.

Spoiled sweet potatoes, infected with a mold *Fusarum solani*, have been demonstrated to produce fatal pulmonary edema and emphysema in cattle. Two toxic compounds have been isolated from these spoiled sweet potatoes: a furanoterpenoid, ipomeanarone, is a hepatoxin in mice; the second compound, 4-ipomeanol, a "lung edema factor" in mice, produces typical signs and lesions of acute pulmonary edema and emphysema when administered per os to cattle. The synthetic compound is also similarly toxic.

It seems likely that other toxic compounds may be demonstrated in connection with this bovine syndrome characterized by acute pulmonary edema and atelectasis.

References

Bradley BJ, Carlson JR, Dickinson EO. 3-Methylindole-induced pulmonary edema and emphysema in sheep. Am J Vet Res 1978;39:1355–1358.

Breeze RG, Pirie HM, Selman IE, et al. Fog fever in cattle: cytology of the hyperplastic alveolar epithelium. J Comp Pathol 1975;85:147–156.

Breeze RG, Pirie HM, Selman IE, et al. Fog fever (acute pulmonary emphysema) in cattle in Britain. Vet Bull 1976;46:243–251.

Carlson JR, Yokoyama MT, Dickinson EO. Tryptophan-induced interstitial pulmonary emphysema in cattle. II. 3-methylindole as a cause of pulmonary edema and emphysema in cattle and goats. Fed Proc 1972;31:681.

Carlson JR, Dickinson EO, Yokoyama MT, et al. Pulmonary edema and emphysema in cattle after intraruminal and intravenous administration of 3-methylindole. Am J Vet Res 1975;36:1341–1348.

Doster AR, Mitchell FE, Farrell RL, et al. Effects of 4-Ipomeanol, a product from mold-damaged sweet potatoes, on the bovine lung. Vet Pathol 1978;15:367–375.

Schiefer B, Jayasekara MU, Mills JHL. Comparison of naturally occurring and tryptophan-induced bovine atypical interstitial pneumonia. Vet Pathol 1974;11:327–339.

Turk MAM, Hank WG, Flory W. 3-methylindole-induced nasal mucosal damage in mice. Vet Pathol 1987;24:400–403.

OSSIFICATION IN THE LUNGS

In cows and in old dogs, cases occur from time to time in which considerable areas of lung are found with spicules or tiny plates of bone extensively distributed in the alveolar walls. These may reach a length of a millimeter or more. They lie entirely within the alveolar septum, which is thickened to accommodate them. Blood vessels are not involved. The bony formations never appear in the pleura nor in the peribronchial areas.

Severe ossification may occur in the lungs of cattle suffering from Manchester wasting disease (Chapter 15).

Neoplasms of the lung

Primary neoplasms of the lung are less frequent than secondary (metastatic) neoplasms in the lung and can usually be distinguished by careful microscopic study. Note that primary tumors are designated as being "of" the lung, secondary tumors are "in" the lung-a tiny detail that is significant to remember. Secondary tumors in the lung may be metastatic from any malignant neoplasm of any part of the body. If malignant cells become detached from a primary growth and are swept into lymphatics or veins, they soon reach the pulmonary circulation. The capillaries of the lung form a fine network through which all of the blood circulates. Tumor cells are readily entrapped and often find the lung a suitable place in which to grow.

Metastatic neoplasms usually maintain some of the histologic features of the primary lesion, which is useful in their identification, particularly when the primary is found and its histologic characteristics are identified. The identity of primary tumors is usually evident from their histologic appearance.

Primary benign and malignant neoplasms of the lung are known to occur in essentially every species that has been adequately studied among domestic, wild, zoo and laboratory animals, including vertebrate and invertebrate species. The observed frequency of these lesions depends upon several factors, including the age and genetic make up of the population, the adequacy of the pathologic examinations and the presence of environmental carcinogens. The most reliable indication of the incidence of neoplasms in a population is found in studies of laboratory animal species (especially rats, mice and hamsters) that are studied for definite periods (2 years, or lifetime) and are compared to suitable control animals kept in an identical environment. Studies of hospitalized animals are of interest but do not usually reflect the frequency of neoplasms in the general population. Species that are allowed to live out their life span (dogs, cats, some laboratory animals)will be found to have more tumors, which develop late in life.

Primary neoplasms of the lung that have been described in one or more animal species are listed and described below:

Adenoma, Adenocarcinoma
(bronchiolar/alveolar carcinoma)
Squamous cell carcinoma
(bronchogenic carcinoma)
Adenosquamous carcinoma
(mucoepidermoid carcinoma)
Chondroma, Chondrosarcoma
Mesenchymal Neoplasms
Lipoma, Liposarcoma
Fibroma, Fibrosarcoma
Hemangiosarcoma
Teratoma
Neuroendocrine tumor
(small cell tumor)
Mesothelioma of the pleura

Adenocarcinoma of the lung apparently arises from the epithelial cells of the alveoli, in some instances from the type II pneumocytes, but in other cases, characteristics of cells of the bronchiolar epithelium are evident in the neoplastic cells. This has led to the use of the term bronchiolar/alveolar carcinoma of the lung (Fig. 20-11). The tumor cells are usually columnar or cuboidal, but may be tall columnar with cilia and protruding cytoplasm. It is clear that these neoplastic cells grow into the alveoli and tend to maintain the structural outline of the alveoli. Acini are formed frequently and cells may become detached but usually remain in contact with adjacent epithelial tumor cells.

Pulmonary adenomatosis of sheep (jaagsiekte) is a disease presumed to be caused by a virus (see Chapter 8). The lesions resemble adenocarcinoma of the lung and may be difficult to distinguish.

Metastasis of adenocarcinoma to bronchial lymph nodes does occur. If the malignant cells get into the efferent lymphatics, they are carried, in turn, to the thoracic duct, the right atrium, right ventricle, and thence, through the pulmonary artery, back to the lungs. Thus metastasis of pulmonary tumors to other parts of the lung is readily accomplished (see Fig 20-11).

Squamous cell carcinoma is much less frequent than adenocarcinoma of the lung in most animal species. This tumor resembles the bronchiogenic carcinoma (squamous cell carcinoma) which is generally associated with cigarette smoking in the human population. The tumor appears to arise from the epithelium of the terminal bronchi which has undergone squamous metaplasia. It extends from its central position peripherally, eventually to involve much of the affected lobule, then the lobe of the lung. The histologic features of this tumor of the lung closely resemble those of sqamous cell carcinomas that originate from squamous epithelium elsewhere in the body.

Chondromas and chondrosarcomas appear to arise from cartilage in the terminal bronchi, and are much less frequent in animals than epithelial tumors.

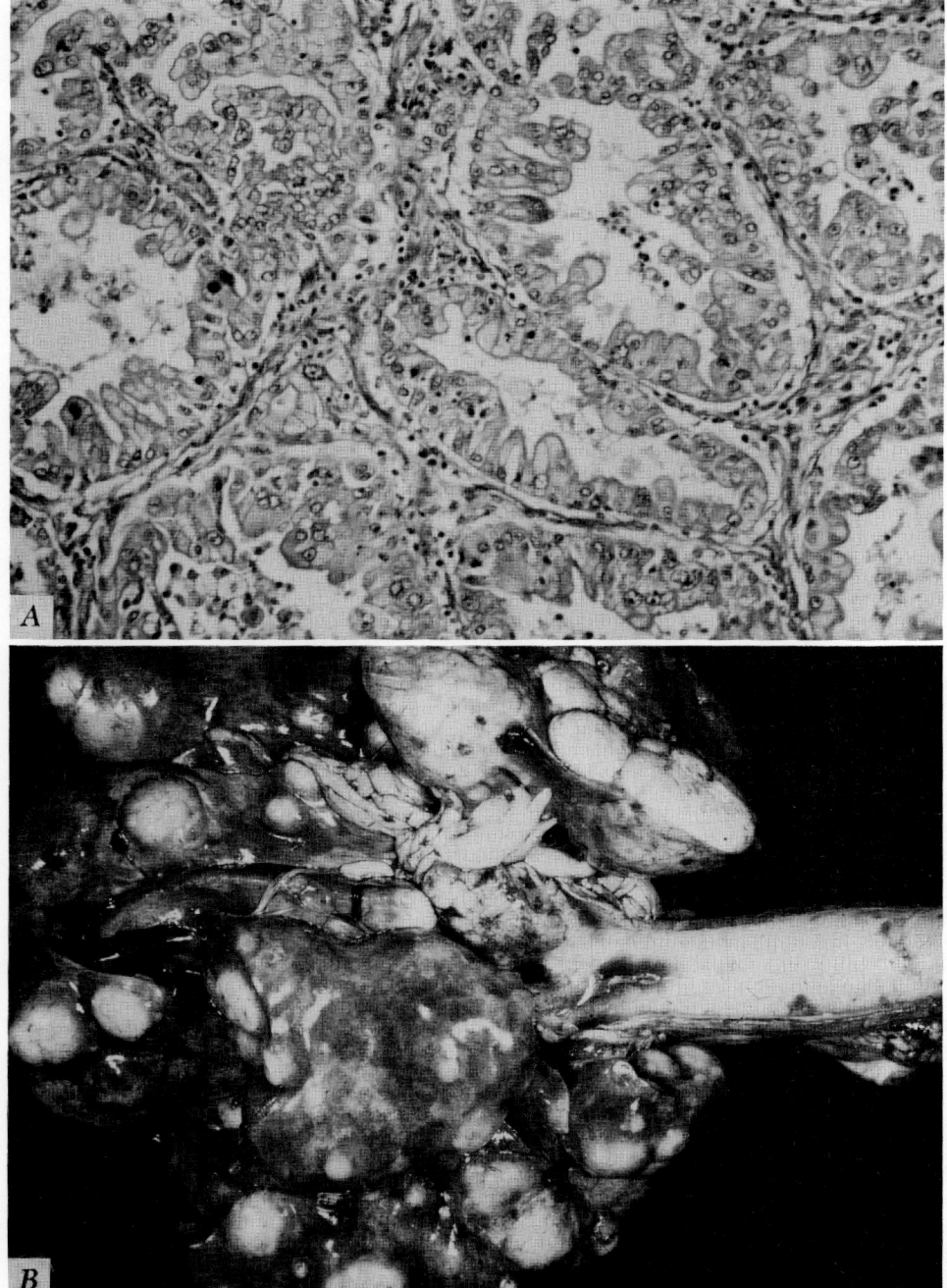

FIG. 20-11 Primary adenocarcinoma or bronchiolar-alveolar carcinoma of the lung of a Cocker-Dachshund, male, nine years old. **A.** Section of one of the tumor nodules. (H & E, ×200.) **B.** The gross lung. Note the large mass in the left lung that is believed to be the primary, and several spherical masses, each of about the same size, and other similar and smaller tumors. These are believed to result from separate metastatic "showers" of cells from the left lung. (Courtesy of Angell Memorial Animal Hospital.)

Other neoplasms arise primarily from the mesenchymal tissues of the lung. These include Lipoma, Liposarcoma, fibroma, fibrosarcoma hemangioma and hemangiosarcoma. These tumors are described elsewhere in this text in association with organ systems in which they are more frequent. **Teratomas,** made up of recognizable tissue from two or more germ cell layers, usually originate in the mediastinum but may involve the lung.

Mesothelioma of the pleura. The pleura may be host to metastatic tumors that reach the lung or arise in the mediastinum, but the only primary tumor is the mesothelioma. This tumor arises from the mesothelial lining of the pleural sac and resembles its parent cells (Fig 20-12). They are usually benign, but may interfere with respiration by their location and by the accompanying hydrothorax. They have been associated with asbestos and other mineral fibers in some laboratory species.

References

Boorman GA, Herbert RA. Alveolar/bronchiolar hyperplasia, adenoma and carcinoma, lung, rat. In: Jones TC, Dungworth DL, Mohr U, eds. Monograph on pathology of laboratory animals,

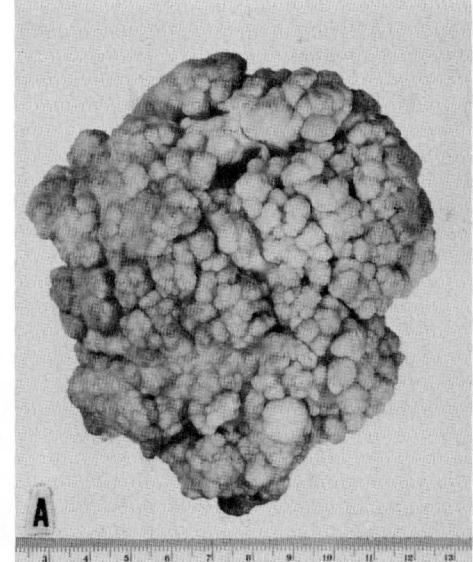
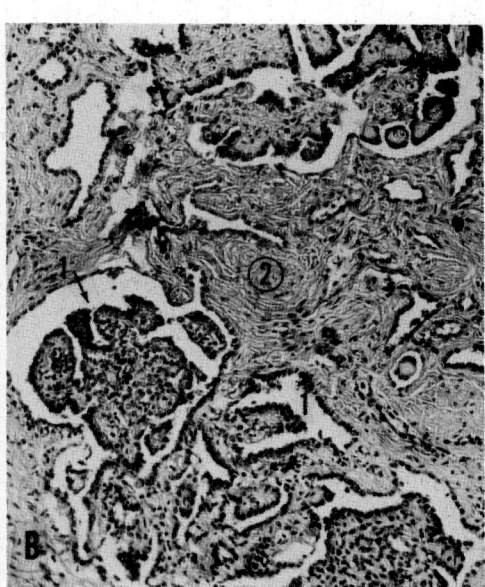

FIG. 20-12 Mesothelioma of the pleura of a six-year-old cow. **A.** Gross appearance of the nodular pleura. **B.** Photomicrograph (×105) showing papillary growth of mesothelium *(1)* and supporting stroma *(2)*. (Courtesy of Armed Forces Institute of Pathology.) Contributor: Dr. C.L. Davis.

respiratory system. 2nd ed. Heidelberg: Springer Verlag, 1996;174–183.

Cardesa A, Bombi JA. Pleural mesothelioma, Syrian hamster. In: Jones TC, Dungworth DL, Mohr U, eds. Monograph on Pathology of laboratory animals, respiratory system 2nd ed. Heidelberg: Springer Verlag, 1996;229–233.

Gould VE, Linnoila I, Memoli VA, et al. Neuroendocrine components of the bronchopulmonary tract: hyperplasia, dysplasia, and neoplasia. Lab Invest 1983;49:519–537.

Hamilton HB, Severin GA, Nold J. Pulmonary squamous cell carcinoma with intraocular metastasis. J Am Vet Med Assoc 1984;185:307–309.

Harrison ML, Godleski JJ. Malignant mesothelioma in urban dogs. Vet Pathol 1983;20:531–540.

Heath JA, Frith CH, Wang P-MM. A morphologic classification and incidence of alveolar-bronchiolar neoplasms in BALB/c female mice. Lab Invest 1982;32:638–647.

Leibelt AG. Metastatic tumors, lung, mouse. In: Jones TC, Dungworth DL, Mohr U, eds. Monograph on Pathology of laboratory animals, respiratory system. 2nd ed. Heidelberg: Springer Verlag, 1996;234–251.

Miller RI, Turk JR, Wells SK, et al. Carcinoma of type II pneumocytes in a striped skunk. Vet Pathol 1985;22:644–645.

Moulton JE, von Tscharmer C. Classification of lung carcinomas in the dog and cat. Vet Pathol 1981;18:513–528.

Palmer KC, Grammas P. Beta-cell adrenergic regulation of secretion from Clara cell adenomas of the mouse lung. Lab Invest 1987;56:329–334.

Rehm S. Comparative aspects of pulmonary carcinogenesis. In: Jones TC, Dungworth DL, Mohr U, eds. Monograph on Pathology of laboratory animals, respiratory system. 2nd ed. Heidelberg: Springer Verlag, 1996;158–173.

Rittinghousen S, Dungworth DL, Ernst H, et al. In: Jones TC, Dungworth DL, Mohr U, eds. Jones TC, Dungworth DL, Mohr U, eds. Monograph on Pathology of laboratory animals, respiratory system 2nd ed. Heidelberg Springer Verlag, 1996;182–206.

Suleman MA, Tarara R, Mandalia KM, et al. Aspontaneous bronchiogenic carcinoma in a Sykes monkey (*Cercopithecus mitis stuhlmani*) J Med Primatol 1984;13:153–157.

Schultze AE, Sonea I, Bell TG. Primary malignant pulmonary neoplasia in two horses. J Am Vet Med Assoc 1988;193:477–480.

21
Cardiovascular system

CONGENITAL CARDIOVASCULAR ANOMALIES

Congenital disorders of the heart and great vessels are among the most frequently encountered and most important anomalies in animals (Figs. 21-1, 21-2, 21-3). The most serious anomalies may not be compatible with fetal life; others, although fully compatible with fetal survival, become apparent with the change from fetal to postnatal circulation. These may lead to rapid development of clinical signs and death due to heart failure early in life: they may at first be inapparent, but slowly lead to heart failure; or they may allow survival into adulthood, although with impaired function. Simplistically, cardiac anomalies can be divided into the following:

(1) Defects that allow shunting of blood from right to left or the reverse;
(2) Defects that lead to obstruction of blood flow;
(3) Valvular defects that may lead to obstruction of flow or regurgitation;
(4) Abnormal arterial and venous connections or positioning; and,
(5) Malposition of the heart.

Many congenital anomalies involve various combinations of this grouping. To a great extent, the consequences of those defects that allow shunting of blood depend upon whether they lead to shunting from left to right or the reverse. Right-to-left shunts lead to inadequate oxygenation of blood and tissue hypoxia. Left-to-right shunts do not have this consequence; however, over time such shunts lead to pulmonary hypertension, right ventricular hypertrophy, and reversal of flow from right to left leading to tissue anoxia. Obstructive defects, when severe, lead to rapid development of heart failure or acute respiratory distress. Valvular diseases allowing back flow have similar consequences.

Although some are inherited as polygenic traits, in general the cause of congenital cardiovascular defects is unknown. They are encountered in all species of animals. Some of the most frequently encountered anomalies are discussed in this section.

DEFECTS THAT ALLOW SHUNTING OF BLOOD: LEFT-TO-RIGHT SHUNTS

Patent ductus arteriosus

In the fetus, one of the mechanisms to divert blood from the lung is by means of the ductus arteriosus, a short blood vessel that leads from the pulmonary artery to the aorta. Following birth, the flow of blood to the lungs through the pulmonary artery is suddenly magnified, and the diversion through the ductus is no longer required. Within a few days after birth, the lumen of the ductus is closed and eventually permanently sealed, the remnant remaining as the ligamentum arteriosum. In this common congenital cardiac defect of humans and animals, the lumen remains open with blood shunted from the aorta to the pulmonary artery (left-to-right shunt), which eventually results in right ventricular hypertrophy and anoxia. Patent ductus arteriosus is characterized by a continuous murmur that sounds like machinery. A review of 532 examples of patent ductus arteriosus in dogs identified the anomaly most frequently in miniature and toy poodles (Ackerman et al., 1978).

ATRIAL SEPTAL DEFECTS

During embryogenesis, the common atrial chamber is divided by the growth of a membranous structure termed the **septum primum.** Initially, this is incomplete with an opening, the **ostium primum,** near the atrioventricular valves. Normally, early in the embryogenesis of the heart, continued growth of the septum primum leads to closure of the ostium primum, but fenestrations that develop in the middle of the septum result in a second opening, the **ostium secundum.** Later a second membrane, the **septum secundum,** formed to the right of the ostium secundum results in an incomplete septum which, along with the lower part of the septum primum, forms a valve overlying the ostium secundum. The septum primum serves as the moving portion of the valve. The channel between the two atria is now termed the **foramen ovale.** In fetal life, oxygenated blood flows through the foramen ovale from the right atrium to the left atrium owing to the greater pressure in the right atrium. After birth, with a reversal of pres-

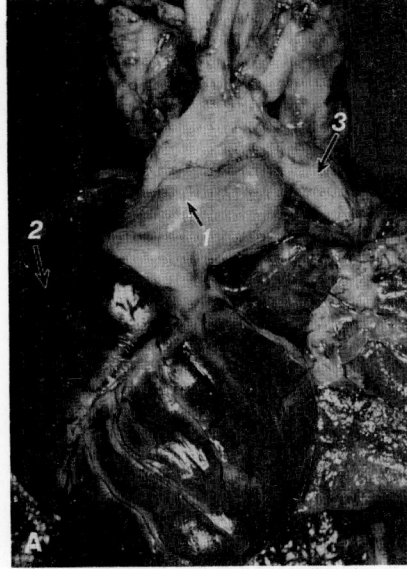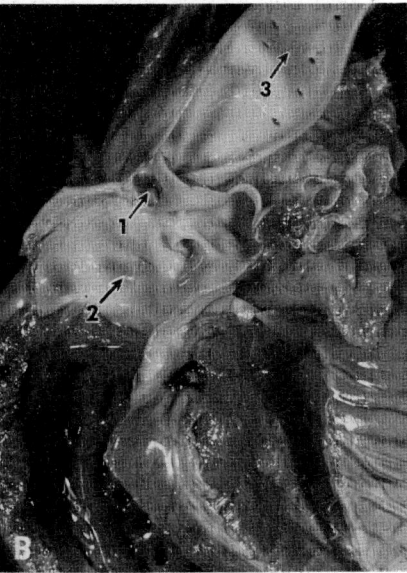

FIG. 21-1 Congenital cardiac anomalies. **A.** Pulmonary stenosis in a seven-month-old German shepherd. 1 The pulmonary artery is dilated due to the "jet effect" of the blood flow through the stenotic aperture at the level of the pulmonary valves. 2 The right atrium is hypertrophied. 3 Aorta. **B.** Aortic-pulmonary communication 1 through a patent ductus arteriosus between 2 the pulmonary artery and 3 aorta. A male Cocker spaniel, 6½ months old. (Courtesy of Angell Memorial Animal Hospital.)

sure gradient, the valvular opening is closed, preventing flow from left to right. The two membranes normally completely fuse, although a small, potential—but functionally closed—orifice often remains and may be detected with a probe at necropsy.

Atrial septal defects can arise from: (1) failure in the closing of the ostium primum; or (2) failure of the septum primum and septum secundum to provide closure of the ostium secundum (patent foramen ovale). A third anomaly that can lead to an atrial septal defect is a failure in the separation of the pulmonary veins and the anterior vena cava, which is referred to as **sinus venosus**. Initially, flow of blood is from the left to the right atrium and does not lead to clinical signs. Small

defects in the septum are well tolerated and may persist into adulthood without significant effect on the health of the animal. With larger defects, the flow of blood from left to right ultimately leads to right ventricular hypertrophy and pulmonary hypertension and a reversal of flow from right to left leading to cyanosis.

VENTRICULAR SEPTAL DEFECTS

Initially in embryonic life, the ventricles consist of a single chamber that is eventually divided into the left and right ventricles by the growth of the interventricular septum. The muscular wall grows upward from the apex of the heart toward the atrioventricular partition. Fusion with the membranous portion of the septum

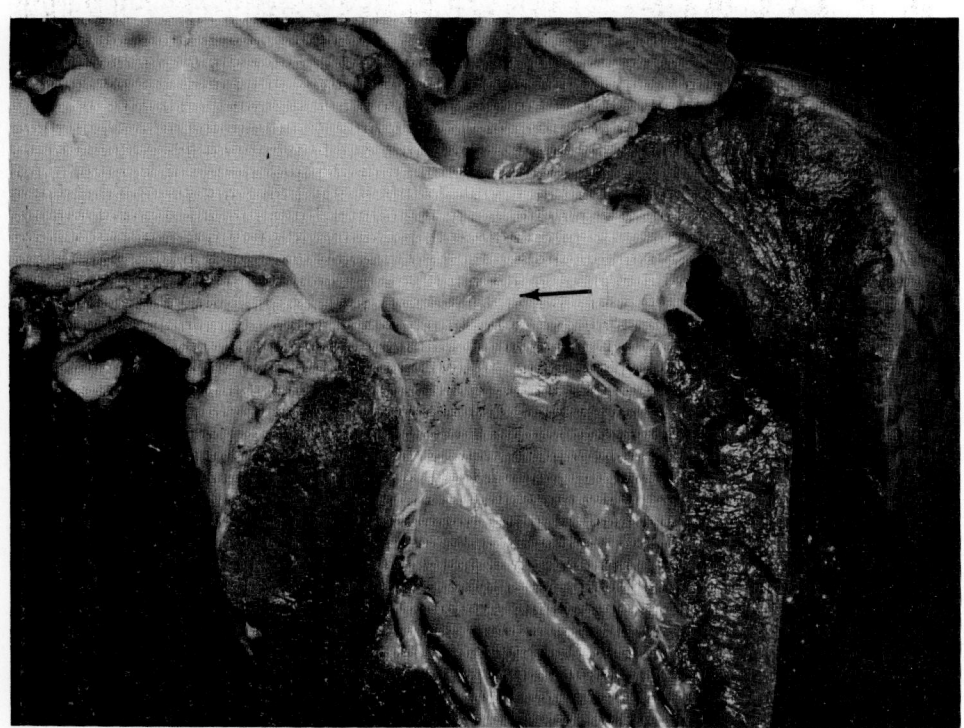

FIG. 21-2 Congenital subaortic stenosis in a six-month-old male German shepherd. Note subaortic constricting band (arrow). (Courtesy of Angell Memorial Animal Hospital.)

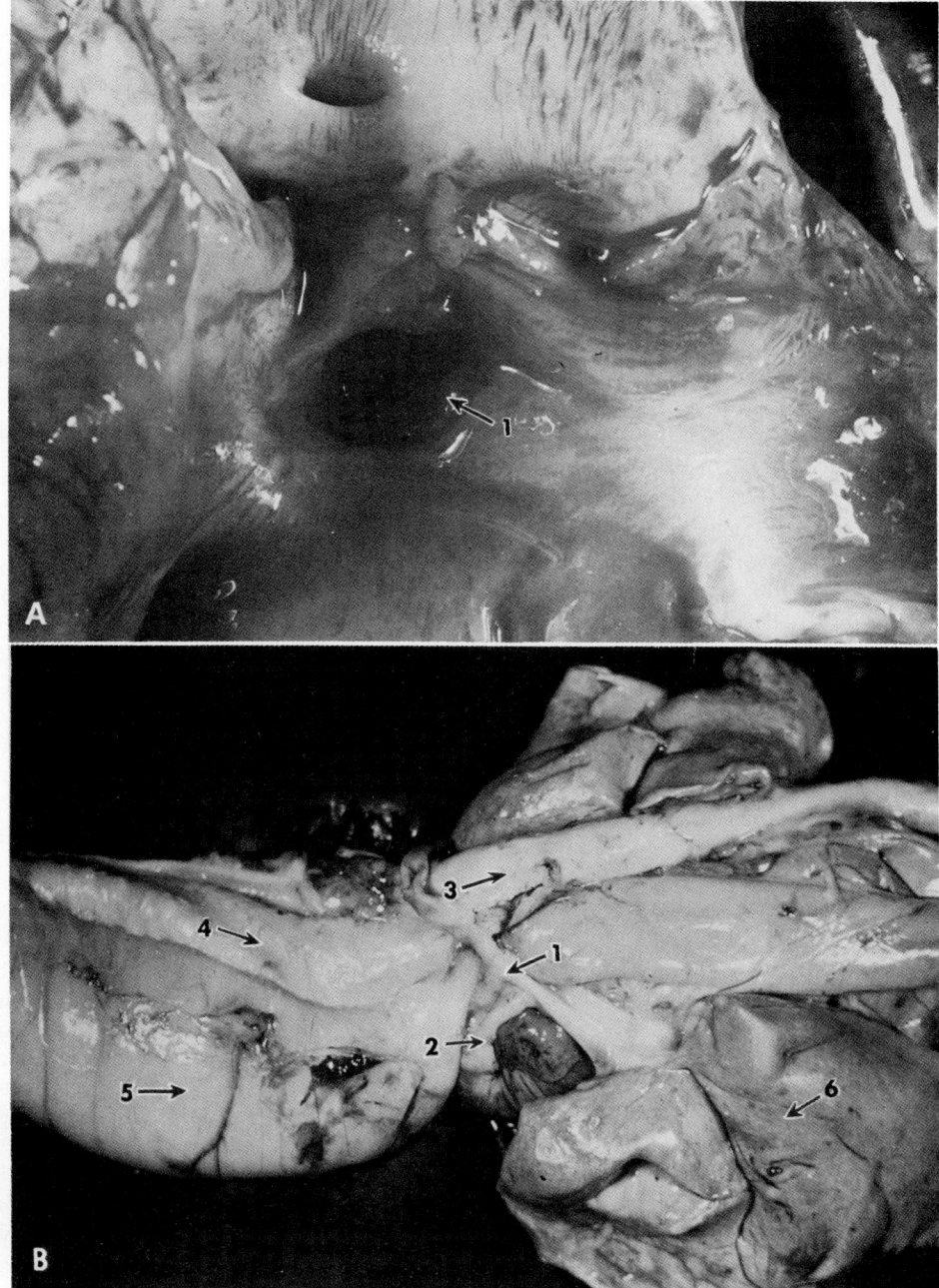

FIG. 21-3 Congenital cardiac anomalies. **A.** Interventricular septal defect 1 in a seven-month-old male German Shepherd puppy (same animal with pulmonary stenosis in Figure 21-1, **A**). **B.** Persistent right aortic arch. 1 The ductus arteriosus completes a vascular ring with 2 the pulmonary artery and 3 aorta. This ring encircles and compresses 4 the trachea and 5 esophagus, which is dilated. 6 The lung is also labeled. This lesion was found in a 10-week-old male German Shepherd. (Courtesy of Angell Memorial Animal Hospital.)

growing downward from the bulbus arteriosus—which eventually divides the aorta and pulmonary artery—results in the closure of communication between ventricles relatively early in embryonic life. Failure of this fusion results in a ventricular septal defect that may be occult (probe patent) or large (Fig. 21-3A). Because of the origin of the membranous part of the interventricular septum, defects in it are often associated with anomalies in the aorta and pulmonary artery.

Small defects in the septum do not significantly impair function and many ultimately repair themselves. Larger and multiple defects result in a left-to-right shunting of blood which, as with other left-to-right shunts, ultimately leads to right ventricular hypertrophy, pulmonary hypertension, and reversal of flow to a right-to-left shunt leading to cyanosis. The endocardium may be thickened and roughened due to the turbulence around the orifice between the ventricles, and the endocardium of the right ventricle opposite the opening may also be thickened as a result of the jet stream of blood from the orifice.

RIGHT TO LEFT SHUNTS
Transposition of the great vessels

Several anomalies in the origin of the aorta and pulmonary artery are possible. The aorta and pulmonary artery may be transposed, the aorta arising from the right ventricle and the pulmonary artery from the left. The right ventricle, thus, becomes the arterial side of the heart, receiving blood from the left atrium, and the left ventricle becomes the venous side, receiving blood from the right atrium. The right ventricle becomes hypertrophic, but in the absence of other anomalies functionally normal circulation is manifest. In another form of transposition, the aorta arises from the right ventricle and the pulmonary artery from the left ventricle; however, the right ventricle remains the venous side and the left ventricle the arterial side, thus resulting in two separate and unconnected circulations which are obviously not compatible with extrauterine life. During fetal life the foramen ovale and ductus arteriosus allow mixing of the two circulations. If these and other communications (such as interventricular septal defect) were to persist postnatally, enough mixing of blood may permit survival, albeit compromised.

The aorta and pulmonary artery may fail to divide, persisting as a large, single blood vessel, the **persistent truncus arteriosus.** This results in mixing of venous and arterial blood and cyanosis, along with right ventricular hypertrophy and pulmonary hypertension. Less severe forms of this anomaly result from partial failure in division of the aorta and pulmonary artery, leaving communication between the two vessels. This has been termed **partial truncus arteriosus** or **aorticopulmonary window.** Rarely, the aorta and pulmonary artery may both arise from either the right or left ventricle (**double outlet right or left ventricle**). A large ventricular septal defect can make this anomaly compatible with life. Transpositions of the arteries are among the most frequent cardiac anomalies in cattle.

Tetralogy of Fallot

The four features of tetralogy of Fallot include:

(1) Ventricular septal defect;
(2) Aorta that overrides the ventricular septal defect (biventricular origin of the aorta, dextraposition of the aortic valve);
(3) Pulmonary or subpulmonic stenosis causing obstruction of right ventricular outflow; and,
(4) Compensatory hypertrophy of the right ventricle.

Tetralogy of Fallot develops from an embryonic failure of development of the interventricular septum and displacement of the conal septum, leading to an overriding aorta and obstruction of right ventricular outflow. It often exists in conjunction with other cardiac anomalies. The extent of each of these anomalies determines the seriousness of tetralogy of Fallot which, however, nearly always leads to cyanosis. It is the degree of pulmonary stenosis that is most critical. In severe pulmonary stenosis, right-to-left shunting of blood occurs with cyanosis. Pulmonary circulation, in part, may be compensated for by persistent ductus arteriosus which lessens the severity of the anomaly. If pulmonary stenosis were not severe and the septal defect large, left-to-right shunting of blood may occur without critical signs. However, even under this circumstance, with growth of the heart pulmonary stenosis increases in severity, ulti-

mately leading to right-to-left shunting. Patterson et al. reported an unusually high frequency of an anomaly resembling the tetralogy of Fallot in Keeshonds (1974).

A related combination of cardiac defects, the **Eisenmenger complex,** has been reported in humans and animals. This complex differs from the tetralogy of Fallot in that pulmonary stenosis is not present. Thus, it consists of interventricular septal defect, overriding aorta (dextraposition), and hypertrophy of the right ventricle. The absence of pulmonary stenosis makes this combination much less serious, and it may exist without cyanosis.

DEFECTS THAT LEAD TO OBSTRUCTION OF BLOOD FLOW

Subaortic stenosis

Subaortic stenosis, a not infrequent congenital cardiac defect in animals results from the formation of a constricting band of dense fibrous connective tissue at a point in the left ventricle just below the aortic semilunar valves (Fig. 21-2). The valves may be essentially normal or slightly distorted by the fibrous band which restricts the outflow of blood into the aorta. The left ventricle undergoes hypertrophy and the aorta above the valves becomes dilated. Thickened and fibrotic intramural arteries in the adjacent myocardium have been described.

Coarctation of the aorta

Coarctation is a narrowing of the aorta which is usually localized to a short segment near or immediately before the attachment of the ductus arteriosus, although longer sections can be involved and coarctation can occur at any point along the aorta. In those examples near the ductus arteriosus, the ductus is often open, which helps supply adequate blood to the systemic circulation. In humans, preductal coarctation (also termed "infantile" coarctation) is usually severe enough to lead to inadequate systemic circulation and congestive heart failure. Postductal coarctation in humans ("adult" coarctation) is usually less severe. Both forms lead to cardiomegaly.

Pulmonary stenosis

In pulmonary stenosis, the lumen of the pulmonary artery is narrowed, most usually below the valve near its origin from the right ventricle, by fibrous connective tissue. The weir or "jet" effect on the blood forced through this narrow orifice results in somewhat bullous distortions of the pulmonary artery (Fig. 21-1). The increased resistance results in hypertrophy of the right ventricle. Pulmonary stenosis is one of the most frequent cardiac anomalies in dogs.

VALVULAR DEFECTS

Congenital defects of various heart valves have much the same functional effects as acquired valvular disease. In domestic animals, they have been most often observed in dogs, cats, and swine. **Anomalous aortic valve with stenosis** resembles subaortic stenosis, but results from an aortic valve that develops as a constrictive ring. The effect is dependent upon the size of the opening. When adequate to permit survival, left ventricular hypertrophy occurs. **Anomalous pulmonary valve** development leads to a narrow opening and much the same consequences as pulmonary stenosis. Abnormal development of the leaflets of the **tricuspid valve** can result in a valve that is misshapen with thickenings, reduced size or absent leaflets, or a valve that is downwardly displaced into the right ventricle, the so called **Ebstein anomaly.** In the latter, the right ventricle is smaller than normal. These disorders of the tricuspid valve lead to incomplete filling of the right ventricle with regurgitation of blood resulting in a significantly enlarged right atrium. In humans, a large atrial septal defect often is present which allows shunting of blood from right to left. Congenitally-deformed **mitral valves** also result in regurgitation of blood with enlargement of the left ventricle and atrium. The endocardium becomes thickened with deposition of fibrous connective tissue.

ABNORMAL ARTERIAL AND VENOUS CONNECTIONS OR POSITIONINGS

Persistent right aortic arch

The aortic arches are formed early in embryonic life as paired structures, some of which atrophy, others which develop to become part of the cardiovascular system of the fetus and matured adult. The aorta normally develops from the left fourth aortic arch. This places the aorta and the ductus arteriosus on the same (left) side of the trachea and esophagus. If the aorta were to develop by persistence of the right fourth arch, the aorta would be on the right side of the trachea and esophagus. The ductus arteriosus (ligamentum arteriosum), by connecting the aorta and pulmonary artery, forms a vascular ring around the trachea and esophagus. As the young animal develops, the esophagus and later the trachea will be partially occluded by the vascular ring (Fig. 21-3B). This anomaly has been observed most frequently in dogs.

Double aortic arch is a condition in which both the right and left aortic arches persist. Usually, the right arch is the larger of the two. The consequences are much the same as in persistent right aortic arch with esophageal and tracheal constriction by the ductus arteriosus (ligamentum arteriosum). Another aortic anomaly is **interruption of the aortic arch** which, in the absence of collateral circulation, is not compatible with life. It has been described in dogs and horses in association with patent ductus arteriosus and ventricular septal defects.

Other examples of major vessel anomalies include: persistent left cranial vena cava; anomalous pulmonary veins; retroesophageal right subclavian artery; anomalous origin of the carotid arteries; arteriovenous fistulae; anomalous origin of the pulmonary arteries; and double renal arteries. Most of these types of anomalies do not interfere with function. **Portocaval (portosystemic) venous shunts,** through persistence of the **ductus venosus** or other congenital anastomoses, are not infrequent in dogs and cats. These allow portal blood to bypass the liver, leading to toxemia, hepatic encephalopathy, and hepatic atrophy.

MALPOSITION OF THE HEART

Ectopia cordis is a rare condition in which the entire heart lies outside the thorax. The most frequent site is under the subcutis in the cervical or pectoral region (Fig. 4-4). The sternum is abnormally shaped and often split. Usually abnormalities in the branching patterns of the major vessels occur from the aorta and often duplication of the cranial vena cava. Rarely, the heart can also be positioned in the abdomen. The condition has been reported most often in cattle. Ectopia cordis is not always fatal.

OTHER CARDIAC AND VASCULAR ANOMALIES

Endocardial fibroelastosis

This rare, congenital malformation has been observed most often in cats, but has also been described in dogs, cattle, sheep, and swine. In cats, it is most common in Siamese and Burmese breeds and appears to be an inherited disorder. As the name implies, the endocardium is thickened by layers of fibrous and elastic tissue, giving the endocardial surface a white to silvery glistening appearance. It usually involves the left atrium and left ventricle to the level of the aortic valves. Left and right ventricular hypertrophy and dilatation of the left atrium occur. Lesions in cats develop in the first few weeks of life and eventually lead to signs and lesions of heart failure. Degeneration of Purkinje fibers is suggested to be of importance to the development of heart failure.

Anomalies of pericardium

Rarely, the pericardium may be totally or partially absent. The most striking anomaly is the presence of an orifice in the pericardium extending through the diaphragm into the peritoneal sac. Herniation of liver and intestines through such an orifice may lead to dramatic clinical consequences. This has occurred in the dog and cat.

CONGENITAL HEREDITARY LYMPHEDEMA

This is a rare disorder resulting from abnormal morphogenesis of the peripheral lymphatic system, resulting in failure to establish connections with the central lymphatic system. It is recognized in humans (Milroy disease), dogs, Ayrshire cattle, and swine. In humans and dogs, the inheritance is an autosomal-dominant trait with variable expression, whereas in cattle and swine, it is an autosomal-recessive trait. Edema may be generalized, in which case neonatal death is the usual outcome, but more usually, edema is restricted to the hind limbs. Other body parts (e.g., ears) may also be affected. In mildly affected pups, edema gradually disappears by about the age of three months. Microscopically, lymphatics in the dermis and subcutis are markedly dilated. In dogs, regional lymph nodes, most often the popliteal and/or axillary, are absent.

FREQUENCY AND ETIOLOGY OF CARDIOVASCULAR ANOMALIES

Although they have been recognized in almost all species of animals, cardiovascular anomalies are reportedly most frequent in dogs, cats, and cattle. The studies of Detweiler et al. (1960) and Patterson (1968) contributed to the understanding of these anomalies in dogs. According to these authors, the prevalence rate of cardiovascular malformations among dogs studied in a large university veterinary clinic was 6.8 per 1000 admissions. Purebred dogs have higher, breed-specific prevalence rates than do mongrels, and patent ductus arteriosus in dogs (as in humans) is more prevalent in females than in males. These authors presented evidence that genetic factors have a bearing on the occurrence of several such cardiovascular anomalies. The frequency of many can be increased by selective matings in certain families of dogs.

Patterson (1968) reported cardiovascular anomalies in 290 dogs studied over a 13-year period. His data are summarized in Table 21-1.

References

Ackerman N, Burk R, Hahn AW, et al. Patent ductus in the dog: a retrospective study of radiographic, epidemiologic, and clinical findings. Am J Vet Res 1978;39:1805–1810.

Anilkumar TV, Sandhyamani S. Atrial septal defect in a bonnet macaque (*Macaca radiata*). J Med Primatol 1990;19:749–752.

Barrett RE, et al. Four cases of congenital portacaval shunt in the dog. J Small Anim Pract 1976;17:71–85.

Bayly WM, et al. Multiple congenital heart anomalies in five Arabian foals. J Am Vet Med Assoc 1982;181:684–689.

Belling TH, Jr. Ventricular septal defect in the bovine heart—report of three cases. J Am Vet Med Assoc 1961;138:595–598.

Bolton GR, Ettinger SJ, Liu S-K. Tetralogy of Fallot in three cats. J Am Vet Med Assoc 1972;160:1622–1631.

Bush M, et al. Tetralogy of Fallot in a cat. J Am Vet Med Assoc 1972;161:1679–1686.

Butterfield AB, Hix WR, Pickrel JC, et al. Acquired peripheral arteriovenous fistula in a dog. J Am Vet Med Assoc 1980;176:445–448.

Cargile J, Lombard C, Wilson JH, et al. Tetralogy of Fallot and segmental uterine aplasia in a three-year-old Morgan filly. Cornell Vet 1991;81:411–418.

Clark ES, Reef VB, Sweeney CR, et al. Aortic valve insufficiency in a one-year-old colt. J Am Vet Med Assoc 1987;191:841–844.

Cordy DR, Ribelin WE. Six congenital cardiac anomalies in animals. Cornell Vet 1950;40:249–256.

Dennis SM, Leipold HW. Congenital cardiac defect in lambs. Am J Vet Res 1968;29:2337–2340.

Detweiler DK, Hubben K, Patterson DF. Survey of cardiovascular disease in dogs. Am J Vet Res 1960;21:329–359.

Easley JC, Carpenter JL. Hepatic arteriovenous fistula in two Saint Bernard pups. J Am Vet Med Assoc 1975;166:167–171.

Eliot TS, et al. First report of the occurrence of neonatal endocardial fibroelastosis in cats and dogs. J Am Vet Med Assoc 1958;133:271–274.

Eyster GE, et al. Ebstein's anomaly: a report of three cases in the dog. J Am Vet Med Assoc 1977;170:709–713.

Eyster GE, et al. Coarctation of the aorta in a dog. J Am Vet Med Assoc 1976;169:426–428.

Feldman EC, Nimmo-Wilkie JS, Pharr JW. Eisenmenger's syndrome in the dog: case reports. J Am Anim Hosp Assoc 1981;17:477–483.

Gaag I, Van Der, Luer RJT, Van Der. Eight cases of pericardial defects in the dog. Vet Pathol 1977;14:14–18.

Gandolfi RC. Hepatoencephalopathy associated with patent ductus venosus in a cat. J Am Vet Med Assoc 1984;185:301–302.

Gopal T, Leipold HW, Dennis SM. Congenital cardiac defects in calves. Am J Vet Res 1986;47:1120–1121.

Gordon B, Trautvetter E, Patterson DF. Pulmonary congestion associated with cor triatriatum in a cat. J Am Vet Med Assoc 1982;180:75–77.

Greene HJ, Wray DD, Greenway JA. Two equine congenital cardiac anomalies. Irish Vet J 1975;29:115–117.

Hadlow WJ, Ward JK. Atresia of the right atrioventricular orifice in an Arabian foal. Vet Pathol 1980;17:622–626.

Hamlin RL, Smetzer DL, Smith RC. Interventricular septal defect (Roger's disease) in the dog. J Am Vet Med Assoc 1964;145:331–340.

Hiraga T, Abe M, Iwasa K, et al. Cervico-pectoral ectopia cordis in two Holstein calves. Vet Pathol 1993;30:529–534.

Hsu FS, Du SJ. Congenital heart disease in swine. Vet Pathol 1982;19:676–686.

Jacobs G, Patterson D, Knight D. Complete interruption of the aortic arch in a dog. J Am Vet Med Assoc 1987;191:1585–1588.

Jeraj K, et al. Double outlet right ventricle in a cat. J Am Vet Med Assoc 1978;173:1356–1360.

Jeraj K, et al. Atrial septal defects (sinus venosus type) in a dog. J Am Vet Med Assoc 1980;177:342–346.

Johnson CA, Armstrong PJ, Hauptman JG. Congenital portosystemic shunts in dogs: 46 cases (1979–1986). J Am Vet Med Assoc 1987;191:1478–1483.

Kemler AG, Martin JE. Incidence of congenital cardiac defects in bovine fetuses. Am J Vet Res 1972;33:249–251.

Linde-Sipman JS, van der. Hypoplasia of the left ventricle in four ruminants. Vet Pathol 1978;15:474–480.

Linde-Sipman JS, van der, Ingh TSGAM van den, Koeman JP. Congenital heart abnormalities in the cat. A description of sixteen cases. Zentralbl Veterinaermed 1973;20A:419–425.

Linton GA. Anomalies of the aortic arches causing strangulation of the esophagus and trachea. J Am Vet Med Assoc 1956;129:1–5.

Liu S-K, Tilley LP. Dysplasia of the tricuspid valve in the dog and cat. J Am Vet Med Assoc 1976;169:623–630.

Ljunggren G, et al. Four cases of congenital malformation of the heart in a litter of eleven dogs. J Small Anim Pract 1966;7:611–623.

Lombard CW, Ackerman N, Berry CR, et al. Pulmonic stenosis and right-to-left atrial shunt in three dogs. J Am Vet Med Assoc 1989;194:71–75.

Luer RJT, van der, Linde-Sipman JS, van der. A rare congenital cardiac anomaly in a foal. Vet Pathol 1978;15:776–778.

Luginbuhl H, Chacko SK, Patterson DF, et al. Congenital hereditary lymphoedema in the dog. II. Pathological studies. J Med Genet 1967;4:153–165.

Martin DG, Ferguson EW, Gunnels RD, et al. Double aortic arch in a dog. J Am Vet Med Assoc 1983;183:697–699.

Martin JE, Gerrity LW, Stein FJ. Anomalous origin of the right subclavian artery in a marmoset (*Callithrix jacchus*). J Med Primatol 1979;8:305–307.

Meyerowitz B. Defectus interventricularis septi in heart of pig. Am J Vet Res 1942;3:368–372.

Milstein JM, deVries PA, Goetzman BW. Persistent truncus arteriosus in a lamb. Am J Vet Res 1982;43:902–903.

Morris B, et al. Congenital lymphatic oedema in Ayrshire calves. Aust J Exp Biol Med Sci 1954;32:265.

Musselman EE, LoGuidice RJ. Hypoplastic left ventricular syndrome in a foal. J Am Vet Med Assoc 1984;185:542–543.

Naylor JR. Regurgitation in pups. I. Persistent aortic arches. J Am Vet Med Assoc 1957;130:283–284.

Nelson AW. Aorticopulmonary window in a dog. J Am Vet Med Assoc 1986;188:1055–1058.

TABLE 21-1 **Cardiovascular malformations in 290 dogs***

Malformation	Number	Percentage of total
Patent ductus arteriosus	82	25.3
Pulmonic stenosis	57	17.5
Subaortic stenosis	40	12.3
Persistent right aortic arch	23	7.1
Ventricular septal defect	20	6.2
Tetralogy of Fallot	11	3.4
Atrial septal defect (ostium secundum inc. patent foramen ovale)	12	3.7
Persistent left cranial vena cava	13	4.0
Mitral insufficiency	9	2.8
Pericardial anomalies:		
Pericardiodiaphragmatic hernia	3	.9
Absent pericardium	1	.3
Incomplete pericardium	1	.3
Arterial anomalies:		
Retro-esophageal right subclavian artery	1	.3
Separate origin of right subclavian artery from ascending aorta	2	.6
Ebstein's anomaly of tricuspid valve	1	.3
Tricuspid insufficiency	1	.3
Double outlet, right ventricle	1	.3
Anomalous pulmonary venous drainage	1	.3
Conduction disturbance—without gross malformations:		
Right bundle branch block	2	.6
Wolff-Parkinson-White syndrome	1	.3
Arteriovenous fistula	1	.3
Incompletely diagnosed	42	12.9
Total	325	100

Note: In 32 dogs, more than one malformation was found.
*(Patterson, 1968)

Nimmo-Wilkie JS, Feldman EC. Pulmonary vascular lesions associated with congenital heart defects in three dogs. J Am Anim Hosp Assoc 1981;17:485–491.

O'Brien SE, Riedesel EA, Myers RK, et al. Right-to-left patent ductus arteriosus with dysplastic left ventricle in a dog. J Am Vet Med Assoc 1988;192:1435–1438.

Olafson P. Congenital cardiac anomalies in animals. J Tech Meth Bull Inter Assn Med Mus 1939;19:129–134.

Paasch LH, Zook BC. The pathogenesis of endocardial fibroelastosis in Burmese cats. Lab Invest 1980;42:197–204.

Patterson DF. Epidemiologic and genetic studies of congenital heart disease in the dog. Circ Res 1968;23:171–202.

Patterson DF, Medway W, Luginbuhl H, et al. Congenital hereditary lymphoedema in the dog. I. Clinical and genetic studies. J Med Genet 1967;4:145.

Patterson DF, et al. Hereditary patent ductus arteriosus and its sequelae in the dog. Circ Res 1971;29:1–13.

Patterson DF, et al. Hereditary defects of the conotruncal septum in Keeshond dogs. Am J Cardiol 1974;34:187–205.

Perkins RL. Multiple congenital cardiovascular anomalies in a kitten. J Am Vet Med Assoc 1972;160:1430–1431.

Prickett ME, Reeves JT, Zent WW. Tetralogy of Fallot in a thoroughbred foal. J Am Vet Med Assoc 1973;162:552–555.

Pyle RL, Patterson DF. Multiple cardiovascular malformation in a family of boxer dogs. J Am Vet Med Assoc 1972;160:965–976.

Roberts SJ, et al. Persistent right aortic arch in a Guernsey bull. Cornell Vet 1953;43:537–543.

Rooney JR, Franks WC. Congenital cardiac anomalies in horses. Path Vet 1964;1:454–464.

Rooney JR II, Watson DF. Persistent right aortic arch in a calf. J Am Vet Med Assoc 1956;129:5–7.

Sass B, Albert TF. A case of Eisenmenger's complex in a calf. Cornell Vet 1970;60:61–65.

Scarratt WK, Sponenberg DP, Welker FH, et al. Endocardial fibroelastosis and tricuspid valve insufficiency in a calf. J Am Vet Med Assoc 1987;190:1435–1436.

Seibold HR, Evans LE. A complex cardiac anomaly in a calf. J Am Vet Med Assoc 1957;130:99–101.

Swindle MM, Kan JS, Adams RJ, et al. Ventricular septal defect in a rhesus monkey. Lab Anim Sci 1986;36:693–695.

Swindle MM, et al. Heritable ventricular septal defect in Yucatan miniature swine. Lab Anim Sci 1990;40:155–161.

Turk JR, Miller LM, Hegreberg GA. Double outlet right ventricle in a dog. J Am Anim Hosp Assoc 1981;17:789–792.

Valentine RW, Carpenter JL. Spleno-mesenteric-renal venous shunt in two dogs. Vet Pathol 1990;27:58–60.

van den Ingh TSGAM, van der Linde-Sipman JS, Berrocal A, et al. Congenital portosystemic shunts in three pigs and one calf. Vet Pathol 1990;27:56–58.

van der Linde-Sipman JS, van der Luer RJT, Stokhof AA, et al. Congenital subvalvular pulmonic stenosis in a cat. Vet Pathol 1980;17:640–643.

van Heerden J, Lourens DC. Tetralogy of Fallot in a two-and-one-half-year old cat. J Am Anim Hosp Assoc 1981;17:129–130.

Van Nie CJ. Congenital malformations of the heart in cattle and swine. A survey of a collection. Acta Morph Neerl Scand 1966;6:387–393.

Van Nie CJ. Anomalous origin of the coronary arteries in animals. Pathol Vet 1968;5:313–326.

van Nie CJ. Atresia of the ostium atrioventriculare dextrum in a pig. Vet Pathol 1980;17:500–502.

Vitums A. Origin of the aorta and pulmonary trunk from the right ventricle in a horse. Pathol Vet 1970;7:482–491.

Vitums A, Bayly WM. Pulmonary atresia with dextraposition of the aorta and ventricular septal defect in three Arabian foals. Vet Pathol 1982;19:160–168.

Vos JH, van der Linde-Sipman JS, Stokhof AA. Double outlet left ventricle in a dog. Vet Pathol 1984;21:174–177.

Ware WA, Montavon P, DiBartola SP, et al. Atypical portosystemic shunt in a cat. J Am Vet Med Assoc 1986;188:187–188.

Wegelius O, von Essen R. Endocardial fibroelastosis in dogs. Acta Pathol Microbiol Scand 1969;77:66–72.

Heart

Cardiac failure

DEFINITION AND CAUSES

Cardiac failure is the inability of the heart to maintain adequate circulation. It is the leading cause of death in adult humans, owing to the high incidence of ischemic heart disease due to coronary atherosclerosis and the high incidence of hypertension. Although they can occur in animals, the frequency and severity of these conditions do not approach the proportions documented in humans. There are, however, other **primary causes** of heart failure that occur in animals (as well as in humans), including: congenital anomalies, cardiomyopathies, infectious myocarditis, valvular disease (congenital and acquired), nutritional deficiencies, certain poisons, conduction disturbances, constrictive pericarditis, volume overload, arrhythmias, and pulmonary disease (cor pulmonale). These various conditions result in one of the following:

(1) Damage to the myocardium and, hence, decreased systolic function with reduced output (myocarditis, myocardial necrosis);
(2) Increased resistance leading to reduced output (cor pulmonale, hypertension);
(3) Decreased output due to inadequate ventricular filling resulting from stenosis or regurgitation caused by defective atrioventricular valves;
(4) Irregular and inadequate rhythm (arrhythmias); or,
(5) Inability of the heart to expand and fill properly leading to reduced output (pericarditis).

PRECIPITATING CAUSES

Although many of the above-mentioned causes of heart failure may lead to acute or chronic cardiac failure, compensatory mechanisms may allow the heart to function adequately without clinical consequences. This situation is referred to as **compensated heart disease.** The compensated heart, however, is more vulnerable to other stresses to which a normal heart can properly adjust. Precipitating causes of heart failure can include a recurrence or superimposition of one of the initial causes of damage cited above, as well as other afflictions. Infections anywhere in the body lead to fever, tachycardia, and an added burden on the heart. When the primary cardiac disease has resulted in pulmonary congestion, pneumonia is particularly common. Anemia causes an added burden to the heart because it requires increased cardiac output. Hyperthyroidism also places an increased demand on the heart to meet increased metabolic requirements. Renal disease, resulting in increased retention of sodium and water, places a volume overload burden on the heart. Increased physical activity is another precipitating cause of heart failure in a compensated heart.

COMPENSATORY MECHANISMS

The effects of these various causes of heart failure on the heart itself and the events that heart failure triggers are complex. Only some of these will be summarized here; the student is referred to textbooks of medicine for details on the pathophysiology of heart failure. In acute heart failure, the patient may die from a sudden halt of cardiac function or from acute pulmonary edema prior to the unfolding of **compensatory responses.** However, when the patient is able to survive the initial insult, several mechanisms help to maintain adequate cardiac output. Although initially beneficial, these compensatory mechanisms over time may further contribute to heart failure. **Cardiac dilatation** leads to an increase in the diastolic volume which, in turn, according to the Frank-Starling law of the heart, results in increased stroke volume. This, along with an increase in heart rate, provides a temporary mechanism to prevent failure. If the demand for increased cardiac output were to continue, **cardiac hypertrophy** with an increase in the size of the individual myocytes would follow, further supporting the increased stroke volume. An increase in sympathetic activity increases the heart rate and ventricular relaxation and filling, all of which also contribute to a compensatory increase in cardiac output. Through decreased renal blood flow and possibly other mechanisms, an increased release of renin and subsequently angiotensin II and aldosterone occurs. Angiotensin II along with increased sympathetic activity causes **generalized vasoconstriction** (to include the kidney) which, although compensatory to decreased cardiac output, actually increases the workload on the heart. Increased tubular reabsorption of sodium and water also is manifest, due to the release of aldosterone which, in turn, leads to **increased blood volume** supporting increased cardiac filling and output. The increased blood volume, although contributing to adequate cardiac output, places an additional burden on the heart. Retention of sodium and water also leads to increased plasma hydrostatic pressure and an increase in interstitial fluid volume, which contributes to the edema of heart failure. The heart controls the deleterious effects of vasoconstriction and volume expansion through the release of the hormone, **atriopeptin** or **atrial natriuretic factor.** This hormone, which is released from myocytes when volume overload occurs, causes an increase in the glomerular filtration rate, diuresis, natriuresis, vasodilation through relaxation of smooth muscle, and inhibition of aldosterone secretion. Each of these contribute to a reduction of extracellular fluid volume and lessening of blood pressure.

CATEGORIES OF HEART FAILURE

Several different descriptive terms are used to categorize heart failure. **Acute** versus **chronic** heart failure are self evident. Chronic heart failure may, however, terminate in an episode of acute failure when precipitated by other insults or as the result of damage to other organs and tissues. The phrases **right-sided** versus **left-sided** heart failure are used to describe the principal clinical and pathologic features of heart failure where the primary disease principally affects one side of the heart. Because the circulatory system is one continuous loop, failure of the entire heart will develop with signs and lesions attributable to **both** right- and left-sided failure over a period of time (months to years), depending on the severity of the disease in the failing side. The terms **backward failure** (venous backup) and **forward failure** (diminished output) explain both the immediate effects of heart failure and the primary mechanism for renal sodium and water retention; however, both increased venous pressure and reduced cardiac output are operable and important. Two other terms sometimes used include **low-output heart failure,** in which cardiac output is reduced, and **high-output heart failure,** in which cardiac output is increased even though the heart is failing. The latter situation occurs in heart failure accompanied by hyperthyroidism or anemia.

ACUTE CARDIAC FAILURE

Acute cardiac failure is the result of a sudden cessation of effective cardiac contraction leading to "brain death" within minutes. In humans, acute cardiac failure is most often the result of ischemic heart disease which, in general, is not common in animals. In animals, it can occur in such disorders as acute myocarditis, dilated or hypertrophic cardiomyopathy (Fig. 21-4), cardiac tamponade (Fig. 21-5), sudden occlusion of the pulmonary artery or aorta, severe electrolyte imbalance, and certain toxicities. Lesions in acute cardiac failure are minimal. The right and/or left ventricles may be acutely dilated, but in the absence of some pre-existing heart disease, the heart may appear normal. Pulmonary and/or systemic congestion may be prominent, but edema is not a feature because of acute failure of circulation. Even when the cause is myocardial necrosis, an insufficient time elapses for the myocytes to be recognized morphologically as necrotic. Should cardiac failure not result in immediate death, but rather extend for one to several days, congestion will be more pronounced and will be accompanied by edema. Degenerative changes may develop in the passively congested organs, particularly the liver where centrilobular necrosis ("nutmeg liver") may be striking. Damaged myocardium will also have had time to become evident grossly and microscopically.

CHRONIC HEART FAILURE

Chronic cardiac failure, often referred to as **congestive heart failure,** is the result of failure of the heart to maintain adequate circulation as a result of diminished output (forward failure) and backing up of blood (backward failure). It is common to divide chronic heart failure into **left-sided heart failure** and **right-sided heart failure,** which may exist independently of one another; however, as previously stated, the circulatory system is one continuous circuit. In time, failure of one side ultimately leads to failure of the other, which results in total heart failure.

Left-sided heart failure may follow damage to the myocardium, aortic and mitral valve disease, various congenital defects, or hypertension. The latter is particularly common in humans, but is much less frequent in animals. Aside from the primary heart disease, dilatation of the left ventricle occurs, except in cases of left-sided failure due to mitral stenosis, when dilatation of the left atrium is evident. Left ventricular hypertrophy also is manifest. **Secondary lesions** of left-sided failure are most striking in the lungs. Alveolar hemorrhage leads to the presence of hemosiderin-laden alveolar macrophages, the so-called "heart failure cells." Alveolar lining cells become hypertrophied and fibrosis develops in alveolar walls. Hydrothorax may also develop. Clinically, dyspnea and shortness of breath occur. Decreased renal circulation leads to increased tubular resorption of sodium and an increase in blood volume, as discussed above.

Right-sided heart failure follows impedance of pulmonary circulation and, therefore, obviously follows left-sided failure. Primary disease of the lungs or pulmonary vasculature may lead to right-sided failure, called **cor pulmonale** (see below). Right-sided failure can also follow disorders of the tricuspid and pulmonary valves. **Secondary lesions** focus on the visceral and portal circulation. Chronic, passive congestion of the **liver** leads to the characteristic "nutmeg" appearance due to centrilobular congestion, hemorrhage, atrophy, necrosis, and fibrosis. Marked congestion of the spleen leads to splenomegaly. Increased venous hydrostatic pressure leads to edema (especially of the subcutis), ascites, and hydrothorax. Increased retention of sodium and water, as discussed above, further contributes to the accumulation of fluids in these sites.

Pulmonary Hypertensive Heart Disease and Cor Pulmonale (High Altitude Disease, Brisket Disease). Any abnormality that restricts the flow of blood through the lungs will lead to hypertension in the pulmonary arterial tree, dilation of the right ventricle, and ultimately right-sided heart failure. Left-sided heart failure and congenital cardiac defects with left-to-right shunts are also causes of pulmonary hypertension and right-sided heart failure. Pulmonary hypertensive heart disease that is not related to left-sided failure or congenital cardiac defects is termed **cor pulmonale.** Cor pulmonale, therefore, is the result of primary disease of the lung, most usually, but not always, the pulmonary vasculature. Many causes of cor pulmonale exist. **Chronic fibrosing pneumonias, pulmonary embolism** (from thromboembolic disease, dead Dirofilaria), and **emphysema** lead to pulmonary hypertension by compression of arterioles and effectively reducing the volume of the pulmonary vascular bed. **Primary arterial disease** of the pulmonary arteries and arterioles from viral arteritis, or poisoning by the pyrrolizidine alkaloid monocrotaline *(Crotalaria spectabilis)* also cause pulmonary hypertension (see Chapter 15). **Hypoxia** is another important cause of pulmonary hypertension. Obviously, primary disease of the lung can lead to hypoxia, but pulmonary hypertension also follows hypoxia from reduced atmospheric oxygen. This occurs in animals and humans residing at high altitudes. This condition is most often reported in cattle—which appear to be particularly sensitive to hypoxia—at altitudes above 7,000 feet and is termed **"high altitude disease"** or **"brisket disease."** In humans, it is seen in individuals residing at much higher elevations (above 12,000 feet) and is termed **Monge disease** or **chronic mountain sickness,** which is common in Peruvian Indians in the Andes. Alveolar hypoxia directly stimulates vasoconstriction of pulmonary arterioles. This vasoconstriction is further augmented by sympathetic nervous stimulation by way of arterial hypoxia. Chronic hypoxia also leads to polycythemia, which increases the viscosity of blood, further augmenting pulmonary hypertension. Acidosis also is a direct cause of vasoconstriction of pulmonary arterioles.

The pathologic effects of cor pulmonale are those of right-sided heart failure, as discussed above. Additionally, left ventricular hypertrophy may be manifest. This is the rule in cor pulmonale induced by high altitude hypoxia, and may develop if the primary pulmonary disease were to lead to marked arterial hypertrophy and intimal fibroelastosis of the pulmonary arteries and arterioles, with a narrowing of the lumens. Medial necrosis and thickening of the adventitia may also occur.

References

Alexander AF, Jensen R. Gross cardiac changes in cattle with high mountain (brisket) disease and in experimental cattle maintained at high altitudes. Am J Vet Res 1959;20:680–689.
Alexander AF, Jensen R. I. Pulmonary arteriographic studies of bovine high mountain disease. II. Pulmonary vascular hypertension in cattle. Am J Vet Res 1963;24:1094–1097, 1112–1122.
Alexander AF, et al. Pulmonary hypertension and right ventricular hypertrophy in cattle at high altitude. Am J Vet Res 1960;21:199–204.
Alpert NR, Hamrell BB. Symposium: cellular and subcellular basis of myocardial hypertrophy. Fed Proc 1986;45:2561–2600.
Angel KL, Tyler JW. Pulmonary hypertension and cardiac insufficiency in three cows with primary lung disease. J Vet Intern Med 1992;6:214–219.
Blaine EH. Symposium: atrial natriuretic factor. Fed Proc 1986;45:2360–2391.
Blake JT. I. Certain hematopathologic conditions associated with brisket disease. II. Cardiac structural changes in cattle with brisket disease. Am J Vet Res 1965;26:68–75, 76–82.
Blake JT——. Etiology of brisket disease. Cornell Vet 1968;58:305–314.
Brewster RD, Benjamin SA, Thomassen RW. Spontaneous cor pulmonale in laboratory beagles. Lab Anim Sci 1983;33:299–302.
Byrne MJ. Coronary thrombosis leading to auricular fibrillation in a thoroughbred gelding. Irish Vet J 1950;4:90–92.
Epling GP. Electron microscopy of bovine cardiac muscle: the transverse sarcotubular system. Am J Vet Res 1965;26:224–238.
Epling GP. Electron microscopy of the bovine heart in congestive failure of high mountain disease. Am J Vet Res 1968;29:97–109.
Gelberg HB, Smetzer DL, Foreman JH. Pulmonary hypertension as a cause of atrial fibrillation in young horses. J Am Vet Med Assoc 1991;198:679–682.

Glover GH, Newsom IE. Brisket disease. Exp Sta Bull 229, Colorado State University, 1933.
Hall JE. Symposium: atrial pressure and body fluid homeostasis. Fed Proc 1986;45:2862–2903.
Hayashi Y, Hussa JF, Lalich JJ. Cor pulmonale in rats. Lab Invest 1967;16:875–881.
Hirano Y, Kitagawa H, Sasaki Y. Relationship between pulmonary arterial pressure and pulmonary thromboembolism associated with dead worms in canine heartworm disease. J Vet Med Sci 1992;54:897–904.
Jacobs G, Hutson C, Dougherty J, Kirmayer A. Congestive heart failure associated with hyperthyroidism in cats. J Am Vet Med Assoc 1986;188:52–56.
Jensen R. Right heart failure. Calif Vet 1952;5:18–19.
Jensen R, et al. Brisket disease in yearling feedlot cattle. J Am Vet Med Assoc 1976;169:515–517.
Katz AM. Cardiomyopathy of overload: a major determinant of prognosis in congestive heart failure. N Engl J Med 1990;322:100–110.
Kitagawa H, Sasaki Y, Ishihara K, et al. Contribution of live heartworms harboring in pulmonary arteries to pulmonary hypertension in dogs with dirofilariasis. Jpn J Vet Sci 1990;52:1211–1217.
Lentz WJ. Canine heart diseases. Vet Ext Quart, Univ Pa, 1948;48:7–17.
Liu S-K. Acquired cardiac lesions leading to congestive heart failure in the cat. Am J Vet Res 1970;31:2071–1088.
Needleman P, Greenwald JE. Atriopeptin: a cardiac hormone intimately involved in fluid, electrolyte, and blood-pressure homeostasis. N Engl J Med 1986;314:828–834.
Oparil S, Haber E. The renin-angiotensin system (parts 1 and 2). N Engl J Med 1974;291:389–401, 446–457.
Oswald GP, Orton EC. Patent ductus arteriosus and pulmonary hypertension in related Pembroke Welsh corgis. J Am Vet Med Assoc 1993;202:761–764.
Pringle JK, et al. Pulmonary hypertension in a group of dairy calves. J Am Vet Med Assoc 1991;198:857–861.
Puntriano GO. Physiological basis of "brisket disease" in cattle. J Am Vet Med Assoc 1954;125:327–329.
Quiring DP, Baker RJ. The equine heart. Am J Vet Res 1953;14:62–67.
Raine AEG, et al. Atrial natriuretic peptide and atrial pressure in patients with congestive heart failure. N Engl J Med 1986;315:533–537.
Rawlings CA, Raynaud JP, Lewis RE, et al. Pulmonary thromboembolism and hypertension after thiacetarsamide vs melarsomine dihydrochloride treatment of Dirofilaria immitis infection in dogs. Am J Vet Res 1993;54:920–925.
Rudofsky UH, Magro AM. Spontaneous hypertension in fawn-hooded rats. Lab Anim Sci 1982;32:389–391.
Rugh KS, Garner HE, Sprouse RF, et al. Left ventricular hypertrophy in chronically hypertensive ponies. Lab Anim Sci 1987;37:335–338.
Ryff JF. Brisket disease syndrome. J Am Vet Med Assoc 1957;131:425–429.
Sheridan JP. The canine heart. Results of 100 random autopsies. J Small Anim Pract 1967;8:373–381.
Vogel JA, et al. Cardiac size and pulmonary hypertension in dogs exposed to high altitude. Am J Vet Res 1971;32:2059–2066.
Wallace CR, Hamilton WF. Study of spontaneous congestive heart failure in the dog. Circ Res 1962;11:301–314.
Will DH, Hicks JL, Card CS, et al. Inherited susceptibility of cattle to high altitude pulmonary hypertension. J Appl Physiol 1975;38:491–494.
Zook BC. Some spontaneous cardiovascular lesions in dogs and cats. Adv Cardiol 1974;13:148–168.

MYOCARDIUM

Hypertrophy

Two forms of myocardial hypertrophy are recognized: **concentric hypertrophy,** in which an increased thickness of the ventricular wall(s) occurs without an increase in the size of the ventricular chamber(s); and **eccentric hy-**

pertrophy, in which an increased thickness of the ventricular walls occurs with a complementary increase in size of the ventricular chamber(s). Hypertrophy of the myocardium is the fundamental adaptive response to situations that place an increased workload on the heart through either volume or pressure overload. These have already been discussed in previous sections on congenital anomalies, heart failure, and cor pulmonale. Other causes include acquired valvular disease, hypertension, and hyperthyroidism. **Systemic hypertension,** the most common cause of hypertrophy in humans, is not nearly as frequent in animals, but does occur in **chronic renal disease** (especially in dogs) and in horses with **equine laminitis.** Idiopathic cardiac hypertrophy is discussed under cardiomyopathy (below). **Microscopically,** individual myofibers in the hypertrophied heart are increased in thickness, often in disarray rather than uniformly parallel, and their nuclei are numerous, enlarged, and tend to be especially plump and square ended.

Cardiomyopathy

Although the term cardiomyopathy implies any disease of the heart, in human medicine the word is used to describe those disorders that result from a primary dysfunction of the myocardium of unknown cause. Most are characterized by dilation and/or hypertrophy. Those diseases of the myocardium of known cause and those secondary to other cardiovascular disorders, such as anomalies, hypertension, valvular disease, which lead to dilation and/or hypertrophy, are termed **secondary cardiomyopathies.**

Three forms of cardiomyopathy are recognized.

(1) **Dilated cardiomyopathy or congestive cardiomyopathy** is a disease in which all four chambers of the heart are dilated, with some degree of either myocardial atrophy or hypertrophy. The outcome is heart failure. In humans, it may occur as an idiopathic disorder as well as a familial disease, is a feature of Duchenne type of progressive muscular dystrophy, and follows other insults to the heart, such as viral myocarditis or alcoholism. Idiopathic dilated cardiomyopathy is occasionally seen in women late in pregnancy or during the first five months after delivery (termed peripartum cardiomyopathy).

(2) **Hypertrophic cardiomyopathy** is a disease in which marked hypertrophy of the myocardium occurs without dilation. All four chambers may be hypertrophic or hypertrophy may be asymmetric. Irregular thickening of the septum may lead to reduced cardiac output (obstructive hypertrophic cardiomyopathy). Microscopically, myofibers are hypertrophied and in disarray; often areas of fibrosis exist and the intima and media of intramural coronary arteries are thickened, narrowing the lumens. Physiologically, reduced distensibility and impaired relaxation of ventricular myocardium occur. In humans, many examples are inherited as an autosomal-dominant trait.

(3) **Restrictive cardiomyopathy,** a disease in which a restriction to ventricular filling occurs and may result from amyloidosis or endocardial fibroelastosis.

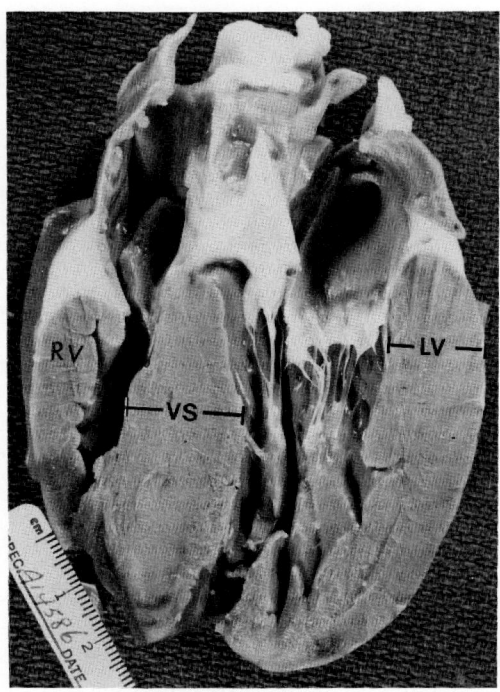

FIG. 21-4 Canine hypertrophic cardiomyopathy. The ventricular septum (VS) is greatly thickened. LV, left ventricular wall; RV, right ventricular wall. (Courtesy of Dr. S. Liu and Journal of the American Veterinary Medical Association.)

Various forms of cardiomyopathy are encountered **in animals,** but with the exception of dogs and cats they are apparently not common. **In dogs,** idiopathic dilated (congestive) cardiomyopathy is found most often in the larger breeds, especially the Doberman pinscher, Great Dane, Irish wolfhound, Saint Bernard, bull mastiff, and Newfoundland. It is more common in males. The principal microscopic findings in the heart include myocardial atrophy and focal necrosis with replacement by adipose cells and fibrous connective tissue. Intimal and medial hyperplasia of intramyocardial arteries has also been noted. Dilated cardiomyopathy is a feature of **Duchenne type muscular** dystrophy, which has been described in golden retrievers and Irish terriers. What appears to be peripartum cardiomyopathy has also been reported to occur in dogs. **Hypertrophic cardiomyopathy** is also seen in dogs, predominantly males, but much less often. German shepherds are among the most frequently affected breeds. Cardiomyopathy, which is believed to result from a genetic defect in **carnitine** metabolism, has been described in boxers (Chapter 16).

In **cats,** dilated (congestive) cardiomyopathy is one of the features of **taurine deficiency** (Chapter 16). Idiopathic hypertrophic cardiomyopathy is also encountered in cats, predominating in males. It is characterized by hypertrophy of both ventricular walls and septum with a reduction in size of the ventricular cavities. Microscopically, disarray of myocytes and fibrosis occurs. Hypertrophic cardiomyopathy is also seen in cats with **hyperthyroidism.**

Restrictive cardiomyopathy is more rarely encountered in animals than in humans. It is a feature of **endocardial fibroelastosis** and may develop in severe myocardial amyloidosis and certain other storage diseases. Endocardial fibroelastosis is most common in cats, and has been reported in rats. In cats, a disorder characterized by an increased number of **moderator bands** in the left ventricle has been described, leading to left atrial dilation, left atrial and ventricular hypertrophy, and left-sided heart failure.

Several conditions termed cardiomyopathies have been described **in cattle.** In Japanese black calves, cardiomyopathy occurs and is believed to be inherited as an autosomal-recessive trait and characterized by extensive myocardial necrosis with cardiomegaly and dilation leading to congestive heart failure. Most affected calves died by 30 days of age. A similar disorder, described in Australian polled Hereford calves with dense, curly (woolly) coats, is also reportedly an autosomal-recessive trait. It is characterized by myocardial necrosis, fibrosis, and mineralization. In Holstein-Friesian cattle, cardiomyopathy has been reported (also believed to be an autosomal trait) and is characterized by dilation without hypertrophy, but accompanied by necrosis and fibrosis.

In any species, **hyperthyroidism** is a cause of secondary hypertrophic cardiomyopathy; however, most reports of cardiomyopathy and heart failure associated with hyperthyroidism have been in cats. Type II **glycogen storage diseases** (Pompe disease; Chapter 2) may result in hypertrophic cardiomyopathy. Cardiomyopathies have also been described in several strains of mice and an hereditary cardiomyopathy that may be secondary to hypertension has been recognized in rats.

Both dilated and hypertrophic cardiomyopathy have been described **in pigs.** Inherited cardiomyopathy exists in certain strains of **Syrian hamsters** that is characterized by myocardial necrosis, fibrosis, calcification, mononuclear infiltration, and mural thrombosis, all associated with dilation and thinning and, on occasion, hypertrophy of the ventricular walls. Degeneration of skeletal muscles also occurs. An increase in calcium-binding sites has been demonstrated, an observation that has also been made in hypertrophic cardiomyopathy in humans. It has been suggested that the associated increased concentrations of calcium in myocytes lead to reduced distensibility and impaired relaxation of the ventricular myocardium, contributing to or causing hypertrophic cardiomyopathy.

Myocardial degenerative changes

Atrophy of the myocardium is recognized by a heart that is smaller than normal and microscopically by a decrease in size of muscle fibers, which may be most apparent by the increase in number of nuclei in proportion to fibers. **Lipofuscin** may be abundant within the myofibers near the poles of nuclei, giving rise to the term, brown atrophy of the heart. Myocardial atrophy is seen in chronic wasting diseases and malnutrition. **Mucoid degeneration** is not rare in the subepicardial fat of the coronary border, and is also seen following cachexia or malnutrition. **Fatty infiltration** is manifest as excessive extension of coronary adipose tissue among cardiac muscle fibers. **Fatty change** leads to the appearance of minute droplets of lipid within muscle fibers. It is detected with certainty only by appropriate stains. **Hyalin degeneration** of muscle fibers occurs as a prenecrotic change. **Calcification** of the myocardium is particularly common in laboratory mice, rats, hamsters, and guinea pigs. In some strains of mice, it is inherited and approaches a 100% incidence. Although usually encountered as an incidental finding, calcification may lead to congestive failure. Myocardial calcification also regularly accompanies many examples of myocardial necrosis.

Myocardial necrosis

Necrosis of the myocardium is the outcome of coronary vascular disease (Fig. 21-5) and a principal cause of acute and chronic heart failure in humans. Although occasionally encountered in animals, this type of necrosis is uncommon; however, other causes of myocardial necrosis in animals exist. The two most common are nutritional deficiencies and various poisonings. **Nutritional deficiencies** of vitamin E/selenium, thiamin, carnitine, potassium, and copper are associated with myocardial necrosis. **Poisonings** by gossypol, coffee senna (Cassia occidentalis), coyotillo (*Karwinskia humboldtiana*), vetch (*Vicia villosa*), gidgee plant (*Acacia georginae*), bracken fern (*Pteridium aquilinum*), lantana (*Lantana camara*), monensin, thallium, selenium, and organomercurials lead to myocardial necrosis. In **uremia,** necrosis of the left atrial myocardium occurs (see endocarditis). Many infectious diseases affect the myocardium and lead to necrosis (see myocarditis).

Myocarditis

Inflammatory diseases of the myocardium in animals are almost always infectious, although examples without an identifiable cause are encountered. Focal areas of myocarditis, myocardial necrosis and fibrosis, whose pathogenesis generally remains unresolved, are encountered with some frequency, particularly in aging animals. **Eosinophilic myositis** in cattle, which can affect the heart, is discussed in the chapter on skeletal muscle. Infectious agents that may cause myocarditis are listed in Table 21-2. Most of these agents also affect other tissues with equal or greater frequency. The nature of the inflammatory reaction is dependent upon the offending organism and resembles that seen in any other tissue. In cases with viral causes of myocarditis, following an initial phase characterized by myocardial necrosis, mononuclear inflammatory reaction may persist even after the virus is undetectable. This is believed to result from altered myocardial antigens leading to **autoimmune myocarditis.** Infectious myocarditis is often as-

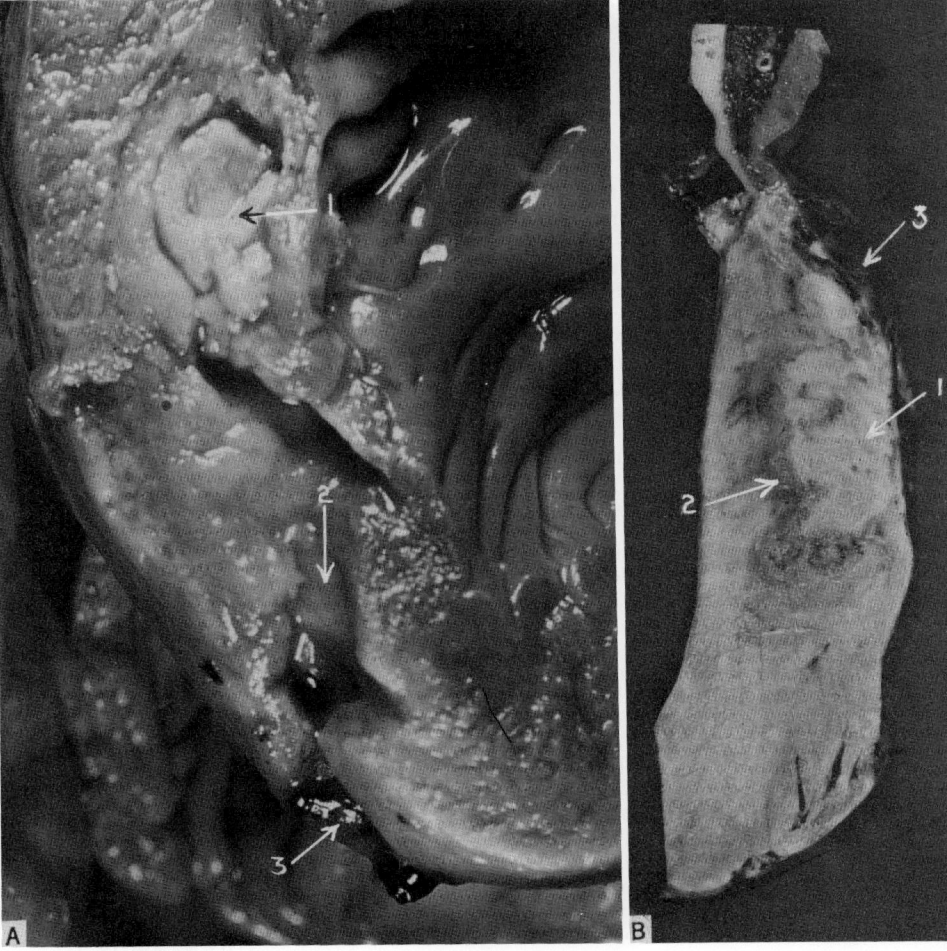

FIG. 21-5 Infarction of the heart. **A.** Infarction of left ventricle of a 12-year-old male mongrel terrier. 1 Necrosis of myocardium has led to 2 formation of a channel in 3 the left ventricle and rupture. Death followed this cardiac tamponade and hemopericardium. **B.** Infarction of the intraventricular septum of a four-year-old spayed female poodle. 1 The gray-colored necrotic myocardium is separated from the normal myocardium by 2 a zone of hemorrhage. 3 Subendocardial hemorrhage is seen. (Courtesy of Angell Memorial Animal Hospital.)

TABLE 21-2 **Some infectious causes of myocarditis**

Viruses

Encephalomyocarditis virus
Canine parvovirus
Foot and mouth disease virus
Canine distemper virus
Canine herpesvirus
Pseudorabies virus
Malignant catarrhal fever virus
Bluetongue virus
Coxsackieviruses
   (rodents, humans)

Protozoa

Toxoplasma gondii
Trypanosoma cruzi
Sarcosporidia spp.

Metazoon parasites

Trichinella spiralis
Echinococcus spp.
Cestode larvae

Bacteria

Mycobacterium spp.
Listeria monocytogenes
Actinobacillus equuli
Clostridium spp.
Haemophilus somnus
Streptococcus spp.
Bacillus piliformis
Rickettsia spp.
Chlamydia spp.

Fungi

Aspergillus spp.
Coccidioides immitis
Cryptococcus neoformans
Blastomyces immitis
Mucor group

---

sociated with hemorrhage and may lead to mural thrombi. The specifics of each disease are discussed in appropriate chapters.

    Scars of white fibrous tissue are occasionally seen in the myocardium. Although such a scar may represent a healed myocardial infarct in humans, in animals, a healed abscess or parasitic lesion is a more likely explanation. The size, shape, and location should afford a clue to previous events.

References

Anversa P, Capasso JM. Cardiac hypertrophy and ventricular remodeling. Lab Invest 1991;64:441–445.

Barlow RM, Smyth JBA, Middleton DJ. Acute cardiomyopathy in heifers. Vet Rec 1990;126:67.

Boorman GA, Zurcher C, Hollander CF, et al. Naturally occurring endocardial disease in the rat. Arch Pathol 1973;96:39–45.

Braunwald E. Hypertrophic cardiomyopathy—continued progress. N Engl J Med 1989;320:800–802.

Brunnert SR, Altman NH. Dystrophic cardiac calcinosis in mice: abnormal myocardial response to freeze-thaw injury. Lab Anim Sci 1990;40:616–619.

Calvert CA, Chapman WL, Toal RL. Congestive cardiomyopathy in Doberman pinscher dogs. J Am Vet Med Assoc 181:598–602.

Cook RW. Cardiomyopathy and woolly hair coat in Poll Hereford calves. Aust Vet Assoc Yearbook 1981;1981:210.

Follis RH JR, et al. Myocardial necrosis in thiamine deficiency in pigs. Am J Pathol 1943;19:341–357.

Finestone AJ, Geschickter CF. Bone formation in the heart. Am J Clin Pathol 1949;19:974–980.

Forbes MS, Sperelakis N. Ultrastructure of cardiac muscle from dystrophic mice. Am J Anat 1972;134:271–290.

Gooding JP, Robinson WF, Wyburn RS, et al. A cardiomyopathy in the English cocker spaniel: a clinicopathological investigation. J Small Anim Pract 1982;23:133–149.

Hazlett MJ, Maxie MG, Allen DG, et al. A retrospective study of heart disease in Doberman pinscher dogs. Can Vet J 1983;24:205–210.

Howell JMcC, Dorling PR, Cook RD. Generalised glycogenosis type II. Comp Pathol Bull 1983;12:2, 4.

Howell JMcC, Dorling PR, Cook RD, et al. Infantile and late onset form of generalised glycogenosis type II in cattle. J Pathol 1981;134:267–277.

Jasmin G, Bajusz E. Myocardial lesions in strain 129 dystrophic mice. Nature 1962;193:181–182.

Kent SP, Diseker M. Early myocardial ischemia: histochemical changes in dogs. Lab Invest 1955;4:398–405.

Lewis DJ. Sub-endocardial fibrosis in the rat: a light and electron microscopical study. J Comp Pathol 1980;90:577–583.

Lipman NS, Murphy JC, Fox JG. Clinical, functional and pathologic changes associated with a case of dilatative cardiomyopathy in a ferret. Lab Invest 1987;37:210–212.

Liu S-K, Fox PR, Tilley LP. Excessive moderator bands in the left ventricle of 21 cats. J Am Vet Med Assoc 1982;180:1215–1219.

Liu S-K, Maron BJ. Comparison of hypertrophic cardiomyopathy in human, cat and dog. Lab Invest 1990;62:58A.

Liu S-K, Maron BJ, Tilley LP. Hypertrophic cardiomyopathy in the dog. Am J Pathol 1979;94:497–508.

Liu S-K, Maron BJ, Tilley LP. Canine cardiac cardiomyopathy. J Am Vet Med Assoc 1979;174:703–713.

Liu S-K, Maron BJ, Tilley LP. Feline hypertrophic cardiomyopathy: gross anatomic and quantitative histologic features. Am J Pathol 1981;102:388–395.

Liu S-K, Peterson ME, Fox PR. Hypertrophic cardiomyopathy and hyperthyroidism in the cat. J Am Vet Med Assoc 1984;185:52–57.

Maron BJ, Bonow RO, Cannon RO III, et al. Hypertrophic cardiomyopathy: interrelations of clinical manifestations, pathophysiology, and therapy (Parts one and two). N Engl J Med 1987;316:780–789, 844–852.

Martig J, Tschudi P, Perritaz C, et al. Gehäufte Fälle von Herzinsuffizienz beim Rind: Vorläufige Mitteilung. [Multiple occurrence of cardiac insufficiency in cattle: preliminary report.] Schweiz Arch Tierheilkd 1982;124:69–82. [Vet Bull 1982;52:4087.]

Martorana PA, van Even P, Wüsten B, et al. Increased myocardial capillary density in dogs with experimental emphysema. Lab Invest 1984;50:592–596.

McLennan MW, Kelly WR. Dilated (congestive) cardiomyopathy in the Friesian heifer. Aust Vet J 1990;67:75–76. [Vet Bull 1990;60:7061.]

Nishi S. A study on animal model for cardiomyopathy: histopathological investigations of the heart in KK mice and dystrophic mice. J Clin Electron Microsc 1977;10:77–108.

Read WK, Pierce KR, O'Hara PJ. Ultrastructural lesions of an acute toxic cardiomyopathy of cattle. Lab Invest 1968;18:227–231.

Robinson WF, Howell JMcC, Dorling PR. Cardiomyopathy in generalised glycogenosis type II in cattle. Cardiovasc Res 1983;17:238–242.

Ruben Z, Miller JE, Rohrbacher E, et al. A potential model for a human disease: spontaneous cardiomyopathy-congestive heart failure in SHR/N-cp rats. Hum Pathol 1984;15:902–903.

Saito K, Nishi S, Kashima T, et al. Histologic and ultrastructural studies on the myocardium in spontaneously diabetic KK mice: a new animal model of cardiomyopathy. Am J Cardiol 1984;53:320–323.

Sandusky GE, Cho D-Y. Congestive cardiomyopathy in a dog associated with pregnancy. Cornell Vet 1984;74:60–64.

Sandusky GE Jr, Capen CC, Kern KM. Histological and ultrastructural evaluation of cardiac lesions in idiopathic cardiomyopathy in dogs. Can J Comp Med 1984;48:81–86.

Schofield FW. Sudden death in calves associated with myocardial degeneration. Can J Comp Med 1947;11:324–329.

Sonoda M, Takahashi K, Kurosawa T, et al. Clinical and clinicopathological studies on idiopathic congestive cardiomyopathy in cattle. Proceedings of the XII World Congress on Diseases of Cattle, held in Amsterdam. Utrecht: World Association of Buiatrics, 1982;1187–1191.

Storie GJ, Gibson JA, Taylor JD. Cardiomyopathy and woolly haircoat syndrome of Hereford cattle. Aust Vet J 1991;68:119. [Vet Bull 1991;61:7332.]

Thomas RE. Congestive cardiac failure in young cocker spaniels (a form of cardiomyopathy?): details of eight cases. J Small Anim Pract 1987;28:265–280.

Tilley LP, Liu S-K. Cardiomyopathy in the dog. Rec Adv Stud Cardiac Struct Metab 1975;10:641–653.

Tilley LP, et al. Primary myocardial disease in the cat. A model for human cardiomyopathy. Am J Pathol 1977;86:493–522.

Valentine BA, Cummings JF, Cooper BJ. Development of Duchenne-type cardiomyopathy. Morphologic studies in a canine model. Am J Pathol 1989;135:671–678.

Van Vleet JF, Ferrans VJ. Review article. Myocardial diseases of animals. Am J Pathol 1986;124:95–178.

Van Vleet JF, Ferrans VJ, Weirich WE. Pathologic alterations in hypertrophic and congestive cardiomyopathy of cats. Am J Vet Res 1980;41:2037–2048.

Van Vleet JF, Ferrans VJ, Weirich WE. Pathologic alterations in congestive cardiomyopathy of dogs. Am J Vet Res 1981;42:416–424.

Wagner JA, et al. Calcium-antagonist receptors in the atrial tissue of patients with hypertrophic cardiomyopathy. N Engl J Med 1989;320:755–761.

Watanabe S, Akita T, Itakura C, et al. Evidence for a new lethal gene causing cardiomyopathy in Japanese black calves. J Hered 1979;70:255–258.

Whittington RJ, Cook RW. Cardiomyopathy and woolly haircoat syndrome of Poll Hereford cattle: electrocardiographic findings in affected and unaffected calves. Aust Vet J 1988;65:341–344. [Vet Bull 1989;59:3479.]

Neoplasms

Primary neoplasms of the myocardium are rare. **Rhabdomyoma** and **rhabdomyosarcoma** are neoplasms of myofibers that are not common in any species. They are usually grayish nodules within the atrial or ventricular myocardium, and often project into the lumen. Microscopically, the neoplastic fibers may resemble normal myocardium, but generally the cells are disorganized and anaplastic with large nuclei and thin cytoplasmic extensions, or so-called strap cells. Multiple cytoplasmic processes may emanate from a single, enlarged hyperchromatic nucleus. Multinucleated tumor cells are frequent. A benign lesion called **congenital rhabdomyoma** has been described in several species, but is most frequent in swine and guinea pigs. It is believed to result from focal arrest of maturation of cardiac muscle and not represent a true neoplasm. These are usually multiple, discrete, nonencapsulated masses of swollen myofibers filled with glycogen.

AORTIC BODY TUMOR-CAROTID BODY TUMOR (PARAGANGLION)

Tumors of the aortic body (Fig. 21-6) or carotid body are not neoplasms of the heart, but are discussed here because those of the aortic body, the more frequent of the two, occur at the base of the heart. They are sometimes called **heart-base tumors.** These bodies are chemoreceptors, sensitive to blood pH, oxygen, and

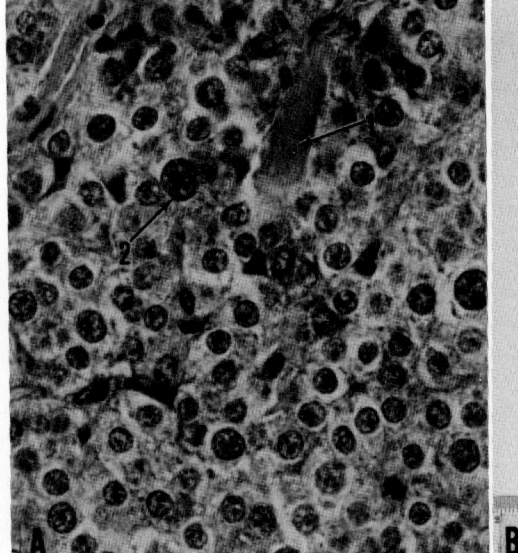 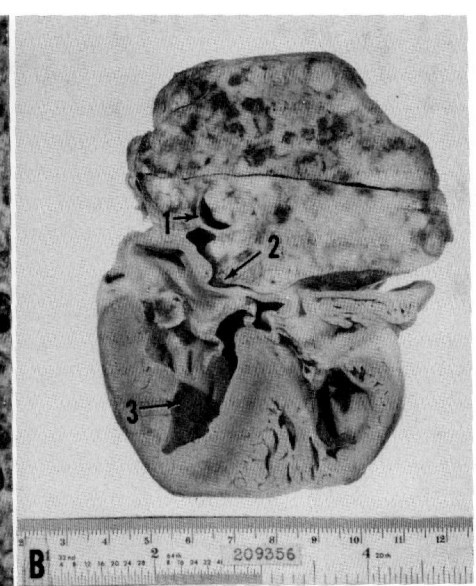

FIG. 21-6 Aortic body tumor. **A.** Photomicrograph (×500). 1 Collagen-rich supporting stroma and 2 polyhedral cells with spherical nuclei, some large and hyperchromatic. **B.** The gross tumor at the base of the heart of a 10-year-old English bulldog. 1 Tumor invades the aorta, and 2 compresses the atrium. 3 Left ventricle. (Courtesy of Armed Forces Institute of Pathology; contributor: Dr. W.H. Riser.)

carbon dioxide, and they help in the regulation of respiration and circulation. Based on this function, neoplasms of the aortic body and carotid body are also known as **chemodectomas.** Both the aortic body and the carotid body are part of the parasympathetic paraganglia network, which is part of the neuroendocrine system, and the preferred nomenclature of these neoplasms is **paraganglioma.** Neoplasms of the aortic and carotid bodies have also been termed **chemodectomas** because they are chemoreceptors, sensitive to blood pH, oxygen, and carbon dioxide, and help in the regulation of respiration and circulation. Rarely, neoplasms may develop from parasympathetic and sympathetic paraganglia at other sites. Other parasympathetic paraganglia are primarily distributed along the glossopharyngeal (tympanic paraganglia of the middle ear) and vagus nerves (jugular and laryngeal paraganglia) and the sympathetic paraganglia along the sympathetic chains.

Neoplasms arise from the neuroendocrine cells (paraneurons) of the paraganglia. These cells, which resemble those of the adrenal medulla, are usually well differentiated, polyhedral in shape, with a lightly stained, vacuolated or granular cytoplasm and spherical, finely stippled nuclei. They are subdivided into small clusters by a highly vascular fibrous stroma. Cells contain dark neurosecretory granules typical of neuroendocrine cells and can be stained with argyrophilic stains, but this reaction is not specific. Granules of paraneurons can be specifically stained with an ultrastructural cytochemical stain termed the uranaffin reaction.

Aortic body tumors are located at the base of the heart, usually intimately related to the aorta or pulmonary artery within the pericardial sac. Most are benign, occurring as solitary and sometimes multiple nodules. Malignant aortic body tumors infiltrate the wall of the

pulmonary artery, aorta, and atria, and may rarely metastasize. Aortic body tumors are most often encountered in dogs, most frequently in brachiocephalic breeds (bulldog, Boston terrier, boxer); however, reports in other species include cats, cattle, and birds.

Carotid body tumors of dogs, much less frequent than aortic body tumors—the opposite is true in humans—also are most frequent in brachiocephalic breeds. They occur at the bifurcation of the common carotid artery, may occur in conjunction with aortic body tumors, and are more often malignant than are aortic body tumors. Carotid body tumors have also been reported in cattle, cats, and mink.

Other neuroendocrine cells, widely dispersed throughout the body, are also subject to neoplastic transformation. The most frequent of these include tumors of argentaffin cells (carcinoid), C cells of the thyroid, and neuroendocrine cells of the lung (carcinoid of Kulchitsky cells).

OTHER NEOPLASMS

Neoplasms at the base of the heart may arise from other tissues as demonstrated by von Bomhard et al. (1974). They studied 69 "heart base tumors" in dogs and found that 45 arose from aberrant thyroid tissue, 20 were true aortic body tumors, and 4 could not be classified. Aberrant parathyroid tumors may also occur at the base of the heart.

What have been termed **epithelial inclusions** are occasionally encountered within the myocardium and can be misinterpreted as metastatic neoplasms. These are composed of acinar or ductular structures lined by cuboidal or columnar nonciliated epithelium. Their exact origin is not known. Often they are at the base of the heart and probably represent ectopic thyroid. In cattle, they may be found in the ventricular myocardium near the apex.

Hemangioendothelioma (hemangiosarcoma) is one of the most frequent primary neoplasms of the heart in dogs. Some surveys indicate that the heart is the most common primary site. German shepherds are the most frequently affected species, followed by other breeds. Tumors usually arise in the right atrium and often metastasize. Hemangioendothelioma is discussed more completely under **Neoplasms of Blood and Lymphatic Vessels,** later in this chapter.

Neurofibromas and **schwannomas,** identical in structure to those described in the chapter on skin (Chapter 19), are relatively common neoplasms of the bovine heart. They occur as single or multiple nodules, usually on the epicardium and may occur in association with neurofibromas at other sites. They are most often encountered as incidental findings, without affecting cardiac function. Schwannomas are also one of the most frequent cardiac neoplasms in certain strains of laboratory rats.

Granular cell myoblastoma has been reported in the atria of a dog. This unusual and rare neoplasm is discussed in Chapter 19.

Fibrosarcomas can arise in the heart, but are rare. Isolated reports describe **chondrosarcomas** arising in the mitral valve, the right atria, and the aortic arch of dogs.

The most frequently encountered neoplasm in the heart is **malignant lymphoma.** A considerable proportion of these neoplasms involve the heart in cattle. Some result in the formation of one or more discrete masses, but many infiltrate among the muscle bundles. An area of faint, white streaks parallel to the course of the muscle fibers should be considered malignant lymphoma until shown to be otherwise (Chapter 22).

References

Alison RH, Elwell MR, Jokinen MP, et al. Morphology and classification of 96 primary cardiac neoplasms in Fischer 344 rats. Vet Pathol 1987;24:488–494.

Anderson WI, Carberry CA, King JM, et al. Primary aortic chondrosarcoma in a dog. Vet Pathol 1988;25:180–181.

Aronsohn M. Cardiac hemangiosarcoma in the dog: a review of 38 cases. J Am Vet Med Assoc 1985;187:922–926.

Baker DC, Schmidt SP, Langheinrich KA, et al. Bovine myocardial epithelial inclusions. Vet Pathol 1993;30:82–88.

Bloom F. Structure and histogenesis of tumors of the aortic bodies in dogs. Arch Pathol 1943;36:1–12.

Buergelt CD, Das KM. Aortic body tumor in a cat: a case report. Pathol Vet 1968;5:84–90.

Cheville NF. Ultrastructure of canine carotid body and aortic body tumors. Comparison with tissues of thyroid and parathyroid origin. Vet Pathol 1972;9:166–189.

Dean MJ, Strafuss AC. Carotid body tumors in the dog: a review and report of four cases. J Am Vet Med Assoc 1975;166:1003–1006.

Frye FL, Knight HD, Brown SI. Hemangiosarcoma in a horse. J Am Vet Med Assoc 1983;182:287–289.

Gliatto JM, Crawford MA, Snider TG III, et al. Multiple organ metastasis of an aortic body tumor in a boxer. J Am Vet Med Assoc 1987;191:1110–1112.

Greenlee PG, Liu SK. Chondrosarcoma of the mitral leaflet in a dog. Vet Pathol 1984;21:540–542.

Hadlow WJ. Carotid body tumor: an incidental finding in older ranch mink. Vet Pathol 1986;23:162–169.

Hoch-Ligeti C, Restrepo C, Stewart HL. Comparative pathology of cardiac neoplasms in humans and in laboratory rodents: a review. JNCI 1986;76:127–142.

Kleine LJ, Zook BC, Munson TO. Primary cardiac hemangiosarcomas in dogs. J Am Vet Med Assoc 1970;157:326–337.

Krotje LJ, Ware WA, Niyo Y. Intracardiac rhabdomyosarcoma in a dog. J Am Vet Med Assoc 1990;197:368–371.

Ladds PW, Daniels PW. Aortic body tumour in an ox. Aust Vet J 1975;51:43.

Montgomery DL, Bendele R, Storts RW. Malignant aortic body tumor with metastasis to bone in a dog. Vet Pathol 1980;17:241–244.

Murray JD, Strafuss AC. Carotid body tumors in the dog: a review and report of four cases. J Am Vet Med Assoc 1975;166:1003–1006.

Nordstoga K. Carotid body tumor in a cow. Pathol Vet 1966;3:412–420.

Nordstoga K, Aleksandersen M. Epithelial inclusions in the bovine myocardium. Vet Pathol 1988;25:525–526.

Patnaik AK, Lord PF, Liu S-K. Chemodectoma of the urinary bladder in a dog. J Am Vet Med Assoc 1974;164:797–800.

Omar A. Congenital cardiac rhabdomyoma in a pig. Pathol Vet 1969;6:469–474.

Robertson JL, Garman RH, Fowler EH. Spontaneous cardiac tumors in eight rats. Vet Pathol 1981;18:30–37.

Sanford SE, Hoover DM, Miller RB. Primary cardiac granular cell tumor in a dog. Vet Pathol 1984;21:489–494.

Scotti TM. The carotid body tumors in dogs. J Am Vet Med Assoc 1958;132:413–419.

Syvurud R. Rhabdomyoma in the cat. West Vet 1959;6:49–50.

Szcsech GM, Blevins WE, Carlton WW, et al. Chemodectoma with metastasis to bone in a dog. J Am Vet Med Assoc 1973;162:376–378.

Trevino GS, Nessmith WB. Aortic body tumor in a white rat. Vet Pathol 1973;9:243–248.

Vicini DS, Didier PJ, Ogilvie GK. Cardiac fibrosarcoma in a dog. J Am Vet Med Assoc 1986;189:1486–1488.

Pericardium

HYDROPERICARDIUM

Hydropericardium or pericardial effusion is the accumulation of fluid in the pericardial sac (Fig. 21-7). It can be distinguished from inflammatory edema or serous pericarditis by the low protein content of the fluid, and the absence of cells and other features of the inflammatory process. The amount of fluid varies greatly. Usually it is not adequate to prevent filling of the heart, but in pronounced examples cardiac function may be compromised (Fig. 21-8). The causes include the usual causes of edema, cardiac and nutritional edema probably being somewhat more important in this respect than renal edema. Hydropericardium is also encountered in African horse sickness, edema disease, and mulberry heart disease of swine.

HEMOPERICARDIUM

In hemopericardium, hemorrhage fills the pericardial sac with blood. The sudden escape of blood into the pericardial sac—perhaps through rupture of the intrapericardial aorta, coronary artery, atrial or myocardial wall, or in the course of traumatic pericarditis—is referred to as **cardiac tamponade.** It leads to interference with cardiac filling and heart failure. Hemopericardium may also be seen in severe forms of pericarditis and secondary to neoplasms. Idiopathic hemopericardium is described in certain large breeds of dogs, particularly the Great Pyrenees, Great Dane, Saint Bernard, and golden retriever.

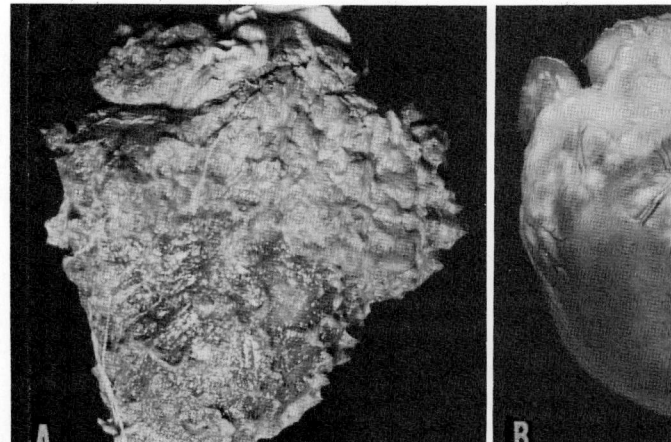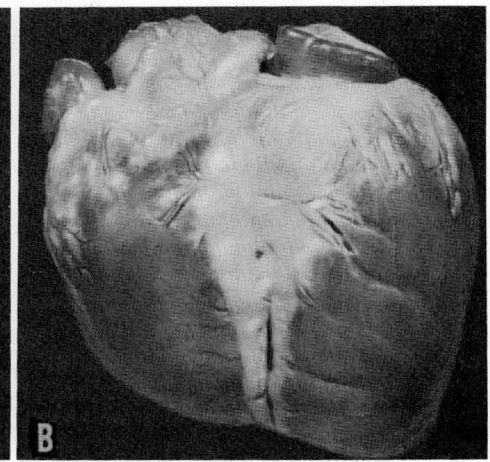

FIG. 21-7 **A.** Chronic organizing fibrinous pericarditis in a sow. **B.** Acute dilatation of the right heart of a young Guernsey cow which died with circulatory collapse following cesarean operation. Note rounded outline of the heart, viewed from the anterior aspect. (Courtesy of College of Veterinary Medicine, Iowa State University.)

PERICARDITIS

Pericarditis includes inflammation of both the parietal and visceral surfaces of the pericardial cavity: in other words, the inner surface of the sac and the outer surface of the heart, the epicardium. It may occur independently of other lesions, but is often seen in association with pleuritis. **Serous pericarditis** is characterized by the accumulation of protein-rich fluid with vary-ing numbers of inflammatory cells in the fluid and pericardium. Hyperemia of pericardial vessels and serous thickening of the pericardium may occur. The amount of fluid is generally less than seen in hydropericardium, from which it may be difficult to differentiate. Pure serous pericarditis is not common, most examples representing the early stages of serofibrinous pericarditis. When seen, the cause is often not identi-

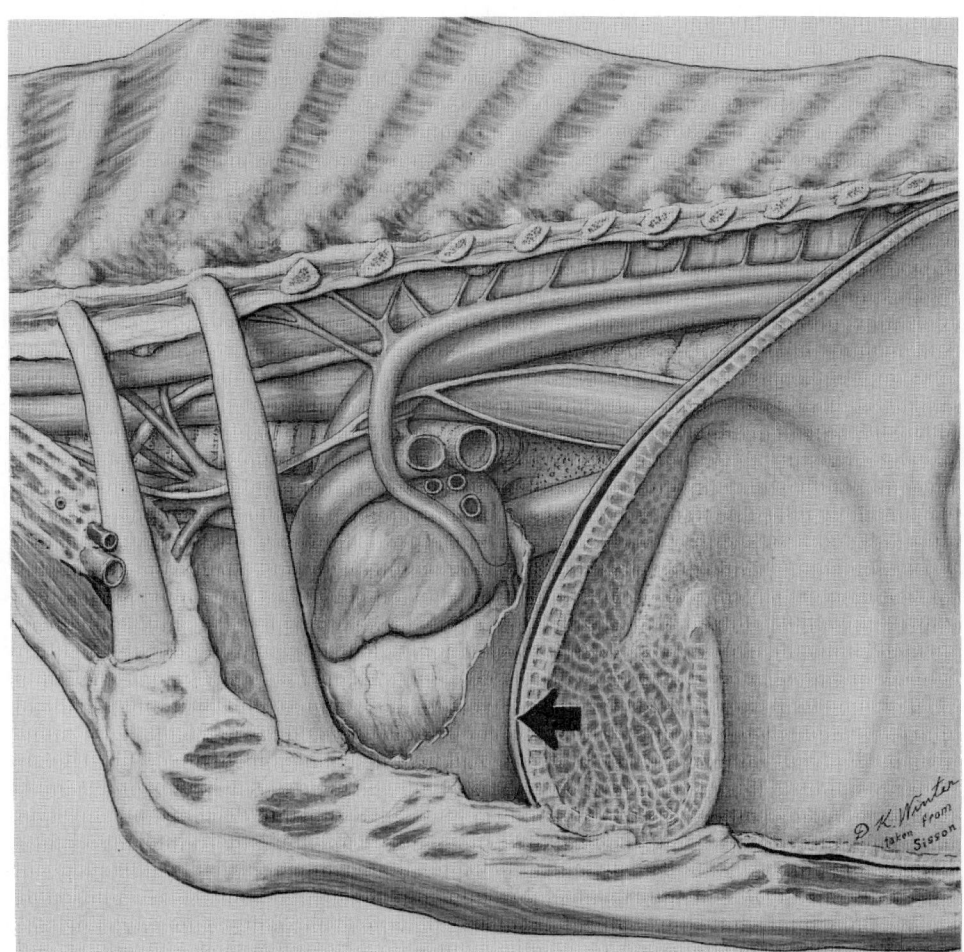

FIG. 21-8 The anatomic relationships in traumatic pericarditis. Foreign bodies penetrate the wall of the reticulum, diaphragm, and pericardium in the direction indicated by the arrow. (Modified after Sisson.)

fied. Uremia is a noninfectious cause of serous pericarditis.

Serofibrinous and **fibrinous pericarditis** are the most frequently encountered forms. It is found in diseases in which fibrinous pleuritis also occurs, including sporadic bovine encephalomyelitis, Glasser disease, pasteurellosis, bovine and caprine pleuropneumonia, porcine enzootic pneumonia, and feline peritonitis, as well as in a variety of primary bacterial infections of the pericardium. The cause is not always identified. It is characterized by varying amounts of serous fluid and extensive deposition of fibrin on the pericardial and epicardial surfaces, which become adherent to one another (adhesive pericarditis). The surface of the heart is covered with a layer of white or blood-stained fibrin several millimeters thick, which is termed "shaggy heart" or **cor rugosum.** If fibrinous exudate were completely resorbed with recovery, no sequelae would occur; however, fibrin often is organized, leaving a layer of fibrous connective tissue (scar). The epicardium and pericardium may become permanently fused, either focally or on occasion completely, leading to what is termed **constrictive pericarditis.** This leads to heart failure because the scar prevents compensatory dilatation and hypertrophy. In dogs, variously sized, papillary projections from the epicardial pericardium are encountered. These consist of fibrous cores lined by mesothelial cells. They are termed epicardial fronds; the cause is not known.

Purulent pericarditis almost always results from pyogenic bacteria which localize in the pericardium. Infections with certain fungi may also cause purulent pericarditis. It is often encountered in association with purulent pleuritis. Frequent causes include *Streptococcus, Klebsiella, Pasteurella, Staphylococcus, Mycoplasma,* and *Nocardia spp.* Purulent exudate, often mixed with fibrin, fills the pericardial space and is present within the epicardium and pericardium. The inflammatory process often extends into the mediastinum. Purulent pericarditis rarely resolves. Healing occurs by organization resulting in adhesive and constrictive fibrosing pericarditis.

Traumatic pericarditis (traumatic reticuloperitonitis, hardware disease) is a disease of cattle resulting from piercing of the reticulum by metal objects. Cattle kept in close proximity to stables and usual farmstead activities often swallow discarded nails, bits of wire, and similar hardware because of their indiscriminate feeding habits. These sharp, metal objects penetrate the wall of the reticulum and slowly move, encompassed in reactive granulation tissue, usually eliciting only localized peritonitis. The direction that the foreign object travels is usually anteroventral, through the diaphragm and pleura, and into the pericardium and heart. Profusely exudative fibrinopurulent pleuritis and pericarditis develops. Rarely, the foreign object perforates a coronary or the heart, leading to fatal hemorrhage. Should the foreign object travel in a different direction, peritonitis surrounding the reticulum, the adjacent forestomachs, and abomasum ensues.

Neoplasms

Neoplasms of the pericardium are infrequent. Fibromas, leiomyomas, and hemangioendotheliomas may arise in the pericardium, but the most frequent primary neoplasms are the mesotheliomas (Fig. 21-9). They resemble mesotheliomas arising in the pleura and peritoneum.

References

Berg RJ, Wingfield WE, Hoopes PJ. Idiopathic hemorrhagic pericardial effusion in eight dogs. J Am Vet Med Assoc 1984;185:988–992.

Bernard W, Reef VB, Clark ES, et al. Pericarditis in horses: six cases (1982–1986). J Am Vet Med Assoc 1990;196:468–471.

Bomhard D von, Luderer M, Hänichen T, et al. Zur histogenese der herzbasistumoren beim hund. Eine histologische, histochemische und elektronenmikroskopische studie. [Histogenesis of heart base tumours in the dog. A histological, histochemical and electron microscope study. Zentralbl Veterinarmed 1974;21A:208–224.

Carnine BL, Schneider G, Cook JE, et al. Pericardial mesothelioma in a horse. Vet Pathol 1977;14:513–515.

Dill SG, et al. Fibrinous pericarditis in the horse. J Am Vet Med Assoc 1982;180:266–271.

de Madron E, Prymak C, Hendricks J. Idiopathic hemorrhagic pericardial effusion with organized thrombi in a dog. J Am Vet Med Assoc 1987;191:324–326.

Mesfin GS. Spontaneous epicardial fibrous fronds on the atria of beagle dogs. Vet Pathol 1990;27:458–461.

Thomas WP, Reed JR, Bauer TG, et al. Constrictive pericardial disease in the dog. J Am Vet Med Assoc 1984;184:546–553.

Endocardium

INFECTIOUS ENDOCARDITIS

Inflammatory lesions of the endocardium are almost always infectious. The lesions, most common on the valves, are termed **valvular endocarditis** (Fig. 21-10). Less frequently, the primary lesion is on the wall of the atrium or ventricle and is termed **mural endocarditis.** The extension of valvular lesions to the mural endocardium or adjacent great vessels is not infrequent. Doubtless because of the greater pressure and mechanical strains to which the structures are subjected, valvular endocarditis is much more frequent on the left side of the heart than on the right, and also more frequent and more extensive on the atrioventricular than the semilunar valves. Bovines are the exception; the right atrioventricular valve is affected more frequently than the left. Infectious endocarditis is also much more prevalent when preexisting cardiac defects exist, either congenital or acquired.

Pathogenesis and lesions Infectious endocarditis can arise from primary adhesion of microorganisms to the endocardium or their adherence to thrombi that have developed on an endocardium damaged for other reasons (e.g., thrombi associated with congenital defects; Figs. 21-11 to 21-13). In the former circumstance, usually a primary infectious process occurs at another site that serves as the source of organisms. The lesions of endocarditis involve the death and disappearance of the endothelium, although this may be preceded by hy-

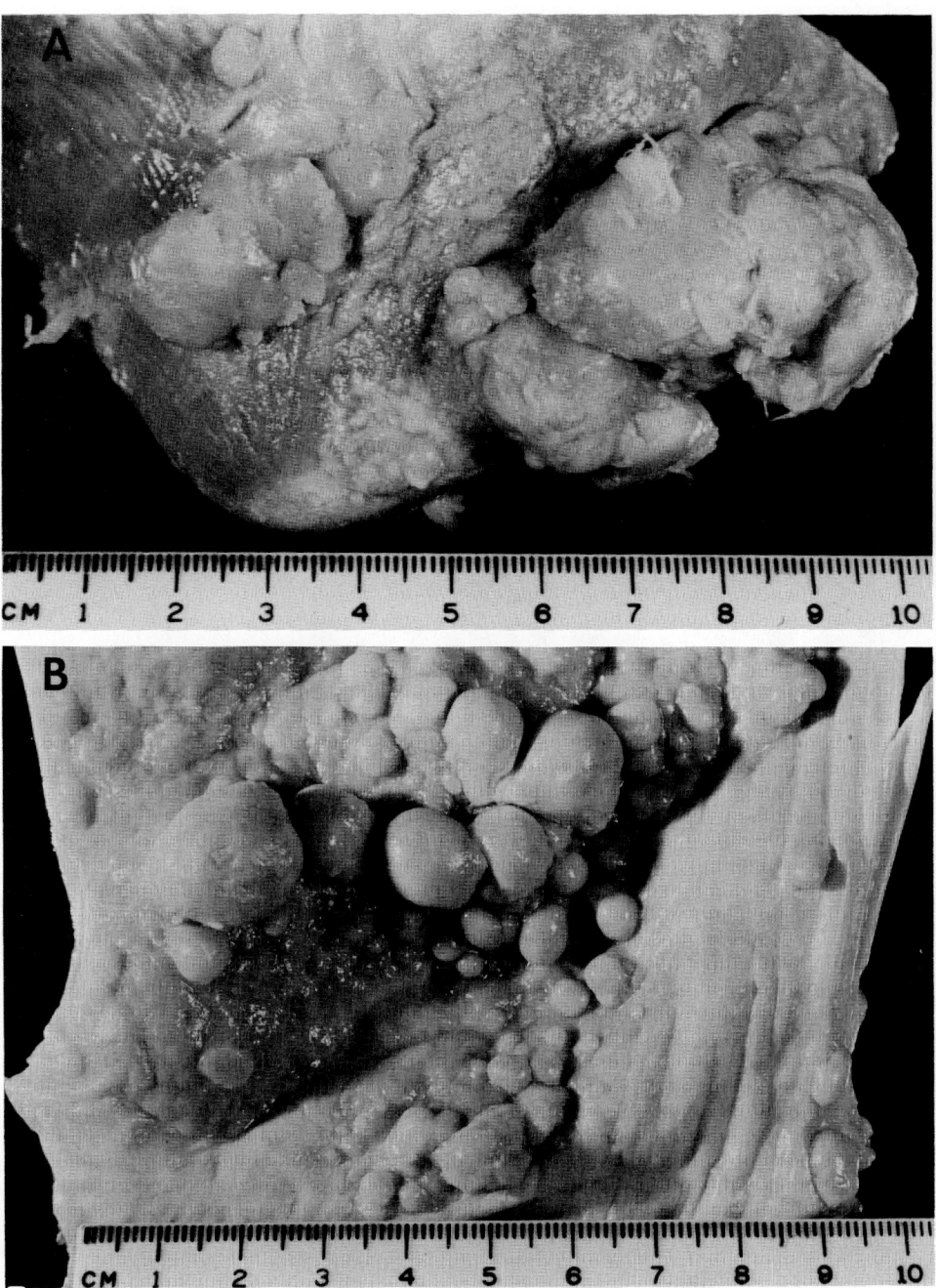

FIG. 21-9 Multiple mesotheliomas of pericardium of a 27-year-old quarter horse mare. **A.** Nodular growth on the epicardium of the apex of the heart. **B.** Multiple mesotheliomas on the pericardial sac of the same horse. (Courtesy of Dr. H.W. Leipold and Veterinary Pathology.)

peremia and infiltration of inflammatory cells in the affected area. On the raw surface left by the destroyed endothelium, a thrombus forms within which large colonies of microorganisms proliferate. The growths increase in size, assuming an irregular and bizarre shape (Fig. 21-11). Such growths are often called "vegetations," presumably because of their similarity in shape to the head of a cauliflower, and the lesion is termed **vegetative endocarditis.** Extension of the infection can lead to such abnormalities as the formation of abscesses in adjacent tissue, necrosis and rupture of chordae tendineae, and interference with conduction. Like other thrombi, the deeper parts are organized by granulation

tissue. In some cases, complete healing is possible, the uneven surface being covered by regenerated endothelium and the thrombus replaced by fibrous connective tissue; this tissue, when on a valve, may still be left with impaired function. As can be readily imagined, the effect of one or more foci of mural endocarditis in the atrium or ventricle may not be serious, but when on a valve—which is most common—important and often disastrous interference in function leads to congestive heart failure.

Another serious sequela to infectious endocarditis is embolization. Variously-sized pieces of the thrombus containing microorganisms detach from the primary le-

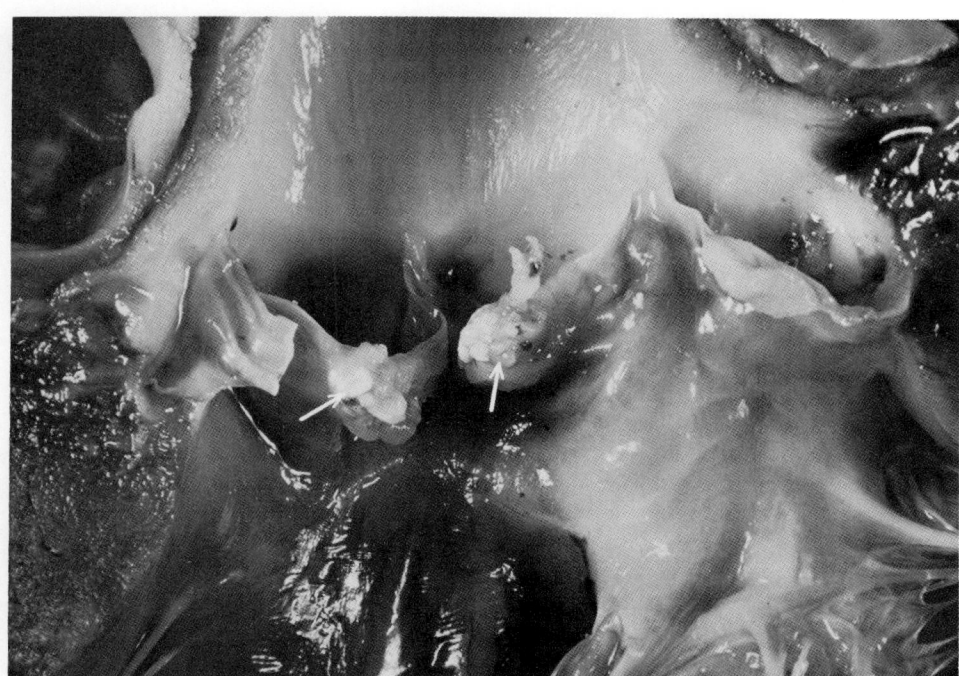

FIG. 21-10 Endocarditis of aortic semilunar valves of an eight-year-old spayed female Dachshund. Nodular lesions (arrows) on margin and surface of valves. (Courtesy of Angell Memorial Animal Hospital.)

sion and enter the systemic or pulmonary circulation. In the lung, these lead to pulmonary abscesses and, rarely, infarction. In the systemic circulation, emboli may lodge almost anywhere, but are most common in the kidney, spleen, and joints.

Causes Most microorganisms may cause endocarditis; however, some are encountered more often than others. In horses, *Streptococcus equi, Actinobacillus equuli,* and other organisms associated with umbilical infec-

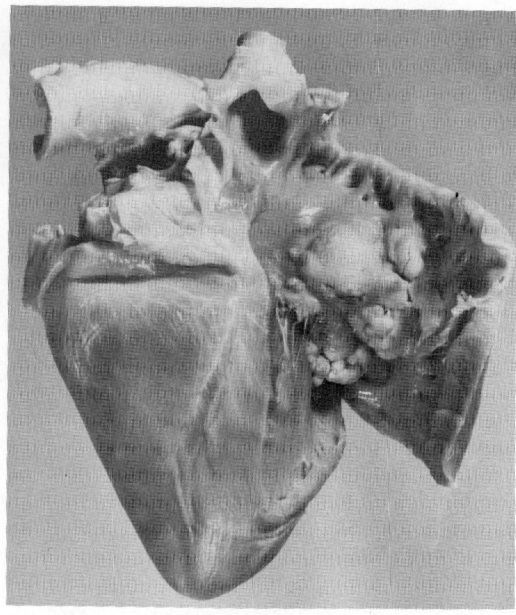

FIG. 21-11 Bacterial endocarditis affecting the tricuspid valve and mural endocardium in a five-year-old white-tailed deer. (Courtesy of Dr. W.J. Hadlow.)

tions of foals are the more recurrent. Migrating strongyle larvae may also lead to endocarditis in horses. In cattle, *Actinomyces pyogenes* is the most frequent isolate, and in swine, *Erysipelothrix rhusiopathiae* and *Streptococcus spp.* are the most frequent. In dogs, *Streptococcus spp., Staphylococcus spp., Corynebacterium spp., Erysipelothrix rhusiopathiae,* and *Escherichia coli* are frequent isolates. Coliforms, staphylococci, and streptococci may affect any species. Bacterial endocarditis is not common in cats. Certain fungi also cause endocarditis. These include Candida, Histoplasma, and fungi that have a predilection for the vascular tree, such as *Aspergillus spp.* and the Mucor group.

NONINFECTIOUS ENDOCARDITIS
Uremic endocarditis Uremia is probably the most common cause of endocarditis (and vasculitis) in dogs. The lesion is usually confined to the left atrium, but may extend into the left ventricle from uremic aortitis. The endocardium becomes edematous, which is followed by endocardial necrosis and thrombosis. Necrosis of the underlying myocardium, infiltration with leukocytes, and mineralization accompany the lesion.

Mural thrombi in the atria and ventricles are also common following other insults to the endocardium: for example, in association with congenital defects and cardiomyopathies.

Valvular endocardiosis (myxomatous or mucoid degeneration of mitral valve) The most common endocardial lesion in dogs is a degenerative lesion of unknown etiology termed, endocardiosis. Although any valve can be affected, it is the **mitral valve** that is usually involved, alone or in combination with the tricuspid valve. Grossly, the valvular cusps are distorted, often nodular and reduced in size, but markedly thickened

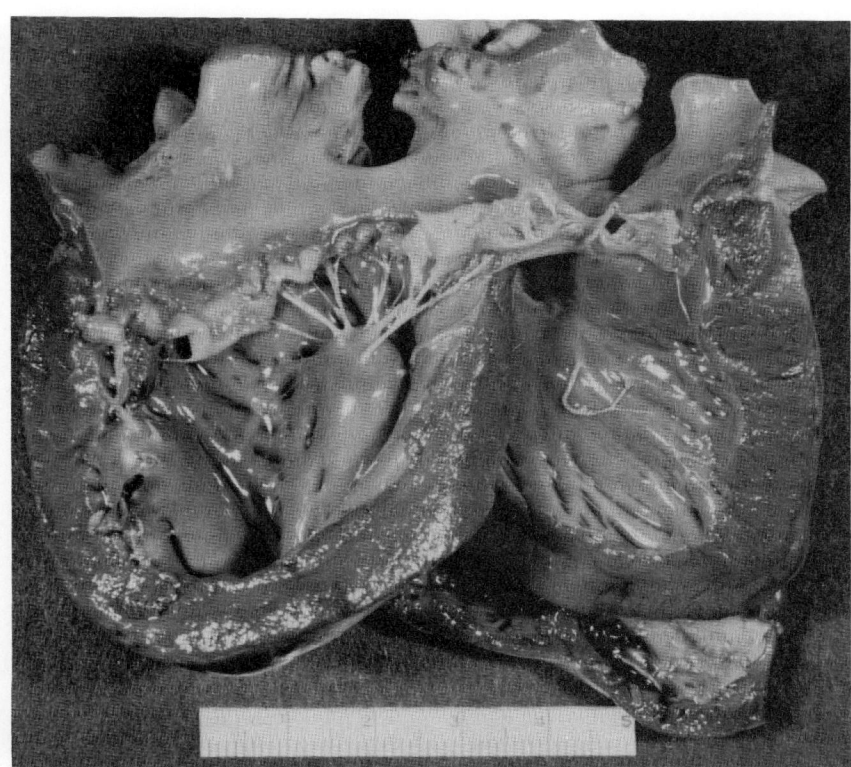

FIG. 21-12 Thickened, nodular left atrioventricular valve. The valve and the left ventricle were also dilated. From a 10-year-old female, crossbreed "Spitz" dog. (Courtesy of Angell Memorial Animal Hospital.)

(Figs. 21-12, 21-13). They are opaque, white, and glistening. Microscopically, the spongiosa layer of the valve is replaced by loose myxomatous connective tissue composed of widely separated stellate cells in a lightly basophilic ground substance composed of mucopolysaccharides, hyaluronic acid, and chondroitin sulfate. Overall, it resembles embryonic mesenchymal tissue. The peripheral fibrosa layer of the valve, which gives it its strength, undergoes hyalin degeneration, becomes disrupted, and ultimately disappears. Proliferation of the overlying endothelium is manifest. These changes may extend into the chordae tendineae, which may rupture. The disorder ultimately leads to failure of the mitral valve and dilatation of the left atrium, hypertrophy of the left ventricle, and congestive heart failure.

This disorder bears some resemblance to a condition in humans referred to as mitral valve prolapse and the aortic changes seen in Marfan syndrome. It is more common in male dogs and the incidence increases with age such that up to 75% of dogs 16 years of age and older are affected. Epidemiologic studies have indicated it to be most common in Cavalier King Charles spaniels, poodles, schnauzers, Doberman pinschers, fox terriers, Boston terriers, and whippets. German shepherds had a lower than expected incidence.

Valvular blood cysts are occasionally encountered on the atrioventricular valves, particularly in cattle and dogs. They appear to originate from valvular blood vessels, which are dilated to the point of becoming cysts resembling hematomas, containing stagnant blood. Smith and Taylor described a second type of blood cyst in cattle that develops from a preexisting invagination at the edge of the valve (1971). Blood cysts heal by replacement with fibrous connective tissue which, in dogs, have been described to contain metaplastic bone. They have not been described as interfering with function.

References

Beardow AW, Buchanan JW. Chronic mitral valve disease in Cavalier King Charles spaniels: 95 cases (1987–1991). J Am Vet Med Assoc 1993;203:1023–1029.

Bobb JRR, et al. Experimental endocarditis and other changes in dogs with arteriovenous fistulas and bacteremia. Am J Pathol 1952;28:523–524.

Buchanan JW. Chronic valvular disease (endocardiosis) in dogs. Adv Vet Sci Comp Med 1977;21:75–106.

Buergelt CD, Cooley AJ, Hines SA, et al. Endocarditis in six horses. Vet Pathol 1985;22:333–337.

Calvert CA. Valvular bacterial endocarditis in the dog. J Am Vet Med Assoc 1982;180:1080–1084.

Cotchin E, Hayward A. Streptococcal endocarditis in a pig following intravenous infection of an organism from a natural case. J Comp Pathol Ther 1953;63:68–73.

Crawshaw GR, et al. Mitral incompetence in the dog. S Afr J Med Sci 1953;18:79–83.

Dick GF, Swartz WB. Experimental endocarditis of dogs. Arch Pathol 1946;42:159–162.

Ernst E, Schneider P, Trautwein G. Aetiology and pathogenesis of endocardiosis and endocarditis of the dog. II. Pathological findings. Dtsch Tierarztl Wochenschr 1973;80:322–328.

Evans ETR. Bacterial endocarditis of cattle. Vet Rec 1957;69:1190–11201.

Hont S, Banks AW. Streptococcal endocarditis in young pigs. Aust Vet J 1944;20:206–210.

Innes JRM, et al. Subacute bacterial endocarditis with pulmonary embolism in a horse associated with Shigella equirulis. Br Vet J 1950;106:245–250.

Jamieson S, Stuart J. Streptococcal endocarditis in lambs. J Pathol Bacteriol 1950;62:235–239.

Johnson CM, Bahn RC, Fass DN. Experimental porcine infective endo-

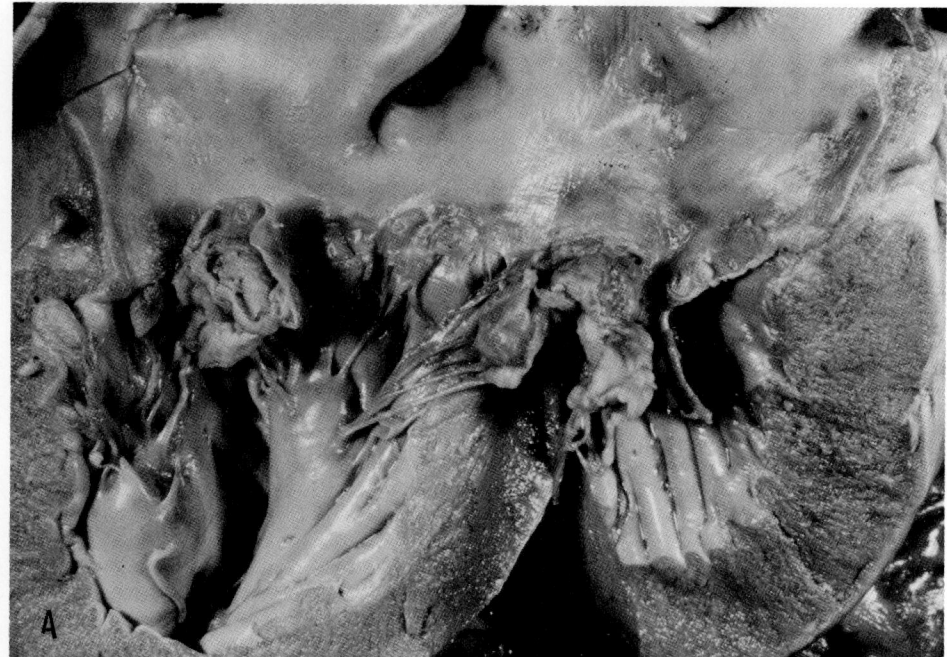

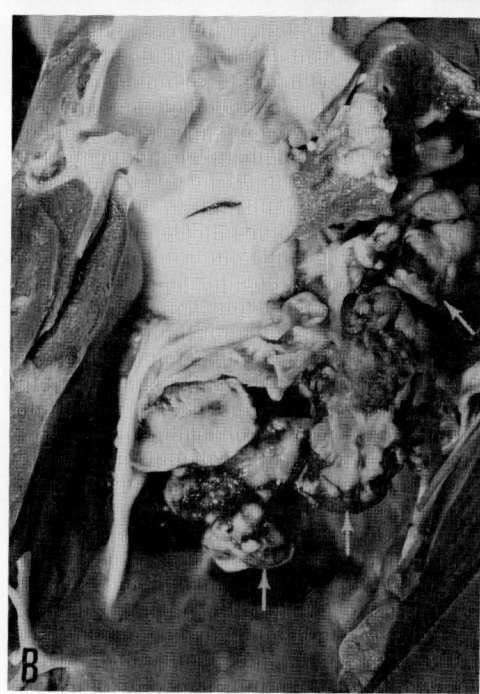

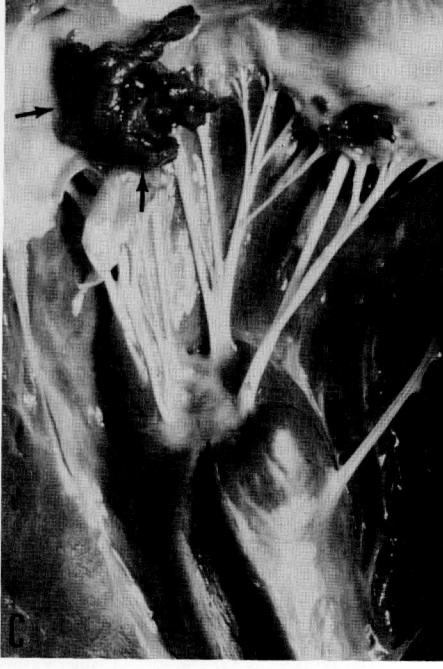

FIG. 21-13 A. Acute bacterial endocarditis involving the left atrioventricular valves of a 15-year-old male crossbreed terrier. (Courtesy of Angell Memorial Animal Hospital.) **B.** Valvular endocarditis in a cow. Note thick, irregular masses firmly attached to the bicuspid valve (arrows). (Courtesy of Armed Forces Institute of Pathology and Dr. C.L. Davis.) **C.** Smaller lesions (arrows) in the bicuspid valve of a cow; *Corynebacterium pyogenes* was isolated from the lesions.

carditis: description of a clinical model. Vet Pathol 1986; 23:780–782.

Kersten U, Brass W. Aetiology and pathogenesis of endocardiosis and endocarditis in dogs. I. Introduction and clinical findings. Dtsch Tierarztl Wochenschr 1973;80:315–322.

Kogure K. Pathology of chronic mitral valvular disease in the dog. Jpn J Vet Sci 1980;42:323–335.

Osebold JW, Cordy DR. Valvular endocarditis associated with Listeria monocytogenes infections of sheep. J Am Vet Med Assoc 1963; 143:990–993.

Peery TM, Belter LF. Brucellosis and heart disease. II. Fatal brucellosis: a review of the literature and report of new cases. Am J Pathol 1960;36:673–679.

Power HT, Rebhun WC. Bacterial endocarditis in adult dairy cattle. J Am Vet Med Assoc 1983;182:806–808.

Schneider P, Ernst E, Trautwein G. Amyloidosis of the heart valves of the dog. Vet Pathol 1971;8:130–145.

Shouse CL, Meier H. Acute vegetative endocarditis in the dog and cat. J Am Vet Med Assoc 1956;129:278–289.

Sisson D, Thomas WP. Endocarditis of the aortic valve in the dog. J Am Vet Med Assoc 1984;184:570–577.

Smith RB, Taylor IM. Blood cysts of the cardiac valves of calves and cattle. Cardovasc Res 1971;5:132–135.

Svenkerud RR, Iversen L. Shigella equirulis (S. viscosum equi) som arsak til klappeendocarditis hos hest. [Shigella equirulis (S. viscosum equi) isolated from a horse with vegetative endocarditis.] Nord Vet Med 1949;1:227–232.

Takeda T, Makita T, Nakamura N, et al. Morphologic aspects and morphogenesis of blood cysts on canine cardiac valves. Vet Pathol 1991;28:16–21.

Whitney JC. Observations on the effect of age on the severity of heart valve lesions in the dog. J Small Anim Pract 1974;15:511–522.

BLOOD VESSELS AND LYMPHATIC VESSELS

Arteries

ARTERIOSCLEROSIS

Arteriosclerosis, which literally means hardening of the arteries, is of infinitely more importance in humans than it is in animals. Under the general term, arteriosclerosis are three different forms: **atherosclerosis, Monckeberg medial sclerosis or calcification,** and **arteriosclerosis.** None of these is common in animals.

Atherosclerosis Atherosclerosis is the most frequent and important vascular disease in humans and is the leading cause of death through myocardial infarction, cerebral infarction, aortic aneurysm, and other complications. It is, however, practically nonexistent in animals, exceptions being the extensive atherosclerosis seen in dogs (Fig. 21-14) with hypothyroidism, and occasional atherosclerotic lesions seen in swine and nonhuman primates. In humans, atherosclerosis chiefly affects large- and medium-sized elastic and muscular arteries, such as the aorta, and coronary and cerebral arteries, but spares smaller branches and arterioles. The basic lesion is referred to as **atheroma,** which is an intimal plaque projecting into the lumen and media. At first, these are small and composed of collections of mononuclear cells whose cytoplasm is filled with lipid droplets. The cells beneath the endothelium in the intima resemble macrophages, but are in fact altered smooth muscle cells (Fig. 21-15). The proliferation of altered smooth muscle cells is believed by many to precede lipid deposition. The accumulated lipids include cholesterol, fatty acids, triglycerides, and phospholipids.

As the lesion progresses, fibrous connective tissue surrounds the lipid-laden cells, prompting the designation **fibrous plaque.** This would appear to be an unsuccessful attempt at healing. With further lipid deposition and fibrosis, the plaques become confluent and may involve the entire arterial wall. Lipids also accumulate outside cells, especially near the centers of plaques. Presumably lipid-filled cells rupture; however, direct extracellular deposition is not ruled out. This is seen as a clear, hazy area, often with cholesterol taking on crystalline form as shown by cholesterol clefts (Fig. 21-16). A number of other features may accompany the advanced lesions including hyalinization of fibrous connective tissue, necrosis of small-to-large areas of plaques, calcification, and osseous metaplasia. The endothelium may be destroyed (ulcerated), exposing the plaque to lumen leading to atheromatous emboli and local thrombosis. The lesion is restricted to the intima, but secondary thinning of the media and fragmentation of the elastica are associated with advanced lesions. The reduced strength of the wall may result in an aneurysm. Al-

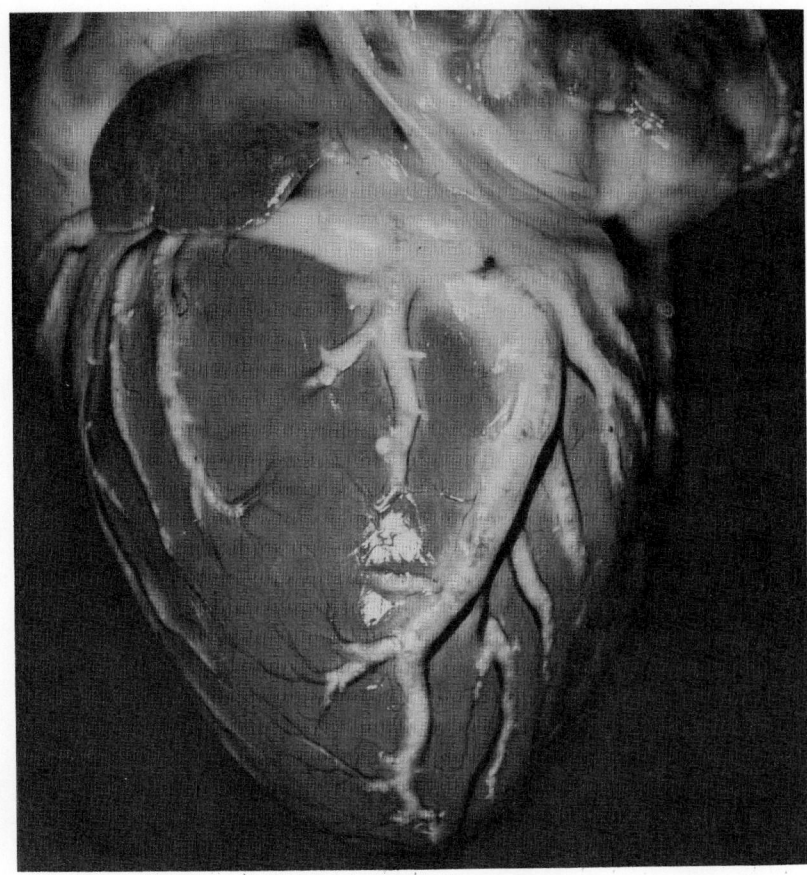

FIG. 21-14 Atherosclerosis of coronary arteries of a nine-year-old German shepherd. The major branches of these arteries are yellowish and thickened due to lipid in the media. (Fig. 21-15 details the microscopic appearance; courtesy of Angell Memorial Animal Hospital.)

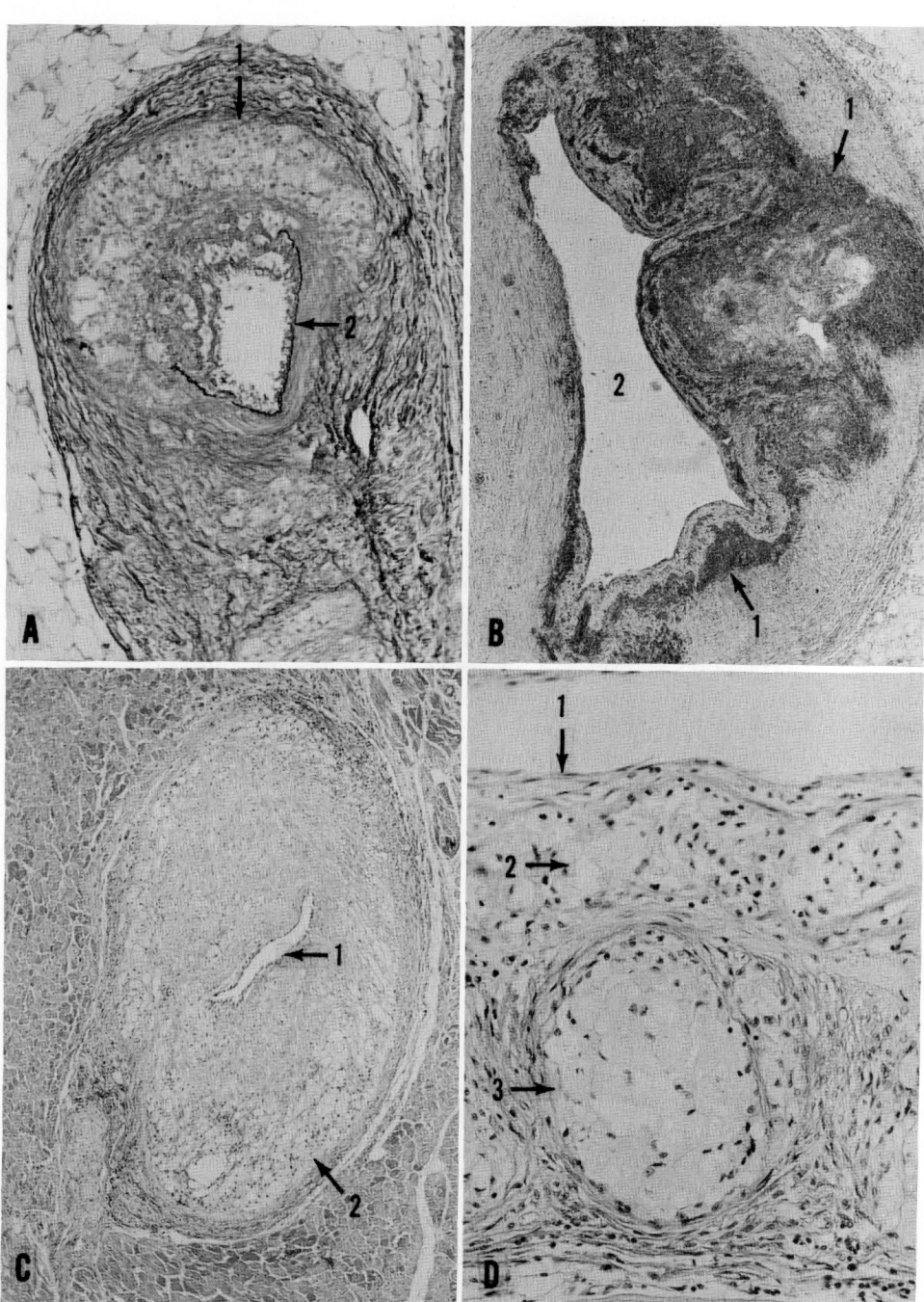

FIG. 21-15 Xanthomatosis or atherosclerosis in the coronary arteries of a dog. **A.** Cross section of a coronary artery (×80). Elastica stain. 1 Lipid-laden cells in media and intima. 2 Note rupture of internal elastic lamina. **B.** A section (×35) of another segment of the same coronary artery, stained for lipid by Sudan III. 1 Note sudanophilic material particularly in the media. 2 The lumen is indicated. **C.** A branch of the coronary artery. 1 Endothelium. 2 Lipid-laden foam cells in media (hematoxylin and eosin stain, ×55.) **D.** Higher magnification (×175) of a wall of a coronary artery. 1 Endothelium, 2 lipid-laden macrophages in subintima, and 3 in media. (Courtesy of Armed Forces Institute of Pathology; and Dr. Wayne H. Riser.)

though the lumen may be narrowed, the most serious consequence of atherosclerosis in humans is thrombosis which often results in myocardial or cerebral ischemia and infarction.

The cause of atherosclerosis is not known. Many theories have been developed, but no single, causative factor has been identified.

Monckeberg medial sclerosis or calcification This is the second of the arteriosclerotic entities. Instead of affecting the large, elastic arteries of the body, it involves the medium-sized, muscular arteries. Hyaline and fatty

degenerative changes occur in the muscular tissue of the media, leading to necrosis. The process is gradual and, as a typical sequence of necrosis, calcification regularly supervenes. Rarely, ossification occurs in the vessel wall. This form of arteriosclerosis is manifest with advancing age but not necessarily with hypertension. It is believed to be related causally to prolonged or habitual overstimulation of the medial musculature by the vasomotor (sympathetic) nerves. Experimentally, a similar calcification has been produced in dogs and rabbits by excessive administration of epinephrine (adrenaline). Nicotine is said to

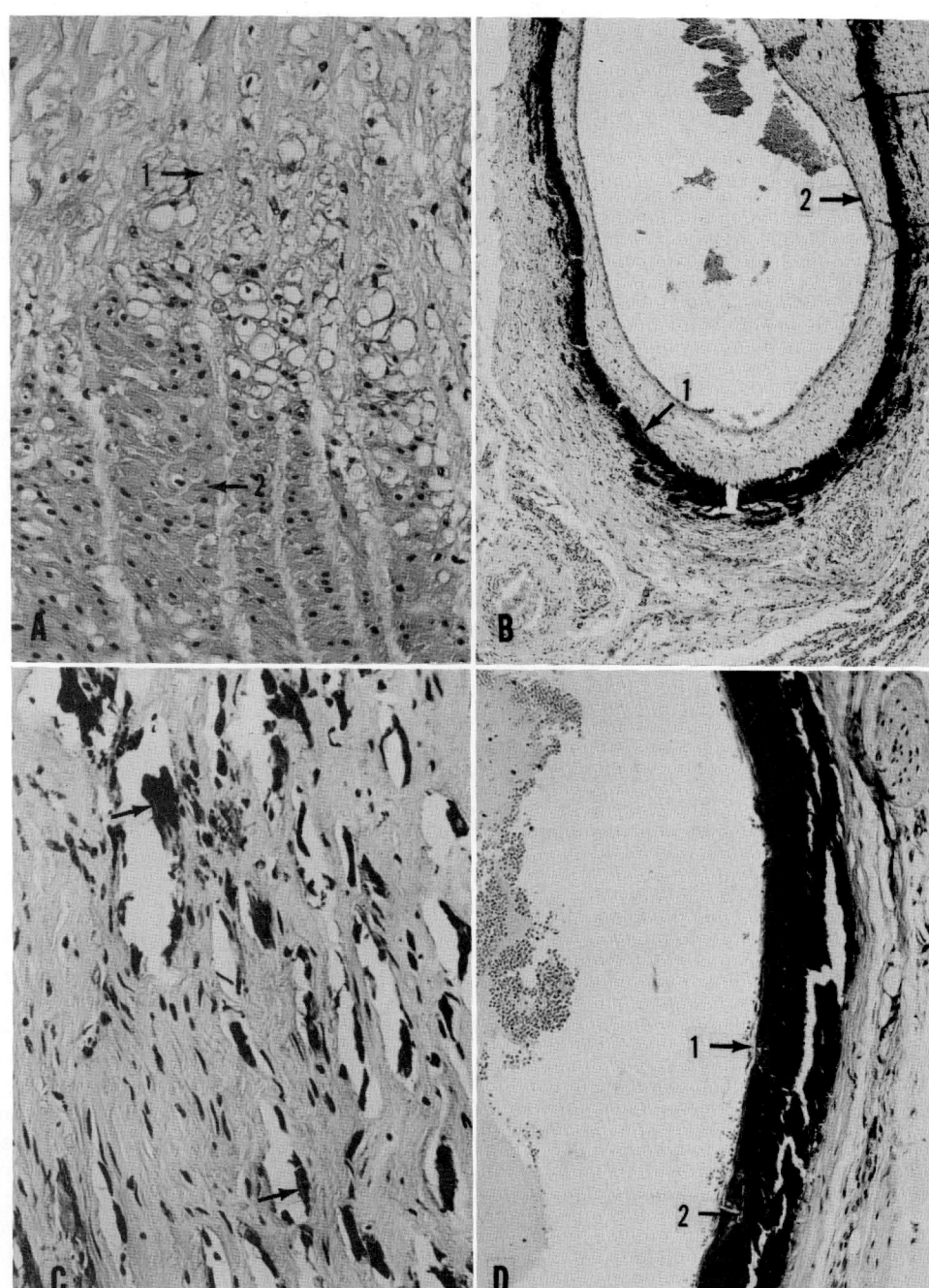

FIG. 21-16 A. Medial sclerosis of aorta (×300) of a cow. 1 Scarred but not yet calcified area is distinguishable from 2 the normal media. (Contributor: Dr. E.L. Stubbs.) **B.** 1 Medial calcification in a bovine pulmonary artery (×45). 2 Intima. (Contributor: Dr. J.F. Ryff.) **C.** Calcification (arrows) of the media of a bovine aorta (×300). (Contributor: Dr. E.L. Stubbs.) **D.** 2 Calcification in an artery (×130) of a cat which died of uremia. 1 Intima. (Courtesy of Armed Forces Institute of Pathology and Dr. Edward Baker.)

have a similar effect. Hyperparathyroidism and vitamin D toxicity are other well-known causes of medial calcification of arteries. Poisoning by *Solanum malacoxylon* and *Cestrum diurnum* also lead to arterial calcification. Deposition of calcium and iron salts in the walls of cerebral arterioles (cerebrovascular siderosis) is occasionally encountered in many species, but is of unknown significance (Fig. 21-16). In horses, small, mineralized bodies, termed **intimal bodies** or **asteroid bodies** are often found in the intima of arterioles, especially in the intestinal submucosa, but their significance is unknown. They stain with toluidine blue and the PAS reaction and react with stains for phosphorus and calcium. They begin to develop early in life and increase in number with age. Extensive calcification of the aorta and large thoracic arteries (media only) has been seen in young cattle, otherwise normal, when slaughtered for beef (Gailiunas, 1958).

Arteriosclerosis This third entity of arteriosclerotic disease is also much more common in humans than in animals. It is subdivided into two major forms, **hyaline arteriosclerosis** and **hyperplastic arteriosclerosis.** Hyaline arteriosclerosis is characterized by replacement of the arteriolar wall with a homogeneous, eosinophilic, hyaline material and narrowing of the lumen. In humans, hyaline arteriosclerosis is a feature of diabetic angiopathy and aging and is more frequent in patients with hypertension. Comparable lesions are encountered sporadically in animals, usually without a known pathogenesis. Vascular lesions of diabetes are less frequent in animals than in humans. Hyperplastic arteriosclerosis is characterized by hyperplasia of arteriolar smooth muscle cells and fibrinoid necrosis. Hypertension is the principal cause in humans. Both of these arteriolar diseases also accentuate hypertension by affecting renal arterioles, leading to **arteriolar nephrocalcinosis** and renal hypertension.

Although it occurs in animals, systemic hypertension is not as important as it is in humans. In animals, it occurs in chronic renal disease, hyperthyroidism, hyperadrenocorticism, and with pheochromocytomas. Pulmonary hypertension (cor pulmonale), as discussed earlier, is a feature of certain congenital anomalies and high altitude disease in cattle. In each of these disorders, arteriolar lesions develop which are characterized by intimal thickening, medial hypertrophy, and medial necrosis.

The most common arteriosclerotic lesions found in animals are incidental findings and essentially unimportant to health. In most species, lesions consisting of varying combinations of irregular thickenings of the intima due to smooth muscle hyperplasia, medial hyperplasia, medial fibrosis, and medial hyalinization can be found, especially in the aorta, large arteries, and coronary arteries. These lesions are seen most frequently in dogs.

HYPERTENSION

Systemic hypertension is one of the most significant and important diseases in humans. Most hypertensive patients are afflicted with what is termed **essential hypertension (primary hypertension, idiopathic hypertension),** for which the cause and pathogenesis are not known. Hypertension can also develop secondarily to other diseases (termed **secondary hypertension**). Hypertension leads to cardiac hypertrophy and changes in small muscular arteries and arterioles, characterized by intimal thickening, smooth muscle hyperplasia, medial hyalinization, and necrosis with narrowing of the lumen.

Essential hypertension in animals is rare, but has been reported in dogs and cats and occurs in horses with laminitis. Secondary hypertension is common in dogs with chronic renal disease. This results from activation of the renin-angiotensin system, as well as expansion of the extracellular fluid volume from retention of sodium and water. Interpretation of hypertension in chronic renal disease requires caution because arteriolar disease secondary to essential hypertension leads to decreased renal perfusion, secondary renal disease, and activation of the renin-angiotensin system and fluid retention. Arteriolar disease in hypertension is generalized and can also lead to ischemic lesions in other organs. Dogs with hypertension often present with blindness due to arteriolar disease of the retina. Other causes of secondary hypertension in animals include hyperadrenocorticism, pheochromocytoma, hyperthyroidism, and hyperparathyroidism.

ARTERITIS

Arteritis is characterized by an inflammatory reaction in the arterial wall, the nature of the inflammation varying with the specific cause. Secondarily, arteritis may occur as part of most any inflammatory disease of other tissues, but is also seen as a primary manifestation in a number of conditions. Arteritis often leads to endothelial damage and thrombosis. Several **metazoan parasites** inhabit or pass part of their life cycle in arteries and elicit varying degrees of inflammation and necrosis. These include: *Strongylus vulgaris* in horses; *Dirofilaria immitis, Spirocerca lupi,* and *Angiostrongylus vasorum* in dogs; *Elaeophora abstrusus* in sheep and elk; *Onchocerca armillata* in cattle; *Aelurostrongylus abstrusus* in cats; and *Angiostrongylus cantonensis* in rats. Arteritis is also a feature of some **viral infections.** These include equine viral arteritis, Border disease, blue tongue, hog cholera, African swine fever, feline infectious peritonitis (also phlebitis), African horse sickness, and cytomegalovirus infections. Arteritis is seen in a number of **bacterial infections,** but with only a few (including *Haemophilus spp.* and *Erysipelothrix rhusiopathiae*) as the primary expression. In **mycotic diseases,** arteritis is commonly seen in conditions caused by *Aspergillus fumigatus* and members of the Mucor group. Additionally, early stages of sarcosporidial **protozoans** invade endothelial cells, leading to arteritis. Many cases of arteritis are due to **hypersensitivity, allergic reactions,** or **immune complex disease.** Examples include serum sickness or the Arthus reaction and equine purpura hemorrhagica, but immune complexes also play a role in several of the infectious forms of arteritis cited above. Hypersensitivity arteritis and arteriolitis are characterized by necrosis and cellular infiltration primarily composed of neutrophils.

In addition to these causes of arteritis, degenerative arteriopathies are encountered in animals as part of other diseases. **Uremic arteriopathy,** often referred to as an arteritis, is one of the most frequently encountered forms in dogs. It is characterized by fibrinoid necrosis and often calcification of the media, intimal edema, and fibrin deposition. Both **edema disease** and **mulberry heart disease** of swine are characterized by fibrinoid or hyaline necrosis of the arterioles. Chronic **selenium poisoning** is characterized by fibrinoid necrosis of arterioles; in some examples of **organomercurial poisoning,** fibrinoid necrosis of arterioles occurs in the leptomininges.

Lesions similar to those described in humans as **polyarteritis nodosa,** sometimes termed periarteritis nodosa or panarteritis nodosa, are occasionally encountered in dogs, cattle, and other animals (Figs. 21-17, 21-18). It affects medium-to-small muscular arteries. One form is particularly frequent in certain strains of laboratory rats. Another has been described as occurring with a relatively high frequency in colonies of beagle dogs, primarily affecting the right coronary artery. Lesions

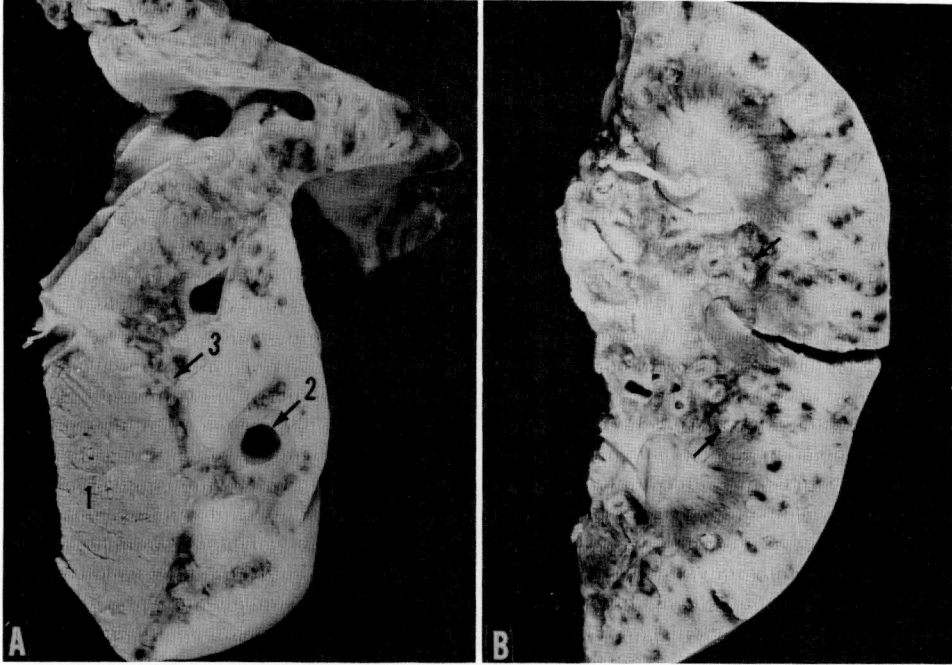

FIG. 21-17 Periarteritis nodosa or generalized arteritis in a bovine. **A.** 1 Myocardium, 2 large, unaffected coronary artery, and 3 many thick-walled arteries in epicardium. **B.** The kidney, with many redundant, thick-walled arteries (arrows). (Courtesy of Armed Forces Institute of Pathology and Dr. C.L. Davis.)

are characterized by segmental arteritis composed of fibrinoid necrosis, extensive infiltration with a mixed population of leukocytes, and intimal and medial fibroplasia.

Aneurysm

Aneurysm is a pathologic dilatation of an artery (or a cardiac chamber), usually, but not invariably, saccular in shape and definitely circumscribed. True aneurysm results from weakening of the vessel wall, which is stretched beyond its capacity to resist, and certain layers, ordinarily the intima and media, have been wholly or partly ruptured. When development has been gradual, replacement of the damaged tissues by an excess of fibrous tissue is the rule.

A second form is the dissecting aneurysm or **false aneurysm.** This is due to fracture or necrosis in the medial layer of the aorta or some other large artery. Through an interruption of the inner coat or sometimes apparently through the vasa vasorum, the blood current gains access to the medial defect. Under consid-

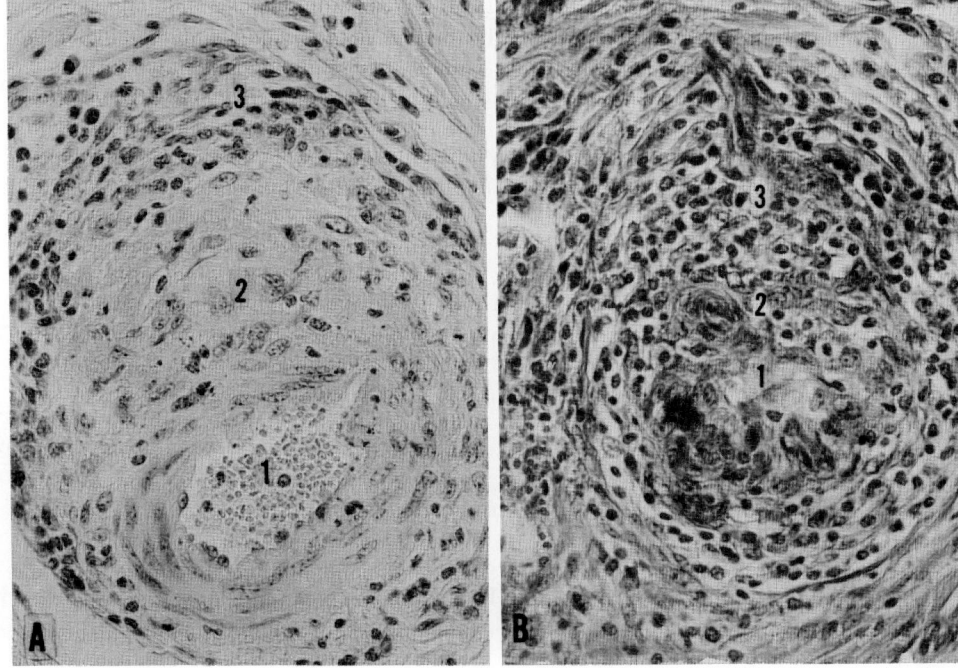

FIG. 21-18 Periarteritis nodosa in bovine arteries. **A.** A mildly affected artery (×330). 1 The arterial lumen, 2 media, and 3 adventitia. **B.** A severely affected artery. 1 Lumen, 2 media, and 3 adventitia. (Courtesy of Armed Forces Institute of Pathology and Dr. C.L. Davis.)

erable arterial pressure, blood splits the inner cylindrical layer from the outer, much as the intact cylinder of bark can sometimes be separated from the inner wood of a twig. Blood, thus, flows in two tubes, one inside the other. Once started, this arrangement may extend for a considerable distance or even for the length of the aorta, the blood returning to its normal channel when one of the main arterial branches is encountered.

The causes of aneurysms are damage done by inflammatory or arteriosclerotic and degenerative disease. Syphilitic aortitis is a classic, but by no means unique cause in humans. However, evidence exists of nutritional causes for dissecting aneurysm in rats, where it accompanies poisoning by the sweet pea *(Lathyrus odoratus)* (Bachhuber and Lalich, 1954), and in turkeys, where a diet containing aflatoxin has appeared to have a causative relationship (Carnaghan, 1955; McSherry et al., 1954; Pritchard et al., 1958). In copper deficiency, the failure to form cross-linking in elastin leads to defective arterial walls, which can result in aneurysms and rupture, especially of the aorta. Aneurysms of the pulmonary artery in cattle may result from infectious emboli lodging at this site and weakening the wall. Emboli originate from thrombi in the vena cava secondary to hepatic abscesses. Injurious effects of aneurysms exist chiefly in the danger of rupture of the vessel or in the formation of a thrombus on the damaged and roughened intimal wall.

Mucoid medial degeneration

Also known as **Erdheim disease** or **idiopathic cystic medionecrosis,** mucoid medial degeneration is a disease of the aorta of unknown cause. It is associated with a genetic defect in Marfan syndrome in humans, but is also seen independently of this disorder. A similar degeneration is occasionally encountered in domestic animals, especially in dogs and cattle, and has been described in poultry. The lesion resembles, in many respects, the aorta in lathyrism. Histopathologically, diffuse or patchy fragmentation occurs, as well as loss of muscle and elastic fibers and a marked increase in mucopolysaccharide ground substance. The resultant weakening of the wall may lead to aneurysms. Comparable lesions may also develop in other major arteries.

Atrophy of arteries

Atrophy of arteries and arterioles occurs in ergotism and the similar poisoning by fescue grass. Continuously contracted, bloodless arteries shrink and accompany the surrounding tissues to gangrenous destruction.

Natural atrophy, which occurs in those vessels that normally change into ligaments with the advent of postnatal life, is a more gradual process than may be expected. For instance, the closing of the umbilical arteries begins when they are severed at birth, but may require as long as two months for completion (e.g., calves). The lumen is contracted, but remains filled with hemolyzed and eventually clotted blood; its slow recession can be followed inch by inch from the umbilicus to the bladder, as a central core of fibrous tissue progresses upward. This

may be viewed as disuse atrophy, similar to the change that occurs when a vessel is ligated.

Hypertrophy

Medial hypertrophy of branches of the pulmonary artery is frequently recognized in the domestic cat. The affected arteries have thick, hyperplastic muscular walls and often intimal fibrosis, which effectively narrows the lumen (Fig. 21-19C). The cause and pathogenesis remain unknown. Evidence indicates that this lesion is related to prior infection with *Aelurostrongylus abstrusus* or *Toxocara cati* (Stunzi et al., 1966; Hamilton, 1966); however, others observed the condition in specific-pathogen-free cats in which no evidence of *A. abstrusus* infection existed (Rogers et al., 1971).

Medial hypertrophy of arteries is a feature of hypertension from any cause. In animals, it is most often encountered in pulmonary arteries following right-sided heart failure. It is also a feature of high altitude disease.

Thrombosis

Coagulation and the causes of thrombosis are reviewed in Chapter 6. Two of the most frequently encountered examples include thrombosis of the anterior mesenteric artery in horses, associated with *Strongylus vulgaris* migration (Fig. 21-19), and aortic saddle thrombosis at the iliac bifurcation in cats and horses. The pathogenesis of saddle thrombi is not clear. In cats, some have been associated with embolisms from cardiac mural thrombi developing in association with cardiomyopathy. Saddle thrombi result in hind leg weakness, paraplegia, loss of femoral pulse, cold rear extremities, pain, and ultimately, muscle atrophy. These signs have been presumed to result from ischemia from inadequate collateral circulation; however, evidence in cats indicates that it is more complicated than simple ischemia.

Butler and others showed that neither single nor double aortic ligation in cats results in paralysis despite loss of femoral pulse (1971). Butler was able to induce paralysis, however, when 5-hydroxytryptamine was injected into the aorta between the double ligatures. He suggested that the release of 5-hydroxytryptamine by platelets in the thrombus interfered with collateral circulation by causing contraction of vascular smooth muscle.

Amyloidosis

Amyloid is often deposited in vessels. Amyloidosis of coronary arteries is not infrequent in aged dogs. Intramural arteries and arterioles are affected, often with obstruction of the lumens and resultant myocardial necrosis and fibrosis.

EQUINE INTIMAL (ASTEROID) BODIES

Mineralized hyaline bodies are a frequent finding in the intima of arterioles of horses (Figs. 21-20 to 21-23). In ordinary paraffin-embedded sections, they appear as pleomorphic, densely-stained bodies in the subendothelial space. They are round to oval, often with projections, and stain with the PAS reaction, toluidine blue, and are positive with stains for calcium and phosphorus. They are most frequently encountered in arterioles of the gastrointestinal tract, affecting all levels with the exception of the esophagus. They are less frequent in other tissues, but also can be found in the liver, lung, heart, kidney, brain, and other organs. Although the etiology and pathogenesis are unknown, mineralized hyaline bodies are believed to originate from smooth muscle cells.

Veins

Phlebitis

PHLEBITIS, THROMBOPHLEBITIS

Phlebitis, inflammation of a vein, is usually accompanied by thrombosis, hence the term, thrombophlebitis. It may be initiated by a primary inflammatory process or by thrombosis accompanied by secondary inflammation. Most frequently neutrophilic leukocytes predominate; in chronic forms, inflammatory fibrous tissue surrounds the vein. These can hardly be expected to be confined within

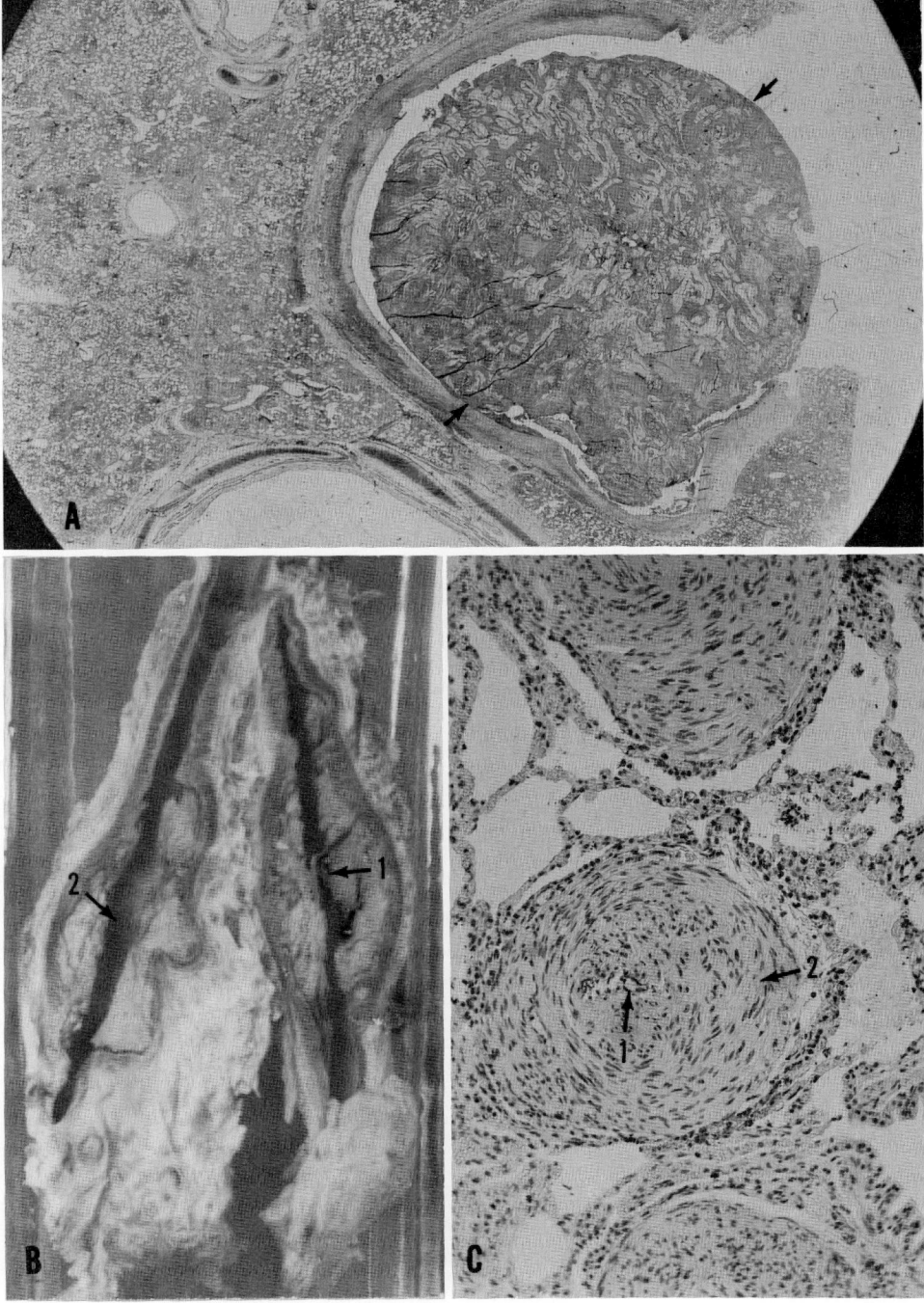

FIG. 21-19 A. Thrombosis of the pulmonary artery (×5) of a horse. (Contributor: Dr. J.R.M. Innes.) **B.** Verminous arteritis, anterior mesenteric artery of a horse. 1 A single larva of *Strongylus vulgaris* is seen; although the wall is necrotic and thickened by inflammation, 2 the lumen appears reasonably patent. (Specimen in Mark Francis Collection, Texas Sch. Vet. Med.) **C.** Medial hypertrophy, branches of the pulmonary artery (×130) of a cat. 1 Intima is surrounded by some sclerosis, 2 but the greatest increase in diameter is due to thickened media. (**A.** and **C.** Courtesy of Armed Forces Institute of Pathology and Dr. Leo L. Lieberman.)

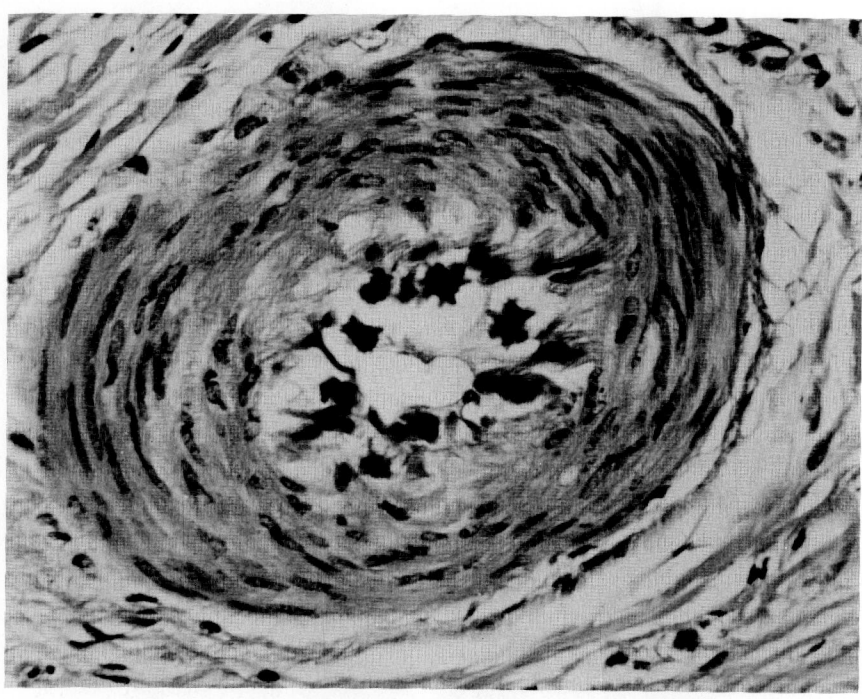

FIG. 21-20 Equine intimal bodies. Irregularly shaped, dense bodies in intima of an arteriole. (Courtesy of Dr. Richard J. Montali and Laboratory Investigation.)

the thin wall of a vein, but phlebitis occurs usually within a more extensively inflamed and infected area through which the vein passes. Or, it may represent spread of the inflammatory process to the wall: for example, the frequent occurrence of thrombophlebitis of the caudal vena cava following hepatic abscesses in cattle. Phlebitis involving the smaller veins is a regular feature of extensively in-

fected wounds, of septic metritis, or of similar processes. The principal dangers from such inflamed (and usually infected) veins include: necrosis resulting in local hemorrhage, and formation of thrombi, parts of which may become detached as emboli.

More specific causes of phlebitis include feline infectious peritonitis and schistosomiasis.

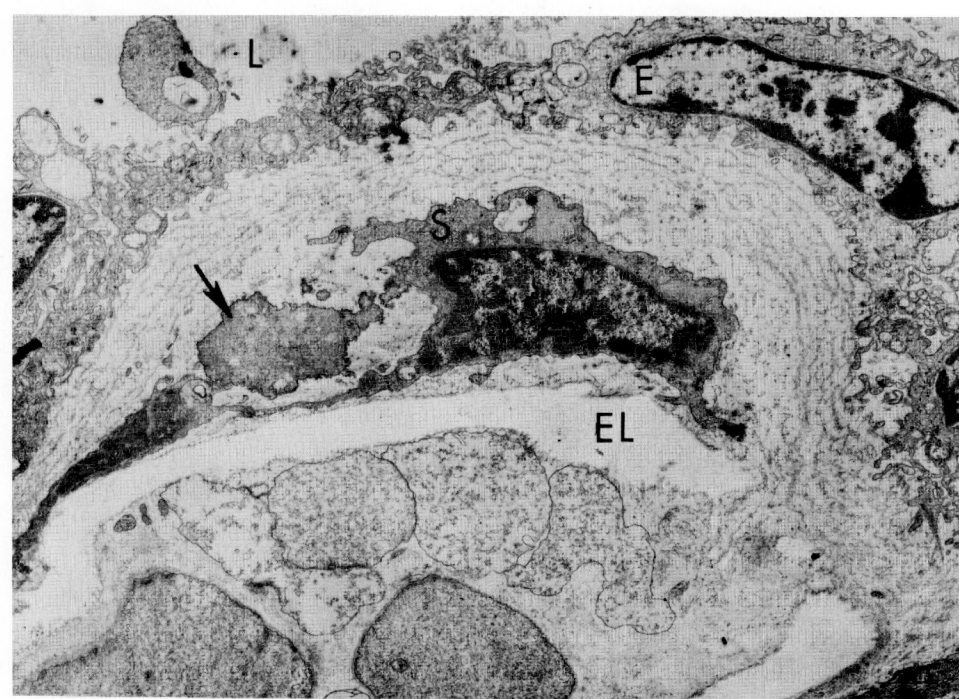

FIG. 21-21 Equine intimal body. Electron micrograph ($\times 8,200$). L, lumen of arteriole; E, nucleus of endothelial cell; EL, internal elastic lamina; S, subendothelial cell; arrow, irregular, dense mass associated with cytoplasm of subendothelial cell. (Courtesy of Dr. Richard J. Montali and Laboratory Investigation.)

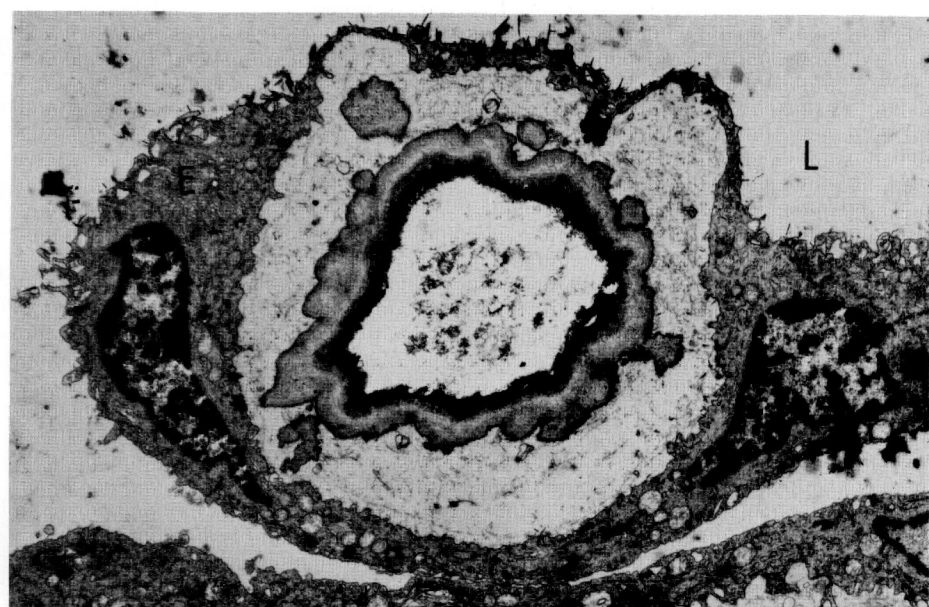

FIG. 21-22 Equine intimal body with a hollow core (×8,000). E, endothelial cell, surrounding central-mass; L, lumen of arteriole. (Courtesy of Dr. Richard J. Montali and Laboratory Investigation.)

Varicose veins

Varicose veins are markedly dilated and, at the same time elongated so that, in order to find a place for the excess length, they follow an irregular, tortuous course. They, thus, hold an abnormal amount of blood, which tends to become static. Local anoxia and malnutrition result, together with a certain amount of pain. The condition also favors thrombosis within the vein, although this is not a frequent complication unless surgery or other intervention is conducted. In animals, they occur chiefly in the hind legs, the saphenous and other superficial veins being involved. The usual cause is trauma or traumatic hindrance of return flow at some point in advance of the varicose area.

Telangiectasis

Telangiectasis is marked dilatation of each of an abnormal cluster of blood vessels which may simulate hemangioma. The structure of their walls usually characterizes

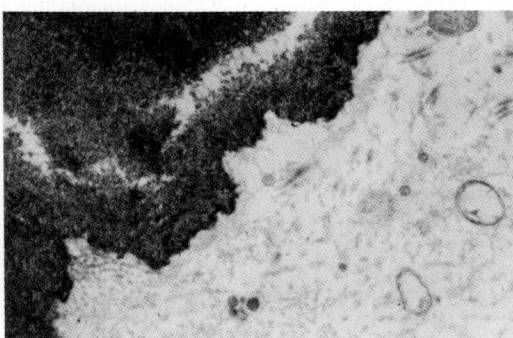

FIG. 21-23 Equine intimal body. Membranous debris, collagen fragments, bits of altered elastica, and basement membrane in light area on right; electron dense central mass on left. (Courtesy of Dr. Richard J. Montali and Laboratory Investigation.)

them as capillaries, although occasionally the more complicated structure of veins may be present. A type occurring beneath the skin or mucous membrane and elsewhere in humans is considered to be hereditary. The most common form of telangiectasis in animals is dilatation of hepatic sinusoids accompanied by hepatocellular atrophy and loss in one or more lobules of the liver. It is most frequent in cattle and cats. The gross appearance is that of a small (one to several millimeters), irregular spot that is slightly depressed and so dark with venous blood as to be almost black. The lesions are often numerous in livers of animals slaughtered for food and cause condemnation of the affected parts. The cause is not known, but it is speculated to result from portal thrombi.

Renal telangiectasis occurs in dogs and may lead to hematuria. Multiple organ telangiectasis with bilateral renal cortical and medullary lesions has been reported in a group of Pembroke Welsh Corgi dogs.

LYMPHATIC VESSELS

Lymphangectasia Dilatation of lymphatics is frequently associated with inflammatory and neoplastic diseases that obstruct the normal lymphatic flow. The parasite *Dracunculus insignis* resides in lymphatics, causing obstruction as well as lymphangitis. Obstruction of lymphatics leads to edema (lymphedema) of the affected organ or tissue. When they are affected by the obstructive process, major lymphatics may rupture leading to chylothorax, chylous ascites, or chylopericardium. Hereditary lymphedema is discussed under congenital anomalies of the cardiovascular system.

Lymphangitis

Lymphangitis is diagnosed under much the same circumstances as phlebitis; that is, when concern exists over an infectious inflammatory process that may spread by the lymphatic vessels. The extremely thin vascular wall is, in itself, scarcely capable of harboring any significant inflammatory exudate; the disease process belongs originally to the surrounding tissues. The specific lymphangitides, such as equine epizootic lymphangitis, cause the subcutaneous and other lymphatic vessels to be visibly distended and somewhat thickened, but the lesions are principally in the contiguous tissues, including the normally microscopic lymphoid aggregates which are interspersed along the vessels. *Corynebacterium ovis*, the cause of caseous lymphadenitis, also causes lymphangitis in horses as does *Sporothrix scheneckii*. Failure of drainage of lymphatics, of course, leads to edema of the part in question.

Lymphatic vessels are regenerated or reinforced by the formation of collateral vessels within a few (4–10) days following operative or traumatic destruction, their function of drainage being only transiently interrupted.

NEOPLASMS OF BLOOD AND LYMPHATIC VESSELS

Nomenclature of neoplasms of blood and lymphatic vessels is somewhat confusing because of the recognition of vascular growths in humans once considered tumors as not being true neoplasms. This has resulted in using the term, capillary hemangioma and cavernous hemangioma in the human literature for benign congenital abnormalities most common in the skin (red birthmarks). Similar clinical and pathologic correlations have not yet been made for animals, but it is wise to bear in mind that some apparent neoplasms of blood vessels may represent anomalous growths.

Hemangioma and hemangioendothelioma

These tumors arise from the endothelial cells that line blood vessels. The tumor consists of a mixture of cellular areas, the endothelial cells resembling short, plump fibroblasts, and of endothelium-lined blood spaces filled with normal, circulating blood. The hemangioma, having small-to-medium-sized blood spaces and no great amount of cellular tissue, is designated as capillary **hemangioma;** the one with large blood spaces, **hemangioma cavernosum;** and the opposite type, with a large amount of cellular tissue and minimal blood spaces, **hemangioma hypertrophicum.** The great majority are benign. In fact, an area of tumor sufficiently anaplastic to be malignant would be unlikely to have any features distinguishing it from other sarcomas, although other areas of the same tumor may be sufficiently well differentiated to identify its origin. Logically or not, those forms considered malignant are usually called **hemangioendotheliomas, malignant hemangiomas,** or **hemangiosarcomas.**

In dogs, hemangioendotheliomas (Fig. 21-24) with malignant potentialities are encountered arising from the spleen, right atrium, and occasionally from the subcutis. These neoplasms consist of ovoid cells with hyperchromatic nuclei and scanty cytoplasm. The cells tend to form many small capillaries, the distinguishing feature of the growth. Cutaneous hemangiomas have

been produced in ducks by the application of methylcholanthrene (Rigdon, 1952), and an association between hemangioendothelioma of the liver and vinyl chloride has been made in humans.

Lymphangioma and lymphangioendothelioma

These tumors are comparable to hemangiomas, except that the vascular spaces are connected to the lymphatic system and contain lymph instead of blood. They are much less frequent than their blood-containing counterparts.

References

Altera KP, Bonasch H. Periarteritis nodosa in a cat. J Am Vet Med Assoc 1966;149:1307–1311.

Andrews EJ, Kelly DF. Naturally occurring aortic medial necrosis in a dog. Am J Vet Res 1970;31:791–795.

Bachhuber TE, Lalich JJ. Production of dissecting aneurysms in rats fed Lathyrus odoratus. Science 1954;120:712–713.

Bevilacqua G, Camici P, L'Abbate A. Spontaneous dissecting aneurysm of the aorta in a dog. Vet Pathol 1981;18:273–275.

Breeze RG, Pirie HM, Selman IE, et al. Thrombosis of the posterior vena cava in cattle. Vet Ann 1976;16:52–59.

Butler HC. An investigation into the relationship of an aortic embolus to posterior paralysis in the cat. J Small Anim Pract 1971; 12:141–158.

Carnaghan RBA. Atheroma of the aorta associated with dissecting aneurysms in turkeys. Vet Rec 1955;67:568–569.

Carpenter JL, Moore FM, Albert DM. Polyarteritis nodosa and rheumatic heart disease in a dog. J Am Vet Med Assoc 1988;192:929–932.

Clarkson TB, et al. Pathogenesis of atherosclerosis: some advances from using animal models. Exp Mol Pathol 1976;24:264–286.

Conklin JW, et al. Necrotizing polyarteritis an aging RF mice. Lab Invest 1967;16:483–487.

Davies AP, et al. Primary lymphedema in three dogs. J Am Vet Med Assoc 1979;174:1316–1320.

Davis JO. Symposium: pathogenic mechanisms in hypertension. Fed Proc 1982;41:2385–2432.

Farrelly BT. Pathogenesis and significance of parasitic endarteritis and thrombosis in the ascending aorta of the horse. Vet Rec 1954; 66:53–61.

French JE, Jennings MA, Florey HW. Morphological studies on atherosclerosis in swine. Ann NY Acad Sci 1965;127:780–799.

Gailiunis P. Calcification of the arteries in young cattle: case report. J Am Vet Med Assoc 1958;132:533.

Gottlieb H, Lalich JJ. Occurrence of arteriosclerosis in the aorta of swine. Am J Pathol 1954;30:851–855.

Hamilton JM. [1] Pulmonary arterial disease of the cat. [2] Experimental lung-worm disease of the cat. Association of the condition with lesions of the pulmonary arteries. J Comp Pathol 1966; 76:133–145, 147–157.

Harding JDJ. A cerebrospinal angiopathy in pigs. Pathol Vet 1966; 3:83–88.

Hartman HA. Idiopathic extramural coronary arteritis in beagle and mongrel dogs. Vet Pathol 1987;24:537–544.

Helmboldt CF, Jungherr EL, Hwang J. Polyarteritis in sheep. J Am Vet Med Assoc 1959;134:556–561.

Hoff EJ, Vandevelde M. Case report: Necrotizing vasculitis in the central nervous system of two dogs. Vet Pathol 1981;18:219–223.

Holzworth J, et al. Aortic thrombosis with posterior paralysis in the cat. Cornell Vet 1955;45:468–487.

Jensen R, et al. Embolic pulmonary aneurysms in yearling feedlot cattle. J Am Vet Med Assoc 1976;169:518–520.

Jensen R, et al. Ischemia: a cause of hepatic telangiectasis in cattle. Am J Vet Res 1982;43:1436–1439.

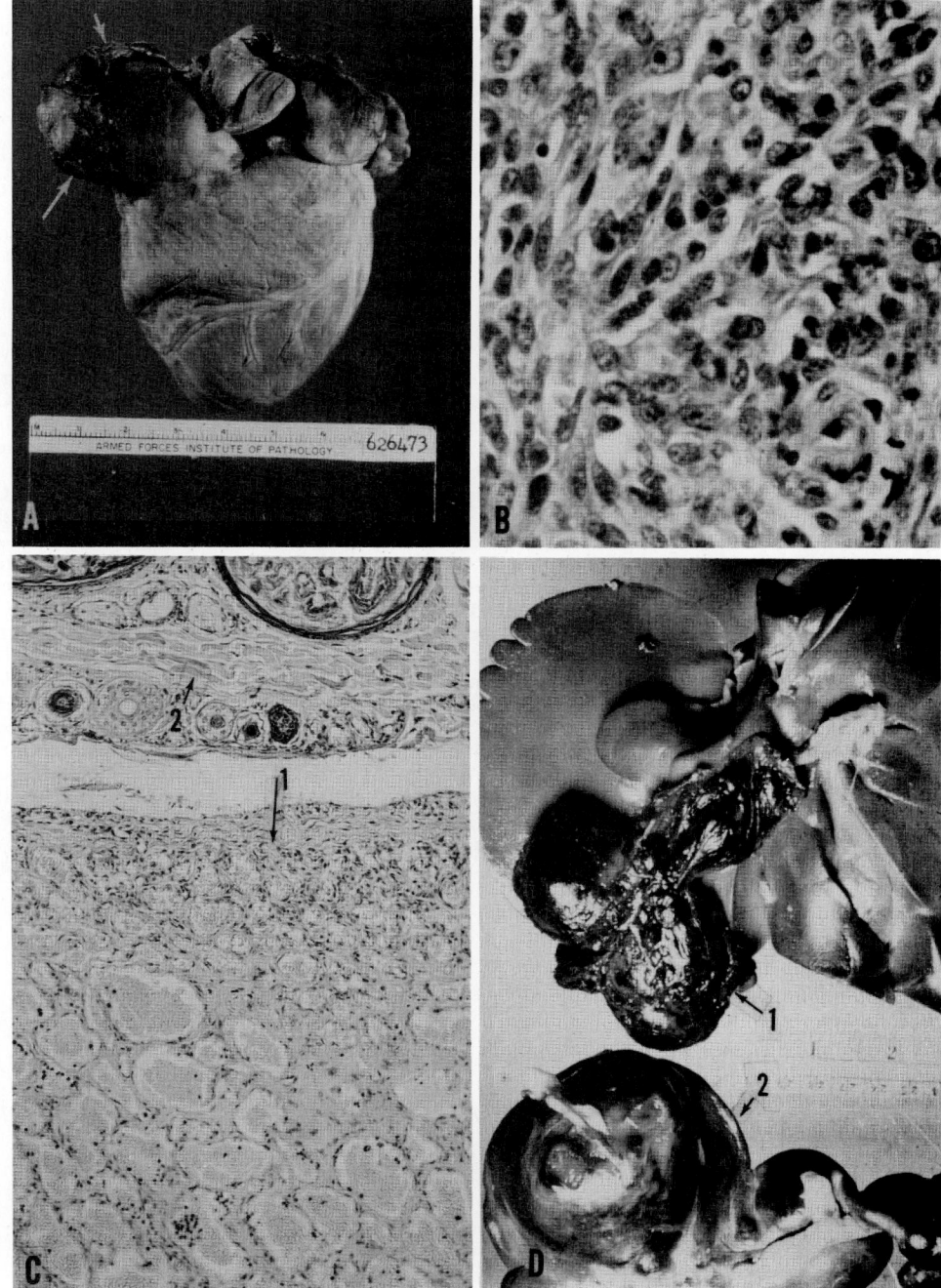

FIG. 21-24 A. Hemangioendothelioma (arrows), primary in the myocardium of the right atrium of a seven-year-old female beagle dog. (Contributor: Dr. Leo L. Lieberman.) **B.** Hemangioendothelioma (×300), primary in spleen of a dog. Tumor cells have elongated nuclei and frequently form vascular channels. **C.** Hemangioma (×75) in the subcutis of tarsal region of a 2½-year-old wire-haired fox terrier. 1 New growth is encapsulated and 2 separated from the dermis. (Courtesy of Armed Forces Institute of Pathology and Dr. Leo L. Lieberman.) **D.** Hemangioendothelioma involving 1 liver and 2 spleen of a dog.

Jones TC, Zook BC. Aging changes in the vascular system of animals. Ann NY Acad Sci 1974;127:671–684.

Jonsson L. Senile cardiac amyloidosis in the dog. Acta Vet Scand 1974;15:206–218.

Kammermann KL, Luginbuhl H, Ratcliffe HL. Intramural coronary arteriosclerosis of normal and dwarfed swine. Vet Pathol 1976;13:104–109.

Keith JC Jr, Rawlings CA, Schaub RG. Histologic examination of selected areas of canine pulmonary arteries. Am J Vet Res 1984;45:751–754.

Kelly WR, Wilkinson GT, Allen PW. Canine angiosarcoma (lymphangiosarcoma): a case report. Vet Pathol 1981;18:224–227.

Knieriem HJ. Electron-microscopic study of bovine arteriosclerotic lesions. Am J Pathol 1967;50:1035–1065.

Likar IN, Robinson RW. Bovine arterial disease. I. Localization of lipids in the abdominal aorta in relation to bovine atherosclerosis. [2] Lipid distribution and pattern in abdominal aorta with and without naturally occurring lesions. Arch Pathol 1966;82:555–560, 561–565.

Lindsay S, Chaikoff IL. Naturally occurring arteriosclerosis in nonhuman primates. J Atheroscler Res 1966;6:36–61.

Lindsay S, Chaikoff IL, Gilmore JW. Arteriosclerosis in the dog: spontaneous lesions in the aorta and coronary arteries. Arch Pathol 1952;53:281–300.

Lindsay S, Chaikoff IL, Gilmore JW. Arteriosclerosis in the cat: spontaneous lesions in the aorta and coronary arteries. Arch Pathol 1955;60:29–38.

Lindsay S, et al. "Arteriosclerosis in the dog." II. Aortic, cardiac, and other vascular lesions in thyroidectomized-hypophysectomized dogs. Arch Pathol 1952;54:573–391.

Littman MP, Robertson JL, Bovée KC. Spontaneous systemic hypertension in dogs: five cases (1981–1983). J Am Vet Med Assoc 1988;193:486–494.

Lucké VM. Renal polyarteritis nodosa in the cat. Vet Rec 1968;82:622–624.

Luginbuhl H, Pauli B, Ratcliffe HL. Atherosclerosis in swine and swine as a model of the study of atherosclerosis. Adv Cardiol 1974;13:119–126.

Luginbuhl H, Rossi GL, Ratcliffe HL, et al. Comparative atherosclerosis. Adv Vet Sci Comp Med 1977;21:421–448.

Lynd FT, et al. Bovine arteriosclerosis in Hawaii. Am J Vet Res 1965;26:1344–1349.

Marcus LC, Ross JN. Microscopic lesions in the hearts of aged horses. Pathol Vet 1967;4:162–185.

Maxie MG, Physick-Sheard PW. Aortic-iliac thrombosis in horses. Vet Pathol 1985;22:238–249.

McSherry BJ, et al. Dissecting aneurysm in internal hemorrhage in turkeys. J Am Vet Med Assoc 1954;124:279–283.

Mohr FC, Carpenter JL. Arteriosclerosis in a cat. Vet Pathol 1987;24:466–469.

Montali EJ, Strandberg JD, Squire RA. A histochemical and ultrastructural study of intimal bodies in horse arterioles. Lab Invest 1970;23:302–306.

Moore FM, Thornton GW. Telangiectasis of Pembroke Welsh Corgi dogs. Vet Pathol 1983;20:203–208.

Moorehead RP, Little JM. Changes in the blood vessels of apparently healthy mongrel dogs. Am J Pathol 1945;21:339–353.

Morris DD. Cutaneous vasculitis in horses: 19 cases (1978–1985). J Am Vet Med Assoc 1987;191:460–464.

Oliveira AC de, Rosenbruch M, Schulz L-CL. Intimal asteroid bodies in horses: light and electron microscopic observations. Vet Pathol 1985;22:226–231.

Prasad MD, Rajya BS, Mohanty GC. Caprine arterial diseases. I. Spontaneous aortic lesions. Exp Mol Pathol 1972;17:14–28.

Pritchard WR, Henderson W, Beall CW. Experimental production of dissecting aneurysm in turkeys. Am J Vet Res 1958;19:696–705.

Randell MG, Hurvitz AI. Immune-mediated vasculitis in five dogs. J Am Vet Med Assoc 1983;183:207–211.

Rebhun WC, Rendano VT, Dill SG, et al. Caudal vena caval thrombosis in four cattle with acute dyspnea. J Am Vet Med Assoc 1980;176:1366–1369.

Rigdon RH. Tumors produced by methylcholanthrene in the duck. Arch Pathol 1952;54:368–377.

Rogers WA, Bishop SP, Rohovsky MW. Pulmonary artery medial hypertrophy and hyperplasia in conventional and specific-pathogen-free cats. Am J Vet Res 1971;32:767–774.

Rooney JR, Prickett ME, Crowe MW. Aortic ring rupture in stallions. Pathol Vet 1967;4:268–274.

Rothwell TLW, et al. Unusual multisystemic vascular lesions in a cat. Vet Pathol 1985;22:510–512.

Schaub RG, Keith JC Jr, Bell FP, et al. A study of atherosclerotic lesion development in the injured pulmonary arteries of dogs with induced hyperlipemia. Lab Invest 1987;56:489–498.

Skold BH, Getty R, Ramsey FK. Spontaneous atherosclerosis in the arterial system of aging swine. Am J Vet Res 1966;27:257–273.

Slavin RE, Gonzalez-Vitale JC. Segmental mediolytic arteritis: a clinical pathologic study. Lab Invest 1976;35:23–29.

Spencer A, Greaves P. Periarteritis in a beagle colony. J Comp Pathol 1987;97:121–128.

Stambaugh JE, Harvey CE, Goldschmidt MH. Lymphangioma in four dogs. J Am Vet Med Assoc 1978;173:759–761.

Strickland HL, Bond MG. Aneurysms in a large colony of squirrel monkeys (Saimiri sciureus). Lab Anim Sci 1983;33:589–592.

Stunzi H, Teuscher E, Pericin-Rauhur D. Die hyperplasia der arteria pulmonalis bei felinen. Pathol Vet 1966;3:461–473.

Vulgamott JC, Clark RG. Arterial hypertension and hypertrophic pulmonary osteopathy associated with aortic valvular endocarditis in a dog. J Am Vet Med Assoc 1980;177:243–246.

Wigley RD, Couchman KC, Maule R. Polyarteritis nodosa: the natural history of a spontaneously occurring model in outbred mice. Aust Ann Med 1970;19:319–327.

Willers EH, et al. Experimental studies of bovine arteriosclerosis in Hawaii. Am J Vet Res 1965;26:1350–1355.

Young YH. Polyarteritis nodosa in lab rats. Lab Invest 1965;14:81–88.

Zeek PM. Periarteritis nodosa and other forms of necrotizing angitis. N Engl J Med 1953;248:764–772.

22

The hemic and lymphatic systems

The hematopoietic system encompasses the bone marrow, thymus, lymph nodes and spleen. The bone marrow's primary function is the production of erythrocytes, granulocytes, monocytes and platelets and is termed myeloid tissue; while the thymus, lymph nodes and spleen are the primary lymphoid tissues. Although certain diseases may be restricted to only one of these tissues, many diseases affect both the myeloid and lymphoid organs and primary disease of one can have secondary effects on the other.

BONE MARROW

The bone marrow is the primary, and usually only, adult organ for hematopoiesis (erythropoiesis and leukopoiesis). Embryologically, hematopoiesis first occurs in the yolk sac and later in the liver and, to a lesser extent, in the spleen, lymph nodes and thymus. In some species, such as rats and mice, hematopoiesis continues in the spleen and, to a lesser degree, other organs into adulthood. In severe anemias, hematopoiesis may be resumed in lymphatic tissues, the liver, adrenal, and even pituitary gland. This is termed extramedullary hematopoiesis. The hematopoietic marrow is often termed red marrow and at birth occupies most of the marrow space. In the adult animal much of the red marrow becomes inactive and is replaced by adipose tissue and is termed fatty marrow. It is the marrow of long bones which becomes most inactive with only a small amount of red marrow at their distal ends and a bit in the epiphyses. In adult animals most of the active marrow is in the flat bones, ribs and vertebrae. Fatty marrow will revert to active marrow with increased demands for hematopoiesis as will occur in such situations as hemorrhagic anemia.

All the circulating cellular elements of blood arise from a common ancestor, the pluripotent hematopoietic stem cell. This cell gives rise to lymphoid stem cells which are the precursors of T and B lymphocytes and myeloid stem cells which in turn proceed to give rise to stem cells destined to produce 1) erythrocytes and megakaryocytes (platelets); 2) neutrophils and monocytes (macrophages); 3) eosinophils; and 4) basophils. The recognition of the various cell types, their various developmental stages and determination of the myeloid:erythroid ratio cannot be made with tissue sections of bone marrow, but requires smears. In tissue sections it is possible to visualize mature granulocytes and their precursors and erythroid precursors, which usually exist in a ratio of about three to one. Tissue sections are generally necessary to evaluate aplasia, hypoplasia, or hyperplasia, as well as to identify focal lesions such as granulomas or metastatic neoplasms. Bone-marrow cells deteriorate rapidly after death, therefore even with tissue sections, analysis is best made from biopsies obtained during life. The complex differentiation of stem cells into mature circulating cells and its control by various regulatory factors such as erythropoietin, interleukins, TNF-α, Granulocyte-macrophage colony stimulating factor (GM-CSF), as well as nutritional factors (iron, vitamins, etc.) can be found in texts of hematology.

Hyperplasia

Hyperplasia of bone marrow is recognized grossly in the form of an increase in the amount of red marrow and a decrease of the fatty marrow, as compared with the normal for a given age. In pronounced hyperplasias which have existed for a considerable time, the red marrow greatly replaces adult fatty marrow of long bones, beginning at the proximal ends of the femur and humerus and extending distally through the extremities. The finer bony trabeculae which reach from the endosteal zone into the marrow cavity tend to disappear before the advancing hyperplastic marrow tissue. In judging the degree of hyperplasia of bone marrows an accurate knowledge of the normal is necessary. In general, at the time a normal animal is half grown there is practically no red marrow in the marrow cavity of the radius, tibia, and bones distal to them. Toward the proximal end of the humerus and femur, a minimal amount of marrow can be expected at this age. As the animal approaches maturity even this disappears. Red marrow, of course, fills the marrow spaces of the spongy, or cancellous, bone of the epiphysis proper at all ages, as well as that of the flat bones, namely the ribs, sternum, and bones of the skull and pelvis. In case a biopsy of bone marrow is to be made, the sternum or iliac crest are the customary sites, although many find the tuber coxae more readily feasible in large animals. There are two principal varieties of myeloid hyperplasia, as the condition is synonymously designated.

Erythroblastic hyperplasia is characterized by red marrow which microscopically is found to consist principally of the precursors of erythrocytes, namely erythroblasts and normoblasts. This occurs in and is a reaction to most of the anemias except toxic aplastic anemia, which owes its existence to inability of the marrow to function. In human pernicious anemia, with its deficient erythrocyte-maturing factor, and in the similar anemia due to the fish tapeworm, *Diphyllobothrium latum,* megaloblasts become numerous, and the terms megaloblastic anemia and megaloblastic hyperplasia are applicable. Very often erythroid hyperplasia is also accompanied by myeloid hyperplasia.

Leukoblastic hyperplasia, on the other hand, is characterized by a predominance of the precursors of leukocytes, usually mature and immature neutrophilic granulocytes and their predecessors, the myelocytes and myeloblasts. This variety of hyperplasia occurs in consequence of those infections which are accompanied by leukocytosis and a vigorous pyogenic reaction. If, however, the pyogenic disease is prolonged for several weeks, the myeloid cells and their progeny become exhausted, leaving little but erythroblastic cells and some lymphoid cells. The leukocytosis is naturally replaced by a leukopenia.

A leukoblastic reaction with large numbers of eosinophilic granulocytes and their predecessors is found in many human cases of ancylostomiasis and trichinosis, and the same may be presumed to be true in animals. In lymphoid leukemia (malignant lymphoma), areas of marrow may be largely replaced by lymphoid cells. In myeloid leukemia, the neoplastic cells take possession of many areas of the marrow. In these cases, as well as in leukoblastic hyperplasia, the marrow grossly tends toward a grayish color without the yellowish tinge of fat.

HYPOPLASIA

Hypoplasia of the bone marrow is seen in toxic aplastic anemias and certain deficiency diseases. The proportion of fatty marrow is greater than normal, and frequently such hematopoietic tissue as remains is scattered in little islands through the fatty marrow (Fig. 22-1) Microscopically, it may be principally the erythropoietic forms of developing cells that are missing or the deficiency may involve all cell types.

Agranulocytosis

Agranulocytosis refers to a more or less complete absence of granulocytes from the circulating blood. This, in turn, is due to a complete aplasia of the leukoblastic cells of the bone marrow. It is thus related to aplastic anemia and is attributable to similar causes. A number of commonly used medicines are known to have a depressant action on the bone marrow and are cited un-

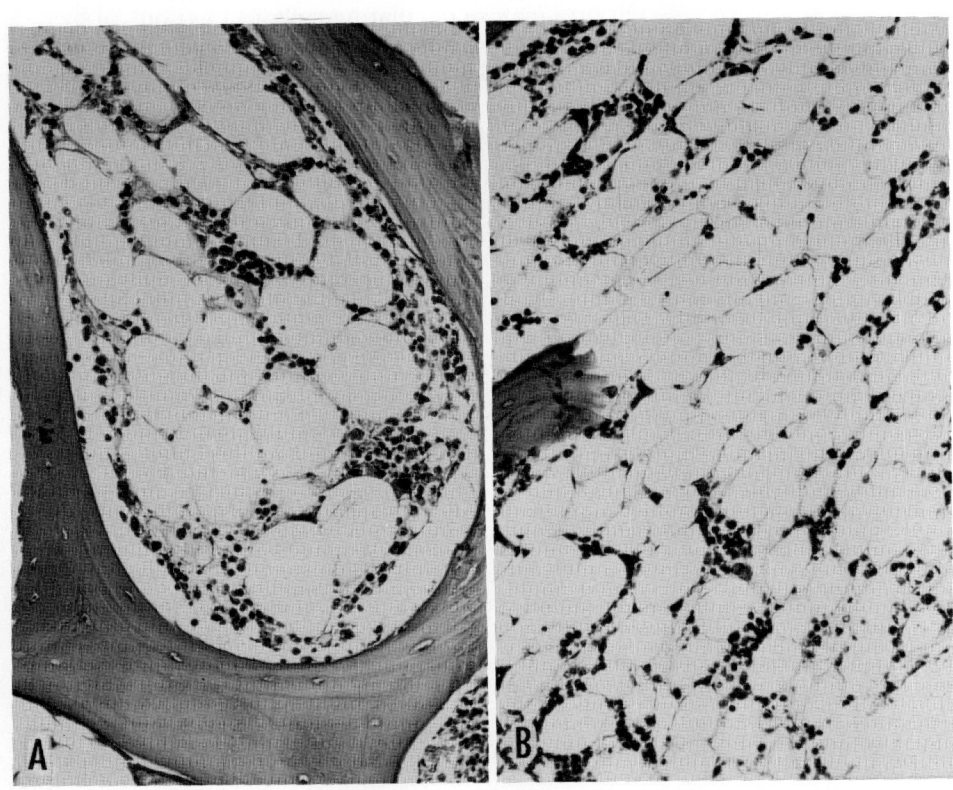

FIG. 22-1 Hypoplasia of the bone marrow in a dog with hypochromic microcytic anemia. **A.** A rib (× 195). **B.** Sternum (× 195) Note paucity of hematopoietic cells as in rib. (**B,** Courtesy of Armed Forces Institute of Pathology.) (Contributor: Dr. E. E. Ruebush)

der the latter type of anemia. Since the tissues are deprived of the protection of leukocytes, the condition is usually fatal in a few weeks at most as the result of some infection which would be trivial in a normal individual.

Osteomyelitis

Osteomyelitis is an inflammatory process in the bone marrow due to infection, which gains access to the marrow through a local wound (fracture, etc.) or by hematogenous metastasis. It is thus a localized process, involving usually a single bone, in contrast to the widespread character of hyperplasia, hypoplasia, and aplasia. The infection is usually pyogenic and the reaction purulent, although specific infections such as tuberculosis, brucellosis and coccidioidomycosis also produce their typical lesions in the bone marrow. Owing to the difficulty of drainage and other anatomic considerations, osteomyelitis was feared prior to the advent of modern antibiotics and is still difficult to treat. The condition is recognized grossly by a painful accumulation of pus, which eventually causes softening and necrosis of the overlying bony wall and makes its way to the body surface. Microscopically, accumulation of neutrophilic polymorphonuclear leukocytes and perhaps fibrin and other inflammatory elements, at times almost to the exclusion of the myeloid cells, reveals the nature of the condition.

Fibrosis

Fibrosis of the bone marrow, with or without myxomatous degeneration, occurs as a rare accompaniment of or sequel to hypoplasia or aplasia. The cause is obscure: possibly some forms represent exhaustion of a previously active marrow. Myxomatous degeneration is prominent in starvation.

References

Golde DW, Martin JC. Regulation of granulopoiesis. N Eng J Med 1975;291:1388–1396.

Goldwasser E. Erythropoietin and the differentiation of red blood cells. Fed Proc 1975;34:2285–2292.

Hillman RS, Finch CA. Erythropoiesis. N Engl J Med 1971;285:99–102.

Latimer KS, Rakich PM. Clinical interpretation of leukocyte responses. Vet Clin North Am Sm Anim Pract 1989;19:637–668.

Louwagie AC. Haemopoietic stem cells. II. Properties, regulation, and identity. Acta Clin Belg 1976;31:136–143.

Prasse KW, Seagrave RC, Kaegerle ML, et al. A model of granulopoiesis in cats. Lab Invest;28:292–299.

Quesenberry MD, Levitt L. Hematopoietic stem cells, Part I. N Engl J Med 1979;301:755–760.

Quesenberry MD, Levitt L. Hematopoietic stem cells, Part II. N Engl J Med 1979;301:818–823.

Quesenberry MD, Levitt L. Hematopoietic stem cells, Part III. N Engl J Med 1979;301:868–892.

Till JE, Price GB, Mak TW, et al. Regulation of blood cell differentiation. Fed Proc 1975;34:2279–2284.

NON-NEOPLASTIC DISORDERS OF ERYTHROCYTES AND MYELOID LEUKOCYTES

Considered here are anemias and congenital disorders of myeloid leukocytes. Bleeding disorders are covered in the chapter on circulation, and changes in myeloid cells in connection with inflammation are also discussed in that chapter. Neoplastic diseases of erythrocytes and leukocytes are presented at the end of this chapter.

Anemia

Anemia is defined as a reduction below normal of the number of erythrocytes and/or hemoglobin concentration per unit volume of blood. With rare exception, anemia is not a primary disease, but rather develops secondary to another disorder. For example, anemia following the rupture of an aortic aneurysm is secondary to the primary disease of the aorta; and anemia following lead poisoning is secondary to the toxic effects of lead and only represents one facet of the primary disease. Anemia, therefore, is usually a sign of another disorder and as such, the term does not represent a specific diagnosis. Anemia does, however, lead to the development of clinical signs which are secondary to the anemia. In chronic anemia, these include pallor of the mucous membranes, cardiac hypertrophy, and dyspnea. Edema may occur secondary to loss of plasma proteins in blood loss anemia. In anemia resulting from acute massive hemorrhage, the clinical signs are referable to those of hemorrhagic shock.

Anemias can be classified as to their cause and on the basis of morphologic characteristics of the erythrocytes. Obviously an etiologic classification is more meaningful and useful in that anemia is a secondary lesion, but morphologic characteristics are often extremely helpful in ascertaining the primary disorder.

MORPHOLOGIC CLASSIFICATION

Two features of red blood cells are used to classify an anemia on a morphologic basis—their size and their hemoglobin content. The size is expressed as **mean corpuscular volume (MCV),** which is determined by dividing the packed cell volume (PCV) in per cent by the erythrocyte count in millions per cubic mm and multiplying by 10. The answer is expressed in cubic micrometers. For example, for a PCV of 42% and an erythrocyte count of 6,000,000/mm3, the MCV is 70 cubic μm

$$\left(\frac{42}{6} \times 10 = 70\right).$$

The hemoglobin content is expressed as the **mean corpuscular hemoglobin concentration (MCHC),** which is determined by dividing the hemoglobin in grams per 100 ml of blood by the PCV in per cent and multiplying by 100. The answer is expressed as per cent hemoglobin per cell. For example, for a hemoglobin of 14 gm% and a PCV of 42, the MCHC is 33.3%

$$\left(\frac{14}{42} \times 100 = 33.3\right).$$

Based on MCV and MCHC, anemias can be classified as macrocytic, normocytic, or microcytic and either normochromic or hypochromic. Hyperchromic anemias do not exist in that there is a limit to the percentage of hemoglobin that can exist in an erythrocyte. This is generally accepted as 33.3% (normochromic). However, an abnormally large erythrocyte in a macrocytic anemia may contain more hemoglobin by weight than a cell of normal size, even though both are normochromic. The amount of hemoglobin in micro-micrograms per erythrocyte is termed **mean corpuscular hemoglobin (MCH)** and is calculated by dividing hemoglobin in grams per 100 ml of blood by erythrocytes in millions per mm3 and multiplying by 10. For example, for a 14 gm% hemoglobin and an erythrocyte count of 6,000,000/mm^3, the MCH is 23.3 micro-micrograms. However, in the classification of anemias MCH is not used to determine hypochromasia or normochromasia.

Macrocytic anemias are most frequent following acute blood loss or acute hemolysis. The outpouring of less mature erythrocytes (reticulocytes) in response to the anemia accounts for the increase in MCV. These cells are usually hypochromic. Macrocytic normochromic anemias result from deficiency of vitamin B$_{12}$, folic acid, and niacin.

Normocytic normochromic anemias are the most frequently encountered anemias in animals. They result from depression of erythrogenesis and are, therefore, often referred to as aplastic anemia. Neoplastic diseases, irradiation, and certain toxicities may produce this form of anemia.

Microcytic hypochromic anemia is the classical iron deficiency anemia or "tired blood." It may follow dietary deficiency of iron or chronic blood loss. Nutritional deficiencies of copper and pyridoxine also produce microcytic hypochromic anemias. Copper is necessary for the utilization of iron in the production of hemoglobin (Fig. 22-2).

OTHER FEATURES OF ANEMIA

While the enumeration of erythrocytes, the determination of hemoglobin, and the calculation of MCV and MCHC are the correct and certain way to establish the presence or absence of anemia, certain other signs afford strong presumptive evidence of the disorder. In the blood film, or smear, stained as for making the white-cell differential count, anemic blood is likely to show one or several of the following changes: In anisocytosis, the erythrocytes are not of sufficiently uniform size, some are markedly larger than others. One should observe by practice how much variation occurs in normal blood, which is not very much. In poikilocytosis, some of the erythrocytes have bizarre and abnormal shapes, being elongated, angular, ovoid or irregularly distorted. The blood film may contain occasional nucleated erythrocytes. These cells, because of the abnormal demand for replenishment of losses in the circulating blood, were hurried out of the bone marrow before they were completely mature. By a somewhat similar mechanism, rubriblasts occasionally are found in the blood smear, although normally they never leave the bone marrow. In basophilic stippling, minute dark specks appear in the erythrocyte, usually several or many in one cell. This feature is especially common following acute blood loss in cattle and sheep. In polychromatophilia, the erythrocytes do not stain uniformly, either as one is compared to another or within the boundaries of the same cell. One should be cautious, however, in attaching significance to paleness in cells which take a weak, but uniform stain. Polychromatophilic erythrocytes are generally reticulocytes which have entered the peripheral blood in response to blood loss and are evidence of active erythrogenesis.

Other evidences of anemia to be found in the tissues include hyperplasia of the bone marrow, a proliferation of red marrow in places where fatty marrow is normal for a given age. Sections of spleen or liver may rarely show erythropoietic centers in severe and prolonged anemia, these organs regaining some of the hematopoietic functions which they had during embryonic life. Such hematopoietic centers consist of a variety of hyperchromatic cells which are essentially myeloblasts, but which may be confused with foci of inflammatory leukocytes. The finding of nucleated erythrocytes in these collections of dark cells is the needed assurance as to their true nature. Megakaryocytes may also be present in these foci. Extramedullary hematopoiesis is not always indicative of a response to anemia. In most species it is normal for varying periods of time in the liver and spleen, and in certain animals such as rodents, hematopoiesis occurs in the spleen throughout life.

In certain hemolytic anemias, denaturation and precipitation of hemoglobin results in the occurrence of supravitally stainable, refractile, purplish granules near the erythrocyte membrane known as Heinz bodies.

Gross appearance The mucous membranes are unusually pale during life. After death, the same is seen to be true of these membranes and the tissues generally. At autopsy, the blood may be noticeably pale and watery, but one's enthusiasm must not be allowed to run away with one's judgment in this observation. Distinct gray dots in the liver may possibly be hematopoietic centers, although they are much more likely to be minute foci of necrosis. The hyperplastic bone marrow is, of course, a gross, as well as a microscopic, observation. With the exception of the last, all these gross indications of anemia are equivocal and have led many observers into error.

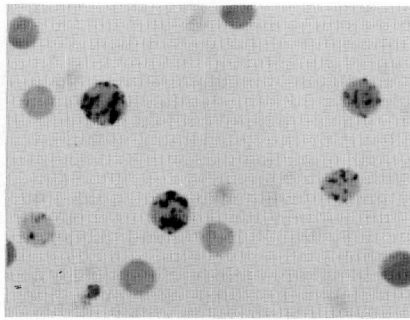

FIG. 22-2 Reticulocytosis following acute blood loss in a rhesus monkey *(Macaca mulatta).* (Courtesy of New England Regional Primate Research Center, Harvard Medical School)

Causes Like our bank accounts, the body's store of erythrocytes can be depleted either because of too heavy withdrawals or through failure of replenishment. Anemia can result from loss or destruction of excessive numbers of circulating erythrocytes or from functional failure of the hematopoietic tissue of the bone marrow. On the basis of the causative mechanism, anemias can be classified under five types.

HEMORRHAGIC ANEMIA

Hemorrhagic anemia results from severe hemorrhages. Acute hemorrhagic anemia is that which follows single or multiple severe hemorrhages. Initially the color and cell volume indices are normal, and the principal effect is due to a sudden drop in blood volume which may lead to shock. Following two to three days with restoration of blood volume anemia will be apparent. The recovery stage is characterized by macrocytosis and a marked reticulocytosis. As stated under the subject of hemorrhage, regeneration is complete in a month or 6 weeks. In addition to traumatic causes, acute bleeding may accompany idiopathic thrombocytopenic purpura, sweet clover and warfarin poisoning, bracken fern poisoning, and poisoning from trichlorethylene-extracted soybean meal.

Chronic hemorrhagic anemia results from continued loss of blood in a series of small hemorrhages. The hemorrhages may be due to unhealed ulcers, such as the human peptic ulcer, but in animals they are much more frequently due to heavy infestations with bloodsucking parasites of which hookworms, the stomach worm of ruminants, *Hemonchus contortus,* and the intestinal strongyles of the horse are outstanding. This type of anemia tends to be hypochromic and slightly macrocytic or normocytic. Poikilocytosis is prominent, as is hyperplasia of the bone marrow. After some time, iron stores of the body approach exhaustion, and this type of anemia becomes the microcytic anemia of iron deficiency. Hemophilia and vitamin C deficiency also result in chronic hemorrhagic anemia.

HEMOLYTIC ANEMIA

Hemolytic anemia results from excessive destruction of the circulating erythrocytes, occurring within the blood stream. Accompanying disturbances which assist in identifying this type of anemia are hemolytic icterus, which may be detected by a high bilirubin level in the blood as well as by the physical signs, hemoglobinemia and hemoglobinuria in the acute forms, and, in more chronic forms, stimulation of the bone marrow, shown in the blood picture by nucleated red cells and reticulocytes. Another form of hemolytic anemia is termed extravascular hemolytic anemia where erythrocytes are phagocytized and destroyed because of their shape or when they are recognized as foreign. In this form of hemolytic anemia there is no hemoglobinemia or hemoglobinuria: there is, however, hemolytic icterus.

The causes of hemolytic anemia are infectious, toxic, and immunologic. They include several infections of the erythrocytes themselves such as piroplasmosis, anaplasmosis, eperythrozoonosis of swine and cattle, hemobartonellosis of dogs and cats, malaria of humans, monkeys, and birds. Among the piroplasmoses are not only the North American tick fever caused by *Babesia (Piroplasma) bigemina,* now extinct in the United States, but also similar tick-borne infections caused by other species of Babesia, and also piroplasmoses in other species of hosts, particularly the dog. Certain viral diseases, such as equine infectious anemia, also destroy erythrocytes. The trypanosomiases destroy large numbers of erythrocytes, presumably by the action of toxins; in dourine the red-cell count is said to reach a figure as low as one-tenth of the normal. Several acute bacterial infections, including those due to *Streptococcus "hemolyticus," Clostridium hemolyticum bovis, Clostridium welchii,* and Leptospirae cause rapid destruction of erythrocytes and severe anemia, although this aspect of the disease is likely to be overshadowed by more startling symptoms and lesions. The same may be said about most snake venoms. Certain chemical poisons have a similar effect, including potassium and sodium chlorate (used to sterilize the soil of weeds and sometimes eaten by cattle), lead, usually as a chronic poisoning, and chronic copper poisoning, formerly known as ictero-hemoglobinuria of sheep. Ricin, the toxic principle of castor beans, phenylhydrazine, and, to a lesser extent, saponin are other strongly hemolytic poisons. The anemia which often accompanies poisoning by kale and rape is believed to be of hemolytic origin.

To this list of causes of hemolytic anemia should be added what is best called hemolytic disease of the newborn, also known as erythroblastosis fetalis, and neonatal isoerythrolysis. This type of hemolytic anemia is discussed further elsewhere in this chapter. Autoimmune hemolytic anemia represents another immunologic hemolytic anemia. Well known for years in humans, and more recently in dogs, this disease results from the failure of an individual to recognize "self" with the formation of antibodies against autogenous tissues. Autoimmune diseases include various genetic defects which render erythrocytes more susceptible to intravascular hemolysis due to membrane defects or shape of the erythrocyte. Mechanical injury to erythrocytes as in disseminated intravascular coagulation.

The hemoglobinemia and hemoglobinuria seen in those hemolytic anemias characterized by intravascular hemolysis must be differentiated from myoglobinuria. Myoglobin, which has a molecular weight of about one-fourth the weight of hemoglobin, appears in the urine when plasma levels reach approximately 20mg/100ml, whereas hemoglobin does not appear in urine until plasma levels approach 100mg/100ml. As a result of this difference, plasma is generally not colored by myoglobin, whereas in those diseases causing hemoglobinuria the plasma is red.

Postparturient hemoglobinuria is an acute hemolytic anemia of dairy cows, which usually is seen in multiparous cows which have given birth a few weeks previously. It is most frequent in western United States and Australia. Hemoglobinemia and hemoglobinuria results from severe hemolysis of circulating erythrocytes with red-cell counts often being less than 1 million. Erythrocytes may contain Heinz bodies. There is icterus, edema and signs and lesions of anoxia, such as labored breathing and centrilobular necrosis of the liver. Lesions of hemoglobinuric nephropathy may be mild to severe. The pathogenesis is not clear, but is related to severe hypophosphatemia. With hypophosphatemia, erythrocyte ATP levels are reduced, which leads to instability of the red blood cell membrane. The cause of the hypophosphatemia is not known. Although dietary deficiency is documented in some examples in others there is no evidence of dietary phosphorous deficiency. Copper deficiency has also been proposed as a cause.

Certain of the toxic hemolytic anemias are designated **Heinz body hemolytic anemias** owing to the presence of refractile bodies within erythrocytes which are precipitates of denatured hemoglobin formed due to oxidative injury. The oxidative damage leads the formation of glutathione and accumulation of hydrogen peroxide with the oxidation of sulfhydryl groups of globin chains. This causes denaturation of hemoglobin which precipitates as Heinz bodies. The best studied example is the X-linked glucose 6 phosphate dehydrogenase deficiency diseases of humans. With G6PD deficiency, regeneration of glutathione to reduced glutathione is impaired. There are reports of G6PD deficiency in a dog, a horse, cats, mice, rats and captive black rhinoceroses. It appears to be very rare with the exception of black rhinoceroses. Heinz bodies cause damage to the erythrocyte membrane, and further are selectively phagocytized by mononuclear cells which leads to further membrane damage. Even in humans with G6PD deficiency, hemolysis is usually only precipitated by exposure to oxidative drugs. Oxidative damage without predisposing G6PD deficiency is the more usual cause of Heinz body formation in animals; cats seem to be uniquely susceptible. The mere presence of Heinz bodies does not necessarily lead to anemia in animals, but when found in cases of unexplained anemia they may help point to the cause. It is a feature of poisoning by rape, kale, onions, phenothiazine, methylene blue, acetaminophen, phenylhydrazine, benzocaine, swamp maple (*Acer rubrum* or red maple), zinc and fava bean. The antimalarials, primaquine and quinacrine and the sulfonamides are causes in humans. Heinz bodies are also seen in postparturient hemoglobinuria in cows and in selenium and copper deficiency. Heinz bodies are often encountered in normal cats. Diets containing nitrites and propylene glycol increase the percentage of Heinz bodies in cats, but do not precipitate hemolytic anemia. Diabetes mellitus, hyperthyroidism and lymphoma also are associated with Heinz body formation. In G6PD deficiency, Heinz body formation can be accentuated *in vitro* by exposure to an oxidant, such as acetylphenylhydrazine.

DEFICIENCY ANEMIAS

These can be caused by deficiencies of several compounds or vitamins.

(1) Iron deficiency can arise from a dietary deficiency, malabsorption or from chronic blood loss. Dietary deficiency of iron is rather frequent in nursing pigs born in the winter in cold climates, for under those circumstances the sow and her litter often spend the first several weeks in a hog house with a concrete or other type of floor. If pigs can have access to the soil their rooting will, in almost any locality, provide the minute amount of iron which is necessary. Swine management systems, designed to prevent infection by helminths and microorganisms, do not allow access to soil and therefore require that some source of iron be provided. Without this or some artificial source of the element, deficiency anemia is likely to develop, for mother's milk, the much heralded "perfect food," does not contain adequate amounts of iron.

This is the traditional example of hypochromic, microcytic anemia. Poikilocytosis is also prominent.

Anemia reported to result from the (experimental) feeding of certain kinds of raw fish (coal-fish, *Gadus virens,* and raw whiting, *G. merlangus,* and not other kinds) to mink was prevented by cooking the fish and cured by feeding 16 mg of organic iron per week.

(2) Deficiency of Copper: Minute traces of copper are also essential to avoid deficiency anemia. Natural deficiency is not common in that most soils contain an adequate amount of this element. However, usual amounts of copper become insufficient in the presence of excessive molybdenum. Copper is necessary for hematopoiesis, as it is required for the proper utilization of iron in the production of hemoglobin. As in iron deficiency, the anemia is microcytic hypochromic.

(3) Deficiency of Cobalt: This deficiency is only of concern in ruminant species. Ruminants enjoy the unique position of not requiring a dietary source of B vitamins including vitamin B_{12}. Instead, they depend upon the rumen flora which synthesize these essential metabolites. Synthesis obviously cannot proceed without certain basic raw ingredients. Cobalt, being an integral component of vitamin B_{12} (cobalamin), is therefore a dietary requirement for the ruminant and deficiency of this mineral is in essence a vitamin B_{12} deficiency.

(4) Vitamin B_{12} Deficiency: This results in a macrocytic normochromic anemia. Deficiency of this vitamin is the basic defect of cobalt deficiency of ruminants. It is required in erythropoiesis for normal development and maturation of erythrocytes, although its exact mechanism of action is not understood. Deficiency is not a commonly encountered clinical problem.

(5) Folic acid deficiency also results in a macrocytic anemia. Although it is essential for maturation of erythrocytes, an understanding of its exact biochemical function is still incomplete. The actions of vitamin B_{12} and folic acid in erythropoiesis are closely related.

(6) Pyridoxine Deficiency: Experimentally induced in dogs, cats, and swine, this deficiency results in a microcytic hypochromic anemia. This is the prototype of sideroblastic anemia, described in animals and men. Siderotic cells are erythroid cells which contain granules of Prussian-blue reactive material recognizable under the light microscope. These granules may be identified in bone marrow in normoblasts (sideroblasts),

reticulocytes (reticulated-siderocytes), and in erythrocytes (siderocytes). Ultrastructurally, these granules may be seen to consist of two types. The first consists of cytoplasmic aggregates of ferritin, usually without a limiting membrane. These are normal structures which occur in metabolic processes involving ferritin. Almost none of these cells reach the circulation except in situations involving rapid blood production.

The second type of siderotic cells, distinguished by electron microscopy, contain granules of iron, not in the form of ferritin, localized within mitochondria. These cells are part of a defective heme synthesis found in sideroblastic anemias of humans and animals. In addition to pyridoxine-deficiency, a natural hereditary anemia of mice is known among the sideroblastic anemias. This disease of mice (Grüneberg, 1941) was the first in which the siderocyte was recognized.

(7) Deficiencies of riboflavin, ascorbic acid, vitamin E (alpha-tocopherol), and selenium may also result in anemia in susceptible species: In the case of ascorbic acid (vitamin C) human and nonhuman primates and guinea pigs are susceptible to scurvy and the associated anemia. Human infants and certain nonhuman primates (*Macaca fascicularis* and *Aotus trivirgatus*) develop anemia due to insufficient selenium and alpha-tocopherol. Both of these substances contribute to the stability of plasma membranes, and their absence is believed to result in disintegration of the membranes of red blood cells.

(8) Pernicious Anemia: While this type of anemia may be chiefly of academic importance in veterinary medicine, the monumental achievements of Whipple (1935), Peabody (1927), and Minot and Murphy (1926), in solving the riddle of human pernicious anemia is worth the attention of anyone in the medical sciences. At this time, a person in need (student) could replenish his or her finances by selling a pint of blood to be used as a transfusion to keep alive some unfortunate person afflicted with pernicious anemia. Then came the discovery that the liver (of human or beast) contained a substance, the "erythrocyte-maturing factor," which, if continuously provided, would relieve the patient of all symptoms. The demand for beef livers became such that liver changed from what was almost a waste-product to one of the more highly priced cuts of meat.

Eating 2 pounds of raw liver a day had its disadvantages but, fortunately, scientists soon learned how to make concentrated extracts, which could be injected at intervals. It was also learned that the mysterious "erythrocyte-maturing factor" in the liver is a storage product made by the action of an unidentified fraction of the gastric juice upon protein (of animal origin) in the food. Vitamin B_{12} is now known to be the essential constituent of the protein, and to become the erythrocyte-maturing factor upon absorption; Pernicious anemia, macrocytic and normochromic, results when this chain is broken. Usually the fault is failure of the stomach to provide its contribution, the "intrinsic factor," in the gastric juice. Many such stomachs have very atrophic glands and secrete almost no gastric juice (achylia gas-

trica); in others, only the hydrochloric acid is demonstrably absent (achlorhydria). The intrinsic factor is a glycoprotein secreted by parietal cells, which binds to vitamin B_{12}, creating a stable complex that is absorbed in the ileum. Occasionally, the chain is broken through shortage of the "extrinsic factor," apparently through failure of assimilation in certain chronic diarrheic diseases such as sprue or an actual dietary lack of animal protein, as in pellagra. Rarely, the liver is so badly damaged, usually cirrhotic, that it fails in its part of the process, which is to serve as a storage reservoir for the finished erythrocyte-maturing substance.

Humans have an anemia of the same macrocytic type when parasitized by the tapeworm *Diphyllobothrium latum*, apparently because of impaired assimilation of the extrinsic factor. Perhaps the anemia which dogs show when harboring this worm represents a parallel condition, although the presence of a hemolytic toxin has been reported. Beyond this, human pernicious anemia appears to have no counterpart in animals.

TOXIC APLASTIC ANEMIAS

In aplastic (meaning no growth) anemia, the hematopoietic tissues of the bone marrow are injured in such a way that their ability to produce erythrocytes is impaired or destroyed. There is nothing remarkable about the size, shape, or color of the cells which remain in the circulating blood during their life span. There is an absence of normoblasts, megaloblasts, reticulated erythrocytes, and polychromasia (basophilic staining of the cytoplasm approaching that of early myeloid cells), all of which are signs of active erythropoiesis in the marrow. The formation of the granulocytic leukocytes is also depressed, leading to more or less severe agranulocytosis. The bone marrow in aplastic anemia is predominantly fatty, with scattered islands of hematopoietic cells, although sometimes it is sclerotic.

Causes To the extent that they are known, the causes are either toxic radiations or toxic substances brought to the marrow cells in the circulating blood. These latter include benzol poisoning (the classical example), trinitrotoluene, and, in at least the case of hypersensitized humans, the sulfonamides. A number of proprietary medicines highly advertised for human self-medication are reported to be almost equally toxic. The Bracken fern owes some of its poisonous effects to production of toxic aplastic anemia, as does poisoning by trichlorethylene-extracted soybean meal. Irradiation, whether by x-rays, radium, or the more recently developed radioactive isotopes, is highly destructive of the hematopoietic tissues and this action is the chief reason that significant dosages are lethal. Neoplastic diseases may also result in a selective depression of erythrogenesis.

Anemia often accompanies nephritis and uremia. While direct toxic action from uremia is possible, the principal mechanism is a reduction in renal production of plasma erythropoietin. In some examples of renal failure, plasma erythropoietin is not detectable. In contrast, plasma erythropoietin is increased in most other forms of anemia.

While not toxic, the anemia seen in some infectious diseases results from hematopoietic stem cell destruction and thus resembles toxic aplastic anemia. Myelopoiesis is utterly destroyed in severe cases of feline panleukopenia. Severe hematopoietic cell destruction also occurs in some forms of East Coast Fever.

MYELOPHTHISIC ANEMIA (MYELO, THE MARROW; PHTHISIS, A WASTING DISEASE)

This type of anemia results from physical destruction of the erythropoietic tissue, usually from its replacement by metastatic tumor tissues. Various carcinomas are prone to fill the marrow cavities with neoplastic tissue in their advanced stages, leaving no room for the normal tissue, which undergoes pressure atrophy and pressure necrosis. This also applies to the anemia which usually accompanies leukemia and malignant lymphoma. Osteopetrosis is similarly destructive to the marrow space.

SIGNIFICANCE AND EFFECT OF ANEMIA

Anoxia of the tissues is the most important product of anemia. This leads to fatty change of the myocardium, liver, and other susceptible organs and even necrosis. It explains the principal symptoms of rapid and perhaps irregular pulse, shortness of breath, and muscular weakness. In hemolytic anemia, the spleen contains much phagocytized hemosiderin. A tendency toward hemorrhage, which is characteristic of anemia, can presumably be explained on the basis of anoxic damage to capillary endothelium. When edema accompanies anemia, it is conceivably related to increased permeability, but in hemorrhagic anemias, protein loss is also contributory and, in those cases which go with helminthiasis, the continued drain of erythrocytes offers some explanation. Removal of the cause cures anemia except in the case of the toxic aplastic anemias, where the changes soon become irreversible.

In perusing the causes of hemolytic anemia, it is noted that they largely duplicate the list given for hemolytic icterus. It is obvious that if erythrocytes are hemolyzed excessively, there tends to be both a shortage of erythrocytes and an accumulation of the products of their destruction. If the rate surpasses the rate at which the liver can eliminate bilirubin, jaundice will result. If the rate of erythrocytic destruction exceeds the capacity of the reticulo-endothelium to convert hemoglobin to bilirubin, hemoglobinemia results, and then hemoglobinuria, as the excess is excreted in the urine.

One characteristic lesion of anoxia in the liver is paracentral necrosis.

Hereditary anemia

Genetically determined defects in erythropoiesis or in viability of red blood cells result in anemias that may be considered as distinct entities. The effects of these anemias are not significantly different from those resulting from anemia due to other causes. A brief description of these anemias will follow, using the gene-designation to identify them.

Hertwig's anemia of the mouse (an, autosomal recessive, chromosome 4, linkage group VIII) is a macrocytic anemia of varying severity, depending upon the genetic background. It results from defective hemopoiesis and is manifest by the twelfth day of gestation. It is accompanied by leukopenia.

Tail short anemia of the mouse (Ts, autosomal dominant, unknown linkage group) is associated with short, kinked tails, and other skeletal anomalies. Deficient hemopoiesis is demonstrable in the yolk sac at 8 days of gestation. The prenatal anemia is thought to result in other abnormalities.

Steel, Steel-Dickie, Grizzle-belly, and **Sooty** are names used to identify four allelic genes in the mouse (Sl, Sl^d, Sl^{ab}, Sl^{so}, autosomal recessive, linkage group IV), each causing similar defects. Homozygotes are white, infertile, black-eyed, and anemic. The hemopoietic cells appear to be normal because they reproduce and differentiate normally when transferred into mice with Dominant, Spotting (W^b). On the other hand neither normal or W cells will cure the anemia of steel mice. The defect appears not to be in the stem cells but in their environment.

Dominant Spotting in the mouse (W, W^c, W^b, W^j, and W^a, chromosome 5, linkage group XVII) is made up of five autosomal recessive alleles at the W locus; any two alleles result in severe macrocytic, hypoplastic anemia. Hemopoiesis is deficient in the liver, and the severity of the anemia depends upon the genetic background and genotype. The mutant mice are sterile and have black eyes and white hair. The names and symbols of these five alleles are: Dominant Spotting (W); Viable Dominant spotting (W^r); Ballantyne's spotting (W^b); Jay's dominant spotting (W^j), and Ames dominant spotting (W^a). Increasing degrees of anemia may be demonstrated in these genotypes: W/+, W^j/+, W^r/W^c, W/W^v, W/W, W/W^j, and W^j/W^j. Transfusion of normal or steel mouse bone marrow cells into mice affected with Dominant Spotting, cures their anemia, indicating that the stem cells are likely to be defective. Erythropoietic cells are not able to respond to erythropoietin stimulation.

Diminutive in the mouse (dm, chromosome 2, linkage group V, autosomal recessive) is a microcytic anemia which occurs in mice with small body size, short kinked tails, accessory ribs, and presacral vertebrae, malformed vertebrae, and fused ribs.

Microcytic in the mouse (mk, autosomal recessive) results in a microcytic, hypochromic anemia and is associated with anomalies of the skin.

Flex-tailed in the mouse (f, autosomal recessive, chromosome 13, linkage group XIV) is associated with siderocytic anemia. This disease led to the identification of siderocytes for the first time (Grüneberg, 1942). The anemia is transient and is associated with axial skeletal deformity and white spotting on the belly. The anemia is most severe on the fifteenth day of gestation, still severe at birth, but absent by 2 weeks of age. The percentage of siderocytes among the red blood cells may reach 80%, significantly higher than in normal mice, which have about 5% siderocytes. The defect is one of fetal hepatic hemopoiesis; the capacity of fetal (f/f) erythroblasts to incorporate iron into hemoglobin is delayed but eventually becomes normal. The capacity of fetal but not adult reticulocytes is impaired. The defect appears to be identified with erythropoietic progenitors, but it is not clear whether the defect in heme synthesis is primary or secondary to abnormal erythroid differentiation.

Sex-linked anemia in the mouse (sla, sex-linked recessive, chromosome X, linkage group XX) is hypochromic anemia with reticulocytosis and apparent deficient marrow. It is manifest in hemizygous males or homozygous females. Growth is retarded in both sexes but the mice usually survive. This anemia results from a deficiency of iron due to faulty absorption from the intestine. Parenteral administration of iron cures the anemia which tends to disappear as the animals become older.

Studies on iron transport in everted intestinal loops indicate that intestinal epithelial cells take up iron but fail to pass it on. The excess iron is held in the epithelial cells in association with rough endoplasmic reticulum and with lysosomes, some of it in the form of ferritin. Other studies indicate a possible transfer defect in the placenta—less iron reaches the fetus in the sla mice than in normal controls.

Belgrade in the rat (b, autosomal recessive, linkage group unknown) is a severe, often lethal anemia of the rat. The red cells are quite hypochromic, containing only 5 μg of hemoglobin compared to 15 μg which is normal for rats and mice. Plasma iron values are usually high, plasma iron clearance is slower than normal, and the electrophoretic pattern of the hemoglobin is normal. Intestinal iron absorption appears to be impaired and red-cell-free erythrocyte protoporphyrin is elevated. Intracellular iron deficiency or a block in hemoglobin synthesis is suspected.

Hemoglobin deficit in the mouse (hbd, autosomal recessive, linkage unknown) identifies a hypochromic macrocytic anemia.

Jaundiced in the mouse (ja, autosomal recessive, linkage group unknown) involves intense hemolysis and is usually lethal. An intrinsic red cell defect is suspected. Anemia is detectable at 14 days gestation; jaundice appears a few hours after birth. Death occurs in the neonatal period with kernicterus, bilirubin toxicity, or anoxia. Microcytic reticulocytes and nucleated erythrocytes appear in the circulation.

Normoblastic in the mouse (nb, autosomal recessive, linkage group unknown) is another hemolytic anemia with an intrinsic red cell defect. Hemoglobinuria may occur.

Pyruvate kinase deficiency (no gene symbol, linkage unknown, autosomal recessive) which leads to a hemolytic anemia has been described in Basenji and Beagle dogs. Known also as congenital hemolytic anemia and familial anemia of Basenjis, this disease is usually recognized during the first year of life, and most dogs succumb before 3 years of age unless treated by repeated blood transfusions. The anemia is hemolytic; the erythrocytes have osmotic fragility and a diminished

life span; severe reticulocytosis is conspicuous as is splenomegaly. Defective erythrocyte pyruvate kinase may be differentiated by any of several chemical methods (Standerfer et al., 1975). Several affinities to the human disease have been described.

Spherocytosis of the mouse (sph, linkage group unknown, autosomal recessive) is manifest as hemolytic anemia, spherocytosis, hyperbilirubinemia, and death shortly after birth. This mutant's effects are suspected to be due to an intrinsic red cell defect.

Spherocytosis occurs in four mutants of common house mouse (*Mus musculus*) (ja/ja; sph/sph; ha/ha; nb/nb) which results from deficiency of the cytoskeletal protein spectrin which causes an erythryocyte membrane defect. Spectrin is entirely lacking in ja/ja mice. The disorder is manifest as hemolytic anemia, spherocytosis, icterus and death shortly after birth.

Elliptocytosis due to membrane protein ban 4.1 deficiency has been described in dogs. The single report described the condition as characterized by elliptocytosis, microcytosis, shortened erythrocyte lifespan, and increased osmotic sensivity. The hemolytic disease was compensated, without anemia. The dog's parents also had decreased band 4.1 and elliptocytosis.

Alaskan Malamute anemia is seen in this breed in association with dwarfism. The dwarfism and anemia are believed to be pleiotrophic effects of one gene. This anemia is characterized by macrocytosis, decreased MCHC, increased osmotic fragility, diminished red cell survival time, reticulocytosis, erythroid hyperplasia, and increased iron turnover. Stomatocytosis is recognized in some red cells by a linear unstained area across their center. This suggested a mouth-like orifice to those who first recognized this feature in human red blood cells. Stomatocytosis has been observed in human erythrocytes in both acquired and inherited anemias. Red blood cell concentration of sodium and water are increased in anemic dogs. Glutathione deficiency is also present. The canine anemia resembles several human hemolytic anemias with similar characteristics.

Hemolytic in the mouse (ha, autosomal recessive, linkage group unknown) identifies a hemolytic anemia which is present on the 14th day of gestation and at birth. Anemic newborn mice have severe neonatal jaundice and hemoglobinuria and usually die within a week. An intrinsic red cell defect is suspected.

Luxoid in the mouse (1st, autosomal recessive, linkage group unknown) is associated with luxation of limbs, polydactyly, and anemia. The anemia is normocytic and hemorrhagic.

Lethal Anemia in the rat (an, autosomal recessive, linkage unknown) identifies a microcytic and spherocytic anemia.

Fetal erythroblastic anemia in the mouse (no gene symbol, linkage group unknown) is lethal in utero and accompanied by hydrops.

Cribriform in the mouse (cri, autosomal recessive, chromosome 4, linkage group VIII) is a gene associated with demyelination and electrolyte disturbance, as well as macrocytic anemia.

IMMUNOHEMOLYTIC ANEMIAS

Immunohemolytic anemias occur in two forms: isoimmune hemolytic anemia and idiopathic immune hemolytic anemia. These anemias are all characterized by the presence of antibodies on the surface of erythrocytes which can be readily detected with the Coomb's antiglobulin test.

Isoimmune hemolytic anemia (erythroblastosis fetalis; hemolytic disease of the newborn) occurs when the fetus inherits erythrocyte antigens from the sire which are foreign to the dam. Leakage of fetal erythrocytes across the placenta in the dam's circulation leads to an immune response to any of the many erythrocytic antigens. In some cases, the mother may be immunized by an incompatible blood transfusion. In humans the most frequent offending antigen are the Rh antigens (factors). Upon exposure of the fetus or newborn to maternal antibodies, an antibody mediated hemolytic anemia (crisis) develops. In humans, nonhuman primates and rabbits, antibody transfer occurs across the placenta, causing hemolysis of erythrocytes in utero or shortly after birth. In most animals however, such as dogs, swine and horses in which the disease occurs, the maternal antibodies are transferred to the newborn only after birth through the colostrum. The animal is born normal, but the anemia is not manifest for several hours to a few days after birth. Isoimmune hemolytic anemia is not common in animals, being most often encountered in foals. In cattle isoimmunization does not appear to occur between fetus and mother, but immunized females have resulted from receiving incompatible blood in certain vaccines (for babesiosis and anaplasmosis). Hemolytic disease has resulted after suckling, in newborn of such animals. Artificial immunization and production of the disease has been demonstrated in dogs and is associated with the blood group CEA-1.

Idiopathic immune hemolytic anemia (autoimmune hemolytic anemia) results from an immune response directed against the animals' own erythrocytes. Most often the reason for the autoimmunity is not known and the disorder is truly idiopathic, but immune mediated hemolytic anemia can be associated with neoplastic disease (most usually lymphoma), viral infection and can be induced by drugs (para-aminosalicylic acid, phenacetin, penicillin). In human patients the disorder is divided into three categories based upon variances in the Coombs antiglobulin test. Warm antibody type is dependent upon an IgG antibody causing erythrocyte agglutination at 37°C; Cold antibody type is dependent upon IgM antibody in which agglutination is most active at 0–4°C; and cold hemolysin type is dependent upon IgG antibody which binds to erythrocytes at cold temperatures and then causes hemolysis at 30°C. In animals, autoimmune hemolytic anemia is not common. It is recognized in dogs with a systemic-lupus-erythematosus-like syndrome and has been described in horses and cats. With the exception of paroxysmal cold hemoglobinuria (cold hemolysin type reaction) in vivo hemolysis does not occur, rather erythrocytes coated with antibody become spherical in shape and become sequestered in the spleen where they are phagocytized and destroyed.

In addition to anemia and spherocytosis, peripheral blood changes consistent with active erythropoiesis are evident as well as thrombocytopenia. Other clinical and pathological features may include splenomegaly, lymphadenopathy, purpura, and glomerulonephritis. Lameness is seen in some affected dogs which may be the result of a "rheumatoid arthritis" (Lewis and Hathaway, 1967). A disease resembling lupus erythematosus also occurs in NZB/BL mice. The disease in mice and humans has been suggested to be a viral infection. Ultrastructural studies of affected mice and men have revealed viral particles in tissue, but their etiological importance has not been established.

Purpura hemorrhagica

Purpura hemorrhagica denotes a syndrome characterized by many hemorrhages, petechial or ecchymotic in size, in the skin and external and internal mucous membranes. It is most common in horses, but also occurs in swine. In the horse, there is usually much subcutaneous edema, perhaps localized about the head or commonly in the form of numerous subcutaneous swellings several centimeters in diameter suggestive of urticaria. The cutaneous hemorrhages frequently bleed into these plaque-like collections of edema fluid. The disease is afebrile throughout most of its stormy course, of variable severity, but frequently fatal. Practically all reported cases have supervened when the patient appeared to be recovering from some infectious or necrotizing disease, such as equine strangles or other respiratory infection, often with streptococcal organisms as the cause.

Classically, purpura hemorrhagica is the result of a severe deficiency of platelets in the circulating blood (thrombocytopenia). This form of purpura is appropriately termed thrombocytopenic purpura and is discussed in chapter 5, but limited studies on horses with purpura hemorrhagica have usually shown no thrombocytopenia, nor defects in coagulation.

That edema and hemorrhage by diapedesis, such as occurs in this disease, could result from injury to the capillaries seems self-evident. The cause of this injury is not known, but thought to be the result of a hypersensitivity reaction, possibly from immune complexes. In that this form of purpura is well established to occur late in infections or to develop during convalescence, this theory has credence.

References

Abe T, et al. A subclinical case of hemolytic disease of newborn pigs caused by anti Ea. Jpn J Vet Sci 1970;32:139–145.

Adachi K, Makimura S. Changes in anti-erythrocyte membrane antibody level of dogs experimentally infected with Babesia gibsoni. J Vet Med Sci 1992;54:1221–1223.

Andrianarivo AG, Muiya P, Opollo M, et al. Trypanosoma congolense: comparative effects of a primary infection on bone marrow progenitor cells from N'Dama and Boran cattle. Exp Parasitol 1995;80:407–418.

Bailey E, Albright DG, Henney PJ. Equine neonatal isoerythrolysis: evidence for prevention by maternal antibodies to the Ca blood group antigen. Am J Vet Res 1988;49:1218–1222..

Bannerman RM, Edwards JA. Hereditary anaemias in laboratory animals. Br J Haematol 1976;32:299–307.

Bannerman RM, Edwards JA, Pinkerton PH. Hereditary disorders of the red cell in animals. Prog Hematol, 1974;8:131–179.

Barker RN, Gruffydd-Jones TJ, Elson CJ. Red cell-bound immunoglobulins and complement measured by an enzyme-linked antiglobulin test in dogs with autoimmune haemolysis or other anaemias. Res Vet Sci 1993;54:170–178.

Bernstein SE. Inherited hemolytic disease in mice: a review and update. Lab Anim Sci 1980;30:197–205..

Cain GR, Suzuki Y. Presumptive neonatal isoerythrolysis in cats. J Am Vet Med Assoc 1985;187:46–48.

Chandler FW Jr., Prasse KW, Callaway CS. Surface ultrastructure of pyruvate kinase-deficient erythrocytes in the Basenji dog. Am J Vet Res, 1975;36:1477–1480.

Christopher MM, Broussard JD, Peterson ME. Heinz body formation associated with ketoacidosis in diabetic cats. J Vet Intern Med, 1995;9:24–31.

Christopher MM, Harvey JW. Specialized hematology tests. [Review]. Semin Vet Med Surg (Small Anim) 1992;7:301–310.

Christopher MM. Relation of endogenous Heinz bodies to disease and anemia in cats: 120 cases (1978–1987). J Am Vet Med Assoc 1989;194:1089–1095.

Cowgill LD. Pathophysiology and management of anemia in chronic progressive renal failure. [Review]. Sem Vet Med Surg (Small Anim) 1992;7:175–182.

Cramer DV, Lewis RM. Reticulocyte response in the cat. J Am Vet Med Assoc 1972;160:61–67.

Dimmock CK, Bell K. Haemolytic disease of the newborn in calves. Aust Vet J 1970;46:44–47.

Edwards JA, Bannerman RM. Hereditary defect of iron transport in mice with sex-lined anemia. J Clin Invest 1970;49:1869–1872.

Ewing GO. Familial nonspherocytic hemolytic anemia of Basenji dogs. J Am Vet Med Assoc 1969;154:503–507.

Farrelly BT, Collins JD, Collins SM. Autoimmune haemolytic anemia (AHA) in the horse. Irish Vet J 1966;20:42–45.

Fletch SM, Brueckner PJ, Pinkerton PH. Hereditary hemolytic anemia and chondrodysplasia in the dog. Fed Proc 1973;32:821.

Groopman JE, Molina JM, Scadden DT. Hematopoietic growth factors. Biology and clinical applications. N Engl J Med 1989; 321:1449–1459.

Grüneberg H. The anemia of flex-tailed mice (Mus musculus). II. Siderocytes. J Genet, 1942;44:246–264.

Hall SA, Rest JR, Linklater KA, et al. Concurrent haemolytic disease of the newborn and thrombocytopenic purpura in piglets without artificial immunization of the dam. Vet Rec 1972;91:677–678.

Harvey JW. Canine hemolytic anemias. J Am Vet Med Assoc 1980; 176:970–974.

Harvey JW, Kornick HP. Phenazopyridine toxicosis in the cat. J Am Vet Med Assoc 1976;169:327–331.

Herbert V. Biology of disease. Megaloblastic anemias. Lab Invest 1985;52:3–19.

Hickman MA, Rogers QR, Morris JG. Effect of diet on Heinz body formation in kittens. Am J Vet Res 1990;51:475–478.

Houston DM, Myers SL. A review of Heinz-body anemia in the dog induced by toxins. [Review]. Vet Hum Toxicol 1993;35:158–161.

Jennings AR, Highet DR. Some cases of purpura haemorrhagica in the horse. Vet J 1947;103:369–376.

Jubb TF, Jerrett IV, Browning JW, et al. Haemoglobinuria and hypophosphataemia in postparturient dairy cows without dietary deficiency of phosphorus. Australian Vet J 1990;67:86–89.

Jubb TF, Jerrett IV, Browning JW, et al. Haemoglobinuria and hypophosphataemia in postparturient dairy cows without dietary deficiency of phosphorus. Aus Vet J 1990;67:86–89.

Katunguka-Rwakishaya E, Murray M, Holmes PH. Pathophysiology of ovine trypanosomiasis: ferrokinetics and erythrocyte survival studies. Res Vet Sci 1992;53:80–86.

King LG, Giger U, Diserens D, et al. Anemia of chronic renal failure in dogs. J Vet Intern Med 1992;6:264–270.

King AS. Studies on equine purpura haemorrhagica: morbid anatomy and histology. Br Vet J 1949;105:35–54.

Langford G, Knott SG, Dimmock CK, et al. Haemolytic disease of newborn calves in a dairy herd in Queensland. Aust Vet J 1971; 47:1–4.

Lavoie JP, Morris DD, Zinkl JG, et al. Pancytopenia caused by bone marrow aplasia in a horse. J Am Vet Med Assoc 1987;191:1462–1464.

Lewis RM, et al. A syndrome of autoimmune hemolytic anemia and thrombocytopenia in dogs. Sci Proc AVMA, pp 1963;140–163.

Lewis RM, Swartz R, Henry WB. Canine systemic lupus erythematosus. Blood 1965;25:143–160.

Linklater KA, Imlah P. Haemolytic disease of the newborn, thrombocytopenic purpura and neutropenia occurring concurrently in a litter of piglets. Br Vet J 1973;129:36–46.

Luttgen PJ, Whitney MS, Wolf AM, et al. Heinz body hemolytic anemia associated with high plasma zinc concentration in a dog. J Am Vet Med Assoc, 1990;197:1347–1350.

Madewell BR, Feldman BF. Characterization of anemias associated with neoplasia in small animals. J Am Vet Med Assoc 1980; 176: 419–425.

Madsen DE, Nielsen HM. Parturient hemoglobinuria of dairy cows. J Am Vet Med Assoc; 1939;94:577–586.

Madsen DE, Nielsen HM. The production of hemoglobinemia by low phosphorus intake. J Am Vet Med Assoc 1944;105:22–25.

Mair TS, Taylor FGR, Hillyer MH. Autoimmune haemolytic anaemia in eight horses. Vet Rec 1990;126:51–53.

Martinovich D, Woodhouse DA. Post-parturient haemoglobinuria in cattle: A Heinz body haemolytic anaemia. NZ Vet J 1971;19:259–263.

Mbassa GK, Balemba O, Maselle RM, et al. Severe anaemia due to haematopoietic precursor cell destruction in field cases of East Coast Fever in Tanzania. Vet Parasitol 1994;52:243–256.

Minot GR, Murphy WP. Treatment of pernicious anemia by a special diet. J Am Med Assoc 1926;87:470–476.

Mullins JC, Ramsay WR. Hemoglobinuria and anaemia associated with aphosphorosis. Aust Vet J 1959;35:140–147.

Noda H, Watanabe Y. Relationships between blood groups and hemolytic disease of newborn foal. Jpn J Zootec Sci 1975;46:180–184.

Ogawa E, Kobayashi K, Yoshiura N, et al. Bovine postparturient hemoglobinuria: hypophosphatemia and metabolic disorder in red blood cells. Am J Vet Res 1987;48:1300–1303.

Oishi A, Sakamoto H, Shimizu R. Canine plasma erythropoietin levels in 124 cases of anemia. J Vet Med Sci 1995;57:747–749.

Osbaldiston GW, Coffman JR, Kruckenbuer SM. Biochemical differentiation of equine anemias. J Am Vet Med Assoc 1970;157:322–325.

Paglia DE. Acute episodic hemolysis in the African black rhinoceros as an analogue of human glucose-6–phosphate dehydrogenase deficiency. Am J Hematol 1993;42:36–45.

Parkinson B, Sutherland AK. Post-parturient haemoglobinuria in dairy cows. Aust Vet J 1954;30:232–236.

Peabody FW. Pathology of the bone marrow in pernicious anemia. Am J Pathol 1927;3:179–202.

Penny RHC, Carlisle CH, Prescott CW, et al. Further observations on the effect of chloramphenicol on the haemopoietic system of the cat. Br Vet J 1970;126:453–458.

Penny RHC. Post-parturient haemoglobinuria (haemoglobinaemia) in cattle. Vet Rec 1956;68:238–241.

Pinkerton PH, Fletch SM, Brueckner PJ, et al. Hereditary stomatocytosis with hemolytic anemia in the dog. Blood 1974;44:557–567.

Pond WG, Walker EF Jr., Kirtland D. Cadmium-induced anemia in growing pigs: protective effect of oral or parenteral iron. J Anim Sci 1973;36:1122–1124.

Ponte CD, Lewis MJ, Rogers JS II. Heinz-body hemolytic anemia associated with phenazopyridine and sulfonamide. DICP 1989 23:140–142.

Prasse KW, et al.: Pyruvate kinase deficiency anemia with terminal myelofibrosis and osteosclerosis in a Beagle. J Am Vet Med Assoc 1975;166:1170–1175.

Schalm OW, Ling GV. Hematologic charcteristics of autoimmune hemolytic anemia in the dog. Calif Vet 1969;23:19–24.

Schechter RD, Schlam OW, Kaneko JJ. Heinz body hemolytic anemia associated with the use of urinary antiseptics containing methylene blue in the cat. J Am Vet Med Assoc 1973;162:37–44.

Searcy GP, Miller DR, Tasker JB. Congenital hemolytic anemia in the Basenji dog due to erythrocyte pyruvate kinase deficiency. Can J Comp Med 1971;35:67–70.

Shull RM, Bunch SE, Maribei J, et al. Spur cell anemia in a dog. J Am Vet Med Assoc 1978;173:978–982.

Sills MR, Zinkham WH. Methylene blue-induced Heinz body hemolytic anemia. Arch Pediat Adoles Med 1994;148:306–310.

Simpson CF. The ultrastructure of Heinz bodies in horse, dog, and turkey erythrocytes. Cornell Vet 1971;61:228–238.

Smith JE, Moore K, Arens M, et al. Hereditary elliptocytosis with protein band 4.1 deficiency in the dog. Blood 1983;61:373–377.

Standerfer RJ, Templeton JW, Black JA. Anomalous pyruvate kinase deficiency in the Basenji dog. Am J Vet Res 1974;35:1541–1544.

Stockham SL, Harvey JW, Kinden DA. Equine Glucose-6–phosphate dehydrogenase deficiency. Vet Pathol 1994;31:518–527.

Stormont CJ. Hemolytic diseases of newborn calves. Fed Proc 1972; 31:761.

Suttle NF, Jones DG, Woolliams C, et al. Heinz body anaemia in lambs with deficiencies of copper or selenium. Brit J Nutr 1987;58:539–548.

Tasker JB, Severin GA, Young S, et al. Familial anemia in the Basenji dog. J Am Vet Med Assoc 1969;154:158–165.

Thompson JC, Pauli JV, Hopcroft DH, et al. An unusual Heinz body anaemia in a cat. J Comp Path 1989;100:343–347.

Venn JAJ, Davies ET. Piglet anaemia. Vet Rec 1965;77:1004–1005.

Weiser MG, Kociba GJ. Sequential changes in erythrocyte volume distribution and microcytosis associated with iron deficiency in kittens. Vet Pathol 1983;20:1–12.

Weiser G, O'Grady M. Erythrocyte volume distribution analysis and hematologic changes in dogs with iron deficiency anemia. Vet Pathol 1983;20:230–241.

Whipple GH. Hemoglobin regeneration as influenced by diet and other factors. Nobel Prize Lecture. J Am Med Assoc 1935;104:791–793.

Chediak-higashi syndrome

Chediak-Higashi syndrome is a hereditary disease which results in abnormally large storage/secretory granules and lysosomes in a variety of cell types. It is described in humans, cattle (Hereford, Japanese black, Brangus), mink, mice (beige), rats, cats, killer whales, white tigers, bison and foxes. In most species it is inherited as a simple autosomal recessive trait and associated with partial albinism. In mink the coat color of this partial albinism is known as Aleutian or "blue" and all Aleutian mink have the Chediak-Higashi syndrome. The syndrome is characterized by the presence of giant granules or cytoplasmic inclusions in neutrophils, eosinophils, basophils, monocytes, lymphocytes, and thrombocytes, as well as in many other cell types, such as hepatocytes, renal tubular epithelium, neurons, endothelial cells and melanocytes. The granules are abnormal lysosomes, secretory or storage granules which tend to locate adjacent to the nucleus. The enlarged granules are thought to mainly result from fusion during cellular maturation. Not all granules in a given cell are abnormal.

Other characteristics of the disease include photophobia, hemorrhagic tendencies, and a marked susceptibility to infections, which usually accounts for the cause of death. In part, increased susceptibility is due to defective mobility and chemotactic response of leukocytes. Phagocytosis may also be impaired. The basis for the partial albinism seems to be the redistribution of melanin granules by the fusion of granules with lysosomes. The melanin deposits are thus in larger granules and farther apart. The hemorrhagic tendency has been related to the reduced uptake and storage of serotonin and adenosine nucleotide by platelets.

References

Amann JF, Prieur DJ. Muscle lesions in beige (Chediak-Higashi syndrome) and heterozygous C57BL/6J mice. Vet Pathol 1986; 23:692–697.

Ayers JR, Leipold HW, Padgett GA. Lesions in Brangus cattle with Chediak-Higashi syndrome. Vet Pathol 1988;25:432–436.

Blume RS, Padgett GA, Wolff SM, et al. Giant neutrophil granules in the Chediak-Higashi Syndrome of man, mink, cattle, and mice. Can J Comp Med 1969;33:271–274.

Burkhardt JK, Wiebel FA, Hester S, et al. The giant organelles in beige and Chediak-Higashi fibroblasts derived from late endosomes and mature lysosomes. J Exp Med 1993;178:1845–1856.

Colgan SP, Blancquaert AM, Thrall MA, et al. Defective in vitro motility of polymorphonuclear leukocytes of homozygote and heterozygote Chediak-Higashi cats. Vet Immunol Immunopathol 1992;31:205–227.

Gallin JI, Klimerman JA, Padgett GA, et al. Defective mononuclear leukocyte chemotaxis in the Chediak-Higashi syndrome of humans, mink, and cattle. Blood 1975;45:863–870.

Hamanaka SC, Gilbert CS, White DA, et al. Ultrastructural morphology, cytochemistry, and morphometry of eosinophil granules in Chediak-Higashi syndrome. Am J Pathol 1993;143:618–627.

Kramer JW, Davis WC, et al. The Chediak-Higashi syndrome of cats. Lab Invest 1977;36:554–562.

Oliver C, Essner E. Formation of anomalous lysosomes in monocytes, neutrophils, and eosinophils from bone marrow of mice with Chediak-Higashi syndrome. Lab Invest 1975;32:17–27.

Osaki K, Maeda H, Nishikawa T, et al. Chediak-Higashi syndrome in rats: light and electron microscopical characterization of abnormal granules in beige rats. J Comp Pathol 1994;110:369–379.

Padgett GA. Comparative studies of the Chediak-Higashi syndrome. Am J Pathol 1967;51:553–571.

Padgett GA. The Chediak-Higashi syndrome. Adv Vet Sci 1968;12:239–284.

Padgett GA, Holland JM, Davis WC, et al. The Chediak-Higashi syndrome: a comparative review. Curr Top Pathol, 1970;51:175–194.

Renshaw HW, Davis WC, Fundenberg HH, et al. Leukocyte dysfunction in the bovine homologue of the Chediak-Higashi syndrome of humans. Infect Immun, 1974;10:928–937.

Robison WG Jr., Kuwabara T, Cogan DG. Lysosomes and melanin granules of the retinal pigment epithelium in a mouse model of the Chediak-Higashi syndrome. Invest Ophthalmol 1975;14:312–317.

Sung JH, Okada K. Neuropathological changes in mink with Chediak-Higashi disease. J Neuropathol Exp Neurol 1971;30:33–62.

Windhorst DB, Padgett GA. The Chediak-Higashi syndrome and the homologous trait in animals. J Invest Dermatol 1973;60:529–537.

Zhao H, Boissy YL, Abdel-Malek Z, et al. On the analysis of the pathophysiology of Chediak-Higashi syndrome. Lab Invest 1994;71:25–34.

CYCLIC NEUTROPENIA

Also known as "gray Collie syndrome," cyclic neutropenia is confined to the collie breed and only occurs in dogs with a gray (dark pewter gray to silver) coat color. A similar cyclic neutropenia has been described in a colony of crossbred research dogs. A comparable disease also occurs in humans. Not all gray collies suffer from cyclic neutropenia, a fact clearly illustrated by the studies of Ford (1969), who demonstrated that at least three types of gray or silver collies exist which are controlled by separate genes. Dominant gray or slate gray is inherited as a dominant gene and only appears if observable in one parent. Dominant gray collies are normal. Maltese gray collie pups appear in litters of nongray parents. The controlling gene is recessive, and the dogs are normal. Lethal gray, which is light silvery gray (almost white), is also inherited as a recessive gene which is apparently not an allele to maltese gray. Lethal gray collies suffer from cyclic neutropenia and generally die before maturity.

As its name suggests, the outstanding characteristic of this disease is a periodic neutropenia occurring at regular intervals of 8 to 12 days. Neutrophils may completely disappear from the peripheral blood at 10.5 to 11.5 day intervals, only to reappear with a "rebound" neutrophilia. The cause of the neutropenia is apparently a failure of maturation of stem cells. The controlling mechanism is not known, nor do we have an explanation for the periodicity of this failure. The dogs are extremely susceptible to infections, which if not controlled lead to their death. Whether other primary abnormalities are associated with the disease and contribute to death has not been determined. Cheville (1968) described fundic ectasia with incomplete pigmentation of the retina, maladsorption, diarrhea, and failure of maturation of the gonads as part of the picture. As a result of study of 8 gray Collies and 5 controls, he further reported (1970) clinical signs in addition to the cyclic neutropenia and gray hair color; these included diarrhea, lameness, and chronic ulceration of oral and genital mucosae.

Microscopic lesions included lymphoid atrophy, amyloidosis, enteritis, aseptic bone necrosis, and acute and chronic purulent inflammation in several organs. Serum albumin and gamma and alpha-2 globulins were elevated. Ultrastructural study of spleen revealed amyloid fibers deposited chiefly at the periphery of the splenic follicle and within the central artery.

The mechanism controlling this phenomenon is not clearly understood. A defect in stem cells is suspected because transplantation of affected bone marrow to a normal recipient will result in cyclic neutropenia in the recipient. Conversely, transplantation of normal marrow into a radiated affected dog results in alleviation of all the clinical signs, including the cyclic neutropenia. Non-cyclic neutropenias which have been described as recurrent or constant have been occasionally described in dogs and cats.

References
Cheville NF. The gray collie syndrome. J Am Vet Med Assoc 1968; 152:620–630.
Cheville NF. Amyloidosis associated with cyclic neutropenia in the dog. Blood. 1968;31:111–114.
Cheville NF, Cutlip RC, Moon HW. Microscopic pathology of the gray collie syndrome. Cyclic neutropenia, amyloidosis, enteritis, and bone necrosis. Pathol Vet, 1970;7:225–245.
Dale DC, Brown CH, Carbone P, et al. Cyclic urinary leukopoietic activity in gray collie dogs. Science. 1971;173:152–153.
Jones JB, Jones ES, Lange RD. Early life hematologic values of dogs affected with cyclic neutropenia. Am J Vet Res, 1974;35:849–852.
Jones JB, Lange RD, Jones ES. Cyclic hematopoiesis in a colony of dogs. J Am Vet Med Assoc 1975;166:365–367.
Lange RD, et al. Erythropoiesis and erythrocytic survival in dogs with cyclic hematopoiesis. Am J Vet Res 1976;37:331–334.
Lund JE, Padgett GA, Ott RL. Cyclic neutropenia in gray collie dogs. Blood 1967;29:452–461.
Lund JE, Padgett GA, Gorham JR. Additional evidence on the inheritance of cyclic neutropenia in the dog. J Hered 1970;61:47–49.
Patt HM, Lund JE, Maloney MA. Cyclic hematopoiesis in gray collie dogs: a stem-cell problem. Blood. 1973;42:873–884.
Swenson CL, Kociba GJ, Arnold P. Chronic idiopathic neutropenia in a cat. J Vet Intern Med 1988;2:100–102.

PELGER-HUËT ANOMALY
This inherited anomaly in the development of granulocytic nuclei has been described in humans, rabbit, and dog. In each species, the gene acts as an automosal dominant, although the effects on the phenotype are varied. The anomaly is recognized in the circulating neutrophilic and eosinophilic granulocytes, which have single, indented, or bilobular nuclei rather than their normal segmented polymorphic nuclei. In humans, the nuclei in the homozygous affected state are predominantly oval, spherical, and indented. In the heterozygote, bilobular nuclei are frequent. These often have the shape of pince-nez glasses. In the human patient, the anomaly has little clinical effect, but is of importance to differentiate affected cells from nonsegmented neutrophils.

Pelger-Huët Anomaly has been recognized particularly in Foxhounds. Approximately 50 to 67% of the neutrophils and eosinophils of heterozygotes have nonsegmented nuclei, and migration of these leukocytes appears to be obstructed. A slight reduction in number of pups weaned (63 versus 81%) in an outbred colony carrying the gene has been recorded. The trait is inherited as a single autosomal dominant gene in dogs, and homozygotes are reported to die at birth. After transfusion to a normal dog, affected neutrophil leukocytes disappear from the circulation in about 5 hours. Eosinophils with the anomaly disappear from the circulation within about 30 minutes.

References
Bowles CA, Alsaker RD, Wolfle TL. Studies of the Pelger-Huët anomaly in foxhounds. Am J Pathol 1979;96:237–248.
Huët GJ. Familial anomaly of leukocytes. Nederl T Geneesk 1931; 75:5956–5959.
Klein A, Hussar AE, Bornstein S. Pelger-Huët anomaly of the leukocytes. N Engl J Med 1955;253:1057–1063.
Nachtsheim H. The Pelger anomaly in man and rabbits. J Hered, 1950;41:131–137.
Pelger K. Demonstratie van een paar zeldzam vorkomende typen van bloedlichamp jes en bespreking der patienten. Nederl T Geneesk 1928;72:1178.

Leukocyte adhesion deficiency

Leukocyte adhesion deficiency is a hereditary disease which is recognized in Holstein-Fresian calves, dogs, and humans. It results from a deficiency or absence of β_2 integrins, or the CD11/CD18 family of glycoproteins which are required for the adhesion of leukocytes to endothelium prior to their extravasation as well as their role in phagocytosis. In cattle and dogs CD11 and CD18 have been found to be deficient. Aleukocyte adhesion deficiency in which CD11 and CD18 are normal but CD16 deficient has been reported in dogs. The disease is characterized by recurrent necrotizing bacterial and fungal infections, particularly of the oral cavity, lung, and gastrointestinal tract. Wound healing is impaired. There is persistent and severe neutrophilia and an absence of neutrophils outside the vascular tree. The disease is fatal before adulthood. The disease can be diagnosed by the polymerase chain reaction for the CD18 allele and the use of monoclonal antibodies for CD18 antigens.

References

Aherholm JS, Houe H, Jorgensen CB, et al. Bovine leukocyte adhesion deficiency in Danish Holstein-Friesian cattle II. Pathoanatomical description of affected calves. Acta Vet Scand 1993;34:237–243.

Etzioni A, Frydman M, Pollack S, et al. Brief report: recurrent severe infections caused by a novel leukocyte adhesion deficiency. N Engl J Med 1992;327:1789–1792.

Gilbert RO, Rebhun WC, Kim CA, et al. Clinical manifestations of leukocyte adhesion deficiency in cattle: 14 cases (1977–1991). J Am Vet Med Assoc 1993;202:445–449.

Jorgensen CB, Agerholm JS, Pederson J, et al. Bovine leukocyte adhesion deficiency in Danish Holstein-Friesian cattle I. PCR screening and allele frequency estimation. Acta Vet Scand 1993;34:231–236.

Muller KE, Bernadina WE, Kalsbeek HC, et al. Bovine leukocyte adhesion deficiency—clinical course and laboratory findings in eight affected animals. Vet Quart 1994;16:27–33.

Nagahata H, Kehrli ME Jr., Murata H, et al. Neutrophil function and pathologic findings in Holstein calves with leukocyte adhesion deficiency. Am J Vet Res 1994;55:40–48.

Nagahata H, Nochi H, Tamoto K, et al. Expression and role of adhesion molecule CD18 on bovine neutrophils. Canad J Vet Res 1995;59:1–7.

Trowald-Wigh G, Johannisson A, Hakansson L. Canine neutrophil adhesion proteins and Fc-receptors in healthy dogs and dogs with adhesion protein deficiency, as studied by flow cytometry. Vet Immunol Immunopathol 1993;38:297–310.

Trowald-Wigh G, Hakansson L, Johannisson A, et al. Leukocyte adhesion protein deficiency in Irish setter dogs. Vet Immunol Immunopathol 1992;32:261–280.

van Garderen E, Muller KE, Wentink GH, et al. Post-mortem findings in calves suffering from bovine leukocyte adhesion deficiency (BLAD). Vet Quart 1994;16:24–26.

THE SPLEEN

By far the most common problem which confronts pathologists as they examine the spleen has to do with its size, for, as with soldiers' uniforms, there appear to be two sizes: too large and too small. While we shall presently mention some pathological enlargements, the great majority of spleens encountered at autopsy are essentially normal. It is well to remember that the spleen is a "great reticulo-endothelial sponge" which holds a large but varying amount of blood. A primary function of the spleen is the filtration of blood to remove foreign elements and erythrocytes which have reached the end of their life span, or have been damaged (extravascular hemolysis). Blood entering the spleen circulates through the splenic sinusoids of the "red pulp" which are lined by a discontinuous endothelium. While most of the circulating blood passes directly through the si-

nusoids to the splenic veins ("closed circulation"), blood may also pass outside the sinusoids to enter the cords of Billroth (splenic cords), the so called "open circulation." The splenic cords are predominantly composed of loose aggregates of macrophages through which the blood is exposed prior to re-entering the sinuoids and continuing on to the splenic veins. Other functions of the spleen include serving as a reserve pool of erythrocytes, an organ of the immune system, a source of lymphocytes, and, under appropriate conditions, a site for hematopoiesis.

The "white pulp" of the spleen or the Malpighian follicles, is composed of T and B lymphocytes and has an intimate relationship to the splenic circulation before the penicillary arterioles empty into the sinusoids. The splenic arteries traversing the splenic trabeculae (which are predominantly smooth muscle in animals) branch to and from what are known as central arteries. These are surrounded by a collar of T lymphocytes. Bulging from and surrounded by this collar is a lymphoid follicle composed of B lymphocytes. If antigenically stimulated this follicle has a germinal center, surrounded by a corona of B lymphocytes and a zone of T lymphocytes continuous with the collar of lymphocytes surrounding the central artery. The central artery and its collar of lymphocytes continue beyond the follicle until it terminates into the penicillary arterioles.

Splenic enlargements, splenomegaly

Enlargement of the spleen can result from several different mechanisms, including circulatory disturbances, inflammatory disease, metabolic disease and neoplastic disease.

Acute congestion of the spleen is seen in acute myocardial failure, and is also seen following euthanasia with Nembutal or similar barbiturates. The acutely congested spleen is enlarged, but not excessively so, and somewhat soft. Its cut surface is dark and bulges moderately, with blood oozing from it. Microscopically, there may be little change beyond a large number of erythrocytes in the sinuses and cords of Billroth. Torsion of the spleen, alone or along with other organs, is sometimes encountered in animals. This results in an acutely congested spleen which, if uncorrected, leads to infarction.

Chronic passive congestion of the spleen results in an enlarged organ that is also filled with blood, but is firm or a little tough because of an increase in fibrous tissue. Microscopically the findings are (1) distention of the sinusoids and cords with blood, (2) often an appreciable hyperplasia of the endothelium of the sinusoids so that the lining cells resemble cuboidal epithelium, (3) marked diffuse fibrosis throughout the pulp, (4) a thickening of the trabeculae, and (5) accumulation of phagocytized hemosiderin from erythrocytes which have been entrapped in the nearly static blood and hemolyzed in excessive numbers. Causes of chronic passive congestion of the spleen include cirrhosis of the liver, congestive heart failure and other disorders which would place increased pressure, or back pressure on the splenic vein.

Hematomas of the spleen are a frequent cause of nodular enlargement, especially in dogs. Depending upon their duration they either are characterized by a pool of blood or a mass of lysed blood and fibrin, surrounded by degenerating granulocytes and a fibrous capsule. Adhesions to the omentum are frequent.

Infections as a cause of splenic enlargement (Acute and Chronic Splenitis) occur in septicemias, anthrax being a classic example. Here the splenic enlargement is due to congestion as well as an influx of neutrophils. There may also be an increase in number of endothelial cells and macrophages as well as an increase in number of lymphocytes. Some septicemias however, lead to destruction of lymphocytes, particularly in the germinal centers. The term "blackberry-jam spleen" has been applied to the severely blood-distended spleen of acute septicemia. Chronic splenitis is seen in many infectious diseases, and may lead to a diffuse enlargement or irregular enlargement (nodular) depending upon the offending organism. Examples of infectious diseases causing chronic splenitis include: brucellosis, tuberculosis, toxoplasmosis, histoplasmosis, tularemia, caseous lymphadenitis, pseudotuberculosis and leishmaniasis. The nature of the inflammatory reaction associated with these various agents is discussed elsewhere. In many of these diseases, there is also lymphoid hyperplasia contributing to the hypersplenism.

Storage diseases and deposition diseases such as Gaucher's disease and amyloidosis lead to splenomegaly.

Anemia is associated with splenic enlargement through two different mechanisms. In hemolytic anemias, especially those characterized by extravascular hemolysis, the spleen is engorged with disintegrating erythrocytes and there is hyperplasia of macrophages. In many chronic anemias, extramedullary hematopoiesis may be extensive enough to lead to enlargement of the organ. Thrombocytopenic purpura is also a cause of splenic enlargement.

Proliferative and neoplastic disease to include hematopoietic neoplasms, hemangioendotheliomas, fibrous histiocytoma and metastatic neoplasms are causes of splenic enlargement.

Hyposplenism, small spleens

Hyposplenism or small spleen is less frequently encountered. Death following acute hemorrhage leads to exhaustion of blood from the spleen leading to a decrease in its size. In hereditary immunodeficiency disease, such as severe combined immunodeficiency as seen in Arabian foals and certain strains of mice, there is marked hypoplasia of the spleen (as well as hypoplasia of lymph nodes and thymus) as a result of an absence of lymphocytes. Rarely, aplasia of the spleen is encountered.

Other disorders of the spleen

Infarctions occur occasionally in the spleen, usually being hemorrhagic but not invariably so. They tend to be conical with the base at the capsule, as explained in the general discussion of infarcts, but may be so large as to occupy a whole end or a considerable segment of the spleen (Fig. 22-3). Infarcted areas in the dog spleen may become quite large, and consist of a mixture of elements, such as necrosis, repeated hemorrhages, blood pigments, and organization by fibrous connective tissue. Some of the hemorrhages may rupture the splenic capsule and cause death by exsanguination into the peritoneal sac.

A lesion consisting of a raised, subcapsular area, almost black in color and usually multiple, occurs in 50% of cases of hog cholera (swine fever). These have been classed as hemorrhagic infarcts, although some have been confused with mere hemorrhages. The obstruction of blood essential to infarction is considered to be due to thickening of capillary walls and minute thrombi in them.

Amyloidosis involves the splenic corpuscles, as previously explained. It is rare except in animals which have been used for the production of hyperimmune serums.

In old dogs, **siderotic plaques** or Gandy-Gamna nodules are frequently found on the splenic capsule. They appear as yellow, dry encrustations. Microscopically yellow-brown, iron positive pigment in trabeculae and capsule is mixed with deep blue (with hematoxy-

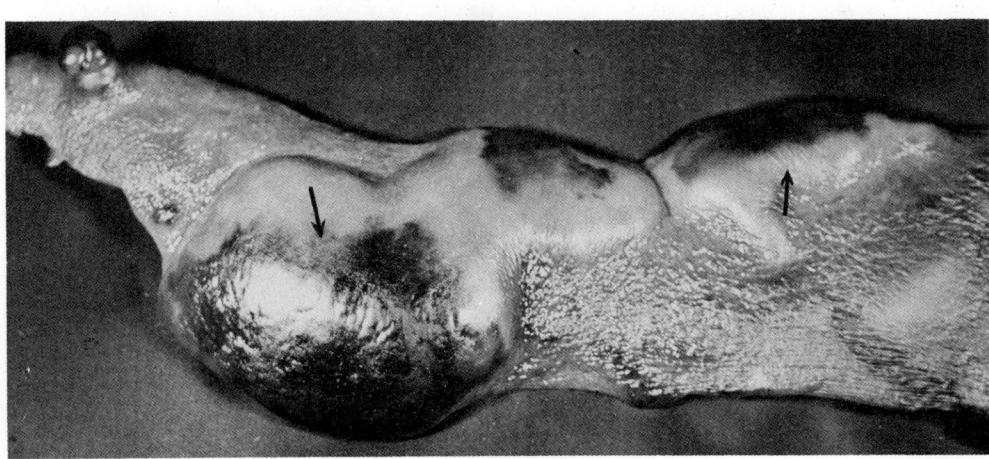

FIG. 22-3 Infarction of the spleen of a ten-year-old female Springer Spaniel. The infarcts (arrows) near the apex are elevated and partially hemorrhagic. (Courtesy of Angell Memorial Animal Hospital).

lin) fibers which react to the usual stains for calcium salts. Although usually considered a senile change, the significance is not known; it may be that they are sites of previous hemorrhages.

Cysts in the spleen may prove to contain the scolices of *Echinococcus granulosus* in the herbivorous and omnivorous species. However, this parasite is practically nonexistent in the United States.

Rupture of the spleen is a not infrequent accident in the dog for reasons which must be evident in a world of automotive transportation (Fig 22-4). A considerable number of dogs so injured survive, and the two or more healed fragments of the spleen are found at autopsy years later. There are even cases in which several small fragments of spleen are spattered over the adjoining areas and become implanted in the mesentery to live and carry on such functions as do not require anatomically normal vascular connections. Infarction of the spleen and malignant tumors (hemangioendothelioma) may also lead to rupture of the capsule and exsanguination. Accessory spleens of varying sizes originate also as congenital malformations, but these are rare.

Neoplasms of the spleen

LYMPHOSARCOMA, MALIGNANT LYMPHOMA

Solitary lesions of lymphosarcoma may occasionally be found in the spleen of many species, but usually such

tumors are present as a part of the generalized neoplastic disease. Sharply demarcated lesions may be seen, made up of lymphocytic cells. In some cases, more diffuse invasion and replacement of the spleen may be evident.

CANINE NODULAR HYPERPLASIA, "SPLENOMA"

Not infrequently in old dogs and occasionally in other species, this lesion may be encountered as an incidental finding at necropsy. The lesion consists of one or more sharply demarcated nodules which elevate the splenic capsule (Fig. 22-5). Microscopically, the lesion is made up of most of the elements of the spleen, except that the lymphocytic cells are quite hyperplastic. Some structures of hyperplastic cells are spherical and resemble splenic corpuscles except that the central artery is absent. The significance of this lesion is unknown. It may or may not be neoplastic but its course is assumed to be benign. Grossly, this lesion may be distinguished by its uniform smooth surface and globoid shape from long standing infarcts of the spleen. Microscopically, the lymphoid nature of the mass is clearly different than the necrosis, hemorrhage, and fibrous organization found in old infarcts.

HEMANGIOENDOTHELIOMA, HEMANGIOSARCOMA

This is among the most frequently encountered primary tumors of the spleen, especially in the dog. The essential feature is the presence of pleomorphic masses of tumor cells resembling endothelial cells. These cells have large, ovoid hyperchromic nuclei and cytoplasm which may be fused with contiguous cells. Mitoses are frequent. The tumor cells may be seen to form blood-filled vascular spaces, a distinguishing characteristic. Sometimes the tumor cells form sheets which suggest the littoral cells and their sinusoids.

Repeated hemorrhages, necrosis, and organization may make this tumor difficult to distinguish from long-standing infarction of the spleen. The critical item in

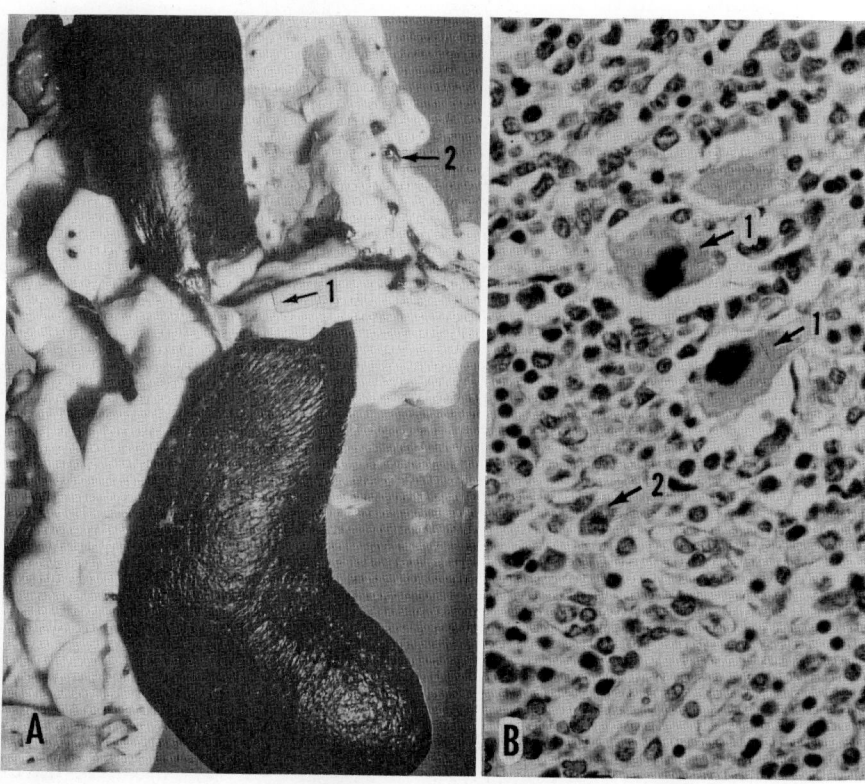

FIG. 22-4 A. Rupture of the spleen (1) of a seven-year-old Scottish Terrier, with implants of spleen (2) in the mesentery. The dog was hit by a car one year prior to necropsy. **B.** Extramedullary hematopoiesis, spleen of a dog. Megakaryocytes (1) and myeloid cells (2) are evident. (**B,** Courtesy of Armed Forces Institute of Pathology.) (Contributor: Dr. John Mills)

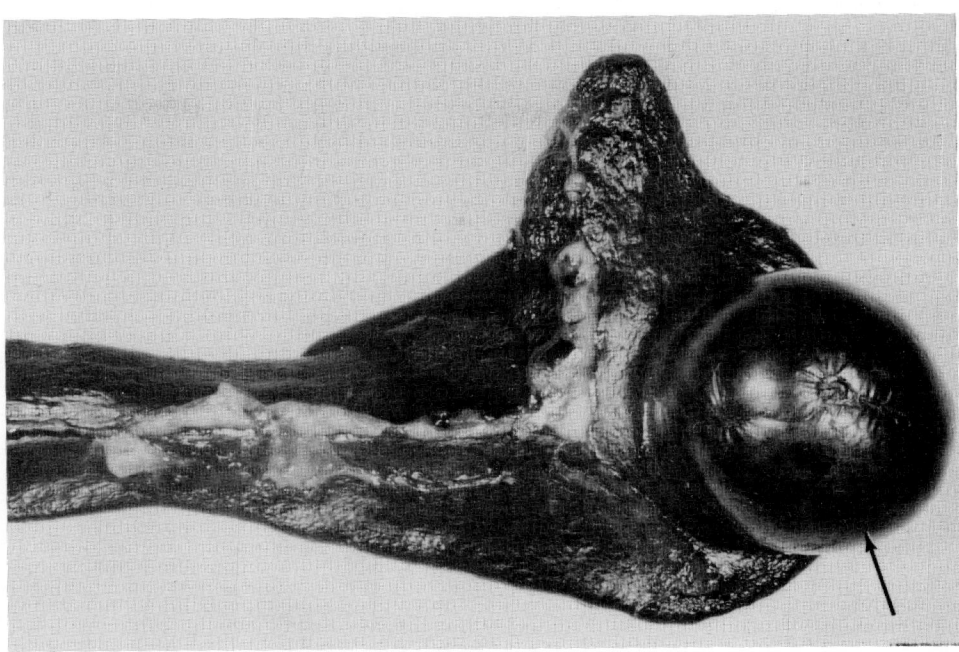

FIG. 22-5 Nodular hyperplasia ("splenoma") of the spleen of a 14-year-old male Collie. (Courtesy of Angell Memorial Animal Hospital)

the diagnosis of hemangioendothelioma is the presence of typical vascular-forming malignant endothelial cells. These are usually found at the periphery of the lesion and sometimes are dwarfed by large amounts of hemorrhage, necrosis, and organization.

These tumors sometimes rupture the splenic capsule and lead to fatal bleeding into the peritoneal sac. If this hemorrhage is not fatal, tumor cells may be seeded and grow on peritoneal surfaces. They may also be associated with multicentric or metastatic hemangioendotheliomas in the liver and atrium of the heart.

LEIOMYOSARCOMA

These tumors presumably arise from the smooth muscle cells of the splenic trabeculae. Light-colored, irregular, single or multiple masses are present in the spleen, often accompanied by hemorrhage. The tumor cells are immature smooth muscle cells with elongated cytoplasm arranged in interwoven sheets and masses with some cells in parallel arrays. The nuclei are ovoid, their long axis parallel to the length of the cells, and mitoses are frequent.

These tumors are considered malignant and may metastasize via the blood stream or become seeded in the peritoneal cavity.

METASTATIC NEOPLASMS

Although not a frequent event, any malignant neoplasm whose cells reach the bloodstream could metastasize to the spleen. It appears that the lung filters out most such circulating malignant cells, but a few are deposited and grow in the spleen. Myeloid leukemia may involve the spleen, presenting a problem in distinguishing it from extramedullary hemopoiesis. A myelolipoma, with myeloid and lipomatous elements, has been described in a cat.

References

Dennis SM. Congenital splenic defects in newborn lambs. Cornell Vet 1972;62:473–476.

Ishmael J, Howell J McC. Neoplasia of the spleen of the dog with a note on nodular hyperplasia. J Comp Path, 1968;78:59–67.

Jacobsen G. Morphological-histochemical comparison of dog and cat splenic ellipsoid sheaths. Anat Rec 1971;169:105–113.

Jolly RD. Nodular hyperplasia of the ovine spleen. N Z Vet J 1967;15:91–94.

Lau DTL. Ectopic splenic nodules in the pancreas of a Capuchin monkey (Cebus albifrons). J Med Primatol 1973;2:67–70.

Prynmak C, McKee LJ, Goldschmidt MH, et al. Epidemiologic, clinical, pathologic, and prognostic characteristics of splenic hemangiosarcoma and splenic hematoma in dogs: 217 cases (1985). J Am Vet Med Assoc 1988;193:706–712.

Sander CH, Langham RF. Myelolipoma of the spleen in a cat. J Am Vet Med Assoc 1972;160:1101–1103.

THE LYMPH NODES

The primary structure of lymph nodes is the lymphoid follicle which is composed of a central area of B lymphocytes surrounded by a perifollicular region of T lymphocytes. These are bathed by lymphatics entering at the cortex and blood vessels entering at the hilus. The intimate association of lymphocytes, lymphatics and blood vessels allows the exchange of lymphocytes from the blood to the follicles and presentation of antigen from lymphatics to the lymphocytes, which occurs by way of follicular dendritic cells and macrophages. Antigenic stimulation leads to reactive hyperplasia which, depending upon the nature of the antigen, is characterized by follicular lymphoid hyperplasia, representing an expansion of B cells, or paracortical lymphoid hyperplasia, representing an expansion of T cells. Marked follicular lymphoid hyperplasia must be differentiated from follicular lymphoma. Generally an immunoreactive node will have an increased population of plasma cells. Lymph nodes can also react to stimulation with a marked hypertrophy and hyperplasia of sinus endothelial cells and their filling with macrophages (histiocytes). This is referred to as sinus histiocytosis. This is a feature of lymph-nodes-draining malignant neoplasms and those which contain metastases (Fig. 22-6).

LYMPHADENITIS

The most common causes of lymphadenitis are infectious agents or their products. In most examples, there is an as-sociated reactive hyperplasia. Although there are many specific diseases which affect lymph nodes, many examples of lymphadenitis are nonspecific. Lymphadenitis is seen in nodes draining primary inflammatory disease of other organs or tissues; for example, the bronchial lymph nodes in the presence of pneumonia, the mandibular and pharyngeal lymph nodes in cases of rhinitis or an infected tooth, or the supramammary nodes in response to mastitis. This is also known as lymph node draining reaction. In **acute nonspecific lymphadenitis,** there is hyperemia and edema with distension of the lymph sinuses.

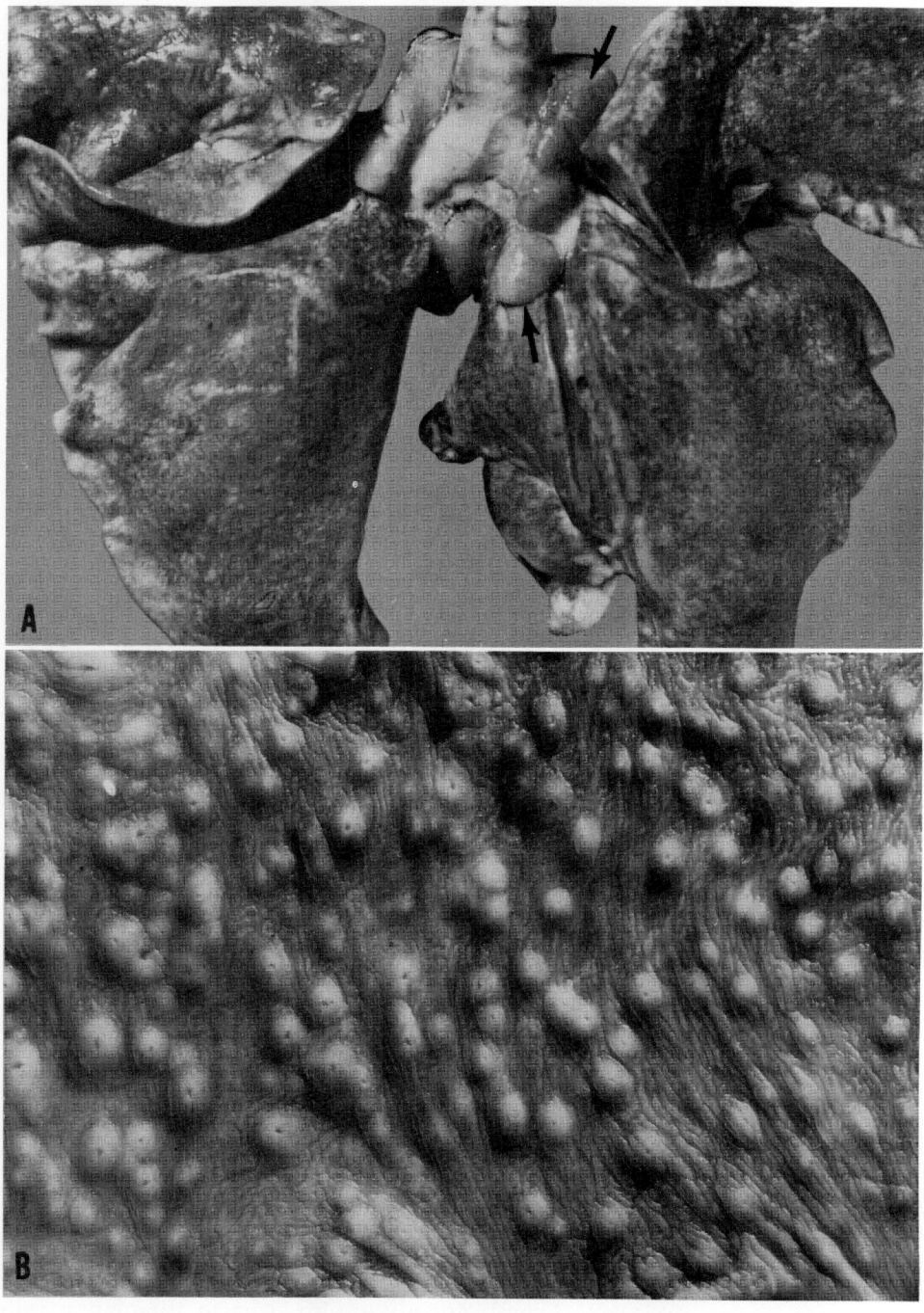

FIG. 22-6 A. Hyperplasia of bronchial lymph nodes (arrows) in a dog with "salmon disease." **B.** Hyperplasia of the lymph nodules in colon of a dog with "salmon disease." (Courtesy of Dr. W. J. Hadlow)

The distended sinuses usually contain a variable number of neutrophils and macrophages. Sometimes there are large numbers of eosinophils present, especially in lymph nodes draining chronic skin disease and hypersensitivity lesions. If bacteria actually become entrapped and established in the node, the reaction becomes clearly purulent, often with abscess formation. The lymphoid follicles become hyperplastic with prominent germinal centers. In some examples of acute lymphadenitis there may also be lysis of lymphocytes(this is particularly true with generalized viral infections, such as canine distemper. Affected nodes are swollen and somewhat soft, and the cut surface is wet and bulges. **Chronic nonspecific lymphadenitis** is characterized by much more marked lymphocytic hyperplasia, which may be predominantly B cell hyperplasia of the follicles or T cell hyperplasia of the paracortical tissue depending upon the nature of the offending antigen. Macrophages and plasma cells are present in the follicles and sinuses and there may be foci of neutrophils. The capsule and septae are thickened with an increase in collagenous connective tissue and, grossly, the nodes are firm and dry.

The specific forms of lymphadenitis exhibit the features of nonspecific lymphadenitis upon which are superimposed the lesions unique to the offending organism. Hemorrhagic lymphadenitis is seen in acute septicemias such as anthrax. Purulent lymphadenitis with formation of abscesses is seen in strangles in puppies and horses and streptococcal lymphadenitis of swine. Granulomatous lymphadenitis is a feature of tuberculosis, pseudotuberculosis, caseous lymphadenitis, tularemia, mycotic infections and various metazoan parasites whose migrations may take them to lymph nodes. The pathological picture in viral induced lymphadenitis varies. In some there is often extensive necrosis of lymphocytes; for example, rinderpest, alpha herpesvirus and parvovirus infections. In others in which there is immunosuppression, the nodes simply look atrophied.

Other disorders of lymph nodes

Hypoplasia of lymph nodes is seen in severe combined immunodeficiency disease in Arabian foals and in comparable syndromes in some strains of laboratory mice. Anthracosis of lymph nodes occurs when carbon pigment is carried to them from the lungs. Black pigment occurs in hepatic lymph nodes of cattle and sheep infested with flukes. Hemosiderosis, hemochromatosis and melanosis may affect the nodes. A brownish discoloration of the medullary portion, especially, seen frequently in bovine lymph nodes does not indicate ill health. It may be related to porphyrinemia. Hyalin is often found within germinal centers.

Neoplasms of the lymph nodes

PRIMARY NEOPLASMS

Primary neoplasms of lymph nodes include lymphosarcoma (malignant lymphoma), hemangioendothelioma, and lymphangiosarcoma. The latter tumor is rare and may arise at other sites, but is usually seen in lymph nodes. The tumor arises from cells of the lymphatic vessels and therefore tends to form cystic spaces lined with endothelium, but not containing blood. Most individual tumors are benign.

Lymphoma and other hematopoietic neoplasms are discussed at the end of this chapter.

METASTATIC NEOPLASMS

Metastatic neoplasms in lymph nodes are a frequent occurrence and present challenges as well as opportunities to the pathologist. All malignant neoplasms have the potential of metastasis to lymph nodes. Those neoplasms most often seen as metastases to lymph nodes of animals include: adenocarcinomas (mammary especially), squamous cell carcinomas, mast cell tumors, hemangiopericytoma, and hemangioendotheliomas. One important point for the histopathologist to remember is that the afferent lymphatics lead to the lymph node's cortex and empty into the cortical sinuses. Malignant cells will initially be seen, therefore, in the cortical sinuses. As the tumor cells proliferate, they involve the cortex of the lymph node. When tumor growth reaches the hilus of the lymph node, malignant cells have the opportunity to metastasize further via the efferent lymphatics. This is true in all domestic animals except the pig in which the cortical and medullary tissues of lymph nodes are reversed. In swine, the afferent lymphatics penetrate deep into the nodes where the lymphatic nodules are located, and the lymph filters to the peripheral sinuses and exits via efferent lymphatics.

If an epithelial neoplasm, such as adenocarcinoma or squamous cell carcinoma, is found in viable state in a lymph node, it is clearly malignant, no matter how differentiated the tumor cells may appear.

Thymus

The Thymus, which is derived from the third pharyngeal pouch, is an epithelial organ in the anterior mediastinum which becomes colonized with T-lymphocytes. The epithelial component is composed of onionskin layers of keratinized cells, the so called Hassall's corpuscles in the medulla, and a loose network in the cortex. These cells contain desmosomes and tonafilaments. Between these are large numbers of lymphocytes (thymocytes), which in the cortex represent immature T cells and, in the medulla, mature T cells. Scattered throughout the organ are myoid cells which bear similarity to smooth muscle cells, both ultrastructurally and antigenically. The thymus is the central organ for T cell production and differentiation. Normally the thymus undergoes involution with age.

Hypoplasia and agenesis of the thymus is seen in severe combined immunodeficiency disease of Arabian foals discussed in Chapter 7. Thymic hypoplasia is also seen in Black Pied Danish cattle. This disorder is related to a failure to absorb zinc and is responsive to zinc supplementation. It is discussed in Chapter 7. Thymic hypoplasia has also been reported in dogs. Branchial cysts, which are from vestiges of the branchial system of the fetus, are sometimes found in the thymus.

Atrophy of the thymus can be difficult to evaluate because of the normal involution of the gland. Most examples result from infectious agents which cause acute or chronic loss of T lymphocytes. Acute destruction is seen in such disorders as alpha herpesvirus infections and parvovirus infections. Evidence of necrosis and an associated inflammatory reaction are often apparent. Chronic loss is seen in feline leukemia virus infection and has been noted in immunodeficiency virus infections.

Thymic hyperplasia is characterized by the formation of typical B-cell lymphoid follicles bearing germinal centers in the medulla and compressing the cortex. Although encountered in animals, its significance is not apparent except in association with myasthenia gravis. This disorder is described in dogs and cats, but best understood in humans. It results from an autoimmune response to the thymic myoid cells.

Neoplasms of the thymus may arise from epithelial cells or lymphocytes. Neoplasms of epithelial cells are termed thymomas and those of lymphocytes, thymic lymphoma. Thymomas are not common tumors and are more frequent in older animals, in contrast to thymic lymphoma which may be encountered in the young. They are seen on occasion in most species, but most often in the dog where there is a predominance in German Shepherd Dogs. Thymomas are composed of epithelial cells which are mixed with of non-neoplastic lymphocytes whose numbers may be few or so extensive as to resemble lymphoma. In dogs, mast cells are also frequently present. The epithelial cells may be polygonal with large pale nuclei, relatively clear cytoplasm and with or without clear cytoplasmic borders. In some examples they take on a spindle shape. Squamous differentiation and Hassall's corpuscles may be prominent, giving the tumor the appearance of squamous cell carcinoma. Epithelial lined cysts are also sometimes present. If, as can be the case, the cells are not clearly epithelial, their origin can be identified by their ultrastructural or immunohistochemical characteristics. The neoplasms are generally confined to the mediastinum. Implantation within the thoracic cavity may occur in some examples, and, rarely, there may be distant metastases. Some examples of thymoma in animals are associated with myasthenia gravis as is true in humans. Polymyositis has also been seen in conduction with thymomas in dogs and cats.

Thymic lymphoma is more common than thymoma. They are most frequent in cats and calves, and in both species the tumors can reach a very large size. Most are believed to be of T-cell origin and consist of a diffuse mass of lymphocytes of uniform size which deface the normal thymic architecture.

References

Abbot DP, Cherry CP. Malignant mixed thymic tumor with metastases in a rat. Vet Pathol 1982;19:721–723.

Aronsohn MG, Schunk KL, Carpenter JL, et al. Clinical and patho-

logic features of thymoma in 15 dogs. J Am Vet Med Assoc 1984;184:1355–1362

Atwater SW, Power BE, Park RD, et al. Thymoma in dogs: 23 cases (1980–1991). J Am Vet Med Assoc 1994;205:1007–1013.

Bellah JR, Stiff ME, Russell RG. Thymoma in the dog: two case reports and review of 20 additional cases. J Am Vet Med Assoc 1983;183:306–311.

Hadlow WJ. High prevalence of thymoma in the dairy goat. Report of seventeen cases. Vet Pathol 1978;15:153–169.

Carpenter JL, Holzworth J. Thymoma in 11 cats. J Am Vet Med Assoc 1982;181:248–251.

Carpenter JL, Valentine BA. Squamous cell carcinoma arising in two feline thymomas. Vet Pathol 1992;29:541–543.

Gores BR, Berg J, Carpenter JL, et al. Surgical treatment of thymoma in cats: 12 cases (1987–1992). J Am Vet Med Assoc 1994; 204:1782–1785.

Hohfeld R. Myasthenia gravis and thymoma: paraneoplastic failure of neuromuscular transmission. Lab Invest 1990;62:241–243.

Loveday RK. Thymoma in a Siamese cat. J So Afr Vet Med Assoc 1959;30:33–34.

Mackey L. Clear-cut thymoma and thymic hyperplasia in a cat. J Comp Pathol 1975;85:367–371.

Robinson M. Malignant thymoma with metastases in a dog. Vet Pathol 1974;11:172–180.

Sandison AT, Anderson LJ. Tumors of the thymus in cattle, sheep and pigs. Cancer Res 1969;29:1146–1150.

Scott JC, Cook JR, Lantz GC. Acquired myasthenia gravis in a cat with thymoma. J Am Vet Med Assoc 1990;196:1291–1293.

Si-kwang L, Patnaik AK, Burk RL. Thymic branchial cysts in the dog and cat. J Am Vet Med Assoc 1983;182:1095–1098.

Thilsted JP, Bolton RG. Thymic lymphosarcoma with bony metaplasia in a cat. Vet Pathol 1985;22:424–425.

Whiteley LO, Leininger JR, Wolf CB, et al. Malignant squamous cell thymoma in a horse. Vet Pathol 1986;23:627–629.

HEMATOPOIETIC NEOPLASMS— LEUKEMIAS—LYMPHOMAS

Neoplasms of the hematopoietic system are amongst the more common of the neoplastic diseases of animals. Within a species and between species there are many different types of hematopoietic neoplasms, based upon their morphologic and clinical presentations. Over the years numerous systems of classification have been developed for the various types of hematopoietic neoplasms, and as newer techniques become available, these classifications continue to evolve. Most systems of classification depend upon morphologic characteristics of the neoplastic cells, however in many examples the cellular identification is difficult at best, and very often not possible with tissue sections. This is particularly true with the acute leukemias. The combined use of enzymatic markers and immunophenotyping provides a more precise confirmation of cell type. Unfortunately immunophenotyping is not readily available to all laboratories, and the monoclonal antibodies used to recognize cellular antigens are in general species specific. A large number of antigens, termed CD antigens (for clusters of differentiation), have been identified for which in some species, monoclonal antibodies have been developed and can be used to specifically identify the various leukocytes. The association of some of these (but by no means all) as well as enzymatic markers are included in Table 22-1.

These diseases can be divided into five broad groups:

1. Leukemias which are neoplasms of hematopoietic stem cells arising in the bone marrow which usually have secondary overflow into the blood.
2. Malignant lymphomas which are neoplasms arising in lymphoid tissue which may overflow into the blood.
3. Plasma cell neoplasms.
4. Histiocytoses which are neoplasms of tissue macrophages or histiocytes.
5. Myeloproliferative disorders which are neoplastic proliferations of hematopoietic stem cells in the bone marrow morphologically distinct from leukemias.

Within these groups there is further subdivision depending on the cell type and its degree of differentiation. The classification presented in Table 22-1 is one of the classifications used for hematopoietic neoplasms in humans, but does not incorporate the many variants of leukemia/lymphoma that have been recognized. Other systems are also in use, and further refinement continues. Most forms of the neoplasms have been identified in animals, but have been less well studied than in humans. Many if not most reports in animals do not precisely identify the exact nature of the neoplastic cells.

LEUKEMIA

Leukemias are malignant neoplasms of hematopoietic stem cells which originate in the bone marrow. The bone marrow becomes diffusely replaced by neoplastic cells, which also usually (but not invariably) enter the peripheral circulation, which gives rise to the designation leukemia. The neoplastic cells may seed and infiltrate other organs and tissues, particularly the liver, spleen and lymph nodes. Replacement of the bone marrow leads to some common clinical findings regardless of the particular form of leukemia. These include anemia, hemorrhage (due to thrombocytopenia) and increased susceptibility to infections. The leukemias are divided into acute leukemias and chronic leukemias, which in turn are further subdivided into several specific forms.

Acute leukemias

The acute leukemias include the acute lymphoblastic leukemias and the myelogenous leukemias, which are classified into seven types (M1 through M7). The differentiation on morphologic grounds can, in many cases, be extremely difficult and diagnosis should include cytochemical and immunophenotyping. Useful differential features are presented in Table 22-2. In general the enzyme myeloperoxidase is the hallmark of myeloid lineage (identified with enzyme histochemistry or by means of monoclonal antibodies against myeloperoxidase which is more sensitive). However, examples of negative myelogenous leukemia negative for myeloper-

TABLE 22-1 **Neoplastic diseases of hemopoietic and lymphopoietic tissues**

Leukemia
  Acute Leukemias
    Acute lymphoblastic leukemia (ALL)
    Acute Myeloblastic leukemia (AML)
      Acute myelocytic leukemia without differentiation
      Acute myelocytic leukemia with differentiation
      Acute promyelocytic leukemia
      Acute myelomonocytic leukemia
      Acute monocytic leukemia
      Acute erythroleukemia
      Acute megakaryocytic leukemia

  Chronic Leukemias
    Chronic lymphocytic leukemia (CLL)
    Chronic myeloid leukemia (CML)
    Chronic myelomonocytic leukemia
    Chronic megakaryocytic leukemia
    Mast cell leukemia

Myeloproliferative Disorders
  Myeloid metaplasia with myelofibrosis
  Polyythemia vera
  Essential thrombocythemia
  Myelodysplasia

Malignant Lymphoma
  Low Grade
    Small lymphocytic
    Follicular, small cleaved cell
    Follicular, mixed small cleaved and large cell
  Intermediate Grade
    Follicular, large cell
    Diffuse, small cleaved cell
    Diffuse, mixed small and large cell
    Diffuse, large cell
  High Grade
    Large cell, immunoblastic
    Lymphoblastic
    Small, noncleaved cell

  Hodgkin's Disease

Plasma Cell Neoplasms
  Multiple myeloma
  Plasmacytoma

Histiocytosis

oxidase can occur, which is why multiple procedures should be applied.

Acute Lymphoblastic Leukemia (ALL) is a rapidly fatal malignant neoplasm of lymphoblasts arising in the bone marrow. In humans, ALL is classified into three morphologic types: L1, composed of a homogeneous population of small round cells, usually without clefts and without visible nucleoli; L2, composed of a heterogeneous population of large cells, often with clefts and visible nucleoli; and L3 composed of a homogeneous population of large cells with prominent nucleoli (con-

TABLE 22-2 **Differentiation of acute leukemias**

Acute lymphoblastic leukemia	PAS + aggregates in cytoplasm Terminal deoxynucleotidyl transferase + Lack azurophilic granules and Auer rods
Non-B Non–T	NK cells/large granular lymphocytes; contain azurophilic granules
B-cell	CD21, CD22 +, CD19 +; surface immunoglobulin
T-cell	CD3 +
Acute myelocytic leukemia	CD13 +, CD33 +, CD19 −, CD22 − (CD3 −)
Myelocytic without differentiation (M1)	Myeloperoxidase + Azurophilic granules, Auer rods Chlor-E neg; ANAE neg
Myelocytic with differentiation (M2)	Myeloperoxidase + + + Azurophilic granules, Auer rods Chlor-E +; ANAE neg, Sudan Black B +
Promyelocytic (M3)	Myeloperoxidase + + +; Chlor-E +; ANAE neg Sudan Black B +
Myelomonocytic (M4)	Myeloperoxidase + +; Chlor-E + *; ANAE + Sudan Black B +
Monocytic leukemia (M5)	Chlor-E Neg; ANAE +;
Erythroleukemia (M6)	Myeloperoxidase +
Megakaryocytic leukemia (M7)	Platelet peroxidase +; CD41 +, CD61 + Myeloperoxidase neg

ChlorE = Naphthol AS-D chloroacetate esterase (granulocyte specific esterase)
ANAE = α-Naphthyl Acetate Esterase (NaF resistant) (monocyte specific esterase)

sidered a leukemic form of Burkitt's lymphoma). This specific classification has not been widely applied to acute lymphoblastic leukemia in animals. However, they are usually classified on the basis of cell size and are distinguished from myeloid leukemias by the lack of cytoplasmic granules. Azurophilic granules are, however, found in NK cells, the so-called large granular lymphocytes. Specific identification can be made by immunophenotyping. Although they may arise from either B-cell or T-cell, most examples studied in animals represent malignancies of B-cell precursors with varying degrees of maturity. Demonstration of CD 19 and 22 expression is a good indication that the cells are of B-lineage. CD 3 is a good marker for T-cells. Most will be positive for terminal deoxynucleotidyl transferase. T-cells are positive for alpha-naphthyl acetate esterase as are mononuclear cells.

In animals, ALL is predominantly a disease of young animals, (particularly dogs, cats, and calves but seen in all species), however malignant lymphoma with leukemia is more common. The cause is not known. Feline leukemia virus is associated with most leukemias

and lymphomas in cats. In contrast, bovine leukemia virus causes lymphoma, but its role in leukemia is less clearly established. Pathologically the bone marrow is diffusely replaced by solid sheets of lymphocytes. Neoplastic lymphocytes also infiltrate the sinuses of lymph nodes and sinusoids of the spleen. They may also flood the cortices of lymph nodes and efface the splenic corpuscles. The liver is also invariably affected with neoplastic cells in the sinusoids and triads. Neoplastic cells can colonize in any organ or tissue. Generally there is invasion of peripheral blood. However, this is not always the case and in some examples there is actually leukopenia.

A disease in cats, first described as reticuloendotheliosis, is included here as it is an acute, rapidly progressive malignancy. It is characterized by proliferation of undifferentiated cells in the bone marrow with their entrance into the peripheral blood and growth in the spleen, liver, and lymph nodes. The cells were originally described as containing large round red-purple eccentric nuclei with fine chromatin, a single pale-blue nucleolus and abundant dull-blue cytoplasm with azurophilic granules. The cells appear to be stem cells with some degree of differentiation. Reports have described differentiation toward the lymphocytic/monocytic lineage, granulocytic lineage and erythrocytic lineage, suggesting that not all examples of what is termed reticulendotheliosis represent the same malignancy. The term reticuloendotheliosis has also been used to describe similar leukemias in dogs.

Acute Myeloblastic Leukemia (AML) (Acute Myelocytic Leukemia) is classified by the French-American-British Study Group into seven different types (M1 through M7) depending upon the degree of cellular maturation and differentiation. Further types have been proposed as well as subdivisions. These are listed in Table 22-1. Differentiation can be towards myeloid cells (neutrophils, eosinophils, basophils), monocytes, erythrocytes (Di Guglielmo's disease) or megakaryocytes. Often there is a mix of cells, with myeloblasts accompanying more differentiated cells (for example, large numbers of myeloblasts with proerythroblasts in erythroleukemia. Those with clearly evident differentiation can be identified with stained smears of bone marrow or peripheral blood. However, many examples cannot be easily classified nor differentiated from ALL. This is particularly true with tissue sections. Acute myelocytic leukemia without differentiation can look exactly like ALL. Morphologic features which are helpful include the presence of azurophilic granules and Auer rods in cells of myelocyte origin and their absence in cells of lymphocytic origin. Auer rods are membrane-bound structures containing longitudinally arranged filamentous material which can be stacked in bundles of faggots (faggot cells). Inclusions resembling Auer rods, however, can be seen in lymphoblastic leukemia, so caution must be exercised. Immunophenotyping with monoclonal antibodies for various myeloid-specific antigens can be very helpful, as can direct staining for myeloperoxidase or its identification with monoclonal antibodies. Not all of the neoplastic cells will react as indicated. Myeloblastic leukemia without differentiation (M1) is characterized by marrow replacement with myeloblasts which may or may not contain azurophilic granules and Auer rods. Some differentiation towards promyelocytes may be evident. If at least 3 to 5% of cells react for myeloperoxidase, it is considered adequate to identify the leukemia as of myeloid origin. The majority of B and T-cell leukemias will be positive for deoxynucleotidyl transferase. However, some leukemias of myeloid origin are also positive for this enzyme. Myeloblastic leukemia with differentiation (M2) is characterized by clearly evident maturation toward granulocytes. Azurophilic granulation is more evident and Auer rods more frequent. In addition to myeloperoxidase, cells will be positive for chloroacetate esterase. Promyelocytic leukemia (M3) is characterized by cells with more intense granulation, more frequent Auer rods and more mature promyelocytes. The enzyme reactions are comparable to myeloblastic leukemia with differentiation. Myelomonocytic leukemia (M4) has indisputable differentiation toward both monocytic and granulocytic cells. Some cells will be positive for Chloroacetate esterase

and some for α-naphthyl acetate esterase. Monocytic leukemia (M5) is characterized by large undifferentiated cells which are myeloperoxidase negative and α-naphthyl acetate esterase positive. Erythroleukemia (M6) which is also known as Di Guglielmo's syndrome, is characterized by proliferation of erythroblasts as well as myeloblasts. The associated leukemia, however, is restricted to erythroid cells. Megakaryocytic leukemia (M7) is characterized by marrow replacement with large irregularly shaped cells with large irregular and often multiple nuclei.

Each of the various types of acute myelogenous leukemia have been recognized in animals, but are reported most frequently in dogs and cats. Acute and chronic lymphocytic leukemia is more frequent. Pathologically, the bone marrow is effaced by diffuse sheets of neoplastic cells which may all be undifferentiated or contain cells recognizable as promyelocytes, monocytes, proerythroblasts and so forth. Azurophilic reticulin fibers are frequently associated with the neoplastic cells. Infiltrates may also be found in lymph nodes, spleen, liver and other organs. These may sometimes form tumor nodules, which may be greenish in color and were once termed chloromas. The morphology of the cells will depend upon their degree of differentiation. Myelodysplasia (see below) is a precursor of AML.

Chronic leukemia

Chronic lymphocytic leukemia (CLL) is a neoplastic proliferation of B-cells (and very rarely T-cells) which arises in the bone marrow and is associated with a severe lymphocytosis. It tends to occur in older animals than ALL. The cells differentiate, but are not functional. They will be CD19 and CD20 positive, but lack CD10 (early B and T cell antigen), are negative for deoxynucleotidyl transferase, and have immunoglobulin on their surface. In contrast to ALL the disease is chronic and may persist for years. The bone marrow is diffusely, or sometimes nodularly, replaced with lymphocytes which vary from large cells with distinct nuclei to small cells with dark nuclei. Cytoplasm is usually minimal. Most circulating cells are small lymphocytes. There is always extensive infiltration of the cords of the spleen and lymph nodes, which become greatly enlarged, and the triads of the liver. CLL must be differentiated from lymphoma with peripheral blood invasion. Large extranodal tumor masses are a feature of many of the lymphomas in animals and the lymph nodes are usually more extensively replaced with neoplastic cells which also efface the cortex. However, it is often impossible to histopathologically distinguish between the two.

Chronic myeloid (myelogenous) leukemia (CML) is a chronic form of the more differentiated forms of AML. In the majority of examples, the differentiation is toward neutrophils, and the predominant cell type in the marrow, tissues, and circulation are mature cells and their precursors. As with the acute forms of myelocytic leukemia, differentiation can proceed along other lines to include monocytic, megakaryocytic and mixed forms. In humans, most examples of CML are associated with a translocation of the long arm of chromosome 22 which is present in all stem cells and their descendants.

Mast cell leukemia (malignant mastocytosis; systemic mast cell disease)

Whether mast cell leukemia should be classified as a leukemia or not is debatable. Although the bone marrow is involved, it is not clear if the disease represents a primary malignant neoplasm of hematopoietic stem cells. The disease is most frequently encountered in cats, although it has been reported in swine. The disease occurs independently of mast cell neoplasms of the skin and gastrointestinal tract. Most often the neoplasm affects the spleen, lymph nodes, liver, bone marrow, lungs, and kidneys. The skin may also be invaded. The spleen is usually greatly enlarged, with a characteristic deep mahogany color and fleshy consistency. Mast cells are usually found in small numbers in the peripheral circulation. The circulating and tissue cells are morphologically identical to mast cells, which stain metachromatically with toluidine blue. An interesting concomitant feature is the presence of small, sharply demarcated ulcers in the mucosa of the pylorus or duodenum. These ulcers are probably the result of excess histamine (or possible serotonin) produced by the mast cells.

MYELOPROLIFERATIVE AND MYELODYSPLASTIC DISORDERS

In classifications of hematopoietic malignancies of humans, four disorders are included under the heading of myeloproliferative disorders: chronic myeloid leukemia (which has been discussed); polycythemia vera; myeloid metaplasia with myelofibrosis; and essential thrombocythemia. The myelodysplastic disorders are characterized by maturation defects.

Polycythemia vera is a rare primary disorder characterized by an absolute excess of circulating erythrocytes. It must be differentiated from hemoconcentration, in which the blood cell count is purely relative, in which the total number of cells is not increased, but the total volume of plasma is decreased. This is the result, ordinarily, of dehydration. It must also be differentiated from secondary polycythemia, also known as erythrocytosis, which occurs secondary to anoxia from such disorders as patent foramen ovale, patent ductus arterosis, heart failure, or pulmonary disease, or from living at a high altitude. Neoplasms have been associated with the production of erythropoietin, which will lead to polycythemia. Polycythemia vera is not associated with increased levels of erythropoietin.

Polycythemia vera is usually accompanied by leukocytosis, thrombocytosis and hypervolemia. It has been described in cattle, horses, dogs and cats. It may also occur in mice infected with the Friend leukemia virus.

In Jersey cattle (Tennant, et al., 1967) the disease was described as an autosomal recessive trait developing in the second month of life, persisting throughout the first year and disappearing at maturity. McGrath (1974) summarized the clinical signs in dogs as polydipsia, polyuria, nocturia, pica, posterior weakness, ataxia, vaginal discharge, enlarged mammary glands, intolerance to heat, and seizures. The consistent hematologic findings include elevated packed cell volume (65 to 82); increased hemoglobin concentration (21.6 to 28.3); elevated red blood cell counts, and total blood volume. Thrombosis of the aorta and other arteries is often encountered, resulting from the increased viscosity of blood. Microscopically, the bone marrow is hypercellular, with increased numbers of erythrocytic, granulocytic, and megakaryocytic elements; however, the erythrocytic cells predominate.

Myeloid metaplasia with myelofibrosis is a rare disorder in which there is marked extramedullary hematopoiesis accompanied by hypocellularity and fibrosis of the bone marrow. Agyrophilic reticulin fibers course between the hematopoietic elements. It is described in dogs and cats and presents with anemia. Extramedullary hematopoiesis is most striking in the spleen, but may also be present in the liver and lymph nodes. All cell types are present. Myelofibrosis is also encountered in animals in the absence of extramedullary hematopoiesis and may also be seen in acute myelogenous leukemia. Fibrosis of the marrow will also follow disorders characterized by bone marrow necrosis.

Essential thrombocythemia is a very rare myeloproliferative disorder of humans which has been described in the dog and cat. It is characterized by marked megakaryocytic proliferation in the bone marrow accompanied by a marked thrombocytosis. The thrombocytes are dysfunctional and clinically the disorder is characterized by bleeding problems. There is usually an anemia. Fibrosis of the bone marrow is another pathologic feature.

Myelodysplasia is an affliction characterized by ineffective hematopoiesis. The bone marrow is hypercellular, with a preponderance of blast cells which fail to properly mature. There is some differentiation along all lines, erythrocytes, granulocytes and platelets but it is disorderly. There is pancytopenia and anemia. In animals, it is described most often in cats and is associated with infection with feline leukemia virus. It is considered a precursor of acute myelogenous leukemia.

References

Abbott DP, Prentice DE, Cherry CP. Mononuclear cell leukemia in aged Sprague-Dawley rats. Vet Pathol 1983;20:434–439.

Alroy J. Basophilic leukemia in a dog. Vet Pathol, 1972;9:90–95.

Baker RJ, Valli VE. Dysmyelopoiesis in the cat: a hematological disorder resembling refractory anemia with excess blasts in man. Canadian J Vet Res 1986;50:3–6.

Barthel CH. Acute myelomonocytic leukemia in a dog. Vet Pathol 1974;11:79–86.

Bean-Knudsen DE, Caldwell CW, Wagner JE, et al. Porcine mast cell leukemia with systemic mastocytosis. Vet Pathol 1989;26:90–92.

Beech J, Bloom JC, Hodge TG. Erythrocytosis in a horse. J Am Vet Med Assoc 1984;184:986–989.

Blatt J, Reaman G, Poplack DG. Biochemical markers in lymphoid malignancy. N Engl J Med 1980;303:918–922.

Blue JT, French TW, Kranz JS. Non-lymphoid hematopoietic neoplasia in cats: a retrospective study of 60 cases. Cornell Vet 1988;78:21–42.

Blue JT. Myelofibrosis in cats with myelodysplastic syndrome: an acute myelogenous leukemia. Vet Pathol 1988;25:154–160.

Brumbaugh GW, Stitzel KA, Zinkl JG, et al. Myelomonocytic myeloproliferative disease in a horse. J Am Vet Med Assoc 1982; 180:313–316.

Buccheri V, Shetty V, Yoshida N, et al. The role of an anti-myeloperoxidase antibody in the diagnosis and classification of acute leukaemia: a comparison with light and electron microscopy cytochemistry. Bri J Haematol 1992;80:62–68.

Burkhardt E, Saldern F, Huskamp B. Monocytic leukemia in a horse. Vet Pathol 19874;21:394–398.

Cain R, Feldman BF, Kawakami TG, et al. Platelet dysplasia associated with megakaryoblastic leukemia in a dog. J Am Vet Med Assoc 1986;188:529–530.

Castoldi GL, Liso V, Specchia G, et al. Acute promyelocytic leukemia: morphological aspects. Review Leukemia 1994;8:S27–32.

Christopher MM, Metz AL, Klausner J, et al. Acute myelomonocytic leukemia with neurologic manifestations in the dog. Vet Pathol 1986;23:140–147.

Cole N. Polycythemia in a dog. North Am Vet 1954;35:601.

Cook SM, Lothrop CD Jr. Serum erythropoietin concentrations measured by radioimmunoassay in normal, polycythemic, and anemic dogs and cats. J Vet Intern Med 1994;8:18–25.

Coons FH, George JW, Appel GO. Reticuloendotheliosis in a dog. Cornell Vet 1976;66:249–257.

Couto CG. Clinicopathologic aspects of acute leukemias in the dog. J Am Vet Med Assoc 1985;186:681–685.

Crow SE, Allen DP, Murphy CJ, et al. Concurrent renal adenocarcinoma and polycythemia in a dog. J Am Anim Hosp Assoc 1995;31:29–33.

Crow SE, Madewell BR, Henness AM. Feline reticuloendotheliosis: a report of four cases. J Am Vet Med Assoc 1977;170:1329–1332.

Donovan EF, Loeb WF. Polycythemia rubra vera in the dog. J Am Vet Med Assoc 1959;134:36–37.

Drach D, Drach J, Glassl H, et al. Flow cytometric detection of cytoplasmic antigens in acute leukemias: implications for lineage assignment. Leukemia Res 1993;17:455–461.

Dunphy CH, Chung D, Dunphy FR. Auer rod-like inclusions in adult common acute lymphoblastic leukemia. Hum Pathol 1994;25: 211–214.

English RV, Breitschwerdt EB, Grindem CB, et al. Zolinger-Ellison syndrome and myelofibrosis in a dog. J Am Vet Med Assoc 1988;192:1430–1434.

Facklam NR, Kociba GJ. Cytochemical characterization of leukemic cells from 20 dogs. Vet Pathol 1985;22:363–369.

Facklam NR, Kociba GJ. Cytochemical characterization of feline leukemia cells. Vet Pathol 1986;23:155–161.

Foster ES, Lothrop CD Jr. Polycythemia vera in a cat with cardiac hypertrophy. J Am Vet Med Assoc 1988;192:1736–1738.

Fowler ME, Cornelius CE, Baker NF. Clinical and erythrokinetic studies on a case of bovine polycythemia vera. Cornell Vet 1964; 54:153–159.

Fraser CJ, Joiner GN, Hardine JH, et al. Acute granulocytic leukemia in cats. J Am Vet Med Assoc 1974;165:355–359.

Gilmore CE, Gilmore VH, Jones TC. Reticulo-endotheliosis, a myeloproliferative disorder of cats: a comparison with lymphocytic leukemia. Pathol Vet 1964;1:161–183.

Goitsuka R, Sunahori S, Ohashi T, et al. Cytochemical and immunologic properties of leukemic cells from a cat with reticuloendotheliosis. J Vet Med Sci 1991;53:327–329.

Grindem CB, Stevens JB, Perman V. Cytochemical reactions in cells from leukemic dogs. Vet Pathol 1986;23:103–109.

Grindem CB. Ultrastructural morphology of leukemic cells from 14 dogs. Vet Pathol 1985;22:456–462.

Grindem CB. Ultrastructural morphology of leukemic cells in the cat. Vet Pathol 1985;22:147–155.

Hardy WD. Hematopoietic tumors of cats. J Am Anim Hosp Assoc 1981;17:921–940.

Harvey JW, Shields RP, Gaskin JM. Feline myeloproliferative disease. Changing manifestations in the peripheral blood. Vet Pathol 1978;15:437–448.

Harvey JW, Terrell TG, Hyde DM, et al. Well-differentiated lymphocytic leukemia in a dog: long-term survival without therapy. Vet Pathol 1981;18:37–47.

Ho FCS, Chan GRC, Todd D. Non-specificity of Sudan Black B in the diagnosis of acute myeloid leukaemia. Bri J Haematology 1983;53:171–172.

Hodgkins EM, Zinkl JG, Madewell BR. Chronic lymphocytic leukemia in the dog. J Am Vet Med Assoc 1980;177:704–707.

Holden AR. Polycythaemia vera in a dog. Vet Rec 1987;120:473–475.

Kajikawa O, Koyama H, Yoshikawa T, et al. Use of alpha-naphthyl acetate esterase staining to identify T lymphocytes in cattle. Am J Vet Res 1983;44:1549–1552.

Keller P, Sager P, Freudiger U, et al. Acute myeloblastic leukaemia in a dog. J Comp Pathol 1985;95:619–632.

Leifer CE, Matus RE, Patnaik AK, et al. Chronic myelogenous leukemia in the dog. J Am Vet Med Assoc 1983;183:686–689.

Loeb WF, Rininger B, Montgomery CA, et al. Myelomonocytic leukemia in a cat. Vet Pathol 1975;12:464–467.

Mackey LJ, Jarrett WFH, Lauder IM. Monocytic leukaemia in the dog. Vet Rec 1975;96:27–30.

Mackey LJ, Jarrett WFH, Wiseman A. Monocytic leukaemia in a cow. Res Vet Sci 1972;13:287–289.

Matus RE, Leifer CE, MacEwen EG. Acute lymphoblastic leukemia in the dog: A review of 30 cases. J Am Vet Med Assoc 1983;183:859–862.

McGrath CJ. Polycythemia vera in dogs. J Am Vet Med Assoc 1974; 164:1117–1122.

Messick J, Carothers M, Wellman M. Identification and characterization of megakaryoblasts in acute megakaryoblastic leukemia in a dog. Vet Pathol 1990;27:212–214.

Michel RL, O'Handley P, Dade AW. Megakaryocytic myelosis in a cat. J Am Vet Med Assoc 1976;168:1021–1025.

Morris DD, Bloom JC, Roby KAW, et al. Eosinophilic myeloproliferative disorder in a horse. J Am Vet Med Assoc 1984;185:993–996.

Ragan HA, Hackett PL, Dagle GE. Acute myelomonocytic leukemia manifested as myelophthisic anemia in a dog. J Am Vet Med Assoc 1976;169:421–425.

Raskin RE, Krehbiel JD. Histopathology of canine bone marrow in malignant lymphoproliferative disorders. Vet Pathol 1988;25:83–88.

Raskin RE, Krehbiel JD. Myelodysplastic changes in a cat with myelomonocytic leukemia. J Am Vet Med Assoc 1985;187:171–174.

Reed C, Ling GV, Gould D, Kaneko JJ, et al. Polycythemia vera in a cat. J Am Vet Med Assoc 1970;157:85–91.

Rohrig KE. Acute myelomonocytic leukemia in a dog. J Am Vet Med Assoc 1983;182:137–141.

Scott CS, Den Ottolander GJ, Swirsky D, et al: Recommended procedures for the classification of acute leukaemias. International Council for Standardization in Haematology (ICSH). Leukemia Lymphoma 1993;11:37–50.

Shimada T, Matsumoto Y, Okuda M, et al: Erythroleukemia in two cats naturally infected with feline leukemia virus in the same household. J Vet Med Sci 1995;57:199–204.

Shull RM, DeNovo RC, McCracken MD. Megakaryoblastic leukemia in a dog. Vet Pathol 1986;23:533–536.

Spier SJ, Madewell BR, Zinkl JG, et al. Acute myelomonocytic leukemia in a horse. J Am Vet Med Assoc 1986;188:861–863.

Steiger R, Feige K. [Case report: polycythemia in a horse]. [German]. Schweizer Archiv fur Tierheilkunde 1995;137:306–311.

Stromberg PC, Vogtsberger LM. Pathology of the mononuclear cell leukemia of Fischer rats. I. Morphologic studies. Vet Pathol 1983;20:698–708.

Stromberg PC, Vogtsberger LM, Marsh LR, et al. Pathology of the mononuclear cell leukemia of Fischer rats. II. Hematology. Vet Pathol 1983;20:709–717.

Tablin F, Jain NC, Mandell CP, et al. Ultrastructural analysis of platelets and megakaryocytes from a dog with probable essential thrombocythemia. Vet Pathol 1989;26:289–293.

Tennant B, Asbury AC, Laben RC, et al. Familial polycythemia in cattle. J Am Vet Med Assoc 1967;150:1493–1509.

Weiss DJ, Armstrong PJ. Secondary myelofibrosis in three dogs. J Am Vet Med Assoc 1985;187:423–425.

Weiss DJ, Raskin R, Zerbe C. Myelodysplastic syndrome in two dogs. J Am Vet Med Assoc 1985;187:1038–1040.

Young KM. Myeloproliferative disorders. [Review]. Vet Clin North Am Sm Anim Pract 1985;15:769–781.

LYMPHOMA (MALIGNANT LYMPHOMA; LYMPHOSARCOMA)

Lymphomas are amongst the most frequent of the neoplastic diseases of animals (Figs. 22-7 through 22-9). They are neoplasms of lymphocytes which originate in lymphoid tissue anywhere in the body. There are many different cytologic forms of lymphoma. Of the many classifications which have evolved, the most recent and widely accepted is termed the working formulation which is presented in Table 22-3 along with the Rappaport Classification and the Luke-Collins Classification which have also been widely used. The low grade lymphomas include those predominantly composed of mature lymphocytes sometimes mixed with a lesser number of large lymphocytes and histiocytes. The lymphocytes in the small lymphocytic form resemble normal lymphocytes, which most often form diffuse masses effacing the architecture of lymph nodes and infiltrating other tissues. In the other two forms of low grade lymphoma (follicular, small cell and follicular mixed cell), the lymphocytes are slightly larger and their nuclei have an abnormal shape which is referred to as cleaved. They tend to form nodules, rather than growing in diffuse sheets. In intermediate grade lymphomas the cells are larger, usually cleaved (or mixed cleaved and noncleaved), and have a higher

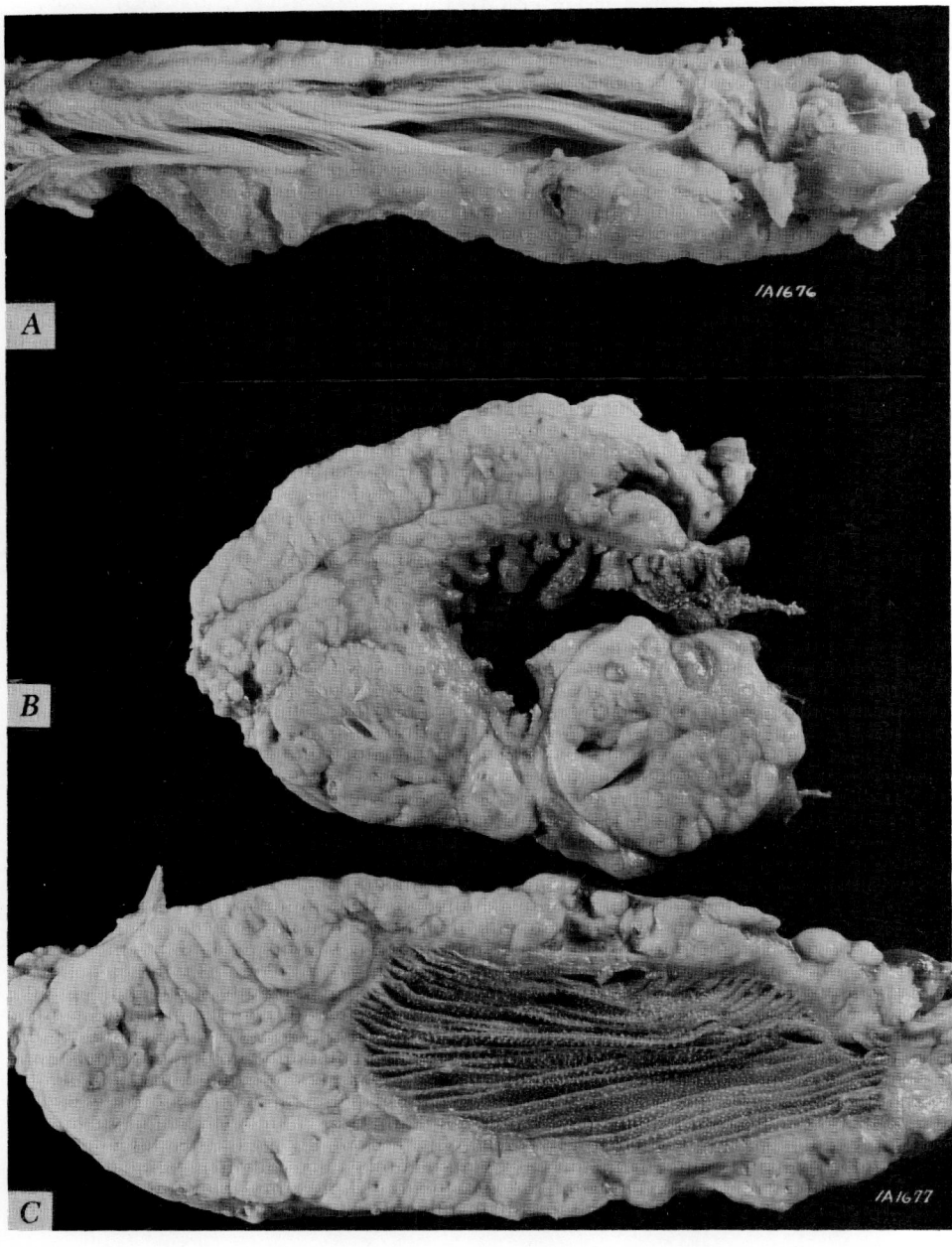

FIG. 22-7 Bovine lymphosarcoma (malignant lymphoma) illustrating neoplastic invasion of cauda equina (**A**), reticulum (**B**), and omasum (**C**) (Courtesy of Dr. M.J. Twiehaus)

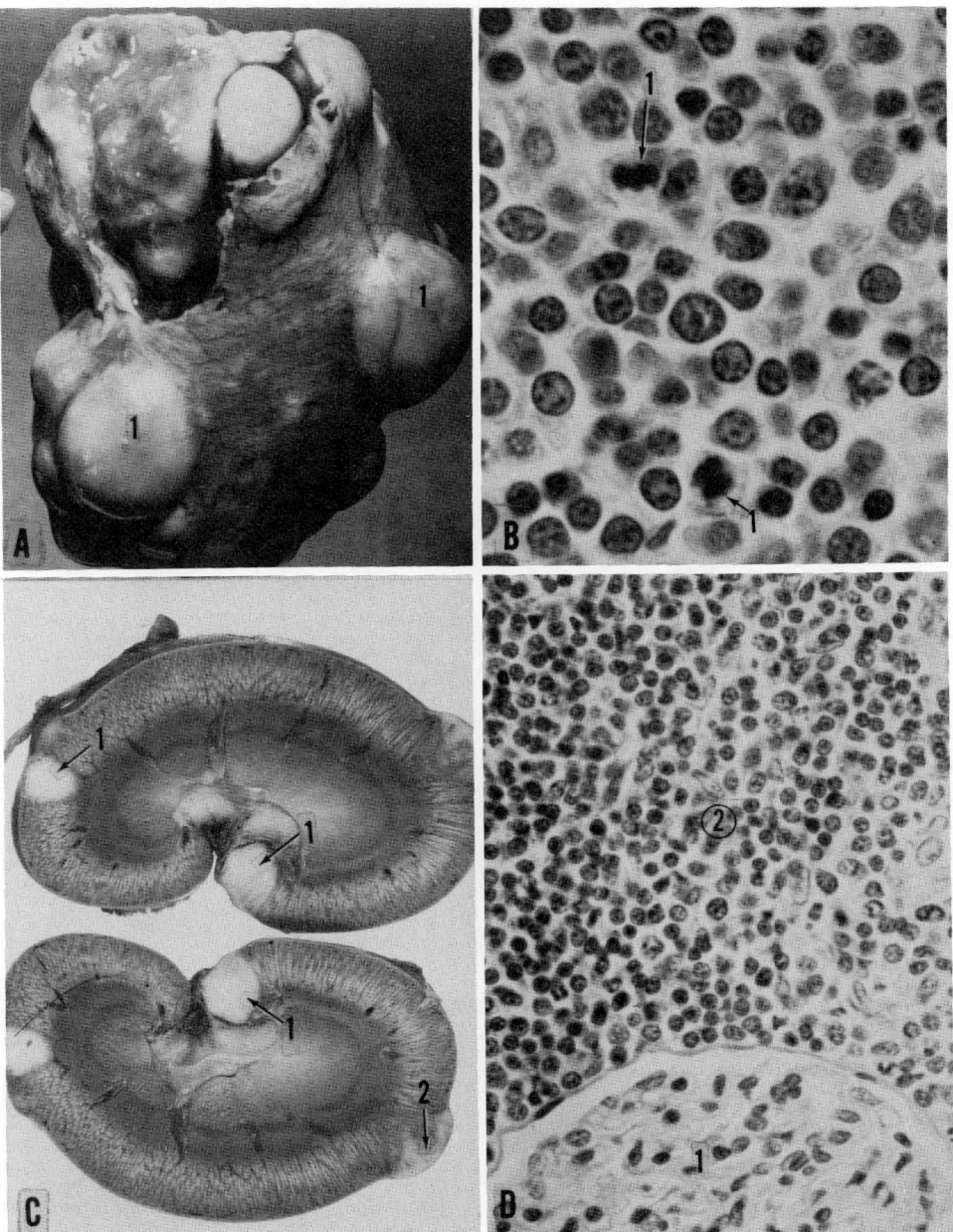

FIG. 22-8 Malignant lymphoma. **A.** Lesions (1) in the kidney of a dog. **B.** Photomicrograph (× 1190) of lesion in **C.** Note individually discrete tumor cells and mitotic figures (1). **C.** Kidney of a five-year-old male German Shepherd. Lymphosarcoma tumor masses (1) and (2) in renal cortex. **D.** Neoplastic cells (× 500); same case as **C.** Note infiltration of renal cortex by tumor cells (2). The glomerulus (1) is not yet invaded by tumor. (Courtesy of Armed Forces Institute of Pathology) (Contributor: Dr. Leo L. Lieberman.)

number of mitotic figures. They can be either diffuse or nodular. High grade lymphomas may be composed of very large lymphoblasts with large vesicular nuclei and abundant amphoteric cytoplasm. The cells of some large cell lymphomas resemble histiocytes and are termed histiocytic lymphoma. The high grade small noncleaved form of lymphoma is in humans designated Burkitt's lymphoma. Most lymphomas in animals are of B-cell origin. Recently a Revised European American Lymphoma Classification has been proposed. This is presented in Table 22-4 along with a comparison to the working formulation. Despite the attempt to develop precise systems of classification, many examples of lymphoma in animals and humans fail to fit existing systems.

The histology (the tissue distribution and site of origin) of lymphomas is also variable within and between species, giving rise to their classification as multicentric,

thymic, alimentary, splenic and cutaneous lymphomas. Multicentric lymphoma generally involves most lymph nodes as well as generalized proliferation in the spleen, liver, bone marrow and other organs and tissues. The other forms are often restricted to the designated site, although regional lymph nodes may become involved. Lymphomas are often aleukemic; however, entrance of neoplastic lymphocytes into the peripheral circulation, resulting in leukemia, may occur, in which case this type of lymphoma must be differentiated from the acute and chronic lymphoid leukemias. In true leukemias, large solid tumor masses are generally not present(the bone marrow is diffusely replaced, in contrast to nodular replacement seen in lymphoma).

Canine lymphoma is most often of the multicentric type and of B-cell origin. It is most frequent in middle-age to older animals. They are characterized by general-

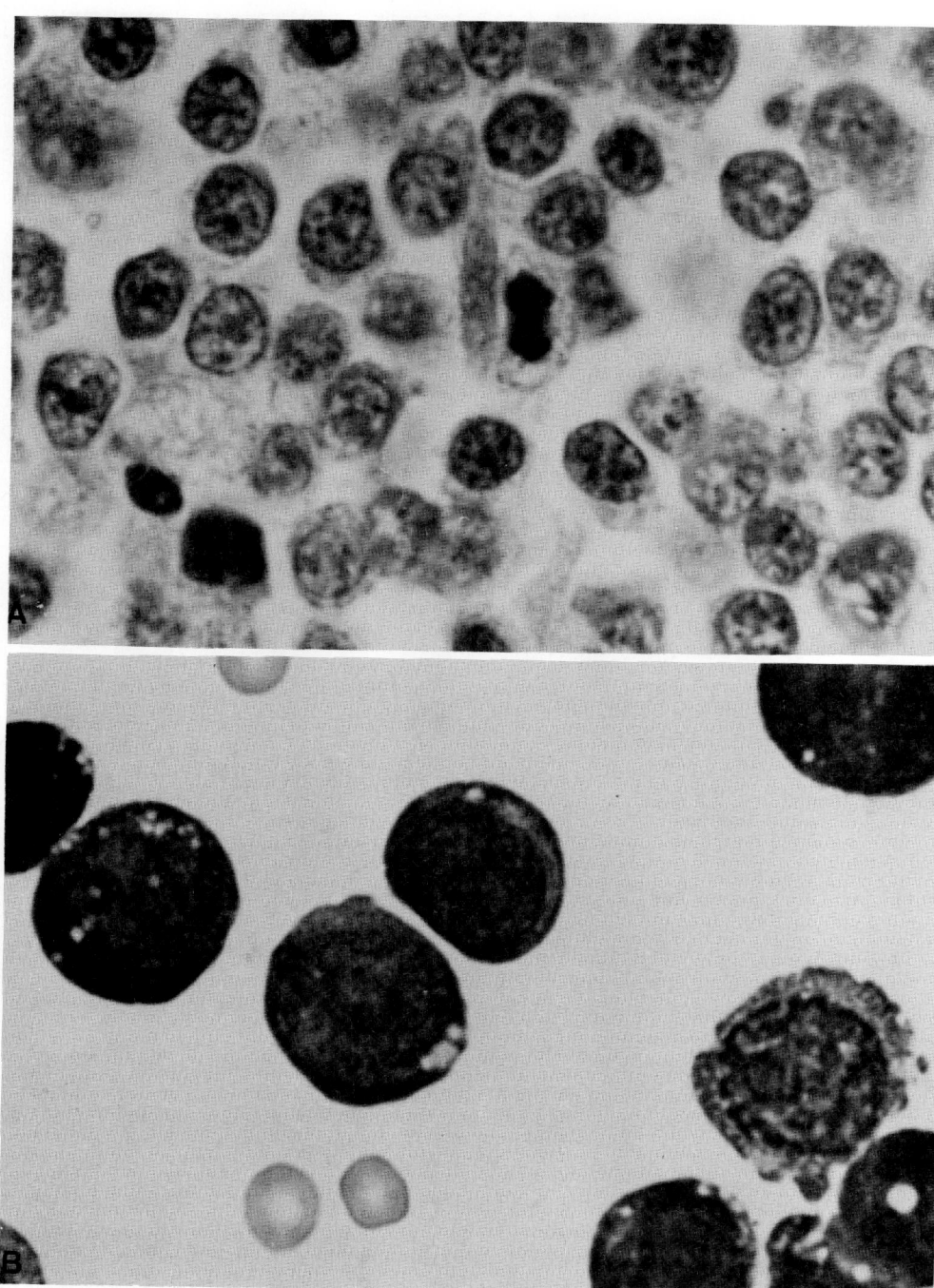

FIG. 22-9 Malignant lymphoma involving thymus and pleura of a cat. **A.** Section of pleura. (H & E, × 1600.) **B.** Smear of fluid aspirated from pleural cavity. (Wright-Giemsa's stain, × 1600.) Note the apparent difference in size of the tumor cells prepared by sectioning and smear techniques.

ized enlargement of lymph nodes, very often with infiltration of the liver, spleen, bone marrow, and other organs. Most lymphomas in dogs are of intermediate to high grade type, with a diffuse pattern of non-cleaved cells. Cleaved cell lymphomas and nodular lymphomas are much less frequent. Primary enteric, thymic, and cutaneous lymphoma are also seen in dogs. One of the cutaneous forms occurs as a chronic disease similar to mycosis fungoides of humans, which is a T-cell lymphoma which may be either CD4+ or CD8+. In dogs, while some examples are of T-cell origin, others are B-cell and some are null-cell. In the classic example,

the cells have a highly convoluted nucleus referred to as a cerebriform nucleus. The lymphoma cells invade the upper dermis and into the epidermis singly and in small clusters termed Pautrier's microabscesses. In humans, mycosis fungoides may progress to lymph node and visceral dissemination and in some cases there is leukemia. Leukemic cells maintain their convoluted shape and are termed Sézary cells, and the disease is termed Sézary syndrome which is characterized by a generalized exfoliative erythroderma. Leukemia has also been noted in dogs with mycosis fungoides.

Feline lymphoma is one of the manifestations of in-

TABLE 22-3 **Comparison of Lymphoma classification schemes**

Working formulation	Rappaport classification	Luke-Collins classification
Low Grade		
Small lymphocytic	Lymphocytic, well differentiated	Small lymphocytic and plasmacytoid lymphocytic
Follicular, small cleaved cell	Nodular, poorly differentiated lymphocytic	Follicular center cell, small cleaved
Follicular, mixed small cleaved and large cell	Nodular, mixed lymphocytic, histiocytic	Follicular center cell, small cleaved and large cleaved
Intermediate Grade		
Follicular, large cell	Nodular, histiocytic	Follicular center cell, large cleaved and or noncleaved
Diffuse, small cleaved cell	Diffuse, poorly differentiated lymphocytic	Follicular center cell, small cleaved diffuse
Diffuse, mixed small and large cell	Diffuse, mixed lymphocytic, histiocytic	Follicular center cell, small cleaved, large cleaved or large noncleaved
Diffuse, large cell	Diffuse histiocytic	Follicular center cell, large cleaved or noncleaved
High Grade		
Large cell, immunoblastic	Diffuse histiocytic	Immunoblastic B or T cell
Lymphoblastic	Lymphoblastic lymphoma	Convoluted T-cell lymphoma
Small, noncleaved cell	Undifferentiated, Burkitt's and non-Burkitt's	Follicular center cell, small noncleaved

fection with feline leukemia virus. Lymphoma is the most frequent of the hematopoietic neoplasms of cats, and cats have a higher incidence than other domestic animals. Most are multicentric, but an almost equal number are enteric or mediastinal (thymic). It is reported that multicentric and enteric lymphomas are of B-cell origin, and mediastinal lymphomas of T-cell origin. Leukemia occurs is over 25% of feline lymphomas. Feline lymphoma can also occur in the kidneys, eyes, skin and other tissues. Most have a diffuse pattern and may be either composed of cleaved or non-cleaved cells. As in dogs, a nodular pattern is infrequent.

Bovine lymphoma is associated with bovine leukemia virus (enzootic bovine lymphoma), although not all examples result from this viral infection (sporadic bovine lymphoma) (Fig. 22-7). **Enzootic bovine lymphoma** is a B-cell lymphoma of adult cattle caused by bovine leukemia virus. It usually involves the lymph nodes, where there may be generalized enlargement, or it may be restricted to certain nodes. Often lymphoma is restricted to mesenteric nodes, pelvic nodes and sublumbar nodes. Extension from sublumbar nodes to the lumbar cord can lead to posterior paralysis. Retrobulbar lymph node enlargement is another common presentation. An alimentary form most often involves the wall of the abomasum and associated lymph nodes. Myocardial invasion, particularly of the right atrium, is frequent, and can lead to signs of heart failures. Bovine leukemia virus can also lead to generalized lymphoma

in sheep and goats. **Sporadic bovine lymphoma** occurs in three forms: juvenile, mediastinal and cutaneous. The juvenile form is seen in young calves, generally before six months of age, but has also been encountered at birth and in fetal cattle. It is a multicentric lymphoma with generalized lymph node enlargement, marrow replacement and peripheral blood invasion. Thymic or mediastinal lymphoma is seen in slightly older calves, up to two years of age. It is restricted to the thymus with extension into adjacent tissues. Cutaneous lymphoma is seen in cattle of about two years of age as a chronic disease characterized by subepithelial lymphoid nodules which are seen as discrete plaques, often ulcerated. The lesions can regress for 1 to 2 years, but usually recur and become generalized.

Lymphomas in cattle are usually of a diffuse pattern and may be composed of either cleaved or non-cleaved cells. Rarely nodular (follicular) lymphoma is encountered.

Equine lymphoma is much less frequent than in other domestic animals, but still one of the more common neoplastic diseases of horse. It may occur as multicentric lymphoma, alimentary lymphoma, splenic lymphoma, cutaneous lymphoma or subcutaneous lymphoma Splenic lymphoma is characterized by a large tumor restricted to the spleen. Cutaneous lymphomas are a chronic disease, as in cattle, some of which are described as histiolymphocytic lymphosarcoma, consisting of a mixture of large histiocytes and

TABLE 22-4 **Classification of human Lymphomas**

Revised European-American classification	*Comparison to working formulation*
B-cell neoplasms	
I. Precursor B-cell Neoplasm	
1. Precursor B-lymphoblastic leukemia/ lymphoma	Lymphoblastic (medium sized cell; round or convoluted nucleus; inconspicuous nucleolus, scant cytoplasm)
II. Peripheral B-cell Neoplasms	
1. B-cell chronic lymphocytic leukemia/ prolymphocytic leukemia/small lymphocytic lymphoma	Small lymphocytic; (prolymphocytes; paraimmunoblasts; pseudofollicles)
2. Lymphoplasmacytoid lymphoma (immunocytoma)	Small lymphocytic; plasmacytoid
3. Mantel cell lymphoma	Diffuse, small cleaved cell
4. Follicle center lymphoma, follicular	
Grade I	Follicular, predominantly small cleaved cell
Grade II	Follicular, mixed small cleaved, and large cell
Grade III	Follicular, predominantly large cell
5. Marginal zone B-cell lymphoma	
a. Extranodal (low grade B-cell lymphoma of mucosa-associated lymphoid tissue type)	Small lymphocytic (Marginal zone cells; perifollicular)
b. Nodal	Small lymphocytic (monocytoid B-cells, sinusoidal pattern)
6. Splenic marginal zone B-cell lymphoma	Small lymphocytic (marginal zone B-cells)
7. Hairy cell leukemia	Small lymphoid cells; abundant cytoplasm; villous cytoplasmic projections; tartrate resistant acid phosphatase +
8. Plasmacytoma/myeloma	Extramedullary plasmacytoma (plasma cells, plasmablasts)
9. Diffuse large B-cell lymphoma	Diffuse large cell (large cells, prominent nucleoli; mutilobated; B-cell; T-cells often present)
10. Burkitt's lymphoma	Small noncleaved cell (medium sized cell; starry sky pattern with macrophages)
11. High grade B-cell lymphoma. Burkitt-like	Small noncleaved cell (large B-cell; starry sky pattern + / −)
T-cell and postulated Natural Killer (NK) cell neoplasms	
I. Precursor T-cell Neoplasm	
1. Precursor T-lymphoblastic lymphoma/ leukemia	Lymphoblastic (medium sized cell; round or convoluted nucleus; inconspicuous nucleolus, scant cytoplasm)
II. Peripheral T-cell and Postulated NK Cell/ Neoplasms	
1. T-cell chronic lymphocytic leukemia/ prolymphocytic leukemia	Small lymphocytic (small lymphocytes; prolymphocytes; moderate cytoplasm)

(continued)

TABLE 22-4 (continued)

Revised European-American classification	Comparison to working formulation
2. Large granular lymphocyte leukemia a. T-cell type	Small lymphocytic (abundant cytoplasm; azurophilic granules; eccentric nucleus)
b. Natural killer cell type	Diffuse small cleaved cell
3. Mycosis fungoides/Sezary syndrome	Small and large cells with cerebriform nuclei
4. Peripheral T-cell lymphomas, unspecified (medium sized cell; mixed medium and large cell; large cell)	Diffuse small and large cell
5. Angioimmunoblastic T-cell lymphoma	Diffuse small and large cell
6. Angiocentric lymphoma	Large cell immunoblastic B; Diffuse small and large cell; (angioinvasive)
7. Intestinal T-cell lymphoma	Diffuse small cleaved; diffuse small and large; diffuse large; Large cell immunoblastic
8. Adult T-cell lymphoma/leukemia, HTLV1 +	Diffuse small cleaved; diffuse small and large cell; diffuse large cell; Large cell immunoblastic
9. Anaplastic large cell lymphoma (T- and null-cell types)	Large cell immunoblastic
10. Anaplastic large cell lymphoma, Hodgkin's like	Large cell immunoblastic; pleomorphic

Hodgkin's Disease

I. Lymphocyte predominance	Lymphocytic and histiocytic cells; usually no classic Reed-Sternberg cells
II. Nodular sclerosis	Nodular pattern; classic Reed-Sternberg cells; mix of lymphocytes histiocytes, granulocytes, plasma cells
III. Mixed cellularity	Mix of lymphocytes, histiocytes, eosinophils, plasma cells; Reed-Sternberg cells; interstitial fibrosis
IV. Lymphocyte depletion	Large lymphocytes, Reed-Sternberg cells, diffuse fibrosis
V. Lymphocyte-rich classical Hodgkin's disease	Predominantly lymphocytes, few Reed-Sternberg cells

Unclassifiable Varieties

B-cell lymphoma unclassifiable (low grade/high grade)
T-cell lymphoma unclassifiable (low grade/high grade)
Hodgkin's disease, unclassifiable
Malignant lymphoma, unclassifiable (low grade/high grade)

small lymphoblasts. Leukemia rarely accompanies lymphoma in horses.

Porcine lymphoma is usually multicentric with extensive replacement of lymph nodes and invasions of the liver, spleen and kidneys. Primary enteric lymphoma also occurs in swine.

In other species, lymphoma and leukemia also generally represent the most common form of neoplastic disease. This includes laboratory rats and mice as well as nonhuman primates. In primates, lymphoma is often associated with immunosuppression and some examples are thought to be due to Epstein-Barr type viruses. The Fisher rat has an unusually high incidence of large granular lymphocyte leukemia (NK cell).

Hodgkin's disease is a complex form of lymphoma which occurs in humans. It is a chronic disease, characterized by slowly enlarging lymph nodes which become replaced by nodular tumors which ultimately effect other organs such as the liver, spleen and bone marrow. More diffuse replacement of lymph nodes can be seen, and the pattern of the tumors can vary from almost pure populations of lymphocytes, to nodules containing large numbers of plasma cells, histiocytes, eosinophils and fibroblasts. Diffuse fibrosis of the lesions occurs in one form of the disease. The histologic picture may be difficult to distinguish from that of a lymphoma or from that of inflammatory granuloma, depending on the predominant cell types. The distinguishing characteristic present in all forms of Hodgkin's disease is the distinctive cell termed the Reed-Sternberg cell. Classically, this is a large cell containing two large nuclei with prominent nucleoli which resemble inclusion bodies. It has been described as a cell with mirror images, or as appearing "owl eyed." Cases in animals are reported from time to time with the proposed diagnosis of Hodgkin's disease, but it is not clear whether they represent the same disease. What appears to be a high incidence of Hodgkin's disease has been described in striped skunks (*Mephitis mephitis*).

PLASMA CELL NEOPLASMS

Multiple myeloma (plasma cell sarcoma) is a malignant neoplasm of plasma cells originating in the bone marrow and often seeding to the liver, spleen, lymph nodes and other viscera. The cell type usually contains an appreciable number of recognizable mature plasma cells, often with Russell bodies, but also less mature cells which may be totally undifferentiated or resembling lymphoblasts. The cells may form discrete masses or may diffusely replace preexisting structures. In humans there is extensive destruction of the skeleton. The cells produce monoclonal immunoglobulins which may be complete or incomplete. This has been termed monoclonal gammopathy, which leads to hyperviscosity of the blood. Owing to their high molecular weight, these proteins are restricted to the plasma, but if incomplete immunoglobulins are produced predominantly of L chains, they will appear in the urine (Bence Jones proteins). Multiple myeloma is also associated with nephrosis, characterized by protein casts in the distal convoluted and collecting tubules associated with tubular atrophy and a cellular infiltrate of plasma cells, lymphocytes, histiocytes and multinucleated giant cells. Amyloidosis is frequently associated with multiple myeloma. Multiple myeloma is occasionally encountered in animals, but infrequently.

Solitary myeloma or plasmacytoma is a tumor mass composed of mostly mature plasma cells. They may occur in bone or soft tissues. They are also associated with monoclonal gammopathy.

Primary Macroglobulinemia (Waldenstrom's macroglobulinemia) is a lymphoproliferative disorder characterized by the production of IgM immunoglobulin. A mixture of plasma cells and lymphocytes are seen replacing the bone marrow, lymph nodes and spleen.

HISTIOCYTOSIS

In this section neoplastic disease of histiocytes, distinct from acute monocytic leukemia, will be considered. Several different types of proliferative disorders of histiocytes exist in animals. The most common is the **cutaneous histiocytoma,** which is the most common tumor of the skin of dogs. It is discussed in the chapter on the skin. What is termed **malignant histiocytosis** occurs in dogs and cats and is characterized by extensive proliferation of large cells in the bone marrow, lymph nodes, spleen, liver, and other tissues. Some examples appear to represent a non-leukemic form of monocytic leukemia, with diffuse replacement of the bone marrow (as well as lymph nodes, liver, spleen, etc.) by neoplastic cells. The cells are pleomorphic with distinct borders, large nuclei with nucleoli, and abundant cytoplasm. Their phagocytic nature is revealed by erythrophagocytosis. Other proliferations of histiocytes are encountered which are less akin to monocytic leukemia. These include two distinct forms of the disease which have been described as familial in Bernese mountain dogs. One, termed **systemic histiocytosis,** which is probably not neoplastic, occurs in young dogs and is characterized by multiple cutaneous nodules over the entire body. These are composed of relatively well-differentiated histiocytes often accompanied by lymphocytes and occasionally neutrophils and eosinophils. The infiltrates tend to concentrate around and invade the walls of small veins and arteries. Rare multinucleated giant cells are present. Similar infiltrates occur in the lung, liver, bone marrow, spleen, lymph nodes and other tissues. The course is chronic with remissions and relapses. This disorder may be similar to histiocytosis X of humans which represents a complex of proliferative diseases of Langerhans cells (Letterer-Siwe syndrome; Hand-Schuller-Christian disease; eosinophilic granuloma). In humans, Langerhans cells contains an inclusion, termed Birbeck granules, which allows their identification. In the original report of systemic histiocytosis in Bernese mountain dogs, the authors state that canine Langerhans cells may not contain such inclusions. The second form of histiocytosis in Bernese mountain dogs has been termed **malignant histiocytosis** which occurs in older male dogs. The disease is rapidly progressive and is characterized by masses of highly pleomorphic histiocytes often with many multinucleated giant cells. The predominant site is the lung and hilar lymph nodes. Masses may also be present in the liver, spleen and lymph nodes may also be affected. In other breeds of dogs multiple histiocytic infiltrates in the skin resembling systemic histiocytosis have been seen and termed cutaneous histiocytosis. These lack systemic lesions.

Another tumor of histiocytes is the **histiocytic sarcoma.** These neoplasms, in contrast to malignant histiocytosis, are solitary tumors. They may be benign or malignant, in which case they may be invasive and may metastasize. Histologically the cell type may be predominantly typical round to polygonal histiocytes to spindle shaped cells resembling fibroblasts. Multinucleated giant cells are present in some of the less differentiated tumors. When predominantly composed of spindle cells, these tumors have been designated malignant fibrous histiocytoma. They must be differentiated from fibrosarcoma. They are most common in the skin and spleen.

Another disease that some have lumped with the histiocytoses is lymphomatoid granulomatosis. It is a disease of humans characterized by granulomatous lesions believed to originate in the lungs, but also present in other tissues, including the kidney, liver, brain, and skin. Some affected patients develop malignant lymphoma. The lesions are composed of lymphocytes, plasma cells, and histiocytes with varying atypia. An example has been reported in the dog.

References

Bostock DE, Owen LN. Porcine and ovine lymphosarcoma: a review. J Natl Cancer Inst 1973;50:933–939.

Calderwood Mays MB, Bergeron JA. Cutaneous histiocytosis in dogs. J Am Vet Med Assoc 1986;188:377–380.

Callanan JJ, Jones BA, Irvine J, et al. Histologic classification and immunophenotype of lymphosarcomas in cats with naturally and experimentally acquired feline immunodeficiency virus infections. Vet Pathol 1996;33:264–272.

Caniatti M, Roccabianca P, Scanziani E, et al. Canine lymphoma: immunocytochemical analysis of fine-needle aspiration biopsy. Vet Pathol 1996;33:204–212.

Chan JKC, Banks PM, Cleary ML, et al. A revised European-American classification of lymphoid neoplasms proposed by the International Lymphoma Study Group. Am J Clin Path 1994;103:543–560.

Cleary ML, Trela MJ, Weiss LM, et al. Most null large cell lymphomas are B lineage neoplasms. Lab Invest 1985;53:521–525.

Day MJ. Immunophenotypic characterization of cutaneous lymphoid neoplasia in the dog and cat. J Comp Pathol 1995;112:79–96.

Detilleux PG, Cheville NF, Sheahan BJ. Ultrastructure and lectin histochemistry of equine cutaneous histiolymphocytic lymphosarcomas. Vet Pathol 1989;26:409–419.

Ferrer JF. Bovine lymphosarcoma. Adv Vet Sci Comp Med 1980;24:1–68.

Fivenson DP, Saed GM, Beck ER, et al. T-cell receptor gene rearrangement in canine mycosis fungoides: further support for a canine model of cutaneous T-cell lymphoma. J Invest Dermatol 1994;102:227–230.

Franks PT, Harvey JW, Calderwood Mays M, et al. Feline large granular lymphoma. Vet Pathol 1986;23:200–202.

Frith CH, Ward JM, Chandra M. The morphology, immunohistochemistry, and incidence of hematopoietic neoplasms in mice and rats. [Review]. Toxicol Pathol 1993;21:206–218.

Glick AD, Holscher M, Campbell GR. Canine cutaneous histiocytoma:

ultrastructural and cytochemical observations. Vet Pathol 1976;13:374–380.

Goitsuka R, Ohno K, Matsumoto Y, et al. Establishment and characterization of a feline large granular lymphoma cell line expressing interleukin 2 receptor alph-chain. J Vet Med Sci 1993;55:863–865.

Grindem CB, Roberts MC, McEntee MF, et al. Large granular lymphocyte tumor in a horse. Vet Pathol 1989;26:86–88.

Haley PJ, Spraker T. Lymphosarcoma in an aborted equine fetus. Vet Pathol 1983;20:647–649.

Hatfield CE, Rebhun WC, Dill SG. Thymic lymphosarcoma in three heifers. J Am Vet Med Assoc 1986;189:1598–1599.

Hawkins EC, Feldman BF, Blanchard PC. Immunoglobulin A myeloma in a cat with pleural effusion and serum hyperviscosity. J Am Vet Med Assoc 1986;188:876–878.

Hoenig M. Multiple myeloma associated with the heavy chains of immunoglobulin A in a dog. J Am Vet Med Assoc 1987;9:1191–1192.

Holmberg CA, Manning JS, Osburn BI. Feline malignant lymphomas: comparison of morphologic and immunologic characteristics. Am J Vet Res 1976;37:1455–1460.

Holmberg CA, Manning JS, Osburn BI. Malignant lymphoma with B-lymphocyte characteristics in dogs. Am J Vet Res 1977;38:1877–1879.

Holmberg CA, Manning JS, Osburn BI. Canine malignant lymphomas: comparison of morphologic and immunologic parameters. J Natl Cancer Inst 1976;56:125–135.

Ishino S, Kadota K, Yoshino T, et al. Pathological and immunohistochemical studies of follicular lymphoma in two calves. J Comp Path 1990;103:265–275.

Johnstone AC, Manktelow BW. The pathology of spontaneously occurring malignant lymphoma in sheep. Vet Pathol 1978;15:301–312.

Lester GD, MacKay RJ, Smith-Meyer B. Primary meningeal lymphoma in a horse. J Am Vet Med Assoc 1992;201:1219–1221.

Lucke VM, Kelly DF, Harrington GA, et al. A lymphomatoid granulomatosis of the lungs in young dogs. Vet Pathol 1979;16:405–412.

MacEwen EG, Patnaik AK, Hurvitz AI, et al. Nonsecretory multiple myeloma in two dogs. J Am Vet Med Assoc 1984;184:1283–1286.

MacEwen EG, Patnaik AK, Johnson GJ, et al. Extramedullary plasmacytoma of the gastrointestinal tract in two dogs. J Am Vet Med Assoc 1984;184:1396–1398.

Madewell BR, Munn RJ. Canine lymphoproliferative disorders. An ultrastructural study of 18 cases. J Vet Int Med 1990;4:63–70.

Mahony OM, Moore AS, Cotter SM, et al. Alimentary lymphoma in cats: 28 cases (1988–1993). J Am Vet Med Assoc 1995;207:1593–1598.

Markel MD, Dorr TE. Multiple myeloma in a horse. J Am Vet Med Assoc 1986;188:621–623.

Moore PF, Olivry T. Cutaneous lymphomas in companion animals. Clin Dermatol 1994;12:499–505.

Moore PF, Rosin A. Malignant histiocytosis of Bernese mountain dogs. Vet Pathol 1986;23:110.

Moore PF. Systemic histiocytosis of Bernese mountain dogs. Vet Pathol 1984;21:554–563.

Morita M. An autopsy case of malignant lymphogranulomatosis (so-called Hodgkin's disease) in Cercopithecus aethiops. Primates 1974;15:47–53.

Morton LD, Barton CL, Elissalde GS, et al. Oral extramedullary plasmacytomas in two dogs. Vet Pathol 1986;23:637–639.

Neufeld JL. Lymphosarcoma in a mare and review of cases at the Ontario Veterinary College. Can Vet J 1973;14:149–153.

Olivry T, Moore PF, Naydan DK, et al. Investigation of epidermotropism in canine mycosis fungoides: expression of intercellular adhesion molecule-1 (ICAM-1) and beta-2 integrins. Arch Dermatol Res 1995;287:186–192.

Onions DE. B and T cells in canine lymphosarcoma. Vet Rec 1975;97:108.

Paterson S, Boydell P, Pike R. Systemic histiocytosis in the Bernese mountain dog. J Sm Anim Prac 1995;36:233–236.

Pileri SA, Leoncini L, Falini B. Revised European-American lymphoma classification. [Review]. Cur Opinion Oncol 1995;7:401–407.

Raich PC, Takashima I, Olson C. Cytochemical reactions in bovine and ovine lymphosarcoma. Vet Pathol 1983;20:322–329.

Rebhun WC, Bertone A. Equine lymphosarcoma. J Am Vet Med Assoc 1984;184:720–721.

Reef VB, Dyson SS, Beech J. Lymphosarcoma and associated immune-mediated hemolytic anemia and thrombocytopenia in horses. J Am Vet Med Assoc 1984;184:313–317.

Rosin A, Moore P, Dubielzig R. Malignant histiocytosis in Bernese Mountain dogs. J Am Vet Med Assoc 1986;188:1041–1045.

Saari S, Jarvien AK. Multicentric lymphoma involving large granular lymphocytes in a cow. Zentralblatt Fur Veterinarmedizin—Reihe A 1994;41:791–794.

Schamber GJ, Olson C, Witt LE. Neoplasms in calves (Bos taurus). Vet Pathol 1982;19:629–637.

Scherlie PH Jr., Smedes SL, Feltz T, et al. Ocular manifestation of systemic histiocytosis in a dog. J Am Vet Med Assoc 1992;201:1229–1232.

Scott DW, Miller WH Jr., Tasker JB, et al. Lymphoreticular neoplasia in a dog resembling malignant histiocytosis (histiocytic medullary reticulosis) in man. Cornell Vet 1979;69:176–197.

Sheahan BJ, Atkins GJ, Russell RJ, et al. Histiolymphocytic lymphosarcoma in the subcutis of two horses. Vet Pathol 1980;17:123–133.

Sheriff D, Newlands RW. A case of foetal leukaemia in a calf. Vet Rec 1976;98:174.

Skavlen PA, Stills HF, Caldwell CW, et al. Malignant lymphoma in a Sinclair miniature pig. Am J Vet Res 1986;47:389–393.

Smith DA, Barker IK. Four cases of Hodgkin's Disease in striped skunks (Mephitis mephitis). Vet Pathol 1983;20:223–229.

Spoknick GJ, Berg J, Moore FM, Cotter SM. Spinal lymphoma in cats: 21 cases (1976–1989). J Am Vet Med Assoc 1992;200:373–376.

Tanimoto T, Minami A, Yano S, et al. Ileal lymphoma in swine. Vet Pathol 1994;31:629–636.

Thrall MA, Macy DW, Snyder SP, et al. Cutaneous lymphosarcoma and leukemia in a dog resembling Sézary syndrome in man. Vet Pathol 1984;21:182–186.

Valli VE, McSherry BJ, Dunham BM, et al. Histocytology of lymphoid tumors in the dog, cat and cow. Vet Pathol 1981;18:494–512.

Weller RE, Holmberg CA, Theilen GH, et al. Histologic classification as a prognostic criterion for canine lymphosarcoma. Am J Vet Res 1980;41:1310–1314.

Wellman ML, Davenport DJ, Morton D, et al. Malignant histiocytosis in four dogs. J Am Vet Med Assoc 1985;187:919–921.

Wells GAH. Hodgkin's disease-like lesions in the dog. J Pathol 1974;112:5–10.

Willemze R, Beljaards RC, Meijer CJ, et al. Classification of primary cutaneous lymphomas. Historical overview and perspectives. [Review]. Dermatology 1994;189:8–15.

23

The Digestive System

MOUTH AND ADNEXA

Developmental abnormalities

CLEFT LIP (CHEILOSCHISIS) AND CLEFT PALATE (PALATOSCHISIS)

These congenital abnormalities occur infrequently in domestic animals. In dogs, brachycephalic breeds are more at risk than other breeds. Factors thought to be involved in their pathogenesis include: hereditary factors, maternal nutritional deficiencies, ingestion of teratogenic drugs, chemicals, or toxic plants during pregnancy, and mechanical interference with the developing embryo. **Cleft lip,** or **cheiloschisis,** affects the upper lip and results from failure of fusion of the maxillary process and the medial nasal process at or near the site known as the philtrum. This condition may occur alone or in association with cleft palate. **Cleft palate** is a longitudinal fusion defect of varying length affecting the bone and mucosa of the midline of the hard palate. This defect in fusion of the lateral palatine shelves from the maxillary processes results in an open cleft between the oral and nasal cavities (See Fig. 4-5). Newborn animals with this abnormality often drip milk from their nostrils during nursing, whereas older animals may develop respiratory infection and pneumonia due to aspiration of food.

Inflammatory processes

EOSINOPHILIC ULCER (INDOLENT OR "RODENT" ULCER)

This is a specific, idiopathic ulcerative lesion of the upper lip of cats. It constitutes one of the three distinctive lesions included in the "feline eosinophilic granuloma complex." Eosinophilic ulcer generally begins as a small plaque on the margin of the upper lip, often adjacent to the lower canine tooth. The lesion gradually increases in size to involve much of the skin between the lip and nose. Persistent licking at the lesion is thought to contribute to its ulcerative nature. When fully developed the lesion has a slightly depressed, granular whitish-yellow center and a slightly elevated, orange-tan

margin. Microscopically, the epidermis is ulcerated and the underlying dermal connective tissue contains scattered foci of intensely eosinophilic degenerate collagen. These foci of altered collagen are surrounded by large numbers of intact and degranulating eosinophils, lesser numbers of histiocytes and mast cells and occasional multinucleated giant cells. The mast cells and degranulating eosinophils probably account for the chronic licking of the lesion in affected cats. Although its cause is not known, the lesion may respond either transiently or permanently to systemic, intralesional or topical steroid therapy or to progestational drug therapy. Cats with labial eosinophilic ulcer may also have concomitant eosinophilic granuloma of the oral cavity and or skin (see Chapter 17).

TRAUMATIC LESIONS

The mucous membranes of the lips, oral cavity, gingiva, tongue, and oropharynx, because of their location at the entrance to the alimentary tract and their role in mastication and conveyance of foodstuffs and other objects of varying consistencies to the lower alimentary tract, are repeatedly subject to varying degrees of trauma. In herbivores, the coarse nature of pasturage and roughage, and foreign objects that may be inadvertently ingested with it, can cause laceration or abrasions of the mucosa. In dogs and cats, sharp bones, splinters, thorns, needles, and string may cause traumatic injury. Burns of chemical, thermal, or electrical origin are seen occasionally in the oral cavity, particularly in young puppies with indiscriminate chewing habits. Such lesions may heal spontaneously or become secondarily infected by a variety of infectious agents, notably bacteria and fungi. Those that fail to heal normally may result in the formation of exuberant masses of **pyogranulation tissue** at the site of injury. This occurs with some frequency on the ventral surface of the tongue of cats and must be distinguished from squamous cell carcinoma.

GINGIVITIS, STOMATITIS, AND PERIODONTITIS

Inflammation of the gingiva is termed **gingivitis.** Most cases of gingivitis result from opportunistic bacterial infections that follow either gingival trauma, poor oral hygiene, or various immunodeficient states. Gingivitis is frequently the first manifestation of feline immunodeficiency virus infection in cats. Grossly, the inflamed gingiva bleeds easily and is erythematous and variably edematous. Microscopically, most of the inflammation is confined to the gingival connective tissue which is infiltrated by variable numbers of neutrophils, lymphocytes, and plasma cells. The overlying gingival epithelium may be ulcerated, or in some cases hyperplastic. The causative agent is often not demonstrable in tissue sections. The gingiva may also be involved as part of a more generalized inflammatory process involving other areas of the oral mucosa, termed stomatitis.

The causes of **stomatitis** and oral ulceration are numerous and include: a variety of bacteria, including fusobacteria and spirochetes; numerous viral agents, fungi *(Candida albican)* and certain parasites; several autoimmune disorders, including systemic lupus erythematosus, pemphigus vulgaris, bullous pemphigoid and occasionally discoid lupus erythematosus; uremia; and deficiency of niacin or vitamin C. These are discussed in detail in the chapters dealing with those topics.

Periodontal disease, or **periodontitis,** is inflammation of the tissues that surround teeth, including the gingival sulcus, the epithelial attachment of the gingiva to the teeth, the periodontal ligament, and the alveolar bone of the tooth socket. It occurs commonly in people, dogs, and cats. Periodontitis begins as a gingivitis resulting from accumulation of bacterial plaque on the lateral surfaces of the tooth. The plaque results from bacterial colonization of food chronically retained in the gingival sulcus surrounding the tooth or in the space between adjacent teeth (Fig. 23-1). Brachycephalic breeds of dogs, because of their high incidence of dental malocclusion, are predisposed to periodontitis. As the disease progresses, the inflammation extends deeper into the gingival sulcus and forms a pocket of inflammation that destroys the attachments of the tooth to the gingiva and surrounding alveolar bone. This results in loosening and eventual loss of the affected tooth. Chronic periodontitis can also serve as a source of chronic bacteremia in the affected host.

Gingival hyperplasia represents a benign proliferative response of the gingival connective tissue and overlying epithelium to chronic gingivitis or periodontitis. It occurs commonly in brachycephalic breeds of dogs, but all breeds of dogs are susceptible. It is rare in cats. In people, a generalized form of reversible gingival hyperplasia involving mainly the gingival epithelium has been associated with anticonvulsant therapy with diphenylhydantoin sodium. Similar lesions have been produced in stump-tail macaque monkeys *(Macaca arctoides)* administered the drug experimentally. Grossly, gingival hyperplasia appears as a solitary or diffuse area of gingival enlargement adjacent to one or more teeth. The enlargement is due to a benign proliferation of the gingival connective tissue and/or overlying gingival epithelium. The hyperplastic tissue in gingival hyperplasia consists of fusiform-shaped fibroblasts and collagen, in contrast to the benign tumor known as fibromatous epulis of the periodontal ligament where the neoplastic fibroblasts are characteristically more stellate.

Oral eosinophilic granuloma is also one of the three distinctive lesions included in the "feline eosinophilic granuloma complex." It commonly involves the ventral

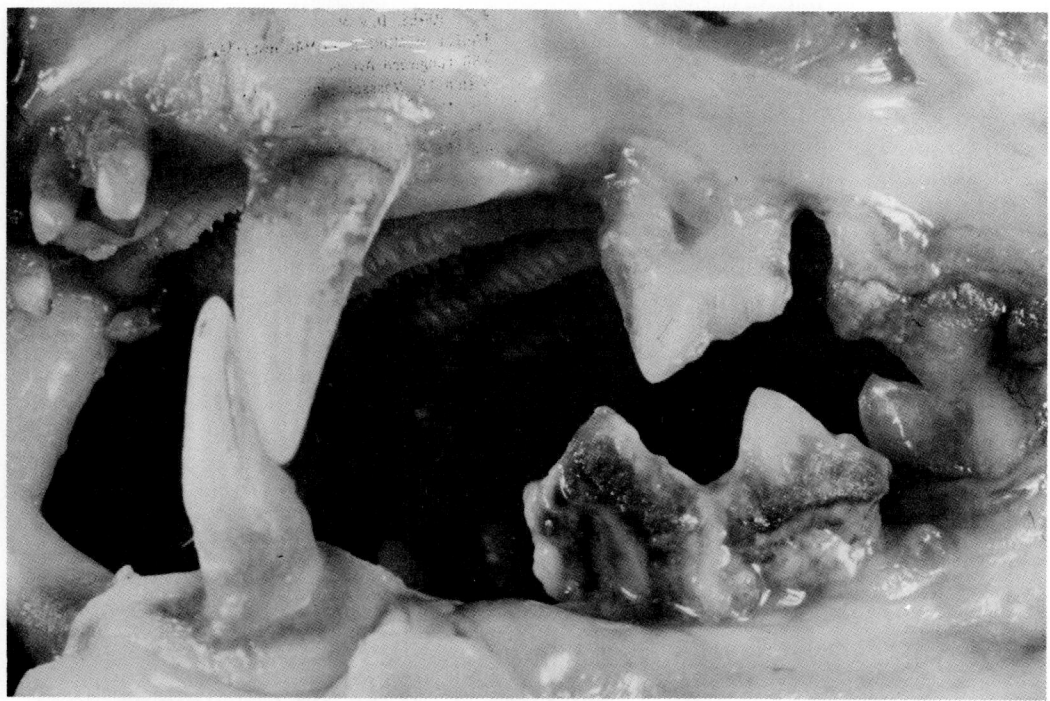

FIG. 23-1. Periodontal disease resulting in receding gums and exposure of roots of teeth of a three-year-old female tortoiseshell and white cat. (Courtesy of Angell Memorial Animal Hospital.)

surface of the tongue, including the frenulum, and the soft palate, but may occur at other sites as well. An identical lesion also occurs occasionally on the ventral surface of the tongue of Siberian Husky dogs. Grossly the lesion appears as a single, or occasionally multiple, firm superficially ulcerated raised nodule within the affected mucosa. Microscopically, the lesion resembles that described above for eosinophilic ulcer. The epithelium overlying the lesion is often ulcerated and the underlying lamina propria contains intensely eosinophilic foci of degenerate collagen surrounded by eosinophils, histioctyes, and occasional multinucleated giant cells. The number of eosinophils present can be highly variable depending upon the duration of the lesion. Older lesions generally contain a lesser number of eosinophils. Interestingly, the collagenolytic foci often contain embedded hair shafts. Whether they constitute an incidental finding or have a role in the evolution of the lesion has not been established. Cats with oral eosinophilic granuloma may also have concomitant cutaneous eosinophilic granuloma ("linear granuloma") or eosinophilic plaque of the skin.

Feline plasmacytic (plasma cell) stomatitis is a distinctive form of stomatitis of the oral cavity of cats, the cause of which is not known. Affected cats often have persistently high concentrations of serum total proteins and serum globulins. Typically, the lesions begin as bilateral, raised, often superficially ulcerated, proliferative masses arising from the mucosa of the glossopalatine arches. With time, the lesions spread to involve the gingiva posterior to the mandibular molars and mucosa of the palatopharyngeal arches. Microscopically, the nodular masses consist of hyperplastic gingival or oral connective tissue containing diffuse infiltrates of mature plasma cells, some of which contain prominent Russell bodies in their cytoplasm. When ulcerated, variable numbers of neutrophils and lymphocytes may be present among the plasma cells. Although its cause is unknown, the condition reportedly responds favorably to steroid therapy, but may recur following its withdrawal.

Actinobacillus lignieresii, a small gram-negative, nonsporulating, coccobacillary bacterium that is a component of the normal oral flora, when introduced into the lamina propria of the oral mucosa, causes multiple abscesses, pyogranulomas, and extensive fibrosis. Infection involves the tongue and to a lesser extent other soft tissues of the oral cavity, neck, and regional lymph nodes of cattle and rarely sheep. In chronic cases, the tongue may be so extensively involved that it becomes enlarged, stiff, and relatively immobile, and cannot be retracted back into the mouth. This has led to the term "woody tongue" for this condition. The microscopic lesions bear a resemblance to and must be distinguished from those caused by the gram-positive *Actinomyces bovis*, the cause of "lumpy jaw" in cattle. The clinical, pathologic, and differentiating features of these two conditions are described in detail in Chapters 10 and 11.

Fusobacterium necrophorum, an anaerobic, gram-negative, filamentous bacterium is a significant cause of necrotic stomatitis in calves, lambs, and piglets. This organism is an opportunsitic pathogen that invades and colonizes mucosal surfaces that have been previously damaged by trauma, viral infection or erupting teeth. **Calf diphtheria,** a disease characterized by necrotic stomatitis, layngitis, and pharyngitis, is caused by this organism. *F. necrophorum* produces a variety of endo- and exotoxins that cause extensive coagulative necrosis of the tissues colonized by it. Grossly, the lesions initially appear as large, well-defined, slightly elevated plaques of yellow-gray, adherent necrotic tissue (diphtheritic membrane) surrounded by a zone of hyperemia. Once the necrotic tissue sloughs, large ulcers undermined by granulation tissue become evident. Microscopically, the lesion consists of a superficial pseudomembrane composed of a mass of eosinophilic, coagulated protein lacking cellular outlines surrounded by a zone of hyperemic granulation tissue containing variable numbers of neutrophils, macrophages, lymphocytes, and plasma cells. The long, filamentous organisms may be found at the interface between necrotic and viable tissue. Affected animals may also develop necrotic lesions in other portions of the alimentary tract and liver. For a discussion of other lesions caused by *F. necrophorum* the reader is referred to Chapter 11.

Noma is a rapidly progressive, gangrenous process that affects the gingiva and underlying bone, and the mucosa of the lips and cheeks. The term noma is derived from the Greek word meaning "to devour" which denotes the aggressive and destructive nature of this disease. It occurs most often in children in underdeveloped parts of Africa, Asia, and South America, and in nonhuman primates. In people and monkeys it has been associated with immunosuppression resulting from chronic malnutrition, malaria, or certain viral diseases. In rhesus monkeys (*Macaca mulatta*) the majority of cases have been associated with concomitant infection with an immunosuppressive type D retrovirus known as simian retrovirus type I (SRV-1), but rarely with infection with the simian lentivirus, simian immunodeficiency virus or SIV. SRV-1 is known to cause a profound neutropenia in some animals, and this may be an important difference between the two immunosuppressive viruses. It has also been reported in Formosan macaques (*M cyclopis*), pig-tailed macaques (*M. nemestrina*), chimpanzees (*Pan troglodytes*) and cotton-top tamarins (*Saguinus oedipus*), but the predisposing factors have not been identified in these species.

A number of aerobic and anaerobic bacteria including *Bacteroides melaningenicus*, *Fusobacterium sp.*, *Shigella flexneri* serotype 4, *Pseudomonas aeruginosa*, coagulase-positive *Staphylococcus*, *Streptococcus* sp. and *Klebsiella sp.* have been isolated from the lesions of noma, but a single etiology has not been identified. Large numbers of spirochetal organisms also are frequently found deep in the lesions in tissue sections stained with the Warthin-Starry silver stain. These organisms may also have an etiologic role in this condition.

Noma begins as a small focal areas of ulceration at the margin of the gingiva that rapidly progresses to involve the surrounding soft tissues and underlying bone. In most cases, the gingival and labial soft tissues slough leaving large areas of necrotic maxillary or mandibular bone exposed. Microscopically, the affected soft tissues and underlying bone are extensively necrotic and blood vessels in the area are frequently thrombosed. The latter finding suggests that at least a part of the tissue damage is due to infarction. Sequestra of necrotic bone may be present in older lesions.

TONSILS

Anatomically, the tonsils consist of either distinct, paired, nodular (dog and cat) or diffuse (pig, cow, and horse) aggregates of lymphoid tissue situated at the opening of the oropharynx. The discrete nodular tonsils of people, dogs, and cats have crypts lined by stratified squamous epithelium that extend into the parenchyma of the organ. Tonsillar lymphoid tissue, whether discrete or diffuse, has a role in immune surveilllance of antigenic substances and microbiologic agents that enter the body through the oropharynx. As with any lymphoid tissue, tonsils are constantly exposed to a wide variety of antigenic stimuli which cause them to undergo varying degrees of physiologic hyperplasia. The crypts of the tonsils are normally inhabited by bacteria that constitute the residential flora of the oropharynx; these are not associated with disease.

Tonsillitis occurs when pathogenic bacteria such as hemolytic streptococci and certain coliforms colonize the tonsillar crypts and incite an acute inflammatory reaction. In such cases, the tonsils will appear swollen and hyperemic, and the crypts will exude a yellow-white purulent exudate. The surface of the tonsil may also be covered with a similar exudate. Fever and painful swelling of the draining mandibular lymph nodes may also accompany tonsillitis.

The tonsils may also be the portal of entry and site of initial replication of a wide variety of lymphotropic viruses that cause systemic disease. The tonsils in such cases will be enlarged and reddened but usually are not covered by a recognizable exudate. Histologically, the lymphoid tissue will exhibit varying degrees of karyorrhexis, lymphocytic depletion, and histiocyte infiltration.

NEOPLASMS OF THE ORAL CAVITY

Viral papillomas

Papillomavirus-induced, benign neoplasms of the squamous epithelium of the oral and labial mucosae occur with some frequency in dogs, cattle and rabbits. The tumors may be single or multiple. Younger animals are generally more susceptible to viral papillomas than older individuals, but age alone does not confer resistance. Papillomaviruses are generally species and site specific, i.e. canine papillomaviruses only infect canines, and those variants that cause oral papillomas generally do not cause cutaneous lesions. Oral papillomas, like those of the skin, may regress spontaneously after several months and leave the host permanently immune. Malignant transformation of a papilloma to a squamous cell carcinoma is an extremely rare event. The molecular basis of papillomavirus-induced neoplastic transformation is discussed in Chapter 4.

Epulis

An epulis (plural: epulides) is a benign neoplasm derived from the periodontal ligament or connective tissue. They occur commonly in dogs and are rare in cats. Three histologic variants of epulides are recog-

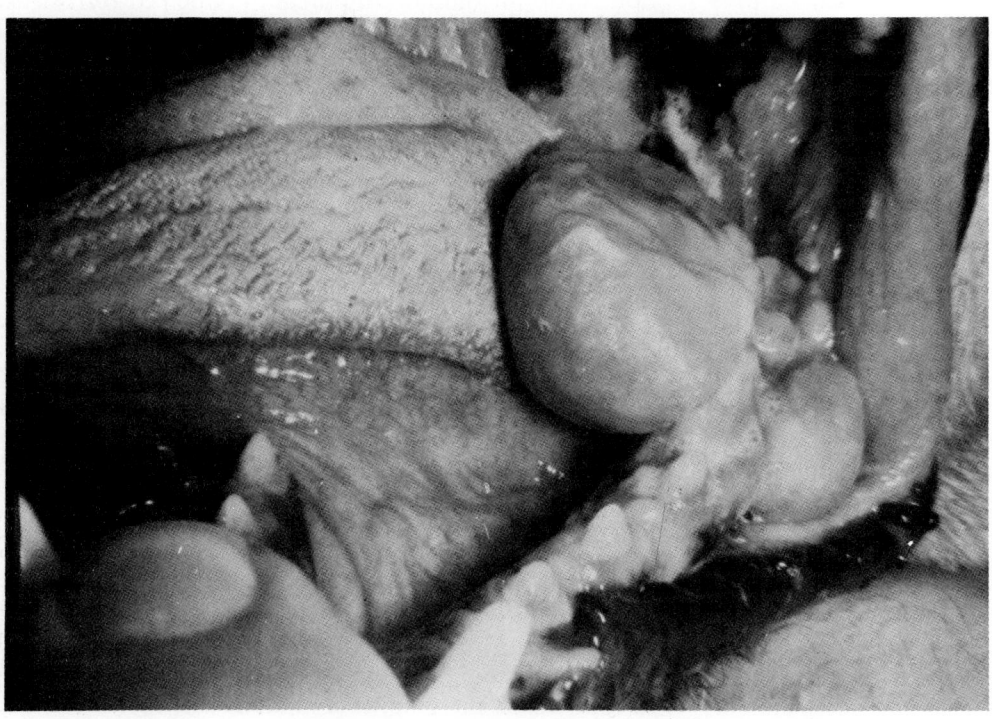

FIG. 23-2. Fibromatous epulis of periodontal origin on mandible. (Courtesy of Dr. R. R. Dubielzig and **Veterinary Pathology.**)

nized based upon their cellular and tissue composition.

A **fibromatous epulis** appears grossly as a single or multiple firm, smooth, sessile-based, pinkish-white, nodule protruding from the gingiva (Fig. 23-2). When large it may cause displacement of the adjacent tooth and interfere with mastication. Fibromatous epulides may become large enough to almost envelope the adjacent tooth, but do not invade the underlying bone. On cut surface, they are solid, firm, and white. Microscopically, they are composed of an expansile mass of stellate fibroblasts surrounded by variable amounts of densely packed, fibrillar collagen (Fig. 23-3). Blood vessels are present throughout the stroma. Mitotic figures are rare. The surface of a fibromatous epulis is generally covered by an intact layer of gingival epithelium that may send long, branching cords of epithelial cells deep into the neoplasm in a manner resembling pseudoepitheliomatous hyperplasia.

An **ossifying** or **cementifying epulis** has all of the features of a fibromatous epulis but in addition contains either irregular islands of osteoid or mineralized bone or acellular, eosinophilic cementum or dentin-like material (Fig. 23-4). These tumors are extremely hard and require decalcification before they can be sectioned.

An **acanthomatous epulis** also has features of a fibromatous epulis but contains broad sheets and cords of stratified squamous epithelium with prominent intercellular bridges. The periphery of these sheets or cords is surrounded by a single layer of tall columnar basal cells oriented perpendicular to the basement membrane (Fig. 23-5). This epithelial component of an acanthomatous epulis may comprise a large portion of the neoplastic mass. Unlike the other forms of epulides, the acanthomatous epulis often invades the underlying bone, and thus must be differentiated from a squamous cell carcinoma. In the older literature this lesion is commonly referred to as an adamantinoma, a term that some investigators feel should be abandoned (Table 23-1).

Squamous cell carcinoma

Primary malignant neoplasms of the stratified squamous epithelium of the oral cavity and oropharynx can occur in any species. It is the most common malignancy of the oral cavity of cats, and in dogs its frequency is only exceeded by malignant melanoma. Squamous cell carcinoma may involve the epithelium of the tonsillar crypts, the gingiva, or the lateral margins and ventral surface of the tongue. At these sites, the tumor appears as an ulcerated, somewhat crateriform lesion surrounded by a rim of firm, slightly elevated tissue (Fig. 23-6). Microscopically, it consists of irregular sheets, cords, and individual nests of pleomorphic squamous cells (Fig. 23-7). These frequently invade the adjacent soft tissues of the affected site, including the connective tissue, lymphoid tissue and skeletal muscle and the alveolar bone of the dental arcades. The pleomorphic nature of the neoplastic cells, their lack of prominent intercellular bridges, and the lack of an associated stellate fibroblastic component serve to distinguish squamous cell carcinoma of the gingival epithelium from an acanthomatous epulis of the periodontium. Squamous cell carcinomas, unlike acanthomatous epulides, may also metastasize to the retropharyngeal and anterior cervical lymph nodes.

Malignant melanoma

Malignant neoplasms derived from melanocytes of the oral cavity occur commonly in dogs, but are rare in other animals. In dogs, it constitutes the most common malignant neoplasm of the oral cavity, and generally has a poorer prognosis than those that arise in skin. They generally arise in partially pigmented mucosa of the gingiva, lips, cheek, palate, oropharynx, and tongue. Typically, they appear as solitary, rapidly-growing, nodular, ulcerated masses that vary considerably in their degree of pigmentation. They tend to be highly invasive and metastasize early. Microscopically, the neoplastic cells are extremely pleomorphic and range from fusiform to round to polygonal. Individual tumor cells also vary in the amount of melanin that is present in their cytoplasm. They may contain so much melanin that all microscopic features of their nuclei and cytoplasm are obscured, contain no melanin at all (amelanotic), or contain amounts between these two extremes. When the nuclei can be seen, they are generally round and pale-staining, and contain a single, large amphophilic nucleolus. Mitotic figures can be highly variable in number. The neoplastic cells exhibit a variety of growth patterns, including small nests in which the cells fit together like slices of an orange, small interlacing bundles, and in solid sheets without a distinctive pattern. Small loosely organized clusters of tumor cells can often be found in the basilar aspect of the overlying epithelium, a lesion termed junctional change. Junctional change is a feature of malignant melanomas, but not benign tumors of melanocytes (melanocytomas). Melanomas of the oral cavity frequently recur following attempts at excision and metastasis is a common complication. Metastasis occurs via hematogenous and lymphatic routes, and the lungs and submandibular lymph nodes are common sites of spread.

Fibrosarcoma

Primary fibrosarcoma can arise from the connective tissue of the oral cavity, with the buccal mucosa being a frequent site. It is the second most frequent malignant neoplasm of the feline oral cavity, being exceeded only by squamous cell carcinoma. They also occur in dogs and other domestic species. Grossly, it appears as a solitary, firm, often ulcerated, multilobulated mass that extends deep into the affected mucosa and underlying tissues. The tumors vary in their degree of cellularity and degree of differentiation with respect to collagen production. The neoplastic fibroblasts are fusiform and are arranged in interlacing fasciculi in which there may be

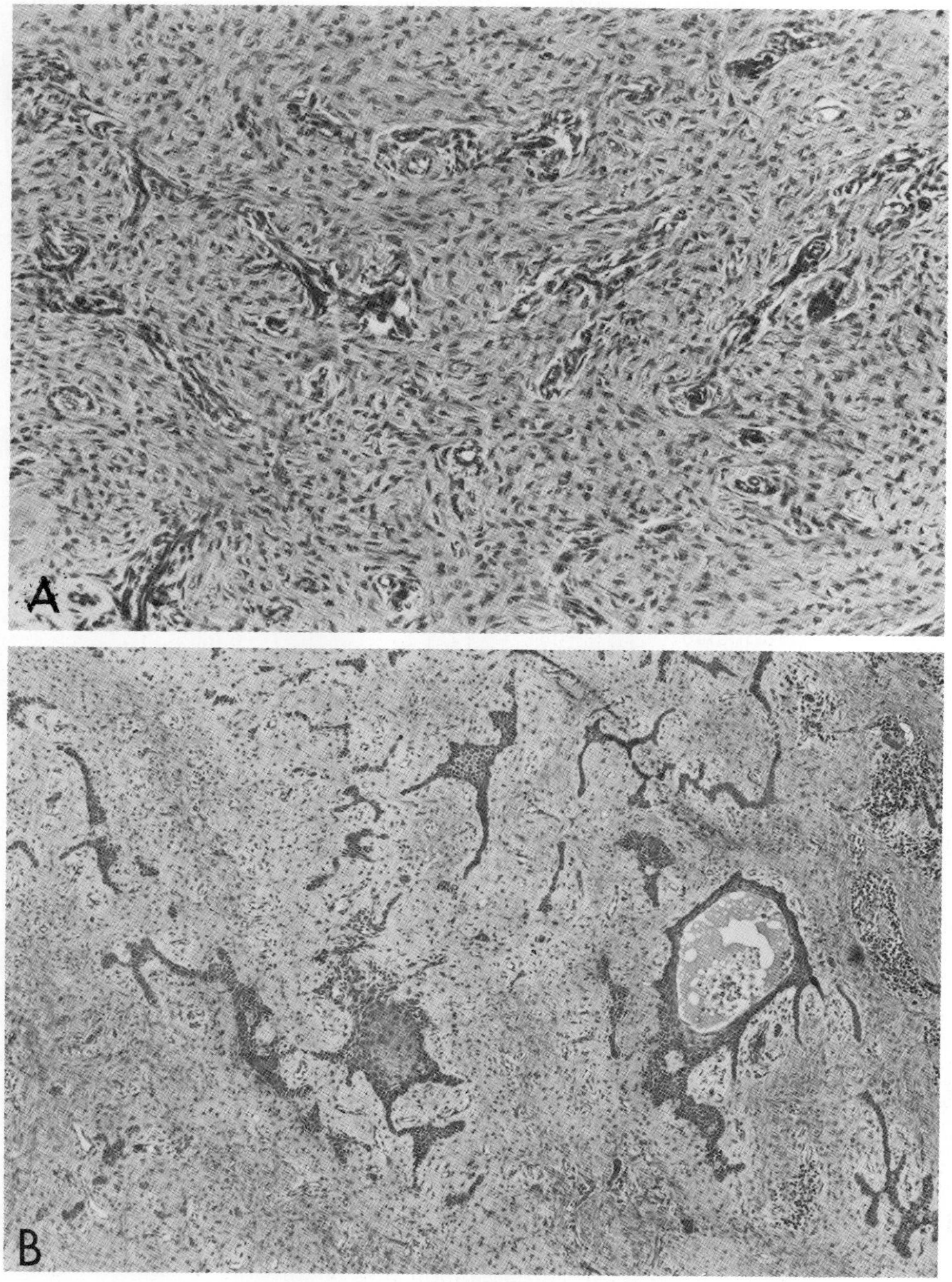

FIG. 23-3. Fibromatous epulis, dog. **A.** Dense fibrillar stroma containing tightly packed stellate cells and blood vessels. **B.** Branching cords of epithelial tissue resembling odontogenic epithelium. (Courtesy of Dr. R.R. Dubielzig and **Veterinary Pathology.**)

varying amounts of necrosis. In poorly differentiated fibrosarcomas, tumor giant cells may be present in the neoplasm. Invasion of the underlying connective tissue, skeletal musculature, and bone at the affected site is a frequent finding. These tumors are capable of widespread metastasis usually via the blood vascular route.

Osteosarcoma

Although more common in the long bones of the axial skeleton, osteosarcoma can occur in the bones of the upper and lower jaws. At these sites, the neoplasm, depending upon its duration, typically causes mild to severe deformity of the affected maxilla or mandible, which radiographically are characterized by areas of lysis and proliferation of the affected bone. Histologically, the neoplasm is composed of stellate to fusiform osteoblastic cells proliferating in solid sheets and nests in which there are irregular islands of osteoid and mineralized bone and/or cartilage. The neoplastic cells can be found invading the bone of the affected jaw. Multinucleated giant cells resembling osteoclasts can be a feature of this type of neoplasm as well. Osteosarcomas

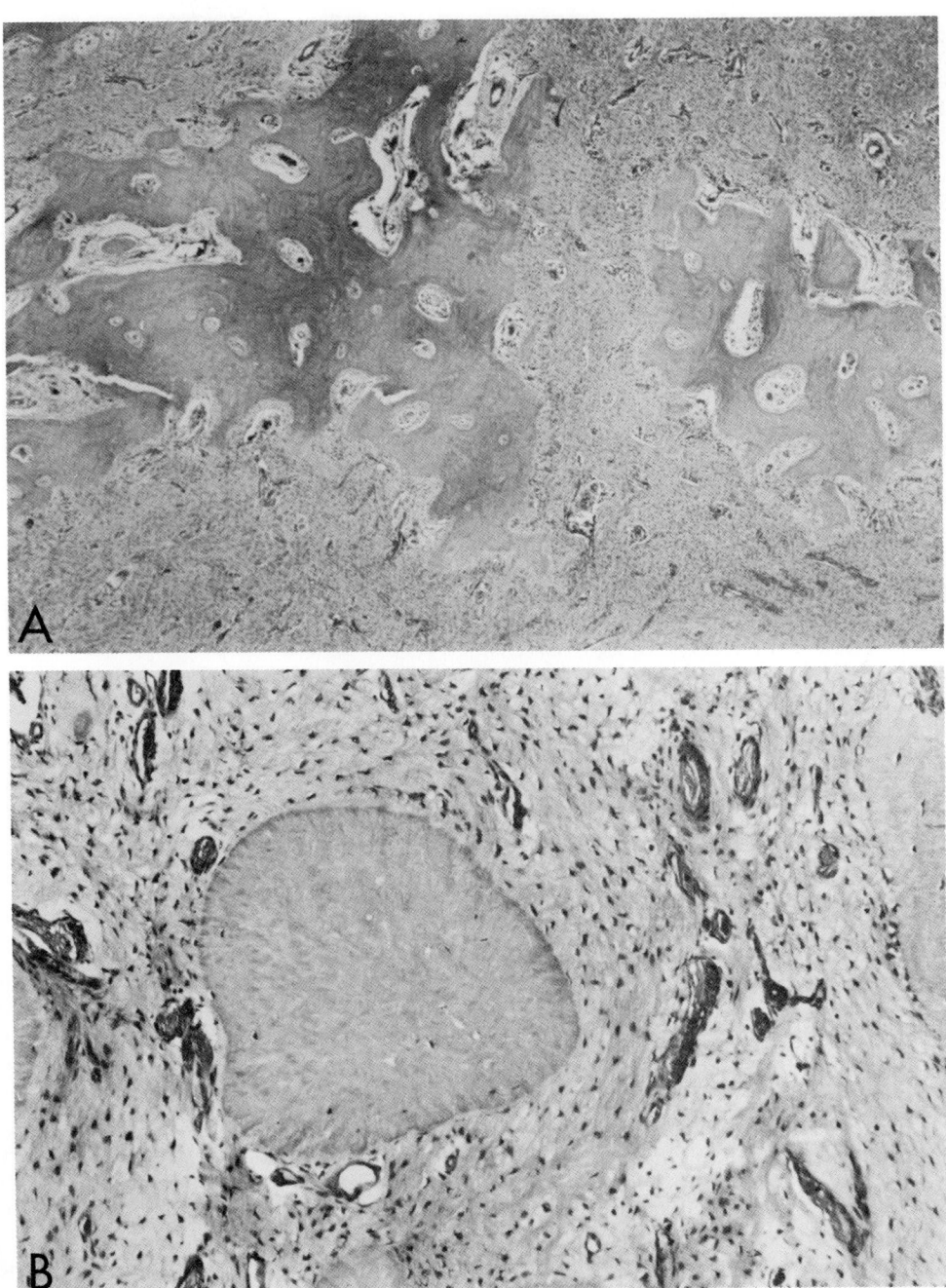

FIG. 23-4. A. Ossifying epulis, dog. Bone within a stroma resembling fibromatous epulis. **B.** Cementum or dentin-like material in a fibromatous epulis. (Courtesy of Dr. R.R. Dubielzig and **Veterinary Pathology.**)

of the jaw, like those of long bones, generally have a relatively poor prognosis because of the high frequency of local recurrence and metastasis.

Odontogenic tumors

This is a category of histologically distinct, usually benign, rare tumors that arise from the epithelial and/or mesenchymal tissues that together give rise to teeth embryologically. Tumors included in this category are: ameloblastoma, ameloblastic fibroma, ameloblastic

odontoma, and complex and compound odontomas. Odontogenic tumors have been described in dogs, cats, laboratory rodents, sheep, and horses.

Ameloblastoma is the most frequently reported of these otherwise rare neoplasms. In animals, it has been best studied in the dog. It is a benign tumor that arises deep within the mandible or maxilla where it appears as a single or multiloculated area of osteolysis surrounding one or more teeth. Osteoblastic activity is also evident in the affected area radiographically. Grossly, the neoplasms appear as solid or cystic masses within the gingiva (Fig. 23-8). The teeth at the affected site are

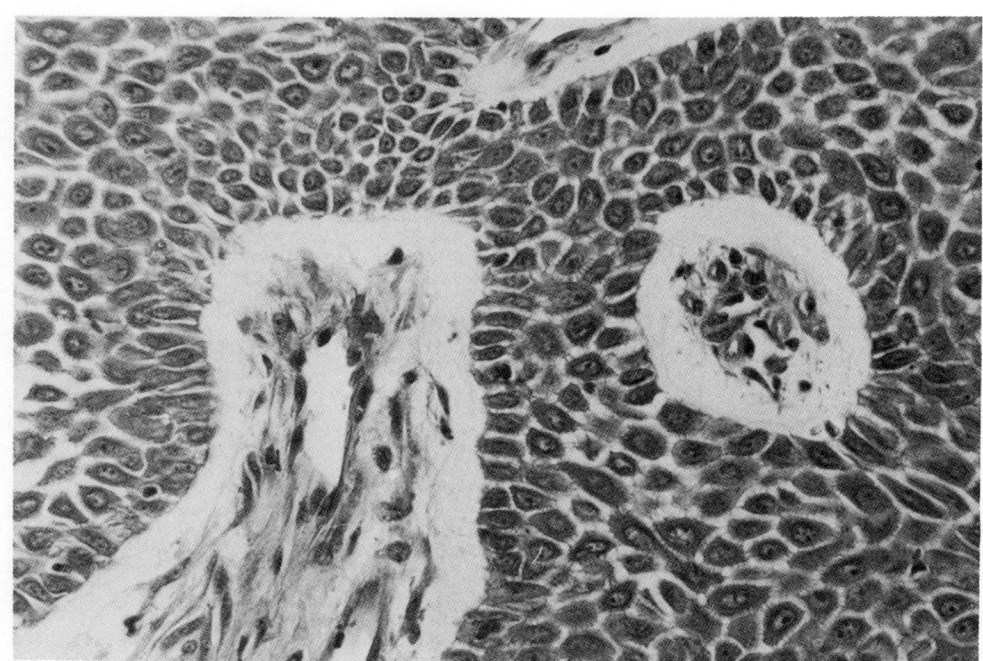

FIG. 23-5. Acanthomatous epulis, dog. The epithelial cells resemble basal or prickle cells with prominent intracellular bridges. (Courtesy of Dr. R.R. Dubielzig and **Veterinary Pathology.**)

often loose or missing. Histologically, ameloblastomas are composed of clusters and sheets of epithelial cells arranged so that the outermost cells closest to the stoma of the tumor form a palisading row aligned perpendicular to the basement membrane. The cells in the center of the sheets or cluster appear more stellate and are separated from one another except for long intercellular attachments. This pattern suggests the appearance of the stellate reticulum of the developing enamel organ. Also present are elongate, branching cords of small epithelial cells, sometimes only two cells thick. A collagenous matrix is usually present in intimate contact with the epithelial structures, a feature that mimics the close association between the epithelial and mesenchymal components of the odontogenic apparatus during embryologic development. The collagenous matrix frequently contains islands of osteoid, cementum or dentin, and enamel inclusions. The latter occur within the sheets of ameloblastic epithelium and vary from small, round eosinophilic deposits between the cells to larger, round or irregular islands with linear radiating streaks. These occlusions often are surrounded by the epithelial cells, a finding suggesting that they are secreted by the latter. Some ameloblastomas also contain areas of keratinization that differs from that seen in squamous cell carcinomas in that the keratinized cells occur in small, round packets sharply demarcated from the nonkeratinized cells. When this feature is prominent the tumor is referred to as a **keratinizing ameloblastoma.**

Ameloblastic fibroma is a variant of ameloblastoma that has been described in maxillae of young cats and in calves. Microscopically, this tumor is composed of elongate cords of epithelial cells that resemble the so-called dental lamina of embryologic development and closely apposed fusiform to stellate-shaped cells that resemble those of the early dental mesenchyme or pulp. In these tumors there is no evidence of more differentiated dental elements. They are benign and behave like an ameloblastoma.

Ameloblastic odontoma can be viewed as a more differentiated form of ameloblastic fibroma because,

TABLE 23-1 **Tumors of mouth and pharynx by tissue of origin**

Oral mucosa	Periodontium	Odontogenic tissues
Squamous cell carcinoma	Fibromatous epulis	Ameloblastoma
Malignant melanoma	Ossifying epulis	Ameloblastic fibroma
Fibrosarcoma	Acanthomatous epulis	Ameloblastic odontoma
Adenocarcinoma of oral salivary glands		Complex odontoma
Granular cell myoblastoma (tongue)		Compound odontoma
Lymphosarcoma (tonsil)		Odontogenic myxoma
Craniopharyngioma		

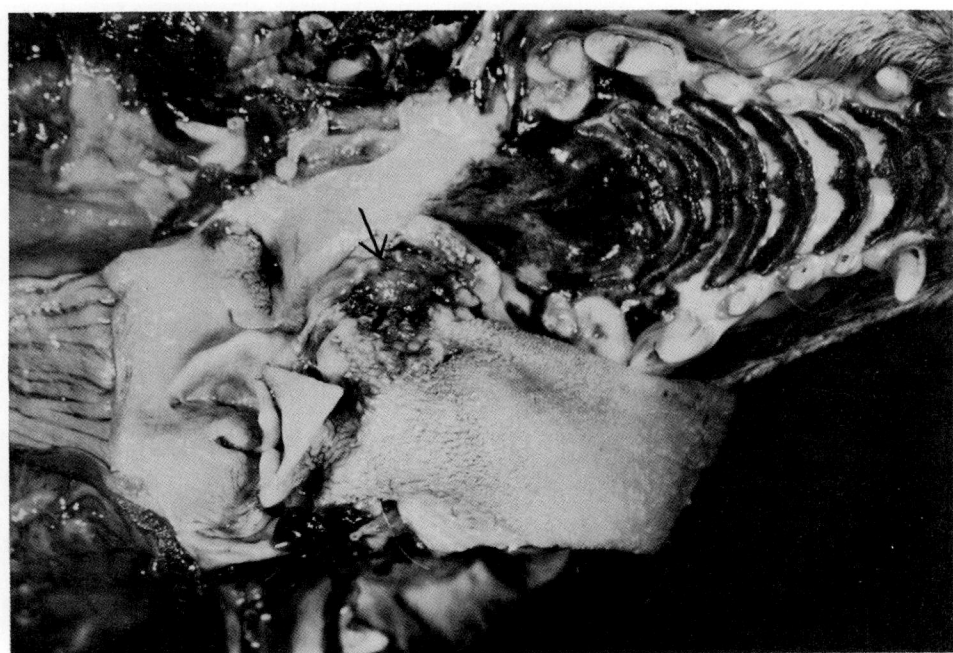

FIG. 23-6. Squamous-cell carcinoma in tonsillar crypt (arrow) of a Spaniel-type dog, aged eight years, spayed female. Note that lesion is eroded and depressed. The left retropharyngeal lymph node was infiltrated by the tumor. (Courtesy of Angell Memorial Animal Hospital.)

in addition to having features of the latter, it also contains islands of dentin and enamel and a more differentiated appearing enamel-producing epithelium. There are rare reports of its occurrence in horses and cattle.

Complex and compound odontomas are regarded as dental malformations rather than true neoplasms. They have been described in dogs, horses, cattle, sheep, and rats. The **complex odontoma** consists of a well-differentiated, but malformed mass of dental tissue in which all of the normal tissue elements are present but not in the form of a normal tooth. **Compound odontomas,** conversely, are characterized by the presence of varying sized masses of tooth-like tissue having enamel, dentin, cementum, and pulp elements but an abnormal arrangement or location within the jaw. Sometimes, they displace the normal tooth at the location.

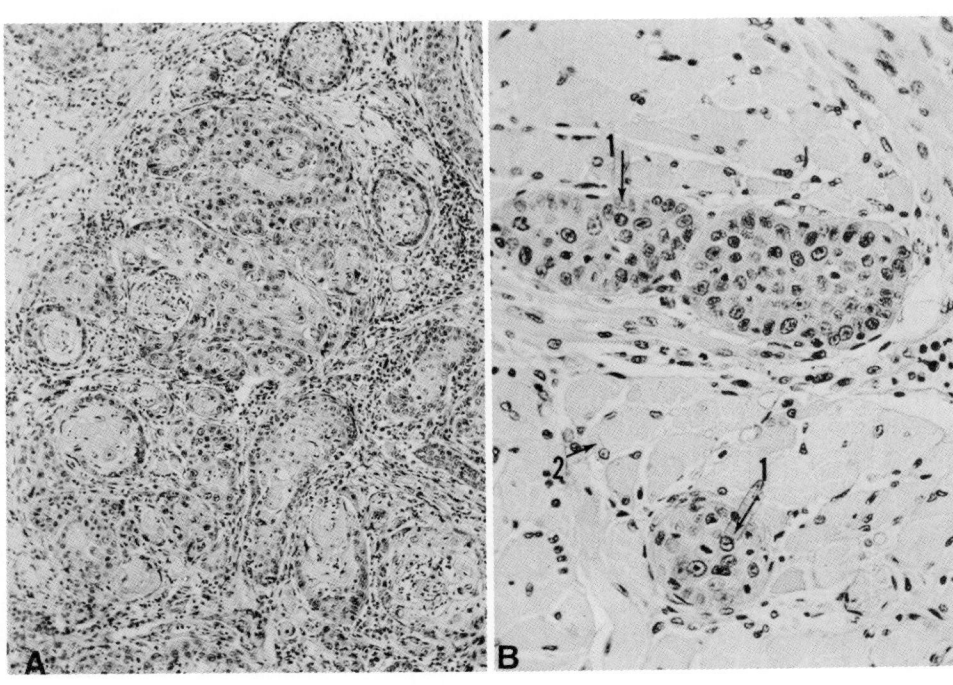

FIG. 23-7. Squamous-cell carcinoma. **A.** Primary tumor (× 90) from epithelium of tongue of a 13-year-old male cat. Note inflammation surrounding irregular nests of tumor cells. **B.** Extension of tumor **(1)** deep into the musculature **(2)** of the tongue. These are probably tumor emboli in lymphatics (× 235). (Courtesy of Armed Forces Institute of Pathology and Dr. Edward Baker.)

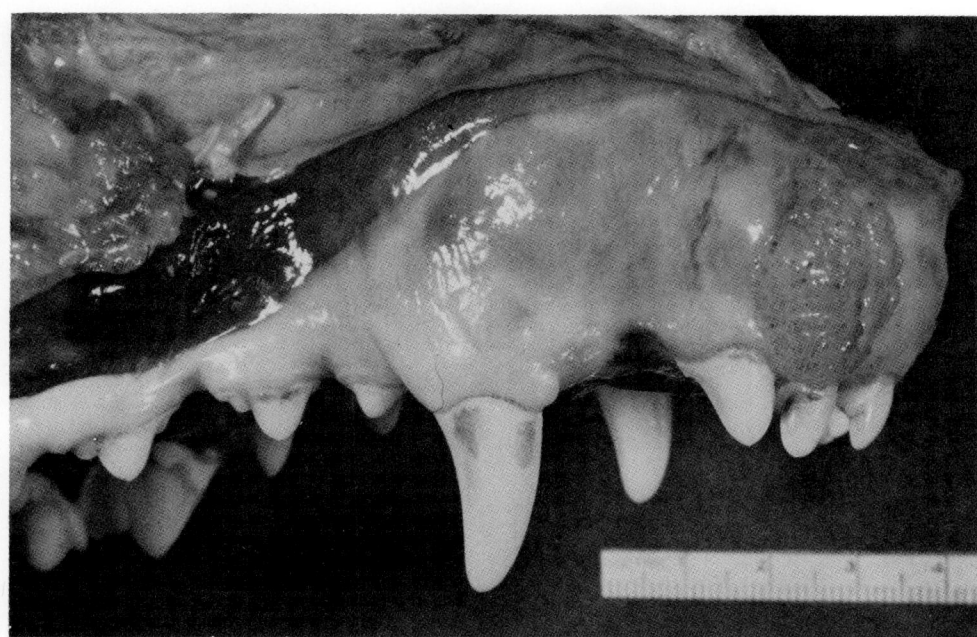

FIG. 23-8. Ameloblastoma of maxilla of a 14-month-old standard poodle. (Courtesy of Angell Memorial Animal Hospital.)

Other tumors of the oral cavity

Lymphosarcoma may involve the lymphoid tissue of the tonsils or pharynx as part of its generalized distribution. One or both tonsils may be involved and grossly enlarged. Histologically, the normal lymphoid tissue of the organ is replaced by solid sheets of neoplastic lymphoid cells.

Mast cell tumors have been reported rarely in the oral cavity of dogs and cats. These may be direct extensions of primary tumors of the skin, of the cheek or lips, or arise de novo from the oral mucosa, particularly the tongue in dogs. Because of the frequent association of this type of tumor and reactive eosinophil infiltration, the lesion must be distinguished from eosinophilic ulcer or granuloma of the oral cavity.

Granular cell tumor, once termed **granular cell myoblastoma,** is a rare, histologically distinct neoplasm of the mucosa of the base of the tongue of dogs. Its cell of origin is controversial, but currently it is thought that it arises from cells having the potential to differentiate into Schwann cells. The neoplasm appears as a solitary, well-circumscribed, nodular mass having a smooth to slightly granular red surface. On cut-section the mass is firm and white. Microscopically, it is composed of large, round to polygonal cells with abundant, coarse, eosinophilic cytoplasmic granules. The granules stain intensely positive with the periodic acid-Schiff (PAS) reaction. The nuclei of the tumor cells are round to oval and contain 1–2 nucleoli. The neoplastic granular cells form nests or cords separated by a thin connective tissue stroma. Mitotic activity is extremely low and the neoplasm grows primarily by expansion rather than invasion. Excision is generally curative, as these tumors do not recur following excision and do not metastasize.

TEETH

Caries

In the past, it has been said that the teeth of animals are much less prone to the development of caries (dental decay, cavities) than the teeth of people. The widespread use of sodium fluoride in municipal drinking water and commercial toothpastes over the last three decades has made human teeth more resistant to dental decay and has drastically reduced the occurrence of caries, particularly in young people. The diet of most animals, unlike that of people, is relatively low in fermentable sugars which are prime substrates for acid-producing cariogenic bacteria of the oral cavity. The pH of the oral secretions of animals is also somewhat higher than that of people; this possibly plays a role in the resistance of animals to dental caries.

Enamel hypoplasia

The enamel of a tooth is produced by specialized cells known as ameloblasts prior to its eruption. Ameloblasts are especially susceptible to injury by certain environmental poisons, such as fluorine (see Chapter 15); drugs, such as tetracycline; and various viral agents, including those of canine distemper and bovine virus diarrhea. Exposure to these agents prior to or during enamel development results in varying degrees of enamel hypoplasia evident after the tooth erupts. Affected teeth have defects in the enamel that may result in exposure of the underlying dentin giving the teeth a mottled appearance.

A more severe disease, termed **amelogenesis imperfecta,** has been described as an autosomal recessive disorder in the SHR-SP strain of rats. The teeth of affected animals remained white (rather than turned yellow by 3 weeks after birth as in unaffected animals), were brittle, lacked hardness, and were easily broken or bent. Microscopically, the enamel organ of affected rats was present but underdeveloped and the teeth lacked enamel.

Dental dysplasia

A form of dental dysplasia recognized only radiographically and histologically has been described in young puppies with uremia. Grossly, the teeth in these pups appeared normal. The lesions consisted of dense areas of mineralization of dysplastic dentin and enamel matrix.

Other abnormalities of tooth development

There are a number of abnormalities that affect tooth development. **Anodontia** is the term for lack of tooth development. It occurs as a sex-linked recessive trait in male calves. **Oligodontia,** or the development of fewer teeth than normal, has been observed in horses, dogs, and cats. In brachycephalic breeds of dogs it is not uncommon for some of the molar teeth to be missing, whereas in toy breeds there may be fewer incisors than normal. **Polyodontia,** the presence of supernumerary teeth, also occurs in brachycephalic dogs and generally involves the incisor teeth. Retention of a deciduous tooth after eruption of the permanent teeth is a form of **pseudopolyodontia.** Finally, **heterotopic polyodontia** refers to the presence of an extra tooth or teeth at sites other than the dental arcades. A common site for such an ectopic tooth is in a branchiogenic cyst found in the parotid region of horses. These cysts are derived from failure of closure of the first branchial cleft with resultant displacement of embryonic tooth germ from the first branchial arch towards the ear. Supernumerary ectopic teeth have been described in horses, cattle, dogs, pigs, and sheep. **Dentigerous cyst** is a tooth-containing cyst derived from a malformed enamel organ.

References

Bjorling DE, Chambers JN, Mahaffey EA. Surgical treatment of epulides in dogs: 25 cases (1974–1984). J Am Vet Med Assoc 1987;190:1315–1322.

Brodey RS. A clinical and pathologic study of 130 neoplasms of the mouth and pharynx in the dog. Am J Vet Res 1960;21:787–812.

Carpenter LG, Withrow BE, Powers BE, et al. Squamous cell carcinoma of the tongue in dogs. J Am Anim Hosp Assoc 1990;29:17–24.

Dillehay DL, Schoeb TR. Complex odontoma in a horse. Vet Pathol 1986;23:341–342.

Dorn CR, Priester WA. Epidemiologic analysis of oral and pharyngeal cancer in dogs, cats, horses and cattle. J Am Vet Med Assoc 1976;169:1202–1206.

Dubielzig RR, Beck KA, Levine S, et al. Complex odontoma in a stallion. Vet Pathol 1986;23:633–635.

Dubielzig RR, Beck KA, Wilson JW, et al. Dental dysplasia in two young uremic dogs. Vet Pathol 1986;23:333–335.

Dubielzig RR, Goldschmidt MH, Brodey RS. The nomenclature of periodontal epulides in dogs. Vet Pathol 1979;16:209–214.

Dubielzig RR, Higgins RJ, Krakowa S. Lesions of the enamel organ of developing dog tooth following experimental inoculation of gnotobiotic puppies with canine distemper virus. Vet Pathol 1981;18:684–689.

Dubielzig RR, Thrall DE. Ameloblastoma and keratinizing ameloblastoma in dogs. Vet Pathol 1982;19:596–607.

Ishibashi K, Iino T, Sekiguchi F. Amelogenesis imperfecta, a new dental mutation in rats. Lab Anim Sci 1990;40:16–20.

Johnessee JS, Hurvitz AI. Feline plasma cell gingivitis-pharyngitis. J Am Anim Hosp Assoc 1983;19:171–181.

Logue DN, Breeze RG, Harvery MJ. Arthrogryposis-palatoschisis and a 1/29 translocation in a Charolais herd. Vet Rec 1977;100:509–510.

Milhaud GE, Barba MA, Krishnaswamy S. Effect of fluoride ingestion on dental fluorosis in sheep. Am J Vet Res 1987;48:873–879.

Morton LD, Barton CL, Elissalde GS, et al. Oral extramedullary plasmacytoma in two dogs. Vet Pathol 1986;23:637–639.

Panter KE, Keeler RF, Buck WB. Induction of cleft palate in newborn pigs by maternal ingestion of poison hemlock (Conium maculatum). Am J Vet Res 1985;46:1368–1371.

Pederson NC. Inflammatory oral cavity diseases of the cat. Vet Clin North Am 1992;22:1323–1345.

Schuh JCL. Squamous cell carcinoma of the oral, pharyngeal and nasal mucosa in the horse. Vet Pathol 1986;23:205–207.

Shupe JL, Christofferson PV, Olson AE, et al. Relationship of cheek tooth abrasion to fluoride-induced permanent incisor lesions in livestock. Am J Vet Res 1987;48:1498–1503.

Stebbins KE, Morse CC, Goldschmidt MH. Feline oral neoplasia: a ten-year survey. Vet Pathol 1989;26:121–128.

Suttie JW, Clay, AB, Shearer TR. Dental fluorosis in bovine temporary teeth. Am J Vet Res 1985;46:404–408.

Todoroff RJ, Brodey RS. Oral and pharyngeal neoplasia in the dog: A retrospective survey of 361 cases. J Am Vet Med Assoc 1979;175:567–645.

Turk MAM, Johnson GC, Gallina AM, et al. Canine granular cell tumor (myoblastoma): A report of four cases and review of the literature. J Small Anim Pract 1983;24:637–645.

Walsh KM, Denholm LJ, Cooper BJ. Epithelial odontogenic tumours in domestic animals. J Comp Pathol 1987;97:503–521.

Williams CA, Aller MS. Gingivitis/stomatitis in cats. Vet Clin North Am Sm Anim Pract 1992;22:1361–1383.

SALIVARY GLANDS

The salivary glands may be affected by infectious inflammatory processes arising in their vicinity, usually from trauma. Inflammation of the salivary gland is referred to as **sialoadenitis.** In domestic animals, there is no specific infection, comparable to mumps, which has a predilection for salivary tissue. It should be recalled that the cytomegaloviruses have a predilection for the salivary gland. However, they rarely induce sialoadenitis. In rats, there are specific forms of transmissible sialoadenitis and sialodacryoadenitis (inflammation of the salivary and lacrimal glands) caused by a coronavirus known as sialodacryadenitis (SDA) virus. It is possible, but quite unusual, for infection to ascend the duct of a parotid or other salivary gland. Foreign bodies, such as kernels of grain or awns of plants, rarely find their way up a parotid or submaxillary duct, causing inflammation and possibly obstruction or dilation of the duct.

Sialoliths, or salivary calculi, form in a duct or in the gland itself as a result of chronic inflammation which provides desquamated cells or consolidated exudate as a minute nidus upon which calcium salts precipitate. Foreign bodies may also initiate the precipitation of salts. Since the salivary secretion contains little dissolved mineral, the process of formation of salivary calculi is possibly more akin to calcification of tissue than it is to the formation of urinary or biliary stones. At any rate, sialoliths may reach astonishing size, parotid calculi several centimeters in diameter and length have been recognized in the horse.

When its duct is occluded for prolonged periods, a salivary gland undergoes atrophy, but before this process is complete, a cyst may form in the obstructed duct due to the dilating effect of the entrapped secretion. Such a cyst in the sublingual duct, located in the frenulum of the tongue, is referred to as a **ranula**. A salivary fistula occasionally forms when an injury creates an opening from the duct to the outside of the body, proper healing being prevented by the flow of saliva through the opening.

Neoplasms of salivary glands

Primary neoplasms of the major (parotid, mandibular, sublingual) and minor (palatine, lingual, labial, gingival) salivary glands are infrequent in animals. However, Koestner and Buerger (1965) assembled and tabulated 43 cases from the literature from 1875 through 1959 and described an additional 30 cases from their own collection. The histologic diagnoses used by these authors will be listed and described briefly.

Three **mucoepidermoid tumors** were described (one mucoepidermoid cystadenoma in the parotid gland of a Hamadryas baboon, and two mucoepidermoid carcinomas—one parotid, one palatine—in dogs). This neoplasm is composed of squamous epithelial elements and mucus-secreting glandular structures. The series included one **squamous cell carcinoma** arising in the sublingual gland of a cat; its possible origin from the oral mucosa could not be excluded. Six tumors were classified as **mixed tumors** characterized by neoplastic epithelial and mesenchymal tissue elements. These neoplasms resemble mixed tumors of the mammary gland in that myoepithelial cells are present along with cartilage, bone, squamous, and glandular epithelium. Two cases occurred in horses and involved the parotid salivary glands. Of three cases in dogs, two arose in the mandibular, and one in the parotid salivary glands. One mixed tumor originated in the sublingual salivary gland of a guinea pig.

Adenoid-cystic carcinoma (**cylindroma**) of the salivary gland is a variant characterized by small dark-staining cells arranged in an adenoid and cystic, as well as a solid pattern. This tumor occurs in human salivary glands but has not been described in animals. **Acinic cell tumor** (**acinic cell carcinoma**) is composed of acinar structures made up of small, rather uniform, neoplastic cells arranged in solid sheets as well as in adenoid and adenoid-cystic patterns. Twelve animal tumors were classified in this category—11 in dogs and 1 in the parotid gland of a horse. All were locally invasive. Of the 11 canine tumors, 7 affected the major salivary glands (5 the parotid, and 2 the mandibular gland) and the remaining 4 arose in minor salivary glands.

Adenocarcinomas were classified as **ductular** (**papillary**) or **trabecular**. In the ductular category, two tumors occurred in dogs; one arose in the parotid, the other in a minor salivary gland of the tongue. Three trabecular adenocarcinomas were identified in a cat, a dog, and a horse. All arose in the parotid gland, were malignant, and metastasized to regional lymph nodes and lung. **Anaplastic** (**undifferentiated carcinomas**) were found in two dogs, one in the mandibular and the other in the sublingual gland. Both metastasized to lymph nodes and other sites. The **papillary cystadenoma lymphomatosum** (Warthin tumor), is a benign neoplasm of the salivary gland of people, consisting of an epithelial and a lymphoid component. This tumor has been reported to have occurred spontaneously in a 2–year old female B$_6$C$_3$F$_1$ hybrid mouse.

In addition to the series of Koestner and Buerger described above, a single, malignant mixed tumor arising in the parotic gland of a 12–year-old neutered female cat has been described by Wells and Robinson (1975). It metastasized to the submandibular lymph nodes and skeletal muscle. The tumor contained epithelial and myoepithelial elements, as well as cartilage, osteoid, and bone.

References

Brunnert SR, Altman NH. Canine lingual acinic cell carcinoma (clear cell variant) of minor salivary gland. Vet Pathol 1990;27:203–205.

Carberry CA, Flanders JA, Harvey HJ, et al. Salivary gland tumors in dogs and cats: a literature and case review. J Am Anim Hosp Assoc 1988;24:561–567.

Glen JB. Canine salivary mucocoeles. Results of sialographic examination and surgical treatment of fifty cases. J Small Anim Pract 1972;3:515–526.

Harrison JD, Garrett JR. An ultrastructural and histochemical study of a naturally occurring salivary mucocele in a cat. J Comp Pathol 1975;85:411–416.

Harrison JD, Garrett JR. Histological effects of ductal ligation of salivary glands of the cat. J Pathol 1976;118:245–254.

Knecht CD, Phares J. Characterization of dogs with salivary cyst. J Am Vet Med Assoc 1971;158:612–613.

Koestner A, Buerger L. Primary neoplasms of the salivary glands in animals compared to similar tumors in man. Pathol Vet 1965;2:201–226.

Mesfin GM, Piper RC. Cystadenoma lymphomatosum-like lesion in the parotid salivary gland of a mouse. Vet Pathol 1986;23:538–539.

Orkin JL, Braswell LD. Sialolithiasis in two chimpanzees. J Am Vet Med Assoc 1990;196:1651–1653.

Spangler WL, Culbertson MR. Salivary gland disease in dogs and cats: 245 cases (1985–1988). J Am Vet Med Assoc 1991;198:465.

Swartz HA, Vogt DW, Kintner LD. Chromosome evaluation of Angus calves with unilateral congenital cleft lip and jaw (cheilognathoschisis). Am J Vet Res 1982;43:729–731.

Wells GAH, Robinson M. Mixed tumour of salivary gland showing histological evidence of malignancy in a cat. J Comp Pathol 1975;85:77–85.

ESOPHAGUS

Disorders of the esophagus can be categorized into one of three types: inflammatory degenerative lesions, obstructive lesions, or motility disorders.

Esophagitis

Inflammation of the esophagus is infrequent but, like that of the mouth, generally results from trauma produced by foreign objects, from caustic chemicals, or from infection.

Reflux esophagitis is a form of chemical esophagitis and occurs when there is reflux of gastric acid and pepsin from the stomach and bile salts and pancreatic enzymes from the duodenum into the lower portion of the esophagus. The stratified squamous epithelium of the esophageal mucosa, unlike the gastrointestinal mucosa, is not protected by a layer of mucus and consequently it may be partially digested by these corrosive juices. Grossly, the affected portion of the esophagus is hyperemic or contains linear erosions or ulcerations which may be covered by a fibrinonecrotic plaque. Microscopically, there are areas of epithelial erosion and/or ulceration with ingrowth of fibroblastic connective tissue, and flattening and proliferation of the adjacent normal epithelium in an attempt to re-epithelialize the denuded surface. The pathogenesis of this condition involves chronic vomiting or transient or permanent loss of integrity of the esophageal sphincter. Reflux esophagitis can be caused by hiatal hernia or can occur as a complication of general anesthesia in dogs and cats.

Any extensive injury, chemical or traumatic, to the esophageal lining is a serious event because of its tendency to produce **stenosis or stricture** of the esophagus. Such lesions result from the formation of excessive scar tissue during the healing process. The contraction of scar tissue as it ages, causes localized constriction of the lumen at the site of injury. Injury from the swallowing of highly irritant or caustic chemicals is a common cause. Surgical procedures on the esophagus may be fraught with similar complications because of contraction of scar tissue at the operative site.

Choke, a complete or partial obstruction or impaction of the esophagus by foreign material, is common in cattle as the result of attempting to swallow large, firm items of food such as beets, turnips, apples, or small ears of corn without first reducing them to small pieces. The horse, on the other hand, practically never makes such a mistake, but does become choked by the gradual accumulation of ground or whole grain or tough grasses that fail to pass through the whole length of the esophagus. Dogs and cats become choked by sharp pieces of bone which lodge usually in the thoracic esophagus. Contrary to popular belief, choking, as long as it only involves the esophagus and not the pharynx or larynx, does not interfere seriously with respiration, although in the cow it does prevent eructation of gas formed in the rumen; this causes rumenal tympanites, which may be fatal within hours. Without this complication, if choke cannot be relieved, death is likely in about 3 days because of pressure necrosis (from compression of local blood vessels), resultant saprophytic organisms entering the blood, toxemia and esophageal rupture.

Sometimes choking on a single foreign body results in only partial obstruction of the esophagus. A common result, especially in the dog, is that food is eaten, but after some minutes is expelled by vomiting, only small amounts if any at all reaching the stomach. In a few weeks, the repeated distention of the wall just above the obstruction produces a sac-like dilatation, usually asymmetric and unilateral, known as an **esophageal diverticulum.** Perforation is a frequent outcome, especially if bones or other sharp objects are the cause.

In dogs, and doubtless in related wild species, the spirurid nematode *Spirocerca lupi* penetrates the mucosa and submucosa of the lower esophagus and causes the formation of submucosal, fibrous nodules as it undergoes development at this site. The smooth-surfaced and sometimes coalescent nodules bulge into the lumen as much as 0.5 cm and usually there is a small fistula connecting the parasite-inhabited center of the nodule to the lumen of the esophagus. Interference with esophageal function appears to be minimal (unless a sarcoma is formed, see below) and the lesions are usually found incidentally postmortem. Other parasites that invade the esophagus include the nematode *Gongylonema spp.* in ruminants and nonhuman primates, larvae of the bot fly *Gastrophilus spp.* in horses, larvae of the warble fly *Hypoderma spp.* in cattle and *Sarcocystis spp.* in sheep, and, rarely, other species.

Cricopharyngeal achalasia has been described in the dog. In this condition, food is retained in the pharynx due to inadequate relaxation of the cricopharyngeal sphincter. According to one report, the signs were relieved by cricopharyngeal myotomy. Microscopic changes in the cricopharyngeal muscle have been inconsistent

References

Amand WB, O'Brien JA, Tucker JA. Dysphagia in a wooly monkey (Lagothrix lagotricha) following a caustic esophageal burn. J Am Vet Med Assoc 1970;57:706–711.

Clifford DH, Soifer FK, Freeman RG. Stricture and dilatation of the esophagus in the cat. J Am Vet Med Assoc 1970;156:1007–1014.

Pearson H, et al, Darke DGG, Gibbs C., et al. Reflux esophagitis and stricture formation after anesthesia; A reveiw of seven cases in dogs and cats. J Small Anim Pract 1978;19:507–519.

Rogers WA, Donovan EF. Peptic esophagitis in a dog. J Am Vet Med Assoc 1973;163:462–464.

Megaesophagus (esophageal achalasia)

Generalized or segmental dilatation of the esophagus results from neuromuscular disorders that impair esophageal motility. The wall of the esophagus in this condition is atonic and flaccid (Fig 23-9). This disorder has been described in dogs, cats, foals, and humans and can be congenital or acquired.

Congenital megaesophagus is an inherited disorder in several breeds of dogs, including the Fox terrier, where it is transmitted as an autosomal recessive trait, and Miniature schnauzers, where it has been shown to be an autosomal dominant in some cases and an autosomal recessive with 60 percent penetance in others. Other breeds with an increased incidence of congenital megaesophagus are the Great Dane, German shepherd, Labrador retriever, Newfoundland, Chinese Shar-Pei and Irish setter. It has also been described in cats, particularly in the Siamese breed. Affected puppies and kittens usually suckle normally but after weaning regurgitate solid food shortly after swallowing it. In some dogs, the condition resolves spontaneously by 6–12 months of age, while in others it persists. The pathogenesis of this condition is poorly understood, but it has been speculated that there is a delay in the maturation of esophageal nervous innervation due to some lesion in the upper motor neurons of the central swallowing center or in the afferent sensory arm of the reflex involved with peristalsis. Microscopically, there is no reduction in the number of myenteric ganglial cells in the wall of the esophagus of dogs and cats with congenital megaesophagus (esophageal achalasia); hence this is not an aganglionic disease.

Acquired megaesophagus occurs spontaneously in adult dogs secondary to any disorder that disrupts the neural reflex involved in swallowing, or the normal function of the esophageal musculature. A variety of central and peripheral nervous system disorders have been associated with the development of megaesophagus. These include canine distemper, other viral encephalitides, neuronal storage diseases, and neoplasia. Peripheral neuropathies including polyradiculoneuritis, polyneuritis, bilateral vagus nerve damage, tetanus, botulism, lead poisoning, anticholinesterase toxicity, myasthenia gravis, dysautonomia, and various forms of myopathy have all been associated with secondary megaesophagus.

Myasthenia gravis is reportedly the most common cause of secondary megaesophagus in the dog. It also occurs in cats with this autoimmune disease. Individuals with this disorder develop autoantibodies to nicotinic acetylcholine receptors which interfere with neuromuscular innervation. Affected dogs may develop generalized muscular weakness preceded or followed by clinical signs of megaesophagus, or in some cases, a localized form of the disease in which there is selective involvement of the esophageal musculature without evidence of generalized muscular weakness.

Dysautonomia is a form of autonomic polyganglionopathy that causes abnormal function of the sympathetic and parasympathetic nervous systems. The condition was originally described in cats in the United Kingdom and Europe and was termed Key-Gaskell syndrome. It has since been described in cats and dogs in the United States and in other parts of the world. Its cause remains unknown. Esophageal hypomotility and megaesophagus constitute major components of this generalized systemic disorder. Clinically, the disease is characterized by depression, anorexia, reduced lacrimation, salivation, bradycardia, pupillary dilatation with delayed pupillary light reflex, megaesophagus, constipation, and sometimes ileal impaction. Microscopically, affected animals have marked reduction in the number of neurons in all autonomic ganglia in the ventral horn of the cervical, thoracic, and lumbar spinal cord. These changes were coupled with proliferation of non-neuronal cells and nodules of proliferating capsule cells. Of the remaining neurons, 30 percent or more had evidence of chromatolytic change with loss of Nissl substance. Similar lesions were also found in the brainstem nuclei of cranial nerves XII, dorsal nucleus of X, VII, V, III, the Edinger-Wesphal nucleus, and nucleus ambiguus (see also chapter 27).

Hypothyroidism and hypoadrenalcorticism have also been associated with megaesophagus in dogs. This condition reportedly is reversible if the hormonal deficiency is corrected.

Congenital vascular ring anomalies that encircle and constrict the esophagus may also lead to the development of secondary megaesophagus. The most com-

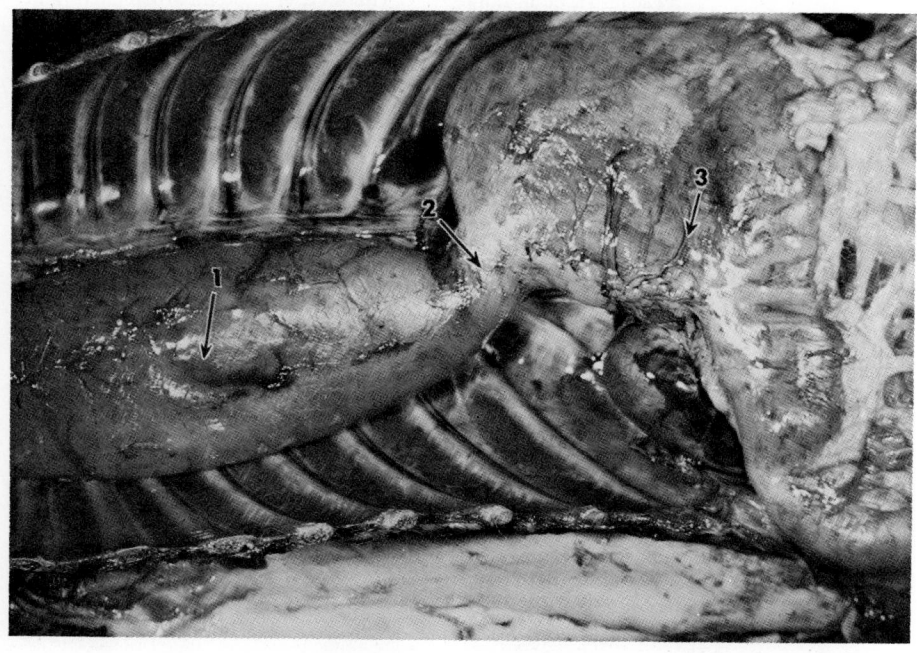

FIG. 23-9. Megaesophagus, nine-month-old female collie, due to unknown cause. The thoracic viscera and diaphragm have been removed, leaving the esophagus and stomach in situ. The esophagus (**1**) was not obstructed at the cardia (**2**) of the stomach (**3**). (Courtesy of Angell Memorial Animal Hospital.)

mon in dogs and cats is the **persistent right aortic arch.** Others include: double aortic arch, left aortic arch and right ligamentum arteriosum, persistent left or right subclavian arteries, ductus arteriosus with normal aortic arch, and others. In dogs, the Irish setter, German shepherd, and Boston terrier breeds are most commonly affected. During normal embryonic development, the right aortic arch disappears and the left becomes the functional aorta. Occasionally, this phenomenon is reversed and the right arch persists and becomes the aorta. When this happens it causes the trachea and esophagus to be incarcerated in a vascular ring composed of the arch of the aorta on the right, the pulmonary artery and base of the heart below, and ligamentum arteriosum (ductus arteriosus) dorsally and to the left. As the growing pup or kitten begins to eat larger quantities of solid food, this vascular ring prevents expansion of the esophagus and causes food to accumulate in the lumen at a point cranial to the base of the heart. This results in distention of the esophagus and with time the development of megaesophagus. The esophaguses of animals with megaesophagus secondary to persistent right aortic arch, in contrast to those with the congenital disease, have a marked reduction in the number of myenteric ganglion cells in their walls.

References

Canton DD, Sharp JH, Aguirre GD. Dysautonomia in a cat. J Am Vet Med Assoc 1988;192:1293–1296.

Clifford DH, Ross JN Jr., Waddell D, et al. Effect of persistent aortic arch on the ganglial cells of the canine esophagus. J Am Vet Med Assoc 1971;158:1401–1410.

Clifford DH, Pirsch JG. Myenteric ganglial cells in dogs with and without hereditary achalasia of the esophagus. Am J Vet Res 1971;32:615–619.

Clifford DH. Myenteric ganglial cells of the esophagus in cats with achalasia of the esophagus. Am J Vet Res 1973;34:1333–1336.

Gray GW. Acute experiments on neuroeffector function in canine esophageal achalasia. Am J Vet Res 1974;35:1075–1082.

Guilford WG, O'Brien DP, Allert A, et al. Diagnosis of dysautonomia in a cat by autonomic nervous system testing. J Am Vet Med Assoc 1988;193:823–828.

Harvey CE, O'Brien JA, Durie VR, et al. Megaesophagus in the dog: a clinical survey of 79 cases. J Am Vet Med Assoc 1974;165:443–446.

Higgs B, Kerr FWL, Ellis FH. The experimental production of esophageal achalasia by electrolytic lesions in the medulla. J Thorac Cardiovasc Surg 1965;50:613–625.

Key TJA, Gaskell CJ. Puzzling syndrome in cats associated with pupillary dilatation. Vet Rec 1982;110:160.

Maddison JE, Allan GS. Megaesophagus attributable to lead toxicosis in a cat. J Am Vet Med Assoc 1990;197:1357–1358.

Nash AS, Griffiths IR, Sharp NJH. The Key-Gaskell syndrome: an autonomic polyganglionopathy. Vet Rec 1982;111:307–308.

Nakayama S, Neya T, Watanabe K, et al. Effects of electrical stimulation and local destruction of the medulla oblongata on swallowing movements in dogs. Rendi Gastroenterol 1974;6:6–11.

Pollin M, Sullivan M. A canine dysautonomia resmbling Key-Gaskell syndrome. Vet Res 1986;118:402–403.

Rosin E, Hanlon GF. Canine cricopharyngeal achalasia. J Am Vet Med Assoc 1972;160:1496–1499.

Schrauwen E, Van Ham L, Maenhaut T, et al. Canine dysautonomia: a case report. Vet Rec 1991;128:524–525.

Shelton GD, Willard MD, Cardinet GH III. Acquired myasthenia gravis. Selective involvement of esophageal, pharyngeal and facial muscles. J Vet Intern Med 1990;4:281–284.

Strombeck DR, Troya L. Evaluation of lower motor neuron function in two dogs with megaesophagus. J Am Vet Med Assoc 1976; 169:411–414.

VanGundy T. Vascular ring anomalies. Compend Cont Ed Pract Vet 1989;11:36–48.

Neoplasms of the esophagus

Papillomas of the oral cavity, pharynx, esophagus, and rumen of cattle are caused by bovine papillomavirus type 4. This virus is related to but distinct from bovine papillomavirus types 3 and 6, which cause cutaneous papillomas, and types 1, 2, and 5, which cause fibropapillomas of the skin. Reports from Kenya and Scotland indicate rather frequent association of **squamous cell carcinomas** with the papillomas of the digestive system. Two causative factors are suspected: first, the bovine **papillomavirus;** second, chronic poisoning resulting from ingestion of bracken fern (*Pteridium aquilinum*). The synergistic effect of these two factors is strongly suspected, but has not been confirmed experimentally. Transitional cell carcinoma of the urinary bladder has also been associated with chronic bracken fern poisoning of cattle.

Osteosarcoma and **fibrosarcoma** of the esophagus of dogs has clearly been associated with long-standing lesions of *Spirocerca lupi*. Interestingly, many dogs with these tumors also have an associated ossifying spondylosis of the cervical and lumbar vertebrae, pulmonary metastasis and hypertrophic osteoarthropathy.

Metastasis of tumors to the esophagus is rare. Tumors of adjacent structures (lymph nodes or thyroid) usually do not invade the esophagus.

References

Jarrett WF. Oesophageal and stomach cancer in cattle: a candidate viral and carcinogen model system and its possible relevance to man. Br J Cancer 1973;28:93.

Pirie HM. Unusual occurrence of squamous carcinoma of the upper alimentary tract in cattle in Britain. Res Vet Sci 1973;15:135–138.

Plowright W. Malignant neoplasia of the esophagus and rumen of cattle in Kenya. J Comp Pathol Therap 1955;65:108–114.

Ribelin WE, Bailey WS. Esophageal sarcoma associated with *Spirocerca lupi* infection in the dog. Cancer 1958;2:1242–1246.

Schutte KH. Esophageal tumors in sheep: some ecological observations. J Natl Cancer Inst 1968;41:821–824.

Seibold HR, Bailey WS, Hoerlein BF, et al. Observations on the possible relation of malignant esophageal tumors and *Spirocerca lupi* lesions in the dog. Am J Vet Res 1955;16:5–14.

Thorsen J, Cooper JE, Warwick GP. Oesophageal papillomata in cattle in Kenya. Trop Anim Health Prod. 1974;6:95–98.

FORESTOMACHS OF RUMINANTS

The rumen, reticulum, and omasum are called stomachs only because of their general shape and size. They have no secretory function comparable to that of a true stomach; the abomasum of ruminants functions as the true glandular stomach where enzymatic breakdown of ingesta occurs. The rumen, reticulum and omasum are lined by keratinized stratified squamous epithelium and function as large fermentation and absorption chambers where symbiotic bacteria and protozoa digest large quantities of plant material, some components of which, such as cellulose, are not digestible by mongastric animals, and convert it into absorbable nutrients. All plant materials are by no means totally digested and absorbed by this process. The fermentation action of ruminal microbial flora produces volatile fatty acids (acetic, proprionic and butyric acids), gases (CO_2 and methane), energy, and water. The relative proportions of these and other byproducts of ruminal fermentation vary considerably with the composition of the diet. Likewise, the composition of the ruminal flora is also markedly influenced by diet and the type and amounts of fermentation byproducts produced as well as the resulting pH. In cattle and sheep the normal pH of the rumen ranges from 5.5 to 7.5. Deviations from this range can drastically alter the composition of the ruminal flora, which in turn can adversely affect ruminal function and the health of the animal.

Abnormalities of the ruminal mucosa

The mucosa of the rumen of adult animals fed adequate amounts of roughage normally has numerous long, slender, gray-white papillae protruding from its surface. These are lined by a thin layer of keratinized, stratified squamous epithelium. The papillae in animals fed rations high in concentrate, barley, or pelleted alfalfa become black, blunted, hard, and club-like, and adhere to one another to form clumps or bundles. Microscopically, the epithelium of these altered papillae is acanthotic, hyperkeratotic, parakeratotic, and hyperpigmented. Secondary papillae may arise from the lateral surfaces of the abnormal papillae and account for the clumping noted grossly. Variable degrees of fibrosis of the lamina propria and submucosa result in thickening of the wall of the rumen. The fibrotic areas may contain a mixed population of inflammatory cells.

The pathogenesis of these mucosal changes involves changes in the concentrations, type, and relative proportions of the volatile fatty acids produced in the rumen; the ruminal pH; and the amount and quality of the roughage being fed. Fermentation of high concentrate feeds produces increased concentrations of proprionic and butyric acids, reduced levels of acetic acid, and a lowered ruminal pH. The hyperkeratosis and parakeratosis of ruminal papillae are thought to represent an adaptive response to the chemical changes in the ruminal contents as a consequence of changes in the diet. This condition does not occur, or is reversible, if the ration contains roughly 15 percent coarse roughage along with the concentrate. The feeding of adequate quantities of roughage increases the concentration of ruminal acetic acid and decreases the quantity of proprionic and butyric acid produced. The abrasive effect of coarse roughage may also prevent the excessive accumulation of keratin on the surface of the ruminal papillae.

Ruminal tympanites or bloat

Tympanites of the rumen, or bloat, consists of the accumulation of excessive quantities of gas in the lumen of the organ, distending it to life-threatening proportions. The gas, which is usually flammable, consists largely of methane, carbon dioxide, carbon monoxide, and smaller amounts of others gases, including the poisonous hydrogen disulfide (H_2S). These gases are the common products of microbiological fermentation of carbohydrates and proteins and result from the action of many kinds of Gram-negative saprophytic bacteria and protozoa present on ingested plant material. The production of these gaseous metabolic by products is normal and goes on continuously, but normally the gas is expelled in the form of frequent belchings or eructations through the esophagus and mouth.

Pathologic bloating can result from any interference with the normal eructations or from the production of gas in quantities that exceed the capacity of esophageal eructations to discharge it. It is not known what mechanisms, if any, limit the amount of gas that can be discharged via the esophagus in a given period of time, but the escape, rather than being a passive process, requires active reverse peristalsis of the esophagus and hence is under the control of the (autonomic) nervous system. The amount of gas produced, of course, depends upon the rate of bacterial fermentation, and this is greatly enhanced when the food ingested is fresh, succulent, green legumes, such as clover and alfalfa.

It is possible that the capacity for repeated eructation is exceeded by the gas production at such times, but this has not been proven. There are other theories regarding its pathogenesis. One is that this green succulent material is very soft and that the initiation of expulsive ruminal contractions requires the mechanical irritation of rough stems and stalks upon the lining of the rumen. This explanation seems only slightly attractive when we consider that when the animal is on a diet of coarse, dry, and largely indigestible straw, the rumen is well-filled yet develops little gas, with few eructations.

Another theory is that the gases arising from the fermentation of fresh green legumes include sufficient amounts of toxic hydrogen disulfide to suppress the function of local nervous structures. It has not been confirmed that important amounts of the gas are absorbed, or that H_2S, if absorbed, has such a toxic effect. It is doubtful that the phenomenon of entrapped gas in the bovine rumen is much different from that in the equine stomach or cecum (see below), where spasmodic contractions of adjacent segments of the alimentary canal are known to exert a sphincter-like action. Certainly in the human experience, excessive gas in the intestine induces a certain degree of spasmodic contraction of the bowel. It is possible that similar reflex spasms of the esophageal tube or orifice are responsible for the retention of ruminal gases, and that the increased pressure is sufficiently irritating to promote further spasm, a vicious cycle thus being established. It is clear, however, that the simple passing of a stomach tube promptly results in the escape of the excess gas.

"Frothy bloat" or **primary bloat** is the most common form of tympanites in cattle and constitutes an exception to the last statement. In this disorder, the gas is dispersed in the form of small bubbles in the somewhat viscous ruminal fluid. The inability of the gas to escape from such a foamy mixture is dependent on the surface tension of the liquid and the colloidal state of dissolved solids. Drugs added to the mixture which reduce its surface tension tend to release the bubbles, but the precise chemical changes responsible for the formation of such bubbles have not been totally elucidated. Chloroplasts and other particulate plant material suspended in ruminal fluid may promote frothy bloat by serving as a medium for colonization by ruminal microorganisms, thereby promoting fermentation and gas formation. Also, chloroplasts of bloat-promoting succulent legumes are known to be rich in soluble proteins which become denatured and insoluble after being released into acidic ruminal fluid by bacterial degradation. These denatured proteins function as a foam-stabilizing agent. Likewise, plant pectins may also increase the surface tension of ruminal fluid and promote the formation of foam. Other factors probably serve to counteract the action of these foam-promoting substances. Plant lipids which may function as antifoaming agents by preventing the soluble proteins from binding metallic ions and becoming denatured. Additionally, factors in saliva are probably also important in the pathogenesis of tympanites. Salivary bicarbonate serves to neutralize ruminal acids and maintain ruminal pH at levels that do not promote the formation of stable foam from soluble proteins. Mucoproteins in saliva tend to increase the viscosity of ruminal fluid, whereas salivary mucins have the opposite effect.

The gas entrapped in the frothy fluid cannot be expelled by eructation and therefore progressively accumulates, causing massive distention of the rumen. Also, if the fluid enters the esophagus, it stimulates the swallowing reflex which in turn prevents normal eructation. Bloating of this kind is acute, occurring suddenly and often causing death in a matter of hours.

The second and less common form of tympanites is termed **secondary bloat** or **"free gas bloat"**. This condition results from some physical obstruction of the esophageal or pharyngeal passageways. Choke resulting from foreign bodies has been mentioned earlier in this chapter as a mechanical cause of such obstruction. Strictures may have the same effect but are rare. Other causes include pressure upon the esophagus by tumors, abscesses, swollen lymph nodes, and other enlargements. Except in the case of a completely obstructing choke, these forms of bloating arise more gradually and often are chronic or intermittent depending upon the cause.

One of the effects of severe bloating is forward displacement of the diaphragm, which severely limits the respiratory capacity. The increased pressure within the rumen causes it to expand and thereby compress the abdominal viscera and occlude the caudal vena cava. This shunts blood from the caudal to the cephalic parts of the body. These mechanisms result in anoxia, which is the immediate cause of death when it occurs. If the excessive pressure is relieved by surgical or other forms of intervention, the above effects promptly subside.

On postmortem examination, animals that die of frothy bloat have marked forward displacement of the diaphram that compresses their lungs into the anterior portion of the thorax. Abdominal viscera appear pale due to compression of their blood vessels by the distended rumen. The ruminal contents will contain small bubbles of entrapped gas. Except for the character of the ruminal contents, animals that die of secondary bloat have similar signs, but in addition may have some form of obstructive lesion involving the pharynx or esophagus.

Sheep, as well as cattle, are susceptible to bloating, but because of their more conservative eating habits, are less commonly affected. Specific types of forage may be incriminated. For example, in Australia, the wild gooseberry plant *(Nicandra physaloides)* has been shown to cause fatal bloat in sheep under certain circumstances.

References

Clarke RTJ, Reid CSW. Foamy bloat of cattle. A review. J Dairy Sci 1974;57:753–785.
Cohen RDH. Bloat in sheep grazing wild gooseberry, *Nicandra physaloides.* Aust Vet J 1970;46:559.
Head MJ. Bloat in cattle. Nature 1959;183:757.
Howarth RE. A review of bloat in cattle. Can Vet J 1975;16:281–294.
Jensen R, Flint JC, Udall RH, et al. Parakeratosis of the rumens of lambs fattened on pelleted feed. Am J Vet Res 1958;19:277–282.
McGavin MD, Morrill JL. Scanning electron microscopy of ruminal papillae in calves fed various amounts and forms of roughage. Am J Vet Res 1976;37:497–508.
Mills JHL, Christian RG. Lesions of bovine ruminal tympany. J Am Vet Med Assoc 1970;157:947–952.
Wright DE, Curtis MW. Bloat in cattle. The action of surface-active chemicals on ciliated protozoa. N Z J Agri Res 1976;19:19–23.

Ruminal acidosis, rumenitis, and ulcers

These conditions represent successive stages of a syndrome often associated with an abrupt change of diet from a low energy ration to one containing large quantities of highly fermentable carbohydrates in the form of grain, beets, turnips, bread, brewery byproducts, or apples. It occurs most often in high production beef and dairy cattle operations, but sheep and goats are also susceptible. Frothy bloat may occur concurrently with this disorder.

The pathogenesis involves the sudden availability of excessive quantities of a highly fermentable carbohydrate substrate for fermentation by the normal ruminal flora and fauna, or what is sometimes referred to as **"carbohydrate or grain overload."** Within hours of ingestion of such a diet, the pH of the rumen begins to decline due to the increased production of volatile fatty acids (acetic, proprionic, and butyric acids). As the pH approaches approximately 5.0, the normal Gram-negative bacteria and protozoa of the rumen die, with a concomitant overgrowth of *Streptococcus bovis* and other streptococci. These organisms, unlike the normal ruminal flora, produce large quantities of lactic acid from the carbohydrate substrate. This results in further decline in ruminal pH to levels less than 5.0 which in turn kills off the streptococci. At this point, the acid-loving *Lactobacillus acidophilus* rapidly proliferate within the ruminal contents. Death may ensue when the pH drops below 4.5.

During the sequence of chemical events described above, the musculature of the rumen and reticulum begins to progressively lose tone and the ability to contract. This phenomenon is mediated by the increasing concentrations of volatile fatty acids in the ruminal contents. These acids interact with epithelial receptors in the ruminal and reticular mucosa to inhibit ruminal and reticular contractions via the vagovagal reflex. The subsequent build-up of lactic acid resulting from overgrowth of streptococci is corrosive to the mucosa of these organs and causes a **chemical rumenitis and reticulitis** leading to damage and loss of epithelium in these organs. Concomitant with these events, there may be cessation of salivation leading to loss of the buffering effect of salivary bicarbonate on ruminal pH. Furthermore, the increased lactic acid concentration in the ruminal and intestinal contents increases the osmotic pressure of the ingesta, which attracts water and electrolytes from the blood, leading to clinical dehydration, hemoconcentration, anuria, and eventually shock. Animals also develop clinical acidosis due to absorption of lactic acid from the rumen.

Postmortem findings in animals dying of ruminal acidosis are not specific, but include signs of dehydration and hemoconcentration. The ruminal contents may have a thick consistency and a distinct odor of fermentation. Microscopically, the ruminal papillae are swollen and the squamous epithelium has prominent cytoplasmic vacuolization, vesiculation with or without erosions, and ulcers. There is generally a variable number of neutrophils present in the lamina propria of papillae. The ruminal erosions and ulcerations resulting from this chemical rumenitis predispose those animals that survive this condition to ruminal infection by opportunistic pathogens, such as *Fusobacterium necrophorum* and fungi in the genera *Mucor*, *Rhizopus*, and *Absidia*. Rumenitis may also be associated with hepatic abscesses.

Necrobacillary rumenitis usually affects the papillated portions of the mucosa of the ventral portion of the rumen and less often the pillars. The early lesion consists of small to large areas where the mucosal papillae appear darker than normal, soft, and covered by an inflammatory exudate. These areas of necrotic papillae eventually slough and become re-epithelialized without regeneration of the papillae. The healed areas may be so small as to be inapparent, or may appear as stellate areas of scar tissue confined mainly to the mucosa (Fig. 23-10).

Mycotic rumenitis, in contrast to necrobacillary rumenitis, tends to extend into the underlying tunica muscularis and may involve the underlying serosa and adjacent peritoneal structures. The mucosal surfaces may contain areas of ulceration, necrosis, and thrombosis because of the tendency of these organisms to invade blood vessels and produce infarction. In addition, in pregnant cows these lesions may serve as a source of infection for mycotic placentitis leading to abortion or stillbirth (see Chapter 25).

Virus-induced ruminal ulceration occurs with numerous generalized epitheliotropic virus infections of domestic animals. These are discussed under the specific etiologic agent in Chapter 8.

References

Allison MJ, Robinson IM, Dougherty RW, et al. Grain overload in cattle and sheep: Changes in microbiological populations in the cecum and rumen. Am J Vet Res 1975;36:181–185.

Chihaya Y, Matsukawa K, Mizushima S, et al. Ruminant forestomach and abomasal mucormycosis under rumen acidosis. Vet Pathol 1988;25:119–123.

Crichlow EC. Ruminal lactic acidosis: Forestomach epithelial receptor activation by undissociated volatile fatty acids and rumen fluids collected during loss of reticuloruminal motility. Res Vet Sci 1988;45:364–368.

Jensen R, Connell WE, Deem AW. Rumenitis and its relation to rate of change of ration and the proportion of concentrate in the ration of cattle. J Anim Sci 1954;15:425–428.

Jensen R, Deane HM, Cooper LJ, et al. Rumenitis-liver abscess complex in beef cattle. Am J Vet Res 1954;15:202–216.

Nichols RE, Penn KE. Simple methods for the detection of unfavorable changes in ruminal ingesta. J Am Vet Med Assoc 1958;133:275–279.

Russell JB, Hino T. Regulation of lactate production in Streptococcus bovis: A spiraling effect that contributes to rumen acidosis. J Dairy Sci 1985;68:1712–1721.

Slyter LL. Influence of acidosis on rumen function. J Anim Sci 1976;43:910–929.

Smith HA. Ulcerative lesions of the bovine rumen and their possible relation to hepatic abscesses. Am J Vet Res 1944;5:234–243.

Vestweber JGE, Leipold HW. Experimentally induced ovine ruminal acidosis: Pathologic changes. Am J Vet Res 1974;35:1537–1540.

Traumatic reticulitis/peritonitis

The bovine species does not have highly sensitive prehensile organs, i.e. lips and tongue, nor a discriminating sense of taste. As a consequence, cattle kept in farmyards, stables, or at other sites close to human mechanical activities are prone to swallow metallic objects such as nails, screws, and pieces of wire that have been carelessly left in their feeding areas. No doubt some of these objects are even picked up from the pasture as the cow wraps its tongue around a choice clump of grass. The incidence of this condition has been significantly reduced by the increased use of twine rather than wire to bind bales of hay, and by the placement of magnets in the reticulum to retain metallic objects in the lumen.

Most foreign bodies almost always remain in the reticulum, being retained there by the baffle-like folds of its mucosal lining (Fig. 23-10A). No particular harm results from the presence of smooth foreign bodies, but sharp ones either become entrapped in perforations they have made in one or more of the mucosal folds or penetrate the wall of the organ. The perforation of a fold alone is a relatively harmless event as shown by the fact that many healthy cattle are slaughtered and found to have nails or pieces of wire embedded horizontally in the reticulated mucosal folds with small white, scarred areas around them. Those that penetrate the wall proper are gradually forced through it by the recurrent peristaltic contractions of the organ.

While migration of the foreign body in any direc-

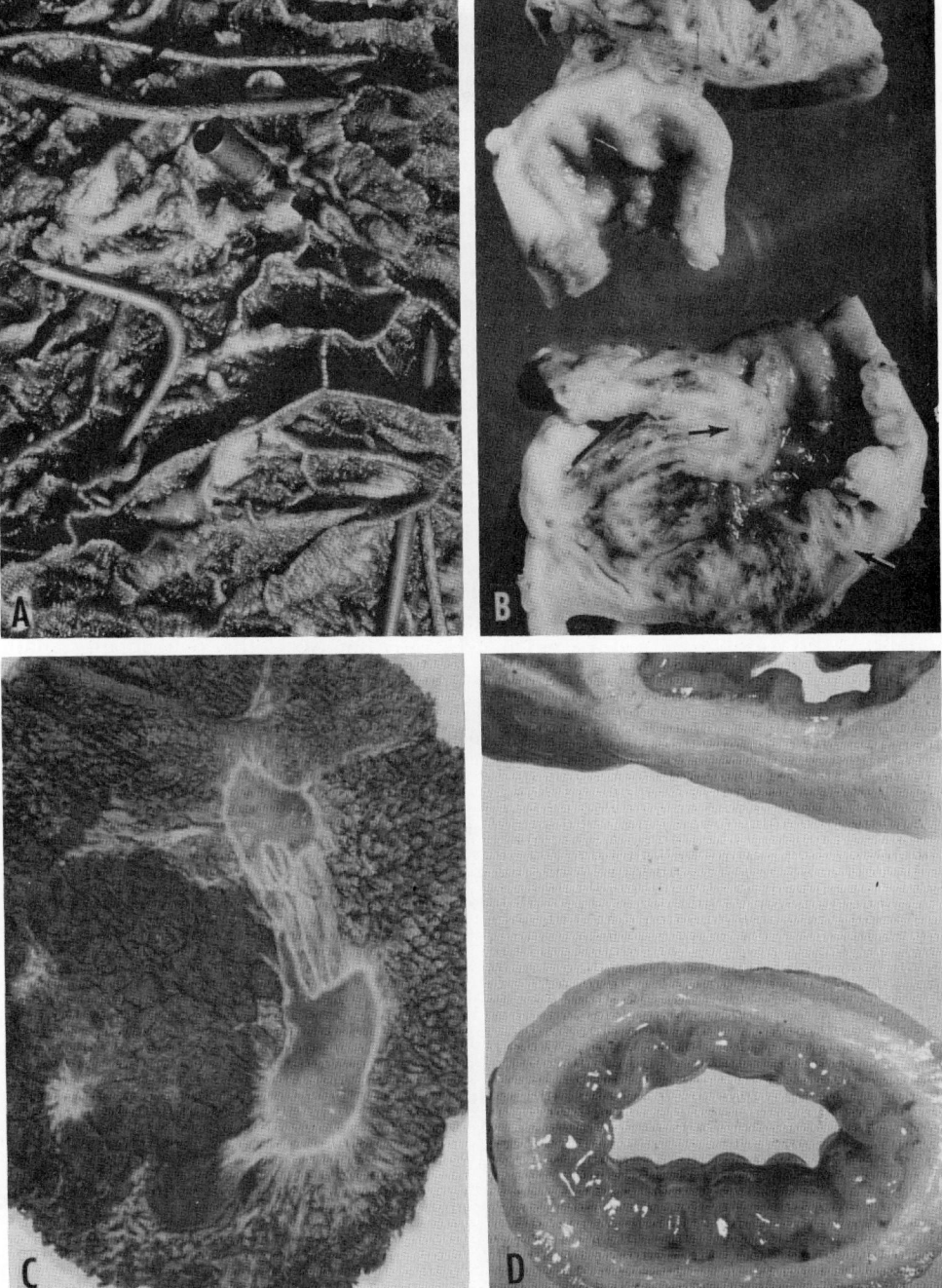

FIG. 23-10. **A.** Foreign bodies in the reticulum of a cow. Note that one nail (lower right) has penetrated the wall. Objects such as these may lead to traumatic gastritis. (Courtesy College of Veterinary Medicine, Iowa State University.) **B.** Regional cicatrizing enterocolitis in a two-year-old dog given euthanasia because of severe diarrhea for six months. (Courtesy Texas A&M School of Veterinary Medicine.) **C.** Ulcers in the rumen of a fattened steer which was slaughtered in apparently normal health. The large dark area at left is undergoing necrosis and would have sloughed. (Courtesy of Colorado State School of Veterinary Medicine.) **D.** Edema of the mucosa and submucosa of the ileum incarcerated in an umbilical hernia in a four-year-old mule. Death followed laparotomy and attempted relief. (Courtesy College of Veterinary Medicine, Iowa State University.)

tion is possible, the vast majority move anterioventrally. They pass through the diaphragm and into the pericardium and heart muscle, carrying ingesta and contaminating bacteria with them, and causing the condition known as **traumatic pericarditis,** or more colorfully **"hardware disease."** There may also be a purulent pleuritis or pneumonia associated with the condition. Movement of the foreign body is usually gradual, so that a dense fibrous wall encircles the path of the wire or penetrating object. Sometimes the foreign object is retracted back into the rumen through the peristaltic movement of this organ and is not found at necropsy.

It is not unusual for iron-containing pieces of wire or nail to become completely rusted out by the time pericardial infection reaches its usually fatal outcome. In such cases, the diagnosis can still be made in the absence of a foreign body in the lesion by finding the dense fibrous encapsulating mass of highly variable size and shape, and containing a slender, blackened tract, usually present along the path created by the penetrating foreign object. The anterior surface of the reticulum is usually adherent to the diaphragm and examination for adhesions in this region should constitute a part of every bovine necropsy. Not infrequently, there are also heavily encapsulated abscesses in the vicinity. If the foreign body penetrates the reticulum in a different direction, there is localized (rarely generalized) peritonitis with intra-abdominal abscesses that may also be present in the liver or spleen. Bacterial organisms commonly contaminating the foreign object and causing the pericarditis, pleuritis, or peritonitis, include, among others, the pyogenic organisms *Actinomyces pyogenes* and *Fusobacterium necrophorum*. If the penetrating foreign body happens to involve the vagus nerves, ruminal atony may lead to failure of reticuloruminal emptying and what has been termed **"vagal indigestion"**.

Omasum

The omasum and the esophageal groove are seldom the site of important pathologic processes. Actinobacillosis rarely localizes in the region, producing the characteristic pyogranulomas. Malignant lymphomas may produce neoplastic masses in any of the local tissues, but are more likely to infiltrate the wall of the rumen or abomasum. Rarely, horn-like growths several millimeters in diameter and some 2 to 4 cm in height occur on the edges of the esophageal groove, on nearby portions of the pillars of the rumen, or at the opening of the omasum. These lesions represent viral-induced papillomas, and are essentially of no clinical significance.

References

Fubini SS, Ducharme NG, Erb HN, et al. Failure of omasal transport attributable to perireticular abscess formation in cattle: 29 cases (1980–1986). J Am Vet Med Assoc 1989;194:811–814.
Misra SS, Angelo SJ. Traumatic reticulopericarditis in bovines. Vet Res J 1981;4:89–113.

Neoplasms of the Forestomachs

The association of bovine papillomavirus type-4 infection and chronic bracken fern poisoning with papillomas and squamous cell carcinomas in the upper digestive tract (esophagus, rumen, reticulum, and omasum) has been discussed. Lymphosarcoma may occasionally involve the wall of the forestomachs.

References

Campo MS. Papillomas and cancer in cattle. Cancer Surv 1987;6:39–54.
Jarrett WFH, Campo MS, Baxter ML, et al. Alimentary fibropapilloma in cattle: A spontaneous tumor nonpermissive for papillomavirus replication. J Natl Cancer Instit 1984;73:499–504.
Plowright W, Linsell CA, Peers FG. A focus of rumenal cancer in Kenyan cattle. Br J Cancer 1971;25:72–80.
Sundberg JP, O'Banion MK. Animal papillomaviruses associated with malignant tumors. Adv Viral Oncol 1989;8:55–71.

STOMACH

The abomasum of ruminants is essentially similar in anatomic structure and physiologic function to the glandular stomach of monogastric mammals. Some animals, such as the rat and horse, have a portion of the stomach lined by stratified squamous epithelium. This is continuous with the squamous epithelium of the esophagus and forms the cardia of the stomach. The fundus is lined by thick glandular epithelium which contains both parietal and chief cells. The pyloric epithelium is continuous with that of the duodenum and is lined by serous and mucus-secreting cells. In each species, the relative size of these distinct anatomic and specialized regions of the stomach is somewhat different and may affect the kind and frequency of lesions in the stomach. In general, however, the stomachs of most nonruminants have similar functions and lesions.

Pyloric stenosis and hypertrophy

Functional pyloric stenosis with or without anatomic lesions occurs with some frequency in young dogs and infrequently in cats and horses. Clinically, it is characterized by delayed gastric emptying, which leads to frequent vomiting and poor growth rate. In some cases, there is grossly visible hypertrophy of the pyloric smooth muscle; whereas in others it appears to be mainly a functional disorder of the gastric sphincter without gross or microscopic lesions. Myomectomy of the pyloric musculature often corrects the functional deficit that characterizes this disorder. Pyloric stenosis may also occur in older animals due to trauma-induced strictures of the pylorus.

In older dogs, a gastric-emptying disorder characterized by intermittent vomition has been termed **hypertrophic pyloric gastropathy**. It is recognized most often in small breeds where it seemingly is an acquired disease. Anatomically, it is characterized by hypertrophy of the pyloric mucosa with or without musculature hypertropy. Its cause is unknown. Grossly, the pyloric mucosa is excessive and thrown up into focal or diffuse folds or rugae. Microscopically, the folds consist of masses of redundant mucosal glands, some of which may be cystic. Lymphocytes and plasma cells are often present in the lamina propria and submucosa. Smooth muscle fibers of the pyloric sphincter may also be hypertrophied.

Gastric dilatation and torsion

Acute distension of the stomach with gas occurs in several species including humans, dogs, horses, swine, rabbits, cats, rhesus monkeys (*Macaca mulatta*), and squirrel monkeys (*Saimiri sciureus*). This life-threatening condition appears to have been studied most extensively in the dog, hence the following remarks will apply especially to the canine disease. The canine disorder is manifested by obvious discomfort, abdominal pain, marked distension of the abdomen, and reluctance to move. Larger breeds of dogs are more often affected, including German shepherds, Great Danes, Irish setters, weimaraners, Doberman pinschers, Saint Bernards, and boxers. Toy and standard-sized breeds are rarely affected.

The cause is generally unknown, although many events have been associated with dilatation, including parturition, overeating, pica, abdominal surgery, and trauma. Most observers are convinced that acute gastric dilatation precedes torsion of the stomach, which is a common sequel. The stomach becomes rotated 190 to 300° around its long axis, resulting in twisting of the gastrosplenic omentum.

The effects of the gastric dilatation have been confirmed by experimental inflation of the stomach with a balloon. This results in mechanical obstruction of the caudal vena cava and portal vein, resulting in shunting of blood into the intervertebral and azygos veins. The common iliac, deep circumflex iliac, and renal veins also are distended by this obstruction. Cardiac output is decreased, arterial hypotension results; cellular catabolism is increased, and renal function is decreased.

Impaired renal function is indicated by rapid elevation of serum urea nitrogen, phosphorus, and creatinine. Serum glucose is elevated, as is serum aspartate aminotransferase (AST), formerly SGOT. Metabolic acidosis is evident from decrease in arterial HCO_3 values.

The principal postmortum findings following sudden death, or death during the night, are the greatly enlarged stomach, distended with gas and variable amounts of ingesta. Torsion may result in twisting of the gastrosplenic omentum. Veins in the caudal aspect of the body are usually severely engorged and the associated tissues congested. The stomach may have ruptured, spilling its contents into the peritoneal cavity. The cranial aspect of the body is usually ischemic and pale. The liver may be pale and friable, and the spleen may be engorged with blood. Petechiae and ecchymoses may be seen in the peritoneum and elsewhere. Sometimes subcutaneous edema is apparent.

Acute dilatation in the horse usually leads to rupture of the stomach. The condition in nonhuman primates closely resembles the canine disease. Rabbits may also be afflicted. The disorder also has been reported in swine, usually in breeding-age sows.

References

Betts CW, Wingfield WE, Greene RW. A retrospective study of gastric dilation-torsion in the dog. J Small Anim Pract 1974;15:727–734.

Blackbum PW, McCrea CT, Randall CJ. Torsion of the stomach in sows. Vet Rec 1974;94:578.

Cedervall A. Gastric torsion in swine. Acta Vet Scand 1971;12:142–144.

Chapman WL Jr. Acute gastric dilation in *Macaca mulatta* and *Macaca speciosa* monkeys. Lab Anim Care 1967;17:130–136.

Hall JA. Canine gastric dilation-volvulus update. Sem Vet Med Surg (Small Anim) 1989;4:188–193.

Horne WA, Gilmore DR, Dietze AE, et al. Effects of gastric distention-volvulus on coronary blood flow and myocardial oxygen consumption in the dog. Am J Vet Res 1985;46:98–104.

Newton WM, Beamer PD, Rhoades HE. Acute bloat syndrome in stumptailed macaques (Macaca arctoides): a report of four cases. Lab Anim Sci 1971;21:193–196.

Turner AE, Cowey A. Bloat syndrome in captive Rhesus monkeys: report on twelve cases. J Inst Anim Tech 1971;22:181–186.

Wingfield WE, Cornelius LM, DeYoung DW. Pathophysiology of the gastric dilation-torsion complex in the dog. J Small Anim Pract 1974;15:735–739.

Wingfield WE, Cornelius LM, DeYoung DW. Experimental acute gastric dilation and torsion in the dog. 1. Changes in biochemical and acid-base parameters. J Small Anim Pract 1975;16:41–53.

Wingfield WE, Cornelius LM, Ackerman N, et al. Experimental acute gastric dilation and torsion in the dog. 2. Venous angiographic

alterations seen in gastric dilation. J Small Anim Pract 1975; 16:55–60.

Displacement of the abomasum

Under certain conditions, as yet poorly defined, the abomasum may be displaced from its ventral and right-sided position in the anterior abdomen to the left side of the abdomen, displacing the rumen to the right. The abomasum moves along the abdominal floor to the left then between the left abdominal wall and the rumen. The cause is unknown although the condition is believed to be preceded by atony and gaseous distention of the abomasum. It is more apt to occur in older dairy cows and is associated with feeding of rations containing high proportions of concentrates rather than roughage. It often follows recent parturition and metritis. Less frequently, the displaced abomasum is found in the right flank rather than the left. More frequent occurrence in certain families has been cited as evidence of predisposing genetic factors.

Clinical signs include anorexia, depression, dehydration, and distended abdomen, particularly protrusion in the left paralumbar fossa. The history often includes recent parturition. Auscultation and percussion are used to detect the abnormal position of the abomasum. If the displacement is not corrected immediately, the condition is fatal.

References

Coppock CE. Displaced abomasum in dairy cattle: etiological factors. J Dairy Sci 1974;57:926–933.

Fubini SL, Grohn YT, Smith DF. Right displacement of the abomasum and abomasal volvulus in dairy cows: 458 cases (1980–1987). J Am Vet Med Assoc 1991;198:460–464.

Jones BEV, Poulsen JSD. Abomasal emptying rate in goats and cows measured by extemal counting of radioactive sodium chromate injected directly into the abomasum. Nord Vet Med 1974;26:13–21.

Martin W. Left abomasal displacement: an epidemiological study. Can Vet J 1972;13:61–68.Poulsen JSD. Clinical chemical examination of a case of left-side abomasal displacement, changing to a right-sided displacement. Nord Vet Med 1974;26:91–96.

Poulsen JSD. Variations in the metabolic acid-base balance and some other clinical chemical parameters in dairy herds during the year. Nord Vet Med 1974;26:1–12.

Poulsen JSD. Right-sided abomasal displacement in dairy cows: Pre- and postoperative clinical chemical findings. Nord Vet Med 1974;26:65–90.

Robertson J. Left displacement of the bovine abomasum: epizootiologic factors. Am J Vet Res 1968;29:421–434.

Smith DF. Right-side torsion of the abomasum in dairy cows: Classification of severity and evaluation of outcome. J Am Vet Med Assoc 1978;173:108–111.

Stober M, Wegner W, Lunebnnk. J. Research on the familial occurrence of left-side displacement of the abomasum in cattle. Bovine Pract 1975;10:59–61.

Impaction

Impaction of the stomach in the horse as the result of rapid ingestion of an excessive amount of ground feed, heavy grains (wheat, corn), or fibrous roughage, without adequate water consumption, is especially serious. Even without gaseous fermentation, which is usual, absorption of toxic products of partial digestion, circulatory disturbances, and shock may be fatal in a few hours or may result in laminitis.

Parasites

A wide variety of parasites may infest the stomach. In horses infestations by *Gastrophilus spp.* larvae, *Habronema spp.*, *Draschia spp.* and *Trichostrongylus axei* are common. In **swine** *Hyostrongylus rubidus*, *Ascarops spp.* *Physocephalus spp.* and *Simondsia spp.* cause gastritis. In **ruminants** stomach worms are a major problem. The more common of these are *Haemonchus spp.*, *Mecistocirrus spp.*, *Ostertagia spp.*, and *Trichostrongylus axei*. **Dogs** occasionally become infested with *Physaloptera spp* and *Gnathostoma spp.* In cats *Physaloptera spp.*, *Cyclicospirura felineus,* and *Ollulanus tricuspis* are associated with inflammatory lesions of the gastric mucosa.

Gastritis

Inflammation of the stomach is essentially a disorder of its mucosal lining. Clinically it is characterized by pain, anorexia, and vomiting. The latter sign is invariably present in gastritis, but may also be induced by reverse peristalsis initiated lower in the gastrointestinal tract, as well as by certain central nervous disorders. Gastritis is usually catarrhal or hemorrhagic in type.

Acute catarrhal gastritis appears as an increased reddening and thickening of the entire surface or parts of the gastric mucosa, the fundic area often being the most severely involved. There is an increase in mucus secretion, which may or may not be discernible grossly. Microscopically, the redness is due to a combination of hyperemia and desquamation of the epithelium. It can be difficult to differentiate the desquamation from that which occurs with postmortem autolysis. These changes may be accompanied by a mild to moderate lymphocytic or, less commonly, neutrophilic infiltration of the mucosa and submucosa. Hyperplasia of the normally minute mucosal lymphoid nodules present in the gastric mucosa is often apparent microscopically, but in chronic cases may even be seen grossly as small white mucosal nodules.

Acute hemorrhagic gastritis is also common and can be distinguished grossly by deeper reddening and by the presence of free blood on the surface or in the gastric contents. It should be noted that blood which has remained for any considerable time exposed to the gastric juice turns brown-black; commonly, it is mixed with mucus and appears as a slimy, viscid, brownish substance, clinging more or less to the gastric surface. In such cases, the hemorrhage is also present within the gastric mucosa microscopically. The presence of free blood in the mucosa and lumen of the stomach without evidence of an accompanying inflammatory reaction should be interpreted as hemorrhage, rather than hemorrhagic gastritis.

Catarrhal or **hemorrhagic gastritis** is a typical effect of various locally destructive poisons, but is also a characteristic lesion of certain infectious diseases, including swine erysipelas. The bites or points of attachment of several kinds of parasitic helminths, especially the trichostrongyles of ruminants, leave tiny hemorrhages or foci of inflammation. With large numbers of parasites, the tiny foci eventually become more or less confluent.

Serous fluid (serous exudate), usually termed inflammatory edema, may be a prominent feature of gastritis, causing marked thickening of the mucosa and submucosa. The other varieties of acute inflammation are unusual in the stomach, although a fibrinous exudate may be formed in response to certain infections of a previously injured mucosa. Certain poisons exert specific effects upon the gastric mucosa when ingested in concentrated form. Mercuric chloride produces coagulative necrosis and at the same time acts as a fixative, preserving the tissue from postmortem changes. Carbolic acid has a similar effect and turns the surface white or gray. Non-steroidal inflammatory drugs, including aspirin, have also been associated with hemorrhagic gastritis and ulceration.

Chronic hypertrophic gastritis ("giant rugal gastritis," "gastritis hypertrophia gigantica") has been described in dogs with a condition resembling Menetrier's protein-losing gastropathy of humans. The disease has been described in boxer, Basenji and Drentse patrijshond (a Dutch breed of setter) dogs. Its etiology is unknown. It is manifested by lethargy, emaciation, vomiting, prolonged anorexia, anemia, hepatic disease, and icterus. Protein is lost, resulting in hypoalbuminemia in late stages of the disease. The lesions consist of marked elevation and folding of the mucosa into prominent rugae due to severe local epithelial hyperplasia, particularly in the fundus around the greater curvature. These gross changes may be associated with progressive loss of parietal cells with compensatory hyperplasia of mucus-secreting goblet cells. Mononuclear inflammatory cells are present in the superficial, variably edematous portions of the lamina propria. Cystic glands are seen at the base of the crypts.

Gastritis glandularis and **gastritis cystica profunda** are terms used to describe a gastropathy observed in nonhuman primates *(Macaca mulatta)* (Scotti, 1973). The gross lesions are diffuse, involving much of the gastric mucosa, but vary in individual cases. The mucosal folds are large in some cases, small and inconspicuous in others. Hyperemia and petechiae are common in the mucosa, and occasional ulcers may be seen. The microscopic lesions include hyperplasia of the mucosa with many mucus-filled cysts in both the mucosa and submucosa. The causes of this lesion are not known but it appears likely that ingestion of some chemical toxins, such as polychlorinated biphenyls, should be considered.

Lymphocytic gastritis of cats, dogs, ferrets, and nonhuman primates has been associated with infection by *Helicobacter felis* and *H. pylori. H. pylori*, formerly known as Campylobacter pylori, is now recognized as a common cause of chronic gastritis and gastric and duodenal ulcers in people.

Eosinophilic gastritis is the term used for severe inflammatory lesions of the stomach, in which eosinophils are a conspicuous component. This chronic gastritis may result in fibrosis of the stomach wall, with fibrinoid necrosis of the wall of muscular arteries. Eosinophilia is usually present in this condition. Polyarteritis may be observed in the omentum and reticuloendothelial hyperplasia may be severe in the spleen. Lymph nodes and liver may contain similar infiltrates. These lesions resemble those described in visceral larva migrans in dogs, except that the helminth larvae are not usually seen. It is possible, but not established, that this lesion may result from repeated infection of a dog with helminth larvae (possibly *Toxocara canis*), after the animal has already been rendered immune by prior infection.

References

Barron CN, Saunders LZ. Visceral larva migrans in a dog. Pathol Vet 1966;3:315–330.
Hayden DW, Van Kruiningen HJ. Eosinophilic gastroenteritis in German shepherd dogs and its relationship to visceral larva migrans. J Am Vet Med Assoc. 1973;162:379–384.
Hayden DW, Fleischman RW. Scirrhous eosinophilic gastritis in dogs with gastric artentis. Vet Pathol 1977;14:441–448.
Kipnis RM. Focal cystic hypertrophic gastropathy in a dog. J Am Vet Med Assoc 1978;173:182–194.
Lee A, Krakowka S, Fox JG, et al. Role of *Helicobacter felis* in chronic canine gastritis. Vet Pathol 1992;29:487–494.
Scotti TM. Simian gastropathy with submucosal glands and cysts. Gastritis glandularis or cystica profunda. Arch Pathol 1973;96:403–408.
Slappendel RJ, van der Gaag I, van Nes JJ et al. Familial stomatocytosis—hypertrophic gastritis (FSHG), a newly recognized disease in the dog (Drentse patrijshond) Vet Quart 1991;13:30–40.
Van Der Gaag I,.Happe RP, Wolvekamp WTC. A boxer dog with chronic hypertrophic gastritis resembling Menetrier's disease in man. Vet Pathol 1976;13:172–185.
Van Kruiningen HJ. Giant hypertrophic gastritis of Basenji dogs. Vet Pathol 1977;14:15–18.

Hemorrhages

Large and small hemorrhages may occur in the gastric mucosa under any of the circumstances listed as causative in the general discussion of hemorrhage, but localized and generalized toxic conditions occupy a prominent place among them. **Uremia** is among the latter, as well as canine "blacktongue." Outstanding among the hemorrhage-producing infections likely to involve the gastric mucosa are hog cholera (swine fever), anthrax, and leptospirosis. Numerous small or punctate hemorrhages, some being old and faded, should lead to a search for helminth parasites, especially for the trichostrongyles of cattle and sheep. On the peritoneal surface, hemorrhages signify either hemorrhage-inducing poisons or infections.

Chronic passive congestion, with or without (noninflammatory) edema, represents the effect upon the stomach of the circulatory impairment which results from cirrhosis or cardiac insufficiency.

Ulcers

Some of the infectious or chemical gastritides are ulcerative, especially in the later stages, and some of the hemorrhages result from erosions or ulcerations, but all of these ulcers are acute and superficial. Ulceration of

the gastric mucosa is now recognized in most domestic species. Some differences between species are apparent, and the etiology may not be the same in each species.

In **cattle**, ulcers in the abomasum occur commonly, expecially in calves, dairy cows and yearling cattle in feedlots. These usually go unrecognized clinically. Necropsies of 1988 yearling cattle in feedlots (Uensen, et al., 1976) revealed 31 (1.6%) cattle in which death was due to perforation or hemorrhage of ulcers. About an equal number of cattle were found to have ulcers which had not perforated. These discrete ulcers were found largely in the pylorus of the abomasum. A study of adult cattle (Aukema and Breukink, 1974) revealed most ulcers to be in the ventral part of the fundus with few in the pylorus. Among 1370 presumed normal cattle, 1% were found at slaughter to have ulcers; in 1200 cows brought in for "emergency slaughter" (due to some illness), 9.1% were found to have abomasal ulcers. In this same study, 141 cows were identified with fatal hemorrhages from abomasal ulcers.

The cause or causes of abomasal ulcers are not known. Several environmental conditions, including stress of transportation and dietary alterations, have been associated with the disease but these have not been unequivocally proven to be causes.

Ulceration of the squamous portion of stomach (pars esophagea) in **swine** is a common and sometimes serious disease. The gastric content of affected swine is usually fluid. The ulcers are irregular in shape and may be single or multiple, varying in size from a few millimeters to several centimeters in diameter, and involve only a small portion, or most of the gastric squamous mucosa. Chronic ulcers appear as punched-out craters surrounded by elevated rolled edges. Histologically, the ulcers extend into the submucosa but rarely beyond, and are associated with edema, arteritis, infiltration of neutrophils and eosinophils, and hyperplasia of submucosal lymphoid follicles. Adjacent epithelium is acanthotic and parakeratotic: changes which are believed to develop prior to erosion and ulceration. Blood in varying quantities may be mixed with the gastric contents. Healed ulcers leave contracted scars. Depending on the degree of ulceration, clinical signs may be inapparent, as death may result from acute gastric hemorrhage without premonitory signs. More often the affected animals are weak, pale (anemic), and dyspneic. Vomiting may occur, and the feces may be tarry. The cause of gastric ulceration in swine is not known. Hyperacidity appears to play an important role in this condition. The feeding of gelatinized corn and finely ground grain rations appears to play an important role in its pathogenesis. Experimentally, animals with this condition have delayed gastric emptying which results in decreased pH of the gastric contents. The squamous portion of the pig's stomach is less resistant to gastric hyperacidity than the glandular portion and thus is more susceptible to its corrosive effect.

Ulceration of the glandular stomach of swine is much less frequent and not associated with ulceration of the nonglandular stomach. Experimental studies have suggested that genetic factors play a significant role in the pathogenesis of gastric ulcers in swine (Grondalen and Vangen, 1974).

Ulceration of the nonglandular portion of the stomach is occasionally encountered in **foals**. Rooney (1964) believes they are related to mechanical trauma by *Gastrophilus intestinalis* larvae, stones, etc. Ulceration of the glandular mucosa also occurs in horses and is common in calves.

Ulcers of the pylorus and proximal duodenum are often associated with solitary, multiple or disseminated mast cell tumors in **dogs** and **cats** (Fig. 23-11). Some of these cases are clinically silent and thus go unrecognized, others are associated with chronic vomiting. These ulcers result from gastric hyperacidity as a result of the hyperhistaminemia associated with these tumors.

In people, chronic gastric ulcers have been associated with ingestion of nonsteroidal anti-inflammatory drugs (NSAIDs) and has been produced experimentally in rats by aspirin administration. The rats develop ulcers in the esophageal (squamous) part of the stomach when given 250 to 500 mg aspirin per day; with slightly smaller doses, multiple erosions appear in the mucosa of the fundus.

References

Angus KW, Bannatyne CC. Abomasal ulceration in adult sheep: a report of two contrasting cases. Vet Rec 1970;86:531–533.

Aukema JJ, Breukink HJ. Abomasal ulcer in adult cattle with fatal haemorrhage. Cornell Vet 1974;64:303–317.

Baustad B, Nafstad I. Gastric ulcers in swine. 4. Effects of dietary particle size and crude fiber contents on ulceration. Pathol Vet 1969;6:546–556.

Berruecos JM, Robison OW. Inheritance of gastric ulcers in swine. J Anim Sci 1972;35:20–24.

Bivin WS, DeBarros CL, DeBarros SS, et al. Gastric ulcers in Brazilian swine. J Am Vet Med Assoc 1974;164:405–407.

Grondalen T, Vangen O. Gastric ulcers in pigs selected for leanness or fatness. Nord Vet Med 1974;26:50–53.

Jensen R, Pierson RE, Braddy PM, et al. Fatal abomasal ulcers in yearling feedlot cattle. J Am Vet Med Assoc 1976;169:524–526.

Norton LP, Nolan JE, Sales L, et al. A swine stress ulcer model. Ann Surg 1972;176:133–138.

Penny RHC, Edwards MJ, Mulley R. Gastric ulcer in the pig: a New South Wales abattoir survey of the incidence of lesions of the pars oesophagea. Br Vet J 1972;128:43–49.

Rooney JR. Gastric ulceration in foals. Pathol Vet 1964;1:497–503.

St. John DJ, Yeomans ND, Deboer WG. Chronic gastric ulcer induced by aspirin: an experimental model. Gastroenterology 1973; 65:634–641.

Tasker JB, Roberts SJ, Fox FH, et al. Abomasal ulcers in cattle—recovery of one cow after surgery. J Am Vet Med Assoc 1958;133:365–368.

Foreign bodies

Foreign bodies are occasionally encountered, for instance, a rubber ball in the stomach of a dog. Hair balls occur commonly in long-haired cats where they may be associated with vomiting. Phytobezoars and trichophytobezoars are occasionally observed in lambs and calves.

Neoplasms of the stomach

The statement is often recorded that tumors of the stomach of animals are rare. While it is true that not many cases have been reported, it appears likely that many cases are either not recognized or, if recognized, simply not reported.

Adenocarcinoma of the stomach has been reported in a variety of species but is most frequently reported in the dog where it is the most common gastric neoplasm (Lingeman, et al., 1971) (Fig. 23-12). Most canine gastric adenocarcinomas arise in the pyloric antrum along the lesser curvature. The tumors tend to aggressively invade the wall of the stomach and often are superficially ulcerated, appearing as a large crater with raised edges. Metastases to lymph nodes, liver, and lung occur with some frequency.

The most frequent type in the dog is described as diffuse with epithelial cells diffusely infiltrating the stomach wall. The tumor cells obviously arise from columnar epithelium of the gastric mucosa, but may, in some species, be papillary, tubular, mucinous, or signet

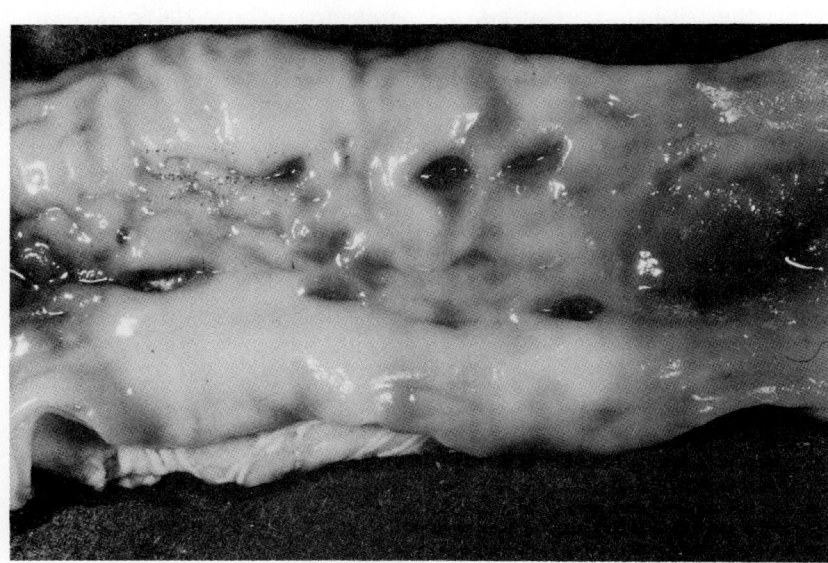

FIG. 23-11. Ulcers in duodenum of a five-year-old spayed female cat. Neoplastic mast cells invaded the spleen. (Courtesy of Angell Memorial Animal Hospital.)

ring cell types (Head, 1976). In the papillary type, the epithelium forms frond-like layers of cells, similar to those seen in papillary adenomas. Tubular structures may predominate in some tumors in other species. The neoplastic cells are mucus-secreting or of the signet-ring configuration in most cases. Signet ring cells get their characteristic shape by the accumulation of mucus in the cytoplasm, which displaces the nucleus to one side of the cell. All of these cells characteristically invade the gastric submucosa and muscularis and eventually metastasize by way of the lymphatics.

Adenomas or benign adenomatous polyps characteristically project from the mucosa into the lumen. They consist of hyperplastic epithelial cells which form elongated villi (papillary or villous form) or irregular tubules (adenomatous polyp). Some tumors may have combined features (papillotubular). Papillomas have been described in the stomach of monkeys (*Macaca fascicularis* and *M. arctoides*) in association with the helminth *(Nochtia nochti)*. The parasites may be seen in microscopic sections, hence should be easily associated with this type of polyp.

Undifferentiated carcinomas (carcinoma simplex, medullary carcinoma, solid carcinoma) are occasionally seen and may be identified by their component of large epithelial cells with many mitoses, in solid nests or masses of cells. Tubules and squamous cells are not present.

Squamous cell carcinomas arise from the squamous epithelium of the cardia of the stomach. In those species which have a large stratifed squamous cardiac component to the stomach (horse, pig, rat), squamous cell carcinoma is more frequent than adenocarcinoma. The tumor is made up of squamous epithelial cells which

have in many places lost their normal polarity in relation to each other and the basement membrane. Mitoses are frequent and may be seen at sites outside the basal cell layer. Invasion of stroma is characteristic, and occasionally tumor cell emboli may be seen in lymphatics. Metastasis occurs by way of the lymphatics.

Leiomyoma and leiomyosarcoma may occasionally originate from the tunica muscularis of the stomach, although more frequently appear in the small or large intestine. The tumor cells resemble those of the muscularis except for irregular arrangement, mitoses, and occasionally very immature cells. The malignant form (leiomyosarcoma) is characteristically composed of more undifferentiated cells, has a higher mitotic index, and has a tendency to invade adjacent tissues. In both benign and malignant types, the tumor cells are arranged in interlacing bundles of parallel cells. Extension to adjacent tissues or organs and metastasis may occur with leiomyosarcoma.

Carcinoid tumors have been reported in the stomach of mastomys *(Mastomys natalensis)* and rarely in the dog. These tumors are composed of epithelial cells in small nests or packets; the cells have a centrally placed vesicular nucleus and finely granular cytoplasm. They are believed to arise from neuroendocrine or enterochromaffin cells which contain acidophilic cytoplasmic granules. In one type, the argentaffin tumor, the cells have the ability to reduce ammoniacal silver to metallic silver. In nonargentaffin tumors, the cells do not give the argentaffin reaction, but are argyrophilic. Neuroendocrine granules may be demonstrated in these cells by silver impregnation techniques with reducers and by electron microscopy.

These tumors arise within the mucosa, but spread

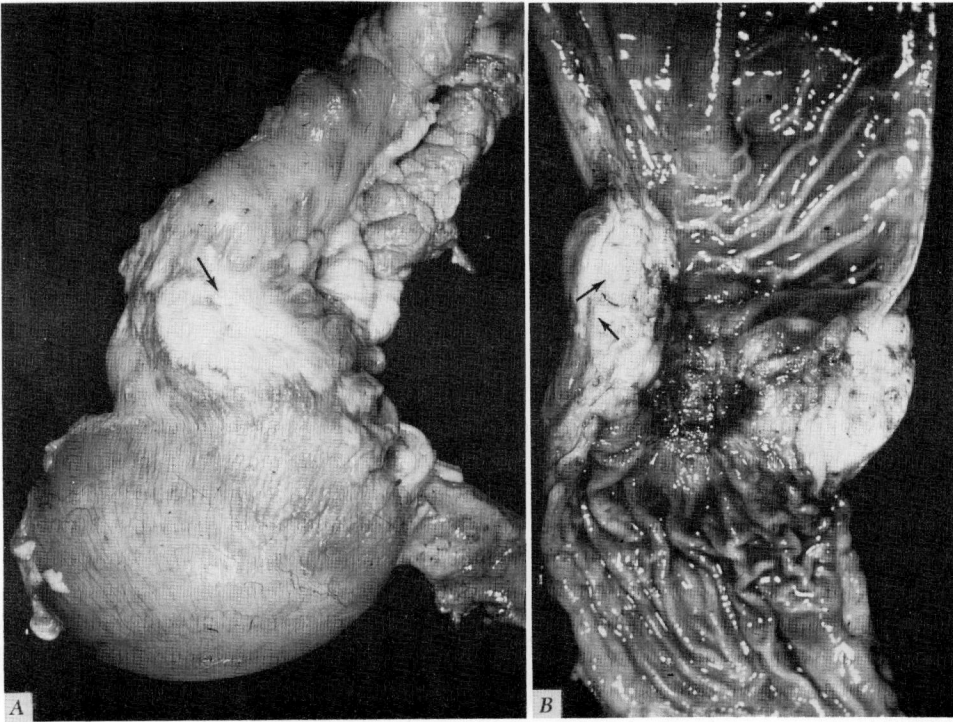

FIG. 23-12. A. Adenocarcinoma of stomach of an Irish setter, female, age 12 years. Note white scar (arrow) on serosal surface. A large ulcer was found on the opposing mucosal surface. **B.** Adenocarcinoma (arrow) of the rectum of an eight-year-old male Springer Spaniel. The tumor encircled the rectal wall, causing partial obstruction. (Courtesy of Angell Memorial Animal Hospital.)

to the submucosa. In the mastomys, these tumors have been shown to produce histamine but not serotonin.

Secondary tumors of the stomach include lymphosarcoma, mast cell tumor, and metastatic tumors from the liver or pancreas. Mesotheliomas of the peritoneum may occasionally involve the stomach wall.

References

Brody RS. Alimentary tract neoplasms in the cat. A clinicopathologic survey of 46 cases. Am J Vet Res 1966;27:74–80.

Conroy JD. Multiple gastric adenomatous polyps in a dog. J Comp Pathol 1969;79:465. Damodaran S, Ramachandran PV. Gastric carcinoma in equines. Indian Vet J 1970;47:118–120.

Davis CL, Naylor JR. Carcinoma in the stomach of a dog. J Am Vet Med Assoc 1943;102:286–288.

Fukushima Y, Kawachi T, Makanishi M. Histamine formation in spontaneous gastric carcinoids of Psamomys (mastomys) natalensis. Gann 1974;65:279–280.

Hayden DW, Nielsen SW. Canine alimentary neoplasia. Zentralbl Veterinaermed 1973;20A:1–22.

Head KW. International histological classification of tumors of domestic animals. XII. Tumors of the lower alimentary tract. Bull WHO 1976;53:167–186.

Krook L. On gastrointestinal carcinoma in the dog. Acta Pathol Microbiol Scand 1956;38:43–57.

Lapin BA, Krylova RI. Gastric polyps in monkeys of Sukhumi Colony. Z Versuchstierkd 1974;16:286–292.

Lingeman CH, Garner FM, Taylor DON. Spontaneous gastric adenocarcinomas of dogs. A review. J Natl Cancer Inst 1971;47:137–153.

Meagher DM, Wheat JD, Tennant B, et al. Squamous cell carcinoma of the equine stomach. J Am Vet Med Assoc 1974;164:81–84.

Murray M, Robinson PB, McKeating FJ, et al. Primary gastric neoplasia in dogs: a clinico-pathological study. Vet Rec 1972;91:474–489.

Patnaik AK, Hurvitz AI, Johnson GF. Canine gastrointestinal neoplasms. Vet Pathol 1977;14:547–555.

Patnaik AK, Hurvitz AI, Johnson GF. Canine gastric adenocarcinoma. Vet Pathol 1978;15:600–607.

Sautter JH, Hanlon GF. Gastric neoplasms in the dog: a report of 20 cases. J Am Vet Med Assoc 1975;168:691–696

Stewart HL. Experimentally induced gastric adenocarcinomas. Lab Invest 1971;25:672–674.

Sullivan M, Lee R, Fisher EW, et al. A study of 31 cases of gastric carcinoma in dogs. Vet Rec 1987;120:79–83.

Titis RS, Leipold HW, Anderson NV. Gastric carcinoma in a mare. J Am Vet Med Assoc 1972;161:270–274.

SMALL INTESTINE

Enteritis

The term enteritis commonly refers to inflammation of any or all parts of the intestinal tract, but most often is used to refer to inflammation of the small intestine only. Other terminology may be used when inflammation involves more than one part of the gastrointestinal tract, such as gastroenteritis (the entire tract), typhlitis or cecitis (involving the cecum), duodenitis, jejunitis, ileitis, colitis, and proctitis. Although in this chapter specific diseases of each part of the tract will be referred to separately, it should be remembered that several parts of the digestive system may be affected simultaneously.

Acute enteritis may conform to any one of the five types of acute exudative inflammation, and subacute lymphocytic and chronic proliferative forms are by no means rare. The whole small intestine may be rather uniformly inflamed, or even the small and large intestines together, but it is more often that the inflamma-

tion be more pronounced toward one end or the other of the small intestine, or perhaps even localized. The location of the inflammation, obviously, coincides with the site of greatest concentration of the inciting agent, be it chemical or infectious. Toxic substances which are ingested may be held for some time in the stomach so that their principal effect is a gastritis. Other toxic substances are of such nature that they are rather quickly propelled from the stomach to the intestine, where most of their effect occurs. Most bacterial enterotoxins are destroyed by gastric juice. Solubility of the initiating agent can also be a factor; those which dissolve slowly may be propelled to the intestine before becoming fully dissolved. The rather high acidity in the stomach and the relative alkalinity of the intestine are also important influences on solubility and absorption. If the agent is of an infectious nature, the time required for adequate replication of the organism may be instrumental in determining where their damage is greatest. A rather common situation is for the upper small intestine to be severely inflamed, with the ileum remaining relatively normal. This is ordinarily attributable to the injurious agent having been destroyed or at least diluted before it reached the lower portions of the small bowel. The length of time during which the ingesta remain in a given location is also important and may be responsible for a cecitis or colitis with little or no damage in the more motile small intestine.

When inflammation is principally confined to the colon, the possibility of its being caused by a toxic substance in the process of being eliminated there should be entertained. Numerous toxic substances of endogenous or exogenous origin are eliminated from the blood into the bowel, some of them principally in the large bowel (mercury, uremic products), causing injury and an inflammatory reaction in the mucosa through which they pass. Lastly, the specific tissue or cellular tropism of a particular infectious agent has to be considered: the coccidia of most mammals confine themselves almost entirely to the last part of the large bowel although certain species localize in the small intestine; the various avian coccidia have different sites of predilection: the cecum or the upper small intestine, depending on the species involved. Some microorganisms depend upon metazoan parasites to provide a portal of entry, and hence localize in the area favored by the metazoan species.

Specific viruses have a particular tropism for specific cell types in the intestinal epithelium. For example, the coronavirus of transmissible gastroenteritis of swine grows in and destroys most of the surface epithelium of the villus; sparing the cells in the crypts; rotaviruses of calf diarrhea and enzootic diarrhea of mice attack the most mature epithelium near the apex of the villus; the parvoviruses of feline panleukopenia and canine parvoviral enteritis have particular tropism for the dividing cells in the crypts of the intestinal mucosa, causing total collapse of the mucosa and impaired regeneration.

In **catarrhal enteritis,** acute or chronic, the changes simulate those of catarrhal gastritis: death of epithelium and perhaps the underlying stroma in the more exposed structures, moderate hyperemia, and moderate lymphocytic infiltration in the deeper portions of the mucosa. Enteritis of this type is a common finding in many infectious diseases, as well as chemical intoxications. The myriad tiny mucosal bites that occur with extensive hookworm infestation in dogs cause confluent hemorrhages and catarrhal or hemorrhagic enteritis in the small intestine. Similar but less conspicuous injury is inflicted on the mucosa of the cecum and large colon of the horse with severe strongylosis.

Occasionally, a truly mucous exudate is encountered, of such intensity that the microscopic section reveals strands of blue-staining epithelial mucin streaming out from the intestinal glands (crypts). Clinically, this type of reaction, occurring in the large bowel, is revealed by broad sheets or strands of white, inspissated mucus on the surface of formed feces. The normally soft stools of cattle are an exception, but in the constipation, which often accompanies benign and transitory enteric disturbances, formed feces flecked with visible clumps of inspissated mucus are seen sometimes even in cattle.

Like its gastric counterpart, **hemorrhagic enteritis** is a more severe form of acute catarrhal enteritis. Its distribution is practically always patchy simply because an animal would not remain alive long enough for the hemorrhagic enteritis to become diffuse and widespread. Hemorrhagic enteritis is usually caused by a locally destructive endo- or exotoxin in concentrated form, or by a highly virulent infection, such as anthrax. Salmonella species, commonly *S. enteritidis* or *S. typhimurium,* cause acute catarrhal, and often hemorrhagic enteritis in cattle, horses, and nonhuman primates. In swine, *Salmonella choleraesuis* is the common cause of acute enteritis, but there are numerous reports of a spirochete *(Treponema hyodysenteriae)* causing severe and fatal enteritis in young pigs. Shigellosis is an important cause of hemorrhagic enteritis in most species of nonhuman primates. Viruses have also been incriminated, especially canine and feline parvovirus infections.

Purulent enteritis is infrequent, but occasionally occurs in association with mechanical injuries from foreign bodies or helminth parasites (e.g., hookworms, nodular worms) that have created mucosal defects that allow secondary invasion by pyogenic bacteria. Chronic mucopurulent enteritis in the dog, apparently of nonspecific origin, is characterized by dense, slightly tenacious, semi-solid, whitish exudate extending to a depth of 2 or 3 mm into the duodenal and jejunal mucosae.

Acute **fibrinous enteritis** is probably observed more often in the large intestine of cattle. The fibrinous exudate is often of the pseudomembranous type, and as the inflammation subsides, the pseudomembrane becomes detached and passes out with the feces in the form of a long, hollow cast bearing a physical resemblance to the lining of a segment of intestine.

A more diphtheritic form of acute fibrinous inflammation sometimes involves either the small or large intestine of the pig. Most observations indicate that it is due to the damage caused by *Salmonella choleraesuis (suipestifer)*.

Lymphocytic-plasmacytic enteritis is the most common idiopathic inflammatory bowel disease of dogs and cats and reportedly is the most common cause of chronic diarrhea and vomiting in these species. The vomiting generally cannot be correlated with consumption of food and often consists only of bile-stained fluid. The diarrhea typically is watery. In severe cases, the intestine may be palpably thickened. Affected animals generally experience progressive weight loss. Clinical manifestations can vary in severity, but reportedly are most severe in the Basenji breed of dogs where the condition has a hereditary basis and is associated with a severe protein-losing enteropathy. Severely affected animals may have hypoproteinemia, ascites, or peripheral edema. Although mixed inflammatory cell infiltrates consisting predominantly of lymphocytes and plasma cells can occur with a wide variety of known enteric infections, in most cases of lymphoplasmacytic enteritis the cause cannot be identified. It has been proposed that it has an immunologic basis, and may represent a localized hypersensitivity reaction to antigens in the diet or to bacterial antigens present in the intestinal flora. Neither of these hypotheses has been proved in any species.

Microscopically, this disorder is characterized by the presence of extensive infiltration of the lamina propria of the small intestine by well-differentiated lymphocytes, plasma cells, and scattered histiocytes. These may extend down to the muscularis mucosa. Intestinal villi, except for the cellular infiltrates, may appear normal in size, blunted, or atrophic, and occasionally are fused. The surface epithelium of affected villi usually remains intact but may be somewhat thinner than normal and contain increased numbers of goblet cells. Crypts may be hyertrophied and dilated by mucus and contain a few exfoliated epithelial cells. There may be varying degrees of lymphangiectasia of central lacteals and the adjacent lamina propria may be edematous. Some patients respond favorably to corticosteroid therapy and diet change again suggesting an immunologic basis for this condition.

References

Hayden DW, Van Kruiningen HJ. Lymphocytic-plasmacytic enteritis in German shepherd dogs. J Am Anim Hosp Assoc 1982;18:89–96.

Jacobs G, Collins-Kelly L, Lappin M, et al. Lymphocytic-plasmacytic enteritis in 24 dogs. J Vet Intern Med 1990;4:45–53.

MacAllister CG, Mosier D, Gualls CW Jr., et al. Lymphocytic-plasmacytic enteritis in two horses. J Am Vet Med Assoc 1990;196: 1995–1998.

MacLachlan NJ, Breitschwerdt EB, Chambers JM, et al. Gastroenteritis of basenji dogs. Vet Pathol 1988;25:36–41.

Tams TR. Chronic feline inflammatory bowel disorders. Part I. Idiopathic inflammatory bowel disease. Comp Contin Ed Pract Vet 1986;8:371–386.

Eosinophilic enteritis

A chronic enteritis or gastroenteritis is recognized in dogs and cats by the occurrence of repeated episodes of diarrhea that may be associated with peripheral eosinophilia. The lesions in the intestinal mucosa consist of diffuse inflammatory cellular infiltrates in which the eosinophil is the predominant cell type. There is generally no villous blunting or atrophy. The gastric mucosa may also be affected in dogs, the colonic mucosa in cats. The cause is unknown, but an immediate type I hypersensitivity reaction to some antigen in the intestinal lumen is suspected. Migration of ascarid larvae in an immune host has been suspected as the cause in some cases of eosinophilic enteritis in dogs.

An idiopathic **eosinophilic enteritis of horses** has been described as part of a generalized systemic disorder in which eosinophils infiltrate many organs including the pancreas, liver, mesenteric lymph nodes, and skin. Affected animals experience progressive weight loss and diarrhea, and have decreased serum albumin levels suggestive of a protein-losing enteropathy. Peripheral eosinophilia is not a feature of this disease. At postmortem, affected animals have mucosal and, occasionally, transmural thickening of the alimentary tract anywhere between the esophagus and rectum. The squamous epithelium of the esophagus and stomach is hyperkeratotic and the mucosa of affected portions of the tract is thrown up into prominent transverse folds. The latter may be marked by areas of ulceration and caseous necrosis. Histologically, the mucosa, submucosa, and sometimes the tunica muscularis are infiltrated by a mixture of eosinophils, mast cells, macrophages, and variable numbers of lymphocytes and plasma cells. The caseous areas consist of a central core of eosinophils surrounded by histiocytes, giant cells, and fibroblastic tissue, i.e. an eosinophilic granuloma. These changes are associated with villous atrophy.

References

Easley JR. Gastroenteritis and associated eosinophilia in a dog. J Am Vet Med Assoc 1972;161:1030–1032.
Hayden DW, Fleischman RW. *Scirrhous* eosinophilic gastritis in dogs with gastric arteritis. Vet Pathol 1977;14:441–448.
Hayden DW, Van Kruiningen HJ. Eosinophilic gastroenteritis in German shepherd dogs and its relationship to visceral larval migrans. J Am Vet Med Assoc 1973;162:377–384.
Hendrick MA. A spectrum of hypereosinophilic syndromes exemplified by six cats with eosinophilic enteritis. Vet Pathol 1981;18:188–200.
Legendre AM, Krehbiel JD. Eosinophilic enteritis in a Chesapeake Bay retriever. J Am Vet Med Assoc 1973;163:258.

Chronic proliferative enteritis

Chronic proliferative enteritis is seen in those granulomatous diseases which involve the intestine, notably paratuberculosis (Johne's disease), tuberculosis, colibacillosis (Hjarre's disease) of fowl, histoplasmosis, and others. The proliferative nature of the intestinal reaction is that which characterizes each disease. Partial obstructions or other mechanical factors occasionally result in localized chronic, inflammatory proliferations of a similar type.

Enteritis caused by specific organisms

Many of the specific infections responsible for enteritis, gastroenteritis, or enterocolitis have been considered elsewhere in this text and will not be considered at length in this chapter. Viral enteritides such as caused by **Rotavirus, Coronavirus,** and **Parvovirus** are discussed in Chapter 8. Bacterial diseases, including colibacillosis, shigellosis, salmonellosis, yersiniosis, pasteurellosis, and infections due to *Clostridium perfringens, Clostridium piliforme* (formerly *Bacillus piliformis*) (Tyzzer's Disease), and **Campylobacter spp.** are described in Chapter 10. Other specific enteric infections, such as paratuberculosis, avian tuberculosis, mucormycosis, and swine dysentery are described in Chapter 11. Protozoal enteric pathogens (coccidiosis, amebiasis, giardiasis, etc.) and the diseases they produce are covered in Chapter 12.

References

Anonymous. Colloquium on selected diarrheal diseases of the young. J Am Vet Med Assoc 1978;173:511–676.
Kent TH, Moon HW. The comparative pathogenesis of some enteric diseases, based on cases presented at the 22nd Annual Seminar of the American College of Veterinary Pathologists. Vet Pathol 1973;10:414–469.
Moon HW. Vacuolated villous epithelium of the small intestine of young pigs. Vet Pathol 1972;9:3–21.
Moon HW, Kohler EM, Whipp SC. Vacuolation: a function of cell age in porcine ileal absorptive cells. Lab Invest 1973;28:23–28.
Moon HW. Mechanisms in the pathogenesis of diarrhea: A review. J Am Vet Med Assoc 1978;172:443–448.
Mottet NK. On animal models for inflammatory bowel disease. Gastroenterol 1972;62:1269–1271.
Mukherjee TM, Williams AW. A comparative study of the ultrastructure of microvilli in the epithelium of small and large intestine of mice. J Cell Biol 1967;34:447–461.
Takeuchi A. Penetration of the intestinal epithelium by various microorganisms. Curr Top Pathol 1971;54:1–27.

Regional transmural granulomatous enterocolitis

Regional cicatrizing enterocolitis, regional ileitis, or Crohn's disease, was established as an entity in humans in 1932. A comparable disease was recognized in the dog by Strande et al. (1954). In the general vicinity of the ileocecal orifice and sometimes both above and below it, the mucosa and submucosa are rather irregularly involved in asymmetrical thickening which may be as great as 6 cm, and grossly is highly suggestive of intestinal neoplasia (Fig 23-10B). Microscopically, the lesion consists of a mass of dense collagenous connective tissue containing numerous epithelioid histiocytes and scattered multinucleated giant cells. The mucosal surface may be focally or diffusely ulcerated and be covered by a purulent exudate. In some cases, the granulomatous inflammation extends to the serosal surface of the intestine. Regional lymph nodes may also contain a similar granulomatous inflammatory process. This expanding inflammatory reaction ultimately leads to partial or complete obstruction of the intestinal lumen. Although the nature of the lesion strongly suggests an infectious etiology, an extensive search for more than 60 years has not identified one in either humans or animals. A similar granulomatous enteritis has also been described in horses and compared to Crohn's disease. The lesions in humans, dogs, and horses are similar, but until the etiologies are identified, the pathogenesis of these disorders will remain unknown.

References

Cave DR, Mitchell DN, Kane SP, et al. Further animal evidence of a transmissible agent in Crohn's disease. Lancet 1973;2:1120–1122.

Cave DR, Mitchell DN, Brooks BN. Exeperimental animal studies of the etiology and pathogenesis of Crohn's disease. Gastroenterol 1975;69:618–624.

Cimprich RE. Equine granulomatous enteritis. Vet Pathol 1974;11:535–547

DiBartola SP, Rogers WA, Boyce JT, et al. Regional enteritis in two dogs. J Am Vet Med Assoc 1982;181:904–908.

Lindberg R. Ultrastructure of granulomatous infiltrates in the small bowel in equine granulomatous enteritis. J Vet Med (A) 1986;33:111–122.

Merritt AM, Cimprich RE, Beech J. Granulomatous enteritis in nine horses. J Am Vet Med Assoc 1976;169:603–609.

Sachar DB, Taub RN, Janowitz HD. A transmissible agent in Crohn's disease? New pursuit of an old concept. N Engl J Med 1975;293:354–355.

Strande A, Sommers SC, Petrak M. Regional enterocolitis in Cocker Spaniel dogs. Arch Pathol 1954;57:357–362.

Porcine intestinal adenomatosis complex

This complex includes four disorders that were once regarded as separate and distinct disease entities, but which now are regarded as different clinicopathologic manifestations or sequelae of a single disease. All four disorders have in common the proliferation of epithelial cells of the glandular crypts of the ileum and proximal colon. In addition, the proliferating cells contain *Campylobacter*-like organisms in their cytoplasm. Moreover, there are similar grossly visible lesions that underly all four conditions. Included in this complex are: 1) porcine intestinal adenomatosis, once termed "regional ileitis", 2) necrotizing (necrotic) enteritis, 3) muscular hypertrophy of the ileum, and 4) proliferative hemorrhagic enteropathy.

Porcine intestinal adenomatosis (formerly regional ileitis or proliferative ileitis of swine)—the adenomatous changes that characterize this component of the porcine intestinal adenomatosis complex also occur to varying degrees in the other three components. It occurs most often in feeder age pigs, but very young piglets and adult swine can be affected. Clinical signs range from mild growth retardation to frank diarrhea and weight loss leading to cachexia and death. Mortality rates vary but can be high. In both experimental and early spontaneous infections the *Campylobacter*-like organisms preferentially invade and actively replicate in the apical cytoplasm of epithelial cells that line the glands near the Peyer's patches of the terminal ileum, cecum, and proximal colon. Goblet cells are rapidly depleted from affected glands and are replaced by undifferentiated, pseudostratied columnar cells with basophilic cytoplasm and a high mitotic index. The glands become long, distorted, branched (in some cases), and dilated. Additionally, they may protrude into the lymphoid tissue of Peyer's patches. Grossly, the mucosa in these areas is thrown up into nodular or ridge-like folds that protrude above areas of non-infected mucosa. As the condition progresses, the folds become more extensive and involve more proximal portions of the il-

eum, the cecum, and proximal colon, where they appear as prominent, raised transverse or longitudinal folds or rugae. The apical portions of these hyperplastic masses of mucosa may be superficially ulcerated and covered by a fibrinous exudate. These mucosal changes impart a rather characteristic cerebriform or gyrate pattern to the serosal surface of the affected segments of bowel. This change is unique and regarded as diagnostic for this disease. Microscopically, there is loss of villi in the affected portions of the severely hyperplastic mucosa, and the mucosa is thrown up into extensive broad folds containing distorted glands lined by poorly differentiated epithelial cells containing numerous *Campylobacter*-like organisms demonstrable with various silver stains. The organisms have the characteristic curved, spiral, or gull-wing profiles. Inflammatory infiltrates in the lamina propria and submucosa at this stage of the disease, except in areas of erosion or ulceration, are relatively mild.

Necrotizing enteritis, also referred to as **"necrotic enteritis"** is a complication or sequel to intestinal adenomatosis. The lesions occur in the large intestine and, to some extent, in the terminal ileum at sites where the hyperplastic mucosal folds develop erosions and ulcerations. Saprophytic anaerobes from the large bowel, such as *Fusobacterium necrophorum*, commonly colonize areas of devitalized mucosa causing extensive areas of coagulative necrosis covered by thick diphtheritic exudate. Grossly, the lesions consist of variable-sized patches of thick, rough, brownish or grayish diphtheritic exudate which is tightly adherent to the underlying necrotic and viable tissue (Fig. 23-13). Typical of diphtheritic exudates, the underlying cells undergo coagulative necrosis, and thin strands of fibrin present in the exudate extend into and around them, anchoring them down in a mat-like membrane. Fecal material becomes mixed with the superficial portions of the exudate. The tenacious exudate may cover a considerable segment of the bowel, or be limited to raised, random patches. At times, they peel off to form almost perfect circular lesions referred to as "button ulcers." Since necrotizing enteritis of this type also occurs commonly in the bowel of pigs with hog cholera, the button ulcer at one time was thought to be diagnostic of that viral disease. However, as has been mentioned previously, *Fusobacterium necrophorum* is an opportunistic saprophyte that can only colonize devitalized tissues that have been previously injured by some other agent—mechanical, chemical, or microbiologic—hence its presence is only an indication of some prior tissue damage. The serosal surface of segments of bowel with necrotizing enteritis complicating intestinal adenomatosis also have the characteristic cerebriform pattern typical of the latter disease.

Muscular hypertrophy of the ileum in swine, once termed **"terminal ileitis,"** is characterized by marked hypertrophic thickening of the tunica muscularis of the last portion of the ileum. Grossly, the condition can be confused with regional granulomatous enteritis described above. The marked thickening of the intestinal wall and stenosis of the lumen of the ileum are similar,

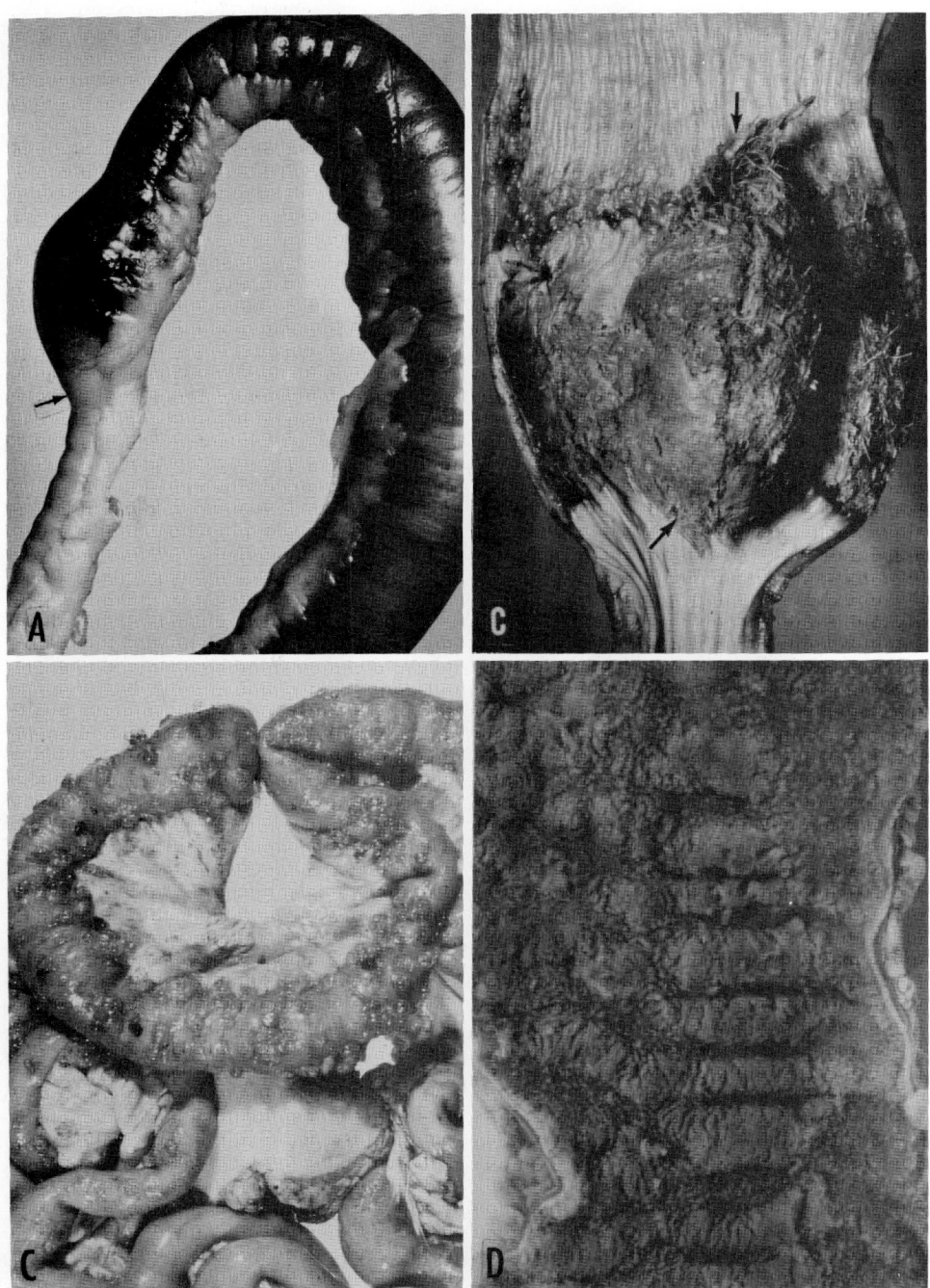

FIG. 23-13. A. Obstruction of the small intestine of a dog. A large peach stone was lodged just above the arrow. **B.** Obstruction of the esophagus (choke) in a horse which died on the third day from severe toxic hepatitis and toxic tubular nephritis. The site of the large obstructing mass of ingesta is indicated by arrows. **C.** Intestinal emphysema, small intestine of swine. Note bubbles of air under serosa. **D.** Necrotizing enteritis of swine. Dark, thick, tenacious exudate consisting largely of fibrin and necrotic cells on intestinal mucosa. (Courtesy of College of Veterinary Medicine, Iowa State University.)

although usually less abrupt. Microscopically, the thickening is not due to granulomatous inflammation but is due to marked hypertrophy of the tunica muscularis of the ileum. This lesion may be associated with areas of ulceration of the overlying mucosa with granulation, tissue infiltration, and residual masses of proliferative mucosa.

There is a single report of segmental hypertrophy of a 5.5 cm length of the transverse colon of a rhesus monkey *(Macaca mulatta)* (Casey et al., 1969). The hypertrophy in this animal also mainly involve the tunica muscularis.

Proliferative hemorrhagic enteropathy. In 1967,

Jones first described an "intestinal haemorrhage syndrome" in pigs in South Wales. This disease sporadically affected young pigs, but did occasionally involve adults. This syndrome or one similar to it was subsequently called "haemorrhagic bowel syndrome" by other authors (O'Neill, 1970; Rowland and Rowntree, 1972; Chu and Hong, 1973). Rowland and Rowntree (1972), Rowland, et al. (1973), and later Rowland and Lawson (1973) described the possible relationship of "porcine intestinal adenomatosis" to "necrotic enteritis," "regional ileitis," and "proliferative haemorrhagic enteropathy."

The principal findings in this hemorrhagic form of

intestinal adenomatosis are the presence of extensive erosions, ulcerations, and massive amounts of hemorrhage involving the ileal, cecal, and colonic mucosa with adenomatous hyperplastic changes. The serosa of these segments of bowel also exhibit the characteristic cerebriform pattern typical of this complex of disorders. Rowland and Lawson (1974) reported the demonstration of unidentified bacteria by electron microscopy and immunologic methods in affected epithelial cells of the ileum.

In addition to the intracellular *Campylobacter*-like organisms that can be readily demonstrated but not cultured from pigs with the various forms of intestinal adenomatosis, *Campylobacter mucosalis* and *C. hyointestinalis* have both been isolated from animals with this condition. These organisms are not related to the intracellular organism and, to date, have not reproduced the disease when pure cultures of them alone or in combination were inoculated into susceptible pigs. Only mucosal tissue from infected animals will transmit the disease. Additional features of campylobacteriosis are described in Chapter 10.

References

Casey HW, Johnson DK, Kupper JL, et al. Segmental hypertrophy of colon in a Rhesus monkey. J Am Vet Med Assoc 1969;155:1245–1248.
Biester HE, Schwarte LH. Intestinal adenoma in swine. Am J Pathol 1931;7:175–185.
Chu RMR, Hong CB. Haemorrhagic bowel syndrome in pigs in Taiwan. Vet Rec 1973;93:562–563.
Crohn B, Ginsburg L, Oppenheimer GD. Regional ileitis, a pathologic and clinical entity. l. Am Med Assoc 1932;99:1323–1329.
Dodd DC. Adenomatous intestinal hyperplasia (proliferative ileitis) of swine. Pathol Vet 1968;5:333–341.
Emsbo P. Terminal or regional ileitis in swine. Nord Vet Med 1951;3:1–28.
Gebhart CJ, Lin GF, McOrist SM, et al. Cloned DNA probes specific for the intracellular Campylobacter-like organism of porcine proliferative enteritis. J Clin Microbiol 1991;29:1011–1015.
Gunnarsson A, Hurvell B, Jonsson L, et al. Regional ileitis in pigs. Isolation of Campylobacter from affected ileal mucosa. Acta Vet Scand 1976;17:267–269.
Jones JET. An intestinal haemorrhage syndrome in pigs. Br Vet J 1967;123:286–294.
Lawson GHK, Rowland AC. Intestinal adenomatosis in the pig: a bacteriological study. Res Vet Sci 1974;17:331–336.
Love DN, Love RJ. Pathology of proliferative haemorrhagic enteropathy in pigs. Vet Pathol 1979;16:41–48.
Nielsen SW. Muscular hypertrophy of the ileum in relation to "terminal ileitis" in pigs. J Am Vet Med Assoc 1955;127:437–441.
O'Hara PJ. Intestinal haemorrhage syndrome in the pig. Vet Rec 1972;91:517–518.
O'Neill PA. Observations on a haemorrhagic bowel syndrome involving pigs on three associated premises. Vet Rec 1970;87:742–747.
Rahko T, Saloniemi H. On the pathology of regional ileitis in the pig. Nord Vet Med 1972;24:132–138.
Rowland AC, Lawson GHK. Intestinal hemorrhage syndrome in the pig. Vet Rec 1973;93:402–404.
Rowland AC, Lawson GHK. Intestinal adenomatosis in the pig: immunofluorescent and electron microscopic studies. Res Vet Sci 1974;17:323–330.
Rowland AC, Lawson GHK. Porcine intestinal adenomatosis: a possible relationship with necrotic enteritis, regional ileitis and proliferative haemorrhagic enteropathy. Vet Rec 1975;97:178–181.
Rowland AC, Lawson GHK. Intestinal adenomatosis in the pig: a possible relationship with a haemorrhagic enteropathy. Res Vet Sci 1975;18:263–268.
Rowland AC, Lawson GHK, Maxwell A. Intestinal adenomatosis in the pig: occurrence of a bacterium in affected cells. Nature 1973;243:417.
Rowland AC, Rowntree PGM. A haemorrhagic bowel syndrome associated with intestinal adenomatosis in the pig. Vet Rec 1972;91:235–241.
Schultheiss PC, Kurtz HJ, Glassman D. Retrospective study of Campylobacter species isolated from porcine diagnostic case material. J Vet Diagn Invest 1989;1:181–182.
Smith WJ, Shanks PL. Intestinal haemorrhage syndrome. Vet Rec 1971;89:55–56.
Ward G, Winkelman NL. Recognizing the three forms of proliferative enteritis in swine. Vet Med 1990;85:197–203.

Proliferative ileitis in hamsters

This disease has been given several names, based on interpretations of its probable cause. It was first called "enzootic intestinal adenocarcinoma" (Jonas, et al. 1965), later "proliferative ileitis" (Boothe and Cheville, 1967), and also "regional enteritis," "atypical ileal hyperplasia," and "hamster enteritis." The diarrhea which occurs in this disease has led some to refer to the condition as "wet tail." Most evidence indicates this is probably an infectious disease. In the report of Boothe and Cheville, the disease spread slowly, had a morbidity rate of 25 to 60% and a mortality rate of 90%. The lesions develop in the ileum, less often in the jejunum, and rarely in the colon. Grossly, the ileum is dilated, thickened, studded with small white subserosal foci, and often adhered to other viscera. Microscopically, there is hyperplasia of the intestinal epithelium, accompanied by purulent inflammation and coagulation necrosis extending into the submucosa. The hyperplastic epithelium impinges on the lumen of the ileum and extends into the submucosa, muscularis, and often to the serosa, forming small glands or cysts which remain after healing. Diffuse and focal collections of large histiocytes occur in the lamina propria, submucosa, muscularis, and serosa as well as in mesenteric lymph nodes.

A bacterial organism identified as *Shigella boydii* has been demonstrated ultrastructurally in hyperplastic intestinal epithelial cells of the hamster, but no other evidence indicates it to be an etiologic agent (Wagner, et al., 1973). Additional electron microscopic studies (Frisk and Wagner, 1977) identified *Escherichia coli* in early lesions and *Campylobacter* species in later lesions in the natural disease. Although the disease can be transmitted with suspensions of tissue from affected ileum, reproduction of the disease with pure cultures of any organism appears not to have been achieved. Hence the disease bears a remarkable similarity to the porcine intestinal adenomatosis in both its pathology and transmissibility.

Similar proliferative enteritides or colitides associated with intracellular *Campylobacter*-like bacteria have been described in ferrets, rabbits, guinea pigs, rats, puppies and blue foxes.

References

Amend NK, Loeffler DG, Ward BC, et al. Transmission of enteritis in the Syrian hamster. Lab Anim Sci 1976;26:566–572.
Boothe AD, Cheville NF. The pathology of proliferative ileitis of the Golden Syrian Hamster. Pathol Vet 1967;4:31–44.

Collins JE, Libal MC. Proliferative enteritis in two pups. J Am Vet Med Assoc 1983;183:886–889.

Elwell MR, Chapman AL, Frenkel JK. Duodenal hyperplasia in a guinea pig. Vet Pathol 1981;18:136–139.

Ericksen K, Landsverk T, Bratberg B. Morphology and immunoperoxidase studies of intestinal adenomatosis in the blue fox, Alopex lagopus. J Comp Pathol 1990;102:265–278.

Frisk CS, Wagner JE. Experimental hamster enteritis: an electron microscopic study. Am J Vet Res 1977;38:1861–1869.

Fox JG, Murphy JC, Ackerman JI, et al. Proliferative colitis in ferrets. Am J Vet Res 1982;43:858–864.

Jacoby RO, Osbaldiston GW, Jonas AM. Experimental transmission of atypical ileal hyperplasia of hamsters. Lab Anim Sci 1975;25:465–473.

Jonas AM, Tomita Y, Wyand DS. Enzootic intestinal adenocarcinoma in hamsters. J Am Vet Med Assoc 1965;147:1102–1108.

Lussier G, Pavilanis V. Presence of intranuclear inclusion bodies in proliferative ileitis of the hamster (Mesocricetus auratus) A preliminary report. Lab Anim Care 1969;19:387–390.

Schoeb TR, Fox JG. *Enterocecocolitis* associated with intraepithelial *Campylobacter-like* bacteria in rabbits *(Oryctolagus cuniculus)*. Vet Pathol 1990;27:73–80.

Stills HF, Hook RR Jr. Experimental production of proliferative ileitis in Syrian hamsters *(Mesocricetus auratus)* by using an ileal homogenate free of *Campylobacter jejuni*. Infect Immun 1989;57:191–195.

Wagner JE, Owens DR, Troutt HF. Proliferative ileitis of hamsters: electron microscopy of bacteria in cells. Am J Vet Res 1973;35:249–252.

Spontaneous ileitis in rats

Also described as "megaloileitis" this disease of unknown cause occurs in young rats less than 2 months of age. Clinically, there is marked distention of the abdomen, rough hair coat, and occasionally diarrhea. Approximately 50% of affected rats die, the others recovering over a period of about a week. At necropsy, the most striking lesion is a severe dilatation of the ileum with 7 to 10 cm segments distended up to 1.5 cm. (Fig. 23-14). The distention generally terminates at or near the ileocecal junction. The contents of the ileum vary from a frothy semi-fluid to a pasty consistency. Microscopically, the lesions are not striking. There is hydropic degeneration and coagulation necrosis of both layers of the tunica muscularis associated with an inflammatory cell infiltration composed of lymphocytes, macrophages, and a lesser number of neutrophils. In the mucosa, a lymphocytic infiltration occurs in the lamina propria, and many of the crypts of Lieberkuhn are occluded with plugs of eosinophilic material. In the healing stages of the condition, fibrovascular proliferation repairs the lesions in the muscularis. Occasionally, the distended ileum becomes adhered to the abdominal wall or other viscera. In some rats with this disease there is also a necrotizing and lymphocytic myocarditis and hepatitis.

References

Geil RG, Davis CL, Thompson SW. Spontaneous ileitis in rats. Am J Vet Res 1961;22:932–936.

Hottendorf GH, Hirth RS, Peer RL. Megaloileitis in rats. J Am Vet Med Assoc 1969;155:1131–1135.

Terminal ileitis in lambs

Terminal ileitis in lambs has been described in one report. The disease involved lambs 4 to 6 months of age which had shown a poor rate of growth. The terminal 50 to 75 mm of the ileum was involved with thickened rugae resulting from hyperplasia of the mucosa. In one lamb, submaxillary edema was also seen. Some of the affected lambs had bleeding ulcers in the ileum. Aerobic and anaerobic cultures failed to yield any bacterial organisms. A similar disease has been described in lambs that survived experimental infection with a noncytopathic biotype of bovine virus diarrhea (BVD) virus, i.e. Border disease, which were superinfected with a homologous, cytopathic strain of the same virus. These findings suggest that terminal ileitis in lambs may be caused by a pestivirus similar to BVD.

References

Cross RF, Smith CK, Parker CF. Terminal ileitis in lambs. J Am Vet Med Assoc 1973;162:564–566.

Chalmers GA, Nation PN, Pritchard J. Border disease—a cause of terminal ileitis in lambs? Can Vet J 1990;31:611.

Diverticulosis of the small intestine

Diverticulosis of the small intestine has been reported in horses, pigs, and sheep. This lesion appears as small, epithelial-lined cavities extending into the muscularis and often reaching the serosa. The serosal surface is elevated by spherical balloonings, which on occasion rupture into the peritoneal cavity, causing peritonitis. This usually results in death from peritonitis. In the horse, the duodenum is most often involved. Hypertrophy of the muscularis often accompanies this diverticulosis, although both may occur independently. Adult horses are usually affected. In young pigs, the site of diverticulosis is the terminal ileum. In swine, its occurrence in certain family groups suggests a possible hereditary origin. However, this has not been confirmed experimentally.

In sheep, adults appear to be most frequently affected, although there are only a few reports in this species. The duodenum and terminal ileum are involved.

References

Cordes DO, Dewes HF. Diverticulosis and muscular hypertrophy of the small intestine of horses, pigs, and sheep. N Z Vet J 1971;19:108–111.

Gill DA. Multiple diverticula of the duodenum in sheep. Vet Rec 1929;9:638.

Hancock JL. Muscular hypertrophy of the ileum in the horse. Vet Rec 1968;83:304.

Hodgson, JL. Animal models in the study of diverticular disease. Clin Gastroenterol 1975;4:201–219.

Rooney JR, Jeffcott LB. Muscular hypertrophy of the ileum in a horse. Vet Rec 1968;83:217–219.

Winter dysentery of cattle

Winter dysentery of cattle is a comparatively mild and transient enteritis of uncertain etiology. *Campylobacter jejuni* and a coronavirus have been suspected as the etiologic agent, but this has not been confirmed experimentally. It is highly contagious, especially in stabled cattle in northern portions of the United States and

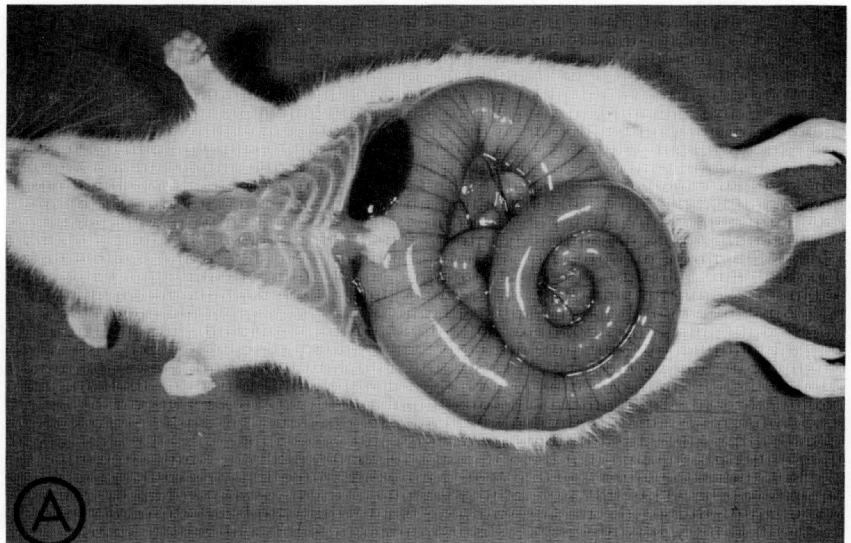

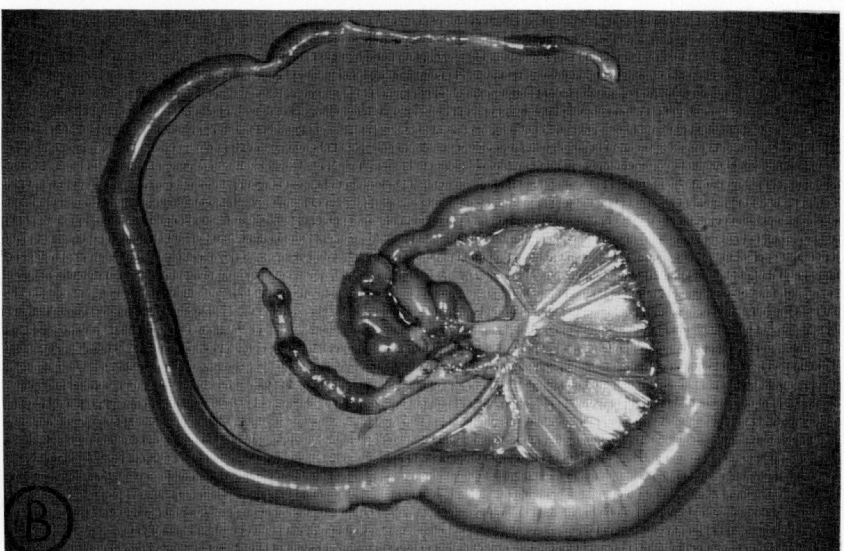

FIG. 23-14. Regional ileitis, rat. There is marked dilation of the ileum. (Courtesy Animal Research Center, Harvard Medical School.)

Canada. The principal postmorten finding is an acute catarrhal ileitis and jejunitis, which in exceptionally severe cases becomes hemorrhagic.

References

Kahrs RF, Scott FW, Hillman RB. Epidemiologic observations on bovine winter dysentery. Bovine Pract 1973;8:36–39.
MacPherson LW. Bovine virus enteritis (winter dysentery). Can J Comp Pathol 1957;21:184–192.
Scott FW, Kahrs RF, Campbell SG, et al. Etiologic studies of bovine winter dysentery. Bovine Pract 1973;8:40–43.
Van Kruiningen HJ, Khairallah LH, Sasseville VG, et al. Calfhood coronavirus enterocolitis: a clue to the etiology of winter dysentery. Vet Pathol 1987;24:564–567.

Staphylococcal enteritis in chinchillas

A severe enteritis in these animals has followed long-term feeding of a mixture containing antibiotics. The normal gram-negative bacterial flora of the intestine were found to have been depleted and replaced by hemolytic *Staphylococcus aureus* in huge numbers. The animals returned to normal when the feeding was changed to more ordinary ingredients. This experience is comparable to staphylococcal infections elsewhere accompanying the indiscriminate use of antibiotics.

Reference

Wood JS, Bennett IL, Yardley, JH. Staphylococcal enterocolitis in chinchillas. Bull Johns Hopkins Hosp 1956;98:454–463.

Edema disease of swine

First reported by Shanks in Ireland in 1938, this disease has been encountered with some frequency in most of the swine-producing countries of the world. It typically occurs during the first few weeks after weaning and is associated with colonization of the gut by certain verotoxin-producing, O–serotypes of hemolytic *Escherichia coli* (O138, O139, O141). The toxin that causes edema disease is a variant of the shiga-like toxin-II (SLT II), referred to as SLTIIv. This neurotoxin is absorbed from the gut and damages the endothelium and the tunica media of small arteries and arterioles throughout the body. The disease strikes previously thrifty animals without warning, produces incoordination and paralysis of the limbs, pain, and coma, and is commonly, but not invariably, fatal within a number of hours or a day or two. It is not highly contagious, but herd morbidity may approach 35%. Mortality may reach 100%. In recent years, this disease appears to be on the decline, possibly due to changes in the ingredients in concentrate rations which in turn affect the composition of the gut flora.

The edema is typically, but not invariably, found in the wall of the stomach, where it may involve the cardiac region, the greater curvature, or the entire organ. The thickness of the gastric wall may be increased just perceptibly or it may reach 3 cm. The coiled portion of the colon, with its mesentery, is another common location of the edema, but these regions are by no means the only sites which may be involved. The body cavities usually contain small or large amounts of fluid; other parts of the intestinal tract sometimes are involved. The face and eyelids are edematous in a high proportion of cases, as can be observed during life. Less frequently, the tarsal and carpal regions and the ventral abdominal wall contain an excess of fluid. The parenchymatous organs of the abdomen usually appear normal, as do the brain and, usually, lungs. Subepicardial hemorrhages sometimes occur, but inflammatory changes are typically absent from all organs, including the gastrointestinal tract. Kurtz and associates (1969) have described lesions in the brain and arterioles which account for the neurologic signs seen in edema disease. They noted a necrotizing arteritis in most all organs and tissues of the body. They also described focal symmetrical encephalomalacia, presumably secondary to arteritis, involving the thalamus, basal ganglia, and nuclei of the brain stem.

References

Bertschinger HU, Pohlenz J. Bacterial colonization and morphology of the intestine in porcine *Escherichia coli* enterotoxemia (edema disease). Vet Pathol 1983;20:99–110.

Gannon VPJ, Gyles CL. Characteristics of the shiga-like toxin produced by *Escherichia coli* associated with porcine edema disease. Vet Microbiol 1990;24:89–100.

Gannon VPJ, Gyles CL, Wilcock BP. Effects of *Escherichia coli* shiga-like toxins (verotoxins) in pigs. Can J Vet Res 1989;53:306–312.

Gitter M, Lloyd MK. Haemolytic *Bact. coli* in the bowel edema syndrome. II. Transmission and protection experiments. Brit Vet J 1957;113:212–218.

Jones JET, Smith HW. Histological studies on weaned pigs suffering diarrhea and oedema disease produced by oral inoculation of *Escherichia coli*. J Pathol 1969;97:168–172.

Kernkamp HCH, Sorensen DK, Hanson LJ, et al. Epizootiology of edema disease in swine. J Am Vet Med Assoc 1965;146:353–357.

Kurtz HJ, Bergeland ME, Barnes DM. Pathologic changes in edema disease of swine. Am J Vet Res 1969;30:791–806.

MacLeod DL, Gyles CL, Wilcock BP. Reproduction of edema disease of swine with purified shiga-like toxin-II variant. Vet Pathol 1991;28:66–73.

Moon HW, Schneider RA, Moseley SL. Comparative prevalences of four enterotoxin genes among Escherichia coli isolated from swine. Am J Vet Res 1986;47:210–212.

Mushin R, Basset CR. Haemolytic *Escherichia coli* and other bacteria in oedema disease of swine. Aust Vet J 1964;40:315–320.

Nielsen NO, Moon HW, Roe WE. Enteric colibacillosis in swine. J Am Vet Med Assoc 1968;153:1590–1606.

Shanks PL. An unusual condition affecting the digestive organs of the pig. Vet Rec 1938;50:356–358.

Smith HW, Halls S. The production of oedema disease and diarrhea in weaned pigs by the oral administration of *E. coli*. Factors that influence the course of the experimental disease. J Med Microbiol 1968;1:45–59.

Underdahl NR, Stair EL, Young GA. Transmission and characterization of edema disease of swine. J Am Vet Med Assoc 1963;142:27–30.

Malabsorption syndrome

Failure of absorption of nutrients from the intestinal tract results in clinical manifestations, collectively called malabsorption syndrome. The clinical signs most evident in humans and animals are: persistent gastrointestinal upset (vomiting, diarrhea), change in eating habits, loss of weight, and steatorrhea (in some cases). Diagnostic laboratory procedures are outlined in Table 23-2. The causal types of malabsorption currently recognized in animals and humans include the conditions covered below.

Pancreatic insufficiency, due to chronic pancreatitis or malignant neoplasia, results in a lack of pancreatic enzymes in the small intestine. Since these (lipase, especially) are involved in the digestion of fats, the appearance of undigested fats in the feces (steatorrhea) is a conspicuous clinical sign. In dogs, chronic pancreatic disease is often accompanied by destruction of pancreatic islets, resulting in an associated diabetes mellitus.

Disease involving the mucosal epithelium of the small intestine may result in defects in transport of glucose, amino acids, or lipids across the epithelial cells. Among the identified entities of this nature is **nontropical sprue** of adult human patients who are sensitized to gluten. The lesions in the small intestine are blunted villi (villous atrophy), elongated crypts, and increased cell turnover (mitoses are increased). These lesions are accompanied by increased permeability of lysosomal membranes and loss of acid hydrolases. The disease in infants is called "coeliac sprue." Removal of gluten from the diet is curative.

Tropical sprue is caused by folic acid deficiency, which leads to macrocytic anemia as well. Dietary supplementation with folic acid is usually curative.

Transmissible gastroenteritis of swine is caused by a coronavirus which attacks mucosal epithelial cells below the apex of the villi and results in villous atrophy and malabsorption. Other viral, bacterial, or toxic enteritides not clearly identified may have a similar effect on intestinal absorption.

Protein-losing enteropathy of unknown cause, associated with dilatation of lymphatics in villi (lymphan-

TABLE 23-2 **Laboratory screening tests in canine malabsorption syndromes***

Types of Lesions	Fat assimilation	Fecal trypsin	Xylose absorption test	Glucose tolerance test	Starch tolerance test	Lactose tolerance test
Pancreatic insufficiency	Severely reduced	Very low	Normal	Abnormal	Abnormal	
Mucosal defect, small intestine	Reduced	Very low or high activity	Reduced	Abnormal	Abnormal	
Lactose or milk intolerance	Normal	Normal	Normal	Normal	Normal	Abnormal
Pancreatic insufficiency and mucosal disease, small intestine	Severely reduced	Very low	Reduced	Abnormal	Abnormal	
Liver disease	Reduced	Normal				

*Adapted after Hill (1972)

giectasia), has also been associated with intestinal malabsorption.

A **combination of pancreatic insufficiency and mucosal malabsorption** may be encountered in animals, especially dogs.

Intolerance to lactose contained in milk may occur in humans or animals due to genetic or acquired deficiency of the enzyme lactase. Removal of lactose from the diet usually relieves the clinical signs of this disorder.

Gastric malfunction, due to neoplasia or chronic gastritis, may also lead to intestinal malabsorption.

Liver malfunction, particularly bile stasis, has also been associated with intestinal malabsorption. Icterus and other evidence of liver dysfunction are present in these cases.

Lesions associated with malabsorption syndrome include chronic pancreatitis and biliary stasis. Lesions found in the small intestine include villous atrophy; the villi are shortened due to loss of epithelium and thickened due to infiltration of leukocytes into the lamina propria. Accelerated proliferation of the epithelial cells in the crypts results in hyperplasia of the epithelium nearest the muscularis mucosa. Increased rate of cell turnover is evidenced by the increased numbers of mitoses in the crypt epithelium.

An essential cellular component involved in the absorption of materials from the intestinal lumen is the brush-border of the mucosal cells of the small intestinal epithelium. This is recognized at the ultrastructural level as made up of myriad microvilli on the lumenal surface. The microvilli project into the lumen about 2 μm in parallel arrays and are covered by the plasma membrane. The interior of each microvillus contains fine parallel contractile fibrils of actin, which extend down into the cell to intertwine and form the terminal web. Contraction of these filaments serves to shorten the microvilli. At the apex of the microvilli on the surface of the brush-border membrane is a mat of material called the glycocalyx. This is a secretory product of the epithelial cells and is rich in neutral and amino sugars. The brush-border contains many hydrolytic enzymes (disaccharidases, peptidases, and phosphatases) as well as nonenzymatic proteins such as the intrinsic-factor-vitamin B_{12} complex and the soluble calcium-binding protein that is dependent upon vitamin D.

Other intestinal lesions which have been associated with malabsorption syndrome in the dog include purulent, eosinophilic, and histiocytic enteritis; lymphosarcoma involving the intestine; and intestinal lymphangiectasia. Lesions in the liver have been described as including fatty change, cirrhosis, proliferation of bile ducts, and intrahepatic cholestasis.

An intriguing malabsorptive effect has been demonstrated in cotton-top tamarins *(Saguinus oedipus)* fed a diet high in cholesterol and coconut oil but otherwise adequate. The result was a jejunal lipodystrophy (accumulation of fat partides in epithelial cells), steatorrhea, and osteomalacia (Dreizen, et al., 1971).

References

Alpers DH, Seetharam B. Pathophysiology of diseases involving intestinal brush-border proteins. N Engl J Med 1977;296:1047–1050.

Carnpbell RSF, Brobst D, Bisgard G. Intestinal lymphangiectasia in a dog. J Am Vet Med Assoc 1968;153:1050–1054.

Dreizen S, Levy BM, Bernick S. Diet-induced jejunal lipodystrophy in the cotton-top marmoset *(Saguinus oedipus)*. Proc Soc Exp Biol Med 1971;138:7–11.

Finco DR, Duncan JR, Schall WD, et al. Chronic enteric disease and hypoproteinemia in 9 dogs. J Am Vet Med Assoc 1973;163:262–271.

Haeltermann EO. On the pathogenesis of transmissible gastroenteritis of swine. J Am Vet Med Assoc 1972;160:534–540.

Hill FWG, Osbome AD, Kidder DE. Pancreatic degenerative atrophy in dogs. J Com Pathol 1971;81:321–330.

Hill FWG. Malabsorption syndrome in the dog: a study of 38 cases. J Small Anim Pract 1972;13:575–594.

Kaneko JJ, Moulton JE, Brodey R, et al. Malabsorption syndrome resembling nontropical sprue in dogs. J Am Vet Med Assoc 1965; 146:463–473.

Maronpot RR, Whitehair CK. Experimental sprue-like intestinal lesions in pigs. Can J Comp Med 1967;31:309–316.

Mouwen JMVM, Schotman AJH. Steatorrhoea in piglets. Vet Rec 1970;87:172–173.

Olson NC, Zimmer JF. Protein-losing enteropathy secondary to intestinal lymphangiectasia in a dog. J Am Vet Med Assoc 1978;173: 271–274.

Robinson JWL. Intestinal malabsorption in the experimental animal. Gut 1972;13:938–945.

Seibold HR, Clewe TH, Wolf RH. Enteropathy resembling sprue in nonhuman primates. Lab Anim Sci 1972;33:353–362.

Strober W, Wochner RD, Carbone PP, et al. Intestinal lymphangiectasia: a protein-losing enteropathy with hypogammaglobulinemia, lymphocytopenia, and impaired homograft rejection. J Clin Invest 1967;46:1643–1656.

Strombeck DR, Guilford WG. Maldigestion, malabsorption, bacterial overgrowth, and protein-losing enteropathy. Chapter 17 (Strombeck WG ed.) In: Small animal gastroenterology. 2nd ed. Davis, CA: Stonegate Publishing, 1990;296–319.

Vernon DG. Idiopathic sprue in a dog. J Am Vet Med Assoc 1962; 140:1062–1067.

Windhorst DB, Lund JE, Decker J, et al. Intestinal malabsorption in the Gray Collie syndrome. Fed Proc 1967;26:260.

Intestinal obstruction

The small intestine, at times, becomes completely obstructed by foreign bodies, such as rubber balls, rubber nipples, nuts, or peach stones in the dog (Fig. 23-14A, Fig. 23-15), or piliconcretions (hairballs) in cats. **Strangulated** **hernias** (usually umbilical or scrotal) cause complete obstruction in any species (Fig. 23-10D), being most frequent in horses and pigs. The long intestine of the horse is subject to obstruction because of accidents stemming from its tortuosity and the length of the mesentery which suspends it. These are **torsions,** or twisting upon itself, or **volvulus,** in which a loop of intestine passes through a tear in the mesentery or similar abnormality.

Intussusceptions occur in any species. In this condition, excessive peristaltic motility forces a segment of the bowel inside the segment just below it, as the smaller tube of a telescope slides into the slightly larger tube just ahead of it. In the intestine, there is actually no difference in the diameters of the outer and inner tubes. As a consequence of this fact, and of the attached mesentery, the outermost of the three layers which make up the intussusception is greatly stretched, the innermost greatly compressed (Fig. 23-16). Interference with the flow of blood being greater in the thin-walled veins than it is in the less compressible arteries, venous stasis and edema promptly develop and lead, in a matter of hours, to adhesive inflammation, which binds the layers together, or to infarction and gangrene of the affected segments. The presence of these features serves to differentiate true pathological intussusceptions, brought about by excessive peristalsis in diarrheic and similar conditions, from those that occur agonally at or near the moment of death, even in slaughtered animals. Because of the pressure, an intussusception is usually completely obstructive to passage of the intestinal contents. **Neoplasms,** especially intestinal carcinomas, tend to cause an annular constriction of the intestinal wall and over time slowly impede the movement of the intestinal contents.

While the effects of a gradually developing obstruction may be mitigated by hypertrophy of the local muscularis (see muscular hypertrophy of the ileum of swine,

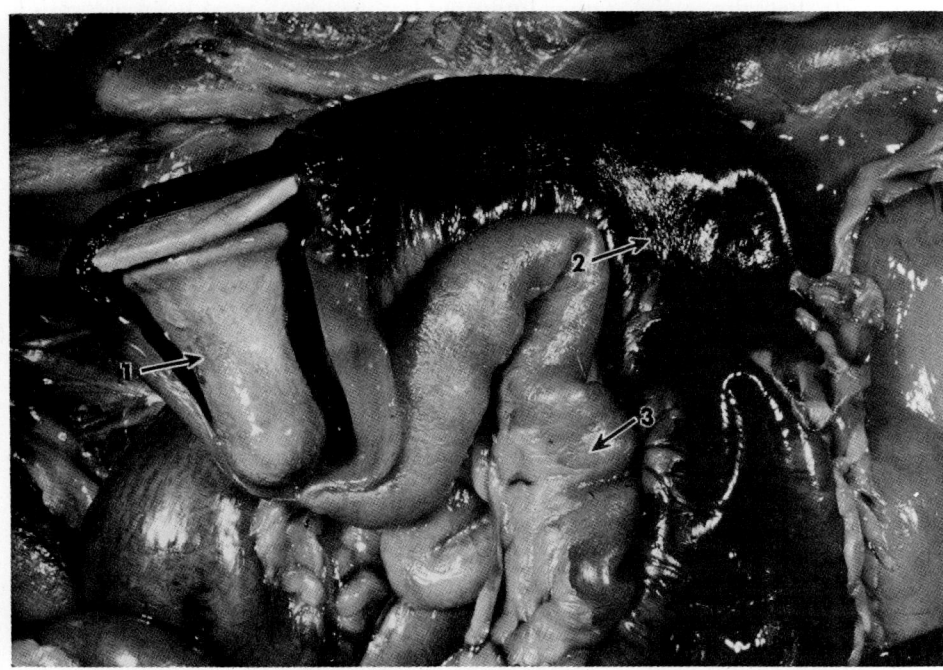

FIG. 23-15. Obstruction of the duodenum of an eight-month-old male Doberman pinscher puppy. The foreign body was a rubber nipple (**1**) from a nursing bottle. Note hemorrhagic wall of duodenum (**2**) proximal to the obstruction, and normal-appearing intestine distal to it (**3**). (Courtesy of Angell Memorial Animal Hospital.)

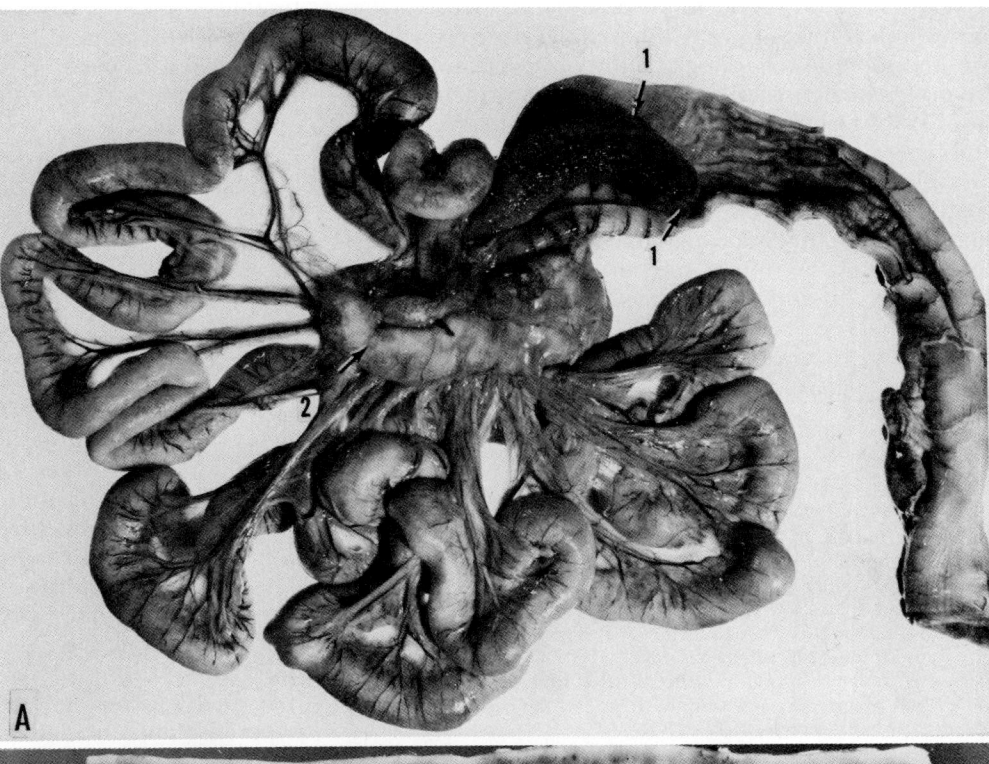

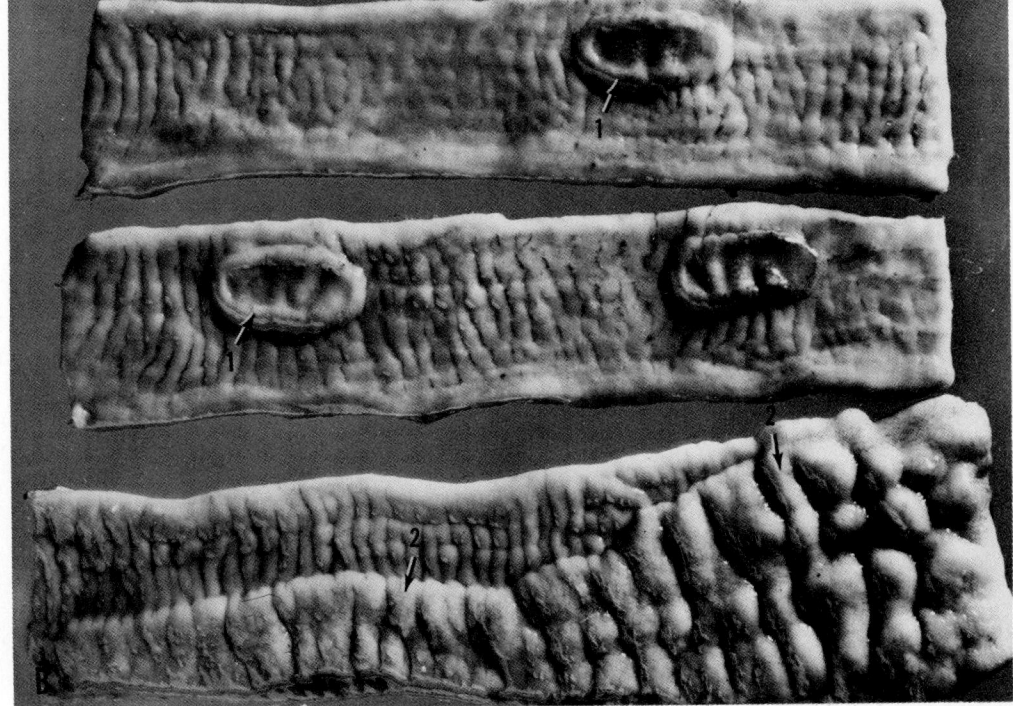

FIG. 23-16. **A.** Intussusception of the ileum (**1**) into the colon of a dog with "salmon disease." Note also hyperplastic lymph node (**2**). **B.** Hyperplasia of Peyer's patches (**1**) and lymphoid tissue in terminal ileum (**2**) in a dog with rickettsiosis of "salmon disease." (Courtesy of Dr. Wm. J. Hadlow.)

above), complete obstruction of the intestinal canal has consistent consequences. The lumen of the bowel for a considerable distance above the obstruction becomes greatly distended with fluid which consists chiefly of inflammatory edema (serous exudate), the accumulated ingesta constituting a minor portion. The wall is not only edematous but red with hyperemia and infiltrated with acute inflammatory cells. These changes are most marked just above (proximal to) the obstruction and gradually decrease in severity with increasing distance proximal from it. Below the obstruction, the bowel is empty and normal. While pathogenic and saprophytic bacteria could conceivably invade and colonize the involved section of the bowel and eventually spread to the peritoneum and cause gangrene (and this sometimes occurs), the usual outcome of complete obstruction of the bowel is death after some hours or, in some species, a day or two unless it is surgically relieved. Death is usually attributed to endotoxic shock. If the obstruction involves the upper small intestine, vomiting is the principal sign, and loss of electrolytes constitutes a significant clinical problem.

Meckel's diverticulum is rarely encountered as a small, 2–4 cm, blind-ended tube protruding from the ileum (Fig. 23-17). It is a congenital anomaly representing persistence of the omphalo-enteric duct of the embryo and has, in a rudimentary way, the histologic appearance of the intestine. Stasis of ingesta occurs in it only exceptionally. This anomaly sometimes forms a nidus for intussusception, and tumors may also originate there.

References

Gaughan EM, Hackett RP. Cecocolic intussusception in horses: 11 cases (1979–1989). J Am Vet Med Assoc 1990;197:1373–1375.
Grant BD, Tennant B. Volvulus associated with Meckel's diverticulum in the horse. J Am Vet Med Assoc 1973;162:550–551.
Harrison IW. Equine large intestinal volvulus—a review of 124 cases. Vet Surg 1988;17:77–81.
Lewis DD, Ellison GW. Intussusception in dogs and cats. Compend Cont Ed Pract Vet 1987;9:523–534.
Pearson H. Intussusception in cattle. Vet Rec 1971;89:426–437.
Pollock WB, Hagan TR. Two cases of torsion of the cecum and ileum in rats. Lab Anim Sci 1972;22:549–551.
Rooney JR. Volvulus, strangulation, and intussusception in the horse. Cornell Vet 1965;55:644–653.
Schoenbaum M, Klopfer U, Egyed MN. Spontaneous intussusception of the small intestine in guinea pigs. Lab Anim 1972;6:327–330.
Wilson GP, Burt JK. Intussusception in the dog and cat: a review of 45 cases. J Am Vet Med Assoc 1974;164:515–519.

Intestinal emphysema

Intestinal emphysema is a rare finding usually encountered in healthy swine at the time of slaughter. It is of no clinical consequence. Numerous small, thin-walled, gas-filled vesicles from 1 mm to 2 cm in diameter are found in the serosa, submucosa, and mucosa of the small intestine and in the mesentery and mesenteric lymph nodes (Fig. 23-14C). Microscopically, the gas bubbles are present within lymphatics. The source of the gas is not known, but it has been speculated that it is produced by bacteria. Occasionally, intestinal emphysema is seen in sheep with enterotoxemia.

References

Meyer RC, Simon J. Intestinal emphysema (pneumatosis cystoides intestinalis) in a gnotobiotic pig. Can J Comp Med 1977;41:302–305.
Sofrenovic D, Matic G, Zigic B. Intestinal emphysema of pigs, in the past and at present. Veterinarski Glasnik 1975;29:119–124.

Neoplasms of the small intestine

The World Health Organization's International Histologic Classification of Tumors of Domestic Animals (Head, 1976) provides a framework for classifying neoplasms of the small intestine on a worldwide basis. For the most part, neoplasms of nonhuman primates, humans, and laboratory animals may also be accommodated by this classification. A brief description of these histologic types follows.

Adenoma, a benign tumor of epithelial cells, is made up of cells that closely resemble those of normal intestinal mucosa, but is more cellular, has generally hyperchromatic nuclei, and is sharply demarcated from the adjacent normal mucosa. Adenomas usually project into the lumen and may be polypoid. They are not readily distinguished from inflammatory polyps, but the increased amount of inflammatory tissue or the presence of foreign bodies or nematodes may be helpful in this regard. The "adenomatosis" of the ileum of swine with the porcine intestinal adenomatosis complex (see above) differs from true adenomas by its diffuse distribution. In all cases, this tumor-like lesion does not invade the submucosa, muscularis mucosa, muscularis, or lymphatics.

Descriptive terms may be used to indicate predominant patterns of growth, such as: papillary (villous), tubular (adenomatous) and papillotubular (tubulovillous)—a combination of the first two.

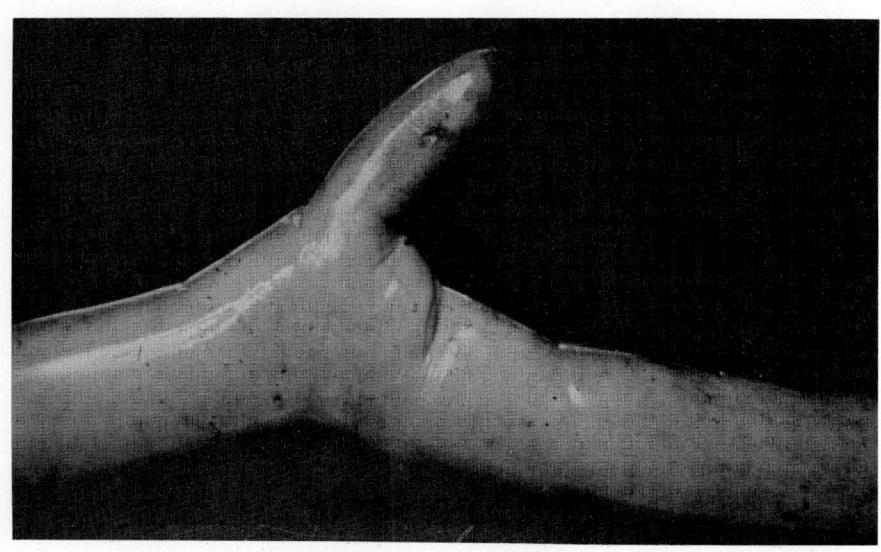

FIG. 23-17. Meckel's diverticulum in the ileum of a pony.

THE DIGESTIVE SYSTEM 1081

Adenocarcinoma is a malignant tumor arising from the epithelial cells of the intestinal mucosa. Although some part of the tumor may project into the lumen, its predominant feature is its growth from the mucosa through the muscularis mucosa into the submucosa and muscularis to the serosa. Invasion of lymphatics is common, as are metastases to regional (mesenteric) lymph nodes and to distant organs (lung, liver, etc.). Adenocarcinomas have a tendency to grow in an annular form around the wall of the intestine. This characteristic as well as the fibrous component of the tumor usually result in constriction and eventually obstruction of the intestinal lumen.

Several morphologic types may be distinguished, sometimes more than one in a single neoplasm, and may be useful in characterizing a specific tumor. **Papillary adenocarcinoma** has finger-shaped fronds of epithelial-covered stroma resembling villi, but more elongated, undifferentiated, and cellular. **Tubular adenocarcinoma** is descriptive of a tumor consisting of branching tubules lined by flattened, cuboidal, or columnar epithelial cells and supported by a fibrous stroma. **Mucinous adenocarcinoma** distinguishes one in which large amounts of mucin are produced by the tumor cells, causing the formation of grossly visible cysts filled with mucin. **Signet ring** cell carcinoma is made up largely of individualized tumor cells with a globule of mucin in their cytoplasm, with a peripherally placed nucleus giving the cell the characteristic appearance of a signet ring.

Adenocarcinoma of the small intestine is an infrequent tumor in most animal species, but nevertheless has been reported as a spontaneous occurrence in many species. A singular exception appears to be its more frequent occurrence in aged sheep in New Zealand, first reported by Dodd (1960) and subsequently documented further by Simpson (1972), Simpson and Jolly (1974), and Webster (1966). This increased frequency in sheep appears to be associated with forage which may be carcinogenic, but experimental reproduction of the disease has not been reported. After sheep, the frequency of reported cases appears to follow in turn: cats, cattle, mice, dogs, hamsters, rats, and other species.

Undifferentiated carcinoma (carcinoma simplex, medullary carcinoma, or solid carcinoma) is made up of epithelial cells which do not form any glandular or papillary structure. This is an even more uncommon type of carcinoma, but may be encountered in domestic, laboratory, or wild animals.

Carcinoid tumors of argentaffin or nonargentaffin types as described in the stomach have been reported in the small intestine of the dog, cat, ox, and elephant. Solid nests of epithelial cells with finely stippled cytoplasm present a characteristic histologic appearance.

Leiomyoma and leiomyosarcoma, the benign and malignant varieties respectively of tumors of smooth muscle, may originate from the tunica muscularis or (rarely) the muscularis mucosa of the small intestine. The tumor cells resemble smooth muscle cells which are elongated, usually in parallel or interlacing bundles.

Their nuclei are elongated with blunt, rounded ends. The malignant variety is distinguished by its lack of cell differentiation, less circumscribed and more irregular borders, more aggressive invasion of neighboring structures, and metastasis. Either tumor may cause intestinal obstruction or serve as initiators of intussusception.

Cavernous hemangioma, a benign lesion composed of blood vascular spaces, has been recorded in the small intestine of most domestic species. The malignant variety, hemangiosarcoma, does not appear to have been reported as primary from the small intestine of domesticated or other species.

Lipomas are benign, circumscribed masses composed of benign, neoplastic lipocytes. They may occur in the wall of the intestine or in the mesentery. In some species, especially the horse, these tumors are pedunculated and may rarely become twisted around the intestine, causing obstruction. Twisting of the pedicle more often leads to infarction of the mass of adipose tissue. The lipoma should be distinguished from lipomatosis or fibrolipomatosis, which is the deposition of normal fat in thick layers in the mesentery, omentum, and retroperitoneum. This may result in as much as 10 cm of fat in the wall of the ileum and colon, between the muscularis and serosa. Fat necrosis and fibrosis may occur, but the effect on the animals appears minimal. Jersey and Guernsey breeds of cattle seem to be most prone to this condition.

Liposarcoma is the malignant variant of lipoma composed of undifferentiated, neoplastic lipocytes. It has been reported on rare occasions in the wall of the small intestine of dogs.

Lymphosarcomas are not infrequent in the wall of the small intestine and presumably arise from gut-associated lymphoid structures (Peyer's patches), but eventually involve the entire wall. The cat is especially prone to this tumor, which may be the presenting lesion in about 20% of feline lymphosarcomas. Single tumors may cause intestinal obstruction or intussusception.

Mast cell tumors may be primary in the small intestine of dog or cat, presumably arising from the mast cells found normally in the subserosa and submucosa of the intestine.

Secondary tumors may involve the small intestine by direct extension from adjacent organs (pancreas), by implantation on the serosa as a consequence of seeding of the peritoneal cavity (for example, hemangiosarcoma from a ruptured splenic neoplasm), or by metastasis via the general circulation (usually in disseminated carcinomatosis or lymphosarcoma). Mesotheliomas of the peritoneum may also extend, rarely, into the wall of the small intestine.

An **osteosarcoma** has been reported (Eckerlin, et al., 1976) in the jejunum of a dog. This tumor, believed to be primary in the jejunum, occurred in a 10–year-old castrated male mongrel.

A single case, designated as **a neoplasm of globular leukocytes,** has been reported in a 12–year-old, castrated, short-haired male cat (Finn and Schwartz, 1972). This tumor was presumed to arise from "globular leukocytes," cells with large non-metachromatic globulin-containing cytoplasmic granules of unknown origin and function, found normally in the wall of the intestine of several species (Takeuchi, et al., 1969).

References

Birchard SJ, Guillermo Couto C, et al. Non-lymphoid intestinal neoplasia in 32 dogs and 14 cats. J Am Anim Hosp Assoc 1986; 22:533–537.

Coop KL, Sharp JG, Osbome JW, et al. An animal model for the study of small bowel tumors. Cancer Res 1974;34:1487–1494.

Cribb AE. Feline gastrointestinal adenocarcinoma: a review and retrospective study. Can Vet J 1988;29:709–712.

Dodd DC. Adenocarcinoma of the small intestine of sheep. NZ Vet J. 1960;8109–112.

Eckerlin RH, Garman RH, Fowler EH. Chondroblastic osteosarcoma in the jejunum of a dog. J Am Vet Med Assoc 1976;168:691–693.

Finn JP, Schwartz LW. A neoplasm of globule leukocytes in the intestine of a cat. J Comp Pathol 1972;82:323–328.

Giles RC Jr, Hildebrandt PK, Montgomery CA Jr. Carcinoid tumor in the small intestine of a dog. Vet Pathol 1974;11:340–349.

Head KW. International histological classification of tumours of domestic animals. XII. Tumours of the lower alimentary tract. Bull WHO 1976;53:137–304.

Kosovsky JE, Matthiesen DT, Patnaik AK. Small intestinal adenocarcinoma in cats; 32 cases (1978–1985). J Am Vet Med Assoc 1988;192:233–235.

Lingeman CH, Garner FM. Comparative study of intestinal adenocarcinomas of animals and man. J Natl Cancer Inst 1972;48:325–346.

McDonald JW, Leaver DO. Adenocarcinoma of the small intestine of Merino sheep. Aust Vet J 1965;41:269–271.

Patnaik AK, Liu SK, Johnson GF. Feline intestinal adenocarcinoma. A clinicopathologic study of 22 cases. Vet Pathol 1976;13:1–10.

Patnaik AK, Hurvitz AI, Johnson GF. Canine gastrointestinal neoplasms. Vet Pathol 1977;14:547–555.

Simpson BH. The geographic distribution of carcinomas of the small intestine in New Zealand sheep. N Z Vet J 1972;20:24–28.

Simpson BH. An epidemiological study of carcinoma of the small intestine in New Zealand sheep. N Z Vet J 1972;20:91–97.

Simpson BH, Jolly RD. Carcinoma of the small intestine in sheep. J Pathol 1974;112:83–92.

Takeuchi A, Jervis HR, Sprinz H. The globule leukocyte in the intestinal mucosa of the cat: A histochemical and electron microscopic study. Anat Rec 1969;164:79–99.

Turk MAM, Gallina AM, Russell TS. Nonhematopoietic gastrointestinal neoplasm in cats: a retrospective study of 44 cases. Vet Pathol 1981;18:614–620.

THE CECUM

Impaction of the cecum

Impactions of the large bowel are often fatal in the horse. Cecal impaction is the most frequent and results when older animals with poor dentition are switched from a soft or lush ration to one consisting of coarse, dry roughage, such as wheat straw. It may be aggravated by periods of water deprivation. The cecum becomes progressively more atonic as it is filled with increasing amounts of undigested stalks and stems, until it is distended to unbelievable dimensions with little chance of recovery. Impaction of segments of the small colon results from one or more unusually large boluses of undigested roughage, frequently coarse alfalfa hay or occasionally from the ingestion of large quantities of sand. The irritated segment of intestine contracts spasmodically around the lodged bolus, tightening the obstruction. This may be complicated by gaseous distention of the more proximal segments of gut (tympanites) and even cecal rupture.

In dogs and cats, the colon may become impacted by inspissated feces (fecoliths), bones, or other foreign bodies.

Tympanites of the cecum is the usual form of alimentary bloating in the horse and is scarcely less formidable than its counterpart in the bovine rumen. Impactions or other disorders that interfere with peristaltic movement through the colon and rectum predispose to this condition without direct relationship to the kind of feed consumed.

Dilatation of the cecum

Dilatation of the cecum is a relatively uncommon abdominal disease in cattle believed to follow atony of the cecum, usually as a consequence of a change to a more concentrated diet. One study (Svendsen and Kristensen, 1970) indicates that change from a ration of hay to one containing 0.5 kg hay and 7.5 kg rolled barley resulted in an increase in concentration of volatile fatty acids and decrease in pH in the cecum. These events led to an increase in the concentration of undissociated ions and a concomitant decrease in frequency of cecal contractions. This study may present a partial explanation of the cecal atony which is believed to precede cecal dilatation.

In germ-free rats, the cecum becomes dilated to about five times the cecal volume of rats with conventional bacterial flora. The dry weight of the cecal contents is increased more than twice. The epithelial cells of the cecum of the germ-free rat are taller and have larger nuclei and microvilli than similar cells in conventional rats. The crypts of Lieberkuhn are more varied in shape than in conventional rats, the lamina propria is almost devoid of plasma cells, but rich in mast cells. The tunica muscularis externa is hypertrophied. The crypts of Lieberkuhn contain what appear to be pure cultures of elongated bacilli in large numbers. The cecal lumen, on the other hand, contains large numbers of varied organisms. This finding led to the postulate that the cecum is important in symbiotic relationships, and the crypts of Lieberkuhn are the sites of this interaction.

Intussusception of the cecum

Rarely in the dog and cat, the cecum becomes inverted into the colon, projecting into the latter for a considerable distance and acting as a partial obstruction. Naturally, a variable degree of edema, inflammation, and perhaps chronic fibrosis results locally, but the disorder is not necessarily fatal.

References

Bertone JJ, Traub-Dargatz JL, Wrigley RW, et al. Diarrhea associated with sand in the gastrointestinal tract of horses. J Am Vet Med Assoc 1988;193:1409–1412.

Boles CL, Kohn CW. Fibrous foreign body impaction in young horses. J Am Vet Med Assoc 1977;171:193–195.

Campbell ML, et al. Cecal impaction in the horse. J Am Vet Med Assoc 1984;184:950–952.

Svendsen P, Kristensen B. Cecal dilatation in cattle. An expenmental study of the etiology. Nord Vet Med 1970;22:578–583.

Neoplasms of the cecum

Neoplasms of the cecum are not often reported, but lymphosarcoma is known to occur, and adenocarcinomas have been recorded in the cecum of the rat, mouse, dog, cat (Fig. 23-18), horse, and genet. Leiomyosarcomas have been reported in the cecum of dogs. These tumors correspond in most respects to those arising in the small intestine.

References

Lingeman CH, Garner FM. Comparative study of intestinal adenocarcinomas of animals and man. J Natl Cancer Inst 1972;48:325–346.

Patnaik AK, Liu SK, Johnson GF. Feline intestinal adenocarcinomas. A clinicopathologic study of 22 cases. Vet Pathol 1976;13:1–10.

Patnaik AK, Hurvitz AI, Johnson GF. Canine gastrointestinal neoplasms. Vet Pathol 1977;14:547–555.

THE COLON

Congenital and hereditary anomalies

Congenital and hereditary anomalies are not numerous in the recorded literature. A few should be mentioned.

Megacolon has been studied in the dog and mice. The lesion is recognized by severe distension of the colon with fecal content, terminating abruptly at the rectum. This lesion appears to be a failure to dilate, the result of absence of myenteric ganglia in the terminal part of the colon distal to the dilated portion. The disease is considered to be inherited in both puppies and young mice. The defect is linked with mutant genes piebald-lethal (**Sl**) and lethal spotting (**ls**) in mice.

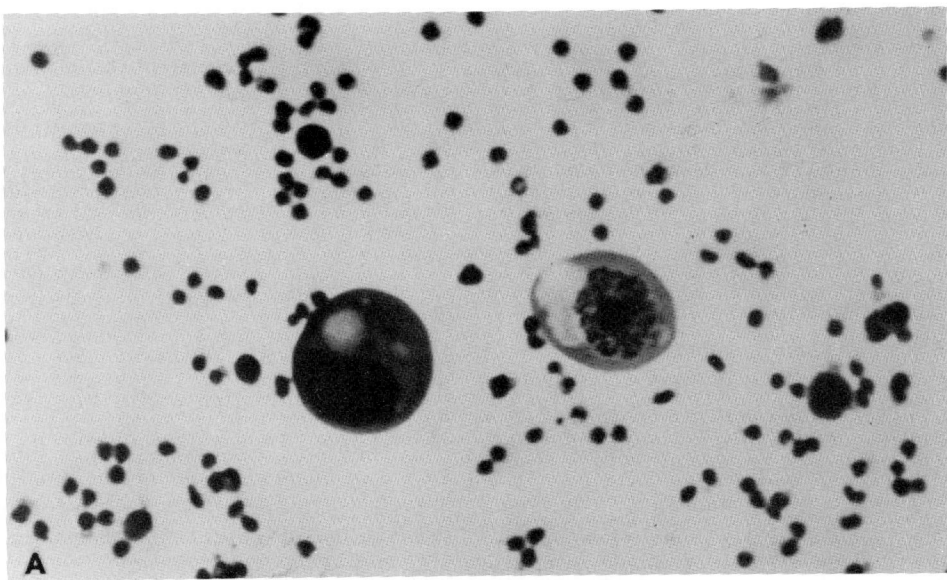

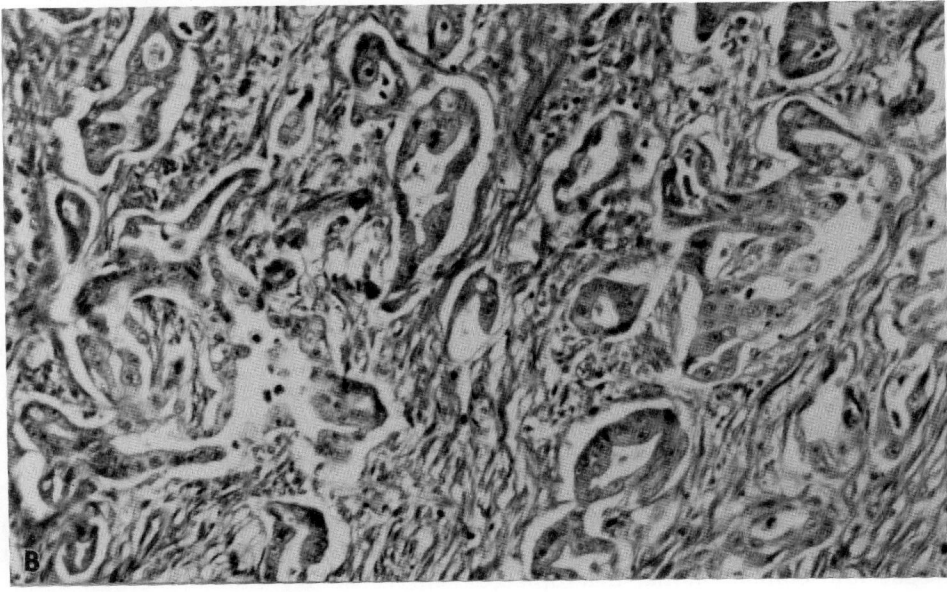

FIG. 23-18. Adenocarcinoma of the cecum of a 14-year-old castrated male cat, with metastases to diaphragm, abdominal wall, liver, and spleen. **A.** Smear of ascitic fluid containing large malignant cells, Giemsa's stain ($\times$ 400). **B.** Section of metastatic tumor in diaphragm. (H & E, $\times$ 250.) (Courtesy of Angell Memorial Animal Hospital.)

Situs inversus viscerum, recognized in rats and humans as a rare, probably polygenic inherited defect, results in transposition of all abdominal viscera from right to left. No functional defect has been identified in association with this transposition.

Duplication of the colon has been described in a dog in association with malformations of the bodies of vertebrae T4 and T5. In this case in a 9–week-old Labrador Retriever, the colon was equally duplicated from the cecum to the rectum, with which the two colons connected.

Atresia coli is another rarely recorded anomaly. In one reported case in an identical twin Simmental calf, the colon was absent, the intestine terminating in a blind cecum. The other identical twin was normal. The monozygosity of these calves was established by identifying identical blood types, electrophoretic patterns, transferrin, and amylase. From this, it was concluded that the atresia coli was not inherited, since each twin should have the same genome.

References

Bolande R., Towler WF. Ultrastructural and histochemical studies of murine megacolon. Am J Pathol 1972;69:139–162.

Hoffsis G, Bruner RR, Jr. Atresia coli in a twin calf. J Am Vet Med Assoc 1977;271:433–434.

Jakowski RM. Duplication of colon in a Labrador Retriever with abnormal spinal column. Vet Pathol 1977;14:256–260.

Webster W. Aganglionic megacolon in piebald-lethal mice. Arch Pathol 1974;97:111–117.

Histiocytic ulcerative colitis of Boxer dogs

Confined to dogs of the Boxer breed, this disorder, also termed granulomatous colitis, is similar in many respects to Whipple's disease of humans. Affected dogs, which are usually less than 2 years of age, pass soft tan feces often mixed with blood, with great frequency (up to 15 times a day). Profuse diarrhea does not occur, and throughout the course of the disease the affected animal is afebrile, and its weight is usually maintained. Significant gross lesions are confined to the colon, cecum, and mesenteric lymph nodes. The wall of the colon and cecum is thickened and the mucosa is ulcerated often to the extent that little intact mucosa remains. Microscopically, the surface of the ulcers is composed of fibrin and neutrophils, but the striking feature throughout the colonic mucosa as well as the submucosa is a marked infiltration by large macrophages, which may be accompanied by lymphocytes, plasma cells, and collagen. The macrophages have pink, foamy cytoplasm which is PAS positive and stains lightly with fat stains. Ultrastructural studies have demonstrated the cells to be filled with packets of phagocytized material composed of membranes often arranged in whorls. In one dog, structures suggesting a psittacoid agent were seen. Enlargement of mesenteric lymph nodes results from lymphocytic hyperplasia and aggregates of macrophages similar to those in the colon and cecum. In advanced cases, peripheral lymph nodes may also be enlarged and contain similar macrophages. The cause of this disease is not known.

References

Cockrell BY, Krehbiel JD. Ultrastructural changes in histiocytic ulcerative colitis in a Boxer. Am J Vet Res 1972;33:453–459.

Russell SW, Gomez JA, Trowbridge JO. Canine histiocytic ulcerative colitis. The early lesion and its progression to ulceration. Lab Invest 1971;25:509–515.

Van Kruiningen HJ, Montali RJ, Strandberg JD, et al. A granulomatous colitis of dogs with histologic resemblance to Whipple's disease. Pathol Vet 1965;2:521–544.

Van Kruiningen HJ. Granulomatous colitis of Boxer dogs. Comparative aspects. Gastroenterol 1967;53:114–122.

Van Kruiningen HJ. Canine colitis comparable to regional enteritis and mucosal colitis of man. Gastroenterol 1972;62:1128–1142.

Van Kruiningen HJ. The ultrastructure of macrophages in granulomatous colitis of Boxer dogs. Vet Pathol 1975;12:446–459.

Infections

Infections of the colon which have been identified with a causal organism are described in other chapters: for example, balantidiasis and amebiasis in Chapter 12; protothecosis and histoplasmosis in Chapter 11; and yersiniosis and salmonellosis in Chapter 10.

Swine dysentery is a highly contagious infectious disease of young, weaned pigs characterized by an acute onset of diarrhea in which there is blood, mucus, and fibrin present in the stool. Affected pigs experience growth retardation. Although it was once thought to caused by *Campylobacter coli,* experimental studies have confirmed that its etiology is an anaerobic spirochete, *Serpula (Treponema) hyodysenteriae.* This organism depends upon the presence of other anaerobic bacteria normally found in the colon to proliferate and cause disease. This disease is described further in Chapter 11.

Ulcerative colitis

An idiopathic ulcerative colitis has been described in many species, including humans. Although the inflammatory and ulcerative features of the disease in the different species bear some similarity, the lack of specific etiology for any of them makes it difficult to make meaningful comparisons.

A spontaneously occurring, idiopathic colitis of laboratory-maintained cotton-top tamarins *Saguinus oedipus* has many features in common with ulcerative colitis of humans. These include: (1) an unknown etiology; (2) lack of a pathognomonic lesion, by which the diagnosis can be made with certainty; (3) a higher prevalence in older individuals, but younger individuals may be affected; (4) sexes are affected equally; (5) characterized by recurrent flares of acute inflammatory activity confined to the mucosa of the colon; (6) repeated episodes of acute inflammatory activity result in structural abnormalities of the colonic mucosa including atrophy and distortion of the colonic crypts and surface epithelium; (7) prominent neutrophilic infiltrates and crypt abscesses characterize the acute flares; (8) there are substantial numbers of lymphocytes, plasma cells, macrophages, and eosinophils present in the lamina propria during periods of remission suggesting an immunologic basis for its pathogenesis; (9) it responds to sulfasalazine or steroid therapy, but relapses occur following cessation of treatment; (10) affected individuals are at increased risk for the development of colonic carcinoma; and (11) the associated colonic carcinoma is multicentric and arises from a flattened rather than a polypoid mucosa.

An ulcerative colitis has been produced in laboratory animals (guinea pigs and rabbits) by addition of pepsin inhibitors (sodium lignosulfonate or sulfated amylopectin) to the drinking water. Carrageenan will also produce ulcerative lesions in the colon of guinea pigs and has been associated with squamous metaplasia of the rectal mucosa of the rat. More recently, an inflammatory bowel disease resembling that of humans has been produced in "knockout" mice in which the genes for the cytokines interleukin-2 (IL-2) or interleukin-10 or the genes for the T cell receptor were deleted. These models hold promise for understanding the immune dysregulation that appears to play a role in the pathogenesis of inflammatory bowel disease.

References

Anver MR, Cohen BJ. Animal model of human disease: ulcerative colitis induced in guinea pigs with degraded carrageenan. Am J Pathol 1976;84:431–434.

Chalifoux LV, Bronson RT. Colonic adenocarcinoma associated with chronic colitis in cotton top marmosets, *Saguinus oedipus.* Gastroenterology 1981;80:942–946.

Fabian RJ, Abraham R, Coulston F, et al. Carrageenan-induced squamous metaplasia of the rectal mucosa in the rat. Gastroenterol. 1973;65:265–276.

Madara JL, Podolsky DK, King NW, et al. Characterization of spontaneous colitis in cotton-top tamarins *(Saguinus oedipus)* and its response to sulfasalazine. Gastroenterology 1985;88:13–19.

Marcus R, Watt J. Ulcerative disease of the colon in laboratory animals induced by pepsin inhibitors. Gastroenterol 1974;67:473–483.

Mullink JWMA. Colitis in the mouse. Z Versuchstierkd 1973;15:217–228.

Scott GBD, Keymer IF. Ulcerative colitis in apes: a comparison with the human disease. J Pathol 1975;115:241–244.

Scotti T. Colitis cystica profunda in Rhesus monkeys. Lab Anim Sci 1975;25:55–61.

Stout LC. Ulcerative colitis-like lesions in siamang gibbons. Digest Dis 1971;16:371–372.

Strober W, Ehrhardt RO. Chronic intestinal inflammation: an unexpected outcome in cytokine or T cell receptor mutant mice. Cell 1993;75:203–205.

Watt J, Marcus R. Experimental ulcerative disease of the colon in animals. Gut 1973;14:506–510.

Murine colonic hyperplasia

Murine colonic hyperplasia is a naturally occurring, transmissible disease of laboratory mice, caused by *Citrobacter freundii.* The signs most often seen in young mice include ruffled fur, retarded growth, soft feces, occasional rectal prolapse, and death of some affected animals. The lesions consist of striking hyperplasia of distal colonic epithelium 2 to 3 weeks after inoculation with cultures of *C. freundii.* The colonic mucosa becomes several times thickened, with great increase in epithelial cells and mitoses, but decrease in number of goblet cells. In young animals, inflammatory and necrotizing changes in the mucosa appear to contribute to higher mortality. In animals destined to recover, the hyperplasia of mucosal epithelium gradually subsides and goblet cells return dramatically, contributing to the formation of mucus-filled cysts deep in the mucosa.

References

Barthold SW, Coleman GL, Jacoby RO, et al. Transmissible murine colonic hyperplasia. Vet Pathol 1978;15:223–236.

Barthold SW, Coleman GL, Bhatt PN, et al. The etiology of transmissible murine colonic hyperplasia. Lab Anim Sci 1978;26:889–894.

Brennan PC, Fritz TE, Flynn RJ, et al. Citrobacter freundii associated with diarrhea in laboratory mice. Lab Anim Care 1965;15:266–275.

Silverman J, Chovannes JM, Rigotty J, et al. A natural outbreak of transmissible murine colonic hyperplasia in A/J mice. Lab Anim Sci 1979;29:209–218.

Neoplasms of the colon

Benign and malignant neoplasms may be classified according to the WHO histologic criteria described for the small intestine. Some rather striking differences in frequency of colonic tumors have been described in different species. Adenocarcinomas of the colon are one of the more important neoplastic diseases of humans. Most animals have a lower frequency of adenocarcinoma of the colon than humans, although several studies have demonstrated that chemical carcinogens (azoxymethane, 1,2–dimethylhydrazine) will induce adenocarcinomas of the colon in a high proportion of animals exposed. Naturally occurring tumors of the colon are generally less frequent than those of the small intestine.

Adenocarcinoma of the colon is recognized in the dog more often than in any other species (Fig. 23-19). Colonic tumors are more common than gastric, but are less frequent than adenocarcinomas of the rectum in this species. Adenocarcinoma in the "W" strain of rats reportedly was seen in 28 out of 3000 necropsies (Miwa et al., 1976). This tumor appears to be much less frequent in cats, hamsters, and mice. In sheep and oxen, the lesions usually involve the spiral colon rather than the rectum and are less frequent than in the dog.

Adenocarcinoma of the colon is quite unusual in most nonhuman primates, but the laboratory-maintained cotton-top tamarin *(Saguinus oedipus)* develops a high incidence of adenocarcinoma of the colon. The neoplasms in these animals always arise in animals with a chronic idiopathic colitis resembling ulcerative colitis of humans. The frequency of this lesion obviously is increasing as animals become older. These adenocarcinomas arise within a flattened mucosa, are typically mucinous and highly invasive, invade the submucosa, tunica muscularis, and lymphatics and metastasize to the colonic and pancreatic lymph nodes. The lungs occasionally are the site of metastases.

References

Chalifoux LV, Bronson RT. Colonic adenocarcinoma associated with chronic colitis in cotton top marmosets, *Saguinus oedipus.* Gastroenterology 1981;80:942–946

Clapp NK, Lushbaugh CC, Humason GL, et al. Natural history and pathology of colon cancer in *Saguinus oedipus.* Dig Dis Sci 1985;30:107S-113S.

Evans JT, Lutman G, Mittleman A. The induction of multiple large bowel neoplasms in mice. J Med 1972;3:212–215.

Head KW. International histological classification of tumours of domestic animals. XII. Tumours of the lower alimentary tract. Bull WHO 1976;53:137–304.

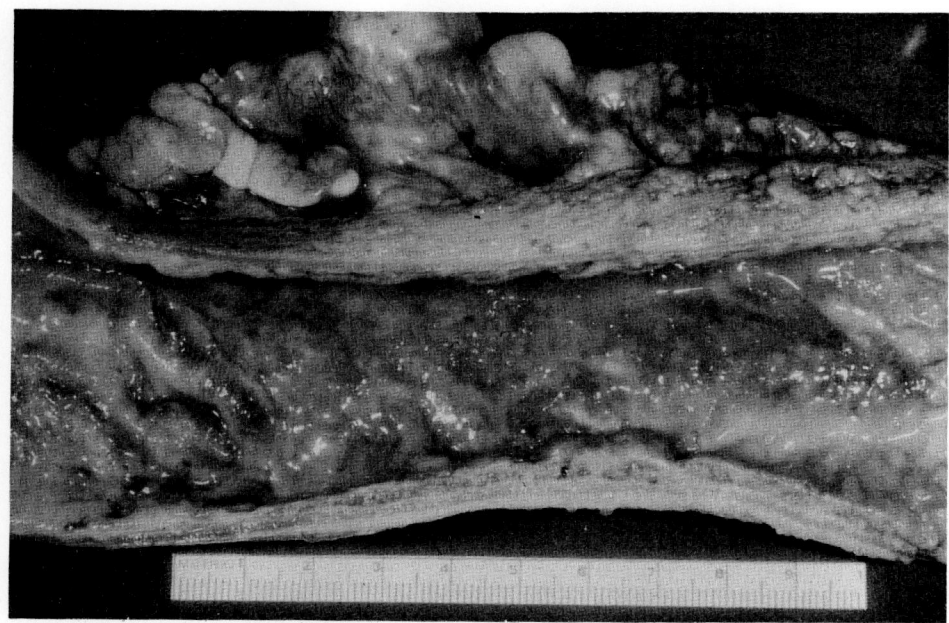

FIG. 23-19. Adenocarcinoma of the colon of a seven-year-old male German shepherd. Note that the mucosa is eroded and the lumen is partially stenotic due to the invasion of the wall by the tumor. (Courtesy of Angell Memorial Animal Hospital.)

Johnson LD, Ausman LM, Sehgal PK, et al. A prospective study of the epidemiology of colitis and colon cancer in cotton-top tamarins (*Saguinus oedipus*). Gastroenterology 1996;110:102–115.

Lushbaugh CC, Humason GL, Swartzendruber DC, et al. Spontaneous colonic adenocarcinoma in marmosets. In: Gengozian N, Deinhardt F, eds. Primates in Medicine. Basel. Karger 1978;10: 119–134.

Madara JL, Podolsky DK, King NW, et al. Characterization of spontaneous colitis in cotton-top tamarins (*Saguinus oedipus*) and its response to sulfasalazine. Gastroenterology 1985;88:13–19.

Martin MS, Martin F, Michiels R, et al. An experimental model for cancer of the colon and rectum. Intestinal carcinoma induced in the rat by 1,2–dimethylhydrazine. Digestion 1973;8:22–34.

Miwa M, Takenaka S, Ito K, et al. Spontaneous colon tumor in rats. J Natl Cancer Inst 1976;56:615–617.

Newberne PM, Rogers AE. Adenocarcinoma of the colon. Animal model. DMH-induced adenocarcinoma of the colon in the rat. Am J Pathol 1973;72:541–544.

Ward JM, Yamamoto RS, Benjamin T, et al. Experimentally induced cancer of the colon in rats and mice. J Am Vet Med Assoc 1975; 164:729–732.

THE RECTUM AND ANUS
Anomalies and infection

Atresia ani is a failure of development of the anal opening. Often there is little more than the skin and subcutis remaining imperforate, and it may be possible to create surgically a satisfactory opening, the muscular sphincter and the rectum being adequately developed.

Prolapse of the rectum probably occurs occasionally in all species, but is seen with some frequency in cattle and swine. The exposed portion of the bowel becomes traumatized, dry and inflamed, as well as filled with venous blood confined there by pressure of the rectal sphincter. Here, as elsewhere, venous flow is often blocked by pressure which permits the arterial circulation to continue. Hemorrhoids, a common condition in people in developed countries, consist of slightly prolapsed hemorrhoidal veins covered by a mucosa; they do not occur in domestic animals.

Stricture of the rectum is a frequent problem in young swine. The natural disease has been associated with salmonellosis and can be reproduced experimentally with pure cultures of *Salmonella typhimurium*. This organism produces an ulcerative fibronecrotic colitis and proctitis in susceptible pigs. The rectum is especially vulnerable to deep ischemic injury due to the restricted source of its blood supply. The cranial hemorrhoidal artery of the pig provides almost the entire blood supply to the rectum. Fibrin thrombi which occasionally develop in the submucosal arterioles of the rectum cause ischemic necrosis of the mucosa and submucosa at this site. At a site 2 to 5 cm proximal to the anorectal junction which still has a blood supply, the deep ulceration eventually heals by scar formation which contracts and forms a constriction that impinges on the lumen of the rectum. The accumulation of feces in the colon as a consequence of this partial occlusion causes severe dilatation of the colon proximal to this site and compression atrophy of abdominal and thoracic viscera. Typically, the affected pig fails to grow and develops a markedly distended abdomen.

Rectal and vaginal constriction in certain herds of Jersey cattle have been described as occurring together, presumably the result of inherited factors (Leipold and Saperstein, 1975).

Acquired inflammatory and neoplastic diseases of the anal sacs are common in dogs. The anal sacs are paired blind pouches lined by stratified squamous epithelium and surrounded by apocrine glands which expel their secretion into the lumens of the sacs. These specialized markings or pheromone secreting glands lie in the subcutis ventrolateral to the anus. These sacs communicate with the lumen of the anus via small ducts, the orifices of which are located at ano-cutaneous junction. Occlusion of the orifices of the ducts of these glands results in distension of the sac by accumulated secretion and predisposes the sac to secondary bacterial infection. This causes considerable local discomfort to the dog until the pressure is relieved either by manual expression, surgical removal, or spontaneous rupture of the sac. Spillage of secretion or exudate from an infected sac into the surrounding subcutis causes an intense localized cellulitis and, at times, the formation of perianal fistulas.

Squamous metaplasia of the rectal mucosa has been recorded in the rat in association with the feeding of degraded carrageenan. The carrageenans are a group of sulfated polysaccharides extracted from seaweeds (*Rhodophyceae*). Native carrageenan is extracted from the seaweed *Chondrus crispus* and used as a suspending agent (suspends particulate materials) in chocolate milk, milk puddings, and infant formulas. The degraded carrageenan is extracted from *Eucheuma spirosum* and has been used in the treatment of ulcers. This latter type has been implicated in the causation of ulcers in the cecum and colon of guinea pigs, rats, and rabbits. The squamous metaplasia induced in rats by carrageenen, is accompanied by severe chronic inflammation in the mucosa and submucosa and occasionally by adenomatous polyps.

Neoplasms of the rectum and anus

Adenocarcinomas of the rectal mucosa are the most frequent gastrointestinal neoplasm in the dog and, in fact, appear more frequently in this species than any other. The canine rectum develops this neoplasm approximately three times more frequently than any other part of the gastrointestinal tract. Some of these rectal adenocarcinomas are thought to arise from benign adenomas in the dog rectum (Fig. 23-12B).

Squamous cell carcinomas occasionally originate at the mucocutaneous junction of the anus. These are most frequently reported in dogs but also occur in other species.

Adenomas and, less frequently, **adenocarcinomas of the circumanal (perianal) glands** are the most frequent neoplasms of the perianal region. These are described in greater detail in Chapter 17 under tumors of the skin.

Adenocarcinomas of apocrine glands of the anal sac occur with some frequency in dogs. Clinically, this neoplasm is almost always associated with hypercalcemia due to its production of a parathormone-like substance. Tumors of this type should always be suspected in dogs in which there is no other explanation for elevated serum calcium concentrations. Metastasis to regional lymph nodes may occur and may be associated with persistent hypercalcemia after excision of the primary neoplasm.

References

Dennis SM, Leipold, HW. Atresia ani in sheep. Vet Rec 1972;91:219–222.
Fabian RJ, Abraham R, Coulston F, et al. Carrageenan-induced squamous metaplasia of the rectal mucosa in the rat. Gastroenterol 1973;65:265–276.
Harvey CE. Incidence and distribution of anal sac disease in the dog. J Am Anim Hosp Assoc 1974;10:573–577.
Head KW. International histological classification of tumours of domestic animals. XII. Tumours of the lower alimentary tract. Bull WHO 1976;53:167–186.
Leipold HW, Saperstein G. Rectal and vaginal constriction in Jersey cattle. J Am Vet Med Assoc 1975;166:231–232.
Lingeman CH, Gamer FM. Comparative study of intestinal adenocarcinomas of animals and man. J Natl Cancer Inst 1972;48:325–346.
Saunders CN. Rectal stricture syndrome in pigs: a case history. Vet Rec 1974;94:61.
Schaffer E, Schiefer B. Incidence and type of canine rectal carcinoma. J Small Anim Pract 1968;9:491–496.
Wilcock BP, Olander HJ. The pathogenesis of porcine rectal stricture. I. The naturally occurring disease and its association with salmonellosis. Vet Pathol 1977;14:36–42.
Wilcock BP, Olander HJ. The pathogenesis of porcine rectal stricture. II.. Experimental salmonellosis and ischemic proctitis. Vet Pathol 1977;14:43–55.

PERITONEUM

Peritonitis

Most cases of peritonitis result from infectious agents. Acute inflammation of the peritoneum may be localized to a given area, or involve the entire peritoneum. This depends upon the mode of entry of the infectious agent and the relative resistance of the host. The latter is largely a matter of species; dogs seldom develop serious peritonitis; on the other hand, the introduction of any appreciable amount of infectious material into the peritoneal cavity of a horse is often fatal, even though antibiotics have substantially reduced the fatality rate of such infections. Cattle may die of generalized peritonitis, but, often have sufficient resistance to keep the infection localized.

The causative organisms of infectious peritonitis are diverse and it is not unusual for more than one agent to be involved. Prominent among the causative bacteria are coliforms, streptococci, staphylococci, corynebacteria and the anaerobic clostridial agents.

The principal routes by which infectious agents enter the peritoneal cavity are (1) surgical incisions through the abdominal wall; (2) rupture or perforation of the stomach, intestine, or uterus (Fig. 23-20); (3) direct extension through the necrotic, ruptured wall of one of these organs when it is chronically infected; (4) via the bloodstream in the case of certain specific agents, such as feline infectious peritonitis. Other routes of infection include ascending infections from the uterine tubes (salpingitis), from an infected umbilicus in the newborn, or by direct extension from an infected kidney or urinary bladder.

The peritoneum constitutes one of the largest absorptive surfaces of the body, even when compared to the gastrointestinal mucosa, or the total area of the pulmonary alveolar or renal tubular surfaces. If its thin, mesothelial lining becomes coated with toxin-producing microorganisms, it results in a serious clinical problem. The infected animal's best chance of survival depends upon keeping the infection localized near its portal of

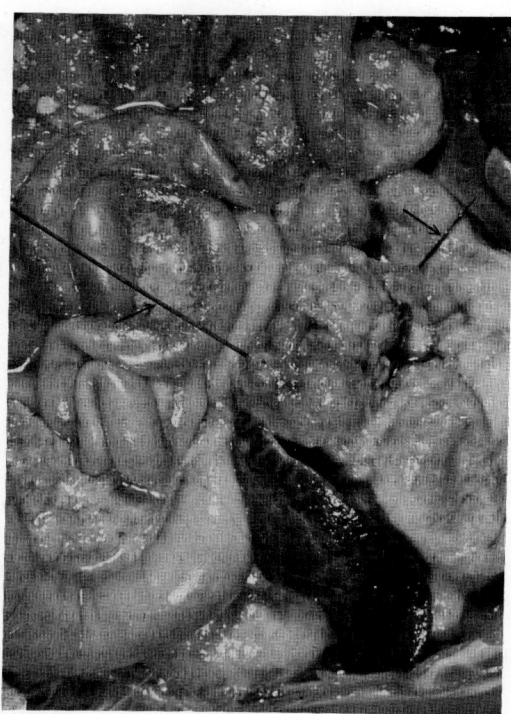

FIG. 23-20. Chronic peritonitis in a cat following ingestion of broom straws (arrows) which penetrated the stomach.

entry, which depends upon the existence of several host mechanisms which are adapted for this purpose. Fibrin tends to seal off infected areas and envelope the invading pathogens, limiting their spread. In those species which have a well-developed omentum, that membrane moves through unknown mechanisms, often within minutes, to cover an infected or injured site, and become adherent to the newly infected surface. The thin-walled omental vessels also facilitate the recruitment and emigration of neutrophils and other inflammatory cells to the site of recent infection. Through reflex, partly the result of pain, bodily movements are minimized; peristalsis ceases, the abdominal wall becomes rigid, and breathing is limited to thoracic movements.

These mechanisms are not without complications. Paralytic ileus may result in a motionless and non-functional intestine. In this condition, the bowel becomes distended with gas and the shock-like accompaniment of intestinal obstruction (see above) may ensue. If the patient survives, the fibrin deposits at most sites, becomes organized by fibroblasts which cause adhesions of contiguous abdominal organs to each other and to the diaphragm and abdominal wall. This process occurs if the inflammation is not resolved within 6 to 10 days. The adhesions that result commonly interfere with peristalsis and the digestive process and may cause further intestinal constriction.

Tuberculous peritonitis, although essentially eliminated from cattle herds in the United States, still occurs in underdeveloped countries where tuberculosis still exists. In cattle, infection of the peritoneum by the tubercle bacillus has been referred to as "pearly disease" because of the large number of shiny gray spherical nodules of individual tubercles on the diaphragmatic or other surfaces of the peritoneum. In those countries where bovine and human tuberculosis is still prevalent, young dogs may contract a severe tuberculous peritonitis.

Actinobacillosis occasionally involves the peritoneum of cattle with a multitude of tiny nodular excrescences of granulation tissue, the mode of entry of the infection being unknown. Diagnosis of this condition depends upon the microscopic features of the lesions and culture of the causative organism from suspect lesions.

Actinobacillosis, as well as tuberculosis, has to be differentiated from **neoplastic transplantations.** Occasionally, a malignant neoplasm, usually a carcinoma arising in the digestive tract, a hemangiosarcoma from a ruptured spleen, or an ovarian adenocarcinoma, ruptures or exfoliates into the peritoneal cavity, and the neoplastic cells become transplanted via movements of the peritoneal surfaces and fluid to numerous sites on the parietal and visceral peritoneum. The tumor cells implant at these sites, proliferate, and form numerous tiny nodular growths.

Feline infectious peritonitis, a viral disease, characterized by extensive fibrinous peritonitis is described in Chapter 8.

Necrosis of abdominal fat regularly accompanies necrotizing pancreatitis, and is occasionally encountered in most animals as small, white plaques or nodules within the abdominal fat. The cause of this condition is not known. A peculiar form of abdominal fat necrosis of unknown cause occurs in cattle, characterized by extremely large masses of necrotic fat in the omentum, mesentery, and retroperitoneal tissues. Casts of necrotic fat may encircle the intestine causing intestinal obstruction.

Hydroperitoneum, ascites

Accumulation of watery fluid in the peritoneal cavity, in its broadest sense, is called hydroperitoneum. If, as is often the case, the fluid represents a true (noninflammatory) edema, the term **ascites** is applicable. Fluid in the peritoneal cavity may, however, represent an inflammatory edema (serous peritonitis) or may result from, especially in male cattle and sheep, a severe acute urinary obstruction with or without rupture of the bladder. With the possible exception of the inflammatory form, the amount of fluid that accumulates within the peritoneal cavity may be tremendous, causing marked distension of the abdomen and all of the symptoms that go with excessive abdominal pressure.

Ascites, or true edema of the peritoneal cavity, may occur as part of a syndrome of generalized edema and be referable to the several causes of that condition. Such cases are manifest by the presence of edema at other sites, which need not be listed here. But, ascites more typically results from chronic passive congestion of the portal venous system. The special causes of that congestion are conditions which incompletely obstruct the flow of blood through the portal vein, most commonly due to hepatic cirrhosis. Other causes of obstruction include pressure of neoplasms, abscesses, granulomas, and enlarged lymph nodes upon the vein, as well as thrombosis within it.

Like all edema fluid, it is a true transudate, with a specific gravity less than 1.017 and with a protein content typically below 3 percent.

Inflammatory accumulation of fluid is distinguished by the presence of other signs of inflammation and by other elements of inflammatory exudation, principally leukocytes and fibrin. The specific gravity and concentration of protein are correspondingly higher in inflammatory exudates.

Peritoneal fluid of urinary tract origin, whether it comes directly from a ruptured bladder as urine, or from a transudate associated with gradual urine infiltration of the tissues of the periurethral region, has the odor and other characteristics of urine. Evidence of urinary obstruction in the form of calculi, cystitis, hydronephrosis, or related lesions is usually present.

The clinical consequences of hydroperitoneum are those of pressure which interferes with the abdominal organs and movement of the diaphragm during respiration. If the fluid is withdrawn by abdominocentesis, more rapidly accumulates. The underlying disorders responsible for its accumulation, of course, produce other characteristic clinical abnormalities, such as uremia in the case of urinary obstruction.

Neoplasms of the peritoneum

Neoplasms of the peritoneum are rare, and only a few primary tumors are known in animals: the mesothelioma, fibrosarcoma, lipoma, and liposarcoma. The mesothelioma arises directly from the mesothelial cells lining the peritoneum. The neoplastic cells are flattened to cuboidal and line numerous thin, papillary projections supported by fibrovascular stroma. In some areas, the neoplastic cells may form tubules or solid masses of tumor cells; in others, the fibrous component dominates, and microscopically must be differentiated from a fibroma or fibrosarcoma. These tumors often become disseminated by exfoliation of tumor cells into the peritoneal cavity with subsequent implantation and proliferation of tumor cells at new sites of implantation. Extensive peritoneal involvement may lead to ascites due to production of excessive peritoneal fluid by the neoplastic cells and occlusion of peritoneal lymphatics by the neoplastic cellular infiltrates. Mesotheliomas of the thoracic and abdominal cavities have been reported in humans, cattle, buffalo, horses, rats, mice, dogs, fowl, sheep, hamsters, and cats.

Lipomas and liposarcomas have been described as tumors involving the mesentery and the wall of the small intestine.

References

Harvey KA, Morris DD, Salk JE, et al. Omental fibrosarcoma in a horse. J Am Vet Med Assoc 1987;191:335–336.
Raflo CP, Nernberger SP. Abdominal mesothelioma in a cat. Vet Pathol 1978;15:781–783.
Ricketts SW, Peace CK. A case of peritoneal mesothelioma in a Thoroughbred mare. Equine Vet J 1976;8:78–80.

Liver

The liver may be seen with the light microscope or even naked eye to be divided into many lobules, about 2.0 mm in diameter, with the shape of an irregular pyramidal hexahedron. These are the classic **anatomic lobules** or **classic lobules.** At the center of anatomic lobules is a central vein, which are the smallest branches of the hepatic vein. Around the periphery of each lobule are four or five portal triads composed of terminal branches of the hepatic artery, portal vein and common bile duct. These are embedded in connective tissue which is ultimately continuous with the hepatic capsule, Glisson's capsule. In swine the connective tissue of the triad extends around each anatomic lobule making each lobule very prominent. The portal vein provides about 40% of the blood to the lobule with the remainder from the hepatic artery. Because the blood supply to each anatomic lobule comes from several different triads and the bile ducts drain only a part of the anatomic lobule, the hepatic lobule has been defined by Rappaport (1973) as a **functional lobule** or **metabolic lobule.** The metabolic lobule, also termed the **hepatic acinus,** has at its center the portal triad and is comprised of pie shaped segments of several adjacent anatomic lobules. The hepatocytes of the metabolic lobule are divided into three zones by the Rappaport system. Those hepatocytes surrounding the triads are termed periportal hepatocytes (Rappaport zone 1); these are surrounded by zone 2 or midzone hepatocytes; and finally by those hepatocytes near the central vein (of the anatomic lobule) which are termed periacinar hepatocytes. The latter are also termed centrilobular hepatocytes based upon the anatomic lobule. The location of hepatocytes within the acinus in part determines their susceptibility to certain forms of injury. Those adjacent to the portal triad are the first to be exposed to toxins arriving via the portal vein or hepatic artery and those at the periphery of the acinus (centrilobular) are the most susceptible to hypoxic injury.

Hepatocytes are arranged in plates which are seen as cords in tissue section. They are large polyhedral cells with abundant cytoplasm, and each has one (or occasionally two) round nucleus containing a fairly prominent nucleolus. There is some variation in nuclear size, often with very large nuclei which are the result of polyploidy. This is particularly apparent in rodent livers. The plates (cords) of hepatocytes are separated from one another by sinusoids which carry portal and arterial blood from the triads to the central vein. Sinusoids are lined by a fenestrated endothelium and phagocytic Kupffer's cells. Plasma can pass through the fenestrations into a space between the endothelium and the plasma membrane of the hepatocytes. This is called the space of Disse. Interspersed between hepatocytes and in contact with the space of Disse are fat-containing cells termed Ito cells or lipocytes. These cells which are thought to be the site of storage of fat-soluble vitamins are of mesodermal origin. They are recognizably conspicuous in vitamin A toxicity.

Between hepatocytes at their poles, opposite the sinusoids, are the smallest divisions of the biliary tree, the bile canaliculi. These canaliculi form an interlacing network that ultimately joins the canals of Hering and thence into bile ductules at the margin of the lobule. Canaliculi are 1 to 2 μm in diameter and lined by the hepatocellular membrane which is thrown into numerous microvilli. The biliary tree becomes lined with its own epithelium at the level of the canals of Hering.

Congenital defects

Congenital defects of the liver are not common. Variation in lobation, including absence of lobes or supernumary lobes, is encountered on occasion, but of no clinical significance. Congenital diaphragmatic hernias may allow displacement of the liver into the thoracic cavity.

Intrahepatic congenital cysts are assumed to represent a congenital malformation in which one or more primitive bile ducts lack an outlet or connection with the main biliary system. They occur more often in dogs, cats, and swine than in other domestic species. They are lined by cuboidal to flattened epithelium and contain clear, serous fluid having little resemblance to bile. Solitary or multiple, they are of varying sizes, even in the same liver, diameters of 2 to 5 cm being common (Fig 23-21). While considered to be congenital, they are not necessarily encountered in the young. Most often they are found incidentally upon death from some other cause. The hepatic parenchyma undergoes pressure atrophy and pressure necrosis when the cysts are numerous and large. In dogs and swine, **congenital polycystic liver disease** accompanied by polycystic kidney disease is described, with an apparent predisposition to the Cairn terrier breed. In humans, a similar disorder is recognized as an inherited dominant trait. **Atresia** of extrahepatic bile ducts can occur and will lead to biliary cirrhosis.

An outbreak of congenital biliary atresia was described in 300 crossbred lambs and 9 crossbred calves in Australia. The affected animals developed jaundice and died within 4 weeks of birth with cholangiohepatopathy and cirrhosis. It was presumed to be the result of a plant toxin. In poisoning by chlorinated naphthalenes, the hyperplastic epithelium of the intrahepatic bile ducts occasionally becomes so irregular as to form a series of cystic spaces as much as 5 or 6 mm in diameter along the wall of the duct.

Congenital portosystemic vascular shunts are seen in dogs and cats, but probably occur, albeit rarely, in other species. They may result from persistence of the ductus venosus or connections between the portal vein and caudal vena cava or the azygous vein. The lack of portal circulation leads to a small liver, with small hepatocytes, small or absent portal veins in the triads, and reduplication of hepatic arterioles in the triads. Affected animals are stunted and may develop hepatic encephalopathy. Portosystemic vascular shunts can also be

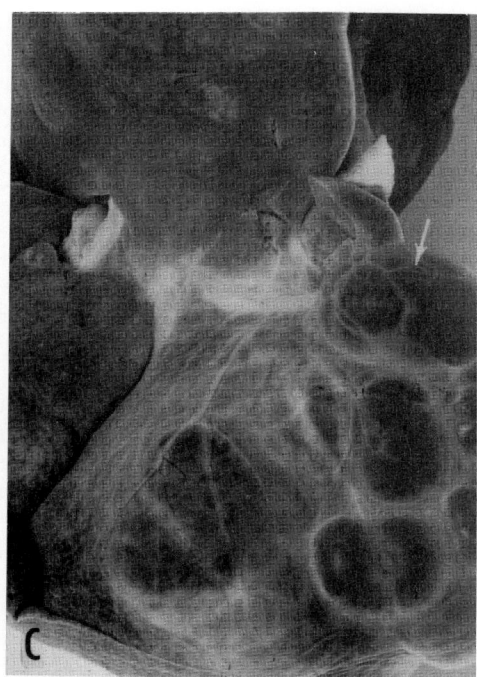

FIG. 23-21. Large cysts in the liver of a ten-year-old female spaniel dog.

acquired. This occurs with portal hypertension most often resulting from chronic liver disease and usually leads to ascites, not seen in congenital portosystemic vascular shunts. Congenital hypoplasia of the portal vein leading to portosystemic shunts has been described in dogs. Intrahepatic portal veins are small or absent, associated with hepatic arteriolar hyperplasia and ductular proliferation. **Arterioportal shunts** (fistulae) are less frequent. These are characterized by connections or fistulae between the hepatic artery and portal vein. The resulting portal hypertension results in the development of acquired portocaval shunts and ascites. There is atrophy of the liver with loss of portal veins and proliferation of hepatic arterioles. Neurologic signs associated with arterioportal shunts result from the coexistence of portocaval shunts.

Hepatic necrosis

Comparable to many other organs and tissues, there are only so many ways the liver responds to injury. One feature common to many different diseases is necrosis of hepatocytes. Often the morphologic features of necrosis are similar in different disease states. However, the pattern of necrosis may provide clues to the etiology of the lesions. Some general explanation of these characteristics is presented here to avoid repetition.

Microscopically, hepatic necrosis is most often coagulative in type, recognized by pyknosis and acidophilic cytoplasm. Disintegration and disappearance of the cells follow. Necrosis may also be preceded by acute cellular swelling. Caseous or liquefactive necrosis may be seen in the liver in granulomatous infections. In hyaline necrosis, affected individual cells become deeply eosinophilic, relatively insoluble, and are most frequently seen in human alcoholic liver disease. They are also referred to as "alcoholic hyaline bodies" or "Mallory's bodies". From the standpoint of location, necrosis may take several different patterns. **Focal necrosis,** in which small necrotic areas, or foci, of sublobular size, appear here and there, occupying any part of any lobule. The focus may consist of one cell to a small group of cells. Necrosis of individual cells or small groups of cells is also sometimes termed **lytic necrosis. Acidophilic necrosis** is used to describe the unicellular death of hepatocytes which become globular and small in size and lose their pyknotic nucleus by extrusion. Such cells are also called "Councilman bodies" or "shrinkage necrosis". They are seen in yellow fever, some forms of human viral hepatitis, and ischemic necrosis. This "Councilman body" may be extruded into the sinusoid and engulfed by Kupffer cells. Focal necrosis is characteristic of disseminated infections. Herpesvirus infections typically produce focal necrosis as does **Toxoplasma gondii.** Focal necrosis characterizes the so called "sawdust" liver of cattle. This descriptive bit of professional slang refers to bovine liver seen frequently (and condemned) by meat inspectors. They come most often from well-fattened young cattle which appear clinically in perfect health. The livers contain several or many minute yellowish foci of necrosis, as if the same number of granules of sawdust had been scattered over them. The necrotic foci, 1 or 2 mm in diameter, are scattered without grossly apparent relation to the lobular architecture. They consist of collections of hepatic epithelial cells in a state of coagulative necrosis or in the process of disappearing, mingled with or surrounded by a thin sprinkling of neutrophils and lymphocytes. They are often concomitant with telangiectasis and hepatic abscesses, and there is at least statistical evidence to link them etiologically with those conditions, however the vast majority of "sawdust" foci certainly do not progress to abscesses.

Zonal necrosis is characterized by hepatocyte necrosis restricted to a particular part of the lobule or acinus. Four patterns are recognized. **Centrilobular necrosis (Periacinar necrosis)** is characterized by necrosis of hepatocytes nearest the central vein. It may entirely circle the central vein or only affect a wedge of the acinus. The necrosis may be restricted to the center of the lobule or in some examples the zones of necrosis may extend from one central vein to another (bridging necrosis), delineating the acinus. Owing to their greater distance from the blood supply, centrilobular necrosis is seen in hypoxic conditions, such as passive congestion and severe anemia. These hepatocytes also are more efficient in oxidizing certain compounds into toxic forms. **Midzonal necrosis** affects the hepatocytes halfway between the periphery and center of the lobule. This form is unusual. **Periportal necrosis** is characterized by necrosis of hepatocytes surrounding the triads. It is also uncommon, but results when strong toxic substances are brought to the lobule, reaching the periph-

eral cells first. It is characteristic of phosphorous poisoning. **Paracentral necrosis** is a form of necrosis in which the entire acinus becomes necrotic. In some disorders, necrotic tissue may extend as a band from the central vein to the periportal areas, or triad to triad, which is termed **bridging necrosis.**

Massive necrosis (diffuse necrosis) is characterized by necrosis of entire lobules and contiguous lobules. It may only affect several lobules or entire lobes of the liver. It can be the outcome of extensive zonal necrosis or circulatory disease (infarction), and is seen in vitamin E/selenium deficiency in pigs (hepatosis dietetica). Infarction of the liver is not common due to its dual blood supply. It is usually associated with occlusion of a major branch of the hepatic artery, but may also follow occlusion of the portal vein. Torsion of the liver leads to ischemic necrosis of an entire lobe. Torsion of lobes of the liver occurs occasionally, especially in dogs, pigs, rats, mice, and rabbits.

Disassociation of liver cells is one characteristic feature of certain diseases, particularly canine leptospirosis, which precedes other evidence of widespread necrosis of liver cells. The liver cells, although still in place, become detached from one another, individualized, and somewhat rounded. Their cytoplasm may become more acidophilic. This striking picture is believed to depict one of the early manifestations of death of hepatocytes.

The **outcome of necrosis**—subsequent to removal of the dead hepatocytes by inflammatory cells there is usually complete resolution with regeneration of hepatocytes. Initially these may appear pleomorphic and disorganized. If, however, the necrosis is so severe as to destroy the reticulum framework of the lobules, the dead tissue is replaced by fibrous connective tissue leading to scarring. The pattern of fibrosis will vary with the nature of the original hepatic injury. If necrosis is primarily centrilobular there is **central fibrosis** or **periacinar fibrosis.** Loss of hepatocytes associated with chronic hepatitis leads to a more diffuse fibrosis which connects portal triads and central veins, or triad to triad, termed **bridging fibrosis.** Following massive necrosis the area of dead tissue is entirely replaced with connective tissue and is termed a **postnecrotic scar.** With chronic hepatitis (see below), necrosis, fibrosis and regeneration often proceed simultaneously. Under this circumstance, regenerating hepatocytes often form nodules, distorting the microscopic and gross appearance of the liver.

Circulatory disorders

Passive congestion of the liver is frequent. It may be either acute or chronic, and with rare exception is traceable to cardiac disease, either myocardial or valvular. Reduction in the flow of blood through the hepatic veins or vena cava through compression from a neoplasm, or the presence of venous thrombosis, are rare causes of hepatic congestion. A striking example of chronic hepatic congestion due to myocardial weakness is the so-called "brisket-disease" which occurs in cattle at high altitudes. Another example exists in gossypol poisoning in swine. Chronic pericarditis, as seen in "traumatic" pericarditis from a penetrating foreign body in cattle, leads to similar congestion of the liver. Rarely, pulmonary emphysema and fibrosis cause similar impairment of the venous circulation. In dogs, endocardiosis of the right atrioventricular valve is a leading cause of chronic passive congestion of the liver. Other mechanisms leading to right sided heart failure are discussed in Chapter 21.

The liver with **acute passive congestion** is dark red and somewhat swollen with rounded edges, and considerable blood escapes when it is incised. The lobular pattern is accentuated, particularly on cut section, a feature described as a "reticulated" pattern. There may be some blood-tinged fluid in the abdominal cavity and often there are fibrin tags on the surface of the liver. Microscopically the central veins and surrounding sinusoids are markedly dilated and filled with erythrocytes. Within a short time the central hepatocytes become smaller and ultimately become necrotic due to hypoxia. Hepatocytes in the remainder of the lobule may undergo fatty change. Hepatic lymphatics within the triads become distended and much more evident.

Chronic passive congestion leaves a liver with a much more pronounced reticular pattern characterized by a fine sprinkling of dark brown and gray reminiscent of nutmeg. Such a liver is called, by professional tradition, a **"nutmeg liver."** The surface of the liver is slightly nodular and rough. There is usually ascites. Chronic congestion also leads to anoxic centrilobular necrosis, the spaces left by the destroyed cells being filled by blood. Fibrous proliferation around the central vein also characterizes chronic congestion. This can become so extensive as to stretch from central vein to central vein forming islands of periportal hepatocytes and triads within an otherwise scarred liver. This is termed **central cirrhosis** or **cardiac cirrhosis.**

Portosystemic shunts have already been mentioned under congenital disorders of the liver. Acquired portosystemic shunts follow chronic liver disease, either secondary to chronic passive congestion or primary liver disease, leading to portal hypertension. Ascites is always present. There are numerous tortuous connections between the portal vein and systemic veins. These may be particularly apparent between the capsule of the liver and the diaphragm.

Telangiectasis denotes a dilatation of functioning blood vessels anywhere. In the liver, the lesion consists of a small group of sinusoids within any part of a lobule which are greatly dilated. The cells of the hepatic cords between the dilated sinusoids have partially or completely disappeared. Grossly, the result is a dark red spot, irregular in shape, from one to several millimeters in diameter. Seen from the surface of the organ these spots tend to be slightly depressed. Telangiectasis is especially common in cattle and of no clinical significance. It has been speculated that telangiectasis may lead to or result from the foci of necrosis termed "sawdust" which is also common in the bovine liver. The two often occur together.

A similar lesion in the liver described under the term **peliosis hepatis** (**pelios** from Greek, meaning blue-black) has been described in cattle in Australia with "St. George disease" or poisoning by plants of the **Pimula** genus. This is discussed in Chapter 16. In human beings, peliosis hepatis is associated with use of anabolic steroids and other drugs. It has been described in cats due to unknown cause, and in rats infected with a specific (9H) virus. Peliotic lesions have also been observed in mice after transplantation of ovarian or testicular tumors. In this species the lesions may be associated with hypervolemia.

Degenerations and depositions

FATTY LIVER.

The accumulation of fat or triglycerides in the cytoplasm of hepatocytes, known as fatty liver, fatty change, or hepatic lipidosis, is one of the most common lesions encountered. The presence of fat, however, does not always indicate a pathologic process. A small amount may be found in normal animals. This is accentuated following a meal high in fat as well as late in pregnancy. Increased hepatic lipid is also a common finding in dairy cows, especially early in lactation. Fasting will also lead to an increased amount of free fat in hepatocytes, long before it reaches the point of starvation. Initially fat is seen as small clear droplets in the cytoplasm. These may be few to numerous. In more severe examples the fat droplets fuse to form several larger globules or a single globule which distends the cell and displaces the nucleus. Hepatocytes may fuse or rupture. Grossly, fatty livers are lighter in color, becoming in some cases almost white or yellow depending upon the species. If, as is often the case, the distribution of fat is primarily confined to a particular portion of the lobule, the liver will have a pronounced reticular pattern. Some of the more common causes in animals are starvation, ketosis, diabetes mellitus, and poisonings. The **pathogenesis** of fatty change in these various disorders is presented in detail in Chapter 2. There are other examples of fatty liver that have been less well studied and less well understood and many examples go unexplained.

Hyperlipidemia is a feature of certain of the disorders leading to fatty liver, and is seen in such diseases as diabetes mellitus, pancreatitis, hypothyroidism, and hyperadrenocorticism, and in animals with high dietary fat intake. There are also examples whose origin is less clear. These are generally viewed as two classes: secondary hyperlipidemia and primary (or idiopathic) hyperlipemia. Miniature horses, ponies, and donkeys are prone to develop hyperlipidemia, hyperlipemia, and fatty liver, which can be rapidly fatal. This has been termed **equine hyperlipemia,** and some examples appear to be congenital. It appears that most cases are secondary to other disorders which lead to a negative energy balance. These include enterocolitis and feed restriction for the treatment of colic. It is also associated with obesity, pregnancy, and lactation. Fatty change in the kidneys and other organs accompanies the syndrome. Studies in ponies have indicated that the hyperlipidemia results from overproduction rather than defective catabolism of lipoproteins. **Feline idiopathic hepatic lipidosis** is a term applied to a syndrome of cats characterized by hyperlipidemia and fatty liver. The pathogenesis is not understood. There is extensive fatty change in the liver which may be associated with centrilobular necrosis. Cats may be icteric. An **inherited hyperlipoproteinemia** due to deficiency of lipoprotein lipase has been described in cats. Fatty change and xanthomas are widespread. Hyperlipidemia is also encountered in dogs. Those examples considered primary are thought to be most likely hereditary. It is encountered most often in miniature schnauzers and beagles in which there is a familial tendency. A genetically determined metabolic disorder leading to hyperlipidemia is seen in a strain of New Zealand White rabbits (Watanabe rabbit).

Ovine white liver disease is a disorder of sheep and goats described in Australia, New Zealand, and Europe in which there are Councilman bodies and there is marked fatty change and ceroid deposition of the liver, especially in the central portions of the lobules. Periportal fibrosis and biliary hyperplasia may also be present. Affected animals are anemic and icteric. Hemosiderosis of the spleen, neuronal necrosis in the brain, and sclerosis of Peyer's patches and germinal centers of mesenteric lymph nodes are also described. The disease is responsive to cobalt and vitamin B_{12} therapy and has been reproduced with cobalt-deficient diets. Affected lambs also have elevated levels of serum copper which may aggravate the disease. The disorder resembles hepatic fatty cirrhosis of sheep seen in the Southwestern United States which is described later.

GLYCOGEN

Hepatocytes normally contain glycogen, which is most pronounced after eating. Abnormal accumulation of glycogen is seen in diabetes mellitus and glycogen storage diseases which are discussed elsewhere. Extreme accumulation of glycogen occurs in **steroid induced hepatopathy** (glucocorticoid induced hepatocellular degeneration) in dogs. Hepatocytes become extremely swollen and distorted due to accumulation of glycogen. They may be enlarged up to ten times normal. The midzone and central portion of the lobule is most affected. Hyperadrenocorticism may lead to the same lesion in dogs. Other species of domestic animals appear to be more resistant to this change, although it has been seen in horses and induced in rats and rabbits. In dogs, even topical use of steroids can lead to the hepatopathy.

PIGMENTS

A number of different pigments may accumulate in the liver. Cholestasis leads to the accumulation of **bile pigments** within distended bile canaliculi and within lysosomes of hepatocytes. It appears yellow to green to brown. Cholestasis is one cause of **icterus** (hyperbilirubinemia), discussed in Chapter 3. Grossly, the liver is yellow-greenish. **Lipofuscin,** the pigment of brown atrophy, is common in the liver, especially in older animals.

It is also increased in vitamin E deficiency. **Ceroid,** a very similar pigment, also accumulates in the liver. Classically it is seen in choline deficiency (which also causes fatty liver and cirrhosis). **Hemosiderin** accumulates in the liver, predominantly within Kupffer's cells, when there is increased destruction of erythrocytes. It is also present in abnormal amounts in hemochromatosis. **Melanosis** is occasionally seen in the liver. A disorder resembling Dubin-Johnson syndrome of humans occurs in Corriedale sheep in which a peculiar pigment accumulates within hepatocytes. A similar disorder has been described in howler monkeys. Infestations with *Fascioloides magna* and schistosomes are associated with the deposition of a black **iron-porphyrin** pigment. All these pigments and conditions are discussed under "Pigments" in Chapter 3.

AMYLOID

The liver is a frequent site of amyloid deposition in both primary and secondary amyloidosis. The amyloid is deposited in the space of Dissé.

NUCLEAR INCLUSIONS

Nuclear inclusions of a crystalline nature called **acidophilic crystalline intranuclear** (ACN) **inclusions** are frequently encountered in hepatocytes and renal tubular epithelium of dogs. They are usually rectangular, up to $15\mu m$ long, and distort the nuclear membrane (Fig. 23-22). Although their significance is not known, they are believed to be crystallized protein and are not related to viral infection. Invagination of cytoplasm into the nucleus produces a peculiar membrane-bound intranuclear inclusion. They are encountered most frequently in aged rodents but may also be found in dogs and monkeys. In addition to the liver, cytoplasmic invaginations are occasionally seen in other tissues, such as corpus luteum, interstitial cell tumors of the testes and adenocarcinoma of the lung. Normal cytoplasmic organelles can be demonstrated within the inclusion with electron microscopy.

Hepatic encephalopathy

The association of hepatic disorders and nervous signs or symptoms has been recorded in medical and nonmedical literature for many years. The offending material was once considered to be retained bile (cholemia), an idea which has not been supported by evidence. Bile seems only to be harmful to the nervous system in neonatal infants and animals (see kernicterus). It is now generally accepted that impaired hepatic function allows various exogenous and endogenous metabolites to enter the circulation which are responsible for the signs and lesions of hepatic encephalopathy. Elevated levels of ammonia and other amines absorbed from the gastrointestinal tract are considered to be the principal offending metabolite. Normally the liver converts ammonia to urea through the urea cycle. Ammonia has been further shown to increase glucagon secretion leading to increased hepatic gluconeogenesis from amino acids, which further contributes to ammonia levels whose con-

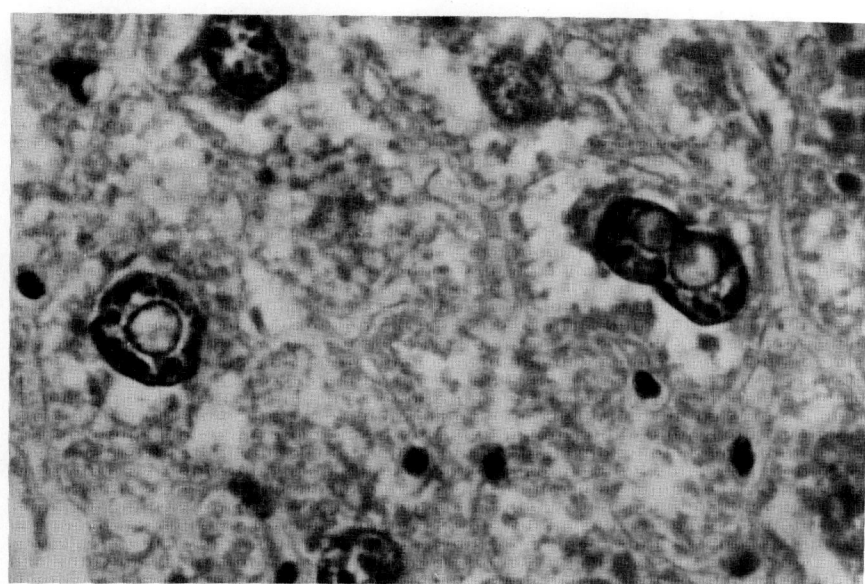

FIG. 23-22. Cytoplasmic invaginations into hepatocyte nuclei in a mouse. (Courtesy of Animal Research Center, Harvard Medical School.)

centration in the brain increases. There are also elevated levels of glutamine, serotonin, and mercaptans in the brain.

Hepatic encephalopathy occurs with severe loss of hepatic function as well as in the presence of portosystemic shunts, which allows portal blood to by-pass the liver. Signs include blindness, abnormal movements, mania, convulsions, coma and death. Lesions within the brain which have been identified in both natural and experimentally induced hepatic encephalopathy include cerebral edema, neuronal necrosis and swelling, and degeneration of astrocytes, particularly of the cerebral cortex and basal ganglia. The changes in astrocytes have been subdivided into two types: Alzheimer type 1 and type 2 (first described by Von Hosslin and Alzheimer in 1912). The type 1 astrocytes are enlarged with multilobed hyperchromatic nuclei and the type 2 astrocytes are enlarged with very pale or vacuolated nuclei which are present in groups of two or more. In some examples of hepatic encephalopathy, however, lesions in the brain have not been present.

References

Andersen AC. The pathogenesis of telangiectasis in the bovine liver. Am J Vet Res 1955;16:27–34.

Bauer JE. Evaluation and dietary considerations in idiopathic hyperlipidemia in dogs. J Am Vet Med Assoc 1995;206:1684–1688.

Bergs W, Scotti TM. Virus-induced peliosis hepatis in rats. Science 1967;158:377–378.

Biourge V, Pion P, Lewis J, et al. Spontaneous occurrence of hepatic lipidosis in a group of laboratory cats. J Vet Intern Med 1993;7:194–197.

Boothe HW, Howe LM, Edwards JF, et al. Multiple extrahepatic portosystemic shunts in dogs: 30 cases (1981–1993). J Am Vet Med Assoc 1996;208:1849–1854.

Butler-Howe LM, Boothe HW Jr, Boothe DM, et al. Effects of vena caval banding in experimentally induced multiple portosystemic shunts in dogs. Am J Vet Res 1993;54:1774–1783.

Center SA, Crawford MA, Guida L, et al. A retrospective study of 77 cats with severe hepatic lipidosis: 1975–1990. J Vet Int Med 1993;7:349–359.

Cohen ND, Carter GK. Steroid hepatopathy in a horse with glucocorticoid-induced hyperadrenocorticism. J Am Vet Med Assoc 1992;200:1682–1684.

Cornelius CE, Gronwall RR. Congenital photosensitivity and hyperbilirubinemia in Southdown sheep in the United States. Am J Vet Res 1968;29:291–295.

Cornelius CE, Arias IM, Osburn BL. Hepatic pigmentation with photosensitivity: a syndrome in Corriedale sheep resembling Dubin-Johnson syndrome in man. J Am Vet Med Assoc 1965;146:709–713.

Cornelius LM, Thrall DE, Halliwell WH, et al. Anomalous portosystemic anastomoses associated with chronic hepatic insufficiency in six young dogs. J Am Vet Med Assoc 1975;167:220–228.

Dimski DS, Taboada J. Feline idiopathic hepatic lipidosis. [Review]. Vet Clin North Am Sm Anim Prac 1995;25:357–373.

Doige CE, Furneaux RW. Liver disease and intrahepatic portal hypertension in the dog. Can Vet J 1975;16:209–214.

Ewing GO, Suter PF, Bailey CS. Hepatic insufficiency associated with congenital anomalies of the portal vein in dogs. J Am Anim Hosp Assoc 1974;10:463–476.

Fischer JE. Hepatic coma in cirrhosis, portal hypertension, and following portacaval shunt: Its etiologies and the current status of its treatment. Arch Surg 1974;108:325–336.

Fittschen C, Bellamy JEC. Prednisone-induced morphologic and chemical changes in the liver of dogs. Vet Pathol 1984;21:399–406.

Fraser CL, Arieff AI. Hepatic encephalopathy. N Engl J Med 1985;31:865–873.

Gerloff BJ, Herdt TH, Emery RS. Relationship of hepatic lipidosis to health and performance in dairy cattle. J Am Vet Med Assoc 1986;188:845–850.

Getty R. The histopathology of a focal hepatitis and of its termination ("sawdust" and "telang") in cattle. Am J Vet Res 1946;7:437–449.

Glaze MB, Crawford MA, Nachreiner RF, et al. Ophthalmic corticosteroid therapy: systemic effects in the dog. J Am Vet Med Assoc 1988;192:73–75.

Godber LM, Brown CM, Mullaney TP. Polycystic hepatic disease, thoracic granular cell tumor and secondary hypertrophic osteopathy in a horse. Cornell Vet 1993;83:227–235.

Harper P, Plant JW, Unger DB. Congenital biliary atresia and jaundice in lambs and calves. Aust Vet J 1990;67:18–22.

Helman RG, Adams LG, Bridges CH. Hepatic fatty cirrhosis in ruminants from western Texas. J Am Vet Med Assoc 1993;202:129–132.

Inoue S, Matsunuma N, Ono K, et al. Five cases of canine peliosis hepatis. Nippon Juigaku Zasshi—Jap J Vet Sci 1988;50:565–567.

Jensen R, Frey PR, Cross F, et al. Telangiectasis, "sawdust," and abscesses in the liver of beef cattle. J Am Vet Med Assoc 1982; 180:1438–1442.

Johnstone AC, Jones BR, Thompson JC, et al. The pathology of an inherited hyperlipoproteinaemia of cats. J Comp Pathol, 1990;102:125–137.

Kennedy DG, Young PB, Blanchflower WJ, et al. Cobalt-vitamin B$_{12}$ deficiency causes lipid accumulation, lipid peroxidation and decreased alpha-tocopherol contractions in the liver of sheep. Int J Vit Nut Res 1994;64:270–276.

Lee KP. Peliosis hepatis-like lesion in aging rats. Vet Pathol 1983;20:410–423.

Mazur A, Ayrault-Jarrier M, Chilliard Y, et al. Lipoprotein metabolism in fatty liver dairy cows. [Review]. Diabete Metabol, 1992;18:145–149.

Mogg TD, Palmer JE. Hyperlipidemia, hyperlipemia, and hepatic lipidosis in American miniature horses: 23 cases (1990–1994). J Am Vet Med Assoc 1995;207:604–607.

Moore PF, Whiting PG. Hepatic lesions associated with intrahepatic arterioportal fistulae in dogs. Vet Pathol 1986;23:57–62.

Rappaport AM. Microcirculatory hepatic units. Microvasc Res 1973; 6:212–228.

Rogers WA, Ruebner BH. A retrospective study of probable glucocorticoid-induced hepatopathy in dogs. J Am Vet Med Assoc 1977; 170:603–606.

Seawright AA, Francis J. Peliosis hepatis(a specific liver lesion in St. George disease of cattle. Aust Vet J 1971;47:91–99.

Seddon AM, Woolf N, LaVille A, et al. Hereditary hyperlipidemia and atherosclerosis in the rabbit due to overproduction of lipoproteins. II. Preliminary report of arterial pathology. Arteriosclerosis 1987;7:113–124.

Stebbins KE. Polycystic disease of the kidney and liver in an adult Persian cat. J Comp Path 1989;100:327–330.

Turner TA, Brown CA, Wilson JH, et al. Hepatic lobe torsion as a cause of colic in a horse. Vet Surg 1993;22:301–304.

Ulvund MJ. Ovine white-liver disease (OWLD). Pathology. Acta Vet Scand 1990;31:309–324.

Ulvund MJ. Ovine white-liver disease (OWLD). Serum copper and effects of copper and selenium supplementation. Acta Vet Scand 1990;31:287–295.

Ulvund MJ. Ovine white-liver disease (OWLD). Trace elements in liver. Acta Vet Scand 1990;31:297–307.

Van den Ingh TS, Routhuizen J. Congenital cystic disease of the liver in seven dogs. J Comp Path 1985;95:405–414.

Van den Ingh TS, Rothuizen J, Meyer HP. Circulatory disorders of the liver in dogs and cats. [Review]. Vet Quart 1995;17:70–76.

Van den Ingh TS, Rothuizen J, Meyer HP. Portal hypertension associated with primary hypoplasia of the hepatic portal vein in dogs. Vet Rec 1995;137:424–427.

Watson TD, Murphy D, Love S. Equine hyperlipaemia in the United Kingdom: clinical features and blood biochemistry in 18 cases. Vet Rec 1992;131:48–51.

Weisbroth SH. Torsion of the caudate lobe of the liver in the domestic rabbit (Oryctolagus). Vet Pathol 1975;12:13–15.

Whitney MS. Evaluation of hyperlipidemias in dogs and cats. Sem Vet Med Surg 1992;7:292–300.

Wilson RB, Holscher MA, Sly DL. Liver lobe torsion in a rabbit. Lab Anim Sci 1987;37:506–507.

Hepatitis

Hepatitis is inflammation of the liver. Usually the term is restricted to those disorders in which acute or chronic inflammatory cells invade the liver, however it is sometimes extended to toxic injuries to the liver (toxic hepatitis) where an inflammatory cell reaction may be minimal or absent. The distinction is blurred because necrosis of hepatocytes may occur in most any injury to the liver, and necrotic cells attract inflammatory cells. There are few generalizations that can be made which encompass all of the various types of hepatitis as there is a broad spectrum of histopathological presentations depending upon the cause. In **acute hepatitis,** vascular features of inflammation, including dilation of arterioles, venules, and lymphatics, and edema may be present in the portal triads. Leukocytes will be present in the periportal connective tissue as well as within the sinusoids. Their makeup is dependent upon the cause— neutrophils predominate in hepatitis of bacterial origin, and mixtures of lymphocytes and plasma cells in viral hepatitis. In most septicemias, increased numbers of leukocytes will be found in the hepatic sinusoids. Kupffer's cells undergo hypertrophy and hyperplasia, a feature termed mobilization of Kupffer's cells. Degenerative changes in hepatocytes include swelling (hydropic degeneration) and increased cytoplasmic acidophilia sometimes leading to dense bodies with or without a nuclear remnant in the sinusoids or space of Dissé (Councilman bodies). Other features of necrosis (karyorrhexis, pyknosis) may also be present. Often hepatocytes will contain bile pigments and canaliculi are distended. Macrophages quickly infiltrate and remove the dead hepatocytes. With most infectious causes of hepatitis, the necrosis is focal. With recovery there is complete resolution, unless the necrosis is extensive in which case there will be scarring. **Chronic hepatitis** is characterized by a predominantly lymphoplasmacytic cellular infiltration, mainly in the portal triads, and is sometimes termed **portal hepatitis.** The amount of fibrous connective tissue in the triads becomes increased and there is proliferation of bile ductules. With progression, the fibrosis extends from the portal triads to the central veins connecting the two, creating a "pseudolobulation", a process known as bridging fibrosis. Chronic hepatitis may also include focal or piecemeal necrosis, with an associated influx of macrophages and some neutrophils, along with fibrosis, intrahepatic cholestasis, and nodules of regenerating hepatocytes. Such a picture is termed **chronic active hepatitis** and is often a progressive disease, which may proceed to cirrhosis. In dogs it is reportedly disproportionately more frequent in Doberman pinschers. Some forms of hepatitis originate within the biliary tree and extend into the portal tissues and ultimately the lobule. These are initially classified as **cholangitis** and with progression **chalangiohepatitis.** This can result from extrahepatic or intrahepatic bile duct obstruction or infectious causes, and progresses to cirrhosis. Superimposed upon these general features there may be, depending upon the cause, fatty change, megalocytosis, granulomas, abscesses, and other degenerative and inflammatory reactions.

CAUSES OF HEPATITIS

Most examples of hepatitis in animals are of infectious or toxic origin. Often, however, the cause is not known. This is especially true with chronic active hepatitis which is a relatively frequent disorder of dogs.

INFECTIOUS HEPATITIS

Infectious hepatitis can be caused by many viral, bacterial, protozoal, fungal, and metazoan organisms. These are discussed in other chapters and will only be mentioned here. With the exception of certain helminths, most causes of infectious hepatitis also affect other organs and tissues. Few are specific for the liver as is the case with several of the causes of viral hepatitis in human beings. One exception is woodchuck hepatitis which is caused by a virus similar to that of hepatitis B of humans (hepadnavirus). Infectious agents can gain access to the liver by several routes. These are the portal vein, the hepatic artery, the umbilical vein in the newborn, the bile-duct system, the hepatic vein, and direct extension. The importance of the portal blood as a carrier of infectious material (as well as toxic) is obvious in view of its large volume and the fact that it drains the extensively exposed intestinal area. Entrance of infective material via the hepatic artery occurs when microorganisms are in the systemic circulation. In farm animals, infection of the umbilical structures by contact soon after birth is by no means unusual. The umbilical vein, filled with partially clotted blood, affords an excellent route of access to the liver. Coming from contaminated soil, the infections entering this way are usually the necrophorus bacillus or the pyogenic organisms, and necrotic abscesses are the usual result. Infections may ascend the biliary passages either through static secretion consequent upon obstruction or by continuous spread of the infectious inflammatory process from the duodenum and up the ductal structures. Usually the two processes are combined. Spread of infection to the liver via the hepatic vein would appear impossible, but it occurs very rarely due to momentary reversal of the current in right-sided valvular disease, the primary source of infection usually being the diseased valve itself. A retrograde thrombus may form, reaching backward into the hepatic vein and its tributaries, the distance involved being really very short. Direct extension of infection from adjoining tissues and organs is, of course, possible. It usually depends upon a traumatic origin, such as that due to foreign bodies in the bovine reticulum.

Viral diseases in which hepatitis is seen include: infectious canine hepatitis; Rift Valley fever, Yellow fever, mouse hepatitis, Wesselbron disease; lymphocytic choriomeningitis, and murine K virus infection. The herpesviruses which cause generalized infection, especially in the neonate or fetus, almost invariably invade the liver (e.g. equine herpesvirus 1, infectious bone rhinotracheitis, canine herpesvirus, feline viral rhinotracheitis; pseudorabies). Hepatic lesions often accompany feline infectious peritonitis virus infection. **Bacterial diseases** in which hepatitis is a prominent feature include black disease *(Clostridium novyi)*, bacillary hemoglobinuria *(Clostridium hemolyticum)*, Tyzzer's disease *(Bacillus piliformis)*, Yersiniosis *(Yersinia pseudotuberculosis* and *Y. enterocolitica)*, Tularemia, Listeriosis, Leptospirosis, Salmonellosis, necrobacillosis *(Fusobacterium necrophorum)*, tuberculosis, nocardiosis, and infections with *Pasteurella hemolytica, Haemophilus agni, Corynebacterium kutscheri,* and *Actinobacillus equuli.* Two species of Helicobacter *(H. hepaticus; H. bilis)* have been associated with hepatitis in mice. **Protozoal infections** which often cause hepatitis include toxoplasmosis, neosporosis, leishmaniasis, hepatic coccidiosis *(Eimeria stiedae)*, and amoebiasis. Many different **fungal diseases** involve the liver, the

most frequent being histoplasmosis. **Metazoan parasites** are important causes of hepatitis in animals. Migration of nematode larvae through the liver as part of their life cycles leads to necrosis, inflammation, and scarring, and, if entrapped there, small abscesses or granulomas. This is encountered with *Ascaris suum* and *Stephanurus dentatus* in swine and strongyles in horses. *Cysticercus tenuicollis* also migrates through the liver prior to becoming the intermediate cyst of *Taenia hydatigenia.* **Capillaria hepatica** resides within the liver within granulomas. Hydatids of **Echinococcus** may occupy the liver often without a significant inflammatory reaction. Adults of *Thysanosoma actinoides* and *Stilesia hepatica* reside within bile ducts and can cause cholangiohepatitis. The various liver flukes constitute an important cause of parasitic hepatitis in ruminants. These include *Fasciola hepatica, F. gigantica, F. magna, Dicrocoelium dendriticum, Platynosomum fastosum, Metorchis conjunctus* and *Opisthorchis (Clonorchis) sinensis* among others. Flukes may damage the liver through both larval migration and the presence of adults within the bile ducts or hepatic parenchyma.

TOXIC HEPATITIS OR TOXIC LIVER DISEASE
A great many drugs and toxins can lead to either acute or chronic injury. In some, the hepatic injury is accompanied by acute or chronic inflammation, hence the term toxic hepatitis. Others lack an inflammatory component, with presentations ranging from fatty change to neoplasia and hence the term toxic liver disease. By way of the portal veins the liver is the first organ to receive substances from the gastrointestinal tract and is therefore the first to be exposed to ingested toxins or toxins formed in the gastrointestinal tract. Indeed one of the functions of the liver is to detoxify and eliminate toxic substances and metabolites. There are two principal mechanisms of toxic liver disease: **direct toxicity** and **hepatic conversion of a xenobiotic to a toxin.** In the latter mechanism the very process of "detoxification" leads to the generation of toxic metabolites. Examples of toxins which are converted to their toxic form in the liver are: pyrrolizidine alkaloids, carbon tetrachloride, and aflatoxins. Toxins can also be subdivided into two classes: **predictable** and **idiosyncratic or unpredictable.** Predictable hepatotoxins have the same effect on all animals within a species whether they are directly toxic or converted to active forms in the liver. Examples include carbon tetrachloride poisoning, phosphorous, and most hepatotoxic plants. The toxicity of idiosyncratic hepatotoxins varies unpredictably between animals. Generally the reason why one animal develops disease and another does not is not known. An example is halothane toxicity. Deficiency of antioxidants, such as selenium and vitamin E, predispose the liver to toxic injury.

The gross and histopathologic features of toxic hepatitis vary with the specific cause. These are presented in Chapter 16 on Poisonings. Some of the specific causes are **chemical poisons, plant poisons, and mycotoxins.** Included among **chemical poisons** are copper, arsenic and arsenical drugs, phosphorus, mercury, iron dextran, ferrous fumarate, chloroform, tannic acid, cincophen, tetrachloroethane, trinitrotoluene, tetrachloroethylene, carbon tetrachloride, phenobarbital, halothane, gossypol and coal tar. With regard to copper, it need not be an exogenous poison to be associated with chronic liver disease. A hereditary copper storage disease occurs in Bedlington and West Highland white terriers which is characterized by chronic active hepatitis progressing to cirrhosis with the occurrence of copper-positive lipofuscin containing lysosomes within hepatocytes. A hereditary defect in copper metabolism also occurs in LEC rats which is analogous to Wilson's disease in human beings. Copper may also accumulate in an already damaged liver and is believed to aggravate the initial disorder. This is particularly true with cholestatic liver disease. Among those **plant poisons** recognized are species of the genera *Senecio, Amsinckia, Crotolaria, Heliotropium, Cynoglossum,* and *Trichodesma,* all of which contain pyrrolizidine alkaloids. Other hepatotoxic plants include species of the genera *Xanthium, Phyllanthus, Tribulus, Cassia, Cestrum, Lantana, Drymaria, Lechuguilla, Vicia,* and *Galenia.* Certain mushrooms are also hepatotoxic as well as some blue green algae. Among the hepatotoxic **mycotoxins** are aflatoxins, phomopsin and sporidesmin.

SERUM HEPATITIS OF HORSES

Serum hepatitis of horses is known by such names as **serum hepatitis, equine viral hepatitis,** and **Theiler's disease,** and is possibly confused with Kimberly horse disease *(Crotolaria retusa).* It is a suddenly occurring and usually fatal disease of horses that has been recognized since as early as 1919 (Theiler). The cause is not known. A virus has been suspected but never proven. The disease occurs in horses which have received a therapeutic agent containing horse serum approximately two months prior to the onset of signs. Among such agents are immunizing sera against several equine infections such as African horse sickness in South Africa and equine encephalomyelitis in North America, as well as tetanus antitoxin. Also occupying a prominent place in the list is the serum of pregnant mares, which is used in the hope of assisting placentation in brood mares. Not all examples, however, have been associated with the injection of horse serum. Also, of the thousands of horses receiving therapeutic sera, only a minute fraction develop this disease. Numerous attempts to produce a hepatitis in horses by the administration of horse serum have given almost uniformly negative results.

The disease is of rapid onset, of short duration and fatal within a day or two. There is marked icterus and signs described as "blind staggers" characterized by aimless walking and pushing, hyperexcitability, and ataxia. Grossly, the liver is swollen with a nutmeg appearance. Microscopically, there is marked centrilobular necrosis with replacement by blood. Often the necrosis is to the extent that only a narrow rim of hepatocytes survives around the periphery of the blood-filled lobule. Even these remaining cells may be swollen. In the portal areas and throughout whatever hepatic parenchyma remains, there is a liberal infiltration of inflammatory cells, chiefly lymphocytes and neutrophils.

The signs of nervous disorder have led to a theory that the supposed virus also attacks the brain. However, convincing lesions have been uniformly lacking.

AUTOIMMUNE HEPATITIS

Autoimmune hepatitis is a chronic active hepatitis resulting from an immune process directed against liver antigens. It is presumed to be precipitated by exposure to an environmental agent which triggers the autoimmune response. The triggering agent, or agents, is not known but viruses are likely candidates. In human beings, measles virus, hepatitis viruses, and Epstein-Barr virus are potential causes. Histopathologically, it is characterized by a portal mononuclear cell infiltrate, often containing many plasma cells, which invades into the lobule. There is piecemeal necrosis of hepatocytes within and adjacent to the expanding infiltrate. There is periportal fibrosis which ultimately extends toward the central vein (bridging fibrosis). The relative importance of autoimmune hepatitis in domestic animals is not established. An immune reaction to persistent infection with infectious canine hepatitis virus is suggested to explain some forms of chronic active hepatitis in dogs.

HEPATIC ABSCESSES

Abscesses occasionally form in the liver of all species as the result of the entrance of microorganisms by any of the routes mentioned under Infectious Hepatitis (Fig. 23-23). Important amongst these in newly born or young animals is the umbilical vein, which affords a route of metastasis or direct extension from the umbilicus. As the metastatic lesions develop in the liver, the primary site of infection at the umbilicus may heal without affecting the hepatic disease. Abscesses also occur in the livers of old dairy cows and others living under barnyard conditions, these being the result of extension from the wounds of penetrating foreign bodies in the reticulum. Abscesses under any of the above circumstances are regularly due to the entrance of pyogenic cocci or other well-recognized pus-producing species. They practically always play a central role in the generalized and fatal disease.

But, the much more frequent and important cause of hepatic abscesses in veterinary medicine is a disease of fattening cattle. These are often encountered in heavily fattened cattle in apparently perfect health. The incidence of these abscesses ranges from 5% up to 100% in some shipments. The liver may contain the "sawdust" foci of necrosis or telangiectasis, and possibly localized diaphragmatic adhesions over certain abscesses. Occasionally, dozens or more of these abscesses are present and can lead to death following acute but vague digestive symptoms. These hepatic abscesses result from ulcerative rumenitis, which was discussed earlier in this chapter, caused by *Fusobacterium necrophorum* and beginning as focal areas of necrosis.

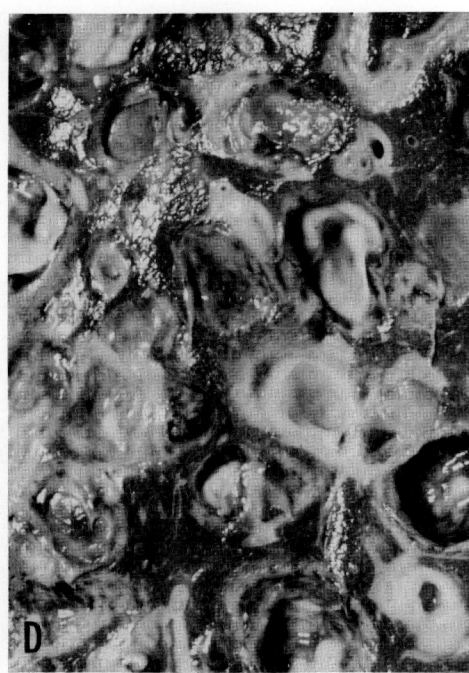

FIG. 23-23. Abscesses in a bovine liver. Ordinarily they are much less numerous. (Courtesy of College of Veterinary Medicine, Iowa State University.)

Cirrhosis

The word cirrhosis comes from the Greek, **kirrhos,** which meant tawny or orange-colored. This relation to the color of the affected liver has over the years lost its meaning. Cirrhosis is not a primary disorder, but rather represents **end stage liver disease** from any of several causes. It is characterized by **diffuse hepatic fibrosis** resulting in altered reconstruction of the lobular parenchyma with widespread connective tissue septae, circumscribed regenerative nodules of hepatocytes and anastomoses between vascular channels linking portal and central vessels (Figs. 23-24–23-26). Depending upon the cause, the fibrous tissue may surround each lobule, run from portal area to portal area, extend from portal area to central vein, or course from central vein to central vein. Collagen is deposited within the space of Disse, which markedly disrupts hepatic function. Fibroblasts within the portal triads serve as a source of the newly formed collagen, but within the lobule most of the new collagen is believed to be derived from Ito cells, whose metabolic function has become altered. With disruption of the hepatic lobule there is attempted regeneration, leading to the nodularity visible grossly. Scarring also disrupts the normal flow of blood, which leads to the development of direct linking of portal veins with the central veins as well as linking of hepatic arterioles with portal veins. With the continuing increase in portal pressure, shunts between the systemic and portal circulation develop elsewhere and there is chronic passive congestion of the spleen and digestive organs and ascites. Cirrhosis is generally considered progressive, non-reversible, and ultimately fatal. True cirrhosis as defined here is not common in domestic animals. **Fibrosis** of the liver in association with healing and with certain forms of chronic injury is, however, encountered with some frequency in animals. It rarely meets the criteria of cirrhosis.

CAUSES OF CIRRHOSIS

Many of the causes of cirrhosis have already been discussed, cirrhosis representing the end stage of various infectious, toxic, and other forms of hepatic injury. Frequently, however, the cause of an individual case of cirrhosis cannot be ascertained as the features of the end stage liver, regardless of cause, may be similar. Indeed most cases of cirrhosis in animals are termed **idiopathic cirrhosis.** What most causes of cirrhosis have in common is that injury is chronic and characterized by chronic active hepatitis.

INFECTIOUS AGENTS AS CAUSES OF CIRRHOSIS

In human beings, chronic infection with hepatitis B virus accounts for between 10 and 20% of all cases of cirrhosis. Although a number of viruses affect the animal liver, no analogous chronic forms of viral hepatitis occur in domestic animals which lead to cirrhosis. Woodchuck hepatitis virus does lead to chronic hepatitis with a high incidence of carcinoma of the liver, however cirrhosis is not the usual outcome. In dogs, persistence of infectious canine hepatitis virus may account for chronic active hepatitis leading to cirrhosis, but its role is uncertain. **Parasitic cirrhosis** is occasionally seen in animals but not with the frequency that hepatic parasitism is encountered. Of greatest significance is the migration of larvae, especially the larvae of the swine kidney worm (*Stephanurus dentatus*) and *Ascaris lumbricoides,* which, if their numbers are great, may result in hepatic necrosis leading to cirrhosis. Migration of liver flukes can have a similar result. Infestation with adult liver flukes rarely causes more than an encircling fibrosis in the immediate vicinity of the invaded ducts.

Central, or **cardiac cirrhosis** refers to hepatic fibrosis concentrated around the central veins resulting from chronic passive congestion due to congestive heart failure. The fibrosis may extend out into the lobule but is only rarely extensive with the formation of bridges to the portal triads.

Postnecrotic cirrhosis can follow extensive hepatic necrosis, whatever the cause. In animals, its relative position as a cause of cirrhosis is unclear. However, many different toxins as well as infectious agents can cause hepatic necrosis.

Pigment cirrhosis refers to the form of cirrhosis which occurs in connection with hemochromatosis. It is not common in animals but is encountered. It can result from metabolic disorders allowing for increased iron absorption or dietary iron overload.

Biliary cirrhosis follows chronic cholangitis which may be due to obstruction somewhere in the extrahepatic ductal system or obstruction of intrahepatic bile ducts. Often it is complicated with bacterial infection of the biliary tree. Initially with extrahepatic obstruction,

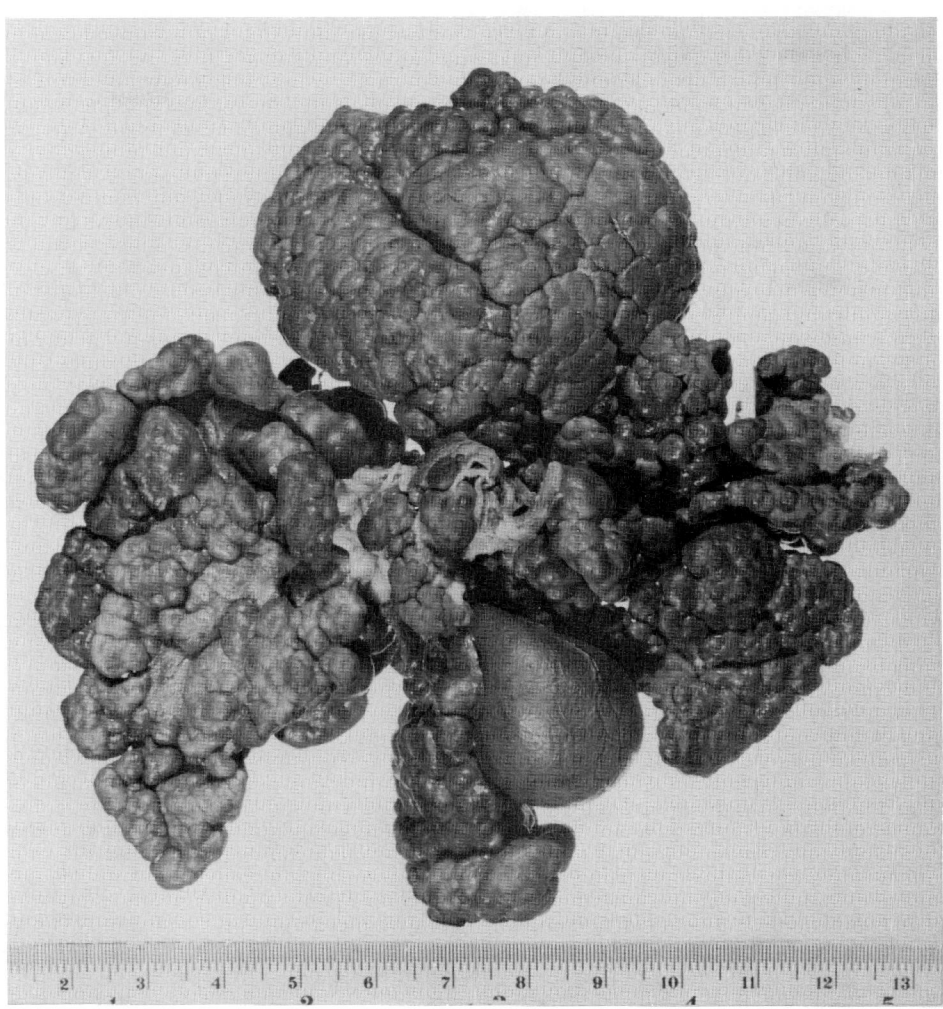

FIG. 23-24. Cirrhosis of liver of a dog. Note extensive nodularity and atrophy. (Courtesy of Armed Forces Institute of Pathology and Dr. Robert Ferber.)

bile ducts become dilated and there is proliferation of ductules. This is followed by fibrosis, which is initially concentrated around the bile ducts but later extends into the hepatic lobules. Newly formed bile ductules (ductular cell reaction) may be prominent and there is usually an infiltration of inflammatory cells which may be predominantly neutrophils if there is secondary bacterial infection. What is termed **primary biliary cirrhosis** (primary sclerosing cholangitis) results from a destructive process of intrahepatic bile ducts, initially characterized by necrosis of ductal epithelium and a mononuclear inflammatory infiltrate. The number of large ducts in the triads decreases with an associated proliferation of small ductules. The bile ducts become surrounded by fibrous connective tissue which ultimately extends from the triads into the lobules and bridges between triads. Immune mechanisms are speculated to be the cause. It has already been mentioned that cholestasis leads to hepatic copper accumulation with may help perpetuate the disease.

TOXIC CAUSES OF CIRRHOSIS

In human beings, alcoholic liver disease is the most common cause of cirrhosis. Comparable poisoning does not occur in animals, but, in farm animals, when cirrhosis is encountered, chronic **poisoning by plants** should be suspected. The most important of those plants contain pyrrolizidine alkaloids, whose chronic consumption leads to extensive fibrosis of the liver (as well as other changes described in Chapter 16. The better known are species of *Senecio* and *Amsinkia* which have a long history of leading to extensive hepatic fibrosis. Also included are species of *Crotolaria*, *Trichodesma*, *Heliotropium*, *Cynoglossum*, and *Echium*. In horses, what was termed "walking disease," described by Van Es in 1929 in Nebraska, proved to be cirrhosis caused by a plant of the *Senecio* genus, while walking disease in the Pacific Northwest resulted from cirrhosis produced by seeds of the plant *Amsinkia intermedia* (tarweed). Hard liver disease of sheep in many parts of the world (Texas, South Africa), Pictous disease of cattle in Canada, and Winton's disease of horses and cattle in New Zealand have been traced to other poisonous senecios. Fibrosis begins at the portal triads and is accompanied by bile ductule proliferation. Fibrosis also occurs beneath the endothelium of hepatic veins, which can obliterate their lumens. This is termed veno-occlusive disease and was first described by Jamaicans who drank bush tea.

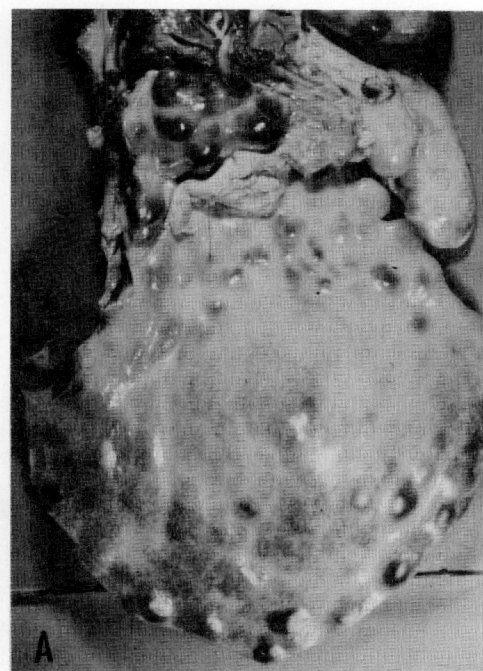

FIG. 23-25. Cirrhosis of the liver of a two-year-old steer.

Certain of the **mycotoxins** lead to hepatic damage characterized by fibrosis. These include the aflatoxins, phomopsin, and sporidesmin. The **copper poisoning** which results from a genetic defect in Bedlington and West Highland white terriers is associated with chronic active hepatitis and extensive fibrosis. Accumulation of copper in the liver has been suggested as a cause of cirrho-

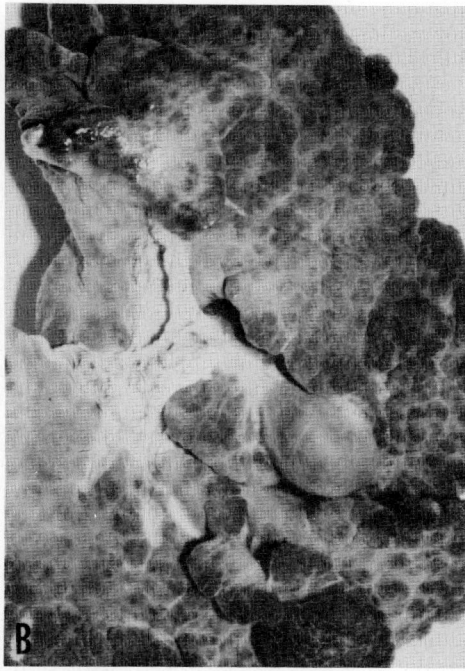

FIG. 23-26. Cirrhosis of the liver of a four-month-old pig.

sis in other breeds of dogs as well as other species of animals. Chronic liver disease itself can lead to the accumulation of copper which may further contribute to injury. Cirrhosis is not a typical feature of copper poisoning as seen in ruminants.

OVINE HEPATIC FATTY CIRRHOSIS

This disorder, which was first described in western Texas in 1932, is primarily a disease of sheep, but what is considered the same entity is also seen in goats, cattle, deer, and pronghorned antelope. In addition to Texas, cases have been described in eastern New Mexico and northeastern Mexico. In sheep, the disorder typically follows a wet winter and a dry summer and morbidity can reach 100% in some flocks with a mortality of 85%. Affected sheep fail to gain or maintain body weight and have signs of hepatic encephalopathy such as head pressing, depression, and coma. The hepatic changes are concentrated in the ventral lobe of the liver, but in advanced examples the entire liver is affected. The disease appears to begin with centrilobular fatty change, which progresses to affect the entire lobule. Fibrosis also commences around the central veins, and ultimately links central veins to central veins, and central veins to the portal areas. There is nodular hyperplasia of hepatocytes trapped between the fibrous septae. The resulting portal hypertension leads to vascular anastomoses between the parietal hepatic capsule and diaphragm, distension of lymphatics, and ascites. There is biliary hyperplasia and deposition of ceroid within the liver and in macrophages in the spleen and mediastinal lymph nodes. The cause of ovine hepatic cirrhosis is not known. Speculation has focused on a mycotoxin from *Phomopsis leptostromigormis* which has been demonstrated in grasses in western Texas, however feeding trials have not reproduced the disease. It has also been compared to nutritional cirrhosis induced in laboratory animals with lipotrope deficiency (methionine, choline), as well as ovine white liver disease which is believed to result from vitamin B_{12}/cobalt deficiency.

References

Acland HM, Mann PC, Robertson JL, et al. Toxic hepatopathy in neonatal foals. Vet Pathol 1984;21:3–9.

Casteel SW, Rottinghaus GE, Johnson GC, et al. Liver disease in cattle induced by consumption of moldy hay. Vet Hum Toxicol 1995;37:248–251.

Center SA, Castleman W, Roth L, et al. Light microscopic and electron microscopic changes in the livers of cats with extrahepatic bile duct obstruction. Am J Vet Res 1986;47:1278–1272.

Dayrell-Hart B, Steinberg SA, Van Winkle TJ, et al. Hepatotoxicity of phenobarbital in dogs: 18 cases (1985–1989). J Am Vet Med Assoc 1991;199:1060–1066.

Dill-Macky E. Chronic hepatitis in dogs. [Review]. Vet Clin North Am Small Anim Pract 1995;25:387–398.

Doige CE, Lester S. Chronic active hepatitis in dogs—A review of fourteen cases. J Am Anim Hosp Assoc 1981;17:725–730.

Fox JG, Yan LL, Dewhirst FE, et al. Lobular dissecting hepatitis in juvenile and young adult dogs. J Vet Internal Med 1994;8:217–220.

Galey FD, Beasley VR, Carmichael WW, et al. Blue-green algae (Microcystis aeruginosa) hepatotoxicosis in dairy cows. Am J Vet Res 1987;48:1415–1420.

Gaunt PS, Meuten DJ, Pecquet-Goad ME. Hepatic necrosis associated with use of halothane in a dog. J Am Vet Med Assoc 1984;184: 478–480.

Haywood S, Rutgers HC, Christian MK. Hepatitis and copper accumulation in Syke terriers. Vet Pathol 1988;25:408–414.

Helman RG, Adams LG, Bridges CH. The lesions of hepatic fatty cirrhosis in sheep. Vet Pathol 1995;32:635–640.

Hultgren BD, Stevens JB, Hardy RM. Inherited, chronic, progressive hepatic degeneration in Bedlington terriers with increased liver copper concentrations: clinical and pathologic observations and comparison with other copper-associated liver diseases. Am J Vet Res 1986;47:365–377.

Johnson GF, Zawie DA, Silbertson SR, et al. Chronic active hepatitis in Doberman pinschers. J Am Vet Med Assoc 1982;180:1438–1442.

Kaplan MM. Primary biliary cirrhosis. N Engl J Med 1987;316:521–528.

Krawitt EL. Autoimmune hepatitis. N Engl J Med 1996;334:897–903.

McCulloch EC. Hepatic cirrhosis of horses, swine, and cattle due to seeds of the tarweed, *Amsinckia intermedia*. J Am Vet Med Assoc 1940;96:5–18.

Messer NT IV, Johnson PJ. Serum hepatitis in two brood mares. J Am Vet Med Assoc 1994;204:1790–1792.

Mori M, Hattori A, Sawaki M, et al. The LEC rat: a model for human hepatitis, liver cancer, and much more. Am J Pathol 1994;144:200–204.

Morrison WB. Cholangitis, choledocholithiasis, and icterus in a cat. Vet Pathol 1985;22:285–286.

Mullaney TP, Brown CM. Iron toxicity in neonatal foals. Equine Vet J 1988;20:119–124.

O'Brien TD, Raffe MR, Cox VS, et al. Hepatic necrosis following halothane anesthesia in goats. J Am Vet Med Assoc 1986;189:1591–1595.

Okudaira M, Atari E, Oubu M. [Liver cirrhosis, its definition and classification—from a morbid anatomical point of view]. [Japanese]. Nippon Rinsho 1994;52:5–10.

Ono T, Fukumoto R, Kondoh Y, et al. Deletion of the Wilson's disease gene in hereditary hepatitis LEC rats. Jpn J Genet 1995;70:25–33.

Ono T, Fukumoto R, Takada S, et al. Responsible gene for hepatitis of the LEC rat (hts) in the homolog of the human Wilson's disease (WD) gene. Transplant Proc 1995;27:1545.

Pearson EG, Hedstrom OR, Poppenga RH. Hepatic cirrhosis and hemochromatosis in three horses. J Am Vet Med Assoc 1994;204:1053–1056.

Prasse KW, Mahaffey EA, DeNovo R, et al. Chronic lymphocytic cholangitis in three cats. Vet Pathol 1982;19:99–108.

Robinson M, Gopinath C, Hughes DL. Histopathology of acute hepatitis in the horse. J Comp Pathol 1975;85:111–118.

Rogers AE, Newberne PM. Animal model: fatty liver and cirrhosis in lipotrope-deficient male rats. Am J Pathol 1973;73:817–820.

Rolfe DS, Twedt DC. Copper-associated hepatopathies in dogs. [Review]. Vet Clin North Am Small Anim Prac 1995;25:399–417.

Rubarth S. Hepatic and subphrenic abscesses in cattle with rupture into vena cava caudalis. Acta Vet Scand 1960;1:363–382.

Rutgers HC, Haywood S, Kelly DF. Idiopathic hepatic fibrosis in 15 dogs. Vet Record 1993;133:155–118.

Scarratt WK, Furr MO, Robertson JL. Hepatoencephalopathy and hypocalcemia in a miniature horse mare. J Am Vet Med Assoc 1991;199:1754–1756.

Smith HA. Ulcerative lesions of the bovine rumen and their possible relation to hepatic abscesses. Am J Vet Res 1944;5:234–243.

Strombeck DR, Meyer DJ, Freedland RA. Hyperammonemia due to a urea cycle enzyme deficiency in two dogs. J Am Vet Med Assoc 1975;166:1109–111.

Taylor NS, Fox JG, Yan L. In vitro hepatotoxic factor in Helicobacter hepaticus, H. pylori and other Helicobacter species. J Med Microbiol 1995;42:48–52.

Theiler A. Acute liver atrophy and parenchymatous hepatitis in horses. Rep Dir Vet Res U S Afr, 1919;5:6–7.

Thornburg LP, Beissenherz M, Dolan M, et al. Histochemical demonstration of copper and copper-associated protein in the canine liver. Vet Pathol 1985;22:327–332.

Thornburg LP, Rottinghaus G, Gage H. Chronic liver disease associated with high hepatic copper concentration in a dog. J Am Vet Med Assoc 1986;188:1190–1191.

Van Es L, Cantwell LR, Martin HM, et al. Nature and cause of the "walking disease" of northwestern Nebraska. Exp Sta Bull No 43, University of Nebraska, Lincoln, 1929.

Wada Y, Kajiwara W, Kato K. Wilson's disease-like lesion in a calf. Vet Pathol 1995;32:538–539.

Ward JM, Anver MR, Haines DC, et al. Chronic active hepatitis in mice caused by Helicobacter hepaticus. Am J Pathol 1994;145:959–968.

Neoplasms of the liver

Primary tumors may arise from any of the cellular elements of the liver, but neoplasms of hepatocytes, biliary epithelium, and endothelium predominate. The liver is also a frequent site for metastatic neoplasms. As with most neoplastic diseases of animals, their cause is not known. In human beings, there is a strong causal relationship with infection with hepatitis B virus. This is substantiated by the near 100% incidence of hepatocellular carcinomas in woodchucks infected with a very similar hepadnavirus. In laboratory animals hepatomas and hepatocellular carcinomas can be induced with a number of chemicals as well as with aflatoxin. Aflatoxin is also considered a potential cause in human beings.

In dogs and cats, neoplasms of bile duct epithelium occur with greater frequency than hepatocellular tumors, whereas in cattle and sheep, hepatocellular tumors, in particular hepatocellular carcinomas, are the most common. Rarely, tumors are seen containing neoplastic elements of hepatocellular and cholangiocellular. In other species they are seen with less frequency.

Hepatocellular adenoma occurs in most domestic animals as well as laboratory rodents and exotic species. These tumors are sharply circumscribed, usually single and tan-colored, and compress, but do not invade, adjacent liver tissue. They may reach a large size but do not metastasize. Most have a trabecular or acinar pattern made up of cells resembling normal hepatocytes, but often contain glycogen and fat droplets. Well differentiated adenomas may be difficult to distinguish from normal liver except that they have no portal triads. In young animals, tumors have been seen in which extramedullary hematopoiesis was a conspicuous feature.

Hepatocellular adenoma must be differentiated from hyperplastic nodules and hepatocellular carcinoma. **Hyperplastic nodules** are common in old dogs and laboratory rodents. These are usually multiple, expanding nodules which compress adjacent tissue. The hepatocytes resemble normal hepatocytes or are slightly smaller or larger. The nodule may stand out because of the presence of lipid or increased amounts of glycogen in the cytoplasm. The only clear way to differentiate this lesion from an adenoma is to identify portal areas. Adenomas do not have portal tracts. In rodents, what have been termed **foci of altered hepatocytes** can resemble a hyperplastic nodule and can be induced with carcinogens. There is, however, no association between hyperplastic nodules and neoplasia in the dog. The histologic differentiation of hepatocellular adenoma from hepatocellular carcinoma can also be difficult. Tumors whose cells "look benign" can metastasize.

Hepatocellular carcinoma is the malignant counterpart of hepatocellular adenoma from which it may be very difficult to differentiate. In some carcinomas the cells may resemble normal hepatocytes without any hint of malignancy. The cells may be arranged in a trabecular or acinar pattern or mixtures of both. Others are solid. In some cases plates of cells may be a few cells thick and separated by sinusoids. In differentiated parts, the tumor cells are polyhedral and clearly resemble hepatocytes, but no portal triads are present. The tumor compresses and may invade adjacent liver. Invasion of portal vessels may be present, which may be the only feature which identifies the tumor as malignant. In some tumors, the cells are undifferentiated with variation in size, tinctorial features, and cytoplasmic content such as fat and glycogen. Mitoses and enlarged nuclei may be frequent. Some are so undifferentiated that the tumor cells are difficult to identify as coming from liver cells as well as to differentiate from cholangiocarcinoma. Some hepatocellular carcinomas are schirrous.

Intrahepatic bile duct adenoma (or cyst-adenoma) is a circumscribed tumor made up of irregular-sized tubules lined with cuboidal epithelium resembling epithelium of intrahepatic bile ducts. The stroma may be conspicuous. The cystic variety is somewhat more frequent. Cysts containing clear fluid may vary in size and the lining cells may be flattened. Mitoses are rarely seen.

Cholangiocarcinoma, or intrahepatic bile duct carcinoma, is a malignant tumor made up of epithelial cells resembling those of the intrahepatic bile ducts (Fig. 23-27). These tumors may occur in any part of the liver and commonly spread along the biliary tract, sometimes into the liver capsule. Metastasis may occur by spread to the liver serosa and via the lymphatics to the lungs. The tumor cells are cuboidal or columnar and have clear or granular cytoplasm. They usually form small acini, but when less differentiated may appear in solid cords with rare formation of lumina. Papillary arrangement of tumor cells may be seen, and mucus secretion in some cases may lead to accumulation of collections of mucin. Bile may occasionally be seen in tumor acini but is not recognizable in cells.

In some cases, accompanying proliferation of connective tissue (desmoplasia) gives the tumors a grossly apparent, dense white fibrous consistency. A few cases containing squamous as well as adenosarcomatous elements are reported, presumably due to metaplasia of adenomatous to squamous epithelial tumor cells.

Hepatoblastoma is an unusual type, made up of granular cells which resemble the smaller hepatocytes of the fetus. Nests of hematopoietic cells always accompany this tumor and are essential to the diagnosis.

In human beings, a second type of hepatoblastoma occurs in which the small fetal cells are admixed with mesenchymal elements, to include osteoid, cartilage and skeletal muscle. Similar neoplasms have been seen in mice.

Hemangiomas may also be primary in the liver, occurring as benign, circumscribed, solitary or multiple nodules of vascular architecture with a fine supporting stroma between endothelial-lined vascular channels. These tumors may compress adjacent liver cells, but do not invade or metastasize.

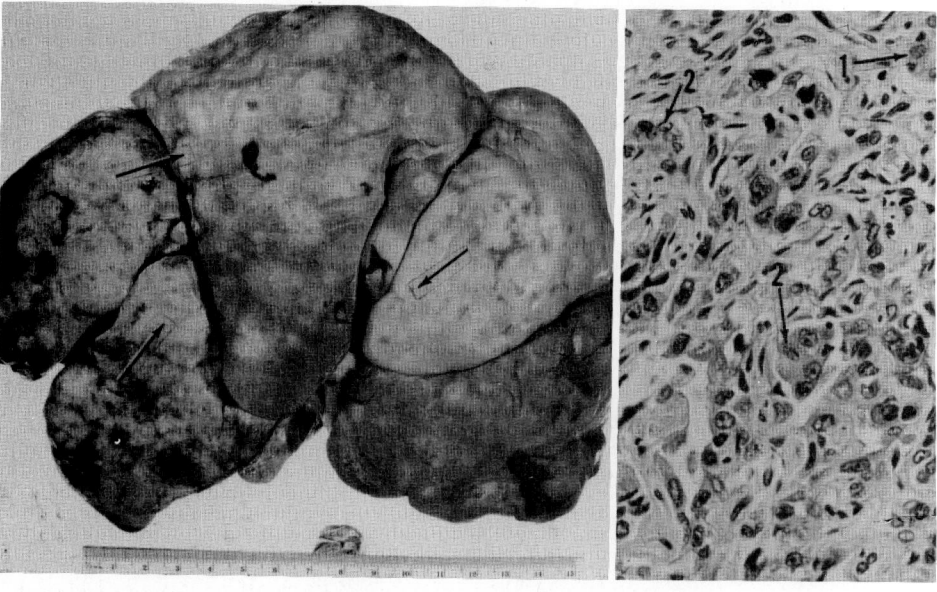

FIG. 23-27. **A.** Adenocarcinoma of intrahepatic bile ducts, liver of a fifteen-year-old male beagle. Masses of tumor (arrows) enlarge the liver and elevate the capsule. **B.** Photomicrograph of the neoplasm in **A** (× 300). The neoplastic cells form structures resembling bile ducts (**1**) in some places, but in others they are undifferentiated (**2**). (Courtesy of Armed Forces Institute of Pathology and Dr. D.N. Bader.

Lymphangioma is a rare primary tumor in the liver.

Hemangiosarcoma (hemangioendothelioma, angiosarcoma) is a malignant vascular tumor with many immature, pleomorphic, endothelial cells which form blood-filled vascular spaces or solid masses of cells. The nuclei are hyperchromatic, often in mitosis, and closely packed. Hemorrhage frequently occurs within these tumors and ischemic necrosis is apt to occur. Hemangiosarcomas are clearly invasive and tend to metastasize to the lung. Rupture into the peritoneal sac may result in implantations of tumor on the peritoneal surface.

Carcinoid tumor of the liver may also occur as a rare primary neoplasm. This tumor is identified by the argentaffin granules in the cells, similar to tumors found in the gastrointestinal tract.

Myelolipoma is a benign lesion of the liver which resembles those seen in the adrenal gland and occasionally at other locations. It is composed of mature lipocytes and erythrocytic and granulocytic myeloid cells. They are often multiple and grossly light in color. They are most frequent in cats, but can be encountered in other species as well.

Fibrosarcoma is rare as a primary tumor of the liver, however they may occur in the liver of rats in association with infestation with *Cysticercus fasciolaris*.

Secondary neoplasms of the liver of animals are in general more frequent than primary. Lymphosarcoma and mast cell tumors may be either primary or metastatic in the liver. The portal vein provides the means for malignant tumors of the intestine and pancreas to metastasize to the liver. A pancreatic adenocarcinoma, metastatic in the liver, may present some difficulties in distinguishing it from a primary adenocarcinoma of intrahepatic bile ducts. The presence of the tumor in the pancreas is helpful, and one can clearly distinguish an adenocarcinoma of acinar pancreas by identifying zymogen granules in the cytoplasm of tumor cells. Tumors, which implant and grow on the peritoneum after escaping from spleen (hemangiosarcoma), intestine (adenocarcinoma), or ovary (adenocarcinoma), may randomly grow on the liver capsule and possibly invade the liver parenchyma.

References

Bergman JR. Nodular hyperplasia in the liver of the dog: an association with changes in the Ito cell population. Vet Pathol 1985; 22:427–438.

Bettini G, Marcato PS. Primary hepatic tumours in cattle. A classification of 66 cases. J Comp Pathol 1992;107:19–34.

Dunning WF, Curtis MR. Malignancy induced by Cysticercus fasciolaris: its dependence on age of the host when infested. Am J Cancer 1939;37:312–328.

Fabry A, Benjamin A, Angleton GM. Nodular hyperplasia of the liver in the beagle dog. Vet Pathol 1982;19:109–119.

Feldman BF, Strafuss AC, Gabbert N. Bile duct carcinoma in the cat: three case reports. Feline Pract 1976;6:33–39.

Hanes MA. Fibrosarcomas in two rats arising from hepatic cysts of Cysticercus fasciolaris. Vet Pathol 1995;32:441–444.

Ivoghli B. Bile duct carcinoma in cattle: three case reports. Am J Vet Res 1973;34:1203–1206.

Kakinuma C, Harada T, Watanabe M, et al. Spontaneous adrenal and hepatic myelolipomas in the common marmoset. Toxicol Pathol 1994;22:440–445.

Krishna L, Chattopadhyay SK, Iyer PKR, et al. A pathological study of hepatocellular carcinoma in sheep. Indian J Anim Sci 1973; 43:34–37.

Ladds PW. Vascular hamartomas of the liver of cattle. Vet Pathol 1983;20:764–767.

Lawler DF, Evans RH. Multiple hepatic cavernous lymphangioma in an aged male cat. J Comp Pathol 1993;109:83–87.

Lawrence HJ, Erb HM, Harvey HJ. Nonlymphomatous hepatobiliary masses in cats: 41 cases (1972 to 1991). Vet Surg 1994;23:365–368.

Manktelow BW. Hepatoblastomas in sheep. J Pathol Bact 1965;89:711–714.

Martin de las Mulas J, Gomez-Villamandos JC, Perez J, et al. Immunohistochemical evaluation of canine primary liver carcinomas: distribution of alpha-fetoprotein, carcinoembryonic antigen, keratins and vimentin. Res Vet Sci 1995;59:124–127.

McCaw DL, da Silva Curiel JMA, Shaw DP. Hepatic myelolipomas in a cat. J Am Vet Med Assoc 1990;197:243–244.

Neu SM. Hepatoblastoma in an equine fetus. J Vet Diag Invest 1993; 5:634–637.

Newberne PM, de Camargo JLV, Clark AJ. Choline deficiency, partial hepatectomy, and liver tumors in rats and mice. Toxicol Pathol 1982;10:95–109.

Newsholme SJ, Fish CJ. Morphology and incidence of hepatic foci of cellular alteration in Sprague-Dawley rats. Toxicol Pathol 1994; 22:524–52.

Nonoyama T, Fullerton F, Reznik G, et al. Mouse hepatoblastomas: a histologic, ultrastructural, and immunohistochemical study. Vet Pathol 1988;25:286–296.

Nonoyama T, Reznik G, Bucci TJ, et al. Hepatoblastoma with squamous differentiation in a B6C3F1 mouse. Vet Pathol 1986; 23:619–622.

Ohfuji S, Kosuda M, Matsui T. Hepatocholangioadenoma in a pig. J Com Pathol 1992;106:89–92.

Orsini JA, Orsini PG, Sepesy L, et al. Intestinal carcinoid in a mare: an etiologic consideration for chronic colic in horses. J Am Vet Med Assoc 1988;193:87–88.

Patnaik AK. A morphologic and immunocytochemical study of hepatic neoplasms in cats. Vet Pathol 1992;29:405–415.

Patnaik AK, Hurvitz AI, Lieberman PH. Canine hepatic neoplasms: a clinicopathologic study. Vet Pathol 1980;17:553–564.

Patnaik AK, Hurvitz AI, Lieberman PH, et al. Canine hepatocellular carcinoma. Vet Pathol 1981;18:427–438.

Patnaik AK, Lieberman PH, Hurvitz AI, et al. Canine hepatic carcinoids. Vet Pathol 1981;18:445–453.

Post G, Patnaik AK. Nonhematopoietic hepatic neoplasms in cats: 21 cases (1983–1988). J Am Vet Med Assoc 1992;201:1080–1082.

Prater PE, Patton CS, Held JP. Pleural effusion resulting from malignant hepatoblastoma in a horse. J Am Med Assoc 1989;194:383–385.

Strafuss AC. Bile duct carcinoma in dogs. J Am Vet Med Assoc 1976; 169:429.

Tanimoto T, Ohtsuki Y. Hepatic haemangioma in a pig. Vet Rec 1992;131:176–177.

Trigo FJ, Thompson H, Breeze RG, et al. The pathology of liver tumors in the dog. J Comp Path 1982;92:21–39.

GALLBLADDER

Cholecystitis and Cholangitis

Inflammation of the gallbladder (cholecystitis) or common bile duct (cholangitis) may result from blood-borne metastasis of infectious organisms or by their ascent from the duodenum. Cholecystitis may also result from the action of retained and concentrated bile or from the presence of choleliths. Experimentally, cholecystitis is claimed to have been produced in poultry and dogs by diets high in fat and low in protein, but this has no known clinical significance. Any of the ordinary types of exudative inflammation are possible, but the usual kinds are mucous (catarrhal), characterized by excessive secretion of the mucous glands, or serous, characterized by inflammatory edema. Leukocytic infiltration is seldom extensive.

More puzzling to the student may be the proper interpretation of the degree of fullness of the organ and the character of its contents. Bile is secreted continually and stored in the gallbladder (except in the horse, rat, and other species that have no gallbladder), to be discharged when a full meal begins to reach the intestine (action of cholecystokinin). Throughout the period of storage, water is resorbed from the bile by the mucosa, and concurrently the mucous glands scattered through the mucous membrane add a small amount of mucus, so that the organ tends slowly to become distended. At the same time, fluid continues to be resorbed, leaving the solids. These, together with the slow accumulation of mucus, make the bile more and more viscous. A catarrhal cholecystitis sometimes coexists, resulting in a markedly increased flow of mucus. With rare exceptions, such as obstruction of the common duct, these mechanisms and failure of the sick animal to eat explain the enlarged gallbladders and viscous, "inspissated bile" so often given prominence in descriptions of disease.

If the ingress of bile to the gallbladder is prevented by swelling of the cystic duct or other obstruction, the epithelium of the gallbladder secretes a clear watery fluid, filling the cavity with what has been called "white bile."

Cystic hyperplasia

Also known as cystic mucinous hypertrophy, papillary adenomatous hypertrophy, and other descriptive phrases, this lesion is frequently encountered in dogs. The mucosa of the gallbladder is thickened by numerous fronds and cysts lined by squamous to columnar epithelium. The epithelial cells and the cysts contain mucin which stains blue in hematoxylin- and eosin-stained tissue sections. Grossly, the wall of the gallbladder is thickened and numerous multilocular, gelatinous, translucent cysts of varying size are evident. The cause and significance of the lesion are not known. Hyperplastic cholecystitis has been observed in the gallbladder of cattle in connection with liver fluke (*Fasciola gigantica* and *F. hepatica*) infestation.

Diverticulosis, probably not related to hyperplasia, has been observed in the Rhesus monkey.

References

Cheema AH. Adenomatous cholecystitis in cattle with chronic fascioliasis. Vet Pathol 1974;11:407–416.

Kovatch RM, Hildebrandt PK, and Marcus LC. Cystic mucinous hypertrophy of the mucosa of the gallbladder in the dog. Pathol Vet 1965;2:574–584.

Rosenquist CJ, Silverman S. Diverticulosis of gallbladder in a Rhesus monkey. J Am Vet Radiol Soc 1978;19:38–40.

Witzleben CL, Buck BE, Schnaufer L, et al. Studies on the pathogenesis of biliary atresia. Lab Invest, 1978;38:525–532.

Yoshida T, Suzuki H, Miki H, et al. Plasma alkaline phosphatase and experimental cholestasis of squirrel monkeys (Saimiri sciureus). Acta Hepat Jpn 1977;18:913–918.

Cholelithiasis

Biliary calculi, gallstones, or choleliths, as they may be called, occur with rarity in all of the usual domestic species, having been reported even in the chicken. They appear to be less rare in cattle than in the other farm or pet animals. They may be of minute size, like grains of sand, several hundred having been found in the bile ducts of a horse, or they may be few or single, a length of 11.5 cm having been reported. Gallstones differ in their chemical composition. The cholesterol stone, is large, white, and light in weight, and contains glistening crystals of cholesterol radially arranged. This cholesterol stone has been seen frequently in squirrel monkeys and baboons maintained on diets containing elevated levels of cholesterol.

The most frequently encountered gallstones in animals are termed "pigment stones" and are yellow to dark brown to black. They vary in weight and fragility depending upon their composition; they are sometime concentrically laminated, and often faceted. These are composed of varying mixtures of materials to include salts of bilirubin, calcium carbonate, calcium phosphate, and glycoproteins.

The cause of this type of gallstone is almost without question cholecystitis of infectious origin. Such infectious processes are by no means frequent in animals and have been studied only occasionally, but the pyocyaneus organism (*Pseudomonas aeruginosa*) has been isolated from cases of cholelithiasis in sheep. The mechanism of formation is doubtless similar to that responsible for urinary calculi, solid particles of dead cells or inspissated material serving as the starting point for a process of crystallization. In the case of gallstones, however, changes in the water content and colloidal state are certainly of considerable importance. It is probable that some constituents of bile are reabsorbed in the event of biliary stasis more easily than others, leaving highly desiccated residues.

Many gallstones are "silent," that is, produce no signs. Others, in humans, cause episodes of severe pain, dyspepsia and nausea, and other gastric symptoms based upon the closely related innervation of both gallbladder and stomach. The accompanying cholecystitis is doubtless more responsible for the symptoms than are the stones themselves. Presumably similar effects occur at times in animal patients, but they have seldom been recognized clinically. Cholelithiasis has more frequently been discovered at autopsy incidental to icterus and hepatic disease of a more general nature. Obstruction of the biliary flow as the result of choleliths is possible but not usual.

Neoplasms of the gallbladder

Primary neoplasms of the gallbladder and common bile duct are uncommon in most animal species. Adenomas and adenocarcinomas appear to be the only such tumors reported in domestic species. Secondary tumors in the liver may occasionally involve the gallbladder by extension.

Adenomas of the gallbladder are benign, localized tumors that occur in most species and originate from the epithelium. The tumor cells form acinar or papillary patterns of tall columnar cells, the tumor mass projects into the lumen and does not infiltrate the deeper parts of the wall. Adenomas or adenomatous polyps (Fig. 23-29) reported in the gallbladder of cattle are distinctive due to the presence of parietal and chief cells similar to those of the gastric mucosa. Mucin-secreting cells are also present.

Adenocarcinoma of the gallbladder is distinguished from its benign counterpart, the adenoma, by its tendency to invade the gallbladder wall, to form incomplete tubules and undifferentiated cells, and to undergo necrosis. Some of these tumors may contain a papillary arrangement in parts of the tumor. Mucin-secreting cells are usually present. Extension to liver and adjacent peritoneum may occur, and metastasis to the lungs and elsewhere can happen in advanced cases. Early evidence of malignancy may be recognized by the invasion of perineural lymphatics.

References

Anderson WA, Monlux AW, Davis CL. Epithelial tumors of the bovine gallbladder. A report of eighteen cases. Am J Vet Res 1988;19:58–65.

Baer JF, Weller RE, Dagle GE, et al. Cholelithiasis in owl monkeys: seven cases. Lab Anim Sci 1990;40:629–633.

Cheema AH. Adenomatous cholecystitis in cattle with chronic fascioliasis. Vet Pathol 1974;11:407–416.

France VM, Wood JR. Gallstones in foetal sheep. J Physiol 1973;233:13–14.

Gurll N, DenBesteu L. Animal models of human cholesterol gallstone disease: a review. Lab Anim Sci 1978;28:428–432.

Ivoghli B, Cheema AH. Bile duct carcinoma in a goat. Vet Pathol 1977;14:538.

Kovatch RM, Hildebrandt PK, Marcus LC. Cystic mucinous hypertrophy of the mucosa of the gallbladder in the dog. Pathol Vet 1965;2:574–584.

O'Brien TR, Mitchum DG. Cholelithiasis in a cat. J Am Vet Med Assoc 1970;156:1015–1017.

Patnaik AK, Hurvitz AI, Lieberman PH, et al. Canine bile duct carcinoma. Vet Pathol 1981;18:439–444.

Redinger RN, Grace DM. Cholesterol gallstones and biliary lipid metabolism in the primate. Gastroenterology 1978;74:201–204.

Rosenquist CJ, Silverman S. Diverticulosis of gallbladder in a Rhesus monkey. J Am Vet Radiol Soc 1978;19:38–40.

Schall WE, Chapman WL, Finco DR, et al. Cholelithiasis in dogs. J Am Vet Med Assoc 1973;163:469–472.

Stalker LK, Schlotthauer CF. Papillary adenoma of the gallbladder in two dogs: intrahepatic gallbladder in one. J Am Vet Med Assoc 1936;89:207–212.

Traub JL, Rantanen N, Reed S, et al. Cholelithiasis in four horses. J Am Vet Med Assoc 1982;181:59–62.

Williard MD, Dunstan RW, Faulkner J. Neuroendocrine carcinoma of the gallbladder in a dog. J Am Vet Med Assoc 1988;192:926–928.

Wood JR, France VM, Sutor DJ. Occurrence of gallstones in foetal sheep. Lab Anim 1974;8:155–159.

PANCREAS

Although a single organ, the pancreas functionally and morphologically is an exocrine gland and an endocrine gland. The endocrine pancreas, and its principal disease diabetes mellitus, is covered in the chapter on the endocrine system. Here we consider those disorders of the exocrine pancreas whose function is the secretion of a number of digestive enzymes (trypsin, chymotrypsin, aminopeptidases, elastase, amylases, lipases, phospholipases). These enzymes (with the exception of amylase and lipase) are synthesized and secreted as inactive proenzymes. Their activation requires the conversion of trypsinogen to trypsin by enterokinase (enteropeptidase) secreted by the duodenum.

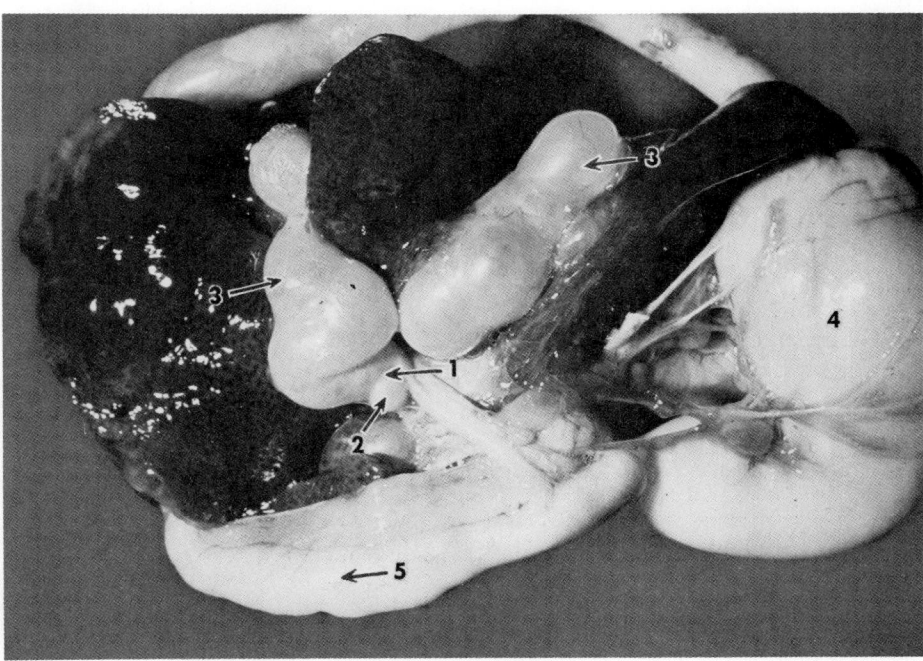

FIG. 23-28. Obstruction of the gallbladder, presumably congenital, in a ten-week-old female Siamese kitten. The obstruction (**1**) was related to a small adenoma (**2**). The distended gallbladder was doubled (**3**) in this animal, an occasional occurrence in Siamese cats. The stomach (**4**) and duodenum (**5**) were not affected. (Courtesy of Angell Memorial Animal Hospital.)

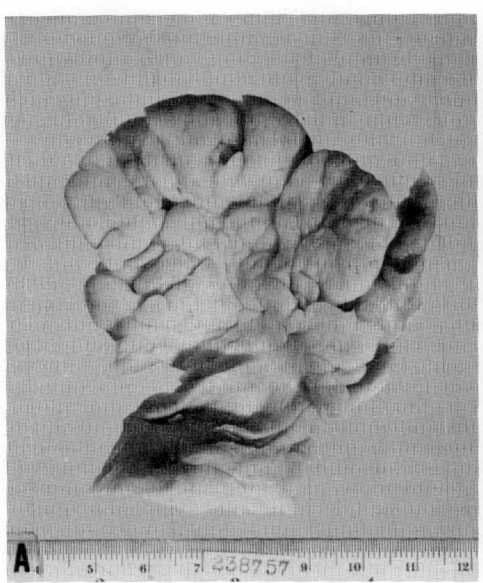
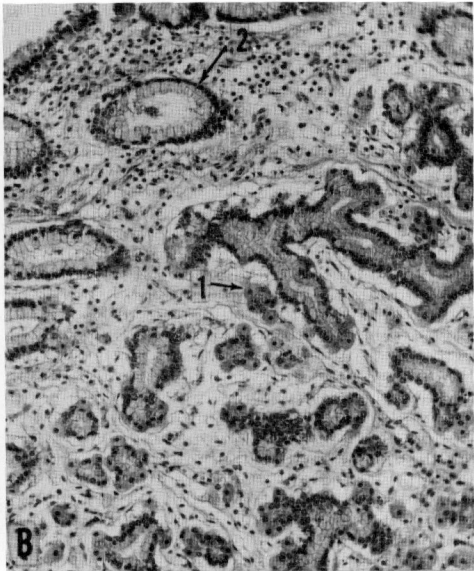

FIG. 23-29. Adenomatous polyp or adenoma in the gallbladder of a seven-year-old cow. **A.** The gross specimen, attached by its sessile stalk (bottom of photograph) in the neck of a gallbladder. **B.** Photomicrograph (× 160) of a tumor. Note "parietal" (**1**) and "chief" (**2**) cells resembling those of the gastric mucosa. These cells are normally present in the neck of the bovine gallbladder. (Courtesy of Armed Forces Institute of Pathology and Dr. C.L. Davis.)

Ectopic pancreatic tissue

Ectopic pancreatic tissue is rarely observed in dogs and other species in the submucosa or muscularis of the gastrointestinal tract and gallbladder or in the mesentery. Rarely it may also be found in the liver or spleen.

Juvenile pancreatic atrophy (or hypoplasia)

This entity is recognized in young dogs (usually less than 13 months old), particularly in German shepherds, although described in other breeds such as the beagle. Clinically, it is characterized by signs of chronic exocrine pancreatic insufficiency. These include some loss of weight in spite of a voracious appetite; increased volume of gray, foul-smelling feces (steatorrhea); and laboratory evidence of decreased pancreatic enzymes in the feces. Signs of diabetes mellitus are not a feature. The disease may be inherited, but definitive evidence is yet to be developed on this point. The condition has been described as pancreatic hypoplasia as well as pancreatic atrophy. In that signs do not develop until the animals are several months of age, it seems most probable that it represents atrophy.

The lesions are characteristic. The glandular pancreas is essentially absent; only pancreatic ducts may be

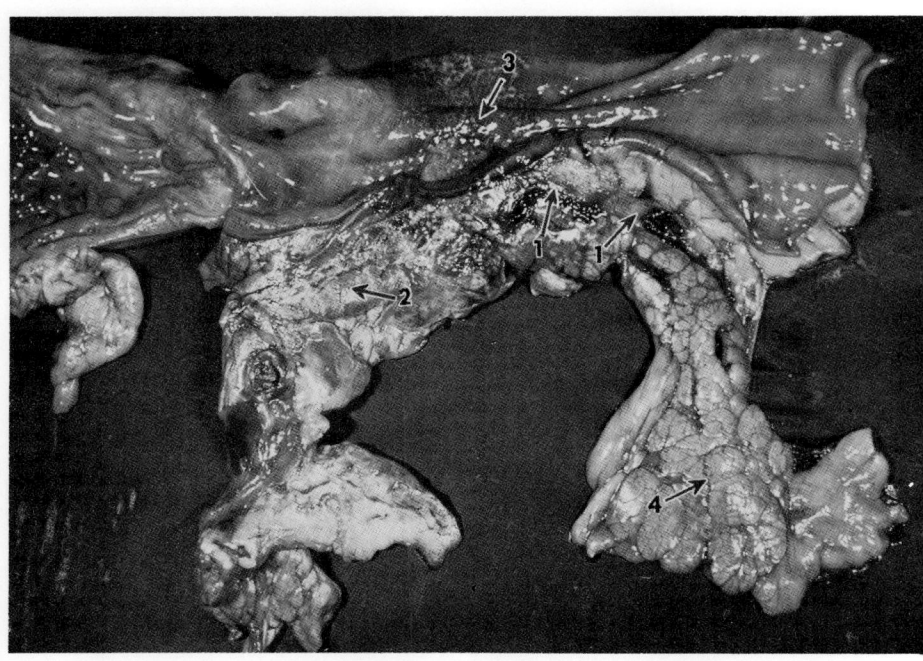

Fig. 23-30. Necrotizing and hemorrhagic pancreatitis in a male beagle dog, age seven years. Interstitial hemorrhage (**1**), gray necrotic areas (**2**), and congestion in duodenal mucosa (**3**). The head of the pancreas (**4**) is not affected. (Courtesy of Angell Memorial Animal Hospital.)

seen in the mesentery at the usual site of the pancreas. Microscopic examination reveals a few poorly formed groups of pancreatic acini along the course of the pancreatic ducts. Islets of Langerhans appear to be unaffected by this massive loss or failure of development of the exocrine pancreas. Inflammation is minimal or absent.

Pancreatitis

Pancreatitis as a specific disease is not frequent in animals with the exception of the dog, however in all species inflammation of the pancreas can occur in association with other diseases. Toxoplasmosis and feline infectious peritonitis may involve the pancreas. In horses, migrating strongyles may cause pancreatitis. Pancreatitis may be seen in systemic adenoviral infections, encephalomyocarditis virus infection, foot and mouth disease, and Coxsackievirus infection. In cats, acute pancreatitis has been seen in conjunction with hepatic lipidosis. Trauma to the organ can initiate necrosis and inflammation. Obstruction of the pancreatic duct will also lead to pancreatitis. This is a frequent cause in human beings and is often the result of gallstones. In animals, a variety of metazoan parasites may inhabit the pancreatic duct and cause obstruction and chronic pancreatitis. Zinc poisoning in sheep and calves can lead to pancreatitis, and has been reproduced in calves, sheep, cats, and birds. Alcoholism is the other major cause of pancreatitis in human beings. The cause of the more frequent forms of pancreatitis, which are acute necrotizing pancreatitis and chronic fibrosing pancreatitis, is not known.

ACUTE NECROTIZING PANCREATITIS (ACUTE PANCREATIC NECROSIS)

Acute necrotizing pancreatitis is an entity which has been observed in dogs, cats, horses, mice, pigs, nonhuman primates, and humans. The dog, however is by far the most commonly affected animal. The clinical signs in the dog are initiated suddenly with decreased appetite, dullness, vomiting, diarrhea, thirst, weak pulse, and severe abdominal pain. The affected dog often has a history of being a scavenger and may have recently eaten a meal rich in fats. It is reportedly more frequent in spayed dogs and castrated male dogs.

Many dogs succumb to this acute disease within days, others may survive and have repeated acute episodes, finally resulting in chronic fibrosing pancreatitis.

The cause of acute pancreatitis in dogs is not known. The lesions, however, result from the release and activation of pancreatic enzymes within the pancreas through undefined mechanisms.

The lesions center around focal necrosis, involving large or small areas and usually starting near the main pancreatic duct and its orifice into the duodenum. The necrosis is accompanied by hemorrhage, thrombosis, and edema, followed by infiltration of leukocytes. Pancreatic necrosis of fat is almost always present and may

extend for some distance into the mesenteric or omental fat. Severe acute pancreatitis leads to almost complete destruction of the pancreas and death within days, probably as a result of shock. Less severe disease either recurs as repeated episodes or continues to smolder, ultimately destroying both exocrine and endocrine tissues of the pancreas. These changes lead to pancreatic insufficiency and diabetes mellitus. The end stage pancreas may be almost entirely absent or replaced by scar tissue.

CHRONIC FIBROSING PANCREATITIS

Severe acute pancreatic necrosis is believed in some cases to be a prelude to chronic fibrosing pancreatitis. The latter is manifest in the dog by loss of body weight; increased volume of foul-smelling, fat laden feces; intermittent diarrhea; and, frequently, diabetes mellitus. Chronic fibrosing pancreatitis is also encountered in horses, cats, and cattle, but with much less frequency, and apparently not as a result of smoldering acute pancreatitis.

The lesions are recognized in the pancreas by it fibrous, nodular, and atrophied appearance grossly and by the fibrous replacement of most exocrine and endocrine cells. Some zones of active necrosis may be identified and are usually accompanied by leukocytic response. Other lesions of diabetes mellitus and malabsorption syndrome may be found.

PARASITES

Small red flukes, *Eurytrema pancreaticum,* usually less than 1 cm in length, may be numerous in the pancreatic ductal system of cattle, buffalo, sheep, and goats, causing chronic fibrosing pancreatitis of mild or minimal nature. They occur commonly in Brazil and Asia. Rarely, *Ascaris lumbricoides* may invade the pancreatic ducts, as well as the bile duct. *E. procyonis* is a pancreatic fluke of carnivores and may also be associated with fibrosing pancreatitis. Other flukes which do not have the pancreatic duct as their primary residence include **Opisthorchis, Dicrocoelium,** and **Metorchis.** A minute spirurid nematode, *Trichospirura leptostoma,* has been found in nearly 30% of necropsied marmosets *(Saguinus spp).* These parasites were associated with inflammation of the pancreatic duct in one marmoset and chronic fibrosing pancreatitis in three others (Cosgrove, et al., 1970).

Pancreatic calculi

Pancreatic calculi are found rarely in the pancreatic ducts of cattle. They are usually hard, white, and numerous, but small. They are reported to consist of carbonates and phosphates of calcium and magnesium, in company with organic substances. In one study in Denmark (Velling, 1975), pancreoliths were found in 279 cattle (0.43%) out of 65,471 examined post mortem at slaughter. No clinical signs or other pathologic changes were found except for some inflammation in the wall of ducts containing calculi. Older cattle were more often affected and the Red Danish breed was more often affected than the Holstein-Friesian or Jersey breeds, based on relation to total populations. The first report of bovine pancreolithiasis is believed to have been made by Furstenberg (1846).

Ectopic pancreatic tissue

Ectopic pancreatic tissue is rarely observed in dogs in the submucosa or muscularis of the gastrointestinal tract and gallbladder, or in the mesentery. Ectopic pancreatic tissue has also been reported in the liver and the duodenal submucosa of two rats, from the principal hepatic canal in a monkey embryo, and from the spleen of a cat.

Neoplasms of the exocrine pancreas

Consideration will be given here to neoplasms primary in the exocrine part of the pancreas. Tumors arising from the pancreatic islets (islets of Langerhans) are discussed in Chapter 26. Neoplasms of the supporting tissues such as hemangiosarcomas, fibrosarcomas, and liposarcomas are quite rare in the pancreas and are described elsewhere. The two neoplasms of the exocrine (zymogen) cells of the pancreas are classified as adenoma and adenocarcinoma of the pancreas.

Adenocarcinoma of the pancreas is the most frequent neoplasm of the pancreas in all species. Reported cases are more numerous from dogs, but this tumor is also recognized in cats, cattle, sheep swine, snakes, rats, mice, and other laboratory and zoo animals. They may arise from either acinar or ductular epithelium, and often have features of both. The neoplastic cells form small or large tubules or acini, or are undifferentiated and hence rarely form tubules. Tumors of tubular cell origin tend to be made up of cells with rather clear cytoplasm, whereas tumors of acinar cell origin tend to be smaller and form acinar structures. The key feature in identification of adenocarcinoma of acinar origin is the presence, in at least a few cells, of zymogen granules characteristic of normal pancreatic exocrine cells. These granules are spherical, eosinophilic in hematoxylin and eosin stain, and acidophilic with Masson's trichrome stain. These tumors may have a dense fibrous stroma in some cases, but usually have a rather delicate connective tissue framework. Invasion of stroma and adjacent normal pancreas is usually extensive, and in advanced cases the pancreas may be essentially destroyed, leading to clinical expression of pancreatic insufficiency. Metastasis to adjacent duodenum, liver, spleen, lymph nodes, mesenteric fat, and lung may be expected rather early in the life of the tumor. Pancreatic adenocarcinomas have been induced with carcinogens (nitrosamines) in mice, rats, and hamsters.

Adenoma of exocrine pancreas is known in several species and is recognized by its ductal or acinar pattern of cells, with an expanding growth pattern and rather complete encapsulation. Cystic spaces may be created by the tumor cells, which may also project in a papillary pattern into the lumen of the cysts. The cytoplasm of the cells near the lumen of tubules may contain zymogen granules which may be less intensely stained than in normal acini.

Hyperplastic nodules may be seen in the pancreas of many older animals. They are usually less well encapsulated than are adenomas, but may be difficult to distinguish with certainty. They are usually multiple.

References

Akol KG, Washabau RJ, Saunders HM, et al. Acute pancreatitis in cats with hepatic lipidosis. J Vet Internal Med 1993;7(4):205–209.

Allen JG, Masters HG, Peet RL, et al. Zinc toxicity in ruminants. J Comp Pathol 1983;93(3):363–377.

Anderson NV, Johnson KH. Pancreatic carcinoma in the dog. J Am Vet Med Assoc 1967;150:286–295.

Banner BF, Alroy J, Kipnis RM. Acinar cell carcinoma of the pancreas in a cat. Vet Pathol 1979;16:543–547.

Bhattacharyya HM, Das SK, Dhar MM, et al. Acute necrotic pancreatitis in pigs. Indian Vet J 1973;50:850–852.

Bockman DE, Schiller WR, Suriyapa C, et al. Fine structure of early experimental acute pancreatitis in dogs. Lab Invest 1973;28:584–592.

Breider MA, Kiely RG, Edwards JF. Chronic eosinophilic pancreatitis and ulcerative colitis in a horse. J Am Vet Med Assoc 1985; 186:809–811.

Cook AK, Breitschwerdt EB, Levine JF, et al. Risk factors associated with acute pancreatitis in dogs: 101 cases (1985–1990). J Am Vet Med Assoc 1994;203(5):673–679.

Cosgrove GE, Humason G, Lushbaugh CC. Trichospirura leptostoma, a nematode of the pancreatic ducts of marmosets (Saguinus spp.). J Am Vet Med Assoc 1970;157:696–698.

Craighead JE. Pathogenicity of the M and E variants of the encephalomyocarditis (EMC) virus: II. Lesions of the pancreas, parotid, and lacrimal glands. Am J Pathol 1966;48:375–386.

Dissin J, Mills LR, Meins DL, et al. Experimental induction of pancreatic adenocarcinoma in rats. J Natl Cancer Inst 1975;55:857–864.

Feldman BF, Attix EA, Strombeck DR, et al. Biochemical and coagulation changes in a canine model of acute necrotizing pancreatitis. Am J Vet Res 1981;42:805–809.

Gans JH. Carcinoma of the pancreas in the dog. Cornell Vet 1958;48:372–377.

Greve T, Dayton AD, Anderson NV. Acute pancreatitis with coexistent diabetes mellitus: an experimental study in the dog. Am J Vet Res 1973;34:939–946.

Hill RC, Van Winkle TJ. Acute necrotizing pancreatitis and acute suppurative pancreatitis in the cat. A retrospective study of 40 cases (1976–1989). J Vet Intern Med 1993;7(1):25–33.

Kitchell BE, Strombeck DR, Cullen J, et al. Clinical and pathologic changes in experimentally induced acute pancreatitis in cats. Am J Vet Res 1986;47:1170–1173.

Lombardi B, Estes LW, Longnecker DS. Acute hemorrhagic pancreatitis (Massive necrosis) with fat necrosis induced in mice by DL4 ethionine fed with a choline-deficient diet. Am J Pathol 1975; 79:465–480.

Longnecker DS. Editorial. Experimental pancreatic carcinogenesis. Lab Invest 1982;46:543–544.

McClure HM, Chandler FW, Hierholzer JC. Necrotizing pancreatitis due to simian adenovirus type 31 in a Rhesus monkey. Arch Pathol Lab Med 1978;102:150–153.

Mia AS, Koger HD, Tierney MM. Serum values of amylase and pancreatic lipase in healthy mature dogs and dogs with experimental pancreatitis. Am J Vet Res 1978;39:965–969.

Murtaugh RJ, Jacobs RM, Sherding RG, et al. Serum pancreatic polypeptide and amylase concentrations in dogs with experimentally induced acute pancreatitis. Am J Vet Res 1985;46:654–656.

Musa BE, Nelson AW, Gillette EL et al. A model to study acute pancreatitis in the dog. J Surg Res 1976;21:51–56.

Prentice DE, James RW, Wadsworth PF. Pancreatic atrophy in young beagle dogs. Vet Pathol 1980;17:575–580.

Priester WA. Data from eleven United States and Canadian colleges of veterinary medicine on pancreatic carcinoma in domestic animals. Cancer Res 1974;34:1372–1375.

Reznik-Schuller H. Ultrastructure of pancreatic tumors induced in syrian hamsters by N-nitroso-2,6–dimethylmorpholine. Vet Pathol 1980;17:352–361.

Roebuck BD, Baumgartner KJ, Thron CD. Characterization of two poopulations of pancreatic atypical acinar cell foci induced by azaserine in the rat. Lab Invest 1984;50:141–146.

Rowlatt U. Spontaneous epithelial neoplasms of the pancreas of mammals. Brit J Cancer 1967;21:82–107.

Strombeck DR, Wheeldon E, Harrold D. Model of chronic pancreatitis in the dog. Am J Vet Res 1984;45:131–136.

Velling K. Bovine pancreaolithiasis in Denmark. Acta Vet Scand 1975;16:327–340.

24

The urinary system

KIDNEYS

Anatomy and physiology

NEPHRON

The essential anatomic and functional unit of the kidney is the nephron. Each kidney contains many nephrons, depending upon the species (the human kidneys are estimated to contain between one and two million, in the rat, 10 to 30 million). Each nephron is made up of the **glomerulus,** a spherical body which is formed by invagination of branching segments of an afferent arteriole into a terminal bud of a **renal tubule.** The renal tubule has distinct segments known as (1) the proximal convoluted tubule, (2) the loop of Henle, with descending and ascending limbs, and (3) the distal convoluted tubule, which connects with a collecting duct, which in turn empties into a duct of Bellini and then to the renal pelvis and ureter.

In the glomerulus, the afferent artery branches and re-anastomoses to form a capillary tuft which is intimately associated with the epithelial cells of the tubule and the visceral layer of Bowman's capsule. The glomerular space surrounds the capillary tuft, communicates with the proximal convoluted tubule, and is surrounded by an epithelial layer and a thin fibrous capsule—the parietal layer of Bowman's capsule.

At light microscopic magnification, the capillary endothelium may be seen to be closely applied to the tubular epithelium, separated only by a basement membrane, which can be best demonstrated with the periodic acid-Schiff reaction or silver-staining methods. Ultrastructurally, the basement membrane is composed of three layers—an electron-dense layer (lamina densa) separating two less compact layers (lamina rara externa, lamina rara interna). The endothelial cell which lines the capillary lumen is stretched out with only a thin layer of cytoplasm over most of the surface of the basement membrane. The endothelial lining is not continuous, but contains multiple fenestrae approximately 1000 Å in diameter where the basement membrane is bare. The cells of the visceral layer of Bowman's capsule are in contact with the basement membrane by means of long extensions of the cytoplasm known as foot processes, giving a name to these cells: **podocytes.** The space between the foot processes is bridged by a thin line called the slit membrane, or diaphragm.

This visceral epithelium of Bowman's capsule is made up of cells which are differentiated in prenatal life in the human and presumably in other species, and are unable to replicate in the adult. If podocytes are destroyed by disease, they are not effectively replaced.

The cell body of the podocyte bulges into the urinary space, has a prominent nucleus, a well-developed Golgi system, abundant smooth and rough endoplasmic reticulum, lysosomes, and mitochondria. Only a few of these organelles are found in the foot processes.

The endothelium, glomerular basement membrane, and the interdigitating foot processes of podocytes function together structurally to form the **filtration barrier.** The function of this barrier is to selectively pass macromolecules, based on size, shape, and charge. Macromolecules, such as plasma proteins, are repelled by an "electromagnetic shield" due to the accumulation of negative charges. Selection for size at the filtration barrier is based on the dense network of extracellular matrices made up by the glomerular basement membrane and the slit diaphragm. Uncharged macromolecules with an effective molecular radius of 1.8 nm pass freely through the filter. Larger components are increasingly restricted with total restriction of elements with an effective radius of more than 4.0 nm. Plasma albumin, with an effective radius of 3.6 nm, would pass through readily except for repulsion due to its negative charge. Proteins of low molecular weight pass through the filter. Water flows through freely.

In addition to the endothelial and epithelial cells, a third cell, the **mesangial** or **intercapillary** cell, is found in the glomerulus. This cell is located centrally within the capillary loops, one side of the capillary always facing the mesangial cell. The cytoplasm of the mesangial cell is similar to that of the epithelial cell, but adjacent extracellular spaces contain fine reticular filaments and material similar to basement membrane (**mesangial matrix**). The function of mesangial cells has received con-

1111

siderable attention, and evidence indicates that they are (1) phagocytic and may clear debris from the mesangium, (2) contractile by virtue of cytoplasmic myofibrillar bundles and may influence glomerular blood flow, and (3) contribute to the formation of glomerular basement membrane.

The **proximal convoluted tubule** leaves the glomerulus as a short segment called the neck piece. The tortuous tubule is lined by a single layer of cuboidal cells which have a brush border on their luminal surface. Under the electron microscope, this brush border is seen to consist of microvilli that increase the absorptive surface of the cells. Infoldings of the cell membrane also extend deep into the cell from the base of the microvilli. Similar membranes extend into these cells from their basal surface. Mitochondria are often found between these membranes.

The major function of the proximal tubule is the resorption of water, inorganic solutes such as sodium, chloride, bicarbonate, potassium, calcium, and organic solutes, including glucose, amino acids, and proteins of low molecular weight. This capacity of high transport is reflected in the predominant occupancy of the renal parenchyma by the proximal convoluted tubules.

Proteins of low molecular weight are absorbed from the lumen by cells of the proximal tubules by endocytosis and pinocytosis. Globules of these proteins become fused with lysosomes and eventually degraded by the lysosomal enzymes, and the end products are discharged into the lumen of the tubule. An excessive amount of these proteins in the proximal tubules or interference with lysosomal enzyme activity (as in human malignant myeloma or in the case of the male rat that produces alpha 2-microglobulin, or in the presence of certain toxic substances) results in accumulation of lysosomal-protein bodies in the cytoplasm of tubular cells. These are recognized with the light microscope as eosinophilic, discrete bodies, that have for many years been designated by pathologists as "hyaline droplet bodies" (See page 1127). The tubule then assumes a straight course, descending toward the medulla, where it becomes the **thin descending limb** of the **loop of Henle,** continuing the renal tubule into the renal medulla. The epithelial cells lining this segment are flattened and contain few mitochondria. The loop is completed, usually in the peripheral medulla, and the lining cells of this ascending limb are cuboidal and contain numerous mitochondria. Their cytoplasm is for this reason usually darker when viewed by light microscopy. The loops of Henle may be **short** or **long,** depending on the position of the glomerulus in the renal cortex. At the point where the ascending limb returns to the cortex, the tubule becomes the **distal convoluted tubule.** The epithelial cells lining this segment are columnar, but have clear cytoplasm and no brush border. A few microvilli may be demonstrated with the electron microscope in these cells. Their basal surface bears deeply infolded cell membranes, which are closely aligned with many mitochondria.

At the point where the ascending limb joins the distal convoluted tubule, the tubule lies in contact with its own afferent arteriole, near the hilus of the glomerulus. The epithelial cells at this point, called the **macula densa,** are uniformly cuboidal and arranged in an easily recognized palisade adjacent to the afferent arteriole. The closely-packed arrangement of these specialized cells give them a distinctive appearance, suggesting the name **macula densa** to early histologists. Cells in the media of the arteriole in this zone are enlarged and resemble cells of the aortic or carotid body. These are believed to be modified smooth muscle cells. Together with the **macula densa,** these cells of the arteriole form the **juxtaglomerular apparatus,** which is the source of **renin.**

Glomeruli, once destroyed, do not regenerate, although those that remain may undergo some compensatory hypertrophy. Fortunately, the total number of nephrons is considerably in excess of requirements, so that many of them, or even a whole kidney, may be lost without fatal effects, providing the remaining renal tissue is uninjured.

Destroyed tubular epithelium regenerates readily. The new cells have hyperchromatic nuclei but may be less columnar than their predecessors. It is not unusual to encounter tubules whose epithelium is flattened and whose lumens are large. These are variously interpreted as dilated because of obstruction, regenerated or hypertrophic with increased functional requirements compensatory to destruction of other tubules, or merely hyperplastic. Although tubular epithelium can undergo hypertrophy and hyperplasia, new nephrons cannot be formed. Thus, hyperplasia of tubular epithelium may repair or enlarge a nephron, but cannot increase the number of nephrons.

In certain species, particularly the dog, rat, and cat, the orifice in Bowman's capsule through which the neck piece of the proximal convoluted tubule passes may be widened under certain circumstances. This permits part of the tubule to protrude into Bowman's space and presents a puzzling feature in histologic sections. This phenomenon has been variously named "protrusions of tubular epithelium" or "infraglomerular epithelial reflux." Mullink and Feron (1967) present evidence that this histologically recognized feature is the result of postmortem change.

Anatomic differences between species are of some consequence in interpreting lesions in the kidneys. A few might be mentioned: Bovine animals have lobulated kidneys, similar to fetal lobulation in other species. Each lobule has multiple calices and a separate ureter, and its blood is supplied through a single artery entering at the hilus. The kidneys of the dog and rat have a single renal ridge which extends the length of the kidney to form what amounts to a single papilla. The capsule is apt to be adherent, and fat is normally present in tubular epithelium. The cat also frequently has fat in renal tubular epithelium and the kidneys are more moveable in the abdomen. The horse has many compound mucous glands in the renal pelvis.

The kidney of newborn and young animals may be recognized histologically by glomeruli which are small with hyperchromic epithelial and endothelial nuclei. The tubules are less well developed than in the adult, and fewer nephrons have tubules which dip into the medulla. The young animal therefore has much less capacity to concentrate urine than does the adult.

BLOOD SUPPLY

The renal vasculature is complex, with two capillary networks, one in the glomeruli and the other surrounding the tubules. As a result of the dual nature of the vasculature, lesions affecting one site ultimately affect the other. After entering the hilus, the renal arteries branch into large segmental arteries, which at the corticomedullary junction give rise to the arcuate arteries. From these, interlobular arteries originate and run parallel to collecting tubules. These tend to lie in groups so that when congested, each group is represented by a red streak, radial in direction, which is readily visible to the naked eye. The interlobular arteries are end arteries with no anastomoses with each other. For this reason, infarction of the renal cortex readily occurs. The infarcted areas take the form of pyramids with their bases at the capsule.

The afferent arteriole originates from the interlobular artery, each one supplying a single glomerulus, where it forms a tuft of capillaries, which in turn join to form the efferent arteriole leaving the glomerulus. The wall of the afferent arteriole is considerably thicker than the efferent arteriole. Small arteries may directly connect afferent and efferent arterioles, bypassing the glomerulus, but they are few in number and apparently insufficiently developed to provide protective anastomoses.

The efferent arteriole then subdivides into a capillary network that surrounds the tubules. The tubular capillary plexus forms venules, which ultimately form intertubular veins, arcuate veins, and ultimately the renal vein. Thus, the delicate epithelial cells of the tubules are dependent for their blood supply upon the free movement of blood through the tortuous passageways of the glomerulus. As will be explained, the glomerulus is, unfortunately, vulnerable to a number of lesions that interfere with this free flow of blood, and death and destruction of tubules as the result of such lesions are of frequent occurrence. The glomeruli are almost equally dependent on proper conditions in the tubular regions, and there are situations, such as swelling of the epithelium of the tubules or other lesions, which will lead to stasis of blood flow with loss of glomerular function.

PHYSIOLOGY

It is computed that about one-third of the cardiac output of blood goes to the kidney at each circuit, and that nearly 10% of blood—equivalent to 16% of the plasma—which passes through the glomerulus filters freely into Bowman's capsule as the "glomerular filtrate." Only about 1% of this is believed to be excreted as urine, the remaining 99% being resorbed through the epithelium of the tubules. Substances with a molecular weight above about 70,000 do not pass into the glomerular filtrate, thus most proteins and, of course, cells, are retained in the blood stream.

Electrolytes such as chlorides, carbonates and bicarbonates, phosphates, silicates (herbivorous animals), and sulfates of ammonium, sodium, potassium, and calcium, as well as various organic substances, including glucose and urea, pass freely into the glomerular filtrate, either to be excreted in the urine or to be resorbed selectively by the epithelial cells of the proximal convoluted tubules. At the same time that many are resorbed, some substances are excreted by the epithelium of the tubules. These include creatinine in humans, but not apparently in the dog.

As indicated, compounds with large molecules, especially the proteins, do not pass through the healthy glomerular filter, which is comparable to a dialyzing membrane, and do not appear in the normal urine. The presence of protein in the urine is a readily determined clinical sign of injury to the glomeruli and a serious renal malfunction.

Glucose is absent from normal urine, because it is completely resorbed in the tubules unless its concentration in the blood is above a certain critical level, called the renal threshold. The latter situation arises in diabetes mellitus, in which the glucose of the blood cannot be utilized, and at times, immediately following an excessively large meal of carbohydrates.

Formation of urine can be prevented completely (anuria) or partially (oliguria) by various lesions in the glomeruli, by renal ischemia, or by the excessive swelling of the tubular epithelium previously mentioned. When this occurs, profound changes appear constituting the condition of uremia.

References

Bachmann S, Kriz W. Nephron and collecting duct structure in the kidney, rat. In: Jones TC, Hard GC, Mohr U, eds. ILSI monograph on pathology of laboratory animals, urinary system. 2nd ed. New York: Springer Verlag, 1997 (in press).

Barajas L, Salido E. Juxtaglomerular apparatus and the renin-angiotensin system. Lab Invest 1986;54:361–364.

Jones DB. Enzymatic dissection of the glomerulus. Lab Invest 1985;52:453–461.

Congenital and hereditary anomalies

Anomalies of the kidney have been reported in humans and many other species. Some are known to be caused by inherited factors, others are of unknown etiology.

APLASIA OR AGENESIS

The most frequently reported anomaly involves aplasia or agenesis of one or both kidneys. Absence of both kidneys, of course, is incompatible with life and would be encountered only in the fetus, newborn, or stillborn animal. On the other hand, aplasia of one kidney results in compensatory hypertrophy of the remaining kidney, and the individual may cope with life quite well. Agenesis of one or both kidneys has been reported in most species of domestic animals. Unilateral agenesis is most common in swine, dogs, and cattle and is less frequent in cats, horses, sheep, and other animals.

RENAL HYPOPLASIA

Renal hypoplasia describes kidneys in newborn or young animals which are markedly smaller than normal with little or no function. Cordes and Dodd (1965) described bilateral renal hypoplasia in 19 swine, 12 of which were born dead or died within 2 days of birth. Varying degrees of hypoplasia were found, from tiny, almost unrecognizable kidneys to bilobate kidneys or kidneys with distinct fetal lobulation. All affected piglets were sired by the same boar, and the evidence indicated probable control of the defect by a single recessive autosomal gene. This condition has also been recognized in the dog and cat.

HORSESHOE KIDNEY

This descriptive name is applied to the appearance of kidneys which are fused at one pole to produce a horseshoe-shaped structure centered roughly in the midline of the abdomen. The ureters are usually intact, and the kidneys function adequately in most instances. This condition has been reported in humans and cats.

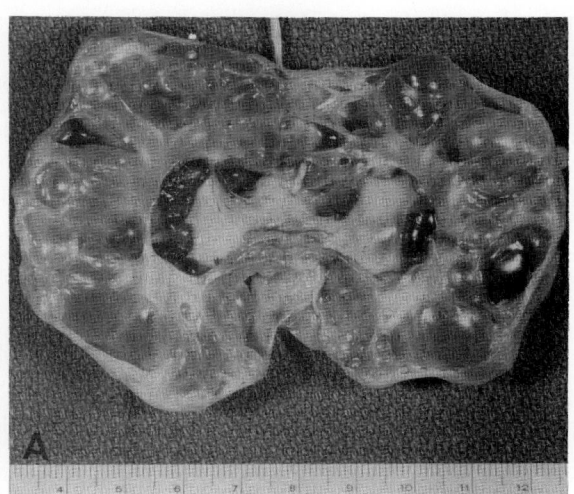

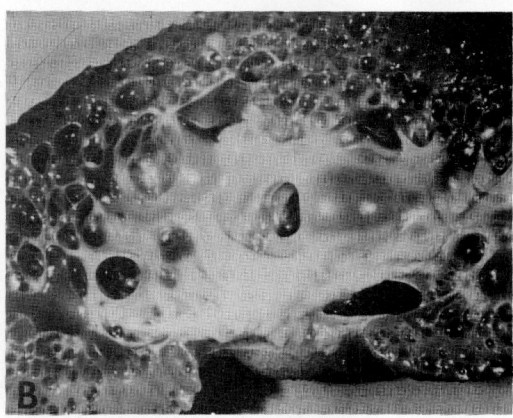

FIG. 24-1. A. Polycystic kidney from an eight-year-old spayed female cat. (Courtesy of Angell Memorial Animal Hospital.) **B.** Polycystic kidney in a hog. (Courtesy of Dr. C. L. Davis.)

VASCULAR ANOMALIES

Congenital variations in origin and course of renal arteries and veins are sometimes observed, usually at the time of necropsy. These have no deleterious effects, except in those instances in which their position partially occludes the ureter. In this instance, hydronephrosis might result.

DISPLACEMENT

The anatomic position of the kidneys is retroperitoneal in all species, but the exact position varies between species and to some extent between individuals. In the cat, for example, the kidneys during life may be quite moveable if the blood vessels are longer than usual. This so-called "floating kidney" appears to have little pathologic significance.

CYSTS IN THE KIDNEY

Simple cysts, presumably acquired, are not infrequently seen in the kidneys of various species, but are considerably more common in swine and dogs than in the other domestic animals. They may be solitary or very numerous, varying in size from those just visible to the eye up to a diameter of about a centimeter in the case of multiple cysts of the pig and dog, or of several centimeters in the case of a single cyst. Their walls are usually thin and transparent, their contents clear and watery, perhaps tinged with yellow. They may bulge from the surface or lie buried in the depths of the parenchyma. Cysts may arise from gradual distention of a nephron whose outlet has been closed, usually by the pressure of exudates or fibrous tissue. But if the kidney contains a considerable number of cysts, the disorder is usually designated as the **congenital polycystic kidney** (Figs. 24-1 A and B). The three most common types of renal cystic disease described in humans have a genetic basis. Similar counterparts have been reported in other species. A brief description of these diseases follow.

Autosomal recessive (childhood or infantile) polycystic kidney disease This disorder commonly referred to as ARPKD affects children and infants at an incidence of 1 in 10,000 live births. It results in high mortality in affected children in their first year of life. A gene associated with this autosomal recessive disorder has been identified on human chromosome 6. Both kidneys are involved, with enlargement and a spongy parenchyma made up of many small cysts in the cortex and medulla. The striking histologic feature is severe dilatation of all collecting tubules. Hepatic cysts and proliferation of portal bile ducts accompany the renal lesion in most cases. Similar disease entities have been reported in the **cpk** (congenital polycystic kidney) and other strains of mice, and also in rabbits, springbok, rats, dogs, and swine. Of these the **cpk** mouse has been best studied. Although the mode of inheritance in this species is similar to the disease of humans, the **cpk** gene mutation is not analagous to the mutated ARPKD gene of human beings.

Autosomal dominant (adult) polycystic kidney disease This is the most prevalent form of polycystic kidney disease of humans. It occurs with a relative frequency of approximately 1 in every 500 people. Renal dysfunction becomes manifest during the third to fifth decade of life and progresses to end-stage renal disease between 55 and 70 years of age. This form of polycystic renal disease is genetically heterogeneous in that at least two distinct mutated genes have been associated with this form of renal disease, one termed PDK1 on chromosome 16 whose product is termed **polycystin,** and the other PDK2 on chromosome 4. Polycystin is thought to play a role in cell to cell or epithelial cell to matrix signaling. The gene product of PDK2 is an integral transmembrane protein that is only partially similar to the amino acid sequence of that of PDK1; it also has a similarity to certain voltage-activated Ca^{2+} and Na^+ α_1 channel proteins. The precise role of these mutated gene products in the pathogenesis of this dominant form of polycystic kidney disease has yet to be determined.

In this group of diseases, cysts occur in any segment of the nephron, interspersed among functional tubules, and are not blind-ended. In advanced disease, the kidneys are essentially replaced by larger cysts. Cysts also occur in other organs: liver, pancreas, lungs, and gonads. Berry aneurysms of cerebral arteries are seen in approximately one fourth of the cases. A polycystic renal disease of cats and dogs, with involvement of the kidney and liver, has been reported and may be analogous to this human disease. These disorders have not been as well studied as the human diseases.

Medullary cystic disease complex This is a group of four progressive renal disorders, the onset of which usually occurs during childhood or adolescence. Of the four, one is non-familial, two are inherited in an autosomal recessive manner, and the fourth as an autosomal dominant trait. The characteristic finding in all of these disorders is the presence of cysts in the medulla associated with secondary atrophy of cortical tubules and interstitial fibrosis. The cysts arise in the collecting ducts within the medulla. Terminal renal failure usually occurs before the age of twenty. The kidneys at autopsy are small and fibrotic with small cysts mainly in the medulla. The closest analagous disease in animals appears to be the experimental disease in rats induced by feeding diphenylamine, diphenylthiazole, or nordihydroguaiaretic acid. This entity is described more fully in the following.

A type of renal cystic disease has been produced experimentally in rats by feeding diphenylamine, diphenylthiazole, or nordihydroguaiaretic acid. This experimental disease most closely resembles the **medullary cystic disease complex** previously described as starting in childhood and resulting in death from renal failure by the age of twenty.

The addition of 1.03 percent of diphenylthiazole to the pelleted feed of rats results, within 2 to 4 weeks, in gross enlargement of the outer medulla of the kidneys due to dilated tubules. The collecting tubules in the outer medulla are initially involved with saccular and fusiform dilations. Cortical collecting and distal convoluted tubules may also be affected. After withdrawal of the drug from the feed, the kidneys return to normal within 4 to 8 weeks.

The microscopic appearance of these induced lesions starts with focal cellular degeneration and necrosis of epithelium of the collecting ducts in the outer medulla. By 8 weeks, the cystic dilation of tubules is marked and the tubular basement membrane (but not the glomerular basement membrane) fail to stain with alcian blue.

The ultrastructural changes are recognized early in the tubular epithelium and later in the basement membranes of the cystic collecting ducts. Smooth endoplasmic reticulum is increased in the tubular epithelium and Golgi's complexes are conspicuous. After 2 to 4 weeks, the rough endoplasmic reticulum and free ribosomes are increased and the cisternae of the endoplasmic reticulum are elongated. By 8 weeks, lysosomes are also enlarged and increased in number. The tubular basement membrane is gradually thickened, and by 8 weeks, greatly thickened and laminated. Ruthenium red staining is reduced and the stainable granules of heparin sulfate protoglycan are lost. All these features return to normal 4 to 8 weeks following withdrawal of the drug.

References

Aziz N. Animal models of polycystic kidney disease. BioEssays 1995;17:703–712.

Biller DS, Chew DJ, DiBartola SP. Polycystic kidney disease in a family of Persian cats. J Am Vet Med Assoc 1990;196:1288–1290.

Brown CA, Crowell WA, Brown SA, et al. Suspected familial renal disease in Chow Chows. J Am Vet Med Assoc 1990;196:1279–1284.

Carone FA, Bacallo R, Kanwar YS. Biology of polycystic disease. Lab Invest 1994;70:437–448.

Carone FA. Diphenylthiazole-induced renal cystic disease, rat. In: Jones TC, Hard GC, Mohr U, eds. ILSI monograph on pathology of laboratory animals, urinary system. 2nd ed. New York: Springer Verlag, 1997 (in press).

Chalifoux LV. Crossed renal ectopia in a Squirrel Monkey (*Saimiri sciureus*) and an Owl Monkey (*Aotus trivirgatus*). J Med Primatol 1986;15:235–239.

Dunham BM, Anderson WI, Steinberg H, et al. Renal dysplasia with multiple urogenital and large intestinal anomalies in a calf. Vet Pathol 1989;26:94–96.

Ebihara I, Killen PD, Laurie GW, et al. Altered mRNA expression of basement membrane components in a murine model of polycystic kidney disease. Lab Invest 1988;58:262–269.

Finco R, Kurtz HJ, Low V, et al. Familial renal disease in Norwegian elkhound dogs. J Am Vet Med Assoc 1970;156:747–760.

Haverty TP, Neilson EG. Basement membrane gene expression in polycystic kidney disease. Lab Invest 1988;58:245–248.

Kaspareit-Rittinghausen J, Rapp K, Deerberg F, et al. Hereditary polycystic kidney disease associated with osteorenal syndrome in rats. Vet Pathol 1989;26:195–201.

Kaufmann ML, Osborne CA, Johnson GR, et al. Renal ectopia in a dog and a cat. J Am Vet Med Assoc 1987;190:73–77.

Kessler MJ, Roberts JA, London WT. Adult polycystic kidney disease in a rhesus monkey (*Macaca mulatta*). J Med Primatol 1984;13:147–152.

Matsell DG, Bennett T, Goodyer P, et al. The pathogenesis of multicystic dysplastic kidney disease: insights from the study of fetal kidneys. Lab Invest 1996;74:883–893.

McKenna SC, Carpenter JL. Polycystic disease of the kidney and liver in the cairn terrier. Vet Pathol 1980;17:436–442.

Mochizuki T, Wu G, Hayashi T, et al. PKD2, a gene for polycystic disease that encodes an integral membrane protein. Science 1996;272:1339–1342.

Morton LD, Sanecki RK, Gordon DE, et al. Juvenile renal disease in miniature schnauzer dogs. Vet Pathol 1990;27:455–458.

Picut CA, Lewis RM. Microscopic features of canine renal dysplasia. Vet Pathol 1987;24:156–163.

Sakakibara I, Honjo S. Spontaneously occurring congenital polycystic kidney in a Cynomologus Monkey (*Macaca fascicularis*). J Med Primatol 1990;19:501–506.

Seier JV, Fincham JE, Taljaard JJF. Horseshoe kidneys in Vervet Monkeys. J Med Primatol 1990;19:595–599.

Diseases of Glomeruli

Glomerulonephritis

The term glomerulonephritis is usually restricted to primary inflammation of the glomeruli. Glomeruli may also suffer damage secondarily to tubular disease or pyelonephritis, but these forms of glomerular disease are not included as primary glomerulonephritis (Fig. 24-3). As indicated earlier, glomerular disease may lead to changes in renal tubules. Several differing systems of classification of glomerulonephritis have appeared over the years and further changes can be anticipated as the causative factors and pathogenesis become better known. We will consider glomerulonephritis under the following headings: acute proliferative glomerulonephritis; membranous glomerulonephritis; membranoproliferative glomerulonephritis; chronic (sclerosing)

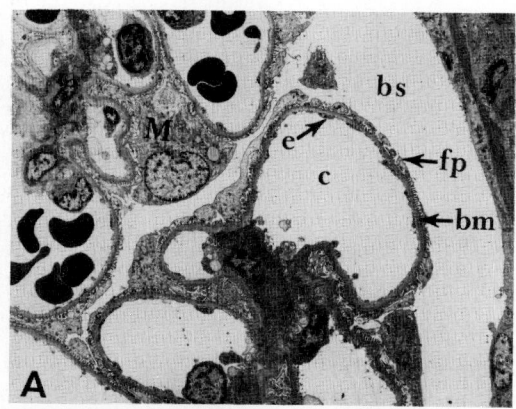

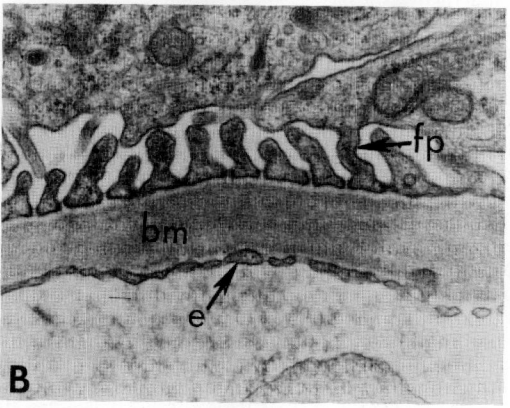

FIG. 24-2. Normal renal glomerulus. **A.** The lumens of glomerular capillaries (**c**) separated from Bowman's space (**bs**) by fenestrated endothelium (**e**), basement membrane (**bm**), and foot processes of epithelial cells (**fp**). **M.** mesangial cell. **B.** Higher magnification illustrating fenestrated endothelium (**e**), the three component laminae of the basement membrane (**bm**), and epithelial foot processes (**fp**). (Courtesy of Dr. N. W. King)

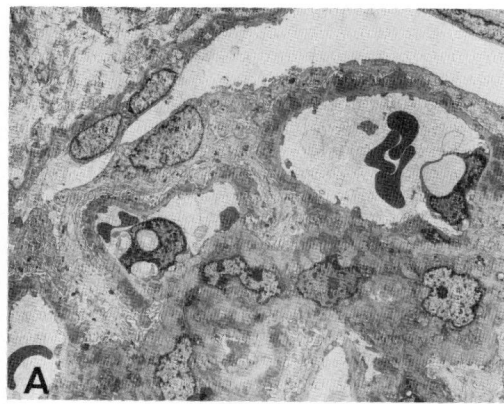

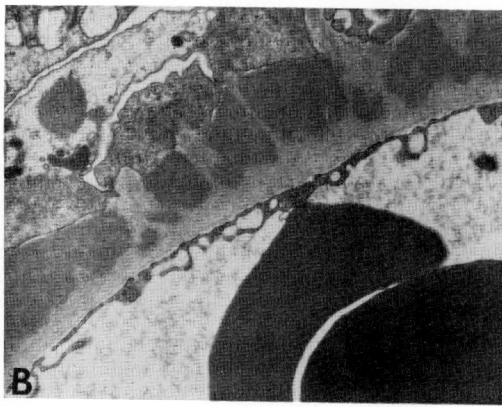

FIG. 24-3. Immune complex glomerulonephritis. **A.** Dense deposits are present in the basement membrane and in an exuberant mesangial matrix. **B.** Higher magnification of a glomerular tuft containing discrete dense deposits in the basement membrane. These correspond to the spikes seen in silver and immunofluorescent preparations. (Courtesy of Dr. N. W. King, Jr.)

glomerulonephritis; and focal embolic glomerulonephritis. The morphologic features of these forms of glomerulonephritis will be described first, and then the immunologic mechanisms of injury will be discussed.

ACUTE PROLIFERATIVE GLOMERULONEPHRITIS

This form of glomerulonephritis is the classic post-streptococcal glomerulonephritis known in children for many years and recently identified as a spontaneous and experimentally induced disease entity in animals (Figs. 24-4–6).

The human disease, which characteristically affects young children, but may appear in adults, typically follows by 2 weeks or more an acute upper respiratory infection by streptococci. The onset of the renal disease is sudden, with fever, nausea, weakness, subcutaneous edema, and excretion of brown or bloody urine in scant amounts. The fever may abate in about a week, but abnormalities in the urine may persist, and some cases may continue as a chronic disease. The lesions may heal or progress to chronic glomerulonephritis.

The lesion in glomeruli is characteristic under the

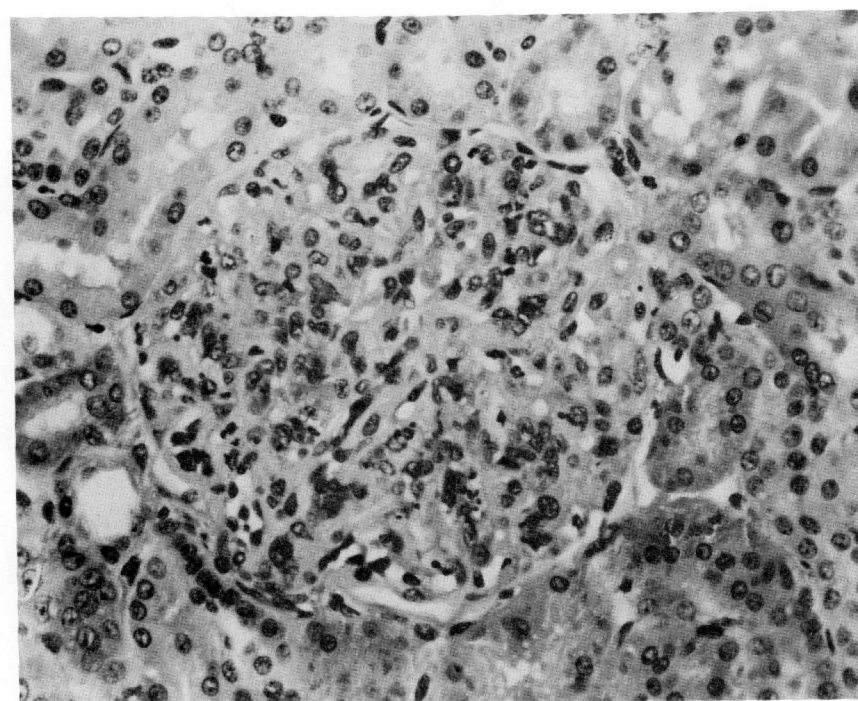

FIG. 24-4. Proliferative glomerulonephritis. Nine-year-old male dog. Glomerulus fills Bowman's space and contains numerous nuclei, including leukocytes. The basement membrane may also be thickened. (Courtesy of Armed Forces Institute of Pathology.)

light microscope. Although not recognizable definitively in the gross specimen, the kidney may be enlarged and pale, with petechiae outlining the glomeruli. The glomeruli are initially congested or edematous and conspicuous at low magnification. The glomerular tufts are increased in size, with increased numbers of endothelial and mesangial cells. In this early stage, leukocytes, particularly neutrophils and monocytes, appear in the glomerulus. This influx and proliferation of cells result in compression of the capillaries and the absence of red blood cells. As the disease progresses, parietal epithelial cells also proliferate, and adhere to the inner surface of Bowman's capsule. These eventually form the epithelial "crescents" seen in subacute or chronic forms. Thrombosis and necrosis of glomerular capillaries may occur, with subsequent hemorrhage into the glomerulus. No obvious thickening of the basement membrane or alteration in the foot processes of epithelial cells is found by examination with the electron microscope.

The most characteristic ultrastructural finding is the presence of deposits or "humps" of immune complex on the epithelial side of the basement membrane. These deposits are usually less than a micron in diame-

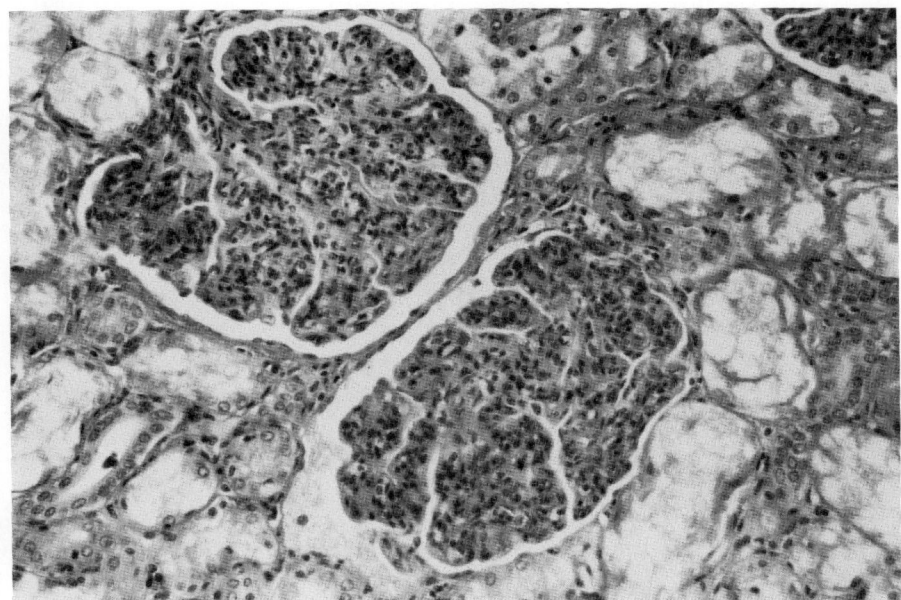

FIG. 24-5. Proliferative glomerulonephritis. Two-year-old Holstein cow. Increased cellularity obscures individual capillary loops. (Courtesy of Drs. R. M. Lewis and D. O. Slauson and **Veterinary Pathology.**)

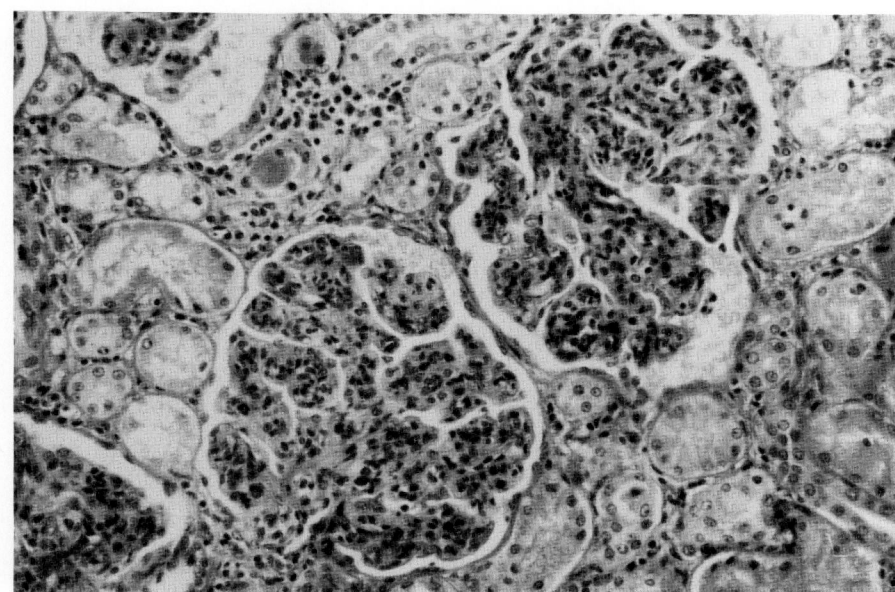

FIG. 24-6. Proliferative glomerulonephritis with a lobular pattern in a horse. There is an increase in overall glomerular cellularity. (Courtesy of Drs. R. M. Lewis and D. O. Slauson and **Veterinary Pathology.**)

ter, but may be large and project between podocytes. Occasionally, the deposits may be present within the lamina densa and in the subendothelial portion of the basement membrane. When stained with silver techniques or the periodic acid-Schiff (PAS) reaction, the basement membrane is disrupted by these deposits, giving it the characteristic "lumpy-bumpy" appearance.

Leukocytic infiltration may occur adjacent to glomeruli or in nearby interstitial tissues. Tubular changes are not pronounced in acute stages of disease aside from proteinaceous casts and red cells in tubular lumens and hyalin droplets in proximal convoluted tubular epithelium.

MEMBRANOUS GLOMERULONEPHRITIS

Rather clearly distinguishable from proliferative glomerulonephritis in humans, membranous glomerulonephritis also occurs naturally as a distinct entity in other animals (Figs. 24-7–10). In individual cases, however, differentiation is not always simple, and it is possible for both forms to occur simultaneously. Membranous glomerulonephritis is distinguished in the final analysis by certain features detected by study of sections with light and electron microscopy, and also by some distinguishing clinical characteristics. It is believed to be the most frequent cause of the nephrotic syndrome in humans and usually has an insidious onset and prolonged course in humans or animals. Early studies in children associated the clinical disease with deposits of lipid in epithelial cells of proximal convoluted tubules, but changes in glomeruli were overlooked, resulting in the application of the now obsolete name "lipoid nephrosis."

The morphologic changes that identify membranous glomerulonephritis are (1) thickening, splitting, and reduplication of the glomerular basement membrane, and (2) loss of the foot processes of the podocytes (epithelial cells) of the glomerulus. With the electron microscope, the earliest detectable lesions appear to be the loss of the foot processes and spaces between glomerular basement membrane and epithelial cells by the application of broad segments of the epithelium to

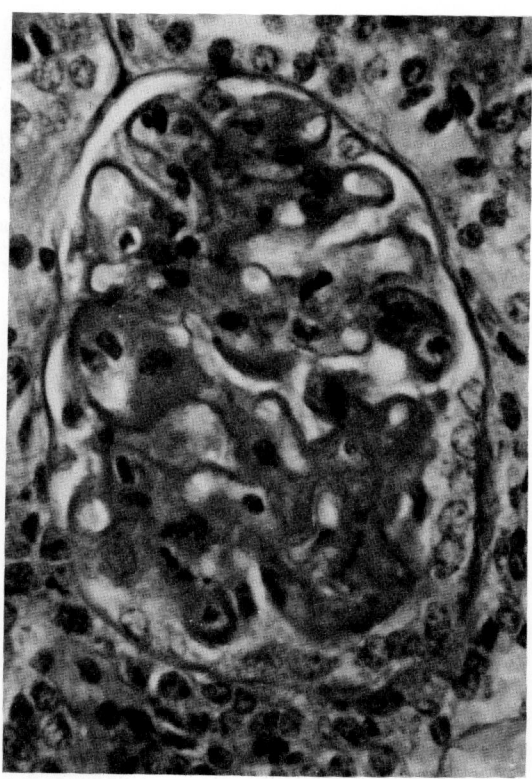

FIG. 24-7. Diffuse membranous glomerulonephritis in mouse with chronic allogeneic disease. Note thickened basement membranes and mesangium. (Courtesy of Dr. Robert M. Lewis and **The Journal of Experimental Medicine.**)

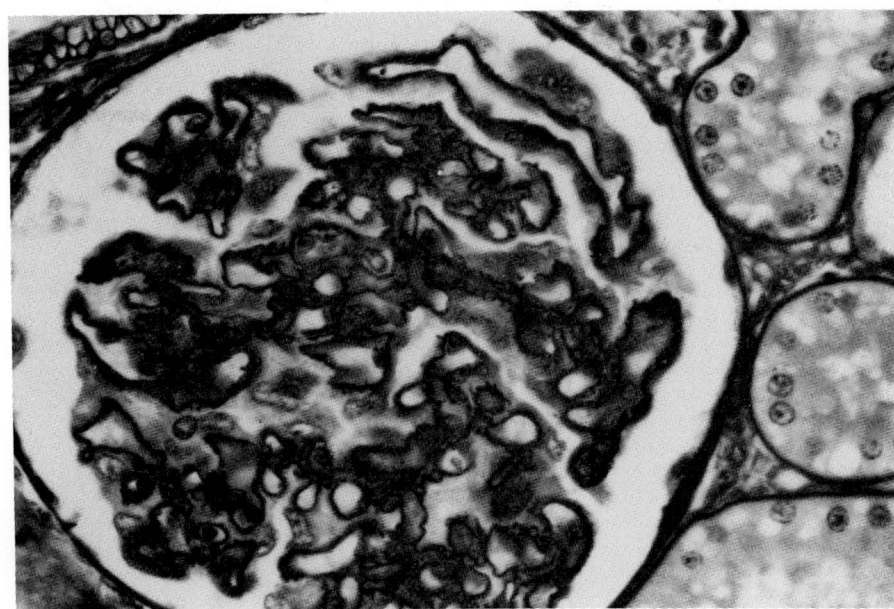

FIG. 24-8. Diffuse membranous glomerulonephritis in a cat. Brushlike "spikes" on outside of basement membranes imply immune complex disease. (PAS-methenamine silver stain.) (Courtesy of Drs. R. M. Lewis and D. O. Slauson and **Veterinary Pathology.**)

the external surface of the basement membrane. Later in the course of the disease, the glomerular basement membrane becomes irregularly thickened with scalloped portions along its external (epithelial) border. This thickening of the basement membrane becomes severe enough to be recognized by light microscopy and is particularly evident in sections stained by PAS and silver impregnation methods. The basement membrane may develop the "lumpy-bumpy" appearance described in the preceding section, and ultrastructurally, dense deposits of immune complex are encountered in the epithelial side of the basement membrane. These deposits are not dissimilar from those described for proliferative glomerulonephritis. The thickened basement membrane is sometimes described as resembling a "wire loop" in microscopic section. The epithelial cells

in the glomerulus may become swollen and laden with fat, giving the glomerulus a hypercellular appearance. Similar lipid vacuoles in the cells of the proximal convoluted tubules may be expected.

After a prolonged course, the glomerulus may become enlarged and hypercellular and distend Bowman's capsule. The glomerular space is rarely obliterated, however, and epithelial crescents and adhesions are not usual. The glomerulus is not only dense and cellular, but is essentially bloodless at this stage.

Grossly, the kidney affected with membranous glomerulonephritis is usually enlarged and pallid ("large pale kidney"), presumably due to the fatty changes and increase in interstitial fluid caused by generalized edema. In some stages, the kidney may become contracted and fibrous as an end stage. The possibility of

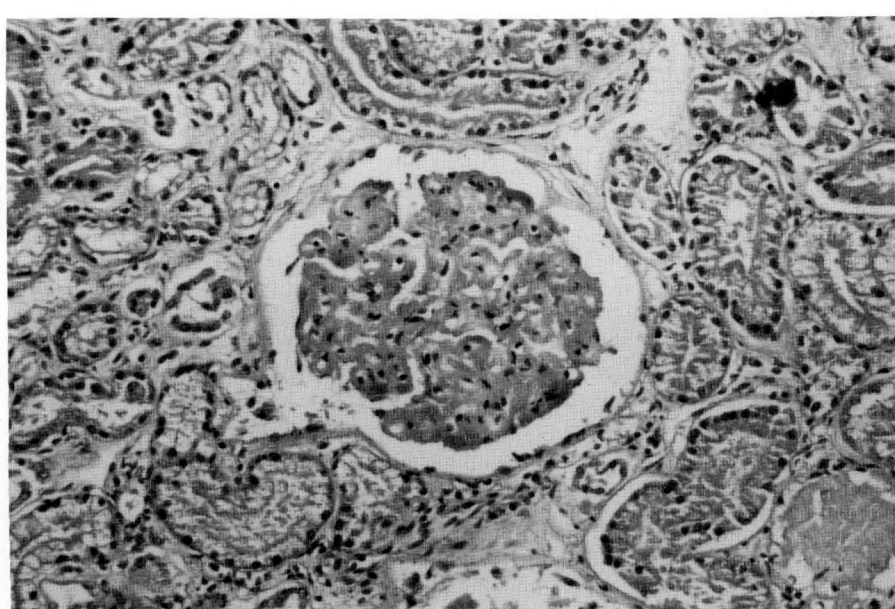

FIG. 24-9. Chronic membranous glomerulonephritis in a dog. The capillary walls are greatly thickened. Note absence of cellular proliferation. (H&E stain.) (Courtesy of Drs. R. M. Lewis and D. O. Slauson and **Veterinary Pathology.**)

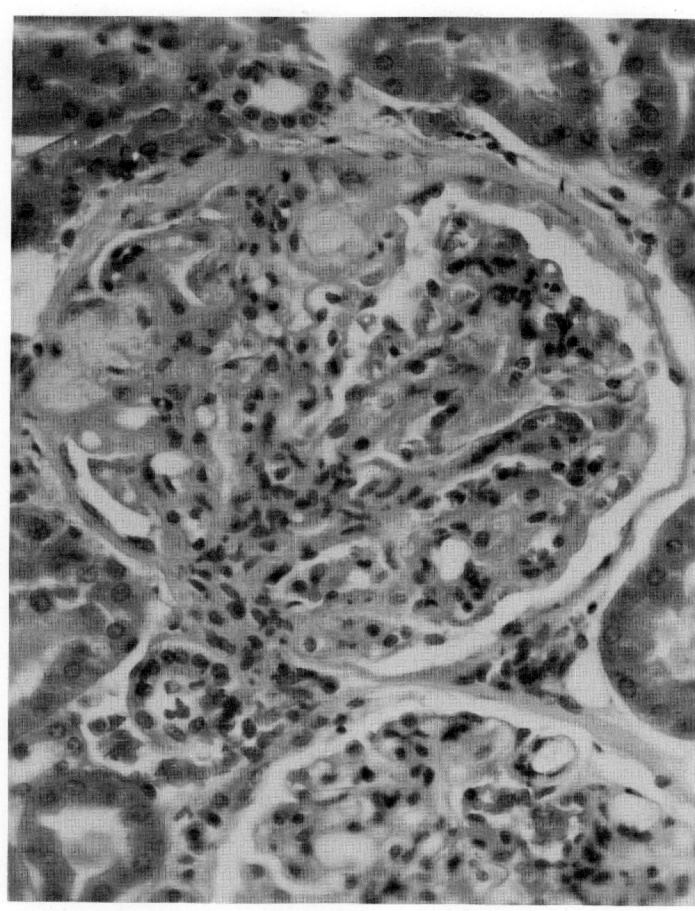

FIG. 24-10. Membranous glomerulonephritis in an aged dog. Basement membranes thickened and adhesions to Bowman's capsule. (Courtesy of Armed Forces Institute of Pathology.)

chronic glomerulonephritis resulting from this entity must also be considered.

MEMBRANOPROLIFERATIVE GLOMERULONEPHRITIS (MESANGIOCAPILLARY GLOMERULONEPHRITIS, MESANGIOPROLIFERATIVE GLOMERULONEPHRITIS)

Often glomerular disease in humans and animals is characterized by both proliferative and membranous changes (Fig. 24-11). The pathologic features represent a combination of the lesions already described, including a marked increase in mesangial cells and mesangial basement membrane substance, thickened basement membranes, and often splitting of basement membranes. It appears to be a distinct entity and not a combination of the other two forms.

The condition has been subgrouped into two types based on two patterns of immunoglobulin deposition. In one, granular deposits of immune globulin are present on the subendothelial side of the basement membrane and in the mesangium, and in the other, a more linear, dense deposit containing little immunoglobulin but significant amounts of complement (see alternate pathway glomerulonephritis) within the basement membrane. A membranoproliferative (mesangiocapillary) glomerulonephritis has been recognized in Finnish Landrace sheep and is believed to resemble the disease as seen in humans. Affected sheep are deficient in

the third component of complement from birth, as are human patients. Glycoprotein deposits, presumably immunoglobulin, are also present in the choroid plexus, associated with focal malacia and edema of the brain.

If the proliferative component is principally mesangial, the term mesangioproliferative glomerulonephritis is applied. This also appears to be a distinct entity and has been associated with mesangial IgM deposition in humans.

CHRONIC GLOMERULONEPHRITIS

This lesion currently appears to be the late stage of one or more of the various forms of glomerulonephritis (Fig. 24-12). At this writing it is not known which forms of glomerular disease are most often responsible for this lesion. This end stage of glomerular disease may be encountered at necropsy and is often the lesion which results in terminal uremia. The clinical manifestations are variable and depend upon the number of glomeruli affected as well as the degree of malfunction in involved glomeruli.

Microscopically, the lesions in glomeruli include increased numbers of cells (endothelial, mesangial, and epithelial) in the glomerulus with disorganization and occlusion of the lumens of glomerular capillaries. The proliferating epithelial cells may accumulate along the parietal layer of Bowman's capsule to form the so-called

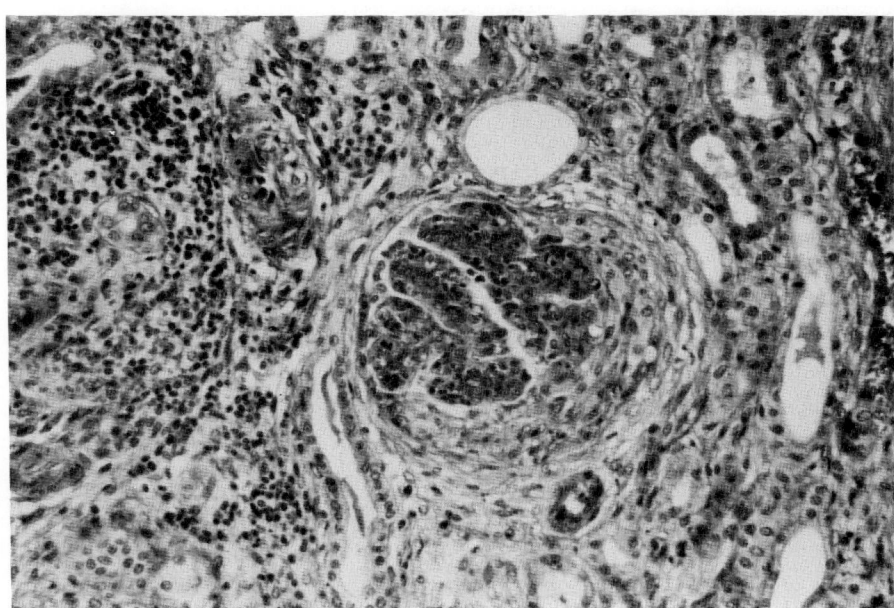

FIG. 24-11. Mesangioproliferative glomerulonephritis in a Finnish Landrace lamb, note proliferative changes in tufts and marked epithelial crescent formation. (Courtesy of Drs. R. M. Lewis and D. O. Slauson and **Veterinary Pathology.**)

epithelial crescents. Adhesions of the glomerulus of Bowman's capsule may occur, and Bowman's space is often obliterated. Electron micrographs confirm the proliferation of epithelial and endothelial cells and disclose reduplication, thickening, and disorganization of the glomerular basement membrane. The lumen of capillaries is usually occluded. In advanced stages, the entire glomerulus is replaced by hyaline connective tissue.

Interference with the circulation through the glomerulus obviously decreases the blood supply to the tubular parts of the nephron and leads to their degeneration. Severe fibrosis of the interstitium results from this ischemia, and many tubules atrophy.

As the fibrous connective tissue contracts, the kidney tends to decrease in size and increase in density. At this end stage it is difficult to reconstruct the events in glomeruli, tubules, or interstitium that may have led to this combination of lesions. Such kidneys are usually smaller than normal, rough or pitted on the surface, and tough to cut, often with a course, granular, or cystic cut surface.

It is evident that chronic glomerulonephritis, from the pathologist's viewpoint, represents a definite combination of lesions which obviously seriously interfered with renal function during life, but whose etiology and pathogenesis cannot be discerned in each individual case. This lesion has been reported in many mammalian and reptilian species. Presumably, it would be found in all mammals by adequate study of these species.

FOCAL EMBOLIC GLOMERULONEPHRITIS

This lesion is most often a sequel to a localized bacterial infection elsewhere in the body (Fig. 24-13). In humans, acute bacterial endocarditis is the most common antecedent—a situation which also occurs in other species, particularly in cattle, swine, and dogs. Other sources of infection may also be possible, such as bacterial pneumonia, reticulitis, and other localized infections. Emboli of infected necrotic tissue are presumed to reach the glomeruli to initiate the lesion, although the presence of organisms is not always demonstrable.

In some instances, however, colonies of bacteria may be demonstrable in glomeruli and some of these may lead to frank abscesses.

The lesion is recognized by light microscopy as a focal zone of necrosis, usually involving part of the glomerulus, with neutrophil infiltration and occasionally hemorrhage. Affected glomeruli are patchily scattered throughout the kidneys. In some, proliferation of epithelial cells and formation of "crescents" may occur, making the lesion difficult to distinguish from proliferative glomerulonephritis. In this latter situation, necrosis is not as conspicuous and larger numbers of glomeruli are involved nearly simultaneously.

Affected kidneys may bear scattered petechiae and occasionally multiple tiny abscesses. In the bovine, one or more renal lobules may be affected with most of the kidney free of gross involvement. Although frank embolism is not demonstrable in each case, it seems expedient to consider this lesion in animals to be most often the result of bacterial embolism.

ETIOLOGY AND PATHOGENESIS

With the exception of embolic glomerulonephritis, the cause (or antigen) involved in glomerulonephritis is generally unknown.

Immunologically mediated glomerulonephritis

The current, most widely held view is that most, but not all, glomerulonephritis is immunologically mediated and under genetic control (Fig. 24-14).

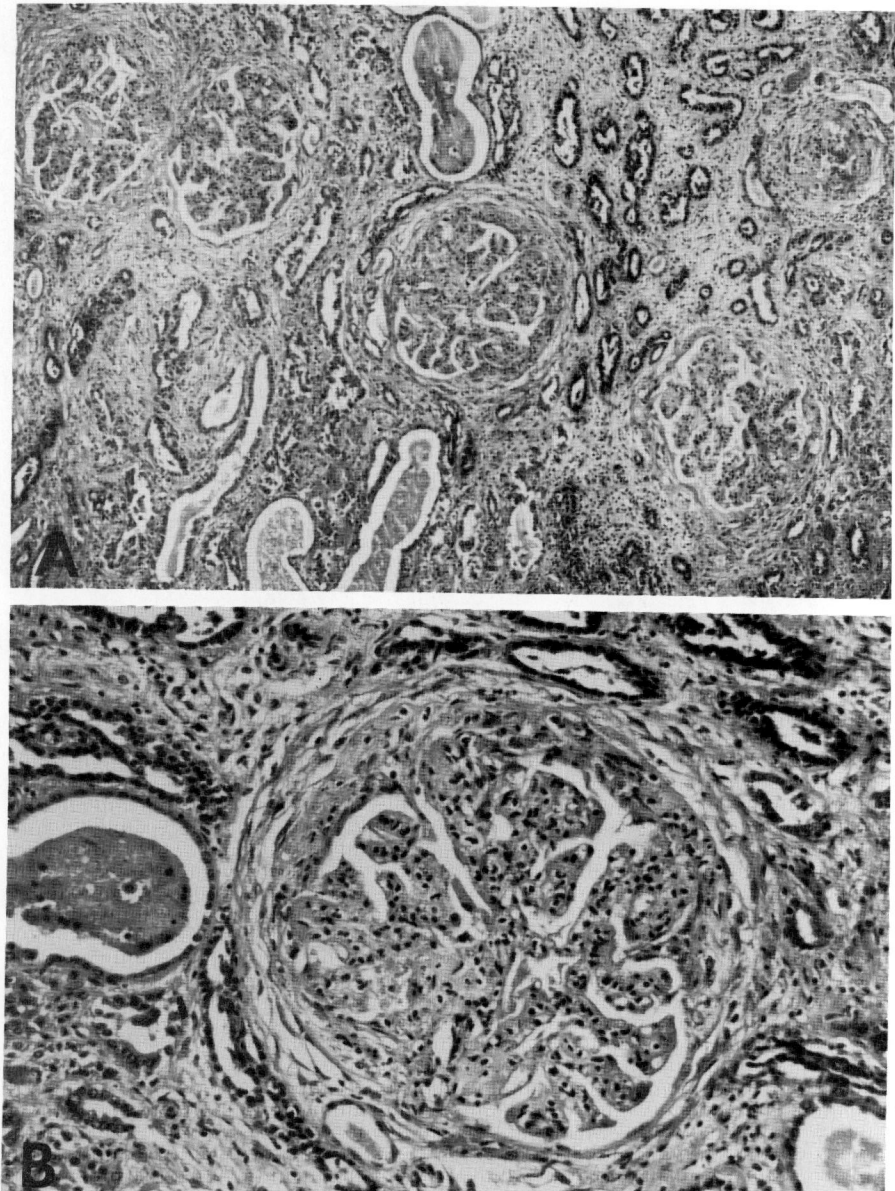

FIG. 24-12. Chronic glomerulonephritis in a dog. **A.** Note proliferative and sclerotic changes within the glomeruli, and concentric periglomerular fibrosis. Tubules are atrophied and replaced by interstitial fibrosis. **B.** Higher magnification of a single glomerulus. (Courtesy of Drs. R. M. Lewis and D. O. Slauson and **Veterinary Pathology.**)

At the time that immunoglobulins were first identified on the epithelial side of the glomerular basement membrane, it was assumed that this disposition was the result of excessive antibody in the circulation. The process now appears much more complicated. Although the offending antigen is not always clearly identified, the presence of immune globulins is usually unequivocal.

The availability of natural and experimentally-induced examples of glomerulonephritis in animals has been very useful in suggesting possible models for study of the pathogenic mechanisms involved in both animals and humans. In this text, it is appropriate to consider the diseases produced or studied in animals, with comparison to human disease when appropriate. Some of the mechanisms involved in these entities will be described in the following.

PASSIVE IMMUNIZATION OF ANIMALS

Nephrotic serum nephritis, (Masugi nephritis) is induced in rats or rabbits by the parenteral injection of heterologous anti-GBM (Glomerular Basement Membrane) antibodies (Fig. 24-15). The lesions include: a linear pattern of binding of antibodies along the glomerular basement membrane, accumulation of leukocytes in the glomeruli, and endothelial cell damage. The antibodies react not only with the glomerular basement membranes but also with basement membranes in placenta, aorta, lung, liver, and brain, affecting these organs as well as glomeruli.

Stebley nephritis is an experimental allergic glomerulonephritis produced by the immunization of sheep with autologous basement membrane preparations, with resultant deposition of antibody on the ovine glomerular basement membrane. The exact na-

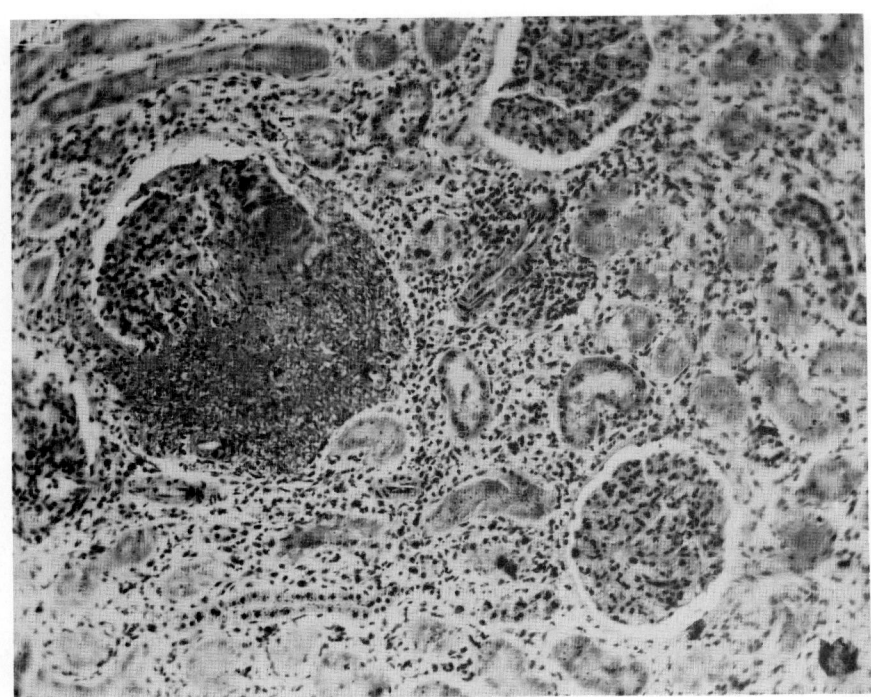

FIG. 24-13. Focal embolic glomerulone-phritis in a dog. (Courtesy of Armed Forces Institute of Pathology.)

ture of the antigen in this case is not known but transfer and absorption studies prove the pathogenic properties of the anti-GBM antibodies. It is now known that the anti-GBM nephritis can be induced by antibodies directed against the non-collagenous 1 (NC 1) domain of the type IV collagen.

Passive Heymann's nephritis in the rat, regarded as a model for human membranous nephritis, is induced by injections of heterologous antibodies directed against rat brush border antigens. Immunoglobulin G (IgG) in a granular pattern is deposited along the glomerular basement membrane under the epithelium, with thickening and formation of "spikes" on the membrane. The aggregates arise from in situ binding of the antibodies to antigen on the surface of the glomerular epithelial cells. The principal pathogenic antigen has been identified as a glycoprotein (gp 330) with molecular weight of 330 kilodaltons (KDs).

ACTIVE IMMUNIZATION OF ANIMALS

Serum sickness is induced in animals by introducing foreign serum proteins, such as bovine serum albumin, parenterally in single or multiple doses. Rabbits are most often used in these studies. Following a single injection of bovine serum albumin, a variable percentage of the rabbits develop diffuse glomerulonephritis with glomerular hypercellularity, due largely to infiltration by macrophages into the glomeruli. Ultrastructural and histochemical findings may differ, depending on the antigen and injection protocol. Granular deposits of IgG, C3, and antigens have been found by some investigators. Electron-dense deposits also have been identified on both sides of the glomerular basement membrane, adjacent to the epithelium or the capillary endothelium. These studies led to the view that the le-

sions in serum sickness are due to the formation of immune complexes in the circulation and deposition in the glomerulus. If antibodies are in excess or equivalence, large immune complexes, formed in the circulation, are either removed by the monocytic/phagocytic system or deposited in the mesangium. If antigen is in excess, small complexes are formed and deposited in the glomerular capillary wall. As mentioned previously, not all of these events apply in all forms of glomerulonephritis.

Active Heymann's nephritis is regarded by many as a model for human membranous nephritis. The lesions of glomerulonephritis appear about six weeks after intraperitoneal injection of rats with homologous kidney homogenates in Freund's adjuvant. This experimental tool has become one of the most extensively investigated models of immunologically mediated glomerular disease.

Chronic serum sickness may be produced in rats or rabbits by giving repeated intravenous injections of a foreign serum protein over a period of 2 to 3 months. Depending on the protocol followed and the level of circulating complexes attained, the animals will develop chronic glomerulonephritis. Early mesangial hypercellularity and mesangial deposition of bovine serum albumin, IgG, and C3 are followed by subendothelial and sub-epithelial aggregates along the glomerular capillary wall, infiltration by neutrophils, and glomerular sclerosis.

POLYCLONAL B-CELL ACTIVATION

Graft versus host reaction may be produced by the injection of lymphocytes from one of the parental strains (usually mice) into an F1 hybrid. A second method is the induction of a host-versus-graft reaction

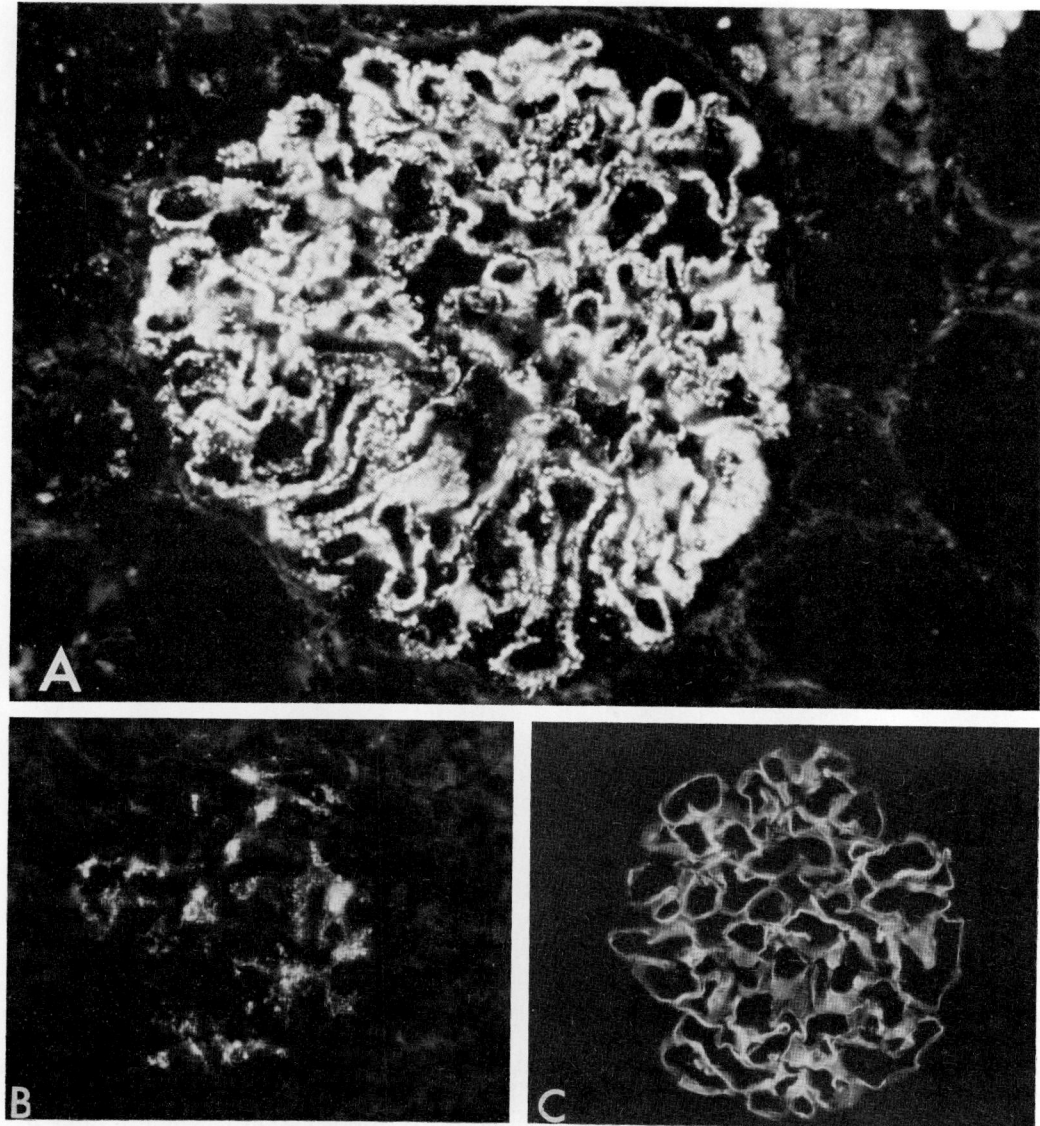

FIG. 24-14. Immunofluorescent patterns in glomerulonephritis. **A.** Chronic membranoproliferative glomerulonephritis in a three-year-old female miniature schnauzer. Focal discrete deposits of canine immunoglobulins and complement along glomerular capillary basement membranes. This is the classic lumpy-bumpy deposition characteristic of immune complex glomerulonephritis. (Courtesy of Dr. R. M. Lewis.) **B.** Granular deposits of immune complexes confined almost exclusively to the mesangial regions. This is from a rat injected four hours earlier with soluble immune complexes. **C.** Anti-GBM disease in a rat following injection of rabbit anti-rat GBM serum. There is a completely continuous smooth (linear) staining for IgG along the glomerular basement membrane. (**B** and **C** courtesy of Dr. A. Bernard Collins, Department of Pathology, Massachusetts General Hospital.)

in chimeras, by neonatal transfer of F1 lymphocytes into a neonate of the parental strain. In the first example, (Balb/c X A/JAX) F1 hybrid mice are injected with a suspension of spleen cells from a Balb/c mouse. One third of the injected mice develop renal lesions resembling human membranous glomerulonephritis. This experimental system illustrates another mechanism which can give rise to glomerulonephritis.

Therapeutic and **toxic agents** may also form the basis for immunological mediated glomerulonephritis.

For example, polyclonal B-cell stimulation may be caused by repeated subcutaneous injection of mercuric chloride into mice, rats, or rabbits. In some strains, an anti-GBM antibody phase precedes the resulting immune complex glomerulonephritis. These experiments have led to the idea that anti-nuclear and anti-basement membrane antibodies may play a pathogenic role in glomerulonephritis.

Infectious organisms are often associated with autoimmunity and immune complex glomerulonephritis in

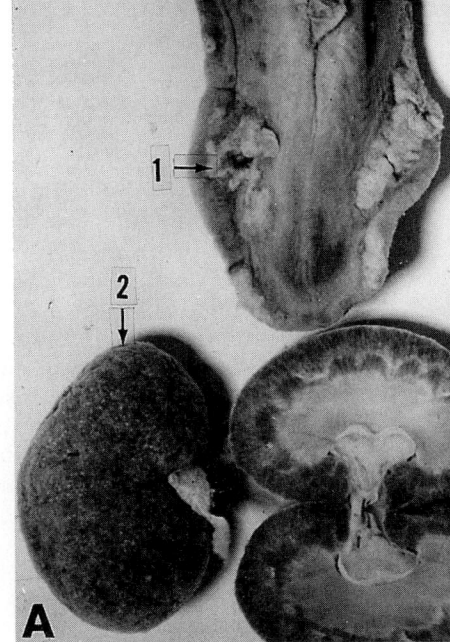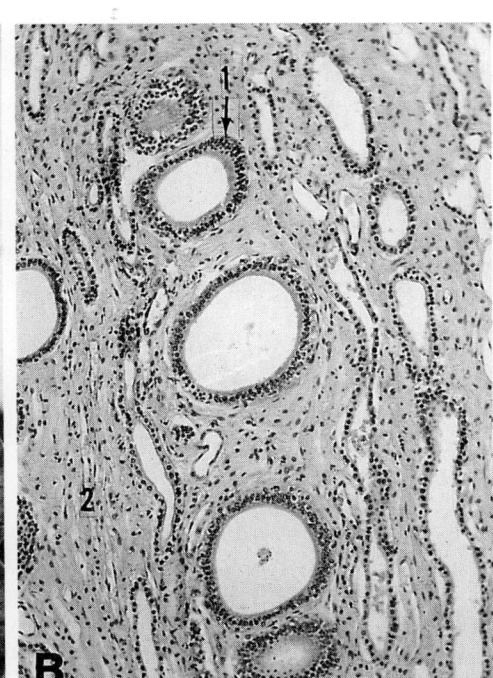

FIG. 24-15. A. Nephrosclerosis, granular contracted kidney of chronic nephritis in a nine-year-old dog. Uremic ulcers of the tongue (**1**) and the pitted, contracted kidney. (**2**) **B.** The renal medulla in same case as **A.** (× 100). Collecting tubules are lined with multiple rows of cells (**1**) and are spherical in outline. Note connective tissue (**2**). Courtesy of Armed Forces Institute of Pathology.) Contributor: Base Veterinarian, Barksdale AFB.

humans and other species. An experimental model has been studied in mice with endogenous leukemia retroviruses and their gene products that may be involved in the pathogenesis of immune mediated nephritis. The retroviral envelope glycoprotein gp 70 has been found in sera of mice with autoimmune diseases, and this gp 70 is deposited in affected glomeruli, along with host immunoglobulin and complement.

Autologous immune complex glomerulonephritis is a much less common cause of immune complex disease, but does represent the major mechanism in two animal diseases: New Zealand Black (NZB) mice disease and canine lupus erythematosus. Autoimmune hemolytic anemia was first described in NZB mice in 1959. Hybrids with a "normal" strain (NZW) were found to have a spontaneous disease in which weight loss, progressive anemia, hepatosplenomegaly, alopecia, positive lupus erythematosus (LE) preparations, and circulating auto-antibody—free and on red blood cells—were conspicuous features. Death occurred from renal failure at 8 to 10 months of age. The glomerular disease is both membranous and proliferative and characterized ultrastructurally by nodular deposits of immune complex within and on either side of the basement membrane. Three antibodies have been recognized in the deposits: antinuclear antibody, antibody to Gross leukemia virus, and antibody directed against erythrocyte antigens. The disease resembles systemic lupus erythematosus of humans but differs in some minute details.

Canine lupus erythematosus is another animal disease complex which closely simulates the human syndrome. The canine disease is manifest by recurring episodes of hemolytic anemia and thrombocytopenia and positive Coombs test and LE preparations; it has an autoimmune basis, the antigen being nuclear deoxyribo-

nucleic acid (DNA). The antinuclear antibody immune complex leads to membranous or membranoproliferative glomerulonephritis. Some canine patients are affected with a type of arthritis typical of the rheumatoid type, and most eventually die from membranous glomerulonephritis. The renal lesions are typical of those described previously in this chapter.

In humans, and to a lesser extent in animals, a third immunologic mechanism has been described called **alternate pathway disease.** In this membranoproliferative glomerulonephritis, immunofluorescence demonstrates deposits of complement and properdin with little immunoglobulin. This mechanism is of interest in membranoproliferative glomerulonephritis.

In human patients a glomerulonephritis is recognized in which large amounts of IgA (with lesser amounts of IgG) are deposited in the mesangium and capillary loops. This **immunoglobulin A glomerulonephritis** is usually focal and nonprogressive.

References

Bruijn JA, Hoedemaeker PJ, Fleuren GJ. Pathogenesis of anti-basement glomerulopathy and immune-complex glomerulonephritis: Dichotomy dissolved. Lab Invest 1989;61:480–488.

Ceol M, Nerlich A, Baggio B, et al. Increased glomerular alpha 1 (IV) collagen expression and deposition in long-term diabetic rats is prevented by chronic glycosaminoglycan treatment. Lab Invest 1996;74:484–495.

Gelberg H, Healy L, Whiteley H, et al. In vivo enzymatic removal of alpha 2–6 linked sialic acid from the glomerular filtration barrier results in podocyte charge alteration and glomerular injury. Lab Invest 1996;74:907–920.

King NW, Baggs RB, Hunt RD, et al. Glomerulonephritis in the Owl Monkey (*Aotus trivirgatus*): Ultrastructural observations. Lab An Sci 1976;26:1093–1103.

Kolaja GJ, Fast PE. Renal lesions in MRL mice. Vet Pathol 1982;19:663–668.

Kopp JB, Factor VM, Mozes M, et al. Transgenic mice with increased plasma levels of TGF-beta 1 develop progressive renal disease. Lab Invest 1996;74:991–1003.

Olson JL, Heptinstall RH. Nonimmunologic mechanisms of glomerular injury. Lab Invest 1988;59:564–578.

Shimizu A, Masuda Y, Kitamura H, et al. Apoptosis in progressive crescentic glomerulonephritis. Lab Invest 1996;74:941–951.

Yang D-H, Goyal M, Sharif K, et al. Glomerular epithelial protein 1 and podocalyxin-like protein 1 in inflammatory glomerular disease (crescentic nephritis) in rabbit and humans. Lab Invest 1996;74:571–584.

Other glomerular lesions

AMYLOID IN THE KIDNEY

The kidney is one of the most frequently affected organs in both primary and secondary amyloidosis described in detail in Chapter 2. The glomeruli are the usual and most important site of deposition in most species, but there is, in addition, usually some deposition in arterial walls and surrounding tubules as well. For reasons unknown, in cats with renal amyloidosis, the glomeruli are usually less affected than are the tubules, especially those in the medulla. The medulla is also frequently affected in bovine renal amyloidosis. Medullary deposits in cats have been associated with papillary necrosis, presumably by interfering with circulation.

Microscopically, the amount of amyloid is seen to be small in the early stages, but eventually many renal corpuscles are almost completely replaced by amyloid. The amyloid usually remains more or less lobulated, however, which facilitates distinguishing amyloidosis from hyaline scarring of glomeruli. Grossly, the change is not easily detected, but the application of an iodine solution such as Lugol's to a slice of fresh kidney which has previously been exposed to a weak acid brings out affected glomeruli as conspicuous brown spots visible to the naked eye.

Extensive glomerular amyloidosis leads to glomerular inefficiency, proteinuria, and renal failure. A high incidence of thrombosis, particularly of pulmonary arteries, has been reported in dogs with renal amyloidosis.

Diseases of renal tubules and the interstitium

In this section, primary degeneration and inflammatory diseases of the renal tubules and interstitium in the absence of glomerular disease will be considered. It has already been stressed that tubular and interstitial disease may be secondary to glomerular damage. Primary tubulointerstitial disease, or interstitial nephritis, is characterized by degeneration and necrosis of tubular epithelium, edema, cellular infiltration, and other components of the inflammatory reaction in the interstitium. Depending on the severity of the insult and its duration, the lesion may progress to chronic interstitial nephritis characterized by marked interstitial fibrosis, absence of tubules, and dilated tubules. The end stage may be a fibrotic kidney containing relatively normal glomeruli. Several systems of classification have evolved for primary tubulointerstitial disease, none of which is completely satisfactory. In part, this results from the diversity of causes.

ACUTE INTERSTITIAL NEPHRITIS

Toxic tubular nephritis In this condition, various irritant toxic substances act directly and without any previous hypersensitization to produce fatty change and necrosis of the delicate epithelial cells lining the tubules, a sequence of degenerative changes which have already been seen to result from the actions of similar toxins on the epithelium of the liver. There is also hyperemia and, somewhat later, limited infiltrations of lymphocytes and neutrophils and proliferation of fibrous tissue. The inflammatory reaction may be minimal, especially if the insult leads to early death. For this reason, the term **nephrosis** (acute toxic tubular nephrosis) is often used to describe the lesion. Toxic tubular nephritis and toxic tubular nephrosis should be considered synonymous.

The proximal convoluted tubules, with their large, highly specialized epithelial cells, suffer most, especially with respect to necrosis, which may, in some toxemias (as poisoning from the budding leaves of certain oaks), leave these tubules as solid, dense-appearing masses of coagulated protoplasm. The lipidosis may be most extensive in these tubules or it may appear chiefly or exclusively in the epithelium of the ascending loops of Henle, especially in the medullary rays. This difference may well have diagnostic significance, but the exact distinctions have not been elucidated. Calcification, usually in the form of granules no larger than one or two cells, is not unusual in tubules which persist after a limited amount of necrosis. The gross appearance of toxic tubular nephrosis is that of the large, pale kidney.

If degeneration and necrosis have not become too extensive, regeneration of the epithelial lining cells is possible upon removal of the cause. Hence, a most important aspect of treatment in the case of acute nephrotoxic poisonings is the adoption of measures (such as dialysis) designed to avoid a fatal uremia before regeneration and restoration of tubular function can occur, a period of 10 days or more. In fatal cases, the proximal tubules, at least, suffer complete destruction; the other parts of the nephron follow the same course less rapidly. In the surviving patient, the fibrous tissue of chronic inflammation partially takes the place of lost tubules, producing the "small, white, granular, contracted kidney." The glomeruli may survive, and, with the loss of most of the intervening tubular structures, they come to lie very close together, giving the erroneous impression that their number has been increased. All of the above changes may advance rapidly in one segment of the kidney, but leave an adjacent part untouched. This is probably because of a physiologic tendency of one group of nephrons to function while another rests, the nonfunctioning group often escaping a transient severe concentration of the blood-borne poison. It is this mechanism which sometimes permits survival of the patient, although with permanent loss of segments of renal parenchyma. In such a case, the remaining tubules tend to undergo a compensatory hypertrophy characterized by increase in size, with or without increase in height of their epithelial linings. Such patients secrete large volumes of poorly concentrated urine of low specific gravity.

A large number of substances are now known to be borne by the circulating blood to the renal tubules where serious effects on the tubular epithelium are recognized under the rubric "toxic tubular nephritis". Some of these substances are described in Chapter 15. Concern about the nature and significance of these nephrotoxins is a driving factor for a significant area of study in toxicologic pathology. This field of study is largely beyond the scope of this text, but an overview of some aspects appear necessary and of interest. One approach to the study of nephrotoxins is to consider them in groups with similar mechanisms by which their effects are produced, namely:

Group 1. Chemicals which exert a direct effect upon the cells of the renal tubules. These include:

a. Aminoglycoside antibiotics
b. Heavy metals: mercury, cadmium, lead

Group 2. Xenobiotics (toxins from the environment) which exert their effects indirectly by their active metabolites that are formed in the body, usually by the action of mixed function oxidases, the same enzyme factors that often function in detoxification. Examples include:

a. Organohalides include organic solvents, synthetic biologic toxins, and chemicals used in the manufacture of resins and plastics. This group includes a number of metabolic products that have a direct toxic effect on the epithelium of the renal tubules—for example, chloroform and phosgene, metabolites of chlorine.
b. Cephalosporins cause injury to epithelial cells of proximal convoluted tubules by achieving a high concentration of their metabolites in these cells through organic anion transport.
c. Mycotoxins, such as ochratoxin A, have been demonstrated to cause nephrotoxicity in human beings and swine. Its metabolism of a reactive intermediate is believed to provide the mechanism of injury.
d. Halogenated alkenes are conjugated with glutathione, an event that decreases the reactivity of the intermediate metabolite but may be subsequently activated to a toxic metabolite by the renal cysteine conjugate beta-lyase. The S-cysteine conjugates are cleaved by beta-lyase to putative toxic thiols, and thereby produce necrosis in the epithelium of proximal tubules.

Group 3. Xenobiotics that affect the tubular epithelial cells by changing the nutritive or endogenous substrata. Included are:

a. Phosphate (see chapter 15)
b. Iron (see chapter 15)
c. Zinc (see chapter 15)
d. Osmotic nephrosis is a term applied to a transitory vacuolated appearance of epithelial cells of proximal convoluted tubules. It can be produced by intravenous injection of sucrose, glucose, mannitol, or dextran. The histologic appearance of vacuolization is due to hydropic swelling of phagolysosomes. Its pathologic significance appears to be minimal.
e. Oxalate nephrosis is manifest by a startling histologic picture of **hydropic degeneration** involving most of the epithelial cells of the kidney. The cytoplasm of these cells contain many clear and apparently empty vacuoles, a change sometimes called **vacuolar degeneration.** The lumina of the renal tubules are distended by doubly refractile crystals of calcium oxalate which can be visualized with polarized light.

Two mechanisms are involved in the etiology of this toxicosis. In the first, calcium or sodium oxalate are ingested by herbivorous animals by eating plants rich in these oxalates (see halogeton poisoning, chapter 15). The second mechanism starts with oral ingestion of ethylene glycol (from automobile "antifreeze"), diethylene glycol (at one time used as a vehicle for sulfonamide drugs), or dioxane (accidentally or experimentally ingested). These chemicals are degraded in the liver by alcohol dehydrogenase to oxalate, which combines with calcium to form calcium oxalate, the active toxin to the renal tubules.
f. Alpha 2-microglobulin nephropathy: Male rats of most strains (excluding the NBR {NCI-BLACK-REITER} strain that lacks the necessary gene) normally produce in the liver a low molecular weight protein (18.7 kDa) called alpha 2-microglobulin. This protein, because of its low molecular weight, passes through the glomerular filter into the proximal convoluted tubules. Here it is taken into the epithelial cells by pinocytosis or endocytic uptake into the form of a membrane-bound vacuole (phagosome). This fuses with a lysosome to form a phagolysosome, which can be observed with the light microscope. For many years, similar membrane-bound bodies have been called "hyaline droplets" by pathologists. Normally, this protein is degraded by hydrolases from the lysosome to its basic components (mostly amino acids) and discharged into the circulation.

Certain xenobiotics (d-limonene, jet fuels, unleaded gasoline, lindane, hexochloroethane, and others, collectively called "chemicals inducing alpha 2-microglobulin accumulation" (CIGA), have been demonstrated to bind to alpha 2-microglobulin and interfere with the lysosomal degradation of this protein. This results in the accumulation of the protein-CIGA complex and enlargement of the phagolysosomes to the point where the epithelial cell undergoes necrosis (apoptosis) and the entire cell contents are discharged into the proximal convoluted tubule. The resulting cell debris is often impeded at the point of narrowing of the lumen at the juncture between the proximal tubule and descending part of Henle's loop. At this point, the tissue debris is seen with the light microscope as granular casts. These casts accumulate in a zone marking the outer stripes of the kidney.

In addition, linear deposits of calcium salts collect in the pre-bend segments of Henle's loops and the renal papilla often undergoes ischemic necrosis. After a prolonged interval, hyperplasia may be evident in regenerating cells in proximal tubules and adenomas or adenocarcinomas develop at these sites. The occurrence of this series of events has come to be called the "alpha 2-microglobulin nephropathy syndrome."

This specific syndrome is limited to male rats of certain strains that produce this specific protein. Other species and female rats do not make this protein, or develop this syndrome, although some do produce and excrete proteins of low molecular weight. Laboratory animals tested so far that do not develop this syndrome include female rats, male rats of the NBR inbred strain, and mice, dogs, and monkeys of both sexes. However, urinary protein of low molecular weight has been detected in mice (mouse urinary protein, MUP) and in human patients with myeloma (Bence-Jones protein) but the syndrome observed in male rats evidently does not occur in mice or humans.

References

Alden CL, Frith CH. Urinary system. In: Haschek WA. Rousseaux CG, eds. Handbook of toxicologic pathology. New York: Academic Press, 1991;315–387.

Swenberg JA, Short B, Borghoff S, et al. The comparative biology of alpha 2u-globulin nephropathy. Toxicol Appl Pharmacol 1989;97:35–46.

Hypoxic (hemoglobinuric, shock, lower nephron) nephrosis A syndrome differing both in tissue changes and in etiology from the ordinary toxic disorders just described exists in the form of the rather poorly understood condition which Lucké has called "lower nephron nephrosis." While this condition has some aspects in common with the toxic tubular nephrosis just discussed, particularly the ultimate necrosis of tubular epithelium, there are two essential characteristics which mark "lower nephron nephrosis" as a different entity. These are (1) that the epithelial damage is primarily in the "lower nephron," that is, the last part of Henle's loop and the distal convoluted tubule, rather than in the usually vulnerable proximal tubule, and (2) the presence of dense and conspicuous casts in many of these lower nephrons. The casts stain a dirty, almost brownish red when submitted to hematoxylin and eosin, a shade quite different from the bright pink of the ordinary hyalin casts of albuminuria. While the exact chemical changes have not been elucidated, the different appearance is due to derivatives of hemoglobin (or myoglobin) and the casts are called **hemoglobin casts.** Lesions which accompany these two pathognomonic changes, at least in the late stages, include cytoplasmic disintegration and necrosis of epithelium in other than the lower parts of the nephron, and localized infiltrations of lymphocytes and other inflammatory cells in the interstitial

tissue. The proximal tubules are often markedly dilated, as if from obstruction lower down in the nephron.

Symptomatically, the syndrome becomes evident with oliguria, anuria, and uremia. Shock or a shock-like condition is a preceding or accompanying derangement contributing to the seriousness of the situation. Obstruction of the lower parts of the nephron by the hemoglobin casts is one postulated cause of the cessation of urinary secretion, but the number of casts is scarcely sufficient to account entirely, or even principally, for the loss of function. The accompanying hypotension and inadequate glomerular hydrostatic pressure are believed to be the principal basis of renal shutdown and ischemic injury to renal tubules. Increased renin excretion further restricts blood supply, augmenting tubular damage.

The extra-renal disorders leading to "lower nephron nephrosis" are numerous and diverse, although the inexact boundaries assigned to this syndrome cause some variations in the list of acceptable causes. Large crushing and bruising injuries, azoturia, and the extensive hemolysis which follows a transfusion with incompatible blood are the most important causes in animals. They all result directly in the accumulation of free hemoglobin or myoglobin in the blood and therefore in the kidneys. Similar renal changes are said to occur in certain rare myoglobinurias resembling azoturia, but affecting other species than the equine. A practically identical syndrome, either histopathologically or clinically, also follows extensive burns and perhaps some other forms of tissue destruction.

The urine in humans suffering this affliction is highly acid, and the suggestion has been made that this acidity is important in precipitating the hemoglobin. Whether the same acidity is present in similar cases in the herbivorous animals, whose urine is normally alkaline, we are not able to say. Lower nephron nephrosis has followed experimental transfusions in dogs, but only when the urine was made highly acidic and the blood was hemolyzed in considerable amounts previous to introduction into the animal's circulation. The disorder was, however, more easily produced in dogs whose renal circulation was already impaired by preexisting chronic nephritis or by the low hydrostatic pressure incident to a state of shock. It may well be that in most naturally occurring cases in humans or animals, both hemoglobinemia and renal ischemia operate synergistically to produce the renal damage and insufficiency.

Reference

Ericsson JLE, Mostofi FK, and Lundgren G. Experimental hemoglobinuric nephropathy. I. Comparative light microscopic, histochemical, and pathophysiologic studies. Virchow's Arch. Abt B Zellpath 1969;3:181–200.

Immunologic tubulointerstitial nephritis Immunologically mediated tubular disease can be induced in experimental animals and is recognized as a rare mechanism in renal disease of human beings. Immune complex disease (foreign and autologous) and antitubular basement membrane disease similar to their glomerular counterparts, as well as injury mediated by cytotoxic antibodies and cell-mediated mechanisms, have been identified. **Immune complex tubular disease** is comparable to immune complex glomerulonephritis, the antigen-antibody complexes being deposited in a granular fashion. Granular immune complex may also be present in the glomeruli. By light microscopy, the lesion is characterized by mononuclear interstitial nephritis and degeneration of tubular epithelial cells.

Antitubular basement membrane nephritis is analogous to antiglomerular basement membrane disease glomerulonephritis, but results from antibodies directed against tubular basement membrane. The disease has been experimentally induced in several laboratory animals, and a similar form of disease has been recognized in humans.

Spontaneous antitubular basement membrane disease has been reported in New Zealand Black/New Zealand White F1 (B/W F1) mice and in a dog with chronic interstitial nephritis. It is reasonable to assume that other cases have occurred. The immunofluorescent findings are characterized by linear accumulation of IgG and, sometimes, C3 along the tubular basement membrane. Histologically, degenerative changes in the tubular epithelium include vacuolation, swelling, increased cytoplasmic acidophilia, and nuclear pyknosis. The cellular infiltrate early in the course of the disease is predominately composed of lymphocytes, macrophages, and multinucleated giant cells with peripheral nuclei. As the disease progresses, tubular necrosis and cellular infiltration become more extensive and accompanied by fibrosis, eventually destroying the overall renal architecture. The relative importance of this autoimmune tubular disease in spontaneous renal disease of animals is not known at present.

In human beings, certain drug-associated tubular damage is recognized as being mediated through immune mechanisms and is not the result of direct toxic action. The toxicity of several antibiotics is believed to result from an immune response to tubular basement membrane (TBM). It is believed that the drugs act like haptens, combining with TBM protein and eliciting the production of anti-TBM antibodies.

References

Mezza LE, Seiler RJ, Smith CA, et al. Antitubular basement membrane autoantibody in a dog with chronic tubulointerstitial nephritis. Vet Pathol 1984;21:178–181.
Rudofsky UH, Dilwith RL, Tung KSK. Susceptibility differences of inbred mice to induction of autoimmune renal tubulointerstitial lesions. Lab Invest 1980;43:463–470.

Infectious interstitial nephritis Many organisms, but most notably the *Leptospira,* cause extensive interstitial nephritis. These organisms are found in renal tubular epithelium, but the inflammatory reaction to their presence is confined to the interstitium. Red blood cells, plasma, and neutrophils make up the exudate in early stages but are gradually replaced by plasma cells, lymphocytes, and epithelioid cells as the disease progresses. Interstitial fibrosis and thickening of Bowman's capsule (periglomerular fibrosis) are also believed to be long-term effects (Fig. 24-16).

Other organisms may also localize in the kidney, resulting in tubular damage and interstitial nephritis. If the organisms are pyogenic, the resulting lesion is acute purulent interstitial nephritis. Certain viruses, such as canine herpesvirus, may also cause tubular damage and interstitial nephritis.

CHRONIC INTERSTITIAL NEPHRITIS

Characterized by marked fibrosis, chronic interstitial nephritis marks the end result of acute interstitial nephritis. Most of the causes of acute interstitial nephritis lead to chronic fibrosing lesions, including chronic bacterial infection, poisons, and immunologic injury. Other mechanisms include ischemia, obstructions, and radiation. The lesion is characterized by marked fibrosis, loss of tubules, and foci of mononuclear cell infiltration. The glomeruli are relatively unaffected.

Chronic interstitial nephritis was once the most common designation for sclerosing nephritis in dogs; however, most evidence indicates this disorder represents the results of chronic glomerulonephritis.

PYELONEPHRITIS

Pyelonephritis represents one of the more frequent and important forms of interstitial and tubular disease. The word signifies inflammation of the renal pelvis and parenchyma of the kidney. Infection is believed to reach the kidney by ascending through the urinary tract or by dissemination through the vasculature. The latter is the so-called descending route of infection, and although feasible, it is not considered the usual mechanism. In human beings as well as animals, most evidence indicates that the ascending route following cystitis is the more usual. This does not imply a progressive inflammatory reaction of the ureters, which indeed is not a regular finding, but rather a **vesicoureteral reflux** which carries organisms from the bladder to the renal pelvis and even into the renal tubules (**intrarenal reflux**). Pyogenic organisms account for most examples of pyelonephritis. *Escherichia coli* and *Staphylococcus aureus* have been incriminated experimentally in dogs, and *Corynebacterium renale* and *Actinomyces pyogenes* are well known pathogens in bovine animals, and *C. suis* in swine. *Actinobacillus equuli* infection of foals is almost always associated with localization in the kidney (hematogenous route). Embolic spread from bacterial endocarditis is another source of infection, but this usually begins as a glomerulitis. In humans, *E. coli* is the most common pathogen; others include: *Enterobacter (Aerobacter) aerogenes, Proteus vulgaris,* alpha hemolytic streptococci, hemolytic staphylococci, *Pseudomonas aeruginosa* and *Klebsiella pneumoniae.*

The lesions in the acute form of pyelonephritis consist of purulent inflammation and necrosis, which involve renal parenchyma and extend into collecting ducts, calyces, and the renal pelvis. Classically, glomeruli and nephrons are spared, but they may become entrapped in the widespread inflammation. The lesions may be focal or diffuse, involving one or both kidneys or a single lobule (in bovines). Some lesions may be sharply circumscribed and consist essentially of ab-

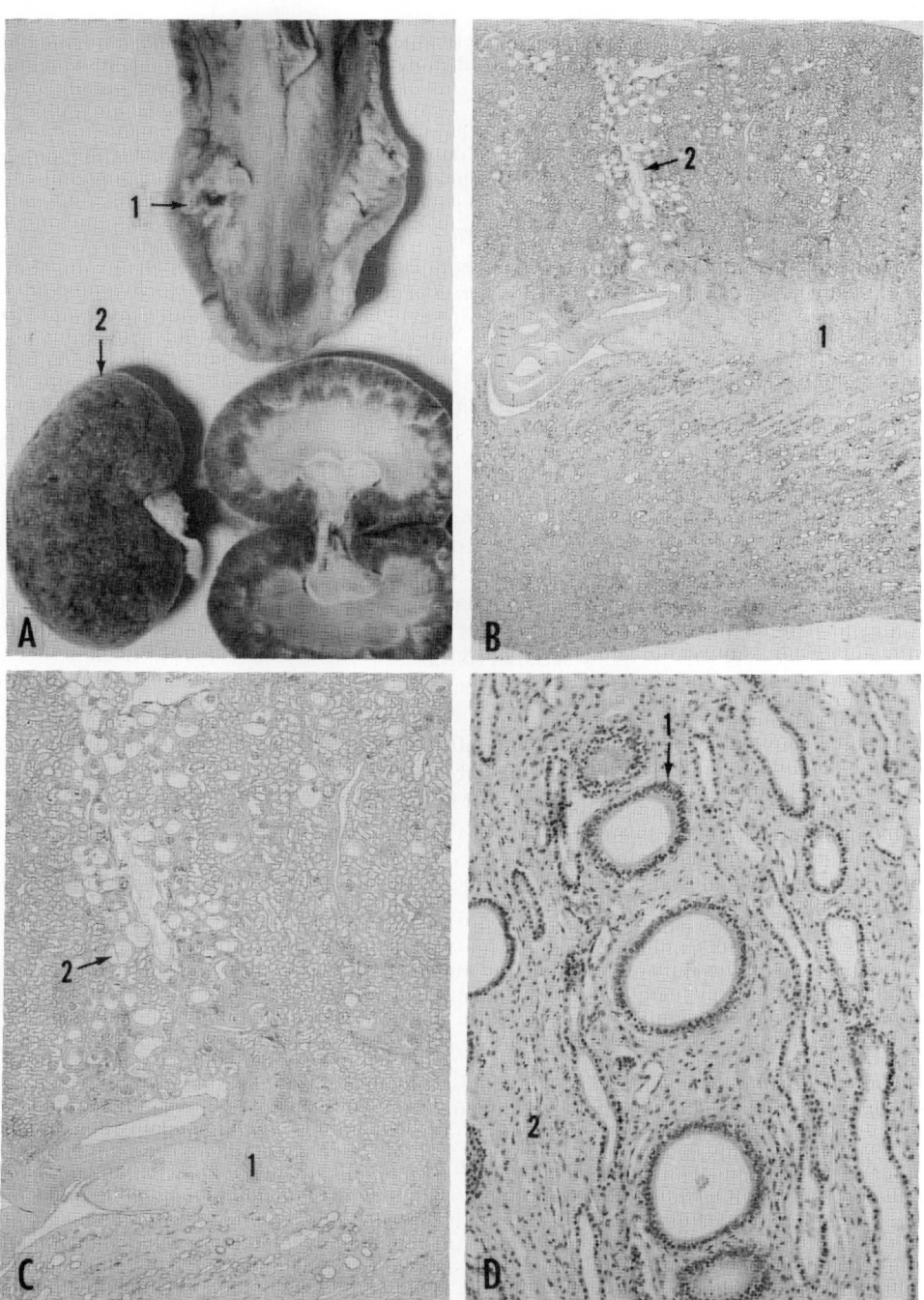

FIG. 24-16. A. Thickened Bowman's capsule (**1**) and lymphoid cells in interstitial stroma (**2**) in kidney (× 450) of a dog with chronic leptospirosis. Contributor: Army Veterinary Research Laboratory. **B.** Dilated Bowman's space (**1**) and renal tubule (**2**) in the kidney (× 100) of a dog with scarring at the cortico-medullary junction. (See Fig. 24-15, **B,C,D.**) **C.** Metastatic abscesses in the kidney of a Jersey cow. The primary lesion was a foreign body reticulitis. *Actinomyces pyogenes* was isolated from lesions of valvularendocarditis. **D.** Depressions of the capsular surface due to old healed infarcts (arrows) in the kidney of a dog. **A** and **D,** courtesy of Armed Forces Institute of Pathology and Dr. Elihu Bond.

scesses. Sometimes the lesions are distributed around a single calyx, suggesting ascending infection from the renal pelvis. Extension of infection into nephrons usually results in neutrophils and granular or leukocytic casts in nephrons or collecting ducts. Purulent exudate may be found in the pelvis or just outside the epithelium of the pelvis.

Grossly, acute pyelonephritis is recognized by congestion, hemorrhages, and sometimes abscesses in the renal cortex, with severe congestion and pus in the pelvis—usually involving the ureters and possibly urethral and bladder mucosae.

Pyelonephritis may be accompanied by fever and malaise and often is preceded by localized or generalized infections (prostatitis, pneumonia). **Pyuria** (pus in the urine) and **bacteriuria** are constant findings, and **dysuria** with frequent urination may occur. Microscopic examination of urine reveals neutrophils, granular and leukocytic casts, red blood cells, and bacteria in large numbers. The acute signs may abate shortly, but persistence of pus and bacteria in the urine indicates active infection which may result in active lesions characteristic of chronic pyelonephritis.

In the chronic form of pyelonephritis, usually but

not always preceded by acute pyelonephritis, the kidneys become grossly scarred and contracted. These scarred areas may be single, with a depressed base located adjacent to the capsule, or may be multiple, giving the kidneys a coarsely nodular appearance. In extreme cases, the kidney may be small, fibrous, and contracted. Microscopically, at this stage, the interstitium contains lymphocytes, plasma cells, and neutrophils; tubules may be atrophic and contain casts and pus (sometimes bacteria); glomerular capsules are thickened by fibrosis (periglomerular fibrosis), and blood vessels may have thickened walls with fibrinous material in the media. In the most advanced stages, fibrous connective tissue replaces the exudate in the interstitium and contraction eventually results. The tubules may be dilated and contain proteinaceous casts. Some lymphocytes and plasma cells usually persist in the interstitium. This stage usually results in death due to uremia.

References

Appleton JA, De Buysscher EV, Kadis S. Antibody formation in Corynebacterium renale-induced experimental pyelonephritis in the rat. Am J Vet Res 1979;40:1757–1761.

Held JP, Wright B, Henton JE. Pyelonephritis associated with renal failure in a horse. J Am Vet Med Assoc 1986;189:688–689.

Mayrer AR, Miniter P, Andriole VT. Immunopathogenesis of chronic pyelonephritis. Am J Med 1983;75:59–70.

MISCELLANEOUS TUBULAR DISORDERS

Tubular transport diseases Excess amounts of inorganic and organic compounds not normally present in appreciable quantity may make their appearance in urine through one of several mechanisms. If there are unusually high levels in the blood, the substance may exceed its normal renal threshold and appear in the urine. Glycosuria of diabetes mellitus is an example. If the integrity of the glomerular filtration mechanism is impaired, larger molecules will enter the filtrate and exceed the ability of the tubules to resorb them. Proteinuria of glomerulonephritis is an example of this mechanism. Tubular damage through poisons, such as mercury or other mechanisms, will result in tubular dysfunction and the appearance of many abnormal urinary constituents. What remains are specific metabolic defects in tubular function which interfere with tubular transport or metabolism of specific compounds.

In humans, a number of specific tubular transport diseases, most of them concerning one or more amino acids or glucose, collectively known as aminoaciduria or glycosuria, have been identified. For some, analogous entities have been recognized in dogs. The best known is uric acid secretion by dogs of the Dalmatian breed. In contrast to other breeds, there is a defect in tubular resorption of uric acid, however, the Dalmatian does possess the enzyme uricase. The defect predisposes to uric acid calculi. Cystinuria has been described in several species of male dogs as a sex-linked hereditary disease in which there is a high incidence of cystine uroliths. In addition to decreased tubular resorption of cystine, the amino acids lysine, arginine and ornithine

are also affected. Aside from calculi, no other renal lesion or other abnormality has been associated with the disease.

A syndrome resembling the Faconi syndrome in human beings has been described in dogs, particularly basenjis. In this condition, there is aminoaciduria, glycosuria, polydipsia, and polyuria.

Cholemic nephrosis Bile pigments may be found in the epithelium of proximal convoluted tubules or loops of Henle in animals with obstructive icterus or severe liver disease. The bile is seen in these tubular cells as yellow granules of irregular size. Formalin-fixed gross specimens of kidney are green in color due to the change of bilirubin to biliverdin. The fresh specimen may be yellow (icteric). Moderate degeneration of tubular epithelium may occur, but severe interference with renal function is not usual. The pathogenesis of this lesion is not clearly understood, although it appears that toxic products released by the liver or not detoxified by the liver may be the cause. Unconjugated bile at elevated levels may be toxic, but bilirubin glucuronide (conjugated bilirubin) does not appear to be injurious to renal cells. Hepatic injury may result in excretion of large amounts of amino acids, such as cystine, arginine, histidine, and tryptophan, which experimentally have been shown to damage renal tubular epithelium.

Uric acid precipitates Extensive deposits of urate crystals may sometimes impart a yellowish color to the renal pyramids. The presence of these crystals in collecting tubules may give a radial pattern to the yellowish streaks. Microscopically, the collecting tubules are seen to be filled with yellow crystals. Urates may also be found (especially in birds) in the interstitial stroma where the crystals have a radial pattern. The urates in tubules presumably result from destruction of cells, particularly erythroblasts in newborn animals, and are most likely to be seen in pigs. This change also may occur in gout.

Cloisonné kidney An interesting pigmented thickening of tubular basement membranes has been described in goats. The pattern of these thickened basement membranes around renal tubules under low magnification suggests the inlay of metal wire in porcelain using the cloisonné technique (cloisonné, Fr. **cloison** = partitioned; Latin, **claudere** = shut, close) (Fig. 24-17). The thickened basement membrane surrounds only the proximal convoluted tubules and has dark brown or grayish-brown color even in unstained sections. The chemical nature of the material in these basement membranes has not been established, although it does not appear to be either hemosiderin or melanin. Iron-positive material has been demonstrated in some places, but for the most part the involved basement membranes do not contain iron. Antecedent hemosiderosis has been postulated as a possible means of staining these basement membranes. The lesion appears to be limited to goats and does not interfere with renal function.

The gross appearance of this change is striking. The renal cortex in both kidneys, in severe cases, is dark brown, almost black. This color extends through

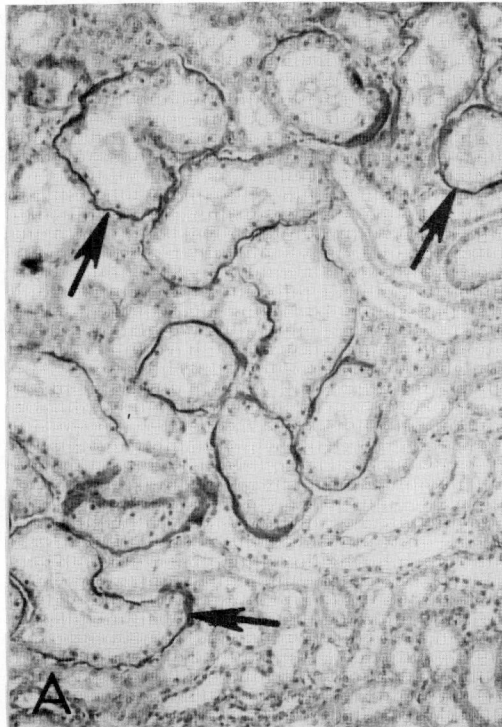
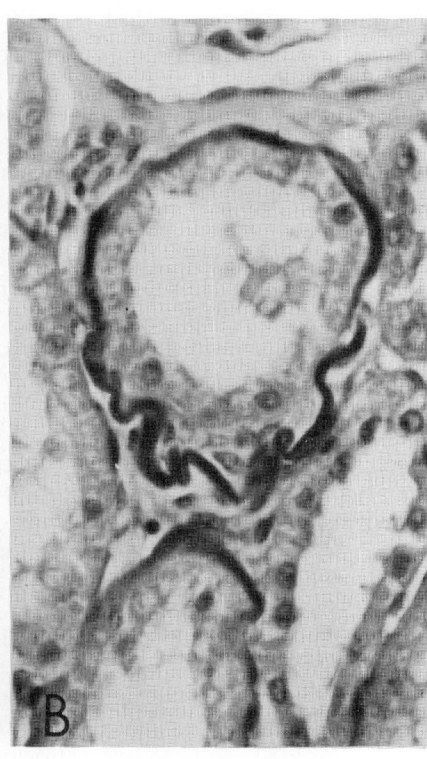

FIG. 24-17. Cloisonné kidney, Angora goat. **A.** Deeply pigmented basement membranes (arrows) encompass renal tubules. **B.** Higher magnification of a single tubule.

the entire cortex, but is abruptly interrupted at the corticomedullary junction.

The lesion has been identified in living goats by histologic examination of specimens of kidney obtained by percutaneous biopsy. Altman confirmed the absence of significant change in renal function and speculated that low levels of erythrocytic glucose-6–phosphate dehydrogenase and glutathione in normal and affected goats, plus elevated serum-iron-binding saturation, predispose to fragility of erythrocytes. The presence of ferritin deposits in affected basement membranes and hemosiderin in tubular epithelial cells in electron micrographs is also presented as evidence for intravascular hemolysis as the antecedent lesion. Further studies are needed to firmly establish the pathogenesis of this lesion.

References

Altman NH. Caprine cloisonne renal lesions. Clinico-pathological observations. Cornell Vet 1968;60:83–90.
Light FW Jr. Pigmented thickening of the basement membranes of the renal tubules of the goat ("cloisonne kidney"). Lab Invest 1960;9:228–238.

Sulfonamides in the kidney Sulfonamide medication, especially if accompanied by a limited intake of water and an acid condition of the urine, may damage the kidney in various ways, often with lethal results. The lesions include toxic tubular degeneration and necrosis, commonly with marked inflammatory infiltrations around the tubules that are involved. As previously stated, the degeneration of tubular epithelium may be of the hydropic type; the changes may also resemble those described for "lower nephron nephrosis." Other changes, apparently based on hypersensitivity, may occur, such as glomerulonephritis, periarteritis nodosa, and necrosis of areas of peripelvic tissue. Some of these changes have been produced experimentally in dogs. The more usual lesion, however, has been, in dogs and cattle, a plugging of the lower collecting tubules with masses of fine crystals, a fatal anuria resulting. The crystals of most of the sulfonamides now in use are elongated, acicular, anisotropic, and yellowish in color. Since they are soluble in water, many or perhaps all of them may be dissolved out in the routine preparation of microscopic sections.

Fat in the kidney Lipids or lipoids stainable by ordinary techniques can be demonstrated in the epithelium of the several parts of the tubules, the glomerular tufts, the walls of Bowman's capsules, the interstitial tissue, the walls of blood vessels, the epithelium of the pelvic lining, and the tubular lumens of the kidneys of the various species of domestic animals and humans. In normal cats, the epithelium of the proximal convoluted tubules contains an abundant amount of neutral lipid (triglycerides), which increases with age. The significance of this species variation is not known.

In all other species, any appreciable amount of lipid in the renal tubular epithelium represents a toxic or anoxic change comparable to that in the liver. As in the liver, lipid is deposited in epithelial cells in diabetes mellitus and ketosis, which characterize ovine toxemia of pregnancy and similar conditions.

The gross appearance of renal lipidosis is pathognomonic only in canine cases of severe fatty change of the ascending arms of Henle's loops. In these instances, the medullary rays stand out as prominent white streaks, radially directed, evenly spaced and reaching from the corticomedullary junction nearly, but not quite, to the capsule. In other species and in other localizations of the fat, little more can be detected grossly than a certain degree of paleness of the cortex and a hazy distinction between the alternating cortical labyrinths and medullary rays, as one views a cut surface traversing the cortex. In many kidneys with the latter appearance, the paler band represents not the medullary ray but the labyrinth, in which the proximal tubules especially have undergone swelling with or without fatty change and necrosis, the picture of toxic tubular nephrosis in general. Microscopically, the fat is in the form of clear cytoplasmic droplets as explained under the general heading of Fatty Change.

Rarely in the dog, a portion of the glomerular area has been taken over by large mononuclear phagocytes cells filled with fat. Other parts of the glomerulus appear normal. The condition has been called glomerular xanthomatosis in some quarters. In some examples of pyelonephritis, large lipid-filled cells may form small nodules, leading to the term xanthogranulomatous pyelonephritis.

Dilated renal tubules The interpretation of this common abnormality deserves a moment of consideration. First of all, the investigator must make sure that the tubules are really dilated. It is possible to mistake enlargement of the tubular lumens resulting from atrophy or flattening of the epithelial lining cells for true enlargement of the whole tubule. Dilatation usually involves a group of tubules, or in some cases, the same nephron is seen several times in cross section, in the same area. They may be either convoluted tubules, the loops of Henle, or collecting tubules, or a combination of these. The degree of dilatation may be slight or the tubule may be enlarged to two or three times its normal diameter. An epithelial-lined space, seen in a single cross section, may give rise to the question of whether it is a greatly dilated tubule or a cyst. The lining cells are most frequently, but not always, flattened; this depends on the cause of the dilatation. In many instances, the condition is due to back pressure caused by closure, from external pressure or otherwise, of the nephron at some lower point in its course. The increased internal pressure naturally tends to compress and flatten the epithelial lining. Such internal pressure must be mild, slowly developed, and prolonged, for sudden and marked increase of intratubular pressure merely stops the filtration process by counterbalancing the "hydrostatic" pressure of the blood within the glomerular capillaries. It appears from careful study, however, that not infrequently, nephrons become dilated through a process of hypertrophy. In such a case, the lining cells may be stretched and flattened or they may be of normal height. If they have recently proliferated or regenerated, the cells tend to be hyperchromatic, like other young cells, even though they have not yet developed to normal height. Such hypertrophy appears to be common in certain nephrons that survive when their neighbors have been destroyed through some pathologic process. It is compensatory hypertrophy, the nephron adding to its own some of the load formerly carried by its departed brethren. Obviously, hypertrophic nephrons of this kind are likely to be located in or near areas of fibrosis. Please refer to Cysts in the Kidney, page 1114.

PERIPELVIC NECROSIS

Peripelvic necrosis, known as **papillitis necroticans,** a necrotizing and at the same time inflammatory change affecting one or, more often, several of the renal papillae, occurs in the human kidney. The distal half or two-thirds of the renal papilla is a yellowish gray and is sharply demarcated from the normal adjacent tissue by a narrow inflammatory zone and, except for its position, resembles an anemic infarct (Figs. 24-18 and 24-19). Microscopically, the tissue is in a state of coagulative necrosis. Some of these lesions occur in connection with pyelonephritis (and concurrent diabetes in the human); others result from urinary obstruction. In the former case, the pressure of intrarenal exudates is thought to compress and close the blood vessels supplying this rather distant and isolated part of the kidney; in the case of urinary obstruction, the back pressure of the urine, acting from several directions on the protruding papilla, is supposed to produce a similar ischemia. The disorder tends to cause anuria and is likely to be fatal. A corresponding change has been seen at least in the dog and rat, in which it involves the renal crest rather than a papilla because of anatomic differences. In one such case, amyloidosis in the basal region of the pyramids appeared to be responsible for compression of the blood vessels.

Papillary necrosis can be produced experimentally in rats by a single intravenous injection of bromoethylamine hydrobromide.

References

Gunson DE, Soma LR. Renal papillary necrosis in horses after phenylbutazone and water deprivation. Vet Pathol 1983;20:603–610.

Gunson DE. Renal papillary necrosis in horses. J Am Vet Med Assoc 1983;182:263–266.

Harper GS, Axelsen RA. Salicylate-induced renal papillary necrosis in the Gunn rat. Lab Invest 1982;47:258–264.

BILATERAL RENAL CORTICAL NECROSIS

Complete or almost complete necrosis of the renal cortices is a rare finding in human beings, which is also rarely seen in dogs, cattle, swine, horses, and cats. In humans, the condition is most frequently associated with complications of pregnancy, but is also associated with various infections and traumatic events. In animals, no clearly established associated illness has been recognized. Microscopically, there is necrosis of all cortical structure with sparing of the medulla. The pathogenesis is not well understood, but believed to result from either vascular spasm or widespread fibrin and platelet thrombi in renal arterioles. It has been induced with injections of bacterial endotoxin, leading to arteriolar thrombi as a component of the generalized Shwartzman reaction. Natural exposure to bacterial toxins is a likely cause, but other conditions which lead

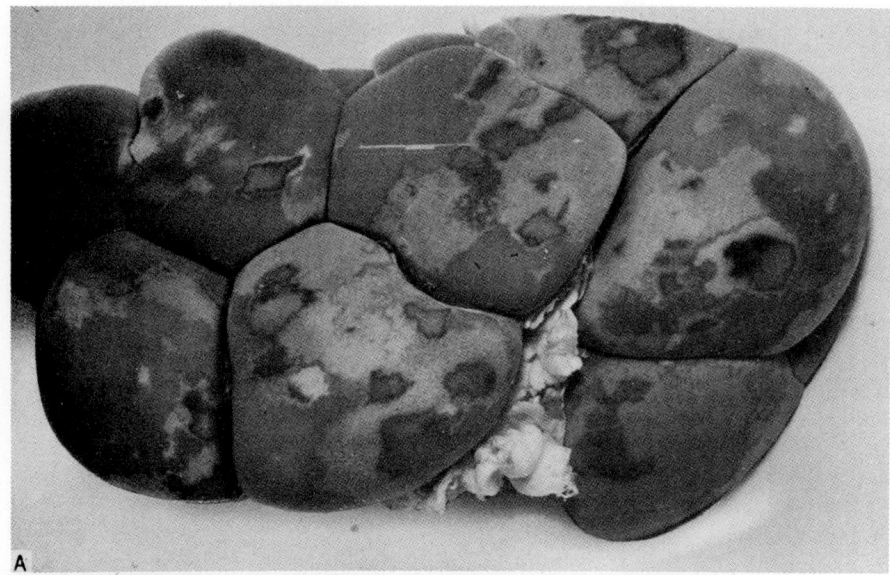

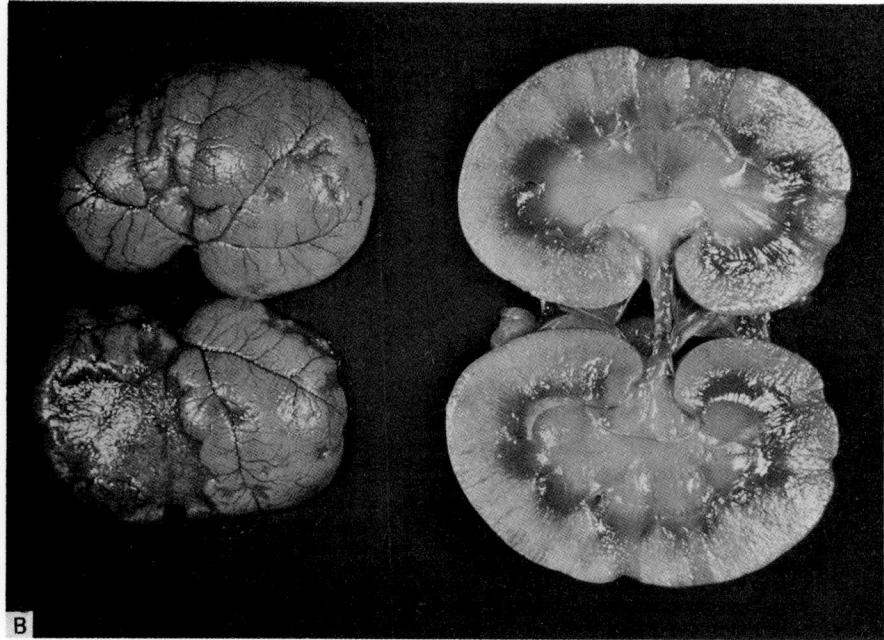

FIG. 24-18. Infarction of the kidney. **A.** Kidney of an 11-year-old cow with septic infarcts secondary to suppurative mastitis and pneumonia. Sharply demarcated anemic gray and hemorrhagic red infarcts are present in this lobulated kidney. **B.** Old infarcts in the kidneys of a seven-year-old castrated male cat. Note depressed zones in cortex in kidney on the left and the wedge-shaped contracted zones which extend from the capsule toward the pelvis of the kidney on the right. (Courtesy of Angell Memorial Animal Hospital.)

to disseminated intravascular coagulation must also be considered. Bilateral renal cortical necrosis in swine with killed *Haemophilus influenza* organisms has been produced and the pathogenesis may be due to a generalized Shwartzman reaction.

NEPHROSCLEROSIS

Whether secondary or primary, the condition of chronic fibrosis of the kidney is often called nephrosclerosis. As discussed earlier, it may result from glomerulonephritis or any of the causes of interstitial nephritis. An important cause in humans, occasionally encountered in animals, is arteriolar sclerosis. Constriction of arteries and arterioles leads to ischemia, tubular atrophy, necrosis and, ultimately, fibrosis. Having developed without a preceding nephritis, this form of nephrosclerosis is known as the **primary contracted kidney.** The distribution of the fibrous tissue often tends to be in the shape of numerous small, healed infarcts—narrow wedges with their base at the capsule. The presence of thick-walled, sclerotic arteries and arterioles is also important in differentiation from the postnephritic secondary contracted kidney. Hindrance of the circulation of blood through the kidneys results in an increase in blood pressure through the release of renin from the juxtaglomerular apparatus. The hypertension accentuates the vascular disease and renal ischemia creating a vicious cycle, known as **malignant hypertension (malignant nephrosclerosis).**

Two sclerosing renal diseases of uncertain classification have been recognized in dogs. In Norwegian elkhound dogs a familial renal disease of uncertain cause and pathogenesis has been described. The pups are born normal, but subsequently develop progressive re-

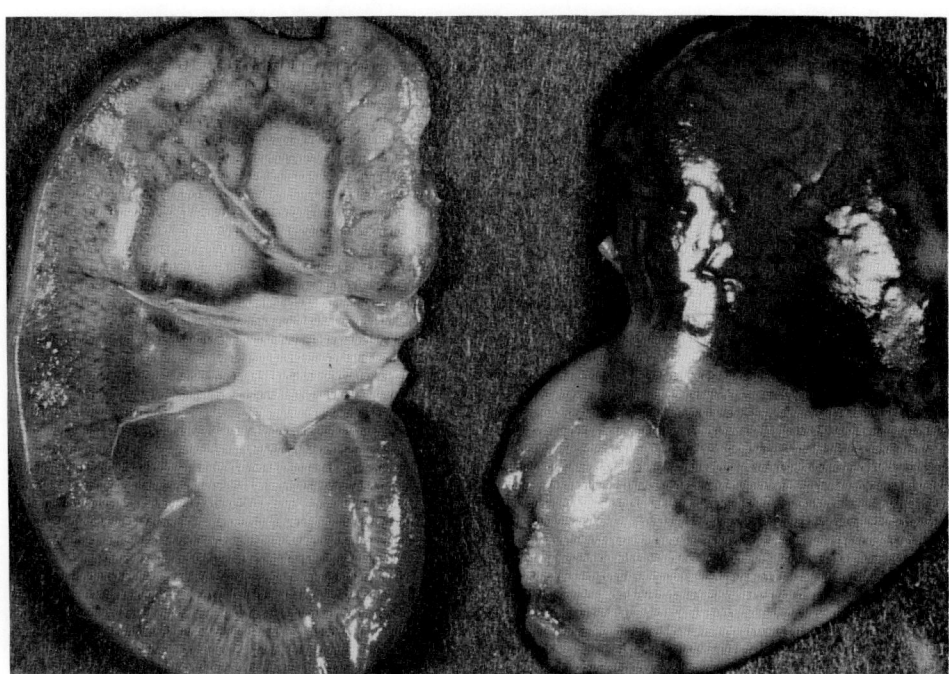

FIG. 24-19. Infarcts of the kidney of a spayed female crossbreed dog, age five years. The light, blanched areas were found to be ischemic and generally necrotic upon microscopic examination. (Courtesy of Angell Memorial Animal Hospital.)

nal disease characterized by loss of glomeruli and tubules and extensive fibrosis in the cortex and medulla. The kidneys ultimately become small, white, and very firm. A renal disease has been reported in Lhasa apso, Pekingese, and similar breeds, characterized by focal to diffuse fibrosis. In contrast to the condition in Norwegian elkhound dogs, there are many small, unperfused glomeruli in the cortex and hyalinized afferent arterioles.

Diseases of the renal vasculature

INFARCTS

Infarcts happen with some frequency in the kidney from the same causes as infarctions elsewhere. Most often, but not invariably, they are of the anemic type and present the picture of one or more sharply outlined wedge-shaped pale—or red, as the case may be—areas with the apex near the zone of the arcuate arteries and the base at the capsule. Given time, they heal with disappearance of the parenchymatous tissue, excepting possibly a few atrophic glomeruli, and with partial replacement by a narrow scar of white fibrous tissue. Due to shrinking of the scar, the capsule comes to be indented at this point. Multiple scarred infarcts of this kind may be indicative of a slowly developing nephrosclerosis but this is very exceptional in animals. Bilateral renal cortical necrosis is discussed earlier.

HEMORRHAGES

Hemorrhages, usually **petechial** in size, located just beneath the capsule and visible through it, or in the intertubular connective tissues, are frequent in septicemic diseases, especially hog cholera, and in many types of poisoning, including those from crotalarias and "oakbuds"(Fig. 24-20). Commonly, death occurs within a

number of hours after their formation so that microscopic examination shows the erythrocytes to be well preserved, but if a few days intervene, the petechiae darken and become indistinct.

Hemorrhages may also open into the glomerular capsules, the tubules, or the renal pelves, producing varying, but usually minor, degrees of hematuria. Extensive hemorrhage into the pelves, or peripherally with separation and distention of the capsule, has occurred, as in poisoning by sweet-clover (coumarin) and lye (NaOH), but ordinarily the hemorrhages are significant as aids in diagnosis rather than for their effect on the patient. Extensive hemorrhage, usually the result of trauma, may occur under the renal capsule. Such hemorrhage may result in ischemia and severe impairment of renal function.

HYPEREMIA

Active hyperemia and passive congestion occur, the former as a feature of acute inflammation, the latter as a part of generalized passive congestion, but neither reaches spectacular proportions in the kidney because of the dense and unyielding character of the organ. Congestion is most evident in the medulla, where the capillaries (venulae rectae) running in groups, produce radial red lines, which are often strikingly conspicuous at autopsy.

ANEMIA

Anemia, general or local, tends to produce a kidney of paler color than normal. This sometimes results in the renal pyramids being practically white. Information is needed on the exact pathogenesis of this latter condition and the reasons for it. Attention may be called here to the fact that without a sufficient blood pressure in the glomeruli, secretion of urine is impossible, a situ-

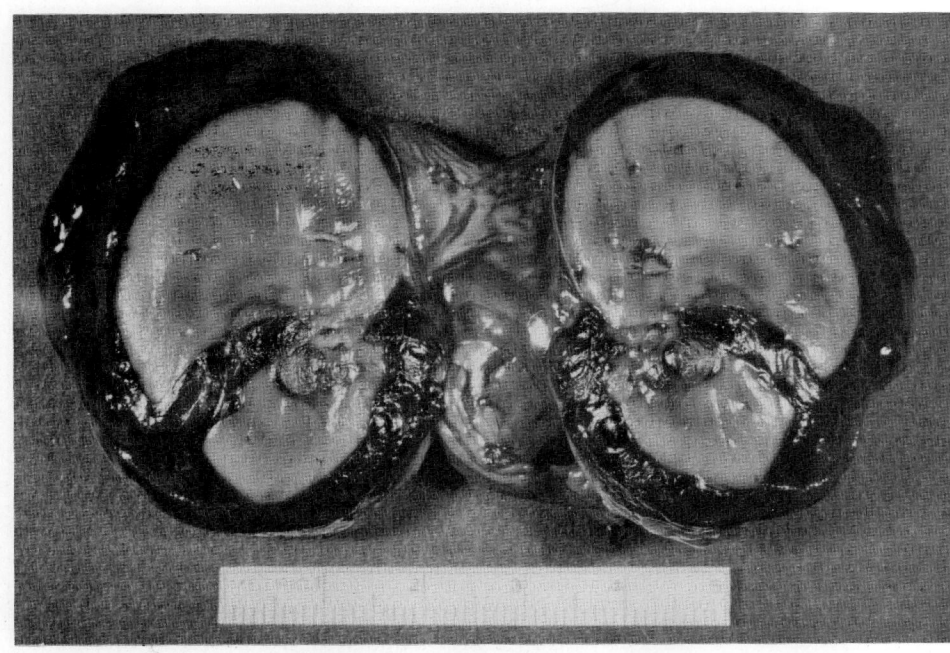

FIG. 24-20. Subscapular hemorrhage, kidney of a four-year-old black cat. Kidney has been incised in the horizontal plane. (Courtesy of Angell Memorial Animal Hospital.)

ation which arises in shock and similar conditions, and which must be considered in therapy.

EDEMA

Edema of the kidney is described, but the kidney takes little part in generalized edema because of the inelastic character of its capsule and firmness of its parenchyma. Since drainage from the kidney is in the form of urine, local edema is represented by hydronephrosis (Figs. 24-21–23).

Urinary obstruction and hydronephrosis

When there is severe or complete obstruction of the outflow of urine at some point below the convergence of the two ureteral streams, as for instance from calculi in the slender penile urethra (common in cattle, sheep, and goats), the result is first a severe and maximal distension of the bladder, which may or may not rupture. There follows in the course of 3 or 4 days a great distension of the abdominal cavity with fluid ("water belly," among stockmen) which has some of the characteristics of dilute urine, but which ultimately contains fibrinogen so that fibrinous deposits develop on the serous surfaces, possibly in some way akin to the fibrin-containing fluid in the pericardial sac in uremia. In some of these cases, the bladder has ruptured, releasing its contents into the peritoneal cavity, but in others no rupture or evidence of previous rupture can be found. Eventually, uriniferous fluid also seeps into the periurethral tissues and urinary region generally, above the point of obstruction. The blood urea nitrogen rises from the normal between 15 and 30 to as high as 400 mg/100 ml of blood, and the animal dies of uremia without sufficient time for extensive gross changes in the kidneys.

Sudden, complete obstruction on one side may

cause rapid atrophy of the corresponding kidney, reducing it almost to the vanishing point without hydronephrosis or other clinical disturbance. Such a change must be distinguished from hypoplasia. On the other hand, when there is partial obstruction, unilateral or bilateral, the patient is usually able to live, and in the course of a few months there develops in the kidney or kidneys subjected to back-pressure the condition known as **hydronephrosis.** In hydronephrosis, the renal pelvis is gradually enlarged at the expense of the parenchyma. A considerable enlargement of the cavity of the renal pelvis can occur without much distortion of the renal parenchyma, but in time (6 months,), the obstructed kidney becomes a mere hollow sac, although distended to larger outside dimensions than formerly. Ridges remain to mark the boundaries of the fetal lobules.

Microscopically, some scattered atrophic glomeruli usually remain in the thin and fibrous mass as the only vestige of kidney structure. Since the glomeruli have first access to the declining blood supply, and since their cells are somewhat less vulnerable than those of the tubules, it is only natural that glomeruli persist in the fibrous remains long after the tubules have disappeared. The fluid in the pelvic space changes from urine to a very watery liquid as the power of selective resorption declines in the dying tubules. Since an obstructed kidney is prone to become infected (see pyelonephritis), the fluid is not infrequently pus at the time of postmortem examination; the condition is then known as **pyonephrosis.** The forms and places of obstruction to the urinary flow are numerous and varied. Calculi are the most frequent, lodging anywhere from the pelvis to the external meatus. A calculus has been observed that fitted the uretero-pelvic orifice as accurately as a stopper fits a bottle, but many start down the ureter or the urethra and lodge in the narrow passage.

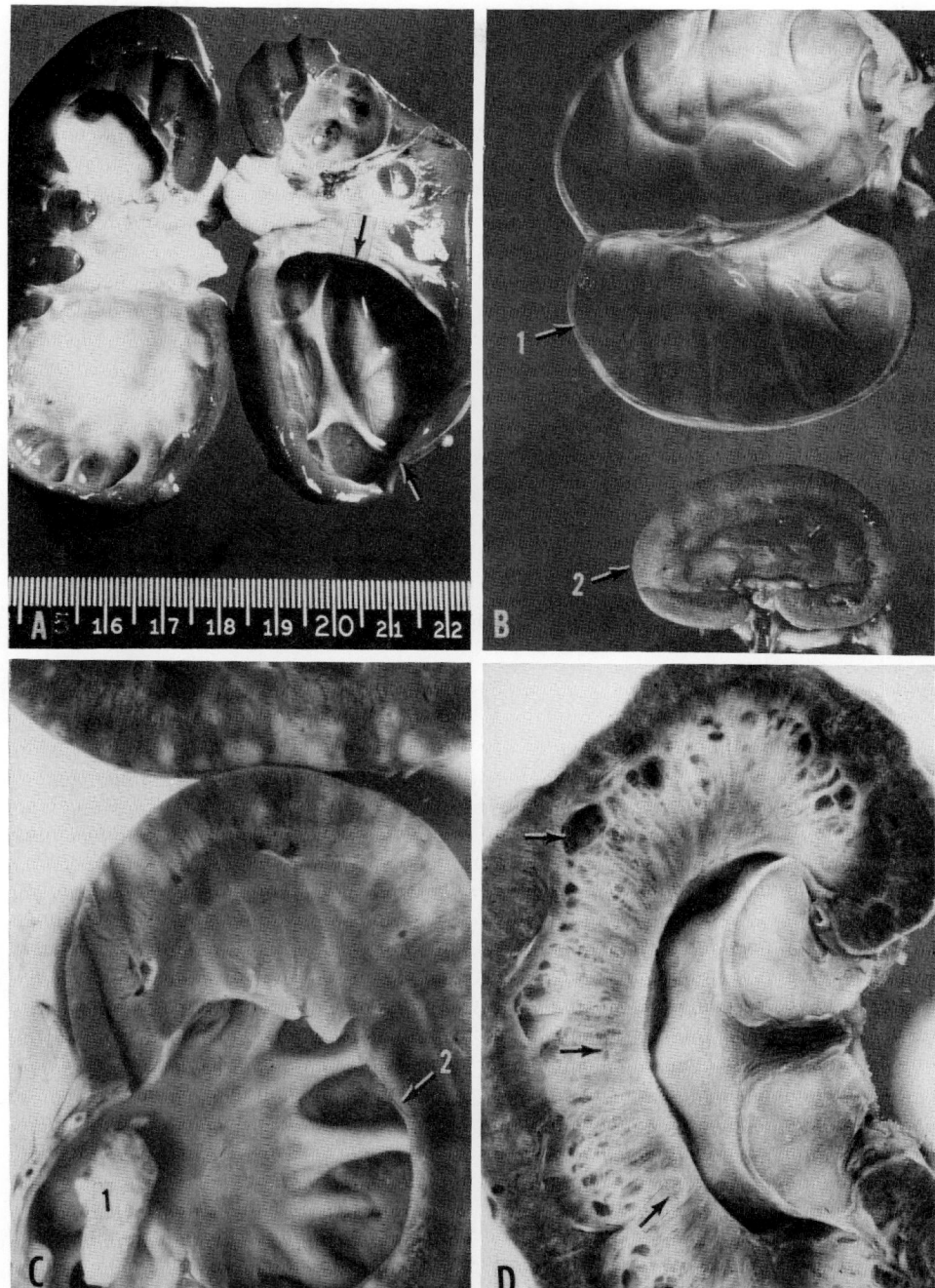

FIG. 24-21. A. Hydronephrosis, kidney of a pig. **B.** Severe hydronephrotic atrophy (**1**), kidney reduced to an empty capsule. Compensatory hypertrophy of the opposite kidney (**2**). One-year-old dog. **C.** Early hydronephrosis, kidney of a ten-year-old female dachshund. Note calculus (**1**) which fitted into the urethral antrum as a stopper fits a bottle. The renal pelvis is dilated (**2**). **D.** Cysts (arrows) in the kidney of a ten-year-old male Chesapeake dog with contracted kidney.

Strictures of either of these tubes are much rarer in animals than in humans, but have been seen. Pressure from the outside of the ureter or urethra can result from a number of things, but neoplasms are the most frequent, particularly growths of malignant lymphoma arising in the lymph nodes of the region. Carcinoma of the bladder and of the canine prostate are also noteworthy in this respect.

In uncomplicated hydronephrosis of one kidney, the other undergoes marked compensatory hypertrophy, and adequate function is usually maintained. **Hypertrophy in the kidney** involves an increase in diameter

and length of the tubules, but no new nephrons are formed.

One of the causes of hydronephrosis is the giant kidney worm, *Dioctophyma renale*. Hydronephrosis, possibly inherited, has been described in rats and inbred mice.

In women and nonhuman primates, the ureter and the renal pelvis undergo a physiologic dilatation referred to as **hydronephrosis of pregnancy.** It results at least in part from endocrine effects, but it is not associated with impaired renal function and disappears after parturition. In women it predisposes to pyelonephritis.

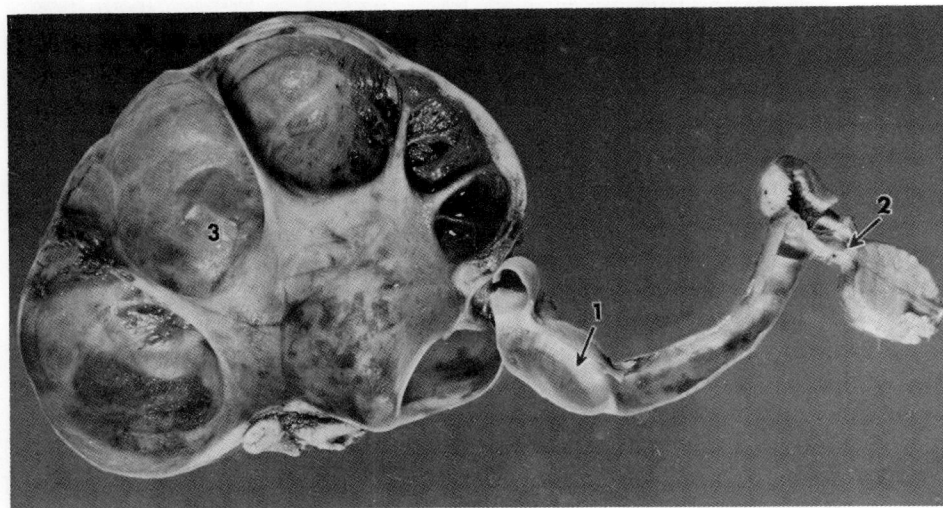

FIG. 24-22. Hydronephrosis of the kidney of a dog. The ureter (**1**) is dilated and tortuous above the obstruction (**2**) and the kidney has become a loculated sac (**3**). (Courtesy of Dr. Wayne H. Riser, Washington, D.C.)

Reference

Gobe GC, Axelsen RA. Genesis of renal tubular atrophy in experimental hydronephrosis in the rat; Role of apoptosis. Lab Invest 1987;56:273–281.

Urolithiasis

The formation of stony precipitates anywhere in the urinary passages is called urolithiasis; the stone is called a urolith or urinary calculus (Fig. 24-24). The calculi are most often found in the bladder, where the name of "cystic calculi" may be applied to them, but in other cases they are in the renal pelvis, or even in distended terminal tubules (the ducts of Bellini). One or more uroliths may lodge in the ureter, producing excruciating pain known as ureteral colic. However, if the calculus is small enough to enter the ureter, it usually is ultimately forced into the bladder, whereupon the colic is relieved. Otherwise, the kidney involved is reduced to negligible size by pressure and disuse atrophy, or it more slowly undergoes hydronephrosis.

Calculi in the bladder are often carried out with the urine and may lodge in the narrow male urethra, usually at the sigmoid flexure in ruminants, the result being fatal obstruction unless relief is obtained. The female usually escapes this trouble because of the larger and shorter urethra.

Uroliths may be of any size from a mere collection of sand-like particles to a single stone practically filling the bladder or renal pelvis. They may be hard or relatively soft, white or yellowish, smooth or rough, and rounded or faceted (that is, with flattened sides). Sili-

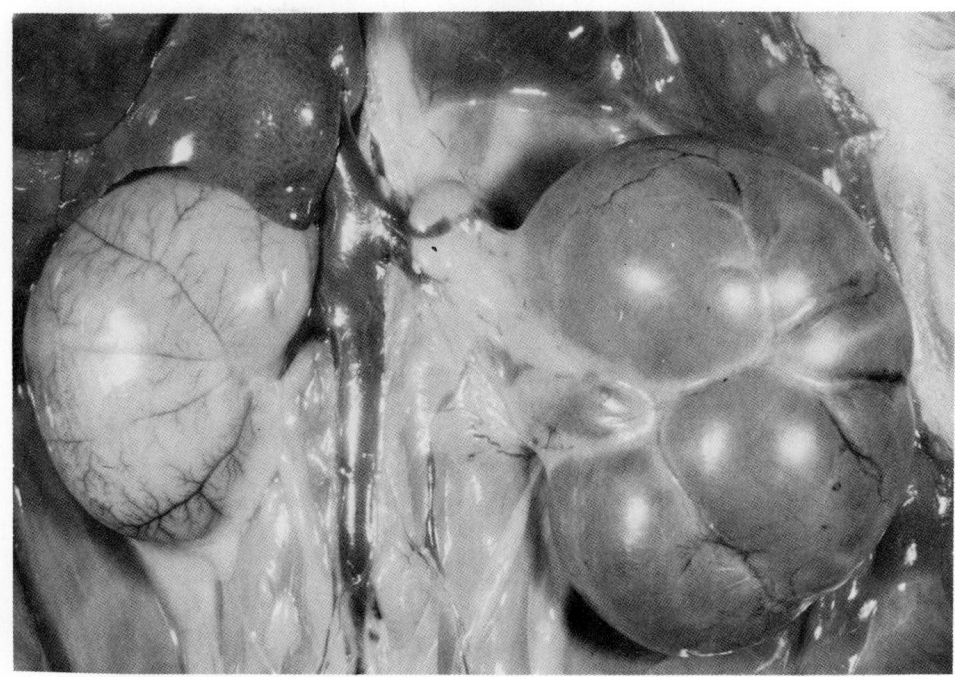

FIG. 24-23. Hydronephrosis of the left kidney of an eight-month-old male cat. (Courtesy of Angell Memorial Animal Hospital.)

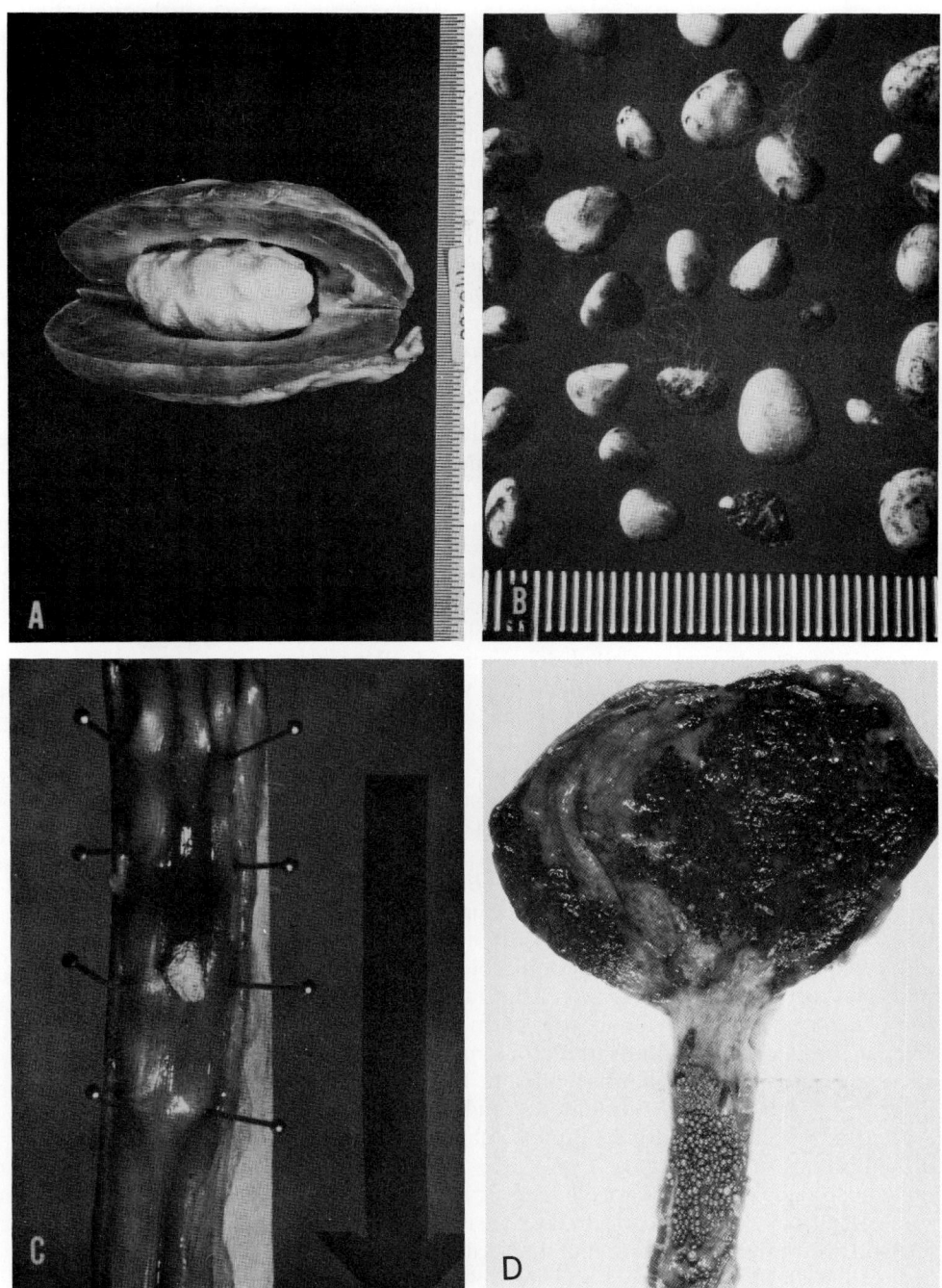

FIG. 24-24. Urolithiasis. **A.** A single large calculus filling the renal pelvis of a dog. (Courtesy of Armed Forces Institute of Pathology and Dr. S. Stern. **B.** Calculi removed from the prostate of a six-year-old cocker spaniel dog. **C.** Calculus in the urethra of a steer. **D.** Cystitis and multiple urethral calculi in a four-year-old wether. (**D.** Courtesy of Dr. W. J. Hadlow.)

ceous stones especially are often fragile or merely collections of sandy material. However, a stone only a few millimeters in diameter is sufficient to obstruct the sigmoid urethra of a steer and must not be overlooked at autopsy.

The composition of calculi varies greatly. Chemically, the usual urinary stone of herbivorous animals contains a predominance of silicates, conjoined in a minority of cases with phosphates, carbonates, or oxalates of calcium, ammonium, and magnesium (Mathams and Sutherland, 1951; Schmidt, 1941; Swingle, 1953). Important amounts of protein are always found with these minerals, a fact which is probably of primary importance, according to the work of Swingle (1953), who analyzed calculi from 63 range steers affected with occluding urolithiasis. He found that the urine of bovine animals kept under the conditions of the western ranges of the United States (where the incidence of urolithiasis is high because of vitamin A deficiency) contains from 50 to 150 ppm of dissolved silica. He concluded that, in all probability, silica is precipitated as an insoluble complex in combination with mucoproteins in the urine. He believed that the aggregation of the dispersed insoluble material into concretions depended upon the presence of particulate nuclei (cellular fragments, organic precipitates) and upon "alterations in the quality and quantity of protective colloids in the urine." The amount of silica in the urine depends upon that in the animal's feed, some plants grown in arid areas being heavily laden with this substance. In other situations, particularly in feedlots, calcium phosphate, calcium carbonate, and triple phosphate calculi occupy a more prominent position in the calculi of herbivora. The usual alkaline pH of the urine of herbivora favors the precipitation of these constituents. Occasionally calculi in herbivora may contain mixtures of both silicates and calcium salts (weddelite). Silicate and phosphate calculi are off-white in color and may be hard or crumbly. In some parts of the world (New Zealand) the nuclein derivative, xanthine (not the xanthin of plants), has been reported as a principal constituent of urinary calculi, especially in sheep. These are brownish and crumbly.

In carnivorous and omnivorous animals, the chemical constituents of uroliths are quite different. The calculi of these animals are much like those of the human, possibly because of the characteristically acid urine which is in contrast to the alkaline urine of herbivora. The **oxalate stone** is a spectacular type, very hard and heavy, white or light yellow, and typically covered with sharp, hard spines. It is usually found as a single stone in the bladder and may reach a diameter of several centimeters. It consists chiefly of calcium oxalate and has sharp edges which may damage the urinary epithelium and cause hemorrhage.

Uric acid calculi consist largely of ammonium (from decomposition of urea) and sodium urates and uric acid. They are of small or medium size, firm or moderately hard, yellow to brown in color, and either spherical or irregular in shape. They are not radiopaque. Like the oxalate calculi, they form in acid urine. They are especially common in Dalmatian dogs, which excrete large amounts of uric acid due to a defect in tubular resorption and subsequent oxidation of uric acid to allantoin, as is done by most mammals except primates.

Phosphate calculi are more like the calculi of herbivora, being white or gray, of chalky consistency, but often soft and friable enough that they can be crushed with little trouble. They are often multiple and may exist merely as sand-like granules. They are the most frequent form of urolithiasis in dogs despite the usual acidity of the urine. Bacterial infection with breakdown of urea to ammonia resulting in elevation of urine pH favors precipitation of phosphates. Magnesium ammonium phosphate (struvite) is the commonest form of phosphate calculi in dogs.

Xanthine stones are brownish red, often concentrically laminated, fragile, and of irregular shape. They are rare.

Cystine stones are small, soft and of variable shape, and have a shiny, greasy appearance. They are yellow and become darker on exposure to air. Cystine, an amino acid, is relatively insoluble and may precipitate in the bladder of animals that excrete an increased amount through the kidneys, which results from failure of tubular resorption of cystine as well as other amino acids. Cystine stones in the dog have a tendency to occlude the urethra at the point where it enters the os penis. Cystine calculi have been reported in men, women, and male dogs. Cystinuria has been recognized in many different breeds of dogs in which the condition is believed to be inherited either as a sex-linked recessive trait or autosomal trait with sex-modified expression.

Siliceous calculi are rare in carnivora, but may develop if the diet contains a large amount of silicic acid.

INCIDENCE

Urinary calculi are common in all species of animals. They are least frequently seen in swine and most often encountered in cattle, dogs, and cats. In dogs, the incidence has been reported to range from 0.6% to 2.8% of all canine illnesses, with strivite calculi accounting for 40 to 85% of all stones; cystine, 7 to 22%; urate, 2 to 8%; and oxalate, 3 to 30%.

CAUSES

While many factors have already been alluded to in the pathogenesis of urinary calculi, many examples go unexplained, as does the underlying mechanism of calculus formation. It is generally believed that an organic matrix, nucleus, or nidus is a necessary requirement for deposition of inorganic crystals and resultant stone formation. This nucleus is usually a mucopolysaccharide or mucoprotein. The nucleus could consist of dead leukocytes, fibrin, cellular debris, or agglutinated bacteria. Crystallization upon or within the nucleus does not necessarily always follow, but results when there is disruption of the colloidal system that supports the supersaturated solution of crystalloids of urine. This may result from an excess of crystalloids overwhelming the protective colloids or the presence of hydrophilic colloids. Some specific conditions associated with urinary calculi include:

1. Bacterial infection of the urinary tract, which allows for nidus formation and alteration of urinary pH. This is the principal cause of phosphate calculi in dogs.
2. Aminoaciduria leading to cystine calculi in male dogs.
3. Metabolic defect in uric acid metabolism in Dalmatian dogs, leading to urate calculi.
4. Vitamin A deficiency, apparently through squamous metaplasia of urinary epithelium and increased nidus formations. Experimentally, urolithiasis has been produced repeatedly in herbivorous animals by the mere expedient of depriving them of adequate amounts of vitamin A. Such experiments have explained the frequent occurrence of urinary calculi in steers, wethers, and male goats fed upon diets of dried sorghums, cottonseed products, bleached hays, straw, corn slaths, and dried pasture grasses, none of which contain any substantial amount of vitamin A.

5. Implantation with diethylstilbestrol or grazing on estrogenic plants may lead to urinary calculi in sheep. The effect of these hormones in causing squamous metaplasia of the genitourinary epithelium is well known, as is their tendency to limit the growth in size of the genitourinary organs.
6. Hyperparathyroidism causes increased excretion of calcium, urolithiasis, and nephrocalcinosis.
7. A picornavirus has been shown to experimentally produce urolithiasis in male cats.
8. Dietary mineral imbalance and diets high in ash are attractive theories as causes of urolithiasis, but are rarely implicated. Diets with imbalances of calcium, phosphate, and magnesium may lead to either urolithiasis or nephrocalcinosis.
9. Inadequate water intake by itself is not a cause of urolithiasis; however, if the diet is high in silicates or other minerals or if other predisposing factors exist, dehydration favors calculus formation. High sodium chloride intake, provided ample water is available, will reduce the incidence of urolithiasis in cattle.

EFFECTS

Calculi are mechanically irritating wherever they may be but only moderately so, as a rule. In the renal pelvis, the stone frequently is molded to fit the calyx or part of a calyx in which it was formed. The principal harm done by uroliths is that of obstruction when they lodge at the uretero-pelvic orifice, in the ureter, or in the urethra. This has been discussed in an earlier paragraph.

References

Abdullah SU, Osborne CA, Leininger JR, et al. Evaluation of a calculolytic diet in female dogs with induced struvite urolithiasis. Am J Vet Res 1984;45:1508–1519.
Bovee KC, Their SO, Rea C, et al. Renal clearance of amino acids in canine cystinuria. Metabolism 1974;23:51–58.
Bovee KC, McGuire T. Qualitative and quantitative analysis of uroliths in dogs: definitive determination of chemical type. J Am Vet Med Assoc 1984;185:983–987.
Finco DR, Barsanti JA, Crowell WA. Characterization of magnesium-induced urinary disease in the cat and comparison with feline urologic syndrome. Am J Vet Res 1985;46:391–400.
Huntington GB, Emerick RJ. Oxalate urinary calculi in beef steers. Am J Vet Res 1984;45:180–182.
Khan SR, Finlayson B, Hackett RL. Scanning electron microscopy of calcium oxalate crystal formation in experimental nephrolithiasis. Lab Invest 1979;41:504–510.
Klausner JS, Osborne CA, O'Leary TP, et al. Struvite urolithiasis in a litter of miniature schnauzer dogs. Am J Vet Res 1980;41:712–719.
Kuhlmann ET, Longnecker DS. Urinary calculi in Lewis and Wistar rats. Lab Anim Sci 1984;34:299–3022.
Ling GV, Franti CE, Ruby AL, et al. Epizootiologic evaluation of urinary calculi from 150 cats. J Am Vet Med Assoc 1990;196:1459–1462.
Lulich JP, Osborne CA, Unger LK, et al. Prevalence of calcium oxalate uroliths in miniature schnauzers. Am J Vet Res 1991;52:1579–1582.
Lulich JP, Osborne CA, Nagode LA, et al. Evaluation of urine and serum metabolites in miniature schnauzers with calcium oxalate urolithiasis. Am J Vet Res 1991;52:1583–1590.
Renlund RC, McGill GE, Cheng PT. Calcite urolith in a Cynomologus monkey. Lab Anim Sci 1986;36:536–537.
Stephens EC, Middleton CC, Thompson LJ. Urinary cystic calculi in a Cynomologus monkey (*Macaca fascicularis*): A case report. Lab Anim Sci 1979;29:797–799.
Taton GF, Hamar DW, Lewis LD. Urinary acidification in the prevention and treatment of feline struvite urolithiasis. J Am Vet Med Assoc 1984;184:437–443.
Tsan M-F, Jones TC, Thornton GW, et al. Canine cystinuria: Its urinary amino acid pattern and genetic analysis. Am J Vet Res 1972;33:2455–2461.
Tsan M-F, Jones TC, Wilson TH. Canine cystinuria: Intestinal renal amino acid transport. Am J Vet Res 1972;33:2463–2468.
Treacher RJ. Intestinal absorption of lysine in cystinuric dogs. J Comp Path 1965;75:309–321.

Neoplasms

EMBRYONAL NEPHROMA, NEPHROBLASTOMA, WILMS' TUMOR

This tumor arises in the kidney or occasionally outside but near it (Figs. 24-25 and 24-26). It is the most common neoplasm in swine and occurs rarely in other species. It arises from the renal blastema, from which kidney is formed, but which in early embryonic stages is not greatly differentiated from the primitive mesenchyme. The latter is pluripotent in its capacity for differentiation into several types of mature tissue, which explains why this embryonal tumor contains more than one kind of tissue. Its structure varies, but typically involves a mixture of a certain number of gland-like acini or tubules, with large masses of cells indistinguishable from those of rather anaplastic fibrosarcoma. This led to the earlier name of **adenosarcoma,** which was in use prior to Feldman's (1932) elucidation of the embryologic origin of the neoplasm.

While the term adenosarcoma is paradoxic, it may be useful in helping the beginning student to fix the microscopic picture of the tumor in mind. It consists typically of what appears to be highly cellular fibroblastic tissue with, here and there, an inexplicable, epithelial-lined glandular acinus resembling a tubule or primitive glomerulus in its midst. In some examples, the glands are scarce and hard to find; at the other extreme are occasional tumors in which many areas consist chiefly of gland-like epithelial structures suggestive of an adenocarcinoma. The tumor is comparable to Wilm's tumor of humans, which typically also contains smooth muscle, but this is seldom seen in the nephroblastomas of animals. Since it has its origin in an anomaly of fetal development, it is essentially a tumor of the young. In humans and animals the tumors are fatal at an early age, but pigs commonly thrive long enough to go to market in the usual way, the tumor being discovered at postmortem inspection. While still rarely seen in most species, this is one of the relatively frequent tumors of swine; it has been reported in cattle and sheep, as well as in chickens, rabbits, and other small mammalian species, becoming evident usually at an early age.

In a study of embryonal nephromas collected from meat-inspection sources, all but two in swine, 77% of these occurred in pigs less than 1 year of age, but since the great majority of pigs encountered in meat inspection are of this age, it may be more significant that one

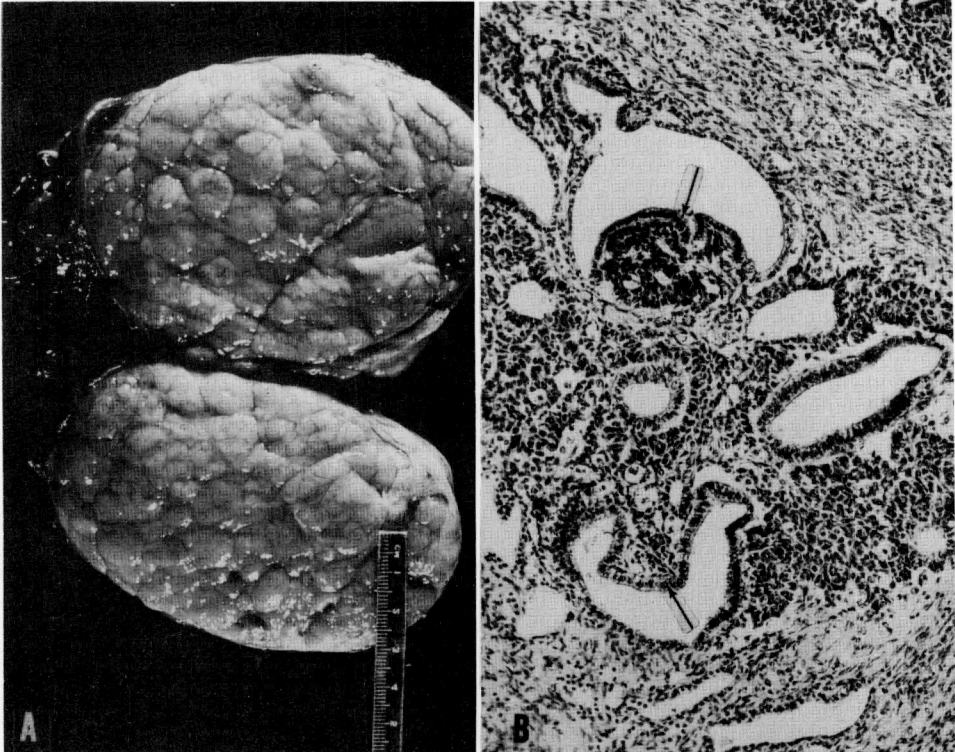

FIG. 24-25. Embryonal nephroma, kidney of a six-month-old male fox terrier. **A.** The gross specimen. **B.** Photomicrograph (× 100). Note structures simulating renal corpuscles. (Courtesy of Armed Forces Institute of Pathology and Dr. H. R. Seibold.

occurred in a sow 6 years old. There were twice as many in females as in males, a finding which has not been explained. The tumors were multiple in 30%, usually bilateral. Most often, but by no means invariably, arising at one pole of the kidney, they ranged from very small up to a diameter of 80 cm and a weight of 27 kg. The typical tumor is a firm, lobulated, light-colored growth with a distinct capsule and numerous trabeculae of dense mature connective tissue. While growth may be described as rapid, metastases are exceptional, being chiefly to the lungs or liver. Striated muscle and partially calcified bone may be demonstrable in a few of these tumors.

Other abattoir surveys have revealed incidence rates from 20/100,000 to 79/100,000 as compared to the occurrence of malignant lymphoma of about 2/100,000. In a report of 161 examples, 93% were in swine under 1 year of age, and of 147 cases, 75 were in barrows, 59 in gilts, 9 in sows, and 2 in stags.

In dogs, embryonal nephroma is not common. Most examples are seen in dogs under 1 year of age, although they have been reported in dogs up to 9 years of age.

References

Bennett BT, Beluhan FZ, Welsh TJ. Malignant nephroblastoma in *Macaca fascicularis.* Lab Anim Sci 1982;32:403–404.

Haenichen T, Stavrou D. Nephroblastoma. Handbook, Animal Models of Human Disease. Registry of Comparative Pathology, Armed Forces Institute of Pathology, November, 1979 Washington DC.

Umeda M, Akashi T, Suzuki H, et al. Cystic nephroblastoma of an aged dog. Vet Pathol 1985;22:84–85.

ADENOMA, ADENOCARCINOMA

These neoplasms arising from renal tubular epithelium usually clearly resemble their tissue of origin in microscopic sections. The tumors are most often encountered in the dog, in which they are usually malignant. An undifferentiated form of this tumor, with large, lipid-laden cells that rarely form tubules, has been called **hypernephroma,** based on an erroneous belief that its origin is in the adrenal cortex. **Undifferentiated renal carcinoma** is a preferable term. The neoplasms blend by imperceptible gradations with "clear-celled adenocarcinomas" and more ordinary adenocarcinomas and adenomas which are known to originate from the renal tubules. Benign or malignant tumors of this general class have been found in the dog, horse, monkey, and laboratory rodent. Although carcinomas of the kidney usually metastasize by way of blood vessels, metastasis may be found in regional lymph nodes in some examples. Occasionally, squamous cell carcinoma may arise from the renal pelvis.

References

Brack M. Renal papillary adenoma in a cotton-topped tamarin (*Saguinus oedipus*) Lab Anim 1985;19:132–133.

Britt JO, Ryan CP, Howard EB. Sarcomatoid renal adenocarcinoma in a cat. Vet Pathol 1985;22:514–515.

Hard GC, Mackay RL, Kochhar OS. Electron microscopic determination of the sequence of acute tubular and vascular injury induced in the rat kidney by a carcinogenic dose of dimethylnitrosamine. Lab Invest 1984;50:659–672.

Jones SR, Casey HW. Primary renal tumors in nonhuman primates. Vet Pathol 1981;18:(Suppl 6)89–104.

Miller RI, Gliatto JM, Casey HW, et al. Renal carcinoma with probable

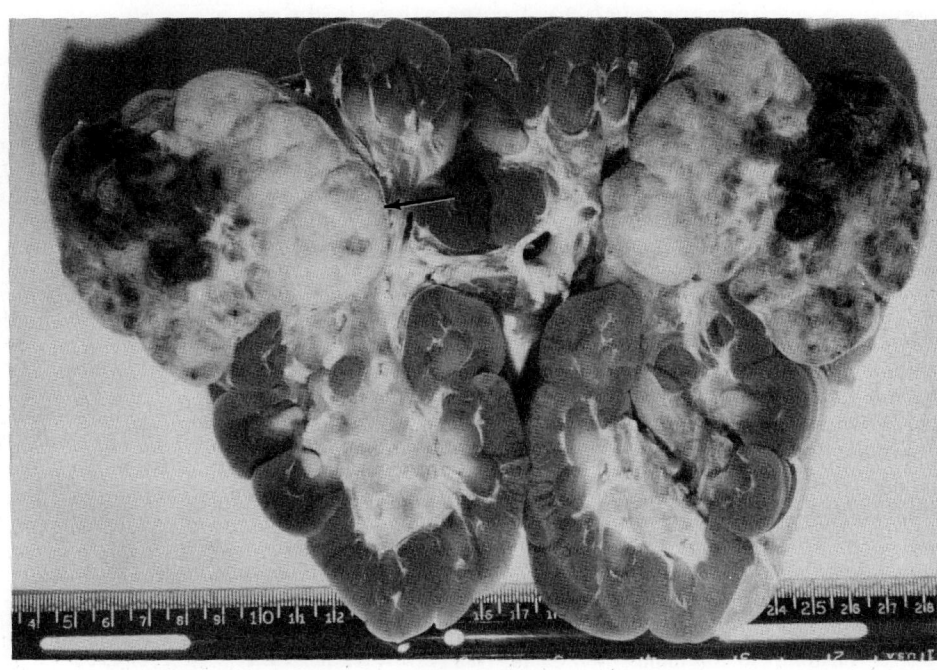

FIG. 24-26. Embryonal nephroma (arrow), kidney of an adult cow.

pulmonary metastasis and chronic interstitial nephritis in a Greater Kudu antelope. Vet Pathol 1985;22:646–647.

Vitovec J. Renal cell carcinoma in a camel (*Camelus dromedarius*). Vet Pathol 1982;19:331–333.

TRANSITIONAL CELL CARCINOMA

Transitional cell carcinoma may originate in the renal pelvis and morphologically is similar to those which develop from the transitional epithelium of the ureter, urethra, or bladder.

Reference

Bell RC, Moeller RB. Transitional cell carcinoma of the renal pelvis in a ferret. Lab Anim Sci 1990;40:537–538.

ONCOCYTOMA

Oncocytoma is an interesting benign tumor in humans and has been experimentally induced in the rat by administration of one of several carcinogens, namely: N-nitrosomorpholine, N-ethyl-N-hydroxyethyl-nitrosamine, cycasin, and N-nitrosodiethylamine, plus lead acetate. The cells from which these tumors arise have been identified as both principal and intercalated cells of the collecting duct system. They usually develop from multiple sites in both kidneys and often accompany other lesions in distal tubules, including other epithelial neoplasms.

The oncocyte is seen with the light microscope as a very large cell with a spherical, centrally located nucleus and abundant densely granular, acidophilic cytoplasm. This distinctive cell and the adenoma formed by them is usually readily seen in H and E sections, but may be differentially stained by PAS reaction, followed with Orange G and iron hematoxylin (the Tri-PAS procedure). The cytoplasm of the oncocytes is a bright yellow with this method, contrasting with the darkexjr tubular epithelium.

The electron microscope reveals the cytoplasm to be stuffed with mitochondria, a few dense osmiophilic bodies and few other organelles, such as beta glycogen particles, Golgi complex, smooth and rough endoplasmic reticulum, and some free polyribosomes. The mitochondria are often greatly distorted in shape, mostly elongated and form stacks with various arrangements. Some cup-shaped mitochondria form complex bodies. The cristae in the elongated mitochondria are often seen in long parallel arrays.

References

Bannasch P, Zerban H, Ahn YS, et al. Oncocytoma, kidney, rat. In: Jones TC, Hard GC, Mohr U, eds. Monograph on pathology of laboratory animals, urinary system. New York: Springer Verlag 1997 (in press).

Krech R, Zerban H, Bannasch P. Mitochondrial anomalies in renal oncocytes induced in rat by N-nitrosomorpholine. Euro J Cell Biol 1981;25:331–339.

Nogueira E, Bannasch P. Cellular origin of rat oncocytoma. Lab Invest 1988;59:337–343.

METASTATIC NEOPLASMS

The kidneys are subject to metastatic invasion by malignant neoplasms of all kinds. However, in proportion to the amount of blood which flows through them, metastases are certainly much less frequent than in the liver and lungs. The most frequent metastatic tumor, by far, is the malignant lymphoma (lymphosarcoma). It may take the form of discrete tumors of large or small size or it may infiltrate insidiously into the intertubular interstitial tissue, with the result that irregular islets of lymphoid cells are seen microscopically here and there. The pathologist must be on guard lest these be mistaken for inflammatory infiltration; if the cells are lymphoid in character, usually somewhat larger than normal lymphocytes, and if leukocytes of other inflammatory types are not recognized, the diagnosis should be malignant lymphoma. If examination of lymph nodes and other structures is possible, the diagnosis can be confirmed. Metastatic tumors reported to occur in the kidney of animals include malignant melanoma, squamous cell carcinoma, hemangioendothelioma lymphosarcoma, and transitional cell carcinoma (from pelvis, ureter, urethra, or bladder).

References

Chrisp CE, Cary C, Rush HG, et al. Bilateral undifferentiated renal sarcomas in a Rhesus monkey. Vet Pathol 1985;22:516–517.

Crow SE, Bell TG, Wortman JA. Hematuria associated with renal hemangiosarcoma in a dog. J Am Vet Med Assoc 1980;176:531–532.

Mooney SC, Hayes AA, Matus RE, et al. Renal lymphoma in cats: 28 cases (1977–1984). J Am Vet Med Assoc 1987;191:1473–1477.

URETERS, URACHUS, BLADDER, AND URETHRA

The ureter

Anomalies of the ureter are rare. These anomalies range from aplasia to complete duplication.

Inflammation of the ureteral mucosa occurs as a part of inflammation of the whole urinary tract. Because of the dense nature of the wall of this small tubular organ, the exudative or proliferative changes are less extensive and attract less attention in the ureter than in the bladder or renal pelvis. The dilatation of the ureteral lumen and the thickening of the wall which occur in ascending pyelonephritis or pyonephrosis have been mentioned. If there is partial obstruction lower in the urinary tract, the gradual dilation of the lumen of one or both ureters (depending on location of the obstruction) can be quite remarkable. Tuberculosis and possibly certain other granulomatous infections occasionally invade the wall of the ureter, producing characteristic lesions.

Strictures in the form of an irregular fold or a gradual narrowing can occur either congenitally or as the result of previous inflammation. Such damage is most likely to be due to the temporary lodgment of calculi somewhere along the tube, although a considerable proportion of strictures are located just at the ureteral inlet.

Neoplasms, usually papillomas or carcinomas, arise from the ureteral mucosa rarely (Fig. 24-27). Metastatic tumors may infiltrate the wall.

References

Hanika C, Rebar AH. Ureteral transitional cell carcinoma in the dog. Vet Pathol 1980;17:643–646.

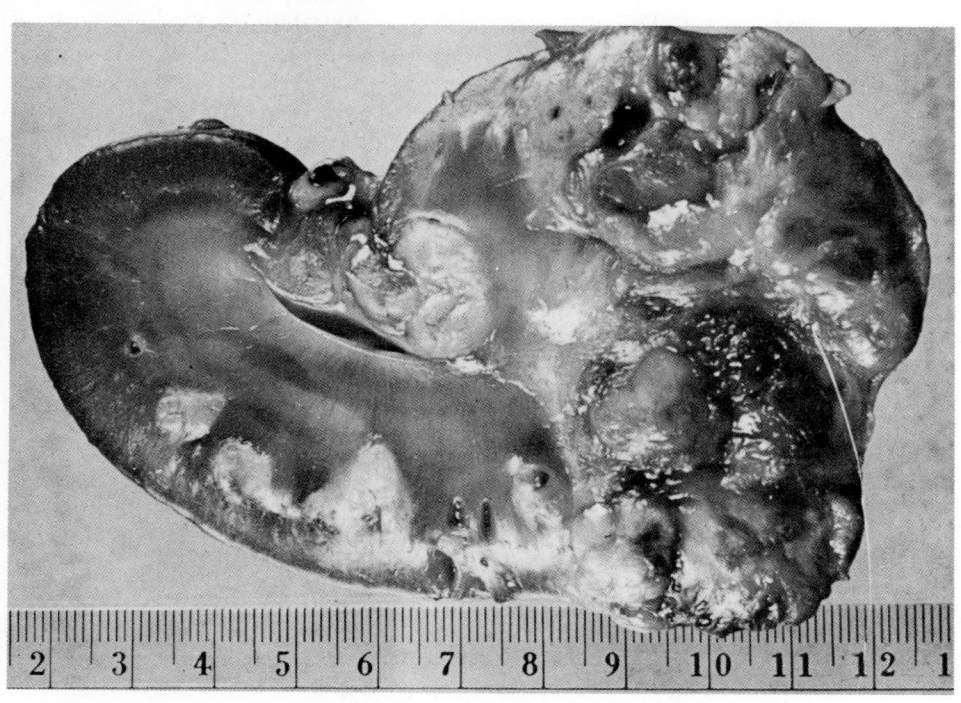

FIG. 24-27. Papillary adenocarcinoma of the kidney of an eight-year-old male springer spaniel.

Hattel AL, Diters RW, Snavely DA. Ureteral fibropapilloma in a dog. J Am Vet Med Assoc 1986;188:873 one page article.
Leib MS, Allen TA, Konde LJ, et al. Bilateral hydronephrosis attributable to bilateral ureteral fibrosis in a cat. J Am Vet Med Assoc 1988;192:795–797.

Bladder

ANOMALIES

"Pervious urachus" is a congenital failure of the fetal urachus to close, and requires surgical intervention. The occasional ascent of infection from a diseased umbilicus to the kidney has been mentioned. Cysts rarely form in the course of a urachus which closes in some parts and not in others, leaving isolated stretches of patent lumen, or they may form in the midline of the bladder. Other congenital anomalies of the urinary bladder such as aplasia, diverticula, and fistula are rare.

CYSTITIS

Especially when there is interference with the normal drainage of urine, the mucosa and deeper layers of the bladder are subject to infectious inflammations of the acute fibrinous, purulent, catarrhal and hemorrhagic types (Fig. 24-28). The purulent form occasionally reaches phlegmonous proportions. Infection with gas-producing bacteria may lead to gas-filled vesicles in the wall of the bladder, a condition known as **emphysematous cystitis.** The latter is most frequent in the presence of glucosuria. Chronicity leads to irregular thickening of the subepithelial connective tissue and mild corrugation of the mucosal side as seen grossly. A form of cystitis occurs rarely in the dog in which numerous epithelial-lined diverticula of uncertain origin become closed at their orifices and form minute cystic spaces in the inflamed and thickened wall.

Involvement by tuberculosis and possibly other infectious granulomas occurs rarely. Tubercles may be small and confined to the submucosa or may form large bulges into the lumen, with or without ulceration. Urolithiasis tends to result from long-continued cystitis of exudative type. Mucinous, adenomatous, and squamous metaplasia of the transitional epithelium is a frequent finding in chronic cystitis. This is especially evident in bovine enzootic hematuria. It is apparently related to chronic inflammation. In swine, mucinous metaplasia of the superficial transitional epithelium, especially of the renal pelvis and ureters, is seen in association with a variety of conditions, particularly exudative epidermitis. It has been called "mucinous degeneration."

OTHER DISORDERS OF THE BLADDER

Hemorrhages, usually petechial, without inflammation are indicative of acute toxemias or septicemias. Petechiae in the mucosa are considered of diagnostic significance in hog cholera.

Hypertrophy of the muscular layer is recognized by raised parallel longitudinal ridges about 2 or 3 mm in width and height (dog) visible on the serosal side. It is a compensatory (or adaptive) hypertrophy designed to provide sufficient force to expel the urine against some partial obstruction, most frequently the periurethral pressure of an enlarged canine prostate.

Two helminth parasites may inhabit the urinary bladder, *Capillaria plica* in cats and *Trichosomoides crassicaudata* in rats. These produce little or no pathologic effect. Certain schistosomes parasitize the vesicular veins, and their eggs may lead to granulomatous lesions in the wall of the urinary bladder.

NEOPLASMS

Papillomas of transitional epithelium are occasionally encountered in any species. They are characterized

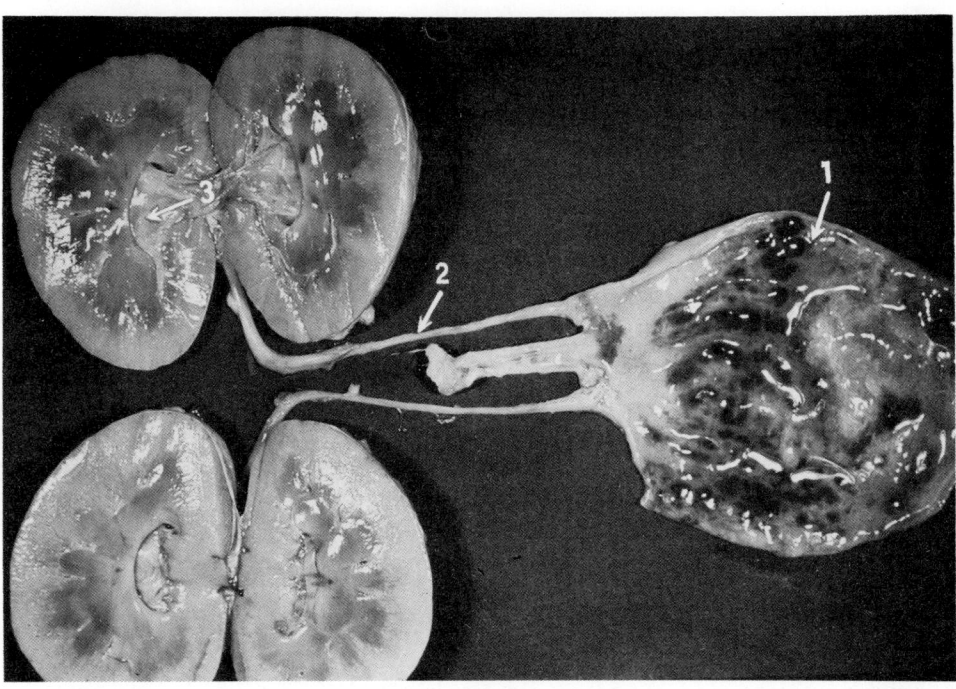

FIG. 24-28. Cystitis, ureteritis and pyelonephritis in a five-year-old male cat. The mucosa of the bladder (**1**) is replaced by hemorrhagic, purulent, and necrotic exudates. The ureters (**2**) and renal pelvis (**3**) were found to be similarly involved when examined microscopically. (Courtesy of Angell Memorial Animal Hospital.)

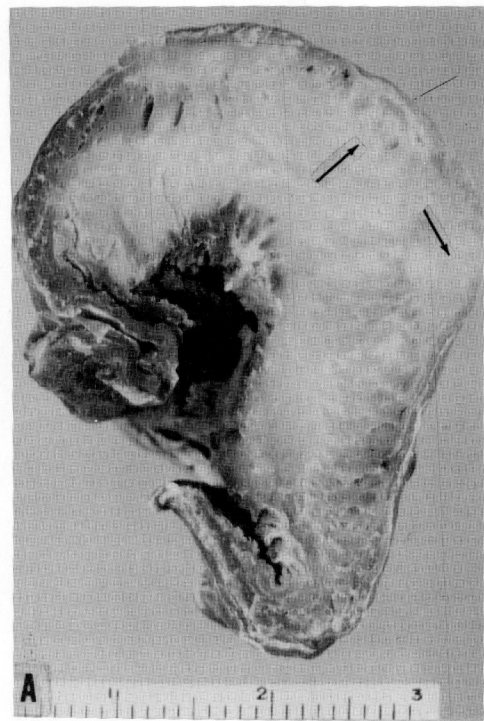
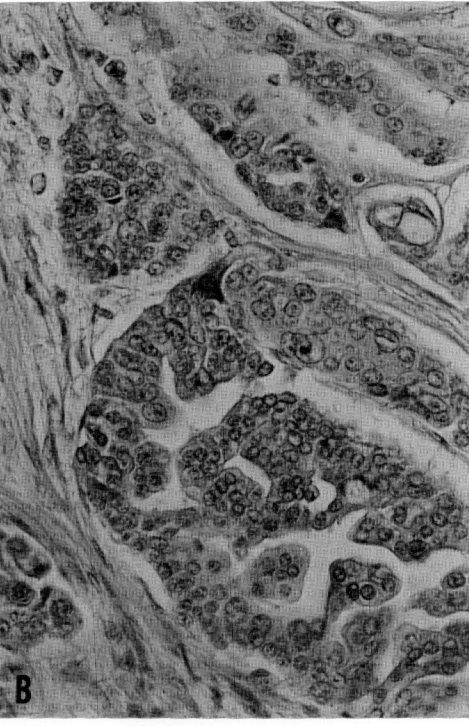

FIG. 24-29. Transitional and squamous-cell carcinoma of the epithelium of the urinary bladder of an 11-year-old male collie-shepherd dog. **A.** The tumor invades and replaces the mucosa as well as the muscular coat and elevates the serosa (arrows). **B.** Photomicrograph (× 305) of a part of the neoplasm in which transitional epithelium is simulated. In other areas squamous cells predominate. (Courtesy of Armed Forces Institute of Pathology and Dr. Leo L. Lieberman.

by numerous and long, stringy papillations which resemble the flower of a dahlia. They are most frequent in cattle as part of the disorder known as bovine enzootic hematuria.

Carcinomas of the urinary bladder may be transitional cell carcinomas, squamous cell carcinomas, or adenocarcinomas (Fig. 24-29). Transitional cell tumors are more frequent, and histologically, may be solid or papillary. They may be sufficiently well differentiated to resemble transitional epithelium, or they may be highly anaplastic with little resemblance to the cells from which they arose. Squamous cell carcinomas and adenocarcinomas, which may secrete mucin, arise in metaplastic epithelium. The cause of the metaplasia is often unknown, but usually ascribed to chronic cystitis or toxicity, such as in bovine enzootic hematuria (Fig. 24-30).

Mesenchymal neoplasms are not common although leiomyomas, leiomyosarcomas, and rhabdomyosarcomas are seen occasionally in dogs.

Metastatic neoplasms, especially malignant lymphomas, may infiltrate the wall of the bladder, usually the submucosa or subserosa. The result is a series of diffuse or nodular thickenings consisting of smoothly homogeneous, white tissue.

Experimentally, papillomas and papillary carcinomas have been produced in the dog's bladder by prolonged administration (over several years) of such compounds as beta-naphthylamine. This was done primarily in connection with the study of certain "aniline tumors" which have developed in people working in aniline industries. There appears, however, to be nothing in the dog's bladder comparable to the human neoplasms which develop in connection with schistosomiasis.

Urethra

The urethra almost never suffers from more than very transient inflammation as long as there is no interference with the drainage of urine. The passing of a catheter usually causes mild injury and inflammation which remains painful for a few days, especially in males. The principal lesion encountered in this organ is the lodgment of calculi. This is especially likely to occur at the sigmoid flexure in male ruminants. There is always a variable degree of hyperemia and inflammation at and above the site of lodgment, none below it. There are in animals no specific infections with a predilection for the urethra, such as gonorrheal infection in the human. The mucosa and probably its tributary glands appear to harbor such organisms as *Tritrochomonas foetus* in the bull, but the condition represents more a symbiosis than a pathogenesis as far as the urethra itself and its glands are concerned. A bull so infected may, however, be a source of contagion to the female, in which the infection is a cause of sterility.

Diverticula (in the female especially) and strictures (in the male chiefly) occur rarely in the urethra, being either congenital or the result of injury by stones, catheters, or compressing injuries from the outside. As in other tubular organs, a dilatation may form above a stricture as the result of pressure of accumulated fluid. The effect of obstruction in the urethra (as elsewhere) in causing hydronephrosis has been discussed.

Obstruction of the urethra of the male cat is a common clinical problem, especially in castrated males. Although uroliths are sometimes demonstrated, in many cases inflammation of the urethra appears to be the underlying factor in the obstruction. Some evidence indicates that a picornavirus may be involved.

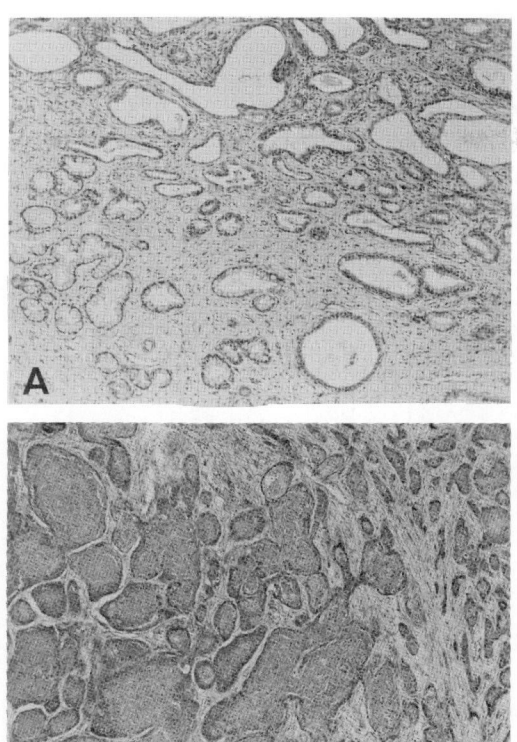

FIG. 24-30. Bovine enzootic hematuria. Mucinous adenocarcinoma, **A.** and squamous cell carcinoma, **B.** of urinary bladder. (Courtesy of Armed Forces Institute of pathology.)

Fistulas

Fistulous tracts can be established between adjacent pelvic organs as a result of necrotizing processes, especially if these are preceded by adhesions between the two surfaces concerned. While all such openings are rare in the domestic animals, it is possible for the rectum to become inflamed and adherent where it passes the bladder and for continuing destruction to lead to perforation into the bladder. Possible causes are trauma from foreign objects, usually surgical, caustic medicaments locally applied, cystic calculi, invasive neoplasms, and some others, conceivably including lesions produced by nodular worms (*Oesophagostomum sp.*).

Rectovaginal fistulas are more frequent than the rectovesical just described. They arise from similar causes and also are at times congenital. The vesicovaginal fistula, rather common in humans, does not occur in the domestic animals to any appreciable extent, since the walls of the two organs are not contiguous as in the human female.

Bovine enzootic hematuria

Reported only from certain sharply limited regions of the world, especially the northwestern United States, western Canada, Japan, New Zealand, and the Black Sea regions of Turkey, Bulgaria, and Yugoslavia, bovine enzootic hematuria is a disease of adult cattle and also water buffalo characterized by persistent hematuria leading to (chronic hemorrhagic) anemia and death. The lesions, which arise most frequently in the bladder, but also occasionally in the ureters or renal pelvis, appear to represent a chronic but violently hyperplastic inflammation with severe hyperemia and recurrent hemorrhage. There is localized proliferation of epithelium with metaplasia either to mucin-forming columnar or to stratified squamous types or a mixture of the two. In certain cases, the hyperplastic epithelium acquires neoplastic properties, developing into a carcinoma (either squamous-cell or adenocarcinoma) which is locally invasive and may metastasize to the regional lymph nodes and the lungs. The capillaries of the inflammatory lesion also participate in the hyperplastic proliferation, sometimes to the extent of forming hemangiomas either in the stroma or projecting from the mucosal surface, and are capable, in themselves, of developing malignant qualities. Two or more different types of neoplasms may be encountered in a given animal. The etiology appears to be well established as one long term effect of poisoning due to bracken fern.

An **epizootic cystitis** in horses has been described in the southwestern United States and Australia. It has been associated with grazing on Sudan or hybrid Sudan grass.

References

Alroy J. Ultrastructure of canine urinary bladder carcinoma. Vet Pathol 1979;16:693–701.

Alroy J, Teramura K, Miller AW III, et al. Isoantigens A, B, and H in urinary bladder carcinomas following radiotherapy. Cancer 1978;41:1739–1745.

Alroy J, Weinstein RS. Intraepithelial asymmetric-unit-membrane plaques in mammalian urinary bladder. Anat Rec 1980;197:75–83.

Brearley MJ, Thatcher C, Cooper JE. Three cases of transitional cell carcinoma in the cat and a review of the literature. Vet Rec 1986;118:91–94.

Lage AL, Gillett NA, Gerlach RF, et al. The prevalence and distribution of proliferative and metaplastic changes in normal appearing canine bladders. J Urol 1989;141:993–997.

Nikula KJ, Benjamin SA, Angleton GM, et al. Transitional cell carcinomas of the urinary tract in a colony of beagle dogs. Vet Pathol 1989;26:455–461.

Pletcher JM, Dalton L. Botryoid rhabdomyosarcoma in the urinary bladder of a dog. Vet Pathol 1981;18:695–697.

Schmidt RE. Transitional cell carcinoma metastatic to the eye of a dog. Vet Pathol 1981;18:832–834.

Trahan CJ, Mitchell WC. Spontaneous transitional cell carcinoma in the urinary bladder of a strain 13 guinea pig. Lab Anim Sci 1986;36:691–693.

25

Genital system

EMBRYOLOGY

During early embryonic development, primitive structures that will become the gonads and other portions of the genital tracts of male and female embryos are morphologically identical. This period is referred to as the indifferent stage of sexual development. At this stage, germ cells, which arise earlier from the endoderm of the yolk sac of the embryo, have migrated to bilateral swellings of pelvic mesoderm (genital ridges) overlying the mesonephroi (primitive kidneys) to form paired bipotential gonads. At about this time, small, mesonephric tubules from the mesonephroi also grow caudally and fuse to form a pair of ducts referred to as the mesonephric (Wolffian) ducts. These continue to grow caudally and eventually fuse with the urogenital sinus. Shortly thereafter, a second pair of ducts, the paramesonephric (müllerian) ducts, emerge from folds in the genital ridges, migrate caudally along the walls of the mesonephric ducts—presumably through some inductive influence of the latter—and fuse for varying lengths along the caudal segment (depending upon the species) before merging with the urogenital sinus.

The next critical stage of genital development involves differentiation of the bipotential gonads into testicles or ovaries. Upon entering the genital ridges after migrating from the yolk sac, the primitive germ cells increase in number by mitosis in the superficial mesenchyme of the bipotential gonads. During this period of active proliferation, the germ cells lose their mobility and become somewhat smaller and thus are transformed into oogonia or spermatogonia. The ridges are covered by a prominent, multilayered coelomic epithelium. Gonadal differentiation is determined genetically and involves the expression, or lack thereof, of a gene normally found on the Y chromosome of the male. This gene is referred to as the SRY gene or "sex determining region of the Y chromosome" and codes for a protein referred to as TDF or "testicular determining factor." In the bipotential gonad, long cordlike masses of coelomic epithelial cells proliferate and burrow radially into the underlying mesenchyme to form primary sex cords. The tips of these cords eventually converge at the center of the gonad to form the rete cords and eventually the rete testis in males and rete ova-

rii in females. In males, the outer portions of the primary sex cords become more compact and prominent to form the primitive seminiferous tubules, whereas in females the outer segments remain relatively undeveloped or regress.

In both sexes, primitive germ cells migrate into the outer mesenchyme between the primary sex cords where they lose their mobility and become smaller, but continue to undergo mitotic division as oogonia. At this stage the number of oogonia in the female greatly exceeds that of the number of spermatogonia in the male; however, this discrepancy is more than compensated for at sexual maturity in postnatal life. At this point the bipotential gonad actually resembles a testicle more than an ovary. Shortly thereafter, however, the coelomic epithelium at the surface of the gonad begins another wave of proliferation and becomes thicker to form a highly cellular outer cortical layer. In males, spermatogonia in this outer cortical region degenerate and the thickened coelomic epithelium eventually becomes transformed into the tunica albuginea, whereas in females the oogonia persist in this zone and continue to divide, eventually becoming the cortex of the fetal ovary. The transformation of this outer layer to the tunica albuginea appears to be a critical event in the formation of a testicle. Subsequently in males, the spermatogonia infiltrate the primitive seminiferous tubules, where they continue to divide mitotically until eventually becoming arrested in the interphase of mitosis where they persist until sexual maturity. The cells comprising these outer segments of the primary sex cords then differentiate into Sertoli cells. The mesenchymal cells surrounding the seminiferous tubules undergo marked hypertrophy to become the interstitial (Leydig) cells of the testicle. At this stage, the interstitial cells comprise a large proportion of the embryonic testicle.

The bipotential gonads of embryos not having the SRY gene (i.e., females with XX genotype) automatically differentiate into ovaries. Ovarian differentiation occurs somewhat later in gestation than that of the testicles and is histologically less striking. This differentiation is not preceded by an accentuation of the outer segments of the primary sex cords as occurs in the testicle to become seminiferous tubules but, instead, by a diminution in the size of these structures referred to in the female as medullary cords.

In females, extensive proliferation of small cells occurs in the outer cortex of the gonad that differentiate from the overlying coelomic epithelium. These cells, which are analogous to those destined to become the tunica albuginea in males, are referred to in females as pregranulosa cells. They comprise a large part of the growing fetal ovary and extend into the underlying mesenchyme as broad masses or clusters separated by thin septa of mesenchyme. As they expand into the deeper portions of the gonad, these cells encapsulate individual and small nests of oogonia. These masses eventually break into smaller nests by outgrowth of mesenchyme tissue (stroma) from the hilum and become the primordial follicles of the ovary. Oogonia that fail to become encapsulated by pregranulosa cells degenerate, particularly those in the medulla of the ovary, whereas those in the cortex persist as primary follicles. Oogonia continue to undergo mitosis until sometime between the midpoint of gestation and the first few weeks of postnatal life, depending upon the species. Once mitotic activity ceases permanently, oogonia enter the first phase (prophase) of meiosis to become oocytes. They remain arrested in this stage of meiosis until postnatal sexual maturity when, with each estrus cycle, a few oocytes complete the first meiotic division to become gametes with the haploid number of chromosomes.

The remaining events in sexual differentiation involving development of the internal and external genital organs are determined by hormonal factors secreted by embryonic gonads. Most evidence suggests that the onset of secretion of hormones by early testicles and ovaries is an autonomous event, whereas later in embryonic development gonadal hormone production is gonadotropin-dependent: chorionic gonadotropin in primates, pregnant mare serum in horses, and luteinizing hormone (LH) or interstitial cell stimulating hormone (ICSH) in other species. In male embryos, Sertoli cells secrete a glycoprotein known as "müllerian inhibitory substance" (MIS) which causes regression of the paramesonephric ducts.

In females, paramesonephric ducts persist and under the influence of estrogen become fully developed uterine tubes, uterus, cervix, and cranial portion of the vagina. In males, gonadectomized before testicular development or males with dysplastic testicles lacking normal Sertoli cell function, the paramesonephric ducts also persist, but as rudimentary female genital organs. In normal males, testosterone secreted by markedly hyperplastic interstitial (Leydig) cells of the embryonic testes induces differentiation of the mesonephric ducts into the epididymides, vas deferens, prostate, seminal vesicles, and bulbourethral glands. It should be noted that carnivores and certain nonhuman primate species (*Daubentonia, Callicebus,* and *Pithecia*) do not develop seminal vesicles, and dogs lack bulbourethral glands.

Later in gestation, fetal interstitial cells undergo physiologic atrophy until sexual maturity in postnatal life when they once again become functional. The ex-

ternal genitalia of males, (penis, prepuce, scrotum) develop from the urogenital sinus, genital tubercle, urethral folds, and labioscrotal swellings, respectively. This event is mediated by 5α-dihydrotestosterone (5α-DHT) rather than by testosterone. The precursor tissues of these organs contain the enzyme, 5α-reductase which converts circulating testosterone to 5α-DHT, which then binds to nuclear receptors in these tissues and causes masculine differentiation. In normal females, the paramesonephric ducts persist in the absence of MIS and become the uterine tubes, uterus, cervix, and cranial portion of the vagina. The caudal segment of vagina and vestibule develop from the urogenital sinus and the vulva from the labioscrotal swellings. This occurs passively in the absence of circulating testosterone because these tissues in females also contain the enzyme, 5α-DHT. With the onset of sexual maturity, the internal and external genitalia of both sexes undergo further growth and development leading to reproductively-competent genital tracts. These final stages of development are largely sex-hormone-dependent.

References

Austin CR, Edwards RG. Mechanisms of sex differentiation in animals and man. New York: Academic Press, 1981.

Bardin CW, Catterall JF. Testosterone: a major determinant of extragenital sexual dimorphism. Science 1981;211:1285–1294.

Byskov AG. Differentiation of mammalian embryonic gonad. Physiol Rev 1986;66:100–147.

Donahue PK, Ito Y, Price JM, Hendren WH. Müllerian-inhibiting activity in bovine fetal, newborn and prepubertal testes. Biol Reprod 1977;16:238–243.

Gier HT, Marion GB. Development of mammalian testes and genital ducts. Biol Reprod Suppl 1969;1:1–23.

Gillman J. The development of the gonads in man, with a consideration of the role of fetal endocrines and the histogenesis of ovarian tumors. Contrib Embryol 1948;32:81–131.

Gordon JW, Ruddle FH. Mammalian gonadal determination and gametogenesis. Science 1981;211:1265–1271.

Gruenwald P. The relation of the growing müllerian duct to the wolffian duct and its importance for the genesis of malformations. Anat Rec 1941;81:1–19.

Gruenwald P. Growth and development of the uterus: the relations of epithelium to mesenchyma. Ann NY Acad Sci 1959;75:436–440.

Haseltine FP, Ohno S. Mechanisms of gonadal differentiation. Science 1981;211:1272–1278.

Johnson CA. The role of the fetal testicle in sexual differentiation. Compend Contin Educ Pract Vet 1983;5:129–132.

Jost A, Vigier B, Prepin J, et al. Studies on sex differentiation in mammals. Recent Prog Horm Res 1973;29:1–35.

Narbaitz R. Embryology, anatomy and histology of the male sex accessory glands. In: Brandes D, ed. Male accessory sex organs. New York: Academic Press, 1974;3–14.

Wilson JD, George FW, Griffin JE. The hormonal control of sexual development. Science 1981;211:1278–1284.

Witchi E. Migration of the germ cells of human embryos from the yolk sac to the primitive gonadal folds. Contrib Embryol 1948;32:67–80.

Witchi E. Embryology of the uterus: normal and experimental. Ann NY Acad Sci 1959;75:412–435.

AMBIGUOUS SEXUAL DIFFERENTIATION

Intersex

This term denotes those developmental abnormalities in which discordance exists between the genetic, gonadal, and/or phenotypic sex; it includes true hermaphrodites, pseudohermaphrodites, and other forms of sex reversal.

True hermaphrodites

True hermaphrodites have both ovarian and testicular tissue either in the form of a combined gonad (**ovotestis**) or as separate organs. True hermaphroditism has been reported in most domestic animal species, but occurs most often in swine and goats. The majority of true hermaphrodites have the XX female genotype, but are positive for the H-Y antigen, a minor histocompatibility antigen normally coded for by a gene located on the Y chromosome of males. Depending upon the nature and location of the gonads, true hermaphrodites are referred to as bilateral (testis and ovary or an ovotestis on each side; Fig. 25-1); unilateral (ovotestis on one side and ovary or testis on the opposite side); or lateral (testis on one side and an ovary on the other). The external genitalia of true hermaphrodites are often ambiguous and exhibit varying degrees of male and female differentiation.

True hermaphrodites with bilateral ovotestes usually have a normal appearing, but hypoplastic, uterus indicating that ovotestes do not secrete adequate quantities of MIS to cause inhibition of paramesonephric duct development. In contrast, unilateral and lateral true hermaphrodites usually lack a uterine tube and horn on the side adjacent to the testis. Varying degrees of development may occur in the epididymis and vas deferens and enlargement of the clitoris in phenotypic female

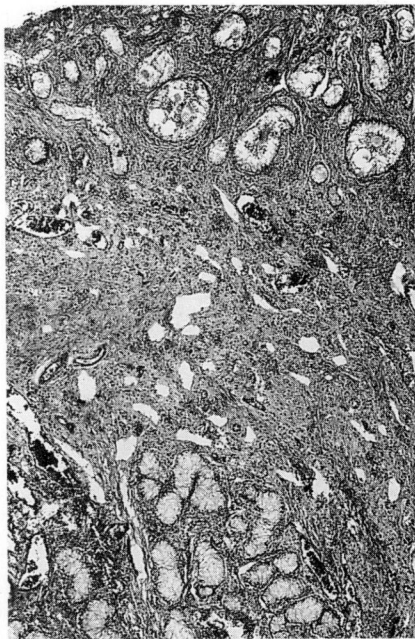

FIG. 25-1 Photomicrograph of a portion of an ovotestis from a canine true hermaphrodite. The cortex (top) consists of ovarian stroma and follicles containing oocytes, whereas the medulla (bottom) contains hypoplastic seminiferous tubules separated by interstitial cells (×100).

true hermaphrodites, indicating that some level of testosterone is produced by these individuals. The gonads of true hermaphrodites are usually retained in the pelvic cavity.

Microscopically, the testicular portion of an ovotestis is always located in the medulla of the gonad, whereas the ovarian portion comprises the cortex. The testicular portion consists of hypoplastic seminiferous tubules lined by Sertoli cells and rare, if any, germ cells. Whether the absence of germ cells is due to hyperthermia from the pelvic location of the ovotestis, or to failure of germ cells to populate the primitive seminiferous tubules during testicular differentiation has not been resolved. Rete tubules are common in the hilar region of ovotestes. Interstitial cells are generally present between the hypoplastic seminiferous tubules. The ovarian portion of an ovotestis contains oogonia, oocytes, and primary and secondary follicles. On rare occasions, true hermaphrodites ovulate and become pregnant.

Pseudohermaphrodites

In contrast to true hermaphrodites, pseudohermaphrodites have the gonads of only one sex, either testes or ovaries, but the external genitalia have features of the opposite sex. They are classified as male or female depending upon the type of gonad present. Several types of pseudohermaphrodites have been described in humans and animals. These include:

XX sex reversal, a form of intersex in which discordance exists between the sex chromosomal composition of the individual and the gonadal and external phenotype. It has been described in an inbred strain of mice (sex reversal gene strain; defined below) where it has been best studied, as well as in dogs, pigs, and goats.

Mice with this disorder develop testicles, male internal genitalia, and exhibit varying degrees of masculinization of external genitalia. It is due to a gene referred to as the **sex reversal gene** (sxr), that is present on the Y chromosome of male sxr mice. These carrier males have abnormal Y chromosomes in which duplication of the sex-determining region occurs (i.e., SRY gene that codes for the protein, testicular determining factor (TDF)). One copy of the SRY gene is frequently translocated from the Y chromosome to the male's own X chromosome during meiosis, or to an autosome during embryogenesis. This has led to its designation as the "sex reversal" or sxr gene. When it is translocated to the male's X chromosome, the condition is transmitted as an X-linked trait, whereas when an autosome is involved it is transmitted as an autosomal-dominant condition. The XX offspring, thus, will develop testicles and a male phenotype because of the presence of the sxr gene on the paternally-derived X chromosome or autosome which produces a product similar, if not identical, to testicular-determining factor (TDF).

The majority of **goats** with sex reversal are male pseudohermaphrodites with XX karyotypes, although some may be true hermaphrodites. The condition in this species has been associated with hornlessness (polledness). In affected goats, a gene that codes for a protein having the effect of TDF is located on an autosome near or linked to the gene for polledness. The gene for polledness is a dominant trait which, in heterozygotes (Pp), produces hornlessness with no effect on sexual differentiation, but in the homozygous state (PP) renders XX carriers hermaphrodites or pseudohermaphrodites. These carriers have testes or ovotestes and exhibit varying degrees of masculinization of the female external genitalia, including clitoromegaly.

In **dogs,** sex reversal occurs most often in the American cocker spaniel breed. These animals have an XX genotype and the sxr gene is located on an autosome. Affected animals may be male pseudohermaphrodites or true hermaphrodites. In both cases the testes or ovotestes are retained within the abdomen and components of the müllerian ducts (uterine tubes and uterus) are often present. Both forms are positive for H-Y antigen. Some true hermaphrodites have functional ovarian tissue in their ovotestes and have given birth to pups with the sxr gene on an autosome. The gene is inherited as an autosomal-recessive trait. The testicular component of pseudohermaphrodites and true hermaphrodites lack germ cells.

XY Gonadal dysgenesis (testicular feminization syndrome; androgen insensitivity)

This condition is a form of male pseudohermaphroditism that is inherited as an X-linked disorder. It has been described in humans, mice, rats, cattle, and horses. Those affected always have the XY genotype and either normal or elevated levels of circulating testosterone. Phenotypically, an individual with this disorder has female external genitalia, a vagina that ends as a blind sac, and no evidence of müllerian-derived internal genitalia. These individuals also either lack or have poorly developed male wolffian-derived structures. The gonads are invariably retained and are clearly testicles. Microscopically, the seminiferous tubules lack germ cells and are lined by a pure population of Sertoli cells. The interstitium of the testicles contains prominent androgen-secreting interstitial cells consistent with normal or elevated, circulating testosterone levels. The lack of müllerian-derived structures internally indicates that the Sertoli cells secreted MIS during embryologic development. The genetic defect in this disorder is either an overall systemic deficiency of, or mutations in, the genes for androgen receptors leading to ineffectiveness. This results in a lack of male differentiation of both internal and external genitalia despite adequate levels of androgens secreted by the testicular interstitial cells.

XY Pseudohermaphrodite syndrome of miniature schnauzers

Unlike male pseudohermaphrodites with androgen insensitivity, dogs with this disorder have male external genitalia, although the penis and prepuce are often hypoplastic. These dogs have retained testes with epididy-mides and vas deferentia, and a normally-formed, albeit hypoplastic, uterus. The cryptorchid testes of these animals, because of their intraabdominal location, are prone to Sertoli cell tumor development, approximately 25% of which become functional and secrete estrogens. The endometrium of the residual uterus often undergoes hyperplasia/mucometra of the estrogen-induced type (see Endometrial Hyperplasia).

The hormonal defect in dogs with this condition has not been determined; however, from the composition of the internal and external genitalia, the defect would appear to involve a deficiency of MIS secretion or a lack of responsiveness of the paramesonephric ducts to the MIS protein being secreted by the Sertoli cells during embryonic development. The presence of epididymides and vas deferentia indicates that testosterone is secreted in sufficient amounts to cause development of the wolffian duct system and because the external genitalia are male there would appear to be adequate quantities of androgen receptors and 5α-reductase activity in the anlage of the external genitalia to achieve masculinization of these structures.

Hormone-induced intersexuality

The administration of androgens and many progestins to pregnant individuals induces masculinization of the genital tract of female offspring of rats, mice, guinea pigs, rabbits, cattle, sheep, dogs, monkeys, and women. These individuals are female pseudohermaphrodites with XX genotype, ovaries, but varying degrees of masculinization of the internal and external genitalia. Conversely, the internal and external genitalia of male rat fetuses can be feminized by the administration of estrogens, certain progestins and antiandrogenic drugs. The extent of genital tract masculinization depends on the stage of development of the genital tract of the fetus at the time of administration of androgen or progestin, as well as the potency of the drug. If androgen is potent enough, the resultant female pseudohermaphrodites will have structures derived from the wolffian ducts if the drug is administered prior to normal regression of these structures. Similarly, the degree of virilization of the external genitalia also depends on the strength of androgen and the stage of development of these structures at fetal exposure.

References

Bardin CW, Bullock LP. Testicular feminization: studies of the molecular basis of a genetic defect. J Invest Dermatol 1974;63:75–84.

Bardin CW, Bullock LP, Sherins RJ, et al. Androgen metabolism and mechanisms of action in male pseudohermaphroditism: a study of testicular feminization. Recent Prog Horm Res 1973;29:65–105.

Benirschke K. Hermaphrodites, freemartins, mosaics and chimaeras in animals. In: Austin CR, Edwards RG, eds. Mechanisms of sex differentiation in animals and man. New York: Academic Press, 1981;421–463.

Brown TT, Burek JD, McEntee K. Male pseudohermaphroditism, cryptorchidism and Sertoli cell neoplasia in three miniature schnauzers. J Am Vet Med Assoc 1976;169:821–825.

Bullock LP, Bardin CW. Androgen receptors in testicular feminization. J Clin Endocrinol Metab 1972;35:935–937.

Curtis EM, Grant RP. Masculinization of female pups by progestogens. J Am Vet Med Assoc 1964;144:395–398.

Eaton ON. The relation between polled and hermaphrodite characters in dairy goats. Genetics 1945;30:51–61.

Lyons MF, Hawkes GS. X-linked gene for testicular feminization in the mouse. Nature 1970;227:1217–1219.

Marshall LS, Oehlert ML, Haskins ME, et al. Persistent müllerian duct syndrome in miniature schnauzers. J Am Vet Med Assoc 1982; 181:798–801.

McEntee K. Reproductive pathology of domestic mammals. New York: Academic Press, 1990.

Myers-Wallen VN, Donahoe PK, Manganaro T, et al. Müllerian inhibiting substance in sex-reversed dogs. Biol Reprod 1987;37:1015–1022.

Myers-Wallen VN, et al. Testicular feminization in a cat. J Am Vet Med Assoc 1989;195:631–634.

Okon E, et al. Male pseudohermaphroditism due to 5–reductase deficiency. Ultrastructure of the gonads. Arch Pathol Lab Med 1980;104:363–367.

Power MM. XY sex reversal in a mare. Equine Vet J 1986;18:233–236.

Reinboth R. Intersexuality in the animal kingdom. Berlin: Springer-Verlag, 1975.

Seldon JR, Wachtel SS, Koo GC, et al. Inherited XX sex reversal in the cocker spaniel dog. Hum Genet 1984;67:62–69.

Thuline HC. Male tortoiseshells, chimerism and true hermaphroditism. J Cat Genet 1964;1:2–3.

Williams G, Gordon I, Edwards J. Observations on the frequency of fused foetal circulations in twin-bearing cattle. Br Vet J 1963;119:467–472.

Winter H, Pfeffer A. Pathogenetic classification of intersex. Vet Rec 1977;100:307–310.

REPRODUCTIVE CYCLE

The permanent pattern of postnatal pituitary gonadotropin secretion that determines the nature of gonadal hormone secretion is established in utero or, in some species, early in postnatal life. This process involves the action of testosterone secreted by testicular interstitial cells on the hypothalamus, a phenomenon known as masculine imprinting. In both sexes, neurons in the hypothalamus secrete a small polypeptide hormone known as **gonadotrophin-releasing hormone (GnRH)** that is responsible for release of **follicle-stimulating hormone (FSH)** and **luteinizing hormone (LH)** or in males **interstitial cell stimulating hormone (ICSH)** from the anterior pituitary (adenohypophysis). These neurons have axons that terminate in the median eminence of the hypothalamus located in the stalk of the pituitary gland (hypophysis) just above the anterior pituitary. GnRH is secreted from these axons directly into vessels in the stalk that supply the anterior pituitary. This vascular arrangement is known as the **hypothalamic-hypophyseal portal system.** In males during this critical period of reproductive development, testosterone in the general circulation causes these neurons to release GnRH in a continuous, noncyclic pattern into the portal system, thereby causing the adenohypophysis to secrete FSH and LH (or ICSH) in a continuous, noncyclic pattern. Female embryos exposed experimentally or inadvertently to testosterone during this critical period will also develop a permanent, noncyclic pattern of GnRH secretion after sexual maturity. In contrast, in the absence of testosterone secretion during this period (i.e., as occurs normally in female embryos or in males

orchiectomized prior to this period), GnRH secretion at sexual maturity occurs in a cyclic pattern that is mediated through positive and negative feedback loops by hormones from the ovary. This results in an **estrous cycle.**

The duration of estrous cycles varies markedly between species from only a few days in rodents to six months or a year in dogs. Moreover, some species cycle year-round, while others (cat, ewe, and mare) do so only during certain seasons (**seasonal polyestrus**). The period of ovarian inactivity between these seasons is referred to as **anestrus.** In these species, **melatonin** secreted by the pineal gland in response to changes in environmental lighting conditions regulates GnRH release thereby imposing seasonality to the reproductive cycle. With the exception of higher primates, including humans, most animals cycle throughout the entire lifespan.

In females, FSH stimulates follicle growth and development during the period of the cycle known as **proestrus,** whereas in males its noncyclic secretion induces maturation of spermatogonia through the secondary spermatocyte stage of spermatogenesis. As they grow under the influence of FSH, ovarian follicles begin to secrete a protein hormone known as **inhibin,** which feeds back on the pituitary to suppress FSH secretion. LH induces the theca cells of the ovarian follicle to convert cholesterol to androgens which, in turn, diffuse into the granulosa cells where they are converted to **estrogens** by the enzyme, aromatase. In males, LH is required for completion of the latter stages of spermatogenesis (maturation of secondary spermatocytes to spermatozoa). Estrogen from the maturing follicles stimulates mitotic activity of the endometrial glands and stroma and increases the concentration of progesterone receptors in the endometrium, an effect known as **estrogen priming.** Estrogen also feeds back on the pituitary to increase LH secretion. Both estrogen and FSH increase the number and concentration of LH receptors in the developing follicles making them more responsive to LH. This positive feed-back mechanism ultimately leads to a surge in LH secretion (LH peak) which results in maturation of the follicle and ovulation.

In most species, ovulation occurs 24–36 hours after LH peak. In other species (cat, rabbit, ferrets, mink, llama) ovulation is induced by cervical stimulation during coitus or by manual manipulation. Following ovulation, granulosa and theca cells lining the follicles undergo marked hypertrophy and hyperplasia to form coarse folds that fill the blood-filled lumen of the ruptured follicle (**corpus hemorrhagicum**). Vessels from the thecal layer rapidly grow into and vascularize the mass of proliferating cells to form the **corpus luteum** (CL). CL begins to secrete increasing amounts of **progesterone** under the influence of decreasing levels of LH. Increasing concentrations of progesterone feed back on the hypothalamus/pituitary to further decrease LH levels and this phase is referred to as **diestrus** or the **luteal phase** of the estrous cycle. Progesterone, acting on the estrogen-primed endometrium, stimulates secretion by the endometrial glands and prepares the uterus for implantation of the blastocyst(s) should fertilization of the ovulated oocyte(s) occur. When pregnancy does not ensue at the end of diestrus, the corpus luteum undergoes lysis and progesterone levels decline. In domestic ungulates (horses, cattle, sheep, goats, pigs), prostaglandin F2α (PGF2α) secreted by the endometrium in response to **oxytocin** secreted by the corpus luteum is responsible for luteolysis and initiation of a new cycle. In these species, PGF2α in the utero-ovarian veins diffuses by countercurrent flow into the adjacent ovarian artery and induces its effect on the corpus luteum. In dogs and cats, which have a long diestrus, lifespan of the corpus luteum is not regulated by PGF2α; the mechanism of luteolysis is not known.

PREGNANCY

Pregnancy interrupts the estrous cycle. Implantation of a blastocyst "rescues" the corpus luteum, allowing it to persist and function as the corpus luteum of pregnancy. In those species where PBF2α is responsible for luteolysis, during implantation the embryo produces protein hormones that block the release of PGF2α from the endometrium or diverts its secretion into the uterine lumen, thereby allowing the corpus luteum to persist. In dogs and cats, which have a long diestrus, the corpus luteum normally persists for almost the length of gestation; hence, rescue is probably not required. Progesterone is required in all species to maintain pregnancy. In some species the rescued corpus luteum secretes progesterone throughout gestation (dogs, cats, goats, swine), whereas in others (cows, mares), it is only secreted for a portion of gestation. In the latter species, progesterone secreted by the placenta is sufficient to maintain pregnancy to term. The syncytiotrophoblastic cells of the chorionic epithelium of the placenta secrete gonadotropins which have luteotropic activity that also assist in maintaining luteal function and pregnancy.

In mares, specialized trophoblastic cells from the chorionic girdle detach from the fetal membranes and invade the endometrium to form what are termed **endometrial cups.** Between days 40–120 of gestation, these structures produce **equine chorionic gonadotropin (eCG),** a substance formerly referred to as **pregnant mare serum gonadotrophin** (PMSG), that has marked LH-like activity (Fig. 25-2). Equine chorionic gonadotropin causes other follicles in the mare's ovary to ovulate and form secondary corpora lutea that assist with maintenance of pregnancy during this period. The endometrial cups degenerate after 120 days of gestation. Pregnancy terminates with **parturition,** during which the fetus(es) and placenta(e) are expelled from the uterus. Factors that initiate and promote parturition are best understood in ruminants; they do not apply to all species.

Adrenocorticotrophic hormone (ACTH) from the pituitary of the term ruminant fetus stimulates the fetal adrenal cortex to secrete a burst of cortisol. This does not occur in equine fetuses. Cortisol, in turn, acts on the placenta to induce enzymes that convert placental progesterone to estrogens. This lowered progesterone

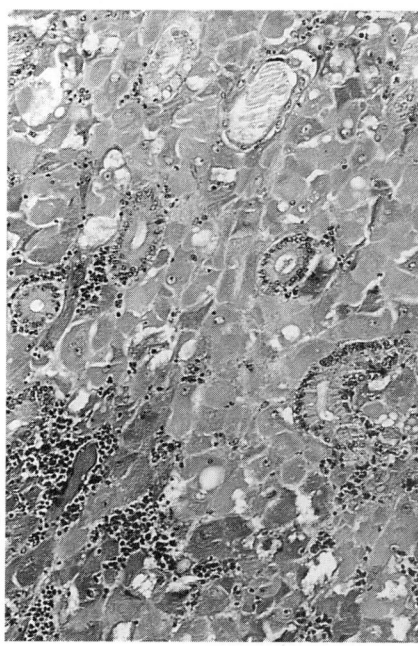

FIG. 25-2 Photomicrograph of a portion of an endometrial cup from a mare at 100 days of gestation. Specialized trophoblastic cells are the source of equine chorionic gonadotropin (eCG), formerly termed pregnant mare serum gonadotropin (PMSG). Note the lymphocytes scattered throughout this tissue which may be responsible for regression at 120 days of gestation (×250).

and elevated estrogen status causes decreased degradation and increased synthesis of PGF2α resulting in elevated levels of PGF2α, increased myometrial tone, and contractility and relaxation of the closed cervix. PGF2α also stimulates the corpus luteum of the cow and placenta of the mare to secrete another hormone, relaxin, which further relaxes the cervix. The elevated levels of estrogen also increase oxytocin receptors in the myometrium. Together, the combination of PGF2α, estrogen, and increased oxytocin activity initiates uterine contractions (labor). As the fetus is forced against the internal os of the cervix, nerve impulses transmitted from this site to the pituitary (Ferguson's reflex) initiate a burst of oxytocin release that intensifies uterine contractions. Finally, the presence of the fetus in the birth canal causes the dam (by spinal reflex), to have forced abdominal contractions that aid in expulsion of the fetus and fetal membranes.

OVARY

Abnormalities of gonadal development

Abnormalities of gonadal development occur infrequently in domestic and laboratory animals. They may be caused by genetic, chromosomal, or hormonal abnormalities, or be unexplained. Such abnormalities may affect one or both gonads and be associated with abnormalities of all or only a portion of the internal and external genitalia, or combinations thereof. These conditions can be divided into three basic categories: gonadal hypoplasia, gonadal dysgenesis, and intersex.

HEREDITARY GONADAL HYPOPLASIA

Hereditary gonadal hypoplasia has been studied most extensively in the Swedish Highland breed of cattle where it affects the gonads of both sexes. It occurs as an autosomal-recessive trait with incomplete penetrance. The condition affects the left gonad of both sexes more often than the right; bilateral involvement is uncommon. The **ovaries** of cattle with this condition have been categorized into three pathologic types depending on the severity and distribution of the germ cell hypoplasia: total, partial, and transitional hypoplasia. Ovaries with **total hypoplasia** (Fig. 25-3) are smaller than normal, fusiform, and have longitudinal grooves on their surfaces.

Microscopically, the ovaries of animals with this form are devoid of germ cells from birth. When both ovaries are equally affected, heifers have infantile uteri and mammary glands. Ovaries with **partial hypoplasia** are small, wrinkled, and lack germ cells and follicles at the uterine extremity of the ovary, but contain these structures as well as corpora lutea at the tubal extremity. Ovaries with transitional hypoplasia are more difficult to recognize grossly because they have smooth surfaces with follicles and corpora lutea protruding from their surfaces. The major difference is their dimensions, which are smaller than a normal ovary of the same age. Other microscopic features that distinguish hypoplastic ovaries from normal ovaries include the presence of increased numbers of anovular cords and follicles, and increased numbers of medullary cords surrounded by connective

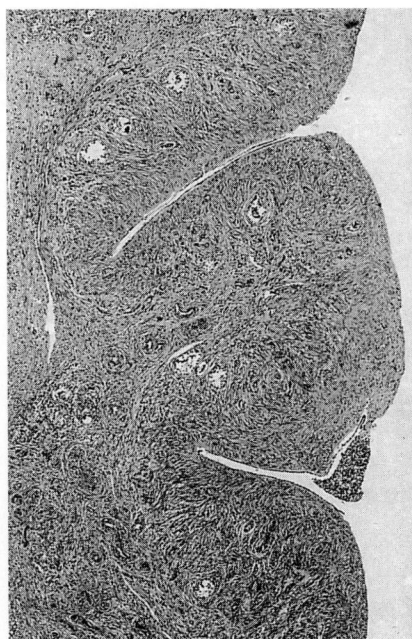

FIG. 25-3 Photomicrograph of the hypoplastic ovary of a calf with congenital gonadal hypoplasia. Note the absence of: germ cells; scattered, small, anovular follicles; and grooved surface of this hypoplastic ovary (×75).

tissue. A similar condition has been seen rarely in other European breeds and zebu cattle.

GONADAL DYSGENESIS

This encompasses conditions in which defective development of the gonads, either male or female, occurs. Some of these conditions have been associated with chromosomal abnormalities, others have not. Those conditions associated with chromosomal abnormalities include:

XO GONADAL DYSGENESIS IN MARES

This condition, analogous to Turner syndrome in women, affects the ovaries and genital organs of mares. It has been described in a number of breeds, including the thoroughbred, standardbred, Arabian, appaloosa, Belgian, and quarter horses, as well as in ponies. The karyotype of affected mares is 63XO, denoting lack of a second X (female) chromosome. Affected mares are sterile, exhibit no signs of estrus, have flaccid, open cervices, hypoplastic uteri, small, smooth ovaries, and smaller than normal vulvas. Microscopically, the ovaries consist predominantly of ovarian stroma containing only a few degenerate germ cells and follicles. An identical syndrome has also been described in mares in which the short arm of the X chromosome is missing.

In addition to mares, XO karyotype with ovarian dysgenesis has also been described in women (Turner syndrome), pigs, cats, rhesus monkeys, and mice. The ovaries of women with Turner syndrome appear as pale, glistening, flat, firm streaks of tissue in the broad ligament laying parallel to and below the uterine tubes. These dysgenetic ovaries are commonly referred to as "streak gonads."

Microscopically, streak gonads consist of solid masses of dense, connective tissue resembling ovarian stroma, but contain no germ cells or follicles. The ovaries of patients with Turner syndrome appear to develop normally until late in gestation when the oogonia and granulosa cells suddenly begin to degenerate. At birth, most, if not all, oogonia have disappeared leaving only the connective tissue stroma. Even though the second X chromosome in normal females is believed to be inactivated and appears in nuclei as the Barr body, the mechanism by which absence of a second X chromosome causes spontaneous degeneration of oogonia is not known.

Those forms of **gonadal dysgenesis** for which no chromosomal or genetic basis exists include:

FREEMARTINISM

Freemartinism is a form of ovarian dysgenesis that has been described only in ungulates. It occurs most often in cattle and is rare in sheep, goats, and swine. A freemartin is the sterile female co-twin of a set of heterosexual twins. The condition results from fusion of placental vessels and the sharing of blood between twins during early embryonic development; such twins are bone marrow chimeras. In cattle, placental anastomosis occurs in approximately 90% of twins, whereas in sheep, goats, and swine the frequency is < 2%. Current knowledge suggests that humoral substances from the blood of the male twin, especially testis-determining factor (TDF) and müllerian-inhibitory substance (MIS) and, to a lesser extent, testosterone are responsible for the ovarian and genital abnormalities that characterize a freemartin.

Phenotyically, freemartins usually have the external genitalia of a normal female with varying degrees of masculinization. They may have long tufts of hair that protrude from the ventral aspect of the vulva, clitoromegaly, and a fold of skin that extends from the groin to the umbilicus. A feature common to all freemartins is the presence of a blind-ended vestibule or vagina that lacks communication with the upper uterus no matter how well the latter is developed. This anomaly results from inhibition of fusion of the paramesonephric ducts with the urogenital sinus due to MIS secreted by the testis of the male twin. Uterine development varies considerably from cordlike remnants of the paramesonephric ducts without lumina to a well-developed uterus. In addition, all freemartins have rudimentary seminal vesicles that arise from vestiges of the male mesonephric duct system. The ovaries of freemartins also exhibit varying degrees of masculine differentiation, both grossly and microscopically. Partial development of the epididymis and vas deferens may occur. The gonads may actually descend through the inguinal canals into the subcutis of the groin in the absence of a scrotum. Microscopically, gonads of a freemartin consist of little more than gonadal stroma containing variable amounts of androgen-secreting interstitial cells and seminiferous cords containing only Sertoli cells. Such gonads lack germ cells.

References

Al-Dahash SYA, David JSE. The incidence of ovarian activity, pregnancy and bovine genital abnormalities shown by an abbatoir study. Vet Rec 1977;101:296–299.

Baylis MS, Wayne DM, Owen JB. An XO/XX mosaic sheep with associated gonadal dysgenesis. Res Vet Sci 1984;36:125–126.

Blue MG, Bruere AN, Dewes HF. The significance of the XO syndrome in infertility of the mare. NZ Vet J 1978;26:137–141.

Buoen LC, Eilts BE, Rushmer A, Weber AF. Sterility associated with an XO karyotype in a Belgian mare. J Am Vet Med Assoc 1983;182:1120–1121.

Chandley AC, et al. Chromosome abnormalities as a cause of infertility in mares. J Reprod Fertil Suppl 1975;23:377–383.

Hughes JP, Benirschke K, Kennedy PC, Trommerhausen-Smith A. Gonadal dysgenesis in the mare. J Reprod Fertil Suppl 1975;23:385–390.

Jones RE, ed. The vertebrate ovary: comparative biology and evolution. New York: Plenum Press, 1978.

Lagerlof N, Boyd H. Ovarian hypoplasia and other abnormal conditions in the sexual organs of cattle of the Swedish Highland breed: results of postmortem examination of over 6000 cows. Cornell Vet 1953;43:64–79.

Lagerlof N, Settergren I. Results of seventeen years' control of hereditary ovarian hypoplasia in cattle of the Swedish Highland breed. Cornell Vet 1953;43:52–64.

Mossman HW, Duke KL. Some comparative aspects of the mammalian ovary. In: Greep RO, Astweed EB, eds. Handbook of physiology. Vol II, Part I. Washington, DC: Am Physiol Soc, 1973;389–402.

Mossman HW, Duke KL. Comparative morphology of the mammalian ovary. Madison: U Wisconsin Press, 1973.

Settergren I. The ovarian morphology in clinical bovine gonadal hypoplasia with some aspects of its endocrine relations. Acta Vet Scand 1964;5(Suppl 1):1–108.

Settergren I, Galloway DB. Studies on the genital malformations in female cattle using slaughterhouse material. Nord Vet Med 1965;17:9–16.

Trommerhausen-Smith A, Hughes JP, Neely DP. Cytogenetic and clinical findings in mares with gonadal dysgenesis. J Reprod Fertil Suppl 1979;27:271–276.

Cysts in ovary and mesovarium

The ovaries and their surrounding supporting ligaments are common sites for the development of cysts of various kinds. Depending on their origin, they may or may not be of clinical significance. These include:

FOLLICULAR CYSTS

Follicular cysts (Fig. 25-4) arise from secondary (antral) follicles of the ovary that fail to ovulate, involute, or luteinize. They occur commonly in cattle and swine, less often in dogs and cats, rarely in sheep and goats, and almost never in mares. Failure of LH release during estrus is believed to be the cause. Because GnRH is effective in treating this condition and affected cows have heavily granulated gonadotrophs in their pituitaries, it is believed that failure of the hypothalamus to respond to positive feedback of increasing levels of circulating estrogens during early estrus may be the underlying basis for this condition.

Others have shown that follicular cysts can be induced by cortisol administration and have suggested that the stress of close confinement and high milk production may contribute to the lack of an LH surge. Follicular cysts are usually > 2.0 cm maximum diameter of a normal graafian follicle. They may secrete estrogens in a noncyclic pattern, presumably under the influence of continuous FSH stimulation, and be associated with continuous estrus or clinical signs of nymphomania. Affected individuals may develop cystic endometrial hyperplasia, hydrometra, or mucometra which, when prolonged, leads to atrophy of the endometrium and myometrium. Cows with chronic cystic follicles eventually undergo permanent anestrus, probably resulting from continuous secretion of progesterone or androgens which prevents GnRH release from the hypothalamus.

Grossly, follicular cysts may be single or multiple, affect one or both ovaries, and arise from within and protrude from the surface of the ovary. Microscopically (Figure 25-5), follicular cysts are lined by single or multiple layers of granulosa cells that may appear normal, degenerate, or partially luteinized. The theca interna is often thickened and may be partially luteinized. Follicular cysts do not contain an ovum.

LUTEINIZED FOLLICLES (LUTEINIZED CYSTS)

Luteinized follicles occur uncommonly in cows and in older nulliparous bitches. The pathogenesis is believed to involve either an insufficient LH surge to cause ovulation, but sufficient amounts of circulating LH to induce luteinization of the anovulatory follicle,

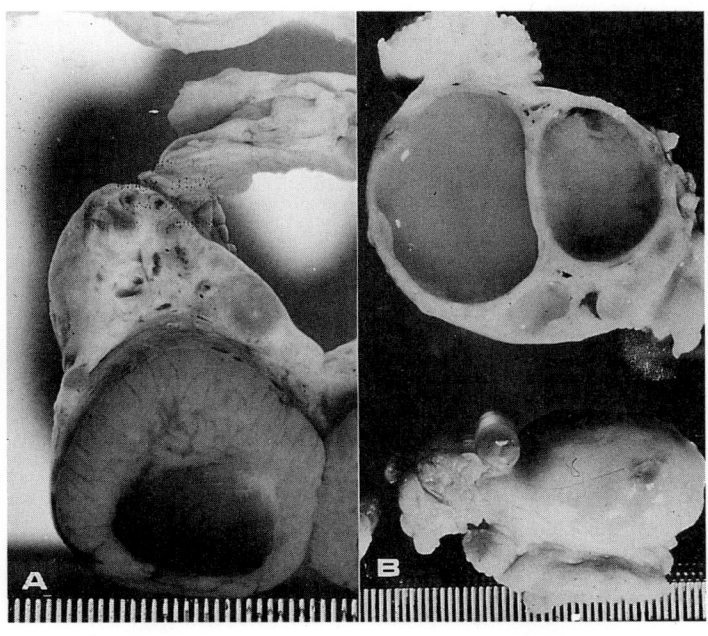

FIG. 25-4 A. Cystic, "retained" corpus luteum from a sterile heifer. **B.** Follicular and parovarian cysts in a bovine ovary.

or possibly immaturity of the follicle at LH surge leading to failure of ovulation. Grossly, luteinized follicles, unlike cystic corpora lutea, lack the ovulatory papilla that occurs with ovulation. Microscopically, lutein cysts differ from follicular cysts in that they are lined by a rim of luteinized cells. This lining is composed of one or more layers of large, luteinized granulosa cells containing fine lipid droplets in cytoplasm and smaller, fusiform theca-lutein cells. Clinical consequences of luteinized follicles are essentially the same as with follicular cysts.

CYSTIC CORPORA LUTEA

Cystic corpora lutea occur frequently in cattle. They result from premature closure of the ovulation site with the formation of a cavity in the center of the developing

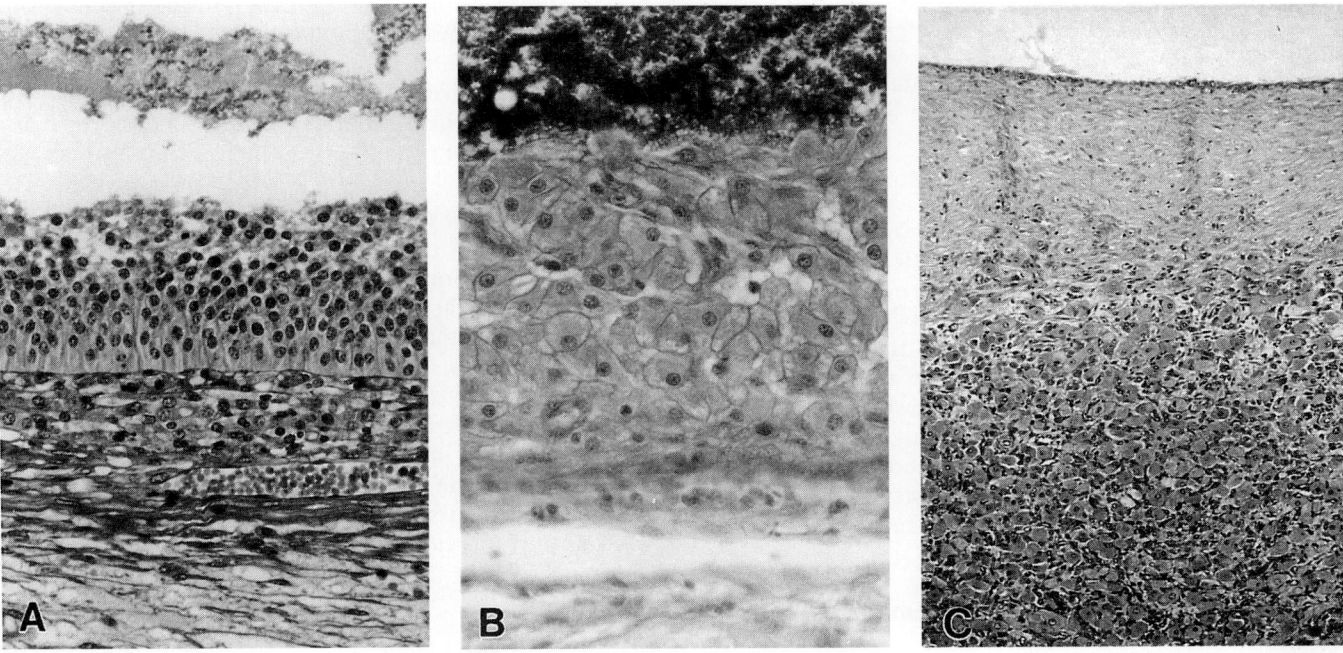

FIG. 25-5 A. Portion of the wall of a bovine ovarian follicular cyst. Note the multiple layers of granulosa cells lining the inner portion of the cyst and the prominent basement membrane that separates the granulosa cell layer from the outer thecal layer of the cyst (×250). **B.** Portion of a bovine ovarian follicular cyst in which granulosa cells have become luteinized (×250). **C.** Cystic corpus lutem in a cow. Note the inner layer of fibrous connective tissue that separates the luteal tissue from the lumen (×125).

corpus luteum. They differ from luteinized follicles in that an obvious ovulatory papilla exists on the surface and the luteal tissue is usually separated from the cyst cavity by a thin layer of fibrous connective tissue.

Cystic corpora lutea have essentially no clinical significance because they usually secrete progesterone in sufficient quantities to maintain pregnancy.

EPITHELIAL INCLUSION CYSTS

Epithelial inclusion cysts arise from small areas near sites of ovulation where the surface epithelium of the ovary become pinched off and embedded in the superficial cortex. These isolated nests of cuboidal to flattened mesothelial cells continue to secrete and form small cysts filled with watery fluid. In most species, epithelial inclusion cysts of the ovary are small and of no clinical significance. In mares, conversely, they occur mainly in and around the ovulation fossa where they are often multiple. With time, these fossa cysts continue to expand and cause atrophy of the adjacent ovarian parenchyma. They may also become so large that they mechanically prevent ovulation. Microscopically, epithelial inclusion cysts in mares may be lined by a single layer of cuboidal mesothelial-like cells or pseudostratified ciliated columnar epithelial cells normally found in the ovulation fossa.

CYSTS OF SUBSURFACE EPITHELIAL STRUCTURES

The ovary of the dog is unusual in that the superficial cortex contains tubules and cords of cells derived from ingrowths of the surface epithelium. These have been termed, subsurface epithelial structures. With increasing age, a greater frequency of cysts is derived from these structures in the canine ovarian cortex. Cysts vary in size, are lined by a single layer of cuboidal epithelium, and contain a clear, watery secretion. Grossly, they can be confused with small follicular cysts, but histologically the character of the lining cells serves to differentiate them.

CYSTIC RETE OVARII

The tubules comprising the rete ovarii of the ovarian medulla occasionally become cystic in most species, but this occurs commonly in dogs and cats. Cysts are usually single, fluid-filled, and lined by a single layer of cuboidal epithelial cells. One or both ovaries may be involved. They may arise during the first year of life, particularly in cats, and enlarge slowly, causing compression and atrophy of the overlying ovarian cortex. Cysts of this type can be distinguished from those derived from adjacent mesonephric ducts (i.e., epoophoron cysts), by the fact that the former are not surrounded by smooth muscle.

CYSTS OF MESONEPHRIC TUBULES AND DUCTS

In females, cysts derived from remnants of the mesonephric tubules and ducts (embryonic male duct system) occur in the mesovarium adjacent to the ovary. Cysts derived from the cranial mesonephric tubules are termed **epoophoron cysts.** They occur in all species of animals and are located in the mesovarium between the ovary and the fimbriated end of the uterine tube. Cysts arising from vestiges of the caudal mesonephric tubules occur much less commonly in domestic animals and are termed, **paroophoron cysts.** They occur in the mesovarium at the uterine pole of the ovary. Cysts derived from the mesonephric duct are located adjacent to the uterine tube. Epoophoron cysts may become large, especially in the mare and bitch, and be mistaken for cystic ovarian follicles. Microscopically, it may not be possible to distinguish epoophoron from paroophoron cysts because both are lined by a single layer of ciliated and nonciliated cuboidal to low columnar epithelial cells and are surrounded by two layers of smooth muscle. Anatomic location is more useful in this regard. **Cysts of mesonephric duct** origin are usually lined by a single layer of nonciliated, low cuboidal epithelium and are surrounded by two layers of smooth muscle that are larger than those surrounding cysts derived from mesonephric tubules.

CYSTS OF PARAMESONEPHRIC (MÜLLERIAN) DUCT: HYDATIDS OF MORGAGNI

During embryogenesis, the ostium of the uterine tube forms from a segment of the paramesonephric duct slightly caudal to the cranial end. The small segment anterior to the tubal ostium occasionally persists and becomes cystic in postnatal life. In women, these cysts have been referred to as hydatids of Morgagni. Grossly, they appear as a pedunculated cyst connected to the uterine tube by a fibromuscular band. Microscopically, they are lined by an epithelum that resembles that of the uterine tube. The epithelium is composed of three cell types: ciliated and nonciliated (secretory) cuboidal to columnar cells and small dark-staining, conical-shaped cells referred to as peg or hobnail cells. The latter cell type represents degenerating or secretorily exhausted secretory cells. The presence of peg cells serves to distinguish cysts of paramesonephric duct origin from those of mesonephric duct origin.

TUBOOVARIAN CYSTS AND OVARIAN BURSAL CYSTS

Total occlusion of the uterine tube due to adhesions of the surface of the ovary to the fimbria occurs rarely in cattle as a consequence of infectious oophoritis or salpingitis. Total obstruction of the outflow of tubal secretion from the ostium leads to distention of the tube and formation of a tuboovarian cyst. When these adhesions involve only a portion of the fimbria such that only the ovarian bursa is occluded, then distention of the bursa by tubal fluid will result in a cystic ovarian bursa without distention of the tube.

References

Al-Dahash SYA, David JSE. Histological examination of ovaries and uteri from cows with cystic ovaries. Vet Rec 1977;101:342–347.

Bierschwal CJ. A clinical study of cystic conditions of the bovine ovary. J Am Vet Med Assoc 1966;149:1591–1595.

Blue MG. A tubo-ovarian cyst, paraovarian cysts and lesions of the oviduct in the mare. NZ Vet J 1985;33:8–10.

Dobson H, Rankin JEF, Ward WR. Bovine cystic ovarian disease:

plasma hormone concentrations and treatment. Vet Rec 1977;101:459–461.

Donaldson LE, Hansel W. Cystic corpora lutea and noram and cystic graafian follicles in the cow. Aust Vet J 1968;44:304–308.

Dow C. Ovarian abnormalities in the bitch. J Comp Pathol 1960;70:59–69.

Eyestone WH, Ax RL. A review of ovarian follicular cysts in cows, with comparisons to the condition in women, rats, and rabbits. Theriogenology 1984;22:109–125.

Hughes JP, Kennedy PC, Stabenfeldt GH. Pathology of the ovary and ovarian disorders in the mare. Proc 9th Int Cong Anim Reprod Artif Insemin 1980;I:203–222.

Kesler DJ, Garverick HA. Ovarian cysts in dairy cattle: a review. J Anim Sci 1982;55:1147–1159.

McEntee K. Cystic corpora lutea in cattle. Int J Fertil 1958;3:120–128.

McEntee K. Reproductive pathology of domestic mammals. New York: Academic Press, 1990.

O'Shea JD. Histochemical observations on mucin secretion by subsurface epithelial structures in the canine ovary. J Morphol 1966;120:347–358.

Saumande J, LeCoustumier J, Marois C. Oestradiol-17β and progesterone in nymphomaniac cows. Theriogenology 1979;12:27–31.

Short RV. Steroid concentrations in normal follicular fluid and ovarian cyst fluid from cows. J Reprod Fertil 1962;4:27–45.

Tsumura J, Sasaki H, Minami S, et al. Cyst formation on mesosalpinx, mesovarium and fimbria in cows and sows. Jpn J Vet Sci 1982;44:1–8.

Infections

OOPHORITIS

Oophoritis (inflammation of the ovary) is rare in domestic animals, but is observed most often in cattle. It generally results from either a direct extension or hematogenous spread of infection in the uterus or uterine tubes to the ovary where it often localizes in the corpus luteum. Agents shown to cause oophoritis include: *Herpesvirus bovis*, *H. suis*, *Akabane virus*, *Mycobacterium tuberculosis var. bovis*, *Brucella spp.*, *Actinomyces pyogenes*, and *Mycoplasma bovis*. Grossly, affected ovaries have varying amounts of fibrin tags, granulation tissue, and fibrous adhesions on the serosal surfaces that may interfere with ovulation or result in the formation of tuboovarian or bursal cysts. Depending on the causative agent and duration of infection, the inflammatory reaction varies from lymphoplasmacytic to neutrophilic to granulomatous with varying degrees of fibrosis and adhesions to fimbria and ovarian bursa.

Neoplasms

PRIMARY NEOPLASMS

Primary neoplasms of the ovary occur in most species of domestic animals, but are reported most often in cows, mares and bitches. They arise from the surface epithelium, including the subsurface epithelial structures in bitches, the sex cord stroma (granulosa-theca cells), the primordial germ cells, and from other supporting stromal elements.

PAPILLARY CYSTADENOMA

Papillary cystadenoma of the ovary is a rare neoplasm of domestic animals, except in bitches. It can arise from the surface epithelium, from the subsurface epithelial structures of the canine ovary, or from the rete ovarii. In bitches, most tumors of this type arise from the subsurface epithelial structures where they can be multicentric and involve both ovaries. Grossly, they appear nodular with smooth surfaces or have a cauliflower-like surface due to compression of papillary projections. On cut surface, they consist of solid, gray-white to yellow masses of tissue containing one or more cysts. Microscopically, papillary cystadenomas begin as blunt-to-papillary projections of fibrovascular stroma lined by a single or pseudostratified layer of cuboidal to columnar, ciliated, and nonciliated epithelial cells. The papillae protrude into the lumens of subsurface epithelial structures initially, but as the tumor grows the papillary structures elongate, and become branched and secretory causing distention of the spaces containing them. Mitotic figures are rare. Papillary cystadenomas arising from the rete ovarii in the medulla of the ovary may cause pressure atrophy of the overlying ovarian cortex.

PAPILLARY CYSTADENOCARCINOMA

Papillary cystadenocarcinoma (Fig. 25-6), the malignant variant of papillary cystadenoma, is a common ovarian neoplasm of older bitches, but is rare in other domestic animals. They also arise most often from the subsurface epithelial structures of the canine ovary and superficially resemble their benign counterpart except that they are larger and often protrude from the ovarian bursa. Histologically, they differ from cystadenomas in that they are invasive, may form solid sheets and masses in some areas, have a higher mitotic index, and frequently exfoliate and implant on the visceral and parietal peritoneum. Invasion and obstruction of lymphatics and venules of the peritoneum and diaphragm may result in ascites. Secretion from the multiple peritoneal implants may also contribute to the ascitic fluid. Metastasis to the lungs, pleura, and bronchial lymph nodes also may occur.

GRANULOSA-THECA CELL TUMORS

Granulosa-theca cell tumors are the most common ovarian neoplasms of cows (Fig. 25-7) and mares, and occur in older bitches with about equal frequency as ovarian papillary cystadenocarcinomas. They arise from the specialized stroma of the ovary and are regarded as sex cord stromal tumors. In cattle and mares, granulosa cell tumors have been described in both young and old animals, with the median age in cattle being seven years and in mares 10.5 years. They are usually unilateral, benign, and may become extremely large. Cows and mares with granulosa cell tumors may develop a variety of sex hormone imbalances characterized by elevated plasma levels of progesterone, estradiol, or testosterone, or all three. Clinically, this may be manifested as signs of nymphomania, masculinization, or no obvious clinical abnormalities. Nymphomania is usually manifested by mounting other animals in the herd; whereas masculinization results in phenotypic changes, such as bull-like thickening of the head and neck, elevation of the tailhead, and development of bull-like vocalization and behavior. Although they occur in nongravid cows, most granulosa cell tumors have been described in pregnant

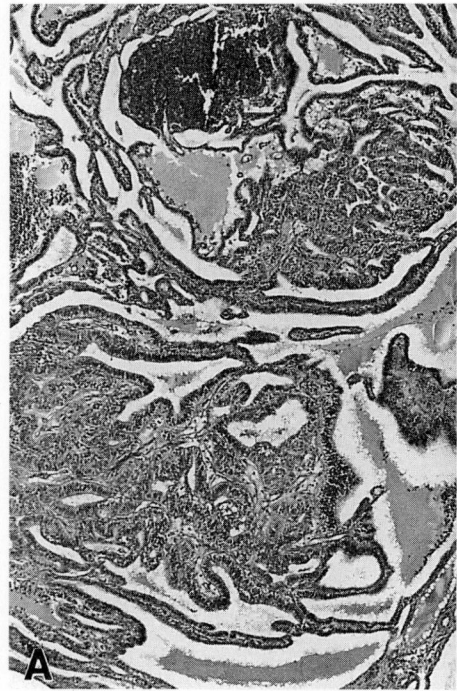
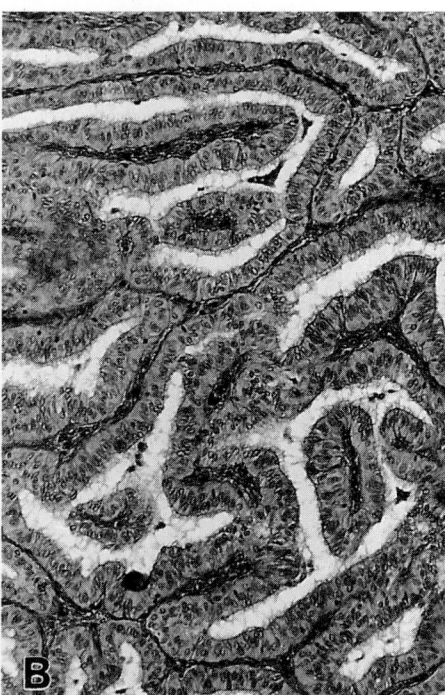

FIG. 25-6 A. Cystadenocarcinoma of the ovary of a dog. Note the papillary projections protruding into cystic spaces filled with fluid (×75). **B.** Higher magnification of one of the compact areas of the same neoplasm (×250).

animals. The gross appearance of ganulosa cell tumors varies considerably. Their surface may be smooth or bossellated and when sectioned may be solid or cystic. The solid portions of the tumor can vary from soft to firm and range from yellow to orange or red. Extensive areas of hemorrhage and necrosis may occur in large tumors.

Microscopically, neoplastic cells proliferate in a variety of patterns, including follicular, trabecular, and Sertoli cell-like patterns, as well as in diffuse sheets surrounding varying sized cystic spaces containing clear fluid or hemorrhage. In most tumors, neoplastic cells resemble normal granulosa cells in being small, polyhedral with scant amounts of eosinophilic cytoplasm and round to ovoid, hyperchromatic nuclei with distinct nucleoli. Within the tumor, neoplastic cells may appear to be more fusiform and theca cell-like; in other areas, they are large and polygonal with abundant eosino-

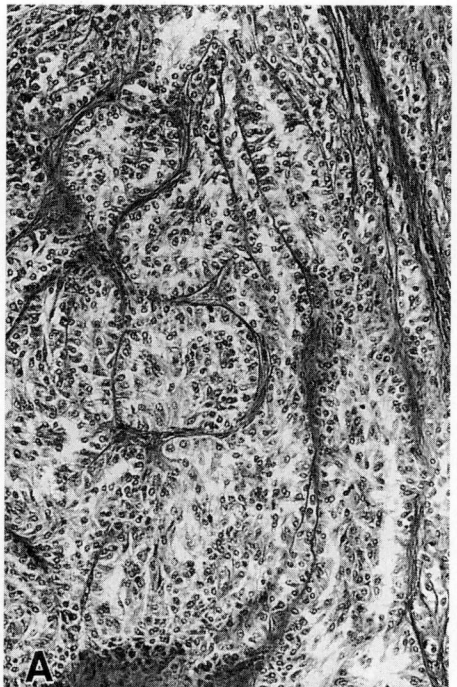
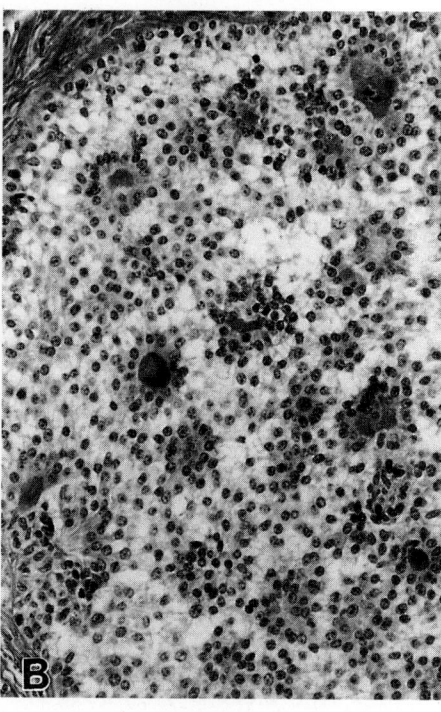

FIG. 25-7 Granulosa cell tumor of a cow. **A.** Note the sertoliform pattern of growth of the neoplastic granulosa cells (×100). **B.** A portion of the same neoplasm in which the neoplastic granulosa cells are forming Call-Exner bodies or rosettes around a central mass of eosinophilic, follicular fluid-like material (×250).

philic cytoplasm and resemble luteinized granulosa or theca cells. Granulosa cell tumors are believed to arise from either anovular follicles in the cortex or from the medullary tubules near the hilum of the ovary. They may form characteristic structures called Call-Exner bodies, which consist of small, central, round to oval space containing eosinophilic follicular fluid surrounded by a collar of radially arranged granulosa cells. When present, these structures are diagnostic of granulosa cell tumors; however, they are not always present, particularly in extremely large tumors.

In dogs and cats, granulosa cell tumors are often associated with clinical signs of hyperestrogenism, including continuous estrus, vulvar swelling, vaginal discharge, endometrial hyperplasia, and pyometra. In addition, the hyperestrogenism may result in bone marrow suppression and nonregenerative anemia and thrombocytopenia. A higher pereentage of canine granulosa cell tumors are malignant and metastasize to regional lymph nodes and other organs. The pattern of growth is similar to that described in cows and mares.

THECA CELL TUMORS

Theca cell tumors (thecomas) differ from granulosa-theca cell tumors in that they are composed of cells with only the theca cell phenotype. They occur much less commonly than granulosa cell tumors and have been described in cows and bitches. Grossly, they are smooth, firm, and composed of solid sheets of white, yellow, or orange tissue that may contain areas of hemorrhage and necrosis. Cysts are generally not a feature of theca cell tumors. Microscopically, these neoplasms are composed of diffuse sheets of fusiform cells arranged in interlacing bundles. Neoplastic cells have long, polar cytoplasmic protrusions that often contain lipid, a feature that distinguishes these tumors from tumors of fibroblastic origin.

INTERSTITIAL CELL TUMOR

Interstitial cell tumor (interstitial gland tumor, luteoma, lipid cell tumor) is a rare neoplasm derived from the so-called interstitial gland cells of the ovary. Interstitial gland cells are believed to arise from luteinized theca internal cells of atretic antral follicles or from hypertrophied granulosa cells of atretic preantral follicles of dogs, cats, rodents, and lagomorphs. Grossly, these tumors tend to have smooth surfaces, are firm, solid, white-yellow to orange with areas of hemorrhage and necrosis. They are usually unilateral and benign. Neoplastic cells are large, polyhedral with prominent cytoplasmic borders, and abundant eosinophilic cytoplasm containing lipid droplets of varying size and sometimes yellow, lipoid pigment. They resemble cells of the corpus luteum (Fig. 25-8). Affected individuals may have abnormal estrous cycles.

DYSGERMINOMAS

Dysgerminomas are neoplasms derived from germ cells of the ovary and are the female counterpart of testicular seminoma in males. They generally occur in aged animals, are usually unilateral, but occasionally bilateral, and up to 20% of them metastasize. They occur most often in bitches, but have been reported in queens, mares, cows, sows, and goats. Most have been reported in older animals. Several reports have described their association with clinical signs of hyperestrogenism, suggesting that a small percentage of them may be hormonally active. Grossly, dysgerminomas vary in size, but may become extremely large before they are detected. They are usually round to ovoid with smooth to lobulated surfaces. On cut surface, the neoplasm varies from soft to firm and is composed of a rather homogeneous gray-white tissue that may be punctuated by areas of hemorrhage and necrosis, particularly in larger tumors.

Microscopically, dysgerminomas are composed of

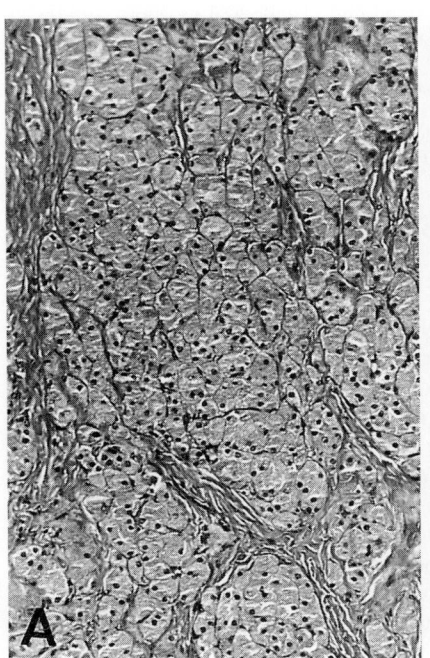
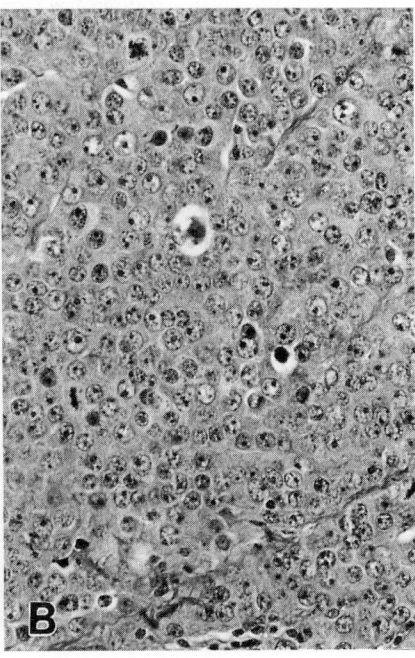

FIG. 25-8 **A.** Luteoma in ovary of a dog. Cells resemble normal luteal cells. **B.** Dysgerminoma in ovary of a dog. This neoplasm resembles the seminoma (Figure 25-31). (Courtesy of Dr. N.W. King, Jr. and Angell Memorial Animal Hospital.)

large, round to polygonal cells with moderate amounts of vesicular to amphophilic cytoplasm and round to ovoid nuclei containing coarsely granular chromatin and one to two nucleoli. Some dysgerminomas contain multinucleated giant cells reminiscent of spermatidic giant cells. Mitoses are frequent and may be abnormal. Tumor cells proliferate in solid sheets and cords with little connective tissue stroma. Necrosis of individual tumor cells or, in some instances, large areas of necrosis and cystic degeneration may be present. Histologically, benign and malignant dysgerminomas may be indistinguishable except for obvious sites of metastasis. Focal aggregates of lymphocytes seen often in the male counterpart of this neoplasm (seminoma) are rare in dysgerminomas.

TERATOMAS

Teratomas, like dysgerminomas, are derived from primitive ovarian germ cells, but differ in that the neoplastic cells rather than being monomorphic, instead exhibit differentiation into a variety of tissues derived from all three embryonic germ cell layers (ectoderm, entoderm, and mesoderm). Current hypotheses regarding their origin center around the parthenogenetic (autofertilization without insemination) theory. Ovarian teratomas occur in two basic types: benign cystic (sometimes referred to as dermoid cysts), and malignant. They are usually unilateral and, in general, occur in younger animals than do other ovarian neoplasms. They have been described in bitches, queens, cows, mares, and various laboratory animal species, including nonhuman primates. Grossly, ovarian teratomas can vary considerably in size and have either a smooth or somewhat lobulated surface. The appearance of the cut surface varies with the tissue components comprising the neoplasm and the degree of necrosis and hemorrhage. Often benign tumors contain large cystic spaces filled with hair and a mixture of keratin and sebaceous secretion. Teeth and bone may also be recognizable in some teratomas.

Microscopically, teratomas may contain varying amounts of virtually any tissue except gonadal tissue. They often contain cystic spaces lined by keratinizing, stratified, squamous epithelium surrounded by dense, collagenous connective tissue containing well-differentiated hair follicles, sebaceous, and apocrine glands typical of skin. Other tissues that may be present include: respiratory epithelium; gastrointestinal epithelium; liver; kidney; spleen; bone containing functional bone marrow; smooth, cardiac, and skeletal muscle; and various types of nervous tissue. Intervening areas of undifferentiated mesenchymal tissue may exist. Metastatic lesions may be widely disseminated and contain all or only a portion of the tissue elements present in the primary neoplasm. Occasionally, metastatic lesions are less differentiated than the primary neoplasm.

References

Andrews EJ, Stookey JL, Helland DR, et al. A histological study of canine and feline ovarian dysgerminomas. Can J Comp Med 1974;38:84–89.

Brandly PJ, Migaki G. Types of tumors found by federal meat inspectors in an eight-year survey. Ann NY Acad Sci 1963;108:872–879.

Cotchin E. Canine ovarian neoplasms. Res Vet Sci 1961;2:133–142.

Cotchin E, Marchant J. Animal tumors of the female reproductive tract. Spontaneous and experimental. In: Blaustein A, ed. Pathology of the female genital tract. New York: Springer-Verlag, 1977;55–56.

Dehner LP, Norris HJ, Garner FM, et al. Comparative pathology of ovarian neoplasms. III. Germ cell tumors of canine, bovine, feline, rodent, and human species. J Comp Pathol 1970;80:299–306.

Gelberg HB, McEntee K. Feline ovarian neoplasms. Vet Pathol 1985;22:572–576.

Greene JA, Richardson RC, Thornill JA, et al. Ovarian papillary cystadenocarcinoma in a bitch: case report and literature review. J Am Anim Hosp Assoc 1979;15:351–356.

Greenlee PG, Patnaik AK. Canine ovarian tumors of germ cell origin. Vet Pathol 1985;22:117–122.

Gruys E, van Dijk JEL, Elsinghorst TAM, et al. Four canine ovarian teratomas and a nonovarian feline teratoma. Vet Pathol 1976;13:455–459.

Hofmann W, Arbiter D, Scheele D. Sex cord stromal tumor in a cat: so-called androblastoma with Sertol-Leydig cell pattern. Vet Pathol 1980;17:508–513.

McEntee K. Reproductive pathology of domestic mammals. New York: Academic Press, 1990.

Meagher DM, Wheat JD, Hughes JP, et al. Granulosa cell tumors in mares—a review of 78 cases. Proc 23rd Annu Convent. Am Assoc Equine Pract 1977;133–143.

Nelson LW, Todd GC, Migaki G. Ovarian neoplasm in swine. J Am Vet Med Assoc 1967;151:1331–1333.

Nielsen SW, Misdorp W, McEntee K. Tumours of the ovary. Bull WHO 1976;53:203–215.

Norris HJ, Garner FM, Taylor HB. Pathology of feline ovarian neoplasms. J Pathol 1969;97:138–143.

Norris HJ, Garner FM, Taylor HB. Comparative pathology of ovarian neoplasm. IV. Gonadal stromal tumors of canine species. J Comp Pathol 1970;80:399–405.

Norris HJ, Taylor HB, Garner FM. Equine ovarian granulosa cell tumours. Vet Rec 1968;82:419–420.

Norris HJ, Taylor HB, Garner FM. Comparative pathology of ovarian neoplasms. II. Gonadal stromal tumors of bovine species. Pathol Vet 1969;6:45–58.

Patnaik AK, Schaer M, Parks J, et al. Metastasizing ovarian teratocarcinoma in dogs. A report of two cases and review of literature. J Small Anim Pract 1976;17:235–246.

Stabenfeldt GH, Hughes JP, Kennedy PC, et al. Clinical findings, pathological changes and endocrinological secretory patterns in mares with ovarian tumors. J Reprod Fertil Suppl 1979;27:277–285.

Stein BS. Tumors of the feline genital tract. J Am Anim Hosp Assoc 1981;17:1077–1085.

Stickle RL, Erb RE, Fessler JF, et al. Equine granulosa cell tumors. J Am Vet Med Assoc 1975;167:148–151.

UTERINE (FALLOPIAN) TUBES
Malformations

CONGENITAL ABNORMALITIES

Congenital abnormalities of the uterine tubes are extremely rare in domestic animal species. They result from faulty development of the paramesonephric (müllerian) ducts during embryogenesis and may also be associated with certain uterine abnormalities, especially when they occur in association with various forms of intersex. Certain anomalies, when bilateral, can result in sterility. These include total and segmental aplasia, atresia of the infundibular or uterine ostia, developmental cysts, and duplication or formation of accessory uterine tubes. These anomalies may go unrecognized clinically unless they result in grossly visible distention of the uterine tube by entrapped secretion, as occurs in **hydrosalpinx,** or are associated with impaired fertility or sterility.

ACQUIRED ABNORMALITIES

Acquired abnormalities of the uterine tubes are much more common, but still relatively rare. These can result from infectious processes, or be a consequence of ovulation, or trauma from manual manipulation of the ovary and adjacent structures. Most acquired structural malformations are characterized by adhesion formation. These may be extraluminal as seen in bursal cysts resulting from adhesion of portions of the ovarian bursa or fimbria of the tube to bleeding ovulation sites or to sites of manually enucleated corpora lutea. When intraluminal, adhesions occur between mucosal folds or plicae, often as a consequence of epithelial damage from an infectious process (e.g., **salpingitis**). These intraluminal scars result in obstruction of the tube and affect fertility (Fig. 25-9). They can also be associated with hydrosalpinx, which results from obstruction of the normal outflow of the watery secretion produced by the tubal epithelium. The resultant distention of the tube may be uniform or irregular, depending on the site and extent of adhesions.

Infections

Most infectious processes that involve the uterine tubes ascend from the uterus and are associated with necrosis and purulent inflammation of the tubal mucosa (**purulent salpingitis**). Affected tubes contain varying amounts

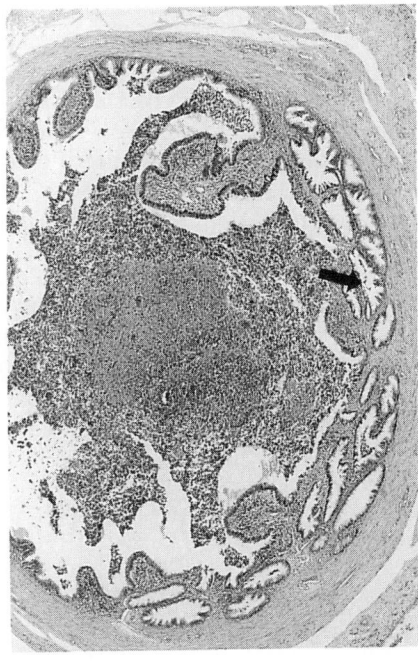

FIG. 25-9 Purulent salpingitis in a cow. Note the distention of the lumen with exudate and the flattening and compression of mucosal folds (arrow; ×75).

of exudate that may cause gross distention of the tube (**pyosalpinx**). Resolution of the inflammatory process may be complicated by intraluminal adhesions. The infectious agents associated with salpingitis are essentially the same as those that cause endometritis and thus will be discussed under that heading. Granulomatous salpingitis was once seen as a complication of bovine tuberculosis, a disease rarely seen in the United States today, but one that still occurs commonly in developing countries.

Neoplasms

Neoplasms of the uterine tubes are extraordinarily rare in domestic animal species. The few that have been described have been either adenomas or adenocarcinomas and have arisen from the epithelial cells of the fimbria or infundibular end of the uterine tube.

References

Archibald LF, Mather EC, McClure JR. Fimbrial cysts as a cause of infertility in the mare. Vet Med Small Anim Clin 1974;69:1163–1165.

Benirschke K. Pathologic processes of the oviduct. In: Hafez ESE, Blandau RJ, eds. The mammalian oviduct: comparative biology and methodology. Chicago: U Chicago Press, 1969;271–307.

Bodemer CW. History of the mammalian oviduct. In: Hafez ESE, Blandau RJ, eds. The mammalian oviduct: comparative biology and methodology. Chicago: U Chicago Press, 1969;3–26.

Carpenter CM, Williams WW, Gilman HL. Salpingitis in the cow. I. The streptococcus as a possible etiological factor. J Am Vet Med Assoc 1921;59:173–183.

Dawson FLM. The incidence of salpingitis and bursitis throughout a series of 200 permanently infertile cows, with notes on its significance and on diagnosis. Proc 3rd Int Congr Anim Reprod Artif Insemin 1956;2:46–48.

Dawson FLM. The diagnosis and significance of bovine endosalpingitis and ovarian bursitis. Vet Rec 1958;70:487–492.

Doig PA, Ruhnke HL, Palmer NC. Experimental bovine genital ureaplasmosis. II. Granular vulvitis, endometritis and salpingitis following uterine inoculation. Can J Comp Med 1980;44:259–266.

Duchateau AB, Whitmore HL. Uterine tube abnormalities in cattle. J Am Vet Med Assoc 1978;172:1308–1309.

Hafez ESE, Blandau RJ, eds. The mammalian oviduct: comparative biology and methodology. Chicago: U Chicago Press, 1969.

Hinrichs K, Kenney RM, Hurtgen JP. Unilateral hydrosalpinx and absence of the infundibulum in a mare. Theriogenology 1984;22:571–577.

Hirth RS, Nielsen SW, Plastridge WM. Bovine salpingo-oophoritis produced with semen containing a Mycoplasma. Pathol Vet 1966;3:616–632.

Johari MP, Sharma SP. Fallopian tube lesions in farm animals: diagnosis. Vet Rec 1964;76:293–294.

Lombard L, Morgan BB, McNutt SH. Some pathologic alterations of the bovine oviduct. Am J Vet Res 1951;12:69–74.

Moberg R. Disease conditions in the fallopian tubes and ovarian bursae of cattle. Vet Rec 1954;66:87–90.

Vandeplassche M, Henry M. Salpingitis in the mare. Proc 23rd Annu Conven. Am Assoc Equine Pract 1977;123–131.

DISEASES OF NONGRAVID UTERUS

General considerations

Anatomically, three basic structural configurations of uteri exist: pyriform (pear-shaped), found in most primate species, pangolins, sloths, and some anteaters; bicornuate (double-horned), found in all domestic animals and numerous other species; and didelphic (double uterus), found mainly in marsupials, lagomorphs, and certain rodents. The size of uteri varies tremendously throughout the class Mammalia. That of the pygmy shrew is approximately 1.0 mm in width and has horns that are approximately 5.0 mm in length. Conversely, the gravid uterus of the world's largest mammal, the blue whale, is approximately 78.0 cm in width and up to 8.0 meters in length.

Congenital developmental abnormalities

CONGENITAL MALFORMATIONS

Congenital malformations of the uteri of domestic animals are not common and are often associated with either inbreeding or intersex. All such anomalies, however, do not necessarily have a genetic basis. With the exception of cattle, the majority of uterine congenital anomalies of domestic animals involve the uterine horns (cornua). These include: **bilateral agenesis, unilateral agenesis (uterus unicornis or hemiuterus),** and **segmental aplasia.** In cattle, the cervix is the most common site of anomalous development of the female reproductive tract. An anomaly affecting mainly the body of the uterus and the cervix is uterus didelphis. A brief description of these congenital uterine anomalies, including their known associations with other disorders, and their effects on reproduction follows.

BILATERAL AGENESIS

Bilateral agenesis of the uterine horns is an extraordinarily rare anomaly and affected individuals are sterile. It occurs in some cases of bilateral true hermaphroditism and freemartinism and results either from primary failure of paramesonephric duct development or more often by inhibition of their development by müllerian inhibitory factor secreted by bilateral ovotestes or dysgenetic gonads.

UNILATERAL AGENESIS

Unilateral agenesis of a uterine horn (sometimes termed uterus unicornis; Fig. 25-10) results from failure of development of a single paramesonephric duct. A small, fibromuscular band may be manifest in place of the normal uterine horn. When this condition affects species with a pyriform uterus, unilateral agenesis is referred to as **hemiuterus.** Uterus unicornis may not affect fertility, but for obvious reasons can affect litter size. This condition can be associated with ipsilateral renal agenesis resulting from failure of mesonephric duct development on the same side. Uterus unicornis has been described in all domestic animal species and has been associated with inbreeding and various forms of intersex. In adult cattle, it often is associated with a persistent corpus luteum on the ipsilateral side, which can predispose the affected animal to pyometra. Persistence of the corpus luteum results from lack of prostaglandin F2α secretion, the luteolytic substance normally secreted by the endometrium in this species.

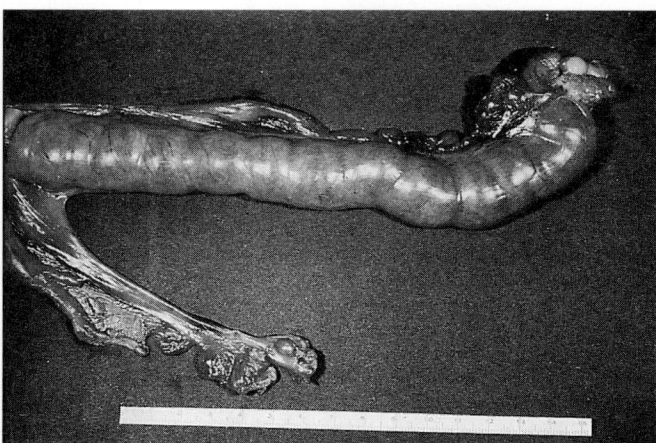

FIG. 25-10 Uterus unicornis in a five-year-old dog. Both ovaries are present. The remaining uterine horn was affected by cystic endometrial hyperplasia. (Courtesy of Drs. C.E. Gilmore and N.W. King, Jr.)

SEGMENTAL APLASIA

Segmental aplasia of a portion of a uterine horn results from segmental defects in paramesonephric duct development. In this condition, portions of the uterine horns may be absent, resulting in isolation of cranial segments from more distal segments and the uterine body. Due to accumulations of secretion in the blind-ended segments, they often become cystic and filled with necrotic cellular debris that becomes inspissated in the form of a putty-like calculus. Clinically, these dilated segments can be mistaken for early pregnancy. This anomaly has been associated with intersex and inbreeding, but can also occur as a nongenetic event. Unless it is bilateral, fertility is not necessarily impaired.

UTERUS DIDELPHYS

Uterus didelphys is the term used to refer to a double uterus. This type of uterus is normal for some species, including marsupials, lagomorphs, and certain rodents. A didelphic uterus has two uterine horns each connected to a separate uterine body and cervix. Two cervical ora communicate with the vagina. In marsupials, double vaginae also exist.

When it occurs as an anomaly, uterus didelphys results from failure of fusion and dissolution of the medial walls of the paramesonephric ducts at the caudal end of the genital tract. Thus, each duct becomes a separate uterus and cervix. Some individuals with this anomaly can have a septate vagina as well, because the cranial portion of the vagina is also of paramesonephric duct origin. Fertility is not impaired in these individuals, but litter size may be reduced as with uterus unicornis.

References

Arthur GH. The functional variability of uterus didelphys. Vet Rec 1958;70:278.

Bennett RC, Olds D, Deaton OW, et al. Nature of white heifer disease (partial genital aplasia) and its mode of inheritance. Am J Vet Res 1973;34:13–19.

Dolby PB. Instance of reproduction with uterus unicornis and uterus didelphys. Vet Med 1951;46:60–61.

Fincher MG, Williams WI. Arrested development of the müllerian ducts associated with inbreeding. Cornell Vet 1926;16:1–19.

Ginther OJ. Segmental aplasia of the müllerian ducts (white heifer disease) in a white shorthorn heifer. J Am Vet Med Assoc 1965;146:133–137.

Gruenwald P. The relationship of the growing müllerian duct to the Wolffian duct and its importance for the genesis of malformations. Anat Rec 1941;81:1–19.

Hunter GL. Life span of the corpora lutea in ewes with one congenitally absent uterine horn. J Reprod Fertil 1970;23:131–133.

Mack CO, McGlothlin JH. Renal agenesis in the female cat. Anat Rec 1949;105:445–450.

Marcella KL, Ramirez M, Hammerslag KL. Segmental aplasia of the uterine horn in a cat. J Am Vet Med Assoc 1985;186:179–181.

Perkins JR, Olds D, Seath DM. A study of 1,000 bovine genitalia. J Dairy Sci 1954;37:1158–1163.

Peterson JE, Parsonson IM, Newsam IDB, et al. Infertility in dairy heifers with particular reference to a high incidence of developmental defects of the paramesonephric duct system. Aust Vet J 1966;42:430–436.

Robinson GW. Uterus unicornis and unilateral renal agenesis in a cat. J Am Vet Med Assoc 1965;147:516–518.

Roine K. Observations on genital abnormalities in dairy cows using slaughterhouse material. Nord Vet Med 1977;29:188–193.

Wiggins EL, Casida LE, Grummer RH. The incidence of female genital abnormalities in swine. J Anim Sci 1950;9:269–276.

Postnatal developmental abnormalities

HYPOPLASIA

Hypoplasia of an otherwise normally formed uterus is a condition resulting from lack of or insufficient ovarian hormonal stimulation. It is usually only recognizable after the normal age of sexual maturity, because before this time the uterus is normally hypoplastic. This condition is found in various forms of intersex, as a consequence of certain forms of hereditary ovarian hypoplasia and as a consequence of ovariectomy prior to sexual maturity. It is characterized by a uterus of infantile proportions in a supposed sexually mature individual. These individuals are sterile.

ATROPHY

Atrophy of a previously normal uterus results from cessation of normal ovarian hormonal stimulation in an individual whose reproductive performance may have been normal previously. It occurs following ovariectomy in sexually mature individuals as a consequence of destructive lesions of the ovaries or following the administration of androgenic substances that counteract the trophic effect of ovarian estrogens. Some degree of physiologic atrophy of the endometrium occurs during periods of anestrus, particularly in the mare. Atrophy is characterized by marked reduction in thickness of both endometrium and myometrium.

Disorders of endometrial growth

ENDOMETRIAL HYPERPLASIA

Endometrial hyperplasia, in contrast to atrophy, occurs as the result of excessive or prolonged female hormonal stimulation. The hormones involved include both estrogens and progestogens, which may be of endogenous or exogenous origin. Among domestic and laboratory animal species, differences occur in the relative importance of estrogens versus progestogens in the pathogenesis of endometrial hyperplasia. In ungulates and rodents, estrogens appear to be the prime offender; whereas in dogs and cats, progesterone acting on an estrogen-primed endometrium is the principal hormone involved.

ESTROGEN-MEDIATED ENDOMETRIAL HYPERPLASIA

Estrogen-mediated endometrial hyperplasia (Fig. 25-11) results from prolonged, noncyclic estrogen stimulation (estrinism) or from excessive levels of circulating estrogens (hyperestrinism). Certain intrinsic lesions of the ovaries are the main sources of endogenous estrogens involved in endometrial hyperplasia, and include single or multiple follicular cysts and granulosa-theca cell tumors. Clinically, individuals with these lesions often exhibit signs of continuous estrus, nymphomania, and persistent vaginal discharge or bleeding. Exogenous sources of estrogens that may result in endometrial hyperplasia include: administration of pharmacologic compounds having estrogenic action; contamination of foodstuffs by estrogenic substances (e.g., diethylstilbestrol when used as a growth promotor in cattle); and ingestion of certain pasture legumes known to contain estrogenic substances, especially subterranean clover, red clover, ladino clover, alfalfa, and birdsfoot trefoil. Weakly estrogenic substances contained in these plants may be converted to more potent estrogens by bacterial metabolism in the rumen. Ewes grazing pastures containing these plants develop temporary infertility that becomes permanent with prolonged exposure. Affected ewes continue to cycle normally and the reduced fertility results from hyperplastic changes in the cervix that impair the passage of spermatozoa. Prolonged exposure may be associated with prolapsed uteri in nonpregnant, as well as postpartum, ewes. Pregnant ewes often experience difficulty during parturition (dystocia).

Regardless of its source, the effects of excessive or prolonged estrogen stimulation on the uterus are twofold: hypertrophy of the myometrium, and hyperplasia of the endometrium (Fig. 25-12). In the early stages, endometrial stroma becomes edematous and frequently contains focal hemorrhage. The glands at all levels increase in size and number. Numerous mitotic figures are present in both glandular and surface epithelium. When stimulation persists, stromal edema and hemorrhage subside, and glands continue to proliferate and become tortuous and dilated. Glandular lumens and uterine cavity become grossly cystic (**cystic endometrial hyperplasia**) and distended by varying amounts of secretion that may be thin and watery (**hydrometra**) or viscous and mucinous (**mucometra**).

Microscopically, glands in bitches become distended along the entire length, a feature that distinguishes estrogen-mediated endometrial hyperplasia from the more common progesterone-mediated endometrial hyperplasia in this species. These markedly hyperplastic changes may be accompanied by downgrowth of the basilar aspect of the glands and adjacent stroma into the myometrium, usually along the paths of myometrial vessels, and may ex-

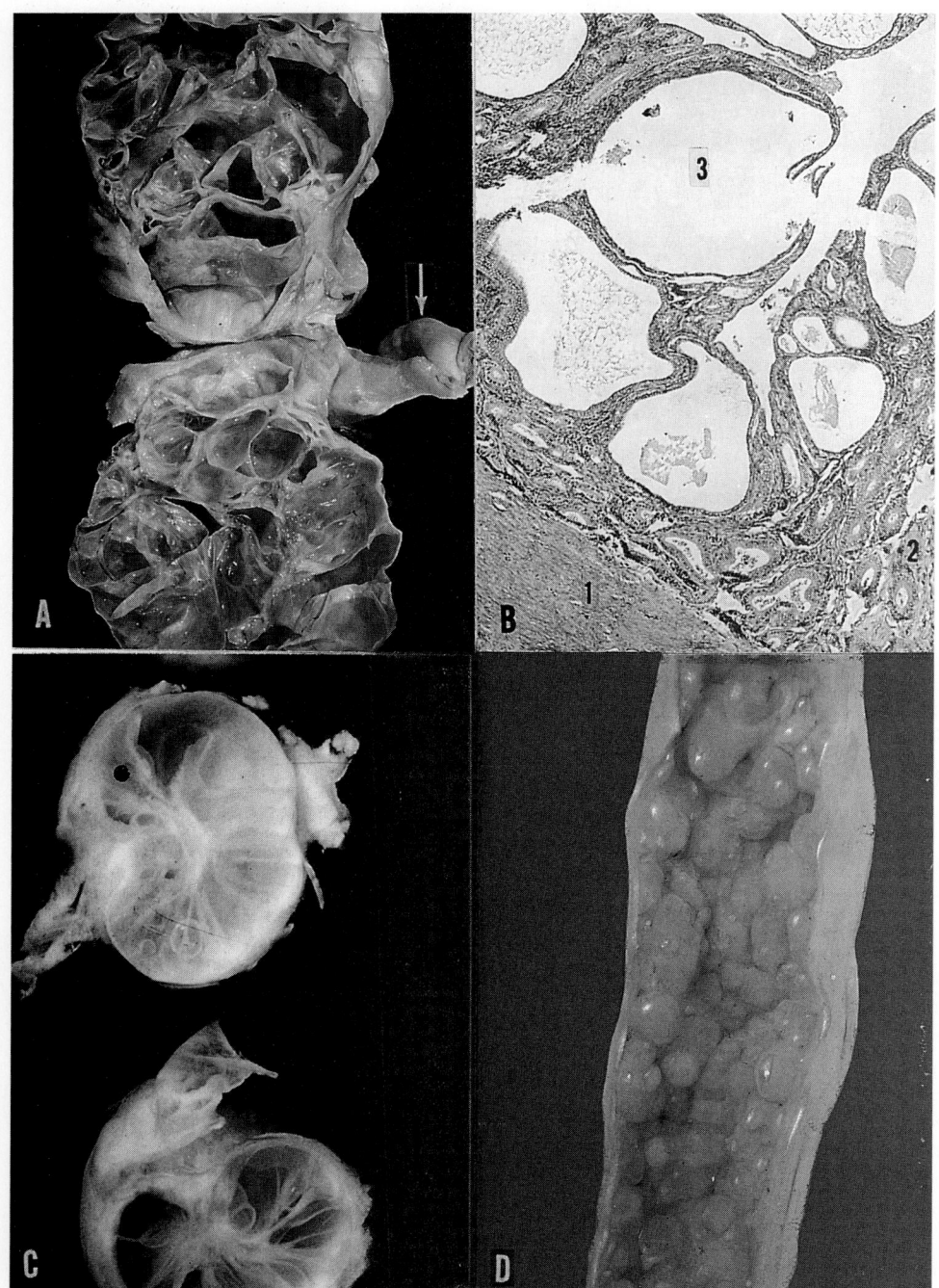

FIG. 25-11 **A.** Multiple cysts in a canine ovary. Uterine horn is indicated by the arrow. (Contributor: Dr. Wayne H. Riser.) **B.** Cystic glandular hyperplasia of the canine uterus (×70), (1) myometrium, (2) endometrium, and (3) cyst of endometrium. (Courtesy of Armed Forces Institute of Pathology; contributor: Dr. C.P. Zepp, Jr.) **C.** Cystic oviduct in a cow. **D.** Cystic glandular hyperplasia in the canine uterus.

tend even to the serosal surface. This condition is referred to as adenomyosis. At this stage, connective tissue begins to appear in appreciable amounts in the endometrium where it replaces stromal cells and between the smooth muscle cells of the myometrium. At this point, the lesion is irreversible.

PROGESTERONE-MEDIATED ENDOMETRIAL HYPERPLASIA

Progesterone-mediated endometrial hyperplasia occurs most often in bitches where it is by far the most common reproductive disorder. Because the resultant hyperplastic changes are usually cystic and often com-

plicated by infection, it is commonly referred to as the **cystic endometrial hyperplasia-pyometra complex.** It also occurs in cattle in association with retained corpora lutea. In both species, it predisposes the affected individual to uterine infection and **pyometra.** Progesterone and progestational compounds stimulate glandular secretion, especially in an estrogen-primed endometrium. Estrogen priming causes increased synthesis of progesterone receptors and thereby enhances the action of progesterone. The normal estrous cycle of the bitch is characterized by a prolonged luteal phase following proestrus and estrus during which estrogen priming occurs. This long luteal phase, referred to as **diestrus**

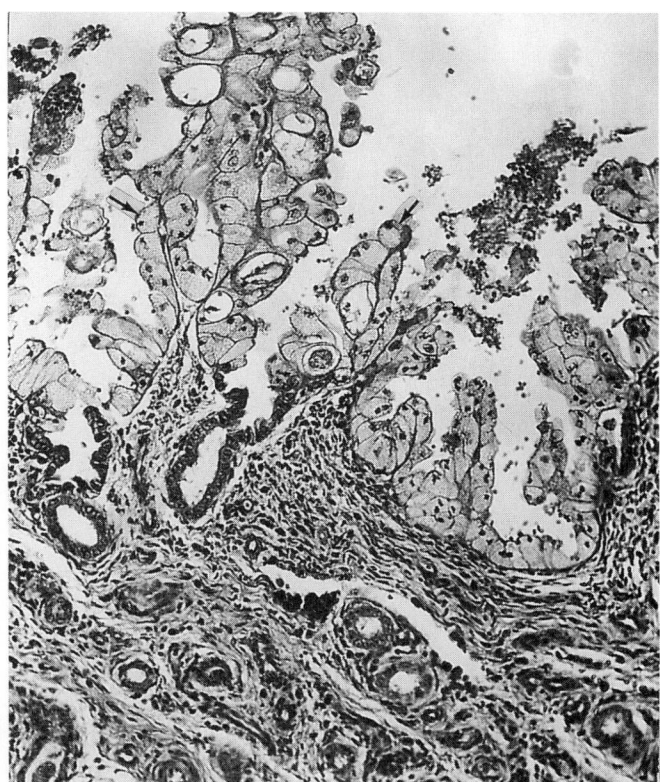

FIG. 25-12 Hypertrophy of the canine endometrium in pseudopregnancy (pseudocyesis). Note large endometrial cells with clear cytoplasm (arrow).

(metestrus) lasts approximately 50–75 days, after which the corpora lutea regress and progesterone secretion ceases. During diestrus, endometrial glands and surface epithelium undergo proliferative and secretory activity even in the absence of pregnancy. Surface epithelial cells and cells surrounding the mouths of endometrial glands become tall and columnar, with finely vacuolated, clear cytoplasm and nuclei that are displaced towards the apical portion of the cell. These findings are the hallmark of progesterone stimulation of the endometrium in bitches. Some nonpregnant bitches at the end of diestrus undergo psychic and physiologic signs of pregnancy, a condition referred to as **pseudopregnancy** or **pseudocyesis.** Clinical signs include weight gain, mammary gland hyperplasia, lactation, mucoid vaginal discharge, inappetence, nesting, and mothering of inanimate objects. This condition results from the decline in progesterone and elevation in **prolactin** concentrations during this period. It is usually self-limiting in one to three weeks. Diestrus is followed by roughly a four-month period of **anestrus** characterized by ovarian inactivity and regression of the proliferative and secretory changes in the uterus.

For reasons that are not well understood, in some bitches, particularly older nulliparous bitches, corpora lutea fail to regress following the normal period of diestrus and continue to secrete progesterone. Proliferative and secretory changes become accentuated and endometrium becomes markedly cystic due to pronounced proliferation of surface epithelium and cells lining the mouths of endometrial glands. These proliferating cells often line long, papillary projections that protrude into multiloculated cysts. The cysts frequently contain either a watery or mucinous secretion (hydrometra or mucometra), and the stroma is infiltrated with large numbers of plasma cells. These proliferative changes may alternate with areas of relatively normal-appearing diestrual endometrium and, thus, mimic implantation sites found during pregnancy. Grossly, uterine horns appear diffusely or, more often, segmentally enlarged and the endometrium contains large numbers of fluid-filled cysts (Figs. 25-13, 25-14).

It is well-established that the uterus is more susceptible to infection while under the influence of progesterone (luteal phase), than it is under the influence of estrogen (follicular phase). Progesterone is mildly immunosuppressive, causes diminished tone and rhythmic contractions of the myometrium, stimulates endometrial secretion, and causes functional closure of the cervix. These phenomena promote colonization of the uterine cavity by bacterial flora from the vagina, urinary, and intestinal tracts; thus, they predispose the uterus to infection (Fig. 25-15). For these reasons, most uterine infections of domestic animals occur either following coitus (i.e., during luteal phase following ovulation); during the prolonged diestrus in bitches and queens; or in most species during pregnancy.

Finally, one should be reminded of the fact that in domestic ungulates (i.e., horses, cows, sheep, goats, pigs), prostaglandin F2α synthesized and secreted by the endometrium is responsible for lysis of the corpus luteum at the end of normal diestrus. Any condition, including infection, that impairs the normal cyclic changes and function of the endometrium of these species may result in impaired secretion of PGF2α, and thus cause retention of corpora lutea. These retained corpora lutea interrupt the normal estrous cycle and, as described above, predispose the uterus to infection; or, when an infection already exists, exacerbate it and can cause **pyometra.** Thus, a vicious cycle becomes established that must be broken for the infection to be resolved.

EXOGENOUS SOURCES OF PROGESTERONE

Exogenous sources of progesterone that have been associated with cystic endometrial hyperplasia-pyometra complex include parenteral administration of a repository form of progesterone (i.e., medroxyprogesterone acetate), when it was temporarily marketed as an inhibitor of estrus in dogs about 30 years ago. It was later withdrawn from the market because of this complication.

Squamous metaplasia of endometrium

Transformation of the normal cuboidal or columnar uterine epithelium to stratified squamous epithelium *(squamous metaplasia)* occurs under several distinct circumstances in different species.

In **sheep** poisoned by highly-chlorinated naphthalenes, the epithelium of endometrial glands is transformed into keratinizing squamous epithelial cells. Plugs of keratin resembling fine hairs may extend from

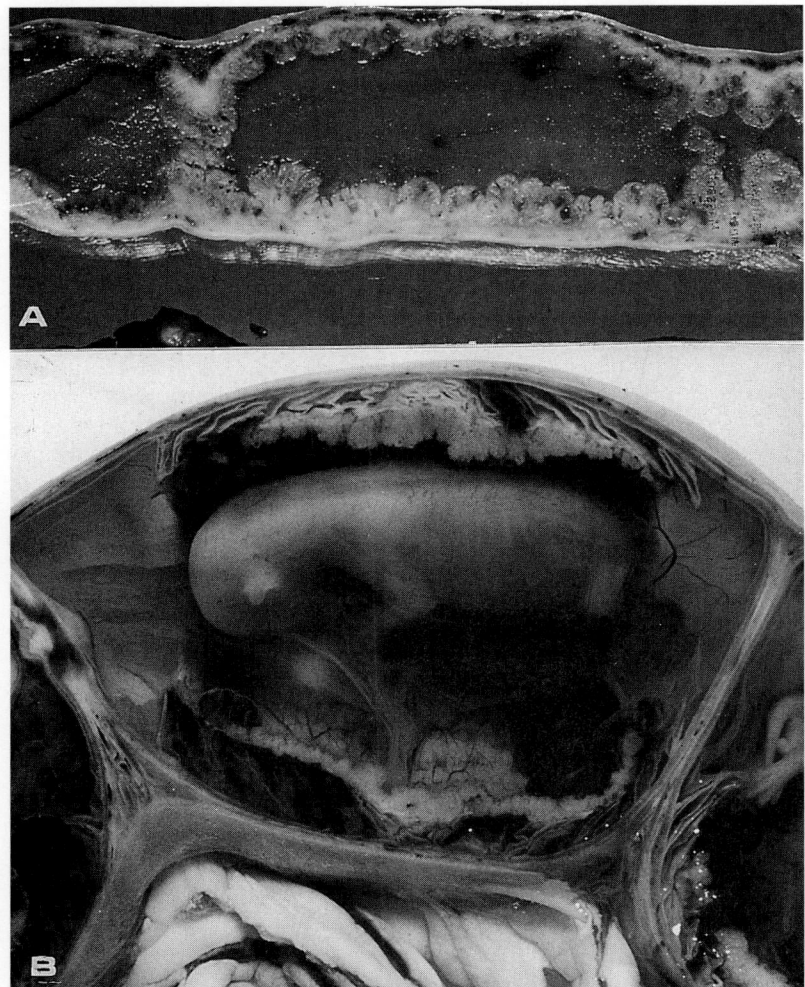

FIG. 25-13 A. Pseudocyesis in a canine uterus (female cocker spaniel, age 12 years). Compare the compartmentation and thickened endometrium with the normal pregnant uterus. **B.** Normal canine fetus in utero four weeks.

the orifices of these severely altered glands into the uterine cavity (Fig. 25-16). Cattle poisoned by the same compounds do not exhibit squamous metaplasia of the endometrium.

Squamous metaplasia of the endometrium has been produced experimentally in laboratory rodents fed diets deficient in vitamin A. The degree of metaplastic change is significantly reduced in ovariectomized animals, suggesting a relationship between estrogen and vitamin A deficiency in the causation of this disorder.

Squamous metaplasia may occur in the surface epithelium of the endometrium of any animal with long-standing pyometra. In these cases, it is believed to result from chronic irritation.

The clinical consequence of squamous metaplasia of the endometrium is infertility or sterility resulting from an inadequately prepared implantation site for the blastocyst.

Endometriosis

Endometriosis is the presence of endometrium outside the uterine cavity (i.e., in ectopic sites). It occurs spontaneously only in those species that menstruate, which include women and most Old World primates. In women, it is an extremely common gynecologic problem and is a frequent cause of dysmenorrhea and infertility. In nonhuman primates, it occurs infrequently as a spontaneous disease, but is a common complication of repeated hysterotomies or cesarean sections. When endometriosis occurs spontaneously, its pathogenesis involves reflux of menstrual fluid from the uterine tubes with subsequent implantation and proliferation of viable fragments of endometrium contained in fluid on the surfaces of pelvic organs.

In laboratory primates, endometriosis is a common complication resulting from spillage of normal endometrium into the pelvic cavity during the course of hysterotomy or cesarean section with subsequent implantation. This ectopic endometrium responds to the normal cyclic ovarian hormonal changes, just as normal endometrium, and undergoes monthly desquamation and bleeding (menstruation) except that it occurs in the pelvic cavity. At this site, the entrapped menstrual fluid provokes an intense inflammatory reaction with resultant fibrosis and adhesion formation between pelvic organs. This results in infertility, abdominal discomfort, and occasionally bowel obstruction.

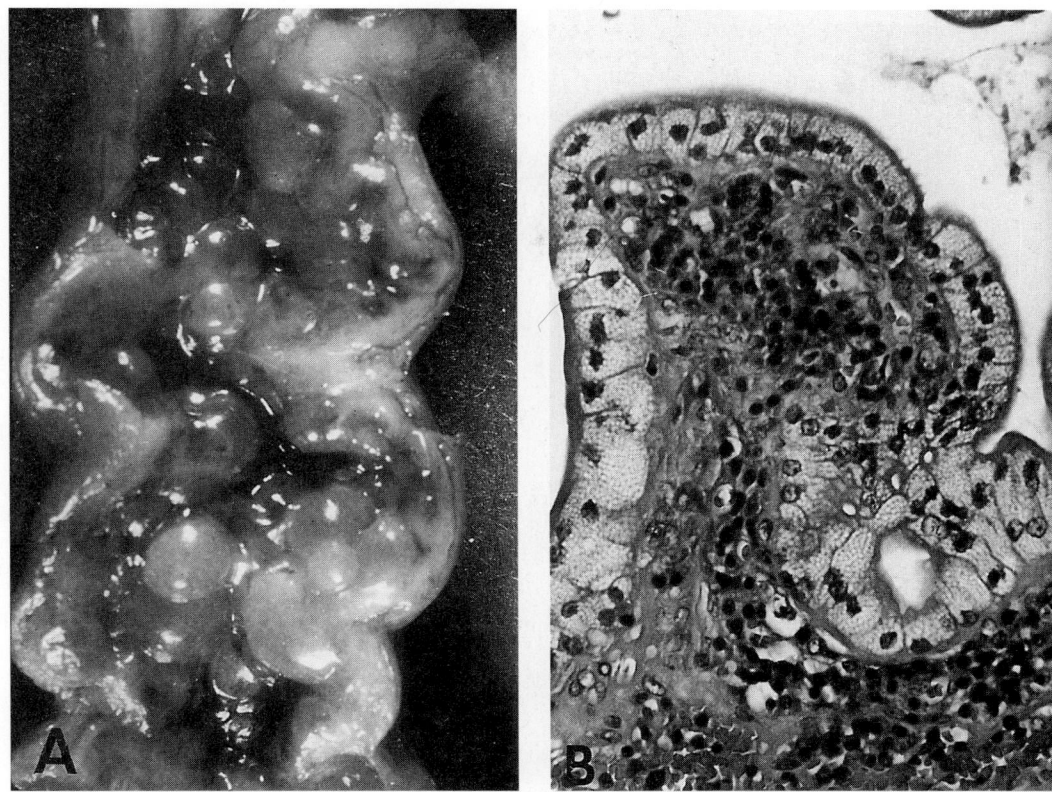

FIG. 25-14 Cystic endometrial hyperplasia in a 12-year-old bitch. **A.** Gross surface of endometrium. **B.** Vacuolated endometrial epithelium typical of progestational endometrium. (Courtesy of Drs. N.W. King, Jr. and C.E. Gilmore.)

Grossly, the ectopic endometrium appears as soft, red-brown, or white polypoid masses of tissue adherent to the serosa of pelvic organs or as large, bosselated masses of connective tissue containing cysts filled with brown menstrual blood. The larger cysts may rupture, spilling their contents into the peritoneal cavity. Commonly, the ovaries, uterine tubes, urinary bladder, and large bowel are involved. Microscopically, (Fig. 25-17), the lesions consist of variable-sized foci of normal-appearing uterine glands surrounded by typical endometrial stroma. Ectopic endometrium may be present as solid masses or lining thick-walled, fibrous cysts filled with blood and cellular debris. Hemosiderin-laden macrophages are often present throughout the dense bands of scar tissue. Infertility results from ovarian and tubal functional impairment.

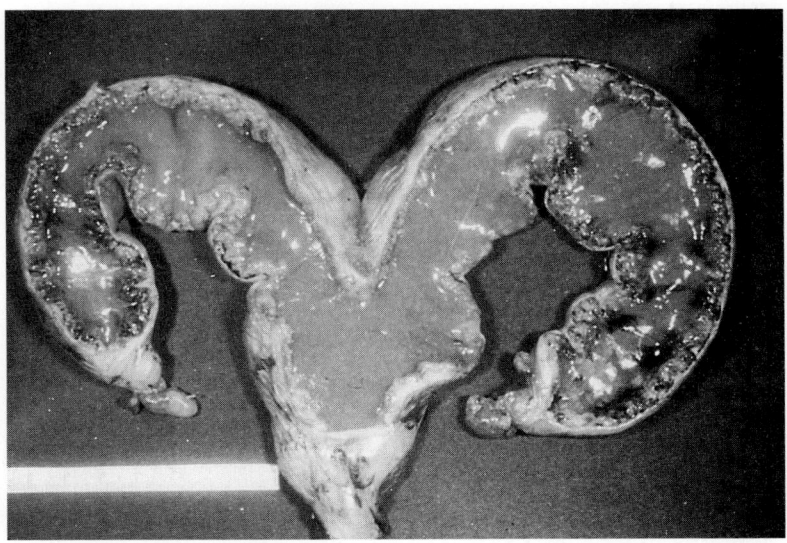

FIG. 25-15 Cystic endometrial hyperplasia and mucometria in a two-year-old bitch. (Courtesy of Drs. C.E. Gilmore and N.W. King, Jr.)

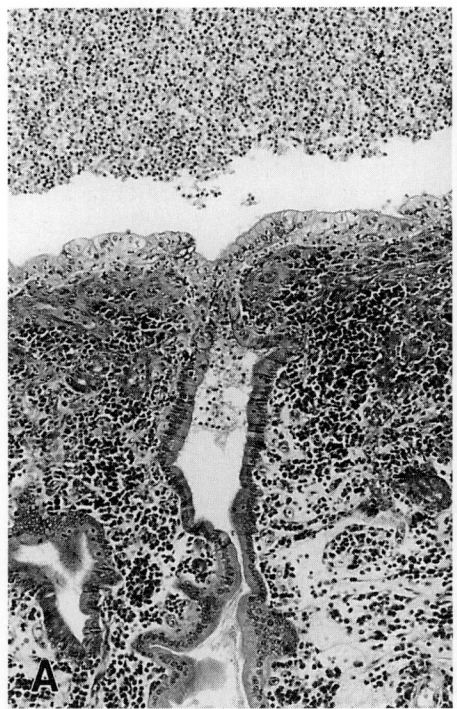
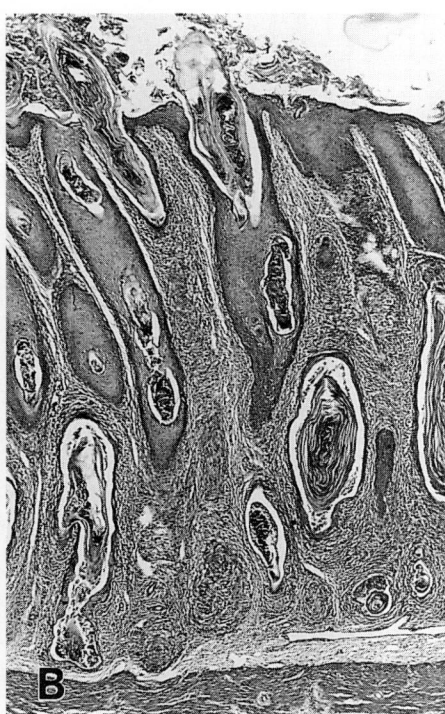

FIG. 25-16 A. Pyometra in a dog. Luminal exudate consists mostly of neutrophils, whereas stromal infiltrate consists mostly of mononuclear cells. Note the vacuolated uterine surface epithelium (×175). **B.** Squamous metaplasia of the uterine glands of a ewe poisoned by chlorinated naphthalenes. Note the plugs of keratin protruding from what formerly were glands (×100).

Neoplasms

Benign endometrial polyps

Benign endometrial polyps are observed occasionally in cats, rats, and mice. They appear as firm, roughly spherical, usually sessile-based masses that protrude from the surface of the endometrium. In cats (Fig. 25-18), the polyps are composed of well-differentiated endometrial glands enmeshed in dense, fibrous connective stroma. In rodents, the amount of glandular component can be highly variable; in some cases, the stroma is the dominant component. In these cases, the polyps are referred to as **endometrial stromal polyps.**

Adenocarcinoma of endometrium

Adenocarcinoma of the endometrium is a disease of older individuals. It is rare in animals, except in rabbits and cattle.

In rabbits, it occurs commonly after two years of age and constitutes the single most common neoplasm in this species. More than 60% of does over four years of age develop spontaneously occurring endometrial adenocarcinoma. The lesions are often multiple, involve one or both horns, and frequently metastasize to distant sites, including liver and lungs.

In cattle, adenocarcinoma of the endometrium occurs much less commonly than in rabbits, but consti-

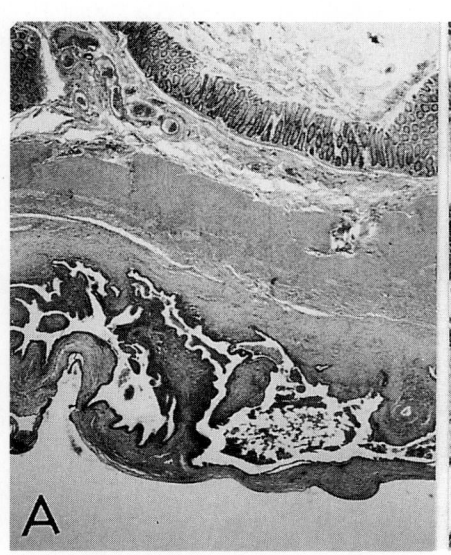
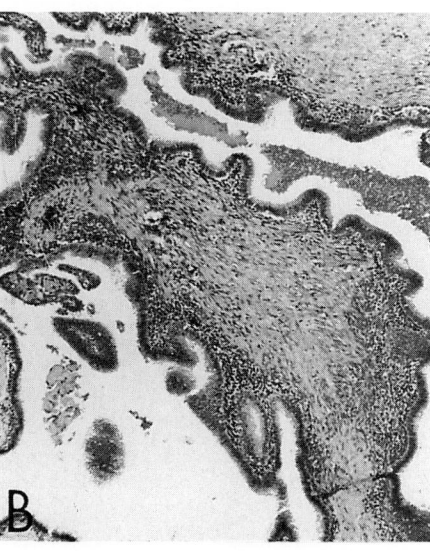

FIG. 25-17 Endometriosis in a rhesus monkey *(Macaca mulatta).* **A.** Endometrium implanted on the wall of the colon. **B.** Uterine columnar epithelium accompanied by endometrial stroma differentiates endometriosis from malignancy. Note detritus which represents evidence of menstruation. Inability of menstrual fluids to escape the body results in toxemia. (Courtesy of New England Regional Primate Research Center, Harvard Medical School.)

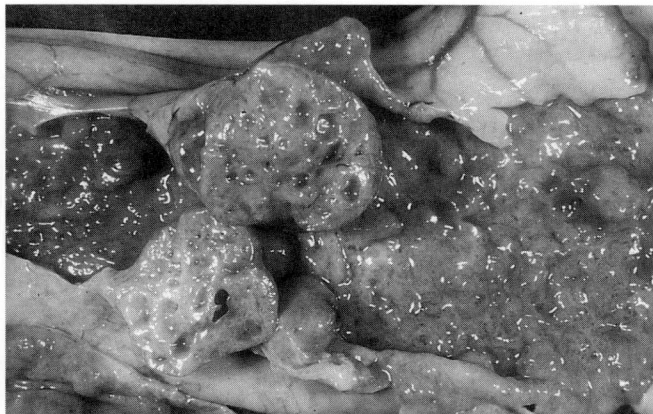

FIG. 25-18 Endometrial polyp arising in hyperplastic endometrium of a 15-year-old cat. (Courtesy of Dr. C.E. Gilmore.)

tutes the third most common spontaneously occurring neoplasm in this species, behind squamous cell carcinoma and lymphoma. It is generally found in cows over six years of age and presents as a solitary, hard, yellow-white mass located in the wall of a uterine horn, often near the body. Its surface is usually contracted. Metastatic lesions occur in the lungs, lymph nodes, and various other organs. Microscopically, endometrial carcinoma in cows is a scirrhous neoplasm, having a prominent dense collagenous connective tissue component. Small islands of neoplastic epithelial cells can be found scattered throughout the dense stromal component where they may form small nests (Fig. 25-19), abortive glands, or undergo calcification. In other domestic animal species, adenocarcinoma of the endometrium is extraordinarily rare.

Leiomyoma and leiomyosarcoma

LEIOMYOMA

Leiomyoma of the uterus arises from smooth muscle cells of the myometrium. Although they occur infrequently in dogs and cats, leiomyomas are the most common uterine neoplasm of these species and are found most often in bitches and queens over 10 years of age. They are also observed in the myometrium of old rodents and nonhuman primates. Grossly, they are round to ovoid and reasonably well-circumscribed. Microscopically, they consist of elongate fasciculi of well-differentiated smooth muscle cells that form a well-circumscribed, expansile rather than an invasive mass. In women, leiomyoma of the myometrium is commonly referred to as a "fibroid."

LEIOMYOSARCOMAS

Leiomyosarcomas of the uterus are extremely rare in most animal species. They have been recognized in cattle, sheep, dogs, cats, rats, and mice. Neoplastic cells are often highly pleomorphic, have a high mitotic index, and may be quite invasive.

Lymphosarcoma

Lymphosarcomas may occur in the uterus of cattle and cats (Fig. 25-20) as part of a generalized disease and must be differentiated from primary tumors of this organ.

References

Adams NR. Pathological changes in the tissues of infertile ewes with clover disease. J Comp Pathol 1976;86:29–35.
Adams NR. Morphological changes in the organs of ewes grazing subterranean clover. Res Vet Sci 1977;22:216–221.

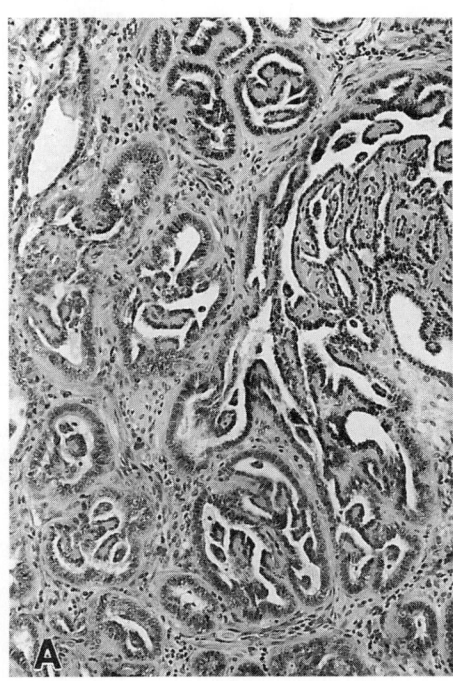
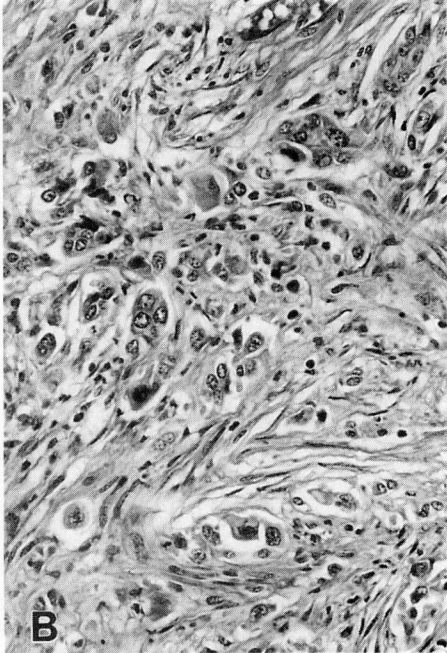

FIG. 25-19 A. Adenocarcinoma in the uterus of a six-year-old New Zealand white rabbit (×100). **B.** Scirrhous adenocarcinoma of the uterus of an eight-year-old cow (×250). Note individual and nests of neoplastic epithelial cells admixed with dense, collagenous, connective tissue stroma.

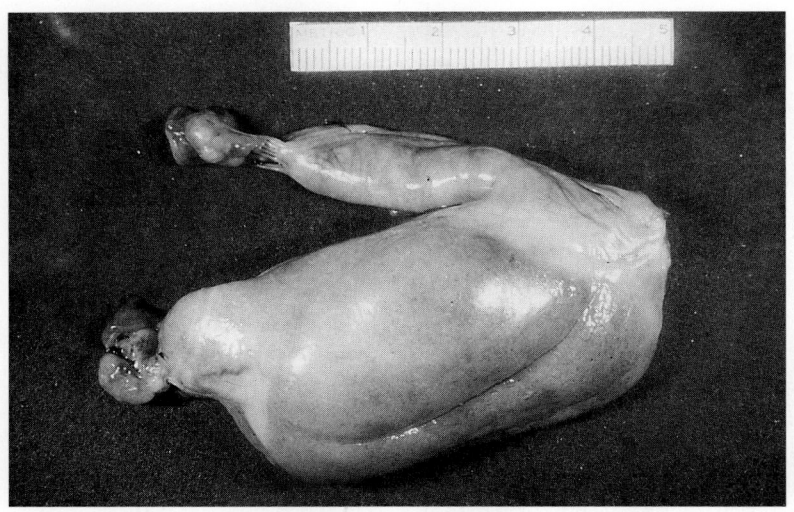

FIG. 25-20 Malignant lymphoma in the uterus of a six-year-old cat. (Courtesy of Dr. C.E. Gilmore.)

Allen WE. Pseudopregnancy in the bitch: the current view on aetiology and treatment. J Small Anim Pract 1986;27:419–424.

Andersen AC. Carcinoma of the uterus in a beagle. J Am Vet Med Assoc 1963;143:500–502.

Anderson LJ, Sandison AT. Tumours of the female genitalia of cattle, sheep and pigs found in a British abattoir survey. J Comp Pathol 1969;79:53–63.

Anderson RK, Gilmore CE, Schnelle GG. Utero-ovarian disorders associated with use of medroxyprogesterone in dogs. J Am Vet Med Assoc 1965;146:1311–1316.

Anderson WA, Davis CL. Neoplasms of the genitalia of the bovine. 3rd Symp Reprod Infertil 1958;41–49.

Austad R, Blom AK, Borreson B. Pyometra in the dog. A pathophysiological investigation. III. Plasma progesterone levels and ovarian morphology. Nord Vet Med 1979;31:258–262.

Beck AB. The oestrogenic isoflavones of subterranean clover. Aust J Agric Res 1964;14:223–230.

Boomsa RA, Jaffee RC, Verhage HG. The uterine progestational response in cats: changes in morphology and progesterone receptors during chronic administration of progesterone to estradiol-primed and nonprimed animals. Biol Reprod 1982;26:511–521.

Borreson B. Pyometra in the dog—a pathophysiological investigation. I. The pyometra syndrome, a review. Nord Vet Med 1975;27:508–517.

Bradley RL, Olson P. Feline pyometra. Feline Pract 1979;9:17–22.

Brandly PJ, Migaki G. Types of tumors found by federal meat inspectors in an eight-year survey. Ann NY Acad Sci 1963;108:862–879.

Brodey RS, Fidler IJ. Clinical and pathologic findings in bitches treated with progestational compounds. J Am Vet Med Assoc 1966;149:1406–1415.

Brodey RS, Roszel JR. Neoplasms of the canine uterus, vagina and vulva: a clinicopathologic survery. J Am Vet Med Assoc 1967;151:1294–1307.

Cotchin E. Spontaneous uterin cancer in animals. Br J Cancer 1964;18:209–227.

Cotchin E, Marchant J. Animal tumors of the female reproductive tract. Spontaneous and experimental. In: Blaustein A, ed. Pathology of the female genital tract. New York: Springer Verlag, 1977.

Davis CL, Leeper RB, Shelton JE. Neoplasms encountered in federally inspected establishments in Denver. J Am Vet Med Assoc 1933;83:229–237.

Dow C. The cystic hyperplasia-pyometra complex in the bitch. Vet Rec 1957;69:1409–1415.

Dow C. The cystic hyperplasia-pyometra complex in the bitch. Vet Rec 1958;70:1102–1110.

Dow C. The cystic hyperplasia-pyometra complex in the bitch. J Comp Pathol 1959;69:237–250.

Dow C. Experimental reproduction of the cystic hyperplasia-pyometra complex in the bitch. J Pathol Bacteriol 1959;78:267–278.

Dow C. The cystic hyperplasia-pyometra complex in the cat. Vet Rec 1962;74:141–147.

Gelberg HB, McEntee K. Hyperplastic endometrial polyps in the dog and cat. Vet Pathol 1984;21:570–573.

Greene RR, Roddick JW Jr, Milligan M. Estrogens, endometrial hyperplasia, and endometrial carcinoma. Ann NY Acad Sci 1959;75:586–600.

Grindley M, Renton JP, Ramsay DH. O-groups of *Escherichia coli* associated with canine pyometra. Res Vet Sci 1973;14:75–77.

Hardy RM, Osborne CA. Canine pyometra: pathophysiology, diagnosis and treatment of uterine and extra-uterine lesions. J Am Anim Hosp Assoc 1974;10:245–268.

Kenney KJ, Matthiesen DT, Brown NO, et al. Pyometra in cats: 183 cases (1979–1984). J Am Vet Med Assoc 191:1130–1132, 1987.

Kenney RM, Ganjam VK. Selected pathological changes of the mare uterus and ovaries. J Reprod Fertil Suppl 1975;23:335–339.

Lagerlof N, Boyd H. Ovarian hypoplasia and other abnormal conditions in the sexual organs of cattle of the Swedish Highland breed: results of postmortem examination of over 6,000 cows. Cornell Vet 1953;43:64–79.

Mawdesley-Thomas LE, Sortwell RJ. Proliferative lesions of the canine uterus associated with high dose oestrogen administration. Vet Rec 1968;82:468–469.

McCann TO, Myers RE. Endometriosis in rhesus monkeys. Am J Obstet Gynecol 1970;106:516–523.

McEntee K, Nielsen SW. Tumours of the female genital tract. Bull WHO 1976;53:217–226.

McEntee K, Olafson P. Reproductive tract pathology in hyperkeratosis of cattle and sheep. Fertil Steril 1953;4:128–136.

Meyers-Wallen VN, Goldschmidt MH, Flickinger GL. Prostaglandin F2a treatment of canine pyometra. J Am Vet Med Assoc 1986; 189:1557–1561.

Migaki G, Carey AM, Turnquist RU, et al. Pathology of bovine uterine adenocarcinoma. J Am Vet Med Assoc 1970;157:1577–1584.

Monlux AW, Anderson WA, Davis CL, et al. Adenocarcinoma of the uterus of the cow—differentiation of its pulmonary metastases from primary lung tumors. Am J Vet Res 1956;17:45–73.

Nelson RW, Feldman EC, Stabenfeldt GH. Treatment of canine pyometra and endometritis with prostaglandin F2a. J Am Vet Med Assoc 1982;181:99–903.

Pack FD. Feline uterine adenomyosis. A case report. Feline Pract 1980;10:45–47.

Papparella S, Roperto F. Spontaneous uterine tumors in three cats. Vet Pathol 1984;21:257–258.

Preiser H. Endometrial adenocarcinoma in a cat. Pathol Vet 1964;1:485–490.

Smith HA. The pathology of malignant lymphoma in cattle. A study of 1113 cases. Pathol Vet 1965;2:68–93.

INFLAMMATION OF NONGRAVID UTERUS

The terms **endometritis, metritis, perimetritis,** and **parametritis** refer to inflammation of the endometrium, endometrium and myometrium, serosal surface of the uterus, and ligamentous structures suspending the uterus, respectively. These terms are useful in that they denote the extent and anatomical distribution of the inflammatory process. Most inflammatory lesions of the nongravid uterus are infectious in origin and result either from ascending infection by organisms that normally inhabit the lower genital tract or infectious agents introduced into the uterine cavity during mating, artificial insemination, or postpartum. The endometrium of the nongravid uterus is relatively resistant to infection even though the vagina contains a variety of bacterial flora. The cervix serves as an effective barrier to ascending infections from the vagina because it is functionally closed during the luteal phase of the estrous cycle when the endometrium is most susceptible to infection. During estrus when the cervix is normally patent, the endometrium is relatively resistant to infection. The mechanism(s) by which estrogen stimulation confers resistance to endometritis is not understood. It has been postulated that increased uterine leukocytosis during estrous plays a role in clearing infectious agents entering the uterus during this time. Heifers with incompletely developed cervical rings and older cows with prolapsed cervical rings due to multiple calvings are prone to chronic endometritis because of an incompetent cervical barrier to ascending infection. Most uterine infections in nongravid individu-

als with normally developed reproductive tracts tend to be transient and self-limiting. Local antibody production to the invading organism may also be important in limiting the course of such infections.

Nonspecific infections of uterus

Nonspecific endometritis results from infection by bacterial organisms that usually are not regarded as specific pathogens of the female reproductive tract but, which under appropriate circumstances, are capable of colonizing the endometrium and causing transient inflammation (Fig. 25-21). Such agents may cause temporary infertility, particularly in young heifers. Nonspecific endometritis occurs frequently in virgin heifers bred to experienced bulls and results from introduction of normal bacterial flora from the heifer's vagina or the bull's penis and prepuce into the uterine cavity. Such infections may also result from artificial insemination with semen not containing antibiotics. With repeated exposure, heifers gradually become resistant to infection by these nonspecific bacteria. Nonspecific endometritis also occurs commonly in the postpartum uterus, especially as a complication of abnormal deliveries, such as abortion, retained placenta, dystocia, twinning, and traumatic injuries of the reproductive tract. In these cases, delayed involution of the uterus, coupled with the accumulation of necrotic placental and endometrial debris in the presence of a open cervix promotes the establishment of infection. In some cases, infection may progress to pyometra.

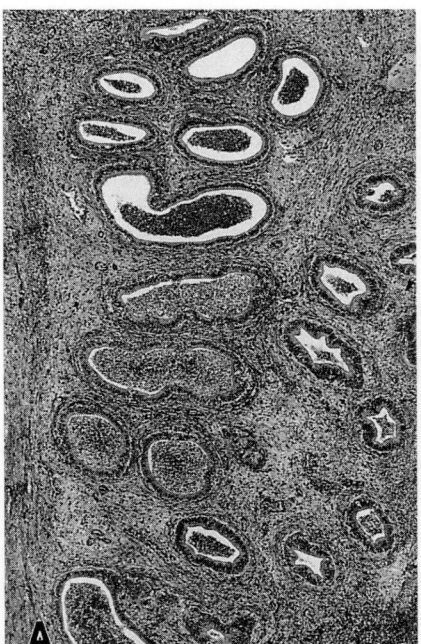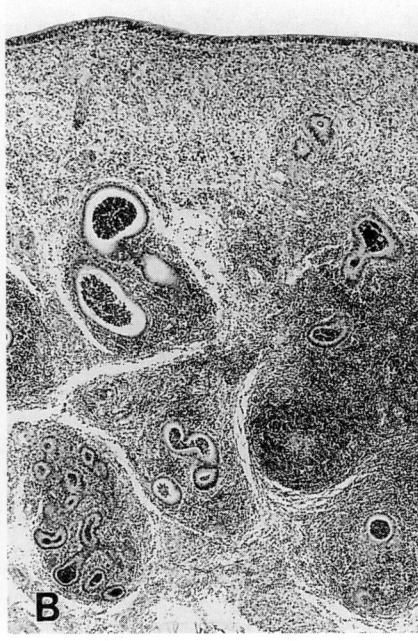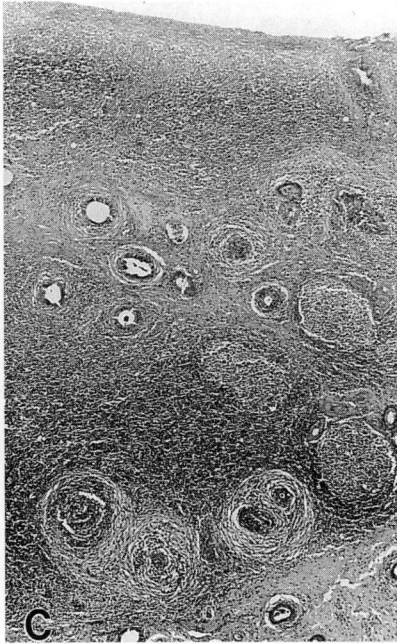

FIG. 25-21 **A.** Acute bacterial endometritis in an infertile heifer. Endometrial glands are distended with purulent exudate but the glandular epithelium is intact. **B.** Subacute endometritis in an infertile heifer. In addition to purulent exudate in glands, focal and diffuse infiltrates of mononuclear cells are present in the stroma along with adenomatous hyperplasia ("nesting") of endometrial glands. **C.** *Tritrichomonas foetus*-induced pyometra in an infertile heifer. Focal and diffuse infiltrates of mononuclear cells occur throughout the zona compacta and zona spongiosa, glandular atrophy, and periglandular fibrosis.

Bacteria isolated from nonspecific endometritis in domestic animal species include: coliforms (*E. coli*) and Proteus; Actinomyces (*Corynebacterium*) pyogenes; β-hemolytic streptococci; *Klebsiella;* gram-positive anaerobes (*Clostridium*); and gram-negative anaerobes (*Fusobacterium* and *Bacteroides*). Grossly in nonspecific endometritis, the endometrium and uterine cavity will contain varying amounts of purulent exudate. The exudate varies from gray-yellow to red-brown depending on the organism involved and the amount of tissue damage present. Postpartum uteri often also contain fragments of necrotic fetal and maternal placental tissue.

Microscopically, mild, nonspecific endometritis of the nongravid uterus is characterized by the presence of many neutrophils in the superficial portions (zona compacta) of the endometrium. These migrate through the glandular and surface epithelium and accumulate as luminal exudate. Frequently, large numbers of lymphocytes and plasma cells are also present in the endometrial stroma. These occur in aggregates around blood vessels and glands and probably reflect an immunologic reaction to infection. With time, neutrophils gradually decrease in number while the mononuclear cells generally persist until the infection is resolved. During the course of infection, varying amounts of necrosis and fibrosis of the endometrium may be manifest, the consequences of which are permanent scarring and dilatation of glands due to obstruction of their openings. When severe, this obviously causes some degree of infertility.

Specific infectious agents causing endometritis

Many of the agents included in this section are transmitted venereally and are well known causes of abortion or stillbirth in pregnant animals. Because they also cause transient endometritis and infertility when introduced into the nongravid uterus during coitus, these agents are briefly mentioned below (*Infections of Gravid Uterus* section provides more details).

BOVINE VENEREAL CAMPYLOBACTERIOSIS
Campylobacter fetus ssp. *venerealis* is a comma-shaped, gram-negative bacillus transmitted by coitus with infected bulls or by artificial insemination with infected semen. The organism multiplies rapidly in the vagina of infected heifers or cows and after about one week invades the endometrium where it causes diffuse, subacute, endometritis that may last 6–12 weeks. The inflamed endometrium is not conducive to blastocyst implantation, thus resulting in infertility. Infected heifers may have prolonged cycles during this period because of the impact of the infection on prostaglandin F2α synthesis and secretion. If pregnancy were to ensue, abortion would be common. Because many cows in a herd may be infected, this disease has been referred to as *enzootic infertility*. Some cows may harbor the organism as a latent infection in their vaginas and, thus, serve as a reservoir of infection for bulls; others become immune.

BRUCELLOSIS
Brucella abortus, a gram-negative coccobacillus, is a primary pathogen of the gravid uterus where it causes abortion. It is mainly transmitted through ingestion. B. abortus causes transient, purulent endometritis when contaminated semen is infused into the nongravid uterus. This is uncommon in the United States because of control measures adopted to eradicate brucellosis.

Brucella suis is primarily transmitted by coitus, but can be transmitted by ingestion as well. It is somewhat unusual among the brucellae in that it regularly colonizes the nongravid uterus where it causes multiple, 2–3 mm granulomas in the endometrium. Microscopically, the lesions consist of central areas of caseous necrosis surrounded by a zone of histiocytes, epithelioid cells, and other mononuclear cells. Scattered neutrophils may be manifest in the lesions as well. These lesions may result in infertility or, when pregnancy occurs, abortion and stillbirth are common.

Brucella canis also has been associated with infertility in bitches. As with bovine brucellosis, it is a major cause of early embryonic death and abortion. Presumably, it can also cause endometritis when introduced into the nongravid uterus, but this has not been well documented.

BOVINE TUBERCULOSIS
Mycobacterium tuberculosis var. *bovis* and *M. avium* are acid-fast bacilli that formerly were responsible for granulomatous endometritis, metritis, and parametritis of the nongravid uterus. Tuberculosis in cattle is extremely rare in the United States because of rigorous control measures taken to eradicate this disease.

BOVINE VENEREAL TRICHOMONIASIS
Tritrichomonas foetus, a piriform flagellated protozoan, is transmitted as a venereal infection by subclinically infected bulls. The organism colonizes the vagina, uterus, and uterine tubes where it causes a purulent endometritis and salpingitis that result in early embryonic death or failure of implantation. Following a variable period of infertility, infected animals may regain their fertility and become resistant to reinfection. Infected heifers may have a mucopurulent vaginal discharge which, when examined microscopically, contains the characteristic motile organisms. T. foetus is also a common cause of pyometra in cattle.

MYCOTIC ENDOMETRITIS
The nongravid uterus is extremely resistant to mycotic infection. However, agents, such as *Aspergillus* and *Mucor*, may occasionally colonize sites of endometrial laceration that occur during parturition. The lesions are typically granulomatous and the fungal hyphae can be seen when special stains are applied. Mycotic endometritis is not a significant cause of infertility, but may result in abortion or stillbirth in both cattle and horses.

CONTAGIOUS EQUINE METRITIS
Hemophilus (*Taylorella*) *equigenitalis*, the etiologic agent of contagious equine metritis, is a nonmotile, gram-negative, coccobacillus. Contagious equine metri-

tis was first recognized in the Newmarket area of England in 1977 and subsequently described in Kentucky in 1978. It has since been shown to occur in other parts of the world. The organism, transmitted primarily by coitus, may persist in the genital tracts of infected horses indefinitely, particularly in the clitoral fossae of mares and the urethral fossae of stallions. Infected mares tend to return to estrus after a shortened diestrus and often develop a mucopurulent vaginal discharge that may be copious. Microscopically, the organism causes severe, purulent, necrotizing endometritis with extensive desquamation of the necrotic endometrial tissue into the uterine lumen. This is most severe during the first two weeks of infection and gradually subsides to a milder, multifocal, lymphoplasmacytic endometritis. At this stage, it is difficult to isolate the organism, probably because of local antibody secretion by plasma cells in the infiltrate. Microscopically, the lesions are not particularly distinctive and, thus, cannot be distinguished from those caused by other pathogenic bacteria. Culture is the only definitive means of diagnosis. No lesions have been reported in infected stallions.

HERPESVIRUS BOVIS

H. bovis infection (infectious bovine rhinotracheitis, pustular vulovaginitis, balanoposthitis) is a venereally-transmitted herpesvirus infection of cattle associated with infertility and abortion. When introduced into the nongravid uterus during coitus or by artificial insemination with contaminated semen, *H. bovis* causes a transient, necrotizing, purulent endometritis associated with temporary infertility.

Pyometra

Pyometra is an acute or chronic suppurative inflammation of the uterus with accumulation of large quantities of pus in the uterine cavity. It is seen with some frequency in bitches, queens, cows, and mares and is rare in ewes and sows. In general, it results from persistence of unresolved, nonspecific bacterial endometritis during periods of prolonged or excessive progesterone stimulation. It occasionally occurs as a consequence of postcoital infection. Its pathogenesis differs among various species affected.

BITCHES AND QUEENS

Pyometra in bitches and queens is a life-threatening condition resulting from bacterial infection of an endometrium that has undergone cystic hyperplasia due to prolonged progesterone stimulation. For this reason the condition is often referred to as **cystic endometrial hyperplasia-pyometra complex.** Bacterial agents responsible for pyometra in these species are generally nonspecific and consist of organisms that normally inhabit the vagina, urinary, or intestinal tracts.

E. coli, Proteus, Staphylococcus, and *Streptococcus* are the most commonly isolated organisms. The uterine horns are variably distended either uniformly or segmentally by accumulation of intraluminal, mucopurulent exudate. The cervix is generally closed preventing escape of the exudate; however, in some cases a small amount of discharge may be evident in the anterior vagina. Microscopically, the endometrium exhibits all of the changes described under progesterone-mediated cystic endometrial hyperplasia in bitches, but in addition has large numbers of neutrophils in the luminal secretion. Moreover, large numbers of plasma cells are usually present in the endometrial stroma. The pathogenesis of pyometra in queens has been less well-studied, but is presumed to be similar to that in bitches.

COWS

Pyometra in cows has a somewhat different pathogenesis than that in bitches, but prolonged progesterone stimulation of the endometrium is a common feature. Infection of the endometrium following coitus, early embryonic death, or as a consequence of retained placenta may cause sufficient damage to the endometrium so that it does not produce sufficient quantities of prostaglandin F2α to cause lysis of the corpus luteum. Hence, the corpus luteum persists. Continued secretion of progesterone by the persistent corpus luteum promotes persistence and progression of the intrauterine infection because it decreases myometrial contractility, causes functional closure of the cervix, and promotes further endometrial secretion; thus, it provides a rich culture medium for the causative agent. The amount of pus that accumulates in the uterus of a cow with pyometra may exceed several liters and is usually thick, mucinous, and yellow or greenish-gray. The wall of the uterus may be thickened and doughy, or thin and fibrotic, depending on the duration of the infection. The condition is generally not life-threatening in cows, but sterility may be a consequence. *Tritrichomonas foetus* is the most common cause of postcoital pyometra, whereas *Actinomyces (Corynebacterium) pyogenes, E. coli, Pseudomonas aeruginosa, Streptococcus,* and *Staphylococcus* are frequently isolated from postpartum pyometra.

MARES

Pyometra in mares may result from postpartum infections, as in cattle, but mares with this condition may continue to cycle indicating that a persistent corpora luteum is not essential for pathogenesis. In most instances, purulent exudate accumulates in the uterine cavity without obvious cervical closure, and discharge of exudate may occur, especially during estrus. In severe cases, mares may have prolonged cycles due to inadequate prostaglandin F2α synthesis and secretion. Organisms commonly isolated from pyometra in mares include *Streptococcus zooepidemicus, E. coli, Pseudomonas aeruginosa, Klebsiella pneumoniae,* and *Pasteurella.*

References

Acland HM, Kenney RM. Lesions of contagious equine metritis in mares. Vet Pathol 1983;20:330–341.

Acland HM, Allen PZ, Kenney RM. Recovery of contagious equine metritis organisms and development of lesions in experimental infection of mares. J Reprod Fertil Suppl 1982;32:187–191.

Acland HM, Allen PZ, Kenney RM. Contagious equine metritis: distribution of organisms in experimental infection of mares. Am J Vet Res 1983;44:1197–1207.

Bartlett DE. Trichomonas foetus infection and bovine reproduction. Am J Vet Res 1947;8:343–352.

Bartlett DE. Bovine venereal trichomoniasis: its nature, recognition, intraherd eradication and intraherd control. Proc 52nd Annu Mtng US Livest Sanit Assoc 1947;170–181.

Berger J. Tuberculosis of the genitalia in bovines and its implications. Vet Rec 1944;56:469–470.

Black WG, et al. Inflammatory response of the bovine endometrium. Am J Vet Res 1953;14:179–183.

Bostedt H. Uterine infections in the postpartum period. Proc Int Congr Anim Reprod Artif Insemin 1984;10:III 25–III 33.

Brewer RA. Contagious equine metritis. Vet Bull 1983;53:881–891.

Broome AWJ, Winter AJ, McNutt SH, et al. Variations in uterine response to experimental infection due to the hormonal state of the ovaries. II The mobilization of leukocytes and their importance in uterine bacteriocidal activity. Am J Vet Res 1960;21:675–681.

Callahan CJ. Postpartum infections of dairy cattle. J Am Vet Med Assoc 1969;155:1963–1967.

Clark WA, Stevenson WG. The bacterial flora of the normal nongravid and gravid bovine uterus. Can J Comp Med 1949;13:92–93.

Corbeil LB, Corbeil RR, Winter AJ. Bovine venereal vibriosis: activity of inflammatory cells in protective immunity. Am J Vet Res 1975;36:403–406.

Crowhurst RC. Genital infection in mares. Vet Rec 1977;100:476.

Dimock WW, Edwards PR. The pathology and bacteriology of the reproductive organs of mares in relation to sterility. Kentucky Agric Exp Sta Res Bull 1928;286:157–237.

Doig PA. Bovine genital mycoplasmosis. Can Vet J 1981;22:339–343.

Elliott L, McMahon KJ, Gier HT, et al. Uterus of the cow after parturition: bacterial content. Am J Vet Res 1968;29:77–81.

Estes PC, Bryner JH, O'Berry PA. Histopathology of bovine vibriosis and the effect of *Vibrio fetus* extracts on the female genital tract. Cornell Vet 1966;57:610–622.

Farin PW, et al. Effect of *Actinomyces pyogenes* and gram-negative anaerobic bacteria on the development of bovine pyometra. Theriogenology 1989;31:979–989.

Fitch CP, Boyd WL, Bishop LM, et al. Localization of *Brucella abortus* in the bovine uterus. Cornell Vet 1939;29:253–260.

Frank AH, Shalkop WT, Bryner JH, et al. Cellular change in the endometrium of *Vibrio fetus*-infected and non-infected heifers. Am J Vet Res 1962;23:1213–1216.

Frank T, Anderson KL, Smith AR, et al. Phagocytosis in the uterus: a review. Theriogenology 1983; 20:103–109.

Griffin JFT, Hartigan PJ, Nunn WR. Non-specific uterine infection and bovine fertility. I. Infection patterns and endometritis during the first seven weeks post-partum. II. Infection patterns and endometritis before and after service. Theriogenology 1974;1: 91–106, 107–116.

Hartigan PJ. The role of non-specific uterine infection in the infertility of clinically normal repeat-breeder cows. Vet Sci Commun 1978;1:307–321.

Hartigan PJ, Griffin JFT, Nunn WR. Some observations on *Corynebacterium pyogenes* infection of the bovine uterus. Theriogenology 1974;1:153–167.

Hartman HA, Tourtellotte ME, Nielsen SW, et al. Experimental bovine uterine mycoplasmosis. Res Vet Sci 1964;5:303–310.

Hoffer MA. Bovine campylobacteriosis: a review. Can Vet J 1981; 22:327–330.

Hughes JP. Contagious equine metritis: a review. Theriogenology 1978;11:209–216.

Hughes JP, et al. Pyometra in the mare. Vet Bull 1979;53:986–1004.

Kendrick JW, McEntee K. The effect of artificial insemination with semen contaminated with IBR-IPV virus. Cornell Vet 1967;57:3–11.

Kopecky KE, Larsen AB, Merkal RS. Uterine infection in bovine tuberculosis. Am J Vet Res 1967;288:1043–1045.

Laing JA, Downe CH. Bovine infertility associated with staphylococcus infection. Vet Rec 1946;58:224–225.

McEntee K, Hughes DE, Gilman HL. Experimentally produced vibriosis in dairy heifers. Cornell Vet 1954;44:376–394.

Miller JM, Van Der Maaten MJ. Reproductive tract lesions in heifers after intrauterine inoculation with infectious bovine rhinotracheitis virus. Am J Vet Res 1984;45:790–794.

Miller RB, Barnum DA, McEntee K. *Hemophilus somnus* in the reproductive tracts of slaughtered cows: location and frequency of isolations and lesions. Vet Pathol 1983;20:515–521.

Miller RB, Lein DL, McEntee K, et al. *Haemophilus somnus* infection of the reproductive tract of cattle: a review. J Am Vet Med Assoc 1983;182:1390–1392.

Parsonson IM, Clarke BL, Dufty JH. Early pathogenesis and pathology of *Tritrichomonas foetus* infection in virgin heifers. J Comp Pathol 1976;86:59–66.

Pierson RE, Sahu SP, Dardiri AH, et al. Contagious equine metritis: clinical description of experimentally induced infection. J Am Vet Med Assoc 1978;173:402–404.

Powell DG, Whitewell K. The epidemiology of contagious equine metritis in England 1977–1978. J Reprod Fertil Suppl 1979;27:331–335.

Sandals WCD, Curtis RA, Cote JF, et al. The effect of retained placenta and metritis complex on reproductive performance in dairy cattle—a case control study. Can Vet J 1982;20:131–135.

Simon J, McNutt SH. Histopathological alterations of the bovine uterus. I. Studies with *Vibrio fetus*. Am J Vet Res 1957;18:43–66.

Smith T. The etiological relation of spiralla (*Vibrio fetus*) to bovine abortion. J Exp Med 1919;30:313–325.

Smith T. Further studies on the etiological significance of *Vibrio fetus*. J Exp Med 1923;37:341–356.

Swerczek TW. The first occurrence of contagious equine metritis in the United States. J Am Vet Med Assoc 1978;173:405–407.

Taylor CED, Rosenthal RO, Brown DFJ, et al. The causative organism of contagious equine metritis 1977: proposal for a new species to be known as *Haemophilus equigenitalis*. Equine Vet J 1978;10: 136–144.

Tennant B, Kendrick JW, Peddicord RG. Uterine involution and ovarian function in the postpartum cow. A retrospective analysis of 2,338 genital organ examinations. Cornell Vet 1967;57:543–557.

Thomsen A. Brucella infection in swine. Acta Pathol Microbiol Scand Suppl 1934;21:11–114.

Winter AJ, Broome AW, McNutt SH, et al. Variations in uterine response to experimental infection due to the hormonal state of the ovaries. I. The role of cervical drainage, leukocyte numbers and noncellular factors in uterine bactericidal activity. Am J Vet Res 1960;21:668–674.

Zafracas AM. *Candida* infection of the genital tract in Throughbred mares. J Reprod Fertil Suppl 1975;23:349–351.

Postpartum involution

The physiologic changes that occur in the uterus during the postpartum period when it is returning to its normal, nongravid functional and anatomic state are referred to as postpartum involution. Because they occur variously among domestic animal species, these changes and durations are described separately.

DOGS

In **bitches,** postpartum involution normally takes approximately 12 weeks. Following whelping, bitches may have mild to moderate serosanguinous vaginal discharge that may persist for four to six weeks. During this period, the myometrium gradually contracts, reducing the size of the uterus; the residual fetal trophoblastic tissue at the placental sites degenerates and desquamates into the uterine lochia, and the endometrium is restored to the normal nongravid state.

COWS

Postpartum involution in cows is generally complete by 40–50 days postpartum. The corpus luteum of pregnancy begins to regress prior to parturition and is in an advanced stage of degeneration within a few days after calving. During the first few days after delivery, the uterus contracts gradually so that by the fourth day it is approximately one-half that during pregnancy and by day 7–8 it is only one-third the size of the gravid uterus. By day 14, the uterus has reached its approximate, non-pregnant size. The normal postpartum uterus is thick-walled and has distinct longitudinal grooves on its serosal surface resulting from contraction of previously distended myometrium. Cows may continue to expel uterine fluid and lochia for up to 18 days postpartum; those that continue to discharge beyond this time should be investigated for abnormality. The character of the discharge also changes during the normal period of involution. Shortly after parturition, the discharge is serosanguinous. As the maternal caruncular material degenerates and desquamates into the uterine lumen, discharge becomes thicker and contains variable amounts of blood which appears red-brown. Necrotic caruncular tissue may appear as white, flocculent material that should not be confused with pus. As long as the discharge does not have a foul odor it is probably normal. Occasionally, caruncles become detached from their stalks without undergoing dissolution. These may persist as puttylike masses in the uterine cavity. The endometrium is normally re-epithelialized by 40–50 days postpartum. Nonspecific bacterial organisms occur commonly in the postpartum uterus, but under normal circumstances these are gradually cleared. Surveys revealed that 93% of uteri in cows 3–15 days postpartum contain bacteria, as compared to 78% of those from 16–30 days postpartum and only 9% of those from 45–60 days postpartum.

HORSES

In mares, postpartum involution proceeds rapidly, as judged by the capacity of some mares to become pregnant during the "foal heat" which occurs approximately nine days after parturition. The conception rate is not high in mares bred during this period; hence, it is likely in most instances that involution is not complete.

References

Al-Bassam MA, Thomson RG, O'Donnell L. Normal postpartum involution of the uterus of the dog. Can J Comp Med 1981;45:217–232.

Archibald LF, Schultz RH, Fahning ML, et al. A sequential histological study of the postpartum bovine uterus. J Reprod Fertil 1972;29:133–136.

Bailey JV, Bristol FM. Uterine involution in the mare after induced parturition. Am J Vet Res 1983;44:793–797.

Baru P, Khar SK, Gupta RC, et al. Uterine involution in goats. J Anim Sci 1983;23:973–980.

Bretzlaff KN, Ott RS. Bacterial flora of postpartum beef cows calving on pasture. Vet Med Small Anim Clin 1983;78:1765–1767.

Elliott L, McMahon KJ, Gier HT, et al. Uterus of the cow after parturition: bacterial content. Am J Vet Res 1968;29:77–81.

Gier HT, Marion GB. Uterus of the cow after parturition. Involutional changes. Am J Vet Res 1968;29:83–96.

Graves WE, Lauderdale JW, Kirkpatrick RL, et al. Tissue changes in the involuting uterus of the postpartum sow. J Anim Sci 1967;26:365–371.

Gygax AP, Ganjam VK, Kenney RM. Clinical, microbiological and histological changes associated with uterine involution in the mare. J Reprod Fertil Suppl 1979;27:571–578.

Morrow DA, Roberts SJ, McEntee K, et al. Postpartum ovarian activity and uterine involution in dairy cattle. J Am Vet Med Assoc 1966;149:1596–1609.

Morrow DA, Roberts SJ, McEntee K, et al. A review of postpartum ovarian activity and involution of the uterus and cervix in cattle. Cornell Vet 1969;59:137–154.

Morrow DA, Roberts SJ, McEntee K, et al. Postpartum ovarian activity and involution of the uterus and cervix in dairy cattle. II. Involution of uterus and cervix. Cornell Vet 1969;59:190–198.

Tennant B, Kendrick JW, Peddicord RG. Uterine involution and ovarian function in the postpartum cow. A retrospective analysis of 2,338 genital organ examinations. Cornell Vet 1967;57:543–557.

Complications of postpartum involution

RETAINED PLACENTA

Retention of the placenta occurs as a complication of the postpartum period in cows more often than in any other species. In cows, fetal membranes are normally expelled from the uterus within 12 hours after delivery. Beyond that period, they are regarded as retained. The pathogenesis of retained fetal membranes is multifactorial and may involve infectious diseases of the placenta, abnormal gestation periods, hormonal imbalances, and mechanical factors. Decomposition of the retained fetal membranes predisposes cows to **postpartum endometritis** caused by either nonspecific bacterial agents from the lower reproductive tract or organisms that may have infected the conceptus during gestation.

SUBINVOLUTION OF PLACENTAL SITES

This is a relatively uncommon condition affecting bitches during the postpartum period. Affected individuals manifest a serosanguinous vaginal discharge that persists beyond the normal four-to-six-week period postpartum. Discharge may contain small fragments of necrotic placental tissue.

Microscopically, the endometrium contains masses of persistent, fetal, trophoblastic tissue at some or all placental sites. The persistent cells consist of both cytotrophoblastic and syncytiotrophoblastic cells. In some cases, this tissue may even invade the myometrium. Bleeding that occurs at these sites is responsible for persistent vaginal discharge. The pathogenesis of this condition is not understood. Circulating estrogen and progesterone levels have been normal in examined cases.

References

Al-Bassam MA, Thomson RG, O'Donnell L. Involution abnormalities in the postpartum uterus of the bitch. Vet Pathol 1981;18:208–218.

Beck AM, McEntee K. Subinvolution of placental sites in a postpartum bitch: a case report. Cornell Vet 1966;56:269–277.

DISEASES OF GRAVID UTERUS
General considerations

For pregnancy to proceed in horses, cattle, sheep, goats, and swine, cessation of the normal cyclic lysis (rescue) of the corpus luteum must occur. This is normally accomplished through implantation of the blastocyst, which inhibits normal synthesis and release of prostaglandin F2α by the endometrium. The rescued corpus luteum (CL), thus, provides all or part of the hormonal support required for maintenance of pregnancy. Early embryonic death, however, may result in resumption of PGF2α synthesis and secretion and restoration of the estrous cycle. Death of the embryo, in these cases, is typically followed by rapid dissolution and expulsion of the embryo from the uterus with no grossly visible evidence that pregnancy had occurred. Although intra-uterine infections may be the cause, the vast majority of early embryonic deaths in most species result from lethal chromosomal abnormalities that occur either during gametogenesis or zygote development. Early embryonic deaths often remain unrecognized in **monotocous species** and frequently are identified only as cases of infertility in which slight prolongation of the estrous cycle occurs. In **multiparous** species, such as swine, death of a single or even multiple embryos may not necessarily interrupt pregnancy; dead embryos may either be resorbed or undergo mummification. When death of the embryo results from infection, as with trichomoniasis in cattle, infection may lead to retention of the corpus luteum and allow progression of the infection to pyometra.

In mares, equine chorionic gonadotropin (eCG) formerly pregnant mare serum gonadotropin (PMSG), is produced by specialized fetal trophoblastic cells that extend from the chorionic girdle on or about day 35 of gestation and invade the endometrium to form the so-called endometrial cups. These are well-defined, pale, elongate, cup-shaped structures that form a horseshoe or ring-shaped band along the endometrial folds of the gravid horn of the uterus. These structures disappear between days 100–120 of gestation, presumably as the result of an immunologic reaction. Their formation and disappearance coincides with the presence of eCG in the mare's blood. Endometrial cups persist and continue to secrete eCG when the fetus dies after 35 days of gestation. This results in the formation of accessory CL, failure of the mare to return to estrous, and pseudopregnancy. During normal pregnancy, endometrial cups slough from the endometrium about day 100 of gestation and lay free in the space between the endometrium and allantochorion. In carnivores (dogs and cats), corpora lutea normally persist and function for approximately the length of gestation following ovulation, whether pregnancy intervenes or not. Therefore, the hormonal milieu required for maintenance of all but the last stages of pregnancy exist even in the absence of pregnancy. In these species, embryonic or fetal death only shortens the length of a gestation cycle slightly. Fetal death prior to the last stages of pregnancy does not result in premature expulsion of dead fetuses but, instead, results in retention, mummification, and expulsion of the remains at or near term.

In swine and goats, corpora lutea are essential for the maintenance of pregnancy throughout gestation, as in dogs and cats. However, in swine and goats, PGF2α will lyse the CL and expulsion of dead fetuses can occur before term. Conversely, in cows, mares, and ewes, corpora lutea are essential only for the first half of pregnancy; hence, death of the fetus during this period can be unpredictable. In those cases in which the corpus luteum is lysed, the fetus may be expelled in a state of maceration; when the corpus luteum persists, the fetus may be either resorbed or mummified. In these species, pregnancy is maintained during the latter half of gestation by hormones from the fetus and placenta. Fetal death during this period results in expulsion after only a few days. Such fetuses usually have undergone moderate autolysis characterized by hemoglobin-stained fluid in the pleural and peritoneal cavities.

Abortion and stillbirth

The terms, abortion and stillbirth, are often used synonymously in veterinary literature, but a semantic difference exists. Abortion refers to expulsion of an embryo or fetus from the uterus prior to an age when it could survive with maximal supportive care in an extra-uterine environment. Stillbirth, conversely, refers to expulsion of a dead fetus from the uterus at an age when it could conceivably survive outside the uterus with minimal supportive care.

Mummification of fetus

Mummification of a fetus occurs in the absence of intra-uterine infection. It results from prolonged retention of a dead fetus in which all of the fluids are resorbed and the fetal membranes collapse around a desiccated, brown-black, leathery mass of dried fetal bones and skin. It occurs most often in multiparous animals, but can occur in monotocous animals when a fetus is retained for long periods.

Maceration and emphysema of fetus

Maceration and emphysema of a fetus result from intra-uterine infection. When an early embryo dies as the result of infection, it undergoes maceration and may be resorbed or expelled from the uterus. This is a frequent occurrence in *Campylobacter fetus* and *Tritrichomonas foetus* infections in cattle. When infection results in death of a fetus, severe endometritis and pyometra may ensue. Emphysema of the fetus results from invasion of the dead fetal tissue by gas-forming, putrefactive bacteria from the vagina, usually as the result of incomplete abortion or dystocia.

Adventitial placentation

Adventitial placentation refers to the development of additional sites of placentation between adjacent placentomes in ruminants, usually as the result of inadequate development of existing placentomes. The condition generally results from an insufficient number of endometrial caruncles resulting either from a congenital disorder or from loss of caruncles due to prior episodes of endometritis. Cows normally have 75–120 caruncles in their uteri, and ewes and goats, 40–125. Adventitial placentation results from fusion of adjacent hypertrophied caruncles with primitive villous attachments between the chorion and the endometrium in intercotlyledonary areas. When adventitial placentation becomes diffuse, pregnancy may not proceed beyond midterm. Hydrallantois is a frequent complication.

Hydramnios and hydrallantois

These conditions, characterized by excessive fluid in the amnion and allantoic sacs, respectively, are infrequent complications of pregnancy, mainly in cattle. At term, cows normally have 15–20 liters of fetal fluid present between the two sacs.

Hydramnios or **hydrops amnion** is generally associated with malformed fetuses, whereas **hydrallantois** is generally associated with adventitial placentation or cows carrying twins. The quantity of fluid present may exceed 150 liters. When the fetus is not aborted early, dystocia, uterine atony with retained fetal membranes, and metritis are common sequelae.

Amniotic plaques and placental calcification

Amniotic plaques consist of focal areas of squamous epithelium on the inner surface of the amnion. They are normal structures that are especially obvious in the bovine placenta and should not be mistaken for lesions.

Calcium deposition occurs normally in the allantois and amnion from the end of the first to the middle of the second trimester, appearing as white streaks or flecks close to small blood vessels. It is assumed that these serve as a reservoir of calcium for the developing fetus. It also should not be misinterpreted as a pathologic finding.

Prolonged gestation

In sheep and cattle, conditions that interfere with the synthesis and release of ACTH by the fetal pituitary and cortisol by the fetal adrenal cortex will result in prolonged gestation. It exists in various hereditary disorders characterized by adrenal hypoplasia and in congenital malformations where the hypothalamus and/or pituitary gland of the fetus are not well-developed.

INFECTIOUS DISEASES OF GRAVID UTERUS

The pregnant uterus and its contents, the placenta and developing embryo or fetus (together referred to as the **conceptus**), are more prone to infection than the nongravid uterus. The reasons for this include: the gravid uterus is normally under the influence of persistent rather than cyclic progesterone stimulation; the chorionic epithelium of the placenta secretes substances that predispose the gravid uterus to certain types of infection; and the placenta and embryo (or fetus) are immunologically-privileged sites not directly protected from infection by the maternal immune system. Two basic sources of infection of the gravid uterus exist: the maternal blood (**hematogenous route),** and the maternal cervix and vagina (**ascending infection).** Certain infectious agents may persist in a latent state and be rela-

tively innocuous in the nonpregnant female, but may become activated during pregnancy and invade the gravid uterus and conceptus resulting in abortion or stillbirth. Infections that characteristically result in abortion or stillbirth are referred to as **abortifacient infections.** Microbiologic agents associated with abortion and stillbirth in domestic animal species include bacteria, fungi, protozoa, rickettsia, chlamydia, and viruses. This discussion concerns bacterial, chlamydial, rickettsial, and mycotic infections of the gravid uterus.

Brucellosis

BRUCELLA ABORTUS INFECTION IN CATTLE

Brucellosis in cattle is distributed worldwide, but has been almost eradicated in the United States due to a strict federal testing and control program. *B. abortus* is a small, gram-negative, coccobacillus that grows best intracellularly. The usual source of infection for cattle is an aborted fetus or placenta or uterine discharges from infected cows. Transmission is generally by ingestion of contaminated tissues or exudates, but can also occur through direct contact of infectious material with vaginal and conjunctival membranes. Sexual transmission is uncommon. Young animals are relatively resistant to infection before sexual maturity, whereas infection is readily established in sexually mature cattle. Following ingestion, the organism colonizes regional lymph nodes where it causes acute lymphadenitis. Typically, infection persists at these sites for months or even years from which it intermittently enters the bloodstream and causes bacteremia that may last for months. *B. abortus* has a special affinity for the gravid uterus, to which it spreads hematogenously during a bacteremic episode and causes lesions in the placenta and fetus. Depending upon the severity of the lesions, the fetus may be aborted typically during the seventh and eighth months of gestation, or the calf may be delivered at term either stillborn or alive. The infection generally clears from the postpartum uterus within two to three weeks.

Grossly, the lesions primarily affect the placenta and fetus. A typical odorless, yellow-gray, pultaceous exudate presents between the chorion and endometrium. Some cotyledons may appear normal, others are variably necrotic. The intercotyledonary membranes are thickened and contain a yellowish, gelatinous fluid that makes them opaque and leathery. Necrotic cotyledons are soft, yellow-gray, and covered by an odorless, brown exudate.

Microscopically, the fetal membranes are edematous and infiltrated with large numbers of mononuclear inflammatory cells and neutrophils. Chorionic epithelial cells are filled with *B. abortus*. These cells synthesize and contain a carbohydrate substance, erythritol, that serves as a strong growth-promoting factor for *B. abortus*. This explains the predilection of this organism for these cells. The infected chorionic epithelial cells become necrotic and desquamate into the uterochorionic space. In the placentome, the chorionic epithelium of the fetal arcade zones are similarly affected and large amounts of exudate accumulate in these areas.

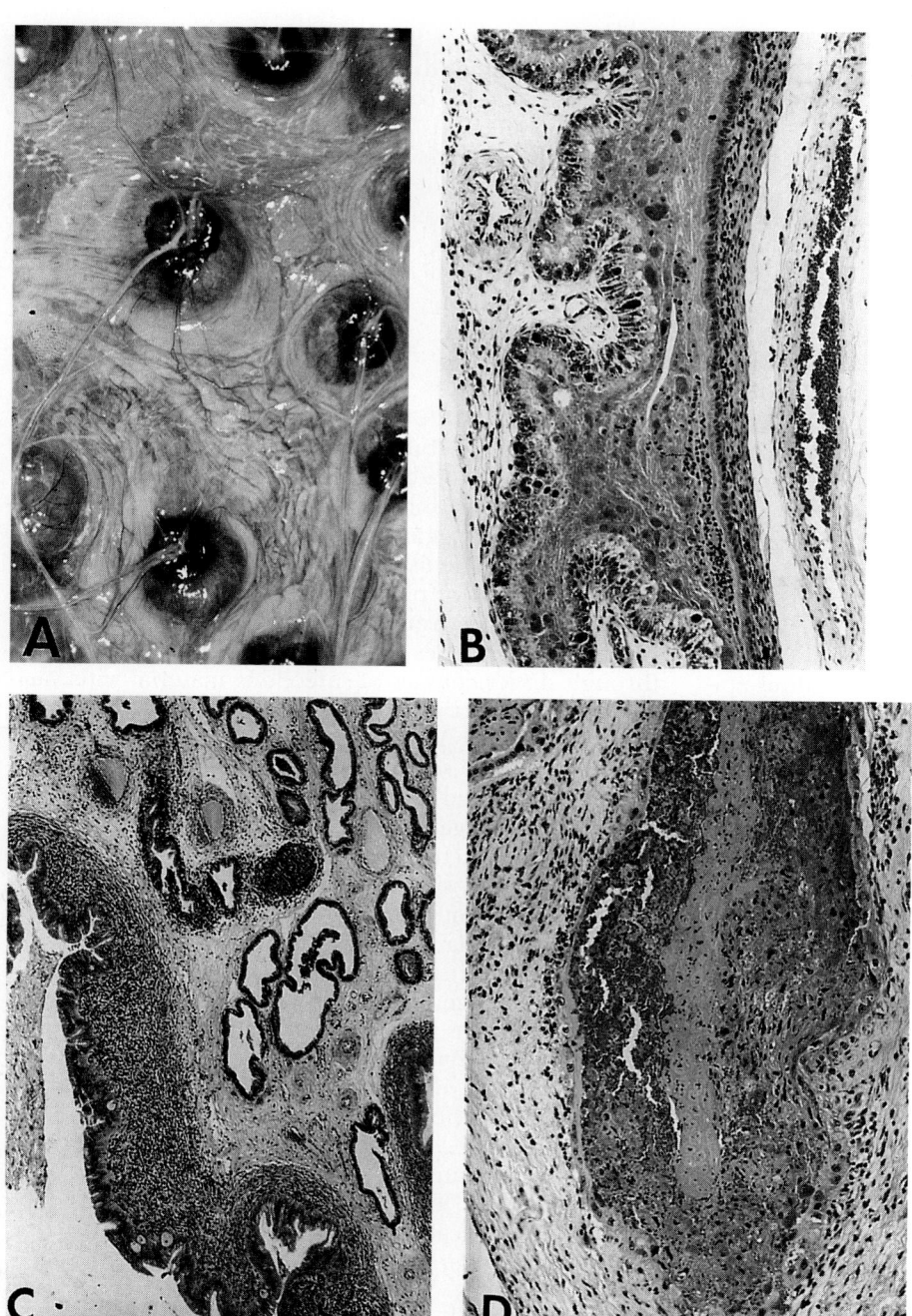

FIG. 25-22 Brucellosis. **A.** Experimental *Brucella ovis* infection in a ewe. Fetal aspect of placenta containing exudate in the periplacentomes and interplacentomes. **B.** Photomicrograph of **A.** Exudate and bacterial colonies occur in the periplacentome. **C.** Experimental *Brucella melitensis* infection in a ewe. There is marked purulent endometritis. **D.** Necrosis of chorionic epithelium in a ewe experimentally infected with *B. melitensis.* (Courtesy of Dr. J.A. Molello.)

The maternal portion of the placentome is relatively uninvolved except for the tips of maternal septa that extend into the arcade zones. These undergo a degree of inflammatory swelling that tends to further lock the fetal and maternal components of the placentome together, thus promoting retention of fetal membranes at abortion or parturition.

The aborted fetus is generally edematous and contains blood-tinged fluid in the subcutis and body cavities. In severe cases, the lungs fail to collapse and have fibrin tags on the pleural surfaces. Microscopically, most fetuses aborted during the last half of gestation have scattered microscopic foci of bronchitis and broncho-

pneumonia. The principal inflammatory cells are mononuclear, but neutrophils may be scattered as well. Characteristic lesions, when present, include: necrotizing arteritis, especially involving pulmonary arteries; and focal areas of necrosis and granulomatous inflammation with giant-cell formation in lymph nodes, liver, spleen, and kidney.

BRUCELLOSIS IN SWINE

Brucellosis in swine is usually caused by *Brucella suis,* although swine are also susceptible to *B. abortus* and *B. melitensis.* Although transmission can occur by ingestion or contamination of mucous membranes, as in cattle, brucellosis in swine is principally transmitted by coitus. Infected boars commonly develop lesions in the testes and accessory sex glands and shed organisms in semen perpetually. As in bovine brucellosis, infected animals develop regional lymphadenitis and intermittent or persistent bacteremia. Unlike bovine brucellosis, *B. suis* commonly infects the nongravid uterus where it causes progressive, caseating granulomas in the endometrium. The gross and microscopic appearance of these lesions have been described previously under the heading, *Infections of Nongravid Uterus*. Infected sows that become pregnant usually abort during the second and third months of gestation, but the incidence of abortion is less than in bovine brucellosis. A high incidence of stillbirths or births of weak piglets may be manifest. Retained placentas are also a frequent complication.

Placentas from aborted fetuses often contain a yellow-gray, mucopurulent exudate on the maternal surfaces; microscopically, numerous bacterial organisms can be found both free and within desquamated chorionic epithelial cells. As in cattle, aborted fetuses have serosanguineous fluid in subcutaneous tissues and body cavities.

BRUCELLOSIS IN SHEEP

Brucella ovis is perhaps the least virulent of all brucellae. Although on some occasions it can invade the gravid uterus and cause abortion and stillbirth, *B. ovis* is more often a cause of epididymitis in rams. The organism can be transmitted via several routes, including coitus. The nongravid uterus is resistant to infection by *B. ovis*. As with other forms of brucellosis, the organism localizes in the chorionic epithelial cells of the placentome and adjacent membranes where it produces necrosis and inflammation. Other than the usual subcutaneous edema and fluid in serous cavities, aborted fetuses have few lesions. Mild pneumonia and lymphadenitis may be present.

BRUCELLA MELITENSIS INFECTION IN SHEEP AND GOATS

B. melitensis is the major cause of brucellosis in sheep and goats. The clinical and pathologic features of the disease in these species are similar to, but less protracted than, those of bovine brucellosis. It is not uncommon for sheep and goats to recover from these infections. Abortion and stillbirth with evidence of placentitis and fetal edema are common pathologic findings.

BRUCELLOSIS IN DOGS

Brucella canis infection in dogs occurs in many parts of the world and is widespread in the United States. Transmission can be by ingestion of infected tissues and exudates, as well as venereally via infected semen. Infected dogs develop bacteremia and localized or generalized lymphadenopathy due to chronic antigenic stimulation. In males, *B. canis* is a common cause of orchitis and epididymitis. Pregnant bitches may abort after 30 days gestation, but it more commonly occurs

after 50 days. Aborted fetuses may be dead, or born alive and die within a few hours or days with evidence of pneumonia, endocarditis, and hepatitis. Placenta has focal necrosis of the chorionic villi with massive accumulations of organisms in the chorionic epithelial cells. It is common for infected bitches to have persistent, gray-green vaginal discharge for several weeks following abortion and to serve as reservoirs of infection for other animals.

Cats are the only domestic animal resistant to natural infection by *Brucella* spp.

References

Christiansen MJ, Thomsen A. Histologische, Untersuchungen über *Brucella suis* infektion bei Schweinen. Acta Pathol Microbiol Scand Suppl 1934;18:64–85.

Molello JA, Flint JC, Collier JR, et al. Placental pathology. II. Placental lesions of sheep experimentally infected with *Brucella melitensis*. Am J Vet Res 1963;24:905–914.

Molello JA, Jensen R, Collier JR, et al. Placental pathology. III. Placental lesions of sheep experimentally infected with *Brucella abortus*. Am J Vet Res 1963;24:915–922.

Molello JA, Jensen R, Flint JC, et al. Placental pathology. I. Placental lesions of sheep experimentally infected with *Brucella ovis*. Am J Vet Res 1963;24:897–904.

Payne JM. The pathogenesis of experimental brucellosis in the pregnant cow. J Pathol Bacteriol 1959;78:447–463.

CAMPYLOBACTERIOSIS

Bacteria in the genus *Campylobacter* are gram-negative, motile, flagellated, comma- or spiral-shaped rods. Two subspecies of *Campylobacter fetus* have been associated with genital tract infections in cattle and sheep. One, *C. fetus* var. *venerealis,* is of bovine origin and is a primary genital pathogen. The other, *C. fetus* var. *intestinalis,* is of ovine origin and is primarily an enteric organism that, under appropriate circumstances, can rarely cause genital infections.

CAMPYLOBACTER FETUS SSP. VENEREALIS INFECTION IN CATTLE

C. fetus ssp. *venerealis,* as its name implies, is a primary venereal disease of cattle transmitted by coitus. It is generally carried by older bulls where it persists as a latent infection in the epithelial crypts that form in the penile mucosa with advancing age. For this reason, it is an uncommon infection in bulls less than four years of age. The organism can also persist for long periods on the surface of the vaginal mucosa without causing lesions. Infected cows gradually become immune to the organism and may eliminate it from the lower genital tracts. The major problem of campylobacteriosis in cattle is not so much the ability of the organism to cause clinically overt abortion but, instead, its ability to cause temporary infertility with prolonged interestrual intervals requiring multiple, repeat breedings. This syndrome results from successful conception and implantation followed by early embryonic death. When abortion occurs, it usually is between the fourth and sixth month of gestation and is generally not associated with retained placenta.

Endometrial lesions resulting in early embryonic

death in repeat breeders consist of mild, focal, and diffuse lymphocytic endometritis with scattered cystic distention of glands. The aborted fetus and placenta are usually autolyzed, indicating death occurred some time before the conceptus was expelled. The placental lesions are not specific, but instead resemble those of brucellosis. The fetal membranes are edematous, thickened and, in some cases, leathery. Microscopically, diffuse infiltration of the stroma occurs by mixed inflammatory cells, including histiocytes. Necrotic cotyledons are yellow, have a puttylike consistency grossly and, microscopically, are necrotic and infiltrated with neutrophils. Numerous organisms are present in chorionic epithelial cells, but as far as is known, the carbohydrate (i.e., erythritol) synthesized by these cells does not exert a trophic influence on *Campylobacter* as it does on *Brucella*. Lesions in the fetus are nonspecific and include the usual edematous changes and effusions in major body cavities as well as diffuse, purulent pneumonia and focal purulent and necrotizing hepatitis.

CAMPYLOBACTER FETUS SSP. INTESTINALIS INFECTION IN SHEEP

C. fetus ssp. *intestinalis* is a primary pathogen of the intestinal tract of sheep which, under appropriate circumstances, may also cause genital infections in ewes and, much less commonly, cows. When it occurs in ewes, *C. fetus* ssp. *intestinalis* results in late abortion, premature birth, and birth of weak lambs. Retention of fetal membranes is not a usual consequence. *C. fetus* ssp. *intestinalis* is generally present in the bile and intestinal tract of infected sheep and may spread hematogenously to the gravid uterus during the course of bacteremia. It is primarily transmitted through ingestion. Immunity may follow infection. In natural outbreaks, 5–70% (average: 25%) of the flock may abort or give birth to dead or weak lambs. As in cattle, fetuses are often edematous and have purulent pneumonia and focal, purulent hepatitis. Placental lesions also resemble those of campylobacteriosis in cattle.

LISTERIOSIS

Listeria monocytogenes is a small, gram-positive, motile rod that can be difficult to isolate from infected tissue. Traditionally, the organism is associated with encephalitis in cattle, sheep, and goats, but may also invade the gravid uterus and cause abortion and stillbirth. For reasons not clearly understood, it is unusual for both clinical manifestations to occur simultaneously in the same flock. Abortions are usually sporadic, but may affect up to 50% of pregnant animals in the herd or flock. Ingestion is believed to be the primary route of transmission. Abortion generally occurs during the last trimester of gestation, but infections acquired early in gestation may also result in early embryonic death. Expelled fetuses, when not severely autolyzed, have numerous gram-positive organisms throughout most organs. The dam usually does not suffer from systemic infection when abortions occur early, but fetal membrane retention may occur due to mild metritis. Infection is rapidly cleared

from the nongravid uterus. Fetuses infected late in gestation may result in abnormal parturition and dystocia with severe metritis and septicemia occurring in the dam. These near-term or term fetuses have gross and microscopic evidence of septicemia consisting of pinpoint yellow-white foci of necrosis and purulent inflammation in liver and spleen. Gram-positive bacilli can be demonstrated in lesions and this distinguishes them from those caused by *Brucella* or *Campylobacter*. Placenta also contains areas of hemorrhage, necrosis, and purulent exudate.

Reference

Molello JA, Jensen R. Placental pathology. IV. Placental lesions of sheep experimentally infected with *Listeria monocytogenes*. Am J Vet Res 1964;25:441–449.

CHLAMYDIAL ABORTIONS IN SHEEP AND GOATS

Chlamydial agents belonging to either the *Chlamydia psittici* or *Chlamydia trachomatis* group are capable of causing abortion in sheep and goats, but their role as abortifacient agents in cattle is not clearly established. In sheep, these agents are responsible for the condition referred to as **enzootic abortion of ewes**. The condition is characterized by late abortion, premature lambing, and retention of fetal membranes. The organism is believed to be transmitted by ingestion of contaminated tissues and exudates and is not spread venereally. Immunity develops following exposure to infection; hence, abortion only occurs in ewes that have not been previously exposed to infection. Aborted fetuses and placentas grossly resemble those described under bovine brucellosis. The cotyledons are variably necrotic and covered by exudate, while the membranes are edematous, thickened, and leathery. Microscopically, the chorionic epithelial cells have large basophilic, granular inclusion bodies in the cytoplasm composed of masses of chlamydial organisms in various stages of maturation. Additionally, intense vasculitis often is present in the edematous chorionic membranes of affected placentas. Fetuses have microscopic evidence of a nonspecific lymphoreticular hyperplasia of lymphoid organs.

RICKETTSIAL ABORTION IN SHEEP AND GOATS

Coxiella burnetti is a rickettsial organism that causes Q fever in humans. The organism commonly causes clinically inapparent infections in dairy cows, sheep, and goats which serve as the reservoir hosts. Infection may occur through inhalation of contaminated dust or ingestion of contaminated milk. Ticks may also perpetuate the infection in animal hosts. Abortion follows initial exposure and may be endemic in certain flocks. They generally occur late in gestation and birth of weak lambs or kids may also occur in infected flocks. The expelled placentas are often thickened, leathery, and covered with thick exudate. Large numbers of organisms can be found in infected chorionic epithelial cells, especially when special stains, such as Ziehl Nielsen or Macchiavello stains, are used. Inflammation is largely confined to the intercotyledonary regions of the placenta and is purulent and necrotizing in character. Although the lesions resemble those seen in chlamydial placentitis, usually no vasculitis occurs. Fetuses have only scattered, focal aggregates of mononuclear cells infiltrating the lungs, liver, and kidneys.

LEPTOSPIRAL ABORTION IN CATTLE AND SWINE

Several serotypes of *Leptospira interrogans* have been associated with abortion in cattle and swine. Infection generally occurs through ingestion of contaminated materials or by direct contact with mucous membranes. In general, abortion occurs late in gestation and results from infection of both the placenta and fetus. Some fetuses are stillborn while others may be born alive but weak. Expelled placentas are edematous and contain numerous spirochetal organisms in the chorionic epithelium that can be demonstrated by silver stains. Aborted fetuses often contain focal, mononuclear inflammatory cellular infiltrates in the kidneys.

OTHER BACTERIA CAUSING ABORTION AND STILLBIRTH IN CATTLE

A number of nonspecific bacterial agents can also cause abortion and stillbirth in cattle under appropriate circumstances. They are, however, not generally regarded as primary abortifacient organisms. These include: *Salmonella dublin, S. typhimurium, Hemophilus somnus, Actinomyces pyogenes, E. coli, Bacillus* spp., *Pasteurella* spp., *Staphylococcus* spp., and *Streptococcus* spp.

BACTERIAL CAUSES OF ABORTION AND STILLBIRTH IN MARES

A number of bacterial organisms commonly associated with septic conditions of the neonatal foal actually may be acquired in utero and, in some instances, result in abortion or stillbirth. They include, in order of frequency: β-hemolytic streptococci, *E. coli, Pseudomonas aeruginosa, Staphylococcus aureus, Klebsiella pneumoniae,* and *Actinobacillus equuli.* These organisms may invade the gravid uterus via the hematogenous route during septicemia in mares, or more commonly occur as ascending infections from the lower genital tract.

MYCOTIC ABORTION

Abortion due to mycotic agents generally occurs sporadically in a herd rather than as an outbreak. *Aspergillus* is the most common cause of mycotic abortion in cattle (Fig. 25-23) and horses, followed by *Absidia, Mucor,* and *Rhizopus* spp. In cattle, infection of the gravid uterus occurs via the hematogenous route, usually by dissemination of the organism from either the respiratory or alimentary tract of the dam to the placen-

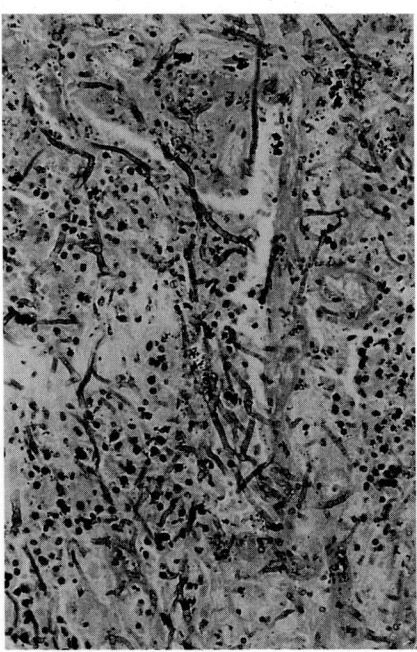

FIG. 25-23 Bovine mycotic abortion. Placental cotyledon is necrotic and contains numerous, branching, septate hyphae of *Aspergillus fumigatus* (×125).

tomes of the gravid uterus. Infected cows commonly have ulcers in the gastrointestinal tracts colonized by the same fungus causing lesions in the placenta. In mares, mycotic placentitis begins in the region of the "placental star," that portion of the placenta covering the internal os of the cervix; thus, it is regarded as an ascending infection from the cervix and vagina. Abortion and stillbirths generally occur late in gestation and are characterized by prominent lesions in the placenta and occasionally in the fetus. The placenta is frequently retained. In advanced cases in cows, a leathery thickening of the placenta is evident and involves both the cotyledonary and intercotyledonary tissues. Edges of the cotyledons are thickened and gray-tan in color. This peripheral thickening is due to a combination of inflammatory cell infiltration and adherence of portions of the necrotic, maternal caruncular tissue to the periphery of the cotyledons. Numerous mycotic hyphae can be demonstrated in the necrotic tissue, especially within and around necrotic and thrombosed blood vessels. These are best demonstrated with silver stains.

Depending upon the severity of the infection, the aborted calf may be small and undernourished due to placental insufficiency or well-developed with or without cutaneous lesions. Systemic lesions in the fetus are variable. Cutaneous lesions consist of raised, gray-white, plaques that occur on the head and neck, as well as on other parts of the body. These result from fungal infection of the fetal skins. Most cows clear the infection from their uteri following abortion and, unless endometrial damage has been severe, fertility is not permanently impaired.

PROTOZOAN INFECTIONS

Toxoplasmosis in sheep and goats

Although it infects many species, *Toxoplasma gondii* is a significant cause of abortion only in sheep and goats and, rarely, affects swine. Abortions generally occur late in gestation and often follow movement of animals late in pregnancy to areas heavily contaminated with cat feces, occurring typically in barns inhabited by infected cats who shed the oocysts in feces.

Infected ewes or does do not exhibit any signs of clinical illness other than abortion, and the aborted fetuses generally have no significant gross lesions. Microscopically, aborted fetuses frequently have focal, nonsuppurative encephalitis and foci of nonsuppurative necrosis in the heart, liver, lungs, and skeletal muscle. Characteristic round to oval, 2–4 mm tachyzoites may be found in the parenchyma immediately adjacent to the necrotic tissue. Characteristic lesions occur in the placenta of aborted animals where the cotyledons are bright red, rather than the normal purple color, and contain multiple, 1–3 mm, yellow-white, sometimes gritty, foci. Microscopically, the chorionic villi are edematous, necrotic, and have desquamated epithelium. Brady- and tachyzoites can be found in the trophoblastic cells, but may be present in small numbers. The intercotyledonary membranes may be edematous.

Neospora caninum infection of dogs, cats, cattle, and sheep

Neospora caninum has only recently been recognized as a pathogen of dogs and cats where it has been associated with neuromuscular and paralytic disease.

Tritrichomonas foetus infection in cattle

Tritrichomonas foetus, as mentioned previously, can infect the nongravid as well as the pregnant uterus. The organism is principally transmitted by coitus where it is usually harbored as a persistent, subclinical infection of the mucosae of the glans penis and prepuce of the bull. Bulls may initially develop a purulent balanoposthitis after acquiring the infection, but this generally subsides despite continued presence of the organism. Young heifers develop an acute vaginitis characterized by vulvar swelling and vaginal discharge several days after being serviced by an infected bull. Vaginal infection subsides shortly, but the organism then colonizes the cervix and uterine cavity. The flagellate organisms can be demonstrated in large numbers in the uterine and cervical discharges that appear during the next estrus. This discharge may be present only in the vagina and not detected on the vulva. The exudate results from the mucopurulent cervicitis and endometritis induced by the organism.

The clinical consequence of this low-grade, persistent endometritis is that heifers frequently become repeat breeders because of early embryonic death. Fertilization and implantation may occur, but are frequently followed by death of the embryo due to infection. In this regard, trichomoniasis somewhat parallels the clinical course of campylobacteriosis. Death of the embryo or fetus may be followed by resorption, abortion, or retention with the development of pyometra. No specific pathologic findings exist in the fetus and the placental lesions are relatively mild, consisting only of variable amounts of yellow, flocculent exudate on the maternal surface, and moderate edema of the membranes. Cotyledons are essentially devoid of lesions. When pyometra develops, the uterine cavity may be distended by several liters of an odorless, watery or gray, flocculent fluid containing massive numbers of motile flagellates.

VIRAL INFECTIONS OF UTERUS AND CONCEPTUS

Herpesviruses

Five herpesviruses of domestic animals have been associated with infertility, abortion, stillbirth, and neonatal infections. Each has also been associated with other forms of clinical disease in young and adult animals of both sexes. The typical herpesvirus infection tends to persist latently in infected hosts after recovery from the primary disease. These agents also tend to be species specific, with the one exception, *Herpesvirus suis.* The lesions produced by all five are characterized by focal areas of necrosis with eosinophilic, intranuclear inclusion body formation, a feature helpful in establishing a specific diagnosis.

HERPESVIRUS EQUI-1 AND H. EQUI-4 INFECTIONS IN MARES

H. equi-1 was formerly described as occurring in two subtypes distinguishable by restriction enzyme cleavage patterns. Subtype 1, now referred to as *H. equi-1* causes a variety of clinical conditions, including **equine viral rhinopneumonitis,** a transient respiratory infection of young horses; abortion; neurologic disease of foals; and enterocolitis. The former subtype 2, now designated *H. equi-4* primarily causes equine viral abortion during the ninth or tenth month of gestation, but does not cause neurologic disease in foals. Mares infected with either of these agents may appear clinically healthy up to the time of abortion. The fetus usually dies at or shortly after abortion.

Aborted fetuses usually have subcutaneous edema and blood-tinged fluid in the body cavities. The lungs are heavy, severely edematous, fail to collapse, and may have impression lines of the ribs on pleural surfaces. The interlobular septa are also edematous. Liver often has multiple, focal, yellow-white areas scattered throughout the parenchyma and spleen may have capsular hemorrhages and prominent lymphoid follicles. Petechial and ecchymotic hemorrhages are usually present throughout the carcass. Histologically, liver, spleen, lungs, and other tissues, including the adrenal, contain focal areas of necrosis with small numbers of eosinophilic, intranuclear inclusion bodies in the adjacent parenchymal cells (Fig. 25-24).

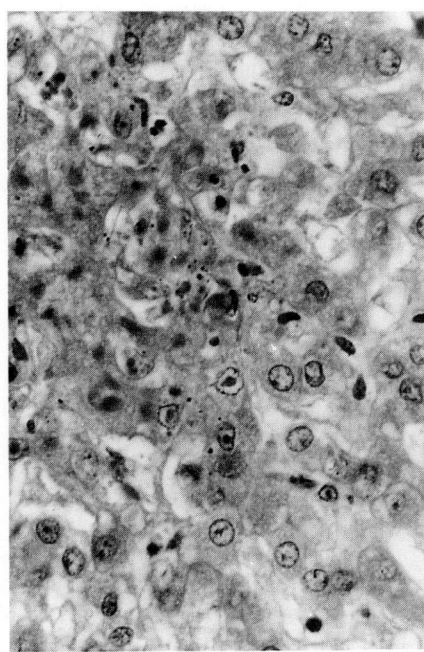

FIG. 25-24 Liver of an equine fetus aborted due to *Herpesvirus equi-1* infection. Eosinophilic, intranuclear inclusion bodies are present in hepatocytes *(arrows)* adjacent to a focus of necrosis (×250).

HERPESVIRUS BOVIS-1 INFECTION IN COWS.

Herpesvirus bovis-1 also causes multiple disease syndromes, including **infectious bovine rhinotracheitis (IBR)**, **infectious pustular vulvovaginitis** (in cows), *infectious pustular balanoposthitis* (in bulls), conjunctivitis, encephalitis, and fetal infection and abortion.

Abortion due to *H. bovis-1* occurs during the second half of gestation and, typically, the fetus dies and undergoes some degree of autolysis before it is expelled. This fact makes recognition of specific lesions somewhat difficult both grossly and microscopically. When autolysis is not severe, focal areas of necrosis containing intranuclear, eosinophilic inclusion bodies can be found in many organs, particularly liver and adrenals.

HERPESVIRUS CANIS INFECTION IN NEONATAL PUPS

H. canis is a significant cause of neonatal mortality in pups, and has been associated with abortion and stillbirth. The virus may be acquired in utero or during the first few days of life from excretions of the dam. Pups that acquire the infection after two weeks of life generally do not develop severe illness. Pups infected in utero or shortly after birth generally die during the first 10 days of life. Before death they refuse to eat, manifest evidence of abdominal pain, may vomit, and have labored breathing.

At autopsy, pups have blood-tinged pleural and peritoneal effusions and petechiae and ecchymoses throughout the body cavities. Lymph nodes are often enlarged and reddened and the spleen is also often enlarged. Lungs are edematous, and frothy fluid may exude from the trachea and bronchi. Liver and, particularly, kidneys frequently contain small focal areas of necrosis and hemorrhage scattered throughout the parenchyma. Microscopically, lungs, liver, kidneys, and spleen contain focal areas of necrosis in which adjacent cells contain intranuclear inclusion bodies that vary from eosinophilic to basophilic in staining reaction. Affected pups may also have focal areas of nonsuppurative meningoencephalomyelitis.

OTHER HERPESVIRUS INFECTIONS CAUSING ABORTION AND STILLBIRTH

Herpesvirus suis (**pseudorabies, Aujesky disease**) and *H. felis* (**feline viral rhinotracheitis**) have also been associated with abortion and stillbirth in sows and queens, respectively. Focal necrotizing lesions containing eosinophilic, intranuclear inclusion bodies may be found in placentas and visceral organs of fetuses provided autolysis is not severe.

References

Baker JA, McEntee K, Gillespie JH. Effects of infectious bovine rhinotracheitis virus-infectious pustular vulvovaginitis virus (IBR-IPV) on newborn calves. Cornell Vet 1960;50:156–170.

Gillespie JH, McEntee K, Kendrick JW, et al. Comparison of infectious pustular vulvovaginitis virus with infectious bovine rhinotracheitis virus. Cornell Vet 1959;49:288–297.

Kendrick JW, Gillespie JH, McEntee K. Infectious pustular vulvovaginitis of cattle. Cornell Vet 1958;48:458–495.

Madin SH, York CJ, McKercher DG. Isolation of bovine rhinotracheitis virus. Science 1956;124:721–722.

Owen NF, Chow TL, Molello JA. Bovine fetal lesions experimentally produced by infectious bovine rhinotracheitis virus. Am J Vet Res 1964;25:1617–1626.

TOGAVIRUSES

The family Togaviridae contains three genera, only one of which, *Arterivirus,* is important as a cause of reproductive failure in animals. The genus *Arterivirus* contains two members, *equine arteritis virus* and *porcine infertility and respiratory syndrome virus* that have been associated with abortion and stillbirth in horses and swine.

Equine arteritis virus infection

Depending on the strain involved, infection with this virus may cause only a mild, sometimes inapparent upper respiratory infection or, rarely, a more severe disease characterized by generalized edema due to virally-induced vascular injury and leakage. In the latter cases, death may result from hypovolemia and hypotension. Infection of pregnant mares with this virus results in abortion or stillbirth in a high percentage of cases. Most fetuses contain no gross or microscopic evidence of virus-induced lesions, but an occasional fetus with necrotizing, lymphocytic arteritis in the myocardium has been described. The uteri of mares aborting due to experimental equine arteritis virus infection have had an acute, multifocal, virally-induced, necrotizing myometritis and interstitial edema. These changes are believed to contribute to abortion, but the mechanism involved has not been defined. Hydropic changes in the endometrium and placenta were regarded as nonspecific and due to ischemia.

References

Coignoul FL, Cheville NF. Pathology of maternal genital tract, placenta, and fetus in equine viral arteritis. Vet Pathol 1984;21:333–340.
Cole JR, et al. Transmissibility and abortigenic effect of equine arteritis in mares. J Am Vet Med Assoc 1986;189:769–771.
Doll ER, et al. Isolation of a filterable agent causing arteritis of horses and abortion in mares. Its differentiation from the equine abortion (influenza) virus. Cornell Vet 1957;47:3–41.

Swine infertility and respiratory syndrome

Since 1987, infection with swine infertility and respiratory syndrome (SIRS; porcine reproductive and respiratory syndrome: PRRS) or related viruses has been recognized as a significant cause of infertility in swine in Europe and the United States. The causative agent, first isolated in the Netherlands, was termed **Lelystad virus.** The syndromes caused by this or related agents have been given a variety of other names, including "mystery swine disease," porcine epidemic abortion, and respiratory syndrome (PEARS), Seuchenhafter Spätabort der Schweine, and "blue ear disease." The reproductive form of this disease is characterized by anorexia, late-term abortions (days 107–112 of gestation), increased numbers of stillbirths, mummified and birth of weak piglets, delayed return to estrus, and increased preweaning mortality. Young pigs with this infection become dyspneic, febrile, and develop acute interstitial pneumonia or sometimes mild, flu-like signs. Infection with this virus causes loss of cilia from respiratory epithelium, profound depletion of alveolar macrophages, and a reduced number of circulating T lymphocytes, all of which predispose piglets to secondary bacterial infections, especially *Pasteurella multocida*, *Haemophilus parasuis*, and *Streptococcus suis*. Virus isolates have been obtained from outbreaks in Europe and the United States, but at present have not been compared. In the United States, sows aborting from experimental SIRS infection had perivascular infiltrates of lymphocytes, plasma cells and macrophages in the myometrium, and myometrial changes somewhat similar to those described for equine arteritis virus infection. Despite the presence of myometrial lesions, the precise mechanisms involved in the abortions caused by arteriviruses have not been established.

References

Benfield DA, et al. Characterization of swine infertility and respiratory syndrome (SIRS) virus (isolate ATCC VR-2332). J Vet Diagn Invest 1992;4:127–133.
Collins JE, et al. Isolation of swine infertility and respiratory syndrome virus (isolate ATCC VR-2332) in North America and experimental reproduction of the disease in gnotobiotic pigs. J Vet Diagn Invest 1992;4:117–126.
Done SH, Paton DJ. Porcine reproductive and respiratory syndrome: clinical disease, pathology and immunosuppression. Vet Rec 1995;136:32–35.
Pol JMA, van Kijk JE, Wensvoort G, et al. Pathological, ultrastructural, and immunohistiochemical changes caused by Lelystad virus in experimentally induced infections of mystery swine disease (synonym: porcine epidemic abortion and respiratory syndrome [PEARS]). Vet Q 1991;13:137–143.
Terpstra C, Wensvoort G, Pol JMA. Experimental reproduction of epidemic abortion and respiratory syndrome (mystery swine disease) by infection with Lelystad virus: Koch's postulates fulfilled. Vet Q 1991;13:131–136.
Wensvoort G, et al. Mystery swine disease in the Netherlands: the isolation of Lelystad virus. Vet Q 1991;13:121–130.

Miscellaneous viral infections of the fetus

Numerous other viral agents cause specific diseases in various domestic animal species which, when they infect a pregnant individual, are capable of invading and causing lesions in the developing embryo or fetus. Some, but not all, of these may be associated with abortion or stillbirth and many are teratogenic, causing various fetal malformations or developmental abnormalities. These are too numerous to be discussed in detail here; most are not primarily genital diseases per se, but merely infect the fetus as a consequence of a systemic infection in the dam. They include: hog cholera virus; bovine virus diarrhea/mucosal disease; border disease of sheep; Japanese B encephalitis in pigs; Wesselsbron disease of sheep and cattle; feline panleukopenia virus; porcine parvovirus; bluetongue virus in sheep and cattle; Akabane virus of sheep, cattle, and goats; and porcine congenital tremor virus.

DISEASES OF UNCERTAIN ETIOLOGY
Epizootic bovine abortion

Epizootic Bovine Abortion (EBA; Foothill Abortion), which occurs primarily in cattle in the brushy foothills of California and adjacent areas of Nevada, Oregon, and northern Mexico, is tick-borne, but its etiology remains unidentified. Over the years, it has been variably attributed to a chlamydial agent, a viral agent, and most recently to a spirochetal bacterium, possibly of the species *Borrelia*. The vector for the disease is the soft tick, *Ornithodoros coriaceus*, which feeds primarily on deer and cattle.

Cattle exposed to these ticks for the first time are primarily at risk. Pregnant cows exhibit no systemic signs of infection, but the infectious agent is transmitted to their fetuses, where a chronic infection is established. Usually, three months elapse between the time that the dam is exposed to the tick and the time that the fetus is aborted. Some calves may be born with the disease, but in a severely weakened state. The placenta is generally passed with no complications. Some apparent immunity is conferred by the first infection; abortion is not a problem in subsequent pregnancies despite further exposure to ticks. Abortion only becomes a major problem when nonexposed pregnant cows are moved to an endemic area.

Abortion occurs most often during the last trimester of pregnancy. Fetuses usually die during delivery or shortly thereafter. Some aborted fetuses have a striking abdominal distention due to ascites. Lymph nodes throughout the fetus are often massively enlarged, as is the spleen. The thymus, conversely, may be slightly smaller than normal and is often surrounded by large areas of hemorrhage and edema. The liver may be massively enlarged and with a coarsely nodular surface, which can be visually striking.

Microscopic findings in the lymphoid organs of fetus aborting due to EBA are dramatic and diagnostic. The massive splenic and lymph node enlargement is due to extensive lymphoid and mononuclear cell hyperplasia. Lymphoid follicles become markedly hyperplastic and expand into the paracortex of the nodes. Sinuses contain large numbers of macrophages that often fill the medullary portions of the nodes. Foci of necrosis may also be present in affected lymphoid organs. The most characteristic lesion is in the thymus where the cortical mantle of lymphocytes is vastly reduced and macrophages diffusely infiltrate the cortex and medulla. Livers contain large, almost granuloma-like accumulations of mononuclear cells; liver cells may be somewhat atrophic due to sinusoidal distention and distention of the central veins. Granulomatous inflammation may be present around blood vessels in a variety of organs, but particularly lung and brain. Placental lesions are mild and nonspecific.

Cervix, Vagina, and Vulva
Congenital Malformations

Congenital malformations of the cervix and vagina result from dysgenesis of the paramesonephric ducts during embryonic development. Cervical anomalies occur most often in cows and result from failure of fusion or dissolution of the medial walls of the paramesonephric ducts during formation of the cervix and cranial portion of the vagina. The most common anomalies include the cervix bifida and double os uteri externa.

CERVIX BIFIDA

This anomaly is characterized by the presence of two separate and distinct cervical canals usually separated by a vertical septum representing persistent portions of the medial walls of the paramesonephric ducts. The anomaly has no effect on fertility, but may result in dystocia.

DOUBLE OS UTERI EXTERNA

This common cervical anomaly in the cow results from persistence of only a small remnant of the medial walls of the paramesonephric ducts at the external os of the cervix. This persistent segment appears as a dense fibromuscular band that divides the normal cervical os into two openings. It also may be a cause of dystocia, but does not affect fertility.

Acquired cervical and vaginal malformations

PROLAPSE OF CERVICAL RINGS

Repeated trauma and inflammation resulting from multiple parturitions in cows predispose them to prolapse of the cervical rings. Generally, the caudal two of the four cervical rings, due to thickening from scar tissue, prolapse into the vaginal canal. This acquired malformation may predispose affected cows to chronic endometritis because of incompetence of the cervical barrier.

CYSTIC GARTNER DUCTS

Vestigial remnants of the mesonephric or wolffian duct system may persist in cows, particularly on the floor of the anterior portion of the vagina. These are usually unrecognized unless they become cystic. Cows poisoned by highly chlorinated naphthalenes or cows experiencing hyperestrogenism from cystic ovaries may develop segmental or diffuse cystic dilatation of these ducts. In some instances, cystic ducts may be 1–2 cm in diameter and tortuous.

CYSTIC BARTHOLIN'S GLANDS

Bartholin's or vestibular glands are the mucus-secreting glands of the female external genital tract. Located on each side of the floor of the vestibule, these glands become cystic and hyperplastic in response to excessive or prolonged estrogen stimulation. They may also become cystic if the excretory ducts were to become obstructed as a result of inflammation.

Inflammatory lesions of the cervix

Virtually all inflammatory lesions of the cervix represent extensions of either an endometritis or vaginitis, and as such do not represent specific disease entities. Specific inflammatory diseases of these organs have already been described.

TRAUMATIC LESIONS OF THE CERVIX AND VAGINA

During parturition in cows, it is common for the cervix and vagina to undergo mild-to-moderate laceration. If the vagina were perforated, death may result from massive hemorrhage. In beef cattle, vaginal lacerations may be complicated by herniation of masses of peripelvic fat into the vaginal canal. These impede the healing process and eventually become surrounded by granulation tissue. In cases where only the cervical or vaginal mucosa is lacerated, the lesions generally heal by scar formation.

VULVAR SWELLING OR TUMEFACTION

The vulva in most domestic animal species undergoes physiologic swelling in response to estrogen stimulation which, under certain circumstances, may be exaggerated, particularly in certain forms of hyperestrogenism.

In swine, marked vulvar swelling is a common consequence of moldy corn poisoning. This condition results from ingestion of moldy grain containing the estrogenic mycotoxin, zearalenone, produced by *Fusarium spp.* Young gilts are mainly affected and their vulvas and vaginas become so swollen that they evert and prolapse. Endometrium also undergoes cystic hyperplasia.

Inflammatory diseases of vagina and vulva

GRANULAR VULVOVAGINITIS

Controversy exists as to whether granular vulvovaginitis (granular venereal disease) represents a specific venereal disease or simply a nonspecific tissue reaction to any infectious agent capable of colonizing the external genital tract for the first time. Although it can occur in virtually any domestic animal species, it is recognized most often in bitches and cows, usually in young animals after having been bred for the first time by natural service. The condition is characterized by development of papular eruptions located primarily on the mucosa of the vulva, especially in the region of the ventral commissure. In some instances, these may extend into the vagina. Grossly, eruptions appear as either pale or pink elevated papules, a few millimeters in diameter, usually covered by intact mucosa. When numerous, they coalesce and become covered by a catarrhal exudate that exudes from the vulva. At this stage, the overlying mucosa may become superficially eroded and bleed. Microscopically (Fig. 25-25A), each papule consists of a hyperplastic lymphoid follicle that often is congested or contains areas of hemorrhage. The germinal centers of these reactive follicles are usually mitotically active. The bull often has similar lesions on its penis and prepuce. These lesions may persist for weeks or months in both sexes. A specific causative agent for this condition has not been definitively identified. Most investigators believe that it is not a specific entity but, instead, represents a nonspecific reaction to a variety of infectious agents capable of being transmitted venereally and col-

onizing the vulva. Others have suggested that ureaplasmal forms of mycoplasma may be the cause. This issue remains unresolved.

INFECTIOUS BOVINE CERVICOVAGINITIS

This condition, a cause of infertility in eastern and southern parts of Africa, is caused by a slow-growing herpesvirus that is serologically distinct from *Herpesvirus bovis-1*, the cause of IBR and infectious bovine pustular vulvovaginitis. The disease is transmitted only by coitus, usually by bulls who have an active epididymitis caused by the same agent. Infected heifers initially develop acute vaginitis characterized by the development of copious amounts of purulent exudate. This condition spreads into the cervix and uterus where similar quantities of the same kind of exudate are produced. Chronic salpingitis and hydrosalpinx with formation of intraluminal tubal adhesions result in sterility of approximately 25% of infected heifers. The condition has not been recognized in the United States.

INFECTIOUS BOVINE PUSTULAR VULVOVAGINITIS

This genital infection is caused by the same herpesvirus that causes IBR, *Herpesvirus bovis-1* (Fig. 25-25B). Although the respiratory and genital disorders can occasionally occur in the same individual, this is generally rare. This disease is highly contagious and, in addition to being transmitted by coitus, can also be transmitted by mechanical vectors and direct contact. Individual or all females in a given herd may be affected within a few days. Recovery usually occurs in approximately 10 days and results in transient immunity.

Lesions develop one to three days after infection

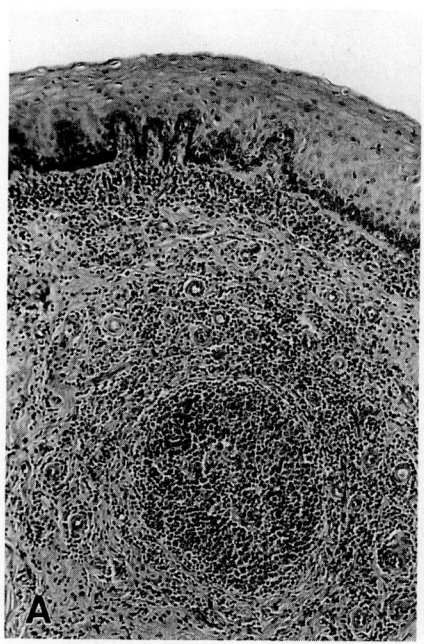 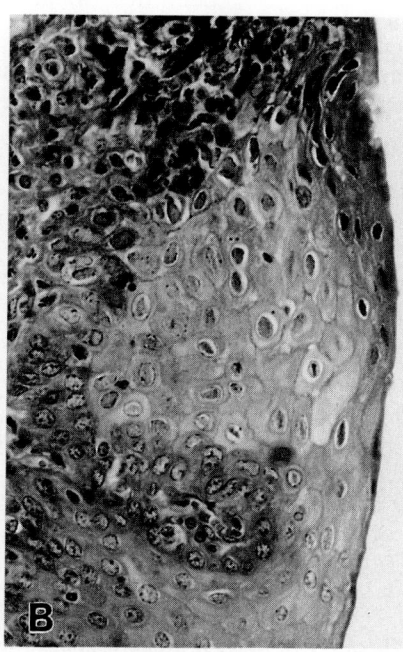 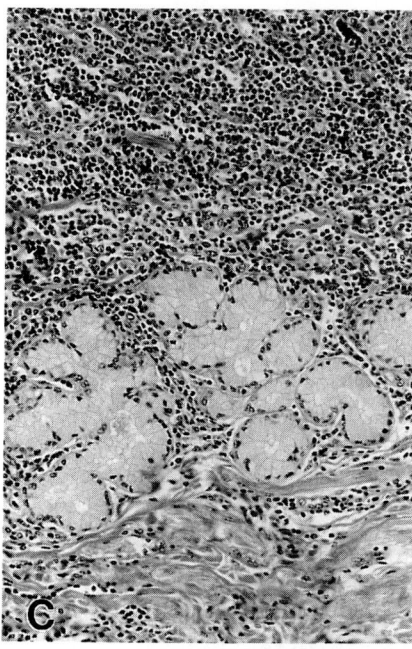

FIG. 25-25 Bovine vulvovaginitis. **A.** Granular vulvovaginitis. Mucosa contains a hyperplastic lymphoid follicle in the lamina propria (×125). **B.** Infectious pustular vulvovaginitis due to *Herpesvirus bovis-1* infection. Vaginal epithelium contains multiple eosinophilic, intranuclear inclusion bodies. (×250) **C.** Chronic inflammation of bovine vestibular (Bartholin's) glands (×250).

and consist of hyperemia of the vaginal and vulvar mucosae with focal hemorrhages occurring over lymphoid follicles. The lesions progress rapidly so that focal lesions soon become raised, necrotic plaques that may reach confluency and be covered by mucopurulent exudate. Microscopically, lesions consist of foci of necrosis of vaginal epithelium with eosinophilic, intranuclear inclusion bodies located in the adjacent, ballooned epithelial cells. Neutrophils are present in large numbers within and adjacent to mucosal lesions. Lymphoid follicles in the mucosa also undergo extensive reactive hyperplasia. Heifers serviced naturally do not experience infertility, but when it is infused into the uterus, semen containing the virus provokes acute endometritis that may lead to temporary infertility.

EQUINE COITAL EXANTHEMA

This disease, caused by *Herpesvirus equi-3*, is a venereal disease of mares that is virtually indistinguishable from infectious pustular vulvovaginitis in cows described above. It also has a transient clinical course.

DOURINE

Dourine is a venereal disease of horses caused by the protozoan, *Trypanosoma equiperdum*. The disease has been eradicated from Europe and North America, but still occurs endemically in Balkan countries, Asia, Africa, and South America. It is transmitted by coitus and both sexes are affected. Following infection, the organism invades the submucosal lymphatics where it proliferates and evokes a purulent vaginal discharge, hyperplasia of lymphoid follicles, and eventually chronic proliferative vaginitis. Its presence in the vaginal exudate waxes and wanes; thus, animals may not always be contagious. Eventually, trypanosomes enter the blood-stream and become disseminated to many parts of the body where they also cause lesions. Large, painless cutaneous swellings often occur as part of the disease. Animals eventually die of degenerative lesions involving the cranial and spinal nerves that lead to paralysis.

NECROTIC VAGINITIS AND VULVITIS

Necrotizing lesions of the vagina and vulva generally result from secondary bacterial infections of devitalized tissue that has been previously traumatized in some way. A significant cause of such trauma is prolonged dystocia, where lacerations may be incurred or tissues of the vagina and vulva are severely traumatized from prolonged pressure during difficult delivery. A variety of bacteria can colonize such devitalized tissue, but *Fusobacterium necrophorus* is most common. This condition may be fatal.

Neoplasms of vagina and vulva

LEIOMYOMA

Leiomyomas of the vagina (Fig. 25-26A) occur most often in middle-aged bitches where they may be single or multiple. Tumor is derived from smooth muscle cells of the wall of the vagina and, in some instances, have occurred more often in association with chronic estrogen stimulation from either cystic ovarian follicles or estrogen-secreting ovarian tumors. They are not seen in females who have been ovariectomized at a young age. They may appear as a globoid, sessile-based mass, or as a pedunculated, polypoid mass that protrudes into the lumen of the vagina or vulva. They may undergo degenerative changes that include intense fibrosis or marked central edema due to compromised circulation. They can usually be completely excised.

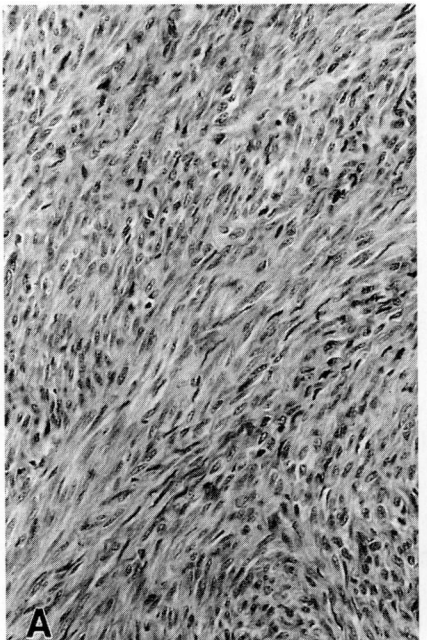 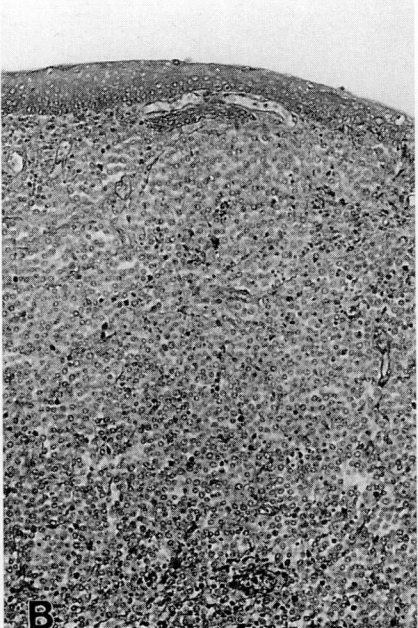 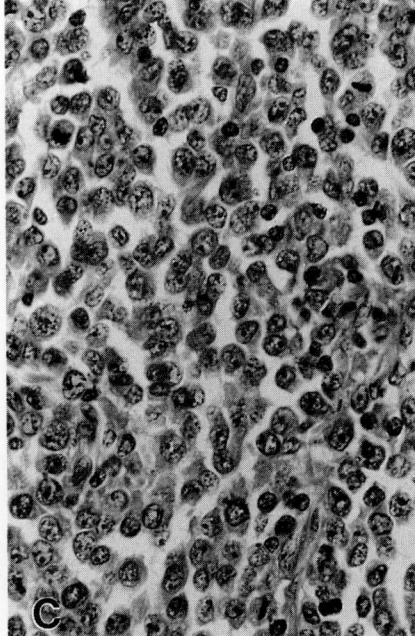

FIG. 25-26 **A.** Leiomyoma of the vagina of a dog (×150). **B.** Transmissible venereal tumor of the vulva of a dog (×125). **C.** Higher magnification of the neoplastic cells in transmissible venereal tumor (×350).

TRANSMISSIBLE VENEREAL TUMOR

Transmissible venereal tumors (Sticker tumor) are unusual in that they are transmitted venereally, but through transplantation of neoplastic cells from affected to unaffected individuals, rather than via an infectious agent. More remarkable is that the cell of origin of this tumor is not known and the neoplastic cells karyotype is 59 rather than the normal 78 for dogs. Tumor can be transmitted to the genital mucosae of either the male or female from the opposite sex or, on some occasions, to the skin. It grows rapidly after transplantation and appears as a highly vascular, friable, polypoid or papillary mass that bleeds easily. Microscopically, tumor cells are round to ovoid with indistinct cell outlines and poorly stained or clear cytoplasm. Considerable variation may occur in the size of the cells and mitoses are frequent. These tumors do occasionally metastasize to regional lymph nodes, but eventually undergo spontaneous regression after several months. Immunity is conferred by previous exposure and presumably this is, at least in part, responsible for spontaneous regression (Fig. 25-26 B & C).

FIBROPAPILLOMA OF VULVA OF CATTLE

Fibropapilloma is a benign neoplasm that arises from the vulva of young heifers as a consequence of infection by **bovine papilloma virus.** The bulk of the tumor is composed of a central mass of fibrovascular connective tissue that protrudes either as a bulbous sessile-based mass or a pedunculated papillary mass covered on its surface by a thin layer of stratified squamous epithelium. These tumors usually regress spontaneously after several months.

TRANSMISSIBLE GENITAL PAPILLOMAS OF PIGS

This rare condition is caused not by a papillomavirus, but instead by a poxvirus. Lesions, which consist of typical papillomas 1–3 cm in size arising from either the vagina or prepuce, have a somewhat acanthomatous epithelial surface and a thin, fibrovascular stroma. Eosinophilic, intracytoplasmic, granular inclusion bodies typical of those caused by poxviruses are present in the epithelium covering the lesions. Underlying connective tissue may have a mononuclear inflammatory reaction. These benign lesions tend to regress spontaneously after several weeks.

SQUAMOUS CELL CARCINOMA OF VULVA

Squamous cell carcinoma occurs with some frequency in mares and cows. High incidences have been reported in cattle from Kenya where they tend to occur more often in lightly pigmented areas and are related to solar radiation.

MALIGNANT MELANOMA OF VULVA

This malignant neoplasm occurs commonly on the skin of the vulva and perianal region of mares, especially gray mares. They often are multiple and may metastasize.

MAMMARY GLAND
Infections of mammary gland (mastitis)

GENERAL CONSIDERATIONS

Although they occur in all mammalian species, infections of the mammary gland are most frequent and cause the most economic loss in dairy cows. Infectious agents known to invade and colonize the mammary gland include: numerous bacterial organisms; certain species of fungi, mycoplasma, and algae; and even a few viral agents. However, the most important of these are bacteria. With few exceptions, identification of the specific cause of mastitis is best made by microbiologic culture of the milk or exudate rather than by histopathology. Most pathogenic organisms enter the mammary gland via the streak canal of the teat, although a few are known to enter via the hematogenous route. In contrast to other species, the mammary glands (udder) of dairy cows, in particular, are predisposed to invasion by pathogenic organisms due to the high incidence of trauma to the orifice, sphincter, or streak canal of the teat. This is not true of beef cows. In cows, the orifices of the teats and streak canals are normally lined by stratified squamous epithelium and are partially occluded by a coagulum consisting of keratin-like material from the epithelial lining and a waxy component of milk which together are referred to as smegma. This waxy plug serves as a natural barrier to ascent of microorganisms into the more vulnerable cistern portion of the gland and its associated ducts and alveoli. The pendulous teats of dairy breeds are easily traumatized by a hoof when a cow is attempting to stand from a recumbent position or more often by faulty operation of milking machines. Trauma to the teats may cause breakdown of this natural barrier and render the cow more susceptible to infections. In cows, susceptibility to *Streptococcus agalactiae* mastitis increases with age. Apparently this is not true of other agents that cause mastitis. Other resistance factors, in addition to the physical barrier imposed by smegma in the streak canal, include humoral and cellular components in milk that inhibit microbial growth or enhance clearance of invading organisms by phagocytosis. These include such substances as lactoferrin (iron-binding protein that inhibits growth of bacteria that require iron), immunoglobulins (enhance opsonization of bacteria for phagocytosis by neutrophils and activate complement-mediated cell lysis), lysozyme (enzymatically degrades components of microorganisms), and lactoperoxidase (generates antibacterial substance hydrogen peroxide during bacterial fermentation of milk products). Perturbations in any or all of these defense mechanisms may increase susceptibility to mastitis.

BOVINE STREPTOCOCCAL MASTITIS

Streptococcus agalactiae, S. dysgalactiae, and *S. uberis,* in decreasing order of frequency, are the common causes of streptococcal mastitis in dairy cows (Fig. 25-27). Other streptococci that sporadically cause mastitis in cattle include: *S. bovis, S. pyogenes,* and *S. pneumoniae.*

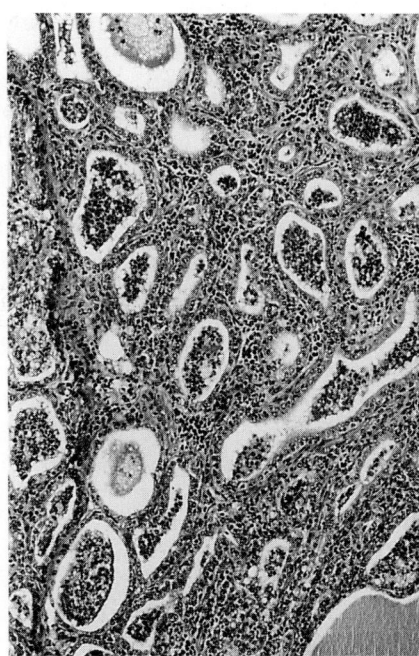

FIG. 25-27 Streptococcal mastitis in a cow. Alveoli are filled with purulent exudate, whereas lymphocytes and plasma cells predominate in the intervening connective tissue (×125).

S. agalactiae is a common cause of an insidious, persistent infection of the bovine mammary gland characterized by flares of inflammatory activity with intervening periods of inflammatory quiescence. The natural habitat of this organism is the mammary gland of cattle and goats and it does not survive long outside the mammae of these species. Approximately half the animals in an average dairy herd in the United States are infected with *S. agalactiae*, yet only 1–2% have clinical signs of mastitis at any given time. *S. agalactiae* remains confined to the lumens and epithelium of the ducts and glands and is not capable of invading the interstitial connective tissue of the gland. During acute flares of mastitis caused by this organism, and presumably in response to chemotactic factors released either from the organism itself or cells damaged by it, the surrounding connective tissue becomes markedly edematous with extravasation of large numbers of neutrophils into the surrounding connective tissue and alveoli. Clinically, this stage may be associated with systemic signs of illness including fever, inappetence, and malaise. With time, this exudative stage subsides and macrophages, lymphocytes, and fibroblasts dominate the residual inflammatory process. At this stage, affected acini and ducts begin to involute, cease secretion, and become distended by static, inspissated plugs of luminal secretion and debris. On clinical examination, affected portions of the gland are swollen, firm, and painful to palpation. Increasing amounts of fibrous connective tissue and collagen begin to be deposited in the periglandular and periductal connective tissue and may also infiltrate and obliterate the lumens of ducts and acini. For reasons that are unknown, *S. agalactiae* is able to persist in the cistern of the teat and ducts despite active phagocytosis by infiltrating neutrophils and the flushing effect of the milking process. Recrudescenses of active inflammation often follow subsequent episodes of trauma to the glands or teats and the gland eventually becomes progressively more atrophic and fibrotic. These atrophic and fibrotic portions of the gland are relatively resistant to reinfection; hence, the organism must spread to uninvolved portions of the gland to persist. This leads to progressive loss of milk production.

S. dysgalactiae typically causes a sudden, acute form of mastitis that may have its origins from a traumatic wound involving the teat. It can be associated with systemic signs of illness, but, unlike *S. agalactiae*, the infection is often self-limiting. The organism can no longer persist after the affected portion of the gland involutes and becomes fibrotic. *S. uberis* typically causes chronic mastitis that is milder than that caused by *S. agalactiae*. Other streptococci associated with sporadic cases of mastitis usually cause acute, self-limiting disease similar to that caused by *S. dysgalactiae*.

BOVINE STAPHYLOCOCCAL MASTITIS

Staphylococcal mastitis occurs more commonly in young dairy cows and susceptibility to infection does not increase with age. Catalase-positive staphylococci are the primary cause of mastitis in cattle. In decreasing order of frequency they include: *Staphylococcus aureus*, *S. intermedius*, and *S. hicus*. *S. epidermidis*, a catalase-negative organism, is a common inhabitant of skin and the mammary gland and is mildly pathogenic for the mammary gland only under unusual conditions.

Other inflammatory lesions of the mammary gland

CHRONIC FIBROSING GALACTOPHORITIS: ECTASIA OF MAMMARY DUCTS

This condition occurs with some frequency in older bitches and clinically may be confused with neoplasia. The major mammary ducts, for unknown reasons, become cystically dilated and surrounded by connective tissue, as well as chronic inflammatory cells. Cystic ducts are often filled with protein-rich fluid which appears clear to reddish-brown grossly. Epithelial cells lining the affected ducts can vary from low cuboidal to squamous in type. Papillary projections containing fusiform myoepithelial cells may extend into the cysts and mimic intraductal inflammatory polyps. A specific cause for this condition has not been identified, but the lesion will often regress following ovariohysterectomy.

Proliferative and neoplastic diseases of the mammary gland

GENERAL CONSIDERATIONS

Tumors of the mammary gland occur commonly in dogs, rats, mice and, somewhat less frequently, in cats. They are rare in other domestic and laboratory animal species. Mammary tumors constitute the most common neoplasm in bitches. The annual rate of incidence is reportedly 198.0 per 100,000 female dogs. Marked variation occurs in the frequency of mammary tumors among different inbred strains of laboratory rats and mice. In some strains (e.g., C3H mouse), virtually 100% of females develop tumors by nine months of age. Most mammary tumors in mice are caused by mouse mammary tumor virus (MMTV), a type B retrovirus (oncornavirus) that replicates in tumor cells and is excreted in milk. Suckling is the principal route of transmission. No firm evidence supports a viral etiology of mammary neoplasia in any other species. In cats, mammary neoplasia constitutes the third most frequently recognized type of neoplasm after those of the skin and hemolymphatic system. Ironically, in cows, where anatomical development and functional activity of the mammary gland are greater than that in any other species, neoplasms of the mammary gland are practically unknown. They are also rare in horses, sheep, and goats.

CANINE

As previously mentioned, mammary tumors constitute the second most common form of neoplasia in dogs, exceeded only by tumors of the skin. They account for 25–50% of all neoplasms in female dogs. The risk for development of mammary neoplasia in bitches increases significantly with age. Mammary tumors are rare in bitches under two years old, but a sharp increase in incidence occurs at approximately six years of age. Ovariohysterectomy (spaying) has a profound sparing effect on the occurrence of mammary neoplasia. It must be done prior to maturity to exert this influence. Bitches neutered prior to the first estrus have 200 times less risk of mammary cancer (0.5%) than do intact bitches. Those neutered after the first cycle have 12 times less risk of mammary cancer (8%) than do intact bitches, whereas those permitted to have two or more cycles have four times less risk of cancer (25%) than do intact bitches. In the latter group, those neutered before 2.5 years of age exhibit a marked sparing effect on the risk of breast cancer not found in those neutered after 2.5 years of age. Neutering has no sparing effect on the risk of mammary cancer development in males which, nevertheless, have a low incidence of mammary neoplasia.

Despite this profound sparing effect of ovariohysterectomy, specific endocrine disorders have not been shown to be associated with increased risk of mammary tumor development in bitches. Administration of exogenous estrogens for prolonged periods has failed to induce mammary neoplasia. Evidence suggests that the pituitaries of bitches with mammary tumors secrete more growth hormone (somatotrophin) and less follicle stimulating hormone (FSH), luteinizing hormone (LH), and thyroid stimulating hormone (TSH) than do normal bitches. This endocrine pattern is also associated with cessation of the estrous cycle (anestrus) and decreased thyroid function. The significance of this observation in the pathogenesis of canine mammary neoplasia, however, has not been established. Certain progestational hormones (megestrol, chlormandinone acetate, and progesterone) tested in dogs prior to use in human oral contraceptives reportedly increase the incidence of nodular (lobular) hyperplasia and mixed tumors.

The subject of mammary neoplasm classification in dogs is one that has been popular but controversial because of its complexity. No single classification of canine mammary neoplasms is universally accepted by all veterinary pathologists; numerous classification schemes have been proposed, but each has its limitations. Some have been overly simplistic, whereas others have been unduly complex and cumbersome. One should be reminded that the primary reason for establishing a classification for any type of neoplasm is to be able to predict the clinical course (render a prognosis) of a patient having a specific histologic type of neoplasm. Such classifications, especially in human medicine, are based on long-term clinical follow-ups of patients with specific morphologic types of neoplasms. In veterinary medicine, long-term, clinical follow-up is often difficult because of the expense of treatment and the owner's option to choose euthanasia. As a result, with few exceptions, studies on dogs generally include relatively small numbers of subjects and often are retrospective rather than prospective analyses of the problem. Other factors contributing to the difficulty of establishing a uniformly acceptable classification of breast tumors in dogs is the fact that such neoplasms are often multicentric and may involve more than one gland. Moreover, within any given neoplasm a variety of histologic patterns or even different neoplastic tissue elements may exist, thus compounding the problem.

PROGNOSTIC CRITERIA

The most useful classification of canine malignant mammary tumors, in terms of prognostic value, is the grading system devised by Gilbertson et al. (1983). This system, based on the biologic behavior of the neoplasm as determined histologically rather than its pattern of growth, recognizes four histologic stages.

Stage 0: Histologically malignant neoplasms that are confined within the borders of the mammary ducts and ductules and for which no evidence of stromal invasion exists (intraductal adenocarcinomas).

Stage I: Histologically malignant neoplasms that have invaded tissues surrounding the mammary duct system, but have not obviously invaded blood vessels or lymphatics (locally invasive adenocarcinomas or carcinomas).

Stage II: Invasive carcinoma with vascular or lymphatic invasion or metastases to regional lymph nodes.

Stage III: Carcinomas with systemic metastases.

Other histologic features that had a positive correlation with poor prognosis in animals with resected mammary carcinomas found by Gilbertson et al. included atypical proliferative changes in the mammary ducts and ductules adjacent to the excised neoplasm and degree of nuclear atypia in the primary neoplasm.

Lobular hyperplasia

Clinically, this condition may be difficult to distinguish from mammary neoplasia in that it presents as one or more palpable nodules within the mammary gland.

During the normal canine estrous cycle, a mild degree of asynchrony often occurs in the development of different mammary lobules. In older intact bitches, this phenomenon may become more evident and one or more lobules of secretory glands may be found in an otherwise inactive gland. The hyperplastic process involves primarily alveolar tissue, not ducts. It is unknown whether these lesions represent preneoplastic nodules (Fig. 25-28).

Mammary adenoma

Adenomas of the mammary gland occur in two basic histologic types, intraductal and lobular.

Intraductal adenomas, sometimes referred to as **intraductal papillomas,** arise from epithelial cells of the large mammary ducts and interlobular ductules. They may be single, but are often multiple and the affected ducts or ductules are often cystic. Grossly, lesions are irregularly nodular, up to 1.0 cm in diameter. On cut section, they are white and obstruct a portion or all of the lumen of the affected duct. Microscopically, they are composed of well-organized papillary or polypoid masses usually lined by a single layer of cuboidal epithelial cells. The cells line long, papillary projections of a delicate, fibrovascular stroma or appear as elongated tubules surrounded by fibrovascular tissue that together form a polypoid mass. Because they tend to be confined to the lumen of the duct, lesions are often completely excised.

Lobular adenomas, also called **acinar or tubular adenomas** depending on the predominant pattern of growth, are benign epithelial neoplasms arising from either the mammary acini or small intralobular ductules. Tumors of this type, especially when secretory, may be difficult to distinguish from lobular hyperplasia (Fig. 25-29). A useful, distinctive feature is the presence or absence of intralobular ducts. These are not found in true adenomas, but are present in hyperplastic lobules. Grossly, these tumors are well-circumscribed and solid,

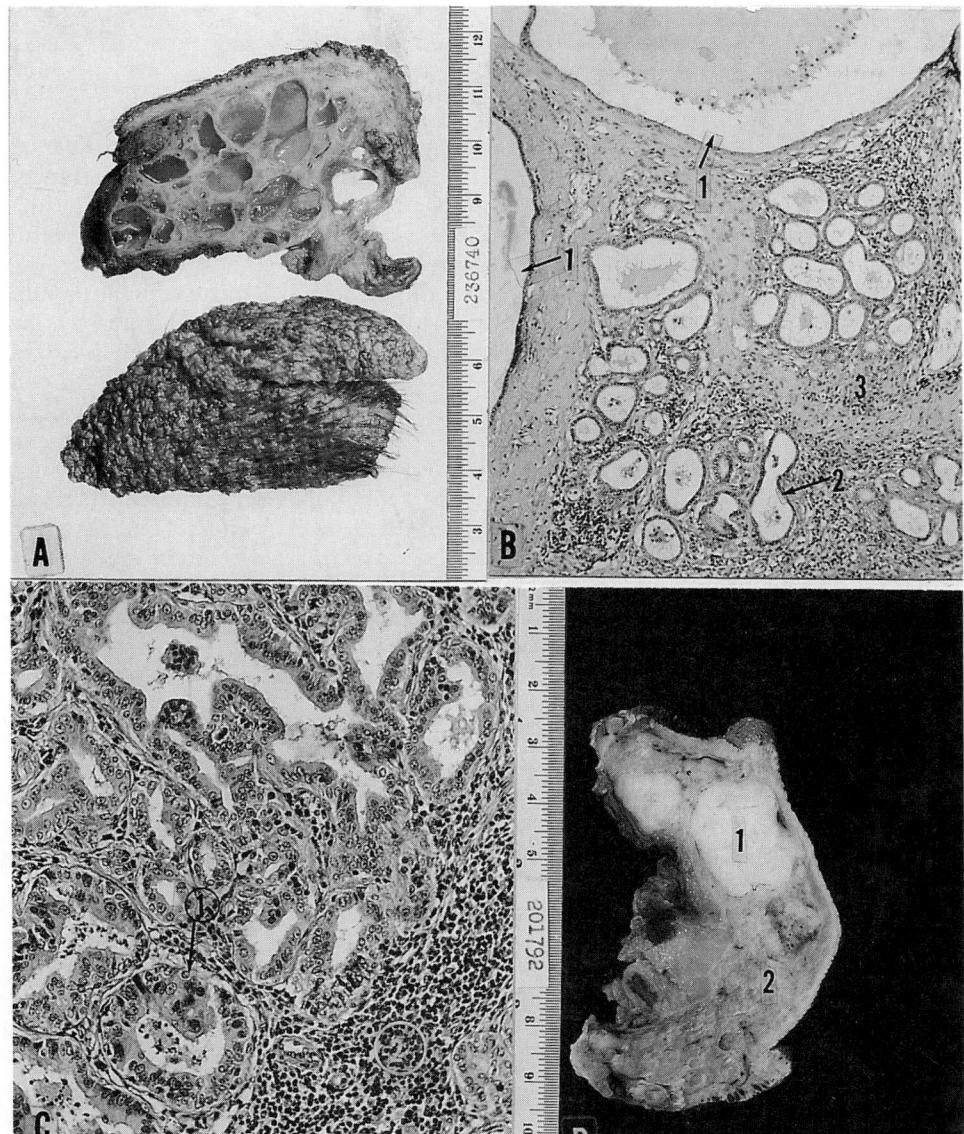

FIG. 25-28 A. Cystic hyperplasia of the mammary gland in a seven-year-old coonhound. **B.** Higher magnification (×80) of the same lesion. (1) Cystic, (2) hyperplastic acini, and (3) dense stroma containing leukocytes. (Contributor: Dr. R.F. Vigue.) **C.** Adenocarcinoma (×150) of the mammary gland of a nine-year-old cocker spaniel. **D.** Gross specimen with (1) solid areas of tumor and (2) diffuse neoplastic infiltration. (Courtesy of Armed Forces Institute of Pathology and Angell Memorial Animal Hospital.)

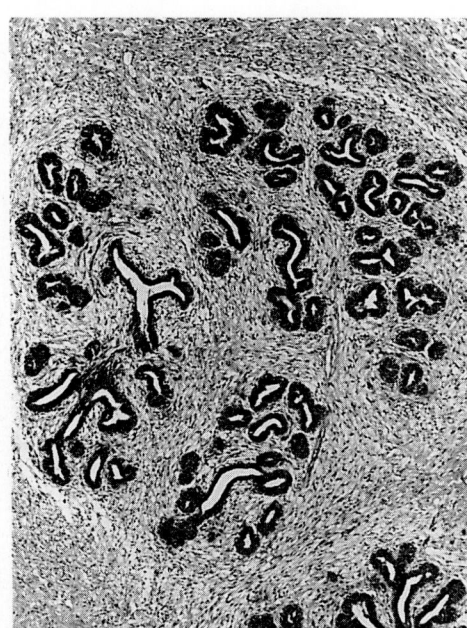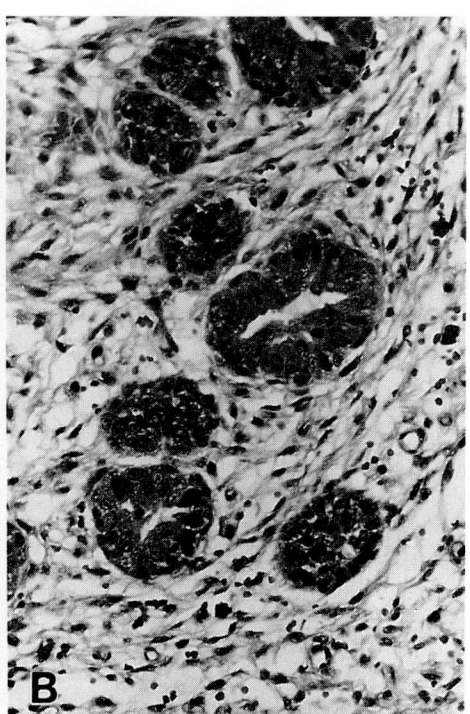

FIG. 25-29 Feline mammary fibroepithelial hyperplasia. **A.** Note the lobules of branching, hyperplastic ducts surrounded by hyperplastic connective tissue (×125). **B.** Higher magnification of hyperplastic ductal epithelial cells and surrounding connective tissue (×400).

but may contain scattered cysts. Microscopically, neoplastic cells are cuboidal and arranged in well-differentiated, closely packed acini of various sizes or in elongated, occasionally branching tubules. Lumens of the neoplastic acini or tubules may contain protein-rich secretion. Margins of the neoplasm are well-defined and adjacent tissues may appear compressed, indicating growth by expansion rather than by invasion.

Adenocarcinoma, carcinoma

Malignant epithelial neoplasms also arise from epithelial cells of the major mammary ducts, the interlobular ducts, the intralobular ductules, and the secretory epithelium of acini (alveoli). In general, three patterns of proliferation occur in mammary adenocarcinomas (i.e., acinar, tubular, and papillary), but in many cases more than one pattern can be found in different regions of the same neoplasm (Fig. 25-30). Each type may also be accompanied by a concomitant proliferation of myoepithelial cells surrounded by a chondromucinous matrix. In the absence of this feature, the neoplasm is referred to as a **simple adenocarcinoma,** but when present as a **complex adenocarcinoma.** Some evidence suggests that the complex varieties are less aggressive clinically than the simple forms. Invasion of the stroma and lymphatics may be found in all histologic types of adenocarcinomas and carcinomas, and in some cases lymphatics may be occluded by tumor cells. As indicated by the Gilbertson et al. classification, tumor cells within venules or lymphatics are a poor prognostic sign because they suggest metastasis to regional lymph nodes and other sites. The following is a description of various histologic patterns of carcinomas recognized in the canine mammary gland.

PAPILLARY ADENOCARCINOMAS

Papillary adenocarcinomas arise from the epithelium of the major and intralobular mammary ducts and grow for a time within their lumens. When it is obvious that the neoplasm is confined to the lumen, it is termed an **intraductal papillary adenocarcinoma.** These appear as papillary projections, but also often contain acinar or tubular elements. They differ from papillary adenomas in that the tumor cells are more pleomorphic and anaplastic and are usually arranged in multiple layers (i.e., piled up, over the papillary projections). The cells may sometimes be arranged in solid nests with necrotic centers (**comedocarcinoma**) or in a seive-like (**cribriform**) pattern. The prognosis is more favorable in those cases where the tumor is confined to the lumen of the duct than in those where it has invaded surrounding tissues. The most distinguishing feature of malignancy is, of course, invasion of the stroma and lymphatics. Small emboli of tumor cells often occlude lymphatics and are difficult to distinguish from neoplastic tubular structures. When myoepithelial proliferation is present, it is termed **complex papillary adenocarcinoma;** when not present, it is termed **simple papillary adenocarcinoma.** If neoplastic tubules were cystic, they would be termed **papillary cystadenocarcinomas.**

TUBULAR ADENOCARCINOMAS

Tubular adenocarcinomas also arise from ducts of the mammary gland, but the pattern of growth is mainly tubular, rather than papillary. They are the most common type of canine mammary gland carcinoma. Microscopically, they consist of uniform-sized, collapsed, or patent tubules lined by single or multiple layers of cuboidal or columnar epithelial cells. In some, tubules may be dilated (tubular cystadenocarcinoma). These tu-

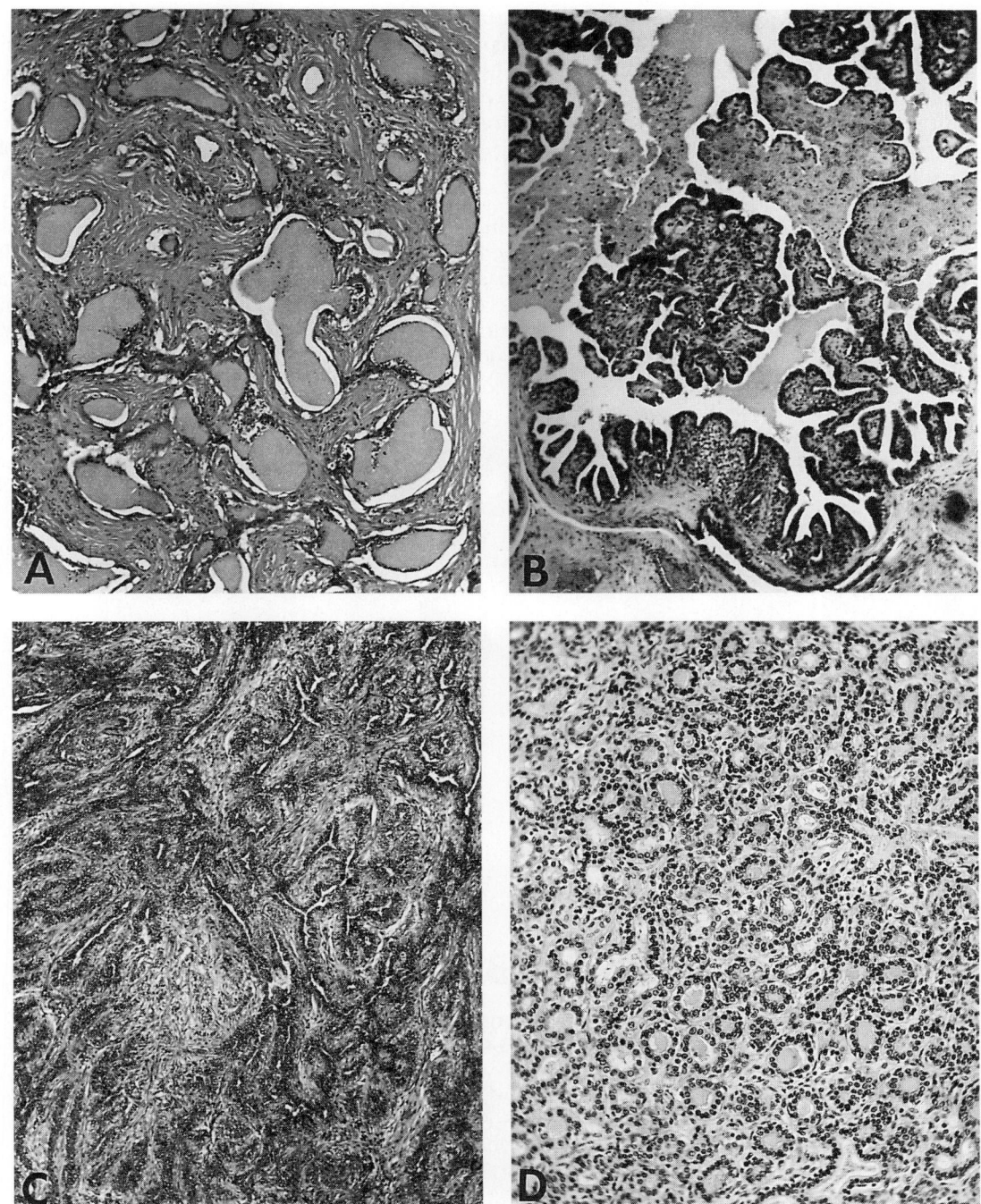

FIG. 25-30 Variations in neoplasms of the mammary gland. **A.** Fibroadenoma in a cat. **B.** Papillary (ductal) adenocarcinoma in a dog. **C.** Tubular (ductal) adenocarcinoma in a dog. **D.** Lobular (acinar) adenocarcinoma in a horse. (Figure 25-30D courtesy of Armed Forces Institute of Pathology; see text for descriptions.)

mors, which may also be of the simple or complex variety with regard to the presence or absence of myoepithelial cells, often invade the stroma and lymphatics as in papillary adenocarcinomas.

LOBULAR (ACINAR) ADENOCARCINOMAS

Lobular (acinar) adenocarcinomas bear some resemblance to tubular adenocarcinomas except that the cells are arranged in distinct acini rather than tubules. Differentiation from tubular adenocarcinomas may be

difficult, and both patterns may coexist. Neoplastic glandular structures are often separated into varying sized lobules by interlacing septa of connective tissue and, for this reason, are also termed lobular adenocarcinomas.

SCIRRHOUS (INFILTRATIVE) ADENOCARCINOMAS

This type may be papillary or tubular, but is accompanied by marked, fibroplastic proliferation which differentiates into mature, dense, collagenous connective tissue (Fig. 25-31). Connective-tissue proliferation represents a desmoplastic response by the host's connective tissue to invasion by neoplastic cells. This response is an apparent attempt to wall off the invading cells. Neoplastic cells, either individually or in nests, are embedded in collagenous connective tissue.

ADENOACANTHOMAS

Adenoacanthomas are adenocarcinomas in which a significant portion of the neoplastic cells have differentiated into squamous cells. Adenoacanthomas should not be confused with a benign tumor because the term lacks the word "carcinoma." They are uncommon and behave as any other adenocarcinoma. Pure squamous

cell carcinomas occur on rare occasions in the canine mammary gland, are highly invasive and, like squamous cell carcinomas arising from other sites, frequently metastasize.

MEDULLARY (SOLID) CARCINOMAS

These carcinomas presumably can arise from either the ductal or glandular epithelium of the mammary gland, but this is rarely determinable. Microscopically, they consist of solid nodules or sheets of neoplastic epithelial cells without evidence of a tubular, papillary, or acinar pattern (Fig. 25-32). Tumor cells are relatively uniform in size and shape. They often invade the surrounding stroma and lymphatics.

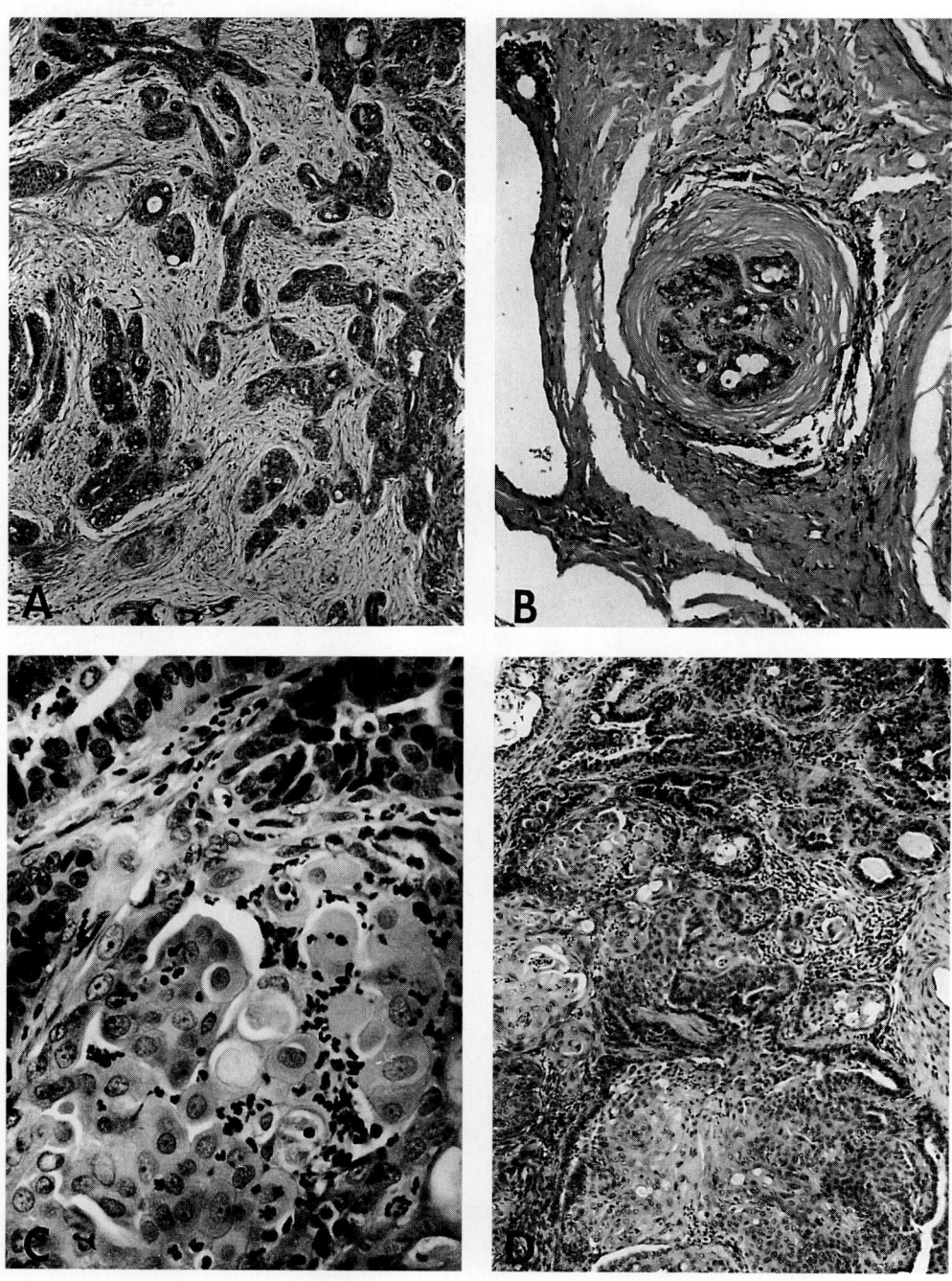

FIG. 25-31 Variations in neoplasms of the mammary gland. **A.** Scirrhous adenocarcinoma in a dog. **B.** Scirrhous adenocarcinoma in a lymphatic, dog. **C.** and **D.** Adenoacanthoma in a cat. (See text for descriptions.)

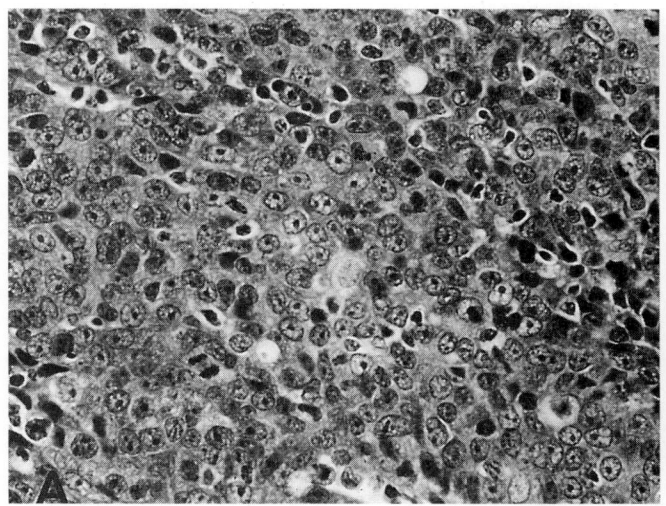

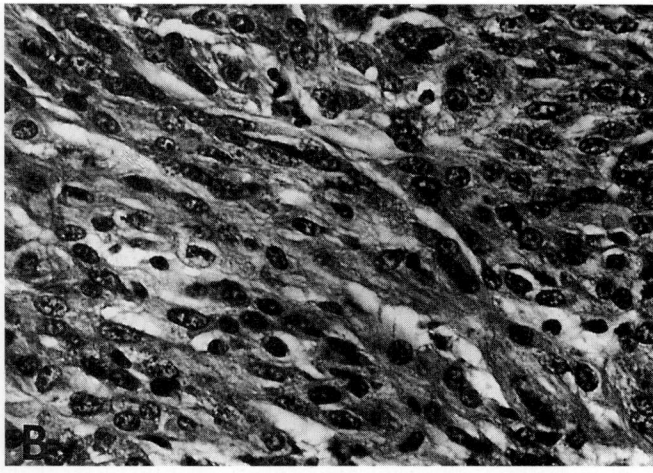

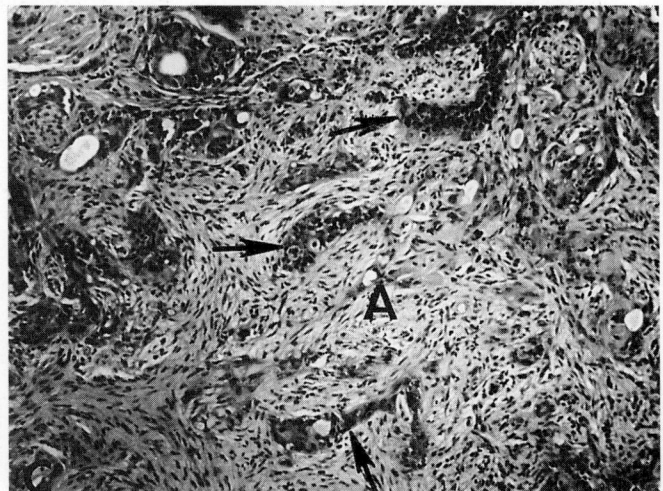

FIG. 25-32 Variations in neoplasms of the mammary gland. **A.** Medullary (solid) carcinoma in a dog. **B.** Myoepithelial tumor (spindle cell carcinoma) in a dog. **C.** Complex tubular adenocarcinoma in a dog. Neoplasms containing **(A)** myoepithelial components, in addition to epithelial proliferation (arrows) are termed complex. (See text for descriptions.)

Anaplastic carcinoma is a rare neoplasm of the mammary gland of the dog that resembles medullary carcinomas in that no differentiation into distinctive mammary structures occurs and neoplastic cells are extremely pleomorphic, varying from round, to polyhedral, to fusiform. Their nuclei are also more hyperchromatic, pleomorphic, and often appear polyploid. Tumor giant cells may also be present. These tumors are highly invasive of both the surrounding tissues and lymphatics.

Mixed tumors of mammary gland

Mixed tumors are the most common neoplasms of the canine mammary gland (Fig. 25-33); however, they are extremely rare in male dogs and in cats. Microscopically, these tumors contain neoplastic proliferation of both epithelial and myoepithelial cells with differentiation of the latter into islands of cartilage and/or bone, sometimes with hematopoietic marrow, thus the designation "mixed." Any of these tissues may constitute the major part of the primary tumor, but when metastasis occurs the epithelial component usually predominates. In many tumors of this type, bone or cartilage com-

prises the predominant neoplastic element and the glandular component may be sparse. Cartilage and bone can be detected clinically by palpation and radiographically. The distinction between benign and malignant mixed tumors can be difficult, but typically is based on the extent of invasion of the surrounding tissues by the epithelial cells or resemblance of the mesenchymal component to osteosarcoma or chondrosarcoma (Fig. 25-34).

Myoepithelioma

The term, myoepithelioma (also termed **spindle cell carcinoma**) denotes neoplasms derived solely from myoepithelial cells of the mammary gland. They are rare. These neoplasms are composed of bundles and whorls of fusiform cells without a lobular pattern and completely lack glandular or tubular differentiation. Tumor cells resemble plump fibroblasts with round or elongated vesicular nuclei and often a vacuolated cytoplasm. Cells are frequently embedded in or surrounded by a pink to light blue chondromucinous matrix, which they presumably secrete. Myoepitheliomas may be benign or malignant.

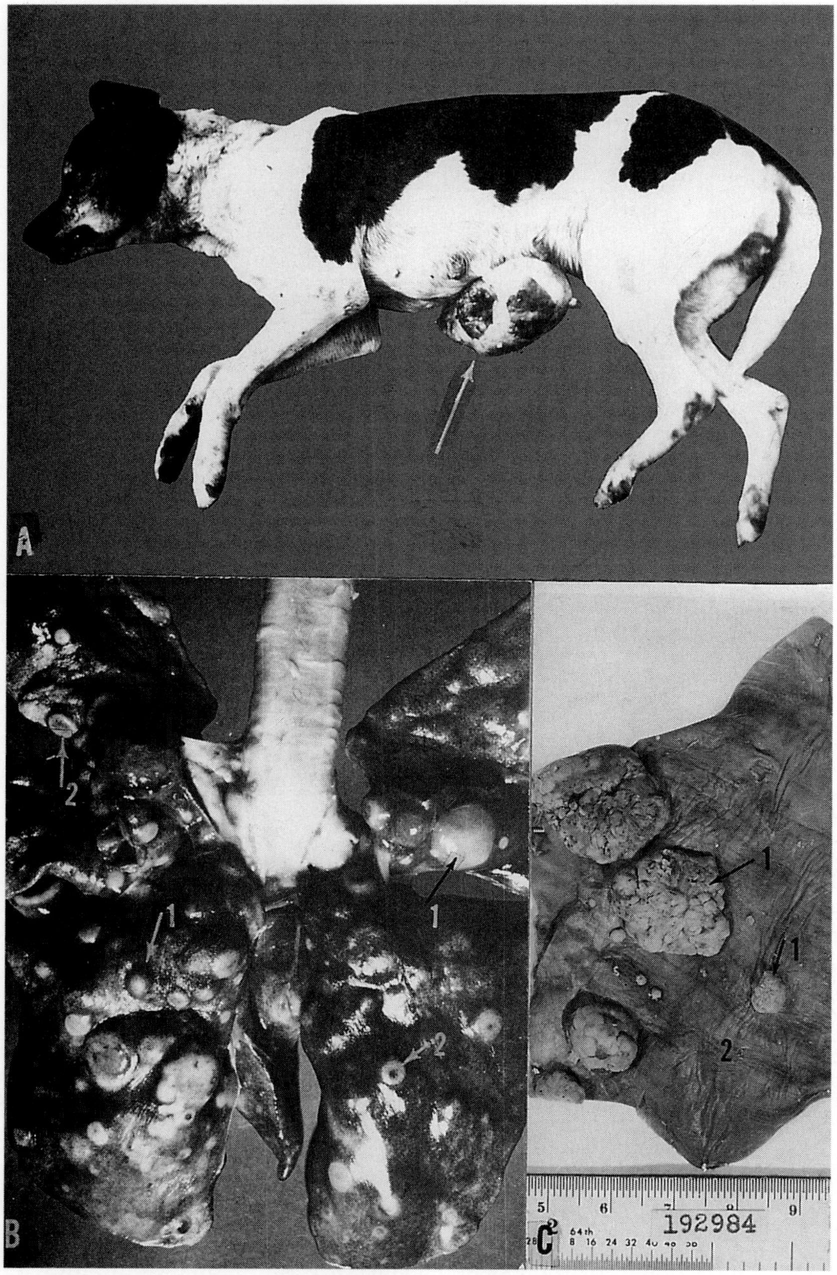

FIG. 25-33 Mixed tumor of the canine mammary gland. **A.** Single tumor of bony hardness in a five-year-old fox terrier. **B.** Metastatic nodules of a malignant mixed tumor from the mammary gland of a 13-year-old female chow. **C.** Metastatic mixed tumor (1) on the diaphragm of a 13-year-old female Dachshund. (Courtesy of Armed Forces Institute of Pathology and Dr. A.M. Berkelhammer.)

Sarcomas

Osteosarcomas, chondrosarcomas, fibrosarcomas, and liposarcomas occur rarely in mammary glands of dogs and other species. These tumors may contain more than one type of neoplastic mesenchymal element, in which case they are termed, **combined sarcomas.** Pathogenesis may be related to that of mixed tumors, but for unknown reasons, epithelial transformation does not occur.

Feline

Mammary neoplasms constitute the third most common type of neoplasia in cats, following those of the skin and hemolymphatic systems. They occur in older,

intact females and in cats spayed at an older age, but are rare in males. As in dogs, early ovariohysterectomy has a marked sparing effect on the risk of mammary cancer in cats. Intact females have a seven-fold higher risk than do spayed cats. Cats generally have four glands in each mammary line and, in contrast to dogs, anterior glands are more frequently affected.

Nearly all mammary neoplasms in cats are carcinomas, mainly of the glandular type; metastasis is frequent. These tumors are characterized by rapid growth, as well as by extensive invasion and ulceration. Benign neoplasms are infrequent in cats and they have been estimated to constitute only 15–20% of feline mammary neoplasms. Histologic classification of mammary neoplasia does not differ greatly from that already pre-

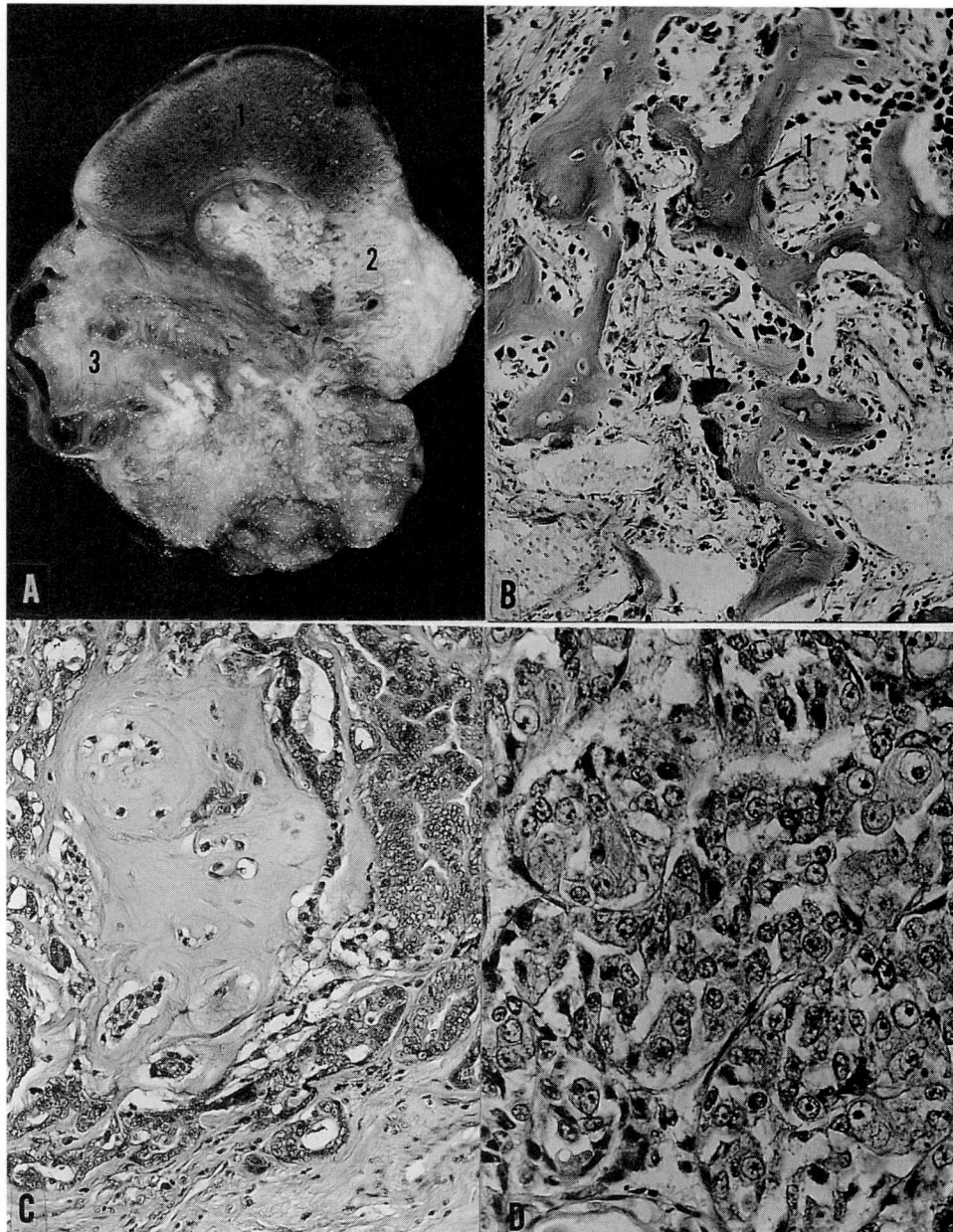

FIG. 25-34 Mixed tumor of the canine mammary gland. **A.** Circumscribed tumor with (1) bone, (2) glandular tissue, and (3) fibrous areas recognizable grossly. **B.** Section of the osseous part in **A** (×130). Spicules of (1) bone surrounded by (2) osteoblasts and some osteoclasts. (Contributor: Major Randall J.J. Foley.) **C.** Cartilage (×145) surrounded by epithelial cells in a malignant mixed tumor (see Figure 25-33C). **D.** Undifferentiated epithelial cells (×350) in the same tumor as **C.** (Courtesy of Armed Forces Institute of Pathology and Dr. A.M. Berkelhammer.)

sented for dogs, except that myoepithelial cell proliferation and mixed tumors are rare. A recently described condition seen in the mammary gland of young cats and often mistaken for a neoplasm is fibroepithelial hyperplasia (feline mammary hypertrophy).

Fibroepithelial hyperplasia (feline mammary hypertrophy)

This condition, referred to in the older literature as adenofibroma or fibroadenoma, is a benign, nonneoplastic proliferation of mammary ducts and periductal connective tissue of young cats, usually less than two years of age. It has also been described in pregnant cats and, on rare occasions, in spayed cats receiving progestogen therapy (Ovaban®). Older intact queens are rarely affected. The condition may involve only a single or all glands and is characterized by sudden, rapid enlargement of the entire gland. Microscopically, the entire breast is uniformly affected and it appears as a well-demarcated, unencapsulated mass composed of branching, epithelial-lined, ductal structures surrounded by prominent, loose, periductal connective tissue in a lobular pattern. Periductal connective tissue often appears edematous, and merges with the more dense connective tissue that separates lobules. Ductal structures are lined by several layers of cuboidal cells with large vesicular nuclei. These cells often lack polarity and have indistinct borders. Mitoses are common in epithelial cells and periductal connective tissue.

Amazingly, this condition regresses spontaneously following ovariohysterectomy. This condition represents an unusual, benign, proliferative response of ductal and periductal tissues to endogenous or exogenous progesterone stimulation. The age of the cat is important in the clinical differentiation of this condition from neoplasia, as is the sudden involvement of the entire gland, which is unlike a true neoplasm that begins as a distinct nodule within a gland and enlarges progressively.

Mice

Mammary tumors are extremely common in certain inbred strains of mice, particularly the C3H strain where 100% of females develop mammary tumors by nine months of age. Tumors are caused by the B-type retrovirus MMTV or Bittner agent, of which several strains exist. MMTV is transmitted via the milk in those strains that carry it. In the GR strain of mice, it may also be transmitted by gametocytes. Mammary tumors caused by MMTV occur at an earlier age and with a much higher incidence than those spontaneous tumors unassociated with a virus. MMTV-associated tumors are also hormonally dependent and require estrogen stimulation for induction. MMTV-infected ovariectomized mice do not develop neoplasms; conversely, castrated males carrying the virus develop a high incidence of neoplasms when treated with estrogens.

Mammary tumors caused by MMTV are preceded by two specific preneoplastic lesions in tissue: hyperplastic alveolar nodules, and plaques, also known as pregnancy-responsive tumors. The first consists of nodules of hyperplastic mammary alveoli and the second of ovoid nodules (plaques) of branching tubular structures surrounding a central core of loose connective tissue. The plaques are dependent on pregnancy hormones and regress after parturition. They reappear with each pregnancy, eventually failing to regress and becoming neoplastic. In mice, mammary tissue extends from the cervical region to the vulva and from the ventral surface to the dorsal midline; hence, mammary tumors may be found almost anywhere in the subcutis.

Mouse mammary tumors are classified by the system devised by Dr. Thelma Dunn of the National Institutes of Health. Her classification recognizes three distinct types of adenocarcinomas designated as A, B, and C, two types of adenoacanthomas (molluscoid and organoid forms), and carcinosarcomas. Others recognized a pale cell carcinoma in the GR strain of mice.

Mammary tumors can also be induced in mice by estrogens, by various chemical carcinogens, and by polyomavirus.

Rats

Mammary neoplasia occurs with an appreciable incidence in all strains of rats. No evidence suggests a viral etiology as in mice. The incidence varies with each strain, but increases with age. Rats 18–30 months of age are most often affected. Rat mammary tumors exhibit marked hormone sensitivity. One to six percent of rat mammary tumors occur in males. Estrogenic substances increase the incidence of carcinomas, whereas growth hormone increases the incidence of fibroadenomas.

By far, the most frequent mammary tumors in rats are benign fibroepithelial tumors (i.e., **fibroadenomas** or **adenofibromas**), depending on the predominant tissue element. They may become large and weigh as much as the affected animal. They do not metastasize. Microscopically, they consist of proliferations of ductular epithelium in the form of tubules surrounded by prominent periductular connective tissue.

Approximately 10% of rat mammary tumors consist of carcinomas. The most common patterns include adenocarcinomas and papillary adenocarcinomas. They are usually well-circumscribed, show little tendency to invade, and rarely metastasize.

References

Allen SW, Mahaffey EA. Canine mammary neoplasia: prognostic indicators and response to surgery. J Am Anim Hosp Assoc 1989;25:540–546.
Bostock DE. The prognosis following the surgical excision of canine mammary neoplasms. Eur J Cancer 1975;11:389–396.
Cameron A, Faulkin L Jr. Hyperplastic and inflammatory nodules in the canine mammary gland. JNCI 1971;47:1277–1287.
Cutler SJ, Black MM, Morki T, et al. Further observations on prognostic factors in cancer of the female breast. Cancer 1969;24:653–667.
Dorn CR, Taylor DON, Schneider R, et al. Survey of animal neoplasms in Alameda and Contra Costa Counties, California. II. Cancer morbidity in dogs and cats from Alameda County. JNCI 1968;40:307–318.
Fidler IJ, Abt DA, Brodey RS. The biological behavior of canine mammary neoplasms. J Am Vet Med Assoc 1967;151:1311–1318.
Fidler IJ, Brodey RS. A necropsy study of canine mammary neoplasms. J Am Vet Med Assoc 1967;151:710–715.
Fowler EH, Wilson GP, Koestner A. Biologic behavior of canine mammary neoplasms based on a histogenetic classification. Vet Pathol 1974;11:212–229.
Gilbertson SR, Kurzman RE, Zachrau RE, et al. Canine mammary epithelial neoplasms: biologic implications of morphologic characteristics assessed in 232 dogs. Vet Pathol 1983;20:127–142.
Giles RC, Kwapien RP, Geil RG, et al. Mammary nodules in beagle dogs administered investigational oral contraceptive steroids. JNCI 1978;60:1351–1364.
Hamilton JM. Comparative aspects of mammary tumors. Adv Cancer Res 1974;19:1–3.
Kurzman ID, Gilbertson SR. Prognostic factors in canine mammary tumors. Semin Vet Med Surg 1986;1:25–28.
Kwapien RP, Giles RC, Geil RG, et al. Malignant mammary tumors in beagle dogs dosed with investigational oral contraceptive steroids. JNCI 1980;65:137–144.
Misdorp W, Cotchin E, Hampe JF, et al. Canine malignant mammary tumors. I. Sarcomas. Vet Pathol 1971;8:99–117.
Misdorp W, Cotchin E, Hampe JF, et al. Canine malignant mammary tumors. II. Adenocarcinomas, solid carcinomas, and spindle cell carcinomas. Vet Pathol 1972;9:447–470.
Misdorp W, Cotchin E, Hampe JF, et al. J. Canine malignant mammary tumors. III. Special types of carcinomas, malignant mixed tumors. Vet Pathol 1973;10:241–256.
Misdorp W, Hart AAM. Prognostic factors in canine mammary cancer. JNCI 1976;56:779–786.
Misdorp W, Hart AAM. Canine mammary cancer. I. Prognosis. II. Therapy and causes of death. J Small Anim Pract 1979;20:385–394, 395–404.
Mitchell L, Delatzlesia FA, Wenkoff MS, et al. Mammary tumors in dogs: survey of clinical and pathological characteristics. Can Vet J 1974;15:131–138.

Monlux AW, Roszel JF, MacVean DW, et al. Classification of epithelial canine mammary tumors in a defined population. Vet Pathol 1975;5:495–506.

Moulton JE. Histological classification of canine mammary tumours: study of 107 cases. Cornell Vet 1954;44:168–180.

Moulton JE, Taylor DON, Dorn CR, et al. Canine mammary tumors. Vet Pathol 1970;7:289–320.

Mulligan RM. Mammary cancer in the dog: a study of 120 cases. Am J Vet Res 1975;36:1391–1396.

Owen LN. A comparative study of canine and human breast cancer. Invest Cell Pathol 1979;2:257–275.

Schneider R. Comparison of age, sex, and incidence rates in human and canine breast cancer. Cancer 1970;26:419–426.

Schneider R, Dorn CR, Taylor DON. Factors influencing canine mammary cancer development and postsurgical survival. JNCI 1969;43:1249–1261.

Strandberg JD, Goodman DG. Animal model of breast cancer. Am J Pathol 1974;75:225–228.

Taylor GN, Shabestari L, Williams J, et al. Mammary neoplasia in a closed beagle colony. Cancer Res 1976;36:2740–2743.

Warner MR. Age, incidence and site distribution of mammary dysplasias in young beagle bitches. JNCI 1976;57:57–61.

TESTIS AND EPIDIDYMIS

Developmental disorders

Unilateral (**monorchism**) or bilateral **agenesis (anorchism)** of the testes and/or epididymis is a rare anomaly in all animal species. Examples of these conditions have been described in dogs and horses. Presumably, it results when embryonic germ cells and/or somatic gonadal primordia fail to develop.

Hypoplasia

Testicular hypoplasia characterized by inadequate development of one or more cellular components of the testis occurs commonly in bulls, rams, boars, and stallions, as well as several laboratory animals, in association with a variety of developmental, genetic, and chromosomal disorders.

Developmental causes of testicular hypoplasia

The most common form of testicular hypoplasia occurs with **cryptorchidism.** Cryptorchidism has a hereditary basis and is characterized by retention of a single or both testes anywhere along the natural course of descent to the scrotum. Bilateral cryptorchid animals are usually sterile, while unilateral cryptorchid animals are fertile but have reduced sperm counts. Common sites for testes to be retained are the sublumbar regions of the abdomen and the inguinal canals. In horses, the mode of inheritance is a dominant trait, whereas in other species it is a single, autosomal-recessive, sex-limited trait. Anatomical causes of cryptorchidism include: shortened spermatic vessels, vas deferens, or cremaster muscle; peritoneal adhesions; poorly developed inguinal rings or canals; and scrotal malformations. Cryptorchidism is an expected finding in male pseudohermaphrodites. Cryptorchidism has been experimentally induced in previously normal rats by feeding them a diet of eggwhites, which contain the antibiotin substance, avidin. Prior to sexual maturity, the gross appearance of a cryptorchid testis does not differ from that of a normal prepuberal testis. After puberty, however, the retained testis appears smaller, is darker in color, and has a softer consistency than a normal, postpuberal testis.

Microscopically (Fig. 25-35), hypoplastic changes are evident primarily in the seminiferous tubules, which are smaller than normal and lined by Sertoli cells and reduced numbers of spermatogonia and spermatocytes. Spermatogenesis is arrested in almost all instances, although one can occasionally find a few spermatozoa present in hypoplastic tubules. Basement membranes of seminiferous tubules are often thickened and hyalinized. The number of interstitial or Leydig cells in the intertubular stroma is variable; they appear reduced in some cryptorchid testes, whereas in others a relative increase occurs. These cells may be present in small, isolated clusters or in diffuse sheets occupying much of the interstitium (Fig. 25-36). Hypoplastic changes evident in retained testes are generally ascribed to hyperthermia resulting from the gonad being located in anatomical sites warmer than the scrotum. Cryptorchid testes, particularly in dogs, are predisposed to the development of neoplasms, more so than scrotal testes. The reason for this is unknown.

Testicular hypoplasia also results from any condition that causes chronic deprivation of fetal pituitary gonadotropins. Although exceedingly rare, the most common such condition is **anencephaly,** in which the pituitary and other portions of the central nervous system fail to develop. Testicular hypoplasia has been produced experimentally in rhesus monkeys (*Macaca mulatta*) by decapitation of the fetus at 80 days gestation followed by continued development in utero until day 150 of gestation. When compared with control fetuses of comparable age, the testes of decapitated fetuses are smaller and weigh only one-tenth the weight of normally developed fetuses. Microscopically, the principal lesion is marked reduction in the number of Leydig (interstitial) cells in the testes of decapitated fetuses. The seminiferous tubules contain spermatogonia and Sertoli cells, but these have evidence of degeneration. Radioimmunoassay of fetal cord blood reveals a marked reduction in androgen production by the testes of such fetuses.

Genetic causes of testicular hypoplasia

GONADAL (TESTICULAR) HYPOPLASIA

Testicular hypoplasia occurs in the Swedish Highland breed of cattle with the hereditary disorder known as gonadal hypoplasia. This condition affects the gonads of both sexes in this breed and is inherited as a single, autosomal-recessive gene with incomplete penetrance. In other breeds of cattle, no definitive evidence that testicular hypoplasia is hereditary exists, although familial trends have been noted. In the Swedish Highland breed, hypoplasia of the left testis occurs in 25% of bulls, both testes are affected in approximately

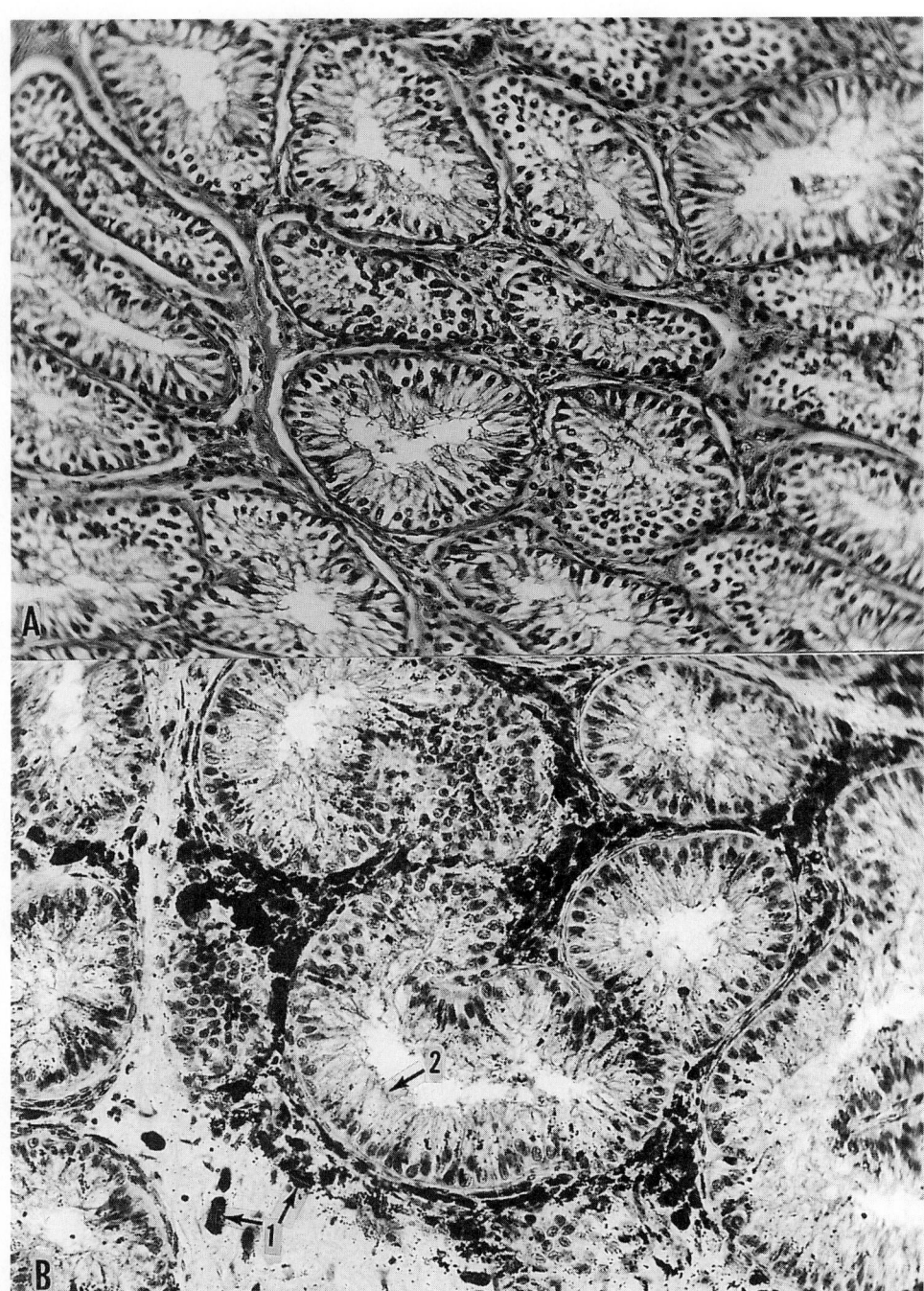

FIG. 25-35 Cryptorchid testis in a dog. **A.** Note tubules are lined completely with tall, columnar Sertoli cells. (hematoxylin-and-eosin stain, ×160.) **B.** Section stained with Sudan III to demonstrate lipid in (1) interstitial cells and (2) Sertoli cells. (Figure 25-35B courtesy of Armed Forces Institute of Pathology; contributor: Dr. Leo L. Lieberman.)

5%, and the right testis is affected only in 1.0%. Hypoplasia generally is only recognizable at puberty or later when affected bulls are found to be sterile or to have reduced fertility. Differing degrees of hypoplasia and fertility result from this genetic disorder and, in some instances, the affected bull may be fertile during its first year of service and become infertile in subsequent years. The defective gene is passed on in this way from affected bulls. These bulls do not generally manifest signs of eunuchism and accessory sex organs develop normally.

Gradations occur in the degree of hypoplasia present in affected bulls. In extreme cases, seminiferous tubules are smaller than normal and are lined mainly by Sertoli cells and scattered spermatogonia with no evidence of mitotic activity. Basement membranes are thickened and hyalinized, and peritubular connective tissue is increased. Interstitial cells appear to be increased in number. In less severe cases, arrested spermatogenesis may occur at the spermatocyte stage. Spermatocytes become vacuolated and degenerate. In mildly affected animals, some tubules may be completely hypo-

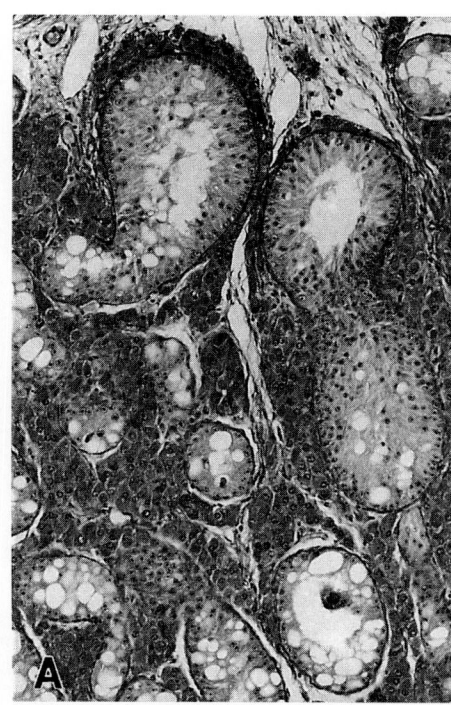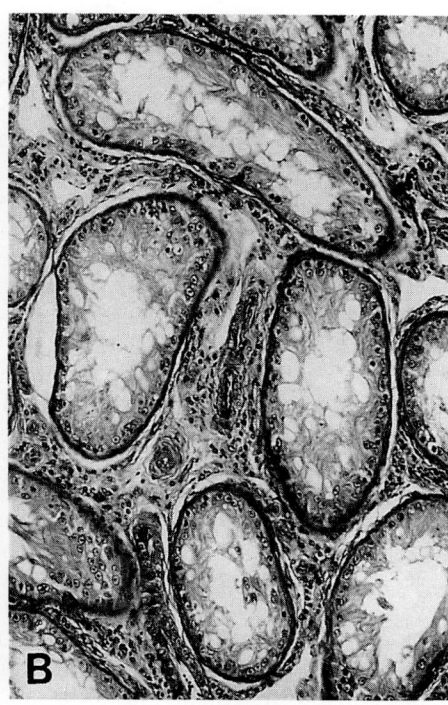

FIG. 25-36 A. Cryptorchid testis of a horse. Note the relative increase in pigmented interstitial cells (×250). **B.** Testicular hypoplasia, Swedish Highland bull. Seminiferous tubules are devoid of germ cells and are lined by Sertoli cells. (×250).

plastic, while others have arrested spermatogenesis at the spermatocyte or spermatid stage. Fusion of spermatids to form **multinucleate spermatidic giant cells** may be seen in affected tubules.

Semen of severely affected bulls is watery and, depending on the degree of involvement, is either **oligospermic** (reduced numbers) or **azoospermic** (devoid of spermatozoa). Multinucleated spermatidic giant cells are often present in the ejaculate.

Testicular hypoplasia has also been described in swine. The pattern of disease is similar to that described in cattle. Sheep affected with testicular hypoplasia usually have shortened spermatic cords and the testes are higher than normal, suggesting that cryptorchism may be responsible for degenerative changes.

A form of testicular hypoplasia described in the ACEP strain of laboratory rabbits is associated with a genetically-determined condition referred to as **hypogonadia.** Hypogonadia in this strain of rabbit is believed to be determined by an autosomal-recessive gene that causes hypoplasia of the gonads in both sexes. The hypoplastic changes in seminiferous tubules of severely affected animals are evident in the late prenatal stages, indicating that this is a congenital, not postnatal, atrophic disorder.

An apparently similar inherited form of testicular hypoplasia has also been described in guinea pigs. This condition is marked by extreme variation in the seminiferous tubule changes. In some animals, complete aplasia of spermatogenic cells is evident, whereas in others the tubules appear normal, but the percentage of fertile matings is reduced.

Chromosomal abnormalities causing testicular hypoplasia

KLINEFELTER SYNDROME

This condition, originally described in men, is a form of male hypogonadism (testicular hypoplasia) that occurs when the patient has two or more X chromosomes and one or more Y chromosomes in his genotype (XXY, XXXY, XXXXY, XXYY). An analogous syndrome has been described in calico and tortoiseshell cats, and in dogs, sheep, swine, cattle, and mice. Affected animals usually have a normal complement of autosomes for the species. In both animals and humans, some individuals with this disorder, rather than having a single genotype, are mosaics or chimeras with some somatic cells having the normal XY male genotype and others containing additional X chromosomes. At the age of sexual maturity, affected males usually develop secondary sex characteristics and behavioral changes associated with testosterone secretion, but their testes remain small. Microscopically, germinal epithelium and Sertoli cells of the seminiferous tubules are severely degenerated and replaced by masses of hyalinized, dense, collagenous connective tissue. The remaining parenchyma consists of diffuse sheets of interstitial cells that appear hyperplastic due to a relative increase brought about by the loss of seminiferous tubules. These individuals are aspermatogenic and sterile.

Male cats with the tortoiseshell (orange and black) or calico (orange, black and white) coat color almost always have an extra X chromosome that renders them sterile due to testicular hypoplasia. In cats, genes for orange and black coat colors are carried on the X chromosome, thus for both colors to be expressed in the same animal at least two X chromosomes must be present in the genotype. Female cats with tortoiseshell or calico coat colors have normal female reproductive tracts.

Testicular hypoplasia also occurs consistently in several species, including humans, in conjunction with aneuploid sex chromosomal abnormality. At least one Y chromosome and two or more X chromosomes (e.g., XXY, XXXY, XXYY) present in at least some of the individual's cells, which implies that the chromosomal anomaly may also occur in mosaic or chimeric genotypes; therefore, it does not have to be present in all affected somatic cells. Affected cells are sex chromatin-positive because they contain at least two X chromosomes. Humans with this chromosomal disorder exhibit characteristic clinical signs, including hypoplastic testes, aspermia, variable degree of gynecomastia, and other signs of abnormal somatic development. In humans, this condition is termed **Klinefelter syndrome.**

The XXY chromosomal abnormality occurring as either a single mode, or as part of a mosaic or chimeric genotype has been reported in rams, dogs, cats, and mice. Affected individuals of these species have testicular hypoplasia and aspermia, but exhibit no other obvious physical abnormalities. Histologically, the testes have a marked reduction in the number of spermatogenic cells and a variable number of interstitial cells. The seminiferous tubules are lined primarily by Sertoli cells.

Recently, testicular hypoplasia and associated sterility have been described in a male mouse in which the X and Y chromosomes failed to maintain an end-to-end association during diakinesis-metaphase of the first meiotic division. As a result, spermatogenesis is arrested after metaphase I; therefore, no secondary spermatocytes or spermatozoa are formed in the testes of these animals. The cause of the failure of the two sex chromosomes to associate during this phase of meiosis is unknown.

Finally, the testes of various, experimentally-produced hybrid animals are often hypoplastic, causing sterility. Several equine hybrids exist: horse (stallion) x donkey (jenny) = hinney; donkey (jack) x horse (mare) = mule; zebra x donkey (jenny) = zebronkey; and zebra x horse (mare) = zebrose. In general, these hybrids are infertile because of the incompatibility of paternal and maternal chromosomes for pairing during meiosis. Germ cells of these hybrids proceed through mitosis, but a block of meiotic division occurs because pairing of homologous chromosomes is impossible due to uneven numbers from the parents. Gonads of these hybrids are generally hypoplastic due to the arrest of gametogenesis. There are isolated reports of fertile, female mules, but these are rare. Other reports of infertile hybrids include the dog x coyote hybrid, and a marmoset (*Saguinus oedipus*) x *Saguinus midas* hybrid. In the latter hybrid, the testes were also retained in the abdomen; hence, the effect of the hybrid state on spermatogenesis could not be unequivocally ascertained.

DYSGENESIS

Congenital malformations of the testis, other than simple hypoplasia, are regarded as forms of dysplasia.

Although extremely rare, the most common dysgenetic lesion of the testis involves it being surrounded by a zone of ovarian cortex to form an **ovotestis.** Ovotestes are almost always retained in the abdomen and are found only in true hermaphrodites.

Spermatoceles are cystic dilatations of the rete testis or epididymal tubules in which large numbers of spermatozoa accumulate (Fig. 25-37). Spermatoceles may be either congenital or acquired, and do not become evident until after spermatogenesis has begun. Pathogenesis of congenitally acquired spermatoceles involves failure of one or more of the rete or mesonephric tubules to connect with the mesonephric duct (future vas deferens). As a result, tubules accumulate spermatozoa from proximal connections with the testes, but cannot expel them because their distal ends are blind or occluded. Impaction and inspissation of spermatozoa in these dilated tubules may cause atrophy of the epithelial lining, as well as rupture of the basement membrane in affected tubules. The latter results in extravasation of spermatozoa into the adjacent interstitial tissues where they incite an intense, foreign-body inflammatory reaction. Microscopically, these **spermatic granulomas** (Fig. 25-38) consist of masses of epithelioid cells, lymphocytes, foreign-body giant cells, and fibrous connective tissue surrounding a central mass of necrotic spermatozoa. Depending on the size and location of the granuloma, retrogressive changes may occur in the seminiferous tubules resulting from stasis of the spermatozoa in the testis.

Although not truly a dysgenetic lesion, small vesicular structures called the **appendix of the testis** are often found on the surface of the upper pole of the testis in the region of the epididymal head. These structures arise from vestiges of the rostral end of the paramesonephric duct. They are extremely common in horses. Histologically, they consist of single or multiple, small, epithelial-lined spaces enmeshed in a mass of connective tissue.

Small nodules of ectopic (accessory) adrenal cortical tissue are frequently present between the head of

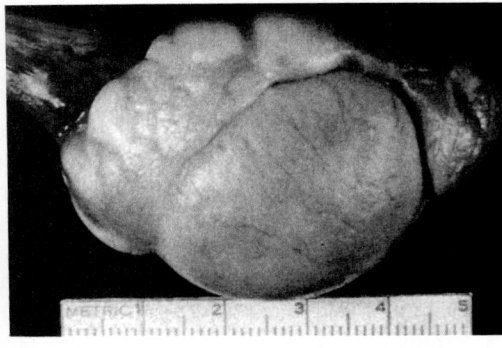

FIG. 25-37 Spermatic granulomas in epididymis of a seven-year-old male beagle. (Courtesy of Angell Memorial Animal Hospital.)

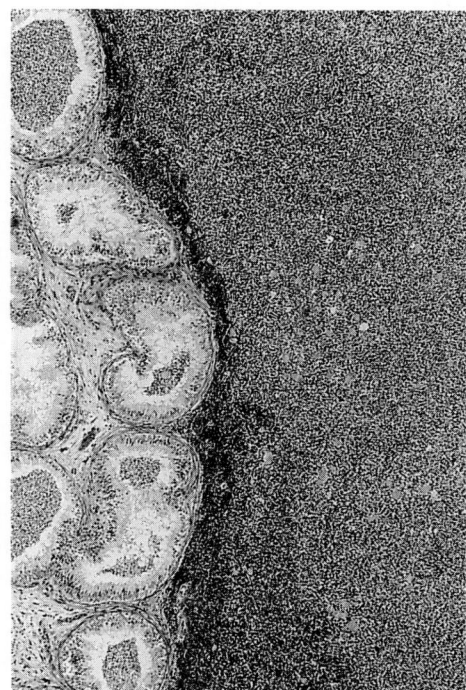

FIG. 25-38 Microscopic section of a spermatic granuloma, canine epididymis. The dark mass consists of inspissated spermatozoa free in the interstitium of the organ (×125).

the epididymis and the testis in the horse. They may also be found in the ligament of the testis and along the spermatic cord. Occasionally, they are located in the mediastinum testis. All three zones of the adrenal cortex may be represented in the nodules. These nodules must be differentiated from neoplastic testicular interstitial cells. In general, adrenal cortical cells are more vacuolated. Adrenal medullary tissue has not been found in these ectopic adrenocortical nodules.

Functional disorders

ATROPHY

Atrophy of previously normal-sized testes can result from a variety of adverse systemic or environmental influences. These include such widely divergent conditions as: deprivation of pituitary gonadotropins; administration of exogenous androgens or estrogens; ionizing radiation; generalized malnutrition; specific vitamin deficiencies (vitamins A and E); prolonged fever or hyperthermia; certain infectious diseases; denervation; occlusion of spermatic vessels; certain genetic disorders; and certain neoplasms.

In general, spermatogenic cells of the testis are the most susceptible to adverse effects of the above-mentioned conditions; consequently, they are the cells most commonly affected in testicular atrophy (Fig. 25-39). Of the spermatogenic series, spermatocytes and their derivatives (spermatids and spermatozoa), are the most vulnerable cells, whereas type A spermatogonia are the

most resistant. At times, Leydig cells also undergo atrophy, but this usually occurs only in certain hormonal imbalances where reduced pituitary gonadotropin secretion is manifest, particularly LH. Sertoli cells are the most stalwart intrinsic cells of the testis, for they seemingly resist the atrophic effects of all but the harshest of noxious stimuli. They are often the only recognizable cells in severely atrophic testes; however, they too may become lost in extreme cases. Depending on the nature and duration of the causative factor, the atrophic process may involve all or only selected cells of the testis.

Atrophy of all principal cellular components of the testis, including germinal, Sertoli and Leydig cells, occurs only under unusual circumstances. It may result from massive doses of ionizing radiation directed at the testis, loss of testicular blood supply due to vascular occlusion, or from torsion of the spermatic cord. Torsion usually occurs only with an excessively long gubernaculum testis. In either case, widespread necrosis of virtually all cells of the testis results. Basement membranes of denuded seminiferous tubules become collapsed and hyalinized and the interstitium is replaced by fibrous connective tissue. Obviously, these changes are irreversible; when both testes are affected, the animal is sterile.

Atrophy of spermatogenic cells represents the most frequent form of testicular atrophy. As mentioned, it results from a variety of systemic and environmental factors, most of which are cited in the first paragraph on

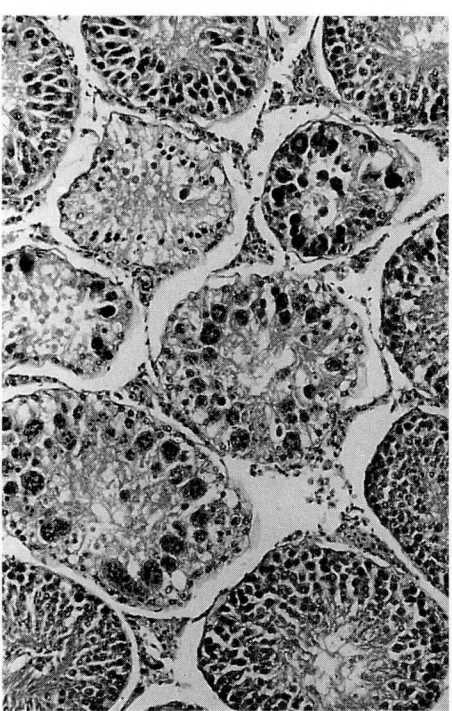

FIG. 25-39 Early changes of testicular atrophy in a vitamin-E-deficient rat. Note the presence of multinucleated spermatidic giant cells in several of the seminiferous tubules (×125).

this subject. Even ionizing radiation—when the dosage is adjusted critically—selectively destroys germ cells and leaves other cell types unaffected. Depending on the nature and duration of the offending influence, atrophic changes may also affect Sertoli and/or Leydig cells; changes in the germinal cells may become irreversible. As a rule, if spermatogonia were completely destroyed, spermatogenesis would cease permanently and the animal would be rendered sterile. Factors known to cause permanent aspermatogenesis include: radiation, denervation, vitamin E deficiency in certain species, and a genetic disorder causing postnatal testicular atrophy in the AsC strain of rat. In most cases, atrophy of spermatogenic cells resulting from other causes is reversible provided the cause is corrected.

In most male animals, pituitary gonadotropins are secreted more or less continuously in approximately the same relative proportions. This is in marked contrast to the cyclic nature of gonadotropin secretion in females which accounts for repeated ovulatory cycles. The pattern of gonadotropin secretion is regulated by the hypothalamus; it is determined for life at a critical period during embryonic or early postnatal life, at least in rodents. In the female rat, mouse, or hamster, a single dose of androgen during the first day or two of life causes continued noncyclic gonadotropin secretion similar to that which occurs normally in males. Such females exhibit continued estrus and, therefore, are sterile. This critical period of masculine imprinting on the hypothalamus appears to coincide with a naturally occurring surge of testosterone secretion by the testes of newborn rats, mice, and hamsters, which sets the pattern for gonadotropin secretion for life. Animals whose gonads fail to secrete testosterone during this period will secrete gonadotropins in a cyclic pattern typical of females. In guinea pigs, this critical period of hypothalamic imprinting occurs midway in gestation instead of immediately after birth.

If a mature male animal were **hypophysectomized** or were **deprived of pituitary gonadotropins,** the testes would atrophy. Microscopically, atrophic changes occur in both germinal and Leydig cells; this varies somewhat with the species. In rats for example, both spermatogonia and spermatocytes persist in appreciable numbers after hypophysectomy, but spermatids and spermatozoa disappear. In guinea pigs and ferrets, spermatogonia persist, but only a few spermatocytes remain; all other germ cells are lost. In other species, including humans, rhesus monkeys, and dogs, only spermatogonia are left following hypophysectomy. Sertoli cells remain essentially unaffected by removal of the pituitary, but Leydig cells in all species except the dog undergo complete atrophy. In dogs, for unknown reasons, Leydig cells become smaller and accumulate lipid, but do not disappear completely as in other species. The changes observed in the testes following hypophysectomy are explicable by the fact that FSH exerts a trophic influence on spermatogenic cells, while LH or ICSH, as it is sometimes called in males, has a similar effect on Leydig cells. This cellular trophism of gonadotropins is not quite this specific, however, for it has been shown that

FSH is effective in promoting spermatogenesis only through the secondary spermatocyte stage. Thereafter, androgens, secreted as the result of LH stimulation of Leydig cells, are essential for spermatid and spermatozoa formation and the completion of spermatogenesis. Moreover, the role of androgens in maintenance of testicular size and function is highly variable and depends on the nature of the androgen, dose and duration of treatment, and age of the animal when administered. For example, testosterone, when administered in small doses to mature rats, causes testicular atrophy as a result of suppression of gonadotropin secretion. Atrophic changes, as would be expected, are found in both the germinal epithelium and Leydig cells. Similar gonadotropin suppression and testicular changes occur following estrogen administration to intact males. Yet, testosterone alone sustains spermatogenesis in mature, hypophysectomized rats, although the testes become smaller than normal and Leydig cells become involuted. The ability of androgens to maintain spermatogenesis is not directly related to the degree of androgenicity. It has been shown that weaker androgens maintain spermatogenesis after hypophysectomy better than stronger ones.

Ionizing radiation, when the dose is adjusted carefully, selectively destroys germ cells and leaves other cells of the testis virtually unscathed. Although androgen secretion and libido are unaffected, the resulting aspermatogenesis causes sterility.

The disastrous consequences of **inanition** or general **malnutrition** on growth and development of various somatic tissues are well known. If nutritional deficiency is prolonged, the testes will also undergo severe atrophic changes. Microscopically, the seminiferous tubules become reduced in size due to marked depletion of germ cells. Severely affected tubules may be lined by only a single layer of Sertoli cells and a few scattered spermatogonia. The tubular lumina contain variable amounts of desquamated cellular debris and, sometimes, multinucleated spermatocytic or spermatidic giant cells. Leydig cells may be reduced in number. Remarkably, the testes are capable of returning to normal and resume spermatogenesis when the dietary deficiency is corrected.

Deficiency of vitamin A in most species and vitamin E in certain species also results in testicular atrophy. Testicular changes associated with vitamin A deficiency are similar to those occurring with inanition. All cells of the spermatogenic series, except spermatogonia, atrophy and disappear from the seminiferous tubules. Because spermatogonia remain, the lesion is reversible if vitamin A is added back to the diet. Testicular atrophy also occurs in rats and guinea pigs with vitamin E deficiency (Fig. 25-39), but unlike the changes seen in general malnutrition and vitamin A deficiency, this type of atrophy is not reversible. Initial changes observed in the testes of vitamin-E-deficient rats and guinea pigs consist of lysis and fusion of spermatozoa with an accumulation of cellular debris in the epididymis. Degenerative changes next appear in the spermatids and spermatocytes, which become vacuolated and desquamate into the tubular lumina. Some of these cells fuse to form multinucleated giant cells which, in some instances, may be numerous. Although the spermatogonia are the last germ cells to manifest morphologic evidence of injury, irreversible injury occurs early in the deficiency state because cells undergo progressive atrophy even when the vitamin is restored in the diet before morphologic changes become apparent. Terminally, all spermatogenic cells disappear from the testes. As a consequence, vitamin E deficiency in rats and guinea pigs results in permanent testicular atrophy and aspermatogenesis. Testicular changes apparently do not occur in vitamin-E-deficient mice and rabbits.

Germinal epithelia of the testes are also remarkably sensitive to **hyperthermia** resulting from **elevations of environmental or body temperatures.** In these instances, the scrotum performs an important thermoregulatory function by constantly altering the position of the testes with respect to the animal's body in response to changes in ambient or body temperature. This compensatory mechanism effectively maintains the gonads at an optimal temperature for normal testicular function. This varies with each species but, in general, it is 1-8°C below normal body temperature. In most species, complex convolutions of the testicular artery, known as the pampiniform plexus, also operate in conjunction with changes in scrotal position to either preheat or cool the blood entering the gonad. Under most circumstances, these homeostatic mechanisms are sufficient to maintain the testes at a fairly constant temperature. However, atrophy occurs when the capacity of this thermoregulatory mechanism is exceeded and the testes become too warm. This occurs as a result of prolonged fever, excessive environmental temperatures, or inguinal-abdominal displacement of a scrotal testis. It also may occur in bulls with excess insulating fat in the scrotum. Atrophic changes affect only germ cells and are characterized by progressive loss of spermatozoa, spermatids, and spermatocytes. If the hyperthermic state is not maintained too long, changes are reversible. Sertoli cells and Leydig cells are not affected. Prolonged inguinal or abdominal displacement of a testis that was formerly in the scrotum (i.e., acquired cryptorchidism) eventually results in atrophy of all germinal epithelia and permanent sterility.

A number of **chemical agents** are known to have antispermatogenic properties. They cause some degree of testicular atrophy when consumed or injected over an appropriate period of time. These include: various alkylating agents (tretamine, busulphone, and isopropyl methanesulfonate); a variety of metals (iron, molybdenum, thallium, lead, cadmium); highly chlorinated naphthalenes; α-chlorohydrin methoxychlor; nitrofurans; thiophenes; dinitropyrroles; diamines; indole-carboxylic acids; deuterium oxide; fluoracetamide; amphotericin B; griseofulvin; chlorcyclizine; and gossypol. The last compound received considerable attention as a potential male contraceptive. Preliminary reports from China indicated that it is 99% effective and is reversible with no permanent side effects.

Testicular atrophy may occur as a sequel to any acute or chronic inflammation of the testis. It has been observed in bulls, rams, boars, and dogs naturally and experimentally infected with respective *Brucella* species. Microscopically, atrophic changes associated with resolving orchitis consist of irregular or diffuse areas of fibrosis and inflammatory cell infiltration replacing the remains of necrotic tubular epithelium and stroma. Inflammatory cellular infiltrate distinguishes it from other forms of testicular atrophy.

Interruption of the sympathetic nerve supply to the testis also causes testicular atrophy. This has been demonstrated in guinea pigs and cats. The decrease in testicular size results from atrophy of germinal epithelium; Sertoli and Leydig cells remain unaffected. Thus, it appears that the sympathetic nerve supply to the testis also provides some trophic influence on the spermatogenic cells. Atrophic changes resulting from denervation are permanent.

Histologic changes produced in the rat testis by **ischemia** resulting from temporary or permanent occlusion of the testicular artery have been studied in great detail. The initial changes occurring during the first hour of ischemia consist of hyperchromasia of spermatogonia and exfoliation of spermatids. As the period of ischemia is prolonged, changes become progressively more severe. Spermatocytes are exfoliated after six hours. By 24 hours, the testis is markedly edematous and many pyknotic, multinucleate cells are present in the tubules. The cytoplasm of Sertoli cells begins to appear vacuolated. By the end of one week, all seminiferous tubules are necrotic. Leydig cells, which appear to be the most resistant to anoxia, do not manifest signs of degeneration until two weeks have passed. After two weeks, they develop cytoplasmic vacuoles and accumulate yellow pigment. After one month, fibroblasts invade the interstitium, and basement membranes of the testicular tubules begin to thicken. By the end of seven months, marked fibrosis is manifest, as well as mild-to-moderate plasma cell infiltration. An occasional Sertoli and Leydig cell may persist in the mass of fibrous connective tissue.

Vascular lesions are seen with some frequency in the equine testis, usually in the vessels of the tunica vaginalis. Lesions consist of arteritis associated with degenerate seminiferous tubules. In some instances, areas of infarction exist. Lesions such as these may be due to migrating strongyle larvae, especially *Strongylus edentatus,* equine viral arteritis, or equine infectious anemia.

Unilateral testicular degeneration and atrophy, probably of ischemic origin, occur congenitally in the left testis of 5% of strain 129 mice. This results from the presence of a congenital hematoma in the testis of these mice. One percent of the males of this strain also develop teratomas in the left testis, but this appears to be unrelated to the ischemic process.

An unusual form of inherited unilateral testicular atrophy has been reported to occur in 20% of male rats of the AxC strain. The condition is characterized by unilateral testicular atrophy and an associated ipsilateral agenesis of the kidney, ureter, ductus deferens, epididymis, and seminal vesicles. The coagulating gland is usually present. Curiously, the testis, which is destined to atrophy, appears normal grossly and histologically as late as 30 days postnatally. After the first month of life, the abnormal testis becomes smaller than its opposite counterpart. At 45–47 days of age, spermatogenesis ceases and the seminiferous tubules become atrophic. Basement membranes of the denuded tubules become thickened and the entire testis becomes fibrotic. Little is known regarding the pathogenesis of this interesting form of testicular atrophy except that it is an inherited disorder.

Testicular atrophy may result from tumors of the pituitary or from an estrogen-secreting neoplasm, such as Sertoli cell tumor of the testis. In either instance, atrophy results from loss of pituitary gonadotropin stimulation. This occurs by either destruction of the pituitary by the neoplasm or the suppression of gonadotropin secretion by elevated levels of circulating estrogens.

Hypertrophy and hyperplasia

Testicular hypertrophy or hyperplasia occurs rarely and is usually a consequence of endocrine imbalance. Following unilateral orchiectomy, the weight of the remaining testis increases slightly. This results principally from hypertrophy and hyperplasia of Leydig cells, which presumably respond to the relatively greater amounts of circulating LH (or ICSH) by secreting more androgens. This increased production of androgens probably serves to diminish gonadotropin secretion via the pituitary-gonad feedback mechanism. One cannot appreciably increase spermatogenesis in the normal testis by administering gonadotropins; the normal testis presumably produces spermatozoa at a maximal rate consistent with the time required for each spermatogenic cell type to mature. It is therefore impossible to accelerate spermatogenesis and still have normal spermatozoa produced.

Inflammation and infection

Orchitis and **epididymitis** occur frequently in most animal species. Such infections may be caused by specific bacterial pathogens that have a predilection for the testis and epididymis in certain species: *Brucella abortus,* including its strain 19 in cattle (Fig. 25-40); *B. ovis* in sheep; *B. suis* in swine; *B. canis* in dogs; and rarely, *Mycobacterium tuberculosis* var. bovis in cattle. Orchitis and epididymitis may also be caused by a variety of ubiquitous bacteria capable of causing tissue damage in any organ to which they are introduced, either hematogenously or via contaminated wound. The latter group of organisms include: *E. coli; Proteus vulgaris; Corynebacterium ovis;* streptococci; and staphylococci. Other bacteria known to cause experimental, but not spontaneous, orchitis in laboratory animals include: *Treponema cuniculi* in rabbits; and *Pseudomonas mallei* and *Pseudomonas pseudomallei,* the causative agents of glanders and melioidosis, respectively, in guinea pigs. The orchitis produced in guinea pigs following intraperitoneal inocula-

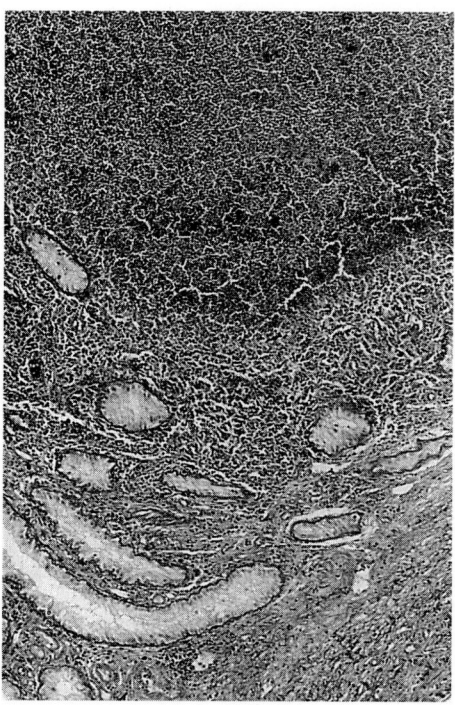

FIG. 25-40 *Brucella-abortus*-induced granulomatous orchitis in a bull (×100).

tion with *P. mallei* and *P. pseudomallei* is called a positive **Strauss reaction.** It has been used in the past for the diagnosis of glanders and melioidosis in other species.

Canine distemper virus may cause orchitis and epididymitis in mature dogs. The lesion differs from other forms of orchitis and epididymitis by the presence of eosinophilic intranuclear and intracytoplasmic inclusion bodies in the Sertoli cells and epididymal epithelium.

In the infectious forms of orchitis or epididymitis, the causative agent enters the testis or epididymis by several routes, including penetrating wounds, blood or lymphatic vessels, other foci of infection, or reflux of exudate through the vas deferens from an infection elsewhere in the genitourinary tract. The earliest changes in the affected organ consists of hemorrhage, edema, and varying amounts of parenchymal necrosis. This is followed by an influx of inflammatory cells. Intensity, distribution, and nature of these inflammatory cells vary according to the virulence of the causative agent. Neutrophils are usually the first inflammatory cells to appear in the infected organ. These are generally scattered diffusely throughout edematous interstitium, but accumulate in great numbers in the lumina of affected seminiferous tubules. Cellular debris from necrotic spermatogenic and Sertoli cells also desquamate into the tubular lumina. This is the type of lesion seen in most cases of *Brucella orchitis* and epididymitis, except in *B. suis* infection where caseous necrosis and granuloma formation are characteristic. If spermatozoa were released into adjacent stroma, intense granulomatous inflammatory reaction would ensue with formation of a spermatic granuloma. This lesion is characterized by an accumulation of large numbers of epithelioid cells around the extravasated sperm. Foreign body giant cells are frequently present in such granulomas. Occasionally, infection penetrates the tunica albuginea of the testis and extends into the scrotal sac. In such cases, the space between the testis and the tunica vaginalis becomes distended with a fibrinopurulent exudate. The healing phase of inflammatory processes in the testis and epididymis is invariably accompanied by varying degrees of fibrosis and mononuclear inflammatory cell infiltration. As a consequence, tubules become obliterated or occluded by fibrous connective tissue. Varying degrees of testicular and/or epididymal atrophy result. Depending on the degree of tubular atrophy and occlusion, fertility may be normal or severely impaired. Leydig cells proliferate to replace those lost; hence, androgen production is not permanently diminished.

Reference

Lambert G, Manthei CA, Deyoe BL. Studies on Brucella abortus in bulls. Am J Vet Res 1963;24:1152–1157.

Testicular neoplasms

GENERAL CONSIDERATIONS

Spontaneous neoplasms of the testis are rare in all species except dogs, bulls, horses, and certain inbred strains of rats and mice. Testicular tumors have also been produced experimentally in rats and certain inbred strains of mice. Naturally occurring primary tumors of the epididymis are rare in all species.

Four types of primary neoplasms arise in the testes of common domestic and laboratory animal species, including Sertoli cell (sustentacular-cell) tumors, interstitial (Leydig) cell tumors, seminomas, and teratomas. Other tumors, including fibromas, hemangiomas, leiomyomas, and their malignant counterparts, may also arise from various cellular components of the testicular stroma, but these are rare.

Testicular neoplasms occur most commonly in older dogs. The testis has been reported to be the third most common site of neoplasia in male dogs, exceeded only by tumors of the skin and connective tissue. In one large survey of 2361 canine neoplasms of all types, testicular tumors comprised 5.8% of the total. The principal tumors of the canine testis are interstitial (Leydig) cell tumors, seminomas, and Sertoli cell tumors; teratomas have not been described in dogs. Discrepancies exist among several published surveys of testicular neoplasms in dogs regarding the relative incidence of the three tumors. Most reports indicate that interstitial cell tumors are the most common, followed by seminomas and Sertoli cell tumors in decreasing frequency. In one survey, however, seminoma was the most common, followed by Sertoli cell and interstitial cell tumors. In still another large series that included 318 canine testicular neoplasms detected mainly in surgical specimens, Sertoli cell tumors comprised 49.4%, seminomas 33.6%, and interstitial cell tumors only 17.0% of the total. Fi-

nally, in a series of 520 canine testicular neoplasms compiled at Angell Memorial Animal Hospital, 38% were interstitial cell tumors, 32% seminomas, and 30% Sertoli cell tumors. These discrepancies may be explained, in part, by differences in the sources of the tumors studied (i.e., whether detected incidentally at autopsy or found in surgical specimens). Because certain testicular neoplasms are more readily detected clinically than others, surgical specimens may represent a somewhat biased sample, not reflecting the true incidence of the three types. It is not uncommon for more than one testicular neoplasm to be present in the same animal. These may be of the same or different cell types and either in the same or opposite testis.

Approximately 25% of dogs with Sertoli cell tumors display signs of feminization (hyperestrinism). These include bilateral alopecia and cutaneous hyperpigmentation, atrophy of the opposite testis, pendulous prepuce, varying degrees of gynecomastia, loss of libido, and a peculiar attraction of male dogs to the affected animal as if it were a bitch in estrus. Affected animals may also develop bone marrow suppression from the excessive estrogens. In addition, the prostate gland often undergoes enlargement due to severe squamous metaplasia of the epithelium. Affected prostates are initially atrophic, but eventually become enlarged. Similar signs of apparent hyperestrinism have rarely been described in dogs with seminomas and interstitial cell tumors. In a large survey of canine testicular neoplasms, Cotchin reported that 16% of 54 animals with interstitial cell tumors displayed clinical evidence of alopecia and/or feminization (1960). This inordinately high incidence of clinical signs—suggestive of a hormonal imbalance associated with interstitial cell tumors—has not been reported in dogs by others. An increased incidence of tumors of the androgen-responsive circumanal glands has been reported in dogs with interstitial cell tumors. It has been shown in humans and rats that interstitial cell tumors may produce androgens, as one may expect, but also occasionally produce estrogens, progesterone, and even corticosteroids. McEntee associated prostatic enlargement, aggressive behavior, and increased volume of ejaculate in dogs and bulls with interstitial cell tumors as presumptive evidence of androgen secretion (1990). Quantitative assays for testosterone have not been done with bovine or canine interstitial cell tumors. Finally, cryptorchidism appears to predispose the testis to neoplasia because Sertoli cell tumors and seminomas occur 10–13 times more frequently in dogs with retained testes than in the general canine population. Interstitial cell tumors do not occur more frequently in cryptorchid testes; the reason for this is unknown.

In bulls, interstitial cell tumors are the most common testicular neoplasm; Sertoli cell tumors are found only occasionally. Testicular neoplasms occur primarily in bulls seven years of age and older. A survey by McEntee reported 20 interstitial cell tumors in a series of 216 (9.2%) bulls over seven years of age (1990). The highest incidence (19%) was in Guernsey bulls and the lowest (4.2%) in the Holstein breed. Sperm production and quality, as well as fertility were somewhat reduced in bulls with interstitial cell tumors. Sertoli cell tumors were found with much less frequency in bulls.

In horses, interstitial cell tumors are also generally found in older animals. Accurate figures on the incidence of this tumor in stallions are not available. Affected stallions may become extremely vicious, suggesting excessive androgen production. Congenital teratomas occur rarely in the testes of young horses and may cause cryptorchidism because of their large size. McEntee reported only one teratoma in the testes of approximately 700 horses.

In rams, hyperplasia of testicular germ cells frequently occurs and is confined to the seminiferous tubules. The lesion is not recognizable grossly and probably does not represent a true neoplasm of germ cells.

The incidence of spontaneous testicular neoplasms in rats varies considerably among different strains. One group of investigators reported only a single seminoma in 31,686 rats from a closed colony. Another group found no testicular tumors in 63 male Sprague-Dawley rats maintained until they died of natural causes. Conversely, 31 (18.6%) of 167 male Wistar rats were reported to have spontaneous interstitial cell tumors of the testis. Similarly, a survey on the incidence of tumors in 279 male rats of the "Rochester strain of Wistar rat" found that 35 (12.5%) had interstitial cell tumors and another report stated that as many as 60% of the Piebald Virol Glaxo (PVG) strain of hooded rats of Wistar origin may have interstitial cell tumors by two years of age. Finally, one other group of investigators observed interstitial tumors of the testis in 68% of 92 aged Fischer rats.

Spontaneous neoplasms of the testis occur rarely in mice except for those of the so-called inbred strain 129. In an early, but extensive survey, only 28 tumors of the testis were found in more than 9000 male mice maintained in a closed colony until they died of natural causes. Although not specifically referred to as such, it appears from the histologic descriptions that most of the tumors were seminomas. All but one occurred in mice of a single strain and its hybrid derivatives. The occurrence of two spontaneous interstitial cell tumors as well as equivocal seminomas in three of 61 hybrid offspring resulting from mating male and female strain A mice with C57 and C3H strains has also been reported. Coincident interstitial cell and Sertoli cell tumors have been described in the testis of a C3H mouse. Conversely, it has been reported that 1% of the males of strain 129 mice develop congenital testicular teratomas; 75–80% of the tumors arise in the left testis. Teratomas have been reported to arise in multiple foci from primordial germ cells of the testis on days 15–17 of gestation. Another interesting, but apparently unrelated, characteristic of this strain is that 5% of the males are also born with atrophic left testes resulting from the presence of a congenital hematoma. Tumors, however, have not been found in the atrophic testes.

Rare reports of testicular neoplasms in other laboratory animal species include: Sertoli cell tumors in two cats, an owl monkey, and a chicken; seminoma in an orangutan and a howler monkey; and testicular adenocarcinoma in a baboon, *Cynocephalus hamadryas*.

Testicular tumors have been experimentally induced in several species by various means. Teratomas have been found in the testes of fowl following intratesticular injection of copper salts. Interstitial (Leydig) cell tumors have been induced in rats by the administration of cadmium salts and ligation of testicular blood vessels and by intrasplenic grafting of infantile rat testis into adult castrate animals. The authors of the latter study concluded that the interstitial cell hyperplasia and neoplasia observed in the transplanted testicular tissue were due to chronic pituitary gonadotropin stimulation. Interstitial cell tumors have been experimentally induced in a variety of mouse strains, as well as in certain hybrids by chronic estrogen administration. The BALB/c strain is reportedly the most susceptible to this means of induction. Similar tumors have been induced in the BALB/c strain of mouse by surgical cryptorchidy.

SERTOLI CELL TUMOR AND TUBULAR ADENOMA

Sertoli cell tumor (sustentacular-cell tumor) occurs most commonly in dogs and occasionally in bulls and horses. These tumors can vary ≤ 1 mm to ≥ 15 cm in diameter. Those arising in retained testes in dogs may become extremely large before they are detected clinically. Enlargement and/or distortion of the affected scrotal testis may be manifest. The tumor is usually a single, firm mass with a smooth, or somewhat bosselated or nodular surface covered by the distended tunica albuginea. These tumors rarely penetrate the fibrous tunic and invade contiguous structures, such as the spermatic cord, epididymis, or scrotum. Metastasis is uncommon, but may occur. Metastatic lesions are most often found in the inguinal, iliac, and sublumbar lymph nodes, and rarely in liver, spleen, lung, or other visceral organs. The cut surface of the Sertoli cell tumor often bulges above the adjacent, atrophic testicular parenchyma and varies from whitish-gray to yellow. Bands of fibrous connective tissue often subdivide the main mass into irregular lobules. Small cysts and areas of necrosis and hemorrhage are occasionally present, particularly in larger tumors.

Microscopically (Fig. 25-41), Sertoli cell tumors consist of masses of elongated, fusiform cells arranged in either variably-sized pseudotubular structures or in diffuse sheets. The pseudotubular pattern may, in some instances, mimic normal testicular architecture. Adjacent neoplastic tubule-like structures are circumscribed and separated by prominent coarse bands of collagenous connective tissue. Neoplastic Sertoli cells are fusiform with long, cytoplasmic protrusions that stream from the opposite poles of a round or ovoid nucleus. Individual cell outlines may be difficult to discern, particularly where the cells are tightly packed. The cytoplasm is homogeneously eosinophilic or variably vacuolated due to the presence of few to many lipid droplets. Cells included in the neoplastic pseudotubules are often arranged in a palisade or picket fencelike pattern in which adjacent tumor cells lay parallel to one another with long axes perpendicular to basement membrane.

In other tumors, the pseudotubular pattern may be

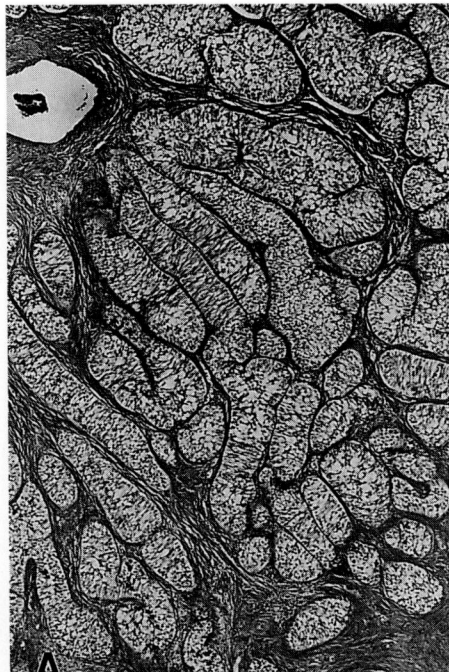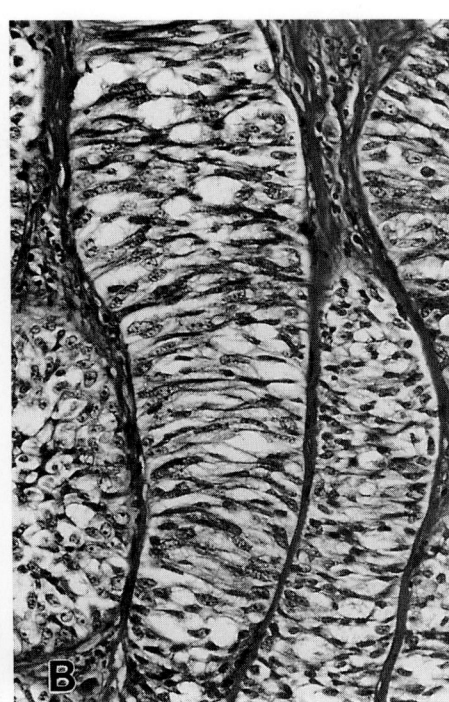

FIG. 25-41 Sertoli cell tumor in a dog (×100). **A.** Neoplastic Sertoli cells are arranged in a palisade pattern within pseudotubular structures resembling seminiferous tubules. Note dense connective tissue stroma. **B.** Higher magnification showing elongated tumor cells arranged perpendicular to the long axes of the pseudotubules (×350).

less evident; instead, neoplastic cells are arranged in diffuse sheets that may be variably traversed by thin bands of connective tissue that subdivide the mass into irregular nests or nodules. Mitotic figures are not generally a prominent feature of these tumors. Seminiferous tubules in the tumor-bearing testis, as well as those in the opposite testis, are often atrophic as a result of estrogen secretion by the tumor. Those tubules adjacent to the neoplasm are also generally compressed due to the expansive nature of the tumor's growth.

INTERSTITIAL CELL TUMOR

Interstitial (Leydig) cell tumors are most common in dogs and bulls, but appear occasionally in stallions and laboratory rodents. These tumors, especially when small, may be difficult to distinguish from the nodular form of interstitial cell hyperplasia observed with some frequency in older animals with senile testicular atrophy. Therefore, this distinction can be somewhat arbitrary and is principally based on size. Interstitial cell tumors are usually discretely round or ovoid and 1–2 cm in diameter. They rarely become large enough to increase the overall size of the testis, although they may cause nodular distortion of the normally smooth contour on the gonad. They may be multiple or solitary and either unilateral or bilateral. On cut surface, this neoplasm is generally well-demarcated, encapsulated, spherical, and commonly bulges above the adjacent testicular parenchyma. Typically, the tumor is soft, yellow to orange, and is somewhat greasy due to the presence of lipids. Those in dogs are often marked by areas of hemorrhage, necrosis, and cystic degeneration.

Histologically, interstitial cell tumors (Fig. 25-42) are composed of large, polyhedral cells with abundant, finely vacuolated, eosinophilic cytoplasm that may also contain yellow-brown lipochrome pigment. Cytoplasmic vacuolization is due to the presence of numerous, small lipid droplets dispersed throughout the cells. Neoplastic interstitial cells in bulls contain few lipids and the vascular supply is not as well developed as that in this type of tumor in dogs. Interstitial cell tumors in stallions are often heavily pigmented and more firm than those in dogs and bulls. The cytoplasm of estrogen-induced testicular interstitial cell tumors of mice, particularly after subsequent transplantation, may contain large inclusion bodies composed of numerous type A, virus-like particles. The significance of these particles and their etiologic relationship, if any, to these tumors is not known.

The pattern of cellular growth varies from tumor to tumor, as well as within the same tumor. Cells are often arranged in diffuse sheets presenting a mosaic pattern. Another common feature is a tendency for tumor cells to be aligned radially around blood vessels in a perithelial- or endocrine-type pattern. These tumors are richly supplied with thin-walled blood vessels, but contain little connective tissue stroma. Considerable hemorrhage, necrosis, and cystic spaces may contain cellular debris in these tumors in dogs. Seminiferous tubules adjacent to the expanding neoplasm commonly exhibit evidence of compression atrophy, whereas those further removed from the mass, as well as those in the unaffected testis, may appear to be normal. Interstitial cell tumors rarely, if ever, metastasize.

SEMINOMA

Seminomas, found most often in dogs (Fig. 25-43), are usually solitary and unilateral, but may be multiple or bilateral. They may arise in scrotal testes, but are re-

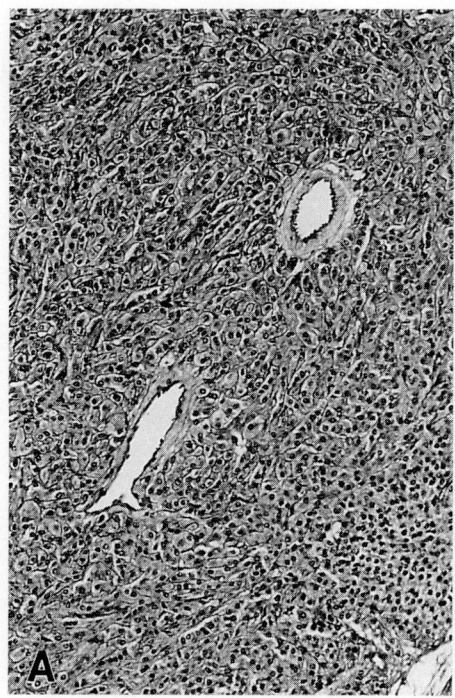

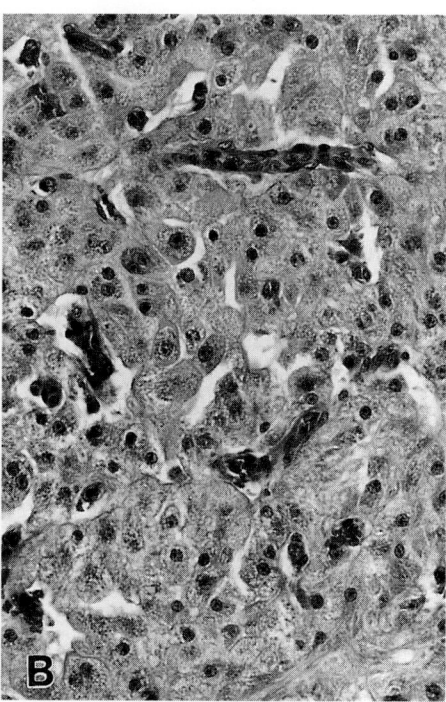

FIG. 25-42 Interstitial cell tumor in a dog. **A.** Diffuse sheets of neoplastic interstitial cells (×125). **B.** Higher magnification of round-to-ovoid neoplastic interstitial cells containing fine-lipid droplets in the cytoplasm. Tumor cells are in close apposition to thin-walled blood vessels (×350).

ported to occur with greater frequency in cryptorchid testes. They may occur simultaneously with either one or both of the two previously described neoplasms, either in the same or opposite testis. Grossly, seminomas can vary from a few millimeters to 5 or more centimeters in diameter and accordingly may cause testicular enlargement. Although they may become quite large, seminomas appear to respect the tunica albuginea and, as a result, they more or less conform to the shape of the normal testis. As with other testicular neoplasms, metastases are rare and usually are found in iliac and sublumbar lymph nodes.

The cut surface (Fig. 25-43A) is generally firm and bulges above the adjacent testicular parenchyma. Color generally varies from white to pale gray, but may be grayish-pink or tan. Delicate fibrous septa may divide the main mass into irregular lobules. Foci of hemorrhage and necrosis may be evident in some tumors.

Microscopically, seminomas are composed of cells that bear a striking resemblance to spermatogonia and spermatocytes. Cells are roughly round or polygonal and can vary somewhat in size. Depending on the density of the tumor cell population, individual cell membranes may be readily discernible. Each cell contains a large, round, centrally placed nucleus with distinctly granular chromatin and a single (sometimes double) prominent nucleolus. Cytoplasm is scant and usually basophilic or amphoteric when stained with hematoxylin and eosin.

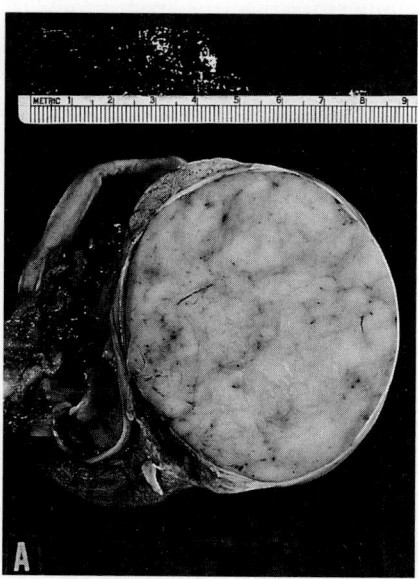

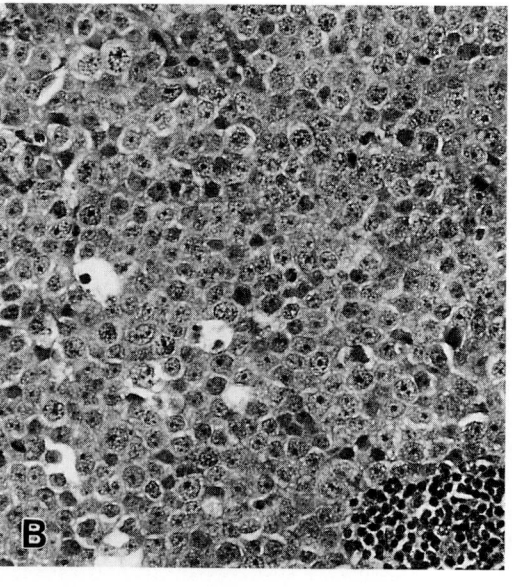

FIG. 25-43 Seminoma. **A.** Spherical mass in the testicle of a 17-year-old chow dog. (Contributor: Dr. Edward Records.) **B.** Seminoma (×355) testicle of a dog. Large spherical cells with hyperchromatic nuclei lymphocytes in lower right. (Courtesy of Armed Forces Institute of Pathology and Angell Memorial Animal Hospital.)

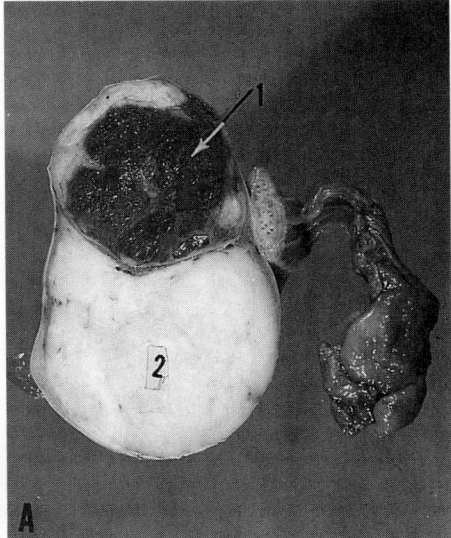
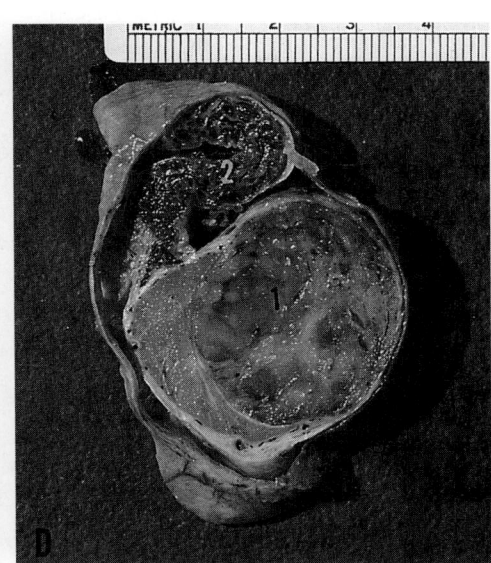

FIG. 25-44 A. (1) Interstitial cell tumor and (2) Sertoli cell tumor in testis of a 12-year-old Dachshund. (Contributor: Dr. Robert Ferber.) **B.** (1) Interstitial cell tumor displacing testicular parenchyma. (2) Epididymis. (Courtesy of Armed Forces Institute of Pathology and Angell Memorial Animal Hospital.)

Tumor is usually multicentric in origin with tumor cells initially proliferating within widely scattered, existing seminiferous tubules. Spermatids and spermatozoa disappear completely from affected tubules. Sertoli cells are either replaced or become severely flattened against the basement membrane by the rapidly expanding mass of neoplastic spermatogenic cells. Within an affected tubule, varying numbers of tumor cells undergo cytoplasmic vacuolization while others manifest early signs of necrosis. Mitotic figures are a prominent feature of this tumor. When an affected tubule becomes filled, tumor cells often penetrate the basement membrane, invade interstitium, and become confluent with those arising in adjacent tubules. This leads to the formation of broad sheets of neoplastic cells which, in later stages, may replace much of the testicular parenchyma. Another fairly consistent feature of seminomas is the focal accumulation of lymphocytes scattered throughout the masses of tumor cells (Fig. 25-43A).

TERATOMA

Testicular teratomas are commonly found in only one mouse strain and rarely in horses. Spontaneous testicular teratomas of strain 129 mice are congenital in origin. Grossly, teratomas do not become apparent until the affected mouse is one week or more of age. Seventy-five to eighty percent of the tumors occur in the left testis, which becomes enlarged and, on cut surface, appears hemorrhagic. With increasing age, the gonad may increase to three to four times normal size and, although it may cause considerable testicular distortion, the tumor never penetrates the tunica albuginea. Such tissues as bone, bone marrow, cartilage, fat, various epithelial-lined cysts, and small masses of twitching or rhythmically pulsating skeletal or cardiac muscle may be seen grossly. In old mice, tumors consist mainly of fluid or blood-filled cysts.

Microscopically, tumors first become evident in the fetal testis at 15 days gestation. At this time, small clusters of cells appear among the germ cells of several seminiferous tubules. These cells differ from primordial germ cells in that they contain a more lucid nucleoplasm and larger nucleoli. Affected tubules are generally continuous and may represent different sections of the same tortuous tubule. By day 16, some tumor cells have become elongated and assume more embryonal features. These may be oriented around a small pool of fluid in a pattern somewhat reminiscent of an "embryoid body" (observed in certain human ovarian and testicular teratomas). By day 17, neoplastic embryonal cells have increased in number. In approximately half of affected animals, cells have penetrated the tubule wall and invaded the interstitium. By day 19, masses of tumor cells from contiguous tubules have coalesced and formed scattered vesicles lined with primitive epithelium. At birth, tumor cells have differentiated into epithelial and mesenchymal cells with an appearance and histogenetic capacity of ectoderm, endoderm, and mesoderm. Curiously, as the affected mouse matures, its tumor also does. Consequently, by 30 days of age, proportionately less embryonic-type tissue is present in the tumor and considerably more well-differentiated tissue of various types is manifest than had appeared immediately after birth. Nervous tissue is present in virtually all such tumors. Epithelial tissue of various types (stratified squamous, columnar, cuboidal, and pseudostratified) may be found with interspersed ciliated and goblet cells in these tumors. Connective tissue elements include fibrous and loose areolar tissue, brown and adult adipose tissue, cartilage, bone, and hematopoietic tissue. Skeletal, cardiac, and smooth muscle cells are present in approximately one-third of tumors. Endocrine tissue including that of the adrenal cortex, anterior pituitary, islets of Langerhans, and thyroid have been observed in a few teratomas. Tissues that have not thus far been recognized in this murine testicular teratoma include pigmented epithelial cells, trophoblastic cells, teeth, hepatic, renal, gonadal, and lung tissues. Hemorrhage and necrosis may be present in some areas of the teratomatous growth. Metastasis does not occur.

OTHER NEOPLASMS

Other neoplasms found rarely in the testis include mesotheliomas fibromas, chondromas, osteomas, hemangiomas, leiomyomas, and malignant counterparts. The testis and epididymis are not common sites of metastasis from other neoplasms. Occasionally, these organs may be infiltrated by neoplastic lymphoid cells in individuals with generalized malignant lymphoma.

References

Becht JL, Thacker HL, Page EH. Malignant seminoma in a stallion. J Am Vet Med Assoc 1979;174:292–293.

Brodey RS, Martin JE. Sertoli cell neoplasms in the dog. The clinicopathological and endocrinological findings in thirty-seven dogs. J Am Vet Med Assoc 1958;133:249–257.

Brown TT, Burek JD, McEntee K. Male pseudohermaphroditism, cryptorchidism and Sertoli cell neoplasia in three miniature schnauzers. J Am Vet Med Assoc 1976;169:821–825.

Cotchin E. Testicular neoplasms in dogs. J Comp Pathol 1960;70:232–248.

Cotchin E. Spontaneous and experimentally-induced testicular tumours in animals. In: Pugh RCB, ed. Pathology of the testis. Oxford: Blackwell, 1976;371–408.

Cullen JM, Whiteside J, Umstead JA, et al. A mixed germ cell-sex cord-stromal neoplasm of the testis in a stallion. Vet Pathol 1987;24:575–577.

Dow C. Testicular tumours in the dog. J Comp Pathol 1962;72:247–265.

Edwards DF. Bone marrow hypoplasia in a feminized dog with a Sertoli cell tumor. J Am Vet Med Assoc 1981;178:494–496.

Fadok VA, Lothrop CD, Coulson P. Hyperprogesteronemia associated with Sertoli cell tumor and alopecia in a dog. J Am Vet Med Assoc 1986;188:1058–1059.

Gelberg HB, McEntee K. Equine testicular interstitial cell tumors. Vet Pathol 1987;24:231–234.

Hayes HM, Pendergrass TW. Canine testicular tumors: epidemiologic features of 410 dogs. Int J Cancer 1976;18:482–487.

Hayes HM, Wilson GP, Pendergrass TW, et al. Canine cryptorchidism and subsequent testicular neoplasia: case-control study with epidemiologic update. Teratology 1985;32:51–56.

Jensen R, Flint JC. Intratubular seminomas in testes of sheep. J Comp Pathol 1963;73:146–149.

Ladds PW, Crane CK. Scrotal mesothelioma in a bull. Aust Vet J 1976;52:534–535.

Ladds PW, Saunders PJ. Sertoli cell tumors in the bull. J Comp Pathol 1976;86:503–508.

McEntee K. Reproductive pathology of domestic mammals. New York: Academic Press, 1990.

Meir H. Sertoli-cell tumor in the cat. Report of two cases. North Am Vet 1956;37:979–981.

Morgan RV. Blood dyscrasias associated with testicular neoplasms in the dog. J Am Anim Hosp Assoc 1982;18:970–974.

Nielsen SW, Lein DH. Tumours of the testis. Bull WHO 1974;50:71–78.

Peterson EE. Equine testicular tumors. J Equine Vet Sci 1984;4:25–27.

Rahaley RS, Gordon BJ, Leipold HW, et al. Sertoli cell tumor in a horse. Equine Vet J 1983;15:68–70.

Rebar AJ, Fessler JF, Erb R. Testicular teratoma in a horse. A case report and endocrinologic study. J Equine Med Surg 1979;3:361–366.

Reif JS, Maguire TG, Kenney RM, et al. A cohort study of canine testicular neoplasia. J Am Vet Med Assoc 1979;175:719–723.

Sherding RG, Wilson GP III, Kociba GJ. Bone marrow hypoplasia in eight dogs with Sertoli cell tumor. J Am Vet Med Assoc 1981;178:497–501.

Shortridge EH, Cordes DO. Seminomas in sheep. J Comp Pathol 1969;79:229–232.

Stevens LC. Testicular teratomas in fetal mice. JNCI 1962;28:247–267.

Stevens LC. Origin of testicular teratomas from primordial germ cells in mice. JNCI 1967;38:549–552.

Thilander G, Lindberg R, Ploen L. Ultrastructural features of the neoplastic Sertoli cells in the dog. Acta Vet Scand 1987;28:445–446.

Trigo FJ, Miller RA, Torbeck RL. Metastatic equine seminoma: report of two cases. Vet Pathol 1984;21:259–260.

Turk JR, Turk MA, Gallina AM. A canine testicular tumor resembling gonadoblastoma. Vet Pathol 1981;18:201–207.

Valentine BA, Weinstock D. Metastatic testicular embryonal carcinoma in a horse. Vet Pathol 1986;23:92–96.

von Bomhard DC, Pukkavesa C, Haenichen T. The ultrastructure of testicular tumours in the dog. III. Sertoli cells and Sertoli cell tumours and general conclusions. J Comp Pathol 1978;88:67–73.

MALE ACCESSORY SEX GLANDS
Prostate

ATROPHY

Atrophy of the prostate gland occurs with any condition that results in cessation of androgen stimulation. The most common causes include castration, estrogen administration, or destructive lesions of the testes. Microscopically, the normal cuboidal to columnar prostatic epithelium become flattened and nonsecretory resulting in collapse of the acini. At this stage, the gland consists primarily of residual fibromuscular tissue with markedly attenuated acini.

CALCULI

Calculi in the prostate gland have been described on rare occasions in dogs. They are often multiple and can range 1–10 mm in diameter. They are generally smooth and white, but may contain mottled-brown streaking and are composed of a combination of triple phosphates, urates, and carbonates often deposited around a central core of organic material, probably degenerate cells. They are usually located within one or more cysts lined by metaplastic stratified squamous epithelium and surrounded by dense collagenous connective tissue containing mononuclear inflamamtory cells.

SQUAMOUS METAPLASIA

Squamous metaplasia of prostatic glandular epithelium occurs with chronic infection or irritation (calculi), prolonged endogenous or exogenous estrogen stimulation, and chlorinated naphthalene poisoning. It occurs most often in dogs with estrogen-secreting Sertoli cell tumors (Fig. 25-45C) and following prolonged estrogen therapy. In advanced stages, prostatic acini become transformed into solid and cystic masses of well-differentiated squamous epithelium, often with central cores of concentrically-laminated keratin. Squamous metaplasia of the prostate is reversible when the offending source of estrogen is eliminated. Its regression following removal of a Sertoli cell tumor can be viewed as a good prognostic sign that metastasis has not occurred.

PROSTATITIS

Prostatitis occurs in all domestic animal species, but appears clinically most often in dogs where it may be associated with hyperplasia of the gland. The causes of prosta-

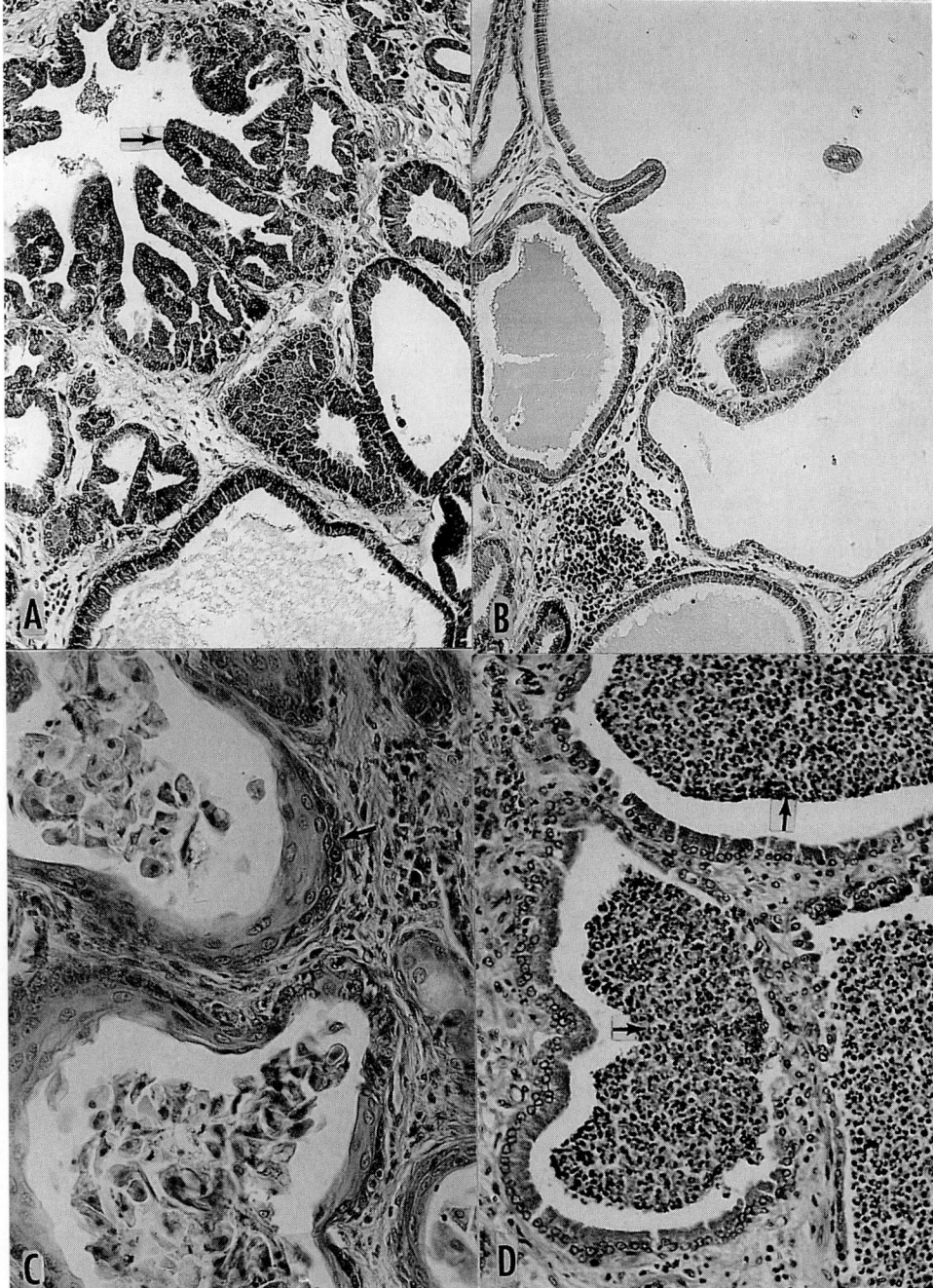

FIG. 25-45 A. Hyperplasia of the canine prostate. Note tall columnar cells (arrows) in long fronds extending into the lumen of prostatic acinus. (Contributor: Dr. S. Pollock.) **B.** Cystic glandular hyperplasia of the canine prostate. Cysts are formed in parts of the gland. (Contributor: Dr. Norman G. Simels.) **C.** Squamous metaplasia (arrow) in the prostate of a dog with Sertoli cell tumor of the testis. (Contributor: Dr. Wayne H. Riser.) **D.** Acute purulent prostatitis in a dog. Note acini filled with neutrophils and cellular debris. (Contributor: Dr. Albert M. Berkelhammer; Figures 25-45A-D: Courtesy of Armed Forces Institute of Pathology.)

titis in dogs include various gram-negative bacteria (*E. coli*, *Proteus spp.*, *Pseudomonas*, and *Brucella canis*), as well as gram-positive bacteria, such as staphylococci, streptococci and *Mycobacterium spp.* Canine distemper virus may also infect prostatic epithelium. Microscopically, the gland may be focally or diffusely affected with accumulation of variable amounts of purulent exudate within the acini. Depending on its duration, variable numbers of lymphocytes, plasma cells, and macrophages may be manifest in the interglandular stroma. With longstanding inflammation, acinar epithelium may undergo focal squamous metaplasia.

BENIGN PROSTATIC HYPERPLASIA

Benign prostatic hyperplasia occurs most often in older dogs and is the most common condition affecting the prostate (Fig. 25-46). The canine prostate continues to grow until approximately 11 years of age. It is not uncommon, however, to find evidence of prostatic hyperplasia within the gland after three years of age. The condition in humans, which mainly affects the central portion of the gland in a nodular fashion, causes compression of the prostatic urethra and difficult urination; in contrast, the condition in dogs affects the gland diffusely with expansion of the prostate dorsally. Most cases of prostatic

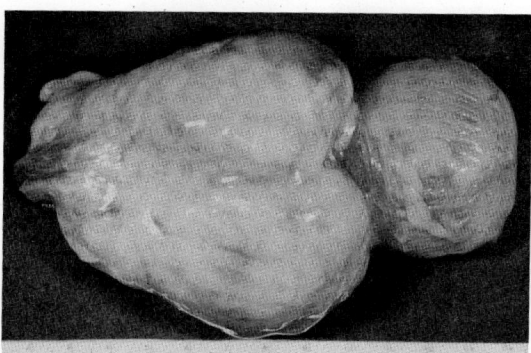

FIG. 25-46 Benign hyperplasia of the prostate of an eight-year-old male German short-haired pointer dog. (Courtesy of Angell Memorial Animal Hospital.)

hyperplasia in dogs are not associated with clinical signs; it is only when the prostate becomes so large as to compress the colon and interfere with defecation that serious effects result. Microscopically, gradual expansion of affected acini occurs with the formation of numerous, branching, papillary infoldings of the prostatic epithelium and associated stroma. Epithelial cells lining these projections may be more columnar than that of unaffected acini and have more intensely eosinophilic cytoplasm. With time, some of the affected acini may become cystic. It is not uncommon for dogs with benign prostatic hyperplasia to develop prostatitis.

Pathogenesis of benign prostatic hyperplasia in older men and dogs involves an increase in the level of the potent androgen, 5α-dihydrotestosterone within affected glands. Experimentally, administration of pharmacologic doses of 5α-dihydrotestosterone to castrated dogs consistently induces benign prostatic hyperplasia. When small quantities of estradiol-17β are administered simultaneously with 5α-dihydrotestosterone, benign prostatic hyperplasia occurs in 100% of castrated dogs. It is believed that estradiol-17β secreted either from the testes or from peripheral conversion of androgens probably has a synergistic effect with 5α-dihydrotestosterone in the induction of benign prostatic hyperplasia by increasing androgen receptors in prostatic tissue.

ADENOCARCINOMA

Adenocarcinoma of the prostate is the third leading cause of death from cancer in men in the United States, but it is rare in other animal species, except dogs and certain strains of rats (Nb and A/C). In dogs, prostatic adenocarcinoma is uncommon and occurs almost exclusively in older animals (average age: 9.9 years). It occurs in castrated dogs almost as frequently as in intact animals; some reports indicate that the risk is even greater in castrated dogs than in intact dogs. This would suggest either that testosterone is not important in the pathogenesis of prostatic cancer or that its effect occurs much earlier in life. This is contrary to what is known about prostatic cancer in men where androgens

are considered important in the etiology. It is possible that in the dog androgens from other sources, such as the adrenal, may be an important etiologic factor.

Clinically, dogs with prostatic cancer often present with difficulty in defecation similar to that seen in benign prostatic hyperplasia. They also may have stranguria, hematuria, and signs of posterior limb weakness or lameness. Rectal palpation of dogs with prostatic adenocarcinoma often reveals an irregularly enlarged, firm, immovable prostate in the pelvic cavity and possibly enlarged, firm, iliac lymph nodes. Radiographically, metastases may be evident in the pelvis and lumbar vertebrae. At autopsy, nodules of tumor often distort the capsule of the gland and may extend into the pelvic fat. The cut surface of the tumor is firm and composed of multiple nodules of yellow-tan tissue with intervening bands of dense gray tissue. Metastasis may occur in the urinary bladder, iliac lymph nodes, pelvic girdle, lumbar vertebrae, and lungs. Histologically (Fig. 25-47), canine prostatic adenocarcinomas proliferate in a variety of patterns, the most frequent of which are the intraalveolar and small acinar types. In the **intraalveolar type,** multiple foci of irregularly-shaped alveoli contain fronds of neoplastic epithelial cells radiating from a dense basal layer towards the center of the alveoli. Neoplastic cells lack polarity and are not located on an obvious basement membrane. Small nests of tumor cells are often present in the stroma adjacent to the larger alveoli. The **small acinar type** is the second most common form of canine prostatic adenocarcinoma. Tumor cells are pleomorphic and arranged in small acini em-

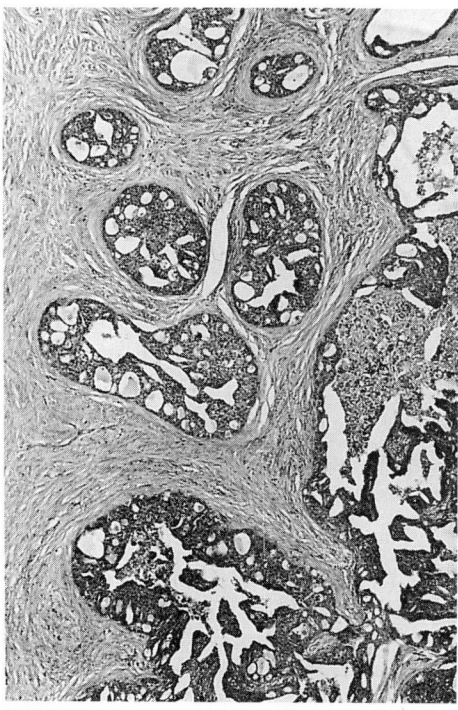

FIG. 25-47 Prostatic adenocarcinoma in a dog. Note alveolar, cribriform, and papillary patterns of growth of neoplastic cells within the prostate (×125).

bedded in a desmoplastic type of fibrous connective tissue. Except for cellular pleomorphism, the pattern somewhat resembles that of an atrophic prostate. Other less common forms of canine prostatic adenocarcinoma include syncytial and discrete epithelial types, which are varieties of less differentiated, prostatic carcinomas.

References

Barsanti JA, Finco DR. Canine bacterial prostatitis. Vet Clin North Am 1979;9:679–700.

Berry SJ, Strandberg JD, Saunders WJ, et al. The development of canine benign prostatic hyperplasia with age. Prostate 1986;9:363–373.

Brendler CB, et al. Spontaneous benign prostatic hyperplasia in the beagle. Age-associated changes in serum hormone levels, and the morphology and secretory function of the canine prostate. J Clin Invest 1983;71:1114–1123.

Clarke L, English PB. Carcinoma of the prostate gland in a dog. Aust Vet J 1966;42:214–218.

DeKlerk DP, et al. Comparison of spontaneous and experimentally induced canine prostatic hyperplasia. J Clin Invest 1979;64:842–849.

Durham SK, Dietz AE. Prostatic adenocarcinoma with and without metastasis to bone in dogs. J Am Vet Med Assoc 1986;188:1432–1436.

Evans JE Jr, Zontine W, Grain E Jr. Prostatic adenocarcinoma in a castrated dog. J Am Vet Med Assoc 1985;186:78–80.

Gloyna RE, Siiteri PK, Wilson JD. Dihydrotestosterone in prostatic hypertrophy. II. The formation and content of dihydrotestosterone in the hypertrophic canine prostate and the effect of dihydrotestosterone on prostatic growth in the dog. J Clin Invest 1970;49:1746–1753.

Hall WC, Neilsen SW, McEntee K. Tumors of the prostate and penis. Bull WHO 1976;53:247–256.

Hieble JP, Caine M. Etiology of benign prostatic hyperplasia and approaches to its pharmacological management. Fed Proc 1986;45:2601–2603.

Hornbuckle WE, MacCoy DM, Allan GS, et al. Prostatic disease in the dog. Cornell Vet 1978;68(Suppl 7):284–305.

Isaacs JT. Common characteristics of human and canine prostatic hyperplasia. Prog Clin Biol Res 1984;145:217–234.

Isaacs JT, Coffey DS. Changes in dihydrotestosterone metabolism associated with the development of canine prostatic hyperplasia. Endocrinology 1981;108:445–453.

Leav I, Cavazos LF. Some morphologic features of normal and pathologic canine prostate. In: Goland M, ed. Normal and abnormal growth of the prostate. Springfield: CC Thomas, 1973.

Leav I, Ling V. Adenocarcinoma of the canine prostate. Cancer 1968;22:1329–1345.

Lumb WV. Prostatic calculi in a dog. J Am Vet Med Assoc 1952;121:14–16.

McEntee M, Isaacs W, Smith C. Adenocarcinoma of the canine prostate: immunohistochemical examination for secretory antigens. Prostate 1987;11:163–170.

Merk FB, et al. Multiple phenotypes of prostatic glandular cells in castrated dogs after individual and combined treatment with androgen and estrogen. Lab Invest 1986;54:442–456.

O'Shea JD. Studies on the canine prostate gland. II. Prostatic neoplasms. J Comp Pathol 1963;73:244–252.

Shain SA, Boesal RB. Androgen receptor content of the normal and hyperplastic canine prostate. J Clin Invest 197861:654–660.

Strandberg JD, Berry SJ. The pathology of prostatic hyperplasia in the dog. In: Rodgers CH, et al., eds. Benign prostatic hyperplasia. Vol 2. Bethesda: National Institutes of Health, 1985;100–117.

Taylor PA. Prostatic adenocarcinoma in a dog and a summary of ten cases. Can Vet J 1973;14:162–166.

Trachtenberg J, Hicks LL, Walsh PC. Androgen and estrogen receptor content in spontaneous and experimentally induced canine prostatic hyperplasia. J Clin Invest 1980;65:1051–1059.

Weaver AD. Fifteen cases of prostatic carcinoma in the dog. Vet Rec 1981;109:71–75.

Seminal vesicles

VESICULITIS

Vesiculitis (seminal vesiculitis) occurs most often in young, sexually mature bulls and rams; it is rare in other domestic animal species. It can be a cause of infertility and poor semen quality in breeding animals. Infection may be acute or chronic depending on the nature of the offending organism and the duration of the disease. The most frequently identified etiologic agent of vesiculitis in bulls is *Actinomyces (Corynebacterium) pyogenes*. Other agents incriminated as causing vesiculitis in bulls either naturally or experimentally include: *E. coli, Actinobacillus actinoides, Corynebacterium renale, Pseudomonas aeruginosa,* staphylococci and streptococci, *Brucella abortus, Mycobacterium bovis, M. paratuberculosis, Candida guilliermondii, Chlamydia* spp., *Mycoplasma bovigenitalium,* and *Ureaplasma* spp. In rams and boars, *Brucella ovis* and *B. suis,* respectively, have been identified as the principal causes of vesiculitis.

Grossly, affected glands are usually enlarged, firmer than normal, and may be adherent to surrounding organs, including rectum and pelvic adipose tissue. Microscopically, the alveoli and stroma of infected glands contain variable amounts of purulent, granulomatous, or nonsuppurative inflammation that, in some cases, extends to the surface of the organ to involve peripelvic tissues. With longstanding inflammation, coarse bands of dense, collagenous connective tissue replace the secretory parenchyma.

References

Ball L, Griner LA, Carroll EJ. The bovine seminal vesiculitis syndrome. Am J Vet Res 1964;25:291–302.

Ball L, Young S, Carroll EJ. Seminal vesiculitis syndrome: lesions in the genital organs of young bulls. Am J Vet Res 1968;29:1173–1184.

Blanchard TL, et al. Bilateral seminal vesiculitis and ampullitis in a stallion. J Am Vet Med Assoc 1988;192:525–526.

Blom E. Studies on seminal vesiculitis in the bull. I. Semen examination methods and post mortem findings. Nord Vet Med 1979;31:193–205.

Blom E, Christensen NO. Seminal vesiculitis in the bull caused by *Corynebacterium pyogenes.* VI. Studies on pathological conditions in the testis, epididymis and accessory sex glands in the bull. Nord Vet Med 1965;17:435–445.

Blom E, Erno H. Mycoplasmosis: infections of the genital organs of bulls. Acta Vet Scand 1967;8:186–188.

Burgess GW, McDonald JW. *Escherichia coli* epididymitis and seminal vesiculitis in a ram. Aust Vet J 1981;57:479–480.

Eugster AK, Ball L, Carroll EJ, et al. Experimental genital infection of bulls and rams with chlamydial (psittacosis) agents. Philadelphia: Proc 6th Int Mtng Dis Cattle (1970). 1971;327–332.

Hancock JL, Kelly R. *Corynebacterium pyogenes* in bull semen. Vet Rec 1948;60:669–670.

Jones TH, Barrett KJ, Greenham LW, et al. Seminal vesiculitis in bulls associated with infection by *Actinobacillus actinoides.* Vet Rec 1964;76:24–28.

LaFaunce NA, McEntee K. Experimental *Mycoplasma bovis* seminal vesiculitis in the bull. Cornell Vet 1982;72:150–167.

Larsen AB, Kopecky KE. *Mycobacterium paratuberculosis* in reproductive organs and semen of bulls. Am J Vet Res 1970;31:244–258.

Larsen AB, et al. *Mycobacterium paratuberculosis* in the semen and genital organs of a semen-donor bull. J Am Vet Med Assoc 1981;179:169–171.

Laws L, Simmons GC, Ludford CG. Experimental *Brucella ovis* infection in rams. Aust Vet J 1972;48:313–317.

Parsonson IM, Al-Aubaidi JM, McEntee K. *Mycoplasma bovigenitalium*: experimental induction of genital disease in bulls. Cornell Vet 1974;64:240–264.

Storz J, Carroll EJ, Ball L, et al. Isolation of a psittacosis agent *(Chlamydia)* from semen and epididymis of bulls with seminal vesiculitis syndrome. Am J Vet Res 1968;29:549–555.

Bulbourethral glands (Cowper's glands)

BULBOURETHRAL ADENITIS

This is a relatively uncommon condition in most domestic animal species. In bulls, it may occur as an extension of vesiculitis and be caused by the same infectious organism.

Penis and prepuce

DEVELOPMENTAL ABNORMALITIES

Developmental abnormalities of the penis and prepuce are rare, except in various forms of intersex where aplasia and hypoplasia of the penis and prepuce may occur.

Diphallus (double penis) occurs rarely as a congenital anomaly of bulls. **Congenital hypoplasia of the preputial orifice** may prevent protrusion of the penis (phimosis) from or retraction of the penis **(paraphimosis)** into the preputial sheath. These conditions also may result from trauma and scarring **(stenosis)** of the preputial orifice. **Hypospadias** (urethral orifice on the ventral aspect of the penis) and **epispadias** (urethral orifice on the dorsal aspect of the penis) are rare developmental anomalies, but have been described in bulls, rams, goats, boars, and dogs. **Persistence of the penile frenulum,** a band of connective tissue that connects the ventral aspect of the penis to the prepuce, has been described in bulls, boars, and dogs. This anomaly may interfere with copulation. **Traumatic lesions** of the penis include contusions, lacerations, hematoma, infarction of the corpus cavernosum, and fracture of the os penis. These may occur during copulation or be inflicted by a nonreceptive mate.

INFECTIOUS DISEASES

Infectious **phalloposthitis** (inflammation of the entire penis and prepuce), sometimes incorrectly referred to by the more restrictive term, **balanoposthitis** (inflammation of the glans penis alone and prepuce) can be caused by a variety of bacterial, viral, and protozoan organisms.

In **bulls,** the penile mucosa undergoes age-associated changes that transform it from a smooth surface in young sexuallly mature bulls to a surface with longitudinal crypts in older bulls. This is an androgen-dependent change that first becomes noticeable at about three years of age and becomes more prominent in five-to–six-year-old bulls. In older bulls, these crypts may become persistently colonized by *Campylobacter fetus* ssp. *venearealis* or *Tritrichomonas foetus* and serve as a source of infection for transmission of these agents to heifers. Young bulls, conversely, may be only transiently infected with these organisms, because they will not persist in the absence of such crypts. In either case, infected bulls rarely exhibit overt clinical signs of infection, even though smears from the crypts may contain mild-to-moderate numbers of inflammatory cells, as well as the organisms. Other bacterial organisms associated with inflammatory lesions of the penis and prepuce in bulls include: *Actinomyces pyogenes,* a common cause of penile and preputial abscesses secondary to trauma; and *Corynebacterium renale,* a bacterium capable of causing a chemically-induced phalloposthitis through the production of ammonia from urea in urine.

The principal viral agent causing phalloposthitis in bulls is ***Herpesvirus bovis-1,*** the venereally-transmitted agent that causes pustular vulvovaginitis in cows. Grossly, early lesions consist of either small vesicles or pustules or, more often, raised yellow-white necrotic plaques that eventually coalesce, slough, and leave areas of erosion and ulceration. In most cases, lesions heal in 10–14 days. Microscopically, lesions consist of focal areas of hydropic degeneration and necrosis and ulceration of the epithelium with the presence of eosinophilic, intranuclear inclusion bodies in the cells in epithelial cells adjacent to necrotic areas.

In **sheep** and **goats,** castration commonly predisposes them to **ulcerative posthitis** (also known as "sheath rot" and "pizzle rot"); however, rams are also occasionally affected. Castration appears to result in an incomplete unfolding of the penis, thus resulting in urination within the sheath. Urea-hydrolyzing bacteria, such as *Corynebacterium renale, Rhodococcus equi,* and *R. hofmanni,* acting on urea-rich urine cause the initial lesion. These organisms are believed to be contracted from contaminated bedding, roughage, and/or insect vectors, as well as venereally. Grossly, the initial lesion appears as an area of necrosis involving the epidermis at the orifice of the prepuce. When this lesion progresses, the preputial orifice becomes constricted and urine accumulates within the sheath, leading to extensive necrosis of the mucosa of the sheath and glans penis.

In **stallions,** chemical disinfection of the penis and prepuce prior to breeding has been shown to predispose them to penile and preputial infections by *Pseudomonas aeruginosa, Klebsiella* spp., and coliform organisms due to loss of normal bacteriocidal flora of the mucosa.

Two viral agents are known to cause lesions of the penis and prepuce of stallions. ***Herpesvirus equi-3,*** the cause of **equine coital exanthema,** produces lesions on the penis and prepuce of stallions that are similar grossly and microscopically to those caused by *Herpesvirus bovis-1* in bulls. As the name implies, it is a venereally-transmitted disease. Stallions and mares that recover from this disease may be left with areas of depigmentation of the affected portions of the external genitalia.

Molluscum contagiosum, a poxvirus-induced disease in humans, has been described on the cutaneous surface of the prepuce of a yearling colt. Grossly, lesions were 2–3 mm in diameter, dome-shaped, and most had smooth, nonpigmented surfaces; a few lesions had roughened surfaces. Microscopically, lesions consisted of well-circumscribed lobulated masses of epidermal proliferation that extended into and compressed the underlying dermal connective tissue, as well as above the surface of the adjacent nonaffected epidermis. As they matured from the stratum geminativum to the surface, epithelial cells became increasingly swollen due to the accumulation of eosinophilic, granular viral inclusion bodies in the cytoplasm that displaced nuclei to the periphery of the cell. These changes are typical of molluscum bodies desribed in human disease. Electron microscopy showed the inclusion bodies to be composed of characteristic poxvirus virions.

In **dogs,** catarrhal phalloposthitis is a common clinical disorder that can be caused by a number of bacterial agents, either alone or in combination. These agents include: *E. coli, Proteus vulgaris,* staphylolocci, and streptococci. Infection may be associated with mild-to-moderate hyperplasia of lymphoid follicles in the penile and preputial mucosa, which imparts a granular appearance to the mucosa. Rarely, in longstanding cases, adhesions develop between the penis and prepuce.

PARASITIC BALANOPOSTHITIS

In **horses,** the common housefly and stable fly, intermediate hosts for the stomach worms in horses, *Draschia megastoma, Habronema muscae,* and *H. microstoma* may deposit larvae on the penis or prepuce where they burrow into the dermis or submucosa causing characteristic granulomas. These granulomas may contain remains of larvae, but characteristically consist of areas of degenerate collagen and cellular debris surrounded by numerous eosinophils. Lesions are commonly referred to as "summer sores."

References

Bartlett DE, Hasson EV, Teeter KG. Occurrence of *Trichomonas foetus* in preputial samples from infected bulls. Relation to, and application in, diagnosis. J Am Vet Med Assoc 1947;110:114–120.

Bier PJ, Hall CE, Duncan R, et al. Experimental infections with *Campylobacter fetus* in bulls of different ages. Vet Microbiol 1977;2:13–27.

Bowen JM, Tobin RB, Simpson B, et al. Effects of washing on the bacterial flora of the stallion's penis. J Reprod Fertil Suppl 1982;32:41–45.

Bull LB. A granulomatous affection of the horse—Habronemic granulomata (cutaneous habronemiasis of Railliet). J Comp Pathol 1916;29:187–199.

Clark BL, White MB, Banfield JC. Diagnosis of *Trichomonas foetus* infection in bulls. Aust Vet J 1971;47:181–183.

Filmer JF. Ovine posthitis and balano-posthitis ("pizzle rot"): some notes on field investigations. Aust Vet J 1938;14:47–52.

Hammond DM, Bartlett DE. The distribution of *Trichomonas foetus* in the preputial cavity of infected bulls. Am J Vet Res 1943;4:143–149.

Huck RA, Millar PG, Evans DH, et al. Penoposthitis associated with infectious bovine rhinotracheitis/infectious pustular vulvovaginitis (I.B.R./I.P.V.) virus in a stud of bulls. Vet Rec 1971;88:292–297.

Humphrey JD, Little PB, Stephens LR, et al. Prevalence and distribution of *Haemophilus somnus* in the male bovine reproductive tract. Am J Vet Res 1982;43:791–795.

Lein D, Erickson I, Winter AJ, et al. Diagnosis, treatment, and control of vibriosis in an artificial insemination center. J Am Vet Med Assoc 1968;153:1574–1580.

Parsonson IM, Clark BL, Dufty J. The pathogenesis of *Tritrichomonas foetus* infection in the bull. Aust Vet J 1974;50:421–423.

Pascoe RR, Bagust TJ, Spradbrow PB. Studies on equine herpesviruses. 4. Infection of horses with a herpesvirus recovered from equine coital exanthema. Aust Vet J 1972;48:99–104.

Rahaley RS, Mueller RE. Molluscum contagiosum in a horse. Vet Pathol 1983;20:247–250.

Roberts SJ. Double penis in a Holstein bull. Cornell Vet 1943;33:388–393.

Southcott WH. Etiology of ovine posthitis: description of a causal organism. Aust Vet J 1965;41:193–200.

Studdert M, Barker CA, Savan M. Infectious pustular vulvovaginitis virus infection of bulls. Am J Vet Res 1964;25:303–314.

Watson RH, Murname D. Non-contagious ovine posthitis ("sheath rot"). Some aspects of its course and etiology. Aust Vet J 1958;34:125–136.

Neoplasms

Neoplasms of the penis and prepuce are rare in most domestic animals. They are observed most often in bulls, stallions, and dogs; the primary neoplasm is different in each species.

In **bulls,** the most common penile or preputial neoplasm is *fibropapilloma.* It occurs most often in young, sexually mature bulls less than three years of age. The causative agent is **bovine papilloma virus type 2,** one of six recognized papillomaviruses of cattle. These tumors may be single or multiple, up to several centimeters in diameter, and may interfere with protrusion of the penis from the prepuce. They are frequently traumatized and bleed during attempts at mating. Surface of the neoplasms is either papillary or nodular and when sectioned is firm, and white-to-pink in color. Microscopically, tumors are composed of a central core of fibroblasts and fibrocytes arranged in prominent interlacing bundles and admixed with varying amounts of collagen. Surface of bovine fibropapillomas is covered by a hyperplastic and often vacuolated, stratified squamous epithelium that may be ulcerated. Reportedly, those occurring in younger bulls are more cellular and have a higher mitotic index than those found in older bulls which has led to misdiagnosis as fibrosarcoma in some cases.

In **stallions, squamous cell papilloma** and **squamous cell carcinoma** are the principal neoplasms of the penis and prepuce (Fig. 25-48). **Squamous cell papillomas** are often multiple and protrude from the mucosal surfaces as variably-sized, cauliflowerlike projections. Histologically, they consist of a central core of fibrovascular connective tissue that has multiple branches covered by a well-differentiated layer of stratified squamous epithelium with normal cellular polarity. Varying degrees of erosion and acute inflammation may be present on surfaces; later, focal infiltrates of lymphocytes are manifest in the stroma of the neoplasm. Although it is a well-documented cause of cutaneous papillomas in horses, no reports exist of equine papillomavirus being incriminated as the cause of genital papillomas in horses. **Squamous cell carcinomas** arise most often from the glans penis of both stallions and geldings. The surface of these tumors is often ulcerated and necrotic. Microscopically, neoplastic cells proliferate in solid sheets, elongate cords, and nests that extend into the penile connective tissue and corpus cavernosum. They frequently exhibit keratinization and keratin pearl forma-

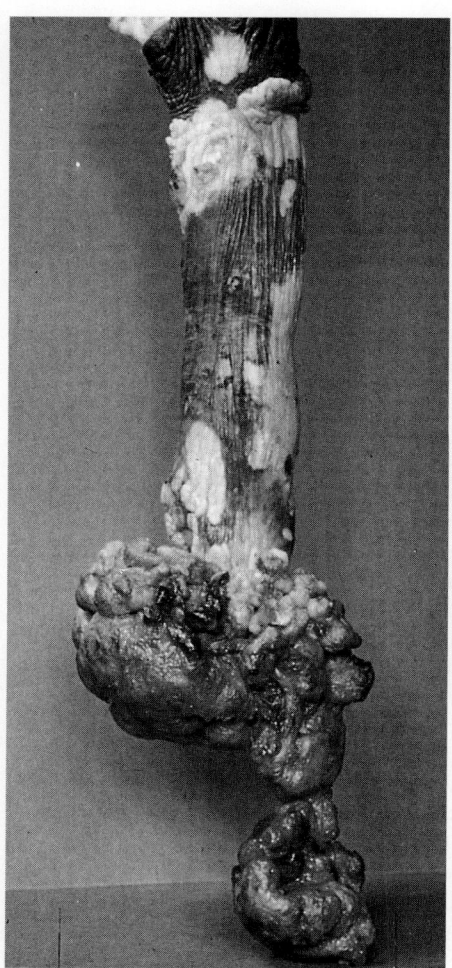

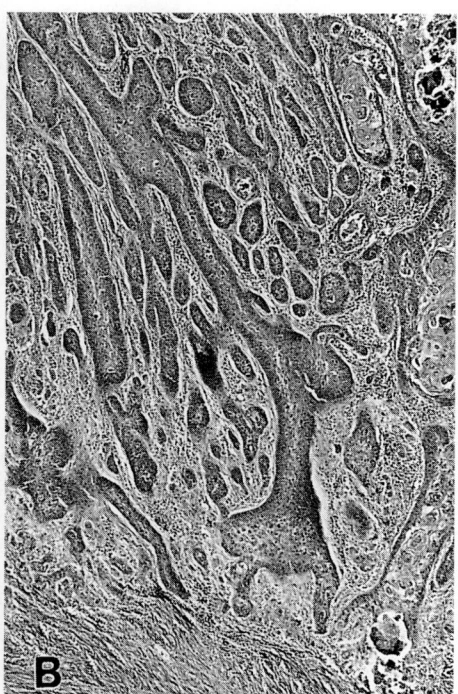

FIG. 25-48 **A.** Squamous cell carcinoma of the penis of a 25-year-old horse. The lower mass was a transplant of tumor to the prepuce. **B.** Long cords and isolated nests of neoplastic squamous cells invading connective tissue of the glans penis (×100).

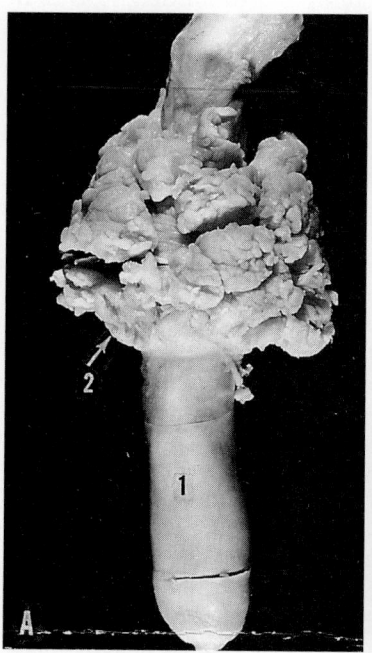

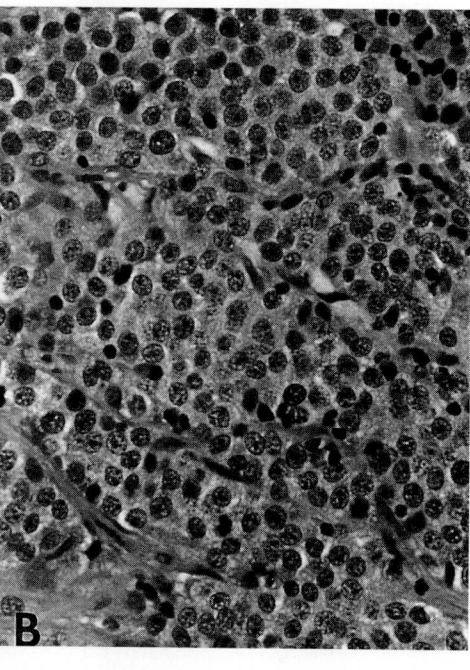

FIG. 25-49 **A.** Canine transmissible venereal tumor. (2) Lesion in the (1) penis of dog. (Courtesy of Armed Forces Institute of Pathology.) **B.** Microscopic appearance of a venereal tumor metastatic to an inguinal lymph node.

tion. Metastasis to inguinal lymph nodes is common, but widespread dissemination is not a frequent finding.

Lesions identical to bovine fibropapillomas, but termed **equine sarcoids** also occur occasionally on the penis and prepuce of stallions. A significant percentage of sarcoids contain bovine papillomavirus genome, and identical tumors have been produced experimentally in horses inoculated with this agent.

In dogs (Fig. 25-49), **transmissible venereal tumor,** also known as **Sticker tumor,** is the most common, spontaneously occurring neoplasm of the penis and prepuce. As its name implies, neoplasm is transmitted naturally from affected to unaffected animals during mating. No infectious agent is involved; tumor cells are mechanically transplanted from neoplasm to genital mucosa or, less often, to abraded skin or other mucous membranes of unaffected dogs, usually during mating. For obvious reasons, neoplasms occur most often in dogs allowed to roam free. Gross, microscopic, and biologic features of this neoplasm have been more completely described under *Neoplasms of Vulva and Vagina.*

References

Bloom F, Paff GH, Noback CR. The transmissible venereal tumor of the dog. Studies indicating that the tumor cells are mature end cells of reticulo-endothelial origin. Am J Pathol 1951;27:119–139.

Danson L, Bierschwal CJ. Fibropapilloma of the bovine penis. Bovine Pract 1983;18:184–187.

Formston C. Fibropapillomas in cattle with special reference to the external genitalia of the bull. Br Vet J 1953;109:244–248.

Hall WC, Nielsen SW, McEntee K. Tumours of the prostate and penis. Bull WHO 1976;53:247–256.

Jarrett WFH, McNeil PE, Laird HM, et al. Papilloma viruses in benign and malignant tumors of cattle. Cold Spring Harbor Conf. Cell Proliferation 1980;7:215–222.

Makino S. Some epidemiological aspects of venereal tumors in dogs as revealed by chromosome and DNA studies. Ann NY Acad Sci 1963;108:1106–1122.

McEntee K. Fibropapillomatosis of the external genitalia of cattle. Cornell Vet 1950;40:304–312.

McLeod CG Jr, Lewis JE. Transmissible venereal tumor with metastasis in three dogs. J Am Vet Med Assoc 1972;161:199–200.

Strafuss AC. Squamous cell carcinoma in horses. J Am Vet Med Assoc 1976;168:61–62.

Yang TJ. Metastatic transmissible venereal sarcoma in a dog. J Am Vet Med Assoc 1987;190:555–556.

26
Endocrine glands

Endocrine glands are specialized organs that produce hormones necessary for homeostasis. Fifty or more hormones are elaborated by a variety of organs and tissues; this chapter, however, will be limited to considering those of the **hypothalamus, hypophysis** (pituitary), **thyroid, parathyroid, adrenal, pancreatic islets,** and **pineal glands.** Other hormone-producing organs and tissues—such as the ovary, testis, placenta, and neuroendocrine cells—are considered elsewhere.

Control mechanisms that regulate hormone synthesis and secretion are complex, but in general each endocrine gland is regulated by a feedback mechanism. In some situations, this is through the circulating level of another hormone, as in the elaboration of several hormones of the anterior pituitary. In other examples, it is the level of various circulating metabolites, such as glucose or calcium, for the release of insulin and parathormone, respectively, or blood pH and oxygen tension in the case of chemoreceptor organs. In addition to these straightforward mechanisms, a variety of other metabolites directly influence hormone release.

For the most part, diseases of the endocrine glands can be simply stated as being caused by an over- or underproduction of hormone. This leads to diverse clinical and pathologic consequences, depending on the hormone involved. Mechanisms vary leading to production imbalance. Neoplasia is the most common cause of **hyperfunction,** where the neoplastic endocrine cells develop an autonomy from usual control mechanisms. Depending on the primary neoplasm, hyperfunction of a target endocrine organ can ensue; for example, excessive secretion of adrenocorticotropic hormone (ACTH) by a neoplasm of the anterior pituitary will lead to hyperplasia and hyperfunction of the adrenal cortex with increased cortisol secretion. Hyperfunction can also follow conditions that alter feedback mechanisms, such as in vitamin D deficiency or chronic renal disease, which lead to hypocalcemia, parathyroid hyperplasia, and increased parathormone secretion. Endocrine **hypofunction** can also result from several other processes. Destruction of an endocrine organ by inflammatory or neoplastic disease interferes with hormone secretion. This can, in some circumstances, lead to hypofunction of a target endocrine organ, such as the adrenal cortex.

Agenesis of an endocrine organ is a rare cause of hypofunction. Persistent viral infections are emerging as another mechanism of altered cell function; such infection, when occuring within endocrine cells, can lead to hypofunction. This has been demonstrated by persistent lymphocytic choriomeningitis virus (LCMV) infection in mice, where the virus can preferentially replicate in somatotrophs and interfere with transcription of the growth hormone gene. This occurs in the absence of any viral lysis of somatotrophs or immune-mediated destruction of the cells. LCMV in mice has been shown to persist in thyroid follicular epithelium and pancreatic islet β cells; this leads to hypothyroidism and diabetes mellitus, again without any morphologic damage to the cells. Venezuelan equine encephalitis virus infection in hamsters has been shown to be capable of interfering with the production of insulin.

Other conditions exist, which are not primary disorders of the endocrine glands themselves, but whose end results are analogous to either primary hyper- or hypofunction. Hormone resistance due to absence of cellular receptors or intracellular metabolism leads to a deficient state; this occurs in the presence of normal or, usually, elevated levels of circulating hormone, coupled with hyperplasia of the primary endocrine organ. A state of hyperfunction can follow the elaboration of hormones by a nonendocrine organ. This is well-exemplified by the secretion of a parathormone-like substance by neoplasms of the apocrine glands of the anal sac in dogs.

PITUITARY (HYPOPHYSIS) AND HYPOTHALAMUS

Structure and development

The pituitary gland and hypothalamus are intimately related to one another. Although the pituitary has been described as the "conductor of the endocrine symphony," it is the hypothalamus that might be thought of as the "board of trustees of the endocrine symphony;" this is because the hypothalamus serves as a higher center for the regulation of pituitary functions. It is the hypothalamus which actually produces the hormones

1223

vasopressin (antidiuretic hormone) and oxytocin for release through the neurohypophysis. Production and release of anterior pituitary hormones are under control of the hypothalamus which, in response to negative feedback mechanisms, produces releasing and inhibiting factors that act on specific cells of the adenohypophysis. This control is accomplished through direct axonal and vascular connections between the two.

The pituitary is divided morphologically into two distinct components, the **anterior pituitary** or **adenohypophysis** and the **posterior pituitary** or **neurohypophysis (pars nervosa).** The adenohypophysis is derived from **Rathke's ,** which grows from the primitive foregut (stomodeum) to make contact with the infundibulum. In the early embryo, a pharyngohypophyseal stalk connects the foregut and pituitary; this attachment is ultimately lost, although remnants sometime remain into adulthood. The anterior wall of Rathke's pouch forms the **pars distalis**—the dominant component of the anterior pituitary—and its upward extension, the **pars tuberalis,** which incompletely surrounds the pituitary stalk **(infundibulum).** The posterior part of Rathke's pouch forms the **pars intermedia,** which is in direct contact with the neurohypophysis and is separated from the pars distalis by a residual lumen of Rathke's pouch. This anatomical arrangement varies among species. In humans, the pars intermedia is essentially nonexistent; in dogs, the pars distalis completely surrounds the pars nervosa. Small cysts of residual Rathke's pouch are often encountered in the pars intermedia. The neurohypophysis develops from the floor of the **diencephalon,** which grows downward to make contact with the posterior wall of Rathke's pouch.

Pituitary hormones and cells of origin

The anterior pituitary secretes six important hormones, as well as several other hormones and metabolically active substances. The six major hormones include: **follicle-stimulating hormone** (FSH), **leutinizing hormone** (LH), **thyroid-stimulating hormone** (TSH), **adrenocorticotropic hormone** (adrenocorticotropin, ACTH), **growth hormone** (GH; somatotropic hormone, STH), and **prolactin** (luteotropic hormone, LTH). The precursor molecule of ACTH—propiomelanocortin (POMC)—produces: **melanocyte-stimulating hormone** (α-, β-, and γ-MSH); **corticotropin-like intermediate peptide** (CLIP); β- and γ-lipotropin (LPH); and α-, β-, and γ-endorphin. Although functionally distinct, these latter compounds and ACTH have functional overlap. In general, a corresponding anterior pituitary cell exists for each hormone. Based on hematoxylin-and-eosin-stained tissue sections, three populations of cells were traditionally recognized: acidophils, basophils, and chromophobes. This, coupled with the PAS and other stains, made possible the rough correlation of cell type with hormone production; however, current immunohistochemical staining procedures enable specific correlatation of cell type with its hormone(s), making the older acidophil-basophil-chromophobe classification obsolete. Five cell types identifiable in the pars distalis are

responsible for secretion of the six major hormones of the anterior pituitary (gonadotrophs secrete both FSH and LH). A sixth cell type, melanotroph—a variant of corticotroph whose products of POMC favor MSH over ACTH—is found in the pars intermedia. In most species, this is the only or predominant cell type of the pars intermedia. In dogs, however, the pars intermedia contains both melanotrophs and corticotrophs typical of those in the pars distalis. The characteristics of these cells are summarized in Table 26-1. Chromophobes are considered inactive basophils or acidophils; however, it should be emphasized that chromophobic neoplasms may be hormonally active. The cell type termed **stellate** or **follicular** sends processes among the above cell types; or, it may line small follicular structures often encountered in the anterior pituitary. This cell is not known to be hormonally active.

Cells of the posterior pituitary are glial cells, termed pituicytes. Their precise function is not clear. They do not synthesize or secrete hormones, but may assist in the transfer of oxytocin and vasopressin (secreted in the hypothalamus) from the neurosecretory axons. Vasopressin release is controlled by osmoreceptors in the hypothalamus as well as by plasma volume, blood pressure, angiotensin II, norepinephrine, and other metabolites. Nipple stimulation serves to release oxytocin.

Hypothalamo-hypophyseal connections: control and release of pituitary hormones

The pituitary and hypothalamus are connected by axons and a vascular portal system that transports hormones, as well as the releasing and inhibiting factors produced within neurons of the hypothalamus. Separate systems exist for the anterior and posterior pituitary. The hormones oxytocin and vasopressin (which differ by only two amino acids) are produced by magnocellular (large) neurons located in the supraoptic and paraventricular nuclei. These hormones and their carrier proteins (neurophysins) are transported—via unmyelinated axons through the supraopticohypophyseal and paraventriculohypophyseal tracts to the posterior pituitary. En route, the hormones are processed to their final form, and are released from nerve terminals in the posterior pituitary. The actual hormones can sometimes be seen in routine tissue sections as eosinophilic globules, termed **Herring bodies.** Vasopressin—whose production and secretion is controlled by the osmolality of blood and other mechanisms—serves to concentrate urine; disorders that interfere with the formation of vasopressin lead to **diabetes insipidus.** Oxytocin is released following nipple stimulation; it serves in milk flow through stimulation of myoepithelial cells in the mammary glands, and in parturition through stimulation of uterine contractions (oxytocic effect).

The adenohypophysis is in communication with the hypothalamus through two components: the tuberoinfundibular tract and the hypophyseal portal system. The releasing and inhibiting factors are produced in

TABLE 26-1 **Endocrine cells and hormones of anterior pituitary**

Cell type	Hormone	Cell characteristics	Primary hypothalamic hormones	Hormone action
Somatotroph* (type 2 acidophil)	Somatotropic or growth hormone	H&E: acidophilic granules PAS: negative Orange G: positive EM: abundant, dense granules 350 nm	Growth hormone releasing hormone Growth hormone inhibiting hormone (somatostatin) ***	Essential for postnatal growth (mediated through somatomedins produced in liver, chondrocytes, kidney, muscle, GI tract etc.)
Lactotrophs* (type 1 acidophil)	Prolactin or lactogenic H.	H&E: acidophilic granules or chromophobic PAS: negative Azocarmine: positive Erythrosine: positive EM: Sparse, dense granules 600–900 nm	Prolactin releasing hormone Prolactin release inhibiting factor (dopamine)	Essential for lactation
Gonadotrophs** (delta or type 2 basophil)	(1) FSH (2) LH	H&E: basophilic PAS: positive Aldehyde fuchsin: negative EM: dense granules 200–250 nm	Luteinizing hormone releasing factor	(1) Stimulates granulosa cells (2) Stimulates Theca cells and Leydig cells
Thyrotrophs (beta-basophil or type 1 basophil)	TSH	H&E: basophilic PAS: positive Aldehyde fuchsin: positive EM: dense granules 150 nm	Thyrotropin releasing hormone (TRH) ****	Stimulates thyroid gland
Corticotrophs (type 3 basophil)	(1) ACTH***** (corticotropin) (2) Gamma lipotropin (3) Beta-endorphin	H&E: basophilic PAS: weakly positive Aldehyde fuchsin: positive EM: variably dense granules 200–400 nm Cytoplasmic filaments	Corticotropin releasing hormone, vasopressin (releasing effect)	(1) Stimulates cortisol release by adrenal cortex (2) Lipolysis and MSH action (3) Opiatelike effects
Melanotrophs	(1) Alpha Melanocyte Stim. H. (MSH) (2) CLIP (3) Beta-endorphin	H&E: basophilic PAS: positive	Melanotroph inhibiting factor	(1) Stimulates melanocyte proliferation, pigmentation, cortisol release and neural growth and regeneration (2) Corticotropin-like (3) Opiatelike effects

*Some cells express both growth hormone and prolactin
**FSH and LH secreting cells cannot be differentiated; both hormones may be secreted by same cell
***Also inhibits TRH and TSH release
****Also stimulates release of prolactin
*****Has some aldosterone stimulating effect

several hypothalamic nuclei by parvicellular (small) neurons, which are located in the tuberal region and in the wall of the third ventricle. These factors are transported by way of axons to the infundibulum. Here, they leave the axons and enter the primary capillary bed of the portal system; they are then transported to the adenohypophysis to act on specific hormone-secreting cells. The portal system arises from the anterior and posterior hypophyseal arteries, some of whose branches—in the infundibulum and pituitary stalk—give rise to specialized vessels, termed **gomotoli.** These are composed of an array of capillaries arising from central arterioles with thick smooth-muscle sphincters. The capillaries join to form portal veins, which join the pituitary stalk to enter the adenohypophysis; there, they branch into capillaries and sinusoids. Although some circulation is supplied directly from the hypophyseal arteries, it is the portal system which provides the bulk of the blood supply to the adenohypophysis.

It is believed that releasing and inhibiting hormones exist for each hormone produced by the anterior pituitary, with the exception of prolactin. The hormones that have been found thus far are peptides and include: **growth hormone-releasing hormone** (GHRH), **gonadotropin-** (luteinizing hormone) **releasing hormone** (GnRH, releases both luteinizing hormone and follicle-stimulating hormone), **thyrotropin-releasing hormone** (TRH), and **corticotropin-releasing hormone** (CRH). Although TRH has a prolactin-releasing effect, a specific prolactin-releasing hormone apparently does not exist. The hypothalamus only exerts an inhibitory control on this hormone; section of the pituitary stalk actually leads to an increased secretion of prolactin, whereas it causes a decreased release of the other anterior pituitary hormones. The inhibiting substances known at present include somatotropin release-inhibiting factor (somatostatin), melanotropin-inhibiting factor and prolactin-inhibiting factor (which may be dopamine or stimulated by dopamine).

Lesions of the anterior pituitary

HYPERPITUITARISM

Excessive secretion of one or more anterior pituitary hormones is almost always the result of a neoplasm that is resistant to the normal suppressive effects of the feedback mechanisms. The types of neoplasms encountered in animals and their morphology is taken up later in this section.

Hypertrophy and hyperplasia of specific anterior-pituitary cell types will follow pathologic and physiologic alterations in target organs. For example, lesions which result in destruction of the thyroid will disrupt the usual feedback mechanisms; this process leads to hypertrophy and hyperplasia of thyrotrophs. Estrogen leads to hyperplasia of lactotrophs during pregnancy. Idiopathic multinodular hyperplasia of specific anterior-pituitary cell types occasionally occurs, and these nodules may be functional. In dogs, the use of progesterone or progestational compounds leads to an increased number and activity of somatotrophs, with excessive elaboration of growth hormone. Acromegaly and diabetes mellitus may result.

Hypopituitarism

This condition may result from any lesion in the pituitary that reduces its production of hormones. One of the frequent causes of pituitary atrophy is the replacement of the gland by any type of cyst or tumor (Fig. 26-1) arising in the pituitary: remnants of Rathke's cleft, craniopharyngeal duct, or pharyngeal hypophysis.

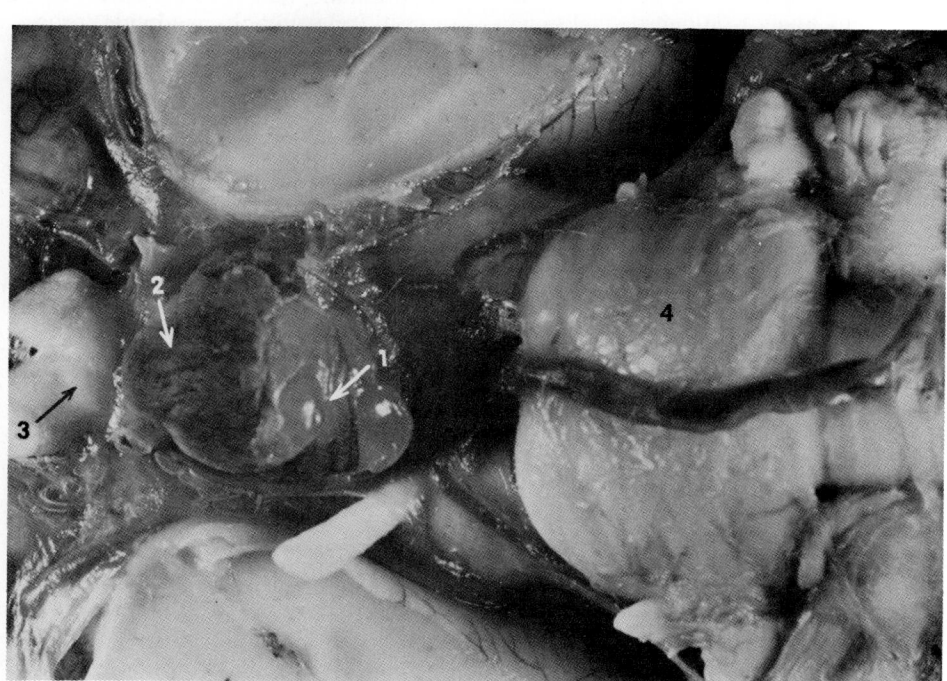

FIG. 26-1 Cyst of the intermediate lobe of the pituitary of a spayed 12-year-old female mongrel terrier. An incidental finding. (1) The cyst; (2) Anterior lobe of pituitary; (3) Optic chiasma; and (4) pons. (Courtesy of Angell Memorial Animal Hospital.)

When the space-occupying lesion replaces the pituitary only, the signs are usually limited to those resulting from pituitary deficiency. When the neoplastic mass replaces the supraoptic nuclei in the thalamus, diabetes insipidus results. Should the optic nerve, optic chiasma, or optic tract be compressed, deficiencies in vision result. Replacement of thalamic nuclei causes signs of behavioral alterations. Secondary tumors in the pituitary have similar effects.

In addition to tumors, cysts or other anomalies may result in loss of pituitary function. Cysts developing from Rathke's cleft are found in cases of pituitary dwarfism: for example, in German shepherds. Other cysts, lined by ciliated columnar epithelium, may originate in the pharyngeal hypophysis—or in the craniopharyngeal duct—and become large enough to cause hypopituitarism.

Aplasia or hypoplasia of the pituitary may occur in association with gross malformations of the head, such as cyclopia and congenital anencephaly (due to poisoning by vitamin A or *Veratrum californicum*). Functional hypoplasia occurs in some gene-controlled situations; examples include underlying aplasia in one type of prolonged gestation in Jersey and Guernsey cattle, and ateliotic dwarfism in mice.

Inflammation and infectious diseases may result in pituitary malfunction; however, the inflammation is usually part of a systemic disease, not limited to the hypophysis. Suppurative and lymphocytic meningitis may rarely involve the pituitary. This may be due to one of several viral, bacterial, helminthic, or mycotic organisms. Hemorrhage and necrosis of the pituitary have been seen in dogs with infectious canine hepatitis (adenovirus), and in swine with hog cholera. *Herpesvirus tamarinus* has produced destructive lesions in the pituitary of marmosets *(Saguinus oedipus)*. It also has been shown that certain viruses can persist in endocrine cells, and can interfere with hormone synthesis without leading to morphologic changes. Lymphocytic choriomeningitis virus infection in mice can persist in somatotrophs and prevent transcription of the growth hormone gene. Septic emboli occasionally lodge in the pituitary (especially in ruminants) and may lead to infarction and necrosis. Urate tophi may be seen in the pituitary of birds and snakes on rare occasions as a part of visceral and articular gout.

PITUITARY DWARFISM

Pituitary dwarfism in dogs has been described in German shepherds, Carelian bear dogs and occasionally other breeds; it is believed to be the result of the same autosomal-recessive gene. Affected dogs have a rudimentary pituitary; the sella turcica is filled with a large multiloculated cystic Rathke's pouch, which is lined by goblet cells and pseudostratified, often-ciliated columnar epithelium. Failure of the oropharyngeal ectoderm to differentiate into the anterior pituitary is believed to initiate pathogenesis. The level of serum somatomedin is decreased in homozygous dwarf dogs, intermediate in heterozygotes, and highest in normal unrelated dogs. Somatomedins are growth-promoting proteins produced in the liver, and are stimulated by growth hormone (somatotropic hormone: STH). A deficiency of somatomedin is considered a reflection of a decreased level of somatotropic hormone (Willeberg et al., 1975).

Affected puppies (gene symbol (**dd**)) are normal at birth, but grow at a rate much lower than that of their normal litter mates. By six months of age, normal dogs weigh six or more times as much as their affected littermates. The homozygous (**dd**) puppy keeps its puppy hair coat for months and fails to develop sexually. It seems likely that the panhypopituitarism in dwarf German shepherds described by Alexander (1962) is the same condition reported by Willeberg et al. (1975) and Jensen (1959), although direct comparisons apparently have not been made.

Pituitary dwarfism has been observed in mutant strains of laboratory mice. Characteristics of the affected mice appear to be similar, but were described at different times and were studied with differing techniques. The Snell dwarf, first described in 1929, is the result of a single recessive gene (**dw**) in the homozygous state. Deficiency of anterior pituitary hormones results in a mouse about one fourth the size of normal littermates. Both males and females are sterile. Secondary myxedema due to thyroid deficiency has also been recognized. Growth at an approximately normal rate may be restored by repeated administration of a fraction of anterior pituitary.

A second pituitary dwarf mutant mouse was originally described by Schaible and Gowen (1961) and named the *Ames dwarf*. The mutant gene (**df**) is located in linkage group VII. The phenotypic characteristics are similar to Snell dwarf. Retardation of growth is recognizable one week after birth; affected mice are significantly reduced in size at adulthood. Early treatment with bovine growth hormone results in approximately normal growth, and at least the males become fertile. The anterior hypophysis (Bartke, 1964) in *df/df* mice lack acidophils, and few thyrotrophs are evident.

A third mutation in mice has been described and named *little* (**lit**) by Eicher and Beamer (1976). This mutant recessive gene is located on chromosome 6 (linkage group XI). The homozygous mouse *(lit/lit)* is recognized by its decreased size at about 15 days of age, and is similar to the Ames *(df/df)* and Snell dwarfs *(dw/dw)* in that the size is reduced (ateliotic) without evidence of gross malformation of bones or other structures, and with body proportions smaller in all systems. Females are fertile and males sire one or two litters, but rarely a third. The anterior pituitary is reduced in size in both sexes; analyses with acrylamide gels reveal significant reduction in growth hormone (STH) and prolactin (LTH). This pituitary dwarfism of mice is believed to be similar to human isolated growth-hormone deficiency, type I.

GENITAL HYPOPLASIA

Associated with a form of hypopituitarism, genital hypoplasia has been described in one of the several mutations that occur at the pink-eyed locus in mice (Johnson and Hunt, 1975). These mice—named "sterile pink-eyed mice"—are homozygous for the p^{25H} gene ($p^{25H}/$ p^{25H}). Males are sterile, small, irritable, and produce abnormal sperm. Females have low fertility; their ovaries are small with few corpora lutea; abnormal follicles contain degenerated ova. The uterus is severely hypoplastic and does not respond to estradiol. Surprisingly, no changes have been detected in the anterior pituitary, but degenerated axons have been reported in the posterior pituitary. The hypothalamus has reduced binding capacity for estradiol-17β, and iodine binding in the thyroid is also decreased.

PROLONGED GESTATION

Prolonged gestation is now recognized as a dysfunction of the fetal pituitary. Abnormally long pregnancies were first recorded in cattle over 75 years ago, but only recently have syndromes in cattle and sheep been characterized and linked to abnormalities of the fetal pituitary. In cattle, two distinct forms of prolonged gestation occur. Both are controlled by a single autosomal-recessive gene. In Holstein-Friesian and Ayrshire cattle, the disease is characterized by a gestation period of up to 380 days; the calf is abnormally large, but lacks obvious deformities. The pituitary is present, but with marked degranulation of the acidophils. Adrenal cortices are hypoplastic, but other endocrine glands are normal. The calf dies in utero and is born dead (if physically possible); or, when delivered by cesarean section, it may be viable but weak; it is unable to nurse, and dies in 6–12 hours. Death is associated with severe hypoglycemia; however, based on the frequent presence of meconium-staining of the skin, other factors associated with intrauterine distress probably contribute.

In Jersey and Guernsey breeds, a second type of prolonged gestation occurs in which the gestation periods may exceed 475 days. Normal parturition does not occur, though a dead fetus may be expelled. Even when delivered by cesarean section, viable calves only survive a few minutes. The calf is small and has hypotrichosis; facial abnormalities are apparent, such as hydrocephalus, anencephalus, and cyclopia. Aplasia of the anterior pituitary occurs, often with hypoplasia of the neurohypophysis. Adrenal and thyroid glands are also hypoplastic.

Types of prolonged gestations have been observed in cattle that do not clearly fit into the two syndromes described; however, the fetuses have not been studied with the detail necessary to reach any conclusion regarding pathogenesis.

In sheep, prolonged pregnancy has been described in Karakul ewes in Southwest Africa. Gestation exceeds 200 days, the lambs are abnormally large, and when delivered they survive only a few hours. The abnormally large lambs resulted in the name Grootlamsiekte (big lamb disease). The anterior pituitary is present, but acidophils are degranulated. The adrenal cortices and thymus are hypoplastic. This form of prolonged gestation is caused by consumption of the plant *Salsola tuberculata* (Joubert et al., 1972). Although the condition most frequently occurs in the Karakul breed (because the plant is common where they are raised), other breeds are also susceptible.

Prolonged gestation has also been described in sheep following ingestion of *Veratrum californicum*. Ingestion of this plant in early pregnancy results in severe cranial malformations (See Chapter 15).

References

Alexander JE. Anomaly of craniopharyngeal duct and hypophysis. Can Vet J 1962;3:83–86.

Andresen E, Willeberg P, Rasmussen PG. Pituitary dwarfism in German shepherd dogs: genetic investigations. Nord Vet Med 1974;26:692–701.

Andresen E, Willeberg P. Pituitary dwarfism in Carelian Bear dogs: evidence of simple, autosomal-recessive inheritance. Hereditas 1976;84:232–234.

Baker E. Congenital hypoplasia of the pituitary and pancreas in the dog. J Am Vet Med Assoc 1955;126:468.

Barr SC. Pituitary tumour causing multiple endocrinopathies in a dog. Aust Vet J 1985;62:127–129.

Bartke A. Histology of the anterior hypophysis, thyroid and gonads of two types of dwarf mice. Anat Rec 1964;149:225–235.

Beyer C, Kaufmann K, Wehner F. Bedeutung des melanozyten-stimulierenden hormons beim malignen melanom: bedeutung von MSH. [Importance and function of the melanocyte-stimulating hormone in malignant melanoma: importance of MSH.] Dermatol Monatsschr 1990;176:589–596.

Bilzer T. Hypophysentumoren als gemeinsame ursache von morbus Cushing und diabetes insipidus des hundes. [Tumors of the hypophysis as the cause of both Cushing's syndrome and diabetes insipidus in dogs.] Tierarztl Prax 1991;19:276–281.

Carsner RL, Rennels EG. Primary site of gene action in anterior pituitary dwarf mice. Science 1960;131:829.

Cutz E, Chan W, Wong V, Conen PE. Endocrine cells in rat lungs: ultrastructural and histochemical study. Lab Invest 1974;30:458–464.

Dores RM. The proopiomelanocortin family. Prog Clin Biol Res 1990;342:22–27.

Eicher EM, Beamer WG. Inherited ateliotic dwarfism in mice: characteristics of the mutation, *little*, on chromosome 6. J Hered 1976;67:87–91.

Eigenmann JE, Venker-van Haagen AJ. Progesterone-induced and spontaneous canine acromegaly due to reversible growth hormone overproduction: clinical picture and pathogenesis. J Am Anim Hosp Assoc 1981;17:813–822.

Ferguson DC, Biery DN. Diabetes insipidus and hyperadrenocorticism associated with high plasma adrenocorticotropin concentration and a hypothalamic/pituitary mass in a dog. J Am Vet Med Assoc 1988;193:835–839.

Halmi NS, Peterson ME, Colurso GJ, et al. Pituitary intermediate lobe in dog: two cell types and high bioactive adrenocorticotropin content. Science 1981;211:72–74.

Holm LW. Prolonged pregnancy. Adv Vet Sci 1967;11:159–205.

Howe A. The mammalian pars intermedia: a review of its structure and function. J Endocrinol 1973;59:385–409.

Huston K, Gier HT. An anatomical description of a hydrocephalic calf from prolonged gestation and the possible relationship of these conditions. Cornell Vet 1958;48:45–53.

Jensen EC. Hypopituitarism associated with cystic Rathke's cleft in a dog. J Am Vet Med Assoc 1959;135:572–575.

Johnson DR, Hunt DM. Endocrinological findings in sterile pink-eyed mice. J Reprod Fertil 1975;42:51–58.

Joubert JPJ, Basson PA, Lucks HJ, et al. "Grootlamsiekte", a specific syndrome of prolonged gestation in sheep: further investigations. Onderstepoort J Vet Res 1972;39:59–70.

Jubb KV, McEntee K. The bovine pituitary gland. I. Adenohypophyseal functional cytology. II. Architecture and cytology with special reference to basophil function. Cornell Vet 1955;45:576–641.

Kennedy PC. Interactions of fetal disease and the onset of labor in cattle and sheep. Fed Proc 1971;30:110–113.

Kennedy PC, Liggins GC, Holm LW. Prolonged gestation. In: Benirschke K, ed. Comparative aspects of reproductive failure. New York: Springer-Verlag, 1967.

Kennedy PC, Kendrick JW, Stormont C. Adenohypophyseal aplasia, an inherited defect associated with abnormal gestation in Guernsey cattle. Cornell Vet 1957;47:161–178.

Lerner AB. The discovery of the melanotropins: a history of pituitary endocrinology. Ann NY Acad Sci 1993;680:1–12.

Lewis UJ. Growth hormone of normal and dwarf mice. Mem Soc Endocrinol 1967;15:179–191.

McGrath P. The pharyngeal hypophysis in some laboratory animals. J Anat 1974;117:95–115.

Melmed S. Acromegaly. N Engl J Med 1990;322:966–977.

Müller-Peddinghaus R, El Etreby MF, Siefert J, et al. Hypophysärer zwergwuchs beim Deutschen Schäferhund. [Pituitary dwarfism in a German shepherd dog.] Vet Pathol 1980;17:406–421.

Phifer RF, Midgley AR, Spicer SS. Immunohistologic evidence that follicle-stimulating hormone and luteinizing hormone are present in the same cell type in the human pars distalis. J Clin Endocrinol 1973;36:125–141.

Roselli-Rehfuss L, et al. Identification of a receptor for gamma melanotropin and other proopiomelanocortin peptides in the hypothalamus and limbic system. Proc Natl Acad Sci USA 1993;90:8856–8860.

Schaible RH, Gowen JW. A new dwarf mouse. Genetics 1961;46:896.

Schteingart DE. Ectopic secretion of peptides of the proopiomelanocortin family. Endocrinol Metab Clin North Am 1991;20:453–471.

Shire JGM, Hambly EA. The adrenal glands of mice with hereditary pituitary dwarfism. Acta Pathol Microbiol Scand 1973;81:226–228.

Snell GD. Dwarf, a new Mendelian recessive character of the house mouse. Proc Natl Acad Sci USA 1929;15:733–734.

Sokol HW, Valtin H. Morphology of the neurosecretory system in rats homozygous and heterozygous for hypothalamic diabetes insipidus (Brattleboro strain). Endocrinology 1965;77:692–700.

Strand FL, et al. Melanotropins as growth factors. Ann NY Acad Sci 1993;680:29–50.

von Lawzewitsch I, Dickmann GH, Amezua L, et al. Cytological and ultrastructural characterization of the human pituitary. Acta Anat 1972;81:286–316.

von Oordt PGWJ. A report of the International Committee for Nomenclature of the Adenohypophysis: nomenclature of the hormone-producing cells in the adenohypophysis. Gen Comp Endocrinol 1965;5:131–134.

Willeberg P, Kastrup KW, Andresen E. Pituitary dwarfism in German shepherd dogs: studies on somatomedin activity. Nord Vet Med 1975;27:448–454.

Zohar M, Salomon Y. Mechanism of action of melanocortin peptides: possible role in astrocyte regulation. J Mol Neurosci 1993;4:55–62.

Lesions of the posterior pituitary

Primary disorders of the posterior pituitary are rare. When they occur, they are reflected as a decrease in antidiuretic hormone (ADH, vasopressin [AVP]); the syndrome of **diabetes insipidus** also manifests. No specific syndrome is associated with the lack of oxytocin. ADH serves to concentrate urine by increasing the movement of water from the lumens of distal tubules and primary collecting ducts to the interstitium of the kidney. Diabetes insipidus is therefore characterized by polydipsia and polyuria of low specific gravity (usually < 1.010).

Several mechanisms can lead to diabetes insipidus. In animals the disease is usually **secondary,** resulting from neoplastic destruction of the pars nervosa or its hypothalmic connections (usually from adenomas of the anterior pituitary). Diabetes insipidus may also be caused by inflammatory lesions and trauma to the posterior pituitary and stalk, or diseases leading to necrosis of neurons in hypothalamic nuclei. Lesions due to nematode larval migration also have been associated with this syndrome.

Primary (central) or **hypothalamic diabetes insipidus** is the result of deficient secretion of ADH, usually of **idiopathic origin.** An example occurs in the Brattleboro strain of rats; an autosomal-recessive genetic trait results in a failure to synthesize ADH and neurophysin. Oxytocin levels are also reduced severely. The supraoptic nuclei and the entire hypothalamo-neurohypophyseal system are hypertrophied in affected rats. It has also been reported in dogs and monkeys.

Nephrogenic diabetes insipidus results from a defect in the renal tubular receptor for ADH. Affected individuals do not respond to the administration of ADH as do those with other forms of the disease. This form of diabetes insipidus has been reported in dogs, horses, and chickens.

Excessive secretion of ADH, described in humans, leads to excessive retention of water and expansion of fluid volume. Most commonly, it results from elaboration of ADH by nonendocrine tumors, particularly oatcell bronchogenic carcinoma.

Neoplasms of the posterior pituitary are rare, but tumors of glial cells have been reported in animals.

References

Authement JM, Boudrieau RJ, Kaplan PM. Transient, traumatically induced, central diabetes insipidus in a dog. J Am Vet Med Assoc 1989;194:683–685.

Boorman GA, Bree MM. Diabetes insipidus syndrome in a rabbit. J Am Vet Med Assoc 1969;155:1218–1220.

Davenport DJ, Chew DJ, Johnson GC. Diabetes insipidus associated with metastatic pancreatic carcinoma in a dog. J Am Vet Med Assoc 1986;189:22–27.

Feldman EC, Nelson RW. Diagnostic approach to polydipsia and polyuria. Vet Clin North Am Amall Anim Pract 1989;19:327–341.

Green RA, Farrow CS. Diabetes insipidus in a cat. J Am Vet Med Assoc 1974;164:524–526.

Grunbaum EG, Moritz A. Zur diagnostik des diabetes insipidus renalis beim hund. [The diagnosis of nephrogenic diabetes insipidus in the dog.] Tierarztl Prax 1991;19:539–544.

Koestner PC, Kendrick JW, Stormont C. Adenohypophyseal aplasia, an inherited defect associated with abnormal gestation in Guernsey cattle. Cornell Vet 1957;47:161–178.

Lage AL. Nephrogenic diabetes insipidus in a dog. J Am Vet Med Assoc 1973;163:251–253.

Moses AM, Miller M. Accumulation and release of pituitary vasopressin in rats heterozygous for hypothalamic diabetes insipidus. Endocrinology 1970;86:34–41.

Perrin IV, Bestetti GE, Zanesco SA, et al. Diabetes insipidus centralis caused by visceral larva migrans of the neurohypophysis in the dog. Schweiz Arch Tierheilkd 1986;128:483–486.

Port CD, Dal Corobbo MD, Kofman S. Idiopathic diabetes insipidus in a rhesus monkey. Lab Anim Sci 1990;40:84–86.

Post J, McNeill JR, Clark EG, et al. Congenital central diabetes insipidus in two sibling Afghan hound pups. J Am Vet Med Assoc 1989;194:1086–1088.

Richards MA, Sloper JC. Hypothalamic involvement by "visceral" larva migrans in a dog suffering from diabetes insipidus. Vet Rec 1964;76:449–451.

Rogers WA, Valdez H, Anderson BC, et al. Partial deficiency of antidiuretic hormone in a cat. J Am Vet Med Assoc 1977;170:545–547.

Saul GB II, Garrity EG, Benirschke K, et al. Inherited hypothalamic diabetes insipidus in the Brattleboro strain of rats. J Hered 1969;57:113–117.

Saunders LZ, Stephenson HC, McEntee K. Diabetes insipidus and adiposogenital syndrome in a dog due to an infundibuloma. Cornell Vet 1951;41:445–458.

Schott HC, Bayly WM, Reed SM, et al. Nephrogenic diabetes insipidus in sibling cats. J Vet Intern Med 1993;7:68–72.

Thomson JR, Anderson DH, Gilmour JS. Neurogenic diabetes insipidus in a sheep. J Comp Pathol 1986;96:119–124.

Valtin H, Schroeder HA, Benirschke K, et al. Familial hypothalamic diabetes insipidus in rats. Nature 1962;196:1109–1110.

Valtin H, Sawyer WH, Sokol HW. Neurohypophyseal principles in rats homozygous and heterozygous for hypothalamic diabetes insipidus (Brattleboro strain). Endocrinology 1965;77:701–706.

Valtin H. Animal model of human disease. Hereditary hypothalamic diabetes insipidus. Am J Pathol 1976;83:633–636.

NEOPLASMS OF PITUITARY

Primary tumors of the pituitary are found in all species of animals, but are most frequent in dogs. They are also frequent in laboratory rats, horses, and cats. Individual case reports concerning other species may be found in the literature.

Traditional methods of classification of pituitary tumors named them—in accordance with the presence of granules detectable by histologic techniques—as acidophilic, basophilic, or chromophobic adenomas or adenocarcinomas. Although still in use, this method of classification does not reliably determine the functional properties of pituitary tumors. Whenever possible, immunoperoxidase techniques should be employed to identify what hormones the neoplastic cell types contain. However, the results of these techniques may not correlate with circulating levels of the hormones involved; therefore, these techniques should be coupled with measures of serum hormones and other functional studies. Although, theoretically, any of the cell types of the anterior pituitary can give rise to hormonally active neoplasms, in animals the most common are adenomas of corticotrophs, which secrete ACTH. Nonfunctional chromophobe adenomas are also frequent. Others are rare.

The vast majority of pituitary tumors are adenomas, which grow by expansion. Because of their space-occupying nature, pituitary adenomas may interfere with the functional integrity of other cells of the anterior pituitary, posterior pituitary, or hypothalamus; thus, they lead to diverse clinical and pathologic pictures. Primary carcinomas of the anterior pituitary occur, but are rare. Their morphology is variable, with marked cellular pleomorphism. They are usually nonfunctional and their cell of origin not definable. They invade the adjacent pituitary, brain, and bone, and may metastasize.

Ectopic secretion of both pituitary hormones and hypothalamic-releasing hormones can mimic hyperpituitarism. Few examples have been reported in animals, but a variety of neoplasms in humans have been shown to produce hormones.

Corticotroph and melanotroph neoplasms Tumors of corticotrophs, which secrete adrenocorticotropin, are the most frequent functional pituitary tumor of animals; they occur most often in dogs. Boxers, Boston terriers and dachshunds seem to have an increased incidence than do other breeds. The tumors are usually adenomas, which arise in the **pars distalis** and grow by expansion, compressing the adjacent pituitary and hy-

pothalamus. Microscopically, the tumor cells are **chromophobic** without demonstrable granules, except by immunohistochemistry or electronmicroscopy. They stain for ACTH, and often MSH and β-lipoprotein. The cytoplasm is usually faintly eosinophilic. In rare examples, basophilic PAS-positive granules may be seen in corticotroph secreting tumors. In humans, these tumors usually have abundant basophilic granules. In dogs, the tumors are composed of either large or small cells. The large type is most frequent, and is polyhedral with a large vesicular nucleus containing one or two conspicuous nucleoli. The small cell type is about half the size of the large, and has a dark nucleus with indistinct nucleoli; the cytoplasm is scant and indistinctly demarcated. Neoplastic cells may form two histologic patterns. The first (**diffuse**) type involves solid sheets of closely packed cells, with few capillaries and little evident stroma. In the second (**sinusoidal**) type, tumor cells are closely arranged in a palisading pattern around many endothelial-lined sinusoids. Fine trabeculae and capillaries or venules separate this tumor into irregularly shaped lobules. Occasionally, tumor cells form small acini and the lumen contains colloid material.

Corticotroph-secreting tumors (adenomas) can arise in the **pars intermedia** of dogs. These, too, are generally chromophobic but immunoreactive for ACTH. They more regularly stain for MSH and β-lipoprotein than do those of the pars distalis, and they differ histologically. These tumors are composed of many colloid-filled acini or follicles, which are lined by tall, often-ciliated, columnar epithelium. Solid arrays of chromophobic cells are scattered among the acini. Chromophobic cells have acidophilic cytoplasm without basophilic granules.

The primary functional impact of corticotroph- or ACTH-secreting tumors—whether arising in the pars distalis or pars intermedia—is the development of adrenocortical hyperplasia and hyperfunction; this condition causes pituitary origin **Cushing disease** (refer to section on the *adrenal cortex*). Larger tumors result in compression of the posterior pituitary and infundibular stalk, leading to diabetes insipidus.

In **horses,** adenomas (and multinodular hyperplasia) of the pars intermedia are the most frequent pituitary neoplasm. We include them here under corticotroph adenomas, however, their secretory products and the associated clinical syndrome are not a simple excess elaboration of ACTH. These tumors are composed of cords of large columnar or polyhedral cells with hyperchromatic nuclei. The cells are arranged in a palisading or nodular fashion, occasionally forming follicular or acinar structures. Ultrastructurally, the cells contain secretory granules. Cells stain strongly for α- and β-MSH, β-lipoprotein, β-endorphin, and POMC, and are thus presumably melanotrophs, not corticotrophs. Reactivity for prolactin and FSH have also been reported. The reaction for ACTH is weak. Circulating levels of these compounds reflect these staining reactions, with increases in POMC, α- and β-MSH, CLIP, and β-endorphin. A variety of clinical findings develop in horses with these tumors: polyphagia, hirsutism, muscle wasting, hyperglycemia, glycosuria, polyuria, polydipsia, diabetes insipidus, polyphagia, progressive debilitation, and an increased incidence of bacterial and fungal infections. These effects are attributed to: compression and damage (by the tumor) to the hypothalamus and the posterior pituitary, and the increased circulating levels of POMC and its non-ACTH derivatives. Hyperglycemia is believed to be related to deranged insulin metabolism due to overeating—possibly similar to insulin resistance which can develop in obese people—and believed to be responsible for the increased incidence of infections. Only a small number of horses with adenomas of the pars intermedia develop adrenocortical hyperplasia. **Multinodular corticotroph hyperplasia** is often seen in conjunction with adenomas of the pars intermedia in horses, and occasionally independently. The cells in these aggregates often stain strongly for ACTH.

Somatotroph neoplasms Tumors of somatotrophs that secrete growth hormone are classic causes of acromegaly and gigantism in humans. They are composed of either acidophilic or chromophobic cells. Rarely, nonsecreting adenomas have been reported in dogs. Growth hormone-secreting acidophil adenomas have been described most frequently in cats, but have also been reported in sheep. In those examples reported, tumors are composed of cells arranged in sheets, columns, or acinar structures. Acidophilic granules are generally clearly visible, although less striking than in normal somatotrophs. Structural changes in the skeleton depend on the age of the animal. In the young, the result is **gigantism** with extremely lengthened long bones. In an adult whose epiphyses are closed, the bones grow heavier and thicker, producing large hands, feet and skull bones. This is called **acromegaly** ("acro" means "extremity"). Gigantism has not been clearly documented in animals, but acromegaly has been reported with enlargement of the skull, mandible, limbs, and feet. These changes result from the production of somatomedins, which stimulate formation of cartilage. Excessive growth-hormone secretion in animals and humans also leads to **diabetes mellitus;** this is caused by interference with tissue glucose uptake and insulin resistance. Blood-glucose concentration is one factor that influences growth-hormone release; hypoglycemia serves as a stimulant and hyperglycemia suppresses growth-hormone release. Other causes of acromegaly in humans include: release of growth hormone from extrapituitary tumors of the pancreas, lung, ovary, and breast; excessive release of growth hormone-releasing hormone from hypothalamic tumors; and tumors of other tissues, including carcinoid, pancreatic-islet cell tumors, adrenal adenoma, and pheochromocytoma.

Adenomas of lactotrophs, gonadotrophs, and thyrotrophs Neoplasms of lactotrophs, gonadotrophs, and thyrotrophs are extremely rare in domestic animals. In laboratory rats, in which pituitary tumors are relatively common, a large percentage of tumors are prolactinomas. Histologically, these appear as chromophobe adenomas. In humans, prolactinomas are the most common of the pituitary adenomas. They lead to amenorrhea and galactorrhea in women, but rarely have overt hormonal effects in men. Schlumberger (1954) reported an increased incidence of chromophobe adenomas and carcinomas in parakeets, some of which appeared to be thyrotropic tumors. Other surveys have not found an increased incidence.

Nonfunctional chromophobe adenomas Nonfunctional adenomas of chromophobes are among the most frequent of pituitary neoplasms. Histologically, these tumors may closely resemble hormonally active pituitary adenomas which, in routine tissue sections, appear to be composed of chromophobes. In the nonsecreting tumors, the cells are polyhedral, arranged in sheets or lobules, and do not stain for any of the anterior pituitary hormones; small granules may be visualized by electron microscopy. These tumors may lead to destruction of the adjacent pituitary, and to hypopituitarism.

Craniopharyngioma Craniopharyngiomas are rare neoplasms arising from remnants of the craniopharyngeal duct or Rathke's pouch. They are composed of an admixture of cords and nests of stratified squamous, cuboidal, and columnar epithelium within a loose fibrous stroma. Cysts lined by one of these epithelial types and containing keratin or colloidal material are common. Areas of necrosis with mineralization usually manifest. These neoplasms resemble adamantinomas or ameloblastomas. Destruction of the anterior and posterior pituitary leads to the expected clinical picture.

Secondary neoplasms in pituitary Although infrequently encountered, metastatic neoplasms reported in the pituitary include lymphosarcoma (dogs, cattle, birds), malignant melanoma (dogs, cats, horses), adenocarcinoma of the mammary gland (dogs), and osteosarcoma and ependymoma (dogs). These metastatic neoplasms may have the same destructive effects on the pituitary, hypothalamus, and thalamus as primary tumors, and therefore produce similar clinical signs.

References

Anderson MP, Capen CC. The endocrine system. In: Benirschke K, Garner FM, Jones TC, eds. Pathology of laboratory animals. New York: Springer-Verlag, 1978;6.

Auer DE, Wilson RG, Groenendyk S, et al. Glucose metabolism in a pony mare with a tumour of the pituitary gland pars intermedia. Aust Vet J 1987;64:379–382.

Barr SC. Pituitary tumour causing multiple endocrinopathies in a dog. Aust Vet J 1985;62:127–129.

Barsoum NJ, Moore JD, Gough AW, et al. Morphofunctional investigations on spontaneous pituitary tumors in Wistar rats. Toxicol Pathol 1985;13:200–208.

Berry PH. Effect of diet or reproductive status on the histology of spontaneous pituitary tumors in female Wistar rats. Vet Pathol 1986;23:610–618.

Bilzer T. Hypophysentumoren als gemeinsame Ursache von Morbus Cushing und Diabetes insipidus der Hundes. [Tumors of the hypophysis as the cause of both Cushing's syndrome and diabetes insipidus in dogs.] Tierarztl Prax 1991;19:276–281.

Boujon CE, Ritz U, Rossi GL, et al. A clinico-pathological study of canine Cushing's disease caused by a pituitary carcinoma. J Comp Pathol 1991;105:353–365.

Boujon CE, Bestetti GE, Meier HP, et al. Equine pituitary adenoma: a functional and morphological study. J Comp Pathol 1993;109:163–178.

Capen CC, Koestner A. Functional chromophobe adenomas of the canine adenohypophysis: an ultrastructural evaluation of a neoplasm of pituitary corticotrophs. Pathol Vet 1967;4:326–347.

Capen CC, Martin SL, Koestner A. [1] Neoplasms in the adenohypophysis of the dog: a clinical and pathologic study. [2] The ultrastructure and histopathology of an acidophil adenoma of the canine adenohypophysis. Pathol Vet 1967;4:301–325, 348–365.

Chalifoux LV, MacKey JJ, King NW. A sparsely granulated, nonsecreting adenoma of the pars intermedia associated with galactorrhea in a male rhesus monkey (*Macaca mulatta*). Vet Pathol 1983;20:541–547.

Dingemans KP. Development of TSH-producing tumours in mouse. Virchows Arch (Cell Pathol) 1973;12:338–359.

Eckersley GN, Geel JK, Kriek NP. A craniopharyngioma in a seven-year-old dog. J S Afr Vet Assoc 1991;62:55–57.

Eckersley GN, Bastianello S, Van Heerden J, et al. An expansile secondary hypophyseal mastocytoma in a dog. J S Afr Vet Assoc 1989;60:113–116.

El Etreby MF, Müller-Peddinghaus R, Bhargava AS, et al. Functional morphology of spontaneous hyperplastic and neoplastic lesions in the canine pituitary gland. Vet Pathol 1980;17:109–122.

Feldman EC. Distinguishing dogs with functional adrenocortical tumors from dogs with pituitary-dependent hyperadrenocorticism. J Am Vet Med Assoc 1983;183:195–200.

Ferguson DC, Biery DN. Diabetes insipidus and hyperadrenocorticism associated with high plasma adrenocorticotropin concentration and a hypothalamic/pituitary mass in a dog. J Am Vet Med Assoc 1988;193:835–839.

Fitzgerald JE, Schardein JL, Kaump DH. Several uncommon pituitary tumors in the rat. Lab Anim Sci 1971;21:581–584.

Furuzawa Y, Une Y, Nomura Y. Pituitary dependent hyperadrenocorticism in a cat. J Vet Med Sci 1992;54:1201–1203.

Guzman-Silva MA, Rossi MI, Guimaraes JS. Craniopharyngioma in the Mongolian gerbil (*Meriones unguiculatus*): a case report. Lab Anim 1988;22:365–368.

Hawkins KL, Diters RW, McGrath JT. Craniopharyngioma in a dog. J Comp Pathol 1985;95:469–474.

Heider K. Spontaneous craniopharyngioma in a mouse. Vet Pathol 1986;23:522–523.

Heinrichs M, Baumgärtner W, Capen CC. Immunocytochemical demonstration of proopiomelanocortin-derived peptides in pituitary adenomas of the pars intermedia in horses. Vet Pathol 1990;27:419–425.

HogenEsch H, Broerse JJ, Zurcher C. Neurohypophyseal astrocytoma (pituicytoma) in a rhesus monkey (*Macaca mulatta*). Vet Pathol 1992;29:359–361.

Horvath CJ, Ames TR, Metz AL, et al. Adrenocorticotropin-containing neoplastic cells in a pars intermedia adenoma in a horse. J Am Vet Med Assoc 1988;192:367–371.

Ito A. Pituitary tumors. In: Jones TC, Hackel DB, Migaki G, eds. Handbook: animal models of human disease. Washington, DC: Registry of Comparative Pathology, AFIP, 1978; No. 121.

Kemppainen RJ, Zenoble RD. Non-dexamethasone-suppressible, pituitary-dependent hyperadrenocorticism in a dog. J Am Vet Med Assoc 1985;187:276–278.

Kipperman BS, Feldman EC, Dybdal NO, et al. Pituitary tumor size, neurologic signs, and relation to endocrine test results in dogs with pituitary-dependent hyperadrenocorticism: 43 cases (1980–1990). J Am Vet Med Assoc 1992;201:762–767.

Kleinberg DL, Noel GL, Frantz AG. Galactorrhea: a study of 235 cases, including 48 with pituitary tumors. N Engl J Med 1977;296:589–600.

Lichtensteiger CA, Wortman JA, Eigenmann JE. Functional pituitary acidophil adenoma in a cat with diabetes mellitus and acromegalic features. Vet Pathol 1986;23:518–521.

Loeb WF, Capen CC, Johnson LE. Adenoma of the pars intermedia associated with hyperglycemia and glycosuria in two horses. Cornell Vet 1966;56:623–639.

Miller WH Jr. Parapituitary meningioma in a dog with pituitary-dependent hyperadrenocorticism. J Am Vet Med Assoc 1991;198:444–446.

Millington WR, Dybdal NO, Dawson R Jr, et al. Equine Cushing's disease: differential regulation of beta-endorphin processing in tumors of the intermediate pituitary. Endocrinology 1988;123:1598–1604.

Nelson RW, Feldman EC, Smith MC. Hyperadrenocorticism in cats: seven cases (1978–1987). J Am Vet Med Assoc 1988;193:245–250.

Nelson RW, Ihle SL, Feldman EC. Pituitary macroadenomas and macroadenocarcinomas in dogs treated with mitotane for pituitary-dependent hyperadrenocorticism: 13 cases (1981–1986). J Am Vet Med Assoc 1989;194:1612–1617.

Olson DP, Ohlson DL, Davis SL, et al. Acidophil adenoma in the pituitary gland of a sheep. Vet Pathol 1981;18:132–135.

Peterson ME, Steele P. Pituitary-dependent hyperadrenocorticism in a cat. J Am Vet Med Assoc 1986;189:680–683.

Peterson ME, et al. Acromegaly in 14 cats. J Vet Intern Med 1990;4:192–201.

Powers RD, Winkler JK. Pituitary carcinoma with extracranial metastasis in a cow. Vet Pathol 1977;14:524–526.

Rijnberk A, Eigenmann JE, Belshaw BE, et al. Acromegaly associated with transient overproduction of growth hormone in a dog. J Am Vet Med Assoc 1980;177:534–537.

Sarfaty D, Carrillo JM, Peterson ME. Neurologic, endocrinologic, and pathologic findings associated with large pituitary tumors in dogs: eight cases (1976–1984). J Am Vet Med Assoc 1988;193:854–856.

Saunders LZ, Rickard CG. Craniopharyngioma in a dog with apparent adiposogenital syndrome and diabetes insipidus. Cornell Vet 1952;42:490–494.

Schlumberger HG. Neoplasia in the parakeet. I. Spontaneous chromophobe pituitary tumors. Cancer Res 1954;14:237–245.

van der Kolk JH, Kalsbeek HC, van Garderen E, et al. Equine pituitary neoplasia: a clinical report of 21 cases (1990–1992). Vet Rec 1993;133:594–597.

Zaki F, Harris J, Budzilovich G. Cystic pituicytoma of the neurohypophysis in a Siamese cat. J Comp Pathol 1975;85:467–471.

THYROID

The thyroid is an endocrine organ found in all vertebrates; in mammals it is usually a bilobed gland located just caudal to the larynx, near the trachea. In some mammals the two lobes are connected by an isthmus that lays across the ventral (anterior) aspect of the trachea. The embryonic development of the thyroid starts from the root of the tongue at the foramen cecum; the thyroid originates as a downward growth of epithelium which forms the thyroglossal duct. The thyroid develops from the end of the duct, with the remainder degenerating before birth. Persistence of portions of the thyroglossal duct into adulthood can give rise to thyroglossal cysts. Should the duct not descend an adequate distance, the thyroid may be placed abnormally high; when it is carried too far, the thyroid may occur within the mediastinum. In addition to vascular, nervous, and connective tissues, the thyroid has two types of endocrine cells. The preponderant epithelial cells are **follicular cells** that are arranged into acini or follicles, and which consist of cells arranged circumferentially around a central mass of colloid material. The epithelial cells may be tall columnar, cuboidal, or flattened, depending upon their secretory activity. These follicular cells concentrate iodide from the circulating blood (Fig. 26-2); in the course of several enzymatic reactions, they form thyroglobulin, which is stored as colloid and then subsequently secreted as thyroxine (T_4) and triiodothyronine (T_3).

The synthesis and release of thyroid hormone involves several steps:

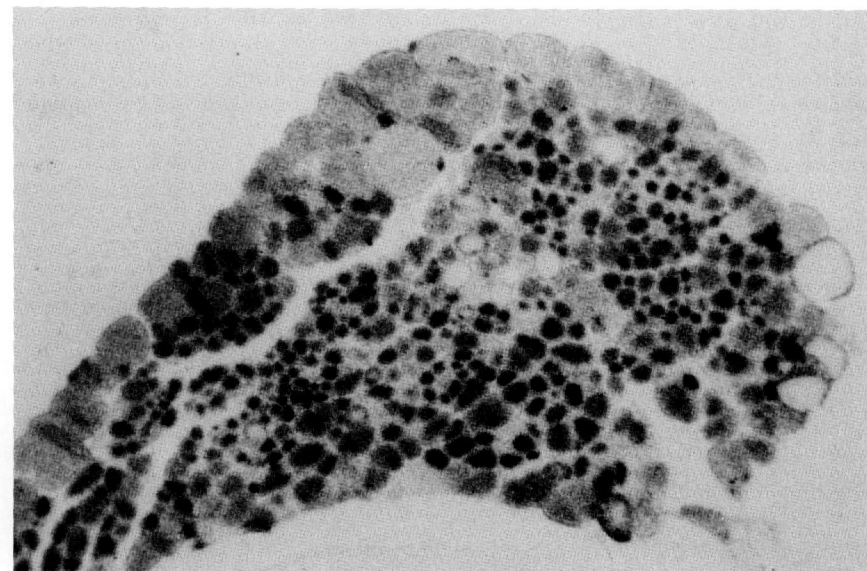

FIG. 26-2 Autoradiograph of normal rat thyroid gland prepared 12 hours following injection of ^{131}I. The radioactive iodine has been concentrated in the thyroid follicles; the radioactive emissions interacted with the photographic emulsion to produce the dark, roughly spherical masses.

1. Circulating iodide is trapped and transported against a gradient toward the follicular lumen;
2. Iodide is oxidized by iodide peroxidase to iodine;
3. At the microvillus border of follicular cell and colloid, iodine binds to the tyrosine residues of thyroglobulin (a glycoprotein synthesized by the follicular cells). The result is the formation of bound monoiodotyrosine (MIT) and diiodotyrosine (DIT) within thyroglobulin;
4. These then undergo a peroxidase-dependent coupling, either as two molecules of DIT (to form thyroxine [T_4]) or one molecule of MIT to one molecule of DIT (to form triiodotyrosine [T_3], the final form of circulating thyroid hormones);
5. Through the process of endocytosis of thyroglobulin and its proteolysis within phagolysosomes, T_3 and T_4 are released from the base of follicular cells into perifollicular capillaries and enter the circulation bound to thyroxin-binding globulin. T_3 is less firmly bound to protein than is T_4 and is therefore more readily available to tissue.

These steps are stimulated by thyroid-stimulating hormone (TSH) which, in turn, is suppressed by an increase in circulating thyroid hormone. In contrast to other hormones, thyroid hormone acts on all cells of the body where it regulates metabolic processes.

The thyroid gland secretes another hormone, **calcitonin** (first identified in dogs by Nonidez, 1923), which is produced by C cells (parafollicular cells, light cells). C cells are derived from the neural crest via the ultimobranchial body which, in most species, fuses with the thyroid gland. In cattle, the ultimobranchial body becomes incorporated into the vasculature and stroma at the hilus of the thyroid. C cells, usually few in number, reside among follicular epithelial cells within or outside the basement membrane (depending upon species), or in small nests between follicles. These cells have a distinct pale or light cytoplasm (hence light cells) in preparations stained with periodic acid Schiff and hematoxylin and eosin. Cytoplasm contains numerous secretory granules of varying size and density, as well as numerous mitochondria and arrays of fine tubules. Secretory granules can be stained with argyrophilic stains—comparable to those used for other neuroendocrine cells—and more specifically identified with the uranaffin reaction. C cells also can be identified immunohistochemically with positive reactions for calcitonin, neuron-specific enolase (NSE), and, in some cells, somatostatin. In most species, immunoreactivity exists for calcitonin gene-related peptide (CGRP), but only a few cells are positive for CGRP in pigs, mice, hamsters, and guinea pigs.

The role of calcitonin in regulation of serum calcium is as an antagonist to parathyroid hormone, acting at the level of bone by inhibiting osteoclast-mediated resorption. It also acts on the kidney by increasing renal clearance of both calcium and phosphate. An increase in serum calcium stimulates the release of calcitonin. Increased secretion of calcitonin is also observed in C cell tumors (medullary adenoma or carcinoma of the thyroid).

Diseases of thyroid

ABERRANT THYROID TISSUE
Aberrant (ectopic) thyroid tissue occurs frequently in most animal species. Most aberrant thyroids result from (1) the failure of all or part of the thyroid anlage to descend from the floor of the pharynx to its normal cervical position, or (2) its descending beyond its normal adult position. In the first case, aberrant thyroid tissue may occur at any median point from the tongue to its normal position; in the second case, it occurs cau-

dal to the normal position—including within the thoracic cavity—and often at the base of the heart. Another form of aberrant thyroid results from anomalous development of fetal tissue in general. Aberrant thyroid responds to the same physiologic stimuli as the cervical gland, including neoplastic transformation.

THYROGLOSSAL CYST

A thyroglossal cyst is a developmental anomaly arising in the thyroglossal duct. In early embryonic life, this duct extends from the lower pharyngeal mucosa to form the primitive thyroid, and normally disappears before birth. When it persists, a sinus tract or a cyst commonly develops. The cyst is always in the midline, and is lined either by stratified squamous or simple columnar epithelium or by a mixture of the two. This is not a frequent anomaly in animals, but developmental anomalies are not reported with a regularity that permits statistical conclusions.

HYPOTHYROIDISM

Hypothyroidism is the condition resulting from a failure to synthesize adequate thyroid hormone, with decreased levels of circulating T_3 and T_4. It is encountered most often in dogs and cats, and can result from any of several different diseases. No consistent pathologic picture exists of the thyroid gland; it can be hypo- or hyperplastic. **Causes** include: aplasia or hypoplasia of the thyroid, thyroiditis, various nontoxic goiters from iodine deficiency or goitrogens, nonfunctional neoplasms that destroy the gland, biosynthetic defects in thyroid hormone synthesis, and diseases that disrupt the hypothalamus or pituitary. Biosynthetic defects resulting in dyshormonogenesis can involve several of the steps in hormone synthesis. In humans, most defects are inherited as autosomal-recessive traits. One form is the result of reduced thyroid peroxidase activity. What appear to be similar recessively inherited defects of thyroid peroxidase have been described in dogs (Giant schnauzers) and cats (Abyssinian). Hereditary hypothyroidism (goiter) has also been recognized in goats, Africaner cattle, and Corriedale, Dorset Horn, Merino, and Romney Marsh sheep; in these cases, the mode of inheritance is as an autosomal-recessive trait. Often, the cause of hypothyroidism is not identifiable (Fig. 26-3).

The essential feature of hypothyroidism occurring at any age is an abnormally low basal metabolic rate. Affected animals are lethargic; they develop muscular weakness and gain weight. Reflexes are slow, and in some cases paresis manifests. The animals seek sources of heat due to their intolerance to cold. Bilaterally symmetric alopecia occurs, with hyperpigmentation, hyperkeratosis, epidermal atrophy, and a thickening of the dermis due to mucin accumulation. Pyoderma is sometimes present. A failure in growth is evident when the animals are affected from birth. In humans, hypothyroidism dating from birth leads to **cretinism,** a condition characterized by marked arrest in both physical and mental growth. When thyroid deficiency arises in an adult human, **myxedema** is the outstanding symptom. This accumulation—in the subcutaneous and other connective tissues of mucin—gives the face and other body surfaces a puffy and edematous appearance. Microscopically, this is seen as blue material disrupting the normal dermal architecture. **Congenital hypothyroidism** occurs when a pregnant animal is hypothyroid. Gestation is prolonged, and the affected fetus may be born dead or die shortly after birth. Newborns have goiter and myxedema, and are frequently hairless.

Animals with hypothyroidism often develop dilated cardiomyopathy. Serum cholesterol levels become elevated above 450 mg/100 ml, which may lead to atherosclerosis. In dogs, acquired von Willebrand disease has been associated with hypothyroidism.

HYPERTHYROIDISM

Hyperthyroidism leads to an increase in metabolic rate. The disorder is most common in cats, but is also seen in other species. The **causes** include: diffuse or multinodular hyperplasia of the thyroid, generally of unknown pathogenesis (i.e., various forms of toxic goiter); adenomas and adenocarcinomas of the thyroid; thyroiditis; and rarely, excessive elaboration of TSH by the pituitary. Each of these usually is associated with cervical swelling, and often coughing and dyspnea. The individual is unusually active and alert, does not store fat in spite of a vigorous appetite, and frequently has an irritable or excitable disposition. Moderate hyperthermia occurs, with heat intolerance, weakness, weight loss, polydipsia, and polyuria. Tachycardia, arrhythmias, and often a hypertrophic cardiomyopathy are also evident. In **humans,** bulging of the eyeballs occurs, known as exophthalmos. In **cats,** hyperthyroidism is the result of multinodular hyperplasia (toxic goiter), follicular cell adenoma, or carcinoma of the thyroid. Multinodular hyperplasia and follicular cell adenoma may be difficult to differentiate. The syndrome appears to have arisen within the past several years and is the most common endocrine disease of cats, appearing in middle-aged to old animals. Some cases appear similar to autoimmune thyrotoxicosis of humans (refer to Graves' disease following).

IDIOPATHIC FOLLICULAR ATROPHY OF DOGS

Hypothyroidism in dogs is generally the result of idiopathic follicular atrophy or lymphocytic thyroiditis. Follicular atrophy is characterized by a small end-stage thyroid; it is predominantly composed of adipose tissue, with a few scattered small follicles containing vacuolated colloid. In the earlier stages of the disorder, the thyroid contains (1) small follicles lined by tall columnar cells, and (2) follicles with degenerate follicular cells containing shrunken nuclei and eosinophilic cytoplasm. Other follicular cells are hypertrophic and ultrastructurally contain colloid-filled vacuoles, termed microfollicles. These microfollicles have been interpreted to be an attempt to continue synthesis of thyroid hormones in the absence of normal follicles (Gosselin et al., 1981). The **cause** of follicular atrophy is not known, but it does not resemble the thyroid atrophy secondary to lack of TSH. In contrast, hypertrophy and hyperplasia of thyrotropic basophils manifest in affected dogs.

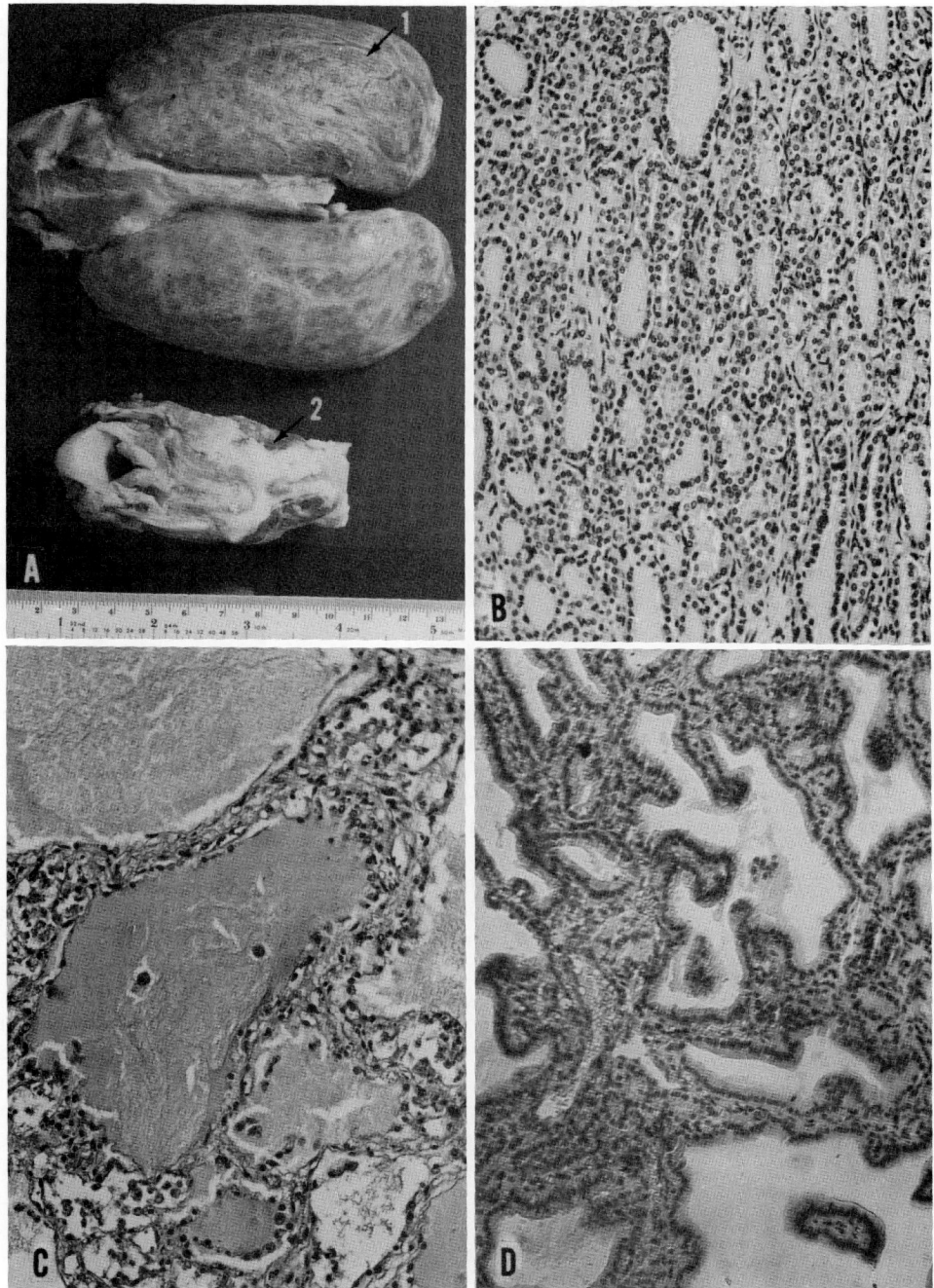

FIG. 26-3 A. Goiter in a newborn lamb. (1) The enlarged thyroid glands; (2) compared with those of a normal lamb. **B.** Normal thyroid (×195) of the newborn lamb, same specimen as a **A2**. **C.** Goitrous thyroid of lamb (×195), same specimen as **A** *(1)*. Note large acini of irregular size. **D.** Thyroid of cretinism in a young calf (×195). Tall cells line large, irregularly shaped acini. (**A-C** Courtesy of Armed Forces Institute of Pathology; contributor: Dr. C. L. Davis.)

LYMPHOCYTIC THYROIDITIS

Spontaneous lymphocytic thyroiditis resulting in hypothyroidism is seen in dogs, laboratory rats, mastomys, and monkeys; it closely resembles Hashimoto thyroiditis in both morphology and pathogenesis. The microscopic features consist of diffuse or nodular infiltration of the gland by lymphocytes, and by lesser numbers of plasma cells, macrophages, and dendritic cells. Lymphocytic nodules may have prominent germinal centers. Displacement and destruction of the follicles may be prominent; colloid gains entrance to the interstitium, where it is engulfed by macrophages and occasionally giant cells. Some follicles are lined by hypertrophied cells that ultrastructurally contain microfollicles. In some examples, follicles are lined by cells— termed oncocytes, Hürthle cells, or oxyphils—containing brightly eosinophilic cytoplasm. These cells do not produce hormones and are believed to represent degenerating cells, which may also be found in other forms of thyroiditis. Nodules of hyperplastic C cells often accompany the lesion. The lesion ultimately progresses to replacement by mature fibrous connective tissue. The pathogenesis of lymphocytic thyroiditis is autoimmune in origin, occurring in animals genetically predisposed. It results from both cytotoxic T cells and autoantibodies directed against TSH receptors, microsomal antigens, thyroglobulin, and follicular cell membranes. In humans, antibodies directed against TSH are of two types: one stimulates hormone synthesis, and another stimulates thyroid growth. In Hashimoto disease, it is mainly the growth-stimulating antibody that predominates. In Graves' disease, which is characterized by hyperthyroidism, both antibodies are expressed.

GOITER

Goiter is the term used for noninflammatory and nonneoplastic enlargement of the thyroid gland. It may be accompanied by either hypo- or hyperthyroidism, or compensated function. Several forms exist in animals, most of which are caused by some interference with the synthesis of thyroid hormone leading to a continued stimulation of the thyroid by TSH from the pituitary; however, circulating levels of TSH may not be elevated. This may allow for adequate T_3 and T_4 synthesis, averting hypothyroidism even though goiter is present.

SIMPLE GOITER (HYPERPLASTIC GOITER, COLLOID GOITER, DIFFUSE NONTOXIC GOITER)

Simple goiter can have many causes and diverse histopathologic features in the thyroid gland. It may be accompanied by hypothyroidism. Three general **causes** exist: (1) **iodine deficiency,** (2) **goitrogens,** and (3) **hereditary biosynthetic defects** of thyroid hormone. In many cases, however, the cause is not identified. **Iodine deficiency** is the classic cause and, despite the long recognition of this association, iodine-deficiency goiter remains a frequent disease throughout the world, especially in developing countries. Selenium deficiency has been shown to aggravate iodine-deficiency goiter, probably through reduced levels of glutathione peroxidase leading to oxidative damage to follicular cells. **Goitrogens** are substances which interfere at various steps in the synthesis of thyroid hormone. Many plants, especially those of the *Brassica* and *Cruciferae* spp., contain goitrogens. Paradoxically, iodine itself can be goitrogenic. The occurrence of iodine-induced goiter has been seen in horses whose diet was supplemented with dried seaweed (kelp). Goitrogens and their mode of action are discussed under *iodine* in chapter 16 on Nutrition. Five different known **biosynthetic defects** exist in thyroid hormone production in humans that lead to what is termed **familial** or **hereditary goiter.** Hereditary goiter has also been recognized in goats, Africaner cattle, and Corriedale, Dorset Horn, Merino, and Romney Marsh sheep, where an autosomal recessive trait is the mode of inheritance. The specific defect appears to be in messenger RNA for thyroglobulin. Affected animals are hypothyroid. Dyshormonogenesis—also recognized in Giant schnauzers and Abyssinian cats—leads to hypothyroidism and goiter. This also appears to be inherited as an autosomal recessive trait, and is believed to result from an organification (peroxidase) defect.

Grossly, the thyroid is uniformly enlarged. **Microscopically,** the initial features are characterized by marked hypertrophy and hyperplasia of the follicular epithelium. The follicles are lined by one or more layers of tall columnar cells, which form papillary projections into the lumens. New follicles, which are small and often lacking in colloid, are formed. It is this stage that is known as **hyperplastic goiter.** For reasons that are not entirely clear, hyperplastic goiter progresses to **colloid goiter;** this condition is characterized by large follicles filled with colloid, which is lined by flattened epithelium. There may be great variation in the size of the follicles, and some may retain papillary projections into the lumens. Mixtures of the features of hyperplastic and colloid goiter may coexist, giving the hyperplastic portions an adenomatous appearance. Colloid goiter is believed to represent an involutional stage of hyperplastic goiter that results when iodine is returned to the diet, or when iodine deficiency is periodic or marginal.

Clinical features of goiter as seen in neonates and adults were presented under hypothyroidism.

Multinodular goiter (adenomatous goiter, nodular thyroid hyperplasia) This form of goiter is characterized by multiple nodules of hyperplastic follicles. They resemble those seen in simple goiter, with one or more layers of tall columnar cells—often with papillary projections into the lumens—and many follicles filled with cells containing little or no colloid. It is a frequent disorder in older cats, and has been seen in dogs and horses. Many examples in animals are euthyroid; however, multinodular goiter in cats is often functional and leads to hyperthyroidism (i.e., toxic goiter). The cause is unknown, although in humans it may develop in cases of long-standing simple goiter. In functional examples in humans, the transition from nontoxic to toxic goiter is believed to result from the development of functional independence of hyperplastic nodules.

Exophthalmic goiter (goiter of hyperthyroidism, toxic goiter, Graves' disease) Exophthalmic goiter or Graves' disease, also known as Basedow disease, is a disorder of humans characterized by hyperthyroidism, marked exophthalmos, and sometimes multifocal edematous dermatopathy. A comparable syndrome has not been clearly documented in animals; however, in some examples of hyperthyroidism in cats, thyroid autoantibodies have been demonstrated and the thyroid contains lymphocytic infiltrates. In humans, goiter is characterized by diffuse hypertrophy and hyperplasia accompanied by lymphocytic infiltration, often with formation of follicles containing germinal centers. Generalized lymphocytic hyperplasia is present in such organs as lymph nodes, spleen, and thymus. Exophthalmos results from a combination of events, including: increased intraocular pressure, lymphocytic infiltration of ocular tissues, and edema and mucopolysaccharide deposition in the orbital tissues. The dermatopathy is also characterized by mucopolysaccharide deposition and has been termed "localized myxedema." The pathogenesis is autoimmune, with the occurrence of antibodies similar to those found in Hashimoto disease. One of the autoantibodies binds to TSH receptors and mimics the action of TSH.

References

Aliapoulios MA, Bernstein DS, Balodimos MC. Thyrocalcitonin: its role in calcium homeostasis. Arch Intern Med 1969;123:88–94.

Avgeris S, Lothrop CD Jr, McDonald TP. Plasma von Willebrand factor concentration and thyroid function in dogs. J Am Vet Med Assoc 1990;196:921–924.

Baker HJ, Lindsey JR. Equine goiter due to excess dietary iodide. J Am Vet Med Assoc 1968;153:1618–1630.

Beierwaltes WH, Nishiyama RH. Dog thyroiditis: occurrence and similarity to Hashimoto's struma. Endocrinology 1968;83:501–508.

Berger AJ. Thyrocalcitonin: a review. Bull Hosp Joint Dis 1971;32:40–49.

Bigazzi PE, Rose NR. Spontaneous autoimmune thyroiditis in animals as models of human disease. Prog Allergy 1975;19:245–274.

Bond BR, Fox PR, Peterson ME, et al. Echocardiographic findings in 103 cats with hyperthyroidism. J Am Vet Med Assoc 1988;192:1546–1549.

Bussolati G, Pearse AGE. Immunofluorescent localization of calcitonin "C" cells of pig and dog thyroid. J Endocrinol 1967;37:205.

Capen CC, Young DM. Thyrocalcitonin: evidence for release in a spontaneous hypocalcemic disorder. Science 1967;157:205–206.

Capen CC, Young DM. The ultrastructure of the parathyroid glands and thyroid parafollicular cells of cows with parturient paresis and hypocalcemia. Lab Invest 1967;17:717–737.

Chan AS, Conen PE. Ultrastructural observations on cytodifferentiation of parafollicular cells in the human fetal thyroid. Lab Invest 1971;25:29–259.

Coffin DL, Munson TO. Endocrine diseases of the dog associated with hair loss. Sertoli-cell tumor of the testis, hypothyroidism, canine Cushing's syndrome. J Am Vet Med Assoc 1953;123:403–408.

Contempre B, Duale NL, Dumont JE, et al. Effect of selenium supplementation on thyroid hormone metabolism in an iodine and selenium deficient population. Clin Endocrinol 1992;36:579–583.

Copp DH, et al. Evidence for calcitonin—a new hormone from the parathyroid that lowers blood calcium. Endocrinology 1962;70:638–644.

DeLellis RA, Nunnemacher G, Wolfe HJ. C cell hyperplasia: an ultrastructural analysis. Lab Invest 1977;36:237–248.

Doi S, et al. Familial goiter in bongo antelope (*Tragelaphus eurycerus*). Endocrinology 1990;127:857–864.

Falconer IR, Roitt IM, Seamark RF, et al. Studies of the congenitally goitrous sheep: iodoproteins of the goitre. Biochem J 1970;117:417–424.

Follis RH. Experimental colloid goiter produced by thiouracil. Nature 1959;183:1817–1818.

Follis RH. Studies on the pathogenesis of colloid goiter. Trans Assoc Am Physicians 1959;72:265–274.

Fritz TE, Zeman RC, Zeele MR. Pathology and familial incidence of thyroiditis in a closed Beagle colony. Exp Mol Pathol 1970;12:14–30.

Gaitan E, Nelson NC, Poole GV. Endemic goiter and endemic thyroid disorders. World J Surg 1991;15:205–215.

Goldwin MC. The early development of the thyroid gland in the dog with especial reference to the origin and position of accessory thyroid tissue within the thoracic cavity. Anat Rec 1936;66:233–251.

Gosselin SJ, Capen CC, Martin SL. Histologic and ultrastructural evaluation of thyroid lesions associated with hypothyroidism in dogs. Vet Pathol 1981;18:299–309.

Gosselin SJ, Capen CC, Martin SL, et al. Induced lymphocytic thyroiditis in dogs: effect of intrathyroidal injection of thyroid autoantibodies. Am J Vet Res 1981;42:1565–1572.

Greco DS, Peterson ME, Cho DY, et al. Juvenile-onset hypothyroidism in a dog. J Am Vet Med Assoc 1985;187:948–950.

Greco DS, Feldman EC, Peterson ME, et al. Congenital hypothyroid dwarfism in a family of Giant schnauzers. J Vet Intern Med 1991;5:57–65, Vet Bull 1991;61:6592.

Hare T. [1] Three cases of heterotopic deposits of thyroid tissue in the dog. [2] Fusion of the thyroid glands in a dog. Proc R Soc Med 1932;25:1496–1499, 1500.

Holzworth J, Theran P, Carpenter JL, et al. Hyperthyroidism in the cat: ten cases. J Am Vet Med Assoc 1980;176:345–353.

Hunt RD. Aberrant thyroid tissue in the mouse. Science 1963;141:1054–1055.

Indrieri RJ, Whalen LR, Cardinet GH, et al. Neuromuscular abnormalities associated with hypothyroidism and lymphocytic thyroiditis in three dogs. J Am Vet Med Assoc 1987;190:544–548.

Jacobs G, Hutson C, Dougherty J, et al. Congestive heart failure with hyperthyroidism in cats. J Am Vet Med Assoc 1986;188:52–56.

Jamieson S, Harbour HE. Congenital goitre in lambs. Vet Rec 1947;59:102.

Jones BR, Gruffydd-Jones TJ, Sparkes AH, et al. Preliminary studies on congenital hypothyroidism in a family of Abyssinian cats. Vet Rec 1992;131:145–148.

Jones HEH, Roitt IM. Experimental autoimmune thyroiditis in the rat. Br J Exp Pathol 1961;42:546–557.

Kameda Y. The accessory thyroid glands of the dog around the intrapericardial aorta. Arch Histol Jpn 1972;34:375–391.

Kennedy RL, Thoday KL. Autoantibodies in feline hyperthyroidism. Res Vet Sci 1988;45:300–306.

Kok K, van Dijk JE, Sterk A, et al. Autosomal recessive inheritance of goiter in Dutch goats. J Hered 1987;78:298–300.

Lucke VM. An histological study of thyroid abnormalities in the domestic cat. J Small Anim Pract 1964;5:351–358.

Mawdesley-Thomas LE, Jolly DW. Autoimmune disease in the beagle. Vet Rec 1967;80:553–554.

Mazzuli GF, Coen G, Bashievi L. Thyrocalcitonin excess syndrome. Lancet 1966;2:1192.

McCauley EH, Linn JG, Goodrich RD. Experimentally induced iodide toxicosis in lambs. Am J Vet Res 1973;34:65–70.

Miller WH Jr, Buerger RG. Cutaneous mucinous vesiculation in a dog with hypothyroidism. J Am Vet Med Assoc 1990;196:757–759.

Mizejewski GJ, Baron J, Poissant G. Immunologic investigations of naturally occurring canine thyroiditis. J Immunol 1971;107:1152–1160.

Musser E, Graham WR. Familial occurrence of thyroiditis in purebred Beagles. Lab Anim Care 1968;18:58–68.

Nesbitt GH, Izzo J, Peterson L, Wilkins RJ. Canine hypothyroidism: a retrospective study of 108 cases. J Am Vet Med Assoc 1980;177:1117–1122.

Nonidez JF. The origin of the "parafollicular" cell, a second epithelial component of the thyroid gland of the dog. Am J Anat 1932;49:479–505.

Nunez EA, et al. Ultrastructure of the parafollicular "C" cells and the parathyroid cell in growing dogs on a high calcium diet. Lab Invest 1974;31:96–108.

Peter HJ, Gerber H, Studer H, et al. Autonomy of growth and of iodine metabolism in hyperthyroid feline goiters transplanted onto nude mice. J Clin Invest 1987;80:491–498.

Peterson ME, Livingston P, Brown RS. Lack of thyroid stimulating immunoglobulins in cats with hyperthyroidism. Vet Immunol Immunopathol 1987;16:277–282.

Rac R, et al. Congenital goitre in Merino sheep due to an inherited defect in the biosynthesis of thyroid hormone. Res Vet Sci 1968;9:209–223.

Rand JS, Levine J, Best SJ, et al. Spontaneous adult-onset hypothyroidism in a cat. J Vet Intern Med 1993;7:272–276.

Ricketts MH, Vandenplas S, van der Walt M, et al. Afrikander cattle congenital goiter: size heterogeneity in thyroglobulin mRNA. Biochem Biophys Res Commun 1985;126:240–246.

Ricketts MH, et al. Autosomal recessive inheritance of congenital goiter in Afrikander cattle. J Hered 1985;76:12–16.

Ricketts MH, et al. Defective splicing of thyroglobulin gene transcripts in the congenital goitre of Afrikander cattle. EMBO J 1985;4:731–737.

Robinson WF, Shaw SE, Stanley B, et al. Congenital hypothyroidism in Scottish deerhound puppies. Aust Vet J 1988;65:386–389.

Sansom BF. Accessory thyroid tissue in the goat. Br Vet J 1967;123:162–169.

Schlotthauer CF. Diseases of the thyroid gland of adult horses. J Am Vet Med Assoc 1931;78:211–218.

Schlotthauer CF, McKenney FD, Caylor HD: The incidence of goiter and other lesions of the thyroid gland in dogs of southern Minnesota. J Am Vet Med Assoc 1930;76:811–819.

Schlumberger HG. Spontaneous goiter and cancer of the thyroid in animals. Ohio J Sci 1955;55:24–43.

Sjollema BE, den Hartog MT, de Vijlder JJ, et al. Congenital hypothyroidism in two cats due to defective organification: data suggesting loosely anchored thyroperoxidase. Acta Endocrinol 1991;125:435–440.

Sreekumaran T, Rajan A. Clinicopathological studies in experimental hypothyroidism in goats. Vet Pathol 1978;15:549–555.

Statham M, Bray AC. Congenital goitre in sheep in southern Tasmania. Aust J Agric Res 1975;26:751–768.

Steyn DG, Sunkel W. Goitre in animals in the Union of South Africa. J S Afr Vet Med Assoc 1954;25:9–18.

Swarts JL, Thompson RL. Accessory thyroid tissue within the pericardium of the dog. J Med Res 1911;24:299–308.

Thoday KL, Mooney CT. Historical, clinical and laboratory features of 126 hyperthyroid cats. Vet Rec 1992;131:257–264.

Vanderpas JB, et al. Selenium deficiency mitigates hypothyroxinemia in iodine-deficient subjects. Am J Clin Nutr 1993;57:271S-275S.

van Jaarsveld P, van der Theron CB, van Zyl A. Congenital goitre in South African Boer goats. J S Afr Vet Med Assoc 1971;42:295–303.

Watson AD. Congenital hyperthyroid dwarfism in a family of Giant schnauzers. J Vet Intern Med 1991;5:306–307.

Wilson JG. Hypothyroidism in ruminants with special reference to foetal goats. Vet Rec 1975;97:161–164.

Wright E, Sinclair DP. The goitrogenic effect of thousand-headed kale (*Brassica oleracea*, var. *acephala*) on adult sheep and rabbits. NZ Vet Agric Res 1958;1:477–485.

NEOPLASMS OF THE THYROID

Neoplasms of the thyroid may originate from follicular cells, C cells, and mesenchymal cells. The majority of thyroid neoplasms are of follicular cell origin and are of several histologic patterns. They may lead to hyperthyroidism—often the case in cats—or hypothyroidism through destruction of the gland. Tumors of C cells are often termed medullary adenomas and medullary carcinomas, and may secrete excessive calcitonin. Neoplasms containing both follicular epithelium and C cells also occur. Often these cells represent the entrapment of either follicular remnants or C cells, but true **mixed thyroid neoplasms** with neoplastic follicular and C-cell components also occur.

Follicular adenoma Follicular adenoma is encountered as single or multiple nodules in one or both lobes of the thyroid. They are most common in cats, followed in order of frequency by dogs and horses. Adenomas are circumscribed masses encapsulated by thin connective tissue; they grow by expansion, compressing adjacent thyroid. Epithelial cells usually form follicles that are smaller than normal thyroid follicles (**microfollicular adenomas**), but may also form solid cords several cells in thickness (**trabecular adenomas**). The resemblance to normal thyroid follicles is usually unmistakable and their presence within the thyroid is characteristic. Cells are usually low-cuboidal and uniform. In some cases, these cells form a papillary pattern and are called "papillary adenoma." Some adenomas contain one or more centrally placed cysts (**cystic adenoma**) filled with mineralized necrotic debris and lined by a fibrous capsule which, in turn, is lined by projecting fronds of epithelial cells forming follicles of a compact cellular pattern. The significance of this difference in growth pattern is not presently understood. Nodular hyperplasia of the thyroid may be difficult, if not impossible, to differentiate from adenoma. Features generally used include the following: when it is solitary, it is an adenoma; and adenomas tend to be well encapsulated, whereas nodular hyperplasia is not.

Carcinomas of follicular cells Carcinomas of follicular cells are most frequent in dogs (Fig. 26-4)—more so than adenomas—and have an increased occurrence of metastasis. Carcinomas in all species occur in several different histologic patterns (Fig. 26-5).

FOLLICULAR ADENOCARCINOMA Follicular adenocarcinoma is composed of cuboidal or columnar cells, which form follicles containing variable amounts of colloid. The follicles are usually microfollicular, but often contain both large and small follicles of various shapes. The follicular pattern is often mixed with papillary zones and the amount of stroma is varied. This appears to be the least malignant histologic type, but local invasion into capsule and blood vessels and metastases to lungs and lymph nodes have been reported, particularly in dogs.

Follicular carcinoma is the usual histologic type in which cells produce thyroxine, which results in clinical signs of thyrotoxicosis or hyperthyroidism.

COMPACT CELLULAR (SOLID) CARCINOMAS Compact cellular, or solid, carcinomas of the thyroid have a gross appearance of firm masses, with a smooth external surface and a uniform creamy, cut surface. The micro-

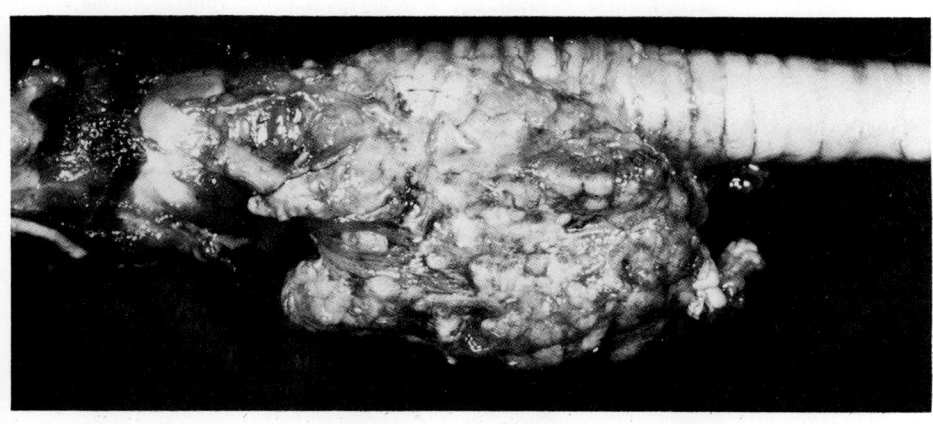

FIG. 26-4 Adenocarcinoma of the left thyroid of a 12-year-old male cocker spaniel. Note the relation of the tumor mass to the larynx and trachea. (Courtesy of Angell Memorial Animal Hospital.)

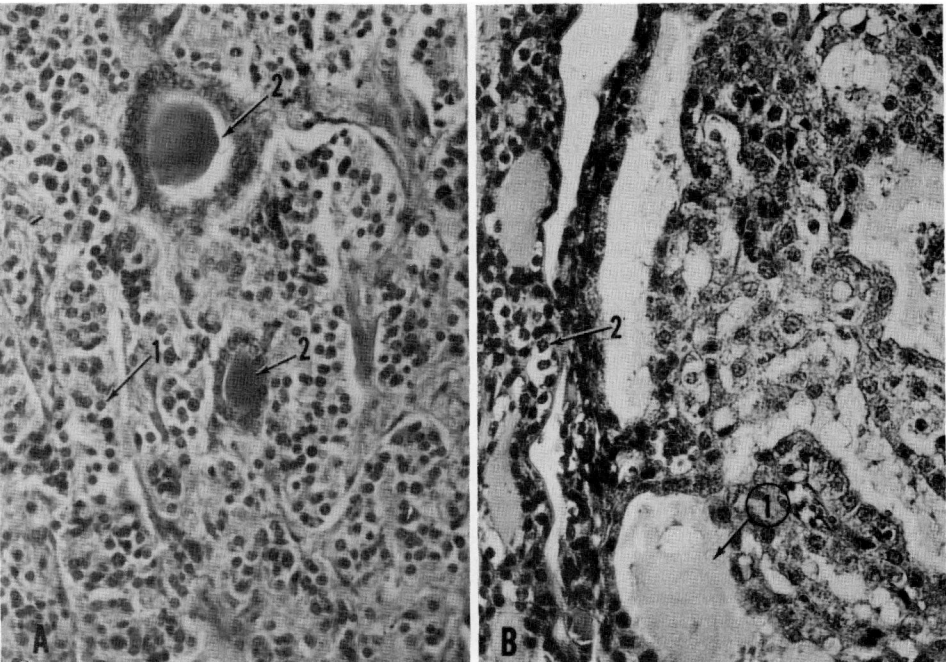

FIG. 26-5 A. Adenocarcinoma of the thyroid of an eight-year-old cow. (1) Solid nests of cells; (2) Acini-containing colloid. (Contributor: Dr. C. L. Davis.) **B.** Adenoma of the thyroid of a ten-year-old male cat. (1) The tumor (×335) is forming large acini; and (2) Compresses the adjacent normal thyroid tissue. (Courtesy of Armed Forces Institute of Pathology; contributor: Dr. Leo L. Lieberman.)

scopic appearance is one of solid sheets of closely packed cells, with a fine stroma dividing the tumor into lobules. Cells are uniform in appearance, with a centrally placed nucleus and granular, lightly eosinophilic cytoplasm. Pleomorphic and large nuclei are not seen often and mitoses are rare. Clusters of cells with somewhat more abundant and dense granular cytoplasm (Hurthle cells) are occasionally evident. Cells often invade the capsule, adjacent thyroid, and blood or lymph vessels. This tumor must be differentiated from medullary carcinoma. **Compact cellular and follicular carcinoma** (solid carcinoma and follicular carcinoma) are terms used to indicate a mixture of these two histologic types.

PAPILLARY CARCINOMA Papillary carcinoma of the thyroid is recognized by the tendency of the epithelial cells to be arranged in fronds of intermixed projections supported by a fine stroma. Nuclei are occasionally pleomorphic and sometimes vesicular; others may have a "ground-glass" appearance. Capsular and vascular invasions are often found. In most cases, the papillary structure is mixed with a follicular pattern in the same tumor. The papillary type is more often seen in the cat than in the dog.

SQUAMOUS CELL CARCINOMA Squamous cell carcinoma of the thyroid is an infrequent tumor in animals, but is occasionally encountered. Cells are similar to those seen in squamous cell carcinoma arising at other sites. Epithelial cells are large and polyhedral; they may form keratin and are often connected by intercellular bridges. These tumors may arise from remnants of the thyroglossal duct or by metaplasia from thyroid epithelium. Squamous cell carcinomas originating in the tonsillar crypt in the dog may reach the thyroid, but are more apt to be found in the nearby lymph nodes.

ANAPLASTIC CARCINOMAS Anaplastic (undifferentiated, giant-cell) carcinomas of the thyroid are so classified on the basis of their cellular pleomorphism and lack of differentiation. The pattern of growth is usually solid, but cells may be individualized and the stroma desmoplastic. Some are made up of small, elongated epithelial cells and are called "spindle-cell carcinoma." Others contain many large multinucleated giant cells ("giant-cell carcinoma") or diffuse small cells ("diffuse small-cell carcinoma").

Disorders of C cells (parafollicular cells)

Disorders of C cells are primarily limited to hyperplastic and neoplastic changes. Among domestic animals, these changes are most commonly encountered in bulls, where they are often part of ultimobranchial tumors. They are, however, also encountered in humans, dogs, sheep, and other species, and are particularly frequent in laboratory rats. Hyperplasia, C-cell adenoma (**medullary adenoma**), C-cell carcinoma (**medullary carcinoma**), and ultimobranchial tumors may represent different stages of a single process initiated by long-standing high dietary calcium intake. Bulls receiving diets high in calcium are prone to developing each of these lesions, which decline in incidence when the animal is returned to a diet lower in calcium. This, however, is not the case with cows; this is believed to be due to an increased demand for dietary calcium, although medullary carcinoma has been reported in cows. C-cell hyperplasia/neoplasia is also encountered in other species, where a relationship to dietary calcium is not clear. In humans, 15–20% of medullary carcinomas are part of a multiple endocrine neoplasia syndrome that is genetically transmitted as an autosomal-dominant trait.

These occur in younger individuals than do the remainder of medullary carcinomas. An increased incidence of hyperplasia/neoplasia of C cells, beginning at an early age in Long-Evans rats, has been suggested to be a similar familial disorder. Reported in rats is an increased incidence of ganglioneuromas of the thyroid, in association with C-cell proliferation. Although hyperplasia and neoplasia of C cells may result in an increased secretion of calcitonin, this ordinarily does not lead to functional abnormalities; however, hypocalcemia has been described in bulls, dogs, and rats.

The differentiation between C-cell and follicular cell tumors is often not obvious in routine tissue sections and requires special staining techniques. C cells contain membrane-bound secretory granules not present in follicular cells. They can be confirmed to be C cells by their reaction to stains for calcitonin, calcitonin gene-related peptide (CGRP), neuron-specific enolase (NSE), and somatostatin; however, species differ in the degree of reaction to these substrates. In the majority of species, calcitonin and NSE are the most reliable; however, CGRP is considered the most reliable identifier in dogs.

HYPERPLASIA OF C CELLS

Hyperplasia of C cells is characterized by a diffuse and sometimes focal increase in the number of C cells surrounding follicles. These cells may fill follicles—producing small clusters of cells—and sometimes form larger discrete nodules that compress adjacent follicles. The latter may be difficult to differentiate from C-cell adenoma, but this may only be academic. Cells are well-differentiated with a central nucleus and abundant pale eosinophilic cytoplasm.

ADENOMA OF C CELLS

Adenoma of C cells is characterized by a single or multifocal nodular collection of well-differentiated C cells. Cells are arranged within the nodules in small clusters where they have filled follicles. Nodules are circumscribed, which is the predominant differentiating feature from hyperplasia of C cells. Deposits of amyloid are often present. In bulls, the tumors are often sclerotic with extensive deposition of collagenous connective tissue.

CARCINOMA OF C CELLS (MEDULLARY CARCINOMA)

Medullary carcinoma usually involves only one lobe of the thyroid; the cut surface is yellow or cream-colored and may be divided into lobules by indistinct septa. In bulls, the tumors appear to arise most often in the hilus of one thyroid lobe. Tumor cells may be large, polygonal cells with foamy or finely granular cytoplasm, or fusiform cells with bright eosinophilic, granular cytoplasm and hyperchromatic, irregular nuclei. Histologically identifiable lobules may have characteristic rows of tall columnar cells with nuclei in rows adjacent to thin fibrous stroma. Several features distinguish carcinoma of C cells from adenoma: cells are less-differentiated with less cytoplasm; they often appear spindle-shaped; and mitotic figures are more numerous. Carcinomas invade within the thyroid and beyond into adjacent tissue. They contain variable amounts of fibrovascular stroma and may be encapsulated. Amyloid is present in some examples. Metastasis to distant sites, usually the lung, is frequent.

MIXED THYROID CARCINOMA (ULTIMOBRANCHIAL TUMORS)

Tumors arising in the ultimobranchial remnants are common in older bulls. They may arise outside or within the thyroid and are often found in conjunction with hyperplasia/neoplasia of C cells in other parts of the thyroid. Ultimobranchial tumors have complex structures of multiple patterns and cell types. They contain follicles often containing colloid which resemble normal thyroid follicles, follicles lined by a tall epithelium, and follicles whose lining forms a cribriform pattern. In addition, there are tubular structures and solid areas composed of small basophilic cells mixed with light polyhedric cells containing abundant cytoplasm. Collections of light cells typical of well-differentiated C cells are present throughout the tumors in variable numbers. Immunohistochemistry demonstrates thyroglobulin immunoreactivity in cells lining follicles, cysts, and tubules. Calcitonin-positive cells are also present within these same structures, as well as within the solid parts of the tumors. These same cells also react for somatostatin.

The occurrence of C-cell hyperplasia, C-cell tumors, and ultimobranchial tumors in bulls receiving high levels of dietary calcium has already been mentioned. In bulls, ultimobranchial neoplasms also often occur in conjunction with pheochromocytomas. In one family of Guernsey bulls, the simultaneous occurrence of both neoplasms has been reported to result from an autosomal-dominant trait. This has been compared to **Sipple syndrome** or **multiple endocrine neoplasia syndrome type 2** in humans.

Mesenchymal tumors

Mesenchymal tumors—such as fibrosarcomas, osteosarcomas, and chondrosarcomas—are occasionally encountered in the thyroid. Their features are described elsewhere.

EPITHELIAL-MESENCHYMAL TUMORS

Epithelial-mesenchymal tumors have been described in the canine thyroid. These tumors may contain both elements of follicular carcinoma and undifferentiated sarcoma in the same primary tumor or in its metastases. When they are found adjacent to one another, these epithelial and mesenchymal elements have been described as "coexistent." Conversely, should these cells be mixed together, the term carcinosarcoma has been applied. Whether this condition involves similar problems and controversies to those surrounding the canine mixed mammary tumor is unknown.

SECONDARY NEOPLASMS

Secondary neoplasms, metastatic to the thyroid, may be observed in animals. Squamous cell carcinoma arising in the tonsillar crypt of the dog may occasionally involve the thyroid as well as the anterior cervical lymph nodes. Lymphosarcoma may also occur as a secondary tumor in the thyroid.

References

Anderson PG, Capen CC. Undifferentiated spindle cell carcinoma of the thyroid in a dog. Vet Pathol 1986;23:203–204.

Bentley JF, Simpson ST, Hathcock JT, et al. Metastatic thyroid solid-follicular carcinoma in the cervical portion of the spine of a dog. J Am Vet Med Assoc 1990;197:1498–1500.

Birchard SJ, Roesel OF. Neoplasia of the thyroid gland in the dog: a retrospective study of 16 cases. J Am Anim Hosp Assoc 1981;17:369–372.

Black HE, Capen CC, Young DM. Ultimobranchial thyroid neoplasms in bulls. A syndrome resembling medullary thyroid carcinoma in man. Cancer 1973;32:865–878.

Boorman GA, van Noord MJ, Hollander CF. Naturally occurring medullary thyroid carcinoma in the rat. Arch Pathol 1972;94:35–41.

Boorman GA, Heersche JNM, Hollander CF. Transplantable calcitonin-secreting medullary carcinomas of the thyroid of the WAG/Rij rat. JNCI 1974;53:1011–1015.

Bundza A, Stead RH. Medullary thyroid carcinoma in two cows. Vet Pathol 1986;23:90–92.

Capen CC, Black HE. Medullary thyroid carcinoma, multiple endocrine neoplasia, Sipple's syndrome. Animal model: ultimobranchial thyroid neoplasm in the bull. Am J Pathol 1974;74:377–380.

Chastain CB, Hill BL, Nichols CE. Excess triiodothyronine production by a thyroid adenocarcinoma in a dog. J Am Vet Med Assoc 1980;177:172–173.

Cheville NF. Ultrastructure of canine carotid body and aortic body tumors: comparison with tissues of thyroid and parathyroid origin. Vet Pathol 1972;9:166–189.

Crissman JW, Valerio MG, Asiedu SA, et al. Ganglioneuromas of the thyroid gland in a colony of Sprague-Dawley rats. Vet Pathol 1991;28:354–362.

Harari J, Patterson JS, Rosenthal RC. Clinical and pathologic features of thyroid tumors in 26 dogs. J Am Vet Med Assoc 1986;188:1160–1164.

Haley PJ, Hahn FF, Muggenburg BA, Griffith WC. Thyroid neoplasms in a colony of beagle dogs. Vet Pathol 1989;26:438–441.

Holm R, Sobrinho-Simoes M, Nesland JM, et al. Medullary thyroid carcinoma with thyroglobulin immunoreactivity. A special entity? Lab Invest 1987;57:28–268.

Holscher MA, Davis BW, Wilson RB, et al. Ectopic thyroid tumor in a dog: thyroglobulin, calcitonin, and neuron-specific enolase immunocytochemical studies. Vet Pathol 1986;23:778–779.

Hovda LR, Shaftoe S, Rose ML, et al. Mediastinal squamous cell carcinoma and thyroid carcinoma in an aged horse. J Am Vet Med Assoc 1990;197:1187–1189.

Johnson KH, Osborne CA. Adenocarcinoma of the thyroid gland in a cat. J Am Vet Med Assoc 1970;156:906–912.

Jones EE, Barker J, Dietrich S. Spontaneous tumors of the thyroid gland in mice. JNCI 1966;36:1–14.

Joyce JR, Thompson RB, Kyzar JR, et al. Thyroid carcinoma in a horse. J Am Vet Med Assoc 1976;168:610–612.

Jubb KV, McEntee K. The relationship of ultimobranchial remnants and derivatives to tumor of the thyroid gland in cattle. Cornell Vet 1958;44:41–69.

Kaspareit-Rittinghausen J, Wiese K, Deerberg F, et al. The incidence and morphology of spontaneous thyroid tumours in different strains of rats. J Comp Pathol 1990;102:421–432.

Krook L, Olsson S, Rooney JR. Thyroid carcinoma in the dog: a case of bone-metastasizing carcinoma simulating secondary hyperparathyroidism. Cornell Vet 1960;50:106–114.

Leav I, Schiller AL, Rijnberk A, et al. Adenomas and carcinomas of the canine and feline thyroid. Am J Pathol 1976;83:61–122.

Leblanc B, Parodi AL, Lagadic M, et al. Immunocytochemistry of canine thyroid tumors. Vet Pathol 1991;28:370–380.

Ljungberg O, Nilsson P-O. Hyperplastic and neoplastic changes in ultimobranchial remnants and in parafollicular "C" cells in bulls: a histologic and immunohistochemical study. Vet Pathol 1985;22:95–103.

Long GG, Clemmons RM, Heath H III. Metastatic canine medullary thyroid carcinoma. Vet Pathol 1980;17:323–330.

McClelland RB. Carcinoma of the thyroid: a report of five cases in dogs. J Am Vet Med Assoc 1941;98:38–40.

Meyers JS, Abdel-Bari W. The syndrome of excessive calcitonin produced by medullary carcinoma of the thyroid gland. N Engl J Med 1968;278:523.

Okada H, Fujimoto Y, Oshima K, et al. C cell hyperplasia and carcinoma developing in sheep with experimentally-induced lymphosarcoma. J Comp Pathol 1991;105:313–322.

Patnaik AK, et al. Canine medullary carcinoma of the thyroid. Vet Pathol 1978;15:590–599.

Patnaik AK, Lieberman PH. Feline anaplastic giant cell adenocarcinoma of the thyroid. Vet Pathol 1979;16:687–692.

Patnaik AK, Lieberman PH. Gross, histologic, cytochemical, and immunocytochemical study of medullary thyroid carcinoma in sixteen dogs. Vet Pathol 1991;28:223–233.

Payne CM, Nagle RB, Borduin V. An ultrastructural cytochemical stain specific for neuroendocrine neoplasms. Lab Invest 1984;51:350–365.

Schlumberger HG. Spontaneous goiter and cancer of the thyroid in animals. Ohio J Sci 1955;55:23–43.

Thake DC, Cheville NF, Sharp RK. Ectopic thyroid adenomas at the base of the heart of the dog: ultrastructural identification of dense tubular structures in endoplasmic reticulum. Vet Pathol 1971;8:421–432.

Turk JR, Nakata YJ, Leathers CW, et al. Ultimobranchial adenoma of the thyroid gland in a horse. Vet Pathol 1983;20:114–117.

Turrel JM, Feldman EC, Nelson RW, et al. Thyroid carcinoma causing hyperthyroidism in cats: 14 cases (1981–1986). J Am Vet Med Assoc 1988;193:359–364.

van der Velden MA, Meulenaar H. Medullary thyroid carcinoma in a horse. Vet Pathol 1986;23:622–624.

Vitovec J. Epithelial thyroid tumors in cows. Vet Pathol 1976;13:401–408.

Wilkie BN, Krook L. Ultimobranchial tumour of the thyroid and pheochromocytoma in the bull. Pathol Vet 1970;7:126–134.

Young DM, Capen CC, Black HE. Calcitonin activity in ultimobranchial neoplasms of bulls. Vet Pathol 1971;8:19–27.

PARATHYROID GLANDS

The parathyroid glands—usually consisting of four glands, two on either side of the midline—occur in the upper cervical region and are often in contact with or embedded within the thyroid. The parathyroids arise embryologically from the III and IV pharyngeal pouches. All air-breathing vertebrates have parathyroids. The functioning cells are called **chief cells,** which are concerned with the secretion of parathyroid hormone (PTH). Chief cells are polygonal with eosinophilic cytoplasm and a central round nucleus. Secretory granules are present in the cytoplasm; their numbers vary with cell activity. At any one time most cells are inactive, with only a few secretory granules. Parathormone is a straight-chain polypeptide, consisting of 84 amino-acid residues, with a molecular weight of 9500. Proparathyroid hormone is synthesized first on ribosomes of the chief cells, from which active parathyroid hormone is then cleaved enzymatically before it is released from the chief cells.

In concert with two other hormones, thyrocalcitonin and vitamin D, parathyroid hormone exercises precise control of the level of calcium ions in the blood. Calcium is involved in key roles in several biologic processes (blood coagulation, muscle contraction, neural excitability, enzyme activity, hormone release, and membrane permeability) and is an essential component of bone structure. The health of humans and animals, therefore, depends upon the precise control of calcium in circulating blood and body fluids. PTH acts at the level of bone, kidney and, indirectly, the intestine. At the level of bone, PTH stimulates the release of calcium into the blood through both an immediate and a delayed effect mediated by osteoclastic bone resorption. The effect on osteoclasts, which do not have receptors for PTH, is mediated through osteoblasts, which do have PTH receptors, by their release of cytokines. PTH also can—under appropriate circumstances, such as periodic administration—have an anabolic effect on bone, leading to increased bone formation. At the level of the kidney, PTH increases tubular resorption of calcium while increasing phosphate excretion; it also increases the tubular synthesis of 1,25-dihydroxy vitamin D, which is required for intestinal absorption of calcium.

Important diseases of the parathyroid glands, as with all endocrines, are those that either decrease or increase the secretion of parathyroid hormone (hypoparathyroidism and hyperparathyroidism, respectively). Normal secretion of parathyroid hormone is regulated by a negative feedback system in which increased blood levels of calcium cause decreased production of parathyroid hormone. Increased production of thyrocalcitonin, stimulated by high levels of blood calcium, acts to decrease blood levels of calcium.

Parathyroid glands contain another cell type termed the **oxyphil cell.** These are larger than chief cells, have more intensely eosinophilic cytoplasm, and contain few to no secretory granules. They are believed to be derived from chief cells; often, cells intermediate between the two are present. Multinucleated **syncytial cells** are frequently present in dogs and humans. These cells, believed to be derived from the fusion of chief cells, contain 2–30 nuclei. Their functional significance is not known.

Important diseases of the parathyroid glands, as with all endocrine organs, are those that either decrease or increase the secretion of parathyroid hormone. Other pathologic findings include **cysts** and **aberrant parathyroids** that may be located in the thymus and serve as a rare site of parathyroid neoplasms.

References

Altenahr E. Ultrastructural pathology of parathyroid glands. Curr Top Pathol 1972;56:1–54.

Bergdahl L, Boquist L. Parathyroid morphology in normal dogs. Pathol Eur 1973;8:95–103.

Boquist L, Lundgren E. Effects of variations in calcium concentration on parathyroid morphology in vitro. Lab Invest 1975;33:638–647.

Capen CC, Koestner A, Cole CR. The ultrastructure and histochemistry of normal parathyroid glands of pregnant and nonpregnant cows. Lab Invest 1965;14:1673–1690.

Capen CC, Rowland GN. The ultrastructure of the parathyroid glands of young cats. Anat Rec 1968;162:327–331.

Capen CC. Functional and fine structural relationships of parathyroid glands. Adv Vet Sci Comp Med 1975;19:249–286.

Fetter AW, Capen CC. The ultrastructure of the parathyroid glands of young pigs. Acta Anat 1970;75:359–372.

Jowsey J, Reiss E, Canterbury JM. Long-term effects of high phosphate intake on parathyroid hormone levels and bone metabolism. Acta Orthop Scand 1974;45:801–808.

Meuten DJ, Capen CC, Thompson KG, et al. Syncytial cells in canine parathyroid glands. Vet Pathol 1984;21:463–468.

Persson J, Luthman J. Some acute metabolic effects of parathyroid hormone in sheep. Acta Vet Scand 1974;15:381–397.

Potts JT, Ambach GD, Sherwood LM, et al. Structural basis of biological and immunological activity of parathyroid hormone. Proc Natl Acad Sci USA 1965;54:1743–1751.

Roth SI, Capen CC. Ultrastructural and functional correlations of the parathyroid gland. Rev Exp Pathol 1974;13:161–221.

Waterhouse C, Heinig RE. Parathormone levels vs. parathormone function. N Engl J Med 1972;294:545–546.

Weisbrode SE, Capen CC, Nagode LA. Effects of parathyroid hormone on bone of thyroparathyroidectomized rats: an ultrastructural and enzymatic study. Am J Pathol 1974;75:529–542.

Hypoparathyroidism

A severely depressed level of parathyroid hormone results in a low concentration of blood calcium and tonic (or tetanic) spasms of muscle known as **parathyroid tetany.** These signs appear within two days following surgical extirpation of all parathyroid glands.

Hypoparathyroidism is not frequent as a spontaneous disease. It may develop subsequent to inflammatory disease of the parathyroids or to their destruction through adjacent neoplasms. PTH secretion is also suppressed following prolonged hypercalcemia. Diets high in calcium fed to cows can result in atrophy of chief cells and concomitant failure of secretion, a mechanism that may be important to **parturient paresis.** High dietary level of vitamin D has the same effect. Increased dietary calcium intake by growing dogs also suppresses PTH secretion (Nunez et al., 1974; Black et al., 1973; Capen, 1975).

End-organ unresponsiveness to PTH occurs in **pseudohypoparathyroidism,** a hereditary disease ocurring in humans. PTH levels are normal or elevated. Hypersecretion of calcitonin by medullary or C-cell adenomas or adenocarcinomas of bulls, rats, and dogs has an inhibiting effect upon parathyroid secretion. Experimental administration of L-asparaginase to rabbits is reported to result in severe hypoparathyroidism with tetany. Experimentally-induced hypoparathyroidism is also reported as a result of production of isoimmune parathyroiditis in dogs (Capen, 1975).

References

Berger B, Feldman EC. Primary hyperparathyroidism in dogs: 21 cases (1976–1986). J Am Vet Med Assoc 1987;191:350–356.

Black HE, Capen CC, Arnaud CD. Ultrastructure of parathyroid glands and plasma immunoreactive parathyroid hormone in pregnant cows fed normal and high calcium diets. Lab Invest 1973;29:173–185.

Capen CC, Koestner A, Cole CR. The ultrastructure, histopathology, and histochemistry of the parathyroid glands of pregnant and nonpregnant cows fed a high level of vitamin D. Lab Invest 1965;14:1809–1825.

Capen CC, Young DM. The ultrastructure of the parathyroid glands and thyroid parafollicular cells of cows with parturient paresis and hypocalcemia. Lab Invest 1967;17:717–737.

Capen CC, Cole CR, Hibbs JW. Influence of vitamin D on calcium metabolism and the parathyroid glands of cattle. Fed Proc 1968;27:141–152.

Forbes S, Nelson RW, Guptill L. Primary hypoparathyroidism in a cat. J Am Vet Med Assoc 1990;196:1285–1287.

Hedhammer A, et al. Overnutrition and skeletal disease: an experimental study in growing Great Dane dogs. Cornell Vet 1974;65:1–160.

Meyer DJ, Terrell TG. Idiopathic hypoparathyroidism in a dog. J Am Vet Med Assoc 1976;168:858–860.

Nunez EA, et al. Ultrastructure of the parafollicular "C" cells and the parathyroid in growing dogs on high calcium diet. Lab Invest 1974;31:96–108.

Tettenborn D, Hobik HP, Luckhaus G. Hypoparathyreoidosmus beim Kaninchen nach Varabreichung von L-asparaginase. Arzneim Forsch 1970;20:1753–1755.

Hyperparathyroidism

Increased synthesis and secretion of parathyroid hormone may result from any of several causes (to be described later). Clinical signs include: weakness, polydipsia, and polyuria associated with hypercalcemia; reduced serum phosphate; increased urinary excretion of inorganic phosphorus; and urinary calculi associated with nephrocalcinosis. Generalized demineralization of the skeleton may lead to bone pain and pathologic fractures. The cortex of long bones becomes thinner and the bones of skull, mandible, and maxilla less radiopaque. Serum levels of alkaline phosphatase elevate and secretion of urinary hydroxyproline increases.

The effect on the skeleton is one of intensified resorption leading to fibrous osteodystrophy. Calcium is also deposited in soft tissues, especially in the elastica of aorta and arteries, pulmonary arteries, cardiac atria, and coronary arteries. Calcification in the kidneys and walls of bronchi and bronchioles may also be conspicuous (refer to section on *metastatic calcification*).

Primary hyperparathyroidism may arise from (1) primary hyperplasia of the parathyroids, (2) functional parathyroid adenoma or adenocarcinoma, or (3) hypersecretion of parathyroids from an unknown cause.

SECONDARY HYPERPARATHYROIDISM

Secondary hyperparathyroidism (Fig. 26-6) results from parathyroid hyperplasia and increased secretion of parathyroid hormone due to renal or nutritional causes. **Renal hyperparathyroidism** (renal osteodystrophy, renal rickets, osteorenal syndrome) is associated with chronic renal insufficiency in humans, rats, and dogs (Fig. 26-7). The secondary hyperparathyroidism associated with renal disease is ascribed to chronic hypocalcemia leading to excessive production of parathyroid hormone. In the progressive renal disease, reduction in glomerular filtration leads to retention of phosphorus and progressive hyperphosphatemia. This decreases the blood calcium. Reduced synthesis of 1,25-dihydrocholecalciferol by diseased kidneys leads to reduced intestinal absorption of calcium.

Skeletal lesions of secondary renal hypoparathyroidism are described in Chapter 19.

Nutritional secondary hyperparathyroidism has been described in humans, horses, cats, dogs, cows, nonhuman primates, domestic and wild birds, and reptiles. The essential deficiency in causal diets is either (1) inadequate amount of calcium, (2) inadequate or inappropriate vitamin D (vitamin D_3 is required by many species), (3) relatively high amounts of phosphorus in the presence of an otherwise adequate amount of calcium, or (4) some combination of the first three factors. Historical examples include all-bran diets fed to miller's horses, the all-meat diets (heart and kidneys) fed to kittens and wild felidae in zoos, and the all-meat diets fed to dogs. Lesions in all these situations are described in Chapter 19.

References

Deluca HF. The kidney as an endocrine organ involved in the function of vitamin D. Am J Med 1975;58:39–47.

Hunt RD, Garcia FG, Hegsted DM. A comparison of vitamin D_2 and D_3 in New World primates. I. Production and regression of osteodystrophy fibrosa. Lab Anim Care 1967;17:222–234.

Ichido S. Pathological studies on the osteorenal syndrome in the dog. Jpn J Vet Sci 1966;28:217–228.

Ingelfinger FJ. Pathogenesis of renal osteodystrophy—a role for calcitonin? N Engl J Med 1977;296:1112–1114.

Itakura C, Iida M, Goto M. Renal secondary hyperparathyroidism in aged Sprague-Dawley rats. Vet Pathol 1977;14:463–469.

Jackson CE, Talbert PC, Caylor HD. Hereditary hyperparathyroidism. J Indiana State Med Assoc 1960;53:1313–1316.

Platt H: The parathyroid glands with particular reference to the "rubber jaw" syndrome. The skeletal system in "rubber jaw". J Comp Pathol Therap 1951;61:188–196, 197–214.

Rowland GN, Capen CC, Nagode LA. Experimental hyperparathyroidism in young cats. Pathol Vet 1968;5:504–509.

Scott PP. Special features of nutrition of cats, with observations on wild felidae nutrition in the London Zoo. Symp Zool Soc Lond 1968;21:21–36.

Thompson KG, et al. Primary hyperparathyroidism in German shepherd dogs: a disorder of probable genetic origin. Vet Pathol 1984;21:370–376.

Weir EC, Norrdin RW, Barthold SW, et al. Primary hyperparathyroidism in a dog: biochemical, bone histomorphometric, and pathologic findings. J Am Vet Med Assoc 1986;189:1471–1474.

Wilson JW, Harris SG, Moore WD, et al. Primary hyperparathyroidism in a dog. J Am Vet Med Assoc 1974;164:942–946.

PSEUDOHYPERPARATHYROIDISM

Pseudohyperparathyroidism is a term applied to a disease that closely resembles hyperparathyroidism, but which occurs in the presence of normal parathyroids. It is also termed **humoral hypercalcemia of malignancy,** and results from the elaboration of factors

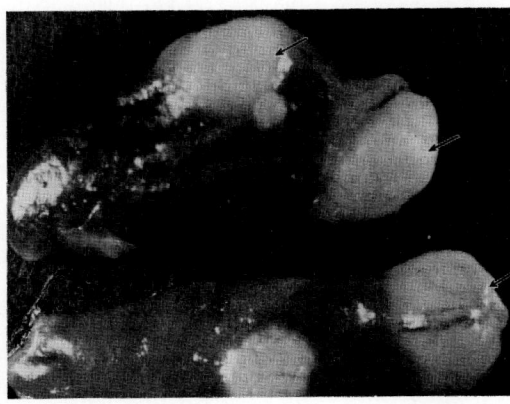

FIG. 26-6 Secondary hyperplasia of parathyroids in a seven-year-old male Airedale with chronic interstitial nephritis. Enlarged gray parathyroids (*arrows*) stand out against the dark-brown thyroids. (Courtesy of Angell Memorial Animal Hospital.)

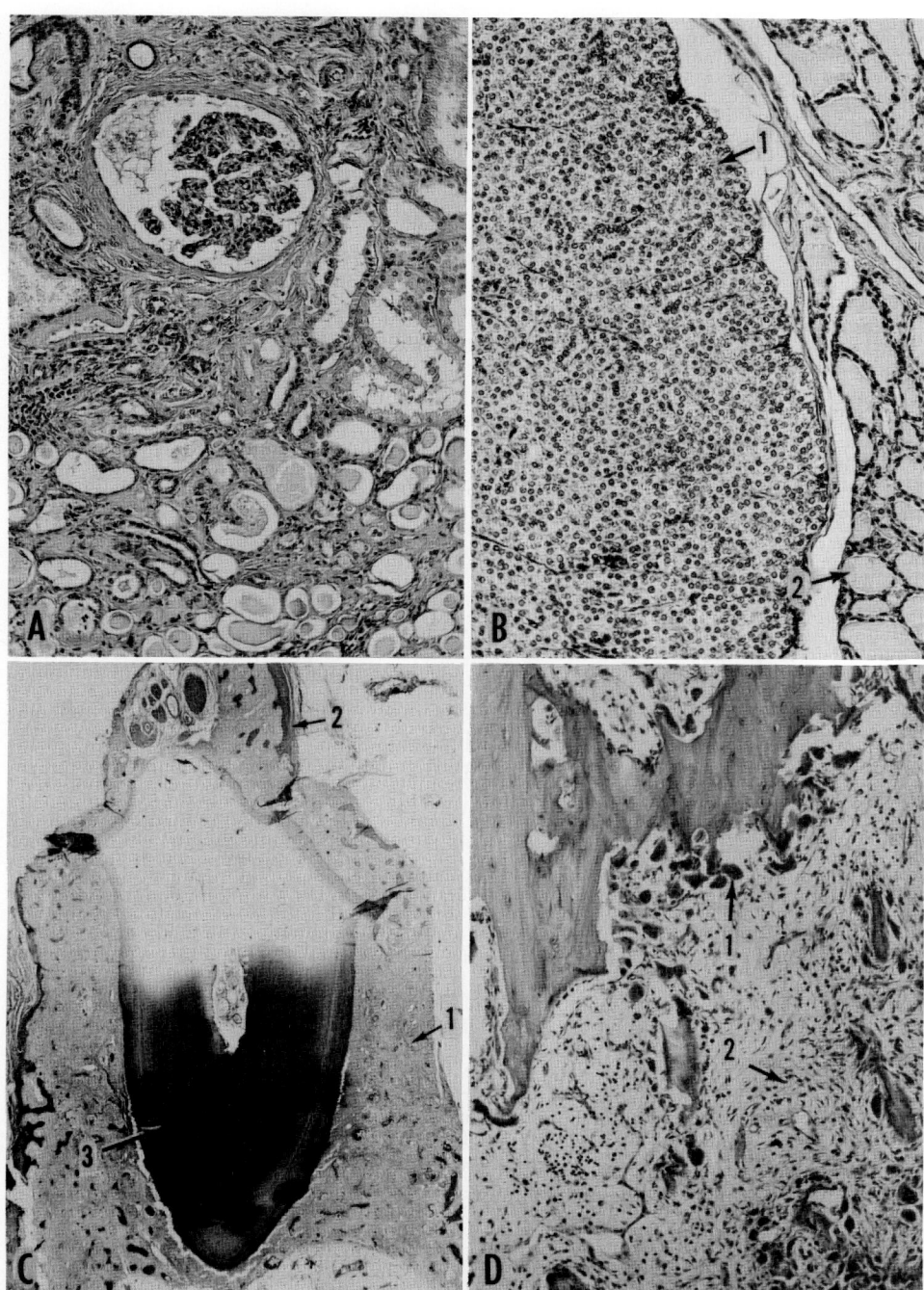

FIG. 26-7 Renal hyperparathyroidism in a dog. **A.** The kidney (×110). **B.** The parathyroid. (1) Enlarged; (2) Compressing adjacent thyroid. **C.** A tooth (×11) poorly supported by soft, spongy bone. (1) Note absence of bone trabeculae; (2) Gingival epithelium; (3) Dentine of the root of the tooth. **D.** The mandible (×145). (1) Note many osteoblasts; (2) Fibrous marrow; and (3) Irregular spicules of bone. (Courtesy of Armed Forces Institute of Pathology; contributor: Dr. Joseph M. Stoyak.)

that mimic the action of parathyroid hormone by neoplasms of other organs and tissues. One of these factors is parathyroid hormone-related protein (PTHrP), which is produced by many cell types, but does not normally enter the circulation. PTHrP binds to parathyroid hormone receptors and induces bone resorption, leading to hypercalcemia. Other factors with hypercalcemic effects include interleukin-1 and tumor necrosis factors (TNF)-α and -β. Tumors of animals most frequently associated with this syndrome are lymphomas and adenocarcinomas of the apocrine glands of the anal sac in dogs. This form of hypercalcemia is also a feature of a rat Leydig cell tumor line and a rat

Walker mammary carcinosarcoma. In humans, squamous cell carcinoma of the lung is the most frequent cause.

References

Engelman RW, Tyler RD, Good RA, et al. Hypercalcemia in cats with feline-leukemia-virus-associated leukemia-lymphoma. Cancer 1985;56:777–781.

Hause WR, Stevenson S, Meuten DJ, et al. Pseudohyperparathyroidism associated with adenocarcinomas of anal sac origin in four dogs. J Am Anim Hosp Assoc 1981;17:373–379.

Knill-Jones RP, et al. Hypercalcemia and increased parathyroid-hormone activity in a primary hepatoma. N Engl J Med 1970; 282:704–708.

Merryman JI, Rosol TJ, Brooks CL, et al. Separation of parathyroid hormone-like activity from transforming growth factor-alpha and -beta in the canine adenocarcinoma (CAC-8) model of humoral hypercalcemia of malignancy. Endocrinology 1989;124:2456–2463.

Merryman JI, Capen CC, McCauley LK, et al. Regulation of parathyroid hormone-related protein production by a squamous carcinoma cell line *in vitro*. Lab Invest 1993;69:347–354.

Osborne CA, Stevens JB. Pseudohyperparathyroidism in the dog. J Am Vet Med Assoc 1973;162:125–135.

Rijnberk A. Pseudohyperparathyroidism in the dog. Tijdschr Diergeneeskd 1970;95:515.

Rosol TJ, Capen CC. Pathogenesis of humoral hypercalcemia of malignancy. Domestic Anim Endocrinol 1988;51:1–21.

Rosol TJ, Capen CC. Tumors of the parathyroid gland and circulating parathyroid hormone-related protein associated with persistent hypercalcemia. Toxicol Pathol 1989;17:346–356.

Rosol TJ, Nagode LA, Robertson JT, et al. Humoral hypercalcemia of malignancy associated with ameloblastoma in a horse. J Am Vet Med Assoc 1994;204:1930–1933.

Suva LJ, et al. A parathyroid hormone-related protein implicated in malignant hypercalcemia: cloning and expression. Science 1987;237:893–896.

Primary hyperplasia and neoplasia of parathyroid glands

PRIMARY PARATHYROID HYPERPLASIA

This rare disorder of animals is characterized by single or multiple nodules of chief cells within one or more of the parathyroids. The nodules compress adjacent tissue; however, in contrast to adenomas, the nodules are not encapsulated. As with nodular hyperplasia of other organs, however, their differentiation from adenomas is not always apparent. Hyperplasia is encountered most often in dogs and laboratory rodents. Rare examples of diffuse hyperplasia have been encountered in puppies. The cause of primary parathyroid hyperplasia is unknown.

Adenoma of parathyroid Adenomas of the parathyroid gland are rare. They have been reported in dogs, laboratory rats, and Syrian hamsters. Among dogs, the incidence in Keeshonds appears to be disproportionally increased in comparison to other breeds. They occur as single nodules composed of well-differentiated chief cells surrounded by a thin, fibrous, connective-tissue capsule. The adjacent parathyroid is compressed and atrophic. Follicular structures occur in some.

Adenocarcinoma of parathyroid Adenocarcinoma of the parathyroid (Fig. 26-8) is also rare. These tumors are less-differentiated and invasive; they metastasize to regional lymph nodes and the lung.

References

Krook L. Spontaneous hyperparathyroidism in the dog. A pathologic-anatomic study. Acta Pathol Microbiol Scand 1957;41:1–88.

Legendre AM, Merkley DF, Carrig CB, et al. Primary hyperparathyroidism in a dog. J Am Vet Med Assoc 1976;168:694–696.

Patnaik AK, et al. Mediastinal parathyroid adenocarcinoma in a dog. Vet Pathol 1978;15:55–63.

Pearson PT, et al. Primary hyperparathyroidism in a beagle. J Am Vet Med Assoc 1965;147:1201–1206.

Stavrou D. Beitrag zum Hyperparathyreoidismus des Hundes. Dtsch Tierärztl Wochenschr 1968;75:117–121.

Warren S, Chute R. Parathyroid carcinoma in parabiont rats. Science 1962;135:927–928.

ADRENAL GLANDS

Adrenal glands are composed of two embryologically and functionally independent endocrine glands: the adrenal cortex, composed of steroid secreting cells; and the adrenal medulla, composed of neuroendocrine cells which secrete catecholamines. The adrenal cortex arises from the urogenital ridge, in common with the several urinary and genital organs; thus, it is of mesodermal origin. The adrenal medulla arises from the neural crest

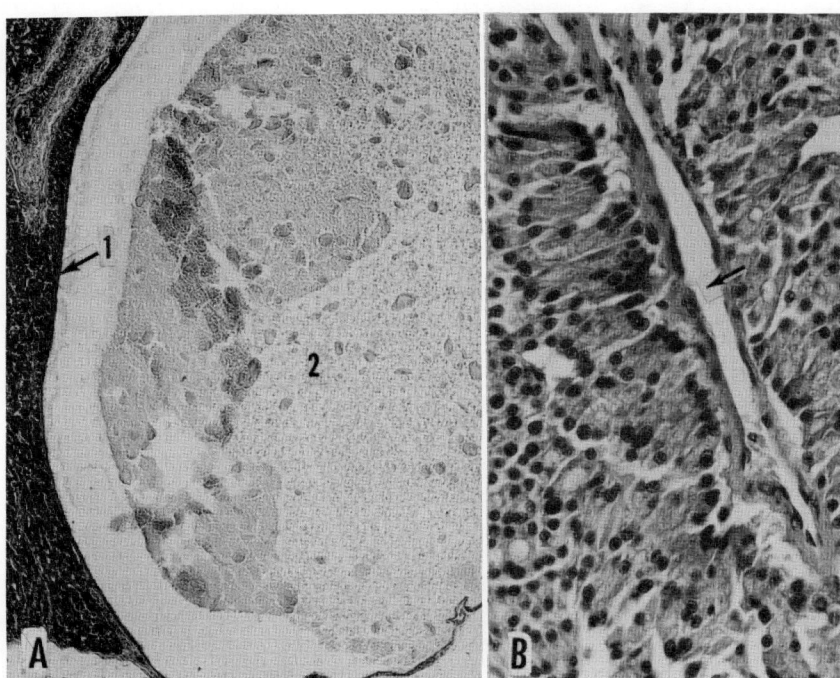

FIG. 26-8 A. Cyst of the parathyroid of a dog (×60), found incidentally. (1) Lined by columnar epithelium; (2) Contains eosinophilic material. (Contributor: Dr. Elihu Bond.) **B.** Adenocarcinoma of parathyroid of a dog (×305). Intimate relationship of cells to blood vessels (arrow) is a feature of neoplasms of endocrine organs. (**A** and **B** Courtesy of Armed Forces Institute of Pathology; contributor: **B.** Dr. M. M. Mason.)

and thus is of ectodermal origin. A functional adrenal cortex is essential for life, whereas the adrenal medulla is not.

Adrenal cortex

Adrenal cortex is divided into three zones that are responsible for the secretion of different hormones. The outer **zona glomerulosa** is composed of groups of cells with a small amount of cytoplasm and centrally placed dark nuclei. These secrete **mineralcorticoids.** The **zona fasciculata** is composed of cords of larger cells with more abundant lipid-laden cytoplasm, giving the cells a vacuolated appearance. This zone is primarily responsible for the secretion of **glucocorticoids.** The inner **zona reticularis** is composed of aggregates of cells which lack cytoplasmic vacuoles. Here, androgens are secreted.

The **mineralcorticoids**—of which **aldosterone** is the principal hormone—promote the retention of sodium, loss of potassium, expansion of extracellular fluid volume, and increased blood pressure. This is principally controlled through the **renin-angiotensin** system. Decreased blood pressure to the kidney, sodium depletion, or potassium excess all increase the release of renin from the juxtaglomerular apparatus. The apparatus converts angiotensin to angiotensin I, which is then converted to angiotensin II. Angiotensin II, in addition to increasing blood pressure through its action on smooth muscle, directly stimulates the production of aldosterone by the zona glomerulosa.

Glucocorticoids—of which cortisol is the principal hormone—favor gluconeogenesis; they raise the level of blood glucose and increase glycogen in the liver. They inhibit the action of insulin, promote hepatic gluconeogenesis, and increase the catabolism of proteins and fat. They are also anti-inflammatory, and lead to an increase in circulating numbers of neutrophils, a decrease in circulating eosinophils, and a decrease in circulating and tissue T-lymphocytes, inhibition of macrophage activation; they also limit the increased vascular permeability of inflammation. Cortisol is released by the action of ACTH from the pituitary.

Androgens from the zona reticularis are produced in the male and female. Their function is the same as those produced in the testicle.

Adrenal medulla

The adrenal medulla is derived embryologically from the neural crest and forms part of the chromaffin system. It is composed of pheochromocytes and a few ganglion cells. Pheochromocytes produce the catecholamines, epinephrine (adrenalin) or norepinephrine. The two functional cell types can be distinguished by characteristics of their secretory granules. Epinephrine granules are about 190 μm in diameter; they are finely granular and dense (but not opaque) and surrounded by a relatively tight fitting membrane. Norepinephrine granules are larger (250 μm), electron opaque, and ec-

centrically located within a space surrounded by a membrane. Both hormones have effects on maintaining or increasing blood pressure. In excessive amounts (as in a functional pheochromocytoma), these hormones produce paroxysmal hypertension. In canine and equine pheochromocytomas, medullary cells also are immunoreactive for leu-enkephalin and somatostatin. Insulin secretion may be suppressed in animals with pheochromocytomas.

Hypoadrenocorticism

Primary adrenal cortical insufficiency, known as **Addison disease,** is a syndrome known since 1855 which was invariably fatal until the discovery and therapeutic use of adrenocortical hormones. In humans, tuberculosis has been the principal cause of Addison disease, but now most cases are idiopathic. In animals, hypoadrenocorticism is not common and is seen most often in dogs. It can result from infectious diseases (usually septicemias, disseminated mycoses, and viral infections), destruction of the cortex by primary or metastatic neoplasms, or from unknown causes. Amyloidosis of the adrenals is not infrequent, but rarely so extensive as to lead to hypoadrenocorticism.

In Addison disease, weakness gradually develops, with feeble heart action, low blood pressure, decrease in blood volume (due to excessive excretion of sodium and chlorides and consequent loss of fluid), hyponatremia, hypokalemia, frequently hypoglycemia (due to failure of gluconeogenesis), and shock. Severe gastrointestinal malfunctions, including vomition, occur. A spectacular symptom regularly present is a marked increase in the pigmentation of the skin. This is believed to be due to an excess of pituitary melanocyte-stimulating hormone that develops reciprocally to a decrease of an inhibitory adrenocortical hormone. Lesions of Addison disease in other organs represent the effects of adrenal insufficiency upon other structures and functions. A compensatory hyperplasia of corticotrophs is evident in the pituitary. Both the thyroid and the heart are often small and atrophic, with areas of atrophic or dying fibers in the myocardium. Lymphoid tissue is often greatly increased in the thyroid and in the lymphoid organs.

IDIOPATHIC CANINE HYPOADRENOCORTICISM

This disorder, now recognized as a spontaneously occurring clinical and pathologic entity in young adult dogs, is characterized by marked atrophy of all three zones of the adrenal cortex. This leads to reduced secretion of all three categories of cortical hormones and the clinical features noted above. The lesion is characterized by marked reduction in size of the cortex, which may be almost completely absent. Small foci of necrosis and foci of lymphocytes and plasma cells may be present. The medulla is unaffected. The **cause** is not known, although immune-mediated destruction of the adrenal cortex has been suggested. A similar entity was reported in a cat.

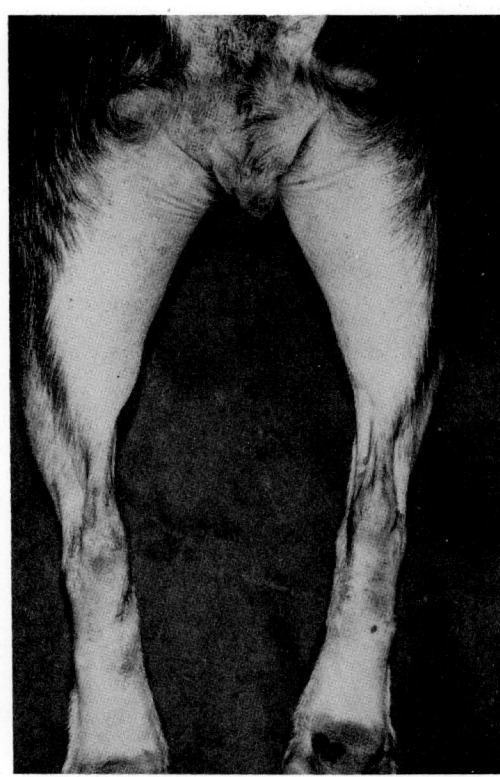

FIG. 26-9 Symmetric alopecia of the thighs of a 10-year-old spayed female Boston terrier with hyperadrenocorticism. (Courtesy of Angell Memorial Animal Hospital.)

TOXIN-INDUCED HYPOADRENOCORTICISM

A few specific toxins have a severe, deleterious effect on the adrenal cortex. The first to be identified as a natural poison and its cytotoxicity demonstrated experimentally is a metabolite of DDT known as DDD or TDE (2,2-bis(parachlorophenyl) 1,1-Dichloroethane). This is an insecticide with such specific toxicity for cells of the adrenal cortex (in dogs and rats) that it has been used to destroy hyperplastic cells of the adrenal in hyperadrenocorticism.

Acryonitrile also has a severe cytotoxic effect on the adrenal cortex and has been used to develop a model for "adrenal apoplexy."

Carbadox and related compounds that have been used as growth-promoting agents in young pigs are toxic to the zona glomerulosa, leading to reduced secretion of aldosterone and its associated effects. The zona glomerulosa becomes disorganized without a clear zonal differentiation.

A **hereditary** form of hypoadrenocorticism occurs in the IIIVO/ahJ strain of rabbit. It results from a hydroxylase deficiency preventing steroidogenesis which, in turn, results in excessive elaboration of ACTH and marked adrenal cortical hyperplasia. The disorder is inherited as an autosomal-recessive trait and affected rabbits die soon after birth. In humans, at least seven defects that prevent adrenal steroidogenesis have been recognized.

BOVINE HYPOADRENOCORTICISM

Congenital hypoplasia of the adrenal cortex, inherited as a recessive trait, is believed to be the underlying lesion in cases of prolonged gestation that occur in Holstein and Ayrshire cattle.

References

Adlersberg C, Schaefer LE, Want CI. Adrenal cortex, lipid metabolism and atherosclerosis: experimental studies in the rabbit. Science 1954;120:319–320.
Anderson MP, Capen CC. The endocrine system. In: Benirschke K, Garner FM, Jones TC, eds. Pathology of laboratory animals. New York: Springer-Verlag, 1978;423–508.
Atkins G, Marotta SF, Hirai K. In vitro studies on distribution of cortisol in dog's blood. Proc Soc Exp Biol Med 1966;122:347–351.
Bowman RE, Wolf RC. Plasma 17–hydroxycorticosteroid response to ACTH in *M. mulatta:* dose, age, weight, sex. Proc Soc Exp Biol Med 1969;130:61–64.
Cameron EHD, Grant JK. Biochemistry of histologically defined zones in the adrenal cortex: cortisol synthesis in the horse. J Endocrinol 1967;37:413–420.
Fox RR, Crary DD. A lethal recessive gene for adrenal hyperplasia in the rabbit. Teratology 1972;5:255.
Frenkel JK. Adrenal infection, necrosis, and hypocorticism. Am J Pathol 1977;86:749–752.
Freudiger U, Lindt S. Beitrage zur Klinik der Nebennierenrinden-Funktions-störungen des Hundes. Schweiz Arch Tierheilkd 1958;100:362–378.
Hadlow WJ. Adrenal cortical atrophy in the dog. Am J Pathol 1953;29:353–361.
Johnessee JS, Peterson ME, Gilbertson SR. Primary hypoadrenocorticism in a cat. J Am Vet Med Assoc 1983;183:881–882.
Marshak RR, Webster GD, Shelley JF. Observations on a case of primary adrenocortical insufficiency in a dog. J Am Vet Med Assoc 1960;136:274–280.
Nabuurs MJ, van der Molen EJ. Clinical signs and performance of pigs during the administration of different levels of carbadox and after withdrawal. Zentrlbl Veterinarmed A 1989;36:209–217.
Nelson AA, Woodward G. Severe adrenal cortical atrophy (cytotoxic) and hepatic damage produced in dogs by feeding 2,2-bis(parachlorophenyl) 1,1–dichloroethane (DDD or TDE). Arch Pathol 1949;48:387–394.
Powers JM, Hennigar GR, Grooms G, et al. Adrenal cortical degeneration and regeneration following administration of DDD. Am J Patho 1974;l75:181–194.
Price PJ, Greef J, Weber HW. Pathological findings in the adrenal gland of Chacma baboons: 160 consecutive cases. J S Afr Vet Med Assoc 1971;42:39–43.
Szabo S, Reynolds ES, Kovacs K. Animal model: Waterhouse-Fredricksen syndrome. Animal Model #101. In: Jones TC, Hackel DB, Migaki G, eds. Handbook: animal models of human disease, Fasc.6. Washington DC: Registry of Comparative Pathology, AFIP, 1977.
van der Molen EJ, de Graaf GJ, Baars AJ. Persistence of carbadox-induced adrenal lesions in pigs following drug withdrawal and recovery of aldosterone plasma concentrations. J Comp Pathol 1989;100:295–304.
Vilar O, Tullner WW. Effects of o,p'-DDD on histology and 17 hydroxycorticosteroid output of the dog adrenal cortex. Endocrinology 1959;65:80–86.
Wassermann D, Wassermann M. Adrenocortical zona fasciculata in rats receiving p,p',-DDT. Environ Physiol Biochem 1973;3:274–280.
White PC. Disorders of aldosterone biosynthesis and action. N Engl J Med 1994;331:250–258.
Willard MD, Schall WD, McCaw DE, et al. Canine hypoadrenocorticism: report of 37 cases and review of 39 previously reported cases. J Am Vet Med Assoc 1982;180:59–62.
Wilson RB, Holscher MA, Kasselberg AG, et al. Leu-enkephalin and somatostatin immunoreactivities in canine and equine pheochromocytomas. Vet Pathol 1986;23:96–98.

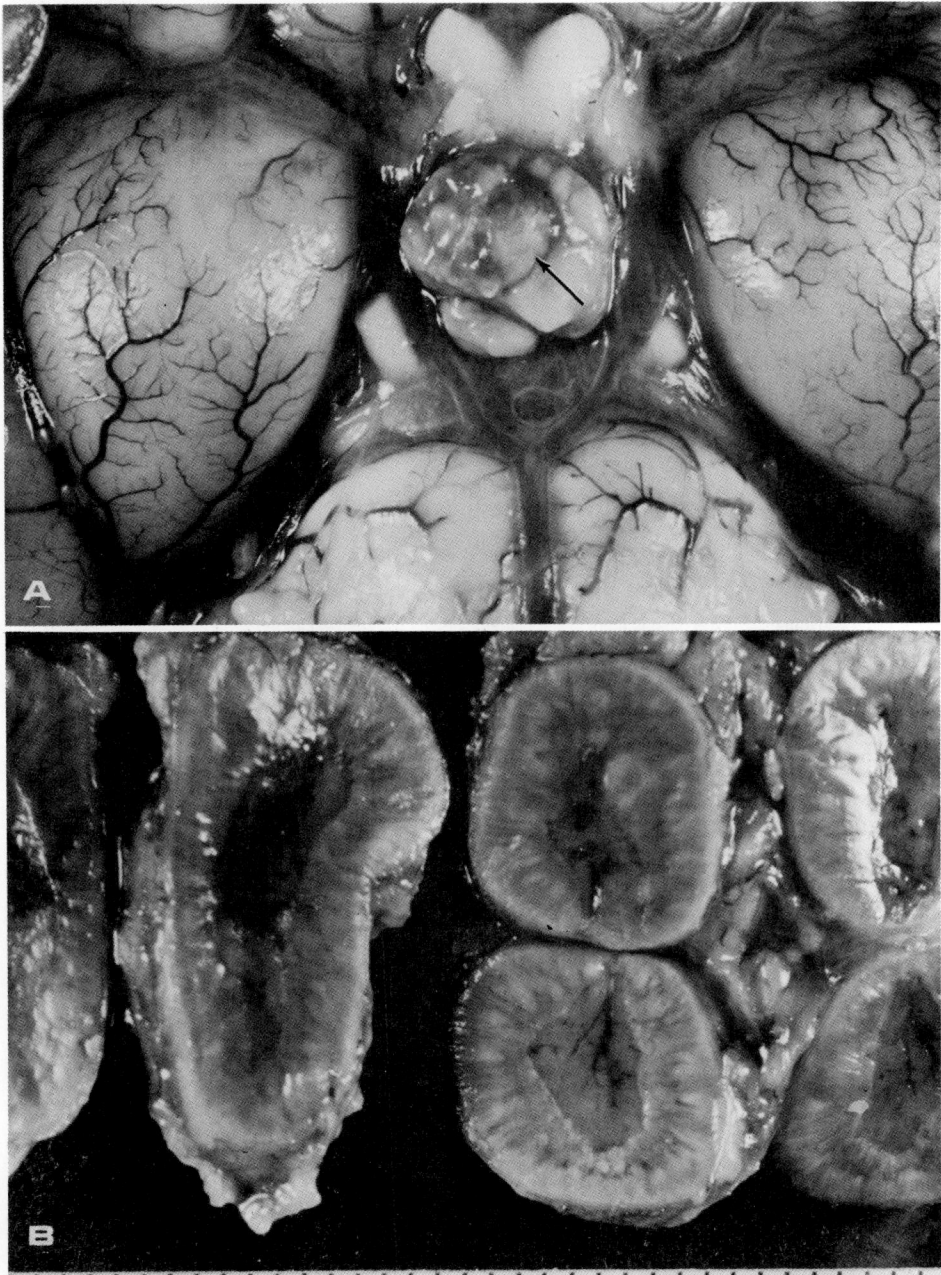

FIG. 26-10 A. Adenoma of the pituitary of a 10-year-old spayed female Boston terrier with canine Cushing disease. **B.** Hyperplasia of adrenal cortices, same dog. (Courtesy of Angell Memorial Animal Hospital.)

Hyperadrenocorticism

Excessive production of hormones by cells of the adrenal cortex, concomitant with hyperplasia or neoplasia, results in clinical manifestations called hyperadrenocorticism (Fig. 26-9) or **Cushing disease**; this condition was first described by Harvey Cushing, a Boston neurosurgeon. The disease is rare, except in the dog (Fig. 26-10). Findings induced by excessive amounts of adrenal cortical hormones include: bilaterally symmetric loss of hair accompanied by marked thinning of the epidermis and hyperkeratosis, muscle weakness, enlarged pendulous abdomen, trembling, obesity, polyuria, and polydipsia. Lymphopenia manifests with eosinopenia and atrophy of lymphoid organs. Serum glucose levels are

elevated and the liver may be enlarged due to increased amounts of glycogen and lipid. Glucocorticoids inhibit the action of insulin. Often, extensive mineralization is evident in the skin (calcinosis cutis), lungs, stomach, and other tissues.

In dogs, Cushing disease can result from two mechanisms. **Pituitary origin Cushing disease** is the result of excess ACTH elaboration by the pituitary from single or multiple corticotroph adenomas. These usually appear as chromophobe adenomas of the pars distalis or pars intermedia, and account for most examples of hyperadrenocorticism in dogs. **Adrenal origin Cushing disease** results from either idiopathic adrenal cortical hyperplasia or functional adrenal cortical neoplasms. Cortisol secreting adrenocortical tumors account for

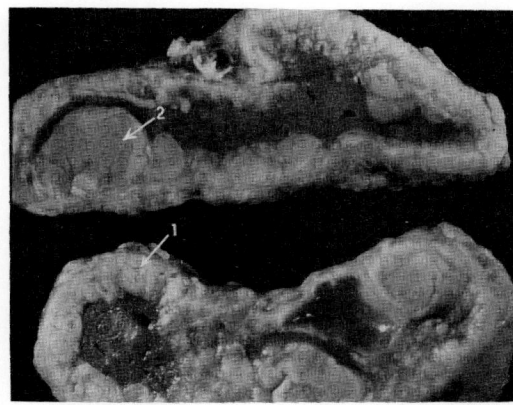

FIG. 26-11 (1) Hyperplasia and (2) adenoma of adrenal cortex of a 12-year-old male English setter. (Courtesy of Angell Memorial Animal Hospital.)

10–15% of hyperadrenocorticism in dogs. Idiopathic hyperadrenocorticism is less frequent. In humans, a third form termed **ectopic Cushing disease** results from the secretion of ACTH by nonendocrine neoplasms. Bronchogenic carcinoma is the most frequent cause. Exogenous administration of corticosteroids for prolonged periods will lead to **iatrogenic Cushing disease.**

ADRENOGENITAL SYNDROME

Excessive secretion of sex hormones, especially androgens, may occur in the adrenal cortex as a result of hyperadrenocorticism from any cause. In humans, deficiency of an enzyme—21-hydroxylase or 11-hydroxylase—leads to excessive production of androgens. Such an excess of androgens in dogs, horses, cattle, and humans results in precocious masculine sexual development and premature closure of epiphyses of the long bones. In females, virilization occurs, including hypertrophy of the clitoris, hirsutism, hypertrophy of the laryngeal muscles, and anestrus; in mares, masculine development of the neck is manifest. The mammary glands and uterus undergo atrophy. The 17-ketosteroid metabolites of androgens may be demonstrable in the urine. This syndrome has been reported in several species, but needs further documentation (Anderson and Capen, 1978).

References

Braun KG, Dillon AR, Mikeal RL, et al. Subclinical myopathy associated with hyperadrenocorticism in the dog. Vet Pathol 1980; 17:134–148.

Capen CC, Martin SL. Cushing's syndrome, hypercortisolism, Cushing's disease, Nelson's syndrome. Model No. 89. In: Jones TC, Hackel DB, Migaki G, eds. Handbook: animal models of human disease, Fasc. 5. Washington DC: Registry of Comparative Pathology, AFIP, 1976.

Coffin DL, Munson TO. Endocrine diseases of the dog associated with hair loss. Sertoli-cell tumor of the testis, hypothyroidism, canine Cushing's syndrome. J Am Vet Med Assoc 1953;123:403–408.

Dunn TB. Normal and pathologic anatomy of the adrenal gland of the mouse, including neoplasms. JNCI 1970;44:1323–1389.

Fox JG, Goad MEP, Garibaldi BA, et al. Hyperadrenocorticism in a ferret. J Am Vet Med Assoc 1987;191:343–344.

Kelley DF, Siegel ET, Berg P. The adrenal gland in dogs with hyperadrenalcorticism: a pathologic study. Vet Pathol 1971;8:385–400.

Rijnberk A, der Kinderen PJ, Thijssen JHH. Spontaneous hyperadrenocorticism in the dog. J Endocrinol 1968;41:397–406.

Ross MA, Gainer JH, Innes JRM. Dystrophic calcification in the adrenal glands of monkeys, cats and dogs. Arch Pathol 1955;60:655–662.

Schulman J, Johnston SD. Hyperadrenocorticism in two related Yorkshire Terriers. J Am Vet Med Assoc 1983;182:524–525.

Siegel ET, Kelly DF, Berg P. Cushing's syndrome in the dog. J Am Vet Med Assoc 1970;157:2081–2090.

Zerbe CA, Nachreiner RF, Dunstan RW, et al. Hyperadrenocorticism in a cat. J Am Vet Med Assoc 1987;190:559–563.

Hyperplasia and neoplasia of adrenal

HYPERPLASIA

Small nodules of hyperplastic cells are often seen within and outside of the adrenal capsule, a condition termed **nodular hyperplasia.** These nodules may be multiple and some are clearly visible with the naked eye (Fig. 26-11). Most of them are believed to be nonfunctional and not neoplastic. The differentiation of such hyperplastic nodules from adenomas is often a problem for the pathologist. Most decisions involving these lesions are arbitrary and perhaps incorrect; however, the clearly functional adenomas usually are larger and contain many large cells with foamy cytoplasm and lipid vacuoles. **Bilateral diffuse cortical hyperplasia** results from hypersecretion of ACTH by the pituitary (refer to *Cushing disease*). This condition is also seen in enzymatic defects which prevent steroidogenesis. Although several enzymatic defects have been described in humans, a similar defect in animals has been described only in laboratory rabbits, in which marked adrenocortical hyperplasia occurs; however, it is hypofunctional, leading to Addison disease. Any circumstances that lead to long-standing production of angiotensin II will lead to hyperplasia of the zona glomerulosa.

NEOPLASIA

Adrenocortical adenoma Adenoma of the adrenal cortex (**adrenocortical adenoma**) is encountered in about every species of mammal and is often functional, producing cortical steroid hormones. These tumors are usually unilateral and arise within the cortex, but may originate from invaginations of cortical cells into the medulla (Fig. 26-9). They may also arise in **ectopic** adrenal cortical tissue, which is most often adjacent to the adrenal; they can also occur as well in other sites, such as the spermatic cord or ovary. They are usually circumscribed and grow by expansion, but are usually incompletely encapsulated. Cells are usually well-differentiated and resemble the cells of one or more zones of the cortex. Most common are those consisting of polyhedral cells in cords or sheets, with or without cytoplasmic lipid, and resembling the cells of the zona fasciculata or zona reticularis. Tumors of the zona glomerulosa are less frequent.

Reliable statistical data are not available concerning the frequency of these adenomas, but they are encountered and reported more frequently in dogs. They are important because they may secrete enough adrenocortical hormones to cause hyperadrenocorticism, a frequent problem in dogs.

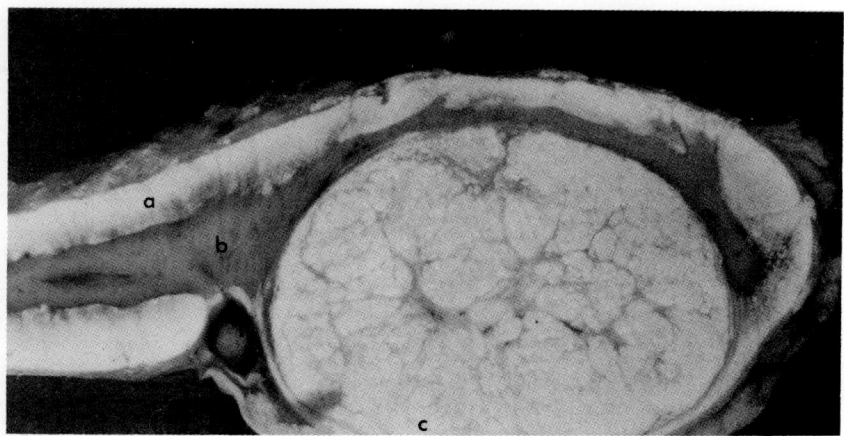

FIG. 26-12 Adenoma of the adrenal cortex of an eight-year-old male hound. (a) Adrenal cortex; (b) Medulla; and (c) Tumor.

Adrenocortical carcinoma Carcinoma of the adrenal cortex (**adrenocortical carcinoma**) is a neoplasm whose cells resemble those of the cortical adenoma (Fig. 26-12), with some differences. Mitoses and less well-differentiated cells are more frequent; necrosis of tumor cells is more apt to be seen; and neoplastic cells invade adjacent adrenal cortex, blood and lymph vessels, and metastasize. Extension into the vena cava and along its intima may occur, and metastatic tumors may be found in lungs or other organs.

Carcinomas may also produce enough corticosteroid hormone to cause hyperadrenocorticism, as discussed elsewhere. Atrophy of the contralateral adrenal cortex occurs with functional adenomas and carcinomas.

Pheochromocytoma Pheochromocytoma is the most frequent tumor of the adrenal medulla (Fig. 26-13) in all species in which it has been reported. Cattle, dogs, and horses are the domestic animals most often affected. Pheochromocytomas and diffuse and nodular hyperplasia of the adrenal medulla are especially common in laboratory rats.

Pheochromocytoma arises in the adrenal medulla from the chromaffin cells and usually keeps a resemblance to them. Tumor cells are large. Their abundant cytoplasm contains granules that can be demonstrated with appropriate technique; Müller, Zenker, Orth, or other dichromate-containing fixative usually help in demonstrating the granules. Tumor cells may be arranged in irregular cords or arcuate arrays, separated by a rich vascular system. Cells are usually elongated, but bovine tumors may also be spherical, giving the impression that two types of cells may be involved.

Grossly, the pheochromocytoma is dark reddish-brown and may be single or multiple, involving one or both adrenals. The surrounding adrenal medulla and cortex may be compressed by the larger tumors. Encapsulation is usually incomplete at best, but some trabeculation may occur in the tumor. Brown pigment (lipofuscin) may be seen at the periphery of the tumor. Poorly differentiated tumor cells may invade the adjacent tissues and grow into the vena cava. Metastasis can be expected in this type.

Some pheochromocytomas have functional effects upon their host as a result of secreting either epinephrine, norepinephrine, or both.

Pheochromocytomas often occur in conjunction with ultimobranchial tumors in bulls (refer to sections on *neoplasms of the thyroid, mixed thyroid carcinoma*).

Neurofibromas Neurofibromas are infrequently recognized in animals, perhaps more frequently in cattle than in other species. These tumors arise in the adrenal medulla, and are believed to originate from precursor cells in the neural crest. Histologically, they are similar to neurofibromas of other sites, consisting of parallel arrays of spindle-shaped cells occasionally arranged in palisades and bizarre patterns.

Ganglioneuroma Ganglioneuroma is a rare tumor, sharing its origin in neural crest with the chromaffin cells of the medulla. It consists of nerve fibers and ganglion cells, and may replace the adrenal medulla but does not metastasize. Although rare, at least three cases have been seen in rats (Todd et al., 1970).

Glanglioneuroblastoma Glanglioneuroblastoma resembles the neuroblastoma, but also contains pleomorphic ganglion cell neurons.

Neuroblastoma Neuroblastoma is a tumor of the adrenal medulla which is most often encountered in young animals. This tumor contains many fine fibrils in which small cells with hyperchromatic nuclei are entangled. Fibrils are more evident in the few places where cell nuclei are sparse. Rosettes and peculiar fan-shaped or "wind-blown" patterns may be seen. This tumor has been reported in dogs, but its natural history and significance are as yet unknown.

Myelolipoma Myelolipoma is not clearly a tumor but consists of collections of myeloid cells in fat, sometimes accompanied by bone. It is a benign lesion, probably not neoplastic. It is seen occasionally as an incidental finding in the adrenal of rats and dogs.

References

Appleby EC. International histological classification of tumours of domestic animals. XVII. Tumours of the adrenal gland and paraganglia. Bull WHO 1976;53:227–235.

Bosland MC, Bär A. Some functional characteristics of adrenal medul-

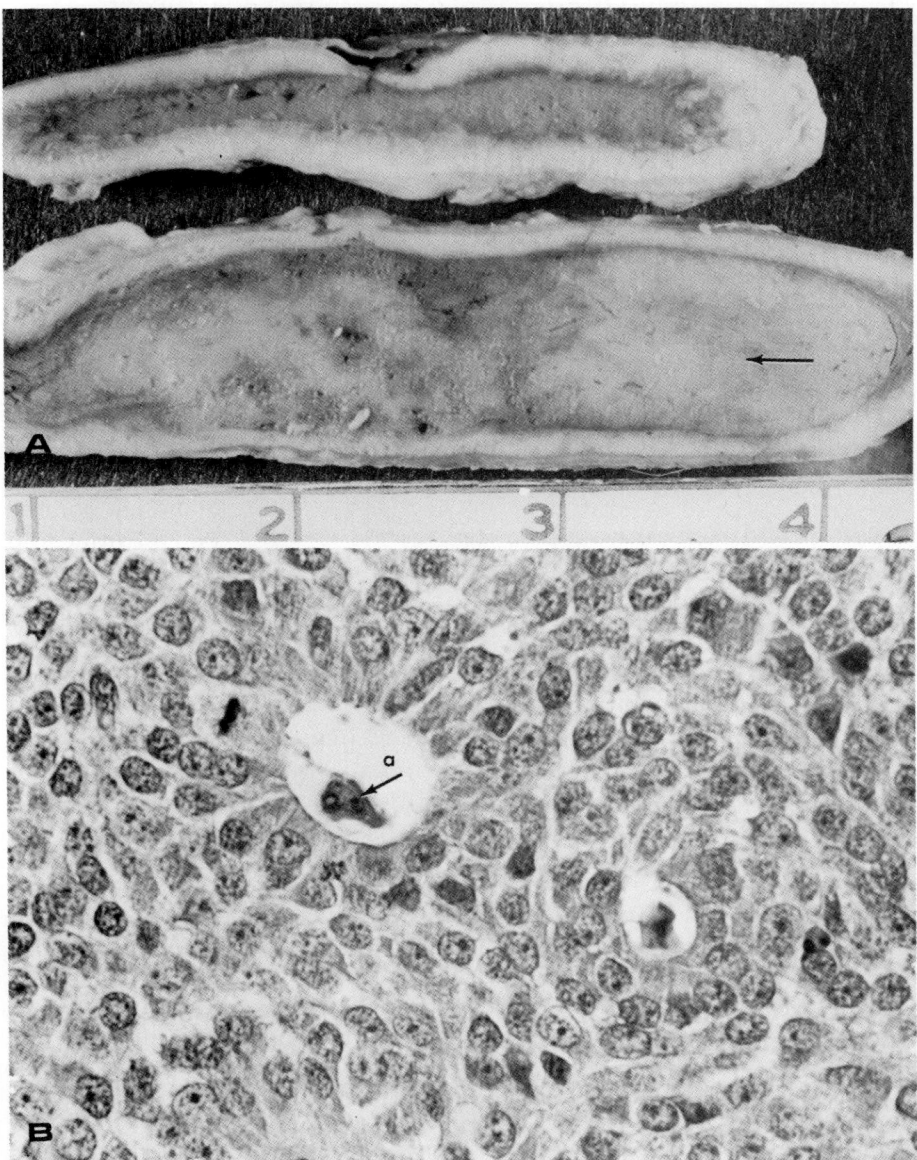

FIG. 26-13 A. Pheochromocytoma (*arrow*), medulla of the adrenal of an eight-year-old male dalmatian. **B.** Same tumor. (hematoxylin-and-eosin-stained, ×1000.) (a) Note intimate relationship of tumor cells to small capillaries, forming "pseudo rosettes" around them. The empty space around the capillary is due to shrinkage artifact. (Courtesy of Angell Memorial Animal Hospital.)

lary tumors in aged male Wistar rats. Vet Pathol 1984;21:129–140.

Bouayad H, Feeney DA, Caywood DD, et al. Pheochromocytoma in dogs: 13 cases (1980–1985). J Am Vet Med Assoc 1987;191:1610–1615.

Chen HHC. Ectopic adrenal cortical nodules in the mesorchium of New Zealand white rabbits. Lab Anim Sci 1986;36:537–538.

Fix AS, Miller LD. Equine adrenocortical carcinoma with hypercalcemia. Vet Pathol 1987;24:190–192.

Fox RR, Crary DD. Genetics and pathology of hereditary adrenal hyperplasia in the rabbit: a model for congenital lipoid adrenal hyperplasia. J Hered 1978;69:251–254.

Froscher BG, Power HT. Malignant pheochromocytoma in a foal. J Am Vet Med Assoc 1982;181:494–496.

Gilman J, Gilbert C, Spence I. Phaeochromocytoma in the rat: pathogenesis and collateral reactions and its relation to comparable tumors in man. Cancer 1953;6:494–511.

Hamburger F, Russfield AB. An inbred line of Syrian hamsters with frequent spontaneous adrenal tumors. Cancer Res 1970;30:305–308.

Howard EB, Nielsen SW. Pheochromocytomas associated with hypertensive lesions in dogs. J Am Vet Med Assoc 1965;147:245–252.

Kintzer PP, Peterson ME. Mitotane treatment of 32 dogs with cortisol-secreting adrenocortical neoplasms. J Am Vet Med Assoc 1994;205:54–61.

Ladds PW, Russell P, Foster RA. Adrenal teratoma in an ox. Aust Vet J 1990;67:464–465, Vet Bull 1991;61:6630.

McClure HM. Tumors in nonhuman primates: observations during a six year period in the Yerkes Primate Research Center. Am J Phys Anthropol 1973;38:425–450.

Reznik G, Ward JM, Reznik-Schüller H. Ganglioneuromas in the adrenal medulla of F344 rats. Vet Pathol 1980;17:614–621.

Ribelin WE, Roloff MV, Houser RM. Minimally functional rat medullary pheochromocytomas. Vet Pathol 1984;21:281–285.

Richter WR. Tubular adenomata of the adrenal of the goat. Cornell Vet 1957;47:558–577.

Richter WR. Adrenal cortical adenomata in the goat. Am J Vet Res 1958;19:895–901.

Sarfaty D, Carrillo JM, Peterson ME. Neurologic, endocrinologic, and pathologic findings associated with large pituitary tumors in dogs: eight cases (1976–1984). J Am Vet Med Assoc 1988;193:854–856.

Seibold HR, Wolf RH. Neoplasms and proliferative lesions in 1065 nonhuman primate necropsies. Lab Anim Sci 1973;23:533–539,

Schardein JL, Fitzgerald JE, Kaump DH. Spontaneous tumors in Holzman-source rats of various ages. Pathol Vet 1968;5:238–252.

Siegel ET, O'Brien JB, Pyle L, et al. Functional adenocortical carcinoma in a dog. J Am Vet Med Assoc 1967;150:760–766.

Sills RC, Dunstan RW, Watson GL, et al. Pheochromocytomas in two raccoon dogs. Vet Pathol 1988;25:178–179.

Skelton-Stroud PN, Ishmael J. Adrenal lesions in the baboon (*Papio* spp). Vet Pathol 1985;22:141–146.

Sponenberg DP, McEntee K. Pheochromocytomas and ultimobranchial (C-cell) neoplasms in the bull: evidence of autosomal dominant inheritance in the Guernsey breed. Vet Pathol 1983;20:396–400.

Tischler AS, et al. Spontaneous proliferative lesions of the adrenal medulla in aging Long-Evans rats. Lab Invest 1985;53:486–498.

Tischler AS, DeLellis RA, Nunnemacher G, et al. Acute stimulation of chromaffin cell proliferation in the adult rat adrenal medulla. Lab Invest 1988;58:733–735.

Todd GC, Pierce EC, Clevinger WG. Ganglioneuroma of the adrenal medulla in rats: a report of three cases. Pathol Vet 1970;7:139–144.

West JL. Bovine pheochromocytoma: case report and review of literature. Am J Vet Res 1975;36:1371–1374.

White PC, New MI, Dupont B. Congenital adrenal hyperplasia. (Parts I and II.) N Engl J Med 1987;316:1519–1524, 1580–1586.

Yarrington JT, Capen CC. Ultrastructural and biochemical evaluation of adrenal medullary hyperplasia and pheochromocytoma in aged bulls. Vet Pathol 1981;18:316–325.

PANCREATIC ISLETS

The pancreatic islets (islets of Langerhans) develop embryonically as tiny buds of epithelial cells arising from the pancreatic ducts. These solid masses of cells become detached from the pancreatic ducts and acquire vasculature by sprouting of capillaries.

The islets are predominantly composed of two principal cell types, beta and alpha; in addition, four other cell types have been identified that may have a different origin, possibly from the neural crest.

Of the six types, the **beta cell** is the most numerous, accounting for 60–70% of the islet cells. They secrete insulin and are concentrated in the central part of the islets. Ultrastructurally, they contain irregularly rectangular granules surrounded by a clear halo enclosed by a membrane. They are distinctively stained by aldehyde fuchsin, which intensifies their granules. **Alpha cells** comprise about 20% of islets and are located peripherally. These cells secrete glucagon and contain granules that are more dense in their centers and are surrounded by a closely applied membrane. They are not stained by aldehyde fuchsin. **Delta cells,** which constitute about 5% of the islets, secrete somatostatin and contain less electron-dense pale granules surrounded by a closely applied membrane. **PP cells** (pancreatic polypeptide cells) secrete a polypeptide that affects gastrointestinal function. They also are present outside the islets and contain small, dark granules. PP cells constitute up to 10% of the islet population. **D1 cells** (delta cells) secrete a substance termed vasoactive intestinal peptide (VIP), and account for only about 1% of the cells. The last cell type, the **enterochromaffin cell,** is a source of serotonin.

References

Cotran RS, Kumar V, Robbins SL. Robbins pathologic basis of disease. 4th ed. The pancreas. Philadelphia: WB Saunders, 1989;981–1010.

Lacy PE, Kissane JM. Pancreas and diabetes mellitus. In: Anderson WAD, Kissane JM, eds. Pathology. 7th ed. St. Louis: CV Mosby, 1977;1457–1482.

Like AA, Chick WL. β-Cell replication in subhuman primates. Am J Pathol 1971;62:77a–78a.

Like AA, Chick WL. Pancreatic beta cell replication induced by glucocorticoids in subhuman primates. Am J Pathol 1975;75:329–348.

Pictet RL, Rall LB, Phelps P, et al. The neural crest and the origin of the insulin-producing and other gastrointestinal hormone-producing cells. Science 1975;191:191–192.

Diabetes mellitus

Diabetes mellitus is a syndrome complex affecting humans and animals; the unifying phenomenon is abnormal or inappropriate metabolism of glucose due to an absolute or relative deficiency of insulin. Diabetes means "siphon" or "to flow through" and mellitus refers to honey. Thus the original concept of an increased flow of urine (polyuria) that was sweet enough to attract bees emphasizes the clinical signs. The primary function of insulin is the transport of glucose into cells, as well as the transmembrane transport of amino acids, formation of glycogen, production of triglycerides, and nucleic acid and protein synthesis. Insulin first binds to cellular receptors and activates tyrosine kinase, which initiates the various metabolic functions (such as the cellular uptake of glucose). Insulin is the major anabolic hormone.

Diabetes mellitus is characterized by fasting hyperglycemia, glycosuria, osmotic polyuria, polydipsia, dehydration, increased appetite, and often ketoacidosis. Susceptibility to infections increases. Affected animals may be either obese or wasted. The student is referred to other texts for details of the complex disruption of the various pathways of intermediary metabolism.

The pathogenesis of diabetes mellitus is complex and, far from being completely understood. The classification scheme for the disease in humans divides diabetes mellitus into **primary** or **idiopathic diabetes mellitus** and **secondary diabetes mellitus. Secondary diabetes mellitus** results from destruction of the islets due to such disorders as acute or chronic pancreatitis or neoplasms. In dogs, acute necrotizing pancreatitis is one of the more common causes of diabetes mellitus. Secondary diabetes mellitus may also occur in association with other endocrinopathies that interfere with insulin secretion or its action. Insulin resistance (due to a decrease in number of receptors or postreceptor defects) develops in Cushing disease, therapeutic steroid use, growth hormone secreting pituitary tumors, and corticotroph pituitary tumors. Excess growth hormone can result from prolonged secretion or exogenous use of progesterone which has been associated with diabetes mellitus in dogs. Pheochromocytomas suppress insulin secretion. Obesity can also lead to insulin resistance and plays a role in some cases of diabetes. **Primary diabetes** is subdivided into **type I** and **type II diabetes mellitus. Type I,** also termed **insulin-dependent diabetes mellitus, juvenile-onset diabetes** and **ketosis-prone diabetes,** results from a reduction in number of beta cells and an absolute decrease in insulin. Such patients require insulin therapy. It accounts for 10–20% of primary diabetes mellitus in humans. Although genetic susceptibility is evident, it is not a simple hereditary disease. The concordance rate among monozygotic twins is about 50%. It is believed to result from an environmental insult that initiates an autoimmune destruction of beta cells in genetically predisposed individuals. Viruses that alter the plasma membrane antigens of beta cells are believed to be one of the major environmental insults. In humans, retroviruses, rubella virus, and cytomegalovirus are possible candidates. A strong association exists among various enteroviruses, particularly Coxsackie B. Infection with these viruses may lead to long-term changes in beta cells, but strong evidence supports that they also induce diabetes by direct lytic destruction of beta cells. Studies with laboratory animals suggest Coxsackie B viruses may actually initiate both mechanisms of beta cell destruction. In rats, autoimmune diabetes can be produced by infection with Kilham's rat virus. Encephalomyocarditis virus type D is another virus that can induce diabetes in laboratory animals. It appears to lead to direct lysis; however, it is associated with lymphocytic insulitis, and the development of diabetes has been shown to be dependent on macrophages. Foot and mouth disease virus is capable of destroying pancreatic islets, leading to diabetes; bovine viral diarrhea-mucosal disease virus has been suggested as a cause of diabetes. A third mechanism allowing viruses to lead to diabetes is their persistence within beta cells, interfering with the production of insulin without causing direct cell lysis or immune-mediated lysis. This has been demonstrated with persistent lymphocytic choriomeningitis virus infection in mice and with Venezuelan equine encephalomyelitis virus infection in hamsters. In neither situation does morphologic evidence of beta cell damage exist.

Type II diabetes mellitus, also known as **noninsulin-dependent diabetes mellitus** or **mature-onset diabetes mellitus,** occurs in two forms in humans: **obese type** and **nonobese type.** Obesity is related to its pathogenesis, but is not essential. This is the most common form of diabetes in humans and has a much stronger genetic influence. Insulin levels are usually normal to high, but are low with respect to the plasma glucose level. Beta cells cannot produce adequate insulin; thus, insulin is relatively deficient. **Insulin resistance** occurs, resulting from a postreceptor defect and a decrease of insulin receptors. Diabetes in such patients can often be controlled by diet, but many do require exogenous insulin.

Several structurally diverse chemicals can damage beta cells, leading to diabetes mellitus. These include Streptozotocin, Alloxan, Chlorozotocin, Vacor, and Cyproheptadine.

In humans, lesions of the islets in diabetes mellitus are characterized by degranulation of beta cells, loss of beta cells with reduction in islet cell size, lymphocytic infiltration (lymphocytic insulitis), fibrosis, and amyloid deposition. The latter two lesions are more common in type II diabetes mellitus.

In animals, diabetes mellitus is most frequent in dogs, cats, and laboratory rodents. It has a reported incidence of 1:200 in dogs and 1:800 in cats. In dogs, many cases are secondary diabetes mellitus due to either pancreatitis or other endocrine abnormalities. Diabetes mellitus resembling types I and II of humans may also occur. Obesity has been associated with these primary forms of diabetes. The disease occurs more frequently in females and castrated males than in intact males. Poodles are reportedly at increased risk. An inherited, early-onset, insulin-dependent form of diabetes mellitus occurs in Keeshond dogs. It results from hypoplasia of beta cells and is therefore different from early-onset diabetes of humans. It is inherited as an autosomal-recessive trait. A similar disorder occurs in golden retrievers and also has been reported in a chow puppy.

In **cats,** the disease is associated with older age, obesity (although affected cats become wasted), and usually results from insular amyloidosis, thus closely resembling the type II disease in humans. Insular amyloidosis occurs in 65% of diabetic cats; it is a localized disease and not part of systemic amyloidosis. The amyloid also has a different chemical composition (it lacks tryptophane and has little tyrosine) and retains congophilia after potassium permanganate treatment. Although it seems evident that amyloidosis is the cause of diabetes mellitus, about 45% of nondiabetic cats over five years of age have insular, but less extensive, amyloidosis. Insular amyloidosis also occurs in several species of monkeys (mostly macaques) and reportedly in raccoons and hyenas.

Diabetes mellitus, both primary and secondary, is occasionally seen in cattle, horses, and other domestic animals. Examples of types I and II diabetes mellitus in laboratory animals that are used as animal models for the human disease include: rats (Cohen, obese/SHR, Wistar fatty, SHR/n-cp, BB), mice (NOD, ob/ob, db/db, KK, KKAy, NZO), sand rats, Chinese hamsters, and a strain of New Zealand rabbits.

Other lesions in diabetes mellitus in animals are neither as pronounced nor as well studied as in humans. Generalized microangiopathic changes occur in capillaries and arterioles of the retina, renal glomeruli, and muscles. This is manifest by thickening of the basement membrane with a homogeneous PAS-positive material. Diffuse thickening of the glomerular mesangium is evident, but generally not to the extent encountered in diabetic nephropathy of humans. Neuropathy characterized by myelin degeneration and axonal damage is described in dogs and cats, but appears to be less common than in humans. Cataracts are frequent in diabetic dogs, but are rarely encountered in cats. Hepatic lipidosis and hepatomegaly are also present.

References

Amankwah KS, Kaufmann RC, Dunaway GA, et al. Animal models of human disease: gestational diabetes. Comp Pathol Bull 1986;18:3–4.

Anderson PG, Braund KG, Dillon AR, et al. Polyneuropathy and hormone profiles in a Chow puppy with hypoplasia of the islets of Langerhans. Vet Pathol 1986;23:528–531.

Baek HS, Yoon JW. Role of macrophages in the pathogenesis of encephalomyocarditis virus-induced diabetes in mice. J Virol 1990;64:5708–5715.

Baek HS, Yoon JW. Direct involvement of macrophages in destruction of beta-cells leading to development of diabetes in virus-infected mice. Diabetes 1991;40:1586–1597.

Baker JR, Ritchie HE. Diabetes mellitus in the horse: a case report and review of the literature. Equine Vet J 1974;6:7–11.

Boquist L. Pancreatic islet morphology in diabetic Chinese hamsters. A light and electron microscopic study. Acta Pathol Microbiol Scand 1969;75:399–414.

Craighead JE. Animal model of human disease. Diabetes mellitus (juvenile- and maturity-onset types). Animal model: mice infected with the M variant of encephalomyocarditis virus. Am J Pathol 1975;78:537–540.

Dixon JB, Sanford J. Pathological features of spontaneous canine diabetes mellitus. J Comp Pathol 1962;72:153–164.

Eigenmann JE. Diabetes mellitus in elderly female dogs: recent findings on pathogenesis and clinical implications. J Am Anim Hosp Assoc 1981;17:805–812.

Farris HE Jr. Spontaneous diabetes in the rabbit: an animal model. Lab Anim 1982;11:40, 42.

Fohlman J, Friman G. Is juvenile diabetes a viral disease? Ann Med 1993;25:569–574.

Guberski DL, et al. Induction of type I diabetes by Kilham's rat virus in diabetes-resistant BB/Wor rats. Science 1991;254:1010–1013. [published erratum appears in Science 1992;255:383.]

Howard CF Jr. Diabetes in *Macaca nigra*: metabolic and histologic changes. Diabetologia 1974;10:671–677.

Howard CF. Basement membrane thickness in muscle capillaries of normal and spontaneously diabetic *Macaca nigra*. Diabetes 1975;24:201–206.

Howard CF. Insular amyloidosis and diabetes mellitus in *Macaca nigra*. Diabetes 1978;27:357–364.

Howard CF. Diabetes and atherosclerosis in *Macaca nigra*. Diabetes 1978;27:447.

Howard CF Jr, Yasuda M. Diabetes mellitus in nonhuman primates: recent research advances and current husbandry practices. J Med Primatol 1990;19:609–625.

Johnson KH, Hayden DW, O'Brien TD, et al. Spontaneous diabetes mellitus-islet amyloid complex in adult cats. Am J Pathol 1986; 125:416–419.

Kaneko JJ, Rhode EA. Diabetes mellitus in a cow. J Am Vet Med Assoc 1964;144:367–373.

Kaptur PE, Thomas DC, Giron DJ. Different attachment of diabetogenic and nondiabetogenic variants of encephalomyocarditis virus to beta cells. Diabetes 1989;38:1103–1108.

Katherman AE, Braund KG. Polyneuropathy associated with diabetes mellitus in a dog. J Am Vet Med Assoc 1983;182:522–524.

Kessler MJ, Howard CF Jr, London WT. Gestational diabetes mellitus and impaired glucose tolerance in an aged *Macaca mulatta*. J Med Primatol 1985;14:237–244.

Kitchen DL, Roussel AJ Jr. Type-I diabetes mellitus in a bull. J Am Vet Med Assoc 1990;197:761–763.

Kramek BA, Moise NS, Cooper B, et al. Neuropathy associated with diabetes mellitus in the cat. J Am Vet Med Assoc 1984;184: 42–45.

Kramer JW, Nottingham S, Robinette J, et al. Inherited, early onset, insulin-requiring diabetes mellitus of Keeshond dogs. Diabetes 1980;29:558–565.

Kramer JW, et al. Inheritance of diabetes mellitus in Keeshond dogs. Am J Vet Res 1988;49:428–431.

Lang CM, Munger BL. Diabetes mellitus in guinea pig. Diabetes 1976;25:434–443.

Leiter EH. The genetics of diabetes susceptibility in mice. FASEB J 1989;3:2231–2241.

Like AA. Spontaneous diabetes in animals. In: Volk BW, Wellmann KF, eds. The diabetic pancreas. New York: Plenum, 1977.

Mattheeuws D, Rottiers R, Kaneko JJ, et al. Diabetes mellitus in dogs: relationship of obesity to glucose tolerance and insulin response. Am J Vet Res 1984;45:98–103.

Munger BL, Lang CM. Spontaneous diabetes mellitus in guinea pigs: the acute cytopathology of the islets of Langerhans. Lab Invest 1973;29:685–702.

Nakagawa C, et al. Retrovirus gag protein p30 in the islets of non-obese diabetic mice: relevance for pathogenesis of diabetes mellitus. Diabetologia 1992;37:614–618.

Nakamura M, Yamada K. Studies on a diabetic (KK) strain of the mouse. Diabetologia 1967;3:212–215.

National Research Council. Special issue: new rat models of obesity and type II diabetes. ILAR News 1990;32:1–38.

Nathan DM. Long-term complications of diabetes mellitus. N Engl J Med 1993;328:1676–1685.

O'Brien TD, Hayden DW, Johnson KH, et al. High dose intravenous glucose tolerance test and serum insulin and glucagon levels in diabetic and non-diabetic cats: relationships to insular amyloidosis. Vet Pathol 1985;22:250–261.

Panciera DL, Thomas CB, Eicker SW, et al. Epizootiologic patterns of diabetes mellitus in cats: 333 cases (1980–1986). J Am Vet Med Assoc 1990;197:1504–1508.

Patz A, et al. Studies on diabetic retinopathy. II. Retinopathy and nephropathy in spontaneous canine diabetes. Diabetes 1965;14: 700–708.

Ricketts HT, et al. Spontaneous diabetes mellitus in the dog: an account of 8 cases. Diabetes 1953;4:288–294.

Szopa TM, Titchener PA, Portwood ND, et al. Diabetes mellitus due to viruses—some recent developments. Diabetologia 1993;36: 687–695.

Taira M, et al. Human diabetes associated with a deletion of the kinase domain of the insulin receptor. Science 1989;245:63–66.

Tajima M, Yazawa T, Hagiwara K, et al. Diabetes mellitus in cattle infected with bovine viral diarrhea-mucosal disease virus. Zentralbl Veterinarmed A 1992;39:616–620.

Taniyama H, Shirakawa T, Furuoka H, et al. Spontaneous diabetes mellitus in young cattle: histologic, immunohistochemical, and electron microscopic studies of the islets of Langerhans. Vet Pathol 1993;30:46–54.

Tasker JB, Whiteman CE, Martin BR. Diabetes mellitus in the horse. J Am Vet Med Assoc 1966;149:393–399.

Velasquez MT, Kimmel PL, Michaelis OE IV. Animal models of spontaneous diabetic kidney disease. FASEB J 1990;4:2850–2859.

Yano BL, Hayden DW, Johnson KH. Feline insular amyloid: ultrastructural evidence for intracellular formation by nonendocrine cells. Lab Invest 1981;45:149–156.

Yano BL, Hayden DW, Johnson KH. Occurrence of secondary systemic amyloid in the pancreatic islets of a cat. Am J Vet Res 1983;44:338–339.

Yasuda M, Takaoka M, Fujiwara T, Mori M. Occurrence of spontaneous diabetes mellitus in a cynomolgus monkey (*Macaca fascicularis*) and impaired glucose tolerance in its descendants. J Med Primatol 1988;17:319–332.

Yoon JW. The role of viruses and environmental factors in the induction of diabetes. Curr Top Microbiol Immunol 1990;164:95–123.

Yoon JW. Induction and prevention of type I diabetes mellitus by viruses. Diabete Metab 1992;18:378–386.

Neoplasms of pancreatic islets

Primary tumors of the pancreatic islets are not common. They have been reported in most domestic animals (Fig. 26-14) as well as in laboratory rodents, but are found most often in dogs. They are usually single nodules, but may be multiple, making their distinction from **hyperplastic islets** difficult. Malignant islet-cell neoplasms are more common than their benign counterpart, and they often metastasize to regional lymph nodes and liver. **Microscopically,** the neoplasms resemble normal islets, with the polyhedral cells forming rows, trabeculae, or small acinar clusters separated by a fine fibrovascular stroma (Fig. 26-15). **Amyloid** is often found within the tumors. Malignant neoplasms are less well-differentiated and they invade the adjacent pancreas. Hormones are identifiable immunohistochemically within the neoplastic cells, but their presence does not always correlate with clinical findings. Although all tumors of pancreatic islets are not

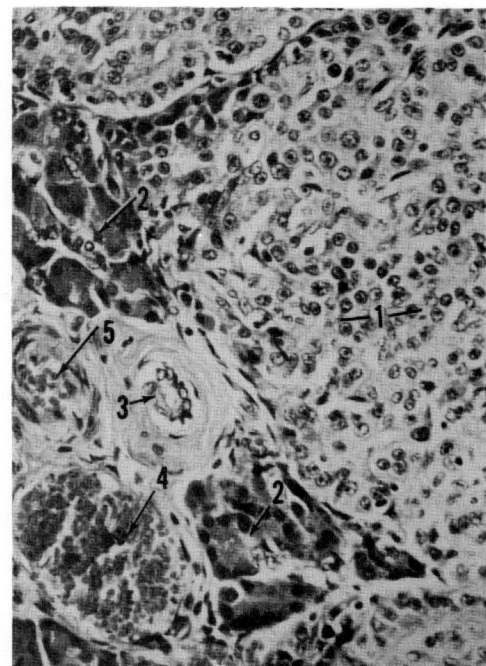

FIG. 26-14 Adenoma of islet cells, pancreas of a ten-year-old female Persian cat (×575). (1) Tumor; (2) Compressing normal pancreatic acini; (3) Pancreatic duct; (4) Vein; and (5) Artery. (Courtesy of Armed Forces Institute of Pathology; contributor: Dr. M. A. Troy.)

functional, their designation is based on their functional status. Most tumors appear to secrete multiple hormones; nevertheless, clinical signs, when present, are usually restricted to only one hormone.

INSULINOMA

Insulinoma, or **beta-cell tumor,** is the most frequently encountered islet-cell neoplasm. When they secrete enough insulin, they lead to hypoglycemia with blood glucose levels usually below 50 mg/dl. Affected dogs suddenly collapse and may go into either convulsions or coma. Insulin is demonstrable in the neoplastic cells; however, many also contain cells that are positive for glucagon, somatostatin, PP, and gastrin.

GASTRINOMA

Gastrinoma—a pancreatic islet-cell tumor that secretes gastrin—is an unusual tumor in that the normal islet does not contain gastrin-secreting cells. Gastrinomas have been reported in dogs, but they are rare. Excessive gastrin leads to what is termed **Zollinger-Ellison syndrome,** a disorder characterized by gastric hypersecretion and peptic ulcer. This condition has been seen in dogs; in humans, gastrinomas also occur in the duodenum.

GLUCAGONOMAS

Glucagonomas are rare tumors of pancreatic-islet alpha cells. Excessive glucagon leads to hyperglycemia. They have been reported in dogs and are associated with a necrotic dermatitis, which is also seen in humans with these tumors.

Tumors of **other** pancreatic cell types occur in humans, but have not been reported in animals. These include **vipomas** (vasoactive intestinal peptide-secreting tumors), **somatostatinoma** and **carcinoid.**

References

Cello RM, Kennedy PC. Hyperinsulism in dogs due to pancreatic islet cell carcinoma. Cornell Vet 1957;47:538–557.

Dahlgren RR, Emerick FM. Pancreatic β-cell carcinoma with renal metastasis in a dog. J Am Vet Med Assoc 1985;187:425–426.

English RV, Breitschwerdt EB, Grindem CB, et al. Zollinger-Ellison syndrome and myelofibrosis in a dog. J Am Vet Med Assoc 1988;192:1430–1434.

Grant CA. Pancreatic insuloma with clinical manifestations in a dog. J Comp Pathol 1960;70:450–456.

Gross TL, O'Brien TD, Davies AP, et al. Glucagon-producing pancreatic endocrine tumors in two dogs with superficial necrolytic dermatitis. J Am Vet Med Assoc 1990;197:1619–1622.

Happé RP, et al. Zollinger-Ellison syndrome in three dogs. Vet Pathol 1980;17:177–186.

Hawkins KL, Summers BA, Kuhadja FP, et al. Immunocytochemistry of normal pancreatic islets and spontaneous islet cell tumors in dogs. Vet Pathol 1987;24:170–179.

Holscher MA, Sly DL, Wilson RB, et al. Multihormonal islet cell carcinoma in a Greater Bushbaby (*Galago crassicaudatus argentatus*). Vet Pathol 1986;23:80–82.

Jones BR, Nicholls MR, Badman R. Peptic ulceration in a dog associated with an islet cell carcinoma of the pancreas and an elevated plasma gastrin level. J Small Anim Pract 1976;17:593–598.

Justus AA. Pancreatic insuloma in a dog. J Am Vet Med Assoc 1963;142:1413–1414.

Kircher CH, Nielsen SW. International histological classification of tumours of domestic animals. XIV. Tumours of the pancreas. Bull WHO 1976;53:195–202.

Kovacs K, Horvath E, Ilse RG, et al. Spontaneous pancreatic beta cell tumor in the rat: a light and electron microscopic study. Vet Pathol 1976;13:286–294.

Kruth SA, Feldman EC, Kennedy PC. Insulin-secreting islet cell tumors: establishing a diagnosis and the clinical course for 25 dogs. J Am Vet Med Assoc 1982;181:54–58.

Leifer CE, Peterson ME, Matus RE. Insulin-secreting tumor: diagnosis and medical and surgical management in 55 dogs. J Am Vet Med Assoc 1986;188:60–64.

O'Brien TD, Hayden DW, O'Leary TP, et al. Canine pancreatic endocrine tumors: immunohistochemical analysis of hormone content and amyloid. Vet Pathol 1987;24:308–314.

Priester WA. Pancreatic islet cell tumors in domestic animals: data from 11 colleges of veterinary medicine in the United States. JNCI 1974;53:227–229.

Shahar R, Rousseaux C, Steiss J. Peripheral polyneuropathy in a dog with functional islet B-cell tumor and widespread metastasis. J Am Vet Med Assoc 1985;187:175–177.

Spencer AJ, Andreu M, Greaves P. Neoplasia and hyperplasia of pancreatic endocrine tissue in the rat: an immunocytochemical study. Vet Pathol 1986;23:11–15.

Strafuss AC, Njoku CO, Blauch B, et al. Islet cell neoplasm in four dogs. J Am Vet Med Assoc 1971;159:1008–1011.

Straus E, Johnson GF, Yalow RS. Canine Zollinger-Ellison syndrome. Gastroenterology 1977;72:380–381.

Stromberg PC, Wilson F, Capen CC. Immunocytochemical demonstration of insulin in spontaneous pancreatic islet cell tumors of Fischer rats. Vet Pathol 1983;20:291–297.

Takarnia CH. Islet cell tumor of the bovine pancreas. J Am Vet Med Assoc 1961;138:541–547.

van der Gaag I, Happé RP. Animal model of human disease: Zollinger-Ellison syndrome. Animal model: non-beta-cell neoplasms of pancreas in the dog. Comp Pathol Bull 1984;16:2,4.

Zollinger RM, Ellison EH. Primary peptic ulceration of the jejunum

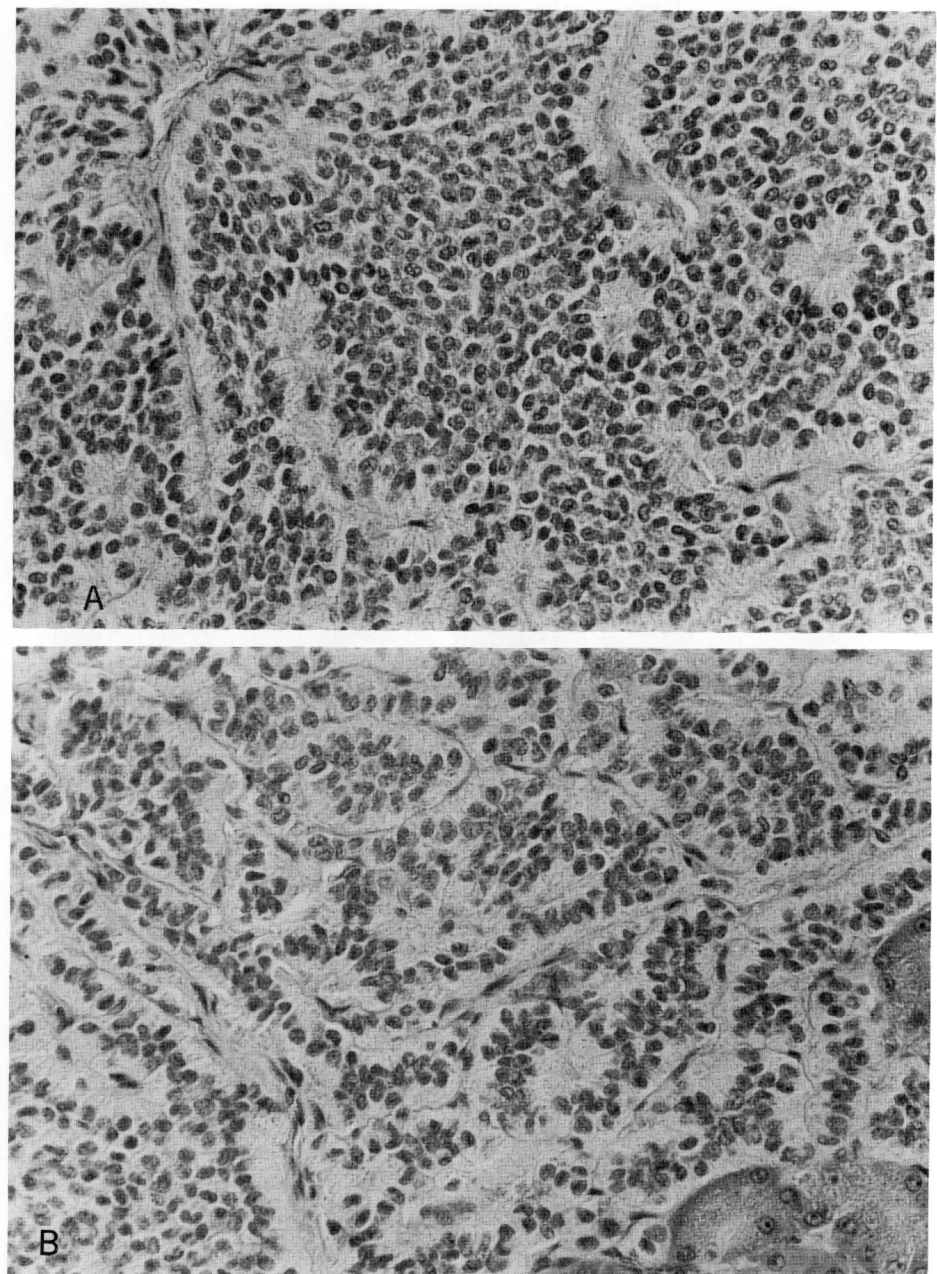

FIG. 26-15 Nonbeta islet cell tumors (Zollinger-Ellison syndrome) in the dog. **A.** Solid masses of cells with ribbon pattern and pseudorosette formation. **B.** Ribbon pattern. (Courtesy of Dr. R. P. Happé and *Veterinary Pathology.*)

associated with islet cell tumors of the pancreas. Ann Surg 1955;142:709–728.

PINEAL GLAND

Although the pineal gland (**pineal body** or **epiphysis cerebri**) has long been believed to have an endocrine function, only recently has evidence been gathered that warrants placing it with the endocrine organs in mammals. Embryologically, the organ is believed to be a vestige of a "third eye" that exists in certain reptiles and amphibians. Indeed, in lower animals such as cyclostomes, the pineal contains cells that resemble the reti-

nal sensory cells. Even in amphibians and birds, the pineal has photoreceptor functions. It has been demonstrated that the amphibian and mammalian pineal secretes a hormone-like compound known as **melatonin.** In amphibians, melatonin synthesis is controlled by photoreceptors within the pineal, and the hormone causes skin-lightening. In mammals, photoreceptor cells are not present and the pineal does not respond directly to light. Instead, the pineal responds to light received by the retina; increased light depresses melatonin synthesis, and decreased light stimulates melatonin synthesis. In mammals, melatonin inhibits gonadotropic hormone synthesis or release by the pituitary, and is believed to play a major role in the seasonal reproductive activity exhibited by many species.

Although knowledge of the ultrastructure and functions of the pineal has increased in recent years, information concerning the pathologic lesions of this interesting organ still remains limited. Necrosis, calcification, cystic degeneration, hyaline degeneration, deposition of hemosiderin, hyperemia, and petechiae have been described in the equine pineal body, but were asymptomatic. Hyperplastic enlargement to four times the normal, with consequent pressure on surrounding nervous structures, has been reported as causing a circling syndrome in a mule.

Pinealoma

This tumor, also known as **pineal adenoma,** is a rare neoplasm derived from the pineal gland. Its histologic appearance is distinctive in that it consists of an indiscriminate mingling of groups of large epithelioid cells with groups of small (neuroglial) cells with small, round nuclei suggestive of lymphocytes. Precocious puberty has been reported in boys with pinealomas. A pine-aloma has been reported in a silver fox, a horse, and a rat (see Chapter 27).

References

Binkley S, Riebman JB, Reilly KB. Time-keeping by the pineal gland. Science 1977;197:1181–1183.

Glass JD, Lynch GR. Melatonin: identification of sites of antigonadal action in mouse brain. Science 1981;214:821–823.

Kerenyi NA, von Westarp C. Post-natal transformation of the pineal gland: effect of constant darkness. Endocrinology 1971;88:1077–1079.

Min K-W, Seo IS, Song J. Postnatal evolution of the human pineal gland: an immunohistochemical study. Lab Invest 1987;57:724–728.

Nobel TA. Circling syndrome in a mule due to hyperplasia of the pineal gland. Cornell Vet 1955;45:570–575.

Reiter FJ, Sorrentino S Jr. Reproductive effects of the mammalian pineal. Am Zoologist 1970;10:247–258.

Roche JF, et al. Effect of pinealectomy on estrus, ovulation and luteinizing hormone in ewes. Biol Reprod 1970;2:251–254.

Santamarina E, Venzke WG. Physiological changes in the mammalian pineal gland correlated with the reproductive system. Am J Vet Res 1953;14:555–562.

Welser JR, Hinsman EJ, Stromberg MW. Fine structure of the canine pinealocyte. Am J Vet Res 1968;29:587–599.

Wurtman RJ, Moskowitz MA. The pineal organ. N Engl J Med 1977;296:1329–1333, 1383–1386.

27

The nervous system

Adalbert Koestner and T.C. Jones

Although the general laws of pathology are by no means abrogated in the nervous system, certain peculiar characteristics of the nervous system have led to a number of names and concepts that need to be added to the list of those encountered in the study of other body systems. At the outset, some structural and functional aspects of the nervous system that are important to understanding pathologic processes in this system need to be explained.

Certain anatomical, histologic, and biochemical features cause reactions in the central nervous system to differ somewhat from lesions of corresponding etiologic basis in other locations. Enclosed in unyielding bony cavities, brain and spinal cord are encompassed by the thin, but dense, fibrous dura mater; in most places, it forms a tough white sheet, suspended with few attachments, between the bony wall and the organ itself. Brain and cord proper are bound by a thin limiting membrane, the pia-arachnoid, whose few cell layers are intimately joined with the underlying soft parenchyma; the pia-arachnoid follows the convolutions of its surface into the depths of the sulci and over the summits of the gyri. In the sulci especially, the pia-arachnoid thickens slightly to form a matrix through which pass most of the blood and lymph vessels. Between the dura and the pia-arachnoid is the subdural space; its surfaces are lined with flat mesenchymal or endothelial cells, according to the terminology used.

With the exception of these membranes, known collectively as the meninges, and of a limited number of adventitial and perivascular fibroblasts accompanying the vessels which ramify into the parenchyma, no fibrous connective tissue exists in brain and spinal cord. Instead, a soft, but densely homogeneous supporting tissue called neuroglia (*glia,* a gluelike substance) constitutes the bulk of these organs and forms a matrix in which nerve cell bodies and dendritic and axonal fibers lay embedded. In this mass two varieties of tissue are grossly recognizable: the **white matter,** which forms the bulk of the inner substance, and the **gray matter,** which constitutes the cortical layer of the cerebrum and cere-

bellum. Gray matter also composes certain islands within the white, called "nuclei," including the basal ganglia. White matter is composed principally of nerve fibers (axons and dendrites) with myelin sheaths and a minimum of supporting tissue comprised of oligodendroglia and astrocytes. Gray matter is composed of neuroglia (principally astrocytes), with numerous nerve cell bodies (neurons) embedded in it. With light microscopy, neurons and glia are embedded in a background of fine, crisscrossing fibrils that stain pink with hematoxylin and eosin. When stained with special methods, such as silver impregnation, fibrils are seen much better and more completely, and predominately represent cytoplasmic processes of astrocytes and neurons.

Neuron

The neuron, functional unit of the nervous system, consists of a nucleus with a large nucleolus surrounded by a relatively abundant amount of cytoplasm, from which projects one or more dendrites and a single axon. Neurons vary in size from no larger than astrocytes (about 5 microns) to large neurons in the cerebellum (Purkinje cells) and cerebral cortex (Betz cells) that exceed 75 microns. Cytoplasm contains basophilic granules called **Nissl substance,** which is uniformly distributed except at the base of the axon (axon hillock). This Nissl substance may be visualized in more detail by electron microscopy and consists of rough endoplasmic reticulum (rER). Its function is to synthesize transport protein; thus, only the nerve cell body and the proximal axon are capable of producing this protein. The distal axon depends on transport of protein from the nerve cell body.

The neuron, as the principal cell for initiation and transportation of stimuli, affects the body as a whole by storage and retrieval of information, cognitive, motor, sensory, and autonomic functions, as well as endocrine and emotional control. After maturation, neurons that are destroyed cannot be replaced, with the exception of those in the nose and tongue involved with smell and taste, respectively.

Three kinds of neuroglial cells can be distinguished. None of the nuclei has visible nucleoli on light microscopy, a fact that distinguishes them from nearly all neurons.

Astrocytes

Astrocytes comprise the bulk of the neuroglia in most regions. Their nuclei are usually elliptical, somewhat pale, and vesicular in tinctorial properties, and of a size somewhat smaller than the nucleus of a monocyte. Special preparations demonstrate that each nucleus has a starlike (**astron,** star) network of branching cytoplasmic processes; at least one of these is connected to a "footpad" at the wall of a nearby blood vessel, while others often extend to the pia mater. Astrocytes with long, thin processes are called **fibrous astrocytes,** and those with shorter, wider, and usually more highly branched processes are called **protoplasmic astrocytes.** In sections stained by ordinary methods, protoplasmic astrocytes are usually distinguishable from smaller nerve cells by the less spherical and more vesicular nuclei—pale, without internal structure, but with a distinct nuclear wall—and from other neuroglial nuclei because the latter are smaller, darker, and denser in appearance. Astrocytes can be identified with certainty by the use of biomarkers, such as monoclonal antibody to glial fibrillary acidic protein (GFAP), under nonneoplastic and many neoplastic conditions. Their fibrils can also be recognized by examination with electron microscopy.

In addition to their role in structural support in the central nervous system, astrocytes have many other functions. They guide migrating neurons in the fetus to their ultimate position in the central nervous system. They maintain a close functional relationship to neurons in adults and are important in neuronal metabolism. They are essential for proper functioning of intracerebral transport because of their integral position in the blood-brain barrier. On the biochemical level, they are involved in neurotransmitter regulation, detoxification of ammonia, and regulation of potassium.

Oligodendroglial cells

Oligodendroglial cells (oligo: few; dendro: branches) have, as just implied, regularly round, darkly-stained nuclei, comparable in size to the nuclei of lymphocytes. The short and scanty fibrils are revealed only by special techniques, but because a majority of these cells occur in the fiber tracts of white matter and appear in straight rows between fibers facilitates recognition. Oligodendroglia found in gray matter line up around neurons in some locations where they are called **satellite cells.** In the white matter in the central nervous system their location is interlaminar and here they form and maintain myelin. In peripheral nerves, cells performing this function with myelin are called Schwann cells. These oligodendroglia surrounding neurons provide nutrients, particularly glucose, which is the sole source of energy for these neurons. Under unfavorable conditions, such as in hypoxia, oligodendrocytes proliferate, resulting in increased numbers of these cells near the neurons, a state called **satellitosis.**

Microglial cells

Microglial cells have small, round, dark nuclei. Fibrils are minimal in both number and length and, as usual, require special techniques for identification. They are of mesodermal rather than neuroectodermal origin, as is the case of the other components of the neuroglia, and in injured tissue become macrophages. Most authorities consider these cells to belong to the mononuclear phagocytic system (formerly called the reticuloendothelial system). They assume two forms as macrophages in the central nervous system. One form consists of cells with voluminous vacuolated cytoplasm, resembling macrophages elsewhere, and are called **gitter cells.** The second form of cells occur around necrotic neurons and have a more compact rod shape.

Ependymal cells

Ependymal cells are cuboidal or columnar cells that line ventricles, choroid plexus, and spinal canal. They may be ciliated and each cilium contains a blepharoplast.

Other cells

Several additional cells that occur in the central and peripheral nervous systems are of interest because they may be involved in inflammation and occasionally cause neoplasms. These include: endothelial, smooth muscle, and perivascular cells (adventitial cells) of the vasculature; cap cells of the meninges; and fibroblasts and histiocytes.

White matter consists essentially of nerve fibers separated from each other by myelin and a small number of neuroglia. Fibers have a tendency to lay evenly spaced and parallel to each other because a number of them follow the same intercommunicating path from one area of gray matter to another. Such parallel groups are called fiber tracts; their particular functions are ascertainable and usually well known to neurologists.

Blood vessels within the central nervous parenchyma have the peculiarity of being surrounded by a zone of appreciable width in which the cells and fibers are so scanty as to be limited to a bare supporting framework. This encircling zone constitutes what is known as the Virchow-Robin space, or, since it serves for the drainage of lymph, as the perivascular lymph space. In infectious inflammations, lymphocytes commonly accumulate in it, constituting perivascular lymphocytic infiltrations ("cuffing").

References

Abbott NJ. Glia and the blood-brain barrier. Nature 1987;325:195.

Goldstein GW, Betz AL. The blood-brain barrier. Sci Amer 1986;255:74–83.

Kimelberg HK, Norenberg MD. Astrocytes. Sci Amer 1989;260:66–76.

Lim RKS, Lie CN, Moffitt RL. A stereotaxic atlas of the dog's brain. Springfield: Thomas, 1960.

Luginbuhl H. Angiopathies of the CNS in animals. Schweiz Arch Tierheilk 1962;104:694–700.

Manuelidis L, Manuelidis EE. Proliferation and response of oligodendrocytes. Lab Invest 1985;52:1–2.

Schelper RL, Adrian EK. Monocytes become macrophages; they do not become microglia: a light and electron microscopic autoradiographic study using 125-iododeoxyuridine. J Neuropathol Neurol 1986;45:1–19.

Spector R, Johanson CE. The mammalian choroid plexus. Sci Amer 1989;261:68–74.

REACTION OF CELLS AND TISSUES TO INJURY

Postmortem autolysis becomes evident early in the central nervous system and, like necrosis, soon leads to liquefaction. It is not unusual for brain to be almost completely liquified in three to four days at mild summer temperatures (70–90°F, 21–32°C). The differentiation between the two forms of death is made according to the principles outlined in Chapter 1.

Necrosis

Necrosis ranges from slow death of an occasional neuron to softening and liquefaction of considerable volumes of central nervous tissue, the former occurring sooner and from milder causes. The usual causes of necrosis in brain or cord are anoxia, chemical and plant poisons, mycotoxins, metabolic disorders, and infectious diseases (Fig. 27-1). Among the poisons are cyanides in repeated small doses, mercury (chronic ingestion), lead (chronic), manganese, carbon monoxide, and alcohol, as well as various other organic and inorganic substances.

Anoxia is a frequent cause of nerve cell death, usually in limited or selected areas. The disorder results from interference with the blood supply, often caused by injury to the microcirculation. Neurons are highly susceptible to anoxia even when transient. Many poisons act through an anoxic mechanism (e.g., lead, sodium chloride, thiamin deficiency). However, massive deprivation of blood through cerebral embolism and infarction, arteriosclerotic changes, or hemorrhage is rare in domestic animals.

Necrosis involves some forms of change that are peculiar to nervous tissue and have not been discussed previously in this text. This is particularly true with respect to necrosis of individual neurons, which can occur upon slight provocation. It is difficult to determine precisely where degenerative and reversible changes become irreversible and must be classified as necrosis. Because the former regularly leads to the latter, the consecutive stages are considered together.

Necrosis of neurons (nerve cell bodies)

Changes in neurons that indicate death or imminent death take several forms. Acute injury is manifest by cellular swelling, as is the case with other kinds of cells. The dendritic processes of multipolar cells tend to disappear, leaving the outline of the cell unduly smooth and rounded. The **Nissl substance** in a normal and perfectly preserved neuron should appear as a sharply granular, basophilic substance in the cytoplasm, giving the latter an appearance like the markings of a tiger, hence the synonym, **tigroid substance.** In a pathogenic environment, such as anoxia, Nissl granules lose sharpness and, in just a few hours, disappear: first centrally (central chromatolysis) and then completely, often by fading, occasionally by a general blackening of the cytoplasm, but more often by increased cytoplasmic eosino-

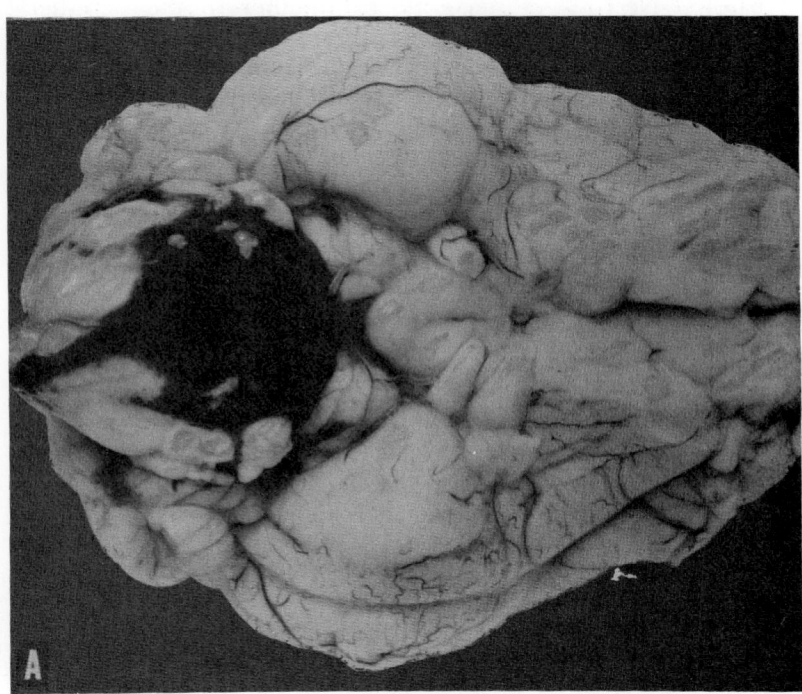

FIG. 27-1 A. Hemorrhage from the basilar artery in brain of a pig that was struck on the forehead.

philia. Concomitantly with the loss of Nissl granules from the cytoplasm and loss of normal cell outlines, the nucleus tends to swell and the nucleolus enlarges even more. The swollen nucleus is commonly displaced from its central to an eccentric position, often to lay against the cell membrane. The nucleus then undergoes karyorrhexis or karyolysis and disappears. The whole neuron tends to swell at first, then shrinks into some angular and unrecognizable form and also disappears. The axon—when it becomes visible—swells, loses its Nissl substance, is distorted into a twisted form, and disappears. All of this transpires in one to two days.

Vacuolization

Vacuolization of neurons, seen under light microscopy, may be demonstrable by electron microscopy to be one of two phenomena:

1. The result of dilatation of the rough endoplastic reticulum profiles and loss of attached ribosomes. At this stage the capacity to produce transport protein is lost. Structural proteins, essential for cell survival, may continue to be synthesized by the ribosomal rosettes, not bound to membranes, as long as they are intact and functioning. This type of vacuolization is characteristic of certain spongiform encephalopathies, such as "scrapie" of sheep, bovine spongiform encephalopathy, kuru, and Creutzfeldt-Jacob disease in humans; and,
2. The term, vacuolization involves a phenomenon in which the lysosomes are distended by the accumulation of degradation products resulting from defective lysosomal enzyme function. This is the basis for the lesions of lysosomal storage diseases (refer to Chapter 2).

Commonly, neurons are observed to be shrunken and angular, with either increased cytoplasmic basophilia or eosinophilia, and distorted dendrites. Such shrunken cells are often encountered in the absence of observable cellular swelling. Although this change may represent a true degenerative process, such cells may be encountered in normal brain, in which case it has been suggested that these shrunken cells are "inactive" neurons. Shrinking of neurons is also a feature of improper fixation. The absence of other reactions in the nervous system or clinical signs of dysfunction must be used to differentiate between artifacts and cell death.

As the neuron enters the final stage of necrosis, it is surrounded by macrophages derived from microglia and monocytes from the blood and the neuronal debris is phagocytized.

These cells are then known as neuronophages and the process is designated as **neuronophagia.** A small collection of microglia is known as a glial nodule. Neuronophagia is an indirect, but no less reliable, sign of neuronal necrosis. Microglial infiltration is reported to develop within a matter of minutes after anoxic injury; neuronophagia occurs within a few hours. These two processes, unlike intracellular regressive changes, do not occur in postmortem autolysis but only in necrosis.

Astrocytes also respond to nerve cell injury. They may increase in number, a condition known as astrocytosis, with many cells containing two and four nuclei, and/or they may increase in size due to an increased amount of eosinophilic cytoplasm, which is ordinarily not visible except as background substance. Such swollen astrocytes are called gemistocytic astrocytes or gemistocytes.

Necrosis in neuroglia

This type of necrosis is also a process of liquefaction, but it develops more slowly; in the case of some of the milder injurious agents, neuroglial necrosis may not occur, even though the nerve cells of the area have been killed. Close observation and precise knowledge of the normal histology of the area are necessary to detect accurately the absence of a few neurons under such circumstances. If an area of neuroglia (and contained nerve cells and fibers) were to undergo necrosis, it at first would soften grossly (at two to five days), a condition known as **encephalomalacia** (or myelomalacia). In one to two weeks, it would disappear through a process of liquefaction, leaving an empty space of no characteristic shape, size, or type except for its frayed and indefinite borders. Such an area may be difficult to distinguish from an artifact caused by imperfect cutting of the section, but the distinctions mentioned in Chapter 1 in connection with liquefactive necrosis apply. When appreciable areas of central nervous tissue undergo necrosis, an increase of neuroglial tissue surrounding the vacant space, called gliosis, and accumulation of macrophagic cells may be manifest after two to three weeks.

Necrosis of nerve fibers

Necrosis of nerve fibers, whether in the peripheral nerves or fiber tracts of brain or spinal cord, involves two processes: (1) **primary demyelination** affects the myelin sheath while the axon remains intact but deficient or unable to conduct impulses; and (2) **axonal degeneration** which involves the axon. Myelin subsequently disappears. The axon degenerates as the result of nerve cell body necrosis or separation by trauma. This results in the change recognized as secondary or Wallerian degeneration. Some toxic substances, such as IDPN (B, B[1] iminodipropionitrile), acrylamide, hexacarbons, and organophosphates, affect axons directly, causing axonal swelling, disruption of axonal transport, and eventually axonal dystrophy which results in dysfunction of the effector organs (e.g., muscles). Such direct axonal injuries are known as proximal and distal axonopathies.

Microglia assume their phagocytic role engulfing axonal fragments and myelin sheaths, converting the myelin to neutral fat. These lipid-containing microglia are known as **gitter cells,** and their presence is indicative of myelin damage that may otherwise be difficult to discern in ordinary hematoxylin-and-eosin-stained tissue sections. In addition to microglia, phagocytes derived from blood monocytes participate in removing necrotic material. Evidence also suggests that oligodendrocytes participate as phagocytes in removing degenerated axoplasmic organelles. The presence of an excessive number and size of holes in an area of white matter is also a morphologic sign of myelin damage. The axon may still be visible in some of them, but difficulty may occur in deciding whether one is dealing with demyelination or spaces due to edema or to excessive shrinkage in tissue preparation.

Because myelin lipid progresses through stages involving the presence of free neutral fats, it is possible to demonstrate demyelination by the usual stains for fats, or more particularly by Marchi's method. However, it is often preferable to demonstrate the disorder by staining methods (myelin-sheath stains) that directly color normal myelin because in the central nervous system, whole fiber tracts usually are affected as well. Demyelination is then detected by a blank area, usually viewed under low magnification, in the midst of the more darkly-stained, healthy tissue. Such areas are usually only relatively colorless, for the remaining neuroglial cells and fibers absorb a minimal amount of stain. Damage to either an individual or group of axons results in these same changes. When isolated axons are affected, they may be recognizable as eosinophilic, spheric masses called spheroids (in cross section), composed of the swollen axon and altered myelin.

In the **peripheral nerves,** destruction of myelin (and of the functioning fiber) may be detected by similar means, but Marchi's method is often used, in spite of a certain reputed inconstancy of action. This involves the use of the oxidizing agent, osmic acid (osmium peroxide) to stain fat separated from the myelin with a deep black color. Because osmic acid would have the same effect on myelin lipids, the tissue is first exposed to a milder oxidizing agent, potassium dichromate, which oxidizes normal myelin without coloring it but leaves the fatty, injured myelin still susceptible to osmic acid. Theoretically, at least, a delicate differentiation is obtainable. About two weeks must elapse between the injury to a peripheral nerve and the possibility of staining injured nerves by this method. Unless the injury is close to the nerve-cell body, the cell body does not die; therefore, this process is not usually necrosis but, rather, degeneration. It is known as **Wallerian degeneration.** The part of the neuron distal to the point of injury—which may be mechanical severance—dies, undergoing Wallerian degeneration throughout its length, and is associated with an influx of macrophages and proliferation of Schwann cells. Macrophages derived from blood monocytes are the principal phagocytic cell, but some believe that Schwann cells may also become phagocytic. Nerve fiber is commonly regenerated by growth from the surviving proximal portion of the neuron, a process requiring a few months. Although it seldom dies because of injury to the axon, the cell body may suffer transiently a certain degree of degeneration, particularly a rounding of the cell, displacement of the nucleus, and fading of the Nissl granules. This is known as **Nissl degeneration.** Recovery usually occurs. Demyelination of nerve fibers results from a variety of types of injury, including mechanical pressure, brief or prolonged, deficiency of thiamin and vitamin-B complex, immune mechanisms, and specific viral infections.

Calcification and, less frequently, some of the other degenerative changes described in Chapter 2, may occur in the central nervous system, but usually in relationship to the vessels or meninges.

Circulatory lesions

Passive congestion of these tissues, most prominent in the pia-arachnoid, accompanies severe, passive congestion of the rest of the body. It is readily recognized by virtue of the dark, distended veins that cover the meningeal surfaces and is usually acute and terminal. **Hyperemia** is part of the process of inflammation. **Hemorrhage** of petechial size is frequent in numerous acute infections and toxemia that injure capillaries in other parts of the body. However, pinpoint spots of blood seen on the cut surface when brain is freshly sliced often mark the cut ends of congested capillaries, not hemorrhage.

Severe blows to the head may result in skull fracture, rupture of one or more branches of the meningeal arteries, and hemorrhage into the space between the dura and bone. **Epidural hemorrhage** is uncommon in the young or old due to close adherence between dura and bone. When it does occur, dura is compressed over brain and may lead rapidly to hemiplegia, convulsions, and death unless relieved surgically. **Subdural hemorrhage,** conversely, usually results from rupture of veins, and blood is mixed with cerebrospinal fluid (CSF). Signs may be delayed as bleeding continues. It is possible for large areas of the cerebrum to be compressed by the resulting hematoma which also could become organized, leading to increased pressure on brain. The location of hemorrhage is not necessarily at the site of impact; it may be on the opposite side from inertia of the brain within the cranium and its elasticity, propensity to rebound strongly, and rupture of vessels on the opposite side (**contrecoup**). If the animal were to survive immediate injury, the effect would be increased pressure, which would depend upon the size of the clot. Death from such impact may then ensue within hours or days.

In humans, massive hemorrhage into brain is an all-too-frequent complication of arteriosclerotic and hypertensive disease. Sudden unconsciousness is known as apoplexy; the result, if the patient were to live, would be paralysis of parts innervated from the portion of brain that undergoes pressure necrosis. Commonly, this occurs on one side of the body, the condition being known popularly as a "paralytic stroke;" infarction from embolism or occlusion also causes such "strokes." Hemorrhage of this nature and stroke, in general, are infrequent in animals, doubtless because arteriosclerotic disease is rare, except in aged swine. (Refer to the discussion on concussion later in this section.)

Edema

Edema of brain is considered to occur in two primary types: **vasogenic edema** (preferentially in white matter) and nonvasogenic or **cytotoxic edema** (preferentially in gray matter). Vasogenic edema is believed to be a consequence of breakdown or impairment of the blood/brain barrier followed by leakage of serum into perivascular parenchyma, such as Virchow-Robin spaces, subarachnoid spaces, and spaces formed around neurons (Figs. 8-50 and 27-15.) Edema fluid in the white matter is extracellular and spreads within extracellular spaces. This fluid in the gray matter is intracellular because there is little extracellular space in this part of brain. The footpads (astrocytic processes) are tightly adherent to the outer wall of vessels, as well as to neuronal membranes unoccupied by synaptic terminals. Fluid escaping from vessels becomes entrapped within astrocytic processes and flows behind membranes, unless these rupture from excessive pressure. Grossly, gyri are swollen, flattened, and the sulci shallow and partly obliterated. The cut surface is moist and shiny; the parenchyma is softened.

Cytotoxic edema is believed to be the result of altered cellular metabolism. Fluid accumulates within intracellular compartments of neurons, neuroglia, and endothelial cells. The blood-brain barrier remains intact. Edema is, therefore, considered nonvasogenic. Gray matter is preferentially involved; however, nonvasogenic edema of white matter has been demonstrated with a number of substances, such as triethyltin and hexachlorophene. In these cases, edema accumulates within the myelin membrane which is split at the interperiod line. The mechanism is believed to be the uncoupling of oxidative phosphorylation resulting in reduced respiration and inhibition of mitochondrial ATPase.

Infarcts are not as frequent in animals as they are in humans, where they are associated with the higher incidence of atherosclerosis. Infarcts may arise from lodged emboli and occur in association with some infectious animal diseases that lead to vasculitis. Focal necrosis of brain unassociated with vascular disease may result from many infectious and noninfectious diseases and are sometimes incorrectly termed, infarcts.

Anoxic (hypoxic) encephalopathy

The central nervous system is particularly susceptible to deprivation of oxygen. Lesions are comparable regardless of cause (e.g., anemia, heart failure, or poisoning by cyanide or carbon monoxide). When death results from acute cerebral anoxia within minutes or up to eight hours, lesions will not be evident. Lesions become evident when survival is prolonged beyond eight hours. The morphologic features, which are not distinctive, include either poliomalacia or leukomalacia. The distribution of lesions, however, is relatively distinctive. There is necrosis of the cerebral cortex, which is usually patchy but may involve the entire cortex. All layers may

be affected or only the deeper lamina, a situation called **laminar necrosis.** The depths of sulci suffer greater damage than the crowns of gyri. Laminar necrosis may also be seen in other conditions, such as polioencephalomalacia of cattle or salt poisoning in swine. There is also selective necrosis of nuclei, with relatively consistent involvement of the globis pallidus, substantia nigra, and thalamus. Focal malacia of cerebral white matter occurs, especially in the corpus callosum and anterior commissure (refer to *porencephaly*). Lesions in the gray and white matter are bilaterally symmetric. Similar neuropathologic changes develop in the fetus from compression of the umbilical cord and other mechanisms.

TRAUMA

Concussion and contusion

Concussion of brain results from nonfatal impact to the head, with possible fracture of the cranial bones. It may produce instant, though transient, unconsciousness. Concussion causes a sudden, violent displacement of the subarachnoid and other fluid in brain and unconsciousness is believed to be due to transient anemia as blood is jarred from the capillaries into larger vessels. The same sudden movement of intravascular blood and perivascular lymph (cerebrospinal fluid) may cause numerous petechiae or lacerations of superficially-placed tissues.

More extensive hemorrhages into brain parenchyma and meningeal spaces are the result of severe trauma and are classified as contusion. In such cases usually two hemorrhagic lesions develop, one at the side of impact (coup lesion) and another, often more severe, at the opposite pole (countercoup lesion). The latter is produced by a sudden stop of a movably suspended brain within the cranial cavity at impact, creating excessive, negative pressure at the opposite pole and resulting in tearing of blood vessels.

The main consequence of mass hemorrhage is diffuse compression, which, when severe or not relieved, may lead to permanent unconsciousness and eventually death. Brain compression with similar consequences may also be caused by space-occupying lesions such as tumors, abscesses, and edema.

The clinical signs may at first be manifest as hyperirritability, perhaps with convulsions; however, as pressure increases, mental depression, somnolence, and coma supervene. Paralysis may occur from the effect of compression on motor centers. Headache is severe in humans and the same is undoubtedly true in animals. This is one, and possibly the principal, reason for the tendency of horses and cattle to press the forehead against objects. It is difficult to evaluate this sign precisely. Vomiting, in the absence of a digestive disorder, is prominent in those species that vomit. The lesions are obviously those that belong to the individual causative disorder. Edematous swelling has been described. In a localized area of compression, softening and liquefaction necrosis would develop if the patient were to survive a few days.

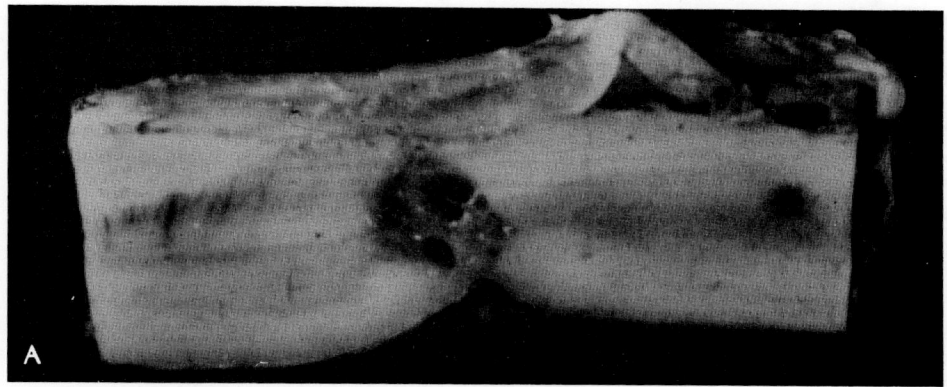

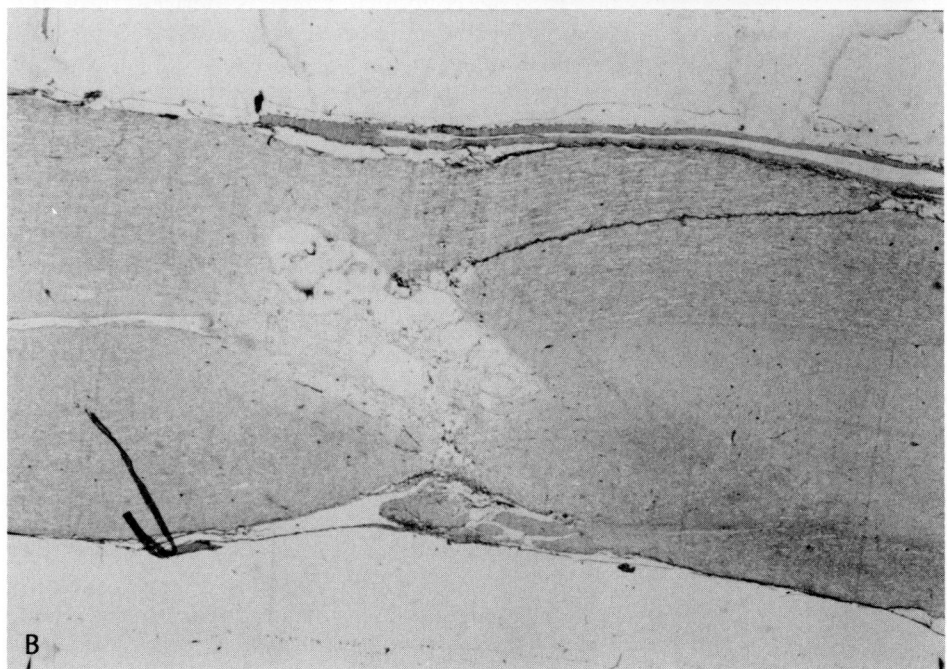

FIG. 27-2 Compression of spinal cord of an eight-month-old female dachshund as result of dislocation of the first and second cervical vertebrae. **A.** Gross specimen incised after formalin fixation. **B.** Low power of a histologic section: hematoxylin-and-eosin-stained, ×4. (Courtesy of Angell Memorial Animal Hospital.)

Stenosis of spinal canal

Stenosis of the spinal canal is the usual proximal cause of traumatic injury to the spinal cord (Fig. 27-2). Several events may contribute to this type of stenosis:

1. Severe trauma to the vertebral column, resulting in vertebral fracture, luxation, or subluxation of vertebrae (e.g., traffic accidents, falls);
2. Dislocation or exostosis of vertebrae (cervical stenotic myelopathy, equine, or canine "wobblers");
3. Protrusion or herniation of nucleus pulposus of intervertebral disc. Rupture of intervertebral ligaments permits most severe herniation (dachshunds and other achondroplastic breeds);
4. Space-occupying mass within the spinal canal impinges on the spinal cord, resulting in a localized necrotic lesion (metastatic or primary neoplasms, granulomas—such as caused by tuberculosis);
5. Proliferation of bone in the thoracolumbar vertebrae, with compression of the spinal cord and paresis, has been observed in cats afflicted with lyso-

somal storage disease, (mucopolysaccharidosis VI: described in Chapter 2); and,
6. Localized ossification and calcification of the meninges (in old German shepherds) may decrease the diameter of the spinal canal enough to cause damaging pressure on the spinal cord.

Pressure upon the cord leads to paralysis of muscles enervated from segments distal to the point of compression (e.g., fractured vertebra), usually initiated with local hyperirritability. Paralysis is of the upper-motor-neuron type (i.e., spastic). Flaccid paralysis involves parts that are enervated directly from the injured segment. Sensation is lost from structures caudal to the lesion. As in brain, softening and liquefaction result from local pressure. Myelin stains indicate demyelination and loss of fibers (Wallerian degeneration) in the motor tracts below and the sensory tracts above the injured segment. The development of this change requires several days.

Descriptions of some syndromes, in which the spinal cord is seriously affected, follow.

Canine ataxia (canine incoordination: "Wobbler Syndrome in Dogs;" cervical stenotic myelopathy: "Wobbler Disease in Dogs")

A neurologic syndrome of dogs, particularly Great Danes and other giant breeds, is remarkably similar to the condition in equines, especially thoroughbred horses, called equine incoordination; it is also called ataxia of fouls, wobbler disease, and other names. The neurologic signs, lesions in cervical vertebrae and spinal cord, and pathogenesis (as far as known) appear to be nearly identical in the canine and equine diseases. The precise initiating cause of lesions in the cervical vertebrae in both species is unknown.

Onset of signs, often insidious but sometimes sudden, is usually detected in young dogs, most under two years of age, and the earliest recorded at three months. Initial ataxia involves the pelvic limbs, eventually extending to the thoracic limbs, and may persist for several years. Loss of limb control results in an insecure gait with the animal wobbling from side to side. Turning the neck to one side or the other side usually accentuates incoordination.

Lesions in the vertebral column are usually limited to the cervical vertebrae and are associated with one or two compression sites in the spinal cord. This compression is most often detected radiographically or at postmortem at the junction of cervical vertebrae C_{5-6} or C_{6-7}. Several abnormalities have been described in the vertebrae, not identical, but each produces stenosis of the spinal canal and thereby focal compression of the spinal cord. One of the common vertebral defects allows one cervical vertebra to override the adjacent caudal one, presumably due to weakness or relaxation of the intervertebral ligament, and to impinge on the spinal cord at that point. This compression of the spinal cord causes trauma at this point that destroys tracts and gray matter, particularly the latter. Wallerian degeneration of ascending tracts cranial to this traumatic lesion and in descending tracts caudal to it may be demonstrated with carefully selected and studied histologic sections.

In some cases, exostosis from the floor of the spinal canal may contribute to the stenosis, but this does not appear to be related to degeneration of the intervertebral disc or protrusion of the nucleus pulposus. Several other factors have been imputed to cause underlying changes in the cervical vertebrae. These include "vertebral instability" (presumably due to defective supporting ligaments), deformation of vertebral arches or articular processes, and malformations or malarticulations of the vertebrae. Thus, several lesions in specific cervical vertebrae have been shown to result in traumatic damage to the spinal cord and to explain the clinical signs, but the underlying nature of the vertebral lesions remains unknown.

References

Olsson SE, Stavenborn M, Hoppe F. Dynamic compression of the cervical spinal cord. A myelographic and pathologic investigation in Great Dane dogs. Acta Vet Scand 1982;23:65–78.

Trotter EJ, DeLahaunta A, Geary JC, et al. Caudal cervical vertebral malformation-malarticulation in Great Danes and Doberman pinschers. J Am Vet Assoc 1976;168:917–930.

Wright F, Rest JR, Palmer AC. Ataxia of the Great Dane caused by stenosis of the cervical vertebral canal: comparison with similar conditions in the basset hound, Doberman pinscher, ridgeback, and thoroughbred horse. Vet Rec 1973;92:1–6.

Equine incoordination (ataxia of foals)

A disease of young horses and mules, in which nonparalytic disturbances of gait are significant features, is referred to as equine incoordination, ataxia of foals, or "wobbles." The colloquial name is derived from the horseman's description of the incoordinated or wobbling gait of affected animals. Horses characteristically display the signs of this disorder during the first four years of life.

The underlying etiology is not known, but the nature of the lesions in spinal column and spinal cord (Figs. 27-3, 27-4) point toward the initial lesion being a transitory or persistent stenosis of the cervical spinal canal. Constriction of the spinal canal with pressure on the adjacent spinal cord is most often believed to be the result of abnormal mobility of one or more vertebrae or due to malformation of these vertebrae. These lesions must be looked for during necropsy (Fig. 27-4). The presence of a traumatic lesion in the cervical spinal cord in relation to pressure from constriction of the spinal canal can be demonstrated to be associated with Wallerian degeneration is ascending tracts cephalic to the injury and similar degeneration in descending tracts caudal to it.

The usual history indicates that severe symptoms become evident suddenly, usually after an accident, such as a fall, but careful clinical observers report that the onset is insidious. In the opinion of Jones, the accident accentuates incoordination, bringing it to the owner's attention, but the usual sequence of events is that the animal's inability to coordinate muscle groups precedes and causes the fall. There is no measurable loss of strength in the muscles, but rather a failure to synchronize their action, causing the animal to weave from side to side as it walks. The pelvic limbs are usually affected first, the incoordination later spreading to the forelimbs. The animal walks with its hind feet spread apart, has difficulty in turning and particularly in backing. The rear quarters sway from side to side during the walk or trot. After falls, which may be frequent, the animal has difficulty in regaining its feet. Early in the course of disease, pressure on the neck in the anterior cervical region or turning the head to one side accentuates the "wobbling" and may cause the horse to fall. Slight excess mobility in the cervical region may be detected early as well. The course is unpredictable. Affected animals may survive, with care, for years, or without warning, be found dead apparently as the result of a fall. Paralysis is not a manifestation except in those singular cases in which subdural hemorrhage occurs in the cervical region. Affected animals are usually sacrificed as incurable.

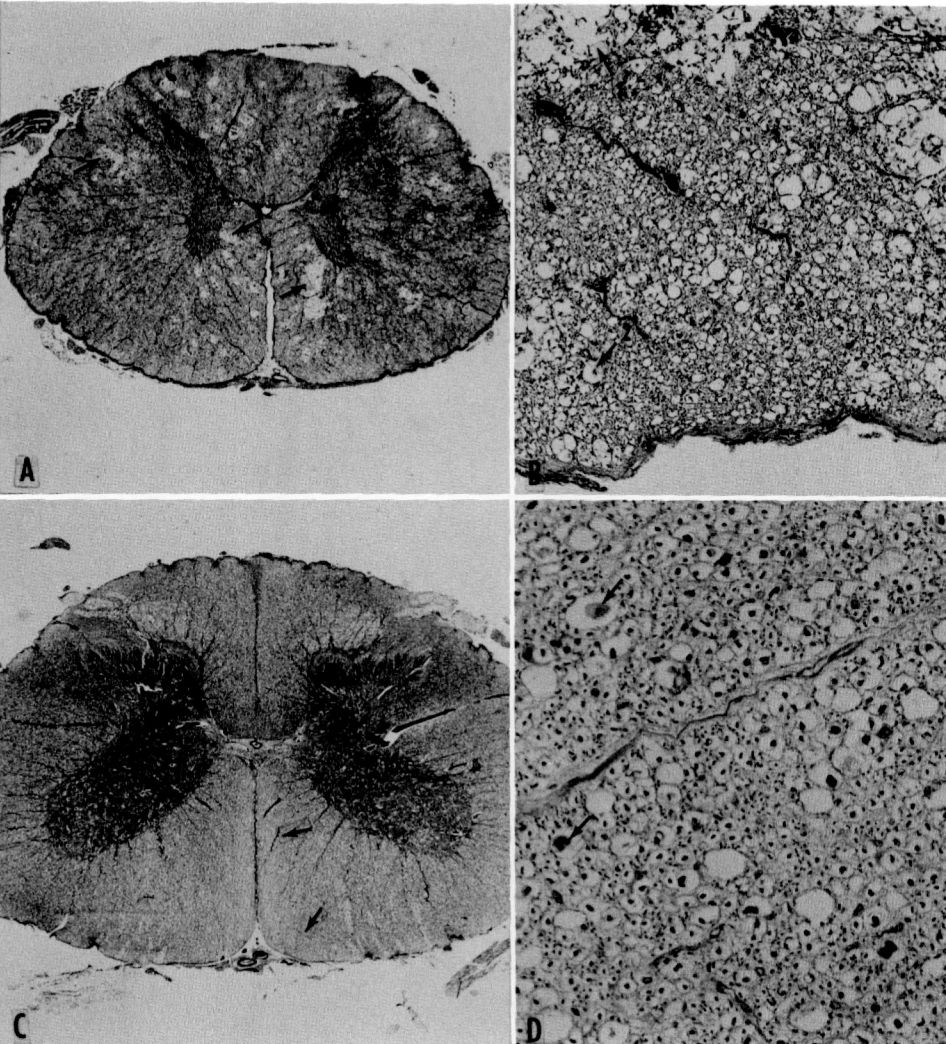

FIG. 27-3 Ataxia of foals (equine incoordination). **A.** Spinal cord (×8) at level of junction of third and fourth cervical vertebrae. Areas of malacia (*arrows*) in several parts of white matter. The primary lesion. **B.** Same section as in **A** (×100). (1) Large irregular spaces and (2) swollen axis sheaths. **C.** Spinal cord of same animal at level of the fifth cervical vertebra (×8). Secondary (Wallerian) degeneration is limited to certain fasciculi (*arrows*) adjacent to the ventral median fissure. **D.** Higher magnification (×205) of secondary degeneration in **C.** Arrows indicate some swollen axons surrounded by a dilated axis sheath. (Courtesy of Armed Forces Institute of Pathology; contributor: Dr. E.R. Doll.)

LESIONS

Lesions in equine incoordination are confined to the spinal column and spinal cord. Distortion of the spinal canal may be seen in most cases at necropsy. Apparent relaxation of the intervertebral ligaments, particularly between the second and third, third and fourth, or fifth and sixth cervical vertebrae, allows them to become misaligned, giving the spinal canal a tortuous course. This kyphoscoliosis in some cases produces obvious constriction of the spinal canal and, hence, causes focal pressure upon the spinal cord. Osteoarthritis involving the vertebral joints may be present, as evidenced by erosion of the joint cartilage and eburnation of the underlying bone. These articular lesions have been explained on the basis of excessive movement of the vertebrae.

In the spinal cord, gross lesions are not evident in most cases, although subdural hemorrhage may be present in the upper cervical region of a few animals dying after a fall or found dead. Microscopic lesions are characteristic but may be overlooked in casual or hurried examinations. Careful examination of many sections usually discloses a primary zone of malacia in the cervical region, usually in relation to a constricted segment of the spinal canal. This primary malacic area in the cord usually is seen as several ragged cavities scattered through various white columns, although sometimes only one cavity exists. Loss of neurons in the gray columns may occur at this site but is not conspicuous, the white matter exhibiting the most severe changes. In these foci of malacia, the large, irregular, empty cavities are presumably the result of pooling of myelin and liquefaction necrosis. Swollen axons may be detected in cross section. Increased numbers of glial cells are present and gitter cells may be evident.

This "primary" focus of malacia in the upper cervical region is sharply delimited and only a few centimeters in length; however, more than one such focus can occur. In cases with only one primary focus, its limits may be clearly defined by microscopic examination of transverse sections of the spinal cord on either side of the lesion. Above (cephalad to) the lesion, Wallerian degeneration is seen in ascending nerve fibers which, for the most part, are located in the dorsal funiculi.

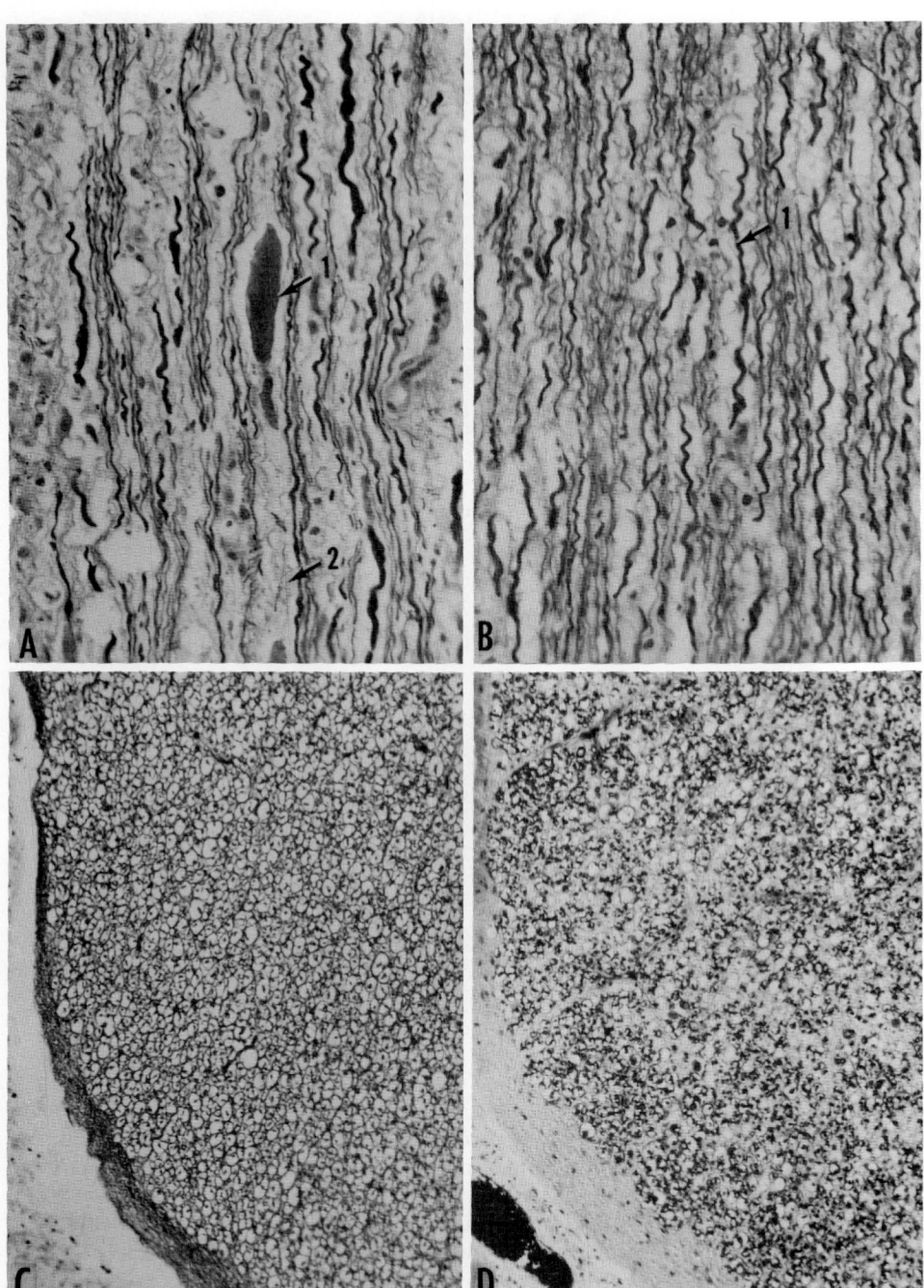

FIG. 27-4 Wallerian degeneration in equine incoordination. **A.** Longitudinal section (×205) of an affected fasciculus in the cervical cord. Weil's stain. (1) Enlarged, fragmented axon and (2) glial fibers. **B.** Normal spinal cord. Weil stain. (1) Axons are of uniform width and surrounded by an intact myelin sheath. **C.** Normal spinal cord (×100). Weil stain. Note uniform size of myelin sheaths. Axons appear as dots within each myelin sheath. **D.** Cross section of an affected spinal cord (×100). Weil stain. Note irregular size of axons, disorganization, and pale areas of glial scarring. (Courtesy of Armed Forces Institute of Pathology; all contributed by Dr. E.R. Doll.)

Caudal to this cervical lesion, Wallerian degeneration occurs in descending fibers. Although they may be found in lateral funiculi, such affected fibers are more constant in ventral funiculi. In the lower cervical region, affected fibers are concentrated in the ventral funiculi on either side of the ventral median fissure. Lesions in these columns may extend well into the thoracic and lumbar cord.

Lesions in ventral funiculi are bilaterally symmetric and typical of Wallerian degeneration of any nerve tract: i.e., resulting from injury to the axon at a point nearer the nerve cell body. Early in the disease, swollen axon sheaths give this tissue a vacuolated, spongy appearance in contrast to the normal white column, in which myelin sheaths are uniform in diameter. Axons are distorted, enlarged to many times their normal dimensions in some segments, and broken off at other points along the course. In transverse sections these affected axons may appear as spherical, darkly-stained structures or may be absent. In sections cut parallel to the length of the tract, axons appear thickened at some points, absent at others. Glial cells increase in number and eventually replace destroyed nerve fibers, giving the affected column a scarred appearance (gliosis).

This change is best demonstrated microscopically by means of Weil stain.

The diagnosis of equine incoordination may be established at necropsy by demonstration of characteristic gross and microscopic lesions in the spinal column and spinal cord.

References

Jones TC, Doll ER, Brown RG. The pathology of equine incoordination (ataxia or "wobbles" of foals). Proc 91st Ann Meeting Am Vet Med Assoc 1954;139–149.

Rooney JR. Equine incoordination. I. Gross morphology. Cornell Vet 1963;53:411–422.

Rooney JR, Prickett ME, Delaney FM, et al. Focal myelitis-encephalitis in horses. Cornell Vet 1970;50:494–501.

INFLAMMATION AND INFLAMMATORY DISEASE

General principles of inflammation can be applied not only to the brain and spinal cord but elsewhere as well; however, manifestations of an inflammatory process are restricted in accordance with the kinds of cells and tissues present and certain anatomical limitations:

1. Because there are no mucous membranes, catarrhal inflammation does not occur;
2. Serous inflammatory reactions probably do not occur; however, if they were to occur, no differentiation from edema would be evident;
3. Hemorrhagic exudates are seldom encountered, although hemorrhages are frequent;
4. Fibrinous inflammation is limited mostly to the meninges and to penetrating wounds; and,
5. Purulent, lymphocytic, and proliferative inflammations are regularly encountered in the central nervous system.

Encephalitis refers to inflammation of the brain. In **encephalomyelitis,** brain and spinal cord are involved in inflammation. In **myelitis,** inflammation is limited to the spinal cord. **Meningitis** indicates inflammatory involvement only of the meninges. **Meningoencephalomyelitis** denotes inflammation of the meninges, brain, and spinal cord. Infection may invade the nervous system by one or more of several routes:

1. By hematogenous route: arborviruses are transmitted by an insect from an infected host, injected through the skin, and carried to brain by the bloodstream;
2. By extension through the nasal or olfactory tissues to brain;
3. Carried along the course of nerves: such as when herpesvirus moves from the oral mucosa via the nerves to reach the brain; and,
4. By direct contact with infection after fracture or penetration of the skull.

A specific infection may have a predilection for particular parts of the nervous tissue. The prefix, **polio-** indicates involvement of the gray matter (e.g., poliomyelitis or polioencephalomyelitis); **leuko-** indicates involvement of the white matter (e.g., leukomalacia); and **pan** as a prefix points to involvement of both white and gray matter (e.g., panencephalitis).

Many infectious diseases are characterized by encephalitis as either the primary manifestation or as part of more generalized diseases. These include inflammations caused by viruses, Mycoplasma, Chlamydia, bacteria, fungi, protozoa, and metazoan parasites, all of which have been discussed in earlier chapters. (Table 27-1).

Infectious thromboembolic meningoencephalitis of cattle caused by a *Haemophilus* organism is characterized by purulent inflammation of brain and meninges, principally within and surrounding vascular walls. A limited amount of purulent exudation accompanies some forms (Eastern strain) of equine encephalomyelitis, although the reaction in this disease is fundamentally lymphocytic. Diffuse suppurative or fibrinopurulent meningitis occurs as a wound infection in the rare event of trauma which pierces the bony covering without being immediately fatal. It does not appear that animals have copiously suppurative meningitis comparable to that caused by meningococcus in humans.

Subacute lymphocytic inflammation is a characteristic type in the central nervous tissues, the cells being trapped in the Virchow-Robin spaces as they leave the vessels and progress further only with difficulty. The cause is usually, but not invariably, one of the neurotropic viruses. Infiltrations of lymphocytes, which may be only perivascular, constitute the most conspicuous lesions in viral infections. They may be accompanied by petechial hemorrhages and notable hyperemia. The primary lesion in most types of viral encephalitis, however, is necrosis of neurons, the morphologic features of which have already been described. In the earlier stages of some viral diseases, such as rabies, practically no visible lesions exist. Such infections as toxoplasmosis and even torulosis (cryptococcosis) also result in limited infiltrations of lymphocytes, usually perivascular, when they involve nervous tissue. Lymphocytic cuffing is also seen adjacent to areas of necrosis (refer to *malacia*), cerebral abscesses, and neoplasms in brain. Practically speaking, however, without the presence of other exudates, and without other apparent explanation, lymphocytic infiltrations may be considered indicative of an infectious disease, quite likely a viral one. The localization of lesions and other features of viral diseases are discussed in Chapter 8.

ENCEPHALOPATHY AND ENCEPHALOMALACIA

Encephalopathy is a general term, used to indicate degeneration of neurons (neuronopathy), axons (axonopathy), myelin (myelinopathy) and vessels (vasculopathy). These degenerations may progress to malacia. Necrosis in the central nervous system is called **malacia; encephalomalacia** occurs in brain and **myelomalacia** in the spinal cord. When gray matter is affected, it is termed **poliomalacia,** and when white matter is affected, **leukomalacia.** Although malacia may be a feature of many infectious forms of encephalitis, necrosis in brain or spinal cord is more apt to accompany many

TABLE 27-1 Inflammatory diseases of the nervous system

Viral infections (Chapter 8)

Herpes simplex	St Louis encephalitis, humans
Herpes B	
Pseudorabies	Japanese B encephalitis, humans
Canine hepatitis (adenovirus)	
African swine fever	Russian tick-borne encephalitis
Feline panleukopenia (cerebellar hypoplasia)	Louping ill, sheep
Poliomyelitis, mice	Kyasanur forest disease
Poliomyelitis, man	Canine distemper encephalitis
Encephalomyocarditis	
Polioencephalomyelitis, porcine	Chronic viral encephalomyelitis, sheep (visna/maedi)
Teschen disease, swine	
Talfan disease, swine	Progressive multifocal leukoencephalitis (measles)
Benign enzootic paresis, swine	
Canada viral encephalomyelitis	Rabies
	Lymphocytic choriomeningitis
Avian encephalomyelitis	Porcine coronaviral encephalitis
New Castle disease, avian	
Malignant catarrhal fever, bovine	Borna disease
	Murine encephalomyelitis
	Equine encephalomyelitis, western, eastern, Venezuelan

Infections due to Chlamydia (Chapter 9)

Sporadic bovine encephalomyelitis
(Chlamydia psittaci)

Bacterial diseases (Chapter 10)

Botulism (Clostridium botulinum)	Tetanus (Clostridium tetani)
Pseudotuberculosis (Corynebacterium pseudotuberculosis)	Listeriosis (Listeria monocytogenes)
	Tuberculosis (M. tuberculosis)
Meningitis (Neisseria meningitidis) (Streptococcus pneumoniae) (Escherichia coli) (Salmonella dublin)	(Haemophilus somnus), bovine (Haemophilus agni), lambs

Fungal infections, Mycoses (Chapter 11)

Actinomycosis (Actinomyces bovis)	Blastomycosis (Blastomyces dermatitides)
Coccidioidomycosis (Coccidioides immitis)	Cryptococcosis (Cryptococcus neoformans)
	Histoplasmosis (Histoplasma capsulatum)

Diseases due to Protozoa (Chapter 12)

Toxoplasmosis (Toxoplasma gondii)	Trypanosomiasis (Trypanosoma cruzi)
Hartmannellosis (Hartmannella sp.)	Encephalitozoonosis (Encephalitozoon cuniculi)

Diseases due to Helminths and Arthropods (Chapter 13)

Cerebrospinal Nematodiasis (Setaria digitata)	Echinococcosis (Echinococcus granulosus)

TABLE 27-1 (continued)

(Angiostrongylus cantonensis)	Cestodiasis
(Odocoileus virginianus)	
(Ascaris columnaris)	(Coenurus cerebralis)
(Strongylus vulgaris)	(Cysticercus cellulosae)

toxic or metabolic disorders. Conditions in which encephalomalacia is a conspicuous finding are listed in Table 27-2.

Toxic, degenerative, and necrotic changes described earlier in this chapter may be accompanied by any of the usual signs of inflammation. A reaction that is both striking and unique, however, does accompany softening and necrosis of appreciable amounts of central nervous tissue. This is the appearance, at the necrotic site, of **scavenger cells,** also known as **compound granular corpuscles, Hortega cells,** or **gitter cells** (German: **gitterzelle**). These are large, lipid-filled phagocytes which, in a few days, infiltrate the injured area in large numbers. Evidence indicates that they arise by proliferation and differentiation of microglial and infiltrating monocytes. They are comparable to monocytes and macrophages found in extraneural organs. Gitter cells phagocytize and assist in the removal of the large amount of lipid which is characteristic of central nervous tissue, slowly disappearing when the task has been completed. Concurrently, oligodendroglial cells swell and remain swollen throughout the period of active reaction.

Within two to three weeks, another proliferative change develops that is comparable to the formation of fibrous granulation tissue. It differs in that the proliferating cells are the fibrillary astrocytes of the neuroglia, and the lesions is named **gliosis.** Unlikely to be detected

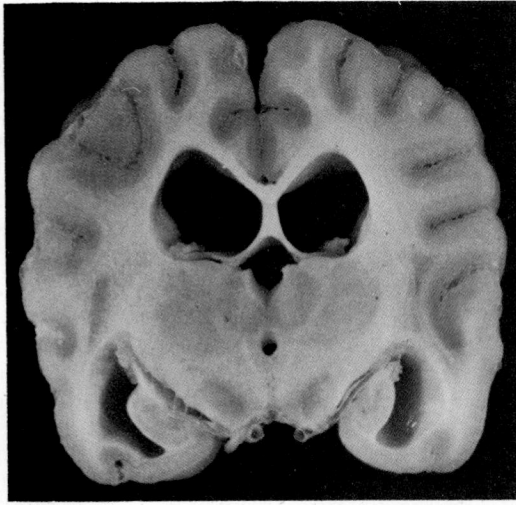

FIG. 27-5 Brain of an 18-year-old dog. Ventricles are enlarged, gyri narrowed, and blood vessels fibrotic. (Courtesy of Dr. H. Wisniewski and *Laboratory Investigation.*)

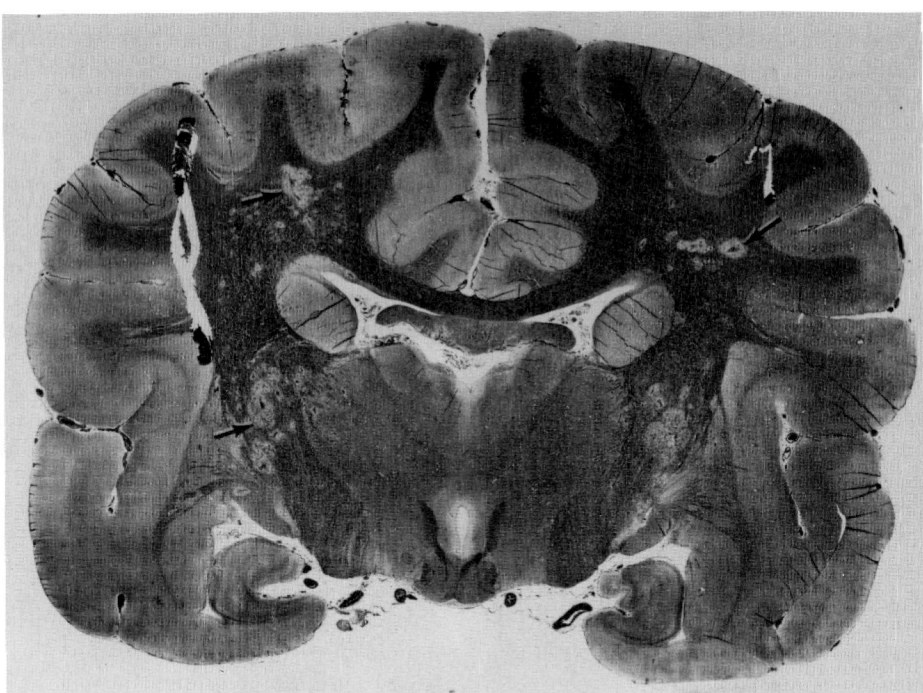

FIG. 27-6 Demyelination in allergic encephalitis in a dog. Transverse section of brain. Weil stain. Arrows indicate pale areas of demyelination in white matter. (Courtesy of Armed Forces Institute of Pathology; contributor: Dr. C.P. Zepp, Jr.)

grossly, gliosis has the appearance microscopically of an area of neuroglia that is denser than the surrounding normal areas, with which it gradually blends. An increase in the number of glial nuclei occurs early, but the increased density is due to the larger number of fibrils per unit of area and also to a somewhat greater diameter of some individual fibrils. The increase of glial tissue is mainly around the perimeter of the defect when a complete loss of substance (liquefaction necrosis) occurred; the new glial tissue does not fill the empty space as would be done by proliferating fibrous granulation tissue. The glia-encircled empty space sometimes remains filled with clear fluid, constituting a cyst.

Proliferation of numerous, small capillaries often accompanies proliferation of the glial cells, or may occur without glial scarring in an area that otherwise is changed little. This constitutes another form of proliferative inflammatory reaction. It first becomes conspic-

uous about one week after an anoxic or toxic injury (Table 27-3).

Sometimes accompanying these several reactive phenomena is a change in the microglia consisting of the formation of "rod cells." These are microglial nuclei that elongate until the length is three to four times that of the diameter; they stain darkly.

Proliferation of fibrous connective tissue is limited to the immediate vicinity of blood vessels (Fig. 27-5) and to the meninges, where a parent fibrous tissue of mesodermal origin exists. This tissue, which proliferates from the perivascular mesenchyme, contributes to healing scars in the nervous system. Astrocytes are currently believed to provide the glial component. Resultant lesions are referred to as glial, mesenchymal, and "mixed glial-mesenchymal" scars. Tissue of this kind is rarely extensive except in the case of traumatic injury to the perivascular and meningeal fibroblastic tissues. Scars—whether glial, mesenchymal, or both—tend to contract as they grow older and, in doing so, place unnatural strains and pressures on the neighboring tissue. In humans, who are more likely than animals to survive after anoxic, toxic, or traumatic injury to brain, malfunction of distorted brain tissue sometimes leads to periodic

---

TABLE 27-2 **Poisons causing nervous manifestations (Chapter 15)**

Anguina	Arsanilic acid
Atropine	Bracken fern
Carbon disulfide	Chlorinated hydrocarbons
Clostridium enterotoxemia	Cycads
Equisetum	Focal spinal poliomyelitis, sheep
Hemlocks	
Larkspur	Lathyrus
Lead	Mercury
Mycotoxins (Chapter 11)	Organic phosphates
Ortho tricresyl phosphates	Phalaris grass
Salt (sodium chloride)	Strychnine
Yellow-star thistle	Vetchlike Astragali

TABLE 27-3 **Deficiency diseases with nervous manifestations (Chapter 16)**

Copper deficiency
Thiamine deficiency
   Polioencephalomalacia of sheep and cattle (Chapter 27)
Vitamin E deficiency in birds
   Mulberry heart disease, swine

convulsive seizures or lapses of consciousness known as traumatic epilepsy. This type of secondary epilepsy is also known in animals, particularly in dogs.

Focal symmetric poliomalacia in sheep

A singular paralytic disease of sheep seen on a farm located in the Rift Valley of Kenya, Africa, was described by Innes and Plowright (1955). The disease was first noticed between February and April 1952, in 10 of 40 lambs two to four months of age. The following year, 60 of 240 animals in the flock died from the disease and this outbreak also involved older animals. The disease apparently did not spread to other farms, but did manifest unusual clinical and pathologic features (Fig. 27-7).

The disease was sudden in onset, only a few sheep exhibiting premonitory signs, such as motor weakness or incoordination of the forelimbs. Flaccid paralysis usually developed rapidly in all limbs, but in some instances spasticity was a feature. Only the forelimbs of some sheep were involved and animals thus affected hopped about on their hind legs like kangaroos during the days or weeks they survived. The muscles of the fixed, adducted front limbs usually underwent atrophy if the animal were to survive for some time, but most died within three weeks. Affected animals were afebrile and the disease apparently was not transmissible from one sheep to another. Cattle in the same pasture did not contract the disease.

LESIONS

Lesions were limited to the spinal cord and could be recognized only upon microscopic examination. Symmetric malacic lesions in the ventral gray columns—never in the dorsal columns—were limited to certain segments in the cervical enlargement, except for a few cases in which lesions were confined to segments of the lumbar enlargement. In a typical case, lesions in the gray columns started at the level of the

fourth cervical vertebra (C4), disappeared at C6 and appeared again at C7 and the first thoracic vertebra (T1). In another case, lesions were found between C4 and C6, as well as in the lumbar enlargement.

Bilateral symmetry was particularly striking, the lesions in one ventral column being a mirror image of those in its opposite. These sharply delimited foci of malacia did not evoke a significant surrounding inflammatory reaction, but a rim of well-preserved gray matter containing neurons was often evident around them and the commissural gray matter was intact. Involved areas of ventral gray matter were sharply demarcated, stained palely, with neurons replaced by a ragged, spongy-appearing lesion in which capillaries and glial fibers were predominant. In early lesions, gitter cells were numerous while, in later stages, astrocytes and newly proliferated capillaries filled the area of softening. Neither vascular lesions nor demyelination was observed in white columns.

The significance of this disease is not known, but it is an interesting addition to the growing list of pathologic entities that result in neurologic disturbances in sheep.

The diagnosis was made upon demonstration of bilaterally symmetric malacic lesions in the spinal cord of sheep which exhibited characteristic signs.

References

Innes JRM, Plowright W. Focal symmetrical poliomalacia of sheep in Kenya. J Neuropathol Exp Neurol 1955;14:185–197.
Pienaar JG, Thornton DJ. Focal symmetrical encephalomalacia in sheep in South Africa. J S Afr Vet Med Assoc 1964;35:351–358. [Vet Bull 1965;35:1051.]

Polioencephalomalacia of cattle and sheep

Lesions of a noninfectious nervous disease in cattle, sheep, and goats known in certain western states as "for-

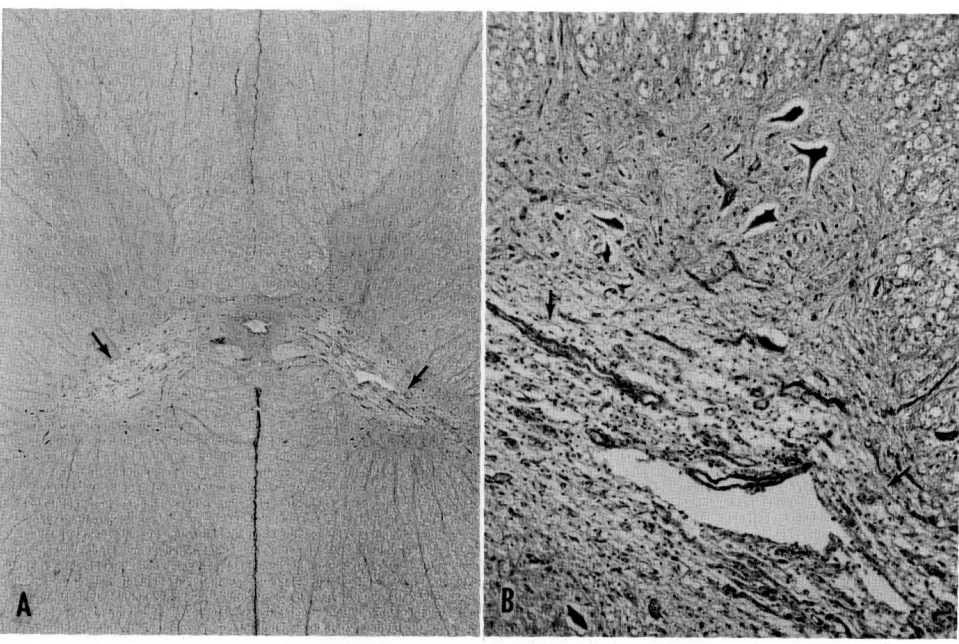

FIG. 27-7 Symmetrical poliomalacia of sheep. **A.** Spinal cord (×16). Note symmetry of lesions in each of the ventral horns of gray matter (*arrows*). **B.** Higher magnification (×110) of the malacic lesion in the gray matter (*arrows*). (**B.** Courtesy of Armed Forces Institute of Pathology; contributor: Dr. J.R.M. Innes.)

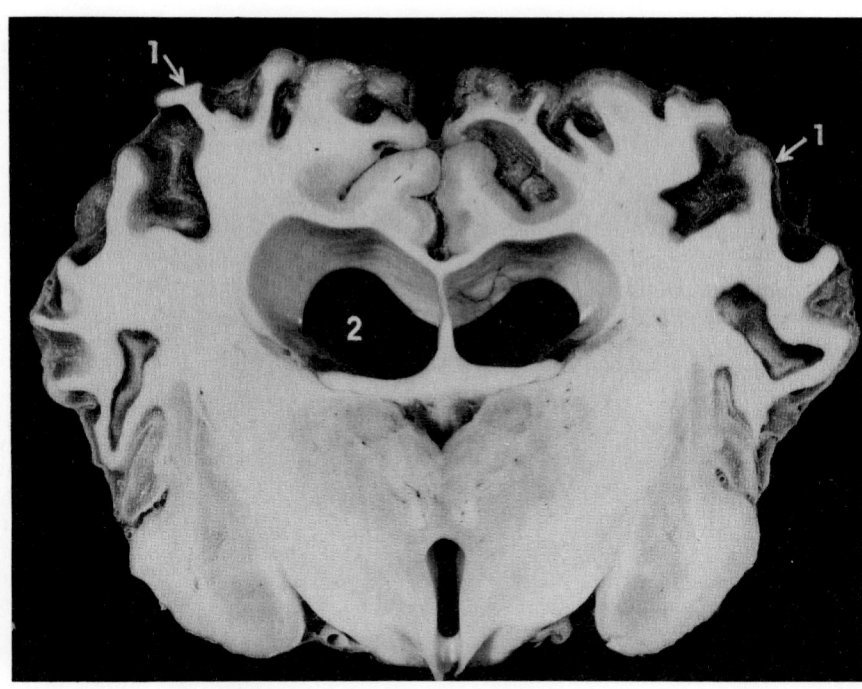

FIG. 27-8 Polioencephalomalacia in brain of a cow. Note loss of (1) cortical gray matter and (2) hydrocephalus. (Courtesy of Drs. Jean C. Flint and Rue Jensen, Colorado State University.)

age poisoning" or "blind staggers," have been characterized by Jensen et al. as necrotizing destruction of cortical gray matter (1956; Fig. 27-8); therefore, the disease was named "polioencephalomalacia." These authors estimated that the incidence of this disease in cattle reached 100 per thousand animals in some regions of Colorado. The disorder was more frequently observed in cattle 12–18 months of age; sheep of all ages were less often affected. The incidence increased during January among cattle in feedlots, while the incidence among those in pasture was highest in July. The disease has been recognized in cattle and sheep in Great Britain, where it is usually referred to as "cerebrocortical necrosis." The disease is also reported in ruminants in Australia and is apparently of worldwide distribution.

The dramatic response of certain clinical cases, diagnosed as having polioencephalomalacia, to the administration of thiamine first suggested that this vitamin may be involved in the etiology. Additional evidence pointing toward thiamine deficiency soon followed. Affected animals have increased levels of blood pyruvate, lactate, creatinine, phosphokinase, and pyruvate kinase, and low levels of thiamine in brain and liver. Thiaminase has been identified in rumen, a thiaminase-producing bacterium has been recovered from it, and the disease has been reproduced by thiamine antagonists. Thiaminase can also cause depletion of nicotinic acid (a cosubstrate), but the possible role of the additional deficiency of this nutrient to the pathogenesis of the disease is uncertain. What appears to be the same entity has been described in Cuba in feedlot cattle fed a molasses-urea-based diet. Pyruvate oxidation was blocked, but brain and liver thiamine concentrations were normal. Thus, the pathogenesis and definite etiologic role of thiamine remains to be incontrovertibly established. Thiamine deficiency diseases are further discussed in Chapter 17 (refer to *Bracken fern* and *Equisetum poisoning*).

CLINICAL MANIFESTATIONS

As originally described, clinical manifestations in severely affected animals begin with muscular tremors, twitching of the ears, eyelids, and facial muscles, followed in some instances by convulsions. Affected animals are unable to see, although no lesions can be detected in the eyes. Visible mucous membranes become injected, respiration and pulse rates accelerated, and temperature sometimes elevated. Mildly affected animals, seen more frequently during the summer months among those in pastures, separate themselves from the herd and occasionally push their heads against solid objects. They are blind, apathetic, and often exhibit purposeless masticatory movements accompanied by excessive salivation and, occasionally, twitching of facial or ear muscles. Death occurs in 50–90% of affected animals, depending upon the severity of the disorder.

Specific lesions are limited to the central nervous system, the changes in the cerebrum being most striking in the cortex, where focal, later diffuse, liquefaction necrosis destroys most of the gray matter. The adjacent white matter is spared. Cerebral convolutions, thus, collapse and appear in cross section to have been sculptured away, appearing in bas relief against the underlying white matter. This gives the impression that brain has decreased in size. Internal hydrocephalus is often recognized in severely affected brain.

This selective malacia is seen microscopically to affect only the gray matter, subcortical white matter showing only vascularization, a few gitter cells, and occasionally perivascular lymphocytic aggregations in regions adjacent to affected gray cortex. In light microscopy neurons appear to become necrotic first, but all cells are eventually involved in areas of necrosis. Ultrastructural studies, however, demonstrated that the earliest lesion is an increase in fluid in the cytoplasm of astrocytes and a perineuronal sponginess or vacuolation (edema) resulting from dilated astrocytic processes (Morgan, 1973). In the cerebellum, necrosis of the granular layer precedes loss of Purkinje cells. Occasionally, cystic cavities are observed, but in most cases debris is removed promptly by gitter cells. Gliosis, with gemistocytic astrocytes predominating, is the usual change adjacent to cortical areas from which all viable tissue has been removed by liquefaction necrosis.

References

Edwin EE, Jackman R. Thiaminase 1 in the development of cerebrocortical necrosis in sheep and cattle. Nature 1970;228:772–774.

Edwin EE, Lewis G, Allcroft R. Cerebrocortical necrosis: a hypothesis for the possible role of thiaminases in its pathogenesis. Vet Rec 1968;83:176–177.

Evans WC, et al. Induction of thiamine deficiency in sheep, with lesions similar to those of cerebrocortical necrosis. J Comp Pathol 1975;85:253–267.

Fenwick DC. Polioencephalomalacia of sheep. Response to thiamine in a single case. Aust Vet J 1967;43:484.

Jensen R, Griner LA, Adams OR. Polioencephalomalacia of cattle and sheep. J Am Vet Med Assoc 1956;129:311–321.

Little, PB. Biochemical and pathologic studies of thiamin deficiency and polioencephalomalacia of cattle. Diss Abstr Int 1970; 30B:4449–4450.

Markson LM, et al. The aetiology of cerebrocortical necrosis: the effects of administering antimetabolites of thiamine to preruminant calves. Br Vet J 1972;128:488–499.

Markson LM, Terlecki S, Lewis G. Cerebrocortical necrosis in calves. Vet Rec 1966;79:578–579.

Markson LM, Terlecki S. The aetiology of cerebrocortical necrosis. Br Vet J 1968;124:309–315.

Morgan KT. An ultrastructural study of ovine polio-encephalomalacia. J Pathol 1973;110:123–130.

Morgan KT, Coop RL, Doxey DL. Amprolium poisoning of preruminant lambs: an investigation of the encephalopathy and the haemorrhagic and diarrhoeic syndromes. J Pathol 1975;116:73–81.

Roberts GW, Boyd JW. Cerebrocortical necrosis in ruminants. Occurrence of thiaminase in the gut of normal and affected animals and its effect on thiamine status. J Comp Pathol 1974;84:365–374.

Smith MC. Polioencephalomalacia in goats. J Am Vet Med Assoc 1979;174:1328–1332.

DISORDERS OF MYELIN

Dysmyelinating and demyelinating diseases

The integrity of the myelin sheath is disrupted in many disorders of the central nervous system that damage nerve fibers and oligodendroglial cells, including infarction, certain poisons, and infectious encephalitis. Demyelination of this type, which is more of a form of necrosis, was discussed previously. There remain two groups of diseases in which the principal lesion focuses on myelin. They are classified as **dysmyelinating diseases** (hypomyelinogenesis), when a defect in myelin formation occurs, and **demyelinating diseases,** when destruction of myelin is manifest. Distinction between the two mechanisms is, however, somewhat arbitrary especially in the case of fetal infections leading to destruc-

---

TABLE 27-4 **Dysmyelination and demyelinating diseases**

Dysmyelination

Hereditary hypomyelinogenesis in swine (congenital tremor) and cattle
Globoid cell leukodystrophy (Chapter 2)
Metachromatic leukodystrophy (Chapter 2)
Sudanophilic leukodystrophy in "quaking" and "jumpy" mice
Hereditary cerebellar ataxia of calves
Feline neuroaxonal dystrophy
Swayback (enzootic ataxia) of lambs

Demyelinating

Allergic encephalomyelitis
  Experimental
  Postrabies vaccination
  Postinfectious
  Postsmallpox vaccination in humans
Polyradiculoneuritis (coonhound paralysis)
Viral encephalomyelitis
  Canine distemper
  Visna
  Mouse hepatitis
  Infectious leukoencephalomyelitis of goats
  Bluetongue (fetal)
  Border disease (bovine virus diarrhea) fetal lambs
  Hog cholera (fetal)
  Subacute sclerosing panencephalitis in humans (measles)
  Progressive multifocal leukoencephalopathy in humans (papovavirus)

Suspected viral origin

Multiple sclerosis of humans
Spinal demyelination in rats

Poisonings

Arsanilic acid
Cicada
Coyotillo
Hexachlorophene
Organic phosphates
Yellow-star thistle

---

tion of myelin-forming cells. Table 27-4 lists diseases that involve disorders of myelin.

CONGENITAL HYPO- OR DYSMYELINOGENESIS

Congenital hypomyelinogenesis is occasionally seen in most species of animals. Certain of the better characterized forms are discussed elsewhere (leukodystrophies, cerebellar ataxia of calves). In swine, two hereditary forms of hypomyelinogenesis are recognized: a sex-linked recessive disease in Landrace pigs and an autosomal-recessive trait in Saddleback pigs. Both are recognized clinically by congenital tremors. In Landrace pigs and a similar disease in dogs, myelin formation in the central nervous system is almost completely absent; however, in the peripheral nervous system, myelin formation is normal because it depends upon Schwann cells. Saddleback pigs appear to have defective synthesis and degeneration of myelin. In Charolais cattle, a condition characterized by slowly progressive ataxia commencing after six months of age is characterized by loss of myelin apparently due to a defect in oligodendrocytes.

References

Blakemore WF, Harding JDJ. Ultrastructural observations on the spinal cord of piglets affected with congenital tremor type AIV. Res Vet Sci 1974;17:248–255.

Blakemore WF, Harding JDJ, Done JT. Ultrastructural observations on the spinal cord of a Landrace pig with congenital tremor type AIII. Res Vet Sci 1974;17:174–178.

Blakemore WF, Palmer AC, Barlow RM. Progressive ataxia of Charolais cattle associated with disordered myelin. Acta Neuropathol 1974;29:127–139.

Herschkowitz N, Vassella F, Bischoff A. Myelin differences in the central and peripheral nervous system in the "Jimpy" mouse. J Neurochem 1971;18:1361–1363.

Kishimoto Y. Abnormality in sphingolipid fatty acids from sciatic nerve and brain of quaking mice. J Neurochem 1971;18:1365–1368.

Palmer AC, Blakemore WF, Barlow RM, et al. Progressive ataxia of Charolais cattle associated with a myelin disorder. Vet Rec 1972;91:592–594.

Patterson DSP, Done JT, Foulkes JA, et al. Neurochemistry of the spinal cord in congenital tremor of piglets (type AII), a spinal dysmyelinogenesis of infectious origin. J Neurochem 1976;26:481–485.

Patton CS. Progressive ataxia in Charolais cattle. Vet Pathol 1977;14:535–537.

Samorajski T, Friede RL, Reimer PR. Hypomyelination in the quaking mouse. A model for the analysis of disturbed myelin formation. J Neuropathol Exp Neurol 1971;29:507–523.

CONGENITAL DEMYELINATING DISEASE OF LAMBS (SWAYBACK, ENZOOTIC ATAXIA)

Newborn or young lambs are frequently affected with a specific demyelinating disease known among shepherds in England, Scotland, and Wales as "swayback." The disease has also been reported from Australia as "enzootic ataxia" and is known colloquially in South Africa as "Lamkruis." It has also been reported in the United States. The disease is manifest in suckling or newborn lambs by severe ataxia: affected animals show incoordinated movements; they are unable to walk but are able to nurse; and they do not exhibit flaccid paralysis. Blindness is sometimes observed; fever is absent, and death usually results from starvation or exposure, frequently accompanied by bronchopneumonia. Generally, affected lambs are sacrificed by the owner.

The disease is most prevalent among lambs born of ewes that have been maintained on a diet low in copper. Many but not all such ewes manifest anemia, some have "stringy" wool, and most have lowered copper levels in blood and liver. It is believed, therefore, that the disease is related to copper deficiency, but the mechanism of action is not known. Chapter 16 provides additional information.

Lesions are limited to the central nervous system and are characterized by diffuse, symmetric destruction of subcortical white matter in the cerebrum accompanied by descending destruction of certain myelinated tracts in the spinal cord. In severe, acute cases the destruction of cerebral white matter leads to grossly visible gelatinous softening in the subcortical white matter with formation of large, symmetric cavities. This cavita-

tion may be followed by secondary internal hydrocephalus. Chromatolysis in neurons of the red nucleus has been observed. Affected myelinated tracts appear spongy microscopically, and in early cases may be bordered by areas containing globules of myelin and collections of gitter cells. All evidence of tissue reaction usually disappears shortly and inflammatory cells are rare in adjacent viable parenchyma.

References

Bennetts HW, Beck AB. Enzootic ataxia and copper deficiency of sheep in Western Australia. Aust Council Sci Indust Res Bull 1942;147:55.

Bennetts HW, Chapman FE. Copper deficiency in sheep in Western Australia: a preliminary account of the aetiology of enzootic ataxia of lambs and anaemia of ewes. Aust Vet J 1937;13:138–149.

Butler EJ, Barlow RM, Smith BSW. Copper deficiency in relation to swayback in sheep. II. Effect of dosing young lambs with molybdate and sulphate. J Comp Pathol 1964;74:419–426.

Cancilla PA, Barlow RM. Structural changes of the central nervous system in swayback (enzootic ataxia) of lambs. IV. Electron microscopy of the white matter of the spinal cord. Acta Neuropathol 1968;11:294–300.

Cancilla PA, Barlow RM. Structural changes of the central nervous system in swayback (enzootic ataxia) of lambs. V. Electron microscopic observations of the corpus callosum. Acta Neuropathol 1969;12:307–313.

Innes JRM, Shearer GD. I. "Swayback": a demyelinating disease of lambs with affinities to Schilder's encephalitis in man. J Comp Pathol Ther 1940;53:1–41.

Jensen R, Maag DD, Flint JC. Enzootic ataxia from copper deficiency in sheep in Colorado. J Am Vet Med Assoc 1958;133:336–340.

Roberts HE, Williams BM, Harvard A. Cerebral oedema in lambs associated with hypocuprosis and its relationship to swayback. I. Field, clinical, gross anatomical and biochemical observations. II. Histopathological findings. J Comp Pathol 1966;76:279–290.

Schulz KCA, van der Merwe PK, van Rensburg PJJ, et al. Studies in demyelinating diseases of sheep associated with copper deficiency. Onderstepoort J Vet Res 1951;25:35–78.

ALLERGIC ENCEPHALOMYELITIS (AUTOIMMUNE ENCEPHALOMYELITIS, AUTOIMMUNE DEMYELINATION, POSTVACCINATION ENCEPHALITIS, DISSEMINATED ENCEPHALOMYELITIS)

Many years ago, after Pasteur introduced the vaccine against rabies, consisting of attenuated rabies virus in suspensions of rabbit brain or spinal cord, it was observed that a few people and animals suddenly exhibited paralytic signs within a few days after receiving the vaccine. This "postvaccinal encephalitis" was reproduced experimentally in monkeys (probably *Macaca mulatta*) by Rivers and Schwenker in 1935 by parenteral injections of suspensions of brain material. This experimental demyelinating disorder has continued to be of intense interest over the years, especially because it has proved to be a useful model for the study of human multiple sclerosis and related disorders.

According to Raine, a study of experimental allergic encephalomyelitis provided a prototype tool for the following (1984): "(a) the dissection of delayed hypersensitivity—type reactions in the central nervous system; (b) biophysical and neurochemical analyses of myelin composition and enzymology; (c) immunologic studies of effector and suppressor mechanisms in demyelination; (d) studies on acute multiple sclerosis, a rare, fatal variant of chronic multiple sclerosis; (e) therapeutic approaches to acute demyelination; and (f) with the development of chronic relapsing models of experimental allergic encephalomyelitis, studies on the pathogenesis and therapy of chronic multiple sclerosis."

Experimental disease may be induced in many species (e.g., nonhuman primates, dogs, rabbits, rats, mice) by repeated injections of suspensions of brain material or myelin basic protein, or by single injections of these substances suspended in or accompanied by Freund's adjuvant (suspension of killed bacteria, such as *Mycobacterium tuberculosis* in mineral oil).

The resulting characteristic destruction of myelin represents a type of induced autoimmune disease and fits into the category of delayed (cellular) hypersensitivity (refer to Chapter 7). The process is mediated by T-lymphocyte lines of cells and will induce the process when such sensitized T lymphocytes are transferred to naive individuals. Transfer of serum alone does not initiate the disease.

Other forms of postvaccination encephalitis with demyelination as a prominent feature are recognized in humans following smallpox vaccination, which does not contain nervous tissue. This reaction, and certain forms of postinfectious encephalitis in humans, such as measles, mumps, and influenza, are believed to represent virus-induced immunologic reactions against myelin.

Signs in this disease usually start with motor paralysis of one or more limbs, which gradually extends to involve most of the body. Death is the usual outcome in animals with a severe form of the disease. Dogs are most commonly affected, presumably because antirabies vaccination is most frequent in this species, but many other species are susceptible.

Lesions are most evident upon microscopic examination of brain and spinal cord. In brain, lesions are sharply limited to white matter, destruction of myelinated tracts being the dominant feature. Tracts of all levels may be involved, although the largest lesions are usually seen in the cerebellar peduncles, internal capsule, and pyramids. Subcortical white matter is often affected and occasionally the corpus callosum is involved. Lesions appear as irregular, nonsymmetrical areas of malacia with destruction of myelin followed by the usual glial and leukocytic responses. Perivascular accumulation of lymphocytes is often intense in regions adjacent to foci of malacia. In the spinal cord, tracts in the myelinated white columns are similarly affected, but accumulation of lymphocytes around blood vessels is a more striking feature. Considerable demyelination in peripheral nerves may also be manifest.

The diagnosis of "allergic encephalitis"(Fig. 27-6) can usually be based upon the history and on the demonstration of characteristic microscopic lesions in brain and spinal cord.

References

Moore GW, McCarron RN, McFarlin DE, et al. Chronic relapsing necrotizing encephalomyelitis produced by myelin basic protein in mice. Lab Invest 1987;57:157–167.

Prud'Homme GJ, Parfrey NA. Role of T helper lymphocytes in autoimmune diseases. Lab Invest 1988;59:158–172.

Raine CS. Analysis of autoimmune demyelination: its impact upon multiple sclerosis. Lab Invest 1984;50:608–635.

Umehara F, Qin Y, Goto M, et al. Experimental autoimmune encephalitis in the maturing central nervous system: transfer of myelin basic protein-specific T line lymphocytes to neonatal Lewis rats. Lab Invest 1990;62:147–155.

Wekerle H. The lesion of acute experimental autoimmune encephalitis: isolation and membrane phenotypes of perivascular infiltrates from encephalic rat brain white matter. Lab Invest 1984;51:199–205.

POLYRADICULONEURITIS

An interesting syndrome in dogs, known colloquially as "coonhound paralysis," has been associated for years with a prior bite or scratch by a raccoon. Coonhounds are most often affected, but other breeds are also susceptible. Lesions consist of inflammation and segmental demyelination of ventral roots and spinal nerves, and resemble those of Landry-Guillain-Barré syndrome in humans. Clinical features involve acute ascending flaccid paralysis starting 7–14 days following the bite of a raccoon. A viral etiology is suspected, perhaps operating on an allergic basis. Attempts to isolate an infectious agent have been unsuccessful; however, an essentially identical condition has been experimentally induced in dogs by inoculation of canine ischiatic nerve and Freund's complete adjuvant, which support the allergic basis of the condition.

Axonal degeneration in the nerve roots and spinal nerves is accompanied by perivascular infiltration of leukocytes, mostly lymphocytes. Plasma cells may predominate in some sections. Peripheral nerves (sciatic) may be affected, but lesions are most consistent in the ventral nerve roots.

References

Cummings JF, Haas DC. Coonhound paralysis. An acute idiopathic polyradiculoneuritis in dogs resembling the Landry-Guillain-Barre syndrome. J Neurol Sci 1947;4:51–81.

Cummings JF, Haas DC. Idiopathic polyneuritis. Guillain-Barre syndrome. Animal model: coonhound paralysis, idiopathic polyradiculoneuritis of coonhounds. Am J Pathol 1972;66:189–192.

Cummings JF, DeLahunta A. Chronic relapsing polyradiculoneuritis in a dog: a clinical, light- and electron-microscopic study. Acta Neuropathol 1974;18:191–204.

Holmes DF, DeLahunta A. Experimental allergic neuritis in the dog and its comparison with the naturally occurring disease: coonhound paralysis. Acta Neuropathol 1974;30:329–337.

Waksman BH, Adams RD. A comparative study of experimental allergic neuritis in the rabbit, guinea pig and mouse. J Neuropathol Exp Neurol 1956;15:293–314.

Viral demyelinating diseases

Certain viral infections are associated with demyelinating encephalitis and some demyelinating diseases are suspected to have a viral cause. The mechanism of viral demyelination is generally unknown, but two basic processes are potentially operable. Destruction of oligodendrogliocytes—and, hence, myelin by direct viral invasion and necrosis—is believed to be the mechanism in neurotropic mouse hepatitis-encephalitis and possibly in canine distemper encephalitis.

The alternative mechanism is analogous to that postulated and just described for allergic encephalomyelitis.

In this case, it is contemplated that viral damage to glial cells releases encephalitogenic peptides, possibly attached to cellular transport proteins, such as chaperonins, which trigger the T-cell-associated autoimmune response. Persistent viral infection perpetuates this process and provides periodic access to sensitized T-cells and antibodies directed to myelin protein and glial cells.

This mechanism is believed to contribute to demyelination in canine distemper and subacute sclerosing panencephalitis in humans, which is associated with measles virus. The mechanism in bluetongue infection in fetal lambs is direct necrosis, as is probably the case in border disease. In visna, the mechanism is unknown. Progressive multifocal leukoencephalopathy in humans is believed to be caused by a papovavirus directly destroying oligodendrogliocytes. Multiple sclerosis is suspected of being caused by a virus, possibly a myxovirus, but is still under investigation.

INFECTIOUS LEUKOENCEPHALOMYELITIS

Infectious leukoencephalomyelitis, a demyelinating disease of young (1–4 months old) dairy goats, which is caused by a virus serologically related to visna virus is also in this category. Demyelination associated with astrocytosis and perivascular lymphocytic cuffing is most severe from the mesencephalon caudally including the spinal cord. This virus also causes pneumonia and arthritis.

Reference

Cork LC, et al. Infectious leukoencephalomyelitis of young goats. J Infect Dis 1974;129:134–141.

SPINAL DEMYELINATION IN RATS

Pappenheimer described a spontaneous demyelinating disease in adult rats exhibiting progressive flaccid paralysis. Lesions are limited to the spinal cord, where ventral and lateral white columns undergo severe demyelination. Lesions are bilaterally symmetric and appear as sharply demarcated, spongy areas replacing most of the white matter. Dorsal columns are generally less severely affected. The cause remains unknown; attempts to transmit the disease or to demonstrate any relationship to viral disease in mice have been unsuccessful. The significance of this disease is unknown; however, if it were reproducible or occurred spontaneously with more frequency, this disease may be useful as a tool for investigation of demyelinating diseases.

Reference

Pappenheimer AM. Spontaneous demyelinating disease of adult rats. Am J Pathol 1952;28:247–255.

Neuroaxonal degeneration or dystrophy

Several other disorders characterized by degeneration of neurons or their processes have been described in animals. Most are not common. Some appear to be hereditary, but infectious agents have not been ruled out for most. Those included in this section are not readily classified with other degenerative diseases, such as leukodystrophies, cerebellar hypoplasias, or disorders of myelin, which are also degenerative diseases. The pathogenesis of these disorders is not understood, but each is characterized by degeneration of neurons or processes called neuroaxonal degeneration or dystrophy. Morphologic features of degenerating neurons and axons have been discussed earlier. Often—especially in dogs—isolated, swollen axons (called spheroids) are encountered as an incidental finding without clinical correlation and unknown pathogenesis.

HEREDITARY NEURONAL ABIOTROPHY IN DOGS

A previously unrecognized disease was described by Sandefeldt et al. in Swedish Lapland dogs as due to a simple autosomal-recessive trait (1973). At five to seven weeks of age, a sudden onset of thoracic or pelvic limb weakening is manifest which progresses rapidly to paralysis of all four limbs (tetraparesis). Muscle atrophy and joint fixation follow and then further progression abates. Movement of the head, tail, and axial musculature is not affected.

Microscopically, neuronal degeneration (or abiotrophy), characterized by central chromatolysis and ultimately neuronophagia, is widespread in spinal lower motor neurons, medullary rays of the cerebellum, Purkinje cells, spinal ganglia, and various nuclei. Wallerian degeneration is present in peripheral nerves in the limbs, especially in the motor nerves. Sandefeldt et al. suggested that nerve cell body degeneration represents a retrograde response to axonal degeneration (1976). The condition is similar to spinal muscular atrophy in humans (Werdnig-Hoffmann disease).

DEGENERATIVE MYELOPATHY IN GERMAN SHEPHERD DOGS

This has been described as a slowly progressive, spastic paralysis of the pelvic limbs in older animals (mean age: 8.2 years). Lesions consist of degeneration of spinal cord myelin and axons in all fasciculi, associated with astrocytosis. Lesions are most extensive in the midthoracic spinal cord. Pathogenesis has not been determined, although intervertebral disc protrusion, spondylosis deformans, or osseous metaplasia of the dura have been excluded.

Myelomalacia affecting the ventromedial spinal cord has been described in Afghan hounds. These dogs, which range 3–13 months of age, developed ataxia and progressive paralysis leading to death or euthanasia. The cause is unknown.

References

Averill DR Jr. Degenerative myelopathy in the aging German shepherd dog. Clinical and pathologic findings. J Am Vet Med Assoc 1973;162:1045–1051.
Cockerell BY, Herigstad RR, Flo GL, Legendre AM. Myelomalacia in Afghan hounds. J Am Vet Med Assoc 1973;162:362–365.

CONGENITAL ANOMALIES

The nervous systems of animals and humans are subject to many anomalies that originate during embryonic life. Any abnormality (Fig. 27-10) that is present at birth is

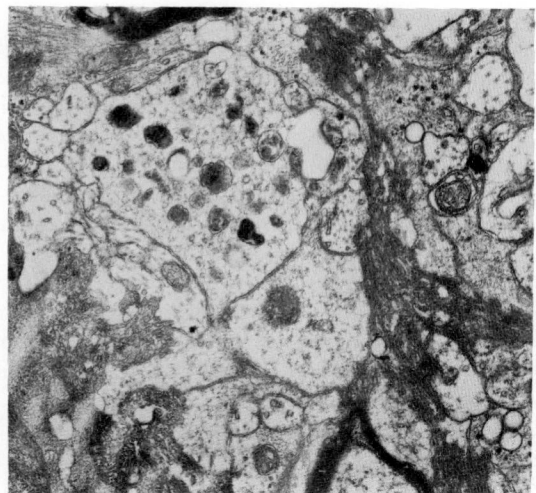

FIG. 27-9 Senile plaque in brain of aged dog, ×16,000. Perimeter of amyloid (left) from a large plaque. (Courtesy of Dr. H. Wisniewski and *Laboratory Investigation*.)

congenital. Contrary to common assumption, congenital anomalies are not necessarily hereditary (Fig. 27-11); however, some anomalies that are congenital will be described in the following pages. Several anomalies may be traced to one of many other causes, including intrauterine infections (especially viruses), nutritional factors (especially deficiencies of vitamin A, folic acid, vitamin B12, hypervitaminosis A), toxins, and trauma. Congenital anomalies have been recognized for centuries and have been given descriptive names (Table 27-5) but their causes are not understood completely.

Some congenital anomalies or syndromes have been clearly established to be the result of nonfatal intrauterine infections (Table 17-6). These are discussed in more detail in Chapter 8.

References

Cho DY, Leipold HW. Congenital defects of the bovine nervous system. Vet Bull 1977;47:489–504.

Cho DY, Leipold HW. Spina bifida and spinal dysraphism in calves. Zbl Vet Med A 1977;24:680–695.

Cho DY, Leipold HW. Agenesis of corpus callosum in calves. Cornell Vet 1978;68:99–105.

Cho DY, Leipold HW. Anencephaly in calves. Cornell Vet 1978;68:60–69.

Gruys E. Dicephalus, spina bifida, Arnold-Chiari malformation and duplication of thoracic organs in a calf. Zbl Vet Med 1973; 20:789–800.

Jerome CP. Craniorachischisis in a squirrel monkey. Lab An Sci 1987;37:76–79.

HYDROCEPHALUS

Hydrocephalus is the slow accumulation of excessive cerebrospinal fluid (CSF) in the lateral and other ventricles and sometimes in the subarachnoid spaces due to obstruction of normal drainage (Fig. 27-11). When confined to the ventricles, this accumulation is termed **internal hydrocephalus,** and when in the subarachnoid space, it is termed **external hydrocephalus.**

Normally, continual secretion of CSF occurs from the choroid plexus of vessels located principally in the lateral ventricles (Fig. 27-12). This drains through the aqueduct of Sylvius into the fourth ventricle. From there, it passes through some minute openings in the roof of that ventricle, known as the foramina of Luschka, into rather indefinite compartments called the basal cisterns in the subarachnoid space. Some fluid drains into the spinal canal as CSF. Overflow continues from the basal cisterns anteriorly through the intercommunicating subarachnoid spaces, where it is reabsorbed into the venous circulation, especially through the arachnoid villi, which project into the venous sinuses to afford increased absorptive surface.

Increased secretion of CSF by a neoplasm of the choroid plexus is a rare cause of hydrocephalus.

The major causes of hydrocephalus are considered to occur from mechanical obstruction of CSF outflow. Such obstruction could occur at one of several obvious sites and a variety of local disorders could initiate the obstruction. The slender aqueduct of Sylvius is easily closed by external pressure, and the foramen of Luschka, which leads from the fourth ventricle (Fig. 27-13), are still more vulnerable. Inflammatory exudates, tumors, parasitic cysts *(Coenurus cerebralis),* and similar structures are possible sources of pressure in these regions. Another potential barrier is the tentorium cerebelli; not only is the cranial cavity sharply narrowed here, facilitating obstruction of the subarachnoid passageways, but the same interference with flow is also achieved by slight displacement of brain either forward or backward. Its soft mass acts as a plug in the narrow incisura tentorii. Such displacement of brain can be produced by inflammation or other swelling in either compartment of the cranial cavity. Brain is occasionally forced backward into the foramen magnum until escape of CSF into the spinal canal is eliminated. The preceding statements on putative causative mechanisms appear to be valid and are widely accepted, but in many cases of hydrocephalus in animals and humans, no obstruction can be demonstrated. Hydrocephalus caused by obstruction is known as noncommunicating hydrocephalus. Other cases are generally classified as communicating hydrocephalus and occur mostly in newborns and infants. This communicating hydrocephalus is attributed to a discrepancy between production and resorption of CSF.

References

Greene HJ, Leipold HW, Vestweber JE. Experimentally induced hydrocephalus in calves. Am J Vet Res 1974;35:945–951.

Higgins RJ, Vandevelde M, Braund KB. Internal hydrocephalus and associated periventricular encephalitis in young dogs. Vet Pathol 1977;14:236–246.

Johnson RT, Johnson KP, Edmonds CJ. Virus-induced hydrocephalus: development of aqueductal stenosis in hamsters after mumps infection. Science 1967;157:1066–1067.

Kilham L, Margolis G. Hydrocephalus in hamsters, ferrets, rats, and mice following inoculations with *Reovirus* type I. I Virologic studies. Lab Invest 1969;21:183–188.

Krous HF, et al. Congenital hydrocephalus produced by attenuated influenza A virus vaccine in Rhesus monkeys. Am J Pathol 1978;92:317–320.

Margolis G, Kilham L. Hydrocephalus in hamsters, ferrets, rats, and

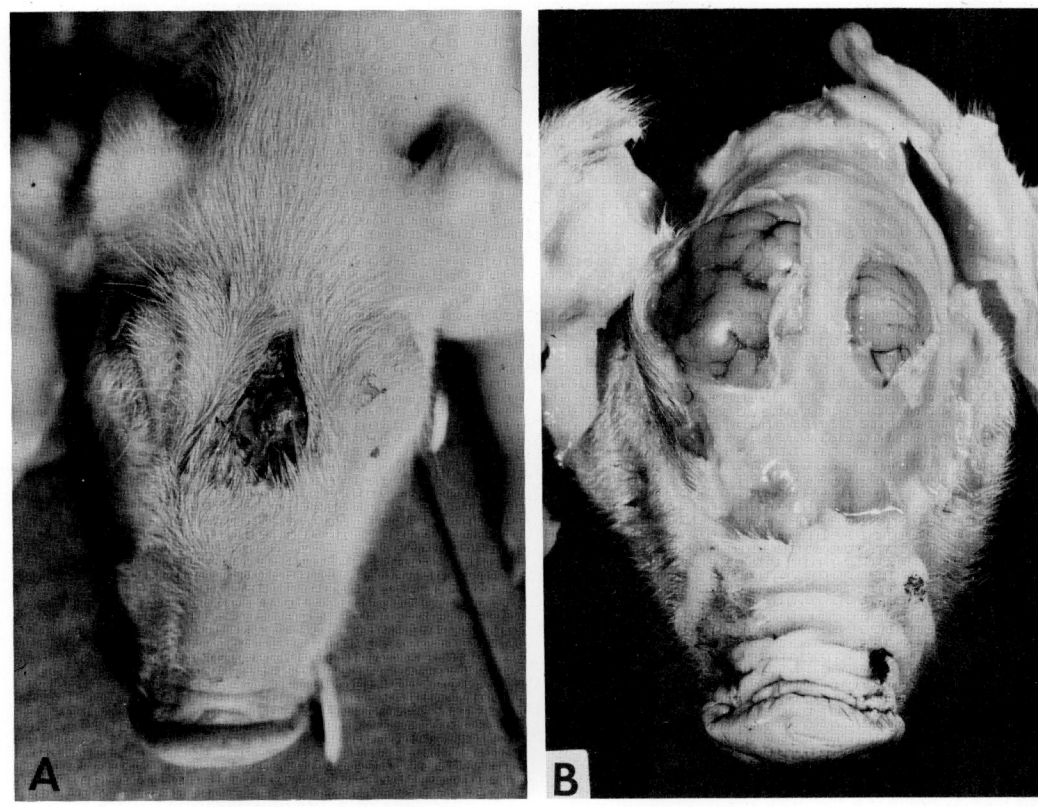

FIG. 27-10 Congenital meningoencephalocele. **A.** Small meningoencephalocele without a covering of skin, in a newborn piglet. **B.** Meningoencephalocele on each side of the frontal suture in a newborn piglet. Skin has been reflected. (Courtesy of Dr. W.S. Wijeratne. Reproduced with permission of *Veterinary Record* and the Controller of Her Britannic Majesty's Stationery Store.)

mice following inoculations with *Reovirus* type I. II. Pathologic studies. Lab Invest 1969;21:189–198.

Margolis G, Kilham L. Experimental virus-induced hydrocephalus. Relation to pathogenesis of the Arnold-Chiari malformation. J Neurosurg 1969;31:1–9.

Weller RO, Wisniewski H, Shulman K, et al. Experimental hydrocephalus in young dogs. Histological and ultrastructural study of the brain tissue damage. J Neuropathol Exp Neurol 1971; 30:613–626.

Wolinsky JS. Mumps virus-induced hydrocephalus in hamsters: ultrastructure of the chronic infection. Lab Invest 1977;37:229–236.

Congenital lesions of cerebellum

Severe destructive lesions of the cerebellum cause marked incoordination of gait, frequently referred to as "cerebellar ataxia." Signs referable to lesions in the cerebellum are characteristic of involvement of this structure but may be the result of any one of several distinct entities. Their cause is often unknown. Some examples appear to be inherited, but others represent destructive lesions from viral infections in utero, as in cerebellar hypoplasia in cats (Fig. 27-14) caused by feline panleukopenia virus, in calves caused by bovine virus diarrhea, and in swine by hog cholera virus—which has also been associated with hypomyelinogenesis. Some of those that have been recognized in animals are described below.

OLIVOPONTOCEREBELLAR HYPOPLASIA

Olivopontocerebellar hypoplasia occurs in cats and has been reported by numerous authors. Signs are not detectable in newborn kittens until normal neonatal ataxia disappears, usually one month after birth. Lesions may be easily recognized in affected animals sacri-

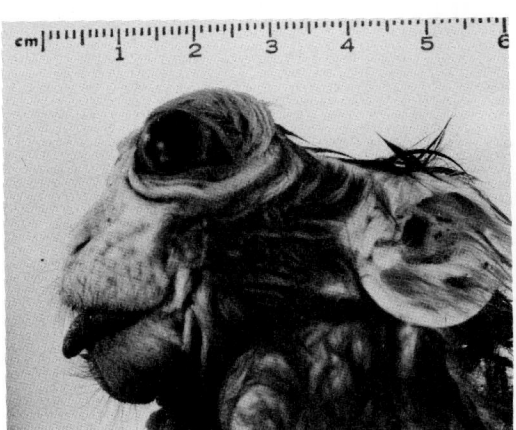

FIG. 27-11 Anencephaly, *Macaca fascicularis.* (Courtesy of New England Regional Primate Research Center. Harvard Medical School.)

TABLE 27-5 Congenital anomalies of the nervous system

Acrania—absence of cranium
Agenesis of corpus callosum—distortion or absence of corpus callosum, sometimes including septum pellucidum and hippocampal commissure
Agyria (lissencephaly)—poor cerebral cytologic organization; too few or no gyri
Amyelia—absence of spinal cord
Anencephaly—absence of brain
Anophthalmos—absence of both eyes
Arnold-Chiari syndrome—caudal shift of medulla and sometimes cerebellum
Arrhinencephaly—absence of rhinencephalon
Cerebellar hypoplasia (aplasia)—failure of cerebellum to develop to normal size and cellularity
Cranioschisis—cranium bifidum, gap in the skull, usually with herniation of brain substance or meninges
Cyclopia—one eye only
Dysraphia (dysraphism)—syringomyelia, midline defect in spinal cord
Encephalocele—herniation of brain through a cranial defect
Exencephaly—brain is outside cranial cavity
Hydranencephaly—cerebral hemispheres are empty sacs due to excessive cerebrospinal fluid, hydrocephalus
Hydrocephalus—ventricles are dilated by excessive cerebrospinal fluid
Hydromyelia—cerebrospinal fluid is retained in dilated central canal of spinal cord
Macroencephaly—brain is enlarged
Macrogyria—cerebral gyri are enlarged
Megaloencephaly—brain is extremely enlarged
Meningocele—herniation of meninges through bony defects in the skull
Microencephaly—small brain
Microgyria—gyri are abnormally small
Myelocele—spinal cord is herniated through a bony defect in vertebral column
Myeloschisis—spinal cord is cleft because of incomplete formation of neural tube
Pachygyria—reduction of number of secondary gyri and increased depth of gray matter
Polygyria—increased number of gyri
Porencephaly—occurrence of cavities in brain
Rachischisis—spina bifida with herniation; spina bifida occulta without herniation
Spina bifida—absence of vertebral arches, producing a defect through which spinal membranes, with or without spinal cord, protrude

TABLE 27-6 Virus-induced congenital anomalies of central nervous system *

Virus	*Anomalies*
Bluetongue (orbivirus)	Hydranencephaly, porencephaly, sheep
Border disease	Hypomyelinogenesis, sheep
Bovine viral diarrhea/mucosal disease (pestivirus)	Cerebellar hypoplasia, cattle, sheep
Feline panleukopenia (parvovirus)	Cerebellar hypoplasia, cats, ferrets
Hog cholera (pestivirus)	Cerebellar hypoplasia, microcephaly, hypomyelinogenesis, swine
Influenza A, Newcastle disease, (influenzavirus)	Microcephaly, myeloschisis, chick embryos
Lymphocytic choriomeningitis (arenavirus)	Cerebellar hypoplasia, rats
Minute virus of mice	Cerebellar hypoplasia, mice
Mumps (paramyxovirus); parainfluenza II; reovirus I; Ross river virus	Aqueductal stenosis, hydrocephalus, hamsters, mice, rats, ferrets

*Refer to Chapter 8 for more information.

penia; Chapter 8 provides additional details. Cerebellar hypoplasia has been reported in kittens in association with dysmyelinogenesis or hypomyelinogenesis. This condition may represent a leukodystrophy.

References

Harding JDJ, Done JT, Darbyshire JH. Congenital tremors in piglets and their relation to swine fever. Vet Rec 1966;79:388–390.
Kilham L, Margolis G. Cerebellar ataxia in hamsters inoculated with rat virus. Science 1964;143:1047–1048.

ficed at this time and occasionally will be detected in adult animals that have exhibited no abnormal signs. The anomaly results in a decided decrease in gross size of the cerebellum with corresponding hypoplasia of the olivary nuclei and pons. In a few cases, the cerebellum is more severely involved on one side than on the other; aplasia in the olive and pons then is limited to the contralateral side. The cerebrum may also be reduced in size, although not as obviously as the cerebellum.

In cats, hypoplasia or agenesis of the cerebellum in most cases is caused by the virus of feline panleuko-

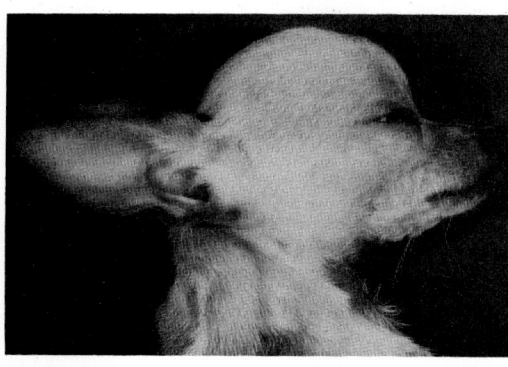

FIG. 27-12 Hydrocephalus in a three-year-old male chihuahua. (Courtesy of Angell Memorial Animal Hospital.)

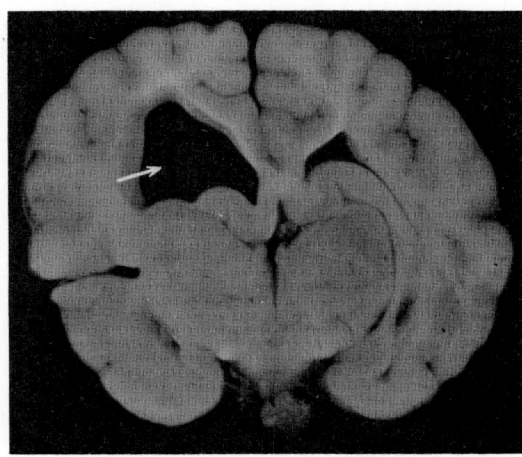

FIG. 27-13 Hydrocephalus involving left lateral ventricle (*arrow*) of a 15-year-old female Boston terrier. An incidental finding at necropsy. (Courtesy of Angell Memorial Animal Hospital.)

INHERITED DISEASES

Inherited or genetically-determined diseases of the nervous system are the result, in progeny, of the recombination of defective genes from the parents (Table 27-7). Expression of the presence of a defective gene depends upon whether the gene is **dominant** or **recessive.** A dominant gene is expressed when one or both chromosomes bear the gene (heterozygous or homozygous). A recessive gene is expressed only when both chromosomes of the pair bear the defective gene (homozygous). Disease appears in the progeny of two parents in numbers determined by this property of the affected gene. Selective breeding is one effective way to demonstrate the inheritance of disease. In some instances, it is possible to demonstrate a defective gene by identification of its product (often an enzyme), or the determination of the nucleotide sequence in its DNA. To establish its inherited nature, the disease must conform to one or more genetic criteria.

References

Chrisman CL, Cork LC, Gamble DA. Neuroaxonal dystrophy of Rottweiler dogs. J Am Vet Med Assoc 1984;184:484–487.

Confer AW, Ward BC. Spinal dysraphism: a congenital myodysplasia in the Weimaraner. J Am Vet Med Assoc 1972;160:1423–1426.

Cordy DR, Richards WPC, Stormont C. Hereditary neuraxial edema in Hereford calves. Pathol Vet 1969;6:487–501.

Cork LC, et al. Hereditary canine spinal muscular atrophy. J Neuropathol Exp Neurol 1979;38:209–221.

DeLaHunta A, Averill DR. Hereditary cerebellar cortical and extrapyramidal nuclear abiotrophy in Kerry blue terriers. J Am Vet Med Assoc 1976;168:1119–1124.

Duffell SJ. Neuraxial oedema of Hereford calves with and without hypomyelinogenesis. Vet Rec 1986;118:95–98.

Innes JRM, Rowlands WT, Parry HB. An inherited form of cortical cerebellar atrophy in ("daft") lambs in Great Britain. Vet Rec 1949;61:225–228.

Lysosomal storage diseases in nervous system

Certain inborn errors of metabolism in humans and animals are unified as a group by several features. They result from inherited lysosomal enzyme defects, have similar morphologic lesions involving excessive accumulation of products of catabolic metabolism in lysosomes of cells, and frequently affect the nervous system. These diseases are discussed in Chapter 2.

Epilepsy (seizure disorders)

Seizure disorders are known to occur in many species but have been most thoroughly studied in humans. Canine epilepsy has many similarities to the human disease. Distinguishing features of this chronic nervous system disease include recurring episodes of convulsions, loss of consciousness, or both. These signs are believed to be associated with episodic synchronous and sustained neuronal discharges that recur periodically with or without typical electroencephalographic (EEG) patterns. These disorders are classified into two categories: primary (idiopathic) and secondary (symptomatic) epilepsy.

PRIMARY (IDIOPATHIC) EPILEPSY

Primary (idiopathic) epilepsy in humans and dogs is defined as being associated with absence of causative morphologic or chemical lesions, such as tumors, inflammatory foci, scars, anomalies, or metabolic disorders. It is clearly inherited in humans and in some breeds of dogs and it may be increased in frequency by inbreeding. However, it is not clear whether only one or several genes are involved. Morphologic lesions have been described in primary epilepsy but the question often lingers as to whether these lesions cause, or are the result of, seizures. In one extensive study, 33 of 68 epileptic beagles had specific lesions consisting of swelling of astrocytic processes, perineuronal basophilic encrustation, and neuronal degeneration evolving to necrosis. Distribution of lesions varied in individual animals but were most frequent in the hippocampus, amygdala, claustrum, basal ganglia, and frontal and pyriform lobes of cerebrum. The nature and distribution of lesions associated with primary epilepsy are consistent with those observed in dogs with spontaneous or experimentally-induced hypoxia and are classified as epileptic brain damage.

SECONDARY (SYMPTOMATIC) EPILEPSY

This type of epilepsy is currently classified on the basis of signs associated with morphologic or biochemical lesions. Precise identification of causal factors has not been achieved at present. Associated lesions considered to be responsible for seizures have been grouped together in seven different categories by Koestner. A brief summary of each of these categories follows:

1. **Temporal lobe epilepsy,** a form of epilepsy singled out in humans based upon clinical features and location of the lesion within or near the temporal lobe, is not clearly recognized in animals. Seizures occur in some dogs with tumors in temporal lobes

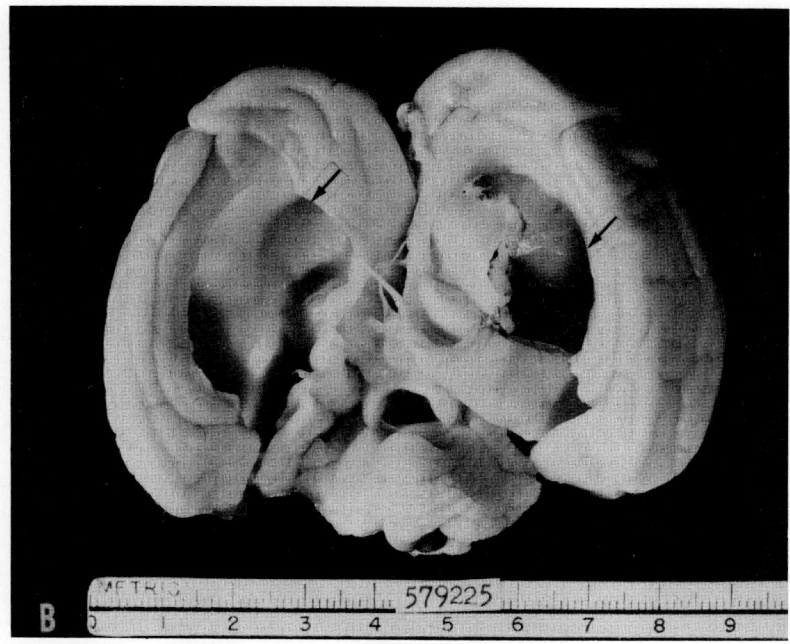

FIG. 27-14 Brain of a newborn puppy with hydrocephalus. Arrows indicate dilated lateral ventricle. (Courtesy of Armed Forces Institute of Pathology; contributor: Dr. Russell B. Oppenheimer.)

of brain, suggesting that more thorough study of these tumors in dogs may be indicated;

2. **Myoclonus epilepsy,** a term used to describe isolated muscular contractions in epileptic patients, also occurs in dogs. Canine disease has been identified with spontaneous cases of inherited glycoproteinosis of the Lafora type. This is described in Chapter 2;

3. **Epilepsy associated with tumors** has been reported in many dogs in association with space-occupying lesions, such as tumors. In McGrath's collection, over 40% of intracranial neoplasms were associated with epilepsy and 80% of these tumors were located in the frontal and temporal lobes. These intracranial tumors, as to be expected, appear with greater frequency in aged dogs;

4. **Posttraumatic epilepsy** may occur as a result of a severe blow to the head in dogs, as it does in some humans;

5. **Epilepsy associated with encephalitis.** Infections of brain may be followed by signs of epilepsy in humans and dogs;

6. **Epilepsy associated with metabolic or toxic injury to brain.** The gamma-aminobutyric-acid (GABA) metabolic pathway is an important factor in seizure disorders. The essential enzyme for formation of GABA is glutamic acid decarboxylase (GAD), which is exclusively active in the gray matter of the central nervous system. Any deficiency that results in loss of GABA may lead to epileptic seizures. Pyridoxine (Vitamin B_6) is a coenzyme of GAD, and essential for synthesis of GABA and its deficiency, natural or experimental, has been shown to cause seizures in infants and young animals. Toxic substances demonstrated to be associated with seizures include unsymmetrical dimethylhydrazine (UDMH), nitrogen trichloride, pentylenetetrazol, bicucculine, organic phosphates, methyl mercury, chlorinated hydrocarbons, strychnine, lead, and cyanide; and,

7. **Congenital and perinatal diseases and epilepsy.** Many congenital anomalies have been associated with epilepsy in children. At present, only one such anomaly, hydrocephalus, has been associated with epilepsy in animals.

References

Anderson B, Olsson SE. Epilepsy in a dog with extensive bilateral damage to the hippocampus. Acta Vet Skand 1959;1:98–104.

Koestner A. Neuropathology of canine epilepsy. Prob Vet Med 1989;1:516–534.

TABLE 27-7 **Transmissible spongiform encephalopathies**

Species affected	Disease
Sheep and goat	Scrapie
Humans	Kuru, Creutzfeldt-Jacob disease, Gerstmann-Sträussler disease
Cattle	Bovine spongiform encephalopathy
Captive mink	Transmissible mink encephalopathy
Captive mule deer and elk	Transmissible spongiform encephalopathy
Cat	Spongiform encephalopathy

Montgomery DL, Lee AC. Brain damage in the epileptic beagle dog. Vet Pathol 1983;20:160–169.

SPONGY DEGENERATION OR VACUOLATION

Several etiologically distinct disorders of the central nervous system are characterized by vacuolation of the gray and/or white matter. The vacuoles are usually within neurons, glial cells, or myelin; in some disorders, a defect in myelin formation occurs. The terms "status spongiosis," "spongy degeneration," and "brain edema" (Fig. 27-15) have been loosely applied to these disorders; however, the occurrence of vacuoles is not a specific change and caution must be used in interpreting their presence. Care must also be exercised in discriminating these diseases from purely demyelinating diseases, although the two groups overlap.

Transmissible spongiform encephalopathy

This includes a group of nervous system diseases in several species, producing similar lesions that are transmissible among species and that are probably caused by similar agents or one agent (Table 27-8). The first disease in this group to be recognized and studied is an ancient disease of sheep, called "scrapie" by shepherds who noted that affected sheep constantly rubbed against objects to the point of losing large amounts of wool. The assumption is that intense pruritus prompted the scratching.

Common lesions in all species, seen under the light microscopy, include the presence of vacuoles in cells of gray matter, that give the tissue a spongy (spongiform) appearance. These vacuoles are actually distended plasma membranes of affected cells that include neurons and their processes, as well as astrocytes and oligodendroglia. This spongy appearance of affected cells is not due to edema, but to coalescing of smaller vacuoles of plasma membranes. Accumulation of plasma membrane fragments within vacuoles may be seen with electron microscopy, and lead to necrosis, loss of neurons, and death of the host. Hypertrophy and proliferation of astrocytes are common manifestations of the disease.

Amyloidosis is frequently present in varying degrees and extent, and has been identified as the scrapie-associated fibril. Another more common feature in all species is the presence of a 27–30 kd protein termed "PrP 27–30," proposed as the major structural component of the scrapie agent or a product induced by the agent. Molecular cloning experiments reveal that PrP 27–30 is derived from a larger precursor (Sp 33–37) encoded by a host gene. PrP messenger RNA is expressed in several cells of the nervous system, such as neurons, ependyma, choroid plexus epithelium, astrocytes, microglia, and endothelial cells in both infected and uninfected animals. The change from the precursor to PrP 27–30 is the consequence of infection by the specific agent. PrP is a unique protein only detected in transmissible spongiform encephalopathies.

More information on the nature of this unique agent may be found in Chapter 8.

INCIDENTAL FINDINGS

Cerebrovascular siderosis

Deposits of iron pigment are common in cerebral blood vessels in horses and are less frequent in cattle. This is apparently a normal process and its significance is unknown, but the amount of iron is believed to increase with age.

Scattered, small granules of yellow-brown pigment are seen in histologic sections with increasing frequency in aged macaque monkeys, particularly in the neutrophil of the globus pallidus and substantia nigra. This pigment is membrane-bound, probably in phagolysosomes and has the staining characteristics associated with lipofuscin. No clinical disease has yet been associated with this finding in macaque monkeys (*Macaca* spp.).

Melanosis

Irregular, brown-to-black-pigmented plaques may be seen with the unaided eye in the meninges of cattle and sheep; Chapter 3 provides additional information in Figs. 3-9 and 3-10. With light microscopy, these plaques are seen to consist of cells filled with granules of brown-to-black pigment, identifiable as melanin. These findings are considered incidental; however, these cells

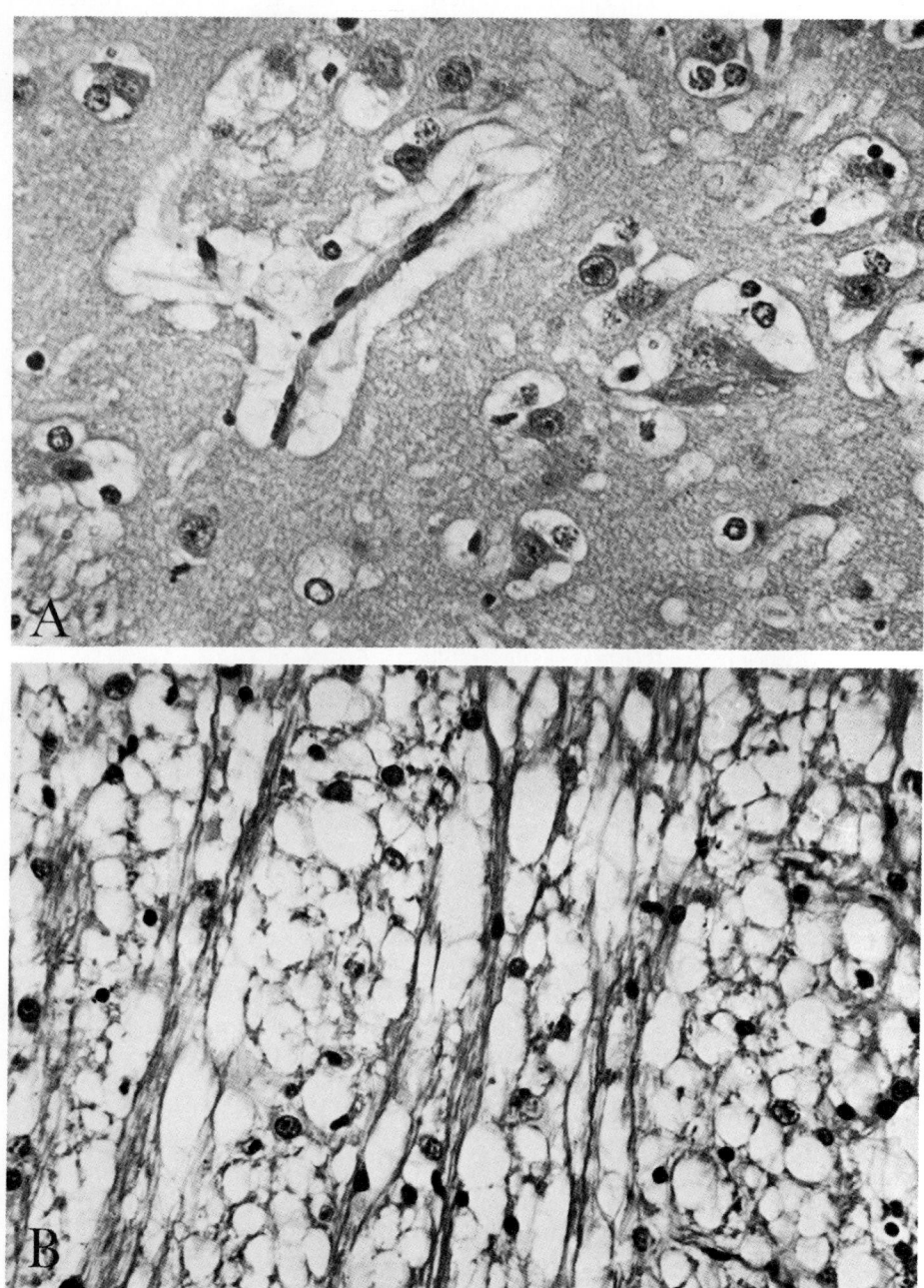

FIG. 27-15 Congenital brain edema of Hereford calves. **A.** Swollen hydropic astrocytes including foot processes around capillaries. **B.** Vacuolation of white matter. (Courtesy of Dr. R.D. Jolly.)

could become the source for malignant melanoma under rare circumstances.

Senile plaques

Focal glial scars have been described in aged dogs and associated with the aging process (Fig. 27-16). Their significance is not clearly understood.

CEREBROVASCULAR AMYLOIDOSIS (CONGOPHILIC ANGIOPATHY, CEREBRAL AMYLOID ANGIOPATHY)

These names have been applied to amyloidosis in brain of aged dogs, squirrels (*Saimiri sciureus*), and macaque (*Macaca mulatta*) monkeys. These changes are

of interest to compare with lesions in Alzheimer's senile dementia and aged human patients.

This lesion is significantly increased in frequency in squirrel monkeys when they reach fifteen or more years of age. This stage is reached by macaques when they arrive at the late twenty years. It has also been demonstrated in a 56-year-old chimpanzee (*Pan troglodytes*). Deposition of amyloid is also more extensive in the brain of squirrel monkeys than in macaques. Cerebrovascular amyloid is distributed as homogenous, eosinophilic deposits in small vessels in the neural parenchyma and in the walls of larger leptomeningeal and penetrating vessels. The amyloid in these monkey species is indistinguishable by tinctorial or immunohistochemical means from human amyloid.

TABLE 27-8 **Examples of inherited diseases, nervous system**

Names	Species, clinical, and pathologic features	References
Ataxia, hereditary	Reported in many species, must be differentiated from congenital viral infections, signs at 2–3 weeks of age: incoordination, leukodysplasia of cerebellum, midbrain, and medulla	Saunders et al., 1952; O'Leary et al., 1962
Cerebellar abiotrophy	Signs in Holstein heifers, starting with incoordination at 3–8 months of age; progresses over several weeks; micro: degeneration of Purkinje cells and neurons of cerebellar nuclei	White and Whitlock, 1975
Cerebellar cortical and extrapyramidal nuclear abiotrophy	In Kerry blue terriers, apparent 9–16 weeks of age, abiotrophy implies degeneration after period of normal development. Cerebellum is normal at outset, gradually decreases, becomes smaller with widened sulci, degeneration of Purkinje cells followed by bilateral degeneration of olivary nuclei, substantia nigra, and caudate nuclei	DeLaHunta and Averill, 1976
Cortical cerebellar atrophy "daft lambs"	In newborn lambs; signs of cerebellar ataxia; occurs in Great Britain and Canada; no gross lesions, microscopic limited to cerebellar cortex: atrophy of individual folia, loss of Purkinje cells following swelling, chromatolysis or basophilia of cytoplasm, and pyknosis of nuclei; empty "basket cells" in silver-impregnated sections	Innes et al., 1949
Canine spinal muscular atrophy Familial motor neuron disease	Rottweiler, brittany spaniels, and other breeds of dogs; autosomal-dominant inheritance; signs at about 6 weeks of age: regurgitation, diminished growth, progressive ataxia, posterior limb weakness, quadriplegia; gross findings: muscle mass reduced, thoracic esophagus dilated; microscopic findings: severe lesions of motor neurons—chromatolysis, swelling of perikarya, Nissl substance diminished, and necrosis	Cork et al., 1979; Cork et al., 1982; Sach et al., 1984; Shell et al., 1987
Lysosomal storage diseases	A large number of rare diseases, many affecting the nervous system*	
Neuroaxonal dystrophy (feline)	Kittens are affected at birth with incoordination that progresses with age; autosomal-recessive inheritance, associated with a dilute coat color; microscopic findings: swelling and ballooning of axons, loss of neurons most severe in olivary and lateral cuneate nuclei, less evident in brainstem, thalamus and cerebellar vermis; loss of Purkinje cells and reduction in granular layer, little or no reduction in cerebellum	Woodard, 1974
Neuroaxonal dystrophy (canine)	Affects dogs, slowly progressive clinical signs of cerebellar disease, membrane-filled bodies, "spheroids" in distal axones	Cork et al., 1983; Chrisman et al., 1984

(continued)

TABLE 27-8 (continued)

Names	Species, clinical, and pathologic features	References
Neuraxial edema Congenital brain edema	Encountered at birth in Herefords, mostly polled breed, calves are unable to stand, have variable tremors, intermittent extensor spasms and hyperesthesia; sometimes severe nystagmus; autosomal-recessive inheritance; gross findings include pale, translucent white matter in cerebellum, cerebellar hypoplasia, and mild hydrocephalus; microscopic findings: severe, widely distributed vacuolization in white matter (Fig. 27-13)	Cordy, 1969; Duffell, 1986; Jolly, 1974
Spinal dysraphism Syringomyelia	Autosomal-recessive trait in young Weimeraner dogs with a "hopping" gait, crouching stance, and abducted pelvic limbs; pathologic findings include anomalies of dorsal septum of spinal cord (absence of septum, rarification of septal and adjacent white matter); anomalies of central canal (hydromelia, syringomyelia, duplication, absence); anomalies of central, dorsal, and ventral horns; anomalies of ventral median fissure	Confer and Ward, 1972; McGrath, 1965

*Chapter 2 provides more details.

CHOLESTEROL GRANULOMA

Evidence of repeated hemorrhage in the choroid plexus is occasionally encountered in aged horses. The lesions sometimes reach rather large size, apparently due to organization of the blood clots following episodes of repeated hemorrhage. Cholesterol clefts are conspicuous in these lesions, in exudate or macrophages, and has prompted the erroneous designation of "cholesteatoma". Large lesions in the choroid may result in internal hydrocephalus and intermittent signs involving the central nervous system.

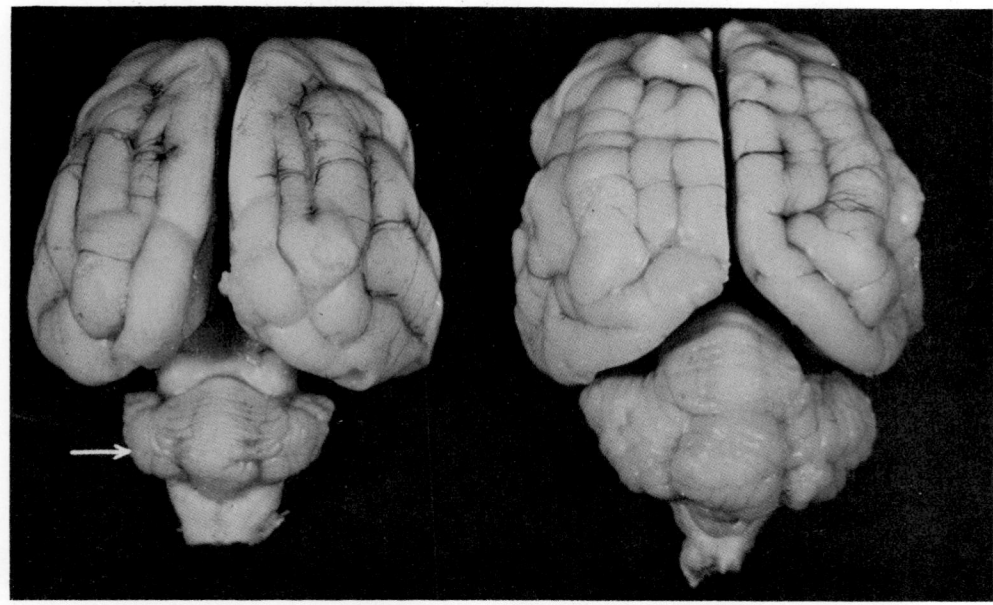

FIG. 27-16 Hypoplasia of cerebellum (*arrow*) in a two-month-old female kitten. Brain of a normal kitten of the same age is on the right for comparison. (Courtesy of Angell Memorial Animal Hospital.)

SPHEROIDS (NEUROAXONAL DYSTROPHY, AXONAL SWELLING)

Spheroids are seen in the globus pallidus and substantia nigra of aged macaque monkeys, in histologic preparations stained with hematoxylin and eosin, as spherical or oblong masses, eosinophilic, homogeneous or slightly granular, 5 to 50 μm in diameter. They have a black, granular appearance when stained with Bodian or Bielschowsky techniques. Some spheroids are argyrophilic and often contain granules which are positive to the periodic acid Schiff (PAS) reagent, but do not contain iron. Immunocytochemical preparations are useful to identify them, using antibodies directed against specific transmitter-related markers or cytoskeletal proteins.

The electron microscope reveals most spheroids to be surrounded by membranes which also intersperse the clumped and granular contents. These spheroids clearly develop from axones.

References

Bronson, R.T., Schoene, E.C.: Spontaneous pallidonigral accumulation of iron pigment and spheroid-like structures in macaque monkeys. J. Neuropathol Exp Neurol 39:181–196, 1980.
Cork, L.C., Walker, L.C.: Age-related lesions, nervous system. In: Jones, T.C., Mohr, U., Hunt, R.D. (eds): ILSi Monograph on pathology of laboratory animals, Nonhuman primates II. Springer, Berlin Heidelberg New York, 1993, pp 173–183.
Gliatto, J.M., Bronson, R.T.: Spontaneous pallidonigral spheroids and iron pigment accumulation, macaques. In: Jones, T.C., Mohr, U., Hunt, R.D. (eds): ILSI Monographs on pathology of laboratory animals, nonhuman primates II. Springer, Berlin Heidelberg New York, 1993, pp 183–187.

AUTONOMIC NERVOUS SYSTEM

Primary dysautonomias

This disease entity has been reported in several species located principally in Great Britain, Scandinavia, and Argentina. Several names have been applied, such as "grass sickness," "mal seco," enteric neuropathy, dysautonomia, and Key-Gaskell syndrome. The syndrome has been described in equine, canine, feline and leporine species, with similar signs and lesions. Etiology is unknown.

Signs include sudden onset of dullness, inappetence, dysphagia, gut stasis, esophageal dysfunction, and bladder atony with straining to urinate or with incontinence. Dogs and cats have dry mucous membranes with inability to swallow, fixed dilatation of pupils, and reduced lacrimation. Death may occur within a few days or be prolonged to several weeks.

Gross lesions usually involve the gastrointestinal tract, with megaesophagus, fluid-distended small intestine and colon, and distended urinary bladder. Microscopic lesions involve the neurons of almost any of the sympathetic ganglia. Cytoplasm of affected neurons lose basophilic granularity (Nissl substance) and take on a homogenous appearance. Affected perikarya become rounded, moderately swollen in early stages, later to become shrunken and irregular in shape. The nuclei are seen as pyknotic and eccentric. Necrotic neurons are

lost, leaving a space or sometimes a small neuronophagic nodule.

The ultrastructure depends upon the stage at which the affected neuron is examined. Findings include a variety of changes involving rough endoplasmic reticulum (RER) which has an unusual distribution. Many cisternae of various sizes and configurations are formed from the RER; some of these are empty, others contain dense, flocculent material or misaligned neurotubules and filaments. Some cisternae contain concentric arrays of membranes. Parallel arrays of smooth endoplasmic reticulum, mitochondria, and lysosomes may be seen in cytoplasm.

References

Griffiths IR, Whitwell KE. Leporine dysautonomia: further evidence that hares suffer from grass sickness. Vet Rec 1993;132:376–377.
Pollin MM, Griffiths IR. A review of the primary dysautonomias of domestic animals. J Comp Pathol 1992;106:99–119.
Scholes SFE, Vaillant C, Peacock P, et al. Enteric neuropathy in horses with grass sickness. Vet Rec 132:647–650.
Schrauwen E, Van Ham L, Maenhout T, et al. Canine dysautonomia: a case report. Vet Rec 1991;128:524–525.
Uzal FA, Robles CA, Olaechea FV. Histopathologic changes in the coeliaco-mesenteric ganglia of horses with "mal seco," a grass sickness-like syndrome, in Argentina. Vet Rec 1992;130:244–246.

NEOPLASMS OF NERVOUS SYSTEM

Study of neoplasms of the nervous system is facilitated by a classification system. Schemata, which have proved most useful over the years, are based upon the morphologic features that permit recognition of the cell or cells from which the lesion originates. The classification depicted in Table 27-9 (central nervous system) and Table 27-10 (peripheral nervous system) are based on the criteria and terminology proposed for animals by Koestner (1994). These proposals follow the WHO classification scheme for human neoplasms with exclusion of variations not yet described in other species.

The most frequently described neoplasms of the central nervous system of animals arise from glial cells and may be grouped together as **gliomas.** The tumor most often encountered in this group is the astrocytoma and will be described, among others, below.

Neoplasms of the central nervous system may grow slowly or rapidly, but rarely metastasize outside the cranium or spinal column. Their effects on the host depend on the interference or destruction of the normal functions of the part of brain involved and, of course, the essential nature of the affected nervous structures.

Reference

Koestner A, Marushiga K. Neurocarcinogenesis. In: Walker MP, Ward JM, eds. Carcinogenesis. New York: Raven Press, 1994;301–337.

Medulloepithelioma

This neoplasm has been encountered rarely in the cerebrum of young children and also in the spinal cord and cerebrum of young animals (dogs and horses). It has also been referred to as "neuroepithelioma" in animals.

TABLE 27-9 **Neoplasms of the central nervous system**

Neoplasm	Origin	Usual location
Neoplasms of neuronal cells and precursors		
Medulloepithelioma	Neural tube	Spinal cord
Medulloblastoma	Primitive granule cell	Cerebellum
Neuroblastoma	Neural precursor	Cerebrum
Gangliocytoma	Neural precursor	Cerebellum
Neoplasms of glia		
Astrocytoma (fibrillary, protoplasmic, gemistocytic, pilocytic, anaplastic)	Astrocyte	Piriform lobe and brainstem
Oligodendroglioma (anaplastic, malignant)	Oligodendrocyte	Cerebrum
Spongioblastoma	Spongioblast	Cerebrum
Mixed glioma (oligoastrocytoma)	Astrocyte and oligodendrocyte	Cerebrum
Anaplastic glioma (glioblastoma)	Precursor cell	Cerebrum
Neoplasms of ependyma and choroid plexus epithelium		
Ependymoma (anaplastic, malignant; glioependymoma)	Ependyma	Ventricles
Papilloma and carcinoma (epithelioma)	Epithelium of choroid plexus	Ventricles
Neoplasms of mesoderm		
Meningioma (malignant)	Meningeal cap cell	Meninges of anterior fossa
Meningeal sarcomatosis	Meningeal mesenchyme	Brainstem, cord
Granular cell tumor (rat)	Meninges	Meninges of anterior fossa
Malignant lymphoma (lymphoreticulosis, microgliomatosis)	Hemopoietic tissue (CNS)	Cerebrum, cord
Special neoplasms of CNS		
Pinealoma (pineocytoma, pineoblastoma, mixed pineocytoma/pineoblastoma)	Pinocyte	Pineal gland
Craniopharyngioma	Endodermal cell	Rathke's pouch
Malignant melanoma (melanocytoma)	Melanocyte	Neural crest

TABLE 27-10 **Neoplasms of the peripheral nervous system**

Neoplasm	Origin	Location
Schwannoma	Schwann Cell	Nerves, roots
Neurofibroma, Neurofibromatosis and Neurofibrosarcoma	Schwann cell and Fibroblast	Subcutis, intestines (many organs)
Neuroblastoma	Neural precursors	Adrenal medulla
Neuroepithelioma (retinoblastoma)	Precursor of receptor cell	Retina
Ganglioneuroma	Neural crest	Sympathetic ganglia, adrenal medulla, thyroid, pituitary
Paraganglioma	Neural crest	Paraganglia

Its origin is inferred from its histologic appearance to be from the embryonal medullary plate and neural tube. Tumor cells are tall columnar to low cuboidal in shape and arranged in single or multiple rows, sometimes forming spherical tubules or elongated ribbons. These rows of cells may have a limiting membrane which is eosinophilic and PAS positive, suggesting a basement membrane. These cells do not bear cilia or have blepharoplasts, features that help to distinguish them from papillomas of the choroid plexus. Vascular fibrous stroma also is not a feature of the medulloepithelioma. Nuclei of the neoplasm are large, hyperchromatic, and often contain mitotic figures.

References

Baumgartner W, Peixoto PV. Immunohistochemical demonstration of keratin in canine neuroepithelioma. Vet Pathol 1987;24:500–503.

Eagle RC, Font RL, Swerczek TW. Malignant medulloepithelioma of the optic nerve in a horse. Vet Pathol 1978;15:488–494.

Kennedy FA, Indrieri RJ, Koestner A. Spinal cord medulloepithelioma in a dog. J Am Vet Med Assoc 1984;185:902–904.

Russell DS, Rubinstein LJ. Pathology of tumors of the nervous system, 5th ed. Baltimore: Williams & Wilkins, 1989.

Medulloblastoma

Although rarely reported, a few cases in the literature indicate that medulloblastoma constitutes a pathologic entity in calves and dogs that may be confused clinically with cerebellar ataxia due to other causes. The lesion has been found in young calves and dogs in which the recorded signs included a high-stepping gait, ataxia, and jerky, uncoordinated movements.

The gross lesion usually consists of a single midline mass affecting the cerebellum with occasional extension to the fourth ventricle, meninges, and brainstem. Tumor typically has a color and consistency resembling brain but may be discolored by areas of hemorrhage and necrosis.

Histologic appearance is uniform because it is made up of densely packed cells, often in parallel arrays, with scant cytoplasm and elongate, hyperchromatic nuclei. Rosette formation is often a feature. Some nests of tumor cells may be seen in the leptomeninges, apart from the main tumor mass. The origin of these cells is not completely understood, but are believed by some to arise from primitive granule cells of the cerebellum. Positive reaction to neuronal biomarkers (neurofilament protein, synaptophysin or neuron-specific enolase) would attest to the neuronal origin of the tumor cells.

References

Crody DR. Medulloblastoma in a steer. Cornell Vet 1953;43:189–193.

Jolly RD, Alley MR. Medulloblastoma in calves. A report of three cases. Pathol Vet 1969;6:463–368.

McGavin MD. A medulloblastoma in calves. A report of three cases. Pathol Vet 1969;6:463–468.

McGavin MD. A medulloblastoma in a calf. Aust Vet J 1961;37:390–393.

NEUROBLASTOMA

These tumors consist of small, round cells of undifferentiated embryonal aspect. Microscopic appearance is similar to that of medulloblastoma, to which neuroblastoma is embryologically related, because both arise from nervous tissue at an early stage of embryonic development. Like medulloblastoma, this tumor also typically forms "rosettes" which are a prime aid in microscopic diagnosis. In neuroblastoma, cells of the rosette are arranged around a small tuft of fibrils of nervous origin.

Neuroblastoma can originate in the central nervous system, but the majority occur in the adrenal medulla; a few arise from sympathetic nervous tissue elsewhere in the abdominal cavity. In the adrenal medulla, tumor sometimes is named **sympathoblastoma.** It occurs in the young and is malignant.

Two additional tumors belong in this group, the retinoblastoma (primitive neoplasm of retinal neuroblasts) and the esthesioblastoma (olfactory neuroblastoma) arising from the olfactory neuroepithelium. Both neoplasms by location are tumors of the peripheral nervous system.

References

Anderson BC, Cordy DR. Olfactory neuroblastoma in a heifer. Vet Pathol 1981;18:536–540.
Helman RG, Adams LG, Hall CL, et al. Metastatic neuroblastoma in a dog. Vet Pathol 1980;17:769–773.

Astrocytoma

This neoplasm has been most frequently reported in brachiocephalic breeds of dogs and often originates in the piriform lobe or brainstem (Fig. 27-17). The cell of origin is the astrocyte, a neuroglial cell with a large cell body with many cytoplasmic processes which, with specific stains, give the cell a stellate configuration. The occurrence of differentiated astrocytes in the tumor is usually helpful in recognizing this tumor in histologic preparations, but immature and variant forms (protoplasmic or gemistocytic types) are frequent and may add difficulties in cytologic identification. Glial fibrillary acidic protein (GFAP) has recently been added as a reliable biomarker for the recognition of the astrocytic derivation of this neoplasm.

References

Hayes KC, Schiefer B. Primary tumors in the CNS of carnivores. Pathol Vet 1969;6:94–116.
Moulton JE. Tumors in domestic animals. 4th ed. Berkeley: Univ Calif Press, 1990.
Russell DS, Rubinstein LJ. Pathology of tumors of the nervous system. 5th ed. Baltimore: Williams & Wilkins, 1989.

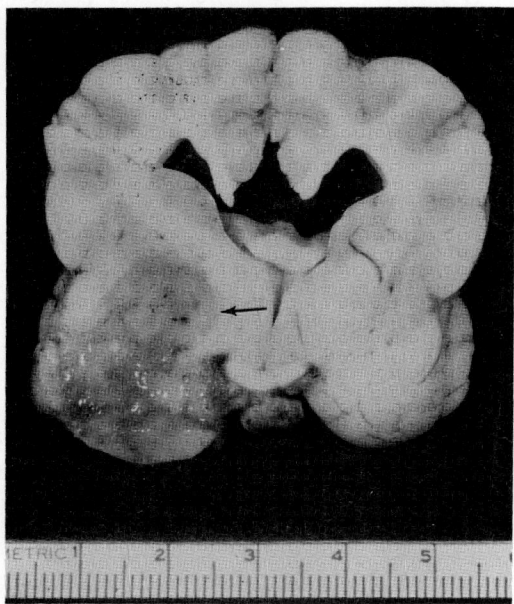

FIG. 27-17 Astrocytoma in right pyriform lobe of cerebrum of a nine-year-old castrated male boxer. (Courtesy of Angell Memorial Animal Hospital.)

Gangliocytoma

This is an extremely rare tumor in humans as well as in animals. The predilection site is the cerebellum. Tumor consists of large, mature nerve cells that can be identified by demonstration of Nissl bodies, argyrophilic axons, and dendrites, as well as by immunohistochemical neuronal biomarkers. Immature nerve cells have been reported to occur occasionally; however, in most cases, neuroblastic elements are not discernible in gangliocytomas at the time of detection. The peripheral counterpart of gangliocytoma is the ganglioneuroma which usually contains a mixture of mature and neuroblastic elements. An astrocytic stroma may be present in gangliocytomas. When present, an astrocytic stroma can be identified by its reaction to GFAP.

Reference

Nyska A, Shamir H, Harmelin A, et al. Intracranial gangliocytoma in a dog. Vet Pathol 1995;32:190–192.

Oligodendroglioma

This tumor arises from glial elements (Fig. 27-18) that differentiate to resemble oligodendrocytes. These cells have small, spherical nuclei that occasionally elongate to rod-shape and cytoplasm that bears short processes. These processes tend to disappear in neoplasms. These glial cells are usually separated into compartments by thin trabeculae. Cytoplasm is not stained by the hematoxylin-and-eosin staining method and thus appears empty in these preparations. As a result, cells that align the trabeculae appear to consist of rows of small nuclei separated from the trabeculae by empty spaces. Calcified granules, equal in size to several cells, often are seen among tumor cells. Mitotic figures are not frequent but tumor cells often infiltrate adjacent tissues. Oligodendrogliomas, in addition to containing oligodendrocytes, often are infiltrated with astrocytes and when these cells are numerous, have led to the diagnostic term "mixed glioma." Oligodendrogliomas occur as frequently as astrocytomas in dogs, especially in brachiocephalic breeds, but also occasionally in cats and cattle.

Reference

Luginbühl HA. A comparative study of neoplasms of the central nervous system in animals. II. Oligodendrogliomas in animals. Acta Neurochir Suppl 1963;10:30–42.

Spongioblastoma

Neoplasms given this name are encountered as rare events in humans during the first or second decade of life. Tumor cells resemble migrating spongioblasts of the developing central nervous system, seen in histologic preparations of the 16–18-week-old human cerebrum. These new growths originate in the vicinity of the ventricular system.

Individual cells are seen microscopically as having thin, tapering bipolar or unipolar shape among many delicate neuroglial fibers. Cells tend to be arranged in compact, parallel rows with the long axis perpendicular

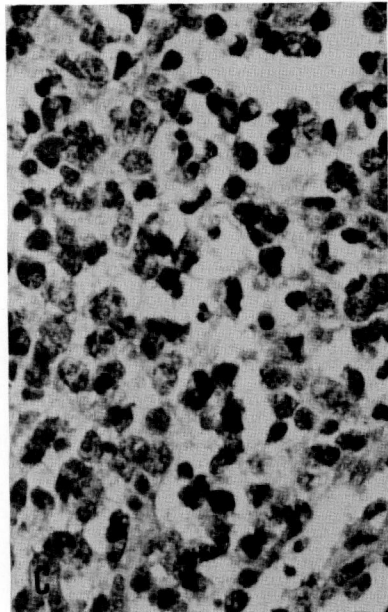
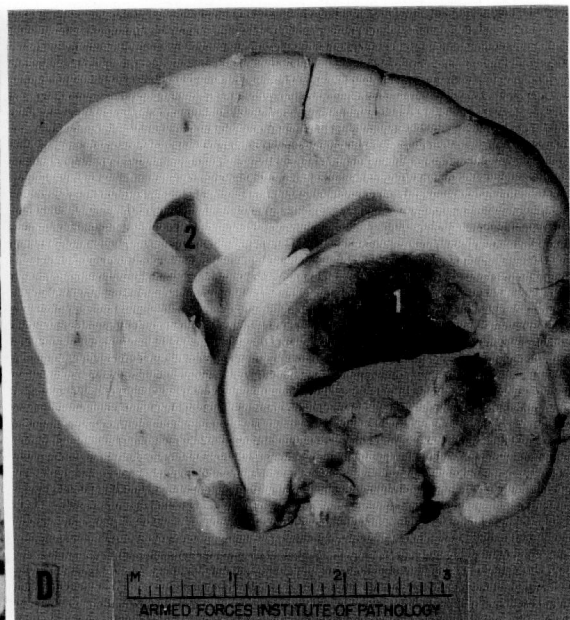

FIG. 27-18 A. Oligodendroglioma in brain of an eight-year-old female boxer. **B.** Gross specimen of same tumor. (1) Tumor displaces the midline. (2) Slight hydrocephalus in lateral ventricle. (Courtesy of Armed Forces Institute of Pathology; contributor: Dr. L.N. Loomis.)

to rows, separated by glial elements. They usually lay at 90° angles to blood vessels, but tapering cells have no footplates of terminal branches. In this respect, cells differ from astroblasts and may be more primitive.

Reference

Russell DS, Rubenstein LJ. Pathology of tumors of the nervous system. 5th ed. Baltimore: Williams and Wilkins, 1989;169–172.

EPENDYMOMA

This neoplasm consists of cells of medium size with irregularly rounded or polyhedral nuclei, which are centrally placed (Fig. 27-19). Nuclei are moderately deep-staining; the cytoplasm is pink. Cells are put together in solid masses, broken at times by thin trabeculae. Occasionally, they reveal the innate tendency to line cavities by forming a tiny opening around which a single zone of cells is radially arranged. Such a structure is called a "rosette." Ependymomas form well-demarcated masses in the region of the fourth or third ventricle, from whose lining they conceivably arise. Ependymomas are rare in all species, although most often are seen in dogs, cats, and cattle.

References

Hayes KC, Schiefer B. Primary tumors in domestic animals in the CNS of carnivores. Pathol Vet 1969;6:94–116.

Nettles VF, Vandevelde M. Thalamic ependymoma as in a white-tailed deer. Vet Pathol 1978;15:133–135.

Saunders GK. Ependymoblastoma in a dairy calf. Vet Pathol 1984; 21:528–529.

Teuscher E, Cherrstrom EC. Ependymoma of the spinal cord in a young dog. Schweiz Arch Tierheilkd 1974;116:461–466.

Neoplasms of choroid plexus

The choroid plexus consists of an irregular mass of tissue consisting of columnar or cuboidal cells, nonciliated, supported in double rows by fibrovascular stroma, and attached to the roof of the lateral, third, or fourth ventricle. Its purpose is to secrete CSF. Neoplasms of this structure have been demonstrated in humans, dogs, and occasionally cats. Signs in dogs are apparently related to hydrocephalus, presumably as a result of excess secretion by new growth. The onset of signs may be sudden or insidious and variously manifested by loss of equilibrium, weakness in pelvic limbs, incoordination, listlessness, aggressive behavior, seizures, staggering, circling, and occasionally, sudden death. Affected males outnumber females in most studies but this may be related to the relatively greater number of males in the population studied. In contrast to the occurrence of gliomas, neoplasms of the choroid plexus are seldom reported in brachiocephalic breeds of dogs.

Gross lesions are restricted to the contents of the cranium and usually limited to one of the ventricles which is dilated and contains one or more cauliflower-shaped masses attached to the choroid plexus but otherwise free within the ventricle. Hemorrhage into brain parenchyma or ventricle is frequent. Tumors occur in the lateral, third, or fourth ventricle with approximately equal frequency.

Histologic examination reveals a papillary growth, clearly resembling and attached to the choroid plexus, consisting usually of fronds of redundant columnar or cuboidal, nonciliated, epithelial cells supported in double rows by congested fibrovascular stroma. This type has often been considered a "papilloma" of the choroid plexus. In other cases, epithelial cells are irregular, sometimes atypical, in multiple rows with frequent foci of necrosis and mitotic figures. Leukocytes and macrophages often fill the stroma in this type. Tumor cells may invade brain and extend into the leptomeninges, but as with most intracranial neoplasms, do not appear outside the cranium, either by extension or metastasis. This second type of new growth is considered by some authors to be a "carcinoma of choroid plexus" and by

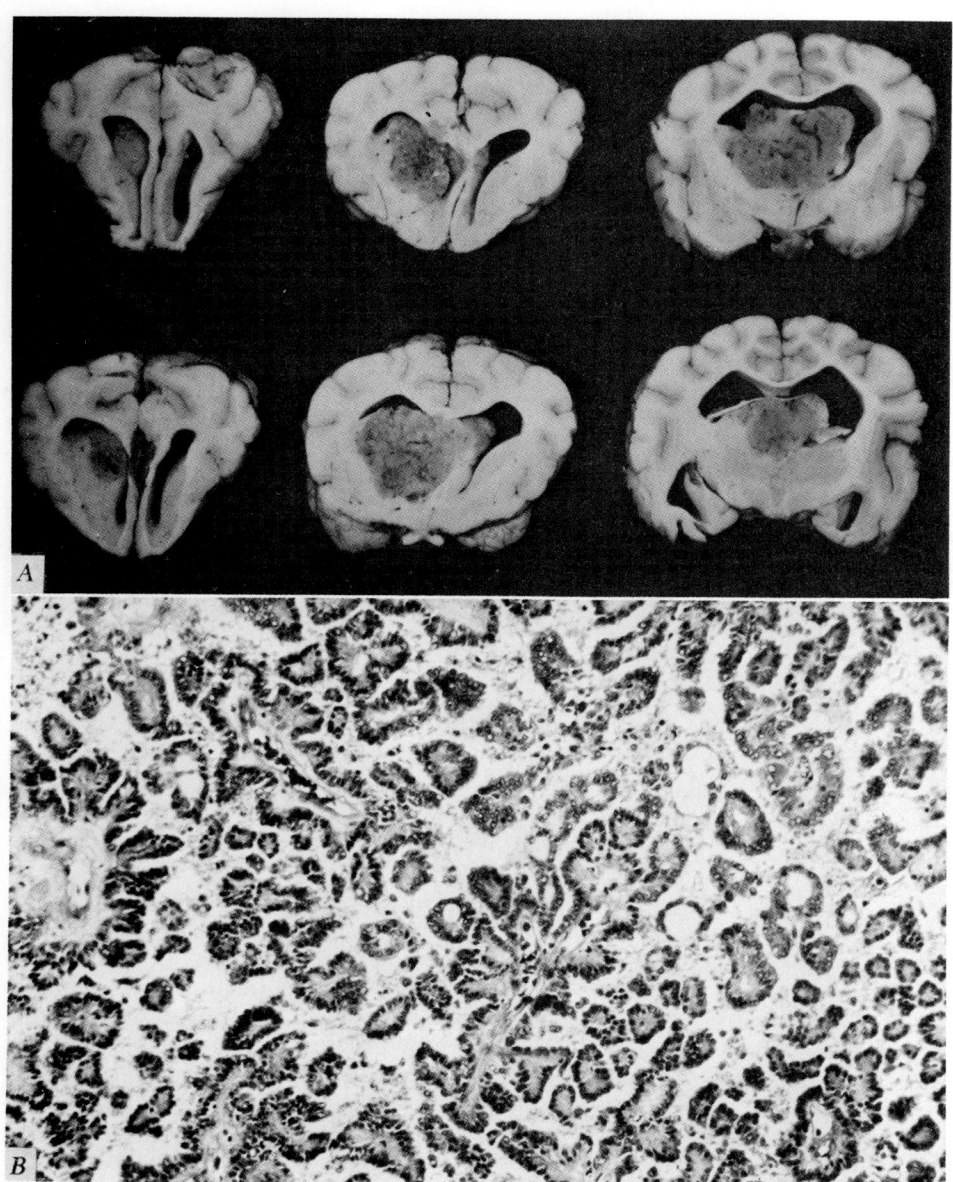

FIG. 27-19 Ependymoma arising in third ventricle of eight-year-old spayed female English bulldog. **A.** Gross brain cut at 1–cm intervals. Note the deviation of the midline and hydrocephalus of the lateral ventricles. **B.** Section of the tumor: hematoxylin-and-eosin-stained, ×200. (Courtesy of Angell Memorial Animal Hospital.)

others as "atypical choroid papilloma." The diagnostic problem is to distinguish these primary lesions from metastatic adenocarcinoma from other organs.

Immunohistochemical staining procedures indicate that these tumors are considered negative for GFAP and epithelial membrane antigen (EMA), but usually stain positively for cytokeratin, and less strongly for pankeratin and carcinoembryonic antigen (CEA).

References

Kurtz HJ, Hanlon GF. Choroid plexus papilloma in a dog. Vet Pathol 1971;8:91–95.

Luginbuhl H, Fankhauser R, McGrath JT. Spontaneous neoplasms of the nervous system in animals. In: Progress in neurological surgery. Vol 2. Chicago: Karger, Basel and Year Book, 1968;85–164.

Ribas JL, Mena H, Braund KG, et al. A histologic and immunocytochemical study of choroid plexus tumors of the dog. Vet Pathol 1989;26:55–64.

Zaki FA, Nafe LA. Choroid plexus tumors in the dog. J Am Vet Med Assoc 1980;176:328–330.

Meningioma

Meningioma is a term applied to a neoplasm that arises in the meninges (pia, arachnoid, dura). These have been reported in significant numbers in humans, cats (Fig. 27-20), dogs, F344 rats, and, less frequently, in other species. Most of these neoplasms occur in the meninges of brain; fewer appear over the spinal cord or adjacent to the nasal cavity. Meningiomas in cats are occasionally found within the lateral or third ventricle. Several diagnostic terms have been developed, based upon histologic features of neoplasms; however, in animals, histologic features are not always significantly reflected in biologic behavior. Nevertheless, histologic

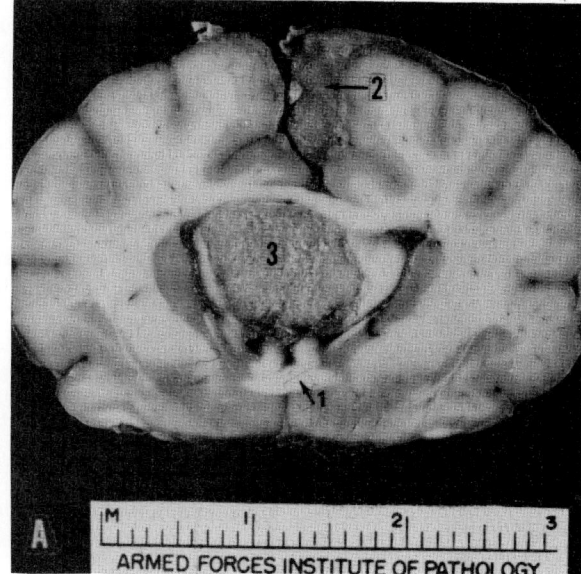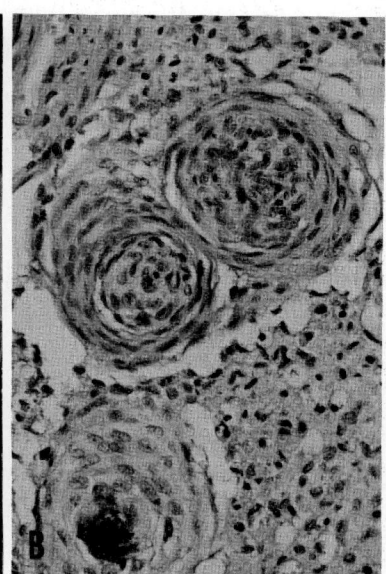

FIG. 27-20 A. Meningioma in brain of a 14-year-old castrated male cat. Section of brain through (1) the anterior commissure, (2) with tumor in pia, and (3) in midline. **B.** Same tumor as **A.** (×210); note concentrically laminated structures. (Contributor: Dr. J. Holzworth.)

ARMED FORCES INSTITUTE OF PATHOLOGY

variants often indicate the tissue of origin and are of interest in the study of these neoplasms. A brief description of the terms applied to these neoplasms in animals follow:

Meningothelial (syncytial, meningotheliomatous, endotheliomatous) **meningioma** consists of tumor cells that are presumed to arise from cells of the pia arachnoid. These cells are polygonal shaped, and often form sheets or sometimes whorls. Nuclei are large, spherical, and centrally placed, with pale nucleoplasm, conspicuous nucleoli, and frequent, clear vacuoles in nuclei.

Fibroblastic (fibrous) **meningioma.** Cells tend to be elongated and spindle-shaped, arranged in interweaving bundles, and contain cytoplasmic fibrils. Reticulum and dense collagen are conspicuous among these cells. Psammoma bodies and whorls of tumor cells may occasionally occur.

Transitional meningioma. In this form, the pattern is dominated by the tendency of the cells to form whorls, a feature of meningothelial cells that tend to wrap around objects, such as calcium granules, capillaries, or other meningothelial cells. Psammoma bodies are frequently encountered.

Granular cell meningioma. This type is seen particularly in F344 rats and consists of large cells with abundant cytoplasm filled with large, eosinophilic, PAS-positive granules which, with electron microscopy, are identifiable as distended lysosomes. Sometimes these granular cells are mixed with meningothelial cells, an observation leading to the idea that these two types of cells have a common origin.

Angioblastic (angiomatous) **meningioma.** Newly-formed and haphazardly-arranged blood vessels form a conspicuous component of this neoplasm.

Papillary meningioma is a form infrequently reported. It contains tumor cells arranged in papillary structure, with distinct stroma supporting tumor cells. Sometimes cells are arranged in a palisade pattern.

Most meningiomas are benign in the conventional sense, but produce serious effects by compressing the underlying parenchyma of brain or spinal cord. Malignant variants are less frequent, their cells are less orderly in arrangement, and their nuclei often hyperchromatic and often in mitosis. Neoplastic cells invade adjacent tissues and metastasize, particularly to the lungs.

References

Luginbühl H. Studies on meningiomas in cats. Review of the literature and report of eight cases. Am J Vet Res 1961;22:1030–1040.

Mitsumori K, Maronpot RR, Boorman GA. Spontaneous tumors of the meninges in rats. Vet Pathol 1987;24:50–58.

Mitsumori K, Stephanski SA, Maronpot RR. Benign and malignant neoplasms, meninges, rat. In: Jones TC, Mohr U, Hunt RD, eds. Pathology of laboratory animals, nervous system. Berlin: Springer-Verlag, 1988;108–117.

Patnaik AK, Kay WJ, Hurwitz AI. Intracranial meningioma: a comparative pathologic study of 28 dogs. Vet Pathol 1986;23:369–373.

Patnaik AK, Lieberman PH, Erlandson RA, et al. Paranasal meningioma in the dog: a clinicopathologic study of ten cases. Vet Pathol 1986;23:362–368.

Ribas JL, Carpenter JL, Mena H, et al. Central nervous system meningiomas in the dog: a review of 50 cases. J Neuropathol Exp Neurol 1991;50:373–379.

Stebbins KE, McGrath JT. Meningioangiomatosis in a dog. Vet Pathol 1988;25:167–168.

SPECIAL NEOPLASMS AFFECTING NERVOUS SYSTEM

Pinealoma

Tumors of the pineal body, pineal gland, or epiphysis cerebri occur infrequently in many species but in spite of their rarity, have been given many names. These include pinealoma, pineal adenoma, pineocytoma, and pineoblastoma. This endocrine organ is located in the cerebral meninges, near the midline of the brain, attached to one of the cerebral hemispheres. The precise location of the pineal gland varies somewhat in different species.

Histologic appearance of the pineal gland and its anatomical location are distinctive. The gland consists of two main cell types, nearly 90% are pinealocytes and the rest are small glial cells, usually considered to be astrocytes. Large pinealocytes are derived from neurosecretory photoreceptor cells still found in primitive forms, such as Anamniotes. In animals in early phylogenic stages these pinealocytes have photoreceptor and secretory functions. Mammals retain only the secretory function. The hormone secreted by the pinealocyte is melatonin.

The pinealocyte is a large cell which in hematoxylin-and-eosin-stained preparations has round, granular nuclei and poorly stained cytoplasm. In sections stained with silver carbonate (Del Rio-Hortega) one to several processes project from the cell membrane and end in a club shape. "Light and dark cells" may be seen, differing by the amount of secretory product in the cytoplasm.

Neoplasms of the pineal are infrequently discovered in animals, except in unusual circumstances, such as may occur in toxicologic pathology studies in laboratory animals or in investigation of other diseases of brain. Adenomatous glands are enlarged, ovoid to spherical, and even more densely cellular and usually consist principally of pinealocytes. Metastases or extensions into nearby organs are rare.

Pineal tumors in humans are encountered in two cytologic forms: in one neoplastic cells closely resemble the principal cells of the normal pineal gland and is called pineocytoma; the second form consists of more primitive cells and is designated as a pineoblastoma. Combinations of these two cell types in the same tumor are referred to as mixed pineocytoma-pineoblastoma. These different types and their combinations have been recognized in pineal tumors in both humans and laboratory rats. The significance of the two cytologic types is yet to be determined.

References

Karasek M, Reiter RJ. Functional morphology of the mammalian pineal gland. In: Jones TC, Capen CC, Mohr U, Hunt RD, eds. ILSI Monograph on pathology of laboratory animals, endocrine system. 2nd ed. 1995; pp 193–204.

Koestner A, Solleveld HA. Tumors of the pineal gland, rat. In: Jones TC, Capen CC, Mohr U, eds. ILSI Monograph on pathology of laboratory animals, endocrine system. 2nd ed. 1995; pp 205–213.

Lerner AB, Case JD, Takahashi, Lee GH, Mori W. Isolation of melatonin, the pineal factor that lightens melanocytes. J Am Chem Soc 1958;82:2587.

Reiter RJ. Pineal melatonin: cell biology of its synthesis and its physiological interactions. Endocrine Rev 1991;12:151–180.

Craniopharyngioma

This new growth arises from Rathke's pouch, the normal outgrowth, in the early embryo, of the foregut that becomes the anterior lobe of the pituitary. The effect of the tumor is to interfere and displace the anterior pituitary, hypothalamus, or thalamus. Clinical signs caused by this lesion include pituitary insufficiency and secondary malfunction of other endocrine organs, resulting in: diabetes insipidus; retardation of growth; and adrenal, sexual, or thyroid insufficiency. This neoplasm is usually considered to come from the endocrine system with severe effects on neuroendocrine function.

Histologic features include invasive growth or squamous epithelium mixed with cells resembling those seen in the anterior pituitary.

References

Carlton WW, Gries CL. Craniopharyngioma, pituitary, rat. In: Jones TC, Capen CC, Mohr U, eds. ILSI Monograph on pathology of laboratory animals, endocrine system. 2nd ed. 1995; pp 86–90.

Heider K. Spontaneous craniopharyngioma in a mouse. Vet Pathol 1985;23:522–523.

Liszczak T, Richardson EP, Phillips SP, et al. Morphological, biochemical, ultrastructural, tissue culture and clinical observations of typical and aggressive craniopharyngiomas. Acta Neuropathol 1978;43:191–203.

Neer TM, Reavis DU. Craniopharyngioma and associated central diabetes insipidus and hypothyroidism in a dog. J Am Vet Med Assoc 1983;182:519–520.

Malignant melanoma

This neoplasm usually originates from cells of the neural crest that have migrated in early embryonic life to the dermis or any other organ. In many species, benign collections of pigmented cells may be found in adult animals in several organs, including brain and spinal cord. These pigment-producing cells may, on rare occasions, give rise to malignant melanoma. A more frequent event is for malignant melanoma to develop in other organs, such as skin, and metastasize elsewhere, including the central nervous system.

Reference

Ackerman AB. Pathology of malignant melanoma. New York: Masson, 1981.

Malignant lymphoma or lymphosarcoma: primary in central nervous system

Certain primary neoplasms of the brain and spinal cord have been recognized in dogs and humans as consisting of individually discrete cells suggesting immature monocytes or lymphocytes. These lesions were classified for many years as "reticuloses" or subdivided into "granulomatous reticulosis," "neoplastic reticulosis," or "microgliomatosis." The older concept of the "reticuloendothelial system" as the origin of these tumors is no longer accepted and immunohistochemical techniques have demonstrated that at least some of these neoplasms in humans and dogs consist of immunoglobulin-producing B-cells. This finding prompted the idea that terms, such as "histiocytic lymphosarcoma" or lymphoma, immunoblastic type are more appropriate. Concepts still evolving await further experimental evidence and study of natural cases in animals.

A controversy exists over the interpretation of this lesion or lesions. Similar lesions have been interpreted differently and called "canine granulomatous meningoencephalomyelitis" by several authors. These observers placed emphasis upon the epithelioid or macrophage nature of some of the cells and interpret others as monocytes. At present, the critical element needed to distinguish two or more similar lesions, namely, the etiologic factor, seems not yet to have been demonstrated.

The characteristic histologic feature depends upon the identification of the cells and their association with the vasculature. Proliferating cells accumulate around vessels, forming concentric laminations in this perivascular location. Some cells are in isolated aggregations, separated by intact nervous parenchyma; others form large, solid-tumor masses. They are most extensive in the white matter of the cerebral hemisphere and in the brainstem. Rarely do cells extend into the cerebral cortex. Leptomeninges are occasionally involved, but in only a few cases are extensive meningeal infiltrations found. Spinal cord may be involved and merits careful attention.

References

Braund KD, Vandevelde M, Walker TL, et al. Granulomatous menin-goencephalitis in six dogs. J Am Vet Assoc 1978;172:1195–1200.

Cordy DR. Canine granulomatous meningoencephalomyelitis. Vet Pathol 1979;16:325–333.

Fankhauser R, Fatzer R, Luginbühl H, et al. Reticulosis of the central nervous system in dogs. Adv Vet Sci Comp Med 1971;16:35–71.

Koestner A, Zeman W. Primary reticulosis of the central nervous system in dogs. Am J Vet Res 1962;23:381–393.

Vandevelde M, Fatzer R, Fankhauser R. Immunohistological studies on primary reticulosis of the canine brain. Vet Pathol 1981;18:577–588.

NEOPLASMS OF PERIPHERAL NERVOUS SYSTEM

Schwannoma and Neurilemmoma

Either of these terms describes a neoplasm, usually benign, which is believed to arise from Schwann cells (neurolemmal cells) surrounding axons of the peripheral nerves (Figs. 27-21, 27-22, Table 27-10). Considerable difference of opinion exists about whether this tumor is distinguishable from neurofibroma, which also may arise from Schwann cells and perhaps from epi- and perineural cell elements. Histologically, however, the tumors are distinct from one another (Fig. 27-23). Studies on biologic behavior are needed to determine whether the continued recognition and separation of these two entities are justified.

Schwannoma is composed of elongated, spindle-shaped cells arranged in a distinctive pattern. Cells, which are similar to those of a neurofibroma and plumper than those of a fibroma, form interlacing fascicles, with clumps of cells lying in windrows. This feature, referred to as palisading of nuclei, is the principal distinctive characteristic of the tumor. Often nodules or lobules of cells exist which are arranged in palisades at either end of a bundle of cytoplasmic processes or parallel fibers. Such a structure is termed a Verocay body. Fasciculi of cells run in wavy or undulating patterns and may also form tight whorls.

As would be expected, growths are located along the course of a nerve or at a plexus or ganglion. These growths occur in most species, but infrequently. They are most common in cattle, in which many have been termed neurofibromas. The term, acoustic neuroma has been applied to schwannomas of the eighth cranial nerve in humans. Schwannomas may also arise from

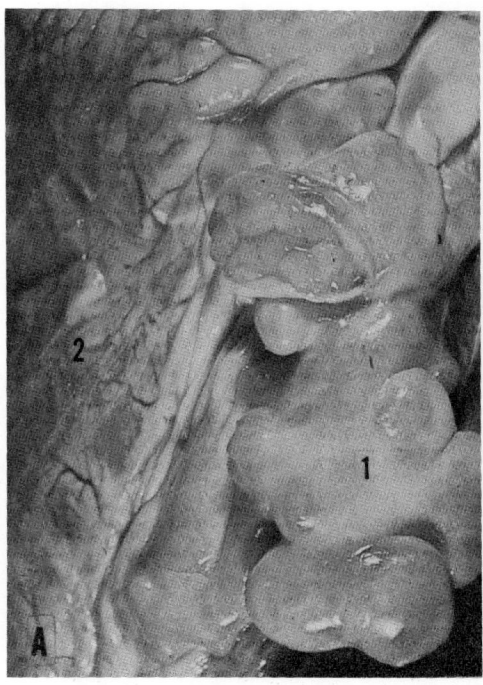
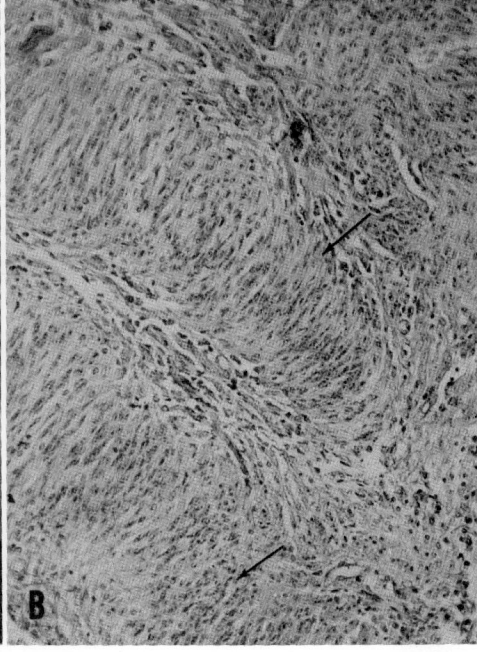

FIG. 27-21   A. (1) Schwannoma of (2) the epicardium in a steer. (Photograph courtesy of Dr. C.L. Davis.) **B.** Neurofibromatosis involving brachial plexus, myocardium, and intercostal nerves of an eight-year-old cow. Section (×150) is from the tumor in the brachial plexus. (Courtesy of Armed Forces Institute of Pathology; contributor: Dr. C.L. Davis.)

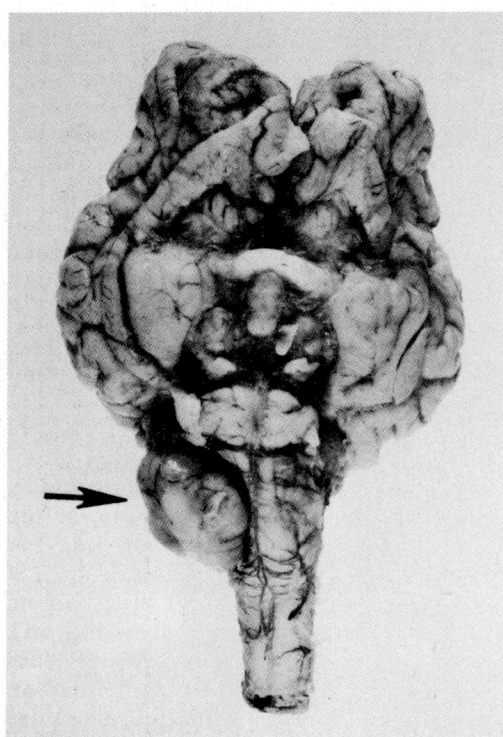

FIG. 27-22 Schwannoma of the eighth cranial nerve in a 14-year-old cow. (Courtesy of Dr. W.J. Hadlow.)

other cranial nerves, excluding olfactory and optic nerves, that do not have Schwann cells. Cranial nerve schwannomas have been reported in dogs.

References

Gough AW, Hanna W, Barsoum NJ, et al. Morphologic and immuno-histochemical features of two spontaneous peripheral nerve tumors in Wistar rats. Vet Pathol 1986;23:68–73.

Patnaik AK, Erlandson RA, Lieberman PH. Canine malignant melanotic schwannomas: a light and electron microscopic study of two cases. Vet Pathol 1984;21:493–488.

Neurofibroma and neurofibrosarcoma

These tumors may arise from Schwann cells and, therefore, represent a histologic variant of schwannomas. Some believe that these tumors arise from "fibroblasts" in the perineurium and are variants of fibromas; however, because Schwann cells cannot be differentiated from perineural cells except by position, this distinction is probably not valid. Neurofibroma is distinct from the ordinary fibroma and lacks the unique architecture of schwannoma. Microscopically, neurofibroma is composed of spindle-shaped cells arranged in circular whorls or wavy fasciculi. Collagen is usually recognized (Fig. 27-23).

Malignant tumors of this class occur rarely and are termed neurofibrosarcomas or neurogenic sarcomas. Microscopically, neurofibrosarcoma may closely resemble a fibrosarcoma, but cells tend to form in plump spindles and retain a whorled or curly arrangement. Neurofibrosarcomas occur in most species but are seen most commonly in cattle, in which they are fairly frequent in the myocardium, sometimes with more than one occurring in a single heart. The tendency to form whorls is sometimes recognizable grossly in the moist, slightly bulging cut surface. In humans, large numbers of cutaneous neurofibromas occur in the same patient in what is known as von Recklinghausen neurofibromatosis. A tumorous condition having similar characteristics has been reported in dogs and neurofibromas are often multiple in cattle.

References

Elling H, Stavrou D. Ueber die Antigenität eines chemisch induzierten neurogenen Sarkoms der Ratte. Vet Pathol 1980;17:477–489.

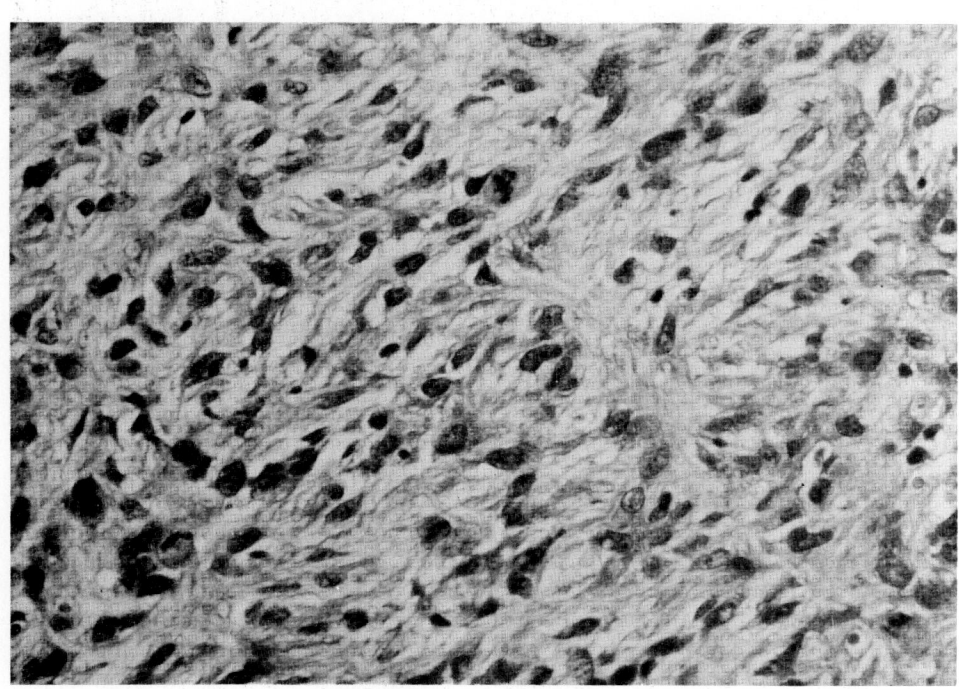

FIG. 27-23 Neurofibrosarcoma from the subcutis of the elbow of a dog. This neoplasm lacks unique architecture of the Schwannoma (Fig. 27-21), and more closely resembles fibrosarcoma. (Courtesy of Dr. N.W. King, Jr.)

Peltonen J, et al. Cellular differentiation and expression of matrix genes in type 1 neurofibromatosis. Lab Invest 1988;59:760–771.

Riccardi VM. Neurofibromatosis: challenges for applied cellular and molecular biology. Lab Invest 1988;59:726–728.

Ganglioneuroma

A distinctive and rare neoplasm in animals, increasingly recognized in several species, including humans, non-human primates, dogs, cats, cattle, horses, and laboratory rats (Fig. 27-24). The location of this lesion in association with tissues and neoplasms originating in the neural crest, such as adrenal medulla (associated with pheochromocytoma), thyroid (with C-cell tumors), intestinal wall (Auerbach's and Meissner's plexuses), is one of its distinguishing features. The neoplasm is made up of haphazardly arranged neuroglia, including astrocytes, Schwann cells, and axons without myelin, and nests of large neurons identifiable as ganglion cells. These cells are conspicuous, with abundant cytoplasm, Nissl substance (sometimes marginated) in the cytoplasm, and axons identifiable with appropriate

TABLE 27-11	Secondary neoplasms in the central nervous system

By extension	
Brain	*Spinal cord*
Pituitary adenoma or carcinoma	Epideremoid cyst
Craniopharyngioma	Synovial cyst
Nasal mucoepithelioma	Chordoma
Nasal esthesioneuroepithelioma	Primitive neuroblastoma
Nasal squamous cell carcinoma	
By metastasis	
Brain or spinal cord	
Lymphosarcoma (Mal. lymphoma)	Carcinoma, squamous cell, adenocarcinoma (any organ)
Myelogenous leukemia	Hemangiosarcoma (any organ)
Malignant melanoma	
Osteosarcoma	

stains. The neuronal nature of tissue can be confirmed by the use of avidin-biotin-complex to demonstrate the presence of neuron-specific enolase or other neuron-specific biomarkers.

The central nervous system counterpart of the ganglioneuroma is the gangliocytoma, as described earlier. It has only recently been reported initially in the cerebellum of a dog. Ganglioneuroma and gangliocytoma differ from neuroblastomas by the considerable degree of maturation. They are believed to arise from neuroblastic elements which undergo progressive maturation. Neuroblastic elements are rarely discernible in gangliocytomas during detection.

References

Cole DE, Migaki G, Leipold HW. Colonic ganglioneuromatosis in a steer. Vet Pathol 1990;27:461–562.

Crissman JW, Valerio MG, Asiedu AA, et al. Ganglioneuroma of the thyroid gland in a colony of Sprague-Dawley rats. Vet Pathol 1991;28:354–362.

Fairley RA, McEntee MD. Colorectal ganglioneuromatosis in a young female dog (lhasa apso). Vet Pathol 1990;27:206–207.

Hawkins KL, Summers BA. Mediastinal ganglioneuroma in a puppy. Vet Pathol 1987;24:283–285.

Nyska A, Shamir MH, Harmelin A, et al. Intracranial gangliocytoma in a dog. Vet Pathol 1995;32:190–192.

Ribas JL, Kwapien KP, Pope ER. Immunohistochemistry and ultrastructure of intestinal ganglioneuroma in a dog. Vet Pathol 1990;27:376–379.

Roth L, Scarratt WK, Shipley CF, et al. Ganglioneuroma of the spinal cord in a calf. Vet Pathol 1987;24:188–189.

Sokale EOA, Ladds PW. Multicentric ganglioneuroma in a steer. Vet Pathol 1983;20:767–770.

SECONDARY TUMORS

Metastatic neoplasms and direct extension of neoplasms from adjacent tissues are common (Table 27-11). Malignant lymphoma is the most frequent secondary tumor. It most often occurs in the spinal canal and is especially frequent in cats and cattle.

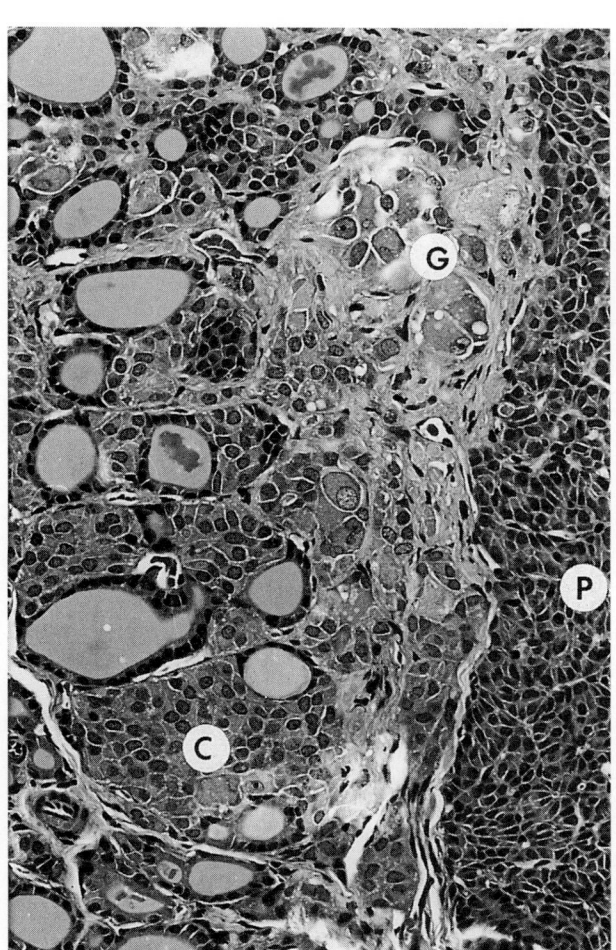

FIG. 27-24 Ganglioneuroma in thyroid gland of a 26-month-old female, Sprague Dawley rat. Ganglioneuroma (*G*) is adjacent to a focus of C-Cell hyperplasia (*C*), and the parathyroid gland (*P*). Hand E Bar = 50 um. (From: Crissman JW, et al. Vet Pathol 1991;28:354–362.)

28
Organs of special sense

EYE

The eye is a wondrously complex structure whose parts perform a function that even the most blasé must consider miraculous. The eyes of each animal or bird are remarkably adapted to its environment and habits. The hawk can spot its tiny prey from fantastic heights and the cat can see its victim on the darkest night. Such functional adaptations depend upon specific structural developments which are different in each species. This alone makes the study of diseased ocular structures in animals both difficult and fascinating.

Not only is the eye the organ of sight, but it also serves as a window through which some disease processes can be observed. With slit-lamp illumination and the corneal microscope, leukocytes or erythrocytes can be seen escaping from the iris, floating in the aqueous, and settling to the bottom of the anterior chamber. Capillaries in the retina can be studied with the ophthalmoscope, and sometimes they yield clues about the condition of capillaries in the rest of the body. It is unfortunate that the general pathologist often avoids the study of the eye, because this organ follows the general laws of biology in its response to injury and can teach much to the observer. This is not to disclaim the necessity for the special knowledge and interest of ophthalmic pathologists, whose contributions are vital, but rather to encourage veterinary pathologists to cultivate a deeper interest in this important organ in their animal patients.

The eye must be studied carefully in the living animal, the gross specimen approached systematically and properly fixed for microscopic examination if the best evaluation is to be made. Some things are best detected in the living animal, including: the luster of the cornea; the size, shape, and response of the pupil to light; opacities in the media-cornea, aqueous, lens and vitreous; intraocular tension; and intraocular masses. The importance of systematic clinical evaluation and recording of findings is especially important to the pathologist in examining this system.

References

Gelatt KN. Veterinary ophthalmology. 2nd ed. Philadelphia: Lea & Febiger, 1991.
Pfeiffer RH. Comparative ophthalmic pathology. Springfield: CC Thomas, 1983.

Adnexa

The **eyelids** have cutaneous and conjunctival surfaces and contain both tear and sebaceous glands (i.e., meibomian glands); lesions may occur in any of these structures. Any lesion of the skin (Chapter 17) may involve the cutaneous part of the eyelid. **Photosensitization** (Chapters 3 and 15) specifically affects unpigmented eyelids and conjunctiva, especially in sheep, cattle, and horses. This is due to circulating photosensitizing substances, resulting from: (1) congenital failure to excrete porphyrins, (2) hepatotoxic interference with the excretion of phylloerythrin, or (3) ingestion of toxic photosensitizing plant material. **Conjunctiva** is frequently subject to nonspecific inflammation, which may at times result in hypertrophy and hyperplasia of subepithelial lymphocytic nodules. This may give the conjunctiva a grossly evident roughened, cobblestone appearance. Congenital inward turning of the eyelids, known as **entropion,** may lead to conjunctivitis and keratitis due to abrasion of the cornea and sclera by the hair of the inverted eyelid. The defect is probably inherited in sheep and is often a serious problem in newborn lambs. Outward eversion of the eyelids, **ectropion,** may also be inherited and presents a cosmetic problem in dogs. Both entropion and ectropion may be alleviated by surgical procedures. A double row of eyelashes, or **distichiasis,** may also cause conjunctivitis; this is reported in dogs. Inflammation or abscesses of sebaceous glands (stye) or meibomian glands (chalazion) are occasionally encountered. Meibomian glands are modified sebaceous glands on the inner surface of the eye. Many of the causes of keratitis, discussed shortly, also cause conjunctivitis.

Neoplasms of sebaceous and meibomian glands are

most often encountered in dogs, where they resemble sebaceous gland tumors of the skin. Neoplasms of the conjunctiva are not infrequent, the most common being squamous cell carcinoma of the bovine eye. This neoplasm most frequently originates in the conjunctiva but may arise from the skin of the eyelid. Basal cell carcinomas, cutaneous horns, and papillomas may also arise from the conjunctival or cutaneous portions of the eyelids.

Membrana nictitans, or nictitating membrane, is particularly well-developed in most domestic animals, but is vestigial in humans. This membrane invests the nasal aspect of the globe and is usually barely visible at the medial canthus. It can be protruded like a "third eyelid" by voluntary or involuntary action to cover most, if not all, of the corneal surface. This is believed to give the eye additional protection and may have a cleansing function. The membrane is covered by conjunctiva and is richly supplied with simple and compound tubular lacrimal glands. Rigidity is given the structure by a central core of cartilage, which is concave to fit the eyeball. Eversion of the membrana nictitans has been reported to be an inherited anomaly in German shorthaired pointers and is sometimes encountered in other breeds at birth.

Inflammation of the lacrimal glands (dacryoadenitis), may come to the attention of the veterinary pathologist. The superficial and deep glands of the membrana nictitans of the dog are most commonly involved. This inflammation results in congestion and enlargement of the gland which, in turn, causes the third eyelid to protrude, usually necessitating its ablation. The microscopic findings in surgical specimens of the third eyelid are usually limited to inflammatory changes in the stroma and the connective tissue surrounding the tubular glands of the eyelid. The ducts of the glands are often dilated and occasionally filled with leukocytes; the acinar elements are hypertrophic. Cysts of lacrimal ducts and glands are occasionally seen. They may be congenital or acquired. Frank neoplastic changes in the glands are rare, but adenomas may occur.

In most species (but not dogs) an accessory lacrimal gland (**harderian gland**) exists at the base of the third eyelid, and may become inflamed or subject to neoplastic disease. In rats, a viral disease of this gland—along with other lacrimal glands and the salivary glands (sialodacryoadenitis)—is a relatively frequent disease; a similar disease is also seen in mice.

References

Gelatt KN. Textbook of veterinary ophthalmology. 2nd ed. Philadelphia: Lea & Febiger, 1991.

Hunt RD. Dacryoadenitis in the Sprague-Dawley rat. Am J Vet Res 1963;24:638–641.

Jacoby RO, Blatt PN, Jonas AM. Pathogenesis of sialodacryoadenitis in gnotobiotic rats. Vet Pathol 1975;12:196–209.

Jonas AM, et al. Sialodacryoadenitis in the rat, a light- and electron-microscopic study. Arch Pathol 1969;88:613–622.

Magrane WG. Canine ophthalmology. 3rd ed. Philadelphia: Lea & Febiger, 1977.

Maronpot RR, Chavannes J-M. Dacryoadenitis, conjunctivitis, and facial dermatitis of the mouse. Lab Anim Sci 1977;27:277–278.

Martin CL, Leach R. Everted membrana nictitans in German shorthaired pointers. J Am Vet Med Assoc 1970;157:1229–1232.

Prince JH, Diesem CD, Eglitis I, et al. Anatomy and histology of the eye and orbit in domestic animals. Springfield: Charles C Thomas, 1960.

Saunders LZ. Pathology of the eye of domestic animals. Berlin: Paul Parey, 1968.

Shively JN, Epling GP. Fine structure of the canine eye. Iris Am J Vet Res 1969;30:13–26.

Shively JN, Epling GP, Jensen R. Fine structure of the canine eye. Am J Vet Res 1970;31:1339–1359.

Wolff E. The anatomy of the eye and orbit. 3rd ed. Philadelphia: Blakiston, 1951.

Wyman M, Donovan EF. The ocular fundus of the normal dog. J Am Vet Med Assoc 1965;147:7–26.

Canine bilateral extraocular polymyositis

Bilateral exophthalmos—protrusion of both ocular globes from the orbit—may occur as the result of hyperthyroidism, bilateral glaucoma, or extraocular neoplasms; however, in this latter case the neoplasm in the orbit and the exophthalmos is apt to be limited to one eye. In the polymyositis syndrome (Fig. 28-1), the eyes protrude from the orbit as a result of swelling of the superior and inferior rectus and oblique muscles of both eyes. The retractor bulbi muscles of the rest of the body do not appear to be involved. Some interference with vision may be evident by the inability of the dog to avoid hitting objects while walking. Intraocular pressure may be increased, but no other effects or lesions are disclosed by ophthalmoscopic examination.

Significant **gross** lesions found at necropsy include enlargement and pallor of the central part of each of the four rectus and oblique muscles in both eyes. The retractor bulbi muscles are not affected. The **microscopic** lesions—demonstrable in biopsy or necropsy specimens of the affected muscles—consist of patchy zones of muscle fiber necrosis, with associated infiltration of lymphocytes, plasma cells, histiocytes, and occasional eosinophils (Fig. 28-1E).

Canine bilateral extraocular polymyositis has been reported in seven dogs: four golden retrievers, one German shepherd, one doberman pinscher, and one mongrel. Three were males and four females (two of which were spayed); their ages ranged 6–18 months. The diagnosis was confirmed by finding polymyositis in extraocular muscle specimens taken by biopsy or necropsy. Most myositis in dogs involves several groups of muscles, with the exception of this disease and canine masticatory myositis, which may also produce exophthalmos (Chapter 18). One hypothesis, applicable to both, is that an immunologic mechanism is directed against specific muscle fiber antigens in these specific muscles. Curative effects of corticosteroid (in the form of dexamethasone) in five clinical cases supports this hypothesis.

References

Carpenter JL, Schmidt GM, Moore FM, et al. Canine bilateral extraocular polymyositis. Vet Pathol 1989;26:510–512.

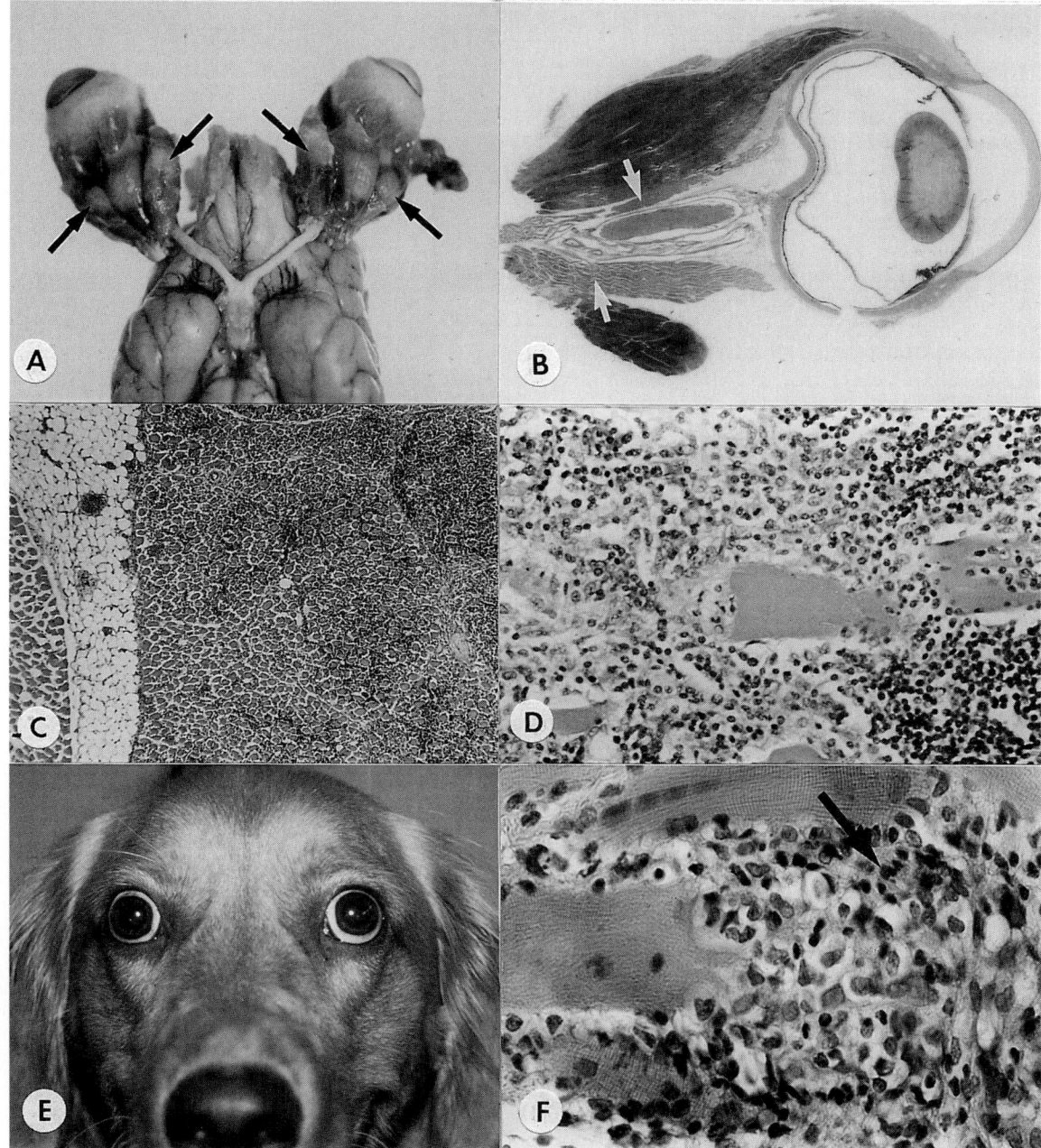

FIG. 28-1 Canine bilateral extraocular polymyositis. **A.** Eight-month-old male golden retriever. Extraocular muscles (arrows) with swollen, pale zones in the mid-bellies and mottled dark and light areas in the tendinous ends. **B.** Section of eye and ocular muscles. Superior and inferior rectus muscles are swollen and dark, retractor oculus muscles *(arrows)* are not affected (hematoxylin and eosin stain). **C.** Retractor oculus muscle (left) is unaffected as is the orbital fat to its right; the superior rectus muscle (center and right) is dark in patches due to inflammatory cell infiltration (hematoxylin and eosin stain). **D.** Medial rectus muscle with segmental necrosis and infiltration by lymphocytes and histiocytes (hematoxylin and eosin stain). **E.** Bilateral exophthalmos, 18-month-old female golden retriever. **F.** Superior rectus oculus from animal in **E.** *Myositis* with necrosis and infiltration with histiocytes, lymphocytes, and a rare eosinophil *(arrow)*. (Courtesy of Dr. James L. Carpenter and *Veterinary Pathology*.)

Cornea and sclera

Some of the important anatomic differences among species will be mentioned as the specific anatomic structure is considered. The sclera is the relatively avascular tunic that gives the globe the structural rigidity to maintain its shape. In birds, it normally contains cartilage, which may ossify to bone.

The cornea of animals of most species is subjected to a variety of harmful influences, but has a good capacity for recovery. Unfortunately, healing of lesions in the cornea may result in scarring, which is not objectionable in other structures, but which may destroy sight by making all or part of the cornea opaque. Wounds—particularly when accompanied by penetrating foreign bodies—are a common cause of inflammation, which may leave opacities in the cornea. Injuries that perforate the cornea are serious, often leading to loss of sight in the involved eye. Perforation of Descemet's membrane permits escape of aqueous humor followed by collapse of the cornea, with prolapse of the iris and dislocation of the lens further possibilities. Secondary infection often causes inflammation of the entire globe (panophthalmitis), which may cause permanent loss of sight.

INFECTIOUS KERATITIS, KERATOCONJUNCTIVITIS

So-called "pink eye," this disease in sheep, goats, and cattle may result in diffuse inflammation of the cornea, producing temporary blindness. Diffuse scarring with loss of transparency is a common sequel of this infection, which often occurs as an outbreak with a relatively high incidence (up to 50%). The cause is often not firmly established, although many organisms have been recovered from infected conjunctival sacs; in some cases, specific organisms have proved to be pathogenic. In cattle, however, *Moraxella bovis* is the principal causative organism. It is recovered from many outbreaks, and instillation of the organism into the conjunctival sac of normal animals is followed by severe keratitis. Solar irradiation augments the disease, with most outbreaks occurring during the summer months. *Mycoplasma* have also been recovered from infected sheep and cattle. The herpesvirus of bovine rhinotracheitis also causes keratoconjunctivitis and is responsible for some outbreaks of pink eye. In sheep, *Rickettsia conjunctivae* is a principal cause of keratoconjunctivitis. Although *Moraxella bovis* has been recovered from affected sheep as well as from horses, its role is uncertain. *Chlamydia* have also been associated with ocular infection in cattle and sheep. The problem of etiologies is still confused; many organisms apparently cause this clinical disease.

Keratitis and keratoconjunctivitis in other species are usually sporadic, with no single cause, except in cats where *Mycoplasma* and *Chlamydia* are common causes. Herpesviruses have a propensity to infect the conjunctiva and should be suspected in any species. Corneal edema and other ocular manifestations of infectious canine hepatitis are discussed elsewhere. In addition to cattle and sheep, *Chlamydia* have also been described as causes of keratitis in swine, guinea pigs, dogs, cats, and humans. Nematodes of the genus *Thelazia* cause conjunctivitis in many different animal species. In horses, larvae of *Habronema* spp. are a common cause. Other causes include vitamin A deficiency, exposure to ultraviolet light, chemical irritants, dust, and trauma. Allergic keratoconjunctivitis is well documented in humans and may account for many examples in animals.

References

Muller RB, Fales WH. Infectious bovine keratoconjunctivitis: an update. Vet Clin North Am Large Anim Pract 1984;6:597–608.
Pugh GW, McDonald TJ, Kopecky KE, et al. Experimental infectious bovine keratoconjunctivitis: effects of feeding colostrum from vaccinated cows on development of pinkeye in calves. Am J Vet Res 1980;41:1611–1614.
Pugh GW, McDonald TJ, Kopecky KE. Infectious bovine keratoconjunctivitis: evidence for genetic modulation of resistance in purebred Hereford cattle. Am J Vet Res 1986;47:885–889.

Keratoconjunctivitis sicca Defective production or function of tears leads to excessive dryness of the corneal surface and soon results in serious pathologic effects. The cornea may become diffusely inflamed, with one or more deep ulcers of the corneal stroma and loss of vision. Many species are subject to this problem, but the disease is best described in humans, dogs, and laboratory rats and mice. Among dogs, a few breeds are more often affected. These include the English bulldog, Cavalier King Charles spaniel, Shih Tzu, and lhaso apso breeds.

The most frequent immediate causes are (1) dacryoadenitis (due to infectious organisms), or (2) toxic reactions to drugs, such as sulfasalazine or phenazopyridine hydrochloride. If untreated, the corneal lesions progress to interstitial keratitis, with deposition of calcium salts in the corneal stroma. Iridocyclitis may follow, with eventual destruction of sight.

References

Kaswan RL, Martin CL, Dawe DL. Rheumatoid factor determination in 50 dogs with keratoconjunctivitis sicca. J Am Vet Med Assoc 1983;183:1073–1075.
Kaswan RL, Martin CL, Chapman WL. Keratoconjunctivitis sicca: histopathologic study of nictitating membrane and lacrimal glands from 28 dogs. Am J Vet Res 1984;45:112–118.
Kaswan RL, Martin CL, Dawe DL. Keratoconjunctivitis sicca: immunological evaluation of 62 canine cases. Am J Vet Res 1985;46:376–383.
Kast A. Keratoconjunctivitis sicca and sequelae, mouse and rat. In: Jones TC, Mohr U, Hunt RD, eds. Monographs on pathology of laboratory animals, eye and ear. Berlin: Springer-Verlag, 1991; 29–37.
Krinke GJ. Atrophy and sclerosis, Harderian gland, rat. In: Jones TC, Mohr U, Hunt RD, eds. Monographs on pathology of laboratory animals, eye and ear. Berlin: Springer-Verlag, 1991;137–140.
Meader VP, Tyler RD, Plunkett ML. Epicardial and corneal mineralization in clinically normal severe combined immunodeficiency (SCID) mice. Vet Pathol 1993;29:247–249.
Morgan RV, Bachrach A. Keratoconjunctivitis sicca associated with sulfonamide therapy in dogs. J Am Vet Med Assoc 1982;180:432–434.

Corneal opacity may also occur in the absence of keratitis as a congenital defect. It has been described in British Friesian cattle as a hereditary disease. It results from edema, but the pathogenesis is uncertain.

Pigmentary keratitis In some instances, for reasons poorly understood, keratitis in dogs not only is accompanied by deep and superficial vascularization of the cornea, but also is followed by deposition of melanin pigment in the corneal epithelium and the underlying stroma. This may involve much of the cornea, giving it a brown or black color and rendering it opaque. Pigmentary keratitis is difficult to treat and often destroys sight in the affected eye.

Vascularization Corneal vascularization may follow trauma to the cornea, especially any injury resulting in ulceration of the corneal epithelium; or, it may be a manifestation of dietary deficiency of certain vitamins (riboflavin) or amino acids (tryptophane). Capillaries that extend into the cornea toward an ulcer usually arise from the vessels in a small zone at the point in the limbus nearest the lesion. **Superficial vascularization,** such as formation of new capillaries in the stroma adjacent to the epithelium, usually occurs first. Proliferation of blood vessels deeper in the stroma (**deep vascularization**) usually follows more prolonged effects on the cornea. Vascularization based upon nutritional deficiency is characterized by proliferation of new capillaries from the corneoscleral junction (limbus) all around the circumference of the cornea. These extend centripetally toward the centrum of the cornea; they may occur in the absence of significant corneal opacity, and do not radiate toward or terminate in an ulcer or opacity of the cornea. **Grossly,** newly formed vessels in the cornea

may appear as vascular arborizations; **microscopically,** however, each blood vessel does not terminate blindly but forms a capillary loop through which the blood can return to the venules at the limbus (Figs. 28-2, 28-3).

References

Burger PC, Chandler DB, Klintworth GK. Corneal neovascularization as studied by scanning electron microscopy of vascular casts. Lab Invest 1983;48:169–180.

McCracken JS, Burger PC, Klintworth GK. Morphologic observations on experimental corneal vascularization in the rat. Lab Invest 1979;41:519–530.

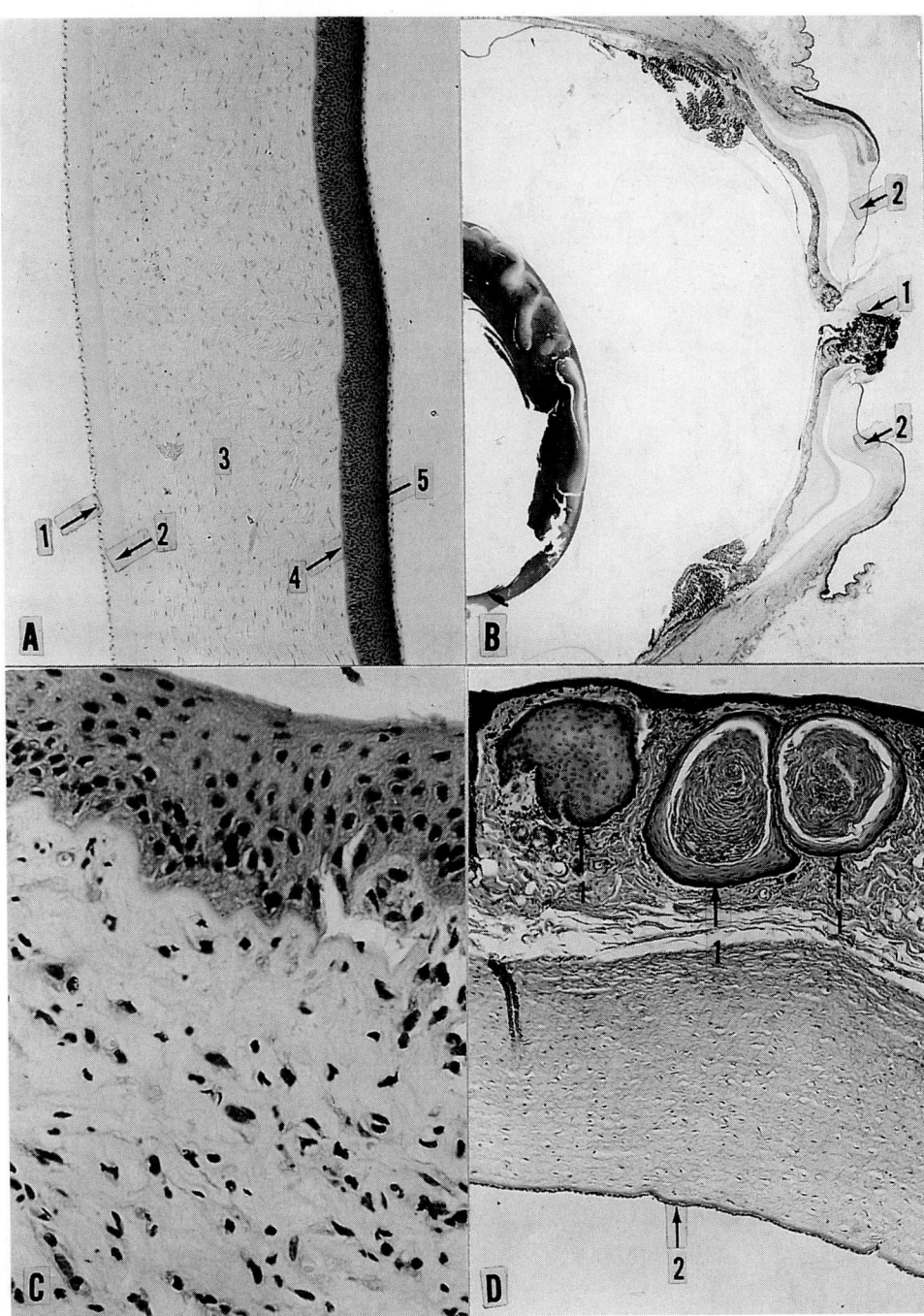

FIG. 28-2 A. Normal equine cornea (×55). (1) Corneal endothelium; (2) Descemet's membrane; (3) Corneal stroma (substantia propria); (4) Bowman's membrane; (5) Corneal epithelium. (Contributor: Army Veterinary Research Laboratory.) **B.** Rupture of the equine cornea following trauma (×2 1/2). (1) The iris has prolapsed; (2) Through the opening in the cornea. (Contributor: Army Veterinary Research Laboratory.) **C.** Keratitis, bovine eye (×330). Note leukocytes in substantia propria of the cornea. (Contributor: Dr. C.L. Davis.) **D.** Corneal dermoid, eye of a lamb (×70). (1) Islands of pigmented epithelium, between the corneal epithelium and stroma; (2) Corneal endothelium. **D,** (Courtesy of Armed Forces Institute of Pathology; contributor: Dr. Robert D. Courter.)

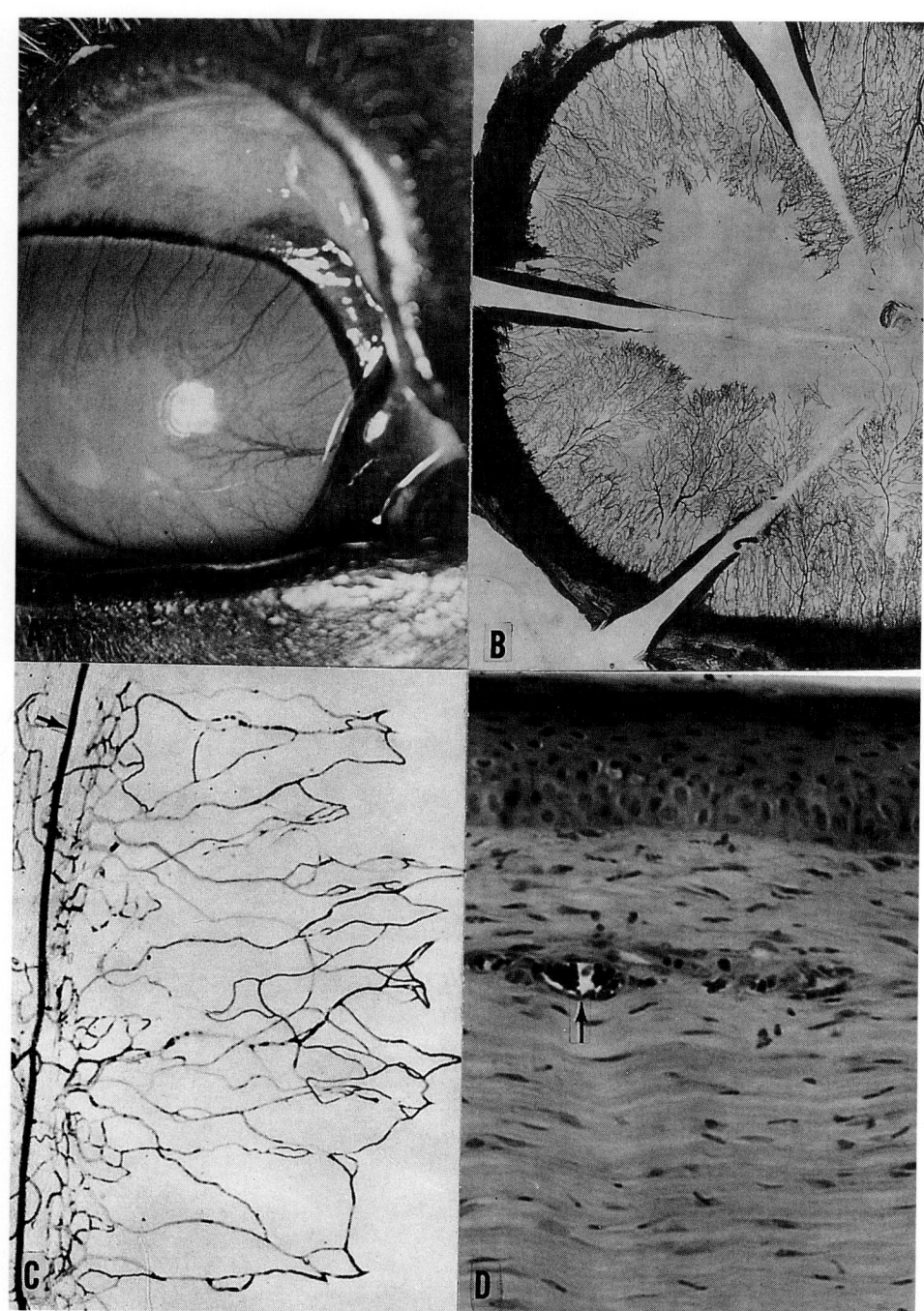

FIG. 28-3 Corneal vascularization. **A.** Eye of a horse during an acute recrudescence of periodic ophthalmia. **B.** Cornea of a horse with periodic ophthalmia. The fixed cornea was mounted flat on a slide. The limbus is black because of its pigment. **C.** Cornea of a rat with riboflavin deficiency (×36). Loops of capillaries extend into the cornea from the vessels at the limbus *(arrow)*. **D.** New blood vessel *(arrow)* in the lamina propria of the cornea of a horse with periodic ophthalmia (×300).

Pannus (pannus degenerativus) Pannus refers to a lesion of the cornea in which vascular granulation tissue extends from the limbus over the cornea. This tissue—often containing leukocytes—is situated between the corneal epithelium and Bowman's membrane, which at times may become duplicated. The granulation tissue may remain as scar tissue and undergo calcification; the overlying corneal epithelium is often disorganized and thickened. This condition is frequently associated with glaucoma. Pannus is especially common in German shepherds. **Anterior corneal dystrophy** is a term applied to specific lesions detected by slit-lamp microscopy as opacities in the anterior cornea of American Dutch belted rabbits. Evidence points toward an inherited anomaly. Microscopic examinations of histologic sections reveal tiny focal lesions involving the loss of epithelial cells overlying irregular thickening of the basement membrane. This entity is important because of its resemblance to a similar one in humans, as well as its possible confusion with induced lesions encountered in the course of studies in toxicologic pathology.

References

Moore CP, Dubielzig R, Glaza SM. Anterior corneal dystrophy of American Dutch Belted rabbits: biomicroscopic and histopathologic findings. Vet Pathol 1987;24:28–33.

Corneal dermoid Corneal dermoid is a congenital lesion observed in newborn animals, and may involve one or both eyes. **Grossly,** the affected cornea appears to be covered over part of its surface with haired, usually pigmented skin. **Microscopically,** the affected part of corneal epithelium is replaced with dermal epithelium having skin adnexa in its underlying stroma. Hair follicles, sebaceous glands, and cysts lined with epithelium and filled with keratin are common. The corneal stroma may be thickened and vascularized but is otherwise unaffected (Fig. 28-2D). Epithelial inclusion cysts may also affect the cornea; they resemble the lesions seen in the skin.

References

Baker JR, Faull WB, Ward WR. Conjunctivitis and keratitis in sheep associated with *Moraxella (Haemophilus)* organisms. Vet Rec 1965;77:402–406.
Hubbert WT, Hermann GJ. A winter epizootic of infectious bovine keratoconjunctivitis. J Am Vet Med Assoc 1970;157:452–454.
Hughes DE, Pugh GW Jr. A five year study of infectious bovine keratoconjunctivitis in a beef herd. J Am Vet Med Assoc 1970;157:443–451.
Hughes DE, Pugh GW Jr, McDonald TJ. Ultraviolet radiation and *Moraxella bovis* in the etiology of bovine infectious keratoconjunctivitis. Am J Vet Res 1965;26:1331–1338.
Hughes DE, Pugh GW Jr, McDonald TJ. Experimental bovine infectious keratoconjunctivitis caused by sunlamp irradiation and *Moraxella bovis* infection: determination of optimal irradiation. Am J Vet Res 1968;29:821–827.
Hughes DE, Pugh GW Jr, McDonald TJ. Experimental bovine infectious keratoconjunctivitis caused by sunlamp irradiation and *Moraxella bovis* infection: resistance to reexposure with homologous and heterologous *Moraxella bovis*. Am J Vet Res 1968;29:829–833.
Hughes DE, Pugh GW Jr. Isolation and description of a *Moraxella* from horses with conjunctivitis. Am J Vet Res 1970;31:457–462.
Monlux AW, Anderson WA, Davis CL. The diagnosis of squamous cell carcinoma of the eye (cancer eye) in cattle. Am J Vet Res 1957;18:5–34.
Moreno G, et al. Infectious keratoconjunctivitis of cattle caused by *Neisseria [Neisseria ovis n. sp.* Lindqvist 1960]. Arqs Irst Biol (Sao Paulo) 1968;35:173–179, Vet Bull 1969;39:2363.
Nichols CW, Yanoff M. Dermoid of a rat cornea. Pathol Vet 1969;6:214–216.
Pugh GW Jr, Hughes DE. Infectious bovine keratoconjunctivitis induced by different experimental methods. Cornell Vet 1971;67:23–45.
Pugh GW Jr, Hughes DE. Bovine infectious keratoconjunctivitis: *Moraxella bovis* as the sole etiologic agent in a winter epizootic. J Am Vet Med Assoc 1972;167:481–486.
Pugh GW Jr, Hughes DE, Packer RA. Bovine infectious keratoconjunctivitis: interactions of *Moraxella bovis* and infectious bovine rhinotracheitis virus. Am J Vet Res 1970;31:653–662.
Pugh GW Jr, Hughes DE, Schulz VD. Infectious bovine keratoconjunctivitis: experimental induction of infection in calves with Mycoplasmas and *Moraxella bovis*. Am J Vet Res 1976;37:493–495.
Wilcox GE. Infectious bovine kerato-conjunctivitis: a review. Vet Bull 1968;38:349–360.
Wilcox GE. Isolation of adenoviruses from cattle with conjunctivitis and keratoconjunctivitis. Aust Vet J 1969;45:265–270.

Iris and ciliary apparatus

Each species has its own peculiar pupillary outline. The contracted pupil of cats is vertically slit-shaped; in horses this slit is horizontal. In both these species the dilated pupil is smoothly circular. In horses, along the dorsal margins of the pupil the iris bears one or more black nodules that may attain a diameter of nearly a centimeter. These structures, the **corpora nigra** or **granula iridis,** are made up of pigmented cells from the epithelium of the iris and have been mistaken for neoplasms. Similar but smaller structures occur in the bovine eye. The amount and distribution of pigment in the iris are highly variable among different species, as well as among individuals. True albinos do not have any pigment in the iris.

Iridal heterochromia and albinism are occasionally seen in cattle, dogs, and cats. In Hereford cattle, it has been associated with incomplete albinism and coloboma (Gelatt et al., 1969).

The iris and ciliary apparatus (**ciliary body** and **ciliary processes**) are intimately associated in structure and function and are frequently involved simultaneously in disease; thus, it is pertinent to consider these structures together. The anterior segment of the vascular tunic, the **uvea,** is formed by the iris and ciliary apparatus; hence, **anterior uvea** is often used as a collective term for these structures. The posterior segment of the uvea consists of the choroid.

PERSISTENT PUPILLARY MEMBRANE
Failure of the pupillary membrane to degenerate results in an absence of the pupil or strands of tissue bridging the pupil. It is seen most often in dogs, cats, cattle, and horses. In the Basenji dog, it may be inherited and associated with other anomalies (Roberts and Bistner, 1968). Remnants may adhere to the lens, causing what have been called capsular cataracts. Persistent pupillary membrane leads to glaucoma.

SYNECHIA
Anterior synechia is the term used to designate adhesion between the anterior surface of the iris and the posterior corneal surface (i.e., the corneal endothelium). This lesion may profoundly affect the movement of the iris; when the iris is completely adherent all around the perimeter of the cornea (peripheral anterior synechia), an increase in intraocular pressure will be the sequel of occlusion of the filtration angle (refer to section on *glaucoma*). Anterior synechia will result from iritis when the anterior chamber is collapsed, or in other situations in which the inflamed iris is forced forward to lie in contact with the posterior corneal surface. In some instances, the causative factors are obscure.

Posterior synechia (Fig. 28-4) refers to adhesion between the posterior surface of the iris and the anterior lens capsule. This is an even more frequent sequel of iritis than anterior synechia, because the iris normally contacts the anterior lens capsule, at least when the pupil is partially or completely closed; thus, the iris has a greater opportunity to adhere. Tenacious posterior synechiae may cause permanent closure of the pupil; or, when adhesions are forcibly torn loose by contraction of the iris, bits of iris pigment may be left clinging to the lens and cause the pupil to appear torn or ragged. Posterior synechia firmly fixed to the lens around the margin of the pupil ("ring synechia") and closing the pupillary orifice block the flow of aqueous from the

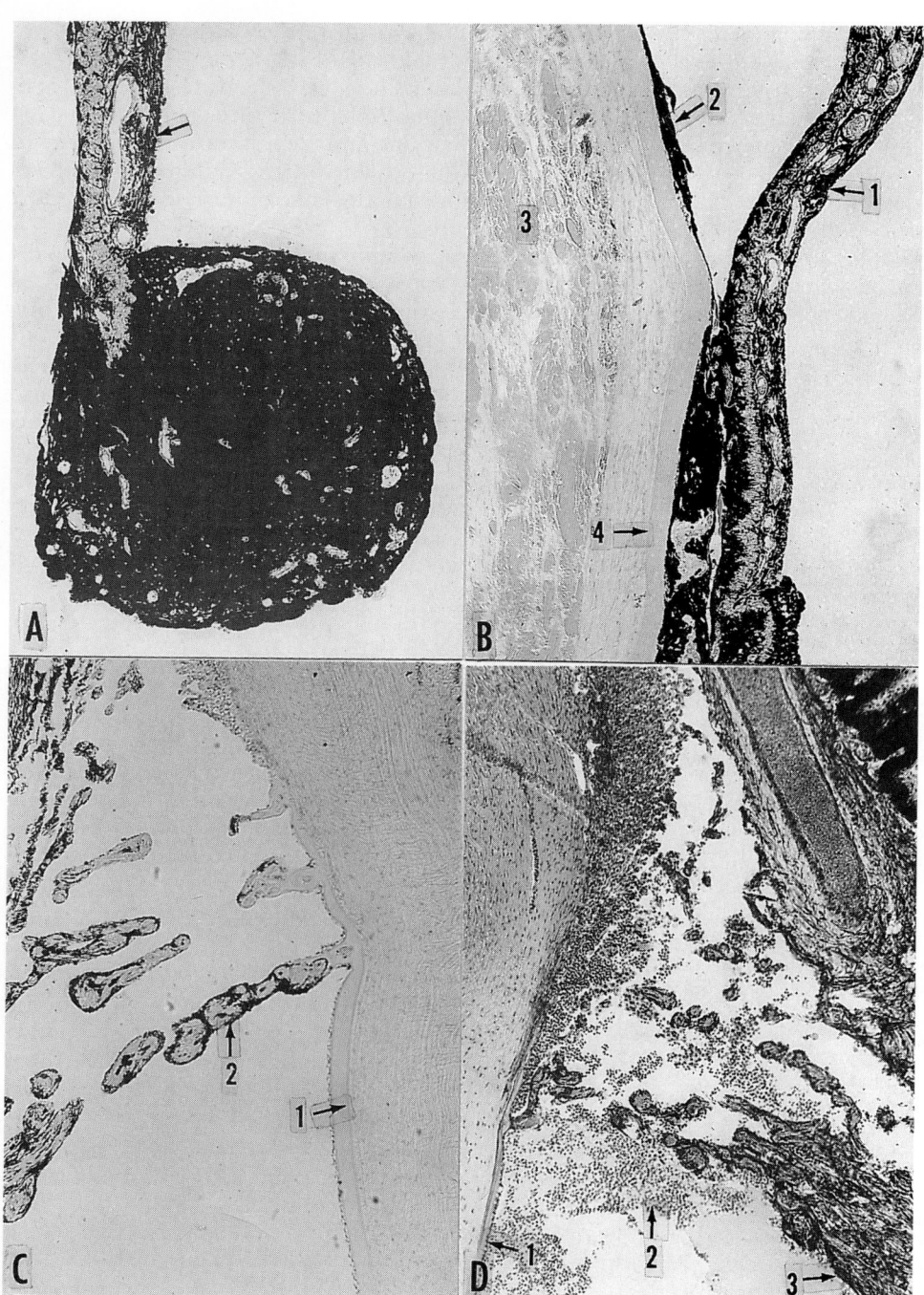

FIG. 28-4 A. Normal iris of the horse (×35) with the large corpora nigra on the dorsal pupillary margin. **B.** Posterior synechia, a sequel of periodic ophthalmia in the horse. (1) The iris is torn away from the lens; (2) Leaves pigment upon it at one point; (3) The cortical lens fibers are disorganized (cataract); (4) The anterior lens capsule is firmly adherent to the iris in one zone. **C.** Normal filtration angle, eye of a horse (×55). (1) Descemet's membrane; and (2) Pectinate ligament may be used as landmarks. **D.** The filtration angle in acute equine periodic ophthalmia (×55). (1) Descemet's membrane; (2) Leukocytes and plasma in anterior chamber; (3) Root of the iris. (**D,** Courtesy of Armed Forces Institute of Pathology; contributor: Army Veterinary Research Laboratory.)

posterior chamber. As a result, aqueous fluid accumulates behind the iris, causing it to bulge forward (**iris bombé**).

Grossly, posterior synechia may be indicated by failure of the pupil to dilate with mydriatics; or, if it does dilate, by the ragged pupil or by iris pigment clinging to the anterior lens capsule. **Microscopically,** the iris is adherent to the lens and some fibrinous or, less often, leukocytic exudate is seen in the zone of adhesion. Usually the anterior lens capsule in this area is thickened, or bits of iris pigment may be tightly fixed to its surface.

IRIDOCYCLITIS

Inflammation of the iris and ciliary apparatus (**anterior uveitis**) is not unusual in animals and may have numerous causes, not all of which are known. The classic example of iridocyclitis in animals is found in recurrent iridocyclitis or periodic ophthalmia of Equidae. The following description of this disease covers all the manifestations of iridocyclitis in any species and from any cause.

Uveitis Inflammation of the iris and ciliary body is termed **anterior uveitis,** and inflammation of the ciliary body and choroid is **posterior uveitis. Chorioretinitis** is inflammation of the choroid and underlying retina. **En-**

dophthalmitis—inflammation of most of the internal portion of the eye—when spread throughout the internal and external structures is termed **panophthalmitis.** The pathologic picture will depend upon the cause, but can take the form of any type of inflammation, from purulent to granulomatous. Causes include many different infectious agents, including bacteria (staphylococci, coliforms), protozoa (toxoplasma), fungi (blastomycosis, histoplasmosis), and viruses (infectious canine hepatitis). Although the pathogenesis is not clear, equine periodic ophthalmia is one of the best-known examples of uveitis in domestic animals.

Equine periodic ophthalmia (recurrent iridocyclitis, **recurrent uveitis)** A specific disease of Equidae, periodic ophthalmia is the most common cause of blindness in horses and mules. Its characteristics include the sudden onset in one or both eyes of severe acute iridocyclitis, which gradually abates in a week or more to become quiescent for a period varying from a few days to many months. Acute exacerbations then follow at irregular intervals, each attack augmenting the damage to the eye. Repeated episodes of acute iridocyclitis usually end in complete loss of vision in the affected eye (Fig. 28-5).

CLINICAL SIGNS Significant clinical signs in the acute stage of the disease include: a tightly contracted pupil (miosis) that fails to dilate in darkness and only

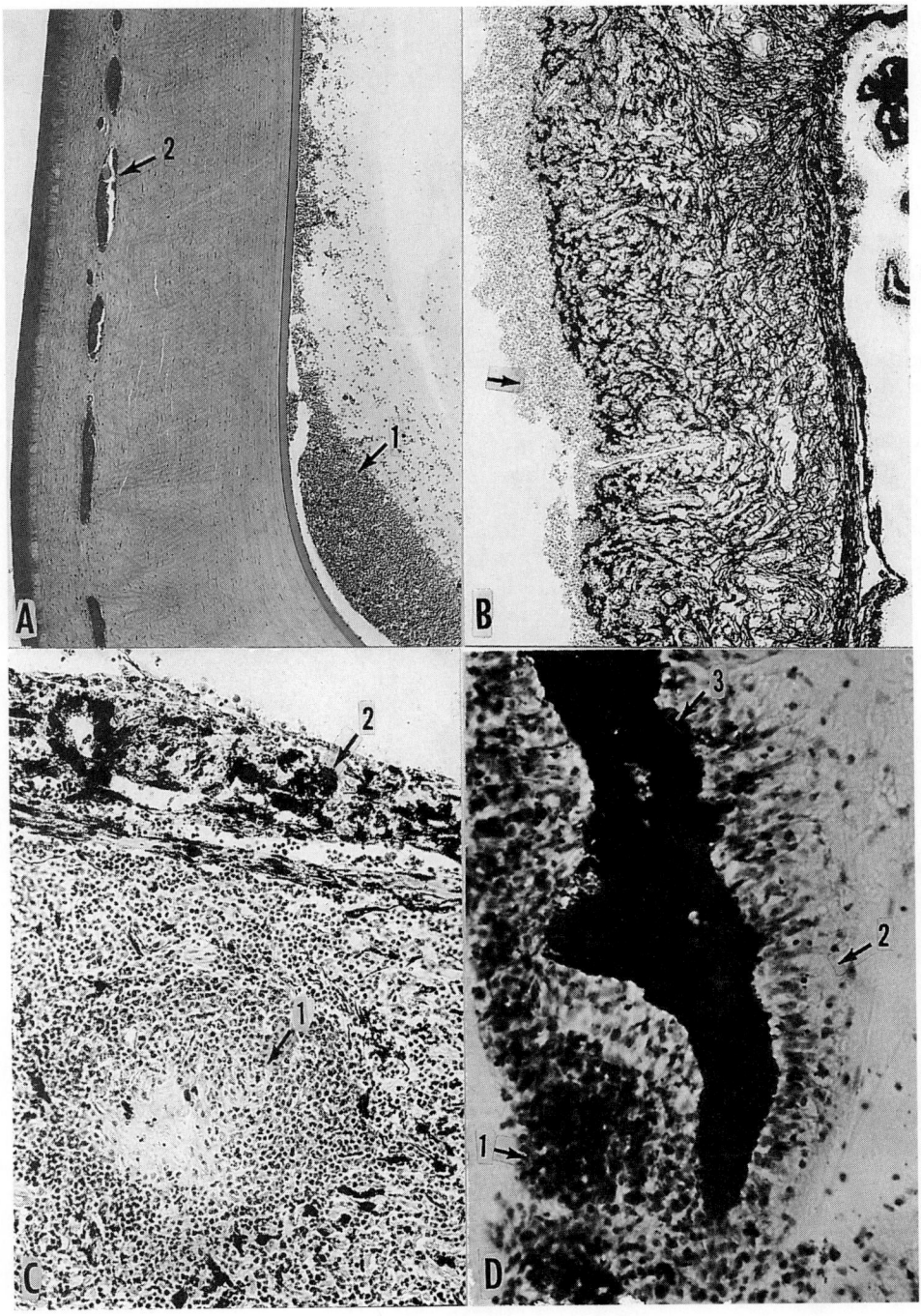

FIG. 28-5 Equine periodic ophthalmia (recurrent iridocyclitis). **A.** The acute stage. (1) Leukocytes in anterior chamber; (2) Corneal vascularization (×45). **B.** Leukocytes in anterior chamber *(arrow)* and iris in the acute stage (×50). **C.** The iris in the acute stage (×150). (1) Circumscribed; and (2) Diffuse collections of leukocytes in the iris. **D.** Ciliary process in the acute stage (×240). (1) Collections of leukocytes; (2) Disorganized ciliary epithelium; and (3) Pigment. (Courtesy of Armed Forces Institute of Pathology; contributor: Army Veterinary Research Laboratory.)

slowly after instillation of mydriatics; an iris that is yellowish instead of the normal brown; filling of the anterior chamber with finely particulate opacities (leukocytes) that usually settle to the ventral half of the chamber; and severe congestion of the sclera and conjunctiva, with tiny capillaries entering the cornea from the limbus (corneal vascularization). This is particularly evident (Fig. 28-3) in acute exacerbations. Photophobia is severe, lacrimation excessive, and intraocular tension diminished.

Acute signs abate quickly, usually within about one week, leaving the disease in a quiescent stage which, however, can be identified by the careful observer. Evidences of the disease during this period are posterior synechiae—indicated by iris pigment clinging to the anterior lens capsule—and tiny opacities in the vitreous humor on ophthalmoscopic examination. The fluorescein test performed at this time reveals increased intraocular vascular permeability.

Repeated acute attacks result in posterior synechiae, subcapsular and diffuse cataracts, extensive corneal vascularization, opacities in the vitreous, detached retina, and decrease in the size of the globe (**phthisis bulbi**).

The etiology of periodic ophthalmia has been a matter of speculation since the fourth century A.D., when the disease was first described by Vegetius. Ancients ascribed the periodic recrudescences of the disease to the lunar cycle; hence, the term "moon blindness."

Studies performed over the years have produced some reliable data relative to the etiology, but many facets remain to be elucidated. Evidence has been obtained to show that affected horses frequently have a high serum titer of agglutinin-lysis antibodies to *Leptospira pomona*.

Experimental infection with *Leptospira pomona* in several studies in horses has been followed by uveitis in 12–24 months. The evidence that *Leptospira* are involved in equine periodic ophthalmia is convincing, although the mechanisms involved are not clearly established.

Infection with microfilaria of *Onchocerca cervicalis* is an event in as many as 60% of horses examined in surveys; it may be incidentally present in animals with equine periodic uveitis, but does not appear to be causal in this disease.

LESIONS Microscopic lesions can be readily correlated with the gross changes, most of which can be seen in the living animal. During the acute stage, the changes are referable largely to the anterior uvea. The iris and ciliary body are severely congested and intensely infiltrated with leukocytes, among which neutrophils predominate at first but are soon replaced by lymphocytes. These cells, along with plasma, escape from the iris and ciliary processes into both the anterior and posterior chambers. A few leukocytes may gain access to the vitreous from the ciliary processes. The anterior choroid and sclera are congested and corneal vascularization is a constant feature. These new vessels start as tiny capillary loops extending from the scleral vessels at the limbus into the lamina propria adjacent to the epithelium, but in later stages well-developed vessels may be demonstrable deeper in the lamina propria of the cornea.

Affected eyes in the quiescent stage have characteristic but subtle microscopic lesions, even after only one acute episode. Nodules of lymphocytes in the ciliary body and iris are the most constant finding. It may be possible to detect some collections of lymphocytes and bits of fibrin on the surface of the ciliary processes, iris, or lens capsules. Similar exudates may sometimes be found in the vitreous humor.

Repeated acute attacks of periodic ophthalmia usually leave the eye partially or completely blind (Fig. 28-6). Posterior synechiae commonly interfere seriously with vision, either by occlusion of the pupil or by leav-

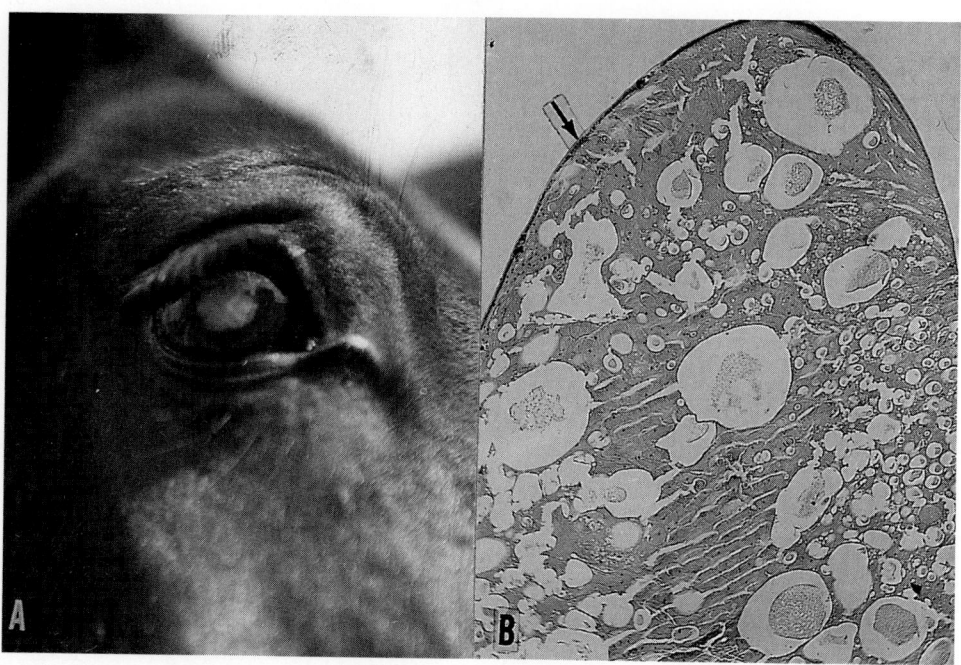

FIG. 28-6 A. Mature cataract in the eye of a horse following several attacks of periodic ophthalmia. **B.** Congenital cataract (×40) in the eye of a newborn puppy. Anterior lens epithelium is indicated by the arrow. Note large vacuoles, disorganization of lens protein and retention of nuclei. (**B,** Courtesy of Armed Forces Institute of Pathology; contributor: Dr. Leo L. Lieberman.)

ing iris pigment and exudates on the anterior lens capsule. Exudates on both the anterior and posterior lens capsule produce capsular opacities that may result in cataracts. Inflammatory changes in the anterior uvea eventually interfere with the nutrition of the lens, which becomes opaque with a fused-quartz appearance. Occasionally, the lens may be luxated. Exudates accumulate in the choroid and retina and eventually cause separation. The pigment layer of the retina usually remains attached to the choroid, while exudate accumulating between it and the layer of rods and cones detaches the retina and forces it into the vitreous. Often, the atrophic retina comes in contact with the posterior lens capsule, but it remains attached at the optic papilla and the ora ciliaris retinae. The entire globe becomes smaller in size (phthisis bulbi) and the sclera thickens. Secondary degeneration may occur in the optic nerve as a consequence of destruction of the neurons in the retina.

Vogt-koyanagi-harada syndrome Vogt-Koyanagi-Harada syndrome is a rare disease in humans, believed to be of autoimmune pathogenesis; it is characterized by uveitis, dermatologic findings (poliosis, vitiligo), and meningoencephalitis. What is believed to be a comparable syndrome has been described in Akita-Inu, Siberian husky, and Samoyed breeds of dogs, although the canine syndrome does not include meningoencephalitis. Granulomatous panuveitis is manifest, particularly of the pigmented uvea, and leads to retinal detachment. Dermal changes consist of depigmentation, crusting, and ulceration associated with a histiocytic and neutrophilic dermatitis.

Lymphocytic uveitis of unknown cause is not infrequent in dogs and cats.

References

Bryans JT. Studies on equine leptospirosis. Cornell Vet 1955;45:16–50.

Heuser H, et al. Die periodische Augenentzundung der Pfrede als Leptospirenerkrankung. Schweiz Med Woschenschr 1948; 78:756–758.

Jones TC. Equine periodic ophthalmia. Am J Vet Res 1942;3:45–71.

Lloyd S, Soulsby EJL. Survey for infection with *Onchocerca cervicalis* in horses in eastern United States. Am J Vet Res 1978;39:1962–1963.

Reusch C, Chang L, Minkus G. Vogt-Koyanagi-Harada Syndrom bei einem Akita-Inu: ein Fallbericht. [Vogt-Koyanagi-Harada syndrome in an Akita-Inu dog: a case report.] Tierarztl Prax 1994;22:398–400.

Ripau W. Leptospira beim Pferde. Tierarztl Umsch 1947;2:177–178.

Trebini F, Appiotti A, Daniele D, et al. Vogt-Koyanagi-Harada syndrome: clinical and instrumental contribution. Ital J Neurol Sci 1991;12:479–484.

Yager RH, Gochenour WS, Wetmore PW. Recurrent iridocyclitis (periodic ophthalmia) of horses. I. Agglutination and lysis of leptospira by serum deriving from horses affected with recurrent iridocyclitis. J Am Vet Med Assoc 1950;117:207–209.

Ectropion uveae A specialized term of ophthalmic pathology, ectropion uveae applies to the extension of the pigmented layer of epithelium from the posterior surface of the iris, around the margin of the pupil, to the anterior surface of the lens. This results from scarring of the iris with eversion of the pupillary margin by contraction of the scars. It is seen following iritis, in glaucoma, and occasionally as a congenital anomaly.

Contraction of the iris—which inverts the pupillary margin—is known as **entropion uveae.**

Neoplasms Primary neoplasms of the iris and ciliary apparatus are seldom recorded, although their incidence is probably higher than published reports indicate. Malignant melanomas may arise from the iris or ciliary body, and hemangiomas have been observed in the iris. Adenomatous new growths (adenomas of ciliary epithelium) apparently arise from the nonpigmented ciliary epithelium; they sometimes displace most of the internal structures of the eyeball. Metastatic neoplasms may occur in the anterior uvea but are rare, with the exception of malignant lymphoma. Ocular neoplasms are discussed more fully later in this chapter.

References

Saunders LZ, Barron CN. Primary pigmented intraocular tumors in animals. Cancer Res 1958;18:234–245.

Vitreous

The vitreous body is that part of the transparent media that occupies the largest chamber of the eye. It may become distorted by luxation of the lens, persistence of the hyaloid artery, or detachment of the retina. As a result of iridocyclitis or retinitis, cells, pigment, and tissue debris may become suspended in the vitreous as opacities. During embryologic development of the lens, the primary vitreous is well-vascularized. This vasculature and the hyaloid artery eventually atrophy under normal circumstances, but may rarely persist, leaving the artery—which terminates in a mass of fibrous, vascular tissue—on the posterior capsule of the lens. Congenital cataract may accompany this anomaly.

References

Grimes TD, Mullaney J. Persistent hyperplastic primary vitreous in a Greyhound. Vet Rec 1969;85:607–611.

Rebhun WC. Persistent hyperplastic primary vitreous in a dog. J Am Vet Med Assoc 1976;169:620–622.

Lens

The adult lens is composed entirely of epithelium, without stroma or vasculature. It receives nourishment from the aqueous humor in which it is bathed. Its simple composition and structure sharply limit the range of morphologic changes that it can experience, regardless of the type of injury to which it may be subjected. It is surrounded by a tough capsule within which is found the growing layer of epithelium (at the poles and on the anterior surface), whose inner layer of cells mature to become the lens fibers. These fibers are laid down in a concentric manner, the oldest being at the center, or nucleus, of the lens.

The morphologic changes that the lens itself can exhibit are limited to (1) abnormal growth changes in the epithelium, (2) deterioration of the lens protein with coagulation and disorganization of the lens fibers, and (3) rupture of the capsule, which exposes the lens substance to external forces that may lead to liquefaction, organization, or dissolution. The lens may be dislocated from its normal position (refer below to *luxation*); however, if still in contact with normal aqueous humor, it may not be significantly altered.

The lens may be damaged by exposure to various toxic substances (naphthalein, ergot) or by nutritive or metabolic disturbances, especially in young animals (riboflavin deficiency, diabetes mellitus). The precise mode of action of substances harmful to the lens is not always clear, although it seems likely that changes in the aqueous probably precede any effect upon the lens.

LUXATION

The lens is held in place by its ligaments, which are attached to the ciliary body. A severe blow to the eyeball, or a less severe one following damage to the suspensory ligaments, may dislocate the lens from its normal position. The luxated lens may be displaced into the anterior chamber, into the ventral part of the posterior chamber, or into the vitreous (Fig. 28-7). The pathologist is sometimes faced with the problem of deciding whether a displaced lens in a specimen is actually luxated, or is an artifact in sectioning the eye. This can usually be determined with certainty by careful gross and microscopic study to determine the status of the ocular tissue adjacent to the lens in its new site. Exudates around the lens, particularly if organized, are indications of luxation.

The luxated lens may be resorbed (**phacolysis**) if its capsule is ruptured, it may remain intact in its new site, or it may become opaque and partially surrounded by leukocytic and fibrinous exudates, which may become organized.

CATARACT

A cataract is an opacity of the lens due to disruption of the lamellar structure of lens fibers. They may be classified on the basis of its morphologic appearance, its etiology, or both. Opacities on the anterior or posterior lens capsule—usually resulting from iridocyclitis—may interfere with transparency of the lens, but are not considered cataracts, nor are they believed to lead, per se, to cataracts.

The principal locations of cataracts include (1) the subcapsular epithelium, (2) the cortex, and (3) the nucleus of the lens. **Subcapsular cataracts** occurring under the anterior capsule (**anterior polar cataract**) are the result of abnormal proliferation of the lens epithelium at this site, often resulting from traumatic injury to the lens capsule. Epithelial cells become redundant, disorganized, or laminated to form an opacity. This lesion may follow prolonged injury to the anterior segment of the lens as the result of a persistent posterior synechia. **Posterior polar cataract,** located under the capsule at the posterior face of the lens, also results from abnormal growth of lens epithelium. However, absence of epithelium on the posterior surface in the normal adult eye indicates that epithelial cells must grow into this area from the equator in order to form a cataract. Damage to the lens capsule at this site can also lead to degeneration of lens fibers and cataract formation. Following damage at the anterior or posterior lens, water may enter the lens, further contributing to the opacity (**intumescent cataract**).

Cortical cataracts result from disorganization of the lens fibers, presumably following altered metabolism of the lens epithelium. Lens fibers lose their normal concentrically laminated structure to become disorganized and aggregated into irregularly spherical masses of material (**morgagnian globules**).

Nuclear cataracts are the result of changes in the transparency of the oldest lens fibers (those at the nucleus). These central fibers apparently become more dense and appear gray or (more often) yellowish in the center of the lens. This type appears most often in, but is not limited to, senile animals. The **morgagnian**

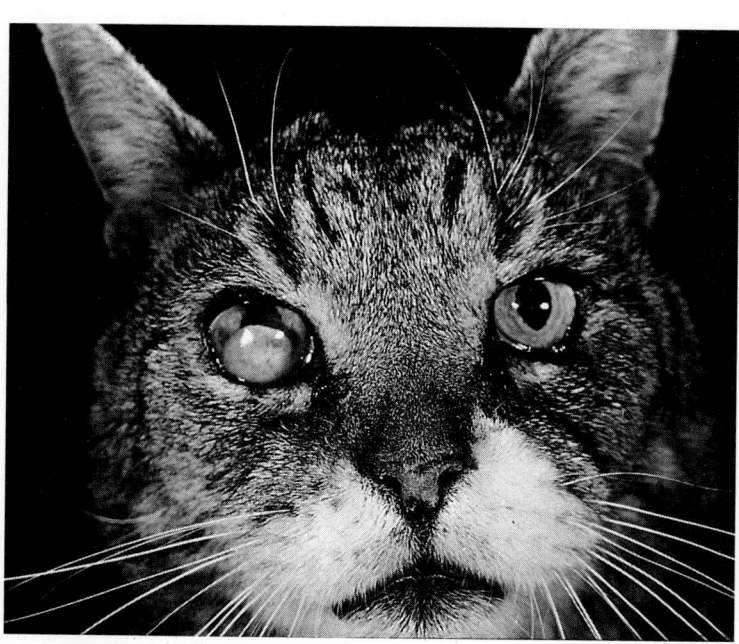

FIG. 28-7 Luxation of the lens into the anterior chamber of a 15-year-old castrated male cat. (Courtesy of Angell Memorial Animal Hospital.)

cataract is characterized by complete liquefaction of cortical substance within which the sclerotic nucleus floats.

Causes Congenital cataracts, observed in most species, are best studied in dogs. The defect is often attributable to failure of closure of the primary lens vesicle; hence, such lesions are most likely to be found near the lens periphery toward the posterior lens surface. Anterior and nuclear congenital cataracts, however, also occur. Genetic factors may be the underlying cause in some congenital cataracts, but other factors may also be important. Many examples of congenital cataracts do, however, represent **hereditary cataracts.** Although most often observed at birth, some hereditary cataracts do not develop until animals are juveniles or adults. The mode of inheritance is not clear in many examples; however, an autosomal-dominant trait exists in Labrador retrievers and beagles. An autosomal-recessive trait is responsible in the miniature schnauzer, standard poodle, afghan hound, cocker spaniel, Old English sheepdog, Holstein-Friesian and Jersey cattle, and certain strains of rats and mice. Congenital cataracts are seen in cats affected with the Chediak-Higashi syndrome, but the relationship between the two is unclear because cataracts are not associated with this disease in cattle, mink, or mice.

Viral infection *in utero* or early in life has been associated with cataracts in several species (rubella in humans, *Herpesvirus canis* in dogs).

Traumatic injury to the lens resulting from a severe blow to the head, penetrating wounds to the eye, or iridocyclitis may lead to cataracts, usually beginning as subcapsular cataracts.

Metabolic disorders, most notably **diabetes mellitus,** may lead to cataracts. These are bilateral and begin with vacuolation of the lens at the equator.

Toxicity Cataracts can also be induced by a variety of experimental manipulations or exposure to certain drugs. Disophenol, an anthelmintic, has been shown to cause cataracts in dogs, as has dimethyl sulfoxide. The association of dinitrophenols and cataracts was first made in the 1930s in humans when these drugs were used in weight control. Oxygen toxicity may lead to cataracts in mice and a variety of other ocular disorders in other species.

CONGENITAL ANOMALIES

Aphakia (absence of the lens) and **microphakia** (small lens) are rare congenital anomalies of the lens, usually associated with other ocular defects. Globular or cone-like protrusion of the posterior lens surface is a congenital defect of the lens known as posterior **lenticonus** and has been reported in dogs, calves, swine, mice, rabbits, and humans. It is often associated with cataract within the protrusion or other areas of the lens. The lesion is believed to result from an overgrowth of lens fibers.

In dogs, anterior capsular cataracts in the center of the lens may result from remnants of the pupillary membrane.

References

Aguirre G, Bistner SI. Posterior lenticonus in the dog. Cornell Vet 1973;63:455–461.
Beech J, Aguirre G, Gross S. Congenital nuclear cataracts in the Morgan horse. J Am Vet Med Assoc 1984;184:1363–1365.
Gelatt KN. Veterinary ophthalmology. 2nd ed. Philadelphia: Lea & Febiger, 1991;429–460.
Gelatt KN, et al. Biometry and clinical characteristics of congenital cataracts and microphthalmia in the Miniature schnauzer. J Am Vet Med Assoc 1983;183:99–102.
Hirth RS, Greenstein ET, Peer RL. Anterior capsular opacities (spurious cataracts) in beagle dogs. Vet Pathol 1974;11:181–194.
Peiffer RL, Gelatt KN. Cataracts in the cat. Feline Pract 1974;4:34–38.
Piatigorsky J. Lens crystallins and their genes: diversity and tissue-specific expression. FASEB J 1989;3:1933–1940.
Rubin LF. Cataract in golden retrievers. J Am Vet Med Assoc 1974;165:457–458.
Rubin LF, Flowers RD. Inherited cataract in a family of Standard poodles. J Am Vet Med Assoc 1972;161:207–208.
Rubin LF, Koch SA, Huber RJ. Hereditary cataracts in Miniature schnauzers. J Am Vet Med Assoc 1969;154:1456–1458.
van Heyningen R. Galactose cataract: a review. Exp Eye Res 1971;11:415–428.
Totter JR, Day PL. Cataract and other ocular changes resulting from tryptophane deficiency. J Nutr 1942;24:159–166.
Warkany J, Schraffenberger E. Congenital malformations of the eyes induced in rats by maternal vitamin A deficiency. Proc Soc Exp Biol Med 1944;57:49–52.

Retina

The retina is the light-sensitive inner coat that lines the posterior segment of the eyeball. Its inner surface is in contact with the vitreous and its outer surface with the choroid. The retina terminates anteriorly near the ciliary body to form a border which, though serrated in humans (**ora serrata**), is usually smooth in most animals (**ora ciliaris retinae**). The retina is firmly attached at this anterior border, as well as around the margin of the optic disc; however, it is more likely to be separated from its pigment epithelium, which coheres closely to the adjacent choroid.

In many animals, a specific laminated structure, the **tapetum,** lies between the retina and choroid; in some species, it is partially pigmented and termed the **tapetum nigrum;** when unpigmented, it is the **tapetum lucidum.** In horses, for example, a horizontal line in the globe just below the level of the optic disc separates the greenish iridescent tapetum lucidum above from the dark-brown, nearly black, tapetum nigrum below. In some species (such as dogs), the tapetum can be detected microscopically or with the ophthalmoscope; the overlying regions of the retina are designated as "tapetal" or "nontapetal." These two areas of the retina sometimes respond differently in disease.

The retinal vessels of each species have distinctive anatomical features that must be understood in order to interpret deviations from normal. In Equidae, for instance, the arteries and veins cannot be distinguished from one another with the ophthalmoscope; they emerge from the margins of the optic disc in a uniform radial manner which gives the disc the appearance of a conventionalized rising sun. In dogs and cats—as in many other species—veins and arteries are readily differentiated as they emerge from the center of the optic disc and follow a tortuous, branching course into the retina. The embryonic hyaloid artery, which extends from the optic disc to the posterior lens capsule, may still be present at birth in vestigial form. This persistence of the hyaloid may be normal in some species (dogs, oxen) and abnormal in others.

The retina may be considered as having two components, the pigment epithelium (which develops from the outer layer of the embryonic cup) and the sensory retina (which develops from the inner layer of the optic cup). The sensory retina has a complex structure consisting of nine layers which, from the innermost toward the outermost, include:

(1) The inner limiting membrane;
(2) Layer of optic nerve fibers;
(3) Layer of ganglion cells;
(4) Inner plexiform layer;
(5) Inner nuclear layer;
(6) Outer plexiform layer;
(7) Outer nuclear layer;
(8) Outer limiting membrane; and,
(9) Layer of rods and cones (photoreceptor layer with inner and outer segments).

These layers vary in thickness in different regions in the retina and among species, but further consideration of these differences lies outside the scope of this book. It is important to recall that the layer of optic nerve fibers contains the axons of the neurons of the layer of ganglion cells (Fig. 28-7); these axons assemble at the optic papilla and continue as the fibers within the optic nerve. Thus, it is apparent that lesions in the layer of ganglion cells or of nerve fibers could easily result in changes in the optic nerve.

The blood supply of the retina comes from two sources: (1) the choriocapillaris, which nourishes the pigment epithelium, the layer of rods and cones, and the outer nuclear layer; and (2) the retinal artery, which emerges within or adjacent to the optic papilla and continues in the retina within the nerve-fiber layer, dividing dichotomously as it spreads out toward the ora ciliaris retinae. Capillaries from this arterial system anastomose only with each other and join only the retinal venous system. The retinal artery supplies the inner layers of the retina (nerve fiber, ganglion cell, inner plexiform, and inner nuclear layers).

The retinal artery extends from the papilla into the retina toward the ora ciliaris retinae during embryonic life. In human fetuses, these vessels start growing from the papilla during the fourth month and reach the ora serrata during the eighth month *in utero*. In some animals (dogs, cats, rats), this development is slower; newborn kittens, puppies, or four-day-old rats have retinal vessels that reach about halfway to the ora ciliaris retinae, a stage of development reached by human fetuses during the seventh month of gestation. This species difference has been used in the experimental reproduction of retrolental fibroplasia or retinopathy of prematurity, by exposing dogs, cats, or rats to excessive oxygen. In an atmosphere increased in oxygen (as in an incubator or oxygen tent), immature retinal vessels of the newborn fail to grow normally. Endothelial cells form nonfunctional nodules resembling glomerular tufts, which lead to retinal detachment, retinal edema and hemorrhages, and vitreous disorganization (features that closely simulate the lesions of retrolental fibroplasia of infants).

The retina is commonly involved in severe cases of iritis, iridocyclitis, and choroiditis; in fact, the retina is so intimately related to the choroid that inflammation of one usually involves the other. **Chorioretinitis** is therefore not an uncommon pathologic finding. Exudates that accumulate in the retina as a consequence of inflammation—especially in recurrent iridocyclitis—are usually found adjacent to the pigment epithelium. The presence of such exudates results in **detachment of the retina.** The accumulation of edema in the retina may dislodge it from its normal position and, in extreme cases, force it into the vitreous; it may occasionally lie in contact with the posterior lens capsule, where it becomes incorporated in an organized **cyclitic membrane.** The recognition of the presence of exudate is essential in order to differentiate between true retinal detachment and detachment as an artifact produced in preparation of the specimen. In either event, the retina remains attached at the optic papilla and ora ciliaris retinae.

RETINAL DISORDERS

Disorders of the retina (**photoreceptor dysplasias**) are difficult to study and classify in an orderly manner. The plethora of diagnostic terms, often indiscriminately used in the present literature, is clearly one of the problems. Although loss of sight is not difficult to recognize in living animals using clinical signs, and lesions in the retina may be detected by ophthalmoscopy and confirmed by electroretinography, not all etiologic factors have been identified (Fig. 28-8). Causative factors established so far include: genetic factors (single or multiple genes), congenital anomalies (intrauterine effects), infectious diseases (canine distemper, coccidioidomycosis, feline panleukopenia, toxoplasmosis), nutritional deficiencies (vitamin A, taurine), radiation (ionizing, phototoxic light), poisoning (bracken fern), and lysosomal storage diseases (also genetic, but not limited to the retina; Chapter 2). Some examples follow of the effects of these etiologies.

Consideration is given in this text to those hereditary retinal disorders most clearly defined at this time. The clinical aspects of many other retinal lesions have been described; however, in the absence of known etiologic factors, they have been identified simply with the breed. This is useful to distinguish these entities, but is not entirely reliable; for example, the same mutant gene may be operating in each of several purebred breeds. The presence of identical mutant genes at the **prcd** locus in miniature poodles, and American and English cocker spaniels clearly illustrates this point. It is evident that much needs to be learned about the etiology and other features of retinopathies in animals before a rational and useful approach can be taken toward their understanding.

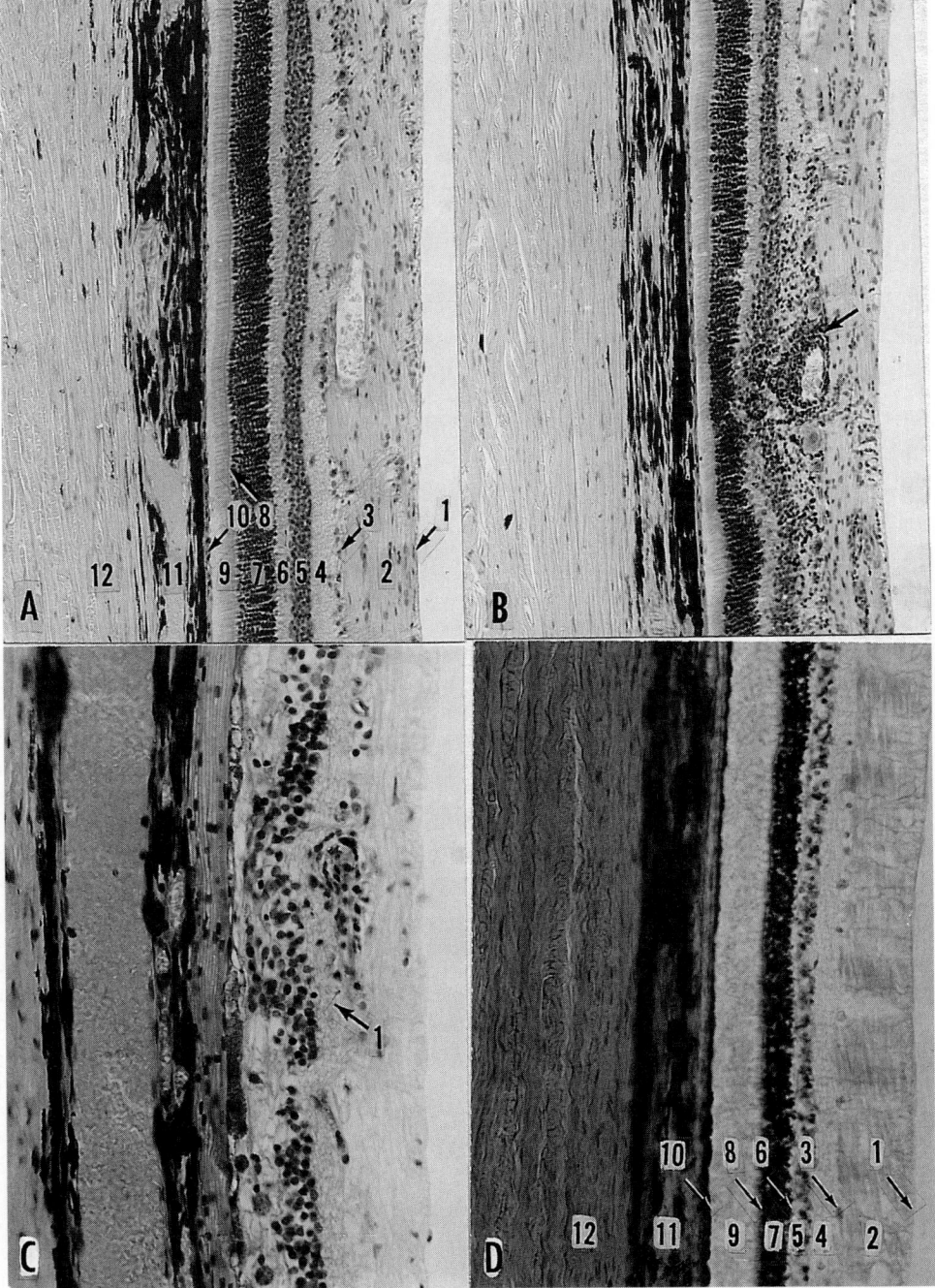

FIG. 28-8. A. Normal canine retina (×130). Section from nontapetal zone. (1) Inner limiting membrane; (2) Layer of optic nerve fibers; (3) Layer of ganglion cells; (4) Inner plexiform layer; (5) Inner nuclear layer; (6) Outer plexiform layer; (7) Outer nuclear layer; (8) Outer limiting membrane; (9) Layer of rods and cones; (10) Pigment epithelium; (11) Choroid; and (12) Sclera. (Contributor: Dr. Claude S. Perry.) **B.** Early retinitis in a dog with toxoplasmosis (×130). Leukocytes around blood vessels *(arrow)*; layers of retina distorted. (Contributor: Dr. Claude S. Perry.) **C.** Retinal atrophy, tapetal zone of retina of a dog. Note atrophy of inner and outer nuclear layers *(arrow)* as well as layer of rods and cones. Note especially swollen cells of pigment epithelium adjacent to the tapetum. **D.** Normal equine retina (×165). Numbers indicate same structures as in **A.** (**A** and **B,** Courtesy of Armed Forces Institute of Pathology.)

Hereditary progressive retinal atrophy in dogs Retinal atrophy (Figs. 28-9 through 28-13), in families of red Irish setters was originally described by Parry. This disease—also called rod-cone dysplasia type 1—has now been shown by mating tests to be initiated by a single autosomal-recessive gene designated as **rcd1.** This gene has been shown to be nonallelic with any of the three other canine genes (**prcd, erd,** or **rcd2**) described in the following text.

By applying certain techniques of molecular biology, Ray et al. demonstrated that a nonsense mutation (guanine to adenine transition at nucleotide position 2420) in the canine cyclic GMP (cGMP) phosphodies-terase beta subunit gene cosegregates with the rod-cone dysplasia 1 disease allele **rcd1** (1994). This mutation only occurs in Irish setters affected with this disease, or in families in which the **rcd1** gene is segregating. It has not been found in dogs carrying or manifesting any other inherited retinal disease. It is now possible to detect and study the mutation in DNA that underlies this disorder.

The underlying biochemical defect is believed to be the result of a cyclic guanosine monophosphate abnormality.

Night-blindness is the first indication of the disease, which may be apparent as early as six weeks of age in

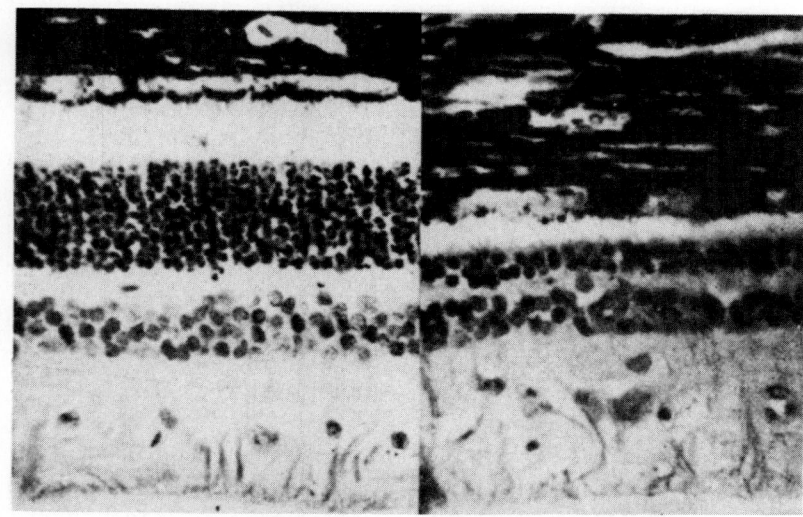

FIG. 28-9 Hereditary progressive retinal atrophy *(rcd1)*. Retina of two 3 1/2-month-old Irish setters, normal on the left (×270). Note reduction in width of outer nuclear and bacillary layers in the affected retina. The rod nuclei are almost completely lost, leaving only cone nuclei. The inner layers are not affected. (Courtesy of Dr. H.B. Parry and *British Journal of Ophthalmology.*)

Irish setters. This progresses to complete blindness over a period of months to years. Lesions are similar in most examples, beginning in the outer layers of the retina with loss of rods, cones, and their nuclei, followed by disappearance of the inner layers. The disease terminates in total sclerosis of the retina, although the ganglion cell layer may be spared. Both the rods and cones in Irish setters are never fully developed.

Three stages of the disease have been recognized and are valuable in studying the lesions. During the first stage—2–9 months in duration—uniform, bilaterally symmetric loss of rods (and their nuclei) occurs, resulting in night-blindness without detectable effect upon day-vision. Although the entire retina is affected, lesions are usually most severe at the periphery. In the second stage—lasting 3–24 months—retinal cones and cone nuclei are lost, causing progressive failure of day-vision. Other layers of the retina remain normal. When the third stage is reached, both day- and night-blindness are complete as a result of the disorganization of all layers of the retina, glial proliferation, and diffuse sclerosis of the retina. The pigment layer of the retina is atrophied and a few pigment-laden cells are dispersed in the sclerotic retina. Accumulations of pigment cells are not seen.

Progressive rod-cone degeneration Progressive rod-cone degeneration in dogs has been studied particularly in miniature poodles, but also occurs with a similar pattern in American and English cocker spaniels (Fig. 28-14). Mating tests involving these three breeds indicate that the same genetic locus (**prcd**) is affected in all three. A single autosomal-recessive gene is evident; matings between affected animals of each of the breeds with the other two result in only affected offspring. One discrepancy has been observed: matings of homozygous (affected) female English cocker spaniels with homozygous (affected) miniature poodle males produce offspring with some phenotypic differences: specifically, the topographic distribution of lesions in the retina, rate of progression of the disease, and ultrastructural variation in the lesions. These phenotypic differences may be ascribed to different genetic backgrounds (effect of modifying genes) in the two breeds, or may result from separate allelic mutations at the same locus.

This retinal disorder has some similarities with human retinitis pigmentosa and has been proposed as a model for the human disease.

Evidence of this disorder may be seen as early as 10 months of age in the form of abnormalities in the electroretinogram. Behavioral signs do not usually appear until ages three to five years, when night-blindness (nyctalopia) may become evident. Signs detected by the

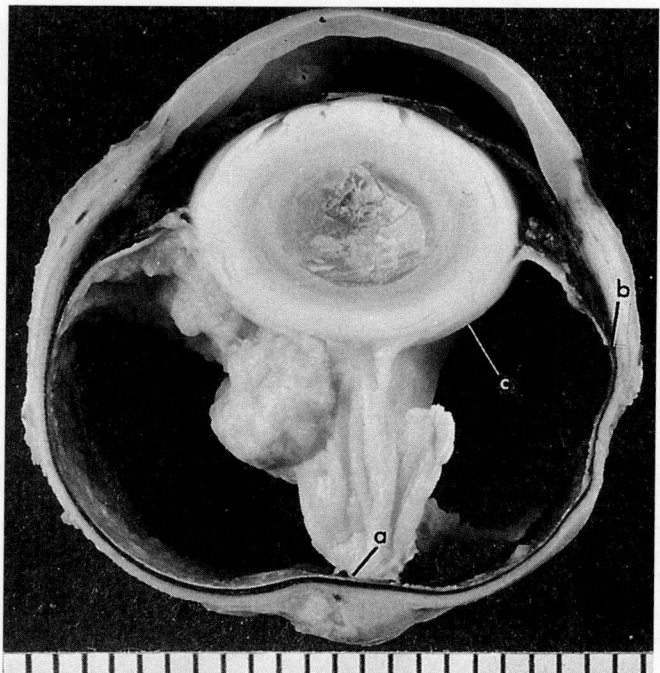

FIG. 28-10 Detachment of the retina, eye of a spayed five-year-old female beagle. Note that the retina remains attached around the margins of the optic disc *(a)* and at the *ora ciliaris retinae (b)*, and is collapsed over the posterior surface of the lens *(c)*. (Courtesy of Angell Memorial Animal Hospital.)

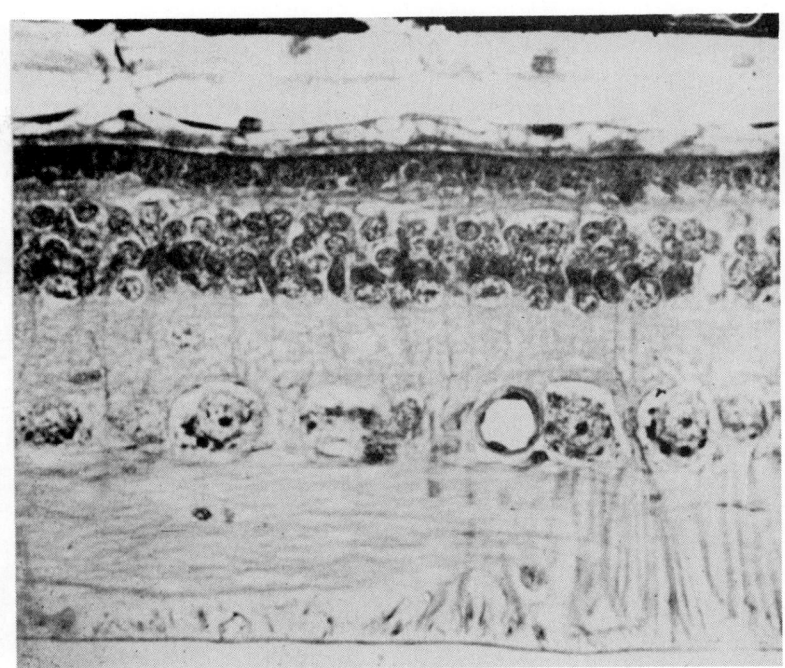

FIG. 28-11 Hereditary progressive retinal atrophy (*rcd1*). Section of retina (×450) of a six-month-old Irish setter with a later stage of atrophy than shown in Figure 28-9. Note complete loss of rod nuclei. Remnants of the cones form a thin layer between the atrophic pigment epithelium and the thickened external limiting membrane. (Courtesy of Dr. H.B. Parry and the *British Journal of Ophthalmology*.)

use of the ophthalmoscope at this stage include alterations in color and increased reflectivity in the tapetal fundus. Loss of retinal pigment may also be detected at this time in the nontapetal fundus, along with mottling of the retina and atrophy of the optic nerve head. Secondary cataracts may be evident in late stages.

Histologic examination of the retina reveals disorganization of the outer segments, with loss of parallel cell borders. Disorganization of the rods is also evident under the electron microscope, with melanin granules and phagosomes present in the pigment epithelium.

Early retinal degeneration Early retinal degeneration—described initially in Norwegian elkhounds—is believed to be caused by an autosomal-recessive gene, **erd**, which is different from the gene loci **prcd, rcd1,** or **rcd2.**

Night-blindness is detectable in affected pups as young as six weeks of age, and blindness is total in 10–18 months. Tapetal hyperreflectivity and attenuation of retinal vessels are seen at about one year of age. In elec-

troretinography, the β-wave is impaired increasingly until only the α-wave response becomes recorded.

At the ultrastructural level, both rod and cone photoreceptors develop abnormally, particularly in relation to the synaptic terminals. Subsequent degeneration of both rods and cones is evident with the light microscope.

Rod dysplasia Rod dysplasia in Norwegian elkhounds is another form of retinal dystrophy in this breed. It has also been termed "photoreceptor abiotrophy" because of the belief that normal photoreceptor development preceded degeneration of photoreceptor cells. Subsequent studies, however, disclosed developmental abnormalities specifically affecting the rod photoreceptors; hence, the term "rod dysplasia." Mating studies confirm the autosomal-recessive mode of inheritance and distinguish this gene locus from that of **rcd1** of Irish setters. Also, the lack of abnormality of cyclic nucleotide metabolism in affected Norwegian elk-

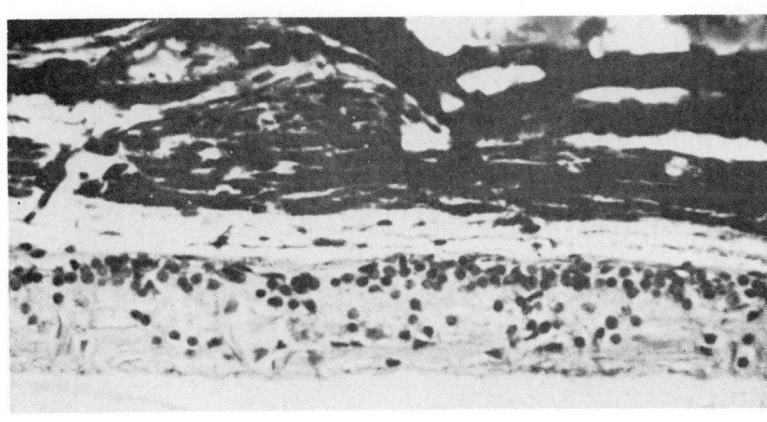

FIG. 28-12 Hereditary progressive retinal atrophy (*rcd1*). Late stage in a six-year-old Irish setter which had been blind for four years (×240). The retina is completely disorganized, most nuclei have disappeared, and the pigment epithelium is missing. The remains of the atrophic retina are in direct contact with the tapetum. (Courtesy of Dr. H.B. Parry and the *British Journal of Ophthalmology*.)

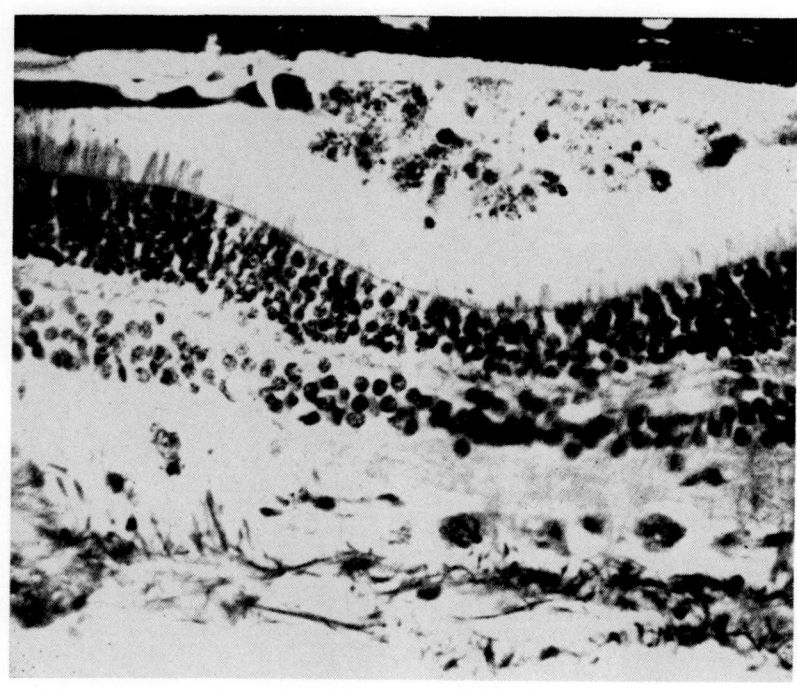

FIG. 28-13 Progressive central retinal atrophy with pigment epithelial dystrophy. Retina of a two-year-old Red Irish setter, (×330). Section from midtapetal fundus near papilla. Note hypertrophied pigment epithelium, which displaces the adjacent layer of rods and cones. Gliosis is apparent in the nerve fiber layer and atrophy in ganglion cells. (Courtesy of Dr. H.B. Parry and *British Journal of Ophthalmology.*)

hounds distinguishes it further from rod-cone dysplasia in Irish setters.

Rod-cone dysplasia type 2 Rod-cone dysplasia type 2 is an inherited retinopathy described in dogs of the Collie breed. The involved gene (**rcd2**) is single, recessively expressed and not allelic, with **rcd1** in Irish setters or **erd** in Norwegian elkhounds, as indicated by mating tests. Night-blindness (**nyctalopia**) is evident in affected Collie puppies by six weeks of age and progresses to near blindness within one year. Signs seen with the ophthalmoscope include tapetal hyperreflectivity, attenuation of retinal vessels, and pallor of the optic disc.

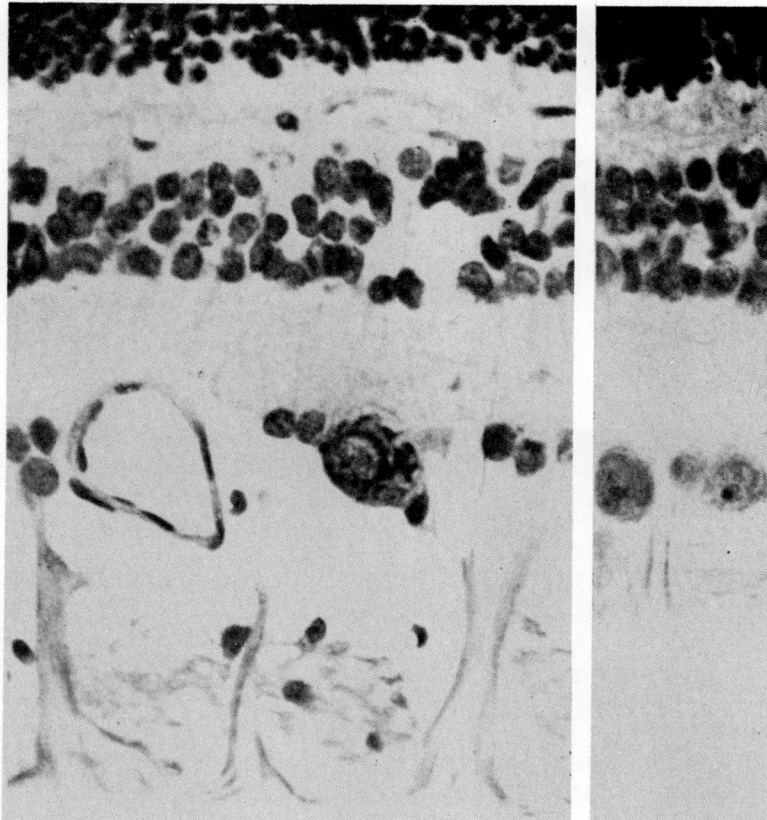

FIG. 28-14 Progressive rod-cone dysplasia (*PRCD*) of the retina. Eight-week-old cocker spaniel (×590) with normal retina on the right for comparison. Note large vacuoles in the outer portion of the optic nerve fiber layer, with only a few fibers near the internal limiting membrane. The conspicuous strands transcending the cavities are Müller's fibers. (Courtesy of Dr. H.B. Parry and *British Journal of Ophthalmology.*)

Markedly reduced retinal response is demonstrable by electroretinography as early as 16 days of age.

Lesions seen by light and electron microscopy involve the outer segments of rods and cones, which fail to develop normally. Changes in retinal pigment epithelium are considered one of the features that suggest a separate disease entity.

Retinal cone atrophy in dogs Retinal cone atrophy in dogs is a degenerative disease of the retina that affects only cones; this condition has been described in Alaskan malamutes. Loss of cones leads to day-blindness (**hemeralopia**). The disease is inherited as a simple autosomal trait. Ultrastructural changes are evident as early as seven weeks of age and progress to lesions visible with light microscopy by six months of age; almost total absence of cones occurs by two years of age.

References

Acland GM, Fletcher RT, Gentleman S, et al. Non-allelism of three genes (rcd1, rcd2, and erd) for early onset hereditary retinal degeneration. Exp Eye Res 1989;49:983–998.

Acland GM, Halloran-Blanton S, Boughman JA, et al. Segregation distortion in inheritance of progressive rod-cone degeneration (prcd) in miniature poodle dogs. Am J Med Genet 1990; 35:354–359.

Acland GM, Aguirre GD. Retinal degenerations in the dog. IV. Early retinal degeneration (erd) in Norwegian Elkhounds. Exp Eye Res 1987;44:491–521.

Aguirre GD, Acland GM. Variations in retinal degeneration phenotype inherited at the prcd locus. Exp Eye Res 1988;46:663–687.

Alvarez RA, Aguirre GD, Acland GM, et al. Docosapentaenoic acid is converted to docosahexaenoic acid in the retinas of normal and prcd-affected miniature poodle dogs. Invest Ophthalmol Vis Sci 1994;35:402–408.

Anderson RE, Maude MB, Alvarez RA, et al. Plasma lipid abnormalities in the miniature poodle with progressive rod-cone degeneration. Exp Eye Res 1991;52:349–355.

Chader GJ, Fletcher RT, Sanyal S, et al. A review of the role of cyclic GMP in neurological mutants with photoreceptor dysplasia. Curr Eye Res 1985;4:811–819.

Mieziewska K, Van Veen T, Aguirre GD. Development and fate of interphotoreceptor matrix components during dysplastic photoreceptor differentiation: a lectin cytochemical study of rod-cone dysplasia 1. Exp Eye Res 1993;56:429–441.

Ray K, Baldwin VJ, Acland GM, et al. Cosegregation of codon 807 mutation of the rod cGMP phosphodiesterase beta gene and rcd1. Invest Ophthalmol Vis Sci 1994;35:4291–4299.

Rubin LF. [1] Clinical features of hemeralopia in the adult Alaskan malamute. [2] Hemeralopia in Alaskan malamute pups. J Am Vet Med Assoc 1971;158:1696–1698, 1699–1701.

Rubin LF, Bourns TKR, Lord LH. Hemeralopia in dogs: heredity of hemeralopia in Alaskan Malamutes. Am J Vet Res 1967;28: 355–357.

Santos-Anderson RM, Tso MO, Wolf ED. An inherited retinopathy in collies: a light and electron microscopic study. Invest Ophthalmol Vis Sci 1980;19:1281–1294.

Wolf ED, Vainisi SJ, Santos-Anderson R. Rod-cone dysplasia in the collie. J Am Vet Med Assoc 1979;173:1331–1333.

Woodford BJ, et al. Cyclic nucleotide metabolism in inherited retinopathy in collies: a biochemical study. Exp Eye Res 1982;34: 703–714.

Central retinal degeneration in cats A central retinal degeneration occurs randomly in cats and apparently is not inherited. The disease is characterized by degeneration and thinning of the outer layers of the central retina and macula, and has also been termed **macular retinal degeneration**. As the disease progresses, loss results of all layers of the central retina, with glial cell proliferation. Hayes et al. showed experimentally that taurine deficiency in the diet leads to an essentially identical central retinal degeneration in cats (1975).

Diffuse retinal atrophy in cats Diffuse retinal atrophy in cats is histologically similar to central degeneration in cats, except that the entire retina is affected. Rods and cones are affected first, and the disease progresses to affect all layers. The condition is considered an inherited disease.

Inherited retinopathies in rodents The best-known in this category in rats is **inherited retinal degeneration** of the RCS (Royal College of Surgeons) hooded rat. The controlling single gene, designated **rdy,** is recessive, autosomal and homozygous in RCS rats. These hooded rats have a white hair coat, except for black hairs over the head and along the midline of the back. Another segregating gene, when homozygous (**pl/pl**), results in a tan color of the black hair and lack of pigment in the iris and retina. This homozygous gene has the effect of accelerating the progress of retinal degeneration.

Ophthalmoscopic examination of affected RCS rats at three to four weeks of age reveals an increasingly dense whitish reflex from the fundus, which obscures the choroidal vessels and details of the retina. At about six weeks of age, the whitish reflex dissipates, revealing the choroidal vessels and a granular appearing retina. About 22 days of age, the stimulus response of electroretinography is increased, but the α- and β-waves decrease progressively at the lower intensity level of light stimulation. The α- and β-waves are both no longer observed in the retinograph by the 80th day of age.

The first observation of abnormality is evident in histologic preparations as early as day 12 after birth. At this time, a distinct zone of disorganized material is evident between the layer of receptor outer segments and the retinal pigment epithelial cells. This zone of disorganization lasts until 21 days of age, when pyknotic nuclei and swollen inner segments may be evident in the photoreceptor layer. By 30 days of age, only a few basal outer segments can be seen in the zone of outer rod segments; the inner segments layer has become thinner and some photoreceptor nuclei are lost. At about 40 days, the outer nuclear layer has been reduced from 11–13 to 2–4 nuclei in width. The rod's inner segment has disappeared and distinct photoreceptor segments can no longer be identified. Abnormal changes in the retinal pigment epithelium also appear. Cells are no longer cuboidal, but flattened along Bruch's membrane; they also are enlarged and irregular in shape. Eventually, the pigment epithelium is invaded by capillaries and gliosis is evident. As the rat ages, the vestiges of photoreceptor cells continue to disappear. By seven months, the inner nuclear layer rests against the pigmented epithelium and the debris has disappeared.

Retinal degeneration is seen in sheep poisoned by bracken fern, and the various storage diseases discussed in Chapter 2 may involve the retina.

References

Barnett KC. Canine retinopathies. I. History and review of the literature. II. The miniature and toy poodle. III. The other breeds. IV. Causes of retinal atrophy. J Small Anim Pract 1965;6:41–55, 93–109, 185–196, 229–242.

Barnett KC. Retinal atrophy. Vet Rec 1965;77:1543–1552.

Bourne MC, Campbell DA, Tansley K. Hereditary degeneration of the rat retina. Br J Ophthalmol 1938;22:613–623.

Cogan, DG, Kuwabara, T. Photoreceptive abiotrophy of the retina in the Elkhound. Pathol Vet 1965;2:101–128.

Dowling JE, Sidman RL. Inherited retinal dystrophy in the rat. J Cell Biol 1962;14:73–109.

Essner E, Pino RM, Griewski RA. Breakdown of blood: retinal barrier in RCS rats with inherited retinal degeneration. Lab Invest 1980;43:418–426.

Gelatt KN. Veterinary ophthalmology. 2nd ed. Philadelphia: Lea & Febiger, 1991;481–496.

Hayes KC, Carey RE, Schmidt SY. Retinal degeneration associated with taurine deficiency in the cat. Science 1975;188:949–951.

Hayes KC, Rabin AR, Berson EL. An ultrastructural study of nutritionally induced and reversed retinal degeneration in cats. Am J Pathol 1975;78:505–524.

Matuk Y. Inherited retinal degeneration, RCS rat. In: Jones TC, Mohr U, Hunt RD, eds. Monographs on pathology of laboratory animals, eye and ear. Berlin: Springer-Verlag, 1991;92–100.

Parry HB. Degenerations of the dog retina. I. Structure and development of the retina of the normal dog. II. Generalized progressive atrophy of hereditary origin. Br J Ophthalmol 1953;37:385–404, 487–502, Vet Rec 1956;68:77.

Retinal dysplasia Retinal dysplasia has been reported in young children, dogs, cattle, and rats as a congenital lesion, apparently present at birth. In children it may be associated with multiple anomalies; in puppies and rats it may be associated with microophthalmia. In dogs it has been reported in Sealyham terriers, Bedlington terriers, beagles, Labrador retrievers, Cocker spaniels and English Springer spaniels as an autosomal-recessive inherited trait. Blindness is usually evident as soon as the behavior of the animal reaches a stage where detection is possible. In microscopic sections, the retina is detached and thrown into disorganized folds and small rosettes. Differentiation of the retina may be incomplete, resulting in lack of definition of its multiple layers. In Herefords and Shorthorn cattle, retinal dysplasia and other ocular anomalies occur in association with hereditary congenital hydrocephalus.

Retinal dysplasia and necrosis have been produced in lambs, with attenuated bluetongue virus vaccine as a component of the neurologic sequelae.

References

Ashton N, Barnett KC, Sachs DD. Retinal dysplasia in the Sealyham terrier. J Pathol Bacteriol 1968;96:269–272.

Barnett KC, Bjorck GR, Kock E. Hereditary retinal dysplasia in the Labrador retriever in England and Sweden. J Small Anim Pract 1970;10:755–759.

Carrig CB, et al. Retinal dysplasia associated with skeletal abnormalities in Labrador retrievers. J Am Vet Med Assoc 1977;170:49–57.

Heywood R, Wells GAH. A retinal dysplasia in the beagle dog. Vet Rec 1970;87:178–180.

Leipold HW, Gelatt KN, Huston K. Multiple ocular anomalies and hydrocephalus in grade beef Shorthorn cattle. Am J Vet Res 1971;32:1019–1026.

Rubin LF. Heredity of retinal dysplasia in Bedlington terriers. J Am Vet Med Assoc 1968;152:260–262.

Schmidt GM, et al. Inheritance of retinal dysplasia in the English Springer spaniel. J Am Vet Med Assoc 1979;174:1089–1090.

Weisse I, Stotzer H, Seitz R. (Neuroepithelial invagination, a form of retinal dysplasia in the beagle.) Zentralbl Veterinaermed 1973;20A:89–99.

Phototoxic retinopathy Injury to the retina by natural or artificial light has been reported in albino rats and mice under laboratory conditions, and in premature human infants in hospital nurseries. The lesions in living rats may be indicated by increased fundic reflexivity and narrowing of retinal vessels, determined with the use of indirect ophthalmoscopy. Affected eyes may also be distinguished by electrophysiologic procedures measuring the amplitude of the β-wave component of an electroretinogram.

Injury to the retina in laboratory rats is dependent upon the intensity and duration of exposure to light as well as upon other factors, such as genetic make up, ocular pigmentation, age, body temperature, and prior history of exposure to light. No effect has been demonstrated in rats exposed to 65 lux or less of light during 12 hour light/dark cycles for three months. Exposure to 270 or 1345 lux under these conditions results in severe damage to the retina. Albino mice housed in cages on top shelves of cage racks, nearer to fluorescent lights, have been shown to be more severely affected than those on lower shelves, further from the light source.

Lesions recognizable by light microscopy include necrosis and loss of cells in the outer and inner layers of photoreceptor segments. Loss of photoreceptor nuclei is particularly intense in the supraoptic region of the retina.

Nutritional retinopathy Nutritional retinopathy, seen with deficiency of vitamins A and E, and taurine, is discussed in Chapter 16.

References

Glass P, et al. Effect of bright light in the hospital nursery on the incidence of retinopathy of prematurity. N Engl J Med 1985;313:401–405.

Greenman DL, Bryant P, Kodell RL, et al. Influence of cage shelf level on retinal atrophy in mice. Lab Anim Sci 1982;32:353–356.

Noell WK, Walker VS, Kang BS, Berman S. Retinal damage by light in rats. Invest Ophthalmol Vis Sci 1966;5:450–473.

Peiffer RL, Porter DP. Light-induced retinal degeneration, rat. In: Jones TC, Mohr U, Hunt RD, eds. Monographs on pathology of laboratory animals, eye and ear. Berlin: Springer-Verlag, 1991;82–86.

Semple-Rowland SL, Dawson WW. Retinal cyclic light damage threshold for albino rats. Lab Anim Sci 1987;37:289–298.

Choroid

The choroid is the posterior part of the middle, vascular tunic of the eye. It occupies the entire posterior part of the globe, lying behind the ora ciliaris retinae, except for the space containing the optic papilla. The retina lies on its inner surface, except in those areas where the two are separated by the tapetum. Sclera surrounds the choroid and gives it support and the entire globe its relative rigidity. Blood vessels of the choroid penetrate the sclera at various points, the locations depending upon the species.

The vascular nature of the choroid determines the kind of lesions to which it is subject. Metastatic neoplasms and bacterial emboli often lodge in the choroid, and leukocytes may readily escape the blood vessels to invade the choroidal stroma. The retina is commonly involved in inflammatory processes of the choroid (**chorioretinitis**). Causes of chorioretinitis in animals are incompletely understood, but some of the infectious agents that have been demonstrated in chorioretinal lesions are *Toxoplasma gondii, Coccidioides immitis,* and *Mycobacterium tuberculosis.* Too few eyes of animals have been studied following or during the course of generalized infections to determine how often the choroid is involved, but it probably is more frequent than the literature indicates.

Optic nerve

ATROPHY

Atrophy of the optic nerve has been reported in animals, usually secondary to retinopathy involving the ganglion cell layer.

CONGENITAL HYPOPLASIA

Congenital hypoplasia of the optic nerve has been reported in purebred Merle blue collie puppies. In these cases, one or both of the optic nerves were grossly atrophic or absent, and the optic nerve layer and ganglion cell layer of the retina were also atrophied. These changes were interpreted as resulting from degeneration in the retina, and no proof was found that they were inherited. Hypoplasia of the optic nerve has also

been reported in cattle, cats, horses, and laboratory rodents. Complete agenesis of the optic nerve has been observed in rats and in swine with congenital anophthalmos; the optic nerve would not develop in the absence of ganglion cells of the retina.

A proliferative optic neuropathy has been described in horses (Saunders et al., 1972). It was characterized by an accumulation of large foamy cells in the nerve and disc. It was believed to represent a storage disease.

PAPILLEDEMA

Papilledema ("choked disc") is the term that denotes edema of the optic papilla and the adjacent retina (Fig. 28-15). This lesion is sometimes associated with internal hydrocephalus, but cannot always be explained on this basis. It has been observed in cattle maintained on vitamin-A-deficient diets, but its pathogenesis in animals is not fully explained.

References

Saunders LZ. Congenital optic nerve hypoplasia in collie dogs. Cornell Vet 1952;42:67–80.

Saunders LZ, Bistner SI, Rubin LF. Proliferative optic neuropathy in horses. Vet Pathol 1972;9:368–378.

Other hereditary and congenital anomalies

A variety of hereditary and congenital defects in addition to those already discussed may be encountered in the eye, either singly or more often as multiple anomalies. They are observed in all species.

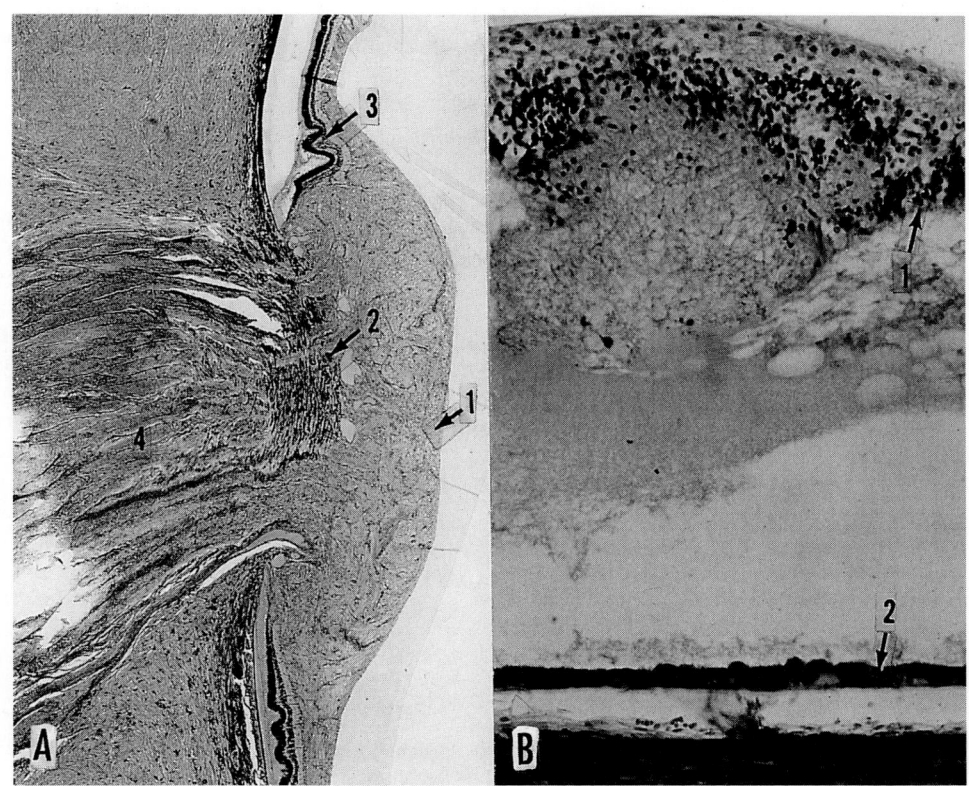

FIG. 28-15 A. Papilledema (×17), eye of a ten-month-old Holstein calf that had been fed a ration low in vitamin A since birth. (1) The optic papilla is elevated; (2) The pigmented cribriform plate is deflected inward; (3) The retina folded; and (4) The optic nerve edematous. (Contributor: Dr. Louis L. Madsen.) **B.** Detachment of the retina in equine periodic ophthalmia (×165). (1) Serous exudate in the layer of rods and cones and outer nuclear layer separates the latter; (2) From the pigment epithelium. (**A,** Courtesy of Armed Forces Institute of Pathology.)

COLOBOMA

Coloboma, as it pertains to the eye, is defined as a congenital defect in the continuity of one of the tunics of the eye, usually the iris. The defect is seen as a cleft in the iris, and is believed to be the result of incomplete fusion of primordial parts in the optic vesicle during embryonic life.

CONGENITAL ANOPHTHALMOS

Congenital anophthalmos—absence of the eye—has been observed in some animals, including swine, foals, dogs, cats, rats, and guinea pigs. This defect has been associated with maternal vitamin A deficiency in swine and is inherited in guinea pigs. Not only are the eyes absent, but also the optic nerve and optic tract. Microscopically, however, remnants of the eye are usually present.

CONGENITAL MICROPHTHALMOS

Congenital microphthalmos—decreased size of the eyes,—has also been observed in dogs, rats, cattle, cats, and swine, and is possibly related to the same factors that result in anophthalmos.

CONGENITAL OPACITY OF CORNEA

Congenital opacity of the cornea is most often encountered in cattle and dogs. The opacity results from edema, but the pathogenesis is unknown. In Holstein-Friesian cattle in Germany and England, it is believed to be inherited as a recessive trait. It has also been described in Aberdeen Angus.

HEMERALOPIA

Hemeralopia (day-blindness) has been reported in two breeds of dogs, Alaskan malamutes, and poodles. Test crosses with clinically identified dogs indicate that this characteristic is inherited under the control of a single autosomal-recessive gene. The lesions have not been reported.

Retinal lesions related to apparent hereditary or congenital factors have been discussed previously. Although such lesions as aplasia of optic nerves, albinism, and other defects have been reported in different species, it is not often that both the anatomic basis for the ocular defect and the evidence for their genetic background are entirely unequivocal.

HEREDITARY OCULAR DISEASE IN MICE

A number of hereditary eye lesions have been identified and studied in detail in laboratory mice. In many instances, the gene has been named, inheritance and linkage established, and the nature of the pathologic lesions described. Constraints of space prevent inclusion of these entities in this text, although they are important and useful to the understanding of ophthalmic pathology. The student is referred to Cook (1991) and Gelatt (1991) for further reading.

References

Cook CS. Microphthalmia and anophthalmia, mouse and rat. In: Jones TC, Mohr U, Hunt RD (eds) Monographs on pathology of laboratory animals, eye and ear. Heidelberg: Springer-Verlag, 1991;125–132.

Gelatt KN. Veterinary ophthalmology. Philadelphia: Lea & Febiger, 1991.

COLLIE EYE ANOMALY

The collie eye anomaly, first reported by Magrane (1953), has been referred to by many names that have resulted from the diverse clinical manifestations of the syndrome: such as, collie ectasia syndrome, congenital anomaly of optic nerve, congenital posterior ectasia of the sclera, ocular fundus anomaly, chorioretinal dysplasia, juxtapapillary staphyloma, retinal detachment, coloboma of optic disc, and excavated optic disc. This syndrome is now recognized as widespread in collies, but less frequent in other breeds, such as Shetland sheepdogs. Evidence indicates that it is controlled by a single autosomal-recessive gene, with some variation in its expression (Yakely et al., 1968).

The lesions vary but may include any one or all of the following: staphyloma or ectasia of the sclera near the optic disc (a defect in the sclera that allows the choroid and retina to dip into it), dysplasia of retina and choroid, detached retina, and intraocular hemorrhage. Some degree of microphthalmos may be present and pigmentary defects in the retina may be associated. Absence of pigment results in the retinal pigment epithelium, which may also degenerate.

References

Magrane WG. Congenital anomaly of the optic nerve in collies. North Am Vet 1953;34:646.

Glaucoma

The term glaucoma appeared in the writings of Hippocrates, but its present meaning has evolved over many centuries and is broader than indicated by its derivation. Glaucoma is not a specific disease entity but a composite of the clinical and pathologic manifestations that result from persistent increase in intraocular pressure.

Glaucoma is classified as **primary** or **secondary glaucoma. Primary glaucoma** may result from defective development of the iridocorneal angle (termed **goniodysgenesis**), in which case it is also termed **primary angle closure glaucoma** or **narrow-angle glaucoma.** Primary glaucoma may also occur, however, in the absence of any morphologic change in the angle, but (for unknown reasons) a poorly functioning filtration angle, in which case it is termed **primary open-angle glaucoma. Secondary glaucoma** follows other abnormalities of the eye, such as anterior synechia following iridocyclitis or trauma to the eye, deformities of the lens, detachment of the retina, intraocular hemorrhage, intraocular neoplasms, or circulatory stasis. The term, **congenital glaucoma** is used to describe glaucoma that is seen at birth or shortly thereafter. It results from goniodysgenesis or other structural abnormalities of the eye.

Both primary and secondary glaucoma occur in animals. Primary glaucoma has been best studied in dogs. Open-angle glaucoma is most common in beagles and toy and miniature poodles. Closed-angle glaucoma is most frequent in cocker spaniels and toy and miniature poodles. Congenital glaucoma is recognized most often in basset hounds. Secondary glaucoma can occur in any species.

Glaucoma may be unilateral or, more often, bilateral (Fig. 28-16); it is recognized in early stages by increased intraocular tension, which eventually enlarges the globe (buphthalmos), sometimes with apparent exophthalmos. Initially, the cornea is edematous and opaque; later, this opacity is accentuated by a degenerative pannus.

The underlying feature usually considered basic to the development of glaucoma is interference with the circulation of the intraocular fluid (aqueous). Aqueous is secreted into the posterior chamber by the ciliary epithelium. From the posterior chamber, this fluid moves through the pupil into the anterior chamber. The aqueous humor drains from the anterior chamber at the filtration angle near the limbus, where it passes through the spaces of Fontana and eventually reaches the veins at the limbus through the canals of Schlemm. If the filtration angle is occluded—for example, by peripheral anterior synechiae—and aqueous continues to enter the posterior chamber, the fluid pressure must increase. If the pupil is occluded for any reason, aqueous will accumulate behind the iris and force it to bulge for-

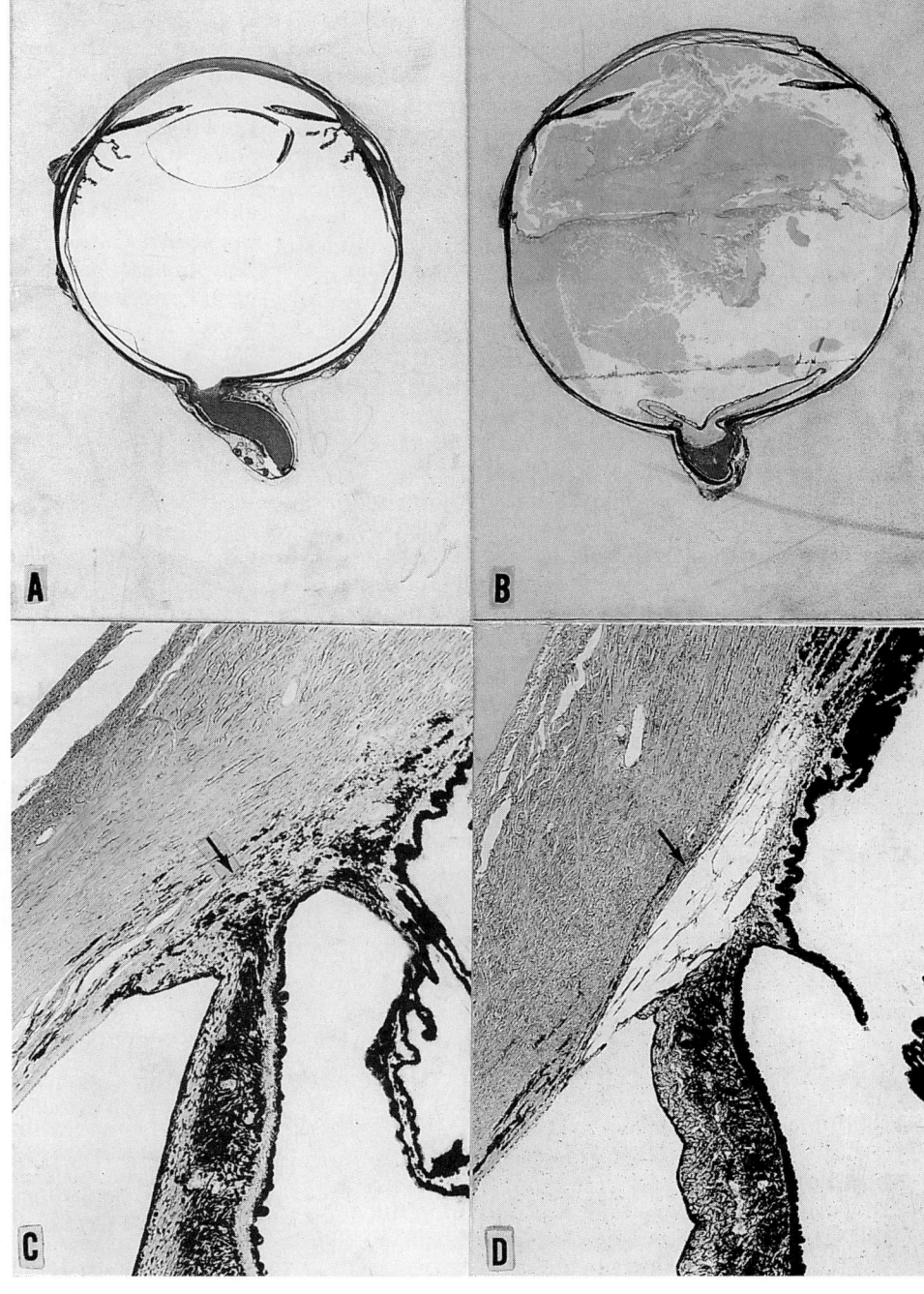

FIG. 28-16 Canine glaucoma. **A.** Section (×2) of the left eye of a dog with moderately severe glaucoma. Note spherical outline of the eye, occlusion of the filtration angle, and cupping of the optic disc. **B.** Absolute glaucoma in the right eye of the same dog as **A** (×2). Buphthalmos, severe cupping of the optic disc, disorganization of contents of globe. **C.** Filtration angle (×35) of same eye as in **A.** Note occlusion *(arrow).* (Contributor: Dr. Leon Z. Saunders.) **D.** Normal filtration angle, eye of a dog (×35). Compare with **C.** (**C,** Courtesy of Armed Forces Institute of Pathology.)

ward into the anterior chamber (refer to section on *iris bombé*).

LESIONS

The findings of pathologic study of the affected eye can be correlated with those of the clinical examination. **Grossly,** the globe is enlarged, increasingly spherical, and turgid. The cornea is opaque, as also may be the lens and vitreous. **Microscopically** evident changes may be found in most of the ocular structures, depending upon the stage in which the eye is studied. Edema in the corneal epithelium is usually seen in the form of small vacuoles that may coalesce to produce small bullae. It is believed that increased pressure in the anterior chamber forces this fluid through the corneal stroma and into the epithelium.

Significant changes are usually found at the filtration angle. Peripheral anterior synechiae may occlude the filtration angle (Fig. 28-16). The iris is usually thin and atrophic, and its blood vessels sometimes are sclerotic. The ciliary processes are thin, compressed, and atrophic. The choroid may be similarly compressed and atrophied, eventually appearing only as a thin pigmented membrane containing some thick-walled hyaline vessels. The retina undergoes degenerative changes after prolonged intraocular hypertension, an effect believed to be due to retinal ischemia.

In dogs, glaucomatous retinopathy—which results in complete blindness and is characterized histologically by atrophy—is more severe in the inner than the outer layers of the retina. Ganglion cells are lost early, followed by disappearance of optic nerve fibers. The bipolar cells of the inner nuclear layer are next to disappear, but the outer nuclear layer and the layer of rods and cones are only slightly damaged. This degeneration is usually more advanced in the nontapetal areas of the retina; the tapetal fundus and central fundus are spared. In the peripheral fundus, the retina usually exhibits the most advanced sclerosis. Retinal pigment is minimally disturbed.

The optic nerve undergoes pathologic changes that are typical for glaucoma. In the advanced stages, the intraocular hypertension causes depression of the optic disc into the characteristic cup shape (cupping of the disc). This change starts with atrophy of the nerve fibers in the area where they go through the lamina cribrosa. The fibers of the lamina cribrosa are also deflected outward to form the cup-shaped space that is usually filled with vitreous. It must be remembered that in some animals (such as elephants) the disc is normally cupped; hence, the normal histologic features must be considered in interpreting this change. Cupping of the disc is usually considered to be the direct result of pressure upon the nerve fibers, but a divergent view holds that the pressure first affects the blood supply to the disc, the neuritic atrophy following secondarily.

DIAGNOSIS

Diagnosis of glaucoma may be based upon the clinical and pathologic evidences of increased intraocular tension that have been described.

References

Barrie KP, Gum GG, Samuelson DA, et al. Morphologic studies of uveoscleral outflow in normotensive and glaucomatous beagles with fluorescein-labeled dextran. Am J Vet Res 1985;46:89–97.

Gelatt KN. The canine glaucoma. In: Gelatt KN, ed. Veterinary ophthalmology. 2nd ed. Philadelphia: Lea & Febiger, 1991;396–428.

Peiffer RL Jr, Gelatt KN. Aqueous humor outflow in beagles with inherited glaucoma: gross and light microscopic observations of the iridocorneal angle. Am J Vet Res 1980;41:861–867.

van der Linde-Sipman JS. Dysplasia of the pectinate ligament and primary glaucoma in the Bouvier des Flandres dog. Vet Pathol 1987;24:201–206.

Wilcock BP, Brooks DE, Latimer CA. Glaucoma in horses. Vet Pathol 1991;28:74–78.

Wilcock BP, Peiffer RL, Davidson MG. The cause of glaucoma in cats. Vet Pathol 1990;27:35–40.

Neoplasms

Many different histologic types of neoplasms have been described as arising from the orbit, ocular adnexa, extraocular tissues, or as metastatic from distal organs. Some have been reported in individual case reports; others have been described from collections of cases and are considered as a group, sometimes with comparisons made among species. Biologic behavior, particularly malignant or benign outcome, has occasionally been considered. Frequency and prevalence have rarely been stated in precise terms because of lack of valid data on the populations from which the affected animals came (Fig. 28-17).

Neoplasms reported most frequently in the eye or adnexa are listed in Table 28-1, where references to the applicable literature are cited.

References

Acland GM, McLean IW, Aguirre GD, et al. Diffuse iris melanoma in cats. J Am Vet Med Assoc 1980;176:52–56.

Bolon B, Calderwood-Mays MB, Hall BJ. Characteristics of canine melanoma and comparison of histology and DNA ploidy to their biologic behavior. Vet Pathol 1990;27:96–102.

Bonny CH, Koch SA, Dice PF, et al. Papillomatosis of conjunctiva and adnexa in dogs. J Am Vet Med Assoc 1980;176:48–51.

Carlton WW, Render JA. Adenoma and adenocarcinoma, Harderian gland, mouse, rat and hamster. In: Jones TC, Mohr U, Hunt RD, eds. Monographs on pathology of laboratory animals, eye and ear. Berlin: Springer-Verlag, 1991;133–137.

Cook CS, Peiffer RL, Stine PE. Metastatic ocular squamous cell carcinoma in a cat. J Am Vet Med Assoc 1984;185:1546–1549.

Cook CS, Rosenkrantz W, Peiffer RL, et al. Malignant melanoma of the conjunctiva in a cat. J Am Vet Med Assoc 1985;186:505–506.

Diters RW, Ryan AM. Canine limbal melanoma. Vet Med Small Anim Clin 1983;178:1529–1534.

Dubielzig RR, Aguirre GD, Gross SL, et al. Choroidal melanomas in dogs. Vet Pathol 1985;22:582–585.

Dubielzig RR, Everitt J, Shadduck JA, et al. Clinical and morphologic features of post-traumatic ocular sarcomas in cats. Vet Pathol 1990;27:62–65.

Dugan SJ, Curtis SR, Roberts SM, et al.: Epidemiologic study of ocular/adnexal squamous cell carcinoma in horses. J Am Vet Med Assoc 1991;198:251–255.

Feeney-Burns L, Burns RP, Gao CL. Ocular pathology in melanomatous Sinclair miniature swine. Am J Pathol 1988;131:62–72.

Friedman DS, Miller L, Dubielzig RR. Malignant canine anterior uveal melanoma. Vet Pathol 1989;26:523–525.

Gallie BL, et al. Mechanism of oncogenesis in retinoblastoma. Lab Invest 1990;62:394–408.

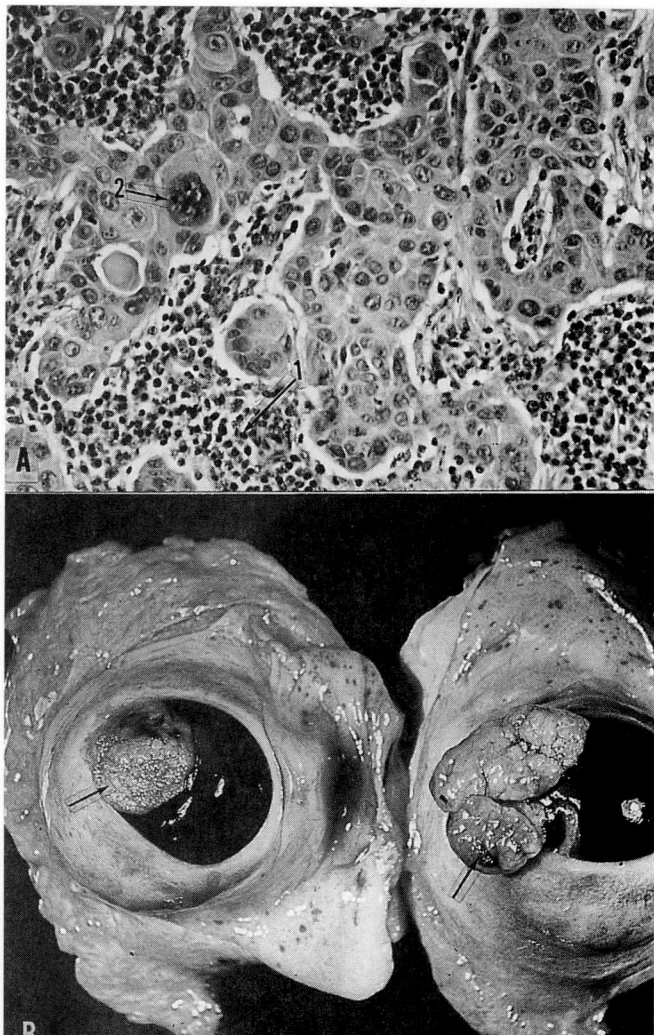

FIG. 28-17 A. Squamous cell carcinoma (×224) arising in corneal epithelium of an 11-year-old Hereford cow. (1) The infiltrating tumor cells are surrounded by leukocytes; and (2) have bizarre giant nuclei. (Courtesy of Armed Forces Institute of Pathology; contributor: Drs. C.N. Barron and G.T. Easley.) **B.** Squamous cell carcinomas in both eyes of a Jersey cow. Note that each is attached at the limbus but extends over the cornea. (Courtesy of Dr. C.L. Davis.)

Gionfriddo JR, Fix AS, Niyo Y, et al. Ocular manifestations of a primary adenocarcinoma in a cat. J Am Vet Med Assoc 1990;197:372–374.

Owen RA, Duprat P. Leiomyoma of the iris in a Sprague-Dawley rat. J Comp Pathol 1987;97:227–229.

Patnaik AK, Mooney S. Feline melanoma: a comparative study of ocular, oral and dermal neoplasms. Vet Pathol 1988;25:105–112.

Rebhun WC. Orbital lymphosarcoma in cattle. J Am Vet Med Assoc 1982;180:149–152.

Render JA, Carlton WW, Vestre WA, et al. Osteosarcoma metastatic to the globes in a dog. Vet Pathol 1982;19:323–326.

Ryan AM, Diters RW. Clinical and pathologic features of canine ocular melanomas. J Am Vet Med Assoc 1984;184:60–67.

Saunders LZ, Rubin LF. Ophthalmic pathology of animals: an atlas and reference book. Basel: Karger, 1975.

Schuh JCL. Congenital intraocular melanoma in a calf. J Comp Pathol 1989;101:113–116.

Szymanski CM. Malignant teratoid medulloepithelioma in a horse. J Am Vet Med Assoc 1987;190:301–302.

Weisse I, Frese K, Meyer D. Benign melanoma of the choroid in a beagle: ophthalmological, light and electron microscopical investigations. Vet Pathol 1985;22:586–591.

Wilcock BP, Peiffer RL. Morphology and behavior of primary ocular melanomas in 91 dogs. Vet Pathol 1986;23:418–424.

Wilcock BP, Peiffer RL. Adenocarcinoma of the gland of the third eyelid in seven dogs. J Am Vet Med Assoc 1988;193:1549–1550.

Williams LW, Gelatt KN, Gwin RM. Ophthalmic neoplasms in the cat. J Am Anim Hosp Assoc 1981;17:999–1008.

Woog J, Albert DM, Gonder JR, et al. Osteosarcoma in a phthisical feline eye. Vet Pathol 1983;20:209–213.

Yoshitomi K, Boorman GA. Spontaneous amelanotic melanomas of the uveal tract in F344 rats. Vet Pathol 1991;28:403–409.

Yoshitomi K, Boorman GA. Palpebral amelanotic melanomas in F344 rats. Vet Pathol 1993;30:280–286.

Systemic infections in eye

Many systemic infectious diseases of animals may affect the eye. Most common infections affect the conjunctiva, but systemic spread to the choroid can be expected, although not always recognized. Uveitis, chorioretinitis, and panophthalmitis may result from ocular involvement due to generalized infections; thus, the retina can become affected. Almost any of the infectious agents considered in previous chapters may spread to the eye. Their identification here depends on recognition of the lesions produced and on the characteristics of each organism. Among the organisms identified in intraocular lesions are the following: canine distemper virus, blue tongue virus, *Herpesvirus canis*, *Toxoplasma gondii*, *Coccidioides immitis*, *Blastomyces canis*, *Brucella* sp., *Histoplasma capsulatum*, and *Ehrlichia canis* (Table 28-2).

Ear

The ears of animals do not often come to the pathologist's attention as separate organs, but are usually studied in connection with generalized lesions or because of some incidental finding. It is desirable to describe the few specific lesions that have been recognized in ears of animals, and to recapitulate briefly some of the systemic diseases in which the ear may become involved. These lesions may be conveniently described in connection with the anatomic divisions of the ear: the external, middle, and inner ear.

External ear

The external ear consists of the external auricular appendage (auricula); this includes the cartilage covered by skin, muscle, and the external auditory meatus which is supported by the cartilage and surrounded by epidermis richly supplied with sebaceous glands, and specialized apocrine glands (ceruminous glands). The external ear is limited in its deepest aspect by the tympanic membrane (**tympanum**). The anatomic details (such as size and position of the auricular appendage, and depth and course of the external auditory meatus) are different in each species; hence, each must be considered individually. However, only those features that influence the nature of lesions are discussed here.

TABLE 28-1 Neoplasms of the eye and adnexa

Neoplasm	Location	Species	Reference
Extraocular			
Squamous cell carcinoma	Eyelids, conjunctiva	Bovine, equine, canine, other	Dugan et al., 1991
Melanoma, malignant (melanotic)	Conjunctiva	Canine, feline, porcine	Cook et al., 1985; Diters and Ryan, 1983; Feeney-Burns et al., 1985, 1988
Melanoma, malignant (amelanotic)	Eyelid	Rodent (rat)	Yoshitomi and Boorman, 1993
Papilloma	Eyelid, conjunctiva	Canine	Bonney et al., 1980
Adenocarcinoma	Glands, 3rd eyelid	Canine, rodents (rat, mouse, hamster)	Wilcock and Peiffer, 1988; Carlton and Render, 1991
Adenoma, adenocarcinoma	Meibomian glands	Canine	Saunders and Rubin, 1975
Melanoma, malignant	Anterior uvea, iris	Canine, equine, bovine, feline, rodent (F344 rat)	Patnaik and Mooney, 1988; Acland et al., 1980; Wilcock and Peiffer, 1986; Bolon et al., 1990; Shuh, 1989; Yoshitomi and Boorman, 1991
Intraocular			
Melanoma, malignant, and benign	Choroid	Canine	Dubielzig et al., 1985; Friedman et al., 1989
Leiomyosarcoma	Iris	Canine, rodent (F344 rat)	Owen and Duprat, 1987
Retinoblastoma (neuroepithelioma)	Retina	Canine, equine	Gallie et al., 1990
Sarcoma "spindle cell" (posttraumatic)	Uvea	Feline	Dubielzig et al., 1990
Metastatic			
Adenocarcinoma	Uvea (lung)	Feline	Gionfriddo et al., 1990
Lymphosarcoma	Orbit (lymphatic system)	Bovine, feline	Rebhun, 1992; Williams et al., 1981
Meningioma	Optic nerve (meninges)	Rodent (F344 rat)	Yoshitomi and Boorman, 1991
Osteosarcoma	Uvea, globe (bone)	Canine	Render et al., 1982; Woog et al., 1983
Squamous cell carcinoma	Uvea (skin)	Feline	Cook et al., 1984

TABLE 28-2 **Intraocular infections**

Species	Etiology	Reference	Lesions
Alpacas, llamas	Equine herpesvirus I	Chapter 8	Optic neuritis, chorioretinitis
Bovine	Malignant catarrhal fever (Alcelaphine herpesvirus-1)	Chapter 8	Anterior uveitis
Canine	Morbillivirus (canine distemper virus)	Chapter 8	Choroiditis, retinopathy
Human	Morbillivirus (measles)	Chapter 8	Retinitis
Canine	*Mycobacterium bovis*	Chapter 10	Choroiditis
Human	*M. tuberculosis*	Chapter 10	Choroiditis
Canine	*Coccidioides immitis*	Chapter 11	Anterior uveitis
Canine	*Toxocara canis* (larvae)	Chapter 13	Granulomatous uveitis and retinitis
Equine	*Leptospira pomona*	Chapter 10	Anterior uveitis
Equine	Equine herpesvirus-1	Slater et al., 1992	Chorioretinitis
Ovine	*Trypanosoma brucei*	Chapter 12	Anterior uveitis
Ovine, canine	*Toxoplasma gondii*	Chapter 12	Anterior uveitis, choroiditis
Ovine	*Mycoplasma agalactia*	Chapter 9	Anterior uveitis
Ovine	*Listeria monocytogenes*	Chapter 10	Chorioretinitis, uveitis
Ovine	*Elaeophora schneideri*	Chapter 13	Anterior uveitis

INFLAMMATION OF EXTERNAL EAR

Inflammation of the external ear, **otitis externa,** is not uncommon in animals and may result from a variety of causes. Among the specific infectious agents is *Actinomyces bovis,* which may produce a specific granulomatous inflammation of the external ear of swine. This infection usually involves the auricular appendage only, giving it a thick, indurated appearance. Histologically, a granulomatous tissue reaction, characteristic of actinomycosis, is found in the subcutis around the cartilage, and sometimes involves the cartilage. In other species, specific infections are uncommon, but nonspecific infections may result from wounds (usually caused by bites) of the external ear.

Parasitic infestations of the external ear are common in most animals and are usually due to parasites that have a specific affinity for the ear. Certain ear mites have an obligate affinity for the external ear: those of rabbits, sheep, cattle, and horses (*Psoroptes communis;* var. *cuniculi, ovis,* etc.); cats *(Notoedres cati);* and dogs *(Otodectes cynotis).* These acarid (mite) parasites are specific for each species; the variety that infests the rabbit is particularly common. These mites burrow into the epidermis lining the external auditory meatus; they cause profuse exudation, with accumulation of tenacious, brown, waxy material in the meatus and, in severe cases, over the inner surface of the external ear. Parasitic otitis externa may in some cases cause rupture of the tympanum and involve the middle ear.

Ticks may also attack the external ear, the most common being the spinose ear tick *(Otobius megnini)* of cattle.

Dermatomycosis is often particularly severe in, or limited to, the external ear. The lesions are not significantly different from those in the skin elsewhere in the body, but the term **otomycosis** may be used to designate infection of this type when limited chiefly to the ear.

Yeasts are often associated with chronic otitis externa in dogs, but it is not known whether these organisms are actually the cause of the inflammation.

Otitis externa is extremely common in dogs. Anatomic peculiarities of the ear, mites, and various other organisms have been incriminated as the cause, but no single theory is universally accepted.

Particularly important among the causes of severe otitis are the awns of certain grasses, particularly *Hordeum* (foxtail grass). These awns may lodge in the fur and occasionally puncture the skin and enter deeper tissues at many sites. They are a hazard when they penetrate the external auditory canal.

Otitis of this etiology is especially frequent in dogs in certain western states. When these bearded grasses penetrate deep into the external meatus, it is difficult to withdraw them. Severe otitis externa develops and the awns may even break through the tympanum to set up severe inflammation in the middle and internal ear.

References

Brennan KE, Ihrke PJ. Grass awn migration in dogs and cats: a retrospective study of 182 cases. J Am Vet Med Assoc 1983;182:1201–1204.

Harvey CE. Ear canal disease in the dog: medical and surgical management. J Am Vet Med Assoc 1980;177:136–139.

Morgan KL. Parasitic ototis in sheep associated with psoroptic infestation: a clinical epidemiological study. Vet Rec 1992;130:530–532.

INFLAMMATORY POLYPS

Inflammatory polyps may occur in cats and sometimes dogs; polyps are attached by a thin pedicle to, or in the region of, the tympanum. These polyps may become relatively large, filling the external auditory meatus; in some cases they may be connected through the eustachian tube with a similar polyp that lies in the nasopharynx (Fig. 20-1). These polyps histologically consist of richly cellular connective tissue; they are liberally supplied with blood vessels and usually infiltrated by leukocytes, particularly when the squamous epithelium covering the mass is eroded. The cause and exact nature of these polyps is unknown. Although they may recur after surgical excision, they do not appear to be neoplastic.

AURICULAR CHONDRITIS IN RATS

A prolonged involvement of the external ear of several strains of laboratory rats appears to be initiated by focal progressive necrosis of the auricular cartilage. The affected cartilage is replaced by large numbers of macrophages and mononuclear cells, including monocytes and plasma cells. This process eventually results in severe destruction of the cartilage and its replacement by immature, hyperplastic, and disorganized cartilaginous tissue. The end result is a grossly thickened, malformed ear with nodular and roughened surfaces. This bears some resemblance to the "cauliflower ear" seen on some professional wrestlers.

Microscopic lesions suggest an immunologic basis for the disease and, further, resemble lesions induced by immunization with type II collagen. The precise etiology is unknown (Fig. 28-18).

References

Chiu T. Auricular chondritis. In: Jones TC, Mohr U, Hunt RD, eds. Monographs on pathology of laboratory animals, eye and ear. Berlin: Springer-Verlag, 1991;149–155.

Chiu T, Lee KP. Auricular chondropathy in aging rats. Vet Pathol 1984;21:500–504.

Prieur DJ, Young DM, Counts DF. Auricular chondritis in fawn hooded rats: a spontaneous disorder resembling that induced by immunization with type II collagen. Am J Pathol 1984;116:69–76.

AURICULAR HEMATOMAS

Auricular hematomas are not infrequent in dogs, especially in long-eared breeds, and often are difficult to treat successfully. The ear (commonly only one at a time) is thickened by extensive hemorrhage into its tissues, making it thick, heavy, and the source of much discomfort. The cause is not always apparent, but vigorous shaking of the head and ears in order to get rid of intense irritation of the external ear is an apparent cause in many instances. Histologic study of some affected ears reveals the hemorrhage to be, in part, within the cartilage and associated with multiple fractures of the cartilage. These fractures contribute to the severity of the injury and delay healing.

References

Dubielzig RR, Wilson JW, Seireg AA. Pathogenesis of canine aural hematomas. J Am Vet Med Assoc 1984;185:873–875.

NEOPLASMS

Neoplasms that are likely to be encountered in the external ear include any new growth of the skin, its adnexa, or the cartilage.

Adenomas and adenocarcinomas of the ceruminous glands Adenomas and adenocarcinomas of the ceruminous glands of the external ear are occasionally encountered in dogs and cats (Fig. 28-19). **Grossly,** they are usually benign, nodular growths, 1 or 2 cm in diameter, which bulge into the auditory canal; however, they may become locally invasive or metastasize to the regional lymph nodes. **Microscopically,** they consist of ordinary glandular acini with lumens of generous size and linings of simple columnar or cuboidal epithelium. These tumors are distinguished by a golden brown, crystalline pigment in the cytoplasm of the epithelial cells.

The specific neoplasm of horses and mules, **equine sarcoid,** appears at the base of the ear, or even on the auricula. **Squamous cell carcinomas** and **rhabdomyomas** have been reported on the pinnae of cats. Aural sebaceous glands in laboratory rats—located under the mucosa of the ear canal or in the subcutis just ventral to the ear—are often called **Zymbal's glands.** Under certain conditions—particularly after long-term administration of specific carcinogens—these glands become the origin of adenomas of sebaceous type or carcinomas of sebaceous or squamous cells.

References

Legendre AM, Krahwinkel DJ Jr. Feline ear tumors. J Am Anim Hosp Assoc 1981;17:1035–1037.

Roth L. Rhabdomyoma of the ear pinna in four cats. J Comp Pathol 1990;103:237–240.

Seely JC. [1] Adenoma of the auditory sebaceous glands, rat. [2] Carcinoma of the auditory sebaceous glands, rat. In: Jones TC, Mohr

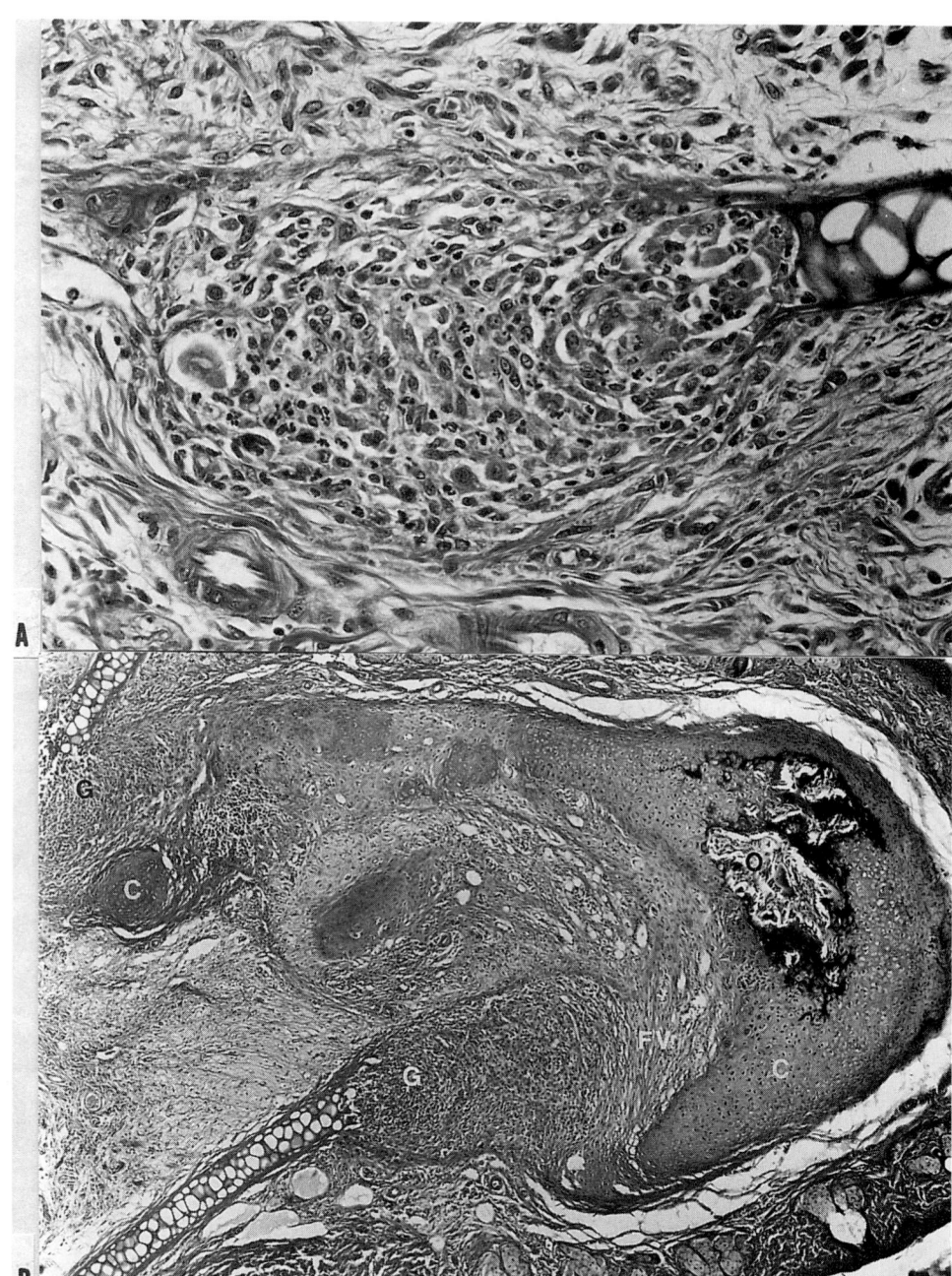

FIG. 28-18 A. Auricular chondritis, male Sprague-Dawley rat. An early lesion with focal granulomatous inflammation involving an otherwise normal cartilage plate. No significant change is present in the surrounding tissues (hematoxylin and eosin stain, ×400.) **B.** An advanced lesion of auricular chondritis, rat. Note the sequential development of various regenerative tissues: fibrovascular *(FV)*, chondrous *(C)*, and osseous *(O)*, next to granulomatous inflammation *(G;* hematoxylin and eosin stain; ×66.) (Courtesy of Dr. Taisan Chiu and Springer Verlag, Heidelberg.)

U, Hunt RD, eds. Monographs on pathology of laboratory animals, eye and ear. Berlin: Springer-Verlag, 1991;143–145, 145–149.

Middle ear

The middle ear includes the tympanic cavity, with its contents, and the auditive (eustachian) tubes. In horses, two large diverticula of the eustachian tubes (the guttural pouches) are also part of the middle ear. The tympanic cavity is lined with epithelium that is continuous with that of the nasal mucosa through the eustachian tubes. The contents include the chain of auditory ossicles (malleus, incus, os lenticulare, and stapes) that communicate vibrations of the tympanum to the inner ear. This tympanic cavity is located within the tympanic and petrous parts of the temporal bone.

Infection of the middle ear (**otitis media**) may reach the tympanic cavity from the external ear by rupture of the tympanum, or may extend from the nasopharynx by way of the eustachian tubes. Extension of otitis externa to involve the middle ear is frequent in ear-mite infestation and with penetrating foreign bodies (grass awns). The inflammation is usually purulent and tends to be chronic. Otitis media is especially frequent in laboratory rats with chronic murine pneumonia and rabbits with pasteurellosis. Occlusion of the eustachian tube predisposes to otitis media.

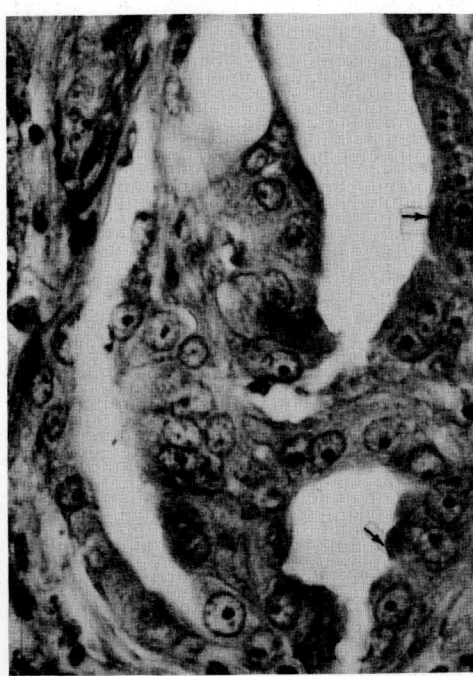

FIG. 28-19 Adenoma of ceruminous gland (×545), ear of an eight-year-old mongrel dog. Tumor contains large columnar cells with granular cytoplasm *(arrows)*. (Courtesy of Armed Forces Institute of Pathology; contributor: Dr. S.W. Stiles.)

References

Boot R, Walvoort HC. Otitis media in guinea pigs. Lab Anim 1986;20:242–249.
Jensen R, Pierson RE, Weibel JL, et al. Middle ear infection in feedlot lambs. J Am Vet Med Assoc 1982;181:805–807.
Jensen R, et al. Cause and pathogenesis of middle ear infection in young feedlot cattle. J Am Vet Med Assoc 1983;182:967–972.
Little CJL, Lane JG, Gibbs C, et al. Inflammatory middle ear disease of the dog: the clinical and pathological features of cholesteatoma, a complication of otitis media. Vet Rec 1991;128:319–322.
Olson LD. Gross and microscopic lesions of middle and inner ear infections in swine. Am J Vet Res 1981;42:1433–1440.
Shimada A, Adachi T, Umemura T, et al. A pathologic and bacteriologic study of otitis media in swine. Vet Pathol 1992;29:337–342.

Inner ear

The inner ear consists of two parts: (1) the membranous labyrinth in which are found the auditory cells and the peripheral ramifications of the auditory nerve; and (2) the osseous labyrinth, a series of cavities in the petrous temporal bone which enclose the membranous labyrinth. The osseous labyrinth is divided into three parts: the vestibule, the cochlea, and the semicircular canals. The membranous labyrinth, which occupies but does not completely fill the osseous labyrinth, is surrounded by the perilymphatic space. The labyrinth contains four divisions: the auricle, the saccule, the semicircular ducts, and the cochlear duct. The inner ear is concerned not only with hearing but also with the sense of equilibrium.

Involvement of the inner ear (**otitis interna, labyrinthitis**) in the presence of otitis media is manifested clinically by disturbances in equilibrium. Examples are the otitis interna of rats and mice, presumably resulting from spread of otitis media caused by *Mycoplasma* sp.

VESTIBULAR SYNDROME (ACUTE VESTIBULAR ATAXIA)

Pathologic involvement of the peripheral vestibular system (utricle, saccule, semicircular canal, vestibular portion of the eighth cranial nerve, and vestibular lobules of the cerebellum) has been observed in dogs, cats and horses, as indicated by several clinical signs. These signs include acute onset of head tilt, asymmetric ataxia without loss of strength, nystagmus, and sometimes facial paralysis or sympathetic ophthalmoplegia. In some cases, otitis externa is present. Some animals recover spontaneously or after a course of antibiotic treatment.

Manifestations indicate involvement of the middle and inner ear, but the precise nature of the lesions is unknown.

References

Burke EE, Moise NS, de Lahunta A, et al. Review of idiopathic feline vestibular syndrome in 75 cats. J Am Vet Med Assoc 1985; 187:941–943.
Powers HT, Watrous BJ, de Lahunta A. Facial and vestibulocochlear nerve disease in six horses. J Am Vet Med Assoc 1983;183:1076–1080.
Schunk KL, Averill DR. Peripheral vestibular syndrome in the dog: a review of 83 cases. J Am Vet Med Assoc 1983;182:1354–1357.

CONGENITAL DEAFNESS

Congenital deafness occurs in several species; cats, mink, dogs, guinea pigs (waltzing), and mice (waltzing). In mink and cats, deafness is the result of degenerative changes in the organ of Corti, which are associated with white coat color. The deaf white cat was observed and commented upon by Darwin more than a hundred years ago, and the histologic features of the affected organ of Corti have been known since the turn of the twentieth century. It appears to be established that the defect is associated with the white coat color (which is due to the dominant white gene [W] in the cat, not albino) and may occur in the presence of blue, yellow, or "odd-eyed" (heterochromia iridis) iris color. The mode of inheritance of the deafness and eye color appears to be complex and is not completely understood. The deafness appears to be more frequent in blue-eyed white cats, but may occur in dominant white cats of any iris color.

The lesions may be seen histologically in kittens after they reach four days of age. Starting with degeneration of the hair cells of the organ of Corti, the lesion progresses to collapse of the tunnel of Corti, contraction of the tectorial membrane, and complete sacculocochlear collapse by 21 days. Ganglion cells decrease in the spiral ganglion, and the ventral cochlear nucleus and the superior olivary complex are reduced in size. The inner ear lesions may be bilateral or unilateral. Hereditary deafness in dalmatians and mink appears to follow the same process as in white cats.

References

Adams EW. Hereditary deafness in a family of foxhounds. J Am Vet Med Assoc 1956;128:302–303.

Altman F. Histologic picture of inherited nerve deafness in man and animals. Arch Otolaryngol 1950;51:852–890.

Anderson H, et al. Genetic hearing impairment in the dalmatian dog. An audiometric, genetic and morphologic study in 53 dogs. Acta Otolaryngol Suppl 1967;232:34.

Bamber RC. Correlation between white coat colour, blue eyes and deafness in cats. J Genet 1927;27:407–413.

Bosher SK, Hallpike CS. Observations on the histogical features, development and pathogenesis of the inner ear degeneration of the deaf white cat. Proc Roy Soc Lond Ser B 1965;162:147–170.

Davis LE, Johnson RT. Experimental viral infections of the inner ear.

I. Acute infections of the newborn hamster labyrinth. Lab Invest 1976;34:349–356.

Getty R, Foust HL, Presley ET, et al. Microscopic anatomy of the ear of the dog. Am J Vet Res 1956;17:364–375.

Hilding DA, Sugiura A, Nakai Y. Deaf white mink: electron microscopic study of the inner ear. Ann Otol Rhinol Laryngol 1967;76:647–663.

Hudson WR, Ruben RJ. Hereditary deafness in dalmatians. Arch Otolaryngol 1962;75:213–216.

Hudspeth AJ. The cellular basis of hearing: the biophysics of hair cells. Science 1985;230:745–752.

Mair IWS. Hereditary deafness in the dalmatian dog. Arch Otol Rhinol Laryngol 1976;212:1–14.

Saunders LZ. The histopathology of hereditary congenital deafness in white mink. Pathol Vet 1965;2:256–263.

Index

Page numbers in *italics* refer to illustrations; those ending in the letter t refer to tables.

Aspergillus niger, 506, 959t
Aspergillus ochraceus, 537t
Aspergillus terreus, 506
Aspergillus versicolor, 537t
Aspicularis tetraptera, 640
Aspiration pneumonia, 962–963, *966*
 air sacs and, 949
Aspirin, toxicity of, 696t, 697t, 779
Asses, *Klossiella equi* in, 573
 parasitic skin diseases in, 846t
Asteroid bodies, 1002–1003, *1004, 1005*
Asthenia, cutaneous dermal, 849–850, *851*
Asthma, allergic, 118
 bronchial, 965
Astragalus, 752
Astragalus lentiginosus, 45
Astrocytes, 1260
Astrocytoma, 1288t, 1290, *1290*
Astrovirus(es), 273, 367
 enteritis, *285*
Ataxia, 1266
 acute vestibular, 1328
 enzootic, 805–806, 1274t, 1275
 hereditary cerebellar, 1274t, 1285t
Atelectasis, 967–968
Atelectasis neonatorum, 968
Ateles, 102t
Ateles geofroyii, 102t
Atheletes foot, 531
Atherosclerosis, *997,* 997–998
Athesmia foxi, 660t
Atlantic bottlenosed dolphins, 529, *529*
Atopic dermatitis, 844
Atopy, 189, 844
Atresia ani, 1086
Atresia coli, 1084
Atrial natriuretic factor, heart failure and, 983
Atrial septal defects, 975–976
Atriopeptin, heart failure and, 983
Atrioventricular valves, endocarditis of, *996*
Atrophic rhinitis, 459t, 950, *951*
Atrophy, 81–82
 arterial, 1002
 brown, 77, *77*
 canine spinal muscular, 1285t
 causes of, 82
 classification of, 82
 cortical cerebellar, 1285t
 epidermal, 835
 fatty, 82
 fibrous, 82
 gross appearance of, 82
 idiopathic follicular, 1234
 juvenile pancreatic, 1106–1107
 microscopic appearance of, 81–82
 of muscle fibers, 882–883, *883*
 myocardial, 987
 numerical, 81
 of optic nerve, 1319
 pancreatic, juvenile, 1106–1107
 pigment, 82
 prostatic, 1214
 quantitative, 81
 retinal cone, 1317
 scirrhous, 82
 serous, of fat, 82
 simple, 82
 testicular, *1205,* 1205–1208
 of uterus, 1165
Atropine, 157, 697t, 755, 1271t
Atypical ileal hyperplasia, 1073
Atypical interstial pneumonia, 537t, 970
Auerbach's plexus, 1297
Aujeszky's disease, 217t, 224

perivascular lymphocytic infiltration of brain in, 148
Auricular chondritis, 1326, *1327*
Australian grass, 76
Autoimmune demyelination, 1275
Autoimmune encephalomyelitis, 193, 1274t, 1275–1276
Autoimmune hemolytic anemia, 193, 1013, 1018
Autoimmune hepatitis, 1097
Autoimmunity, 192–193
 disease and, 193–196
 viral infections and, 195–196
Autologous immune complex glomerulone- phritis, 1125
Autolysis, 9–10
 postmortem, 10, *15,* 15–16
Autonomic nervous system, 1287
Autophagic vacuoles, 6
Autotransplantation, 252
Avian borreliosis, 476t, 478
Avian encephalomyelitis, 265t
Avian erythroblastosis virus, 98t, 107t
Avian herpesvirus, 217
Avian lymphomatosis, 218t
Avian myeloblastosis, 107t
Avian myelocytoma virus, 98t
Avian myelocytomatosis virus, 107t
Avian sarcoma virus, 98t
Avian schistosomiasis, 662t
Avian spirochaetosis, 476t
Avian trichomoniasis, 583
Avian tuberculosis, 490t, 491–492, *497*
Avian type C oncoviruses, 330t
Avian viruses, oncogenic, 107t
Avipoxvirus(es), diseases caused by, 203t, 206
Axonal degeneration, 789t, 1262
Axonal swelling, 1287
Ayrshire cattle, 885
Azo dyes, 100t
Azoturia, 889
Azurophil granules, 115

B cell(s), 122–123
 deficiency of, 187
 neoplasms of, 1038t
 polyclonal activation, 1123–1125
 T cell interactions with, *179*
B-virus, 217t
Babes' nodules, 326
Babesia, 549, 550t, 595
Babesia argentina, 595, 596t
Babesia bigemina, 595, 596t, 597
Babesia bovis, 595, 596t, 597
Babesia caballi, 595, 596t, 597
Babesia canis, 595, 596t, 597
Babesia divergens, 595, 596t, 597
Babesia equi, 595, 596t, 597
Babesia felis, 595, 596t
Babesia gibsoni, 595, 596t, 597
Babesia major, 595, 596t
Babesia motasi, 595, 596t
Babesia ovis, 595, 596t
Babesia pullorum, 396t
Babesia trautmanni, 595, 596t
Babesiosis, 595, 596t, 597
 bovine, 595, 596t, 597
 canine, 595, 596t, 597
 equine, 595, 596t, 597
 in humans, 595, 597
Baboon(s), 219
 Hamadryas, 1054
 Hepatocystis in, 594, *594*

measles in, 319
 schistosomiasis in, 662t
Baboon type C oncovirus, 330t
Bacillary dysentery, 458
Bacillary hemoglobinuria, bovine, 417t, *418,* 418–419
Bacillus, 414–416
 filamentaous cilia-associated respiratory, 465
Bacillus anthracis, 71, 177
Bacillus mallei, 450, 451
Bacillus piliformis, 463
 in enteritis, 1070
 in myocarditis, 987t
Back muscle necrosis, 890
Bacteria, in endometritis, 1173, *1173,* 1174
 pneumonia and, 959t
 pyogenic, 145
 radiation of, 684
Bacterial diseases. *See also specific bacterium, eg., Staphylococcus.*
 hepatitis and, 1096
 of nervous system, 1270t
Bacterial endocarditis, *996*
Bacterium aerugineum, 452
Bacterium aeruginosum, 452
Bacterium pyocyaneum, 452
Bacterium pyocyaneus, 452
Bacteriuria, 1130
Bacteroides melaningenicus, 1045
Badger, 311
 lungworm in, 632t
Baileya, toxicity of, 696t, 731
Baileya multiradiata, 731
Balanoposthitis, 439t
 infectious, 215, 217t, 1185
 parasitic, 1219
Balansia, 537t
Balantidiasis, 583
Balantidium, 550t
Balantidium coli, 549, 583
Balantidium suis, 583
Balbiani gigantea, 565t
Ballooning degeneration, epidermal injury and, 823
Balouria anserina, 396t
Balouria gallinarum, 396t
Bangkok hemorrhagic disease, 570
Bang's disease, 444
Barber's itch, 532
Bare lymphocyte syndrome, 187
Barr body, 7
*Bartholin's glands, cystic, 1187
Bartonella, 372t, 394, *395*
Bartonella bacilliformis, 394t
Bartonella canis, 396t
Bartonella muris, 396t
Bartonellaceae, 372t
 diseases caused by, 394, 394t
Bartonellosis, 394t
Basal cell tumor, 854–855, *855, 856*
 ribbon-type, 855
 trabecular variant of, 855
Basedow's disease, 1236
Basement membrane, 1112
Basic multicellular units, of bone, 900, *901*
Basidiobolus, 524
Basidiobolus haptosporus, 523t
Basidiobolus ranarum, 523t
Basophils, 118
Basset hounds, glaucoma in, 1321
 nonlysosomal storage disease in, 46
Bat(s), fruit, 593
 Klossiella in, 573
Bat virus, 324t, 325